The Autoimmune Diseases

The Autoimmune Diseases

Fifth Edition

Edited by

Noel R. Rose
Departments of Pathology and of Molecular
Microbiology and Immunology
The Johns Hopkins University
Baltimore, Maryland
USA

and

Ian R. Mackay
Department of Biochemistry and Molecular Biology
Monash University
Clayton, Victoria
Australia

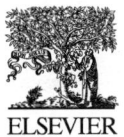

AMSTERDAM • BOSTON • HEIDELBERG • LONDON
NEW YORK • OXFORD • PARIS • SAN DIEGO
SAN FRANCISCO • SINGAPORE • SYDNEY • TOKYO
Academic Press is an imprint of Elsevier

Academic Press is an imprint of Elsevier
525 B Street, Suite 1800, San Diego, CA 92101-4495, USA
32 Jamestown Road, London NW1 7BY, UK
225 Wyman Street, Waltham, MA 02451, USA

Fifth edition 2014

Notice
No responsibility is assumed by the publisher for any injury and/or damage to persons, or property as a matter
of products liability, negligence or otherwise, or from any use or, operation of any methods, products, instructions
or ideas contained in the material herein. Because of rapid advances in the medical sciences, in particular,
independent verification of diagnoses and drug dosages should be made.

Front cover image:
Necrotizing arteritis in a small artery in the dermis of a mouse 6 days after intravenous injection of mouse antimyelo-
peroxidase IgG. There is a central area of deeply eosinophilic fibrinoid necrosis surrounded by leukocytes with leuko-
cytoclasia (H&E stain). From Jennette, J.C. and Falk, R.J. Necrotizing Arteritis and Small Vessel Vasculitis In: The
Autoimmune Diseases. (Rose, N.R. and Mackay, I.R., eds.) Fifth Edition. pp. 1065-1084. Oxford, Elsevier Academic
Press, with permission.

British Library Cataloguing-in-Publication Data
A catalogue record for this book is available from the British Library

Library of Congress Cataloging-in-Publication Data
A catalog record for this book is available from the Library of Congress

ISBN: 978-0-12-384929-8

For information on all Academic Press publications
visit our website at elsevierdirect.com

Typeset by MPS Limited, Chennai, India
www.adi-mps.com

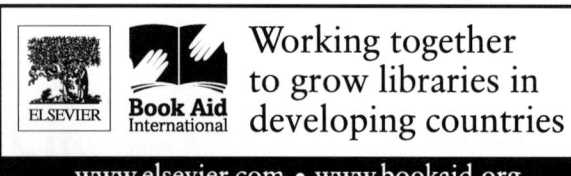

Working together
to grow libraries in
developing countries

www.elsevier.com • www.bookaid.org

Contents

List of Contributors   xxvii
Preface   xxxiii

Part 1
Immunologic Basis of Autoimmunity

1. Autoimmune Disease: The Consequence of Disturbed Homeostasis

Noel R. Rose and Ian R. Mackay

Evolution of the Autoimmune Response	3
A Phylogenetic Perspective	4
The Innate Immune System	4
The Adaptive Immune System	4
Self and Non-Self, and the Nature of Autoantigens	5
Autoimmunity and Autoimmune Disease	5
The Common Threads	5
The "Proper Study…"	6
Towards the Future	8
The Last Word	8
References	9

2. Autoimmunity: A History of the Early Struggle for Recognition

Arthur M. Silverstein

The Search for Autoantibodies	12
Horror Autotoxicus	12
The Nature of Ehrlich's "Contrivances"	12
Challenges to the Thesis	13
Lens Autoantibodies	13
Paroxysmal Cold Hemoglobinuria	13
Sympathetic Ophthalmia	13
The Wassermann Antibody	13
The Shift to Immunochemistry	14
The Return of Immunobiology	15
Concluding Remarks	16
References	16

3. General Features of Autoimmune Disease

Anne Davidson and Betty Diamond

Innate Immune Activation	19
Cells of the Adaptive Immune System	20
Defining Autoimmune Disease	21
Prevalence of Autoimmunity	21
Genetics of Autoimmunity	22
Association of Single Gene Defects with Autoimmunity	22
Genome-wide Association Studies (GWAS) Identify Multiple Gene Loci that are Associated with Autoimmunity	22
Hormones and Autoimmunity	24
Autoimmunity and Central Tolerance	24
Autoimmunity and Peripheral Tolerance	25
Triggers of Autommunity	25
Activation of the Immune System	26
Role of Antigen as a Driver of Autoimmunity	27
Defective Downregulation of an Immune Response	28
Regulatory Lymphocytes	28
The Role of the Gut Microbiota in Autoimmunity	29
Mechanisms of Tissue Damage	29
Flares and Remissions During Disease	30
Therapeutic Advances	30
Goals for the Future	31
Concluding Remarks	31
Acknowledgments	32
References	32

4. The Concept of Autoinflammatory Diseases

Monique Stoffels and Anna Simon

Historical Perspective	39
Definition	40
Spectrum from Autoimmune to Autoinflammatory Disease	40
Mechanisms in Autoinflammation	40

Classical Hereditary Autoinflammatory
   Disorders   41
   Common Phenotype   41
   Cryopyrin-Associated Periodic Syndrome   43
   Familial Mediterranean Fever   44
   TNF Receptor-Associated Periodic Syndrome   44
   HIDS (also Known as Mevalonate Kinase
     Deficiency)   45
Polygenic or Acquired Autoinflammatory
   Disorders   46
Autoinflammatory Mechanisms of Disease
   in Common Disorders   46
   Type 2 Diabetes Mellitus   46
   Atherosclerosis   46
Newest Developments: Rare Hereditary
   Disorders with Autoinflammatory Aspects   46
   Proteasome Defects   47
   PLCγ2 Deficiency   47
   Heme-Oxidized IRP2 Ubiquitin Ligase   47
Conclusion   48
References   48

Part 2
Immune Cells and Immune Responses

5. Innate and Adaptive Systems of Immunity

Peter J. Delves

Introduction   53
The Innate and Adaptive Responses   53
Innate Responses   54
   Cellular Components   54
   Soluble Mediators   57
Adaptive Immune Responses   58
   T Cell Development   59
   Functional Activities of T Cells   60
   B Cell Development and Functions   62
   Antibodies   63
   Secondary Lymphoid Tissues   64
   Resolution of the Immune Response   66
References   66

6. T Cells and their Subsets in Autoimmunity

*Patrick R. Burkett, Youjin Lee, Anneli Peters,
and Vijay K. Kuchroo*

Introduction   69
TH1 Cells   70
TH17 Cells   71
   Discovery and Differentiation   71
   Function   72
   Reciprocal Relationship with Tregs   72
   The Role of IL-23 in the Generation
     of Th17 Cells   73
   Th17 Pathogenicity and Plasticity   73
   Th17 Regulation in the Intestine   74
Regulatory CD4$^+$ T Cells   74
Tr1 Cells   76
TFH Cells   77
Th2 Cells   78
Th9 Cells   78
Concluding Remarks   78
References   79

7. Immunological Tolerance—T Cells

*Sara R. Hamilton, Sarah Q. Crome,
and Pamela S. Ohashi*

Early Studies Supporting the Induction of
   Tolerance   87
Thymic Tolerance   87
   Brief Overview of Thymocyte Development   87
   Mechanisms of Thymic Tolerance   88
   Expression of Tissue-Restricted Antigens
     in the Thymus   90
Peripheral Tolerance   90
   Impact of Dendritic Cells   91
   Mechanisms of Peripheral Tolerance   93
   Expression of Tissue-Specific Antigens
     by Lymph Node Stromal Cells   96
Concluding Remarks   97
Acknowledgments   97
References   97

8. The Role of Invariant Natural Killer T Cells in Autoimmune Diseases

Gerhard Wingender and Mitchell Kronenberg

The Curious Case of iNKT Cells   103
   The Many Names of NKT Cells   103
   The Many Faces of iNKT Cells   104
   The Many Effector Functions of iNKT Cells   105
   The Many Kinds of iNKT Cells   106
   Technical Problems and the Species Divide   107
The Janus-Like Character of iNKT Cells in
   Autoimmunity   108
   Too Much of a Good Thing: Detrimental
     Roles of iNKT Cells   108
   Missed so Sadly: Beneficial Roles
     of iNKT Cells   113
Good or Bad Performers?   116
   The Far End of the Question?   116
Conclusion   118
Acknowledgments   118
Abbreviations   118
References   118

9. **B Cell Development: How to Become One of the Chosen Ones**

Fritz Melchers

Introduction—What has to be Generated in B Cell Development to Make it to Maturity? 131
Follicular B Cells 132
Intraepithelial B Cells 132
Two Types of Memory B Cells 133
B Lymphopoiesis Before Ig Repertoire Generation—Development of Progenitor and Precursor Cells 134
Development in Waves During Ontogeny, and in Niches Throughout Life 134
Cellular Environments of the First Phase of Early, Antigen-Independent B Cell Development 134
Early Commitments to Antigen-Independent B Cell Development 135
The Second, Eventually Autoantigen-Sensitive, Phase of B Cell Development to sIgM⁺ Immature B Cells 136
The First Checkpoint for the Emerging B Cell Repertoire—Probing the Fitness for a Good BCR 137
Expression of IgL Chains 138
The Second Checkpoint: Sites and Mechanisms of Selection of Newly Generated sIgM⁺ B Cells 139
Future Approaches to Understanding Central B Cell Tolerance 140
Acknowledgments 142
References 142

10. **B Cell Activation and B Cell Tolerance**

Claudia Mauri, Venkat Reddy, and Paul A. Blair

B Cell Activation 147
Antigen-Triggered Activation 147
Secondary Signals for B Cell Activation 148
The Immediate Consequences of B Cell Activation 148
B Cell Activation Requires Interaction with Helper T cells 148
Cell Surface Molecules Involved in B Cell–T Cell Interactions 148
Cytokines Involved in B Cell–T Cell Interactions 149
Activation and Maturation of B Cells Occurs in Lymphoid Organs 149
Where Do B Cells become Antigen Activated? 149
Antigen Activation of B Cells Leads to the Selection of High Affinity Class-Switched Antibody 150
The Germinal Center 150

T Cell-Independent Antibody Responses 150
B Cell Tolerance: A Traditional and New Concept 151
B Cell Tolerance is Acquired by at Least Three Different Processes 151
Receptor Editing and Clonal Deletion 151
Defective Receptor Editing Can Promote Autoimmunity 153
Anergy 153
Characteristics of Anergic B Cells 153
Survival Factors and Tonic Signals Modulate B Cell Tolerance 154
Tonic Signaling in B Cell Development 154
Tonic Signaling and Autoimmunity 154
BAFF and Autoimmunity 154
Regulatory T cells 155
Antibody-Independent Activity of B cells in Tolerance 155
Cytokine Production by B Cells 155
Regulatory B Cells 155
Future Directions 156
References 156

Part 3
Non-Antigen-Specific Recognition

11. **Role of Macrophages in Autoimmunity**

Siamon Gordon and Annette Plüddemann

Introduction 161
Origin and Distribution of Monocytes and Macrophages 162
Recognition, Sensing, and Responses 163
Phagocytosis, Antigen Presentation, and Secretion 166
Activation and Downregulation: Interactions with T and B Lymphocytes 167
Role of Macrophages in Adaptive Immunity and Tolerance 168
Role of Macrophages in Autoimmune Models and Diseases 168
Generation of Autoantigens 169
Modulation of Macrophage Activation 169
Conclusions and Questions 171
Acknowledgments 171
References 171

12. **Dendritic Cells in Autoimmune Disease**

Kristen Radford, Ken Shortman, and Meredith O'Keeffe

Antigen Processing by Dendritic Cells 175
Pattern Recognition Receptors 176
Dendritic Cell Activation 176

Dendritic Cell Subsets   176
Mouse Dendritic Cells   176
Dendritic Cells in the Mouse Thymus   179
Dendritic Cell Subsets and Tolerance   179
Human Dendritic Cell Subsets in
    Steady State   180
Dendritic Cell Subsets in Human Skin:
    Epidermal Langerhans Cells and dermal
    Dendritic Cells   180
Dendritic Cells and Autoimmune Disease   181
    Systemic Lupus Erythematosus   181
    IBD—Crohn's Disease and Ulcerative
        Colitis   182
Dendritic Cell Immunotherapy as a
    Treatment for Autoimmune Diseases   182
Targeting of Dendritic Cells in Autoimmune
    Disease   182
Conclusions and Future Prospects   183
References   183

13. Natural Killer Cells

Yenan T. Bryceson, Niklas K. Björkström, Jenny
Mjösberg, and Hans-Gustaf Ljunggren

Introduction to NK Cells   187
NK Cell Development and Differentiation   188
Phenotype and Tissue Localization
    of NK Cells   189
Functional Responses by NK Cells   189
NK Cell Receptor Signaling and Effector
    Functions   190
    NK Cell Contact and Adhesion to Target
        Cells   190
    NK Cell Lytic Granule Polarization and
        Maturation   191
    NK Cell Cytolytic Granule Exocytosis   192
    NK Cell Chemokine and Cytokine
        Production   192
NK Cells and Human Autoimmunity   193
    Defective Control of other Immune Cells Links
        NK Cells to Autoimmune Diseases   193
    Genetic Association Studies Revealing Links
        between NK Cells and Autoimmune
        Diseases   194
Conclusions   195
References   195

14. Granulocytes: Neutrophils, Basophils, Eosinophils

Xavier Bosch and Manuel Ramos-Casals

Neutrophils   201
    Basic Biology and Role in Immunity   201
    Neutrophil Extracellular Traps and NETosis:
        A Novel Form of Cell Death   202
    Pathogenic Role of Neutrophils in
        Autoimmune Diseases   202
Basophils   206
    Basic Biology and Role in Immunity   206
    Basophils in Autoimmune Diseases   207
Eosinophils   208
    Basic Biology and Role in Immunity   208
    Eosinophils in Churg—Strauss
        Syndrome   209
Conclusions and Therapeutic
    Implications   210
References   211

15. The Roles and Contributions of the Complement System in the Pathophysiology of Autoimmune Diseases

Wilhelm J. Schwaeble, Youssif M. Ali, and
Robert B. Sim

The Complement System and Complement
    Activation Pathways   217
    The Classical Pathway   218
    The Lectin Pathway   218
    The Alternative Pathway   219
    The Membrane Attack Complex   219
Control of Complement Activation   219
    Fluid Phase Regulators   220
    Membrane-Bound Regulators   220
The Biological Effects of Complement
    Activation   220
Complement Involvement in the
    Pathophysiology of Diverse Autoimmune
    Diseases   221
References   224

16. Cytokines, their Receptors and Signals

Joost J. Oppenheim

Historical Perspective   229
Cytokines and Immunity   230
Cytokine Receptor Subsets   232
    The Common γc Chain Subset   232
    The βc Utilizing Subset   233
    The gp130 Utilizing Subset (IL-6 Family)   233
    Cytokines Sharing either a p35 or p40
        Ligand Chain   234
    Th17 Cytokines and Receptors   235
Class II Cytokine Receptor Family   235
    Type I Interferons α and β   235
    Type II Interferon Gamma   235
    Type III Interferon Lambda   236
    Non-Interferon Members   236
TNF Receptor Family   236
The IL-1/TLR Family of Receptors   237

Immunosuppressive Cytokines/Growth
   Factors   239
Chemokines   239
Alarmins   239
Conclusions   239
Acknowledgments   240
References   240

Part 4
Initiation of Autoimmunity

17. Cellular Injury and Apoptosis

Stefania Gallucci, Roberto Caricchio and Philip L. Cohen

Apoptosis   245
  History of Apoptosis   245
  Molecular Pathways of Apoptosis   245
  Apoptotic Cell Morphology   246
Apoptosis in Autoimmunity   246
  Defective Apoptosis   246
  Excessive Apoptosis and Apoptotic Cells as
    Sources of Autoantigen   247
  Apotopes   247
  NETosis   248
Necrosis   248
  Necroptosis   248
  Parthanatos {Par[poly(ADP-ribosyl)ation]
    and thanatos (death)}   248
Clearance of Dead Cells   249
  Find-me Signals   249
  Eat-me Signals and their Receptors   249
  Receptors for Necrotic Cells   251
Anti-Inflammatory Effects of Apoptotic
  Cells   251
Immuno-Stimulatory Effects of Necrotic
  Cells   251
A Glimpse into the Future   252
References   252

18. Autophagy in Autoimmunity

Jan Lünemann and Christian Münz

Autophagy Pathways   257
Autophagy in Innate Immunity   258
Autophagy in Lymphocyte Development
  and Activation   258
Antigen Presentation for CD4$^+$ and CD8$^+$
  T Cell Recognition   259
Autophagy in Tolerance and Autoimmunity   260
Future Prospects   260
References   261

19. Infectious Triggers of T Cell Autoimmunity

Daniel R. Getts, Meghann Teague Getts, Nicholas J.C. King, and Stephen D. Miller

Introduction   263
Role of Infections in Priming of Autoreactive
  Immune Responses   263
Potential Mechanisms of Infection Triggering
  Autoimmunity   264
  Molecular Mimicry   264
  Bystander Activation of Autoreactive Cells
    and Epitope Spreading   268
  Emerging Mechanisms of Infection-Induced
    Autoimmune Disease   268
  Reciprocal Relationships of
    Pathogen-Derived Mechanisms of
    Autoimmunity   269
How do these Mechanisms Lead to
  Autoimmune Disease?   269
  Autoimmunity Can Occur at a Site Distal
    to the Initiating Infection   270
Conclusions   270
Acknowledgments   271
References   271

20. Autoimmune Diseases: The Role for Vaccines

S. Sohail Ahmed and Paul-Henri Lambert

Introduction   275
Theoretical Concerns for Autoimmune
  Diseases in the Context of Vaccination   276
Crossfire and Coincidence   276
Challenges using Animal Models   277
  One Size does "not" Fit All   277
  Induced Autoimmune Disease in
    Animals   278
  Spontaneous Autoimmune Disease
    in Animals   278
  "Of Mice and Men"—The Correct
    Application of Human Epidemiology
    and Translation of Human Immunology
    to Rodent Immunology   279
Practical Approach to Vaccination in
  Patients with Autoimmune Disease   279
  The Reality Facing Clinicians Currently   280
  Certainty about Vaccines, Uncertainty about
    Compatibility of Administration in Certain
    Settings   280
  Search and You Will Find   281
Conclusion   281
References   281

21. Non-infectious Environmental Agents and Autoimmunity

Frederick W. Miller

Introduction	283
Evidence Supporting the Role of Environmental Agents in Autoimmune Disease	284
Identifying and Defining Environmentally Associated Autoimmune Diseases	285
Non-Infectious Agents Associated with Autoimmune Diseases	286
Drugs	286
Occupational Exposures	288
Others	289
Possible Mechanisms by Which Environmental Agents May Induce Autoimmune Diseases	291
Overview and Future Directions	291
References	293

22. Adhesion Molecules and Chemoattractants in Autoimmunity

Charles R. Mackay and Ulrich H. von Andrian

Microvascular Determinants of T Cell Recruitment	297
Adhesion Molecules	297
Chemoattractants and their Receptors	299
Multistep Adhesion Cascades	302
Organized Lymphoid Tissues: Venues for Naïve T Cell Homing and Dendritic Cell Interactions	302
Effector T Cell Migration	303
Homing to Non-Lymphoid Tissues	303
Some Clinical Applications	304
Conclusions and Future Directions	306
Acknowledgments	306
References	306

Part 5
Facilitation of Autoimmunity

23. Effector Mechanisms in Autoimmunity

Arian Laurence and Martin Aringer

Introduction	311
Autoantibodies	311
Direct Antibody-Mediated Disease	311
Immune Complex Disease	312
Complement Cascades	313
Macrophages	313
Neutrophils	313
Mast Cells	314

Natural Killer Cells and Cytotoxic T Cells	314
Effector T Helper Cell-Mediated Autoimmune Disease	314
Effector Cytokines and their Targets	315
Conclusions	316
References	317

24. Sexual Dimorphism in the Immune System

Pamela A. McCombe and Judith M. Greer

Introduction	319
Overview of Sexual Dimorphism	319
Sexual Dimorphism in the Immune System	319
Effects of Hormones on the Immune System	321
Estrogens	321
Progesterone	322
Androgens	322
Role of the Sex Chromosomes in Immunity	323
X Chromosome	323
Y Chromosome	323
Environmental Effects on Sex Differences in Immunity	324
Consequences for Autoimmunity of Sexual Dimorphism in the Immune System	324
Concluding Remarks	325
References	325

25. Microbiome and Autoimmunity

Jean-François Bach and Alicia Perez-Arroyo

Introduction	329
The Intestinal Microbiome	330
Intestinal Microbiome Composition and Genotyping Techniques	330
The Microbiome Changes Over a Lifetime	330
The Intestinal Microbiome Depends on the Environment	330
Germ-Free (GF) Animals	331
Effect of a GF Environment on Experimental Diseases	331
Non-Obese Diabetic Mouse	331
Experimental Allergic Encephalomyelitis	332
Experimental Arthritis	332
Murine Lupus	332
Microbiome Composition and Autoimmune Diseases	333
Type 1 Diabetes	333
Rheumatoid Arthritis	333
Effect of Probiotics on Autoimmune Diseases	333
Probiotic Mixtures	334
Specific Probiotics	334
Role of Toll-like Receptor Stimulation	334

The Relationship Between the Intestinal
Microbiome and the Hygiene Hypothesis 334
Brief Overview of the Hygiene Hypothesis 334
A Clean Environment Promotes the Onset
of Autoimmune Diabetes 335
Autoimmune Diseases Can be Prevented by
Infections With a Pathogen 335
Synthesis and Conclusions 336
The Strength of the Protective Effect of
Pathogens 336
The Ambiguous Effect on Autoimmune
Disease of the GF or Axenic Status 337
The Delicate Interpretation of the Reduction
in the Diversity of the Intestinal
Microbiome 337
Perspectives 337
Acknowledgments 338
References 338

26. Genetic Predisposition, Humans

*Margaret A. Jordan, Judith Field, Helmut
Butzkueven, and Alan G. Baxter*

Introduction 342
Diseases of Interest 342
Type 1 Diabetes 342
Multiple Sclerosis 342
Systemic Lupus Erythematosus 342
Human Leukocyte Antigen (*HLA*) Complex
and other Candidate genes 343
Association of Type 1 Diabetes with HLA
and other Candidate Genes 343
Association of Multiple Sclerosis with HLA
and other Candidate Genes 344
Association of Lupus with HLA and other
Candidate Genes 345
Mechanisms of Complement and Fc
Associations with Autoimmunity 346
Mechanisms of HLA Association with
Autoimmunity 347
Gene Linkage Studies of Autoimmunity 347
Linkage Studies of Type 1 Diabetes 347
Linkage Studies in Multiple Sclerosis 349
Linkage Studies in Lupus 349
Genome-Wide Association Studies of
Autoimmunity 351
Genome-Wide Association Studies of Type 1
Diabetes 351
Genome-Wide Association Studies
of Multiple Sclerosis 352
Genome-Wide Association Studies of
Systemic Lupus Erythematosus 354
From Location to Molecular Mechanisms 355
Concluding Comments 356
Acknowledgments 356
References 356

27. Genetic Predisposition to Autoimmune Diseases Conferred by the Major Histocompatibility Complex: Utility of Animal Models

*Veena Taneja, Ashutosh Mangalam, and
Chella S. David*

Major Histocompatibility Complex 365
MHC and Autoimmunity 366
The Mystery of HLA-B27 and
Spondyloarthropathies 366
HLA Class II Association with Autoimmune
Diseases 368
Predisposition 368
Onset 369
Environmental Factors 369
Infectious Agent 369
Porphyromonas Gingivalis and Rheumatoid
Arthritis 370
Smoking and Autoimmunity 370
Vitamin D in Autoimmune Diseases 370
Post-Translational Modifications in
Autoimmunity 371
Deimination 371
Deamidation 372
Humanized Animal Models of
Autoimmunity 372
Collagen-Induced Arthritis 373
Non-RA-Associated HLA Alleles Can
Predispose to Autoimmunity 374
HLA-DR Transgenic Mice with EAE as an
Animal Model of MS 374
Role of DQ Molecules in Predisposition
to MS 375
Animal Model of Celiac Disease 375
Animal Model for Type 1 Diabetes 376
HLA Class II Molecules Regulate Infection
Through Modulation of Cytokine
Networks 376
Concluding Remarks 377
References 377

28. Epigenetics and Autoimmune Diseases

Moncef Zouali

Epigenetic Modifications 382
DNA Methylation 382
Histone Post-Translational Modifications 382
Acetylation and Deacetylation 383
Histone Methylation 383
Arginine Methylation 383
Ubiquitination 384
MicroRNAs 384
Epigenetic Stability 384

Epigenetics of Immune Tolerance to Self   384
  Epigenetic Regulators of Tolerant T Cells   384
  Role of CpG DNA Methylation in Treg
    Development and Function   385
  Impacts of Histone Acetylation on
    Development and Function of Tregs   385
  Epigenetic Modulation of Treg Stability   386
Systemic Lupus Erythematosus   386
  DNA Methylation   386
  DNA Methylation Control by miRNA   387
  Histone Acetylation   388
  Environmental Epigenetics in SLE   388
  Epigenetic Disruption of B Cell Tolerance
    in SLE   388
Rheumatoid Arthritis   389
  Acetylation Marks   389
  Genomic DNA Hypomethylation and the
    Activated Phenotype of RASFs   389
  miRNA and the Destructive Potential
    of RASFs   390
  Aberrant SUMOylation   390
Systemic Sclerosis   390
Sjögren's Syndrome   390
Antineutrophil Cytoplasmic Autoantibodies-
  Associated Vasculitis   391
Type 1 Diabetes   391
  DNA Methylation Profiling   392
  Chromatin Remodeling and Histone
    Acetylation   392
  Histone Deacetylase Inhibitors in
    Preclinical Studies   392
Multiple Sclerosis   393
  Generation of Neo-Epitopes   393
  DNA Hypomethylation   393
  Deregulation of Acetylation Homeostasis   394
Epigenetic Therapy   394
  Targeting DNA Methylation   395
  Histone Deacetylase Inhibitors   395
  Epigenetic Generation of Tregs   396
Future Prospects   396
References   396

29. Autoimmunity in Primary
    Immunodeficiency Disorders

Thomas A. Fleisher and Arnold I. Levinson

Introduction   403
T Cell Developmental Defects   403
  Severe Combined Immunodeficiency   403
  Combined Immune Deficiencies   404
  DiGeorge Syndrome   405
  Wiskott–Aldrich Syndrome   405
Antibody Production Defects   406
  X-Linked Agammaglobulinemia   406
  Common Variable Immunodeficiency   406
  Selective IgA Deficiency   408

  Immunodeficiency with Hyper-IgM
    Syndrome   409
Innate Immune Defects   411
  Chronic Granulomatous Disease   411
  Early Complement Component Deficiency   411
  Toll-Like Receptor 3 (TLR3) Polymorphism
    and Autoimmunity   412
Monogenic Defects Affecting Immune
  Homeostasis and/or Tolerance   412
  Autoimmune Polyendocrinopathy,
    Candidiasis, Ectodermal Dystrophy   412
  Immunodysregulation, Polyendocrinopathy,
    Enteropathy X-Linked   413
  Autoimmune Lymphoproliferative
    Syndrome   414
Conclusion   414
Acknowledgment   416
References   416

Part 6
Experimental Models of Autoimmunity

30. Animal Models: Systemic Autoimmune Diseases

Masayuki Mizui and George C. Tsokos

Introduction   421
Spontaneous Models of Systemic
  Autoimmunity   421
Genetically Manipulated Models of
  Systemic Autoimmunity   423
  Lymphocyte Activation Molecules   423
  Ubiquitination-Protein Ligases   424
  Cytokines and their Receptors   425
  Complement and Complement Receptor
    Proteins   426
  Clearance of Dead Cells   426
  Innate Immune Cell Signaling   427
Induced Models of Systemic Autoimmunity   427
Concluding Comments   428
References   430

31. Animal Models of Organ-Specific Autoimmune Disease

Ken Coppieters and Matthias von Herrath

What Can Animal Models Teach us about
  Organ-Specific Autoimmunity?   435
  The Inciting Autoantigen   435
  Antigen-specific Tolerization Strategies   436
  Other Immune Therapies   436
  Gene Function   436
  Understanding the Complexity of
    Organ-Specific Autoimmunity   436

Animal Models—Advantages and
Disadvantages   437
Animal Models for Organ-Specific
Autoimmune diseases   438
Spontaneous Models of Organ-Specific
Autoimmunity   438
Genetically Engineered Animal Models
for Organ-Specific Autoimmunity   439
Induced Animal Models for Organ-Specific
Autoimmune Diseases   439
Protein/Peptide and Adjuvant   440
Cell Transfer or Depletion   442
Comparison of Organ-Specific Autoimmune
Disease in Animal Models and Humans   444
Conclusions   444
References   444

Part 7
Multisystem Autoimmune Diseases

32. Systemic Lupus Erythematosus

Robert G. Lahita

Introduction   451
Pathogenesis   451
Genetics   452
Epidemiology   452
Autoantibody   452
Clinical   453
Measurement of Clinical Activity   454
Musculoskeletal   454
Renal   455
Neuropsychiatric   455
Cardiac   456
Pulmonary   457
Hematology   457
Dermatology   457
Gastroenterological   458
ENT and Eye   458
Lupus Therapeutics   458
References   459

33. Systemic Sclerosis, Scleroderma

Nabeel H. Borazan and Daniel E. Furst

Introduction   463
Clinical, Pathologic, and Epidemiologic
Features   463
Clinical Features   463
Pathologic Features   464
Epidemiologic Features   464
Autoimmune Features and Immunologic
Markers in Disease   465
Potential Pathogenetic Antibodies   465
Diagnostic and Prognostic Antibodies   465
Genetic Features   466
Environmental Influences   466
Animal Models of SSc   467
UCD200 Chickens   467
Tsk1 and Tsk2 Mice   468
Scl-GvHD   468
TGF-β, CTGF, and bFGF   468
Bleomycin-Induced Fibrosis   468
Fra2-Transgenic Mice   469
TβRIIΔk Mice   469
Wnt-10b-Transgenic Mice   469
Pathogenic Mechanisms   469
Vasculopathy   469
Immunological Abnormalities   470
Fibrosis   472
Concluding Remarks and Future Prospects   473
References   473

34. Antiphospholipid Syndrome

*Nancy Agmon-Levin, Angela Tincani,
and Yehuda Shoenfeld*

Introduction   481
The Clinical Spectrum of Antiphospholipid
Syndrome   482
Obstetric APS   482
Thrombotic APS   482
Neurological APS   483
Hematologic APS   483
Dermatologic APS   483
Cardiac APS   483
Pulmonary APS   484
Renal APS   484
Catastrophic Antiphospholipid Syndrome   484
The Antiphospholipid Antibodies   484
The b2GPI—Anti-b2GPI Complex in APS   485
Non-Criteria aPL Antibodies   485
aPL of the IGA Isotype   485
Low-level aPL   486
The Mechanisms of aPL-Mediated Disease
Expressions   486
Thrombotic Manifestations   487
Obstetric Manifestations   488
Neurologic Manifestations   488
The Complement System in APS   489
Treatment of APS   489
Conclusions and Future Aspects   490
References   490

35. Sjögren's Syndrome

*Clio P. Mavragani, George E. Fragoulis, and
Haralampos M. Moutsopoulos*

Introduction   495
Clinical Features   496
Local Manifestations (Salivary and
Lachrymal Glands)   496

Systemic Manifestations (Beyond Salivary
and Lachrymal Glands) 496
Overlapping Autoimmune Entities 498
Diagnosis and Differential Diagnosis 498
**Autoimmune Features and Pathogenic
Mechanisms** 498
Immunopathology 498
Autoantibodies 502
Etiopathogenesis 502
Genetics 502
Epigenetics 503
Environmental Factors 503
Exocrine Gland Dysfunction 504
Apoptosis 504
Neurotransmission 504
Aquaporins 504
Structural Abnormalities 504
Therapy 504
Future Prospects 505
References 505

36. Rheumatoid Arthritis

Josef S. Smolen and Kurt Redlich

Introduction 511
**Clinical, Pathologic, and Epidemiologic
Features** 511
Autoimmune Features 512
Genetic Features 514
***In Vivo* Models** 515
Pathologic Effector Mechanisms 516
**Autoantibodies as Potential Immunologic
Markers** 517
Concluding Remarks—Future Prospects 519
Acknowledgment 519
References 519

37. Juvenile Idiopathic Arthritis

Clara Malattia and Alberto Martini

Epidemiology 525
Clinical Features 525
Systemic Arthritis 525
Rheumatoid Factor-Positive Polyarthritis 526
Enthesitis-Related Arthritis 526
Oligoarthritis 527
Rheumatoid Factor-Negative Polyarthritis 527
Psoriatic Arthritis 527
Undifferentiated Arthritis 527
Perspectives 527
Etiology and Pathogenesis 528
Systemic Juvenile Idiopathic Arthritis 528
Oligoarticular Juvenile Idiopathic Arthritis 531
Treatment 532
References 533

38. Spondyloarthritides

Uta Syrbe and Joachim Sieper

**Definition, Epidemiology, Clinical Manifestations,
and Treatment** 537
Reactive Arthritis 538
Arthritis with IBD 538
Psoriatic Arthritis 538
**The Role of HLA-B27 in the Pathogenesis
of Spondyloarthritis** 538
Arthritogenic Peptide Hypothesis 538
Misfolded HLA-B27 Hypothesis 539
**The Role of Non-MHC Genes in
Spondyloarthritis** 540
**Bacterial Trigger and Autoimmunity in the
Pathogenesis of the Spondyloarthritides** 541
**Cytokines in the Pathogenesis of Reactive
Arthritis** 541
**Cytokines in the Pathogenesis of Ankylosing
Spondylitis** 542
**What is the Immune Target in Ankylosing
Spondylitis?** 542
Inflammation and Bone Formation 542
Concluding Remarks—Future Prospects 543
References 543

39. The Autoimmune Myopathies

Livia Casciola-Rosen and Antony Rosen

Defining Autoimmune Myopathies 547
**Clinical and Pathological Descriptions
of Different Phenotypes, including IMNM** 547
**Characteristic Pathology, but Significant
Overlap between Phenotypes** 548
Epidemiological Clues into Mechanism 548
**Specific Autoantibodies are Strongly
Associated with Phenotype, Making
them Useful Probes of Disease
Mechanism** 549
Myositis-Specific Autoantibodies 549
HMG CoA Reductase Autoantibodies
in Statin-Associated Immune-Mediated
Necrotizing Myopathy 550
Mechanisms of Disease 551
The Association of Malignancy with
Myositis: Insights into Disease Initiation 551
Enhanced Expression of Myositis Autoantigens
in Regenerating Muscle Cells to Focus
Propagation on Muscle 551
Modification of Autoantigen Expression or
Structure by Immune Effector Pathways
to Generate a Self-Sustaining Phenotype 552
Therapeutic Insights 552
Concluding Remarks 553
References 553

Part 8
Endocrine System

40. Thyroid Disease

Anthony P. Weetman

Autoimmune Thyroiditis	557
Historic Background	557
Clinical, Pathologic, and Epidemiologic Features	557
Autoimmune Features	558
Genetic Features	560
Environmental Influences	560
In Vivo Models	561
Pathologic Effector Mechanisms	562
Autoantibodies as Potential Immunological Markers	563
Treatment and Outcome	563
Concluding Remarks—Future Prospects	564
Graves' Disease	564
Historic Background	564
Clinical, Pathologic, and Epidemiologic Features	564
Autoimmune Features	565
Genetic Features	565
Environmental Influences	566
In Vivo Models	566
Pathologic Effector Mechanisms	567
Autoantibodies as Potential Immunological Markers	568
Treatment and Outcome	568
Thyroid-Associated Ophthalmopathy and Dermopathy	568
Concluding Remarks—Future Prospects	568
References	569

41. Autoimmune (Type 1) Diabetes

Ahmed J. Delli and Åke Lernmark

Introduction	575
Clinical and Pathologic Features	575
Epidemiologic Features	577
Genetic Features	578
HLA Genetic Factors: The *DR-DQ* Alleles	578
Non-HLA Genetic Factors	578
Autoimmune Features	580
Pathologic Effector Mechanisms	580
Triggering Autoimmunity	580
APCs in Genetically Predisposed Subjects	581
In Vivo and In Vitro Models	581
Autoantibodies as Potential Immunologic Markers	582
Concluding Remarks—Future Prospects	582
References	583

42. Adrenalitis

Corrado Betterle and Renato Zanchetta

Introduction	587
Anatomy and Physiology of the Adrenals	588
Epidemiology of Addison's Disease and Autoimmune Adrenalitis	588
Autoimmune Addison's Disease (AAD)	589
Histopathology	589
Focal Lymphocytic Adrenalitis	589
Diffuse Lymphocytic Adrenalitis	590
Animal Models	590
Induced Immunity	590
Spontaneous Animal Models of AD	590
Immunologic Studies	591
Genetic Predisposition	591
Cellular Immunity	591
Humoral Immunity	591
Natural History of AAD	594
Diagnosis of AAD	595
Clinical Manifestations	595
Hormonal Tests	595
Imaging	596
Different Clinical Presentations of AAD	596
Association with other Autoimmune Disorders	596
Therapy	597
General Information	597
Acknowledgments	599
References	599

43. Polyendocrine Syndromes

Pärt Peterson and Eystein S. Husebye

Historical Background	605
Clinical, Pathologic and Epidemiologic Features	606
Autoimmune Features	608
Genetic Features	608
Environmental Features	610
Animal Models	611
AIRE-Deficient Mouse as a Model for APS-1	611
Spontaneous Animal Models	611
Thymectomy Animal Model	611
Pathogenic Mechanisms	612
Immunologic Markers in Diagnosis	612
Treatment and Outcome	613
Concluding Remarks—Future Prospects	613
Acknowledgments	613
References	614

44. Autoimmune Gastritis and Pernicious Anemia

Ian R. van Driel, Eric Tu, and Paul A. Gleeson

Clinical, Pathologic, and Epidemiologic Features	620
Autoimmune Features	622
Autoantibodies	622
T Cell Immunity	623
Genetic Features	623
In Vivo and *In Vitro* Models	624
Pathologic Effector Mechanisms	626
Autoantibodies as Potential Immunologic Markers	626
Concluding Remarks—Future Prospects	626
References	627

45. Autoimmune Hypophysitis

Patrizio Caturegli, Isabella Lupi, and Angelika Gutenberg

Definition and Classification of Autoimmune Hypophysitis	633
Historical Background	633
Epidemiology and Body of Literature	634
Clinical Features	635
Pathological Features	637
Autoimmune Features	639
Genetic and Environmental Influences	640
Animal Models	640
Diagnosis	641
Treatment	641
Outcome	642
Hypophysitis Secondary to CTLA-4 Blockade	642
Concluding Remarks—Future Perspectives	644
Acknowledgments	644
References	644

Part 9
Blood Disorders

46. Autoimmune Hemolytic Anemia

Mark A. Vickers and Robert N. Barker

Historical Background	649
Classification of AIHA	649
Animal Models of AIHA	650
Mechanisms of RBC Destruction in AIHA	650
Cold Reactive Antibodies	650
Warm Reactive Antibodies	651
Pathogenicity of Warm Reactive IgG Antibodies	651
Additional Mechanisms of Hemolysis by Warm Antibodies	652
RBC Autoantigens	653

Clinical Signs of AIHA	653
Laboratory Diagnosis of AIHA	654
Treatment of AIHA	654
Etiology of AIHA and Predisposing Factors	654
Genetic Predisposition	654
Gender and Age	655
Infectious Agents	655
Drugs	655
Neoplasia	655
Immune Mechanisms Underlying Loss of Self Tolerance in Warm AIHA	655
B Cells and Tolerance	655
T Helper (Th) Cells and Tolerance	656
Concluding Remarks	657
References	657

47. Immune Thrombocytopenia

Berengere Gruson and James B. Bussel

Clinical, Pathologic, and Epidemiologic Features	663
General Features and Definitions	663
Diagnosis	664
Epidemiology and Clinical Presentation in Children	664
Epidemiology and Clinical Presentation in Adults	665
Autoimmune Features	665
Autoimmune Markers in Primary ITP	665
Evans Syndrome	666
ITP Secondary to Systemic Lupus Erythematosus	666
ITP Secondary to Primary Immunodeficiencies	666
Genetics Features	667
Familial ITP	667
Genetic Markers of ITP	667
In Vivo Models	668
Pathologic Effector Mechanisms	668
Increased Platelet Destruction	668
Insufficient Platelet Production	669
Infection-related Thrombocytopenia	670
Autoantibodies as Potential Immunologic Markers	670
Concluding Remarks—Future Prospects	671
References	672

48. Autoimmune Neutropenia

Parviz Lalezari

Historical Background	677
Clinical and Pathologic Features	677
Autoimmune Neutropenia of Infancy	678
Primary Autoimmune Neutropenia in Adolescents and Adults	678
Neutrophil-Specific Antigens in Primary Autoimmune Neutropenias	678
Secondary Autoimmune Neutropenias	679

Differential Diagnosis 679
   Mechanisms of Cell Destruction 680
Laboratory Diagnosis 680
Treatment 681
Perspectives and Future Directions 681
References 681

49. Acquired Aplastic Anemia

Robert A. Brodsky and Richard J. Jones

Historical Background 685
Genetic Features 685
Clinical, Pathologic, and Epidemiologic
   Features 685
Autoimmune Features and Pathogenic
   Mechanisms 687
Environmental Features 687
Animal Models 687
Therapy for Aplastic Anemia 688
   Bone Marrow Transplantation (BMT) 688
   BMT from Unrelated Donors 688
Immunosuppressive Therapy 689
High-Dose Cyclophosphamide without
   BMT 689
Aplastic Anemia and Clonality 690
Concluding Remarks—Future Prospects 691
References 692

50. Monogenic Autoimmune Lymphoproliferative Syndromes

Joao Bosco Oliveira, V. Koneti Rao, Helen Su, and Michael Lenardo

Introduction—Apoptosis and the Immune
   System 695
Clinical and Pathological Features 696
   Autoimmune Lymphoproliferative
     Syndrome 696
   Clinical Presentation 697
   Laboratory Evaluation 698
   Imaging Studies 699
   Treatment 699
   Prognosis 700
ALPS-Related Disorders 700
   Caspase-8 and FADD Deficiencies 700
   RAS-Associated Autoimmune
     Leukoproliferative Disorder 702
   Genetic Features 702
Autoimmune Lymphoproliferative
   Syndrome (ALPS) 702
   Germline *FAS* Mutations 702
   Somatic *FAS* Mutations 703
   Additional Genetic Etiologies 703
RAS-Associated Autoimmune
   Leukoproliferative Disorder 704
   In Vivo and *In Vitro* Models of Disease 704
   Pathogenic Effector Mechanisms 705

Conclusion 707
Acknowledgments 707
References 707

51. Autoimmune Clotting Dysfunction

Christoph Königs

Introduction 711
Procoagulant Thrombotic Diseases 712
   Autoimmune Inhibitors to ADAMTS13 713
Anticoagulant (Bleeding) Diseases 714
   Autoimmune Antibody Inhibitors to
     Fibrinogen (Factor I) and Fibrin 714
   Autoimmune Inhibitors to Prothrombin
     (Factor II) and Thrombin 714
   Autoimmune Inhibitors to Factor V 716
   Autoimmune Inhibitors to Factor VII 717
   Autoimmune Inhibitors to Factor VIII 717
   Autoimmune Inhibitors to Factor IX 720
   Autoimmune Inhibitors to Factor X 720
   Autoimmune Inhibitors to Factor XI 720
   Autoimmune Inhibitors to Factor XII 721
   Autoimmune Inhibitors to Factor XIII 721
   Autoimmune Inhibitors to Von
     Willebrand Factor 722
   Autoimmune Inhibitors to Further Proteins 722
Conclusions and Future Prospects 722
Acknowledgments 723
References 723

Part 10
Central and Peripheral Nervous System

52. Multiple Sclerosis

Amanda L. Hernandez, Kevin C. O'Connor, and David A. Hafler

Historical Background 735
Clinical Features 736
   Imaging 737
Immunological Markers in Diagnosis 738
Pathology 738
Epidemiology of MS 739
   Genetic Factors 739
   Environmental Factors 740
Immune Pathogenesis 742
   T Cell Pathogenesis 743
   Immune Dysregulation 744
   Autoantigens 745
   Meningeal Ectopic B Cell Follicles 745
Treatment 745
   Interferons 746
   Glatiramer Acetate (Copaxone®) 747
   Natalizumab (Tysabri®) 747

Mitoxantrone (Novantrone®) 748
Fingolimod (Gilenya®) 748
Teriflunomide (Aubagio®) 748
Dimethyl Fumarate, BG-12 (Tecfidera®) 748
Concluding Remarks 749
References 749

53. **Peripheral Neuropathies**

Michael P.T. Lunn and Kazim A. Sheikh

Introduction 757
Acute Neuropathies: The Guillain–Barré
Syndrome 757
Historical Background 757
Epidemiology 758
Clinical Features and Subtypes of GBS 758
Autoimmune Features 759
Environmental Effects 762
Animal Models of Disease 763
Cellular Mechanisms 763
Cellular and Humoral Immune Elements
are Synergistic 765
Genetic Aspects of GBS 765
Treatment and Outcomes 766
Chronic Neuropathies: Chronic
Inflammatory Demyelinating
Polyradiculoneuropathy 766
History 766
Epidemiology and Clinical Features 766
Autoimmune Features 768
Immunogenetic Features 768
Environmental Influences 768
Animal Models 768
Pathogenic Mechanisms 769
Treatment and Outcome 769
Concluding Remarks and Future Prospects 770
Acknowledgments 770
References 770

54. **Myasthenia Gravis and Related**
Disorders

Stuart Viegas and Angela Vincent

Introduction 777
The Neuromuscular Junction 777
AChR, MuSK, and Lrp4 778
Neuromuscular Transmission 779
Myasthenia Gravis 779
Epidemiology 779
Etiology 779
General Aspects 780
Clinical Heterogeneity 780
Early-onset AChR Antibody Positive MG
(AChRab⁺ MG) 780
Late-onset AChR Antibody Positive MG
(AChRab⁺ MG) 781

Thymoma-Associated MG (Thymoma MG) 781
MuSK Antibody-Positive MG
(MuSKab⁺ MG) 781
Neonatal MG 781
Antibodies in Myasthenia 782
Serological Testing 782
AChR Antibody Characteristics 782
MuSK and Other Antibodies 783
Pathogenic Mechanisms 783
Evidence for Pathogenicity of AChR
and MuSK Antibodies 783
AChR Antibody-Positive MG 783
MuSK Antibody-Positive MG 784
The Thymus and Cellular Immunity in MG 784
Role of T Lymphocytes in MG 784
The Thymus and MG 785
Lambert–Eaton Myasthenic Syndrome 785
Epidemiology and Etiology 786
Clinical Features 786
Investigation and Treatment 786
Pathophysiology 786
Conclusions and Future Prospects 786
References 787

55. **Ocular Disease**

Monica D. Dalal, H. Nida Sen, and
Robert B. Nussenblatt

Historical Background 793
Clinical Features 793
Pathologic Features 795
Epidemiologic Features 795
Autoimmune Features 796
Hormonal Influences 797
Genetic Factors 797
Animal Models 798
Pathogenic Mechanisms 798
Ocular Immune Responses 799
Tissue Destruction 799
Immunologic Markers 799
Treatment and Outcomes 800
Concluding Remarks and Future
Prospects 801
References 801

56. **Immune-Mediated Inner Ear Disease**

Claudio Lunardi and Antonio Puccetti

Introduction 805
Clinical Features 805
IMIED Associated with Systemic
Autoimmune Diseases 806
IMIED Associated with Primary
Vasculitides 807
Evidence of Autoimmunity 808
Genetic Susceptibility 810
Animal Models 810

Treatment 811
Concluding Remarks and Future
    Perspectives 812
Acknowledgments 812
References 812

57. Encephalomyelopathies

Eric Lancaster

Introduction 817
Neurological Syndromes of Autoimmune
    Causation 818
    Cerebral Syndromes 818
    Ataxia 818
    Spinal Myelitis 818
    Stiff Person Syndrome 818
Systemic Immunopathic Disorders with
    Encephalitis and Myelitis 818
    Systemic Lupus Erythematosus 818
    Sarcoidosis 819
    Sjögren's Syndrome 819
    Behçet's Disease 820
Diseases with Autoantibodies to
    Cell-surface Channels, Receptors 820
    Neuromyelitis Optica (NMO; Devic's
        disease) 820
    Encephalitis with Antibodies to
        N-methyl-d-aspartate receptor (NMDAR) 821
    Anti-AMPAR 822
    Anti-GABA-B-R 822
    Group 1 Metabotropic Glutamate Receptors
        (mGluR1, mGluR5) 822
    Glycine Receptor (GlyR) 822
    Voltage-Gated Potassium Channel
        Complex (VGKC) 823
    LGI1 823
    Caspr2 824
    PCA-Tr 824
CNS Diseases with Autoantibodies to
    Intracellular Antigens 824
    GAD65 824
    Amphiphysin I 824
    Neuronal nuclear antigens (NNA) 825
Conclusions and Future Prospects 826
Acknowledgments 827
Abbreviations 827
References 827

58. Paraneoplastic Neurologic Syndromes

Paula K. Rauschkolb and Jerome B. Posner

Introduction 835
Pathogenesis 836
Diagnosis 837
Antibodies 838
    Nuclear/Nucleolar Antibodies 838
    Cytoplasmic Antibodies 841

Synaptic/Cell Surface Antibodies 842
Ion Channel Antibodies 843
Treatment 844
Clinical Syndromes 844
    Paraneoplastic Cerebellar
        Degeneration 844
    Paraneoplastic Encephalomyelitis 845
    Paraneoplastic Limbic Encephalitis 845
    Brainstem Encephalitis 846
    Myelitis 846
    Subacute Sensory Neuronopathy 846
    Autonomic Neuropathy 846
    Vision Loss 847
    Retinopathy 847
    Optic Neuropathy 847
    Stiff Person Syndrome 847
    Lambert–Eaton Myasthenic Syndrome 847
References 848

Part 11
Gastrointestinal System

59. Celiac Disease

Ludvig M. Sollid and Knut E.A. Lundin

Clinical, Pathologic, and Epidemiologic
    Features 855
    Clinical Features and Associated Disorders 855
    Pathology of the Intestinal Lesion 856
    Epidemiology 856
Autoimmune Features 857
    Autoantibodies 857
    Autoreactive Intraepithelial
        Lymphocytes (IELs) 859
Genetic Features 859
    HLA Genes 859
    Non-HLA Genes 859
Environmental Influences 860
    Gluten Proteins 860
    Other Environmental Factors 860
In Vivo and *In Vitro* Models 861
    Animal Models 861
    Organ Culture Assays 861
Pathogenic Mechanisms 861
    Gluten-reactive CD4$^+$ T Cells 861
    Role of Transglutaminase 2 861
    Gluten Antigen Presentation by
        Disease-associated DQ Molecules 862
    Mucosal Antigen-presenting Cells 864
    Effector Mechanisms Leading to Mucosal
        Alterations 864
Autoantibodies as Potential Immunologic
    Markers 864
    Serology 864
    Staining of Immune Complexes 865

Treatment and Outcome   865
  Current Treatment and Outcome   865
  Novel Therapeutic Options   865
Concluding Remarks—Future Prospects   866
Acknowledgments   866
References   866

60. Inflammatory Bowel Diseases

Vera Kandror Denmark and Lloyd Mayer

Introduction   873
History   873
Epidemiology and Environmental Factors   874
Clinical and Pathologic Features   874
  Disease Presentation   874
  Pathology   875
Genetics   875
Immunopathogenesis   876
  Epithelial Barrier and Innate Immunity   877
  Adaptive Immunity   877
  Host—Microbial Interactions   878
Biomarkers   878
  Fecal Markers   878
  Serologic Markers   879
Treatment   879
  Medical   879
  Surgical   881
Future Prospects   882
References   882

61. Hepatitis

*Diego Vergani, Ian R. Mackay, and Giorgina
Mieli-Vergani*

Clinical, Pathologic, and Epidemiologic
  Features   890
  Clinical Features   890
  Pathologic Features   891
  Epidemiologic Features   892
Autoimmune Features   892
Autoantibodies as Potential Immunologic
  Markers   893
Genetic Features   896
Animal Models   897
Pathologic Effector Mechanisms   898
Treatment and Outcome   900
  Standard Treatment   900
  Alternative Treatments   901
  Duration of Treatment   902
  Liver Transplantation   902
  Future Treatment Approaches   902
Concluding Remarks—Future Prospects   903
References   903

62. Primary Biliary Cirrhosis

Carlo Selmi, Ian R. Mackay, and M. Eric Gershwin

Clinical, Pathologic, and Epidemiologic
  Features   909
  History   909
  Diagnosis   909
  Pathology   910
  Clinical Features   910
  Epidemiology and Natural History   910
  Treatment   913
Autoimmune Features   913
Genetic Features   914
  Familial PBC: Twins and Relatives   914
  HLA Association   915
  Genome-wide Association Studies (GWAS)   915
  Epigenetic Effects   915
  Fetal Microchimerism   916
  Genes on the X Chromosome   916
Environmental Provocation of PBC   916
  Infections   916
  Xenobiotics   916
Experimental Animal Models   916
Pathologic Effector Mechanisms   917
Autoantibodies as Potential Immunologic
  Markers   918
Concluding Remarks—Future Prospects   919
References   920

63. Primary Sclerosing Cholangitis

*John E. Eaton, Jayant A. Talwalkar, and
Keith D. Lindor*

Epidemiology and Risk Factors   925
  Epidemiologic Features   925
  Risk Factors   925
Natural History, Clinical Features, and
  PSC-IBD   926
  Natural History and Clinical Features   926
  PSC-IBD   926
Diagnosis   926
  Biochemical Features   926
  Cholangiography   927
  Histology   927
PSC Subtypes and Pediatric PSC   927
  Small Duct PSC   927
  PSC-AIH   928
  Pediatric PSC   928
PSC-Associated Malignancies   929
  Colorectal Neoplasia   929
  Cholangiocarcinoma (CCA)   929
  Gallbladder Neoplasia   929
  Hepatocellular Carcinoma   929
Genetics   929

Animal Models 930
  Overview 930
  Summary of PSC Models 930
Potential Pathogenic Mechanisms 930
  Overview 930
  Bacterial Translocation, Pathogen-associated
    Molecular Patterns, and Innate Immune
    Response 930
  Adhesion Molecules, Lymphocyte Homing,
    and the Liver–Gut Axis 931
  Antibodies, Memory, and Regulatory
    T cells 931
  Transporter Defects and Bile Acids 931
  Autoimmune Features 932
Treatment 932
  Medical Therapy 932
  Therapeutic Endoscopy 932
  Liver Transplantation 932
Concluding Remarks 933
References 933

64. Autoimmune Pancreatitis and IgG4-related Disease

Shigeyuki Kawa, Hideaki Hamano, and Kendo Kiyosawa

Historical Background 937
Autoimmune Pancreatitis – Clinical,
  Pathologic, and Epidemiological Features 938
  Clinical Features 938
  Extra-pancreatic Lesions 939
  Pathological Features 939
  Epidemiologic Features 940
  Autoimmune Features 940
  Genetic Features 941
Animal Models 942
Pathological Mechanisms 942
Immunological Markers in Diagnosis 944
Treatment and Outcome 944
IgG4-related Disease 944
  Definition 944
  Historical Background 945
  Epidemiology 945
  Clinical Features of IgG4-related Disease 945
  Definite IgG4-related Diseases 945
  Possible IgG4-related Diseases 946
  Pathological Features 947
  Autoimmune Features, Genetic Features,
    Animal Models, and Pathological
    Mechanisms 947
  Diagnosis 947
  Treatment 947
Concluding Remarks: Future Prospects 948
References 948

Part 12
Skin Diseases

65. Autoimmune Bullous Skin Diseases— Pemphigus and Pemphigoid

Donna A. Culton, Zhi Liu, and Luis A. Diaz

Introduction 955
Pemphigus Vulgaris 956
  Clinical, Pathologic, and Epidemiologic
    Features 956
  Autoimmune Features 956
  Genetic Features 959
  In Vivo and In Vitro Models 959
  Pathologic Effector Mechanisms 959
  Autoantibodies as Potential Immunologic
    Markers 960
Pemphigus Foliaceus 960
  Clinical, Pathologic, and Epidemiologic
    Features 960
  Autoimmune Features 960
  Genetic Features 961
  In Vivo and In Vitro Models 961
  Pathologic Effector Mechanisms 961
  Autoantibodies as Potential Immunologic
    Markers 961
  Environmental Factors involved in Fogo
    Selvagem 961
Other Types of Pemphigus 962
  Paraneoplastic Pemphigus 962
  Drug-induced Pemphigus 962
  IgA Pemphigus 962
Bullous Pemphigoid 963
  Clinical, Pathologic, and Epidemiologic
    Features 963
  Autoimmune Features 963
  Genetic Features 963
  In Vivo and In Vitro Models 963
  Pathologic Effector Mechanisms 964
  Autoantibodies as Potential Immunologic
    Markers 964
Other Subepidermal Bullous
  Diseases 964
  Herpes Gestationis (Pemphigoid
    Gestationis) 964
  Cicatricial Pemphigoid 964
  Linear IgA Disease 965
  Epidermolysis Bullosa Acquisita 965
  Dermatitis Herpetiformis 965
Treatment of Autoimmune Bullous
  Diseases 965
Concluding Remarks 966
References 966

66. Non-bullous Skin Diseases: Alopecia Areata, Vitiligo, Psoriasis, and Urticaria

Stanca A. Birlea, Marc Serota, and David A. Norris

Alopecia Areata	971
Clinical, Pathologic, and Epidemiologic Features	971
Autoimmune Features	972
Genetic Features	973
In Vivo and *In Vitro* Models	973
Pathologic Effector Mechanisms	973
Autoantibodies as Potential Immunologic Markers	974
Concluding Remarks— Future Prospects	974
Vitiligo	974
Clinical, Pathologic, and Epidemiologic Features	974
Autoimmune Features	975
Genetic Features	976
In Vivo and *In Vitro* Models	976
Pathogenetic Mechanism	977
Autoantibodies as Potential Immunologic Markers	977
Concluding Remarks—Future Prospects	978
Psoriasis	978
Clinical, Pathologic, and Epidemiologic Features	978
Autoimmune Features	978
Genetic Features	980
In Vivo and *In Vitro* Models	980
Pathogenic Mechanism	981
Autoantibodies as Potential Immunologic Markers	981
Concluding Remarks—Future Prospects	982
Chronic Urticaria	982
Clinical, Pathologic, and Epidemiologic Features	982
Autoimmune Features	982
Genetic Features	983
In Vivo and *In Vitro* Models	983
Pathologic Effector Mechanisms	983
Autoantibodies as Potential Immunologic Markers	984
Concluding Remarks—Future Prospects	984
References	984

Part 13
Nephropathies and Reproductive System

67. Autoimmune Disease in the Kidney

Gloria A. Preston and Ronald J. Falk

Introduction	993
Are there Hallmarks of Autoimmune Disease?	993
Autoantibodies and Their Antigens	993
Hallmarks of Autoimmune Diseases of the Kidney	994
Autoreactive T and B Cells Evade Deletion	994
Pre-existence of Asymptomatic "Normal" Autoantibodies	996
Hyperactivity of Fc–FcR Pathway	997
Antigenic Alterations of "Self" Proteins	997
Susceptibility to Environmental Impacts	999
Microbial Infections	999
Summary	1001
Future Directions	1001
References	1001

68. Autoimmune Orchitis and Autoimmune Oophoritis

Livia Lustig, Claudia Rival, and Kenneth S.K. Tung

Introduction	1007
Experimental Autoimmune Disease of the Testis	1008
Autoimmune Orchitis in the Dark Mink	1008
Autoimmune Orchitis in Rats Expressing Transgenic Human HLA B27 and Human β2 Microglobulin	1008
Post-vasectomy Autoimmune Orchitis in Mice with Treg Depletion and Post-vasectomy Tolerance to Testis Antigens	1008
Autoimmune Orchitis Associated with Viral Infection	1009
Autoimmune Orchitis in Day 3 Thymectomized (d3tx) Mice	1009
Classical Experimental Autoimmune Orchitis Induced by Immunization with Testis Antigen in Adjuvant	1009
Clinical Autoimmune Disease of the Testis	1011
Idiopathic Male Infertility	1011
Infertility and ASA Coexist with Other Autoimmune Diseases	1012
Vasectomy, Sperm Granuloma, and Cystic Fibrosis	1012
Orchitis Associated with Virus Infections	1012
Experimental Autoimmune Disease of the Ovary	1013
Spontaneous Autoimmune Ovarian Disease (AOD) in AIRE Null Mice	1013
AOD in Day 3 Thymectomized (d3tx) Mice	1013
AOD in Neonatal Mice by Maternal Antibody to Murine ZP3	1014
Classical Experimental Autoimmune Oophoritis	1014

Clinical Autoimmune Disease of the Ovary   1015
Concluding Remarks   1016
Acknowledgments   1016
References   1016

Part 14
Cardiovascular System and Lungs

69. Rheumatic Fever and Rheumatic Heart Disease

L. Guilherme and J. Kalil

Clinical, Pathological, and Epidemiologic
   Features   1023
Autoimmune Features   1024
Genetic Features   1024
   Innate Immune Response   1024
   Adaptive Immune Response   1025
   Both Innate and Adaptive Immune
      Response   1027
In Vivo and *In Vitro* Models   1027
   In Vivo Model of Myocarditis and
      Valvulitis   1027
   In Vitro Model of Rheumatic Heart
      Disease Autoimmune Reactions   1028
Pathologic Effector Mechanisms   1028
Autoantibodies as Potential Immunologic
   Markers   1029
Concluding Remarks—Future Prospects   1030
References   1030

70. Myocarditis and Dilated Cardiomyopathy

Noel R. Rose and Ziya Kaya

Historical Background   1033
Clinical, Pathologic, and Epidemiologic
   Features   1033
   Myocarditis   1033
   Dilated Cardiomyopathy   1035
Autoimmune Features and Immunologic
   Markers   1037
   Circulating Antibodies   1037
   Immunofluorescence   1037
   Western Immunoblot   1038
   Immunoassay with Defined Antigens   1038
   Immunologic Assessment of Biopsies   1038
Genetic Features   1039
Environmental Features   1039
Animal Models and Pathogenic
   Mechanisms   1040
Treatment and Outcome   1043
Personal Thoughts   1044
Acknowledgments   1044
References   1044

71. Atherosclerosis

*Ban-Hock Toh, Tin Kyaw, Peter Tipping,
and Alex Bobik*

Introduction   1049
Development of Atherosclerotic Lesions   1050
Mouse Models of Atherosclerosis   1050
Culprit Autoantigens   1050
   Oxidized Low-density Lipoprotein
      (oxLDL)   1050
   Heat Shock Protein 60 (HSP60)   1050
   β2 Glycoprotein 1 (β2-GP1)   1050
Immune Responses in Atherosclerosis   1051
   Innate Immunity in Atherosclerosis   1051
   Adaptive Immunity in Atherosclerosis   1054
   Other Key Cellular Players   1056
   Immune System Activation   1056
   Experimental Therapeutics: A Protective
      "Vaccine" for Atherosclerosis   1059
   Implications for Clinical Translation   1060
References   1061

72. Necrotizing Arteritis and Small Vessel Vasculitis

J. Charles Jennette and Ronald J. Falk

Historical Background   1067
   Necrotizing Arteritis   1067
   Purpura and Small Vessel Vasculitis   1069
Polyarteritis Nodosa   1070
   Clinical, Epidemiologic, and Pathologic
      Features   1070
   Autoimmune Features   1070
   Genetic Features and Environmental
      Influences   1070
   In Vivo Models   1071
   Pathologic Effector Mechanisms   1071
   Autoantibodies as Potential Immunologic
      Markers   1071
Kawasaki's Disease   1071
   Clinical, Pathologic, and Epidemiologic
      Features   1071
   Autoimmune Features   1072
   Genetic Features and Environmental
      Influences   1072
   In Vivo Models   1072
   Pathologic Effector Mechanisms   1072
   Autoantibodies as Potential Immunologic
      Markers   1073
ANCA-Associated Vasculitis (AAV)   1073
   Clinical, Pathologic, and Epidemiologic
      Features   1073
   Autoimmune Features   1074
   Genetic Features   1075
   Environmental Influences   1075
   In Vivo Models   1076

Pathologic Effector Mechanisms 1076
Autoantibodies as Immunologic Markers 1077
Cryoglobulinemic Vasculitis 1079
Clinical, Pathologic, and Epidemiologic
Features 1079
Autoimmune Features 1079
Genetic Features and Environmental
Influences 1079
In Vivo Models 1080
Pathologic Effector Mechanisms 1080
Autoantibodies as Immunologic Markers 1080
IgA Vasculitis (Henoch–Schönlein Purpura) 1080
Clinical, Pathologic, and Epidemiologic
Features 1080
Autoimmune Features 1081
Genetic Features and Environmental
Influences 1081
In Vivo Models 1081
Pathologic Effector Mechanisms 1081
Autoantibodies as Potential Immunologic
Markers 1081
Concluding Remarks—Future Prospects 1082
References 1082

73. Large and Medium Vessel Vasculitides

Cornelia M. Weyand and Jörg J. Goronzy

**Vasculitides of Large and Medium-sized
Blood Vessels** 1087
Giant Cell Arteritis 1087
Historical Background 1088
Clinical, Pathologic, and Epidemiologic
Features 1089
The Vascular Lesion 1091
Epidemiology 1091
Genetic Features 1091
Pathogenic Mechanisms 1091
T Cells and Antigen-Presenting Cells in
Giant Cell Arteritis 1092
Macrophages in Giant Cell Arteritis 1093
Intimal Hyperplasia 1094
Immuno-stromal Interactions Promoting
Vasculitis 1094
The Systemic Inflammatory Syndrome 1094
Treatment, Monitoring, and Outcome 1095
Takayasu's Arteritis 1096
Historical Background 1096
Clinical, Pathologic, and Epidemiologic
Features 1096
Genetic Features 1098
Pathogenic Mechanisms 1098
Treatment and Outcome 1098
Concluding Remarks—Future Perspectives 1099
Acknowledgment 1100
References 1100

**74. Idiopathic and Autoimmune Interstitial
Lung Disease**

Brian Gelbman and Ronald G. Crystal

Introduction 1105
History 1105
Cryptogenic Organizing Pneumonia 1105
Idiopathic Pulmonary Fibrosis 1106
**Clinical, Pathological, and Epidemiological
Features** 1106
Cryptogenic Organizing Pneumonia 1106
Idiopathic Pulmonary Fibrosis 1107
Autoimmune Features 1109
Cryptogenic Organizing Pneumonia 1109
Idiopathic Pulmonary Fibrosis 1110
Genetic Features 1112
Cryptogenic Organizing Pneumonia 1112
Idiopathic Pulmonary Fibrosis 1112
In Vivo and *In Vitro* **Models** 1113
Cryptogenic Organizing Pneumonia 1113
Idiopathic Pulmonary Fibrosis 1113
Pathologic Effector Mechanisms 1113
Cryptogenic Organizing Pneumonia 1113
Idiopathic Pulmonary Fibrosis 1114
Treatment and Outcome 1116
Cryptogenic Organizing Pneumonia 1116
Idiopathic Pulmonary Fibrosis 1116
Conclusions 1117
Acknowledgments 1118
References 1118

Part 15
Unclassified Expressions of Autoimmunity

75. Cameos: Candidates and Curiosities

Ian R. Mackay

Introduction 1127
**Autoimmune/Inflammatory Syndrome
Induced by Adjuvants** 1127
Autonomic Neuropathy 1128
Birdshot Retinopathy 1129
Cystitis, Interstitial 1129
Endometriosis 1130
Epilepsy 1131
Fatigue Syndrome 1131
Folate Deficiency 1132
Lichen Sclerosus 1132
Lymphocytic Mastitis 1133
Metabolic–Genetic Storage Diseases 1133
Movement Disorders 1133
Narcolepsy 1134
Osteoarthritis 1134

Contents

Parathyroid Disease 1135
Polychondritis, Relapsing 1136
Prostatitis 1136
Sarcoidosis 1137
References 1137

76. Autoantibodies Against Cytokines

John W. Schrader and James W. Goding

Introduction 1142
Autoantibodies Against Cytokines
  in Humans 1142
  Autoantibodies Against Type I and Type II
    Interferon 1142
  Autoantibodies Against IL-1α 1142
  Autoantibodies Against Tumor Necrosis
    Factor (TNF) 1142
  Autoantibodies Against IL-6 1142
  Autoantibodies against Granulocyte-
    Macrophage Colony-Stimulating
    Factor 1143
Pathogenicity of Autoantibodies Against
  Cytokines—General Comments 1143
  Autoantibodies Against GM-CSF Cause
    Idiopathic Pulmonary Alveolar
    Proteinosis 1143
  Autoantibodies Against Erythropoietin
    Cause Pure Red Cell Aplasia 1144
  Autoantibodies Against IFN-γ Cause
    Mycobacteria Infections 1144
  Autoantibodies Against IL-17A, IL-17F,
    and IL-22 Correlate with Mucocutaneous
    Candidiasis in Autoimmune-
    Polyendocrinopathy-Candidiasis-
    Ectodermal Dystrophy 1144
  Opportunistic Infections in Patients
    with a Thymoma 1144
  Autoantibodies Against the Bioactivity
    of Osteoprotegerin 1144
  Autoantibodies Against IL-8 1145
  Autoantibodies Against IL-1α 1145
  Autoantibodies Against IL-6 1145
  What Is the Therapeutic Benefit of
    Autoantibodies against Cytokines from
    Pharmaceutically Prepared
    Immunoglobulin? 1145
Are Anti-Cytokine Autoantibodies Against
  a Range of Cytokines in all Healthy
  Humans? 1145
Analysis of a Panel of Neutralizing
  Monoclonal Antibodies to GM-CSF 1146
  The Advantage of Studying Monoclonal
    Autoantibodies with Natural and
    Authentic H and L Chain Pairing 1146
  The Autoantibodies Against GM-CSF
    Were all Polyclonal, Excluding a
    "Forbidden B Cell Clone" 1146
No Preferred V-gene Usage in
    Autoantibodies to GM-CSF 1147
  Multiple Epitopes Recognized by
    Pathogenic Monoclonal Autoantibodies
    to GM-CSF 1147
  Mechanism of Pathogenicity of
    Monoclonal Autoantibodies to GM-CSF 1147
  Inhibitory Activity Is Strengthened by
    Formation of Stable High-avidity
    Complexes Comprising Multiple
    Antibodies Binding to Multiple
    Epitopes 1147
  Somatic Mutation of Autoantibodies to
    GM-CSF 1148
  Is Antibody Autoreactivity a Consequence
    of Somatic Mutation? 1148
  Could Autoantibodies Arise in Response
    to a B Cell Epitope on a Pathogen
    Antigen that Mimics a Self-antigen
    GM-CSF? 1148
Autoantibodies to GM-CSF: Implications
  for B Cell Tolerance to Cytokines 1149
  General B Cell Tolerance 1149
  Antibodies Binding to Multiple Epitopes
    on GM-CSF Suggest that B Cells Lack
    Tolerance to Cytokines 1149
Role of T Cells and the Thymus in
  Pathogenesis of Autoantibodies
  to Cytokines 1150
  General T Cell Tolerance 1150
  Role of the AIRE Gene in T Cell Tolerance 1150
  T Cell Tolerance to Cytokines 1150
  T Cell Tolerance Is Incomplete and
    Breakable 1150
  Autoantibodies against Cytokines in
    APECED 1151
  Autoantibodies against Cytokines in
    Patients with Thymoma 1152
Induction of Autoantibodies as a
  Consequence of Therapy with
  Recombinant Cytokines 1152
Conclusions and Future Prospects 1153
References 1154

Part 16
Diagnosis, Prevention, and Therapy

77. Autoantibody Assays: Performance, Interpretation, and Standardization

Marvin J. Fritzler

Introduction 1161
Spectrum of Autoantibodies 1163
Assays and Technologies for Autoantibody
  Testing 1165

Clinical Interpretation and Application of
    Autoantibody Testing   1166
Clinical Practice Guidelines   1167
Laboratory Reports, Electronic Medical
    Records, and Cost Analysis   1167
Standardization and Quality Assurance   1170
Conclusions and Future Prospects   1170
References   1170

78. Prediction of Autoimmune Disease

*George S. Eisenbarth, Jennifer Barker,
and Roberto Gianani*

Type 1 Diabetes Mellitus as a Model for
    Prediction of Autoimmune Disease   1177
The Pancreatic Pathology in Type 1
    Diabetes Mellitus and Islet
    Autoimmunity   1177
    Genetics   1179
Laboratory Markers of Autoimmunity
    (Including Autoantibodies and T Cell
    Assays)   1179
    Metabolic Studies   1181
Organ-Specific Autoimmune Diseases   1182
    Thyroid   1182
    Addison's Disease   1183
    Celiac Disease   1183
    Multiple Sclerosis   1184
Non-Organ Specific Disease   1184
    Rheumatoid Arthritis   1184
    Systemic Lupus Erythematosus   1185
Conclusions   1185
Acknowledgments   1186
References   1186

79. Prevention of Autoimmune Disease: The Type 1 Diabetes Paradigm

Leonard C. Harrison and John M. Wentworth

Introduction   1191
People at Risk for Type 1 Diabetes   1196
Primary Prevention   1198
    Diet and the Intestinal Environment   1198
    Viruses   1199
Secondary Prevention   1199
    Mucosa-mediated Antigen-specific
        Tolerance   1200
    Trials of Islet Autoantigen-specific
        Vaccination in Humans   1200

Epilogue   1203
Acknowledgments   1203
References   1203

80. Treatment of Autoimmune Disease: Established Therapies

Bevra H. Hahn and Jennifer K. King

Principles of Immune Suppression   1209
General Considerations   1211
Non-Specific Anti-Inflammatory Drugs   1211
    NSAIDs   1211
    Glucocorticoids   1212
Established Treatments of Rheumatic
    Diseases   1212
    Antimalarials   1212
    Sulfasalazine   1213
    Leflunomide   1213
    Methotrexate   1213
    Cyclophosphamide   1214
    Mycophenolate Mofetil (Cellcept)   1214
    Azathioprine (Imuran)   1215
    Cyclosporin A   1215
Other Treatment Options   1216
    B Cell Suppressive Therapies   1216
    IVIG   1216
Moving Towards Biological and Molecular
    Therapies   1216
References   1217

81. Treatment of Autoimmune Disease: Biological and Molecular Therapies

Lucienne Chatenoud

Introduction   1221
The Therapeutic Armamentarium Derived
    from Biotechnology   1221
    Monoclonal Antibodies (mAbs)   1221
    Other Soluble Receptors and Protein
        Fusion Conjugates   1232
Soluble Autoantigens   1232
Bone Marrow Transplantation   1232
Cell Therapy and Gene Therapy   1234
    Cell Therapy   1234
    Gene Therapy   1235
Perspectives for the Future   1235
References   1235

Index   1247

Nancy Agmon-Levin, The Zabludowicz Center for Autoimmune Diseases, Sheba Medical Center, Tel-Hashomer, affiliated to Tel Aviv University, Israel

S. Sohail Ahmed, Global Clinical Sciences, Vaccines Research, Novartis Vaccines & Diagnostics, Siena, Italy

Youssif M. Ali, Department of Infection, Immunity and Inflammation, Faculty of Medicine, University of Leicester, Leicester, UK

Martin Aringer, University Clinical Center Carl Gustav Carus, Dresden, Germany

Jean-François Bach, Institut National de la Santé et de la Recherché Médicale, Paris, France

Jennifer Barker, Barbara Davis Center for Childhood Diabetes, Denver, CO, USA

Robert N. Barker, Section of Immunology and Infection, Division of Applied Medicine, Institute of Medical Sciences, University of Aberdeen, Foresterhill, Aberdeen, UK

Alan G. Baxter, Comparative Genomics Centre, James Cook University, Townsville, Queensland, Australia

Corrado Betterle, Endocrine Unit, Department of Medicine, University of Padova, Padova, Italy

Stanca A. Birlea, Department of Dermatology, University of Colorado School of Medicine, Anschutz Medical Campus, University of Colorado Denver, CO, USA

Niklas K. Björkström, Center for Infectious Medicine, Department of Medicine, Karolinska Institutet, Karolinska University Hospital, Stockholm, Sweden; Liver Immunology Laboratory, Department of Medicine, Karolinska Institutet, Karolinska University Hospital, Stockholm, Sweden

Paul A. Blair, Centre for Rheumatology, Division of Medicine, University College London, London, UK

Alex Bobik, Vascular Biology and Atherosclerosis Laboratory, Baker IDI Heart and Diabetes Institute, Victoria, Australia

Nabeel H. Borazan, Division of Rheumatology, University of California, Los Angeles, CA, USA

Xavier Bosch, Department of Internal Medicine, Hospital Clinic, Institut d'Investigacions Biomèdiques August Pi i Sunyer, University of Barcelona, Barcelona, Spain; Sjögren's Syndrome Research Group, Laboratory of Autoimmune Diseases Josep Font, Department of Autoimmune Diseases, Hospital Clinic, Institut d'Investigacions Biomèdiques August Pi i Sunyer, University of Barcelona, Barcelona, Spain

Robert A. Brodsky, Division of Hematology, Department of Medicine and The Sidney Kimmel Comprehensive Cancer Center at Johns Hopkins, Baltimore, MD, USA

Yenan T. Bryceson, Center for Infectious Medicine, Department of Medicine, Karolinska Institutet, Karolinska University Hospital, Stockholm, Sweden

Patrick R. Burkett, Center for Neurologic Diseases, Brigham and Women's Hospital, Harvard Medical School, Boston, MA, USA; Pulmonary and Critical Care Division, Department of Medicine, Brigham and Women's Hospital, Boston, MA, USA

James B. Bussel, Departments of Pediatrics, Medicine, and Obstetrics and Gynecology, New York Presbyterian Hospital, Weill Cornell Medical Center, New York, NY, USA

Helmut Butzkueven, Department of Medicine, Royal Melbourne, Parkville, Victoria, Australia

Roberto Caricchio, Department of Medicine, Rheumatology Section, Temple University School of Medicine, Philadelphia, PA, USA

Livia Casciola-Rosen, Johns Hopkins University School of Medicine, Division of Rheumatology, Mason Lord Building Center Tower, Baltimore, MD, USA

Patrizio Caturegli, Department of Pathology, The Johns Hopkins University, Baltimore, MD, USA

Lucienne Chatenoud, Université Paris Descartes, Sorbonne Paris Cité, Paris, France, INSERM U1013, Necker Hospital, Paris, France

Philip L. Cohen, Department of Medicine, Rheumatology Section, Temple University School of Medicine, Philadelphia, PA, USA

Ken Coppieters, Type 1 Diabetes Research and Development Center, Novo Nordisk, Seattle, WA, USA

Sarah Q. Crome, Campbell Family Institute, Ontario Cancer Institute, Departments of Medical Biophysics and Immunology, Toronto, ON, Canada

Ronald G. Crystal, Department of Genetic Medicine, Weill Medical College of Cornell University, New York, NY, USA; Division of Pulmonary and Critical Care Medicine, Weill Medical College of Cornell University, New York, NY, USA

Donna A. Culton, Department of Dermatology, University of North Carolina at Chapel Hill, Chapel Hill, NC, USA

Monica D. Dalal, The Laboratory of Immunology, National Eye Institute, National Institutes of Health, Bethesda, MD, USA

Chella S. David, Department of Immunology and Rheumatology, Mayo Clinic, Rochester, MN, USA

Anne Davidson, Center for Autoimmunity and Musculoskeletal Diseases, Feinstein Institute for Medical Research, Manhasset, NY, USA

Ahmed J. Delli, Lund University, Clinical Research Center, Department of Clinical Sciences, Skåne University Hospital SUS, Malmö, Sweden

Peter J. Delves, Department of Immunology, Division of Infection and Immunity, University College London, London, UK

Vera Kandror Denmark, Newton Wellesley Hospital, Newton, MA, USA

Betty Diamond, Center for Autoimmunity and Musculoskeletal Diseases, Feinstein Institute for Medical Research, Manhasset, NY, USA

Luis A. Diaz, Department of Dermatology, University of North Carolina at Chapel Hill, Chapel Hill, NC, USA

John E. Eaton, Mayo Clinic, Rochester, MN, USA

George S. Eisenbarth, Barbara Davis Center for Childhood Diabetes, Denver, CO, USA

Ronald J. Falk, UNC Kidney Center, Division of Nephrology and Hypertension, Department of Medicine, University of North Carolina at Chapel Hill, Chapel Hill, NC, USA

Judith Field, Florey Institute of Neuroscience and Mental Health, Melbourne Brain Centre, The University of Melbourne, Parkville, Victoria, Australia

Thomas A. Fleisher, Department of Laboratory Medicine, NIH Clinical Center, National Institutes of Health, Bethesda, MD, USA

George E. Fragoulis, Department of Pathophysiology, University of Athens, Athens, Greece

Marvin J. Fritzler, Faculty of Medicine, University of Calgary, Calgary, Canada

Daniel E. Furst, Division of Rheumatology, University of California, Los Angeles, CA, USA

Stefania Gallucci, Department of Microbiology and Immunology, Temple University School of Medicine, Philadelphia, PA, USA

Brian Gelbman, Division of Pulmonary and Critical Care Medicine, Weill Medical College of Cornell University, New York, NY, USA

M. Eric Gershwin, Division of Rheumatology, Allergy, and Clinical Immunology, University of California at Davis, Davis, CA, USA

Daniel R. Getts, Department of Microbiology-Immunology and Interdepartmental Immunobiology Center, Northwestern University, Feinberg School of Medicine, Chicago, IL, USA

Meghann Teague Getts, Department of Microbiology-Immunology and Interdepartmental Immunobiology Center, Northwestern University, Feinberg School of Medicine, Chicago, IL, USA

Roberto Gianani, Barbara Davis Center for Childhood Diabetes, Denver, CO, USA

Paul A. Gleeson, Department of Biochemistry and Molecular Biology, Bio21 Molecular Science and Biotechnology Institute, The University of Melbourne, Parkville, Victoria, Australia

James W. Goding, Department of Physiology, Monash University, Victoria, Australia

Siamon Gordon, Sir William Dunn School of Pathology, University of Oxford, Oxford, UK,

Jörg J. Goronzy, Department of Medicine, Division of Immunology and Rheumatology, Stanford University School of Medicine, Stanford, CA, USA

Judith M. Greer, The University of Queensland, UQ Centre for Clinical Research, Royal Brisbane and Women's Hospital, Brisbane, Queensland, Australia

Berengere Gruson, Department of Hematology, Centre Hospitalier Universitaire d'Amiens, Amiens, France

L. Guilherme, Heart Institute (InCor), School of Medicine, University of São Paulo, São Paulo, Brazil; Immunology Investigation Institute, National Institute for Science and Technology, University of São Paulo, São Paulo, Brazil

Angelika Gutenberg, Department of Neurosurgery, Medical University of Mainz, Mainz, Germany

David A. Hafler, Department of Neurology, Yale University School of Medicine, New Haven CT, USA

Bevra H. Hahn, University of California, Los Angeles, Division of Rheumatology, Rehab Center, Los Angeles, CA, USA

Hideaki Hamano, Department of Medical Information, Shinshu University School of Medicine, Matsumoto, Japan

Sara R. Hamilton, Campbell Family Institute, Ontario Cancer Institute, Departments of Medical Biophysics and Immunology, Toronto, ON, Canada

Leonard C. Harrison, Walter & Eliza Hall Institute of Medical Research, Royal Parade, Parkville, Victoria, Australia

Amanda L. Hernandez, Department of Neurology, Interdepartmental Neuroscience Program, Yale University School of Medicine, New Haven CT, USA

Eystein Husebye, Department of Clinical Science, University of Bergen, Bergen, Norway; Department of Medicine, Haukeland University Hospital, Bergen, Norway

J. Charles Jennette, Department of Pathology and Laboratory Medicine, University of North Carolina, Chapel Hill, NC, USA

Richard J. Jones, Division of Hematology, Department of Medicine and The Sidney Kimmel Comprehensive Cancer Center at Johns Hopkins, Baltimore, MD, USA

Margaret A. Jordan, Comparative Genomics Centre, James Cook University, Townsville, Queensland, Australia

J. Kalil, Clinical Immunology and Allergy Division, School of Medicine, University of São Paulo, São Paulo, Brazil; Heart Institute (InCor), School of Medicine, University of São Paulo, São Paulo, Brazil; Immunology Investigation Institute, National Institute for Science and Technology, University of São Paulo, São Paulo, Brazil

Christoph Königs, J.W. Goethe University, Department of Pediatrics, Clinical and Molecular Hemostasis, Frankfurt am Main, Germany

Shigeyuki Kawa, Center for Health, Safety and Environmental Management, Shinshu University, Matsumoto, Japan

Ziya Kaya, Department of Cardiology, University of Heidelberg, Heidelberg, Germany

Jennifer K. King, University of California, Los Angeles, Division of Rheumatology, Rehab Center, Los Angeles, CA, USA

Nicholas J.C. King, The Discipline of Pathology, School of Medical Sciences, Bosch Institute, The University of Sydney, Sydney, NSW, Australia

Kendo Kiyosawa, Department of Medicine, Nagano Red Cross Hospital, Nagano, Japan

Mitchell Kronenberg, La Jolla Institute for Allergy and Immunology (LIAI), San Diego, CA, USA

Vijay K. Kuchroo, Center for Neurologic Diseases, Brigham and Women's Hospital, Harvard Medical School, Boston, MA, USA

Tin Kyaw, Centre for Inflammatory Diseases, Department of Medicine, Southern Clinical School, Faculty of Medicine, Nursing and Health Sciences, Monash University, Victoria, Australia

Jan Lünemann, Institute of Experimental Immunology, University of Zürich, Switzerland

Robert G. Lahita, Newark Beth Israel Medical Center, University of Medicine and Dentistry, Newark, NJ, USA

Parviz Lalezari, Montefiore Medical Center and Department of Medicine and Pathology, Albert Einstein College of Medicine, New York, NY, USA

Paul-Henri Lambert, Center of Vaccinology, University of Geneva, Switzerland

Eric Lancaster, The Hospital of the University of Pennsylvania, Department of Neurology, Philadelphia, PA, USA

Arian Laurence, National Institute for Arthritis and Musculoskeletal and Skin Diseases, NIH, Bethesda, MD, USA

Youjin Lee, Center for Neurologic Diseases, Brigham and Women's Hospital, Harvard Medical School, Boston, MA, USA

Michael Lenardo, Molecular Development Section, Laboratory of Immunology, National Institute of Allergy and Infectious Diseases, National Institutes of Health, Bethesda, MD, USA

Åke Lernmark, Lund University, Clinical Research Center, Department of Clinical Sciences, Skåne University Hospital SUS, Malmö, Sweden

Arnold I. Levinson, Associate Dean for Research, Perelman School of Medicine, University of Pennsylvania, Philadelphia, PA, USA

Keith D. Lindor, Arizona State University, Phoenix, AZ, USA

Zhi Liu, Department of Dermatology, University of North Carolina at Chapel Hill, Chapel Hill, NC, USA

Hans-Gustaf Ljunggren, Center for Infectious Medicine, Department of Medicine, Karolinska Institutet, Karolinska University Hospital, Stockholm, Sweden

Claudio Lunardi, Department of Medicine, University Hospital, Verona, Italy

Knut E.A. Lundin, Centre for Immune Regulation and Department of Immunology, Department of Medicine, University of Oslo and Oslo University Hospital, Oslo, Norway; Department of Gastroenterology, Oslo University Hospital-Rikshospitalet, Oslo, Norway

Jan Lünemann, Institute of Experimental Immunology, University of Zürich, Switzerland

Michael P.T. Lunn, National Hospital for Neurology and Neurosurgery, Queen Square, London, UK

Isabella Lupi, Department of Endocrinology and Metabolism, University of Pisa, Pisa, Italy

Livia Lustig, Instituto de Investigaciones Biomédicas, Facultad de Medicina, Universidad de Buenos Aires, Paraguay, Argentina

Christian Münz, Institute of Experimental Immunology, University of Zürich, Switzerland

Charles R. Mackay, School of Biological Sciences, Monash University, Clayton, Victoria, Australia

Ian R. Mackay, Department of Biochemistry and Molecular Biology, Monash University, Clayton, Victoria, Australia

Clara Malattia, Pediatria II, Reumatologia, Istituto Giannina Gaslini, Genova e Dipartimento di Pediatria, Università of Genova, Genova, Italy

Ashutosh Mangalam, Department of Immunology and Rheumatology, Mayo Clinic, Rochester, MN, USA

Alberto Martini, Pediatria II, Reumatologia, Istituto Giannina Gaslini, Genova e Dipartimento di Pediatria, Università of Genova, Genova, Italy

Claudia Mauri, Centre for Rheumatology, Division of Medicine, University College London, London, UK

Clio P. Mavragani, Department of Experimental Physiology, University of Athens, Athens, Greece

Lloyd Mayer, Immunology Institute, Mount Sinai School of Medicine, New York, NY, USA

Pamela A. McCombe, The University of Queensland, UQ Centre for Clinical Research, Royal Brisbane and Women's Hospital, Brisbane, Queensland, Australia

Fritz Melchers, Max Planck Institute for Infection Biology, Berlin, Germany

Giorgina Mieli-Vergani, Paediatric Liver, GI & Nutrition Centre, King's College London School of Medicine at King's College Hospital, London, UK

Frederick W. Miller, Environmental Autoimmunity Group, Office of Clinical Research, National Institute of Environmental Health Sciences, National Institutes of Health, Bethesda, MD, USA

Stephen D. Miller, Department of Microbiology-Immunology and Interdepartmental Immunobiology Center, Northwestern University, Feinberg School of Medicine, Chicago, IL, USA

Masayuki Mizui, Division of Rheumatology, Beth Israel Deaconess Medical Center, Harvard Medical School, Boston, MA, USA

Jenny Mjösberg, Center for Infectious Medicine, Department of Medicine, Karolinska Institutet, Karolinska University Hospital, Stockholm, Sweden

Haralampos M. Moutsopoulos, Department of Pathophysiology, University of Athens, Athens, Greece

David A. Norris, Department of Dermatology, University of Colorado School of Medicine, Anschutz Medical Campus, University of Colorado Denver, CO, USA

Robert B. Nussenblatt, The Laboratory of Immunology, National Eye Institute, National Institutes of Health, Bethesda, MD, USA

Kevin C. O'Connor, Department of Neurology, Human and Translational Immunology Program, Yale University School of Medicine, New Haven CT, USA

Pamela S. Ohashi, Campbell Family Institute, Ontario Cancer Institute, Departments of Medical Biophysics and Immunology, Toronto, ON, Canada

Meredith O'Keeffe, Centre for Immunology, Burnet Institute, Melbourne, Victoria, Australia, Department of Immunology, Monash University, Clayton, Victoria, Australia

Joao Bosco Oliveira, Instituto de Medicina Integral Prof. Fernando Figueira- IMIP, Recife, PE Brazil

Joost J. Oppenheim, Laboratory of Molecular Immunoregulation, Cancer and Inflammation, National Cancer Institute, National Institutes of Health, Frederick, MD, USA

Alicia Perez-Arroyo, Université Paris Descartes, Sorbonne Paris Cité, Faculté de Médecine, Paris, France

Anneli Peters, Center for Neurologic Diseases, Brigham and Women's Hospital, Harvard Medical School, Boston, MA, USA

Pärt Peterson, Molecular Pathology, University of Tartu, Tartu, Estonia

Annette Plüddemann, Department of Primary Care Health Sciences, University of Oxford, Oxford, UK

Jerome B. Posner, Department of Neurology, Memorial Sloan-Kettering Cancer Center, New York, NY, USA

Gloria A. Preston, UNC Kidney Center, Division of Nephrology and Hypertension, Department of Medicine, University of North Carolina at Chapel Hill, Chapel Hill, NC, USA

Antonio Puccetti, Institute Giannina Gaslini and Department of Experimental Medicine, University of Genova, Genova, Italy

Kristen Radford, Cancer Immunotherapies Group, Mater Medical Research Institute, South Brisbane, Australia

Manuel Ramos-Casals, Sjögren's Syndrome Research Group, Laboratory of Autoimmune Diseases Josep Font, Department of Autoimmune Diseases, Hospital Clinic, Institut d'Investigacions Biomèdiques August Pi i Sunyer, University of Barcelona, Barcelona, Spain

V. Koneti Rao, Molecular Development Section, Laboratory of Immunology, National Institute of Allergy and Infectious Diseases, National Institutes of Health, Bethesda, MD, USA

Paula K. Rauschkolb, Department of Neurology, Memorial Sloan-Kettering Cancer Center, New York, NY, USA

Venkat Reddy, Centre for Rheumatology, Division of Medicine, University College London, London, UK

Kurt Redlich, Division of Rheumatology, Department of Medicine 3, Medical University of Vienna, Austria

Claudia Rival, Beirne Carter Center for Immunology Research and Department of Pathology, University of Virginia, Charlottesville, VA, USA

Noel R. Rose, Departments of Pathology and of Molecular Microbiology and Immunology, The Johns Hopkins Schools of Medicine and Public Health, Baltimore, MD, USA

Antony Rosen, Johns Hopkins University School of Medicine, Division of Rheumatology, Mason Lord Building Center Tower, Baltimore, MD, USA

John W. Schrader, The Biomedical Research Centre, University of British Columbia, Vancouver, Canada

Wilhelm J. Schwaeble, Department of Infection, Immunity and Inflammation, Faculty of Medicine, University of Leicester, Leicester, UK

Carlo Selmi, Division of Rheumatology and Clinical Immunology, Humanitas Clinical and Research Center, University of Milan, Italy; Division of Rheumatology, Allergy, and Clinical Immunology, University of California at Davis, Davis, CA, USA

H. Nida Sen, The Laboratory of Immunology, National Eye Institute, National Institutes of Health, Bethesda, MD, USA

Marc Serota, Department of Dermatology, University of Colorado School of Medicine, Anschutz Medical Campus, University of Colorado Denver, CO, USA

Kazim A. Sheikh, University of Texas Medical School at Houston, TX, USA

Yehuda Shoenfeld, Incumbent of the Laura Schwarz-Kipp Chair for Research of Autoimmune Diseases, Sackler Faculty of Medicine, Tel Aviv University, Israel; The Zabludowicz Center for Autoimmune Diseases, Sheba Medical Center, Tel-Hashomer, affiliated to Tel Aviv University, Israel

Ken Shortman, Immunology Division, The Walter and Eliza Hall Institute, Parkville, Australia and Centre for Immunology, Burnet Institute, Melbourne, Victoria, Australia; Centre for Biomedical Research, Burnet Institute, Melbourne, Victoria, Australia

Joachim Sieper, Department of Gastroenterology, Infection Medicine and Rheumatology, Charité Campus Benjamin Franklin; Charité University Medicine Berlin, Berlin, Germany

Arthur M. Silverstein, Institute of the History of Medicine, Johns Hopkins Medical School, Baltimore, MD, USA

Robert B. Sim, Department of Infection, Immunity and Inflammation, Faculty of Medicine, University of Leicester, Leicester, UK

Anna Simon, Department of Medicine, Radboud University Nijmegen Medical Centre; Nijmegen Centre for Infection, Inflammation and Immunity Centre for Immunodeficiency and Autoinflammation; Nijmegen Centre for Molecular Life Sciences, Nijmegen, The Netherlands

Josef S. Smolen, Division of Rheumatology, Department of Medicine 3, Medical University of Vienna, Austria; Second Department of Medicine, Hietzing Hospital, Vienna, Austria

Ludvig M. Sollid, Centre for Immune Regulation and Department of Immunology, University of Oslo and Oslo University Hospital-Rikshospitalet, Oslo, Norway

Monique Stoffels, Department of Medicine, Radboud University Nijmegen Medical Centre; Nijmegen Centre for Infection, Inflammation and Immunity Centre for Immunodeficiency and Autoinflammation; Nijmegen Centre for Molecular Life Sciences, Nijmegen, The Netherlands

Helen Su, Human Immunological Diseases Unit, Laboratory of Host Defenses, National Institute of Allergy and Infectious Diseases, National Institutes of Health, Bethesda, MD, USA

Uta Syrbe, Department of Gastroenterology, Infection Medicine and Rheumatology, Charité Campus Benjamin Franklin; Charité University Medicine Berlin, Humboldt University, Berlin, Germany

Jayant A. Talwalkar, Mayo Clinic, Rochester, MN, USA

Veena Taneja, Department of Immunology and Rheumatology, Mayo Clinic, Rochester, MN, USA

Angela Tincani, Rheumatology and Clinical Immunology, Spedali Civili and University of Brescia, Brescia, Italy

Peter Tipping, Prince Henry's Institute of Medical Research, Clayton, Victoria, Australia

Ban-Hock Toh, Centre for Inflammatory Diseases, Department of Medicine, Southern Clinical School, Faculty of Medicine, Nursing and Health Sciences, Monash University, Victoria, Australia

George C. Tsokos, Division of Rheumatology, Beth Israel Deaconess Medical Center, Harvard Medical School, Boston, MA, USA

Eric Tu, Department of Biochemistry and Molecular Biology, Bio21 Molecular Science and Biotechnology Institute, The University of Melbourne, Parkville, Victoria, Australia

Kenneth S.K. Tung, Beirne Carter Center for Immunology Research and Department of Pathology, University of Virginia, Charlottesville, VA, USA

Ian R. van Driel, Department of Biochemistry and Molecular Biology, Bio21 Molecular Science and Biotechnology Institute, The University of Melbourne, Parkville, Victoria, Australia

Diego Vergani, Institute of Liver Studies, King's College London School of Medicine at King's College Hospital, London, UK

Mark A. Vickers, Academic Transfusion Medicine Unit, Scottish National Blood Transfusion Service, Aberdeen, UK

Stuart Viegas, Nuffield Department of Clinical Neurosciences, Oxford University, Oxford, UK

Angela Vincent, Department of Neurology, St Mary's Hospital, Imperial College NHS Trust, London, UK

Ulrich H. von Andrian, CBR Institute for Biomedical Research, Harvard Medical School, Boston, MA, USA

Matthias von Herrath, Type 1 Diabetes Research and Development Center, Novo Nordisk, Seattle, WA, USA

Anthony P. Weetman, The Medical School, University of Sheffield, Sheffield, UK

John M. Wentworth, Walter & Eliza Hall Institute of Medical Research, Royal Parade, Parkville, Victoria, Australia

Cornelia M. Weyand, Department of Medicine, Division of Immunology and Rheumatology, Stanford University School of Medicine, Stanford, CA, USA

Gerhard Wingender, La Jolla Institute for Allergy and Immunology, San Diego, CA, USA

Renato Zanchetta, Endocrine Unit, Department of Medicine, University of Padova, Padova, Italy

Moncef Zouali, University Paris Diderot, Sorbone Paris Cité, Paris, France

PRESENT AT THE BEGINNING

Both editors of *The Autoimmune Diseases*, 5th edition, were present when it happened in the mid-1950s. The topic of autoimmune disease emerged from the "dark ages," as Silverstein characterizes it in Chapter 2. One of us (I.R.M.) was collaborating with F.M. Burnet as the current foundations of modern immunity were laid, based on the requirements for self-recognition and cellular selection of immune repertoires. The other editor (N.R.R.) studied with Ernest Witebsky, who devoted a lifetime to delineating the antigenic characteristics of differing normal and malignant cells. If some of the wisdom and vision of these giants, on whose shoulder the editors stood, is evident in this book, they will be especially pleased. In a foreword to *The Autoimmune Diseases*, 1st edition, in 1985, Burnet concluded: "Every chapter of this book represents a fusion of acts and ideas from both the clinical and experimental fields. It is both inevitable and essential that this cooperation go on indefinitely."

Grateful acknowledgments go to a number of individuals who made completion of this volume possible. On the side of the publisher, Elsevier, Mary Preap has been a critical member of the team from the beginning. More recently, Melissa Read and Marion Stockton provided the final touches. It was indeed an international team effort. Each of the editors received editorial support from skilled secretarial administrators including Kathleen Spinnato and Starlene Murray at Johns Hopkins, and Elaine Pearson at Monash University. As in previous editions, the Editors record that successful completion of this fifth edition depended upon the encouragement, forbearance, and keen sense of humor of our wives. I.R.M. thanks Monash University through the Dean of the Faculty of Medicine, Professor Christina Mitchell, for ongoing provision of full academic and scholarly facilities via an appointment as Adjunct Professor. Most of all, the editors thank the many contributors. They not only submitted learned chapters but graciously withstood the rigor of editorial review. Many chapters were revised multiple times before the "picky" editors released them to the publisher.

The editors have the sad need to tender particular tribute to two of the authors, highly esteemed colleagues and huge contributors to knowledge of autoimmune diseases George Eisenbarth and Lloyd Mayer. Both died during the later stages of preparing this book. George's last communication to the editors, sent a few weeks before his death, was to reassure them that his contribution would be submitted in due time. Lloyd's chapter was completed before his untimely death, but his co-author took on the challenges of editorial corrections. Their energy and insights will be greatly missed by all who strive to reduce the burden of autoimmune disease.

Noel R. Rose
Ian R. Mackay

Part 1

Immunologic Basis of Autoimmunity

Autoimmune Disease: The Consequence of Disturbed Homeostasis

Noel R. Rose[1] and Ian R. Mackay[2]

[1]*Departments of Pathology and Molecular Microbiology and Immunology, The Johns Hopkins Schools of Medicine and Public Health, Baltimore, MD, USA,* [2]*Department of Biochemistry & Molecular Biology, Monash University, Clayton, Victoria, Australia*

Chapter Outline

Evolution of the Autoimmune Response	3	The Common Threads	5
A Phylogenetic Perspective	4	The "Proper Study…"	6
The Innate Immune System	4	Towards the Future	8
The Adaptive Immune System	4	The Last Word	8
Self and Non-Self, and the Nature of Autoantigens	5	References	9
Autoimmunity and Autoimmune Disease	5		

"…the best test of a physiological concept is its application to pathological conditions"

F.M. Burnet, 1959

EVOLUTION OF THE AUTOIMMUNE RESPONSE

The goal of this book, like the previous editions, is to promote and promulgate newer knowledge and deeper understanding of the family of autoimmune diseases. Progress towards that goal is enhanced by considering the evolution of immunity itself. Diverse as they are in their clinical manifestations, all of the autoimmune diseases are related by the fact that host-directed immune responses play a significant role in their etiology and pathogenesis. The proper function of the immune response entails maintaining a careful balance between vital effector activities with judicious regulation. As challenges, both internal and external, arise continuously, the immune system must be highly adaptable. An understanding of the physiology of the immune system presupposes recognition of its evolution over the long term and its plasticity in the short term.

A century and a half ago, Charles Darwin and Alfred Russel Wallace taught us that survival of life depends upon adaptation of an organism to its ever-changing environment. On a populational level, successful adaptation leads to natural selection and permits propagation of a species. Among individuals, successful adaptation is measured as survival and reproduction. On both individual and population levels, the immune system needs to distinguish components of the environment that promote survival from those that threaten it. For example, an evolutionary connection between nutrition, the ability to recognize and take in substances needed but not manufactured by the host, and protection of the host, based on recognition and disposal of pathogenic agents, was described by Metchnikoff in Darwinian terms (Tauber and Chernyak, 1991) and liberal use was made by F.M. Burnet (1959) of the concepts of variation and survival of the fittest, and homeostatic processes, in formulating his clonal selection theory of acquired immunity.

Throughout evolutionary time, organisms have devised more and more mechanisms that fit them for survival, devices that must be robust enough yet flexible enough to facilitate survival despite internal changes and external threats. The term homeostasis was foreshadowed by use of *milieu interne* by Claude Bernard (1865), and further developed by Walter Cannon (1932) who described homeostasis as the requirement for a harmonious interaction among these many devices, ultimately providing the optimal conditions for various physiologic

N. Rose & I. Mackay (Eds): The Autoimmune Diseases, Fifth edition. DOI: http://dx.doi.org/10.1016/B978-0-12-384929-8.00001-0

functions. Continued existence of an individual organism or propagation of a population depends upon maintaining and adjusting homeostasis, even in the presence of a hostile environment. "Normality" of any organism, including members of our own species, can be defined as the condition at that moment when the homeostatic requirements imposed by evolution are best satisfied.

Among all of the agents of the external environment that may adversely affect human survival, microorganisms are among the most common threats. Highly diverse and ever changing, they surround and cohabit our bodies and thrive in a symbiotic relationship in the intestinal tract. Consequently, the immune system in fulfilling its core function for providing protection has developed multiple strategies to recognize and manage microorganisms that may enter the body, especially the pathogenic ones that have the ability to upset normal homeostasis, yet tolerate others that confer benefit on the host.

A PHYLOGENETIC PERSPECTIVE

The tools employed by the human immune system for recognition have been increasingly refined, specialized, and expanded during the long evolution of multicellular organisms. Many of the elements of the human immune system have been reshaped from invertebrate predecessors. Some immunologic devices recognize the broad array of potential pathogens. Among these are barriers such as skin and mucous membranes which daily present the most effective protective measures available to the host. If they are disrupted, invasion of the body by microorganisms is a common, but unwelcome outcome.

The Innate Immune System

If these covering barriers fail in their function, the immune system draws on additional resources defined collectively as the innate immune system (Chapter 5). A limited number of pattern recognition receptors (PRRs), accumulated during evolution, are inherited to some extent by all members of our species. The PRRs of the innate immune system, capable of acting immediately, are designed to recognize a broad array of molecules present on or secreted by different invading microorganisms. The receptors are hard wired to signaling pathways that drive cell metabolism to produce mediators affording host protection. Included among the generators of these prompt responses are specialized cells such as granulocytes (Chapter 14), monocytes (Chapter 11), natural killer (NK) cells (Chapter 13), soluble products such as the complement system (Chapter 15), and naturally occurring polyreactive antibodies secreted by the special B1 subset of B cells (Chapters 9 and 10). The components of the innate immune system, resulting from many eons of

evolution, are borrowed in one form or another from the many species lower on the evolutionary timescale.

Our long evolutionary history has seen the components of the innate immune system capable of injuring tissues of the host selected against and effectively silenced. However, the cells of the innate immune system, like any other rapidly multiplying cells, are subject to the vicissitudes of mutation which, if not lethal, can become established in the germline. Some of these genetic traits can result in products like IL-1β that induce inflammation after exposure, not only to unwanted intruders, but as well to native cells of the host. These increasingly recognized genetically determined deviations in inflammation are now well described as autoinflammatory diseases (Chapter 4). Some hitherto have been considered as genuine examples of autoimmunity, but they lack evidence of an adaptive autoimmune response. Because these diseases also share inflammatory mediators with the autoimmune diseases, they may lend themselves to similar modes of treatment.

The Adaptive Immune System

In its strategy to produce such a broad, all-encompassing recognition system, the innate immune response sacrifices potency, precise specificity, and memory for breadth and immediacy. The more recently evolved adaptive immune system seen in jawed vertebrates builds upon many of the same constituent cells and cell products represented in the innate immune system. For example, inflammatory processes that accompany innate immunity may provide the costimulatory signals that act as adjuvants for the adaptive response (Nhu and Rose, 2013). The adaptive response has developed a strategy of focusing recognition on specified, molecular structures such that the outcome of an adaptive response is highly directed reactivity. The generation of this huge diversity of specific receptors is the job of the lymphocytes and their antigen receptors. To recognize a virtually infinite number of potential antigens, the lymphocyte population depends upon the well-studied post-genetic mechanisms, including hyper-mutation and recombination activating genes (RAG)-dependent recombination (Chapters 6 and 10). Finally, there has evolved a very necessary guidance system to position the appropriate defensive lymphocyte to exactly where it is needed to fulfill its particular purpose—this is the task of the adressins and chemokine receptors that engage chemokine ligands (Chapter 22).

Random recombinations inevitably lead to receptors on some lymphocytes that recognize antigens of the host. Such lymphocytes represent a clear and present danger, and must be carefully regulated. Some of these lymphocytes are eliminated during their birth and others are controlled later by the active and passive processes that jointly contribute to "self tolerance" (Chapters 7, 9, and 10). When the controlling measures fail, diseases caused by the adaptive immune system—the classical autoimmune diseases—ensue. These represent prototypic examples of homeostatic dysregulation within the adaptive immune system and point to a need to be rebalanced repeatedly through the lifespan as environmental changes occur.

SELF AND NON-SELF, AND THE NATURE OF AUTOANTIGENS

Any discussion on autoimmunity necessarily raises the issue of distinction of self–non-self, and the structure and nature of autoimmune epitopes. Historically "self" was regarded as an entity fixed during early development and responsible for imposing and maintaining natural immune tolerance in the primary lymphoid tissues, thymus (Chapter 7) or bone marrow (Chapter 9), "central tolerance." It depended on precise processes that entailed physical deletion of lymphocytes capable of autoimmune reactivity. These theoretical ideas were made real, in the case of T cell tolerance, by the discovery of the *AIRE* genes, which encode an autoimmune regulator protein that facilitates the deletion of autoreactive lymphocytes in the thymus and possibly in peripheral lymphoid tissues too (Kyewski, 2008). The "immunologic self," then, represents all host antigens presented in the thymus, or otherwise inducing unresponsiveness. However, over recent years self–non-self distinctions have become blurred. Can immunologic self include the intestinal microbiota, thereby justifying "autoimmune" for the colonic inflammatory diseases (Chapter 60)? Products derived from aberrant apoptotic cell death can induce systemic autoimmunity (Chapter 17), while tumor-derived autoantigens from primary neoplasms of ovary, breast, or lung (which are also represented in normal brain tissue) can evoke devastating neurological syndromes (Chapters 57 and 58). Self-tolerance clearly needs to be redefined.

A related issue is the nature of reactive sites—epitopes—for antibodies and T cells on autoantigenic molecules. In the case of thyroglobulin, a large glycoprotein produced and stored in the thyroid glands, patients with autoimmune thyroid disease react with epitopes that differ from the many recognized by normal individuals (Caturegli et al., 1994). Taking the example of glutamic acid decarboxylase, a pancreatic islet autoantigen, epitope sites, identifiable by use of specifically reactive monoclonal antibodies and crystallographic data, are quite limited in number, with most of the surface-exposed sites being immunologically silent (Fenalti et al., 2008). The degree to which such information can clarify how autoimmune disease is initiated remains to be seen.

AUTOIMMUNITY AND AUTOIMMUNE DISEASE

In the decade since the publication of the fourth edition of *The Autoimmune Diseases* in 2006, our understanding of the homeostatic regulation of the adaptive immune system has expanded greatly. These changes have required that most of the chapters on underlying immunologic principles be extensively rewritten. Some topics are entirely new. For example, we now recognize a population of large lymphocytes that bear the signature markers of NK cells, but produce the T cell receptors of very limited variability. These receptor-invariant NKT cells, like other cell systems of the immune response, are becoming subclassifiable, as described in Chapter 8. A greater understanding of the pathways that carry the signals from antigen-specific binding of receptors to induce nuclear changes has begun to explain the concurrence of events that leads to an escalating autoimmune response. The role of epigenetic changes (heritable or non-heritable) in the immune process continues to provide fresh understandings of how the immune system operates (Chapter 28), including how substances in the environment can actually lead to immune dysregulation and autoimmune disease (Chapter 21). The distinction between autoimmunity as the everyday consequence of ongoing clonal diversification and autoimmune disease as an exceptional pathologic outcome has been greatly advanced by investigating the various nuances of antigen presentation by differing subtypes of dendritic cells and macrophages (Chapters 11 and 12). Investigations of effector mechanisms dependent on infiltrating cells and their products provide clues for potential biologic therapies (Chapters 23 and 81). The progression from autoimmunity to autoimmune disease also follows the chance accumulation of particular genetic alleles, many of which help to maintain immunologic homeostasis on a day-to-day basis. The coincidence of these genetic traits leads to a wide spectrum of autoimmune disease susceptibility (Chapters 26 and 27). On the brighter side, however, greater knowledge of these genetic traits combined with functional early warnings such as appearance of multiple autoantibodies and presence of key cytokine or other mediators in the blood provide the first hope for earlier diagnosis, more effective interventions and a real possibility for prediction and prevention (Chapters 78 and 79).

THE COMMON THREADS

The reader will note that the number of diseases included in the current edition of the book exceeds that in previous editions. In fact, that number has increased with each succeeding edition since the first in 1985 as more diseases are seen as sharing the common threads of autoimmune pathogenesis. Broadly, we define an autoimmune disease as one in which autoimmunity demonstrated by self-reactive T cells or antibodies plays a causative or a significant contributory role (Rose and Bona, 1993). In humans, the evidence to support autoimmunity as a pathogenetic agent can be determined with varying degrees of certainty. In a few instances, there is direct evidence that a human disease is caused by autoimmunity based on disease transfer. At this time, T cell transfers between humans are not feasible and this metric pertains to instances where transfer of antibody is possible. The situation prevails mainly in cases of maternal to fetal exchange, as in neonatal lupus (Chapter 35), myasthenia gravis (Chapter 54), and Graves' disease (Chapter 40). Pertinent here as well is transient autoantibody-mediated thrombocytopenia in human volunteers after serum from a patient with immune-mediated thrombocytopenia, as in Harrington's classic experiment in 1951 (Chapter 47). In some instances a human pathogenic autoantibody can transfer features of a particular disease to a rodent recipient (Chapter 57).

If no evidence is available to show a direct causative effect of autoantibodies, indirect evidence can be marshaled. It depends on the creation or identification of a model in experimental animals where the appropriate antibody or adoptive cell transfers can be carried out. The availability of a genetically engineered rodent has opened new opportunities to explore mechanisms of induction and pathogenesis (Chapters 30 and 31). The great majority of autoimmune diseases are defined on the basis of such indirect evidence, even though the model may not completely mimic the human condition.

In many other instances, only inferential or circumstantial evidence is available based on the appearance of the common features of autoimmune diseases such as the presence of relevant autoantibodies at an unquestionable level, co-occurrence (clustering) with better established autoimmune disorders and shared genetic traits. Genetic markers are becoming more informative with widening applicability of genome-wide searches that are increasingly showing single-nucleotide polymorphisms (SNPs) common to autoimmune diseases as well those that are disease unique (Chapters 26 and 27). In some situations, regrettably, the now-appealing concept of autoimmunity is becoming applied to odd diseases that actually fail to qualify, perhaps furthered by a lack of stringency of results for autoantibodies reported by immuno-diagnostic laboratories (Chapter 77). Some of these diseases are described in a special chapter by Mackay (Chapter 75).

In reviewing the human diseases attributable to effects of autoimmunity, our emphasis has been placed heavily on the common features that underlie these clinically varied disorders (Rose, 1997). The common threads uniting the autoimmune diseases represent shared maladaptations of the adaptive immune response to changes in internal or external environments. The common threads often represent particular inadequacies in the homeostatic control measures that normally prevent the progression of benign autoimmune responses to the far less common pathogenic autoimmunity. These maladaptations can sometimes be traced to specific genetic traits (Chapter 26), to environmental stresses, or to hormonal changes (Chapters 21 and 24), but most often result from all of them combined.

There is an intimate relationship between the endocrine system and the immune system based on their co-evolution (Chapter 3). They even share some mediators and signaling messengers. Hormonal changes explain much of the sex bias and the age dependence of autoimmune diseases. Although the autoimmune diseases predominantly occur in females, a few such diseases are seen mainly in males. This finding supports the view, now well established, that multiple mechanisms come into play in determining the female to male ratio (Chapter 24). Another set of common threads characteristic of the family of autoimmune diseases is their dependence on an environmental initiator. With a few striking exceptions, (Chapter 29) heritability alone is insufficient to explain the occurrence or expression of an autoimmune disorder. In outbred humans autoimmune disease depends on exposure to some endogenous or exogenous influence, be it infection or some chemical or physical agent. The importance of greater study of environmental triggers rests on the demonstration in a few instances that an autoimmune disease can be arrested or actually prevented even in a genetically disposed individual if separated from that environmental agent. A telling example is the virtual disappearance in developed countries of rheumatic carditis associated with elimination of endemic beta-hemolytic streptococcal infections (Chapter 69).

The internal environment, represented in part by the microbiome, is acquired at or soon after birth and their "pattern" tends to remain throughout life (Chapter 25). These microorganisms, especially bacteria, live harmoniously and may even benefit the host. For reasons only partly understood, the pattern may become "destabilized" and changes in the microbial population can have great impact on the host immune response. But allowing for effects of physical or chemical agents in some cases, infection with a microorganism is in general seldom out of the picture and can influence the immune response in almost countless ways to incite autoimmune disease (Chapter 19).

THE "PROPER STUDY…"

Accepting that the "proper study of mankind is man," an appropriate investigation of autoimmune disease begins with a careful assessment of the disease itself, starting with a patient's present illness, its history, social setting, and familial occurrences (Rose, 2013). A large array of immunologic tests and radiologic imaging procedures is presently available. As individuals with similar histories and exposures are collected, epidemiologic studies reveal common environmental and genetic risks. These population-based investigations are now being expanded by multinational consortia, allowing for the assembly of many thousands of cases for valid statistical analysis. Clinical presentation and epidemiologic aspects are dealt with in each disease-related chapter of the book. Sometimes patient-based information obtained from carefully studied patients is sufficient in itself to identify the pathogenetic mechanisms underlying an autoimmune disease, especially if there are laboratory procedures that can reproduce the essence of the pathology outside of the body. Examples are seen in the hematologic cytopenias (Chapters 46—48) and antireceptor diseases such as myasthenia gravis (Chapter 54) or cerebral neuroreceptor diseases that are attracting increasing interest among neurologists and neuropathologists (Chapters 57 and 58). As mentioned above, experimental models have proved to be of great value in determining the precise effector mechanisms of disease, even though the initiation of the disease in the model can be quite different from the human counterpart. For this reason, as well as the well-known intrinsic differences in the physiologic basis of immunity in different species, the principal findings obtained from experimental models need to be referred back to the human equivalents often in the form of immunologic comparisons and clinical trials. Importantly, particular interventions devised in animal models form the basis of preclinical data needed before undertaking clinical trials.

Data emerging from extensive studies in animals provide a template for understanding the steps leading to human autoimmune disease; specifically its initiation, progression, and injury. With respect to initiation in experimental animals, studies have informed us how the delicate normal balance of the immune response—homeostasis—can be perverted by a multitude of influences. In broad terms, an autoimmune response can exceed the bounds of the normal homeostatic controls because it is too strongly induced, too long maintained, or too inadequately regulated, singly or in combination. An autoimmune response may be strengthened by an external antigenic mimic, by an agent with the properties of an adjuvant, or by one of the many non-antigenic-specific costimulators of immune responses. Very likely, both antigen-specific and non-antigen-specific regulatory pathways are needed for an autoimmune disease to get started.

Once the threshold of homeostatic adaptation has been exceeded, an autoimmune response can progress on to its pathologic outcome. That process may—in fact usually does—take weeks or even years, well recognized in the extensively studied example of autoimmune diabetes mellitus in humans and in rodent models (Chapter 41). During that time it is often characterized by an escalation or augmentation of the autoimmune response. This may involve spread of the response from a single to multiple epitopes (designated as epitope spreading) on an original antigenic molecule or, in the case of inflammatory diseases, production of additional autoantibodies to different organ-specific antigens (Chapter 78). This escalation of the autoimmune response is often the first clinical clue that a well-regulated autoimmune reaction has progressed to a dysregulated immune reaction in the form of overt autoimmune disease (Rose, 2007).

In recent years, much progress has been made in studies of cellular injury during autoimmune responses (Chapter 17). For instance, defects in processes of apoptosis can allow emergence of autoimmunogenic derivatives of nuclear or cytoplasmic constituents of the cell. Ironically, the damaging effector mechanisms during autoimmune disease are generally the same ones as those that confer protective immunity in infections. Many new specifically targeted modes of treatment of autoimmune disease are based on careful dissection of the various effector mechanisms. Thus, blocking particular cytokines or their receptors promises winning strategies for treating the deleterious effects of an autoimmune response (Chapter 76). The recent prodigious progress in this area is comprehensively described by Chatenoud (Chapter 81).

Important as these advances have been in benefiting patients by arresting and even reversing progression and so providing symptomatic relief, they do not necessarily change the underlying cause(s). The expectation is that as homeostasis is re-established, the sufferer becomes separated from some of the exogenous causal factors, perhaps "a triumph of hope over experience." Thus cures or elimination of autoimmune disease mostly remain in the future excepting, perhaps, instances like celiac disease (Chapter 59) and rheumatic carditis (see above) where the initiating agent can be confidently determined.

A requirement for homeostasis in the immune system was envisioned early on by Burnet (1959, p. 122) while recognizing that 'there was no experimental evidence whatever on the point'. This has changed, with homeostasis now becoming more widely understood by immunologists to describe various functional activities of the immune system. One example is seen in the fine balance between the "positive" effector processes mediated by autoantibody-producing B lymphocytes and Th1/Th17 $CD4^+$ T lymphocytes counterbalanced by the "negative" effector processes mediated by B lymphocytes (Chapter 10) and maybe by anti-idiotypic antibody, and by T lymphocytes with regulation by several T cell types among which we see the CD4$^+$ CD25$^+$ Fox p3 Treg subset as being the one of major prominence.

TOWARDS THE FUTURE

Much of the research on the autoimmune diseases conducted during the latter part of the 20th century has been based on the reductionist principle of isolating a single variable within a complex background. The overall success of this approach is evident in the remarkable advances described in this and prior editions of the book. Yet, all biologists realize that evolution has produced a highly integrated and interactive immunologic network: changes in any one component alter the entire network. The availability of new tools based on microarray platforms with capabilities for managing large amounts of biologic data have made it possible to construct an image of such complex physiologic system. The fruits of a systems approach are already visible in looking at large panels of autoantibodies (Chapter 77). Combining an initial systems analysis with subsequent reductionist research on precise mechanisms promises fresh visions into the complex biologic reactions underlying autoimmune responses.

Progress in research on the autoimmune diseases will certainly accelerate over the next decade. One major imperative of the numerous population studies in progress is explaining the striking temporal increase in incidence of many of the autoimmune diseases, in particular autoimmune diabetes, multiple sclerosis, celiac disease, and Crohn's disease, as analyzed in the corresponding Chapters 41, 52, 59, and 60. Better recognition could be only a partial explanation. It is unlikely that most of the rise can be assigned to an accumulation of genetic susceptibilities, leaving environmental pressures as the main drivers of the increase. One popular but still hotly debated idea is that the current overly hygienic lifestyle in developed countries is not conducive to optimal development for an "under-challenged" maturing immune system. However, there are many alternative possibilities such as the so-called "Western" diet with its relatively low fiber content, which yields an insufficiency of diet-derived ligands; this is exemplified by short-chain fatty acids to engage "metabolite sensing receptors" such as G protein-coupled receptor (GPR) 43 situated on immune (and other) cell types so favorably modulating immune homeostasis and the character of the intestinal microbiome (Maslowski et al., 2009; Maslowski and Mackay, 2011).

Whatever the case, environmental changes may be induced within the immune system itself, in interrelated physiologic systems, or to the microbiome. Since the changes operative through the environment still rest on the foundation of host genetics, they will be highly personal. Thus, knowledge of a person's genome and microbiome may be critical in explaining the diversity of individual responses to changing environmental provocations. As it broadens to meet the changing environment, medicine in general and immunology in particular will have to become more individualized.

Another lesson gained from 20th century research is the likelihood that there is a long incubation period in the development of many of the autoimmune diseases as judged by the presence of signal autoantibodies in archived sera. So, when does an autoimmune disease actually begin? What happens on "day 1?" This information is of the greatest importance in devising a cure or attaining the ultimate goal of prevention. Animal models have clearly shown that in most cases it is considerably easier to arrest or even reverse an injurious autoimmune response by intervening before the immune response is fully under way and "memory" populations of effector lymphocytes have settled in. Later interventions are more problematic and associated with much greater risk of adverse outcomes, particularly after novel interventions. Given sufficient personal, quantitative information on risk based on genetic data combined with early immunologic and biochemical signs, it may well become acceptable practice to intervene actively to primarily prevent autoimmune disease before it is clinically evident or has secondarily extended to avoid recurrence.

THE LAST WORD

We are far from writing the last word on the pathways to autoimmune disease. An immune system, charged with sensing an ever-changing environment and making appropriate modifications, requires constant recalibration. Environmental changes needed to sustain life on this planet (and perhaps other planets) are likely to increase. It will be the task of the ever-evolving immune system to gather new tools to accommodate new demands. The risk of biologic errors will remain even in the best regulated system. Accordingly, autoimmune disease will remain a problem as long as variation and natural selection remain laws of nature. Our continuing goal remains to nullify the destructive effects of immunity while maintaining its vital protective functions.

We face the future with cautious optimism. In a forthcoming work on the historical foundations of autoimmunity (Anderson and Mackay, 2014) there is cited the apt phrase of the English historian of science J.W.N. Sullivan (1921): "This spirit is chiefly a sense of unlimited possibilities."

Autoimmunity as a cause of human disease is well established as a clinical reality, shifting so many formerly enigmatic diseases out of the idiopathic category. The clinical laboratory has given us remarkable tools for earlier, more precise diagnosis and the research laboratory has provided rational targets for intervening successfully in many formerly unmanageable diseases. By considering the autoimmune diseases as a category of related disorders and concentrating on their core causes, possibilities of true cures and eventual preventions are slowly emerging. Most important, the size of the autoimmune disease problem is gaining increasing attention from the medical profession and, ultimately, from the public, the best prognostic for future progress.

REFERENCES

Anderson, W., Mackay, I.R., 2014. Intolerant Bodies: Autoimmune Disease and the Modern Self. Johns Hopkins University Press, Baltimore, MD.

Bernard, C., 1865. Introduction a la Medicine Experimentale. 1927. An Introduction to the Study of Experimental Medicine. Macmillan Company, New York, NY, USA.

Burnet, F.M., 1959. The Clonal Selection Theory of Acquired Immunity. Cambridge University Press, London.

Cannon, W.B., 1932. The Wisdom of the Body. W.W. Norton & Co., New York, USA.

Caturegli, P., Mariotti, S., Kuppers, R.D., Burek, C.L., Pinchera, A., Rose, N.R., 1994. Epitopes on thyroglobulin: a study of patients with thyroid disease. Autoimmunity. 18, 41–49.

Fenalti, G., Hampe, C.S., Arafat, Y., Law, R.H.P., Banga, J.P., Mackay, I.R., et al., 2008. COOH-terminal clustering of autoantibody and T-cell determinants on the structure of GAD65 provide insights into the molecular basis of autoreactivity. Diabetes. 57, 1293–1301.

Kyewski, B., 2008. A breath of Aire for the periphery. Science. 321, 776–777.

Maslowski, K.M., Mackay, C.R. 2011. Diet, gut microbiota and immune responses. Nat Immunol 12, 5–9.

Maslowski, K.M., Viera, A.T., Ng, A., Kranich, J., Sierro, F., Yu, D., et al., 2009. Regulation of inflammatory responses by gut microbiota and chemoattractant receptor GPR43. Nature. 461, 1282–1286.

Nhu, Q., Rose, N.R., 2013. Infections as adjuvants for autoimmunity: The adjuvant effect. In: Textbook of Vaccines and Autoimmunity, Eds: Yehuda Shoenfeld and Nancy Agmon-Levin. Wiley, in press

Rose, N.R., 1997. Autoimmune diseases: tracing the shared threads. Hosp. Pract. 32, 147–154.

Rose, N.R., 2007. Autoimmune escalation: through the crystal ball. Clin. Exp. Immunol. 147, 9.

Rose, N.R., 2013. The proper study. Ann. N. Y. Acad. Sci. 1285, v–vii.

Rose, N.R., Bona, C., 1993. Defining criteria for autoimmune diseases (Witebsky's postulates revisited). Immunol. Today. 14, 426–430.

Sullivan, J.W.N., 1921. The new scientific horizon. Nation Athenaeum. 29, 722.

Tauber, A.I., Chernyak, L., 1991. Metchnikoff and the Origins of Immunology. Oxford University Press, New York.

Chapter 2

Autoimmunity: A History of the Early Struggle for Recognition

Arthur M. Silverstein

Institute of the History of Medicine, Johns Hopkins Medical School, Baltimore, MD, USA

Chapter Outline

The Search for Autoantibodies 12
  Horror Autotoxicus 12
  The Nature of Ehrlich's "Contrivances" 12
Challenges to the Thesis 13
  Lens Autoantibodies 13
  Paroxysmal Cold Hemoglobinuria 13

Sympathetic Ophthalmia 13
The Wassermann Antibody 13
The Shift to Immunochemistry 14
The Return of Immunobiology 15
Concluding Remarks 16
References 16

"...1955—1965 [was] the decade marked by the question, Does autoimmunity exist?"

(Rose and Mackay, 1985)

It is one of the curious situations in science that certain well-demonstrated facts are refused entry into the body of accepted knowledge, and may become so effaced from the collective memory that they must be rediscovered many years later in order to gain acceptance. Such was the case in immunology with Donath and Landsteiner's (1904) discovery that paroxysmal cold hemoglobinuria (PKH) is an autoimmune disease, or with Clemens von Pirquet's (1910) explanation of immune complex disease. The cause of this selective amnesia may merely be an earlier contradictory pronouncement by a respected leader in the field; sometimes it lies in an inability to fit the new finding into the working paradigm that guides thought in the field, as the historian of science Thomas Kuhn (1970) has suggested. In the end, it may be that Ludwik Fleck (1979) was right when he proposed that acceptance of a fact in science depends less upon its truth than upon its acknowledgment by the leaders in the discipline (whom Fleck called the *Denkkollektiv*). Ultimately the truth in science will emerge, although sometimes it takes a very long time.

The earliest discoveries in immunology were made in the context of the battle to ward off infectious diseases. These included Louis Pasteur's (1880) preventive vaccines, Ilya Metchnikoff's (1884) bacteria-eating phagocytes, and Behring and Kitasato's (1890) curative antidiphtheria and antitetanus sera. It seemed evident that these efficient mechanisms for the protection of the body were Darwinian adaptations designed to prevent or control infectious disease, a widespread view in the 1890s even after it was demonstrated that specific antibodies might be formed against such innocuous antigens as egg albumin, bovine serum proteins, and sheep red cells. It seemed unthinkable at the time that a grand mechanism designed to prevent disease might turn the tables and cause disease. This concept of a benign immune system became so well established that demonstrations that antibodies might cause disease were either disregarded entirely, or else ascribed to "aberrant" antibodies acting under the influence of a "misdirected" immunity (Silverstein, 2009). This was how the early discoveries of serum sickness, hay fever, asthma, and a variety of immunopathological phenomena were treated by mainstream immunology during the first half of the twentieth century.

It is beyond the scope of this chapter to discuss the entire history of the unwillingness to accept that the

N. Rose & I. Mackay (Eds): The Autoimmune Diseases, Fifth edition. DOI: http://dx.doi.org/10.1016/B978-0-12-384929-8.00002-2

immune response might lead to a variety of harmful outcomes (which we now describe under the rubric "immunopathology"). We shall limit the present discussion to the way in which a subset of the whole, autoimmune diseases, was regarded (or rather disregarded) during the first half of the twentieth century. This sample should provide a quite adequate representation of the way that early immunologists dealt with the paradox presented by the almost oxymoronic word *immunopathology*.

THE SEARCH FOR AUTOANTIBODIES

Horror Autotoxicus

It was Richard Pfeiffer (1894) who discovered a new mechanism that functions to mediate immunity—the destruction of bacteria by humoral antibodies. Jules Bordet (1899) showed that not only were bacteria lysed by thermostable antibody and a thermolabile substance that he called *alexine* (later termed *Komplement* by Paul Ehrlich), but that mammalian erythrocytes could be hemolyzed specifically by two similar agents. Here was a technique that would see broad application in many areas of immunology (Silverstein, 1994), not least in connection with the question of whether an individual could form antibodies against its own self.

Two consequences of Bordet's report were immediately apparent. Karl Landsteiner (1900) became interested in red cells and discovered blood groups in humans (for which he received the Nobel Prize in 1930). Then Paul Ehrlich and Julius Morgenroth (1900, 1901) launched a series of studies of immune hemolysis in order to develop additional support for Ehrlich's (1897, 1900) side-chain theory of how antibodies are produced and how they function. It was Ehrlich's interpretation of his hemolysis experiments that would play a major role in the early history of autoimmunity. These hemolysis experiments are described and analyzed in detail by Silverstein (2002).

During the course of these experiments, Ehrlich and Morgenroth immunized many different species with the red cells of other species. They also immunized animals with the red cells of other members of their own species, and even tried to immunize animals with their own red cells. In every case, they were able to demonstrate the production of xenohemolysins and isohemolysins, but autohemolysins were never observed. This led inexorably and logically to the conclusion that animals could not make autotoxic antibodies to any self-antigens, a postulate that Ehrlich named *horror autotoxicus*. Indeed, he would conclude that, "It would be dysteleological in the highest degree, if under these circumstances self-poisons of the parenchyma—autotoxins—were formed" (Ehrlich, 1902).

But Ehrlich was not the only one who responded to Bordet's publication on immune hemolysis. If red cells could stimulate an immune response, why not other tissues and organs? In no time, attempts were undertaken to immunize animals with all types of cells and tissue extracts, especially at the Pasteur Institute in Paris where Bordet had worked. As expected, cytotoxic xenoantibodies against a variety of tissues were reported; indeed, volume 14 of the *Annales de l'Institut Pasteur* was largely devoted to these studies, including a review of antitissue antibodies by Metchnikoff (1900). Most surprising was a report by Metalnikoff (1900) that some animals were able to form antibodies against their own spermatozoa. But while these autoantibodies could destroy the sperm *in vitro*, they seemed to have no effect *in vivo* on the viable sperm in the immunized animal.

Ehrlich was not impressed! These are not "autocytotoxins within our meaning" said he, since they do not cause disease (Ehrlich and Morgenroth, 1901). Here was the true meaning of *horror autotoxicus*: not that autoantibodies cannot be formed, but that they are prevented "by certain contrivances" from exerting any destructive action (Goltz, 1980). Due in part to Ehrlich's worldwide prestige and to the fact that an autoantibody seemed so obviously counter-intuitive, *horror autotoxicus* found broad acceptance as a guiding principle. Indeed, so firm was the conviction that autoimmune disease was impossible that everyone soon forgot Ehrlich's suggestion that an autoantibody might exist without causing disease. It would be some 80 years before the important distinction would be made between autoimmunity and autoimmune disease (Rose and Mackay, 1985).

The Nature of Ehrlich's "Contrivances"

Paul Ehrlich was nothing if not logical. He proposed one of his typical thought-experiments to examine the possible outcomes (Ehrlich and Morgenroth, 1900). Suppose the existence of a self-antigen α. Then, since antibody formation results from the interaction of antigen with preformed cell receptors according to the side-chain theory (the first selection theory!), two possibilities are seen:

- The host possesses no anti-α cell receptors. Therefore no autoantibody response and thus no disease can occur. (Here is, in embryo, Burnet's later clonal deletion idea!)
- The host does possess anti-α cell receptors on its cells. Therefore autoanti-α is formed. But the host also possesses the self-antigen α on its cells, with which the anti-α may react to stimulate the formation of anti-anti-α. (Remember, Ehrlich knew nothing about lymphocytes, and conceived that all cells possess receptors, and thus may be stimulated to form antibodies.) But the specific site on the anti-antibody should be identical with that on the original antigen, since they are both able to react specifically with the

antibody combining site! Ehrlich therefore concluded that a self-regulating equilibrium would be established between autoantibody and antigen (= anti-antibody) to suppress the development of autoimmune disease. (Here was a regulatory network theory 70 years before Niels Jerne's (1974) idiotype—anti-idiotype theory!)

CHALLENGES TO THE THESIS

Lens Autoantibodies

The initial flurry of interest in antitissue antibodies quickly subsided as the implications of *horror autotoxicus* gained broad acceptance. In 1903, however, Paul Uhlenhuth (1903) demonstrated the existence of organ-specific antigens by showing that the proteins of the lens are unique to that tissue; they are found nowhere else in the body. Moreover, these antigens are shared by the lenses of different species. Ophthalmologists seized upon this finding to suggest that an immune response to one's own lens might be responsible for the development of senile cataract (Römer, 1905). They showed further that an intraocular inflammation may be induced by the experimental rupture of the lens in the eye of a lens-immunized animal (Krusius, 1910).

Here were observations that would fascinate both ophthalmic clinicians and a later generation of immunopathologists interested in the possible workings of autoimmune disease. First, there was this early preview of what would later be called the "sequestered antigen" concept. Since "self" antigens by definition cannot elicit an immune response, then such antigens as do must be "foreign"—in this case isolated from the immunologic apparatus of the host, like sperm and lens. Secondly, Römer and Gebb (1912) concluded that if indeed disease does result from the formation of autoantibodies, this would represent a most unusual occurrence and must be considered as an aberration due to a malfunction of Ehrlich's "contrivances." Here they showed that unlike a future generation, they understood Ehrlich's "law of immunity research" completely.

Interest in the possibility that autoimmunity to lens might lead to disease did not disappear in the years that followed. But whereas the initial studies had been done in the context of the new immunology and was known to all workers in the field, further work was restricted to ophthalmologists and eye departments. Thus, a broad clinical study led Verhoeff and Lemoine (1922) to identify numerous cases of lens-induced inflammatory disease, to which they gave the name phacoanaphylaxis, a process which would later be accepted as a true autoimmune disease. Thenceforth, the description would appear routinely in textbooks of ophthalmic pathology, and clinical diagnoses would be made.

Paroxysmal Cold Hemoglobinuria

Fast on the heels of the lens antigen demonstration came an even more convincing case involving erythrocyte antigens. PKH was a rare disease presenting with signs of intravascular red cell lysis and a resulting hemoglobinuria, following exposure of the patient to the cold. Donath and Landsteiner (1904, 1906) published reports that reproduced *in vitro* all features of the disease. They demonstrated beyond question that it was due to a peculiar autoantibody in the patient's serum that affixes to his own red cells only in the cold, and mediates hemolysis with complement when the sensitized cells are rewarmed.

It was clear from the outset that Landsteiner fully understood the implications of this discovery and its meaning for Ehrlich's *horror autotoxicus*. Indeed, even Ehrlich's student Hans Sachs gave a somewhat grudging acceptance of the phenomenon and its interpretation (Sachs, 1909). But again, the implication seemed to be that this was an unusual exception to the regular scheme, and the implications of PKH as the prototypical autoimmune disease soon vanished almost completely from view.

Sympathetic Ophthalmia

It had always seemed odd to clinicians that after traumatic injury to one eye, the second eye might spontaneously develop a blinding inflammatory disease even years later. Soon after the discovery of cytotoxic antibodies, the proposal was advanced that sympathetic ophthalmia might be caused by the formation of "autocytotoxins" (Santucci, 1906). The concept was picked up and given broad currency by one of the foremost ophthalmologists of the day, Elschnig of Prague (1910a, b). As with autoimmunity to lens, work on the immunology of sympathetic ophthalmia continued, but only in ophthalmology departments. Woods (1921, 1933) reported the presence of antiuveal antibodies in patients with perforating injuries of the globe, and uveal pigment was implicated as the causative antigen (Woods, 1925; Friedenwald, 1934).

The Wassermann Antibody

The discovery of the role of complement in immune hemolysis was soon followed by the finding that *any* antigen—antibody interaction would fix complement nonspecifically (Bordet and Gengou, 1901). The ability to measure this uptake using a hemolytic assay meant that antibody could be titered if specific antigen were available. With the recent identification of *Treponema pallidum* as the cause of syphilis, a serological test for this disease was sought. But since the organism could not be grown in culture, Wassermann and colleagues (1906) and, independently, Detré (1906) used extracts of tissues from syphilitic patients as the antigen, and a valuable diagnostic test was born.

Most perplexing, however, was the report from many laboratories that positive tests for syphilis might be obtained as well, using extracts of normal tissues as antigens. This ran counter to the prevailing view that only *specific* antigens can interact with antibodies to fix complement. It appeared necessary to conclude, therefore, that the "Wassermann antigen," being native, must be measuring an autoantibody rather than an anti-treponemal antibody. This suggestion was made, in fact, by Weil and Braun (1909) who speculated that the Wassermann antibody is an autoantibody specific for the tissue breakdown products generated in the syphilitic lesions. They suggested further that these autoantibodies exacerbate the disease, and that the brain lesions in tertiary syphilis (paresis) may represent an autoimmune disease directed against neural antigens. (A century later, the antigen involved in the Wassermann reaction has been identified as a lipid named cardiolipin, but why these antibodies are formed is still a mystery, as is their role in the disease process!)

THE SHIFT TO IMMUNOCHEMISTRY

Despite all these hints that autoimmune diseases might exist, interest in the question waned in mainstream immunology—indeed almost disappeared—for some 40 years, from just before the First World War to the mid to late 1950s. This was due in part to the continuing sway of Ehrlich's *horror autotoxicus*. But there was another factor at play—the change in the overall direction of the field of immunology.

During the quarter-century prior to the First World War, immunology had been concerned chiefly with medical problems, and was pursued almost exclusively by physician-researchers. It had achieved notable successes in the prevention of some infectious diseases (vaccine development), their cure (serotherapy), and their diagnosis (serology). It had even begun to define several immunogenic diseases (anaphylaxis, serum sickness, hay fever, and asthma). But most of the easy problems had been solved, and further successes in these areas became disappointingly rare. Vaccines were sought, generally unsuccessfully, for the remaining great scourges of mankind: syphilis, tuberculosis, typhus, and the many serious tropical diseases. Few diseases were caused by exotoxins like diphtheria and tetanus, and thus new serotherapeutic approaches were rare. Yet other forces were at work. The Wassermann test and its offshoots became so widespread for the diagnosis of disease that it moved from the immunological research laboratory to the clinic. A new discipline, serology, arose that soon became independent of the mother discipline, immunology. In the same way, experimental anaphylaxis and its human

disease relations, hay fever and asthma, stimulated the interest of clinicians, who soon took over work in this field and called their new discipline "allergy."

When in a science one research direction reaches the point of severely diminishing returns, its practitioners will usually move to more productive pursuits. So it was with immunology, beginning shortly after the end of the First World War. Karl Landsteiner started working with haptens, and soon devoted himself almost entirely to a chemically-oriented study of the structural basis of immunological specificity and crossreactions (Landsteiner, 1962). Then Michael Heidelberger (Heidelberger and Avery, 1923) studied the immunochemistry of pneumococcal polysaccharides and introduced a variety of quantitative methods for the estimation of antigens and antibodies, best typified by the popular text written by his students, *Quantitative Immunochemistry* (Kabat and Mayer, 1949). For more than three decades, the field was devoted largely to studies of structure, specificity, and the thermodynamics of antigen–antibody interactions. The texts and monographs were primarily chemically oriented, and the practitioners were either chemically trained or at least chemically oriented. Even the theories of antibody formation that guided the field, Breinl and Haurowitz's (1930) and Pauling's (1940) antigen-instruction concept, were chemical (i.e., nonbiological and non-Darwinian) in spirit. It was easy to assume that a protein might be synthesized according to external instruction; for the chemist, molecules have no evolutionary history.

Given the continuing influence of Ehrlich's dictum, and the generally nonmedical orientation of the most prominent immunological investigators, it is not surprising that autoantibodies and autoimmune diseases were not among the most popular topics in the research laboratory. This is not to say, however, that there was absolutely no work along these lines. As we have seen, ophthalmologists reported findings in lens-induced disease and in sympathetic ophthalmia, but these were published in specialty ophthalmic journals. In the early 1930s, Rivers and coworkers published a series of papers on the production of an experimental encephalomyelitis (Rivers et al., 1933; Rivers and Schwentker, 1935) that only later would be shown to represent an autoimmune process. While these studies are viewed today as important milestones in autoimmunity research, they attracted little attention at the time among immunologists.

The contemporary view of autoimmunity during the 1940s and early 1950s is perhaps best exemplified by the position of Ernest Witebsky, trained in immunology by Ehrlich's student Hans Sachs and himself a disease-oriented physician. He could say as late as 1954 at the celebration of the centenary of the birth of Ehrlich that, "The validity of the law (sic!) of *horror autotoxicus* certainly should be evident to anyone interested in blood transfusion and blood disease. Autoantibodies—namely, antibodies directed against receptors of the same individual—are not formed" (Witebsky, 1954). This from the individual who, only two years later with his student Noel Rose, would help refocus interest on autoimmunity with the demonstration of the production of experimental autoimmune thyroiditis! (Rose and Witebsky, 1956; Witebsky et al., 1957).

THE RETURN OF IMMUNOBIOLOGY

During the late 1930s and 1940s, a series of observations began to question the assumptions that had guided recent thought and experiment in immunology. How could one explain in chemical terms the enhanced booster antibody response, or the change with time in the specificity and affinity of the antibodies formed? How to explain the persistence of antibody formation in the apparent absence of antigen? Even more troubling was the lack of relationship between immunity to certain viral diseases and the titer of antiviral antibodies, or the absence of a correlation between antibodies and "delayed" hypersensitivity skin tests. Here were basic biological questions that demanded answers—questions with which current theory was unable to cope, and for which it could not even provide experimental approaches. But even more difficult questions arising from biology and medicine would pose further challenges.

Peter Medawar's (1945) experiments showed that the rejection of tissue grafts was somehow mediated by immunological mechanisms. Then Ray Owen (1945) described the paradoxical situation in which dizygotic twin cattle might share one another's red cells without being able to mount an immune response to these foreign antigens. Macfarlane Burnet, biologist *par excellence*, called attention to all of these inexplicable phenomena and hypothesized the existence of a fundamental biological mechanism to explain Owen's finding—an embryonic interaction that

would suppress the ability to respond to one's own native antigens (Burnet and Fenner, 1949). This was soon confirmed by Medawar's group (Billingham et al., 1953), and would be termed immunological tolerance. Yet other observations would emphasize the awakening biomedical movement in immunology—the description of a group of immune deficiency diseases. Taken together, these new questions and phenomena foretokened a radical change of direction—what I have termed elsewhere as the "immuno-biological revolution" (Silverstein, 1991). Not only did these questions challenge the accepted dogma but they also served to stimulate the entry into the field of a new group of investigators. These were basic scientists from such fields as genetics and physiology, and clinicians from a variety of medical disciplines. They were unfettered by any allegiance to earlier ideas and techniques, and thus could entertain iconoclastic ideas and design novel experiments.

Perhaps the best illustration we may provide of the long period during which immunologists showed little interest in disease may be seen in Table 2.1. Here we list for each organ or disease entity the interval between the last significant study during the "classical" period and the first significant contribution of the "modern" era. The average hiatus, for those for which both ending and restarting dates can be identified, is about 44 years! This is an extremely long interlude for a field that was only some 70 years old in 1950.

In the context of a growing interest in the more biomedical aspects of the immune response, work on autoimmunity thus became respectable. This was also due to the increasing use of Freund's adjuvant, which made animal models of the various autoimmune diseases more readily available and more reproducible. Advances came rapidly. Coombs, Mourant, and Race (1945) showed with the antiglobulin test that many cases of

TABLE 2.1 The "Dark Ages" of Autoimmunity

Disease/Organ	Last "classical" contribution	First "modern" contribution
Hemolytic disease	1909	1945 (Coombs et al., 1945)
Sperm and testicular	1900	1951 (Voisin et al., 1951)
Encephalomyelitis	1905	1947 (Kabat et al., 1947)
Sympathetic ophthalmia	1912	1949 (Collins, 1949)
Phacoanaphylaxis	1911	1957 (Halbert et al., 1957)
Thyroid	1910	1956 (Rose and Witebsky, 1956; Roitt et al., 1956)
Wassermann antibody	1909	—
Platelet disease	—	1949 (Ackroyd, 1949)

Adapted from Silverstein (2009).

acquired hemolytic anemia were due to "incomplete" (non-agglutinating) antibodies. Kabat, Wolfe, and Bezer (1947) refocused attention on the immunopathogenesis of "allergic" encephalomyelitis. Collins (1949) introduced a reproducible animal model of sympathetic ophthalmia. Voisin, Delaunay, and Barber (1951) showed how to produce an experimental allergic orchitis. Finally, Rose and Witebsky (1956) demonstrated in experimental animals and Roitt et al. (1956) in human Hashimoto's disease that some forms of thyroid disease might be based upon autoimmune processes. In addition, an understanding of the pathogenesis of some of these diseases was made easier by the increasing appreciation of the fact that not all were mediated by circulating antibodies; some involved the action of subclasses of lymphocytes that originate in the thymus.

These new findings not only opened wide the floodgates of autoimmunity studies, but stimulated further interest in the more general field of immunopathology as well. This new movement was provided with a theoretical base with Talmage's (1957) suggestion and Burnet's Clonal Selection Theory (Burnet, 1959), which emphasized for the first time the biologically important role of cell dynamics in the antibody response. It is no accident that the late 1950s saw the first international conferences on immunopathology (Miescher and Vorlaender, 1958; Grabar and Miescher, 1959) and on the fundamentals of hypersensitivity (Lawrence, 1959; Shaffer et al., 1959). For the first time, in 1963, there appeared a textbook aimed at medical students (Humphrey and White, 1963), and then two comprehensive descriptions of immunological diseases aimed at clinicians (Gell and Coombs, 1963; Samter et al., 1965). It was in the spirit of the new immunology that Mackay and Burnet (1963) could summarize contemporary knowledge in the increasingly active field of the autoimmune diseases.

CONCLUDING REMARKS

This, then, is the story of the early stirrings of interest in the possibility that disease might result from an immune response to one's own autochthonous antigens. Perhaps the initial reports were too premature to be incorporated into the received wisdom of the young field of immunology, just as the discovery of the several allergic diseases could not at first be integrated. Certainly Paul Ehrlich's dictum of *horror autotoxicus* contributed to an unwillingness to recognize the full significance of the initial findings of a response to spermatozoa, erythrocytes, and retina. But the mounting challenges to the dogma would eventually prove irresistible and the field of autoimmunity would finally flourish. The more modern history of autoimmunity, resulting from the remarkable modern advances in our understanding of the cellular, molecular,

and genetic contributions to the field, will be found in the accompanying chapters in this volume.

REFERENCES

Ackroyd, J.F., 1949. The pathogenesis of thrombocytopenic purpura due to hypersensitivity to sedormid. Clin. Sci. 8, 267−287.

Behring, E., Kitasato, S., 1890. Ueber das Zustandekommen der Diphtherie-immunität und der Tetanus-immunität bei Thieren. Dtsch. Med. Wochenschr. 16, 1113−1114.

Billingham, R.E., Brent, L., Medawar, P.B., 1953. Actively acquired tolerance of foreign cells. Nature (London). 172, 603−606.

Bordet, J., 1899. Sur l'gglutination et la dissolution des globules rouges par le sérum d'animaux imjectés de sang défibriné. Ann. Inst. Pasteur. 12, 688−695.

Bordet, J., Gengou, O., 1901. Sur l'existence des substances sensibilisatrices dans la plupart des sérums anti-microbiens. Ann. Inst. Pasteur. 15, 289−302.

Breinl, F., Haurowitz, F., 1930. Chemische Untersuchung des Präzipitates aus Hämoglobin und Anti-Hämoglobin und Bemerkungen über die Natur des Antikörpers. Z. Physiol. Chem. 192, 45−57.

Burnet, F.M., 1959. The Clonal Selection Theory of Acquired Immunity. Cambridge University Press, London.

Burnet, F.M., Fenner, F., 1949. The Production of Antibodies. second ed. Macmillan, New York.

Collins, R.C., 1949. Experimental studies on sympathetic ophthalmia. Am. J. Ophthalmol. 32, 1687−1699.

Coombs, R.R.A., Mourant, A.E., Race, R.R., 1945. A new test for the detection of weak and "incomplete" Rh agglutinins. Brit. J. Exp. Pathol. 26, 255−266.

Detré, L., 1906. Ueber den Nachweis von spezifischen Syphilis Antisubstanzen und deren Antigenen bei Luetikern. Wien. Klin. Wochenschr. 19, 619.

Donath, J., Landsteiner, K., 1904. Ueber paroxysmale Hämoglobinurie. Münch. Med. Wochenschr. 51, 1590−1593.

Donath, J., Landsteiner, K., 1906. Ueber paroxysmale Hämoglobinurie. Z. Klin. Med. 58, 173−189.

Ehrlich, P., 1897. Die Wertbemessung des Diphtherieheilserums und deren theoretischen Grundlagen. Kinische Jahrb. 6, 299−326.

Ehrlich, P., 1900. On immunity with special reference to cell life: Croonian Lecture. Proc. Roy. Soc. London. 66, 424−448.

Ehrlich, P., 1902. Die Schutzstoffe des Blutes. Verh. Ges. Dtsch. Naturforsch. Aerzte. 1, 250−275.

Ehrlich, P., Morgenroth, J., 1900. Ueber Hämolysine: Dritte Mittheilung. Berlin Klin. Wochenschr. 37, 453−458.

Ehrlich, P., Morgenroth, J., 1901. Ueber Hämolysine: Fünfte Mittheilung. Berlin Klin. Wochenschr. 38, 251−255.

Elschnig, A., 1910a. Studien zur sympatischen Ophthalmie. von Graefes Arch. Ophthalmol. 75, 459−474.

Elschnig, A., 1910b. Studien zur sympatischen Ophthalmie: Die Antigene Wirkung des Augenpigmentes. von Graefes Arch. Opthalmol. 76, 509−546.

Fleck, L., 1979. Genesis and Development of a Scientific Fact. University of Chicago Press, Chicago.

Friedenwald, J.S., 1934. Notes on the allergy theory of sympathetic ophthalmia. J. Am. Med. Assoc. 17, 1008−1018.

Gell, P.G.H., Coombs, R.R.A., 1963. Clinical Aspects of Immunology. Blackwell Scientific, Oxford.

Goltz, D. 1980. Horror Autotoxicus: Ein Beitrag zur Geschichte und Theorie der Autoimmunpathologie im Spiegel eines vielzitierten Begriffes. Thesis, University of Münster.

Grabar, P., Miescher, P., 1959. Immunopathology-Immunopathologie. Benno Schwabe, Basel.

Halbert, S.P., et al., 1957. Homologous immunological studies of ocular lens II. Biological aspects. J. Exp. Med. 105, 453–462.

Heidelberger, M., Avery, O.T., 1923. The soluble specific substances of pneumococcus. J. Exp. Med. 38, 73–79.

Humphrey, J.H., White, R.G., 1963. Immunology for Students of Medicine. Blackwell Scientific, Oxford.

Jerne, N.K., 1974. Towards a network theory of the immune system. Ann. Immunol. (Paris). 125C, 373–389.

Kabat, E.A., Mayer, M.M., 1949. Quantitative Immunochemistry. Charles C. Thomas, Springfield, Ill.

Kabat, E.A., Wolfe, A., Bezer, A.E., 1947. The rapid production of acute encephalomyelitis in Rhesus monkeys by injection of heterologous and homologous brain tissue with adjuvants. J. Exp. Med. 85, 117–130.

Krusius, F.F., 1910. Ueberempfindlichkeitsversuche vom Auge aus. Arch. Augenheilk. 67, 6–35.

Kuhn, T., 1970. The Structure of Scientific Revolutions. second ed. University of Chicago Press, Chicago.

Landsteiner, K., 1900. Zur Kenntnis der antifermentativen, lytischen und agglutinierenden Wirkung des Blutserums und der Lymphe. Centralbl. Bakteriol. 27, 357–362.

Landsteiner, K. 1962. The Specificity of Serological Reactions, reprint of second ed., 1945. Dover, New York.

Lawrence, H.S., 1959. Cellular and Humoral Aspects of Hypersensitivity States. Hoeber-Harper, New York.

Mackay, I.A., Burnet, F.M., 1963. Autoimmune Diseases. Charles C. Thomas, Springfield, Ill.

Medawar, P.B., 1945. The behaviour and fate of skin autografts and skin homografts in rabbits. J. Anat. 78, 176–199.

Metalnikoff, S., 1900. Etudes sur la spermotoxine. Ann. Inst. Pasteur. 14, 577–589.

Metchnikoff, I.I., 1884. Ueber eine Sprosspilzkrankheit der Daphnien: Beitrag zur Lehre ueber den Kampf des Phagozyten gegen Krankheitserreger. Arch. Pathol. Anat. 86, 177–195.

Metchnikoff, E., 1900. Sur les cytotoxines. Ann. Inst. Pasteur. 14, 369–377.

Miescher, P., Vorlaender, K.O., 1958. Immunpathologie in Klinik und Forschung. Georg Thieme, Stuttgart.

Owen, R.D., 1945. Immunogenetic consequences of vascular anastomoses between bovine twins. Science. 102, 400–401.

Pasteur, L., 1880. Sur les maladies virulentes et en particulier sur la maladie appelée vulgairement choléra des poules. Compt. Rend. Acad. Sci. 90, 239–248.

Pauling, L., 1940. A theory of the structure and process of formation of antibodies. J. Am. Chem. Soc. 62, 2643–2657.

Pfeiffer, R., 1894. Weitere Untersuchungen über das Wesen der Choleraimmunität und über spezifische bactericide Prozesse. Z. Hygiene. 18, 1–16.

Rivers, T.M., Sprunt, D.H., Berry, G.P., 1933. Observations on attempts to produce acute disseminated encephalomyelitis in monkeys. J. Exp. Med. 58, 39–54.

Rivers, T.M., Schwentker, F.F., 1935. Encephalitis accompanied by myelin destruction experimentally produced in monkeys. J. Exp. Med. 61, 689–702.

Roitt, I.M., Doniach, D., Campbell, P.N., Vaughan-Hudson, R., 1956. Auto-antibodies in Hashimoto's disease (lymphadenoid goiter). Lancet. 2, 820–821.

Römer, P., 1905. Die Pathogenese der Cataracta senilis vom Standpunkt der Serumforschung. von Graefes Arch. Ophthalmol. 60, 175–186.

Römer, P., Gebb, H., 1912. Beitrag zur Frage der Anaphylaxie durch Linseneiweiss und Eiweiss aus andern Geweben des Auges. von Graefes Arch. Ophthalmol. 81, 367–402.

Rose, N.R., Mackay, I.R., 1985. Autoimmunity versus autoimmune disease. In: Rose, N.R., Mackay, I.R. (Eds.), The Autoimmune Diseases. Academic Press, New York, pp. xxv–xxvi.

Rose, N.R., Witebsky, E., 1956. Studies on organ specificity V. Changes in the thyroid gland of rabbits following active immunization with rabbit thyroid extracts. J. Immunol. 76, 417–427.

Sachs, H., 1909. Hämolysine und Cytotoxine des Blutserums, Handbuch der Technik und Methodik der Immunitätsforschung, vol. 2. Fischer, Jena, pp. 896–897.

Samter, M., et al., 1965. Immunological Diseases. Little Brown, Boston.

Santucci, S., 1906. Citotossine. Riv. Ital. Ottal. Roma. 2, 213–221.

Shaffer, J.H., LoGrippo, G.A., Chase, M.W. (Eds.), 1959. Mechanisms of Hypersensitivity. Little, Brown, Boston.

Silverstein, A.M., 1991. The dynamics of conceptual change in twentieth century immunology. Cell. Immunol. 132, 515–531.

Silverstein, A.M., 1994. The heuristic value of experimental systems: the case of immune hemolysis. J. Hist. Biol. 27, 437–447.

Silverstein, A.M., 2002. Paul Ehrlich's Receptor Immunology. Academic Press, New York, pp. 95–122.

Silverstein, A.M., 2009. Allergy and immunopathology: the price of immunity, A History of Immunology. second ed. Elsevier, New York, pp. 177–209.

Talmage, D.W., 1957. Allergy and immunology. Annu. Rev. Med. 8, 239–256.

Uhlenhuth, P., 1903. Zur Lehre von der Unterscheidung verschiedener Eiweissarten mit Hilfe spezifischer Sera. Festschrift zum 60 Geburtstag von Robert Koch. Fischer, Jena, p. 49.

Verhoeff, F.H., Lemoine, A.N., 1922. Endophthalmitis phacoanaphylactica. Am. J. Ophthalmol. 5, 737–745.

Voisin, G., Delaunay, A., Barber, M., 1951. Sur des lésions testiculaires provoquées chez le cobaye par iso- et auto-sensibilisation. Ann. Inst. Pasteur. 81, 48–63.

von Pirquet, C., 1910. Allergie. Springer, Berlin (English transl., Allergy. American Medical Association, Chicago, 1911).

von Wassermann, A., Neisser, A., Bruck, C., 1906. Eine Serodiagnostische Reaktion bei Syphilis. Dtsch. med. Wochenschr. 32, 745–746.

Weil, E., Braun, H., 1909. Ueber das Wesen der luetischen Erkrankung auf Grund der neueren Forschungen. Wien. Klin. Wochenschr. 22, 372–374.

Witebsky, E., 1954. Ehrlich's side-chain theory in light of present immunology. Ann. N.Y. Acad. Sci. 59 (168–181), 173.

Witebsky, E., et al., 1957. Chronic thyroiditis and autoimmunization. J. Am. Med. Assoc. 164, 1439–1447.

Woods, A.C., 1921. Immune reactions following injuries to the uveal tract. J. Am. Med. Assoc. 77, 1217–1222.

Woods, A.C., 1925. Sympathetic ophthalmia: the use of uveal pigment in diagnosis and treatment. Trans. Ophth. Soc. UK. 45, 208–249.

Woods, A.C., 1933. Allergy and Immunity in Ophthalmology. Johns Hopkins University Press, Baltimore.

Chapter 3

General Features of Autoimmune Disease

Anne Davidson and Betty Diamond

Center for Autoimmunity and Musculoskeletal Diseases, Feinstein Institute for Medical Research, Manhasset, NY, USA

Chapter Outline

Innate Immune Activation	19
Cells of the Adaptive Immune System	20
Defining Autoimmune Disease	21
Prevalence of Autoimmunity	21
Genetics of Autoimmunity	22
Association of Single Gene Defects with Autoimmunity	22
Genome-wide Association Studies (GWAS)	
Identify Multiple Gene Loci that are Associated	
with Autoimmunity	22
MHC Associations with Autoimmunity	22
Other Genes Identified by GWAS Studies	22
GWAS Studies Identify Common Pathways for	
Autoimmmunity	23
Application of Data from GWAS Studies to	
Clinical Practice	23
Epigenetic Alterations Associated with Autoimmunity	23
Hormones and Autoimmunity	24
Autoimmunity and Central Tolerance	24
Autoimmunity and Peripheral Tolerance	25
Triggers of Autommunity	25
Activation of the Immune System	26
Role of Antigen as a Driver of Autoimmunity	27
Defective Downregulation of an Immune Response	28
Regulatory Lymphocytes	28
The Role of the Gut Microbiota in Autoimmunity	29
Mechanisms of Tissue Damage	29
Flares and Remissions During Disease	30
Therapeutic Advances	30
Goals for the Future	31
Concluding Remarks	31
Acknowledgments	32
References	32

A host of diseases are characterized by activation of the immune system in the absence of an external threat to the organism. In these diseases, inflammation and tissue damage occur in the absence of infection, toxin exposure, or tumor growth. These diseases can be characterized as those that display activation of the innate immune system and an excess of inflammatory mediators, but no evidence of an antigen-specific immune response; familial Mediterranean fever and other inflammasome diseases, Behçet disease, even atherosclerosis, can be considered to fall within this category. Alternatively, there are diseases characterized by an activation of the adaptive immune response with T and B lymphocytes responding to self-antigen in the absence of any detectable microbial assault or tumor invasion. These diseases constitute the vast majority of diseases considered to be autoimmune in origin. There are over 80 defined autoimmune diseases in composite affecting 5−7% of the population. Moreover, their incidence is increasing (Patterson et al., 2009).

INNATE IMMUNE ACTIVATION

Activation of the innate immune response is a feature of many, perhaps all, autoimmune diseases (Mills, 2011). This activation may be the primary event involved in triggering the disease process. One example is activation of the innate immune system in systemic lupus due to complement deficiencies that permit excess accumulation of proinflammatory apoptotic debris (Manderson et al., 2004). Increased production of type 1 interferon is present in first degree relatives of some lupus patients, suggesting that this enhanced innate immune activation may be a triggering immune abnormality in these patients (Niewold, 2011). Likewise, inflammatory bowel disease (IBD) is associated with genetic alterations in the inflammasome pathway, leading to increased production of proinflammatory cytokines (Hamilton et al., 2012; Zaki et al., 2011). It is also apparent that the innate immune system can be activated secondarily in autoimmune disease. Immune

N. Rose & I. Mackay (Eds): The Autoimmune Diseases, Fifth edition. DOI: http://dx.doi.org/10.1016/B978-0-12-384929-8.00003-4

complexes containing endogenous Toll-like receptor (TLR) ligands such as DNA, RNA, or citrullinated proteins can activate dendritic cells and other myeloid cells to amplify inflammatory pathways (Green and Marshak-Rothstein, 2011; Sokolove et al., 2011). Tissue injury also leads to activation of innate immune cell networks (Kawai and Akira, 2010; Miyake and Yamasaki, 2012); thus, once autoimmune-triggered tissue injury is ongoing, the innate as well as the adaptive immune system is always engaged.

A low threshold for activation of myeloid cells and differentiation of monocytes to dendritic cells predisposes to autoimmune disease in animal models, and blockade of pathways of the innate immune system can ameliorate many autoimmune diseases. In particular, TLR signaling seems to be a critical feature of many autoimmune diseases as deletion of MyD88, a common component of the signaling cascade for several TLRs, and neutralization of high mobility group protein B1 (HMGB1), a cytokine which synergizes with many TLR agonists, can prevent or treat murine models of diabetes, rheumatoid arthritis, systemic lupus, IBD, and more (Andersson and Tracey, 2011; Herlands et al., 2008; Pagni et al., 2010; Rivas et al., 2012). The success of IL-1 and more recently IL-6 inhibition in rheumatoid arthritis and IL-12 inhibition in IBD also attest to the involvement of the innate immune response in autoimmune diseases.

Interestingly, the innate immune response, and more specifically monocyte activation, is under the control of the cholinergic anti-inflammatory pathway. This pathway is initiated in the central nervous system, is mediated through the vagus nerve (cholinergic) and the splenic nerve (adrenergic), and culminates in the induction of acetylcholine production by splenic T cells that then inhibits the production of inflammatory cytokines by monocytes that express an α7 cholinergic receptor (Rosas-Ballina and Tracey, 2009). The identification of this pathway has provided a potential therapeutic target that regulates multiple cytokines simultaneously.

CELLS OF THE ADAPTIVE IMMUNE SYSTEM

There is a coordinated interplay among the cells of the adaptive immune system with dendritic cells (DCs), T cells, and B cells interacting to generate the effector response of the immune system. DCs activate T cells and B cells. T cells activate DCs and B cells. B cells activate T cells. This cascade leads to an immune response that recognizes a broad spectrum of epitopes of microbial pathogens and enlists multiple effector mechanisms (Blanco et al., 2008; Goodnow et al., 2010; O'Shea and Paul, 2010; Shlomchik, 2008; Steinman, 2007).

DCs are antigen-presenting cells (APCs) that are the intermediary between the innate and the adaptive immune systems. DCs can be tolerogenic in their resting state (Kalantari et al., 2011; Morel and Turner, 2011), but when activated they are critical in initiating an immune response. Similarly, monocytes clear the apoptotic debris generated from the billions of cells that die daily in a tolerogenic fashion but, when exposed to inflammatory mediators, they differentiate into macrophages or DCs (Dominguez and Ardavin, 2010). Activation of the innate immune system, therefore, can establish a population of immunogenic DCs for activation of the adaptive immune system. Like essentially all cells, monocytes and DCs display surface expression of class I major histocompatibility complex (MHC) molecules, which permit the presentation of intracellular antigens to T cells. DCs and some macrophage subsets also express class II MHC molecules, which are present on a much more restricted set of cells and permit the presentation of extracellular antigens (Banchereau and Steinman, 1998). Multiple alleles of class I and II molecules exist and thus each individual has a unique set of MHC molecules (Beck and Trowsdale, 2000). DCs also express an array of nonpolymorphic receptors, such as TLRs, and pattern-recognition receptors that bind microbial antigens, products of tissue injury, and nucleic acids (Kawai and Akira, 2010, 2011). Engagement of these receptors causes the DCs to upregulate expression of costimulatory molecules and to deliver an obligatory second signal for activation (Dzopalic et al., 2012; Engels and Wienands, 2011; Vincenti and Luggen, 2007). It is important to note that each DC can recognize and respond to a broad spectrum of microbial antigens.

Each T cell and each B cell express a single receptor for antigen. These antigen receptors are acquired by gene rearrangements that occur in somatic cells (Gellert, 2002); thus, there is no inheritance of the T or B cell repertoire. T cells mature in the thymus (Stritesky et al., 2012). Each T cell expresses a unique receptor (TCR) that recognizes a molecular complex on the surface of an APC consisting of a class I or class II MHC molecule associated with a small peptide derived from an intra- or extra-cellular protein antigen, respectively. Signaling through both the TCR and costimulatory molecules is needed to effect activation of mature T cells (Engels and Wienands, 2011; Vincenti and Luggen, 2007; Weinstein et al., 2012). B cells also express a single receptor for antigen, but the B cell receptor (BCR) recognizes native antigen rather than processed antigen. B cell activation also requires signaling through both the BCR and costimulatory molecules (Crow, 2004). Activated B cells not only secrete antibody, but can also function as APCs to engage a greater number of T cells in the immune response. B cells also secrete molecules that are essential for lymphoid organization, and can secrete a variety of cytokines (Leon et al., 2012; Lipsky, 2001; Marino and Grey, 2012).

A critical feature of both T and B cells is that they proliferate in response to antigenic stimulation to create clonal expansions of cells with a unique antigenic specificity and to develop cells with a memory phenotype (Bishop et al., 2003; Grossman et al., 2004; McKinstry et al., 2010). Memory cells have an accelerated and enhanced response following re-exposure to antigen. B cells have the added feature of undergoing class switching of the immunoglobulin heavy chain gene and random somatic mutation of the BCR followed by selection of those B cells with improved affinity for the eliciting antigen (Li et al., 2004; Victora and Nussenzweig, 2012). Thus, there is a progression from low-affinity IgM antibodies to high-affinity IgG antibodies during the course of an immune response. The memory response reactivates the high-affinity IgG-producing B cells, whose repertoire is unique to each individual.

For the immune system to function effectively there must be a sufficient number in both the naïve and memory repertoires of T and B cells that can respond to an enormous diversity of microbial antigens, and a means of regulating those cells that respond to self-antigen.

DEFINING AUTOIMMUNE DISEASE

An autoimmune disease is a condition in which tissue injury is caused by T cell or antibody reactivity to self. The immune activation may be initiated by infection, but then persists in the absence of any detectable microbial antigen (Davidson and Diamond, 2001). It is important to state that although many diseases considered autoimmune display anti-self-reactivity, evidence may still be lacking that the self-reactivity is, in fact, responsible for tissue damage. It is sometimes possible to determine whether autoantibodies are pathogenic by transferring them to a rodent host; however, T cell reactivity is not transferable from humans to rodents because T cell activation and T cell effector function occur only in the context of self-MHC molecules. Thus, demonstrating the pathogenicity of the autoimmune response has not been accomplished in all autoimmune diseases. In some instances, a disease is presumed to be of autoimmune origin only because B and T cells are present in affected tissue.

Animal models of autoimmune disease have been enormously useful in aiding our understanding of both disease inception and disease pathogenesis (Bar-Or et al., 2011; Billiau and Matthys, 2011; Howell, 2002; King, 2012; Lam-Tse et al., 2002; Mandik-Nayak and Allen, 2005; Peutz-Kootstra et al., 2001; Wooley, 2004). Some models develop spontaneous disease. Others represent genetically modified mice that target a particular pathway in the immune response. Finally, some autoimmune diseases can be triggered in animals by immunization with self-antigen. While all these animal models have been very important in informing our understanding of autoimmunity, it is important to recognize that we do not know how closely they reflect human disease (Bodaghi and Rao, 2008; Kollias et al., 2011). Some of these models may be more similar to human disease in the effector mechanisms of tissue injury than in the mechanisms of induction of autoreactivity. Indeed, autoantibody-mediated tissue damage is probably most alike in human disease and animal models (Monach et al., 2004). It is also important to consider that there may be extensive heterogeneity in human disease and that the animal models we study intensively may reflect only a subset of individuals with a given disease. A challenge that confronts us is to understand which animal models are most similar to human disease, and can teach us most about the genetic predisposition to disease, disease pathogenesis, and effective therapy.

PREVALENCE OF AUTOIMMUNITY

It is striking that while each autoimmune disease individually affects only a small number of people, the prevalence of all autoimmune diseases is approximately 5–7% (Jacobson et al., 1997). Two critical facts about autoimmune disease are important in understanding the high frequency of these diseases. First, autoreactivity is an aspect of every normal immune system. In fact, the repertoire of immunocompetent lymphocytes that provides protective immunity is selected based on autoreactivity (Gu et al., 1991; Nobrega et al., 2002; Vallejo et al., 2004). Regulation of autoreactivity helps shape the immune system so that it does not become the pathogenic autoreactivity associated with tissue damage: this requires constant vigilance. The immune system maintains a precarious balance between the two: too little response leads to potential neglect of danger, while an overexuberant response can potentially lead to autoreactivity. How this balance is maintained is discussed below. Second, there is a genetic predisposition to autoimmunity and aspects of this predisposition may be similar for many different autoimmune diseases (Cho and Gregersen, 2011). Autoimmune disease requires not just autoreactivity, but may also be influenced by target-organ vulnerability (Liao et al., 1995; Liu et al., 2009). Some of the recent studies of the genetic basis of autoimmunity show that the genetic factors governing specific organ vulnerability are distinct from those governing autoreactivity. Thus, individuals may share pathways promoting autoreactivity, yet present with different autoimmune diseases (Cho and Gregersen, 2011; Cotsapas et al., 2011).

GENETICS OF AUTOIMMUNITY

Association of Single Gene Defects with Autoimmunity

It is clear from epidemiologic studies and studies of animal models of autoimmune disease that there is a genetic component to essentially every autoimmune disease. A few autoimmune diseases appear to be monogenic diseases (Chapters 29 and 50). The human disease autoimmune-polyendocrinopathy-candidiasis-ectodermal-dystrophy (APECED), an autoimmune disease of multiple endocrine organs, is a consequence of a deletion in the AIRE gene that encodes a protein that causes tissue-specific genes to be expressed in medullary epithelial cells in the thymus (Akirav et al., 2011; Anderson and Su, 2011). These cells mediate negative selection of T cells reactive with peptides that derive from tissue-specific proteins. In the absence of AIRE expression, a spectrum of autoreactive T cells fails to be deleted; these cells mature to immunocompetence and mediate an immune attack on various organs. The absence of the AIRE gene appears sufficient for autoimmunity, although the phenotype of the disease that emerges, even within a single family, can be quite variable. Similarly, a defect in the Fas gene can also lead to autoimmunity. The Fas protein is expressed on activated lymphocytes. Engagement of Fas by Fas ligand leads to the death of the Fas-expressing cell, a process critical for downregulating the immune response. Individuals deficient in Fas expression have a disease called autoimmune lymphoproliferative syndrome (ALPS) characterized by an excess of T and B cells and by autoantibody production (Fleisher et al., 2001; Grodzicky and Elkon, 2002; Madkaikar et al., 2011). Of note, not all individuals with deficient Fas expression display ALPS; thus, even in this disease other genes must modulate disease phenotype. Deficiency in certain complement components also results in a high incidence of the autoimmune disease systemic lupus erythematosus (SLE). In this case the mechanism is thought to be a failure of clearance of immune complexes and apoptotic material, resulting in an overload of immunogenic necrotic material that can activate the immune system through engagement of TLRs and other innate receptors (Lewis and Botto, 2006; Pettigrew et al., 2009). Finally, deficiency in Foxp3 that is required for the development of regulatory T cells is associated with severe autoimmunity affecting the bowel and endocrine organs (Ochs et al., 2007).

Genome-wide Association Studies (GWAS) Identify Multiple Gene Loci that are Associated with Autoimmunity

For most autoimmune diseases, multiple susceptibility loci contribute to the disease phenotype. Studies from mouse models of autoimmune disease have also revealed the presence of loci that suppress the autoimmune phenotype (Wakeland et al., 2001). Thus, an individual's risk of developing an autoimmune disease depends on a summation of susceptibility and resistance loci. A major advance in the last 5 years has been the application of genome-wide association scans (GWAS) that evaluate large numbers of common single nucleotide polymorphisms (SNPs) as genomic markers to type increasingly large datasets of well-defined patient and control populations. Studies in multiple autoimmune diseases have definitively linked a number of genetic variants to disease susceptibility (Deng and Tsao, 2010; Flesher et al., 2010; Harley et al., 2008).

MHC Associations with Autoimmunity

Despite the identification of a large number of autoimmunity associated genes using the GWAS approach, the polymorphic locus most closely linked to autoimmunity in studies of virtually every autoimmune disease is the MHC locus, an association that has long been known. For example, anti-cyclic citrullinated protein (CCP) positive rheumatoid arthritis in the white population is highly associated with the expression of a set of DR4 alleles that have a particular structural motif, called the "shared epitope" (Winchester, 2004). Reactive arthritis occurs in individuals expressing B27 or, less commonly, B7 class I MHC molecules. In type 1 diabetes both pathogenic and protective DR and DQ alleles have been identified and the *trans*-complementing heterodimer encoded by DQA1*0501 and DQB1*0302 confers very high risk. In celiac disease, 98−99% of affected individuals bear a susceptibility DQ allele—thus DQ testing can be used clinically to exclude disease with a high degree of certainty (Wolters and Wijmenga, 2008). Multiple sclerosis and systemic lupus display particular human leukocyte antigen (HLA) associations, as do many other autoimmune diseases (Fernando et al., 2008; Tomlinson and Bodmer, 1995; Winchester, 2004; Wong and Wen, 2003). The basis for the association of MHC polymorphisms with autoimmune disease is still for the most part unknown but might be due to T cell recognition of particular pathogenic peptides that can bind within the peptide binding cleft of certain MHC molecules, cross-reactivity of peptides derived from infectious organisms with self-peptides, or alterations in the T cell repertoire that result in a decrease in regulatory T cells.

Other Genes Identified by GWAS Studies

A number of non-MHC genes within or in linkage disequilibrium with the MHC locus could help regulate the immune response and may also contribute to a genetic predisposition to autoimmunity. Genetic studies are allowing an exploration of this question. In rheumatoid arthritis, for example, virtually all the risk for CCP positive disease within the MHC locus is attributable to variations within the peptide binding groove of HLA DR with a lesser contribution from two MHC class I alleles and virtually none from non-MHC genes (Raychaudhuri et al., 2012).

With the exception of the MHC, the other genetic risk loci for autoimmunity that have been identified by GWAS involve a conglomeration of approximately 150–200 relatively common alleles (Cho and Gregersen, 2011), each of which confers only a modest risk, with odds ratios <1.5–2. Some of these polymorphisms are shared between autoimmune disorders and some, but not all, cross major racial groups. In mouse models there is evidence that genetic susceptibility can be a consequence of combinations of genes within each gene locus, and not the consequence of a single gene in each locus. For example, a region on chromosome 1 that is implicated in autoimmunity in SLE has several sub-loci which contribute to various aspects of the disease (Morel, 2010; Morel et al., 2001).

Clinically, it has long been appreciated that autoimmune diseases cluster in families. The biologic basis for this observation is now clear; the same susceptibility genes can influence many different autoimmune diseases. For example, a polymorphism of CTLA-4, an inhibitory costimulatory molecule present on activated T cells, conveys risk for insulin-dependent diabetes, autoimmune hemolytic anemia, and Graves' disease (Ueda et al., 2003), while the CARD15 (NOD-2) gene is associated with both IBD and psoriasis (Bene et al., 2011; Rahman et al., 2003; Russell et al., 2004; Zaki et al., 2011). Similarly, polymorphisms in PTPN22, a molecule that regulates lymphocyte receptor signaling, is associated with type 1 diabetes, SLE, RA, and Crohn's disease but not multiple sclerosis (Burn et al., 2011). The differences in disease phenotype may lie in associated genes, those governing target organ susceptibility or those that modulate disease severity (Russell et al., 2004) or in different environmental exposures. Indeed, the genetic association of HLA and Ptpn22 with CCP-positive rheumatoid arthritis is considerably magnified in smokers, leading to a postulated pathogenetic mechanism whereby damage to the lung by cigarette smoke induces autoimmunity to citrullinated proteins specifically in genetically susceptible individuals (Mahdi et al., 2009).

GWAS Studies Identify Common Pathways for Autoimmmunity

One of the most striking advances made as a result of the GWAS analyses has been the identification of immune pathways associated with autoimmune tendencies, some

of which are shared across diseases. A meta-analysis of the autoimmunity associated genes identified thus far suggests that individual diseases can be clustered in groups that share pathogenetic mechanisms. For example, using this type of methodology, disease associations with polymorphisms in IL-2 can be distinguished from those associated with IL-21 that are within the same genetic locus (Cotsapas et al., 2011). The genetic studies in sum suggest that autoimmunity can result from a defect in almost any pathway of immune homeostasis and affect thresholds for innate immune cell activation and for selection and activation of autoreactive lymphocytes.

Application of Data from GWAS Studies to Clinical Practice

Applying this new information to individual patients represents a major challenge since attribution of an SNP identified by GWAS to a single gene often requires extensive resequencing of large regions of DNA from many patients. Furthermore, since the GWAS approach (Cantor et al., 2010) identifies only common polymorphisms with frequencies within the population of >1–5%, the risk variants identified by this method account for only a small proportion of the overall heritability of the disease (Deng and Tsao, 2010). New methodologies to identify rare variants or copy number variations are being developed, but these variations will only be seen in a small fraction of those who are affected. Finally, establishing a link between genetic variations, gene function, and disease pathogenesis has not been easy. Many of the risk alleles identified by GWAS are common variants with subtle effects that are compatible with normal immunological function; in many cases the variation is not even within the gene coding region. Even for genes with coding region mutations such as Ptpn22, functional studies may yield conflicting results (Rieck et al., 2007; Zhang et al., 2011). More studies will be required to understand how the disease-associated variants affect immune responses and interact with each other to contribute to the risk of a particular disease. Nevertheless, as the function of the variants is clarified and potentially pathogenic pathways are identified, personalized interventions may become possible.

Epigenetic Alterations Associated with Autoimmunity

Despite the advances in understanding the genetics of autoimmunity, concordance in monozygotic twins remains below 50% for most diseases, indicating a contribution from random and/or environmental factors. Epigenetic alterations that change the access of DNA regions to the transcriptional machinery through methylation or acetylation, or silence transcription through inhibitor miRNAs, or alter protein longevity or processing within the cell through ubiquitination or citrullination, may all influence immune system function. T cell differentiation, for example, is influenced by epigenetic mechanisms that reinforce the T cell cytokine-producing phenotype (Nakayamada et al., 2012). While it is clear that epigenetic alterations may profoundly influence cell phenotype, the application of this concept to autoimmunity is in its early phases (Chapter 28). Abnormalities of methylation or acetylation or of expression of particular miRNAs has been demonstrated among peripheral blood cells of patients with several autoimmune diseases (Ceribelli et al., 2011a, b; Ghosh et al., 2012) and there are several examples of deficiencies of particular enzymes or miRNA species causing spontaneous autoimmune disease in mice (Glasmacher et al., 2010; Namjou et al., 2011).

HORMONES AND AUTOIMMUNITY

Since many autoimmune diseases occur more commonly in women than in men, and autoimmunity in general is almost three times more common in women than in men, there have been several investigations of the role of sex hormones in autoimmune disease (Chapter 24). Animal studies have shown multiple effects of sex steroids on the immune system (Rubtsov et al., 2010); studies in mice lacking an estrogen receptor have clearly attributed estrogen effects to signaling through the estrogen receptor α. However, it has been difficult to extrapolate the conclusions from these studies to autoimmunity. Not all autoimmune diseases are more common in women. Some, such as ankylosing spondylitis, have a much higher incidence in men. Furthermore, the predisposition to autoimmunity can be sex determined or hormonally modulated; thus, the higher incidence of disease in women may not always reflect the influence of female hormones on the immune system. The X chromosome in fact harbors many genes of immunologic interest. In gonad matched mice the presence of XX confers a greater susceptibility to pristane induced lupus than does XY (Smith-Bouvier et al., 2008). Similarly, in humans, the XXY phenotype is associated with an increased prevalence of SLE. Nevertheless, the genetic components of the XX chromosome complement associated with lupus risk are not yet clear. The evidence also shows that the effects of sex hormones differ in different diseases. While there is significant evidence that estrogen can exacerbate systemic lupus, estrogen seems to protect against rheumatoid arthritis. Additionally, estrogen or other sex hormones might affect target-organ antigen display or target-organ susceptibility to immune-mediated damage. Thus, there is no simple paradigm to explain the relationship between sex and autoimmunity (Grimaldi et al., 2005).

AUTOIMMUNITY AND CENTRAL TOLERANCE

The hallmark of autoimmune disease is the activation of self-reactive T and B lymphocytes. A major mechanism of self-tolerance is the elimination of self-reactive immature lymphocytes by antigen ligation of the T cell receptor (TCR) or BCR at critical stages of development. For autoimmunity to develop there must be a lack of stringency in the elimination of autoreactive cells. Because TCRs and BCRs are generated by random gene rearrangements that occur within the nucleus of the cell and are not determined by knowledge of the world of self or foreign antigen, autoreactive T and B cells arise routinely. To eliminate autoreactive cells and maintain self-tolerance, T and B cells routinely undergo a selection process during their maturation in primary lymphoid organs, the thymus and bone marrow, respectively (Alexandropoulos and Danzl, 2012; Goodnow et al., 2010; Rajewsky, 1996; Vallejo et al., 2004; von Boehmer and Melchers, 2010). B cells again undergo a second process of selection after somatic mutation of immunoglobulin genes, as somatic mutation routinely generates autoreactivity (Goodnow et al., 2010; Shlomchik, 2008).

T cells that mature in the thymus and enter peripheral lymphoid organs must display TCRs with some affinity for self-peptide—self-MHC complexes in order to receive the necessary signals for survival, termed positive selection. T cells arising in the thymus that express TCRs lacking any affinity for the self-peptide—self-MHC complexes fail to undergo positive selection and die. T cells that are strongly reactive to self-peptide—self-MHC complexes are eliminated in a process termed negative selection. The threshold for both positive and negative selection represents a continuum. As the peptide—MHC complexes present in the thymus differ in each individual and the threshold for negative selection varies from individual to individual, each individual releases a different repertoire of antimicrobial and antiself reactive T cells to the periphery, each reflecting a different spectrum of foreign and self-peptide specificities (Bommhardt et al., 2004; Vallejo et al., 2004; Werlen et al., 2003). It is also probable that certain stimuli can rescue T cells.

B cells similarly undergo a process of negative selection prior to achieving immunocompetence. This process occurs in the bone marrow and continues in the spleen where B cells migrate as transitional cells after exiting the bone marrow. Whether B cells require positive selection on self-antigen for survival and need to display some degree of autoreactivity remains an area of active investigation. It is clear, however, that highly autoreactive B cells are negatively selected on self-antigens encountered during early maturation, and again the threshold for deletion is different for each individual (Monroe et al.,

2003). Deletion occurs with the highest extent of BCR cross-linking; anergy occurs with less cross-linking. Thus, the degree of autoreactivity in the B cell repertoire is also variable. B cell selection is influenced not only by the strength of the signal received through the BCR but also by the availability of the tumor necrosis factor (TNF) like cytokine BAFF. In late transitional B cells the interaction of BAFF with BAFF-R cooperates with signals received though the BCR to promote B cell survival and metabolic fitness. Since the availability of BAFF depends to a large extent on the number of B cells, B cell depletion can result in high levels of BAFF leading to relaxation in the stringency of selection and the escape of autoreactive B cells to the periphery (Liu and Davidson, 2011; Mackay and Schneider, 2009). Anergic autoreactive B cells may also be rescued in a proinflammatory setting by engagement of costimulatory molecules on the B cell membrane or by signaling through TLRs (Monroe and Keir, 2008). Thus, the repertoire of naïve B cells will vary over time within an individual, with higher-affinity autoreactive B cells present during times of infection, inflammation or lymphopenia, and fewer, lower-affinity autoreactive cells present during times of immunologic quiescence (Goodnow et al., 2010; Liu and Davidson, 2011; Shlomchik, 2008).

This paradigm must be understood in the context of our knowledge that autoimmunity is often accompanied by some degree of immunodeficiency. A failure of proper selection may lead to a repertoire that includes too many antigen-reactive T or B cells. This might result in a secondary failure to focus on those clones that mediate protective immunity. The presence of autoreactivity in individuals who are immunosuppressed is more straightforward. For example, the increased levels of BAFF that result from B cell lymphopenia will lead to a failure to appropriately select the B cell repertoire. Some defects that affect T cell activation also impair expansion of regulatory cells or T cell apoptosis and may therefore impair both responses to pathogens and self-tolerance. In the presence of T cell lymphopenia, homeostatic expansion of self-reactive cells can occur.

AUTOIMMUNITY AND PERIPHERAL TOLERANCE

Negative selection of T and B cells occurs in the periphery as well as in primary lymphoid organs, permitting the removal of autoreactive cells that do not encounter autoantigen in the thymus or bone marrow. This process of negative selection is termed peripheral tolerance. Like central tolerance, it is mediated by engagement of the TCR or BCR in a noninflammatory setting (Goodnow et al., 2010; Walker and Abbas, 2002). Although it has

been traditional to debate whether autoimmunity results from a defect in central tolerance in the thymus or bone marrow, or in peripheral tolerance in secondary lymphoid organs, current knowledge of tolerance induction suggests that this may be an artificial distinction. Engagement of the antigen receptor is critical to both central and peripheral tolerance, although there are some differences in antigen receptor signaling pathways, expression of co-receptors and costimulatory molecules that exist between immature T or B cells and their mature counterparts. Mouse models of autoimmunity suggest that defects in negative selection can be limited to central or peripheral tolerance (Anderson and Su, 2011; Linterman et al., 2009; Vinuesa et al., 2005) whereas others may paradoxically impair central tolerance and enhance peripheral activation (Seo et al., 2003). Thus, some autoimmune-prone individuals might exhibit a general lack of stringency in B or T cell tolerance while others might have a defect that is stage specific. This distinction has important therapeutic implications; learning to subset patients based on their tolerance impairment mechanism might permit a better pairing of patient with therapy, in short more personalized medicine. In summary, the thresholds for survival and deletion need to be set within appropriate limits at multiple times in the maturation and activation of a lymphoid cell (Goodnow et al., 2010; Liu and Davidson, 2011; von Boehmer and Melchers, 2010). Too little deletion at any stage and autoreactivity ensues; too much deletion and the protective repertoire may be compromised. Any genetic change that reduces deletion or enhances activation may be a risk factor for autoimmunity.

TRIGGERS OF AUTOMMUNITY

Environmental factors are important triggers for expression of autoimmunity. Autoimmunity may develop following sterile tissue damage. Smoking, drug exposure, diet, chemical exposure, and sunlight have all been implicated as risk factors for particular diseases (D'Cruz, 2000; Debandt et al., 2003; Knip and Akerblom, 1999; Moriyama and Eisenbarth, 2002; Price and Venables, 1995; Steen, 1999; Vaarala, 2012). Molecular pathways for some of these have been established (Chapter 21). Smoking and periodontal disease lead to the generation of citrullinated proteins; these are a target of autoantibodies in rheumatoid arthritis (Klareskog et al., 2011; Routsias et al., 2011). Notably, PAD, the gene encoding petidyl arginine deiminase involved in the citrullination of proteins, contains a susceptibility allele for rheumatoid arthritis (Bang et al., 2010; Kochi et al., 2011). UV light causes apoptosis of keratinocytes, liberating cellular debris which is then bound by SLE-associated autoantibodies, initiating an inflammatory response in the skin

(Bijl and Kallenberg, 2006; Kuhn and Beissert, 2005). It is now appreciated that pattern recognition receptors for microbial pathogen-associated molecular patterns (PAMPs) also bind to endogenous ligands, DAMPs, or damage-associated molecular patterns. The release of DAMPs in damaged tissue can establish a proinflammatory milieu leading to immunogenic presentation of self-antigens that are normally sequestered from the immune system, such as many intracellular antigens (Zhang et al., 2010). Once these become targets of an immune response, ongoing inflammation may be sustained. For example, the ongoing inflammation in some diseases, such as autoimmune myositis, targets regenerating tissue, preventing tissue repair and resolution of inflammation (Mammen et al., 2011; Suber et al., 2008).

Clearly, infection can also precipitate autoimmune disease. It has even been suggested that most autoimmune diseases represent the late sequelae of an infectious process (Christen et al., 2012; James and Robertson, 2012) (Chapter 19). Proving this hypothesis has, however, been difficult. For some diseases, such as rheumatic fever, the causal connection between microbial infection, the antimicrobial response, and autoimmune disease is clearly established (Cunningham, 2003; Guilherme and Kalil, 2004). For other diseases, there is suggestive epidemiologic evidence in humans or evidence from animal models that autoimmunity can follow microbial infection, or T cell or antibody cross-reactivity with both microbial and self-antigen has been identified (James and Robertson, 2012; Kuon and Sieper, 2003; Strassburg et al., 2003). In general, researchers have sought to implicate particular infections in the pathogenesis of particular autoimmune diseases, but it is possible that for some autoimmune diseases there is more than one possible microbial trigger. Importantly, the interaction of the TCR with a peptide–MHC complex must be of higher affinity to activate a naïve T cell than a memory T cell. Thus, a microbial peptide may initiate a response that can then be sustained by self-peptide. Moreover, once a response to self-antigen is initiated, epitope spreading to other epitopes on the same protein or on associated proteins occurs, often through B cell-mediated antigen presentation (Shlomchik et al., 2001).

Recent studies have provided remarkable information on the progression of autoimmunity, demonstrating that the autoantibodies characteristic of a given autoimmune disease are present as long as 10 years before the onset of clinical disease (Arbuckle et al., 2003). Moreover, cytokine abnormalities can also be observed before the onset of clinical symptomatology (Deane et al., 2010). These observations suggest there may be an opportunity to abort or retard the progression to disease in predisposed individuals.

Finally, the adipocyte has joined the ranks of immunomodulatory cells. It can secrete a variety of cytokines that promote a proinflammatory, proimmunogenic milieu (de Heredia et al., 2012). Thus, increasing obesity may be one contributor to the increasing incidence of autoimmune disease.

ACTIVATION OF THE IMMUNE SYSTEM

Activation of both T and B cells in the periphery requires that the cells receive two signals, one derived by ligation of the antigen receptor and the other by engagement of a costimulatory receptor. In general, when antigen enters the system, there is an activation of DCs, the critical APC in a primary immune response. This occurs because microbes express molecules that bind to pattern-recognition receptors or TLRs on the DC. The consequence of this binding is upregulation of the costimulatory molecules CD80 (B7.1) and CD86 (B7.2) on DCs, and transformation of the DC from resting, or tolerogenic to activated, or immunogenic. T cells recognizing microbial peptide in either class I or class II MHC molecules on the immunogenic DC will be activated. Because some degree of autoreactivity is present in all T cells, each time a T cell is activated by a foreign-peptide–self-MHC complex, that activated T cell may also recognize a self-peptide–self-MHC complex. It is a feature of memory T cells that they can be activated by a lower-affinity interaction with the TCR than is required to activate primary T cells; this is due to epigenetic changes and alterations in the structure of lipid rafts in the membrane that facilitate rapid receptor cross-linking with much less requirement for costimulatory signals (Weng et al., 2012). Thus, a T cell that is not activated by a self-peptide–self-MHC complex while still a naïve cell may be activated self-antigen once it becomes a memory T cell. Memory T cells may therefore be autoreactive in a proinflammatory setting. In addition, the signaling cascades within activated lymphocytes may differ in autoimmune vs. healthy individuals. For example, peripheral T cells from SLE patients have altered signaling and a faster T cell calcium flux than those of healthy individuals due to replacement of the principal signaling molecule of the TCR complex, CD3ζ, by the FcRγ chain (Moulton and Tsokos, 2011). This results in use of the adaptor molecule Syk rather than the usual ZAP70 and activation of the downstream kinase calcium/calmodulin-dependent protein kinase type IV (CaMK4) that, via the transcription factor Cremα, enhances production of IL-17 and blocks production of IL-2. B cells activated in an inflammatory setting may also recruit aberrant signaling pathways that amplify the inflammatory phenotype of the cell (Doreau et al., 2009).

There are many examples in the literature of a T cell derived from an individual with autoimmune disease that recognizes both a microbial peptide and a self-peptide. This cross-reactivity is termed molecular mimicry, and represents a mechanism by which autoimmunity can be triggered by infection (Cusick et al., 2012). The hypothesis that molecular mimicry predisposes to autoimmunity clearly has validity in rodent models of autoimmune disease, and suggests that laxity in selection of the naïve T cell repertoire can be a major contributor to autoimmunity. Those individuals with less stringent negative selection will have multiple T cells that can be activated by foreign antigen and will also display pathogenic autoreactivity.

The activated T cell provides T cell help or costimulatory signals to B cells that are encountering microbial antigen. B cells that bind both microbial antigen and self-antigen will ingest, process, and present epitopes of self-antigen, which can then be recognized by T cells. Because B cells often process antigen to different peptides than do DCs, the B cells can present novel epitopes of self-antigen and activate T cells with novel autospecificities (Bockenstedt et al., 1995; Sercarz et al., 1993; Yan et al., 2006). These cross-reactive B cells will, therefore, contribute to a cascade of autoreactivity, as they activate an expanded repertoire of T cells. Memory B cells are also potent antigen presenting cells that can activate naïve T cells. The B cell repertoire, therefore, critically influences the T cell repertoire (Whitmire et al., 2009). The fewer autoreactive B cells present, the less presentation of self-antigen to T cells.

There is much complexity in the cytokine expression patterns of activated T cells with at least four subsets of well-described helper T cells (Th1, Th2, Th17, and T_{FH}) as well as regulatory cells that help to restrain immune responses. The balance of transcriptional regulators expressed in each T cell will help determine its precise function, whereas epigenetic changes will help to reinforce a particular phenotype through subsequent rounds of proliferation. Nevertheless, there is emerging evidence that helper T cells have a substantial amount of flexibility with respect to their phenotype. Signals from the innate immune system can be drivers of T cell reprogramming, suggesting that inflammation or infection may have a profound effect on T cell function, converting T cells with a protective phenotype to those that amplify inflammation (Nakayamada et al., 2012).

Much is now known about the signaling pathways that are downstream of receptor and costimulatory molecule mediated stimulation and that are required for B and T cell activation and cytokine production. Since activated lymphocytes are major mediators of the effector inflammatory response, some of these pathways are targets for immune interventions with small molecules. Both inhibitors of Syk and of Jak3 have been used clinically in autoimmune diseases and other kinase inhibitors are in development (Kontzias et al., 2012). In addition, because

the high rate of cell growth and proliferation occurring in expanding clones requires a large amount of energy, there is increasing recognition that immune responses are linked to metabolism and that different types of effector and regulatory T cells have different metabolic requirements (Gerriets and Rathmell, 2012).

ROLE OF ANTIGEN AS A DRIVER OF AUTOIMMUNITY

A major question in autoimmune disease is whether the process is autonomous or driven by antigen, and, if the latter, whether the antigen is self-antigen or foreign antigen. Animal models of disease definitively show that molecular mimicry following activation by microbial antigen can initiate autoreactivity (Cunningham, 2003; Cusick et al., 2012; Kuwabara, 2004).

There are also data suggesting that self-antigen drives the autoimmune response. First, in animal models of systemic lupus, it appears that an excess of apoptotic cells or a problem in their clearance can result in a lupus-like serology with antichromatin reactivity (Peng and Elkon, 2011; Peng et al., 2007). Current understanding would suggest that an excess of apoptotic debris can activate TLRs and transform tolerogenic DCs into immunogenic APCs, as well as activate B cells (Filardy et al., 2010).

Second, extensive tissue damage can lead to the presentation of normally sequestered self-antigen in a proinflammatory setting (Bratton and Henson, 2011; Horwitz et al., 2002; Vezys and Lefrancois, 2002) or post-translational alteration of self-antigen such that it is now immunogenic (Doyle and Mamula, 2012). The proinflammatory setting may be enhanced by apoptosis of cells following tissue insult. This can clearly lead to an autoimmune response. Whether in some individuals this response is perpetuated because of a lack of appropriate restoration to homeostasis is an important question.

Finally, polymorphisms in autoantigens may also constitute risk factors for autoimmune disease (Pauza et al., 2004; Suzuki et al., 2003). As the genetic susceptibility to autoimmune disease is further explored, the degree to which molecular mimicry, aberrant expression of autoantigens, or exposure to previously sequestered antigen in an immunogenic setting contributes to disease will become more apparent.

A variety of environmental exposures might also nonspecifically accelerate disease by activating the innate immune system resulting in the release of proinflammatory cytokines that initiate autoimmunity. In mice, for example, type I interferons can initiate SLE in susceptible strains (Koutouzov et al., 2006) and may be responsible for the Koebner phenomenon observed in psoriasis. Tissue damage also results in the release of soluble mediators such as HMGB1, defensins and heat shock proteins that can activate DAMPs and TLRs and further amplify immune activation pathways.

DEFECTIVE DOWNREGULATION OF AN IMMUNE RESPONSE

The induction of an immune response needs to be followed by a downregulation or elimination of most of the cells that have undergone clonal expansion. A major observation of recent studies of autoimmune disease is that a defect in the restoration of immune homeostasis, or in downregulation of an immune response, can be a risk factor for autoimmunity. Since all reactivity with foreign antigen includes reactivity to self-antigen, anti-self-responses are routinely generated in the process of mounting an immune response to foreign antigen. The potential pathogenicity of the autoimmune response will vary from individual to individual. In general, however, the mechanisms that exist to dampen the immune response also diminish the autoreactivity, and even potentially pathogenic autoreactivity is downregulated. B and T cells are routinely downregulated as soon as they are activated. For the B cell, this occurs, in part, by cross-linking of the BCR and FcRIIB by antigen−antibody complexes. When FcRIIB is absent or deficient on B cells, as occurs in many individuals with SLE, autoantibody production is poorly controlled (Bolland and Ravetch, 2000; Fukuyama et al., 2005). Multiple coinhibitory molecules are expressed on activated T cells. Interaction with their receptors either within lymphoid organs or in the peripheral site of inflammation transduces an inhibitory signal to the T cells, signaling them to downmodulate their response (Francisco et al., 2010; Scandiuzzi et al., 2011). There is also some evidence that engagement of CD80 (B7) on the APC by the T cell coinhibitory molecule CTLA-4 transduces an inhibitory signal to the APCs. Mutations in two coinhibitory molecules, PD1 and CTLA-4, are associated with several autoimmune diseases (Chen, 2004; Khoury and Sayegh, 2004). Both B and T cells are also susceptible to activation-induced cell death mediated through Fas−Fas ligand interactions (Brunner et al., 2003; Li-Weber and Krammer, 2003). Defects in this process can lead to autoimmunity.

Thus, controlling the immune response is critical to normal homeostasis of the immune system and is mediated by multiple inhibitory pathways. A major component of autoimmune disease in some individuals may be a defect in the suppression of immune activation.

REGULATORY LYMPHOCYTES

Another area of intensive study is the characterization and mechanisms of action of CD4- positive T regulatory cells, some of which arise during thymic development and others after antigen exposure in the periphery (Wing and Sakaguchi, 2010). These cells regulate immune responses in a variety of ways that include secretion of inhibitory cytokines, promotion of apoptosis of effector lymphocytes, depriving effector T cells of cytokines or essential amino acids leading to apoptosis, or inhibition of dendritic cell function. Absence of Tregs in mice results in lymphoproliferation and fatal multi-organ autoimmunity, demonstrating the need for the ongoing regulation of pathogenic self-reactive cells that escape into the periphery. A population of $CD4^+/CD25^{hi}$ (γ chain of the IL-2 receptor) naturally occurring T regulatory cells (nTregs) arises in the thymus in response to TCR encounter with self-antigens with an avidity lower than that required for negative selection; their development depends on both CD28 and IL-2. Tregs can also be generated after antigen exposure in the periphery from naïve T cells in a manner that is dependent on IL-2 and TGFβ and may be enhanced by the vitamin A metabolite retinoic acid. Both these types of Tregs express the master transcriptional regulator Foxp3; its expression is stabilized by epigenetic modifications of DNA that reinforce the transcriptional availability of suppressive cytokines while preventing access of transcription factors to DNA encoding inflammatory cytokines (Hsieh et al., 2012; Josefowicz et al., 2012a).

Cells expressing immunosuppressive cytokines such as transforming growth factor (TGF)-β or IL-10 (Tr1 cells) (Pot et al., 2011) arise under particular conditions of antigen exposure and once activated, mediate suppression through both cytokine secretion and contact mediated lysis of effector cells. Tr1 cells are present in large numbers in the gut where they help to protect from colitis and they can also protect against multiple sclerosis in mice. Tr1 cells are Foxp3 negative and can be induced by IL-27 (Wojno and Hunter, 2012) but have been difficult to study due to lack of a clear phenotype. Nevertheless, the transcriptional program of these cells is being unraveled and recent studies have suggested that both IFNβ and galectin 1 induce DCs to produce IL-27, suggesting a way in which Tr1 cells can be induced therapeutically.

Other studies have identified a population of CD8 suppressor cells that may directly lyse autoreactive cells or may secrete immunosuppressive cytokines (Cortesini et al., 2001; Jiang et al., 2010). In lupus models these cells can be induced by autoantigen or by idiotype peptides (Sawla et al., 2012). $CD8^+$ regulatory T cells have recently been described during adaptive immune responses where they serve to regulate humoral responses in the germinal center by lysing B cells (Kim and Cantor, 2011). Another group of Tregs expresses neither CD4 nor CD8 and its function is dependent on IFNγ.

The balance between effector cells and regulatory cells may determine whether an autoreactive response that arises in the course of microbial exposure is terminated or perpetuated. However, application of this new knowledge to the treatment of autoimmunity is still in its earliest stages. One approach has been to use inhibitors of the mammalian target of rapamycin (mTOR) to induce or stabilize Foxp3 expression (Chinen and Rudensky, 2012; Josefowicz et al., 2012b). Another is to use low-dose IL-2 or IL-2 anti-IL-2 complexes to enhance Treg development. This strategy has recently been successfully applied to the treatment of graft versus host disease (GVHD) and cryoglobulinemic vasculitis in humans in which an increase in Tregs was associated with a therapeutic response (Oo et al., 2012). *In vitro* expansion and delivery of a stable population of Tregs or *in vivo* activation of antigen-specific Tregs by tolerogenic self-peptides have been problematic since the precise TCR affinity or antigen dose required for Treg generation are not known and many factors in the microenvironment may influence the survival or stability of transferred Tregs or the outcome of TCR peptide encountered *in vivo*. Clinical trials directed at tolerance induction in new onset type 1 diabetes by manipulation of Tregs have failed to cure disease despite an increase in Treg numbers, although several approaches have had partial effects (Gallagher et al., 2011).

B cells may also have regulatory functions (Klinker and Lundy, 2012). One such B cell subset produces IL-10 and can regulate autoimmunity in mice. The phenotype of these cells has not been fully elucidated but they may derive from immature or innate B cell populations (B1). The human counterpart of these cells and an understanding of how and where these cells regulate autoimmunity remains to be clarified. Another way in which B cells can regulate immune responses is by post-transcriptional modification of antibodies. Alterations in galactosylation and sialylation of the Fc region of Ig molecules may have a profound effect on immune responses. Sialylated immunoglobulin suppresses immune responses by binding to DC-SIGN on macrophages and DCs and initiating a suppressive program that results in upregulation of the suppressive Fc receptor FcRII on macrophages (Anthony et al., 2011). Specific IgM antibodies that have low affinity autoreactivity can also suppress immune responses by promoting opsonization of apoptotic material and promoting non-inflammatory clearance (Chen et al., 2009).

Since intense immunosuppression may inactivate both effector and regulatory T cells and B cell depletion may deplete both effector and regulatory B cells, improved strategies to inhibit effector cells, while allowing regulatory cells to expand, are being actively pursued. The success of this strategy will depend on a better understanding of the origins and growth requirements of the various regulatory cell types and the development of mechanisms to target them specifically and reinforce their stability *in vivo*.

THE ROLE OF THE GUT MICROBIOTA IN AUTOIMMUNITY

An emerging theme in autoimmunity is the heretofore unrecognized role of the gut microbiota in regulating immune responses (Atarashi and Honda, 2011) (Chapter 25). A vast colony of bacteria of multiple species is found in the human gut and can be changed by diet and other environmental exposures. One of the most important observations in this field is that the induction of TH17 cells in mice requires segmented filamentous bacteria; absence of these bacteria prevents the induction of experimental forms of arthritis and multiple sclerosis in normal mice and the spontaneous onset of type 1 diabetes in a susceptible mouse strain (Romano-Keeler et al., 2012). The bacteria provide TLR ligands and induce other inflammatory genes that trigger DCs and are also a source of ATP that helps to activate TH17 cells. The precise function of these cells, either as pathogenic cells, or as regulatory cells that also produce IL-10, will depend on other factors in the gut environment. Pathogenic bacteria may be found in some types of autoimmunity. For example, transfer of commensal bacteria from diseased to normal mice can transmit inflammatory bowel disease, suggesting that the initiating trigger for this disease may be communicable (Garrett et al., 2007). Importantly, susceptibility to colitis may be altered by dietary changes that prevent the emergence of the pathogenic bacteria suggesting that fecal transplants or probiotics are therapeutic strategies that should be tested. Gut microbiota also appear to be required for the generation of gut Tr1 cells and this may be mediated by different bacterial species than those that induce TH17 cells. Conversely, the absence of regulatory T cells can affect the composition of the gut microbiota (Chinen and Rudensky, 2012; Josefowicz et al., 2012b). How the balance of pro- and anti-inflammatory gut microbiota is maintained and how this might be manipulated for the prevention or treatment of autoimmunity remains an important question.

MECHANISMS OF TISSUE DAMAGE

Studies over the past decade have clearly demonstrated that the mechanisms that incite autoimmune disease may differ substantially from the mechanisms that propagate tissue damage. Autoreactive T and B cells that are activated in secondary lymphoid organs and initiate disease may be activated in a different microenvironment and may have a different cytokine profile from the effector cells that migrate into target organs and cause tissue fibrosis (Campbell et al., 2001; Gerriets and Rathmell, 2012; Katzman et al., 2011). Thus, it is clear that at each stage of autoimmune disease, induction of autoreactivity and tissue destruction need to be separately explored, and that the previous characterization of certain cytokines as proinflammatory and others as anti-inflammatory may be misleading. While TGF-β may dampen the induction of autoreactivity, it may hasten tissue fibrosis (Valluru et al., 2011). Similarly, IL-10 is anti-inflammatory during disease initiation through its inhibitory effects on APCs, but may lose its anti-inflammatory properties (Herrero et al., 2003) and even drive T cell proliferation, immunoglobulin class switching, and antibody production later in disease (Mocellin et al., 2004). Even the proinflammatory cyto-kine interferon-γ can have anti-inflammatory properties in the early stages of some autoimmune diseases (Billiau, 1996; Grohmann and Puccetti, 2002; Rosloniec et al., 2002) perhaps by antagonizing the differentiation of T cells secreting IL-17. It is important, as we move forward in studies of autoimmune disease, to consider the mechanism of both immune activation and tissue destruc-tion, and to be aware that cytokines, hormones, or other mediators may exhibit differential effects in each process. Studies of animal models have now clearly shown that it is possible to intervene in disease progression to protect organs from immune-mediated destruction, even while autoreactivity continues unabated (Clynes et al., 1998; Schiffer et al., 2003).

Recent studies emphasize the role of innate immune cells in tissue injury, particularly neutrophils and macro-phages that are recruited to sites of ischemic injury. Macrophages have a complex program in which they first release proinflammatory mediators to fight pathogens but may then initiate programs to help in the clearance of dead tissue and tissue repair. While the latter response is beneficial if short-lived, continued activation of the repair program may be detrimental if it becomes chronic (Bethunaickan et al., 2011).

FLARES AND REMISSIONS DURING DISEASE

The vast majority of animal models of autoimmune disease develop chronic progressive disease activity. Once the autoimmune disease becomes manifest, it progresses to organ failure or death. Much human autoimmune disease, in contrast, is characterized by periods of disease remission and flare. Little is known in human disease about the cellu-lar events that lead to disease remission. It is also true that little is known regarding the cause of disease flares. In mouse models of multiple sclerosis, disease flares can result from epitope spreading with sequential recruitment of T cell populations that recognize different epitopes of myelin (Mallone et al., 2011; Vanderlugt et al., 1998). Similarly in humans, epitope spreading has been observed among cohorts of lupus patients from whom pre-diseased serum was available (Arbuckle et al., 2003; Deshmukh et al., 2003). Nevertheless, a major area of ignorance

concerns the cell type responsible for disease flares. It is not known for most autoimmune diseases whether flares represent a *de novo* activation of naïve autoreactive cells or a reactivation of quiescent memory cells and whether these flares are due to a new environmental exposure or to failure of regulation, or both. Our ignorance in this regard derives largely from the difficulty of sampling a large enough repertoire of autoreactive T or B cells. Often, these cells are poorly represented in peripheral blood (Bischof et al., 2004; Newman et al., 2003; Reddy et al., 2003). The development of MHC class I and class II tetramers containing peptides of known autoantigens is beginning to facilitate analysis of pathogenic T cells in human autoimmune diseases and animal models in which the autoantigens are known (Mallone et al., 2011; Massilamany et al., 2011). Similarly, the development of single cell PCR technology is allowing the analysis of the frequency and binding specificity of autoreactive B cells from peripheral blood (Meffre and Wardemann, 2008). These studies have shed light on how autoreactiv-ity is regulated in human B cells during B cell develop-ment and have demonstrated abnormalities in regulation of the B cell repertoire in individuals with a variety of immune deficiencies and autoimmunity related genetic polymorphisms (Isnardi et al., 2010; Meffre and Wardemann, 2008; Menard et al., 2011).

THERAPEUTIC ADVANCES

A major advance in the last decade has been the applica-tion of new knowledge about immune system function to the treatment of autoimmune diseases (Chapter 81). New therapies target innate immunity, adaptive immunity and even tissue injury. As these new drugs have entered clinical practice it has become clear that the pleiomorphic and stage-specific functions of particular molecules can result in both beneficial and adverse therapeutic effects of the drugs that target them. TNF inhibitors, for example, while highly therapeutic in RA and IBD, can induce SLE, multiple sclerosis, and vasculitis (Kollias, 2005). Another important lesson has been that some therapies are highly effective for some diseases but not others. These responses have, however, been difficult to predict based on our current understanding of disease pathogenesis. For example, global B cell depletion using an antibody to CD20 is therapeutic in RA and multiple sclerosis (Barun and Bar-Or, 2012; Buch et al., 2011), diseases that were initially thought to be T cell dependent, but has much less, if any, effect in SLE, a prototypic B cell disease (Merrill et al., 2010). Variability among patients results in response rates that rarely reach more than 70% even for the best of the new therapies. Finding ways to identify responders and non-responders before initiating an expen-sive and potentially toxic new therapy is a task that is being actively pursued using large patient databases and genetic and "omics" studies.

New drugs to treat autoimmune disease are constantly in development. Many of the current approaches are based on a perceived need to institute immunosuppression and anti-inflammatory therapy at the time of autoimmune tissue destruction. Multiple pathways of immune activation, including innate TLR and pattern-recognition receptor signaling pathways, costimulatory pathways and T and B cell activation and cytokine signaling pathways are being targeted to reduce activation of the immune system (Rosenblum et al., 2012). Our most updated understanding of autoimmunity would suggest that it might also be appropriate to consider treating disease during times of disease quiescence. The goal of this therapeutic approach would be to alter T and B cell repertoire selection or to drive the expansion of regulatory cells and enhance regulation (Daniel and von Boehmer, 2011). Currently, antigen-specific therapies remain a dream even for those diseases in which causative antigens have been identified (Michels and Eisenbarth, 2011).

Protecting target organs and preventing irreversible tissue damage will require different therapeutic strategies from blocking systemic autoreactivity (Katschke et al., 2007; Sica et al., 2011; Szekanecz et al., 2009). These new therapeutic approaches offer the hope of maintaining immunocompetence while eliminating the consequences of pathogenic autoreactivity.

Finally, the observation that autoimmunity and immunodeficiency can be linked suggests that effective treatment of autoimmunity will lead to enhanced immunocompetence, and the reversal of developmental defects in lymphoid cells should reduce autoreactivity. This is the metric against which therapeutic interventions should be judged.

GOALS FOR THE FUTURE

Over the past several years, new technologies have been developed that will substantially increase our understanding of autoimmune disease. High-throughput technologies to examine genetic polymorphisms, epigenetic changes, gene expression and protein expression and modifications, linked with the collection of well-characterized databases of patients make it possible to determine the level of expression of a very large number of genes or proteins in defined populations of patients and subpopulations of cells. These data may provide new insights into disease pathogenesis and new ways to phenotype patients with autoimmune disease. These technologies may also provide sets of biomarkers that will help determine risk for developing a particular disease, characterize current activity of the disease and disease prognosis, and assess response to therapy at an earlier time point than current

clinical endpoints. It is reasonable to predict that patterns of gene and protein expression will reveal differences and similarities among autoimmune diseases.

The development of biomarkers will, undoubtedly, improve the therapy of autoimmune disease. It may be possible to identify early those patients whose disease is likely to be severe and to monitor disease activity without waiting for clinical symptomatology. Furthermore, the recognition that autoimmunity can be detected before clinical symptomatology and that the likelihood of development of disease in individual patients can be predicted with more certainty will allow testing of therapies that have the potential to prevent or cure autoimmune disease before tissue damage occurs. Ultimately, it may be possible to customize therapy for each patient, thereby enhancing efficacy and avoiding unnecessary toxicities and expense.

CONCLUDING REMARKS

The past several years have witnessed a change in our understanding of autoimmunity and a clear new direction in our approach to the study of autoimmunity. Multiple genetic polymorphisms contribute to autoimmunity risk and more remain to be identified. The complexity of regulation of gene expression suggests several other mechanisms by which gene expression may be aberrantly regulated in autoimmunity. It is clear that activation of the innate immune system can act as a trigger for the initiation of autoimmunity in susceptible individuals and can amplify tissue damage in target organs. Autoimmunity can result from either a failure in T and B cell repertoire selection or a failure in the regulation of activated T and B cells. Autoimmune B and T cells can be identified years before the emergence of clinical disease, suggesting that multiple triggers act sequentially to precipitate disease. It is also clear that autoimmunity needs to be coupled to target-organ vulnerability to immune attack for autoimmune disease to be present and that inflammatory cascades can be interrupted or regulated in the periphery. This understanding suggests new therapeutic targets and new therapeutic strategies.

The focus on new technologies to provide biomarkers of immune function represents an exciting opportunity to treat disease prior to tissue damage and to customize therapy for each patient. Furthermore, studies of gene and protein expression will help elucidate those mechanisms of immune dysfunction that are shared among multiple autoimmune diseases and those that are unique to a particular disease. Thus, there are reasons to be optimistic, but acquiring the necessary new knowledge and translating that knowledge to therapy will take time and will require more clinical trials.

ACKNOWLEDGMENTS

Supported by grants R01 DK085241-01 and R01AI083901-01A1 (to AD) and PO1 AI073693 and RO1 AR057084 (to BD).

REFERENCES

Akirav, E.M., Ruddle, N.H., Herold, K.C., 2011. The role of AIRE in human autoimmune disease. Nat. Rev. Endocrinol. 7, 25–33.

Alexandropoulos, K., Danzl, N.M., 2012. Thymic epithelial cells: antigen presenting cells that regulate T cell repertoire and tolerance development. Immunol. Res. 54 (1–3), 177–190.

Anderson, M.S., Su, M.A., 2011. Aire and T cell development. Curr. Opin. Immunol. 23, 198–206.

Andersson, U., Tracey, K.J., 2011. HMGB1 is a therapeutic target for sterile inflammation and infection. Annu. Rev. Immunol. 29, 139–162.

Anthony, R.M., Kobayashi, T., Wermeling, F., Ravetch, J.V., 2011. Intravenous gammaglobulin suppresses inflammation through a novel T(H)2 pathway. Nature. 475, 110–113.

Arbuckle, M.R., McClain, M.T., Rubertone, M.V., Scofield, R.H., Dennis, G.J., James, J.A., et al., 2003. Development of autoantibodies before the clinical onset of systemic lupus erythematosus. N. Engl. J. Med. 349, 1526–1533.

Atarashi, K., Honda, K., 2011. Microbiota in autoimmunity and tolerance. Curr. Opin. Immunol. 23, 761–768.

Bancherau, J., Steinman, R.M., 1998. Dendritic cells and the control of immunity. Nature. 392, 245–252.

Bang, S.Y., Han, T.U., Choi, C.B., Sung, Y.K., Bae, S.C., Kang, C., 2010. Peptidyl arginine deiminase type IV (PADI4) haplotypes interact with shared epitope regardless of anti-cyclic citrullinated peptide antibody or erosive joint status in rheumatoid arthritis: a case control study. Arthritis Res. Ther. 12, R115.

Bar-Or, A., Rieckmann, P., Traboulsee, A., Yong, V.W., 2011. Targeting progressive neuroaxonal injury: lessons from multiple sclerosis. CNS Drugs. 25, 783–799.

Barun, B., Bar-Or, A., 2012. Treatment of multiple sclerosis with anti-CD20 antibodies. Clin. Immunol. 142, 31–37.

Beck, S., Trowsdale, J., 2000. The human major histocompatability complex: lessons from the DNA sequence. Annu. Rev. Genomics Hum. Genet. 1, 117–137.

Bene, L., Falus, A., Baffy, N., Fulop, A.K., 2011. Cellular and molecular mechanisms in the two major forms of inflammatory bowel disease. Pathol. Oncol. Res. 17, 463–472.

Bethunaickan, R., Berthier, C.C., Ramanujam, M., Sahu, R., Zhang, W., Sun, Y., et al., 2011. A unique hybrid renal mononuclear phagocyte activation phenotype in murine systemic lupus erythematosus nephritis. J. Immunol. 186, 4994–5003.

Bijl, M., Kallenberg, C.G., 2006. Ultraviolet light and cutaneous lupus. Lupus. 15, 724–727.

Billiau, A., 1996. Interferon-gamma in autoimmunity. Cytokine Growth Factor Rev. 7, 25–34.

Billiau, A., Matthys, P., 2011. Collagen-induced arthritis and related animal models: how much of their pathogenesis is auto-immune, how much is auto-inflammatory? Cytokine Growth Factor Rev. 22, 339–344.

Bischof, F., Hofmann, M., Schumacher, T.N., Vyth-Dreese, F.A., Weissert, R., Schild, H., et al., 2004. Analysis of autoreactive CD4 T cells in experimental autoimmune encephalomyelitis after primary and secondary challenge using MHC class II tetramers. J. Immunol. 172, 2878–2884.

Bishop, G.A., Haxhinasto, S.A., Stunz, L.L., Hostager, B.S., 2003. Antigen-specific B-lymphocyte activation. Crit. Rev. Immunol. 23, 149–197.

Blanco, P., Palucka, A.K., Pascual, V., Banchereau, J., 2008. Dendritic cells and cytokines in human inflammatory and autoimmune diseases. Cytokine Growth Factor Rev. 19, 41–52.

Bockenstedt, L.K., Gee, R.J., Mamula, M.J., 1995. Self-peptides in the initiation of lupus autoimmunity. J Immunol. 154, 3516–3524.

Bodaghi, B., Rao, N., 2008. Relevance of animal models to human uveitis. Ophthalmic Res. 40, 200–202.

Bolland, S., Ravetch, J.V., 2000. Spontaneous autoimmune disease in Fc(gamma)RIIB-deficient mice results from strain-specific epistasis. Immunity. 13, 277–285.

Bommhardt, U., Beyer, M., Hunig, T., Reichardt, H.M., 2004. Molecular and cellular mechanisms of T cell development. Cell Mol. Life Sci. 61, 263–280.

Bratton, D.L., Henson, P.M., 2011. Neutrophil clearance: when the party is over, clean-up begins. Trends Immunol. 32, 350–357.

Brunner, T., Wasem, C., Torgler, R., Cima, I., Jakob, S., Corazza, N., 2003. Fas (CD95/Apo-1) ligand regulation in T cell homeostasis, cell-mediated cytotoxicity and immune pathology. Semin. Immunol. 15, 167–176.

Buch, M.H., Smolen, J.S., Betteridge, N., Breedveld, F.C., Burmester, G., Dorner, T., et al., 2011. Updated consensus statement on the use of rituximab in patients with rheumatoid arthritis. Ann. Rheum. Dis. 70, 909–920.

Burn, G.L., Svensson, L., Sanchez-Blanco, C., Saini, M., Cope, A.P., 2011. Why is PTPN22 a good candidate susceptibility gene for autoimmune disease? FEBS Lett. 585, 3689–3698.

Campbell, D.J., Kim, C.H., Butcher, E.C., 2001. Separable effector T cell populations specialized for B cell help or tissue inflammation. Nat. Immunol. 2, 876–881.

Cantor, R.M., Lange, K., Sinsheimer, J.S., 2010. Prioritizing GWAS results: a review of statistical methods and recommendations for their application. Am. J. Hum. Genet. 86, 6–22.

Ceribelli, A., Yao, B., Dominguez-Gutierrez, P.R., Chan, E.K., 2011a. Lupus T cells switched on by DNA hypomethylation via microRNA? Arthritis Rheum. 63, 1177–1181.

Ceribelli, A., Yao, B., Dominguez-Gutierrez, P.R., Nahid, M.A., Satoh, M., Chan, E.K., 2011b. MicroRNAs in systemic rheumatic diseases. Arthritis Res. Ther. 13, 229.

Chen, L., 2004. Co-inhibitory molecules of the B7-CD28 family in the control of T-cell immunity. Nat. Rev. Immunol. 4, 336–347.

Chen, Y., Park, Y.B., Patel, E., Silverman, G.J., 2009. IgM antibodies to apoptosis-associated determinants recruit C1q and enhance dendritic cell phagocytosis of apoptotic cells. J. Immunol. 182, 6031–6043.

Chinen, T., Rudensky, A.Y., 2012. The effects of commensal microbiota on immune cell subsets and inflammatory responses. Immunol. Rev. 245, 45–55.

Cho, J.H., Gregersen, P.K., 2011. Genomics and the multifactorial nature of human autoimmune disease. N. Engl. J. Med. 365, 1612–1623.

Christen, U., Bender, C., von Herrath, M.G., 2012. Infection as a cause of type 1 diabetes? Curr. Opin. Rheumatol. 24 (4), 417–423.

Clynes, R., Dumitru, C., Ravetch, J.V., 1998. Uncoupling of immune complex formation and kidney damage in autoimmune glomerulonephritis. Science. 279, 1052–1054.

Cortesini, R., LeMaoult, J., Ciubotariu, R., Cortesini, N.S., 2001. CD8 + CD28 − T suppressor cells and the induction of antigen-specific, antigen-presenting cell-mediated suppression of Th reactivity. Immunol. Rev. 182, 201–206.

Cotsapas, C., Voight, B.F., Rossin, E., Lage, K., Neale, B.M., Wallace, C., et al., 2011. Pervasive sharing of genetic effects in autoimmune disease. PLoS Genet. 7, e1002254.

Crow, M.K., 2004. Costimulatory molecules and T-cell–B-cell interactions. Rheum. Dis. Clin. North Am. 30, 175–191, vii–viii.

Cunningham, M.W., 2003. Autoimmunity and molecular mimicry in the pathogenesis of post-streptococcal heart disease. Front. Biosci. 8, s533–s543.

Cusick, M.F., Libbey, J.E., Fujinami, R.S., 2012. Molecular mimicry as a mechanism of autoimmune disease. Clin. Rev. Allergy Immunol. 42, 102–111.

D'Cruz, D., 2000. Autoimmune diseases associated with drugs, chemicals and environmental factors. Toxicol. Lett. 112–113, 421–432.

Daniel, C., von Boehmer, H., 2011. Extrathymic generation of regulatory T cells—chances and challenges for prevention of autoimmune disease. Adv. Immunol. 112, 177–213.

Davidson, A., Diamond, B., 2001. Autoimmune diseases. N. Eng. J. Med. 345 (5), 340–350.

de Heredia, F.P., Gomez-Martinez, S., Marcos, A., 2012. Obesity, inflammation and the immune system. Proc. Nutr. Soc.1–7.

Deane, K.D., O'Donnell, C.I., Hueber, W., Majka, D.S., Lazar, A.A., Derber, L.A., et al., 2010. The number of elevated cytokines and chemokines in preclinical seropositive rheumatoid arthritis predicts time to diagnosis in an age-dependent manner. Arthritis Rheum. 62, 3161–3172.

Debandt, M., Vittecoq, O., Descamps, V., Le Loet, X., Meyer, O., 2003. Anti-TNF-alpha-induced systemic lupus syndrome. Clin. Rheumatol. 22, 56–61.

Deng, Y., Tsao, B.P., 2010. Genetic susceptibility to systemic lupus erythematosus in the genomic era. Nat. Rev. Rheumatol. 6, 683–692.

Deshmukh, U.S., Gaskin, F., Lewis, J.E., Kannapell, C.C., Fu, S.M., 2003. Mechanisms of autoantibody diversification to SLE-related autoantigens. Ann. N.Y. Acad. Sci. 987, 91–98.

Dominguez, P.M., Ardavin, C., 2010. Differentiation and function of mouse monocyte-derived dendritic cells in steady state and inflammation. Immunol. Rev. 234, 90–104.

Doreau, A., Belot, A., Bastid, J., Riche, B., Trescol-Biemont, M.C., Ranchin, B., et al., 2009. Interleukin 17 acts in synergy with B cell-activating factor to influence B cell biology and the pathophysiology of systemic lupus erythematosus. Nat. Immunol. 10, 778–785.

Doyle, H.A., Mamula, M.J., 2012. Autoantigenesis: the evolution of protein modifications in autoimmune disease. Curr. Opin. Immunol. 24, 112–118.

Dzopalic, T., Rajkovic, I., Dragicevic, A., Colic, M., 2012. The response of human dendritic cells to co-ligation of pattern-recognition receptors. Immunol. Res. 52, 20–33.

Engels, N., Wienands, J., 2011. The signaling tool box for tyrosine-based costimulation of lymphocytes. Curr. Opin. Immunol. 23, 324–329.

Fernando, M.M., Stevens, C.R., Walsh, E.C., De Jager, P.L., Goyette, P., Plenge, R.M., et al., 2008. Defining the role of the MHC in autoimmunity: a review and pooled analysis. PLoS Genet. 4, e1000024.

Filardy, A.A., Pires, D.R., Nunes, M.P., Takiya, C.M., Freire-de-Lima, C.G., Ribeiro-Gomes, F.L., et al., 2010. Proinflammatory clearance of apoptotic neutrophils induces an IL-12(low)IL-10(high) regulatory phenotype in macrophages. J. Immunol. 185, 2044–2050.

Fleisher, T.A., Straus, S.E., Bleesing, J.J., 2001. A genetic disorder of lymphocyte apoptosis involving the fas pathway: the autoimmune lymphoproliferative syndrome. Curr. Allergy Asthma Rep. 1, 534–540.

Flesher, D.L., Sun, X., Behrens, T.W., Graham, R.R., Criswell, L.A., 2010. Recent advances in the genetics of systemic lupus erythematosus. Expert Rev. Clin. Immunol. 6, 461–479.

Francisco, L.M., Sage, P.T., Sharpe, A.H., 2010. The PD-1 pathway in tolerance and autoimmunity. Immunol. Rev. 236, 219–242.

Fukuyama, H., Nimmerjahn, F., Ravetch, J.V., 2005. The inhibitory Fcgamma receptor modulates autoimmunity by limiting the accumulation of immunoglobulin G + anti-DNA plasma cells. Nat. Immunol. 6, 99–106.

Gallagher, M.P., Goland, R.S., Greenbaum, C.J., 2011. Making progress: preserving beta cells in type 1 diabetes. Ann. N.Y. Acad. Sci. 1243, 119–134.

Garrett, W.S., Lord, G.M., Punit, S., Lugo-Villarino, G., Mazmanian, S.K., Ito, S., et al., 2007. Communicable ulcerative colitis induced by T-bet deficiency in the innate immune system. Cell. 131, 33–45.

Gellert, M., 2002. V(D)J recombination: RAG proteins, repair factors, and regulation. Annu. Rev. Biochem. 71, 101–132.

Gerriets, V.A., Rathmell, J.C., 2012. Metabolic pathways in T cell fate and function. Trends Immunol. 33, 168–173.

Ghosh, D., Kis-Toth, K., Juang, Y.T., Tsokos, G.C., 2012. CREMalpha suppresses spleen tyrosine kinase expression in normal but not systemic lupus erythematosus T cells. Arthritis Rheum. 64, 799–807.

Glasmacher, E., Hoefig, K.P., Vogel, K.U., Rath, N., Du, L., Wolf, C., et al., 2010. Roquin binds inducible costimulator mRNA and effectors of mRNA decay to induce microRNA-independent post-transcriptional repression. Nat. Immunol. 11, 725–733.

Goodnow, C.C., Vinuesa, C.G., Randall, K.L., Mackay, F., Brink, R., 2010. Control systems and decision making for antibody production. Nat. Immunol. 11, 681–688.

Green, N.M., Marshak-Rothstein, A., 2011. Toll-like receptor driven B cell activation in the induction of systemic autoimmunity. Semin. Immunol. 23, 106–112.

Grimaldi, C.M., Hill, L., Xu, X., Peeva, E., Diamond, B., 2005. Hormonal modulation of B cell development and repertoire selection. Mol. Immunol. 42, 811–820.

Grodzicky, T., Elkon, K.B., 2002. Apoptosis: a case where too much or too little can lead to autoimmunity. Mt Sinai J. Med. 69, 208–219.

Grohmann, U., Puccetti, P., 2002. The immunosuppressive activity of proinflammatory cytokines in experimental models: potential for therapeutic intervention in autoimmunity. Curr. Drug Targets Inflamm. Allergy. 1, 77–87.

Grossman, Z., Min, B., Meier-Schellersheim, M., Paul, W.E., 2004. Concomitant regulation of T-cell activation and homeostasis. Nat. Rev. Immunol. 4, 387–395.

Gu, H., Tarlinton, D., Muller, W., Rajewsky, K., Forster, I., 1991. Most peripheral B cells in mice are ligand selected. J. Exp. Med. 173, 1357–1371.

Guilherme, L., Kalil, J., 2004. Rheumatic fever: from sore throat to autoimmune heart lesions. Int. Arch. Allergy Immunol. 134, 56–64.

Hamilton, M.J., Snapper, S.B., Blumberg, R.S., 2012. Update on biologic pathways in inflammatory bowel disease and their therapeutic relevance. J. Gastroenterol. 47, 1–8.

Harley, J.B., Alarcon-Riquelme, M.E., Criswell, L.A., Jacob, C.O., Kimberly, R.P., Moser, K.L., et al., 2008. Genome-wide association scan in women with systemic lupus erythematosus identifies susceptibility variants in ITGAM, PXK, KIAA1542 and other loci. Nat. Genet. 40, 204–210.

Herlands, R.A., Christensen, S.R., Sweet, R.A., Hershberg, U., Shlomchik, M.J., 2008. T cell-independent and toll-like receptor-dependent antigen-driven activation of autoreactive B cells. Immunity. 29, 249–260.

Herrero, C., Hu, X., Li, W.P., Samuels, S., Sharif, M.N., Kotenko, S., et al., 2003. Reprogramming of IL-10 activity and signaling by IFN-gamma. J. Immunol. 171, 5034–5041.

Horwitz, M.S., Ilic, A., Fine, C., Rodriguez, E., Sarvetnick, N., 2002. Presented antigen from damaged pancreatic beta cells activates autoreactive T cells in virus-mediated autoimmune diabetes. J. Clin. Invest. 109, 79–87.

Howell, C.D., 2002. Animal models of autoimmunity. Clin. Liver Dis. 6, 487–495.

Hsieh, C.S., Lee, H.M., Lio, C.W., 2012. Selection of regulatory T cells in the thymus. Nat. Rev. Immunol. 12, 157–167.

Isnardi, I., Ng, Y.S., Menard, L., Meyers, G., Saadoun, D., Srdanovic, I., et al., 2010. Complement receptor 2/CD21 − human naive B cells contain mostly autoreactive unresponsive clones. Blood. 115, 5026–5036.

Jacobson, D.L., Gange, S.J., Rose, N.R., Graham, N.M., 1997. Epidemiology and estimated population burden of selected autoimmune diseases in the United States. Clin. Immunol. Immunopathol. 84, 223–243.

James, J.A., Robertson, J.M., 2012. Lupus and Epstein–Barr. Curr. Opin. Rheumatol. 24 (4), 383–388.

Jiang, H., Canfield, S.M., Gallagher, M.P., Jiang, H.H., Jiang, Y., Zheng, Z., et al., 2010. HLA-E-restricted regulatory CD8(+) T cells are involved in development and control of human autoimmune type 1 diabetes. J. Clin. Invest. 120, 3641–3650.

Josefowicz, S.Z., Lu, L.F., Rudensky, A.Y., 2012a. Regulatory T cells: mechanisms of differentiation and function. Annu. Rev. Immunol. 30, 531–564.

Josefowicz, S.Z., Niec, R.E., Kim, H.Y., Treuting, P., Chinen, T., Zheng, Y., et al., 2012b. Extrathymically generated regulatory T cells control mucosal TH2 inflammation. Nature. 482, 395–399.

Kalantari, T., Kamali-Sarvestani, E., Ciric, B., Karimi, M.H., Kalantari, M., Faridar, A., et al., 2011. Generation of immunogenic and tolerogenic clinical-grade dendritic cells. Immunol. Res. 51, 153–160.

Katschke Jr., K.J., Helmy, K.Y., Steffek, M., Xi, H., Yin, J., Lee, W.P., et al., 2007. A novel inhibitor of the alternative pathway of complement reverses inflammation and bone destruction in experimental arthritis. J. Exp. Med. 204, 1319–1325.

Katzman, S.D., Hoyer, K.K., Dooms, H., Gratz, I.K., Rosenblum, M.D., Paw, J.S., et al., 2011. Opposing functions of IL-2 and IL-7 in the regulation of immune responses. Cytokine. 56, 116–121.

Kawai, T., Akira, S., 2010. The role of pattern-recognition receptors in innate immunity: update on Toll-like receptors. Nat. Immunol. 11, 373–384.

Kawai, T., Akira, S., 2011. Toll-like receptors and their crosstalk with other innate receptors in infection and immunity. Immunity. 34, 637–650.

Khoury, S.J., Sayegh, M.H., 2004. The roles of the new negative T cell costimulatory pathways in regulating autoimmunity. Immunity. 20, 529–538.

Kim, H.J., Cantor, H., 2011. Regulation of self-tolerance by Qa-1-restricted CD8(+) regulatory T cells. Semin. Immunol. 23, 446–452.

King, A., 2012. The use of animal models in diabetes research. Br. J. Pharmacol. 166 (3), 877–894.

Klareskog, L., Malmstrom, V., Lundberg, K., Padyukov, L., Alfredsson, L., 2011. Smoking, citrullination and genetic variability in the immunopathogenesis of rheumatoid arthritis. Semin. Immunol. 23, 92–98.

Klinker, M.W., Lundy, S.K., 2012. Multiple mechanisms of immune suppression by B lymphocytes. Mol. Med. 18, 123–137.

Knip, M., Akerblom, H.K., 1999. Environmental factors in the pathogenesis of type 1 diabetes mellitus. Exp. Clin. Endocrinol. Diabetes. 107 (Suppl. 3), S93–S100.

Kochi, Y., Thabet, M.M., Suzuki, A., Okada, Y., Daha, N.A., Toes, R.E., et al., 2011. PADI4 polymorphism predisposes male smokers to rheumatoid arthritis. Ann. Rheum. Dis. 70, 512–515.

Kollias, G., 2005. TNF pathophysiology in murine models of chronic inflammation and autoimmunity. Semin. Arthritis Rheum. 34, 3–6.

Kollias, G., Papadaki, P., Apparailly, F., Vervoordeldonk, M.J., Holmdahl, R., Baumans, V., et al., 2011. Animal models for arthritis: innovative tools for prevention and treatment. Ann. Rheum. Dis. 70, 1357–1362.

Kontzias, A., Laurence, A., Gadina, M., O'Shea, J.J., 2012. Kinase inhibitors in the treatment of immune-mediated disease. F1000 Med. Rep. 4, 5.

Koutouzov, S., Mathian, A., Dalloul, A., 2006. Type-I interferons and systemic lupus erythematosus. Autoimmun. Rev. 5, 554–562.

Kuhn, A., Beissert, S., 2005. Photosensitivity in lupus erythematosus. Autoimmunity. 38, 519–529.

Kuon, W., Sieper, J., 2003. Identification of HLA-B27-restricted peptides in reactive arthritis and other spondyloarthropathies: computer algorithms and fluorescent activated cell sorting analysis as tools for hunting of HLA-B27-restricted chlamydial and autologous crossreactive peptides involved in reactive arthritis and ankylosing spondylitis. Rheum. Dis. Clin. North Am. 29, 595–611.

Kuwabara, S., 2004. Guillain–Barre syndrome: epidemiology, pathophysiology and management. Drugs. 64, 597–610.

Lam-Tse, W.K., Lernmark, A., Drexhage, H.A., 2002. Animal models of endocrine/organ-specific autoimmune diseases: do they really help us to understand human autoimmunity? Springer Semin. Immunopathol. 24, 297–321.

Leon, B., Ballesteros-Tato, A., Misra, R.S., Wojciechowski, W., Lund, F.E., 2012. Unraveling effector functions of B cells during infection: the hidden world beyond antibody production. Infect. Disord. Drug Targets. 12 (3), 213–221.

Lewis, M.J., Botto, M., 2006. Complement deficiencies in humans and animals: links to autoimmunity. Autoimmunity. 39, 367–378.

Li-Weber, M., Krammer, P.H., 2003. Function and regulation of the CD95 (APO-1/Fas) ligand in the immune system. Semin. Immunol. 15, 145–157.

Li, Z., Woo, C.J., Iglesias-Ussel, M.D., Ronai, D., Scharff, M.D., 2004. The generation of antibody diversity through somatic hypermutation and class switch recombination. Genes Dev. 18, 1–11.

Liao, L., Sindhwani, R., Rojkind, M., Factor, S., Leinwand, L., Diamond, B., 1995. Antibody-mediated autoimmune myocarditis depends on genetically determined target organ sensitivity. J. Exp. Med. 181, 1123–1131.

Linterman, M.A., Rigby, R.J., Wong, R., Silva, D., Withers, D., Anderson, G., et al., 2009. Roquin differentiates the specialized functions of duplicated T cell costimulatory receptor genes CD28 and ICOS. Immunity. 30, 228–241.

Lipsky, P.E., 2001. Systemic lupus erythematosus: an autoimmune disease of B cell hyperactivity. Nat. Immunol. 2, 764–766.

Liu, K., Li, Q.Z., Delgado-Vega, A.M., Abelson, A.K., Sanchez, E., Kelly, J.A., et al., 2009. Kallikrein genes are associated with lupus and glomerular basement membrane-specific antibody-induced nephritis in mice and humans. J. Clin. Invest. 119, 911–923.

Liu, Z., Davidson, A., 2011. BAFF and selection of autoreactive B cells. Trends Immunol. 32, 388–394.

Mackay, F., Schneider, P., 2009. Cracking the BAFF code. Nat. Rev. Immunol. 9, 491–502.

Madkaikar, M., Mhatre, S., Gupta, M., Ghosh, K., 2011. Advances in autoimmune lymphoproliferative syndromes. Eur. J. Haematol. 87, 1–9.

Mahdi, H., Fisher, B.A., Kallberg, H., Plant, D., Malmstrom, V., Ronnelid, J., et al., 2009. Specific interaction between genotype, smoking and autoimmunity to citrullinated alpha-enolase in the etiology of rheumatoid arthritis. Nat. Genet. 41, 1319–1324.

Mallone, R., Scotto, M., Janicki, C.N., James, E.A., Fitzgerald-Miller, L., Wagner, R., et al., 2011. Immunology of Diabetes Society T-Cell Workshop: HLA class I tetramer-directed epitope validation initiative T-Cell Workshop Report-HLA Class I Tetramer Validation Initiative. Diabetes Metab. Res. Rev. 27, 720–726.

Mammen, A.L., Chung, T., Christopher-Stine, L., Rosen, P., Rosen, A., Doering, K.R., et al., 2011. Autoantibodies against 3-hydroxy-3-methylglutaryl-coenzyme A reductase in patients with statin-associated autoimmune myopathy. Arthritis Rheum. 63, 713–721.

Manderson, A.P., Botto, M., Walport, M.J., 2004. The role of complement in the development of systemic lupus erythematosus. Annu. Rev. Immunol. 22, 431–456.

Mandik-Nayak, L., Allen, P.M., 2005. Initiation of an autoimmune response: insights from a transgenic model of rheumatoid arthritis. Immunol. Res. 32, 5–13.

Marino, E., Grey, S.T., 2012. B cells as effectors and regulators of autoimmunity. Autoimmunity. 45 (5), 377–387.

Massilamany, C., Upadhyaya, B., Gangaplara, A., Kuszynski, C., Reddy, J., 2011. Detection of autoreactive CD4 T cells using major histocompatibility complex class II dextramers. BMC Immunol. 12, 40.

McKinstry, K.K., Strutt, T.M., Swain, S.L., 2010. The potential of CD4 T-cell memory. Immunology. 130, 1–9.

Meffre, E., Wardemann, H., 2008. B-cell tolerance checkpoints in health and autoimmunity. Curr. Opin. Immunol. 20, 632–638.

Menard, L., Saadoun, D., Isnardi, I., Ng, Y.S., Meyers, G., Massad, C., et al., 2011. The PTPN22 allele encoding an R620W variant interferes with the removal of developing autoreactive B cells in humans. J. Clin. Invest. 121, 3635–3644.

Merrill, J.T., Neuwelt, C.M., Wallace, D.J., Shanahan, J.C., Latinis, K.M., Oates, J.C., et al., 2010. Efficacy and safety of rituximab in moderately-to-severely active systemic lupus erythematosus: the randomized, double-blind, phase II/III systemic lupus erythematosus evaluation of rituximab trial. Arthritis Rheum. 62, 222–233.

Michels, A.W., Eisenbarth, G.S., 2011. Immune intervention in type 1 diabetes. Semin. Immunol. 23, 214–219.

Mills, K.H., 2011. TLR-dependent T cell activation in autoimmunity. Nat. Rev. Immunol. 11, 807–822.

Miyake, Y., Yamasaki, S., 2012. Sensing necrotic cells. Adv. Exp. Med. Biol. 738, 144–152.

Mocellin, S., Marincola, F., Rossi, C.R., Nitti, D., Lise, M., 2004. The multifaceted relationship between IL-10 and adaptive immunity: putting together the pieces of a puzzle. Cytokine Growth Factor Rev. 15, 61–76.

Monach, P.A., Benoist, C., Mathis, D., 2004. The role of antibodies in mouse models of rheumatoid arthritis, and relevance to human disease. Adv. Immunol. 82, 217–248.

Monroe, J.G., Bannish, G., Fuentes-Panana, E.M., King, L.B., Sandel, P.C., Chung, J., et al., 2003. Positive and negative selection during B lymphocyte development. Immunol. Res. 27, 427–442.

Monroe, J.G., Keir, M.E., 2008. Bridging Toll-like- and B cell-receptor signaling: meet me at the autophagosome. Immunity. 28, 729–731.

Morel, L., 2010. Genetics of SLE: evidence from mouse models. Nat. Rev. Rheumatol. 6, 348–357.

Morel, L., Blenman, K.R., Croker, B.P., Wakeland, E.K., 2001. The major murine systemic lupus erythematosus susceptibility locus, Sle1, is a cluster of functionally related genes. Proc. Natl. Acad. Sci. U.S.A. 98, 1787–1792.

Morel, P.A., Turner, M.S., 2011. Dendritic cells and the maintenance of self-tolerance. Immunol. Res. 50, 124–129.

Moriyama, H., Eisenbarth, G.S., 2002. Genetics and environmental factors in endocrine/organ-specific autoimmunity: have there been any major advances? Springer Semin. Immunopathol. 24, 231–242.

Moulton, V.R., Tsokos, G.C., 2011. Abnormalities of T cell signaling in systemic lupus erythematosus. Arthritis Res. Ther. 13, 207.

Nakayamada, S., Takahashi, H., Kanno, Y., O'Shea, J.J., 2012. Helper T cell diversity and plasticity. Curr. Opin. Immunol. 24 (3), 297–302.

Namjou, B., Kothari, P.H., Kelly, J.A., Glenn, S.B., Ojwang, J.O., Adler, A., et al., 2011. Evaluation of the TREX1 gene in a large multi-ancestral lupus cohort. Genes Immun. 12, 270–279.

Newman, J., Rice, J.S., Wang, C., Harris, S.L., Diamond, B., 2003. Identification of an antigen-specific B cell population. J. Immunol. Methods. 272, 177–187.

Niewold, T.B., 2011. Interferon alpha as a primary pathogenic factor in human lupus. J. Interferon Cytokine Res. 31, 887–892.

Nobrega, A., Stransky, B., Nicolas, N., Coutinho, A., 2002. Regeneration of natural antibody repertoire after massive ablation of lymphoid system: robust selection mechanisms preserve antigen binding specificities. J. Immunol. 169, 2971–2978.

O'Shea, J.J., Paul, W.E., 2010. Mechanisms underlying lineage commitment and plasticity of helper CD4 + T cells. Science. 327, 1098–1102.

Ochs, H.D., Gambineri, E., Torgerson, T.R., 2007. IPEX, FOXP3 and regulatory T-cells: a model for autoimmunity. Immunol. Res. 38, 112–121.

Oo, Y.H., Mutimer, D., Adams, D.H., 2012. Low-dose interleukin-2 and HCV-induced vasculitis. N. Engl. J. Med. 366, , 1353–1354; author reply1354.

Pagni, P.P., Traub, S., Demaria, O., Chasson, L., Alexopoulou, L., 2010. Contribution of TLR7 and TLR9 signaling to the susceptibility of MyD88-deficient mice to myocarditis. Autoimmunity. 43, 275–287.

Patterson, C.C., Dahlquist, G.G., Gyurus, E., Green, A., Soltesz, G., 2009. Incidence trends for childhood type 1 diabetes in Europe during 1989–2003 and predicted new cases 2005–20: a multicentre prospective registration study. Lancet. 373, 2027–2033.

Pauza, M.E., Dobbs, C.M., He, J., Patterson, T., Wagner, S., Anobile, B.S., et al., 2004. T-cell receptor transgenic response to an endogenous polymorphic autoantigen determines susceptibility to diabetes. Diabetes. 53, 978–988.

Peng, Y., Elkon, K.B., 2011. Autoimmunity in MFG-E8-deficient mice is associated with altered trafficking and enhanced cross-presentation of apoptotic cell antigens. J. Clin. Invest. 121, 2221–2241.

Peng, Y., Martin, D.A., Kenkel, J., Zhang, K., Ogden, C.A., Elkon, K. B., 2007. Innate and adaptive immune response to apoptotic cells. J. Autoimmun. 29, 303–309.

Pettigrew, H.D., Teuber, S.S., Gershwin, M.E., 2009. Clinical significance of complement deficiencies. Ann. N.Y. Acad. Sci. 1173, 108–123.

Peutz-Kootstra, C.J., de Heer, E., Hoedemaeker, P.J., Abrass, C.K., Bruijn, J.A., 2001. Lupus nephritis: lessons from experimental animal models. J. Lab. Clin. Med. 137, 244–260.

Pot, C., Apetoh, L., Kuchroo, V.K., 2011. Type 1 regulatory T cells (Tr1) in autoimmunity. Semin. Immunol. 23, 202–208.

Price, E.J., Venables, P.J., 1995. Drug-induced lupus. Drug Saf. 12, 283–290.

Rahman, P., Bartlett, S., Siannis, F., Pellett, F.J., Farewell, V.T., Peddle, L., et al., 2003. CARD15: a pleiotropic autoimmune gene that confers susceptibility to psoriatic arthritis. Am. J. Hum. Genet. 73, 677–681.

Rajewsky, K., 1996. Clonal selection and learning in the antibody system. Nature. 381, 751–758.

Raychaudhuri, S., Sandor, C., Stahl, E.A., Freudenberg, J., Lee, H.S., Jia, X., et al., 2012. Five amino acids in three HLA proteins explain most of the association between MHC and seropositive rheumatoid arthritis. Nat. Genet. 44, 291–296.

Reddy, J., Bettelli, E., Nicholson, L., Waldner, H., Jang, M.H., Wucherpfennig, K.W., et al., 2003. Detection of autoreactive myelin proteolipid protein 139–151-specific T cells by using MHC II (IAs) tetramers. J. Immunol. 170, 870–877.

Rieck, M., Arechiga, A., Onengut-Gumuscu, S., Greenbaum, C., Concannon, P., Buckner, J.H., 2007. Genetic variation in PTPN22 corresponds to altered function of T and B lymphocytes. J. Immunol. 179, 4704–4710.

Rivas, M.N., Koh, Y.T., Chen, A., Nguyen, A., Lee, Y.H., Lawson, G., et al., 2012. MyD88 is critically involved in immune tolerance breakdown at environmental interfaces of Foxp3-deficient mice. J. Clin. Invest. 122 (5), 1933–1947.

Romano-Keeler, J., Weitkamp, J.H., Moore, D.J., 2012. Regulatory properties of the intestinal microbiome effecting the development and treatment of diabetes. Curr. Opin. Endocrinol. Diabetes Obes. 19, 73–80.

Rosas-Ballina, M., Tracey, K.J., 2009. The neurology of the immune system: neural reflexes regulate immunity. Neuron. 64, 28–32.

Rosenblum, M.D., Gratz, I.K., Paw, J.S., Abbas, A.K., 2012. Treating human autoimmunity: current practice and future prospects. Sci. Transl. Med. 4, 125sr121.

Rosloniec, E.F., Latham, K., Guedez, Y.B., 2002. Paradoxical roles of IFN-gamma in models of Th1-mediated autoimmunity. Arthritis Res. 4, 333–336.

Routsias, J.G., Goules, J.D., Goules, A., Charalampakis, G., Pikazis, D., 2011. Autopathogenic correlation of periodontitis and rheumatoid arthritis. Rheumatology (Oxford). 50, 1189–1193.

Rubtsov, A.V., Rubtsova, K., Kappler, J.W., Marrack, P., 2010. Genetic and hormonal factors in female-biased autoimmunity. Autoimmun. Rev. 9, 494–498.

Russell, R.K., Nimmo, E.R., Satsangi, J., 2004. Molecular genetics of Crohn's disease. Curr. Opin. Genet. Dev. 14, 264–270.

Sawla, P., Hossain, A., Hahn, B.H., Singh, R.P., 2012. Regulatory T cells in systemic lupus erythematosus (SLE); role of peptide tolerance. Autoimmun. Rev. 11, 611–614.

Scandiuzzi, L., Ghosh, K., Zang, X., 2011. T cell costimulation and coinhibition: genetics and disease. Discov. Med. 12, 119–128.

Schiffer, L., Sinha, J., Wang, X., Huang, W., von Gersdorff, G., Schiffer, M., et al., 2003. Short term administration of costimulatory blockade and cyclophosphamide induces remission of systemic lupus erythematosus nephritis in NZB/W F1 mice by a mechanism downstream of renal immune complex deposition. J. Immunol. 171, 489–497.

Seo, S.J., Mandik-Nayak, L., Erikson, J., 2003. B cell anergy and systemic lupus erythematosus. Curr. Dir. Autoimmun. 6, 1–20.

Sercarz, E.E., Lehmann, P.V., Ametani, A., Benichou, G., Miller, A., Moudgil, K., 1993. Dominance and crypticity of T cell antigenic determinants. Annu. Rev. Immunol. 11, 729–766.

Shlomchik, M.J., 2008. Sites and stages of autoreactive B cell activation and regulation. Immunity. 28, 18–28.

Shlomchik, M.J., Craft, J.E., Mamula, M.J., 2001. From T to B and back again: positive feedback in systemic autoimmune disease. Nat. Rev. Immunol. 1, 147–153.

Sica, A., Melillo, G., Varesio, L., 2011. Hypoxia: a double-edged sword of immunity. J. Mol. Med. (Berl.). 89, 657–665.

Smith-Bouvier, D.L., Divekar, A.A., Sasidhar, M., Du, S., Tiwari-Woodruff, S.K., King, J.K., et al., 2008. A role for sex chromosome complement in the female bias in autoimmune disease. J. Exp. Med. 205, 1099–1108.

Sokolove, J., Zhao, X., Chandra, P.E., Robinson, W.H., 2011. Immune complexes containing citrullinated fibrinogen costimulate macrophages via Toll-like receptor 4 and Fcgamma receptor. Arthritis Rheum. 63, 53–62.

Steen, V.D., 1999. Occupational scleroderma. Curr. Opin. Rheumatol. 11, 490–494.

Steinman, R.M., 2007. Dendritic cells: understanding immunogenicity. Eur. J. Immunol. 37 (Suppl. 1), S53–S60.

Strassburg, C.P., Vogel, A., Manns, M.P., 2003. Autoimmunity and hepatitis C. Autoimmun. Rev. 2, 322–331.

Stritesky, G.L., Jameson, S.C., Hogquist, K.A., 2012. Selection of self-reactive T cells in the thymus. Annu. Rev. Immunol. 30, 95–114.

Suber, T.L., Casciola-Rosen, L., Rosen, A., 2008. Mechanisms of disease: autoantigens as clues to the pathogenesis of myositis. Nat. Clin. Pract. Rheumatol. 4, 201–209.

Suzuki, A., Yamada, R., Chang, X., Tokuhiro, S., Sawada, T., Suzuki, M., et al., 2003. Functional haplotypes of PADI4, encoding citrullinating enzyme peptidylarginine deiminase 4, are associated with rheumatoid arthritis. Nat. Genet. 34, 395–402.

Szekanecz, Z., Besenyei, T., Paragh, G., Koch, A.E., 2009. Angiogenesis in rheumatoid arthritis. Autoimmunity. 42, 563–573.

Tomlinson, I.P., Bodmer, W.F., 1995. The HLA system and the analysis of multifactorial genetic disease. Trends Genet. 11, 493–498.

Ueda, H., Howson, J.M., Esposito, L., Heward, J., Snook, H., Chamberlain, G., et al., 2003. Association of the T-cell regulatory gene CTLA4 with susceptibility to autoimmune disease. Nature. 423, 506–511.

Vaarala, O., 2012. Is the origin of type 1 diabetes in the gut? Immunol. Cell Biol. 90, 271–276.

Vallejo, A.N., Davila, E., Weyand, C.M., Goronzy, J.J., 2004. Biology of T lymphocytes. Rheum. Dis. Clin. North Am. 30, 135–157.

Valluru, M., Staton, C.A., Reed, M.W., Brown, N.J., 2011. Transforming growth factor-beta and endoglin signaling orchestrate wound healing. Front. Physiol. 2, 89.

Vanderlugt, C.L., Begolka, W.S., Neville, K.L., Katz-Levy, Y., Howard, L.M., Eagar, T.N., et al., 1998. The functional significance of epitope spreading and its regulation by co-stimulatory molecules. Immunol. Rev. 164, 63−72.

Vezys, V., Lefrancois, L., 2002. Cutting edge: inflammatory signals drive organ-specific autoimmunity to normally cross-tolerizing endogenous antigen. J. Immunol. 169, 6677−6680.

Victora, G.D., Nussenzweig, M.C., 2012. Germinal centers. Annu. Rev. Immunol. 30, 429−457.

Vincenti, F., Luggen, M., 2007. T cell costimulation: a rational target in the therapeutic armamentarium for autoimmune diseases and transplantation. Annu. Rev. Med. 58, 347−358.

Vinuesa, C.G., Cook, M.C., Angelucci, C., Athanasopoulos, V., Rui, L., Hill, K.M., et al., 2005. A RING-type ubiquitin ligase family member required to repress follicular helper T cells and autoimmunity. Nature. 435, 452−458.

von Boehmer, H., Melchers, F., 2010. Checkpoints in lymphocyte development and autoimmune disease. Nat. Immunol. 11, 14−20.

Wakeland, E.K., Liu, K., Graham, R.R., Behrens, T.W., 2001. Delineating the genetic basis of systemic lupus erythematosus. Immunity. 15, 397−408.

Walker, L.S., Abbas, A.K., 2002. The enemy within: keeping self-reactive T cells at bay in the periphery. Nat. Rev. Immunol. 2, 11−19.

Weinstein, J.S., Hernandez, S.G., Craft, J., 2012. T cells that promote B-cell maturation in systemic autoimmunity. Immunol. Rev. 247, 160−171.

Weng, N.P., Araki, Y., Subedi, K., 2012. The molecular basis of the memory T cell response: differential gene expression and its epigenetic regulation. Nat. Rev. Immunol. 12, 306−315.

Werlen, G., Hausmann, B., Naeher, D., Palmer, E., 2003. Signaling life and death in the thymus: timing is everything. Science. 299, 1859−1863.

Whitmire, J.K., Asano, M.S., Kaech, S.M., Sarkar, S., Hannum, L.G., Shlomchik, M.J., et al., 2009. Requirement of B cells for generating CD4 + T cell memory. J. Immunol. 182, 1868−1876.

Winchester, R., 2004. The genetics of autoimmune-mediated rheumatic diseases: clinical and biologic implications. Rheum. Dis. Clin. North Am. 30, 213−227, viii.

Wing, K., Sakaguchi, S., 2010. Regulatory T cells exert checks and balances on self tolerance and autoimmunity. Nat. Immunol. 11, 7−13.

Wojno, E.D., Hunter, C.A., 2012. New directions in the basic and translational biology of interleukin-27. Trends Immunol. 33, 91−97.

Wolters, V.M., Wijmenga, C., 2008. Genetic background of celiac disease and its clinical implications. Am. J. Gastroenterol. 103, 190−195.

Wong, F.S., Wen, L., 2003. The study of HLA class II and autoimmune diabetes. Curr. Mol. Med. 3, 1−15.

Wooley, P.H., 2004. The usefulness and the limitations of animal models in identifying targets for therapy in arthritis. Best Pract. Res. Clin. Rheumatol. 18, 47−58.

Yan, J., Harvey, B.P., Gee, R.J., Shlomchik, M.J., Mamula, M.J., 2006. B cells drive early T cell autoimmunity in vivo prior to dendritic cell-mediated autoantigen presentation. J. Immunol. 177, 4481−4487.

Zaki, M.H., Lamkanfi, M., Kanneganti, T.D., 2011. The Nlrp3 inflammasome: contributions to intestinal homeostasis. Trends Immunol. 32, 171−179.

Zhang, J., Zahir, N., Jiang, Q., Miliotis, H., Heyraud, S., Meng, X., et al., 2011. The autoimmune disease-associated PTPN22 variant promotes calpain-mediated Lyp/Pep degradation associated with lymphocyte and dendritic cell hyperresponsiveness. Nat. Genet. 43, 902−907.

Zhang, Q., Raoof, M., Chen, Y., Sumi, Y., Sursal, T., Junger, W., et al., 2010. Circulating mitochondrial DAMPs cause inflammatory responses to injury. Nature. 464, 104−107.

Chapter 4

The Concept of Autoinflammatory Diseases

Monique Stoffels and Anna Simon

Department of Medicine, Radboud University Nijmegen Medical Centre; Nijmegen Centre for Infection, Inflammation and Immunity Centre for Immunodeficiency and Autoinflammation; Nijmegen Centre for Molecular Life Sciences, Nijmegen, The Netherlands

Chapter Outline

Historical Perspective	39	**Polygenic or Acquired Autoinflammatory Disorders**	46
Definition	40	**Autoinflammatory Mechanisms of Disease in Common**	
Spectrum from Autoimmune to Autoinflammatory		**Disorders**	46
Disease	40	Type 2 Diabetes Mellitus	46
Mechanisms in Autoinflammation	40	Atherosclerosis	46
Classical Hereditary Autoinflammatory Disorders	41	**Newest Developments: Rare Hereditary Disorders with**	
Common Phenotype	41	**Autoinflammatory Aspects**	46
Cryopyrin-Associated Periodic Syndrome	43	Proteasome Defects	47
Familial Mediterranean Fever	44	PLCg2 Deficiency	47
TNF Receptor-Associated Periodic Syndrome	44	HOIL	47
HIDS (also Known as Mevalonate Kinase		**Conclusion**	48
Deficiency)	45	**References**	48

Autoinflammation is increasingly recognized as a distinct mechanism of disease, not only in rare monogenic syndromes, but also in more heterogeneous inflammatory disease as well as in common disorders such as atherosclerosis. This chapter will give an overview of autoinflammation with a focus on pathophysiology.

HISTORICAL PERSPECTIVE

The term "autoinflammatory syndrome" was first coined in 1999, in connection with the discovery of the genetic background of an autosomal dominantly inherited disorder that subsequently became known as tumor necrosis factor (TNF) receptor-associated periodic syndrome (TRAPS) (McDermott et al., 1999). Starting off in the niche group of so-called "hereditary periodic fever syndromes," concerning relatively few patients and physicians, it has in the past decade gained more interest and a bigger audience. This is partly due to the advent of biologicals inhibiting specific cytokines, particularly interleukin-1β (IL-1β). Before, these diseases were curiosities with no treatment options and as such there was no great incentive for a correct diagnosis. When very effective treatment became available, diagnosis became of new importance (and pharmaceutical companies suddenly began to show interest as well).

At the same time, this increasing interest has paralleled the increasing interest and insight into innate immunity in general (Medzhitov and Janeway, 2000), which revealed a much more important role for the innate immune system than had previously been thought. With the discovery of multiple receptors for recognition of pathogens and endogenous danger signals, as well as newly recognized innate immune cell types and intricate effector mechanisms, their role in human disease (either when too active or too inactive) could quickly be recognized.

By now, "autoinflammatory disease" has become established as a recognized category of disease, and is used in daily clinical practice—and even abused, as most

N. Rose & I. Mackay (Eds): The Autoimmune Diseases, Fifth edition. DOI: http://dx.doi.org/10.1016/B978-0-12-384929-8.00004-6

medical terms will be, just as "autoimmune disease" became the mantra for many immunological disorders. However, some degree of inflammation can be detected in almost any disease. So what defines a disease as "autoinflammatory"?

DEFINITION

The original 1999 definition for an autoinflammatory disease from the group of Daniel Kastner was: "seemingly unprovoked inflammation without high-titer autoantibodies or antigen-specific T-lymphocytes" (McDermott et al., 1999). This is useful to distinguish the group of diseases from autoimmune disorders, but consists mainly of negative definition: prescribing what is not part of it (no provocation, no autoantibodies), and not what is. Also, with our greater understanding of autoinflammatory disorders, we are able to recognize factors that can provoke the inflammatory episodes of these diseases, such as vaccination in hyper-IgD syndrome (HIDS) or cold in cryopyrin-associated periodic syndrome (CAPS), thus "seemingly unprovoked" became misleading.

Therefore, 11 years later, Kastner et al. proposed a new formulation: "abnormally increased inflammation, mediated predominantly by the cells and molecules of the innate immune system, with a significant host predisposition" (Kastner et al., 2010). This definition is broad enough to encompass both the original Mendelian-inherited fever syndromes, as well as the more complex polygenic or acquired disorders (Kastner et al., 2010). It again distinguishes these disorders from autoimmune disorders because of the focus on the innate immune system versus the adaptive immune system. Also, the latter part of this definition implies that there should be some intrinsic defect in the innate immune system underlying the disease. This is important because increased inflammation can of course be seen in many diseases. A pneumococcal pneumonia (in a previously healthy person) will be accompanied by a lot of inflammation but will not fall under this definition, since the inflammation is an adequate response to the infection. A systemic inflammatory reaction upon exposure to cold is not an adequate response, and occurs in CAPS because of an intrinsic defect in the innate immune system—and therefore does fall under this definition.

Despite the difficulty of definition, recognizing auto-inflammatory disease as a category in clinical medicine has its clear usefulness. First, it can be used when working on the differential diagnosis in a complex patient. Many of these disorders are rare, and patients go undiagnosed for years, due to lack of awareness about these disorders. Recognizing the possibility of a category of disease increases the chances of reaching a definite diagnosis. Second, it increases the chances of finding an

effective treatment, even in cases where the specific diagnosis remains elusive. Recognition of an autoimmune clinical phenotype will warrant treatment with prednisone or other immune suppressive therapy directed against T cell immunity. In the same way, recognition of an autoinflammatory phenotype will make treatment with an inhibitor of cytokines or innate immune cells more rational. Third, the recognition of autoinflammatory disorders, or autoinflammatory aspects of disorders, supports the existence of common features in the underlying pathogenesis. This facilitates research into the pathogenic background of these diseases, which will in future support diagnosis and treatment.

Several classifications within the group of autoinflammatory disorders have been proposed in recent years (Masters et al., 2009; Kastner et al., 2010), based on pathogenic mechanism or clinical phenotype or a combination of these.

SPECTRUM FROM AUTOIMMUNE TO AUTOINFLAMMATORY DISEASE

The innate and the adaptive immune system can of course not be seen as two completely separate entities. There are many areas in which the distinction is hard to make, for example in several types of regulatory T cells. In the same way, the disease categories "autoimmune" and "autoinflammatory" should in many cases not be seen as completely separate. McGonagle and McDermott (McGonagle and McDermott, 2006) suggested the idea of a spectrum of disease, ranging from autoimmune to autoinflammatory, in which many of the disorders have some aspects of both (Figure 4.1). The relative importance of the innate versus the adaptive immune system in the pathogenesis of a disorder determines its place on the spectrum. To fully comprehend this categorization, it is important to understand the mechanisms that play a role in innate immunity. In the ensuing paragraphs, we will first give a general overview of pathophysiological mechanisms in autoinflammation, followed by a number of examples from this spectrum.

MECHANISMS IN AUTOINFLAMMATION

As per the definition, the pathogenic defect in autoinflammation is located in the innate immune system. A key step in the innate immune response is the processing of the proinflammatory cytokines IL-1β and IL-18. In many diseases in this category, the defect is primarily located in the regulation of IL-1β.

IL-1β is an extremely potent inflammatory cytokine. Therefore, its production, secretion and signaling need to be tightly regulated at multiple levels (Figure 4.2). IL-1β signaling is controlled by means of expression of multiple

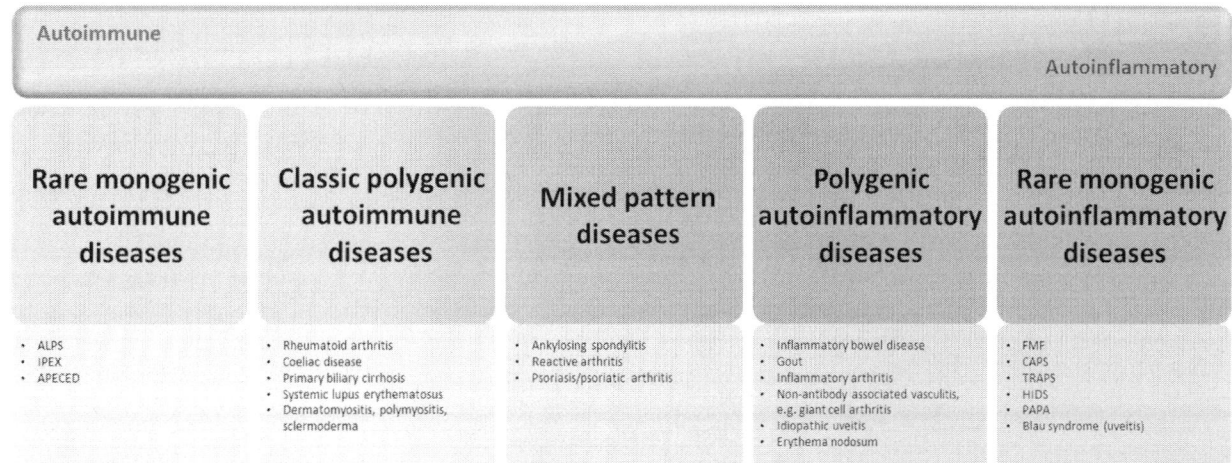

FIGURE 4.1 Spectrum from autoimmune to autoinflammatory disease. In between the two extremes of monogenic autoimmune and autoinflammatory disorders is a continuum of disease phenotypes comprising, to a different degree, characteristics from both autoimmune and autoinflammatory disease. This list serves as an example and is not complete. *Figure adapted from McGonagle and McDermott (2006).*

IL-1 receptors and the existence of an IL-1 receptor antagonist (IL-1Ra). For IL-1β production and secretion two distinct signals are required. The first is triggered by Toll-like receptor (TLR) activation. This leads to the production of pro-IL-1β. In the presence of the second signal, mediated by ionic pertubations, pro-IL-1β can be cleaved into active IL-1β by the so-called inflammasome. This is a concept first coined by Jurg Tschopp (Martinon et al., 2002), which holds that a scaffold of multiple proteins is formed to activate pro-caspase-1 into caspase-1, which in turn can cleave and activate pro-IL-1β. The existence of this inflammasome as an actual multi-protein complex has only definitely been demonstrated in overexpression models; but it has been shown that the components of this complex are at least all required for intracellular IL-1β activation *in vivo*. Several types of inflammasome have been described so far; the main function of each of these appears to be activation of IL-1β. The most studied inflammasome is the so-called NLRP3 inflammasome (for clarity reasons, only this is depicted in Figure 4.2, for more details on other inflammasomes we refer to Box 4.1). Several proteins and mechanisms can either directly or indirectly modify inflammasome activation. Some of these will be detailed in the following paragraphs about the associated diseases. There are also inflammasome-independent ways of activating IL-1β, but these fall outside the scope of this chapter.

IL-1β is mainly a paracrine and autocrine acting cytokine. Serum concentrations of IL-1β are always very low, and are therefore not a good indicator of its importance in the pathogenesis of a disease. For example, the IL-1β serum concentration is not always clearly increased in CAPS, despite its hereditary defect in the inflammasome. The role of IL-1β can be better examined by *ex-vivo*

stimulation of relevant cell types (especially peripheral blood mononuclear cells (PBMCs)), or by the therapeutic effect of inhibitors of IL-1.

Some authors almost equate autoinflammation with IL-1-related disease, maintaining that this inflammatory cytokine is always at the heart of the pathogenesis. However, defects in other parts of the innate immune system have been described, such as NF-κB and NOD2. And although inhibition of IL-1 is a good therapeutic option in many autoinflammatory diseases, it is not true for all of them.

CLASSICAL HEREDITARY AUTOINFLAMMATORY DISORDERS

Common Phenotype

At the far extreme of the spectrum are the monogenic hereditary autoinflammatory disorders, previously known as hereditary periodic fever syndromes. The genetic defect in each of these disorders is directly located in a protein of the innate immune system. Familial Mediterranean Fever (FMF) is the hallmark example of a classic hereditary autoinflammatory syndrome, but several others exist (Table 4.1) (Lachmann, 2011; Park et al., 2012). The common phenotype of these disorders is a lifelong recurrence of systemic inflammation, which can manifest itself as fever and/or various skin lesions, serositis, abdominal pain, myalgia, arthralgia or arthritis, lymphadenopathy, aphthous ulcers, and more. In some of these disorders, the inflammatory episodes are clearly demarcated by symptom-free intervals, in others the inflammation is fluctuating in severity but almost continuously present. In all of these, the systemic inflammation

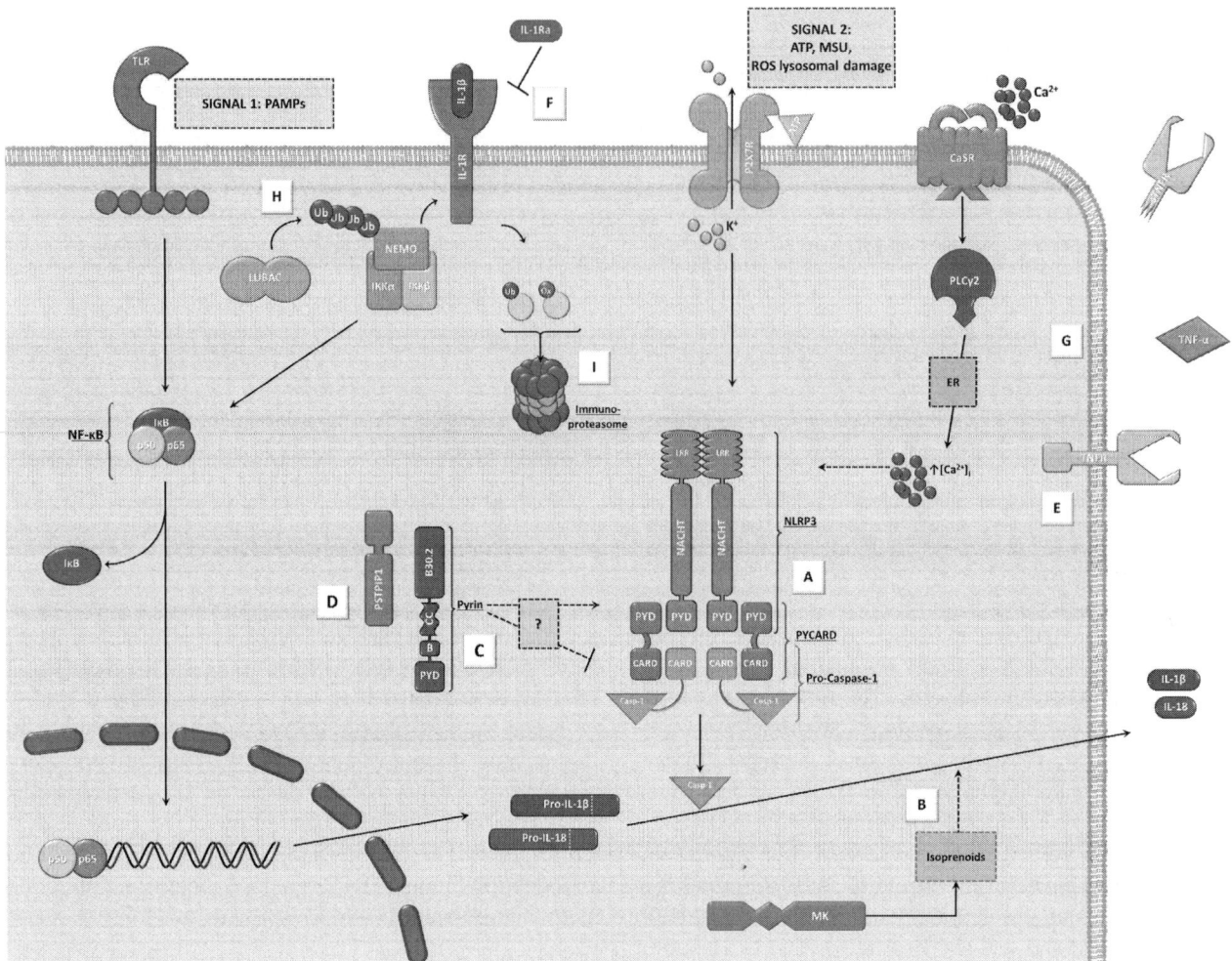

FIGURE 4.2   Schematic overview of mechanisms that play a role in autoinflammation.   For detailed description of these mechanisms the reader is referred to the text and to the references in Box 4.1. Briefly, upon TLR signaling in combination with a second stimulus, the inflammasome (A) is formed, pro-IL-1β is activated and IL-1β will be secreted (B). Pyrin (C) can interact with and influence the activation of the inflammasome. In its turn, PSTPIP1 (D) binds to pyrin, thereby indirectly influencing activation of the inflammasome. IL-1β secretion can, through autocrine or paracrine binding of IL-1 receptor, stimulate more cytokine secretion, including TNF and IL-1β itself. (E) Upon TNF secretion, the extracellular domain of the TNFR is shed to prevent overstimulation of the cell. The IL-1R is inhibited when IL-1Ra (F) binds to it. PLCγ2 activation (G) leads to increased [Ca²⁺]ᵢ and as a consequence increased inflammasome activation. NEMO is a modulator of NF-κB, and a complex called LUBAC targets it via ubiquitination to signalosomes of IL-1R1, TNFR, and TLRs (H).

Location of disease pathology in this schematic overview: (A) in CAPS, mutations in NLRP3 cause an overactivation of the inflammasome, (B) in HIDS, MK activity is drastically decreased and leads to increased IL-1β secretion, (C) in FMF, mutations in pyrin result in more IL-1 secretion, (D) in PAPA (pyogenic arthritis, pyoderma gangrenosum, and acne) mutations in PSTPIP1 change its binding properties to pyrin, thereby indirectly influencing inflammasome activation, (E) in TRAPS, mutations in TNFR1 result in distorted TNF signaling, and consequently disturbed IL-1 signaling, (F) in DIRA, the absence of (functional) IL-1Ra leads to overstimulation of the IL-1 signaling route, (G) in (A)PLAID, deletions in PLCγ2 result in failure of autoinhibition and thus constitutive phospholipase activity, (H) in HOIL, mutations in one of the LUBAC components impair this process, and dependent on the cell type result in diminished NF-κB activation or hyper-responsiveness to IL-1β, (I) in PSMB8 related disorders, immunoproteasome activity is compromised, leading to accumulation of ubiquitinated and oxidized proteins.

is always accompanied by an acute phase response (e.g., raised C-reactive protein or erythrocyte sedimentation rate). They have a varying risk for the development of AA-type amyloidosis. All have an autosomal inheritance pattern and almost all are directly or indirectly caused by a relative surplus of IL-1β.

Apart from this common phenotype, these disorders each have their own characteristics (Table 4.1).

A physician with experience in these disorders can generally make a preliminary diagnosis based on the clinical phenotype, although not in all cases. The four most common and well described of these syndromes will be briefly discussed in the following paragraphs, focusing on symptoms and signs distinguishing them from the common phenotype, and on pathophysiology.

Box 4.1 Suggested Further Reading

Touitou (2013)	Genetic point of view on current knowledge on autoinflammatory diseases. Addresses issues concerning nomenclature and the increased discovery rate of new diseases.
Park et al. (2012)	Recent advances in the genetic and cell biological basis of inflammation (not limited to IL-1) in Mendelian autoinflammatory diseases as well as in more common rheumatic diseases.
Masters et al. (2009)	Detailed and complete overview of autoinflammatory diseases.
Dinarello et al. (2012)	Elaborate review on IL-1 blockade in treatment of a broad range of inflammatory diseases.
Lamkanfi and Dixit (2012)	Reviews current knowledge on inflammasome types and their relevance in health and disease.
Mankan et al. (2012)	This review elaborates on the currently known inflammasome complexes with a special focus on their activation mechanisms.

TABLE 4.1 Major Monogenic Autoinflammatory Disorders: Molecular Pathology and Features

Disease	Gene	Protein	Inheritance	Mechanism	Distinctive symptoms	Duration and frequency of attacks
FMF	MEFV	Pyrin	AR	Gene-dosage and ASC dependent, NLRP3-independent, inflammasome activation	Colchicine responsive, erysipelas-like erythema, serositis	1−3 days, variable
TRAPS	TNFRSF1A	Tumor necrosis factor receptor 1	AD	Abnormal aggregation and intracellular accumulation of TNFR1, ligand-independent signaling; mitochondrial ROS, MAPK activation	Prolonged symptoms, migrating skin rash and severe myalgia	>week, may be very prolonged
MKD	MVK	Mevalonate kinase	AR	Reduced geranylgeranylation of proteins leading to increased IL-1β secretion	Diarrhoea, lymphadenopathy, aphthous ulcers	3−7 days, 1−2 monthly
CAPS	NLRP3	NLRP3	AD	Abnormal oligomerization, sponteneous activation of caspase-1 activity	Cold-induced fever, urticarial rash, sensorineural deafness, aseptic meningitis, deforming arthropathy, mental retardation	24−48 h, depending on environmental factors (FCAS) continuous
PAPA	PSTPIP1	PSTPIP1	AD	Distorted pyrin function due to PSTPIP1 binding	Pyogenic arthritis, pyoderma gangrenosum, cystic acne	Intermittent attacks with migratory arthritis, may be continuous
Blau syndrome	NOD2	NOD2	AD	Affected nucleotide binding domain might cause increased NF-κB activation	Granulomatous polyarthritis, iritis, dermatitis	+/− continuous
DIRA	IL-1RN	IL-1 receptor antagonist	AR	Absence of or non-functional IL-1 Ra leads to unregulated IL-1 signaling	Sterile multi-focal osteomyelitis, periostitis and pustulosis	continuous

FMF: familial Mediteranean fever, TRAPS: TNF receptor-associated periodic syndrome, MKD: mevalonate kinase deficiency, CAPS: cryopyrin-associated periodic syndrome, PAPA: pyoderma gangrenosum, acne and pyogenic arthritis, DIRA: deficiency of IL-1ra, NLRP3: NACHT, LRR and PYD domains-containing protein 3, PSTPIP1: proline-serine-threonine phosphatase-interacting protein 1, NOD2: nucleotide-binding oligomerization domain-containing protein 2, AD: autosomal dominant, AR: autosomal recessive, ASC: apoptosis-associated speck-like protein containing a CARD, ROS: reactive oxygen species, MAPK: mitogen-activated protein kinase.
Adapted from Lachmann et al. (2011), Park et al. (2012).

Cryopyrin-Associated Periodic Syndrome

One of the clearest examples of dysregulation of IL-1β is CAPS, a hereditary disorder caused by mutations in the NLRP3 protein which lead to easier NLRP3 inflammasome activation and secretion of IL-1β (Hoffman et al., 2001; Aksentijevich et al., 2002; Feldmann et al., 2002; Goldbach-Mansky, 2012). CAPS is the current name for three previously recognized clinical syndromes with an autosomal dominant inheritance pattern: the relatively mild Familial Cold Autoinflammatory Syndrome (FCAS); the intermediate Muckle−Wells syndrome (MWS); and the far more severe NOMID (also known as CINCA). Distinguishing clinical features of these disorders include an urticaria-like skin rash, progressive perceptive hearing loss, inflammatory episodes provoked by systemic exposure to cold, and in severe cases joint deformations and aseptic meningitis, resulting in developmental delay and significant disability. Genetic studies revealed a common genetic background in these patients, i.e., an activating mutation in the gene for NLRP3 (upon discovery, this protein was named cryopyrin, resulting in the name of the disorder CAPS; but NLRP3 is now recognized as the official name for the protein) (Bertin and DiStefano, 2000; Fairbrother et al., 2001; Martinon et al., 2001; Ting et al., 2008). NLRP3 is the central protein in the most important inflammasome, and mutations result in an increased production of active IL-1β (Figure 4.2A) (Agostini et al. 2004). Since the discovery of the common genetic background, it has been recognized that rather than three separate entities, the clinical phenotype should be seen as a continuous spectrum ranging from mild to very severe disease. There is no conclusive phenotype−genotype correlation, and disease severity can even vary within families—so it is likely that there are other contributing (genetic) factors. Treatment with inhibitors of IL-1 is very effective and has dramatically improved quality of life for these patients in recent years (Dinarello et al., 2012).

Familial Mediterranean Fever

The most prevalent of these rare disorders, and the one which has been recognized for the longest time, is FMF. This was already recognized as a distinct familial syndrome with autosomal recessive inheritance more than a century ago. Patients suffer from recurring episodes of serositis. A classic FMF attack presents as peritonitis, with or without fever, lasting for 2−3 days. Before the patient is diagnosed as having FMF, these episodes are frequently mistaken for appendicitis or other acute abdomen, resulting in unnecessary abdominal surgery. Other presentations of the FMF-associated serositis can be pleuritis, pericarditis, arthritis, and more rarely meningitis or acute scrotal inflammation (Masters et al., 2009).

The name FMF is derived from the epidemiological observation that many patients have an ethnic background originating from the countries around the Mediterranean Sea (Sohar et al., 1967). Until the 1970s, FMF was considered a disease with a significantly reduced life expectancy, mainly due to the high prevalence of renal failure due to AA-type amyloidosis. This changed with the

discovery of the high efficacy of prophylactic use of colchicine. In more than 90% of FMF patients, chronic use of a sufficiently high dose of colchicine (1−2 mg per day) will either prevent the occurrence of inflammatory attacks or greatly reduce their severity and frequency. It also prevents the occurrence of AA-type amyloidosis, and renal failure is now very rare in patients who are compliant with therapy (Ozturk et al., 2011).

In 1997, two groups practically simultaneously discovered the genetic background of FMF, and raced each other for publication and for the naming of the protein involved, which was previously unknown (International FMF Consortium, 1997; French FMF Consortium, 1997). The gene was named *MEFV* (Mediterranean FeVer gene), and the protein is now known as pyrin. Pyrin has a regulatory function; mutations in pyrin affect the function of the NLRP3 inflammasome, leading to increased IL-1β (see Figure 4.2C) (Masters et al., 2009; Stoffels et al., 2013). Most mutations are missense mutations, and most patients are compound heterozygous for two different missense mutations. There is some information on phenotype−genotype correlations; the mutation associated with most severe disease and the highest prevalence of amyloidosis is M694V (Masters et al., 2006). A clear founder effect has been proven for this mutation, which explains its prevalence in communities around the Mediterranean Sea and Jewish populations. There has been some speculation on a survivor advantage for carriers of one *MEFV* gene mutation, such as increased survival of certain infectious diseases, to explain the relatively high prevalence in some areas, but this is hard to prove (Masters et al., 2009).

TNF Receptor-Associated Periodic Syndrome

Distinguishing clinical features of TRAPS are a migrating painful erythematous skin rash, severe myalgia, and particularly prolonged inflammatory episodes, of weeks rather than days (Masters et al., 2009; Cantarini et al., 2012).

TRAPS is one of the autoinflammatory disorders that is not caused by a direct effect of IL-1β signaling. It is caused by autosomal dominant heterozygous mutations in TNFRSF1A, which encodes the TNF-α receptor 1, a transmembrane protein and member of the TNFR superfamily. The ligand for this receptor is TNF-α, which is produced mainly by monocytes and macrophages, and is involved in systemic inflammation, apoptosis, and cell proliferation (Bazzoni and Beutler, 1996). The intracellular signaling subsequent on binding of TNF-α to its receptor is complicated, and can include activation of NF-κB, c-Jun/activator protein 1 (AP-1), apoptosis, and protein−kinase pathways activated by mitogens (Wajant et al., 2003).

TRAPS mutations almost exclusively affect the extracellular domain of TNFRSF1A. Initially, it was hypothesized that the mutations would have an activating effect. However, there is no increased binding of TNF-α, no spontaneous activation of the receptor, and no increased receptor expression (McDermott et al., 1999). Another hypothesis was that TNFR mutations would lead to a defect in receptor shedding (Mullberg et al., 1995), the process in which a receptor is cleaved off the membrane to prevent constitutive signaling, and to act as a decoy for excess extracellular ligand. But this shedding hypothesis could not hold true, because shedding defects could only be detected in some TRAPS-associated TNFR1 mutations and only in certain cell types (Aksentijevich et al., 2001; Huggins et al., 2004).

Recent studies have shed new light on the pathophysiology. TRAPS-related mutations actually have several characteristics of function inhibiting mutations: impaired membrane trafficking, and as a consequence retainment of the receptor in the endoplasmic reticulum (ER) (Todd et al., 2004, 2007; Lobito et al., 2006); no oligomerization of mutant- with WT-receptors (Lobito et al., 2006), and decreased binding of TNF-α (Todd et al., 2004). It was shown that accumulated mutant receptors result in increased spontaneous activation of mitogen-activated protein kinase (MAPKs), thereby priming the TRAPS cells to become more susceptible to low doses of inflammatory stimuli and responding by secreting more proinflammatory cytokines, in particular IL-1β (Simon et al., 2010). This effect is mediated by increased mitochondrial-derived reactive oxygen species (ROS) (Bulua et al., 2011).

Initially, treating patients with etanercept, a synthetic version of soluble TNF receptor (sTNFR), seemed most appropriate, to substitute the deficiency of sTNFR. However, the clinical efficacy of etanercept in TRAPS can be disappointing, and actually the inhibition of IL-1 is more effective than the inhibition of TNF—supporting the observation that even TRAPS symptomatology is mediated more by increased IL-1β than TNF-α.

HIDS (also Known as Mevalonate Kinase Deficiency)

In 1984, van der Meer et al. described an autoinflammatory disease that was different from FMF, and named the disease after the high serum IgD concentrations that were found in these patients: hyperimmunoglobulinemia D and periodic fever (HIDS) (van der Meer et al., 1984). The common clinical phenotype as described above is seen, distinguished by an age of onset around 3 months, with characteristic accompanying symptoms such as lymphadenopathy, hepatosplenomegaly and aphthous ulcers, and the fact that any vaccination can trigger an inflammatory attack.

In the early days, the diagnosis was made solely based on careful clinical observation. Elevated serum IgD concentrations are characteristic, but not related to disease severity, presence or absence of a fever attack and it is not present in all patients; therefore the original name can be misleading.

In 1999, the genetic defect causing this rare disorder was found: mutations in the MVK gene lead to amino acid substitutions in mevalonate kinase, an enzyme in the isoprenoid pathway (Drenth et al., 1999; Houten et al., 1999). Patients with the far more severe mevalonic aciduria (MA) also have a defect in mevalonate kinase (Berger et al., 1985). These patients have the same symptoms as HIDS patients, but in addition suffer from growth retardation, dysmorphic features, and neurological symptoms such as ataxia and mental retardation. There is a spectrum of clinical phenotypes related to mevalonate kinase deficiency (MKD), with HIDS at the mild end of the spectrum and MA at the other end (Simon et al., 2004). Recently, Zhang et al. found MVK mutations in disseminated superficial actinic porokeratosis (Zhang et al., 2012), and we have found them in patients with isolated retinitis pigmentosa (Siemiatkowska et al., in press), diversifying this spectrum even further. There is some correlation between residual MK enzyme activity and disease severity, and some correlation between enzyme activity and certain MVK mutations, but the genotype–phenotype correlation is not perfect.

It is intriguing how an enzyme defect in a pathway that seemingly has nothing to do with inflammation can cause these phenotypes. MK is a major enzyme in the mevalonate pathway (also called isoprenoid pathway), from which the end products are, for example, cholesterol and isoprenoids. The enzyme 3-hydroxyl-3-methylglutaryl-coenzyme A (HMG-CoA) reductase converts HMG-CoA to mevalonate, which is then phosphorylated by mevalonate kinase. Further down in the pathway the end products are formed; these metabolites are important for various cellular functions. For example, protein prenylation can regulate the activation status of proteins, such as some small GTPases of the Ras super family (Henneman et al., 2010). Mutations in MVK result in decreased enzyme activity, sometimes even below detection level, and therefore the formation of end products, including isoprenoids, is compromised. The exact link between MKD and inflammation is at present still unknown (Figure 4.2B), although it is likely to be the defect or dysregulation of protein isoprenylation. *In vitro* studies showed that shortage of isoprenoids, mainly geranyl-geranyl, induced increased caspase-1 activation and hypersecretion of IL-1β in monocytes (Mandey et al., 2006; Stoffels and Simon, 2011).

POLYGENIC OR ACQUIRED AUTOINFLAMMATORY DISORDERS

This can encompass a large and very diverse group of disorders, similar to the autoimmune diseases (see Figure 4.1).

For some of these, the designation autoinflammatory is clearly more apt than the term "autoimmune." Examples of these include gout, in which the pathogenic role of IL-1β and the NLRP3 inflammasome has become clear. A rare disorder with a clear autoinflammatory background is the syndrome of periodic fever with aphthous stomatitis, pharyngitis, and cervical adenitis (PFAPA), a childhood disease characterized by episodes of the symptoms described in its name, which is often self-limiting within a number of years. PFAPA is suspected to have a polygenic background (Stojanov et al., 2011).

It could also be argued that the inflammatory bowel diseases are part of this group of polygenic autoinflammatory disorders. Although many aspects of the etiology are still unclear, there are certainly features of increased inflammation. This is also supported by the link with mutations in the NOD2 gene. For a more detailed discussion of the pathophysiology of these diseases, see Chapter 60.

More to the middle of the spectrum are the disorders for which an approximately equal contribution of innate and adaptive immunity is suspected in the pathophysiology. For example, IL-17 dysregulation is important in the pathophysiology of psoriasis, leading to dysregulation of both innate and adaptive immunity. The importance of the innate immune system is underscored by the recent finding of mutations in the IL-36 receptor antagonist as the cause of a rare hereditary subgroup termed generalized pustular psoriasis (Marrakchi et al., 2011; Onoufriadis et al., 2011).

AUTOINFLAMMATORY MECHANISMS OF DISEASE IN COMMON DISORDERS

The effects of IL-1β are not restricted to a small group of rare autoinflammatory diseases. In some common diseases there is also an autoinflammatory component. Below we will describe two of those examples: type 2 diabetes and atherosclerosis.

Type 2 Diabetes Mellitus

Obesity and inactivity are high risk factors for acquiring type 2 diabetes, leading to insulin resistance, where the insulin-producing β cells cannot adapt to increasing insulin demands. A role for IL-1β has been suggested in this pathophysiology. Low IL-1β concentrations have been shown to be selectively toxic for insulin-producing pancreatic β-cells, supporting a causative role for IL-1β in the loss of β cell mass (Dinarello et al., 2010) (see Chapter 66). The autoinflammation is driven by glucose, free fatty acids, leptin, and IL-1β itself; caspase-1 is also required for the release of free fatty acids from the adipocyte. Treatment with IL-1 receptor antagonist in patients with type 2 diabetes in clinical trials resulted in improved glycemia and β cell function (without effect on weight or insulin sensitivity). These data show potential for long-term glycemic control and reduced risk for cardiovascular events (Dinarello et al., 2012).

Atherosclerosis

It is clear that atherosclerosis can be viewed as an inflammatory disease; inflammatory lesions in arteries result in vascular plaques, and rupture of these plaques can result in the complications associated with this common disorder. Chapter 71 of this book deals in great detail with the current knowledge on the pathophysiology of atherosclerosis; the authors argue that this fits with an autoimmune basis for the disease. However, as they show in their Table 71.1, a large role is played by cells of the innate immune system. A direct role for the NLRP3 inflammasome in atherosclerosis has also been suggested by numerous studies: e.g., NLRP3 inflammasome activation is required for vascular smooth muscle cell calcification (Wen et al., 2013), apolipoprotein E deficient mice, a model for vascular inflammation, developed significantly less atherosclerosis when crossed with caspase-1 deficient mice (Usui et al., 2012), and cholesterol crystals, as found in atherosclerotic plaques, activate NLRP3 in primed immune cells (Duewell et al., 2010), resulting in IL-1β secretion (Grebe and Latz, 2013). Thus, atherosclerosis is likely located more to the right of the autoimmune–autoinflammatory spectrum (Figure 4.1), with increasing evidence for autoinflammatory mechanisms of disease.

NEWEST DEVELOPMENTS: RARE HEREDITARY DISORDERS WITH AUTOINFLAMMATORY ASPECTS

With the rise of next generation sequencing techniques, disease discovery has significantly speeded up. Diseases that previously could not be distinguished or of unknown origin are now being unraveled at a higher rate. Some of these newly discovered syndromes belong somewhere in the middle of the autoinflammation–autoimmunity spectrum. Others combine aspects of both autoinflammation and immunodeficiency, or other defects such as lipodystrophy, which were not recognized as part of these disorders before. Below we discuss a few of the recently discovered syndromes, which are not only worthy of mention because they are new, but even more because they extend the range of mechanisms that are involved in autoinflammation.

Proteasome Defects

From the 1980s, several hereditary syndromes have been described with largely similar phenotype, although with small variations. These each received their own name, and became known as Nakajo–Nishimura syndrome (NNS (Kitano et al., 1985; Tanaka et al., 1993; Kasagi et al., 2008), recently named JASL (Kitamura et al., 2011)), JMP (Megarbane et al., 2002; Garg et al., 2010), and CANDLE (Torrelo et al., 2010; Ramot et al., 2011). They are characterized by marked lipodystrophy, which seems to be induced by panniculitis, and muscular atrophy, as well as episodes of fever and inflammation, skin rash, violaceous swollen eyelids, hypochromic or normocytic anemia and joint contractures.

More or less at the same time, several groups discovered that autosomal recessive mutations in PSMB8, encoding the inducible proteasome subunit beta-type-8, are the cause of all of these syndromes (Agarwal et al., 2010; Arima et al., 2011; Kitamura et al., 2011; Liu et al., 2012). The different mutations result in a reduced activity of the immunoproteasome. Consequently, ubiquitinated and oxidized proteins accumulate in cells expressing these immunoproteasomes, instead of being degraded (Figure 4.2I). This also results in an increase of IL-6 and IFN-γ inducible protein (IP)-10 serum concentrations.

These high concentrations of IP-10 and a prominent IFN-γ signature distinguish these disorders from IL-1-mediated disorders (Agarwal et al., 2010; Arima et al., 2011; Liu et al., 2012). It remains to be seen whether these provide a link to pathogenesis and whether this can point to effective treatment strategies (Goldbach-Mansky, 2012).

PLCγ2 Deficiency

In 2012, two groups reported defects in the PLCG2 gene, encoding a signaling molecule expressed in B cells, natural killer cells, and mast cells: phospholipase Cγ2. Its activation leads to increased intracellular [Ca^{2+}], which turn can activate the inflammasome (Brough et al., 2003; Lee et al., 2012; Murakami et al., 2012; Rossol et al., 2012; Haneklaus et al., 2013). PLCG2 mutations lead to a spectrum of PLCγ2-related phenotypes that combine both autoinflammatory and immunodeficiency properties.

Initially, three families with a dominantly inherited complex of cold-induced urticaria, antibody deficiency, and susceptibility to infection and autoimmunity were described, and the phenotype was coined as PLAID (Ombrello et al., 2012b). Affected family members suffered from atopy, granulomatous rash, autoimmune thyroiditis (with the presence of antinuclear antibodies), sinopulmonary infections, and hypogammaglobulinemia (including reduced serum concentrations of IgA and IgM). This was accompanied by reduced circulating natural killer cells and class-switched memory B cells. Genetic analysis in these families revealed PLCG2 deletions of exon 19, and exons 20–22, located in the autoinhibitory domain, rendering PLCγ2 constitutively activated. At physiologic temperatures, cells had diminished signaling; however, at subphysiologic temperatures, signaling was enhanced. So PLCG2 deletions can lead to gain of PLCγ2 function, causing signaling abnormalities in multiple leukocyte subsets, and a phenotype that consists of both excessive and deficient immune function.

In the same year, a missense mutation in PLCγ2, p.Ser707Tyr, located in an autoinhibitory SH2 domain, causing enhanced PLCγ2 activation, was found in another patient (Zhou et al., 2012). The p.Ser707Tyr substitution is responsible for a phenotype that is not provoked by cold, and includes recurrent blistering skin lesions, bronchiolitis, arthralgia, ocular inflammation, enterocolitis, absence of autoantibodies, and mild immunodeficiency. The authors considered this to be a very distinct phenotype and suggested their own name for the disease: APLAID (autoinflammation and PLCγ2-associated antibody deficiency and immune dysregulation). Very likely, PLAID and APLAID are part of a continuum of inflammatory diseases related to PLCγ2 defects.

Heme-Oxidized IRP2 Ubiquitin Ligase

Recently, Boisson et al. provided the clinical molecular description of a new fatal human disorder, characterized by chronic autoinflammation, invasive bacterial infections, and muscular amylopectinosis (Boisson et al., 2012; Ombrello et al., 2012a). Patients combine symptoms of both autoinflammation and immunodeficiency, and very early in life develop recurrent episodes of fever and systemic inflammation with an acute-phase response, hepatosplenomegaly and lymphadenopathy.

Again, the underlying pathophysiology turned out to be surprising. Loss-of-expression and loss-of-function mutations in heme-oxidized IRP2 ubiquitin ligase-1 (HOIL-1), a component of the linear ubiquitin chain assembly complex (LUBAC), are responsible for this disease. LUBAC is a multiprotein complex that attaches linear chains of ubiquitin molecules to protein substrates (Kirisako et al., 2006), which is important for targeting proteins for proteasomal degradation, protein-protein interactions, and protein trafficking to cellular locations (Tokunaga et al., 2009). An example is targeting NEMO (modulator of NF-κB) to signalosomes of IL-1R1, TNFR, and TLRs.

The described mutations in HOIL1 resulted in impaired LUBAC stability, and as a consequence NF-κB activation in response to IL-1β was diminished in patient fibroblasts. On the other hand, monocytes were hyperresponsive to IL-1β, explaining the appearance of both autoinflammation and immunodeficiency in the patients. These data show that LUBAC differentially regulates NF-κB-dependent IL-1β responses in different cell types (Figure 4.2H). It remains to be elucidated which mechanisms underlie the diversity in effects observed.

CONCLUSION

Autoinflammation and autoimmunity are part of a spectrum of immunological diseases, in the same way that innate and adaptive immunity are part of an immunological continuum. Recognizing autoinflammation as a distinct mechanism of disease helps in unraveling the pathophysiology, and also in finding the right therapeutic approach. It is likely that the definition of "autoinflammatory disease" will continue to evolve over the next decades, just as that of autoimmune disease has done, to match our increased insight.

REFERENCES

Agarwal, A.K., Xing, C., DeMartino, G.N., Mizrachi, D., Hernandez, M. D., Sousa, A.B., et al., 2010. PSMB8 encoding the beta5i proteasome subunit is mutated in joint contractures, muscle atrophy, microcytic anemia, and panniculitis-induced lipodystrophy syndrome. Am. J. Hum. Genet. 87, 866–872.

Agostini, L., Martinon, F., Burns, K., McDermott, M.F., Hawkins, P.N., Tschopp, J., 2004. NALP3 forms an IL-1beta-processing inflammasome with increased activity in Muckle-Wells autoinflammatory disorder. Immunity. 20, 319–325.

Aksentijevich, I., Galon, J., Soares, M., Mansfield, E., Hull, K., Oh, H.H., et al., 2001. The tumor-necrosis-factor receptor-associated periodic syndrome, new mutations in TNFRSF1A, ancestral origins, genotype-phenotype studies, and evidence for further genetic heterogeneity of periodic fevers. Am. J. Hum. Genet. 69, 301–314.

Aksentijevich, I., Nowak, M., Mallah, M., Chae, J.J., Watford, W.T., Hofmann, S.R., et al., 2002. De novo CIAS1 mutations, cytokine activation, and evidence for genetic heterogeneity in patients with neonatal-onset multisystem inflammatory disease (NOMID). A new member of the expanding family of pyrin-associated autoinflammatory diseases. Arthritis Rheum. 46, 3340–3348.

Arima, K., Kinoshita, A., Mishima, H., Kanazawa, N., Kaneko, T., Mizushima, T., et al., 2011. Proteasome assembly defect due to a proteasome subunit beta type 8 (PSMB8) mutation causes the autoinflammatory disorder, Nakajo–Nishimura syndrome. Proc. Natl. Acad. Sci. U.S.A. 108, 14914–14919.

Bazzoni, F., Beutler, B., 1996. The tumor necrosis factor ligand and receptor families. N. Engl. J. Med. 334, 1717–1725.

Berger, R., Smit, G.P., Schierbeek, H., Bijsterveld, K., le Coultre, R., 1985. Mevalonic aciduria, an inborn error of cholesterol biosynthesis? Clin. Chim. Acta. 152, 219–222.

Bertin, J., DiStefano, P.S., 2000. The PYRIN domain, a novel motif found in apoptosis and inflammation proteins. Cell Death Differ. 7, 1273–1274.

Boisson, B., Laplantine, E., Prando, C., Giliani, S., Israelsson, E., Xu, Z., et al., 2012. Immunodeficiency, autoinflammation and amylopectinosis in humans with inherited HOIL-1 and LUBAC deficiency. Nat. Immunol. 13, 1178–1186.

Brough, D., Le Feuvre, R.A., Wheeler, R.D., Solovyova, N., Hilfiker, S., Rothwell, N.J., et al., 2003. Ca2 + stores and Ca2 + entry differentially contribute to the release of IL-1 beta and IL-1 alpha from murine macrophages. J. Immunol. 170 (6), 3029–3036.

Bulua, A.C., Simon, A., Maddipati, R., Pelletier, M., Park, H., Kim, K.Y., et al., 2011. Mitochondrial reactive oxygen species promote production of proinflammatory cytokines and are elevated in TNFR1-associated periodic syndrome (TRAPS). J. Exp. Med. 208, 519–533.

Cantarini, L., Lucherini, O.M., Muscari, I., Frediani, B., Galeazzi, M., Brizi, M.G., et al., 2012. Tumour necrosis factor receptor-associated periodic syndrome (TRAPS), state of the art and future perspectives. Autoimmun. Rev. 12, 38–43.

Dinarello, C.A., Donath, M.Y., Mandrup-Poulsen, T., 2010. Role of IL-1beta in type 2 diabetes. Curr. Opin. Endocrinol. Diabetes Obes. 17, 314–321.

Dinarello, C.A., Simon, A., van der Meer, J.W., 2012. Treating inflammation by blocking interleukin-1 in a broad spectrum of diseases. Nat. Rev. Drug Discov. 11, 633–652.

Drenth, J.P., Cuisset, L., Grateau, G., Vasseur, C., van de Velde-Visser, S.D., de Jong, J.G., et al., 1999. Mutations in the gene encoding mevalonate kinase cause hyper-IgD and periodic fever syndrome. International Hyper-IgD study group. Nat. Genet. 22, 178–181.

Duewell, P., Kono, H., Rayner, K.J., Sirois, C.M., Vladimer, G., Bauernfeind, F.G., et al., 2010. NLRP3 inflammasomes are required for atherogenesis and activated by cholesterol crystals. Nature. 464, 1357–1361.

Fairbrother, W.J., Gordon, N.C., Humke, E.W., O'Rourke, K.M., Starovasnik, M.A., Yin, J.P., et al., 2001. The PYRIN domain, a member of the death domain-fold superfamily. Protein Sci. 10, 1911–1918.

Feldmann, J., Prieur, A.M., Quartier, P., Berquin, P., Certain, S., Cortis, E., et al., 2002. Chronic infantile neurological cutaneous and articular syndrome is caused by mutations in CIAS1, a gene highly expressed in polymorphonuclear cells and chondrocytes. Am. J. Hum. Genet. 71, 198–203.

Garg, A., Hernandez, M.D., Sousa, A.B., Subramanyam, L., Martínez de Villarreal, L., dos Santos, H.G., et al., 2010. An autosomal recessive syndrome of joint contractures, muscular atrophy, microcytic anemia, and panniculitis-associated lipodystrophy. J. Clin. Endocrinol. Metab. 95, E58–E63.

Goldbach-Mansky, R., 2012. Immunology in clinic review series; focus on autoinflammatory diseases, update on monogenic autoinflammatory diseases, the role of interleukin (IL)-1 and an emerging role for cytokines beyond IL-1. Clin. Exp. Immunol. 167, 391–404.

Grebe, A., Latz, E., 2013. Cholesterol crystals and inflammation. Curr. Rheumatol. Rep. 15, 313.

Haneklaus, M., O'Neill, L.A., Coll, R.C., 2013. Modulatory mechanisms controlling the NLRP3 inflammasome in inflammation, recent developments. Curr. Opin. Immunol. 25, 40–45.

Henneman, L., Schneiders, M.S., Turkenburg, M., Waterham, H.R., 2010. Compromised geranylgeranylation of RhoA and Rac1 in mevalonate kinase deficiency. J. Inherit. Metab. Dis. 33, 625–632.

Hoffman, H.M., Mueller, J.L., Broide, D.H., Wanderer, A.A., Kolodner, R.D., 2001. Mutation of a new gene encoding a putative pyrin-like protein causes familial cold autoinflammatory syndrome and Muckle–Wells syndrome. Nat. Genet. 29, 301–305.

Houten, S.M., Kuis, W., Duran, M., de Koning, T.J., van Royen-Kerkhof, A., Romeijn, G.J., et al., 1999. Mutations in MVK, encoding mevalonate kinase, cause hyperimmunoglobulinaemia D and periodic fever syndrome. Nat. Genet. 22, 175–177.

Huggins, M.L., Radford, P.M., McIntosh, R.S., Bainbridge, S.E., Dickinson, P., Draper-Morgan, K.A., et al., 2004. Shedding of mutant tumor necrosis factor receptor superfamily 1A associated with tumor necrosis factor receptor-associated periodic syndrome, differences between cell types. Arthritis Rheum. 50, 2651–2659.

Kasagi, S., Kawano, S., Nakazawa, T., Sugino, H., Koshiba, M., Ichinose, K., et al., 2008. A case of periodic-fever-syndrome-like disorder with lipodystrophy, myositis, and autoimmune abnormalities. Mod. Rheumatol. 18, 203–207.

Kastner, D.L., Aksentijevich, I., Goldbach-Mansky, R., 2010. Autoinflammatory disease reloaded, a clinical perspective. Cell. 140, 784–790.

Kirisako, T., Kamei, K., Murata, S., Kato, M., Fukumoto, H., Kanie, M., et al., 2006. A ubiquitin ligase complex assembles linear polyubiquitin chains. EMBO J. 25, 4877–4887.

Kitamura, A., Maekawa, Y., Uehara, H., Izumi, K., Kawachi, I., Nishizawa, M., et al., 2011. A mutation in the immunoproteasome subunit PSMB8 causes autoinflammation and lipodystrophy in humans. J. Clin. Invest. 121, 4150–4160.

Kitano, Y., Matsunaga, E., Morimoto, T., Okada, N., Sano, S., 1985. A syndrome with nodular erythema, elongated and thickened fingers, and emaciation. Arch. Dermatol. 121, 1053–1056.

Lachmann, H.J., 2011. Clinical Immunology Review Series, An approach to the patient with a periodic fever syndrome. Clin. Exp. Immunol. 165, 301–309.

Lamkanfi, M., Dixit, V.M., 2012. Inflammasomes and their roles in health and disease. Annu. Rev. Cell Dev. Biol. 28, 137–161.

Lee, G.S., Subramanian, N., Kim, A.I., Aksentijevich, I., Goldbach-Mansky, R., Sacks, D.B., et al., 2012. The calcium-sensing receptor regulates the NLRP3 inflammasome through Ca2+ and cAMP. Nature. 492, 123–127.

Liu, Y., Ramot, Y., Torrelo, A., Paller, A.S., Si, N., Babay, S., et al., 2012. Mutations in proteasome subunit beta type 8 cause chronic atypical neutrophilic dermatosis with lipodystrophy and elevated temperature with evidence of genetic and phenotypic heterogeneity. Arthritis Rheum. 64, 895–907.

Lobito, A.A., Kimberley, F.C., Muppidi, J.R., Komarow, H., Jackson, A.J., Hull, K.M., et al., 2006. Abnormal disulfide-linked oligomerization results in ER retention and altered signaling by TNFR1 mutants in TNFR1-associated periodic fever syndrome (TRAPS). Blood. 108, 1320–1327.

Mandey, S.H., Kuijk, L.M., Frenkel, J., Waterham, H.R., 2006. A role for geranylgeranylation in interleukin-1beta secretion. Arthritis and Rheum. 54, 3690–3695.

Mankan, A., Kubarenko, A., Hornung, V., 2012. Immunology in clinic review series; focus on autoinflammatory diseases, inflammasomes, mechanisms of activation. Clin. Exp. Immunol. 167, 369–381.

Marrakchi, S., Guigue, P., Renshaw, B.R., Puel, A., Pei, X.Y., Fraitag, S., et al., 2011. Interleukin-36-receptor antagonist deficiency and generalized pustular psoriasis. N. Engl. J. Med. 365, 620–628.

Martinon, F., Burns, K., Tschopp, J., 2002. The inflammasome, a molecular platform triggering activation of inflammatory caspases and processing of proIL-beta. Mol. Cell. 10, 417–426.

Martinon, F., Hofmann, K., Tschopp, J., 2001. The pyrin domain, a possible member of the death domain-fold family implicated in apoptosis and inflammation. Curr. Biol. 11, R118–R120.

Masters, S.L., Simon, A., Aksentijevich, I., Kastner, D.L., 2009. Horror autoinflammaticus, the molecular pathophysiology of autoinflammatory disease. Annu. Rev. Immunol. 27, 621–668.

Masters, S.L., Yao, S., Willson, T.A., Zhang, J.G., Palmer, K.R., Smith, B.J., et al., 2006. The SPRY domain of SSB-2 adopts a novel fold that presents conserved Par-4-binding residues. Nat. Struct. Mol. Biol. 13, 77–84.

McDermott, M.F., Aksentijevich, I., Galon, J., McDermott, E.M., Ogunkolade, B.W., Centola, M., et al., 1999. Germline mutations in the extracellular domains of the 55 kDa TNF receptor, TNFR1, define a family of dominantly inherited autoinflammatory syndromes. Cell. 97, 133–144.

McGonagle, D., McDermott, M.F., 2006. A proposed classification of the immunological diseases. PLoS Med. 3 (8), e297.

Medzhitov, R., Janeway Jr., C., 2000. Innate immunity. N. Engl. J. Med. 343 (5), 338–344.

Megarbane, A., Sanders, A., Chouery, E., Delague, V., Medlej-Hashim, M., Torbey, P.H., 2002. An unknown autoinflammatory syndrome associated with short stature and dysmorphic features in a young boy. J. Rheumatol. 29, 1084–1087.

Mullberg, J., Durie, F.H., Otten-Evans, C., Alderson, M.R., Rose-John, S., Cosman, D., et al., 1995. A metalloprotease inhibitor blocks shedding of the IL-6 receptor and the p60 TNF receptor. J. Immunol. 155, 5198–5205.

Murakami, T., Ockinger, J., Yu, J., Byles, V., McColl, A., Hofer, A.M., et al., 2012. Critical role for calcium mobilization in activation of the NLRP3 inflammasome. Proc. Natl. Acad. Sci. U.S.A. 109, 11282–11287.

Ombrello, M., Kastner, D.L., Milner, J.D., 2012a. HOIL and water, the two faces of HOIL-1 deficiency. Nat. Immunol. 13, 1133–1135.

Ombrello, M., Remmers, E.F., Sun, G., Freeman, A.F., Datta, S., Torabi-Parizi, P., et al., 2012b. Cold urticaria, immunodeficiency, and autoimmunity related to PLCG2 deletions. N. Engl. J. Med. 366, 330–338.

Onoufriadis, A., Simpson, M.A., Pink, A.E., Di Meglio, P., Smith, C.H., Pullabhatla, V., et al., 2011. Mutations in IL36RN/IL1F5 are associated with the severe episodic inflammatory skin disease known as generalized pustular psoriasis. Am. J. Hum. Genet. 89, 432–437.

Ozturk, M.A., Kanbay, M., Kasapoglu, B., Onat, A.M., Guz, G., Furst, D.E., et al., 2011. Therapeutic approach to familial Mediterranean fever, a review update. Clin. Exp. Rheumatol. 29, S77–S86.

Park, H., Bourla, A.B., Kastner, D.L., Colbert, R.A., Siegel, R.M., 2012. Lighting the fires within, the cell biology of autoinflammatory diseases. Nat. Rev. Immunol. 12, 570–580.

Ramot, Y., Czarnowicki, T., Maly, A., Navon-Elkan, P., Zlotogorski, A., 2011. Chronic atypical neutrophilic dermatosis with lipodystrophy and elevated temperature syndrome, a case report. Pediatr. Dermatol. 28, 538–541.

Rossol, M., Pierer, M., Raulien, N., Quandt, D., Meusch, U., Rothe, K., et al., 2012. Extracellular Ca2 + is a danger signal activating the NLRP3 inflammasome through G protein-coupled calcium sensing receptors. Nat. Commun. 3, 1329.

Simon, A., Kremer, H.P., Wevers, R.A., Scheffer, H., De Jong, J.G., Van Der Meer, J.W., et al., 2004. Mevalonate kinase deficiency. Evidence for a phenotypic continuum. Neurology. 62, 994–997.

Simon, A., Park, H., Maddipati, R., Lobito, A.A., Bulua, A.C., Jackson, A.J., et al., 2010. Concerted action of wild-type and mutant TNF receptors enhances inflammation in TNF receptor 1-associated periodic fever syndrome. Proc. Nat. Acad. Sci. U.S.A. 107, 9801–9806.

Sohar, E., Gafni, J., Pras, M., Heller, H., 1967. Familial Mediterranean fever. A survey of 470 cases and review of the literature. Am. J. Med. 43 (2), 227–253.

Stoffels, M., Simon, A., 2011. Hyper-IgD syndrome or mevalonate kinase deficiency. Curr. Opin. Rheumatol. 23, 419–423.

Stoffels, M., Szperl, A., Simon, A., Netea, M.G., Plantinga, T.S., van Deuren, M., et al., 2013. MEFV mutations affecting pyrin amino acid 577 cause autosomal dominant autoinflammatory disease. Ann. Rheum. Dis. (Epub ahead of print).

Stojanov, S., Lapidus, S., Chitkara, P., Feder, H., Salazar, J.C., Fleisher, T.A., et al., 2011. Periodic fever, aphthous stomatitis, pharyngitis, and adenitis (PFAPA) is a disorder of innate immunity and Th1 activation responsive to IL-1 blockade. Proc. Natl. Acad. Sci. U.S.A. 108, 7148–7153.

Tanaka, M., Miyatani, N., Yamada, S., Miyashita, K., Toyoshima, I., Sakuma, K., et al., 1993. Hereditary lipo-muscular atrophy with joint contracture, skin eruptions and hyper-gamma-globulinemia, a new syndrome. Intern. Med. 32, 42–45.

The French FMF Consortium, 1997. A candidate gene for familial Mediterranean fever. Nat. Genet. 17, 25–31.

The International FMF Consortium, 1997. Ancient missense mutations in a new member of the RoRet gene family are likely to cause familial Mediterranean fever. Cell. 90, 797–807.

Ting, J.P., Lovering, R.C., Alnemri, E.S., Bertin, J., Boss, J.M., Davis, B.K., et al., 2008. The NLR gene family, a standard nomenclature. Immunity. 28, 285–287.

Todd, I., Radford, P.M., Daffa, N., Bainbridge, S.E., Powell, R.J., Tighe, P.J., 2007. Mutant tumor necrosis factor receptor associated with tumor necrosis factor receptor-associated periodic syndrome is altered antigenically and is retained within patients' leukocytes. Arthritis Rheum. 56, 2765–2773.

Todd, I., Radford, P.M., Draper-Morgan, K.A., McIntosh, R., Bainbridge, S., Dickinson, P., et al., 2004. Mutant forms of tumour necrosis factor receptor I that occur in TNF-receptor-associated periodic syndrome retain signalling functions but show abnormal behaviour. Immunology. 113 (1), 65–79.

Tokunaga, F., Sakata, S., Saeki, Y., Satomi, Y., Kirisako, T., Kamei, K., et al., 2009. Involvement of linear polyubiquitylation of NEMO in NF-kappaB activation. Nat. Cell Biol. 11, 123–132.

Torrelo, A., Patel, S., Colmenero, I., Gurbindo, D., Lendínez, F., Hernández, A., et al., 2010. Chronic atypical neutrophilic dermatosis with lipodystrophy and elevated temperature (CANDLE) syndrome. J. Am. Acad. Dermatol. 62, 489–495.

Touitou, I., 2013. Inheritance of autoinflammatory diseases, shifting paradigms and nomenclature. J. Med. Genet. 50, 349–359.

Usui, F., Shirasuna, K., Kimura, H., Tatsumi, K., Kawashima, A., Karasawa, T., et al., 2012. Critical role of caspase-1 in vascular inflammation and development of atherosclerosis in Western diet-fed apolipoprotein E-deficient mice. Biochem. Biophys. Res. Commun. 425, 162–168.

van der Meer, Vossen, J.M., Radl, J., van Nieuwkoop, J.A., Meyer, C.J., Lobatto, S., et al., 1984. Hyperimmunoglobulinaemia D and periodic fever, a new syndrome. Lancet. 1, 1087–1090.

Wajant, H., Pfizenmaier, K., Scheurich, P., 2003. Tumor necrosis factor signaling. Cell Death Differ. 10, 45–65.

Wen, C., Yang, X., Yan, Z., Zhao, M., Yue, X., Cheng, X., et al., 2013. Nalp3 inflammasome is activated and required for vascular smooth muscle cell calcification. Int. J. Cardiol.. 10.1016/j.ijcard.2013.01.211.

Zhang, S.Q., Jiang, T., Li, M., Zhang, X., Ren, Y.Q., Wei, S.C., et al., 2012. Exome sequencing identifies MVK mutations in disseminated superficial actinic porokeratosis. Nat. Genet. 44, 1156–1160.

Zhou, Q., Lee, G.S., Brady, J., Datta, S., Katan, M., Sheikh, A., et al., 2012. A hypermorphic missense mutation in PLCG2, encoding phospholipase Cgamma2, causes a dominantly inherited autoinflammatory disease with immunodeficiency. Am. J. Hum. Genet. 91, 713–720.

Part 2

Immune Cells and Immune Responses

Innate and Adaptive Systems of Immunity

Peter J. Delves

Department of Immunology, Division of Infection and Immunity, University College London, London, UK

Chapter Outline

Introduction	53	Functional Activities of T Cells	60
The Innate and Adaptive Responses	53	B Cell Development and Functions	62
Innate Responses	54	Antibodies	63
Cellular Components	54	Secondary Lymphoid Tissues	64
Soluble Mediators	57	Resolution of the Immune Response	66
Adaptive Immune Responses	58	**References**	66
T Cell Development	59		

INTRODUCTION

The cells of the immune system are derived from self-renewing hematopoietic stem cells (HSCs) which give rise to multipotent progenitors (MPPs) that are no longer able to self renew (Boisset and Robin, 2012). Cytokines and other signals lead to the expression of different patterns of transcription factors (Sarrazin and Sieweke, 2011) which drive the MPPs down particular differentiation pathways, ultimately leading to the generation of lymphocytes, natural killer (NK) cells, dendritic cells (DCs), neutrophils, eosinophils, basophils, mast cells, monocytes, macrophages, megakaryocytes, and erythrocytes.

THE INNATE AND ADAPTIVE RESPONSES

The immune system can mount innate responses that occur to the same extent, however many times the antigen is encountered, and adaptive (acquired) responses that generate immunologic memory leading to quantitatively and qualitatively enhanced responses upon re-encounter with the antigen. Both types of response detect a threat using receptors that recognize molecules associated with pathogens (Table 5.1). Innate responses exhibit broad specificity based upon detection of pathogen-associated molecular patterns (PAMPs) and damage-associated molecular patterns (DAMPs) by pattern recognition receptors (PRRs) (de Wet and Gordon, 2007; Moresco et al.,

2011), and the binding to complement receptors and Fc receptors of opsonized antigens coated with complement or antibody. Only the lymphocytes, the dedicated cells of the adaptive response, bear antigen-specific receptors which permit exquisitely refined recognition of individual antigens. Each lymphocyte possesses approximately 10^5 antigen receptors of identical specificity. While the B cell receptor (BCR) recognizes structures (epitopes) on the surface of native antigen, the epitopes recognized by the T cell receptor (TCR) are short peptides (Figure 5.1). The peptides are produced by proteolytic processing of antigen within cells and are presented to T cells by highly polymorphic major histocompatibility complex (MHC) class I and class II cell surface molecules. The main human class I molecules are HLA-A, B, and C and the class II comprise HLA-DP, DQ, and DR. Thus an individual who is heterozygous at each locus will express 12 variants, although cross-pairing of some class II chains can increase this number. MHC class II, which presents 8–30 amino acid long peptides to the TCR on CD4$^+$ helper T cells, is expressed on DCs, macrophages, B cells, activated human (but not mouse) T cells, thymic epithelial cells, and can be induced on a variety of other cell types. In contrast, MHC class I molecules, which present peptides of 8–9 amino acids in length, are ubiquitously expressed on nearly all nucleated cells in the body and are concerned with alerting CD8$^+$ cytotoxic T lymphocytes (CTL) to the presence of intracellular infection.

N. Rose & I. Mackay (Eds): The Autoimmune Diseases, Fifth edition. DOI: http://dx.doi.org/10.1016/B978-0-12-384929-8.00005-8

TABLE 5.1 Innate and Adaptive (Acquired) Responses Detect a Threat using Receptors that Recognize Molecules Associated with Pathogens

Receptor	PRR	MHC	TCR	Antibody (BCR)
Location	Cell surface, cytoplasmic, secreted	Cell surface	Cell surface	Cell surface, secreted
Recognition	PAMPs and DAMPs	Each MHC variant can bind many different peptide sequences	Highly peptide-MHC specific	Highly antigen specific
Protein diversity in an individual	10 s–100 s	~12 for classical MHC	Millions	Millions
Genes	Each protein individually encoded. Low polymorphism	Each protein individually encoded. Extremely polymorphic	Genetic recombination creates diversity	Genetic recombination creates diversity

The cells of the immune system need to detect a threat and do so using four main groups of receptors. Pattern recognition receptors (PRR) are predominantly employed by cells of the innate response (although they are also present on lymphocytes) and collectively are found on cell surfaces, intracellularly or as secreted molecules. They recognize pathogen-associated molecular patterns (PAMPs) and danger-associated molecular patterns (DAMPs). MHC class I is present on all nucleated cells in the body although MHC class II is highly restricted in its expression. The TCR is restricted to T lymphocytes. The transmembrane version of antibody, the BCR, is only present on the surface of B lymphocytes, but antibody is also present throughout the body both as a soluble molecule and held on the surface of cells by Fc receptors.

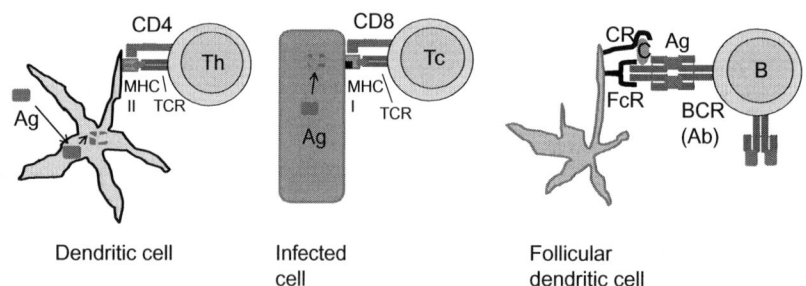

Dendritic cell   Infected cell   Follicular dendritic cell

FIGURE 5.1 **Antigen recognition by lymphocytes.** Dendritic cells take up external (exogenous) antigen (Ag), process it, and then present it on their cell surface in the form of a peptide fragment bound to MHC class II molecules. This peptide–MHC complex is recognized by the T cell receptor (TCR) on CD4⁺ helper T cells (Th). Antigens lurking inside cells (endogenous antigens, e.g., viruses) can be processed within the cell and then presented on the surface of the infected cell in the form of a peptide fragment bound to MHC class I molecules. This peptide–MHC complex is recognized by the TCR on CD8⁺ cytotoxic T cells (Tc). Cross-presentation can also occur whereby exogenous antigens are presented by MHC class I and endogenous antigens by MHC class II. The B cell receptor (BCR) is a transmembrane version of the antibody (Ab) molecule. This directly detects intact antigen, a process which can be assisted by follicular dendritic cells holding complexes of Ab-Ag and complement (C) bound to their surface by Fc receptors (FcR) and complement receptors (CR).

INNATE RESPONSES

Cellular Components

Cells of the innate immune response include neutrophils, eosinophils, monocytes, macrophages, and DCs, all of which to varying degrees can act as phagocytic cells, together with the non-phagocytic basophils, mast cells, and NK cells. All of these cell types are capable of producing inflammatory mediators. Detection of infection or tissue injury can result in the activation of intracellular molecular complexes referred to as inflammasomes (Figure 5.2), leading to the secretion of proinflammatory mediators such as the cytokines interleukin (IL)-1β and

IL-18 (Strowig et al., 2012). The immediate consequence of an encounter with an entity that is deemed to pose a threat is the generation of an acute inflammatory response in which cells and molecules of the immune system are rapidly recruited to the site of the stimulus. Inflammatory mediators and microbial products cause the upregulation of adhesion molecules on vascular endothelium, thereby alerting inflammatory cells to the presence of a local infection (Figure 5.3). Histamine released from mast cells causes smooth muscle contraction and an increase in local vascular permeability, facilitating the passage of neutrophils from the blood to the tissues. Activation of the complement system (Chapter 15) plays a pivotal role in this

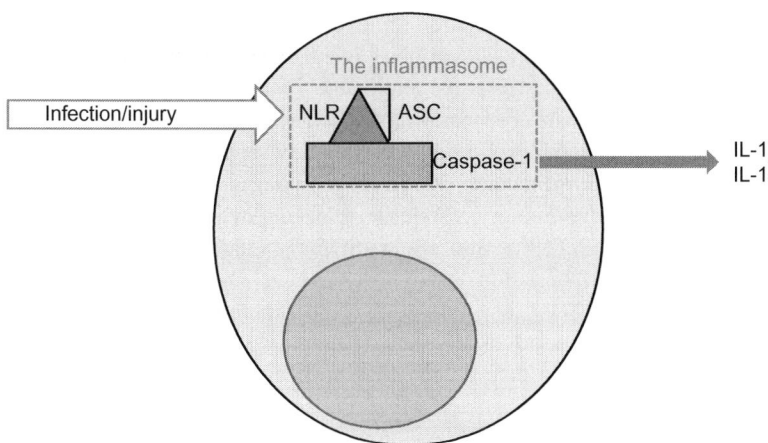

FIGURE 5.2 **The inflammasome.** Inflammasomes comprise multi-protein cytoplasmic complexes that promote inflammation by converting the IL-1β precursor into active IL-1β, and additionally by stimulating the generation of IL-18. The proinflammatory caspase-1, complexed with NOD-like receptors (NLR) such as NLRP3 and with the apoptosis-associated speck-like (ASC) adaptor protein, becomes activated in response to danger signals resulting from infection or tissue damage.

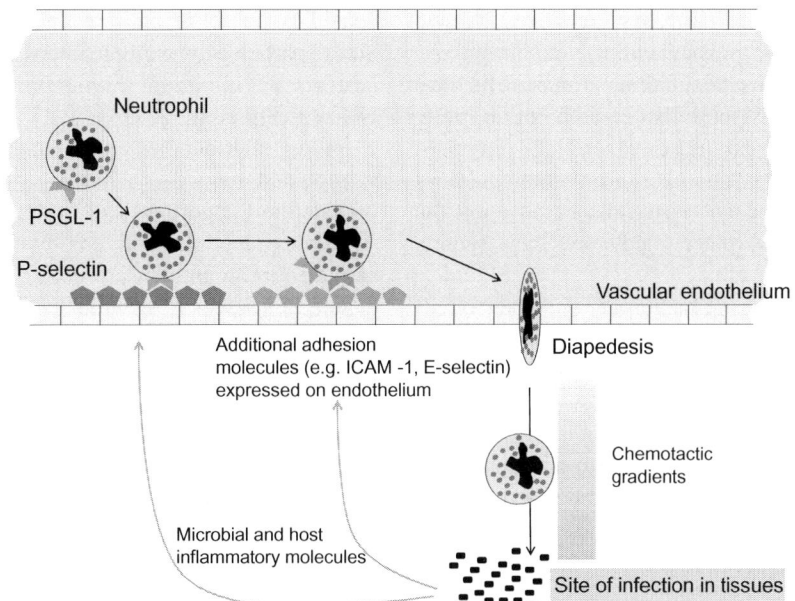

FIGURE 5.3 **Entry of neutrophils into tissue during an inflammatory response.** Microbial products such as lipopolysaccharide (LPS), together with inflammatory mediators such as histamine, thrombin, and the cytokines IL-1β, IL-17 and tumor necrosis factor (TNF)-α, lead to the increased expression of vascular endothelial adhesion molecules. This alerts neutrophils and other inflammatory cells to the presence of an infection in the underlying tissues. P-selectin becomes expressed on the surface of the endothelium and captures neutrophils due to their possession of PSGL-1 (P-selectin glycoprotein ligand-1). Initially the neutrophils are slowed down and roll along the blood vessel wall. Signaling through PSGL-1 causes the neutrophils to activate β_2 integrins. Additional vascular endothelial adhesion molecules become expressed such as ICAM-1, which binds to the β_2 integrins LFA-1 and/or CR3, and E-selectin which binds to ESL-1 (E-selectin ligand-1), PSGP-1 and CD44 on the neutrophils (Zarbock et al., 2011; Muller, 2011). Eventually the neutrophils are brought to a halt and squeezed out of the blood vessels, a process known as diapedesis which is greatly facilitated by the deformable nature of the multi-lobed nucleus in these polymorphonuclear leukocytes.

process, triggering mast cell degranulation and chemotactically attracting the neutrophils (Chapter 14). Chemotactic cytokines (chemokines) help guide the neutrophils to the site of the infection (Sanz and Kubes, 2012). The presence on the neutrophil cell surface of both Fc receptors for antibodies and complement receptors greatly facilitates phagocytosis if the antigen is opsonized

with these agents (Underhill and Ozinsky, 2002). Engulfed microorganisms are killed within the neutrophil by a plethora of toxic molecules including superoxide anions, hydroxyl radicals, hypochlorous acid, nitric oxide, proteases, defensins, and lysozyme. Neutrophil extracellular traps (NETs) prevent microbial spreading and focus released microbicidal substances onto any non-phagocytosed pathogens in the immediate vicinity of the neutrophil (Borregaard, 2010; Remijsen et al., 2011).

Although eosinophils (Chapter 14) are able to phagocytose microorganisms, their role in protection against infection is perhaps more specialized towards the release of granules containing cationic proteins in order to destroy extracellular parasites such as helminths. Eosinophils are also involved in immune regulation, secrete leukotriene C4, platelet-activating factor and an array of cytokines, and can be induced to express MHC class II and thereby act as antigen-presenting cells for T cell activation (Rothenberg and Hogan, 2006; Kita, 2011). Blood basophils and tissue mast cells are not phagocytic and share many features. They become sensitized with IgE antibodies bound to their high affinity Fcε receptors (FcεRI) and, when antigen cross-links the IgE, release preformed inflammatory mediators including histamine, platelet-activating factor, and many different cytokines. Newly synthesized leukotrienes, prostaglandins, and thromboxanes are also released. Two populations of mast cells have been described in humans, those that contain both tryptase and chymase (MC_{TC}) and those which lack chymase (MC_T) (Galli et al., 2011). A number of immunoregulatory roles have been proposed for mast cells based upon the particular cytokines and other mediators they secrete (Galli et al., 2011).

The tissue macrophages (Chapter 11) and their circulating precursors, the blood monocytes, possess both Fc receptors and complement receptors, and contain similar microbicidal substances to neutrophils. However, they live much longer than neutrophils and are able to process antigens for presentation to helper T cells. An additional role of the macrophage is the removal of the body's own dead or dying cells. While tissue damage associated with necrotic cell death triggers inflammation, cells dying due

to apoptosis are removed much more quietly. Loss of membrane symmetry is a feature of apoptotic cell death and exposes the molecule phosphatidylserine on the cell surface, marking the cell for phagocytosis by macrophages expressing phosphatidylserine receptors (Devitt and Marshall, 2011). Macrophages are key players in inflammatory responses, releasing cytokines such as IL-1β and TNFα, and are particularly characteristic of chronic inflammation.

Sets of activating and inhibitory receptors are expressed on NK cells (Chapter 13). They enable the NK cells to detect cells that have either lost or altered their expression of self MHC molecules as a result of infection or oncogenesis. A dominant signal through the activating receptors will lead to the induction of apoptosis in the target cell (Figure 5.4). NK cells can also mediate antibody-dependent cellular cytotoxicity (ADCC) of antibody-coated target cells, and are a rich source of certain cytokines, particularly gamma interferon. This latter activity bestows an important immunoregulatory role upon the NK cell (Shi et al., 2011).

A key interface between innate and adaptive responses is provided by DCs, a heterogeneous population which include the Langerhans cell in the skin. DCs (Chapter 12) sample extracellular antigens by endocytosis and become activated to an antigen-presenting mode when their PRRs (Table 5.1), which include Toll-like receptors (TLRs), NOD-like receptors (NLRs), and various C-type lectin receptors, recognize PAMPs such as LPS, terminal mannose, and microbial CpG motifs (unmethylated cytosine-guanosine dinucleotide sequence flanked by two 5′ purines and two 3′ pyrimidines). Endogenous DAMPs such as uric acid and heat shock proteins can also activate these cells (Ueno et al., 2007). The activated DCs travel to the local draining lymph node where they present antigen

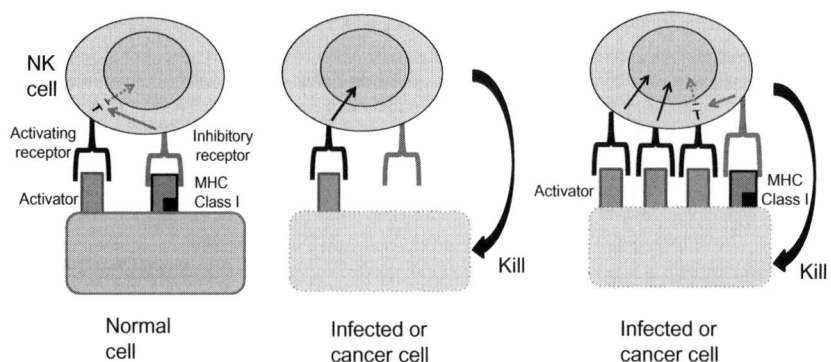

FIGURE 5.4   **Natural killer (NK) cells possess both activating and inhibitory receptors.**   The activating receptors recognize a number of different activator ligands constitutively expressed on many cells in the body (e.g., CD112) or expressed in response to factors such as cell stress (e.g., MICA). Activation of killing is usually blocked by the engagement of inhibitory receptors that recognize the MHC class I molecules normally expressed on all nucleated cells in the body. Cells lacking MHC class I are not able to engage the inhibitory receptors, are therefore deemed abnormal, and are killed by the NK cells. Even in the presence of MHC class I, if sufficient activating signals are received (because infection, cancer, or other types of cell stress has caused the cell to express higher levels of activators), the inhibitory signal is subdominant and the target cell will be killed.

to T cells. During their migration through the afferent lymphatics, they upregulate their cell surface MHC class II molecules and the CD80 (B7.1) and CD86 (B7.2) costimulatory ligands for CD28 on the T cell (Ueno et al., 2007). Such costimulation is required, together with antigen, for T cell activation (Figure 5.5). Within the DC the antigen is processed into short peptides and then expressed on the cell surface together with the MHC class II molecules for presentation to CD4$^+$ helper T cells and regulatory T cells (Tregs). DCs are also able to cross-present exogenous antigens by transferring them into the MHC class I processing and presentation pathway for recognition by CD8$^+$, mostly cytotoxic, T cells (Amigorena and Savina, 2010). Conversely, cytoplasmic antigens can undergo autophagy and be cross-presented to CD4$^+$ (mostly helper) T cells following delivery to the MHC class II presentation pathway (Pierdominici et al., 2012).

DCs can also act to limit immune responses. T cell interactions with DCs lacking the expression of the crucial CD80/CD86 costimulatory molecules induce anergy (functional inactivation) in the T cell. Immunosuppression by DCs can be mediated via their production of the tryptophan-depleting enzyme indoleamine 2,3-dioxygenase (tryptophan being required for T cell proliferation) or by

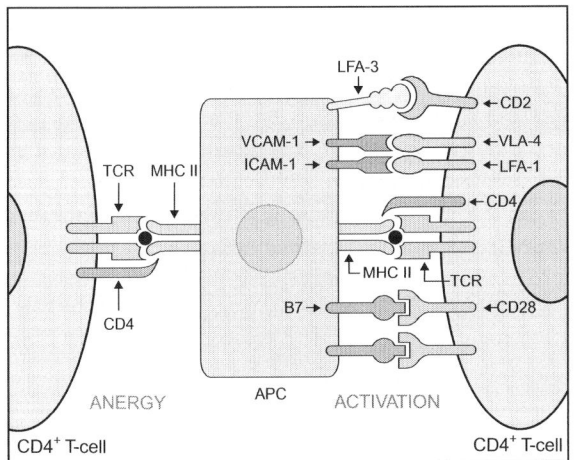

FIGURE 5.5 T cell activation. Interaction of costimulatory molecules leads to activation of resting T lymphocytes by antigen-presenting cells (APC) on engagement of the T cell receptor (TCR) with its cognate antigen–MHC complex. Engagement of the TCR without accompanying costimulatory signals leads to anergy (functional inactivation). Note, a cytotoxic rather than a helper T cell would involve coupling of CD8 to MHC class I. Costimulation is delivered to a resting T cell primarily through engagement of CD28 on the T cell by B7.1 (CD80) or B7.2 (CD86) on the APC. Other molecules involved can include intercellular adhesion molecule-1 (ICAM-1), lymphocyte function-associated molecules-1/3 (LFA-1/3), vascular cell adhesion molecule-1 (VCAM-1), and very late antigen-4 (VLA-4). *Modified from Delves, P.J., Martin, S.J., Burton, D.R., Roitt I.M. 2011. Roitt's Essential Immunology, 12th ed. Wiley-Blackwell.*

the preferential stimulation of Tregs (Maldonado and von Andrian, 2010).

Although B cells are able to recognize antigen without the intervention of any other cell type, recognition is more efficient if multiple copies of the antigen are "presented" to the B cell in the form of immune complexes held on the surface of follicular dendritic cells (FDCs) (Aguzzi and Krautler, 2010). These are an entirely different cell type to the DCs discussed above. Unlike DCs they are not phagocytic, and they lack MHC class II molecules. Furthermore, they appear not to be bone marrow derived, probably arising from fibroblastic reticular cells in the B cell areas of lymphoid tissues. They can present immune complexes to B cells very efficiently by virtue of their FcγRIIB receptors for IgG and CR1 and CR2 receptors for complement.

The role that erythrocytes perform in immune responses should not be overlooked. Their possession of CR1 complement receptors for C3b, C4b, and iC3b confers on these cells an important role in clearing immune complexes from the circulation, rapidly transporting them to the liver and spleen where they are destroyed by Küpffer cells and splenic macrophages (Birmingham, 1995).

Soluble Mediators

The complement system (Chapter 15) is based upon an enzymic amplification cascade which can be triggered using one of three pathways; classical, lectin, and alternative (Ehrnthaller et al., 2011). These all lead to the cleavage of complement component C3 by a C3 convertase which "converts" C3 into C3a and C3b (Figure 5.6). The classical pathway is activated by IgG and IgM antibodies when they bind antigen, thereby creating an array of closely associated immunoglobulin Fc regions to which complement component C1q binds, followed by C1r and C1s. This event initiates a series of enzymic reactions leading to the generation of the classical pathway C3 convertase, $\overline{C4b2a}$. The lectin pathway, which is essentially an antibody-independent variant of the classical pathway, leads to the generation of the same C3 convertase when microbial carbohydrates interact with mannose binding protein (MBP) which then binds to the two MBP-associated serine proteases MASP-1 and MASP-2. The initially quite separate alternative pathway is activated when complement component C3b becomes stabilized by binding to microbial cell walls. The C3b then combines with factor B which is cleaved by factor D, generating a different C3 convertase, $\overline{C3bBb}$. This C3 convertase is further stabilized by properdin. Both proteolysis and thiolester hydrolysis of C3 constitutively generate very low levels of C3b. However, in the alternative pathway, it is only when $\overline{C3bBb}$ is generated that there is substantial splitting of C3

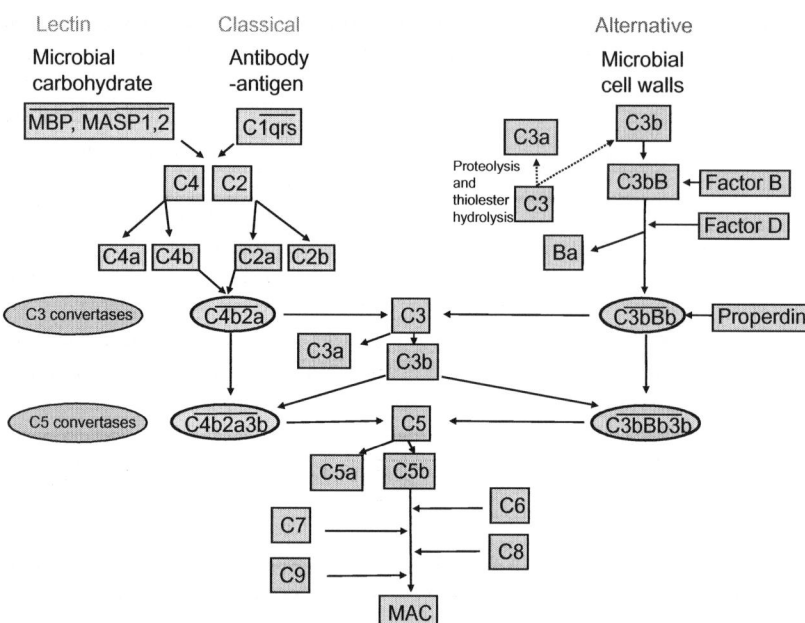

FIGURE 5.6 **The complement system.** For simplicity complement regulatory proteins have been omitted. The classical and lectin pathways (pale blue) are very similar. Like the alternative pathway (pink), these pathways generate C3 and C5 convertases, leading to shared post-C3 events (yellow). For details see text.

into C3a and C3b. Subsequently, a C5 convertase, either C4b2a3b (from the classical and lectin pathways) or C3bBb3b (from the alternative pathway), is produced by addition of C3b to the C3 convertase. This splits C5 into C5a and C5b, ultimately leading to the generation of the membrane attack complex (MAC) composed of complement components C5b, C6, C7, C8, and C9. Because complement activation consists of a series of sequential enzyme reactions, there is a tremendous amplification of the initial response and along the way a number of complement components with potent immunologic activities are generated.

A major function of C3b (and its cleavage products iC3b and C3d) and of C4b is to enhance the engulfment of antigens by phagocytic cells bearing the complement receptors CR1 and CR3. The C3a, C4a, and C5a components act as anaphylatoxins triggering the release of inflammatory mediators from mast cells. C5a is also a potent neutrophil chemoattractant. The MAC generates pores in cell membranes, ultimately leading to the demise of the target cell by apoptosis. Because of these many potent activities, the complement cascades are tightly controlled by a number of complement regulatory proteins including C1 inhibitor (which dissociates the C1qrs complex), factor H and factor I (which cooperate to break down C3b in the alternative pathway), CD46 (membrane cofactor protein) and CD55 (decay accelerating factor) both of which limit the formation and function of the C3 convertases, and CD59 (homologous restriction factor, an inhibitor of MAC formation) (Kim and Song, 2006).

Complement components C3, C9, and factor B are classed as acute phase proteins. This diverse group of mediators, which also include C-reactive protein, serum amyloid A protein, proteinase inhibitors and coagulation proteins, share an ability to undergo a rapid change in plasma concentration in response to infection, inflammation, and tissue injury. Collectively the acute phase proteins facilitate host resistance to infection and promote the resolution of tissue damage (Gabay and Kushner, 1999).

Another group of proteins, which function in both the innate and adaptive response, are the cytokines (Fitzgerald et al., 2001) (Chapter 16). These soluble mediators facilitate communication both within the immune system and between the immune system and other cells of the body. In order to respond to a given cytokine a cell must express the relevant cytokine receptor. One subset of cytokines, the chemokines (Juan and Colobran, 2009), are important in ensuring that immune system cells end up in the correct location as already mentioned in the context of an acute inflammatory response. In addition to acting as communication molecules, some cytokines play a more direct role in immune defense. For example, the interferons produced by virally-infected cells establish a state of viral resistance in surrounding non-infected cells, thereby acting as a "firebreak" against the spread of the infection (Randall and Goodbourn, 2008).

ADAPTIVE IMMUNE RESPONSES

The adaptive responses involve the clonal expansion of antigen-specific B and T lymphocytes. B cells differentiate into plasma cells which secrete the antigen-specific antibodies responsible for the elimination of extracellular antigens. T cells help other cells in the immune response, kill infected cells, or suppress undesirable immune responses.

T Cell Development

T cell precursors migrate from the bone marrow to the thymus, an organ essential for their production. T cell development occurs in the thymus throughout life, despite the fact that it undergoes significant atrophy during aging (Dooley and Liston, 2012). The TCR on T cells comes in two different versions, either a αβ or a γδ heterodimer; each chain of the dimer having one variable domain and one constant domain. Collectively, T lymphocytes are capable of producing vast numbers of different TCR variable regions by recombining variable (V) and joining (J) gene segments from the pools of α and γ TCR genes and V, diversity (D) and J gene segments from the pools of β and δ TCR genes (Ciofani and Zúñiga-Pflücker, 2010). There are a number of different sequences for each segment and one out of each V(D)J set is utilized in the rearrangement event (Figure 5.7). Recombination-activating

genes encode the enzymes RAG-1 and RAG-2 which mediate these processes following the recognition of the recombination signal sequence (RSS) nucleotide motifs flanking the V, D, and J gene segments (Jung et al., 2006). Splicing inaccuracies and the insertion of additional nucleotides around the V(D)J junctions by the enzyme terminal deoxynucleotidyl transferase (TdT) further increase diversity (Benedict et al., 2000).

Recombination, and subsequent expression, of the TCR genes does not occur until the precursor T cells reach the thymus. Developing αβ T cells switch on expression of both CD4 and CD8 cell surface molecules and are therefore referred to as "double positive" T cells. This dual expression permits αβ T cells to potentially interact with both MHC class I and MHC class II molecules. CD4 binds to conserved (nonpolymorphic) residues on the MHC class II molecule, whilst CD8 binds to conserved residues on MHC class I. Positive and negative selection of the αβ T cells then occurs (Starr et al., 2003). At this relatively early stage in their differentiation αβ T cells are programmed to undergo apoptosis (Chapter 17) and are only rescued from this default "death by neglect" if their

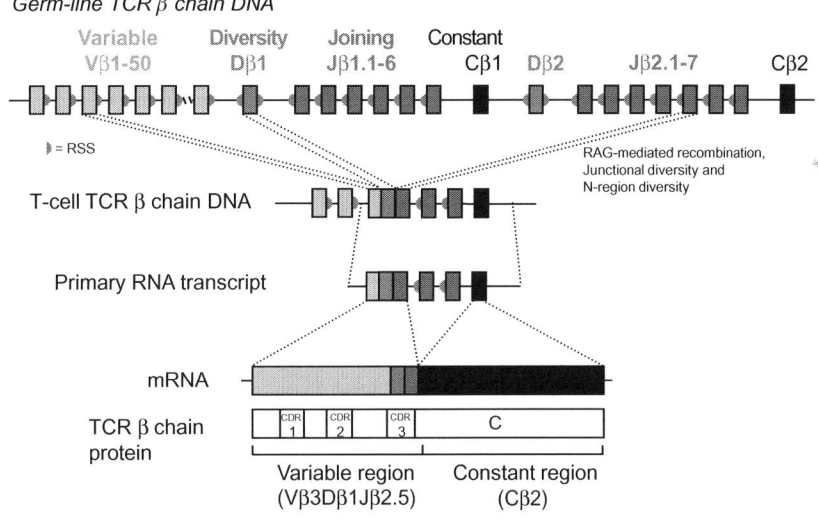

FIGURE 5.7   Diversity of antigen receptors.   As an example, the recombination of the TCR β chain genes is shown. Early in T cell development the recombination-activating genes RAG-1 and RAG-2 are expressed. Random rearrangement of either the diversity (D) β2 gene segment next to any one of the seven joining (J) β2 gene segments, or of the Dβ1 gene segment to any one of the 13 Jβ1 or Jβ2 gene segments, is followed by recombination of any one out of approximately 50 variable (V) gene segments next to the already rearranged DJ segment. The RAG enzymes recognize recombination signal sequences (RSS) found 3′ of each V gene segment, both 5′ and 3′ of each D gene segment, and 5′ of each J gene segment. Different T cells will recombine a different segment out of each pool, thereby creating one level of diversity. Additional heterogeneity is brought about by junctional diversity due to splicing inaccuracies and by the fairly random incorporation of nucleotides (N-region diversity) mediated by the enzyme terminal deoxynucleotidyl transferase (TdT). The primary RNA transcript is processed into messenger RNA (mRNA), with splicing of the rearranged VDJ next to the downstream Cβ constant region gene. This mRNA will encode a TCR β chain which is placed on the surface of the pre-T cell together with an invariant pre-Tα chain. As the pre-T cell undergoes further maturation the TCR α gene segments (for simplicity not shown in the figure) rearrange to produce the TCR α chain. This replaces the pre-Tα chain in order to produce a mature αβ TCR on the cell surface. The complementarity-determining regions CDR1 and CDR2 within the α and β chain variable regions bind to MHC while CDR3 binds to the peptide. Although the detailed organization of the germ-line genes for the TCR α chain, Ig heavy chain, Ig κ light chain and Ig λ light chain are somewhat different to each other, they all consist of pools of V, J, and, for IgH as well as TCR β-chain and TCR δ-chain, D gene segments that undergo recombination to create antigen receptor diversity. The same general principles regarding the rearrangement process therefore apply to the generation of the γδ TCR on γδ T cells and to the BCR on B cells.

TCR is capable of binding to self peptide + self MHC on the thymic epithelial cells (Figure 5.8). Positive selection ensures that the randomly generated αβ TCR is able to interact with self MHC molecules (i.e., those allelic variants of the MHC that are present in the individual). The T cells lose expression of either CD4 or CD8 to become "single positive" CD4 or CD8 cells during positive selection. The majority of the αβ T cells fail at this first hurdle and are therefore eliminated. For the remaining cells apoptosis is induced in any lymphocytes capable of high affinity binding to self peptide + self MHC on DCs, macrophages, and thymic epithelial cells. Negative selection by clonal deletion in the thymus constitutes central tolerance of self-reactive T cells (Chapter 7). Peptides are generated from a number of organ- and tissue-restricted self antigens ectopically expressed in the thymus and peripheral lymph nodes under the transcriptional control of the autoimmune regulator (AIRE) protein (Metzger and Anderson, 2011). Negative selection, like failure to be positively selected, results in extensive T cell death within the thymus. T cells that successfully pass through these hurdles exit the thymus and enter the periphery, a term used to denote any location outside of the primary lymphoid organs (bone marrow and thymus). These mature naive αβ T cells will be capable of recognizing foreign peptides presented by self MHC. Generally, γδ T cells, although also arising in the thymus, do not express either CD4 or CD8 and they recognize antigen directly rather than in the form of peptide−MHC.

Functional Activities of T Cells

The αβ and γδ TCRs are not by themselves able to transmit activation signals into the cell, this function being

assigned to the CD3 molecules (CD3γ, CD3δ, CD3ε) and the CD3-associated ζ chains. Receptor aggregation occurs within lipid rafts which also incorporate a number of adhesion and costimulatory molecules including LFA-1, CD2, CD28, and CD45 to form the immunological synapse (Fooksman et al., 2010). Stimulation through the synapse results in the phosphorylation of tyrosines within immunoreceptor tyrosine-based activation motifs (ITAMs) present on the cytoplasmic tails of the CD3 complex and the ζ chains. A number of protein kinases including Lck, Fyn, and ZAP-70, together with the adaptor proteins SLP-76 and LAT, are involved in initiating the signaling cascade (Smith-Garvin et al., 2009). The CD45 phosphatase also plays a critical role in both T and B cell activation by its ability to act as both a positive and negative regulator of Lck and Fyn (Saunders and Johnson, 2010).

Broadly speaking, CD4$^+$ T cells act as helper or regulatory T lymphocytes, while CD8$^+$ T cells are usually cytotoxic (Chapter 6). However, some CD4$^+$ cells can exhibit cytotoxic activity (van de Berg et al., 2008), while CD8$^+$ cells secrete cytokines that can help in the generation of immune responses, be cytotoxic, or be immunosuppressive (Woodland and Dutton, 2003).

The TCR on CD8$^+$ CTL binds to peptide−MHC class I on target cells. Endogenous antigens, including self antigens and viral proteins, are broken down into peptides by a proteolytic structure known as the immunoproteasome (Krüger and Kloetzel, 2012). If the TCR recognizes the peptide−MHC combination and receives costimulation then the CTL becomes activated to kill the target cell, for example a cell infected with a virus or a tumor cell (Dustin and Long, 2010). It does this by inducing apoptosis in the target via engaging the Fas molecule on the

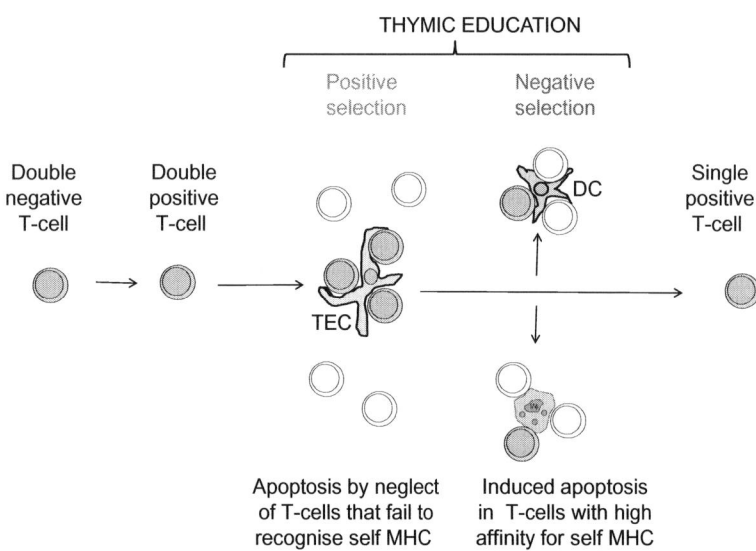

FIGURE 5.8 Positive and negative selection in the thymus. Following a productive recombination of their TCR α-chain and TCR β-chain genes T cells express a cell surface TCR together with both CD4 and CD8 to become double-positive T cells. Positive selection on thymic epithelial cells (TEC) that express both MHC class I and MHC class II will rescue T cells from a default pathway of apoptosis which occurs if these cells are neglected. As long as they have generated a TCR able to recognize self MHC they are saved from neglect. The rescued cells are then protected from apoptosis unless they actively undergo negative selection due to high affinity interaction of their TCR with self MHC or self MHC + self peptides present on DCs and macrophages. The CD4$^+$ CD8$^-$ and CD4$^-$ CD8$^+$ single-positive T cells that exit the thymus therefore possess an αβ TCR with the potential to detect foreign peptides presented by self MHC. *Modified from Delves, P.J., Martin, S.J., Burton, D.R., Roitt I.M. 2011. Roitt's Essential Immunology, 12th ed. Wiley-Blackwell.*

target cell with Fas ligand on the CTL or by using the perforin/granzyme pathway (Figure 5.9).

In contrast to the ubiquitously expressed MHC class I, MHC class II is only present on a few specialized cells, including DCs, macrophages and B cells ("professional antigen-presenting cells"). These cells generate peptides by proteolytic cleavage of engulfed antigens within endosomal vesicles and then present the peptide—MHC class II combination to CD4$^+$ T cells. Helper T cells can be divided into different populations based upon the cytokines they produce. Cells secreting IL-2, interferon-γ (IFNγ) and tumor necrosis factor β (TNFβ, lymphotoxin) but not IL-4 and IL-5 are designated Th1 cells, those secreting IL-4, IL-5, IL-10, and IL-13 but not IL-2 and IFNγ are classified as Th2 cells, and those secreting IL-17 and IL-22 are termed Th17 cells (Mosmann and Sad, 1996; Littman and Rudensky, 2010) (Figure 5.10). In general, cytokine production by Th1 cells facilitates cell-mediated immunity, involving macrophage activation and T cell mediated cytotoxicity, and assists in the production of some humoral responses. Cytokines produced by Th2 cells are mostly involved in humoral immunity, particularly involving IgE and IgA responses, and cytokines from Th17 cells mediate inflammatory and a variety of other

responses (Fitzgerald et al., 2001; Peters et al., 2011). IL-12 from DCs drives T cells towards a Th1 phenotype (Moser and Murphy, 2000) and Th1/Th2 responses tend to become polarized because the IFN-γ from Th1 cells downregulates Th2 activity, whereas IL-4 and IL-10 from Th2 cells downregulates Th1 cells.

A population of CD4 lymphocytes exist which have some properties of NK cells and some properties of T cells. Many of these NKT cells (Chapter 8) express an invariant TCR which recognizes lipid antigen presented by the non-classical MHC molecule CD1d. NKT cells are multifunctional and secrete a range of cytokines (Godfrey and Berzins, 2007; Godfrey et al., 2010).

The antigen specificities and functions of $\gamma\delta$ T cells are less well characterized than that of $\alpha\beta$ T cells (Chapter 6), but some $\gamma\delta$ TCRs recognize molecules that are upregulated in response to cellular infection or stress. $\gamma\delta$ T cells take up residence throughout the body, being particularly prevalent in epithelia including the mucosal tissues. They can function as cytotoxic cells, and mediate both inflammatory and suppressive activity via their ability to secrete a diverse range of cytokines including TNFα, IFNγ, TGFβ, IL-4, IL-5, IL-10, IL-13, and IL-17 (Bonneville et al., 2010).

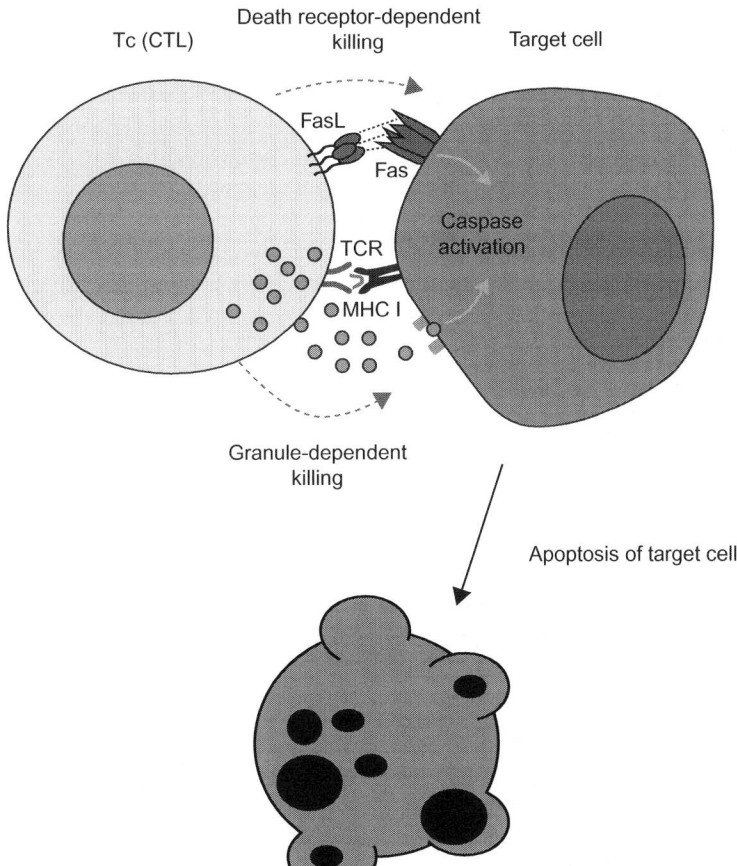

FIGURE 5.9 Cytotoxic T lymphocytes. Cytotoxic T cells (Tc or CTL) can kill target cells by the granule-dependent pathway in which the CTL inserts perforin into the target cell membrane to act as a channel for the passage of granzyme B and other serine proteases into the target cell. They can also kill target cells by engaging Fas on the target using their cell surface Fas ligand (FasL). Both pathways result in the activation of caspases leading to apoptotic cell death in the target cell. *Modified from Delves, P.J., Martin, S.J., Burton, D.R., Roitt I.M. 2011. Roitt's Essential Immunology, 12th ed. Wiley-Blackwell.*

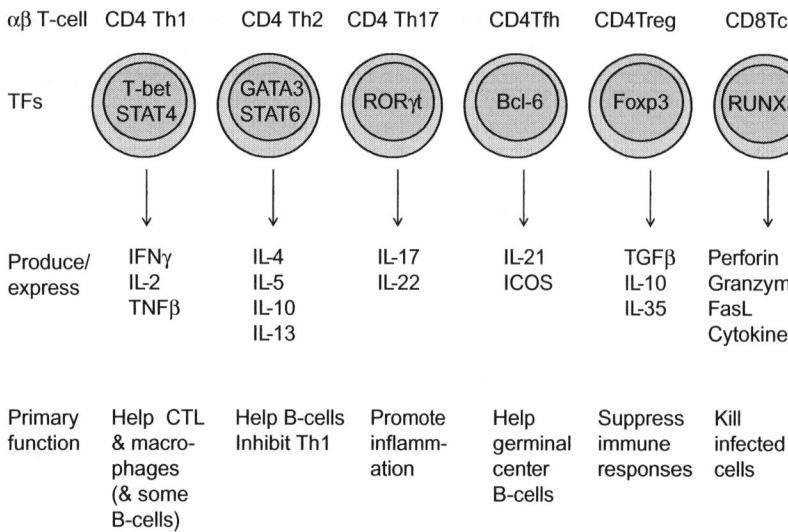

FIGURE 5.10 T cell subpopulations. The major subpopulations of αβ T lymphocytes are shown with key transcription factors, characteristic secreted or cell surface molecules and functional attributes that distinguish them. Note that cytotoxic T cells can also be subdivided on the basis of cytokine production into Tc1, Tc2, etc. Abbreviations: ICOS, inducible T cell costimulator (cell surface molecule); Tc, cytotoxic T cell, TFs, transcription factors; Tfh, follicular helper T cell; Th, helper T cell; Treg, regulatory T cell.

B Cell Development and Functions

A minor population of B cells (Chapter 9), B1 cells, develops early during ontogeny and often expresses the CD5 cell surface molecule (Berland and Wortis, 2002). These cells secrete low to moderate affinity IgM antibodies which can exhibit polyreactivity, i.e., recognize several different antigens, often including common pathogens and autoantigens. Such antibodies are often referred to as natural antibodies because of their existence in the absence of an obvious antigenic stimulus. The majority of B cells, B2 cells, lack CD5 and develop slightly later in ontogeny. Like T cells, these B cells are collectively capable of producing a huge number of different variable regions on their antigen receptors. They achieve this by recombining the immunoglobulin heavy and light chain gene loci in a process analogous to the rearrangement of TCR genes in T cells.

Early in B cell development, pro-B cells mature into pre-B cells, at which stage they express RAG-1 and RAG-2. Random rearrangement of any one of 25 D gene segments next to any one of six J gene segments is followed by rearrangement of any one out of approximately 50 V gene segments next to the already recombined DJ segment. As with the TCR in T cells, additional diversity is brought about by splicing inaccuracies and the action of terminal deoxynucleotidyl transferase (TdT). The heavy chain primary RNA transcript is processed into mRNA, with splicing of the rearranged VDJ next to the Cμ constant region gene. This mRNA will encode a μ heavy chain which is placed on the surface of the pre-B cell together with the surrogate light chain Vpre-B λ5 encoded by two non-recombining genes termed VpreB and λ5. Expression of this pre-BCR on the immature B

cell leads to ligand-independent signaling which drives B cell differentiation towards the mature naïve B cell coexpressing conventional IgM and IgD antibodies on the cell surface (Geier and Schlissel, 2006). As the pre-B cell undergoes maturation the immunoglobulin light chain V (which number about 40 for Vκ and 30 for Vλ) and J (of which there are five for each light chain isotype) gene segments rearrange to produce a κ or λ light chain. This light chain replaces the surrogate light chain in order to produce a mature IgM BCR the cell surface. Expression of RAG-1 and RAG-2 is now switched off. Once the B cells express a mature antigen receptor their survival and further differentiation becomes antigen dependent. The BCR at this stage also comprises IgD antibodies of the same specificity, produced by alternative splicing of the rearranged VDJ to either the Cμ or Cδ constant region genes.

The cell surface immunoglobulin is associated with several molecules including Igα (CD79a), Igβ (CD79b), CD19, CD21 (the CR2 complement receptor), CD81 (TAPA-1), and CD225 (Leu13), which collectively transmit activation signals into the cell when receptor aggregation occurs following cross-linking of the antibody by antigen (Chapter 10). This signaling initially involves phosphorylation of ITAM sequences on Igα and Igβ by the protein tyrosine kinase Lyn with subsequent recruitment of additional kinases including Syk and Btk (Harwood and Batista, 2010). Upon binding to the BCR, the antigen is endocytosed and then processed within acidified endosomes for presentation by MHC class II to CD4$^+$ helper T cells (Clark et al., 2004). In addition to an antigen-presenting role, B cells secrete a variety of cytokines including IL-10, IL-12, IL-13, TNFα, TNFβ (lymphotoxin), transforming growth factor-β (TGFβ), and granulocyte-macrophage colony-stimulating factor (GM-CSF) (Fitzgerald et al., 2001). Following an encounter with the antigen in the presence of costimulatory signals the B cells undergo rounds of proliferation and then differentiate into memory cells or alternatively into plasma cells which produce high levels of soluble antibody. Many plasma cells are short-lived, but others survive for long periods of time, particularly in the bone marrow (Oracki et al., 2010).

Antibodies

The immunoglobulin antibody molecules are composed of two identical heavy polypeptide chains and two identical light polypeptide chains, held together by interchain disulfide bonds. All immunoglobulins are glycoproteins, containing between 2 and 14% carbohydrate depending on the antibody class (Arnold et al., 2007). The N-termini of the light and heavy chains are each folded into a variable domain containing three hypervariable loops, constituting the complementarity determining regions (CDRs) responsible for non-covalent binding to the antigen. Most epitopes recognized by antibodies are discontinuous, comprising amino acids that are only brought together upon protein folding (Muller and Jacoby, 2009). The heavy chain C-terminal domains form the constant region which specifies the class/subclass of antibody. The light chain constant domain determines the κ or λ isotype. The human antibody classes are IgG, IgA, IgM, IgD, and IgE, with four IgG (IgG1−4) and two IgA (IgA1−2) subclasses (Schroeder and Cavacini, 2010) (Table 5.2). Each antibody can be produced either with a hydrophobic transmembrane sequence to anchor the molecule in the B cell membrane where it functions as the BCR or as a secreted molecule lacking the transmembrane sequence.

The basic antibody monomer (biochemically a tetramer) is bivalent with two antigen-binding arms of identical specificity. Secretory IgA at mucosal surfaces is a tetravalent dimer, whereas circulating IgM is most frequently a decavalent pentamer with a minor proportion of hexamers and tetramers. IgA and IgM polymerization is stabilized by a polypeptide J chain (Johansen et al., 2000).

Antibodies that are capable of inhibiting the binding of microorganisms or biological molecules (toxins, hormones, cytokines, and so forth) to their cellular receptors exert their effect independently of other immune system components and are referred to as neutralizing antibodies. Usually, however, antibodies do not function in isolation but are employed to activate the classical complement pathway and/or link antigen to Fc receptor-bearing cells. Antigens opsonized with IgG, IgA, or IgE bind to the appropriate Fc receptors (FcγR, FcαR, or FcϵR) on phagocytic cells (Powell and Hogarth, 2008). Alternatively, both IgG and IgE can mediate ADCC in which NK cells, monocytes, macrophages, and neutrophils bearing Fcγ receptors or macrophages, eosinophils, and platelets bearing Fcϵ receptors are focused onto antibody-coated target cells or parasites (Graziano and Guyre, 2006). The target is destroyed by apoptosis using perforin and granzymes. IgE antibodies are also able to sensitize mast cells and basophils via the high affinity IgE receptor FcϵRI and if cross-linked by antigen will trigger the release of inflammatory mediators.

The epithelial cell poly-Ig receptor transports dimeric secretory IgA produced by plasma cells underlying

TABLE 5.2 The Main Properties and Approximate Serum Concentration of Human Antibodies

Antibody class/subclass	Serum conc. (approx.)	Major features include:
IgM	1.5 mg/ml	Constitutes, together with IgD, the BCR on naïve B-cells. Secreted IgM acts mainly in the circulation and is the first antibody class to be produced in an immune response. Activates complement. Powerful agglutinin
IgG1	9 mg/ml	Most abundant antibody in the blood. Activates complement and enhances phagocytosis. Can cross the placenta
IgG2	3 mg/ml	Activates complement. Poorly transported across placenta
IgG3	1 mg/ml	Activates complement and enhances phagocytosis. Can cross the placenta
IgG4	0.5 mg/ml	Main effector function unclear. Can cross the placenta
IgA1	3 mg/ml	In secretory form protects mucosal surfaces
IgA2	0.5 mg/ml	In secretory form protects mucosal surfaces
IgD	30 μg/ml	Constitutes, together with IgM, the BCR on naïve B cells
IgE	0.05 μg/ml	In presence of antigen triggers release of inflammatory mediators from mast cells and basophils

mucosal surfaces (Johansen and Brandtzaeg, 2004). On the luminal side of the epithelium the IgA is released by proteolytic cleavage of the receptor, leaving a fragment called secretory component still attached to the IgA. Secretory IgA acts to prevent microbial adhesion to the epithelial cell surface (Corthésy, 2010).

Another type of receptor, FcRn, is expressed on vascular endothelium where it is involved throughout life in the recycling of IgG in order to increase the circulating half-life of this class of immunoglobulin. It is also present in the placenta, where it transports IgG from the maternal to the fetal circulation, and on the intestinal epithelium of the neonate where it is involved in the uptake of IgG from maternal milk (Roopenian and Akilesh, 2007).

Secondary Lymphoid Tissues

The primary lymphoid organs, the bone marrow and thymus, are where fully differentiated mature naïve T and B cells are generated. However, activation of lymphocytes occurs in structurally organized B and T cell compartments in the secondary lymphoid tissues; the mucosa-associated lymphoid tissues (MALT), lymph nodes, and spleen. Large numbers of lymphoid cells are also present throughout the lung (Bienenstock and McDermott, 2005) and in the lamina propria of the intestinal wall (Dahan et al., 2007). Because only a handful of lymphocytes will be specific for a given antigen, T and B cells recirculate through the different lymphoid tissues in order to increase the chances of encountering antigen. While responses to blood-borne antigens are usually initiated in the spleen, those to antigens in the tissues are stimulated in the local draining lymph nodes.

Lymphoid follicles within the secondary lymphoid tissues contain germinal centers where B cell activation occurs within a meshwork of FDCs displaying immune complexes on their surface (Figure 5.11). T follicular helper cells are specialized for providing help to germinal center B cells (Vinuesa and Cyster, 2011). Germinal centers are at the heart of the generation of adaptive responses for it is here that B cells proliferate, class switch, undergo affinity maturation, and differentiate into memory cells and into plasma cell precursors (Gatto and Brink, 2010). B cells can increase the binding affinity of their BCR by somatic hypermutation of the V(D)J genes. Higher affinity clones will then be preferentially selected by antigen. Class switching from IgM to IgG, IgA, and IgE involves switch sequences composed of highly repetitive nucleotide motifs present immediately upstream of each constant region gene (except Cδ, IgM and IgD being co-expressed as the BCR on naïve B cells). Both somatic hypermutation and class switching require the expression of activation-induced cytidine deaminase (AID) and the utilization of the nonhomologous DNA end-joining (NHEJ) machinery (Lieber, 2010; Stavnezer, 2011). A process referred to as receptor editing enables self-reactive B cells to replace the variable region gene in the recombined VDJ heavy or VJ light chain sequence with a different variable region gene in order to eliminate auto-reactivity (von Boehmer and Melchers, 2010).

Most pathogens enter the body through mucosal surfaces. The palatine tonsils and adenoids are the sites for the induction of responses to intranasal and inhaled antigens (Brandtzaeg, 2011). Antigens from the gut are taken up by specialized epithelial microfold (M) cells which transport the antigens across the epithelium for access to the Peyer's patches where mucosal responses are initiated (Corr et al., 2008). Activated lymphocytes exit the Peyer's patches via the efferent lymphatics, traffic through the blood, and then home to the lamina propria and other mucosal effector sites (Brandtzaeg, 2009) (Chapter 22). Intraepithelial lymphocytes (IEL) are interspersed between the gut epithelial cells, have a diverse phenotype, and can be either cytotoxic or immunoregulatory (Cheroutre et al., 2011).

Lymphocytes enter lymph nodes, tonsils, and Peyer's patches either via the afferent lymphatics or from the blood via high endothelial venules (HEV). L-selectin is constitutively expressed on lymphocytes and constitutes a ligand for adhesion molecules referred to as peripheral lymph node addressins (Rosen, 2004). If increased expression of LFA-1 (lymphocyte function-associated antigen-1) is induced on the lymphocytes their adhesion to HEV is enhanced and they migrate across the HEV into these lymphoid tissues. Lymphocytes leave the lymph nodes via the efferent lymphatics. Although the spleen lacks HEV, circulating lymphocytes can directly access the marginal zone of this organ from the blood vessels. T cells locate mostly to the periarteriolar lymphoid sheaths, while B cells enter the lymphoid follicles. Lymphocytes exit the spleen via the splenic vein.

When naïve lymphocytes first encounter antigen in the secondary lymphoid tissues they mount a primary immune response, generating both effector and memory cells. The memory cells are responsible for the quantitatively and qualitatively superior secondary immune response that occurs upon any subsequent encounters with the same antigen (Zielinski et al., 2011). Memory cells have a lower activation threshold than naïve cells and the secondary response is more rapid, involves larger numbers of lymphocytes, and, for B cells, produces higher levels of antibody with a superior affinity for antigen.

The term T-independent antigen is used to refer to antigens which are capable of generating an antibody response without a requirement for helper T cells. Polysaccharides, polymerized flagellin, and a number of other antigens have repetitive determinants which can extensively cross-link the BCR and thereby directly activate the B cell (Möller, 2001). Because they do not

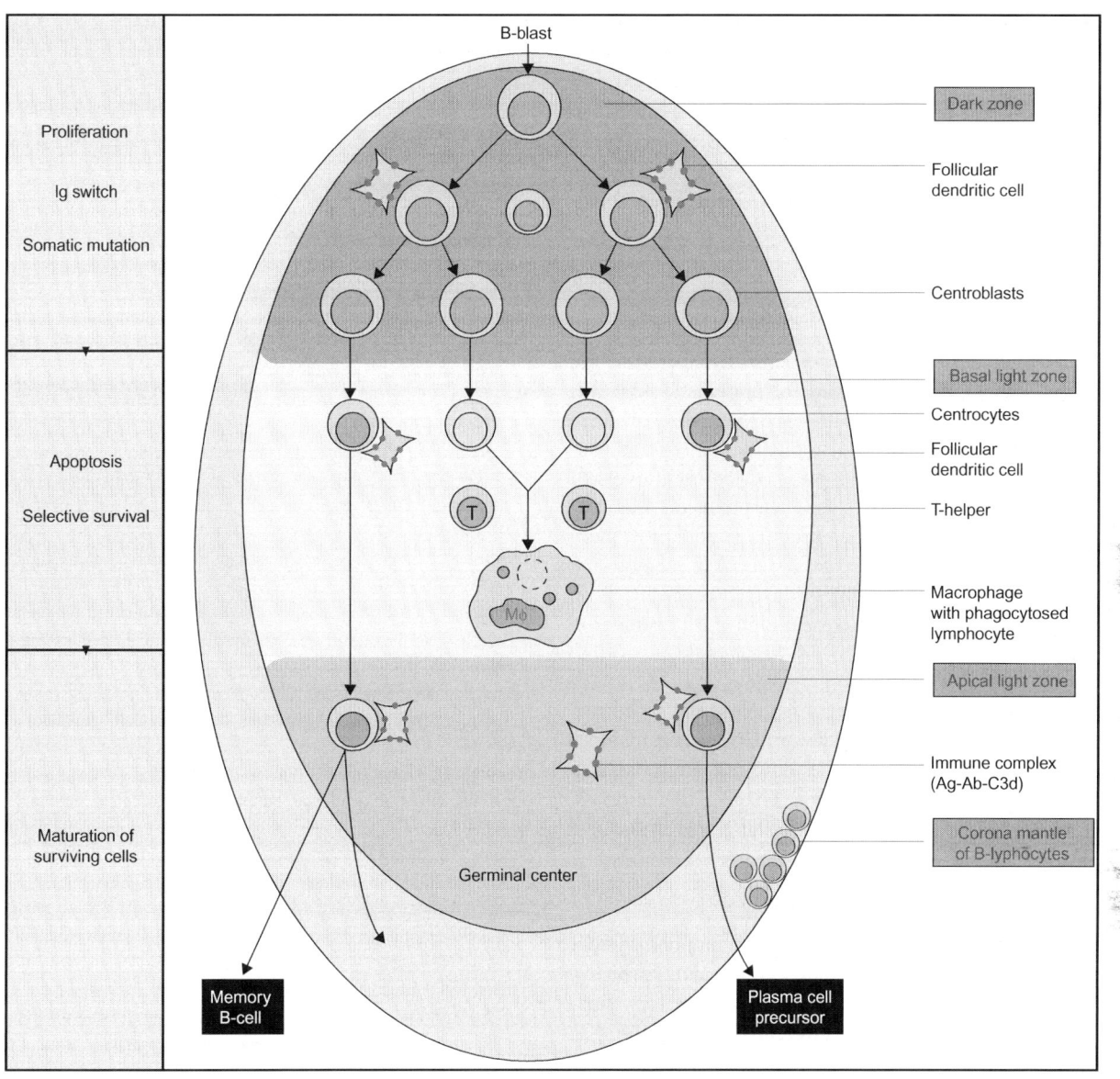

FIGURE 5.11 The germinal center. During the initiation of the acquired immune response, these structures form in the secondary lymphoid tissues in order to generate a microenvironment where all the necessary antigen-specific and innate antigen-presenting cells can interact. Antigen-stimulated B cell proliferation occurs in the dark zone and is accompanied by affinity maturation, due to somatic hypermutation (SHM) of the immunoglobulin V(D)J genes, and class switch recombination (CSR). Both SHM and CSR are associated with the expression of activation-induced cytidine deaminase (AID) in the B cell. Upon passage into the basal light zone, high affinity antigen-specific B cells are positively selected by interaction with antigen, which is present in the form of immune complexes on the surface of follicular dendritic cells. B cells which fail to be positively selected undergo apoptosis and are phagocytosed by macrophages. The positively selected cells migrate to the apical light zone where proliferation continues, and memory cells and plasma cell precursors are generated. *From Delves, P.J., Martin, S.J., Burton, D.R., Roitt I.M. 2011. Roitt's Essential Immunology, 12th ed. Wiley-Blackwell.*

recruit T cells, T-independent antigens fail to provoke the formation of germinal centers and therefore are unable to induce B cell memory, class switching, or significant amounts of affinity maturation. Thus, low affinity IgM antibodies are produced in response to T-independent antigens and, although involving B cells, the response does not go on to exhibit the characteristics of adaptive immunity. The majority of antigens that stimulate B cells are, however, T cell dependent in that the B cell response requires help from T cells. As mentioned earlier, the BCR on the surface of the B cell internalizes bound antigen which is then processed into peptides for presentation by MHC class II molecules. Upon recognition of the peptide—MHC complex by the T cells in the secondary lymphoid tissues, the costimulatory molecule CD154 (CD40 ligand) on the T cell engages CD40 on the B cell, leading to class switching (Ford and Larsen, 2009). In addition to cell surface molecules, cytokines play a key role in the mutual activation of the T and B lymphocytes. T cell help can also be recruited by DCs and macrophages presenting the relevant peptide–MHC class II combination to the helper T cell.

Resolution of the Immune Response

Antigen stimulates the immune response and therefore, for a foreign antigen, its clearance by the immune system will naturally lead to a waning of the response. However, there are additional mechanisms which initially amplify and subsequently downregulate the response. Once high levels of class-switched antigen-specific IgG are produced, the antibody can inactivate the antigen-specific B cells in a manner reminiscent of classical negative feedback loops in the endocrine system. Cross-linking of the BCR to FcγRIIB on B cells by immune complexes results in the transmission of inhibitory signals into the B cell (Smith and Clatworthy, 2010). A number of signals from cytokines and cell surface molecules can also be inhibitory. Ligation of the T cell surface molecule CTLA-4 by CD80 and CD86, and of PD-1 by PD-L1 and PD-L2, provide downregulating signals (Bour-Jordan et al., 2011). Some Foxp3^{+} regulatory T cells secrete IL-10, IL-35 and transforming growth factor β (TGFβ) which can act in an immunosuppressive capacity, while others suppress responses by cell-contact-dependent mechanisms (Josefowicz et al., 2012).

Neuroendocrine interactions with the immune system provide a further level of regulation (Butts and Sternberg, 2008). For example, TLR ligands and inflammatory mediators such as IL-1β result in efferent nerve signaling in the spleen, triggering the release of acetylcholine from splenic T cells which in turn inhibits the release of proinflammatory cytokines from macrophages in order to maintain immune homeostasis and thereby avoid an excessive inflammatory response (Andersson and Tracey, 2012).

REFERENCES

Aguzzi, A., Krautler, N.J., 2010. Characterizing follicular dendritic cells: a progress report. Eur. J. Immunol. 40, 2134–2138.

Amigorena, S., Savina, A., 2010. Intracellular mechanisms of antigen cross presentation in dendritic cells. Curr. Opin. Immunol. 22, 109–117.

Andersson, U., Tracey, K.J., 2012. Reflex principles of immunological homeostasis. Annu. Rev. Immunol. 30, 313–335.

Arnold, J.N., Wormald, M.R., Sim, R.B., Rudd, P.M., Dwek, R.A., 2007. The impact of glycosylation on the biological function and structure of human immunoglobulins. Annu. Rev. Immunol. 25, 21–50.

Benedict, C.L., Gilfillan, S., Thai, T.H., Kearney, J.F., 2000. Terminal deoxynucleotidyl transferase and repertoire development. Immunol. Rev. 175, 150–157.

Berland, R., Wortis, H.H., 2002. Origins and functions of B-1 cells with notes on the role of CD5. Ann. Rev. Immunol. 20, 253–300.

Bienenstock, J., McDermott, M.R., 2005. Bronchus- and nasal-associated lymphoid tissues. Immunol. Rev. 206, 22–31.

Birmingham, D.J., 1995. Erythrocyte complement receptors. Crit. Rev. Immunol. 15, 133–154.

Boisset, J.C., Robin, C., 2012. On the origin of hematopoietic stem cells: progress and controversy. Stem Cell Res. 8, 1–13.

Bonneville, M., O'Brien, R.L., Born, W.K., 2010. Gammadelta T cell effector functions: a blend of innate programming and acquired plasticity. Nat. Rev. Immunol. 10, 467–478.

Borregaard, N., 2010. Neutrophils, from marrow to microbes. Immunity. 33, 657–670.

Bour-Jordan, H., Esensten, J.H., Martinez-Llordella, M., Penaranda, C., Stumpf, M., Bluestone, J.A., 2011. Intrinsic and extrinsic control of peripheral T-cell tolerance by costimulatory molecules of the CD28/B7 family. Immunol. Rev. 241, 180–205.

Brandtzaeg, P., 2009. Mucosal immunity: induction, dissemination, and effector functions. Scand. J. Immunol. 70, 505–515.

Brandtzaeg, P., 2011. Potential of nasopharynx-associated lymphoid tissue for vaccine responses in the airways. Am. J. Respir. Crit. Care Med. 183, 1595–1604.

Butts, C.L., Sternberg, E.M., 2008. Neuroendocrine factors alter host defense by modulating immune function. Cell. Immunol. 252, 7–15.

Cheroutre, H., Lambolez, F., Mucida, D., 2011. The light and dark sides of intestinal intraepithelial lymphocytes. Nat. Rev. Immunol. 11, 445–456.

Ciofani, M., Zúñiga-Pflücker, J.C., 2010. Determining $\gamma\delta$ versus $\alpha\beta$ T cell development. Nat. Rev. Immunol. 10, 657–663.

Clark, M.R., Massenburg, D., Siemasko, K., Hou, P., Zhang, M., 2004. B-cell antigen receptor signaling requirements for targeting antigen to the MHC class II presentation pathway. Curr. Opin. Immunol. 16, 382–387.

Corr, S.C., Gahan, C.C., Hill, C., 2008. M-cells: origin, morphology and role in mucosal immunity and microbial pathogenesis. FEMS Immunol. Med. Microbiol. 52, 2–12.

Corthésy, B., 2010. Role of secretory immunoglobulin A and secretory component in the protection of mucosal surfaces. Future Microbiol. 5, 817–829.

Dahan, S., Roth-Walter, F., Arnaboldi, P., Agarwal, S., Mayer, L., 2007. Epithelia: lymphocyte interactions in the gut. Immunol. Rev. 215, 243–253.

de Wet, B.J.M., Gordon, S., 2007. Pattern Recognition Receptor. Encyclopedia of Life Sciences. 10.1002/9780470015902.a0020175.

Devitt, A., Marshall, L.J., 2011. The innate immune system and the clearance of apoptotic cells. J. Leukoc. Biol. 90, 447–457.

Dooley, J., Liston, A., 2012. Molecular control over thymic involution: from cytokines and microRNA to aging and adipose tissue. Eur. J. Immunol. 42, 1073–1079.

Dustin, M.L., Long, E.O., 2010. Cytotoxic immunological synapses. Immunol. Rev. 235, 24–34.

Ehrnthaller, C., Ignatius, A., Gebhard, F., Huber-Lang, M., 2011. New insights of an old defense system: structure, function, and clinical relevance of the complement system. Mol. Med. 17, 317–329.

Fitzgerald, K.A., O'Neill, L.A.J., Gearing, A.J.H., Callard, R.E., 2001. The Cytokine Factsbook. 2nd ed. Academic Press, London.

Fooksman, D.R., Vardhana, S., Vasiliver-Shamis, G., Liese, J., Blair, D.A., Waite, J., et al., 2010. Functional anatomy of T cell activation and synapse formation. Annu. Rev. Immunol. 28, 79—105.

Ford, M.L., Larsen, C.P., 2009. Translating costimulation blockade to the clinic: lessons learned from three pathways. Immunol. Rev. 229, 294—306.

Gabay, C., Kushner, I., 1999. Acute-phase proteins and other systemic responses to inflammation. New Eng. J. Med. 340, 448—454.

Galli, S.J., Borregaard, N., Wynn, T.A., 2011. Phenotypic and functional plasticity of cells of innate immunity: macrophages, mast cells and neutrophils. Nat. Immunol. 12, 1035—1044.

Gatto, D., Brink, R., 2010. The germinal center reaction. J. Allergy Clin. Immunol. 126, 898—907.

Geier, J.K., Schlissel, M.S., 2006. Pre-BCR signals and the control of Ig gene rearrangements. Semin. Immunol. 18, 31—39.

Godfrey, D.I., Berzins, S.P., 2007. Control points in NKT-cell development. Nat. Rev. Immunol. 7, 505—518.

Godfrey, D.I., Stankovic, S., Baxter, A.G., 2010. Raising the NKT cell family. Nat. Immunol. 11, 197—206.

Graziano, R.F., Guyre, P.M., 2006. Antibody-dependent cell-mediated cytotoxicity (ADCC). eLS. John Wiley & Sons Ltd, Chichester. Available from: http://dx.doi.org/10.1038/npg.els.0000498, <http://www.els.net>.

Harwood, N.E., Batista, F.D., 2010. Early events in B cell activation. Annu. Rev. Immunol. 28, 185—210.

Johansen, F.E., Braathen, R., Brandtzaeg, P., 2000. Role of J chain in secretory immunoglobulin formation. Scand. J. Immunol. 52, 240—248.

Johansen, F.E., Brandtzaeg, P., 2004. Transcriptional regulation of the mucosal IgA system. Trends Immunol. 25, 150—157.

Josefowicz, S.Z., Lu, L.F., Rudensky, A.Y., 2012. Regulatory T cells: mechanisms of differentiation and function. Annu. Rev. Immunol. 30, 531—564.

Juan, M., Colobran, R., 2009. Chemokines and chemokine receptors. eLS. John Wiley & Sons Ltd, Chichester. Available from: http://dx.doi.org/10.1002/9780470015902.a0000933.pub2, <http://www.els.net>.

Jung, D., Giallourakis, C., Mostoslavsky, R., Alt, F.W., 2006. Mechanism and control of V(D)J recombination at the immunoglobulin heavy chain locus. Annu. Rev. Immunol. 24, 541—570.

Kim, D.D., Song, W.C., 2006. Membrane complement regulatory proteins. Clin. Immunol. 118, 127—136.

Kita, H., 2011. Eosinophils: multifaceted biological properties and roles in health and disease. Immunol. Rev. 242, 161—177.

Krüger, E., Kloetzel, P.M., 2012. Immunoproteasomes at the interface of innate and adaptive immune responses: two faces of one enzyme. Curr. Opin. Immunol. 24, 77—83.

Lieber, M.R., 2010. The mechanism of double-strand DNA break repair by the nonhomologous DNA end-joining pathway. Annu. Rev. Biochem. 79, 181—211.

Littman, D.R., Rudensky, A.Y., 2010. Th17 and regulatory T cells in mediating and restraining inflammation. Cell. 140, 845—858.

Maldonado, R.A, von Andrian, U.H., 2010. How tolerogenic dendritic cells induce regulatory T cells. Adv. Immunol. 108, 111—165.

Metzger, T.C., Anderson, M.S., 2011. Control of central and peripheral tolerance by Aire. Immunol. Rev. 241, 89—103.

Möller, G., 2001. Antigens: thymus independent. eLS. John Wiley & Sons Ltd, Chichester. Available from: http://dx.doi.org/10.1038/npg.els.0000504, <http://www.els.net>.

Moresco, E.M., LaVine, D., Beutler, B., 2011. Toll-like receptors. Curr. Biol. 21, R488—493.

Moser, M., Murphy, K.M., 2000. Dendritic cell regulation of TH1—TH2 development. Nat. Immunol. 1, 199—205.

Mosmann, T.R., Sad, S., 1996. The expanding universe of T-cell subsets: Th1, Th2 and more. Immunol. Today. 17, 138—146.

Muller, C.P., Jacoby, M., 2009. Epitopes. eLS. John Wiley & Sons Ltd, Chichester. Available from: http://dx.doi.org/10.1002/9780470015902.a0000514.pub2, <http://www.els.net>.

Muller, W.A., 2011. Mechanisms of leukocyte transendothelial migration. Annu. Rev. Pathol. 6, 323—344.

Oracki, S.A., Walker, J.A., Hibbs, M.L., Corcoran, L.M., Tarlinton, D.M., 2010. Plasma cell development and survival. Immunol. Rev. 237, 140—159.

Peters, A., Lee, Y., Kuchroo, V.K., 2011. The many faces of Th17 cells. Curr. Opin. Immunol. 23, 702—706.

Pierdominici, M., Vomero, M., Barbati, C., Colasanti, T., Maselli, A., Vacirca, D., et al., 2012. Role of autophagy in immunity and autoimmunity, with a special focus on systemic lupus erythematosus. FASEB J. 26, 1400—1412.

Powell, M.S., Hogarth, P.M., 2008. Fc receptors. Adv. Exp. Med. Biol. 64, 22—34.

Randall, R.E., Goodbourn, S., 2008. Interferons and viruses: an interplay between induction, signalling, antiviral responses and virus countermeasures. J. Gen. Virol. 89, 1—47.

Remijsen, Q., Kuijpers, T.W., Wirawan, E., Lippens, S., Vandenabeele, P., Vanden Berghe, T., 2011. Dying for a cause: NETosis, mechanisms behind an antimicrobial cell death modality. Cell Death Differ. 18, 581—588.

Roopenian, D.C., Akilesh, S., 2007. FcRn: the neonatal Fc receptor comes of age. Nat. Rev. Immunol. 7, 715—725.

Rosen, S.D., 2004. Ligands for L-selectin: homing, inflammation, and beyond. Annu. Rev. Immunol. 22, 129—156.

Rothenberg, M.E., Hogan, S.P., 2006. The eosinophil. Ann. Rev. Immunol. 24, 147—174.

Sanz, M.J., Kubes, P., 2012. Neutrophil-active chemokines in in vivo imaging of neutrophil trafficking. Eur. J. Immunol. 42, 278—283.

Sarrazin, S, Sieweke, M., 2011. Integration of cytokine and transcription factor signals in hematopoietic stem cell commitment. Semin. Immunol. 23, 326—334.

Saunders, A.E., Johnson, P., 2010. Modulation of immune cell signalling by the leukocyte common tyrosine phosphatase, CD45. Cell Signal. 22, 339—348.

Schroeder Jr., H.W., Cavacini, L., 2010. Structure and function of immunoglobulins. J. Allergy Clin. Immunol. 125, S41—52.

Shi, F.D., Ljunggren, H-G., La Cava, A., Van Kaer, L., 2011. Organ-specific features of natural killer cells. Nature Rev. Immunol. 11, 658—671.

Smith, K.G., Clatworthy, M.R., 2010. FcgRIIB in autoimmunity and infection: evolutionary and therapeutic implications. Nat. Rev. Immunol. 10, 328—343.

Smith-Garvin, J.E., Koretzky, G.A., Jordan, M.S., 2009. T cell activation. Annu. Rev. Immunol. 27, 591—619.

Starr, T.K., Jameson, S.C., Hogquist, K.A., 2003. Positive and negative selection of T cells. Ann. Rev. Immunol. 21, 139—176.

Stavnezer, J., 2011. Complex regulation and function of activation-induced cytidine deaminase. Trends Immunol. 32, 194–201.

Strowig, T., Henao-Mejia, J., Elinav, E., Flavell, R., 2012. Inflammasomes in health and disease. Nature. 481, 278–286.

Ueno, H., Klechevsky, E., Morita, R., Aspord, C., Cao, T., Matsui, T., et al., 2007. Dendritic cell subsets in health and disease. Immunol. Rev. 219, 118–142.

Underhill, D.M., Ozinsky, A., 2002. Phagocytosis of microbes: complexity in action. Ann. Rev. Immunol. 20, 825–852.

van de Berg, P.J., van Leeuwen, E.M., ten Berge, I.J., van Lier, R., 2008. Cytotoxic human CD4 + T cells. Curr. Opin. Immunol. 20, 339–343.

Vinuesa, C.G., Cyster, J.G., 2011. How T cells earn the follicular rite of passage. Immunity. 35, 671–680.

von Boehmer, H., Melchers, F., 2010. Checkpoints in lymphocyte development and autoimmune disease. Nat. Immunol. 11, 14–20.

Woodland, D.L., Dutton, R.W., 2003. Heterogeneity of CD4+ and CD8+ T cells. Curr. Opin. Immunol. 15, 336–342.

Zarbock, A., Ley, K., McEver, R.P., Hidalgo, A., 2011. Leukocyte ligands for endothelial selectins: specialized glycoconjugates that mediate rolling and signaling under flow. Blood. 118, 6743–6751.

Zielinski, C.E., Corti, D., Mele, F., Pinto, D., Lanzavecchia, A., Sallusto, F., 2011. Dissecting the human immunologic memory for pathogens. Immunol. Rev. 240, 40–51.

Chapter 6

T Cells and their Subsets in Autoimmunity

Patrick R. Burkett[1,2], Youjin Lee[1], Anneli Peters[1], and Vijay K. Kuchroo[1]

[1]Center for Neurologic Diseases, Brigham and Women's Hospital, Harvard Medical School, Boston, MA, USA

[2]Pulmonary and Critical Care Division, Department of Medicine, Brigham and Women's Hospital, Boston, MA, USA

Chapter Outline

Introduction   69
TH1 Cells   70
TH17 Cells   71
  Discovery and Differentiation   71
  Function   72
  Reciprocal Relationship with Tregs   72
  The Role of IL-23 in the Generation of Th17 Cells   73
  Th17 Pathogenicity and Plasticity   73
Th17 Regulation in the Intestine   74
Regulatory CD4[+] T Cells   74
Tr1 Cells   76
TFH Cells   77
Th2 Cells   78
Th9 Cells   78
Concluding Remarks   78
References   79

INTRODUCTION

The immune system has evolved to defend against a wide array of pathogens, and optimal immune function requires coordinated responses from both the innate and adaptive systems. While the innate immune system utilizes a relatively small number of invariant receptors specific for conserved microbial products, such as the cell wall components of bacteria, the adaptive immune system makes use of a nearly unlimited repertoire of receptors generated by random recombination of the T and B cell receptor loci. Although random recombination allows for incredible lymphocyte receptor diversity, it comes at the price of generating potentially autoreactive receptors. The risk for self-reactivity is in part mitigated by checkpoints during lymphocyte development that eliminate most self-reactive clones (referred to as central tolerance) as well as mechanisms that limit the ability of self-reactive clones to mount responses in the periphery (referred to as peripheral tolerance). However, the existence of lymphocyte-dependent autoimmune disease is a clear indication that these mechanisms are imperfect and some self-reactive lymphocytes are able to initiate destructive autoimmune inflammation.

Self-reactive CD4[+] T helper cells (Th) play a crucial role in the pathogenesis of many human autoimmune diseases. This is in part due to the unique ability of Th cells to undergo further differentiation into distinct subsets that are specialized at recruiting and coordinating different immune effector mechanisms, largely via the secretion of particular sets of cytokines and chemokines (Figure 6.1). The differentiation of naïve Th cells into distinct subsets is dependent both upon recognition of cognate antigen–major histocompatibility complexes (MHC) as well as environmental cues, particularly cytokines, that drive different transcriptional modules. Although multiple factors are important for Th differentiation, in many cases a single transcription factor is crucial for initiating and stabilizing expression of the transcriptional module that defines a given Th subset (Figure 6.1). Additionally, there is a complicated interplay between the different Th subsets, as factors that are produced by one subset may inhibit the differentiation of another. Thus, understanding the factors that drive differentiation of Th subsets and the

N. Rose & I. Mackay (Eds): The Autoimmune Diseases, Fifth edition. DOI: http://dx.doi.org/10.1016/B978-0-12-384929-8.00006-X

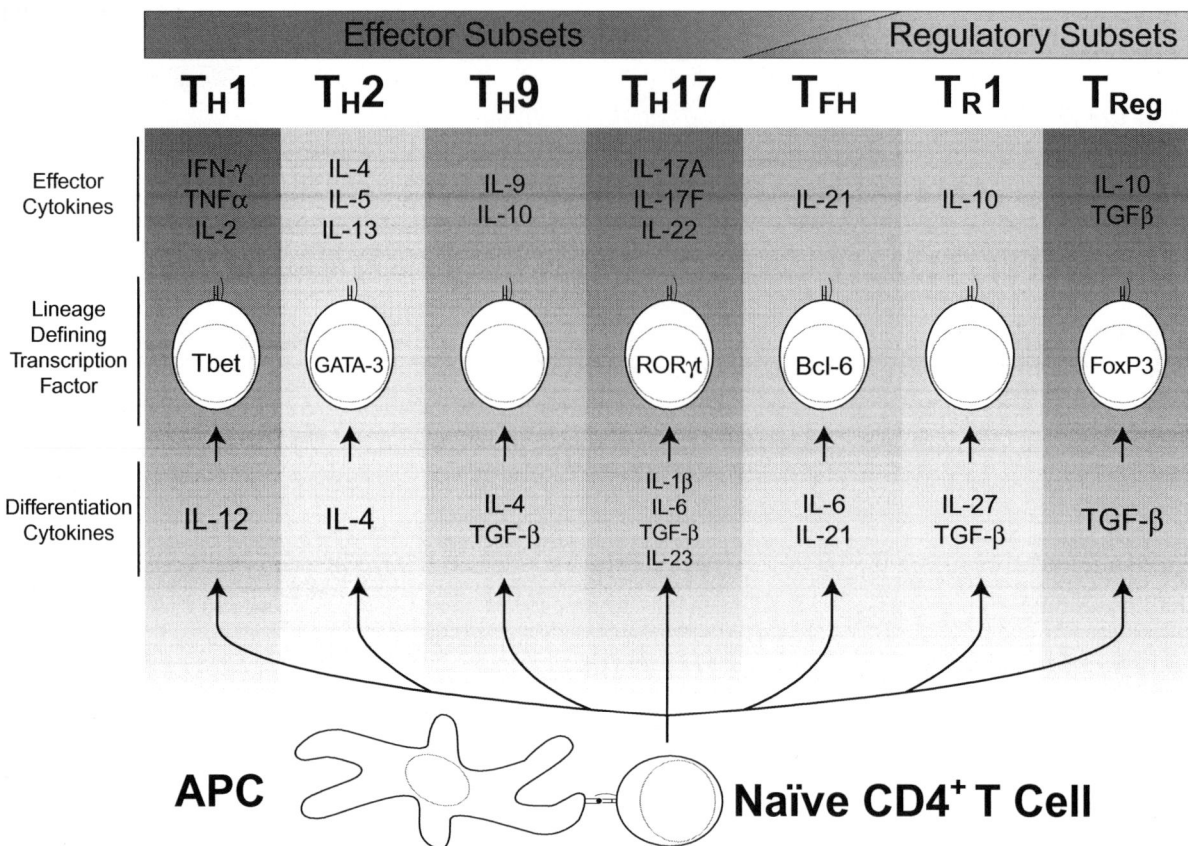

FIGURE 6.1   Generation and function of Th subsets.   Naïve CD4$^+$ T cells are capable of differentiating into various effector and regulatory subsets. Th subsets are shown, along with the cytokines critical for differentiation, lineage-defining transcription factors, and effector cytokines.

effector mechanisms those Th subsets utilize to promote or inhibit tissue inflammation is important for understanding the pathophysiology of autoimmune disease.

TH1 CELLS

Approximately 20 years ago, Tim Mosmann and Robert Coffman (1986) published a seminal paper describing the heterogeneity of the effector CD4$^+$ T cells that can be divided into two distinct subsets, Th1 and Th2 cells, so named because they were the first two to be described. Th1 cells play a critical role in inducing protective immune responses to extracellular pathogens such as *Mycobacterium tuberculosis* or intracellular pathogens like *Listeria monocytogenes* (Mosmann and Coffman, 1989a, b; Geginat et al., 1998; Neighbors et al., 2001; Viegas et al., 2007; Wan and Flavell, 2009). In response to certain microbial stimuli, dendritic cells and macrophages produce cytokines, including interleukin (IL)-12, IL-18, and type 1 interferons, that promote Th1 development by inducing expression of the transcription factor T-bet, the key transcriptional regulator of Th1 cells(Nakanishi et al., 2001; Szabo et al., 2003;

Wan and Flavell, 2009). While multiple cytokines are important for Th1 differentiation, IL-12 is particularly crucial. Thus, mice deficient for either IL-12 or the IL-12 receptor (IL-12R) chains have impaired Th1 differentiation and are extremely susceptible to intracellular pathogens (Mosmann and Coffman, 1989a, b). Upon binding to its receptor, IL-12 promotes Th1 lineage commitment by activating STAT4, which then enhances production of interferon (IFN)-γ, the hallmark cytokine of Th1 cells (Mucida and Cheroutre, 2010; Oh and Ghosh, 2013; Yamane and Paul, 2013). IFN-γ feeds back in an autocrine manner via activation of STAT1 to enhance T-bet expression thus further promoting Th1 polarization. T-bet then promotes further IFN-γ production by inducing chromatin remodeling of the IFN-γ locus (Szabo et al., 2003; Mucida and Cheroutre, 2010; Oh and Ghosh, 2013; Yamane and Paul, 2013). Finally, IFN-γ also inhibits the differentiation of naïve CD4$^+$ T cells into other subsets, such as Th2 or Th17 cells (Schoenborn and Wilson, 2007). Thus, Th1 differentiation can be viewed as a feed forward loop, in which IFN-γ is first induced and then stabilizes lineage commitment.

The role of Th1 cells in inflammation and autoimmune pathology has been extensively studied and Th1 cells have been shown to play an important role in many organ-specific autoimmune diseases, including type 1 diabetes, multiple sclerosis (MS), inflammatory bowel disease (IBD), and rheumatoid arthritis (RA) (Szabo et al., 2003). Prior to the discovery of Th17 cells, an imbalance between Th1/Th2 subsets was proposed to be a key driver of autoimmunity, with skewing towards a Th2 phenotype being considered protective while Th1 predominance was felt to be pathogenic (Adorini et al., 1996a, b). For instance, animal studies revealed that transgenic expression of IL-4 on the pancreatic islets protected non-obese diabetic (NOD) mice from developing insulin-dependent diabetes mellitus (IDDM), while adoptive transfer of Th1 cell clones promoted diabetes (Katz et al., 1995; Mueller et al., 1996). IFN-γ producing Th cells were often found within the target tissue in multiple other organ-specific human autoimmune diseases, thereby implicating Th1 cells in disease pathogenesis. Subsequent studies in animal models of human diseases have further validated the importance of Th1 cells in causing immunopathology (Kuchroo et al., 1993; Lafaille, 1998; Oppmann et al., 2000; Neurath et al., 2002; Szabo et al., 2003).

In an animal model of MS, experimental autoimmune encephalomyelitis (EAE), Th1 cells have been shown to induce disease and play an important role in propagating epitope spreading, whereby infiltrating Th1 cells in the CNS induce inflammation and demyelination causing the release of new, previously sequestered antigens (Katz-Levy et al., 2000; Yin et al., 2001; Mack et al., 2003). Newly released antigens are then picked up and presented by antigen presenting cells (APCs) to induce activation of additional autoreactive T cells (Mcmahon et al., 2005). It is unknown how myelin-specific T cells are initially activated, particularly as myelin-associated antigens are sequestered within the CNS by the blood−brain barrier. One potential mechanism is that a viral infection may induce the activation of T cells that cross-react with myelin, a mechanism termed molecular mimicry. These cross-reactive T cells then attain a pathogenic effector phenotype, traffic to the target organ, and induce inflammation and tissue destruction, resulting in CNS autoimmunity (Schreiner et al., 2007; Chastain and Miller, 2012). Furthermore, IFN-γ has been shown to enhance effector function of scavenger APCs which may promote molecular mimicry as well as epitope spreading by the auto-reactive T cells and enhance autoimmune pathology (Karni et al., 2006; Smith and Miller, 2006; Schoenborn and Wilson, 2007). However, there is evidence to support that IFN-γ may not be the key cytokine responsible for pathogenic effector functions of Th1 cells in many autoimmune

conditions Matthys et al., 1999; Chu et al., 2000; Trembleau et al., 2003; Zhang et al., 2012).

TH17 CELLS

Discovery and Differentiation

Although Th1 cells were thought to be the main drivers of organ-specific autoimmunity, animals lacking the Th1 signature cytokine IFN-γ or other molecules involved in the Th1 differentiation pathway, including IFN-γR and STAT-1, are not resistant, but more susceptible to multiple autoimmune diseases including experimental autoimmune encephalomyelitis (EAE), experimental autoimmune uveitis (EAU), and collagen-induced arthritis (CIA) (Ferber et al., 1996; Jones et al., 1997; Matthys et al., 1998). Even more surprising, mice deficient for the IL-12 chain p35 were also more susceptible to EAE, whereas loss of the other chain of IL-12, p40, made mice highly resistant to EAE. This conundrum was solved when it was shown that p40 does not only pair with p35 to form IL-12, but can also pair up with another cytokine chain p19 to form a novel cytokine called IL-23 (Oppmann et al., 2000). In a seminal study, Cua and colleagues showed that loss of both p40 and p19 (IL-23) protected animals from EAE, whereas IL-12-p35-deficient animals, which lacked IL-12 and Th1 responses, remained susceptible to EAE (Cua et al., 2003; Langrish et al., 2005). These data provided the foundation for the hypothesis that IL-23 rather than IL-12 is crucial for the development of autoimmunity. It was later revealed that IL-23 is involved in the generation of a unique T cell subset, named Th17 cells, owing to their production of the effector cytokine IL-17.

Although generation of Th17 cells was initially thought to be driven by IL-23, naïve T cells do not express the receptor for IL-23 (IL-23R); rather, Th17 differentiation requires the presence of the cytokines TGF-β and IL-6 (Bettelli et al., 2006; Mangan et al., 2006 Veldhoen et al., 2006). In addition, IL-21 also induces Th17 differentiation, particularly in the absence of IL-6, and promotes self-amplification of Th17 cells in a feed-forward loop (Korn et al., 2007; Nurieva et al., 2007; Zhou et al., 2007). Finally, IL-1β can synergize with IL-6 to induce murine Th17 cell differentiation (Chung et al., 2009), and, in conjunction with TGF-β, IL-6, and IL-21, has also been described as a critical differentiation factor for human Th17 cells (Manel et al., 2008; Yang et al., 2008a).

Upon engagement with their respective receptors both IL-6 and IL-21 induce phosphorylation of STAT3, which is crucial for proper Th17 differentiation (Yang et al., 2007). IL-6 and TGF-β signals ultimately lead to the expression of the Th17 lineage-specific transcription factors RORγt and RORα, which transactivate many Th17 signature genes including IL-17A and IL-17F, IL-23R, and the Th17-specific chemokine receptor CCR6 (Zhou and Littman, 2009; Yang et al., 2008b; Ciofani et al., 2012). In addition, the transcription factors IRF4 and BATF mediate the effects of IL-21 on Th17 differentiation and self-amplification and are required for the induction of RORγt (Huber et al., 2008; Schraml et al., 2009; Brüstle et al., 2007). A recent study demonstrated that BATF and IRF4 cooperatively bind to DNA and regulate chromatin accessibility, allowing subsequent binding of pSTAT3 and RORγt and initiation of the Th17-specific transcriptional program (Ciofani et al., 2012). Another factor that is involved in certain aspects of Th17 cell differentiation and regulation is c-Maf, which both enhances the production of IL-21 in Th17 cells, thereby contributing to the amplification of Th17 cells (Bauquet et al., 2009), and also increases production of IL-10 and represses production of IL-22, thus modulating Th17 effector functions (Rutz et al., 2011). The identification of RORγt as the Th17-lineage-specific transcription factor, together with the observation that transcription factors of other lineages, including T-bet and GATA-3, are dispensable for Th17 cell differentiation, established Th17 cells as an independent lineage (Bettelli et al., 2008). Moreover, recent studies examining transcriptional networks induced during Th17 differentiation have shown that antagonist transcriptional modules promote Th17 differentiation while at the same time suppressing development of other T cell subsets (Ciofani et al., 2012; Yosef et al., 2013).

Function

The Th17 signature cytokines IL-17A and IL-17F can form homo- or heterodimers and are partly redundant in their effector functions. They signal through a receptor complex composed of IL-17RA and IL-17RC, which is expressed on both hematopoietic cells and non-hematopoietic cells. IL-17 receptor signaling induces production of proinflammatory cytokines and chemokines, including IL-6, IL-1, TNF, CXCL1, CCL20, GCP-2, and IL-8, as well as anti-microbial peptides and matrix-metalloproteinases. Thus, Th17 cells promote tissue inflammation and neutrophil recruitment (Bettelli et al., 2008). Th17 cells are important for host defense against a variety of pathogens, most notably bacteria like *Citrobacter*, *Klebsiella pneumoniae*, and *Staphylococcus aureus*, as well as fungi such as *Candida albicans* (Bettelli et al., 2008). In humans, the critical role of IL-17 and Th17 cells in host defense is evident in the susceptibility of patients with genetic defects in the *IL17RA*, *IL17F*, or in the *STAT3* gene to *C. albicans* and *S. aureus* infections (Cypowyj et al., 2012).

Aside from host defense, Th17 cells have been primarily associated with autoimmune tissue inflammation. Thus, elevated levels of IL-17 were detected in several autoimmune diseases including MS (Matusevicius et al., 1999), RA (Aarvak et al., 1999), and psoriasis (Teunissen et al., 1998). In EAE, treatment with IL-17 neutralizing antibodies ameliorated disease (Hofstetter et al., 2005) and IL-17 deficient animals developed attenuated CIA and EAE (Nakae et al., 2003; Ishigame et al., 2009). Furthermore, therapies targeting Th17 cells or Th17 effector cytokines in humans have yielded positive results as ustekinumab, a human anti-p40 antibody, ameliorates both Crohn's disease and psoriasis (Papp et al., 2008; Sandborn et al., 2008), and anti-IL-17A antibodies were shown to be effective in the treatment of psoriasis, RA, and uveitis (Genovese et al., 2010; Hueber et al., 2010; Leonardi et al., 2012). In addition, proof-of-concept studies indicate that anti-IL-17 antibody may also be effective in reducing gadolinium-enhancing lesions in MS patients (Havrdová et al., 168, 28th ECTRIMS congress, Lyon, 2012). These studies established the importance of Th17 cells as a therapeutic target in several human autoimmune diseases.

Reciprocal Relationship with Tregs

Exposure of naïve T cells to TGF-β leads to expression of the transcription factor Foxp3 and differentiation into immunosuppressive regulatory T cells (Tregs). However, in combination with the proinflammatory cytokine IL-6, TGF-β induces RORγt and promotes Th17 differentiation (Bettelli et al., 2006; Veldhoen et al., 2006). The molecular basis for the reciprocal relationship between Tregs and Th17 cells lies in the ability of RORγt/RORα and Foxp3 to physically bind to each other and antagonize each other's function (Zhou et al., 2008; Du et al., 2008). Thus, many factors have been shown to have opposite effects on Tregs and Th17 cells and modulate immune responses by shifting the balance between Tregs and Th17 cells. For example, IL-2 acts as a growth factor for Tregs while inhibiting Th17 cell differentiation, whereas IL-21 amplifies Th17 responses, but inhibits Treg expansion (Laurence et al., 2007; Liu et al., 2011). Similarly, retinoic acid promotes Treg differentiation, but inhibits Th17 cells (Mucida et al., 2007). Another example is the aryl hydrocarbon receptor (AhR), which promotes Th17 differentiation upon engagement with the natural ligand FICZ (Veldhoen et al., 2008a), but upon interaction with TCDD, a synthetic ligand, seems to primarily expand Tregs by enhancing Foxp3 expression (Quintana et al., 2008). Finally, recent studies reported that Hif-1α, a metabolic sensor of hypoxia, enhances Th17 differentiation on a transcriptional level, while simultaneously attenuating Treg development by targeting Foxp3 for proteasomal degradation (Dang et al., 2011; Shi et al., 2011). Importantly, the reciprocal relationship of Th17 cells and Tregs offers attractive opportunities for therapeutic interventions in autoimmunity, as future therapies may be able to simultaneously weaken Th17 and strengthen Treg responses.

The Role of IL-23 in the Generation of Th17 Cells

Although initial *in vitro* and *in vivo* differentiation of naïve T cells into Th17 cells does not require IL-23, generation of pathogenic Th17 responses *in vivo* is impaired in both IL-23 and IL-23R deficient mice (Langrish et al., 2005; Awasthi et al., 2009; McGeachy et al., 2009). Furthermore, several studies have demonstrated genetic linkage of *IL23R* to susceptibility to human autoimmune diseases including psoriasis, ankylosing spondylitis, and Crohn's disease (Duerr et al., 2006; Burton et al., 2007; Cargill et al., 2007; Liu et al., 2008), suggesting that IL-23 is also crucial for autopathogenic T cell responses in humans. Expression of the receptor for IL-23, which is composed of IL-12Rβ1 and the specific chain IL-23R (Parham et al., 2002), is induced by IL-6 and TGF-β during Th17 differentiation and is further upregulated by IL-23 itself (Awasthi et al., 2009). IL-23 induces pSTAT3 and thus enhances IL-17 production and reinforces the Th17 transcriptional program. In addition, IL-23 also induces *de novo* production of the Th17 effector cytokine IL-22 (Liang et al., 2006; Zheng et al., 2007), which promotes epithelial growth and induces expression of acute-phase reactants and β-defensins, thus promoting barrier function (Wolk et al., 2010). Recent data also show that IL-23 drives re-expression of IL-7Rα on Th17 cells (McGeachy et al., 2009), thus rendering Th17 cells responsive to IL-7, which may be important for terminal differentiation and survival/expansion of pathogenic Th17 cells (Liu et al., 2010). In addition to expanding and stabilizing Th17 cells, IL-23 is essential for inducing pathogenic effector functions in Th17 cells (see below). However, to date the signaling network downstream of IL-23R is not completely understood.

Th17 Pathogenicity and Plasticity

Numerous studies indicate that Th17 cells may come in different flavors and vary in terms of gene expression, effector functions and pathogenicity. Thus, adoptive transfer studies in EAE have shown that Th17 cells generated with TGF-β1/IL-6 in the absence of IL-23 are non-pathogenic despite their production of IL-17 (McGeachy et al., 2007; Ghoreschi et al., 2010). In contrast, Th17 cells generated in the presence of TGF-β1/IL-6/IL-23 or IL-1β/IL-6/IL-23 or TGF-β3/IL-6 are capable of inducing severe autoimmune tissue inflammation (McGeachy et al., 2007; Jäger et al., 2009; Ghoreschi et al., 2010; Lee et al., 2012), indicating that abundance of TGF-β1 together with relative lack of IL-23 during differentiation favors the generation of non-pathogenic Th17 cells, while the presence of IL-23 promotes the generation of pathogenic Th17 cells. In addition, other factors like IL-1β fine-tune the effector phenotype of Th17 cells: thus, it was shown recently that IL-1β enhances IL-23R expression via MyD88 and mTOR and thus promotes responsiveness of Th17 cells to IL-23 (Gulen et al., 2012; Chang et al., 2013). At the molecular level, the Th17 effector phenotype is a result of transcription factors that are differentially expressed in pathogenic vs. non-pathogenic Th17 cells. Thus, a recent study has identified pathogenic signature and non-pathogenic signature genes in Th17 cells, which determine the pathogenic properties of Th17 cells (Lee et al., 2012).

A prominent example for a pathogenic signature gene is *Csf2*, which encodes the cytokine GM-CSF. Importantly, GM-CSF has been associated with Th17 pathogenicity during EAE in two independent studies, and IL-23 and IL-1β were shown to drive GM-CSF production in Th17 cells (Codarri et al., 2011; El-Behi et al., 2011). GM-CSF prompts antigen presenting cells to produce proinflammatory cytokines including IL-6 and IL-23, which amplify Th17 responses, and it also attracts a wave of secondary cells, primarily macrophages, which further propagate tissue inflammation (Codarri et al., 2011; El-Behi et al., 2011). In contrast, important examples for non-pathogenic signature genes are *cMaf* and *Il10*. Consistent with the role of IL-23 in promoting pathogenicity, expression of c-Maf and IL-10 is diminished by IL-23 and enhanced by TGF-β1 (McGeachy et al., 2007; Ahern et al., 2010). IL-10 can limit autoimmune tissue inflammation by enabling Tregs to suppress Th17-induced inflammation (Chaudhry et al., 2011) and also by directly inhibiting proliferation of Th17 cells (Huber et al., 2011).

The Th1 transcription factor Tbet, which controls expression of IFN-γ, is also part of the pathogenic signature in Th17 cells. Although Th17 cells do not produce much IFN-γ *in vitro*, IL-17⁺IFN-γ⁺ double producers are commonly seen in target organs of various autoimmune disease models, including the CNS during EAE (Ivanov et al., 2006; Abromson-Leeman et al., 2009) and the colon during colitis (Hue et al., 2006; Kullberg et al., 2006). Whether these cells arise from Th1 or Th17 cells has been much debated; however, fate-mapping experiments now indicate that IL-17⁺IFN-γ⁺ double producers are derived from Th17 cells in an IL-23-dependent fashion (Hirota et al., 2011). Additionally, Th17 cells generated in the absence of IL-23 lose expression of IL-17 relatively easily and switch over/dedifferentiate into IFN-γ producers (Shi et al., 2008; Bending et al., 2009;

Lee et al., 2009 Jäger et al., 2009), while Th17 cells generated in the presence of IL-23 maintain stable IL-17 production, but often co-produce IFN-γ in the target organ (Mangan et al., 2006; Jäger et al., 2009; McGeachy et al., 2009; Liu et al., 2010). The co-production of the Th1 cytokine IFN-γ by Th17 cells emphasizes that Th17 cells are potentially more plastic than other Th subsets. However, whether production of IFN-γ by Th17 cells is beneficial or detrimental for the development of tissue inflammation and autoimmunity remains unclear. Analogous to the variety of Th17 effector phenotypes described in mice, human Th17 cells also show different effector phenotypes depending on the microenvironment. For instance, *C. albicans* infection generated an IL-1β-rich cytokine milieu that prompted Th17 cells to co-produce IL-17 and IFN-γ, whereas *S. aureus* infection primed Th17 cells to produce IL-17 together with IL-10 (Zielinski et al., 2012). Similarly, different microenvironments in different tissues and target organs may cause Th17 cells to have slightly different cytokine profiles and effector functions in the various human autoimmune diseases.

Th17 Regulation in the Intestine

Under non-pathologic conditions, a population of Th17 cells exists in the small intestine, where they protect the organism from infections. Th17 cell differentiation in the intestine is triggered by certain commensal microbiota, especially by segmented filamentous bacteria (Ivanov et al., 2009; Huber et al., 2012), and under steady-state conditions Th17 populations in the intestine are kept in check by Tregs and immunosuppressive cytokines such as IL-10 (Huber et al., 2012). However, if not controlled, Th17 cells in the intestine may induce autoimmune tissue inflammation both directly in the intestine (Huber et al., 2012) as well as in distant organs. Indeed, recent studies demonstrated that Th17 differentiation triggered in the intestine by commensals can promote autoimmune tissue inflammation in the CNS during EAE and in the joints during arthritis (Wu et al., 2010; Berer et al., 2011). These data suggest that environmental factors such as diet can influence Th17 differentiation in the gut either directly or by modulating the composition of microbiota and and thereby increase susceptibility to autoimmune diseases. In support of this hypothesis, two recent studies showed that a high salt diet increases Th17 differentiation in the gut and exacerbates development of autoimmune tissue inflammation during EAE (Kleinewietfeld et al., 2013; Wu et al., 2013). Importantly, the strong connection of Th17 cells with the gut also offers attractive therapeutic opportunities, as it might be possible to manipulate the effector phenotype of Th17 cells and reduce their pathogenicity with enterally targeted

therapeutics. Indeed, a recent study suggested that proinflammatory Th17 cells can be redirected to the gut and tolerized (Esplugues et al., 2011). A similar approach could potentially be beneficial in the therapy for human autoimmune diseases.

REGULATORY CD4$^+$ T CELLS

While Th1 and Th17 CD4$^+$ T cell subsets have been implicated in inducing autoimmune disease, regulatory CD4$^+$ T cells (Tregs) represent a distinct Th cell subset that maintains self-tolerance and controls immune responses. The importance of T cells for controlling autoimmunity was first suggested by neonatal thymectomy experiments carried out by Nishizuka & Sakakura (1969), who found that thymectomy prior to day 7 of life led to the development of multi-organ autoimmune disease. Subsequent adoptive transfer studies found that transfer of purified populations of CD4$^+$ T cells (CD45RB^{hi} or CD5^{lo}) into lymphopenic rodents led to the development of T cell-mediated autoimmunity that could be mitigated by co-transfer of CD45RB^{lo} or CD5^{hi} CD4$^+$ T cells, suggesting the existence of a subset of CD4$^+$ T cells with regulatory properties (Sakaguchi, et al., 1985; Powrie and Mason, 1990). Sakaguchi and colleagues further demonstrated that within the CD5^{hi} CD45RB^{lo} CD4$^+$ T cell population the CD25$^+$ subset was uniquely able to inhibit the development of organ-specific autoimmunity, whereas depletion of CD25$^+$ cells was sufficient to cause multi-organ autoimmune disease (Sakaguchi et al., 1995). Subsequently, it was demonstrated that CD4$^+$CD25$^+$ T cells express Foxp3, the lineage defining transcription factor for Tregs (Hori et al., 2003), and spontaneous mutations in Foxp3 lead to the development of severe, multi-organ autoimmunity in both mice (*scurfy*) and humans (immunodysregulation polyendocrinopathy enteropathy X-linked syndrome) (Bennett et al., 2001; Wildin et al., 2001; Khattri et al., 2003). Thus, Foxp3-expressing CD4$^+$CD25$^+$ Treg cells are critical for maintaining peripheral self-tolerance in both mice and humans.

The number of genes directly regulated by Foxp3 is relatively small and does not encompass the majority of the genes that regulate Treg development, suggesting that other factors are equally critical to maintaining the Treg transcriptional program (Hill et al., 2007). Additionally, naïve human Th cells can upregulate Foxp3 upon activation without acquiring regulatory function (Gavin et al., 2006). Fate-mapping experiments in mice have also demonstrated a population of "ex-Tregs" that once expressed Foxp3, but no longer do so and readily produce effector cytokines such as IFN-γ and IL-17 (Zhou et al., 2009). Intriguingly, adoptive transfer of such "ex-Tregs" leads to rapid development of autoimmune disease, consistent with loss of regulatory and acquisition of effector function. Thus, while expression of Foxp3 is a defining characteristic of Tregs, Foxp3 expression alone is not sufficient for stable regulatory function. Several groups have recently shown that Tregs possess a unique epigenetic pattern of DNA methylation (Floess et al., 2007; Schmidl et al., 2009; Wei et al., 2009; Ohkura et al., 2012). Acquisition of this methylation pattern begins during thymic development and does not require Foxp3 expression, although it does help to maintain Foxp3 expression and regulatory function *in vivo* and *in vitro* (Ohkura et al., 2012). Therefore, stable Treg differentiation depends upon both Foxp3 expression and a unique pattern of DNA methylation.

Tregs can develop both in the thymus (tTregs, formerly natural, or nTregs) and in the periphery (pTregs, formerly induced, or iTregs). While tTregs appear to primarily maintain peripheral tolerance to organ-specific antigens, pTregs are thought to be important in maintaining tolerance to exogenous but innocuous antigens the immune system encounters at mucosal sites. The neonatal thymectomy studies of Nishizuka and Sakakura highlighted the importance of thymus-derived tTregs in preventing organ-specific autoimmunity and raised the question of what drives their development in the thymus. One clear factor appears to be some degree of self-reactivity, as demonstrated by studies utilizing mice engineered to transgenically express T cell receptors (TCRs) of defined antigen specificity. On a recombination activating gene (RAG)-deficient background, foreign antigen-specific TCR transgenic mice had no tTregs, whereas on a RAG-sufficient background, tTregs were present and showed evidence of endogenous TCRα chain rearrangement (Itoh et al., 1999). Moreover, ectopic thymic expression of cognate foreign antigen was sufficient to allow tTreg differentiation in RAG-deficient TCR transgenic mice (Kawahata et al., 2002). Finally, the unique DNA methylation pattern seen in Tregs depended on TCR recognition of cognate peptide (Ohkura et al., 2012). These data therefore suggest a model in which tTreg development requires recognition of self-peptide/MHC complexes.

While specificity for self-antigen appears to be a critical factor in tTreg development and differentiation in the thymus, pTreg differentiation is controlled by the molecular context in which T cells are activated. Thus, the cytokine TGF-β has been shown to be important for development of pTregs both *in vivo* and *in vitro* via activation of SMAD3, which in turn binds to the CNS1 regulatory element within the Foxp3 gene and promotes pTreg differentiation in concert with other factors (Chen et al., 2003; Fantini et al., 2004; Kim and Leonard, 2007; Zheng et al., 2010). Interestingly, TGF-β can also promote Th17 differentiation in conjunction with inflammatory cytokines such as IL-6 (Bettelli et al., 2006).

Therefore, depending on the context in which the antigen is encountered, a T cell may be driven to differentiate into either a potentially inflammatory Th17 cell or a tolerogenic pTreg.

Treg expression of CD25, which along with CD122 and the common γ-chain (γ_c), makes up the high-affinity IL-2 receptor complex, highlights the importance of IL-2 in Treg biology. Because IL-2 was initially described as a growth factor for activated T cells, the finding that mice deficient in IL-2, CD25, or CD122 developed autoimmune and lymphoproliferative disorders was initially quite surprising (Schorle et al., 1991; Kramer et al., 1995; Suzuki et al., 1995). This apparent conundrum was resolved when mice deficient in IL-2 or its receptor components were found to have markedly reduced numbers of Foxp3^{+} Tregs in the periphery (Papiernik et al., 1998; Almeida et al., 2002; Malek et al., 2002). Subsequent studies clarified a critical role for IL-2 in supporting the peripheral survival and function of Tregs (Thornton et al., 2004; Fontenot et al., 2005). Administration of blocking antibodies to IL-2 or CD25 resulted in a marked decline in Treg cell numbers, whereas administration of IL-2 at low doses augmented Treg numbers (Setoguchi et al., 2005; Grinberg-Bleyer et al., 2010). This strategy has been extended to clinical trials, where administration of low dose IL-2 led to increased Treg frequency and clinical improvement in both graft versus host disease and hepatitis C-associated vasculitis (Koreth et al., 2011; Saadoun et al., 2011). Thus, IL-2 functions to support the peripheral homeostasis and function of Tregs, and is amenable to therapeutic modulation in T cell mediated inflammatory conditions.

The means by which Tregs control effector T cell responses is an area of active inquiry. *In vitro* proliferation suppression assays have demonstrated that Tregs can control effector responses both by acting directly on the responding effector T cell as well as indirectly, by modifying APC function. Regardless of the mechanism of action, Tregs require cell−cell interaction in order to exert their suppressive function *in vitro*. *In vitro* direct suppressive mechanisms include release of inhibitory cytokines, such as IL-10 and IL-35, restricting the bioavailability of IL-2, either by decreasing IL-2 transcription or by preferentially consuming IL-2, and direct granzyme-mediated cytolysis (Thornton and Shevach, 1998; Grossman et al., 2004; Collison et al., 2007; Pandiyan et al., 2007). In contrast, Tregs indirectly reduce effector T cell proliferation by altering APC function, either by inhibiting APC maturation (such as via LAG-3/MHCII interactions or catabolizing ATP released on tissue damage via CD39), or by reducing expression of B7-1 or B7-2 (Borsellino et al., 2007; Liang et al., 2008; Onishi et al., 2008). B7-1 and B7-2 downregulation is dependent upon Treg expression of CTLA-4, which binds B7-1 and B7-2 and physically removes them from the APC via transendocytosis (Wing et al., 2008; Qureshi et al., 2011). Thus, Tregs are able to utilize a variety of molecular mechanisms to both directly and indirectly regulate effector T cell activation and expansion *in vitro*.

An intriguing finding is that while Foxp3-mutant *scurfy* mice uniformly develop spontaneous autoimmune disease, the nature of the pathogenic effector response varies depending upon the genetic background of the mice (Lin et al., 2005; Suscovich et al., 2012). Thus, modifier genes can exert significant influence on the ability of Tregs to control immune responses *in vivo* and suggests that Tregs may utilize distinct molecular mechanisms to control distinct effector responses. The hypothesis that Treg control of different effector subsets requires additional factors has been bolstered by the finding that Tregs can be induced to express transcription factors associated with these subsets and expression of these transcription factors is important for proper *in vivo* regulation of the associated effector subset. For instance, Tregs upregulate Tbet in response to either IFN-γ or IL-27, and Tbet in turn drives expression of CXCR3, facilitating Treg responsiveness to IFN-γ-dependent chemokines, such as CXCL10 (Koch et al., 2009, 2012; Hall et al., 2012a). Interestingly, while Tbet-deficient Tregs had normal *in vitro* suppressive activity (Bettelli et al., 2004), they failed to prevent lethal Th1-mediated autoimmune disease upon adoptive transfer into *scurfy* mice (Koch et al., 2009), suggesting that Treg-specific Tbet expression is crucial for proper regulation of Th1 responses *in vivo*. Similarly, expression of IRF4 or STAT3 appears to be critical for Tregs to properly regulate Th2 or Th17 responses *in vivo* (Chaudhry et al., 2009; Zheng et al., 2009). These findings support the idea that Tregs possess both a core module of regulatory factors that are generally required for their suppressive function, including Foxp3 and CTLA-4, as well as inducible modules specific for control of distinct effector Th subsets (Wing and Sakaguchi, 2012).

The multi-organ autoimmunity seen in both mice and humans with spontaneous mutations in Foxp3 shows that Tregs are vital in restraining potentially autoreactive Th cells and suggests that defects in Treg function may underlie the development of other autoimmune diseases. Supporting this, single nucleotide polymorphisms in multiple genes important for Treg function, including CTLA-4, IL-2, IL-2Ra, and IL-10, have been found to be risk alleles in genome-wide association screens for a number of autoimmune diseases, such as type 1 diabetes, RA, IBD, and MS (Howson et al., 2012; Vandenbroeck, 2012). Moreover, there is evidence for some autoimmune diseases that the frequency of Tregs is altered, such as the finding that in IBD Treg frequency in the peripheral blood inversely correlates with disease activity (Takahashi et al., 2006; Saruta et al., 2007). Similarly, by

the careful immunophenotyping of circulating Tregs, Miyara et al. (2009) were able to distinguish resting and activated Treg populations and observed altered population dynamics in patients with active systemic lupus erythematosus (SLE). Finally, impaired Treg-mediated suppression of effector T cell proliferation has been demonstrated in some patients with MS, SLE, and diabetes mellitus (DM) (Viglietta et al., 2004; Alvarado-Sanchez et al., 2006; Kumar et al., 2006; Ferraro et al., 2011). Thus, alterations in Treg frequency and function are observed in human autoimmune disease, and pathways regulating Treg survival and function may represent promising therapeutic targets for treatment of human autoimmune diseases.

TR1 CELLS

Type 1 T regulatory (Tr1) cells are a recently identified Th subset that possesses regulatory function in the absence of Foxp3 expression, in large part via production of IL-10. Tr1 cell differentiation is dependent upon IL-27, a heterodimeric cytokine composed of EBI3 and p28, and additionally Tr1 cell differentiation can be amplified by TGF-β (Pot et al., 2011a; Hall et al., 2012a) IL-27 induces activation of STAT1 and STAT3, which have been shown to be essential for Tr1 differentiation (Hall et al., 2012b). Exogenous IL-27 also promotes transcription of c-Maf, IL-21, and ICOS, and subsequently IL-21 acts as an autocrine growth factor (Pot et al., 2009, 2011a, b; Hall et al., 2012b) indicating that IL-27 and IL-21 cooperate in the generation of Tr1 cells. To date, detailed functional characterization of Tr1 cells has been hampered by lack of specific markers that can reliably differentiate Tr1 cells from other IL-10 producing regulatory and effector T cell subsets. In addition, it is unclear whether Tr1 cells are only generated in the periphery or whether Tr1 cells are also generated through thymic selection, analogous to tTregs (Fujio et al., 2010).

Functionally, IL-27 treatment ameliorated EAE by increasing the frequency of IL-10 producing T cells and thereby suppressing IL-17 producing Th17 cells, suggesting it may be useful therapeutically (Kastelein et al., 2007). Furthermore, IL-27Rα deficient mice were shown to develop exacerbated EAE (Batten et al., 2006). Intriguingly, recent clinical trials suggested that IFN-β, which is widely used as a first line treatment for MS, increased serum IL-27 levels (Sweeney et al., 2011). Some MS patients have been reported to have decreased IL-10 production (Ozenci et al., 1999), thus, the clinical efficacy of IFN-β in MS has been attributed to the induction of IL-27, consequently promoting an increased frequency of IL-10 producing Tr1 cells which can then potentially control auto-pathogenic T effector cells (Guo et al., 2008; Ramgolam et al., 2009; Sweeney et al., 2011). Another area where regulatory cells are of high therapeutic value is organ transplants, such as pancreatic islet transplants in insulin-dependent diabetes mellitus (IDDM), where inadequate immunosuppression gives rise to graft rejection. A strong correlation has been described between transplant acceptance and frequency of circulating tTregs (Berney et al., 2009), as well as IL-10 production by peripheral blood mononuclear cells (Huurman et al., 2009), suggesting that tTregs play an important role in maintaining long-term tolerance. However, generation, expansion, and stability of antigen-specific Tregs remains a major challenge (Sagoo et al., 2008). Thus, an alternative to tTreg therapy is the adoptive transfer of *in vitro* generated IL-10 producing Tr1 cells that can sustain long-term survival *in vivo*. Indeed, the transfer of antigen-specific Tr1 cells prevented islet graft rejection in mouse models of islet transplant (Gagliani et al., 2010). Additionally, preliminary data indicate that adoptive transfer of host-specific Tr1 cells may prevent graft versus host disease (GvHD) in leukemia patients who underwent stem cell transplant (Allan et al., 2008; Bacchetta et al., 2010; Hippen et al., 2011; Roncarolo et al., 2011) supporting the potential value of Tr1 therapy in generating tolerance.

TFH CELLS

T cell-dependent antibody responses occur in germinal centers (GC) of lymphoid follicles and require interaction between antigen-specific B cells and Th cells (MacLennan et al., 1997; Garside et al., 1998). Recent evidence suggests that this interaction is mediated by a distinct Th subset, termed follicular T helper cells (TFH). These TFH cells are activated by antigen in the T cell zone of lymphoid tissues, and then migrate specifically to the outer edge of the B cell follicles in order to encounter antigen-specific B cells that have also migrated to this location (Vinuesa and Cook, 2011). The homing of the TFH cells to the GC is dependent on a two-step chemotactic process that begins with the downregulation of CCR7, the receptor for the chemokines CCL19 and CCL21, which are produced in the T cell zone of the lymphoid tissue (Gunn et al., 1998; Ansel et al., 2000; Luther et al., 2000), followed by the induction of CXCR5, which allows TFH cells to migrate into the GCs (Breitfeld et al., 2000; Haynes et al., 2007). The downregulation of CCR7 and upregulation of CXCR5 is driven by the B cell lymphoma 6 protein (Bcl6), the master transcription factor regulating TFH cell differentiation. The stable induction of Bcl6 is also critically dependent on the physical interaction of T and B cells (Liu et al., 2012, 2013). In addition to CXCR5, TFH cells express the costimulatory molecule ICOS (inducible costimulator) and interaction of ICOS with ICOS ligand on B cells promotes the

differentiation of T cells to TFH cells (Ramiscal and Vinuesa, 2013). TFH cell development also requires expression of the signaling molecule SAP and SLAM, an adaptor protein, as these are crucial for the induction of Bcl6 (Ramiscal and Vinuesa, 2013). Deletion of Bcl6 prevents the generation of TFH cells and inhibits GC reactions, including affinity maturation, isotype switching, B cell proliferation, and generation of memory B cells and plasma cells (Nurieva et al., 2009a). The differentiation of TFH cells is mediated by IL-21 and IL-6, and TFH cells require STAT3 (Nurieva et al., 2008) and c-Maf for their generation (Bauquet et al., 2009). With the activation of Bcl6, TFH cells begin secreting their signature cytokine, IL-21, which has been shown to be essential for B cell survival and promoting germinal center reactions (Nurieva et al., 2008; Nurieva et al., 2009b). While other T helper subsets also produce IL-21, the amount of IL-21 produced by TFH cells is far greater compared to both Th1 and Th2 cells (Chtanova et al., 2004).

Immune responses that drive differentiation of other Th subsets may also give rise to distinct subtypes of TFH cells (King et al., 2008). For example, *in vitro* generated Th1 and Th2 cells have been shown to develop into TFH cells upon adoptive transfer. Consistent with the important role of cytokines in regulating isotype switching, TFH cells can secrete IFN-γ, IL-4, and IL-17, though at levels lower than conventional Th1, Th2, or Th17 cells. Thus, during the early stages of TFH cell development some cells may have upregulated CXCR5 but not yet turned on Bcl6 (Crotty, 2011). However, with entry into the follicle and upon interaction with B cells, Bcl6 expression increases, and TFH lineage commitment stabilizes, commensurate with downregulation of the Th1, Th2, and Th17 associated genes (Crotty, 2011). Thus, the ability of other Th subsets to give rise to TFH cells is likely crucial to appropriately coordinate humoral and cellular immune responses (Crotty, 2011). Collectively, TFH cells have emerged as a distinct T helper subset that provides critical help to B cells and regulates GC reactions, and as a result ultimately controls humoral immune responses.

A number of autoimmune diseases are characterized by the presence of self-reactive autoantibodies. It has been suggested that GCs may the drive the pathogenic generation of autoantibodies. In animal models for SLE, for example, spontaneous generation of GCs correlated with increased serum concentration of autoantibodies (Luzina et al., 2001; Hsu et al., 2008). Cognate help from TFH cells has been demonstrated to promote the survival, expansion, and differentiation of self-reactive B cells, which ultimately resulted in autoantibody production and promoted tissue injury (Zhang et al., 2013). In addition, aberrant TFH cell function has been shown to promote development of disease in animal models of SLE and

RA, and is characterized by GC expansion, increased IL-21, and TFH cell expansion in extra-follicular sites (Zhang et al., 2013). In human autoimmune diseases, expansion of circulating TFH cells in patients with juvenile dermatomyositis, RA, SLE, and Sjögren's syndrome has been observed to strongly correlate with increased plasmablasts and serum concentrations of anti-dsDNA and antinuclear antibodies (Morita et al., 2011; Ma et al., 2012; Zhang et al., 2013). These observations are highly suggestive of the role that aberrant TFH cells may play in the pathogenesis of autoimmunity.

TH2 CELLS

Initially described for their distinct pattern of cytokine expression and their ability to promote IgE class-switching (Mosmann et al., 1986), Th2 cells are critical for amplifying and sustaining inflammation marked by eosinophil recruitment and mast cell activation. Th2 responses may be either protective, in the case of host defense against helminthes and other extracellular parasites, or detrimental and lead to the development of asthma and environmental allergies (Paul and Zhu, 2010; Pulendran and Artis, 2012). Th2 differentiation is induced by IL-4, which, upon binding a heterodimeric receptor consisting of IL-4Rα and the γ_c-chain, results in the phosphorylation and activation of STAT6 and in turn induces expression of GATA-3. GATA-3 then transactivates many Th2-specific cytokines, most notably IL-4, IL-5, and IL-13, all of which share a common genetic locus (Zheng and Flavell, 1997). Th2 development results in significant chromatin remodeling at the *Il4* gene locus, such that IL-4 production by established Th2 cells can be seen even after the conditional deletion of GATA-3 (Baguet and Bix, 2004; Zhu et al., 2004). The same molecular pathways that promote Th2 differentiation simultaneously counter-regulate the development of other effector Th subsets, particularly Th1 cells. For instance, GATA-3 can downregulate expression of Th1-promoting genes such as STAT4 and IL-12Rβ2 (Zheng and Flavell, 1997). Additionally, the transcription factor c-Maf both transactivates the *Il4* locus and induces downregulation of IFN-γ (Ho et al., 1996, 1998). Th2 differentiation is thus a powerful counter-regulator of Th1 differentiation.

The role of Th2 cells in autoimmune disease is complex. They have been implicated in facilitating isotype switching in SLE (Singh et al., 2003) and high levels of IL-4 and IL-13 are commonly seen in patients with systemic sclerosis, although the role of these cytokines in the pathogenesis of this disease is still unclear (O'Reilly et al., 2012). In contrast, many inflammatory autoimmune diseases show marked bias towards Th1 and Th17 responses and prior infection with a Th2 skewing pathogen can ameliorate EAE in mice (Sewell et al., 2003).

Moreover, many inflammatory autoimmune diseases have lower incidences in areas where parasitic infections are more common and longitudinal studies of MS patients with asymptomatic intestinal parasitemia suggest these patients have milder disease than uninfected controls (Correale and Farez, 2007). These observations have been extended to clinical trials assessing the efficacy and safety of administering ova from *Trichuris suis*, a pig nematode that is unable to productively infect humans, to patients with ulcerative colitis. Early studies showed clinically significant improvement in over 40% of patients with severe ulcerative colitis, compared to a placebo response rate of 17% (Summers et al., 2005), and larger scale trials are underway (Weinstock and Elliott, 2013). Additionally, glatiramer acetate, an immunomodulatory agent approved for use in MS, appears to be efficacious in part due to skewing the immune response towards a Th2-biased response (Arnon and Aharoni, 2004). Thus, Th2 counter-regulation of other Th effector subsets can be utilized clinically in inflammatory autoimmune disorders.

TH9 CELLS

Th9 cells, a recently identified Th subset generated by activating naïve Th cells in the presence of TGF-β and IL-4, produce both IL-9 and IL-10 (Dardalhon et al., 2008; Veldhoen et al., 2008b). The requirement for IL-4 in Th9 differentiation raises the question of whether Th9 cells represent a distinct lineage or are a subset of specialized Th2 cells, particularly given that both Th2 and Th9 cells can readily induce allergic airway inflammation (Chang et al., 2010; Staudt et al., 2010). Similar to Th2 cells, Th9 cells also require the transcription factors IRF4 and STAT6; however, IL-9 production is uniquely dependent upon the TGF-β-induced transcription factor PU.1, which, although expressed by other Th subsets, is not required for Th2 differentiation (Chang et al., 2010; Staudt et al., 2010; Goswami et al., 2012). Moreover, while myelin-specific *in vitro* differentiated Th2 cells failed to induce EAE upon adoptive transfer, transfer of Th9 cells resulted in robust disease, suggesting Th9 cells have distinct functional properties from Th2 cells (Jäger et al., 2009). However, Th9 cells do show considerable plasticity after adoptive transfer (Dardalhon et al., 2008; Jäger et al., 2009), leaving open the question of whether they represent a truly terminally differentiated Th subset.

CONCLUDING REMARKS

The functional diversity and plasticity of CD4$^+$ T cells is crucial for successful host defense against diverse environmental pathogens but can also go dangerously awry in the setting of autoimmune disease. Recent years have seen the identification of novel Th subsets as well as a remarkable growth in our understanding of the molecular mechanisms that underlie Th cell differentiation. In particular, the identification of Th17 cells and Tregs as distinct lineages has greatly furthered our knowledge of the pathobiology of a variety of autoimmune disorders and allowed the identification and development of novel therapeutic approaches. Recent work investigating the complex transcriptional networks involved in Th17 differentiation clearly illustrates the dynamic tension between transcriptional modules that enhance Th17 cell differentiation and inhibit development of other T cell subsets, thus providing the molecular basis for counter-regulation between Th subsets (Ciofani et al., 2012; Yosef et al., 2013). Although impairment of counter-regulatory mechanisms may lead to autoimmune tissue inflammation, these same pathways are amenable to modulation and offer opportunities for the development of novel immunomodulatory therapies for autoimmune diseases.

REFERENCES

Aarvak, T., Chabaud, M., Miossec, P., Natvig, J.B., 1999. IL-17 is produced by some proinflammatory Th1/Th0 cells but not by Th2 cells. J. Immunol. 162, 1246–1251.

Abromson-Leeman, S., Bronson, R.T., Dorf, M.E., 2009. Encephalitogenic T cells that stably express both T-bet and ROR gamma t consistently produce IFNgamma but have a spectrum of IL-17 profiles. J. Neuroimmunol. 215, 10–24.

Adorini, L., Gregori, S., Magram, J., Trembleau, S., 1996a. The role of IL-12 in the pathogenesis of Th1 cell-mediated autoimmune diseases. Ann. N.Y. Acad. Sci. 795, 208–215.

Adorini, L., Guery, J.C., Trembleau, S., 1996b. Manipulation of the Th1/Th2 cell balance: an approach to treat human autoimmune diseases? Autoimmunity 23, 53–68.

Ahern, P.P., Schiering, C., Buonocore, S., McGeachy, M.J., Cua, D. J., Maloy, K.J., et al., 2010. Interleukin-23 drives intestinal inflammation through direct activity on T cells. Immunity 33, 279–288.

Allan, S.E., Broady, R., Gregori, S., Himmel, M.E., Locke, N., Roncarolo, M.G., et al., 2008. CD4+ T-regulatory cells: toward therapy for human diseases. Immunol. Rev. 223, 391–421.

Almeida, A.R., Legrand, N., Papiernik, M., Freitas, A.A., 2002. Homeostasis of peripheral CD4+ T cells: IL-2R alpha and IL-2 shape a population of regulatory cells that controls CD4+ T cell numbers. J. Immunol. 169, 4850–4860.

Alvarado-Sanchez, B., Hernandez-Castro, B., Portales-Perez, D., Baranda, L., Layseca-Espinosa, E., Abud-Mendoza, C., et al., 2006. Regulatory T cells in patients with systemic lupus erythematosus. J. Autoimmun. 27, 110–118.

Ansel, K.M., Ngo, V.N., Hyman, P.L., Luther, S.A., Forster, R., Sedgwick, J.D., et al., 2000. A chemokine-driven positive feedback loop organizes lymphoid follicles. Nature 406, 309–314.

Arnon, R., Aharoni, R., 2004. Mechanism of action of glatiramer acetate in multiple sclerosis and its potential for the development of new

applications. Proc. Natl. Acad. Sci. U.S.A. 101 (Suppl. 2), 14593–14598.

Awasthi, A., Riol-Blanco, L., Jäger, A., Korn, T., Pot, C., Galileos, G., et al., 2009. Cutting edge: IL-23 receptor gfp reporter mice reveal distinct populations of IL-17-producing cells. J. Immunol. 182, 5904–5908.

Bacchetta, R., Gregori, S., Serafini, G., Sartirana, C., Schulz, U., Zino, E., et al., 2010. Molecular and functional characterization of alloantigen-specific anergic T cells suitable for cell therapy. Haematologica. 95, 2134–2143.

Baguet, A., Bix, M., 2004. Chromatin landscape dynamics of the Il4–Il13 locus during T helper 1 and 2 development. Proc. Natl. Acad. Sci. USA 101, 11410–11415.

Batten, M., Li, J., Yi, S., Kljavin, N.M., Danilenko, D.M., Lucas, S., et al., 2006. Interleukin 27 limits autoimmune encephalomyelitis by suppressing the development of interleukin 17-producing T cells. Nat. Immunol. 7, 929–936.

Bauquet, A.T., Jin, H., Paterson, A.M., Mitsdoerffer, M., Ho, I.C., Sharpe, A.H., et al., 2009. The costimulatory molecule ICOS regulates the expression of c-Maf and IL-21 in the development of follicular T helper cells and TH-17 cells. Nat. Immunol. 10, 167–175.

Bending, D., De la Peña, H., Veldhoen, M., Phillips, J.M., Uyttenhove, C., Stockinger, B., et al., 2009. Highly purified Th17 cells from BDC2.5NOD mice convert Th1-like cells in NOD/SCID recipient mice. J. Clin. Invest. 119, 565–572.

Bennett, C.L., Christie, J., Ramsdell, F., Brunkow, M.E., Ferguson, P.J., Whitesell, L., et al., 2001. The immune dysregulation, polyendocrinopathy, enteropathy, X-linked syndrome (IPEX) is caused by mutations of FOXP3. Nat. Genet. 27, 20–21.

Berer, K., Mues, M., Koutrolos, M., Rasbi, Z.A., Boziki, M., Johner, C., et al., 2011. Commensal microbiota and myelin autoantigen cooperate to trigger autoimmune demyelination. Nature 479, 538–541.

Berney, T., Ferrari-Lacraz, S., Buhler, L., Oberholzer, J., Marangon, N., Philippe, J., et al., 2009. Long-term insulin-independence after allogeneic islet transplantation for type 1 diabetes: over the 10-year mark. Am. J. Transplant. 9, 419–423.

Bettelli, E., Carrier, Y., Gao, W., Korn, T., Strom, T.B., Oukka, M., et al., 2006. Reciprocal developmental pathways for the generation of pathogenic effector TH17 and regulatory T cells. Nature 441, 235–238.

Bettelli, E., Korn, T., Oukka, M., Kuchroo, V.K., 2008. Induction and effector functions of T(H)17 cells. Nature. 453, 1051–1057.

Bettelli, E., Sullivan, B., Szabo, S.J., Sobel, R.A., Glimcher, L.H., Kuchroo, V.K., 2004. Loss of T-bet, but not STAT1, prevents the development of experimental autoimmune encephalomyelitis. J. Exp. Med. 200, 79–87.

Borsellino, G., Kleinewietfeld, M., Di Mitri, D., Sternjak, A., Diamantini, A., Giometto, R., et al., 2007. Expression of ectonucleotidase CD39 by Foxp3 + Treg cells: hydrolysis of extracellular ATP and immune suppression. Blood. 110, 1225–1232.

Breitfeld, D., Ohl, L., Kremmer, E., Ellwart, J., Sallusto, F., Lipp, M., et al., 2000. Follicular B helper T cells express CXC chemokine receptor 5, localize to B cell follicles, and support immunoglobulin production. J. Exp. Med. 192, 1545–1552.

Brüstle, A., Heink, S., Huber, M., Rosenplänter, C., Stadelmann, C., Yu, P., et al., 2007. The development of inflammatory T(H)-17 cells requires interferon-regulatory factor 4. Nat. Immunol. 8, 958–966.

Burton, P.R., Clayton, D.G., Cardon, L.R., Craddock, N., Deloukas, P., Duncanson, A., et al., 2007. Association scan of 14,500 nonsynonymous SNPs in four diseases identifies autoimmunity variants. Nat. Genet. 39, 1329–1337.

Cargill, M., Schrodi, S.J., Chang, M., Garcia, V.E., Brandon, R., Callis, K.P., et al., 2007. A large-scale genetic association study confirms IL12B and leads to the identification of IL23R as psoriasis-risk genes. Am. J. Hum. Genet. 80, 273–290.

Chang, H.C., Sehra, S., Goswami, R., Yao, W., Yu, Q., Stritesky, G.L., et al., 2010. The transcription factor PU.1 is required for the development of IL-9-producing T cells and allergic inflammation. Nat. Immunol. 11, 527–534.

Chang, J., Burkett, P.R., Borges, C.M., Kuchroo, V.K., Turka, L.A., Chang, C.H., 2013. MyD88 is essential to sustain mTOR activation necessary to promote T helper 17 cell proliferation by linking IL-1 and IL-23 signaling. Proc. Natl. Acad. Sci. USA 110, 2270–2275.

Chastain, E.M., Miller, S.D., 2012. Molecular mimicry as an inducing trigger for CNS autoimmune demyelinating disease. Immunol. Rev. 245, 227–238.

Chaudhry, A., Rudra, D., Treuting, P., Samstein, R.M., Liang, Y., Kas, A., et al., 2009. CD4 + regulatory T cells control TH17 responses in a Stat3-dependent manner. Science 326, 986–991.

Chaudhry, A., Samstein, R.M., Treuting, P., Liang, Y., Pils, M.C., Heinrich, J.M., et al., 2011. Interleukin-10 signaling in regulatory T cells is required for suppression of Th17 cell-mediated inflammation. Immunity. 34, 566–578.

Chen, W., Jin, W., Hardegen, N., Lei, K.J., Li, L., Marinos, N., et al., 2003. Conversion of peripheral CD4 + CD25− naïve T cells to CD4+ CD25+ regulatory T cells by TGF-beta induction of transcription factor Foxp3. J. Exp. Med. 198, 1875–1886.

Chtanova, T., Tangye, S.G., Newton, R., Frank, N., Hodge, M.R., Rolph, M.S., et al., 2004. T follicular helper cells express a distinctive transcriptional profile, reflecting their role as non-Th1/Th2 effector cells that provide help for B cells. J. Immunol. 173, 68–78.

Chu, C.Q., Wittmer, S., Dalton, D.K., 2000. Failure to suppress the expansion of the activated CD4 T cell population in interferon gamma-deficient mice leads to exacerbation of experimental autoimmune encephalomyelitis. J. Exp. Med. 192, 123–128.

Chung, Y., Chang, S.H., Martinez, G.J., Yang, X.O., Nurieva, R., Kang, H.S., et al., 2009. Critical regulation of early Th17 cell differentiation by interleukin-1 signaling. Immunity 30, 576–587.

Ciofani, M., Madar, A., Galan, C., Sellars, M., Mace, K., Pauli, F., et al., 2012. A validated regulatory network for Th17 cell specification. Cell 151, 289–303.

Codarri, L., Gyulveszi, G., Tosevski, V., Hesske, L., Fontana, A., Magnenat, L., et al., 2011. RORgammat drives production of the cytokine GM-CSF in helper T cells, which is essential for the effector phase of autoimmune neuroinflammation. Nat. Immunol. 12, 560–567.

Collison, L.W., Workman, C.J., Kuo, T.T., Boyd, K., Wang, Y., Vignali, K.M., et al., 2007. The inhibitory cytokine IL-35 contributes to regulatory T-cell function. Nature 450, 566–569.

Correale, J., Farez, M., 2007. Association between parasite infection and immune responses in multiple sclerosis. Ann. Neurol. 61, 97–108.

Crotty, S., 2011. Follicular helper CD4 T cells (TFH). Annu. Rev. Immunol. 29, 621–663.

Cua, D.J., Sherlock, J., Chen, Y., Murphy, C.A., Joyce, B., Seymour, B., et al., 2003. Interleukin-23 rather than interleukin-12 is the critical cytokine for autoimmune inflammation of the brain. Nature 421, 744–748.

Cypowyj, S., Picard, C., Marodi, L., Casanova, J.L., Puel, A., 2012. Immunity to infection in IL-17-deficient mice and humans. Eur. J. Immunol. 42, 2246–2254.

Dang, E.V., Barbi, J., Yang, H.Y., Jinasena, D., Yu, H., Zheng, Y., et al., 2011. Control of T(H)17/T(reg) balance by hypoxia-inducible factor 1. Cell 146, 772–784.

Dardalhon, V., Awasthi, A., Kwon, H., Galileos, G., Gao, W., Sobel, R.A., et al., 2008. IL-4 inhibits TGF-beta-induced Foxp3+ T cells and, together with TGF-beta, generates IL-9+ IL-10+ Foxp3(−) effector T cells. Nat. Immunol. 9, 1347–1355.

Du, J., Huang, C., Zhou, B., Ziegler, S.F., 2008. Isoform-specific inhibition of ROR alpha-mediated transcriptional activation by human FOXP3. J. Immunol. 180, 4785–4792.

Duerr, R.H., Taylor, K.D., Brant, S.R., Rioux, J.D., Silverberg, M.S., Daly, M.J., et al., 2006. A genome-wide association study identifies IL23R as an inflammatory bowel disease gene. Science 314, 1461–1463.

El-Behi, M., Ciric, B., Dai, H., Yan, Y., Cullimore, M., Safavi, F., et al., 2011. The encephalitogenicity of T(H)17 cells is dependent on IL-1- and IL-23-induced production of the cytokine GM-CSF. Nat. Immunol. 12, 568–575.

Esplugues, E., Huber, S., Gagliani, N., Hauser, A.E., Town, T., Wan, Y.Y., et al., 2011. Control of TH17 cells occurs in the small intestine. Nature 475, 514–518.

Fantini, M.C., Becker, C., Monteleone, G., Pallone, F., Galle, P.R., Neurath, M.F., 2004. Cutting edge: TGF-beta induces a regulatory phenotype in CD4 + CD25 − T cells through Foxp3 induction and down-regulation of Smad7. J. Immunol. 172, 5149–5153.

Ferber, I.A., Brocke, S., Taylor-Edwards, C., Ridgway, W., Dinisco, C., Steinman, L., et al., 1996. Mice with a disrupted IFN-gamma gene are susceptible to the induction of experimental autoimmune encephalomyelitis (EAE). J. Immunol. 156, 5–7.

Ferraro, A., Socci, C., Stabilini, A., Valle, A., Monti, P., Piemonti, L., et al., 2011. Expansion of Th17 cells and functional defects in T regulatory cells are key features of the pancreatic lymph nodes in patients with type 1 diabetes. Diabetes 60, 2903–2913.

Floess, S., Freyer, J., Siewert, C., Baron, U., Olek, S., Polansky, J., et al., 2007. Epigenetic control of the foxp3 locus in regulatory T cells. PLoS Biol. 5, e38.

Fontenot, J.D., Rasmussen, J.P., Gavin, M.A., Rudensky, A.Y., 2005. A function for interleukin 2 in Foxp3-expressing regulatory T cells. Nat. Immunol. 6, 1142–1151.

Fujio, K., Okamura, T., Yamamoto, K., 2010. The family of IL-10-secreting CD4+ T cells. Adv. Immunol. 105, 99–130.

Gagliani, N., Jofra, T., Stabilini, A., Valle, A., Atkinson, M., Roncarolo, M.G., et al., 2010. Antigen-specific dependence of Tr1-cell therapy in preclinical models of islet transplant. Diabetes 59, 433–439.

Garside, P., Ingulli, E., Merica, R.R., Johnson, J.G., Noelle, R.J., Jenkins, M.K., 1998. Visualization of specific B and T lymphocyte interactions in the lymph node. Science 281, 96–99.

Gavin, M.A., Torgerson, T.R., Houston, E., Deroos, P., Ho, W.Y., Stray-Pedersen, A., et al., 2006. Single-cell analysis of normal and FOXP3-mutant human T cells: FOXP3 expression without regulatory T cell development. Proc. Natl. Acad. Sci. USA 103, 6659–6664.

Geginat, G., Lalic, M., Kretschmar, M., Goebel, W., Hof, H., Palm, D., et al., 1998. Th1 cells specific for a secreted protein of Listeria monocytogenes are protective in vivo. J. Immunol. 160, 6046–6055.

Genovese, M.C., Van Den Bosch, F., Roberson, S.A., Bojin, S., Biagini, I.M., Ryan, P., et al., 2010. LY2439821, a humanized anti-interleukin-17 monoclonal antibody, in the treatment of patients with rheumatoid arthritis: A phase I randomized, double-blind, placebo-controlled, proof-of-concept study. Arthritis Rheum. 62, 929–939.

Ghoreschi, K., Laurence, A., Yang, X.P., Tato, C.M., McGeachy, M.J., et al., 2010. Generation of pathogenic T(H)17 cells in the absence of TGF-beta signalling. Nature 467, 967–971.

Goswami, R., Jabeen, R., Yagi, R., Pham, D., Zhu, J., Goenka, S., et al., 2012. STAT6-dependent regulation of Th9 development. J. Immunol. 188, 968–975.

Grinberg-Bleyer, Y., Baeyens, A., You, S., Elhage, R., Fourcade, G., Gregoire, S., et al., 2010. IL-2 reverses established type 1 diabetes in NOD mice by a local effect on pancreatic regulatory T cells. J. Exp. Med. 207, 1871–1878.

Grossman, W.J., Verbsky, J.W., Barchet, W., Colonna, M., Atkinson, J.P., Ley, T.J., 2004. Human T regulatory cells can use the perforin pathway to cause autologous target cell death. Immunity 21, 589–601.

Gulen, M.F., Bulek, K., Xiao, H., Yu, M., Gao, J., Sun, L., et al., 2012. Inactivation of the enzyme GSK3alpha by the kinase IKKi promotes AKT-mTOR signaling pathway that mediates interleukin-1-induced Th17 cell maintenance. Immunity 37, 800–812.

Gunn, M.D., Tangemann, K., Tam, C., Cyster, J.G., Rosen, S.D., Williams, L.T., 1998. A chemokine expressed in lymphoid high endothelial venules promotes the adhesion and chemotaxis of naive T lymphocytes. Proc. Natl. Acad. Sci. USA 95, 258–263.

Guo, B., Chang, E.Y., Cheng, G., 2008. The type I IFN induction pathway constrains Th17-mediated autoimmune inflammation in mice. J. Clin. Invest. 118, 1680–1690.

Hall, A.O., Beiting, D.P., Tato, C., John, B., Oldenhove, G., Lombana, C.G., et al., 2012a. The cytokines interleukin 27 and interferon-gamma promote distinct Treg cell populations required to limit infection-induced pathology. Immunity 37, 511–523.

Hall, A.O., Silver, J.S., Hunter, C.A., 2012b. The immunobiology of IL-27. Adv. Immunol. 115, 1–44.

Havrdová, E. et al. Positive Proof of Concept of AIN457 (Secukinumab), an Antibody Against Interleukin-17A, in Relapsing-Remitting Multiple Sclerosis. In: 28th ECTRIMS Congress, Lyon, October, 2012. Abstract 168.

Haynes, N.M., Allen, C.D., Lesley, R., Ansel, K.M., Killeen, N., Cyster, J.G., 2007. Role of CXCR5 and CCR7 in follicular Th cell positioning and appearance of a programmed cell death gene-1high germinal center-associated subpopulation. J. Immunol. 179, 5099–5108.

Hill, J.A., Feuerer, M., Tash, K., Haxhinasto, S., Perez, J., Melamed, R., et al., 2007. Foxp3 transcription-factor-dependent and -independent regulation of the regulatory T cell transcriptional signature. Immunity 27, 786–800.

Hippen, K.L., Riley, J.L., June, C.H., Blazar, B.R., 2011. Clinical perspectives for regulatory T cells in transplantation tolerance. Semin. Immunol. 23, 462–468.

Hirota, K., Duarte, J.H., Veldhoen, M., Hornsby, E., Li, Y., Cua, D.J., et al., 2011. Fate mapping of IL-17-producing T cells in inflammatory responses. Nat. Immunol. 12, 255–263.

Ho, I.C., Hodge, M.R., Rooney, J.W., Glimcher, L.H., 1996. The proto-oncogene c-maf is responsible for tissue-specific expression of interleukin-4. Cell 85, 973–983.

Ho, I.C., Lo, D., Glimcher, L.H., 1998. C-maf promotes T helper cell type 2 (Th2) and attenuates Th1 differentiation by both interleukin 4-dependent and -independent mechanisms. J. Exp. Med. 188, 1859–1866.

Hofstetter, H.H., Ibrahim, S.M., Koczan, D., Kruse, N., Weishaupt, A., Toyka, K.V., et al., 2005. Therapeutic efficacy of IL-17 neutralization in murine experimental autoimmune encephalomyelitis. Cell Immunol. 237, 123–130.

Hori, S., Nomura, T., Sakaguchi, S., 2003. Control of regulatory T cell development by the transcription factor Foxp3. Science 299, 1057–1061.

Howson, J.M., Cooper, J.D., Smyth, D.J., Walker, N.M., Stevens, H., She, J.X., et al., 2012. Evidence of gene–gene interaction and age-at-diagnosis effects in type 1 diabetes. Diabetes 61, 3012–3017.

Hsu, H.C., Yang, P., Wang, J., Wu, Q., Myers, R., Chen, J., et al., 2008. Interleukin 17-producing T helper cells and interleukin 17 orchestrate autoreactive germinal center development in autoimmune BXD2 mice. Nat. Immunol. 9, 166–175.

Huber, M., Brüstle, A., Reinhard, K., Guralnik, A., Walter, G., Mahiny, A., et al., 2008. IRF4 is essential for IL-21-mediated induction, amplification, and stabilization of the Th17 phenotype. Proc. Natl. Acad. Sci. U.S.A. 105, 29846–29851.

Huber, S., Gagliani, N., Esplugues, E., O'Connor Jr., W., Huber, F.J., Chaudhry, A., et al., 2011. Th17 cells express interleukin-10 receptor and are controlled by Foxp3 and Foxp3+ regulatory CD4+ T cells in an interleukin-10-dependent manner. Immunity 34, 554–565.

Huber, S., Gagliani, N., Flavell, R.A., 2012. Life, death, and miracles: Th17 cells in the intestine. Eur. J. Immunol. 42, 2238–2245.

Hue, S., Ahern, P., Buonocore, S., Kullberg, M.C., Cua, D.J., McKenzie, B.S., et al., 2006. Interleukin-23 drives innate and T cell-mediated intestinal inflammation. J. Exp. Med. 203, 2473–2483.

Hueber, W., Patel, D.D., Dryja, T., Wright, A.M., Koroleva, I., Bruin, G., et al., 2010. Effects of AIN457, a fully human antibody to interleukin-17A, on psoriasis, rheumatoid arthritis, and uveitis. Sci. Transl. Med. 2, 52–72.

Huurman, V.A., Velthuis, J.H., Hilbrands, R., Tree, T.I., Gillard, P., Van Der Meer-Prins, P.M., et al., 2009. Allograft-specific cytokine profiles associate with clinical outcome after islet cell transplantation. Am. J. Transplant. 9, 382–388.

Ishigame, H., Kakuta, S., Nagai, T., Kadoki, M., Nambu, A., Komiyama, Y., et al., 2009. Differential roles of interleukin-17A and -17F in host defense against mucoepithelial bacterial infection and allergic responses. Immunity 30, 108–119.

Itoh, M., Takahashi, T., Sakaguchi, N., Kuniyasu, Y., Shimizu, J., Otsuka, F., et al., 1999. Thymus and autoimmunity: production of CD25+ CD4+ naturally anergic and suppressive T cells as a key function of the thymus in maintaining immunologic self-tolerance. J. Immunol. 162, 5317–5326.

Ivanov, I.i., Atarashi, K., Manel, N., Brodie, E.L., Shima, T., Karaoz, U., et al., 2009. Induction of intestinal Th17 cells by segmented filamentous bacteria. Cell 139, 485–498.

Ivanov, I.i., Mckenzie, B.S., Zhou, L., Tadokoro, C.E., Lepelley, A., Lafaille, J.J., et al., 2006. The orphan nuclear receptor RORgammat directs the differentiation program of proinflammatory IL-17(+) T helper cells. Cell 126, 1121–1133.

Jäger, A., Dardalhon, V., Sobel, R.A., Bettelli, E., Kuchroo, V.K., 2009. Th1, Th17, and Th9 effector cells induce experimental autoimmune encephalomyelitis with different pathological phenotypes. J. Immunol. 183, 7169–7177.

Jones, L.S., Rizzo, L.V., Agarwal, R.K., Tarrant, T.K., Chan, C.C., Wiggert, B., et al., 1997. IFN-gamma-deficient mice develop experimental autoimmune uveitis in the context of a deviant effector response. J. Immunol. 158, 5997–6005.

Karni, A., Abraham, M., Monsonego, A., Cai, G., Freeman, G.J., Hafler, D., et al., 2006. Innate immunity in multiple sclerosis: myeloid dendritic cells in secondary progressive multiple sclerosis are activated and drive a proinflammatory immune response. J. Immunol. 177, 4196–4202.

Kastelein, R.A., Hunter, C.A., Cua, D.J., 2007. Discovery and biology of IL-23 and IL-27: related but functionally distinct regulators of inflammation. Annu. Rev. Immunol. 25, 221–242.

Katz, J.D., Benoist, C., Mathis, D., 1995. T helper cell subsets in insulin-dependent diabetes. Science 268, 1185–1188.

Katz-Levy, Y., Neville, K.L., Padilla, J., Rahbe, S., Begolka, W.S., Girvin, A.M., et al., 2000. Temporal development of autoreactive Th1 responses and endogenous presentation of self myelin epitopes by central nervous system-resident APCs in Theiler's virus-infected mice. J. Immunol. 165, 5304–5314.

Kawahata, K., Misaki, Y., Yamauchi, M., Tsunekawa, S., Setoguchi, K., Miyazaki, J., et al., 2002. Generation of CD4(+)CD25(+) regulatory T cells from autoreactive T cells simultaneously with their negative selection in the thymus and from nonautoreactive T cells by endogenous TCR expression. J. Immunol. 168, 4399–4405.

Khattri, R., Cox, T., Yasayko, S.A., Ramsdell, F., 2003. An essential role for Scurfin in CD4+CD25+ T regulatory cells. Nat. Immunol. 4, 337–342.

Kim, H.P., Leonard, W.J., 2007. CREB/ATF-dependent T cell receptor-induced FoxP3 gene expression: a role for DNA methylation. J. Exp. Med. 204, 1543–1551.

King, C., Tangye, S.G., Mackay, C.R., 2008. T follicular helper (TFH) cells in normal and dysregulated immune responses. Annu. Rev. Immunol. 26, 741–766.

Kleinewietfeld, M., Manzel, A., Titze, J., Kvakan, H., Yosef, N., Linker, R.A., et al., 2013. Sodium chloride drives autoimmune disease by the induction of pathogenic TH17 cells. Nature 496, 518–522.

Koch, M.A., Thomas, K.R., Perdue, N.R., Smigiel, K.S., Srivastava, S., Campbell, D.J., 2012. T-bet(+) Treg cells undergo abortive Th1 cell differentiation due to impaired expression of IL-12 receptor beta2. Immunity 37, 501–510.

Koch, M.A., Tucker-Heard, G., Perdue, N.R., Killebrew, J.R., Urdahl, K.B., Campbell, D.J., 2009. The transcription factor T-bet controls regulatory T cell homeostasis and function during type 1 inflammation. Nat. Immunol. 10, 595–602.

Koreth, J., Matsuoka, K., Kim, H.T., McDonough, S.M., Bindra, B., Alyea 3rd, E.P., et al., 2011. Interleukin-2 and regulatory T cells in graft-versus-host disease. N. Engl. J. Med. 365, 2055–2066.

Korn, T., Bettelli, E., Awasthi, A., Jäger, A., Strom, T.B., Oukka, M., et al., 2007. IL-21 initiates an alternative pathway to induce proinflammatory T(H)17 cells. Nature. 448, 484–487.

Kramer, S., Schimpl, A., Hunig, T., 1995. Immunopathology of interleukin (IL) 2-deficient mice: thymus dependence and suppression by thymus-dependent cells with an intact IL-2 gene. J. Exp. Med. 182, 1769–1776.

Kuchroo, V.K., Martin, C.A., Greer, J.M., Ju, S.T., Sobel, R.A., Dorf, M.E., 1993. Cytokines and adhesion molecules contribute to the ability of myelin proteolipid protein-specific T cell clones to mediate experimental allergic encephalomyelitis. J. Immunol. 151, 4371–4382.

Kullberg, M.C., Jankovic, D., Feng, C.G., Hue, S., Gorelick, P.L., McKenzie, B.S., et al., 2006. IL-23 plays a key role in Helicobacter hepaticus-induced T cell-dependent colitis. J. Exp. Med. 203, 2485–2494.

Kumar, M., Putzki, N., Limmroth, V., Remus, R., Lindemann, M., Knop, D., et al., 2006. CD4+CD25+FoxP3+ T lymphocytes fail to suppress myelin basic protein-induced proliferation in patients with multiple sclerosis. J. Neuroimmunol. 180, 178–184.

Lafaille, J.J., 1998. The role of helper T cell subsets in autoimmune diseases. Cytokine Growth Factor Rev. 9, 139–151.

Langrish, C.L., Chen, Y., Blumenschein, W.M., Mattson, J., Basham, B., Sedgwick, J.D., et al., 2005. IL-23 drives a pathogenic T cell population that induces autoimmune inflammation. J. Exp. Med. 201, 233–240.

Laurence, A., Tato, C.M., Davidson, T.S., Kanno, Y., Chen, Z., Yao, Z., et al., 2007. Interleukin-2 signaling via STAT5 constrains T helper 17 cell generation. Immunity 26, 371–381.

Lee, Y.K., Turner, H., Maynard, C.L., Oliver, J.R., Chen, D., Elson, C. O., et al., 2009. Late developmental plasticity in the T helper 17 lineage. Immunity. 30, 92–107.

Lee, Y., Awasthi, A., Yosef, N., Quintana, F.J., Xiao, S., Peters, A., et al., 2012. Induction and molecular signature of pathogenic T(H) 17 cells. Nat. Immunol 13, 991–999.

Leonardi, C., Matheson, R., Zachariae, C., Cameron, G., Li, L., Edson-Heredia, E., et al., 2012. Anti-interleukin-17 monoclonal antibody ixekizumab in chronic plaque psoriasis. N. Engl. J. Med. 366, 1190–1199.

Liang, B., Workman, C., Lee, J., Chew, C., Dale, B.M., Colonna, L., et al., 2008. Regulatory T cells inhibit dendritic cells by lymphocyte activation gene-3 engagement of MHC class II. J. Immunol. 180, 5916–5926.

Liang, S.C., Tan, X.Y., Luxenberg, D.P., Karim, R., Dunussi-Joannopoulos, K., Collins, M., et al., 2006. Interleukin (IL)-22 and IL-17 are coexpressed by Th17 cells and cooperatively enhance expression of antimicrobial peptides. J. Exp. Med. 203, 2271–2279.

Lin, W., Truong, N., Grossman, W.J., Haribhai, D., Williams, C.B., Wang, J., et al., 2005. Allergic dysregulation and hyperimmunoglobulinemia E in Foxp3 mutant mice. J. Allergy Clin. Immunol. 116, 1106–1115.

Liu, S.M., Lee, D.H., Sullivan, J.M., Chung, D., Jager, A., Shum, B. O., et al., 2011. Differential IL-21 signaling in APCs leads to disparate Th17 differentiation in diabetes-susceptible NOD and diabetes-resistant NOD.Idd3 mice. J. Clin. Invest. 121, 4303–4310.

Liu, X., Leung, S., Wang, C., Tan, Z., Wang, J., Guo, T.B., et al., 2010. Crucial role of interleukin-7 in T helper type 17 survival and expansion in autoimmune disease. Nat. Med. 16, 191–197.

Liu, X., Nurieva, R.I., Dong, C., 2013. Transcriptional regulation of follicular T-helper (Tfh) cells. Immunol. Rev. 252, 139–145.

Liu, X., Yan, X., Zhong, B., Nurieva, R.I., Wang, A., Wang, X., et al., 2012. Bcl6 expression specifies the T follicular helper cell program in vivo. J. Exp. Med. 209 (1841–1852), S1–S24.

Liu, Y., Helms, C., Liao, W., Zaba, L.C., Duan, S., Gardner, J., et al., 2008. A genome-wide association study of psoriasis and psoriatic arthritis identifies new disease loci. PLoS Genet. 4, e1000041.

Luther, S.A., Tang, H.L., Hyman, P.L., Farr, A.G., Cyster, J.G., 2000. Coexpression of the chemokines ELC and SLC by T zone stromal cells and deletion of the ELC gene in the plt/plt mouse. Proc. Natl. Acad. Sci. USA 97, 12694–12699.

Luzina, I.G., Atamas, S.P., Storrer, C.E., Dasilva, L.C., Kelsoe, G., Papadimitriou, J.C., et al., 2001. Spontaneous formation of germinal centers in autoimmune mice. J. Leukoc. Biol. 70, 578–584.

Ma, J., Zhu, C., Ma, B., Tian, J., Baidoo, S.E., Mao, C., et al., 2012. Increased frequency of circulating follicular helper T cells in patients with rheumatoid arthritis. Clin. Dev. Immunol. 2012, 827480.

Mack, C.L., Vanderlugt-Castaneda, C.L., Neville, K.L., Miller, S.D., 2003. Microglia are activated to become competent antigen presenting and effector cells in the inflammatory environment of the Theiler's virus model of multiple sclerosis. J. Neuroimmunol. 144, 68–79.

MacLennan, I.C., Gulbranson-Judge, A., Toellner, K.M., Casamayor-Palleja, M., Chan, E., Sze, D.M., et al., 1997. The changing preference of T and B cells for partners as T-dependent antibody responses develop. Immunol. Rev. 156, 53–66.

Malek, T.R., Yu, A., Vincek, V., Scibelli, P., Kong, L., 2002. CD4 regulatory T cells prevent lethal autoimmunity in IL-2Rbeta-deficient mice. Implications for the nonredundant function of IL-2. Immunity 17, 167–178.

Manel, N., Unutmaz, D., Littman, D.R., 2008. The differentiation of human T(H)-17 cells requires transforming growth factor-beta and induction of the nuclear receptor RORgammat. Nat. Immunol. 9, 641–649.

Mangan, P.R., Harrington, L.E., O'Quinn, D.B., Helms, W.S., Bullard, D.C., Elson, C.O., et al., 2006. Transforming growth factor-b induces development of Th17 lineage. Nature 441, 231–234.

Matthys, P., Vermeire, K., Mitera, T., Heremans, H., Huang, S., Billiau, A., 1998. Anti-IL-12 antibody prevents the development and progression of collagen-induced arthritis in IFN-gamma receptor-deficient mice. Eur. J. Immunol. 28, 2143–2151.

Matthys, P., Vermeire, K., Mitera, T., Heremans, H., Huang, S., Schols, D., et al., 1999. Enhanced autoimmune arthritis in IFN-gamma receptor-deficient mice is conditioned by mycobacteria in Freund's adjuvant and by increased expansion of Mac-1+ myeloid cells. J. Immunol. 163, 3503–3510.

Matusevicius, D., Kivisakk, P., He, B., Kostulas, N., Ozenci, V., Fredrikson, S., et al., 1999. Interleukin-17 mRNA expression in blood and CSF mononuclear cells is augmented in multiple sclerosis. Mult. Scler. 5, 101–104.

McGeachy, M.J., Bak-Jensen, K.S., Chen, Y., Tato, C.M., Blumenschein, W., McClanahan, T., et al., 2007. TGF-beta and IL-6 drive the production of IL-17 and IL-10 by T cells and restrain T(H)-17 cell-mediated pathology. Nat. Immunol. 8, 1390–1397.

McGeachy, M.J., Chen, Y., Tato, C.M., Laurence, A., Joyce-Shaikh, B., Blumenschein, W.M., et al., 2009. The interleukin 23 receptor is essential for the terminal differentiation of interleukin 17-producing effector T helper cells in vivo. Nat. Immunol. 10, 314–324.

Mcmahon, E.J., Bailey, S.L., Castenada, C.V., Waldner, H., Miller, S.D., 2005. Epitope spreading initiates in the CNS in two mouse models of multiple sclerosis. Nat. Med. 11, 335–339.

Miyara, M., Yoshioka, Y., Kitoh, A., Shima, T., Wing, K., Niwa, A., et al., 2009. Functional delineation and differentiation dynamics of human CD4 T cells expressing the FoxP3 transcription factor. Immunity. 30, 899–911.

Morita, R., Schmitt, N., Bentebibel, S.E., Ranganathan, R., Bourdery, L., Zurawski, G., et al., 2011. Human blood CXCR5(+)CD4(+) T cells are counterparts of T follicular cells and contain specific subsets that differentially support antibody secretion. Immunity 34, 108–121.

Mosmann, T.R., Cherwinski, H., Bond, M.W., Giedlin, M.A., Coffman, R.L., 1986. Two types of murine helper T cell clone. I. Definition according to profiles of lymphokine activities and secreted proteins. J. Immunol. 136, 2348–2357.

Mosmann, T.R., Coffman, R.L., 1989a. Heterogeneity of cytokine secretion patterns and functions of helper T cells. Adv. Immunol. 46, 111–1147.

Mosmann, T.R., Coffman, R.L., 1989b. TH1 and TH2 cells: different patterns of lymphokine secretion lead to different functional properties. Annu. Rev. Immunol. 7, 145–173.

Mucida, D., Cheroutre, H., 2010. The many face-lifts of CD4 T helper cells. Adv. Immunol. 107, 139–152.

Mucida, D., Park, Y., Kim, G., Turovskaya, O., Scott, I., Kronenberg, M., et al., 2007. Reciprocal TH17 and regulatory T cell differentiation mediated by retinoic acid. Science 317, 256–260.

Mueller, R., Krahl, T., Sarvetnick, N., 1996. Pancreatic expression of interleukin-4 abrogates insulitis and autoimmune diabetes in nonobese diabetic (NOD) mice. J. Exp. Med. 184, 1093–1099.

Nakae, S., Nambu, A., Sudo, K., Iwakura, Y., 2003. Suppression of immune induction of collagen-induced arthritis in IL-17-deficient mice. J. Immunol. 171, 6173–6177.

Nakanishi, K., Yoshimoto, T., Tsutsui, H., Okamura, H., 2001. Interleukin-18 regulates both Th1 and Th2 responses. Annu. Rev. Immunol. 19, 423–474.

Neighbors, M., Xu, X., Barrat, F.J., Ruuls, S.R., Churakova, T., Debets, R., et al., 2001. A critical role for interleukin 18 in primary and memory effector responses to Listeria monocytogenes that extends beyond its effects on Interferon gamma production. J. Exp. Med. 194, 343–354.

Neurath, M.F., Finotto, S., Glimcher, L.H., 2002. The role of Th1/Th2 polarization in mucosal immunity. Nat. Med. 8, 567–573.

Nishizuka, Y., Sakakura, T., 1969. Thymus and reproduction: sex-linked dysgenesia of the gonad after neonatal thymectomy in mice. Science. 166, 753–755.

Nurieva, R., Yang, X.O., Martinez, G., Zhang, Y., Panopoulos, A.D., Ma, L., et al., 2007. Essential autocrine regulation by IL-21 in the generation of inflammatory T cells. Nature. 448, 480–483.

Nurieva, R.I., Chung, Y., Hwang, D., Yang, X.O., Kang, H.S., Ma, L., et al., 2008. Generation of T follicular helper cells is mediated by interleukin-21 but independent of T helper 1, 2, or 17 cell lineages. Immunity 29, 138−149.

Nurieva, R.I., Chung, Y., Martinez, G.J., Yang, X.O., Tanaka, S., Matskevitch, T.D., et al., 2009a. Bcl6 mediates the development of T follicular helper cells. Science 325, 1001−1005.

Nurieva, R.I., Liu, X., Dong, C., 2009b. Yin-Yang of costimulation: crucial controls of immune tolerance and function. Immunol. Rev. 229, 88−100.

O'Reilly, S., Hugle, T., Van Laar, J.M., 2012. T cells in systemic sclerosis: a reappraisal. Rheumatology (Oxford). 51, 1540−1549.

Oh, H., Ghosh, S., 2013. NF-kappaB: roles and regulation in different CD4(+) T-cell subsets. Immunol. Rev. 252, 41−51.

Ohkura, N., Hamaguchi, M., Morikawa, H., Sugimura, K., Tanaka, A., Ito, Y., et al., 2012. T cell receptor stimulation-induced epigenetic changes and Foxp3 expression are independent and complementary events required for Treg cell development. Immunity. 37, 785−799.

Onishi, Y., Fehervari, Z., Yamaguchi, T., Sakaguchi, S., 2008. Foxp3+ natural regulatory T cells preferentially form aggregates on dendritic cells in vitro and actively inhibit their maturation. Proc. Natl. Acad. Sci. USA 105, 10113−10118.

Oppmann, B., Lesley, R., Blom, B., Timans, J.C., Xu, Y., Hunte, B., et al., 2000. Novel p19 protein engages IL-12p40 to form a cytokine, IL-23, with biological activities similar as well as distinct from IL-12. Immunity 13, 715−725.

Ozenci, V., Kouwenhoven, M., Huang, Y.M., Xiao, B., Kivisakk, P., Fredrikson, S., et al., 1999. Multiple sclerosis: levels of interleukin-10-secreting blood mononuclear cells are low in untreated patients but augmented during interferon-beta-1b treatment. Scand. J. Immunol. 49, 554−561.

Pandiyan, P., Zheng, L., Ishihara, S., Reed, J., Lenardo, M.J., 2007. CD4 + CD25 + Foxp3 + regulatory T cells induce cytokine deprivation-mediated apoptosis of effector CD4+ T cells. Nat. Immunol. 8, 1353−1362.

Papiernik, M., De Moraes, M.L., Pontoux, C., Vasseur, F., Penit, C., 1998. Regulatory CD4 T cells: expression of IL-2R alpha chain, resistance to clonal deletion and IL-2 dependency. Int. Immunol. 10, 371−378.

Papp, K.A., Langley, R.G., Lebwohl, M., Krueger, G.G., Szapary, P., Yeilding, N., et al., 2008. Efficacy and safety of ustekinumab, a human interleukin-12/23 monoclonal antibody, in patients with psoriasis: 52-week results from a randomised, double-blind, placebo-controlled trial (PHOENIX 2). Lancet. 371, 1675−1684.

Parham, C., Chirica, M., Timans, J., Vaisberg, E., Travis, M., Cheung, J., et al., 2002. A receptor for the heterodimeric cytokine IL-23 is composed of IL-12Rbeta1 and a novel cytokine receptor subunit, IL-23R. J. Immunol. 168, 5699−5708.

Paul, W.E., Zhu, J., 2010. How are T(H)2-type immune responses initiated and amplified? Nat. Rev. Immunol. 10, 225−235.

Pot, C., Apetoh, L., Awasthi, A., Kuchroo, V.K., 2011a. Induction of regulatory Tr1 cells and inhibition of T(H)17 cells by IL-27. Semin. Immunol. 23, 438−445.

Pot, C., Apetoh, L., Kuchroo, V.K., 2011b. Type 1 regulatory T cells (Tr1) in autoimmunity. Semin. Immunol. 23, 202−208.

Pot, C., Jin, H., Awasthi, A., Liu, S.M., Lai, C.Y., Madan, R., et al., 2009. Cutting edge: IL-27 induces the transcription factor c-Maf, cytokine IL-21, and the costimulatory receptor ICOS that coordinately act together to promote differentiation of IL-10-producing Tr1 cells. J. Immunol. 183, 797−801.

Powrie, F., Mason, D., 1990. OX-22high CD4 + T cells induce wasting disease with multiple organ pathology: prevention by the OX-22low subset. J. Exp. Med. 172, 1701−1708.

Pulendran, B., Artis, D., 2012. New paradigms in type 2 immunity. Science 337, 431−435.

Quintana, F.J., Basso, A.S., Iglesias, A.H., Korn, T., Farez, M.F., Bettelli, E., et al., 2008. Control of T(reg) and T(H)17 cell differentiation by the aryl hydrocarbon receptor. Nature 453, 65−71.

Qureshi, O.S., Zheng, Y., Nakamura, K., Attridge, K., Manzotti, C., Schmidt, E.M., et al., 2011. Trans-endocytosis of CD80 and CD86: a molecular basis for the cell-extrinsic function of CTLA-4. Science 332, 600−603.

Ramgolam, V.S., Sha, Y., Jin, J., Zhang, X., Markovic-Plese, S., 2009. IFN-beta inhibits human Th17 cell differentiation. J. Immunol. 183, 5418−5427.

Ramiscal, R.R., Vinuesa, C.G., 2013. T-cell subsets in the germinal center. Immunol. Rev. 252, 146−155.

Roncarolo, M.G., Gregori, S., Lucarelli, B., Ciceri, F., Bacchetta, R., 2011. Clinical tolerance in allogeneic hematopoietic stem cell transplantation. Immunol. Rev. 241, 145−163.

Rutz, S., Noubade, R., Eidenschenk, C., Ota, N., Zeng, W., Zheng, Y., et al., 2011. Transcription factor c-Maf mediates the TGF-beta-dependent suppression of IL-22 production in T(H)17 cells. Nat. Immunol. 12, 1238−1245.

Saadoun, D., Rosenzwajg, M., Joly, F., Six, A., Carrat, F., Thibault, V., et al., 2011. Regulatory T-cell responses to low-dose interleukin-2 in HCV-induced vasculitis. N. Engl. J. Med. 365, 2067−2077.

Sagoo, P., Lombardi, G., Lechler, R.I., 2008. Regulatory T cells as therapeutic cells. Curr. Opin. Organ Transplant. 13, 645−653.

Sakaguchi, S., Fukuma, K., Kuribayashi, K., Masuda, T., 1985. Organ-specific autoimmune diseases induced in mice by elimination of T cell subset. I. Evidence for the active participation of T cells in natural self-tolerance; deficit of a T cell subset as a possible cause of autoimmune disease. J. Exp. Med. 161, 72−87.

Sakaguchi, S., Sakaguchi, N., Asano, M., Itoh, M., Toda, M., 1995. Immunologic self-tolerance maintained by activated T cells expressing IL-2 receptor alpha-chains (CD25). Breakdown of a single mechanism of self-tolerance causes various autoimmune diseases. J. Immunol. 155, 1151−1164.

Sandborn, W.J., Feagan, B.G., Fedorak, R.N., Scherl, E., Fleisher, M.R., Katz, S., et al., 2008. A randomized trial of Ustekinumab, a human interleukin-12/23 monoclonal antibody, in patients with moderate-to-severe Crohn's disease. Gastroenterology 135, 1130−1141.

Saruta, M., Yu, Q.T., Fleshner, P.R., Mantel, P.Y., Schmidt-Weber, C.B., Banham, A.H., et al., 2007. Characterization of FOXP3 + CD4 + regulatory T cells in Crohn's disease. Clin. Immunol. 125, 281−290.

Schmidl, C., Klug, M., Boeld, T.J., Andreesen, R., Hoffmann, P., Edinger, M., et al., 2009. Lineage-specific DNA methylation in T cells correlates with histone methylation and enhancer activity. Genome Res. 19, 1165−1174.

Schoenborn, J.R., Wilson, C.B., 2007. Regulation of interferon-gamma during innate and adaptive immune responses. Adv. Immunol. 96, 41−101.

Schorle, H., Holtschke, T., Hunig, T., Schimpl, A., Horak, I., 1991. Development and function of T cells in mice rendered interleukin-2 deficient by gene targeting. Nature 352, 621–624.

Schreiner, B., Bailey, S.L., Miller, S.D., 2007. T-cell response dynamics in animal models of multiple sclerosis: implications for immunotherapies. Exp. Rev. Clin. Immunol. 3, 57–72.

Schraml, B.U., Hildner, K., Ise, W.L., Lee, W.L., Smith, W.A., Solomon, B., et al., 2009. The AP-1 transcription factor Batf controls T(H)17 differentiation. Nature. 460, 405–409.

Setoguchi, R., Hori, S., Takahashi, T., Sakaguchi, S., 2005. Homeostatic maintenance of natural Foxp3(+) CD25(+) CD4(+) regulatory T cells by interleukin (IL)-2 and induction of autoimmune disease by IL-2 neutralization. J. Exp. Med. 201, 723–735.

Sewell, D., Qing, Z., Reinke, E., Elliot, D., Weinstock, J., Sandor, M., et al., 2003. Immunomodulation of experimental autoimmune encephalomyelitis by helminth ova immunization. Int. Immunol. 15, 59–69.

Shi, G., Cox, C.A., Vistica, B.P., Tan, C., Wawrousek, E.F., Gery, I., 2008. Phenotype switching by inflammation-inducing polarized Th17 cells, but not by Th1 cells. J. Immunol. 181, 7205–7213.

Shi, L.Z., Wang, R., Huang, G., Vogel, P., Neale, G., Green, D.R., et al., 2011. HIF1alpha-dependent glycolytic pathway orchestrates a metabolic checkpoint for the differentiation of TH17 and Treg cells. J. Exp. Med. 208, 1367–1376.

Singh, R.R., Saxena, V., Zang, S., Li, L., Finkelman, F.D., Witte, D. P., et al., 2003. Differential contribution of IL-4 and STAT6 vs STAT4 to the development of lupus nephritis. J. Immunol. 170, 4818–4825.

Smith, C.E., Miller, S.D., 2006. Multi-peptide coupled-cell tolerance ameliorates ongoing relapsing EAE associated with multiple pathogenic autoreactivities. J. Autoimmun. 27, 218–231.

Staudt, V., Bothur, E., Klein, M., Lingnau, K., Reuter, S., Grebe, N., et al., 2010. Interferon-regulatory factor 4 is essential for the developmental program of T helper 9 cells. Immunity. 33, 192–202.

Summers, R.W., Elliott, D.E., Urban Jr., J.F., Thompson, R.A., Weinstock, J.V., 2005. Trichuris suis therapy for active ulcerative colitis: a randomized controlled trial. Gastroenterology. 128, 825–832.

Suscovich, T.J., Perdue, N.R., Campbell, D.J., 2012. Type-1 immunity drives early lethality in scurfy mice. Eur. J. Immunol. 42, 2305–2310.

Suzuki, H., Kundig, T.M., Furlonger, C., Wakeham, A., Timms, E., Matsuyama, T., et al., 1995. Deregulated T cell activation and autoimmunity in mice lacking interleukin-2 receptor beta. Science 268, 1472–1476.

Sweeney, C.M., Lonergan, R., Basdeo, S.A., Kinsella, K., Dungan, L.S., Higgins, S.C., et al., 2011. IL-27 mediates the response to IFN-beta therapy in multiple sclerosis patients by inhibiting Th17 cells. Brain Behav. Immun. 25, 1170–1181.

Szabo, S.J., Sullivan, B.M., Peng, S.L., Glimcher, L.H., 2003. Molecular mechanisms regulating Th1 immune responses. Annu. Rev. Immunol. 21, 713–758.

Takahashi, M., Nakamura, K., Honda, K., Kitamura, Y., Mizutani, T., Araki, Y., et al., 2006. An inverse correlation of human peripheral blood regulatory T cell frequency with the disease activity of ulcerative colitis. Dig. Dis. Sci. 51, 677–686.

Teunissen, M.B., Koomen, C.W., Malefyt, D.e.W.a.a.l., Wierenga, R., Bos, J.D., E.A., 1998. Interleukin-17 and interferon-gamma synergize in the enhancement of proinflammatory cytokine production by human keratinocytes. J. Invest. Dermatol. 111, 645–649.

Thornton, A.M., Donovan, E.E., Piccirillo, C.A., Shevach, E.M., 2004. Cutting edge: IL-2 is critically required for the in vitro activation of CD4+ CD25+ T cell suppressor function. J. Immunol. 172, 6519–6523.

Thornton, A.M., Shevach, E.M., 1998. CD4 + CD25 + immunoregulatory T cells suppress polyclonal T cell activation in vitro by inhibiting interleukin 2 production. J. Exp. Med. 188, 287–296.

Trembleau, S., Penna, G., Gregori, S., Giarratana, N., Adorini, L., 2003. IL-12 administration accelerates autoimmune diabetes in both wild-type and IFN-gamma-deficient nonobese diabetic mice, revealing pathogenic and protective effects of IL-12-induced IFN-gamma. J. Immunol. 170, 5491–5501.

Vandenbroeck, K., 2012. Cytokine gene polymorphisms and human autoimmune disease in the era of genome-wide association studies. J. Interferon Cytokine Res. 32, 139–151.

Veldhoen, M., Hirota, K., Westendorf, A.M., Buer, J., Dumoutier, L., Renauld, J.C., et al., 2008a. The aryl hydrocarbon receptor links TH17-cell-mediated autoimmunity to environmental toxins. Nature 453, 106–109.

Veldhoen, M., Hocking, R.J., Atkins, C.J., Locksley, R.M., Stockinger, B., 2006. TGFbeta in the context of an inflammatory cytokine milieu supports de novo differentiation of IL-17-producing T cells. Immunity 24, 179–189.

Veldhoen, M., Uyttenhove, C., Van Snick, J., Helmby, H., Westendorf, A., Buer, J., et al., 2008b. Transforming growth factor-beta "reprograms" the differentiation of T helper 2 cells and promotes an interleukin 9-producing subset. Nat. Immunol. 9, 1341–1346.

Viegas, M.S., Do Carmo, A., Silva, T., Seco, F., Serra, V., Lacerda, M., et al., 2007. CD38 plays a role in effective containment of mycobacteria within granulomata and polarization of Th1 immune responses against Mycobacterium avium. Microbes Infect. 9, 847–854.

Viglietta, V., Baecher-Allan, C., Weiner, H.L., Hafler, D.A., 2004. Loss of functional suppression by CD4+ CD25+ regulatory T cells in patients with multiple sclerosis. J. Exp. Med. 199, 971–979.

Vinuesa, C.G., Cook, M.C., 2011. Blood relatives of follicular helper T cells. Immunity 34, 10–12.

Wan, Y.Y., Flavell, R.A., 2009. How diverse-CD4 effector T cells and their functions. J. Mol. Cell Biol. 1, 20–36.

Wei, G., Wei, L., Zhu, J., Zang, C., Hu-Li, J., Yao, Z., et al., 2009. Global mapping of H3K4me3 and H3K27me3 reveals specificity and plasticity in lineage fate determination of differentiating CD4 + T cells. Immunity 30, 155–167.

Weinstock, J.V., Elliott, D.E., 2013. Translatability of helminth therapy in inflammatory bowel diseases. Int. J. Parasitol. 43, 245–251.

Wildin, R.S., Ramsdell, F., Peake, J., Faravelli, F., Casanova, J.L., Buist, N., et al., 2001. X-linked neonatal diabetes mellitus, enteropathy and endocrinopathy syndrome is the human equivalent of mouse scurfy. Nat. Genet. 27, 18–20.

Wing, J.B., Sakaguchi, S., 2012. Multiple treg suppressive modules and their adaptability. Front. Immunol. 3, 178.

Wing, K., Onishi, Y., Prieto-Martin, P., Yamaguchi, T., Miyara, M., Fehervari, Z., et al., 2008. CTLA-4 control over Foxp3 + regulatory T cell function. Science 322, 271–275.

Wolk, K., Witte, E., Witte, K., Warszawska, K., Sabat, R., 2010. Biology of interleukin-22. Semin. Immunopathol. 32, 17–31.

Wu, C., Yosef, N., Thalhamer, T., Zhu, C., Xiao, S., Kishi, Y., et al., 2013. Induction of pathogenic Th17 cells by inducible salt-sensing kinase SGK1. Nature 496, 513—517.

Wu, H.J., Ivanov, I.i., Darce, J., Hattori, K., Shima, T., Umesaki, Y., et al., 2010. Gut-residing segmented filamentous bacteria drive autoimmune arthritis via T helper 17 cells. Immunity 32, 815—827.

Yamane, H., Paul, W.E., 2013. Early signaling events that underlie fate decisions of naive CD4(+) T cells toward distinct T-helper cell subsets. Immunol. Rev. 252, 12—23.

Yang, L., Anderson, D.E., Baecher-Allan, C., Hastings, W.D., Bettelli, E., Oukka, M., et al., 2008a. IL-21 and TGF-beta are required for differentiation of human T(H)17 cells. Nature 454, 350—352.

Yang, X.O., Panopoulos, A.D., Nurieva, R., Chang, S.H., Wang, D., Watowich, S.S., et al., 2007. STAT3 regulates cytokine-mediated generation of inflammatory helper T cells. J. Biol. Chem. 282, 9358—9363.

Yang, X.O., Pappu, B.P., Nurieva, R., Akimzhanov, A., Kang, H.S., Chung, Y., et al., 2008b. T helper 17 lineage differentiation is programmed by orphan nuclear receptors ROR alpha and ROR gamma. Immunity 28, 29—39.

Yin, L., Yu, M., Edling, A.E., Kawczak, J.A., Mathisen, P.M., Nanavati, T., et al., 2001. Pre-emptive targeting of the epitope spreading cascade with genetically modified regulatory T cells during autoimmune demyelinating disease. J. Immunol. 167, 6105—6112.

Yosef, N., Shalek, A.K., Gaublomme, J.T., Jin, H., Lee, Y., Awasthi, A., et al., 2013. Dynamic regulatory network controlling T17 cell differentiation. Nature 496, 461—468.

Zhang, H.L., Azimullah, S., Zheng, X.Y., Wang, X.K., Amir, N., Mensah-Brown, E.P., et al., 2012. IFN-gamma deficiency exacerbates experimental autoimmune neuritis in mice despite a mitigated systemic Th1 immune response. J. Neuroimmunol. 246, 18—26.

Zhang, X., Ing, S., Fraser, A., Chen, M., Khan, O., Zakem, J., et al., 2013. Follicular helper T cells: new insights into mechanisms of autoimmune diseases. Ochsner J. 13, 131—139.

Zheng, W., Flavell, R.A., 1997. The transcription factor GATA-3 is necessary and sufficient for Th2 cytokine gene expression in CD4 T cells. Cell 89, 587—596.

Zheng, Y., Chaudhry, A., Kas, A., Deroos, P., Kim, J.M., Chu, T.T., et al., 2009. Regulatory T-cell suppressor program co-opts transcription factor IRF4 to control T(H)2 responses. Nature. 458, 351—356.

Zheng, Y., Danilenko, D.M., Valdez, P., Kasman, I., Eastham-Anderson, J., Wu, J., et al., 2007. Interleukin-22, a T(H)17 cytokine, mediates IL-23-induced dermal inflammation and acanthosis. Nature 445, 648—651.

Zheng, Y., Josefowicz, S., Chaudhry, A., Peng, X.P., Forbush, K., Rudensky, A.Y., 2010. Role of conserved non-coding DNA elements in the Foxp3 gene in regulatory T-cell fate. Nature. 463, 808—812.

Zhou, L., Littman, D.R., 2009. Transcriptional regulatory networks in Th17 cell differentiation. Curr. Opin. Immunol. 21, 146—152.

Zhou, L., Ivanov, I.I., Spolski, R., Min, R., Shenderov, K., Egawa, T., et al., 2007. IL-6 programs T(H)-17 cell differentiation by promoting sequential engagement of the IL-21 and IL-23 pathways. Nat. Immunol. 8, 967—974.

Zhou, L., Lopes, J.E., Chong, M.M., Ivanov, I.i., Min, R., Victora, G.D., et al., 2008. TGF-beta-induced Foxp3 inhibits T(H)17 cell differentiation by antagonizing RORgammat function. Nature 453, 236—240.

Zhou, X., Bailey-Bucktrout, S.L., Jeker, L.T., Penaranda, C., Martinez-Llordella, M., Ashby, M., et al., 2009. Instability of the transcription factor Foxp3 leads to the generation of pathogenic memory T cells in vivo. Nat. Immunol. 10, 1000—1007.

Zhu, J., Min, B., Hu-Li, J., Watson, C.J., Grinberg, A., Wang, Q., et al., 2004. Conditional deletion of Gata3 shows its essential function in T(H)1-T(H)2 responses. Nat. Immunol. 5, 1157—1165.

Zielinski, C.E., Mele, F., Aschenbrenner, D., Jarrossay, D., Ronchi, F., Gattorno, M., et al., 2012. Pathogen-induced human TH17 cells produce IFN-gamma or IL-10 and are regulated by IL-1beta. Nature 484, 514—518.

Chapter 7

Immunological Tolerance—T Cells

Sara R. Hamilton, Sarah Q. Crome, and Pamela S. Ohashi

Campbell Family Institute, Ontario Cancer Institute, Departments of Medical Biophysics and Immunology, Toronto, ON, Canada

Chapter Outline

Early Studies Supporting the Induction of Tolerance 87
Thymic Tolerance 87
    Brief Overview of Thymocyte Development 87
    Mechanisms of Thymic Tolerance 88
        Clonal Deletion 88
        Anergy as a Mechanism for Self-Tolerance 89
        Thymic Development of Regulatory T Cells Maintain Tolerance 89
    Expression of Tissue-Restricted Antigens in the Thymus 90
Peripheral Tolerance 90
    Impact of Dendritic Cells 91
        Dendritic Cells: Directors of Peripheral Immune Tolerance 91
        Molecular Programming of Resting DCs is Critical for Preventing Autoimmunity 92
    Mechanisms of Peripheral Tolerance 93
        Clonal Deletion 93
        Anergy as a Mechanism of Peripheral Tolerance 94
        Ignorance 94
        Induced Regulatory T Cells and the Maintenance of Peripheral Tolerance 94
        Negative Regulatory Mechanisms that Impact Tolerance 96
    Expression of Tissue-Specific Antigens by Lymph Node Stromal Cells 96
Concluding Remarks 97
Acknowledgments 97
References 97

EARLY STUDIES SUPPORTING THE INDUCTION OF TOLERANCE

Some of the earliest evidence for immune tolerance came from studies examining the epidemiology of lymphochoriomeningitis virus (LCMV), a natural, non-cytopathic mouse pathogen. Traub observed that mice infected with LCMV *in utero* became lifelong carriers of the virus without producing significant quantities of anti-virus neutralizing antibodies (Traub, 1936, 1938). This observation suggested that a host could become tolerant to foreign antigens, as long as they had been "seen" early enough in development. A study published by Ray Owen in 1945 supported this idea. He found that non-identical twins became hematopoietic chimeras *in utero* and, as a result, they remained tolerant to antigens expressed on the other's red blood cells (Owen, 1945). In 1953, a transplant surgeon by the name of Peter Medawar extended Owen's observations by noting that non-identical twin cattle could also accept skin grafts from each other, suggesting that this tolerance was maintained throughout the life of the non-identical twins. In 1953, Medawar et al. provided the most compelling evidence for immunological tolerance to date. In this study they injected allogeneic blood cells from one inbred mouse strain into newborn mice from a different inbred strain. They found that the donor blood cells engrafted, resulting in lifelong chimerism such that the recipient mice demonstrated significant tolerance to skin grafts that was specific for the foreign tissue antigens encountered neonatally (Billingham et al., 1953). Medawar went on to describe this phenomenon as actively acquired tolerance. The importance of actively acquired tolerance was highlighted in 1960 when Medawar shared the Nobel Prize in medicine with Frank MacFarlane Burnet for their collective work in acquired tolerance.

THYMIC TOLERANCE

Brief Overview of Thymocyte Development

The development of immature thymocytes into mature T cells can be followed by the expression of the cell surface

N. Rose & I. Mackay (Eds): The Autoimmune Diseases, Fifth edition. DOI: http://dx.doi.org/10.1016/B978-0-12-384929-8.00007-1

proteins CD4 and CD8 (Figure 7.1a). Initially, bone marrow-derived progenitors that enter the thymus do not express CD4 or CD8 and are referred to as CD4⁻CD8⁻ double negative (DN) thymocytes. Following T cell receptor (TCR) β chain rearrangement, only thymocytes expressing a functionally rearranged TCRβ chain continue to mature. These thymocytes then upregulate both CD4 and CD8 to become CD4⁺CD8⁺ double positive (DP) thymocytes. At this DP stage, TCRα chain rearrangement is initiated and functionally rearranged TCRα chains are expressed on the cell surface with the TCRβ chain. The production of TCRα and TCRβ chains involves random rearrangement of gene segments, and, together with the additional diversity created by the rearrangement process, gives rise to thymocytes that have the potential to recognize a wide array of antigens including self-molecules (Starr et al., 2003). Thymocytes expressing TCRs that are unable to productively engage self-major histocompatibility complex (MHC) molecules die within a few days (death by neglect). Thymocytes expressing a TCR that is able to interact with low to intermediate affinity with self-MHC molecules are rescued from death and instead undergo positive selection (Shearer, 1974; Zinkernagel & Doherty, 1974). However, a strong interaction between the TCR and self-MHC molecules leads to the elimination of self-reactive thymocytes by a process referred to as negative selection (clonal deletion) (Werlen et al., 2003).

Mechanisms of Thymic Tolerance

Several events that occur in the thymus are critical for establishing and maintaining tolerance. Thymocytes that express receptors that are capable of recognizing self-antigens may undergo clonal deletion or clonal inactivation (anergy). In addition, an important subset of T cells known as regulatory T cells (Tregs) are selected in the thymus. These cells are essential for limiting the function of autoreactive cells and preventing the onset of autoimmunity.

Clonal Deletion

One of the major processes that occurs during thymocyte development is the elimination of many autoreactive T cells via clonal deletion. While clonal deletion had long been proposed to be a mechanism of self-tolerance, it wasn't until the generation of TCR-specific antibodies that Kappler et al. were able to provide the first definitive evidence of this (Kappler et al., 1987). Using a monoclonal antibody specific for the Vβ17 segment of the TCR, they showed that Vβ17⁺ T cells react with the class II MHC molecule I-E and are not present in the periphery of mice expressing I-E. They further found that immature DP thymocytes expressing the Vβ17⁺ I-E reactive TCR were present in the

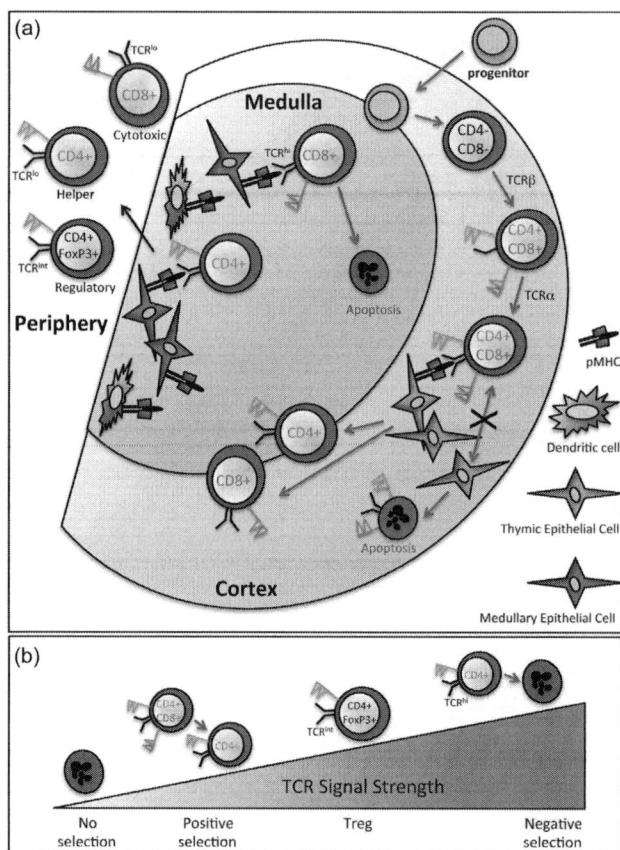

FIGURE 7.1 Thymocyte development in the thymus. (a) The development of thymocytes into mature T cells can be followed by the expression of surface markers including CD4 and CD8. Bone marrow-derived progenitors that enter the thymus do not express either CD4 or CD8 and are referred to as CD4⁻CD8⁻ double negative cells. Thymocytes expressing a functionally rearranged TCRβ chain upregulate both CD4 and CD8 to become CD4⁺CD8⁺ double positive thymocytes. At this CD4⁺CD8⁺ DP stage, TCRα chain rearrangement is initiated and functionally arranged TCRα chains are expressed on the cell surface with the TCRβ chain. The diverse array of TCRs now expressed by the developing thymocytes interact with self-MHC molecules expressed by thymic epithelial cells in a process referred to as positive selection. During this stage of development, thymocytes that do not interact with self-MHC molecules undergo apoptosis within a few days (death by neglect), while thymocytes that express TCRs able to functionally interact with self-MHC molecules with low to intermediate affinity are rescued from death and instead continue on in development to become CD4⁺ or CD8⁺ single positive thymocytes. However, thymocytes that bind to self-MHC molecules with high affinity are deleted in a process called negative selection. (b) The random rearrangements resulting in the TCRα and β chains result in a TCR repertoire with an array of specificities, and the affinity of the TCR with self-MHC determines the fate of the developing thymocytes. Those with TCRs not able to recognize or bind to self-peptides presented by self-MHC (pMHC) do not receive any signal through their TCR and die within a few days via apoptosis (death by neglect). Cells that receive extremely strong signals through their TCR due to high affinity interactions with self-MHC are deleted during negative selection so as to eliminate potentially autoreactive T cells. Thymocytes with TCRs that can recognize and bind to self-MHC with low to intermediate affinities (do not recognize "self") during positive selection finish development and enter the periphery as mature, naïve T cells. T cells with high affinity TCRs that survive negative selection differentiate into CD4⁺FoxP3⁺ regulatory T cells (Tregs).

thymus of I-E$^+$ mice suggesting that the I-E reactive thymocytes were deleted at later stages of development.

Further evidence for clonal deletion was provided by the use of TCR transgenic mice (Kisielow et al., 1988). In this model, the TCRα and β chains were taken from a CD8$^+$ T cell clone that was specific for the male antigen H-Y presented by the MHC class I molecule H-2D^b. In female transgenic mice, the H-Y specific CD8$^+$ T cells were positively selected by H-2D^b. However, there was a striking reduction in the number of DP thymocytes and mature CD8$^+$ T cells in the male mice suggesting that H-Y-specific thymocytes were negatively selected during the DP stage of development. Many subsequent studies using monoclonal antibodies and TCR transgenic models supported the principle of clonal deletion as a key mechanism of tolerance (MacDonald et al., 1988; Sha et al., 1988; Pircher et al., 1989).

Anergy as a Mechanism for Self-Tolerance

In addition to clonal deletion, anergy has been proposed as an alternative mechanism of self-tolerance. The term anergy describes a T cell that is present but unable to respond to its cognate antigen because of earlier exposure to the same antigen (Nossal, 1983). Ramsdell et al. developed a novel model that supported anergy as a mechanism of thymic tolerance *in vivo* by following the induction of T cell tolerance to a minor antigen known as Mls-1^a. The Mls (minor lymphocyte stimulating) group of molecules was originally described by Hilliard Festenstein and these antigens were later shown to be derived from endogenous retroviruses (Festenstein and Kimura, 1988; Frankel et al., 1991; Marrack et al., 1991). Fowlkes' group generated chimeric mice in which Mls-1^b bone marrow was transplanted into irradiated Mls-1^a/Mls-1^b hybrid recipients (Ramsdell et al., 1989). The recipient bone marrow cells are sensitive to irradiation while the thymic epithelial cells are resistant, leading to the selective depletion of the bone marrow in the irradiated recipient. Thus, in the resulting chimeras, expression of the tolerizing Mls-1^a was limited to the thymic stroma. They found that the Mls-1^a reactive Vβ6$^+$ T cells, which were normally deleted in an Mls-1^a host, could mature and were found in the periphery. However, these mature Vβ6$^+$ T cells were unresponsive to activation by either Mls-1^a antigen or activating monoclonal antibodies, therefore demonstrating that T cells could be rendered unresponsive to antigen in the thymus and that anergy could be an alternative mechanism of self-tolerance.

Thymic Development of Regulatory T Cells Maintain Tolerance

Early work by many groups supported the presence of a population of cells known as the suppressor T cell that could inhibit immune responses. However, in-depth molecular studies disputed the existence of this subset (Shevach, 2002). Nonetheless, strong evidence remained that a population of cells existed that could negatively regulate immunity, and this population was "reborn" as the Treg. Tregs (Figure 7.1a, b) develop in the thymus when CD4$^+$ T cells receive a relatively strong signal that is below the threshold required to induce deletion (Feuerer et al., 2009). Thymus-derived Tregs are a cell population that prevents autoimmunity and plays an important role in modulating inflammatory immune responses. Early work found that neonatal thymectomy of some inbred lab rodent strains led to the development of autoimmunity (Nishizuka & Sakakura, 1969; Penhale et al., 1973), which eventually led to the identification of a subset of cells that could protect against autoimmunity. These studies showed that transfer of naïve CD4$^+$ T cells into immunodeficient rats resulted in autoimmune diabetes and inflammatory bowel disease but that this autoimmunity could be blocked by the co-transfer of CD4$^+$ T cells that expressed memory T cell surface markers (Powrie & Mason, 1990). This work was extended to mice when it was found that transfer of CD4$^+$CD25$^-$ T cells into young BALB/c mice resulted in autoimmune inflammation in several tissues, which could be suppressed with co-transfer of CD4$^+$CD25$^+$ T cells (Sakaguchi et al., 1995).

One key discovery in the field identified a gene that was critical for the development of Tregs by studying autoimmune disorders of mice and humans. FoxP3 was identified as the essential transcription factor required for the differentiation of CD4$^+$CD25$^+$ Tregs (Brunkow et al., 2001), and was shown to be the mutation that drives an autoimmune phenotype in scurfy mice. Importantly, FoxP3 mutations were also identified in patients with the severe and potentially fatal inflammatory disorder Immune dysregulation, Polyendocrinopathy, Enteropathy, X-linked (IPEX) syndrome (Chatila et al., 2000; Bennett et al., 2001; Wildin et al., 2001). Clinical symptoms vary between patients but commonly include type 1 diabetes, enteropathy, and eczema (Ochs et al., 2005). Subsequently, FoxP3$^+$ thymus-derived Tregs, referred to as natural Tregs (nTregs), have been shown to suppress autoimmunity, allergy, and inflammation (Fontenot et al., 2003; Hori et al., 2003; Allan et al., 2005).

During T cell selection in the thymus, variations in TCR signaling events are central for T cell lineage fate determinations. It is therefore not surprising that there are particular requirements in TCR signaling for the induction of FoxP3 expression and Treg lineage commitment. Direct evidence indicating that Tregs are exposed to high affinity TCR signals came from studies using transgenic mice expressing a TCR specific for myelin basic protein in the absence of any endogenous TCR rearrangements

(RAG deficient). These mice developed inflammatory lesions in the brain, while a subset of T cell expressing endogenous TCRs was able to prevent this inflammatory disease in RAG-sufficient mice (Lafaille et al., 1994; Olivares-Villagomez et al., 1998). These studies and others point to a critical role of TCR specificity in the development of nTregs. In addition to TCR stimulation, CD28 costimulation is important for the differentiation and peripheral survival of nTregs as Treg frequencies are significantly reduced in CD28 or CD80/CD86-deficient mice (Salomon et al., 2000).

Expression of Tissue-Restricted Antigens in the Thymus

Negative selection of T cells in the thymus is essential for the elimination of self-reactive T cells during development. However, one of the conceptual caveats associated with negative selection was how T cells could be tolerized in the thymus to self-antigens expressed by tissues outside the thymus. This led to the possibility that negative selection would be incapable of establishing tolerance to self-antigens that are expressed only in peripheral tissues; for example, insulin in the pancreas. However, it has become increasingly clear that cells of the thymic stroma, originally dubbed "peripheral antigen expressing cells" (Jolicoeur et al., 1994; Smith et al., 1997), can express tissue-specific antigens (TSAs) to facilitate negative selection of autoreactive T cells. While it has since been shown that the thymic medullary epithelial cells (mTECs) express a wide array of self-antigens (Derbinski et al., 2001, 2005), it was still not known how this was regulated.

Work done by human molecular geneticists led to the discovery of a novel gene called the autoimmune regulator (AIRE). Mutations in this gene were responsible for a disorder called autoimmune polyendocrinopathy-candidiasis ectodermal dystrophy (APECED) or autoimmune polyendocrinopathy syndrome (APS-1), which is characterized by the progressive development of multiple, organ-specific autoimmune diseases (Aaltonen & Consortium, 1997; Nagamine et al., 1997). Initial analyses of AIRE indicated that it functioned by binding DNA based on the presence of conserved domains and clustering of disease-inducing mutations within those domains (Aaltonen & Consortium, 1997; Nagamine et al., 1997; Bjorses et al., 2000). Later, AIRE expression was shown in mTECs, suggesting a role for AIRE in regulating tolerance in the thymus, either by maintaining normal thymic architecture or by regulating interactions with T cells undergoing negative selection (Heino et al., 1999). Finally, studies showed that AIRE existed primarily as a nuclear protein in the mTECs (Aaltonen & Consortium, 1997; Nagamine et al., 1997; Heino et al., 1999), suggesting that it may ultimately be functioning as a transcription factor. Since both AIRE and peripheral tissue antigens were expressed in mTECs, it was speculated and later confirmed that AIRE is a transcription factor that controls the expression of many TSAs.

To further study the function of AIRE and its role in tolerance, two independent groups generated AIRE-deficient mice (Anderson et al., 2002; Ramsey et al., 2002). Similar to what was seen in the human disease setting, these mice developed spontaneous, organ-specific autoimmune disease, characterized by lymphocytic infiltrates and autoantibodies directed against a variety of peripheral organs and tissues including the salivary gland, retina, stomach, thyroid, and ovaries. These mice had no defects in T cell subsets or T cell function and the use of bone marrow chimeras and thymus grafts demonstrated that while AIRE expression in the radio-resistant cells of the thymic stroma was crucial for negative selection, loss of AIRE in the hematopoietic compartment did not significantly affect autoimmunity (Anderson et al., 2002). Having demonstrated that AIRE expression in the thymus was critical for the prevention of autoimmunity, Anderson et al. went on to show that AIRE promotes the expression of a multitude of TSAs in the mTECs. Accordingly, AIRE-deficient mice were shown to have severely disrupted expression of a variety of tissue-restricted antigens in the mTECs, which resulted in defective negative selection of tissue-specific T cells (Liston et al., 2003). However, it is also worth noting that the AIRE does not control the expression of all TSAs.

More recently, a transgenic mouse was made where AIRE expression can be repressed with the administration of doxycycline (Guerau-de-Arellano et al., 2009). This study found that perinatal expression of AIRE was crucial for its role in tolerance as these mice only developed autoimmunity if AIRE expression was repressed before the pups were weaned. Conversely, loss of AIRE expression after 21 days of age did not result in autoimmunity.

Therefore, AIRE can contribute to central tolerance by driving the expression of tissue-specific antigens to provide negatively selecting ligands to developing self-reactive thymocytes.

PERIPHERAL TOLERANCE

Not all self-reactive thymocytes are deleted during development and, as a consequence, various peripheral tolerance mechanisms are in place to control self-reactive T cells (Figure 7.2a, b). Perhaps the most compelling evidence for peripheral tolerance comes from studies exploring the importance of Tregs. Elimination of Tregs results in autoimmune disease demonstrating that there are a multitude of self-reactive T cells that must be kept in

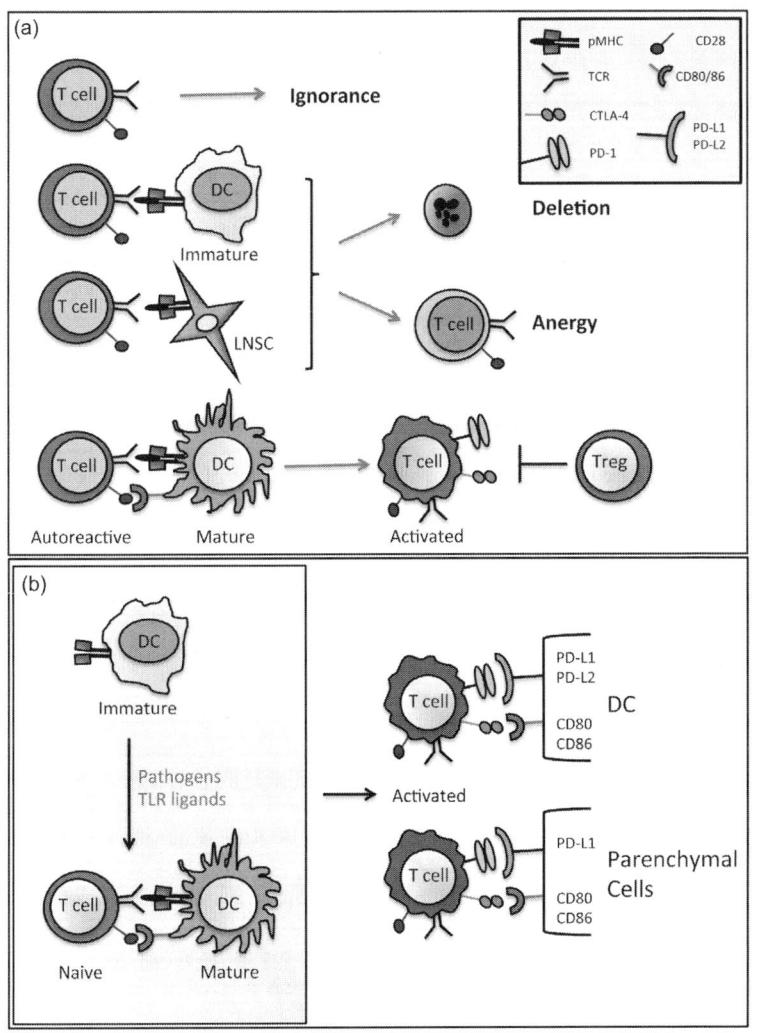

FIGURE 7.2 Mechanisms of peripheral tolerance. (a) Not all self-reactive thymocytes are deleted in the thymus during central tolerance and as a consequence, peripheral tolerance mechanisms have evolved that allow mature T cells to be eliminated or rendered unresponsive to self-antigens to avoid autoimmunity. CD4$^+$FoxP3$^+$ Tregs can inhibit the activation or activity of activated, autoreactive T cells via a variety of mechanisms. Alternatively, if a T cell encounters antigen presented on a resting dendritic cell (DCs) or TSAs presented on lymph node stromal cells, the autoreactive T cells can be deleted or rendered unresponsive or anergic. If naïve, autoreactive T cells do not encounter antigen then they remain ignorant. (b) Interactions between naïve T cells and mature DCs is essential for both the initiation of an effective immune response as well as inducing tolerance. Engagement of Toll-like receptors, for example, on DCs leads to their maturation, which includes the upregulation of B7 family members such as B7-1/CD80 and B7-2/CD86. These are able to bind to the costimulatory receptor CD28 expressed on the surface of naïve T cells, leading to T cell activation. Coinhibitory receptors such as CTLA-4 and PD-1 are upregulated on the surface of activated T cells. CTLA-4 competitively binds to the B7-1 and B7-2 with higher affinity than CD28, thus contributing to the inhibition of active T cells. PD-1 binds to PD-L1 (B7-H1) and PD-L2 (B7-DC), which also sends an inhibitory signal to activated T cells. B7 family members are expressed on a variety of cells to contribute to immune homeostasis including DCs and tissue parenchymal cells.

check. This section will describe the various mechanisms that maintain self-tolerance, including deletion, anergy, ignorance, as well as control by suppressor cell populations such as Tregs. Importantly, one of the pivotal cells that regulates the decision between T cell tolerance and activation is the dendritic cell (DC). Therefore, DC biology plays a critical role in the induction and maintenance of tolerance.

Impact of Dendritic Cells

Dendritic Cells: Directors of Peripheral Immune Tolerance

In the thymus, engagement of high affinity TCR and peptide/MHC (pMHC) interactions generally lead to clonal deletion or anergy, while strong TCR signals in mature T cells are required to induce an effective immune response. How, then, can a mature T cell distinguish between a TCR-specific interaction that leads to activation vs.

tolerance? Solving this problem holds tremendous potential for solving clinical problems such as transplant rejection, autoimmunity, and tumor immunology.

Early work suggested that the induction of an immune response required the presence of adjuvants such as lipopolysaccharide (LPS). When LPS (a component from Gram-negative bacteria) was given with antigen *in vivo*, a functional immune response was induced, while antigen administered in the absence of LPS resulted in tolerance induction (Dresser, 1961; Claman, 1963). Further work studying allograft rejection and tolerance led to the "passenger leukocyte concept," which suggested that APCs from the donor were critical for eliciting graft rejection (Lafferty & Cunningham, 1975; Talmage et al., 1976; Lafferty et al., 1983). Other models proposed that the adaptive immune system is induced by two signals, an antigen-specific signal 1 with a costimulatory signal 2. This model predicted that signal 1 alone led to the induction of tolerance. The discovery of CD28, a T cell costimulatory receptor constitutively expressed on the surface of most T cells, fulfilled the role of signal 2 (Linsley et al., 1990; Harding et al., 1992).

DCs have been shown to be the key APC that can activate T cells (Steinman & Cohn, 1973). Groundbreaking work by many groups has demonstrated that adjuvants such as LPS can cause DCs to mature, via receptors known as the Toll-like receptors (TLRs) (Medzhitov et al., 1997; Poltorak et al., 1998; Akira et al., 2006). DC maturation is now known to occur downstream of many stimuli, such as NOD-like receptor (NLR) or RIG-like receptor stimulation. Various studies subsequently demonstrated that the maturation state of the DC determines the outcome of T cell tolerance vs. activation (Figure 7.2a, b) (Garza et al., 2000; Dhodapkar et al., 2001; Hawiger et al., 2001). TCR-specific interactions between resting DCs and T cells result in tolerance (anergy and/or deletion), while antigens encountered on mature DCs induce immunity. Importantly, upon DC maturation, a number of molecules including the ligands for CD28, CD80 (B7-1), and CD86 (B7-2), are upregulated, which contributes to optimal T cell activation (Figure 7.2b) (Linsley et al., 1990; Azuma et al., 1993; Freeman et al., 1993; Steinman et al., 2003). Additionally, DC maturation invokes the upregulation of other costimulatory and coinhibitory ligands that control T cell activation, as well as the induction of proinflammatory cytokines such as IL-12, IFNs, TNF, and chemokines, which all impact the function, survival, and migration of cells of the adaptive immune response (Reis e Sousa, 2006; Iwasaki & Medzhitov, 2010; Kawai & Akira, 2010).

Molecular Programming of Resting DCs is Critical for Preventing Autoimmunity

Previous evidence suggested that resting DCs were a default state and that adaptive immunity was controlled by various signals that led to DC maturation. However, recent studies have provided compelling evidence that the resting or immature DC state is programmed by molecular pathways. Perturbing these pathways by removing negative regulatory molecules leads to an altered DC state that is able to activate T cell responses and contribute to autoimmunity *in vivo* (Figure 7.3).

The first evidence that DCs are not tolerogenic by default, but are instead actively maintained in a resting state, came from a study investigating the functions of NF-κB1 in DCs (Dissanayake et al., 2011). NF-κB1 belongs to a family of transcription factors that are critical regulators of both the innate and adaptive immune systems (Vallabhapurapu & Karin, 2009). This family is composed of homo- and heterodimeric protein complexes containing RelA, RelB, c-Rel, as well as p50 and p52 which are processed by the proteasome from the precursor proteins NF-κB1 and NF-κB2, respectively. In unstimulated cells, NF-κB complexes are sequestered in the cytoplasm by inhibitory IκB proteins. NF-κB activating signals trigger the degradation of IκB allowing NF-κB to translocate to the nucleus. The function of NF-κB1 in DCs was of particular interest as it has linked to both the initiation and inhibition of gene transcription. Upon TLR stimulation, NF-κB1 p50 can heterodimerize with p65 to promote the transcription of proinflammatory genes

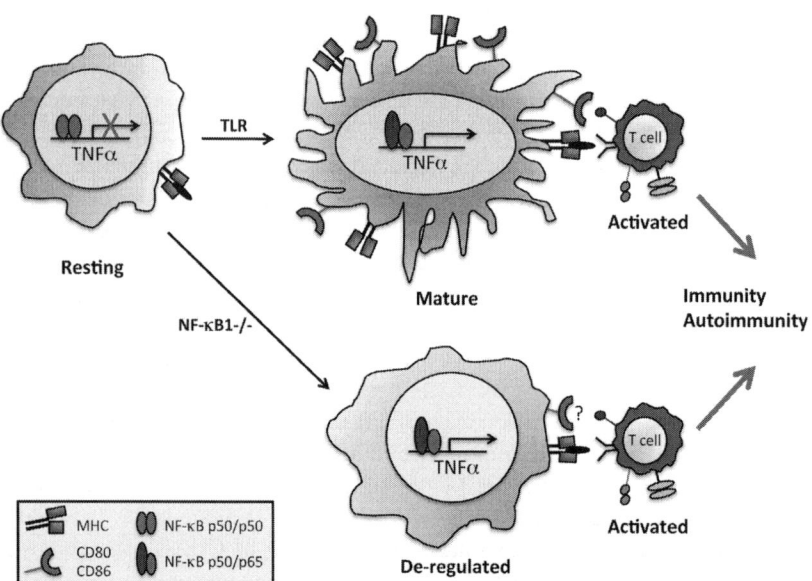

Resting   TLR   **Mature**   **Activated**

NF-κB1-/-   **De-regulated**   **Activated**

Immunity Autoimmunity

MHC   NF-κB p50/p50
CD80 CD86   NF-κB p50/p65

FIGURE 7.3 **Molecular programming of resting DCs.** Resting DCs can mature in response to a variety of stimuli including pathogens or other TLR ligands. After maturation, DCs upregulate several cell surface receptors including MHC and B7 family members such as CD80 and CD86. Mature DCs can contribute to autoimmunity, in part through the activation of autoreactive T cells. Alternatively, if the molecular programs that normally maintain DCs in their resting state are perturbed then these deregulated DCs can also interact with autoreactive T cells to induce autoimmunity. An example of this is NF-κB1. In normal, resting DCs, the p50–p50 homodimers act as transcriptional repressors and prevent the expression of proinflammatory cytokines such as TNF-α. However, in the absence of NF-κB1, the repressive p50 homodimers are lost and p50–p65 heterodimers are now able to bind the TNF-α promoter to induce its expression, ultimately resulting in the induction of autoimmunity.

(Sha et al., 1995). Conversely, p50 is also found in transcriptionally repressive homodimers in many unstimulated cells, including DCs (Carmody et al., 2007).

Ohashi et al. developed a novel *in vivo* system that can evaluate the role of defined pathways and genes in DC function in which the induction of CD8$^+$ T cell-mediated autoimmunity is dependent upon self-antigen presentation by DCs that have been matured by TLR stimulation (Dissanayake et al., 2011). Using this model they found that NFκ-B1-deficient DCs do not require TLR-induced maturation to initiate self-reactive CTL activity *in vivo*. These "immature" NF-κB1-deficient DCs did not express increased levels of classic DC maturation markers (CD80/CD86/CD40) or IL-12. Furthermore, the immature NF-κB1-deficient DCs spontaneously expressed TNF-α, which is normally seen only after maturation. Ultimately, these DCs were able to induce autoimmunity *in vivo*, suggesting that NF-κB1 is required to maintain DCs in a quiescent state. The importance of these findings may be highlighted by an identified polymorphism in the NF-κB binding site on the TNF promoter region (Udalova et al., 2000) that results in reduced binding by p50 homodimers. This polymorphism has been linked to autoimmune disease in humans including type 1 diabetes (Seki et al., 1999; Li et al., 2008; Stayoussef et al., 2010) and may be the result of aberrant DC maturation leading to activation of autoreactive T cells.

The idea that DCs are actively maintained in a resting state was supported by other studies that found that the absence of the ubiquitin-editing molecule A20 in DCs also resulted in spontaneous DC maturation resulting in activation and expansion of CD8$^+$ T cells and autoimmunity (Hammer et al., 2011; Kool et al., 2011).

A20 is an ubiquitin-binding protein that also has deubiquitinating and E3 ligase activity. It is upregulated in most cell types in response to proinflammatory cytokines and can inhibit the activation of NF-κB in response to TNF-α or IL-1 (Jaattela et al., 1996; Song et al., 1996). In addition to TNF-α-mediated inflammation, A20 can restrict activating signals from TLRs and NLRs, as well as from CD40, by limiting NF-κB signaling (Lee et al., 2000; Wertz et al., 2004). A20-deficient mice spontaneously develop a lethal, multi-organ inflammatory condition and die perinatally (Lee et al., 2000). Additionally, these mice were extremely sensitive to other inflammatory stimuli, as well as sub-lethal doses of TNF-α, IL-1, or LPS. These studies have clearly established A20 as a critical negative regulator of NF-κB that is essential in the maintenance of immune homeostasis. Given the critical role for A20 in restricting diverse activating signals that are important for DC maturation, a conditional knockout in which only the DCs are A20 deficient was generated to determine if DC-derived A20 was important for regulating immune homeostasis (Hammer et al., 2011).

This study demonstrated spontaneous maturation and activation of A20-deficient DCs, as well as the spontaneous development of lymphocyte-dependent colitis, seronegative ankylosing arthritis, and enthesitis, conditions that mimic inflammatory bowel disease (IBD) in humans, suggesting that A20 in DCs is required to retain them in their quiescent state, preventing spontaneous autoimmunity. Again, the importance of these findings may be highlighted by the identification of single-nucleotide polymorphisms (SNPs) in the human A20 gene, which have been associated with several human autoimmune diseases, including systemic lupus erythematosus, rheumatoid arthritis, psoriasis, and celiac disease (Plenge et al., 2007; Musone et al., 2008; Elder, 2009; Trynka et al., 2009). The identification of these mutations suggests that altered A20 function contributes to autoimmunity.

Collectively, these studies identify intrinsic factors within DCs that are programmed to inhibit the ability of the DC to activate the adaptive immune system. They further demonstrate that the functions of DCs are regulated even in the absence of external stimulation and that the removal of these repressive mechanisms can result in the activation of autoreactive T lymphocytes.

Mechanisms of Peripheral Tolerance

Clonal Deletion

If T cells recognize antigens presented by resting DCs, tolerance may occur by clonal deletion (Figure 7.2a). This mechanism of peripheral tolerance was demonstrated *in vivo* by a number of different groups. Collectively, these studies showed that TCR stimulation of mature, peripheral T cells in the absence of costimulatory and proinflammatory signals results in several rounds of proliferation. This proliferative burst is short-lived, however, and tolerance is ultimately induced. Either the daughter cells were deleted or they failed to form into fully functional helper, cytotoxic T cells or memory cells.

In one of the earliest studies analyzing peripheral T cell tolerance, Mls-1^a-expressing splenocytes were infused into thymectomized Mls-1^b mice (Webb et al., 1990). The Mls-1^a reactive Vβ6$^+$ T cells initially expanded but were eliminated from the T cell repertoire. Studies looking at T cell responses to exogenous antigens such as Staphylococcal enterotoxin B (SEB) found similar observations (Kawabe & Ochi, 1990). Collectively, these studies suggested that while exposure of T cells to exogenous antigens in the absence of microbial or adjuvant costimulation resulted in limited T cell activation, the response was generally aborted and ultimately led to the deletion of reactive cells.

Further studies using transgenic models showed that self-antigen specific T cells were tolerized by presentation of self-antigen in lymph nodes that drain particular tissues. For example, in a study by Kurts et al., OVA-specific CD8$^+$ T cells were transferred into recipients expressing a membrane-bound form of the OVA antigen on their pancreatic islet cells and in the kidneys (Kurts et al., 1997, 1998). The OVA-specific T cells underwent expansion in the pancreatic and kidney draining lymph nodes where they had encountered antigen cross-presented by immature DCs. Additionally, the expanded OVA-specific CD8$^+$ T cells displayed an active phenotype and had CTL activity. Nevertheless, the OVA-specific T cells were subsequently almost entirely deleted from the T cell repertoire, demonstrating deletion as a mechanism of peripheral tolerance. Importantly, these studies demonstrated that cross-presentation of self-antigens *in vivo* leads to cross-tolerance.

Anergy as a Mechanism of Peripheral Tolerance

While engagement of the TCR on mature T cells with cognate antigen in the periphery can result in deletion, some antigen-specific T cells remain in the peripheral T cell repertoire in a hyporesponsive state (Figure 7.2a). The first direct evidence for anergy as a tolerance mechanism came from *in vitro* studies in which antigens expressed on chemically fixed APCs were used to induce T cell anergy. These studies found that when T cells were incubated with high concentrations of their cognate peptide antigens in the absence of APCs, the T cells became unresponsive to restimulation with the same antigen presented by stimulatory APCs. However, these hyporesponsive T cells could be rescued through the addition of exogenous IL-2, a cytokine known to drive T cell proliferation (Jenkins & Schwartz, 1987; Mueller et al., 1989).

This *in vitro* work was extended to *in vivo* models by a number of groups. Rammensee et al. transferred Mls-1^a-expressing cells into Mls-1^b positive recipients (Rammensee et al., 1989). After the initial expansion and deletion of the Mls-1^a-reactive Vβ6$^+$ T cells, the authors noted that Vβ6$^+$ T cells remained in the periphery but were unable to respond to restimulation by Mls-1^a antigen. In the early 1990s, Rocha et al. furthered this work by utilizing the male-specific antigen (H-Y). Rocha et al. transferred H-Y-specific CD8$^+$ T cells isolated from female TCR transgenic mice into nude male mice (Rocha and von Boehmer, 1991). After deletion of most of these cells in the male recipients, the authors noted that any H-Y-specific T cells that remained in the peripheral repertoire failed to respond to restimulation with male cells or anti-H-Y TCR antibodies, suggesting that they had been inactivated. They also noted that if these anergic T cells were transferred into female mice that do not express the H-Y antigen, the anergic T cells recovered and could now

respond to and proliferate in response to antigen. This suggested that anergy induced during tolerance requires persistent exposure to antigen.

Ignorance

Not all autoreactive T cells are deleted or inactivated in the thymus or in the periphery. Instead, if T cells are unable to detect self-antigen then they may remain in the peripheral repertoire in an "ignorant" state (Figure 7.2a) (Ohashi et al., 1991; Oldstone et al., 1991).

Ignorance was first clearly demonstrated by Ohashi et al., in which a viral glycoprotein (LCMV-gp) was expressed in the pancreatic islet cells under the control of the rat insulin promoter (RIP-gp) (Ohashi et al., 1991). These mice were crossed to the P14 TCR transgenic mice, expressing a TCR specific for the LCMV-gp. Examination of the mature T cell repertoire in both the RIP-gp and P14/RIP-gp mice clearly showed that the islet-specific T cells were not deleted in the thymus or tolerized in the periphery. Despite the presence of mature, islet-specific T cells in these mice, they did not develop spontaneous autoimmunity. However, LCMV infection of either RIP-gp or P14/RIP-gp mice resulted in the induction of diabetes, due to the activation and cytotoxic activity of the LCMV-gp-specific CD8$^+$ T cells. Other studies have shown similar results in which autoimmunity can be induced by immunizing animals with tissue-specific antigens in the presence of adjuvant, leading to the activation of autoreactive T cells (Kuchroo et al., 2002). Collectively, these studies suggest that T cells are not all tolerized in the presence of antigen and instead may remain "ignorant." Immunological ignorance may be a consequence of undetectable or low levels of self-antigen presentation (Kurts et al., 1999).

Induced Regulatory T Cells and the Maintenance of Peripheral Tolerance

FoxP3$^+$ Tregs were originally identified as a population of cells that arise in the thymus. However, it is now appreciated that Tregs also develop in the periphery from naïve CD4$^+$ T cells and are commonly referred to as induced Tregs (iTregs) (Josefowicz et al., 2012). While the essential role for nTregs in the control of dysregulated immune responses has been well characterized, the role of iTregs has been harder to understand, in part due to the existence of subsets of iTregs that are distinct in both their development and mechanisms of action. While both nTregs and iTregs limit inflammation, several key differences have been reported.

Several specialized subsets of iTregs have been identified, the best characterized of which are FoxP3$^+$ iTregs and the IL-10-producing type 1 Tregs (Tr1). Tr1 cells were first described in severe combined immunode-ficient SCID patients who had long-term tolerance to stem cell allografts but have since been described in a variety of settings (Battaglia et al., 2006) and their importance in tolerance is well appreciated. Tr1 cells develop when a naïve T cell encounters a tolerogenic APC in the presence of IL-10 (Levings et al., 2005) and function through the inhibition of T cells and other immune cells in an IL-10 and TGF-β-dependent manner. Currently Tr1 cells are defined by their cytokine pro-files. These cells express exceptionally high levels of IL-10, an immunosuppressive cytokine that is critical in the maintenance of tolerance, and are a central mediator of cytokine-dependent immune regulation in both humans and mice (Bacchetta et al., 1994; Groux et al., 1997; Roncarolo et al., 2006). In addition to IL-10 and TGF-β, Tr1 cells express low levels of IL-2 and variable levels of IL-5 and IFN-γ (Gregori et al., 2012). In con-trast to FOXP3$^+$ iTregs, Tr1 cells only transiently express FOXP3 following activation (Allan et al., 2008), a phenomenon observed in all human CD4$^+$ T cells (Allan et al., 2007). Although Tr1 cells require TCR activation to acquire suppressive function, they are able to mediate "bystander suppression" against cells that recognize other antigens. Tr1 cells specific for self-antigens can be isolated in a variety of settings including desmoglein3 in pemphigus patients (Veldman et al., 2004) and islet antigens in diabetes patients (Tree et al., 2010). Foreign antigen-specific Tr1 cells have also been observed in celiac disease and allergy patients (Cavani et al., 2000; Akdis et al., 2004; Gianfrani et al., 2006; Meiler et al., 2008).

FoxP3$^+$ iTregs are phenotypically and functionally similar to thymus-derived nTregs. While they may only contribute minimally to peripheral tolerance under homeostatic conditions (Almeida et al., 2006; Wong et al., 2007), FoxP3$^+$ iTregs are a natural consequence of protective immunity and develop in parallel to that of effector CD4$^+$ T cells. The resulting FoxP3$^+$ iTregs likely control the escalating T effector cell responses and limit damage to tissues (Kang et al., 2007). These cells express typical nTreg markers including FoxP3, CD25 and TGF-β (Tran et al., 2007; Horwitz et al., 2008). However, surface expression of Helios on nTregs may differentiate them from FoxP3$^+$ iTregs (Thornton et al., 2010). FoxP3$^+$ iTregs suppress a wide variety of immune cells including naïve and memory CD4$^+$ and CD8$^+$ T cells, B cells, monocytes, and DCs (Lin et al., 2002, Lim et al., 2005; Miyara & Sakaguchi, 2007; Tiemessen et al., 2007). Therefore, while many different subsets of Tregs have been described, they likely work together to maintain immune homeostasis. It is also clear that both nTregs and iTregs contribute to the induction and mainte-nance of tolerance.

FoxP3 expression appears to be induced at particularly high levels at mucosal sites, possibly due to the presence of specialized tolerogenic DCs and cytokines. CTLA-4, which is not required for nTreg differentiation, is required for TGF-β-mediated induction of FoxP3 expression in vitro (Zheng et al., 2006). Conversely, CD28 cross-linking was shown to inhibit FoxP3 expression (Kim & Rudensky, 2006; Benson et al., 2007). Collectively, these studies indicate that high-affinity TCR signaling, in con-junction with suboptimal costimulation, favors induction of FoxP3 expression and conversion of peripheral CD4$^+$ T cells into iTregs.

The cytokine environment is also important for devel-opment of iTregs. TGF-β is able to induce FoxP3 expres-sion in CD4$^+$ T cells in vitro and in vivo (Chen et al., 2003; Selvaraj & Geiger, 2007). However, there is debate as to whether TGF-β alone converts naïve CD4$^+$ T cells into stable iTregs. There is also a subset of peripheral CD4$^+$FoxP3-negative cells that upregulate FoxP3 in response to IL-2 alone (Schallenberg et al., 2010) and many studies have determined that IL-2 cooperation with TGF-β promotes the differentiation of stable iTregs in vitro (Davidson et al., 2007; Horwitz et al., 2008). Additionally, retinoic acid, in conjunction with TGF-β and chronic antigen exposure in some tissues promotes iTreg development (Benson et al., 2007). Clearly, the microenvironment is an important contributor to iTreg differentiation.

While the importance of Tregs to immune homeosta-sis is clear, the mechanisms whereby they suppress immune responses have been widely debated (Schmidt et al., 2012). Tregs inhibit the proliferation and inflam-matory cytokine production of effector T cells by both direct and indirect mechanisms and can suppress the activation and maturation of APCs (Allan et al., 2008). While suppression of T cells requires cell contact in vitro, in vivo many mechanisms have been reported including the production of immunoregulatory cytokines IL-10, IL-35, and TGF-β (Ostroukhova et al., 2004; Von Boehmer, 2005; Uhlig et al., 2006; Collison et al., 2007), induction of indoleamine 2,3-dioxygenase in tar-get cells (Fallarino et al., 2003), adenosine (Bopp et al., 2007; Deaglio et al., 2007), and by inducing apoptosis in target cells (Grossman et al., 2004). Additionally, studies have proposed that Tregs consume IL-2 in the local microenvironment, thus depriving effector T cells of IL-2 (Pandiyan et al., 2007). While various molecular mechanisms of suppression have been described, there is so far no agreement on a universal mechanism. It is likely that there are multiple suppressive mechanisms that can be employed by Tregs and will depend on the local microenvironment, the site of the immune reaction, as well as the type and/or activation status of both the Treg and the target cell.

Despite the difficulties in defining their precise mechanism of suppression, the ability of Tregs to dampen harmful immune responses is clear and has led to great interest in utilizing them in cell-based therapies for transplantation and autoimmunity.

Negative Regulatory Mechanisms that Impact Tolerance

Studies have clearly shown that costimulatory and coinhibitory molecules play important roles in both T cell activation and in maintaining peripheral tolerance (Figure 7.2b). CTLA-4, PD-1, and PD-L1-deficient mice all develop spontaneous autoimmune diseases to varying degrees and have been proposed to regulate tolerance through the control of autoreactive T cells (Tivol et al., 1995; Waterhouse et al., 1995; Nishimura et al., 2001; Probst et al., 2005; Schmidt et al., 2009).

Similar to CTLA-4, PD-1 is expressed on mature T cells after activation and is constitutively expressed on Tregs. It has two known ligands, PD-L1 (B7-H1) and PD-L2 (B7-DC). PD-L1 has broad expression and is found on T cells, B cells, DCs, macrophages, as well as non-hematopoietic parenchymal cells. Conversely, PD-L2 expression is limited to macrophages and DCs. Tregs have been shown to express both PD-1 and PD-L1 (Fife & Bluestone, 2008). Signaling through PD-1 blocks the function and survival of effector T cells and expression of PD-L1 on parenchymal cells has been suggested to be important for maintenance of tolerance (Keir et al., 2006). Collectively, these studies suggest that tolerance is maintained, in part, by negative regulation of the immune system.

Figures 7.2 and 7.3 summarize the different mechanisms of peripheral tolerance. If T cells detect antigen, then tolerance may occur through deletion or anergy. If T cells are unable to detect TSAs then T cells may remain ignorant. Therefore, the level of self-antigen can determine the fate of autoreactive T cells. However, tissue-specific T cells can escape both central and peripheral tolerance and can potentially cause autoimmune disease. Autoimmunity may be prevented through the function of Tregs and DCs.

Expression of Tissue-Specific Antigens by Lymph Node Stromal Cells

Peripheral tolerance has been shown to result from cross-presentation of tissue antigens to naïve, self-reactive lymphocytes by quiescent, tissue-resident DCs that migrate to the local lymph node (LN), leading to anergy or deletion (Lukacs-Kornek & Turley, 2011). The prevailing models of peripheral tolerance therefore rely on both resident and incoming DCs to provide the signals for determining activation vs. tolerance and requires trafficking of DCs to peripheral tissue draining LNs or cell-independent transfer of TSAs from organ to LN (Allan et al., 2006; Lukacs-Kornek et al., 2008). However, recent studies have suggested an alternate mechanism of peripheral tolerance in which, similar to the mTECs, the non-hematopoietic stromal cells in secondary lymphoid tissues can present TSAs to induce tolerance (Fletcher et al., 2011).

Like many stromal populations, lymph node stromal cells (LNSCs) were assumed to primarily provide parenchymal support. However in 2007, Lee et al. provided the first evidence of peripheral tolerance mediated by LNSCs (Lee et al., 2007). In this study they used a transgenic model with a truncated OVA protein expressed in the intestinal epithelia under the control of the intestinal fatty acid-binding protein (iFABP) promoter. This study demonstrated that the gut-restricted OVA was ectopically expressed by the LNSCs in non-draining lymph nodes. It further showed that transfer of OVA-specific TCR transgenic CD8$^+$ T cells into these mice resulted in a proliferative burst of the transferred cells followed by their eventual deletion from the peripheral T cell pool. This "activation" of the OVA-specific T cells occurred even in the absence of functional hematopoietic APCs, such as DCs, suggesting that the LNSCs could directly present the OVA antigen to CD8$^+$ T cells. These results were confirmed and extended in subsequent studies (Nichols et al., 2007; Gardner et al., 2008; Cohen et al., 2010). While these earlier studies relied on transgenic antigens expressed under the control of tissue-specific promoters, Cohen et al. went on to evaluate tolerance in response to an endogenous tissue antigen (Cohen et al., 2010). This study examined tolerance to the melanocyte-specific antigen tyrosinase and found that tolerance depended on expression of tyrosinase in non-hematopoietic LNSCs. While tyrosinase mRNA was detected in the thymus, autoreactive T cells were not deleted efficiently when tyrosinase-sufficient thymi were transplanted into tyrosinase-deficient albino mice. Furthermore, tyrosinase was expressed in peripheral LNs, where CD8$^+$ T cell deletion occurred, but not in the spleen. Tyrosinase-specific CD8$^+$ TCR transgenic T cells that were adoptively transferred into tyrosinase-sufficient mice were shown to traffic to LNs, where they were initially activated and subsequently tolerized by LNSCs directly presenting antigen. This study therefore supported the previous conclusions that peripheral tolerance can be induced by expression and direct presentation of TSAs by the LNSCs to CD8$^+$ T cells. This study further demonstrated that tyrosinase-derived antigens were not cross-presented by either radiosensitive DCs or radio-resistant Langerhans cells under steady-state conditions, suggesting that unlike the thymus, classical APCs are not able to cross-present tissue antigens to induce tolerance.

While it is increasingly clear that peripheral tolerance can be induced by LNSCs, the tolerogenic cell type within the LNSC population had not been clearly identified. It was initially assumed that a single, specialized cell type was responsible but collectively these studies have instead demonstrated that this is not the case. For example, in the iFABP-OVA transgenic model, only fibroblastic reticular cells expressed OVA (Lee et al., 2007), whereas Cohen et al. found that only lymphatic endothelial cells directly expressed tyrosinase-derived antigens (Cohen et al., 2010), suggesting that there is no specialized tolerogenic cell type in the LNs. Instead, tolerance induction is a function shared between cells of various lineages that can interact directly with T cells (Fletcher et al., 2011).

LNSCs can express a wide array of tissue antigens but little was known about how their expression was regulated. As was discussed previously, AIRE regulates expression of peripheral tissue antigens in the thymus and as AIRE has also been detected in peripheral tissues (Heino et al., 2000; Kogawa et al., 2002), it was assumed that it was regulating expression of TSAs in the LNSCs. This was initially supported by Gardner et al. who developed a mouse model in which a GFP-fused pancreatic protein (IGRP) was expressed in the *AIRE* locus in a bacterial artificial chromosome (BAC) (Gardner et al., 2008). The authors found expression of AIRE in a population of LNSCs (EpCAM$^+$MHCII$^+$UEA-1-gp38 stromal cells) that did not express costimulatory markers such as CD80 and CD86 but could induce tolerance of transgenic T cells specific for IGRP. Interestingly, this study also demonstrated that AIRE-induced TSAs expressed in mTECs and in extrathymic AIRE-expressing cells are largely distinct, suggesting that AIRE-induced tolerance in the thymus and periphery are not redundant (Gardner et al., 2008; Fletcher et al., 2011). While there is clearly a role for AIRE in driving expression of TSAs in LNSCs, it is increasingly clear that it does not drive expression of all TSAs in the periphery. For example, tolerance to tyrosinase is AIRE-independent (Cohen et al., 2010). In addition to AIRE, deformed epidermal autoregulatory factor 1 (DF1) has also been linked to the expression of tissue antigens in the pancreatic draining LN of aged NOD mice (Yip et al., 2009). Furthermore, DF1 transcripts have been identified in each of the different LNSC populations suggesting a role for it in driving peripheral tolerance (Fletcher et al., 2010).

In addition to mediating deletion of autoreactive T cells through the AIRE-dependent and -independent expression of TSAs, there is also evidence that LNSCs can contribute to peripheral tolerance through the induction of Tregs. For example, LNSCs present in the mesenteric LNs produce retinoic acid, which is known to promote the differentiation of Tregs (Coombes et al., 2007).

Several groups have reported expression of TSAs in peripheral cells other than LNSCs. For example, initial studies on the role of AIRE in tolerance had noted that epithelial cells from tissues other than the thymus can constitutively express tissue-associated antigens and may be tolerogenic (Heino et al., 2000; Kogawa et al., 2002). Furthermore, there is evidence for a tolerogenic role of stromal cell populations outside of the secondary lymphoid compartments. For example, cancer associated fibroblasts (CAFs) are phenotypically similar to gp38$^+$ FRCs found in LNs and are functionally associated with an immunosuppressive microenvironment (Egeblad et al., 2005). Mesenchymal stromal cells, which are found in most tissues, can induce tolerance and reduce inflammation seen in inflammation-associated pathologies such as graft versus host disease (GVHD) and colitis (Tyndall & Uccelli, 2009). Additionally, myofibroblasts found in the colon exhibit a suppressive phenotype in the absence of inflammation (Pinchuk et al., 2008). These cells express PD-L1, PD-L2, and MHCII but lack expression of costimulatory molecules and have been shown *in vitro* to suppress the proliferation of CD4$^+$ T cells (Pinchuk et al., 2008).

Collectively, these studies clearly demonstrate that tolerance can be induced when autoreactive T cells encounter their cognate antigen presented by various LNSC populations and that expression of TSAs by LNSCs was both necessary and sufficient for tolerance induction. They further suggest that induction of peripheral tolerance is a complex process that involves many different cell types.

CONCLUDING REMARKS

While research over the last decades has led to a better understanding of how T cell tolerance is regulated in the thymus and periphery, much remains unknown. As we benefit from the genomics era, a clearer understanding of the molecular pathways that regulate the cellular functions that keep tolerance in check will undoubtedly lead to a detailed understanding of human autoimmunity. Ideally, key discoveries will provide novel strategies to utilize the physiological processes of immunological tolerance to prevent transplant rejection, allergies, and autoimmunity and to promote rejection of tumor cells.

ACKNOWLEDGMENTS

We would like to thank Dylan Johnson and Anne Brüstle for their critical reading of this manuscript. PSO holds a Canada Research Chair in Autoimmunity and Tumor Immunity.

REFERENCES

Aaltonen, J., Consortium, T.F.-G.A., 1997. An autoimmune disease, APECED, caused by mutations in a novel gene featuring two PHD-type zinc-finger domains. Nat. Genet. 17, 399—403.

Akdis, M., Verhagen, J., Taylor, A., Karamloo, F., Karagiannidis, C., Crameri, R., et al., 2004. Immune responses in healthy and allergic individuals are characterized by a fine balance between allergen-specific T regulatory 1 and T helper 2 cells. J. Exp. Med. 199, 1567–1575.

Akira, S., Uematsu, S., Takeuchi, O., 2006. Pathogen recognition and innate immunity. Cell 124, 783–801.

Allan, R.S., Waithman, J., Bedoui, S., Jones, C.M., Villadangos, J.A., Zhan, Y., et al., 2006. Migratory dendritic cells transfer antigen to a lymph node-resident dendritic cell population for efficient CTL priming. Immunity 25, 153–162.

Allan, S.E., Broady, R., Gregori, S., Himmel, M.E., Locke, N., Roncarolo, M.G., et al., 2008. CD4+ T-regulatory cells: toward therapy for human diseases. Immunol. Rev. 223, 391–421.

Allan, S.E., Crome, S.Q., Crellin, N.K., Passerini, L., Steiner, T.S., Bacchetta, R., et al., 2007. Activation-induced FOXP3 in human T effector cells does not suppress proliferation or cytokine production. Int. Immunol. 19, 345–354.

Allan, S.E., Passerini, L., Bacchetta, R., Crellin, N., Dai, M., Orban, P. C., et al., 2005. The role of 2 FOXP3 isoforms in the generation of human CD4+ Tregs. J. Clin. Invest. 115, 3276–3284.

Almeida, A.R., Zaragoza, B., Freitas, A.A., 2006. Competition controls the rate of transition between the peripheral pools of CD4+CD25– and CD4+CD25+ T cells. Int. Immunol. 18, 1607–1613.

Anderson, M.S., Venanzi, E.S., Klein, L., Chen, Z., Berzins, S., Turley, S.J., et al., 2002. Projection of an immunological self-shadow within the thymus by the AIRE protein. Science 298, 1395–1403.

Azuma, M., Ito, D., Yagita, H., Okumura, K., Phillips, J.H., Lanier, L.L., et al., 1993. B70 antigen is a second ligand for CTLA-4 and CD28. Nature 366, 76–79.

Bacchetta, R., Bigler, M., Touraine, J.L., Parkman, R., Tovo, P.A., Abrams, J., et al., 1994. High levels of interleukin 10 production in vivo are associated with tolerance in SCID patients transplanted with HLA mismatched hematopoietic stem cells. J. Exp. Med. 179, 493–502.

Battaglia, M., Gregori, S., Bacchetta, R., Roncarolo, M.G., 2006. Tr1 cells: from discovery to their clinical application. Semin. Immunol. 18, 120–127.

Bennett, C.L., Christie, J., Ramsdell, F., Brunkow, M.E., Ferguson, P.J., Whitesell, L., et al., 2001. The immune dysregulation, polyendocrinopathy, enteropathy, X-linked syndrome (IPEX) is caused by mutations of FOXP3. Nat. Genet. 27, 20–21.

Benson, M.J., Pino-Lagos, K., Rosemblatt, M., Noelle, R.J., 2007. All-trans retinoic acid mediates enhanced T reg cell growth, differentiation, and gut homing in the face of high levels of co-stimulation. J. Exp. Med. 204, 1765–1774.

Billingham, R.E., Brent, L., Medawar, P.B., 1953. Actively acquired tolerance of foreign cells. Nature 172, 603–606.

Bjorses, P., Halonen, M., Palvimo, J.J., Kolmer, M., Aaltonen, J., Ellonen, P., et al., 2000. Mutations in the AIRE gene: effects on subcellular location and transactivation function of the autoimmune polyendocrinopathy-candidiasis-ectodermal dystrophy protein. Am. J. Hum. Genet. 66, 378–392.

Bopp, T., Becker, C., Klein, M., Klein-Hessling, S., Palmetshofer, A., Serfling, E., et al., 2007. Cyclic adenosine monophosphate is a key component of regulatory T cell-mediated suppression. J. Exp. Med. 204, 1303–1310.

Brunkow, M.E., Jeffery, E.W., Hjerrild, K.A., Paeper, B., Clark, L.B., Yasayko, S.A., et al., 2001. Disruption of a new forkhead/winged-helix protein, scurfin, results in the fatal lymphoproliferative disorder of the scurfy mouse. Nat. Genet. 27, 68–73.

Carmody, R.J., Ruan, Q., Palmer, S., Hilliard, B., Chen, Y.H., 2007. Negative regulation of toll-like receptor signaling by NF-kappaB p50 ubiquitination blockade. Science 317, 675–678.

Cavani, A., Nasorri, F., Prezzi, C., Sebastiani, S., Albanesi, C., Girolomoni, G., 2000. Human CD4+ T lymphocytes with remarkable regulatory functions on dendritic cells and nickel-specific Th1 immune responses. J. Invest. Dermatol. 114, 295–302.

Chatila, T.A., Blaeser, F., Ho, N., Lederman, H.M., Voulgaropoulos, C., Helms, C., et al., 2000. JM2, encoding a fork head-related protein, is mutated in X-linked autoimmunity-allergic disregulation syndrome. J. Clin. Invest. 106, R75–R81.

Chen, W., Jin, W., Hardegen, N., Lei, K.J., Li, L., Marinos, N., et al., 2003. Conversion of peripheral CD4+CD25– naive T cells to CD4+CD25+ regulatory T cells by TGF-beta induction of transcription factor Foxp3. J. Exp. Med. 198, 1875–1886.

Claman, H.N., 1963. Tolerance to a protein antigen in adult mice and the effect of nonspecific factors. J. Immunol. 91, 833–839.

Cohen, J.N., Guidi, C.J., Tewalt, E.F., Qiao, H., Rouhani, S.J., Ruddell, A., et al., 2010. Lymph node-resident lymphatic endothelial cells mediate peripheral tolerance via AIRE-independent direct antigen presentation. J. Exp. Med. 207, 681–688.

Collison, L.W., Workman, C.J., Kuo, T.T., Boyd, K., Wang, Y., Vignali, K.M., et al., 2007. The inhibitory cytokine IL-35 contributes to regulatory T-cell function. Nature 450, 566–569.

Coombes, J.L., Siddiqui, K.R., Arancibia-Carcamo, C.V., Hall, J., Sun, C.M., Belkaid, Y., et al., 2007. A functionally specialized population of mucosal CD103+ DCs induces Foxp3+ regulatory T cells via a TGF-beta and retinoic acid-dependent mechanism. J. Exp. Med. 204, 1757–1764.

Davidson, T.S., Dipaolo, R.J., Andersson, J., Shevach, E.M., 2007. Cutting edge: IL-2 is essential for TGF-beta-mediated induction of Foxp3+ T regulatory cells. J. Immunol. 178, 4022402–4022406.

Deaglio, S., Dwyer, K.M., Gao, W., Friedman, D., Usheva, A., Erat, A., et al., 2007. Adenosine generation catalyzed by CD39 and CD73 expressed on regulatory T cells mediates immune suppression. J. Exp. Med. 204, 1257–1265.

Derbinski, J., Gabler, J., Brors, B., Tierling, S., Jonnakuty, S., Hergenhahn, M., et al., 2005. Promiscuous gene expression in thymic epithelial cells is regulated at multiple levels. J. Exp. Med. 202, 33–45.

Derbinski, J., Schulte, A., Kyewski, B., Klein, L., 2001. Promiscuous gene expression in medullary thymic epithelial cells mirrors the peripheral self. Nat. Immunol. 2, 1032–1039.

Dhodapkar, M.V., Steinman, R.M., Krasovsky, J., Munz, C., Bhardwaj, N., 2001. Antigen-specific inhibition of effector T cell function in humans after injection of immature dendritic cells. J. Exp. Med. 193, 233–238.

Dissanayake, D., Hall, H., Berg-Brown, N., Elford, A.R., Hamilton, S.R., Murakami, K., et al., 2011. Nuclear factor-kappaB1 controls the functional maturation of dendritic cells and prevents the activation of autoreactive T cells. Nat. Med. 17, 1663–1667.

Dresser, D.W., 1961. Effectiveness of lipid and lipidophilic substances as adjuvants. Nature 191, 1169–1171.

Egeblad, M., Littlepage, L.E., Werb, Z., 2005. The fibroblastic coconspirator in cancer progression. Cold Spring Harb. Symp. Quant. Biol. 70, 383–388.

Elder, J.T., 2009. Genome-wide association scan yields new insights into the immunopathogenesis of psoriasis. Genes Immun. 10, 201–209.

Fallarino, F., Grohmann, U., Hwang, K.W., Orabona, C., Vacca, C., Bianchi, R., et al., 2003. Modulation of tryptophan catabolism by regulatory T cells. Nat. Immunol. 4, 1206–1212.

Festenstein, H., Kimura, S., 1988. The Mls system: past and present. J. Immunogenet. 15, 183–196.

Feuerer, M., Hill, J.A., Mathis, D., Benoist, C., 2009. Foxp3+ regulatory T cells: differentiation, specification, subphenotypes. Nat. Immunol. 10, 689–695.

Fife, B.T., Bluestone, J.A., 2008. Control of peripheral T-cell tolerance and autoimmunity via the CTLA-4 and PD-1 pathways. Immunol. Rev. 224, 166–182.

Fletcher, A.L., Lukacs-Kornek, V., Reynoso, E.D., Pinner, S.E., Bellemare-Pelletier, A., Curry, M.S., et al., 2010. Lymph node fibroblastic reticular cells directly present peripheral tissue antigen under steady-state and inflammatory conditions. J. Exp. Med. 207, 689–697.

Fletcher, A.L., Malhotra, D., Turley, S.J., 2011. Lymph node stroma broaden the peripheral tolerance paradigm. Trends Immunol. 32, 12–18.

Fontenot, J.D., Gavin, M.A., Rudensky, A.Y., 2003. Foxp3 programs the development and function of CD4+CD25+ regulatory T cells. Nat. Immunol. 4, 330–336.

Frankel, W.N., Rudy, C., Coffin, J.M., Huber, B.T., 1991. Linkage of Mls genes to endogenous mammary tumour viruses of inbred mice. Nature 349, 526–528.

Freeman, G.J., Gribben, J.G., Boussiotis, V.A., Ng, J.W., Restivo Jr., V.A., Lombard, L.A., et al., 1993. Cloning of B7-2: a CTLA-4 counter-receptor that costimulates human T cell proliferation. Science 262, 909–911.

Gardner, J.M., Devoss, J.J., Friedman, R.S., Wong, D.J., Tan, Y.X., Zhou, X., et al., 2008. Deletional tolerance mediated by extrathymic AIRE-expressing cells. Science 321, 843–847.

Garza, K.M., Chan, S.M., Suri, R., Nguyen, L.T., Odermatt, B., Schoenberger, S.P., et al., 2000. Role of antigen presenting cells in mediating tolerance and autoimmunity. J. Exp. Med. 191, 2021–2027.

Gianfrani, C., Levings, M.K., Sartirana, C., Mazzarella, G., Barba, G., Zanzi, D., et al., 2006. Gliadin-specific type 1 regulatory T cells from the intestinal mucosa of treated celiac patients inhibit pathogenic T cells. J. Immunol. 177, 4178–4186.

Gregori, S., Goudy, K.S., Roncarolo, M.G., 2012. The cellular and molecular mechanisms of immuno-suppression by human type 1 regulatory T cells. Front. Immunol. 3, 30.

Grossman, W.J., Verbsky, J.W., Barchet, W., Colonna, M., Atkinson, J.P., Ley, T.J., 2004. Human T regulatory cells can use the perforin pathway to cause autologous target cell death. Immunity. 21, 589–601.

Groux, H., O'Garra, A., Bigler, M., Rouleau, M., Antonenko, S., De Vries, J.E., et al., 1997. A CD4+ T-cell subset inhibits antigen-specific T-cell responses and prevents colitis. Nature 389, 737–742.

Guerau-De-Arellano, M., Martinic, M., Benoist, C., Mathis, D., 2009. Neonatal tolerance revisited: a perinatal window for AIRE control of autoimmunity. J. Exp. Med. 206, 1245–1252.

Hammer, G.E., Turer, E.E., Taylor, K.E., Fang, C.J., Advincula, R., Oshima, S., et al., 2011. Expression of A20 by dendritic cells preserves immune homeostasis and prevents colitis and spondyloarthritis. Nat. Immunol. 12, 1184–1193.

Harding, F.A., McArthur, J.G., Gross, J.A., Raulet, D.H., Allison, J.P., 1992. CD28-mediated signalling co-stimulates murine T cells and prevents induction of anergy in T-cell clones. Nature 356, 607–609.

Hawiger, D., Inaba, K., Dorsett, Y., Guo, M., Mahnke, K., Rivera, M., et al., 2001. Dendritic cells induce peripheral T cell unresponsiveness under steady state conditions in vivo. J. Exp. Med. 194, 769–779.

Heino, M., Peterson, P., Kudoh, J., Nagamine, K., Lagerstedt, A., Ovod, V., et al., 1999. Autoimmune regulator is expressed in the cells regulating immune tolerance in thymus medulla. Biochem. Biophys. Res. Commun. 257, 821–825.

Heino, M., Peterson, P., Sillanpaa, N., Guerin, S., Wu, L., Anderson, G., et al., 2000. RNA and protein expression of the murine autoimmune regulator gene (AIRE) in normal, RelB-deficient and in NOD mouse. Eur. J. Immunol. 30, 1884–1893.

Hori, S., Nomura, T., Sakaguchi, S., 2003. Control of regulatory T cell development by the transcription factor Foxp3. Science 299, 1057–1061.

Horwitz, D.A., Zheng, S.G., Wang, J., Gray, J.D., 2008. Critical role of IL-2 and TGF-beta in generation, function and stabilization of Foxp3+CD4+ Treg. Eur. J. Immunol. 38, 912–915.

Iwasaki, A., Medzhitov, R., 2010. Regulation of adaptive immunity by the innate immune system. Science 327, 291–295.

Jaattela, M., Mouritzen, H., Elling, F., Bastholm, L., 1996. A20 zinc finger protein inhibits TNF and IL-1 signaling. J. Immunol. 156, 1166–1173.

Jenkins, M.K., Schwartz, R.H., 1987. Antigen presentation by chemically modified splenocytes induces antigen-specific T cell unresponsiveness in vitro and in vivo. J. Exp. Med. 165, 302–319.

Jolicoeur, C., Hanahan, D., Smith, K.M., 1994. T-cell tolerance toward a transgenic beta-cell antigen and transcription of endogenous pancreatic genes in thymus. Proc. Natl. Acad. Sci. USA 91, 6707–6711.

Josefowicz, S.Z., Lu, L.F., Rudensky, A.Y., 2012. Regulatory T cells: mechanisms of differentiation and function. Annu. Rev. Immunol. 30, 531–564.

Kang, S.M., Tang, Q., Bluestone, J.A., 2007. CD4+CD25+ regulatory T cells in transplantation: progress, challenges and prospects. Am. J. Transplant. 7, 1457–1463.

Kappler, J.W., Roehm, N., Marrack, P., 1987. T cell tolerance by clonal elimination in the thymus. Cell 49, 273–280.

Kawabe, Y., Ochi, A., 1990. Selective anergy of V beta 8+,CD4+ T cells in Staphylococcus enterotoxin B-primed mice. J. Exp. Med. 172, 1065–1070.

Kawai, T., Akira, S., 2010. The role of pattern-recognition receptors in innate immunity: update on Toll-like receptors. Nat. Immunol. 11, 373–384.

Keir, M.E., Liang, S.C., Guleria, I., Latchman, Y.E., Qipo, A., Albacker, L.A., et al., 2006. Tissue expression of PD-L1 mediates peripheral T cell tolerance. J. Exp. Med. 203, 883–895.

Kim, J.M., Rudensky, A., 2006. The role of the transcription factor Foxp3 in the development of regulatory T cells. Immunol. Rev. 212, 86–98.

Kisielow, P., Blåthmann, H., Staerz, U.D., Steinmetz, M., Von Boehmer, H., 1988. Tolerance in T cell receptor transgenic mice involves deletion of nonmature CD4+ 8+ thymocytes Nature. 333, 742−746.

Kogawa, K., Nagafuchi, S., Katsuta, H., Kudoh, J., Tamiya, S., Sakai, Y., et al., 2002. Expression of AIRE gene in peripheral monocyte/ dendritic cell lineage. Immunol. Lett. 80, 195−198.

Kool, M., Van Loo, G., Waelput, W., De Prijck, S., Muskens, F., Sze, M., et al., 2011. The ubiquitin-editing protein A20 prevents dendritic cell activation, recognition of apoptotic cells, and systemic autoimmunity. Immunity 35, 82−96.

Kuchroo, V.K., Anderson, A.C., Waldner, H., Munder, M., Bettelli, E., Nicholson, L.B., 2002. T cell response in experimental autoimmune encephalomyelitis (EAE): role of self and cross-reactive antigens in shaping, tuning, and regulating the autopathogenic T cell repertoire. Annu. Rev. Immunol. 20, 101−123.

Kurts, C., Carbone, F.R., Barnden, M., Blanas, E., Allison, J., Heath, W. R., et al., 1997. CD4 + T cell help impairs CD8+ T cell deletion induced by cross-presentation of self-antigens and favors autoimmunity. J. Exp. Med. 186, 2057−2062.

Kurts, C., Heath, W.R., Kosaka, H., Miller, J.F., Carbone, F.R., 1998. The peripheral deletion of autoreactive CD8 + T cells induced by cross-presentation of self-antigens involves signaling through CD95 (Fas, Apo-1). J. Exp. Med. 188, 415−420.

Kurts, C., Sutherland, R.M., Davey, G., Li, M., Lew, A.M., Blanas, E., et al., 1999. CD8 T cell ignorance or tolerance to islet antigens depends on antigen dose. Proc. Natl. Acad. Sci. USA 96, 12703−12707.

Lafaille, J.J., Nagashima, K., Katsuki, M., Tonegawa, S., 1994. High incidence of spontaneous autoimmune encephalomyelitis in immunodeficient anti-myelin basic protein T cell receptor transgenic mice. Cell 78, 399−408.

Lafferty, K.J., Cunningham, A.J., 1975. A new analysis of allogeneic interactions. Aust. J. Exp. Biol. Med. Sci. 53, 27−42.

Lafferty, K.J., Prowse, S.J., Simeonovic, C.J., Warren, H.S., 1983. Immunobiology of tissue transplantation: a return to the passenger leukocyte concept. Annu. Rev. Immunol. 1, 143−173.

Lee, E.G., Boone, D.L., Chai, S., Libby, S.L., Chien, M., Lodolce, J.P., et al., 2000. Failure to regulate TNF-induced NF-kappaB and cell death responses in A20-deficient mice. Science 289, 2350−2354.

Lee, J.W., Epardaud, M., Sun, J., Becker, J.E., Cheng, A.C., Yonekura, A. R., et al., 2007. Peripheral antigen display by lymph node stroma promotes T cell tolerance to intestinal self. Nat. Immunol. 8, 181−190.

Levings, M.K., Gregori, S., Tresoldi, E., Cazzaniga, S., Bonini, C., Roncarolo, M.G., 2005. Differentiation of Tr1 cells by immature dendritic cells requires IL-10 but not CD25 + CD4 + Tr cells. Blood 105, 1162−1169.

Li, N., Zhou, Z., Liu, X., Liu, Y., Zhang, J., Du, L., et al., 2008. Association of tumour necrosis factor alpha (TNF-alpha) polymorphisms with Graves' disease: a meta-analysis. Clin. Biochem. 41, 881−886.

Lim, H.W., Hillsamer, P., Banham, A.H., Kim, C.H., 2005. Cutting edge: direct suppression of B cells by CD4 + CD25 + regulatory T cells. J. Immunol. 175, 4180−4183.

Lin, C.Y., Graca, L., Cobbold, S.P., Waldmann, H., 2002. Dominant transplantation tolerance impairs CD8 + T cell function but not expansion. Nat. Immunol. 3, 1208−1213.

Linsley, P.S., Clark, E.A., Ledbetter, J.A., 1990. T-cell antigen CD28 mediates adhesion with B cells by interacting with activation antigen B7/BB-1. Proc. Natl. Acad. Sci. USA 87, 5031−5035.

Liston, A., Lesage, S., Wilson, J., Peltonen, L., Goodnow, C.C., 2003. AIRE regulates negative selection of organ-specific T cells. Nature Immunol. 4, 350−354.

Lukacs-Kornek, V., Burgdorf, S., Diehl, L., Specht, S., Kornek, M., Kurts, C., 2008. The kidney-renal lymph node-system contributes to cross-tolerance against innocuous circulating antigen. J. Immunol. 180, 706−715.

Lukacs-Kornek, V., Turley, S.J., 2011. Self-antigen presentation by dendritic cells and lymphoid stroma and its implications for autoimmunity. Curr. Opin. Immunol. 23, 138−145.

MacDonald, H.R., Schneider, R., Lees, R.K., Howe, R.C., Acha-Orbea, H., Festenstein, H., et al., 1988. T cell receptor V_β use predicts reactivity and tolerance to Mlsa-encoded antigens. Nature 332, 40−45.

Marrack, P., Kushnir, E., Kappler, J., 1991. A maternally inherited superantigen encoded by a mammary tumour virus. Nature. 349, 524−526.

Medzhitov, R., Preston-Hurlburt, P., Janeway Jr., C.A., 1997. A human homologue of the Drosophila Toll protein signals activation of adaptive immunity. Nature 388, 394−397.

Meiler, F., Zumkehr, J., Klunker, S., Ruckert, B., Akdis, C.A., Akdis, M., 2008. In vivo switch to IL-10-secreting T regulatory cells in high dose allergen exposure. J. Exp. Med. 205, 2887−2898.

Miyara, M., Sakaguchi, S., 2007. Natural regulatory T cells: mechanisms of suppression. Trends Mol Med. 13, 108−116.

Mueller, D.L., Jenkins, M.K., Schwartz, R.H., 1989. Clonal expansion versus functional clonal inactivation: a costimulatory signalling pathway determines the outcome of T cell antigen receptor occupancy. Annu. Rev. Immunol. 7, 445−480.

Musone, S.L., Taylor, K.E., Lu, T.T., Nititham, J., Ferreira, R.C., Ortmann, W., et al., 2008. Multiple polymorphisms in the TNFAIP3 region are independently associated with systemic lupus erythematosus. Nat. Genet. 40, 1062−1064.

Nagamine, K., Peterson, P., Scott, H.S., Kudoh, J., Minoshima, S., Heino, M., et al., 1997. Positional cloning of the APECED gene. Nat. Genet. 17, 393−398.

Nichols, L.A., Chen, Y., Colella, T.A., Bennett, C.L., Clausen, B.E., Engelhard, V.H., 2007. Deletional self-tolerance to a melanocyte/ melanoma antigen derived from tyrosinase is mediated by a radioresistant cell in peripheral and mesenteric lymph nodes. J. Immunol. 179, 993−1003.

Nishimura, H., Okazaki, T., Tanaka, Y., Nakatani, K., Hara, M., Matsumori, A., et al., 2001. Autoimmune dilated cardiomyopathy in PD-1 receptor deficient mice. Science 291, 319−322.

Nishizuka, Y., Sakakura, T., 1969. Thymus and reproduction: sex-linked dysgenesia of the gonad after neonatal thymectomy in mice. Science 166, 753−755.

Nossal, G.J.V., 1983. Cellular mechanisms of immunologic tolerance. Ann. Rev. Immunol. 1, 33−62.

Ochs, H.D., Ziegler, S.F., Torgerson, T.R., 2005. FOXP3 acts as a rheostat of the immune response. Immunol. Rev. 203, 156−164.

Ohashi, P.S., Oehen, S., Bårki, K., Pircher, H., Ohashi, C.T., Odermatt, B., et al., 1991. Ablation of "tolerance" and induction of diabetes by virus infection in viral antigen transgenic mice. Cell 65, 305−317.

Oldstone, M.B.A., Nerenberg, M., Southern, P., Price, J., Lewicki, H., 1991. Virus infection triggers insulin-dependent diabetes mellitus in a transgenic model: role of anti-self (virus) immune response. Cell 65, 319−331.

Olivares-Villagomez, D., Wang, Y., Lafaille, J.J., 1998. Regulatory CD4 (+) T cells expressing endogenous T cell receptor chains protect myelin basic protein-specific transgenic mice from spontaneous autoimmune encephalomyelitis. J. Exp. Med. 188, 1883–1894.

Ostroukhova, M., Seguin-Devaux, C., Oriss, T.B., Dixon-McCarthy, B., Yang, L., Ameredes, B.T., et al., 2004. Tolerance induced by inhaled antigen involves CD4(+) T cells expressing membrane-bound TGF-beta and FOXP3. J. Clin. Invest. 114, 28–38.

Owen, R.D., 1945. Immunogenetic consequences of vascular anastomoses between bovine twins. Science 102, 400–401.

Pandiyan, P., Zheng, L., Ishihara, S., Reed, J., Lenardo, M.J., 2007. CD4 + CD25 + Foxp3 + regulatory T cells induce cytokine deprivation-mediated apoptosis of effector CD4 + T cells. Nat. Immunol. 8, 1353–1362.

Penhale, W.J., Farmer, A., McKenna, R.P., Irvine, W.J., 1973. Spontaneous thyroiditis in thymectomized and irradiated Wistar rats. Clinical and Experimental Immunology. 15, 225–236.

Pinchuk, I.V., Saada, J.I., Beswick, E.J., Boya, G., Qiu, S.M., Mifflin, R. C., et al., 2008. PD-1 ligand expression by human colonic myofibroblasts/fibroblasts regulates CD4 + T-cell activity. Gastroenterology 135, 1228–1237, 1237 e1–e2.

Pircher, H., Bårki, K., Lang, R., Hengartner, H., Zinkernagel, R., 1989. Tolerance induction in double specific T-cell receptor transgenic mice varies with antigen. Nature. 342, 559–561.

Plenge, R.M., Cotsapas, C., Davies, L., Price, A.L., De Bakker, P.I., Maller, J., et al., 2007. Two independent alleles at 6q23 associated with risk of rheumatoid arthritis. Nat. Genet. 39, 1477–1482.

Poltorak, A., He, X., Smirnova, I., Liu, M.Y., Van Huffel, C., Du, X., et al., 1998. Defective LPS signaling in C3H/HeJ and C57BL/10ScCr mice: mutations in Tlr4 gene. Science 282, 2085–2088.

Powrie, F., Mason, D., 1990. OX-22high CD4 + T cells induce wasting disease with multiple organ pathology: prevention by the OX-22low subset. J. Exp. Med. 172, 1701–1708.

Probst, H.C., McCoy, K., Okazaki, T., Honjo, T., Van Den, B.M., 2005. Resting dendritic cells induce peripheral CD8 + T cell tolerance through PD-1 and CTLA-4. Nat. Immunol. 6, 280–286.

Rammensee, H.G., Kroschewski, R., Frangoulis, B., 1989. Clonal anergy induced in mature $V_\beta6 +$ T lymphocytes on immunizing Mls-1 b mice with Mls-1 a expressing cells. Nature 339, 541–544.

Ramsdell, F., Lantz, T., Fowlkes, B.J., 1989. A nondeletional mechanism of thymic self tolerance. Science 246, 1038–1041.

Ramsey, C., Winqvist, O., Puhakka, L., Halonen, M., Moro, A., Kämpe, O., et al., 2002. AIRE deficient mice develop multiple features of APECED phenotype and show altered immune response. Hum. Mol. Genet. 11, 397–409.

Reis e Sousa, C., 2006. Dendritic cells in a mature age. Nat. Rev. Immunol. 6, 476–483.

Rocha, B., Von Boehmer, H., 1991. Peripheral selection of the T cell repertoire. Science 251, 1225–1228.

Roncarolo, M.G., Gregori, S., Battaglia, M., Bacchetta, R., Fleischhauer, K., Levings, M.K., 2006. Interleukin-10-secreting type 1 regulatory T cells in rodents and humans. Immunol. Rev. 212, 28–50.

Sakaguchi, S., Sakaguchi, N., Asano, M., Itoh, M., Toda, M., 1995. Immunologic self-tolerance maintained by activated T cells expressing IL-2 receptor α-chains (CD25). J. Immunol. 155, 1151–1164.

Salomon, B., Lenschow, D.J., Rhee, L., Ashourian, N., Singh, B., Sharpe, A., et al., 2000. B7/CD28 costimulation is essential for the homeostasis of the CD4 + CD25 + immunoregulatory T cells that control autoimmune diabetes. Immunity 12, 431–440.

Schallenberg, S., Tsai, P.Y., Riewaldt, J., Kretschmer, K., 2010. Identification of an immediate Foxp3(−) precursor to Foxp3(+) regulatory T cells in peripheral lymphoid organs of nonmanipulated mice. J. Exp. Med. 207, 1393–1407.

Schmidt, A., Oberle, N., Krammer, P.H., 2012. Molecular mechanisms of treg-mediated T cell suppression. Front. Immunol. 3, 51.

Schmidt, E.M., Wang, C.J., Ryan, G.A., Clough, L.E., Qureshi, O.S., Goodall, M., et al., 2009. Ctla-4 controls regulatory T cell peripheral homeostasis and is required for suppression of pancreatic islet autoimmunity. J. Immunol. 182, 274–282.

Seki, N., Kamizono, S., Yamada, A., Higuchi, T., Matsumoto, H., Niiya, F., et al., 1999. Polymorphisms in the 5′-flanking region of tumor necrosis factor-alpha gene in patients with rheumatoid arthritis. Tissue Antigens 54, 194–197.

Selvaraj, R.K., Geiger, T.L., 2007. A kinetic and dynamic analysis of Foxp3 induced in T cells by TGF-beta. J. Immunol. 179, (11p following 1390).

Sha, W.C., Liou, H.C., Tuomanen, E.I., Baltimore, D., 1995. Targeted disruption of the p50 subunit of NF-kappa B leads to multifocal defects in immune responses. Cell 80, 321–330.

Sha, W.C., Nelson, C.A., Newberry, R.D., Kranz, D.M., Russell, J.H., Loh, D.Y., 1988. Positive and negative selection of an antigen receptor on T cells in transgenic mice. Nature 336, 73–76.

Shearer, G.M., 1974. Cell mediated cytotoxicity to trinitrophenyl-modified syngeneic lymphocytes. Eur. J. Immunol. 4, 257.

Shevach, E.M., 2002. CD4+ CD25+ suppressor T cells: more questions than answers. Nat. Rev. Immunol. 2, 389–400.

Smith, K.M., Olson, D.C., Hirose, R., Hanahan, D., 1997. Pancreatic gene expression in rare cells of thymic medulla: evidence for functional contribution to T cell tolerance. Int. Immunol. 9, 1355–1365.

Song, H.Y., Rothe, M., Goeddel, D.V., 1996. The tumor necrosis factor-inducible zinc finger protein A20 interacts with TRAF1/TRAF2 and inhibits NF-kappaB activation. Proc. Natl. Acad. Sci. USA 93, 6721–6725.

Starr, T.K., Jameson, S.C., Hogquist, K.A., 2003. Positive and negative selection of T cells. Annu. Rev. Immunol. 21, 139–176.

Stayoussef, M., Benmansour, J., Al-Jenaidi, F.A., Rajab, M.H., Said, H. B., Ourtani, M., et al., 2010. Identification of specific tumor necrosis factor-alpha-susceptible and -protective haplotypes associated with the risk of type 1 diabetes. Eur. Cytokine Netw. 21, 285–291.

Steinman, R.M., Cohn, Z.A., 1973. Identification of a novel cell type in peripheral lymphoid organs of mice: I. Morphology, quantitation, tissue distribution. Journal of Experimental Medicine. 137, 1142–1162.

Steinman, R.M., Hawiger, D., Nussenzweig, M.C., 2003. Tolerogenic dendritic cells. Annu. Rev. Immunol. 21, 685–711.

Talmage, D.W., Dart, G., Radovich, J., Lafferty, K.J., 1976. Activation of transplant immunity: effect of donor leukocytes on thyroid allograft rejection. Science 191, 385–388.

Thornton, A.M., Korty, P.E., Tran, D.Q., Wohlfert, E.A., Murray, P.E., Belkaid, Y., et al., 2010. Expression of Helios, an Ikaros transcription factor family member, differentiates thymic-derived from peripherally induced Foxp3 + T regulatory cells. J. Immunol. 184, 3433–3441.

Tiemessen, M.M., Jagger, A.L., Evans, H.G., Van Herwijnen, M.J., John, S., et al., 2007. CD4 + CD25 + Foxp3 + regulatory T cells induce alternative activation of human monocytes/macrophages. Proc. Natl. Acad. Sci. USA 104, 19446–19451.

Tivol, E.A., Boriello, F., Schweitzer, A.N., Lynch, W.P., Bluestone, J.A., Sharpe, A.H., 1995. Loss of CTLA-4 leads to massive lymphoproliferation and fatal multiorgan tissue destruction. Immunity 3, 541–547.

Tran, D.Q., Ramsey, H., Shevach, E.M., 2007. Induction of FOXP3 expression in naive human CD4 + FOXP3 T cells by T-cell receptor stimulation is transforming growth factor-beta dependent but does not confer a regulatory phenotype. Blood 110, 2983–2990.

Traub, E., 1936. An epidemic in a mouse colony due to the virus of acute lymphocytic choriomeningitis. J. Exp. Med. 63, 533–546.

Traub, E., 1938. Factors influencing the persistence of choriomeningitis virus in the blood after clinical recovery. J. Exp. Med. 68, 229–251.

Tree, T.I., Lawson, J., Edwards, H., Skowera, A., Arif, S., Roep, B.O., et al., 2010. Naturally arising human CD4 T-cells that recognize islet autoantigens and secrete interleukin-10 regulate proinflammatory T-cell responses via linked suppression. Diabetes 59, 1451–1460.

Trynka, G., Zhernakova, A., Romanos, J., Franke, L., Hunt, K.A., Turner, G., et al., 2009. Coeliac disease-associated risk variants in TNFAIP3 and REL implicate altered NF-kappaB signalling. Gut. 58, 1078–1083.

Tyndall, A., Uccelli, A., 2009. Multipotent mesenchymal stromal cells for autoimmune diseases: teaching new dogs old tricks. Bone Marrow Transplant. 43, 821–828.

Udalova, I.A., Richardson, A., Denys, A., Smith, C., Ackerman, H., Foxwell, B., et al., 2000. Functional consequences of a polymorphism affecting NF-kappaB p50–p50 binding to the TNF promoter region. Mol. Cell. Biol. 20, 9113–9119.

Uhlig, H.H., Coombes, J., Mottet, C., Izcue, A., Thompson, C., Fanger, A., et al., 2006. Characterization of Foxp3 + CD4 + CD25 + and IL-10-secreting CD4 + CD25 + T cells during cure of colitis. J. Immunol. 177, 5852–5860.

Vallabhapurapu, S., Karin, M., 2009. Regulation and function of NF-kappaB transcription factors in the immune system. Annu. Rev. Immunol. 27, 693–733.

Veldman, C., Hohne, A., Dieckmann, D., Schuler, G., Hertl, M., 2004. Type I regulatory T cells specific for desmoglein 3 are more frequently detected in healthy individuals than in patients with pemphigus vulgaris. J. Immunol. 172, 6468–6475.

Von Boehmer, H., 2005. Mechanisms of suppression by suppressor T cells. Nat. Immunol. 6, 338–344.

Waterhouse, P., Penninger, J.M., Timms, E., Wakeham, A., Shahinian, A., Lee, K.P., et al., 1995. Lymphoproliferative disorders with early lethality in mice deficient in Ctla-4. Science 270, 985–988.

Webb, S., Morris, C., Sprent, J., 1990. Extrathymic tolerance of mature T cells: clonal elimination as a consequence of immunity. Cell 63, 1249–1256.

Werlen, G., Hausmann, B., Naeher, D., Palmer, E., 2003. Signaling life and death in the thymus: timing is everything. Science 299, 1859–1863.

Wertz, I.E., O'Rourke, K.M., Zhou, H., Eby, M., Aravind, L., Seshagiri, S., et al., 2004. De-ubiquitination and ubiquitin ligase domains of A20 downregulate NF-kappaB signalling. Nature 430, 694–699.

Wildin, R.S., Ramsdell, F., Peake, J., Faravelli, F., Casanova, J.L., Buist, N., et al., 2001. X-linked neonatal diabetes mellitus, enteropathy and endocrinopathy syndrome is the human equivalent of mouse scurfy. Nat. Genet. 27, 18–20.

Wong, J., Mathis, D., Benoist, C., 2007. TCR-based lineage tracing: no evidence for conversion of conventional into regulatory T cells in response to a natural self-antigen in pancreatic islets. J. Exp. Med. 204, 2039–2045.

Yip, L., Su, L., Sheng, D., Chang, P., Atkinson, M., Czesak, M., et al., 2009. Deaf1 isoforms control the expression of genes encoding peripheral tissue antigens in the pancreatic lymph nodes during type 1 diabetes. Nat. Immunol. 10, 1026–1033.

Zheng, S.G., Wang, J.H., Stohl, W., Kim, K.S., Gray, J.D., Horwitz, D.A., 2006. TGF-beta requires CTLA-4 early after T cell activation to induce FoxP3 and generate adaptive CD4 + CD25 + regulatory cells. J. Immunol. 176, 3321–3329.

Zinkernagel, R.M., Doherty, P.C., 1974. Restriction of in vitro T cell mediated cytotoxicity in lymphocytic choriomeningitis within a syngeneic or semiallogeneic system. Nature 248, 701–702.

Chapter 8

The Role of Invariant Natural Killer T Cells in Autoimmune Diseases

Gerhard Wingender and Mitchell Kronenberg

La Jolla Institute for Allergy and Immunology, San Diego, CA, USA

Chapter Outline

The Curious Case of *i*NKT Cells	**103**	Rheumatoid Arthritis	111
The Many Names of NKT Cells	103	Skin Disorders	112
The Many Faces of *i*NKT Cells	104	Missed so Sadly: Beneficial Roles of	
Phenotype	104	*i*NKT Cells	**113**
Distribution	104	Diabetes	113
The Many Effector Functions of *i*NKT Cells	105	IBD/Crohn's Disease	115
Activation	105	Multiple Sclerosis/EAE	115
Cytokine Production	106	Systemic Lupus Erythematosus (SLE)	115
Downstream Effects	106	**Good or Bad Performers?**	**116**
The Many Kinds of *i*NKT Cells	106	The Far End of the Question?	116
Technical Problems and the Species Divide	107	What Activates *i*NKT Cells During Autoimmune	
The Species Divide	108	Responses?	116
The Janus-Like Character of *i*NKT Cells in Autoimmunity	**108**	Which *i*NKT Cell Effector Functions	
Too Much of a Good Thing: Detrimental		Orchestrate the Development of Autoimmune	
Roles of *i*NKT Cells	108	Responses?	117
Atherosclerosis	108	**Conclusion**	**118**
Asthma	110	**Acknowledgments**	**118**
IBD/Colitis	111	**Abbreviations**	**118**
Primary Biliary Cirrhosis (PBC)	111	**References**	**118**

THE CURIOUS CASE OF *i*NKT CELLS

The Many Names of NKT Cells

Natural killer T (NKT) cells are a unique subset of T lymphocytes found in mice, humans, and other mammals that phenotypically and functionally resemble NK cells as well as T cells, and thereby exhibiting features of the innate as well as the adaptive immune system (Kronenberg and Gapin, 2002; Taniguchi et al., 2003; Godfrey and Kronenberg, 2004; Kronenberg, 2005; Wingender and Kronenberg, 2006; Bendelac et al., 2007; Tupin et al., 2007; Cerundolo et al., 2009; Godfrey et al., 2010).

They were originally defined by co-expression of a T cell antigen receptor (TCR) and NK cell receptors, especially NK1.1 (NKR-P1C) in certain mouse strains (Watanabe et al., 1995) and CD56 or CD161 (NKR-P1A) in human (Lanier et al., 1994; Exley et al., 1998; Doherty et al., 1999). This classification, however, is an oversimplification, as conventional T cells can express NK receptors, especially after activation (Hammond et al., 1999; Assarsson et al., 2000; Slifka et al., 2000; McMahon et al., 2002) and the expression of NK markers by NKT cells varies with their maturity, activation state, and in mice, with the genetic background (Kronenberg and Gapin, 2002; Kronenberg, 2005; Bendelac et al., 2007).

Although the term "NKT cell" is still sometimes used in this broad sense, nowadays it usually refers to T cells expressing an αβ TCR that are reactive to antigens presented by CD1d, a non-polymorphic major

N. Rose & I. Mackay (Eds): The Autoimmune Diseases, Fifth edition. DOI: http://dx.doi.org/10.1016/B978-0-12-384929-8.00008-3

histocompatibility complex (MHC) class I-like antigen-presenting molecule. CD1d reactive αβ T cells are often divided into Type I and II NKT cells, based on the TCR they express (for reviews see Kronenberg and Gapin, 2002; Taniguchi et al., 2003; Godfrey and Kronenberg, 2004; Kronenberg, 2005; Wingender and Kronenberg, 2006; Bendelac et al., 2007; Tupin et al., 2007).

Type I NKT cells are the largest and best-studied fraction of NKT cells and they carry a canonical Vα14 to Jα18 TCR rearrangement (Vα14i) in mice and an orthologous Vα24-Jα18 TCR chain (Vα24i) in humans. This invariant TCR α chain (iTCR) pairs predominantly with Vβ8, Vβ7 or Vβ2 in mice, and almost exclusively with Vβ11 in human, although these β chains have highly diverse rearrangements to Jβ segments (Matsuda et al., 2001; Ronet et al., 2001;). Considering the β chain variability, and the near complete absence of variability in the α chain, in reality these cells have a semi-invariant TCR. However, they are typically referred to as invariant NKT (iNKT) cells, a designation we will use herein. The specificity of iNKT cells is remarkably conserved over at least 50 million years of evolution, since the divergence of hominids and rodents. In fact, there is a surprising degree of interspecies cross-reactivity, with mouse iNKT cells recognizing human CD1d and vice versa (Brossay et al., 1998; Brossay and Kronenberg, 1999; Kronenberg, 2005). This conservation suggests an important function for these cells in the mammalian immune system.

In contrast to iNKT cells, type II NKT cells, also termed variant NKT (vNKT) cells, encompass all other CD1d reactive T lymphocytes that utilize a more variable TCR (Wingender and Kronenberg, 2008). However, there is a degree of oligoclonality in these cells, with enrichment for some TCRs such as: Vα3.2 and Vα8 (Park et al., 2001). The specificity of these cells is largely unknown, although some recognize sulfatide, a self glycolipid antigen (Jahng et al., 2004; Blomqvist et al., 2009).

Sometimes, especially in earlier literature, a third group (type III) of NKT cells is listed. This group is more heterogeneous, as it subsumes all non-CD1d reactive T lymphocytes that express NK receptors (Kronenberg and Gapin, 2002; Taniguchi et al., 2003; Wingender and Kronenberg, 2006; Wingender et al., 2006). Furthermore, it should be noted that several other non-conventional T cell subsets have been defined based on their TCR α chain repertoire. Mucosal NKT (mNKT) or mucosal associated invariant T (MAIT) cells express a fixed Vα19i TCR in mice, and a homologous Vα7.2i in humans (Shimamura and Huang, 2002; Treiner et al., 2003; Wingender and Kronenberg, 2008; Le Bourhis et al., 2010, 2011). They are reactive to MR1, a highly conserved MHC class I homologue (Treiner et al., 2003; Le Bourhis et al., 2011). Additionally, Vα10

expressing NKT cells have recently been described (Pellicci et al., 2011). These cells are also CD1d reactive, and have a specificity similar to iNKT cells, although the CDR3 regions of their α chains are not invariant (Pellicci et al., 2011).

The focus of this review is exclusively iNKT cells in rodents, non-human primates (NHP) and humans and their roles in autoimmune disease pathogenesis and prevention.

The Many Faces of iNKT Cells

Phenotype

Even as they differentiate in the thymus (for reviews see Das et al., 2010; Hu et al., 2011; Engel and Kronenberg, 2012), iNKT cells begin to express a pattern of surface markers (CD69$^+$, CD44^{high}, CD11a^{high}, CD62L^{low}, CD122$^+$) typically associated with activated or memory T cells (Bendelac et al., 1997; Dutton et al., 1998; Godfrey et al., 2000; Kronenberg and Gapin, 2002; Sprent and Surh, 2002). This effector/memory phenotype is also displayed by iNKT cells that are derived from umbilical cord blood (van der Vliet et al., 2000; D'Andrea et al., 2000) or from germ-free animals (Park et al., 2000; Wingender et al., 2012b), and they maintain this pattern as mature cells.

Additionally, these cells constitutively express detectable mRNA for IL-4 and IFNγ (Matsuda et al., 2003; Stetson et al., 2003), although these transcripts increase dramatically following activation. Taken together, these data suggest that iNKT cells undergo a strong antigenic stimulation during their differentiation, consistent with the hypothesis that true TCR agonists mediate their positive selection (Kronenberg, 2005). However, two reports indicated that peripheral TCR-CD1d interactions aid the full maturation and reactivity of iNKT cells (McNab et al., 2005; Wingender et al., 2012b).

Distribution

Vα14i NKT cells have the highest representation within the total T cell population in the liver and the bone marrow ($>$10%), followed by significant numbers in thymus, peripheral blood, and spleen (1−3%), whereas they are relatively rare in all other organs ($<$0.5%), including sites where conventional T lymphocytes are numerous, such as the lymph nodes and intestinal tissue (Kronenberg and Gapin, 2002; Kronenberg, 2005; Bendelac et al., 2007). Interestingly, in humans the frequency of iNKT cells is generally much lower, although a high degree of inter-individual variability in peripheral blood mononuclear cells (PBMC) has been reported (Prussin and Foster, 1997; van der Vliet et al., 2001; Gumperz et al., 2002; Kita et al., 2002). Although the reason for this variability is unknown, nonetheless, the frequency of iNKT cells in the PBMC of an individual appears to be stable over time (Lee et al., 2002b; Wither et al., 2008). *i*NKT cells are also relatively infrequent, compared to mice, in human intrahepatic lymphocytes (Kita et al., 2002; Kenna et al., 2003), but recent evidence indicates they may be much more abundant in adipose tissue (Lynch et al., 2009) and also to some extent, in peritoneal fluid (Wingender et al., 2012a).

The Many Effector Functions of *i*NKT Cells

Activation

*i*NKT cells recognize glycolipid antigens presented by CD1d (Bendelac, 1995; Bendelac et al., 1995; Kawano et al., 1997; Zeng et al., 1997), and one of the best-studied antigens is the glycolipid α-galactosylceramide (αGalCer). αGalCer is a synthetic glycosphingolipid, a category of glycolipids that contains ceramide as the lipid portion. Glycosphingolipids are natural compounds found in many organisms, including mammals. αGalCer was originally purified from a marine sponge, and was optimized by medicinal chemistry to yield its exceptionally strong agonistic potential (Morita et al., 1995). αGalCer contains an unusual α-anomeric linkage of the sugar to the ceramide lipid, unlike mammalian glycosphingolipids (Morita et al., 1995) and this α-linkage is crucial for its great stimulatory capacity (Bendelac et al., 1997; Kawano et al., 1997). Numerous synthetic derivates of αGalCer have been studied (East et al., 2012), and natural antigens that can stimulate the majority of *i*NKT cells have been characterized from a few bacteria as well, including glycosphingolipids from environmental bacteria *Sphingomonas* spp. (Kinjo et al., 2005; Mattner et al., 2005). Because the *Sphingomonas*-derived antigens are similar to αGalCer, and *Sphingomonas* bacteria are found in aqueous environments (White et al., 1996), it is widely believed that the original αGalCer compound derived from a bacterium associated with the sponge. Antigens from pathogenic microbes include diacylglycerols from *Borrelia burgdorferi*, the causative agent of Lyme disease (Kinjo et al., 2006), and diacylglycerols from *Streptococcus pneumonia* and group B *Streptococcus* (Kinjo et al., 2011). The biochemistry of lipid antigen binding to CD1d and recognition of the antigen CD1d complex by the TCR is very well understood as a result of biophysical and X-ray crystallographic studies. This topic has been reviewed recently (Zajonc and Kronenberg 2009; Pei et al., 2012; Rossjohn et al., 2012).

Activation of *i*NKT cells by TCR-mediated recognition of antigen bound to CD1d has been referred to as direct or antigen-dependent activation (Kinjo and Kronenberg, 2005; Parekh et al., 2005). It is known,

however, that memory T cells can be activated by cytokines alone in a TCR-independent manner (Berg and Forman, 2006). Considering their constitutively activated phenotype, it therefore is not surprising that a similar cytokine-dependent activation was reported for *i*NKT cells as well (Nagarajan and Kronenberg, 2007; Tyznik et al., 2008). This so-called indirect or antigen-independent activation (Kinjo and Kronenberg, 2005; Parekh et al., 2005) can be induced by several proinflammatory cytokines, such as IFNα, IFNβ, IL-12, and IL-18, alone (Leite-de-Moraes et al., 1999; Biron and Brossay, 2001) or more effectively, in combination (Dao et al., 1998; Ogasawara et al., 1998; Leite-de-Moraes et al., 1999, 2001). Dendritic cells (DCs) and macrophages produce these cytokines following the engagement of Toll-like receptors (TLR) or other stimuli for the innate immune system, like early after bacterial or viral infections.

One has to keep in mind, however, that the direct, TCR-driven and the indirect, cytokine-driven pathways of *i*NKT cell activation are not exclusive. The innate cell-derived cytokines IL-12 and IFNα/β have been reported to augment CD1d-dependent *i*NKT cell activation (Brigl et al., 2003; Mattner et al., 2005; Mallevaey et al., 2006; Paget et al., 2007), which was especially crucial for stimulation with presumably weak antigens.

Furthermore, in some cases, it has been shown that *i*NKT cells require the recognition of endogenous or self-ligands presented by CD1d for activation in a cytokine-dependent context (Brigl et al., 2003). This is exemplified by the activation of *i*NKT cells following *Salmonella* infection, which is not only dependent on IL-12, but also on CD1d (Brigl et al., 2003; Mattner et al., 2005; Mallevaey et al., 2006). As *Salmonella* is not known to express antigens that activate *i*NKT cells, these data demonstrate that self-antigens presented by CD1d acted in concert with IL-12 to activate *i*NKT cells. In line with the idea of recognition of "self" by *i*NKT cells is the observation that mature *i*NKT cells can under some circumstances display autoreactivity (Salio and Cerundolo 2009; Hegde et al., 2010). Additionally, data with tumor-derived glycolipids suggest (Behar et al., 1999; Gumperz et al., 2000; Metelitsa et al., 2003; Rauch et al., 2003; Wu et al., 2003; Metelitsa, 2010) such self-antigens could provide an "altered-self" for *i*NKT cell activation.

The structure of such self-antigens important for the activation of mature *i*NKT cells is still controversially debated, and there could be several types, but currently the best candidates are lysophospholipids (Fox et al., 2009), at least for human *i*NKT cells and β-D-glucopyranosylceramide (Brennan et al., 2011). A lysophosphatidylethanolamine with an ether bond or plasmalogen has been suggested to be important for *i*NKT cell positive selection (Facciotti et al., 2012).

Cytokine Production

In accordance with their constitutively activated phenotype is the remarkable ability of *i*NKT cells to rapidly (<1 hour) exert effector functions such as cytokine production and cytotoxicity (Wingender et al., 2010). After antigenic, TCR-driven activation they rapidly produce copious amounts of various cytokines such as T helper type 1 (Th1; e.g., IFNγ, TNF) and Th2 cytokines (e.g., IL-4, IL-10, IL-13) (Kronenberg, 2005; Wingender and Kronenberg, 2006; Bendelac et al., 2007), with a subset capable of producing IL-17 A (Michel et al., 2007, 2008; Coquet et al., 2008; Pichavant et al., 2008; Doisne et al., 2009, 2011; Milpied et al., 2011) and IL-22 (Paget et al., 2012). This explosive production of cytokines is more similar to innate immune cells or a memory T cell response, as a conventional naïve T lymphocyte would take days of stimulation to produce these cytokines. In contrast to naïve T cells, *i*NKT cells are somewhat resistant to cytokine polarization (Matsuda et al., 2003) and the response towards a strong TCR agonist is always a mixed IFNγ/IL-4 or Th0 response (Sullivan et al., 2010).

In contrast to this manifold array of cytokines following TCR-driven activation, the indirect, cytokine-driven activation, for example by IL-12 and IL-18, leads exclusively to the production of IFNγ by the stimulated *i*NKT cells (Nagarajan and Kronenberg, 2007; Tyznik et al., 2008). Similarly, IL-1β and IL-23 stimulate the IL-17 A producing subset to secrete IL-17 (Moreira-Teixeira et al., 2011; Doisne et al., 2011), and some *i*NKT cells are stimulated by IL-25 to produce IL-13 (Terashima et al., 2008).

Downstream Effects

Due to their cytokine production, *i*NKT cells have a pronounced impact on other lymphocytes, amplifying responses of DCs (Kitamura et al., 1999; Chen et al., 2005; Kojo et al., 2005), macrophages (Flesch et al., 1997; Denney et al., 2012), neutrophils (Li et al., 2007; Michel et al., 2007; Wintermeyer et al., 2009; De Santo et al., 2010; Emoto et al., 2010), NK cells (Eberl and MacDonald, 2000; Smyth et al., 2000a,b), B and T cells. However, in some cases the interaction has been shown to be in part cell−cell contact dependent (Novak et al., 2005; Baev et al., 2008; Caielli et al., 2010; Yang et al., 2011).

Moreover, activated *i*NKT cells can skew or polarize the character of the entire immune response either towards a Th1- (Denkers et al., 1996; Cui et al., 1999; Kitamura et al., 1999; Gonzalez-Aseguinolaza et al., 2002) or a Th2- (Yoshimoto et al., 1995a,b; Bendelac et al., 1996; Burdin et al., 1999; Singh et al., 1999; Hong et al., 2001; Sharif et al., 2001) direction. This can be

promoted by the stimulating antigen utilized, with some synthetic glycolipids, like C-glycoside (Schmieg et al., 2003), leading to a Th1 bias and others like OCH (Miyamoto et al., 2001) and C:20 (Yu et al., 2005), leading to a Th2 bias (East et al., 2012; Pei et al., 2012). Interestingly, this bias is not reflected in the initial *i*NKT cell cytokine response, which remains Th0 (Sullivan et al., 2010), but instead reflects the interactions between networks of cells including the presentation of the antigen on antigen-presenting cells (APC) (Im et al., 2009; Arora et al., 2011). For example, Th1 skewing of the cytokine response reflects enhanced IFNγ production by NK cells (East et al., 2012; Pei et al., 2012).

Consequently, by orchestrating the ensuing immune response, with regard to its strength and properties, *i*NKT cells can act as a bridge between innate and adaptive immune responses. Therefore, it is not surprising that *i*NKT cells have been reported to be crucially involved in the early phases of a dazzling variety of different immune reactions, ranging from self-tolerance and autoimmunity to include responses to pathogens and tumors (Bendelac et al., 1997; Kronenberg and Gapin, 2002; Godfrey and Kronenberg, 2004; Kronenberg, 2005; Kinjo and Kronenberg, 2005; Parekh et al., 2005; Godfrey et al., 2010).

The Many Kinds of *i*NKT Cells

There is increasing evidence that the functionally diverse roles of *i*NKT cells are partly due to functional *i*NKT cells subsets with distinct homing properties and cytokine profiles. These may be pre-programmed in the thymus, or induced in the periphery under the influence of particular stimulatory conditions. At first, *i*NKT cells subsets were defined by the expression of surface molecules, such as CD4 (Gumperz et al., 2002; Kim et al., 2002; Lee et al., 2002a), NK1.1 (McNab et al., 2007), IL17RB$^+$ (Terashima et al., 2008), Ly49 receptors (Hammond et al., 1999; Skold and Cardell, 2000) and CD49b/DX5 (Hammond et al., 1999; Pellicci et al., 2005), among others.

However, with very recent advances, it now seems feasible, at least in the mouse, to attempt to define some *i*NKT cell subsets based on transcription factor usage (Table 8.1): (a) NKT1 are Tbet^{high}, PLZF^{low}, GATA3^{low}, RORγt^{neg} and they characteristically produce IFNγ. (b) NKT2 are PLZF^{high}, GATA3^{high}, Tbet^{low}, RORγt^{low} and produce IL-4. (c) NKT17 are RORγt^{pos}, GATA3^{high}, PLZF^{int}, Tbet^{low} and are characterized by IL-17A production (Michel et al., 2007, 2008; Coquet et al., 2008; Pichavant et al., 2008; Doisne et al., 2009, 2011; Milpied et al., 2011) (transcription factor usage in (a−c) based on Kristin A. Hogquist, personal communication). These subsets can be identified in the thymus and therefore may

TABLE 8.1 Features of CD1d-reactive NKT Cell Subsets

Name	Invariant (*i*)NKT							Variable (*v*)NKT	
Alternative names	Vα14*i* NKT type I or classical NKT cells					Vα24*i* NKT type I or classical NKT cells		Type II or non-classical NKT cells	
Species	mouse					human		mouse/human	
TCR repertoire	invariant Vα14-Jα18					invariant Vα24-Jα18		diverse or semi-diverse (Vα3, Vα8)	
Reactivity	CD1d					CD1d		CD1d	
Antigens	αGalCer and others					αGalCer and others		sulfatide	nd
Positive selection	DP thymocytes					DP thymocytes		thymus, cell unknown	
Subset	NKT1	NKT2	NKT17	T$_{FH}$	FoxP3$^+$	CD4^{pos}	CD4^{neg}	sulfatide-reactive	nd
Differentiation requirement	nd	nd	nd	strong TCR trigger	strong TCR trigger + TGFβ	nd	nd	nd	nd
Defining transcription factor	T-bet^{high} PLZF^{low}	GATA3^{high} PLZF^{high}	RORγt^{pos} PLZF^{int}	Bcl6^{pos}	FoxP3^{pos}	nd	nd	nd	nd
Peripheral phenotype	CD4 or DN, NK1.1$^+$ CD122$^+$ CD27$^+$	CD4$^+$ NK1.1^{neg} CD122^{neg} CD27$^+$	DN NK1.1^{neg} CD122^{neg} CD27$^{+/-}$ CD103$^+$ CD121a$^+$ CD196$^+$	CD4$^+$ NK1.1^{neg} PD−1$^+$ CXCR5$^+$	CD4$^{+/-}$ NK1.1^{neg} CD25$^+$ GITR$^+$ CD103$^+$	CD4$^+$ CD56$^{+/-}$ CD161$^{+/-}$	DN or CD8αα$^{+/-}$ CD56$^{+/-}$ CD161$^{+/-}$	CD4$^+$ or DN NK1.1$^+$	CD4$^+$ or DN NK1.1$^{+/-}$
Prominent location	liver, thymus, spleen, bone marrow	liver, thymus, spleen,	LN, skin	spleen, LN	intestine	liver, thymus, spleen, bone marrow	liver, thymus, spleen, bone marrow	liver, spleen	liver, spleen
Key cytokine/ function	IFNγ	IL-4	IL-17A	IL-21	IL-10?	Th0/Th2	Th1	nd	nd

The table does not include the Vα10$^+$ NKT cells or other non-conventional T cells. nd = not determined or not clear.

be considered preprogrammed. (d) T$_{FH}$-NKT cells are induced by strong antigenic stimulation and are characterized by the expression of the transcription factor Bcl6 and the surface markers CXCR5 and PD-1 (Chang et al., 2011; King et al., 2011; Tonti et al., 2012). (f) FoxP3$^+$ iNKT cells acquire FoxP3 expression following strong antigenic stimulation in the presence of high amounts of TGFβ (Moreira-Teixeira et al., 2011, 2012).

In contrast, in humans *i*NKT cell subsets are not yet as well defined. However, expression of CD4 has been correlated with functional differences. Following antigenic stimulation the cytokine production of CD4$^+$ Vα24*i* NKT cells follows a Th0-pattern, whereas CD4^{neg} *i*NKT cells are biased towards to a Th1-pattern (Gumperz et al., 2002; Lee et al., 2002a). Furthermore, an IL-17 producing subset of human *i*NKT cells exists, but unlike in mice, it requires exposure to inflammatory cytokines as well as TCR activation for IL-17 production (Moreira-Teixeira et al., 2011).

Altogether, these data demonstrate that *i*NKT cells are heterogeneous. Because the prevalence of functional *i*NKT cell subsets may differ between inbred mouse strains or individuals, some of the current controversies regarding the roles of *i*NKT cells could depend on subset prevalence or selective activation of subsets under certain conditions.

Technical Problems and the Species Divide

Several technical problems complicate the interpretation of the reported human data on *i*NKT cells and autoimmunity that we summarize below. Human *i*NKT cells can be identified by CD1d/αGalCer tetramers, which may be the most inclusive and accurate method. A clonotype-specific antibody that recognizes the CDR3α region formed by the invariant Vα24-Jα18 rearrangement is also available (Montoya et al., 2007), but may miss some human αGalCer and CD1d reactive cells that do not use Vα24 (Gadola et al., 2002; Brigl et al., 2006). In one study, these αGalCer reactive cells with this non-canonical TCR α chain were up to 20% of the tetramer binding population (Brigl et al., 2006). Interestingly, the TCRs expressed by these cells are related to the canonical TCR, as they express Vβ11 and the predominant Vα-segments they express (Vα3.1 and Vα10.1) are rearranged to the same Jα18 expressed by Vα24i NKT cells (Gadola et al., 2002; Brigl et al., 2006). The combination of Vα24 and Vβ11 antibodies is also sometimes used, but this might leave out some Vα24 negative iNKT cells, as well as including some non-iNKT cells. However, frequently less accurate methods to define iNKT cells are used, including: (a) Vα24-specific antibodies alone, (b) αβTCR and expression of one of several NK cell markers (e.g., CD161, CD56, CD16), (c) CD4⁻CD8⁻ (DN) αβT cells, and (d) RT-PCR for the iTCR, which does not allow for a direct assessment of cell frequency. Altogether, this means that different human studies are difficult to compare, as different populations may have been investigated. Here we will focus on reports using CD1d/αGalCer tetramers, the 6B11 antibody or Vα24⁺Vβ11⁺ cells. Furthermore, the depths of the characterization of iNKT cells in humans remains limited, especially regarding functional subsets, as analysis is usually confined to CD4 expression, one of the NK receptors, IFNγ, and IL-4. However, a "global" look at iNKT cells might miss important phenotypic and functional changes by a so far overlooked subset, which might be relevant in a particular disease. Also, most information about human iNKT cells is, for obvious reasons, derived from PBMCs. How human iNKT cells in peripheral blood relate to tissue iNKT cells, especially in affected organs, is largely unknown. For mice it has been reported that iNKT cells in blood poorly reflect the cells in other tissues regarding frequency, phenotype, and function (Berzins et al., 2004). Finally, when the frequency or function of iNKT cells during autoimmune diseases was reported, this was usually done at a single time in an individual, rather than longitudinally, which could be misleading in cases wherein the relevance of iNKT cells changes at different stages during disease progression.

The Species Divide

Most of the work on iNKT cells has been done in mouse models. Apart from the quip that "mice are not humans," and the obvious fact that the genetic background in human subjects is much more varied than in the few

inbred mice strains commonly used, there are a few other aspects worth noting that complicate the translation of findings from mice to humans. A striking difference is in the relative distribution of iNKT cells in different organs. In mice the highest frequency of iNKT cells is found in liver, followed in descending order by adipose tissue, thymus/spleen/bone marrow/PBMCs, and lymph nodes. In humans iNKT cells are abundant in adipose tissue, but not especially abundant in liver/peritoneum and generally lower in frequency than in the commonly studied inbred mouse strains. Additionally, in human mNKT and type II NKT cells are more frequent than in mice and they contain additional non-conventional T lymphocytes reactive to CD1a, CD1b, and CD1c (Kronenberg and Gapin, 2002; Kronenberg, 2005; Bendelac et al., 2007). So, whereas in many cases the role of iNKT cells in animal models of autoimmunity is well established, controversy to varying degrees remains with regard to their role in human autoimmunity.

THE JANUS-LIKE CHARACTER OF iNKT CELLS IN AUTOIMMUNITY

In line with the diversity of iNKT cells, cytokine and effector responses, and their involvement in shaping immune responses, it is not surprising that iNKT cells have also been reported to participate in autoimmune disease pathogenesis (for earlier reviews on this topic see Ronchi and Falcone, 2008; Balato et al., 2009; Wu and Van Kaer, 2009; Berzins et al., 2011; Novak and Lehuen, 2011; Simoni et al., 2012). Despite conflicting data, we try here to distinguish those autoimmune diseases is in which iNKT cells seem to promote pathogenesis in the majority of reports from those in which they tend to prevent it. Given the vast literature in the field, not all details can be described here, but rather we summarize the major findings, emphasizing the underlying mechanisms and focusing on recent developments.

Too Much of a Good Thing: Detrimental Roles of iNKT Cells

For diseases in this section, the data are most consistent with roles for iNKT cells in initiating and/or aggravating pathogenesis (Table 8.2).

Atherosclerosis

Atherosclerosis is a chronic inflammatory disease within the vessels, driven by responses to accumulated lipids in the arterial intima. A contribution of the adaptive as well as the innate immune system, and an autoimmune component, has recently become apparent (Shi, 2010; Grundtman and Wick, 2011; for earlier reviews on the

TABLE 8.2 Detrimental Involvement of Human *i*NKT Cells in Selected Autoimmune Diseases

Disease	*i*NKT cell frequency*	*i*NKT cell cytokines	Effects of treatment	Etc.
Atherosclerosis	• decreased in PBMCs: Kyriakakis et al. (2010).	*i*NKT cell lines derived from atherosclerotic plaques were more sensitive to antigen stimulation than lines derived from PBMCs (Kyriakakis et al., 2010).		CD1d expression is enhanced in the atherosclerotic plaques (Melián et al., 1999; Bobryshev, 2005; Chan et al., 2005; Kyriakakis et al., 2010). [1]
Crohn's disease	• decreased in PBMCs: van der Vliet et al. (2001); Grose et al. (2007b). • Vα24 mRNA and the numbers of Vα24+ T cells are reduced in the intestine: Grose et al. (2007b)			
Diabetes mellitus	Frequency in PBMCs: • decreased: Wilson et al. (1998); Kukreja et al. (2002); Kis et al. (2007); Montoya et al. (2007). • unchanged: Lee et al. (2002b); Michalek et al. (2006); Tsutsumi et al. (2006); Oling et al. (2007); Zhang et al. (2011). • increased: Oikawa et al. (2002).	• The cytokine production from PBMC derived *i*NKT cell (lines) was: (a) less and/or Th2 bias in Wilson et al. (1998); Wilson et al. (2000); Kukreja et al. (2002); Kis et al. (2007). (b) no difference: Lee et al. (2002b); Roman-Gonzalez et al. (2009). • Less IL-4 production by pancreatic lymph node derived *i*NKT cell lines (Kent et al., 2005).		
Multiple sclerosis	Frequency in PBMCs: • decreased:Illes et al. (2000); van der Vliet et al. (2001); Araki et al. (2003); Demoulins et al. (2003). • unchanged: Gigli et al. (2007); O'Keeffe et al. (2008).	• The cytokine production from PBMC derived *i*NKT cell lines displayed: (a) a Th2-bias: Araki et al. (2003); O'Keeffe et al. (2008). (b) no difference: Gigli et al. (2007). (c) a Th1-bias: Gausling et al. (2001).	*i*NKT cell frequency increased in PBMCs from patients under treatment (IFNβ, Gigli et al., 2007) or patients in remission (Araki et al., 2003).	The frequency of *i*NKT cells in PBMCs was especially decreased in patients under remission (Illes et al., 2000; Araki et al., 2003).
Systemic lupus erythematosus	• decreased in PBMCs: Sumida et al. (1995, 1998); Kojo et al. (2001); van der Vliet et al. (2001); Wither et al. (2008); Wong et al. (2009); Parietti et al. (2010); Cho et al. (2011); Yu and Wang (2011); Bosma et al. (2012).	*i*NKT cell lines (Kojo et al., 2001; Cho et al., 2011; Yu and Wang, 2011; Bosma et al., 2012) or fresh *i*NKT cells from PBMCs (Bosma et al., 2012) displayed a Th2-bias but produced less cytokines overall.	The frequency of *i*NKT cells in PBMCs increased following therapy (Oishi et al., 2001; Bosma et al., 2012).	The frequency of *i*NKT cells in PBMCs correlated with (a) disease severity (Cho et al., 2011; Parietti et al., 2010) [2] and (b) serum levels of autoreactive IgGs (Green et al., 2007; Wither et al., 2008).

*The table only lists reports in which iNKT cells were identified by CD1d/αGalCer tetramers or 6B11 antibodies or the combination of Vα24+Vβ11+. Comments: [1] NKT-cell like (CD3+CD161+) cells are found in atherosclerotic plaques (Bobryshev, 2005; Chan et al., 2005). [2] Differing results by Wither et al. (2008).

role of *i*NKT cell in atherosclerosis see Braun et al., 2010; Getz et al., 2011, see also Chapter 71).

In PBMCs of human patients, *i*NKT cell numbers were decreased (Kyriakakis et al., 2010) and NKT cell-like (CD3⁺CD161⁺) cells were found in atherosclerotic plaques, where they represented up to 2% of the lymphocytes (Bobryshev, 2005; Chan et al., 2005). Interestingly, CD1d expression was enhanced in the atherosclerotic plaques (Melián et al., 1999; Bobryshev, 2005; Chan et al., 2005; Kyriakakis et al., 2010). *i*NKT cell lines derived from atherosclerotic plaques produced proinflammatory cytokines following αGalCer stimulation and did this with an approximately 10-fold higher antigenic sensitivity than PBMC-derived cell lines (Kyriakakis et al., 2010).

In mouse models of atherosclerosis, *i*NKT cells could also be found in the atherosclerotic lesions (Tupin et al., 2004; Nakai et al., 2004; Aslanian et al., 2005) and data with reporter mice suggest that CXCR6 signaling might be required for this accumulation (Galkina et al., 2007). Interestingly, when serum lipids from atherosclerosis-prone LDL-receptor deficient mice were fed to DCs, this led to a CD1d-dependent stimulation of *i*NKT cell hybridomas (VanderLaan et al., 2007). *i*NKT cell deficient mice developed a greatly ameliorated disease (Major et al., 2004; Nakai et al., 2004; Tupin et al., 2004; Aslanian et al., 2005; Ström et al., 2007; Rogers et al., 2008; To et al., 2009) and transfer of CD4⁺*i*NKT cells could transfer susceptibility (VanderLaan et al., 2007; To et al., 2009). The reduced plaque formation in *i*NKT cell deficient animals correlated with an approximately 90% decrease in IFNγ mRNA in the atherosclerotic lesions (Rogers et al., 2008). Consequently, activation of *i*NKT cells either by antigens (Tupin et al., 2004; Nakai et al., 2004; Major et al., 2004) or with lipopolysaccharide (LPS) (Ostos et al., 2002; Andoh et al., 2012) aggravated disease. This is in line with the observation that microbial infections enhance the development of atherosclerosis in both human and animal models (Hansson et al., 2006). Despite this, one study reported a protective effect of *i*NKT cell stimulation on atherosclerosis (van Puijvelde et al., 2009). Several proteins involved in lipid metabolism have also been shown to be involved in CD1d lipid antigen loading and *i*NKT cell development, including apoE (Elzen et al., 2005), sphingolipid activator protein (SAP) (Zhou et al., 2004), microsomal triglyceride transfer protein (MTTP) (Brozovic et al., 2004), and ABCG1 (Sag et al., 2012). For example, apoE can bind αGalCer and aid in its uptake (Elzen et al., 2005; Allan et al., 2009).

Asthma

Asthma is multi-factorial disease that could in some cases have an autoimmune component. Several studies have

implicated Vα24*i* NKT cells in the pathogenesis of asthma in humans (Matangkasombut et al., 2009b; Rijavec et al., 2011; Thomas et al., 2010; Umetsu and DeKruyff, 2010). A decreased frequency in PBMCs from asthmatic patients, at least in the CD4⁺ subset of *i*NKT cells, has been reported by some (Koh et al., 2010; Yan-ming et al., 2012), but not by others (Magnan et al., 2000; Akbari et al., 2006). Interestingly, upper respiratory tract infections, which often exacerbate asthma, were correlated with a decrease of *i*NKT cells in PBMC (Koh et al., 2012), suggesting potential recruitment to the lung. In line with this notion, *i*NKT cells are almost undetectable in the airways of healthy controls, either in lung biopsies (Akbari et al., 2006; Vijayanand et al., 2007; Reynolds et al., 2009) or in the bronchoalveolar lavage fluid (BALF) (Akbari et al., 2006; Thomas et al., 2007; Matangkasombut et al., 2009a), but can be detected in samples from asthmatic patients. However, controversy remains about the magnitude of this increase within the lungs of asthmatics. For BALF only two studies reported a frequency of more than 2.5% of *i*NKT cells within total T cells (Akbari et al., 2006; Matangkasombut et al., 2009a) with most studies reporting frequencies between 0.6 and 2.5% (Thomas et al., 2006, 2007; Vijayanand et al., 2007; Bratke et al., 2007; Heron et al., 2007; Mutalithas et al., 2007; Matangkasombut et al., 2009a; Brooks et al., 2010). For lung biopsies the values ranged from 1.7 (Vijayanand et al., 2007) to 9.8 (Reynolds et al., 2009) to over 50% (Akbari et al., 2006). Importantly, it was noted that the frequency of *i*NKT cells in the lung increases with the severity of symptoms (Akbari et al., 2006; Hamzaoui et al., 2006; Matangkasombut et al., 2009a; Reynolds et al., 2009; Koh and Shim, 2010). Most forms of asthma are associated with Th2 cytokine profile, but conflicting data were reported regarding the presence of a Th2 skewed cytokine production by restimulated *i*NKT cells from PBMC of asthma patients (Sen et al., 2005; Yan-ming et al., 2012). However, antigen stimulated *i*NKT cells from BALF of asthmatic patients produced IL-4 and IL-13, but hardly any IFNγ (Akbari et al., 2006), in line with the hypothesized Th2 bias.

In mouse airway inflammation models, the evidence is strong for a major pathogenic role for *i*NKT cells in airway hypersensitivity. The potency of *i*NKT cells in airway inflammation is illustrated by the fact that airway challenge with *i*NKT cell glycolipid antigens alone, like αGalCer, induces many of the pathological features of asthma, even in MHC class II deficient mice that lack conventional CD4⁺ T cells (Meyer et al., 2006). This suggests that asthma might be induced directly by airway exposures to *i*NKT cell antigens present in inspired air. Clearly, weak environmental *i*NKT cell antigens found in house dust can act as potent adjuvant in the sensitization to a model antigen (Wingender et al., 2011). Even in the

absence of known *i*NKT cells antigens, several groups
have found that *i*NKT cells are required in mouse models
of asthma initiated by ovalbumin (OVA) sensitization
(Akbari et al., 2003; Lisbonne et al., 2003; Kim et al.,
2004, 2009), ragweed (Bilenki et al., 2004), or ozone
(Pichavant et al., 2008). This is best illustrated by the
clearly reduced airway inflammation in *i*NKT cell deficient animals in several models, and the restoration of
susceptibility by *i*NKT cell transfer (Cui et al., 1999;
Akbari et al., 2003; Lisbonne et al., 2003; Pichavant
et al., 2008; Wingender et al., 2011; Kim et al., 2012).

In the allergen-induced model of airway hypersensitivity, IL-4 and IL-13 secretion by *i*NKT cells has been
implicated (Akbari et al., 2003; Meyer et al., 2006;
Terashima et al., 2008), while the ozone-induced model
depended upon IL-17A as well as IL-4 and IL-13
(Pichavant et al., 2008).

Two studies in macaques were in line with the findings in mouse models in showing that a glycolipid antigen
for *i*NKT cells could induce hypersensitivity and that an
allergen challenge could lead to *i*NKT cell infiltration
into the lung (Matangkasombut et al., 2008; Ayanoglu
et al., 2011).

IBD/Colitis

Inflammatory bowel disease (IBD) denotes a spectrum of
T cell-dependent chronic disorders of different parts of
the gastrointestinal tract. The inflammatory response is
triggered by antigens derived from the gut lumen, which
may follow a perturbation of the epithelial layer, caused
either through genetic alterations or the administration of
exogenous agents. Several reviews on the role of *i*NKT
cells in colitis models have been published (Zeissig et al.,
2007; Wingender and Kronenberg, 2008). Some types of
intestinal bacteria are probiotic, in that they prevent
inflammation of the intestine. It is therefore of note that
*i*NKT cells can influence the microbial colonization and
the composition of intestinal bacteria (Nieuwenhuis et al.,
2009). Furthermore, the activation state of *i*NKT cells,
and their influence on the mucosal immune response, is
highly altered in germ-free mice (Olszak et al., 2012;
Wingender et al., 2012b).

Ulcerative colitis is an inflammation of the superficial
layers of the colon that has been attributed in some studies to an exaggerated Th2 response. *i*NKT cells were
decreased in the PBMCs of ulcerative colitis patients (van
der Vliet et al., 2001; Grose et al., 2007b). Additionally,
there was a reduction in Vα24 mRNA in the intestine of
colitis patients (Grose et al., 2007a), but the majority of
these Vα24+ cells might not be *i*NKT cells, as judged by
Vβ11 expression (O'Keeffe et al., 2004). Interestingly, in
ulcerative colitis patients, it was found that *v*NKT cells,
rather than *i*NKT cells, were the major CD1d-dependent

producers of the deleterious IL-13 (Fuss et al., 2004). This
is in contrast to results obtained using the oxazolone-
induced mouse model of colitis, where it was shown that
the pathogenic IL-13 was derived from *i*NKT cells (Heller
et al., 2002). In this model, interfering with *i*NKT cell activation prevented disease development (Heller et al., 2002;
Brozovic et al., 2004; Camelo et al., 2012).

Primary Biliary Cirrhosis (PBC)

PBC is characterized by portal inflammation and
immune-mediated chronic destruction of intrahepatic
small bile duct epithelial cells (i.e., cholangitis) (for earlier reviews on *i*NKT cell activity in this disease see
Camelo et al., 2012; Uibo et al., 2012).

*i*NKT cells are increased in PBMCs as well as in the
liver of PBC patients (Kita et al., 2002) and these livers
contain higher IFNγ levels (Omenetti et al., 2009). The
increase of *i*NKT cells in the liver coincided with an
increase of CD1d expression levels on epithelial cells of
the small bile duct of PBC patients (Tsuneyama et al.,
1998; Kita et al., 2002). The cross-reactivity of antibodies
to several bacteria with the lipidated mitochondrial protein PDC-E2 has been implicated in the genesis of PBC
(Selmi et al., 2003; Bogdanos et al., 2004; Bogdanos and
Vergani, 2009; Yanagisawa et al., 2011).

One bacterium in particular that is the target of
these cross-reactive antibodies from PBC patients is
Novosphingobium aromaticivorans (Selmi et al., 2003;
Olafsson et al., 2004). This bacterium is of interest
because of its relation to *Sphingomonas* bacteria, which
bear known *i*NKT cell antigens (Kinjo et al., 2005;
Mattner et al., 2005). Most importantly, *N. aromaticivorans* can induce a PBC-like disease in a mouse model
in an *i*NKT cell-dependent fashion (Mattner et al.,
2008; Mohammed et al., 2011). The crucial role for
*i*NKT cells in initiating PBC-like disease in mice has
been supported by other reports (Chuang et al., 2008;
Wu et al., 2011).

Rheumatoid Arthritis

In rheumatoid arthritis (RA) autoreactive Th1 and Th17
T cells cause inflammation of small and large synovial
joints, leading to joint deformation and loss of movement
(for earlier reviews on the role of *i*NKT cells in RA see
Coppieters et al., 2007a; Drennan et al., 2010; Sowden
and Ng, 2012).

Human RA patients display reduced *i*NKT cell frequencies in PBMCs (Kojo et al., 2001; van der Vliet et al.,
2004; Parietti et al., 2010; Tudhope et al., 2010) and the
rheumatoid synovium (Maeda et al., 1999; Linsen et al.,
2005). Although the *i*NKT cell frequency did not correlate with clinical disease severity (Parietti et al., 2010;

Tudhope et al., 2010) it was noted that the frequency increased following treatment (Parietti et al., 2010; Tudhope et al., 2010). *i*NKT cell lines derived from RA patient PBMCs expanded less *in vitro* following αGalCer stimulation (Kojo et al., 2001; Linsen et al., 2005; Tudhope et al., 2010) and produced reduced cytokines, although with a Th1 bias (Kojo et al., 2001; Linsen et al., 2005), when compared to control lines. In contrast to PBMCs, no impairment of *i*NKT cell expansion and function was observed in synovial derived *i*NKT cell lines (Linsen et al., 2005). Even though the expression levels of CD1d on PBMCs might not be altered (no change: Kojo et al., 2003; higher on DCs: Jacques et al., 2010) it was reported that RA patients have decreased levels of soluble CD1d in the serum (Kojo et al., 2003; Segawa et al., 2009).

Without delineating the details of the different mouse models for RA that have been studied, the role of *i*NKT cells overall is pathogenic. The frequency of *i*NKT cells increased with disease progression (Chiba et al., 2005; Postigo et al., 2012), they upregulated activation markers (Kim, 2006; Jung et al., 2009; Miellot-Gafsou et al., 2010) and they were recruited to the joints (Kim et al., 2005) where they could be activated directly by aggregated antibodies (Kim et al., 2005). Furthermore, the percentage of IL-17A$^+$*i*NKT cells increased with disease progression (Jung et al., 2009). Injection of blocking αCD1d antibodies ameliorated arthritis (Chiba et al., 2005; Miellot-Gafsou et al., 2010) and in *i*NKT cell deficient mice the disease was less severe (Jα18$^{-/-}$: Chiba et al., 2005; Ohnishi et al., 2005; Yoshiga et al., 2008; CD1d$^{-/-}$: Ohnishi et al., 2005; Kim et al., 2005; Kim, 2006; Jung et al., 2009; Teige et al., 2010). Such diseased *i*NKT cell deficient animals had higher IL-10 production by collagen-specific T cells (Chiba et al., 2005; Jung et al., 2009) and proinflammatory cytokines tended to be lower (Chiba et al., 2005; Ohnishi et al., 2005; Yoshiga et al., 2008; Jung et al., 2009). Additionally, they had reduced antigen-specific antibody titers (Jung et al., 2009; Ohnishi et al., 2005) with an elevated IgG1/IgG2a ratio (Chiba et al., 2005), suggesting a Th2 deviation. Furthermore, injection of *i*NKT cell antigens generally ameliorated disease (Chiba et al., 2004; Miellot et al., 2005; Takagi et al., 2006; Coppieters et al., 2007b; Kaieda et al., 2007; Yoshiga et al., 2011). The disease amelioration could be attributed to the impairment of the pathogenic Th17 response, rather than to a Th2 cytokine deviation (Chiba et al., 2004; Kaieda et al., 2007; Yoshiga et al., 2011). By contrast, only two studies implied a beneficial role of *i*NKT cells in mouse models of RA. In one, tolerogenic DCs were only effective ameliorating arthritis when they were CD1d$^+$ (Jung et al., 2010), suggesting a role for type I and/or type II NKT cells. Also, Teige et al. (2010) reported a protective role

of *i*NKT cells. Intriguingly, it has recently been suggested, that Vα14*i* NKT cells might recognize a mouse collagen II derived peptide (mCII$_{707-721}$) in a CD1d-dependent manner (Liu et al., 2011). This report is one of very few indicating that peptides, in addition to lipids, can be presented by CD1d (Castano et al., 1995; Zeng et al., 1997; Lee et al., 1998; Tangri et al., 1998). Further studies will be required to understand the mechanism of peptide binding into the hydrophobic CD1d groove, and to confirm that *i*NKT cells are in fact reactive to a peptide bound to CD1d.

Skin Disorders

Psoriasis is a local inflammation of the skin driven by a mixed Th1/Th17 T cell response (Lowes et al., 2008; Zaba et al., 2009) leading to abnormal proliferation and differentiation of keratinocytes (for earlier *i*NKT cell reviews see Balato et al., 2009; Peternel and Kastelan, 2009; Tobin et al., 2011). There are numerous reports of T cells expressing NK cell markers in skin (Bonish et al., 2000; Nickoloff, 2000; Cameron et al., 2002; Gilhar et al., 2002; Koreck et al., 2002; Curry et al., 2003; Langewouters et al., 2007) and increases in these cells in psoriatic plaques (Zhao et al., 2008). For *i*NKT cells, one report showed a decreased frequency in PBMCs from psoriasis patients (van der Vliet et al., 2004). Furthermore, CD1d expression is upregulated in the inflamed skin (Gober et al., 2008; Zhao et al., 2008). Specifically, IFNγ pre-treated keratinocytes upregulate CD1d and can induce IFNγ, but not IL-4, production by *i*NKT cell lines (Bonish et al., 2000).

In systemic sclerosis NKT cells from patient PBMCs have been reported to be decreased (Kojo et al., 2001; van der Vliet et al., 2001) and to display a Th1-bias (Kojo et al., 2001).

Similarly, in contact dermatitis NKT cells from patient PBMCs, especially the DN subset, were decreased in most (Oishi et al., 2000; Takahashi et al., 2003; Ilhan et al., 2007; Gyimesi et al., 2011), but not all (Magnan et al., 2000; Prell et al., 2003; Wu et al., 2010) reports. Whereas skin from control subjects did not contain detectable *i*NKT cells, they could be found in patient skin biopsies (Gober et al., 2008; Simon et al., 2009; Wu et al., 2010; Balato et al., 2012), consistent with a possible migration from the blood to the site of inflammation. *i*NKT cells, all CD4$^+$, were found within the dermal infiltrating cells and made up 6–9% of the T cells, although none were found in the epidermis (Gober et al., 2008; Simon et al., 2009). After stimulation of PBMC *i*NKT cells two reports noted a Th2 bias (IL-4 > IFNγ) of the cytokine response in patient *i*NKT cells (Takahashi et al., 2003; Gyimesi et al., 2011), whereas one report observed a Th1 bias (Oishi et al., 2000).

Furthermore, production of IFNγ and IL-4 by iNKT cells was also detected within the affected skin of patients (Gober et al., 2008; Simon et al., 2009). Interestingly, thymic stromal lymphopoietin (TSLP), a cytokine that is produced by activated keratinocytes (Soumelis et al., 2002) and is elevated in patient lesions (Nakamura et al., 2008; Wu et al., 2010) can bias cytokine production by activated iNKT cells towards a Th2 pattern (IL-4, IL-13) (Wu et al., 2010; Jariwala et al., 2011).

In an animal model of contact hypersensitivity (CHS), the majority of studies demonstrated the involvement of iNKT cells (Campos et al., 2003, 2006a,b; Nieuwenhuis et al., 2005; Dey et al., 2011; Askenase et al., 2011), although two reports did not (Elkhal et al., 2006; Goubier et al., 2012). Furthermore, iNKT cell deficient animals showed an impaired CHS response (Nieuwenhuis et al., 2005; Askenase et al., 2011). Interestingly, topical application of a CD1d-binding non-stimulatory glycolipid reduced the severity of the CHS response, likely by blocking the presentation of antigenic lipids by CD1d (Nieuwenhuis et al., 2005). The pathogenic role of iNKT cells could be attributed to their rapid production of IL-4 (Campos et al., 2003, 2006b).

Missed so Sadly: Beneficial Roles of iNKT Cells

Here we outline cases where the current consensus points to a beneficial role of iNKT cells in preventing disease development (Table 8.3).

Diabetes

Type 1 diabetes mellitus (T1D), also called insulin-dependent diabetes mellitus, is a Th1 autoimmune disease caused by the selective destruction of insulin-producing β-cells in the islets of Langerhans in the pancreas, leading ultimately to the loss of glucose homeostasis (for earlier iNKT cell reviews see Fletcher and Baxter, 2009; Wu and Van Kaer, 2009; Lehuen et al., 2010; Berzins et al., 2011; Novak and Lehuen, 2011).

Conflicting data on the frequency and function of iNKT cells from patient PBMC have been reported. Whereas some reports observed lower iNKT cell frequencies, at least of the CD4+ cells (Wilson et al., 1998; Kukreja et al., 2002; Kis et al., 2007; Montoya et al., 2007), others found equal (Lee et al., 2002b; Michalek et al., 2006; Tsutsumi et al., 2006; Oling et al., 2007; Zhang et al., 2011) or even more iNKT cells (Oikawa et al., 2002) in patient PBMCs compared to healthy controls. Furthermore, whereas some authors noted reduced cytokine production of iNKT cell (lines) and/or a Th2 bias (Wilson et al., 1998, 2000; Kukreja et al., 2002; Kis et al., 2007), others did not find such differences (Lee et al., 2002b; Roman-Gonzalez et al.,

2009). Importantly, one study analyzed iNKT cell lines derived from the draining pancreatic lymph node and observed reduced IL-4 production following antigen stimulation (Kent et al., 2005).

Non-obese diabetic (NOD) mice develop spontaneous T1D and have been studied extensively. iNKT cells in NOD mice are reduced in frequency (Berzins et al., 2004; Chen et al., 2011) and produce fewer cytokines following αGalCer (Gombert et al., 1996; Lehuen et al., 1998; Falcone et al., 1999; Hong et al., 2001; Sharif et al., 2001) or after stimulation of the innate immune system (Falcone et al., 1999). Increasing the iNKT cell frequency in NOD mice, either by cell transfer (Baxter et al., 1997; Hammond et al., 1998; Lehuen et al., 1998; Beaudoin et al., 2002; Chen et al., 2005; Cain et al., 2006; Simoni et al., 2011) or by overexpression of the iTCR (Lehuen et al., 1998), or by overexpression of CD1d on pancreatic island cells (Falcone et al., 2004), prevented or ameliorated symptoms. Consequently, iNKT cell deficient NOD mice showed increased frequency and earlier onset of disease (Naumov et al., 2001; Shi et al., 2001; Wang et al., 2001; Fletcher and Baxter, 2009). Furthermore, the repetitive injection of αGalCer ameliorated disease progression, even when treatment was started after the onset of insulitis (Hong et al., 2001; Naumov et al., 2001; Sharif et al., 2001; Wang et al., 2001). Other αGalCer derivatives were similarly effective (Mizuno et al., 2004; Forestier et al., 2007; Ly et al., 2010). The original explanation for the therapeutic effect of αGalCer was the shift to a Th2 reponse (Hong et al., 2001; Naumov et al., 2001; Sharif et al., 2001), but not all studies observed such a shift (Shi et al., 2001; Wang et al., 2001; Beaudoin et al., 2002) and work with congenic NOD lines demonstrated that such a shift is not required for protection (Rocha-Campos et al., 2006; Jordan et al., 2007). Furthermore, the results from a number of papers are not in agreement as to which cytokine is essential for the protection from diabetes. IL-10 (Hammond et al., 1998; Hong et al., 2001; Naumov et al., 2001; Sharif et al., 2001) and/or IL-4 (Hong et al., 2001; Naumov et al., 2001; Sharif et al., 2001) were claimed to be important, but not in every case (Beaudoin et al., 2002; Mi et al., 2004; Novak et al., 2005; Chen et al., 2006), and even IFNγ elicited by iNKT cell activation was implicated as protective in one study (Cain et al., 2006). However, it was shown that activated iNKT cells can directly interact and influence T cells and DCs in multiple ways. Activated iNKTs were reported to impair the differentiation of pathogenic islet-specific CD4+ T cells, leading to T cell anergy (Beaudoin et al., 2002; Hugues et al., 2002; Novak et al., 2005). This was dependent on cell–cell contact between the iNKT and CD4+ T cells (Novak et al., 2005) and independent of CD4 T cell CD1d expression (Novak et al., 2007). Although overall numbers of regulatory T (Treg) cells in the NOD/αGalCer model did not differ

TABLE 8.3 Beneficial Involvement of Human iNKT Cells in Selected Autoimmune Diseases

Disease	iNKT cell frequency*	iNKT cell cytokines	Effects of treatment	Etc.
Asthma	• decreased in PBMCs? (a) yes: Koh et al. (2010); Yan-ming et al. (2012). (b) no: Magnan et al. (2000); Akbari et al. (2006). • present in the BALF of asthmatic patients: Akbari et al. (2006); Phamthi et al. (2006); Thomas et al. (2006); Bratke et al. (2007); Heron et al. (2007); Mutalithas et al. (2007);Thomas et al. (2007); Vijayanand et al. (2007); Matangkasombut et al. (2009a); Brooks et al. (2010). • present in the lung of asthmatic patients: Akbari et al. (2006); Vijayanand et al. (2007); Reynolds et al. (2009).	iNKT cells from BALF of asthmatic patients produced IL-4 and IL-13, but hardly any IFNγ (Akbari et al., 2006).		The frequency of iNKT cells in the lung increases with the severity of symptoms (Akbari et al., 2006; Hamzaoui et al., 2006; Matangkasombut et al., 2009a; Reynolds et al., 2009; Koh and Shim, 2010).
Dermatitis	• decreased in PBMCs: Oishi et al. (2000) [1]; Takahashi et al. (2003); Ilhan et al. (2007); Gyimesi et al. (2011). • increased in the skin: Gober et al. (2008); Simon et al. (2009); Wu et al. (2010); Balato et al. (2012).	Skin iNKT cells in patient lesions produce IFNγ and IL-4 (Gober et al., 2008; Simon et al., 2009).		
Primary biliary cirrhosis	• increased in PBMCs and the liver: Kita et al. (2002).			Livers contain higher IFNγ mRNA levels (Omenetti et al., 2009) [2].
Psoriasis	• decreased in PBMCs: van der Vliet et al. (2004). • increased in psoriatic plaques Zhao et al. (2008).		IFNγ pre-treated keratinocytes upregulated CD1d and could induce IFNγ, but not IL-4, production by iNKT cell lines (Bonish et al., 2000).	CD1d is upregulated in the inflamed skin (Bonish et al., 2000, Gober et al., 2008; Zhao et al., 2008).
Rheumatoid arthritis	• decreased in PBMCs: Kojo et al. (2001); van der Vliet et al. (2004); Parietti et al. (2010); Tudhope et al. (2010). • decrease in synovium: Maeda et al. (1999); Linsen et al. (2005).	Less cytokines and Th1 bias in iNKT cell lines derived from PBMCs (Kojo et al., 2001; Linsen et al., 2005; Tudhope et al., 2010), but not from synovial derived cell lines (Linsen et al., 2005).	iNKT cell frequency increased in PBMCs (Parietti et al., 2010, αCD20-Ab (rituximab) positive correlation with clinical outcome; Tudhope et al., 2010 (methotraxate therapy) no correlation)).	RA patients have decreased levels of soluble CD1d in the serum (Kojo et al., 2003; Segawa et al., 2009).
Systemic sclerosis	• decreased in PBMCs: Kojo et al. (2001); van der Vliet et al. (2004).	Th1 bias in iNKT cell lines derived from PBMCs (Kojo et al., 2001).		
Ulcerative colitis	• decrease in PBMCs: van der Vliet et al. (2001); Grose et al. (2007). • less Vα24 mRNA in the intestine of colitis patients: Grose et al. (2007).			

*The table only lists reports in which iNKT cells were identified by CD1d/αGalCer tetramers or 6B11 antibodies or the combination of Vα24+Vβ11+.
Comments: [1] differing results in Magnan et al. (2000); Prell et al. (2003); Wu et al. (2010); [2] NKT-like (CD3+ CD57+) cells accumulated in the bile ducts of PBC patients (Harada et al., 2003).
Reference: Harada, K. et al. 2003. Accumulating CD57+ CD3+ natural killer T cells are related to intrahepatic bile duct lesions in primary biliary cirrhosis. Liver Int. 23(2), 94–100.

(Sharif et al., 2001; Ly et al., 2006; Forestier et al., 2007) their activity has been implicated by some (Ly et al., 2006; Diana et al., 2011), but not by others (Beaudoin et al., 2002; Cain et al., 2006). Tolerogenic effects on CD8$^+$ T cells have been reported too (Chuang et al., 2011). Furthermore, *i*NKT cells in NOD mice treated with αGalCer could affect several DC populations leading to a tolerogenic outcome (Naumov et al., 2001; Chen et al., 2005; Saxena et al., 2007; Driver et al., 2010; Diana et al., 2011). Interestingly, this also required cell–cell contact (Baev et al., 2008; Caielli et al., 2010) but required CD1d expression on the DCs as well (Caielli et al., 2010). These tolerogenic DC were reported to induce Tregs (Diana et al., 2011) and migrate to the pancreatic lymph node to tolerize T cells locally (Chen et al., 2005). The diverse outcomes in the NOD mouse could reflect the different experimental systems used, for example, the transfer of different NOD mouse cell populations to recipients.

IBD/Crohn's Disease

Crohn's disease is characterized by a chronic and discontinuous inflammation deep in the tissues of both the small and large intestines, with high levels of Th1 cytokines. *i*NKT cells are reduced in PBMCs of affected patients (van der Vliet et al., 2001; Grose et al., 2007b). Additionally, Vα24 mRNA and the numbers of Vα24$^+$ cells were reduced in the intestine (Grose et al., 2007b).

In Th1 cytokine-mediated mouse colitis models, stimulation of *i*NKT cells could ameliorate disease (Saubermann et al., 2000; Numata et al., 2005; Ueno et al., 2005). The data are consistent with the conclusion that this activation shifted the immune response from the deleterious Th1 cytokine pattern to a protective Th2 response (Saubermann et al., 2000; Numata et al., 2005; Ueno et al., 2005).

Multiple Sclerosis/EAE

Multiple sclerosis (MS) is a chronic, Th1/Th17 T cell-driven inflammatory disease directed against myelin antigens in the central nervous system (CNS), leading to progressive paralysis.

The frequency of *i*NKT cells was reduced in patient PBMCs in most (Illes et al., 2000; van der Vliet et al., 2001; Araki et al., 2003; Demoulins et al., 2003), but not all studies (Gigli et al., 2007; O'Keeffe et al., 2008). This reduction was especially prominent in patients under remission (Illes et al., 2000; Araki et al., 2003). Furthermore, when *i*NKT cell lines derived from patient PBMCs were analyzed for cytokine production, one study found no difference (Gigli et al., 2007), one study observed a Th1 bias (Gausling et al., 2001), whereas two studies noticed a Th2 bias

of the *i*NKT cell lines (Araki et al., 2003; O'Keeffe et al., 2008;). Interestingly, MS patients under treatment (IFNβ: Gigli et al., 2007) or patients in remission (Araki et al., 2003) displayed an increased frequency of *i*NKT cells in PBMCs and increased cytokine production by them.

MS-like features can be replicated in mice by immunization with CNS peptides creating a model now called experimental autoimmune encephalomyelitis (EAE). Most (Jahng et al., 2001; Teige et al., 2004; Oh and Chung, 2011), but not all studies (Singh et al., 2001; Furlan et al., 2003) reported that *i*NKT cell deficient animals display exacerbated disease. Additionally, an increased *i*NKT cell frequency, due to expression of a Vα14*i* transgene, ameliorated disease (Mars et al., 2002, 2008). Importantly, activation of *i*NKT cells with αGalCer or Th2 biasing glycolipids related to αGalCer (Miyamoto et al., 2001; Zhang et al., 2008) protected mice against EAE. Protection correlated with a Th1 to Th2 cytokine diversion (Jahng et al., 2001; Miyamoto et al., 2001; Pal et al., 2001; Singh et al., 2001; Furlan et al., 2003; Zhang et al., 2008; Oh and Chung 2011) and a reduction of the Th17 T cell response (Mars et al., 2009; Yokote et al., 2010; Oh and Chung, 2011). However, which *i*NKT cell cytokines are important for these changes is not known. IL-4 and/or IL-10 have been suggested (Jahng et al., 2001; Miyamoto et al., 2001; Singh et al., 2001; Oh and Chung, 2011), but some data contradict this (Mars et al., 2002; Furlan et al., 2003); similarly divergent results have been reported role for IFNγ (Pro: Furlan et al., 2003; Mars et al., 2009 Con: Jahng et al., 2001; Oh and Chung, 2011). Although, *i*NKT cells can enter the CNS (Jahng et al., 2001; Mars et al., 2008; Oh and Chung, 2011) it is not certain if this is required for protection. Likewise, the importance of CD1d, beyond the primary *i*NKT cell stimulation, has been disputed (Wiethe et al., 2007; Mars et al., 2008). Recently, it was shown that *i*NKT cells activated by αGalCer in an EAE model skewed the CNS-infiltrating macrophage population towards a protective M2 type (Denney et al., 2012).

Systemic Lupus Erythematosus (SLE)

SLE is characterized by the production and deposition of autoantibodies against multiple nuclear antigens, leading to chronic inflammation of various tissues. The autoantigens are thought to derive from a defective clearance of apoptotic cells (see Chapter 17). According to one hypothesis, *i*NKT cells suppress autoreactive B cells in a CD1d-dependent fashion (for earlier *i*NKT cell reviews see Ronchi and Falcone, 2008; Gabriel et al., 2009; Chuang et al., 2012).

*i*NKT cells from patient PBMCs were reduced in frequency (Sumida et al., 1995, 1998; Kojo et al., 2001; van der Vliet et al., 2001; Wither et al., 2008; Wong et al., 2009; Parietti et al., 2010; Cho et al., 2011; Yu and Wang, 2011; Bosma et al., 2012) and proliferated less after stimulation *in vitro* with αGalCer (Kojo et al., 2001; Cho et al., 2011; Yu and Wang, 2011). Furthermore, resulting *i*NKT cell lines (Kojo et al., 2001; Cho et al., 2011; Yu and Wang, 2011; Bosma et al., 2012) or fresh *i*NKT cells from PBMCs (Bosma et al., 2012) displayed a Th2 bias but produced fewer cytokines overall. The frequency of *i*NKT cells in PBMCs correlated in most studies with disease severity (yes: Parietti et al., 2010; Cho et al., 2011; no: Wither et al., 2008) and serum levels of autoreactive IgGs (Green et al., 2007; Wither et al., 2008). Interestingly, the frequency of *i*NKT cells in peripheral blood increased following therapy (Oishi et al., 2001; Bosma et al., 2012). Whereas CD1d expression levels on APCs from patient PBMCs and healthy subjects did not differ, a decrease of CD1d surface expression was observed on patient B cells (Cho et al., 2011), and it was suggested that B cells in SLE patients were responsible for most of the *i*NKT cell defects (Bosma et al., 2012).

SLE in mice is studied either with mouse lines genetically prone to develop lupus-like diseases spontaneously, or in induced models by injection of either the hydrocarbon oil pristane, LPS, or apoptotic bodies in selected mouse strains (see Chapter 30). Most data are in line with the idea of a protective role of *i*NKT cells. Crossing lupus-prone mouse lines onto an *i*NKT cell deficient background led to exacerbated disease (Chan et al., 2001; Yang et al., 2004, 2007), although this was more pronounced for some organs than others (Chan et al., 2001; Yang et al., 2004). Interestingly, aged Jα18$^{-/-}$ mice by themselves have been shown to develop lupus-like symptoms (Sireci et al., 2007). Similarly, in the induced lupus models *i*NKT cell deficiency exacerbated symptoms (Yang et al., 2003, 2011; Wermeling et al., 2010). However, the effect of antigenic stimulation of *i*NKT cells led to conflicting outcomes in the different models. In the (NZB/NZW)F1 mouse model of spontaneous SLE, injection of αGalCer into young mice was beneficial, but detrimental in aged animals (Zeng et al., 2003; Major et al., 2006; Yang et al., 2007). In line with a switch to a pathogenic role later in the disease is the observation that *i*NKT cells numbers increased with lupus progression in these (NZB/NZW)F1 mice (Morshed et al., 2002; Forestier et al., 2005; Yang et al., 2007). Furthermore, in aged mice *i*NKT cells become hyperactive (Forestier et al., 2005) and interfering with their activation by means of blocking glycolipids (Morshed et al., 2009) or anti-CD1d antibodies (Zeng et al., 2000, 2003; Takahashi and Strober, 2008) ameliorated disease. Not surprisingly, strain differences are also important as the effects of

αGalCer treatment in the spontaneous models affected lupus nephritis in one mouse line, but not the other (Zeng et al., 2003; Forestier et al., 2005), and likewise a strain dependence was observed for the induced models (Singh et al., 2005).

GOOD OR BAD PERFORMERS?

In some autoimmune diseases, *i*NKT cell number and/or function are altered, but it is much less certain if they play a role in pathogenesis or in regulation/prevention of disease. We consider two examples here.

Sjögren's syndrome is mediated by an autoimmune destruction of exocrine glands and *i*NKT cells in PBMCs from patients are reduced in numbers (Kojo et al., 2001; van der Vliet et al., 2001) and tend to show a Th1 cytokine bias following antigen stimulation (Kojo et al., 2001).

Celiac disease (CeD) is a chronic inflammation of the small intestine driven by the adaptive immune system and triggered by dietary gluten (Stepniak and Koning, 2006). As there is to date no animal model, data on the role of *i*NKT cells are still very limited. In PBMCs from CeD patients a decrease of *i*NKT cells has been reported in three out of four studies (yes: Grose et al., 2007a; Cseh et al., 2011; Calleja et al., 2011; no: van der Vliet et al., 2001). Additionally, fewer Vα24$^+$ T cells were found in the intestine of CeD patients (Grose et al., 2007a), but again, it is uncertain how much of this expression was derived from *i*NKT cells (O'Keeffe et al., 2004). Furthermore, it has been suggested that patient *i*NKT cells produced less cytokine following *in vitro* stimulation (Grose et al., 2007a). In patients the adherence to a gluten-free diet normalizes symptoms and, interestingly, this improvement correlates with a normalization of the *i*NKT cell numbers in PBMCs (Bernardo et al., 2008; Calleja et al., 2011; Cseh et al., 2011).

The Far End of the Question?

What emerges from this survey is that unlike some other T lymphocyte subsets, for example Foxp3$^+$ Tregs, *i*NKT cells have diverse effects on autoimmune disease pathogenesis. How can we account for this, considering their limited TCR diversity and essentially clonal specificity? Two main questions capture the potential involvement of *i*NKT cells during autoimmune diseases: What draws *i*NKT cells in, and what effect do they initiate?

What Activates iNKT Cells During Autoimmune Responses?

It is likely that *i*NKT cells need some form of activation to be involved in disease progression and like conventional T cells this could be modulated by differences in signal 1 (TCR), signal 2 (costimulation), and signal 3 (cytokines).

- Signal 1 (TCR): Beyond the inherent autoreactivity of *i*NKT cells, CD1d-mediated activation of *i*NKT cells could conceivably be augmented in inflammatory settings by several means: (a) upregulation of CD1d on APCs, (b) the increased presentation of stimulatory self-antigens, e.g., following metabolic changes in activated APCs, (c) the presentation of stimulatory neo-antigen, and (d) so far unknown foreign antigens, e.g., from commensals or opportunistic pathogens. Furthermore, heterogeneity in the outcome of *i*NKT cell activation could arise from the fact that different glycolipids can elicit divergent cytokine responses and also different *i*NKT cell subsets respond differently to the same antigen.
- Signal 2 (costimulation): Besides these "classical" means of *i*NKT cell activation, additional pathways of activation have been described, some of which are known to be important for T cell costimulation. Well-known costimulatory molecules like CD28 (Kawano et al., 1997; Hayakawa et al., 2001; Wang et al., 2009) and CD154 (CD40L) (Kawano et al., 1997; Hayakawa et al., 2001) can affect *i*NKT cell activation, but so can other members of the TNF superfamily such as 4-1BB (Kim et al., 2008) and OX40 (Diana et al., 2009). The Ig superfamily molecule PD-1, known as a coinhibitory molecule, plays a role in modulating *i*NKT cells in mouse asthma models (Akbari et al., 2010). In addition, there are other receptors that can modulate *i*NKT cell stimulation, including NK receptors (Arase et al., 1996; Exley et al., 1998; Ortaldo et al., 2006), FcγRIII during arthritis (Kim 2006), adenosine receptors (Lappas et al., 2006), and β-adrenergic receptors (Wong et al., 2011). Some of these, such as the NK receptors, can act independently of TCR stimulation, while others apparently act in concert with the TCR. Although there is still limited information, as different subsets will likely express a different set of these receptors, they will respond differently. As these affects are cell−cell contact dependent, they are also dependent on migratory behavior of *i*NKT cells, which allows them to interact with a given APC.
- Signal 3 (cytokines): Activation of *i*NKT cells by cytokine combinations like IL-12/IL-18, IL-1β/IL-23, IL-25, and TGFβ have been outlined above. Additional cytokines have been suggested to modulate *i*NKT cell responses, including IL-2 (Sakuishi et al., 2007), IL-7 (Hameg et al., 1999), IL-15 (Li et al., 2006), IL-33 (Smithgall et al., 2008), GM-CSF (Crough et al., 2004), the prostaglandin D$_2$ (PGD2) (Torres et al., 2008), and TSLP (Wu et al., 2010;

Jariwala et al., 2011). Many of these cytokines can be secreted in affected tissues during autoimmune-mediated inflammation. Therefore, different combinations of local cytokines could induce diverse responses from *i*NKT cell subsets that express the appropriate cytokine receptors.

Therefore, the *i*NKT cell-mediated influence on the immune response depends on the means by which a particular *i*NKT cell gets activated. This reflects a complex "information input" that depends on the subset characteristics of the *i*NKT cell, the particulars of the local cytokine milieu, and the type and activation status of the APC they interact with.

Which iNKT Cell Effector Functions Orchestrate the Development of Autoimmune Responses?

The different "inputs" causing the activation of *i*NKT cells lead to different "outputs" or *i*NKT cell responses that will affect autoimmune disease pathogenesis in different ways. Whereas the bias towards Th2 cytokines imparted by *i*NKT cells seems to be most often raised as the mechanism for the effects of *i*NKT cells in autoimmune diseases, newer data paint a more complex picture. *i*NKT cells can impact the Th1/2 balance via their cytokine production, whereby IL-4 and IL-13 promote Th2; IFNγ and TNF promote a Th1 response; IL-10 and TGFβ suppress pathogenic Th1 responses; and under some circumstances even IFNγ has been shown to contribute to the development of Th2 responses (Bocek, 2004). However, the Th2 bias is clearly not sufficient to explain all observations and other factors play a role, dependent on the particular disease, its stage, and many other circumstances. Importantly, beyond the Th1/2 paradigm Th17 responses can be pathogenic (Weaver et al., 2007) and *i*NKT cells have shown to be effective at suppressing Th17 responses, as exemplified by their role in rheumatoid arthritis.

Additional *i*NKT cell-driven mechanisms have been suggested. For example, IFNγ can aid in the induction of anergy or apoptosis in antigen-specific Th1 T cells and this was suggested to be important in diabetes (Beaudoin et al., 2002; Hugues et al., 2002; Novak et al., 2005). Furthermore, IL-4, IL-10, and/or GM-CSF can promote the differentiation/recruitment of tolerogenic DCs. In addition, *i*NKT cells can under some circumstances aid in the induction of Tregs, either via tolerogenic DCs or via cytokines like IL-2, IL-10, and TGFβ (Kojo et al., 2005; Liu et al., 2005; Cava et al., 2006; Ly et al., 2006). Furthermore, cell−cell contact-dependent mechanisms are important, and the activation of the above outlined receptor/ligand pairs is often mutual. Additionally, the timing of *i*NKT cell action might be critical, as there are indications, for example in rheumatoid arthritis (Coppieters et al., 2007b; Kim et al., 2005), that the impact of *i*NKT cell activation can be beneficial and detrimental at different stages of the disease. Also, the diverse means by which distinct *i*NKT cell subsets are activated, and the different responses they make, are of course not mutually exclusive. This complexity surely contributes to some of the contradictory results on the role of *i*NKT cells in particular autoimmune diseases.

CONCLUSION

As outlined here, *i*NKT cells have been shown to be crucially involved in a wide range of autoimmune responses. Whereas it seems at first puzzling that a relatively small population has so many effects, one should keep in mind that even if present at less than a 1% frequency, *i*NKT cells are as abundant as typical CD4 memory cell populations, and they can exert their pivotal role due to their clonal specificity and explosive cytokine production. However, despite the vast literature on the role of *i*NKT cells in autoimmune diseases, much remains to be learned.

One important question, of course, is the extent to which the knowledge gained from animal models can be applied to humans. Although data from human patients are still relatively scarce, in several contexts they do suggest roles for *i*NKT cells that are comparable to the ones observed in mice. This is indeed very promising. Furthermore, we expect that soon functionally distinct *i*NKT cell subsets will be better characterized in humans, which most likely will help to readdress more specifically the role of *i*NKT cells in autoimmune diseases. A related issue is the potential of stimulating or inhibiting *i*NKT cells for therapeutic purposes. Despite the fact that αGalCer is already used in clinical trials for cancer, and other glycolipids and approaches for manipulating *i*NKT cells are in trial or are being planned, the therapeutic potential of *i*NKT cells remains to be validated.

ACKNOWLEDGMENTS

The authors would like to thank Kristin A. Hogquist and her colleagues for sharing unpublished data, and Isaac Engel for his critical reading of parts of the manuscript. Supported by NIH grants AI 71922 and AI 45053 (MK).

ABBREVIATIONS

αGalCer	α-galactosylceramide
APC	antigen presenting cell
BALF	bronchoalveolar lavage fluid
Bcl6	B-cell lymphoma 6 protein
c	canonical
CDR	complementarity determining regions
Celiac disease	CeD
CHS	contact hypersensitivity
CNS	central nervous system
CXCR	chemokine (C-X-C motif) receptor
DC	dendritic cell
DN	double negative (CD4$^-$CD8$^-$)
DP	double positive (CD4$^+$CD8$^+$)
EAE	experimental allergic encephalomyelitis
FoxP3	forkhead box P3
GATA3	GATA binding protein 3
i	invariant
IBD	inflammatory bowel disease
IFN	interferon
Ig	immunoglobulin
IL	interleukin
LN	lymph node
int	intermediate
LPS	lipopolysaccharide
m	mucosal
MAIT	mucosal associated invariant T cell
*m*NKT	mucosal NKT
MS	multiple sclerosis
MTTP	microsomal triglyceride transfer protein
NHP	non-human-primate
NK	natural killer
NKT	natural killer T
NOD	non-obese diabetic
OVA	ovalbumin
PBC	primary biliary cirrhosis
PBMC	peripheral blood mononuclear cells
PD-1	programmed cell death 1
PGD2	prostaglandin D$_2$
PLZF	promyelocytic leukemia zinc finger
RA	rheumatoid arthritis
ROR-γt	RAR-related orphan receptor gamma
SAP	sphingolipid activator protein
SLE	systemic lupus erythematosus
T1D	Type 1 diabetes mellitus
Tbet	T-cell-specific T-box transcription factor
TCR	T cell antigen receptor
T$_{FH}$	follicular helper T cells
tg	transgenic
TGF	transforming growth factor
Th	T helper type
TLR	Toll-like receptors
Treg	regulatory T
TSLP	thymic stromal lymphopoietin
v	variable repertoire
V	antigen receptor variable region.

REFERENCES

Akbari, O., et al., 2006. CD4+ invariant T-cell-receptor + natural killer T cells in bronchial asthma. New England Journal of Medicine. 354, 1117–1129.

Akbari, O., et al., 2003. Essential role of NKT cells producing IL-4 and IL-13 in the development of allergen-induced airway hyperreactivity. Nat. Med. 9, 582–588.

Akbari, O., et al., 2010. PD-L1 and PD-L2 modulate airway inflammation and iNKT-cell-dependent airway hyperreactivity in opposing directions. Mucosal Immunol. 3, 81–91.

Allan, L.L., et al., 2009. Apolipoprotein-mediated lipid antigen presentation in B cells provides a pathway for innate help by NKT cells. Blood. 114, 2411–2416.

Andoh, Y., et al., 2012. Natural killer T cells are required for lipopolysaccharide-mediated enhancement of atherosclerosis in apolipoprotein E-deficient mice. Immunobiology 218, 561–569.

Araki, M., et al., 2003. Th2 bias of CD4 + NKT cells derived from multiple sclerosis in remission. Int. Immunol. 15, 279–288.

Arase, H., Arase, N., Saito, T., 1996. Interferon gamma production by natural killer (NK) cells and NK1.1 + T cells upon NKR-P1 cross-linking. J. Exp. Med. 183, 2391–2396.

Arora, P., et al., 2011. A rapid fluorescence-based assay for classification of iNKT cell activating glycolipids. J. Am. Chem. Soc. 133, 5198–5201.

Askenase, P.W., et al., 2011. Participation of iNKT cells in the early and late components of Tc1-mediated DNFB contact sensitivity: cooperative role of γδ-T cells. Scand. J. Immunol. 73, 465–477.

Aslanian, A.M., Chapman, H.A., Charo, I.F., 2005. Transient role for CD1d-restricted natural killer T cells in the formation of atherosclerotic lesions. Arterioscler. Thromb. Vasc. Biol. 25, 628–632.

Assarsson, E., et al., 2000. CD8+ T cells rapidly acquire NK1.1 and NK cell-associated molecules upon stimulation in vitro and in vivo. J. Immunol. (Baltimore, Md.: 1950). 165, 3673–3679.

Ayanoglu, G., et al., 2011. Modelling asthma in macaques: longitudinal changes in cellular and molecular markers. Eur. Respir. J. 37, 541–552.

Baev, D.V., et al., 2008. Impaired SLAM-SLAM homotypic interaction between invariant NKT cells and dendritic cells affects differentiation of IL-4/IL-10-secreting NKT2 cells in nonobese diabetic mice. J. Immunol. 181, 869–877.

Balato, A., et al., 2012. CD1d-dependent, iNKT-cell cytotoxicity against keratinocytes in allergic contact dermatitis. Exp. Dermatol. 21, 915–920.

Balato, A., Unutmaz, D., Gaspari, A.A., 2009. Natural killer T cells: an unconventional T-cell subset with diverse effector and regulatory functions. J. Invest. Dermatol. 129, 1628–1642.

Baxter, A.G., et al., 1997. Association between alphabetaTCR + CD4− CD8− T-cell deficiency and IDDM in NOD/Lt mice. Diabetes 46, 572–582.

Beaudoin, L., et al., 2002. NKT cells inhibit the onset of diabetes by impairing the development of pathogenic T cells specific for pancreatic beta cells. Immunity 17, 725–736.

Behar, S.M., et al., 1999. Diverse TCRs recognize murine CD1. J. Immunol. (Baltimore, Md.: 1950). 162, 161–167.

Bendelac, A., 1995. Positive selection of mouse NK1 + T cells by CD1-expressing cortical thymocytes. J. Exp. Med. 182, 2091–2096.

Bendelac, A., et al., 1995. CD1 recognition by mouse NK1 + T lymphocytes. Science 268, 863–865.

Bendelac, A., et al., 1997. Mouse CD1-specific NK1 T cells: development, specificity, and function. Annu. Rev. Immunol. 15, 535–562.

Bendelac, A., Hunziker, R.D., Lantz, O., 1996. Increased interleukin 4 and immunoglobulin E production in transgenic mice overexpressing NK1 T cells. J. Exp. Med. 184, 1285–1293.

Bendelac, A., Savage, P.B., Teyton, L., 2007. The biology of NKT cells. Annu. Rev. Immunol. 25, 297–336.

Berg, R.E., Forman, J., 2006. The role of CD8 T cells in innate immunity and in antigen non-specific protection. Curr. Opin. Immunol. 18, 338–343.

Bernardo, D., et al., 2008. Decreased circulating iNKT cell numbers in refractory coeliac disease. Clin. Immunol. 126, 172–179.

Berzins, S.P., et al., 2004. Systemic NKT cell deficiency in NOD mice is not detected in peripheral blood: implications for human studies. Immunol. Cell Biol. 82, 247–252.

Berzins, S.P., Smyth, M.J., Baxter, A.G., 2011. Presumed guilty: natural killer T cell defects and human disease. Nat. Rev. Immunol. 11, 131–142.

Bilenki, L., et al., 2004. Natural killer T cells contribute to airway eosinophilic inflammation induced by ragweed through enhanced IL-4 and eotaxin production. Eur. J. Immunol. 34, 345–354.

Biron, C.A., Brossay, L., 2001. NK cells and NKT cells in innate defense against viral infections. Curr. Opin. Immunol. 13, 458–464.

Blomqvist, M., et al., 2009. Multiple tissue-specific isoforms of sulfatide activate CD1d-restricted type II NKT cells. Eur. J. Immunol. 39, 1726–1735.

Bobryshev, Y.V., 2005. Natural killer T cells in atherosclerosis. Arteriosclerosis, Thrombosis, and Vascular Biol. 25, (e40—author reply e40).

Bocek, P., 2004. Interferon enhances both in vitro and in vivo priming of CD4 + T cells for IL-4 production. J. Exp. Med. 199, 1619–1630.

Bogdanos, D.-P., et al., 2004. Microbial mimics are major targets of crossreactivity with human pyruvate dehydrogenase in primary biliary cirrhosis. J. Hepatology. 40, 31–39.

Bogdanos, D.P., Vergani, D., 2009. Bacteria and primary biliary cirrhosis. Clin. Rev. Allergy and Immunol. 36, 30–39.

Bonish, B., et al., 2000. Overexpression of CD1d by keratinocytes in psoriasis and CD1d-dependent IFN-gamma production by NK-T cells. J. Immunol. (Baltimore, Md.: 1950). 165, 4076–4085.

Bosma, A., et al., 2012. Lipid-antigen presentation by CD1d + B cells is essential for the maintenance of invariant natural killer T cells. Immunity. 36, 477–490.

Bratke, K., Julius, P., Virchow, J.C., 2007. Invariant natural killer T cells in obstructive pulmonary diseases. New England J. Med. 357, (194—author reply 194–195).

Braun, N.A., Covarrubias, R., Major, A.S., 2010. Natural killer T cells and atherosclerosis: form and function meet pathogenesis. J. Innate Immun. 2, 316–324.

Brennan, P.J., et al., 2011. Invariant natural killer T cells recognize lipid self antigen induced by microbial danger signals. Nat. Immunol. 12, 1202–1211.

Brigl, M., et al., 2006. Conserved and heterogeneous lipid antigen specificities of CD1d-restricted NKT cell receptors. J. Immunol. (Baltimore, Md.: 1950). 176, 3625–3634.

Brigl, M., et al., 2003. Mechanism of CD1d-restricted natural killer T cell activation during microbial infection. Nat. Immunol. 4, 1230–1237.

Brooks, C.R., et al., 2010. Invariant natural killer T cells and asthma: immunologic reality or methodologic artifact? J. Allergy Clin. Immunol. 126, 882–885.

Brossay, L., Kronenberg, M., 1999. Highly conserved antigen-presenting function of CD1d molecules. Immunogenetics 50, 146–151.

Brossay, L., et al., 1998. CD1d-mediated recognition of an alpha-galactosylceramide by natural killer T cells is highly conserved through mammalian evolution. J. Exp. Med. 188, 1521–1528.

Brozovic, S., et al., 2004. CD1d function is regulated by microsomal triglyceride transfer protein. Nat. Med. 10, 535–539.

Burdin, N., Brossay, L., Kronenberg, M., 1999. Immunization with alpha-galactosylceramide polarizes CD1-reactive NK T cells towards Th2 cytokine synthesis. Eur. J. Immunol. 29, 2014–2025.

Caielli, S., et al., 2010. On/off TLR signaling decides proinflammatory or tolerogenic dendritic cell maturation upon CD1d-mediated interaction with invariant NKT cells. J. Immunol. (Baltimore, Md.: 1950). 185, 7317–7329.

Cain, J.A., et al., 2006. NKT cells and IFN-gamma establish the regulatory environment for the control of diabetogenic T cells in the non-obese diabetic mouse. J. Immunol. (Baltimore, Md.: 1950). 176, 1645–1654.

Calleja, S., et al., 2011. Dynamics of non-conventional intraepithelial lymphocytes—NK, NKT, and γδT—in celiac disease: relationship with age, diet, and histopathology. Dig. Dis. Sci. 56, 2042–2049.

Camelo, A., et al., 2012. Blocking IL-25 signalling protects against gut inflammation in a type-2 model of colitis by suppressing nuocyte and NKT derived IL-13. J. Gastroenterology. 47, 1198–1211.

Cameron, A.L., et al., 2002. Natural killer and natural killer-T cells in psoriasis. Arch. Dermatological Res. 294, 363–369.

Campos, R.A., et al., 2003. Cutaneous immunization rapidly activates liver invariant Valpha14 NKT cells stimulating B-1 B cells to initiate T cell recruitment for elicitation of contact sensitivity. J. Exp. Med. 198, 1785–1796.

Campos, R.A., et al., 2006a. Interleukin-4-dependent innate collaboration between iNKT cells and B-1 B cells controls adaptive contact sensitivity. Immunology 117, 536–547.

Campos, R.A., et al., 2006b. Invariant NKT cells rapidly activated via immunization with diverse contact antigens collaborate in vitro with B-1 cells to initiate contact sensitivity. J. Immunol. (Baltimore, Md.: 1950). 177, 3686–3694.

Castano, A.R., et al., 1995. Peptide binding and presentation by mouse CD1. Science 269, 223–226.

Cava, A.L., Kaer, L.V., Fu Dong, S., 2006. CD4(+)CD25(+) Tregs and NKT cells: regulators regulating regulators. Trends Immunol. 27, 322–327.

Cerundolo, V., et al., 2009. Harnessing invariant NKT cells in vaccination strategies. Nat. Rev. Immunol. 9, 28–38.

Chan, O.T., et al., 2001. Deficiency in beta(2)-microglobulin, but not CD1, accelerates spontaneous lupus skin disease while inhibiting nephritis in MRL-Fas(lpr) nice: an example of disease regulation at the organ level. J. Immunol. (Baltimore, Md.: 1950). 167, 2985–2990.

Chan, W.L., et al., 2005. Atherosclerotic abdominal aortic aneurysm and the interaction between autologous human plaque-derived vascular smooth muscle cells, type 1 NKT, and helper T cells. Circ. Res. 96, 675–683.

Chang, P.-P., et al., 2011. Identification of Bcl-6-dependent follicular helper NKT cells that provide cognate help for B cell responses. Nat. Immunol. 13, 35–43.

Chen, Y.-G., et al., 2006. CD38 is required for the peripheral survival of immunotolerogenic CD4+ invariant NK T cells in nonobese diabetic mice. J. Immunol. (Baltimore, Md.: 1950). 177, 2939–2947.

Chen, Y.G., et al., 2005. Activated NKT cells inhibit autoimmune diabetes through tolerogenic recruitment of dendritic cells to pancreatic lymph nodes. J. Immunol. (Baltimore, Md.: 1950). 174, 1196–1204.

Chen, Y.G., Tsaih, S.-W., Serreze, D.V., 2011. Genetic control of murine invariant natural killer T-cell development dynamically differs dependent on the examined tissue type. Genes and Immunity 13, 164–174.

Chiba, A., et al., 2004. Suppression of collagen-induced arthritis by natural killer T cell activation with OCH, a sphingosine-truncated analog of alpha-galactosylceramide. Arthritis Rheum. 50, 305–313.

Chiba, A., et al., 2005. The involvement of V(alpha)14 natural killer T cells in the pathogenesis of arthritis in murine models. Arthritis Rheum. 52, 1941–1948.

Cho, Y.N., et al., 2011. Numerical and functional deficiencies of natural killer T cells in systemic lupus erythematosus: their deficiency related to disease activity. Rheumatology (Oxford).

Chuang, Y.-H., et al., 2008. Natural killer T cells exacerbate liver injury in a transforming growth factor beta receptor II dominant-negative mouse model of primary biliary cirrhosis. Hepatology 47, 571–580.

Chuang, Y.-P., et al., 2012. Modulatory function of invariant natural killer T cells in systemic lupus erythematosus. Clin. Dev. Immunol. 2012, 478429.

Chuang, Y.-P., Lin, Y.-C., Sytwu, H.-K., 2011. α-Galactosylceramide ameliorates autoimmune diabetes in non-obese diabetic mice through a suppressive effect mediated by CD8 + T cells. Immunol. Lett. 138, 54–62.

Coppieters, K., et al., 2007a. NKT cells: manipulable managers of joint inflammation. Rheumatology (Oxford). 46, 565–571.

Coppieters, K., et al., 2007b. A single early activation of invariant NK T cells confers long-term protection against collagen-induced arthritis in a ligand-specific manner. J. Immunol. (Baltimore, Md.: 1950). 179, 2300–2309.

Coquet, J.M., et al., 2008. Diverse cytokine production by NKT cell subsets and identification of an IL-17-producing CD4-NK1.1- NKT cell population. Proc. Nat. Acad. Sci. USA 105, 11287–11292.

Crough, T., Nieda, M., Nicol, A.J., 2004. Granulocyte colony-stimulating factor modulates alpha-galactosylceramide-responsive human Valpha24 + Vbeta11 + NKT cells. J. Immunol. (Baltimore, Md.: 1950). 173, 4960–4966.

Cseh, A., et al., 2011. Immune phenotype of children with newly diagnosed and gluten-free diet-treated celiac disease. Dig. Dis. Sci. 56, 792–798.

Cui, J., et al., 1999. Inhibition of T helper cell type 2 cell differentiation and immunoglobulin E response by ligand-activated Valpha14 natural killer T cells. J. Exp. Med. 190, 783–792.

Curry, J.L., et al., 2003. Reactivity of resident immunocytes in normal and prepsoriatic skin using an ex vivo skin-explant model system. Arch. Pathol. Lab. Med. 127, 289–296.

D'Andrea, A., et al., 2000. Neonatal invariant Valpha24 + NKT lymphocytes are activated memory cells. Eur. J. Immunol. 30, 1544–1550.

Dao, T., Mehal, W.Z., Crispe, I.N., 1998. IL-18 augments perforin-dependent cytotoxicity of liver NK-T cells. J. Immunol. (Baltimore, Md.: 1950). 161, 2217–2222.

Das, R., Sant'angelo, D.B., Nichols, K.E., 2010. Transcriptional control of invariant NKT cell development. Immunol. Rev. 238, 195–215.

De Santo, C., et al., 2010. Invariant NKT cells modulate the suppressive activity of IL-10-secreting neutrophils differentiated with serum amyloid A. Nat. Immunol. 11, 1039–1046.

Demoulins, T., et al., 2003. A biased Valpha24 + T-cell repertoire leads to circulating NKT-cell defects in a multiple sclerosis patient at the onset of his disease. Immunol. Lett. 90, 223–228.

Denkers, E.Y., et al., 1996. A role for CD4 + NK1.1 + T lymphocytes as major histocompatibility complex class II independent helper cells in the generation of CD8 + effector function against intracellular infection. J. Exp. Med. 184, 131–139.

Denney, L., et al., 2012. Activation of invariant NKT cells in early phase of experimental autoimmune encephalomyelitis results in differentiation of Ly6Chi inflammatory monocyte to M2 macrophages and improved outcome. J. Immunol. 189, 551–557.

Dey, N., et al., 2011. Stimulatory lipids accumulate in the mouse liver within 30 min of contact sensitization to facilitate the activation of naïve iNKT cells in a CD1d-dependent fashion. Scand. J. Immunol. 74, 52–61.

Diana, J., et al., 2009. NKT cell-plasmacytoid dendritic cell cooperation via OX40 controls viral infection in a tissue-specific manner. Immunity 30, 289–299.

Diana, J., et al., 2011. Viral infection prevents diabetes by inducing regulatory T cells through NKT cell-plasmacytoid dendritic cell interplay. J. Exp. Med. 208, 729–745.

Doherty, D.G., et al., 1999. The human liver contains multiple populations of NK cells, T cells, and CD3 + CD56 + natural T cells with distinct cytotoxic activities and Th1, Th2, and Th0 cytokine secretion patterns. J. Immunol. (Baltimore, Md.: 1950). 163, 2314–2321.

Doisne, J.M., et al., 2011. Cutting edge: crucial role of IL-1 and IL-23 in the innate IL-17 response of peripheral lymph node NK1.1- invariant NKT cells to bacteria. J. Immunol. (Baltimore, Md.: 1950). 186, 662–666.

Doisne, J.M., et al., 2009. Skin and peripheral lymph node invariant NKT cells are mainly retinoic acid receptor-related orphan receptor (gamma)t + and respond preferentially under inflammatory conditions. J. Immunol. (Baltimore, Md.: 1950). 183, 2142–2149.

Drennan, M.B., Aspeslagh, S., Elewaut, D., 2010. Invariant natural killer T cells in rheumatic disease: a joint dilemma. Nat. Rev. Rheumatol. 6, 90–98.

Driver, J.P., et al., 2010. Invariant natural killer T-cell control of type 1 diabetes: a dendritic cell genetic decision of a silver bullet or Russian roulette. Diabetes 59, 423–432.

Dutton, R.W., Bradley, L.M., Swain, S.L., 1998. T cell memory. Annu. Rev. Immunol. 16, 201–223.

East, J.E., Kennedy, A.J., Webb, T.J., 2012. Raising the roof: the preferential pharmacological stimulation of Th1 and Th2 responses mediated by NKT cells. Med. Res. Rev. Available from: http://dx.doi.org/10.1002/med.21276.

Eberl, G., MacDonald, H.R., 2000. Selective induction of NK cell proliferation and cytotoxicity by activated NKT cells. Eur. J. Immunol. 30, 985–992.

Elkhal, A., et al., 2006. CD1d restricted natural killer T cells are not required for allergic skin inflammation. J. Allergy Clin. Immunol. 118, 1363–1368.

Elzen, P.V.D., et al., 2005. Apolipoprotein-mediated pathways of lipid antigen presentation. Nature 437, 906–910.

Emoto, M., et al., 2010. Alpha-GalCer ameliorates listeriosis by accelerating infiltration of Gr-1 + cells into the liver. Eur. J. Immunol. 40, 1328–1341.

Engel, I., Kronenberg, M., 2012. Making memory at birth: understanding the differentiation of natural killer T cells. Curr. Opin. Immunol. 24, 184–190.

Exley, M., et al., 1998. CD161 (NKR-P1A) costimulation of CD1d-dependent activation of human T cells expressing invariant V alpha 24 J alpha Q T cell receptor alpha chains. J. Exp. Med. 188, 867–876.

Facciotti, F., et al., 2012. Peroxisome-derived lipids are self antigens that stimulate invariant natural killer T cells in the thymus. Nat. Immunol. 13, 474–480.

Falcone, M., et al., 1999. A defect in interleukin 12-induced activation and interferon gamma secretion of peripheral natural killer T cells in nonobese diabetic mice suggests new pathogenic mechanisms for insulin-dependent diabetes mellitus. J. Exp. Med. 190, 963–972.

Falcone, M., et al., 2004. Up-regulation of CD1d expression restores the immunoregulatory function of NKT cells and prevents autoimmune diabetes in nonobese diabetic mice. J. Immunol. (Baltimore, Md.: 1950). 172, 5908–5916.

Flesch, I.E., Wandersee, A., Kaufmann, S.H., 1997. IL-4 secretion by CD4 + NK1 + T cells induces monocyte chemoattractant protein-1 in early listeriosis. J. Immunol. (Baltimore, Md.: 1950). 159, 7–10.

Fletcher, M.T., Baxter, A.G., 2009. Clinical application of NKT cell biology in type I (autoimmune) diabetes mellitus. Immunol. Cell Biol. 87, 315–323.

Forestier, C., et al., 2005. Expansion and hyperactivity of CD1d-restricted NKT cells during the progression of systemic lupus erythematosus in (New Zealand Black × New Zealand White)F1 mice. J. Immunol. (Baltimore, Md.: 1950). 175, 763–770.

Forestier, C., et al., 2007. Improved outcomes in NOD mice treated with a novel Th2 cytokine-biasing NKT cell activator. J. Immunol. (Baltimore, Md.: 1950). 178, 1415–1425.

Fox, L.M., et al., 2009. Recognition of lyso-phospholipids by human natural killer T lymphocytes. PLoS Biol. 7, e1000228.

Furlan, R., et al., 2003. Activation of invariant NKT cells by alphaGalCer administration protects mice from MOG35-55-induced EAE: critical roles for administration route and IFN-gamma. Eur. J. Immunol. 33, 1830–1838.

Fuss, I.J., et al., 2004. Nonclassical CD1d-restricted NK T cells that produce IL-13 characterize an atypical Th2 response in ulcerative colitis. J. Clin. Invest. 113, 1490–1497 (Available at: <http://www.jci.org/cgi/doi/10.1172/JCI200419836>).

Gabriel, L., Morley, B.J., Rogers, N.J., 2009. The role of iNKT cells in the immunopathology of systemic lupus erythematosus. Ann. N.Y. Acad. Sci. 1173, 435–441.

Gadola, S.D., et al., 2002. Valpha24-JalphaQ-independent, CD1d-restricted recognition of alpha-galactosylceramide by human CD4 (+) and CD8alphabeta(+) T lymphocytes. J. Immunol. (Baltimore, Md.: 1950). 168, 5514–5520.

Galkina, E., et al., 2007. CXCR6 promotes atherosclerosis by supporting T-cell homing, interferon production, and macrophage accumulation in the aortic wall. Circulation. 116, 1801–1811.

Gausling, R., Trollmo, C., Hafler, D.A., 2001. Decreases in interleukin-4 secretion by invariant CD4−CD8−Vα24JαQ T Cells in peripheral blood of patients with relapsing–remitting multiple sclerosis. Clin. Immunol. 98, 11–17.

Getz, G.S., VanderLaan, P.A., Reardon, C.A., 2011. Natural killer T cells in lipoprotein metabolism and atherosclerosis. Thromb. Haemost. 106, 814–819.

Gigli, G., et al., 2007. Innate immunity modulates autoimmunity: type 1 interferon-beta treatment in multiple sclerosis promotes growth and function of regulatory invariant natural killer T cells through dendritic cell maturation. Immunology 122, 409–417.

Gilhar, A., et al., 2002. Psoriasis is mediated by a cutaneous defect triggered by activated immunocytes: induction of psoriasis by cells with natural killer receptors. J. Invest. Dermatol. 119, 384−391.

Gober, M.D., et al., 2008. Human natural killer T cells infiltrate into the skin at elicitation sites of allergic contact dermatitis. J. Invest. Dermatol. 128, 1460−1469.

Godfrey, D.I., Kronenberg, M., 2004. Going both ways: immune regulation via CD1d-dependent NKT cells. J. Clin. Invest. 114, 1379−1388 (Available at: <http://www.jci.org/cgi/doi/10.1172/JCI200423594>).

Godfrey, D.I., et al., 2000. NKT cells: facts, functions and fallacies. Immunol. Today 21, 573−583.

Godfrey, D.I., Stankovic, S., Baxter, A.G., 2010. Raising the NKT Cell Family. Nat. Immunol. 11, 197−206.

Gombert, J.M., et al., 1996. Early quantitative and functional deficiency of NK1 + -like thymocytes in the NOD mouse. Eur. J. Immunol. 26, 2989−2998.

Gonzalez-Aseguinolaza, G., et al., 2002. Natural killer T cell ligand alpha-galactosylceramide enhances protective immunity induced by malaria vaccines. J. Exp. Med. 195, 617−624.

Goubier, A., et al., 2012. Invariant NKT cells suppress CD8(+) T-cell-mediated allergic contact dermatitis independently of regulatory CD4(+) T cells. J. Invest. Dermatol. 133, 980−987

Green, M.R., et al., 2007. Natural killer T cells in families of patients with systemic lupus erythematosus: their possible role in regulation of IGG production. Arthritis Rheum. 56, 303−310.

Grose, R.H., Cummins, A.G., Thompson, F.M., 2007a. Deficiency of invariant natural killer T cells in coeliac disease. Gut. 56, 790−795.

Grose, R.H., et al., 2007b. Deficiency of invariant NK T cells in Crohn's disease and ulcerative colitis. Dig. Dis. Sci. 52, 1415−1422 (Available at: <http://www.springerlink.com/index/10.1007/s10620-006-9261-7>).

Grundtman, C., Wick, G., 2011. The autoimmune concept of atherosclerosis. Curr. Opin. Lipidol. 22, 327−334.

Gumperz, J.E., et al., 2002. Functionally distinct subsets of CD1d-restricted natural killer T cells revealed by CD1d tetramer staining. J. Exp. Med. 195, 625−636.

Gumperz, J.E., et al., 2000. Murine CD1d-restricted T cell recognition of cellular lipids. Immunity 12, 211−221.

Gyimesi, E., et al., 2011. Altered peripheral invariant natural killer T cells in atopic dermatitis. J. Clin. Immunol. 31, 864−872.

Hameg, A., et al., 1999. IL-7 up-regulates IL-4 production by splenic NK1.1 + and NK1.1 − MHC class I-like/CD1-dependent CD4 + T cells. J. Immunol. (Baltimore, Md.: 1950). 162, 7067−7074.

Hammond, K.J., et al., 1998. Alpha/beta-T cell receptor (TCR) + CD4 − CD8 − (NKT) thymocytes prevent insulin-dependent diabetes mellitus in nonobese diabetic (NOD)/Lt mice by the influence of interleukin (IL)-4 and/or IL-10. J. Exp. Med. 187, 1047−1056.

Hammond, K.J., et al., 1999. NKT cells are phenotypically and functionally diverse. Eur. J. Immunol. 29, 3768−3781.

Hamzaoui, A., et al., 2006. NKT cells in the induced sputum of severe asthmatics. Mediators Inflamm. 2006, 71214.

Hansson, G.K., Robertson, A.-K.L., Söderberg-Nauclér, C., 2006. Inflammation and atherosclerosis. Annu. Rev. Pathol. 1, 297−329.

Hayakawa, Y., et al., 2001. Differential regulation of Th1 and Th2 functions of NKT cells by CD28 and CD40 costimulatory pathways. J. Immunol. (Baltimore, Md.: 1950). 166, 6012−6018 (Available at: <http://eutils.ncbi.nlm.nih.gov/entrez/eutils/elink.fcgi?dbfrom = pubmed&id = 11342617&retmode = ref&cmd = prlinks>).

Hegde, S., et al., 2010. Autoreactive natural killer T cells: promoting immune protection and immune tolerance through varied interactions with myeloid antigen-presenting cells. Immunology 130, 471−483.

Heller, F., et al., 2002. Oxazolone colitis, a Th2 colitis model resembling ulcerative colitis, is mediated by IL-13-producing NK-T cells. Immunity 17, 629−638.

Heron, M., Claessen, A.M.E., Grutters, J.C., 2007. Invariant natural killer T cells in obstructive pulmonary diseases. New England J. Med. 357, (194—author reply 194−195).

Hong, S., et al., 2001. The natural killer T-cell ligand alpha-galactosylceramide prevents autoimmune diabetes in non-obese diabetic mice. Nat. Med. 7, 1052−1056.

Hu, T., Gimferrer, I., Alberola-Ila, J., 2011. Control of early stages in invariant natural killer T-cell development. Immunology 134, 1−7.

Hugues, S., et al., 2002. Tolerance to islet antigens and prevention from diabetes induced by limited apoptosis of pancreatic beta cells. Immunity 16, 169−181.

Ilhan, F., et al., 2007. Atopic dermatitis and Valpha24 + natural killer T cells. Skinmed. 6, 218−220.

Illes, Z., et al., 2000. Differential expression of NK T cell V alpha 24J alpha Q invariant TCR chain in the lesions of multiple sclerosis and chronic inflammatory demyelinating polyneuropathy. J. Immunol. (Baltimore, Md.: 1950). 164, 4375−4381.

Im, J.S., et al., 2009. Kinetics and cellular site of glycolipid loading control the outcome of natural killer T cell activation. Immunity. 30, 888−898.

Jacques, P., et al., 2010. Invariant natural killer T cells are natural regulators of murine spondylarthritis. Arthritis Rheum. 62, 988−999.

Jahng, A., et al., 2004. Prevention of autoimmunity by targeting a distinct, noninvariant CD1d-reactive T cell population reactive to sulfatide. J. Exp. Med. 199, 947−957.

Jahng, A.W., et al., 2001. Activation of natural killer T cells potentiates or prevents experimental autoimmune encephalomyelitis. J. Exp. Med. 194, 1789−1799.

Jariwala, S.P., et al., 2011. The role of thymic stromal lymphopoietin in the immunopathogenesis of atopic dermatitis. Clin. Exp. Allergy 41, 1515−1520.

Jordan, M.A., et al., 2007. Slamf1, the NKT cell control gene Nkt1. J. Immunol. (Baltimore, Md.: 1950). 178, 1618−1627.

Jung, S., et al., 2009. Natural killer T cells promote collagen-induced arthritis in DBA/1 mice. Biochem. Biophys. Res. Commun. 390, 399−403.

Jung, S., et al., 2010. The requirement of natural killer T-cells in tolerogenic APCs-mediated suppression of collagen-induced arthritis. Exp. Mol. Med. 42, 547−554.

Kaieda, S., et al., 2007. Activation of invariant natural killer T cells by synthetic glycolipid ligands suppresses autoantibody-induced arthritis. Arthritis Rheum. 56, 1836−1845.

Kawano, T., et al., 1997. CD1d-restricted and TCR-mediated activation of valpha14 NKT cells by glycosylceramides. Science 278, 1626−1629.

Kenna, T., et al., 2003. NKT cells from normal and tumor-bearing human livers are phenotypically and functionally distinct from murine NKT cells. J. Immunol. (Baltimore, Md.: 1950). 171, 1775−1779.

Kent, S.C., et al., 2005. Loss of IL-4 secretion from human type 1a diabetic pancreatic draining lymph node NKT cells. J. Immunol. (Baltimore, Md.: 1950). 175, 4458−4464.

Kim, C.H., Butcher, E.C., Johnston, B., 2002. Distinct subsets of human Valpha24-invariant NKT cells: cytokine responses and chemokine receptor expression. Trends Immunol. 23, 516−519.

Kim, D.-H., et al., 2008. 4-1BB engagement costimulates NKT cell activation and exacerbates NKT cell ligand-induced airway hyperresponsiveness and inflammation. J. Immunol. (Baltimore, Md.: 1950). 180, 2062−2068.

Kim, H.Y., Kim, S., Chung, D.H., 2006. FcgRIII engagement provides activating signals to NKT cells in antibody-induced joint inflammation. J. Clin. Invest 116, 2484−2492.

Kim, H.Y., et al., 2012. Innate lymphoid cells responding to IL-33 mediate airway hyperreactivity independently of adaptive immunity. J. Allergy Clin. Immunol. 129, 216−27; e1−e6.

Kim, H.Y., et al., 2005. NKT cells promote antibody-induced joint inflammation by suppressing transforming growth factor {beta}1 production. J. Exp. Med. 201, 41−47.

Kim, H.Y., et al., 2009. The development of airway hyperreactivity in T-bet-deficient mice requires CD1d-restricted NKT cells. J. Immunol. (Baltimore, Md.: 1950). 182, 3252−3261.

Kim, J.-O., et al., 2004. Asthma is induced by intranasal coadministration of allergen and natural killer T-cell ligand in a mouse model. J. Allergy Clin. Immunol. 114, 1332−1338.

King, I.L., et al., 2011. Invariant natural killer T cells direct B cell responses to cognate lipid antigen in an IL-21-dependent manner. Nat. Immunol. 13, 44−50.

Kinjo, Y., Kronenberg, M., 2005. Vα14i NKT cells are innate lymphocytes that participate in the immune response to diverse microbes. J. Clin. Immunol. 25, 522−533.

Kinjo, Y., et al., 2011. Invariant natural killer T cells recognize glycolipids from pathogenic Gram-positive bacteria. Nat. Immunol. 12, 966−974.

Kinjo, Y., et al., 2006. Natural killer T cells recognize diacylglycerol antigens from pathogenic bacteria. Nat. Immunol. 7, 978−986.

Kinjo, Y., et al., 2005. Recognition of bacterial glycosphingolipids by natural killer T cells. Nature 434, 520−525.

Kis, J., et al., 2007. Reduced CD4 + subset and Th1 bias of the human iNKT cells in Type 1 diabetes mellitus. J. Leukoc. Biol. 81, 654−662.

Kita, H., et al., 2002. Quantitation and phenotypic analysis of natural killer T cells in primary biliary cirrhosis using a human CD1d tetramer. Gastroenterology 123, 1031−1043 (Available at: <http://linkinghub.elsevier.com/retrieve/pii/S0016508502002081>).

Kitamura, H., et al., 1999. The natural killer T (NKT) cell ligand alpha-galactosylceramide demonstrates its immunopotentiating effect by inducing interleukin (IL)-12 production by dendritic cells and IL-12 receptor expression on NKT cells. J. Exp. Med. 189, 1121−1128.

Koh, Y.-I., et al., 2010. Inverse association of peripheral blood CD4(+) invariant natural killer T cells with atopy in human asthma. Hum. Immunol. 71, 186−191.

Koh, Y.-I., et al., 2012. The role of natural killer T cells in the pathogenesis of acute exacerbation of human asthma. Int. Arch. Allergy Immunol. 158, 131−141.

Koh, Y.I., Shim, J.U., 2010. Association between sputum natural killer T cells and eosinophilic airway inflammation in human asthma. Int. Arch. Allergy Immunol. 153, 239−248.

Kojo, S., et al., 2001. Dysfunction of T cell receptor AV24AJ18 +, BV11 + double-negative regulatory natural killer T cells in autoimmune diseases. Arthritis Rheum. 44, 1127−1138.

Kojo, S., et al., 2005. Induction of regulatory properties in dendritic cells by Valpha14 NKT cells. J. Immunol. (Baltimore, Md.: 1950). 175, 3648−3655.

Kojo, S., et al., 2003. Low expression levels of soluble CD1d gene in patients with rheumatoid arthritis. J. Rheumatol. 30, 2524−2528.

Koreck, A., et al., 2002. CD3 + CD56 + NK T cells are significantly decreased in the peripheral blood of patients with psoriasis. Clin. Exp. Immunol. 127, 176−182.

Kronenberg, M., 2005. Toward an understanding of NKT cell biology: progress and pparadoxes. Annu. Rev. Immunol. 23, 877−900.

Kronenberg, M., Gapin, L., 2002. The unconventional lifestyle of NKT cells. Nat. Rev. Immunol. 2, 557−568.

Kukreja, A., et al., 2002. Multiple immuno-regulatory defects in type-1 diabetes. J. Clin. Invest. 109, 131−140.

Kyriakakis, E., et al., 2010. Invariant natural killer T cells: linking inflammation and neovascularization in human atherosclerosis. Eur. J. Immunol. 40, 3268−3279

Langewouters, A.M.G., et al., 2007. The effect of topical corticosteroids in combination with alefacept on circulating T-cell subsets in psoriasis. J. Dermatological Treat. 18, 279−285.

Lanier, L.L., Chang, C., Phillips, J.H., 1994. Human NKR-P1A. A disulfide-linked homodimer of the C-type lectin superfamily expressed by a subset of NK and T lymphocytes. J. Immunol. (Baltimore, Md.: 1950). 153, 2417−2428.

Lappas, C.M., et al., 2006. Adenosine A2A receptor activation reduces hepatic ischemia reperfusion injury by inhibiting CD1d-dependent NKT cell activation. J. Exp. Med. 203, 2639−2648.

Le Bourhis, L., et al., 2010. Antimicrobial activity of mucosal-associated invariant T cells. Nat. Immunol. 11, 701−708.

Le Bourhis, L., et al., 2011. Mucosal-associated invariant T cells: unconventional development and function. Trends Immunol. 32, 212−218.

Lee, D.J., et al., 1998. Induction of an antigen-specific, CD1-restricted cytotoxic T lymphocyte response in vivo. J. Exp. Med. 187, 433−438.

Lee, P.T., et al., 2002a. Distinct functional lineages of human V(alpha) 24 natural killer T cells. J. Exp. Med. 195, 637−641.

Lee, P.T., et al., 2002b. Testing the NKT cell hypothesis of human IDDM pathogenesis. J. Clin. Invest. 110, 793−800.

Lehuen, A., et al., 2010. Immune cell crosstalk in type 1 diabetes. Nat. Rev. Immunol. 10, 501−513.

Lehuen, A., et al., 1998. Overexpression of natural killer T cells protects Valpha14- Jalpha281 transgenic nonobese diabetic mice against diabetes. J. Exp. Med. 188, 1831−1839.

Leite-de-Moraes, M.C., et al., 1999. A distinct IL-18-induced pathway to fully activate NK T lymphocytes independently from TCR engagement. J. Immunol. (Baltimore, Md.: 1950). 163, 5871−5876.

Leite-de-Moraes, M.C., et al., 2001. IL-18 enhances IL-4 production by ligand-activated NKT lymphocytes: a pro-Th2 effect of IL-18 exerted through NKT cells. J. Immunol. (Baltimore, Md.: 1950). 166, 945−951.

Li, B., et al., 2006. Interleukin-15 prevents concanavalin A-induced liver injury in mice via NKT cell-dependent mechanism. Hepatology 43, 1211−1219.

Li, L., et al., 2007. NKT cell activation mediates neutrophil IFN-gamma production and renal ischemia-reperfusion injury. J. Immunol. (Baltimore, Md.: 1950). 178, 5899−5911.

Linsen, L., et al., 2005. Peripheral blood but not synovial fluid natural killer T cells are biased towards a Th1-like phenotype in rheumatoid arthritis. Arthritis Res. Ther. 7, R493–R502.

Lisbonne, M., et al., 2003. Cutting edge: invariant V alpha 14 NKT cells are required for allergen-induced airway inflammation and hyperreactivity in an experimental asthma model. J. Immunol. (Baltimore, Md.: 1950). 171, 1637–1641.

Liu, R., et al., 2005. Cooperation of invariant NKT Cells and CD4 + CD25 + T regulatory cells in the prevention of autoimmune Myasthenia. J. Immunol. (Baltimore, Md.: 1950). 175, 7898–7904.

Liu, Y., et al., 2011. Endogenous collagen peptide activation of CD1d-restricted NKT cells ameliorates tissue-specific inflammation in mice. J. Clin. Invest. 121, 249–264.

Lowes, M.A., et al., 2008. Psoriasis vulgaris lesions contain discrete populations of Th1 and Th17 T cells. J. Investi. Dermatol. 128, 1207–1211.

Ly, D., et al., 2010. An alpha-galactosylceramide C20:2 N-acyl variant enhances anti-inflammatory and regulatory T cell-independent responses that prevent type 1 diabetes. Clin. Exp. Immunol. 160, 185–198.

Ly, D., et al., 2006. Protection from type 1 diabetes by invariant NK T cells requires the activity of CD4 + CD25 + regulatory T cells. J. Immunol. (Baltimore, Md.: 1950). 177, 3695–3704.

Lynch, L., et al., 2009. Invariant NKT cells and CD1d(+) cells amass in human omentum and are depleted in patients with cancer and obesity. Eur. J. Immunol. 39, 1893–1901.

Maeda, T., et al., 1999. Decreased TCR AV24AJ18 + double-negative T cells in rheumatoid synovium. Rheumatology (Oxford). 38, 186–188.

Magnan, A., et al., 2000. Relationships between natural T cells, atopy, IgE levels, and IL-4 production. Allergy 55, 286–290.

Major, A.S., et al., 2004. Quantitative and qualitative differences in proatherogenic NKT cells in apolipoprotein E-deficient mice. Arterioscler. Thromb. Vasc. Biol. 24, 2351–2357.

Major, A.S., et al., 2006. The role of invariant natural killer T cells in lupus and atherogenesis. Immunol. Res. 34, 49–66.

Mallevaey, T., et al., 2006. Activation of invariant NKT cells by the helminth parasite schistosoma mansoni. J. Immunol. (Baltimore, Md.: 1950). 176, 2476–2485.

Mars, L.T., et al., 2002. Cutting edge: V alpha 14-J alpha 281 NKT cells naturally regulate experimental autoimmune encephalomyelitis in nonobese diabetic mice. J. Immunol. (Baltimore, Md.: 1950). 168, 6007–6011.

Mars, L.T., et al., 2009. Invariant NKT cells inhibit development of the Th17 lineage. Proc. Nat. Acad. Sci. USA 106, 6238–6243.

Mars, L.T., et al., 2008. Invariant NKT cells regulate experimental autoimmune encephalomyelitis and infiltrate the central nervous system in a CD1d-independent manner. J. Immunol. 181, 2321–2329.

Matangkasombut, P., et al., 2008. Direct activation of natural killer T cells induces airway hyperreactivity in nonhuman primates. J. Allergy Clin. Immunol. 121, 1287–1289.

Matangkasombut, P., et al., 2009a. Natural killer T cells in the lungs of patients with asthma. J. Allergy Clin. Immunol. 123, 1181–1185. e1.

Matangkasombut, P., et al., 2009b. Natural killer T cells and the regulation of asthma. Mucosal Immunol. 2, 383–392.

Matsuda, J.L., et al., 2003. Mouse V alpha 14i natural killer T cells are resistant to cytokine polarization in vivo. Proc. Nat. Acad. Sci. USA 100, 8395–8400.

Matsuda, J.L., et al., 2001. Natural killer T cells reactive to a single glycolipid exhibit a highly diverse T cell receptor beta repertoire and small clone size. Proc. Nat. Acad. Sci. USA 98, 12636–12641.

Mattner, J., et al., 2005. Exogenous and endogenous glycolipid antigens activate NKT cells during microbial infections. Nature 434, 525–529.

Mattner, J., et al., 2008. Liver autoimmunity triggered by microbial activation of natural killer T cells. Cell Host and Microbe. 3, 304–315.

McMahon, C.W., et al., 2002. Viral and bacterial infections induce expression of multiple NK cell receptors in responding CD8(+) T cells. J. Immunol. (Baltimore, Md.: 1950). 169, 1444–1452.

McNab, F.W., et al., 2007. Peripheral NK1.1 NKT cells are mature and functionally distinct from their thymic counterparts. J. Immunol. (Baltimore, Md.: 1950). 179, 6630–6637.

McNab, F.W., et al., 2005. The influence of CD1d in postselection NKT cell maturation and homeostasis. J. Immunol. (Baltimore, Md.: 1950). 175, 3762–3768.

Melián, A., et al., 1999. CD1 expression in human atherosclerosis. A potential mechanism for T cell activation by foam cells. Am. J. Pathol. 155, 775–786.

Metelitsa, L.S., 2010. Anti-tumor potential of type-I NKT cells against CD1d-positive and CD1d-negative tumors in humans. Clin. Immunol 140, 119–129.

Metelitsa, L.S., et al., 2003. Expression of CD1d by myelomonocytic leukemias provides a target for cytotoxic NKT cells. Leukemia 17, 1068–1077.

Meyer, E.H., et al., 2006. Glycolipid activation of invariant T cell receptor + NK T cells is sufficient to induce airway hyperreactivity independent of conventional CD4 + T cells. Proc. Nat. Acad. Sci. USA 103, 2782–2787.

Mi, Q.-S., et al., 2004. Interleukin-4 but not interleukin-10 protects against spontaneous and recurrent type 1 diabetes by activated CD1d-restricted invariant natural killer T-cells. Diabetes 53, 1303–1310.

Michalek, J., et al., 2006. Immune regulatory T cells in siblings of children suffering from type 1 diabetes mellitus. Scand. J. Immunol. 64, 531–535.

Michel, M.-L., et al., 2008. Critical role of ROR-γt in a new thymic pathway leading to IL-17-producing invariant NKT cell differentiation. Proc. Nat. Acad. Sci. 105, 19845–19850.

Michel, M.L., et al., 2007. Identification of an IL-17-producing NK1.1neg iNKT cell population involved in airway neutrophilia. J. Exp. Med. 204, 995–1001.

Miellot, A., et al., 2005. Activation of invariant NK T cells protects against experimental rheumatoid arthritis by an IL-10-dependent pathway. Eur. J. Immunol. 35, 3704–3713.

Miellot-Gafsou, A., et al., 2010. Early activation of invariant natural killer T cells in a rheumatoid arthritis model and application to disease treatment. Immunology 130, 296–306.

Milpied, P., et al., 2011. IL-17-producing invariant NKT cells in lymphoid organs are recent thymic emigrants identified by neuropilin-1 expression. Blood 118, 2993–3002.

Miyamoto, K., Miyake, S., Yamamura, T., 2001. A synthetic glycolipid prevents autoimmune encephalomyelitis by inducing TH2 bias of natural killer T cells. Nature 413, 531–534.

Mizuno, M., et al., 2004. Synthetic glycolipid OCH prevents insulitis and diabetes in NOD mice. J. Autoimmunity 23, 293–300.

Mohammed, J.P., et al., 2011. Identification of Cd101 as a susceptibility gene for Novosphingobium aromaticivorans-induced liver autoimmunity. J. Immunol. 187, 337–349.

Montoya, C.J., et al., 2007. Characterization of human invariant natural killer T subsets in health and disease using a novel invariant natural killer T cell-clonotypic monoclonal antibody, 6B11. Immunology 122, 1–14.

Moreira-Teixeira, L., et al., 2011. Proinflammatory environment dictates the IL-17-producing capacity of human invariant NKT cells. J. Immunology 186, 5758–5765.

Moreira-Teixeira, L., et al., 2012. Rapamycin combined with TGF⁻ converts human invariant nkt cells into suppressive Foxp3 + regulatory cells. J. Immunol. 188, 624–631.

Morita, M., et al., 1995. Structure-activity relationship of alpha-galactosylceramides against B16-bearing mice. J. Med. Chem. 38, 2176–2187.

Morshed, S.R., et al., 2009. Beta-galactosylceramide alters invariant natural killer T cell function and is effective treatment for lupus. Clin. Immunol. 132, 321–333.

Morshed, S.R., et al., 2002. Tissue-specific expansion of NKT and CD5 + B cells at the onset of autoimmune disease in (NZBxNZW) F1 mice. Eur. J. Immunol. 32, 2551–2561.

Mutalithas, K., et al., 2007. Bronchoalveolar lavage invariant natural killer T cells are not increased in asthma. J. Allergy Clin. Immunol. 119, 1274–1276.

Nagarajan, N.A., Kronenberg, M., 2007. Invariant NKT cells amplify the innate immune response to lipopolysaccharide. J. Immunol. (Baltimore, Md.: 1950). 178, 2706–2713.

Nakai, Y., et al., 2004. Natural killer T cells accelerate atherogenesis in mice. Blood 104, 2051–2059.

Nakamura, K., et al., 2008. Serum thymic stromal lymphopoietin levels are not elevated in patients with atopic dermatitis. J. Dermatol. 35, 546–547.

Naumov, Y.N., et al., 2001. Activation of CD1d-restricted T cells protects NOD mice from developing diabetes by regulating dendritic cell subsets. Proc. Nat. Acad. Sci. USA 98, 13838–13843.

Nickoloff, B.J., 2000. Characterization of lymphocyte-dependent angiogenesis using a SCID mouse: human skin model of psoriasis. J. Invest. Dermatol. Symposium Proceedings/the Society for Investigative Dermatology, Inc. [and] European Society for Dermatological Research. 5, 67–73.

Nieuwenhuis, E.E., et al., 2009. Cd1d-dependent regulation of bacterial colonization in the intestine of mice. J. Clin. Invest. 119, 1241–1250.

Nieuwenhuis, E.E.S., et al., 2005. CD1d and CD1d-restricted iNKT-cells play a pivotal role in contact hypersensitivity. Exp. Dermatol. 14, 250–258.

Novak, J., Lehuen, A., 2011. Mechanism of regulation of autoimmunity by iNKT cells. Cytokine 53, 263–270.

Novak, J., et al., 2005. Inhibition of T cell differentiation into effectors by NKT cells requires cell contacts. J. Immunol. (Baltimore, Md.: 1950). 174, 1954–1961.

Novak, J., et al., 2007. Prevention of type 1 diabetes by invariant NKT cells is independent of peripheral CD1d expression. J. Immunol. (Baltimore, Md.: 1950). 178, 1332–1340.

Numata, Y., et al., 2005. Therapeutic effect of repeated natural killer T cell stimulation in mouse cholangitis complicated by colitis. Dig. Dis. Sci. 50, 1844–1851.

O'Keeffe, J., et al., 2004. Diverse populations of T cells with NK cell receptors accumulate in the human intestine in health and in colorectal cancer. Eur. J. Immunol. 34, 2110–2119.

O'Keeffe, J., et al., 2008. T-cells expressing natural killer (NK) receptors are altered in multiple sclerosis and responses to alpha-galactosylceramide are impaired. J. Neurological Sci. 275, 22–28.

Ogasawara, K., et al., 1998. Involvement of NK1 + T cells and their IFN-gamma production in the generalized Shwartzman reaction. J. Immunol. (Baltimore, Md.: 1950). 160, 3522–3527.

Oh, S.J., Chung, D.H., 2011. Invariant NKT cells producing IL-4 or IL-10, but not IFN-{gamma}, inhibit the Th1 response in experimental autoimmune encephalomyelitis, whereas none of these cells inhibits the Th17 response. J. Immunol. (Baltimore, Md.: 1950). 186, 6815–6821.

Ohnishi, Y., et al., 2005. TCR Valpha14 natural killer T cells function as effector T cells in mice with collagen-induced arthritis. Clin. Exp. Immunol. 141, 47–53.

Oikawa, Y., et al., 2002. High frequency of valpha24(+) vbeta11(+) T-cells observed in type 1 diabetes. Diabetes Care 25, 1818–1823.

Oishi, Y., et al., 2000. CD4 − CD8 − T cells bearing invariant Valpha24JalphaQ TCR alpha-chain are decreased in patients with atopic diseases. Clin. Exp. Immunol. 119, 404–411.

Oishi, Y., et al., 2001. Selective reduction and recovery of invariant Valpha24JalphaQ T cell receptor T cells in correlation with disease activity in patients with systemic lupus erythematosus. J. Rheumatol. 28, 275–283.

Olafsson, S., et al., 2004. Antimitochondrial antibodies and reactivity to N. Aromaticivorans proteins in Icelandic patients with primary biliary cirrhosis and their relatives. Am. J. Gastroenterol. 99, 2143–2146.

Oling, V., et al., 2007. Circulating CD4 + CD25 high regulatory T cells and natural killer T cells in children with newly diagnosed type 1 diabetes or with diabetes-associated autoantibodies. Ann. N.Y. Acad. Sci. 1107, 363–372.

Olszak, T., et al., 2012. Microbial exposure during early life has persistent effects on natural killer T cell function. Science 336, 489–493.

Omenetti, A., et al., 2009. Repair-related activation of hedgehog signaling promotes cholangiocyte chemokine production. Hepatology 50, 518–527.

Ortaldo, J.R., et al., 2006. Regulation of ITAM-positive receptors: role of IL-12 and IL-18. Blood. 107, 1468–1475 (Available at: <http://eutils.ncbi.nlm.nih.gov/entrez/eutils/elink.fcgi?dbfrom = pubmed&id = 16249390&retmode = ref&cmd = prlinks>).

Ostos, M.A., et al., 2002. Implication of natural killer T cells in atherosclerosis development during a LPS-induced chronic inflammation. FEBS Lett. 519, 23–29.

Paget, C., et al., 2007. Activation of invariant NKT cells by toll-like receptor 9-stimulated dendritic cells requires type I interferon and charged glycosphingolipids. Immunity 27, 597–609.

Paget, C., et al., 2012. Interleukin-22 is produced by invariant natural killer T lymphocytes during influenza A virus infection: potential role in protection against lung epithelial damages. J. Biol. Chem. 287, 8816–8829.

Pal, E., et al., 2001. Costimulation-dependent modulation of experimental autoimmune encephalomyelitis by ligand stimulation of V alpha 14 NK T cells. J. Immunol. (Baltimore, Md.: 1950). 166, 662–668.

Parekh, V.V., Wilson, M.T., Van Kaer, L., 2005. iNKT-cell responses to glycolipids. Crit. Rev. Immunol. 25, 183–213.

Parietti, V., et al., 2010. Rituximab treatment overcomes reduction of regulatory iNKT cells in patients with rheumatoid arthritis. Clin. Immunol. 134, 331–339.

Park, S.H., et al., 2000. Unaltered phenotype, tissue distribution and function of Valpha14(+) NKT cells in germ-free mice. Eur. J. Immunol. 30, 620–625.

Park, S.H., et al., 2001. The mouse CD1d-restricted repertoire is dominated by a few autoreactive T cell receptor families. J. Exp. Med. 193, 893–904.

Pei, B., et al., 2012. Interplay between carbohydrate and lipid in recognition of glycolipid antigens by natural killer T cells. Ann. N.Y. Acad. Sci. 1253, 68–79.

Pellicci, D.G., et al., 2005. DX5/CD49b-positive T cells are not synonymous with CD1d-dependent NKT cells. J. Immunol. (Baltimore, Md.: 1950). 175, 4416–4425.

Pellicci, D.G., et al., 2011. Recognition of β-linked self glycolipids mediated by natural killer T cell antigen receptors. Nat. Immunol. 12, 827–833.

Peternel, S., Kastelan, M., 2009. Immunopathogenesis of psoriasis: focus on natural killer T cells. J. Eur. Acad. Dermatol. Venereol. 23, 1123–1127.

Pichavant, M., et al., 2008. Ozone exposure in a mouse model induces airway hyperreactivity that requires the presence of natural killer T cells and IL-17. J. Exp. Med. 205, 385–393.

Postigo, J., et al., 2012. Mice deficient in CD38 develop an attenuated form of collagen type II-induced arthritis. PLoS One. 7, e33534.

Prell, C., et al., 2003. Frequency of Valpha24 + CD161 + natural killer T cells and invariant TCRAV24-AJ18 transcripts in atopic and nonatopic individuals. Immunobiology 208, 367–380.

Prussin, C., Foster, B., 1997. TCR V alpha 24 and V beta 11 coexpression defines a human NK1 T cell analog containing a unique Th0 subpopulation. J. Immunol. (Baltimore, Md.: 1950). 159, 5862–5870.

Rauch, J., et al., 2003. Structural features of the acyl chain determine self-phospholipid antigen recognition by a CD1d-restricted invariant NKT (iNKT) cell. J. Biol. Chem. 278, 47508–47515.

Reynolds, C., et al., 2009. Natural killer T cells in bronchial biopsies from human allergen challenge model of allergic asthma. J. Allergy Clin. Immunol. 124, 860–862, —author reply 862.

Rijavec, M., et al., 2011. Natural killer T cells in pulmonary disorders. Respir. Med. 105, S20–S25.

Rocha-Campos, A.C., et al., 2006. Genetic and functional analysis of the Nkt1 locus using congenic NOD mice: improved V{alpha}14-NKT cell performance but failure to protect against type 1 diabetes. Diabetes 55, 1163–1170.

Rogers, L., et al., 2008. Deficiency of invariant V 14 natural killer T cells decreases atherosclerosis in LDL receptor null mice. Cardiovascular Res. 78, 167–174.

Roman-Gonzalez, A., et al., 2009. Frequency and function of circulating invariant NKT cells in autoimmune diabetes mellitus and thyroid diseases in Colombian patients. Hum. Immunol. 70, 262–268.

Ronchi, F., Falcone, M., 2008. Immune regulation by invariant NKT cells in autoimmunity. Front. Biosci. 13, 4827–4837.

Ronet, C., et al., 2001. Role of the complementarity-determining region 3 (CDR3) of the TCR-beta chains associated with the V alpha 14 semi-invariant TCR alpha-chain in the selection of CD4 + NK T Cells. J. Immunol. (Baltimore, Md.: 1950). 166, 1755–1762.

Rossjohn, J., et al., 2012. Recognition of CD1d-restricted antigens by natural killer T cells. Nat. Rev. Immunol. 12, 845–857.

Sag, D., et al., 2012. ATP-Binding Cassette Transporter G1 Intrinsically Regulates Invariant NKT Cell Development. J. Immunol. 189, 5129–5138.

Sakuishi, K., et al., 2007. Invariant NKT cells biased for IL-5 production act as crucial regulators of inflammation. J. Immunol. (Baltimore, Md.: 1950). 179, 3452–3462.

Salio, M., Cerundolo, V., 2009. Linking inflammation to natural killer T cell activation. PLoS Biol. 7, e1000226.

Saubermann, L.J., et al., 2000. Activation of natural killer T cells by alpha-galactosylceramide in the presence of CD1d provides protection against colitis in mice. Gastroenterology 119, 119–128.

Saxena, V., et al., 2007. The countervailing actions of myeloid and plasmacytoid dendritic cells control autoimmune diabetes in the nonobese diabetic mouse. J. Immunol. (Baltimore, Md.: 1950). 179, 5041–5053.

Schmieg, J., et al., 2003. Superior protection against malaria and melanoma metastases by a C-glycoside analogue of the natural killer T cell ligand alpha-Galactosylceramide. J. Exp. Med. 198, 1631–1641.

Segawa, S., et al., 2009. Low levels of soluble CD1d protein alters NKT cell function in patients with rheumatoid arthritis. Int. J. Mol. Med. 24, 481–486.

Selmi, C., et al., 2003. Patients with primary biliary cirrhosis react against a ubiquitous xenobiotic-metabolizing bacterium. Hepatology 38, 1250–1257.

Sen, Y., et al., 2005. V alpha 24-invariant NKT cells from patients with allergic asthma express CCR9 at high frequency and induce Th2 bias of CD3 + T cells upon CD226 engagement. J. Immunol. (Baltimore, Md.: 1950). 175, 4914–4926.

Sharif, S., et al., 2001. Activation of natural killer T cells by alpha-galactosylceramide treatment prevents the onset and recurrence of autoimmune Type 1 diabetes. Nat. Med. 7, 1057–1062.

Shi, F.D., et al., 2001. Germ line deletion of the CD1 locus exacerbates diabetes in the NOD mouse. Proc. Nat. Acad. Sci. USA 98, 6777–6782.

Shi, G.P., 2010. Immunomodulation of vascular diseases: atherosclerosis and autoimmunity. Eur. J. Vasc. Endovascul. Surg. 39, 485–494.

Shimamura, M., Huang, Y.-Y., 2002. Presence of a novel subset of NKT cells bearing an invariant V(alpha)19.1-J(alpha)26 TCR alpha chain. FEBS Lett. 516, 97–100.

Simon, D., Kozlowski, E., Simon, H., 2009. Natural killer T cells expressing IFN-gamma and IL-4 in lesional skin of atopic eczema. Allergy 64, 1681–1684.

Simoni, Y., et al., 2011. NOD mice contain an elevated frequency of iNKT17 cells that exacerbate diabetes. Eur. J. Immunol. 41, 3574–3585.

Simoni, Y., et al., 2012. Therapeutic manipulation of natural killer (NK) T cells in autoimmunity: are we close to reality? Clin. Exp. Immunol. 171, 8–19.

Singh, A.K., et al., 2001. Natural killer T cell activation protects mice against experimental autoimmune encephalomyelitis. J. Exp. Med. 194, 1801–1811.

Singh, A.K., et al., 2005. The natural killer T cell ligand alpha-galactosylceramide prevents or promotes pristane-induced lupus in mice. Eur. J. Immunol. 35, 1143–1154.

Singh, N., et al., 1999. Cutting edge: activation of NK T cells by CD1d and alpha-galactosylceramide directs conventional T cells to the acquisition of a Th2 phenotype. J. Immunol. (Baltimore, Md.: 1950). 163, 2373–2377.

Sireci, G., et al., 2007. Immunoregulatory role of Jalpha281 T cells in aged mice developing lupus-like nephritis. Eur. J. Immunol. 37, 425–433.

Skold, M., Cardell, S., 2000. Differential regulation of Ly49 expression on CD4 + and CD4 − CD8 − (double negative) NK1.1 + T cells. Eur. J. Immunol. 30, 2488–2496.

Slifka, M.K., Pagarigan, R.R., Whitton, J.L., 2000. NK markers are expressed on a high percentage of virus-specific CD8 + and CD4 + T cells. J. Immunol. (Baltimore, Md.: 1950). 164, 2009–2015.

Smithgall, M.D., et al., 2008. IL-33 amplifies both Th1- and Th2-type responses through its activity on human basophils, allergen-reactive Th2 cells, iNKT and NK cells. Int. Immunol. 20, 1019–1030.

Smyth, M.J., Taniguchi, M., Street, S.E., 2000a. The anti-tumor activity of IL-12: mechanisms of innate immunity that are model and dose dependent. J. Immunol. (Baltimore, Md.: 1950). 165, 2665–2670.

Smyth, M.J., et al., 2000b. Differential tumor surveillance by natural killer (NK) and NKT cells. J. Exp. Med. 191, 661–668.

Soumelis, V., et al. 2002. Human epithelial cells trigger dendritic cell–mediated allergic inflammation by producing TSLP. Nat. Immunol 3, 673-680.

Sowden, E., Ng, W.F., 2012. Invariant natural killer T cells in rheumatoid arthritis and other inflammatory arthritides. In: Andrew Lemmey (Ed.), Rheumatoid Arthritis - Etiology, Consequences and Co-Morbidities, pp. 19–40.

Sprent, J., Surh, C.D., 2002. T cell memory. Annu. Rev. Immunol. 20, 551–579.

Stepniak, D., Koning, F., 2006. Celiac disease—sandwiched between innate and adaptive immunity. Human Immunol. 67, 460–468.

Stetson, D.B., et al., 2003. Constitutive cytokine mRNAs mark natural killer (NK) and NK T cells poised for rapid effector function. J. Exp. Med. 198, 1069–1076.

Ström, A., et al., 2007. Involvement of the CD1d-natural killer T cell pathway in neointima formation after vascular injury. Circ. Res. 101, e83–e89.

Sullivan, B.A., et al., 2010. Mechanisms for glycolipid antigen-driven cytokine polarization by Valpha14i NKT cells. J. Immunol. (Baltimore, Md.: 1950). 184, 141–153.

Sumida, T., et al., 1995. Selective reduction of T cells bearing invariant V alpha 24J alpha Q antigen receptor in patients with systemic sclerosis. J. Exp. Med. 182, 1163–1168.

Sumida, T., et al., 1998. TCR AV24 gene expression in double negative T cells in systemic lupus erythematosus. Lupus. 7, 565–568.

Takagi, D., et al., 2006. Natural killer T cells ameliorate antibody-induced arthritis in macrophage migration inhibitory factor transgenic mice. Int. J. Mol. Med. 18, 829–836.

Takahashi, T., Strober, S., 2008. Natural killer T cells and innate immune B cells from lupus-prone NZB/W mice interact to generate IgM and IgG autoantibodies. Eur. J. Immunol. 38, 156–165.

Takahashi, T., et al., 2003. V alpha 24 + natural killer T cells are markedly decreased in atopic dermatitis patients. Hum. Immunol. 64, 586–592.

Tangri, S., et al., 1998. Presentation of peptide antigens by mouse CD1 requires endosomal localization and protein antigen processing. Proc. Nat. Acad. Sci. USA 95, 14314–14319.

Taniguchi, M., et al., 2003. The regulatory role of Vα14 NKT cells ininnate and acquired immune response. Annu. Rev. Immunol. 21, 483–513.

Teige, A., et al., 2004. CD1-dependent regulation of chronic central nervous system inflammation in experimental autoimmune encephalomyelitis. J. Immunol. (Baltimore, Md.: 1950). 172, 186–194.

Teige, A., et al., 2010. CD1d-dependent NKT cells play a protective role in acute and chronic arthritis models by ameliorating antigen-specific Th1 responses. J. Immunol. (Baltimore, Md.: 1950). 185, 345–356.

Terashima, A., et al., 2008. A novel subset of mouse NKT cells bearing the IL-17 receptor B responds to IL-25 and contributes to airway hyperreactivity. J. Exp. Med. 205, 2727–2733.

Thomas, S.Y., et al., 2007. Multiple chemokine receptors, including CCR6 and CXCR3, regulate antigen-induced T cell homing to the human asthmatic airway. J. Immunol. (Baltimore, Md.: 1950). 179, 1901–1912.

Thomas, S.Y., Chyung, Y.H., Luster, A.D., 2010. Natural killer T cells are not the predominant T cell in asthma and likely modulate, not cause, asthma. J. Allergy Clin. Immunol. 125, 980–984.

Thomas, S.Y., Lilly, C.M., Luster, A.D., 2006. Invariant natural killer T cells in bronchial asthma. New England J. Med. 354, 2613–2616, —author reply 2613–2616.

To, K., et al., 2009. NKT cell subsets mediate differential proatherogenic effects in ApoE$^{-/-}$ mice. Arteriosclerosis, Thrombosis, and Vascular Biol. 29, 671–677.

Tobin, A.-M., et al., 2011. Natural killer cells in psoriasis. J. Innate Immun. 3, 403–410.

Tonti, E., et al., 2012. Follicular helper NKT cells induce limited B cell responses and germinal center formation in the absence of CD4+ T cell help. J. Immunol. 188, 3217–3222.

Torres, D., et al., 2008. Prostaglandin D2 inhibits the production of IFN-gamma by invariant NK T cells: consequences in the control of B16 melanoma. J. Immunol. (Baltimore, Md.: 1950). 180, 783–792.

Treiner, E., et al., 2003. Selection of evolutionarily conserved mucosal-associated invariant T cells by MR1. Nature 422, 164–169.

Tsuneyama, K., et al., 1998. Increased CD1d expression on small bile duct epithelium and epithelioid granuloma in livers in primary biliary cirrhosis. Hepatology 28, 620–623.

Tsutsumi, Y., et al., 2006. Phenotypic and genetic analyses of T-cell-mediated immunoregulation in patients with Type 1 diabetes. Diabet. Med. 23, 1145–1150.

Tudhope, S.J., et al., 2010. Profound invariant natural killer T-cell deficiency in inflammatory arthritis. Ann. Rheumatic Diseases. 69, 1873–1879.

Tupin, E., et al., 2004. CD1d-dependent activation of NKT cells aggravates atherosclerosis. J. Exp. Med. 199, 417–422.

Tupin, E., Kinjo, Y., Kronenberg, M., 2007. The unique role of natural killer T cells in the response to microorganisms. Nat. Rev. Microbiol. 5, 405–417.

Tyznik, A.J., et al., 2008. Cutting edge: the mechanism of invariant NKT cell responses to viral danger signals. J. Immunol. (Baltimore, Md.: 1950). 181, 4452–4456.

Ueno, Y., et al., 2005. Single dose of OCH improves mucosal T helper type 1/T helper type 2 cytokine balance and prevents experimental colitis in the presence of valpha14 natural killer T cells in mice. Inflamm. Bowel Dis. 11, 35—41.

Uibo, R., et al., 2012. Primary biliary cirrhosis: a multi-faced interactive disease involving genetics, environment and the immune response. APMIS. 120, 857—871.

Umetsu, D.T., DeKruyff, R.H., 2010. Natural killer T cells are important in the pathogenesis of asthma: the many pathways to asthma. J. Allergy Clin. Immunol. 125, 975—979.

van der Vliet, H.J., et al., 2000. Human natural killer T cells acquire a memory-activated phenotype before birth. Blood 95, 2440—2442.

van der Vliet, H.J.J., et al., 2001. Circulating Vα24+ Vβ11+ NKT cell numbers are decreased in a wide variety of diseases that are characterized by autoreactive tissue damage. Clin. Immunol. 100, 144—148.

van der Vliet, H.J.J., et al., 2004. The immunoregulatory role of CD1d-restricted natural killer T cells in disease. Clin. Immunol. 112, 8—23.

van Puijvelde, G.H., et al., 2009. Effect of natural killer T cell activation on the initiation of atherosclerosis. Thromb. Haemost. 102, 223—230.

VanderLaan, P.A., et al., 2007. Characterization of the natural killer T-cell response in an adoptive transfer model of atherosclerosis. Am. J. Pathol. 170, 1100—1107.

Vijayanand, P., et al., 2007. Invariant natural killer T cells in asthma and chronic obstructive pulmonary disease. New England J. Med. 356, 1410—1422.

Wang, B., Geng, Y.B., Wang, C.R., 2001. CD1-restricted NK T cells protect nonobese diabetic mice from developing diabetes. J. Exp. Med. 194, 313—320.

Wang, J., et al., 2009. Cutting edge: CD28 engagement releases antigen-activated invariant NKT cells from the inhibitory effects of PD-1. J. Immunol. (Baltimore, Md.: 1950). 182, 6644—6647.

Watanabe, H., et al., 1995. Relationships between intermediate TCR cells and NK1.1+ T cells in various immune organs. NK1.1+ T cells are present within a population of intermediate TCR cells. J. Immunol. (Baltimore, Md.: 1950). 155, 2972—2983.

Weaver, C.T., et al., 2007. IL-17 family cytokines and the expanding diversity of effector T cell lineages. Annu. Rev. Immunol. 25, 821—852.

Wermeling, F., et al., 2010. Invariant NKT cells limit activation of autoreactive CD1d-positive B cells. J. Exp. Med. 207, 943—952.

White, D.C., Sutton, S.D., Ringelberg, D.B., 1996. The genus Sphingomonas: physiology and ecology. Curr. Opin. Biotechnol. 7, 301—306.

Wiethe, C., et al., 2007. Interdependency of MHC class II/self-peptide and CD1d/self-glycolipid presentation by TNF-matured dendritic cells for protection from autoimmunity. J. Immunol. (Baltimore, Md.: 1950). 178, 4908—4916.

Wilson, S.B., et al., 1998. Extreme Th1 bias of invariant Valpha24JalphaQ T cells in type 1 diabetes. Nature 391, 177—181.

Wilson, S.B., et al., 2000. Multiple differences in gene expression in regulatory Valpha 24Jalpha Q T cells from identical twins discordant for type I diabetes. Proc. Nat. Acad. Sci. USA 97, 7411—7416.

Wingender, G., Kronenberg, M., 2006. Invariant natural killer cells in the response to bacteria: the advent of specific antigens. Future Microbiol. 1, 325—340.

Wingender, G., Kronenberg, M., 2008. Role of NKT cells in the digestive system. IV. The role of canonical natural killer T cells in mucosal immunity and inflammation. Am. J. Physiol. Gastrointestinal and Liver Physiol. 294, G1—G8.

Wingender, G., et al., 2010. Antigen-specific cytotoxicity by invariant NKT cells in vivo is CD95/CD178-dependent and is correlated with antigenic potency. J. Immunol. (Baltimore, Md.: 1950). 185, 2721—2729.

Wingender, G., et al., 2006. Immediate antigen-specific effector functions by TCR-transgenic CD8+ NKT cells. Eur. J. Immunol. 36, 570—582.

Wingender, G., et al., 2011. Invariant NKT cells are required for airway inflammation induced by environmental antigens. J. Exp. Med. 208, 1151—1162.

Wingender, G., et al., 2012a. Neutrophilic granulocytes modulate invariant NKT cell function in mice and humans. J. Immunol. 188, 3000—3008.

Wingender, G., et al., 2012b. Intestinal microbes affect phenotypes and functions of invariant natural killer T cells in mice. Gastroenterology 143, 418—428.

Wintermeyer, P., et al., 2009. Invariant natural killer T cells suppress the neutrophil inflammatory response in a mouse model of cholestatic liver damage. Gastroenterology 136, 1048—1059.

Wither, J., et al., 2008. Reduced proportions of natural killer T cells are present in the relatives of lupus patients and are associated with autoimmunity. Arthritis Res. Ther. 10, R108.

Wong, C.H.Y., et al., 2011. Functional innervation of hepatic iNKT cells is immunosuppressive following stroke. Science 334, 101—105.

Wong, P.T.Y., et al., 2009. Decreased expression of T lymphocyte co-stimulatory molecule CD26 on invariant natural killer T cells in systemic lupus erythematosus. Immunol. Invest. 38, 350—364.

Wu, D.Y., et al., 2003. Cross-presentation of disialoganglioside GD3 to natural killer T cells. J. Exp. Med. 198, 173—181.

Wu, L., Van Kaer, L., 2009. Natural killer T cells and autoimmune disease. Curr. Mol. Med. 9, 4—14.

Wu, S.-J., et al., 2011. Innate immunity and primary biliary cirrhosis: activated invariant natural killer T cells exacerbate murine autoimmune cholangitis and fibrosis. Hepatology 53, 915—925.

Wu, W.H., et al., 2010. Thymic stromal lymphopoietin-activated invariant natural killer T cells trigger an innate allergic immune response in atopic dermatitis. J. Allergy Clin. Immunol. 126, 290—299.e.

Yan-ming, L., et al., 2012. The effect of specific immunotherapy on natural killer T cells in peripheral blood of house dust mite-sensitized children with asthma. Clin. Dev. Immunol. 2012, 148262.

Yanagisawa, N., et al., 2011. Are dysregulated inflammatory responses to commensal bacteria involved in the pathogenesis of hepatobiliary-pancreatic autoimmune disease? An analysis using mice models of primary biliary cirrhosis and autoimmune pancreatitis. ISRN Gastroenterol. 2011, 513—514.

Yang, J.-Q., et al., 2004. CD1d deficiency exacerbates inflammatory dermatitis in MRL-lpr/lpr mice. Eur. J. Immunol. 34, 1723—1732.

Yang, J.-Q., et al., 2003. Immunoregulatory role of CD1d in the hydrocarbon oil-induced model of lupus nephritis. J. Immunol. (Baltimore, Md.: 1950). 171, 2142—2153.

Yang, J.Q., et al., 2007. Examining the role of CD1d and natural killer T cells in the development of nephritis in a genetically susceptible lupus model. Arthritis Rheum. 56, 1219—1233.

Yang, J.Q., et al., 2011. Invariant NKT cells inhibit autoreactive B cells in a contact- and CD1d-dependent manner. J. Immunol. (Baltimore, Md.: 1950). 186, 1512–1520.

Yokote, H., et al., 2010. NKT Cell-dependent amelioration of a mouse model of multiple sclerosis by altering gut flora. Am. J. Pathol. 173, 1714–1723.

Yoshiga, Y., et al., 2011. Activation of natural killer T cells by α-carba-GalCer (RCAI-56), a novel synthetic glycolipid ligand, suppresses murine collagen-induced arthritis. Clin. Exp. Immunol. 164, 236–247.

Yoshiga, Y., et al., 2008. Invariant NKT cells produce IL-17 through IL-23-dependent and -independent pathways with potential modulation of Th17 response in collagen-induced arthritis. Int. J. Mol. Med. 22, 369–374.

Yoshimoto, T., et al., 1995a. Defective IgE production by SJL mice is linked to the absence of CD4 + , NK1.1 + T cells that promptly produce interleukin 4. Proc. Nat. Acad. Sci. USA 92, 11931–11934.

Yoshimoto, T., et al., 1995b. Role of NK1.1 + T cells in a TH2 response and in immunoglobulin E production. Science 270, 1845–1847.

Yu, K.O.A., et al., 2005. Modulation of CD1d-restricted NKT cell responses by using N-acyl variants of alpha-galactosylceramides. Proc. Nat. Acad. Sci. USA 102, 3383–3388.

Yu, X.M., Wang, X.F., 2011. The in vitro proliferation and cytokine production of Valpha24 + Vbeta11 + natural killer T cells in patients with systemic lupus erythematosus. Chin. Med. J. (Engl.). 124, 61–65.

Zaba, L.C., et al., 2009. Psoriasis is characterized by accumulation of immunostimulatory and Th1/Th17 cell-polarizing myeloid dendritic cells. J. Invest. Dermatol. 129, 79–88.

Zajonc, D.M., Kronenberg, M., 2009. Carbohydrate specificity of the recognition of diverse glycolipids by natural killer T cells. Immunol. Rev. 230, 188–200.

Zeissig, S., et al., 2007. Role of NKT cells in the digestive system. III. Role of NKT cells in intestinal immunity. Am. J. Physiol. Gastrointestinal and Liver Physiol. 293, G1101–G1105.

Zeng, D., et al., 2003. Activation of natural killer T cells in NZB/W mice induces Th1-type immune responses exacerbating lupus. J. Clin. Invest. 112, 1211–1222.

Zeng, D., et al., 2000. Cutting edge: a role for CD1 in the pathogenesis of lupus in NZB/NZW mice. J. Immunol. (Baltimore, Md.: 1950). 164, 5000–5004.

Zeng, Z., et al., 1997. Crystal structure of mouse CD1: an MHC-like fold with a large hydrophobic binding groove. Science 277, 339–345.

Zhang, Q., et al., 2011. Significant increase in natural-killer T cells in patients with tuberculosis complicated by type 2 diabetes mellitus. J. Int. Med. Res. 39, 105–111.

Zhang, W., et al., 2008. Alpha-lactosylceramide as a novel "sugar-capped" CD1d ligand for natural killer T cells: biased cytokine profile and therapeutic activities. Chembiochem. 9, 1423–1430.

Zhao, Y., et al., 2008. Activation of keratinocyte protein kinase C zeta in psoriasis plaques. J. Invest. Dermatology. 128, 2190–2197.

Zhou, D., et al., 2004. Lysosomal glycosphingolipid recognition by NKT cells. Science 306, 1786–1789.

Chapter 9

B Cell Development: How to Become One of the Chosen Ones

Fritz Melchers

Max Planck Institute for Infection Biology, Berlin, Germany

Chapter Outline

Introduction—What Has to be Generated in B Cell
Development to Make it to Maturity? 131
Follicular B Cells 132
Intraepithelial B Cells 132
Two Types of Memory B Cells 133
B Lymphopoiesis Before Ig Repertoire Generation—
Development of Progenitor and Precursor Cells 134
Development in Waves During Ontogeny, and in Niches
Throughout Life 134
Cellular Environments of the First Phase of Early, Antigen-
Independent B Cell Development 134
Early Commitments to Antigen-Independent B Cell
Development 135
The Second, Eventually Autoantigen-Sensitive, Phase of
B Cell Development to sIgM⁺ Immature B Cells 136
The First Checkpoint for the Emerging B Cell Repertoire—
Probing the Fitness for a Good BCR 137
Expression of IgL Chains 138
The Second Checkpoint: Sites and Mechanisms of Selection of
Newly Generated sIgM⁺ B Cells 139
Future Approaches to Understanding Central B Cell
Tolerance 140
Acknowledgments 142
References 142

INTRODUCTION—WHAT HAS TO BE GENERATED IN B CELL DEVELOPMENT TO MAKE IT TO MATURITY?

One B lymphocyte makes one antibody, which it displays on the cell surface in 10^4 to 10^5 copies as antigen-recognizing B cell receptors (BCRs). This central dogma of immunology (Jerne, 1955; Burnet, 1959) is observed in 98–99% of all B cells for the immunoglobulin heavy (IgH) chain locus, and in 95–97% of all Ig light (L) chain loci. Hence, in the majority of all B cells only one of two IgH, and only one of four (in the mouse), or six (in humans) IgL loci are expressed. This choice of only one IgH and one IgL allele for expression of protein is called "allelic exclusion" (for reviews see Melchers and Rolink, 1999, 2006).

The repertoires of different antigen-specific BCRs can maximally contain the number of Ig-producing B lymphocyte-lineage cells that produce one Ig heavy (H) and one light (L) chain. From the cellular dynamics of B cell development one can try to estimate how many B lineage cells are generated in the lifetime of a mouse or a human, how many of these B lineage cells make it to a successful, Ig-producing B cell, and how many of these Ig$^+$ B cells make it into the pools of peripheral, mature, antigen-reactive B cells. The antibody repertoire which is generated from progenitor cells by V(D)J rearrangements in the IgH and IgL chain gene loci is so diverse that many of the developing B cells can recognize autoantigens, and some are even polyreactive to several antigens (Zhou et al., 2007). At a first, immature stage of B cell development these autoreactive B cells are eliminated (Lederberg, 1959) in the primary lymphoid organ in a process termed "negative selection" (during adult life in bone marrow), at cellular sites yet to be discovered, before they can reach the peripheral sites of mature B cells. Pools of mature B lymphocytes are found at different sites in the body in different numbers and at different stages of differentiation from newly generated cells to antigen-experienced memory cells and

N. Rose & I. Mackay (Eds): The Autoimmune Diseases, Fifth edition. DOI: http://dx.doi.org/10.1016/B978-0-12-384929-8.00009-5

antibody-secreting plasma cells. In a 6- to 8-month-old inbred strain of mice, such as C57BL/6, such mature cells are predominantly found at two types of sites of the body that accommodate either B1 or B2 B cells.

FOLLICULAR B CELLS

In the follicular regions of spleen and lymph nodes, B cells aggregate in "B cell-rich" areas (Pillai and Cariappa, 2009), and find themselves surrounded, in the neighborhood of follicular helper T lymphocytes (King, 2009), ready to react to foreign antigen, but—in the absence of foreign antigen—over 98% are in a non-stimulated, resting, G0 cell cycle state. Clearly, they are not stimulated by autoantigens present in their neighborhood. Newly generated B cells are short-lived, with half-lives of less than a week. Experience by exposure to stimulation (e.g., by antigen) induces a longer half-life, in some cases of weeks and months. T cell-dependent stimulation in expanding germinal centers (Klein and Dalla-Favera 2008) at the interphase between T cell- and B cell-rich regions induces not only longevity, but also hypermutations of V regions of IgH and L chain genes at rates of 10^{-3} per base pair per division of the proliferating B cells, so that every cell division generates a somatic mutant in the variable regions of IgH and IgL chain genes. Hypermutating B cells in the dark zone of germinal centers divide at least once every 18 hours, and maybe even more rapidly, e.g., with cell cycle times of 6 hours, a finding that is paradoxical if DNA replication during the S phase of the cell cycle takes 8 hours and needs further investigation. Therefore, this proliferative expansion generates at least 1000 V region mutant B cells from one antigen-stimulated B cell in a week.

It is not the subject of this review, but should be noted that such hypermutations are likely to generate long-lived, autoantigen-reactive mature B cells that need to be silenced, not to elicit an autoaggressive response. It is also clear that the antigen-driven expansion of mutant B cells increasingly contributes to the total B cell repertoires as life goes on.

T cell-dependent stimulation of follicular B cells also induces IgH class switching and B cell differentiation to Ig-secreting plasma cells, followed by the migration of resting, long-lived, hypermutated, and Ig class-switched "memory" B cells and Ig-secreting plasma cells (Shapiro-Shelef and Calame, 2005) out of the follicular regions of spleen and lymph nodes, maybe even out of the secondary lymphoid organ and into specific sites ("niches") within spleen and bone marrow (Tokoyoda et al., 2010; Weill et al., 2013). It has been estimated that a 6- to 8-week-old C57BL/6 mouse has around 5×10^8 of these B2 cells, but a more detailed quantitation of the sizes of

these different B cell subpopulations with age is missing for mice and humans.

INTRAEPITHELIAL B CELLS

In the gut- (and lung-associated) epithelia B lymphocytes are located at two distinct sites: in the gut they are found in follicular structures, surrounded by T lymphocytes not unlike in spleen and lymph nodes, near flat epithelial cells which are suspected to allow permeation of food- and commensal bacteria-derived antigens from the lumen into these lymphoid cell aggregations. Separate from these aggregations single B lymphocytes and Ig (predominantly M and A)-secreting plasma cells are dispersed in the lamina propia of the gut, from where their secreted IgA can traverse the epithelium and the mucous membranes into the lumen to interact with antigens of food and with commensal bacteria. Many of these so-called B1 lymphocytes (Tung and Herzenberg, 2006; Baumgarth, 2011; Montecino-Rodriguez and Dorshkind, 2012) appear somehow activated (as they are slightly larger and, occasionally, enter cell cycle), and it has been suggested that these B cells are reactive, or at least crossreactive, to autoantigens and such "quasi-autoantigens" as food and commensal bacteria. B1 cells need the spleen to develop (Wardemann et al., 2002). It is, therefore, possible that these B1 cells are positively selected by autoantigens by a low affinity reaction of their BCRs with these autoantigens present at these sites. Many of them can respond to antigens in the absence of helper T cells and, hence, to T cell-independent antigens. Many of them can activate activation-induced cytidine deaminase (AID) (Muramatsu et al., 2000; Revy et al., 2000) for Ig class switch recombination, again apparently without the help of T cells, but this class switch is almost entirely to IgA, and their capacity to hypermutate their V regions is very limited. It is not clear whether both populations of B cells in the gut, those organized in aggregates and surrounded by T cells near flat epithelium, and the others, the single B cells in the lamina propia, are B1-type cells.

Furthermore, and in contrast to conventional, B2-type B cells, B1 cells are able to repopulate their compartments after adoptive transfers and show strong clonal persistence *in vivo*. Thus, they can be considered to have "stem cell"-like properties, e.g., the capacity of migration to the right sites (e.g., gut) and the property of long-term self-renewal. Many of the B lymphocytes at these sites can be characterized as B1-type cells. In a 6- to 8-week-old C57BL/6 mouse around 5×10^8 cells may be found, i.e., as many as there are conventional B2-type cells in follicular regions of spleen and lymph nodes, but these numbers vary considerably with the health of the animal. B1 cells are considered to be the main source of so-called "natural antibodies" (Hooijkaas et al., 1984; Bos and Meeuwesen, 1989; Bos et al., 1989). Again, a more precise quantitative analysis of the sizes of these B1 compartments with time is missing.

All these B cell sites are connected by blood and lymph vessels. Hence, when B lymphocytes are first generated in primary lymphoid organs, they enter the peripheral immune system via the blood, mainly through the central artery in the spleen from where they distribute themselves via the marginal zone to the different locations. Some marginal zone B cells probably continue their travel to gut- and lung-associated lyphoid regions where many of them establish themselves as B1-type B cells. Other marginal zone B cells begin to migrate continuously from the marginal zone into the follicular regions of spleen and back (Arnon et al., 2013). Eventually they also emigrate from the marginal zone to peripheral lymphoid organs, such as lymph nodes. In the peripheral lymphoid organs B cells can become experienced by antigenic stimulation, then circulate back, and reappear in the marginal zone of the spleen. This may, on rare and ill-understood circumstances, even allow them to change their preimposed preference to circulate back to the peripheral lymphoid site from whence they came, and redistribute themselves into another site in the system. For a site-specific distribution into B1- or B2-rich areas they need to be directed by specific chemokines, but it remains unclear whether (low affinity) recognition by autoantigens influences their choice of the B1 compartments, and whether ignorance (lack of any affinity) of autoantigens allows their aggregation in follicular B2 zones in spleen and lymph nodes. In addition, autoantigen recognition at non-lymphoid sites (such as, for example, in the articular synovial fluid of joints during active phases of rheumatoid arthritis) may contribute to the formation of lymphoid follicular structures capable of performing germinal center reactions at unusual, normally non-lymphoid sites in the body.

TWO TYPES OF MEMORY B CELLS

The distinction between B1 and B2 cells is particularly striking in the way memory is maintained in antibody-producing B cells. Longevity in the B1 compartment appears to be connected to continuous presence of the antigen, and to its stimulation to maintain an antigen-specific, long-lived, modestly activated state. Whenever such B1 cells show long-term repopulation potential upon transplantation, with longevity and persistence in the areas of the gut-associated lymphoid tissues, continued low-level antigenic stimulation via the BCR is suspected to be the selecting and survival-inducing signaling force. Food- or commensal bacterially-derived antigens, maybe with low level cross-reactivity with autoantigens, could

be such B cell receptor-mediated selecting forces. It is suspected that this cross-reactivity to autoantigens is beneficial to positively selecting and expanding a first line of B cells that encounter microbes which colonize the body after birth.

Memory B2 (classical) B cells and long-lived plasma cells have properties of long-term repopulating hematopoietic stem cells (LT-pHSCs) (Wagers and Weissman 2004; Luckey et al., 2006; Eliasson and Jönsson, 2010; Lesinski et al., 2012). They can migrate to, and become resident in, "niches" of spleen and bone marrow as long-term resting cells for long, in some cases life-long, periods of time. They retain this property when they are transplanted. We expect memory B2 cells not to rely on continuous low level stimulation via B cell receptors for survival. Their long-term resting persistence should be independent of the presence and continuous stimulation by antigen. Antigen-dependent restimulation mobilizes these resting B2 cells to leave their "niches," and it remains to be seen how antigen specific this mobilization really is, i.e., whether memory cells specific for other, unrelated antigens are co-mobilized. Once the mobilized B2 memory cells have arrived at a peripheral lymphoid organ (e.g., a lymph node), the rechallenging antigen will activate the antigen-specific memory B2 cells to a memory-type B cell response, while those mobilized memory cells that are not specific for the challenging antigen may remain resting, and may return to their sites of rest in spleen and bone marrow.

Once the peripheral, mature, B lymphoid sites in the body have been formed and filled, a constant number of cells appear to maintain a given size by (largely unknown) mechanisms of homeostasis. Since the large majority of B cells are expected to turn over within days, weeks, or months, it follows that these B cell populations must be continuously replenished during life. However, the relative, and even the absolute, sizes of different B cell compartments change with age.

The description of the different B cell compartments, restricted to a few inbred strains of mice at a restricted time in their life, is far more detailed than that of humans—not to mention other species such as other mammals, fish, or birds. B1 and conventional B2 compartments, comparable but not necessarily identical to mouse, have been found and defined in humans (Descatoire et al., 2011). Very generally summarized, humans with a thousand-fold higher body size than mice have a thousand times more B cells with similar sites of cellular organization of similar subpopulations with similar functions. However, we lack a more systematic comparison with age and immunological experience of the two species, as these are studied for different reasons—mice, because of the tremendous experimental opportunities to study and interfere with its immune system, and humans, often because of self-centered, health-minded interests.

The limitations of the description of B cell development that follows should be seen in this light.

B LYMPHOPOIESIS BEFORE IG REPERTOIRE GENERATION— DEVELOPMENT OF PROGENITOR AND PRECURSOR CELLS

Lymphocyte development occurs in two phases. In the first phase cells are developed in sufficient numbers to the stage at which they first express an antigen receptor. Obviously, this phase is independent of any influence by antigen, because the antigen receptors have not yet been made. Developing hematopoietic cells on their way to B lineage cells enter a series of decisions which are influenced by their interactions with an inductive microenvironment. Once they are committed to the B lineage cells they begin the second phase when they begin to express BCRs.

DEVELOPMENT IN WAVES DURING ONTOGENY, AND IN NICHES THROUGHOUT LIFE

Three waves of hematopoietic cell developments colonize the mouse embryo (Cumano et al., 2001; Godin and Cumano, 2002; Ling and Dzierzak, 2002). The first wave (primitive hematopoiesis) begins at embryonic day (E) 7.5 in yolk sac, i.e., extra-embryonically. This wave does not develop B lymphocytes, but only fetal-type hemoglobin-expressing erythrocytes, megakaryocytes, platelets, and special types of myeloid cells—the latter with unusual longevity (Irion et al., 2010; Schulz et al., 2012). The second and third waves of (now definitive) hematopoiesis originate intra-embryonically at E10.5 from the aorta–gonad–mesonephros area (Cumano et al., 1996; Medvinsky and Dzierzak, 1996), from where undifferentiated pHSCs (Ohmura et al., 2001; Huber et al., 2004; Cumano and Godin, 2007; Yokomizo et al., 2011) migrate through embryonic blood to developing rudiments of fetal liver, omentum, thymus, and bone marrow.

B cells develop in fetal liver, omentum, and bone marrow, probably in a process involving the transmigration of pHSCs from inside the blood vessels through vascular endothelium, to further differentiate on the other side in contact with mesenchymal and epithelial microenvironments (Tsuneto et al., 2013). Since B1 cell development in fetal liver occurs in one wave between E12.5 and birth of a mouse this organ never establishes a niche for long-term residing pHSCs.

By contrast, bone and its marrow—which generates B1 and B2 cells throughout life—is capable of developing "niches" of long-term resting pHSCs in the neighborhood of, and in close contact with, non-hematopoietic stromal cells. It secures continuous, life-long generation of new hematopoietic cells, hence also B lymphocytes (Lu et al., 2011). The niches for pHSCs appear localized at subendosteal sites near intra-bone surfaces that allow the long-term residence of pHSCs with the capacity to long-term (LT) reconstitute a lethally irradiated host with all lineages of hematopoietic cells, including B lymphocytes. LT-pHSCs exist in different states of the cell cycle. In one state they are activated into cell cycle, i.e., they divide. One of the two asymmetrically dividing daughter pHSCs keep their stem cell status, hence they self-renew, while the other daughter cell differentiates to short-term (ST) repopulating HSCs that retain hematopoietic pluripotency, i.e., capacity to differentiate to multipotent myeloid/lymphoid progenitors (MPP), to common myeloid progenitors (CMP), and to common lymphoid progenitors (CLP), from which B lineage cells develop (Akashi et al., 1999).

In the other state they are resting in a G0 state of the cell cycle, and consume low levels of energy in a subosteal, hypoxic microenvironment. From this resting state a small number of cells can be mobilized (stem cell mobilization) to enter the cycling state. However, cycling LT-pHSCs might also revert back to a long-term resting state. Bone marrow microenvironments appear uniquely specialized to harbor resting, long-time residing cell types, such as long-term repopulating pHSCs, memory lymphocytes, and plasma cells. Among all LT-pHSCs in the resting cell population, only a minor subfraction of cells is "mobilized" at any time to enter asymmetric cell divisions and, because of this, only a part of all long-term resting pHSCs participate in hematopoiesis at any given time. This might allow the hematopoietic cell system to continuously refresh its pHSC pools by new, unused pHSCs, thereby preserving its genetic integrity and protecting itself from adverse somatic mutations in actively proliferating pHSCs—mutations that could contribute to breaking tolerance to autoantigens. On the other hand, if cycling LT-pHSCs can revert back to the G0 long-term resting state their somatically mutated genetic constitution might increase the chances for abnormal hematopoiesis and B lymphopoiesis with age (Rossi et al., 2007).

CELLULAR ENVIRONMENTS OF THE FIRST PHASE OF EARLY, ANTIGEN-INDEPENDENT B CELL DEVELOPMENT

Early embryonic phases of the first wave of B cell development in fetal liver of the mouse can be studied *in situ* in histological sections as the organ develops with time. Attracted by the chemokine ligands CXCL10 and CXCL12, produced by non-hematopoietic vascular endothelial cells and mesenchymally-derived stromal cells, CXCR3 and CXCR4-expressing pHSCs and other early progenitors transit from embryonic blood through vascular endothelium into the developing fetal liver and migrate inside to mesenchymally-derived stromal cells. These non-hematopoietic cells provide the hematopoietic and B-lymphopoietic progenitors with interleukin-7 (IL-7), the cytokine which is mandatory to interact with IL-7 receptors (IL-7 R) on the hematopoietic progenitors to induce the early, antigen-independent stages of B1 cell development (Tsuneto et al., 2013). Thymic stromal lymphopoietin (TSLP) has been implied as an alternative stimulating cytokine in fetal liver (Montecino-Rodriguez et al., 2006).

Microenvironmental influences of these early phases of B cell development during the second, continuous wave of B cell development in developing bone are mostly yet to be discovered, but it appears reasonable to expect that, by similar modes, pHSCs will have to transit from embryonic blood into the environment of developing bone and marrow, and that IL-7, again, is the major force that drives the early phases of B cell development. While fetal liver generates almost exclusively B1a cells, bone marrow develops B1- and B2-type B lymphocytes, but the B1 cells, called B1b, differ from the embryonically developed B1a cells. Transplantation of E13.5 fetal liver pHSC-like cells repopulate the host preferentially with B1 cells, while transplantations of pHSCs and progenitors from adult mice repopulate the host preferentially with B2 lymphocytes. Bone marrow retains this capacity, though the numbers of pHSCs decrease with increasing age by at least 100-fold in 1 year of the life of a mouse.

B1a cells generated in fetal liver also differ in some properties from B1b and B2 cells generated in bone marrow. Since the enzyme terminal desoxynucleotidyl transferase (TdT)—which inserts N-region nucleotides at VDJ joints during Ig gene rearrangements—is not expressed in fetal liver (but only in bone marrow) the repertoires of newly generated B cell receptors are less diverse. How much that influences the capacities of these early embryonic repertoires to recognize and distinguish foreign from autoantigens is still not clear. B1a cells from fetal liver express CD5, a cell surface marker indicating cell activation, while most bone marrow-derived B1b cells do not. Furthermore, micro-RNAs play regulatory roles in the development of fetal liver-derived B1a and bone marrow-derived B cells. Thus the gene Lin28b is selectively expressed in hematopoietic progenitors of fetal liver, but not of adult bone marrow. It downregulates the expression of a family of miRNAs, the let7 miRNA cluster. Ectopic expression of Lin28 in bone marrow-derived pHSCs and progenitors reprograms B cell development, so that B1a cells are generated. These results argue for the existence of two B cell lineages, B1a and B2 (including, maybe, B1b), that are developed as two consecutive layers of B

cell repertoires (Tung et al., 2006; Montecino-Rodriguez and Dorshkind, 2012).

EARLY COMMITMENTS TO ANTIGEN-INDEPENDENT B CELL DEVELOPMENT

The initiation and maintenance of the development of B lymphoid lineage cells from pHSCs, MPP, CLP, and pro-/pre-B cells to pre-BI cells, before the generation of sIgM + immature and mature B cells, is controlled externally by a microenvironment of non-hematopoietic (and maybe also hematopoietic) cells that provide cell contacts, cytokines, and chemokines for their mutual attraction, proliferation, and differentiation. After ST-pHSCs have been induced from LT-pHSCs by the action of FLT3 ligand, acting on flt3, to become MPPs, and after IL-7 has induced IL-7 R-expressing progenitors to enter the lymphoid pathway of differentiation. Inside the hematopoietic cells signal transducing and gene transcription-controlling factors regulate these processes of proliferation, cell survival, and differentiation. Three transcription factors, E2A, EBF, and Pax5 (Bain et al., 1994; Zhuang et al., 1994; Sigvardsson et al., 1997; Kee and Murre, 1998; Roessler and Grosschedl, 2006; Kwon et al., 2008), control B cell development from CLP. By contrast, little is known how microenvironments influence the choices of a multipotent progenitor to become myeloid or lymphoid, and how an oligopotent commom lymphoid progenitor is influenced to become either a natural killer (NK) lineage, T lineage, or B lineage cell. While these decisions should have no influence on the repertoires of IgH and IgL chains that are generated, they may well be important for the efficiencies with which B cells are provided among the mature pools of cells. Over- or underproduction of B lineage cells could well have an influence on the functions of these B cell pools.

The molecular details of the transcriptional activation of B cell development have been clarified in remarkable detail (Decker et al., 2009; Ebert et al., 2011; Medvedovic et al., 2011; Revilla-I-Domingo et al., 2012; Vilagos et al., 2012). First, E2A begins to be transcribed as early in hematopoiesis as in pHSCs. In these cells the promotor of Pax5 remains silenced while its enhancer is activated. One developmental stage later, in MPP, E2A directly activates the expression of early B cell factor (EBF). This remains the pattern of gene activation, until the Pax5 promoter is activated in pro-/pre-B cells. This allows EBF to bind to the Pax5 promoter, and PU.1, IRF-4, IRF-8, and nFkB to bind to the activated Pax5 enhancer. EBF-complexed promoter and PU.1/IRF-4/IRF-8/nFkB-complexed enhancer form a supercomplex that allows the expression of Pax5. Pax5 then induces a large number of genes involved in early and late steps of B cell development, while downregulating the expression of genes involved in myelo-poiesis (Schebesta et al., 2007). Finally, Pax5 expression is terminated when differentiation to Ig-secreting plasma cells is induced (Shapiro-Shelef and Calame, 2005; Delogu et al., 2006; Ochiai et al., 2013).

Targeted deletions of the genes encoding these tran-scription factors result in blocking of B cell development at different developmental stages. E2A-deficient progeni-tor B cells have not yet entered DH to JH rearrangements at the IgH chain locus (Ikawa et al., 2004), whereas EBF-deficient and Pax5-deficient progenitors have done so, the latter on both alleles (Rolink et al., 1999). Both EBF- and Pax5-deficient CLP-like pro-/pre-B cells from bone mar-row can be established as stable cell lines proliferating for long periods of time, like pre-BI cell lines (Rolink et al., 1991), identifiable as clones of cells by their indi-vidual sets of DHJH-rearranged IgH chain alleles on stro-mal cells (providing stem cell factor (SCF), the ligand of c-kit, and IL-7), added in sufficient quantities *in vitro* by the recombinant cytokine.

The Pax5-deficient progenitors are remarkably flexible cells. Clones of these cells, genetically marked by individ-ual sets of DHJH/DHJH rearrangements at their IgH chain alleles, respond to different cell contacts and cytokines by different differentiation programs. Thus, *in vitro* they can be induced to macrophages by macrophage colony-stimulating factor (M-CSF), to dendritic cells by granulo-cyte-macrophage colony-stimulating factor (GM-CSF) and M-CSF, to granulocytes by GM-CSF and G-CSF, to natural killer cells by IL-2 and IL-15, to osteoclasts by TRANCE expressed on mesenchymally-derived stromal cells, and to thymocytes by mesenchymally-derived stro-mal cells expressing the NOTCH ligand DELTA1 in the presence of FLT3 ligand and IL-7, while their develop-ment to B cells—which is induced by stromal cells in the presence of FLT3 ligand and IL-7 in Pax5$^{+/+}$ cells—is blocked by the Pax5 deficiency (Nutt et al., 1999; Rolink et al., 1999; Höflinger et al., 2004; Radtke et al., 2004).

Removal of the cytokine IL-7 *in vitro*, or transplanta-tion into suitable recipient mice *in vivo*, induces the differ-entiation to VHDHJH/VLJL-rearranged, sIgM + immature B cells—however, only of wild-type-, but not of EBF- or Pax5-deficient cells. *In vivo* mature B1 cells (Hayakawa et al., 1985) develop from fetal liver- as well as bone marrow-derived wild-type cell lines, detectable in spleen and peritoneum of recombination activating gene (RAG)-deficient recipient mice. From fetal liver cell lines, B1a cells develop, while bone marrow-derived cells generate B1b cells (Hayakawa et al., 1985; Vegh et al., 2010).

In the presence of T cells, as in JH-T mice, or in RAG-deficient mice co-transplanted with CD4$^+$ (and CD4$^+$25$^+$ T cells), there are also formed B2-type follicular B cells, mainly in spleen. These wild-type-, fetal liver-, or bone marrow-derived, wild-type Pax5-expressing cells do not

repopulate the bone marrow. By contrast, Pax5-deficient pro-/pre-B cells do migrate and reside after transplanta-tion to bone marrow (Schaniel et al., 2002a,b), and this homing to bone marrow, also characteristic of earlier cellular stages of hematopoiesis (including pHSCs), is controlled by miR221 (Knoll et al., 2013). Expression of externally added, i.e., retrovirally transduced Pax5 induces B cell differentiation to CD19$^+$ pre-BI cells, but not beyond, since the Pax5-deficient pro-/pre-B cell lines express an endogenously VH(7183)DHJH-rear-ranged IgH chain that apparently affects allelic exclu-sion (Simmons et al., 2012). It is still not clear whether such premature IgH chain rearrangements also occur during normal B cell development *in vivo*, and, if so, how such cells overcome the arrest due to allelic exclu-sion—maybe by VH gene replacements.

The long-term proliferating pro-/pre-B and pre-BI cell lines have been successfully used in experiments that have investigated the transgenic expression of genes active in B cell development and their functions *in vivo*, such as graded Pax5 expression in Pax5$^{-/-}$ cells to bi-phenotypic myeloid/lymphoid cells, or miR221 expression in pre-BI cells, inducing cell migration to bone marrow, or the synergistic transforming activities of two onco-genes, one, pim-1, inhibiting apoptosis, the other, c-myc, inducing proliferation of pre-B cells to form pre-B lymphomas (Bouquet and Melchers, 2012). Unfortunately, such transduced expression of individual antibody genes has not yet been achieved, because the IgH chain gene cannot be expressed at the appropriate stage of B cell development, but is induced too early, blocking normal B cell development due to allelic exclusion.

THE SECOND, EVENTUALLY AUTOANTIGEN-SENSITIVE, PHASE OF B CELL DEVELOPMENT TO SIGM$^+$ IMMATURE B CELLS

In the second phase of B cell development, Ig genes are rearranged, Ig H and L chains are made, deposited as pre-BCRs and BCRs on the cell surface and molecularly linked to intracellular signaling pathways. V(D)J rearran-gements at the Ig loci occur stepwise at different cellular stages of B cell development. The emerging repertoires of IgH and L chains are screened successively at two check-points, at the first for their fitness by pre-BCR formation, and at the second for autoantigen recognition after BCR formation.

After IL-7 has induced IL-7R-expressing lymphoid/myeloid progenitors to enter the lymphoid pathway of dif-ferentiation, the rearrangement-active genes RAG1 and 2 and TdT (the latter only in bone marrow, not in fetal liver), as well as the genes encoding the Ig membrane anchoring molecules Ig alpha and beta, and the components of the surrogate light chain (SLC), Vpre-B and lambda5, become expressed in CLPs. Vpre-B and lambda5 associate non-covalently to form an IgL chain-like structure in pro-/pre-B cells.

As soon as IgH chains become expressed, this SLC can form, between the IgL chain constant region domain-like lambda5 and the first cμH domain, S-S-bonded Ig-(BCR)-like structures, called pre-B cell receptors (pre-BCR) (Melchers, 2005).

In SLC a carboxy-terminal peptide of Vpre-B and an amino-terminal peptide of lambda5 protrude at the location of the third complementarity-determining region of a normal VL domain. These non-Ig parts control the turnover of pre-BCRs with opposite effects on the cell surface: Vpre-B stabilizes surface deposition, while lambda5 downregulates pre-BCR by internalization. As pre-BCR signaling is dependent on the quantity of molecules on the surface, they appear to modulate pre-BCR signaling in opposite ways (Knoll et al., 2012).

When CLPs enter the B lymphoid pathway they open the IgH chain loci for DH to JH rearrangements and become c-kit flt3$^+$CD19-pro-/pre-B cells, not yet expressing Pax5. Pax5$^{-/-}$ pro-/pre-B cells appear arrested in B cell development at that stage.

In pro-/pre-B cells of mice, but not of humans, B cell development with DHJH rearrangements in reading frame 2 results in the expression of a DJ-cμ protein that can assemble with SLC to form a VH-deficient pre-B cell receptor (pre-BCR)-like molecule on the surface of such cells. This appears to result in negative signaling to induce the deletion of these pre-BCR-like expressing cells (Haasner et al., 1994). This state of negative selection may extend into that phase of development when VH to DHJH rearrangements are initiated. In Pax5$^{-/-}$ pro-/pre-B cell lines we have found VHDHJH-rearranged IgH loci, expressing IgH chains containing VH segments within the 7183-VH cluster (most frequently the VH81X segment), which are located at the 3' end of the clusters of VH segments in the IgH locus, but which cannot pair with SLC, thereby apparently evading this negative signaling by a pre-BRR (Wolf, I. and Melchers, F., unpublished). If IgH chains were made that could pair with SLC, such IgH chain loci might enter VH replacement reactions to generate an SLC non-pairing H chain to evade this negative selection (Nakajima et al., 2009). It has been estimated that, in the mouse, between 1 and 7% of all VHDHJH-rearranged IgH loci result from such editing of VH replacements (Davila et al., 2007). It is not known whether a possible specificity of the VH to autoantigens influences this negative selection, but an autoreactive (transgenic) IgH chain has been shown to induce VH editing in pro-/pre-B cells without having to form a functional pre-BCR (Nakajima et al., 2009).

At the chromosomal level of organization the IgH locus is controlled by contractions of large regions (Feeney et al., 2011; Guo et al., 2011a,b). In cells not yet expressing Pax5 the parts of the regions of the IgH locus containing DH segments are brought into proximity to the JH region for rearrangements.

Once these Pax5-negative cells have undergone DH to JH rearrangements, DH proximal VH regions (VH7183 and Q52) can also be brought near to the DHJH-rearranged regions, and rearranged, even before Pax5 is expressed. Strikingly, one VH segment, VH81x, is rearranged as the first VH segment most frequently. When rearranged "in-frame" with N-region insertions in bone marrow μH chains are made which, in the vast majority of instances, cannot pair with SLC. Hence, in the adult, the B2 repertoire is selected against inclusion of these VH81x-expressing pre-B and B cells. By contrast, VH81x-containing μH chains, produced in fetal liver without N-region insertions, can pair with SLC and appear in the peripheral, mature B1a cell repertoire. This "useless" function of the earliest VDJ rearrangements for the developing adult B cell repertoire in bone marrow has long been an enigma. However, the recent discovery that the IgH locus is further subdivided for additional control of VH rearrangements suggests a more differential usage of VH segments for the total process of VDJ rearrangements at the IgH locus. In the chromosomal region of the IgH locus between the DH and the JH segments a CTCF-cohesin binding site is located that further regulates the order of VH to DHJH rearrangements. Deletion of this site on the IgH locus increases proximal (VH7183, especially VH81x) over distal (VH J558) rearrangements (Giallourakis et al., 2010). As the 3'-located VH segments have been found to be used preferentially, as B cells begin VHDHJH rearrangements, we can speculate that the VH regions of the IgH locus are opened in a step-wise fashion. In the first step, accessibility of the locus may be more important than productivity for μH chains.

THE FIRST CHECKPOINT FOR THE EMERGING B CELL REPERTOIRE—PROBING THE FITNESS FOR A GOOD BCR

Once the locus is open at all VH regions, distal VH rearrangements induced by Pax5 can be made. They are induced when Pax5-negative flt3$^+$CD19-pro-/pre-B cells differentiate to Pax5-expressing flt3$^-$CD19$^+$ pre-BI cells (Ebert et al., 2011). At this first checkpoint the emerging repertoire of μH chains is probed for fitness of pairing with SLC. Pre-B cells expressing an SLC-fitting μH chain can display the resulting pre-BCR on the surface. Cross-linking of the pre-BCRs by ligands provided either by the microenvironment or by the pre-B cells themselves induce proliferation of large pre-BII cells, signal downregulation of the rearrangement machinery (RAG1 and 2) and of SLC expression, thereby limiting the supply of SLCs for pre-BCR formation, and hence limiting pre-BCR-induced proliferation. The VH repertoires of early pre-B cells before SLC-mediated proliferative expansion and of large pre-BII cells during proliferative expansion have been found to use VH segments at different frequencies, suggesting that the fitness for SLC pairing may be different for different VH families. This VH repertoire shift is delayed in surrogate light chain-deficient bone marrow (ten Boekel et al., 1997).

Only between 20 and 50% of all IgH chains can pair to form a pre-BCR on the surface of pre-BII cells, and they do so with varying degrees of fitness (ten Boekel et al., 1997, 1998; Kawano et al., 2006). The better they fit, the longer they proliferate. Cross-linking of pre-BCRs through positively charged arginine residues in the non-immunoglobulin portion of λ5, possibly mediated by repetitive negative charges on molecules such as nucleic acids and other molecules on stromal cells, or by molecules expressed in pre-B cells themselves (Bradl et al., 2003; Ohnishi and Melchers, 2003), initiates pre-BCR signaling. Some μH chains have been found that enter proliferation as large pre-BII cells even in the absence of a functional SLC. They carry charged amino acids (arginines, lysines) in the CDR3 regions of their VH domains, not unlike the carriage of non-Ig parts of SLC. This suggests that the charged amino acids in CDR3s can function in place of SLC to signal proliferative expansion of pre-BII cells. It remains to be seen what terminates this proliferation that is normally limited by SLC expression.

Pre-BII cells also close the second, often DHJH-rearranged IgH allele for further rearrangements, thereby securing allelic exclusion at the IgH locus. Since triple-deficient $V_{pre-B1}^{-/-}$, $V_{pre-B2}^{-/-}$, $\lambda5^{-/-}$ B lineage cells still show allelic exclusion of expression of their IgH loci, pre-BCRs cannot be involved in signaling for allelic exclusion, leaving it open just how the successful expression of an IgH chain mediates allelic exclusion in such situations (Shimizu et al., 2002). Since double productively VHDHJH-rearranged B lineage cells have been found in numbers expected from a random process of in- and out-of-frame rearrangements at the IgH alleles, and since in all these cases only one of the two productively rearranged alleles could form a pairing IgH chain (ten Boekel et al., 1998), it remains to be seen just which is the SLC analogous partner to sense the pairing capacity of a newly made IgH chain.

Those heavy chains unfit to pair with surrogate light chains do not induce proliferation of pre-BII cells through pre-BCRs. In situations where pre-BCRs cannot be formed, such nonproliferating pre-BII cells nevertheless proceed towards differentiation (Grawunder et al., 1993,

1995; Rolink et al., 1996). However, because such pre-BCR-defective pre-B cells do not proliferate, their contribution to the developing B cell compartment should be at least 20- to 40-fold lower than that of their pre-BCR-expressing counterparts (Rolink et al., 1993).

In conclusion, the pre-BCRs do not use the classical complementarity-determining regions (CDRs) of the V_H domain of their IgH chains to bind ligands that could induce proliferation. Therefore, the newly generated V_H domain repertoire is not screened for antigen, i.e., autoantigen binding, but merely for fitness to pair, first with SLC and eventually with conventional IgL chains. In this way, there is exclusion of unfit H chains that may have other unwanted deleterious properties, such as the formation of self-aggregating immune complexes that might confer the danger of glomerulonephritis and vasculitis (Melchers, 2005).

EXPRESSION OF IgL CHAINS

When large pre-BII cells have terminated their proliferative expansion, they become resting, small pre-BII cells, just as the SLC non-pairing, non-proliferating pre-BII cells do. The IgL loci are opened, RAG1 and 2 become re-expressed and VL to JL rearrangements are initiated, in the mouse five times more frequently at the kL locus than the λL loci, whereas in the human equally frequently at the kL and λL loci. Only 10% of all potentially rearrangeable Vk segments, spread over the entire Vk region, are used in these first rearrangements, and they use the most 5′-located Jk most frequently. Vk segments, which are located in both orientations in the locus, are equally frequently rearranged by deletions and inversions. Two-thirds of the emerging in-frame rearranged immature sIgM$^+$ B cells are immediately selected, such that further IgL loci rearrangements are terminated by downregulation of the RAG genes, the second kL allele remains in germ-line, non-rearranged form, and all λL loci remain non-rearranged (Melchers et al., 2007). The immature B cell is likely to sense the production and surface deposition of a BCR, probably by "tonic" signaling and without recognition by an autoantigen binding to the VH/VL domains of the BCRs.

In the remaining pre-BII cells secondary and even subsequent rearrangements occur, probably for two reasons. One reason is that two of three VL to JL rearrangements end up out of frame, and hence do not allow translation into IgL chains. Hence the cell remains in the pre-BII stage, does not express BCRs, keeps the RAG genes expressed and all IgL alleles open for secondary and subsequent rearrangements, until it either manages a productive rearrangement to produce an IgL chain and, hence, a BCR and becomes an immature sIgM$^+$ B cell, or until it runs out of opportunities to rearrange, when all JL segments have been used up.

The other reason is that, either after the first, or after any subsequent productive VL to JL rearrangement, the resulting BCR is autoantigen reactive. This immature autoreactive B cell is then recognized at the second checkpoint by autoantigens existing in bone marrow, and presented by a specialized microenvironment. It has been found that such autoantigen recognition keeps RAG expression upregulated, giving the immature B cell the opportunity to "edit" its BCR by secondary and subsequent VL to JL rearrangements, in an attempt to abrogate the recognition of autoantigen and enter the resting, immature sIgM$^+$ B cell compartment, ready for exit from the bone marrow to the periphery, through blood via the central artery into the spleen. Hence, "edited" B cells contain signs of secondary rearrangements, as circles of DNA containing the excised intervening sequences between the VL and the JL segment used in the rearrangement, and by an increased frequency of Vλ to Jλ-rearranged alleles.

In human B cell development, most of the polyreactive cells (Wardemann and Nussenzweig, 2007) and some, but not all, autoreactive cells are lost during the transition from pre-B2 to immature B cells. In patients with systemic lupus erythematosus (SLE) and rheumatoid arthritis, however, these autoreactive and polyreactive BCRs are not lost at this checkpoint (Witsch et al., 2006), pointing to a role of this checkpoint in preventing autoimmune disease. By contrast, Köhler et al. (2008) found a subset of polyreactive pre-BCRs, expressed in pre-B2-like cells, to induce proliferation *in vitro*, suggesting positive selection by polyreactive pre-BCRs. However, other experiments indicate that pre-BCR cross-linking in fetal liver organ culture does not boost pre-B cell proliferation (Ceredig et al., 1998).

During the process of light chain editing, evolutionarily selected "editor" immunoglobulin light chains with low isoelectric points can "neutralize" the DNA-binding properties of certain heavy chains. Such IgL chains may preclude diseases, e.g., SLE that is mediated by antibody–DNA complexes (Li et al., 2001). Continued VL to JL rearrangement can also lead to the expression of two or even more different light chains in a single immature B cell (Gerdes and Wabl, 2004; Doyle et al., 2006; Khan et al., 2008). Immature B cells with one autoreactive and one non-autoreactive BCR can become unreactive to autoantigen because of dilution of the autoreactive with the non-autoreactive BCR. Dual-IgL-expressor B cells can enter the mature B cell pool while remaining potentially autoreactive. Light chain replacement can also lead to polyreactivity (Witsch et al., 2006). Interestingly, some human B cells co-express Vpre-B and conventional light chains together with μ chains containing CDR3 regions enriched in positively

charged and/or aromatic amino acids. Two-thirds of these cells are autoreactive and appear to have escaped central tolerance. Although human Vpre-B, which has an isoelectric point of 5.67, may act as an "editor" by neutralizing positively charged CDR3 regions, mouse Vpre-B proteins have an isoelectric point of 9.37 and thus may not be able to perform this function (Meffre et al., 2004).

THE SECOND CHECKPOINT: SITES AND MECHANISMS OF SELECTION OF NEWLY GENERATED SIGM$^+$ B CELLS

While V_H repertoires expressed in immature B cells in the bone marrow and in immature and mature B cells in spleen are not significantly different, almost 90% of the newly formed immature B cells never leave the bone marrow (Rolink et al., 1999). They have half-lives of less than a week, probably for two reasons: they might have an intrinsic cellular program to enter apoptosis, unless selected to transit out of bone marrow into the periphery, and they might be subject to autoantigen-induced mechanisms of cellular deletion. In essence, a 6–8-week-old mouse continuously generates from around 10^4 pHSCs over 2.5×10^6 pre-BI cells, and 5×10^7 small pre-BII 2×10^7 immature sIgM$^+$ B cells, into a pool of around 10^8 such immature B cells, only to discard 9×10^7, i.e., the vast majority of them, mostly in fear of autoreactivity. The invention of nature to generate diversity of recognition by V(D)J rearrangements must have been an accident in evolution that was developed as the adaptive branch of the immune system to be advantageous for the defense of the individual against unexpected aggressors, yet a dangerous weapon that could destroy this individual. No wonder, then, that most of the BCRs on immature B cells ever made have to be eliminated.

In this establishment of "central" tolerance in B cell repertoires by negative selection, neither the cellular microenvironments in the bone marrow nor the molecular mechanisms of deletion are well known. This is all the more remarkable since the processes of negative selection to establish central tolerance for the T cell repertoires in the thymus have been so well investigated. While the studies in the thymus have been aided by the realization that autoantigens should be presented by major histocompatibility complex (MHC) I and II molecules, nothing comparable is evident from the genetics of B cell development that would guide the search for the autoantigen-presenting modes that establish central B cell tolerance. However, the rapidly expanding cases of genetically identified immunodeficiencies leading to early blockages of B cell development should help to clarify the means whereby central B cell tolerance is established. Thus, it has been realized for some time that the complement components C1q, C4, serum amyloid protein, complement receptor-2, or secreted natural serum IgM could be involved, as deficiencies of any one of these lead to SLE.

Two models for the selection of the emerging B cell repertoires have been proposed. In one model (Carroll, 2004), the maturing B cells are protected from the stimulatory influence of autoantigens released from apoptosing, blebbing cells in the primary lymphoid organ because macrophages expressing complement receptors (CIqR for CIq, CRI for C4) efficiently take up, and thereby remove, apoptosing cells bound by natural serum IgM and complexed with CIq and C4b. This model, however, does not explain how the developing repertoire of immature B cells is purged of autoreactive cells, nor does it take into account that immature B cells are sensitive to induction of apoptosis rather than to proliferation and development of Ig-secreting plasma cells and memory B cells.

In contrast, the second model (Melchers and Rolink, 2006) (Figure 9.1, redrawn from Figure 2 in von Boehmer and Melchers, 2010) proposes that autoantigens from dying cells are presented to the emerging repertoire of B cells by stromal cells in the primary lymphoid organ, i.e., bone marrow. The presenting cells are expected to express receptors for natural serum IgM that can bind via its Fc to IgM-Fc receptors. IgM via its variable regions could bind to autoantigens, possibly even in solution, then fix CIq and create a bridge between the CIqR, CRI, and FcR on the presenting cells. In this way autoreactive BCR on the immature B cell would then be brought together by CIq, C4, serum IgM, and autoantigens. Depending on the strength of the interaction of the BCRs with autoantigens, and possibly also on the nature of the presenting stroma cell, this autoantigen-induced signaling can have different outcomes. It can lead to apoptosis of the B cell, if the avidity of autoantigen-BCR binding is high, leading to negative selection of the B cell repertoire. Such negative selection has been documented in a variety of experimental settings. If BCR downregulation and re-expression of a secondary BCR due to editing of a new L chain, thus leading to a new, nonautoreactive BCR, occurs fast enough, this apoptosis may be avoided. Since approximately 90% of the 2×10^7 sIgM$^+$ immature B cells that are made each day in the bone marrow of a mouse never arrive at the immature sIgM$^+$ B cell pool of the spleen, it is likely that this negative selection engages the vast majority of the newly generated immature sIgM$^+$ B cell repertoires in bone marrow, and before their transit to spleen (Rolink et al., 1999).

Alternatively, the interaction of the newly generated immature B cells can lead to positive selection, maybe into the B1b compartment, if the avidity of BCR-mediated interaction is low. Those B cells expressing BCRs with no avidity to autoantigens present in bone marrow will be "ignored," and will be allowed to exit to the periphery, as long as they show their "passport" specifying an unrecognized BCR on their surface. It is truly remarkable that, despite this extensive effort to avoid autoimmunity, the peripheral, mature B cells continue to be an autoimmune threat.

Further, it remains equally remarkable just how many cells are made, and then discarded, to generate the few that are finally allowed to leave the bone marrow to face the world of foreign antigens. This fate of the majority of all newly generated B cells reminds me of a fable, told by Anatole France (1893), of a young Persian king who asked his academicians to write the history of mankind—as this article is written to describe the history of B cells. Their initial rendition was carried to the king on 20 camels with 500 books each. The king complained that he would not have the time to read it all, and asked for a shorter version. Even the shorter versions were always too long to be read by the king in his remaining lifetime. Finally, a lone academician arrived with only one book, but the king responded by saying: "So I will die without knowing human history." To which the academician replied: "I can summarize it for you in three words: 'Ils naquirent, ils souffrirent, ils moururent' ('They are born, they suffer, they die')."

FUTURE APPROACHES TO UNDERSTANDING CENTRAL B CELL TOLERANCE

A better understanding of the modes of central tolerance induced by apoptosis, editing, anergy, and ignorance still requires an identification of all of the relevant antigen-presenting cell populations. A strikingly similar model has been proposed for the establishment of peripheral B cell tolerance, i.e., negative selection of autoreactive B cells which are randomly, hence accidentally, generated by somatic hypermutation and class switching of a follicular helper T cell-driven immune response within germinal centers (Vinuesa et al., 2010). In this model the hypermutated, autoantigen-recognizing IgG takes the role of the natural IgM antibody proposed in our model (above) for the establishment of central tolerance of B cells.

In contrast to T cell development, in which only MHC-restricted, i.e., self MHC I- or II- plus autoantigen peptide-recognizing, T cells that recognize self MHC-I or MHC-II are allowed to exit the thymus and enter the periphery, B cells just need to show surface-bound IgM that does not recognize any autoantigen in bone marrow, and that has been "ignored" by the selecting environment to gain exit from the bone marrow. Once in the periphery, particularly the spleen, hardly any further cell loss is detected during the transition from immature (including transitional T1 and T2 B cells) to mature B cells in the spleen. In humans

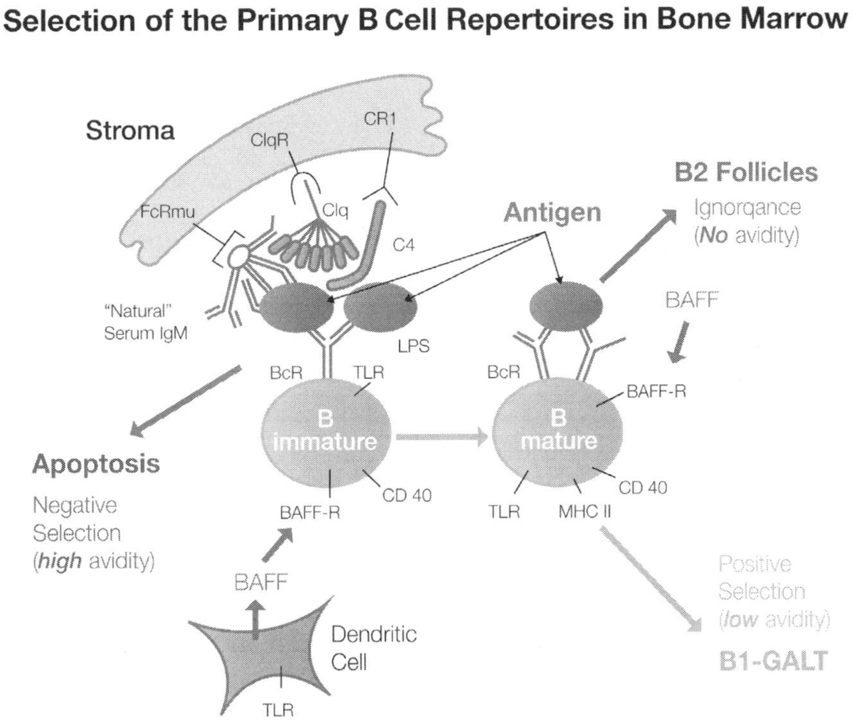

Selection of the Primary B Cell Repertoires in Bone Marrow

FIGURE 9.1 **Proposed Site for Autoantigen-Mediated Selection of Immature B Cells.** A hypothetical microenvironmental cell, non-hematopoietic?, follicular dendritic?, expresses Fc-μ-receptors, C1q receptors, and complement receptor 1 (CR1). Note that several cells close to each other could also express these different receptors. Fc-μ-R bind natural IgM antibodies, which bind C1q when complexed with autoantigen. That allows binding of C1q to C1qR. C4 bridges the immune complexes with CR1. Newly generated immature sIgM⁺ B cells bind autoantigens with different avidities. High avidity binding induces apoptosis (negative selection), possibly aided by signaling from unknown cytokines. Low avidity binding induces survival and selection into B1 pools (not aided by BAFF). No avidity (ignorance) induces BAFF-mediated transfer into the periphery of mature follicular B2 cell pools (via T1 and T2 intermediates) expressing MHC II and CD40. *Adapted from von Boehmer and Melchers (2010), and redrawn by Justin Hewlett, MNHS Multimedia Unit, Monash University.*

there is a further reduction of the percentage of autoreactive cells (40 to 20%) across this transition, whereas the percentage of polyreactive cells remains at the low level (6%) already achieved during the transition from pre-B to immature B cells (Wardemann and Nussenzweig, 2007). Patients with, say, SLE or rheumatoid arthritis fail to establish recessive tolerance even at this second checkpoint, indicating that failure of several mechanisms for establishing tolerance likely contributes to these diseases (Yurasov et al., 2005). The genetics of autoimmune diseases and immunodeficiencies are now investigated by full genome analyses (Mackay et al., 1999; Rolink et al., 2002; Kumar et al., 2006; Deane et al., 2007; Liu et al., 2007; Xie et al., 2007; Shlomchik, 2008). It is predictable that an ever-increasing number of mutant molecules involved in (often also epigenetic) regulation of gene expression, of signal transductions from a variety of receptors involved in the interactions of B lineage cells with their inducing microenvironments, controlling proliferation, differentiation, migration and survival on their way to mature B cells will be found to change the normal course of B cell development.

Finally, it is unclear how the affinity for antigen of a BCR decides what it signals to either the immature or later the mature B cell. Of relevance here, a monoclonal, autoreactive, dsDNA-binding, SLE-propagating, hypermutated IgG autoantibody was isolated from an SLE patient. The corresponding VH and VL domains of the IgH and IgL chain genes were then "back-mutated" to the germline-encoded VH/VL sequence, and expressed as an antibody (Schroeder et al., 2013). In this back-mutated form, the antibody remarkably failed to bind to dsDNA any longer. The corresponding immature B cell expressing this antibody as a BCR was evidently not negatively selected by dsDNA, which is abundantly present in bone marrow throughout life. How, then, did the mature BCR⁺ B cell ever become autoreactive? Possibly the cell entered a germinal center reaction, hypermutated, and that a dsDNA-binding somatic mutant B cell then evaded negative selection in the process of peripheral tolerance induction—but who or what triggered it?

It is fully possible that we do not understand how a cell surface-bound BCR establishes contact with the autoantigen (in bone marrow) or antigen (in the periphery), possibly presented (as occurs for T cells in thymus and periphery) by antigen-presenting cells. To quote Huppa and Davis (Huppa et al., 2010; Huppa and Davis, 2013) on their studies of the interaction of T cells with antigen-presenting cells in immunological synapses: "There is increasing evidence that the molecular dynamics of receptor–ligand interactions are not only dependent on the intrinsic properties of the binding partners but also become transformed by cell biological parameters such as the geometrical constraints within the immune synapse, mechanical forces, and local molecular crowding. To appreciate the complete picture, we think a multidisciplinary approach is imperative, which includes genetics, biochemistry, and structure determination and also biophysical analyses and the latest molecular imaging techniques." It seems therefore not unreasonable to expect that similar dynamics of antigen recognition by BCRs on immature and on mature B cells, and of costimulatory or co-inhibitory surface-bound ligands and receptors will become evident, which will lead to redefinitions of the distinction between "self" and "non-self" in B cell repertoires at different stages of development.

All these examples should make it clear that we are merely at the very beginning of a vision of the control of autoimmunity, or better, the lack of it , in the genetic variants of nearly 7×10^9 human individuals with a functional immune system. Moreover, it will not only be the genetics of B cells, but also their environment, that will be found to exert control. Kurt Tucholsky (1890–1935), German journalist and satirical writer, unwillingly but farsightedly defined what appears to become so important to understand about the functioning of the immune system of lymphocytes in their environments: "Ein Loch ist da, wo etwas nicht ist...Das Merkwürdigste an einem Loch ist der Rand. Er gehört noch zum Etwas, sieht aber beständig in das Nichts, eine Grenzwache der Materie. Das Nichts hat keine Grenzwache: während den Molekülen am Rande schwindlig wird, weil sie das Loch sehen, wird den Molekülen des Lochs 'fest-lig'?" (Zur soziologischen Psycholgie der Löcher, 1931). (Translated: "A hole is there where something is not...The most remarkable thing about the hole is its rim. It belongs to the something, but looks into the nothing, as a border control of the material. The nothing has no border control, while the molecules at the rim of the hole get dizzy, because they see the hole, do the molecules of the hole get 'stabilized'?" (The Sociological Psychology of the Holes, 1931).

ACKNOWLEDGMENTS

It should be clear to the reader that my description of B cell development is highly personal, often biased, and incomplete in the quotation of relevant literature, particularly of opposing views. I apologize to all those whom I might have disappointed or even offended. During my attempts to assemble it, I was often ready to give up. Only the patient persistence of the editors has brought this article to its present status. To once more quote Anatole France (as I was alerted to him by one of the editors, I.M.): my article is less than 500 books in size, and more than the final format of the one sentence quoted above, in the hope that the king does have the time to read it.

I thank my long-time scientific friends, especially Jan Andersson and Ton Rolink at the no-longer-existing Basel Institute for Immunology, for the never-ending discussions of the scientific subject that has united us for so many years. Finally, I thank the Max Planck Society and its Institute for Infection Biology in Berlin for the many years of support as a Max Planck Fellow, well beyond the limits of my official retirement from the Basel Institute for Immunology.

REFERENCES

Akashi, K., Kondo, M., Cheshier, S., Shizuru, J., Gandy, K., Domen, J., et al., 1999. Lymphoid development from stem cells and the common lymphocyte progenitors. Cold Spring Harb. Symp. Quant. Biol. 64, 1–12.

Arnon, T.I., Horton, R.M., Grigorova, I.L., Cyster, J.G., 2013. Visualization of splenic marginal zone B-cell shuttling and follicular B-cell egress. Nature. 493, 684–688.

Bain, G., Maandag, E.C., Izon, D.J., Amsen, D., Kruisbeek, A.M., Weintraub, B.C., et al., 1994. E2A proteins are required for proper B cell development and initiation of immunoglobulin gene rearrangements. Cell. 79, 885–892.

Baumgarth, N., 2011. The double life of a B-1 cell: self-reactivity selects for protective effector functions. Nat. Rev. Immunol. 11, 34–46.

von Boehmer, H., Melchers, F., 2010. Checkpoints in lymphocyte development and autoimmune disease. Nat. Immunol. 11, 14–20.

ten Boekel, E., Melchers, F., Rolink, A.G., 1997. Changes in the V(H) gene repertoire of developing precursor B lymphocytes in mouse bone marrow mediated by the pre-B cell receptor. Immunity. 7, 357–368.

ten Boekel, E., Melchers, F., Rolink, A.G., 1998. Precursor B cells showing H chain allelic inclusion display allelic exclusion at the level of pre-B cell receptor surface expression. Immunity. 8, 199–207.

Bos, N.A., Meeuwsen, C.G., 1989. B cell repertoire in adult antigen-free and conventional neonatal BALB/c mice. I. Preferential utilization of the CH-proximal VH gene family PC7183. Eur. J. Immunol. 19, 1811–1815.

Bos, N.A., Kimura, H., Meeuwsen, C.G., De Visser, H., Hazenberg, M.P., Wostmann, B.S., et al., 1989. Serum immunoglobulin levels and naturally occurring antibodies against carbohydrate antigens in germ-free BALB/c mice fed chemically defined ultrafiltered diet. Eur. J. Immunol. 19, 2335–2339.

Bouquet, C., Melchers, F., 2012. Pim1 and Myc reversibly transform murine precursor B lymphocytes but not mature B lymphocytes. Eur. J. Immunol. 42, 522–532.

Bradl, H., Wittmann, J., Milius, D., Vettermann, C., Jäck, H.-M., 2003. Interaction of murine precursor B cell receptor with stroma cells is controlled by the unique tail of lambda 5 and stroma cell-associated heparan sulfate. J. Immunol. 171, 2338–2348.

Burnet, F.M., 1959. The Clonal Selection Theory of Acquired Immunity. Cambridge Univ. Press, London.

Carroll, M.C., 2004. A protective role for innate immunity in systemic lupus erythematosus. Nat. Rev. Immunol. 4, 825–831.

Ceredig, R., ten Boekel, E., Rolink, A., Melchers, F., Andersson, J., 1998. Fetal liver organ cultures allow the proliferative expansion of pre-B receptor-expressing pre B-II cells and the differentiation of immature and mature B cells in vitro. Int. Immunol. 10, 49–59.

Cumano, A., Godin, I., 2007. Ontogeny of the hematopoietic system. Annu. Rev. Immunol. 25, 745–785.

Cumano, A., Ferraz, J.C., Klaine, M., Di Santo, J.P., Godin, I., 2001. Intraembryonic, but not yolk sac hematopoietic precursors, isolated before circulation, provide long-term multilineage reconstitution. Immunity. 15, 477–485.

Davila, M., Liu, F., Cowell, L.G., Lieberman, A.E., Heikamp, E., Patel, A., et al., 2007. Multiple, conserved cryptic recombination signals in VH gene segments, detection of cleavage products only in pro B cells. J. Exp. Med. 204, 3195–3208.

Deane, J.A., Pisitkun, P., Barrett, R.S., Feigenbaum, L., Town, T., Ward, J.M., et al., 2007. Control of toll-like receptor 7 expression is essential to restrict autoimmunity and dendritic cell proliferation. Immunity. 27, 801–810.

Decker, T., Pasca di Magliano, M., McManus, S., Sun, Q., Bonifer, C., Tagoh, H., et al., 2009. Stepwise activation of enhancer and promoter regions of the B cell commitment gene Pax5 in early lymphopoiesis. Immunity. 30, 508–520.

Delogu, A., Schebesta, A., Sun, Q., Aschenbrenner, K., Perlot, T., Busslinger, M., 2006. Gene repression by Pax5 in B cells is essential for blood cell homeostasis and is reversed in plasma cells. Immunity. 24, 269–281.

Descatoire, M., Weill, J.C., Reynaud, C.A., Weller, S., 2011. A human equivalent of mouse B-1 cells?. J. Exp. Med. 208, 2563–2564.

Doyle, C.M., Han, J., Weigert, M.G., Prak, E.T., 2006. Consequences of receptor editing at the lambda locus, multireactivity and light chain secretion. Proc. Natl. Acad. Sci. U.S.A. 103, 11264–11269.

Ebert, A., McManus, S., Tagoh, H., Medvedovic, J., Salvagiotto, G., Novatchkova, M., et al., 2011. The distal V(H) gene cluster of the Igh locus contains distinct regulatory elements with Pax5 transcription factor-dependent activity in pro-B cells. Immunity. 34, 175–187.

Eliasson, P., Jönsson, J.I., 2010. The hematopoietic stem cell niche: low in oxygen but a nice place to be. J. Cell Physiol. 222, 17–22.

Feeney, A.J., 2011. Epigenetic regulation of antigen receptor gene rearrangement. Curr. Opin. Immunol. 23, 171–177.

France, A., 1893. L'Histoire, Chapter XVI, Les Opinions de M. Jerome Coignard.

Giallourakis, C.C., Franklin, A., Guo, C., Cheng, H.L., Yoon, H.S., Gallagher, M., et al., 2010. Elements between the IgH variable (V) and diversity (D) clusters influence antisense transcription and lineage-specific V(D)J recombination. Proc. Natl. Acad. Sci. U.S.A. 107, 22207–22212.

Godin, I., Cumano, A., 2002. The hare and the tortoise: an embryonic haematopoietic race. Nat. Rev. Immunol. 2, 593–604.

Grawunder, U., Haasner, D., Melchers, F., Rolink, A., 1993. Rearrangement and expression of kappa light chain genes can occur without mu heavy chain expression during differentiation of pre-B cells. Int. Immunol. 5, 1609–1618.

Grawunder, U., Leu, T.M., Schatz, D.G., Werner, A., Rolink, A.G., Melchers, F., et al., 1995. Down-regulation of RAG1 and RAG2 gene expression in preB cells after functional immunoglobulin heavy chain rearrangement. Immunity. 3, 601–608.

Guo, C., Alt, F.W., Giallourakis, C., 2011a. PAIRing for distal Igh locus V(D)J recombination. Immunity. 34, 139–141.

Guo, C., Yoon, H.S., Franklin, A., Jain, S., Ebert, A., Cheng, H.L., et al., 2011b. CTCF-binding elements mediate control of V(D)J recombination. Nature. 477, 424–430.

Haasner, D., Rolink, A., Melchers, F., 1994. Influence of surrogate L chain on DHJH-reading frame 2 suppression in mouse precursor B cells. Int. Immunol. 6, 21–30.

Hayakawa, K., Hardy, R.R., Herzenberg, L.A., Herzenberg, L.A., 1985. Progenitors for Ly-1 B cells are distinct from progenitors for other B cells. J. Exp. Med. 161, 1554–1568.

Höflinger, S., Kesavan, K., Fuxa, M., Hutter, C., Heavey, B., Radtke, F., et al., 2004. Analysis of Notch1 function by in vitro T cell differentiation of Pax5 mutant lymphoid progenitors. J. Immunol. 173, 3935–3944.

Hooijkaas, H., Benner, R., Pleasants, J.R., Wostmann, B.S., 1984. Isotypes and specificities of immunoglobulins produced by germ-free mice fed chemically defined ultrafiltered "antigen-free" diet. Eur. J. Immunol. 14, 1127–1130.

Huppa, J.B., Davis, M.M., 2013. The interdisciplinary science of T-cell recognition. Adv. Immunol. 119, 1–50.

Huppa, J.B., Axmann, M., Mörtelmaier, M.A., Lillemeier, B.F., Newell, E.W., Brameshuber, M., et al., 2010. TCR-peptide-MHC interactions in situ show accelerated kinetics and increased affinity. Nature. 463, 963–967.

Ikawa, T., Kawamoto, H., Wright, L.Y., Murre, C., 2004. Long-term cultured E2A-deficient hematopoietic progenitor cells are pluripotent. Immunity. 20, 349–360.

Irion, S., Clarke, R.L., Luche, H., Kim, I., Morrison, S.J., Fehling, H.J., et al., 2010. Temporal specification of blood progenitors from mouse embryonic stem cells and induced pluripotent stem cells. Development. 137, 2829–2839.

Jerne, N.K., 1955. The natural-selection theory of antibody formation. Proc. Natl. Acad. Sci. U.S.A. 41, 849–857.

Kawano, Y., Yoshikawa, S., Minegishi, Y., Karasuyama, H., 2006. Pre-B cell receptor assesses the quality of IgH chains and tunes the pre-B cell repertoire by delivering differential signals. J. Immunol. 177, 2242–2249.

Kee, B.L., Murre, C.J., 1998. Induction of early B cell factor (EBF) and multiple B lineage genes by the basic helix-loop helix transcription factor E12. Exp. Med. 188, 699–713.

Khan, S.N., Witsch, E.J., Goodman, N.G., Panigrahi, A.K., Chen, C., Jiang, Y., et al., 2008. Editing and escape from editing in anti-DNA B cells. Proc. Natl. Acad. Sci. U.S.A. 105, 3861–3866.

King, C., 2009. New insights into the differentiation and function of T follicular helper cells. Nat. Rev. Immunol. 9, 757–766.

Klein, U., Dalla-Favera, R., 2008. Germinal centres, role in B-cell physiology and malignancy. Nat. Rev. Immunol. 8, 22–33.

Knoll, M., Yanagisawa, Y., Simmons, S., Engels, N., Wienands, J., Melchers, F., et al., 2012. The non-Ig parts of the VpreB and λ5 proteins of the surrogate light chain play opposite roles in the surface representation of the precursor B cell receptor. J. Immunol. 188, 6010–6017.

Knoll, M., Simmons, S., Bouquet, C., Grün, J.R., Melchers, F., 2013. miR-221 redirects precursor B cells to the BM and regulates their residence. Eur. J. Immunol.. 10.1002/eji.201343367.

Köhler, F., Hug, E., Eschbach, C., Meixlsperger, S., Hobeika, E., Kofer, J., et al., 2008. Autoreactive B cell receptors mimic autonomous pre-B cell receptor signaling and induce proliferation of early B cells. Immunity. 29, 912–921.

Kumar, K.R., Li, L., Yan, M., Bhaskarabhatla, M., Mobley, A.B., Nguyen, C., et al., 2006. Regulation of B cell tolerance by the lupus susceptibility gene Ly108. Science. 312, 1665–1669.

Kwon, K., Hutter, C., Sun, Q., Bilic, I., Cobaleda, C., Malin, S., et al., 2008. Instructive role of the transcription factor E2A in early B lymphopoiesis and germinal center B cell development. Immunity. 28, 751–762.

Lederberg, J., 1959. Genes and antibodies: do antigens bear instructions for antibody specificity or do they select cell lines that arise by mutation? Science. 129, 1649–1653.

Lesinski, D.A., Heinz, N., Pilat-Carotta, S., Rudolph, C., Jacobs, R., Schlegelberger, B., et al., 2012. Serum- and stromal cell-free hypoxic generation of embryonic stem cell-derived hematopoietic cells in vitro, capable of multilineage repopulation of immunocompetent mice. Stem. Cells Transl. Med. 1, 581–591.

Li, H., Jiang, Y., Prak, E.L., Radic, M., Weigert, M., 2001. Editors and editing of anti-DNA receptors. Immunity. 15, 947–957.

Ling, K.W., Dzierzak, E., 2002. Ontogeny and genetics of the hemato/lymphopoietic system. Curr. Opin. Immunol. 14, 186–191.

Liu, Y., Li, L., Kumar, K.R., Xie, C., Lightfoot, S., Zhou, X.J., et al., 2007. Lupus susceptibility genes may breach tolerance to DNA by impairing receptor editing of nuclear antigen-reactive B cells. J. Immunol. 179, 1340–1352.

Lu, R., Neff, N.F., Quake, S.R., Weissman, I.L., 2011. Tracking single hematopoietic stem cells in vivo using high-throughput sequencing in conjunction with viral genetic barcoding. Nat. Biotechnol. 29, 928–933.

Luckey, C.J., Bhattacharya, D., Goldrath, A.W., Weissman, I.L., Benoist, C., Mathis, D., 2006. Memory T and memory B cells share a transcriptional program of self-renewal with long-term hematopoietic stem cells. Proc. Natl. Acad. Sci. U.S.A. 103, 3304–3309.

Mackay, F., Woodcock, S.A., Lawton, P., Ambrose, C., Baetscher, M., Schneider, P., et al., 1999. Mice transgenic for BAFF develop lymphocytic disorders along with autoimmune manifestations. J. Exp. Med. 190, 1697–1710.

Medvedovic, J., Ebert, A., Tagoh, H., Busslinger, M., 2011. Pax5: a master regulator of B cell development and leukemogenesis. Adv. Immunol. 111, 179–206.

Medvinsky, A., Dzierzak, E., 1996. Definitive hematopoiesis is autonomously initiated by the AGM region. Cell. 86, 897–906.

Meffre, E., Schaefer, A., Wardemann, H., Wilson, P., Davis, E., Nussenzweig, M.C., 2004. Surrogate light chain expressing human peripheral B cells produce self-reactive antibodies. J. Exp. Med. 199, 145–150.

Melchers, F., 2005. The pre-B-cell receptor, selector of fitting immunoglobulin heavy chains for the B-cell repertoire. Nat. Rev. Immunol. 5, 578–584.

Melchers, F., Rolink, A., 1999. B lymphocyte development and biology. In: Paul, W.E. (Ed.), Fundamental Immunology, fourth ed. Lippincott-Raven, Philadelphia, pp. 183–224.

Melchers, F., Rolink, A.R., 2006. B cell tolerance—how to make it and how to break it. Curr. Top. Microbiol. Immunol. 305, 1–23.

Melchers, F., Yamagami, T., Rolink, A., Andersson, J., 2007. Rules for the rearrangement events at the L chain gene loci of the mouse. Adv. Exp. Med. Biol. 596, 63–70.

Montecino-Rodriguez, E., Dorshkind, K., 2012. B-1 B cell development in the fetus and adult. Immunity. 36, 13–21.

Montecino-Rodriguez, E., Leathers, H., Dorshkind, K., 2006. Identification of a B-1 B cell-specified progenitor. Nat. Immunol. 7, 293–301.

Muramatsu, M., Kinoshita, K., Fagarasan, S., Yamada, S., Shinkai, Y., Honjo, T. 2000. Class switch recombination and hypermutation require activation-induced cytidine deaminase (AID), a potential RNA editing enzyme. Cell. 102, 553–63

Nakajima, P.B., Kiefer, K., Price, A., Bosma, G.C., Bosma, M.J., 2009. Two distinct populations of H chain-edited B cells show differential surrogate L chain dependence. J. Immunol. 182, 3583–3596.

Nat Gerdes, T., Wabl, M., 2004. Autoreactivity and allelic inclusion in a B cell nuclear transfer mouse. Immunology. 5, 1282–1287.

Nutt, S.L., Heavey, B., Rolink, A.G., Busslinger, M., 1999. Commitment to the B-lymphoid lineage depends on the transcription factor Pax5. Nature. 401, 556–562.

Ochiai, K., Maienschein-Cline, M., Simonetti, G., Chen, J., Rosenthal, R., Brink, R., et al., 2013. Transcriptional regulation of germinal center B and plasma cell fates by dynamical control of IRF4. Immunity. 38, 918–929.

Ohmura, K., Kawamoto, H., Lu, M., Ikawa, T., Ozaki, S., Nakao, K., et al., 2001. Immature multipotent hemopoietic progenitors lacking long-term bone marrow-reconstituting activity in the aorta-gonad-mesonephros region of murine day 10 fetuses. J. Immunol. 166, 3290–3296.

Ohnishi, K., Melchers, F., 2003. The nonimmunoglobulin portion of lambda5 mediates cell-autonomous pre-B cell receptor signaling. Nat. Immunol. 4, 849–856.

Pillai, S., Cariappa, A., Pirnie, S.P., 2009. Esterases and autoimmunity: the sialic acid acetylesterase pathway and the regulation of peripheral B cell tolerance. Trends. Immunol. 30, 488–493.

Radtke, F., Wilson, A., MacDonald, H.R., 2004. Notch signaling in T- and B-cell development. Curr. Opin. Immunol. 16, 174–179.

Revilla-I-Domingo, R., Bilic, I., Vilagos, B., Tagoh, H., Ebert, A., et al., 2012. The B-cell identity factor Pax5 regulates distinct transcriptional programmes in early and late B lymphopoiesis. EMBO J. 31, 3130–3146.

Revy, P., Muto, T., Levy, Y., Geissmann, F., Plebani, A., Sanal, O., et al. 2000. Activation-induced cytidine deaminase (AID) deficiency causes the autosomal recessive form of the Hyper-IgM syndrome (HIGM2). Cell. 102, 565–575

Roessler, S., Grosschedl, R., 2006. Role of transcription factors in commitment and differentiation of early B lymphoid cells. Semin. Immunol. 18, 12–19.

Rolink, A., Kudo, A., Karasuyama, H., Kikuchi, Y., Melchers, F., 1991. Long-term proliferating early pre B cell lines and clones with the potential to develop to surface Ig-positive, mitogen reactive B cells in vitro and in vivo. EMBO J. 10, 327–336.

Rolink, A., Karasuyama, H., Grawunder, U., Haasner, D., Kudo, A., Melchers, F., 1993. B cell development in mice with a defective lambda 5 gene. Eur. J. Immunol. 23, 1284–1288.

Rolink, A., Melchers, F., Andersson, J., 1996. The SCID but not the RAG-2 gene product is required for S mu-S epsilon heavy chain class switching. Immunity. 5, 319–330.

Rolink, A.G., Nutt, S.L., Melchers, F., Busslinger, M., 1999. Long-term in vivo reconstitution of T-cell development by Pax5-deficient B-cell progenitors. Nature. 401, 603–606.

Rolink, A.G., Tschopp, J., Schneider, P., Melchers, F., 2002. BAFF is a survival and maturation factor for mouse B cells. Eur. J. Immunol. 32, 2004–2010.

Rossi, D.J., Seita, J., Czechowicz, A., Bhattacharya, D., Bryder, D., Weissman, I.L., 2007. Hematopoietic stem cell quiescence attenuates DNA damage response and permits DNA damage accumulation during aging. Cell Cycle. 6, 2371–2376.

Schaniel, C., Bruno, L., Melchers, F., Rolink, A.G., 2002a. Multiple hematopoietic cell lineages develop in vivo from transplanted Pax5-deficient pre-B I cell clones. Blood. 99, 472–478.

Schaniel, C., Gottar, M., Roosnek, E., Melchers, F., Rolink, A.G., 2002b. Extensive in vivo self-renewal, long-term reconstitution capacity, and hematopoietic multipotency of Pax5-deficient precursor B-cell clones. Blood. 99, 2760–2766.

Schebesta, A., McManus, S., Salvagiotto, G., Delogu, A., Busslinger, G. A., Busslinger, M., 2007. Transcription factor Pax5 activates the chromatin of key genes involved in B cell signaling, adhesion, migration, and immune function. Immunity. 27, 49–63.

Schroeder, K., Herrmann, M., Winkler, T.H., 2013. The role of somatic hypermutation in the generation of pathogenic antibodies in SLE. Autoimmunity. 46, 121–127.

Schulz, C., Gomez Perdiguero, E., Chorro, L., Szabo-Rogers, H., Cagnard, N., Kierdorf, K., et al., 2012. A lineage of myeloid cells independent of Myb and hematopoietic stem cells. Science. 336, 86–90.

Shapiro-Shelef, M., Calame, K., 2005. Regulation of plasma-cell development. Nat. Rev. Immunol. 5, 230–242.

Shimizu, T., Mundt, C., Licence, S., Melchers, F., Mårtensson, I.L., 2002. VpreB1/VpreB2/lambda 5 triple-deficient mice show impaired B cell development but functional allelic exclusion of the IgH locus. J. Immunol. 168, 6286–6293.

Shlomchik, M.J., 2008. Sites and stages of autoreactive B cell activation and regulation. Immunity. 28, 18–28.

Sigvardsson, M., O'Riordan, M., Grosschedl, R., 1997. EBF and E47 collaborate to induce expression of the endogenous immunoglobulin surrogate light chain genes. Immunity. 7, 25–36.

Simmons, S., Knoll, M., Drewell, C., Wolf, I., Mollenkopf, H.J., Bouquet, C., et al., 2012. Biphenotypic B-lymphoid/myeloid cells expressing low levels of Pax5, potential targets of BAL development. Blood. 120, 3688–3698.

Tokoyoda, K., Hauser, A.E., Nakayama, T., Radbruch, A., 2010. Organization of immunological memory by bone marrow stroma. Nat. Rev. Immunol. 10, 193–200.

Tsuneto, M., Tokoyoda, K., Kajikhina, E., Hauser, A.E., Hara, T., Tani-Ichi, S., et al., 2013. B cell progenitors and precursors change their microenvironment in fetal liver during early development. Stem Cells. 10.1002/stem.1421.

Tucholsky, K., 1931. Zwischen Gestern und Morgen. Eine Auswahl aus seinen Schriften und Gedichten. Herausgegeben von Mary Gerold-Tucholsky Rowohld Taschenbuch Verlag, 60. Auflage. 2012, 42–43.

Tung, J.W., Mrazek, M.D., Yang, Y., Herzenberg, L.A., Herzenberg, L. A., 2006. Phenotypically distinct B cell development pathways map to the three B cell lineages in the mouse. Proc. Natl. Acad. Sci. U.S. A. 103, 6293–6298.

Vegh, P., Winckler, J., Melchers, F., 2010. Long-term "in vitro" proliferating mouse hematopoietic progenitor cell lines. Immunol. Lett. 130, 32–35.

Vilagos, B., Hoffmann, M., Souabni, A., Sun, Q., Werner, B., Medvedovic, J., et al., 2012. Essential role of EBF1 in the generation and function of distinct mature B cell types. J. Exp. Med. 209, 775–792.

Vinuesa, C.G., Linterman, M.A., Goodnow, C.C., Randall, K.L., 2010. T cells and follicular dendritic cells in germinal center B-cell formation and selection. Immunol. Rev. 237, 72–89.

Wagers, A.J., Weissman, I.L., 2004. Plasticity of adult stem cells. Cell. 116, 639–648.

Wardemann, H., Nussenzweig, M.C., 2007. B-cell self-tolerance in humans. Adv. Immunol. 95, 83–110.

Wardemann, H., Boehm, T., Dear, N., Carsetti, R., 2002. B-1a B cells that link the innate and adaptive immune responses are lacking in the absence of the spleen. J. Exp. Med. 195, 771–780.

Weill, J.C., Le Gallou, S., Hao, Y., Reynaud, C.A., 2013. Multiple players in mouse B cell memory. Curr. Opin. Immunol. 25, 334–338.

Witsch, E.J., Cao, H., Fukuyama, H., Weigert, M., 2006. Light chain editing generates polyreactive antibodies in chronic graft-versus-host reaction. J. Exp. Med. 203, 1761–1772.

Xie, C., Patel, R., Wu, T., Zhu, J., Henry, T., Bhaskarabhatla, M., et al., 2007. PI3K/AKT/mTOR hypersignaling in autoimmune lymphoproliferative disease engendered by the epistatic interplay of Sle1b and FASlpr. Int. Immunol. 19, 509–522.

Yokomizo, T., Ng, C.E., Osato, M., Dzierzak, E., 2011. Three-dimensional imaging of whole midgestation murine embryos shows an intravascular localization for all hematopoietic clusters. Blood. 117, 6132–6134.

Yurasov, S., Wardemann, H., Hammersen, J., Tsuiji, M., Meffre, E., Pascual, V., et al., 2005. Defective B cell tolerance checkpoints in systemic lupus erythematosus. J. Exp. Med. 201, 703–711.

Zhou, Z.H., Tzioufas, A.G., Notkins, A.L., 2007. Properties and function of polyreactive antibodies and polyreactive antigen-binding B cells. Autoimmun. 29, 219–228.

Zhuang, Y., Soriano, P., Weintraub, H., 1994. The helix-loop-helix gene E2A is required for B cell formation. Cell. 79, 875–884.

B Cell Activation and B Cell Tolerance

Claudia Mauri, Venkat Reddy, and Paul A. Blair

Centre for Rheumatology, Division of Medicine, University College London, London, UK

Chapter Outline

B Cell Activation	**147**
Antigen-Triggered Activation	147
Secondary Signals for B Cell Activation	148
The Immediate Consequences of B Cell Activation	148
B Cell Activation Requires Interaction with	
Helper T Cells	**148**
Cell Surface Molecules Involved in B Cell–T Cell Interactions	148
Cytolkines Involved in B Cell–T Cell Interactions	149
Activation and Maturation of B Cells Occurs in Lymphoid	
Organs	**149**
Where Do B Cells become Antigen Activated?	149
Antigen Activation of B Cells Leads to the Selection of High Affinity Class-	
Switched Antibody	150
The Germinal Center	150
T Cell-Independent Antibody Responses	**150**
B Cell Tolerance: A Traditional and New Concept	**151**

B Cell Tolerance is Acquired by at Least Three Different	
Processes	151
Receptor Editing and Clonal Deletion	151
Defective Receptor Editing Can Promote	
Autoimmunity	153
Anergy	153
Characteristics of Anergic B Cells	153
Survival Factors and Tonic Signals Modulate	
B Cell Tolerance	**154**
Tonic Signaling in B Cell Development	154
Tonic Signaling and Autoimmunity	154
BAFF and Autoimmunity	154
Regulatory T cells	**155**
Antibody-Independent Activity of B Cells in Tolerance	**155**
Cytokine Production by B Cells	155
Regulatory B Cells	155
Future Directions	**156**
References	**156**

B CELL ACTIVATION

B cells form an important part of the immune system by helping the host to fight against pathogens. In pursuit of their mission of surveillance for foreign antigens, B cells must: (1) gain access to the area where antigens are available (migration); (2) recognize and bind to antigen (antigen specificity); (3) increase antigen-specific cell numbers (proliferate); and (4) mature into terminally differentiated cells including *plasma cells* that secrete antibodies to neutralize antigen and *memory cells* that remember previous encounters with antigen and aid subsequent recognition of the same antigen during future infections. The process controlling this series of events is referred to as B cell activation.

T-dependent activation of B cells occurs in two distinct phases: first, B cells are activated by foreign protein antigen, and second, antigen-specific B cells interact with activated helper T cells with the same antigen specificity.

Antigen-Triggered Activation

Engagement of the B cell antigen receptor (BCR) initiates two interdependent processes, signaling and receptor internalization (information on the mechanisms driving the assembly of the BCR is provided in Box 10.1). Cross-linking B cell surface receptors (IgD or monomeric IgM on naïve B cells) leads to a cascade of reactions, comprising the first step of B cell activation. When two or more receptor molecules are cross-linked by multivalent antigens, the cytosolic subunit Igα-Igβ dimers, which are covalently linked to the BCRs, initiate intracellular signaling. The conserved signaling motifs (immunoreceptor tyrosine-based activation motifs or ITAMs) contained within the cytosolic tails of Igα-Igβ are tyrosine phosphorylated by Src-family tyrosine kinases (Lyn, Fyn, and Btk). These initial events lead to the activation of intracellular signaling molecules and transcription of genes involved in the regulation of B cell activation (Harwood & Batista, 2010).

N. Rose & I. Mackay (Eds): The Autoimmune Diseases, Fifth edition. DOI: http://dx.doi.org/10.1016/B978-0-12-384929-8.00010-1

- B cells share with T cells the ability to recognize specific antigens through their expression of antigen receptors that are expressed early in B cell development through the rearrangement of immunoglobulin genes.
- Diversity in BCRs is achieved through the random recombination of the Ig heavy and light chain genes that encode the BCR and the antibody produced.
- Rearrangement of Ig genes to bring heavy chain variable region genes into proximity with different heavy chain constant region genes also determines the isotype of antibody the B cells produce, either IgM, IgG, IgA, or IgE.
- The isotype of antibody produced, and the nature of the constant region of the BCR, can change over the course of an immune response, allowing the B cell to make the appropriate antibody response for the particular threat.

Secondary Signals for B Cell Activation

However, since BCR cross-linking by antigen alone is not sufficient to fully activate B cells, several pathways exist to deliver additional signals that boost the BCR activation signal. A second set of signals is delivered when the BCR becomes closely associated with the BCR–coreceptor complex (Harwood & Batista, 2010). This complex comprises three main components: CD19 (containing the cytoplasmic signaling domain of the BCR), CD81 (of unknown function), and CD21 (complement receptor CR2 which binds to iC3b, an inactive derivative of C3b, C3dg, or C3d) (Carroll, 1998). Microbes possess antigens rich in polysaccharides that activate the complement system directly through binding C3b. Despite further degradation of C3b its derivative C3d continues to bind to the microbial surface. The BCR–coreceptor complex will bind to complement components on microbial surfaces via CD21, leading to further receptor clustering which significantly enhances the BCR activation signal in response to antigen.

The importance of complement-mediated activation of B cells is shown in mice with a disrupted CR2 gene. These mice display a reduced number of B cells in the spleen, a defect that is reversed upon reconstitution with bone marrow from CR2 expressing wild-type mice (Ahearn et al., 1996). Similarly, mice lacking CR2 expression are unable to generate antigen-specific plasma cells, or to maintain antibody production, in response to viral infection, as CR2 mediated costimulation is required to induce the transcriptional regulators Blimp-1 and XBP-1, molecules driving plasma cell differentiation (Gatto et al., 2005).

The Immediate Consequences of B Cell Activation

B cells process antigen through a series of orderly steps. The endocytosis of receptor-bound antigen is the first in a series of signaling-mediated events that ensures that antigens are efficiently captured, processed, and presented to cognate T cells. These include the prompt transfer of internalized antigens to the endosome and then to the lysosome where the BCR–antigen complex is degraded into peptides. Peptides coupled with major histocompatibility complex (MHC) class II molecules are transported to the cell membrane for presentation to T-helper cells. The intracellular trafficking of BCR–Ag complexes is mediated via the reorganization of actin cytoskeleton and involves the synergistic action of small proteins that promote cell contraction (e.g., Myosin II), and "chaperone molecules" that escort the BCR–Ag complexes to lysosomes (Vascotto et al., 2007). Signaling via the BCR enhances the synthesis of MHC class II molecules and increases expression of costimulatory molecules CD80, 86 (B7-1, B7-2). Any defects in the molecules or mechanisms involved with the transport of antigen or its degradation, or involved in the coupling with MHC class II, result in impaired antigen presentation to T cells and consequently abnormal B cell activation.

B CELL ACTIVATION REQUIRES INTERACTION WITH HELPER T CELLS

The process of mutual stimulation between B and T cells is known as costimulation and requires specificity of both B and T cells for the same antigen. It is possible that B and T cells will recognize different epitopes on the same antigen. Nevertheless, although B cells recognize intact antigen and T cells recognize antigen-derived peptides presented in MHC, the antibody produced by the B cells will be specific for the same antigen as the T cells recognize. T cells activate B cells both by direct contact and indirectly through secretion of cytokines (Guy & Hodes, 1989).

Cell Surface Molecules Involved in B Cell–T Cell Interactions

Activated T cells express high levels of CD154 that binds to CD40, a molecule constitutively expressed on the surface of B cells. The engagement of CD40 by CD154 leads to a further upregulation of CD80/86 on B cells, which in turn bind to CD28 on T cells, resulting in further activation of T cells. The interaction between CD40 and CD154 is also important for class switch recombination (CSR) (discussed later), the clinical relevance of which became apparent when defects in the CD40 (*CD154L*) gene were found to be associated with the development of X-linked hyper IgM syndrome type 1. These patients present with excessive production of IgM at the expense of IgG, IgA, and IgE, and have increased susceptibility to common infections including pneumonia, sinusitis, and otitis (Noelle, 1996). Blocking the CD40—CD154 pathway using an anti-CD154 monoclonal antibody has been shown to be effective in reducing the severity of autoimmune diseases such as experimental collagen-induced arthritis in rodents (Durie et al., 1993) and immune thrombocytopenia in humans (Kuwana et al., 2004), further reinforcing the importance of this pathway in B cell activation.

Cytokines Involved in B Cell—T Cell Interactions

Activation of costimulatory pathways not only stabilizes and strengthens the communication between T and B cells but also leads to the transcription of several genes by both B and T cells, including the upregulation of cytokine receptors on the surface of B cells. Activated T cells will release several cytokines including IL-2, lymphotoxin, interferon-γ, and IL-10. IL-2 induces proliferation of B cells, whereas IL-4 and IL-10 are needed for their further differentiation into mature B cells (Mingari et al., 1984; Rousset et al., 1992). These accumulated signals will activate the transcription of immunoglobulin (Ig) genes and at this stage some of the B cells will differentiate into plasma cells producing antibodies.

It is important to note that the profile of cytokines secreted by T cells also influences the isotype of antibody produced. For example, abundant IL-4 induces production of predominantly IgG1 and IgE, whereas IFN-γ favors IgG2a production, and TGF-β favors IgA production (McHeyzer-Williams & McHeyzer-Williams, 2005).

Therefore, interaction with a specific antigen of high affinity and effective cross-linking of the BCR, followed by cognate interaction with activated cytokine-producing helper T cells, is required for full activation of B cells. The absence of any of these signals during T—B cell interactions results in B cell anergy. As discussed in more detail later in this chapter, anergic B cells in the periphery are unable to proliferate or to develop further into mature B cells.

A better understanding of the costimulation pathways involved in the activation of B cells and their further maturation to antibody producing plasma cells (or autoreactive antibody) has led to the development of therapeutic agents to treat autoimmune diseases. For example, abatacept, a CTLA4-Ig fusion protein, was developed to block costimulation of B and T cells and its safety and therapeutic efficacy have been demonstrated in the treatment of rheumatoid arthritis (Genovese et al., 2012).

ACTIVATION AND MATURATION OF B CELLS OCCURS IN LYMPHOID ORGANS

In the previous section we learned how activation of B cells requires highly synchronized processes initiated by the recognition of antigen and by interaction with T cells. But where do B cells encounter T cells with the same antigen specificity?

Where Do B Cells become Antigen Activated?

In the bone marrow, B cells carrying an antigen receptor develop from pluripotent stem cells. Only cells that do not react against self-antigens progress through distinct developmental stages. Immature B cells migrate from the bone marrow and through the blood and lymphatic system to a designated location (primary lymphoid follicle) in the spleen or lymph nodes where they mature into naïve B cells (B cells that are yet to encounter a foreign antigen). In addition to B cells, this area is enriched with follicular dendritic cells (FDC), which are cells of mesenchymal origin that help organize lymphoid architecture. FDCs capture opsonized antigen (antigen bound with antibody and complement components) on their cell surfaces via the expression of complement and Fc receptors, which facilitates B cell antigen recognition. Naïve B cell migration through the lymph nodes is guided by the release of chemokines by both FDCs and stromal reticular cells. The chemokine molecules CCL21 (expressed by stromal cells) and CXCL13 (expressed by stromal cells and FDCs) guide CCR7 and CXCR5 expressing B cells through the follicles (Cyster, 2010). The expression of the chemoattractant-type receptor Epstein-Barr virus-induced G-protein coupled receptor 2 (EBI2) by naïve B cells is also important for their migration through lymph nodes; however, the ligand for EBI2 is not yet established (Cyster, 2010). This is a dynamic process as B cells that have not been primed within the initial 24 hours of arriving in the lymphoid tissue recirculate back to the blood in search of cognate antigen (Gonzalez et al., 2011).

To facilitate an encounter with antigen, naïve B cells travel among the FDCs to the outer follicle attracted by CXCL13 and EBI2L. After eventual encounter with their specific antigen, B cells upregulate the expression of adhesion molecules promoting interaction with FDCs, and of integrins that drive their migration towards the T cell zone (Spaargaren et al., 2003). Similarly, CCL21 and CCL19 expression by fibroblastic reticular cells in the T cell zone encourages the B cells to recirculate to the interface between the B and T cell zones. Subsequent upregulation of chemokine receptors (e.g., CCR7, a receptor for CCL19 and CCL21) traps the B cells in this area.

Antigen Activation of B Cells Leads to the Selection of High Affinity Class-Switched Antibody

Once in the T cell zone, some B cells further proliferate and differentiate directly into plasma-blasts, the direct precursor of antibody producing plasma cells. This provides for a "quick fix" to control the spread of infection and is usually referred to as the primary response. However, some of the antigen-activated B cells migrate into the primary lymphoid follicle and form germinal centers (GC). GCs comprise dividing B cells and a small proportion of antigen-specific T cells that provide help to B cells (Cyster, 2010). Several important events related to activation occur in GCs, including *somatic hypermutation*, a process altering the V-regions of Ig genes; *affinity maturation*, which involves selecting the B cells with high antigen specificity; and *class switching*, whereby the selected B cells change the classes of antibodies they secrete to exert their distinct functions.

Somatic hypermutation (SHM) is the initial step. Here site-directed point mutations are induced in the variable (V) regions of the Ig genes of activated B cells, resulting in the expression of BCRs with potentially altered specificities. The mutated B cells are selected based on their affinity for the antigen. If SHM results in a BCR with a high affinity for the original antigen, the B cell expressing this BCR will outcompete antigen-specific B cells with lower BCR antigen affinities for cognate interactions with helper T cells. The B cells with higher affinity BCRs will then receive survival signals provided either by CD154 (CD40L) expressed on the helper T cells or by FDCs. This process, called affinity maturation, will lead to a pool of antigen-specific B cells secreting higher affinity antibody than those secreted by the initial antigen-specific B cell pool (Di Noia and Neuberger, 2007).

CSR occurs after SHM and affinity maturation have taken place (Muramatsu et al., 2000). Transcriptional gene rearrangements lead to the recombination of the Ig genes so that the IgM heavy chain gene is excised from the Ig locus and the constant region for another Ig heavy chain is joined to the heavy chain Ig variable region. The variable region of the Ig heavy chain remains unchanged. As a result of these processes (SHM and affinity maturation), cells switch the class of Igs they secrete from low affinity IgM to a high affinity IgG isotype (Di Noia and Neuberger, 2007). A genetic defect in any gene involved in CSR results in the development of hyper IgM syndrome type 2. These immune-deficient patients are characterized by the absence of immunoglobulin CSR, the lack of immunoglobulin somatic hypermutations, and lymph node hyperplasia caused by the presence of enlarged GCs (Revy et al., 2000). These events occurring

in the GCs prepare the B cell for the production of a long-term targeted response to a foreign antigen.

The Germinal Center

The GC can be divided into three zones: the dark zone, the light zone, and the mantle zone. Within the dark zone of the GC, antigen-activated B cells evolve to form large rapidly dividing cells, the centroblasts (Figure 10.1(2)). It is at this stage and in this location that centroblasts diversify their IgV genes by SHM. Centroblasts move out from the densely packed dark zone and enter the light zone (FDC area) where they differentiate into centrocytes, which then form the outer rim or mantle zone of the GC. Although most centrocytes die *in situ*, those receiving appropriate help from surrounding T cells will differentiate into memory or plasma cells. The end result of GC formation is the production of antigen-specific plasma cells that secrete high affinity antigen-specific Igs, and generate memory cells to counteract any subsequent infection with the same antigen. Memory B cells are long-lived cells, surviving sometimes for up to many years, as also is the case for some plasma cells (Klein & Dalla-Favera, 2008).

T CELL-INDEPENDENT ANTIBODY RESPONSES

B cell responses to non-protein antigens, including polysaccharides and lipids, do not require T cell help and are defined as T-independent responses. Such responses are of two types, 1 and 2. The type-1 response (TI-1) involves engagement by antigens of additional receptors expressed by B cells that regulate innate immune responses, e.g., Toll-like receptors (TLR). TLRs play an important role in regulating the innate immune response and recognize highly conserved molecules expressed by microorganisms. Type-2 responses (TI-2) are against antigens that contain repeating epitopes, such as the cell wall polysaccharides of *Streptococcus*, which simultaneously cross-link multiple BCRs and deliver prolonged signals to the B cells. The cumulative intracellular signaling following engagement of BCRs, TLRs, and B cell coreceptors provides the necessary signal strength to promote B cell activation, proliferation, and plasma cell differentiation in the absence of T cell help. B cells express varying levels and types of TLRs, among which TLR9 is the most highly expressed. TLR9 recognizes CpG motifs in bacterial DNA. The expression of TLR9 by B cells is particularly relevant in the context of autoimmune diseases such as systemic lupus erythematosus (SLE). TLR9 and TLR7 bind to endogenous DNA and RNA respectively and, following BCR recognition and internalization of these auto-antigens, there is enhanced release of autoantibodies

Chapter | 10   B Cell Activation and B Cell Tolerance

151

Box 10.2 Pathways of Breakdown in Self-Tolerance Leading to Autoimmune Diseases due to a Primary Defect of B Cells (A, B, and C) or Secondary Immune Dysregulation (D and E)

- T-independent antigens such as lipopolysaccharides and DNA CpG motifs can activate autoreactive B cells through TLR 4 and 9 to secrete rheumatoid factors and anti-DNA antibodies.
- Foreign antigen, modified by infection or drugs, can activate "ignorant" autoreactive B cells. Examples include rheumatic fever following streptococcal infection and autoimmune hemolytic anemia associated with α-methyldopa.
- Tonic signals and intrinsic B cell defects and/or polymorphisms of BCR, FcγRIIb, Lyn, CD22, and CD45 might influence B cell activation and tolerance and lead to the development of systemic autoimmune diseases.
- Impaired extrinsic regulatory mechanisms such as defective complement pathways and regulatory T cells are associated with systemic autoimmune diseases, rheumatoid arthritis and SLE.
- Autoreactive B cells present self-antigens to T cells, with the same antigen specificity, leading to multiple organ-specific autoimmune disease.

against nuclear components, a hallmark of SLE (Green & Marshak-Rothstein, 2011) (summarized in Box 10.2).

B CELL TOLERANCE: A TRADITIONAL AND NEW CONCEPT

The immune system is highly efficient in defending the host against continuous exposure to foreign antigens while halting the maturation of B cells that recognize self-antigens—autoreactive B cells. This latter process (among others) provides for B cell tolerance. Defects in any of the component parts of this process contribute to the development of a group of diseases wherein various organs in the body come under misguided attack from its own defense system. The profound discrepancy between the frequency of autoreactive cells generated in the thymus or bone marrow, some 90% of all new cells, and the rarity of autoimmune diseases highlights the efficacy of tolerance mechanisms for purging the immune system of autoreactive B cells. Tolerance acquired during the development of B cells in the bone marrow constitutes "central tolerance," whereas mechanisms halting the maturation of autoreactive B cells in the peripheral lymphoid tissues constitute "peripheral tolerance." Fifty to seventy-five percent of antibodies produced by early immature B cells isolated from human bone marrow are autoreactive or polyreactive (Wardemann et al., 2003); however, multiple checkpoints throughout B cell development

usually prevent mature B cells from producing autoantibody. In addition to the classical view of B cell tolerance as a process that has evolved to prevent production of autoantibodies, we will introduce a new concept in which B cells can serve as effector cells that actively suppress autoimmune responses.

B Cell Tolerance is Acquired by at Least Three Different Processes

First, if a B cell expresses an autoreactive BCR, particularly at an early stage of development, then the B cell can alter its BCR genes in order to express a non-autoreactive version, a process called "receptor editing." Second, if "receptor editing" fails, autoreactive B cells can be removed while still in the bone marrow by a process termed "clonal deletion." Third, autoreactive B cells that nevertheless escape to the periphery may acquire tolerance by entering a state of unresponsiveness to antigen, termed "anergy" (Figure 10.1).

Receptor Editing and Clonal Deletion

The generation of adaptive immune responses relies on the random rearrangement of antigen receptor genes to produce a diverse repertoire of antigen receptor specificities. Successful in frame V, (D) J recombination leads to the expression of a productive BCR, followed by suppression of RAG 1 and 2 genes to prevent further rearrangements (Nussenzweig et al., 1987). However, if these rearrangements produce an autoreactive BCR, the B cells may undergo receptor editing. Receptor editing is a second rearrangement of the VJ genes encoding the Ig light chains that results in the expression of a BCR with a new specificity and has been reported to be the main mechanism of B cell central tolerance towards high avidity membrane bound antigens. If rearrangement of the light chain genes results in the expression of a productive BCR with no autoreactive specificity then B cells are allowed to survive and reach maturity (Halverson et al., 2004). For instance, Gay et al. generated mice that were transgenic for Ig heavy and light chain genes that encoded a BCR that was specific for dsDNA, an autoantigen in murine and human lupus. As these genes were already rearranged they would be the first heavy and light chains to be transcribed and, in the absence of receptor editing, all B cells should have been clonally deleted due to their autoreactive BCRs. However, the adult mice had a normal number of mature B cells due to the fact that, while all their B cells expressed the heavy chain transgene, all mature B cells expressed an endogenous light chain, demonstrating that receptor editing had taken place to produce a non-autoreactive BCR (Gay et al., 1993).

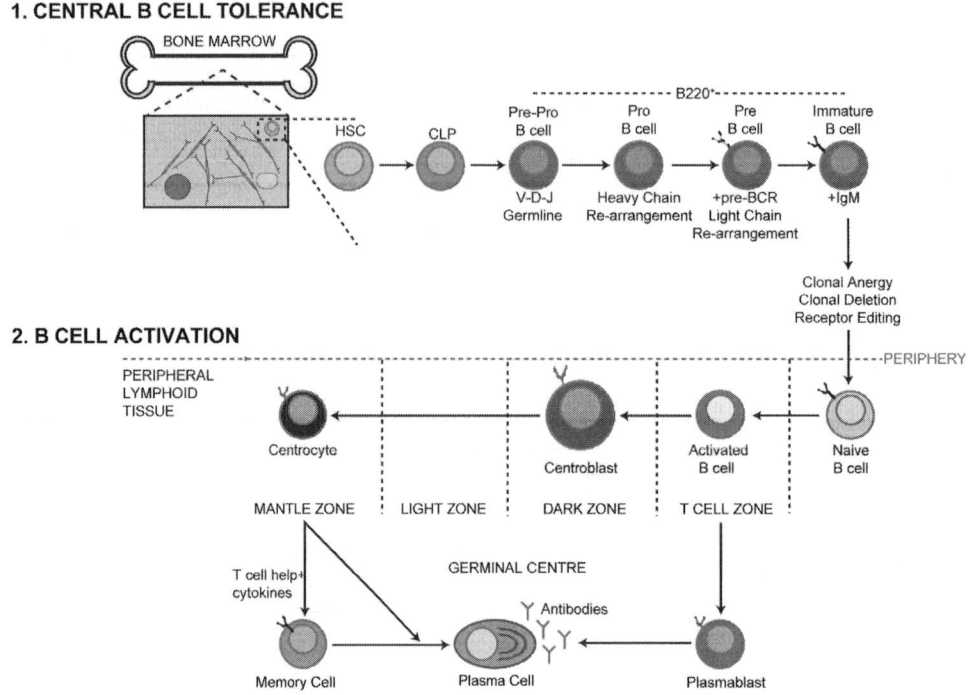

FIGURE 10.1   Following the journey of B cell from the bone marrow to the periphery.   (1) In the bone marrow, B cells develop from common lymphocyte progenitor (CLP) cells that originate from hematopoietic stem cells (HSC). The random rearrangement of Ig genes results in expression of the B cell receptor (BCR). Immature B cells bearing non-self-reactive BCR (IgM) survive and emigrate from the bone marrow. Clones of autoreactive cells that recognize multivalent membrane bound self-antigen may be deleted or undergo receptor editing in an attempt to express non-autoreactive BCRs. Autoreactive B cells that bind monovalent or oligovalent soluble antigen become anergic. (2) Naïve B cells reach the peripheral lymphoid tissues (lymph nodes and spleen) via the blood and lymphatic systems, where they migrate, following chemo-attractant gradients, to areas where they can interact with follicular dendritic cells and T cells. Interaction with antigen results in B cell activation. In the absence of T cell help antigen-activated B cells undergo apoptotic death. However, if the antigen-activated B cells receive T cell help then some will give rise to short-lived IgM plasma blasts and plasma cells, while others will become rapidly dividing centroblasts (found in the dark zone) that proliferate to become centrocytes (found in the mantle zone). With further T cell help B cells may mature to become memory cells and plasma cells. (3) Additional regulatory systems exist to control the potential damage that maturation of autoreactive B cells may have on the immune system. In response to activation with autoantigen, and/or upon interaction with lipopolysaccharides (LPS), some B cells may differentiate into regulatory B cells (Bregs). Bregs limit tissue damage in certain autoimmune conditions by dampening inflammatory responses. This is achieved by the secretion of anti-inflammatory cytokines such as interleukin (IL)-10 and Transforming Growth Factor (TGF)-β, and/or via inhibition of the development of proinflammatory T cells (T helper-1/T helper-17), and/or by promoting the development of regulatory T cells (Tregs) which in turn inhibit the production of autoantibody.

Receptor editing usually occurs early during B cell development and predominantly, although not exclusively, in the bone marrow. Secondary rearrangements may also occur in the periphery although their importance in maintaining tolerance remains to be fully defined. RAG genes are re-expressed in germinal centers, and it

has been demonstrated in mice that mature follicular B cells that are autoreactive and anti-dsDNA specific can undergo receptor editing in germinal centers following antigen activation, which removes dsDNA specificity (Rice et al., 2005). However, receptor editing, or revision of light chains at this stage of development may have a role in the generation of high affinity antibodies rather than a role in B cell tolerance (Wang et al., 2007).

If receptor editing in the bone marrow fails to produce B cells with functional BCRs that are not autoreactive then the B cells may be eliminated by apoptosis, a process termed "clonal deletion." Clonal deletion was originally thought to be the major mechanism of B cell central tolerance to high avidity membrane bound or multivalent self-antigens; however, later studies have suggested that receptor editing is the primary mechanism for removing autoreactive B cells. Clonal deletion provides a final failsafe when receptor editing fails (Pelanda & Torres, 2012).

Defective Receptor Editing Can Promote Autoimmunity

Although receptor editing is the main process contributing to the removal of autoreactive B cells, this system is not perfect. The Ig heavy chain often has the dominant contribution to BCR specificity and if the heavy chain is autoreactive the rearrangement of the light chain may not fully remove the autoreactivity (Luning Prak et al., 2011). In addition, light chain rearrangement does not always lead to the abrogation of expression of the initial light chain and when the B cells reach the periphery the initial autoreactive light chain may be re-expressed (Li et al., 2002b).

Defective receptor editing has been associated with autoimmunity in both mice and humans. Both excessive and inadequate receptor editing can be seen in mice with autoimmune conditions, extensively reviewed by Luning Prak et al. (2011). Excessive receptor editing can result in the generation of B cells with autoreactive BCRs. For example, lupus-prone MRL/*lpr.56*R mice that are transgenic for an autoreactive Ig heavy chain have an increased production of autoantibodies compared to nontransgenic MRL/*lpr* mice. However, the majority of the autoantibodies in the transgenic mouse do not use the transgenic Ig heavy chain, suggesting that excessive receptor editing has led to the generation of autoreactive BCR (Li et al., 2002a). Nevertheless, inadequate editing can allow the escape to the periphery of autoreactive B cells; lupus-prone non-transgenic MRL/*lpr* mice display less efficient receptor editing compared to non-lupus-prone controls (Lamoureux et al., 2007). Furthermore, it has been hypothesized that inefficient receptor editing in autoimmune-prone mice might allow the escape to the periphery of B cells with two types of Ig heavy or light chain. These dual reactive B cells are rare in healthy mice but increased in number in autoimmune strains and are frequently more autoreactive than B cells expressing only one heavy and light chain (Fournier et al., 2012).

Anergy

Despite the efficiency of receptor editing and clonal deletion, B cells carrying self-reactive BCRs may still escape central tolerance and reach the periphery. Here, tolerance can be achieved by inducing a state of unresponsiveness to antigen, known as anergy, in the autoreactive B cells. Anergy results from B cell binding to low avidity or soluble antigen without receiving adequate additional signals to support their activation. Anergic B cells are unable to interact effectively with helper T cells and do not participate in immune responses against their cognate antigen. It was initially demonstrated that B cell tolerance to antigens could arise through anergy rather than clonal deletion (Nossal & Pike, 1980), as follows. Treatment of newborn mice with a soluble molecule, fluorescein-human gamma globulin (Flu-HGG), resulted in tolerance to this molecule in the adult mice. After treatment, adult mice were tolerant to Flu-HGG but unexpectedly this was not as a result of clonal deletion, rather the mice retained normal numbers of Flu-HGG-specific B cells, but these B cells were unable to respond to the antigen. Subsequently, Hartley et al. elegantly demonstrated that it is the nature of the antigen, rather than the affinity of BCR−antigen interactions, that is responsible for whether tolerance comes from clonal deletion or anergy (Hartley et al., 1991). Hartley et al. generated two transgenic mouse models with both carrying B cell receptors that were specific for hen egg lysozyme (HEL); the first expressed membrane-bound HEL as well as the transgenic BCR, and the second expressed soluble HEL as well as the transgenic BCR. The results demonstrated that clonal deletion of the HEL-specific transgenic B cells occurred when mice expressed membrane-bound HEL, whereas clonal anergy occurred in mice expressing soluble HEL. Thus, immature B cell binding to high avidity multivalent membrane-bound antigen mainly leads to receptor editing, or clonal deletion, while binding to low avidity monovalent, or oligovalent, soluble antigen mainly leads to anergy.

Characteristics of Anergic B Cells

Anergic B cells are characterized by a low expression of BCR on their cell surface due to reduced BCR recirculation from the endoplasmic reticulum. This low expression of the BCR is an important feature of anergic B cells. First, it prevents signaling through the autoreactive BCRs. Second, anergic B cells show an increased recruitment of negative signaling regulators, including SHP1 and SHIP, to the BCR complex. Increased SHP1 and SHIP expression can inhibit BCR-mediated B cell activation by the dephosphorylation of signaling molecules downstream of the BCR and Igα/Igβ. Defects in SHP1 or SHIP are associated with increased autoantibody production (Huang et al., 2003). Third, anergic B cells have a half-life of 1−5 days in contrast to non-autoreactive naïve B cells with a half-life of around 40 days (Fulcher & Basten, 1994). The short half-life of anergic B cells adds an additional brake to B cell autoreactivity.

SURVIVAL FACTORS AND TONIC SIGNALS MODULATE B CELL TOLERANCE

Tonic Signaling in B Cell Development

Immature B cells with fully functional BCRs leave the bone marrow and emigrate to the periphery where they further mature into transitional 1 (T1) and transitional 2 (T2) B cells. Transitional B cells survive for around 3.5 days, and only 10–30% of them will become mature marginal zone (MZ) or follicular (FO) B cells. Two factors are critical for this transition: tonic BCR signaling, and stimulation by the B lymphocyte activating factor (BAFF) (Pelanda & Torres, 2012). Signaling that occurs in the absence of antigen engagement with the pre-BCR or BCR is called tonic BCR signaling (Monroe, 2006). Stochastic interactions between CD45 in the BCR signaling complex and SRC family protein tyrosine kinases (PTKs) lead to the phosphorylation of ITAMS associated with Igα and Igβ and initiate signaling downstream of the BCR (Monroe, 2006). Tonic BCR signaling is held in a dynamic equilibrium with negative signals from BCR coreceptors such as CD5, CD22, and CD72. SRC PTKs that are activated by tonic BCR signals also phosphorylate inhibitory immunoreceptor tyrosine-based inhibitory motifs (ITIMs) on molecules such as CD22, which in turn recruit protein tyrosine phosphatases that dephosphorylate the ITAMs on Igα/β to inhibit BCR signals. Thus, tonic signaling does not in itself lead to full B cell activation but for immature B cells plays a role in development and survival (Rowland et al., 2012). Tonic signaling positively regulates the expression of BAFF receptor (BAFF-R), and the combination of tonic signaling and BAFF/BAFF-R signaling drives immature B cell maturation to transitional and mature B cells (Rowland et al., 2012). The requirement for both BAFF-R expression and tonic signaling for immature B cell maturation provides a checkpoint for preventing the escape of autoreactive B cells into the periphery; binding of autoantigen by autoreactive B cells leads to the internalization of the BCR and thus a loss of both tonic signaling and BAFF-R expression (Rowland et al., 2010; Pelanda & Torres, 2012).

Tonic Signaling and Autoimmunity

Defects or deficiencies in tonic signaling can lead to autoimmunity. A failure of tonic signaling at an immature B cell stage leads to a developmental regression that can restart the process of Ig gene recombination and potentially break allelic exclusion (Tze et al., 2005). This may result in B cells that express both autoreactive and non-autoreactive BCRs; the tonic signals from the non-autoreactive BCR provide the developmental and survival signals that allow the escape of dual specific autoreactive B cells (Pelanda & Torres, 2012). Deficiencies in the molecules that negatively regulate tonic, and antigen-dependent, BCR signaling can also lead to autoimmunity. CD22 deficient mice produce high affinity anti-dsDNA antibodies suggesting that defects in CD22 function may support B cell-mediated autoimmunity (O'Keefe et al., 1999). FcγRIIb, an inhibitory Fc receptor, which also contains an ITIM on its intracellular domain, plays a role in regulating BCR signals through the recruitment of tyrosine phosphatases. Mice deficient in this receptor develop spontaneous autoimmune disease characterized by fatal glomerulonephritis and accumulate anti-dsDNA plasma cells (Fukuyama et al., 2005). In humans, polymorphsims in the FcγRIIb gene that encode molecules with reduced regulatory activity have been associated with SLE (Niederer et al., 2010). In lupus-prone mice, overexpression of FcγRIIb restored B cell tolerance (McGaha et al., 2005).

BAFF and Autoimmunity

B cell survival depends on the presence of several key chemical mediators. One such mediator is BAFF, which belongs to the tumor necrosis factor (TNF) ligand family, also known as B lymphocyte survival factor (BLyS). As well as its role in promoting B cell maturation, it promotes mature B cell proliferation and differentiation (Schneider et al., 1999). The major sources of BAFF for normal B cell homeostasis are stromal cells in the bone marrow and spleen; however, at sites of inflammation it is mainly produced by monocytes (Gorelik et al., 2003). BAFF binds to three different receptors expressed on B cells at different stages of maturation: BAFF-receptor, BCMA (B cell maturation antigen), and TACI (transmembrane activator and calcium modulator and cyclophilin ligand interactor). The predominant receptor expressed on human peripheral blood B cells is BAFF-R, while BCMA and TACI appear to be preferentially expressed on plasma cells and transitional B cells, respectively (Ng et al., 2004). The importance of BAFF in B cell maturation was elegantly demonstrated by work from the Mackay group. B cells in BAFF and BAFF-receptor-deficient mice were developmentally arrested at the transitional 1 stage of B cell development (Mackay et al., 2002); this group also demonstrated that B cells from BAFF transgenic mice secreted unusually high amounts of rheumatoid factor (RF) antibody and the mice developed lupus-like disease (Mackay et al., 1999). BAFF overexpression rescued autoreactive B cells from deletion in the periphery, but not from the bone marrow, and favored their migration to follicular and marginal zone areas of lymphoid organs (Thien et al., 2004). Patients with autoimmune diseases such as Sjögren's syndrome and SLE have high levels of BAFF, which may contribute to altered differentiation of B cells (Pillai et al., 2011). Treatment with Belimumab (an anti-BAFF monoclonal antibody) leads to an improvement in symptoms in patients with SLE (Navarra et al., 2011). Thus, whereas BAFF signaling is critical in normal B cell development, when dysregulated it can provoke a breakdown in B cell tolerance leading to systemic autoimmunity.

REGULATORY T CELLS

B cell peripheral tolerance is also maintained by regulatory T cell (Treg) suppression of autoantibody production by B cells. Tregs can suppress autoantibody production indirectly by preventing the maturation of the humoral response by suppression of the T helper cells that would support B cell antibody production (Fields et al., 2005), or directly by inducing apoptosis of autoreactive B cells (Gotot et al., 2012). However, the exact mechanisms by which Tregs suppress autoantibody production remain elusive.

ANTIBODY-INDEPENDENT ACTIVITY OF B CELLS IN TOLERANCE

Cytokine Production by B Cells

As discussed earlier, the generation of B cell tolerance is shaped during the development of B lymphocytes, by receptor editing, clonal deletion, and anergy. However, evidence has emerged for an antibody-independent role for B cells in the maintenance and breakdown and of tolerance. B cells can produce a polarized array of cytokines depending on their primary encounter with antigen and T cells so, as for T cells, B cells can be distinguished based on the cytokines that they produce. Naïve B cells that differentiate in the presence of T helper 1 cells release high levels of IFNγ, IL-12, and TNFα and contribute to the clearance of infection, or contribute to the pathogenesis of Th1-mediated autoimmune diseases. In contrast, naïve B cells that differentiate in the presence of T helper 2 cells predominantly produce IL-2, IL-4, and IL-6 and so may play a pathogenic role in allergic reactions (Harris et al., 2000). The contribution of the cytokines released by B cells in the pathogenesis of autoimmune disease is yet to be clearly defined, but recent findings have shown that IL-6 producing B cells promote Th17 responses and contribute to the pathogenesis of experimental autoimmune encephalomyelitis (EAE), and multiple sclerosis (Barr et al., 2012).

Regulatory B Cells

B cells can also produce the cytokines IL-10 and TGF-β, known to restrain the excessive inflammation associated with autoimmunity. Over the last decade, numerous studies have confirmed the importance of IL-10 producing regulatory B cells (Bregs) in the maintenance of tolerance (Mauri & Bosma, 2012). Studies utilizing chimeric mice, whose B cells alone are IL-10 deficient, have revealed that B cell derived IL-10 limits the severity of inflammation in several autoimmune disorders (Carter et al., 2011; Fillatreau et al., 2002). In the absence of IL-10 producing B cells, chimeric mice present a reduction in the number of Tr1 and Foxp3$^+$ Tregs, and an increase in inflammatory Th1 and Th17 cells compared to mice with IL-10 sufficient B cells. Thus, Bregs contribute to the maintenance of peripheral tolerance by production of potent anti-inflammatory cytokines (IL-10 and/or TGFβ), directly by inhibiting the differentiation of Th1 and Th17 cells, and indirectly by converting targeted effector T cells into Tregs (Carter et al., 2011). BCR activation, which is crucial in dictating the specificity of antibody responses and the function of B cells as antigen presenting cells, may also have a role in Breg function. Research has revealed that exposure to an autoantigen leads to an increased IL-10 production by Bregs and an enhanced ability to suppress the pathogenesis of autoimmune disease (Mauri et al., 2003). Similarly, in the field of transplantation, it has been reported that TIM-1$^+$ Bregs prolonged pancreatic islet allograft survival, but only when the TIM-1$^+$ B cells are specific for the MHC expressed by the transplanted islet cells, suggesting a role for specific BCR signaling (Ding et al., 2011).

Bregs also play a role in the maintenance of tolerance in healthy individuals. Immature B cells isolated from healthy volunteers produce a higher amount of IL-10 than any other human peripheral blood B cell subset, and can suppress proinflammatory cytokine production by CD4$^+$ T cells following polyclonal activation with anti-CD3 *in vitro*. Interestingly, in patients with SLE, isolated Bregs failed to upregulate IL-10 in response to CD40 engagement, and failed to suppress the production of proinflammatory cytokine by T cells (Blair et al., 2010). Accordingly rituximab, a B cell depleting anti-CD20 monoclonal antibody which has proved successful in treating some autoimmune conditions, may function not only by depleting autoantibody producing B cells, but also by resetting the balance between pathogenic and regulatory B cells following B cell repopulation (Manjarrez-Orduno et al., 2009; Bosma et al., 2012).

The immune system has several checkpoints to curtail the escape of autoreactive B cells in the periphery and hence prevent autoimmunity. Among these checkpoints are receptor editing, clonal deletion, and anergy. However, it is becoming clearer that in the periphery tolerance is also maintained by regulatory subsets of cells, including Bregs and Tregs, that control the production of inflammatory cytokines and limit autoreactive responses (Figure 10.1(3)).

FUTURE DIRECTIONS

Knowledge of the mechanisms of B cell tolerance is as yet incomplete. Until recently clonal deletion was thought to be the major mechanism of B cell tolerance; however, it is now clear that receptor editing has a greater influence. Similarly, the exact nature and location of the events that decide whether an autoreactive B cell undergoes receptor editing or becomes anergic warrants further study. Moreover, the majority of the work done to elucidate B cell tolerance has been performed in mice and these results need to be extended to humans.

Whether defects in particular mechanisms of B cell tolerance result in clinically different autoimmune diseases is as yet unanswered. For instance, could defects in receptor editing that lead to the expression of two distinct B cell receptors by mature B cells, one autoreactive and one reactive to a microbial antigen, be important in generating autoantibody to autoantigens that the B cells might otherwise not see? B cells expressing dual BCRs may be activated by the microbial antigen to produce autoreactive antibody and contribute to the pathogenesis of autoimmune diseases despite the offending autoantigen not being generally subject to immune surveillance, e.g., antigens in the central nervous system. Similarly, it is not currently clear what effect the presence of a constantly renewing niche of anergic B cells in healthy humans has on B cell-driven immune responses (Palanichamy et al., 2009). Assuming a large proportion of these anergic B cells are autoreactive they may compete with non-anergic B cells for autoantigen, and thus their presence could prevent the activation of autoreactive T cells. Defects in the generation of anergic B cells may thus lead to autoreactive T cell-mediated autoimmunity. Or indeed an excessively large anergic B cell pool may prevent non-anergic B cells from activating T cells. Defects in individual tolerance checkpoints may thus characterize individual autoimmune diseases.

REFERENCES

Ahearn, J.M., Fischer, M.B., Croix, D., Goerg, S., Ma, M., Xia, J., et al., 1996. Disruption of the Cr2 locus results in a reduction in B-1a cells and in an impaired B cell response to T-dependent antigen. Immunity 4, 251–262.

Barr, T.A., Shen, P., Brown, S., Lampropoulou, V., Roch, T., Lawrie, S., et al., 2012. B cell depletion therapy ameliorates autoimmune disease through ablation of IL-6-producing B cells. J. Exp. Med. 209, 1001–1010.

Blair, P.A., Norena, L.Y., Flores-Borja, F., Rawlings, D.J., Isenberg, D.A., Ehrenstein, M.R., et al., 2010. CD19(+)CD24 (hi)CD38(hi) B cells exhibit regulatory capacity in healthy individuals but are functionally impaired in systemic lupus erythematosus patients. Immunity 32, 129–140.

Bosma, A., Abdel-Gadir, A., Isenberg, D.A., Jury, E.C., Mauri, C., 2012. Lipid-antigen presentation by CD1d(+) B cells is essential for the maintenance of invariant natural killer T cells. Immunity 36, 477–490.

Carroll, M.C., 1998. CD21/CD35 in B cell activation. Semin. Immunol. 10, 279–286.

Carter, N.A., Vasconcellos, R., Rosser, E.C., Tulone, C., Munoz-Suano, A., Kamanaka, M., et al., 2011. Mice lacking endogenous IL-10-producing regulatory B cells develop exacerbated disease and present with an increased frequency of Th1/Th17 but a decrease in regulatory T cells. J. Immunol. 186, 5569–5579.

Cyster, J.G., 2010. B cell follicles and antigen encounters of the third kind. Nat. Immunol. 11, 989–996.

Di Noia, J.M., Neuberger, M.S., 2007. Molecular mechanisms of antibody somatic hypermutation. Annu. Rev. Biochem. 76, 1–22.

Ding, Q., Yeung, M., Camirand, G., Zeng, Q., Akiba, H., Yagita, H., et al., 2011. Regulatory B cells are identified by expression of TIM-1 and can be induced through TIM-1 ligation to promote tolerance in mice. J. Clin. Invest. 121, 3645–3656.

Durie, F.H., Fava, R.A., Foy, T.M., Aruffo, A., Ledbetter, J.A., Noelle, R.J., 1993. Prevention of collagen-induced arthritis with an antibody to gp39, the ligand for CD40. Science 261, 1328–1330.

Fields, M.L., Hondowicz, B.D., Metzgar, M.H., Nish, S.A., Wharton, G. N., Picca, C.C., et al., 2005. CD4+ CD25+ regulatory T cells inhibit the maturation but not the initiation of an autoantibody response. J. Immunol. 175, 4255–4264.

Fillatreau, S., Sweenie, C.H., McGeachy, M.J., Gray, D., Anderton, S.M., 2002. B cells regulate autoimmunity by provision of IL-10. Nat. Immunol. 3, 944–950.

Fournier, E.M., Velez, M.G., Leahy, K., Swanson, C.L., Rubtsov, A.V., Torres, R.M., et al., 2012. Dual-reactive B cells are autoreactive and highly enriched in the plasmablast and memory B cell subsets of autoimmune mice. J. Exp. Med. 209, 1797–1812.

Fukuyama, H., Nimmerjahn, F., Ravetch, J.V., 2005. The inhibitory Fcgamma receptor modulates autoimmunity by limiting the accumulation of immunoglobulin G+ anti-DNA plasma cells. Nat. Immunol. 6, 99–106.

Fulcher, D.A., Basten, A., 1994. Reduced life span of anergic self-reactive B cells in a double-transgenic model. J. Exp. Med. 179, 125–134.

Gatto, D., Pfister, T., Jegerlehner, A., Martin, S.W., Kopf, M., Bachmann, M.F., 2005. Complement receptors regulate differentiation of bone marrow plasma cell precursors expressing transcription factors Blimp-1 and XBP-1. J. Exp. Med. 201, 993–1005.

Gay, D., Saunders, T., Camper, S., Weigert, M., 1993. Receptor editing: an approach by autoreactive B cells to escape tolerance. J. Exp. Med. 177, 999–1008.

Genovese, M.C., Schiff, M., Luggen, M., Le Bars, M., Aranda, R., Elegbe, A., et al., 2012. Longterm safety and efficacy of abatacept through 5 years of treatment in patients with rheumatoid arthritis and an inadequate response to tumor necrosis factor inhibitor therapy. J. Rheumatol. 39, 1546–1554.

Gonzalez, S.F., Degn, S.E., Pitcher, L.A., Woodruff, M., Heesters, B.A., Carroll, M.C., 2011. Trafficking of B cell antigen in lymph nodes. Annu. Rev. Immunol. 29, 215–233.

Gorelik, L., Gilbride, K., Dobles, M., Kalled, S.L., Zandman, D., Scott, M.L., 2003. Normal B cell homeostasis requires B cell activation factor production by radiation-resistant cells. J. Exp. Med. 198, 937–945.

Gotot, J., Gottschalk, C., Leopold, S., Knolle, P.A., Yagita, H., Kurts, C., et al., 2012. Regulatory T cells use programmed death 1 ligands to directly suppress autoreactive B cells in vivo. Proc. Natl. Acad. Sci. USA 109, 10468–10473.

Green, N.M., Marshak-Rothstein, A., 2011. Toll-like receptor driven B cell activation in the induction of systemic autoimmunity. Semin. Immunol. 23, 106–112.

Guy, R., Hodes, R.J., 1989. Antigen-specific, MHC-restricted B cell activation by cell-free Th2 cell products. Synergy between antigen-specific helper factors and IL-4. J. Immunol. 143, 1433–1440.

Halverson, R., Torres, R.M., Pelanda, R., 2004. Receptor editing is the main mechanism of B cell tolerance toward membrane antigens. Nat. Immunol. 5, 645–650.

Harris, D.P., Haynes, L., Sayles, P.C., Duso, D.K., Eaton, S.M., Lepak, N.M., et al., 2000. Reciprocal regulation of polarized cytokine production by effector B and T cells. Nat. Immunol. 1, 475–482.

Hartley, S.B., Crosbie, J., Brink, R., Kantor, A.B., Basten, A., Goodnow, C.C., 1991. Elimination from peripheral lymphoid tissues of self-reactive B lymphocytes recognizing membrane-bound antigens. Nature 353, 765–769.

Harwood, N.E., Batista, F.D., 2010. Early events in B cell activation. Annu. Rev. Immunol. 28, 185–210.

Huang, Z.Y., Hunter, S., Kim, M.K., Indik, Z.K., Schreiber, A.D., 2003. The effect of phosphatases SHP-1 and SHIP-1 on signaling by the ITIM- and ITAM-containing Fcgamma receptors FcgammaRIIB and FcgammaRIIA. J. Leukoc. Biol. 73, 823–829.

Klein, U., Dalla-Favera, R., 2008. Germinal centres: role in B-cell physiology and malignancy. Nat. Rev. Immunol. 8, 22–33.

Kuwana, M., Nomura, S., Fujimura, K., Nagasawa, T., Muto, Y., Kurata, Y., et al., 2004. Effect of a single injection of humanized anti-CD154 monoclonal antibody on the platelet-specific autoimmune response in patients with immune thrombocytopenic purpura. Blood 103, 1229–1236.

Lamoureux, J.L., Watson, L.C., Cherrier, M., Skog, P., Nemazee, D., Feeney, A.J., 2007. Reduced receptor editing in lupus-prone MRL/lpr mice. J. Exp. Med. 204, 2853–2864.

Li, Y., Li, H., Ni, D., Weigert, M., 2002a. Anti-DNA B cells in MRL/lpr mice show altered differentiation and editing pattern. J. Exp. Med. 196, 1543–1552.

Li, Y., Li, H., Weigert, M., 2002b. Autoreactive B cells in the marginal zone that express dual receptors. J. Exp. Med. 195, 181–188.

Luning Prak, E.T., Monestier, M., Eisenberg, R.A., 2011. B cell receptor editing in tolerance and autoimmunity. Ann. N.Y. Acad. Sci. 1217, 96–121.

Mackay, F., Woodcock, S.A., Lawton, P., Ambrose, C., Baetscher, M., Schneider, P., et al., 1999. Mice transgenic for BAFF develop lymphocytic disorders along with autoimmune manifestations. J. Exp. Med. 190, 1697–1710.

Mackay, I.R., Groom, J., Mackay, C.R., 2002. Levels of BAFF in serum in primary biliary cirrhosis and autoimmune diabetes. Autoimmunity 35, 551–553.

Manjarrez-Orduno, N., Quach, T.D., Sanz, I., 2009. B cells and immunological tolerance. J. Invest. Dermatol. 129, 278–288.

Mauri, C., Bosma, A., 2012. Immune regulatory function of B cells. Annu. Rev. Immunol. 30, 221–241.

Mauri, C., Gray, D., Mushtaq, N., Londei, M., 2003. Prevention of arthritis by interleukin 10-producing B cells. J. Exp. Med. 197, 489–501.

McGaha, T.L., Sorrentino, B., Ravetch, J.V., 2005. Restoration of tolerance in lupus by targeted inhibitory receptor expression. Science. 307, 590–593.

McHeyzer-Williams, L.J., McHeyzer-Williams, M.G., 2005. Antigen-specific memory B cell development. Annu. Rev. Immunol. 23, 487–513.

Mingari, M.C., Gerosa, F., Carra, G., Accolla, R.S., Moretta, A., Zubler, R.H., et al., 1984. Human interleukin-2 promotes proliferation of activated B cells via surface receptors similar to those of activated T cells. Nature 312, 641–643.

Monroe, J.G., 2006. ITAM-mediated tonic signalling through pre-BCR and BCR complexes. Nat. Rev. Immunol. 6, 283–294.

Muramatsu, M., Kinoshita, K., Fagarasan, S., Yamada, S., Shinkai, Y., Honjo, T., 2000. Class switch recombination and hypermutation require activation-induced cytidine deaminase (AID), a potential RNA editing enzyme. Cell 102, 553–563.

Navarra, S.V., Guzman, R.M., Gallacher, A.E., Hall, S., Levy, R.A., Jimenez, R.E., et al., 2011. Efficacy and safety of belimumab in patients with active systemic lupus erythematosus: a randomised, placebo-controlled, phase 3 trial. Lancet. 377, 721–731.

Ng, L.G., Sutherland, A.P., Newton, R., Qian, F., Cachero, T.G., Scott, M.L., et al., 2004. B cell-activating factor belonging to the TNF family (BAFF)-R is the principal BAFF receptor facilitating BAFF costimulation of circulating T and B cells. J. Immunol. 173, 807–817.

Niederer, H.A., Clatworthy, M.R., Willcocks, L.C., Smith, K.G., 2010. FcgammaRIIB, FcgammaRIIIB, and systemic lupus erythematosus. Ann. N.Y. Acad. Sci. 1183, 69–88.

Noelle, R.J., 1996. CD40 and its ligand in host defense. Immunity 4, 415–419.

Nossal, G.J., Pike, B.L., 1980. Clonal anergy: persistence in tolerant mice of antigen-binding B lymphocytes incapable of responding to antigen or mitogen. Proc. Natl. Acad. Sci. USA 77, 1602–1606.

Nussenzweig, M.C., Shaw, A.C., Sinn, E., Danner, D.B., Holmes, K.L., Morse 3rd, H.C., et al., 1987. Allelic exclusion in transgenic mice that express the membrane form of immunoglobulin mu. Science 236, 816–819.

O'Keefe, T.L., Williams, G.T., Batista, F.D., Neuberger, M.S., 1999. Deficiency in CD22, a B cell-specific inhibitory receptor, is sufficient to predispose to development of high affinity autoantibodies. J. Exp. Med. 189, 1307–1313.

Palanichamy, A., Barnard, J., Zheng, B., Owen, T., Quach, T., Wei, C., et al., 2009. Novel human transitional B cell populations revealed by B cell depletion therapy. J. Immunol. 182, 5982–5993.

Pelanda, R., Torres, R.M., 2012. Central B-cell tolerance: where selection begins. Cold Spring Harb. Perspect. Biol. 4, a007146.

Pillai, S., Mattoo, H., Cariappa, A., 2011. B cells and autoimmunity. Curr. Opin. Immunol. 23, 721–731.

Revy, P., Muto, T., Levy, Y., Geissmann, F., Plebani, A., Sanal, O., et al., 2000. Activation-induced cytidine deaminase (AID) deficiency causes the autosomal recessive form of the Hyper-IgM syndrome (HIGM2). Cell 102, 565–575.

Rice, J.S., Newman, J., Wang, C., Michael, D.J., Diamond, B., 2005. Receptor editing in peripheral B cell tolerance. Proc. Natl. Acad. Sci. USA 102, 1608–1613.

Rousset, F., Garcia, E., Defrance, T., Peronne, C., Vezzio, N., Hsu, D. H., et al., 1992. Interleukin 10 is a potent growth and differentiation factor for activated human B lymphocytes. Proc. Natl. Acad. Sci. USA 89, 1890–1893.

Rowland, S.L., Leahy, K.F., Halverson, R., Torres, R.M., Pelanda, R., 2010. BAFF receptor signaling aids the differentiation of immature B cells into transitional B cells following tonic BCR signaling. J. Immunol. 185, 4570–4581.

Rowland, S.L., Tuttle, K., Torres, R.M., Pelanda, R., 2012. Antigen and cytokine receptor signals guide the development of the naive mature B cell repertoire. Immunol. Res. 55, 231–240.

Schneider, P., Mackay, F., Steiner, V., Hofmann, K., Bodmer, J.L., Holler, N., et al., 1999. BAFF, a novel ligand of the tumor necrosis factor family, stimulates B cell growth. J. Exp. Med. 189, 1747–1756.

Spaargaren, M., Beuling, E.A., Rurup, M.L., Meijer, H.P., Klok, M.D., Middendorp, S., et al., 2003. The B cell antigen receptor controls integrin activity through Btk and PLCgamma2. J. Exp. Med. 198, 1539–1550.

Thien, M., Phan, T.G., Gardam, S., Amesbury, M., Basten, A., Mackay, F., et al., 2004. Excess BAFF rescues self-reactive B cells from peripheral deletion and allows them to enter forbidden follicular and marginal zone niches. Immunity 20, 785–798.

Tze, L.E., Schram, B.R., Lam, K.P., Hogquist, K.A., Hippen, K.L., Liu, J., et al., 2005. Basal immunoglobulin signaling actively maintains developmental stage in immature B cells. PLoS Biol. 3, e82.

Vascotto, F., Lankar, D., Faure-Andre, G., Vargas, P., Diaz, J., Le Roux, D., et al., 2007. The actin-based motor protein myosin II regulates MHC class II trafficking and BCR-driven antigen presentation. J. Cell Biol. 176, 1007–1019.

Wang, H., Feng, J., Qi, C.F., Li, Z., Morse 3rd, H.C., Clarke, S.H., 2007. Transitional B cells lose their ability to receptor edit but retain their potential for positive and negative selection. J. Immunol. 179, 7544–7552.

Wardemann, H., Yurasov, S., Schaefer, A., Young, J.W., Meffre, E., Nussenzweig, M.C., 2003. Predominant autoantibody production by early human B cell precursors. Science 301, 1374–1377.

Part 3

Non-Antigen-Specific Recognition

Role of Macrophages in Autoimmunity

Siamon Gordon[1] and Annette Plüddemann[2]

[1]Sir William Dunn School of Pathology, University of Oxford, Oxford, UK, [2]Department of Primary Care Health Sciences, University of Oxford, Oxford, UK

Chapter Outline

Introduction 161
Origin and Distribution of Monocytes and
Macrophages 162
Recognition, Sensing, and Responses 163
Phagocytosis, Antigen Presentation, and Secretion 166
Activation and Downregulation: Interactions
with T and B lymphocytes 167
Role of Macrophages in Adaptive Immunity and
Tolerance 168
Role of Macrophages in Autoimmune Models
and Diseases 168
Generation of Autoantigens 169
Modulation of Macrophage
Activation 169
Conclusions and Questions 171
Acknowledgments 171
References 171

INTRODUCTION

Although the role of macrophages in innate immunity, and of closely related dendritic cells (DCs) as the bridge to adaptive immunity, has been amply recognized, most recently through the award of Nobel Prizes, their contribution to autoimmunity has been strangely neglected, often reduced to a secondary role in inflammation and tissue injury. A primary role for macrophages in the initiation and perpetuation of autoimmune diseases remains elusive. This is partly due to semantics, if autoimmunity is restricted to antigen-specific drivers of T and B lymphocytes, whereas in many instances the pathogenic role of antigen-activated T and B cells cannot be ascribed only to their own effector cytokines and antibodies, which may themselves be secondary to dysregulated antigen presentation. Moreover, in many classic autoimmune diseases it has not been possible to identify specific autoantigens. The recent delineation of rare but instructive autoinflammatory syndromes, their attribution to genetic abnormalities in intracellular sensing pathways of macrophages, and the dramatic benefits of IL-1 receptor antagonist treatment indicate that there may be a continuous spectrum of genetic and environmental inflammatory diseases that are not strictly autoimmune, but which cannot be easily distinguished from demonstrably antigen-driven conditions. Furthermore, it is invidious to separate the contributions of myeloid antigen presenting cells (APC, DC, and macrophages), from B and T cell subpopulations, as well as humoral mediators, even interactions with tissue-specific non-hematopoietic stromal cells in the pathogenesis of "autoimmune" tissue injury. In this chapter we review, concisely, the properties of macrophages, and, to a lesser extent DC, which can give rise to autoimmune diseases, and consider particular examples in which macrophage molecules and functions could contribute substantially. We focus on human disease where known. More detailed reviews can be consulted for an overview of macrophage immunobiology (Gordon, 2012).

The classic problem of innate and adaptive immunity is to recognize and discriminate between "self" and "nonself," such as microbial constituents. This question remains open; the multicellular organism has to distinguish altered/modified self from self to maintain homeostasis, for example by the safe, non-inflammatory removal of dying cells and their products, a major function of specialized phagocytes. Toll-like receptors (TLR) sense ligands of exogenous origin, but also react to endogenous stimuli. Although additional plasma membrane and cytoplasmic sensors and receptors have now

N. Rose & I. Mackay (Eds): The Autoimmune Diseases, Fifth edition. DOI: http://dx.doi.org/10.1016/B978-0-12-384929-8.00011-3

been identified, the structural determinants of their selectivity are not sufficient to account for self/non-self recognition. The answer presumably lies in the complex interactions of receptors, signaling pathways, and gene expression.

From the macrophage viewpoint, their primary function is to maintain systemic homeostasis; in addition to host defense against infection, a range of mechanisms exist to limit potentially deleterious effector responses below a disease threshold; when such a threshold is exceeded, the host response becomes pathological and can give rise to acute or chronic inflammation, especially if the stimulus persists. We therefore pay particular attention to known mechanisms of sensing a threat or abnormality, and the regulation of activation, both by macrophages themselves and in combination with other cells and mediators of inflammation.

Mouse models of genetic manipulation, microbial and sterile host stimulation have been particularly useful in studying autoimmune diseases, including diabetes, colitis, arthritis, multiple sclerosis, and glomerulonephritis, but translation to naturally occurring human autoimmune diseases remains problematic. Recent studies on human genomics, identification of inborn errors and polymorphisms, combined with improved definition of lymphocyte subsets, gene expression and cytokines, have made it possible to gain insights into diseases such as rheumatoid arthritis, systemic lupus erythematosus (SLE), and uveitis. However, while the macrophage effector mechanisms clearly are integral to these diseases, their study within human tissue, normally and in a range of conditions, remains limited.

ORIGIN AND DISTRIBUTION OF MONOCYTES AND MACROPHAGES

Traditional views of the mononuclear phagocytic system, derived mainly from studies in the mouse, are undergoing change, with current emphasis on the distinct origins of Langerhans cells and microglia, for example, even in the adult, from yolk sac, fetal liver, and bone marrow (Hoeffel et al., 2012). Antigen markers and chemokine receptors are differentially expressed on distinct subsets of blood monocytes, in humans as well as mice (Figure 11.1) (Ziegler-Heitbrock et al., 2010). Macrophages and closely related DC, which share progenitors and overlapping markers, are widely distributed in lymphohematopoietic and non-hematopoietic tissues throughout life, in the absence of inflammation, as so-called resident cells. Recent studies have reported a novel DC-specific transcription factor zDC which is not

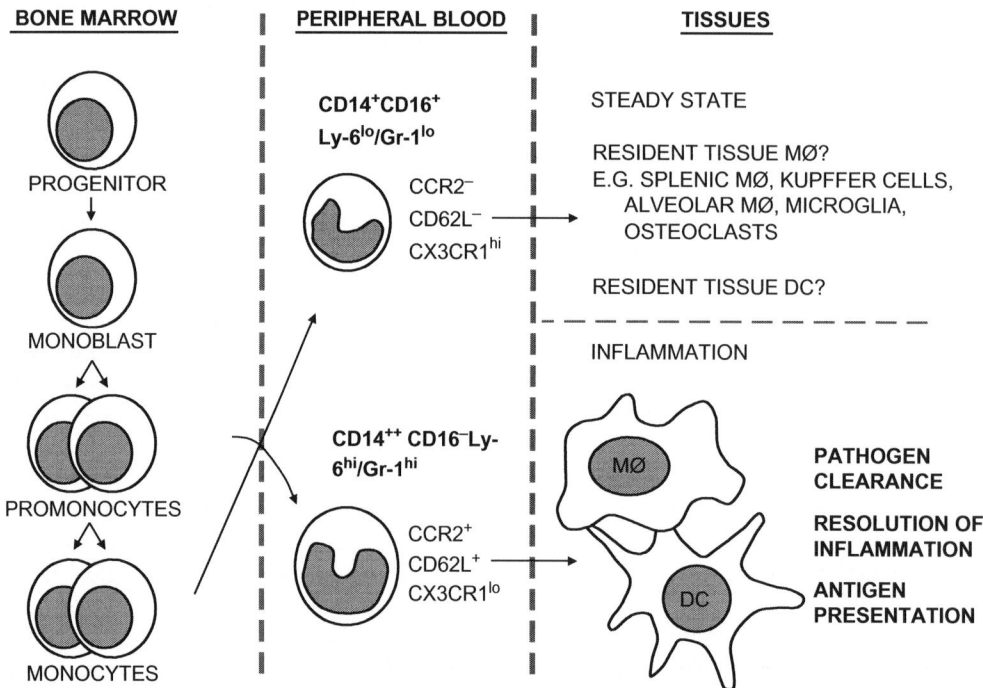

FIGURE 11.1 Schematic presentation of monocyte heterogeneity. Monocytes are present as two distinct subsets which express different surface antigens and chemokine receptors, corresponding to the origin of distinct resident and recruited tissue macrophages. See text for further details.

expressed by monocytes or macrophages (Meredith et al., 2012; Satpathy et al., 2012). Resident macrophages perform phagocytic, clearance, and poorly understood trophic functions; they act as tissue sentinels, able to initiate inflammation and contribute to repair, following injury and infection. A great deal remains unknown concerning their particular functions in different tissues. They arise from hematopoietic progenitors, respond to growth factors such as CSF-1 and GM-CSF, circulate as monocytes, and can be constitutively recruited to tissues such as lung, gut, and brain from early on in development, by poorly understood mechanisms.

In response to injury and infection, a selected monocyte inflammatory subpopulation can be recruited by chemokines and well-defined adhesion molecules to tissues, where they adapt to their local microenvironment. Such recruited cells acquire a new phenotype, including the ability to generate proinflammatory cytokines, to generate a respiratory burst, with release of oxidative radicals, and to serve as APC. Another subpopulation of monocytes appears to patrol the intravascular compartment (Cros et al., 2010).

Apoptosis plays an important part in macrophage turnover especially in an inflammatory milieu, including granulomata, infections such as tuberculosis, and in atherosclerosis. Fas/fas ligand interactions are important as shown in mouse strains that are susceptible to lymphoproliferative as well as myelodysplastic syndromes (Strasser et al., 2009).

The relationship of macrophages to myeloid-derived classical DC is not entirely clear; many genes are expressed in common (Moberg, 2011; Miller et al., 2012), but the mature cells acquire distinct functions; plasmacytoid DC (PDC) differ with regard to marker expression and specialized functions (Hanabuchi and Liu, 2011). Human monocytes can be differentiated by cultivation in different growth factor-containing media to become DC-like APC or acquire macrophage functions. While macrophages and DCs are terminally differentiated, non-proliferating, relatively radio-resistant cells, selected resident and inflammatory recruited macrophages are capable of renewal and local expansion (Jenkins et al., 2011).

Much remains to be learnt about particular resident and newly recruited tissue macrophage populations in humans. The use of marker antigens, F4/80 (Gordon et al., 2011) in the mouse and CD68 in humans as well as the mouse, has made it possible to identify tissue macrophages by immunocytochemistry (Gordon, 2012), and to a lesser extent by FACS analysis. Once within tissues, macrophages are modulated by their local environment, neighboring cells and extracellular matrix, cytokines, and through cell–cell interactions. In mice it is possible to distinguish different phenotypes of activated macrophages as innate, classically activated, or alternatively activated

(Gordon and Martinez, 2010). The signature markers derive mainly from in vitro studies with interferon gamma and IL-4/13, respectively, as well as immune complexes (Fleming and Mosser, 2011), which yield distinct regulatory-type macrophages, discussed further below. Markers to identify different forms of activated human macrophages in tissue are still poorly defined.

Granuloma formation is associated with selected infections, e.g., tuberculosis and schistosome egg deposition, and other chronic, persistent inflammatory lesions, such as Crohn's disease. They contain abundant activated, often fused macrophages, as well as lymphoid and other myeloid cells. The determinants of macrophage fusion and giant cell formation have been studied mainly in vitro (Helming and Gordon, 2009). In situ analysis of phenotype and intravital studies of cell motility (Germain et al., 2012), granuloma formation, and function in mice suggest containment of infection, and promotion of healing. The possible role of macrophages in fibrosis is still obscure (Wynn and Ramalingam, 2012).

Concomitant with activation, a range of deactivating cytokines and arachidonate metabolites downregulate (IL-10) or modulate macrophages (TGF-β, prostaglandin E), thus limiting potentially deleterious inflammatory effects, e.g., after uptake of apoptotic cells, and promoting repair. Plasma membrane glycoproteins, such as CD200/CD200R (Mukhopadhyay et al., 2011) and SIRPα/CD47 (Han et al., 2012), downregulate a range of macrophage responses. Other negative regulators include TLR-related antagonists and the SOCS cytoplasmic proteins.

RECOGNITION, SENSING, AND RESPONSES

Macrophages express a wide range of receptors recognizing pathogenic and host-derived ligands (Figure 11.2). These include opsonic Fc receptors (Nimmerjahn and Ravetch, 2008) and complement receptors (Carroll, 2004); and non-opsonic receptors, such as lectins (e.g., DC-SIGN, Mannose Receptor, Dectin-1), and scavenger receptors (e.g., SR-A I/II, MARCO) (Taylor et al., 2005b). We place particular emphasis on the non-opsonic receptors since their potential role in autoimmune disease is less appreciated, compared with the contribution of Fc and complement receptors.

Fc and complement receptors are heterogeneous in structure and expression, and function by either activating or inhibiting macrophage responses, depending on the receptor and ligand (Carroll, 2004; Nimmerjahn and Ravetch, 2008). Opsonins which promote uptake by these receptors include antibody, IgG complexed with antigens, complement molecules, fibronectin, or milk fat globulins. Macrophages

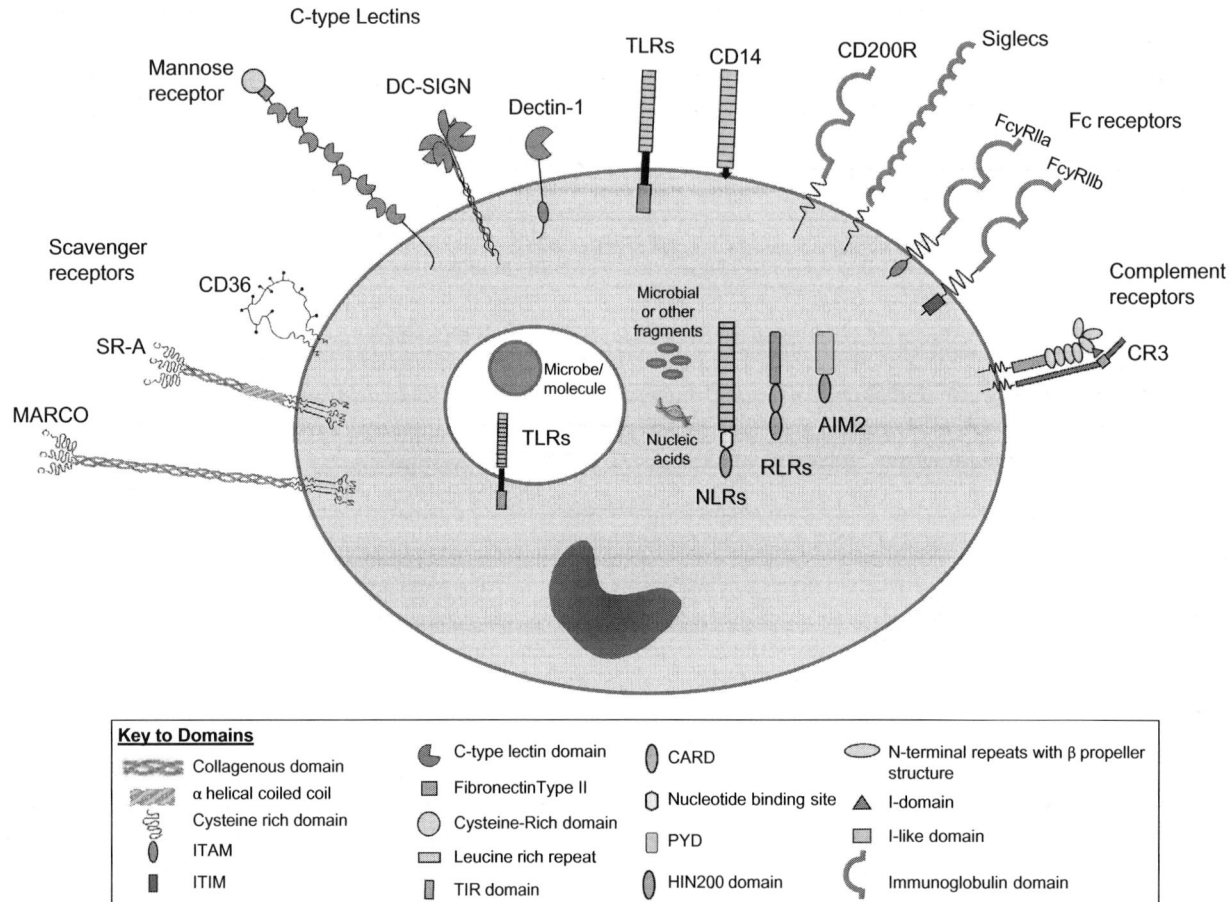

FIGURE 11.2   Schematic structures of selected macrophage receptors.   Macrophages express a wide variety of receptors which mediate recognition of self and non-self molecules. Phagocytic surface receptors include non-opsonic receptors (e.g., C-type lectins and scavenger receptors), as well as opsonic receptors (e.g., complement receptors and Fc receptors). Toll-like receptors (TLRs) are sensors, of which some are expressed on the surface (e.g., TLR4), while others are vacuolar (e.g., TLR9). Sensing receptors are also found in the cytoplasm and these include the NOD-like receptors (NLRs), RIG-like receptors (RLRs) and DNA sensors (e.g., AIM2). Abbreviations: AIM2, absent in melanoma 2; CARD, caspase recruitment and activation domain; CR3, complement receptor 3; FcγR, Fc gamma receptor; ITAM/ITIM; immunoreceptor tyrosine-based activation/inhibition motif; MARCO, macrophage receptor with collagenous structure; NLRs, NOD-like receptors; PYD, pyrin domain; RLRs, RIG-like receptors; SR-A, scavenger receptor A; Siglecs, sialic acid-binding Ig-like lectins; TLRs, Toll-like receptors.

express a range of receptors recognizing complement cleavage products, e.g., CR3, which also has a role in the clearance of apoptotic cells. Resident macrophages in liver and pancreas express a newly described CRIg which plays a protective role in autoimmune diabetes (Fu et al., 2012). Fc receptors belong to the immunoglobulin superfamily and have immunoreceptor tyrosine-based activation or inhibitory motifs (ITAMs and ITIMs), which interact with other membrane molecules and cytoplasmic kinases to regulate complex signaling pathways.

The macrophage *scavenger receptors* are a large family of structurally diverse receptors, which recognize a range of ligands including modified low density lipoproteins (LDL), selected polyanionic ligands, and microbial structures (Pluddemann et al., 2007). The Class A scavenger receptor I (SR-AI) was the first to be identified in studies by Brown

and Goldstein who investigated the accumulation of cholesterol from LDL in atherosclerotic plaques. Other Class A scavenger receptors expressed on macrophages include two alternative splice variants of the SR-AI gene, SR-AII, and the distinct macrophage receptor with collagenous structure (MARCO). The receptors are all trimeric type II transmembrane glycoproteins generally consisting of several domains including an α helical coiled-coil domain, collagenous domain, and C-terminal cysteine-rich domain, although MARCO lacks the coiled—coil domain and has a longer collagenous domain. For SR-AI and SR-AII the collagenous domain has been shown to be the ligand-binding domain, whereas for MARCO this may lie within the cysteine-rich domain. SR-A are expressed on tissue macrophages and selected endothelia, but not resting monocytes, while MARCO is constitutively expressed on subpopulations of tissue macrophages (resident peritoneal, spleen marginal zone, and medullary lymph node macrophages). For Class B scavenger receptors CD36 and SR-B, ligand binding is likely mediated via the central part of the extracellular loop structure and these receptors recognize not only modified LDL, but also native lipoproteins (VLDL, LDL, and HDL), and play an important role in cholesterol transport, metabolism, and homeostasis. Other scavenger receptors expressed by macrophages include CD68 and FEEL-1 (predominantly expressed intracellularly), SREC, and SR-PSOX. SREC receptors have been shown to bind molecular chaperones (e. g., calreticulin, gp96, and heat shock protein 70), playing a role in the transport of ligands to the major histocompatibility complex (MHC) Class-I antigen presentation pathway (Berwin et al., 2004). SR-PSOX is the chemokine ligand for a G protein-coupled CXC chemokine receptor 6 (CXCR6) expressed on activated T cells and NKT cells, supporting adhesion of these cells to DCs (Shimaoka et al., 2004).

C-type lectin receptors expressed on macrophages include the mannose receptor (MR), DC-SIGN, SIGNR1, Dectin-1, and Dectin-2 (Gazi and Martinez-Pomares, 2009; Kerrigan and Brown, 2010). These receptors generally have one or more carbohydrate recognition domains and bind ligands in a Ca^{2+}-dependent manner recognizing either mannose- or galactose-type ligands (McGreal et al., 2005). In some cases recognition is independent of the carbohydrate recognition domain or Ca^{2+}. Dectin-1, a β-glucan receptor, bears a cytoplasmic hemi-ITAM, which is coupled to Syk kinase and signals via CARD9, resulting in activation of NF-κB, thereby contributing to induction of innate and adaptive immunity (Drummond et al., 2011). Collectively, these receptors do not only play a role in pathogen recognition (fungi, bacteria, and viruses), but also recognize endogenous ligands. MR can bind to sulfated carbohydrates found on endogenous glycoproteins (e.g., sialoadhesin and CD45) via a cysteine-rich domain (Fiete et al., 1998) and has been shown to play an important role in the clearance of self-antigens. This receptor has been implicated in controlling levels of the pituitary hormone lutropin, thereby playing a role in fertility (Mi et al., 2002). Dectin-1 also interacts with an endogenous ligand on activated T cells, contributing to T cell proliferation, and can stimulate both $CD4^+$ and $CD8^+$ T cells (Ariizumi et al., 2000; Willment et al., 2001). Dectin-1 agonists have been shown to activate DCs, promoting Th1/Th17 differentiation and initiating IL-17 expression by Treg cells (Drummond et al., 2011).

Macrophage receptor recognition of endogenous ligands has been implicated in several *disease processes*. Class A scavenger receptors SR-A and MARCO recognize oxidized and acetylated LDL and play a role in vascular disease by mediating uptake of these modified lipoproteins, leading to the formation of lipid laden foam cells in atherosclerotic lesions (Krieger and Herz,

1994). SR-A and CD36 have also been implicated in the pathology of Alzheimer's disease, where microglia bind β-amyloid fibrils via SR-A and CD36, which stimulates production of cytotoxic reactive oxygen molecules (Santiago-Garcia et al., 2001). Macrophages bind and endocytose advanced glycation end products (AGE) via several receptors including the scavenger receptors SR-AII and CD36, and the AGE receptors 1, 2, and 3 (Lu et al., 2004). AGE are found in many tissues during oxidative stress and inflammation, such as atherosclerotic lesions of arterial walls and kidneys of diabetic patients with chronic renal failure (Nagai et al., 2000), as well as during ageing. Recently, dietary AGE (e.g., from processed food) have also been linked to chronic kidney injury, for example by suppressing AGER1 and inducing oxidative stress and inflammatory responses, thus contributing to pathogenesis and complications of diabetes mellitus (Vlassara and Striker, 2011).

Macrophages play a role in tissue *maintenance and homeostasis*, for example the involvement of several macrophage receptors (e.g., SR-A, CD36, CD14) in the clearance of apoptotic cells, such as apoptotic thymocytes and olfactory sensory neurons, via recognition of cell surface-exposed oxidized phosphatidylserine and phosphatidylcholine (Taylor et al., 2005b). TAM receptor tyrosine kinases Tyro3, Axl, and Mer and their ligands (Gas6 and Protein S) are essential for the phagocytosis of apoptotic cells and membranes. TAM signaling is normally activated by TLR and type I interferon signaling, as part of the innate inflammatory response in macrophages and DCs (Rothlin and Lemke, 2010). The recognition of apoptotic cells by CD36 has been shown to contribute to peripheral tolerance and prevention of autoimmunity by impairing DC maturation (e.g., ligation of cell surface CD36 negatively regulates DC maturation by enhancing IL-10 secretion and reducing the secretion of TNF-α and IL-1β) (Puig-Kroger et al., 2006). The mannose receptor (MR) is mostly localized intracellularly and is involved in endocytosis, contributing to clearance of mannose-terminal lysosomal hydrolases, neutrophil granule glycoproteins (e.g., myeloperoxidase), hormones (e.g., thyroglobulin), and exocrine secretion products (e.g., amylase) (Gazi and Martinez-Pomares, 2009). Some receptors are specific for recognition of markers of tissue damage and initiate sterile inflammation, for example, the DC-restricted receptor DNGR-1 (Clec9A), a receptor for necrotic cells, recognizes the F-actin component of the cellular cytoskeleton (Ahrens et al., 2012; Zhang et al., 2012).

Some lectins expressed by macrophages, such as Siglec-1, recognize sialic acid molecules and are involved in *cell–cell interactions* (Taylor et al., 2005b). The scavenger receptor CD36 has been shown to mediate adhesion between macrophages and activated platelets via interaction with the platelet glycoprotein, thrombospondin (Silverstein et al., 1989). This adhesion may, for example, play a role in macrophage recruitment to areas of vascular injury. Ligands for MARCO have been reported on subsets of splenic marginal zone B cells and disruption of these cell–cell interactions was shown to be critical for development and maintenance of the rodent spleen marginal zone microarchitecture (Karlsson et al., 2003; Chen et al., 2005). DCs express high levels of MARCO in response to tumor lysate, inducing specific antitumor responses (Grolleau et al., 2003).

Receptor expression depends on the cell type (monocyte, macrophage, or DC), tissue micro-environment and activation state. For these receptors, ligand recognition generally triggers endocytosis or phagocytosis, depending on the size and nature of the ligand, and receptors can cooperate in the recognition of complex ligands. Phagocytosis/endocytosis triggers complex signaling pathways, membrane and cytoskeleton remodeling, and fusion of phagosomes/endosomes with other intracellular vesicles. Depending on the ligand, secretion of low molecular weight metabolites and pro- and/or anti-inflammatory molecules is triggered. Upon phagocytosis of pathogens, killing mechanisms are initiated, which include oxidative (e.g., the respiratory burst) and non-oxidative methods (e.g., antimicrobial peptides). The ability to activate host immune defense pathways varies among receptors.

Sensing is mediated via TLRs expressed on the macrophage plasma membrane or within endocytic compartments, and cytosolic NOD-like (NLR) and RIG-I helicase (RLR) families of receptors, which form part of multiprotein complexes called inflammasomes (Kanneganti et al., 2007; Kawai and Akira, 2011; Loo and Gale, 2011). The *TLRs* are a family of type I transmembrane receptors with an extracellular domain containing leucine-rich repeats (LRRs) and a cytoplasmic portion homologous to the interleukin-1 receptor family (IL-1R) (O'Neill, 2008). The cytoplasmic domain interacts with adaptor molecules MyD88 ("myeloid differentiation primary response protein 88"), TRAM ("Toll-like receptor adaptor molecule"), TRIF ["Toll-interleukin-1 receptor (TIR)-domain-containing adaptor inducing IFN-β"], and TIRAP/Mal ("TIR-domain containing adaptor protein") and the adaptor molecules vary between different TLRs. Interaction with the adaptor molecules induces signal transduction pathways leading to the activation of the transcription factor NF-κB, MAP kinases p38, and Jun N-terminal kinase (JNK), as well as interferon regulatory factors. Apart from bacterial ligands, TLRs can recognize endogenous ligands, such as heat-shock proteins. TLR signaling has been shown to play a role in the initiation and progression of non-infectious inflammatory processes, e.g., rheumatoid arthritis, experimental autoimmune encephalitis

(EAE), and others (Lin et al., 2011). Recently, an endogenous TLR ligand has been identified, which may play a role in persistent activation of macrophages in chronic inflammatory diseases such as rheumatoid arthritis (Shi et al., 2012). TLR stimulation may also promote inflammatory macrophages in atherosclerosis (Seneviratne et al., 2012) and genome-wide association studies have linked TLR7 and TLR8 to the genetic susceptibility to coeliac disease, a common autoimmune disorder (Netea et al., 2012).

The *NLR family* of receptors consist of a combination of domains, including a central nucleotide-binding and oligomerization (NACHT) domain, which is commonly flanked by C-terminal leucine-rich repeats (LRRs) and N-terminal caspase recruitment (CARD) or pyrin (PYD) domains (Schroder and Tschopp, 2010). Within the NLRs there are three distinct subfamilies, namely the NODs, the NLRPs, and the IPAFs. The carboxy-terminal leucine-rich repeats are thought to sense different microbial and endogenous damage stimuli. Intracellular nucleic acid sensors include the RIG-like helicases RIG-I and MDA5, and the DNA sensor, DAI and AIM2. Recognition of microbial molecules, such as microbial nucleic acids, by these receptors mediates inflammasome activation, which involves assembly of procaspase-1 with different members of the nucleotide-binding domain, leucine-rich repeat (LRR) protein family (NLRs), or absent in melanoma 2 (AIM2)-like receptors (ALRs), or, as recently demonstrated, guanylate-binding protein 5 (GBP5) (Shenoy et al., 2012). This results in caspase cleavage and production of IL-1β and IL-18 (Schroder and Tschopp, 2010).

PHAGOCYTOSIS, ANTIGEN PRESENTATION, AND SECRETION

Macrophages play an important role in the recognition, phagocytosis, and endocytosis, not only of microbes and foreign particles, but also of modified host components. Macrophages can initiate and perpetuate chronic and acute inflammation, but depending on the ligand and receptors involved, uptake may be silent (clearance) or even suppress inflammation [e.g., uptake of apoptotic cells by macrophages (Henson and Bratton, 2009)]. In general, phagocytosis consists of formation of a phagocytic synapse (Goodridge et al., 2011), phagosome formation, fusion with secretory vesicles from the Golgi, lowering of pH and digestion, and maturation to lysosomes/phagolysosomes (Fairn et al., 2009; Mukherjee and Maxfield, 2009; Swanson, 2009). PI3-kinase and phosphoinositides play a role in the initial fusion and association between cellular membranes and cytoskeleton, while membrane trafficking is controlled by small GTPases (Ridley and Hall, 2004; Swanson, 2008). Uptake may lead to antigen processing and presentation, e.g., SR-A has been shown to mediate uptake of modified antigens for presentation to antigen-specific T cells (Nicoletti et al., 1999). Macrophage cellular responses include inflammasome activation, autophagy, apoptosis, and necrosis. The secretion pathways of pro- and anti-inflammatory cytokines have been extensively described (Kaiser and O'Garra, 2009). Proinflammatory cytokines (e.g., IL-6, TNF) can activate the macrophage itself, recruit other inflammatory cells, or mediate T cell and natural killer cell activation. They induce acute phase proteins, which act as opsonins and pyrogens. Anti-inflammatory cytokines (e.g., IL-4, IL-10, TGF-β) downregulate macrophages and reduce inflammation, affecting different cellular processes, such as proliferation, differentiation, and apoptosis, among others. Interferons (IFNs) inhibit viral replication and cell proliferation, upregulate MHC class I expression, and downregulate MHC class II expression. Recently, interferons have been shown to play a role in autoimmunity, for example SLE and diabetes (Gough et al., 2012). Macrophages also secrete other important growth and differentiation factors, such as enzymes and pro-enzymes, which regulate angiogenesis, as well as antimicrobial peptides, lytic agents, and inhibitory proteins. Resolution of acute inflammation is mediated by specialized proresolving mediators (SPMs), such as lipoxins, resolvins, protectins, and maresins, which are produced by macrophages from the endogenous essential fatty acid, docosahexaenoic acid (DHA) (Campbell et al., 2011). Activated macrophages can exert effector functions by inducing apoptosis in other cells via Fas-ligand and nitric oxide (Strasser et al., 2009). Mutations in Fas have been shown to lead to the development of lymphoproliferation and autoimmune disease and normal expression of Fas in inflammatory macrophages plays an important role in maintaining systemic immune homeostasis (Cuda et al., 2012).

Recognition of cytosolic proteins, nucleic acids, and breakdown products is mediated by inflammasome complexes. As outlined above, these are multiprotein complexes which mediate caspase-1 activation, proteolytic maturation, and secretion of interleukin-1β (IL-1β) and IL-18 (Gross et al., 2011). RIG-I-like receptors recognize viral nucleic acids and interact with an adaptor protein located on the mitochondrial membrane, triggering production of type I interferon and induction of NF-κB (Kato et al., 2011). Apart from microbial molecules, NLRs recognize molecules released during tissue injury, such as recognition of extracellular ATP, hyaluronan, amyloid-β fibrils, and uric acid crystals by NLRP3 (Rathinam et al., 2012). They have been implicated in autoimmune disease, e.g., the association of Nod2 with Crohn's disease (Werts et al., 2011) and the link between polymorphisms in

NLRP1 and SLE (Pontillo et al., 2012). Blocking of IL-1, particularly IL-1β, is now standard therapy for many auto-inflammatory diseases, such as rheumatoid arthritis, osteoarthritis, Blau syndrome, familial Mediterranean fever (FMF), and type 2 diabetes, among others (Dinarello, 2011).

Autophagy is a mechanism which macrophages can use to capture cytoplasmic components in a double-membrane vacuole for degradation in lysosomes. Autophagy is induced by different families of receptors (e.g., TLRs, NOD-like receptors) and is not only a host defense mechanism against intracellular pathogens, but can also be used as a source of nutrients during starvation. Alterations in the functions of autophagy proteins can lead to enhanced susceptibility to disease and have also been implicated in chronic inflammatory and autoimmune disease processes. For example, mutations in regulators of autophagy have been linked to Crohn's disease (Levine et al., 2011).

ACTIVATION AND DOWNREGULATION: INTERACTIONS WITH T AND B LYMPHOCYTES

Macrophages and DC interact with other hematopoietic cells as well as non-hematopoietic cells in all compartments of the body. In the bone marrow, in addition to developing monocytes, macrophages form a part of the hematopoietic stroma, performing a poorly understood trophic role during hematopoiesis, in addition to clearing erythroid nuclei (Crocker et al., 1991). Specialized adhesion molecules, including Siglec1 (CD169), a sialic acid-binding lectin, and another poorly characterized divalent cation-dependent adhesion receptor, contribute to non-phagocytic interactions with erythroblasts, myeloblasts, and possibly plasma cells (Klaas et al., 2012). In the blood or as sinus-lining cells in liver, spleen, and lymph nodes, monocyte/macrophages interact with endothelium and other circulating cells including erythrocytes, neutrophils, platelets, as well as apoptotic and senescent cells.

The marginal zone in rodent spleen (Martinez-Pomares and Gordon, 2012) and the subcapsular sinus of lymph nodes (Gray and Cyster, 2012) represent important interfaces of blood and lymph-borne circulating cells, antigens, and microorganisms with resident lymphoid populations (den Haan and Kraal, 2012). The marginal zone metallophils are macrophage-like and CD169[+], but lack F4/80; the outer marginal zone macrophages are phagocytic, express DC-SIGN as well as MARCO, an adhesion receptor for B1 lymphocytes. Red pulp macrophages are responsible for the clearance of senescent erythrocytes and neutrophils, and in rodents provide a reservoir of monocyte/macrophages for recruitment to peripheral sites of injury, infection, or disturbed metabolism as in atherosclerosis (Swirski et al., 2009). CD68$^+$ macrophages are present in the white pulp of spleen, in T cell-dependent areas, but lack the F4/80 antigen; DCs migrate into such areas after antigenic stimulation. In lymph nodes CD169$^+$ subcapsular macrophages play a role in antigen capture, interactions with DC and, subsequently, B cells. In germinal centers, tingible body and monocyte-derived macrophages play a role in the activation and affinity maturation of B cells and the phagocytosis of apoptotic cells.

Macrophages and DC are present in thymus, where the DCs contribute to thymocyte selection, whereas F4/80$^+$ macrophages remove apoptotic thymocytes. They also associate with viable thymocytes, which are not phagocytosed.

Granulomata contain numerous F4/80$^+$ macrophages, which associate with T lymphocytes, other myeloid cells, and connective tissue stroma. The interactions between macrophages, DC, and lymphocytes in granuloma and other lymphoid tissues are still poorly understood, and involve direct cell–cell contact, release, and capture of exosomes and other secretory products.

ROLE OF MACROPHAGES IN ADAPTIVE IMMUNITY AND TOLERANCE

Study of the phagocytic and non-phagocytic interactions of various macrophages with innate and adaptive lymphoid cells is surprisingly neglected, in spite of the clear evidence that cell surface and secreted cytokines, as well as direct contact through plasma membrane receptors and ligands, profoundly, selectively, and reciprocally modulate macrophage and lymphocyte gene expression, cytokine production, and plasma membrane expression of costimulatory and coinhibitory plasma membrane glycoproteins. Particular attention has been paid to the heterogeneity of T cell subsets, Th1, Th2, Th17, and regulatory T cells (Tregs), and their possible macrophage counterparts. Much remains to be done to define the interplay between macrophages and Tregs (Pearson et al., 2012), and with various cytokine producing innate lymphocytes, such as nuocytes (Barlow and McKenzie, 2011). Macrophage activation syndromes, genetic and acquired, e.g., after viral infection, are poorly understood, compared with primary immunodeficiency of T and B cells. This situation may be changing, with the description of a fas/ligand primary defect involving macrophages (Cuda et al., 2012), and the discovery of a novel oncogene mutation in Langerhans histiocytosis.

Apart from their role in phagocytic removal of apoptotic T and B cells, macrophages clear necrotic cell debris, chromatin, etc. from all dying cells, including those killed by CD8$^+$ cytotoxic T cells. The DCs (Coquerelle and Moser, 2010) are uniquely able to activate naïve, resting CD4$^+$ T helper cells, through their response to maturation stimuli, e.g., adjuvants, potent antigen capture, processing, and presentation in association with MHC molecules, as well as by MHC I-dependent cross-presentation (Joffre et al., 2012). The role of plasmacytoid DC in antigen presentation is less clear. Macrophages, which may express more labile and lower levels of MHCII, degrade potential macromolecular antigens more completely through their arsenal of digestive hydrolases and can activate primed but not naïve lymphocytes. Resting and activated macrophages are also potent suppressors of T cell activation, e.g., through PGE2. Macrophages are a prime source of important Th1 and Th2 activating cytokines, IL12, IL18, IL23, as well as of TNFα, IL-10, TGF-β, and IL-6, an important survival and growth factor for B lymphocytes and plasma cells (Kaiser and O'Garra, 2009). Macrophages may regulate antigen access to DC by phagocytosis, digestion, or release of antigen fragments, for cross-presentation, and influence DC maturation by soluble mediators and surface contact.

DCs pay an important role in central and peripheral tolerance, as well as in immune activation. Macrophages have no known role in central tolerance in the thymus, unlike DC; the autoimmune regulator (AIRE) protein is expressed by ill-defined cells (Metzger and Anderson, 2011), possibly APC, in peripheral tissues. In the periphery, the F4/80 antigen, possibly expressed by a subset of DC rather than macrophages, plays a role in the ACAID tolerance model of the eye (Lin et al., 2005), and also in low dose oral tolerance. Further studies are needed to extend these findings to other mouse models of tolerance and to humans.

The marginal zone of spleen, in particular the MARCO scavenger receptor, has been proposed as a regulator of autoantibody formation (McGaha et al., 2011).

ROLE OF MACROPHAGES IN AUTOIMMUNE MODELS AND DISEASES

From the above overview it is evident that macrophages are an integral component of the innate and adaptive cellular and humoral elements of immunity and hence in autoimmunity and autoinflammatory diseases. Evidence for a primary pathogenic role in autoimmunity will depend on implicating molecules that are myeloid, if not macrophage restricted, or disease models in which myeloid-selective gene knockout, e.g., of fas, excludes primary lymphoid cell functions. The efficacy of anti-TNF and IL-1β treatment indicates that primarily macrophage-derived inflammatory products are major factors in tissue damage, even if part of a more complex immune network. Figure 11.3 and Table 11.1 illustrate

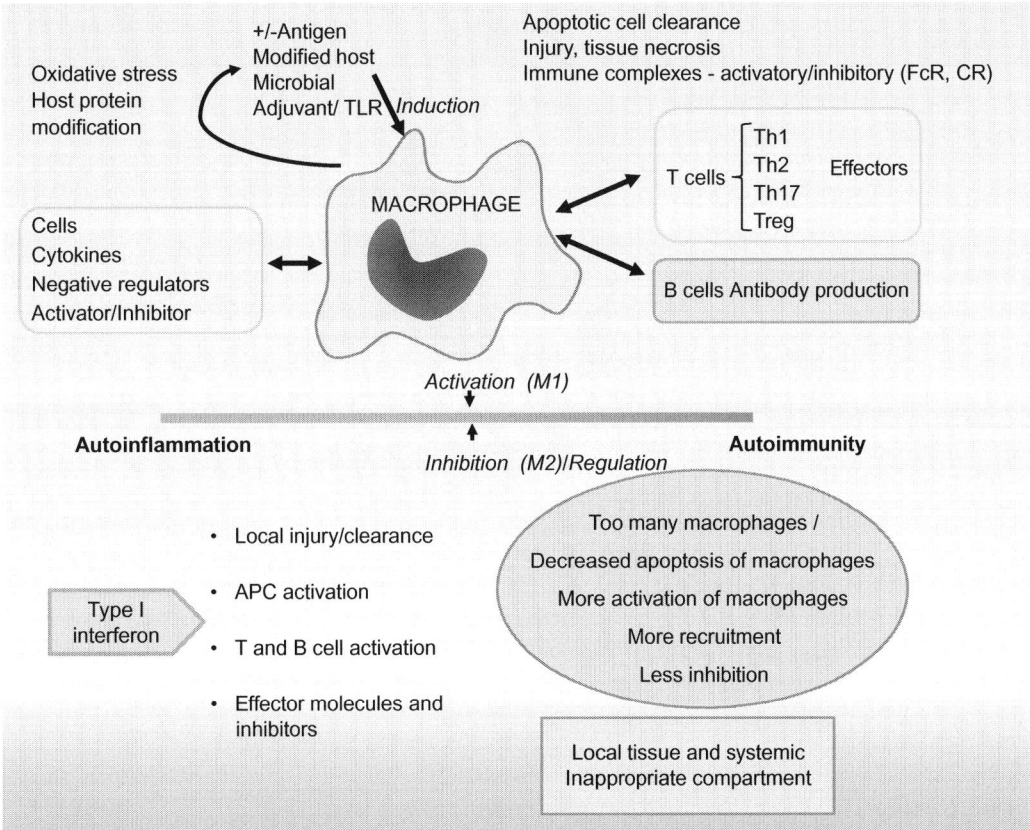

FIGURE 11.3 Overview of macrophage functions which are able to initiate, regulate, and perpetuate autoimmune pathology. Details are discussed in the text.

examples of macrophage function which can initiate and perpetuate autoimmune pathology.

Generation of Autoantigens

Macrophages play a major role in homeostatic clearance of cell debris, and apoptotic bodies generated during cell turnover, physiologically, and in disease. A range of myeloid opsonic and non-opsonic receptors contribute to efficient phagocytosis, endocytosis, and controlled removal, including SR and the family of TAM receptors. C1q deficiency provided an early example of the importance of complement in apoptotic cell clearance (Taylor et al., 2000). A newly described CRIg receptor, expressed by resident macrophages in the pancreas, is protective in the development of early disease in NOD mice (Fu et al., 2012). Host proteins modified by myeloid-induced oxidative injury or amino acid modification, e.g., by citrullination, can give rise to autoantigenicity (Wegner et al., 2010); cross-reaction of host molecules with microbes, for example selected streptococci, contributes to rheumatic fever and heart disease (Cunningham, 2012). The TLR pathway is important in

sensing microbial, adjuvant, and altered host ligands, and interacts with other plasma membrane, endosomal, and cytosolic sensors. Immune complexes, acting via FcR through ITAM/ITIM activatory and inhibitory signaling motifs, have been implicated in SLE (Ivashkiv, 2011).

DC play a major role in uptake, processing, and presentation of peptide antigens in association with MHC molecules and the activation of naïve and primed T and B lymphocytes, as well as of Th17 and Tregs. Macrophages can present antigen to primed T lymphocytes, directly and indirectly, through production of cytokines and autocrine amplification, especially type I interferon. However, we still know little about the intracellular proteolytic hydrolases in APC which limit degradation of proteins, and the actual peptide antigens associated with MHC molecules from macrophages and DC have not been characterized.

Modulation of Macrophage Activation

Recent studies have drawn attention to the balance between M1 (classically activated) and M2 (alternatively

TABLE 11.1 Examples of Macrophage Functions and their Role in Autoimmune Disease

Molecule	Role of molecule	Example disease(s)	Reference
Complement C1q	C1q deficiency—importance of complement in apoptotic cell clearance	Systemic lupus erythematosus (SLE)	(Taylor et al., 2000)
TAM receptors	Apoptotic cell recognition	SLE	(Rothlin and Lemke, 2010)
Toll-like receptors (TLRs)	Sensing receptors—induction of innate immune responses	Type 1 and Type 2 diabetes; SLE, coeliac disease, rheumatoid arthritis	(Lin et al., 2011; Netea et al., 2012)
Nod-like receptors (NLRs)	Cytosolic sensors—induction of immune responses, maintenance of homeostasis	Crohn's disease	(Werts et al., 2011)
Citrullination and oxidative modification	Autoantigenicity	Rheumatoid arthritis	(Wegner et al., 2010)
MARCO	Adhesion, recognition, autoantigen	SLE	(Wermeling et al., 2007; McGaha et al., 2011)
Complement receptor of the immunoglobulin superfamily (CRIg)	Inhibition of activation, proliferation, cytokine production	Protective role in autoimmune diabetes	(Fu et al., 2012)
Fas	Induction of apoptosis	Autoimmune and lymphoproliferative disorders	(Takahashi et al., 1994; Cuda et al., 2012)
Immune complexes	cDC-B cell interactions	SLE	(Joo et al., 2012)
	Defect in rho GTPase activity	SLE	(Fan et al., 2006)
CD200/CD200R interactions	Negative regulation of cell activation by TLR, NLR, and inflammasome	Autoimmune uveitis	(Taylor et al., 2005a)
CD47	Regulation of cell activation	Experimental autoimmune encephalomyelitis (EAE)	(Han et al., 2012)
Indoleamine 2,3-dioxygenase (IDO)	Regulation of immune response to apoptotic cells	SLE	(Ravishankar et al., 2012)
Macrophage inhibitory factor (MIF)	Innate immune response regulation—mediates recruitment and retention of monocytes	SLE	(Leng et al., 2011)
Colony stimulating factor 1 (CSF-1)	Macrophage growth factor—promotes macrophage survival and maturation	SLE/Lupus nephritis	(Menke et al., 2011; Iwata et al., 2012)

activated, regulatory macrophages), its importance in dysregulation, and opportunity for therapeutic manipulation of autoimmunity (Fleming and Mosser, 2011; Parsa et al., 2012). This assessment is likely to be simplistic. The heterogeneity of macrophage gene expression and functions is only beginning to be revealed by *in vitro* and *ex vivo* analysis, and the actual phenotypic markers and functions need to be validated *in situ*, taking due regard of the contribution of the local microbiome (Mathis and Benoist, 2012). Activated macrophages often express a mixed phenotype, requiring further population as well as single cell analysis. The studies of Mosser and colleagues (Fleming and Mosser, 2011) have revealed a striking role for immune complexes in modulating the balance between

IL-12/IL-10, and exploited this in the treatment of autoimmune paralysis in mice. Uptake of autoimmune haematopoietic cells, e.g., platelets and erythrocytes, may contribute to dysregulation of pro- and anti-inflammatory cytokine balance in macrophage activation syndromes.

In principle, macrophages can be increased in number, recruitment, activation, fail to undergo apoptosis, or be inadequately inhibited, tilting the balance between tolerance and immune/inflammatory activation. Indoleamine 2,3-dioxygenase (IDO) has been implicated in the maintenance of peripheral tolerance (Ravishankar et al., 2012). Further studies, including models of autoimmunity, are required to extend our knowledge of the F4/80 molecule in immune tolerance. M-CSF has been implicated in mouse models of renal tubular epithelial injury (Menke et al., 2011; Iwata et al., 2012). Bucala and co-workers have demonstrated a critical role for macrophage inhibitory factor (MIF), a cytokine produced and acting on macrophages, in systemic and local regulation of macrophages (Bucala, 2006; Leng et al., 2011). An intriguing possibility is that anatomic dysregulation of marginal zone macrophages can result in autoimmune activation of B cells, through their interactions with MARCO (Wermeling et al., 2007).

CONCLUSIONS AND QUESTIONS

In order to progress, technical challenges have to be overcome; in humans, improved cell phenotyping and population analysis in tissues, e.g., by laser capture microscopy and immunocytochemistry, before, early, as well as late in the development of autoimmune diseases. Analysis of macrophage-expressed gene polymorphisms in disease-prone individuals should emphasize negative as well as positive controls of macrophage growth, recruitment, activation, and turnover. The identification of biomarkers on readily accessible blood monocytes could improve diagnosis and be used to follow the natural history of systemic autoimmune diseases; a recent example has indicated a correlation between monocyte subsets and Th17 responses (Rossol et al., 2012). In mouse models, better methods are required for selective and efficient macrophage depletion, silencing, and conditional genetic manipulation, distinct from dendritic and other myeloid cells.

The clearance functions of macrophages are mediated by a growing list of plasma membrane receptors. Lectins, such as the macrophage mannose receptor, contribute to the removal of lysosomal hydrolases and degranulation products from the circulation and extracellular space. The proteolytic processing by macrophages and DC and modification of macromolecules by phagocyte oxidation and secretory activities may profoundly affect antigenicity and adjuvanticity.

The balance of activation and inhibition of tissue macrophage phenotypes determines the outcome of many autoimmune diseases, and provides targets for treatment. While the role of macrophage activities and products in diseases like rheumatoid arthritis is established, their possible contribution to systemic autoimmune diseases such as scleroderma, for example, is obscure. The relevance of mouse models to human disease is often problematic. Above all, the predilection of many autoimmune diseases to affect selected tissues such as eyes, joints, and endocrine organs remains obscure. The presence of resident macrophages and possibly organ-specific stromal cells (McGettrick et al., 2012) at these sites and their response to many types of local injury, make them attractive targets for further investigation.

ACKNOWLEDGMENTS

The authors would like to thank Diane Mathis, Christophe Benoist, Richard Bucala, and Vicki Kelley for their help, and the Medical Research Council (United Kingdom) for financial support.

REFERENCES

Ahrens, S., Zelenay, S., Sancho, D., Hanc, P., Kjaer, S., Feest, C., et al., 2012. F-actin is an evolutionarily conserved damage-associated molecular pattern recognized by DNGR-1, a receptor for dead cells. Immunity. 36, 635–645.

Ariizumi, K., Shen, G.L., Shikano, S., XU, S., Ritter 3rd, R., Kumamoto, T., et al., 2000. Identification of a novel, dendritic cell-associated molecule, dectin-1, by subtractive cDNA cloning. J. Biol. Chem. 275, 20157–20167.

Barlow, J.L., McKenzie, A.N., 2011. Nuocytes: expanding the innate cell repertoire in type-2 immunity. J. Leukoc. Biol. 90, 867–874.

Berwin, B., Delneste, Y., Lovingood, R.V., Post, S.R., Pizzo, S.V., 2004. SREC-I, a type F scavenger receptor, is an endocytic receptor for calreticulin. J. Biol. Chem. 279, 51250–51257.

Bucala, R., 2006. MIF and the genetic basis of macrophage responsiveness. Curr. Immunol. Rev. 2, 217–223.

Campbell, E.L., Serhan, C.N., Colgan, S.P., 2011. Antimicrobial aspects of inflammatory resolution in the mucosa: a role for proresolving mediators. J. Immunol. 187, 3475–3481.

Carroll, M.C., 2004. The complement system in regulation of adaptive immunity. Nat. Immunol. 5, 981–986.

Chen, Y., Pikkarainen, T., Elomaa, O., Soininen, R., Kodama, T., Kraal, G., et al., 2005. Defective microarchitecture of the spleen marginal zone and impaired response to a thymus-independent type 2 antigen in mice lacking scavenger receptors MARCO and SR-A. J. Immunol. 175, 8173–8180.

Coquerelle, C., Moser, M., 2010. DC subsets in positive and negative regulation of immunity. Immunol. Rev. 234, 317–334.

Crocker, P.R., Morris, L., Gordon, S., 1991. Adhesion receptors involved in the erythroblastic island. Blood Cells. 17, 83–91 (discussion 91–96).

Cros, J., Cagnard, N., Woollard, K., Patey, N., Zhang, S.Y., Senechal, B., et al., 2010. Human CD14dim monocytes patrol and sense nucleic acids and viruses via TLR7 and TLR8 receptors. Immunity 33, 375–386.

Cuda, C.M., Agrawal, H., Misharin, A.V., Haines 3rd, G.K., Hutcheson, J., Weber, E., et al., 2012. Requirement of myeloid cell-specific Fas expression for prevention of systemic autoimmunity in mice. Arthritis Rheum. 64, 808–820.

Cunningham, M.W., 2012. Streptococcus and rheumatic fever. Curr. Opin. Rheumatol. 24, 408–416.

Den Haan, J.M., Kraal, G., 2012. Innate immune functions of macrophage subpopulations in the spleen. J. Innate Immun. 4, 437–445.

Dinarello, C.A., 2011. Interleukin-1 in the pathogenesis and treatment of inflammatory diseases. Blood 117, 3720–3732.

Drummond, R.A., Saijo, S., Iwakura, Y., Brown, G.D., 2011. The role of Syk/CARD9 coupled C-type lectins in antifungal immunity. Eur. J. Immunol. 41, 276–281.

Fairn, G.D., Gershenzon, E., Grinstein, S., 2009. Membrane trafficking during phagosome formation and maturation. In: Russell, D.G., Gordon, S. (Eds.), Phagocyte—Pathogen Interactions: Macrophages and the Host Response to Infection. ASM Press, Washington, DC.

Fan, H., Patel, V.A., Longacre, A., Levine, J.S., 2006. Abnormal regulation of the cytoskeletal regulator Rho typifies macrophages of the major murine models of spontaneous autoimmunity. J. Leukoc. Biol. 79, 155—165.

Fiete, D.J., Beranek, M.C., Baenziger, J.U., 1998. A cysteine-rich domain of the "mannose" receptor mediates GalNAc-4-SO4 binding. Proc. Natl. Acad. Sci. USA 95, 2089—2093.

Fleming, B.D., Mosser, D.M., 2011. Regulatory macrophages: setting the threshold for therapy. Eur. J. Immunol. 41, 2498—2502.

Fu, W., Wojtkiewicz, G., Weissleder, R., Benoist, C., Mathis, D., 2012. Early window of diabetes determinism in NOD mice, dependent on the complement receptor CRIg, identified by noninvasive imaging. Nat. Immunol. 13, 361—368.

Gazi, U., Martinez-Pomares, L., 2009. Influence of the mannose receptor in host immune responses. Immunobiology. 214, 554—561.

Germain, R.N., Robey, E.A., Cahalan, M.D., 2012. A decade of imaging cellular motility and interaction dynamics in the immune system. Science 336, 1676—1681.

Goodridge, H.S., Reyes, C.N., Becker, C.A., Katsumoto, T.R., Ma, J., Wolf, A.J., et al., 2011. Activation of the innate immune receptor Dectin-1 upon formation of a "phagocytic synapse." Nature 472, 471—475.

Gordon, S., 2012. Macrophages and phagocytosis. In: Paul, W.E. (Ed.), Fundamental Immunology, 7th ed. Lippincott, Williams and Wilkins, Philadelphia, USA.

Gordon, S., Hamann, J., Lin, H.H., Stacey, M., 2011. F4/80 and the related adhesion-GPCRs. Eur. J. Immunol. 41, 2472—2476.

Gordon, S., Martinez, F.O., 2010. Alternative activation of macrophages: mechanism and functions. Immunity 32, 593—604.

Gough, D.J., Messina, N.L., Clarke, C.J., Johnstone, R.W., Levy, D.E., 2012. Constitutive type I interferon modulates homeostatic balance through tonic signaling. Immunity 36, 166—174.

Gray, E.E., Cyster, J.G., 2012. Lymph node macrophages. J. Innate Immun. 4, 424—436.

Grolleau, A., Misek, D.E., Kuick, R., Hanash, S., Mule, J.J., 2003. Inducible expression of macrophage receptor Marco by dendritic cells following phagocytic uptake of dead cells uncovered by oligonucleotide arrays. J. Immunol. 171, 2879—2888.

Gross, O., Thomas, C.J., Guarda, G., Tschopp, J., 2011. The inflammasome: an integrated view. Immunol. Rev. 243, 136—151.

Han, M.H., Lundgren, D.H., Jaiswal, S., Chao, M., Graham, K.L., Garris, C.S., et al., 2012. Janus-like opposing roles of CD47 in autoimmune brain inflammation in humans and mice. J. Exp. Med. 209, 1325—1334.

Hanabuchi, S., Liu, Y.J., 2011. In vivo role of pDCs in regulating adaptive immunity. Immunity. 35, 851—853.

Helming, L., Gordon, S., 2009. Molecular mediators of macrophage fusion. Trends Cell Biol. 19, 514—522.

Henson, P.M., Bratton, D.L., 2009. Recognition and removal of apoptotic cells. In: Russell, D.G., Gordon, S. (Eds.), Phagocyte—Pathogen Interactions: Macrophages and the Host Response to Infection. ASM Press, Washington, DC.

Hoeffel, G., Wang, Y., Greter, M., See, P., Teo, P., Malleret, B., et al., 2012. Adult Langerhans cells derive predominantly from embryonic fetal liver monocytes with a minor contribution of yolk sac-derived macrophages. J. Exp. Med. 209, 1167—1181.

Ivashkiv, L.B., 2011. Inflammatory signaling in macrophages: transitions from acute to tolerant and alternative activation states. Eur. J. Immunol. 41, 2477—2481.

Iwata, Y., Bostrom, E.A., Menke, J., Rabacal, W.A., Morel, L., Wada, T., et al., 2012. Aberrant macrophages mediate defective kidney repair that triggers nephritis in lupus-susceptible mice. J. Immunol. 188, 4568—4580.

Jenkins, S.J., Ruckerl, D., Cook, P.C., Jones, L.H., Finkelman, F.D., Van Rooijen, N., et al., 2011. Local macrophage proliferation, rather than recruitment from the blood, is a signature of TH2 inflammation. Science 332, 1284—1288.

Joffre, O.P., Segura, E., Savina, A., Amigorena, S., 2012. Cross-presentation by dendritic cells. Nat. Rev. Immunol. 12, 557—569.

Joo, H., Coquery, C., Xue, Y., Gayet, I., Dillon, S.R., Punaro, M., et al., 2012. Serum from patients with SLE instructs monocytes to promote IgG and IgA plasmablast differentiation. J. Exp. Med. 209, 1335—1348.

Kaiser, F., O'Garra, A., 2009. Cytokines and macrophages and dendritic cells: key modulators of immune response. In: Russell, D.G., Gordon, S. (Eds.), Phagocyte—Pathogen Interactions: Macrophages and the Host Response to Infection. ASM Press, Washington, DC.

Kanneganti, T.D., Lamkanfi, M., Nunez, G., 2007. Intracellular NOD-like receptors in host defense and disease. Immunity 27, 549—559.

Karlsson, M.C., Guinamard, R., Bolland, S., Sankala, M., Steinman, R. M., Ravetch, J.V., 2003. Macrophages control the retention and trafficking of B lymphocytes in the splenic marginal zone. J. Exp. Med. 198, 333—340.

Kato, H., Takahasi, K., Fujita, T., 2011. RIG-I-like receptors: cytoplasmic sensors for non-self RNA. Immunol. Rev. 243, 91—98.

Kawai, T., Akira, S., 2011. Toll-like receptors and their crosstalk with other innate receptors in infection and immunity. Immunity 34, 637—650.

Kerrigan, A.M., Brown, G.D., 2010. Syk-coupled C-type lectin receptors that mediate cellular activation via single tyrosine based activation motifs. Immunol. Rev. 234, 335—352.

Klaas, M., Oetke, C., Lewis, L.E., Erwig, L.P., Heikema, A.P., Easton, A., et al., 2012. Sialoadhesin promotes rapid proinflammatory and type I IFN responses to a sialylated pathogen, Campylobacter jejuni. J. Immunol. 189, 2414—2422.

Krieger, M., Herz, J., 1994. Structures and functions of multiligand lipoprotein receptors: macrophage scavenger receptors and LDL receptor-related protein (LRP). Annu. Rev. Biochem. 63, 601—637.

Leng, L., Chen, L., Fan, J., Greven, D., Arjona, A., Du, X., et al., 2011. A small-molecule macrophage migration inhibitory factor antagonist protects against glomerulonephritis in lupus-prone NZB/NZW F1 and MRL/lpr mice. J. Immunol. 186, 527—538.

Levine, B., Mizushima, N., Virgin, H.W., 2011. Autophagy in immunity and inflammation. Nature. 469, 323—335.

Lin, H.H., Faunce, D.E., Stacey, M., Terajewicz, A., Nakamura, T., Zhang-Hoover, J., et al., 2005. The macrophage F4/80 receptor is required for the induction of antigen-specific efferent regulatory T cells in peripheral tolerance. J. Exp. Med. 201, 1615—1625.

Lin, Q., Li, M., Fang, D., Fang, J., Su, S.B., 2011. The essential roles of Toll-like receptor signaling pathways in sterile inflammatory diseases. Int. Immunopharmacol. 11, 1422—1432.

Loo, Y.M., Gale Jr., M., 2011. Immune signaling by RIG-I-like receptors. Immunity. 34, 680–692.

Lu, C., He, J.C., Cai, W., Liu, H., Zhu, L., Vlassara, H., 2004. Advanced glycation endproduct (AGE) receptor 1 is a negative regulator of the inflammatory response to AGE in mesangial cells. Proc. Natl. Acad. Sci. USA 101, 11767–11772.

Martinez-Pomares, L., Gordon, S., 2012. CD169+ macrophages at the crossroads of antigen presentation. Trends Immunol. 33, 66–70.

Mathis, D., Benoist, C., 2012. The influence of the microbiota on type-1 diabetes: on the threshold of a leap forward in our understanding. Immunol. Rev. 245, 239–249.

McGaha, T.L., Chen, Y., Ravishankar, B., Van Rooijen, N., Karlsson, M.C., 2011. Marginal zone macrophages suppress innate and adaptive immunity to apoptotic cells in the spleen. Blood 117, 5403–5412.

McGettrick, H.M., Butler, L.M., Buckley, C.D., Rainger, G.E., Nash, G.B., 2012. Tissue stroma as a regulator of leukocyte recruitment in inflammation. J. Leukoc. Biol. 91, 385–400.

McGreal, E.P., Miller, J.L., Gordon, S., 2005. Ligand recognition by antigen-presenting cell C-type lectin receptors. Curr. Opin. Immunol. 17, 18–24.

Menke, J., Iwata, Y., Rabacal, W.A., Basu, R., Stanley, E.R., Kelley, V. R., 2011. Distinct roles of CSF-1 isoforms in lupus nephritis. J. Am. Soc. Nephrol. 22, 1821–1833.

Meredith, M.M., Liu, K., Darrasse-Jeze, G., Kamphorst, A.O., Schreiber, H.A., Guermonprez, P., et al., 2012. Expression of the zinc finger transcription factor zDC (Zbtb46, Btbd4) defines the classical dendritic cell lineage. J. Exp. Med. 209, 1153–1165.

Metzger, T.C., Anderson, M.S., 2011. Control of central and peripheral tolerance by Aire. Immunol. Rev. 241, 89–103.

Mi, Y., Shapiro, S.D., Baenziger, J.U., 2002. Regulation of lutropin circulatory half-life by the mannose/N-acetylgalactosamine-4-SO4 receptor is critical for implantation in vivo. J. Clin. Invest. 109, 269–276.

Miller, J.C., Brown, B.D., Shay, T., Gautier, E.L., Jojic, V., Cohain, A., et al., 2012. Deciphering the transcriptional network of the dendritic cell lineage. Nat. Immunol. 13, 888–899.

Moberg, C.L., 2011. An appreciation of Ralph Marvin Steinman (1943–2011). J. Exp. Med. 208, 2337–2342.

Mukherjee, S., Maxfield, F.R., 2009. Acidification of endosomes and phagosomes. In: Russell, D.G., Gordon, S. (Eds.), Phagocyte–Pathogen Interactions: Macrophages and the Host Response to Infection. ASM Press, Washington, DC.

Mukhopadhyay, S., Varin, A., Chen, Y., Liu, B., Tryggvason, K., Gordon, S., 2011. SR-A/MARCO-mediated ligand delivery enhances intracellular TLR and NLR function, but ligand scavenging from cell surface limits TLR4 response to pathogens. Blood 117, 1319–1328.

Nagai, R., Matsumoto, K., Ling, X., Suzuki, H., Araki, T., Horiuchi, S., 2000. Glycolaldehyde, a reactive intermediate for advanced glycation end products, plays an important role in the generation of an active ligand for the macrophage scavenger receptor. Diabetes 49, 1714–1723.

Netea, M.G., Wijmenga, C., O'Neill, L.A., 2012. Genetic variation in Toll-like receptors and disease susceptibility. Nat. Immunol. 13, 535–542.

Nicoletti, A., Caligiuri, G., Tornberg, I., Kodama, T., Stemme, S., Hansson, G.K., 1999. The macrophage scavenger receptor type A

directs modified proteins to antigen presentation. Eur. J. Immunol. 29, 512–521.

Nimmerjahn, F., Ravetch, J.V., 2008. Fcgamma receptors as regulators of immune responses. Nat. Rev. Immunol. 8, 34–47.

O'Neill, L.A., 2008. The interleukin-1 receptor/Toll-like receptor superfamily: 10 years of progress. Immunol. Rev. 226, 10–18.

Parsa, R., Andresen, P., Gillett, A., Mia, S., Zhang, X.M., Mayans, S., et al., 2012. Adoptive transfer of immunomodulatory M2 macrophages prevents type 1 diabetes in NOD mice. Diabetes. 61, 2881–2892.

Pearson, C., Uhlig, H.H., Powrie, F., 2012. Lymphoid microenvironments and innate lymphoid cells in the gut. Trends Immunol. 33, 289–296.

Pluddemann, A., Neyen, C., Gordon, S., 2007. Macrophage scavenger receptors and host-derived ligands. Methods 43, 207–217.

Pontillo, A., Girardelli, M., Kamada, A.J., Pancotto, J.A., Donadi, E.A., Crovella, S., et al., 2012. Polymorphisms in inflammasome genes are involved in the predisposition to systemic lupus erythematosus. Autoimmunity 45, 271–278.

Puig-Kroger, A., Dominguez-Soto, A., Martinez-Munoz, L., Serrano-Gomez, D., Lopez-Bravo, M., Sierra-Filardi, E., et al., 2006. RUNX3 negatively regulates CD36 expression in myeloid cell lines. J. Immunol. 177, 2107–2114.

Rathinam, V.A., Vanaja, S.K., Fitzgerald, K.A., 2012. Regulation of inflammasome signaling. Nat. Immunol. 13, 333–342.

Ravishankar, B., Liu, H., Shinde, R., Chandler, P., Baban, B., Tanaka, M., et al., 2012. Tolerance to apoptotic cells is regulated by indoleamine 2,3-dioxygenase. Proc. Natl. Acad. Sci. USA 109, 3909–3914.

Ridley, A.J., Hall, A., 2004. Snails, Swiss, and serum: the solution for Rac 'n' Rho. Cell. 116 (S23–S25), (2p following S25).

Rossol, M., Kraus, S., Pierer, M., Baerwald, C., Wagner, U., 2012. The CD14(bright) CD16+ monocyte subset is expanded in rheumatoid arthritis and promotes expansion of the Th17 cell population. Arthritis Rheum. 64, 671–677.

Rothlin, C.V., Lemke, G., 2010. TAM receptor signaling and autoimmune disease. Curr. Opin. Immunol. 22, 740–746.

Santiago-Garcia, J., Mas-Oliva, J., Innerarity, T.L., Pitas, R.E., 2001. Secreted forms of the amyloid-beta precursor protein are ligands for the class A scavenger receptor. J. Biol. Chem. 276, 30655–30661.

Satpathy, A.T., Kc, W., Albring, J.C., Edelson, B.T., Kretzer, N.M., Bhattacharya, D., et al., 2012. Zbtb46 expression distinguishes classical dendritic cells and their committed progenitors from other immune lineages. J. Exp. Med. 209, 1135–1152.

Schroder, K., Tschopp, J., 2010. The inflammasomes. Cell. 140, 821–832.

Seneviratne, A.N., Sivagurunathan, B., Monaco, C., 2012. Toll-like receptors and macrophage activation in atherosclerosis. Clin. Chim. Acta. 413, 3–14.

Shenoy, A.R., Wellington, D.A., Kumar, P., Kassa, H., Booth, C.J., Cresswell, P., et al., 2012. GBP5 promotes NLRP3 inflammasome assembly and immunity in mammals. Science 336, 481–485.

Shi, B., Huang, Q., Tak, P.P., Vervoordeldonk, M.J., Huang, C.C., Dorfleutner, A., et al., 2012. SNAPIN: an endogenous toll-like receptor ligand in rheumatoid arthritis. Ann Rheum. Dis. 71, 1411–1417.

Shimaoka, T., Nakayama, T., Fukumoto, N., Kume, N., Takahashi, S., Yamaguchi, J., et al., 2004. Cell surface-anchored SR-PSOX/CXC chemokine ligand 16 mediates firm adhesion of CXC chemokine receptor 6-expressing cells. J. Leukoc. Biol. 75, 267–274.

Silverstein, R.L., Asch, A.S., Nachman, R.L., 1989. Glycoprotein IV mediates thrombospondin-dependent platelet-monocyte and platelet-U937 cell adhesion. J. Clin. Invest. 84, 546–552.

Strasser, A., Jost, P.J., Nagata, S., 2009. The many roles of FAS receptor signaling in the immune system. Immunity. 30, 180–192.

Swanson, J.A., 2008. Shaping cups into phagosomes and macropinosomes. Nat. Rev. Mol. Cell Biol. 9, 639–649.

Swanson, J.A., 2009. Signaling for phagocytosis. In: Russell, D.G., Gordon, S. (Eds.), Phagocyte–Pathogen Interactions: Macrophages and the Host Response to Infection. ASM Press, Washington, DC.

Swirski, F.K., Nahrendorf, M., Etzrodt, M., Wildgruber, M., Cortez-Retamozo, V., Panizzi, P., et al., 2009. Identification of splenic reservoir monocytes and their deployment to inflammatory sites. Science 325, 612–616.

Takahashi, T., Tanaka, M., Brannan, C.I., Jenkins, N.A., Copeland, N.G., Suda, T., et al., 1994. Generalized lymphoproliferative disease in mice, caused by a point mutation in the Fas ligand. Cell 76, 969–976.

Taylor, N., McConachie, K., Calder, C., Dawson, R., Dick, A., Sedgwick, J.D., et al., 2005a. Enhanced tolerance to autoimmune uveitis in CD200-deficient mice correlates with a pronounced Th2 switch in response to antigen challenge. J. Immunol. 174, 143–154.

Taylor, P.R., Carugati, A., Fadok, V.A., Cook, H.T., Andrews, M., Carroll, M.C., et al., 2000. A hierarchical role for classical pathway complement proteins in the clearance of apoptotic cells in vivo. J. Exp. Med. 192, 359–366.

Taylor, P.R., Martinez-Pomares, L., Stacey, M., Lin, H.H., Brown, G.D., Gordon, S., 2005b. Macrophage receptors and immune recognition. Annu. Rev. Immunol. 23, 901–944.

Vlassara, H., Striker, G.E., 2011. AGE restriction in diabetes mellitus: a paradigm shift. Nat. Rev. Endocrinol. 7, 526–539.

Wegner, N., Lundberg, K., Kinloch, A., Fisher, B., Malmstrom, V., Feldmann, M., et al., 2010. Autoimmunity to specific citrullinated proteins gives the first clues to the etiology of rheumatoid arthritis. Immunol. Rev. 233, 34–54.

Wermeling, F., Chen, Y., Pikkarainen, T., Scheynius, A., Winqvist, O., Izui, S., et al., 2007. Class A scavenger receptors regulate tolerance against apoptotic cells, and autoantibodies against these receptors are predictive of systemic lupus. J. Exp. Med. 204, 2259–2265.

Werts, C., Rubino, S., Ling, A., Girardin, S.E., Philpott, D.J., 2011. Nod-like receptors in intestinal homeostasis, inflammation, and cancer. J. Leukoc. Biol. 90, 471–482.

Willment, J.A., Gordon, S., Brown, G.D., 2001. Characterization of the human beta -glucan receptor and its alternatively spliced isoforms. J. Biol. Chem. 276, 43818–43823.

Wynn, T.A., Ramalingam, T.R., 2012. Mechanisms of fibrosis: therapeutic translation for fibrotic disease. Nat. Med. 18, 1028–1040.

Zhang, J.G., Czabotar, P.E., Policheni, A.N., Caminschi, I., Wan, S.S., Kitsoulis, S., et al., 2012. The dendritic cell receptor Clec9A binds damaged cells via exposed actin filaments. Immunity 36, 646–657.

Ziegler-Heitbrock, L., Ancuta, P., Crowe, S., Dalod, M., Grau, V., Hart, D.N., et al., 2010. Nomenclature of monocytes and dendritic cells in blood. Blood 116, e74–e80.

Chapter 12

Dendritic Cells in Autoimmune Disease

Kristen Radford[1], Ken Shortman[2,3], and Meredith O'Keeffe[3,4]

[1]Cancer Immunotherapies Group, Mater Medical Research Institute, South Brisbane, Australia, [2]Immunology Division, The Walter and Eliza Hall Institute, Parkville, Australia and Centre for Immunology, Burnet Institute, Melbourne, Victoria, Australia, [3]Centre for Biomedical Research, Burnet Institute, Melbourne, Victoria, Australia, [4]Department of Immunology, Monash University, Clayton, Victoria, Australia

Chapter Outline

Antigen Processing by Dendritic Cells 175
Pattern Recognition Receptors 176
Dendritic Cell Activation 176
Dendritic Cell Subsets 176
Mouse Dendritic Cells 176
Dendritic Cells in the Mouse Thymus 179
DC Subsets and Tolerance 179
Human DC subsets in Steady State 180
DC subsets in Human Skin: Epidermal
Langerhans Cells and Dermal DC 180
DC and Autoimmune Disease 181
Systemic Lupus Erythematosus 181
IBD—Crohn's Disease and Ulcerative
Colitis 182
DC Immunotherapy as a Treatment for
Autoimmune Diseases 182
Targeting of DC in Autoimmune Disease 182
Conclusions and Future Prospects 183
References 183

ANTIGEN PROCESSING BY DENDRITIC CELLS

Dendritic cells (DC) take up antigenic material, soluble and particulate, self and foreign, by a variety of processes including phagocytosis, pinocytosis and receptor mediated endocytosis. Some DC are equipped with receptors for recognition of apoptotic or necrotic cells of the body (Sancho et al., 2009; Zhang et al., 2012). Non-activated ("immature") DC are especially active in antigen uptake; some uptake processes are shut off once the DC become activated ("mature"). In contrast to other phagocytic cells such as macrophages that rapidly and completely degrade phagocytosed material, DC conserve antigenic material for a prolonged period, allowing continuous processing and presentation of antigen. There are several antigen-processing routes in DC (Trombetta and Mellman, 2005; Wilson and Villadangos, 2005). Exogenous antigens are usually processed in endocytic vesicles, leading to appropriate peptides being loaded onto major histocompatibility complex (MHC) class II molecules. The MHC class II associated antigens then presented to CD4 T cells will include peptides from exogenous foreign antigens, along with peptides from self components such as recycling DC surface molecules. When conventional DC are activated, the MHC class II—peptide complexes all shift to the cell surface and are no longer recycled, so for their limited lifespan the mature DC present a "snapshot" of the antigenic environment at the time of activation.

DC, along with most other cells, produce, as a by-product of protein synthesis, peptides that are loaded onto MHC class I for presentation to CD8 T cells. Such endogenously derived "self" antigens will include viral antigens if the DC are infected with a virus. Some DC have the additional ability to take up and shuttle exogenous antigens into the MHC class I presentation pathway. This specialized function is only performed efficiently by particular DC subtypes, and has been termed "cross-presentation" (Heath et al., 2004). Cross-presentation of exogenous antigens, including material from dead cells, is important for the generation of cytotoxic T cell responses to intracellular pathogens that do not infect the DC themselves. The pathways of cross-presentation are still being determined, but involve movement of antigen from the endocytic vesicles through the cytosol into the endoplasmic reticulum to join the MHC class I loading pathway.

N. Rose & I. Mackay (Eds): The Autoimmune Diseases, Fifth edition. DOI: http://dx.doi.org/10.1016/B978-0-12-384929-8.00012-5

Only some DC subsets cross-present antigens efficiently and this capacity is induced as a late step in their development (Shortman and Heath, 2010).

PATTERN RECOGNITION RECEPTORS

A unifying feature of all DC is the expression of receptors that recognize microbial products or damaged cells, aspects of the environment often generalized as "danger." These receptors, collectively called pattern recognition receptors (PRR) are not all expressed on all DC subsets and indeed the differential expression of PRR is a major functional discriminator of DC subsets (Hochrein and O'Keeffe, 2008; Table 12.1).

PRRs exist on the plasma membrane, in the cytoplasm, and on endosomal membranes of cells. They belong to four major families: Toll-like receptors (TLR) 1–13; Rig-like helicases (RLH); C-type lectin receptors; and nucleotide-binding domain, leucine-rich repeat containing (NLR) receptors.

The PRRs recognize a variety of pathogen-derived and self molecules. For recent reviews see: TLR (Uematsu and Akira, 2008; Kawai and Akira, 2010, 2011); NLR (Martinon and Tschopp, 2005, Davis et al., 2011; Elinav et al., 2011); RLH (Barbalat et al., 2011; Loo and Gale Jr., 2011); C-type lectin receptors (Robinson et al., 2006; Diebold, 2009; Kerrigan and Brown, 2009; Osorio and Reis e Sousa, 2011). Most importantly, not all DC express all receptors and in fact there is heterogeneity in the expression of the different receptor families. Particularly relevant for vaccine design, adjuvants induce different immune responses and this is mediated at least in part by the fact that different adjuvants work through different PRR and target different subsets of immune cells such as DC. Likewise, PRR activation in autoimmune disease may involve activation of discrete DC subsets exemplified by the activation of plasmacytoid DC (pDC) in patients with lupus (see below).

It is important to note that the pattern of expression of PRR is not always the same between similar cells of different species and thus caution must be taken in interpreting effects of ligation of different PRR in animal models of disease and their relevance to human disease settings.

DENDRITIC CELL ACTIVATION

The engagement of PRR provides signals that are needed to activate DC to full immunogenic function. The signaling pathways downstream of PRR all converge on the activation of the transcription factor family NF-κB, leading to the production of cytokines and the upregulation of costimulator molecules and MHC molecules on the DC surface (Kawai and Akira, 2007; Diebold, 2009).

DENDRITIC CELL SUBSETS

DC can be divided into two major categories; conventional (c) DC (sometimes termed myeloid DC) and plasmacytoid (p) DC (sometimes termed lymphoid DC). The cDC can be further divided into migratory and resident subsets based upon tissue location and surface phenotype (Table 12.1: DC subsets, location, PRR expression, known cytokine production). The migratory DC collect antigen in peripheral tissues then migrate to lymph nodes for presentation to T cells. The lymphoid tissue resident DC collect antigen within the lymphoid organs, either directly or as antigen acquired from other cell types including migratory DC. It is also useful to distinguish the DC found in normal, healthy "steady-state" from activated "inflammatory" DC that are generated, sometimes in substantial numbers, in response to inflammation or infection. Inflammatory DC can develop from monocytes; they are modeled by the development of DC in culture when monocytes are cultured with cytokines including GM-CSF, although recent reports suggest that M-CSF may actually be the crucial growth factor required by these DC (Greter et al., 2012). The most detailed information on individual DC subsets comes from studies on laboratory mice. Although the general picture translates to the human immune system, many of the details of surface markers and specialized functions differ, so mouse and human DC subsets will be discussed separately.

MOUSE DENDRITIC CELLS

Mouse spleen, lacking input from the lymphatics, serves as an enriched source of resident DC (Table 12.1). CD8α has been a useful marker in mice for distinguishing resident cDC subsets, although its function is unknown and it is not expressed on human DC. The CD8α$^+$ cDC, as well as having the unifying DC function of presenting exogenous antigens on MHC class II, have the additional capacity for "cross-presentation," i.e., the ability to present exogenous antigen in the context of MHC class I (Villadangos and Schnorrer, 2007). Accordingly, CD8$^+$ cDC are particularly efficient at inducing CD8$^+$ T cells in response to exogenous antigens. High IL-12p70 production on activation via PRR is another hallmark of CD8α$^+$ cDC (Reis e Sousa et al., 1997; Maldonado-Lopez et al., 1999; Hochrein et al., 2001) and this leads to a capacity to bias activated T cells to an inflammatory Th1 response. The CD8$^+$ DC express high levels of TLR3, recognizing dsRNA, and TLR9, recognizing ssDNA, both located in intracellular endosomes. These PRR equip the CD8$^+$ DC to respond to viral and bacterial nucleic acids. The CD8$^+$ cDC are also especially efficient in the uptake of dead and dying cells. One PRR involved in dead cell recognition by

TABLE 12.1 Pattern Recognition Receptors Expressed by Mouse DC

				Conventional DC		pDC
				CD8$^+$	CD8$^-$	
Toll-like Receptors						
TLR1	Plasma membrane	Triacyl lipoprotein	Bacteria	✓	✓	✓
TLR2	Plasma membrane	Lipoprotein	Bacteria, viruses, parasites	✓	✓	✓
TLR3	Endolysosome	dsRNA	Virus, mammals	✓	+/-	X
TLR4	Plasma membrane	LPS	Bacteria, viruses	✓	✓	X
TLR5	Plasma membrane	Flagellin	Bacteria	X	✓ subset	X
TLR6	Plasma membrane	Diacyl lipoprotein	Bacteria, viruses	✓	✓	✓
TLR7	Endolysosome	ssRNA	Virus, bacteria, mammals	X	✓	✓
TLR9	Endolysosome	CpG DNA	Virus, bacteria, protozoa, mammals	✓	✓	✓
TLR11	Plasma membrane	Profilin-like molecule	Protozoa	✓	X	X
Rig-like Helicases						
RIG-1	Cytoplasm	Short ds RNA	RNA viruses, DNA virus	X	✓	+/-
MDA5	Cytoplasm	Long ds RNA	RNA viruses	X	✓	+/-
NOD-like Receptors						
NOD-1	Cytoplasm	g-D-glutamyl-meso-diaminopimelic acid (iE-DAP)	Bacteria	+/-	✓	+/-
C-type Lectins						
CD205	Plasma membrane	Unknown but used successfully for DC targeting		X	X	✓
Clec9A	Plasma membrane	Dead cells of self origin		✓	X	✓

Selected pattern recognition receptors, their cellular location, and specificity are shown along with their pattern of expression in the DC subsets of mouse spleen. +/- depicts low or weak expression.

$CD8^+$ DC is Clec9A, which recognizes the filamentous form of actin (F actin), exposed when the membrane of a cell is disrupted (Sancho et al., 2009; Zhang et al., 2012). With the dual functions of cross-presentation and dead cell uptake, the $CD8^+$ DC are perfectly equipped to present viral and bacterial antigens from infected dead and dying cells. Moreover, it is not hard to imagine that in an autoimmune setting the $CD8^+$ DC could be particularly detrimental as they may be activated by self nucleic acids taken up in dead cells and present self peptides present in these cells, leading to activation of cytotoxic T cells.

The $CD8^-$ lymphoid tissue resident cDC are more numerous than the $CD8^+$ cDC, but recent evidence indicates they consist of two distinct DC subsets separable by expression of several markers including Clec12A, DCIR2, and CD4 (Kasahara and Clark, 2012). However, most functional data so far relate to the unseparated $CD8^-$ DC population. All cDC are capable of presenting antigen to $CD4^+$ T cells via MHC class II but the $CD8^-$ cDC are the most efficient. T cell activation driven by activated $CD8^-$ DC may lead to a Th2 response, possibly due to the DCIR2 DC subset. The $CD8^-$ cDC express TLR7 (recognizes ssRNA), TLR9, and very high levels of intracellular Rig-like helicase receptors (RLR) that recognize dsRNA in the cytoplasm (Luber et al., 2010). The high expression of RLR and some NLR (Luber et al., 2010), suggests that the $CD8^-$ cDC are particularly primed to rapidly respond to intracellular viral and bacterial infection. The $CD8^-$ cDC express high levels of chemokines including CCL5 (RANTES), CCL3 (MIP-1α), and CCL4 (MIP-1β). These chemokines are elevated upon PRR activation but are also expressed constitutively by $CD8^-$ cDC (Proietto et al., 2004).

Lymph nodes, as well as containing similar resident cDC to spleen, also contain migratory DC even in steady state, but the input from peripheral tissues increases markedly on infection or inflammation. These DC that have migrated in from peripheral tissues are more mature than the resident DC in terms of costimulator molecule expression even in the steady state, but are not necessarily immunogenic and do not produce cytokines unless they have received the appropriate PRR signals. Three basic types of migratory DC have been identified (Bursch et al., 2007; Poulin et al., 2007). Langerhans cells in the skin epidermis were identified long before their function as DC was recognized (Merad et al., 2008). They have an exceptionally long lifespan in the epidermis, but turn over rapidly post migration. Recent work suggests they have a predominantly tolerogenic role, even in an activated state (Shklovskaya et al., 2011). DC resembling Langerhans cells also occur in other epithelial tissues. A more rapidly migrating DC population occurs in the skin dermis

and as interstitial DC in other tissues. Recently a minor but important migratory DC subset was discovered in the skin dermis and in other tissues, first distinguished by expression of CD103 and sharing with Langerhans cells the expression of langerin, a pathogen recognition molecule expressed at high levels in Langerhans cells but also at lower levels in some other DC (Nagao et al., 2009). However, this numerically minor DC subset, although not expressing CD8, is similar in functional properties to the resident $CD8^+$ DC subset in expressing Clec9A, in processing material from dead cells and in a marked capacity for cross-presentation. It may be considered as the migratory counterpart of the resident $CD8^+$ cDC.

The pDC are generally considered as part of the DC "family" but in many respects have similarities to B cells. pDC circulate through the bloodstream much like lymphocytes and have a lymphocyte-like morphology. pDC also normally lack the ability to stimulate naïve T cells (O'Keeffe et al., 2002). The categorization of the pDC as a member of the DC "family" rests upon morphological and phenotypical features that they display upon activation, when the pDC upregulate costimulation markers and MHC molecules to levels resembling the cDC and rapidly acquire the typical stellate morphology of cDC.

The pDC express high levels of TLR7 and TLR9. If given specific PRR stimuli they can induce some T cell division, more than B cells or macrophages but typically in the order of 10-fold or less that of the cDC (Villadangos and Young, 2008). Unlike cDC the pDC continually present antigens on MHC class II molecules once they are activated and as a result can continue to present new viral antigens during the course of infection (Young et al., 2008). The importance of this function of pDC during an ongoing infection is not yet elucidated. Instead the pDC, also referred to as natural interferon-producing cells (NIPC), are renowned for their production of Type I interferons (IFN-I) in response to viral or bacterial stimuli and mimics thereof (Gilliet et al., 2008; Kadowaki, 2009). The pDC of both mouse and humans recognize ssDNA via TLR9. As a consequence of endoplasmic reticulum to lysosome internal trafficking of TLR9 and differential expression of molecules that are involved in the TLR9 signaling complex, such as high constitutive expression of IRF7, the pDC have the ability to produce extremely high levels of IFN-I upon TLR9 ligation (Gilliet et al., 2008). Synthetic CpG-containing oligonucleotides (ODN), without addition of transfection reagent, are sufficient for the triggering of IFN-I from pDC. The pDC and a recently identified DC in bone marrow (miDC) (O'Keeffe et al., 2012) are the only cell types known to produce IFN-I in response to CpG-ODN alone.

DENDRITIC CELLS IN THE MOUSE THYMUS

Although thymic DC may serve the same sentinel role as in other tissues, their main role is likely to be in the selection of the specificity repertoire of developing T cells, so ensuring tolerance to self components (Ardavin, 1997). Although thymic epithelial cells are the major source of self antigens for thymocyte selection, DC appear to contribute to negative selection and can collect and present antigens originally produced by the epithelial component (Klein et al., 2011). Thymic DC are of two distinct origins. The CD8$^+$ thymic DC are produced endogenously, possibly from the same early precursors that give rise to T cells. They resemble the CD8$^+$ conventional DC in peripheral lymphoid organs and, being in the immature state, are likely to induce tolerance. However, their cross-presentation capacity is fully developed and this may be important for presentation of self antigens derived from other thymic cells (Gallegos and Bevan, 2004). In contrast, the thymic CD8$^-$ conventional DC appear to be a little more mature than the CD8$^+$ thymic DC and they enter the thymus preformed from the bloodstream; this may enable them to carry into the thymus peripheral self antigens for induction of central tolerance. These thymic CD8$^-$ DC may also contribute to negative selection, but are particularly effective at generation of regulatory T cells (Proietto et al., 2008). The plasmacytoid cells in the thymus also enter the organ directly from the bloodstream. It is not known whether they play any role in thymic T cell selection, or whether they are simply on patrol in case of a viral infection.

DENDRITIC CELL SUBSETS AND TOLERANCE

As discussed above, the CD8$^-$ migratory cDC in thymus are particularly efficient in the induction of regulatory T cells (Tregs) in the thymus. This function, together with their ability to carry peripheral tissue antigens into the thymus and to play an important role in the deletion of thymocytes reactive to these self antigens (Bonasio et al., 2006; Proietto et al., 2008) contributes to central tolerance (Proietto et al., 2008).

Migratory DC in the gut also play a major role in inducing tolerance, specifically to oral and commensal bacterial antigens. The CD103$^+$ DC in the lamina propria migrate to mesenteric lymph nodes where they produce retinoic acid from dietary vitamin A and induce gut-homing Tregs (reviewed in Scott et al., 2011).

The CD8$^+$ cDC of both spleen and lymph nodes can present self-antigen by endocytosis of apoptotic cells *in vivo* in the steady state and tolerize self-reactive T cells in the periphery (Iyoda et al., 2002). This ability to cross-present exogenous antigen on MHC class I (den Haan et al., 2000) is probably also responsible for the ability of CD8$^+$ cDC to induce peripheral tolerance to tissue associated antigens (Belz et al., 2002). Moreover, CD8$^+$ cDC produce TGF-β in the steady state and induce antigen-specific Treg cells, further contributing to peripheral tolerance (Yamazaki et al., 2008).

Although the pDC have a remarkable proinflammatory function based on their IFN-I production, they have also been credited with protection from allergy (Lambrecht and Hammad, 2008) and determining oral (Goubier et al., 2008) and transplant tolerance (Abe et al., 2005; Ochando et al., 2006). Mechanisms of tolerance induction and/or immunosuppression by non-activated pDC probably include, but are not limited to, their ability to produce indoleamine-pyrrole 2,3-dioxygenase (IDO, the enzyme catalyzing L-tryptophan to N-formylkynurenine breakdown; Fallarino et al., 2007) and to induce Tregs (Ochando et al., 2006; Hadeiba et al., 2008).

DC differentiated from human monocytes or mouse bone marrow *in vitro* can be rendered tolerogenic by a variety of mechanisms including culture with IL-10 or TGF-β, treatment with drugs such as dexamethasone or BAY 11-7085 that inhibit NF-κB signaling, vitamin D3 or genetic modification by transduction of IL-4, IDO or treatment with antisense oligonucleotides for costimulatory molecules CD80, CD86, and CD40 (Steinman et al., 2003; Thomson and Robbins, 2008; Stoop et al., 2011). Tolerogenic DC differentiated by these mechanisms are characterized by low expression of costimulatory molecules, low production of proinflammatory cytokines, and high production of IL-10. They can induce tolerance by a variety of mechanisms including promotion of T cell death or anergy, the induction of Tregs, diversion of Th1 and Th17 responses towards a Th2 phenotype, and secretion of immunosuppressive molecules such as IDO (Thomson and Robbins, 2008). Vaccination with tolerogenic DC can prevent disease onset and limit disease severity in the collagen-induced arthritis mouse model, a commonly used model of rheumatoid arthritis. Similarly in NOD mice, transfer of tolerogenic DC prevents the onset of diabetes (Giannoukakis et al., 2008; Mukherjee and Dilorenzo, 2010). Several studies have shown a requirement for DC loading with specific autoantigen, e.g., type II collagen for collagen-induced arthritis, or islet beta cell antigens for diabetes, while others have demonstrated better efficacy if DC are not loaded with specific antigen. In the latter case it is presumed that DC acquire autoantigen *in vivo*. These promising preclinical studies in animal models have provided the impetus for the initiation of a number of Phase I studies in humans using tolerogenic DC as a treatment for rheumatoid arthritis or type 1 diabetes (Thomson and Robbins, 2008). Although the main endpoint of these Phase I trials is safety, results based on defined secondary

TABLE 12.2 Human DC Subsets of Mouse Blood Showing their Expression of C-type Lectins and TLRs and the Mouse DC Subsets to which they Align

	Human blood DC subsets			
	CD141	CD1c	PDC	MoDC
C-type lectins	Clec9A, DEC-205	DEC-205	CD303 (BDCA-2), DEC-205	CD206 (mannose receptor), CD209 (DC-SIGN), DEC-205
Toll-like receptors	TLR3, TLR10	TLR2 (TLR3, 4, 7 weak)	TLR7, TLR9, TLR10	TLR2, TLR4, TLR8
Putative *ex vivo* Mouse DC counterpart	CD8$^+$ DC and CD8$^-$Clec9A$^+$ migratory DC subsets	CD8$^-$CD11b$^+$ DC subsets	pDC	*In vitro* generated DC from monocytes with GM-CSF

endpoints are promising in a Phase I rheumatoid arthritis trial, where a decrease in general hyperinflammatory responses was observed in tolerogenic DC-treated patients (Nel et al., 2012) and in a diabetes trial where DC-treated patients showed some evidence of the induction of tolerogenic B cells (Giannoukakis et al., 2011).

HUMAN DENDRITIC CELL SUBSETS IN STEADY STATE

The study of human DC subsets is still in its infancy due to their rarity and lack of distinguishing markers and constraints on accessing human tissue. Most human studies have focused on DC differentiated from blood monocytes after *in vitro* culture in the presence of GM-CSF and IL-4 (MoDC). Their *in vivo* counterparts are currently unclear, but they most likely resemble the mouse inflammatory DC subtype.

Human blood DC comprise approximately 1% of circulating peripheral blood mononuclear cells (PBMC) and are classically defined as Ag-presenting leukocytes that lack other leukocyte lineage markers (CD3, 14, 15, 19, 20, 56) and express high levels of MHC class II (HLA-DR) molecules (lineage$^-$HLA-DR$^+$). Like mouse DC, these can be broadly categorized into pDC (defined as CD11c$^-$CD123$^+$ in humans) and cDC (defined as CD11c$^+$CD123$^-$). Human pDC are functionally aligned with their mouse counterparts and are characterized by expression of TLR7 and TLR9 and their ability to rapidly produce high levels of IFN-I.

Conventional DC in human blood comprise the CD141 (BDCA-3)$^+$ and CD1c (BDCA-1)$^+$ DC subsets. These have unique gene expression profiles that are distinct from monocytes and MoDC and this predicts that they have different functions (Lindstedt et al., 2005; Robbins et al., 2008).

Human CD141$^+$ DC and mouse CD8$^+$ DC share features that are essential for the induction of CTL responses against viruses and tumors (Bachem et al., 2010; Crozat et al., 2010; Jongbloed et al., 2010; Poulin et al., 2010). They express TLR3 (Edwards et al., 2003; Lindstedt et al., 2005), the C-type lectin Clec9A (Caminschi et al., 2008; Huysamen et al., 2008; Sancho et al., 2008), nectin-like protein 2 (Necl2) (Galibert et al., 2005), and chemokine receptor XCR1 (Bachem et al., 2010; Crozat et al., 2010). Human CD141$^+$ DC and mouse CD8$^+$ DC subsets produce IFN-β and IFN-λ in response to poly I:C (Scheu et al., 2008; Jongbloed et al., 2010; Lauterbach et al., 2010) and are specialized in their capacity to cross-present exogenous Ag from necrotic cells on MHC class I for the induction of antiviral and antitumor CD8$^+$ T cell responses (den Haan et al., 2000; Iyoda et al., 2002; Schnorrer et al., 2006; Crozat et al., 2010; Jongbloed et al., 2010). However, a key difference is that TLR9 is expressed by mouse CD8$^+$ DC but not by human CD141$^+$ DC and this would predict interspecies differences in the capacity of DC to respond to ssDNA.

The function of the human CD1c$^+$ DC subset, and whether it aligns with the mouse CD11b$^+$CD8$^-$ DC subset as predicted by their transcriptomes, has not been defined. Human CD1c$^+$ DC and CD141$^+$ DC are also found in lymph nodes, tonsil, spleen, skin, liver, gut, and lung. Table 12.2 shows human DC subsets, aligned with putative mouse equivalents.

DENDRITIC CELL SUBSETS IN HUMAN SKIN: EPIDERMAL LANGERHANS CELLS AND DERMAL DENDRITIC CELLS

Langerhans cells (LCs) are the main DC subset located in the epidermis of human skin. LCs are considered as the classical sentinels that are at the forefront of contact with invading microbial pathogens in the epidermis. They are characterized by expression of langerin (CD207) that functions as a receptor for microbial pathogens, and E-cadherin which facilitates adhesion with nearby keratinocytes (Cunningham et al., 2010). Human LCs are powerful stimulators of CD4$^+$ T cell proliferation and induce polarization towards a Th2 phenotype characterized by production of IL-4, IL-5, and IL-13 (Klechevsky et al., 2008). Human LCs can cross-present antigens and are potent stimulators of naïve CD8$^+$ T cell whereas most studies in mice do not support a role for LC in cross-presentation and the induction of antiviral CD8$^+$ T cell responses. Although LCs have been implicated in the inhibition of inflammation and the induction of tolerance in mice, these functions are yet to be addressed in humans.

Three separate populations of DC have been found in human dermis (Klechevsky et al., 2008; Nestle et al., 2009; Zaba et al., 2009; Haniffa et al., 2012). The first subset of dermal DC can be defined by expression of CD14. These DC play a specialized role in the development of humoral B cell responses by promoting the differentiation of CD4$^+$ T cells into follicular Th cells that prime naïve B cells to become plasma cells (Klechevsky et al., 2008). A subpopulation of CD14$^+$ dermal DC constitutively expresses IL-10 and induces Tregs that inhibit skin inflammation (Chu et al., 2012). The CD14$^-$ dermal DC can be further subdivided into two populations based on reciprocally high expression of CD141 or CD1c. Like human blood CD141$^+$ DC and the mouse lymphoid resident CD8$^+$ and migratory CD103$^+$ DC, human dermal CD141^{hi} DC share expression of TLR3, Clec9A, XCR1, Necl2, and are superior to other dermal DC and epidermal LC in their capacity to cross-present Ag to CD8$^+$ T cells (Haniffa et al., 2012). pDC are rare in healthy human skin but accumulate in inflamed tissue and facilitate disease pathogenesis in systemic lupus erythematosus (SLE) and psoriasis (Blanco et al., 2001; Nestle et al., 2005). Inflammatory myeloid DC infiltrate both epidermis and dermis of psoriatic lesions and are proposed to play a major role in psoriasis pathogenesis by production of the inflammatory mediators, inducible nitric oxide synthase (iNOS), and TNF-α (Lowes et al., 2005; Zaba et al., 2009).

DENDRITIC CELLS AND AUTOIMMUNE DISEASE

The DC subsets show a remarkable dichotomy in function relating to the induction of thymic and peripheral tolerance, as well as the induction of potent inflammatory responses to activation stimuli. Many factors, still mostly unknown, must control this finely tuned balance. Likewise, many factors contribute to autoimmune disease but clearly an imbalance in the tolerizing versus activation states of DC would lead to or enhance autoimmune disease. Two examples of this are discussed below.

Systemic Lupus Erythematosus

B cells and T cells in SLE are autoreactive to self nucleic acids (dsDNA, ssDNA, and RNA) and nuclear proteins, particularly nuclear antigens, including RNA-binding proteins such as those associated with U1-RNA (Migliorini et al., 2005). The exact mechanisms that drive development and activation of these autoreactive lymphocytes in SLE remain unknown but genetic influences play a major role in determining susceptibility (see Chapter 26). HLA loci have been linked to SLE, as have more than 30 additional genes, including many involved in proinflammatory cascades, e.g., genes encoding Fcγ receptors, TNFSF4, IRAK1, STAT4 (Delgado-Vega et al., 2010; Deng and Tsao, 2010; Sestak et al., 2011). Many of these genes are involved in pathways leading to production of type I interferons (IFN-I) or responses to IFN-I (Deng and Tsao, 2010).

Indeed many patients with SLE typically carry an "IFN signature" (Rönnblom and Pascual, 2008) as evidence of the expression of genes that are dependent on IFN-I for transcription. IFN-I in SLE is predominantly produced by pDC that respond to nucleic acid/autoantibody complexes via signaling through TLR7 and TLR9 (Means et al., 2005; Rönnblom and Pascual, 2008). Delivery of nucleic acid complexes to pDC in SLE depends on FcR that bind antinucleic acid immune complexes (Means et al., 2005) or nucleic acid complexes associated with neutrophils. Dying neutrophils in SLE patients release neutrophil extracellular traps (NETs); these neutrophils die from "netosis," thereby releasing large amounts of DNA/DNA-binding antimicrobial protein complexes that allow increased uptake of DNA by pDC and subsequent IFN-I production by TLR9-induced activation (Garcia-Romo et al., 2011; see Chapter 11).

IFN-I production in SLE is seen as a major contributor to the etiology of this disease since it greatly enhances activation of DC, self-reactive B cells and T cells, and the production of many other proinflammatory cytokines. Although studies of IFN-I in SLE suggest this as a therapeutic target, it is important to recognize that the same IFN signature can be induced by another family of IFNs produced by pDC, the type III IFNs, also called IFN-lambda (IFN-λ).

As for type I IFNs (particularly IFN-α), pDC are a major source of IFN-λ in response to TLR9 signaling in mice, and to both TLR7 and 9 in humans; pDC also produce large amounts of IFN-λ in response to viral stimulation (Ank and Paludan, 2009). Apart from pDC, the human CD141$^+$ DC and mouse CD8$^+$ DC also produce large amounts of IFN-λ in response to dsRNA via TLR3. Our unpublished data indicate that, similarly to IFN-I, IFN-λ enhances DC activation and it is thus very likely that IFN-λ production by DC subsets, like IFN-α, will play a role in enhancing proinflammatory responses in autoimmune diseases like SLE and also psoriasis where self nucleic acids are major immunogens.

IBD—Crohn's Disease and Ulcerative Colitis

Inflammatory bowel diseases (IBD) ulcerative colitis (UC) and Crohn's disease (CrD) are not initiated by an endogenous autoimmune event, but the pathology is autoimmune in nature. These diseases are presumed to manifest as a result of dysregulated immune responses to the intestinal microbiota. Mutations in NLR family members NOD2 and NLRP3 are highly associated with CrD (Cho, 2008; Villani et al., 2009). These PRR are mainly expressed by DC and macrophages and emerging evidence suggests they play a crucial role in maintaining immunological homeostasis in the intestine (Strober et al., 2006; Zaki et al., 2011). NOD2 functions as a receptor for the bacterial cell wall component muramyl dipeptide (MDP). Triggering of NOD2 in human MoDC *in vitro* stimulates processing and presentation of bacterial antigens to $CD4^+$ T cells, so generating an antibacterial response due to an increased production of antibacterial IL-17 (Cooney et al., 2010; van Beelen et al., 2007). NLRP3 is activated by a wide variety of microbial agonists and drives IL-1β secretion that activates the antimicrobial functions of innate immune cells such as macrophages and DC, and induces $CD4^+$ Th17 immune responses (Schroder et al., 2010). Thus, abnormal signaling by DC in response to the intestinal microbiota, consequent to mutations in these PRR, likely contributes to the pathogenesis of CrD.

Further evidence derived from mice and humans suggests that an imbalance in intestinal DC subsets, distribution, and function plays a crucial role driving inflammation and disease pathogenesis (Ng et al., 2011; Varol et al., 2010). Depletion of DC in mouse models of colitis leads to increased or decreased disease severity depending on the time-point, demonstrating a crucial role for DC in both the downregulation and exacerbation of intestinal inflammation. The balance between the functions of mouse intestinal $CD103^+$ and $CX3CR1^+$ DC subsets regulates immune homeostasis and controls inflammatory responses. $CD103^+$ DC are migratory DC that reside in the lamina propria and transport microbial antigens to the lymph nodes where they play an essential role in the induction of peripheral Tregs and the generation of oral tolerance. In contrast, the levels of $CX3CR1^+$ DC are dramatically increased in mouse colitis models and augment the severity of disease. pDC also accumulate in intestinal tissue in mouse colitis models (Karlis et al., 2004) and are contributors to the protective effects of GM-CSF treatment on colitis (Sainathan et al., 2008).

DC (defined as lacking the markers of other cell lineages and having high levels of MHC class II) can be found in the lamina propria of the human colonic mucosa (Ng et al., 2010). They comprise mostly $CD11c^+$ cDC

and few pDC, but their phenotype, function, and degree of alignment with mouse DC subsets is poorly characterized. Increased numbers of activated cDC are found in inflamed tissue in CrD compared to non-inflamed tissue, supporting a role for DC in disease pathogenesis (Ng et al., 2011). These DC express CD40 and CD83, TLR2 and TLR4, and produce proinflammatory cytokines including IL-6, TNF, and IL-12. An increased number of pDC are also present in the colonic mucosa and mesenteric lymph nodes of patients with CrD and ulcerative colitis (Baumgart et al., 2011). However, pDC infiltration in the lamina propria is associated with a clinical response and remission in patients with CrD following G-CSF treatment (Mannon et al., 2009). Thus the contribution of pDC to IBD pathogenesis remains unclear.

DENDRITIC CELL IMMUNOTHERAPY AS A TREATMENT FOR AUTOIMMUNE DISEASES

The essential role of DC in inducing immune responses makes them attractive targets for the development of immunomodulatory vaccines. DC loaded *ex vivo* with antigen and activators and administered as vaccines have been used as a treatment for a variety of malignancies (Vulink et al., 2008; Palucka and Banchereau, 2012) and some infectious diseases (García and Routy, 2011). These studies have demonstrated that DC vaccination is safe and to a degree efficacious. While vaccination with activated DC induces proinflammatory B cell and T cell adaptive immune responses, vaccination with immature DC results in the expansion of IL-10-secreting, Tregs (Dhodapkar et al., 2001). These studies provide some rationale for the adaptation of DC immunotherapy to induce a tolerogenic immune response for the treatment of autoimmune diseases.

TARGETING OF DENDRITIC CELLS IN AUTOIMMUNE DISEASE

Ex vivo manipulation of DC is expensive, logistically impractical, complicated by regulations, and needs to be tailored specifically for individual patients. Delivering antigen to DC directly *in vivo* using antibodies specific for DC-associated molecules such as DEC-205 can overcome many of the current limitations of DC therapy (Tacken et al., 2007). This approach is currently in early phase clinical trials for cancer and is just beginning to be explored in preclinical experimental models for autoimmune diseases. In the absence of adjuvant, targeting antigen to DC *in vivo* using antibodies to DEC-205 induces antigen-specific T cell deletion and unresponsiveness to oligodendrocyte glycoprotein (MOG) in a model of autoimmune experimental acute

encephalomyelitis and to model antigens including oval-
bumin (Bonifaz et al., 2002; Hawiger et al., 2004).
Furthermore, DEC-205 targeting of autoantigens in the
NOD and other mouse models of type 1 diabetes pre-
vents disease onset and progression (Bruder et al., 2005;
Mukhopadhaya et al., 2008).

An alternative approach being developed is microspheres carrying CD40, CD80, and CD86 antisense oligonucleotides. Vaccination with these microspheres can
prevent and reverse new-onset type 1 diabetes in NOD
mice, presumably via uptake by DC *in vivo* and the
expansion of Tregs (Phillips et al., 2008).

Targeting the innate functions of DC, such as cytokine
production, is also likely to be successful in autoimmune
diseases that are known to have a detrimental DC functional component. The example of SLE cited above is a
key candidate for pDC targeting. Targeting strategies that
block TLR7 and 9, for example, would extinguish the
IFN-I production by pDC in response to self-nucleic acids
in SLE.

CONCLUSIONS AND FUTURE PROSPECTS

The roles of DC subsets in mice, and mouse models of
disease, are steadily being deciphered. The field has really
only just begun to understand the complexity of function
of different DC subsets in humans and how they may
contribute to disease. Unraveling the functions of DC subsets in different anatomical locations will continue to lend
insight into their potential roles in disease states. There is
a real possibility that directly targeting DC either through
harnessing or dampening their specific functions may
lead to novel tailored therapies for autoimmune diseases.

It will be a great challenge to induce tolerogenic DC
in humans. DC will be targeted with antibodies to specific
surface receptors that are directly conjugated either to
drugs or to the surface of nanocomplexes. As described
above, drugs such as those that inhibit NF-κB signaling
can freeze DC in a tolerogenic state. Drugs that inhibit
TLR-7 or 9 signaling would prevent pDC activation in
SLE. The combination of antibody, drug, and antigen,
delivered in a nanocomplex, will perhaps ultimately create the perfect tolerogenic, DC-targeting vaccine. The
challenge is to determine what is the best antibody, the
best anti-inflammatory drug, the best antigen, and how
best to complex these in a nanoparticle-like delivery system, for different types of autoimmune disease.

In addition, DC may be increased *in vivo* using growth
factors, such as Flt-3 ligand, that we know are safe and
induce high numbers of DC (Maraskovsky et al., 2000).
These DC would then be targeted by a tolerizing vaccine.
Large numbers of tolerogenic DC may be extremely efficient at maintaining a tolerogenic state. The challenge
here would be in the timing, since any increase in DC

that are amenable to activation in an inflammatory state
would presumably only exacerbate disease.

REFERENCES

Abe, M., Wang, Z., de Creus, A., Thomson, A.W., 2005. Plasmacytoid
dendritic cell precursors induce allogeneic T-cell hyporesponsiveness and prolong heart graft survival. Am. J. Transplant. 5,
1808–1819.

Ank, N., Paludan, S.R., 2009. Type III IFNs: new layers of complexity
in innate antiviral immunity. Biofactors. 35, 82–87.

Ardavin, C., 1997. Thymic dendritic cells. Immunol Today. 18,
350–361.

Bachem, A., Guttler, S., Hartung, E., Ebstein, F., Schaefer, M., Tannert,
A., et al., 2010. Superior antigen cross-presentation and XCR1
expression define human CD11c+ CD141+ cells as homologues of
mouse CD8+ dendritic cells. J. Exp. Med. 207, 1273–1281.

Bancereau, J., Steinman, R.M., 1998. Dendritic cells and the control of
immunity. Nature. 392, 245–252.

Barbalat, R., Ewald, S.E., Mouchess, M.L., Barton, G.M., 2011. Nucleic
acid recognition by the innate immune system. Annu. Rev.
Immunol. 29, 185–214.

Baumgart, D.C., Metzke, D., Guckelberger, O., Pascher, A., Grotzinger,
C., Przesdzing, I., et al., 2011. Aberrant plasmacytoid dendritic cell
distribution and function in patients with Crohn's disease and ulcerative colitis. Clin. Exp. Immunol. 166, 46–54.

Belz, G.T., Behrens, G.M., Smith, C.M., Miller, J.F., Jones, C., Lejon,
K., et al., 2002. The CD8alpha(+) dendritic cell is responsible for
inducing peripheral self-tolerance to tissue-associated antigens.
J. Exp. Med. 196, 1099–1104.

Blanco, P., Palucka, A.K., Gill, M., Pascual, V., Bancereau, J., 2001.
Induction of dendritic cell differentiation by IFN-alpha in systemic
lupus erythematosus. Science. 294, 1540–1543.

Bonasio, R., Scimone, M.L., Schaerli, P., Grabie, N., Lichtman, A.H.,
von Andrian, U.H., 2006. Clonal deletion of thymocytes by circulating dendritic cells homing to the thymus. Nat. Immunol. 7,
1092–1100.

Bonifaz, L., Bonnyay, D., Mahnke, K., Rivera, M., Nussenzweig, M.C.,
Steinman, R.M., 2002. Efficient targeting of protein antigen to the
dendritic cell receptor DEC-205 in the steady state leads to antigen
presentation on major histocompatibility complex class I products
and peripheral CD8+ T cell tolerance. J. Exp. Med. 196,
1627–1638.

Bruder, D., Westendorf, A.M., Hansen, W., Prettin, S., Gruber, A.D.,
Qian, Y., et al., 2005. On the edge of autoimmunity: T-cell stimula-
tion by steady-state dendritic cells prevents autoimmune diabetes.
Diabetes. 54, 3395–3401.

Bursch, L.S., Wang, L., Igyarto, B., Kissenpfennig, A., Malissen, B.,
Kaplan, D.H., et al., 2007. Identification of a novel population of
Langerin+ dendritic cells. J. Exp. Med. 204, 3147–3156.

Caminschi, I., Proietto, A.I., Ahmet, F., Kitsoulis, S., Shin Teh, J., Lo,
J.C., et al., 2008. The dendritic cell subtype-restricted C-type lectin
Clec9A is a target for vaccine enhancement. Blood. 112,
3264–3273.

Cho, J.H., 2008. The genetics and immunopathogenesis of inflammatory
bowel disease. Nat. Rev. Immunol. 8, 458–466.

Chu, C.C., Ali, N., Karagiannis, P., Di Meglio, P., Skowera, A.,
Napolitano, L., et al., 2012. Resident CD141 (BDCA3)+ dendritic

cells in human skin produce IL-10 and induce regulatory T cells that suppress skin inflammation. J. Exp. Med. 209, 935—945.

Cooney, R., Baker, J., Brain, O., Danis, B., Pichulik, T., Allan, P., et al., 2010. NOD2 stimulation induces autophagy in dendritic cells influencing bacterial handling and antigen presentation. Nat. Med. 16, 90—97.

Crozat, K., Guiton, R., Contreras, V., Feuillet, V., Dutertre, C.A., Ventre, E., et al., 2010. The XC chemokine receptor 1 is a conserved selective marker of mammalian cells homologous to mouse CD8alpha + dendritic cells. J. Exp. Med. 207, 1283—1292.

Cunningham, A.L., Abendroth, A., Jones, C., Nasr, N., Turville, S., 2010. Viruses and Langerhans cells. Immunol. Cell Biol. 88, 416—423.

Davis, B.K., Wen, H., Ting, J.P.Y., 2011. The inflammasome NLRs in immunity, inflammation, and associated diseases. Annu. Rev. Immunol. 29, 707—735.

Delgado-Vega, A., Sanchez, E., Lofgren, S., Castillejo-Lopez, C., Alarcon-Riquelme, M.E., 2010. Recent findings on genetics of systemic autoimmune diseases. Curr. Opin. Immunol. 22, 698—705.

den Haan, J.M., Lehar, S.M., Bevan, M.J., 2000. CD8(+) but not CD8 (−) dendritic cells cross-prime cytotoxic T cells in vivo. J. Exp. Med. 192, 1685—1696.

Deng, Y., Tsao, B.P., 2010. Genetic susceptibility to systemic lupus erythematosus in the genomic era. Nat. Rev. Rheumatol. 6, 683—692.

Dhodapkar, M.V., Steinman, R.M., Krasovsky, J., Munz, C., Bhardwaj, N., 2001. Antigen-specific inhibition of effector T cell function in humans after injection of immature dendritic cells. J. Exp. Med. 193, 233—238.

Diebold, S.S., 2009. Activation of dendritic cells by toll-like receptors and C-type lectins. Handb. Exp. Pharmacol. 3—30.

Edwards, A.D., Chaussabel, D., Tomlinson, S., Schulz, O., Sher, A., Reis e Sousa, C., 2003. Relationships among murine CD11c(high) dendritic cell subsets as revealed by baseline gene expression patterns. J. Immunol. 171, 47—60.

Elinav, E., Strowig, T., Henao-Mejia, J., Flavell, Richard, A., 2011. Regulation of the Antimicrobial Response by NLR Proteins. Immunity 34, 665—679.

Fallarino, F., Gizzi, S., Mosci, P., Grohmann, U., Puccetti, P., 2007. Tryptophan catabolism in IDO + plasmacytoid dendritic cells. Curr. Drug Metab. 8, 209—216.

Galibert, L., Diemer, G.S., Liu, Z., Johnson, R.S., Smith, J.L., Walzer, T., et al., 2005. Nectin-like protein 2 defines a subset of T-cell zone dendritic cells and is a ligand for class-I-restricted T-cell-associated molecule. J. Biol. Chem. 280, 21955—21964.

Gallegos, A.M., Bevan, M.J., 2004. Central tolerance to tissue-specific antigens mediated by direct and indirect antigen presentation. J. Exp. Med. 200, 1039—1049.

Garcia-Romo, G.S., Caielli, S., Vega, B., Connolly, J., Allantaz, F., Xu, Z., et al., 2011. Netting neutrophils are major inducers of type i ifn production in pediatric systemic lupus erythematosus. Sci. Translational Med. 3, 73ra20.

García, F., Routy, J.-P., 2011. Challenges in dendritic cells-based therapeutic vaccination in HIV-1 infection: Workshop in dendritic cell-based vaccine clinical trials in HIV-1. Vaccine 29, 6454—6463.

Giannoukakis, N., Phillips, B., Finegold, D., Harnaha, J., Trucco, M., 2011. Phase I (safety) study of autologous tolerogenic dendritic cells in type 1 diabetic patients. Diabetes Care 34, 2026—2032.

Giannoukakis, N., Phillips, B., Trucco, M., 2008. Toward a cure for type 1 diabetes mellitus: diabetes-suppressive dendritic cells and beyond. Pediatr. Diabetes 9, 4—13.

Gilliet, M., Cao, W., Liu, Y.J., 2008. Plasmacytoid dendritic cells: sensing nucleic acids in viral infection and autoimmune diseases. Nat. Rev. Immunol. 8, 594—606.

Goubier, A., Dubois, B., Gheit, H., Joubert, G., Villard-Truc, F., Asselin-Paturel, C., et al., 2008. Plasmacytoid dendritic cells mediate oral tolerance. Immunity 29, 464—475.

Greter, M., Helft, J., Chow, A., Hashimoto, D., Mortha, A., Agudo-Cantero, J., et al., 2012. GM-CSF controls nonlymphoid tissue dendritic cell homeostasis but is dispensable for the differentiation of inflammatory dendritic cells. Immunity. 36, 1031—1046.

Hadeiba, H., Sato, T., Habtezion, A., Oderup, C., Pan, J., Butcher, E.C., 2008. CCR9 expression defines tolerogenic plasmacytoid dendritic cells able to suppress acute graft-versus-host disease. Nat. Immunol. 9, 1253—1260.

Haniffa, M., Shin, A., Bigley, V., McGovern, N., Teo, P., See, P., et al., 2012. Human tissues contain CD141hi cross-presenting dendritic cells with functional homology to mouse CD103 + nonlymphoid dendritic cells. Immunity 37, 60—73.

Hawiger, D., Masilamani, R.F., Bettelli, E., Kuchroo, V.K., Nussenzweig, M.C., 2004. Immunological unresponsiveness characterized by increased expression of CD5 on peripheral T cells induced by dendritic cells in vivo. Immunity. 20, 695—705.

Heath, W.R., Belz, G.T., Behrens, G.M., Smith, C.M., Forehan, S.P., Parish, I.A., et al., 2004. Cross-presentation, dendritic cell subsets, and the generation of immunity to cellular antigens. Immunol. Rev. 199, 9—26.

Hochrein, H., O'Keeffe, M., 2008. Dendritic cell subsets and toll-like receptors. Handb. Exp. Pharmacol. 153—179.

Hochrein, H., Shortman, K., Vremec, D., Scott, B., Hertzog, P., O'Keeffe, M., 2001. Differential production of IL-12, IFN-alpha, and IFN-gamma by mouse dendritic cell subsets. J. Immunol. 166, 5448—5455.

Huysamen, C., Willment, J.A., Dennehy, K.M., Brown, G.D., 2008. CLEC9A is a novel activation C-type lectin-like receptor expressed on BDCA3 + dendritic cells and a subset of monocytes. J. Biol. Chem. 283, 16693—16701.

Iyoda, T., Shimoyama, S., Liu, K., Omatsu, Y., Akiyama, Y., Maeda, Y., et al., 2002. The CD8 + dendritic cell subset selectively endocytoses dying cells in culture and in vivo. J. Exp. Med. 195, 1289—1302.

Jongbloed, S.L., Kassianos, A.J., McDonald, K.J., Clark, G.J., Ju, X., Angel, C.E., et al., 2010. Human CD141 + (BDCA-3) + dendritic cells (DCs) represent a unique myeloid DC subset that cross-presents necrotic cell antigens. J. Exp. Med. 207, 1247—1260.

Kadowaki, N., 2009. The divergence and interplay between pDC and mDC in humans. Front Biosci. 14, 808—817.

Karlis, J., Penttila, I., Tran, T.B., Jones, B., Nobbs, S., Zola, H., et al., 2004. Characterization of colonic and mesenteric lymph node dendritic cell subpopulations in a murine adoptive transfer model of inflammatory bowel disease. Inflamm. Bowel. Dis. 10, 834—847.

Kasahara, S., Clark, E.A., 2012. Dendritic cell-associated lectin 2 (DCAL2) defines a distinct CD8alpha- dendritic cell subset. J. Leukoc. Biol. 91, 437—448.

Kawai, T., Akira, S., 2007. Antiviral signaling through pattern recognition receptors. J. Biochem. 141, 137—145.

Kawai, T., Akira, S., 2010. The role of pattern-recognition receptors in innate immunity: update on Toll-like receptors. Nat. Immunol. 11, 373–384.

Kawai, T., Akira, S., 2011. Toll-like receptors and their crosstalk with other innate receptors in infection and immunity. Immunity 34, 637–650.

Kerrigan, A.M., Brown, G.D., 2009. C-type lectins and phagocytosis. Immunobiology. 182, 4150–4157.

Klechevsky, E., Morita, R., Liu, M., Cao, Y., Coquery, S., Thompson-Snipes, L., et al., 2008. Functional specializations of human epidermal Langerhans cells and CD14 + dermal dendritic cells. Immunity 29, 497–510.

Klein, L., Hinterberger, M., von Rohrscheidt, J., Aichinger, M., 2011. Autonomous versus dendritic cell-dependent contributions of medullary thymic epithelial cells to central tolerance. Trends Immunol. 32, 188–193.

Lambrecht, B.N., Hammad, H., 2008. Lung dendritic cells: targets for therapy in allergic disease. Chem. Immunol. Allergy 94, 189–200.

Lauterbach, H., Bathke, B., Gilles, S., Traidl-Hoffmann, C., Luber, C.A., Fejer, G., et al., 2010. Mouse CD8α + DCs and human BDCA3 + DCs are major producers of IFN-λ in response to poly IC. J. Exp. Med. 207, 2703–2717.

Lindstedt, M., Lundberg, K., Borrebaeck, C.A., 2005. Gene family clustering identifies functionally associated subsets of human in vivo blood and tonsillar dendritic cells. J. Immunol. 175, 4839–4846.

Loo, Y.-M., Gale Jr., M., 2011. Immune signaling by RIG-I-like receptors. Immunity 34, 680–692.

Lowes, M.A., Chamian, F., Abello, M.V., Fuentes-Duculan, J., Lin, S.L., Nussbaum, R., et al., 2005. Increase in TNF-alpha and inducible nitric oxide synthase-expressing dendritic cells in psoriasis and reduction with efalizumab (anti-CD11a). Proc. Natl. Acad. Sci. USA 102, 19057–19062.

Luber, C.A., Cox, J., Lauterbach, H., Fancke, B., Selbach, M., Tschopp, J., et al., 2010. Quantitative proteomics reveals subset-specific viral recognition in dendritic cells. Immunity 32, 279–289.

Maldonado-Lopez, R., De Smedt, T., Michel, P., Godfroid, J., Pajak, B., Heirman, C., et al., 1999. CD8alpha + and CD8alpha − subclasses of dendritic cells direct the development of distinct T helper cells in vivo. J. Exp. Med. 189, 587–592.

Mannon, P.J., Leon, F., Fuss, I.J., Walter, B.A., Begnami, M., Quezado, M., et al., 2009. Successful granulocyte-colony stimulating factor treatment of Crohn's disease is associated with the appearance of circulating interleukin-10-producing T cells and increased lamina propria plasmacytoid dendritic cells. Clin. Exp. Immunol. 155, 447–456.

Maraskovsky, E., Daro, E., Roux, E., Teepe, M., Maliszewski, C.R., Hoek, J., et al., 2000. In vivo generation of human dendritic cell subsets by Flt3 ligand. Blood 96, 878–884.

Martinon, F., Tschopp, J., 2005. NLRs join TLRs as innate sensors of pathogens. Trends Immunol. 26, 447–454.

Means, T.K., Latz, E., Hayashi, F., Murali, M.R., Golenbock, D.T., Luster, A.D., 2005. Human lupus autoantibody-DNA complexes activate DCs through cooperation of CD32 and TLR9. J. Clin. Invest. 115, 407–417.

Merad, M., Ginhoux, F., Collin, M., 2008. Origin, homeostasis and function of Langerhans cells and other langerin-expressing dendritic cells. Nat. Rev. Immunol. 8, 935–947.

Migliorini, P., Baldini, C., Rocchi, V., Bombardieri, S., 2005. Anti-Sm and anti-RNP antibodies. Autoimmunity 38, 47–54.

Mukherjee, G., Dilorenzo, T.P., 2010. The immunotherapeutic potential of dendritic cells in type 1 diabetes. Clin. Exp. Immunol. 161, 197–207.

Mukhopadhaya, A., Hanafusa, T., Jarchum, I., Chen, Y.G., Iwai, Y., Serreze, D.V., et al., 2008. Selective delivery of beta cell antigen to dendritic cells in vivo leads to deletion and tolerance of autoreactive CD8 + T cells in NOD mice. Proc. Natl. Acad. Sci. USA 105, 6374–6379.

Nagao, K., Ginhoux, F., Leitner, W.W., Motegi, S., Bennett, C.L., Clausen, B.E., et al., 2009. Murine epidermal Langerhans cells and langerin-expressing dermal dendritic cells are unrelated and exhibit distinct functions. Proc. Natl. Acad. Sci. U. S. A. 106, 3312–3317.

Nel, H., Law, S., Street, S., Ramnoruth, N., Shams, R., Pahau, H., et al., 2012. ARA scientific posters, ARA-P6. Outcome of a phase I trial of Rheumavax in patients with rheumatoid arthritis. Internal Med. J. 42, 9–35.

Nestle, F.O., Conrad, C., Tun-Kyi, A., Homey, B., Gombert, M., Boyman, O., et al., 2005. Plasmacytoid predendritic cells initiate psoriasis through interferon-α production. J. Exp. Med. 202, 135–143.

Nestle, F.O., Di Meglio, P., Qin, J.Z., Nickoloff, B.J., 2009. Skin immune sentinels in health and disease. Nat. Rev. Immunol. 9, 679–691.

Ng, S.C., Kamm, M.A., Stagg, A.J., Knight, S.C., 2010. Intestinal dendritic cells: their role in bacterial recognition, lymphocyte homing, and intestinal inflammation. Inflamm. Bowel Dis. 16, 1787–1807.

Ng, S.C., Benjamin, J.L., McCarthy, N.E., Hedin, C.R., Koutsoumpas, A., Plamondon, S., et al., 2011. Relationship between human intestinal dendritic cells, gut microbiota, and disease activity in Crohn's disease. Inflamm. Bowel Dis. 17, 2027–2037.

O'Keeffe, M., Fancke, B., Suter, M., Ramm, G., Clark, J., Wu, L., et al., 2012. Nonplasmacytoid, high IFN-alpha-producing, bone marrow dendritic cells. J. Immunol. 188, 3774–3783.

O'Keeffe, M., Hochrein, H., Vremec, D., Caminschi, I., Miller, J.L., Anders, E.M., et al., 2002. Mouse plasmacytoid cells: long-lived cells, heterogeneous in surface phenotype and function, that differentiate into CD8(+) dendritic cells only after microbial stimulus. J. Exp. Med. 196, 1307–1319.

Ochando, J.C., Homma, C., Yang, Y., Hidalgo, A., Garin, A., Tacke, F., et al., 2006. Alloantigen-presenting plasmacytoid dendritic cells mediate tolerance to vascularized grafts. Nat. Immunol. 7, 652–662.

Osorio, F., Reis e Sousa, C., 2011. Myeloid C-type lectin receptors in pathogen recognition and host defense. Immunity 34, 651–664.

Palucka, K., Banchereau, J., 2012. Cancer immunotherapy via dendritic cells. Nat. Rev. Cancer 12, 265–277.

Phillips, B., Nylander, K., Harnaha, J., Machen, J., Lakomy, R., Styche, A., et al., 2008. A microsphere-based vaccine prevents and reverses new-onset autoimmune diabetes. Diabetes 57, 1544–1555.

Poulin, L.F., Henri, S., de Bovis, B., Devilard, E., Kissenpfennig, A., Malissen, B., 2007. The dermis contains langerin + dendritic cells that develop and function independently of epidermal Langerhans cells. J. Exp. Med. 204, 3119–3131.

Poulin, L.F., Salio, M., Griessinger, E., Anjos-Afonso, F., Craciun, L., Chen, J.L., et al., 2010. Characterization of human DNGR-1 + BDCA3 + leukocytes as putative equivalents of mouse CD8alpha + dendritic cells. J. Exp. Med. 207, 1261–1271.

Proietto, A.I., O'Keeffe, M., Gartlan, K., Wright, M.D., Shortman, K., Wu, L., et al., 2004. Differential production of inflammatory chemokines by murine dendritic cell subsets. Immunobiology 209, 163–172.

Proietto, A.I., van Dommelen, S., Zhou, P., Rizzitelli, A., D'Amico, A., Steptoe, R.J., et al., 2008. Dendritic cells in the thymus contribute to T-regulatory cell induction. Proc. Natl. Acad. Sci. USA 105, 19869–19874.

Reis e Sousa, C., Hieny, S., Scharton-Kersten, T., Jankovic, D., Charest, H., Germain, R.N., et al., 1997. In vivo microbial stimulation induces rapid CD40 ligand-independent production of interleukin 12 by dendritic cells and their redistribution to T cell areas. J. Exp. Med. 186, 1819–1829.

Robbins, S.H., Walzer, T., Dembele, D., Thibault, C., Defays, A., Bessou, G., et al., 2008. Novel insights into the relationships between dendritic cell subsets in human and mouse revealed by genome-wide expression profiling. Genome Biol. 9, R17.

Robinson, M.J., Sancho, D., Slack, E.C., LeibundGut-Landmann, S., Reis e Sousa, C., 2006. Myeloid C-type lectins in innate immunity. Nat. Immunol. 7, 1258–1265.

Rönnblom, L., Pascual, V., 2008. The innate immune system in SLE: type I interferons and dendritic cells. Lupus. 17, 394–399.

Sainathan, S.K., Hanna, E.M., Gong, Q., Bishnupuri, K.S., Luo, Q., Colonna, M., et al., 2008. Granulocyte macrophage colony-stimulating factor ameliorates DSS-induced experimental colitis. Inflamm. Bowel Dis. 14, 88–99.

Sancho, D., Joffre, O.P., Keller, A.M., Rogers, N.C., Martinez, D., Hernanz-Falcon, P., et al., 2009. Identification of a dendritic cell receptor that couples sensing of necrosis to immunity. Nature 458, 899–903.

Sancho, D., Mourao-Sa, D., Joffre, O.P., Schulz, O., Rogers, N.C., Pennington, D.J., et al., 2008. Tumor therapy in mice via antigen targeting to a novel, DC-restricted C-type lectin. J. Clin. Invest. 118, 2098–2110.

Scheu, S., Dresing, P., Locksley, R.M., 2008. Visualization of IFNbeta production by plasmacytoid versus conventional dendritic cells under specific stimulation conditions in vivo. Proc. Natl. Acad. Sci. USA 105, 20416–20421.

Schnorrer, P., Behrens, G.M., Wilson, N.S., Pooley, J.L., Smith, C.M., El-Sukkari, D., et al., 2006. The dominant role of CD8 + dendritic cells in cross-presentation is not dictated by antigen capture. Proc. Natl. Acad. Sci. USA 103, 10729–10734.

Schroder, K., Zhou, R., Tschopp, J., 2010. The NLRP3 inflammasome: a sensor for metabolic danger? Science. 327, 296–300.

Scott, C.L., Aumeunier, A.M., Mowat, A.M., 2011. Intestinal CD103 + dendritic cells: master regulators of tolerance? Trends in Immunol. 32, 412–419.

Sestak, A.L., Furnrohr, B.G., Harley, J.B., Merrill, J.T., Namjou, B., 2011. The genetics of systemic lupus erythematosus and implications for targeted therapy. Ann. Rheum. Dis. 70 (Suppl. 1), i37–i43.

Shklovskaya, E., O'Sullivan, B.J., Ng, L.G., Roediger, B., Thomas, R., Weninger, W., et al., 2011. Langerhans cells are precommitted to immune tolerance induction. Proc. Natl. Acad. Sci. USA 108, 18049–18054.

Shortman, K., Heath, W.R., 2010. The CD8 + dendritic cell subset. Immunol. Rev. 234, 18–31.

Steinman, R.M., Cohn, Z.A., 1973. Identification of a novel cell type in peripheral lymphoid organs of mice. I. Morphology, quantitation, tissue distribution. J. Exp. Med. 137, 1142–1162.

Steinman, R.M., Hawiger, D., Nussenzweig, M.C., 2003. Tolerogenic dendritic cells. Annu. Rev. Immunol. 21, 685–711.

Stoop, J.N., Robinson, J.H., Hilkens, C.M., 2011. Developing tolerogenic dendritic cell therapy for rheumatoid arthritis: what can we learn from mouse models? Ann. Rheum. Dis. 70, 1526–1533.

Strober, W., Murray, P.J., Kitani, A., Watanabe, T., 2006. Signalling pathways and molecular interactions of NOD1 and NOD2. Nat. Rev. Immunol. 6, 9–20.

Tacken, P.J., de Vries, I.J., Torensma, R., Figdor, C.G., 2007. Dendritic-cell immunotherapy: from ex vivo loading to in vivo targeting. Nat. Rev. Immunol. 7, 790–802.

Thomson, A.W., Robbins, P.D., 2008. Tolerogenic dendritic cells for autoimmune disease and transplantation. Ann. Rheum. Dis. 67 (Suppl. 3), iii90–iii96.

Trombetta, E.S., Mellman, I., 2005. Cell biology of antigen processing in vitro and in vivo. Annu. Rev. Immunol. 23, 975–1028.

Uematsu, S., Akira, S., 2008. Toll-Like receptors (TLRs) and their ligands 8. Handb. Exp. Pharmacol. 1–20.

van Beelen, A.J., Zelinkova, Z., Taanman-Kueter, E.W., Muller, F.J., Hommes, D.W., Zaat, S.A., et al., 2007. Stimulation of the intracellular bacterial sensor NOD2 programs dendritic cells to promote interleukin-17 production in human memory T cells. Immunity 27, 660–669.

Varol, C., Zigmond, E., Jung, S., 2010. Securing the immune tightrope: mononuclear phagocytes in the intestinal lamina propria. Nat. Rev. Immunol. 10, 415–426.

Villadangos, J.A., Schnorrer, P., 2007. Intrinsic and cooperative antigen-presenting functions of dendritic-cell subsets in vivo. Nat. Rev. Immunol. 7, 543–555.

Villadangos, J.A., Young, L., 2008. Antigen-presentation properties of plasmacytoid dendritic cells. Immunity 29, 352–361.

Villani, A.C., Lemire, M., Fortin, G., Louis, E., Silverberg, M.S., Collette, C., et al., 2009. Common variants in the NLRP3 region contribute to Crohn's disease susceptibility. Nat Genet. 41, 71–76.

Vulink, A., Radford, K.J., Melief, C., Hart, D.N., 2008. Dendritic cells in cancer immunotherapy. Adv. Cancer Res. 99, 363–407.

Wilson, N.S., Villadangos, J.A., 2005. Regulation of antigen presentation and cross-presentation in the dendritic cell network: facts, hypothesis, and immunological implications. Adv. Immunol. 86, 241–305.

Yamazaki, S., Dudziak, D., Heidkamp, G.F., Fiorese, C., Bonito, A.J., Inaba, K., et al., 2008. CD8 + CD205 + splenic dendritic cells are specialized to induce Foxp3 + regulatory T cells. J. Immunol. 181, 6923–6933.

Young, L.J., Wilson, N.S., Schnorrer, P., Proietto, A., ten Broeke, T., Matsuki, Y., et al., 2008. Differential MHC class II synthesis and ubiquitination confers distinct antigen-presenting properties on conventional and plasmacytoid dendritic cells. Nat. Immunol. 9, 1244–1252.

Zaba, L.C., Krueger, J.G., Lowes, M.A., 2009. Resident and "inflammatory" dendritic cells in human skin. J. Invest. Dermatol. 129, 302–308.

Zaki, M.H., Lamkanfi, M., Kanneganti, T.D., 2011. The Nlrp3 inflammasome: contributions to intestinal homeostasis. Trends Immunol. 32, 171–179.

Zhang, J.G., Czabotar, P.E., Policheni, A.N., Caminschi, I., Wan, S.S., Kitsoulis, S., et al., 2012. The dendritic cell receptor Clec9A binds damaged cells via exposed actin filaments. Immunity 36, 646–657.

Chapter 13

Natural Killer Cells

Yenan T. Bryceson[1], Niklas K. Björkström[1,2], Jenny Mjösberg[1], and Hans-Gustaf Ljunggren[1]

[1]*Center for Infectious Medicine, Department of Medicine, Karolinska Institutet, Karolinska University Hospital, Stockholm, Sweden,* [2]*Liver Immunology Laboratory, Department of Medicine, Karolinska Institutet, Karolinska University Hospital, Stockholm, Sweden*

Chapter Outline

Introduction to NK Cells	187
NK Cell Development and Differentiation	188
Phenotype and Tissue Localization of NK Cells	189
Functional Responses by NK Cells	189
NK Cell Receptor Signaling and Effector Functions	190
NK Cell Contact and Adhesion to Target Cells	190
NK Cell Lytic Granule Polarization and Maturation	191
NK Cell Cytolytic Granule Exocytosis	192
NK Cell Chemokine and Cytokine Production	192
NK Cells and Human Autoimmunity	193
Defective Control of other Immune Cells Links NK Cells to Autoimmune Diseases	193
Genetic Association Studies Revealing Links between NK Cells and Autoimmune Diseases	194
Conclusions	195
References	195

INTRODUCTION TO NK CELLS

Natural killer (NK) cells were described in the 1970s as large granular lymphocytes exhibiting "natural cytotoxicity" against several types of tumor cells (Kiessling et al., 1975). Significant progress has been made since then in the dissection of additional functional traits of NK cells. By their cytotoxic potential they can kill many more types of cells than tumor cells, e.g., virus infected cells and several types of activated immune cells (Vivier et al., 2008). To carry out these functions, and to discriminate target cells from non-activated "normal" cells, NK cells are equipped with a molecular detection system that includes a variety of cell surface activating and inhibitory receptors (Lanier, 2005). Activating NK cell receptors can detect the presence of ligands on cells in "distress," such as stress-induced self-ligands (Bryceson et al., 2006a). In parallel, NK cells use inhibitory receptors to monitor the presence of constitutively expressed self-major histocompatibility complex (MHC) class I molecules (Long, 2008); MHC class I expressing cells are normally spared while cells lacking these molecules can be targeted by NK cells, a recognition strategy originally referred to as "missing-self" recognition (Ljunggren and

Kärre, 1990). NK cells are also critical components of the innate immune response, because of their ability to produce a variety of cytokines and chemokines (Vivier et al., 2008). Thus, NK cells may drive, shape, and regulate the activities of other immune cells and by these means affect the development of adaptive immune responses. NK cells respond to initial cues from myeloid cells including myeloid-derived dendritic cells (DC), as well as macrophages and plasmacytoid DC. This response is possible because NK cells express receptors for several myeloid-derived cytokines (Caligiuri, 2008; Vivier et al., 2008). Thus, secondary to triggering of myeloid cells by pattern recognition receptors, NK cells can relay and amplify key cytokine signals. Perhaps the best-characterized cytokine produced by NK cells is interferon (IFN)-γ. However, NK cells also secrete a number of other additional cytokines and other factors, including tumor necrosis factor (TNF)-α and immunoregulatory cytokines such as interleukin (IL)-5, IL-10, IL-13, the growth factor GM-CSF, and chemokines CCL3 (MIP-1α), CCL4 (MIP-1β), CCL5 (RANTES), and CXCL8 (IL-8). The ability to respond to a variety of cytokines suggests that the local microenvironment in which NK cells exist may shape and modulate

N. Rose & I. Mackay (Eds): The Autoimmune Diseases, Fifth edition. DOI: http://dx.doi.org/10.1016/B978-0-12-384929-8.00013-7

their function (Caligiuri, 2008; Vivier et al., 2008). Consistent with their functions as innate sentinels, NK cells are spread throughout lymphoid and non-lymphoid tissues. In many tissues, they represent a minor fraction of total lymphocytes. However, in other tissues like the liver and pregnant uterus they are abundant (Vivier et al., 2008).

Although important aspects of NK cell biology have been revealed using mice as a model organism, it should be noted that many central NK cell receptors are rapidly evolving in evolutionary terms. Thus, significant differences between the mouse and human immune systems exist, particularly with respect to NK cells (Mestas and Hughes, 2004). Our review is focused on the phenotype and function of human NK cells, highlighting recent advances in understanding their role in autoimmune diseases.

NK CELL DEVELOPMENT AND DIFFERENTIATION

NK cells belong to the hematopoietic system. They are derived from $CD34^+$ hematopoietic precursor cells (HPCs). In transcriptional terms, NK cells are most closely related to cytotoxic T lymphocytes (Sun and Lanier, 2011) and in humans typically defined as $CD3^- CD56^+$ lymphocytes. According to a newly proposed nomenclature, NK cells have been categorized as belonging to the family of innate lymphoid cells (ILCs) and more specifically the group 1 innate lymphoid cells (ILC1s) (Spits et al., 2013). In addition to differential transcriptional regulation, NK cells are distinguishable from other ILCs as NK cells do not express CD127. Furthermore, ILCs lack cytotoxic function as well as several functional NK cell markers including NKG2A and NKG2D. However, the exact relationships and plasticity between the NK cells and other ILCs remains to be further elucidated, especially in humans (Spits et al., 2013).

During fetal development, NK cells are among the first immune cells to appear. It is generally accepted that most NK cells develop in the bone marrow, based on evidence from early studies of bone marrow ablation in mice (Haller and Wigzell, 1977). Bone marrow-derived human $CD34^+$ HPCs can also be manipulated to differentiate *in vitro* into NK cells (Miller et al., 1992). In this setting, NK cell development is dependent on bone marrow stroma (Miller et al., 1994). Furthermore, it requires IL-2 and/or IL-15 (Miller et al. 1992, 1994) and is potentiated by flt3-ligands (Yu et al., 1998). One important question is: do NK cell precursors, formed in the bone marrow, traffic to distinct peripheral anatomical locations for their final stages of development? Several lines of research support this notion; for example, immune precursor cells with NK cell developmental potential are selectively enriched in human secondary lymphoid tissues (SLT),

such as lymph nodes and tonsil (Freud et al., 2005). These $CD34^+ CD45RA^+$ cells represent more than 95% of all HPCs in SLT, but are infrequent in bone marrow and blood.

Based on this, and other insights, a continuous SLT NK cell developmental pathway has been proposed (Freud et al., 2006; Freud and Caligiuri, 2006). In this pathway, "stage 1" NK cells (pro-NK cells) are characterized by a $CD34^+ CD117^- CD94^-$ phenotype, the lack of expression and transcription of CD122 (IL-2/15 receptor β-chain) and unresponsiveness to IL-15. Upon stimulation with flt3-ligand, IL-3, and IL-7, possibly in a stroma cell-dependent manner, these pro-NK cells acquire a "stage 2" NK cell (pre-NK cells) phenotype characterized by upregulation of CD122 that provides responsiveness to IL-15 (Freud et al., 2006). $CD34^+ CD117^+ CD94^-$ pre-NK cells are not fully committed to the NK cell lineage and can also give rise to other immune cells such as T cells and myeloid DCs. Furthermore, they lack characteristic NK cell functions, such as cytotoxicity and the capacity to produce IFN-γ. However, with IL-15 stimulation, pre-NK cells develop into "stage 3" NK cells (immature NK cells, iNK cells) characterized by loss of CD34 and a step-wise acquisition of CD56 together with a functional commitment to the NK cell linage. Finally, these iNK cells progress into "stage 4" NK cells characterized by bright expression of CD56 ($CD56^{bright}$ NK cells). This progression is marked by the acquisition of the inhibitory receptor CD94/NKG2A and such NK cell-associated activating receptors as NKp46 and NKG2D, as well as by the capacity to produce IFN-γ and to release perforin and granzyme-containing granules (Freud et al., 2006). NK cell expression of killer cell immunoglobulin-like receptors (KIR) for self-MHC class I confers NK cells with effector potential in a yet molecularly poorly defined process termed "education" or "licensing" (Kim et al., 2005; Anfossi et al., 2006; Elliott and Yokoyama, 2011). At present, many open questions remain with respect to how NK cell function relates to development and to what extent NK cell differentiation can be regarded as linear or branched.

Key transcription factors that regulate NK cell development and differentiation have recently been characterized (Klose et al., 2012; Cichocki et al., 2013). STAT5B has been implicated in the early stages of NK cell differentiation, alongside E4BP4 that induces ID2 and GATA3. Without any one of these transcription factors, NK cell development is grossly impaired with a block at the pre-NK to iNK stage. Similarly, but in an apparently parallel pathway, TOX is required for the pre-NK to iNK transition. TBX21 (T-bet) is also required for early NK cell development, while expression of EOMES is required for sustenance of NK cells in a mature stage. Importantly, NK cell selective deficiencies have been associated with autosomal dominant mutations in *GATA2* and *MCM4* (Gineau et al.,

2012; Mace et al., 2013). Much more information is needed to get a better view of how transcription factors program NK cell development and differentiation.

PHENOTYPE AND TISSUE LOCALIZATION OF NK CELLS

In humans, "mature" NK cells are divided into $CD56^{bright}$ and $CD56^{dim}$ subsets, defined by expression levels of CD56 (Lanier et al., 1986; Jacobs et al., 1992; Cooper et al., 2001; Caligiuri, 2008). These two subsets are present at varying proportions in different compartments of the human body. In blood, bone marrow, and spleen, $CD56^{dim}$ NK cells dominate, representing around 90% of all NK cells. On the other hand, in tonsils and other SLT $CD56^{bright}$ NK cells dominate. The liver, in contrast, contains nearly equal proportions of $CD56^{dim}$ and $CD56^{bright}$ NK cells. The $CD56^{bright}$ and $CD56^{dim}$ NK cell subsets differ in phenotype and function. In brief, $CD56^{bright}$ NK cells are negative for, or express only low levels of, the low affinity Fc-receptor CD16, express few inhibitory killer cell immunoglobulin-like receptors (KIRs), or cytotoxic molecules such as perforin and different granzymes (Cooper et al., 2001). On the other hand, $CD56^{bright}$ NK cells uniformly express the inhibitory CD94/NKG2A receptor, as well as CD62L and the high affinity IL-2 receptor α chain (CD25). $CD56^{dim}$ NK cells display a variegated expression of KIRs, NKG2A, and CD62L, express high levels of CD16 on their surface, and contain intracellular granules with large amounts of perforin and granzymes (Cooper et al., 2001). With respect to function, $CD56^{bright}$ NK cells were generally believed to produce large amounts of cytokines but have little capacity to perform cytotoxicity, whereas $CD56^{dim}$ NK cells were believed to be efficient killers but poor at producing cytokines (Fehniger et al., 2003; Ferlazzo et al., 2004; Morandi et al., 2006; Burt et al., 2009). However, recent work suggests that $CD56^{bright}$ NK cells also can mediate some cytotoxicity and produce cytokines in response to exogenous cytokine stimuli, whereas $CD56^{dim}$ NK cells both have efficient capacities for performing cytotoxicity and producing cytokines upon specific target cell recognition (Fauriat et al., 2010).

$CD56^{bright}$ and $CD56^{dim}$ NK cell subsets might represent two sequential stages of NK cell differentiation, with $CD56^{bright}$ cells being less mature (Lanier et al., 1986; Caligiuri, 2008). Several lines of (sometimes indirect) evidence support this hypothesis. First, $CD56^{bright}$ NK cells appear earlier in immune reconstitution settings than do $CD56^{dim}$ NK cells, and the former can represent up to 70−80% of all peripheral blood NK cells a few months after hematopoietic stem cell transplantation (Jacobs et al., 2001; Shilling et al., 2003). Second, $CD56^{bright}$ NK cells

have a more immature phenotype compared to $CD56^{dim}$ NK cells with, for instance, expression of CD117 (c-kit) (Matos et al., 1993), which is typically expressed by immature HPCs. $CD56^{bright}$ NK cells also display longer telomeres (25) and, morphologically, constitute both granular and agranular cells, whereas all $CD56^{dim}$ NK cells are granular (Romagnani et al., 2007). Furthermore, in humanized mice purified $CD56^{bright}$ NK cells were recently shown to differentiate into $CD56^{dim}$ NK cells (Huntington et al., 2009). Hence, a substantial amount of evidence suggests $CD56^{bright}$ ("stage 4") NK cells to be precursors of $CD56^{dim}$ ("stage 5") NK cells. Until recently, $CD56^{dim}$ NK cells were considered an "end stage" of human NK cell differentiation. However, recent data have demonstrated that even $CD56^{dim}$ NK cells undergo a continuous differentiation process, the latter characterized by a gradual shift from $NKG2A^{+}CD62L^{+}CD57^{-}KIR^{-}$ cells towards more terminally differentiated $NKG2A^{-}CD62L^{-}CD57^{+}KIR^{+}$ cells (Björkström et al., 2010).

Besides $CD56^{bright}$ and $CD56^{dim}$ NK cells, which constitute the majority of NK cells in human peripheral blood and tissues at variable relative frequencies, a distinct population of $CD56^{superbright}$ NK cells has been characterized in the endometrium which becomes the dominant lymphocyte population in the decidua of pregnant women (Manaster and Mandelboim 2010). Such uterine NK cells may represent relatively immature NK cells and display a unique phenotype, expressing the tetraspanin CD9, high frequencies of activation markers CD69 and HLA-DR, as well as inhibitory NKG2A and KIR. Interestingly, they do not express CD16 or CD57.

FUNCTIONAL RESPONSES BY NK CELLS

NK cells and cytotoxic T cells (CTLs) are thought to share mechanisms for target cell elimination. Cytotoxicity by both NK cells and CTLs relies on directed release of their lytic granule contents. These lytic granules are specialized secretory lysosomes that contain perforin, granzymes, and Fas ligand that all contribute to target cell killing (Dustin and Long, 2010; Griffiths et al., 2010). Imaging studies comparing target cell recognition by NK cells and CTLs *in vitro* and *in vivo* suggest some noteworthy distinctions. *In vitro*, CTLs rapidly establish cytoskeletal polarity, whereas NK cells are more tentative in their interactions with target cells (Wulfing et al., 2003). *In vivo*, CTLs form stable contacts with tumor cells expressing cognate antigen, whereas NK cells establish mainly dynamic contacts (Deguine et al., 2010). These observations suggest differences in the molecular machinery underlying NK cell and CTL recognition and elimination of target cells.

Recent studies of NK cell responses have also highlighted considerable heterogeneity among human peripheral blood NK cells, including hierarchies that govern the strength of activation stimuli needed for induction of specific responses (Bryceson et al., 2005, 2009, 2011). For example, induction of inside-out signals for leukocyte functional antigen (LFA)-1-mediated adhesion exhibits a markedly low threshold for activation. Induction of chemokines such as MIP-1β requires stronger activating stimuli, whereas degranulation and production of cytokines such as TNF-α and IFN-γ display the most stringent requirements for induction (Bryceson et al., 2011). Some of the functional heterogeneity in different NK cell populations can be accounted for by differences in cellular differentiation (Björkström et al., 2010; Juelke et al., 2010; Lopez-Verges et al., 2010). For example, relatively immature CD56^bright NK cells excel at cytokine production in response to exogenous cytokines such as IL-2, IL-12, IL-15, and IL-18. The same cells, however, express low levels of perforin and are, consequentially, less cytotoxic than CD56^dim NK cells and do not produce cytokines as readily in response to target cell recognition. In contrast, relatively more differentiated (NKG2A⁺CD62L⁺CD57⁻KIR⁻) CD56^dim NK cells produce significant amounts of IFN-γ in response to exogenous cytokines, express higher levels of perforin, and have a stronger ability to mediate cytotoxicity. They can also produce ample amounts of cytokines in response to target cell recognition. Finally, highly differentiated (NKG2A⁻CD62L⁻CD57⁺KIR⁺) CD56^dim NK cells express high levels of perforin and display potent cytotoxic capacity. These cells are also strong producers of cytokines in response to target cell recognition. However, the response of these NK cells to exogenous cytokines is comparatively blunted.

In parallel to the continuous maturation process, recognition of self-MHC class I molecules by inhibitory receptors potentiates the NK cell's ability to respond functionally, a process referred to as "education" or "licensing" (Kim et al., 2005; Anfossi et al., 2006; Elliott and Yokoyama, 2011). Superimposing differentiation and education processes on NK cell functionality does not, however, fully explain the heterogeneity in NK cell responses. Studies have revealed that the thresholds for effector responses are highly dynamic. For example, different molecular pathways are likely used depending on activation by different cytokines and triggering of different (combinations of) cellular receptors, and gives rise to differences in response rates (Bryceson et al., 2009, 2011).

NK CELL RECEPTOR SIGNALING AND EFFECTOR FUNCTIONS

A multitude of activating NK cell receptors that belong to different receptor families have been described (Table 13.1). They contain highly divergent cytoplasmic signaling domains. The signaling pathways orchestrated by some activating NK cell receptors are known whereas others are significantly less well characterized (Bryceson et al., 2006a; Watzl and Long, 2010). In contrast, structurally distinct inhibitory NK cell receptors all contain immunoreceptor tyrosine-based inhibition motifs (ITIMs). The signaling by such motifs has been extensively studied and is mainly mediated through activation of tyrosine phosphatases such as SHP-1 as well as the tyrosine kinase c-Abl (Long, 2008; Peterson and Long, 2008). Some inhibitory receptors engage other negative regulators such as SHIP, an inositol 5-phosphatase, and the Src family tyrosine kinase CSK. Taken together, today's knowledge suggests that potent NK cell effector functions such as cytotoxicity and cytokine production require dynamic integration of signals derived from multiple receptors (Liu et al., 2009). The following sections will focus on advances in our understanding of the molecular processes underlying NK cell effector responses.

NK Cell Contact and Adhesion to Target Cells

A first step in NK cell responses to pathogen-infected target cells or tumor cells involves recruitment of NK cells to the site of inflammation/infection or to the tumor. NK cells express several chemokine receptors. The mechanism of NK cell trafficking to inflamed tissues is fairly well understood and has recently been reviewed elsewhere (Gregoire et al., 2007). During inflammation, NK cells can be recruited by chemokines that bind the CCR2, CCR5, CXCR3, and CX3CR1 chemokine receptors. However, the degree to which NK cells constitutively traffic in normal tissues is relatively less well understood. How NK cells detect and discriminate target cells has recently been studied quite extensively. The initial contact between NK cells and target cells may involve any of a number of different receptors, leading to adhesion mediated by the integrin leukocyte functional antigen (LFA)-1. Activating receptors, including CD16, 2B4, NKG2D, DNAM-1, as well as LFA-1 itself, can rapidly induce necessary inside-out signals for the activation of LFA-1 in freshly isolated human NK cells, promoting the initial signals required for adhesion (Bryceson et al., 2009). As opposed to activating receptors, inhibitory receptor signals can abrogate adhesion to target cells (Burshtyn et al., 2000; Bryceson et al., 2009). The signals for induction of inside-out activation of LFA-1 are not well defined. As the activating NK cell receptors have distinct cytoplasmic domains, their signaling cascades differ. Live cell imaging of NK cells on supported planar lipid bilayers carrying ligands for LFA-1, NKG2D, 2B4, and CD16 has shown that, indeed, these receptors induce quite diverse behaviors by NK cells (Liu et al., 2009). In regards to signals for

TABLE 13.1 Specificity and Signaling of Human NK Cell Receptors

Receptor	Signaling	Cellular ligand	Function
FcgRIIIa (CD16)	Activation (ITAM)	IgG	Elimination of antibody coated cells (ADCC)
NKp30 (CD337)	Co-activation (ITAM)	B7-H6	NK cell–myeloid cell cross-talk, tumor recognition
NKp44 (CD336)	Activation (ITAM)	?	?
NKp46 (CD335)	Co-activation (ITAM)	?	Surveillance of mitotic cells
KIR (CD158a, b, etc.)	Activation (ITAM)	HLA class I	?
CD94/NKG2C (CD159c)	Activation (ITAM)	HLA-E	?
NKG2D (CD314)	Co-activation (YxNM)	ULBP, MICA, MICB	Surveillance of tumor cells and genotoxic stress
NKp80	? (hemi-ITAM)	AICL	NK cell–myeloid cell cross-talk
DNAM-1 (CD226)	Co-activation	CD112, CD155	Surveillance of tissue integrity
2B4 (CD244)	Co-activation (ITSM)	CD48	Interaction with hematopoetic cells
CRACC (CD319)	Co-activation (ITSM)	CRACC (CD319)	Interaction with hematopoetic cells
NTB-A	Co-activation (ITSM)	NTB-A	Interaction with hematopoetic cells
CD2	Co-activation	CD58	Interaction with hematopoetic and endothelial cells
KIR2DL4 (CD158d)	?	HLA-G (soluble)	Trophoblast-induced vascular remodeling?
LFA-1 (CD11a/CD18)	Granule polarization	ICAM	Recruitment and activation during inflammation, efficient cytotoxicity
KIR (CD158)	Inhibition (ITIM)	HLA class I alleles	Assess loss of MHC class I alleles
LIR1, LILR1 (CD85j)	Inhibition (ITIM)	HLA class I	Assess loss of MHC class I expression
CD94/NKG2A (CD159a)	Inhibition (ITIM)	HLA-E	Gauge MHC class I expression
KLRG1	Inhibition (ITIM)	E-cadherin	Assess loss of tissue integrity
NKR-P1 (CD161)	Inhibition (ITIM)	LLT1	?
LAIR-1 (CD305)	Inhibition (ITIM)	Collagen	Control activation in extracellular matrix
Siglec-7 (CD328)	Inhibition (ITIM)	Sialic acid	?
Siglec-9 (CD329)	Inhibition (ITIM)	Sialic acid	?
IRp60 (CD300a)	Inhibition (ITIM)	?	?

inside-out activation of LFA-1, phosphorylation and activation of VAV1 has been postulated to be a common denominator of signaling pathways downstream of activating receptors including LFA-1 itself. Concomitantly, VAV1 phosphorylation provides a point at which inhibitory receptor signals can oppose signals from activating receptors. Specifically, phosphorylated VAV1 is a substrate of SHP-1 that is recruited by inhibitory NK cell receptors and acts to prevent NK activation (Stebbins et al., 2003). Several other signaling proteins, including

WASP, Cdc42, Ras, Rap1, CrkL, and HS1, have been implicated in signaling for adhesion.

NK Cell Lytic Granule Polarization and Maturation

Besides adhesion, LFA-1 has a key role in promoting perforin-containing granule polarization towards the target cell, facilitating efficient cytotoxicity (Barber et al., 2004; Bryceson et al., 2005). Moreover, such granule polarization towards the immune synapse is the result of two different molecular processes. First, granules rapidly converge in dynein-dependent, minus-end directed motion to the microtubule-organizing center (MTOC) (Mentlik et al., 2010). In the NK cell line YTS, antibody-mediated blockade of LFA-1 impairs granule convergence at the MTOC upon target cell contact, suggesting that LFA-1-mediated signals facilitate this process (Mentlik et al., 2010). Second, following convergence of the granules and within minutes, the MTOC and granules polarize towards the interaction site in an LFA-1-dependent manner (Bryceson et al., 2005; Mentlik et al., 2010). In regards to the signaling pathways involved in LFA-1-mediated polarization, several key proteins have been identified. Talin, binding to the cytoplasmic tail of LFA-1, is required for the recruitment of WASP, Arp2/3, vinculin, and actin (Mace et al., 2009, 2010). Furthermore, WASP is required for the accumulation of F-actin at the synapse. Moreover, silencing of WASP interacting protein (WIP) in the human NK cell line YTS impaired lytic granule polarization but had no effect on the formation of conjugates with target cells (Krzewski et al., 2008). The second messenger, diacylglycerol, was required for MTOC polarization and cytotoxicity by CTL (Quann et al., 2009); however, the extent to which diacylglycerol regulates LFA-1-mediated MTOC polarization in NK cells remains to be established. Recent evidence indicated that signaling for granule polarization by LFA-1 in IL-2-expanded human NK cells also involved CD3ζ-chain phosphorylation, SYK recruitment and activation, and PLC-γ activation (March and Long 2011). Activation of PLC-γ resulted in hydrolysis of phosphatidylinositol (4,5)-bisphosphate (PIP$_2$) to generate the second messengers, diacylglycerol and inositol (1,4,5)-trisphosphate (IP$_3$). Downstream of LFA-1, PLC-γ activation led to PKC activation, and pharmacological inhibition of PLC-γ abrogated granule polarization (March and Long 2011). Upon recognition of susceptible target cells, the tyrosine kinase PYK2 was also recruited to the immune synapse, and transfection of dominant negative PYK2 blocked MTOC and paxillin movement to the synapse (Sancho et al., 2000). In summary, a number of studies suggest pathways involving talin, WASP, WIP, PYK, JNK, and paxillin, as well as CD3ζ, SYK, and PLC-γ for granule polarization.

NK Cell Cytolytic Granule Exocytosis

Vesicle exocytosis is a requirement for NK cell cytotoxicity (Bryceson et al., 2006b). Studies of knockout mice have demonstrated an essential role for PLC-γ in granule exocytosis (Tassi et al., 2005; Caraux et al., 2006). Following the activation of PLC-γ, IP$_3$ can trigger cytoplasmic release of Ca^{2+} from the endoplasmic reticulum (ER). Engagement of

CD16 is sufficient to induce robust intracellular Ca^{2+} mobilization, whereas several other receptors do not. Rather, co-activation receptors trigger intracellular Ca^{2+} mobilization when engaged in specific pair-wise combinations (Bryceson et al., 2006b). Additional data suggest that the molecular basis for such co-activation involves complementary phosphorylation of SLP-76 as well as overcoming a threshold for activation of VAV1 that is set by the ubiquitin ligase c-Cbl (Kim et al., 2010). PLC-γ activation leads to IP$_3$-mediated Ca^{2+} release from the ER, which ultimately results in depletion of intracellular Ca^{2+} stores and induction of store-operated Ca^{2+} entry (SOCE). NK cells from patients with mutations in either STIM1 or ORAI1 display defective degranulation, demonstrating a requirement for ORAI1 channel-mediated SOCE for lytic granule exocytosis (Maul-Pavicic et al., 2011). Notably, the ORAI1 deficiency does not affect signals for adhesion or granule polarization (Maul-Pavicic et al., 2011). Further downstream, several proteins required for NK cell exocytosis have been identified through studies of patients with hyperinflammatory syndromes caused by defective lymphocyte cytotoxicity. These proteins include Rab27a that facilitates terminal trafficking of lytic granules to sites of exocytosis, Munc13-4 that primes lytic granule exocytosis, as well as syntaxin-11 and Munc18-2 that facilitate membrane fusion (Stinchcombe et al., 2001; Feldmann et al., 2003; Bryceson et al., 2007; Wood et al., 2011). Furthermore, results suggest that distinct endosomal compartments fuse prior to lytic granule fusion with the plasma membrane, facilitating the exocytic process (Menager et al., 2007; Wood et al., 2009). Finally, for efficient cytotoxicity, lytic granules must traverse the actin-rich immunological synapse to enable exocytosis. The adenosine triphosphate (ATP)-dependent actin motor protein myosin IIA has been shown to associate with lytic granules in NK cells and play a role in mediating lytic granule traversation for exocytosis (Sanborn et al., 2009).

NK Cell Chemokine and Cytokine Production

Target cell recognition by freshly isolated human NK cells induces a set of chemokines, including CCL3, CCL4, CCL5, as well as the cytokines TNF-α and IFN-γ (Fauriat et al., 2010). Chemokines are induced within one hour of stimulation, whereas secretion occurs several hours after activation. Importantly, experiments varying the signaling input for NK cell activation have revealed a hierarchy in requirements for the induction of chemokines and cytokines, with chemokines induced by weakly activating signals, degranulation induced by intermediate levels of activating stimuli, and cytokines requiring the strongest activation. This hierarchy is reflected in the requirements for induction of different effector responses. PLC-γ is required for all responses (Tassi et al., 2005; Caraux et al., 2006). A deficiency in SOCE, as seen in NK cells from humans with autosomal recessive STIM1 and ORAI1 mutations, results in defective degranulation and cytokine production induced upon target cell recognition, but only partially impairs chemokine production (Maul-Pavicic et al., 2011). Notably, NK cells from PI3K p110δ-deficient mice displayed selectively impaired cytokine production, whereas knockout of both p110δ and p110γ was required to impair cytotoxicity (Kim et al., 2007; Tassi et al., 2007). Moreover, PKCθ-deficient mice had defects in IFN-γ transcription and secretion due to impaired JNK, AP-1, and NFAT activation (Tassi et al., 2008). Yet, NK cell-mediated cytotoxicity was not impaired in PKCθ-deficient mice. Curiously, a Rap1b deficiency in mice selectively deters NK cell chemokine and cytokine production, but not cytotoxicity (Awasthi et al., 2010). Thus, a few proteins, including PI3K p110δ and PKCθ may be specifically required for transcription of cytokine genes. Further studies are required to understand how these proteins are integrated in the signaling pathways for NK cell activation and how the engagement of different activating receptor controls their function.

NK CELLS AND HUMAN AUTOIMMUNITY

Classically, autoimmune diseases typify syndromes caused by an inappropriate activation of cells of the adaptive immune system; i.e., T cells and B cells, resulting in cell-specific, organ-specific, or systemic tissue damage. Typical examples of such diseases include multiple sclerosis, rheumatoid arthritis, and insulin-dependent type 1 diabetes. Autoimmune diseases often display sexual bias. In this respect, several studies indicate somewhat higher NK cell numbers and activity in men than in women, but these differences often do not reach statistical significance with studies of relatively small sample sizes. Autoimmune diseases have been thought to be initiated in steps, including release of self-antigens from the target organ, a priming step in secondary lymphoid organs, and finally immune cell homing to the target organ/tissue and subsequent tissue destruction (Ji et al., 1999). NK cells can likely act at all these steps; i.e., as mediators of initial target damage leading to release of self-antigens, at the level of T cell priming in secondary lymphoid organs, and at the level of the target organ as immunomodulatory or effector cells (Pazmany, 2005; Shi & van Kaer, 2006; Perricone et al., 2008; Flodström-Tullberg et al., 2009) (Figure 13.1).

Most research results pointing towards a role for NK cells in human autoimmune diseases are, obviously, correlative. Associations between NK cell activity and autoimmune conditions appear in several reports, including

Promotion of autoimmune disease

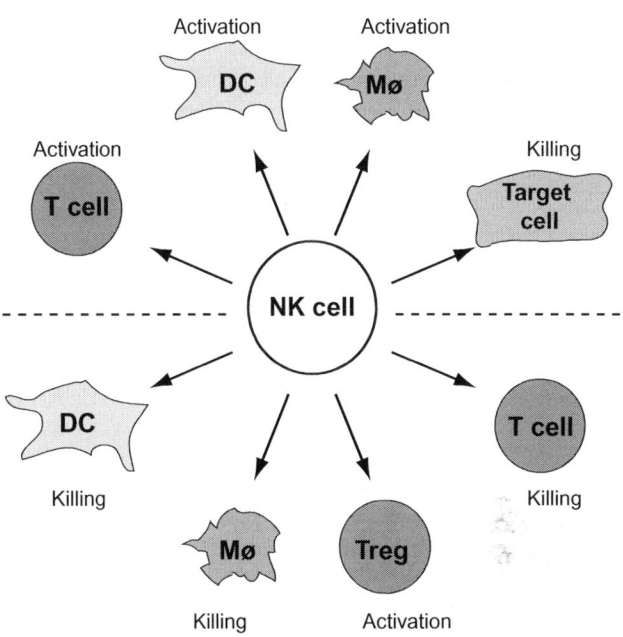

Protection from autoimmune disease

FIGURE 13.1   NK cells may affect autoimmune diseases in many different ways, for example by promoting or preventing functions of other cells, or by killing them. The figure illustrates possible interactions between NK cells and other cells as well as their outcomes. *Figure modified from Flodstrom-Tullberg et al., 2009.*

those describing studies finding altered numbers, phenotypes, and functions of NK cells (Shi & van Kaer, 2001; Pazmany, 2005; Perricone et al., 2008; Flodström-Tullberg et al., 2009). Some older studies are, however, difficult to interpret since they fail to distinguish NK cells from regulatory NKT cells or T cells expressing NK cell-associated receptors. An additional problem is determining if abnormalities in NK cell populations are a cause and/or an effect of a given disease state. Finally, most studies rely on assessment of NK cells from peripheral blood, not from appropriate secondary lymphoid organs or affected tissues. Despite these shortcomings, a substantial amount of evidence supports a direct involvement of NK cells in human autoimmunity.

Defective Control of other Immune Cells Links NK Cells to Autoimmune Diseases

The impaired NK cell cytotoxic function frequently observed in some humans with autoimmune diseases and/or other inflammatory conditions highlights the role of NK cells in controlling other cells, e.g., macrophages. Macrophage activation syndrome (MAS) is associated with several rheumatic diseases, most commonly with systemic juvenile idiopathic arthritis (sJIA) (Villanueva et al., 2005; Kelly and Ramanan, 2007) (Chapter 37). Clinically, this syndrome closely resembles familial hemophagocytic lymphohistiocytosis (FHL), a life-threatening genetic disorder in which NK cell function is absent or depressed (Bryceson and Ljunggren, 2007; Wood et al., 2011). As in FHL, patients with MAS have profoundly decreased NK cell cytotoxic activity (Ravelli et al., 2012). Therefore, impaired NK cell cytotoxicity might be, at least in part, causative of MAS. Supporting this notion, an sJIA patient with low NK cell cytotoxic function was found to harbor compound heterozygous splice-site and missense mutations in *UNC13D*, a gene associated with FHL (Hazen et al., 2008). Another link between NK cells and macrophages comes from studies showing that CD56^{bright} NK cells accumulate in certain inflammatory lesions and, in the appropriate cytokine environment, can engage with monocytes in a reciprocal activation fashion, thereby amplifying the inflammatory response. Moreover, CD56^{bright} NK cells can trigger the differentiation of monocytes into DCs (Zhang et al., 2007). Such positive feedback loops could well promote the pathogenesis of chronic inflammatory conditions such as rheumatoid arthritis (Dalbeth et al., 2004). Moreover, naturally occurring mutations in genes that cause a defect in NK cells are found in patients with abnormalities in TAP-peptide transporters, who typically suffer from chronic infections in childhood and autoimmune manifestations later in life. Notably, although interactions with macrophages are particularly relevant to organ-specific autoimmunity, NK cells also modulate innate and adaptive immunity by interacting with many other cell types, e.g., other lymphocytes including NKT cells as well as effector and regulatory T cells (Carnaud et al., 1999; Assarsson et al., 2004; Ferlazzo et al., 2004; Martín-Fontecha et al., 2004; Ghiringhelli et al., 2006; Shanker et al., 2007).

A specific point at which NK cells cytotoxicity can act to modify immune responses is through killing of activated T cells. Interestingly, upon cytomegalovirus infection in mice, NK cells can kill activated CD4$^+$ T cells, thereby affecting CD8$^+$ T cell function and exhaustion (Waggoner et al., 2011). In a mouse model of arthritis, blockade of the NK cell receptor NKG2A facilitated NK cell elimination of pathogenic CD4$^+$ T cells, arresting disease progression (Leavenworth et al., 2011). Such NK cell-mediated modulation of immune responses may well have implications for human autoimmunity. Moreover, NK cells may limit responses through modes other than cellular cytotoxicity. In studies of lupus, at least *in vitro*, NK cells can potentiate IFN-α production by plasmacytoid DC by up to a thousand-fold. IFN-α is a key cytokine involved in driving the pathogenesis of the disease

(Eloranta et al., 2009). The NK cell-mediated enhancement of IFN-α production by plasmacytoid DC is contact dependent and partially relies on secretion of the chemokine CCL4 (MIP-1β) by NK cells (Hagberg et al., 2011). Thus, NK cell immunoregulatory interactions may also exacerbate autoimmune responses.

Although less is known in contexts of autoimmunity, roles for NK cells as inducers of organ-specific and systemic tissue damage have also recently been suggested in certain acute and chronic viral infections. For instance, during flares of chronic hepatitis B virus infection, NK cells have been implicated to mediate liver damage via the apoptosis-inducing molecule TRAIL (Dunn et al., 2007). During acute human hantavirus infection, a hemorrhagic fever-inducing virus infection with high mortality, NK cells are highly activated and damage arises to the vasculature system long after the virus has been cleared from the body (Björkström et al., 2011).

Genetic Association Studies Revealing Links between NK Cells and Autoimmune Diseases

Linkage analysis in several autoimmune disease conditions has implicated various NK cell receptors in pathogenesis (Kulkarni et al., 2008). For example, certain *KIR* receptor genes, the products of which are expressed on NK cells and some T cell subsets, have been associated with the development of autoimmune diseases. *KIR* genes are polymorphic and the *KIR* gene complex is polygenic, encoding varying numbers of inhibitory and activating receptors. Interactions of the independently segregating KIR and HLA loci are important for NK cell education/licensing and target cell recognition (Jonsson and Yokoyama, 2009). The existence of KIR-HLA genotypes that tune NK cells towards activation are favorable in some infectious diseases, but might also predispose to autoimmunity (Kulkarni et al., 2008). A number of associations predisposing to autoimmune diseases have been identified in which activating KIR or KIR/HLA genotypes are accompanied by lack of inhibition. For example, scleroderma, a disease of tissue fibrosis, inflammation, and vascular injury, has been linked to the presence of activating *KIR2DS2*, in the absence of a corresponding inhibitory *KIR2DL2* (Momot et al., 2004). Likewise, the risk of psoriatic arthritis is enhanced in patients carrying *KIR2DS1* and/or *KIR2DS2*, and this effect is augmented in the absence of ligands for the inhibitory *KIR2DL1* and *KIR2DL2/3*, respectively (Nelson et al., 2004). Similarly, for rheumatoid arthritis, increased risk is associated with a presence of the *KIR2DS2* gene (Yen et al., 2001). Type 1 diabetes is associated with the expression of KIR2DS2/HLA ligand pairs in an environment of weak inhibitory interactions (van der Slik et al., 2003, 2007). In primary sclerosing cholangitis, a claimed autoimmune liver disease characterized by progressive destruction of the biliary tract, homozygosity for HLA-C1, a ligand for KIR2DL3, is associated with increased susceptibility for disease (Karlsen et al., 2007; Hov et al., 2010). Finally, ankylosing spondylitis shows a strong relationship to *HLA-B27*, a ligand for KIR3DL2; NK cells from patients with this disease have predominant KIR3DL2 expression and show an activated phenotype as measured by CD38 expression (Chan et al., 2005). Thus, the interplay between human NK cell inhibitory and activating receptor-MHC class I ligand pairs has provided significant evidence with respect to the involvement of NK cells in human autoimmunity. Noteworthy, however, the function of KIR may in some instances also be exerted at the level of autoimmune T cells, e.g., through augmentation of low affinity activation signals (Björkström et al., 2012).

In addition to receptors that bind MHC class I molecules, a number of other receptors that bind stress-induced ligands or regulate interactions with other immune cells may dictate NK cell specificity. Inappropriate expression of activating receptor NKG2D ligands can lead to detrimental NK cell activation, which in turn may trigger or exacerbate autoimmunity. The best-characterized NKG2D ligands are the MICA/B cellular stress-induced molecules that act as danger signals to alert NK cells and CD8 T lymphocytes (Bauer et al., 1999). Acquisition of MICA/B ligands on the surfaces of potential target cells may cause the breakdown of tolerance. MICA/B molecules, when inappropriately expressed, may thus trigger or worsen an autoimmune response. The involvement of NKG2D and its ligands in autoimmunity was first revealed in patients with rheumatoid arthritis (Groh et al., 2003). It has also been demonstrated that MICA/B are overexpressed on gut epithelium during active celiac disease (Hüe et al., 2004). However, in situations of MICA/B upregulation, these molecules may be targets not only for NK cells but also for T cells, as demonstrated in several studies (Meresse et al., 2004). Polymorphisms of human *MICA* have been associated with a variety of autoimmune disorders. One such example is patients with primary sclerosing cholangitis in whom several studies have identified the *MICA*008* allele in association with increased disease susceptibility (Norris et al., 2001; Wiencke et al., 2001). The functional implications of such polymorphism are, however, far from clear, and *MICA* associations frequently reflect a linkage disequilibrium with *HLA-B* alleles (Field et al., 2008). Still to be established is whether mutations in the NKG2D gene (*KLRK1*) might underlie some autoimmune diseases. Recently, however, a single nucleotide polymorphism (SNP) in *CD226*, conferring an amino acid substitution in the DNAM-1 receptor, was linked to the development of multiple sclerosis, rheumatoid arthritis, type 1 diabetes, and autoimmune thyroid disease (Hafler et al., 2009). In addition, two intronic SNPs in *CD244*, that likely increase 2B4 receptor surface expression, have been connected with the development of rheumatoid arthritis in a Japanese cohort (Suzuki et al., 2008). However, in a mouse model of lupus, *Cd224*-deficiency exacerbated autoantibody production in an NK cell-independent manner (Brown et al., 2011). Together, these data implicate activating NK cell receptors in susceptibility to multiple autoimmune diseases. We should note, however, that despite the often-used term "NK cell receptors," these receptors are also expressed on other lymphocyte populations, and it remains to be established to what degree genetic associations are conferred by alterations specifically in NK cell function.

CONCLUSIONS

With the exception of genetic linkage analysis, relatively few studies have been undertaken to explore the role of NK cells in human autoimmunity compared to other diseases where NK cells are more directly implicated. Much knowledge on the role of NK cells in autoimmunity still comes from studies in experimental animal models, and caution must be taken before translating those results directly to human conditions. The emerging view, however, is that NK cells may function as important regulatory cells during the priming phase of adaptive immune responses and as regulatory and effector cells at the sites of target organ during inflammation. NK cell control of macrophage activation may be one important checkpoint at the level of the target organ in the development of autoimmunity. The ability of NK cells to influence adaptive immune responses and to control immune cell homeostasis in humans clearly deserves further attention. Improved comprehension of how NK cells affect numerous autoimmune conditions may furthermore pave the way for new immunotherapeutic approaches towards alleviating or preventing such diseases.

REFERENCES

Anfossi, N., Andre, P., Guia, S., Falk, C.S., Roetynck, S., Stewart, C.A., et al., 2006. Human NK cell education by inhibitory receptors for MHC class I. Immunity. 25, 331–342.

Assarsson, E., Kambayashi, T., Schatzle, J.D., Cramer, S.O., von Bonin, A., Jensen, P.E., et al., 2004. NK cells stimulate proliferation of T and NK cells through 2B4/CD48 interactions. J. Immunol. 173, 174–180.

Awasthi, A., Samarakoon, A., Chu, H., Kamalakannan, R., Quilliam, L.A., Chrzanowska-Wodnicka, M., et al., 2010. Rap1b facilitates NK cell functions via IQGAP1-mediated signalosomes. J. Exp. Med. 207, 1923–1938.

Barber, D.F., Faure, M., Long, E.O., 2004. LFA-1 contributes an early signal for NK cell cytotoxicity. J. Immunol. 173, 3653–3659.

Bauer, S., Groh, V., Wu, J., Steinle, A., Phillips, J.H., Lanier, L.L., et al., 1999. Activation of NK cells and T cells by NKG2D, a receptor for stress-inducible MICA. Science. 285, 727–729.

Björkström, N.K., Beziat, V., Chihocki, F., Liu, L.L., Levine, J., Larsson, S., et al., 2012. CD8 T cells express randomly selected KIRs with distinct specificities compared with NK cells. Blood. 120, 3455–3465.

Björkström, N.K., Lindgren, T., Stoltz, M., Fauriat, C., Braun, M., Evander, M., et al., 2011. Rapid expansion and long-term persistence of elevated NK cell numbers in humans infected with hantavirus. J. Exp. Med. 208, 13–21.

Björkström, N.K., Riese, P., Heuts, F., Andersson, S., Fauriat, C., Ivarsson, M.A., et al., 2010. Expression patterns of NKG2A, KIR, and CD57 define a process of CD56dim NK cell differentiation uncoupled from NK cell eduction. Blood. 116, 3853–3864.

Brown, D.R., Calpe, S., Keszei, M., Wang, N., McArdel, S., Terhorst, C., et al., 2011. Cutting edge: an NK cell-independent role for Slamf4 in controlling humoral autoimmunity. J. Immunol. 187, 21–25.

Bryceson, Y.T., Chiang, S.C., Darmanin, S., Fauriat, C., Schlums, H., Theorell, J., et al., 2011. Molecular mechanisms of natural killer cell activation. J. Innate Immun. 3, 216–226.

Bryceson, Y.T., Ljunggren, H.G., 2007. Lymphocyte effector functions: armed for destruction? Curr. Opin. Immunol. 19, 337–338.

Bryceson, Y.T., Ljunggren, H.G., Long, E.O., 2009. Minimal requirement for induction of natural cytotoxicity and intersection of activation signals by inhibitory receptors. Blood. 114, 2657–2666.

Bryceson, Y.T., March, M.E., Barber, D.F., Ljunggren, H.G., Long, E.O., 2005. Cytolytic granule polarization and degranulation controlled by different receptors in resting NK cells. J. Exp. Med. 202, 1001–1012.

Bryceson, Y.T., March, M.E., Ljunggren, H.G., Long, E.O., 2006a. Activation, coactivation, and costimulation of resting human natural killer cells. Immunol. Rev. 214, 73–91.

Bryceson, Y.T., March, M.E., Ljunggren, H.G., Long, E.O., 2006b. Synergy among receptors on resting NK cells for the activation of natural cytotoxicity and cytokine secretion. Blood. 107, 159–166.

Bryceson, Y.T., Rudd, E., Zheng, C., Edner, J., Ma, D., Wood, S.M., et al., 2007. Defective cytotoxic lymphocyte degranulation in syntaxin-11 deficient familial hemophagocytic lymphohistiocytosis 4 (FHL4) patients. Blood. 110, 1906–1915.

Burshtyn, D.N., Shin, J., Stebbins, C., Long, E.O., 2000. Adhesion to target cells is disrupted by the killer cell inhibitory receptor. Curr. Biol. 10, 777–780.

Burt, B.M., Plitas, G., Zhao, Z., Bamboat, Z.M., Nguyen, H.M., Dupont, B., et al., 2009. The lytic potential of human liver NK cells is restricted by their limited expression of inhibitory killer Ig-like receptors. J. Immunol. 183, 1789–1796.

Caligiuri, M.A., 2008. Human natural killer cells. Blood. 112, 461–469.

Caraux, A., Kim, N., Bell, S.E., Zompi, S., Ranson, T., Lesjean-Pottier, S., et al., 2006. Phospholipase C-gamma2 is essential for NK cell cytotoxicity and innate immunity to malignant and virally infected cells. Blood. 107, 994–1002.

Carnaud, C., Lee, D., Donnars, O., Park, S.H., Beavis, A., Koezuka, Y., et al., 1999. Cutting edge: Cross-talk between cells of the innate immune system: NKT cells rapidly activate NK cells. J. Immunol. 163, 4647–4650.

Chan, A.T., Kollnberger, S.D., Wedderburn, L.R., Bowness, P., 2005. Expansion and enhanced survival of natural killer cells expressing the killer immunoglobulin-like receptor KIR3DL2 in spondylarthritis. Arthritis Rheum. 52, 3586–3595.

Cichocki, F., Miller, J.S., Anderson, S.K., Bryceson, Y.T., 2013. Epigenetic regulation of NK cell differentiation and effector functions. Front. Immunol. 4, 55.

Cooper, M.A., Fehniger, T.A., Turner, S.C., Chen, K.S., Ghaheri, B.A., Ghayur, T., et al., 2001. Human natural killer cells: a unique innate immunoregulatory role for the CD56 (bright) subset. Blood. 97, 3146–3151.

Dalbeth, N., Gundle, R., Davies, R.J., Lee, Y.C., McMichael, A.J., Callan, M.F., 2004. CD56bright NK cells are enriched at inflammatory sites and can engage with monocytes in a reciprocal program of activation. J. Immunol. 173, 6418–6426.

Deguine, J., Breart, B., Lemaitre, F., Di Santo, J.P., Bousso, P., 2010. Intravital imaging reveals distinct dynamics for natural killer and CD8(+) T cells during tumor regression. Immunity. 33, 632–644.

Dunn, C., Brunetto, M., Reynolds, G., Christophides, T., Kennedy, P.T., Lampertico, P., et al., 2007. Cytokines induced during chronic hepatitis B virus infection promote a pathway for NK cell-mediated liver damage. J. Exp. Med. 204, 667–680.

Dustin, M.L., Long, E.O., 2010. Cytotoxic immunological synapses. Immunol. Rev. 235, 24–34.

Elliott, J.M., Yokoyama, W.M., 2011. Unifying concepts of MHC-dependent natural killer cell education. Trends Immunol. 32, 364–372.

Eloranta, M.L., Lövgren, T., Finke, D., Mathsson, L., Rönnelid, J., Kastner, B., et al., 2009. Regulation of the interferon-alpha production induced by RNA-containing immune complexes in plasmacytoid dendritic cells. Arthritis Rheum. 60, 2418–2427.

Fauriat, C., Long, E.O., Ljunggren, H.G., Bryceson, Y.T., 2010. Regulation of human NK-cell cytokine and chemokine production by target cell recognition. Blood. 115, 2167–2176.

Fehniger, T.A., Cooper, M.A., Nuovo, G.J., Cella, M., Facchetti, F., Colonna, M., et al., 2003. CD56bright natural killer cells are present in human lymph nodes and are activated by T cell-derived IL-2: a potential new link between adaptive and innate immunity. Blood. 101, 3052–3057.

Feldmann, J., Callebaut, I., Raposo, G., Certain, S., Bacq, D., Dumont, C., et al., 2003. Munc13-4 is essential for cytolytic granules fusion and is mutated in a form of familial hemophagocytic lymphohistiocytosis (FHL3). Cell. 115, 461–473.

Ferlazzo, G., Pack, M., Thomas, D., Paludan, C., Schmid, D., Strowig, T., et al., 2004. Distinct roles of IL-12 and IL-15 in human natural killer cell activation by dendritic cells from secondary lymphoid organs. Proc. Natl. Acad. Sci. U.S.A. 101, 16606–16611.

Ferlazzo, G., Thomas, D., Lin, S.L., Goodman, K., Morandi, B., Muller, W.A., et al., 2004. The abundant NK cells in human secondary lymphoid tissues require activation to express killer cell Ig-like receptors and become cytolytic. J. Immunol. 172, 1455–1462.

Field, S.F., Nejentsev, S., Walker, N.M., Howson, J.M., Godfrey, L.M., Jolley, J.D., et al., 2008. Sequencing-based genotyping and association analysis of the MICA and MICB genes in type 1 diabetes. Diabetes. 57, 1753–1756.

Flodström-Tullberg, M., Bryceson, Y.T., Shi, F.D., Höglund, P.H., Ljunggren, H.G., 2009. Natural killer cells in human autoimmunity. Curr. Op. Immunol. 21, 634–640.

Freud, A.G., Becknell, B., Roychowdhury, S., Mao, H.C., Ferketich, A.K., Nuovo, G.J., et al., 2005. A human CD34(+) subset resides in lymph nodes and differentiates into CD56bright natural killer cells. Immunity. 22, 295–304.

Freud, A.G., Caligiuri, M.A., 2006. Human natural killer cell development. Immunol. Rev. 214, 56–72.

Freud, A.G., Yokohama, A., Becknell, B., Lee, M.T., Mao, H.C., Ferketich, A.K., et al., 2006. Evidence for discrete stages of human natural killer cell differentiation in vivo. J. Exp. Med. 203, 1033–1043.

Ghiringhelli, F., Ménard, C., Martin, F., Zitvogel, L., 2006. The role of regulatory T cells in the control of natural killer cells: relevance during tumor progression. Immunol. Rev. 214, 229–238.

Gineau, L., Cognet, C., Kara, N., Lach, F.P., Dunne, J., Veturi, U., et al., 2012. Partial MCM4 deficiency in patients with growth retardation, adrenal insufficiency, and natural killer cell deficiency. J Clin. Invest. 122, 821–832.

Gregoire, C., Chasson, L., Luci, C., Tomasello, E., Geissmann, F., Vivier, E., et al., 2007. The trafficking of natural killer cells. Immunol. Rev. 220, 169–182.

Griffiths, G.M., Tsun, A., Stinchcombe, J.C., 2010. The immunological synapse: a focal point for endocytosis and exocytosis. J. Cell Biol. 189, 399–406.

Groh, V., Bruhl, A., El-Gabalawy, H., Nelson, J.L., Spies, T., 2003. Stimulation of T cell autoreactivity by anomalous expression of NKG2D and its MIC ligands in rheumatoid arthritis. Proc. Natl. Acad. Sci. U.S.A. 100, 9452–9457.

Hafler, J.P., Maier, L.M., Cooper, J.D., Plagnol, V., Hinks, A., Simmonds, M.J., et al., 2009. CD226 Gly307Ser association with multiple autoimmune diseases. Genes Immun. 10, 5–10.

Haller, O., Wigzell, H., 1977. Suppression of natural killer cell activity with radioactive strontium: effector cells are marrow dependent. J. Immunol. 118, 1503–1506.

Hagberg, J.I., Berggren, O., Leonard, D., Weber, G., Bryceson, Y.T., Alm, G.V., et al., 2011. IFN-a production by plasmacytoid dendritic cells stimulated with RNA-containing immune complexes is promoted by NK cells via MIP-1b and LFA-1. J. Immunol. 186, 5085–5094.

Hazen, M.M., Woodward, A.L., Hofmann, I., Degar, B.A., Grom, A., Filipovich, A.H., et al., 2008. Mutations of the hemophagocytic lymphohistiocytosis-associated gene UNC13D in a patient with systemic juvenile idiopathic arthritis. Arthritis Rheum. 58, 567–570.

Hov, J.R., Lleo, A., Selmi, C., Woldseth, B., Fabris, L., Strazzabosco, M., et al., 2010. Genetic associations in Italian primary sclerosing cholangitis: heterogeneity across Europe defines a critical role for HLA-C. J. Hepatol. 52, 712–717.

Hüe, S., Mention, J.J., Monteiro, R.C., Zhang, S., Cellier, C., Schmitz, J., et al., 2004. A direct role for NKG2D/MICA interaction in villous atrophy during celiac disease. Immunity. 21, 367–377.

Huntington, N.D., Legrand, N., Alves, N.L., Jaron, B., Weijer, K., Plet, A., et al., 2009. IL-15 trans-presentation promotes human NK cell development and differentiation in vivo. J. Exp. Med. 206, 25–34.

Jacobs, R., Stoll, M., Stratmann, G., Leo, R., Link, H., Schmidt, R.E., 1992. CD16 − CD56 + natural killer cells after bone marrow transplantation. Blood. 79, 3239–3244.

Ji, H., Korganow, A.S., Mangialaio, S., Höglund, P., André, I., Lühder, F., et al., 1999. Different modes of pathogenesis in T-cell-dependent autoimmunity: clues from two TCR transgenic systems. Immunol. Rev. 169, 139–146.

Jonsson, A.H., Yokoyama, W.M., 2009. Natural killer cell tolerance licensing and other mechanisms. Adv. Immunol. 101, 27–79.

Juelke, K., Killig, M., Luetke-Eversloh, M., Parente, E., Gruen, J., Morandi, B., et al., 2010. CD62L expression identifies a unique subset of polyfunctional CD56dim NK cells. Blood. 116, 1299–1307.

Karlsen, T.H., Boberg, K.M., Olsson, M., Sun, J.Y., Senitzer, D., Bergquist, A., et al., 2007. J. Hepatol. 46, 899–906.

Kelly, A., Ramanan, A.V., 2007. Recognition and management of macrophage activation syndrome in juvenile arthritis. Curr. Opin. Rheumatol. 19, 477–481.

Kiessling, R., Klein, E., Wigzell, H., 1975. "Natural" killer cells in the mouse. I. Cytotoxic cells with specificity for mouse Moloney leukemia cells. Specificity and distribution according to genotype. Eur. J. Immunol. 5, 112–117.

Kim, H.S., Das, A., Gross, C.C., Bryceson, Y.T., Long, E.O., 2010. Synergistic signals for natural cytotoxicity are required to overcome inhibition by c-Cbl ubiquitin ligase. Immunity. 32, 175–186.

Kim, N., Saudemont, A., Webb, L., Camps, M., Ruckle, T., Hirsch, E., et al., 2007. The p110delta catalytic isoform of PI3K is a key player in NK-cell development and cytokine secretion. Blood. 110, 3202–3208.

Kim, S., Poursine-Laurent, J., Truscott, S.M., Lybarger, L., Song, Y.J., Yang, L., et al., 2005. Licensing of natural killer cells by host major histocompatibility complex class I molecules. Nature. 436, 709–713.

Klose, C.S., Hoyler, T., Kiss, E.A., Tanriver, Y., Diefenbach, A., 2012. Transcriptional control of innate lymphocyte fate decisions. Curr. Opin. Immunol. 24, 290–296.

Krzewski, K., Chen, X., Strominger, J.L., 2008. WIP is essential for lytic granule polarization and NK cell cytotoxicity. Proc. Natl. Acad. Sci. U.S.A. 105, 2568–2573.

Kulkarni, S., Martin, M.P., Carrington, M., 2008. The Yin and Yang of HLA and KIR in human disease. Semin. Immunol. 20, 343–352.

Lanier, L.L., 2005. NK cell recognition. Ann. Rev. Immunol. 23, 225–274.

Lanier, L.L., Le, A.M., Civin, C.I., Loken, M.R., Phillips, J.H., 1986. The relationship of CD16 (Leu-11) and Leu-19 (NKH-1) antigen expression on human peripheral blood NK cells and cytotoxic T lymphocytes. J. Immunol. 136, 4480–4486.

Leavenworth, J.W., Wang, X., Wenander, C.S., Spee, P., Cantor, H., 2011. Mobilization of natural killer cells inhibits development of collagen-induced arthritis. Proc. Natl. Acad. Sci. U.S.A. 108, 14584–14589.

Ljunggren, H.G., Kärre, K., 1990. In search of the "missing self": MHC molecules and NK cell recognition. Immunol. Today. 11, 237–244.

Liu, D., Bryceson, Y.T., Meckel, T., Vasiliver-Shamis, G., Dustin, M.L., Long, E.O., 2009. Integrin-dependent organization and bidirectional vesicular traffic at cytotoxic immune synapses. Immunity. 31, 99–109.

Long, E.O., 2008. Negative signaling by inhibitory receptors: the NK cell paradigm. Immunol. Rev. 224, 70–84.

Lopez-Verges, S., Milush, J.M., Pandey, S., York, V.A., Arakawa-Hoyt, J., Pircher, H., et al., 2010. CD57 defines a functionally distinct population of mature NK cells in the human CD56dimCD16 + NK-cell subset. Blood. 116, 3865–3874.

Mace, E.M., Hsu, A.P., Monaco-Shawver, L., Makedonas, G., Rosen, J.B., Dropulic, L., et al., 2013. Mutations in GATA2 cause human NK cell deficiency with specific loss of the CD56(bright) subset. Blood. 121, 2669–2677.

Mace, E.M., Monkley, S.J., Critchley, D.R., Takei, F., 2009. A dual role for talin in NK cell cytotoxicity: activation of LFA-1-mediated cell adhesion and polarization of NK cells. J. Immunol. 182, 948–956.

Mace, E.M., Zhang, J., Siminovitch, K.A., Takei, F., 2010. Elucidation of the integrin LFA-1-mediated signaling pathway of actin polarization in natural killer cells. Blood. 116, 1272–1279.

Manaster, I., Mandelboim, O., 2010. The unique properties of uterine NK cells. Am. J. Reprod. Immunol. 63, 434–444.

March, M.E., Long, E.O., 2011. b2 Integrin induces TCRz–Syk–phospholipase C-g phosphorylation and paxillin-dependent granule polarization in human NK cells. J. Immunol. 186, 2998–3005.

Martín-Fontecha, A., Thomsen, L.L., Brett, S., Gerard, C., Lipp, M., Lanzavecchia, A., et al., 2004. Induced recruitment of NK cells to lymph nodes provides IFN-gamma for Th1 priming. Nat. Immunol. 5, 1260–1265.

Matos, M.E., Schnier, G.S., Beecher, M.S., Ashman, L.K., William, D.E., Caligiuri, M.A., 1993. Expression of a functional c-kit receptor on a subset of natural killer cells. J. Exp. Med. 178, 1079–1084.

Maul-Pavicic, A., Chiang, S.C.C., Rensing-Ehl, A., Jessen, B., Fauriat, C., Wood, S.M., et al., 2011. ORAI1-mediated calcium influx is required for human cytotoxic lymphocyte degranulation and target cell lysis. Proc. Natl. Acad. Sci. U.S.A. 108, 3324–3329.

Menager, M.M., Menasche, G., Romao, M., Knapnougel, P., Ho, C.H., Garfa, M., et al., 2007. Secretory cytotoxic granule maturation and exocytosis require the effector protein hMunc13-4. Nat. Immunol. 8, 257–267.

Mentlik, A.N., Sanborn, K.B., Holzbaur, E.L., Orange, J.S., 2010. Rapid lytic granule convergence to the MTOC in natural killer cells is dependent on dynein but not cytolytic commitment. Mol. Biol. Cell. 21, 2241–2256.

Meresse, B., Chen, Z., Ciszewski, C., Tretiakova, M., Bhagat, G., Krausz, T.N., et al., 2004. Coordinated induction by IL15 of a TCR-independent NKG2D signaling pathway converts CTL into lymphokine-activated killer cells in celiac disease. Immunity. 21, 357–366.

Mestas, J., Hughes, C.C., 2004. Of mice and not men: differences between mouse and human immunology. J. Immunol. 172, 2731–2738.

Miller, J.S., Alley, K.A., McGlave, P., 1994. Differentiation of natural killer (NK) cells from human primitive marrow progenitors in a stroma-based long-term culture system: identification of a CD34 + 7 + NK progenitor. Blood. 83, 2594–2601.

Miller, J.S., Verfaillie, C., McGlave, P., 1992. The generation of human natural killer cells from CD34 + /DR − primitive progenitors in long-term bone marrow culture. Blood. 80, 2182–2187.

Momot, T., Koch, S., Hunzelmann, N., Krieg, T., Ulbricht, K., Schmidt, R.E., et al., 2004. Association of killer cell immunoglobulin-like receptors with scleroderma. Arthritis Rheum. 50, 1561–1565.

Morandi, B., Bougras, G., Muller, W.A., Ferlazzo, G., Münz, C., 2006. NK cells of human secondary lymphoid tissues enhance T cell polarization via IFN-gamma secretion. Eur. J. Immunol. 36, 2394–2400.

Nelson, G.W., Martin, M.P., Gladman, D., Wade, J., Trowsdale, J., Carrington, M., 2004. Cutting edge: heterozygote advantage in autoimmune disease: hierarchy of protection/susceptibility conferred by HLA and killer Ig-like receptor combinations in psoriatic arthritis. J. Immunol. 173, 4273–4276.

Norris, S., Kondeatis, E., Collins, R., Satsangi, J., Clare, M., Chapman, R., et al., 2001. Mapping the MHC-encoded susceptibility and resistance in primary sclerosing cholangitis: the role of MICA polymorphism. Gastroenterology. 120, 1475–1482.

Pazmany, L., 2005. Do NK cells regulate human autoimmunity? Cytokine. 32, 76–80.

Perricone, R., Perricone, C., De Carolis, C., Shoenfeld, Y., 2008. NK cells in autoimmunity: a two-edged weapon of the immune system. Autoimmun. Rev. 7, 384–390.

Peterson, M.E., Long, E.O., 2008. Inhibitory receptor signaling via tyrosine phosphorylation of the adaptor Crk. Immunity. 29, 578–588.

Quann, E.J., Merino, E., Furuta, T., Huse, M., 2009. Localized diacylglycerol drives the polarization of the microtubule-organizing center in T cells. Nat. Immunol. 10, 627–635.

Ravelli, A., Grom, A.A., Behrens, E.M., Cron, R.Q., 2012. Macrophage activation syndrome as part of systemic juvenile idiopathic arthritis: diagnosis, genetics, pathophysiology and treatment. Genes Immun. 13, 289–298.

Romagnani, C., Juelke, K., Falco, M., Morandi, B., D'Agostino, A., Costa, R., et al., 2007. CD56brightCD16- killer Ig-like receptor-NK cells display longer telomeres and acquire features of CD56dim NK cells upon activation. J. Immunol. 178, 4947–4955.

Sanborn, K.B., Rak, G.D., Maru, S.Y., Demers, K., Difeo, A., Martignetti, J.A., et al., 2009. Myosin IIA associates with NK cell lytic granules to enable their interaction with F-actin and function at the immunological synapse. J. Immunol. 182, 6969–6984.

Sancho, D., Nieto, M., Llano, M., Rodriguez-Fernandez, J.L., Tejedor, R., Avraham, S., et al., 2000. The tyrosine kinase PYK-2/RAFTK regulates natural killer (NK) cell cytotoxic response, and is translocated and activated upon specific target cell recognition and killing. J. Cell. Biol. 149, 1249–1262.

Shanker, A., Verdeil, G., Buferne, M., Inderberg-Suso, E.M., Puthier, D., Joly, F., et al., 2007. CD8 T cell help for innate antitumor immunity. J. Immunol. 179, 6651–6662.

Shi, F.D., van Kaer, L., 2006. Reciprocal regulation between natural killer cells and autoreactive T cells. Nat. Rev. Immunol. 6, 751–760.

Shilling, H.G., McQueen, K.L., Cheng, N.W., Shizuru, J.A., Negrin, R.S., Parham, P., 2003. Reconstitution of NK cell receptor repertoire following HLA-matched hematopoietic cell transplantation. Blood. 101, 3730–3740.

Spits, H., Artis, D., Colonna, M., Diefenbach, A., Di Santo, J.P., Eberl, G., et al., 2013. Innate lymphoid cells – a proposal for uniform nomenclature. Nat. Rev. Immunol. 13, 145–149.

Stebbins, C.C., Watzl, C., Billadeau, D.D., Leibson, P.J., Burshtyn, D.N., Long, E.O., 2003. Vav1 dephosphorylation by the tyrosine phosphatase SHP-1 as a mechanism for inhibition of cellular cytotoxicity. Mol. Cell. Biol. 23, 6291–6299.

Stinchcombe, J.C., Barral, D.C., Mules, E.H., Booth, S., Hume, A.N., Machesky, L.M., et al., 2001. Rab27a is required for regulated secretion in cytotoxic T lymphocytes. J. Cell. Biol. 152, 825–834.

Sun, J.C., Lanier, L.L., 2011. NK cell development, homeostasis and function: parallels with CD8 + T cells. Nat. Rev. Immunol. 11, 645–657.

Suzuki, A., Yamada, R., Kochi, Y., Sawada, T., Okada, Y., Matsuda, K., et al., 2008. Functional SNPs in CD244 increase the risk of rheumatoid arthritis in a Japanese population. Nat. Genet. 40, 1224—1229.

Tassi, I., Cella, M., Gilfillan, S., Turnbull, I., Diacovo, T.G., Penninger, J.M., et al., 2007. p110gamma and p110delta phosphoinositide 3-kinase signaling pathways synergize to control development and functions of murine NK cells. Immunity. 27, 214—227.

Tassi, I., Cella, M., Presti, R., Colucci, A., Gilfillan, S., Littman, D.R., et al., 2008. NK cell-activating receptors require PKC-theta for sustained signaling, transcriptional activation, and IFN-gamma secretion. Blood. 112, 4109—4116.

Tassi, I., Presti, R., Kim, S., Yokoyama, W.M., Gilfillan, S., Colonna, M., 2005. Phospholipase C-γ2 is a critical signaling mediator for murine NK cell activating receptors. J. Immunol. 175, 749—754.

van der Slik, A.R., Alizadeh, B.Z., Koeleman, B.P., Roep, B.O., Giphart, M.J., 2007. Modelling KIR-HLA genotype disparities in type 1 diabetes. Tissue Antigens. 1, 101—105.

van der Slik, A.R., Koeleman, B.P., Verduijn, W., Bruining, G.J., Roep, B.O., Giphart, M.J., 2003. KIR in type 1 diabetes: disparate distribution of activating and inhibitory natural killer cell receptors in patients versus HLA-matched control subjects. Diabetes. 52, 2639—2642.

Villanueva, J., Lee, S., Giannini, E.H., Graham, T.B., Passo, M.H., Filipovich, A., et al., 2005. Natural killer cell dysfunction is a distinguishing feature of systemic onset juvenile rheumatoid arthritis and macrophage activation syndrome. Arthritis Res. Ther. 7, R30—R37.

Vivier, E., Tomasello, E., Baratin, M., Waltzer, T., Ugolini, S., 2008. Functions of natural killer cells. Nat. Immunol. 9, 503—510.

Waggoner, S.N., Cornberg, M., Selin, L.K., Welsh, R.M., 2011. Natural killer cells act as rheostats modulating antiviral T cells. Nature. 481, 394—398.

Watzl, C., Long, E.O., 2010. Signal transduction during activation and inhibition of natural killer cells. Curr. Protoc. Immunol. (Chapter 11: Unit 11 19B).

Wiencke, K., Spurkland, A., Schrumpf, E., Boberg, K.M., 2001. Primary sclerosing cholangitis is associated to an extended B8-DR3 haplotype including particular MICA and MICB alleles. Hepatology. 34, 625—630.

Wood, S.M., Ljunggren, H.G., Bryceson, Y.T., 2011. Insights into NK cell biology from human genetics and disease associations. Cell. Mol. Life Sci. 68, 3479—3493.

Wood, S.M., Meeths, M., Chiang, S.C., Bechensteen, A.G., Boelens, J.J., Heilmann, C., et al., 2009. Different NK cell-activating receptors preferentially recruit Rab27a or Munc13-4 to perforin-containing granules for cytotoxicity. Blood. 114, 4117—4127.

Wulfing, C., Purtic, B., Klem, J., Schatzle, J.D., 2003. Stepwise cytoskeletal polarization as a series of checkpoints in innate but not adaptive cytolytic killing. Proc. Natl. Acad. Sci. U.S.A. 100, 7767—7772.

Yen, J.H., Moore, B.E., Nakajima, T., Scholl, D., Schaid, D.J., Weyand, C.M., et al., 2001. Major histocompatibility complex class I-recognizing receptors are disease risk genes in rheumatoid arthritis. J. Exp. Med. 193, 1159—1167.

Chapter 14

Granulocytes: Neutrophils, Basophils, Eosinophils

Xavier Bosch[1,2] and Manuel Ramos-Casals[2]

[1]*Department of Internal Medicine, Hospital Clinic, Institut d'Investigacions Biomèdiques August Pi i Sunyer, University of Barcelona, Barcelona,*

Spain, [2]*Sjögren's Syndrome Research Group, Laboratory of Autoimmune Diseases Josep Font, Department of Autoimmune Diseases, Hospital Clinic,*

Institut d'Investigacions Biomèdiques August Pi i Sunyer, University of Barcelona, Barcelona, Spain

Chapter Outline

Neutrophils	**201**	Basic Biology and Role in Immunity	206
Basic Biology and Role in Immunity	201	Basophils in Autoimmune Diseases	207
Neutrophil Extracellular Traps and NETosis:		Role of IgE in Systemic Autoimmune	
A Novel Form of Cell Death	202	Diseases	207
Pathogenic Role of Neutrophils in		Basophils in Lupus Nephritis	207
Autoimmune Diseases	202	Basophils in Rheumatoid Arthritis and	
Systemic Lupus Erythematosus	202	Vasculitides	208
Systemic Vasculitides	204	Basophils in Autoinflammatory	
Rheumatoid Arthritis	205	Diseases	208
Primary Sjögren Syndrome	206	**Eosinophils**	**208**
Systemic Sclerosis	206	Basic Biology and Role in Immunity	208
Antiphospholipid Syndrome	206	Eosinophils in Churg–Strauss Syndrome	209
Autoimmune Skin Diseases	206	**Conclusions and Therapeutic Implications**	**210**
Basophils	**206**	**References**	**211**

NEUTROPHILS

Basic Biology and Role in Immunity

Neutrophils, the most abundant leukocytes in the human body, have a short lifespan which is balanced by their continuous release from the bone marrow. Neutrophils form part of the innate immune system, the first line of defense against invading pathogens. Neutrophil-mediated inflammatory responses are a complex process, with initial adhesion of circulating cells to the activated vascular endothelium followed by their extravasation and migration towards inflammatory foci and, finally, *in situ* destruction of pathogens (Kaplan, 2011). Microbes are eliminated through various processes including phagocytosis, reactive oxygen species (ROS) generated via the respiratory burst, release of microbiocidal substances from cytoplasmic granules (Kobayashi and DeLeo, 2009),

and NETosis, a process characterized by the formation of neutrophil extracellular traps (NETs) (Brinkmann et al., 2004) (see below).

Neutrophils contain various types of granules, enabling the sequential release of hundreds of constitutively expressed proteins into the extracellular environment, including proinflammatory mediators that have effects on antigen-presenting cells and induce dendritic cell maturation (Faurschou and Borregaard, 2003). The proteins contained in primary (azurophilic) neutrophil granules include alarmins, molecules that activate antigen-presenting cells and trigger innate and adaptive immune responses (Kobayashi and DeLeo, 2009). These alarmins include antimicrobial peptides such as α-defensins, lactoferrin, and cathelicidin peptides, such as LL-37, which are chemotactic to various leukocytes. Together with self-DNA release by NETosis, LL-37 also promotes

N. Rose & I. Mackay (Eds): The Autoimmune Diseases, Fifth edition. DOI: http://dx.doi.org/10.1016/B978-0-12-384929-8.00014-9

Box 14.1 Antimicrobial Peptides of NETs
- Neutrophil elastase
- Myleoperoxidase
- Cathepsin G
- Proteinase 3
- Lactoferrin
- Bacterial permeability increasing protein (BPI)
- Cathelicidin (LL-37)
- Tryptase
- Gelatinase
- Human neutrophil peptides
- Histones (nucleosome histones, H1)
- Calprotectin

activation of plasmacytoid dendritic cells, increasing their expression of costimulatory molecules and production of type I interferon (IFN) (Lande et al., 2007). Other molecules released by neutrophils, including myeloperoxidase, neutrophil elastase, and cathepsin G, also play a role in activating innate immunity (Box 14.1). Neutrophils also produce inflammatory cytokines and eicosanoids, regulate vascular permeability, and may induce endothelial damage (Murphy et al., 1998; Marzocchi-Machado et al., 2002). They also express toll-like receptors (TLRs) 1–10, with the exception of TLR3, facilitating the initiation of potentially important immune responses when pathogen-associated molecular patterns are recognized.

Neutrophil Extracellular Traps and NETosis: A Novel Form of Cell Death

Stimulated neutrophils may suffer NETosis, an active form of cell death resulting in the release of decondensed chromatin into the extracellular space (Brinkmann et al., 2004; Fuchs et al., 2007). NETs are fibrous chromatin-based structures containing DNA, histones, and granular proteins, including neutrophil elastase and myeloperoxidase (Urban et al., 2009), which are expelled into the extracellular matrix during neutrophil death from NETosis and may immobilize and kill pathogens.

NETs trap many types of microbes *ex vivo*, have been identified in *in vivo* disease models, and are thought to kill pathogens by exposing them to elevated local antimicrobial concentrations (Papayannopoulos and Zychlinsky, 2009). It is not clear how NETs are formed, although the reactive oxygen pathway is involved, as nicotinamide adenine dinucleotide phosphate (NADPH) oxidase and myeloperoxidase are required for NET formation in response to chemical and biological stimuli (Fuchs et al., 2007; Patel et al., 2010; Metzler et al., 2011). Nitric oxide donors can induce NETs via a mechanism that also requires ROS production (Patel et al., 2010), like all

activators of NET formation discovered to date. Upstream of NADPH oxidase, the Raf-MEK-ERK pathway is implicated in NET formation (Hakkim et al., 2011), but later in the process, neutrophil elastase translocates from the granules to the nucleus and degrades histones, leading to chromatin decondensation (Papayannopoulos et al., 2010).

Excess NET formation or impaired NET removal is suggested to be linked to autoimmune diseases, including small-vessel necrotizing vasculitis and systemic lupus erythematosus (SLE) (see below). A recent study found that the cell destructive effect of neutrophils is due to NET components and not to other secreted neutrophil components (Saffarzadeh et al., 2012). NETs induce dose-dependent cytotoxic effects on direct interaction with epithelial and endothelial cells, with NET-mediated cytotoxicity probably being due to histones and myeloperoxidase.

Pathogenic Role of Neutrophils in Autoimmune Diseases

Systemic Lupus Erythematosus

Neutrophil actions normally successfully sequester and resolve inflammatory damage, although their recruitment and activation may provoke disease, resulting in substantial tissue damage. In autoimmune diseases, a potential role for neutrophils in the pathogenesis and associated organ damage of SLE, including description of the LE cell, was described many years ago (Holman, 1960).

Neutropenia and Abnormal Neutrophil Function in SLE

Nearly half the patients with SLE may have neutropenia (Hepburn et al., 2010). The mechanisms driving neutropenia in SLE include: neutrophil-reactive autoantibody-driven cell removal; neutralizing autoantibodies against growth factors that act on neutrophils such as granulocyte colony-stimulating factor; bone marrow suppression; increased neutrophil apoptosis and secondary necrosis; and, possibly, death by NETosis (Arenas et al., 1992). In addition, there is evidence of qualitative abnormalities in some neutrophil functions in SLE. Serum from SLE patients induces increased neutrophil aggregation and impairs phagocytosis and lysosomal enzyme release by normal neutrophils *in vitro* (Brandt and Hedberg, 1969; Abramson et al., 1983). It is suggested that aberrant clearance of apoptotic products by phagocytes, including neutrophils, may play a role in the pathogenesis of SLE (Courtney et al., 1999). Likewise, reduced responsiveness to cytokines such as interleukin (IL)-8 has been reported in SLE-derived neutrophils (Hsieh et al., 2008), as has premature telomere shortening indicative of enhanced senescence (Wu et al., 2007). Evidence suggests that intravascularly activated neutrophils in SLE patients over-express various adhesion molecules and tend to form aggregates (Abramson et al., 1983; Molad et al., 1994). Various autoantibodies, including anti-β_2-glycoprotein I, are involved in neutrophil activation (Arvieux et al., 1995). Likewise, it is suggested that nucleosomes, which are probably major SLE autoantigens, are putative activators and recruiters of neutrophils in SLE, although the mechanisms remain unclear (Rönnefarth et al., 2006). Increased neutrophil apoptosis and aberrant clearance of apoptotic bodies are associated with SLE disease activity (Ren et al., 2003; Donnelly et al., 2006), and the *in vitro* rate of neutrophil secondary necrosis is increased in SLE-derived samples (Ren et al., 2003).

Low-Density Granulocytes in SLE

Low-density granulocytes are a specific subset of aberrant neutrophils that have recently been identified in peripheral blood mononuclear cell (PBMC) preparations from pediatric and adult SLE patients (Kaplan, 2011). Low-density granulocytes display phenotypic characteristics of immature neutrophils with nonsegmented nuclei and greater expression of myeloperoxidase, neutrophil elastase, and defensin-3 (Hacbarth and Kajdacsy-Balla, 1986; Bennett et al., 2003). Low-density granulocytes have a proinflammatory phenotype characterized by augmented secretion of tumor necrosis factor (TNF) and type I and II IFNs after stimulation, which could promote and increase tissue damage. They also have a markedly increased ability to kill endothelial cells upon cell—cell contact (Denny

et al., 2010), and to form NETs compared with normal density SLE-derived neutrophils and control neutrophils (Villanueva et al., 2011) (Figure 14.1). Low-density granulocytes are suggested to account for the increased type I IFN production that leads to abnormal function of endothelial progenitor cells and/or circulating myeloid angiogenic cells *in vitro* and, possibly, *in vivo* in SLE. This aberrant subset of neutrophils has an increased propensity to undergo NETosis (Knight and Kaplan, 2012), and SLE patients with cutaneous involvement and vasculitis have a higher percentage of low-density granulocytes.

NETosis in SLE

As mentioned, NETs may have detrimental effects on the host. They result in autoimmunity by extracellular exposure of self-molecules. In some SLE patients, NET degradation is impaired due to DNase I inhibitors or antibodies to NETs. Recent studies by Lande and colleagues (2011) and Garcia-Romo and colleagues (2011) suggest that NETs and NETosis are the link between INF-α production and neutrophil death through the implication of some peptides such as LL-37 (an antimicrobial peptide that is a key mediator of plasmacytoid dendritic cell activation) and human neutrophil peptide (Bosch, 2011). The hypothesis is that these peptides, in combination with extracellular DNA, are pivotal components of NETs in SLE, and recent studies have suggested that they may be involved in the immunogenicity of self nucleic acids in immune complexes. Lande and colleagues (2011) found high levels of expression of LL-37 in the blood of SLE patients, and suggested that LL-37, together with human

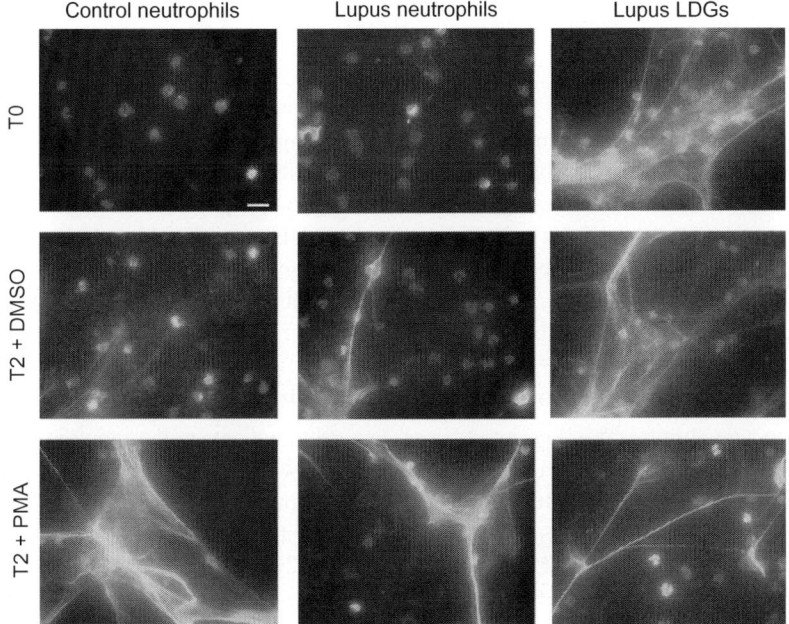

FIGURE 14.1 Circulating low-density granulocytes (LDGs) from SLE undergo increased NETosis. Characteristic images of control neutrophils, SLE-derived neutrophils, and SLE-derived LDGs isolated from peripheral blood and studied at baseline (T0) or after 2 hours' (T2) stimulation with DMSO or PMA. Top panels show merged immunofluorescence images of NETs, which were identified by neutrophil elastase (green). DNA was labeled with Hoechst 33342 (blue). Original magnification, ×40. Scale bar, 20 μm. Abbreviations: DMSO, dimethyl sulfoxide; LDGs, low-density granulocytes; NETs, neutrophil extracellular traps; PMA, phorbol 12-myristate 13-acetate. *Permission to reproduce this figure was obtained from The American Association of Immunologists, Inc. © Villanueva et al. (2011).*

neutrophil peptide, is essential for the immunogenicity of DNA-containing immune complexes in SLE, because free human DNA entered and activated plasmacytoid dendritic cells through TLR9 when complexed with LL-37. Both anti-LL-37 and anti-human neutrophil peptide antibodies activate neutrophils to release NETs; exposure of neutrophils to INF-α *in vitro* is followed by expression of LL-37 and human neutrophil peptide. Lande and colleagues (2007) found a significant correlation between high levels of anti-LL-37, anti-human neutrophil peptide antibodies, and anti-DNA antibody titers, suggesting that neutrophil-derived antimicrobial peptides act as B cell autoantigens in conjunction with DNA. Likewise, autoantibodies in immune complexes interacted with the Fcγ surface receptor II (FcγRII) on plasmacytoid dendritic cells and triggered receptor-mediated endocytosis of self DNA. Garcia-Romo and colleagues (2011) also showed that NETs in SLE contain LL-37 and that immune complexes harboring antiribonucleoprotein autoantibodies bonded with FcγRIIA on neutrophils suffering death by NETosis, resulting in ROS production. Although the molecular basis of NET formation remains unclear, it is known that ROS trigger activation of neutrophil enzymes and their relocation to the nucleus to initiate the DNA unwinding on which NET formation depends. Increased production of ROS, such as the superoxide anion and hydrogen peroxide, is associated with SLE, as shown by oxidative protein modifications, lipid peroxidation, and lipoprotein oxidation. Ultimately, these events led to plasmacytoid dendritic cell activation and, therefore, the secretion of INF-α. This suggests that, in SLE, anti-self antibodies activate neutrophils, which then release NETs containing DNA−antimicrobial peptide complexes that activate plasmacytoid dendritic cells, leading to INF-α release and worsening or perpetuation of inflammation and disease. Finally, Leffler et al. (2012) have recently found that NETs are a potent complement activator in SLE, and that patients who fail to degrade NETs had a more active disease and lower serum levels of C3 and C4.

Neutrophils and Organ Damage in SLE

A probable etiopathogenic role of neutrophils in SLE-related organ damage has principally been postulated for cardiovascular, renal, and cutaneous involvement. Type I IFNs are reported to play a vital role in the abnormal vascular repair that occurs in SLE through harmful effects on endothelial progenitor cells and circulating myeloid angiogenic cells (Denny et al., 2007; Lee et al., 2007). Depleting low-density granulocytes from SLE proangiogenic cultures restores the ability of endothelial progenitor cells and/or circulating myeloid angiogenic cells to differentiate into mature endothelium (Denny et al., 2010). Thus, low-density granulocytes might play a dual

role in inducing premature cardiovascular damage in SLE patients by promoting endothelial damage and inflammation while inhibiting vascular repair. This hypothesis is bolstered by evidence that high levels of low-density granulocytes correlate with vascular inflammation in SLE (Denny et al., 2010). The probable contribution of neutrophils to the pathogenesis of antibody-mediated lupus nephritis, and especially to acute flares, is confirmed by depletion studies (selective removal of neutrophils from wild-type animals) and adoptive transfer studies (reintroduction of neutrophils into deficient animals) (Cochrane et al., 1965). In several types of glomerulonephritis, neutrophils are predominantly located in the glomerular tuft (Hotta et al., 1996), and release enzymes, including neutrophil elastase, myeloperoxidase and various cathepsins, which can destroy glomerular structures (Camussi et al., 1980; Johnson et al., 1988). Likewise, proinflammatory mediators elicit secretion of B lymphocyte stimulator, which is stored in activated neutrophils (Scapini et al., 2005). Neutrophil infiltration has been associated with some types of cutaneous involvement in SLE. Infiltration of neutrophils and neutrophilic debris beneath the basement membrane zone occurs in acute cutaneous lupus erythematosus (Obermoser et al., 2010). The neutrophilic component is most prominent in bullous lupus erythematosus (an autoantibody-mediated subepidermal blistering disease affecting SLE patients), in which affected skin is infiltrated by neutrophils that then suffer death from NETosis, exposing LL-37, dsDNA, and IL-17 at the tissue level. Furthermore, cutaneous NETosis is associated with increased levels of serum anti-dsDNA (Hacbarth and Kajdacsy-Balla, 1986), while high low-density granulocyte levels in peripheral blood have been associated with skin involvement in SLE patients (Rönnefarth et al., 2006).

Systemic Vasculitides

Antineutrophil cytoplasmic antibody (ANCA) positivity is a hallmark of ANCA-associated vasculitis, which includes granulomatosis with polyangiitis (Wegener), microscopic polyangiitis, and Churg−Strauss syndrome. Myeloperoxidase and proteinase 3 are the main targets of ANCA, which are directed against antigens in the neutrophil cytoplasm.

Neutrophils and Vasculitic Organ Damage

The severity of organ damage in patients with granulomatosis with polyangiitis correlates with the polymorphonuclear infiltrate rather than with other parameters of autoimmunity such as T cell activation or autoantibody titers (Brouwer et al., 1994; Amulic et al., 2012). In addition, ANCA bind myeloperoxidase and proteinase 3 expressed on the surface of activated neutrophils, promoting degranulation and release of chemoattractants and ROS, which together lead to cyclical tissue damage and inflammation (Gómez-Puerta et al., 2012). In 1990, Falk and colleagues demonstrated that ANCA stimulate respiratory bursts in neutrophils and trigger the release of primary granule constituents (Falk et al., 1990). They also provoke vascular damage *in vitro* by inducing neutrophil effector functions, including cytokine and chemokine release, and produce lysis through adhesion to cultured endothelial cells (Bosch et al., 2006).

NETs in ANCA-Associated Vasculitis

NETs, rather than apoptosis, have been implicated in NETosis in ANCA-associated vasculitis, where they seem to make myeloperoxidase and proteinase 3 available to initiate an autoimmune response. Kessenbrock and colleagues (2009) demonstrated that NET formation could result in endothelial damage and might maintain autoimmune responses against neutrophil components in ANCA-associated vasculitis. After priming neutrophils with purified IgG, they observed that 23% of neutrophils incubated with ANCA-IgG produced NETs after 3 h compared with 11% of IgG-treated neutrophils from healthy controls. Induction of NETs with proteinase 3-specific mouse monoclonal antibodies showed that both proteinase 3 and myeloperoxidase localized with extracellular chromatin fibers and interacted directly with NET-DNA. The finding of NET components near to neutrophil infiltrates in affected glomeruli from renal biopsies of patients with ANCA-associated vasculitis with acutely worsened renal function provides *in vivo* evidence of NET formation. NETs were prominent in samples with strong neutrophil infiltration, suggesting NET formation may occur mainly during active disease. Using myeloperoxidase-specific capture and subsequent DNA-specific detection antibodies, the study identified circulating myeloperoxidase−DNA complexes in patients with ANCA-associated vasculitis but not in healthy controls. NET production resulted in raised levels of proteinase 3 and myeloperoxidase, which are components of NETs, thus providing additional autoantigens to further the autoimmune response. The authors concluded that ANCA might perpetuate cyclical NET production, sustaining the delivery of antigen−chromatin complexes to the immune system.

Rheumatoid Arthritis

Neutrophils are the most abundant leukocytes found in rheumatoid arthritis synovial fluid and show an activated phenotype, suggesting they have undergone activation and have probably released inflammatory mediators (Németh and Mócsai, 2012). Their pathogenetic role has also been demonstrated in animal models of arthritis. In

the K/BxN transgenic mouse model of inflammatory arthritis, neutrophil recruitment into the joints is promoted by the chemotactic lipid leukotriene B4 (LTB4) through its receptor BLT1, both of which are expressed by neutrophils (Chou et al., 2010). Neutrophil activation by immune complexes in the joints promotes IL-1β production, which then stimulates synovial cells to produce chemokines, thus amplifying neutrophil recruitment into the joints (Chou et al., 2010). Likewise, IL-8 receptor beta [(IL8RB or C-X-C chemokine receptor type 2 (CXCR2)]-dependent neutrophil activation and consequent induction of inflammation is demonstrated in two murine models of multiple sclerosis (Carlson et al., 2008; Liu et al., 2010).

Notably, the K/BxN model of arthritis is critically reliant on spleen tyrosine kinase-mediated FcγR signaling, yet the specific cells needed for the signaling events were unknown. Elliott et al. (2011) have recently reported that specific deletion of spleen tyrosine kinase in neutrophils halts the inception of arthritis in the K/BxN model, suggesting that signaling dependent on this enzyme in neutrophils alone is the chief mediator of arthritis in this model.

Studies have recently shown that neutrophils are a major source of cytokines involved in maturation, survival, and differentiation of B cells, including B cell activating factor (BAFF) (Kessenbrock et al., 2009) and the proliferation-inducing ligand APRIL (the molecule most closely related to BAFF) (Mantovani et al., 2011). Neutrophils in rheumatoid arthritis synovial fluid (Gabay et al., 2009) and in various neoplasms including B cell malignancies express and secrete high APRIL levels. Since APRIL promotes the survival and proliferation of normal and malignant B cells, neutrophil-derived APRIL might maintain autoantibody production, as in rheumatoid arthritis (Roosnek et al., 2009), or malignant growth, as in B cell lymphoma (Roosnek et al., 2009).

Neutrophil-derived cytokines are also involved in bone resorption. Human and murine neutrophils upregulate the expression of functionally active, membrane-bound receptor activator of nuclear factor kappa-B ligand (RANKL) following activation *in vitro* and *in vivo* (Chakravarti et al., 2009). Neutrophils from synovial fluid of patients with exacerbated rheumatoid arthritis express high levels of RANKL (Chakravarti et al., 2009), which, after interaction with osteoclasts, activate osteoclastogenesis in a RANKL-dependent manner (Chakravarti et al., 2009). As there are elevated amounts of neutrophils at sites of inflammatory bone loss that express other regulatory factors involved in bone remodeling, including RANK and osteoprotegerin [also known as tumor necrosis factor receptor superfamily, member 11b (TNFRSF11B)] (Poubelle et al., 2007; Chakravarti et al., 2009), neutrophils could, potentially, orchestrate bone resorption in rheumatoid arthritis.

Primary Sjögren Syndrome

Neutropenia is a relevant hematologic finding in primary Sjögren syndrome, with nearly 30% of patients having autoimmune neutropenia (Brito-Zerón et al., 2009), a percentage substantially higher than that for other cytopenias (e.g., leukopenia or thrombocytopenia). Neutropenia is associated with a higher rate of hospital admission due to infection. Agranulocytosis is rare in primary Sjögren syndrome (only about 2% of patients), and is found especially in patients with an underlying hematologic neoplasia (mainly B cell lymphoma). The etiopathogenic role of anti-neutrophil antibodies in these patients, if any, is unclear. Two studies have found no association between autoantibodies to surface neutrophil antigens and agranulocytosis in Sjögren syndrome patients (Lamour et al., 1995; Coppo et al., 2003).

Systemic Sclerosis

Some studies have suggested a possible role of neutrophils in the etiopathogenesis of systemic sclerosis. Activated neutrophils have the potential to release agents capable of endothelial injury, including ROS and proteases, and the ability to affect cytokine signaling. Barnes et al. (2011) have recently demonstrated that serum from patients with systemic sclerosis induces endothelial cell activation and apoptosis in endothelial cell−neutrophil co-cultures, mediated largely by IL-6 and dependent on the presence of neutrophils, suggesting that IL-6 might be a potential therapeutic target in systemic sclerosis. Hussein et al. (2005) have reported increased neutrophilic infiltration in cutaneous biopsies of patients with systemic sclerosis in comparison with controls. Other studies have explored neutrophil function in systemic sclerosis, in particular their ability to contribute to oxidative stress by producing ROS, although the results were contradictory (Maslen et al., 1987; Stevens et al., 1992). However, recent studies have found that neutrophils from patients with systemic sclerosis produce less ROS *in vitro* than unstimulated control neutrophils (Foerster et al., 2006), and that neutrophils from patients with systemic sclerosis are hypofunctional in tests of ROS generation and chemotaxis (Barnes et al., 2011). In addition, proteomic studies show that neutrophils from systemic sclerosis have increased expression of proteins that are also increased on stimulation with lipopolysaccharide or TNF, again indicative of neutrophil activation *in vivo* (Barnes et al., 2011).

Antiphospholipid Syndrome

Women with antiphospholipid syndrome, a systemic autoimmune disease characterized by recurrent thrombosis associated with the presence of antiphospholipid antibodies, often suffer pregnancy-related complications, including miscarriage. Samarkos et al., 2012 have suggested a close association between neutrophils and complement activation in the fetal losses of patients with antiphospholipid syndrome. Studies have found that C5a induction of tissue factor expression in neutrophils contributed to respiratory burst and trophoblast injury (Redecha et al., 2008; Seshan et al., 2009). Neutrophils from antiphospholipid antibody-treated mice expressed protease-activated receptor 2, whose stimulation led to neutrophil activation, trophoblast injury, and fetal death. Furthermore, simvastatin and pravastatin were found to decrease tissue factor and protease-activated receptor 2 expression on neutrophils and prevent pregnancy loss, suggesting that tissue factor/factor VIIa/protease-activated receptor 2 signaling mediates neutrophil activation and fetal death in antiphospholipid syndrome and that statins might be tested in women with antiphospholipid syndrome-related pregnancy complications.

Autoimmune Skin Diseases

Bullous pemphigoid is a subepidermal blistering skin disease characterized by an autoimmune response against epidermal/dermal proteins. The major autoantigens in bullous pemphigoid are hemidesmosomal proteins such as BP180 or BP230. Sera and purified IgG from patients with bullous pemphigoid are able to recruit neutrophils to the dermal−epidermal junction and to induce *ex vivo* subepidermal separation in human skin cryosections (Sitaru et al., 2002). This response was completely dependent on the Fc portion of the autoantibodies (Sitaru et al., 2002), suggesting a pathogenic role of Fc-receptor-mediated neutrophil activation by bullous pemphigoid-related autoantibodies. Psoriasis is another chronic autoimmune skin disease characterized by hyperplasia of epidermal keratinocytes. Neutrophils are found in skin lesions of psoriatic patients and drug-induced agranulocytosis causes the disappearance of psoriasis vulgaris (Toichi et al., 2000).

BASOPHILS

Basic Biology and Role in Immunity

Basophils, the scarcest circulatory granulocytes, account for 0.3% of nucleated bone marrow cells (Bosch et al., 2011). In the 1990s, it was discovered that human and murine basophils rapidly secrete large quantities of T helper 2 (Th2)-type cytokines, including IL-4 and IL-13, in response to stimuli, including FcεRI mediated signaling (Piccinni et al., 1991; Seder et al., 1991; Schroeder et al., 2001). The number of known factors that positively or negatively regulate basophil activation continues to increase. IL-3 aids differentiation of early precursors into fully mature basophils in the bone marrow and spleen (Arinobu et al., 2005; Ohmori et al., 2009), and enhances IL-4 production in mature basophils (Le Gros et al., 1990; Lantz et al., 2008; Hida et al., 2009). IL-4 plays a fundamental role in driving naïve T cell differentiation to Th2 cells, which produce Th2 cytokines and contribute to antiparasitic immunity and allergic inflammatory responses (Zhu et al., 2010; Paul and Zhu, 2010).

Basophils also enhance B cell IgE production *in vitro* by producing Th2 cytokines and expressing CD40 ligand (Gauchat et al., 1993; Yanagihara et al., 1998). Basophils efficiently capture intact antigens and enhance B cell activation, particularly B cell proliferation and immunoglobulin production (Denzel et al., 2008). IL-4 and IL-6 produced by basophils optimize CD4 T cell-dependent B cell help (Denzel et al., 2008). *In vivo*, basophil-mediated effects on B cells are vital in providing humoral immunity against bacteria (Chen et al., 2009). Circulating human IgD binds to basophils and induces B cell-stimulating factors, including BAFF, IL-1, and IL-4, as well as antimicrobial and opsonizing factors (Chen et al., 2009).

Basophils in Autoimmune Diseases

Basophils play an immunomodulatory role by provoking Th2 cell differentiation *in vivo*, and therefore may be hypothesized to play a role in immune diseases other than allergies. In addition to evidence of peripheral basophilia and constitutive Th2 skewing of CD4 T cells in lyn (a tyrosine-protein kinase) deficient mice [lyn $(-/-)$ mice], basophil involvement is also reported in autoimmune urticaria, where autoantibodies to the high affinity receptor FcεRIα induce basophil activation (Bischoff et al., 1996; Grattan, 2001). Autoimmune urticaria is known to have a Th2 component, and the immunomodulatory and effector responses of basophils contribute to the development of autoimmune symptoms. Th1 and Th2 cell subsets are suggested to be the primary effector cells involved in chronic inflammation in models of multiple sclerosis (experimental autoimmune encephalomyelitis), human posterior uveitis (experimental autoimmune uveitis), and rheumatoid arthritis (murine collagen-induced arthritis) (Damsker et al., 2010).

Role of IgE in Systemic Autoimmune Diseases

Although IgE is recognized as a human Th2 marker, some studies have found increased levels of IgE in Th1 and Th17 responses in autoimmune diseases (Sekigawa et al., 2003; Veldhoen, 2009). Allergy and autoimmunity share features, including those related to autoantibody production and circulating immune complex formation (Martin and Chan, 2004). Studies suggest that some allergens, including many environmental allergens, and

autoantigens have a common structure (Valenta et al., 2000), which might explain autoimmune diseases such as chronic urticaria. However, increased IgE levels are not associated with increased allergic disease in other autoimmune diseases, such as SLE (Morton et al., 1998).

The pathogenetic mechanisms of lupus nephritis include Th1- and Th17-mediated mechanisms (Crispín et al., 2010). In addition to Th1, Th17, and regulatory T cells, Th2 cells may play a role in SLE (Zeng et al., 2003; Valencia et al., 2007; Pernis, 2009), as suggested by the marked humoral response. Studies show increased IgE and the presence of self-reactive IgE in sera from some SLE patients, without increases in allergy (Tsuiji et al., 2006; Tiller et al., 2007). Patients with SLE without allergy have elevated total IgE and anti-nuclear IgE autoantibody levels, which seem to be linked to disease severity (Charles and Rivera, 2011). In addition, the presence of IgE in glomerular immune complex deposits in renal biopsies of SLE patients and a murine model of systemic autoimmune disease suggests that IgE plays a role in lupus nephritis (Atta et al., 2010). A study of anti-nuclear IgE antibody specificity and cytokine involvement found IgE antibodies against cell autoantigens implicated in protein expression, cell proliferation, and apoptosis in SLE and suggested that IL-10 may downregulate IgE autoimmune responses in SLE (Atta et al., 2010). Charles and colleagues (2010) showed that IgE immune complexes activate basophils and that removing self-reactive IgEs forming functional circulating immune complexes prevents renal disease. As circulating IgE levels are reduced, omalizumab, a monoclonal antibody binding to human IgE and reducing FcεRI expression on basophils (Lin et al., 2004), which is currently used as therapy for asthma and allergic rhinitis (Asai et al., 2001; Charles et al., 2010), may be of therapeutic interest in SLE patients with elevated IgE levels.

Basophils in Lupus Nephritis

Lyn, a Src kinase family member involved in B cell activation, dampens basophil expression of the trans-acting T cell-specific transcription factor GATA-3 (Charles et al., 2009), and B cells from some SLE patients express reduced levels of lyn kinase (Liossis et al., 2001). The lyn $(-/-)$ mouse develops an SLE-like autoimmune disease (Yu et al., 2001), with the production of circulating antinuclear and anti-dsDNA antibodies, and glomerular damage caused by deposition of circulating immune complexes that may result in renal failure and death. Lyn $(-/-)$ mice develop early, strong, constitutive Th2 skewing and exacerbated responses to Th2 challenges (Odom et al., 2004; Beavitt et al., 2005) and present basophilia and constitutive Th2 effector CD4 T cells (Charles et al., 2009). Th2-prone immune responses found in these mice require both basophils and IL-4, further highlighting the importance of IL-4-dependent immune modulation by basophils.

Therefore, lyn ($-/-$) mice may be a good model to study the effects of the Th2 environment on lupus-like nephritis. Charles et al. (2010) have demonstrated that basophils can promote antibody production and aggravate lupus nephritis, and that a Th2 phenotype contributes to lupus-like nephritis in lyn ($-/-$) mice and is associated with lupus nephritis in human SLE. Lupus-like disease in lyn ($-/-$) mice has been related to the presence of IL-4 and IgE, whose absence reversed Th2 skewing. IgG anti-dsDNA and anti-nuclear antibody titers and circulating immune complex levels were also reduced in mice deficient for IgE and lyn, and IL-4 and lyn, respectively, showing that autoantibody production in lyn ($-/-$) mice was, at least partly, dependent on the Th2 environment. Therefore, the study showed that basophils contribute to self-reactive antibody production in SLE and could enhance pre-existing loss of B cell tolerance. However, the identification of basophils is problematic owing to the lack of specific basophil markers. Since basophils may be found together with plasmacytoid dendritic cells in lesional tissues of SLE patients, these two cellular types share the same forward and sideward scatter properties in flow cytometry, as remarked by Dijkstra et al. (2012), who suggested that, due to their similarities, it may be difficult to analyze either cell type separately or to clearly differentiate between the two.

Basophils in Rheumatoid Arthritis and Vasculitides

Basophils have various immunoregulatory functions, explaining why research into pharmacological modulation by specific inhibitors or regulators is ongoing, particularly in allergic processes and, possibly, soon in autoimmune conditions, as demonstrated by the recent finding of basophil activation by anti-citrullinated protein antibodies (ACPAs) in sera from patients with rheumatoid arthritis (Schuerwegh et al., 2010). Schuerwegh and colleagues (2010) showed that IgE-bearing basophils from patients with ACPA are activated directly on exposure to citrullinated antigens, probably due to FcεRI-bound IgE—ACPAs on basophil surfaces. Identification of this activation pathway mediated by IgE—ACPAs in basophils might lead to new therapies for rheumatoid arthritis. Basophils should also be assessed in diseases driven by immunoglobulins directed against defined renal structures (e.g., anti-glomerular basement membrane disease), deposited in the glomeruli (e.g., membranous nephropathy) or driven by systemic vasculitis (e.g., ANCA-associated vasculitis), as they may help to generate and maintain high specific immunoglobulin levels and disease progression (Bosch et al., 2011).

Basophils in Autoinflammatory Diseases

Autoinflammatory diseases such as hyper-IgD syndrome are characterized by periodic fever associated with an abnormal release of IL-1 and TNF (Ryan and Kastner, 2008). Human basophils release IL-1β and TNF upon the cross-linking of surface-bound IgD, but not IgE (Chen et al., 2009). These disorders are characterized by elevated amounts of both circulating and mucosal IgD (+) IgM (−) B cells, and more IgD-armed basophils in the mucosa (Chen et al., 2009). Dysregulation of IgD-mediated basophil activation may contribute to the pathogenesis of autoinflammation.

EOSINOPHILS

Basic Biology and Role in Immunity

Eosinophils, although formed elements of the peripheral circulation, are primarily tissue-dwelling cells, of which gastrointestinal eosinophils predominate (Mishra et al., 1999). Eosinophil levels in the gastrointestinal tract are regulated by the constitutive expression of eotaxin-1 and eosinophil chemokine receptor-3 (Humbles et al., 2002; Pope et al., 2005). The eosinophil life cycle has bone marrow, blood, and tissue phases. Eosinophils are produced in bone marrow from pluripotent stem cells. Hematopoietic factors (IL-3, granulocyte-macrophage colony stimulating factor, and IL-5) are important for eosinophil proliferation and differentiation. IL-3 and granulocyte-macrophage colony stimulating factor stimulate proliferation of neutrophils, basophils, and eosinophils. In contrast, IL-5 specifically stimulates eosinophil production (Sanderson, 1992) and synergistically enhances the chemotactic response of eosinophils to chemokines or lipid mediators (Warringa et al., 1992; Schweizer et al., 1994). In addition to producing a number of regulatory or proinflammatory cytokines and chemokines (Hogan et al., 2008; Moqbel and Lacy, 2000), eosinophils secrete mediators that potentially promote Th2-type immune responses.

Identification of key eosinophil regulatory cytokines such as IL-5 and the eotaxin subfamily of chemokines have revealed mechanisms that selectively regulate eosinophil production and localization at baseline and during inflammatory responses. Specifically, an integrated mechanism involving Th2 cell-derived IL-5 regulating eosinophil expansion in the bone marrow and blood and Th2 cell-derived IL-13 regulating eotaxin production explains how T cells regulate eosinophils (Rothenberg and Hogan, 2006).

Eosinophils in Churg–Strauss Syndrome

There is mounting evidence suggesting that eosinophils play a key etiopathogenic role in Churg–Strauss syndrome (CSS), a systemic inflammatory disease characterized by adult-onset asthma, peripheral eosinophilia, and eosinophilic tissue infiltration. Because of the common positivity of ANCAs (30–40% of cases), and the main involvement of small vessels, CSS has been categorized as an ANCA-associated vasculitis together with granulomatosis with polyangiitis and microscopic polyangiitis (Pagnoux et al., 2007). The immunopathogenesis of CSS is complex, involving B cells, T cells, eosinophils, and resident epithelial and endothelial cells. Dense eosinophilic tissue infiltration, eosinophilic granulomas, and eosinophilia are characteristic of CSS (Terrier et al., 2010; Vaglio et al., 2012). Infiltrating eosinophils are frequently found in vasculitic lesions (Masi et al., 1990), and peripheral blood eosinophils correlate with the disease course, suggesting they play a role in CSS pathogenesis, although T cells are also involved (Lanham et al., 1984; Masi et al., 1990). Cellular immunity has been inferred from various findings, including the presence of memory T cells in vasculitic lesions (Hattori et al., 1999), increased T cell activation as reflected by cellular and soluble T cell activation markers (Schmitt et al., 1998), and responsiveness of disease activity to treatment with suppressors of cellular immunity (Guillevin et al., 1999).

On a cellular level, a strong shift toward a Th2-like response with massive T cell activation is evident in CSS (Dallos et al., 2010). *In vitro*, T cell lines from CSS patients produce significant amounts of IL-4 and IL-13 (Kiene et al., 2001), as shown by the high serum levels of IgE and IgE-containing immune complexes usually found in patients with active CSS (Manger et al., 1985). Th2 cytokines contribute to eosinophil recruitment, activation, and survival (Romagnani, 1991) and biopsy reveals granulomatous vasculitic lesions filled with eosinophils, macrophages, and lymphocytes (Koss et al., 1981). Chemokines mainly belonging to Th2-skewed pathways are secreted by epithelial and endothelial cells, a mechanism which amplifies CSS-associated inflammation. The chemokine eotaxin 3 [chemokine (C-C motif) ligand 26 (CCL26)] is strongly expressed in affected tissue from CSS patients and is also specifically related to disease activity and eosinophilia (Polzer et al., 2008).

Chemokine (C-C motif) ligand 17 (CCL17)/thymus and activation-related chemokine (TARC) is a CC chemokine secreted by PBMCs and various subsets of monocyte-derived dendritic cells, including thymic dendritic cells and endothelial cells (Imai et al., 1996). Recently, marked CCL17/TARC elevation was found in sera from patients with the lymphocytic subtype of idiopathic hypereosinophilic syndrome, which is characterized by circulating IL-5-producing clonal Th2 cells (de Lavareille et al., 2002). CCL17/TARC selectively recruits and migrates activated Th2 lymphocytes to affected tissue. Production of CCL17/TARC by dendritic cells is stimulated by Th2 cytokines, providing additional chemoattraction for Th2 cells (de Lavareille et al., 2001). CCL17/TARC expression has been demonstrated in Langerhans cells and keratinocytes in the skin of patients with atopic dermatitis (Kakinuma et al., 2001), considered to be a Th2-dominated disease in its acute phase. CCL17/TARC plays a vital role in Th2-mediated experimental allergen-induced asthma in mice, which may be inhibited by a monoclonal antibody against CCL17/TARC (Kawasaki et al., 2001). Dallos et al. (2010) hypothesized that CCL17/TARC may play a role in recruiting Th2 cells to sites of inflammation in CSS-affected tissue, finding expression of CCL17/TARC by infiltrating cells and occasionally the respiratory epithelium, as in a previous study (Kakinuma et al., 2001). Thus, CCL17/TARC may contribute to trafficking of Th2 cells and eosinophils to affected tissue in CSS. Th2 infiltration may promote activation and degranulation of eosinophils, resulting in tissue damage. In this study, infiltration of Th2 cells in active CSS lesions was demonstrated, as evidenced by the presence of CD294[+] lymphocytes. Moreover, Dallos et al. (2010) found increased serum levels of CCL17/TARC in patients with untreated CSS compared with healthy controls, although on commencement of therapy, CCL17/TARC concentrations decreased to a level not significantly different from that of controls. Concentrations of CCL17/TARC paralleled the disease course in patients in whom sequential serum samples were obtained. Accordingly, CCL17/TARC concentrations correlated well with IgE levels and eosinophil counts.

A recent study by Terrier et al. (2010) was the first to demonstrate the involvement of IL-25 and its receptor IL-17RB in the pathogenesis of CSS and its correlation with disease activity, suggesting that IL-25 production by eosinophils may play an essential role in promoting Th2 responses in CSS target tissues. IL-25 produced by epithelial cells, eosinophils, basophils, and mast cells enables innate and adaptive immunity by enhancing Th2 cytokine production (Angkasekwinai et al., 2007; Saenz et al., 2008; Wang and Liu, 2009). Elevated expression of IL-25 and IL-17RB was observed in tissues from patients with chronic asthma and atopic dermatitis (Wang et al., 2007), suggesting that IL-25 plays a role in evoking Th2 cell-mediated inflammation that features the infiltration of eosinophils and Th2 memory cells, and may increase allergic inflammation by enhancing the maintenance and functions of adaptive Th2 memory cells. Terrier et al. (2010) found higher levels of IL-25 in the serum of active CSS patients compared with atopic and patients with hypereosinophilic syndrome and with healthy donors.

IL-25 serum level was correlated with CSS clinical activity and the eosinophil count and was more than 10-fold higher in CSS patients than that observed in hypereosinophilic syndrome and atopy. Although the eosinophil count was elevated in patients with hypereosinophilic syndrome, their serum IL-25 level was low. Thus, increased levels of IL-25 in CSS patients may depend on specific priming and differentiation of activated eosinophils. IL-25 was mainly produced in the peripheral blood of CSS patients by eosinophils but not by neutrophils, monocytes, or T cells. IL-25 and IL-17RB were observed within the vasculitic lesions of CSS patients, and IL-17RB colocalized with T cells. Analysis of T cell differentiation in CSS patients pointed toward a polarized type 2 immune response with increased production of IL-4.

CONCLUSIONS AND THERAPEUTIC IMPLICATIONS

Lymphocytes are the white blood cells overwhelmingly implicated in the etiopathogenesis of most systemic autoimmune diseases. However, recent studies have increasingly focused on granulocytes, especially in SLE and systemic vasculitides, and neutrophils are currently under intensive investigation. The dysregulated neutrophil cell death and/or clearance often found in autoimmune diseases (Harper et al., 2001; Ren et al., 2003; Raza et al., 2006) may play a leading role in the pathogenesis of these diseases, as neutrophils release proteolytic and cytotoxic molecules that can trigger organ damage. Neutrophil products act as both targets and mediators of autoimmunity. Self DNA–antimicrobial peptide complexes, LL-37 and human neutrophil peptide, which would seem to be pivotal components of NETs, activate plasmacytoid dendritic cells to produce INF. It is unclear whether NETosis could serve as a biomarker or predictor of tissue damage in SLE or whether enhanced NETosis, which occurs in some vasculitides, could play a role in other autoimmune diseases associated with autoantibody production, INF signatures, or vascular damage, such as Sjögren syndrome, rheumatoid arthritis, or inflammatory myopathies. An attractive hypothesis is that inhibition of NETosis could be a potential therapeutic target in SLE (Knight and Kaplan, 2012). Suppression of NET formation due to ROS scavenging might stop chronic autoimmunity in SLE. Diphenylene iodonium (a potent inhibitor of NADPH oxidase that prevents oxygen-derived free-radical generation in neutrophils) severely impairs NET formation. Glutathione, a hydrogen peroxide scavenger, inhibits neutrophil death; catalase, which reduces hydrogen peroxide to water, delays normal neutrophil apoptosis (Bosch, 2011). Antioxidants such as N-acetyl-cysteine have been shown to block NET formation *in vitro*

(Patel et al., 2010), and N-acetyl-cysteine has been used to treat patients with SLE, Sjögren syndrome, and systemic sclerosis. In addition, antimalarial drugs, a key therapeutic option in SLE (Ruiz-Irastorza et al., 2010), are hypothesized to play a role as endosomal antagonists, and might have the potential to block the processing of NETs through TLR9 in plasmacytoid dendritic cells (Kuznik et al., 2011). Anti-IFN-α drugs are also under development in a phase I trial whose objective is to alter the IFN signature in SLE patients through administration of an anti-IFN monoclonal antibody (Yao et al., 2009), and a phase II study that is underway. The therapeutic hypothesis is that the blockade of IFN-α might help break the aforementioned cycle of NETosis (Knight and Kaplan, 2012). Finally, as activated neutrophils are one of the major sources of the pathogenic soluble IL-6 receptor (Kuznik et al., 2011), the monoclonal antibody tocilizumab may be shown to affect the contribution of neutrophils to autoimmune disease pathogenesis (Németh and Mócsai, 2012).

With respect to basophils, studies show that basophils, IgE, and IL-4 participate in maintaining autoantibody production in lyn ($-/-$) mice and suggest the Th2 environment contributes to autoimmunity. Basophils seem to amplify lupus nephritis rather than initiate the disease. The essential requirements are self-reactive IgE-dependent basophil activation, IL-4 production by basophils, and promotion of Th2 cell differentiation. Therefore, reducing circulating levels of self-reactive IgE or dampening basophil activity could have therapeutic benefits in lupus nephritis and determining whether basophil reduction or inactivation in early disease could defer or rescue the early development of lupus nephritis is of interest. A recent phase 3 multicenter, placebo-controlled trial in patients with active SLE found that belimumab, a monoclonal antibody against BAFF, is safe and efficacious (Kaveri et al., 2010; Navarra et al., 2011). Belimumab, besides affecting B cells, might deplete basophils (which contain membrane-bound BAFF), and thus could be useful in some patients with lupus nephritis, perhaps combined with treatments suppressing IgE production.

The pathogenic role of eosinophils in CSS is increasingly becoming clearer. As outlined above, IL-5 is a major survival factor for eosinophils, and targeted therapies using monoclonal antibodies directed against IL-5 (e.g., mepolizumab, resilizumab) are now used to treat eosinophilic asthma (Rosenwasser and Rothenberg, 2010). The IL-5-neutralizing antibody mepolizumab is proven to be an effective steroid-sparing agent in patients with hypereosinophilic syndrome negative for the FIP1L1-PDGFRA fusion gene (Rothenberg et al., 2008), and also demonstrated some efficacy in refractory CSS (Kahn et al., 2010). The anti-human IgE monoclonal antibody omalizumab, now used for asthma, has been trialed in CSS but has also been suspected of causing the development of full-blown CSS, perhaps because it allows (as do leukotriene receptor antagonists) steroid tapering (Wechsler et al., 2009). This may limit a more widespread use of omalizumab for CSS. Finally, IL-25/IL-17RB may be a key molecular pair in the maintenance of inflammation in CSS and therefore could be a potential target for the development of novel therapies.

REFERENCES

Abramson, S.B., Given, W.P., Edelson, H.S., Weissmann, G., 1983. Neutrophil aggregation induced by sera from patients with active systemic lupus erythematosus. Arthritis Rheum. 26, 630−636.

Amulic, B., Cazalet, C., Hayes, G.L., Metzler, K.D., Zychlinsky, A., 2012. Neutrophil function: from mechanisms to disease. Annu. Rev. Immunol. 30, 459−489.

Angkasekwinai, P., Park, H., Wang, Y.H., Wang, Y.H., Chang, S.H., Corry, D.B., et al., 2007. Interleukin 25 promotes the initiation of proallergic type 2 responses. J. Exp. Med. 204, 1509−1517.

Arenas, M., Abad, A., Valverde, V., Ferriz, P., Pascual, R., 1992. Selective inhibition of granulopoiesis with severe neutropenia in systemic lupus erythematosus. Arthritis Rheum. 35, 979−980.

Arinobu, Y., Iwasaki, H., Gurish, M.F., Mizuno, S., Shigematsu, H., Ozawa, H., et al., 2005. Developmental checkpoints of the basophil/mast cell lineages in adult murine hematopoiesis. Proc. Natl. Acad. Sci. U.S.A. 102, 18105−18110.

Arvieux, J., Jacob, M.C., Roussel, B., Bensa, J.C., Colomb, M.G., 1995. Neutrophil activation by anti-β2 glycoprotein I monoclonal antibodies via Fcγ receptor II. J. Leukoc. Biol. 57, 387−394.

Asai, K., Kitaura, J., Kawakami, Y., Yamagata, N., Tsai, M., Carbone, D.P., et al., 2001. Regulation of mast cell survival by IgE. Immunity. 14, 791−800.

Atta, A.M., Santiago, M.B., Guerra, F.G., Pereira, M.M., Sousa Atta, M.L., 2010. Autoimmune response of IgE antibodies to cellular self-antigens in systemic lupus erythematosus. Int. Arch. Allergy Immunol. 152, 401−406.

Barnes, T.C., Spiller, D.G., Anderson, M.E., Edwards, S.W., Moots, R.J., 2011. Endothelial activation and apoptosis mediated by neutrophil-dependent interleukin 6 trans-signalling: a novel target for systemic sclerosis?. Ann. Rheum. Dis. 70, 366−372.

Beavitt, S.J., Harder, K.W., Kemp, J.M., Jones, J., Quilici, C., Casagranda, F., et al., 2005. Lyn-deficient mice develop severe, persistent asthma: Lyn is a critical negative regulator of Th2 immunity. J. Immunol. 175, 1867−1875.

Bennett, L., Palucka, A.K., Arce, E., Cantrell, V., Borvak, J., Banchereau, J., et al., 2003. Interferon and granulopoiesis signatures in systemic lupus erythematosus blood. J. Exp. Med. 197, 711−723.

Bischoff, S.C., Zwahlen, R., Stucki, M., Müllner, G., de Weck, A.L., Stadler, B.M., et al., 1996. Basophil histamine release and leukotriene production in response to anti-IgE and anti-IgE receptor antibodies. Comparison of normal subjects and patients with urticaria, atopic dermatitis or bronchial asthma. Int. Arch. Allergy Immunol. 110, 261−271.

Bosch, X., Guilabert, A., Font, J., 2006. Antineutrophil cytoplasmic antibodies. Lancet. 368, 404−418.

Bosch, X., Lozano, F., Cervera, R., Ramos-Casals, M., Min, B., 2011. Basophils, IgE, and autoantibody-mediated kidney disease. J. Immunol. 186, 6083−6090.

Bosch, X., 2011. Systemic lupus erythematosus and the neutrophil. N. Engl. J. Med. 365, 758−760.

Brandt, L., Hedberg, H., 1969. Impaired phagocytosis by peripheral blood granulocytes in systemic lupus erythematosus. Scand. J. Haematol. 6, 348−353.

Brinkmann, V., Reichard, U., Goosmann, C., Fauler, B., Uhlemann, Y., Weiss, D.S., et al., 2004. Neutrophil extracellular traps kill bacteria. Science. 303, 1532−1535.

Brito-Zerón, P., Soria, N., Muñoz, S., Bové, A., Akasbi, M., Belenguer, R., et al., 2009. Prevalence and clinical relevance of autoimmune neutropenia in patients with primary Sjögren's syndrome. Semin. Arthritis Rheum. 38, 389−395.

Brouwer, E., Huitema, M.G., Mulder, A.H., Heeringa, P., van Goor, H., Tervaert, J.W., et al., 1994. Neutrophil activation in vitro and in vivo in Wegener's granulomatosis. Kidney Int. 45, 1120−1131.

Camussi, G., Cappio, F.C., Messina, M., Coppo, R., Stratta, P., Vercellone, A., 1980. The polymorphonuclear neutrophil (PMN) immunohistological technique: detection of immune complexes bound to the PMN membrane in acute poststreptococcal and lupus nephritis. Clin. Nephrol. 14, 280−287.

Charles, N., Watford, W.T., Ramos, H.L., Hellman, L., Oettgen, H.C., Gomez, G., et al., 2009. Lyn kinase controls basophil GATA-3 transcription factor expression and induction of Th2 cell differentiation. Immunity. 30, 533−543.

Charles, N., Hardwick, D., Daugas, E., Illei, G.G., Rivera, J., 2010. Basophils and the T helper 2 environment can promote the development of lupus nephritis. Nat. Med. 16, 701−707.

Charles, N., Rivera, J., 2011. Basophils and autoreactive IgE in the pathogenesis of systemic lupus erythematosus. Curr. Allergy Asthma Rep. 11, 378−387.

Carlson, T., Kroenke, M., Rao, P., Lane, T.E., Segal, B., 2008. The Th17 − ELR + CXC chemokine pathway is essential for the development of central nervous system autoimmune disease. J. Exp. Med. 205, 811−823.

Chakravarti, A., Raquil, M.A., Tessier, P., Poubelle, P.E., 2009. Surface RANKL of Toll-like receptor 4-stimulated human neutrophils activates osteoclastic bone resorption. Blood. 114, 1633−1644.

Chen, K., Xu, W., Wilson, M., He, B., Miller, N.W., Bengtén, E., et al., 2009. Immunoglobulin D enhances immune surveillance by activating antimicrobial, proinflammatory and B cell-stimulating programs in basophils. Nat. Immunol. 10, 889−898.

Chou, R.C., Kim, N.D., Sadik, C.D., Seung, E., Lan, Y., Byrne, M.H., et al., 2010. Lipid-cytokine-chemokine cascade drives neutrophil recruitment in a murine model of inflammatory arthritis. Immunity. 33, 266−278.

Cochrane, C.G., Unanue, E.R., Dixon, F.J., 1965. A role of polymorphonuclear leukocytes and complement in nephrotoxic nephritis. J. Exp. Med. 122, 99−116.

Coppo, P., Sibilia, J., Maloisel, F., Schlageter, M.H., Voyer, A.L., Gouilleux-Gruart, V., et al., 2003. Primary Sjögren's syndrome associated agranulocytosis: a benign disorder? Ann. Rheum. Dis. 62, 476−478.

Courtney, P.A., Crockard, A.D., Williamson, K., Irvine, A.E., Kennedy, R.J., Bell, A.L., 1999. Increased apoptotic peripheral blood neutrophils in systemic lupus erythematosus: relations with disease activity, antibodies to double stranded DNA, and neutropenia. Ann. Rheum. Dis. 58, 309–314.

Crispín, J.C., Liossis, S.N., Kis-Toth, K., Lieberman, L.A., Kyttaris, V.C., Juang, Y.T., et al., 2010. Pathogenesis of human systemic lupus erythematosus: recent advances. Trends Mol. Med. 16, 47–57.

Dallos, T., Heiland, G.R., Strehl, J., Karonitsch, T., Gross, W.L., Moosig, F., et al., 2010. CCL17/thymus and activation-related chemokine in Churg–Strauss syndrome. Arthritis Rheum. 62, 3496–3503.

Damsker, J.M., Hansen, A.M., Caspi, R.R., 2010. Th1 and Th17 cells: adversaries and collaborators. Ann. N.Y. Acad. Sci. 1183, 211–221.

de Lavareille, A., Roufosse, F., Schandené, L., Stordeur, P., Cogan, E., Goldman, M., 2001. Clonal Th2 cells associated with chronic hypereosinophilia: TARC-induced CCR4 down-regulation in vivo. Eur. J. Immunol. 31, 1037–1046.

de Lavareille, A., Roufosse, F., Schmid-Grendelmeier, P., Roumier, A.S., Schandené, L., Cogan, E., et al., 2002. High serum thymus and activation-regulated chemokine levels in the lymphocytic variant of the hypereosinophilic syndrome. J. Allergy Clin. Immunol. 110, 476–479.

Denny, M.F., Thacker, S., Mehta, H., Somers, E.C., Dodick, T., Barrat, F.J., et al., 2007. Interferon-α promotes abnormal vasculogenesis in lupus: a potential pathway for premature atherosclerosis. Blood. 110, 2907–2915.

Denny, M.F., Yalavarthi, S., Zhao, W., Thacker, S.G., Anderson, M., Sandy, A.R., 2010. A distinct subset of proinflammatory neutrophils isolated from patients with systemic lupus erythematosus induces vascular damage and synthesizes type I IFNs. J. Immunol. 184, 3284–3297.

Denzel, A., Maus, U.A., Rodriguez Gomez, M., Moll, C., Niedermeier, M., Winter, C., et al., 2008. Basophils enhance immunological memory responses. Nat. Immunol. 9, 733–742.

Dijkstra, D., Hennig, C., Witte, T., Hansen, G., 2012. Basophils from humans with systemic lupus erythematosus do not express MHC-II. Nat. Med. 18, 488–489 (author reply 489–490).

Donnelly, S., Roake, W., Brown, S., Young, P., Naik, H., Wordsworth, P., et al., 2006. Impaired recognition of apoptotic neutrophils by the C1q/calreticulin and CD91 pathway in systemic lupus erythematosus. Arthritis Rheum. 54, 1543–1556.

Elliott, E.R., Van Ziffle, J.A., Scapini, P., Sullivan, B.M., Locksley, R.M., Lowell, C.A., 2011. Deletion of Syk in neutrophils prevents immune complex arthritis. J. Immunol. 187, 4319–4330.

Falk, R.J., Terrell, R.S., Charles, L.A., Jennette, J.C., 1990. Antineutrophil cytoplasmic autoantibodies induce neutrophils to degranulate and produce oxygen radicals in vitro. Proc. Natl. Acad. Sci. U.S.A. 87, 4115–4119.

Faurschou, M., Borregaard, N., 2003. Neutrophil granules and secretory vesicles in inflammation. Microbes Infect. 5, 1317–1327.

Foerster, J., Storch, A., Fleischanderl, S., Wittstock, S., Pfeiffer, S., Riemekasten, G., et al., 2006. Neutrophil respiratory burst is decreased in scleroderma and normalized by near-infrared mediated hyperthermia. Clin. Exp. Dermatol. 31, 799–806.

Fuchs, T.A., Abed, U., Goosmann, C., Hurwitz, R., Schulze, I., Wahn, V., et al., 2007. Novel cell death program leads to neutrophil extracellular traps. J. Cell Biol. 176, 231–241.

Gabay, C., Krenn, V., Bosshard, C., Seemayer, C.A., Chizzolini, C., Huard, B., 2009. Synovial tissues concentrate secreted APRIL. Arthritis Res. Ther. 11, R144.

Garcia-Romo, G.S., Caielli, S., Vega, B., Connolly, J., Allantaz, F., Xu, Z., et al., 2011. Netting neutrophils are major inducers of type I IFN production in pediatric systemic lupus erythematosus. Sci. Transl. Med. 3, 73ra20.

Grattan, C.E., 2001. Basophils in chronic urticaria. J. Investig. Dermatol. Symp. Proc. 6, 139–140.

Gauchat, J.F., Henchoz, S., Mazzei, G., Aubry, J.P., Brunner, T., Blasey, H., et al., 1993. Induction of human IgE synthesis in B cells by mast cells and basophils. Nature. 365, 340–343.

Gómez-Puerta, J.A., Quintana, L.F., Stone, J.H., Ramos-Casals, M., Bosch, X., 2012. B-cell depleting agents for ANCA vasculitides: A new therapeutic approach. Autoimmun. Rev. 11, 646–652.

Guillevin, L., Cohen, P., Gayraud, M., Lhote, F., Jarrousse, B., Casassus, P., 1999. Churg–Strauss syndrome. Clinical study and long-term follow-up of 96 patients. Medicine (Baltimore). 78, 26–37.

Hacbarth, E., Kajdacsy-Balla, A., 1986. Low density neutrophils in patients with systemic lupus erythematosus, rheumatoid arthritis, and acute rheumatic fever. Arthritis Rheum. 29, 1334–1342.

Hakkim, A., Fuchs, T.A., Martinez, N.E., Hess, S., Prinz, H., Zychlinsky, A., et al., 2011. Activation of the Raf-MEK-ERK pathway is required for neutrophil extracellular trap formation. Nat. Chem. Biol. 7, 75–77.

Harper, L., Cockwell, P., Adu, D., Savage, C.O., 2001. Neutrophil priming and apoptosis in anti-neutrophil cytoplasmic autoantibody-associated vasculitis. Kidney Int. 59, 1729–1738.

Hattori, N., Ichimura, M., Nagamatsu, M., Li, M., Yamamoto, K., Kumazawa, K., et al., 1999. Clinicopathological features of Churg Strauss syndrome-associated neuropathy. Brain. 122, 427–439.

Hepburn, A.L., Narat, S., Mason, J.C., 2010. The management of peripheral blood cytopenias in systemic lupus erythematosus. Rheumatology (Oxford). 49, 2243–2254.

Hida, S., Yamasaki, S., Sakamoto, Y., Takamoto, M., Obata, K., Takai, T., et al., 2009. Fc receptor gamma-chain, a constitutive component of the IL-3 receptor, is required for IL-3-induced IL-4 production in basophils. Nat. Immunol. 10, 214–222.

Hogan, S.P., Rosenberg, H.F., Moqbel, R., Phipps, S., Foster, P.S., Lacy, P., et al., 2008. Eosinophils: biologicalproperties and role in health and disease. Clin. Exp. Allergy. 38, 709–750.

Holman, H.R., 1960. The L. E. cell phenomenon. Annu. Rev. Med. 11, 231–242.

Hotta, O., Oda, T., Taguma, Y., Kitamura, H., Chiba, S., et al., 1996. Role of neutrophil elastase in the development of renal necrotizing vasculitis. Clin. Nephrol. 45, 211–216.

Hsieh, S.C., Wu, T.H., Tsai, C.Y., Li, K.J., Lu, M.C., Wu, C.H., et al., 2008. Abnormal in vitro CXCR2 modulation and defective cationic ion transporter expression on polymorphonuclear neutrophils responsible for hyporesponsiveness to IL-8 stimulation in patients with active systemic lupus erythematosus. Rheumatology (Oxford). 47, 150–157.

Humbles, A.A., Lu, B., Friend, D.S., Okinaga, S., Lora, J., Al-Garawi, A., et al., 2002. The murine CCR3 receptor regulates both the role of eosinophils and mast cells in allergen-induced airway inflammation and hyperresponsiveness. Proc. Natl. Acad. Sci. USA 99, 1479–1484.

Hussein, M.R., Hassan, H.I., Hofny, E.R., Elkholy, M., Fatehy, N.A., Abd Elmoniem, A.E., et al., 2005. Alterations of mononuclear inflammatory cells, CD4/CD8 + T cells, interleukin 1beta, and tumour necrosis factor alpha in the bronchoalveolar lavage fluid, peripheral blood, and skin of patients with systemic sclerosis. J. Clin. Pathol. 58, 178—184.

Imai, T., Yoshida, T., Baba, M., Nishimura, M., Kakizaki, M., Yoshie, O., 1996. Molecular cloning of a novel T cell-directed CC chemokine expressed in thymus by signal sequence trap using Epstein-Barr virus vector. J. Biol. Chem. 271, 21514—21521.

Johnson, R.J., Couser, W.G., Alpers, C.E., Vissers, M., Schulze, M., Klebanoff, S.J., 1988. The human neutrophil serine proteinases, elastase and cathepsin G, can mediate glomerular injury in vivo. J. Exp. Med. 168, 1169—1174.

Kahn, J.E., Grandpeix-Guyodo, C., Marroun, I., Catherinot, E., Mellot, F., Roufosse, F., et al., 2010. Sustained response to mepolizumab in refractory Churg—Strauss syndrome. J. Allergy Clin. Immunol. 125, 267—270.

Kakinuma, T., Nakamura, K., Wakugawa, M., Mitsui, H., Tada, Y., Saeki, H., et al., 2001. Thymus and activation-regulated chemokine in atopic dermatitis: serum thymus and activation-regulated chemokine level is closely related with disease activity. J. Allergy Clin. Immunol. 107, 535—541.

Kaplan, M.J., 2011. Neutrophils in the pathogenesis and manifestations of SLE. Nat. Rev. Rheumatol. 7, 691—699.

Kaveri, S.V., Mouthon, L., Bayry, J., 2010. Basophils and nephritis in lupus. N. Engl. J. Med. 363, 1080—1082.

Kawasaki, S., Takizawa, H., Yoneyama, H., Nakayama, T., Fujisawa, R., Izumizaki, M., et al., 2001. Intervention of thymus and activation-regulated chemokine attenuates the development of allergic airway inflammation and hyperresponsiveness in mice. J. Immunol. 166, 2055—2062.

Kessenbrock, K., Krumbholz, M., Schönermarck, U., Back, W., Gross, W.L., Werb, Z., et al., 2009. Netting neutrophils in autoimmune small-vessel vasculitis. Nat. Med. 15, 623—625.

Kiene, M., Csernok, E., Müller, A., Metzler, C., Trabandt, A., Gross, W.L., 2001. Elevated interleukin-4 and interleukin-13 production by T cell lines from patients with Churg—Strauss syndrome. Arthritis Rheum. 44, 469—473.

Knight, J.S., Kaplan, M.J., 2012. Lupus neutrophils: "NET" gain in understanding lupus pathogenesis. Curr. Opin. Rheumatol.. 10.1097/BOR.0b013e3283546703.

Kobayashi, S.D., DeLeo, F.R., 2009. Role of neutrophils in innate immunity: a systems biology-level approach. Wiley Interdiscip. Rev. Syst. Biol. Med. 1, 309—333.

Koss, M.N., Antonovych, T., Hochholzer, L., 1981. Allergic granulomatosis (Churg—Strauss syndrome): pulmonary and renal morphologic findings. Am. J. Surg. Pathol. 5, 21—28.

Kuznik, A., Bencina, M., Svajger, U., Jeras, M., Rozman, B., Jerala, R., 2011. Mechanism of endosomal TLR inhibition by antimalarial drugs and imidazoquinolines. J. Immunol. 186, 4794—4804.

Lamour, A., Le Corre, R., Pennec, Y.L., Cartron, J., Youinou, P., 1995. Heterogeneity of neutrophil antibodies in patients with primary Sjögren's syndrome. Blood. 86, 3553—3559.

Lande, R., Gregorio, J., Facchinetti, V., Chatterjee, B., Wang, Y.H., Homey, B., et al., 2007. Plasmacytoid dendritic cells sense self-DNA coupled with antimicrobial peptide. Nature. 449, 564—569.

Lande, R., Ganguly, D., Facchinetti, V., Frasca, L., Conrad, C., Gregorio, J., et al., 2011. Neutrophils activate plasmacytoid dendritic cells by releasing self-DNA-peptide complexes in systemic lupus erythematosus. Sci. Transl. Med. 3, 73ra19.

Lanham, J.G., Elkon, K.B., Pusey, C.D., Hughes, G.R., 1984. Systemic vasculitis with asthma and eosinophilia: a clinical approach to the Churg—Strauss syndrome. Medicine (Baltimore). 63, 65—81.

Lantz, C.S., Min, B., Tsai, M., Chatterjea, D., Dranoff, G., Galli, S.J., 2008. IL-3 is required for increases in blood basophils in nematode infection in mice and can enhance IgE-dependent IL-4 production by basophils in vitro. Lab. Invest. 88, 1134—1142.

Le Gros, G., Ben-Sasson, S.Z., Conrad, D.H., Clark-Lewis, I., Finkelman, F.D., Plaut, M., et al., 1990. IL-3 promotes production of IL-4 by splenic non-B, non-T cells in response to Fc receptor cross-linkage. J. Immunol. 145, 2500—2506.

Lee, P.Y., Li, Y., Richards, H.B., Chan, F.S., Zhuang, H., Narain, S., et al., 2007. Type I interferon as a novel risk factor for endothelial progenitor cell depletion and endothelial dysfunction in systemic lupus erythematosus. Arthritis Rheum. 56, 3759—3769.

Leffler, J., Martin, M., Gullstrand, B., Tydén, H., Lood, C., Truedsson, L., et al., 2012. Neutrophil extracellular traps that are not degraded in systemic lupus erythematosus activate complement exacerbating the disease. J. Immunol. 188, 3522—3531.

Lin, H., Boesel, K.M., Griffith, D.T., Prussin, C., Foster, B., Romero, F. A., et al., 2004. Omalizumab rapidly decreases nasal allergic response and Fc epsilon RI on basophils. J. Allergy Clin. Immunol. 113, 297—302.

Liossis, S.N., Solomou, E.E., Dimopoulos, M.A., Panayiotidis, P., Mavrikakis, M.M., Sfikakis, P.P., 2001. B-cell kinase lyn deficiency in patients with systemic lupus erythematosus. J. Investig. Med. 49, 157—165.

Liu, L., Belkadi, A., Darnall, L., Hu, T., Drescher, C., Cotleur, A.C., et al., 2010. CXCR2-positive neutrophils are essential for cuprizone-induced demyelination: relevance to multiple sclerosis. Nat. Neurosci. 13, 319—326.

Manger, B.J., Krapf, F.E., Gramatzki, M., Nüsslein, H.G., Burmester, G.R., Krauledat, P.B., et al., 1985. IgE-containing circulating immune complexes in Churg—Strauss vasculitis. Scand. J. Immunol. 21, 369—373.

Mantovani, A., Cassatella, M.A., Costantini, C., Jaillon, S., 2011. Neutrophils in the activation and regulation of innate and adaptive immunity. Nat. Rev. Immunol. 11, 519—531.

Martin, F., Chan, A.C., 2004. Pathogenic roles of B cells in human autoimmunity; insights from the clinic. Immunity. 20, 517—527.

Marzocchi-Machado, C.M., Alves, C.M., Azzolini, A.E., Polizello, A.C., Carvalho, I.F., Lucisano-Valim, Y.M., 2002. Fcgamma and complement receptors: expression, role and co-operation in mediating the oxidative burst and degranulation of neutrophils of Brazilian systemic lupus erythematosus patients. Lupus. 11, 240—248.

Masi, A.T., Hunder, G.G., Lie, J.T., Michel, B.A., Bloch, D.A., Arend, W.P., et al., 1990. The American College of Rheumatology 1990 criteria for the classification of Churg—Strauss syndrome (allergic granulomatosis and angiitis). Arthritis Rheum. 33, 1094—1100.

Maslen, C.L., Hall, N.D., Woolf, A.D., Maddison, P.J., 1987. Enhanced oxidative metabolism of neutrophils from patients with systemic sclerosis. Br. J. Rheumatol. 26, 113—117.

Metzler, K.D., Fuchs, T.A., Nauseef, W.M., Reumaux, D., Roesler, J., Schulze, I., et al., 2011. Myeloperoxidase is required for neutrophil extracellular trap formation: implications for innate immunity. Blood. 117, 953—959.

Mishra, A., Hogan, S.P., Lee, J.J., Foster, P.S., Rothenberg, M.E., 1999. Fundamental signals that regulate eosinophil homing to the gastrointestinal tract. J. Clin. Invest. 103, 1719–1727.

Molad, Y., Buyon, J., Anderson, D.C., Abramson, S.B., Cronstein, B.N., 1994. Intravascular neutrophil activation in systemic lupus erythematosus (SLE): dissociation between increased expression of CD11b/CD18 and diminished expression of L-selectin on neutrophils from patients with active SLE. Clin. Immunol. Immunopathol. 71, 281–286.

Moqbel, R., Lacy, P., 2000. New concepts in effector functions of eosinophil cytokines. Clin. Exp. Allergy. 30, 1667–1671.

Morton, S., Palmer, B., Muir, K., Powell, R.J., 1998. IgE and non-IgE mediated allergic disorders in systemic lupus erythematosus. Ann. Rheum Dis. 57, 660–663.

Murphy, H.S., Bakopoulos, N., Dame, M.K., Varani, J., Ward, P.A., 1998. Heterogeneity of vascular endothelial cells: differences in susceptibility to neutrophil-mediated injury. Microvasc. Res. 56, 203–211.

Navarra, S.V., Guzmán, R.M., Gallacher, A.E., Hall, S., Levy, R.A., Jimenez, R.E., et al., 2011. Efficacy and safety of belimumab in patients with active systemic lupus erythematosus: a randomised, placebo-controlled, phase 3 trial. Lancet. 377, 721–731.

Németh, T., Mócsai, A., 2012. The role of neutrophils in autoimmune diseases. Immunol. Lett. 143, 9–19.

Obermoser, G., Sontheimer, R.D., Zelger, B., 2010. Overview of common, rare and atypical manifestations of cutaneous lupus erythematosus and histopathological correlates. Lupus. 19, 1050–1070.

Odom, S., Gomez, G., Kovarova, M., Furumoto, Y., Ryan, J.J., Wright, H.V., et al., 2004. Negative regulation of immunoglobulin E-dependent allergic responses by Lyn kinase. J. Exp. Med. 199, 1491–1502.

Ohmori, K., Luo, Y., Jia, Y., Nishida, J., Wang, Z., Bunting, K.D., et al., 2009. IL-3 induces basophil expansion in vivo by directing granulocyte- monocyte progenitors to differentiate into basophil lineage-restricted progenitors in the bone marrow and by increasing the number of basophil/mast cell progenitors in the spleen. J. Immunol. 182, 2835–2841.

Pagnoux, C., Guilpain, P., Guillevin, L., 2007. Churg–Strauss syndrome. Curr. Opin. Rheumatol. 19, 25–32.

Papayannopoulos, V., Metzler, K.D., Hakkim, A., Zychlinsky, A., 2010. Neutrophil elastase and myeloperoxidase regulate the formation of neutrophil extracellular traps. J. Cell Biol. 191, 677–691.

Papayannopoulos, V., Zychlinsky, A., 2009. NETs: a new strategy for using old weapons. Trends Immunol. 30, 513–521.

Patel, S., Kumar, S., Jyoti, A., Srinag, B.S., Keshari, R.S., Saluja, R., et al., 2010. Nitric oxide donors release extracellular traps from human neutrophils by augmenting free radical generation. Nitric Oxide. 22, 226–234.

Paul, W.E., Zhu, J., 2010. How are T(H)2-type immune responses initiated and amplified? Nat. Rev. Immunol. 10, 225–235.

Pernis, A.B., 2009. Th17 cells in rheumatoid arthritis and systemic lupus erythematosus. J. Intern. Med. 265, 644–652.

Piccinni, M.P., Macchia, D., Parronchi, P., Giudizi, M.G., Bani, D., Alterini, R., et al., 1991. Human bone marrow non-B, non-T cells produce interleukin 4 in response to cross-linkage of Fcε and Fcγ receptors. Proc. Natl. Acad. Sci. U.S.A. 88, 8656–8660.

Polzer, K., Karonitsch, T., Neumann, T., Eger, G., Haberler, C., Soleiman, A., et al., 2008. Eotaxin-3 is involved in Churg–Strauss

syndrome: a serum marker closely correlating with disease activity. Rheumatology (Oxford). 47, 804–808.

Pope, S.M., Fulkerson, P.C., Blanchard, C., Akei, H.S., Nikolaidis, N.M., Zimmermann, N., et al., 2005. Identification of a cooperative mechanism involving interleukin-13 and eotaxin-2 in experimental allergic lung inflammation. J. Biol. Chem. 280, 13952–13961.

Poubelle, P.E., Chakravarti, A., Fernandes, M.J., Doiron, K., Marceau, A.A., 2007. Differential expression of RANK, RANK-L, and osteoprotegerin by synovial fluid neutrophils from patients with rheumatoid arthritis and by healthy human blood neutrophils. Arthritis Res. Ther. 9, R25.

Raza, K., Scheel-Toellner, D., Lee, C.Y., Pilling, D., Curnow, S.J., Falciani, F., et al., 2006. Synovial fluid leukocyte apoptosis is inhibited in patients with very early rheumatoid arthritis. Arthritis Res. Ther. 8, R120.

Redecha, P., Franzke, C.W., Ruf, W., Mackman, N., Girardi, G., 2008. Neutrophil activation by the tissue factor/factor VIIa/PAR2 axis mediates fetal death in a mouse model of antiphospholipid syndrome. J. Clin. Invest. 118, 3453–3461.

Ren, Y., Tang, J., Mok, M.Y., Chan, A.W., Wu, A., Lau, C.S., 2003. Increased apoptotic neutrophils and macrophages and impaired macrophage phagocytic clearance of apoptotic neutrophils in systemic lupus erythematosus. Arthritis Rheum. 48, 2888–2897.

Romagnani, S., 1991. Human TH1 and TH2 subsets: doubt no more. Immunol. Today. 12, 256–257.

Rönnefarth, V.M., Erbacher, A.I., Lamkemeyer, T., Madlung, J., Nordheim, A., Rammensee, H.G., et al., 2006. TLR2/TLR4-independent neutrophil activation and recruitment upon endocytosis of nucleosomes reveals a new pathway of innate immunity in systemic lupus erythematosus. J. Immunol. 177, 7740–7749.

Roosnek, E., Burjanadze, M., Dietrich, P.Y., Matthes, T., Passweg, J., Huard, B., 2009. Tumors that look for their springtime in APRIL. Crit. Rev. Oncol. Hematol. 72, 91–97.

Rosenwasser, L.J., Rothenberg, M.E., 2010. IL-5 pathway inhibition in the treatment of asthma and Churg–Strauss syndrome. J. Allergy Clin. Immunol. 125, 1245–1246.

Rothenberg, M.E., Hogan, S.P., 2006. The eosinophil. Annu. Rev. Immunol. 24, 147–174.

Rothenberg, M.E., Klion, A.D., Roufosse, F.E., Kahn, J.E., Weller, P.F., Simon, H.U., et al., 2008. Treatment of patients with the hypereosinophilic syndrome with mepolizumab. N. Engl. J. Med. 358, 1215–1228.

Ruiz-Irastorza, G., Ramos-Casals, M., Brito-Zeron, P., Khamashta, M.A., 2010. Clinical efficacy and side effects of antimalarials in systemic lupus erythematosus: a systematic review. Ann. Rheum. Dis. 69, 20–28.

Ryan, J.G., Kastner, D.L., 2008. Fevers, genes, and innate immunity. Curr. Top Microbiol. Immunol. 321, 169–184.

Saenz, S.A., Taylor, B.C., Artis, D., 2008. Welcome to the neighborhood: epithelial cell-derived cytokines license innate and adaptive immune responses at mucosal sites. Immunol. Rev. 226, 172–190.

Saffarzadeh, M., Juenemann, C., Queisser, M.A., Lochnit, G., Barreto, G., Galuska, S.P., et al., 2012. Neutrophil extracellular traps directly induce epithelial and endothelial cell death: a predominant role of histones. PLoS One. 7, e32366.

Samarkos, M., Mylona, E., Kapsimali, V., 2012. The role of complement in the antiphospholipid syndrome: a novel mechanism for pregnancy morbidity. Semin. Arthritis Rheum. 42, 66–69.

Sanderson, C.J., 1992. Interleukin-5, eosinophils, and disease. Blood. 79, 3101–3109.

Scapini, P., Carletto, A., Nardelli, B., Calzetti, F., Roschke, V., Merigo, F., et al., 2005. Proinflammatory mediators elicit secretion of the intracellular B-lymphocyte stimulator pool (BLyS) that is stored in activated neutrophils: implications for inflammatory diseases. Blood. 105, 830–837.

Schmitt, W.H., Csernok, E., Kobayashi, S., Klinkenborg, A., Reinhold-Keller, E., Gross, W.L., 1998. Churg–Strauss syndrome: serum markers of lymphocyte activation and endothelial damage. Arthritis Rheum. 41, 445–452.

Schroeder, J.T., MacGlashan Jr., D.W., Lichtenstein, L.M., 2001. Human basophils: mediator release and cytokine production. Adv. Immunol. 77, 93–122.

Schuerwegh, A.J., Ioan-Facsinay, A., Dorjée, A.L., Roos, J., Bajema, I.M., van der Voort, E.I., et al., 2010. Evidence for a functional role of IgE anticitrullinated protein antibodies in rheumatoid arthritis. Proc. Natl. Acad. Sci. U.S.A. 107, 2586–2591.

Schweizer, R.C., Welmers, B.A., Raaijmakers, J.A., Zanen, P., Lammers, J.W., Koenderman, L., 1994. RANTES- and interleukin-8-induced responses in normal human eosinophils: effects of priming with interleukin-5. Blood. 83, 3697–3704.

Seder, R.A., Paul, W.E., Dvorak, A.M., Sharkis, S.J., Kagey-Sobotka, A., Niv, Y., et al., 1991. Mouse splenic and bone marrow cell populations that express high-affinity Fcε receptors and produce interleukin 4 are highly enriched in basophils. Proc. Natl. Acad. Sci. U.S.A. 88, 2835–2839.

Sekigawa, I., Yoshiike, T., Iida, N., Hashimoto, H., Ogawa, H., 2003. Allergic diseases in systemic lupus erythematosus: prevalence and immunological considerations. Clin. Exp. Rheumatol. 21, 117–121.

Seshan, S.V., Franzke, C.W., Redecha, P., Monestier, M., Mackman, N., Girardi, G., 2009. Role of tissue factor in a mouse model of thrombotic microangiopathy induced by antiphospholipid antibodies. Blood. 114, 1675–1683.

Sitaru, C., Schmidt, E., Petermann, S., Munteanu, L.S., Bröcker, E.B., Zillikens, D., 2002. Autoantibodies to bullous pemphigoid antigen 180 induce dermal-epidermal separation in cryosections of human skin. J. Invest. Dermatol. 118, 664–671.

Stevens, T.R., Hall, N.D., McHugh, N.J., Maddison, P.J., 1992. Spontaneous neutrophil activation in patients with primary Raynaud's phenomenon and systemic sclerosis. Br. J. Rheumatol. 31, 856.

Terrier, B., Bièche, I., Maisonobe, T., Laurendeau, I., Rosenzwajg, M., Kahn, J.E., et al., 2010. Interleukin-25: a cytokine linking eosinophils and adaptive immunity in Churg–Strauss syndrome. Blood. 116, 4523–4531.

Tiller, T., Tsuiji, M., Yurasov, S., Velinzon, K., Nussenzweig, M.C., Wardemann, H., 2007. Autoreactivity in human IgG + memory B cells. Immunity. 26, 205–213.

Toichi, E., Tachibana, T., Furukawa, F., 2000. Rapid improvement of psoriasis vulgaris during drug-induced agranulocytosis. J. Am. Acad. Dermatol. 43, 391–395.

Tsuiji, M., Yurasov, S., Velinzon, K., Thomas, S., Nussenzweig, M.C., Wardemann, H., 2006. A checkpoint for autoreactivity in human IgM + memory B cell development. J. Exp. Med. 203, 393–400.

Urban, C.F., Ermert, D., Schmid, M., Abu-Abed, U., Goosmann, C., Nacken, W., et al., 2009. Neutrophil extracellular traps contain calprotectin, a cytosolic protein complex involved in host defense against Candida albicans. PLoS Pathog. 5, e1000639.

Vaglio, A., Moosig, F., Zwerina, J., 2012. Churg–Strauss syndrome: update on pathophysiology and treatment. Curr. Opin. Rheumatol. 24, 24–30.

Valencia, X., Yarboro, C., Illei, G., Lipsky, P.E., 2007. Deficient CD4 + CD25high T regulatory cell function in patients with active systemic lupus erythematosus. J. Immunol. 178, 2579–2588.

Valenta, R., Seiberler, S., Natter, S., Mahler, V., Mossabeb, R., Ring, J., et al., 2000. Autoallergy: a pathogenetic factor in atopic dermatitis? J. Allergy Clin. Immunol. 105, 432–437.

Veldhoen, M., 2009. The role of T helper subsets in autoimmunity and allergy. Curr. Opin. Immunol. 21, 606–611.

Villanueva, E., Yalavarthi, S., Berthier, C.C., Hodgin, J.B., Khandpur, R., Lin, A.M., et al., 2011. Netting neutrophils induce endothelial damage, infiltrate tissues, and expose immunostimulatory molecules in systemic lupus erythematosus. J. Immunol. 187, 538–552.

Wang, Y.H., Angkasekwinai, P., Lu, N., Voo, K.S., Arima, K., Hanabuchi, S., et al., 2007. IL-25 augments type 2 immune responses by enhancing the expansion and functions of TSLP-DC-activated Th2 memory cells. J. Exp. Med. 204, 1837–1847.

Wang, Y.H., Liu, Y.J., 2009. Thymic stromal lymphopoietin, OX40-ligand, and interleukin-25 in allergic responses. Clin. Exp. Allergy. 39, 798–806.

Warringa, R.A., Schweizer, R.C., Maikoe, T., Kuijper, P.H., Bruijnzeel, P.L., Koendermann, L., 1992. Modulation of eosinophil chemotaxis by interleukin-5. Am. J. Respir. Cell Mol. Biol. 7, 631–636.

Wechsler, M.E., Wong, D.A., Miller, M.K., Lawrence-Miyasaki, L., 2009. Churg–Strauss syndrome in patients treated with omalizumab. Chest. 136, 507–518.

Wu, C.H., Hsieh, S.C., Li, K.J., Lu, M.C., Yu, C.L., 2007. Premature telomere shortening in polymorphonuclear neutrophils from patients with systemic lupus erythematosus is related to the lupus disease activity. Lupus. 16, 265–272.

Yanagihara, Y., Kajiwara, K., Basaki, Y., Ikizawa, K., Ebisawa, M., Ra, C., et al., 1998. Cultured basophils but not cultured mast cells induce human IgE synthesis in B cells after immunologic stimulation. Clin. Exp. Immunol. 111, 136–143.

Yao, Y., Richman, L., Higgs, B.W., Morehouse, C.A., de los Reyes, M., Brohawn, P., et al., 2009. Neutralization of interferon-alpha/beta inducible genes and downstream effect in a phase I trial of an antiinterferonalpha monoclonal antibody in systemic lupus erythematosus. Arthritis Rheum. 60, 1785–1796.

Yu, C.C., Yen, T.S., Lowell, C.A., DeFranco, A.L., 2001. Lupus-like kidney disease in mice deficient in the Src family tyrosine kinases Lyn and Fyn. Curr. Biol. 11, 34–38.

Zeng, D., Liu, Y., Sidobre, S., Kronenberg, M., Strober, S., 2003. Activation of natural killer T cells in NZB/W mice induces Th1-type immune responses exacerbating lupus. J. Clin. Invest. 112, 1211–1222.

Zhu, J., Yamane, H., Paul, W.E., 2010. Differentiation of effector CD4 T cell populations. Annu. Rev. Immunol. 28, 445–489.

Chapter 15

The Roles and Contributions of the Complement System in the Pathophysiology of Autoimmune Diseases

Wilhelm J. Schwaeble, Youssif M. Ali, and Robert B. Sim

Department of Infection, Immunity and Inflammation, Faculty of Medicine, University of Leicester, Leicester, UK

Chapter Outline

The Complement System and Complement Activation
Pathways   217
  The Classical Pathway   218
  The Lectin Pathway   218
  The Alternative Pathway   219
  The Membrane Attack Complex   219
Control of Complement Activation   219
  Fluid Phase Regulators   220
  Membrane-Bound Regulators   220
The Biological Effects of Complement Activation   220
Complement Involvement in the Pathophysiology of Diverse
Autoimmune Diseases   221
References   224

THE COMPLEMENT SYSTEM AND COMPLEMENT ACTIVATION PATHWAYS

In the 1890s, Jules Bordet observed that bactericidal activity of serum essentially requires two components, one which is present prior to immunization and heat-labile that he named Alexin (from Greek *alexein*: to ward off) and the other component, which is heat-stabile and generated by immunization. He demonstrated in 1898 that the same basic mechanisms that compose the bacteriolytic activity of immune sera are responsible for the hemolytic activity of serum towards erythrocytes of other species, a methodology that was used to analyze the biological activities of complement for decades to come. The prevailing name "complement" for this bacteriolytic plasma component was coined by Paul Ehrlich at about the same time to underline that this component was essential for "amboceptors" (the name he proposed for antibodies) to lyse cells and thereby "complement" their function (Dunkelberger and Song, 2010; Schmalstieg and Goldman, 2010). Up to the present day, the bactericidal (or hemolytic) activity of complement mediated through the formation of a lytic membrane attack complex

(formed following the activation of the terminal complement components C5b–C9) is still the most widely known biological activity of the complement system.

Complement is composed of a very complex system of zymogen precursor components, their substrates, fluid phase or cell surface resident regulators/cofactors and receptors for complement activation products comprising altogether more than 40 components (Whaley and Schwaeble, 1997; Carroll and Sim, 2011). Cell surface resident receptors for complement activation products continuously sense the activation state of the complement system and coordinate cellular responses of both the innate and the adaptive immune system. As such, complement activation is involved in the initiation and maintenance of numerous inflammatory reactions and inappropriate control of complement activation can predispose to a wide spectrum of infectious or inflammatory pathologies.

Although the bactericidal or hemolytic activity of complement elicited through the formation of membrane attack complexes is the most popular and widely known function of complement, it is only effective against some bacterial species, while complement-mediated

N. Rose & I. Mackay (Eds): The Autoimmune Diseases, Fifth edition. DOI: http://dx.doi.org/10.1016/B978-0-12-384929-8.00015-0

opsonization which targets bacteria, viruses, yeast, host cellular and bacterial debris and eukaryotic parasites for phagocytosis and elimination through the various phagocytes of the reticulo-endothelial system (via their receptors either for C3b, iC3b, C3d, C4b, or C1q/MBL/ficolins). The cellular receptors on phagocytes responsible for the enhanced uptake of opsonized particles and cells include complement receptors type 1 (CR1 also known as CD35), type 3 (CR3, alias of CD11b/CD18), and type 4 (CR4 CD11c/CD18) (Wagner and Frank, 2010). Phagocytes are directed to the location of complement activation by chemotaxis sensing the release of the potent complement chemotactic factor and anaphylatoxin C5a and the anaphylotoxin C3a, through the receptors C3aR and C5aR (alias CD88) (Van Beek et al., 2003; Wallis, 2007). Complement anaphylatoxins C3a and C5a can also increase vascular permeability aiding the transmigration and extravasation of leukocytes into tissue (Williams, 1983). Various complement deficiencies result in a defective recruitment of leukocytes to the site of damage or infection.

Complement activation products also facilitate transport of antigens to the lymphoid follicles and critical interactions between follicular dendritic cells and B cells in order to promote both B cell memory and the production of specific antibodies (Barrington et al., 2002; Le Friec and Kemper, 2009; Gonzalez et al., 2010). Moreover, complement activation also modulates T cell responses by coordinating the necessary interactions between antigen-presenting cells (APC) and T cells (Zhou et al., 2006; Le Friec and Kemper, 2009; Kwan et al., 2012). The complement system is activated via three activation pathways which all converge through the formation of C3 and C5 convertase complexes and the subsequent formation of the membrane attack complex (MAC).

The Classical Pathway

The first component of the complement C1 is composed of a multimolecular initiation complex that triggers complement activation.

The 790 kDa C1 complex consists of a recognition protein, C1q, and a heterotetramer of C1r and C1s zymogens to form the C1q:C1s:C1r$_2$:C1s complex (Figure 15.1). C1q is composed of six identical subunits joined together through their collagen-like stalks that end in globular heads. Each subunit consists of three homologous polypeptide chains (Arlaud et al., 2002). Classical pathway activation is initiated either by direct binding of C1q to a target (e.g., bacterial) surface or indirectly by binding of C1q to antibodies deposited on the target (immune complexes). IgM, IgG1, IgG2, and IgG3 bind C1q (Arlaud et al., 2002). Binding of C1q to complement activators leads to a conformational change in the

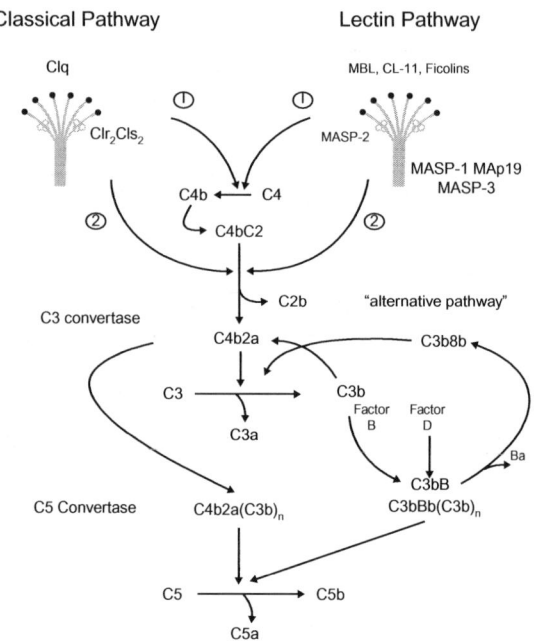

FIGURE 15.1 Flow diagram of the three activation pathways of complement. Activation step 1 depicts the C1s and MASP-2-mediated cleavage of complement C4 to C4a and C4b, activation step 2 depicts the subsequent C1s and MASP-2-mediated cleavage of C4bC2 to form the C3 convertase of the classical and lectin pathway C4bC2a. With the conversion of C5 into C5a and C5b, all enzymatic steps of complement activation are completed. Both the classical as well as the alternative pathways are thought to correspond with the alternative pathway activation loop through provision of C3b.

collagenous region of C1q which in turn leads to the auto-activation of C1r, which cleaves its only substrate, C1s. C1s in turn cleaves C4 into C4a and C4b and then cleaves C2 bound to the C4b, resulting in the formation of the classical pathway C3 convertase (C4b2a) (Arlaud et al., 2002; Carroll and Sim, 2011).

C4b2a is a protease which activates C3 to form C3a and C3b. C3b, like C4b, can bind covalently to the complement activator, and hundreds of molecules of C3b can be deposited in close proximity to the C3 convertase complex. C3b can bind directly to C4b2a, forming the classical pathway C5 convertaseC4b2a3b, in which C4b and C3b form a binding site for C5, orienting it for cleavage by C2a.

The Lectin Pathway

In evolutionary terms, the lectin pathway (LP) of complement activation seems to be the oldest of the three (Dodds, 2002; Wallis, 2007). The LP is initiated by the binding of a multimolecular LP activation complex, similar in structure to the classical pathway C1, to pathogen-associated molecular patterns (PAMPs), mainly carbohydrate structures present on microorganisms, or DAMPS (damage-associated molecular patterns) on damaged host tissue. The LP recognition molecules are mannose binding lectin (MBL), an MBL-like collectin called CL-11, and ficolins. Like C1q, they are made up of subunits with globular heads and collagenous stalks. Activation is initiated by the binding of the globular heads to carbohydrate structures present on microorganisms or aberrant glycocalyx patterns on apoptotic, necrotic, malignant, or oxygen-deprived cells (Fujita, 2002; Schwaeble et al., 2002). Rodents have at least four circulating LP recognition molecules, with differing, but overlapping, carbohydrate specificities; two mannan-binding lectins (MBL-A and MBL-C), collectin-11 (CL-11), and ficolin A (Fcna) (Schwaeble et al., 2011; Ali et al. 2012). A second murine ficolin, Fcnb, associated with monocyte and macrophage cell surfaces does not activate complement in mice, but may act as a lectin pathway recognition molecule in rats (Girija et al., 2011). Humans have a single MBL (the product of *MBL2*; *MBL1* is a pseudogene), CL-11 (collectin kidney 1, CL-K1), and three ficolins, FCN1 (M-ficolin), FCN2 (L-ficolin), and FCN3 (H-ficolin) (Fujita, 2002; Liu et al., 2005; Hansen et al., 2010). These recognition molecules form complexes with the serine proteases called MASP-1, -2, and -3 (MBL-associated serine proteases 1, 2, and 3). These are homologous to C1r and C1s, and form homodimers (and perhaps some heterodimers). The serine proteases in the CP and LP activation complexes all interact with a highly conserved binding motif within the collagenous region of the recognition subunit, i.e., C1q for the CP and MBL, ficolins or CL-11 for the LP (Wallis et al., 2004). Each recognition molecule can bind one protease dimer. The recognition molecules also interact with MAp19 and MAp44 (alias MBL/ficolin-associated protein 1), which are non-enzymatic, truncated alternative splice products of the *MASP2* and *MASP1/3* genes, respectively. Both truncated gene products lack the serine protease domain and may regulate LP activation by competing for the binding of MASPs to the carbohydrate recognition molecules (Thiel et al., 1997; Stover et al., 1999; Takahashi et al., 1999; Schwaeble et al., 2002; Iwaki et al., 2006; Degn et al., 2009; Skjoedt et al., 2010). Of the three MASPs, only MASP-2 is required and essential to form the LP C3 and C5 convertases (C4b2a and C4b2a3b) (Thiel et al., 1997; Vorup-Jensen et al., 2000; Rossi et al., 2001; Schwaeble et al., 2011).

Like C1s, activated MASP-2 cleaves C4 and C4b-bound C2, generating C4b2a. Neither MASP-1 nor MASP-3 can cleave C4 (Schwaeble et al., 2011). The function of MASP-1 is still uncertain. It may facilitate LP activation by either direct cleavage of complex-bound MASP-2 or cleavage of C4b-bound C2 (Takahashi et al., 2008; Kocsis et al., 2010; Schwaeble et al., 2011). Recent work demonstrated that MASP-1 (and possibly MASP-3) plays a key role in the maturation and initiation of the alternative activation pathway (Takahashi et al., 2008; Iwaki et al., 2011). The LP is probably mainly activated by charge-neutral sugar structures and clusters of acetyl moieties, whereas in the classical pathway,

C1q recognizes mainly charge clusters. The lectin pathway can also respond to immunoglobulins deposited on targets, by binding to glycans on some human IgG, IgA glycoforms, and to the glycans on mouse (but not human) IgM (Carroll and Sim, 2011).

The Alternative Pathway

Factor B, factor D, and properdin (factor P) are specific components of the alternative pathway of complement activation. Unlike the classical and lectin pathways (which are initiated via specific recognition proteins such as C1q or MBL) the alternative pathway is initiated through a spontaneous steady-state hydrolysis of C3 to form C3 (H_2O) which in turn binds to factor B to form a C3(H_2O)B zymogen complex. In this complex, factor B is cleaved by factor D releasing a Ba fragment while Bb remains attached to the complex. The newly formed complex C3 (H_2O)Bb is a C3 convertase enzyme and cleaves C3 into C3a and C3b. Once C3b is generated, it will bind covalently to the surface of pathogens where it can bind to another molecule of factor B and form a new alternative pathway C3 convertase C3bBb (Carroll and Sim, 2011). The alternative pathway also acts as an amplification loop where C3b generated by either the classical or the LP binds to factor B to generate the convertase C3bBb (Schwaeble and Reid, 1999). The C3bBb is homologous to C4b2a (C3 is a homologue of C4, and factor B of C2) and like C4b2a will switch its substrate specificity from cleaving C3 to cleaving C5 upon binding of C3b to the convertase, forming C3bBb3b, the C5 convertase.

The Membrane Attack Complex

The C5 convertases C4b2a3b and C3bBb3b cleave C5 into C5b and C5a. C5b then binds to C6, C7, and C8 to form a C5b-8 complex that can bind to cell surfaces and initiate cell lysis by inserting into the lipid bilayer. Multiple C9 molecules can bind to C5b-8, accelerating lysis and forming the MAC, or C5b-9 (Podack et al., 1982).

CONTROL OF COMPLEMENT ACTIVATION

The complement system is tightly regulated to avoid runaway activation of the enzymatic cascade that would otherwise lead to excess host tissue damage and inflammation. Key events at the center of the cascade are carefully controlled by five closely related complement control proteins, all of which are encoded by genes located in the RCA (regulator of complement activation) cluster on chromosome 1q32 in man. Complement regulatory components include membrane-bound regulators and fluid phase regulators (Kirschfink and Mollnes, 2003; Carroll and Sim, 2011).

Two host membrane proteins, complement receptor type 1 (CR1) and membrane cofactor protein (MCP or CD46), and two fluid-phase regulators, factor H and C4-binding protein (C4bp), act as cofactors for factor I, which inactivates C3b and C4b, preventing formation of the C3 and C5 convertases. C4bp also shortens the half-life of the classical pathway C3 and C5 convertases, while factor H has the same effect on the alternative pathway C3 and C5 convertases. CR1 and another host membrane protein, decay accelerating factor (DAF), act on both the classical and alternative pathway convertases. A truncated splice variant of factor H, factor H-like protein 1 (FHL-1), is also found in serum and has regulatory activity similar to that of factor H (Schwaeble et al., 1987). Prevention of factor H binding results in an increased half-life of C3b containing convertase complexes and overshooting activation of the alternative pathway leading to FHR-C3GN (Ramaglia et al., 2012).

Fluid Phase Regulators

C1 inhibitor (C1 inh), also known as Serpin G1, is a serine protease inhibitor which irreversibly inhibits C1r, C1s, MASP-1, and MASP-2 by forming a covalent complex with the protease active site (Chen et al., 1998; Presanis et al., 2004; Cicardi et al., 2005). Besides complement regulation Serpin G1 can also inactivate serine proteases of the coagulation cascade (FXIa and FXIIa), and of the contact system (kallikrein) (Cicardi et al., 2005; Wagner and Frank, 2010).

Factor I is a protease and a fluid phase regulator of all three pathways. It converts hemolytically active C3b into hemolytically inactive iC3b, in a cofactor-dependent manner. In the fluid phase, factor H, an abundant plasma component, binds to free and complex-bound C3b to allow factor I to convert C3b to iC3b. A further conversion of iC3b to C3c and C3dg by factor I is also cofactor dependent. In a similar fashion, factor I inactivates C4b in the presence of the cofactor C4-binding protein (C4BP) (Seya et al., 1995). Binding of C4BP to C4b inhibits C4b−C2a binding, preventing the formation of the C3 convertase (Blom et al., 2004). Subsequent factor I-dependent conversion of C4b generates the fragments iC4b, C4c, and C4d. Conversion of C3b to iC3b is important in another function: iC3b is a powerful opsonin, recognized by CR3 and CR4, while C3b is a less effective opsonin, recognized by CR1.

Factor H is an important alternative pathway regulator, the main activity of which, besides mediating C3b inactivation by factor I, is to destabilize and also accelerate the decay of the alternative pathway C3 convertase (C3bBb) and C5 convertase (C3bBb3b) (Whaley and Ruddy; 1976, Weiler et al., 1976). Factor H destabilizes the C3 convertase by competitive binding to C3b, which

dislodges Bb from the convertase (C3bBb). Factor H is important for the discrimination of self from non-self cells and therefore preventing autoimmunity. Binding of factor H, for example on sialic acid or glycosaminoglycans of host cells, inhibits alternative pathway activation on the surface of host cells (Pangburn et al., 2000). Carboxypeptidase N (CPN) is an inactivating regulator of the C3a and C5a anaphylatoxins (Bokisch and Muller-Eberhard 1970). Clusterin and S protein are regulators for the terminal activation cascade of complement. They bind to C5b-7 complex and prevent the insertion of C8 and C9 leading to the inhibition of the MAC formation (Jenne and Tschopp, 1989; Wagner and Frank, 2010).

Properdin is the only known and essential positive regulator of the complement system. It is essential for alternative pathway activation as properdin depleted sera lack the ability to activate the alternative pathway (Schwaeble and Reid, 1999). Properdin is produced by monocytes/macrophages, peripheral T lymphocytes and granulocytes (i.e., neutrophils) (Wirthmueller et al., 1997) and acts as a positive regulator by stabilizing the alternative pathway C3 and C5 convertases (Schwaeble and Reid, 1999; Stover et al., 2008).

Membrane-Bound Regulators

Complement activation is also controlled by at least four characterized membrane-bound proteins or receptors, which protect host cells from attack by complement. These comprise the decay-accelerating factor (DAF, also known as CD55), the complement receptor 1 (CR1, also known as CD35), the membrane cofactor protein (MCP, also known as CD46), and CD59 (also known as protectin) (Wagner and Frank, 2010). Like factor H, DAF regulates complement activation by accelerating the decay (dissociation of the convertases) of the C3 convertases (C3b2a and C3bBb) (Lublin and Atkinson, 1989). CR1 and MCP act as cofactors for the cleavage of C3b and C4b by factor I (Wagner and Frank, 2010). CD59 is a regulator of the MAC complex. CD59 binds the nascent MAC complex (C5b-8) inhibiting C9 polymerization and subsequent pore formation on the surface of a cell (Lehto et al., 1997; Farkas et al., 2002). DAF, MCP, and CD59 are found on most cell types, but CR1 has more restricted distribution (erythrocytes, lymphocytes, dendritic cells, and kidney podocytes).

THE BIOLOGICAL EFFECTS OF COMPLEMENT ACTIVATION

Complement activation leads to a multitude of biological activities including opsonization, initiation of a proinflammatory response, immune complex clearance, and direct killing of cells via the membrane attack complex.

Opsonization of pathogens is mediated by the major opsonin C3b or iC3b and C4b to a lesser extent. C3b coats the surface of microorganisms and enhances their phagocytosis by leukocyte via binding to complement receptor type 1 (CR1). iC3b binds to CR3 and CR4. L-ficolin, MBL, and C1q have been reported to initiate phagocytosis directly by binding to pathogens and enhancing phagocytosis by binding to collectin receptors on the surface of the phagocytes (Jack et al., 2001; Aoyagi et al., 2005). In other instances complement can mediate direct killing of bacteria, especially Gram-negative bacteria via the formation of the membrane attack complex which form pores in the cell membrane leading to cell lysis (Nauta et al., 2004). During complement activation, proinflammatory cleavage products anaphylatoxins C4a, C5a, and C3a are released. The release of anaphylatoxins increases vascular permeability and formation of inflammatory exudates. These inflammatory exudates enhance the recruitment of inflammatory mediators and inflammatory cells to the site of injury and efficient elimination of invading pathogens or other inflammatory factors. Increased vascular permeability leads to extravasation of leukocytes to the site of inflammation, which helps in clearing invading pathogens. C5a acts as a potent chemotactic factor that stimulates leukocyte migration. In addition, C5a was found to increase the synthesis of other chemotactic agents like ecosanoids and chemokines. Schindler et al. reported that C5a stimulates the expression of interleukin-1 (IL-1) and tumor necrosis factor (TNF) (Schindler et al., 1990). Complement also plays a major role in the clearance of apoptotic and necrotic cells in addition to immune complexes and microorganisms. The globular head of C1q binds to the surface of apoptotic cells and facilitates the uptake of the cells by macrophages (Taylor et al., 2000). In addition, opsonization of apoptotic cells with iC3b leads to recognition of these cells by CR3 and CR4 on the surface of phagocytes with subsequent engulfment of these cells (Mevorach et al., 1998).

Complement also inhibits the precipitation of immune complexes and enhances their solubility by binding of C1q, C3b, and C4b. This binding inhibits further increase in the aggregation of the immune complex. These complexes bind to CR1 on the surface of erythrocytes which transfer them into the liver and the spleen where they are cleared from the circulation by the resident macrophages (Manderson et al., 2004).

COMPLEMENT INVOLVEMENT IN THE PATHOPHYSIOLOGY OF DIVERSE AUTOIMMUNE DISEASES

As a powerful effector system of both the innate and the adaptive immune response, uncontrolled complement activation can lead to the loss of antimicrobial immune protection, but can also initiate, feed, and perpetuate inflammatory conditions leading to tissue destruction and autoimmune disease. Uncontrolled, dysregulated complement activation can be caused by inherited or acquired deficiencies of complement components as well as through gain of function or loss of function mutations in complement genes or genes encoding enzymes that further process complement components. An example for the latter is the X-linked phosphatidylinositol glycan class A (PIG-A) gene encoding an enzyme necessary for the synthesis of N-acetylglucosaminyl-phosphatidol, an intermediate required for the membrane anchoring of the membrane protective complement regulatory components decay accelerating factor (i.e., DAF or CD55) and protectin (i.e., CD59) which are attached to the outer cell surface through glycosyl-phosphatidylinositol (GPI) anchoring. A rare inherited or acquired deficiency of the PIG-A leads to the loss of the membrane localization of CD55 and CD59 which in turn renders in particular erythrocytes susceptible to autologous complement lysis cells and presents as a hematological disorder named paroxysmal nocturnal hemoglobinuria (PNH) or Marchiafava–Micheli syndrome. In most cases, PNH is a consequence of a non-malignant clonal expansion of one or more hematopoetic stem cells with an acquired somatic mutation in the PIG-A gene. PNH clinically presents as a chronic hemolytic anemia with both intravascular and extravascular lysis of erythrocytes leading to hemoglobin in the urine and a predisposition of thrombosis. The severity of disease is predicted by the degree of loss of CD55 and CD59 anchoring on blood cells, which can vary between partial loss (PNH type II) and total loss (PNH type III). The condition is potentially life-threatening due to the high risk of thrombotic disease and is presently treated with high-dose applications of a recombinant humanized anti-C5 monoclonal antibody, eculizumab, which prevents C5 activation and MAC formation (Risitano, 2013). This treatment effectively reduces the intravascular lysis, but anemia with the need for blood transfusion persists due to the continuous opsonization of PNH erythrocytes by complement C3 activation products, which makes these erythrocytes susceptible to opsonophagocytosis and extravascular hemolysis. A more effective treatment would be to block complement activation further upstream to avoid C3 deposition. In PNH plasma, the direct antiglobulin test (DAT, or direct Coombs' test) is usually negative, as the hemolysis of PNH is not caused by antibodies. This sets PNH apart from another autoimmune disorder, called autoimmune hemolytic anemia (AIHA), where antibody-mediated complement activation lyses erythrocytes. In most cases of AIHA, the autoantibody is of the IgM class. Treating AIHA with red blood cell transfusions is often ineffective, since the autoantibodies attach to recipient and donor cells alike. Therapeutic application of C1-esterase inhibitor concentrate was recently shown to protect from complement-induced red blood cell destruction and may offer a safe and effective treatment of AIHA (Wouters et al., 2013).

An extremely strong association has been established between deficiencies of the classical pathway of complement activation and systemic lupus erythematosus (SLE).

The first description of an acquired deficiency of the first component of complement in the serum of an SLE patient was published more than 40 years ago showing the presence of anti-C1q autoantibodies by gel diffusion chromatography (Agnello et al., 1971). The hereditary deficiency of C1q and the predisposition for autoimmune SLE or SLE-like disease represents one of the most powerful associations with over 90% of C1q deficient individuals developing severe SLE. The disease manifestations such as rash, glomerulonephritis, and central nervous system (CNS) disease can vary, but the severity of disease invariably progresses and requires extensive medical care (Walport et al., 1998). A recent report described the successful long-term replacement of C1q through fresh frozen plasma infusions in a young C1q deficient patient for over 9 years (Mehta et al., 2010). Bone marrow transplantation was successfully conducted replacing the bone marrow of a C1q deficient mouse with bone marrow of a syngenic WT mouse (Cortes-Hernandez et al., 2004), restoring normal C1q levels. Interestingly, both inherited or acquired deficiency of each of the classical pathway components C1, C4, C2, and C3 predisposes to lupus-like autoimmune disease (Carroll et al., 2004; Pradhan et al., 2012).

This strongly implies a critical role of the classical pathway in the maintenance of immune tolerance and prevention of autoimmune disease. The present understanding points to the conclusion that the classical pathway fulfills an important scavenger function in removing immune complexes as well as cellular debris and that in the absence of this scavenger system, the clearance of debris is significantly impaired which in turn results in continuous presentation of autoantigens (Arlaud et al., 2002).

A rare but invariably severe autoimmune pathology is caused by an IgG autoantibody directed against the alternative pathway C3, convertase C3bBb. This autoantibody binds to C3bBb and protects this complex from decay by factor H and subsequent inactivation by factor I and thereby increases the half-life of the alternative pathway C3 convertase leading to a continuous activation of the alternative pathway and secondary hypocomplemetemia. This perpetual activation of the alternative pathway clinically presents as a form of membranoproliferative glomerulonephritis (i.e., mesangiocapillary glomerulonephritis type II), which earned this autoantibody the name nephritic factor (NeF). Patients suffering from this rare autoimmune disease frequently show abnormalities in the distribution of their adipose tissue, named partial lipodystrophy (PLD). A recent report provided a plausible explanation showing that NeF can also stabilize the C3 convertase on the surface of fat cells and lyse fat cells through perpetual generation of membrane attack complexes (Mathieson et al., 1993). An even rarer variant of NeF presents as an autoantibody directed against the classical/LP C3 convertase (i.e., C4b2a), called C4 nephritic factor, which stabilizes this convertase causing hypocomplementemia by continuous consumption of C3 (Miller et al., 2012). The majority of the C4-NeF cases were identified in a cohort of lupus nephritis patients. Dysregulated alternative pathway activation caused by deficiencies of the alternative pathway regulators factor H, factor I, membrane cofactor protein and the factor H-related genes (FHR5 and FHR1) predisposes to C3 glomerulopathies (C3GN). The predisposing mutations in the factor H-related genes lead to the formation of FHR dimers which effectively bind and compete with factor H for the binding to C3b. Prevention of factor H binding results in an increased half-life of C3b containing convertase complexes and overshooting activation of the alternative pathway (Ramaglia et al., 2012).

The commonest cause of C3GN is complement factor H-related 5 (CFHR5) nephropathy, which is endemic in Greek Cypriots. Other C3GNs include membranoproliferative glomerulonephritis 1 (MPGN1), fMPGN3, and dense deposit disease (DDD), a rare form of glomerulonephritis characterized by the presence of electron dense deposits within the glomerular basement membrane (GBM) with intense deposition of C3 fragments (De Cordoba et al., 2012).

Hemolytic uremic syndrome (HUS) is a life-threatening condition often following infections with Shiga toxin-producing *Escherichia coli* strains (STEC-HUS; EHEC-HUS). It presents as Coombs' test-negative microangiopathic anemia with severe diarrhea. An atypical form of HUS (aHUS) does not present with diarrhea. It has a poor long-term prognosis as it is recurrent and results in a fatality rate of up to 30%. aHUS can develop in individuals with inherited or acquired predispositions for poorly controlled complement activation, either through mutations in the complement regulatory components factor H, or MCP, factor I or through gain-of-function mutations in factor B and complement C3 (Goicoechea de Jorge et al., 2007), or have autoantibodies against factor H or disease promoting mutations in factor H-related proteins CFHR1 and CFHR5 (see above). Another thrombotic microangiopathy called thrombotic thrombocytopenic purpura (TTP) is pathologically very similar to HUS as it presents with an autoantibody-induced consumption of complement and thrombi in the microcirculation of many organs, including kidney, brain, heart, lung, liver, and gut (Noris et al., 2012). A majority of TTP patients present with acquired autoantibodies that inhibit a plasma metalloprotease called ADAMTS13 that cleave von Willebrand factor. Inherited forms of TTP are caused by ADAMTS13 gene deficiencies.

In 2005, several independent reports identified a loss-of-function mutation (CHF$_{Y402H}$) in the complement regulatory component factor H to be a major predisposing factor for age-related macular degeneration (AMD), a degenerative disorder of the retinal pigment epithelium (RPE) and the most common cause of blindness in the Western world (Klein et al., 2005). Interestingly, retinal drusen, the hallmark of AMD, stain positive for complement activation products, indicating that complement activation is involved in drusen formation. *In vitro* models of complement activation on retinal pigmented epithelial monolayers have demonstrated that oxidative stress significantly induced complement activation on the surface of these cells and initiated complement activation in a LP-dependent fashion (Joseph et al., 2013). The sublytic deposition of complement on RPE required the presence of MASP-2 to initiate complement activation, while reduced functional activity of alternative pathway regulators may be critical for the disease process to establish and therefore predispose for the severity and the time of onset of AMD pathology. Most recent work also identified that the loss-of-function mutation (CHF$_{Y402H}$) of factor H also as a high risk polymorphism for other diseases with autoimmune characteristics such as ocular sarcoidosis, atherosclerosis, and a subgroup of Alzheimer patients (i.e., ApoE4 risk allele carriers) (Thompson et al., 2013).

Complement has also been identified as a critical player in the pathophysiology of diverse autoimmune diseases of the CNS caused by autoantibody-mediated destruction of cells where activation of complement by either the classical or the LP plays a critical role. These diseases include myasthenia gravis (MG) (Romi et al., 2005), Guillain—Barré syndrome (GBS) (Kaida and Kusunoki, 2009), and neuromyelitis optica (NMO) (Asgari et al., 2013). MG is caused by an autoantibody directed against the acetylcholine receptor (AChR), which strongly activates complement and blocks signal transduction at the motor neuron synapse to muscle cells causing muscle weakness and loss of muscle control. In an animal model of MG, experimental autoimmune myasthenia gravis (EAMG) was shown that complement activation is required for the disease to develop, since the disease cannot be induced in absence of C3, C4, or C5 and the application of complement inhibitors ameliorates the severity of established disease (Tuzun and Christadoss 2013). In GBS antiganglioside autoantibodies trigger complement activation leading to a complement-dependent disruption of voltage-gated sodium channel clusters, while in NMO anti-aquaporin-4 autoantibodies trigger complement

activation through the classical and/or the lectin activation pathway.

In other autoimmune pathologies of the CNS, such as multiple sclerosis (MS) (a condition caused by autoimmune destruction of the myelin sheets around the axon of neurons), motor neuron disease (MND) (describing a group of neurological disorders selectively affecting motor neurons), and Alzheimer's disease (AD) (which was recently defined as an autoimmune disorder triggered by herpes simplex (Wozniak et al., 2007), the involvement of complement in the pathophysiology is somewhat more complex. In experimental autoimmune encephalomyelitis (EAE), a mouse model for MS, the alternative complement activation pathway is essential for the priming of microglial cells. Mice deficient in the C3 convertase regulator complement receptor 1-related protein y (Crry) show an accelerated onset of EAE signs and early microglial priming, but no disease develops in mice deficient in both Crry and C3 and Crry and factor B (Donev et al., 2013). Classical pathway deficiency, however, does not protect from developing EAE. Therapeutic inhibition of factor B in a mouse model does not prevent the onset of EAE, but ameliorates the severity of disease once it is established (Hu et al., 2013). In MND, local complement biosynthesis is increased and therapeutic inhibition of the complement anaphylatoxin C5a reduces inflammatory pathology and survival in a rat model of amyotrophic lateral sclerosis, but at present too little is known to define a definite role of complement in this devastating autoimmune pathology (Woodruff et al., 2008).

In AD the classical pathway recognition component C1q co-localizes with the amyloid-β depositions in the disease lesion areas. In a mouse model of AD, C1q deficient mice show a faster progression of AD neurodegeneration and most recent work demonstrated that C1q is neuroprotective against amyloid-β toxicity (Benoit et al., 2013).

Rheumatoid arthritis (RA) is a highly disabling systemic autoimmune disease characterized by a persistent inflammation of the synovial membrane lining the joint, with associated infiltration of macrophages, granulocytes, T cells, and B cells. Local complement activation is critically involved in the onset and maintenance of this inflammatory disease with a preponderant role of the alternative activation pathway in a mouse model (Dimitrova et al., 2012). Deficiencies of C5 and C6 also protect from RA indicating that the terminal activation cascade essentially contributes to the severity of disease while deficiency of an early component like C2 is a predisposing factor (Jonsson et al., 2005).

Complement-mediated cytotoxicity plays a critical role in the pathophysiology of vitiligo, a common depigmenting autoimmune disorder. Autoimmune antibodies lyse melanocytes through both complement activation and antibody-dependent cellular cytotoxicity (ADCC) (Norris et al., 1988).

Pernicious anemia (PA) is the most common cause of vitamin B12 deficiency. PA patients have complement activating autoantibodies against parietal cells in serum and gastric fluid, but since the antigen H^+/K^+-ATPase is not expressed on the surface of the target cell, cytotoxicity in PA is unlikely to be complement mediated (De Aizpurua et al., 1983).

Complement does not appear to be involved in the pathophysiology of primary Sjögren's syndrome. It is likely that complement consumption in Sjörgen's syndrome patients is caused by concomitant and secondary systemic disease (Lindgren et al., 1993).

Hashimoto's thyroiditis (HT) and Graves' disease (GD) share many common features including the presence of autoantibodies against thyroperoxidase and thyroid stimulating hormone (TSH) receptor. In GD, a subset of TSH receptor antibodies stimulates this receptor and causes the phenotype of hyperthyroidism, the hallmark of GD. The role of the other autoantibodies, however, remains unclear. In HT, immune complexes on the thyroid follicular membrane are often associated with complement deposition indicating a role of complement in the tissue destruction. Previous studies claim that thyrocytes are usually resistant to direct complement lysis as these cells are expressing high levels of membrane-associated complement regulators such as CD59 (Tandon et al., 1992). Non-lytic activation of complement generates soluble membrane attack complexes during the acute phase of HT (Weetman et al., 1989). A more recent study claims that thyroperoxidase on the surface of thyrocytes can also initiate complement activation through the binding of C4 and C4b to a complement control module in the ectodomain of thyroperoxidase leading to direct complement-mediated killing of thyrocytes *in vitro* (Blanchin et al., 2003). This proposed activation mechanism, however, has not been confirmed.

Ischemia/reperfusion injury (IRI) is a complement-mediated post-inflammatory condition leading to major tissue loss. IRI was first thought to be mediated through the classical pathway, since it is less pronounced in IgM deficiency, but more recent work identified that it is predominantly driven by the LP of complement in a MASP-2-dependent fashion (Schwaeble et al., 2011). In experimental models of stroke and myocardial infarction, therapeutic inhibition of MASP-2 reduces infarct sizes by up to 40% and may offer a promising new avenue of treatment to reduce morbidity and mortality in these major ischemic pathologies.

REFERENCES

Agnello, V., Koffler, D., Eisenberg, J.W., et al., 1971. C1q precipitins in the sera of patients with systemic lupus erythematosus and other hypocomplementemic states: characterization of high and low molecular weight types. J. Exp. Med. 134, 228–241.

Ali, Y.M., Lynch, N.J., Haleem, K.S., Fujita, T., Endo, Y., Hansen, S., et al., 2012. The lectin pathway of complement activation is a critical component of the innate immune response to pneumococcal infection. PLoS Pathogens. 8, e1002793.

Aoyagi, Y., Adderson, E.E., Min, J.G., Matsushita, M., Fujita, T., Takahashi, S., et al., 2005. Role of L-ficolin/mannose-binding lectin-associated serine protease complexes in the opsonophagocytosis of type III group B streptococci. J. Immunol. 174, 418–425.

Arlaud, G.J., Gaboriaud, C., Thielens, N.M., Budayova-Spano, M., Rossi, V., Fontecilla-Camps, J.C., 2002. Structural biology of the C1 complex of complement unveils the mechanisms of its activation and proteolytic activity. Mol. Immunol. 39, 383–394.

Asgari, N., Khorooshi, R., Lillevang, S.T., Owens, T., 2013. Complement-dependent pathogenicity of brain-specific antibodies in cerebrospinal fluid. J. Neuroimmunol. 254, 76–82.

Barrington, R.A., Pozdnyakova, O., Zafari, M.R., Benjamin, C.D., Carroll, M.C., 2002. B lymphocyte memory: role of stromal cell complement and FcgammaRIIB receptors. J. Exp. Med. 196, 1189–1199.

Benoit, M.E., Hernandez, M.X., Dinh, M.L., Benavente, F., Vasquez, O., Tenner, A.J., 2013. C1q-induced LRP1B and GPR6 proteins expressed early in Alzheimer disease mouse models, are essential for the C1q-mediated protection against amyloid-beta neurotoxicity. J. Biol. Chem. 288, 654–665.

Blanchin, S., Estienne, V., Durand-Gorde, J.M., Carayon, P., Ruf, J., 2003. Complement activation by direct C4 binding to thyroperoxidase in Hashimoto's thyroiditis. Endocrinology 144, 5422–5429.

Blom, A.M., Villoutreix, B.O., Dahlback, B., 2004. Complement inhibitor C4b-binding protein-friend or foe in the innate immune system?. Mol. Immunol. 40 (18), 1333–1346.

Bokisch, V.A., Muller-Eberhard, H.J., 1970. Anaphylatoxin inactivator of human plasma: its isolation and characterization as a carboxypeptidase. J. Clin. Invest. 49 (12), 2427–2436.

Carroll, M.C., 2004. A protective role for innate immunity in systemic lupus erythematosus. Nature Reviews. Immunology 4 (10), 825–831.

Carroll, M.V., Sim, R.B., 2011. Complement in health and disease. Adv. Drug Delivery Rev. 63 (12), 965–975.

Chen, C.H., Lam, C.F., Boackle, R.J., 1998. C1 inhibitor removes the entire C1qr2s2 complex from anti-C1Q monoclonal antibodies with low binding affinities. Immunology 95, 648–654.

Cicardi, M., Zingale, L., Zanichelli, A., Pappalardo, E., Cicardi, B., 2005. C1 inhibitor: molecular and clinical aspects. Springer Semin. Immunopathol. 27, 286–298.

Cortes-Hernandez, J., Fossati-Jimack, L., Petry, F., Loos, M., Izui, S., Walport, M.J., et al., 2004. Restoration of C1q levels by bone marrow transplantation attenuates autoimmune disease associated with C1q deficiency in mice. Eur. J. Immunol. 34, 3713–3722.

De Aizpurua, H.J., Cosgrove, L.J., Ungar, B., Toh, B.H., 1983. Autoantibodies cytotoxic to gastric parietal cells in serum of patients with pernicious anemia. New Engl. J. Med. 309, 625–629.

De Cordoba, S.R., Tortajada, A., Harris, C.L., Morgan, B.P., 2012. Complement dysregulation and disease: from genes and proteins to diagnostics and drugs. Immunobiology 217, 1034–1046.

Degn, S.E., Hansen, A.G., Steffensen, R., Jacobsen, C., Jensenius, J.C., Thiel, S., 2009. MAp44, a human protein associated with pattern recognition molecules of the complement system and regulating the lectin pathway of complement activation. J. Immunol. (Baltimore). 183, 7371–7378.

Dimitrova, P., Ivanovska, N., Belenska, L., Milanova, V., Schwaeble, W., Stover, C., 2012. Abrogated RANKL expression in properdin-deficient mice is associated with better outcome from collagen-antibody-induced arthritis. Arthritis Res. Ther. 14, R173.

Dodds, A.W., 2002. Which came first, the lectin/classical pathway or the alternative pathway of complement? Immunobiology 205 (4–5), 340–354.

Dunkelberger, J.R., Song, W.C., 2010. Complement and its role in innate and adaptive immune responses. Cell Res. 20, 34–50.

Farkas, I., Baranyi, L., Ishikawa, Y., Okada, N., Bohata, C., Budai, D., et al., 2002. CD59 blocks not only the insertion of C9 into MAC but inhibits ion channel formation by homologous C5b-8 as well as C5b-9. J. Physiol. 539 (Pt 2), 537–545.

Fujita, T., 2002. Evolution of the lectin-complement pathway and its role in innate immunity. Nature Reviews. Immunology. 2, 346–353.

Girija, U.V., Mitchell, D.A., Roscher, S., Wallis, R., 2011. Carbohydrate recognition and complement activation by rat ficolin-B. Eur. J. Immunol. 41, 214–223.

Goicoechea De Jorge, E., Harris, C.L., Esparza-Gordillo, J., Carreras, L., Arranz, E.A., Garrido, C.A., et al., 2007. Gain-of-function mutations in complement factor B are associated with atypical hemolytic uremic syndrome. Proc. Nat. Acad. Sci. USA 104, 240–245.

Hansen, S., Selman, L., Palaniyar, N., Ziegler, K., Brandt, J., Kliem, A., et al., 2010. Collectin 11 (CL-11, CL-K1) is a MASP-1/3-associated plasma collectin with microbial-binding activity. J. Immunol. (Baltimore, Md.: 1950). 185 (10), 6096–6104.

Hu, X., Holers, V.M., Thurman, J.M., Schoeb, T.R., Ramos, T.N., Barnum, S.R., 2013. Therapeutic inhibition of the alternative complement pathway attenuates chronic EAE. Mol. Immunol. 54 (3–4), 302–308.

Iwaki, D., Kanno, K., Takahashi, M., Endo, Y., Lynch, N.J., Schwaeble, W.J., et al., 2006. Small mannose-binding lectin-associated protein plays a regulatory role in the lectin complement pathway. J. Immunol. (Baltimore, Md.: 1950). 177 (12), 8626–8632.

Iwaki, D., Kanno, K., Takahashi, M., Endo, Y., Matsushita, M., Fujita, T., 2011. The role of mannose-binding lectin-associated serine protease-3 in activation of the alternative complement pathway. J. Immunol. 187, 3751–3758.

Jack, D.L., Klein, N.J., Turner, M.W., 2001. Mannose-binding lectin: targeting the microbial world for complement attack and opsonophagocytosis. Immunol. Rev. 180, 86–99.

Jenne, D.E., Tschopp, J., 1989. Molecular structure and functional characterization of a human complement cytolysis inhibitor found in blood and seminal plasma: identity to sulfated glycoprotein 2, a constituent of rat testis fluid. Proc. Nat. Acad. Sci. USA 86 (18), 7123–7127.

Jonsson, G., Truedsson, L., Sturfelt, G., Oxelius, V.A., Braconier, J.H., Sjoholm, A.G., 2005. Hereditary C2 deficiency in Sweden: frequent occurrence of invasive infection, atherosclerosis, and rheumatic disease. Medicine 84, 23–34.

Joseph, K., Kulik, L., Coughlin, B., Kunchithapautham, K., Bandyopadhyay, M., Thiel, S., et al., 2013. Oxidative Stress Sensitizes RPE Cells to Complement-Mediated Injury in a Natural Antibody-, Lectin Pathway- and Phospholipid Epitope-Dependent Manner. J. Biol. Chem 288, 12753–12765.

Kaida, K., Kusunoki, S., 2009. Guillain–Barre syndrome: update on immunobiology and treatment. Exp. Rev. Neurotherapeutics 9, 1307–1319.

Kirschfink, M., Mollnes, T.E., 2003. Modern complement analysis. Clin. Diagn. Lab. Immunol. 10, 982–989.

Klein, R.J., Zeiss, C., Chew, E.Y., Tsai, J.Y., Sackler, R.S., Haynes, C., et al., 2005. Complement factor H polymorphism in age-related macular degeneration. Science (New York, N.Y.). 308 (5720), 385–389.

Kocsis, A., Kekesi, K.A., Szasz, R., Vegh, B.M., Balczer, J., Dobo, J., et al., 2010. Selective inhibition of the lectin pathway of complement with phage display selected peptides against mannose-binding lectin-associated serine protease (MASP)-1 and -2: significant contribution of MASP-1 to lectin pathway activation. J. Immunol. (Baltimore, Md.: 1950) 185.4169–4178.

Kwan, W.H., Van Der Touw, W., Heeger, P.S., 2012. Complement regulation of T cell immunity. Immunol. Res. 54 (1–3), 247–253.

Le Friec, G., Kemper, C., 2009. Complement: coming full circle. Arch. Immunol. Ther. Exp. 57, 393–407.

Lehto, T., Morgan, B.P., Meri, S., 1997. Binding of human and rat CD59 to the terminal complement complexes. Immunology 90, 121–128.

Lindgren, S., Hansen, B., Sjoholm, A.G., Manthorpe, R., 1993. Complement activation in patients with primary Sjogren's syndrome: an indicator of systemic disease. Autoimmunity 16, 297–300.

Liu, Y., Endo, Y., Iwaki, D., Nakata, M., Matsushita, M., Wada, I., et al., 2005. Human M-ficolin is a secretory protein that activates the lectin complement pathway. J. Immunol. (Baltimore, Md.: 1950). 175, 3150–3156.

Manderson, A.P., Botto, M., Walport, M.J., 2004. The role of complement in the development of systemic lupus erythematosus. Annu. Rev. Immunol. 22, 431–456.

Mathieson, P.W., Wurzner, R., Oliveria, D.B., Lachmann, P.J., Peters, D.K., 1993. Complement-mediated adipocyte lysis by nephritic factor sera. J. Exp. Med. 177, 1827–1831.

Mehta, P., Norsworthy, P.J., Hall, A.E., Kelly, S.J., Walport, M.J., Botto, M., et al., 2010. SLE with C1q deficiency treated with fresh frozen plasma: a 10-year experience. Rheumatology (Oxford, England). 49, 823–824.

Mevorach, D., Mascarenhas, J.O., Gershov, D., Elkon, K.B., 1998. Complement-dependent clearance of apoptotic cells by human macrophages. J. Exp. Med. 188 (12), 2313–2320.

Miller, E.C., Chase, N.M., Densen, P., Hintermeyer, M.K., Casper, J.T., Atkinson, J.P., 2012. Autoantibody stabilization of the classical pathway C3 convertase leading to C3 deficiency and Neisserial sepsis: C4 nephritic factor revisited. Clin. Immunol. (Orlando, Fla.). 145, 241–250.

Nauta, A.J., Castellano, G., Xu, W., Woltman, A.M., Borrias, M.C., Daha, M.R., et al., 2004. Opsonization with C1q and mannose-binding lectin targets apoptotic cells to dendritic cells. J. Immunol. (Baltimore, Md.: 1950). 173, 3044–3050.

Noris, M., Mescia, F., Remuzzi, G., 2012. STEC-HUS, atypical HUS and TTP are all diseases of complement activation. Nature Reviews. Nephrology. 8 (11), 622–633.

Norris, D.A., Kissinger, R.M., Naughton, G.M., Bystryn, J.C., 1988. Evidence for immunologic mechanisms in human vitiligo: patients' sera induce damage to human melanocytes in vitro by complement-mediated damage and antibody-dependent cellular cytotoxicity. J. Invest. Dermatol. 90, 783–789.

Podack, E.R., Muller-Eberhard, H.J., Horst, H., Hoppe, W., 1982. Membrane attach complex of complement (MAC): three-dimensional analysis of MAC-phospholipid vesicle recombinants. J. Immunol. (Baltimore, Md.: 1950). 128, 2353–2357.

Pradhan, V., Rajadhyaksha, A., Mahant, G., Surve, P., Patwardhan, M., Dighe, S., et al., 2012. Anti-C1q antibodies and their association with complement components in Indian systemic lupus erythematosus patients. Indian J. Nephrol. 22, 353–357.

Presanis, J.S., Hajela, K., Ambrus, G., Gal, P., Sim, R.B., 2004. Differential substrate and inhibitor profiles for human MASP-1 and MASP-2. Mol. Immunol. 40 (13), 921–929.

Ramaglia, V., Hughes, T.R., Donev, R.M., Ruseva, M.M., Wu, X., Huitinga, I., et al., 2012. C3-dependent mechanism of microglial priming relevant to multiple sclerosis. Proc. Nat. Acad. Sci. USA 109, 965–970.

Risitano, A.M., 2013. Paroxysmal nocturnal hemoglobinuria and the complement system: recent insights and novel anticomplement strategies. Adv. Exp. Med. Biol. 735, 155–172.

Romi, F., Kristoffersen, E.K., Aarli, J.A., Gilhus, N.E., 2005. The role of complement in myasthenia gravis: serological evidence of complement consumption in vivo. J. Neuroimmunol. 158 (1–2), 191–194.

Rossi, V., Cseh, S., Bally, I., Thielens, N.M., Jensenius, J.C., Arlaud, G. J., 2001. Substrate specificities of recombinant mannan-binding lectin-associated serine proteases-1 and -2. J. Biol. Chem. 276 (44), 40880–40887.

Schindler, R., Lonnemann, G., Shaldon, S., Koch, K.M., Dinarello, C.A., 1990. Transcription, not synthesis, of interleukin-1 and tumor necrosis factor by complement. Kidney Int. 37, 85–93.

Schmalstieg Jr., F.C., Goldman, A.S., 2010. Birth of the science of immunology. J. Med. Biography. 18, 88–98.

Schwaeble, W., Dahl, M.R., Thiel, S., Stover, C., Jensenius, J.C., 2002. The mannan-binding lectin-associated serine proteases (MASPs) and MAp19: four components of the lectin pathway activation complex encoded by two genes. Immunobiology 205 (4–5), 455–466.

Schwaeble, W., Zwirner, J., Schulz, T.F., Linke, R.P., Dierich, M.P., Weiss, E.H., 1987. Human complement factor H: expression of an additional truncated gene product of 43 kDa in human liver. Eur. J. Immunol. 17 (10), 1485–1489.

Schwaeble, W.J., Lynch, N.J., Clark, J.E., Marber, M., Samani, N.J., Ali, Y.M., et al., 2011. Targeting of mannan-binding lectin-associated serine protease-2 confers protection from myocardial and gastrointestinal ischemia/reperfusion injury. Proc. Nat. Acad. Sci. USA 108 (18), 7523–7528.

Schwaeble, W.J., Reid, K.B., 1999. Does properdin crosslink the cellular and the humoral immune response? Immunol. Today. 20, 17–21.

Seya, T., Nakamura, K., Masaki, T., Ichihara-Itoh, C., Matsumoto, M., Nagasawa, S., 1995. Human factor H and C4b-binding protein serve as factor I-cofactors both encompassing inactivation of C3b and C4b. Molecular Immunol. 32, 355–360.

Skjoedt, M.O., Hummelshoj, T., Palarasah, Y., Honore, C., Koch, C., Skjodt, K., et al., 2010. A novel mannose-binding lectin/ficolin-associated protein is highly expressed in heart and skeletal muscle tissues and inhibits complement activation. J. Biol. Chem. 285 (11), 8234–8243.

Stover, C.M., Luckett, J.C., Echtenacher, B., Dupont, A., Figgitt, S.E., Brown, J., et al., 2008. Properdin plays a protective role in polymicrobial septic peritonitis. J. Immunol. (Baltimore, Md.: 1950). 180, 3313–3318.

Stover, C.M., Thiel, S., Thelen, M., Lynch, N.J., Vorup-Jensen, T., Jensenius, J.C., et al., 1999. Two constituents of the initiation complex of the mannan-binding lectin activation pathway of complement are encoded by a single structural gene. J. Immunol. (Baltimore, Md.: 1950). 162, 3481–3490.

Takahashi, M., Endo, Y., Fujita, T., Matsushita, M., 1999. A truncated form of mannose-binding lectin-associated serine protease (MASP)-2 expressed by alternative polyadenylation is a component of the lectin complement pathway. Int. Immunol. 11, 859–863.

Takahashi, M., Iwaki, D., Kanno, K., Ishida, Y., Xiong, J., Matsushita, M., et al., 2008. Mannose-binding lectin (MBL)-associated serine protease (MASP)-1 contributes to activation of the lectin complement pathway. J. Immunol. (Baltimore, Md.: 1950). 180, 6132–6138.

Tandon, N., Morgan, B.P., Weetman, A.P., 1992. Expression and function of membrane attack complex inhibitory proteins on thyroid follicular cells. Immunology. 75, 372–377.

Taylor, P.R., Carugati, A., Fadok, V.A., Cook, H.T., Andrews, M., Carroll, M.C., et al., 2000. A hierarchical role for classical pathway complement proteins in the clearance of apoptotic cells in vivo. J. Exp. Med. 192, 359–366.

Thiel, S., Vorup-Jensen, T., Stover, C.M., Schwaeble, W., Laursen, S.B., Poulsen, K., et al., 1997. A second serine protease associated with mannan-binding lectin that activates complement. Nature 386 (6624), 506–510.

Thompson, I.A., Liu, B., Sen, H.N., Jiao, X., Katamay, R., Li, Z., et al., 2013. Association of Complement Factor H Tyrosine 402 Histidine Genotype with Posterior Involvement in Sarcoid-Related Uveitis. Am. J. Ophthalmol 155, 1068–1074.

Tuzun, E., Christadoss, P., 2013. Complement Associated Pathogenic Mechanisms in Myasthenia Gravis. Autoimmun. Rev 12, 904–911.

Van Beek, J., Elward, K., Gasque, P., 2003. Activation of complement in the central nervous system: roles in neurodegeneration and neuroprotection. Ann. N. Y. Acad. Sci. 992, 56–71.

Vorup-Jensen, T., Petersen, S.V., Hansen, A.G., Poulsen, K., Schwaeble, W., Sim, R.B., et al., 2000. Distinct pathways of mannan-binding lectin (MBL)- and C1-complex autoactivation revealed by reconstitution of MBL with recombinant MBL-associated serine protease-2. J. Immunol. (Baltimore, Md.: 1950). 165, 2093–2100.

Wagner, E., Frank, M.M., 2010. Therapeutic potential of complement modulation. Nat. Rev. Drug Discovery. 9, 43–56.

Wallis, R., 2007. Interactions between mannose-binding lectin and MASPs during complement activation by the lectin pathway. Immunobiology 212 (4–5), 289–299.

Wallis, R., Shaw, J.M., Uitdehaag, J., Chen, C.B., Torgersen, D., Drickamer, K., 2004. Localization of the serine protease-binding sites in the collagen-like domain of mannose-binding protein: indirect effects of naturally occurring mutations on protease binding and activation. J. Biol. Chem. 279 (14), 14065–14073.

Walport, M.J., Davies, K.A., Botto, M., 1998. C1q and systemic lupus erythematosus. Immunobiology 199, 265–285.

Weetman, A.P., Cohen, S.B., Oleesky, D.A., Morgan, B.P., 1989. Terminal complement complexes and C1/C1 inhibitor complexes in autoimmune thyroid disease. Clin. Exp. Immunol. 77, 25–30.

Weiler, J.M., Daha, M.R., Austen, K.F., Fearon, D.T., 1976. Control of the amplification convertase of complement by the plasma protein beta1H. Proc. Nat. Acad. Sci. USA 73, 3268–3272.

Whaley, K., Ruddy, S., 1976. Modulation of the alternative complement pathways by beta 1 H globulin. J. Exp. Med. 144, 1147–1163.

Whaley, K., Schwaeble, W., 1997. Complement and complement deficiencies. Semin. Liver Dis. 17, 297−310.

Williams, T.J., 1983. Vascular permeability changes induced by complement-derived peptides. Agents Actions. 13 (5−6), 451−455.

Wirthmueller, U., Dewald, B., Thelen, M., Schafer, M.K., Stover, C., Whaley, K., et al., 1997. Properdin, a positive regulator of complement activation, is released from secondary granules of stimulated peripheral blood neutrophils. J. Immunol. (Baltimore, Md.: 1950). 158, 4444−4451.

Woodruff, T.M., Costantini, K.J., Crane, J.W., Atkin, J.D., Monk, P.N., Taylor, S.M., et al., 2008. The complement factor C5a contributes to pathology in a rat model of amyotrophic lateral sclerosis. J. Immunol. (Baltimore, Md.: 1950). 181 (12), 8727−8734.

Wouters, D., Stephan, F., Strengers, P., De Haas, M., Brouwer, C., Hagenbeek, A., et al., 2013. C1-esterase inhibitor concentrate rescues erythrocytes from complement-mediated destruction in autoimmune hemolytic anemia. Blood 121, 1242−1244.

Wozniak, M.A., Itzhaki, R.F., Shipley, S.J., Dobson, C.B., 2007. Herpes simplex virus infection causes cellular beta-amyloid accumulation and secretase upregulation. Neurosci. Lett. 429 (2−3), 95−100.

Zhou, W., Patel, H., Li, K., Peng, Q., Villiers, M.B., Sacks, S.H., 2006. Macrophages from C3-deficient mice have impaired potency to stimulate alloreactive T cells. Blood 107, 2461−2469.

Chapter 16

Cytokines, their Receptors and Signals

Joost J. Oppenheim

Laboratory of Molecular Immunoregulation, Cancer and Inflammation, National Cancer Institute, National Institutes of Health, Frederick, MD, USA

Chapter Outline

Historical Perspective	229	Type III Interferon Lambda	236
Cytokines and Immunity	230	Non-Interferon Members	236
Cytokine Receptor Subsets	232	TNF Receptor Family	236
The Common γc Chain Subset	232	The IL-1/TLR Family of Receptors	237
The βc Utilizing Subset	233	Immunosuppressive Cytokines/Growth Factors	239
The gp130 Utilizing Subset (IL-6 Family)	233	Chemokines	239
Cytokines Sharing either a p35 or p40 Ligand Chain	234	Alarmins	239
Th17 Cytokines and Receptors	235	Conclusions	239
Class II Cytokine Receptor Family	235	Acknowledgments	240
Type I Interferons α and β	235	References	240
Type II Interferon Gamma	235		

HISTORICAL PERSPECTIVE

Although cytokines are the intermediary intercellular protein signals of the immune system, overproduction of proinflammatory cytokines or deficient production of immunosuppressive cytokine mediators can be a direct cause of autoimmune conditions. Cytokines have been the focus of research for over 60 years and over 500,000 articles have reported on cytokines. This chapter will highlight in brief only those cytokines contributing to autoimmune and autoinflammatory diseases. Fortunately, there are only 27,000 plus references to autoimmunity and only about 6000 relating cytokines to autoimmunity.

The history of cytokine studies was initiated by the report of Menkin (1944) which was the first to propose that "soluble pyrexins" might be responsible for fever by purifying them from inflammatory exudates. However, these pyrexins survived boiling and were contaminated by pyrogenic bacterial endotoxins. Bennett and Beeson (1953) were the first to extract endotoxin-free endogenous pyrogenic from peripheral blood leukocytes. At the same time nerve growth factors were discovered (Levi-Montalcini and Hamburger, 1953). Thereafter, interferons with antiviral activities were distinguished from antibodies (Isaacs and Lindenmann, 1957).

Several reports initiated the studies of lymphocyte-derived factors. Mitogenic factors for lymphocytes were first detected in the supernatants of antigen or alloantigen stimulated mixed leukocyte cultures (Kasakura and Lowenstein, 1965). This was rapidly followed by the detection of immunologically nonspecific macrophage migration inhibitory factors (MIF) in such supernatants (Bloom and Bennett, 1966). The MIF activity was subsequently also found to have macrophage activating activity (MAF) (Nathan et al., 1971) that was subsequently attributed to interferon-gamma (IFNγ). The historic MIF activity is distinct from the more recently discovered MIF, which is produced by the anterior pituitary and is present at detectable levels in normal human serum. This MIF is hormone-like and counters the immunosuppressive effects of corticosteroids as reviewed by Metz and Bucala (2001). These lymphocyte-derived factors were termed lymphokines (Dumonde et al., 1969). Subsequently, it was shown that nonlymphocytes such as macrophages could also produce a thymocyte and lymphocyte activating factor (LAF) (Gery et al., 1971). It was subsequently observed that even fibroblast cell lines could produce factors promoting inflammatory reactions and the term "cytokines" was coined (Cohen et al., 1974). Cytokines serve as signals between every nucleated cell type and

N. Rose & I. Mackay (Eds): The Autoimmune Diseases, Fifth edition. DOI: http://dx.doi.org/10.1016/B978-0-12-384929-8.00016-2

regulate the survival, growth, activation, differentiation, and suppression of both innate and adaptive immune responses involved in host defense and restoration of homeostasis. Although by 1978 over 100 cytokine activities had been reported, in 1979 at a meeting of "cytokinologists" it was decided to call all monocyte/macrophage-derived cytokines interleukin-1 (IL-1) and the lymphocyte-derived ones interleukin-2 (IL-2) (Mizel and Farrar, 1979). This was based on the simplistic presumption that all the activities could be attributed to two molecules. Today we are up to interleukin 38 and there are many more cytokines with idiosyncratic names. For example, over 40 chemotactic cytokines called "chemokines" have been discovered that promote the directional migration of many cell types.

Immunologists at the time were enamored with specific antibodies, and initially considered these nonspecific factors to be "lymphodrek" and to have little merit. However, the advent of the molecular age led to the identification of these molecules as gene products with distinct functions, forever changing immunology research. The first cytokine to be cloned was IFNβ1 (Taniguchi et al., 1980), followed by IFNα1 (Nagata et al., 1980), and IFNγ (Gray et al., 1982). IL-2 was the first interleukin to be cloned (Taniguchi et al., 1983). The era of "receptorology" was initiated when the first of the three chains of the receptor for IL-2 (IL-2 Rα) was identified and cloned (Leonard et al., 1984). We now have hundreds of cloned cytokines.

Thus, cytokines, like hormones, are intercellular regulators of immune cell reactions, but unlike hormones they are more prominent at local inflammatory sites rather than in the serum. Unlike hormones which are usually produced by glands, cytokines are produced at lower (nanomolar) concentrations by a great variety of cells and tissues. Cytokines, like hormones, also interact with selective cell receptors inducing an intracellular signal transduction cascade culminating in gene activation. Cytokines usually have localized "paracrine" effects on neighboring cells or "autocrine" effects on the producing cells, but less often have "endocrine" systemic effects of hormones. The appearance of elevated levels of cytokines in the serum actually has systemic effects such as pyrexia, hypotension, muscle aches and pains, and malaise and is responsible for the systemic symptoms of infections and injury. In the most severe inflammatory states, as in sepsis, this is called a "cytokine storm," which can be lethal.

Development of technology to delete or modify gene expression yielded "knockout" mice lacking selected cytokine gene activities. This revealed surprising *in vivo* roles and redefined the functions of a number of cytokines. For example, tumor necrosis factor (TNF), which had cytotoxic antitumor activity in tissue culture (Carswell et al., 1975), was identified as a key proinflammatory host defense cytokine (Nedospasov et al., 2003). IL-2 based on its *in vitro* effects was considered a mitogenic factor, but knockout mice often developed lymphoproliferative autoimmune syndromes based on the absence of the stimulating effects of IL-2 on immunosuppressive T regulatory cells (Tregs) (Hunig and Schimpl, 2003). Thus, studies of knockout mice often revealed specialized and unique roles for many cytokines. Ironically, the advent of knockout mice highlighted the primacy of "*in vivo* veritas" and drove immunologists and molecular biologists from tissue culture studies back to investigating *in vivo* models.

Today we are confronted by a plethora of cytokines, with apparent overlapping redundant activities, in part based on the sharing of receptors. The close interrelationship and apparent overlap in cytokine activities is accentuated by their capacity to induce one another and by their receptors to cross-talk and thus to "trans-activate" each other. Thus, cytokines and their receptors operate in a linked network and inhibition of one often downregulates the effects of other cytokines. It has become apparent over the past two decades that many cytokines mediate inflammatory responses aimed at eliminating invasive organisms and eliminating tissue debris generated by traumatic injuries. However, the identification of Tregs and their immunosuppressive mediators IL-10, transforming growth factor β (TGFβ) and CTLA4 have identified a number of anti-inflammatory cytokines that aim to restore homeostasis and mediate tissue repair. Thus, cytokines mediate the immunological balancing act between pro- and anti-inflammatory reactions to pathogenic organisms and tissue damage. They also mediate the discrimination between self and non-self and can enhance or suppress inappropriate reactions to self.

CYTOKINES AND IMMUNITY

The initial "innate" immune responses are preprogrammed in the genome and are based on the induction of proinflammatory cytokine and chemokine production. These signals result in recruiting a rapid inflammatory response to invasive pathogenic organisms or tissue injury by phagocytic neutrophils followed by monocytes, macrophages, and dendritic cells (DC). This cytokine-driven innate immune response is initiated by the interaction of exogenous "pathogen associated molecular patterns" (PAMPs) or so-called stored endogenous "alarmins" with Toll-like receptors (TLRs), nucleotide binding oligomerization domain 2 (NOD2), RIG-like helicases (RLHs), DNA sensors absent in melanoma2 (AIM2), or cell surface c-type lectin receptors (CLRs) present on or in many somatic cell types including inflammatory cells. These pattern recognition receptors (PRRs) enable host cells to respond to PAMPs and damaged self-proteins (as reviewed in Bellanti et al., 2012).

The receptors on phagocytic DC internalize, digest, and process the antigens derived from PAMPs yielding peptide fragments that are then presented in conjunction with major histocompatibility complex (MHC) cell surface molecules to T lymphocytes. The presented MHC−peptide complexes activate CD4$^+$ T cells that express the appropriate receptors to divide, multiply, and produce lymphokines, thus initiating the adaptive immune response with the capacity to mount specific reactions to invasive organisms and/or damaged cell products. The nature of the stimulant and cytokine response is crucial in determining the type of adaptive response that is generated. The activated CD4$^+$ T cells differentiate into subsets that exhibit Th1, Th2, Th17, or Treg cell responses as reviewed by Zhu et al. (2010). As shown in Figure 16.1 (O'Shea and Paul, 2010), the Th1 lymphocytes producing IFNγ favor the production of cellular immune delayed hypersensitivity reactions. Th2 lymphocyte-derived cytokines such as IL-4, 5, 9, and 13 favor humoral antibody-mediated immunity to parasites and allergic reactions. Furthermore, these cytokines reciprocally downregulate the other subset. Thus, IFNγ suppresses the Th2 pathway and IL-4 and IL-13 suppress the Th1 pathway. The lymphocyte-derived Th17 type of cytokines (IL-17, IL-22, IL-23) favor acute inflammatory and autoimmune reactions. Treg cells consist of four subsets known as Th3, cell contact-dependent natural or induced Tregs, or Tr1 subsets which mediate their suppressive effects by expressing cell associated TGFβ, CTLA4, and secreting IL-10, respectively. They are all engaged as feedback downregulators of inflammation and adaptive immunity and function to promote tissue repair by reducing inflammation and maintaining tolerance.

Lymphocyte subsets also express lineage specific transcription factors called "master regulators," such as Tbet, GATA3, RORγt, and FoxP3 for Th 1, 2, 17, and Tregs, respectively, that are responsible for the production of the characteristic cytokines. The CD4$^+$ T cell commitment to the production of those cytokines in the case of Th1 and Th2 subsets is largely stable, but the Th17 and Treg subsets do show considerable plasticity and interconvertibility. Despite the fact that cytokines are mediators or "intermediaries," they can play pivotal direct or indirect roles in the capacity of the immune system to distinguish between self and non-self. Overactivity of cytokines or of their receptors such as members of the IL-17 pathway that play a proinflammatory role can lead to excessive immune responses and decreases in the ability to differentiate between self and non-self. Conversely, failure to produce anti-inflammatory cytokines or defective responses by cytokine receptors such as the IL-10 pathway can result in autoimmune or autoinflammatory conditions, since this usually also results in upregulation and overproduction of proinflammatory cytokines.

The interaction of activated "matured" DC and naïve CD4 T lymphocytes in various cytokine milieus results in phosphorylation of lineage-specific transcription factors and master regulators as follows: The Th1 subset is induced by DC-derived IL-12 and this is markedly augmented by IL-18 and by a positive feedback loop involving IFNγ. IL-4 derived from mast cells and basophils initiates the induction of the Th2 lineage. This can be augmented by IL-33 and thymic stromal-derived lymphopoietin (TSLP). TGFβ with the help of IL-6 and/or IL-21 induces Th17 lineage cells. This lineage is augmented by IL-1 and maintained by IL-23. TGFβ converts naïve CD4$^+$ cells to induced Tregs. Their survival requires IL-2 and they are expanded in numbers by ligands such as TNF interacting with TNFR2. The "augmenting" cytokine ligands upregulate expression of selected cytokine receptors on the subsets enabling them to expand and maintain

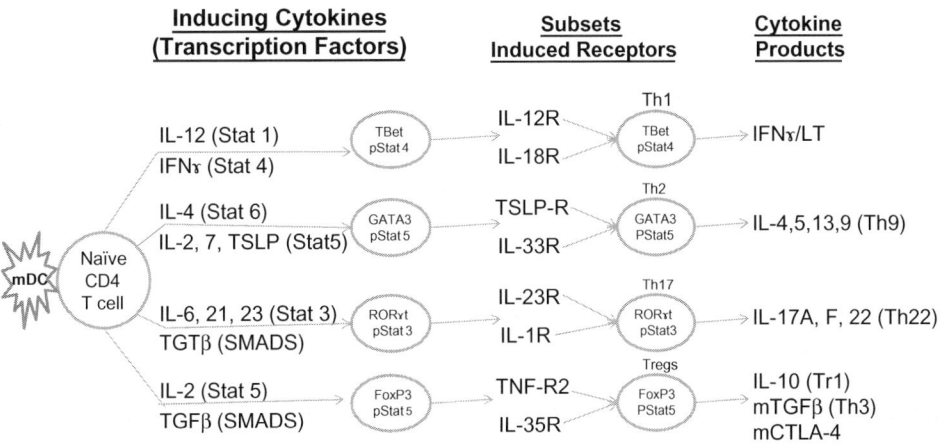

FIGURE 16.1 Helper T cell "differentiation" and Master Regulators. *Adapted from O'Shea and Paul (2010).*

the lineage and its production of additional characteristic cytokine products. The Th1 and Th2 lineages are largely stable, but the Th17 lineage can develop into dual Tbet and Rorγt expressing cells that produce both IL-17A and IFNγ. Some of the Th2 subset can become IL-9 producing cells (Th9), while some of the Th17 cells or naïve CD4$^+$ T cells can go on to produce IL-22 and have been termed Th22. Some Tregs secrete the immunosuppressive IL-10 cytokine (Tr1 subset), while others express TGFβ on their cell membranes (Th3 subset) or membrane associated CTLA4. The Treg subset is the most plastic and can develop into FoxP3 expressing cells that also express Tbet, GATA3, or Rorγt resulting in effector cells that are no longer suppressive, but function as Th1, Th2, or Th17 cells.

CYTOKINE RECEPTOR SUBSETS

The Common γc Chain Subset

Cytokines can be classified based on their structure, functions, gene locations, cells of origin, or targets, but such groupings leads to difficulties because of their pleomorphic overlapping effects. Although some cytokines exhibit homologous amino acid sequences, they can best be categorized based on their utilization of related members of receptor families which determines their target cells and effects.

The class I (hematopoietin) family of cytokines includes the common γc utilizing subfamily of cytokines including IL-2, 4, 7, 9, 15, and 21 as well as the TSLP "stepbrother" of IL-7. Mice with defective γ common chain genes develop severe combined immune deficiency (SCID) syndrome and lack T and B cell immune host defenses against infectious agents (as reviewed in Liao et al., 2011).

IL-2 was initially discovered as a mitogenic factor for T and B cells, but subsequently also figured prominently in mediating the process of apoptosis (AICD) of lymphocytes. IL-2 is produced by CD4$^+$ T cells and uses a receptor consisting of three chains IL-2Rα, β, and γ as reviewed by Akdis et al. (2011). The development of IL-2 deficient mice unexpectantly results in hyperplastic lymphadenopathy associated with autoimmune hemolytic anemia. This subsequently was attributed to the crucial role of IL-2 in maintaining the survival and expansion of CD25$^+$ (IL-2Rα) expressing Tregs. Scurfy mice based on defective Foxp3 genes also lack CD25$^+$ Tregs. Consequently, they have hyperactive CD4$^+$ T cells and overproduce proinflammatory cytokines. The homologous human autoimmune disease is known as "immune dysregulation, polyendocrinopathy, enteropathy, and X-linked" (IPEX). Thus, the IL-2 function of supporting Tregs is crucial in preventing autoimmune disease.

IL-15 is structurally homologous to IL-2, but is produced by non-lymphoid cells (Di Sabatino et al., 2011). IL-15 interacts with a heterotrimeric receptor consisting of IL-2 15Rβ, γc, and a unique IL-15Rα chain. IL15 is a more effective stimulant of natural killer (NK) cells, but less active in stimulating Treg cells than IL-2. Deletion of IL-15 or IL-15Rα results in mice deficient in DC, NK cells, and DC8$^+$ memory T cells. Defective IL-15 production in mice has also been associated with increased susceptibility to infectious challenges. Conversely, IL-15 overproduction has been shown to play a crucial pathogenic role in a number of autoimmune diseases. Neutralizing antibodies to IL-15 have been shown to decrease inflammation in mouse models of rheumatoid arthritis (RA), psoriasis, and experimental autoimmune encephalomyelitis (EAE).

Another γc cytokine is IL-7 which serves to maintain a stable number of T and pre-B lymphocytes. This product of stromal cells thus maintains lymphocyte homeostasis by interacting with a receptor consisting of an IL-7 Rα and the γc chains. The absence of a functional IL-7 ligand or IL-7Rα chain in mice and humans also yields a SCID phenotype, since IL-7 is required for the generation as well as maturation and survival of all T and B cells. Human polymorphisms of IL7R resulting in excessive inflammatory and immune reactions are a risk factor for a variety of autoimmune diseases. Another gain of function mutation of IL7R is associated with acute lymphoblastic leukemia (Mazzucchelli et al., 2012).

The deletion of IL-7 Rα in mice also inhibits the functions of TSLP, which is produced by epithelial cells and uses a heterodimeric receptor consisting of TSLP-R and IL7Rα chains (Ziegler, 2010). TSLP is a potent inducer of Th2 responses and production of pro-allergic cytokines such as IL-4 and 13 by T and B cells, DC, mast cells, eosinophils, and macrophages. Mutations causing overproduction of TSLP result in mice with severe atopic dermatitis, and TSLP is necessary and sufficient to produce airway inflammatory disease in mice. Although they share a receptor chain, IL-7 functions to maintain the normal level of lymphocytes, while its stepbrother TSLP promotes Th2 immune responses.

IL-21 is a pleiotropic type I cytokine that is a product of CD4$^+$ T cells belonging to Th17 and T follicular helper (Tfh) subsets and NK T cells (Spolski and Leonard, 2010). The Tfh subset of cells has been reported to originate from naïve CD4 T cells by stimulation of Stat 5 and to express Bcl-6 as its master regulator. These T cells express CD4$^+$ CXCR5$^+$ ICOS$^+$ markers and are located in germinal centers (GC) of lymph nodes. Tfh cells produce high levels of IL-21 and B cell antibody production and exhibit considerable plasticity. IL-21 is a potent inducer of proliferation and differentiation of CD4$^+$ and CD8$^+$ T cells, NK T cells, B cells, DC, macrophages, and epithelial cells including terminal differentiation and apoptosis. IL-21 interacts with the IL-21 R/γ_c heterodimer. IL-21 stimulates a wide variety of target cells and contributes to the development of both innate and adaptive immunity. IL-21 does this in part by priming Th17 cells and by upregulating their IL-23R expression. IL-21 can also have feedback downregulatory effects by inducing Tr1 cells to produce IL-10 and by arresting DC in an immature state.

IL-21 along with TGFβ and IL-4 may also induce Th9 cells to produce IL-10. IL-21 stimulated B cells also are a rich source of IL-10. Despite these anti-inflammatory effects, studies of IL-21 and IL-21R knockout mice show markedly reduced IL-17 production and reduced development and progression of EAE and systemic lupus erythematosus (SLE). Although IL-21 effects may be tempered by IL-10, overall IL-21 is a proinflammatory effector cytokine.

IL-9 is another pleiotropic cytokine that is produced by a distinct subset of T lymphocytes and mast cells and has therefore been termed a selective product of a unique Th9 pathway (Noelle and Nowak, 2011). However, it is unclear whether IL-9 is a product of stably differentiated cells or whether they exhibit plasticity. IL-9 can also be produced by the Th17 subset and can be co-expressed by IL-17A and by "redifferentiated" Tregs. TGFβ in the presence of IL-4 induces stat 6-dependent IL-9 production by GATA3 rather than by Fox3 expressing cells. The PU.1 transcription factor is also essential for the development of Th9 cells. IL-9 utilizes a heterodimeric receptor with IL-9R and γc chains. IL-9 behaves like a Th2 cytokine. Mice deficient in IL-9 or IL-9Rα are deficient in generating mast cells. In contrast, IL-9 induces mast cells to produce IL-1β, IL-5, IL-6, IL-9, IL-10, and IL-13. IL-9 is associated with allergic inflammation and immunity to extracellular parasites. Furthermore, adoptive transfer of Th9 polarized cells can promote the development of EAE and experimental autoimmune uveitis (EAU). Conversely, IL-9Rα deficiency or neutralizing anti-IL-9 partially ameliorates EAE.

The βc Utilizing Subset

Another class I subset of cytokines, including GM-CSF, IL-3, and IL-5, interacts with heterodimeric receptors including a βc chain (Bellanti et al., 2012). In addition, each of these cytokine ligands uses a distinctive receptor chain. GM-CSF is produced not only by T cells and macrophages, but also by endothelial cells and fibroblasts. GM-CSF is a colony stimulating factor that induces progenitor cells in the bone marrow to differentiate into granulocytic and myelocytic lineage cells. Transgenic mice overproducing GM-CSF developed increases in neutrophils, eosinophils, macrophages, and committed

precursors of erythroid and megakaryocytes, which proved lethal because of the excessive inflammatory consequences. *In vitro* culture of monocytes with GM-CSF results in the development of DC, while *in vivo* local injections of GM-CSF or of tumor cells transfected to produce GM-CSF results in the *in situ* accumulation of DC and enhances tumor immunity.

Surprisingly, GM-CSF deficient mice exhibited normal hematopoiesis and myelopoiesis. Only infectious challenge revealed modest defects in granulocyte and macrophage responses. However, GM-CSF deficient mice do develop pulmonary alveolar proteinosis (PAP) and humans with PAP have high titers of anti-βc antibodies or anti-GM-CSF. Since treatment with GM-CSF benefits such patients, PAP may be due to GM-CSF deficiency, which results in dysfunctional macrophages that fail to clear and metabolize surfactant lipoproteins. The GM-CSF deficient mice did accumulate lymphoid and mononuclear cells around their airways and pulmonary blood vessels. They also developed T cells deficient in IFNγ production and cytotoxicity and decreases in B cell antibody production. GM-CSF knockout mice were resistant to lipopolysaccharide (LPS) challenge and resisted induction of autoimmune arthritis and EAE. Although the hematopoietic effects of GM-CSF appear to be redundant, GM-CSF has considerable proinflammatory cytokine functions.

IL-5, a Th2 cytokine produced by T cells and mast cells, is a critical regulator of eosinophil expansion in the bone marrow and peripheral blood and tissues in response to allergic and parasitic stimuli (Akdis et al., 2011). However, eosinophil migration is regulated by eotaxin (CCL11) and other chemokines and its development by hematopoietic growth factors. IL-5 deficient mice develop reduced numbers of mature functional eosinophils, but there is partial redundancy with other cytokines such as GM-CSF and IL-3.

IL-3 is a product of activated T cells that stimulates the proliferation, differentiation, and activation of multiple hematopoietic progenitor cells, mast cells, basophils, neutrophils, macrophages, eosinophils, and DC. IL-3 thus promotes antigen presentation to T cells and enhances macrophage cytotoxicity. IL-3 deficient mice, however, are normal and its functions are redundant except for a reduced mast cell production in response to stem cell factor (SCF) and parasitic challenge. They also produce fewer basophils in response to parasitic infections and their contact hypersensitivity responses were also diminished.

The gp130 Utilizing Subset (IL-6 Family)

A third subfamily of class I cytokines utilizes a signal transducing gp130 receptor chain in common with a unique binding chain for each of the nine cytokine ligands in the family. They include IL-6, IL-11, IL-27, IL-31, leukemia inhibiting factor (LIF), oncostatin M (OSM), ciliary neurotrophic factor (CNTF), cardiotropin-1 (CT-1), and cardiotropin-like cytokine (CLC) (Akdis et al., 2011). Although these cytokines share one signaling chain, they have widely divergent functions depending on the cellular location of their unique binding chains.

IL-6 is one of the most important pleomorphic proinflammatory cytokines. IL-6 is produced by macrophages and activated T lymphocytes, but also by fibroblasts, endothelial cells, and other somatic cells. IL-6 interacts with IL-6Rα, which is restricted to certain tissues. However, IL-6Rα is frequently shed and available in a soluble form that complexes IL-6. These complexes can trigger the widely expressed gp130 receptor and initiate signal transduction by JAK and STAT transcription factors. This enables IL-6 to activate T and B cells, macrophages, megakaryocytes, hepatocytes, endothelial cells neuronal cells, and fibroblasts. This can result in local inflammation, but IL-6 often becomes available in the serum resulting in fever and acute phase responses. IL-6 is a potent inducer of B cell proliferation with the potential of developing plasma cell tumors (multiple myeloma), and growth of neuronal cells. Stimulation by the two other major proinflammatory cytokines, IL-1 and TNF, can induce IL-6 production and IL-6 can synergize with these cytokines. Consequently, IL-6 is a major exacerbator of autoimmune inflammatory diseases (Barr et al., 2012). Neutralizing anti-IL-6 antibodies have been used with therapeutic success to treat Castleman's disease, a form of plasma cell leukemia, but also juvenile idiopathic arthritis (JIA) and rheumatoid arthritis (RA). Anti-IL-6 has been used successfully in some RA patients that were unresponsive to inhibitors of TNF.

Cytokines Sharing either a p35 or p40 Ligand Chain

The so-called IL-12 cytokine family consists of cytokines with an α chain (p19, p28, or p35) and a β chain (p40 or EBI3) as follows: IL-12 (p35 and p40), IL-23 (p19 and p40), IL-27 (p28 and EBI3), and IL-35 (EBI3 and p35) (Akdis et al., 2011).

IL-12 is produced mostly by myeloid DC and macrophages, but also by activated B lymphocytes and neutrophils. IL-12 utilizes a heterodimeric receptor formed by IL-12Rβ1 and IL-12Rβ2. IL-12Rβ2 appears to be the signaling component of the receptor on Th1 lymphocytes and NK cells that becomes tyrosine phosphorylated and activates Tyk2 and JAK2 and subsequently Stat 4. This enables IL-12 to play a crucial role in promoting Th1-dependent cytotoxicity of T cells and NK cells and their

production of IFNγ. IL-2 promotes this pathway by enhancing expression of the IL-12R, while IFNγ promotes the production of more of the IL-12 cytokine; resulting in a positive loop. IL-12 has anti-angiogenic effects by inducing IFNγ, which in turn produces an angiostatic chemokine known as IP-10 CXCL10. Mice defective in IL-12 p40 or IL-12R become much more susceptible to infections by intracellular pathogens such as mycobacteria and even non-pathologenic Bacille Calmette-Guerin (BCG) organisms. Such knockout mice are much more resistant to the induction of autoimmunity, while administration of IL-12 exacerbates autoimmune conditions (Adorini, 2003). These results point out the important contribution of Th1 immune responses to various autoimmune states including EAE, EAU, RA, autoimmune myasthenia gravis, and autoimmune thyroiditis.

An anti-IL-12 antibody has induced clinical responses and remissions in patients with Crohn's disease (Mannon et al., 2004).

IL-23 is a heterodimeric cytokine, which shares a p40 chain with IL-12. Like IL-12, IL-23 is produced by antigen presenting cells such as DCs and macrophages and synovial fibroblasts. IL-23, however, has unique functions of stimulating committed Th17 memory cells that express the heterodimeric receptor for IL-23 consisting of IL-23R and IL-12 Rβ1. IL-23 serves to maintain Th17 responses by inducing the production of IL-17A, IL-17F, TNF, IL-6, GM-CSF, IL-22, and some chemokines (CXCL1 and CCL20). Knockout mice with deficiencies in either p19 or IL-23R develop less severe autoimmune inflammatory bowel disease (IBD) and EAE. This presumably is based on the reduced production of Th17 cytokines, which are important contributors to autoimmune inflammatory states. An anti-p40 antibody, which inhibits both IL-12 and IL-23, has therapeutic efficacy in psoriasis (Krueger et al., 2007).

IL-27 is reported to be a product of DC and macrophages as well as epithelial cells that interact with a receptor consisting of an IL-27R and the gp130 chains. Consequently, IL-27 belongs to both IL-6 and IL-12 subfamilies. IL-27 synergizes with IL-12 in activating T cells to produce IFNγ with consequent Th1, antiangiogenic, and antitumor effects. IL-27 also suppresses the development of Th17 cells and can induce considerable IL-10 production with its anti-inflammatory effects (Pot et al., 2011). IL-27 gene deletion results in mice with hyperreactive Th2 inflammatory responses to challenges with pathogenic parasitic organisms. Oral administration of IL-27 expressing lactococci by inducing mucosal IL-10 production suppresses IBD in mice. Thus, the suppressive functions of IL-27 may be less redundant.

IL-35 is reported to be a product of Treg cells and has suppressive effects on Th17 cells and CD4$^+$ CD25$^-$ T cells. IL-35 is reported to stimulate the proliferation of

Treg cells. It is therefore said to be an immunosuppressive product contributing to the effects of Tregs. However, this cytokine has recently been reported to be produced by TEK factor cells.

Th17 Cytokines and Receptors

It was recently recognized that in addition to the Th1 IFNγ cytokine, a family of IL-17 cytokines is a major contributor to autoimmune reactions; especially IL-17A and IL-17-F, which show 50% homology (Iwakura et al., 2011). IL-17 is induced by the combination of TGFβ and IL-6 and is maintained by IL-23 and/or IL-1. IL-17 is produced mainly by Th17 CD4$^+$ and CD8$^+$ T cells and by NK cells. IL-17 activates neutrophils, T cells, antigen presenting cells (APCs), and fibroblasts, endothelial cells, and stromal cells expressing various IL-17 receptors. IL17A and IL-17F utilize IL-17RA and IL-17RD receptors, respectively, while IL-17B, C, and D use IL-17RB. IL-17 induces many other inflammatory cytokines, chemokines, and prostaglandins. Consequently, IL-17 is important in driving acute inflammatory as well as allergic and autoimmune responses. IL-17 actually has suppressive effects on the Th1 pathway and the production of IFNγ. Nevertheless, T cells producing both IL-17 and IFNγ have been detected. IL-17 promotes the production of proinflammatory cytokines such as IL-6, GM-CSF, G-CSF, IL-1β, TNF, IL-21, IL-22, IL-26, IL-11 various chemokines, and even TGFβ. Deletion of IL-17A and/or IL-17F or their receptors results in mice with markedly reduced resistance to infectious challenges. Airway hypersensitivity and T cell-dependent antibody production are also considerably reduced. These IL-17A and F knockout mice develop less severe collagen-induced arthritis (CIA) and resist induction of EAE. Attempts to suppress autoimmune diseases in mouse models with neutralizing anti-IL-17 antibodies have not met with resounding success, perhaps because multiple redundant Th1 and Th2 cytokines all are involved in exacerbating the inflammation in these diseases. A humanized anti-IL-17 antibody has been effective in the treatment of RA (Genovese et al., 2010).

IL-25 (IL-17E) is produced by Th2 lymphocytes, mast cells, basophils, eosinophils, and epithelial cells (Akdis et al., 2011). IL-25 utilizes a receptor consisting of IL-17RA and IL-17RB chains. Receptor deleted mice fail to produce IL-5 or IL-13 in response to IL-25. Consequently, IL-25 is an inducer of Th2 and Th9 responses (IL-4, 5, and 13) and actually suppresses Th1 and IL-17 production. In particular, IL-25 is prominently involved in chronic inflammation of the gastrointestinal (GI) tract, including in IBD. IL25 knockout mice show reduced eosinophil infiltration in allergic states due to reduction in Th2 and Th9 responses.

CLASS II CYTOKINE RECEPTOR FAMILY

The class II receptors are utilized by the interferon family (IFN-α, β, γ) and also by IL-10, 19, 20, 22, 24, 26, 28, 29, and 30. The receptors consist of one ligand binding and one signal transducing chain. The interferons are the major host defense cytokines directed against viruses, bacteria, parasites, and fungi. They include IFN-α, β, γ, and λ (consisting of IL-28 and IL-29). The other family members have a diversity of functions.

Type I Interferons α and β

There are actually 13 subtypes of IFN-α and two subtypes of IFN-β (Huber and Farrar, 2011). IFNα/β both interact with the type I IFN receptor, which consists of two subunits IFNAR1 and IFNAR2 and are widely expressed by all nucleated cells. The type I IFN-α/β are induced by a wide variety of exogenous and endogenous proinflammatory stimulants (especially viral infections) in many cell types. Plasmacytoid DCs are major producers of IFN-α and IFN-α is particularly elevated in patients with SLE and psoriasis. Fibroblasts are a greater source of IFN-β. Although many functions have been ascribed to IFN-α/β, mice knocked out for IFNAR1 exhibit predominantly reduced antiviral host defenses and some reduction in their responses to LPS and CSF-1. However, genetic polymorphisms resulting in the elevation of IFN-α predispose to the development of human SLE (Niewold, 2011) IFN-α/β are potent stimulators of the maturation of myeloid DC and thus promote adaptive immunity, but this is a redundant function. IFN-α is used in the treatment of hepatitis B and C. IFN-β is used to treat multiple sclerosis, but the mechanism by which IFN-β suppresses symptoms and signs of MS may be based on suppression of IL-17 producing T cells. IFN-α/β therapy is associated with unpleasant flu-like side effects.

Type II Interferon Gamma

IFN-γ actually has minimal antiviral activity and is the major immunoregulatory product and co-inducer of the Th1 cytokine pathway. IFN-γ enhances autoimmunity (Akdis et al., 2011). It is selectively produced by T lymphocytes, NK cells, and NKT cells. There are reports claiming that IFN-γ is also produced by macrophages, neutrophils and B cells, but their contribution, if any, is minor. IFN-γ utilizes a receptor consisting of IFNGR1 and IFNGR2 expressed by NK cells, macrophages, Th1 lymphocytes, CD8$^+$ CTL, and B cells. IFN-γ has a major role in protecting against intracellular bacteria, based on its macrophage activating effects. Humans with gene defects in the IFNγ pathway and mice lacking IFN-γ or the IFNGR exhibit markedly reduced resistance to mycobacteria and other intracellular bacterial, fungal, and parasitic infections. Macrophage production of nitric oxide, TNF, IL-1, IL-12, and IL-6 is impaired. Unexpectedly, the knockout mice were not more resistant to the induction of EAE or uveitis, but more readily developed arthritis. Instead, IFN-γ was found to be critical in suppressing chronic inflammation and restoring T cell homeostasis by promoting T cell apoptosis. Administration of IFN-γ exacerbates multiple sclerosis (MS). IFN-γ is used therapeutically to treat infections in patients with chronic granulomatous disease.

Type III Interferon Lambda

The recently identified subgroup of IFN-λ 1, 2, and 3 are also termed as IL-29, IL-28A, and IL-28B, respectively (Donnelly and Kotenko, 2010). These cytokines utilize a heterodimeric receptor consisting of an IL-28R chain and IL-10R2 chain. The IFN-λs have both antiviral and immunostimulatory activities. Since the receptors for the IFN-λ are selectively expressed on epithelial cells, they may have fewer undesirable side effects than IFN-α and have demonstrated initial efficacy in the treatment of hepatitis. IL-28 may also have a protective role in EAE and is being investigated as a therapy for autoimmunity.

Non-Interferon Members

IL-10, another family member, has no antiviral activity, but is an active immunodulatory mediator that uses a heterodimeric receptor consisting of IL-10R1 and IL-10R2 chains (Saraiva and O'Garra, 2010). IL-10, a homodimeric cytokine, is produced by many cell types including Th1, Th2 lymphocytes, cytotoxic T cells, B lymphocytes, mast cells, monocytes, DCs, and the Tr1 subset of Tregs. IL-10 has many suppressive effects by inhibiting proinflammatory cytokine production and activities of T cells, NK cells, mononuclear phagocytes, and DC. However, IL-10 also has stimulatory effects particularly for B cells and promotes B cell proliferation, differentiation, and antibody production and induces isotype switching.

By capturing and sequestering antigens, antibodies may suppress inflammation and cellular immune responses, thus further supporting the anti-inflammatory role of IL-10. Stat 3 is essential for the suppressive effects of IL-10 on cytokines, since IL-10 fails to have such an effect on Stat 3 knockout mice. Stat 3 depleted mice become hypersensitive to endotoxic shock and develop chronic enterocolitis (IBD). The suppressive effects of IL-10 also involve the induction of inhibitory SOCS 1 and 3 signal transducers. IL-10 immunosuppressive effects, thus, protect the host from excessive inflammatory responses including allergic reactions. IL-10 knockout mice show normal lymphocyte development and

antibody responses, but they develop runting, anemia, and chronic colitis (IBD) due to excessive production of proinflammatory cytokines in response to enteric bacterial antigens. Polymorphisms reducing the effectiveness of IL-10 have resulted in a variety of human autoimmune diseases. IL-10 has a protective role in autoimmune diseases such as SLE, RA, and type 1 diabetes.

The other members of the class II cytokine receptor family have distinct nonimmunosuppressive functions (Akdis et al., 2011). IL-22 is usually considered a product of the Th17 pathways, although it is also induced by IL-9. IL-22 interacts with receptors consisting of IL-22R1 and IL-10R2. IL-22 is produced by Th17 and NK-22 cells and acts primarily on keratinocytes and epithelial lining cells, which express IL-22R1. IL-22 deficient and IL-22R-deficient mice have increased intestinal epithelial damage and become much more susceptible to *C. rodentium* infection. Thus, IL-22 plays a major role in maintenance and repair of epithelial lining tissues. IL-22 levels are elevated in psoriasis and IBD.

IL-19 shares the IL-20R receptor with IL-24 and IL-26. Since it augments IL-4, but decreases IFNγ production, IL-19 favors Th2 responses. IL-19 is elevated and IL-19 polymorphisms have been associated with psoriasis. IL-20 is also elevated in psoriasis and RA and IL-20 polymorphisms are associated with psoriasis. IL-20 is pro-angiogenic and a keratinocyte stimulant. IL-24 promotes wound healing and is apoptotic for some tumor cells. IL-24 is elevated in melanomas and psoriasis. IL-26 is a proinflammatory cytokine, which is absent in mice and difficult to study. IL-26 is elevated in IBD and polymorphisms of IL-26 are protective of MS and RA.

TNF RECEPTOR FAMILY

The TNF family consists of 19 cytokines, which use 29 structurally related receptors that share intracellular signaling pathways (Aggarwal et al., 2012; Croft et al., 2012). Tumor necrosis factor (TNF) was discovered as a factor in serum that was cytotoxic for tumors (Carswell et al., 1975). TNF is produced by T and B cells, NK cells, and macrophages. Although it interacts with the widely expressed TNFR1 receptor that contains a death domain, TNF acts on immune, endothelial, and other cell types as a major proinflammatory cytokine that mediates acute and chronic inflammatory responses to bacterial infections. TNF stimulates the hypothalamic—pituitary axis to release numerous hormones, induces liver-derived acute phase proteins, activates endothelial cells to express adhesion molecules, and results in egress of TNF activated leukocytes out of blood vessels. Thus, systemic TNF can cause fever, myalgias, malaise, hypotension, vascular leakage, cachexia, osteoporosis, and other signs of inflammation. Nevertheless, studies of mice with deletion of

TNF or TNFR1 receptors showed increased resistance to development of endotoxin shock, resistance to carcinogenesis, reduced resistance to infectious challenges, and partial resistance to induction of EAE. A number of polymorphisms of human TNF gene resulting in excessive activity have been associated with a variety of autoimmune diseases. TNF promotes inflammation and exacerbates autoimmune disorders such as RA, ankylosing spondylitis, Crohn's disease, and psoriasis. This can be countered by treating patients with these disorders with inhibitors of TNF such as anti-TNF antibodies or soluble receptors for TNF. Such immuno-therapies do reduce host resistance and can result in activating latent tuberculosis infections. Despite this TNF blockade has benefited millions of autoimmune patients.

The second receptor for TNF, TNFR2, is expressed only on T lymphocytes and NK cells. TNFR2 is predominantly expressed on all naturally occurring Tregs and activated-induced Tregs (iTregs). Consequently, ligand-induced signals from TNFR2 provide a means of downregulating TNF−TNFR1 proinflammatory effects.

Lymphotoxin (LTα) is the closest relative of TNF and also utilizes TNFR1 and 2. LTβ also utilizes two other receptors (LTβR and HVEM). The lymphotoxin name also represents a misnomer based on their initial discovery as in vitro cytotoxic activities (Ruddle and Waksman (1967)). LT is produced by activated T cells, NK cells, mast cells, fibroblasts, and endothelial and epithelial cells. Studies of knockout mice yielded the surprising revelation that LT was crucial for the organogenesis and maintenance of peripheral lymphoid tissues. Mice deficient in LT had only rudimentary lymph nodes and Peyer's patches and a disorganized splenic lymphoid architecture. Although LTα also uses TNFR1 and TNFR2, the unique effects of LT are based on the fact that LTα forms heterotrimeric complexes with lymphocyte membrane associated LTβ, which then act on LT-βR. In contrast, LTα homotrimers by acting on TNFR1 can mimic the effects of TNF. Consequently, double TNF/LTα knockout mice become even more susceptible to bacterial challenge than single knockout mice. Although the antibody responses and immunoglobulin switching by such mice are defective, their cellular immune responses remain fairly intact based on redundant pathways.

Some of the other members of the TNF superfamily contribute to autoimmune disorders. Humans with disabling heterozygous mutations in the "fragment apoptosis stimulating" (Fas/CD95) receptor develop a disease called autoimmune lymphoproliferative syndrome (ALS) with lymphadenopathy, splenomegaly, and the production of autoantibodies (Lobito et al., 2011). This is based on failure to remove long-lived lymphocytes by the usual Fas-dependent apoptotic mechanism (Strasser et al., 2009). The homotrimeric FasL triggers the Fas receptor, which contains a death domain, and results in the elimination of senescent lymphocytes. In the absence of normal Fas or FasL functions humans and mice develop B cell lymphomas and autoimmune syndromes based on the accumulation of senescent and defective lymphocytes.

Another family member, "TNF-related apoptosis inducing ligand" (TRAIL), similarly acts on death domain expressing DR4 and DR5 receptors. In addition to mediating antitumor effects, mice with deletion of TRAIL or its receptors develop autoimmune diseases. Analogous to Fas deletion, the absence of TRAIL results in failure to eliminate senescent and defective lymphocytes by apoptosis.

A number of the TNF family of cytokines are potent stimulants of B cells and have been implicated in causing or exacerbating SLE. This is true of the B cell activating factor member of the TNF family known as BAFF or BLYS or BLVS (Vincent et al., 2012). BAFF is a product of activated T cells, macrophages and DCs. BAFF interacts with two receptors known as TACI and BR3 expressed by B and T cells. In addition, BAFF heterotrimerizes with another TNF family member known as APRIL, which interacts with TACI and BCMA receptors (Cancro et al., 2009). Mice with deletion of a functional BAFF show impaired development of B cells, while mice with defective APRIL expression show impaired development of more mature plasma cells. Conversely, transgenic mice that overexpress BAFF have B cell hyperplasia and develop a lupus-like phenotype. Both BAFF and APRIL are elevated in SLE patients and other autoimmune diseases. A monoclonal anti-BAFF antibody that depletes B cells and shows therapeutic benefit has therefore been approved for use in SLE.

Several other TNF family members appear to function as costimulators, which, depending on the context, can enhance inflammatory responses or promote Treg cell activities. These include OX40−OX40L interactions (Ishii et al., 2010), TL1A−DR3 interactions (Ishii et al., 2010; Meylan et al., 2011), and 4-1BBL−4-1BB interactions (Hamano et al., 2011). These interactions can thus either promote autoimmune reactions or can prevent or dampen autoimmune disorders by augmenting Treg activities.

THE IL-1/TLR FAMILY OF RECEPTORS

The IL-1 family has expanded to 11 members, but the three initial members have been most thoroughly studied (Sims and Smith, 2010). They consist of agonistic IL1α, which is usually cell membrane associated, the soluble IL-1β, and the soluble IL-1 receptor antagonist (IL-1RA). These ligands interact with the ubiquitously expressed type I IL-1R, which transduces signals that result in proinflammatory effects similar to those of TNF, except they do not induce apoptosis. IL-1RA acts as an antagonist of IL-1α and IL-1β by binding tightly to type I IL-1R and competes with the agonist ligands for this receptor. The type II IL-1R also binds IL-1β and IL-1α with high affinity, but fails to signal and is therefore considered a "decoy" receptor, which traps the ligands. Thus, IL-1 is downregulated by these two mechanisms. Furthermore, IL-1α and β are generated with pro-domains. IL-1β and IL-18 are generally, but not always, cleaved by caspase-1. This enzyme is generated by the "inflammasome" pathway, which is activated by microbial-derived ligands that interact with nucleotide-binding oligomerization domains (NOD-like receptors NLRs). This provides another means of regulating the activity of IL-1β as evidenced from the fact that genetically heritable gain of function mutations in the inflammasome pathway result in autoinflammatory periodic fever syndromes such as Muckle Wells syndrome, familial Mediterranean fever, hyper-IgD syndrome, familial cold autoinflammatory syndrome, and others (e.g., NOMID, CINCA). IL-1α is usually cleaved by calpain and other enzymes, rather than by inflammasome-derived caspase-1. IL-1RA contains a classical signal peptide and is secreted by the endoplasmic reticulum and Golgi apparatus like most other cytokines. The other IL-1 family members all are biologically active as full-length molecules, but enzymatic processing at their N-terminal ends increases their activities. The IL-1 family members all interact with closely related receptors containing extracellular immunoglobulin domains, and they signal through cytoplasmic Toll/IL-1R (TIR) domains using a transduction pathway similar to that of the TLR.

There is another IL-1 family inhibitory receptor, SIGIRR, expressed largely on epithelial cells that decreases the inflammatory responses to IL-1, IL-18, IL-33, IL-36α, β, γ, and to TLR ligands. This is based on observations showing that SIGIRR deficient mice have enhanced responses to these ligands and develop more severe IBD, asthma, and colon cancer. Thus, SIGIRR also downregulates responses to most of the IL-1 family members.

Despite the plethora of IL-1 activities, deletion of IL-1α and/or β or of the type I IL-1R has limited deleterious effects on mice with only a modest decrease in cellular and humoral immune responses and decreased resistance to infectious challenges. IL-1/IL-1R deleted mice exhibit greater resistance to induction of autoimmune diseases. In contrast, deletion of IL1-RA yielded dramatic phenotypic effects with hyperinflammatory reactions due to overproduction of inflammatory cytokines, enhanced delayed type hypersensitivity (DTH), humoral immunity, increased resistance to infection, and enhanced induction of autoimmune states including spontaneous development of arthritis. These findings have led to the development of IL-1RA (anakinra) and other inhibitors of IL-1 as therapeutics.

These antagonists are having dramatic benefits in patients with autoinflammatory diseases. They are also benefiting patients with gain of function mutations in TNFR1 (TRAPS syndrome), Behçet's syndrome, gout, and are being investigated for their utility in type 2 diabetes, congestive heart failure, and other conditions (Dinarello, 2011).

IL-18 also is a member of the IL-1 family that is expressed by a wide range of cell types as an inactive precursor that requires cleavage by caspase-1 generated by the inflammasome pathway. IL-18 interacts with widely expressed heterodimeric IL-18R in which the α chain binds and the β chain signals in response to IL-18. The IL-18 ligand by itself is a weak stimulant of IFNγ (Th1) or IL-13 (Th2) responses, but IL-18 synergizes with IL-12 to produce high levels of IFNγ, or with IL-2 to produce more IL-13. A neutralizing IL-18 binding protein (IL-18BP) has been isolated from the urine of Italian nuns, which binds and inhibits IL-18 with high affinity. IFNγ is a potent inducer of IL-18BP, thus it functions as a negative feedback inhibitor.

IL-18 promotes the development of Th1 responses and functions of NK cells in host defense against bacterial infections. Consequently, IL-18 deficient mice show reduced resistance to parasitic, viral, and bacterial infections. IL-18 is usually elevated in autoimmune diseases and IL-18 deficient mice develop less severe CIA and resist induction of IBD. Moreover, polymorphisms in the promoter regions of the human IL-18 gene have been associated with RA.

IL-33 functions as a nuclear binding transcriptional factor as well as an extracellular cytokine, like IL-1α. Full-length IL-33, like IL1α, is also active, but it can be cleaved by caspase-1 from a 30 kDa to an active 18 kDa cytokine. IL-33 interacts with the ST2 receptor expressed on T helper cells, dendritic cells, and mast cells. Although initially reported as an inducer of Th2 responses, more recent data indicated that IL-33 also can be a potent inducer of Th1 polarized cytotoxic CD8 T cells. A soluble shed form of ST2 has the capacity to bind and inhibit IL-33. Thus, administration of sST2 reduces inflammation in an asthma model in mice and sST2 levels are elevated in autoimmune disorders such as SLE and RA. Mice with defective ST2 receptors have reduced Th2 responses, increased sensitivity to endotoxin challenge, and increased susceptibility to streptozotocin-induced diabetes.

There are some even newer members of the IL-1 family which are proinflammatory, namely IL36α, β, and γ (previously named IL-1F6, F8, and F9). Overproduction of IL-36 is reported to induce a psoriatic-like skin disease in mice. IL-1F5, now known as IL-36Ra, is an antagonist of IL-36. IL-37 appears to be an immune suppressive cytokine. It is elevated in tissues of RA patients, where it presumably has an inhibitory feedback effect.

IMMUNOSUPPRESSIVE CYTOKINES/ GROWTH FACTORS

We have already discussed immunosuppresive cytokines that play pivotal roles in preventing exuberant inflammatory reactions against non-self and self antigens such as IL-10, IL-25, and IL-37. The other cytokine that plays a major suppressive role is TGFβ. TGFβ belongs to a family of over 40 cytokines that utilize serine threonine kinase receptors. Tregs and the subset of Th3 cells, as well as platelets, macrophages, NK cells, epithelial cells, and glial cells, are major sources of TGFβ. It is usually classified as a growth factor because it promotes wound healing and fibrosis. Concomitantly, TGFβ has antiproliferative and suppressive effects on T and B cells, macrophages, endothelial cells, hematopoiesis, and suppresses inflammatory reactions which interfere with wound healing. Tumor cells often produce considerable TGFβ and thus have anti-inflammatory and anti-immune effects supporting Virchow's idea that "tumors are wounds that fail to heal."

Deletion of TGFβ in mice is lethal for neonatal mice. They exhibit uncontrolled T cell activation with excessive production of cytokines and die of a "cytokine storm" resembling the effects of "septic endotoxic shock." Conversely, overexpression of TGFβ results in renal fibrosis and diabetes. TGFβ is crucial in the generation of Treg cells from naïve T cells and in preventing the maturation of DC, which are crucial in preventing the development of autoimmunity. We will not discuss the other growth factors because they are not known to have direct effects on autoimmune responses.

CHEMOKINES

There are over 40 chemoattractant cytokines (chemokines) that interact with over 20 different Gi protein coupled receptors (GiPCR). These chemokines play a major role in the trafficking of inflammatory and noninflammatory cells and are responsible for organogenesis of lymphoid and other tissues. Chemokines generally have minimal immune cell activating effects. Deletion of various chemokine or chemokine receptor genes have diverse effects depending on the distribution of their receptors. However, although elevated in autoimmune diseases, chemokines are not directly responsible for any autoimmune disorders. Nevertheless, as key mediators in the pathogenesis of inflammatory, autoimmune, and neoplastic disorders, polymorphisms of various chemokine genes have been associated with a variety of diseases (Colobran et al., 2007). For example, SDF1/CXCL-12 and IL-8/CXCL-8 polymorphisms have been associated with SLE (Wu et al., 2012; Sandling et al., 2011), while defective CCR5 expression has a protective effect on RA.

ALARMINS

There are a number of preformed constitutively available molecules residing in cell granules, cytoplasm, or binding to chromatin that are released by cellular degranulation or necrotic cell death (Yang et al., 2009). These "alarmins" have chemotactic/recruiting activity and also activating effects on mononuclear phagocytes and on dendritic cells resulting in cytokine production and promotion of antigen presentation and adaptive immunity. Thus, alarmins are proinflammatory and enhance both innate and adaptive immunity. Alarmins are produced by a wide variety of leukocytes and non-leukocytes and interact with some GiPCR as well as Toll-like receptors (TLR) to yield chemotactic and activating effects, respectively. Some alarmins such as histamine, IL-33, and eosinophil-derived neurotoxin (EDN) polarize Th2 responses, while others such as HMGB1 and HMGN1 are potent polarizers of Th1 responses. Most other alarmins such as defensins, cathelicidins, IL-1α, and granulysin promote both Th1 and Th2 responses. IL-1α and IL-33 as well as HMGB1 and HMGN1 are nuclear binding proteins as well as cytokines with proinflammatory recruiting and activating effects. Many of these alarmins have been experimentally deleted in mice. Deletion of various antimicrobial defensins and cathelicidin results in reduced resistance to bacterial challenges. Deletion of HMGB1 has embryonic lethal effects, while deletion of HMGN1 results in immunodeficient mice with reduced tumor immunity. Studies of the role of alarmins in autoimmunity are limited. Defects in NOD2 with consequent defensin deficiency are associated with enhanced susceptibility to IBD in humans. This NOD2 defect results in overreactive inflammatory responses to gastrointestinal flora in the microbiome. The levels of HMGB1 have been found to be elevated in a number of autoimmune conditions and are correlated with the degree of inflammation. HMGB1 is present in the nucleosomes of SLE serum and autoantibodies to HMGB1 have been detected in SLE sera. However, alarmins have not been implicated as directly causative of autoimmune disorders.

CONCLUSIONS

Cytokines play important roles as either mediators or suppressors of inflammation in autoimmunity. They can, therefore, be targeted therapeutically with beneficial, although non-curative effects. This brief chapter is of necessity incomplete based on our ignorance and on the enormity of the topic. More cytokines and receptors remain to be discovered and some may play central roles in autoimmune processes. More detailed information concerning the role of cytokines in various autoimmune diseases is to be found in many of the chapters in this textbook.

ACKNOWLEDGMENTS

I am grateful to Drs. Scott Durum, Howard Young, O.M. Zack Howard, and Dennis Klinman for their helpful constructive comments and for the secretarial help of Ms. Sondra Sheriff.

REFERENCES

Adorini, L., 2003. IL-12 deficient mice. In: Fantuzzi, G. (Ed.), Cytokine Knockouts. Humana Press, Totowa NJ, pp. 253–268.

Aggarwal, B.B., Gupta, S.C., Kim, J.H., 2012. Historical perspectives on tumor necrosis factor and its superfamily: 25 years later, a golden journey. Blood. 119, 651–665.

Akdis, M., Burgler, S., Crameri, R., Eiwegger, T., Fujita, H., Gomez, E., et al., 2011. Interleukins, from 1 to 37, and interferon-gamma: receptors, functions, and roles in diseases. J. Allergy Clin. Immunol. 127, 701–721.

Barr, T.A., Shen, P., Brown, S., Lampropoulou, V., Roch, T., Lawrie, S., et al., 2012. B cell depletion therapy ameliorates autoimmune disease through ablation of IL-6-producing B cells. J. Exp. Med. 209, 1001–1010.

Bellanti, J.A., Escobar-Gutierrez, A., Oppenheim, J.J., 2012. Cytokines, chemokines and the immune system. In: Bellanti, J.A. (Ed.), Immunology IV Clinical Applications in Health and Disease. I Care Press, Bethesda, MD, pp. 287–366.

Bennett I.L.Jnr, Beeson, P.B. 1953. Studies of pathogenesis of fever: II. Characterization of fever-producing substances from polymorphonuclear leukocytes and from the fluid of sterile exudates. J Exp Med. 98, 493–508.

Bloom, B.R., Bennett, B., 1966. Mechanism of a reaction in vitro associated with delayed-type hypersensitivity. Science 153, 80–82.

Cancro, M.P., D'Cruz, D.P., Khamashta, M.A., 2009. The role of B lymphocyte stimulator (BLyS) in systemic lupus erythematosus. J. Clin. Invest. 119, 1066–1073.

Carswell, E.A., Old, L.J., Kassel, R.L., Green, S., Fiore, N., Williamson, B., 1975. An endotoxin-induced serum factor that causes necrosis of tumors. Proc. Natl. Acad. Sci. USA 72, 3666–3670.

Cohen, S., Bigazzi, P.E., Yoshida, T., 1974. Commentary. Similarities of T cell function in cell-mediated immunity and antibody production. Cell. Immunol. 12, 150–159.

Colobran, R., Pujol-Borrell, R., Armengol, M.P., Juan, M., 2007. The chemokine network. II. On how polymorphisms and alternative splicing increase the number of molecular species and configure intricate patterns of disease susceptibility. Clin. Exp. Immunol. 150, 1–12.

Croft, M., Duan, W., Choi, H., Eun, S.Y., Madireddi, S., Mehta, A., 2012. TNF superfamily in inflammatory disease: translating basic insights. Trends Immunol. 33, 144–152.

Di Sabatino, A., Calarota, S.A., Vidali, F., MacDonald, T.T., Corazza, G.R., 2011. Role of IL-15 in immune-mediated and infectious diseases. Cytokine Growth Factor Rev. 22, 19–33.

Dinarello, C.A., 2011. Interleukin-1 in the pathogenesis and treatment of inflammatory diseases. Blood 117, 3720–3732.

Donnelly, R.P., Kotenko, S.V., 2010. Interferon-lambda: a new addition to an old family. J. Interferon Cytokine Res. 30, 555–564.

Dumonde, D.C., Wolstencroft, R.A., Panayi, G.S., Matthew, M., Morley, J., Howson, W.T., 1969. "Lymphokines": non-antibody mediators of cellular immunity generated by lymphocyte activation. Nature 224, 38–42.

Genovese, M.C., Van Den Bosch, F., Roberson, S.A., Bojin, S., Biagini, I.M., Ryan, P., et al., 2010. LY2439821, a humanized anti-interleukin-17 monoclonal antibody, in the treatment of patients with rheumatoid arthritis: a phase I randomized, double-blind, placebo-controlled, proof-of-concept study. Arthritis Rheum. 62, 929–939.

Gery, I., Gershon, R.K., Waksman, B.H., 1971. Potentiation of cultured mouse thymocyte responses by factors released by peripheral leucocytes. J. Immunol. 107, 1778–1780.

Gray, P.W., Leung, D.W., Pennica, D., Yelverton, E., Najarian, R., Simonsen, C.C., et al., 1982. Expression of human immune interferon cDNA in E. coli and monkey cells. Nature 295, 503–508.

Hamano, R., Huang, J., Yoshimura, T., Oppenheim, J.J., Chen, X., 2011. TNF optimally activatives regulatory T cells by inducing TNF receptor superfamily members TNFR2, 4-1BB and OX40. Eur. J. Immunol. 41, 2010–2020.

Huber, J.P., Farrar, J.D., 2011. Regulation of effector and memory T-cell functions by type I interferon. Immunology 132, 466–474.

Hunig, T., Schimpl, A., 2003. A unique role for IL-2 in self-tolerance. In: Fantuzzi, G. (Ed.), Cytokine Knockouts. Humana Press, Totowa, NJ, pp. 135–150.

Isaacs, A., Lindenmann, J., 1957. Virus interference. I. The interferon. Proc. R. Soc. Lond. B. Biol. Sci. 147, 258–267.

Ishii, N., Takahashi, T., Soroosh, P., Sugamura, K., 2010. OX40–OX40 ligand interaction in T-cell-mediated immunity and immunopathology. Adv. Immunol. 105, 63–98.

Iwakura, Y., Ishigame, H., Saijo, S., Nakae, S., 2011. Functional specialization of interleukin-17 family members. Immunity. 34, 149–162.

Kasakura, S., Lowenstein, L., 1965. A factor stimulating DNA synthesis derived from the medium of leukocyte cultures. Nature 208, 794–795.

Krueger, G.G., Langley, R.G., Leonardi, C., Yeilding, N., Guzzo, C., Wang, Y., et al., 2007. A human interleukin-12/23 monoclonal antibody for the treatment of psoriasis. N. Engl. J. Med. 356, 580–592.

Leonard, W.J., Depper, J.M., Crabtree, G.R., Rudikoff, S., Pumphrey, J., Robb, R.J., et al., 1984. Molecular cloning and expression of cDNAs for the human interleukin-2 receptor. Nature 311, 626–631.

Levi-Montalcini, R., Hamburger, V., 1953. A diffusible agent of mouse sarcoma producing hyperplasia of sympathetic ganglia and hyerneurotization of the chick embryo. J. Exp. Zool. 123, 233–288.

Liao, W., Lin, J.X., Leonard, W.J., 2011. IL-2 family cytokines: new insights into the complex roles of IL-2 as a broad regulator of T helper cell differentiation. Curr. Opin. Immunol. 23, 598–604.

Lobito, A.A., Gabriel, T.L., Medema, J.P., Kimberley, F.C., 2011. Disease causing mutations in the TNF and TNFR superfamilies: Focus on molecular mechanisms driving disease. Trends Mol. Med. 17, 494–505.

Mannon, P.J., Fuss, I.J., Mayer, L., Elson, C.O., Sandborn, W.J., Present, D., et al., 2004. Anti-interleukin-12 antibody for active Crohn's disease. N. Engl. J. Med. 351, 2069–2079.

Mazzucchelli, R.I., Riva, A., Durum, S.K., 2012. The human IL-7 receptor gene: deletions, polymorphisms and mutations. Semin. Immunol. 24, 225–230.

Menkin V. 1944. Chemical basis of fever. Science 100, 337–338.

Meylan, F., Richard, A.C., Siegel, R.M., 2011. TL1A and DR3, a TNF family ligand-receptor pair that promotes lymphocyte costimulation, mucosal hyperplasia, and autoimmune inflammation. Immunol. Rev. 244, 188–196.

Mizel, S.B., Farrar, J.J., 1979. Revised nomenclature for antigen-nonspecific T-cell proliferation and helper factors. Cell. Immunol. 48, 433–436.

Nagata, S., Taira, H., Hall, A., Johnsrud, L., Streuli, M., Ecsodi, J., et al., 1980. Synthesis in E. coli of a polypeptide with human leukocyte interferon activity. Nature 284, 316–320.

Nathan, C.F., Karnovsky, M.L., David, J.R., 1971. Alterations of macrophage functions by mediators from lymphocytes. J. Exp. Med. 133, 1356–1376.

Nedospasov, S.A., Grivennikov, S.I., Kuprash, D.V., 2003. Physiological roles of members of the TNF and TNF receptor families as revealed by knockout models. In: Fantuzzi, G. (Ed.), Cytokine Knockouts. Humana Press, Totowa NJ, pp. 439–460.

Niewold, T.B., 2011. Interferon alpha as a primary pathogenic factor in human lupus. J. Interferon Cytokine Res. 31, 887–892.

Noelle, R.J., Nowak, E.C., 2011. Cellular sources and immune functions of interleukin-9. Nat. Rev. Immunol. 10, 683–687.

O'Shea, J.J., Paul, W.E., 2010. Mechanisms underlying lineage commitment and plasticity of helper CD4+ T cells. Science 327, 1098–1102.

Pot, C., Apetoh, L., Awasthi, A., Kuchroo, V.K., 2011. Induction of regulatory Tr1 cells and inhibition of T(H)17 cells by IL-27. Semin. Immunol. 23, 438–445.

Ruddle, N.H., Waksman, B.H., 1967. Cytotoxic effect of lymphocyte-antigen interaction in delayed hypersensitivity. Science 157, 1060–1062.

Sandling, J.K., Garnier, S., Sigurdsson, S., Wang, C., Nordmark, G., Gunnarsson, I., et al., 2011. A candidate gene study of the type I interferon pathway implicates IKBKE and IL8 as risk loci for SLE. Eur. J. Hum. Genet. 19, 479–484.

Saraiva, M., O'Garra, A., 2010. The regulation of IL-10 production by immune cells. Nat. Rev. Immunol. 10, 170–181.

Sims, J.E., Smith, D.E., 2010. The IL-1 family: regulators of immunity. Nat. Rev. Immunol. 10, 89–102.

Spolski, R., Leonard, W.J., 2010. IL-21 is an immune activator that also mediates suppression via IL-10. Crit. Rev. Immunol. 30, 559–570.

Strasser, A., Jost, P.J., Nagata, S., 2009. The many roles of FAS receptor signaling in the immune system. Immunity 30, 180–192.

Taniguchi, T., Matsui, H., Fujita, T., Takaoka, C., Kashima, N., Yoshimoto, R., et al., 1983. Structure and expression of a cloned cDNA for human interleukin-2. Nature 302, 305–310.

Taniguchi, T., Ohno, S., Fujii-Kuriyama, Y., Muramatsu, M., 1980. The nucleotide sequence of human fibroblast interferon cDNA. Gene. 10, 11–15.

Vincent, F.B., Morand E.F., Mackay, F., 2012. BAFF and innate immunity: new therapeutic targets for systemic lupus erythematosus. Immunol. Cell Biol, 90, 293–303.

Wu, F.X., Luo, X.Y., Wu, L.J., Yang, M.H., Long, L., Liu, N.T., et al., 2012. Association of chemokine CXCL12-3′G801A polymorphism with systemic lupus erythematosus in a Han Chinese population. Lupus. 21, 604–610.

Yang, D., De La Rosa, G., Tewary, P., Oppenheim, J.J., 2009. Alarmins link neutrophils and dendritic cells. Trends Immunol. 30, 531–537.

Zhu, J., Yamane, H., Paul, W.E., 2010. Differentiation of effector CD4 T cell populations. Annu. Rev. Immunol. 28, 445–489.

Ziegler, S.F., 2010. The role of thymic stromal lymphopoietin (TSLP) in allergic disorders. Curr. Opin. Immunol. 22, 795–799.

Part 4

Initiation of Autoimmunity

Cellular Injury and Apoptosis

Stefania Gallucci[1], Roberto Caricchio[2], and Philip L. Cohen[2]

[1]Department of Microbiology and Immunology, Temple University School of Medicine, Philadelphia, PA, USA, [2]Department of Medicine, Rheumatology Section, Temple University School of Medicine, Philadelphia, PA, USA

Chapter Outline

Apoptosis	245
History of Apoptosis	245
Molecular Pathways of Apoptosis	245
Apoptotic Cell Morphology	246
Apoptosis in Autoimmunity	246
Defective Apoptosis	246
Excessive Apoptosis and Apoptotic Cells as Sources of Autoantigen	247
Apotopes	247
NETosis	248
Necrosis	248
Necroptosis	248
Necroptosis in Autoimmunity	248

Parthanatos {Par[poly(ADP-ribosyl)ation] and thanatos (death)}	248
Parthanatos in Autoimmunity	249
Clearance of Dead Cells	249
Find-me Signals	249
Eat-me Signals and their Receptors	249
Phosphatidylserine	249
Other Eat-me Signals	250
Receptors for Necrotic Cells	251
Anti-Inflammatory Effects of Apoptotic Cells	251
Immuno-Stimulatory Effects of Necrotic Cells	251
A Glimpse into the Future	252
References	252

APOPTOSIS

History of Apoptosis

In 400 BC Hippocrates used the word "apoptosis" in the book of *Mochlicon* to describe the resulting gangrene from treatment of fractures with bandages (Andre, 2003). Two millennia went by and in the mid-19th century Carl Vogt described cell death for the first time. Shortly after, Rudolf Virchow and Walther Flemming reported two types of cell death and demonstrated that they were the consequence of mechanical or chemical damage (Diamantis et al., 2008). In the early 20th century the seminal work in embryology of several investigators such as Charles Perez and Alfred Glucksmann led to a detailed histological description of cellular death (Diamantis et al., 2008). It was only in 1972 that John F. Kerr coined the word "apoptosis" independently from Hippocrates and after a suggestion from a Greek professor (Kerr et al., 1972). Kerr, along with Andrew Wyllie and Alastair Currie, not only described the "shrinkage necrosis" as a defined pattern and sequence of events during cell death but also intended to make apoptosis an integral part of cell biology such as mitosis, necessary to the maintenance of life (Kerr et al., 1972). Indeed today, four decades later, this form of cell death has become a fundamental mechanism in all fields of biology. The genetics of cell death had a breakthrough in the late 1970s with the work of John Sulston and Robert Horvitz in the *Caenorhabditis elegans*, a nematode in which a fixed percentage of somatic cells die predictably (Sulston and Horvitz, 1977). This model gave the opportunity to geneticists to dissect the pathways to cell death and to clone several genes called *CED* (*C. elegans* Death). The *CED* genes were eventually shown to be highly preserved in mammalians (Lockshin and Zakeri, 2001). Today apoptosis and necrosis are fundamental parts of physiological and pathological processes and are explored as therapeutic venues.

Molecular Pathways of Apoptosis

Two essential components characterize an apoptotic cell: its morphology and the activation of a programmed molecular cascade (reviewed by Kroemer et al. (2009) and Galluzzi

N. Rose & I. Mackay (Eds): The Autoimmune Diseases, Fifth edition. DOI: http://dx.doi.org/10.1016/B978-0-12-384929-8.00017-4

et al. (2012)). Both components can be triggered by *extrinsic* and *intrinsic* mechanisms, hence the concept of extrinsic and intrinsic apoptosis (Riedl and Salvesen, 2007).

Initiation of *extrinsic apoptosis* requires the triggering of a trans-membrane receptor. In the presence of their ligands, such as FasL, TNF-α, or TNF-related apoptosis-inducing ligand (TRAIL) (Takahashi et al., 1994; Wiley et al., 1995), these death receptors (FAS, TNFR1, and TRAILR 1 and 2) trimerize to form the "death-inducing signaling complex" (DISC) (Lavrik and Krammer, 2011). DISC formation depends on a conserved death domain (DD), which can recruit receptor-interacting protein kinase 1 (RIP1) (Varfolomeev et al., 2005), FAS-associated protein with a DD (FADD) (Chinnaiyan et al., 1995), multiple isoforms of c-FLIP, and pro-caspase-8. The triggering of TNFR1 may also lead to activation of NF-κB or to necrotic death. Once the DISC is formed, activation of caspase-8 ensues (Scaffidi et al., 1999).

In apoptotic lymphocytes (also called type I cells) (Barnhart et al., 2003) caspase-8 activates caspase-3, which initiates proteolytic cleavage of cytoplasmic and nuclear proteins, and the activation of caspase-activated DNase (CAD), which cleaves internucleosomal chromatin (Enari et al., 1998). There is cross-talk between extrinsic and intrinsic pathways. For example, in apoptotic hepatocytes (also referred to as type II cells) there is involvement of the mitochondrial pathway, and caspase-8 instead of activating caspase-3 cleaves BH3-interacting domain death agonist, inducing mitochondrial outer membrane permeabilization (MOMP) and reduction of the transmembrane potential ($\Delta\psi_m$) (Kroemer et al., 2007). The resulting release of cytochrome c (CYTC) triggers assembly of the apoptosome (CYTC, the cytoplasmic adaptor protein APAF1 and dATP), activation of caspase-9, and finally the initiation of the executioner phase by cleavage of caspase-3 (Bratton et al., 2001).

Intrinsic apoptosis can be triggered by DNA damage, reactive oxygen species, and accumulation of unfolded proteins in the endoplasmic reticulum (ER) (Galluzzi et al., 2012). The pathways that lead to cellular demise share mechanisms intrinsic to mitochondria. Anti-apoptotic pathways are simultaneously engaged, and the fate of a cell depends on which pathway prevailed. As for intrinsic apoptosis, MOMP dramatically reduces adenosine triphosphate (ATP) synthesis, thereby boosting reactive oxygen species (ROS) production (Aon et al., 2006). MOMP also triggers the release of CYTC, DIABLO, apoptosis-inducing factor (AIF), and endonuclease G (ENDOG) (Leibowitz and Yu, 2010). The assembly of the apoptosome leads to the activation of caspase-9 and cleavage of caspase-3, with subsequent cytoplasmic demise and nuclear fragmentation (Bratton et al., 2001). In some circumstances, AIF and ENDOG translocate to the nucleus and initiate chromatin fragmentation in a caspase-independent manner (Lartigue et al., 2009). Therefore, the mandatory involvement of mitochondria, the dispensable role of caspases and the bioenergetics and metabolic catastrophe are major characteristics of this form of apoptosis.

Apoptotic Cell Morphology

Once an extrinsic or intrinsic trigger has been delivered, the cell starts to round up, mostly due to retraction of pseudopods and reduction of cellular and nuclear volume (pyknosis), accompanied by modification of cytoplasmic organelles and plasma membrane blebbing (Mills et al., 1999). There is preservation of plasma membrane integrity and exposure of phospholipids, a fundamental "eat-me" signal (Darzynkiewicz et al., 1992; Martin et al., 1995). The executioner phase is characterized by nuclear fragmentation (karyorrhexis) and its disintegration into micronuclei surrounded by plasma membrane, called apoptotic bodies and microparticles (Nagata, 2005). An important last step is the engulfment of the apoptotic cell by resident phagocytes (Wang et al., 2003).

APOPTOSIS IN AUTOIMMUNITY

Abnormalities in the apoptotic process have been linked to a variety of autoimmune diseases, both systemic such as systemic lupus erythematosus (SLE) and organ specific such as primary biliary cirrhosis (PBC).

Defective Apoptosis

The inability to control the immune response via cell death can result in autoimmunity; for example, defects in the extrinsic pathway, such as the lack of Fas in MRL/lpr mice renders lymphocytes resistant to cell death with marked lymphadenopathy and lupus-like disease (Cohen and Eisenberg, 1991). MRL/lpr mice succumb prematurely to severe lupus-like disease and accumulate large numbers of lymphocytes, mostly unusual T cells but also B cells (Kono and Theofilopoulos, 2000). Interestingly, the lack of Fas (or caspase-8) in dendritic cells also leads to lupus-like autoimmunity (Chen et al., 2006; Stranges et al., 2007). Human autoimmune lymphoproliferative syndrome, caused by mutations in the Fas death pathway, is a parallel condition (Drappa et al., 1996; Oliveira et al., 2010). Abnormal expression of apoptotic genes in the intrinsic pathway also results in autoimmunity. Overexpression of the anti-apoptotic Bcl-2 gene or deletion of the pro-apoptotic Bim gene lead to accelerated autoimmunity, due to uncontrolled T and B cell proliferation (Tischner et al., 2011; Strasser et al., 1991; Hutcheson et al., 2008). These findings demonstrate the tight control of autoimmunity by cell death.

Excessive Apoptosis and Apoptotic Cells as Sources of Autoantigen

Apoptotic cell excess can result in systemic autoimmunity or in flares of pre-existing disease, presumably by supplying immunogenic nuclear antigens. Injection of UV-irradiated apoptotic cells induces a rise in antinuclear antibodies in normal mice without glomerulonephritis (Mevorach et al., 1998). Injection of dendritic cells that had phagocytosed apoptotic cells accelerates disease onset in lupus-prone mice while inducing transient expression of autoantibodies in normal mice (Bondanza et al., 2003). These and other studies suggest that apoptotic cells may serve as a source of autoantigens.

Generally, an apoptotic cell is non-inflammatory and induces tolerance; nevertheless there are circumstances during which this type of cell death triggers inflammation and amplifies autoimmune response (Green et al., 2009). For example, the redistribution of nuclear contents into membrane blebs and microparticles allows opsonization by autoantibodies. Uptake via proinflammatory Fc receptors and autoantigen presentation may in turn amplify the autoimmune response (Frisoni et al., 2005). Further, during conditions of excessive apoptosis, dying cells may progress into secondary necrosis due to delayed clearance (Munoz et al., 2009). Secondary necrosis allows the release of proinflammatory "danger signals" (Wu et al., 2001).

Autoimmunity toward nuclear components such as chromatin and ribonucleoprotein (RNPs) complexes is one of the most striking characteristics of systemic lupus erythematosus (Rahman and Isenberg, 2008). Yet these autoantigens are generally protected by the nuclear and the cytoplasm membrane, which shield them from the adaptive immune system. Apoptotic cells redistribute their nuclear material into membrane blebs (Casciola-Rosen et al., 1994; Radic et al., 2004), and these apoptotic cell autoantigens, when engulfed by dendritic cells, may be presented to T lymphocytes (Frisoni et al., 2005).

The cellular components released from dead cells, notably nucleic acids, may further stimulate the autoimmune reaction. Indeed lack of toll-like receptors (TLR) TLR7 or TLR9, receptors for ssRNA and dsDNA, abolishes the production of autoantibodies in several models of lupus-like autoimmunity (Green and Marshak-Rothstein, 2011).

Apotopes

Modifications of antigens on apoptotic cells such as cleavage and post-translational modifications (Rosen and Casciola-Rosen, 1997; Utz et al., 1997) lead to the generation of "apotopes," a term used to designate epitopes displayed on the surface of early or late apoptotic cells and derived from the translocation of intracellular

autoantigens (Reed et al., 2007). Apotopes are recognized by specific autoantibodies, leading to the formation of pathogenic immune complexes such as IgG-apoptotic cells (Cocca et al., 2002), IgG-blebs (Frisoni et al., 2005), or IgG-microparticles (Beyer and Pisetsky, 2010). The recognition of apotopes by autoimmune IgG can also impair clearance of apoptotic cells by neighboring cells (Reed et al., 2008). Primary biliary cirrhosis (PBC), Sjögren syndrome, neonatal lupus (NL) and systemic lupus erythematosus (SLE) are major autoimmune diseases in which this concept has been demonstrated. In PBC, the E2 component of the pyruvate dehydrogenase complex (PDC-E2) is considered a major autoantigen and biliary epithelial cells (BECs) display PDC-E2 as an apotope on blebs during cell death (Lleo et al., 2011). Importantly, PDC-E2 maintains its antigenicity after it translocates to the cell membrane and is recognized by anti-mitochondrial antibodies (AMA). Subsequently, these complexes activate the innate immune system in multiple ways, resulting in increased TNF-alpha production and autoantigen presentation (Lleo et al., 2009). Apotopes have been also demonstrated in NL, a condition in which the passive transfer of anti-SS-A/SS-B (anti-Ro/anti-La) from the mother to the fetus induces congenital heart block (Buyon et al., 2009). Fetal cardiomyocytes expose these antigens during early and late phases of apoptosis, and they are recognized by anti-SS-A/SS-B, inducing further apoptosis (Tran et al., 2002). The apotope of SS-A is normally masked by cytoplasmic Y RNAs, but during apoptosis Y RNA is cleaved and SS-A translocates to blebs and can be recognized by autoantibodies (Reed et al., 2010).

Lupus autoimmunity is arguably the most diverse; nevertheless autoantibodies are usually directed toward chromatin and its individual components (i.e., DNA and histones), making the nucleosome, the basic unit of chromatin, the most frequent target (Arbuckle et al., 2003).

During apoptosis, chromatin undergoes dramatic changes, with fragmentation into the nucleosomes and polynucleosomes (Nagata et al., 2003). These apotope-bearing fragments also redistribute to the cell membrane into blebs and microparticles and may form complexes with antinuclear antibodies (Frisoni et al., 2005; Radic et al., 2004). These complexes may induce and sustain the autoimmune response and may activate TLRs, the best known receptors that activate innate immunity (Marshak-Rothstein and Rifkin, 2007). Apoptotic blebbing requires rho-associated coil-containing protein kinase 1 (ROCK1) (Orlando et al., 2006). Inhibition of ROCK1 inhibits the redistribution of nucleosomes and the binding of autoantibodies (Frisoni et al., 2005). Inhibition of apoptotic nuclear and chromatin fragmentation leads to milder lupus-like disease in inducible models but to worsened autoimmunity in genetically predisposed ones

(Frisoni et al., 2007; Jog et al., 2012). The results suggest that apoptotic autoantigens might serve both as immunogens but also as tolerogens.

NETosis

The formation and release of neutrophil extracellular traps (NETs) may play a key role in stimulating systemic autoimmunity (Knight and Kaplan, 2012; see Chapter 14). These extracellular structures are made of chromatin, histones, and microbicidal granular proteins and are triggered in neutrophils in response to lipopolysaccharides, granulocyte—macrophage colony-stimulating factor (GMCSF), and IL-8 (Yousefi et al., 2008). NETosis is caspase independent and depends on the production of NAPDH oxidase and ROS.

NETs are triggered by granulomatous vasculitis-associated anti-neutrophil cytoplasmic antibodies (ANCA), and contain their target antigens proteinase-3 (PR3) and myeloperoxidase (MPO) (Kessenbrock et al., 2009). Excess NETosis may play a role in SLE (Knight and Kaplan, 2012). They contain histones and DNA, two major lupus autoantigens, and also danger signals such as HMGB1 and proinflammatory cytokines like IL-17 (Garcia-Romo et al., 2011). Moreover LL37, a neutrophil-derived antimicrobial peptide present in NETs, has been found in complexes with anti-DNA and DNA, and its presence triggers type I interferon (IFN-I) production by plasmacytoid dendritic cells (pDC) (Garcia-Romo et al., 2011). Therefore, in SLE, NETs may provide autoantigens and the milieu necessary to amplify the autoimmune response and tissue damage.

NECROSIS

Swelling of the cytoplasm and intracellular organelles, early loss of membrane integrity, and moderate chromatin condensation are the typical morphological changes of a necrotic cell (Kroemer et al., 2009). Molecular steps regulating this process have led to the term programmed necrosis. Two major examples relevant to autoimmunity are described below.

Necroptosis

This necrotic molecular cascade is dependent on the activation of receptor interacting protein kinase (RIP)-1 and/or its homologous RIP-3 (Degterev et al., 2008; Feng et al., 2007). The best-described trigger of necroptosis is TNFR engagement. Trimerization of TNFR triggers the formation of DISC in which RIP-1/RIP-3 phosphorylation is inhibited by caspase-8; in this setting the molecular cascade proceeds toward apoptosis. In contrast, in the absence or inhibition of FADD or caspase-8, there is

reciprocal phosphorylation of RIP-1 and RIP-3, which stimulates oxidative metabolism via activation of NADPH oxidase (NOX1), with production of ROS and consumption of ATP (He et al., 2009). Excess of ROS and decreased availability of ATP lead to energy collapse and necroptosis (Declercq et al., 2009).

Necroptosis in Autoimmunity

Necroptosis plays a role in sterile inflammation such as ischemia/reperfusion injury and neurological disorders (Rosenbaum et al., 2010). Its inhibition benefits models of stroke, myocardial infarction and Parkinson's disease (Vandenabeele et al., 2010). Nevertheless, necroptosis causes release of damage associated molecular patterns (DAMPs), danger signals derived from dead or damaged cells that activate the innate immune system. Necrotic cells stimulate proinflammatory cytokines in SLE and in inflammatory bowel disease (IBD) (Caricchio et al., 2003; Welz et al., 2011). In mice in which caspase-8 was conditionally eliminated, TNFα-induced Crohn's-like lesions with intestinal mucosal destruction and increased expression of RIP-3 kinase (Welz et al., 2011). The lesions were reversed by pretreatment with Necrostatin-1, a RIP-1 inhibitor (Gunther et al., 2011). Similar lesions in patients with Crohn's disease, especially in Paneth cells, demonstrate necroptosis features, without caspase-3 activation and with increased RIP-3 expression (Gunther et al., 2011). This death pathway is likely to be relevant in both activating the immune system and inducing tissue damage, for example in small-vessel vasculitis and glomerulonephritis.

Parthanatos {*Par*[poly(ADP-ribosyl)ation] and *thanatos* (death)}

Poly(ADP-ribosyl)ation of nuclear proteins is an early response to DNA damage in eukaryotic cells (Schreiber et al., 2006). Upon DNA damage, often induced during inflammation by ROS, PARP-1 is selectively activated and uses NAD^+ to catalyze nuclear protein poly(ribosyl)ation (Luo and Kraus, 2012). If the repair is completed, cells survive, while if DNA damage is extensive, PARP-1 is overactivated, resulting in excessive consumption of NAD^+. As the cell attempts to resynthesize this substrate, it depletes available ATP, resulting in a sudden reduction of cellular energy and necrosis (Bouchard et al., 2003). PARP-1 also induces a forward loop by poly(ribosyl)ation of AIF which translocates to the nucleus and induces DNA damage and further PARP-1 activation (Moubarak et al., 2007). Interestingly, PARP-1 is also part of necroptosis and contributes to the energy collapse (Jouan-Lanhouet et al., 2012).

Parthanatos in Autoimmunity

Parthanatos is characterized by the release of DAMPs, including HMGB1 (Ditsworth et al., 2007). PARP-1 activation and consequent necrosis participates in the pathogenesis of acute and chronic inflammation by facilitating NFκB activation and production of TNFα, IL6, and iNOS (Krishnakumar and Kraus, 2010). If PARP-1 is absent or inhibited, there is reduced NFκB activation and disease severity during septic shock, ischemia/reperfusion injury or collagen-induced arthritis (Eliasson et al., 1997; Soriano et al., 2002; Gonzalez-Rey et al., 2007). Because necrotic lesions are often a key feature of immune-mediated nephropathies, parthanatos may be important in inducing tissue damage. Absence of PARP-1 protects from spontaneous and inducible mouse models of lupus nephritis by decreasing necrotic cell death and *in situ* production of TNFα. As the protection only applies to males, females may use a different necrotic pathway, possibly necroptosis (Jog et al., 2009).

CLEARANCE OF DEAD CELLS

One of the most important tasks of the immune system is the removal of the large number of cells that die every day (Ravichandran, 2011). Efferocytosis (decathelineau and Henson, 2003), from the latin root *effero* for "take to the grave," is the process of phagocytosis and digestion of dying cells that most cell types can perform, including epithelial cells and fibroblasts, although in mammals efferocytosis is also a primary function of "professional" phagocytes, such as macrophages. Efferocytosis removes apoptotic cells before they release harmful intracellular components and stimulates anti-inflammatory factors to preserve a healthy non-inflammatory environment (Erwig and Henson, 2007). Apoptotic cells are normally cleared with extreme efficiency and rapidity, so their detection *in vivo* is usually possible only when there are defects in their clearance (Scott et al., 2001). Failure to remove dead cells promptly has been shown to predispose to inflammation and autoimmunity in a variety of models and in human lupus, where uningested apoptotic cells are evident in lymphoid tissue (Baumann et al., 2002; Cohen and Caricchio, 2004). Deficient phagocytosis may lead to autoimmunity by allowing the apoptotic cells to undergo secondary necrosis and to release autoantigens and DAMPs activating innate immune cells (Ren et al., 2003). In order to accomplish efficient efferocytosis, phagocytes need to be in close proximity to apoptotic cells and to be able to distinguish apoptotic cells from live or necrotic cells. These two functions are promoted by the find-me signals and the eat-me signals, respectively.

Find-me Signals

Macrophages and dendritic cells are recruited by "find-me" signals released by apoptotic cells that promote the directional migration of phagocytes by establishing a chemical gradient (Nagata et al., 2010; Ravichandran, 2011). Lysophosphatidylcholine (LPC) is released by dying cells upon activation of phospholipase A2 in a caspase-3-dependent way. LPC binds the G protein-coupled receptor G2A on phagocytes; mice lacking G2A develop late-onset autoimmunity (Lauber et al., 2003). Another find-me signal is sphingosine 1-phosphate (S1P), an important sphingolipid involved in several biological processes, from lymphocyte trafficking to immunity and cancer (Orr Gandy and Obeid, 2013). S1P is released by apoptotic cells, and its inhibitor FTY720 is attracting interest in various autoimmune diseases like multiple sclerosis and thyroiditis.

Another chemotactic factor is the soluble fragment of the chemokine fractalkine (CX3CL1), which is cleaved in a caspase-dependent way from the plasma membranes of apoptotic cells. Mice lacking fractalkine receptor CX3CR1 have defective migration of macrophages in germinal centers, where many B cells undergo apoptosis (Truman et al., 2008). The latest molecules proposed as find-me signals are ATP and UTP. These nucleotides are released by early apoptotic cells and recruit monocytes upon triggering P2Y2 receptors (Elliott et al., 2009); mice enzymatically depleted of nucleotides or lacking P2Y2 receptors show deficient phagocyte migration and uncleared apoptotic cells. Early apoptotic cells employ the pannexin family of plasma membrane channels to secrete about 2% of the cellular content of ATP and UTP as a find-me signal, much less than the fraction of these nucleotides released by necrotic cells as DAMP upon loss of plasma membrane integrity. Thus, nucleotides either attract non-inflammatory phagocytes or recruit neutrophils and activate dendritic cells, depending on the amount released. Apoptotic cells may also release "keep-out" signals, like lactoferrin, to avoid the recruitment of proinflammatory cells (Bournazou et al., 2009).

Eat-me Signals and their Receptors

Phosphatidylserine

Phagocytes engulf apoptotic cells because they can recognize specific "eat-me" signals expressed by the apoptotic cells. The anionic phospholipid phosphatidylserine is the best known eat-me signal (Fadok et al., 1992). Healthy cells maintain phosphatidylserine hidden in the inner leaflet of the plasma membrane, while apoptotic cells flip the phospholipid content of their membrane through the inhibition of translocases (flippases) and the activation of scramblases, and thereby expose phosphatidylserine in the outer leaflet (Nagata et al., 2010). Professional phagocytes and neighboring cells can recognize phosphatidylserine through a number of receptors and engage in phagocytosis. The exposure of phosphatidylserine in the outer membrane is a universal marker of early apoptosis, occurring within 1−2 hours from the apoptotic insult, and is detected experimentally by staining with the soluble molecule annexin V (Ravichandran, 2011). The insertion of phosphatidylserine into the plasma membrane of erythrocytes leads to their phagocytosis by macrophages (Tanaka and Schroit, 1983), and the masking of phosphatidylserine with specific antibodies impairs the clearance of apoptotic cells *in vitro* and *in vivo* (Asano et al., 2004). It is still debated whether phosphatidylserine is *per se* sufficient to induce phagocytosis: indeed, contrary to what was observed in erythrocytes, living cells artificially exposing phosphatidylserine are not efficiently phagocytosed, suggesting that either other still unknown eat-me signals are necessary, or that "don't eat-me" signals, such as CD31 and CD47, protect living cells from removal (Devitt and Marshall, 2011; Ravichandran, 2011). Moreover, phosphatidylserine can be chemically modified during apoptosis and indeed some phosphatidylserine receptors preferentially bind oxidized molecules.

The binding of phagocytes to apoptotic cells requires cooperation with adhesion molecules for firmer binding, a process defined as "tethering and tickling" (Henson et al., 2001); this has been compared to the immunological synapse and therefore termed the "phagocytic synapse" (Devitt and Marshall, 2011). The molecules able to recognize phosphatidylserine can be divided into two categories: receptors on the plasma membrane of the phagocytes that directly recognize phosphatidylserine and those that instead recognize a bridge, i.e., a soluble molecule that opsonizes apoptotic cells. The first category includes the members of the T cell immunoglobulin and mucin (TIM) family. TIM4 is expressed by macrophages and dendritic cells, while TIM3 is expressed in the spleen by CD8a$^+$ dendritic cells, which are antigen presenting cells specialized in cross-priming. TIM receptors may allow dendritic cells to engulf dead cells and present their antigens for immunity. TIM4 deficient mice show persistence of apoptotic bodies, hyperactivated T and B cells, and systemic autoimmunity (Rodriguez-Manzanet et al., 2010). Other possible direct phosphatidylserine receptors are the brain angiogenesis inhibitor 1, expressed in neurons, and Stabilin-2, expressed by endothelial cells in lymphoid organs (Nagata et al., 2010).

The second category of receptors for phosphatidylserine includes receptors that recognize soluble molecules bridging phagocytes and apoptotic cells. Milk fat globule EGF factor 8 (MFG-E8) is expressed by most phagocytes, including tingible-body macrophages, by follicular dendritic cells in germinal centers, and by epidermal Langerhans cells. MFG-E8 binds phosphatidylserine on the apoptotic cells using its two factor-VIII-homologous C-terminal C1 and C2 domains, and to the integrins a_vb_3 or a_vb_5 on the phagocytes using an N-terminal EGF domain carrying an RGD motif (Arg-Gly-Asp) (Nagata et al., 2010). During an immune response, mice deficient for MFG-E8 show accumulation of uncleared apoptotic cells in germinal centers, indicating a non-redundant role for MFG-E8 in the removal of apoptotic cells by tingible-body macrophages *in vivo*. MFG-E8 deficient mice also develop spontaneous lupus-like autoimmune disease, with anti-dsDNA and glomerulonephritis (Hanayama et al., 2004).

Gas-6 and Protein S are two other examples of molecular bridges that opsonize apoptotic cells by recognizing phosphatidylserine and promote their phagocytosis. Gas-6 and Protein S bind to members of the TAM family of tyrosine kinases: Tyro3, Axl, and Mer on phagocytes (Rothlin and Lemke, 2010). These kinases are involved in phagocytosis and in the modulation of the immune function of the phagocytes. Mer is expressed by macrophages, dendritic cells, natural killer (NK) cells, and NK T cells (Behrens et al., 2003). Mer-deficient mice show accumulation of apoptotic cells upon a strong apoptotic stimulus and spontaneously develop SLE-like autoimmunity, characterized by anti-DNA, anti-chromatin, antiphospholipid antibodies, and a mild glomerulonephritis (Cohen et al., 2002). This autoimmune phenotype is more severe in mice lacking all three members of the TAMs, with more intense macrophage activation, swollen joints, and glomerular immune complex deposition (Lu and Lemke, 2001; Cohen and Caricchio, 2004). As seen in MFG-E8 deficient mice and other knockout mice (Cohen and Caricchio, 2004), Mer-deficient mice develop severe autoimmunity in the genetic background of the strain 129, while the phenotype is less striking on the C57BL/6 background, presumably reflecting the allelic polymorphisms carried by the 129 strain that promote autoimmunity (Heidari et al., 2006).

Other Eat-me Signals

Many receptors, such as CD14, CD36, CD68, the LDL-receptor-related protein, the oxidized low density lipoprotein recognizing receptors, and the scavenger receptors, bind dead cells independently from phosphatidylserine (Ravichandran, 2011). Natural IgM antibodies can bind phosphatidylcholine exposed by apoptotic cells and enhance the uptake of apoptotic cells by phagocytes by recruiting C1q and mannose binding lectin (MBL). Studies suggest that these natural IgMs protect against autoimmunity and atherosclerosis by promoting clearance of apoptotic cells and regulating immune activation

(Gronwall et al., 2012). Some receptors for apoptotic cells are organ specific, like surfactant A and D, which may be important in the lung: surfactant D deficient mice spontaneously develop emphysema, possibly because the accumulation of intrapulmonary apoptotic cells promotes inflammation and destruction of the pulmonary parenchyma (Vandivier et al., 2002).

Receptors for Necrotic Cells

The C-type lectins are a large family of proteins and some of them are expressed by innate immune cells and recognize damaged and necrotic cells and pathogens (Sancho and Reis e Sousa, 2012). DNGR-1 is a C-type lectin that is expressed by $CD8a^+$ dendritic cells and binds a self-protein, the F-actin component of the cellular cytoskeleton, which, like phosphatidylserine, is normally hidden in the cytoplasm of healthy cells and is exposed extracellularly upon necrotic death. Triggering of DNGR-1 marks the phagocytosed cargo as necrotic and shuttles it for cross-presentation (Sancho and Reis e Sousa, 2012).

LOX-1 is another C-type lectin that recognizes molecules from injured or dead cells such as modified LDL and heat shock proteins, and also facilitates other dead cell recognition receptors such as C-reactive protein and C1q. LOX-1 deficient mice show delayed atherosclerosis and reduced ischemia-induced organ damage, possibly because of decreased inflammation (Sawamura et al., 2012).

Complement is an important player in the recognition of necrotic cells. C1q binds to cells in the late stage of apoptosis and possibly to primary necrotic cells and C1q deficient mice develop a lupus-like disease, with anti-DNA and immune complex-dependent renal disease on the 129 genetic background (Mitchell et al., 2002). Furthermore, C1q deficiency in humans leads to lupus-like disease in nearly all homozygous individuals. Autoantibodies against C1q may also cause a functional deficiency of C1q and may block its binding to dead cells and thus exacerbate SLE disease (Cohen and Caricchio, 2004).

Another class of receptors involved in the recognition of dead cells, either apoptotic or necrotic, is the pentraxins (Bottazzi et al., 2010). The short pentraxins, C-reactive protein (CRP) and serum amyloid P (SAP), are acute phase proteins induced by IL-6 in hepatocytes during inflammation, while the long pentraxin PTX3 is expressed by macrophages, myeloid dendritic cells, neutrophils, and some non-immune cells in response to inflammatory cytokines and TLR ligands. CRP, SAP, and PTX3 bind pathogens and dead cells and promote their complement-mediated killing and phagocytosis. Mice deficient in pentraxins show defective clearance of dead cells and develop lupus (Munoz et al., 2010).

ANTI-INFLAMMATORY EFFECTS OF APOPTOTIC CELLS

Apoptotic cells are normally considered anti-inflammatory not only because they preserve their membrane integrity and so do not release DAMPs but also because they actively provide anti-inflammatory signals to the phagocytes (Erwig and Henson, 2007). Apoptotic cells inhibit phagocyte production of proinflammatory cytokines like TNFa and IL-12 and increase the production of the anti-inflammatory cytokines IL-10 (Voll et al., 1997), TGF-beta, prostaglandin E2, and platelet-activating factor (PAF) (Fadok et al., 1998). Phagocytosis of apoptotic cells polarizes macrophages toward the "alternatively-activated" M2 differentiation state, which is reparative and nonphlogistic, through the production of the anti-inflammatory cytokines TGF-beta and IL-10 (Sica and Mantovani, 2012). Many receptors may mediate this anti-inflammatory effect of apoptotic cells.

Indeed, ligation of Mer by apoptotic cells can suppress the response of the innate immune cells to TLR stimulation and proinflammatory cytokines, through the autocrine production of type I interferons and the induction of suppressors of cytokine signaling (SOCS) molecules, dampening the innate and adaptive immune response (Rothlin et al., 2007). Therefore, the autoimmunity in Mer-deficient mice could be ascribed to an excess of autoantigens because of their impaired clearance, with these being presented immunogenically because of the DAMPs released by secondary necrotic cells, and also because of the absence of the anti-inflammatory function of Mer on innate immune cells (Rothlin and Lemke, 2010).

CR3, also known as CD11b or Mac-1, is expressed by macrophages and myeloid dendritic cells and, upon binding apoptotic cells opsonized by the complement component iC3b, it signals anti-inflammatory effects in phagocytes (Behrens et al., 2007). CR3 deficient mice have no defects in apoptotic cell clearance or autoimmunity possibly due to the redundancy of anti-inflammatory signals from apoptotic cells.

Some forms of apoptotic cells are instead proinflammatory, such as those killed by ultraviolet irradiation: such cells express IL-1a (Caricchio et al., 2003) and activate dendritic cells (Rovere et al., 1998).

IMMUNO-STIMULATORY EFFECTS OF NECROTIC CELLS

Necrotic cells activate dendritic cells and stimulate immune responses *in vitro* and *in vivo* (Gallucci et al., 1999; Matzinger, 2002) through the release of endogenous "danger signals" or DAMPs (Miyake and Yamasaki, 2012; Gallo and Gullucci, 2013). Among these signals, nucleic acids are crucial in lupus pathogenesis because they are important self-antigens and, either in immune complexes with autoantibodies (Leadbetter et al., 2002) or carried by other chaperones (heat shock proteins, HMGB-1, etc.), they activate innate immunity through TLR7 and TLR9 stimulation (Marshak-Rothstein and Rifkin, 2007). Other DAMPs released by necrotic cells include heat shock proteins, uric acid, and degradation products of the extracellular matrix (ECM). These ECM products, such as hyaluronic acid, fibrinogen, and tenascin-C, are upregulated after tissue injury. Their levels are increased in rheumatoid arthritis (RA) tissues, and their administration induces joint inflammation in mice. Mice deficient in tenascin-C show rapid resolution of inflammation (Goh and Midwood, 2011), suggesting a pathogenetic role for ECM molecules in RA.

Finally, HMGB1 is a DNA-binding protein that stabilizes the nucleosome and regulates transcription (Andersson and Tracey, 2011). It is released by necrotic cells and activates innate immune cells by triggering RAGE, TLR2, and TLR4. Necrotic cells lacking HMGB1 are less stimulatory, and neutralizing antibodies ameliorate inflammation (Bianchi and Manfredi, 2007). HMGB1 can participate in the pathogenesis of RA, SLE, experimental autoimmune encephalomyelitis (EAE), and autoimmune diabetes in NOD mice (Andersson and Tracey, 2011). Inhibition of HMGB1 ameliorates arthritis in animals, while its administration into the joints induces arthritis (Kokkola et al., 2003). In RA patients, HMGB1 levels are increased in serum and synovial fluid, and decrease upon therapies that ameliorate joint inflammation (Zetterstrom et al., 2008). SLE patients have anti-HMGB1 autoantibodies and their levels of serum HMGB1 correlate with disease activity; in animals, the injection of HMGB1—nucleosome complexes induces lupus-like autoantibodies.

A GLIMPSE INTO THE FUTURE

The last 20 years have been pivotal in the investigation of the role of apoptosis and clearance of apoptotic cells in the pathogenesis of autoimmune diseases, while only very recently has necrosis been considered a form of programmed cell death with pathogenic relevance in autoimmunity. The discovery of novel kinds of cell death mediated by novel molecular cascades or programs will certainly advance our understanding of the association between programmed cell death and autoimmunity, and may identify therapeutic targets. Next generation deep sequencing studies will indicate the genetic links between novel forms of cell death and disease and identify the subgroups of patients in the affected human population. This chapter will expand to reflect the complex interactions between death, clearance, and recognition of damage by the immune system.

REFERENCES

Andersson, U., Tracey, K.J., 2011. HMGB1 is a therapeutic target for sterile inflammation and infection. Annu. Rev. Immunol. 29, 139–162.

Andre, N., 2003. Hippocrates of Cos and apoptosis. Lancet. 361, 1306.

Aon, M.A., Cortassa, S., Akar, F.G., O'Rourke, B., 2006. Mitochondrial criticality: a new concept at the turning point of life or death. Biochim. Biophys. Acta. 1762, 232–240.

Arbuckle, M.R., Mcclain, M.T., Rubertone, M.V., Scofield, R.H., Dennis, G.J., et al., 2003. Development of autoantibodies before the clinical onset of systemic lupus erythematosus. N. Engl. J. Med. 349, 1526–1533.

Asano, K., Miwa, M., Miwa, K., Hanayama, R., Nagase, H., Nagata, S., et al., 2004. Masking of phosphatidylserine inhibits apoptotic cell engulfment and induces autoantibody production in mice. J. Exp. Med. 200, 459–467.

Barnhart, B.C., Alappat, E.C., Peter, M.E., 2003. The CD95 type I/type II model. Semin Immunol. 15, 185–193.

Baumann, I., Kolowos, W., Voll, R.E., Manger, B., Gaipl, U., Neuhuber, W.L., et al., 2002. Impaired uptake of apoptotic cells into tingible body macrophages in germinal centers of patients with systemic lupus erythematosus. Arthritis Rheum. 46, 191–201.

Behrens, E.M., Gadue, P., Gong, S.Y., Garrett, S., Stein, P.L., Cohen, P. L., 2003. The mer receptor tyrosine kinase: expression and function suggest a role in innate immunity. Eur. J. Immunol. 33, 2160–2167.

Behrens, E.M., Sriram, U., Shivers, D.K., Gallucci, M., Ma, Z., Finkel, T.H., et al., 2007. Complement receptor 3 ligation of dendritic cells suppresses their stimulatory capacity. J. Immunol. 178, 6268–6279.

Beyer, C., Pisetsky, D.S., 2010. The role of microparticles in the pathogenesis of rheumatic diseases. Nat. Rev. Rheumatol. 6, 21–29.

Bianchi, M.E., Manfredi, A.A., 2007. High-mobility group box 1 (HMGB1) protein at the crossroads between innate and adaptive immunity. Immunol. Rev. 220, 35–46.

Bondanza, A., Zimmermann, V.S., Dell'antonio, G., Dal Cin, E., Capobianco, A., Sabbadini, M., et al., 2003. Cutting edge: dissociation between autoimmune response and clinical disease after vaccination with dendritic cells. J. Immunol. 170, 24–27.

Bottazzi, B., Doni, A., Garlanda, C., Mantovani, A., 2010. An integrated view of humoral innate immunity: pentraxins as a paradigm. Annu. Rev. Immunol. 28, 157–183.

Bouchard, V.J., Rouleau, M., Poirier, G.G., 2003. PARP-1, a determinant of cell survival in response to DNA damage. Exp. Hematol. 31, 446–454.

Bournazou, I., Pound, J.D., Duffin, R., Bournazos, S., Melville, L.A., Brown, S.B., et al., 2009. Apoptotic human cells inhibit migration of granulocytes via release of lactoferrin. J. Clin. Invest. 119, 20–32.

Bratton, S.B., Walker, G., Srinivasula, S.M., Sun, X.M., Butterworth, M., Alnemri, E.S., et al., 2001. Recruitment, activation and retention of caspases-9 and -3 by Apaf-1 apoptosome and associated XIAP complexes. EMBO J. 20, 998–1009.

Buyon, J.P., Clancy, R.M., Friedman, D.M., 2009. Cardiac manifestations of neonatal lupus erythematosus: guidelines to management, integrating clues from the bench and bedside. Nat. Clin. Pract. Rheumatol. 5, 139–148.

Caricchio, R., McPhie, L., Cohen, P.L., 2003. Ultraviolet B radiation-induced cell death: critical role of ultraviolet dose in inflammation and lupus autoantigen redistribution. J. Immunol. 171, 5778–5786.

Casciola-Rosen, L.A., Anhalt, G., Rosen, A., 1994. Autoantigens targeted in systemic lupus erythematosus are clustered in two populations of surface structures on apoptotic keratinocytes. J. Exp. Med. 179, 1317–1330.

Chen, M., Wang, Y.H., Wang, Y., Huang, L., Sandoval, H., Liu, Y.J., et al., 2006. Dendritic cell apoptosis in the maintenance of immune tolerance. Science 311, 1160–1164.

Chinnaiyan, A.M., O'Rourke, K., Tewari, M., Dixit, V.M., 1995. FADD, a novel death domain-containing protein, interacts with the death domain of Fas and initiates apoptosis. Cell 81, 505–512.

Cocca, B.A., Cline, A.M., Radic, M.Z., 2002. Blebs and apoptotic bodies are B cell autoantigens. J. Immunol. 169, 159–166.

Cohen, P.L., Caricchio, R., 2004. Genetic models for the clearance of apoptotic cells. Rheum. Dis. Clin. North Am. 30, 473–486, viii.

Cohen, P.L., Caricchio, R., Abraham, V., Camenisch, T.D., Jennette, J.C., Roubey, R.A., et al., 2002. Delayed apoptotic cell clearance and lupus-like autoimmunity in mice lacking the c-mer membrane tyrosine kinase. J. Exp. Med. 196, 135–140.

Cohen, P.L., Eisenberg, R.A., 1991. Lpr and gld: single gene models of systemic autoimmunity and lymphoproliferative disease. Annu. Rev. Immunol. 9, 243–269.

Darzynkiewicz, Z., Bruno, S., Del Bino, G., Gorczyca, W., Hotz, M.A., Lassota, P., et al., 1992. Features of apoptotic cells measured by flow cytometry. Cytometry 13, 795–808.

decathelineau, A.M., Henson, P.M., 2003. The final step in programmed cell death: phagocytes carry apoptotic cells to the grave. Essays Biochem. 39, 105–117.

Declercq, W., Vanden Berghe, T., Vandenabeele, P., 2009. RIP kinases at the crossroads of cell death and survival. Cell 138, 229–232.

Degterev, A., Hitomi, J., Germscheid, M., Ch'en, I.L., Korkina, O., Teng, X., et al., 2008. Identification of RIP1 kinase as a specific cellular target of necrostatins. Nat. Chem. Biol. 4, 313–321.

Devitt, A., Marshall, L.J., 2011. The innate immune system and the clearance of apoptotic cells. J. Leukoc. Biol. 90, 447–457.

Diamantis, A., Magiorkinis, E., Sakorafas, G.H., Androutsos, G., 2008. A brief history of apoptosis: from ancient to modern times. Onkologie. 31, 702–706.

Ditsworth, D., Zong, W.X., Thompson, C.B., 2007. Activation of poly (ADP)-ribose polymerase (PARP-1) induces release of the pro-inflammatory mediator HMGB1 from the nucleus. J. Biol. Chem. 282, 17845–17854.

Drappa, J., Vaishnaw, A.K., Sullivan, K.E., Chu, J.L., Elkon, K.B., 1996. Fas gene mutations in the Canale–Smith syndrome, an inherited lymphoproliferative disorder associated with autoimmunity. N. Engl. J. Med. 335, 1643–1649.

Eliasson, M.J., Sampei, K., Mandir, A.S., Hurn, P.D., Traystman, R.J., Bao, J., et al., 1997. Poly(ADP-ribose) polymerase gene disruption renders mice resistant to cerebral ischemia. Nat. Med. 3, 1089–1095.

Elliott, M.R., Chekeni, F.B., Trampont, P.C., Lazarowski, E.R., Kadl, A., Walk, S.F., et al., 2009. Nucleotides released by apoptotic cells act as a find-me signal to promote phagocytic clearance. Nature 461, 282–286.

Enari, M., Sakahira, H., Yokoyama, H., Okawa, K., Iwamatsu, A., Nagata, S., 1998. A caspase-activated DNase that degrades DNA during apoptosis, and its inhibitor ICAD. Nature 391, 43–50.

Erwig, L.P., Henson, P.M., 2007. Immunological consequences of apoptotic cell phagocytosis. Am. J. Pathol. 171, 2–8.

Fadok, V.A., Bratton, D.L., Konowal, A., Freed, P.W., Westcott, J.Y., Henson, P.M., 1998. Macrophages that have ingested apoptotic cells in vitro inhibit proinflammatory cytokine production through autocrine/paracrine mechanisms involving TGF-beta, PGE2, and PAF. J. Clin. Invest. 101, 890–898.

Fadok, V.A., Voelker, D.R., Campbell, P.A., Cohen, J.J., Bratton, D.L., Henson, P.M., 1992. Exposure of phosphatidylserine on the surface of apoptotic lymphocytes triggers specific recognition and removal by macrophages. J. Immunol. 148, 2207–2216.

Feng, S., Yang, Y., Mei, Y., Ma, L., Zhu, D.E., Hoti, N., et al., 2007. Cleavage of RIP3 inactivates its caspase-independent apoptosis pathway by removal of kinase domain. Cell Signal. 19, 2056–2067.

Frisoni, L., McPhie, L., Colonna, L., Sriram, U., Monestier, M., Gallucci, S., et al., 2005. Nuclear autoantigen translocation and autoantibody opsonization lead to increased dendritic cell phagocytosis and presentation of nuclear antigens: a novel pathogenic pathway for autoimmunity? J. Immunol. 175, 2692–2701.

Frisoni, L., McPhie, L., Kang, S.A., Monestier, M., Madaio, M., Satoh, M., et al., 2007. Lack of chromatin and nuclear fragmentation in vivo impairs the production of lupus anti-nuclear antibodies. J. Immunol. 179, 7959–7966.

Gallucci, S., Lolkema, M., Matzinger, P., 1999. Natural adjuvants: endogenous activators of dendritic cells. Nat. Med. 5, 1249–1255.

Galluzzi, L., Vitale, I., Abrams, J.M., Alnemri, E.S., Baehrecke, E.H., Blagosklonny, M.V., et al., 2012. Molecular definitions of cell death subroutines: recommendations of the Nomenclature Committee on Cell Death 2012. Cell Death Differ. 19, 107–120.

Garcia-Romo, G.S., Caielli, S., Vega, B., Connolly, J., Allantaz, F., Xu, Z., et al., 2011. Netting neutrophils are major inducers of type I IFN production in pediatric systemic lupus erythematosus. Sci. Transl. Med. 3, 73ra20.

Goh, F.G., Midwood, K.S., 2011. Intrinsic danger: activation of Toll-like receptors in rheumatoid arthritis. Rheumatology (Oxford). 51, 7–23.

Gonzalez-Rey, E., Martinez-Romero, R., O'Valle, F., Aguilar-Quesada, R., Conde, C., Delgado, M., et al., 2007. Therapeutic effect of a poly(ADP-ribose) polymerase-1 inhibitor on experimental arthritis by downregulating inflammation and Th1 response. PLoS One. 2, e1071.

Green, D.R., Ferguson, T., Zitvogel, L., Kroemer, G., 2009. Immunogenic and tolerogenic cell death. Nat. Rev. Immunol. 9, 353–363.

Green, N.M., Marshak-Rothstein, A., 2011. Toll-like receptor driven B cell activation in the induction of systemic autoimmunity. Semin Immunol. 23, 106–112.

Gronwall, C., Vas, J., Silverman, G.J., 2012. Protective roles of natural IgM antibodies. Front Immunol. 3, 66.

Gunther, C., Martini, E., Wittkopf, N., Amann, K., Weigmann, B., Neumann, H., et al., 2011. Caspase-8 regulates TNF-alpha-induced epithelial necroptosis and terminal ileitis. Nature 477, 335–339.

Hanayama, R., Tanaka, M., Miyasaka, K., Aozasa, K., Koike, M., Uchiyama, Y., et al., 2004. Autoimmune disease and impaired uptake of apoptotic cells in MFG-E8-deficient mice. Science 304, 1147–1150.

He, S., Wang, L., Miao, L., Wang, T., Du, F., Zhao, L., et al., 2009. Receptor interacting protein kinase-3 determines cellular necrotic response to TNF-alpha. Cell 137, 1100–1111.

Heidari, Y., Bygrave, A.E., Rigby, R.J., Rose, K.L., Walport, M.J., Cook, H.T., et al., 2006. Identification of chromosome intervals from 129 and C57BL/6 mouse strains linked to the development of systemic lupus erythematosus. Genes Immun. 7, 592–599.

Henson, P.M., Bratton, D.L., Fadok, V.A., 2001. The phosphatidylserine receptor: a crucial molecular switch? Nat. Rev. Mol. Cell Biol. 2, 627–633.

Hutcheson, J., Scatizzi, J.C., Siddiqui, A.M., Haines 3rd, G.K., Wu, T., Li, Q.Z., et al., 2008. Combined deficiency of proapoptotic regulators Bim and Fas results in the early onset of systemic autoimmunity. Immunity. 28, 206–217.

Jog, N.R., Dinnall, J.A., Gallucci, S., Madaio, M.P., Caricchio, R., 2009. Poly(ADP-ribose) polymerase-1 regulates the progression of autoimmune nephritis in males by inducing necrotic cell death and modulating inflammation. J. Immunol. 182, 7297–7306.

Jog, N.R., Frisoni, L., Shi, Q., Monestier, M., Hernandez, S., Craft, J., et al., 2012. Caspase-activated DNase is required for maintenance of tolerance to lupus nuclear autoantigens. Arthritis Rheum. 64, 1247–1256.

Jouan-Lanhouet, S., Arshad, M.I., Piquet-Pellorce, C., Martin-Chouly, C., Le Moigne-Muller, G., Van Herreweghe, F., et al., 2012. TRAIL induces necroptosis involving RIPK1/RIPK3-dependent PARP-1 activation. Cell Death Differ. 19, 2003–2014.

Kerr, J.F., Wyllie, A.H., Currie, A.R., 1972. Apoptosis: a basic biological phenomenon with wide-ranging implications in tissue kinetics. Br. J. Cancer. 26, 239–257.

Kessenbrock, K., Krumbholz, M., Schonermarck, U., Back, W., Gross, W.L., Werb, Z., et al., 2009. Netting neutrophils in autoimmune small-vessel vasculitis. Nat. Med. 15, 623–625.

Knight, J.S., Kaplan, M.J., 2012. Lupus neutrophils: "NET" gain in understanding lupus pathogenesis. Curr. Opin. Rheumatol. 24, 441–450.

Kokkola, R., Li, J., Sundberg, E., Aveberger, A.C., Palmblad, K., Yang, H., et al., 2003. Successful treatment of collagen-induced arthritis in mice and rats by targeting extracellular high mobility group box chromosomal protein 1 activity. Arthritis Rheum. 48, 2052–2058.

Kono, D.H., Theofilopoulos, A.N., 2000. Genetics of systemic autoimmunity in mouse models of lupus. Int. Rev. Immunol. 19, 367–387.

Krishnakumar, R., Kraus, W.L., 2010. The PARP side of the nucleus: molecular actions, physiological outcomes, and clinical targets. Mol. Cell. 39, 8–24.

Kroemer, G., Galluzzi, L., Brenner, C., 2007. Mitochondrial membrane permeabilization in cell death. Physiol. Rev. 87, 99–163.

Kroemer, G., Galluzzi, L., Vandenabeele, P., Abrams, J., Alnemri, E.S., Baehrecke, E.H., et al., 2009. Classification of cell death: recommendations of the Nomenclature Committee on Cell Death 2009. Cell Death Differ. 16, 3–11.

Lartigue, L., Kushnareva, Y., Seong, Y., Lin, H., Faustin, B., Newmeyer, D.D., 2009. Caspase-independent mitochondrial cell death results from loss of respiration, not cytotoxic protein release. Mol. Biol. Cell. 20, 4871–4884.

Lauber, K., Bohn, E., Krober, S.M., Xiao, Y.J., Blumenthal, S.G., Lindemann, R.K., et al., 2003. Apoptotic cells induce migration of phagocytes via caspase-3-mediated release of a lipid attraction signal. Cell. 113, 717–730.

Lavrik, I.N., Krammer, P.H., 2011. Regulation of CD95/Fas signaling at the DISC. Cell Death Differ. 19, 36–41.

Leadbetter, E.A., Rifkin, I.R., Hohlbaum, A.M., Beaudette, B.C., Shlomchik, M.J., Marshak-Rothstein, A., 2002. Chromatin-IgG complexes activate B cells by dual engagement of IgM and Toll-like receptors. Nature 416, 603–607.

Leibowitz, B., Yu, J., 2010. Mitochondrial signaling in cell death via the Bcl-2 family. Cancer Biol. Ther. 9, 417–422.

Lleo, A., Selmi, C., Invernizzi, P., Podda, M., Coppel, R.L., Mackay, I. R., et al., 2009. Apotopes and the biliary specificity of primary biliary cirrhosis. Hepatology 49, 871–879.

Lleo, A., Shimoda, S., Ishibashi, H., Gershwin, M.E., 2011. Primary biliary cirrhosis and autoimmune hepatitis: apotopes and epitopes. J. Gastroenterol. 46 (Suppl. 1), 29–38.

Lockshin, R.A., Zakeri, Z., 2001. Programmed cell death and apoptosis: origins of the theory. Nat. Rev. Mol. Cell Biol. 2, 545–550.

Lu, Q., Lemke, G., 2001. Homeostatic regulation of the immune system by receptor tyrosine kinases of the Tyro 3 family. Science 293, 306–311.

Luo, X., Kraus, W.L., 2012. On PAR with PARP: cellular stress signaling through poly(ADP-ribose) and PARP-1. Genes Dev. 26, 417–432.

Marshak-Rothstein, A., Rifkin, I.R., 2007. Immunologically active autoantigens: the role of toll-like receptors in the development of chronic inflammatory disease. Annu. Rev. Immunol. 25, 419–441.

Martin, S.J., Reutelingsperger, C.P., Mcgahon, A.J., Rader, J.A., Van Schie, R.C., Laface, D.M., et al., 1995. Early redistribution of plasma membrane phosphatidylserine is a general feature of apoptosis regardless of the initiating stimulus: inhibition by overexpression of Bcl-2 and Abl. J. Exp. Med. 182, 1545–1556.

Matzinger, P., 2002. The danger model: a renewed sense of self. Science 296, 301–305.

Mevorach, D., Zhou, J.L., Song, X., Elkon, K.B., 1998. Systemic exposure to irradiated apoptotic cells induces autoantibody production. J. Exp. Med. 188, 387–392.

Mills, J.C., Stone, N.L., Pittman, R.N., 1999. Extranuclear apoptosis. The role of the cytoplasm in the execution phase. J. Cell Biol. 146, 703–708.

Mitchell, D.A., Pickering, M.C., Warren, J., Fossati-Jimack, L., Cortes-Hernandez, J., Cook, H.T., et al., 2002. C1q deficiency and autoimmunity: the effects of genetic background on disease expression. J. Immunol. 168, 2538–2543.

Miyake, Y., Yamasaki, S., 2012. Sensing necrotic cells. Adv. Exp. Med. Biol. 738, 144–152.

Moubarak, R.S., Yuste, V.J., Artus, C., Bouharrour, A., Greer, P.A., Menissier-De, M., et al., 2007. Sequential activation of poly(ADP-ribose) polymerase 1, Calpains, and Bax is essential in apoptosis-inducing factor-mediated programmed necrosis. Mol. Cell. Biol. 27, 4844–4862.

Munoz, L.E., Janko, C., Grossmayer, G.E., Frey, B., Voll, R.E., Kern, P., et al., 2009. Remnants of secondarily necrotic cells fuel inflammation in systemic lupus erythematosus. Arthritis Rheum. 60, 1733–1742.

Munoz, L.E., Lauber, K., Schiller, M., Manfredi, A.A., Herrmann, M., 2010. The role of defective clearance of apoptotic cells in systemic autoimmunity. Nat. Rev. Rheumatol. 6, 280–289.

Nagata, S., 2005. DNA degradation in development and programmed cell death. Annu. Rev. Immunol. 23, 853–875.

Nagata, S., Hanayama, R., Kawane, K., 2010. Autoimmunity and the clearance of dead cells. Cell. 140, 619–630.

Nagata, S., Nagase, H., Kawane, K., Mukae, N., Fukuyama, H., 2003. Degradation of chromosomal DNA during apoptosis. Cell Death Differ. 10, 108–116.

Oliveira, J.B., Bleesing, J.J., Dianzani, U., Fleisher, T.A., Jaffe, E.S., Lenardo, M.J., et al., 2010. Revised diagnostic criteria and classification for the autoimmune lymphoproliferative syndrome (ALPS): report from the 2009 NIH International Workshop. Blood 116, e35—e40.

Orlando, K.A., Stone, N.L., Pittman, R.N., 2006. Rho kinase regulates fragmentation and phagocytosis of apoptotic cells. Exp. Cell Res. 312, 5—15.

Orr Gandy, K.A., Obeid, L.M., 2013. Targeting the sphingosine kinase/sphingosine 1-phosphate pathway in disease: review of sphingosine kinase inhibitors. Biochim. Biophys. Acta. 1831, 157—166.

Radic, M., Marion, T., Monestier, M., 2004. Nucleosomes are exposed at the cell surface in apoptosis. J. Immunol. 172, 6692—6700.

Rahman, A., Isenberg, D.A., 2008. Systemic lupus erythematosus. N. Engl. J. Med. 358, 929—939.

Ravichandran, K.S., 2011. Beginnings of a good apoptotic meal: the find-me and eat-me signaling pathways. Immunity 35, 445—455.

Reed, J.H., Jackson, M.W., Gordon, T.P., 2008. B cell apotopes of the 60-kDa Ro/SSA and La/SSB autoantigens. J. Autoimmun. 31, 263—267.

Reed, J.H., Jackson, M.W., Gordon, T.P., 2010. A Ro60 apotope is cryptic on the intracellular autoantigen. Lupus. 19, 107—108.

Reed, J.H., Neufing, P.J., Jackson, M.W., Clancy, R.M., Macardle, P.J., Buyon, J.P., et al., 2007. Different temporal expression of immunodominant Ro60/60 kDa-SSA and La/SSB apotopes. Clin. Exp. Immunol. 148, 153—160.

Ren, Y., Tang, J., Mok, M.Y., Chan, A.W., Wu, A., Lau, C.S., 2003. Increased apoptotic neutrophils and macrophages and impaired macrophage phagocytic clearance of apoptotic neutrophils in systemic lupus erythematosus. Arthritis Rheum. 48, 2888—2897.

Riedl, S.J., Salvesen, G.S., 2007. The apoptosome: signalling platform of cell death. Nat. Rev. Mol. Cell Biol. 8, 405—413.

Rodriguez-Manzanet, R., Sanjuan, M.A., Wu, H.Y., Quintana, F.J., Xiao, S., Anderson, A.C., et al., 2010. T and B cell hyperactivity and autoimmunity associated with niche-specific defects in apoptotic body clearance in TIM-4-deficient mice. Proc. Natl. Acad. Sci. USA 107, 8706—8711.

Rosen, A., Casciola-Rosen, L., 1997. Macromolecular substrates for the ICE-like proteases during apoptosis. J. Cell Biochem. 64, 50—54.

Rosenbaum, D.M., Degterev, A., David, J., Rosenbaum, P.S., Roth, S., Grotta, J.C., et al., 2010. Necroptosis, a novel form of caspase-independent cell death, contributes to neuronal damage in a retinal ischemia-reperfusion injury model. J. Neurosci. Res. 88, 1569—1576.

Rothlin, C.V., Lemke, G., 2010. TAM receptor signaling and autoimmune disease. Curr. Opin. Immunol. 22, 740—746.

Rothlin, C.V., Ghosh, S., Zuniga, E.I., Oldstone, M.B., Lemke, G., 2007. TAM receptors are pleiotropic inhibitors of the innate immune response. Cell. 131, 1124—1136.

Rovere, P., Vallinoto, C., Bondanza, A., Crosti, M.C., Rescigno, M., Ricciardi-Castagnoli, P., et al., 1998. Bystander apoptosis triggers dendritic cell maturation and antigen-presenting function. J. Immunol. 161, 4467—4471.

Sancho, D., Reis e Sousa, C., 2012. Signaling by myeloid C-type lectin receptors in immunity and homeostasis. Annu. Rev. Immunol. 30, 491—529.

Sawamura, T., Kakino, A., Fujita, Y., 2012. LOX-1: a multiligand receptor at the crossroads of response to danger signals. Curr. Opin. Lipidol. 23, 439—445.

Scaffidi, C., Schmitz, I., Krammer, P.H., Peter, M.E., 1999. The role of c-FLIP in modulation of CD95-induced apoptosis. J. Biol. Chem. 274, 1541—1548.

Schreiber, V., Dantzer, F., Ame, J.C., De Murcia, G., 2006. Poly(ADP-ribose): novel functions for an old molecule. Nat. Rev. Mol. Cell Biol. 7, 517—528.

Scott, R.S., Mcmahon, E.J., Pop, S.M., Reap, E.A., Caricchio, R., Cohen, P.L., et al., 2001. Phagocytosis and clearance of apoptotic cells is mediated by MER. Nature 411, 207—211.

Sica, A., Mantovani, A., 2012. Macrophage plasticity and polarization: in vivo veritas. J. Clin. Invest. 122, 787—795.

Soriano, F.G., Liaudet, L., Szabo, E., Virag, L., Mabley, J.G., Pacher, P., et al., 2002. Resistance to acute septic peritonitis in poly(ADP-ribose) polymerase-1-deficient mice. Shock 17, 286—292.

Stranges, P.B., Watson, J., Cooper, C.J., Choisy-Rossi, C.M., Stonebraker, A.C., Beighton, R.A., et al., 2007. Elimination of antigen-presenting cells and autoreactive T cells by Fas contributes to prevention of autoimmunity. Immunity 26, 629—641.

Strasser, A., Whittingham, S., Vaux, D.L., Bath, M.L., Adams, J.M., Cory, S., et al., 1991. Enforced BCL2 expression in B-lymphoid cells prolongs antibody responses and elicits autoimmune disease. Proc. Natl. Acad. Sci. USA 88, 8661—8665.

Sulston, J.E., Horvitz, H.R., 1977. Post-embryonic cell lineages of the nematode, Caenorhabditis elegans. Dev. Biol. 56, 110—156.

Takahashi, T., Tanaka, M., Brannan, C.I., Jenkins, N.A., Copeland, N.G., Suda, T., et al., 1994. Generalized lymphoproliferative disease in mice, caused by a point mutation in the Fas ligand. Cell 76, 969—976.

Tanaka, Y., Schroit, A.J., 1983. Insertion of fluorescent phosphatidylserine into the plasma membrane of red blood cells. Recognition by autologous macrophages. J. Biol. Chem. 258, 11335—11343.

Tischner, D., Woess, C., Ottina, E., Villunger, A., 2011. Bcl-2-regulated cell death signalling in the prevention of autoimmunity. Cell Death Dis. 1, e48.

Tran, H.B., Macardle, P.J., Hiscock, J., Cavill, D., Bradley, J., Buyon, J.P., et al., 2002. Anti-La/SSB antibodies transported across the placenta bind apoptotic cells in fetal organs targeted in neonatal lupus. Arthritis Rheum. 46, 1572—1579.

Truman, L.A., Ford, C.A., Pasikowska, M., Pound, J.D., Wilkinson, S.J., Dumitriu, I.E., et al., 2008. CX3CL1/fractalkine is released from apoptotic lymphocytes to stimulate macrophage chemotaxis. Blood 112, 5026—5036.

Utz, P.J., Hottelet, M., Schur, P.H., Anderson, P., 1997. Proteins phosphorylated during stress-induced apoptosis are common targets for autoantibody production in patients with systemic lupus erythematosus. J. Exp. Med. 185, 843—854.

Vandenabeele, P., Galluzzi, L., Vanden Berghe, T., Kroemer, G., 2010. Molecular mechanisms of necroptosis: an ordered cellular explosion. Nat. Rev. Mol. Cell Biol. 11, 700—714.

Vandivier, R.W., Ogden, C.A., Fadok, V.A., Hoffmann, P.R., Brown, K.K., Botto, M., et al., 2002. Role of surfactant proteins A, D, and C1q in the clearance of apoptotic cells in vivo and in vitro: calreticulin and CD91 as a common collectin receptor complex. J. Immunol. 169, 3978—3986.

Varfolomeev, E., Maecker, H., Sharp, D., Lawrence, D., Renz, M., Vucic, D., et al., 2005. Molecular determinants of kinase pathway activation by Apo2 ligand/tumor necrosis factor-related apoptosis-inducing ligand. J. Biol. Chem. 280, 40599—40608.

Voll, R.E., Herrmann, M., Roth, E.A., Stach, C., Kalden, J.R., Girkontaite, I., 1997. Immunosuppressive effects of apoptotic cells. Nature 390, 350–351.

Wang, X., Wu, Y.C., Fadok, V.A., Lee, M.C., Gengyo-Ando, K., Cheng, L.C., et al., 2003. Cell corpse engulfment mediated by C. elegans phosphatidylserine receptor through CED-5 and CED-12. Science 302, 1563–1566.

Welz, P.S., Wullaert, A., Vlantis, K., Kondylis, V., Fernandez-Majada, V., Ermolaeva, M., et al., 2011. FADD prevents RIP3-mediated epithelial cell necrosis and chronic intestinal inflammation. Nature 477, 330–334.

Wiley, S.R., Schooley, K., Smolak, P.J., Din, W.S., Huang, C.P., Nicholl, J.K., et al., 1995. Identification and characterization of a new member of the TNF family that induces apoptosis. Immunity 3, 673–682.

Wu, X., Molinaro, C., Johnson, N., Casiano, C.A., 2001. Secondary necrosis is a source of proteolytically modified forms of specific intracellular autoantigens: implications for systemic autoimmunity. Arthritis Rheum. 44, 2642–2652.

Yousefi, S., Gold, J.A., Andina, N., Lee, J.J., Kelly, A.M., Kozlowski, E., et al., 2008. Catapult-like release of mitochondrial DNA by eosinophils contributes to antibacterial defense. Nat. Med. 14, 949–953.

Zetterstrom, C.K., Jiang, W., Wahamaa, H., Ostberg, T., Aveberger, A.C., Schierbeck, H., et al., 2008. Pivotal advance: inhibition of HMGB1 nuclear translocation as a mechanism for the anti-rheumatic effects of gold sodium thiomalate. J. Leukoc. Biol. 83, 31–38.

Chapter 18

Autophagy in Autoimmunity

Jan Lünemann and Christian Münz

Institute of Experimental Immunology, University of Zürich, Switzerland

Chapter Outline

Autophagy Pathways	257	Autophagy in Tolerance and Autoimmunity	260
Autophagy in Innate Immunity	258	Future Prospects	260
Autophagy in Lymphocyte Development and Activation	258	References	261
Antigen Presentation for CD4+ and CD8+ T Cell Recognition	259		

Autophagy is a homeostatic process that enables eukaryotic cells to deliver cytoplasmic constituents for lysosomal degradation, to recycle nutrients, and to survive during starvation (Klionsky, 2007; Levine and Kroemer, 2008). The term autophagy, derived from Greek and meaning "eating of self," was first coined by Christian de Duve over 40 years ago to explain earlier electron microscopic observations of mitochondrial degradation in double-membrane vesicles, a process that had been named autolysis. In keeping with this clearance function, at least one of the autophagic pathways, called macroautophagy, assists in the restriction and elimination of intracellular pathogens as an innate immune response to viral and microbial infection. In addition, macroautophagy regulates CD4+ T cell-mediated immune responses to intracellular self and pathogen-derived proteins by delivering intracellular and extracellular antigens major histocompatibility complex (MHC) class II antigen-loading compartments (MIIC) (Schmid et al., 2007b; Nedjic et al., 2008). Here, we provide an introduction to autophagy as an innate immune defense mechanism, highlight its role in the initiation and execution of adaptive immune responses, and discuss its possible role in the development of autoimmune tissue inflammation.

AUTOPHAGY PATHWAYS

Today, three separate pathways have been identified that transport cytoplasmic content into lysosomes for degradation: microautophagy, chaperone-mediated autophagy (CMA), and macroautophagy which has more particular relevance to autoimmunity and so is the type given attention in this chapter. Microautophagy is characterized by the uptake of cytoplasmic components at the lysosomal membrane via budding into the lysosome, through poorly defined mechanisms. During CMA, proteins are directly imported into lysosomes through the lysosomal-associated membrane protein 2a (LAMP-2a) transporter (Cuervo and Dice, 1996, 2000) assisted by cytosolic and lysosomal heat shock cognate protein 70 (HSC70) chaperones. Substrates of chaperone-mediated autophagy carry signal peptides for sorting into lysosomes, similar to other protein transport mechanisms across membranes (Agarraberes and Dice, 2001). Macroautophagy is the major route of degradation of cytoplasmic constituents; macroautophagy assembles a vesicle around the cargo, which is destined for degradation. This vesicle, called the autophagosome, envelops its substrate with two membranes. The autophagsosome fuses with late endosomes and lysosomes to amphisomes and autolysosomes, respectively. In these fusion vesicles, the inner autophagosome membrane and the autophagosome cargo are degraded by lysosomal hydrolysis.

Two ubiquitin-like systems participate in this process which is mediated by evolutionary conserved proteins known as autophagy-related (Atg) proteins. These ubiquitin-like systems can be monitored as well as targeted to investigate the function of macroautophagy in innate and adaptive immune responses. One of these systems, Atg8/LC3, is processed by the cytosolic protease Atg4 to cleave off five C-terminal amino acids and to make a C-terminal glycine residue (G120) accessible. Atg8/LC3 is then activated by the E1-like enzyme Atg7

N. Rose & I. Mackay (Eds): The Autoimmune Diseases, Fifth edition. DOI: http://dx.doi.org/10.1016/B978-0-12-384929-8.00018-6

and conjugated by the E2-like enzyme Atg3 to phosphatidylethanolamine (PE) on the outside and inside of the assembling autophagosome membrane. Whereas Atg8/LC3 gets recycled from the outer membrane after completion of the autophagosome by Atg4, Atg8/LC3, which is coupled to the inner membrane, stays associated with the autophagic vesicle and is degraded with this membrane by lysosomal hydrolysis. This conjugation of Atg8/LC3 to the autophagosomal membrane might serve two purposes. It facilitates membrane fusion during the elongation of the autophagosome membrane (Nakatogawa et al., 2007; Weidberg et al., 2011). In addition, it allows for recruitment of substrates into autophagosomes via Atg8/LC3 binding anchor proteins (Kirkin et al., 2009). In the other ubiquitin-like system, Atg12 gets coupled through its C-terminal glycine residue (G140) to a lysine residue of Atg5 by the E1- and E2-like enzymes Atg7 and Atg10. The Atg12—Atg5 complex associates with Atg16 and then binds to the outer surface of the isolation membrane. This complex mediates Atg8/LC3 conjugation to the autophagosome membrane as an E3-like enzyme (Fujita et al., 2008). Upon completion of the autophagosome, the Atg5—Atg12—Atg16 complex dissociates from the outer autophagosomal membrane and only Atg8/LC3 remains associated with the completed autophagosome. Autophagosomes then fuse with late endosomes and lysosomes for degradation of their cargo and their intravesicular membranes.

AUTOPHAGY IN INNATE IMMUNITY

As an innate immune response to viral and microbial pathogens, macroautophagy participates in limiting pathogen replication in host cells. Bacteria and parasites that either escape from endosomes and replicate in the cytosol or condition the phagosome to serve as their replication niche—by preventing fusion with lysosomes—have been found to be delivered for lysosomal degradation via macroautophagy (Gutierrez et al., 2004; Nakagawa et al., 2004; Singh et al., 2006). Innate immune responses to microbial antigens are mediated through stimulation of pattern-recognition receptors (PRRs) which include Toll-like receptors, nucleotide-binding and oligomerization domain (NOD)-like receptors, retinoic-acid-inducible gene I (RIG-I)-like helicases, and a subset of C-type lectin receptors which endow cells of the innate immune system with the ability to recognize a large number of molecular patterns expressed by bacteria, viruses, or fungi. Recent data have revealed an intricate, mutual interplay between PRRs and macroautophagy, whereby macroautophagy on the one hand facilitates the recognition of cognate ligands by PRRs by fostering their physical interaction, and on the other hand serves as an immune effector mechanism downstream of PRR stimulation. For example, cytosolic viral replication intermediates of single-stranded RNA (ssRNA) viruses, recognized by PRRs, are delivered to endosomally located TLR7 by macroautophagy, which results in robust type I interferon-dependent innate immune responses by plasmacytoid dendritic cells (pDCs) (Lee et al., 2007). PRR signaling and cytokines such as interferons (IFNs) and members of the tumor necrosis factor (TNF) family can induce or augment macroautophagy, which might represent a feedback mechanism by which activated T cells augment macroautophagy under inflammatory conditions (Orvedahl et al., 2007; Xu et al., 2007; Delgado et al., 2008).

AUTOPHAGY IN LYMPHOCYTE DEVELOPMENT AND ACTIVATION

In addition to mediating innate, cell intrinsic immunity, the pro-survival function of macroautophagy also contributes to the shaping of immune system components. Most of these immune cells originate from hematopoietic progenitor cells (HPCs). This precursor cell population depends on macroautophagy for its survival (Mortensen et al., 2011; Salemi et al., 2012). Not only HPC cell numbers were not maintained upon targeted deletion of the essential macroautophagy gene Atg7 in HPCs, but also myeloproliferations were observed in the affected mice *in vivo* (Mortensen et al., 2011). This expanded myeloid compartment was probably also responsible for the increased reactive oxygen species (ROS) production, resulting in DNA damage and possibly originating from elevated mitochondria numbers. The decreased lymphocyte compartment in mice with deficient macroautophagy in HPCs already indicated that primarily the lymphocyte compartment among the immune system components is affected by macroautophagy loss. Indeed T and B cell development is compromised when macroautophagy deficiency is targeted to these lineages (Pua et al., 2007, 2009; Miller et al., 2008; Arsov et al., 2011). In mice with Atg6/Beclin-1 deficiency in the hematopoietic lineage, T and B cell precursors are diminished in thymus and bone marrow, respectively, while peripheral T and B cell compartments are largely normal (Arsov et al., 2011). The susceptibility of lymphocyte precursors could result from the biphasic expression of Atg6/Beclin-1 and resulting macroautophagic activity during development, while non-activated T and B cells then again seem to have low macroautophagy levels (Arsov et al., 2008). Upon activation, macroautophagy is then upregulated in peripheral lymphocytes, including T cells (Pua et al., 2007; Arsov et al., 2008). Part of the sensitivity of T cell development towards macroautophagy deletion is due to a requirement for mitochondria clearance (Pua et al., 2009). In absence of this clearance during the transition from thymocytes to mature T cells, elevated ROS levels and an imbalance in pro- and anti-apoptotic protein expression can be observed. The requirement during T cell activation, however, results at least in part from impaired Ca2$^+$ mobilization upon T cell receptors engagement (Jia et al., 2011). While the Ca2$^+$ storing endoplasmic reticulum is enlarged, influx of this secondary messenger upon T cell activation is impaired, resulting in reduced immune responses. While in developing B cells the transition from pro- to pre-B cells is affected by macroautophagy loss (Miller et al., 2008; Arsov et al., 2011), among mature B cells only the mostly innate B-1a subset is affected (Miller et al., 2008). In contrast to lymphocyte populations myeloid and DCs seem to be much less affected by macroautophagy deficiency. Along these lines conventional and plasmacytoid DCs are found at normal frequencies, if macroautophagy deficiency is selectively targeted to these leucocyte subsets (Lee et al., 2007, 2010). Therefore, primarily lymphocyte development and their activation are compromised upon downregulation of macroautophagy, which could, for example, result from half-life shortening or partial loss-of-function mutations in essential autophagy genes. The resulting changes in immune system responsiveness could also affect tolerizing mechanisms like regulatory T cell populations.

ANTIGEN PRESENTATION FOR CD4$^+$ AND CD8$^+$ T CELL RECOGNITION

In addition to regulating T cell development and activation, macroautophagy also contributes to the shaping of the T cell repertoire via self-protein processing for MHC class II presentation. T cells recognize proteolytic fragments of proteins that are presented on MHC molecules. MHC class I molecules present primarily proteasomal products to CD8$^+$ T cells, while MHC class II molecules present ligands generated by lysosomal degradation to CD4$^+$ T cells (Trombetta and Mellman, 2005). Among those peptides that can be eluted from affinity purified MHC class II molecules around 20–30% originate from cytosolic and nuclear antigens (Dengjel et al., 2005), which possibly reach lysosomes by an intracellular route. Interestingly, two mammalian Atg8 homologues of higher eukaryotes LC3 and GABARAP are among the source proteins for natural MHC class II ligands (Dengjel et al., 2005; Suri et al., 2008). MHC class II presentation of these peptides derived from cytosolic and nuclear antigens can be increased by 50% upon starvation, a process that also induces macroautophagy (Dengjel et al., 2005). In contrast, starvation did not affect loading of ligands from membrane bound proteins. Indeed, autophagosomes, which could deliver these self-ligands, frequently fuse with MHC class II containing compartments (MIICs),

which are used for antigen loading (Schmid et al., 2007a; van den Boorn et al., 2011). Furthermore, proteins that are incorporated into autophagosomes due to their fusion with Atg8/LC3 are up to 10-fold better presented on MHC class II molecules than their unmodified counterparts (Schmid et al., 2007a; Comber et al., 2011). These studies indicate that cytosolic and nuclear proteins gain access to MHC class II loading via macroautophagy.

The best characterized among these are the nuclear antigen 1 of the Epstein–Barr virus (EBNA1) and the bacterial transposon-derived neomycin phosphotransferase II (NeoR). EBNA1 is intracellularly processed for MHC class II presentation by Epstein–Barr virus infected B cells (Münz et al., 2000). This processing is executed by lysosomes, because EBNA1 accumulates in cytosolic vesicles upon inhibition of lysosomal proteolysis (Paludan et al., 2005). Furthermore, CD4$^+$ T cell recognition of EBNA1 expressing B cells is compromised upon RNA silencing of essential macroautophagy genes (Paludan et al., 2005; Leung et al., 2010). Inhibition of nuclear import of EBNA1 increases macroautophagy-dependent MHC class II presentation of this antigen (Leung et al., 2010). NeoR on the other hand is a cytosolic antigen, whose processing for MHC class II presentation is sensitive to macroautophagy inhibition (Nimmerjahn et al., 2003). Vice versa, antigens that are fused to NeoR are more efficiently presented to CD4$^+$ T cells via macroautophagy (Comber et al., 2011). However, in contrast to EBNA1, nuclear import of NeoR does not compromise its presentation on MHC class II molecules after macroautophagic antigen processing (Riedel et al., 2008). Therefore, nuclear localization by itself does not necessarily protect antigens from processing for MHC class II presentation via macroautophagy, suggesting that the subcompartimentalization of the antigen in the nucleus could dictate if this antigen gains access to the cytosol after nuclear envelope dissociation during mitosis and falls prey to macroautophagy.

Recent studies suggest that macroautophagy also seems to contribute to extracellular antigen processing. Atg5 deficient DCs were found to process pulsed antigen less efficiently onto MHC class II, but equally well onto MHC class I molecules when compared to their wild-type counterparts (Lee et al., 2010). This defect correlated with slower phagosome maturation, possibly due to less efficient fusion with lysosomes. Indeed, Atg8/LC3 recruitment to phagosomes has been suggested to facilitate their fusion with lysosomes (Sanjuan et al., 2007; Florey et al., 2011). Alternatively, autophagosomes could also directly deliver processing enzymes to phagosomes to increase antigenic peptide formation. Along these lines it was reported that peptidylarginine deiminase (PAD), which citrunillates endocytosed proteins and thereby gives rise to autoantigens that are recognized in some autoimmune diseases, like rheumatoid arthritis, reaches phagosomes via macroautophagy (Ireland and Unanue, 2011). Thus, support of extracellular antigen processing by the molecular machinery of macroautophagy could result from Atg8/LC-assisted fusion with lysosomes or processing enzyme delivery to phagosomes by autophagosomes.

While most of the available information points towards a role of macroautophagy for antigen processing towards MHC class II presentation, few studies also implicate this pathway in MHC class I-mediated antigen presentation to CD8$^+$ T cells. Along these lines, late during herpes simplex virus (HSV) infection of macroautophages it was observed that autophagosomes engulf viral capsids at the outer nuclear membrane (English et al., 2009). Inhibition of macroautophagy in these cells diminished MHC class I-mediated recognition of these HSV-infected cells by CD8$^+$ T cells. Furthermore, antigen donor cells seem to more efficiently package antigen for cross-presentation onto MHC class I molecules via macroautophagy (Li et al., 2008; Uhl et al., 2009). Moreover, aggregated proteins are redirected towards proteasomal degradation and MHC class I antigen processing in the absence of macroautophagy (Wenger et al., 2012). And finally, macroautophagy seems to promote the formation of cross-presenting compartments in macrophages and DCs (Luca et al., 2012). Therefore, macroautophagy seems to contribute to compartments which are beneficial for antigen processing onto MHC class I, namely nuclear membrane-derived autophagosomes, cross-presentation compartments, or exosomes for antigen transfer. Which of these pathways significantly contributes to antigen presentation to CD8$^+$ T cells *in vivo* will be an interesting topic for future studies.

AUTOPHAGY IN TOLERANCE AND AUTOIMMUNITY

The first *in vivo* situation that was identified to involve macroautophagy-mediated antigen processing for MHC class II presentation is thymic T cell selection. Recognition of self-antigen-derived epitopes presented by MHC class II molecules on thymic epithelial cells (TECs) is critical for the generation of a functional and self-tolerant CD4$^+$ T cell repertoire. TECs shape the T cell repertoire to recognize self-peptide/MHC complexes with low affinity by a process called positive selection and weed out T cells that react to these self-structures with high affinity by negative selection (Kyewski and Klein, 2006). Even though they express MHC class II molecules to fulfill these functions for CD4$^+$ T cells, their endocytic capacity is low, but autophagosomes also fuse in these cells frequently with MIICs (Kasai et al., 2009). Indeed,

when positive selection of TCR transgenic T cells through macroautophagy deficient thymi was investigated, only some T cell specificities were correctly selected, while others were deleted and loss of macroautophagy in TECs resulted in severe colitis and multi-organ inflammation (Nedjic et al., 2008). Changes in the MHC class II-presented peptide repertoire were visualized by an elevated presentation of a membrane bound protein in the absence of macroautophagy. In contrast, positive selection of CD8$^+$ T cells was not macroautophagy dependent. These data suggest that macroautophagy processes some self-ligands for MHC class II presentation that are involved in positive T cell selection in the thymus and thereby contributes to the generation of a self-tolerant T cell repertoire. In addition to its function in central tolerance induction, we find considerable macroautophagy in immature DCs (Schmid et al., 2007a), which have been implicated in peripheral tolerance induction (Steinman et al., 2003).

Another possible link between macroautophagy and autoimmune tissue inflammation independent from antigen presentation is the role of macroautophagy in the removal of apoptotic cell corpses. Rapid removal of apoptotic cell material is thought to be crucial for the prevention of tissue inflammation. Efficient elimination of apoptotic bodies during programmed cell death involves exposure of phosphatidylserine (PS) on the surface and release of lysophosphatidylcholine (LPC) by apoptotic cells. Apoptotic cells, which did not express Atg5 or Beclin-1 genes, failed to expose PS at the cell surface, and produced lower levels of LPC compared to the wild-type counterpart (Qu et al., 2007). Defective clearance of apoptotic cells has long been suggested to drive autoimmunity in patients with systemic lupus erythematosus and other autoimmune diseases (Bratton and Henson, 2005, and see Chapter 17). Therefore, macroautophagy might prevent inflammatory tissue damage and the generation of autoimmune effector responses owing to sensitization of dying cells for early recognition and non-inflammatory removal. In addition, macroautophagy might be crucial in the induction and maintenance of CD4$^+$ T cell tolerance through thymic T cell repertoire selection and by mediating peripheral CD4$^+$ T cell tolerance toward self-antigens.

FUTURE PROSPECTS

Macroautophagy in thymic epithelial cells contributes to CD4$^+$ T cell selection and is essential for the generation of a self-tolerant T cell repertoire. However, some autoreactive lymphocytes escape central tolerance induction, exit the thymus and enter the periphery as mature T cells. These circulating autoantigen-specific T cells are thought to play a key role in the initiation and perpetuation of many autoimmune diseases. Peripheral mechanisms of self-tolerance include deletion or abortive activation of autoreactive lymphocytes by APCs that express low levels of costimulators. It is currently not known whether autophagy, in addition to its function in thymic T cell selection, is involved in peripheral tolerance maintenance and which types of APCs preferentially use autophagy to regulate T cell responses.

Recent studies also suggested a role for macroautophagy in regulating intracellular antigen processing for MHC class I presentation and in packaging antigens for optimal cross-presentation on MHC class I molecules. While these additional pathways require further investigation to understand the underlying mechanisms, autophagy-mediated antigen delivery to both MHC class II and MHC class I molecules should be explored for its potential to limit inflammatory tissue damage in T cell-driven autoimmune disease and to increase the efficacy of antigen-specific tolerization strategies. Future studies might provide a more precise understanding of how and by which mechanisms autophagy regulates T cell immunity and tolerance during health and disease *in vivo* and how this pathway could be harnessed for immunotherapy.

REFERENCES

Agarraberes, F.A., Dice, J.F., 2001. A molecular chaperone complex at the lysosomal membrane is required for protein translocation. J. Cell Sci. 114, 2491–2499.

Arsov, I., Adebayo, A., Kucerova-Levisohn, M., Haye, J., MacNeil, M., Papavasiliou, F.N., et al., 2011. A role for autophagic protein Beclin 1 early in lymphocyte development. J. Immunol. 186, 2201–2209.

Arsov, I., Li, X., Matthews, G., Coradin, J., Hartmann, B., Simon, A.K., et al., 2008. BAC-mediated transgenic expression of fluorescent autophagic protein Beclin 1 reveals a role for Beclin 1 in lymphocyte development. Cell Death Differ. 15, 1385–1395.

Bratton, D.L., Henson, P.M., 2005. Autoimmunity and apoptosis, refusing to go quietly. Nat. Med. 11, 26–27.

Comber, J.D., Robinson, T.M., Siciliano, N.A., Snook, A.E., Eisenlohr, L.C., 2011. Functional macroautophagy induction by influenza a virus without a contribution to MHC-class II restricted presentation. J Virol 85, 6453–6463.

Cuervo, A.M., Dice, J.F., 1996. A receptor for the selective uptake and degradation of proteins by lysosomes. Science 273, 501–503.

Cuervo, A.M., Dice, J.F., 2000. Unique properties of lamp2a compared to other lamp2 isoforms. J. Cell Sci. 113 (Pt 24), 4441–4450.

Delgado, M.A., Elmaoued, R.A., Davis, A.S., Kyei, G., Deretic, V., 2008. Toll-like receptors control autophagy. Embo J. 27, 1110–1121.

Dengjel, J., Schoor, O., Fischer, R., Reich, M., Kraus, M., Muller, M., et al., 2005. Autophagy promotes MHC class II presentation of peptides from intracellular source proteins. Proc. Natl. Acad. Sci. USA 102, 7922–7927.

English, L., Chemali, M., Duron, J., Rondeau, C., Laplante, A., Gingras, D., et al., 2009. Autophagy enhances the presentation of endogenous viral antigens on MHC class I molecules during HSV-1 infection. Nat. Immunol. 10, 480–487.

Florey, O., Kim, S.E., Sandoval, C.P., Haynes, C.M., Overholtzer, M., 2011. Autophagy machinery mediates macroendocytic processing and entotic cell death by targeting single membranes. Nat. Cell Biol. 13, 1335–1343.

Fujita, N., Itoh, T., Omori, H., Fukuda, M., Noda, T., Yoshimori, T., 2008. The Atg16L complex specifies the site of LC3 lipidation for membrane biogenesis in autophagy. Mol. Biol. Cell. 19, 2092–2100.

Gutierrez, M.G., Master, S.S., Singh, S.B., Taylor, G.A., Colombo, M.I., Deretic, V., 2004. Autophagy is a defense mechanism inhibiting BCG and mycobacterium tuberculosis survival in infected macrophages. Cell (119), 753–766.

Ireland, J.M., Unanue, E.R., 2011. Autophagy in antigen-presenting cells results in presentation of citrullinated peptides to CD4 T cells. J. Exp. Med. 208, 2625–2632.

Jia, W., Pua, H.H., Li, Q.J., He, Y.W., 2011. Autophagy regulates endoplasmic reticulum homeostasis and calcium mobilization in T lymphocytes. J. Immunol. 186, 1564–1574.

Kasai, M., Tanida, I., Ueno, T., Kominami, E., Seki, S., Ikeda, T., et al., 2009. Autophagic compartments gain access to the MHC class II compartments in thymic epithelium. J. Immunol. 183, 7278–7285.

Kirkin, V., McEwan, D.G., Novak, I., Dikic, I., 2009. A role for ubiquitin in selective autophagy. Mol. Cell. 34, 259–269.

Klionsky, D.J., 2007. Autophagy, from phenomenology to molecular understanding in less than a decade. Nat. Rev. Mol. Cell Biol. 8, 931–937.

Kyewski, B., Klein, L., 2006. A central role for central tolerance. Annu. Rev. Immunol. 24, 571–606.

Lee, H.K., Lund, J.M., Ramanathan, B., Mizushima, N., Iwasaki, A., 2007. Autophagy-dependent viral recognition by plasmacytoid dendritic cells. Science 315, 1398–1401.

Lee, H.K., Mattei, L.M., Steinberg, B.E., Alberts, P., Lee, Y.H., Chervonsky, A., et al., 2010. In vivo requirement for Atg5 in antigen presentation by dendritic cells. Immunity 32, 227–239.

Leung, C.S., Haigh, T.A., Mackay, L.K., Rickinson, A.B., Taylor, G.S., 2010. Nuclear location of an endogenously expressed antigen, EBNA1, restricts access to macroautophagy and the range of CD4 epitope display. Proc. Natl. Acad. Sci. USA 107, 2165–2170.

Levine, B., Kroemer, G., 2008. Autophagy in the pathogenesis of disease. Cell 132, 27–42.

Li, Y., Wang, L.X., Yang, G., Hao, F., Urba, W.J., Hu, H.M., 2008. Efficient cross-presentation depends on autophagy in tumor cells. Cancer Res. 68, 6889–6895.

Luca, A.D., Iannitti, R.G., Bozza, S., Beau, R., Casagrande, A., D'Angelo, C., et al., 2012. CD4+ T cell vaccination overcomes defective cross-presentation of fungal antigens in a mouse model of chronic granulomatous disease. J. Clin. Invest. 122, 1816–1831.

Miller, B.C., Zhao, Z., Stephenson, L.M., Cadwell, K., Pua, H.H., Lee, H.K., et al., 2008. The autophagy gene ATG5 plays an essential role in B lymphocyte development. Autophagy 4, 309–314.

Mortensen, M., Soilleux, E.J., Djordjevic, G., Tripp, R., Lutteropp, M., Sadighi-Akha, E., et al., 2011. The autophagy protein Atg7 is essential for hematopoietic stem cell maintenance. J. Exp. Med. 208, 455–467.

Münz, C., Bickham, K.L., Subklewe, M., Tsang, M.L., Chahroudi, A., Kurilla, M.G., et al., 2000. Human CD4(+) T lymphocytes consistently respond to the latent Epstein-Barr virus nuclear antigen EBNA1. J. Exp. Med. 191, 1649–1660.

Nakagawa, I., Amano, A., Mizushima, N., Yamamoto, A., Yamaguchi, H., Kamimoto, T., et al., 2004. Autophagy defends cells against invading group A Streptococcus. Science 306, 1037–1040.

Nakatogawa, H., Ichimura, Y., Ohsumi, Y., 2007. Atg8, a ubiquitin-like protein required for autophagosome formation, mediates membrane tethering and hemifusion. Cell 130, 165–178.

Nedjic, J., Aichinger, M., Emmerich, J., Mizushima, N., Klein, L., 2008. Autophagy in thymic epithelium shapes the T-cell repertoire and is essential for tolerance. Nature 455, 396–400.

Nimmerjahn, F., Milosevic, S., Behrends, U., Jaffee, E.M., Pardoll, D. M., Bornkamm, G.W., et al., 2003. Major histocompatibility complex class II-restricted presentation of a cytosolic antigen by autophagy. Eur. J. Immunol. 33, 1250–1259.

Orvedahl, A., Alexander, D., Talloczy, Z., Sun, Q., Wei, Y., Zhang, W., et al., 2007. HSV-1 ICP34.5 confers neurovirulence by targeting the Beclin 1 autophagy protein. Cell Host & Microbe. 1, 23–35.

Paludan, C., Schmid, D., Landthaler, M., Vockerodt, M., Kube, D., Tuschl, T., et al., 2005. Endogenous MHC class II processing of a viral nuclear antigen after autophagy. Science 307, 593–596.

Pua, H.H., Dzhagalov, I., Chuck, M., Mizushima, N., He, Y.W., 2007. A critical role for the autophagy gene Atg5 in T cell survival and proliferation. J. Exp. Med. 204, 25–31.

Pua, H.H., Guo, J., Komatsu, M., He, Y.W., 2009. Autophagy is essential for mitochondrial clearance in mature T lymphocytes. J. Immunol. 182, 4046–4055.

Qu, X., Zou, Z., Sun, Q., Luby-Phelps, K., Cheng, P., Hogan, R.N., et al., 2007. Autophagy gene-dependent clearance of apoptotic cells during embryonic development. Cell 128, 931–946.

Riedel, A., Nimmerjahn, F., Burdach, S., Behrends, U., Bornkamm, G. W., Mautner, J., 2008. Endogenous presentation of a nuclear antigen on MHC class II by autophagy in the absence of CRM1-mediated nuclear export. Eur. J. Immunol. 38, 2090–2095.

Salemi, S., Yousefi, S., Constantinescu, M.A., Fey, M.F., Simon, H.U., 2012. Autophagy is required for self-renewal and differentiation of adult human stem cells. Cell Res. 22, 432–435.

Sanjuan, M.A., Dillon, C.P., Tait, S.W., Moshiach, S., Dorsey, F., Connell, S., et al., 2007. Toll-like receptor signalling in macrophages links the autophagy pathway to phagocytosis. Nature 450, 1253–1257.

Schmid, D., Pypaert, M., Munz, C., 2007a. Antigen-loading compartments for major histocompatibility complex class II molecules continuously receive input from autophagosomes. Immunity 26, 79–92.

Schmid, D., Pypaert, M., Münz, C., 2007b. MHC class II antigen loading compartments continuously receive input from autophagosomes. Immunity 26, 79–92.

Singh, S.B., Davis, A.S., Taylor, G.A., Deretic, V., 2006. Human IRGM induces autophagy to eliminate intracellular mycobacteria. Science. 313, 1438–1441.

Steinman, R.M., Hawiger, D., Nussenzweig, M.C., 2003. Tolerogenic dendritic cells. Annu. Rev. Immunol. 21, 685–711.

Suri, A., Walters, J.J., Rohrs, H.W., Gross, M.L., Unanue, E.R., 2008. First signature of islet β-cell-derived naturally processed peptides selected by diabetogenic class II MHC molecules. J. Immunol. 180, 3849–3856.

Trombetta, E.S., Mellman, I., 2005. Cell biology of antigen processing in vitro and in vivo. Annu. Rev. Immunol. 23, 975–1028.

Uhl, M., Kepp, O., Jusforgues-Saklani, H., Vicencio, J.M., Kroemer, G., Albert, M.L., 2009. Autophagy within the antigen donor cell facilitates efficient antigen cross-priming of virus-specific CD8+ T cells. Cell Death Differ. 16, 991–1005.

van den Boorn, J.G., Picavet, D.I., van Swieten, P.F., van Veen, H.A., Konijnenberg, D., van Veelen, P.A., et al., 2011. Skin-depigmenting agent monobenzone induces potent T-cell autoimmunity toward pigmented cells by tyrosinase haptenation and melanosome autophagy. J. Invest. Dermatol. 131, 1240–1251.

Weidberg, H., Shpilka, T., Shvets, E., Abada, A., Shimron, F., Elazar, Z., 2011. LC3 and GATE-16N termini mediate membrane fusion processes required for autophagosome biogenesis. Dev. Cell. 20, 444–454.

Wenger, T., Terawaki, S., Camosseto, V., Abdelrassoul, R., Mies, A., Catalan, N., et al., 2012. Autophagy inhibition promotes defective neosynthesized proteins storage in ALIS, and induces redirection toward proteasome processing and MHCI-restricted presentation. Autophagy 8.

Xu, Y., Jagannath, C., Liu, X.D., Sharafkhaneh, A., Kolodziejska, K.E., Eissa, N.T., 2007. Toll-like receptor 4 is a sensor for autophagy associated with innate immunity. Immunity 27, 135–144.

Chapter 19

Infectious Triggers of T Cell Autoimmunity

Daniel R. Getts[1], Meghann Teague Getts[1], Nicholas J.C. King[2], and Stephen D. Miller[1]

[1]*Department of Microbiology-Immunology and Interdepartmental Immunobiology Center, Northwestern University, Feinberg School of Medicine, Chicago, IL, USA,* [2]*The Discipline of Pathology, School of Medical Sciences, Bosch Institute, The University of Sydney, Sydney, NSW, Australia*

Chapter Outline

Introduction   263
Role of Infections in Priming of Autoreactive Immune
Responses   263
Potential Mechanisms of Infection Triggering Autoimmunity   264
   Molecular Mimicry   264
   Bystander Activation of Autoreactive Cells and Epitope
   Spreading   268
   Emerging Mechanisms of Infection-Induced Autoimmune
   Disease   268

Reciprocal Relationships of Pathogen-Derived
   Mechanisms of Autoimmunity   269
How Do these Mechanisms Lead to Autoimmune Disease?   269
   Autoimmunity Can Occur at a Site Distal to the Initiating
   Infection   270
Conclusions   270
Acknowledgments   271
References   271

INTRODUCTION

The immune system has evolved multiple mechanisms over millennia that allow it to distinguish between self- and non-self-recognition, which are critical for host preservation. Deficits in self-/non-self-discrimination can result in opportunistic infections or, on the other side of the coin, immunological overreactivity resulting in immunopathology and autoimmunity. It is therefore not surprising that multiple genetic loci that influence activation and regulation of the immune system are associated with triggering autoimmune diseases; however, clinical symptom development may only manifest after viral infections. How infection triggers autoimmunity is likely to involve multiple pathways that converge to trigger overt disease. Unfortunately, this also implies that self-reactive immune responses may be triggered by one or more pathogens. Together these factors make it difficult to associate distinct pathogens and immune response pathways with particular autoimmune diseases. Therefore, this review will discuss mechanisms through which host–pathogen interactions may trigger autoimmune disease and the mechanisms by which autoimmune disease could alter the ability of the host to control infections and regulate the immune system.

ROLE OF INFECTIONS IN PRIMING OF AUTOREACTIVE IMMUNE RESPONSES

At the level of the innate immune response, defense against invading pathogens is initially mediated by the activation of germline-encoded receptors known as pattern recognition receptors (PRR). These molecules, expressed by various cells of the innate immune system, recognize a multitude of pathogen-associated molecular patterns (PAMPS) and include Toll-like receptors (TLRs), nucleotide-binding and oligomerization domain (NOD)-like receptors (NLRs), (RIG-I)-like helicases (RLH), and a subset of C-type lectin receptors (CLR) (reviewed in Ishii et al., 2008). The signaling pathways triggered by engagement of these molecules culminate in cellular activation, the production of type I interferons, costimulatory molecules, inflammatory cytokines, and chemokines, all of which combine to initiate and direct the antimicrobial immune response. Both pathogenic antigens and

N. Rose & I. Mackay (Eds): The Autoimmune Diseases, Fifth edition. DOI: http://dx.doi.org/10.1016/B978-0-12-384929-8.00019-8

PRR-triggered inflammatory molecules drive the expansion of pathogen-specific T and B cells. Thus, by triggering PRRs, stimulating early cytokine responses by the innate immune system and enhancing the function of antigen presenting cells (APCs), pathogens act as adjuvants for the immune response, while at the same time providing an antigen source to drive T cell activation and effector function. Within this highly inflammatory environment, regulation is critical, with the failure of immune checkpoint regulation potentially resulting in bystander tissue damage and even death. It has been shown that overactive immune responses can cause fatal immune-mediated pathology in viral infections such as those caused by West Nile Virus (WNV) (Terry et al., 2012), or the generation of myelin-specific autoimmunity as observed in mice with cerebral Theiler's murine encephalomyelitis virus (TMEV) infection (Munz et al., 2009). Excluding pathogenic mechanisms driving immune pathology that do not have an antigen-specific component, there are several postulated mechanisms by which pathogenic infections can trigger autoimmune disease, most of which are supported by substantial evidence from animal models.

POTENTIAL MECHANISMS OF INFECTION TRIGGERING AUTOIMMUNITY

Molecular Mimicry

The idea that T cell receptors (TCRs) specific for microbes may cross-react with other self antigens was a concept originally brought forth by Fujinami and Oldstone (Fujinami and Oldstone, 1985, 1989). The degeneracy of antigen recognition by the TCR is now well understood, and the ability of foreign antigens to subsequently stimulate T cells that are also cross-reactive with (mimic) self antigens is very likely (Figure 19.1A). T cells have the capacity to respond to a variety of different peptides that are quite distinct from each other and peptides bound to different major histocompatibility complex (MHC) molecules can lead to cross-reactivity by the same TCR as long as the complexes share similarity in charge distribution and overall shape (Hammer et al., 1993; Gautam et al., 1994; Wucherpfennig et al., 1994; Wucherpfennig and Strominger, 1995; Hemmer et al., 1999; Lang et al., 2002; Gregersen et al., 2006). This has been further highlighted in the transplant setting where allogeneic T cell responses are stimulated by regions of the MHC molecule outside of classical peptide binding motifs critical for TCR restriction. While potentially detrimental, with respect to allograft and autoantigen recognition, this flexibility is central to many homeostatic immunologic processes, including thymic selection and the ability to generate a broad TCR repertoire capable of recognizing pathogen-derived peptides. Notwithstanding, *in vitro* studies have shown that viral peptides having some degree of

homology with self peptides can stimulate autoreactive T cells (Wucherpfennig and Strominger, 1995).

Animal models in which molecular mimicry may be a trigger of autoimmune disease are abundant. These include: Theiler's murine encephalomyelitis virus-induced demyelinating disease (TMEV-IDD), a model of human multiple sclerosis (MS) in which intracerebral TMEV infection of mice leads to an autoimmune demyelinating disorder 30–40 days post-infection (Croxford et al., 2002); *Acanthamoeba castellanii*-induced experimental autoimmune encephalomyelitis (EAE) in Swiss James Lambert (SJL) mice (Massilamany et al., 2010, 2011); herpes simplex virus (HSV) stromal keratitis, in which HSV infection leads to T cell-mediated blindness in both humans and mice; diabetes model(s); autoimmune demyelinating disease and Semliki forest virus (SFV) (Mokhtarian et al., 1999); autoimmune myocarditis associated with coxsackievirus infection (Gauntt et al., 1995); and others (Lawson, 2000). Furthermore, there exist multiple less physiological scenarios that do not necessarily aim to closely model a particular disease but highlight the potential mechanisms through which immune responses to infections could lead to autoimmunity through molecular mimicry (Table 19.1).

Multiple investigations have employed models of molecular identity, in which an exact microbial protein/epitope is transgenically expressed in a particular tissue. Under these conditions, animals are not generally susceptible to development of spontaneous autoimmune disease. Upon infection with the microbe containing the protein, however, autoimmunity in the transgenic protein-expressing organ ensues (Ohashi et al., 1991; Oldstone et al., 1991; von Herrath et al., 1994 Evans et al., 1996). Though some aspects of these approaches are perhaps predictable, they clearly indicate that T cells specific for a "self" antigen can become activated by infection with a microbe containing an identical antigen and which provides appropriate innate immune signals resulting and subsequently results in overt autoimmune disease. Even when the transgene-expressed antigen is also expressed within the thymus, so that normal mechanisms of negative selection significantly diminish the number of high affinity T cells specific for the viral/self antigen, infection eventually results in autoimmunity (von Herrath et al., 1994). These experiments indicate that even T cells with low affinity for a self antigen, as would be the case for many self antigen-specific responses, can be activated through molecular mimicry with a microbial antigen and cause disease. Similarly, in the TMEV-IDD model of MS, a severe rapid-onset central nervous system (CNS) demyelinating disease is induced by intracerebral or peripheral infection with TMEV that has been engineered to express the immunodominant myelin proteolipid protein (PLP)139–151 epitope (Olson et al., 2001).

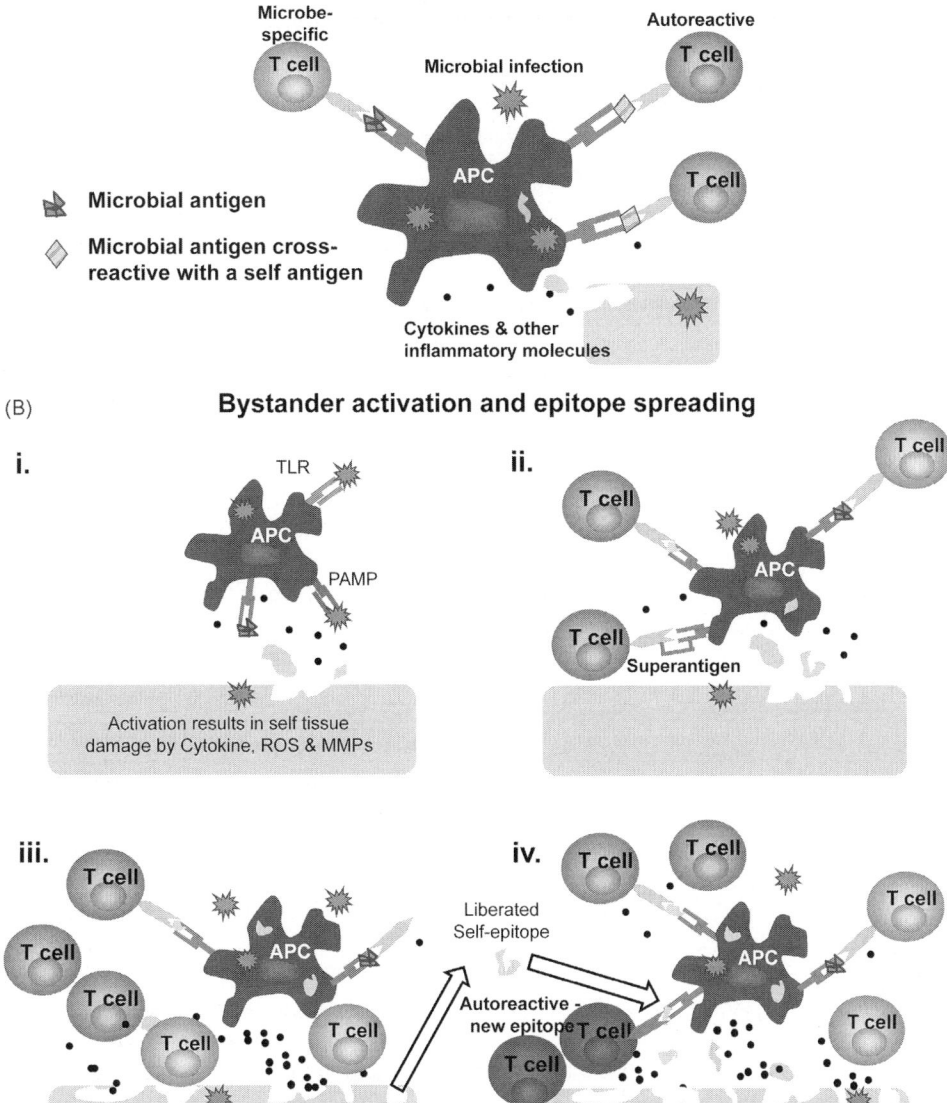

(A)

Molecular mimicry

Microbe-specific T cell

Microbial infection

Autoreactive T cell

T cell

APC

🡒 Microbial antigen

◇ Microbial antigen cross-reactive with a self antigen

Cytokines & other inflammatory molecules

(B)

Bystander activation and epitope spreading

i.

TLR

APC

PAMP

Activation results in self tissue damage by Cytokine, ROS & MMPs

ii.

T cell

T cell

T cell

APC

Superantigen

iii.

T cell

T cell

T cell

T cell

APC

T cell

iv.

T cell

T cell

T cell

APC

T cell

Liberated Self-epitope

Autoreactive new epitope T cell

T cell

FIGURE 19.1 **Mechanisms of infection-induced autoimmunity.** (A) *Molecular mimicry* occurs through cross-reactive recognition between a microbial antigen/self MHC complex and a self antigen/self MHC complex. (B) i, Microbial pathogen associated molecular patterns (PAMPs) stimulate an immune response leading to tissue destruction via inflammatory mediators originating from cells of the innate immune system. ii, During *bystander activation*, engulfment of self tissue debris leads to self antigen presentation to autoreactive T cells (concomitant with presentation of virus antigen to virus-specific T cells). Alternatively an infection can lead to microbial *superantigen*-induced activation of a subset of T cells, some of which are specific for self antigen. iii, T cell-mediated tissue destruction along with innate immune cell-derived inflammatory molecule-mediated destruction leads to release of endogenous self epitopes from tissue. iv, During *epitope spreading*, the response spreads to T cells specific for additional endogenous self antigens. TLR—Toll-like receptor; PAMP—pathogen-associated molecular pattern; ROS—reactive oxygen species; MMP—matrix metalloproteinase.

Several bacterially- and virally-derived peptides that mimic PLP$_{139-151}$ have been identified (Carrizosa et al., 1998), and these have been used in models that more directly address the possibility of molecular mimicry-induced autoimmune disease. TMEV engineered to express peptides derived from *Haemophilus influenzae* (TMEV-HI—sharing 6/13 amino acids) or murine hepatitis virus (TMEV-MHV—sharing only 3/13 amino acids), induces a rapid onset, severe demyelinating disease that is similar to that induced by infection with TMEV containing PLP$_{139-151}$ itself (Olson et al., 2001; Croxford et al., 2006). The *H. influenzae* mimic can also be processed and presented out of its own native flanking sequences

when larger portions of the bacterial protein are expressed in TMEV, more rigorously supporting a potential role for molecular mimicry in a natural infection (Croxford et al., 2005). Relevant to human disease, bacterially-derived peptide mimics of the myelin basic protein (MBP) 85−99 epitope induce demyelinating disease in mice that transgenically express a human MBP$_{85-99}$-specific TCR as well as a humanized MHC class II molecule (Greene et al., 2008). Molecular mimicry was also demonstrated in a model of diabetes in which lymphocytic choriomeningitis virus (LCMV) nucleoprotein (NP) was expressed under the rat insulin promoter (RIP). Infection with Pichinde virus, which contains an epitope that mimics a

TABLE 19.1 Selected Pathogen-Induced Murine Models of Human Autoimmune Disease

Relevant Human Disease	Mouse Model/Infectious Agent	Proposed Mechanism(s) of Autoimmunity	Comment	References
MS	TMEV-IDD	Bystander activation/ Epitope spreading	Natural virus-induced autoimmune disease of mice	(Miller et al., 1997)
	TMEV transgenically expressing PLP$_{139-151}$	Molecular identity		(Olson et al., 2001)
	TMEV transgenically expressing PLP$_{139-151}$ mimics	Molecular mimicry		(Croxford et al., 2005, 2006)
	Coxsackievirus B4 transgenically expressing PLP$_{139-151}$	Molecular identity	Infection can be at a site distant from where autoimmunity occurs	In preparation (S.D. Miller)
	LCMV infection of mice expressing LCMV proteins in the CNS	Molecular identity		(Evans et al., 1996)
	Semliki forest virus (SFV) infection	Molecular mimicry	Immunization with ACA specific peptides NAD 108–120 results in EAE	(Mokhtarian et al., 1999)
	Acanthamoeba castellanii	Molecular mimicry		(Massilamany et al., 2011)
T1D	Coxsackie B4 virus infection	Bystander activation		(Horwitz et al., 1998)
	LCMV infection of mice expressing LCMV protein in the pancreas	Molecular identity	TCR affinity for the LCMV peptide determines rapidity and severity of autoimmune disease	(Ohashi et al., 1991; Oldstone et al., 1991; von Herrath et al., 1994)
	Pichinde virus infection of mice expressing LCMV protein in the pancreas	Molecular mimicry	Autoimmunity can only be accelerated, not initiated *de novo*, in this model	(Christen et al., 2004)
Myocarditis	Mouse cytomegalovirus infection	Bystander activation or molecular mimicry	Circumstantial evidence points to molecular mimicry, but does not exclude bystander activation	(Lawson et al., 1992; Lawson, 2000; Fairweather et al., 2001)
	Coxsackievirus B3 infection	Molecular mimicry		(Gauntt et al., 1995; Lawson, 2000; Fairweather et al., 2001)
Stromal keratitis	Corneal HSV infection—induced stromal keratitis (HSK)	Molecular mimicry/ bystander activation	Some controversy over which mechanism is responsible	(Zhao et al., 1998; Benoist and Mathis, 2001; Deshpande et al., 2001)

subdominant epitope within the LCMV NP, accelerated autoimmune disease that had already been established by previous infection with LCMV (Christen et al., 2004). HSV-induced stromal keratitis is mediated by anti-corneal antigen-specific T cell responses that are induced upon corneal HSV infection. This is a non-synthetic, natural model of autoimmune disease in which molecular mimicry can occur in the absence of genetic manipulation (Zhao et al., 1998). Though the results from these experiments were called into question by a later study in which HSV-induced stromal keratitis could be induced in mice in the absence of T cell responses against HSV (Deshpande et al., 2001), since different model systems were used, the strong case for molecular mimicry put forth by the former study, in particular the genetic contribution to it, has yet to be ruled out (Benoist and Mathis, 2001).

In addition to these animal models, patients with autoimmune diseases such as systemic lupus erythematosus (SLE), rheumatoid arthritis (RA), and multiple sclerosis (MS) show higher frequencies, activation states and/or less costimulatory requirements of self-reactive lymphocytes (Lovett-Racke et al., 1998; Markovic-Plese et al., 2001; Bielekova et al., 2004; Samuels et al., 2005; Yurasov et al., 2005). In MS, receptor analysis of T and B cells in CNS tissue and cerebrospinal fluid (CSF) demonstrated

TABLE 19.2 Virus Pathogens Implicated in Human Autoimmune Diseases

Pathogen	Autoimmune Disease	Evidence	Selected References
RNA viruses			
Coxsackievirus	T1D	• Altered immune responses • Enterovirus positive beta cells detected in pancreata from T1D subjects • Experimental infection causes T1D	(Horwitz et al., 1998, 2002; Jones and Crosby, 1996; Ylipaasto et al., 2004)
Rubella virus	T1D	• Tropism for pancreatic beta cells • Molecular mimicry	(Menser et al., 1978; Ou et al., 2000)
HTLV-1	HTLV-1 associated myelopathy	• Molecular mimicry	(Levin et al., 2002)
Measles virus	MS	• Infection can result in demyelination, higher titers of virus-specific IgG and increased frequencies of virus-specific T cells in the CSF	(Jarius et al., 2009; Johnson et al., 1984; Link et al., 1992)
DNA viruses			
HHV1/HSV1	Autoimmune stromal keratitis	• Molecular mimicry	(Zhao et al., 1998)
HHV4/EBV	MS	• Increased risk to develop MS after primary symptomatic infection • Increased antibody responses in healthy individuals who will develop MS • Increased seroprevalence • Altered T cell and humoral immune responses • Molecular mimicry • Localization in diseased tissue	(Ascherio and Munch, 2000; Levin et al., 2005; Lunemann et al., 2006, 2008b, c; Nielsen et al., 2007; Serafini et al., 2007; Sundstrom et al., 2004; Thacker et al., 2006)
	RA	• Altered immune responses • Higher viral loads in circulating blood cells • Localization in diseased tissues	(Alspaugh et al., 1981; Balandraud et al., 2003; Lunemann et al., 2008a; Scotet et al., 1996; Tosato et al., 1981, 1984)
	SLE	• Increased seroprevalence • Altered immune responses • Increased viral load • Molecular mimicry	(Gross et al., 2005; Kang et al., 2004; McClain et al., 2005)
HHV6	MS	• Localization in diseased tissue • Heightened immune responses	(Challoner et al., 1995; Soldan et al., 1997)
Torque Teno virus	MS	• Localization in diseased tissue • Clonally expanded CSF-infiltrating T cells recognize virus-encoded antigen	(Sospedra et al., 2005)
Parvovirus B19	RA	• Phenotype of acute infection can mimic early RA • Detection of viral DNA in synovial tissue	(Kozireva et al., 2008; Saal et al., 1992)
	SLE	• Phenotype of acute infection can mimic early SLE • SLE patients. Increased frequency of virus carriers	(Seve et al., 2005)

clonal expansions in both populations, indicating clonal reactivity to a restricted number of disease-relevant antigens (Baranzini et al., 1999; Babbe et al., 2000; Skulina et al., 2004) and longitudinal studies provided evidence for long-term persistence of individual myelin-specific T cell clones tracked over several years in the blood of patients with MS (Meinl et al., 1993; Goebels et al., 2000; Muraro et al., 2003), indicating a strong, persisting memory response and/or ongoing autoantigen exposure at least for a subset of myelin-reactive T cells in MS.

These memory responses may reflect, at least in part, persisting clonal expansions of poly-specific T cells recognizing both self and virus antigens that have been found associated with human autoimmune diseases (Table 19.2). For example, the high viral loads that occur during symptomatic primary Epstein-Barr virus (EBV) infection, infectious mononucleosis (IM), are associated with an increased risk of developing MS (Thacker et al., 2006; Nielsen et al., 2007), and could prime these poly-specific T cell responses. Viral titers in circulating blood cells from patients with MS are, however, similar to those detectable in healthy virus carriers (Lunemann et al., 2006) and patients with MS do not differ from healthy EBV carriers in the rate of EBV-induced B cell transformation or in their ability to control outgrowth of EBV-infected B cells *in vitro* (Lunemann et al., 2008c). This argues against an increased viral replication or impaired immune control of chronic EBV infection in MS. Yet, patients with MS show predominant expansions of T cells specific for the EBV-encoded nuclear antigen 1 (EBNA1), the most consistently recognized EBV-derived CD4$^+$ T cell antigen in healthy virus carriers, and EBNA1-specific T cells recognize myelin antigens more frequently than other autoantigens not associated with MS (Lunemann et al., 2008c). Notably, myelin cross-reactive T cells produce IFN-γ but differ from EBNA1-monospecific cells in their capability to produce interleukin-2, indicative of poly-functional T cells, which are thought to be particularly important under conditions of antigen persistence and high antigen load because they are less susceptible to exhaustion or activation-induced cell death (Harari et al., 2007). Consistent with these considerations, a more extensive priming of poly-functional cross-reactive T cells during symptomatic primary EBV infection with high viral loads, and continuous restimulation caused by autoimmune tissue inflammation could potentially establish and maintain a distinct repertoire of myelin-reactive virus-specific T cells, which could predispose to MS.

Bystander Activation of Autoreactive Cells and Epitope Spreading

APCs activated within the inflammatory milieu of a pathogenic infection can stimulate activation and expansion of auto-reactive T or B cells in a process known as bystander activation. In this case, APCs present self antigen, obtained subsequent to tissue destruction and/or uptake of local dying cells, to autoreactive cells (Walker and Abbas, 2002; Zipris et al., 2005) (Figure 19.1B). Related to this concept is the mechanism of epitope spreading, a situation in which an immune response, initiated by any number of stimuli including microbial infection, trauma, transplanted tissue, antitumor responses, or autoimmunity, spreads to include responses directed against a different antigen on the same protein (intramolecular spreading) or on a different protein (intermolecular spreading) (Figure 19.1B). Activating a broader set of T cells through epitope spreading is helpful in an antipathogen or antitumor response, but disease may potentially arise when spread to and within self proteins occurs subsequent to self tissue destruction. Epitope spreading in animal models

proceeds in an orderly, directed, and hierarchical manner, such that more immunodominant epitopes elicit responses first, followed by less dominant responses. This type of spreading has been shown in EAE, a non-infectious model of MS (McRae et al., 1995; Yu et al., 1996), as well as in TMEV-IDD (Miller et al., 1997; Borrow et al., 1998; Katz-Levy et al., 1999, 2000), and in the non-obese diabetic (NOD) mouse model of type 1 diabetes (Kaufman et al., 1993; Prasad et al., 2012).

An even broader bystander activation is achieved by cross-linking T cell receptors of a given Vβ domain with microbial-derived superantigens presented by MHC class II molecules on APCs. The polyclonal population of T cells stimulated in this fashion could potentially contain a subset of T cells specific for a self antigen (Wucherpfennig, 2001). This mechanism is potentially highly relevant in the human context, where, unlike mice, T cells express human leukocyte antigen (HLA) and can present antigen to each other. In addition, there are multiple examples where superantigens have been shown to influence pathogenesis of diseases such as EAE, arthritis, and inflammatory bowel disease, making superantigens another mechanism by which bystander activation can initiate, or minimally exacerbate, autoimmunity in mouse models (Brocke et al., 1993; Cole and Griffiths, 1993; Dalwadi et al., 2001) (Table 19.1). Furthermore, association of certain genotypes of the superantigen-encoding endogenous retrovirus HERV-K18, which is transactivated by EBV (Sutkowski et al., 2001), with MS has been reported (Tai et al., 2008). However, Vβ7 and Vβ13 positive T cells, which are stimulated by the retroviral superantigen, do not seem to be selectively expanded in MS patients. Nevertheless, viral antigen-specific and/or superantigen-expanded T cells might participate in the development or maintenance of autoimmune disease.

Emerging Mechanisms of Infection-Induced Autoimmune Disease

Infections affect the immune response in many ways, and mechanisms such as molecular mimicry and bystander activation are certainly not the only ways in which pathogens trigger or accelerate autoimmune disease. A recent study showed that in a spontaneous animal model of SLE, lipid raft aggregation on T cells, which was induced by cholera toxin B from *Vibrio cholerae* in the study but could be induced by a number of microbes or toxins, enhanced T cell signaling and exacerbated SLE (Deng and Tsokos, 2008; James and Robertson, 2012). Furthermore, viral infections could also directly maintain autoreactive effector cells or autoantigen presenting cells (Pender, 2003). For example, EBV immortalizes B cells and assists in their differentiation to long-lived memory B cells (Thorley-Lawson and Gross, 2004). In addition, even in infected memory B cells that usually do not express latent EBV proteins, non-translated viral RNAs contribute to resistance to cell death (Nanbo et al., 2002). These mechanisms could preserve autoreactive B cells or a reservoir of APCs capable of presenting autoantigens to promote autoimmunity. The reservoir of EBV-infected B cells that were recently described in submeningeal aggregates of MS brains could fulfill these functions (Serafini et al., 2007).

An important consideration is the fact that in most cases viruses and other microbes can infect a host without triggering any clear clinical symptoms. This has further hampered direct linkage of infection with specific autoimmune disease development. This fact, combined with the ever-increasing number of pathways through which pathogens have been shown to be capable of hijacking a host immune response, certainly suggests that consideration of other viral infections and changes in pathogen–host interactions should be considered. One potential pathogen that has spread significantly in the last decade is WNV (King et al., 2007). WNV employs some unusual host evasion strategies that, while designed to circumvent the immune response, may indirectly result in bystander self-reactive T cell activation. WNV replicates about 10-fold greater in cycling cells, but seemingly paradoxically increases MHC expression as well as expression of adhesion molecules like ICAM in quiescent cells (King et al., 2007). This decoy mechanism is thought to promote immune-mediated killing of low virus yielding G_0 cells rather than infected proliferating cells, which support virus replication better. Along the lines invoked for EBV infection, therefore, this raises the possibility that WNV infection generates poly-specific T cells, by increasing the avidity of interaction between T cells and infected cells via increased MHC expression, and that infection activates an array of T cell clones that range from those with high affinity for MHC/virus peptide to those with significant cross-reactivity for self. In the case of WNV, this cross-reactivity of low affinity anti-viral T cells with self has been demonstrated in a mouse model (King et al., 1989; Mullbacher et al., 1991). A direct link between WNV and autoimmunity in humans remains to be made, and is complicated by the fact that over 90% of WNV cases are asymptomatic. Notwithstanding, the WNV example serves to show that there are numerous potential mechanisms through which immune responses to infections result in or accelerate autoimmune diseases. Since evidence of autoimmunity is likely to become clinically apparent only after a considerable period of subclinical autoimmune responses, pathogen-derived triggers may be difficult to identify.

Reciprocal Relationships of Pathogen-Derived Mechanisms of Autoimmunity

All of the above described mechanisms are interrelated, non-mutually exclusive, and dynamic, so the idea of microbial infection eliciting autoimmunity must be viewed not as a defined event that occurs via a particular mechanism, but as a process that can occur through many pathways simultaneously and/or sequentially. For example, epitope spreading can be initiated via molecular mimicry, as illustrated by the activation of $PLP_{178-191}$-specific T cells in SJL mice in which autoimmunity was induced by infection with TMEV expressing $PLP_{139-151}$ (Olson et al., 2001), or following bystander damage. Molecular mimicry can initially activate autoreactive T cells that then expand and become pathogenic via bystander activation, or vice versa. As a result, it can be difficult to distinguish among all of the postulated mechanisms, even in seemingly simple animal models (Fujinami and Oldstone, 1985; Benoist and Mathis, 2001; Deshpande et al., 2001 Fujinami et al., 2006).

HOW DO THESE MECHANISMS LEAD TO AUTOIMMUNE DISEASE?

Animal model studies have made it clear that, in principle, infections can trigger autoimmune responses. This must be distinguished, however, from the elicitation of overt autoimmune disease as a direct result of microbial infection, which may be more difficult to establish.

Autoreactive adaptive immune cells are unavoidably present in the periphery in humans and animals. These cells may exist because their cognate self antigen was not expressed in the thymus and will therefore only become apparent to the immune system following tissue destruction as a result of infection or trauma. Alternatively, while many autoreactive T cells are deleted in the thymus during development, some T cells that make their way to the periphery may be highly specific for a microbial antigen, but also have lesser affinity for a self antigen. The presence of autoreactive cells in the periphery, however, does not necessarily predispose to clinical autoimmune disease.

It is clear that in many cases an infection is necessary for the development of overt disease, even when abundant autoreactive T cells are present. This is cogently exemplified by the following. Although both priming with $PLP_{139-151}$ peptide in complete Freund's adjuvant (CFA) and infection with TMEV expressing a $PLP_{139-151}$ mimic readily induce demyelinating disease, priming with $PLP_{139-151}$ mimics in CFA does not induce overt disease, despite the fact that T cells from these mice robustly respond to $PLP_{139-151}$ (Carrizosa et al., 1998; Croxford et al., 2006; Walker and Abbas, 2002). Presumably, TLR engagement and other innate immune stimuli that are present upon infection with TMEV expressing the mimic peptide allow APC to provide the necessary signals for full-blown activation and optimal migration of pathogenic Th1 and Th17 autoreactive T cells (Olson and Miller, 2004). However, the nature of a pathogen, which directs the type of immune response elicited, profoundly influences the potential for development of autoimmune disease, and could in fact enhance *or* inhibit the likelihood of autoimmunity in the presence of autoreactive cells. Also, in the case of molecular mimicry, the virus-encoded mimic itself plays an important role, as a peptide that partially mimics a self antigen (altered peptide ligand), depending on the context of the infection, could have a tolerizing rather than an immunizing effect (Olson and Miller, 2004).

Even the presence of autoreactive T cells along with the presence of an appropriate infection may not lead to autoimmune disease. In the Pichinde virus infection of RIP-LCMV-NP mice, while the mimic-encoding Pichinde virus was not sufficient to initiate overt autoimmunity, it was able to accelerate autoimmune disease that had already been established by infection with LCMV (Christen et al., 2004). Thus, viral "adjuvant" and self mimics may in some cases be able to trigger autoimmune disease only if autoreactive cells are already "primed" to some degree, such that autoreactive T cells that have been previously activated exist at a higher precursor frequency (Hamilton-Williams et al., 2005). The affinity of T cell receptors for various self peptide/MHC complexes may also play a key role in the development of autoimmune disease. Indeed, a threshold level of TCR affinity has been shown to be important for the establishment of autoimmunity (Gronski et al., 2004). In RIP-LCMV mice, whether or not the self antigen was expressed in the thymus during development (thus affecting T cell affinity) has a significant impact on the speed with which autoimmune disease develops (von Herrath et al., 1994). TLR engagement alone can be sufficient for the development of autoimmune disease if autoreactive T cells are of high enough affinity for self antigen (von Herrath et al., 1994; Lang et al., 2005). However, since most T cells will have low affinity for self, studies in which TCR affinity for self antigen is low may have greater relevance to human autoimmune disease.

Thus, the potential for the development of overt disease is dependent on the presence of autoreactive T cells. However, whether overt disease actually occurs may depend on various other coincident events, including the number, avidity, and affinity of autoreactive T cells, and the presence of innate inflammatory signals required for activation and differentiation of those T cells to a pathogenic phenotype. Despite the requirement for all of these elements, it is apparent that these events do not necessarily need to happen at the same time or in the same place to elicit autoimmune disease.

Autoimmunity Can Occur at a Site Distal to the Initiating Infection

In many animal models, autoimmune responses are triggered during the initial or acute response to an infection, and autoimmune disease occurs exclusively in the infected organ. Along these lines, submeningeal reservoirs of EBV infected B cells have been reported in the brains of patients with MS (Serafini et al., 2007), but it remains unclear if these focus the pathogenic immune response on the diseased tissue. Models, in which infection directs autoreactive responses to distinct tissues, provide a simple system in which to study the pathologic mechanisms of infection-induced autoimmunity. However, in most cases a robust immune response to a pathogenic infection within the target organ is usually not easily associated with the development of autoimmunity in humans. None of the proposed mechanisms for the development of infection-induced autoimmunity exclude the possibility that disease can occur temporally and/or spatially distal from the site of the initiating infection. Animal models that allow study of this aspect of infection-induced autoimmune disease are few, but may provide important insights relative to human disease.

Autoimmune CNS demyelinating disease can be triggered via molecular mimicry when the pathogen containing the mimic epitope does not infect the CNS itself. When mice that express an LCMV protein within the CNS were peripherally infected with LCMV, autoimmune responses occurred within the CNS despite the fact that LCMV was not detectable in that organ (Evans et al., 1996). In non-transgenically manipulated mice, pancreas-tropic coxsackievirus engineered to express $PLP_{139-151}$, induces CNS demyelinating disease associated with $PLP_{139-151}$-specific T cell responses, also in the absence of any infection within the CNS itself (S.D. Miller, in preparation).

The fact that the various mechanisms for infection-induced autoimmunity discussed here are non-mutually exclusive make them both more complicated and more plausible as potential causes for human autoimmune disease. As we consider the potentially multi-mechanistic nature of autoimmunity, it is important to remember that an established autoimmune response can also have effects on pathogen-directed immune responses occurring in the same organ or elsewhere in the body.

CONCLUSIONS

Inherent genetic susceptibility plays a major role indetermining susceptibility to the development of autoimmune diseases; however, epidemiological and animal studies have clearly shown that infection is an equally important factor in the generation of autoimmune disease. Potential mechanisms by which infections can induce autoimmune disease include molecular mimicry, bystander T cell activation culminating in epitope spreading, as well as potential roles for microbial toxins and virus-induced decoy of the immune system.

ACKNOWLEDGMENTS

The authors thank other members of the Miller Lab for advice and commentary.

REFERENCES

Alspaugh, M.A., Henle, G., Lennette, E.T., Henle, W., 1981. Elevated levels of antibodies to Epstein−Barr virus antigens in sera and synovial fluids of patients with rheumatoid arthritis. J. Clin. Invest. 67, 1134−1140.

Ascherio, A., Munch, M., 2000. Epstein−Barr virus and multiple sclerosis. Epidemiology 11, 220−224.

Babbe, H., Roers, A., Waisman, A., Lassmann, H., Goebels, N., Hohlfeld, R., et al., 2000. Clonal expansions of CD8(+) T cells dominate the T cell infiltrate in active multiple sclerosis lesions as shown by micromanipulation and single cell polymerase chain reaction. J. Exp. Med. 192, 393−404.

Balandraud, N., Meynard, J.B., Auger, I., Sovran, H., Mugnier, B., Reviron, D., et al., 2003. Epstein−Barr virus load in the peripheral blood of patients with rheumatoid arthritis: accurate quantification using real-time polymerase chain reaction. Arthritis Rheum. 48, 1223−1228.

Baranzini, S.E., Jeong, M.C., Butunoi, C., Murray, R.S., Bernard, C.C., Oksenberg, J.R., 1999. B cell repertoire diversity and clonal expansion in multiple sclerosis brain lesions. J. Immunol. 163, 5133−5144.

Benoist, C., Mathis, D., 2001. Autoimmunity provoked by infection: how good is the case for T cell epitope mimicry? Nat. Immunol. 2, 797−801.

Bielekova, B., Sung, M.H., Kadom, N., Simon, R., McFarland, H., Martin, R., 2004. Expansion and functional relevance of high-avidity myelin-specific CD4+ T cells in multiple sclerosis. J. Immunol. 172, 3893−3904.

Borrow, P., Welsh, C.J., Tonks, P., Dean, D., Blakemore, W.F., Nash, A.A., 1998. Investigation of the role of delayed-type-hypersensitivity responses to myelin in the pathogenesis of Theiler's virus-induced demyelinating disease. Immunology 93, 478−484.

Brocke, S., Gaur, A., Piercy, C., Gautam, A., Gijbels, K., Fathman, C. G., et al., 1993. Induction of relapsing paralysis in experimental autoimmune encephalomyelitis by bacterial superantigen. Nature 365, 642−644.

Carrizosa, A.M., Nicholson, L.B., Farzan, M., Southwood, S., Sette, A., Sobel, R.A., et al., 1998. Expansion by self antigen is necessary for the induction of experimental autoimmune encephalomyelitis by T cells primed with a cross-reactive environmental antigen. J. Immunol. 161, 3307−3314.

Challoner, P.B., Smith, K.T., Parker, J.D., MacLeod, D.L., Coulter, S.N., Rose, T.M., et al., 1995. Plaque-associated expression of human herpesvirus 6 in multiple sclerosis. Proc. Natl. Acad. Sci. USA 92, 7440−7444.

Christen, U., Edelmann, K.H., McGavern, D.B., Wolfe, T., Coon, B., Teague, M.K., et al., 2004. A viral epitope that mimics a self antigen can accelerate but not initiate autoimmune diabetes. J. Clin. Invest. 114, 1290−1298.

Cole, B.C., Griffiths, M.M., 1993. Triggering and exacerbation of autoimmune arthritis by the Mycoplasma arthritidis superantigen MAM. Arthritis Rheum. 36, 994−1002.

Croxford, J.L., Anger, H.A., Miller, S.D., 2005. Viral delivery of an epitope from *Haemophilus influenzae* induces central nervous system autoimmune disease by molecular mimicry. J. Immunol. 174, 907−917.

Croxford, J.L., Ercolini, A.M., Degutes, M., Miller, S.D., 2006. Structural requirements for initiation of cross-reactivity and CNS autoimmunity with a PLP139-151 mimic peptide derived from murine hepatitis virus. Eur. J. Immunol. 36, 2671−2680.

Croxford, J.L., Olson, J.K., Miller, S.D., 2002. Epitope spreading and molecular mimicry as triggers of autoimmunity in the Theiler's virus-induced demyelinating disease model of multiple sclerosis. Autoimmun. Rev. 1, 251−260.

Dalwadi, H., Wei, B., Kronenberg, M., Sutton, C.L., Braun, J., 2001. The Crohn's disease-associated bacterial protein I2 is a novel enteric T cell superantigen. Immunity 15, 149−158.

Deng, G.M., Tsokos, G.C., 2008. Cholera toxin B accelerates disease progression in lupus-prone mice by promoting lipid raft aggregation. J. Immunol. 181, 4019−4026.

Deshpande, S.P., Lee, S., Zheng, M., Song, B., Knipe, D., Kapp, J.A., et al., 2001. Herpes simplex virus-induced keratitis: evaluation of the role of molecular mimicry in lesion pathogenesis. J. Virol. 75, 3077−3088.

Evans, C.F., Horwitz, M.S., Hobbs, M.V., Oldstone, M.B., 1996. Viral infection of transgenic mice expressing a viral protein in oligodendrocytes leads to chronic central nervous system autoimmune disease. J. Exp. Med. 184, 2371−2384.

Fairweather, D., Kaya, Z., Shellam, G.R., Lawson, C.M., Rose, N.R., 2001. From infection to autoimmunity. J. Autoimm. 16, 175−186.

Fujinami, R.S., Oldstone, M.B., 1985. Amino acid homology between the encephalitogenic site of myelin basic protein and virus: mechanism for autoimmunity. Science 230, 1043−1045.

Fujinami, R.S., Oldstone, M.B., 1989. Molecular mimicry as a mechanism for virus-induced autoimmunity. Immunol. Res. 8, 3−15.

Fujinami, R.S., von Herrath, M.G., Christen, U., Whitton, J.L., 2006. Molecular mimicry, bystander activation, or viral persistence: infections and autoimmune disease. Clin. Microbiol. Rev. 19, 80−94.

Gauntt, C.J., Arizpe, H.M., Higdon, A.L., Wood, H.J., Bowers, D.F., Rozek, M.M., et al., 1995. Molecular mimicry, anti-coxsackievirus B3 neutralizing monoclonal antibodies, and myocarditis. J. Immunol. 154, 2983−2995.

Gautam, A.M., Lock, C.B., Smilek, D.E., Pearson, C.I., Steinman, L., McDevitt, H.O., 1994. Minimum structural requirements for peptide presentation by major histocompatibility complex class II molecules: implications in induction of autoimmunity. Proc. Natl. Acad. Sci. USA 91, 767−771.

Goebels, N., Hofstetter, H., Schmidt, S., Brunner, C., Wekerle, H., Hohlfeld, R., 2000. Repertoire dynamics of autoreactive T cells in multiple sclerosis patients and healthy subjects: epitope spreading versus clonal persistence. Brain 123, 508—518.

Greene, M.T., Ercolini, A.M., Degutes, M., Miller, S.D., 2008. Differential induction of experimental autoimmune encephalomyelitis by myelin basic protein molecular mimics in mice humanized for HLA-DR2 and an MBP(85-99)-specific T cell receptor. J. Autoimmun. 31, 399—407.

Gregersen, J.W., Kranc, K.R., Ke, X., Svendsen, P., Madsen, L.S., Thomsen, A.R., et al., 2006. Functional epistasis on a common MHC haplotype associated with multiple sclerosis. Nature 443, 574—577.

Gronski, M.A., Boulter, J.M., Moskophidis, D., Nguyen, L.T., Holmberg, K., Elford, A.R., et al., 2004. TCR affinity and negative regulation limit autoimmunity. Nat. Med. 10, 1234—1239.

Gross, A.J., Hochberg, D., Rand, W.M., Thorley-Lawson, D.A., 2005. EBV and systemic lupus erythematosus: a new perspective. J. Immunol. 174, 6599—6607.

Hamilton-Williams, E.E., Lang, A., Benke, D., Davey, G.M., Wiesmuller, K.H., Kurts, C., 2005. Cutting edge: TLR ligands are not sufficient to break cross-tolerance to self-antigens. J. Immunol. 174, 1159—1163.

Hammer, J., Valsasnini, P., Tolba, K., Bolin, D., Higelin, J., Takacs, B., et al., 1993. Promiscuous and allele-specific anchors in HLA-DR-binding peptides. Cell 74, 197—203.

Harari, A., Cellerai, C., Enders, F.B., Kostler, J., Codarri, L., Tapia, G., et al., 2007. Skewed association of polyfunctional antigen-specific CD8 T cell populations with HLA-B genotype. Proc. Natl. Acad. Sci. USA 104, 16233—16238.

Hemmer, B., Gran, B., Zhao, Y., Marques, A., Pascal, J., Tzou, A., et al., 1999. Identification of candidate T-cell epitopes and molecular mimics in chronic Lyme disease. Nat. Med. 5, 1375—1382.

Horwitz, M.S., Bradley, L.M., Harbetson, J., Krahl, T., Lee, J., Sarvetnick, N., 1998. Diabetes induced by Coxsackie virus: initiation by bystander damage and not molecular mimicry. Nat. Med. 4, 781—786.

Horwitz, M.S., Ilic, A., Fine, C., Rodriguez, E., Sarvetnick, N., 2002. Presented antigen from damaged pancreatic beta cells activates autoreactive T cells in virus-mediated autoimmune diabetes. J. Clin. Invest. 109, 79—87.

Ishii, K.J., Koyama, S., Nakagawa, A., Coban, C., Akira, S., 2008. Host innate immune receptors and beyond: making sense of microbial infections. Cell Host Microbe 3, 352—363.

James, J.A., Robertson, J.M., 2012. Lupus and Epstein—Barr. Curr. Opin. Rheumatol. 24, 383—388.

Jarius, S., Eichhorn, P., Jacobi, C., Wildemann, B., Wick, M., Voltz, R., 2009. The intrathecal, polyspecific antiviral immune response: specific for MS or a general marker of CNS autoimmunity? J. Neurol. Sci. 280, 98—100.

Johnson, R.T., Griffin, D.E., Hirsch, R.L., Wolinsky, J.S., Roedenbeck, S., Lindo de Soriano, I., et al., 1984. Measles encephalomyelitis—clinical and immunologic studies. New Engl. J. Med. 310, 137—141.

Jones, D.B., Crosby, I., 1996. Proliferative lymphocyte responses to virus antigens homologous to GAD65 in IDDM. Diabetologia. 39, 1318—1324.

Kang, I., Quan, T., Nolasco, H., Park, S.H., Hong, M.S., Crouch, J., et al., 2004. Defective control of latent Epstein—Barr virus infection in systemic lupus erythematosus. J. Immunol. 172, 1287—1294.

Katz-Levy, Y., Neville, K.L., Girvin, A.M., Vanderlugt, C.L., Pope, J. G., Tan, L.J., et al., 1999. Endogenous presentation of self myelin epitopes by CNS-resident APCs in Theiler's virus-infected mice. J. Clin. Invest. 104, 599—610.

Katz-Levy, Y., Neville, K.L., Padilla, J., Rahbe, S.M., Begolka, W.S., Girvin, A.M., et al., 2000. Temporal development of autoreactive Th1 responses and endogenous antigen presentation of self myelin epitopes by CNS-resident APCs in Theiler's virus-infected mice. J. Immunol. 165, 5304—5314.

Kaufman, D.L., Clare-Salzler, M., Tian, J., Forsthuber, T., Ting, G.S., Robinson, P., et al., 1993. Spontaneous loss of T-cell tolerance to glutamic acid decarboxylase in murine insulin-dependent diabetes. Nature 366, 69—72.

King, N.J., Getts, D.R., Getts, M.T., Rana, S., Shrestha, B., Kesson, A. M., 2007. Immunopathology of flavivirus infections. Immunol. Cell Biol. 85, 33—42.

King, N.J., Maxwell, L.E., Kesson, A.M., 1989. Induction of class I major histocompatibility complex antigen expression by West Nile virus on gamma interferon-refractory early murine trophoblast cells. Proc. Natl. Acad. Sci. USA 86, 911—915.

Kozireva, S.V., Zestkova, J.V., Mikazane, H.J., Kadisa, A.L., Kakurina, N.A., Lejnieks, A.A., et al., 2008. Incidence and clinical significance of parvovirus B19 infection in patients with rheumatoid arthritis. J. Rheumatol. 35, 1265—1270.

Lang, H.L., Jacobsen, H., Ikemizu, S., Andersson, C., Harlos, K., Madsen, L., et al., 2002. A functional and structural basis for TCR cross-reactivity in multiple sclerosis. Nat. Immunol. 3, 940—943.

Lang, K.S., Recher, M., Junt, T., Navarini, A.A., Harris, N.L., Freigang, S., et al., 2005. Toll-like receptor engagement converts T-cell autoreactivity into overt autoimmune disease. Nat. Med. 11, 138—145.

Lawson, C.M., 2000. Evidence for mimicry by viral antigens in animal models of autoimmune disease including myocarditis. Cell Mol. Life Sci. 57, 552—560.

Lawson, C.M., O'Donoghue, H.L., Reed, W.D., 1992. Mouse cytomegalovirus infection induces antibodies which cross-react with virus and cardiac myosin: a model for the study of molecular mimicry in the pathogenesis of viral myocarditis. Immunology 75, 513—519.

Levin, L.I., Munger, K.L., Rubertone, M.V., Peck, C.A., Lennette, E.T., Spiegelman, D., et al., 2005. Temporal relationship between elevation of epstein-barr virus antibody titers and initial onset of neurological symptoms in multiple sclerosis. J. Am. Med. Assoc. 293, 2496—2500.

Levin, M.C., Lee, S.M., Kalume, F., Morcos, Y., Dohan Jr., F.C., Hasty, K.A., et al., 2002. Autoimmunity due to molecular mimicry as a cause of neurological disease. Nat. Med. 8, 509—513.

Link, H., Sun, J.B., Wang, Z., Xu, Z., Love, A., Fredrikson, S., et al., 1992. Virus-reactive and autoreactive T cells are accumulated in cerebrospinal fluid in multiple sclerosis. J. Neuroimmunol. 38, 63—73.

Lovett-Racke, A.E., Trotter, J.L., Lauber, J., Perrin, P.J., June, C.H., Racke, M.K., 1998. Decreased dependence of myelin basic protein-reactive T cells on CD28-mediated costimulation in multiple sclerosis patients. A marker of activated/memory T cells. J. Clin. Invest. 101, 725—730.

Lunemann, J.D., Edwards, N., Muraro, P.A., Hayashi, S., Cohen, J.I., Munz, C., et al., 2006. Increased frequency and broadened specificity of latent EBV nuclear antigen-1-specific T cells in multiple sclerosis. Brain 129, 1493—1506.

Lunemann, J.D., Frey, O., Eidner, T., Baier, M., Roberts, S., Sashihara, J., et al., 2008a. Increased frequency of EBV-specific effector memory CD8+ T cells correlates with higher viral load in rheumatoid arthritis. J. Immunol. 181, 991–1000.

Lunemann, J.D., Huppke, P., Roberts, S., Bruck, W., Gartner, J., Munz, C., 2008b. Broadened and elevated humoral immune response to EBNA1 in pediatric multiple sclerosis. Neurology 71, 1033–1035.

Lunemann, J.D., Jelcic, I., Roberts, S., Lutterotti, A., Tackenberg, B., Martin, R., et al., 2008c. EBNA1-specific T cells from patients with multiple sclerosis cross react with myelin antigens and co-produce IFN-gamma and IL-2. J. Exp. Med. 205, 1763–1773.

Markovic-Plese, S., Cortese, I., Wandinger, K.P., McFarland, H.F., Martin, R., 2001. CD4 + CD28 − costimulation-independent T cells in multiple sclerosis. J. Clin. Invest. 108, 1185–1194.

Massilamany, C., Asojo, O.A., Gangaplara, A., Steffen, D., Reddy, J., 2011. Identification of a second mimicry epitope from Acanthamoeba castellanii that induces CNS autoimmunity by generating cross-reactive T cells for MBP 89-101 in SJL mice. Int. Immunol. 23, 729–739.

Massilamany, C., Steffen, D., Reddy, J., 2010. An epitope from Acanthamoeba castellanii that cross-react with proteolipid protein 139-151-reactive T cells induces autoimmune encephalomyelitis in SJL mice. J. Neuroimmunol. 219, 17–24.

McClain, M.T., Heinlen, L.D., Dennis, G.J., Roebuck, J., Harley, J.B., James, J.A., 2005. Early events in lupus humoral autoimmunity suggest initiation through molecular mimicry. Nat. Med. 11, 85–89.

McRae, B.L., Vanderlugt, C.L., Dal Canto, M.C., Miller, S.D., 1995. Functional evidence for epitope spreading in the relapsing pathology of experimental autoimmune encephalomyelitis. J. Exp. Med. 182, 75–85.

Meinl, E., Weber, F., Drexler, K., Morelle, C., Ott, M., Saruhan-Direskeneli, G., et al., 1993. Myelin basic protein-specific T lymphocyte repertoire in multiple sclerosis. Complexity of the response and dominance of nested epitopes due to recruitment of multiple T cell clones. J. Clin. Invest. 92, 2633–2643.

Menser, M.A., Forrest, J.M., Bransby, R.D., 1978. Rubella infection and diabetes mellitus. Lancet. 1, 57–60.

Miller, S.D., Vanderlugt, C.L., Begolka, W.S., Pao, W., Yauch, R.L., Neville, K.L., et al., 1997. Persistent infection with Theiler's virus leads to CNS autoimmunity via epitope spreading. Nat. Med. 3, 1133–1136.

Mokhtarian, F., Zhang, Z., Shi, Y., Gonzales, E., Sobel, R.A., 1999. Molecular mimicry between a viral peptide and a myelin oligodendrocyte glycoprotein peptide induces autoimmune demyelinating disease in mice. J. Neuroimmunol. 95, 43–54.

Mullbacher, A., Hill, A.B., Blanden, R.V., Cowden, W.B., King, N.J., Hla, R.T., 1991. Alloreactive cytotoxic T cells recognize MHC class I antigen without peptide specificity. J. Immunol. 147, 1765–1772.

Munz, C., Lunemann, J.D., Getts, M.T., Miller, S.D., 2009. Antiviral immune responses: triggers of or triggered by autoimmunity? Nat. Rev. Immunol. 9, 246–258.

Muraro, P.A., Wandinger, K.P., Bielekova, B., Gran, B., Marques, A., Utz, U., et al., 2003. Molecular tracking of antigen-specific T cell clones in neurological immune-mediated disorders. Brain. 126, 20–31.

Nanbo, A., Inoue, K., Adachi-Takasawa, K., Takada, K., 2002. Epstein−Barr virus RNA confers resistance to interferon-alpha-induced apoptosis in Burkitt's lymphoma. EMBO J. 21, 954–965.

Nielsen, T.R., Rostgaard, K., Nielsen, N.M., Koch-Henriksen, N., Haahr, S., Sorensen, P.S., et al., 2007. Multiple sclerosis after infectious mononucleosis. Arch. Neurol. 64, 72–75.

Ohashi, P.S., Oehen, S., Buerki, K., Pircher, H., Ohashi, C.T., Odermatt, B., et al., 1991. Ablation of "tolerance" and induction of diabetes by virus infection in viral antigen transgenic mice. Cell 65, 305–317.

Oldstone, M.B., Nerenberg, M., Southern, P., Price, J., Lewicki, H., 1991. Virus infection triggers insulin-dependent diabetes mellitus in a transgenic model: role of anti-self (virus) immune response. Cell 65, 319–331.

Olson, J.K., Croxford, J.L., Calenoff, M., Dal Canto, M.C., Miller, S.D., 2001. A virus-induced molecular mimicry model of multiple sclerosis. J. Clin. Invest. 108, 311–318.

Olson, J.K., Miller, S.D., 2004. Microglia initiate central nervous system innate and adaptive immune responses through multiple TLRs. J. Immunol. 173, 3916–3924.

Ou, D., Mitchell, L.A., Metzger, D.L., Gillam, S., Tingle, A.J., 2000. Cross-reactive rubella virus and glutamic acid decarboxylase (65 and 67) protein determinants recognised by T cells of patients with type I diabetes mellitus. Diabetologia. 43, 750–762.

Pender, M.P., 2003. Infection of autoreactive B lymphocytes with EBV, causing chronic autoimmune diseases. Trends Immunol. 24, 584–588.

Prasad, S., Kohm, A.P., McMahon, J.S., Luo, X., Miller, S.D., 2012. Pathogenesis of NOD diabetes is initiated by reactivity to the insulin B chain 9-23 epitope and involves functional epitope spreading. J. Autoimm. 39, 347–353.

Saal, J.G., Steidle, M., Einsele, H., Muller, C.A., Fritz, P., Zacher, J., 1992. Persistence of B19 parvovirus in synovial membranes of patients with rheumatoid arthritis. Rheumatol. Int. 12, 147–151.

Samuels, J., Ng, Y.S., Coupillaud, C., Paget, D., Meffre, E., 2005. Impaired early B cell tolerance in patients with rheumatoid arthritis. J. Exp. Med. 201, 1659–1667.

Scotet, E., David-Ameline, J., Peyrat, M.A., Moreau-Aubry, A., Pinczon, D., Lim, A., et al., 1996. T cell response to Epstein−Barr virus transactivators in chronic rheumatoid arthritis. J. Exp. Med. 184, 1791–1800.

Serafini, B., Rosicarelli, B., Franciotta, D., Magliozzi, R., Reynolds, R., Cinque, P., et al., 2007. Dysregulated Epstein−Barr virus infection in the multiple sclerosis brain. J. Exp. Med. 204, 2899–2912.

Seve, P., Ferry, T., Koenig, M., Cathebras, P., Rousset, H., Broussolle, C., 2005. Lupus-like presentation of parvovirus B19 infection. Sem. Arth. Rheum. 34, 642–648.

Skulina, C., Schmidt, S., Dornmair, K., Babbe, H., Roers, A., Rajewsky, K., et al., 2004. Multiple sclerosis: brain-infiltrating CD8 + T cells persist as clonal expansions in the cerebrospinal fluid and blood. Proc. Natl. Acad. Sci. USA 101, 2428–2433.

Soldan, S.S., Berti, R., Salem, N., Secchiero, P., Flamand, L., Calabresi, P.A., et al., 1997. Association of human herpes virus 6 (HHV-6) with multiple sclerosis: increased IgM response to HHV-6 early antigen and detection of serum HHV-6 DNA. Nat. Med.1394–1397.

Sospedra, M., Zhao, Y., zur Hausen, H., Muraro, P.A., Hamashin, C., de Villiers, E.M., et al., 2005. Recognition of conserved amino acid motifs of common viruses and its role in autoimmunity. PLoS Pathog. 1, e41.

Sundstrom, P., Juto, P., Wadell, G., Hallmans, G., Svenningsson, A., Nystrom, L., et al., 2004. An altered immune response to Epstein−Barr virus in multiple sclerosis: a prospective study. Neurology 62, 2277–2282.

Sutkowski, N., Conrad, B., Thorley-Lawson, D.A., Huber, B.T., 2001. Epstein–Barr virus transactivates the human endogenous retrovirus HERV-K18 that encodes a superantigen. Immunity 15, 579–589.

Tai, A.K., O'Reilly, E.J., Alroy, K.A., Simon, K.C., Munger, K.L., Huber, B.T., et al., 2008. Human endogenous retrovirus-K18 Env as a risk factor in multiple sclerosis. Mult. Scler. 14, 1175–1180.

Terry, R.L., Getts, D.R., Deffrasnes, C., van Vreden, C., Campbell, I.L., King, N.J., 2012. Inflammatory monocytes and the pathogenesis of viral encephalitis. J. Neuroinflamm. 9, 270.

Thacker, E.L., Mirzaei, F., Ascherio, A., 2006. Infectious mononucleosis and risk for multiple sclerosis: a meta-analysis. Ann. Neurol. 59, 499–503.

Thorley-Lawson, D.A., Gross, A., 2004. Persistence of the Epstein–Barr virus and the origins of associated lymphomas. New Engl. J. Med. 350, 1328–1337.

Tosato, G., Steinberg, A.D., Blaese, R.M., 1981. Defective EBV-specific suppressor T-cell function in rheumatoid arthritis. New Engl. J. Med. 305, 1238–1243.

Tosato, G., Steinberg, A.D., Yarchoan, R., Heilman, C.A., Pike, S.E., De Seau, V., et al., 1984. Abnormally elevated frequency of Epstein–Barr virus-infected B cells in the blood of patients with rheumatoid arthritis. J. Clin. Invest. 73, 1789–1795.

von Herrath, M.G., Dockter, J., Oldstone, M.B., 1994. How virus induces a rapid or slow onset insulin-dependent diabetes mellitus in a transgenic model. Immunity 1, 231–242.

Walker, L.S., Abbas, A.K., 2002. The enemy within: keeping self-reactive T cells at bay in the periphery. Nat. Rev. Immunol. 2, 11–19.

Wucherpfennig, K.W., 2001. Mechanisms for the induction of autoimmunity by infectious agents. J. Clin. Invest. 108, 1097–1104.

Wucherpfennig, K.W., Sette, A., Southwood, S., Oseroff, C., Matsui, M., Strominger, J.L., et al., 1994. Structural requirements for binding of an immunodominant myelin basic protein peptide to DR2 isotypes and for its recognition by human T cell clones. J. Exp. Med. 179, 279–290.

Wucherpfennig, K.W., Strominger, J.L., 1995. Molecular mimicry in T cell-mediated autoimmunity: viral peptides activate human T cell clones specific for myelin basic protein. Cell 80, 695–705.

Ylipaasto, P., Klingel, K., Lindberg, A.M., Otonkoski, T., Kandolf, R., Hovi, T., et al., 2004. Enterovirus infection in human pancreatic islet cells, islet tropism in vivo and receptor involvement in cultured islet beta cells. Diabetologia. 47, 225–239.

Yu, M., Johnson, J.M., Tuohy, V.K., 1996. A predictable sequential determinant spreading cascade invariably accompanies progression of experimental autoimmune encephalomyelitis: a basis for peptide-specific therapy after onset of clinical disease. J. Exp. Med. 183, 1777–1788.

Yurasov, S., Wardemann, H., Hammersen, J., Tsuiji, M., Meffre, E., Pascual, V., et al., 2005. Defective B cell tolerance checkpoints in systemic lupus erythematosus. J. Exp. Med. 201, 703–711.

Zhao, Z.S., Granucci, F., Yeh, L., Schaffer, P.A., Cantor, H., 1998. Molecular mimicry by herpes simplex virus-type 1: autoimmune disease after viral infection. Science 279, 1344–1347.

Zipris, D., Lien, E., Xie, J.X., Greiner, D.L., Mordes, J.P., Rossini, A.A., 2005. TLR activation synergizes with Kilham rat virus infection to induce diabetes in BBDR rats. J. Immunol. 174, 131–142.

Chapter 20

Autoimmune Diseases: The Role for Vaccines

S.Sohail Ahmed[1] and Paul-Henri Lambert[2]

[1]Global Clinical Sciences, Vaccines Research, Novartis Vaccines & Diagnostics, Siena, Italy, [2]Center of Vaccinology, University of Geneva, Switzerland

Chapter Outline

Introduction	275
Theoretical Concerns for Autoimmune Diseases in the Context of Vaccination	276
Crossfire and Coincidence	276
Challenges using Animal Models	277
One Size does "not" Fit All	277
Induced Autoimmune Disease in Animals	278
Spontaneous Autoimmune Disease in Animals	278
"Of Mice and Men"—The Correct Application of Human Epidemiology and Translation of Human Immunology to Rodent Immunology	279
Practical Approach to Vaccination in Patients with Autoimmune Disease	279
The Reality Facing Clinicians Currently	280
Certainty about Vaccines, Uncertainty about Compatibility of Administration in Certain Settings	280
Search and You will Find	281
Conclusion	281
References	281

INTRODUCTION

Vaccines are essential components of any public health program. Their beneficial effects have been largely recognized and vaccination is generally considered as the most cost-effective approach in preventive medicine. Therefore vaccines are used extensively and coverage can reach over 90% in a given population. Since autoimmune diseases affect approximately 5—10% of the population in Europe and North America, most people that develop an autoimmune disease are likely to be exposed to some vaccines at some time before or after the onset of the disease process. While earlier vaccines were mainly targeted for pediatric age groups, the development of recent vaccines for adolescents (e.g., human papillomavirus vaccine (HPV)) and older individuals (e.g., pneumococcus and influenza) has increased the probability of coincidental associations of vaccination with autoimmune diseases.

Two major questions are of particular relevance to vaccination and autoimmune diseases. First, can vaccination trigger or enhance autoimmune responses? This frequently expressed concern is based either on a putative mimicry between vaccines and host antigens or on the fact that vaccination is associated with a transitory and variable activation of innate immunity. The use of adjuvants exploiting the immunostimulatory effect of Toll-like receptors (TLRs) has triggered concerns related to their possible role in autoimmune disease development. Indeed, TLR-related pathways are being independently studied by investigators for their role in autoimmune disease modulation. Second, should patients with chronic autoimmune diseases be routinely vaccinated? Since several infections are known to enhance disease activity in some autoimmune diseases, one can expect that their prevention, when feasible, would be beneficial. However, activation of innate immunity with some vaccines may also bear a theoretical risk of enhancing disease activity. Numerous allegations have been made and it is essential to restrict oneself to evidence-based conclusions rather than focusing on isolated case reports of coincidental events. Therefore it is of importance to define guidelines regarding the use of essential vaccines in patients with autoimmune diseases. Such

N. Rose & I. Mackay (Eds): The Autoimmune Diseases, Fifth edition. DOI: http://dx.doi.org/10.1016/B978-0-12-384929-8.00020-4

guidelines have been proposed by the American College of Rheumatology and the European League Against Rheumatism and will be discussed in subsequent sections in this chapter.

THEORETICAL CONCERNS FOR AUTOIMMUNE DISEASES IN THE CONTEXT OF VACCINATION

Under the generic term of "vaccines," there is a whole range of products that include complex live attenuated microorganisms as well as purified proteins or polysaccharides. The common purpose of vaccination is to trigger a protective immune response in the host (similar to that seen with naturally acquired infection) but without the host becoming sick. Both in the previous decades for live or non-adjuvanted vaccines and more recently for adjuvanted vaccines, a major safety concern has centered on the possibility of potent stimulators of the immune response increasing the risk of developing an autoimmune disease. In fact, very few cases of vaccine-induced autoimmunity have been clearly demonstrated with past vaccines. The old rabies vaccine that was produced using rabbit brain tissue was associated with the occasional (0.33/1000) development of immune-mediated encephalitis and anti-myelin T cell responses (Swaddiwuthipong et al., 1998). This is no longer observed with modern rabies vaccines produced on cell lines. Measles vaccination is also occasionally associated with a transitory ITP-like thrombocytopenia. However, this syndrome is observed 6–10 times more frequently after natural measles infection (Beeler et al., 1996; Wraith et al., 2003). More recently, an epidemiological association of narcolepsy with the use of an AS03-adjuvanted H1N1 vaccine has been reported in Finland in a group 4–19 years of age representing over 900,000 people (National Narcolepsy Task Force Interim Report, 2011; Statement on Narcolepsy and Vaccination, 2011). The incidence of narcolepsy was 9.0 in the vaccinated as compared to 0.7/100,000 person years in the unvaccinated individuals, the rate ratio being 12.7. However, the pathogenesis of this adverse event is still ill-defined and the respective role of the vaccine and of the concomitant exposure to pandemic influenza remains unclear. This pandemic wave was shown in China to be associated with a 3–4 rise of narcolepsy in the absence of vaccination (Han et al., 2011). The swine influenza vaccine that was used in 1976 was associated with a significant increase in the frequency (incidence of 1 in 100,000) of Guillain–Barré syndrome in the weeks following vaccination (Wraith et al. 2003) but this is not seen after seasonal vaccines (risk of Guillain–Barré reduced to 1 in 1,000,000) (Schonberger et al., 1979; Chen et al., 2001).

CROSSFIRE AND COINCIDENCE

The historical associations described previously remind us of the extent of our current capabilities in identifying risks associated with vaccines—that is, through statistical associations. While identifying causation would be ideal (e.g., a clear and unequivocal link between vaccination and rare adverse events such as autoimmune disease), this is difficult given the individual, environmental, and temporal variables that occur during the window of immunization. While disease incidence in the setting of vaccination can be identified using statistical tools, this analysis can be confounded by the occurrence of "coincidental" associations. There is a background rate of these events that occur despite vaccination and a risk of such event occurring at the same time as the vaccine, by chance alone, which can confound the interpretation of vaccine safety.

One possible but not always practical solution is to collect autoimmune disease prevalence and incidence data in a given population before vaccination to illustrate these coincidental associations. Such an approach was utilized prior to the large-scale introduction of the HPV vaccine where a cohort study of 214,896 female adolescents and 221,472 young adults was carried out to monitor the prevalence of autoimmune disease before vaccine introduction (Siegrist et al., 2007). This elegant approach collected data on the frequency of immune-mediated conditions leading to outpatient visits, the number of women hospitalized, and the most frequently diagnosed autoimmune disease. These data were then used to model temporal associations that would have occurred theoretically had the vaccine been used with 80% coverage. One can quickly appreciate how such population-based efforts enable one to identify, in advance, confounding issues affecting safety perception to avoid a negative impression of an inherently safe vaccine. This approach emphasizes that without better incidence data on autoimmune diseases, the increased large-scale surveillance in vaccine studies may make it incorrectly appear that all vaccines increase the risk of autoimmune diseases.

Table 20.1 has been adapted primarily from autoimmune disease epidemiological data reported in a systematic review (Jacobson et al., 1997) in which four additional categories were added from a study published in 2003 (Cooper and Stroehla, 2003). These combined data represent, to our knowledge, the most comprehensive and conservative estimates to date. Table 20.1 intentionally focuses on the incidence of autoimmune diseases more commonly occurring in adults because the adult population is traditionally enrolled in first-in-human clinical trials with vaccines (the rates of autoimmunity in pediatric patients, though limited, suggest that they are quite different and reflect the contributions of time and

TABLE 20.1 Autoimmune Disease Epidemiological Data Reported in a Systematic Review

Autoimmune Disease[a]	Incidence[a] (per 100,000 persons per year)	Expected New Diagnoses[a] (persons >18 years of age)
Adult rheumatoid arthritis	23.7	55,092
Thyroiditis (hypothyroidism)	21.8	50,675
Graves' disease (hyperthyroidism)	13.9	32,311
Type 1 diabetes (age >20 years)	8.1	18,829
Systemic lupus erythematosus	7.3	16,969
Sjögren disease	3.9	9,065
Multiple sclerosis	3.2	7,438
Primary systemic vasculitis	2.0	4,649
Polymyositis/Dermatomyositis	1.8	4,184
Systemic sclerosis	1.4	3,254
Addison disease	0.6	1,394
Myasthenia gravis	0.4	929
Total		204,789

[a]Table obtained with permission from Ahmed, S., Plotkin, S.A., Black, S., Coffman, R.L. 2011. Assessing the safety of adjuvanted vaccines. Sci. Transl. Med. 3, 93rv2.

environmental exposure to disease development). These autoimmune diseases, based on previously reported estimates of incidence (Jacobson et al., 1997; Cooper and Stroehla, 2003), would have been responsible for 204,789 new cases of autoimmune disease in a population >18 years of age in the United States based on the 2010 US Census (US Census Bureau, 2011). With this extrapolated table, one rapidly gains a perspective on the risk of coincidental association that can occur when an autoimmune disease is diagnosed in a subject immunized during a vaccine clinical trial (independent of the vaccine's effect). Table 20.2 uses the incidence data from these autoimmune diseases and calculates the probability of observing at least one case of autoimmune disease in clinical trials ranging from 200 to 10,000 subjects. As demonstrated, there is an increase in the probability of observing one patient with autoimmune disease when examining a trial with 200 subjects (15%) versus 3000 subjects (91%) which illustrates why coincidental associations occasionally occur during large phase III vaccine studies and even more during post-licensure monitoring of vaccination adverse events.

CHALLENGES USING ANIMAL MODELS

The existence of animal models in which autoimmune disease is triggered using autoantigen preparations that contain adjuvants may also lead to the misperception that adjuvanted vaccines will trigger autoimmune disease in

subjects. However, one must keep in mind that the adjuvants used in these studies are typically strong adjuvants (e.g., complete Freund's adjuvant (CFA)), and are used on purpose with self or self-mimetic antigen to break immunological tolerance in animals. Furthermore, CFA, which is a mixture containing an antigen and inactivated and dried mycobacteria emulsified in mineral oil, is not approved for use in people because of its local toxicity. What needs to be emphasized here is that vaccine preparations that prevent infectious diseases in humans use adjuvants that are formulated to specifically promote immune responsiveness of vaccine antigens, not break immunological tolerance. Moreover, vaccine antigens are screened for molecular mimicry to exclude autoantigens, using in silico and in vitro studies, and thus are missing the necessary ingredient to potentially enable breaking of tolerance in the presence of a strong adjuvant.

One Size does "not" Fit All

Thus, suitable preclinical models for predicting relatively rare and delayed adverse events, such as an increase in the incidence of a specific autoimmune disease, have proven elusive. Human autoimmune diseases are diverse and complex, and the nature of the trigger cannot be simplified to the point that one "model" can be reliably expected to predict autoimmune disease induction. For example, many animal models exist for autoimmune

TABLE 20.2 Incidence Data from Autoimmune Diseases

	Study Sample Size				
	N = 200	N = 1000	N = 2000	N = 3000	N = 10,000
	Probability to Observe at Least One Case[a]				
Autoimmune disease[a]					
Adult rheumatoid arthritis	4.6%	21.1%	37.8%	50.9%	90.7%
Thyroiditis (hypothyroidism)	4.3%	19.6%	35.3%	48.0%	88.7%
Graves' disease (hyperthyroidism)	2.7%	13.0%	24.3%	34.1%	75.1%
Type 1 diabetes (age >20 years)	1.6%	7.8%	15.0%	21.6%	55.5%
Systemic lupus erythematosus	1.4%	7.0%	13.6%	19.7%	51.8%
Sjögren disease	0.8%	3.8%	7.5%	11.0%	32.3%
Multiple sclerosis	0.6%	3.1%	6.2%	9.2%	27.4%
Primary systemic vasculitis	0.4%	2.0%	3.9%	5.8%	18.1%
Polymyositis/Dermatomyositis	0.4%	1.8%	3.5%	5.3%	16.5%
Systemic sclerosis	0.3%	1.4%	2.8%	4.1%	13.1%
Addison disease	0.1%	0.6%	1.2%	1.8%	5.8%
Myasthenia gravis	0.1%	0.4%	0.8%	1.2%	3.9%
Total	15.0%	55.5%	80.2%	91.2%	100.0%

[a]Table obtained with permission from Ahmed, S., Plotkin, S.A., Black, S., Coffman, R.L. 2011. Assessing the safety of adjuvanted vaccines. Sci. Transl. Med. 3, 93rv2.

disease mimicking certain features of a human disease. However, most of these models have been developed on the basis of similarities to end-stage pathology of the human disease instead of similarities in the etiology or pathogenic mechanisms. The widely used mouse models of lupus including (NZBxNZW)F1 and MRL-Fas[lpr] mouse strains (Kono and Theofilopoulos, 2006) mirror the high levels of autoantibody and consequent lupus nephritis but do not reflect the musculoskeletal or neurological symptoms commonly seen in systematic lupus erythematosus (SLE). Evaluating the effects of a vaccine or adjuvant on one or two disease models would provide no information about the effects on other disease models. Difficulties and limitations with this approach include the differences between animal disease models and human disease clinical manifestations, fundamental genetic and physiological differences between humans and commonly used laboratory animals, and finally the poorly understood etiology of human autoimmune diseases in general. The following section will address these differences in greater detail.

Induced Autoimmune Disease in Animals

So what about animal models of autoimmune disease that are induced experimentally? Given that the etiologies of

human autoimmune diseases remain a mystery, factors that initiate disease in animal models may not be relevant to human disease development. For example, models in which disease is induced by immunization with high doses of autoantigens and adjuvants might reflect the downstream stage of organ pathology, but the upstream induction phase in these models may have little, if any, relevance to disease development in humans. A widely used rodent model for multiple sclerosis, experimental autoimmune encephalomyelitis, is induced by immunizing animals with a homogenate of spinal cords emulsified in CFA (Hemmer et al., 2006). The relevance of these models for shedding light on the potential of a candidate vaccine or adjuvant to influence onset or severity of autoimmune diseases in humans is very little if none. The take home message: the incomplete correlation with human disease and the divergent mechanisms of disease initiation limit the relevance of even the "best" inducible animal models to specific human autoimmune diseases.

Spontaneous Autoimmune Disease in Animals

What about animal models of autoimmune disease that occur spontaneously? Spontaneous models of autoimmunity may be more relevant to human disease development than induced models, but these models are not without their limitations. Rodent models in which autoimmune disease develops spontaneously reflect a combination of genetic and environmental factors analogous to those thought to determine human autoimmune disease. A good example is autoimmune diabetes in nonobese diabetic (NOD) mice which may be the most similar to its human counterpart in antigenic components, genetic contributions, and pathological features (Kikutani and Makino, 1992). While one could envision using NOD mice to test agents for their potential to accelerate disease development or increase the severity of autoimmune diabetes, one needs to consider that CFA, which typically is used to *trigger* disease in autoimmune models, unexpectedly confers protection against diabetes development in NOD mice (Sadelain et al., 1990; Qin et al., 1993) questioning the utility of data generated in such an animal model. The same holds true for a number of TLR ligands being evaluated as adjuvants for vaccines against human diseases (Aumeunier et al., 2010). Other realities that need to be considered with animal models that spontaneously develop autoimmune disease are that while there may be pathological similarities to human autoimmune disease, the genetic associations and pathogenic mechanism may be quite different. The MRL-Fas^{lpr} mouse is a model known to spontaneously develop renal disease resembling lupus nephritis. A null mutation in the gene encoding Fas is the key element in this model and leads to defective lymphocyte apoptosis (Kono and Theofilopoulos, 2006). However, when attempting to translate these findings to human disease, one will see that genome-wide association studies in systemic lupus erythematosus patients have not demonstrated a link in polymorphisms in Fas to disease susceptibility (Crow, 2008; Graham et al., 2009).

"Of Mice and Men"—The Correct Application of Human Epidemiology and Translation of Human Immunology to Rodent Immunology

The reader should also consider the artificial nature of animal models regarding disease frequency compared to the real-life incidence of autoimmune diseases which, when compared to other medical diseases, are rare! Scientists using animal models to evaluate what in humans is considered a delayed vaccine adverse event (e.g., subsequent triggering of autoimmune disease) are cognizant of the fact that animal models developing autoimmune disease at high frequency ($>50\%$) are not designed to evaluate factors that increase the incidence of rare events in humans. For example, in well-characterized

animal models of autoimmune disease, there is an artificial optimization of the genetic background and immunization conditions to reproducibly generate disease at high frequency. This disease in human populations may occur at a frequency of only 1 in 10,000 to 1 in 100,000 per year. Therefore, current animal models cannot predict an increased incidence in humans due to this artificial optimization. Clinical trials, therefore, may be the only modality to test such risks in that a vaccine that increases the annual incidence of a disease in humans from 1 in 100,000 to 10 in 100,000 (a 10-fold increase) would be considered unacceptable. Furthermore, species-specific differences between rodents and human immunology complicate the utility of preclinical observations for human disease. For example, TLR9 is expressed in human B cells and plasmacytoid dendritic cells (Hornung et al., 2002; Bernasconi et al., 2003; Rothenfusser et al., 2003) but in mice has been demonstrated additionally in macrophages, myeloid dendritic cells, and activated T cells (Gilliet et al., 2002; Gelman et al., 2004; Martin-Orozco et al., 1999; Suzuki et al., 2005). These differences are reflected in the safety and tolerability of inhaled or injected CpG-ODN (a TLR9-dependent agonist) in human and nonhuman primates (Creticos et al., 2006; Fanucchi et al., 2004; Gauvreau et al., 2006; Krieg et al., 2004; Simons et al., 2004; Tulic et al., 2004) and highlight the challenges in interpreting preclinical toxicology studies of CpG-ODN-containing vaccines.

While the development of more appropriate animal models including transgenic, humanized, and nonrodent animal models is warranted, this will need to be balanced with the Animal Welfare Act's focus of reducing, refining, or replacing animal tests (National Institutes of Health Revitalization Act of 1993 and the Interagency Coordinating Committee on the Validation of Alternative Methods Authorization Act of 2000). Clearly, such a focus on animal welfare when juxtaposed with the limited applicability of animal models of autoimmune disease for recapitulating or even predicting human autoimmune disease is likely to limit preclinical studies on rare serious adverse events (e.g., autoimmune disease).

PRACTICAL APPROACH TO VACCINATION IN PATIENTS WITH AUTOIMMUNE DISEASE

What is frequently forgotten, but is commonly observed by clinicians managing patients with autoimmune diseases, is that natural infection, unlike vaccination, is a *more likely and proven risk factor* for triggering ("flare") and augmenting severity of autoimmune diseases. For example, an influenza vaccine study with 69 patients with SLE and 54 patients with rheumatoid arthritis (RA) demonstrated that every viral and bacterial infection (seen predominantly in the non-vaccinated cohort) resulted in worsening of the main disease (Stojanovich, 2006). Similarly, a case report described a severe flare of SLE in a patient infected with parvovirus B19 (Hemauer et al., 1999). A recent meta-analysis arrived at a similar conclusion that several vaccine-preventable infections occurred more often in patients with autoimmune disease, that vaccines were efficacious in these patients, and that there did not appear to be an increase in vaccination-related harm compared to nonvaccinated patients (van Assen et al., 2011). Influenza and other acute respiratory infections are also commonly associated with an increased frequency of relapses in patients with relapsing multiple sclerosis (Oikonen et al., 2011). This risk is markedly reduced in patients that received the seasonal influenza vaccine (De Keyser et al., 1998).

The Reality Facing Clinicians Currently

The last 10 years has ushered in several new vaccines which rheumatologists caring for their patients should be familiar with. Some of these vaccines are relevant for the age groups being targeted by vaccination, while others may be live-attenuated vs. being inactivated (thus not capable of replication) and thus need to be considered carefully depending on the clinical interventions being considered for the patient. These new vaccines include those for meningitis (quadrivalent conjugate), pneumococcus (conjugate), papillomavirus (alum and TLR4 adjuvanted), rotavirus, and, lastly, the tetanus, diphtheria, and acellular pertussis vaccine (e.g., DTaP). Yet despite evidence of the impact and benefits of vaccinations, clinicians are not adequately vaccinating their patients according to established guidelines with the most significant barrier to vaccination identified by the Centers for Disease Control being *lack of knowledge* about these vaccines among adult patients and providers (Kroger et al., 2011). This section will provide guidance to the practicing rheumatologist regarding the role for vaccines in the patients that they treat based on 2011 guidelines published by the Advisory Committee on Immunization Practices (ACIP) and detailed guidelines that have been proposed by the American College of Rheumatology and the European League Against Rheumatism (to be discussed below).

Certainty about Vaccines, Uncertainty about Compatibility of Administration in Certain Settings

For those physicians that are aware of the vaccines currently available and recommended for their patients, questions are sometimes raised regarding what to do where patients are being treated with immunomodulators or the efficacy of vaccines in patients that are immunosuppressed. This concern is based on the observation that immunosuppression resulting from primary or secondarily altered immunocompetence creates the greatest risk for infections in patients. Most patients being managed by rheumatologists are immunosuppressed by drugs prescribed to control their autoimmune disease and, thus, the immunodeficiency is a function of dose and type of therapy. A recent publication from the American College of Rheumatology Drug Safety Committee succinctly addresses this challenge and is the source of the recommendations highlighted in the following sections (Dao and Cush, 2012).

Distinguishing those vaccines that are live from those that are inactivated is critical when considering immunization of patients with autoimmune diseases on immunomodulatory treatments. Examples of live vaccines include the following: smallpox, adenovirus type 4 and 7, Bacille Calmette-Guérin, typhoid (oral), rotavirus, yellow fever, herpes zoster, influenza (live attenuated), varicella zoster, and measles-mumps-rubella. In the case of live vaccines, therapy with low doses of methotrexate and azathioprine are not considered sufficiently immunosuppressive and corticosteroid therapy is not usually a contraindication in the following cases: duration of treatment is less than 2 weeks, use of a dose less than 20 mg per day, duration of >2 weeks but with alternate-day treatment of short-acting formulations, doses that are physiologic, or route of administration is topical or injected within joints, tendons, or bursae. However, the ACIP identifies patients receiving tumor necrosis factor (TNF) inhibitors or doses of prednisone greater than 20 mg/day for longer than 2 weeks sufficiently immunosuppressed to contradict the use of live attenuated vaccines due to the concern for uncontrolled replication of the viral/bacterial microorganism in the host. If higher doses of steroids are used (>20 mg/day for more than 2 weeks), it is recommended to wait a month after immunosuppression before a live vaccine is given as severe complications have been reported following vaccinations with live vaccines. Such concerns do not apply to inactivated vaccines (whether killed whole-organism, subunit, recombinant, polysaccharide, or toxoid vaccines). Examples of inactivated vaccines include the following: typhoid (polysaccharide), tetanus-diphtheria/acellular pertussis, hepatitis A, hepatitis B, human papilloma, influenza (A/B/H1N1), pneumococcal, polio, rabies, and meningococcal. The reader should be aware that some vaccines licensed for immunization and distribution in the United States (e.g., influenza and typhoid) have been developed by different manufacturers as distinct live or inactivated products. A complete list may be found at the following website: http://www.fda.gov/BiologicsBloodVaccines/Vaccines/ApprovedProducts/UCM093833.

Search and You Will Find

Guidance has been published for the use of vaccination in patients with autoimmune diseases. This has been in part due to the increasing awareness of the importance of vaccines in healthy populations and, ironically, also due to the perceived risk with newer vaccines containing adjuvants. Furthermore, more studies are being conducted and published on the value of vaccinations in patients with autoimmune diseases. Recent data obtained from patients with inflammatory rheumatic diseases that were immunized against pH1N1 influenza with an adjuvanted vaccine indicated a lower immunogenicity in RA patients treated with disease-modifying antirheumatic drugs (DMARDs) (Gabay et al., 2011). One should note that in the same study, there were no significant differences between baseline findings and follow-up findings for any of the disease parameters in 82 RA, 28 spondylarthritis, and 18 SLE patients. While studies such as these confirm the safety of vaccination in such patients, they raise questions about immunogenicity in this patient population. However, one should realize that lower "immunogenicity" does not imply lower "efficacy." Indeed, this is supported by a recent meta-analysis that emphasizes that vaccines are effective in these patients (van Assen et al., 2011). As a result of this meta-analysis, several new recommendations have been published to guide the vaccination of adults with autoimmune disease (Meyer-Olson and Witte, 2011) and the reader is also referred to a web-based article ("How and when to administer inactivated vaccines" at the following website: www.cdc.gov/vaccines/recs/schedules/downloads/adult/adult-schedule.pdf).

CONCLUSION

The primary focus of this chapter is to update clinicians treating patients with autoimmune disease with a concise overview of the challenges facing vaccine development and the best application of this health intervention for their patient population. Those familiar with autoimmune diseases and those involved with vaccine development may already be aware of the common thread to both fields—that is, the triggering of the immune response. However, for those not familiar with these specialties, this common thread has also led to unjustified speculations regarding the relationship between this disease state and this disease intervention. Because this chapter is dedicated to vaccines and their use in patients with autoimmune diseases, the authors thought it would be relevant to mention a few points related to a recently coined syndrome called ASIA. ASIA stands for autoimmune/inflammatory syndrome induced by adjuvants and was first reported in 2011 (Shoenfeld and Agmon-Levin, 2011). While this syndrome attempts to associate a spectrum of immune-mediated diseases with an adjuvant stimulus, the authors coining the term correctly emphasized recently that the clinical proof of causality remains a challenge (Agmon-Levin et al., 2012). There are

some animal models that are being used to try to better understand this rare association (Agmon-Levin et al., 2012) but, in the end, may still be inconclusive for the reasons cited previously on the pitfalls of using animal models for understanding autoimmune disease etiology.

While it is critical to have a high level of scrutiny for the benefit/risk ratio of any prophylactic or therapeutic intervention in human subjects, one needs to keep in mind that vaccines have been responsible for preventing more deaths than virtually any other medicinal product. The value and impact of vaccinations for human health is undeniable—this is the most cost-effective intervention in preventive medicine. Those clinicians not utilizing vaccines routinely in their practices are requested to familiarize themselves in detail regarding vaccines (those with and without adjuvants, live vs. inactivated), the patient populations likely to benefit from such interventions (e.g., young girls and HPV vaccination), and their correct use in patients undergoing immunosuppressive treatments. It is hoped that this review has provided a concise overview that will serve as the basis for more detailed study and prepare the clinicians for the questions posed by their patients about the safety of vaccines.

REFERENCES

Agmon-Levin, N., Hughes, G.R.V., Shoenfeld, Y., 2012. The spectrum of ASIA: "Autoimmune (Auto-inflammatory) Syndrome induced by Adjuvants." Lupus. 21, 118.

Aumeunier, A., Grela, F., Ramadan, A., Pham Van, L., Bardel, E., Gomez Alcala, A., et al., 2010. Systemic Toll-like receptor stimulation suppresses experimental allergic asthma and autoimmune diabetes in NOD mice. PloS One. 5, e11484.

Beeler, J., Varricchio, F., Wise, R., 1996. Thrombocytopenia after immunization with measles vaccines: review of the vaccine adverse events reporting system (1990 to 1994). Pediatr. Infect. Dis. J. 15, 88–90.

Bernasconi, N.L., Onai, N., Lanzavecchia, A., 2003. A role for Toll-like receptors in acquired immunity: up-regulation of TLR9 by BCR triggering in naive B cells and constitutive expression in memory B cells. Blood 101, 4500–4504.

Chen, R.T., Pless, R., Destefano, F., 2001. Epidemiology of autoimmune reactions induced by vaccination. J. Autoimmun. 16, 309–318.

Cooper, G.S., Stroehla, B.C., 2003. The epidemiology of autoimmune diseases. Autoimmun. Rev. 2, 119–125.

Creticos, P.S., Schroeder, J.T., Hamilton, R.G., Balcer-Whaley, S.L., Khattignavong, A.P., Lindblad, R., et al., 2006. Immune Tolerance Network Group, immunotherapy with a ragweed–Toll-like receptor 9 agonist vaccine for allergic rhinitis. N. Engl. J. Med. 355, 1445–1455.

Crow, M.K., 2008. Collaboration, genetic associations, and lupus erythematosus. N. Engl. J. Med. 358, 956–961.

Dao, K., Cush, J.J., 2012. A vaccination primer for rheumatologists. DSQ (Drug Safety Quarterly). 4 (1), 1–4.

De Keyser, J., Zwanikken, C., Boon, M., 1998. Effects of influenza vaccination and influenza illness on exacerbations in multiple sclerosis. J. Neurol. Sci. 159 (1), 51–53.

Fanucchi, M.V., Schelegle, E.S., Baker, G.L., Evans, M.J., McDonald, R.J., Gershwin, L.J., et al., 2004. Immunostimulatory oligonucleotides attenuate airways remodeling in allergic monkeys. Am. J. Respir. Crit. Care Med. 170, 1153–1157.

Gabay, C., Bel, M., Combescure, C., Ribi, C., Meier, S., Posfay-Barbe, K., et al., 2011. H1N1 Study Group. Impact of synthetic and biologic disease-modifying antirheumatic drugs on antibody responses to the AS03-adjuvanted pandemic influenza vaccine: a prospective, open-label, parallel-cohort, single-center study. Arthritis Rheum. 63 (6), 1486–1496.

Gauvreau, G.M., Hessel, E.M., Boulet, L.P., Coffman, R.L., O'Byrne, P.M., 2006. Immunostimulatory sequences regulate interferon-inducible genes but not allergic airway responses. Am. J. Respir. Crit. Care Med. 174, 15–20.

Gelman, A.E., Zhang, J., Choi, Y., Turka, L.A., 2004. Toll-like receptor ligands directly promote activated CD4+ T cell survival. J. Immunol. 172, 6065–6073.

Gilliet, M., Boonstra, A., Paturel, C., Antonenko, S., Xu, X.L., Trinchieri, G., et al., 2002. The development of murine plasmacytoid dendritic cell precursors is differentially regulated by FLT3-ligand and granulocyte/macrophage colony-stimulating factor. J. Exp. Med. 195, 953–958.

Graham, R.R., Hom, G., Ortmann, W., Behrens, T.W., 2009. Review of recent genome-wide association scans in lupus. J. Intern. Med. 265, 680–688.

Han, F., Lin, L., Warby, S.C., Faraco, J., Li, J., Dong, S.X., et al., 2011. Narcolepsy onset is seasonal and increased following the 2009 H1N1 pandemic in China. Ann. Neurol. 70 (3), 410–417.

Hemauer, A., Beckenlehner, K., Wolf, H., Lang, B., Modrow, S., 1999. Acute parvovirus B19 infection in connection with a flare of systemic lupus erythematodes in a female patient. J. Clin. Virol. 14, 73–77.

Hemmer, B., Nessler, S., Zhou, D., Kieseier, B., Hartung, H.P., 2006. Immunopathogenesis and immunotherapy of multiple sclerosis. Nat. Clin. Pract. Neurol. 2, 201–211.

Hornung, V., Rothenfusser, S., Britsch, S., Krug, A., Jahrsdörfer, B., Giese, T., et al., 2002. Quantitative expression of Toll-like receptor 1–10 mRNA in cellular subsets of human peripheral blood mononuclear cells and sensitivity to CpG oligodeoxynucleotides. J. Immunol. 168, 4531–4537.

Jacobson, D.L., Gange, S.J., Rose, N.R., Graham, N.M., 1997. Epidemiology and estimated population burden of selected autoimmune diseases in the United States. Clin. Immunol. Immunopathol. 84, 223–243.

Kikutani, H., Makino, S., 1992. The murine autoimmune diabetes model: NOD and related strains. Adv. Immunol. 51, 285–322.

Kono, D.H., Theofilopoulos, A.N., 2006. Genetics of SLE in mice. Springer Semin. Immunopathol. 28, 83–96.

Krieg, A.M., Efler, S.M., Wittpoth, M., Al Adhami, M.J., Davis, H.L., 2004. Induction of systemic TH1-like innate immunity in normal volunteers following subcutaneous but not intravenous administration of CpG 7909, a synthetic B-class CpG oligodeoxynucleotide TLR9 agonist. J. Immunother. 27, 460–471.

Martin-Orozco, E., Kobayashi, H., Van Uden, J., Nguyen, M.D., Kornbluth, R.S., Raz, E., 1999. Enhancement of antigen-presenting cell surface molecules involved in cognate interactions by immunostimulatory DNA sequences. Int. Immunol. 11, 1111–1118.

Meyer-Olson, D., Witte, T., 2011. Immunology: prevention of infections in patients with autoimmune diseases. Nat. Rev. Rheumatol. 7, 198–200.

Kroger, A.T., Sumaya, C.V., Pickering, L.K., Atkinson, W.L., 2011. Recommendations of the advisory committee on immunization practices (ACIP). MMWR 60, 1–60.

National Narcolepsy Task Force Interim Report (National Institute for Health and Welfare), 2011. Helsinki, Finland.

Oikonen, M., Laaksonen, M., Aalto, V., Ilonen, J., Salonen, R., Erälinna, J.P., et al., 2011. Temporal relationship between environmental influenza A and Epstein-Barr viral infections and high multiple sclerosis relapse occurrence. Mult. Scler. 17 (6), 672–680.

Qin, H.Y., Sadelain, M.W., Hitchon, C., Lauzon, J., Singh, B., 1993. Complete Freund's adjuvant-induced T cells prevent the development and adoptive transfer of diabetes in nonobese diabetic mice. J. Immunol. 150, 2072–2080.

Rothenfusser, S., Tuma, E., Endres, S., Hartmann, G., 2002. Plasmacytoid dendritic cells: the key to CpG. Hum. Immunol. 63, 1111–1119.

Sadelain, M.W., Qin, H.Y., Lauzon, J., Singh, B., 1990. Prevention of type I diabetes in NOD mice by adjuvant immunotherapy. Diabetes. 39, 583–589.

Schonberger, L.B., Bregman, D.J., Sullivan-Bolyai, J.Z., Keenlyside, R. A., Ziegler, D.W., Retailliau, H.F., et al., 1979. Guillain-Barre syndrome following vaccination in the National Influenza Immunization Program, United States, 1976–1977. Am. J. Epidemiol. 110, 105–123.

Shoenfeld, Y., Agmon-Levin, N., 2011. ASIA—Autoimmune/inflammatory syndrome induced by adjuvants. J. Autoimmun. 36, 4–8.

Siegrist, C.A., Lewis, E.M., Eskola, J., Evans, S.J., Black, S.B., 2007. Human papilloma virus immunization in adolescent and young adults: a cohort study to illustrate what events might be mistaken for adverse reactions. Pediatr. Infect. Dis. J. 26, 979–984.

Simons, F.E., Shikishima, Y., Van Nest, G., Eiden, J.J., HayGlass, K.T., 2004. Selective immune redirection in humans with ragweed allergy by injecting Amb a 1 linked to immunostimulatory DNA. J. Allergy Clin. Immunol. 113, 1144–1151.

Statement on Narcolepsy and Vaccination (Global Advisory Committee on Vaccine Safety), 2011. World Health Organization, Geneva, Switzerland.

Stojanovich, L., 2006. Influenza vaccination of patients with systemic lupus erythematosus (SLE) and rheumatoid arthritis (RA). Clin. Dev. Immunol. 13, 373–375.

Suzuki, K., Suda, T., Naito, T., Ide, K., Chida, K., Nakamura, H., 2005. Impaired Toll-like receptor 9 expression in alveolar macrophages with no sensitivity to CpG DNA. Am. J. Respir. Crit. Care Med. 171, 707–713.

Swaddiwuthipong, W., Weniger, B.G., Wattanasri, S., Warrell, M.J., 1998. A high rate of neurological complications following Semple anti-rabies vaccine. Trans. R. Soc. Trop. Med. Hyg. 82 (3), 472–475.

Tulic, M.K., Fiset, P.O., Chistodoulopoulos, P., Vaillancourt, P., Desrosiers, M., Lavigne, et al., 2004. Amb a 1-immunostimulatory oligodeoxynucleotide conjugate immunotherapy decreases the nasal inflammatory response. J. Allergy Clin. Immunol. 113, 235–241.

US Census Bureau, 2011. Statistical Abstract of the United States, Table 7. Resident Population by Sex and Age: 1980 to 2009. US Government Printing Office, Washington, DC, <http://www.census. gov/compendia/statab/2011/tables/11s0007.pdf>.

van Assen, S., Elkayam, O., Agmon-Levin, N., Cervera, R., Doran, M. F., Dougados, M., et al., 2011. Vaccination in adult patients with auto-immune inflammatory rheumatic diseases: A systematic literature review for the European League Against Rheumatism evidence-based recommendations for vaccination in adult patients with auto-immune inflammatory rheumatic diseases. Autoimmun. Rev. 10, 341–352.

Wraith, D.C., Goldman, M., Lambert, P.H., 2003. Vaccination and autoimmune disease: What is the evidence? Lancet. 362, 1659–1666.

Chapter 21

Non-infectious Environmental Agents and Autoimmunity

Frederick W. Miller

Environmental Autoimmunity Group, Office of Clinical Research, National Institute of Environmental Health Sciences, National Institutes of Health, Bethesda, MD, USA

Chapter Outline

Introduction	283	Tobacco Smoke	290
Evidence Supporting the Role of Environmental Agents in		Heavy Metals	290
Autoimmune Disease	284	Microchimerism	290
Identifying and Defining Environmentally Associated		Vaccines	290
Autoimmune Diseases	285	Implants	290
Non-Infectious Agents Associated with Autoimmune Diseases	286	Stress	291
Drugs	286	Possible Mechanisms by Which Environmental Agents May	
Occupational Exposures	288	Induce Autoimmune Diseases	291
Others	289	Overview and Future Directions	291
Foods	289	References	293

INTRODUCTION

Although the mechanisms for the development of autoimmune diseases remain obscure, accumulating evidence suggests that these increasingly recognized disorders result from environmental exposures in genetically susceptible individuals (Luppi et al., 1995; Cooper et al., 1999; Miller, 1999; Gourley and Miller, 2007; Miller et al., 2012; Pollard et al., 2010). Despite the great progress that has been made in understanding a number of major histocompatibility complex (MHC) and non-MHC genetic risk factors for autoimmune diseases (see Chapters 26 and 28), relatively little information is now available regarding the role of specific environmental agents in the development of these disorders. This is partly the result of the lack of validated exposure biomarkers and environmental assessment tools, difficulties inherent in defining which of the many environmental exposures are related to disease, the little formal training in environmental medicine, the few resources dedicated to this area, and the lack of consensus approaches for the definition of environmentally associated diseases. As a result, in the case of most autoimmune conditions, the specific environmental triggers remain unknown.

Just as there are likely to be multiple genes needed to induce autoimmune disease, multiple environmental exposures may need to occur in a particular sequence, or in tandem, to provoke the chronic immune activation that leads to autoimmunity. It is also possible that epigenetics, referring to modifications in gene expression that are controlled by heritable but potentially reversible changes in DNA methylation and/or chromatin structure, may be influenced by environmental exposures (Javierre et al., 2011). In this regard, many lessons might be learned from studies and registries of cancers, which like autoimmune diseases are multifactorial disorders in which multiple genetic and environmental risk factors must interact in a correct sequence, with occasional long latencies, before development of disease (Sarasin, 2003). Thus, in some cases, a change induced by one exposure may be necessary before a subsequent exposure can have its effect. Alternatively, mixtures of exposures, including possible infectious and non-infectious agents, perhaps occurring during critical windows when persons may be more

N. Rose & I. Mackay (Eds): The Autoimmune Diseases, Fifth edition. DOI: http://dx.doi.org/10.1016/B978-0-12-384929-8.00021-6

susceptible to them (i.e., *in utero*, in childhood, during puberty, pregnancy, or lactation) may be necessary in order to overcome tolerance. Other general principles from cancer that might be relevant to autoimmunity include the pathogenetic heterogeneity of currently defined disorders, the likely low effect sizes from many environmental exposures, and the possible requirement for inducers, promoters, and sustainers of disease at different points in the pathogenetic process (Cooper et al., 2002). This is particularly borne out by investigations suggesting that autoantibodies precede the development of clinical disease by months to years and are antigen-driven (Dotta and Eisenbarth, 1989; Miller et al., 1990; Leslie et al., 2001; Arbuckle et al., 2003; Klareskog et al., 2004; Hirschfield and Gershwin, 2013). This suggests that certain environmental exposures may be necessary to overcome tolerance in genetically susceptible individuals and induce autoantibody formation, while other agents may be necessary to promote expression of clinical disease.

If one defines environmental agents as everything outside the genome, then the many exposures that have been suspected of being involved in the pathogenesis of autoimmunity may be divided into two general categories: infectious and non-infectious agents. This chapter will focus on the evidence for the role of non-infectious environmental agents in the pathogenesis of human autoimmune diseases, while infectious agents are reviewed in Chapter 19.

EVIDENCE SUPPORTING THE ROLE OF ENVIRONMENTAL AGENTS IN AUTOIMMUNE DISEASE

Evidence for the role of environmental agents in autoimmune disease comes from a variety of investigative approaches (Box 21.1). Although many of these methods are indirect, anecdotal, or may be only applicable to single patients, taken together these diverse findings strongly support the contention that most autoimmune diseases do have an important environmental component (Cooper et al., 1999; Smyk et al., 2012).

One line of evidence for the role of the environment is that for autoimmune diseases studied to date there is generally less than 50% disease concordance in monozygotic twins (Leslie and Hawa, 1994; Cooper et al., 1999; Bogdanos et al., 2012). These findings also hint that even if all the genetic risk factors for a given autoimmune disease could be fully identified, this would not allow for prediction of disease with any greater accuracy than the flip of a coin without the incorporation of environmental or other factors.

For certain agents it can be relatively clear when a given exposure is inducing a disease in an individual patient. The definition of an environmental disease in an individual can be accomplished by identifying a new clinical disorder, which develops soon after a novel exposure, resolves when the exposure is removed (dechallenge), and then recurs after reintroduction of the same exposure (rechallenge). This approach is most easily applied in the case of exposures to defined chemical entities such as drugs, foods, topical, or inhaled toxicants. Unfortunately, many xenobiotics (compounds not naturally found in the body) cannot easily be removed from an organism after exposure, and therefore for these agents this approach is not usually helpful. Exposures in this category include inhaled silica, vaccines, fat-soluble oils, and collagen or silicone implants.

The nonrandom distribution in time and space of some autoimmune illnesses also implies that non-genetic factors are important in disease development (Moroni et al., 2012). Studies in these areas are preliminary, and sometimes have not been reproduced, leading critics to posit that referral or other biases might explain some of the findings. Nonetheless, intriguing investigations have

---

Box 21.1 Lines of Evidence Supporting the Role of Environmental Agents in the Development of Autoimmune Disease

1. Less than 50% disease concordance in monozygotic twins
2. Strong temporal associations with some environmental exposures and disease onset
3. Dechallenge (disease resolution or improvement in an individual after removal of the suspect agent)
4. Rechallenge (disease recurrence or worsening in an individual after re-exposure to the suspect agent)
5. Seasonality in birth dates and disease onset
6. Geographic clustering in disease incidence or prevalence
7. Changes in the prevalence or incidence of disease over time and when genetically similar cohorts move to different geographic locations
8. Major genetic risk factors for autoimmune diseases are polymorphic genes that influence responses to environmental exposures
9. Strong biologic plausibility from animal models
10. Epidemiologic associations between particular exposures and certain diseases

suggested that certain autoimmune disorders have a seasonal onset or that there is a seasonal association with subsets of patients based upon disease-specific autoantibodies. The diseases reported to have seasonal associations include autoimmune myositis (Leff et al., 1991; Miller, 1993; Sarkar et al., 2005), juvenile rheumatoid arthritis (Feldman et al., 1996), type 1 diabetes (Weinberg et al., 1984; Willis et al., 2002), narcolepsy (Han et al., 2011), Wegener's granulomatosis, anti-neutrophil cytoplasmic antibodies associated glomerulonephritis, and systemic vasculitis (Schlesinger and Schlesinger, 2005). Furthermore, studies of type 1 diabetes, myositis, and other diseases have found significant associations with birth dates (Ursic-Bratina et al., 2001; Willis et al., 2002; Vegosen et al., 2007) implying that certain exposures at certain times of the year may alter the target tissues or immune systems of fetuses or neonates resulting in later autoimmunity. While infectious agents are often presumed to be the source of such seasonal or geographic associations, the immune system, like other organ systems, appears to have cyclic or rhythmic patterns (Haus and Smolensky, 1999), possibly related to light exposure and mediated by melatonin or other neurohormones (Nelson and Drazen, 2000). Additionally, many occupational or other exposures are seasonal, including exposures to certain pesticides, chemicals in sunscreens, and some air or water pollutants, so it is possible that non-infectious agents could account for some of these data in ways that have not been accounted for. Geographic clustering or gradients in disease prevalence or incidence have also been found for some autoimmune diseases. These investigations have primarily shown associations with latitude, suggesting a role of ultraviolet radiation in inducing disease, as may be the case for dermatomyositis (Okada et al., 2003; Love et al., 2009), altering mortality, as may be the case in lupus (Grant, 2004), or protecting from disease, as may be the case in multiple sclerosis and type 1 diabetes (Ponsonby et al., 2002).

Measurable increases or decreases in the incidence or prevalence of disease over time imply a non-genetic etiology given the slow rate of genetic change in a population. Although data are limited in this area—and several studies are possibly confounded as a result of improvements in the ability to diagnose some conditions over time—it appears that type 1 diabetes, multiple sclerosis, lupus, and myositis are becoming increasingly prevalent, while rheumatoid arthritis in adults and children may be decreasing in frequency in some populations (Oddis et al., 1990; Onkamo et al., 1999; Uramoto et al., 1999; Cooper and Stroehla, 2003). Changes in living standards and treatment approaches may also have an impact on disease frequency, as in the case of decreasing rheumatic heart disease (Johnson et al., 1975). Some authors believe that as our exposure to microbial agents has decreased in our modern urban environments, the development of our immune systems has been altered to result in greater frequencies of autoimmune disorders, a concept known as the "hygiene hypothesis" (Rook, 2012).

Studies of genetically similar populations living under different conditions are also illuminating. The incidences of both multiple sclerosis and type 1 diabetes have changed as members of a population move to new regions (Dahlquist, 1998; Noseworthy et al., 2000).

Epidemiologic studies linking specific exposures to autoimmunity are limited and usually consist of relatively small, often underpowered investigations resulting in low effect sizes and large confidence limits. Much larger, well-designed, multicentered, and sometimes international studies, using appropriate controls and collecting adequate information to minimize confounding, will be needed in the future to more fully define the specific environmental risk factors for disease (Miller et al., 2012).

IDENTIFYING AND DEFINING ENVIRONMENTALLY ASSOCIATED AUTOIMMUNE DISEASES

One of the limitations in making progress towards identifying and defining environmental triggers for autoimmune disorders has been the lack of general consensus on the necessary and sufficient evidence needed to define an environmentally associated condition. Medical—legal issues that surround many environmental exposures have further complicated this area. A group of experts in the field—members of the American College of Rheumatology Environmentally Associated Rheumatic Disease Study Group—developed consensus on a general approach to overcome this problem (Miller et al., 2000). In their scheme, the overall process, from the identification of the first possible patient who developed a disease after an exposure, to the refinement of classification criteria for the disease, is divided into four stages (Table 21.1).

The first stage begins with the identification of a single case, or a series of cases, which is suspected of resulting from a given exposure. The consensus proposal is that these cases need to meet certain criteria to assure a minimum number of attribution elements are present (Miller et al., 2000). A total of at least four of all eight possible attribution elements need to be present, including at least three of five primary elements. The five primary elements are: temporal plausibility (taking into account the pharmacokinetics/pharmacodynamics of the agent, minimum induction time, and maximum latency); exclusion of other likely causes for the syndrome; dechallenge (if possible); rechallenge (if appropriate); and biologic plausibility. The additional three secondary elements are: identification of

TABLE 21.1 Proposed Stages for Identifying and Defining Environmentally-Associated Autoimmune Diseases[a].

Stage	Description	Nomenclature (example)
Stage 1—Proposing the association	Case reports, defined by ascertainment criteria, propose a possible association of a specific clinical syndrome with a given exposure	Syndrome following exposure (rheumatoid arthritis following hepatitis B vaccination)
Stage 2—Testing the association	After a number of such cases are reported, surveillance criteria are proposed and epidemiologic and laboratory studies test that hypothesis	Cardinal signs, symptoms and labs but without the putative exposure (eosinophilia myalgia syndrome)
Stage 3—Defining criteria for the condition	If studies above are positive, then specific preliminary classification and other criteria are defined for that specific environmental disease	Exposure-associated disorder (L tryptophan-associated eosinophilia myalgia syndrome)
Stage 4—Refining criteria for the condition	Criteria are reassessed and refined as additional data are obtained about the disease	Exposure-induced disorder (hydralazine-induced lupus-like disorder)

[a]Modified from Miller et al. (2000).

prior reports of similar cases (analogy); identification of prior reports of nearly identical cases (specificity); and evidence for a dose–response effect. In addition to meeting these criteria, it is suggested that complete information regarding the history and examination, laboratory reports, core demographic data, family history, prior infections, or physiology-altering exposures, all prior diagnoses, and the type/route/ dose/duration of the exposure are detailed in the report.

The second stage involves testing the possible association. This should include epidemiologic studies, using surveillance criteria, to evaluate the relationship between a given exposure and a given syndrome. *In vitro*, *in vivo*, and animal studies should also assess the biologic effects of the agent and plausibility of the development of the syndrome. Other approaches—such as clinical, laboratory, or genetic risk factor studies—could determine in case–control settings if cases of environmental disease differ from those with similar diseases without the exposure or differ from subjects similarly exposed who do not develop disease.

If data from the second stage results in convincing evidence that the assocation is real, then the third stage will develop preliminary criteria for that environmentally associated disease. Classification criteria will define, with reasonable sensitivity and specificity, groups of patients with one disorder from closely related diseases. Expert committee consensus, mathematical algorithms or other approaches could develop these criteria. Symptom, sign, and laboratory criteria should be expressed in clinically sensible and practical formats with precise definitions of constituent elements. Diagnostic, prognostic, and outcome criteria, and disease activity and damage indexes, should be considered when adequate data exist. The fourth stage repeats the same processes used in the

third stage if new information is collected to warrant a redefinition of the disease.

Although this proposed staging structure has limitations, in that the decisions as to when to progress to the next stage remain somewhat subjective, it nonetheless provides an overall framework to plan for future studies and it allows the classification of the current environmental agents into groups with different levels of evidence for their association with specific syndromes. Unfortunately, most environmental agents suspected of being associated with autoimmune diseases today remain in Stages 1 or 2.

NON-INFECTIOUS AGENTS ASSOCIATED WITH AUTOIMMUNE DISEASES

Drugs

Of all the non-infectious environmental exposures associated with autoimmunity, drugs are the best recognized and most often reported (Table 21.2). This is partly due to their widespread use and careful monitoring by clinicians, the strict regulatory oversight and adverse event reporting systems in many countries, and the ease of collection of dechallenge and rechallnge evidence to make associations in individual patients. Despite the fact that several hundred drugs have been associated in case reports or case series with a number of immune-mediated or autoimmune illnesses, few of the publications have met the consensus criteria described above to allow exclusion of confounding factors and few have been studied in epidemiologic investigations. Chemical agents have been the most often reported drugs preceding the development of autoimmunity, although the increasing use of biologic agents has resulted in more focus on these in recent years.

TABLE 21.2 Selected Drugs Associated in Case Reports or Case Series with Autoimmune Disorders[a].

Drug	Associated Autoimmune Disorders
α-methyldopa	lupus-like syndrome, hemolytic anemia, thrombocytopenia
allopurinol	lupus-like syndrome, vasculitis
bleomycin	scleroderma
captropril	lupus-like syndrome, vasculitis, membranous glomerulopathy
chlorpromazine	lupus-like syndrome, hemolytic anemia
D-penicillamine	lupus-like syndrome, myositis, hypothyroidism, Goodpasture's
erythromycins	lupus-like syndrome, myositis, hepatitis
estrogens	lupus-like syndrome, myositis
gold salts	lupus-like syndrome, membranous glomerulopathy
halothane	hepatitis
hydralazines	lupus-like syndrome, vasculitis, hepatitis
interferon-alpha	lupus-like syndrome, anti-phospholipid syndrome, arthritis, hemolytic anemia, thrombocytopenia, hepatitis, hypothyroidism
interferon-gamma	lupus-like syndrome, myositis, arthritis, hypothyroidism
interleukin-2	scleroderma, anti-phospholipid syndrome, arthritis, hypothyroidism
iodine	hypothyroidism
isoniazid	lupus-like syndrome, arthritis, hepatitis, vasculitis, hypothyroidism
L-tryptophan	EMS, scleroderma, myositis, neuropathies
lipid-lowering agents	lupus-like syndrome, myositis, hepatitis
penicillins	anemia, lupus-like syndrome, hepatitis
phenytoin	scleroderma, lupus-like syndrome, hepatitis, thrombocytopenia
procainamide	lupus-like syndrome
propylthiouracil	lupus-like syndrome, ANCA + vasculitis, myositis
quinidine	lupus-like syndrome, arthritis, thrombocytopenia
rifampicin	thrombocytopenia, vasculitis
sulphonamides	lupus-like syndrome, vasculitis
tetracyclines	lupus-like syndrome, arthritis, vasculitis
TNF-inhibitors	lupus-like syndrome

[a]Reviewed in Love and Miller (1993); Bigazzi (1997); Mackay (1999); D'Cruz (2000); Hess (2002); Liu and Kaplowitz (2002); Chang and Gershwin (2011); abbreviations: ANCA, antineutrophil cytoplasmic antibodies; EMS, eosinophilia myalgia syndrome; TNF, tumor necrosis factor.

The most commonly recognized drug-related syndromes are lupus-like disorders (Hess and Mongey, 1991). These are characterized by autoantibodies to histones and single-stranded DNA, rather than autoantibodies to double-stranded DNA as are found more often in non-drug-related lupus. Drug-related lupus also differs from non-drug-related lupus in having more frequent arthritis and less frequent neurologic and renal involvement, as well as having possibly different genetic risk factors. Virtually all of the 80 or more autoimmune diseases have been anecdotally reported to be associated with one or more drugs. In some of these cases drug-linked disorders differ from the non-drug-related forms in clinical, serologic, or genetic features, while in other cases they do not.

It is noteworthy that although some drugs appear to be associated with a number of autoimmune conditions (Table 21.2), there are no common structures, mechanisms of action, metabolites, or other features among them that consistently allow prediction of their toxicity or a

TABLE 21.3 Occupational Exposures Associated with Autoimmune Diseases via Epidemiologic Studies[a].

Exposure	Disease	Summary of Results
Silica	Scleroderma	Three-fold increased risk in four occupational cohort studies; mixed results in five population-based case–control studies
	Rheumatoid arthritis	Three-fold (or higher) increased risk in five occupational cohort studies
	Lupus	>10-fold increased risk in three occupational cohort studies
	ANCA + vasculitis	Four-fold increased risk in three case–control studies
Solvents	Scleroderma	Mixed results, but some evidence of two to three-fold increased risk with specific solvents (e.g., paint thinners and removers, trichloroethylene) and with "any" solvent
	Undifferentiated multisystem rheumatic diseases	Two-fold increased risk with paint thinners and removers, mineral spirits; three-fold increased risk with specific solvent-related occupations
	Rheumatoid arthritis	Weak or no association with specific solvents, but two-fold increased risk among spray painters and lacquer workers
	Multiple sclerosis	Two to three-fold increased risk with solvent exposures in most studies
Pesticides	Rheumatoid arthritis, lupus	Weak associations (relative risks <2.0) seen with pesticide exposure and in farmers and horticultural workers
Ultraviolet radiation	Multiple sclerosis	Reduced risk (OR 0.74) of multiple sclerosis and mortality with increased occupational exposure to sunlight
	Dermatomyositis	Positive correlation of the proportion of dermatomyositis with global surface sunlight intensity in international and US studies

[a]Data from Cooper et al. (2002, 2010); Love et al. (2009); McCormic et al. (2010); Parks et al. (2011); abbreviations: OR, odds ratio; ANCA, antineutrophil cytoplasmic antibodies.

current understanding of the pathogenesis of these syndromes. The challenge today is to begin to decipher the genetic and other risk factors that interact with exposure to these drugs that result in disease so that they can someday be predicted and prevented.

Occupational Exposures

Limited but growing epidemiologic and experimental data have linked a number of occupational exposures to autoimmune diseases (Table 21.3). The most studied of these include silica, solvents, pesticides, and ultraviolet radiation (Westberg et al., 2009; Cooper et al., 2002, 2010; Parks et al., 2011). One of the first occupationally associated rheumatic diseases identified was Caplan's syndrome, which is seropositive rheumatoid arthritis associated with a specific form of pneumoconiosis that develops in anthracite coal-miners and in persons exposed to silica and asbestos (Williams, 1991). The strongest occupational associations with autoimmune disease (i.e., relative risks of 3.0 and higher) have been documented in investigations of silica dust and rheumatoid arthritis, lupus, scleroderma and antineutrophil cytoplasmic autoantibody (ANCA) associated glomerulonephritis (Parks et al., 1999; Khuder et al., 2002). Weaker associations are seen, however, for solvent exposures (in scleroderma, undifferentiated multisystem rheumatic disease, and

multiple sclerosis) and for farming or pesticide exposures (in rheumatoid arthritis). Vinyl chloride has been linked to the development of a scleroderma-like disease characterized by skin thickening, Raynaud's phenomenon, acroosteolysis, and pulmonary involvement. This observation, and the publication of several case reports, stimulated research into associations between scleroderma and other chlorinated solvents (e.g., trichloroethylene and trichloroethane) with varying results (Cooper et al., 2002, 2009).

There are many difficulties in assessing the role of occupational exposures in disease. First, there are few biomarkers for such exposures and essentially none that allow an estimate of lifetime cumulative exposure. Second, there are few validated occupational exposure questionnaires and those that do exist are awkward and costly to apply. Third, most studies in this area have been underpowered given the rarity of the diseases, the likely effects of different genotypes, and the occupations of interest, resulting in imprecise risk estimates. And finally, there is possible confounding from multiple concurrent exposures that makes it difficult to ascertain whether different effects can be attributed to different chemicals. Thus, it may not be surprising that in some cases discrepancies exist in different investigations, making it difficult to assess the true overall risks of most occupational exposures.

TABLE 21.4 Other Exposures Proposed as Possible Risk Factors for Autoimmune Diseases[a].

Exposure	Disease	Comments (Reference)
Foods (gluten)	Celiac disease	Celiac disease develops after ingestion of foods containing gluten and related proteins in some genetically susceptible persons (Alaedini and Green, 2005)
Cigarette smoking	Rheumatoid arthritis	Studies suggest relative risks of 1.5–3 with a greater effect in men, seropositive disease and those with the HLA shared epitope (Krishnan, 2003; Stolt et al., 2003; Kallberg et al., 2011)
	Autoimmune thyroid disease	Meta-analyses suggest two to three-fold increased risks of Graves' and Hashimoto's (Vestergaard, 2002)
	Inflammatory bowel disease	Smoking increases risks for Crohn's disease but decreases risks for ulcerative colitis (Timmer, 2003)
Heavy metals	Multiple syndromes	"Pink disease" (acrodynia) and glomerulopathy from mercury toxicity; related syndromes with elements of autoimmunity from cadmium and gold salt toxicity; granulomatous pneumonitis from beryllium exposure; support for genetic risk factors in animal models (Bigazzi, 1994; Dally, 1997; Fontenot and Kotzin 2003)
Microchimerism	Scleroderma, lupus, primary biliary cirrhosis, autoimmune thyroid disease	Fetal cells detected in maternal blood or target tissue specimens years after pregnancy—not all findings have been reproduced, possibly due to different methodologies with different sensitivities to detect rare microchimeric cells (Sarkar and Miller 2004)
	Juvenile myositis	Maternal cells detected in children who developed myositis (Artlett et al., 2000)
Vaccines	Multiple syndromes	Arthritis after rubella virus vaccines; thrombocytopenia after measles vaccines; Guillain–Barre syndrome after swine flu vaccine and tetanus; controversy remains over others (Wraith et al., 2003)
Collagen implants	Myositis	In one study, OR = 5.05; 95% CI, 2.31 to 9.59 for all forms of myositis (Cukier et al., 1993)
Silicone implants	Multiple syndromes	Most studies do not find associations with common autoimmune diseases (Janowsky et al., 2000; Tugwell et al., 2001); rare or atypical multisystem rheumatic diseases and fibromyalgia remain inadequately studied (Brown et al., 1998; Brown, 2002).
Stress	Graves' disease	Stressful life events in the 12 months preceding the diagnosis were significantly higher than controls (OR = 6.3, CI = 2.7–14.7 (Winsa et al., 1991); other diseases poorly studied

[a]*Abbreviations: OR, odds ratio; CI, 95% confidence interval; ANCA, antineutrophil cytoplasmic antibodies.*

Others

A wide variety of other exposures with greatly different properties have been proposed to be associated with auto-immune diseases (Table 21.4). The evidence supporting these proposed associations range from case reports to epidemiologic studies and many are speculative at this time. These are listed below under the major categories into which they may be classified.

Foods

Foods represent some of the better examples of environmental agents associated with autoimmune diseases. The best example is celiac disease, which is characterized by an immune response to ingested wheat gluten and related proteins of rye and barley that leads to autoantibodies to transglutaminase and inflammation, villous atrophy, and crypt hyperplasia in the intestine (Alaedini and Green, 2005). These is also good evidence for gene–environment interaction in celiac disease with human leukocyte antigens DQ2 and DQ8 being the major known genetic risk factors. Celiac disease is one of the few medical conditions for which dietary intervention is the main treatment modality and a gluten-free diet markedly decreases symptoms in most individuals. Although there is less support for an autoimmune etiology of other food-associated inflammatory disorders—including the L-tryptophan-associated eosinophilia myalgia syndrome (Sullivan et al., 1996) and the contaminated rapeseed oil-associated toxic oil syndrome (Gelpi et al., 2002)—it is possible that some of these represent cases of food-associated autoimmunity given their frequent autoantibodies and immunogenetic associations (Okada et al., 2009).

Tobacco Smoke

Tobacco smoke has been associated epidemiologically with an increased risk of seropositive rheumatoid arthritis, in which a gene–environment interaction is clear (Bang et al., 2010), autoimmune thyroid disease, and Crohn's disease in several studies, but inconsistent results were found in studies of smoking and systemic lupus erythematosus, multiple sclerosis, and Hashimoto's thyroiditis (Miller et al., 2012).

Smoking may be associated with a reduced risk of ulcerative colitis, an inflammatory bowel disease implying that the complex mix of chemicals in tobacco smoke may have different effects in different genetic backgrounds.

Heavy Metals

Exposures to heavy metals, including mercury, cadmium, gold salts, and beryllium, have been associated with a variety of pathologic syndromes, some of which have features of autoimmunity. A recent study of communities in Amazonian Brazil with well-characterized exposures to mercury was the first to document immunologic changes, indicative of autoimmune dysfunction, in persons exposed to mercury (Silva et al., 2004). Additionally, many animal models have documented inflammatory and sometimes highly specific autoimmune responses to the heavy metals, even at subtoxic doses, which appear to differ in different genetic backgrounds (Bagenstose et al., 1999). The mechanisms for these many effects remain unclear, but possibilities include changing the response repertoire by direct and indirect means via changes in cytokine profiles, influencing expression of new antigens, new peptides, and/or antigen presentation by modifying the antigen-presenting complex (Rowley and Monestier, 2005), as has been reported for Abacavir loading of novel self-peptides into HLA-B*57: 01 (Norcross et al., 2012).

Microchimerism

Microchimerism is the persistence of a low level of non-host stem cells or their progeny in an individual. A possible role of microchimerism in the pathogenesis of some (systemic sclerosis, systemic lupus erythematosus, primary biliary cirrhosis, autoimmune thyroid diseases, and juvenile myositis) but not all autoimmune diseases has been suggested by recent studies (Sarkar and Miller,

2004). The initial impetus to explore this exposure was that many of the diseases associated with microchimerism have features that are shared with graft-versus-host disease suggesting a possible mechanism. Although an appealing hypothesis, controversy in the area continues due to the lack of reproducible studies to date and the lack of proof of the role of microchimeric cells in the pathogenesis of these disorders. That cells of multiple origins and different genetic backgrounds may combine to result in functional organ systems, both in mothers and their offspring, requires a re-evaluation of many current paradigms. It is possible that such chimeric mixtures play a role in autoimmunity, tissue repair, and other areas (Fugazzola et al., 2011). Further research—using standardized, sensitive, and validated methods—is needed to address the many questions that the early findings in this field have raised.

Vaccines

Because vaccines are foreign proteins often injected with adjuvants into muscle to induce immune responses, it may not be surprising that immune-mediated adverse events have been reported after a wide variety of immunizations. Although a number of autoimmune diseases have been found to develop following vaccinations, only a few have been deemed to be associated with disease by the Advisory Committee on Immunization Practices (Advisory Committee on Immunization Practices, 1996) and are now compensated by the National Vaccine Injury Compensation Program (http://www.hrsa.gov/vaccinecompensation/index.html). These include cases of chronic arthritis after rubella virus vaccines and thrombocytopenic purpura after measles vaccines. There remains significant controversy over other illnesses possibly caused by immunizations, but most of the epidemiologic studies in this area have not shown significant associations (Wraith et al., 2003).

Implants

Bovine collagen implants are biomaterials used for the correction of dermal contour deformities. The use of bovine collagen implants in patients with a personal history of autoimmune diseases is contraindicated by the manufacturer due to concerns that they might induce adverse immune responses, since anti-collagen autoantibodies are present in some patients with multisystem rheumatic diseases. Few epidemiologic studies have been performed in this area, although one study has evaluated the development of myositis in nine patients following collagen implants (Cukier et al., 1993). Eight of the nine patients had a delayed-type hypersensitivity response at the test or treatment sites, and five of six patients tested were found to have increased serum

TABLE 21.5 Possible Mechanisms by which Environmental Agents May Induce Autoimmunity and Promote and Sustain Autoimmune Diseases (Possible Examples in Parentheses)[a].

1. Alteration of target tissue autoantigen structure (bystander drugs, heavy metals)
2. Upregulation or altered locations of normally sequestered autoantigens (UV radiation)
3. Cytotoxic, inhibitory, or stimulatory effects on components of the immune system (interferons, interleukins)
4. Molecular mimicry—structures shared between environmental agent and self (infectious agents)
5. Other effects and combinations of the above

[a]Initiators of autoimmunity may differ in action from promoters and sustainers of autoimmune disease.

antibodies to collagen. Compared with the general population, the incidence of dermatomyositis or polymyositis among collagen-treated patients was significantly increased.

Silicone implants remain some of the most controversial environmental agents proposed to be associated with connective tissue disorders. Studies in this area have been hampered by the extensive litigation involved in adverse events following silicone breast implants and the lack of adequate regulatory review prior to their initial use. Most studies have not found associations with common autoimmune diseases (Janowsky et al., 2000; Tugwell et al., 2001); however, some investigators believe that rare or atypical multisystem rheumatic diseases and fibromyalgia remain inadequately studied (Brown et al., 1998; Brown, 2002). Of interest, women who develop myositis after silicone implants appear to be an immunogenetically distinct subgroup with different allelic associations than are seen in women who develop myositis without implants (O'Hanlon et al., 2004).

Stress

Anecdotes have been reported that stressful life events have preceded the development of many autoimmune diseases. A large population-based, case–control study of Graves' disease showed that patients had more negative life events in the 12 months preceding the diagnosis of Graves', and negative life-event scores were also significantly higher (Winsa et al., 1991). Other diseases have not been adequately studied. Although the mechanisms for how stress may play a role remain unclear, it has been hypothesized that, under certain conditions, stress hormones may boost immune responses through induction of tumor necrosis factor (TNF)-alpha, interleukin (IL)-1, and IL-8 and by inhibiting transforming growth factor (TGF)-beta production (Elenkov and Chrousos, 1999). Therefore, conditions that are associated with significant changes in stress system activity may modulate the neuroendocrine–immune axis and perturb systemic cytokine balances resulting in proinflammatory changes and disease induction.

POSSIBLE MECHANISMS BY WHICH ENVIRONMENTAL AGENTS MAY INDUCE AUTOIMMUNE DISEASES

Although the mechanisms for the development of autoimmune diseases associated with non-infectious agent exposures remain poorly understood, a variety of theories have been postulated to explain how xenobiotics may induce disease (Table 21.5). The wide range of these theories emphasizes the lack of understanding of mechanisms even for the most carefully defined environmentally associated diseases. This also suggests that different pathogenic mechanisms are likely at work in different syndromes.

Whatever the specific mechanisms for the development of an autoimmune disease, it has been suggested that an overall framework should include the concept of heterogeneity within the currently defined diseases. A working hypothesis that addresses this issue has been termed the "elemental disorder hypothesis," which posits that each autoimmune disease as currently recognized contains many elemental disorders (Shamim and Miller, 2000; Gourley and Miller, 2007). In this scenario, an elemental disorder is defined as a unique sign–symptom–laboratory complex (syndrome) that results from a distinct pathogenesis as a result of the interaction of the necessary and sufficient genetic and environmental risk factors. If this concept is true, elemental disorders are likely confounding most studies of disease today by inducing "comparisons of apples and oranges." If identified, elemental disorders should greatly increase the homogeneity of populations under study and thus decrease the numbers of individuals needed for genetic, environmental, and therapeutic studies. In the future, elemental disorder identification could allow for the prevention of some illnesses by avoidance of environmental risk factors or via gene therapy to correct deleterious genetic risk factors.

OVERVIEW AND FUTURE DIRECTIONS

The multifactorial nature of autoimmune diseases has inhibited understanding of the mechanisms that initiate and sustain them. Autoimmune syndromes are believed to arise, however, from a complex and ill-understood interplay of predisposing genetic and environmental risk factors. While some progress is being made in defining the multiple genetic risk factors, we are in our infancy in the identification of the environmental risk factors for autoimmune illnesses. Understanding the interactions of those elements that are necessary for disease development offers the promise of preventing or treating autoimmune diseases in novel ways. But before that can be accomplished important questions remain to be answered. Which specific gene–environment interactions lead to which specific clinical syndromes? What are the pathogenic mechanisms involved? Is every autoimmune disease, as currently understood, actually composed of many subsets or "elemental disorders," each of which may be defined by a unique pathogenesis resulting from interactions of the necessary and sufficient risk factors? Can selected autoimmune diseases be better treated, cured, or even prevented through answers to some of the above questions?

We live in an increasingly complex sea of xenobiotics, which complicates exposure assessments. More than 80,000 chemicals are registered for use in commerce in the United States, and an estimated 2000 new ones are introduced annually to be included in our foods, personal care products, drugs, household cleaners, and a host of industrial processes. The long-term effects of most of these chemicals on human health are unknown, yet we may be exposed to them during the manufacture, distribution, use, and disposal of products or as pollutants in our air, water, or soil. As a result, none of us knows the full range of environmental agents we are exposed to on a daily basis.

The concept of the exposome, which would be all the exposures that an individual has experienced during their lifetime, has been proposed to be a useful construct to focus attention on the critical need for more comprehensive environmental exposure assessments. Currently we are not able to simultaneously measure the many important components of the exposome—including xenobiotics approved in commerce, the additional thousands of compounds not approved but to which we are exposed in our foods, air and water supplies, plus stressful life events, cigarette smoke or alcoholic drink compositions, drugs and dietary supplements, nanoparticles, biotoxins, cosmetics, hair dyes, ultraviolet and other radiation and climatic factors, electric and magnetic fields—at any single time point in an individual, let alone over a lifetime. Much more work is needed to develop the novel assessment tools that could begin to evaluate these multiple exposures, either directly or indirectly, via their effects on gene expression or epigenetic modification, microRNA levels, or protein composition of various matrices in the body, both in real time and in summation over time.

To summarize, many challenges have prevented further understanding of the environmental risk factors that might trigger autoimmune diseases in genetically susceptible individuals. These include: inadequate validated exposure assessment tools and bioassays; poor training in the evaluation of environmental exposures; the lack of population-based incidence, prevalence, demographic information, and databases or repositories for most diseases; inadequate funding; and the lack of accepted and standardized approaches for defining the minimal criteria for an environmental disease. A number of coordinated initiatives may be useful in overcoming these obstacles and making more progress in the future (Box 21.2). Central to all these efforts are greater attention to and funding for understanding the essential environmental exposures that initiate, promote, or sustain autoimmune disorders. Such investments are likely to be very cost effective since they would have important clinical and financial implications for improving the public health.

REFERENCES

Advisory Committee on Immunization Practices, 1996. Update: Vaccine Side Effects, Adverse Reactions, Contraindications, and Precautions Recommendations of the Advisory Committee on Immunization Practices (ACIP). MMWR Morb Mortal Wkly Rep, 45 (RR-12), 1–35 available from: <http://www.cdc.gov/epo/mmwr/preview/mmwrhtml/00046738.htm>

Alaedini, A., Green, P.H., 2005. Narrative review: celiac disease: understanding a complex autoimmune disorder. Ann. Intern. Med. 142, 289–298.

Arbuckle, M.R., McClain, M.T., Rubertone, M.V., Scofield, R.H., Dennis, G.J., James, J.A., et al., 2003. Development of autoantibodies before the clinical onset of systemic lupus erythematosus. N. Engl. J. Med. 349, 1526–1533.

Artlett, C.M., Ramos, R., Jiminez, S.A., Patterson, K., Miller, F.W., Rider, L.G., 2000. Chimeric cells of maternal origin in juvenile idiopathic inflammatory myopathies. Childhood Myositis Heterogeneity Collaborative Group. Lancet. 356, 2155–2156.

Bagenstose, L.M., Salgame, P., Monestier, M., 1999. Murine mercury-induced autoimmunity: a model of chemically related autoimmunity in humans. Immunol. Res. 20, 67–78.

Bang, S.Y., Lee, K.H., Cho, S.K., Lee, H.S., Lee, K.W., Bae, S.C., 2010. Smoking increases rheumatoid arthritis susceptibility in individuals carrying the HLA-DRB1 shared epitope, regardless of rheumatoid factor or anti-cyclic citrullinated peptide antibody status. Arthritis Rheum. 62, 369–377.

Bigazzi, P.E., 1994. Autoimmunity and heavy metals. Lupus. 3, 449–453.

Bigazzi, P.E., 1997. Autoimmunity caused by xenobiotics. Toxicology. 119, 1–21.

Bogdanos, D.P., Smyk, D.S., Rigopoulou, E.I., Mytilinaiou, M.G., Heneghan, M.A., Selmi, C., et al., 2012. Twin studies in autoimmune disease: genetics, gender and environment. J. Autoimmun. 38, J156–J169.

Brown, S.L., 2002. Epidemiology of silicone-gel breast implants. Epidemiology. 13, S34–S39.

Brown, S.L., Langone, J.J., Brinton, L.A., 1998. Silicone breast implants and autoimmune disease. J. Am. Med. Womens Assoc. 53 (21–24), 40.

Chang, C., Gershwin, M.E., 2011. Drug-induced lupus erythematosus: incidence, management and prevention. Drug. Saf. 34, 357–374.

Cooper, G.S., Stroehla, B.C., 2003. The epidemiology of autoimmune diseases. Autoimmun. Rev. 2, 119–125.

Cooper, G.S., Miller, F.W., Pandey, J.P., 1999. The Role of Genetic Factors in Autoimmune Disease: Implications for Environmental Research. Environ. Health Perspect. 107, 693–700.

Cooper, G.S., Miller, F.W., Germolec, D.R., 2002. Occupational exposures and autoimmune diseases. Int. Immunopharmacol. 2, 303–313.

Cooper, G.S., Makris, S.L., Nietert, P.J., Jinot, J., 2009. Evidence of autoimmune-related effects of trichloroethylene exposure from studies in mice and humans. Environ. Health Perspect. 117, 696–702.

Cooper, G.S., Wither, J., Bernatsky, S., Claudio, J.O., Clarke, A., Rioux, J.D., et al., 2010. Occupational and environmental exposures and risk of systemic lupus erythematosus: silica, sunlight, solvents. Rheumatology (Oxford). 49, 2172–2180.

Cukier, J., Beauchamp, R.A., Spindler, J.S., Spindler, S., Lorenzo, C., Trentham, D.E., 1993. Association between bovine collagen dermal implants and a dermatomyositis or a polymyositis-like syndrome. Ann. Intern. Med. 118, 920–928.

Dahlquist, G., 1998. The aetiology of type 1 diabetes: an epidemiological perspective. Acta. Paediatr. Suppl. 425, 5–10.

Dally, A., 1997. The rise and fall of pink disease. Soc. Hist. Med. 10, 291–304.

Dotta, F., Eisenbarth, G.S., 1989. Type I diabetes mellitus: a predictable autoimmune disease with interindividual variation in the rate of beta cell destruction. Clin. Immunol. Immunopathol. 50, S85–S95.

D'Cruz, D., 2000. Autoimmune diseases associated with drugs, chemicals and environmental factors. Toxicol. Lett. 112–113, 421–432.

Elenkov, I.J., Chrousos, G.P., 1999. Stress, cytokine patterns and susceptibility to disease. Baillieres Best. Pract. Res. Clin. Endocrinol. Metab. 13, 583–595.

Feldman, B.M., Birdi, N., Boone, J.E., Dent, P.B., Duffy, C.M., Ellsworth, J.E., et al., 1996. Seasonal onset of systemic-onset juvenile rheumatoid arthritis. J. Pediatr. 129, 513–518.

Fontenot, A.P., Kotzin, B.L., 2003. Chronic beryllium disease: immune-mediated destruction with implications for organ-specific autoimmunity. Tissue Antigens. 62, 449–458.

Fugazzola, L., Cirello, V., Beck-Peccoz, P., 2011. Fetal microchimerism as an explanation of disease. Nat. Rev. Endocrinol. 7, 89–97.

Gelpi, E., de la Paz, M.P., Terracini, B., Abaitua, I., de la Camara, A.G., Kilbourne, E.M., et al., 2002. The Spanish toxic oil syndrome 20 years after its onset: a multidisciplinary review of scientific knowledge. Environ. Health Perspect. 110, 457–464.

Gourley, M., Miller, F.W., 2007. Mechanisms of disease: environmental factors in the pathogenesis of rheumatic disease. Nat. Clin. Pract. Rheumatol. 3, 172–180.

Grant, W.B., 2004. Solar UV-B radiation is linked to the geographic variation of mortality from systemic lupus erythematosus in the USA. Lupus. 13, 281–282.

Han, F., Lin, L., Warby, S.C., Faraco, J., Li, J., Dong, S.X., et al., 2011. Narcolepsy onset is seasonal and increased following the 2009 H1N1 pandemic in China. Ann. Neurol. 70, 410–417.

Haus, E., Smolensky, M.H., 1999. Biologic rhythms in the immune system. Chronobiol. Int. 16, 581–622.

Hess, E.V., 2002. Environmental chemicals and autoimmune disease: cause and effect. Toxicology. 181–182, 65–70.

Hess, E.V., Mongey, A.B., 1991. Drug-related lupus. Bull. Rheum. Dis. 40, 1–8.

Hirschfield, G.M., Gershwin, M.E., 2013. The immunobiology and pathophysiology of primary biliary cirrhosis. Annu. Rev. Pathol. 8, 303–330.

Janowsky, E.C., Kupper, L.L., Hulka, B.S., 2000. Meta-analyses of the relation between silicone breast implants and the risk of connective-tissue diseases. N. Engl. J. Med. 342, 781–790.

Javierre, B.M., Hernando, H., Ballestar, E., 2011. Environmental triggers and epigenetic deregulation in autoimmune disease. Discov. Med. 12, 535–545.

Johnson, D.H., Rosenthal, A., Nadas, A.S., 1975. A forty-year review of bacterial endocarditis in infancy and childhood. Circulation. 51, 581–588.

Kallberg, H., Ding, B., Padyukov, L., Bengtsson, C., Ronnelid, J., Klareskog, L., et al., 2011. Smoking is a major preventable risk factor for rheumatoid arthritis: estimations of risks after various exposures to cigarette smoke. Ann. Rheum. Dis. 70, 508–511.

Khuder, S.A., Peshimam, A.Z., Agraharam, S., 2002. Environmental risk factors for rheumatoid arthritis. Rev. Environ. Health. 17, 307–315.

Klareskog, L., Alfredsson, L., Rantapaa-Dahlqvist, S., Berglin, E., Stolt, P. and Padyukov, L. 2004. What precedes development of rheumatoid arthritis? Ann. Rheum. Dis. 63, ii28–ii31.

Krishnan, E., 2003. Smoking, gender and rheumatoid arthritis—epidemiological clues to etiology. Results from the behavioral risk factor surveillance system. Joint. Bone. Spine. 70, 496–502.

Leff, R.L., Burgess, S.H., Miller, F.W., Love, L.A., Targoff, I.N., Dalakas, M.C., et al., 1991. Distinct seasonal patterns in the onset of adult idiopathic inflammatory myopathy in patients with anti-Jo-1 and anti-signal recognition particle autoantibodies. Arthritis Rheum. 34, 1391–1396.

Leslie, D., Lipsky, P., Notkins, A.L., 2001. Autoantibodies as pr edictors of disease. J. Clin. Invest. 108, 1417–1422.

Leslie, R.D., Hawa, M., 1994. Twin studies in auto-immune disease. Acta. Genet. Med. Gemellol. (Roma). 43, 71–81.

Liu, Z.X., Kaplowitz, N., 2002. Immune-mediated drug-induced liver disease. Clin. Liver Dis. 6, 755–774.

Love, L.A., Miller, F.W., 1993. Noninfectious environmental agents associated with myopathies. Curr. Opin. Rheumatol. 5, 712–718.

Love, L.A., Weinberg, C.R., McConnaughey, D.R., Oddis, C.V., Medsger Jr., T.A., Reveille, J.D., et al., 2009. Ultraviolet radiation intensity predicts the relative distribution of dermatomyositis and anti-Mi-2 autoantibodies in women. Arthritis Rheum. 60, 2499–2504.

Luppi, P., Rossiello, M.R., Faas, S., Trucco, M., 1995. Genetic background and environment contribute synergistically to the onset of autoimmune diseases. J. Mol. Med. 73, 381–393.

Mackay, I.R., 1999. Immunological perspectives on chronic hepatitis: virus infection, autoimmunity and xenobiotics. Hepatogastroenterology. 46, 3021–3033.

McCormic, Z.D., Khuder, S.S., Aryal, B.K., Ames, A.L., Khuder, S.A., 2010. Occupational silica exposure as a risk factor for scleroderma: a meta-analysis. Int. Arch. Occup. Environ. Health. 83, 763–769.

Miller, F.W., 1993. In: Serratrice, G. (Ed.), Seasonal, Geographic, Clinical and Immunogenetic Associations of the Myositis Specific Autoantibodies. Francaise, Paris.

Miller, F.W., 1999. Genetics of environmentally-associated rheumatic disease. In: Kaufman, L.D., Varga, J. (Eds.), Rheumatic Diseases and the Environment. Arnold Publishers, London, pp. 33–45.

Miller, F.W., Waite, K.A., Biswas, T., Plotz, P.H., 1990. The role of an autoantigen, histidyl-tRNA synthetase, in the induction and maintenance of autoimmunity. Proc. Natl. Acad. Sci. U.S.A. 87, 9933–9937.

Miller, F.W., Hess, E.V., Clauw, D.J., Hertzman, P.A., Pincus, T., Silver, R.M., et al., 2000. Approaches for identifying and defining environmentally associated rheumatic disorders. Arthritis Rheum. 43, 243–249.

Miller, F.W., Alfredsson, L., Costenbader, K.H., Kamen, D.L., Nelson, L.M., Norris, J.M., et al., 2012. Epidemiology of environmental exposures and human autoimmune diseases: findings from a National Institute of Environmental Health Sciences Expert Panel Workshop. J. Autoimmun. 39, 259–271.

Moroni, L., Bianchi, I., Lleo, A., 2012. Geoepidemiology, gender and autoimmune disease. Autoimmun. Rev. 11, A386–A392.

Nelson, R.J., Drazen, D.L., 2000. Melatonin mediates seasonal changes in immune function. Ann. N.Y. Acad. Sci. 917, 404–415.

Norcross, M.A., Luo, S., Lu, L., Boyne, M.T., Gomarteli, M., Rennels, A.D., et al., 2012. Abacavir induces loading of novel self-peptides into HLA-B*57: 01: an autoimmune model for HLA-associated drug hypersensitivity. AIDS. 26, F21–F29.

Noseworthy, J.H., Lucchinetti, C., Rodriguez, M., Weinshenker, B.G., 2000. Multiple sclerosis. N. Engl. J. Med. 343, 938–952.

Oddis, C.V., Conte, C.G., Steen, V.D., Medsger Jr., T.A., 1990. Incidence of polymyositis-dermatomyositis: a 20-year study of hospital diagnosed cases in Allegheny County, PA 1963–1982. J. Rheumatol. 17, 1329–1334.

Okada, S., Weatherhead, E., Targoff, I.N., Wesley, R., Miller, F.W., 2003. Global surface ultraviolet radiation intensity may modulate the clinical and immunologic expression of autoimmune muscle disease. Arthritis Rheum. 48, 2285–2293.

Okada, S., Kamb, M.L., Pandey, J.P., Philen, R.M., Love, L.A., Miller, F.W., 2009. Immunogenetic risk and protective factors for the development of L-tryptophan-associated eosinophilia-myalgia syndrome and associated symptoms. Arthritis Rheum. 61, 1305–1311.

Onkamo, P., Vaananen, S., Karvonen, M., Tuomilehto, J., 1999. Worldwide increase in incidence of Type I diabetes—the analysis of the data on published incidence trends. Diabetologia. 42, 1395–1403.

O'Hanlon, T., Koneru, B., Bayat, E., Love, L., Targoff, I., Malley, J., et al., 2004. Immunogenetic differences between Caucasian women with and those without silicone implants in whom myositis develops. Arthritis Rheum. 50, 3646–3650.

Parks, C.G., Conrad, K., Cooper, G.S., 1999. Occupational exposure to crystalline silica and autoimmune disease. Environ. Health. Perspect. 107 (Suppl. 5), 793–802.

Parks, C.G., Walitt, B.T., Pettinger, M., Chen, J.C., De Roos, A.J., Hunt, J., et al., 2011. Insecticide use and risk of rheumatoid arthritis and systemic lupus erythematosus in the Women's Health Initiative Observational Study. Arthritis Care Res. (Hoboken). 63, 184–194.

Pollard, K.M., Hultman, P., Kono, D.H., 2010. Toxicology of Autoimmune Diseases. Chem. Res. Toxicol..

Ponsonby, A.L., McMichael, A., van der Mei, I., 2002. Ultraviolet radiation and autoimmune disease: insights from epidemiological research. Toxicology. 181–182, 71–78.

Rook, G.A., 2012. Hygiene hypothesis and autoimmune diseases. Clin. Rev. Allergy Immunol. 42, 5–15.

Rowley, B., Monestier, M., 2005. Mechanisms of heavy metal-induced autoimmunity. Mol. Immunol. 42, 833–838.

Sarasin, A., 2003. An overview of the mechanisms of mutagenesis and carcinogenesis. Mutat. Res. 544, 99–106.

Sarkar, K., Miller, F.W., 2004. Possible roles and determinants of microchimerism in autoimmune and other disorders. Autoimmun. Rev. 37, 291–294.

Sarkar, K., Weinberg, C.R., Oddis, C.V., Medsger Jr., T.A., Plotz, P.H., Reveille, J.D., et al., 2005. Seasonal influence on the onset of idiopathic inflammatory myopathies in serologically defined groups. Arthritis Rheum. 52, 2433–2438.

Schlesinger, N., Schlesinger, M., 2005. Seasonal variation of rheumatic diseases. Discov. Med. 5, 64–69.

Shamim, E.A., Miller, F.W., 2000. Familial autoimmunity and the idiopathic inflammatory myopathies. Curr. Rheumatol. Rep. 2, 201–211.

Silva, I.A., Nyland, J.F., Gorman, A., Perisse, A., Ventura, A.M., Santos, E.C., et al., 2004. Mercury exposure, malaria, and serum antinuclear/antinucleolar antibodies in amazon populations in Brazil: a cross-sectional study. Environ. Health. 3, 11.

Smyk, D., Rigopoulou, E.I., Baum, H., Burroughs, A.K., Vergani, D., Bogdanos, D.P., 2012. Autoimmunity and environment: am I at risk? Clin. Rev. Allergy Immunol. 42, 199–212.

Stolt, P., Bengtsson, C., Nordmark, B., Lindblad, S., Lundberg, I., Klareskog, L., et al., 2003. Quantification of the influence of ciga-rette smoking on rheumatoid arthritis: results from a population based case-control study, using incident cases. Ann. Rheum. Dis. 62, 835–841.

Sullivan, E.A., Kamb, M.L., Jones, J.L., Meyer, P., Philen, R.M., Falk, H., et al., 1996. The natural history of eosinophilia-myalgia syndrome in a tryptophan-exposed cohort in South Carolina. Arch. Intern. Med. 156, 973–979.

Timmer, A., 2003. Environmental influences on inflammatory bowel disease manifestations. Lessons from epidemiology. Dig. Dis. 21, 91–104.

Tugwell, P., Wells, G., Peterson, J., Welch, V., Page, J., Davison, C., et al., 2001. Do silicone breast implants cause rheumatologic disor-ders? A systematic review for a court-appointed national science panel. Arthritis Rheum. 44, 2477–2484.

Uramoto, K.M., Michet Jr., C.J., Thumboo, J., Sunku, J., O'Fallon, W. M., Gabriel, S.E., 1999. Trends in the incidence and mortality of systemic lupus erythematosus, 1950–1992. Arthritis Rheum. 42, 46–50.

Ursic-Bratina, N., Battelino, T., Krzisnik, C., Laron-Kenet, T., Ashkenazi, I., Laron, Z., 2001. Seasonality of birth in children

(0–14 years) with type 1 diabetes mellitus in Slovenia. J. Pediatr. Endocrinol. Metab. 14, 47–52.

Vegosen, L.J., Weinberg, C.R., O'Hanlon, T.P., Targoff, I.N., Miller, F. W., Rider, L.G., 2007. Seasonal birth patterns in myositis subgroups suggest an etiologic role of early environmental exposures. Arthritis Rheum. 56, 2719–2728.

Vestergaard, P., 2002. Smoking and thyroid disorders—a meta-analysis. Eur. J. Endocrinol. 146, 153–161.

Weinberg, C.R., Dornan, T.L., Hansen, J.A., Raghu, P.K., Palmer, J.P., 1984. HLA-related heterogeneity in seasonal patterns of diagnosis in Type 1 (insulin-dependent) diabetes. Diabetologia. 26, 199–202.

Westberg, M., Feychting, M., Jonsson, F., Nise, G., Gustavsson, P., 2009. Occupational exposure to UV light and mortality from multi-ple sclerosis. Am. J. Ind. Med. 52, 353–357.

Williams, W.J., 1991. Caplan's syndrome. Br. J. Clin. Pract. 45, 285–288.

Willis, J.A., Scott, R.S., Darlow, B.A., Lewy, H., Ashkenazi, I., Laron, Z., 2002. Seasonality of birth and onset of clinical disease in chil-dren and adolescents (0–19 years) with type 1 diabetes mellitus in Canterbury, New Zealand. J. Pediatr. Endocrinol. Metab. 15, 645–647.

Winsa, B., Adami, H.O., Bergstrom, R., Gamstedt, A., Dahlberg, P.A., Adamson, U., et al., 1991. Stressful life events and Graves' disease. Lancet. 338, 1475–1479.

Wraith, D.C., Goldman, M., Lambert, P.H., 2003. Vaccination and autoimmune disease: what is the evidence? Lancet. 362, 1659–1666.

Chapter 22

Adhesion Molecules and Chemoattractants in Autoimmunity

Charles R. Mackay[1] and Ulrich H. von Andrian[2]

[1]*School of Biological Sciences, Monash University, Clayton, Victoria, Australia,* [2]*CBR Institute for Biomedical Research, Harvard Medical School, Boston, MA, USA*

Chapter Outline

Microvascular Determinants of T Cell Recruitment	297	Effector T Cell Migration	303
Adhesion Molecules	297	Homing to Non-Lymphoid Tissues	303
Chemoattractants and Their Receptors	299	Some Clinical Applications	304
Multistep Adhesion Cascades	302	Conclusions and Future Directions	306
Organized Lymphoid Tissues: Venues for Naïve T Cell		Acknowledgments	306
Homing and Dendritic Cell Interactions	302	References	306

MICROVASCULAR DETERMINANTS OF T CELL RECRUITMENT

Specialized microvessels control T cell migration from blood into tissues. In microvascular beds of most tissues except the spleen, lung, and liver, postcapillary venules, but not arterioles or capillaries, bind leukocytes. Because intravascular leukocytes are subjected to extreme physical conditions (sheer stress), cells use specialized adhesion receptors, the selectins, which form stable bonds with counter-receptors in the vascular wall (Table 22.1) (Carlos and Harlan, 1994; Springer, 1994). Adhesion receptors on leukocytes and on vascular endothelial cells also function as tissue-specific recognition molecules. For example, the specialized high endothelial venules (HEVs) in lymph nodes and Peyer's patches constitutively express vascular addressins, which support a considerable rate of traffic of "resting" lymphocytes, i.e., naïve T and B cells and some memory T cells, whereas endothelial cells elsewhere permit only minimal leukocyte binding unless they are exposed to inflammatory mediators. Thus, two vascular beds can be distinguished, which support fundamentally different types of leukocyte traffic: those in lymphoid organs which recruit lymphocytes constitutively, and those in normal or inflamed tissues which recruit effector leukocytes whose job is to combat pathogens (Figure 22.1). The same anti-pathogen effector leukocytes also can mediate tissue damage in autoimmune disease settings.

ADHESION MOLECULES

A central paradigm that underpins leukocyte extravasation is the multistep model of leukocyte binding to endothelium (Springer, 1994). Leukocytes must engage several sequential adhesion steps in order to leave the circulation (Figure 22.2). Initially, tethers are formed by adhesion receptors that are specialized to engage rapidly and with high tensile strength. The most important initiators of adhesion are the three selectins, expressed on leukocytes (L-selectin), endothelial cells (P- and E-selectin), and activated platelets (P-selectin) (Kansas, 1996). All selectins bind oligosaccharides related to sialyl-Lewis[X]. The most relevant selectin-binding sugars are components of sialomucin-like glycoproteins (Vestweber and Blanks, 1999). Selectin-mediated binding of leukocytes to endothelium results in a characteristic rolling motion. To stop rolling, cells must engage additional (secondary) receptors (Lawrence and Springer, 1991; von Andrian et al., 1991), members of the integrin family, specifically LFA-1 (CD11a/CD18, aLb2), and the two a4 integrins, a4b1 (VLA-4) and a4b7. a4 integrins can also mediate

N. Rose & I. Mackay (Eds): The Autoimmune Diseases, Fifth edition. DOI: http://dx.doi.org/10.1016/B978-0-12-384929-8.00022-8

TABLE 22.1 Selectings, Integrins, and Their Ligands.

Adhesion Molecule	Distribution	Ligand(s), Receptor(s)	Role in T-cell Migration
Selectins			
L-selectin (CD62L)	Most leukocytes	PNAd, PSGL-1, MAdCAM-1, E-selectin, others	Homing to lymph nodes and Peyer patches
E-selectin (CD62E)	Endothelial cells	PSGL-1, ESL-1, CLA, sLe^{X+} glycol-proteins and -lipids	Memory/effector cell homing to skin and sites of inflammation
P-selectin (CD62P)	Endothelial cells, platelets	PSGL-1, CD24, PNAd	Memory/effector (Th1) cell homing to sites of inflammation; platelet-mediated interaction with PNAd$^+$ venules
Selectin Ligands			
Sialyl-Lewis^X (sCD15)	Myeloid cells; some memory (Th1) cells; HEVs; other cell types	All selectins	Function depends on presentation molecule
PSGL-1	All leukocytes	P-selectin; also binds L-/E-selectin	Effector cell homing to inflamed tissues
Peripheral node addressin (PNAd)	HEVs in LNs and inflamed tissues	L-selectin, P-selectin	Naïve/central memory T-cell homing to LNs
Cutaneous lymphocyte antigen (CLA)	Skin-homing T cells, dendritic cells, granulocytes	E-selectin	Memory/effector T-cell homing to inflamed skin
b2 Integrins[a]			
aLb2 (LFA-1, CD11a/CD18)	All leukocytes	ICAM-1, -2, -3, -4 and -5	Homing; inflammation; adhesion to APCs
aMb2 (Mac-1, CD11b/CD18)	Myeloid cells, some activated T cells	ICAM-1, factor X, fibrinogen, C3b$_i$	Unknown
aXb2 (p150/95, CD11c/CD18)	Dendritic cells	Fibrinogen, C3b$_i$	Unknown
aDb2 (CD11d/CD18)	Monocytes, macrophages, eosinophils	VCAM-1, ICAM-1 and -3	Unknown
a4 Integrins[a]			
a4b1 (VLA-4)	Most leukocytes except neutrophils	VCAM-1, fibronectin, a4 integrin	Memory/effector cell homing to inflamed tissues, esp. lung
a4b7	Lymphocytes, NK, mast cells, basophils, monocytes	MAdCAM-1, fibronectin, weak binding to VCAM-1	Homing to gut and associated lymphoid tissues
Immunoglobulin Superfamily			
ICAM-1 (CD54)	Most cell types	LFA-1, Mac-1, fibrinogen	Critical endothelial ligand for b2 integrins
ICAM-2 (CD102)	Endothelial cells, platelets	LFA-1	Unknown
VCAM-1 (CD106)	Endothelial cells, BM stroma, FDC, osteoblasts, mesothelium	a4b1, a4b7, aDb2	Memory/effector cell homing to inflamed tissues
MAdCAM-1	HEVs in gut-associated lymphoid tissues; lamina propria	a4b7, L-selectin	T-cell homing to gut-associated lymphoid tissues

[a]*The integrins are named according to the composition of their constituent a and b protein chains, which are each identified by a number or letter (e.g., a4b1 or aDb2), but some integrins are often referred to by alternative names, e.g., LFA-1, shown in parenthesis.*
APC, antigen-presenting cell; BM, bone marrow; CD, cluster of differentiation; CLA, cutaneous lymphocyte antigen; ESL-1, E-selectin ligand-1; FucT-VII, fucosyltransferase-VII; GlyCAM-1, glycosylation-dependent cell adhesion molecule-1; HEV, high endothelial venule; ICAM, intercellular cell adhesion molecule; IL-1, interleukin-1; LFA-1, leukocyte function-associated antigen-1; LPS, lipopolysaccharide; Mac-1, macrophage antigen-1; MAdCAM-1, mucosal addressin cell adhesion molecule-1; NK, natural killer cell; p150/95, protein with 150kDa and 95kDa subunits; PNAd, peripheral node addressin; PSGL-1, P-selectin glycoprotein ligand-1; sgp200, sialylated glycoprotein of 200kD; sLeX, sialyl-LewisX; Th, T-helper; TNF-a, tumor necrosis factor a; VCAM-1, vascular cell adhesion molecule-1; VLA-4, very late antigen-4.

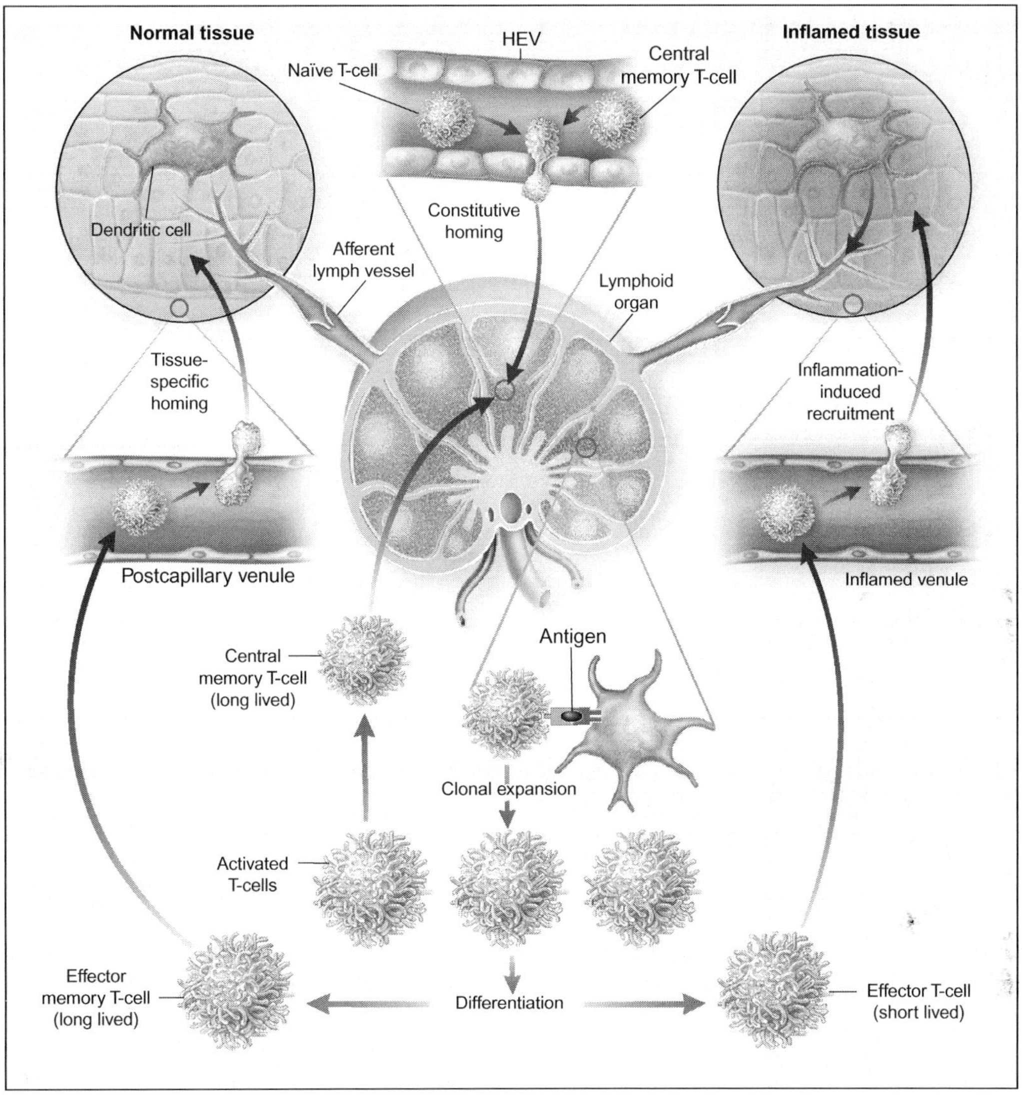

FIGURE 22.1 Migratory routes of T cells. Naïve T cells "home" continuously from the blood to lymph nodes and other secondary lymphoid tissues. Homing to lymph nodes occurs across high endothelial venules (HEVs), which express traffic molecules for constitutive lymphocyte recruitment. Lymph nodes are percolated by lymph fluid that is channeled to them from peripheral tissues, where dendritic cells (DCs) collect antigenic material. In inflamed tissues, DCs are mobilized to carry antigen to lymph nodes, where they stimulate antigen-specific T cells. Upon stimulation, T cells proliferate and differentiate into effector cells, which express receptors that enable them to migrate to sites of inflammation. While most effector cells are short lived, a few antigen-experienced cells survive for a long time. These memory cells are subdivided into two populations based on their migratory ability (Sallusto et al., 1999): one subset is termed *effector memory* T cells and is localized to peripheral tissues, and the other *central memory* T cells that express a similar repertoire of homing molecules as do naïve T cells and migrate preferentially to lymphoid organs. The traffic signals that direct effector and memory cells to peripheral tissues are organ specific; for example, molecules required for migration to the skin are different from those to the gut; they are modulated by inflammatory mediators and are distinct for different T cell subsets, e.g., Th1 and Th2 cells show differences in their responses to various chemoattractants. *Reproduced from von Andrian and Mackay (2000), with permission.*

tethering and rolling, albeit less efficiently than selectins (Alon et al., 1995; Berlin et al., 1995).

CHEMOATTRACTANTS AND THEIR RECEPTORS

Selectins are constitutively active whereas integrins are activated by signals from chemoattractant receptors

(Cyster, 1999; Kim and Broxmeyer, 1999). Just like adhesion molecules, chemoattractant receptors can be upregulated or lost as cells differentiate, allowing leukocytes to coordinate their migratory routes with their immunologic function. The most extensive family of chemoattractants, particularly for adaptive immune responses, are the chemokines (Table 22.2). While some chemokines trigger intravascular adhesion (Campbell et al., 1998), others

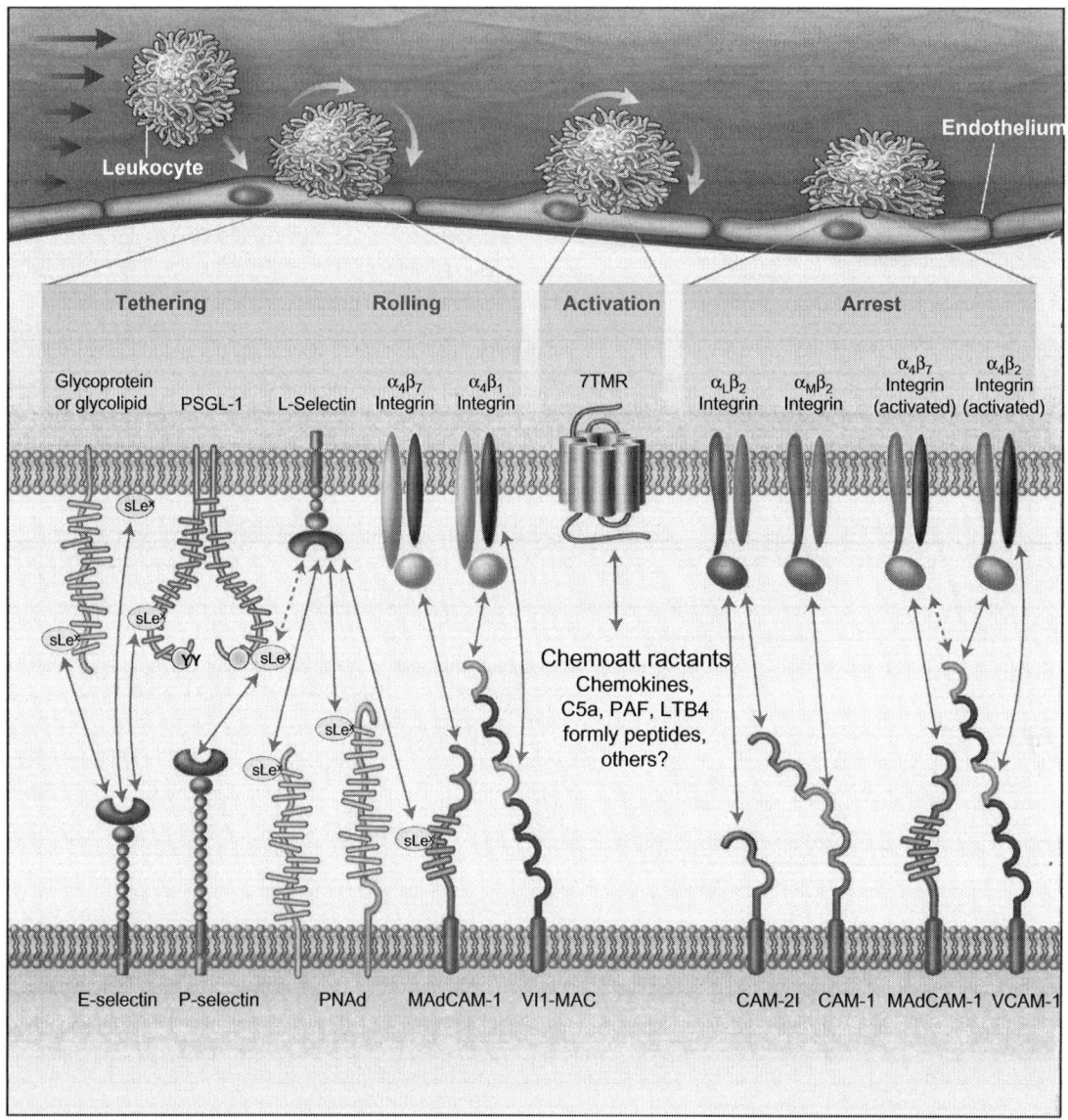

FIGURE 22.2 Essential molecular players in the multistep adhesion cascade.   The top of this schematic diagram depicts the four distinct adhesion steps that leukocytes must undergo to accumulate in a blood vessel. Also shown are the predominant molecular determinants of each step with respect to leukocytes (middle of the diagram) and endothelial cells (bottom). A number of molecules can interact with more than one partner, symbolized by arrows. Leukocytes in the bloodstream (arrows at left symbolize the laminar flow profile) tether to endothelial cells and roll slowly downstream. Tethering is greatly facilitated by leukocyte receptors that occur at high density on the tips of microvillous surface protrusions (L-selectin, PSGL-1, and a4 integrins), whereas subsequent rolling is not influenced by the topography of adhesion receptors (Stein et al., 1999). The most efficient tethering molecules are L- and P-selectin. L-selectin recognizes sulfated sialyl-Lewis^X (sLe^X)-like sugars (PNAd) in high endothelial venules. It may also interact with other ligands on inflamed endothelial cells (not shown) and with PSGL-1 on adherent leukocytes (broken arrow). PSGL-1 binding to L- and P-selectin requires decoration with an sLe^X-like sugar in close vicinity to an N-terminal motif containing three tyrosines (Y) that must be sulfated. E-selectin can also interact with PSGL-1, but does not require sulfation and also recognizes other sLe^X-bearing glycoconjugates. E-selectin and the a4 integrins can tether some leukocytes, but their predominant function is to reduce rolling velocities. Rolling leukocytes respond to chemoattractants on endothelial cells because they express specific receptors with seven transmembrane domains (7TMR), which transmit intracellular signals through G proteins. The activating signal induces rapid activation of b2 and/or a4 integrins, which bind to endothelial immunoglobulin superfamily members. Note that a4 integrins can mediate activation-independent rolling interactions as well as firm arrest. However, the latter function requires integrin activation, symbolized by the open conformation of the integrin heterodimer. For a list of abbreviations, see Table 22.1. *Reproduced from von Andrian and Mackay (2000), with permission.*

TABLE 22.2 Chemoattractant Receptors and Their Ligands in Leukocyte Migration.

Biologic Activity	Chemoattractant Receptor(s)	Predominant ligands[a,b]
Naïve T-cell Migration		
To LN and Peyer patch	CCR7	CCL21 (SLC); CCL19 (Mip-3b)
Within lymphoid tissues	CXCR4	CXCL12 (SDF-1a)
Memory T-cell Migration		
To lymphoid tissues	CCR7	CCL21 (SLC); CCL19 (Mip-3b)
To the skin	CCR4,	CCL17 (TARC); CCL22 (MDC-1)
	CCR10	CCL27 (CTACK)
To the gut	CCR9	CCL25 (TECK)
To sites of inflammation	CCR2	CCL2 (MCP-1)
	CCR5	CCL5 (RANTES), CCL4 (MIP-1b)
Effector T-cell Migration		
Th1 cells	CCR2	CCL2 (MCP-1)
	CCR5	CCL5, CCL4 (MIP-1b)
	CXCR3	CXCL9, 10, 11
Th2 cells	CCR3	CCL11 (Eotaxin)
	CCR4	CCL17 (TARC); CCL22 (MDC-1)
	CCR8	CCL1 (I-309)
	CXCR4	CXCL12 (SDF-1a)
B-cell migration	CCR7	CCL21 (SLC); CCL19 (Mip-3b)
	CXCR4	CXCL12 (SDF-1a)
	CXCR5	CXCL13 (BLC)
Dendritic Cell Migration		
To lymphoid tissues	CCR7	CCL21 (SLC); CCL19 (Mip-3b)
To normal skin	CCR6	CCL20 (MIP-3a)
To sites of inflammation	CCR1	CCL5, CCL3
	CCR2	CCL2 (MCP-1)
	CCR5	CCL5, CCL4 (MIP-1b)
	CXCR1	CXCL8 (IL-8)
Monocyte recruitment	CCR1	CCL5, CCL3
	CCR2	CCL2 (MCP-1)
	CCR5	CCL5, CCL4 (MIP-1b)
	CCR8	CCL1 (I-309)
	CXCR1	CXCL8 (IL-8)
	CX3CR1	
	C5aR	C5a
Neutrophil recruitment	CXCR1	CXCL8 (IL-8)
	CXCR2	CXCL8 (IL-8); Groa, b, g
	C5aR	C5a
	fmlpR	fmlp
Eosinophil recruitment	CCR3	CCL11 (Eotaxin)
	C5aR	C5a

[a]The physiologic function of several chemokine receptors are multiple, since CCR9 promotes prothymocyte homing to the thymus, and T-cell migration to the gut; CXCR4 is widely expressed and appears to have multiple roles.
[b]An established nomenclature for chemokines (Zlotnik and Yoshie, 2000) has superseded older and in many cases duplicate names for a single chemokine. Frequently used alternative names are shown in parenthesis.
CCR, receptor for CC chemokine; CXCR, receptor for CXC chemokine; LN, lymph node, Th, helper T cell.

direct leukocyte migration into and within extravascular spaces. Since lymphocytes must be positioned correctly to interact with other cells, the pattern of chemokine receptors and the type and distribution of chemokines in tissues critically influence immune responses (Cyster, 1999; Sallusto et al., 1999; Syrbe et al., 1999). Over 50 chemokines and some 18 chemokine receptors have been identified (Kim and Broxmeyer, 1999; Zlotnik and Yoshie, 2000). This multitude ensures robust recruitment of inflammatory cells, even if individual pathways are disabled by genetic defects or through subversion by pathogens (Mantovani, 1999). Also, the multitude of chemokines is consistent with the complex nature of the mammalian immune system, the numerous leukocyte cell types, and the distinct microenvironments wherein migration must be regulated. For instance, neutrophils may use different chemoattractant receptors sequentially, to travel from a to b to c, in a process termed *multistep navigation* (Foxman et al., 1997).

Chemokines are divided into four subfamilies based on the position of N-terminal cysteine residues, and are also classified as inflammatory or lymphoid. *Inflammatory chemokines* primarily attract neutrophils, monocytes, and other effector leukocytes. The major sources of these chemokines are activated endothelial cells, epithelial cells, and leukocytes, although virtually any cell has the potential to produce chemokines (and attract leukocytes) when stimulated by lipopolysaccharides (endotoxin) or inflammatory cytokines. *Lymphoid chemokines* are primarily produced in lymphoid tissues. They maintain constitutive leukocyte traffic and compartmentalization within the lymphoid tissue (Cyster, 1999; Jung and Littman, 1999). In addition to the chemokine receptors, the closely related "classical" chemoattractant receptors such as C5aR serve similar functions particularly during inflammatory responses. The very large number of chemokines, and patterns of chemokine receptor expression on subsets of T cells, suggest that this system of chemoattractants evolved to meet the elaborate demands of the adaptive immune system.

MULTISTEP ADHESION CASCADES

A general consideration for drug development is how selective or broad acting an antagonist should be. Chemokine and chemokine-receptor redundancy, and the expression of multiple receptors by cell types such as monocytes, questions whether any single receptor antagonist will always be effective (Mayadas et al., 1993; Arbones et al., 1994; Bullard et al., 1996; Frenette et al., 1996; Wagner et al., 1996; Andrew et al., 1998; Berlin-Rufenach et al., 1999; Forster et al., 1999; Robinson et al., 1999; Stein et al., 2000; Warnock et al., 2000). Deficiencies in any one of the steps, i.e., selectin binding, chemoattractant signaling, or integrin binding, can derail

cell migration. The numerous leukocyte adhesion receptors, endothelial counter-receptor(s), chemokines, and chemokine receptors means that there are hundreds of possible three-step combinations, and thus great flexibility in the regulation of leukocyte migration (Butcher, 1991; Springer, 1994). Indeed, several multistep combinations occur uniquely in specialized tissues and serve to attract very distinct subsets of blood-borne leukocytes (Springer, 1994; Butcher and Picker, 1996; Robert and Kupper, 1999; Stein et al., 2000; Warnock et al., 2000). In considering whether a single receptor antagonist will always be effective, studies *in vivo* using single-receptor antagonists, or with monoclonal antibodies (mAb) to individual chemokine ligands, have actually proved very effective in animal models (Gong et al., 1997; Gonzalo et al., 1998; Ulbrich et al., 2003; Szekanecz and Koch, 2004). Yet, despite this, emergence of effective drugs for human use remains slow. However, we can mention the considerable interest in targeting chemoattractant receptor signaling pathways wherein numerous receptors would be affected: the phosphoinositide 3-kinases (PI3K) are a good example (Ward, 2004). Mice lacking one of the four isoforms, PI3Kg, are viable, but their neutrophils and macrophages show impaired activation through chemoattractant receptors (Hirsch et al., 2000; Li et al., 2000), and poor chemotactic responses.

Organized Lymphoid Tissues: Venues for Naïve T Cell Homing and Dendritic Cell Interactions

The adhesion cascades that mediate homing of naïve T cells to lymph nodes and Peyer's patches have become well understood (Bargatze et al., 1995; Warnock et al., 1998, 2000; Stein et al., 2000). Circulating lymphocytes gain access to both of these tissues by crossing HEVs (Marchesi and Gowans, 1964; Girard and Springer, 1995). A characteristic feature of HEVs in lymph nodes is the expression of the peripheral node addressin (PNAd), whereas HEVs in Peyer's patches express mucosal addressin cell adhesion molecule (MAdCAM)-1. L-Selectin binds both of these addressins, but it sustains rolling only on PNAd in lymph nodes, whereas in Peyer's patches additional binding of a4b7 integrin to MAdCAM-1 is required (Bargatze et al., 1995; Warnock et al., 1998). Cells expressing high levels of a4b7, such as gut-homing effector T cells, tether directly to MAdCAM-1, whereas naïve T cells first engage L-selectin (Bargatze et al., 1995; Kunkel et al., 1998). The chemokines and chemokine receptors important for lymphocyte entry to lymphoid tissues are CCL19 and CCL21 binding to CCR7. CCR7 is expressed at high levels by naïve T cells and central memory T cells, but not effector memory T cells. CCR7 and another chemokine receptor, CXCR4, are expressed in a reciprocal manner with inflammatory chemokine receptors, such as CCR5 (Bleul et al., 1997), which marks mainly effector memory T cells.

Naïve T cells are normally restricted in their migration to lymphoid tissues. It is here where naïve T cells and other cells necessary for a primary immune response must gather and interact. Dendritic cells (DCs) in lymphoid tissues are usually derived from monocytes, which enter tissues and differentiate to "immature" DCs (see Chapter 12). Both monocytes and immature DCs express receptors for inflammatory chemokines and other chemoattractants that are released during inflammatory responses (Dieu et al., 1998; Sallusto et al., 1998). Langerhans cells in skin also express CCR6 which promotes their constitutive migration through normal skin. Immature DCs patrol tissues and engulf microorganisms, dead cells, and cellular debris. Exposure to inflammatory products stimulates their movement to regional lymph nodes via afferent lymph vessels, with loss of their receptors for inflammatory chemokines, and upregulation of receptors for lymphoid chemokines (Sallusto and Lanzavecchia, 1999). CCR7 expression allows maturing DCs to home to the T cell area of lymph nodes. While in transit, DCs also alter their functional role to that of antigen presentation, and begin producing chemokines that attract subsets of T cells (Sallusto and Lanzavecchia, 1999).

There is a rationale for naïve T cells being restricted in their migration to lymphoid tissues: that is, that the large-scale percolation of naïve lymphocytes, all with different antigen receptors, allows the very rare antigen-specific cell to encounter its cognate antigen. Moreover, lymphoid tissues are the venue for T cell−DC interactions, T−B cell interactions including the germinal center (GC) reaction, and are also a place to which antigen drains and is captured and retained. Perhaps the restriction of naïve T cells to lymphoid tissues facilitates immune tolerance by limiting exposure of naïve T cells to self-antigens in the periphery.

EFFECTOR T CELL MIGRATION

Naïve T cells differentiate to effector cells in lymphoid organs (Figure 22.1). However, the principal sites where effector cells are needed are peripheral tissues, wherein pathogens are encountered. Thus, effector cells upregulate receptors for inflammation-induced endothelial adhesion molecules and inflammatory chemoattractants (Butcher and Picker, 1996). However, different pathogens require different effector responses, e.g., by Th1, Th2, Th17 cells, and Th1, Th2 and Th17 cells express distinct receptors and obey different traffic signals (Syrbe et al., 1999). Tfh cells are another type of effector T cell that provides help to B cells and drives GC reaction. Distinctive chemokine

receptors on Th1 cells include CCR5 and CXCR3 (Bonecchi et al., 1998; Sallusto et al., 1998), which bind inflammatory chemokines (see Table 22.1). In rheumatoid arthritis and multiple sclerosis (both often thought of as Th1/Th17 related), virtually all infiltrating T cells express CCR5 and CXCR3 (Qin et al., 1998). People with a homozygous mutation that disrupts the CCR5 gene (Paxton and Kang, 1998) may also be less susceptible to some inflammatory disorders, including rheumatoid arthritis (Gomez-Reino et al., 1999). Tfh cells express the chemokine receptor CXCR5, as do B cells, and this expression facilitates their co-location and interaction in follicles where the ligand CXCL13 is expressed. Adhesion molecules also play a role; Th1 cells express abundant selectin ligands. P- and E-selectin, which occur on inflamed endothelium, and their ligand, PSGL-1, are critical for Th1 cell migration to inflamed skin (Austrup et al., 1997; Borges et al., 1997) and peritoneum (Xie et al., 1999). Expression of fucosyltransferase-VII is necessary for cells to synthesize selectin ligands (Maly et al., 1996). This enzyme is induced by interleukin (IL)-12, which drives Th1 differentiation, whereas T cell exposure to the Th2 cytokine IL-4 downmodulates selectin ligand expression (Wagers et al., 1998; Lim et al., 1999).

Th2 cells also express distinctive chemoattractant receptors, including CRTh2 and CCR3 (Sallusto et al., 1997). Eotaxin, a ligand of CCR3, has been implicated in eosinophil recruitment into hyperreactive airways and is prominent in mucosal tissues undergoing allergic and anti-parasitic responses (Jose et al., 1994). Eotaxin production is stimulated by Th2 cytokines, such as IL-4 or IL-13, and is absent from Th1-mediated lesions (Ponath et al., 1996). CCR3 is also expressed on basophils and mast cells, which presumably allows these allergy-related leukocytes to co-localize and interact at sites of allergic inflammation (Gutierrez-Ramos et al., 1999). CrTh2 is another chemoattractant receptor also preferentially expressed on Th2 cells.

The trafficking of regulatory T cells (Tregs), now regarded as crucial contributors to immunological homeostasis, is governed by lineage-distinct expressions of chemokines and integrins that facilitate their movement to, and retention at sites where their selective activities are required (Wei et al., 2008).

Homing to Non-Lymphoid Tissues

Antigen-experienced effector T cells often display a bias in their tissue migration patterns in order to enhance their chances for re-encountering antigen. T cells that respond to cutaneous pathogens in skin-draining lymph nodes migrate preferentially to the skin, whereas effector cells that arise in Peyer's patches in response to enteroviral infections migrate preferentially to the gut (Butcher and

Picker, 1996). Indeed, lymphocytes express different homing receptors when they respond to orally administered antigen, compared to when the same antigen is given parenterally (Kantele et al., 1999). The best understood tissue-selective homing pathways are in the skin and intestine (Butcher and Picker, 1996; Robert and Kupper, 1999), but other selective migration streams may well exist, such as to the lung, joints, and central nervous system (Salmi et al., 1992). Thus, tissue-selective migration streams offer the prospect of selectively inhibiting cell migration through a diseased tissue, such as the gut, and leaving other tissues unaffected. For instance, mAb inhibitors of $\alpha4\beta7$ integrin and MadCam have been trialed in patients with inflammatory bowel disease and this pathway remains attractive for the emergence of a new migration inhibitor for inflammatory diseases.

Some Clinical Applications

Chemoattractant receptors and adhesion molecules have long been promising targets for anti-inflammatory therapies (Carlos and Harlan, 1994; Oppenheimer-Marks and Lipsky, 1998; Homey and Zlotnik, 1999; Mackay, 2001; von Andrian and Engelhardt, 2003; Szekanecz and Koch, 2004), and possible antagonists have been pursued vigorously by the biotechnology and pharmaceutical industries (Table 22.3). Numerous antibodies, recombinant soluble adhesion molecules, receptor-blocking mutant chemokines, and small molecules have been tested for clinical application in multiple sclerosis, inflammatory bowel disease, chronic arthropathies, and psoriasis. In general, studies on experimental animals have validated various receptors or ligands in inflammatory disease models, including asthma, rheumatoid arthritis, multiple sclerosis, sepsis, and transplantation (Grant et al., 2002; Haskell et al., 2002; Miller et al., 2003; von Andrian and Engelhardt, 2003; Mackay, 2008). Subversion of immune responses by pathogens also provides a pointer to the best anti-inflammatory strategies. A telling feature of many pathogens is their subversion of host responses through the chemokine system (Alcami, 2003). Chemoattractant receptors probably offer the most promise because the known seven-transmembrane structure of these receptors would favor recognition of agents leading to inhibition with organic small molecules.

Natalizumab (Tysabri) requires particular mention. This mAb to α_4 integrin developed by Biogen-Idec and Elan for the treatment of multiple sclerosis and Crohn's disease, together with the LFA-1 integrin inhibitor, Efaluzimab (Raptiva), validate the effectiveness of migration inhibitors for human inflammatory diseases. Natalizumab binds to both $\alpha4\beta1$ (VLA-4) and $\alpha4\beta7$. Studies in rodents, indicating that an $\alpha4$-integrin inhibitor should be highly effective for human multiple sclerosis

and inflammatory bowel disease, were borne out by results of phase 3 clinical trials, as well as experience from some years of clinical use showing that natalizumab greatly reduced the number of relapses in multiple sclerosis (see Chapter 52). However, a worrisome adverse effect was the development of JC virus-induced progressive multifocal leukoencephalopathy (PML), attributed to the otherwise weakly pathogenic effect of this virus, and resulting in restrictions on the type of patient that can receive this therapy. However, the Food and Drug Administration (FDA) did not require withdrawal of natalizumab from marketing because its clinical benefits appeared to outweigh the risks involved. For efaluzimab, however, the risk of PML did result in the European Medicines Agency and the FDA recommending suspension of the drug in the European Union and the USA.

Fingolimod (Gilenya, FTY720, Novartis) is another interesting new anti-inflammatory agent (Brinkman et al., 2010) which, after natalizumab, is the most established migration inhibitor for use in human autoimmune disease, particularly in multiple sclerosis. Fingolimod works by increasing lymphocyte retention in lymph nodes, with a consequent lymphopenia in blood. This drug is phosphorylated *in vivo* to yield a molecule that mimics sphingosine-1-phosphate (S1P) and acts as an agonist for four of the five members of the S1P family of G-protein coupled receptors (see Chapter 52). The physiological role of S1P receptors on lymphocytes is to control their exit from lymphoid tissues. This exit is very much an active and regulated process, and certain stimuli, particularly antigen challenge, can reduce lymphocyte exit from lymph nodes to almost zero. In two Phase III clinical trials, fingolimod reduced the rate of relapses in multiple sclerosis patients by over one-half compared to a placebo or interferon beta. Fingolimod is now approved by regulatory agencies for use in the USA and in Europe. A potential side effect of fingolimod treatment is bradycardia due to expression of certain S1P receptors, particularly S1P3, in the heart.

Potent small molecule antagonists have been developed for a number of the chemoattractant receptors (Table 22.3), especially CCR1, CCR3, CCR5, CXCR3, and CXCR4 (Haringman et al., 2003; Szekanecz and Koch, 2004; Mackay, 2008). Chemokine receptor antagonists have proven highly efficacious in animal models, particularly in models of rheumatoid arthritis according to Szekanecz and Koch (2004). One noteworthy example is a small molecule antagonist of both CCR5 and CXCR3, TAK-779, which inhibits ligand binding of these two Th1-type chemokine receptors (Gao et al., 2003), and also inhibits the development of arthritis by interfering with T cell migration to joint lesions (Yang et al., 2002). Effector T cells in the synovium of patients with rheumatoid arthritis express high levels of CCR5 and CXCR3

TABLE 22.3 Adhesion Molecules and Chemoattractant Receptors as Targets for the Treatment of Inflammatory Diseases.

Target Pathway/ Receptor	Involved in Leukocyte or T-cell Migration to these Sites[a]	Potential Clinical Applications[b]	Comments, Examples of Drug Development[b]
Adhesion Pathways			
a4b1–VCAM-1	Numerous inflamed tissues, Th2 lesions	Asthma, MS, vasculitis	Promising phase II data in MS (Miller et al., 2003; von Andrian and Engelhardt, 2003)
a4b7–MAdCAM-1	Non-pulmonary mucosal tissues	IBD using anti-a4b7 mAb	Promising mouse data, disappointing phase II data
Mac-1–ICAM-1	Inflamed tissues?	Ischemia–reperfusion	Anti-ICAM mAb discontinued in phase III
LFA-1–ICAM-1	Most inflamed tissues, T-cell interactions with APCs	Numerous	Promising phase III data with efazulimab for psoriasis
Selectins–PSGL-1	Acute inflammation, Th1 lesions, esp. in the skin	Numerous	Disappointing phase II data, mixed data with various antagonists (Ulbrich et al., 2003)
Fucosyltransferase-VII	Acutely inflamed tissues, Th1 lesions	Numerous	Requires intracellular inhibitors, none described
Chemokine Receptors/Ligands			
CXCR1,2–numerous CXC chemokines	Some inflamed tissues, esp. skin	Psoriasis, RA, reperfusion injuries	Efficacy of antagonists not determined in humans
CCR1–CCL3, 5	Numerous inflamed tissues	RA, others	Promising phase Ib data (Haringman et al., 2003)
CCR2–CCL2 (MCP-1)	Numerous inflamed tissues	RA, MS	Promising animal data (Gong et al., 1997)
CCR3–CCL11 (Eotaxin)	Th2 lesions, allergic inflammation	Asthma, allergies	Promising phenotypes in knock-out mice, but possible redundancy issues
CCR4–CCL17, 22	Skin, Th2 lesions	Asthma, psoriasis, atopic dermatitis	Importance not established *in vivo*
CCR5–CCL3, 4, 5	Th1 lesions	RA, HIV infection	Promising small molecule antagonists (Baba et al., 1999; Gao et al., 2003)
CCR9–CCL25	Intestine	IBD	Importance not yet established *in vivo*
CXCR3–CXCL9, 10, 11	Th1 lesions	RA, MS, transplantation	Possible redundancy of Th1 chemokine pathways Promising data with CXCR3 knock-out mice
SDF-1a–CXCR4	Numerous tissues	HIV infection	Critical for embryogenesis; inhibitors may alter hematopoiesis
Classical and other Chemoattractant Receptors			
C5aR–C5a	Neutrophil, mast cells	RA, sepsis, reperfusion injuries	Ongoing clinical trial in RA
BLR–LTB4	Mast-cell initiated inflammatory lesions	RA, asthma	Potent small molecule drugs developed, effectiveness in autoimmune disease unclear
S1P receptors (esp. S1P1) i.e., FTY720, effective	Lymphocyte egress from tissues	Numerous	S1P receptor agonist drugs, in animal models of disease (Goetzl and Graler, 2004; Ward, 2004)

[a]Most of these molecular pathways have been targeted with either small molecule antagonists or blocking mAbs, and are currently in clinical trials for various indications. In addition, a substantial amount of animal experimentation has validated these pathways for various diseases.
[b]For reviews of adhesion molecule or chemoattractant receptor antagonists, and their use in preclinical and clinical trials, see Ulbrich et al. (2003), Szekanecz and Koch (2004) and Mackay (2008).
APC, antigen-presenting cell; CCR, receptor for CC chemokine; CXCR, receptor for CXC chemokine; HIV, human immune deficiency virus; IBD, inflammatory bowel disease; ICAM-1, intercellular cell adhesion molecule-1; IL-8, interleukin-8; LAD, leukocyte adhesion deficiency syndrome; LFA-1, leukocyte function-associated antigen-1; Mac-1, macrophage antigen-1; MAdCAM-1, mucosal addressin cell adhesion molecule-1; MS, multiple sclerosis; PSGL-1, P-selectin glycoprotein ligand-1; RA, rheumatoid arthritis; Th, T-helper; VCAM-1, vascular cell adhesion molecule-1.

(Qin et al., 1998), so it is expected that some of these drugs will succeed in clinical trials and prove useful in the treatment of autoimmune diseases. Interactions involving integrins or selectins are more difficult to inhibit with small molecules, but there are promising results with antagonists of α4β1–VCAM-1 and LFA-1–ICAM-1 interactions (Kelly et al., 1999; Lin et al., 1999). As a general conclusion, cell-migration inhibitors could greatly alleviate the disabling effects of autoimmune inflammation well before the basic nature of autoimmunity is finally understood.

CONCLUSIONS AND FUTURE DIRECTIONS

The disruption of cell-migration pathways has emerged as a new approach to the treatment of inflammatory autoimmune diseases. Well-established examples include multiple sclerosis, rheumatoid arthritis, Crohn's disease, psoriasis, and various others (see Chapter 81). The wealth of data available on trafficking molecules now calls for a more precise understanding of their physiologic and pathologic relevance to human health and disease, with this requiring new experimental and therapeutic entities such as antibodies, recombinant proteins, small molecule inhibitors, screening assays, and, certainly not least, expertly conducted and meaningful clinical trials. One pivotal question is whether to treat autoimmune diseases with broad inhibitors (the sledgehammer approach) using, for instance, an inhibitor of a common signaling pathway of chemoattractant receptors, or whether to treat such diseases with much more specific inhibitors, for instance inflammatory bowel disease with a CCR9 or an α4β7 inhibitor? Further experience should see this question answered.

ACKNOWLEDGMENTS

CRM is supported by grants from the National Health and Medical Research Council of Australia UvA.

REFERENCES

Alcami, A., 2003. Viral mimicry of cytokines, chemokines and their receptors. Nat. Rev. Immunol. 3, 36–50.

Alon, R., Kassner, P.D., Carr, M.W., Finger, E.B., Hemler, M.E., Springer, T.A., 1995. The integrin VLA-4 supports tethering and rolling in flow on VCAM-1. J. Cell Biol. 128, 1243–1253.

Andrew, D.P., Spellberg, J.P., Takimoto, H., Schmits, R., Mak, T.W., Zukowski, M.M., 1998. Transendothelial migration and trafficking of leukocytes in LFA-1-deficient mice. Eur. J. Immunol. 28, 1959–1969.

von Andrian, U.H., Engelhardt, B., 2003. Alpha4 integrins as therapeutic targets in autoimmune disease. N. Engl. J. Med. 348, 68–72.

von Andrian, U.H., Mackay, C.R., 2000. T-cell function and migration. Two sides of the same coin. N. Engl. J. Med. 343, 1020–1034.

von Andrian, U.H., Chambers, J.D., McEvoy, L.M., Bargatze, R.F., Arfors, K.E., Butcher, E.C., 1991. Two-step model of leukocyte-endothelial cell interaction in inflammation: Distinct roles for LECAM-1 and the leukocyte b2 integrins in vivo. Proc. Natl. Acad. Sci. U.S.A. 88, 7538–7542.

Arbones, M.L., Ord, D.C., Ley, K., Ratech, H., Maynard-Curry, C., Otten, G., et al., 1994. Lymphocyte homing and leukocyte rolling and migration are impaired in L-selectin-deficient mice. Immunity. 1, 247–260.

Austrup, F., Vestweber, D., Borges, E., Lohning, M., Brauer, R., Herz, U., et al., 1997. P- and E-selectin mediate recruitment of T-helper-1 but not T-helper-2 cells into inflamed tissues. Nature. 385, 81–83.

Baba, M., Nishimura, O., Kanzaki, N., Okamoto, M., Sawada, H., Iizawa, Y., et al., 1999. A small-molecule, nonpeptide CCR5 antagonist with highly potent and selective anti-HIV-1 activity. Proc. Natl. Acad. Sci. U.S.A. 96, 5698–5703.

Bargatze, R.F., Jutila, M.A., Butcher, E.C., 1995. Distinct roles of L-selectin and integrins a4b7 and LFA-1 in lymphocyte homing to Peyer's patch-HEV in situ: the multistep model confirmed and refined. Immunity. 3, 99–108.

Berlin, C., Bargatze, R.F., von Andrian, U.H., Szabo, M.C., Hasslen, S.R., Nelson, R.D., et al., 1995. a4 integrins mediate lymphocyte attachment and rolling under physiologic flow. Cell. 80, 413–422.

Berlin-Rufenach, C., Otto, F., Mathies, M., Westermann, J., Owen, M.J., Hamann, A., et al., 1999. Lymphocyte migration in lymphocyte function-associated antigen (LFA)-1-deficient mice. J. Exp. Med. 189, 1467–1478.

Bleul, C.C., Wu, L., Hoxie, J.A., Springer, T.A., Mackay, C.R., 1997. The HIV coreceptors CXCR4 and CCR5 are differentially expressed and regulated on human T lymphocytes. Proc. Natl. Acad. Sci. U.S.A. 94, 1925–1930.

Bonecchi, R., Bianchi, G., Bordignon, P.P., D'Ambrosio, D., Lang, R., Borsatti, A., Sozzani, S., et al., 1998. Differential expression of chemokine receptors and chemotactic responsiveness of type 1 T helper cells (Th1s) and Th2s. J. Exp. Med. 187, 129–134.

Borges, E., Tietz, W., Steegmaier, M., Moll, T., Hallmann, R., Hamann, A., et al., 1997. P-selectin glycoprotein ligand-1 (PSGL-1) on T helper 1 but not on T helper 2 cells binds to P-selectin and supports migration into inflamed skin. J. Exp. Med. 185, 573–578.

Brinkman, V., Billich, A., Baumruker, T., Heining, P., Schmouder, R., Francis, G., et al., 2010. Fingolimod (FTY720): discovery and development of an oral drug to treat multiple sclerosis. Nat. Rev. Drug. Discov. 9, 883–897.

Bullard, D.C., Kunkel, E.J., Kubo, H., Hicks, M.J., Lorenzo, I., Doyle, N.A., et al., 1996. Infectious susceptibility and severe deficiency of leukocyte rolling and recruitment in E-selectin and P-selectin double mutant mice. J. Exp. Med. 183, 2329–2336.

Butcher, E.C., 1991. Leukocyte-endothelial cell recognition: three (or more) steps to specificity and diversity. Cell. 67, 1033–1036.

Butcher, E.C., Picker, L.J., 1996. Lymphocyte homing and homeostasis. Science. 272, 60–66.

Campbell, J.J., Hedrick, J., Zlotnik, A., Siani, M.A., Thompson, D.A., Butcher, E.C., 1998. Chemokines and the arrest of lymphoyctes rolling under flow conditions. Science. 279, 381–384.

Carlos, T.M., Harlan, J.M., 1994. Leukocyte-endothelial adhesion molecules. Blood. 84, 2068–2101.

Cyster, J.G., 1999. Chemokines and cell migration in secondary lymphoid organs. Science. 286, 2098–2102.

Dieu, M.C., Vanbervliet, B., Vicari, A., Bridon, J.M., Oldham, E., Ait-Yahia, S., et al., 1998. Selective recruitment of immature and mature dendritic cells by distinct chemokines expressed in different anatomic sites. J. Exp. Med. 188, 373–386.

Forster, R., Schubel, A., Breitfeld, D., Kremmer, E., Renner-Muller, I., Wolf, E., et al., 1999. CCR7 coordinates the primary immune response by establishing functional microenvironments in secondary lymphoid organs. Cell. 99, 23–33.

Foxman, E.F., Campbell, J.J., Butcher, E.C., 1997. Multistep navigation and the combinatorial control of leukocyte chemotaxis. J. Cell Biol. 139, 1349–1360.

Frenette, P.S., Mayadas, T.N., Rayburn, H., Hynes, R.O., Wagner, D.D., 1996. Susceptibility to infection and altered hematopoiesis in mice deficient in both P- and E-selectins. Cell. 84, 563–574.

Gao, P., Zhou, X.Y., Yashiro-Ohtani, Y., Yang, Y.F., Sugimoto, N., Ono, S., et al., 2003. The unique target specificity of a nonpeptide chemokine receptor antagonist: selective blockade of two Th1 chemokine receptors CCR5 and CXCR3. J. Leukoc. Biol. 73, 273–280.

Girard, J.-P., Springer, T.A., 1995. High endothelial venules (HEVs): specialized endothelium for lymphocyte migration. Immunol. Today. 16, 449–457.

Goetzl, E.J., Graler, M.H., 2004. Sphingosine 1-phosphate and its type 1 G protein-coupled receptor: trophic support and functional regulation of T lymphocytes. J. Leukoc. Biol. 76, 30–35.

Gomez-Reino, J.J., Pablos, J.L., Carreira, P.E., Santiago, B., Serrano, L., Vicario, J.L., et al., 1999. Association of rheumatoid arthritis with a functional chemokine receptor, CCR5. Arthritis Rheum. 42, 989–992.

Gong, J.-H., Ratkay, L.G., Waterfield, J.D., Clark-Lewis, I., 1997. An antagonist of monocyte chemoattractant protein1 (MCP-1) inhibits arthritis in the MRL-lpr mouse model. J. Exp. Med. 186, 131–137.

Gonzalo, J.A., Lloyd, C.M., Wen, D., Albar, J.P., Wells, T.N., Proudfoot, A., et al., 1998. The coordinated action of CC chemokines in the lung orchestrates allergic inflammation and airway hyperresponsiveness. J. Exp. Med. 188, 157–167.

Grant, E.P., Picarella, D., Burwell, T., Delaney, T., Croci, A., Avitahl, N., et al., 2002. Essential role for the C5a receptor in regulating the effector phase of synovial infiltration and joint destruction in experimental arthritis. J. Exp. Med. 196, 1461–1471.

Gutierrez-Ramos, J.C., Lloyd, C., Gonzalo, J.A., 1999. Eotaxin: from an eosinophilic chemokine to a major regulator of allergic reactions. Immunol. Today. 20, 500–504.

Haringman, J.J., Kraan, M.C., Smeets, T.J., Zwinderman, K.H., Tak, P.P., 2003. Chemokine blockade and chronic inflammatory disease: proof of concept in patients with rheumatoid arthritis. Ann. Rheum. Dis. 62, 715–721.

Haskell, C.A., Ribeiro, S., Horuk, R., 2002. Chemokines in transplant rejection. Curr. Opin. Investig. Drugs. 3, 399–405.

Hirsch, E., Katanaev, V.L., Garlanda, C., Azzolino, O., Pirola, L., Silengo, L., et al., 2000. Central role for G protein-coupled phosphoinositide 3-kinase gamma in inflammation. Science. 287, 1049–1053.

Homey, B., Zlotnik, A., 1999. Chemokines in allergy. Curr. Opin. Immunol. 11, 626–634.

Jose, P.J., Griffiths-Johnson, D.A., Collins, P.D., Walsh, D.T., Moqbel, R., Totty, N.F., et al., 1994. Eotaxin: a potent eosinophil chemoattractant cytokine detected in a guinea pig model of allergic airways inflammation. J. Exp. Med. 179, 881–887.

Jung, S., Littman, D.R., 1999. Chemokine receptors in lymphoid organ homeostasis. Curr. Opin. Immunol. 11, 319–325.

Kansas, G.S., 1996. Selectins and their ligands: current concepts and controversies. Blood. 88, 3259–3287.

Kantele, A., Zivny, J., Hakkinen, M., Elson, C.O., Mestecky, J., 1999. Differential homing commitments of antigen-specific T cells after oral or parenteral immunization in humans. J. Immunol. 162, 5173–5177.

Kelly, T.A., Jeanfavre, D.D., McNeil, D.W., Woska Jr., J.R., Reilly, P.L., Mainolfi, E.A., et al., 1999. Cutting edge: a small molecule antagonist of LFA-1-mediated cell adhesion. J. Immunol. 163, 5173–5177.

Kim, C.H., Broxmeyer, H.E., 1999. Chemokines: signal lamps for trafficking of T and B cells for development and effector function. J. Leukoc. Biol. 65, 6–15.

Kunkel, E.J., Ramos, C.L., Steeber, D.A., Muller, W., Wagner, N., Tedder, T.F., et al., 1998. The roles of L-selectin, beta 7 integrins, and P-selectin in leukocyte rolling and adhesion in high endothelial venules of Peyer's patches. J. Immunol. 161, 2449–2456.

Lawrence, M.B., Springer, T.A., 1991. Leukocytes roll on a selectin at physiologic flow rates: distinction from and prerequisite for adhesion through integrins. Cell. 65, 859–873.

Li, Z., Jiang, H., Xie, W., Zhang, Z., Smrcka, A.V., Wu, D., 2000. Roles of PLC-beta2 and -beta3 and PI3Kgamma in chemoattractant-mediated signal transduction. Science. 287, 1046–1049.

Lim, Y.C., Henault, L., Wagers, A.J., Kansas, G.S., Luscinskas, F.W., Lichtman, A.H., 1999. Expression of functional selectin ligands on Th cells is differentially regulated by IL-12 and IL-4. J. Immunol. 162, 3193–3201.

Lin, K., Ateeq, H.S., Hsiung, S.H., Chong, L.T., Zimmerman, C.N., Castro, A., et al., 1999. Selective, tight-binding inhibitors of integrin alpha4beta1 that inhibit allergic airway responses. J. Med. Chem. 42, 920–934.

Mackay, C.R., 2001. Chemokines: immunology's high impact factors. Nat. Immunol. 2, 95–101.

Mackay, C.R., 2008. Moving targets: cell migration inhibitors as new anti-inflammatory therapies. Nat. Immunol. 9, 988–998.

Maly, P., Thall, A.D., Petryniak, B., Rogers, C.E., Smith, P.L., Marks, R.M., et al., 1996. The a(1,3) fucosyltransferase Fuc-TVII controls leukocyte trafficking through an essential role in L-, E-, and P-selectin ligand biosynthesis. Cell. 86, 643–653.

Mantovani, A., 1999. The chemokine system: redundancy for robust outputs. Immunol. Today. 20, 254–257.

Marchesi, V.T., Gowans, J.L., 1964. The migration of lymphocytes through the endothelium of venules in lymph nodes: an electron microscope study. Proc. R. Soc. B. 159, 283–290.

Mayadas, T.N., Johnson, R.C., Rayburn, H., Hynes, R.O., Wagner, D.D., 1993. Leukocyte rolling and extravasation are severely compromised in P-selectin-deficient mice. Cell. 74, 541–554.

Miller, D.H., Khan, O.A., Sheremata, W.A., Blumhardt, L.D., Rice, G., Libonati, M.A., et al., 2003. A controlled trial of Natalizumab in relapsing multiple sclerosis. N. Engl. J. Med. 348, 15–23.

Oppenheimer-Marks, N., Lipsky, P.E., 1998. Adhesion molecules in rheumatoid arthritis. Springer Semin. Immunopathol. 20, 95–114.

Paxton, W.A., Kang, S., 1998. Chemokine receptor allelic polymorphisms: relationships to HIV resistance and disease progression. Semin. Immunol. 10, 187–194.

Ponath, P.D., Qin, S., Ringler, D.J., Clark-Lewis, I., Wang, J., Kassam, N., et al., 1996. Cloning of the human eosinophil chemoattractant, eotaxin. Expression, receptor binding, and functional properties suggest a mechanism for the selective recruitment of eosinophils. J. Clin. Invest. 97, 604–612.

Qin, S., Rottman, J.B., Myers, P., Kassam, N., Weinblatt, M., Loetscher, M., et al., 1998. The chemokine receptors CXCR3 and CCR5 mark subsets of T cells associated with certain inflammatory reactions. J. Clin. Invest. 101, 746–754.

Robert, C., Kupper, T.S., 1999. Inflammatory skin diseases, T cells, and immune surveillance. N. Engl. J. Med. 341, 1817–1828.

Robinson, S.D., Frenette, P.S., Rayburn, H., Cummiskey, M., Ullman-Cullere, M., Wagner, D.D., et al., 1999. Multiple, targeted deficiencies in selectins reveal a predominant role for P-selectin in leukocyte recruitment. Proc. Natl. Acad. Sci. U.S.A. 96, 11452–11457.

Sallusto, F., Lanzavecchia, A., 1999. Mobilizing dendritic cells for tolerance, priming, and chronic inflammation. J. Exp. Med. 189, 611–614.

Sallusto, F., Mackay, C.R., Lanzavecchia, A., 1997. Selective expression of the eotaxin receptor CCR3 by human T helper 2 cells. Science. 277, 2005–2007.

Sallusto, F., Lanzavecchia, A., Mackay, C.R., 1998. Chemokines and chemokine receptors in T-cell priming and Th1/Th2-mediated responses. Immunol. Today. 19, 568–574.

Sallusto, F., Lenig, D., Mackay, C.R., Lanzavecchia, A., 1998. Flexible programs of chemokine receptor expression on human polarized T helper 1 and 2 lymphocytes. J. Exp. Med. 187, 875–883.

Sallusto, F., Schaerli, P., Loetscher, P., Schaniel, C., Lenig, D., Mackay, C.R., et al., 1998. Rapid and coordinated switch in chemokine receptor expression during dendritic cell maturation. Eur. J. Immunol. 28, 2760–2769.

Sallusto, F., Lenig, D., Forster, R., Lipp, M., Lanzavecchia, A., 1999. Two subsets of memory T lymphocytes with distinct homing potentials and effector functions. Nature. 401, 708–712.

Sallusto, F., Palermo, B., Hoy, A., Lanzavecchia, A., 1999. The role of chemokine receptors in directing traffic of naïve, type 1 and type 2 T cells. Curr. Top. Microbiol. Immunol. 246, 123–128.

Salmi, M., Granfors, K., Leirisalo-Repo, M., Hamalainen, M., MacDermott, R., Leino, R., et al., 1992. Selective endothelial binding of interleukin-2-dependent human T-cell lines derived from different tissues. Proc. Natl. Acad. Sci. USA. 89, 11436–11440.

Springer, T.A., 1994. Traffic signals for lymphocyte recirculation and leukocyte emigration: the multi-step paradigm. Cell. 76, 301–314.

Stein, J.V., Cheng, G., Stockton, B.M., Fors, B.P., Butcher, E.C., von Andrian, U.H., 1999. L-selectin-mediated leukocyte adhesion in vivo: microvillous distribution determines tethering efficiency, but not rolling velocity. J. Exp. Med. 189, 37–50.

Stein, J.V., Rot, A., Luo, Y., Narasimhaswamy, M., Nakano, H., Gunn, M.D., et al., 2000. The CC chemokine thymus-derived chemotactic agent 4 (TCA-4, secondary lymphoid tissue chemokine, 6Ckine, exodus-2) triggers lymphocyte function-associated antigen 1-mediated arrest of rolling T lymphocytes in peripheral lymph node high endothelial venules. J. Exp. Med. 191, 61–76.

Syrbe, U., Siveke, J., Hamann, A., 1999. Th1/Th2 subsets: distinct differences in homing and chemokine receptor expression? Springer Semin. Immunopathol. 21, 263–285.

Szekanecz, Z., Koch, A.E., 2004. Therapeutic inhibition of leukocyte recruitment in inflammatory diseases. Curr. Opin. Pharmacol. 4, 423–428.

Ulbrich, H., Eriksson, E.E., Lindbom, L., 2003. Leukocyte and endothelial cell adhesion molecules as targets for therapeutic interventions in inflammatory disease. Trends Pharmacol. Sci. 24, 640–647.

Vestweber, D., Blanks, J.E., 1999. Mechanisms that regulate the function of the selectins and their ligands. Physiol. Rev. 79, 181–213.

Wagers, A.J., Waters, C.M., Stoolman, L.M., Kansas, G.S., 1998. Interleukin 12 and interleukin 4 control T cell adhesion to endothelial selectins through opposite effects on alpha1, 3-fucosyltransferase VII gene expression. J. Exp. Med. 188, 2225–2231.

Wagner, N., Lohler, J., Kunkel, E.J., Ley, K., Leung, E., Krissansen, G., et al., 1996. Critical role for b7 integrins in formation of the gut-associated lymphoid tissue. Nature. 382, 366–370.

Ward, S.G., 2004. Do phosphoinositide 3-kinases direct lymphocyte navigation?. Trends Immunol. 25, 67–74.

Warnock, R.A., Askari, S., Butcher, E.C., von Andrian, U.H., 1998. Molecular mechanisms of lymphocyte homing to peripheral lymph nodes. J. Exp. Med. 187, 205–216.

Warnock, R.A., Campbell, J.J., Dorf, M.E., Matsuzawa, A., McEvoy, L.M., Butcher, E.C., 2000. The role of chemokines in the microenvironmental control of T versus B cell arrest in Peyer's patch high endothelial venules. J. Exp. Med. 191, 77–88.

Wei, S., Kyczek, I., Zou, W., 2008. Regulatory T-lymphocyte compartmentalization and trafficking. Blood. 108, 426–431.

Xie, H., Lim, Y.C., Luscinskas, F.W., Lichtman, A.H., 1999. Acquisition of selectin binding and peripheral homing properties by CD4(+) and CD8(+) T cells. J. Exp. Med. 189, 1765–1776.

Yang, Y.F., Mukai, T., Gao, P., Yamaguchi, N., Ono, S., Iwaki, H., et al., 2002. A non-peptide CCR5 antagonist inhibits collagen-induced arthritis by modulating T cell migration without affecting anti-collagen T cell responses. Eur. J. Immunol. 32, 2124–2132.

Zlotnik, A., Yoshie, O., 2000. Chemokines: a new classification system and their role in immunity. Immunity. 12, 121–127.

Part 5

Facilitation of Autoimmunity

Effector Mechanisms in Autoimmunity

Arian Laurence[1] and Martin Aringer[2]

[1]*National Institute for Arthritis and Musculoskeletal and Skin Diseases, NIH, Bethesda, MD, USA,* [2]*University Clinical Center Carl Gustav Carus, Dresden, Germany*

Chapter Outline

Introduction	311	Mast Cells	314
Autoantibodies	311	Natural Killer Cells and Cytotoxic T Cells	314
Direct Antibody-Mediated Disease	311	Effector T Helper Cell-Mediated Autoimmune Disease	314
Immune Complex Disease	312	Effector Cytokines and their Targets	315
Complement Cascades	313	Conclusions	316
Macrophages	313	References	317
Neutrophils	313		

INTRODUCTION

In the 1960s, pathological reactions produced by an otherwise healthy immune system were subdivided into four groups on the basis of the effector mechanism initiated. More recent advances in our understanding of cellular immunology have led to less prominent use, and critique, of the Gell and Coombs classification system (Rajan, 2003), which cannot be upheld as such in the light of today's knowledge. Nevertheless, it remains a useful introductory way of characterizing some aspects of autoimmune effector mechanisms. Of the four types of "hypersensitivity reactions," type I represented "conventional" allergic and anaphylactic responses, while the other three contribute to *bona fide* autoimmune pathology.

AUTOANTIBODIES

Autoantibodies are a hallmark of autoimmune disease (Tan, 1991). In fact, their presence is so common in autoimmunity that autoinflammatory disease, which does not involve specific immune recognition, is principally defined by the absence of autoantibodies (Ombrello and Kastner, 2011) (see Chapter 4). In most cases, autoantibodies are important for diagnostic purposes and may not directly influence the outcome of the disease. However, an increasing number of autoantibodies have been directly linked to inflammation,

cell death, or functional problems. Antibody-mediated autoimmune disease is distinguished into two groups by the Gell–Coombs classification system. Type II hypersensitivity reactions that are mediated by a direct effect of the antibody binding its target antigen; examples of pathogenic autoantibody effects are listed in Table 23.1. By contrast, type III hypersensitivity reactions are mediated by the deposition of immune complexes in affected tissues that will almost always result in inflammation, as discussed below.

DIRECT ANTIBODY-MEDIATED DISEASE

Type II hypersensitivity reactions mainly lead to cell death and removal, or disturb physiological functions (Table 23.1).

Autoantibodies leading to cell death include those against thrombocyte membranes in autoimmune thrombocytopenia, to erythrocyte membranes in hemolytic anemia, to various, mostly uncharacterized, antigens in SLE (systemic lupus erythematosus) cytopenias, or, presumably, to endothelial cell antigens in systemic sclerosis. These autoantibodies follow typical antibody function patterns that include antibody-dependent cell cytotoxicity (ADCC) where the antibody recruits an immune (natural killer, NK) cell to induce cells to kill or phagocytose any target that is marked by an antibody. Alternatively, antibodies may destroy their target by recruiting components of the complement system. Essentially all these antibodies are of particular IgG subclasses, and the

N. Rose & I. Mackay (Eds): The Autoimmune Diseases, Fifth edition. DOI: http://dx.doi.org/10.1016/B978-0-12-384929-8.00023-X

TABLE 23.1 Variable Effects of Well-Defined Autoantibodies.

Antibody to	Disease	Function of Antibody
Acetylcholine receptors	Myasthenia gravis	Receptor blockade
Aquaporin-4	Neuromyelitis optica	Cytotoxicity
Beta-2 glycoprotein I	Anti-phospholipid syndrome	Activation of coagulation
Desmogleins	Pemphigus vulgaris	Binding function blocked
Factor VIII	Acquired hemophilia	Coagulation factor removal
Glycoprotein IIb/IIIa	Immune thrombocytopenic purpura	Thrombocyte clearance
Thyrotropin receptor	Graves' disease	Receptor stimulation

specific IgG subclass is relevant for their properties. For example, IgG1 and IgG3 activate complement, while IgG2 is a poor complement activator, and IgG4 does not activate complement at all (Daha et al., 2011). The same classes that activate complement, i.e., IgG1 and IgG3, also avidly bind the activating Fc receptor FcγR1 (Nimmerjahn and Ravetch, 2010) and mediate ADCC.

Blood cells marked by antibodies will be phagocytosed in the spleen (and liver), and cleared (Cines and Blanchette, 2002; Gehrs and Friedberg, 2002), while immobile cells, such as endothelial cells to which antibodies bind in systemic sclerosis, may be killed by cytotoxic cells (Sgonc et al., 1996). While the former mechanism is usually obvious and can be easily proven, for example by recording clinical improvement following removal of autoantibodies (American College of Rheumatology Ad Hoc Committee, 2004), ADCC often cannot be proven *in vivo*, and is even difficult to prove in an *in vitro* situation. Nevertheless, the latter most probably is the more common process.

In addition to marking cells for ADCC or phagocytosis, autoantibodies can also cause significant pathology by functionally disturbing physiological processes. Important examples of this type of autoantibody-induced mechanism are antibodies to proteins and glycoproteins, such as to factor VIII (Zeitler et al., 2013) in acquired hemophilia or to β2-glycoprotein I, which induce thrombotic events in the antiphospholipid antibody syndrome (Giannakopoulos and Krilis, 2013) (see Chapters 51 and 34). Autoantibodies may engage cell receptors, such as the TSH receptor in Graves' disease (Dalan and Leow, 2012), triggering their activation and so leading to thyrotoxicosis or neuromuscular acetylcholine receptors in myasthenia gravis (Levinson, 2013) preventing their activation leading to muscle weakness, or to channel proteins, such as aquaporin 4, which is targeted in neuromyelitis optica/Devic's disease (see Chapter 57 and Papadopoulos and Verkman, 2012). Other examples of antibodies impairing functions are those to desmogleins in the autoimmune blistering disease pemphigus (Stanley and Amagai, 2006), or those mediating psychosis in SLE (Fong and Thumboo, 2010).

IMMUNE COMPLEX DISEASE

Commonly, pathology is not induced by IgG monomers, but by immune complexes consisting of autoantigen and autoantibodies resulting in a type III hypersensitivity reaction. In this case, other antibody classes also play a major role. In particular, this is relevant to the pentameric IgM and the dimeric IgA, due to their cross-linking capabilities. Immune complexes will strongly activate complement, and will be recognized by Fc receptors, thus causing inflammation.

IgM and IgA rheumatoid factors (RF) are characteristic for active seropositive rheumatoid arthritis (RA). RF bind to the Fc portion of IgG, and in this way induce immune complexes, which likely play a major role in RA pathophysiology. In fact, the complement system is clearly activated in rheumatic joints (Olmez et al., 1991). Moreover, beyond disease activity, high titer rheumatoid factors are associated with incurring damage (Aletaha et al., 2013).

Immune complexes also play a major role in organ inflammation in systemic autoimmune diseases, and in SLE in particular. For example, immune complexes of double-stranded DNA (dsDNA) and anti-dsDNA antibodies lead to proliferative glomerulonephritis. These antibodies can directly be detected in glomeruli. However, rather than being deposited from the blood, they may form locally, by antibodies to nucleosomes being caught at the negatively charged glomerular basement membrane (Yung and Chan, 2008; Mjelle et al., 2011).

Similarly, antibodies to the nuclear antigen Ro/SS-A are associated with subacute cutaneous lupus erythematosus (SCLE) (Sontheimer, 2005), where, likewise, immune complexes can be directly detected in the affected skin. While ANCA-associated vasculitides are not immune complex driven, lupus vasculitis is, as are RA vasculitis, cryoglobulinemic vasculitis, IgA vasculitis (Henoch—Schönlein disease), or hypocomplementemic urticarial vasculitis (Jennette et al., 2013).

COMPLEMENT CASCADES

Immune complexes, as well as most antibodies binding to surfaces, activate the complement cascade via the classical pathway (see Chapter 15 and Daha et al., 2011). Binding occurs via complement component C1, leading to cleavage of C4 and C2 (Walport, 2001). The activated larger cleavage products C4b and C2a form the convertase for C3, the central complement of the downstream complement cascade, which then leads to the activation of C5 and the membrane attack complex consisting of C5b, C6, 7, 8, and 9. In addition to formation of the membrane attack complex, C1q, C3b, and C4b bound to immune complexes facilitate phagocytosis, a process called opsonization. Mannose binding lectins form an initiating event similar to that of C1, which is not known to play a role in autoimmunity.

In contrast, the alternative complement pathway is commonly involved in autoimmune disease. This amplification pathway is started by cleavage of C3, upon which C3b has to bind to a membrane. Membrane bound C3b then binds to factor B, and together they activate the alternative C3 convertase C3bBb. Antibodies stabilizing the C3bBb complex, called nephritic factor, are associated with type II dense deposit membranoproliferative glomerulonephritis as well as with partial lipodystrophy (Walport, 2001).

Cells have mechanisms to defend against occasional deposition of C3b. CD59 (membrane inhibitor of reactive lysis) protects autologous cells against the membrane attack complex, and its deficiency leads to paroxysmal nocturnal hemoglobinuria (Yamashina et al., 1990), where erythrocytes are slowly but continuously destroyed by unrestrained activation of the alternate complement pathway. In addition, the inhibitory plasma protein factor H binds to C3b, leading to its inactivation by factor I (Walport, 2001). Two membrane proteins, namely CD35 (complement receptor type I) and CD46 (membrane cofactor protein), also play a role in complement inactivation. As another option, cells may be able to eject complement bound membrane by forming microparticles, albeit at the risk of inducing immune complex disease elsewhere (Pisetsky, 2012).

The classical complement pathway is checked by C1 inhibitor, the deficiency of which causes angioedema. This is related to yet another function of the complement system: The smaller fragments C3a, C5a, and C4a act as anaphylatoxins, inducing the chemotaxis and activation of leukocytes (Walport, 2001). This may play a role in the kidney disease of ANCA-associated vasculitides, since C5a receptor deficient animals are resistant to this disease (Schreiber et al., 2009).

Finally, complement may play a role in limiting immune complex disease by aiding the clearance of immune complexes—or of apoptotic cells. Inherited deficiencies of C1–C4 are all associated with an increased incidence of SLE (Aringer et al., 2012).

MACROPHAGES

Monocytes and macrophages are the main cells to deal with immune complexes (see Chapter 11). They are equipped with both Fc receptors and complement receptors, thus simultaneously recognizing immune complexes and C5a (Karsten and Kohl, 2012). Under such circumstances, removal of immune complexes (and attached particles) becomes a highly inflammatory process. Not only will these M1 macrophages then present antigen, they will also produce a variety of proinflammatory cytokines. Immune complex recognition leads to the release of tumor necrosis factor (TNF) (Aringer and Smolen, 2012), but also of other cytokines, including IL-6, IL-1, IL-8, and GM-CSF (Jarvis et al., 1997). In this way, macrophages link between immune complex deposition and inflammation. Indeed, Fc receptor deficiency was illustrated by uncoupling of immune complex deposition from glomerulonephritis in a lupus mouse model (Clynes et al., 1998). In addition to their role as essential promoters of inflammation in autoimmune complex disease, macrophages are also an important effector in autoimmune thrombocytopenia and hemolytic anemia, where antibody-loaded cells are cleared in spleen and kidney (Cines and Blanchette, 2002; Gehrs and Friedberg, 2002).

NEUTROPHILS

As the most common leukocytes, neutrophils are prototypical effector cells of the immune system (Amulic et al., 2012). In addition to phagocytosis and degranulation, NETosis has more recently been investigated. NETosis is a form of "aggressive" neutrophil cell death that constrains and kills pathogens; in the end it is the physiological background of what has long been known as pus. Neutrophil extracellular traps (NETs) consist of fibrous structures that contain decondensed chromatin, histones, and antimicrobial proteins (Amulic et al., 2012). NETosis may be importantly involved in autoimmune tissue inflammation, such as in SLE (Kaplan, 2011) or in ANCA-associated vasculitides (Kessenbrock et al., 2009). Neutrophils also produce cytokines, including IL-8, IL-1, IL-17, and TNF, as well as chemokines (Hoshino et al., 2008; Amulic et al., 2012).

Like macrophages, neutrophils carry both Fc and complement receptors, and accordingly react to antibodies and immune complexes (Hoshino et al., 2008; Nemeth and Mocsai, 2012). In addition, neutrophils are activated by high concentrations of IL-8, which in lower concentrations acts as a chemoattractant (Amulic et al., 2012). Activated platelets can also activate neutrophils (Caudrillier et al., 2012). In other inflammatory situations, Toll-like and nonobese diabetic (NOD)-like receptors recognizing pathogen-associated molecular patterns (PAMPs) and danger-associated molecular patterns (DAMPs) play a major role (Amulic et al., 2012).

MAST CELLS

Principal players in allergic or type I hypersensitivity reactions, there are indications that mast cells also act as effectors in autoimmune diseases. In addition to histamine and serotonin, mast cells also produce the proinflammatory cytokines IL-6 and TNF (Wesolowski and Paumet, 2011). In rheumatoid arthritis, mast cells have been found within the synovitic joint (Kiener et al., 1998), and mast cell deficient mice are protected against arthritis in the K/BxN model (Lee et al., 2002). Antibodies to citrullinated peptides, which are fairly specific for rheumatoid arthritis, also exist as IgE antibodies, and are then associated with synovial histamine release (Schuerwegh et al., 2010). Mast cells are also activated by IgG immune complexes, a process that is potentiated by the presence of the inflammatory cytokine, IL-33 (Kaieda et al., 2012).

NATURAL KILLER CELLS AND CYTOTOXIC T CELLS

To protect the organism, virally infected and transformed cells are actively eliminated by NK cells and $CD8^+$ cytotoxic T lymphocytes. Cytotoxicity is principally mediated via membrane bound ligands of death receptors, such as Fas ligand, and Granzyme B (Afonina et al., 2010), all of which induce apoptosis in the target cell. Extracellular Granzyme B also has proinflammatory effects in that it enhances IL-1α activity by processing this cytokine (Afonina et al., 2011). Conversely, IFNγ and TNF made by either cell type increase Fas (CD95) expression on target cells that facilitates their destruction (Bergman and D'Elios, 2010).

Cytotoxic T cells require priming by myeloid cell-dependent antigen presentation in order to be able to kill (Sigal et al., 1999), and recognize specific peptides presented by autologous major histocompatibility complex (MHC) I molecules. These cells are implicated in *H. pylori*-related gastric autoimmunity (Bergman and D'Elios, 2010), type 1 diabetes mellitus (Coppieters and von Herrath, 2011), and autoimmune central nervous system (CNS) disease (Melzer et al., 2009).

In contrast to cytotoxic T lymphocytes, NK cells need no previous activation. NK cells have receptors that have evolved in parallel with the MHC class I proteins they recognize (Parham and Moffett, 2013). This points to their function in recognizing small changes in MHC class I, which may herald an important safety issue with the afflicted cell. In addition, NK cells kill cells targeted by autoantibodies, a process termed ADCC. Whereas circulating cells covered by autoantibodies are removed in spleen and liver, ADCC is the deadly effector pathway of IgG autoantibodies that bind non-circulating cells, such as endothelial cells in systemic sclerosis (Sgonc et al., 1996). This process may thus induce tissue damage anywhere in the body, but this will be difficult to prove *in vivo*.

EFFECTOR T HELPER CELL-MEDIATED AUTOIMMUNE DISEASE

Whereas $CD8^+$ cytotoxic T cells act directly to damage target tissues, $CD4^+$ helper T cells (Th cells) drive a specific immune attack by employing a variety of additional mechanisms. For any specific immune reaction these cells are of the utmost importance, and need to be addressed when investigating effector mechanisms in autoimmune disease.

A priori, the immune system does not know which kind of pathogens to expect next. Therefore, naïve T cells are entirely flexible. This flexibility changes for determination in the process of activation. Like cytotoxic T cells, naïve Th cells need antigen presentation by myeloid cells in order to be able to mature into effector Th cells. These two groups of T cells mediate delayed type (type IV) hypersensitivity responses; the 24–48 hour delay is due to the required period of antigen presentation. During this process of antigen presentation, the presence of cytokines secreted by the myeloid cell or other nearby immune cell will determine what lineage of effector Th cell will be generated. These include Th1 cells, Th2 cells, and Th17 cells (Tato and O'Shea, 2006; Reiner, 2007).

Th1 cells are important for the clearance of intracellular pathogens (Infante-Duarte and Kamradt, 1999). They are induced by activation in the presence of IL-12 and are characterized by the ability to secrete IFN-γ (Table 23.2), which activates macrophages to kill such organisms and activates NK cells and cytotoxic T lymphocytes, as well as the ability to enhance MHC expression.

Th2 cells are essential for defending mucosal and epithelial barriers against worms and parasites (Paul and Zhu, 2010; Maizels et al., 2012). They are induced in the presence of IL-4 and are characterized by the ability to secrete IL-4, IL-13, and IL-5 when activated. IL-4 stimulates IgG class switching to IgG4 and IgE, and together with IL-13 alternatively activates macrophages towards the M2 phenotype. IL-9 mobilizes mast cells, and IL-5 plays the same role for eosinophils. Together, IL-4, IL-13, and IL-5 increase mucus secretion, which helps eliminate pathogens such as helminths and other parasites. The related, newly identified lineage, Th9 cells, mainly produce IL-9, but do not produce IL-4 (Dardalhon et al., 2008). They emerge in situations where both IL-4 and TGF-β are present.

Th17 cells are highly relevant for the defense against extracellular bacteria, such as *Staphylococcus* or *Klebsiella*, as well as against *Candida* (Annunziato et al., 2009; Peters et al., 2011). They are induced in the presence of TGFβ, IL-6, and IL-23 and are characterized by the secretion of IL-17 when activated, which leads to increased neutrophil formation via G-CSF and GM-CSF, and to increased neutrophil recruitment via IL-8 and other chemokines (Zuniga et al., 2013). In addition, IL-17 stimulates the production of defensins and other antimicrobial substances. While Th17 cells also produce IL-22 that induces expression of defensin proteins in target cells,

TABLE 23.2 Characterization of Important Effector Cells by their Receptors and their Mediators.

Effector Cell	Important Receptors (Receptor Chains)	Important Cytokines and Mediators
Monocyte	FcγRI, IIa, IIb; CR1, 3, 4, C5aR	TNF, IL-6, IL-8, GM-CSF
Macrophage	FcγRI, IIa, IIb, RIIIa; CR1, 3, 4, C5aR	TNF, IL-6, IL-8, GM-CSF
Neutrophil	FcγRI, IIa; CR1, C3aR, C4aR, C5aR	TNF, IL-1, IL8
Mast cell	FcεR, FcγRIII; C3aR, C4aR, C5aR	Histamine, serotonin, IL-6, TNF
NK cell	NCRs; FcγRIIIa; CR3, 4; KIRs	IFNγ, TNF, GM-CSF, IL-8, granzyme B
Cytotoxic T cell	TCR; KIRs; CTLA-4	IFNγ, TNF, granzyme B, perforin
Th1	TCR; IL-12R (β1 + β2), IL-18R	IFNγ, IL-2, TNF
Th2	TCR; IL-4R (α + γc)	IL-4, IL-5, IL-9, IL-13, IL-25
Th17	TCR; IL-23 R (IL-12 Rβ1 + IL-23 R)	IL-17, GM-CSF, TGF-β, TNF

FcγRI = CD64, FcγRIIa = CD32, FcγRIIIa = CD16 activating Fcγ receptors, FcγRIIb inhibitory Fcγ receptor; CR1 (complement receptor 1) = CD35, CR2 = CD21, CR3 = CD11b + CD18, CR4 = CD11c + CD18; NCRs natural cytotoxicity receptors; KIRs killer cell immunoglobulin-like receptors; TCR T cell receptor.

there are cells that produce IL-22, but not IL-17, and are therefore termed Th22 cells (Duhen et al., 2009). This subset is particularly prevalent among skin homing cells.

After exposure, the immune system tries to completely eliminate any foreign invader; this process may become protracted. It is therefore not surprising that the T helper phenotype is largely stable. This is achieved by combining several mechanisms. First, lineage-specific transcription factors are stably expressed that drive differentiation. For Th1 cells the critical transcription factor is T-bet, for Th-2 cells it is GATA-3, and for Th17 cells RORγt.

The Th1 transcription factor T-bet is induced by Stat1 and Stat4 homodimers, activated by IFNγ and IL-12, respectively. T-bet in turn promotes IFNγ production and represses IL-4 production, among many other effects essential for the maturation of Th1 cells (Miller and Weinmann, 2010). The Th2 transcription factor GATA-3 is induced by homodimers of Stat6, the principal signaling molecule of IL-4 and IL-13. GATA-3 induces IL-4, IL-5, IL-13, and GATA-3 itself (Wei et al., 2011). RORγt is induced by homodimers of Stat3, the principal signaling molecule of IL-6, IL-21, and IL-23; at the same time T-bet and IFNγ production are inhibited, whether by (low concentrations of) TGFβ or by other means (Hirahara et al., 2010; Peters et al., 2011). RORγt in a protein complex that includes STAT3 induces the expression of IL-17 and the IL-23R.

In addition, there is a second level of control, namely epigenetic regulation, whereby chromatin accessibility is regulated, further restricting gene expression. Global DNA methylation mapping has demonstrated that the IFNγ locus is open in Th1, but not Th2 or Th17 cells; the IL-4 locus is exclusively open in Th2 cells, and the IL-17 locus is open in Th17 cells only (Wei et al., 2009). Thus epigenetic modifications are one means by which cell differentiation is kept stable during T cell expansion, or, less fortunately, in autoimmune disease or allergy.

EFFECTOR CYTOKINES AND THEIR TARGETS

Essentially all of the immune cells discussed produce significant amounts of cytokines. These are essential for shaping the immune system at any given time. However, some of these cytokines also have important effects on other tissues (Table 23.3), thereby directly contributing to tissue pathology in autoimmune disease. The importance of individual cytokines is highlighted by the success of anti-cytokine antibodies in the treatment of a number of autoimmune diseases.

TNF is a particularly well-known example in this regard. TNF is produced by many immune cells (Table 23.2), and by monocytes and macrophages in particular. Mice transgenic for, and thus overexpressing, human TNF display peripheral and sacroiliac joint pathology indistinguishable from RA and ankylosing spondylitis, respectively (Keffer et al., 1991; Redlich et al., 2004). TNF fosters the development of osteoclast precursors from monocytes and enhances osteoclast activity, which is essential in that osteoclasts are the only cells able to digest bone (Redlich et al., 2002). Conversely, pharmacological TNF blockade blocks radiographic progression in RA even when disease activity is not adequately controlled (Smolen et al., 2006). TNF also activates fibroblasts (Vasilopoulos et al., 2007) and endothelial cells and leads to vascular leakage (Bradley, 2008).

Since both TNF and IL-1 signal via NF-κB and mitogen-activated protein kinases (MAPKs), it is not surprising that IL-1 in part reduplicates and further enhances such effects, leading to pronounced inflammatory reactions (Dinarello et al., 2012). Unchecked IL-1 effects in infants lacking IL-1 receptor antagonist (IL-1RA) leads to a fatal, highly inflammatory disease with pronounced skin and bone involvement, which can be effectively treated with recombinant IL-1RA (Aksentijevich et al., 2009).

TABLE 23.3 Important Examples of Cytokines Targeting Cells Outside the Immune System.

Cytokine (Signaling Pathways)	Target Cell	Effects
TNF (NF-κB, MAPK)	Monocytes	Osteoclast formation
	Osteoclasts	Bone resorption
	Fibroblasts	Activation
IL-1 (NF-κB, MAPK)	Hypothalamic cells	Fever
	Pancreatic islet cells	Cell death, diabetes
IL-6 (Stat3)	Osteoblasts	Reduced bone formation
	Hepatocytes	CRP and hepcidin production
IL-17 (NF-κB)	Epithelial cells	Chemokine production
	Osteoblasts	RANKL expression
TGFβ (Smads, MAPK)	Fibroblasts	Extracellular matrix deposition
	Podocytes	GBM thickening

NF-κB, nuclear factor-κB; MAPK, mitogen activated protein kinase; Stat3, signal transducer and activator of transcription 3; GBM, glomerular basement membrane.

Acting systemically, IL-1 is essential for inducing fever by switching on cyclooxygenase in hypothalamic cells. Acting locally, IL-1 may also be key to the death of islet cells in diabetes (Dinarello et al., 2012).

IL-6 is the third highly inflammatory cytokine that is currently targeted in the clinic. While the full IL-6 receptor is only expressed on leukocytes and hepatocytes, all other cells are able to recruit IL-6 bound soluble IL-6 receptor to the gp130 chain they express (Rose-John et al., 2006). This process is termed trans-signaling. Although IL-6 signals via STAT3, which is distinct from TNF and IL-1 signaling, its *in vivo* effects are less obviously different (Nishimoto and Kishimoto, 2006). Nevertheless, IL-6 has many unique actions including the induction of C-reactive protein (CRP) and other acute phase reactants, the inhibition of iron uptake and use via hepcidin, and is critical for the maturation of Th17 cells. Finally IL-6 is known to influence sleep and fatigue (Rohleder et al., 2012).

IL-17 receptors are found on a variety of non-immune cells, including epithelial cells, endothelial cells, fibroblasts, and adipocytes (Pappu et al., 2011) as well as osteoblasts (Onishi and Gaffen, 2010). Signaling via NF-κB, albeit less effectively than TNF (Sonder et al., 2011), IL-17 induces epithelial cells to secrete chemokines, a process likely to be of importance in psoriasis (Onishi and Gaffen, 2010), where IL-17 blockade apparently works well (Miossec and Kolls, 2012). On osteoblasts, IL-17 is able to induce the expression of RANKL, which stimulates osteoclast differentiation (Onishi and Gaffen, 2010). IL-17 may also reduce cartilage matrix synthesis by chondrocytes (Hu et al., 2011).

TGFβ has a complex role, exerting both anti-inflammatory and profibrotic effects within the immune system. It is able to inhibit the expression of a number of other inflammatory cytokines and is known to inhibit Th1 and Th2 polarization, and, conversely, in the presence of IL-6, it is known to induce Th17 cells in both mice and humans and in the presence of IL-4 can induce Th9 cells. Furthermore it acts on fibroblasts to produce extracellular matrix, and thus tissue fibrosis in many organs (Pohlers et al., 2009). TGFβ has therefore been suggested as a therapeutic target for systemic sclerosis (Varga and Pasche, 2009). Similarly, TGFβ may stimulate podocytes to produce extracellular matrix, leading to glomerular basal membrane thickening (Lee, 2012).

CONCLUSIONS

As to be expected given the time the immune system has had to evolve in an environment where pathogens of various kinds threaten the organism, its effector mechanisms are impressive and have the potential to constrain all current and future pathogens. The adaptive immune system, in particular, has developed highly specialized cells and mechanisms for a differential response. Unfortunately, all of these cells and mechanisms can in some way damage the organism when the immune system makes the error of mistaking self for a dangerous intruder. While our understanding on the mechanisms involved has deepened, and while biological and apheresis methods have become more successful in arresting autoimmune disease while preserving immune function, effective non-toxic cures for many autoimmune diseases remain elusive. We hope that further advances in our understanding of the immune system will continue to improve the situation in years to come.

REFERENCES

Afonina, I.S., Cullen, S.P., Martin, S.J., 2010. Cytotoxic and non-cytotoxic roles of the CTL/NK protease granzyme B. Immunol. Rev. 235, 105–116.

Afonina, I.S., Tynan, G.A., Logue, S.E., Cullen, S.P., Bots, M., Luthi, A.U., et al., 2011. Granzyme B-dependent proteolysis acts as a switch to enhance the proinflammatory activity of IL-1alpha. Mol. Cell. 44, 265–278.

Aksentijevich, I., Masters, S.L., Ferguson, P.J., Dancey, P., Frenkel, J., van Royen-Kerkhoff, A., et al., 2009. An autoinflammatory disease with deficiency of the interleukin-1-receptor antagonist. N. Engl. J. Med. 360, 2426–2437.

Aletaha, D, Alasti, F., Smolen, J.S., 2013. Rheumatoid factor determines structural progression of rheumatoid arthritis dependent and independent of disease activity. Ann. Rheum. Dis. 72, 875–880.

American College of Rheumatology Ad Hoc Committee, 2004. The American College of Rheumatology response criteria for systemic lupus erythematosus clinical trials: measures of overall disease activity. Arthritis Rheum. 50, 3418–3426.

Amulic, B., Cazalet, C., Hayes, G.L., Metzler, K.D., Zychlinsky, A., 2012. Neutrophil function: from mechanisms to disease. Annu. Rev. Immunol. 30, 459–489.

Annunziato, F., Cosmi, L., Liotta, F., Maggi, E., Romagnani, S., 2009. Type 17 T helper cells-origins, features and possible roles in rheumatic disease. Nat. Rev. Rheumatol. 5, 325–331.

Aringer, M., Smolen, J.S., 2012. Therapeutic blockade of TNF in patients with SLE-promising or crazy?. Autoimmun. Rev. 11, 321–325.

Aringer, M., Gunther, C., Lee-Kirsch, M.A., 2012. Innate immune processes in lupus erythematosus. Clin. Immunol..

Bergman, M.P., D'Elios, M.M., 2010. Cytotoxic T cells in H. pylori-related gastric autoimmunity and gastric lymphoma. J. Biomed. Biotechnol. 2010, 104918.

Bradley, J.R., 2008. TNF-mediated inflammatory disease. J. Pathol. 214, 149–160.

Caudrillier, A., Kessenbrock, K., Gilliss, B.M., Nguyen, J.X., Marques, M.B., Monestier, M., et al., 2012. Platelets induce neutrophil extracellular traps in transfusion-related acute lung injury. J. Clin. Invest. 122, 2661–2671.

Cines, D.B., Blanchette, V.S., 2002. Immune thrombocytopenic purpura. N. Engl. J. Med. 346, 995–1008.

Clynes, R., Dumitru, C., Ravetch, J.V., 1998. Uncoupling of immune complex formation and kidney damage in autoimmune glomerulonephritis. Science. 279, 1052–1054.

Coppieters, K.T., von Herrath, M.G., 2011. Viruses and cytotoxic T lymphocytes in type 1 diabetes. Clin. Rev. Allergy Immunol. 41, 169–178.

Daha, N.A., Banda, N.K., Roos, A., Beurskens, F.J., Bakker, J.M., Daha, M.R., et al., 2011. Complement activation by (auto-) antibodies. Mol. Immunol. 48, 1656–1665.

Dalan, R., Leow, M.K., 2012. Immune manipulation for Graves' disease: re-exploring an unfulfilled promise with modern translational research. Eur. J. Intern. Med. 23, 682–691.

Dardalhon, V, Awasthi, A, Kwon, H., Galileos, G., Gao, W., Sobel, R. A., et al., 2008. IL-4 inhibits TGF-beta-induced Foxp3 + T cells and, together with TGF-beta, generates IL-9 + IL-10 + Foxp3(−) effector T cells. Nat. Immunol. 9, 1347–1355.

Dinarello, C.A., Simon, A., Van der Meer, J.W., 2012. Treating inflammation by blocking interleukin-1 in a broad spectrum of diseases. Nat. Rev. Drug Discov. 11, 633–652.

Duhen, T., Geiger, R., Jarrossay, D., Lanzavecchia, A., Sallusto, F., 2009. Production of interleukin 22 but not interleukin 17 by a subset of human skin-homing memory T cells. Nat. Immunol. 10, 857–863.

Fong, K.Y., Thumboo, J., 2010. Neuropsychiatric lupus: clinical challenges, brain-reactive autoantibodies and treatment strategies. Lupus. 19, 1399–1403.

Gehrs, B.C., Friedberg, R.C., 2002. Autoimmune hemolytic anemia. Am. J. Hematol. 69, 258–271.

Giannakopoulos, B., Krilis, S.A., 2013. The pathogenesis of the antiphospholipid syndrome. N. Engl. J. Med. 368, 1033–1044.

Hirahara, K., Ghoreschi, K., Laurence, A., Yang, X.P., Kanno, Y., O'Shea, J.J., 2010. Signal transduction pathways and transcriptional regulation in Th17 cell differentiation. Cytokine Growth Factor Rev. 21, 425–434.

Hoshino, A., Nagao, T., Nagi-Miura, N., Ohno, N., Yasuhara, M., Yamamoto, K., et al., 2008. MPO-ANCA induces IL-17 production by activated neutrophils in vitro via classical complement pathway-dependent manner. J. Autoimmun. 31, 79–89.

Hu, Y., Shen, F., Crellin, N.K., Ouyang, W., 2011. The IL-17 pathway as a major therapeutic target in autoimmune diseases. Ann. N.Y. Acad. Sci. 1217, 60–76.

Infante-Duarte, C., Kamradt, T., 1999. Th1/Th2 balance in infection. Springer Semin. Immunopathol. 21, 317–338.

Jarvis, J.N., Wang, W., Moore, H.T., Zhao, L., Xu, C., 1997. In vitro induction of proinflammatory cytokine secretion by juvenile rheumatoid arthritis synovial fluid immune complexes. Arthritis Rheum. 40, 2039–2046.

Jennette, J.C., Falk, R.J., Bacon, P.A., Basu, N., Cid, M.C., Ferrario, F., et al., 2013. 2012 revised International chapel hill consensus conference nomenclature of vasculitides. Arthritis Rheum. 65, 1–11.

Kaieda, S., Wang, J.X., Shnayder, R., Fishgal, N., Hei, H., Lee, R.T., et al., 2012. Interleukin-33 primes mast cells for activation by IgG immune complexes. PLoS One 7 (e47252), .

Kaplan, M.J., 2011. Neutrophils in the pathogenesis and manifestations of SLE. Nat. Rev. Rheumatol. 7, 691–699.

Karsten, C.M., Kohl, J., 2012. The immunoglobulin, IgG Fc receptor and complement triangle in autoimmune diseases. Immunobiology. 217, 1067–1079.

Keffer, J., Probert, L., Cazlaris, H., Georgopoulos, S., Kaslaris, E., Kioussis, D., et al., 1991. Transgenic mice expressing human tumour necrosis factor: a predictive genetic model of arthritis. EMBO J. 10, 4025–4031.

Kessenbrock, K., Krumholz, M., Schonermarck, U., Back, W., Gross, W.L., Werb, Z., et al., 2009. Netting neutrophils in autoimmune small-vessel vasculitis. Nat. Med. 15, 623–625.

Kiener, H.P., Baghestanian, M., Dominkus, M., Walchshofer, S., Ghannadan, M., Willheim, M., et al., 1998. Expression of the C5a receptor (CD88) on synovial mast cells in patients with rheumatoid arthritis. Arthritis Rheum. 41, 233–245.

Lee, D.M., Friend, D.S., Gurish, M.F., Benoist, C., Mathis, D., Brenner, M.B., 2002. Mast cells: a cellular link between autoantibodies and inflammatory arthritis. Science. 297, 1689–1692.

Lee, H.S., 2012. Mechanisms and consequences of TGF-ss overexpression by podocytes in progressive podocyte disease. Cell Tissue Res. 347, 129–140.

Levinson, A.I., 2013. Modeling the intrathymic pathogenesis of myasthenia gravis. J. Neurol. Sci. 333, 60–67.

Maizels, R.M., Hewitson, J.P., Smith, K.A., 2012. Susceptibility and immunity to helminth parasites. Curr. Opin. Immunol. 24, 459–466.

Melzer, N., Meuth, S.G., Wiendl, H., 2009. CD8 + T cells and neuronal damage: direct and collateral mechanisms of cytotoxicity and impaired electrical excitability. FASEB J. 23, 3659–3673.

Miller, S.A., Weinmann, A.S., 2010. Molecular mechanisms by which T-bet regulates T-helper cell commitment. Immunol. Rev. 238, 233–246.

Miossec, P., Kolls, J.K., 2012. Targeting IL-17 and TH17 cells in chronic inflammation. Nat. Rev. Drug Discov. 11, 763–776.

Mjelle, J.E., Rekvig, O.P., van der Vlag, J., Fenton, K.A., 2011. Nephritogenic antibodies bind in glomeruli through interaction with exposed chromatin fragments and not with renal cross-reactive antigens. Autoimmunity. 44, 373–383.

Nemeth, T., Mocsai, A., 2012. The role of neutrophils in autoimmune diseases. Immunol. Lett. 143, 9–19.

Nimmerjahn, F., Ravetch, J.V., 2010. Antibody-mediated modulation of immune responses. Immunol. Rev. 236, 265–275.

Nishimoto, N., Kishimoto, T., 2006. Interleukin 6: from bench to bedside. Nat. Clin. Pract. Rheumatol. 2, 619–626.

Olmez, U., Garred, P., Mollnes, T.E., Harboe, M., Berntzen, H.B., Munthe, E., 1991. C3 activation products, C3 containing immune complexes, the terminal complement complex and native C9 in patients with rheumatoid arthritis. Scand. J. Rheumatol. 20, 183–189.

Ombrello, M.J., Kastner, D.L., 2011. Autoinflammation in 2010: expanding clinical spectrum and broadening therapeutic horizons. Nat. Rev. Rheumatol. 7, 82–84.

Onishi, R.M., Gaffen, S.L., 2010. Interleukin-17 and its target genes: mechanisms of interleukin-17 function in disease. Immunology. 129, 311–321.

Papadopoulos, M.C., Verkman, A.S., 2012. Aquaporin 4 and neuromyelitis optica. Lancet Neurol. 11, 535–544.

Pappu, R., Ramirez-Carrozzi, V., Sambandam, A., 2011. The interleukin-17 cytokine family: critical players in host defence and inflammatory diseases. Immunology. 134, 8–16.

Parham, P., Moffett, A., 2013. Variable NK cell receptors and their MHC class I ligands in immunity, reproduction and human evolution. Nat. Rev. Immunol. 13, 133–144.

Paul, W.E., Zhu, J., 2010. How are T(H)2-type immune responses initiated and amplified? Nat. Rev. Immunol. 10, 225–235.

Peters, A., Lee, Y., Kuchroo, V.K., 2011. The many faces of Th17 cells. Curr. Opin. Immunol. 23, 702–706.

Pisetsky, D.S., 2012. Microparticles as autoantigens: making immune complexes big. Arthritis Rheum. 64, 958–961.

Pohlers, D., Brenmoehl, J., Loffler, I., Muller, C.K., Leipner, C., Schultze-Mosgau, S., et al., 2009. TGF-beta and fibrosis in different organs—molecular pathway imprints. Biochim. Biophys. Acta. 1792, 746–756.

Rajan, T.V., 2003. The Gell–Coombs classification of hypersensitivity reactions: a re-interpretation. Trends Immunol. 24, 376–379.

Redlich, K., Hayer, S., Ricci, R., David, J.P., Tohidast-Akrad, M., Kollias, G., et al., 2002. Osteoclasts are essential for TNF-alpha-mediated joint destruction. J. Clin. Invest. 110, 1419–1427.

Redlich, K., Görtz, B., Hayer, S., Zwerina, J., Kollias, G., Steiner, G., et al., 2004. Overexpression of TNF causes bilateral sacroiliitis. Arthritis Rheum. 50, 1001–1005.

Reiner, S.L., 2007. Development in motion: helper T cells at work. Cell. 129, 33–36.

Rohleder, N., Aringer, M., Boentert, M., 2012. Role of interleukin-6 in stress, sleep, and fatigue. Ann. N.Y. Acad. Sci. 1261, 88–96.

Rose-John, S., Scheller, J., Elson, G., Jones, S.A., 2006. Interleukin-6 biology is coordinated by membrane-bound and soluble receptors: role in inflammation and cancer. J. Leukoc. Biol. 80, 227–236.

Schreiber, A., Xiao, H., Jennette, J.C., Schneider, W., Luft, F.C., Kettritz, R., 2009. C5a receptor mediates neutrophil activation and ANCA-induced glomerulonephritis. J. Am. Soc. Nephrol. 20, 289–298.

Schuerwegh, A.J., Ioan-Facsinay, A., Dorjee, A.L., Roos, J., Bajema, I.M., van der Voort, E.I., et al., 2010. Evidence for a functional role of IgE anticitrullinated protein antibodies in rheumatoid arthritis. Proc. Natl. Acad. Sci. U.S.A. 107, 2586–2591.

Sgonc, R., Gruschwitz, M.S., Dietrich, H., Recheis, H., Gershwin, M.E., Wick, G., 1996. Endothelial cell apoptosis is a primary pathogenetic event underlying skin lesions in avian and human scleroderma. J. Clin. Invest. 98, 785–792.

Sigal, L.J., Crotty, S., Andino, R., Rock, K.L., 1999. Cytotoxic T-cell immunity to virus-infected non-haematopoietic cells requires presentation of exogenous antigen. Nature. 398, 77–80.

Smolen, J.S., van der Heijde St, D.M., Clair, E.W., Emery, P., Bathon, J.M., Keystone, E., et al., 2006. Predictors of joint damage in patients with early rheumatoid arthritis treated with high-dose methotrexate with or without concomitant infliximab: results from the ASPIRE trial. Arthritis Rheum. 54, 702–710.

Sonder, S.U., Saret, S., Tang, W., Sturdevant, D.E., Porcella, S.F., Siebenlist, U., 2011. IL-17-induced NF-kappaB activation via CIKS/Act1: physiologic significance and signaling mechanisms. J. Biol. Chem. 286, 12881–12890.

Sontheimer, R.D., 2005. Subacute cutaneous lupus erythematosus: 25-year evolution of a prototypic subset (subphenotype) of lupus erythematosus defined by characteristic cutaneous, pathological, immunological, and genetic findings. Autoimmun. Rev. 4, 253–263.

Stanley, J.R., Amagai, M., 2006. Pemphigus, bullous impetigo, and the staphylococcal scalded-skin syndrome. N. Engl. J. Med. 355, 1800–1810.

Tan, E.M., 1991. Autoantibodies in pathology and cell biology. Cell. 67, 841–842.

Tato, C.M., O'Shea, J.J., 2006. Immunology: what does it mean to be just 17? Nature. 441, 166–168.

Varga, J., Pasche, B., 2009. Transforming growth factor beta as a therapeutic target in systemic sclerosis. Nat. Rev. Rheumatol. 5, 200–206.

Vasilopoulos, Y., Gkretsi, V., Armaka, M., Aidinis, V., Kollias, G., 2007. Actin cytoskeleton dynamics linked to synovial fibroblast activation as a novel pathogenic principle in TNF-driven arthritis. Ann. Rheum. Dis. 66 (Suppl. 3), iii23–iii28.

Walport, M.J., 2001. Complement. First of two parts. N. Engl. J. Med. 344, 1058–1066.

Wei, G., Wei, L., Zhu, J., Zang, C., Hu-Li, J., Yao, Z., et al., 2009. Global mapping of H3K4me3 and H3K27me3 reveals specificity and plasticity in lineage fate determination of differentiating CD4 + T cells. Immunity. 30, 155–167.

Wei, G., Abraham, B.J., Yagi, R., Jothi, R., Cui, K., Sharma, S., et al., 2011. Genome-wide analyses of transcription factor GATA3-mediated gene regulation in distinct T cell types. Immunity. 35, 299–311.

Wesolowski, J., Paumet, F., 2011. The impact of bacterial infection on mast cell degranulation. Immunol. Res. 51, 215–226.

Yamashina, M., Ueda, E., Kinoshita, T., Takami, T., Ojima, A., Ono, H., et al., 1990. Inherited complete deficiency of 20-kilodalton homologous restriction factor (CD59) as a cause of paroxysmal nocturnal hemoglobinuria. N. Engl. J. Med. 323, 1184–1189.

Yung, S., Chan, T.M., 2008. Anti-DNA antibodies in the pathogenesis of lupus nephritis—the emerging mechanisms. Autoimmun. Rev. 7, 317–321.

Zeitler, H., Goldmann, G., Marquardt, N., Ulrich-Merzenich, G., 2013. Long term outcome of patients with acquired hemophilia—a monocenter interim analysis of 82 patients. Atheroscler.(Suppl. 13), 223–228.

Zuniga, L.A., Jain, R., Haines, C., Cua, D.J., 2013. Th17 cell development: from the cradle to the grave. Immunol. Rev. 252, 78–88.

Chapter 24

Sexual Dimorphism in the Immune System

Pamela A. McCombe and Judith M. Greer

The University of Queensland, UQ Centre for Clinical Research, Royal Brisbane and Women's Hospital, Brisbane, Queensland, Australia

Chapter Outline

Introduction   319
Overview of Sexual Dimorphism   319
Sexual Dimorphism in the Immune System   319
Effects of Hormones on the Immune System   321
  Estrogens   321
  Progesterone   322
  Androgens   322
Role of the Sex Chromosomes in Immunity   323

X Chromosome   323
Y Chromosome   323
Environmental Effects on Sex Differences in Immunity   324
Consequences for Autoimmunity of Sexual Dimorphism in the Immune System   324
Concluding Remarks   325
References   325

INTRODUCTION

Sexual dimorphism is the term that refers to differences between males and females of the same species, and is most obvious as differences in external appearances. However, there can also be sexual dimorphism of internal organs and biological functions, including the immune system. Sexual dimorphism in the immune system is important in medicine because it can lead to sex differences in the responses to infection and vaccination and sex differences in the development of autoimmune disease (McCombe et al., 2009). This chapter focuses on the effects of sexual dimorphism on immunocompetence, and on some of the possible mechanisms underlying these effects, including the effects of the sex hormones, sex chromosomes, and sexually-dimorphic cultural and environmental effects on immunity. The possible consequences for autoimmunity of sexual dimorphism in the immune system are also considered.

OVERVIEW OF SEXUAL DIMORPHISM

The sex chromosomes evolved many millions of years ago (Livernois et al., 2012). In humans, most males have X and Y chromosomes and most females have two X chromosomes. In humans, other combinations of sex chromosomes are found, with the most common being a single X chromosome (Turner's syndrome) or XXY (Klinefelter's syndrome). Sexual dimorphism was noted by Darwin (Darwin, 1871) who thought it was due to sexual selection, as, for example, larger, stronger males might have a reproductive advantage. Other possibilities for the evolution of sexual dimorphism include intersexual competition for food (Hedrick and Temeles, 1989). Overall, in humans, males are larger than females, with greater strength, but shorter life expectancy. In medicine, there are sex differences in the prevalence of many diseases, and there can be sex differences in the response to medications.

Sexual dimorphism is related to the sex chromosome complement of an individual (Wijchers and Festenstein, 2011). Many genes show sex-specific differences in expression (Ellegren and Parsch, 2007; Mank, 2009). Sex differences in the immune system are discussed below.

SEXUAL DIMORPHISM IN THE IMMUNE SYSTEM

Immunocompetence is a word used to describe the overall level of function of the immune system, and is a complex

N. Rose & I. Mackay (Eds): The Autoimmune Diseases, Fifth edition. DOI: http://dx.doi.org/10.1016/B978-0-12-384929-8.00024-1

genetic trait (Flori et al., 2011). It has been recognized that females have increased immunoreactivity (immuno-competence) compared to males and it is suggested that this leads to increased autoimmune disease in females (Zandman-Goddard et al., 2007). In the past it has been suggested that the expression of male sexual traits is inversely related to immunocompetence (the immuno-competence handicap hypothesis) (Folstad, and Karter 1992). However, further studies have not confirmed this (Roberts et al., 2004) and others have suggested that the differences in overall immunocompetence between males and females are related to the pressures of selection on the basis of fitness. It is thought that fitness in females is maximized by lengthening the lifespan through greater investment in immune defenses; in contrast, males require fitness early in life to maximize sexual mating, and so do not need to invest in immune defenses to prolong the life-span (Nunn et al., 2009). There are also differences between males and females in immunosenescence, which is the decline in immune function in later life, with greater decline in males (Das et al., 2008; Yan et al., 2010) (Table 24.1).

Overall immunocompetence is the sum of the ele-ments of the immune system. There is sexual dimorphism of many of the components of the immune system. In terms of cell counts, there are numerical differences between the males and females. In males the total lym-phocyte count is similar to that in females (Giltay et al., 2000; Bouman et al., 2004), but the percentage of T cells within the lymphocyte population is lower (Bouman et al., 2004). The ratio of CD4$^+$:CD8$^+$ T cells is greater in females than in males (Das et al., 2008; Wikby et al., 2008). There are no reports of differences in B cell counts between females and males; however, there are long-recognized differences in levels of IgM but not in other immunoglobulin isotypes, with females showing increased levels for all ages >6 years (Butterworth et al., 1967; Lichtman et al., 1967).

The reproductive phase of females also influences the immune system, as post-menopausal women, compared to fertile women, have fewer total lymphocytes (as a conse-quence of decreased numbers of B and helper T cells (Th cells)) (Giglio et al., 1994; Yang et al., 2000). During the reproductive years, there is an increase in the suppressive activity of CD4$^+$CD25$^+$Foxp3$^+$ regulatory T cells (Tregs) during the late follicular and luteal phase of each menstrual cycle, whereas after menopause there is a drop in the per-cell activity of Tregs (Trzonkowski et al., 2001; Prieto and Rosenstein, 2006; Arruvito et al., 2007). The greatest expansion in numbers and per-cell activity of Tregs occurs during pregnancy, both in humans and experimental animals (Aluvihare et al., 2004; Somerset et al., 2004), presumably in order to tolerate the allogenic fetal tissues.

In laboratory animals, there are also sex differences in the structure of primary immune organs: in male rats the thymus is heavier, has a greater yield of cells, and contains a higher percentage of double negative CD4$^-$ CD8$^-$ cells (Leposavic et al., 1996) and catecholamine-containing cells (Pilipovic et al., 2008) than thymi of female rats. However, in humans, in autopsy studies, no difference was found between the weight of adult thymi from females or males, after correction for body weight (Narongchai and Narongchai, 2008). The differ-ences are possibly more clear-cut in inbred laboratory animals.

TABLE 24.1 Summary of Sexual Dimorphism of Immune Functions

Immune Functions that Show Sexual Dimorphism	Difference Between Males and Females
Percentage of lymphocytes in total leukocyte population	Lower in males (Bouman et al., 2004)
Immunosenescence	Greater in males
IgM levels	Greater in females (Butterworth et al., 1967; Lichtman et al., 1967).
Allograft rejection	Greater in females (Kongshavn and Bliss, 1970)
In vitro response to mitogens	Greater in females (Santoli et al., 1976; Weinstein et al., 1984)
Resistance to the induction of immune tolerance	Greater in females (Bebo et al., 1999)
Ability to combat infection	Greater in females (Dos Santos et al., 2005; Lotter et al., 2006).
Response to vaccination	Greater in women (Klein et al., 2010)
CD4:CD8 ratio	Greater in women (Das et al., 2008; Wikby et al., 2008)
Th1 responses	Greater in females (Huygen and Palfliet, 1984).
Treg number and per-cell activity	Increased in females during reproductive years

There are differences in the function of the immune system of males and females. Generally, females produce more vigorous humoral and cellular immune responses than males (Weinstein et al., 1984; Ansar et al., 1985), shown in female mice by an augmented response to a variety of antigens (Terres et al., 1968), the ability to reject allografts more rapidly than males (Kongshavn and Bliss, 1970), and in female mice and humans by better *in vitro* responses to mitogens (Santoli et al., 1976; Weinstein et al., 1984) and relative resistance to the induction of immune tolerance (Bebo et al., 1999). Following trauma-hemorrhage, immune function is severely depressed in young male mice and ovariectomized and aged females, but is maintained in proestrus females (Kahlke et al., 2000; Choudhry et al., 2007). The survival rate in proestrus females following trauma-hemorrhage and the induction of subsequent sepsis is significantly higher than in age-matched males and ovariectomized females.

Furthermore, females are more successful than males in resisting a variety of bacterial, viral, and parasitic infestations and this enhanced immune capability might explain, in part at least, why the life expectancy of females exceeds that of males. For example, female mice have a greater ability than male mice to combat various infections, including leishmaniasis and amebic infection with liver abscess (Lotter et al., 2006), which is thought to be due to sex differences in Th1 and Th2 responses (Mock and Nacy, 1988). Moreover, in Wistar rats infected with *Trypanosoma cruzi*, there is less parasitemia in females than males (dos Santos et al., 2005). Of relevance to autoimmunity, there are gender differences in resistance to inflammation of the heart after coxsackievirus infection, which are inferior in males and related to poorer Treg responses in males than females (Frisancho-Kiss et al., 2007). In immunized mice, females show greater production of the Th1 cytokine interferon (IFN)-γ than males (Huygen and Palfliet, 1984). These differences in Th1 and Th2 response are mediated in part through IL-13 (Sinha et al., 2008).

In humans, the antibody response to a variety of vaccines and test antigens, including flagellin protein (Rowley and Mackay, 1969), influenza, hepatitis B, rubella and tetanus (Cook, 2008) and a variety of other viral vaccines (Klein et al., 2010), is more vigorous in females than in males. In women, the innate immune response is also stronger.

Another, less quantifiable, functional difference between females and males is seen in the immune response to injury, according to reports on greater degrees of immunosuppression in men than in women after physical trauma (Choudhry et al., 2005) and after abdominal surgery (Wichmann et al., 2003), as measured by B lymphocyte, T lymphocyte, T helper cell counts, and natural killer (NK) cell counts and circulating levels of IL-6.

There are many examples of sex differences in biochemical pathways involved in immunity. Sexual dimorphism is also expressed at a cellular level, since stimulation of invariant NKT (iNKT) cells with α-galactosylceramide leads to higher concentrations of interferon gamma in the serum of female mice (Gourdy et al., 2005) and the concentration of serotonin and histamine in white blood cells and mast cells is greater in female than in male rats (Csaba et al., 2003) (see Table 24.1).

EFFECTS OF HORMONES ON THE IMMUNE SYSTEM

Sexual dimorphism in the immune system could be due to the effects of sex and reproductive hormones. These hormones have cognate receptors that are widely expressed on many cell types, including cells of the immune system. There is evidence that sexual dimorphism in immune functions in C57Bl/6 mice are dependent on puberty, which suggests that the effects of the sex hormones are important (Lamason et al., 2006). There are numerous effects of the sex hormones in human immunity (Bouman et al., 2005). The effects of the various sex hormones on immune function are summarized below.

Estrogens

There are three estrogenic hormones, estrogen (E1), estradiol (E2), and estriol (E3), with E3 being produced only in pregnancy. As well as being present at high levels in females, estrogens are also present in males, in whom they have widespread effects (Sharpe, 1998). Estrogens act on intracellular estrogen receptors (ER). The best-known ERs (ERα and ERβ) belong to the class known as ligand regulated nuclear transcription factors (Matthews and Gustafsson, 2003). There is also a membrane bound G-protein coupled estrogen receptor (Prossnitz et al., 2007), which is prominent on vascular tissue and has rapid "non-genomic" effects (Simoncini et al., 2004). ER are widespread, and have important effects on the growth of cells. ERα and ERβ are expressed on antigen presenting cells (APCs) (Nalbandian and Kovats, 2005), and at higher levels in CD4$^+$ T cells and B cells than in CD8$^+$ T cells; however, whereas B cells express higher levels of ERβ than ERα, CD4$^+$ T cells show higher levels of ERα than ERβ (Pernis, 2007).

The results of many experiments indicate that estrogen can affect immune function: for example, T lymphocytes from patients with SLE, but not from healthy controls, can be activated via ERα and ERβ to increase expression of the T cell activation markers CD154 and calcineurin (Rider et al., 2006). Furthermore, different types of estrogens can have differential effects (Ding and Zhu, 2008). Estrogen induces thymic atrophy by preventing proliferation of early thymic progenitor cells (Zoller and Kersh, 2006), and this is due in part to the effects of estrogen on the membrane bound estrogen receptor (Wang et al., 2008). Estrogen has effects on dendritic cells (DCs) (Ding and Zhu, 2008), modulates the effects of lipopolysaccharide (LPS) on monocytes (Pioli et al., 2007), and inhibits monocyte adhesion to endothelium (Nilsson, 2007). Such results, however, may not relate to the role of estrogens at physiologic levels. Much of what has been observed *in vitro* is likely to be what occurs in high estrogen states, such as pregnancy, rather than in non-pregnant women.

Estrogen has numerous effects on the function of $CD4^+$ T cells (Pernis, 2007). Low doses of estrogen, as would occur in non-pregnant women, enhance Th1 responses whereas high levels, as would occur in pregnancy, enhance Th2 responses. Estrogen also influences chemokine production by activated splenocytes (Lengi et al., 2007) and influences T cell trafficking. E2 can convert $CD25^-$ cells to $CD25^+$ Treg cells (Tai et al., 2008). Thus enhancement of Th2 responses and induction of Treg cells by high doses of estrogens could ameliorate Th1-mediated autoimmune diseases. It is thought that the drop in Treg activity around the time of menopause is related to estrogen-mediated changes in levels of IL-6 (Rachon et al., 2002). Estrogen enhances antibody production in response to antigen immunization (da Silva, 1999). This effect differs between E3 and E2 (Ding and Zhu, 2008), with E3 strongly stimulating antibody response to bacteria (da Silva, 1999).

There is some evidence that estrogens are more directly involved in autoimmunity. Thus, in patients with myasthenia gravis, there is alteration of expression of ER in the thymus (Nancy and Berrih-Aknin, 2005), a site wherein the disease may be generated (Hill et al., 2008). In SLE, estrogen promotes the survival of B cells with affinity for DNA (as does prolactin) (Grimaldi, 2006). Genetic studies among Japanese show that there are associations with polymorphisms in the ER in rheumatoid arthritis (Takagi et al., 2000), although not in autoimmune diabetes (Ban et al., 2000). In females with multiple sclerosis (MS) who carry HLA-DR2, carriage of an $ER\alpha4$ polymorphism conveys the additional risk of developing disease (Mattila et al., 2001).

Progesterone

Progesterone is a steroid hormone that is present in the blood during the menstrual cycle and in high levels in pregnancy. Adult males have levels similar to those in women during the follicular phase of the menstrual cycle. In women, progesterone is produced in the ovary as well as the placenta during pregnancy. In males, progesterone is produced by the adrenal gland and testes. The action of progesterone is mediated through cytosolic progesterone

receptors, of which there are three isoforms, belonging to the nuclear hormone receptor superfamily of transcription factors. The different isoforms are widely distributed and have specific tissue expression patterns that can be modified following exposure to hormones. Ligand binding induces changes in gene expression through direct binding to promoter elements or through protein—protein interactions with other transcription factors (Tait et al., 2008). In some cells, including T cells (Dosiou et al., 2008), progesterone may also act via membrane G-coupled protein receptors that rapidly transduce hormone-induced signals across the cell membrane (Boonyaratanakornkit et al., 2008). Since these additional phenomena do not depend on the genome, these actions are called nongenomic or extranuclear effects (Wehling and Losel, 2006).

Progesterone has immunomodulatory effects (Tait et al., 2008) which are generally anti-inflammatory, including inhibition of glucocorticoid-mediated thymocyte apoptosis (McMurray et al., 2000), reduction of nitric oxide production (Miller et al., 1996), and expression of Toll-like receptors (TLR) (Jones et al., 2008) by macrophages. Progesterone promotes Th2 differentiation *in vitro* (Piccinni et al., 1995) and also influences antibody production, especially production of antibodies that are asymmetrically glycosylated in such a way that they fail to trigger immune effector mechanisms. Such antibodies are thought to be self-protective (Canellada et al., 2002). High doses of progesterone enhance differentiation of human and mouse DCs *in vitro* and expression of the costimulatory molecules CD80, CD86, and CD40, as well as major histocompatibility complex (MHC) II (Ivanova et al., 2005; Liang et al., 2006).

Androgens

Androgens, the best known of which is testosterone, stimulate or control the development and maintenance of masculine characteristics; however, they have other functions, including maintenance of bone mass in both women and men. Androgens are also the precursors of all estrogens. In males, androgens, primarily testosterone, are present at high levels, but these decline with increasing age (Mitchell et al., 1995). In contrast, in females, lower levels of androgens (particularly the adrenal-derived androgens DHEA and DHEA-S) persist throughout life (Davison et al., 2005). The best-known androgen receptors are nuclear receptors, but non-genomic signaling also occurs (Lutz et al., 2003).

The potent and rapidly occurring immunosuppressive effects of testosterone in mice occur at least in part by induction of thymic atrophy, and cessation of testosterone production by castration of males results in thymic hypertrophy; these effects occur via interaction of sex hormones with receptors on thymic stromal cells (Hince et al., 2008). Testosterone also impairs thymocyte proliferation in response to the mitogen Con A (Yao and Shang, 2005). In men treated with medical castration, there is a reduction in levels of $CD4^+CD25^+$ Tregs and in IFN-γ production following mitogen-induced activation of $CD8^+$ T cells (Page et al., 2006). Intriguingly, recent studies using non-obese diabetic (NOD) mice suggest that changing the gut microbial environment can change testosterone levels in these mice, thereby modifying progression to autoimmunity (Markle et al., 2013).

ROLE OF THE SEX CHROMOSOMES IN IMMUNITY

The differences between males and females are due to differences in sex chromosomes. People with a Y chromosome show masculinization, due largely to the effects of the testis forming gene, *Sry*, on the Y chromosome, and the effects of high levels of testosterone. However, the *Sry* gene also has effects other than testis formation, such as controlling concentrations of dopamine (which may explain why there is a higher incidence of dopamine-related disorders such as Parkinson's disease in males) (Wijchers et al., 2010) and other genes on the sex chromosomes play a role in sexual dimorphism, largely through epigenetic effects. Some of the effects of sex chromosomes in immunity are examined below.

X Chromosome

The increased prevalence of autoimmunity in females has generated considerable interest in the X chromosome in immunity, particularly since there was shown to be a direct influence of the overall complement of X chromosomes to the female bias toward autoimmune disease (Smith-Bouvier et al., 2008). Typically, the X chromosome in men is active, whereas women have one active and one inactive copy of each X chromosome, although some genes on the "inactive" chromosome can escape inactivation through the action of epigenetic modifiers. Consequently, females exposed to these modifying agents can have elevated levels of expression of some molecules encoded on the X chromosome. For example, exposure of $CD4^+$ T cells to the drug 5-azacytidine leads to elevated levels of CD40 ligand (CD154—which is encoded on the X chromosome) on T cells from females but not males (Lu et al., 2007). There are observations of elevated levels of CD154 in a multitude of autoimmune disorders, including SLE, autoimmune thyroid disease, type 1 diabetes, inflammatory bowel disease, psoriasis, MS, and rheumatoid arthritis (Toubi and Shoenfeld, 2004).

Other genes on the X chromosome are also of potential relevance for autoimmunity, including those encoding

the IL-2 Rγ chain (also known as the common γ chain because it is shared by receptors for IL-2, IL-7, IL-15, and IL-21) (Alves et al., 2007), and Foxp3, which is important in the development and function of Tregs (Zheng and Rudensky, 2007). Mutations of these genes lead to X-linked severe combined immune deficiency (SCID) (Leonard et al., 1994) and IPEX (immune dysregulation, polyendocrinopathy, enteropathy, X-linked) syndrome (Bennett et al., 2001), respectively. Additional molecules encoded by genes on the X chromosome that might be important for autoimmunity are: tissue inhibitors of metalloproteinases (TIMPs) 1–4, which are important in inflammation (Anderson and Brown, 2002); the X-linked inhibitor of apoptosis that regulates T cell function (Zehntner et al., 2007); and the pattern recognition receptors TLR 7 and TLR8, both of which are important in the recognition of single-stranded RNA and which have also been associated with asthma and other inflammatory diseases (Fish, 2008; Moller-Larsen et al., 2008). There are also many X-linked genes encoding possible target antigens of autoimmune disease: changes in dosage of these autoantigens could also provide an initiating event for the development of autoimmunity.

Women with Turner's syndrome have one normal X chromosome, but the other X is either missing or structurally altered; these women also have an increased incidence of autoimmune disease overall, and especially thyroid autoimmunity (Wilson et al., 1996). Interestingly, the thyroid disease is associated with the presence of an X isochromosome, in which the short distal arm of one X chromosome (X_p) is deleted and replaced with a copy of the long distal arm (X_q) from the sister chromosome. This suggests that a gene on X_q may play an important pathogenetic role in the development of autoimmune thyroid disease (Elsheikh et al., 2001), or alternatively that genetic elements on X_p help protect against disease.

Males who have SLE in addition to Klinefelter's syndrome (wherein they have at least two X chromosomes and at least one Y chromosome) share many characteristics of the female with SLE (Lahita, 1999), including increased oxidation of androgens, suggesting that there is some role for the two X chromosomes in this process, although exactly what this role is is not yet known.

Y Chromosome

The Y chromosome contains few genes. Most of the DNA is male specific and the remainder is autosomal. The Y chromosome encodes at least 27 proteins, some of which are confined to testis and some of which are more widely expressed (Skaletsky et al., 2003). The most important Y chromosome gene is *Sry*, which is the gene responsible for the formation of testes and masculine features.

There is some effect of Y chromosome genes on the development of experimental autoimmune encephalomyelitis (EAE), the animal model of MS, since female offspring of backcross strains carrying the susceptible SJL/J Y chromosome behaved more like their male siblings than like the female mice from three other birth crosses carrying the resistant C57BL/6 Y chromosome, both in lesion severity (reduced) and clinical sensitivity to central nervous system (CNS) damage (increased) (Teuscher et al., 2006). With increased age, male SJL/J mice show increased susceptibility to EAE, and this has been shown to be due to a polymorphism on the Y chromosome (Spach et al., 2009). Y chromosome candidate genes potentially responsible for these effects in mice include *Hya*, *Yaa*, and *Sry* (Teuscher et al., 2006).

Interestingly, *Yaa*, which predisposes to autoimmunity in mice, is actually a translocation of a cluster of X chromosome genes, including the gene encoding TLR7 (Subramanian et al., 2006). It has been demonstrated that even relatively modest increases in the expression of TLR7 can result in dramatic lymphocyte activation and autoimmunity in mice (Deane et al., 2007). It has been suggested that a similar effect in humans could dictate susceptibility to SLE. However, a study of 190 male and female SLE patients and controls found no lupus-related difference in copy number of the *TLR7* gene, suggesting that human lupus is not commonly due to a *Yaa*-like mutation (Kelley et al., 2007).

ENVIRONMENTAL EFFECTS ON SEX DIFFERENCES IN IMMUNITY

As with many issues in biology, there can be an interaction between genes and the environment. The sex differences noted above are what are observed in humans living in natural conditions, and it is possible that there is plasticity in the immune responses in response to the environment. It is theorized that the sex differences are a result of the pressures of the environment (availability of food, availability of sexual partners), and that the males and females differ in traits that limit their fitness so the response to the environment will differ. It is possible that alteration of the environment could alter the sexual dimorphism in the immune system. In experiments with *Drosophila*, increased availability of food led to increased female immune function, and increased availability of mates led to decreased male immune function (McKean and Nunney, 2005). It is possible that gender differences in human immune function could be affected by environmental and social factors. For example, caloric restriction in humans has anti-inflammatory effects (Morgan et al., 2007).

Some environmental effects on sex differences in immunity may relate to differences in the likelihood of exposure of males and females to those effects. For example, recent evidence has implicated UV-induced vitamin D in immune function and protection from development of autoimmunity. Generally, males have more sun exposure and use less sun protection than females, which could help to explain some of the sexual dimorphism in susceptibility to many autoimmune diseases. Similarly, it has been suggested that chemicals in cosmetics act as a trigger for primary biliary cirrhosis (Rieger et al., 2006), which has an overwhelming female predominance.

CONSEQUENCES FOR AUTOIMMUNITY OF SEXUAL DIMORPHISM IN THE IMMUNE SYSTEM

There is a marked sexual dimorphism in the incidence of many autoimmune diseases, ranging from those with a

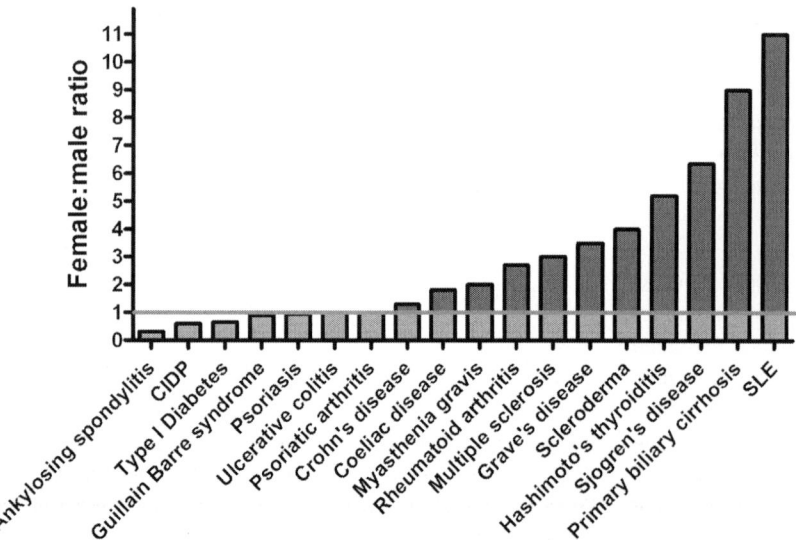

FIGURE 24.1 **Some Human Autoimmune Diseases have a Strong Female Preponderance.** The ratio of females to males for a variety of autoimmune diseases is shown. The green line represents a 1:1 ratio. A pink colored top to the bar indicates that the disease is more common in females than in males. CIDP—chronic inflammatory demyelinating polyradiculoneuropathy. SLE—systemic lupus erythematosus.

strong female preponderance (e.g., SLE and primary biliary cirrhosis) to those that show a modest increase in females (e.g., MS and rheumatoid arthritis) to those that are actually male dominated, such as type 1 diabetes, some types of vasculitis and ankylosing spondylitis (Figure 24.1). It is likely that the overall increase in autoimmune disease in females is due, at least in part, to the stronger female immune system. When autoimmune disease occurs in males, this could mean that these individuals have immune systems that are particularly vulnerable to disease. This theory, which is known as the Carter effect (Carter, 1969), is applicable to polygenic disorders and suggests that if a subject has an innate biological resistance to a particular disease then there will be a greater burden of genetic risk factors required to overcome that resistance for disease to occur. Thus, for a male to develop a true autoimmune disorder would require a much heavier load of other contributing elements, be they genetic or environmental: males who do present with diseases such as autoimmune thyroid disorder, primary biliary cirrhosis, or lupus may warrant particular scrutiny, as non-sex-related causal elements might be more readily identifiable.

There may also be other gender-specific differences that indirectly affect immune reactivity and contribute to skewing of susceptibility to autoimmune disease in females (McCombe et al., 2009; Greer and McCombe, 2011, 2012; Borchers and Gershwin, 2012; Nussinovitch and Shoenfeld, 2012; Pan and Chang, 2012; Pollard, 2012; Quintero et al., 2012). These differences could include: sexual dimorphism in the vulnerability of the target organ to autoimmune attack; epigenetic effects of the sex hormones or gender-specific environmental or lifestyle exposures on genetic risk factors; differences in genomic imprinting in males and females; and effects related to female reproduction. The future challenge is to determine which of these differences between males and females is most important in the development of autoimmunity, since understanding the influences of sexual dimorphism in autoimmune diseases is likely to provide opportunities for better therapies.

CONCLUDING REMARKS

Sexual dimorphism in the immune system affects the relative immunocompetence of males and females. While the greater immunocompetence of females, as a result of hormonal and X-linked effects, leads to an enhanced ability to fight infection and a lengthening of lifespan, it also increases the risk to females of developing autoimmune disease. Improving our understanding of the underlying causes of sexual dimorphism in the immune system will ultimately improve the potential to successfully treat autoimmune disease.

REFERENCES

Aluvihare, V.R., Kallikourdis, M., Betz, A.G., 2004. Regulatory T cells mediate maternal tolerance to the fetus. Nat. Immunol. 5, 266–271.

Alves, N.L., Arosa, F.A., Van Lier, R.A., 2007. Common gamma chain cytokines: dissidence in the details. Immunol. Lett. 108, 113–120.

Anderson, C.L., Brown, C.J., 2002. Variability of X chromosome inactivation: effect on levels of TIMP1 RNA and role of DNA methylation. Hum. Genet. 110, 271–278.

Ansar, A.S., Penhale, W.J., Talal, N., 1985. Sex hormones, immune responses, and autoimmune diseases. Mechanisms of sex hormone action. Am. J. Pathol. 121, 531–551.

Arruvito, L., Sanz, M., Banham, A.H., Fainboim, L., 2007. Expansion of CD4 + CD25 + and FOXP3 + regulatory T cells during the follicular phase of the menstrual cycle: implications for human reproduction. J. Immunol. 178, 2572–2578.

Ban, Y., Taniyama, M., Tozaki, T., Tomita, M., 2000. Estrogen receptor alpha dinucleotide repeat polymorphism in Japanese patients with autoimmune thyroid diseases. BMC Med. Genet. 1, 1.

Bebo Jr., B.F., Adlard, K., Schuster, J.C., Unsicker, L., Vandenbark, A.A., Offner, H., 1999. Gender differences in protection from EAE induced by oral tolerance with a peptide analogue of MBP-Ac1-11. J. Neurosci. Res. 55, 432–440.

Bennett, C.L., Christie, J., Ramsdell, F., Brunkow, M.E., Ferguson, P.J., Whitesell, L., et al., 2001. The immune dysregulation, polyendocrinopathy, enteropathy, X-linked syndrome (IPEX) is caused by mutations of FOXP3. Nat. Genet. 27, 20–21.

Boonyaratanakornkit, V., Bi, Y., Rudd, M., Edwards, D.P., 2008. The role and mechanism of progesterone receptor activation of extranuclear signaling pathways in regulating gene transcription and cell cycle progression. Steroids. 73, 922–928.

Borchers, A.T., Gershwin, M.E., 2012. Sociological differences between women and men: implications for autoimmunity. Autoimmun. Rev. 11, A413–A421.

Bouman, A., Schipper, M., Heineman, M.J., Faas, M.M., 2004. Gender difference in the non-specific and specific immune response in humans. Am. J. Reprod. Immunol. 52, 19–26.

Bouman, A., Heineman, M.J., Faas, M.M., 2005. Sex hormones and the immune response in humans. Hum. Reprod. Update. 11, 411–423.

Butterworth, M., McClellan, B., Allansmith, M., 1967. Influence of sex in immunoglobulin levels. Nature. 214, 1224–1225.

Canellada, A., Blois, S., Gentile, T., Margni Idehu, R.A., 2002. In vitro modulation of protective antibody responses by estrogen, progesterone and interleukin-6. Am. J. Reprod. Immunol. 48, 334–343.

Carter, C.O., 1969. Genetics of common disorders. Br. Med. Bull. 25, 52–57.

Choudhry, M.A., Schwacha, M.G., Hubbard, W.J., Kerby, J.D., Rue, L.W., Bland, K.I., et al., 2005. Gender differences in acute response to trauma-hemorrhage. Shock. 24 (Suppl. 1), 101–106.

Choudhry, M.A., Bland, K.I., Chaudry, I.H., 2007. Trauma and immune response—effect of gender differences. Injury. 38, 1382–1391.

Cook, I.F., 2008. Sexual dimorphism of humoral immunity with human vaccines. Vaccine. 26, 3551–3555.

Csaba, G., Kovacs, P., Pallinger, E., 2003. Gender differences in the histamine and serotonin content of blood, peritoneal and thymic cells: a comparison with mast cells. Cell Biol. Int. 27, 387–389.

Da Silva, J.A., 1999. Sex hormones and glucocorticoids: interactions with the immune system. Ann. N.Y. Acad. Sci. 876, 102–118.

Darwin, C., 1871. The Sescent of Man and Selection in Relation to Sex. John Murray.

Das, B.R., Bhanushali, A.A., Khadapkar, R., Jeswani, K.D., Bhavsar, M., Dasgupta, A., 2008. Reference ranges for lymphocyte subsets in adults from western India: influence of sex, age and method of enumeration. Indian J. Med. Sci. 62, 397–406.

Davison, S.L., Bell, R., Donath, S., Montalto, J.G., Davis, S.R., 2005. Androgen levels in adult females: changes with age, menopause, and oophorectomy. J. Clin. Endocrinol. Metab. 90, 3847–3853.

Deane, J.A., Pisitkun, P., Barrett, R.S., Feigenbaum, L., Town, T., Ward, M., Jerrold, M., et al., 2007. Control of toll-like receptor 7 expression is essential to restrict autoimmunity and dendritic cell proliferation.. Immunity. 27, 801–810.

Ding, J., Zhu, B.T., 2008. Unique effect of the pregnancy hormone estriol on antigen-induced production of specific antibodies in female BALB/c mice. Steroids. 73, 289–298.

Dos Santos, C.D., Toldo, M.P., Do Prado Junior, J.C., 2005. Trypanosoma cruzi: the effects of dehydroepiandrosterone (DHEA) treatment during experimental infection.. Acta Trop. 95, 109–115.

Dosiou, C., Hamilton, A.E., Pang, Y., Overgaard, M.T., Tulac, S., Dong, J., et al., 2008. Expression of membrane progesterone receptors on human T lymphocytes and Jurkat cells and activation of G-proteins by progesterone. J. Endocrinol. 196, 67–77.

Ellegren, H., Parsch, J., 2007. The evolution of sex-biased genes and sex-biased gene expression. Nature reviews. Genetics. 8, 689–698.

Elsheikh, M., Wass, J.A., Conway, G.S., 2001. Autoimmune thyroid syndrome in women with Turner's syndrome—the association with karyotype. Clin. Endocrinol. (Oxf). 55, 223–226.

Fish, E.N., 2008. The X-files in immunity: sex-based differences predispose immune responses. Nature reviews. Immunology. 8, 737–744.

Flori, L., Gao, Y., Laloe, D., Lemonnier, G., Leplat, J.J., Teillaud, A., et al., 2011. Immunity traits in pigs: substantial genetic variation and limited covariation. PloS One. 6, e22717.

Folstad, I., Karter, A.J., 1992. Parasites, bright males, and the immunocompetence handicap. Am. Nat. 139, 603–622.

Frisancho-Kiss, S., Davis, S.E., Nyland, J.F., Frisancho, J.A., Cihakova, D., Barrett, M.A., et al., 2007. Cutting edge: cross-regulation by TLR4 and T cell Ig mucin-3 determines sex differences in inflammatory heart disease. J. Immunol. 178, 6710–6714.

Giglio, T., Imro, M.A., Filaci, G., Scudeletti, M., Puppo, F., De Cecco, L., et al., 1994. Immune cell circulating subsets are affected by gonadal function. Life Sci. 54, 1305–1312.

Giltay, E.J., Fonk, J.C., Von Blomberg, B.M., Drexhage, H.A., Schalkwijk, C., Gooren, L.J., 2000. In vivo effects of sex steroids on lymphocyte responsiveness and immunoglobulin levels in humans. J. Clin. Endocrinol. Metab. 85, 1648–1657.

Gourdy, P., Araujo, L.M., Zhu, R., Garmy-Susini, B., Diem, S., Laurell, H., et al., 2005. Relevance of sexual dimorphism to regulatory T cells: estradiol promotes IFN-gamma production by invariant natural killer T cells. Blood. 105, 2415–2420.

Greer, J.M., McCombe, P.A., 2011. Role of gender in multiple sclerosis: clinical effects and potential molecular mechanisms. J. Neuroimmunol. 234, 7–18.

Greer, J.M., McCombe, P.A., 2012. The role of epigenetic mechanisms and processes in autoimmune disorders. Biologics: Targets and Therapy. 6, 307–327.

Grimaldi, C.M., 2006. Sex and systemic lupus erythematosus: the role of the sex hormones estrogen and prolactin on the regulation of autoreactive B cells. Curr. Opin. Rheumatol. 18, 456–461.

Hedrick, A.V., Temeles, E.J., 1989. The evolution of sexual dimorphism in animals: hypotheses and tests. Trends Ecol. Evol. 4, 136–138.

Hill, M.E., Shiono, H., Newsom-Davis, J., Willcox, N., 2008. The myasthenia gravis thymus: a rare source of human autoantibody-secreting plasma cells for testing potential therapeutics. J. Neuroimmunol. 201–202, 50–56.

Hince, M., Sakkal, S., Vlahos, K., Dudakov, J., Boyd, R., Chidgey, A., 2008. The role of sex steroids and gonadectomy in the control of thymic involution. Cell Immunol. 252, 122–138.

Huygen, K., Palfliet, K., 1984. Strain variation in interferon gamma production of BCG-sensitized mice challenged with PPD II. Importance of one major autosomal locus and additional sexual influences. Cell Immunol. 85, 75–81.

Ivanova, E., Kyurkchiev, D., Altankova, I., Dimitrov, J., Binakova, E., Kyurkchiev, S., 2005. CD83 monocyte-derived dendritic cells are present in human decidua and progesterone induces their differentiation in vitro. Am. J. Reprod. Immunol. 53, 199–205.

Jones, L.A., Anthony, J.P., Henriquez, F.L., Lyons, R.E., Nickdel, M.B., Carter, K.C., et al., 2008. Toll-like receptor-4-mediated macrophage activation is differentially regulated by progesterone via the glucocorticoid and progesterone receptors. Immunology. 125, 59–69.

Kahlke, V., Angele, M.K., Schwacha, M.G., Ayala, A., Cioffi, W.G., Bland, K.I., et al., 2000. Reversal of sexual dimorphism in splenic T lymphocyte responses after trauma-hemorrhage with aging. Am. J. Physiol. Cell Physiol. 278, C509–C516.

Kelley, J., Johnson, M.R., Alarcón, G.S., Kimberly, R.P., Edberg, J.C., 2007. Variation in the relative copy number of the TLR7 gene in patients with systemic lupus erythematosus and healthy control subjects. Arthritis Rheum. 56, 3375–3378.

Klein, S.L., Jedlicka, A., Pekosz, A., 2010. The Xs and Y of immune responses to viral vaccines. Lancet Infect. Dis. 10, 338–349.

Kongshavn, P.A., Bliss, J.Q., 1970. Sex differences in survival of H-2 incompatible skin grafts in mice treated with antithymocyte serum. Nature. 226, 451.

Lahita, R.G., 1999. Emerging concepts for sexual predilection in the disease systemic lupus erythematosus. Ann. N.Y. Acad. Sci. 876, 64–70.

Lamason, R., Zhao, P., Rawat, R., Davis, A., Hall, J.C., Chae, J.J., et al., 2006. Sexual dimorphism in immune response genes as a function of puberty. BMC Immunol. 7, 2.

Lengi, A.J., Phillips, R.A., Karpuzoglu, E., Ahmed, S.A., 2007. Estrogen selectively regulates chemokines in murine splenocytes. J. Leukoc. Biol. 81, 1065–1074.

Leonard, W.J., Noguchi, M., Russell, S.M., McBride, O.W., 1994. The molecular basis of X-linked severe combined immunodeficiency: the role of the interleukin-2 receptor gamma chain as a common gamma chain, gamma c. Immunol. Rev. 138, 61–86.

Leposavic, G., Karapetrovic, B., Obradovic, S., Vidiic, D.B., Kosec, D., 1996. Differential effects of gonadectomy on the thymocyte phenotypic profile in male and female rats. Pharmacol. Biochem. Behav. 54, 269–276.

Liang, J., Sun, L., Wang, Q., Hou, Y., 2006. Progesterone regulates mouse dendritic cells differentiation and maturation. Int. Immunopharmacol. 6, 830–838.

Lichtman, M.A., Vaughan, J.H., Hames, C.G., 1967. The distribution of serum immunoglobulins, anti-gamma-G globulins ("rheumatoid factors") and antinuclear antibodies in White and Negro subjects in Evans County, Georgia. Arthritis Rheum. 10, 204–215.

Livernois, A.M., Graves, J.A., Waters, P.D., 2012. The origin and evolution of vertebrate sex chromosomes and dosage compensation. Heredity. 108, 50–58.

Lotter, H., Jacobs, T., Gaworski, I., Tannich, E., 2006. Sexual dimorphism in the control of amebic liver abscess in a mouse model of disease. Infect. Immun. 74, 118–124.

Lu, Q., Wu, A., Tesmer, L., Ray, D., Yousif, N., Richardson, B., 2007. Demethylation of CD40LG on the inactive X in T cells from women with lupus. J. Immunol. 179, 6352–6358.

Lutz, L.B., Jamnongjit, M., Yang, W.H., Jahani, D., Gill, A., Hammes, S.R., 2003. Selective modulation of genomic and nongenomic androgen responses by androgen receptor ligands. Mol. Endocrinol. 17, 1106–1116.

Mank, J.E., 2009. Sex chromosomes and the evolution of sexual dimorphism: lessons from the genome. Am. Nat. 173, 141–150.

Markle, J.G., Frank, D.N., Mortin-Toth, S., Robertson, C.E., Feazel, L.M., Rolle-Kampczyk, U., et al., 2013. Sex differences in the gut microbiome drive hormone-dependent regulation of autoimmunity. Science. 339, 1084–1088.

Matthews, J., Gustafsson, J.A., 2003. Estrogen signaling: a subtle balance between ER alpha and ER beta. Mol. Interv. 3, 281–292.

Mattila, K.M., Luomala, M., Lehtimaki, T., Laippala, P., Koivula, T., Elovaara, I., 2001. Interaction between ESR1 and HLA-DR2 may contribute to the development of MS in women. Neurology. 56, 1246–1247.

McCombe, P.A., Greer, J.M., Mackay, I.R., 2009. Sexual dimorphism in autoimmune disease. Curr. Mol. Med. 9, 1058–1079.

McKean, K.A., Nunney, L., 2005. Bateman's principle and immunity: phenotypically plastic reproductive strategies predict changes in immunological sex differences. Evolution. 59, 1510–1517.

McMurray, R.W., Wilson, J.G., Bigler, L., Xiang, L., Lagoo, A., 2000. Progesterone inhibits glucocorticoid-induced murine thymocyte apoptosis. Int. J. Immunopharmacol. 22, 955–965.

Miller, L., Alley, E.W., Murphy, W.J., Russell, S.W., Hunt, J.S., 1996. Progesterone inhibits inducible nitric oxide synthase gene expression and nitric oxide production in murine macrophages. J. Leukoc. Bsiol. 59, 442–450.

Mitchell, R., Hollis, S., Rothwell, C., Robertson, W.R., 1995. Age related changes in the pituitary-testicular axis in normal men; lower serum testosterone results from decreased bioactive LH drive. Clin. Endocrinol. (Oxf.). 42, 501–507.

Mock, B.A., Nacy, C.A., 1988. Hormonal modulation of sex differences in resistance to Leishmania major systemic infections. Infect. Immun. 56, 3316–3319.

Moller-Larsen, S., Nyegaard, M., Haagerup, A., Vestbo, J., Kruse, T.A., Borglum, A.D., 2008. Association analysis identifies TLR7 and TLR8 as novel risk genes in asthma and related disorders. Thorax. 63, 1064–1069.

Morgan, T.E., Wong, A.M., Finch, C.E., 2007. Anti-inflammatory mechanisms of dietary restriction in slowing aging processes. Interdiscip. Top. Gerontol. 35, 83–97.

Nalbandian, G., Kovats, S., 2005. Understanding sex biases in immunity: effects of estrogen on the differentiation and function of antigen-presenting cells. Immunol. Res. 31, 91–106.

Nancy, P., Berrih-Aknin, S., 2005. Differential estrogen receptor expression in autoimmune myasthenia gravis. Endocrinology. 146, 2345–2353.

Narongchai, P., Narongchai, S., 2008. Study of the normal internal organ weights in Thai population. J. Med. Assoc. Thai. 91, 747–753.

Nilsson, B.O., 2007. Modulation of the inflammatory response by estrogens with focus on the endothelium and its interactions with leukocytes. Inflamm. Res. 56, 269–273.

Nunn, C.L., Lindenfors, P., Pursall, E.R., Rolff, J., 2009. On sexual dimorphism in immune function. Philos. Trans. R. Soc. London, Ser. B, Biol. Sci. 364, 61–69.

Nussinovitch, U., Shoenfeld, Y., 2012. The role of gender and organ specific autoimmunity. Autoimmun. Rev. 11, A377–A385.

Page, S.T., Plymate, S.R., Bremner, W.J., Matsumoto, A.M., Hess, D.L., Lin, D.W., et al., 2006. Effect of medical castration on CD4 + CD25 + T cells, CD8 + T cell IFN-gamma expression, and NK cells: a physiological role for testosterone and/or its metabolites. Am. J. Physiol. Endocrinol. Metab. 290, E856–E863.

Pan, Z., Chang, C., 2012. Gender and the regulation of longevity: implications for autoimmunity. Autoimmun. Rev. 11, A393–A403.

Pernis, A.B., 2007. Estrogen and CD4 + T cells. Curr. Opin. Rheumatol. 19, 414–420.

Piccinni, M.P., Giudizi, M.G., Biagiotti, R., Beloni, L., Giannarini, L., Sampognaro, S., et al., 1995. Progesterone favors the development of human T helper cells producing Th2-type cytokines and promotes both IL-4 production and membrane CD30 expression in established Th1 cell clones. J. Immunol. 155, 128–133.

Pilipovic, I., Vidic-Dankovic, B., Perisic, M., Radojevic, K., Colic, M., Todorovic, V., et al., 2008. Sexual dimorphism in the catecholamine-containing thymus microenvironment: a role for gonadal hormones. J. Neuroimmunol. 195, 7–20.

Pioli, P.A., Jensen, A.L., Weaver, L.K., Amiel, E., Shen, Z., Shen, L., et al., 2007. Estradiol attenuates lipopolysaccharide-induced CXC chemokine ligand 8 production by human peripheral blood monocytes. J. Immunol. 179, 6284–6290.

Pollard, K.M., 2012. Gender differences in autoimmunity associated with exposure to environmental factors. J. Autoimmun. 38, J177–J186.

Prieto, G.A., Rosenstein, Y., 2006. Oestradiol potentiates the suppressive function of human CD4 CD25 regulatory T cells by promoting their proliferation. Immunology. 118, 58–65.

Prossnitz, E.R., Arterburn, J.B., Sklar, L.A., 2007. GPR30: a G protein-coupled receptor for estrogen. Mol. Cell Endocrinol. 265–266, 138–142.

Quintero, O.L., Amador-Patarroyo, M.J., Montoya-Ortiz, G., Rojas-Villarraga, A., Anaya, J.M., 2012. Autoimmune disease and gender: plausible mechanisms for the female predominance of autoimmunity. J. Autoimmun. 38, J109–J119.

Rachon, D., Mysliwska, J., Suchecka-Rachon, K., Wieckiewicz, J., Mysliwski, A., 2002. Effects of oestrogen deprivation on interleukin-6 production by peripheral blood mononuclear cells of postmenopausal women. J. Endocrinol. 172, 387–395.

Rider, V., Li, X., Peterson, G., Dawson, J., Kimler, B.F., Abdou, N.I., 2006. Differential expression of estrogen receptors in women with systemic lupus erythematosus. J. Rheumatol. 33, 1093–1101.

Rieger, R., Leung, P.S., Jeddeloh, M.R., Kurth, M.J., Nantz, M.H., Lam, K.S., et al., 2006. Identification of 2-nonynoic acid, a cosmetic component, as a potential trigger of primary biliary cirrhosis. J. Autoimmun. 27, 7–16.

Roberts, M.L., Buchanan, K.L., Evans, M.R., 2004. Testing the immuno-competence handicap hypothesis: a review of the evidence. Anim. Behav. 68, 227–239.

Rowley, M.J., Mackay, I.R., 1969. Measurement of antibody-producing capacity in man. I. The normal response to flagellin from *Salmonella adelaide*. Clin. Exp. Immunol. 5, 407–418.

Santoli, D., Trinchieri, G., Zmijewski, C.M., Koprowski, H., 1976. HLA-related control of spontaneous and antibody-dependent cell-mediated cytotoxic activity in humans. J. Immunol. 117, 765–770.

Sharpe, R.M., 1998. The roles of oestrogen in the male. Trends Endocrinol. Metab. 9, 371–377.

Simoncini, T., Mannella, P., Fornari, L., Caruso, A., Varone, G., Genazzani, A.R., 2004. Genomic and non-genomic effects of estrogens on endothelial cells. Steroids. 69, 537–542.

Sinha, S., Kaler, L.J., Proctor, T.M., Teuscher, C., Vandenbark, A.A., Offner, H., 2008. IL-13-mediated gender difference in susceptibility to autoimmune encephalomyelitis. J. Immunol. 180, 2679–2685.

Skaletsky, H., Kuroda-Kawaguchi, T., Minx, P.J., Cordum, H.S., Hillier, L., Brown, L.G., et al., 2003. The male-specific region of the human Y chromosome is a mosaic of discrete sequence classes. Nature. 423, 825–837.

Smith-Bouvier, D.L., Divekar, A.A., Sasidhar, M., Du, S., Tiwari-Woodruff, S.K., King, J.K., et al., 2008. A role for sex chromosome complement in the female bias in autoimmune disease. J. Exp. Med. 205, 1099–1108.

Somerset, D.A., Zheng, Y., Kilby, M.D., Sansom, D.M., Drayson, M.T., 2004. Normal human pregnancy is associated with an elevation in the immune suppressive CD25 + CD4 + regulatory T-cell subset. Immunology. 112, 38–43.

Spach, K.M., Blake, M., Bunn, J.Y., McElvany, B., Noubade, R., Blankenhorn, E.P., et al., 2009. Cutting edge: the Y chromosome controls the age-dependent experimental allergic encephalomyelitis sexual dimorphism in SJL/J mice. J. Immunol. 182, 1789–1793.

Subramanian, S., Tus, K., Li, Q.Z., Wang, A., Tian, X.H., Zhou, J., et al., 2006. A Tlr7 translocation accelerates systemic autoimmunity in murine lupus. Proc. Natl. Acad. Sci. U.S.A. 103, 9970–9975.

Tai, P., Wang, J., Jin, H., Song, X., Yan, J., Kang, Y., et al., 2008. Induction of regulatory T cells by physiological level estrogen. J. Cell Physiol. 214, 456–464.

Tait, A.S., Butts, C.L., Sternberg, E.M., 2008. The role of glucocorticoids and progestins in inflammatory, autoimmune, and infectious disease. J. Leukoc. Biol. 84, 924–931.

Takagi, H., Ishiguro, N., Iwata, H., Kanamono, T., 2000. Genetic association between rheumatoid arthritis and estrogen receptor microsatellite polymorphism. J. Rheumatol. 27, 1638–1642.

Terres, G., Morrison, S.L., Habicht, G.S., 1968. A quantitative difference in the immune response between male and female mice. Proc. Soc. Exp. Biol. Med. 127, 664–667.

Teuscher, C., Noubade, R., Spach, K., McElvany, B., Bunn, J.Y., Fillmore, P.D., et al., 2006. Evidence that the Y chromosome influences autoimmune disease in male and female mice. Proc. Natl. Acad. Sci. U.S.A. 103, 8024–8029.

Toubi, E., Shoenfeld, Y., 2004. The role of CD40-CD154 interactions in autoimmunity and the benefit of disrupting this pathway. Autoimmunity. 37, 457–464.

Trzonkowski, P., Mysliwska, J., Tukaszuk, K., Szmit, E., Bryl, E., Mysliwski, A., 2001. Luteal phase of the menstrual cycle in young healthy women is associated with decline in interleukin 2 levels. Horm. Metab. Res. 33, 348–353.

Wang, C., Dehghani, B., Magrisso, I.J., Rick, E.A., Bonhomme, E., Cody, D.B., et al., 2008. GPR30 contributes to estrogen-induced thymic atrophy. Mol. Endocrinol. 22, 636–648.

Wehling, M., Losel, R., 2006. Non-genomic steroid hormone effects: membrane or intracellular receptors? J. Steroid Biochem. Mol. Biol. 102, 180–183.

Weinstein, Y., Ran, S., Segal, S., 1984. Sex-associated differences in the regulation of immune responses controlled by the MHC of the mouse. J. Immunol. 132, 656–661.

Wichmann, M.W., Muller, C., Meyer, G., Adam, M., Angele, M.K., Eisenmenger, S.J., et al., 2003. Different immune responses to abdominal surgery in men and women. Langenbecks Arch. Surg. 387, 397–401.

Wijchers, P.J., Festenstein, R.J., 2011. Epigenetic regulation of autosomal gene expression by sex chromosomes. Trends Genet. 27, 132–140.

Wijchers, P.J., Yandim, C., Panousopoulou, E., Ahmad, M., Harker, N., Saveliev, A., et al., 2010. Sexual dimorphism in mammalian autosomal gene regulation is determined not only by Sry but by sex chromosome complement as well. Dev. Cell. 19, 477–484.

Wikby, A., Mansson, I.A., Johansson, B., Strindhall, J., Nilsson, S.E., 2008. The immune risk profile is associated with age and gender: findings from three Swedish population studies of individuals 20–100 years of age. Biogerontology. 9, 299–308.

Wilson, R., Chu, C.E., Donaldson, M.D., Thomson, J.A., McKillop, J.H., Connor, J.M., 1996. An increased incidence of thyroid antibodies in patients with Turner's syndrome and their first degree relatives. Autoimmunity. 25, 47–52.

Yan, J., Greer, J.M., Hull, R., O'Sullivan, J.D., Henderson, R.D., Read, S.J., et al., 2010. The effect of ageing on human lymphocyte subsets: comparison of males and females. Immunity Ageing. 7, 4.

Yang, J.H., Chen, C.D., Wu, M.Y., Chao, K.H., Yang, Y.S., Ho, H.N., 2000. Hormone replacement therapy reverses the decrease in natural killer cytotoxicity but does not reverse the decreases in the T-cell subpopulation or interferon-gamma production in postmenopausal women. Fertil. Steril. 74, 261–267.

Yao, G., Shang, X.J., 2005. A comparison of modulation of proliferation of thymocyte by testosterone, dehydroisoandrosterone and androstenedione in vitro. Arch. Androl. 51, 257–265.

Zandman-Goddard, G., Peeva, E., Shoenfeld, Y., 2007. Gender and autoimmunity. Autoimmun. Rev. 6, 366–372.

Zehntner, S.P., Bourbonniere, L., Moore, C.S., Morris, S.J., Methot, D., St Jean, M., et al., 2007. X-linked inhibitor of apoptosis regulates T cell effector function. J. Immunol. 179, 7553–7560.

Zheng, Y., Rudensky, A.Y., 2007. Foxp3 in control of the regulatory T cell lineage. Nat. Immunol. 8, 457–462.

Zoller, A.L., Kersh, G.J., 2006. Estrogen induces thymic atrophy by eliminating early thymic progenitors and inhibiting proliferation of beta-selected thymocytes. J. Immunol. 176, 7371–7378.

Chapter 25

Microbiome and Autoimmunity

Jean-François Bach[1] and Alicia Perez-Arroyo[2]

[1]*Institut National de la Santé et de la Recherche Médicale, Paris, France,* [2]*Université Paris Descartes, Sorbonne Paris Cité, Faculté de Médecine, Paris, France*

Chapter Outline

Introduction	329
The Intestinal Microbiome	330
Intestinal Microbiome Composition and Genotyping Techniques	330
The Microbiome Changes Over a Lifetime	330
The Intestinal Microbiome Depends on the Environment	330
Germ-Free (GF) Animals	331
Effect of a GF Environment on Experimental Diseases	331
Non-Obese Diabetic Mouse	331
Experimental Allergic Encephalomyelitis	332
Experimental Arthritis	332
Murine Lupus	332
Microbiome Composition and Autoimmune Diseases	333
Type 1 Diabetes	333
Rheumatoid Arthritis	333
Effect of Probiotics on Autoimmune Diseases	333
Probiotic Mixtures	334
Specific Probiotics	334
Role of Toll-like Receptor Stimulation	334

The Relationship Between the Intestinal Microbiome and the Hygiene Hypothesis	334
Brief Overview of the Hygiene Hypothesis	334
A Clean Environment Promotes the Onset of Autoimmune Diabetes	335
Experimental Data	335
Human Data	335
Autoimmune Diseases Can be Prevented by Infections With a Pathogen	335
Experimental Data	335
Human Data	335
Synthesis and Conclusions	336
The Strength of the Protective Effect of Pathogens	336
The Ambiguous Effect on Autoimmune Disease of the GF or Axenic Status	337
The Delicate Interpretation of the Reduction in the Diversity of the Intestinal Microbiome	337
Perspectives	337
Acknowledgments	338
References	338

INTRODUCTION

As soon as the concept of autoimmune diseases emerged, it was suggested that infectious agents have a role in their etiology. In fact, we now know that certain autoimmune diseases, such as rheumatic fever (streptococci) and certain cases of the Guillain–Barré syndrome (*Campilobacter jejuni*), are directly caused by bacterial infection through molecular mimicry.

New insight was gained unexpectedly when it was proposed that the decrease in infectious diseases observed in industrialized countries over the past four decades might cause a parallel increase in the frequency of autoimmune and allergic diseases, suggesting a new role for infectious agents (Bach, 2002). The problem reached an additional level of complexity when it was found that lifestyle changes associated with socioeconomic progress, which largely explained the decreased frequency of infectious diseases, also contributed to modifying the intestinal flora (Pflughoeft and Versalovic, 2012). Furthermore, gut flora itself is known to have an effect on the onset of dysimmune diseases such as autoimmune, inflammatory bowel and allergic diseases (Proal et al., 2009; Round and Mazmanian, 2009; Mathis and Benoist, 2011; Cho and Blaser, 2012; Chervonsky, 2013; Shanahan, 2013).

Thus, presently one may wonder, what is the respective role of infectious pathogenic agents and of commensal bacteria in the protection from autoimmune diseases?

N. Rose & I. Mackay (Eds): The Autoimmune Diseases, Fifth edition. DOI: http://dx.doi.org/10.1016/B978-0-12-384929-8.00025-3

THE INTESTINAL MICROBIOME

The expression "intestinal microbiome" is generally understood today as meaning the commensal bacteria of the gut flora.

In addition to intestinal commensal bacteria, every individual is confronted with or lives in symbiosis with many commensal bacteria located outside the intestine (for example, the skin and vaginal microbioma which are discussed below) that are part of the host environment. Innate immunity and, often also, adaptive immunity are continuously challenged by this environment.

Intestinal Microbiome Composition and Genotyping Techniques

Each human being harbors in his or her gut more than 10 trillion bacteria amounting to a weight of over 1.5 kg. They represent a wide diversity of species (200 main species and globally probably more than 1000) (Reid et al., 2011; Molloy et al., 2012). It has become relatively easy to analyze gut flora composition using genetic techniques strongly supported by bioinformatic methods.

Access to modern genetic techniques has opened considerable opportunities in terms of our inventory capacity regarding the intestinal microbiome. The classical techniques of bacterial culture and identification were labor-intensive and not very efficient because many commensal bacteria could not be grown *in vitro*. Gut bacteria are now defined by their genes and designated collectively as "microbiota." They are referenced by their genetic makeup under the general term "metagenome."

Two main techniques based on DNA sequencing are used to genotype the gut microbiome:

*   The Shotgun sequencing can generate in parallel over 100 million gene sequences (50 to 75 bases) and makes it possible to sequence any given segment of DNA from its two ends (Li et al., 2010). DNA is broken-up randomly into numerous small segments, which are sequenced using the chain termination method to obtain *reads*. Multiple overlapping reads for the target DNA are obtained by performing several rounds of this fragmentation and sequencing. Computer programs then use the overlapping ends of different reads to assemble them into a continuous sequence. The main challenge of using this technique to create a gene catalogue is the assembling of a sufficient number of small sequences of adequate length to obtain contiguous portions of the DNA sequence of interest, the length of which needs to be at least equal to that of a typical bacterial gene.
*   The 16S bacterial rRNA gene sequencing generates longer sequences (300–800 bases) and is widely used

for metagenomics analysis (Marguiles et al., 2005). It has been established as the "gold standard" for identification and taxonomic classification of bacterial species mainly due to the lower technical and cost issues. However, the limitation of this technique lies in the sequencing of only one gene for all the samples, with a lower identity percentage than for the whole genome sequencing.

For the two techniques the sequencing can be performed by different technologies, the most largely used being the Illumina dye sequencing and the 454 Pyrosequencing, which differ in the way of detection of the added nucleotides into the sequence.

Several hundred human metagenomes have already been studied, mainly by big international consortiums (such as MetaHit consortium in Europe). A limited number of different profiles (enterotypes) have been identified but the significance of this categorization is not yet clear (Dusko Ehrlich, 2010).

The Microbiome Changes Over a Lifetime

The intestinal flora appears in the days following birth as a consequence of the first intestinal colonization, usually by the mother's vaginal microbiome in children born through natural delivery (Martin et al., 2010). For those children, and also, of course, also for those born through cesarean section, the initial intestinal microbiome is acquired through feeding, whether the mother breast feeds or not.

Most of the microbiome is fixed in humans as early as the first week of life and is nearly completed by the end of the infant's first months. Its composition may vary in cases of intestinal infection or antibiotic treatment but reverts to its initial composition with small variations after recovering from illness or the treatment.

The Intestinal Microbiome Depends on the Environment

The composition of the microbiome depends on the host's environment. Thus sanitary conditions, hygiene, and the medical and nutritional context can have a considerable role on the composition of the microbiome (Pflughoeft and Versalovic, 2012). It has been shown in pigs that rearing animals in sanitary and controlled conditions after delivery by cesarean section significantly altered the composition of the gut microbiome (Mulder et al., 2009). Interestingly, similar results were observed when pigs born by natural delivery were placed in a clean environment by the third day of life, once the first intestinal colonization, mainly of vaginal origin, had occurred (Schmidt et al., 2011).

In humans studies were carried on Italian children living in the Florence region and African children from Burkina Faso. It was found that a number of well-defined bacteria were present in very different amounts in the two groups of children studied (DeFilippo et al., 2010). It is interesting to note in this example the difficulty of knowing which environmental factor is responsible for the observed difference in the composition of the microbiome—diet or hygiene—both of which are very different in these two countries.

Germ-Free (GF) Animals

Several techniques are available to raise germ-free (GF) (also termed axenic) animals throughout their first weeks of life. The first technique consists in raising animals in sterile conditions, in a GF atmosphere in terms of environment and food. The second technique consists of administering at birth, or even to the mother during pregnancy, antibiotics to eliminate most (but not necessarily all) commensal bacteria. Various protocols have been used to successfully eliminate commensal bacteria. Specific antibiotics such as vancomycin or streptomycin have been used, as well as antibiotic cocktails. The results have been different depending on the type of treatment, as determined from microbiome analyses.

Raising animals in a GF environment leads to modifications in the development of the immune system since the intestinal microbiome plays an important role in its maturation (Tlaskalova-Hogenova et al., 2011). It has been known for a long time, in particular from Sterzel's experiments in Prague in the 1980s, that GF animals display severe immune deficiency (Tlaskalova-Hogenova et al., 1983). How intestinal microbiome influences this maturation is still unknown. This partial immunodeficiency essentially affects antibody production and also probably (but this has been less well studied) cellular immunity. Furthermore, a decrease has been observed in intestinal responses to infections that are associated with lymphoid atrophy affecting Peyer's patches (Chinen et al., 2010).

Recently, many studies have focused on identifying the cellular mechanisms underlying this immune deficiency. Particular attention was given to several species of commensal bacteria that can induce regulatory T cells or Th17 cells.

Various studies have shown that commensal bacteria of the Clostridium genus can induce regulatory CD4$^+$CD25$^+$FoxP3$^+$ T cells affecting both cell number and function. In particular, the oral administration to GF animals of a bacterial mixture of several Clostridium species induced these regulatory T lymphocytes in the colonic lamina propria (Atarashi et al., 2011; Nagano et al., 2012). Simultaneously, a preventive effect on the

induction of inflammatory colitis and the production of IgE was observed.

Similarly, it was shown that the commensal bacterium Bacteroides fragilis belonging to the Clostridium genus was particularly effective at inducting regulatory T cells that produce interleukin (IL)-10 (Round and Mazmanian, 2010). Kasper and collaborators have shown that in GF animals the same effect could be achieved by replacing the commensal bacterium with one of its polysaccharide constituents, namely polysaccharide A or PSA (Ochoa-Repáraz et al., 2010). It appears that the regulatory T cells induced in the intestine by these bacteria represent a very specific subpopulation of regulatory T cells which, interestingly enough, are not induced in mice invalidated for the IL-10 gene (Ochoa-Repáraz et al., 2010).

It has been observed that GF mice display a deficit of IL-17 producing Th17 cells. Interestingly, it is possible to restore the ability to produce IL-17 in GF mice by colonization with a single bacterium, the segmented filamentous bacterium (SFB) (Ivanov et al., 2009; Gaboriau-Routhiau et al., 2009). In spite of its importance, this observation should not overshadow the fact that other commensal bacteria can also induce Th17 cells in GF mice, in particular Citrobacter rodentium and Salmonella typhimurium infection (Geddes et al., 2011). These observations have led to important applications in the field of autoimmunity, especially results showing that pathologies involving Th17 cells could be induced by SFB. Thus, the arthritis observed in K/NxB mice (see below) described by D. Mathis et al. could be induced in GF mice, which normally do not develop this disease, after monocolonization by SFB (Wu et al., 2010). Similar results have been observed in experimental allergic encephalomyelitis (EAE) (Ochoa-Reparaz et al., 2009; Lee et al., 2011). Inversely, it has been shown that the presence of SBF in the intestine is positively correlated with protection against autoimmune diabetes in female non-obese diabetic (NOD) mice (but not in male NOD mice) (Kriegel et al., 2011).

EFFECT OF A GF ENVIRONMENT ON EXPERIMENTAL DISEASES

The effect of a GF environment on experimental autoimmune diseases has been mainly studied in four types of models: autoimmune diabetes in NOD mice, EAE, experimental arthritis, and murine lupus.

Non-Obese Diabetic Mouse

Contradictory results were obtained from the study of germ-free NOD mice. The first study led to a significant increase in the incidence of the disease (Suzuki et al., 1985), while other studies could not find any difference between GF and specific pathogen-free (SPF) housing conditions (Taniguchi et al., 2007; Wen et al., 2008; King and Sarvetnick, 2011). Another study showed increased insulitis without any worsening of diabetes (Alam et al., 2011). Lastly, recent data showed a major increase in disease incidence in NOD males but not in females with the additional interesting but intriguing observation that transplanting gut microbiome from SPF male mice to SPF females decreased the incidence of diabetes in the recipients, an effect associated with an elevation of testosterone levels (Markle et al., 2013). These different outcomes can be explained by the different GF conditions used in the studies, or more subtly by differences in the sanitary conditions of the control animals. Whatever the cause may be, the important point is that there is a difference between "clean" and less clean animals. Thus, the analysis of GF NOD mice is not very informative. As will be seen below, more information can be obtained by comparing SPF mice and mice raised in fully conventional sanitary conditions.

The question remains open as to when during the life of an animal (at birth or later) bacteria present in the environment have an effect. The involvement of the intestinal microbiome is all the more likely if the effect of the infections occurs early.

Experimental Allergic Encephalomyelitis

The effect of a GF environment on EAE was studied on two types of models:

- Conventional EAE induced by immunization against myelin proteins in normal animals and
- The spontaneous (or antigen-boosted) development of EAE in transgenic mice carrying a T cell receptor that recognizes a myelin protein.

For the first model, it was shown by Ochoa-Reparaz et al. that oral antibiotic treatment can prevent EAE development after immunization against myelin basic protein (MBP) (Ochoa-Reparaz et al., 2009). This study also showed that the antibiotic treatment induced a simultaneous decrease in proinflammatory cytokines and an increase in IL-10 and IL-13 production. The fact that, contrary to orally administered antibiotics, antibiotics administered intraperitoneally did not decrease EAE suggested that oral antibiotics acted on the microbiota (Ochoa-Reparaz et al., 2009).

Two studies involving transgenic mouse models have been published: the first concerned transgenic mice carrying a T cell receptor that recognized MBP (Goverman, 2009) and the second concerned transgenic mice carrying a T cell receptor that recognized myelin oligodendrocyte protein (MOG) (Berer et al., 2011; Lee et al., 2011). In both cases, the mice spontaneously developed EAE when

they were raised under SPF conditions but not when raised in a GF environment. We mentioned earlier that GF mice are deficient in Th17 cells that play a key role for the development of EAE. Transgenic mice carrying an anti-MOG transgenic T cell receptor were shown to have reduced levels of intestinal Th17 cells and increased levels of CD4$^+$CD25$^+$FoxP3$^+$ regulatory T cells (Berer et al., 2011; Lee et al., 2011).

Interestingly, there are no cross-reactions between MOG receptors and commensal bacteria, which suggest that these bacteria induce Th17 cells via an activation signal that is independent of the cognate antigen.

One can consider that EAE onset requires the presence of Th17 cells, itself contingent upon the presence of certain commensal bacteria. This would explain the different effects of the GF status on this autoimmune disease compared to other models such as diabetes where Th17 cells do not appear to be directly involved.

Experimental Arthritis

As early as 1979 it was shown that GF rats developed collagen-induced arthritis at a higher frequency than SPF rats while rats raised under conventional sanitary conditions did not develop the disease (Kohashi et al., 1979). It was confirmed in 1993 that the GF status increased the frequency of collagen-induced arthritis in rats along with an increased level of collagen autoantibodies (Breban et al., 1993).

These results seemed to be in apparent contradiction with the observation mentioned above made by the group of D. Mathis that K/BxN mice that developed a spontaneous arthritis in SPF conditions did not do so in GF conditions (Wu et al., 2010). This inflammatory arthritis model was based on the serendipitous observation of polyarthritis development in K/BxN mice bred from a cross between transgenic KRN-C57BL/6 mice, carrying a transgenic T cell receptor recognizing a bovine ribonuclease peptide, and NOD mice. The mice suffered from a polyarthritis that was, in many aspects, similar to human rheumatoid arthritis. Most interestingly, the pathophysiology of the disease involved autoantibodies, as proved by the fact that the disease could be induced in other mice by transfer of serum. Furthermore, the ability to develop arthritis in GF K/BxN mice was restored after colonization by SFB, which is known for its capacity to induce TH17 cells. Thus, as in the EAE model discussed above, the fact that this arthritis model is dependent on IL-17 might explain the absence of disease in the GF mice.

Murine Lupus

Two articles published years ago showed that the production of anti-nuclear antibodies and the development of lupus disease in NZB mice were inhibited under GF conditions (Unni et al., 1975; Mizutani et al., 2005). Why the production of antibodies is inhibited is not yet clearly understood. It can be hypothesized that the presence of commensal bacteria in this particular case could act to stimulate autoantibody production.

MICROBIOME COMPOSITION AND AUTOIMMUNE DISEASES

Metagenomics studies were applied to several diseases other than autoimmune diseases with interesting results. This subject is now the focus of intense research, especially within the last 2 years, as evident from the large number of recent publications.

The numerous data obtained for allergic and inflammatory bowel diseases will not be discussed here, even though some of them might help clarify the role of the microbiome in autoimmune diseases. Nor will we discuss type 2 diabetes, obesity, and the effect on the functioning of the central nervous system, which appear also to be affected by the intestinal microbiome. We shall concentrate herein on observations made within the context of autoimmune diseases. Although the number of patients analyzed is still limited, yet the information is valuable and deserves to be presented. Data are available mainly for two diseases, insulin-dependent (type 1) diabetes and rheumatoid arthritis. Overall, these studies converge on the idea that these two diseases are associated with decreased metagenome diversity.

Type 1 Diabetes

There has been only limited data published on the metagenome in NOD mice (Wen et al., 2008; Markle et al., 2013). None of these studies present a systematic comparison with normal control (non-autoimmune) mice. One article has been published on BB rats. This rat strain is known to develop insulin-dependent diabetes (designated DP rats, for diabetes prone) and is usually compared to genetically similar rats that are diabetes resistant (DR rats). A number of differences were found between the two rat strains; in particular a higher abundance of *Lactobacillus* and *Bifidobacterium* was observed in BB-DR rats (Roesch et al., 2009). The administration of two species of commensal bacteria isolated from the gut of BB-DR rats to BB-DP rats slowed or even inhibited the onset of autoimmune diabetes (Valladares et al., 2010). Interestingly, preliminary data suggested that an inhibition of indoleamine 2,3-dioxygenase (IDO), an enzyme involved in tryptophan catabolism and immune tolerance (Munn and Mellor, 2013), could be involved in the protective effect observed (Valladares et al., 2013). However, these experimental results should be interpreted cautiously since DR rats are

significantly genetically different from DP rats regarding genes other than those involved in diabetes susceptibility.

Four studies have been published on this topic in humans. All of them have found a lower Firmicutes/Bacteroidetes ratio in patients as compared to healthy control subjects. The first study (Brown et al., 2011) found that diabetic patients had a smaller quantity of butyrate-producing bacteria and more short chain fatty acid-producing bacteria resulting in non-optimal mucin synthesis. In another study (Giongo et al., 2011), the same group established a relationship between the composition of microbiota in children at high genetic risk for autoimmune diabetes and the development of the disease over time. The children who developed autoimmune diabetes had a less diverse and stable micobiome. A third study (Murri et al., 2013) showed a correlation between a decrease in the Firmicutes/Bacteroidetes ratio, in the *Bifidobacteria* and *Lactobacillus* species and an increase in plasma glucose levels in children with autoimmune diabetes. In the last study (deGoffau et al., 2013), Vaarala's group found that a smaller quantity of butyrate-producing bacteria such as *Bifidobacterium* was associated with changes in the intestinal epithelial barrier function in recently diagnosed diabetic children.

Rheumatoid Arthritis

Very few studies have examined the composition of the gut microbiota in rheumatoid arthritis (RA) patients. One study published in 2008 found that adult RA patients had fewer *Bifidobacteria* and *Bacteroides* than patients with fibromyalgia used as "controls"; however, the techniques used at the time were less sensitive than those available today (Vaahtovuo et al., 2008). A recent study by Liu et al. found that in patients with early RA the diversity and quantity of some *Lactobacillus* species were lower (Liu et al., 2013).

EFFECT OF PROBIOTICS ON AUTOIMMUNE DISEASES

We discussed in detail above that in some animal models, a GF environment accelerates the onset of an autoimmune disease. Moreover, autoimmune diseases are in some cases associated with a reduced diversity of the gut microbiome. It was therefore logical to study the protective effect of the "preventive/therapeutic" administration of commensal intestinal bacteria, designated as probiotics (by reference to their potential effect), in several experimental models of autoimmune disease. A distinction will be made between studies that use probiotic mixtures, such as those used in a clinical context, and those using a single well-defined probiotic species. This section will refer only to studies carried out on animals raised under physiological (SPF or conventional) sanitary conditions.

Studies involving GF animals, which for obvious reasons are outside the scope of translational approaches, have been discussed in a preceding section.

Probiotic Mixtures

The effect of probiotic mixtures administered orally to 4- to 6-week-old NOD mice was studied by several groups. Calcinaro et al. have shown that such a treatment prevents the onset of insulitis and diabetes (Calcinaro et al., 2005). Interestingly, this prevention was associated with an increased expression of IL-10 in the intestine and pancreas. Furthermore, the protective effect was shown to be of the active type since it could be transferred to untreated mice using spleen cells of protected treated mice. We ourselves have reported that the administration of probiotics (different from the ones used by Calcinaro et al.) induced an IL-10-dependent diabetes prevention in NOD mice (the prevention was no longer seen in mice treated with antibodies against the IL-10 receptor) (Aumeunier et al., 2010).

Several studies have shown that probiotics have a preventive effect on EAE. The best result was observed with a mixture of probiotics. The presence of several lactobacilli was necessary in this model. When used in isolation, none of the microorganisms was efficient in spite of the fact that some lactobacilli can stimulate certain regulatory IL-10 producing CD4$^+$CD25$^+$FoxP3$^+$ T cells (Lavasani et al., 2010). Another study confirmed the ability of a mixture of lactobacilli to prevent EAE with the added result that this prevention depended on the lactobacillus strains (Maasen and Claasen, 2008).

Specific Probiotics

Several studies recently demonstrated the beneficial effect of some commensal bacteria in the prevention or treatment of several autoimmune diseases.

As mentioned above, in BB rats, a delay in the onset of diabetes was observed when they were orally administered *Lactobacillus johnsonii N6.2*. There was concomitant suppression of some inflammation markers (like IDO) (Valladares et al., 2010, 2013).

In the EAE model, the administration of *Pediococcus acidilactici*, a lactic acid bacterium, reduced the severity of EAE when administered both prophylactically and therapeutically, mainly by increasing CD4$^+$FoxP3$^+$ IL-10-producing regulatory T cells in the mesenteric lymph nodes and spleens of treated mice (Takata et al., 2011).

In the collagen-induced arthritis model, two species of lactobacillus reduced the symptoms of the disease, mainly by inhibiting the proinflammatory environment (Amdekar et al., 2011; Nowak et al., 2012).

Inversely, the importance of commensal bacteria contribution to the onset of an autoimmune disease is yet to be determined. Two examples were mentioned in the previous section, EAE and arthritis in K/BxN mice. Their special characteristics compared to the models just discussed are that they involve IL-17-producing Th17 cells. In spontaneous diabetes models and collagen-induced arthritis, the involvement of Th17 cells does not seem to be so prominent, if at all significant. It is relevant to highlight, as we discussed in detail above, that both in EAE and K/BxN mice, probiotics are efficient essentially in GF mice.

Role of Toll-like Receptor Stimulation

A limited number of experimental data show that the probiotic protective effect is not found in mice genetically deficient for Toll-like receptors. Thus, a probiotic mixture lost its therapeutic efficacy in ovalbumine-induced allergy when administered to MyD88-/- NOD mice (Aumeunier et al., 2010). Data in autoimmune diseases are more difficult to collect because of the potential inhibition of the development of these diseases upon blockade of Toll-like receptor signaling, an effect probably due to opportunistic infections in these mice (Wen et al., 2008; Aumeunier et al., 2010).

THE RELATIONSHIP BETWEEN THE INTESTINAL MICROBIOME AND THE HYGIENE HYPOTHESIS

Brief Overview of the Hygiene Hypothesis

The frequency of infectious diseases has significantly diminished in the last four decades in Western countries. In parallel, during the same period of time, the frequency of allergic and autoimmune diseases has considerably increased, more than two-fold in the case of some allergic diseases. It has been tempting to correlate the two observations. This forms the basis of the hygiene hypothesis. According to this hypothesis, improved hygiene and advances in medicine in industrialized countries contributed to a reduction in infectious diseases that resulted in an increase in allergic and autoimmune diseases (Bach, 2002). The hypothesis was substantiated by many epidemiological data that showed in particular the existence of a geographical (north–south) gradient for allergic and autoimmune diseases correlated with socioeconomic conditions. It was also supported by experimental data in spontaneous or induced autoimmune disease models and induced allergy models.

In fact, the hypothesis is essentially based on two types of evidence, which we will discuss below in the case of autoimmune diseases, taking the example of insulin-dependent diabetes. These two types of data are:

the effect of hygiene on the onset of diabetes and the prevention of the disease by infections.

A Clean Environment Promotes the Onset of Autoimmune Diabetes

Experimental Data

The basic observation is well established. NOD SPF mice with a good health status, showing negative results for common microbiological tests, display a very high incidence (over 90%) of autoimmune diabetes, especially in females. The frequency rarely exceeds 50% in males but can reach 60 to 70% in some colonies. However, when mice are not raised in a "clean" (SPF) environment, the frequency of the disease is reduced to levels as low as 10% (Pozzilli et al., 1993; Bach, 2002). An essential point is that when animals are decontaminated at birth by cesarean section and then raised in an isolator, the frequency of the disease shoots up again to 90% in females as early as the first generation (Bach, 2002).

Data are less clear concerning GF mice that immediately after birth by cesarean section are maintained for a prolonged period of time in an isolator and fed a sterile diet. As discussed above in greater detail, depending on the study, a disease frequency comparable to that of SPF mice or higher has been reported (Suzuki et al., 1985; Wen et al., 2008; Alam et al., 2011; King and Sarvetnick, 2011; Markle et al., 2013). This variation in results is not really surprising since the GF status is heterogeneous and depends on the technical details pertaining to the handling of the mice. Furthermore, the GF status significantly affects the development of the immune system, as we discussed. This resulting immaturity of the immune system may interfere with the development of the disease.

Little data are available concerning the effect of antibiotics on the onset of diabetes in NOD mice. The first study published showed, paradoxically in the light of this chapter, a protective effect of vancomycin: However the treatment was applied at the late prediabetic stage (8 weeks), no effect in diabetes incidence was observed (Hansen et al., 2012). Nonetheless, the article published by Chervonsky's group showed that there was an increase in the frequency of diabetes in NOD MyD88$^{+/+}$ mice, a genetically modified mouse strain that normally does not develop the disease unless they were administered an antibiotic cocktail (Wen et al., 2008).

Human Data

There is a high frequency of the disease in populations with good hygiene.

A north–south gradient is observed for autoimmune diabetes, with a higher prevalence in northern countries, especially in Europe where epidemiological data are well documented (Bach, 2002). Some regional studies, in particular those carried out in the United Kingdom, have shown that the frequency of diabetes was directly linked to sanitary conditions (Patterson et al., 1996). Of particular interest is a study comparing disease frequency in the Karelian Republic of Russia and neighboring Finland. Although the two populations studied belong to the same ethnic group, the frequency of type 1 diabetes (and allergic diseases) is much lower in Karelian compared to Finnish people who enjoy a much higher social and economic level (Kondrashova et al., 2005). Interestingly, this difference in prevalence of type 1 diabetes is not associated with a different frequency of autoantibodies to β cells (Kondrashova et al., 2007).

In the same vein, data studying the incidence of disease according to the birth order points to the same conclusion. Insulin-dependent diabetes is more frequent in first-borns, who are less exposed to infections, than in the second, third, or fourth child who is, for obvious reasons, more exposed to intercurrent infections (Cardwell et al., 2005). These studies took into consideration the confounding factor represented by the increased diabetes incidence in off siblings (Bingley et al, 2000; Cardwell et al., 2005). The disease is also more frequent in children born by cesarean section than those born by natural birth which exposes them to an immediate contact with the vaginal microbiome of their mother (Cardwell et al., 2008).

Autoimmune Diseases Can be Prevented by Infections With a Pathogen

Experimental Data

Numerous articles have reported prevention of insulin-dependent diabetes in NOD mice by early administration of pathogens (Bach, 2002; Shoda et al., 2005). The pathogens can be bacteria but also viruses and parasites, an important point concerning the intestinal microbiome. Among the bacteria, some are enteric and others not, such as mycobacteria (Sadelain et al., 1990; Qin and Singh, 1997).

The protective effect of infectious agents, in particular bacteria, does not require the administration of live agents. It can be observed using bacterial extracts. In the latter case, it has been shown that protection is maintained in IL-4 genetically deficient mice but not in mice where transforming growth factor (TGF)β has been neutralized by a specific antibody (Alyanakian et al., 2006). Protection can also be observed when using bacterial ligands for many Toll-like receptors (Aumeunier et al., 2010).

Human Data

Prevention of type 1 diabetes by infection with pathogens has not been documented in humans for obvious reasons.

The issue is compounded by the fact that in humans, the onset of the disease is sudden whereas in mice and rats, the natural course of the disease can be monitored and early intervention is possible. Furthermore, an infection can temporarily increase insulin needs and give the impression that diabetes has been triggered when what is revealed is an already existing deficit in insulin production by β cells.

The only data available on humans regarding type 1 diabetes are preliminary. They concern the BCG and Q-fever vaccinations (Elliott et al., 1998; Allen et al., 1999; Faustman et al., 2012). No tangible results were reported in spite of a significant effect observed in NOD mice (Qin and Singh, 1997; Silva et al., 2003). The discrepancy can be explained by differences in the protocols used in humans and mice.

More convincing results have been obtained for other immune diseases in the context of the hygiene hypothesis, in particular for allergic diseases, multiple sclerosis, and inflammatory bowel diseases. Several studies have demonstrated the protective effect of certain porcine parasites (*Trichuris suis*) (Benzel et al., 2012) and probiotic preparations used mostly in the treatment of inflammatory intestinal diseases, atopic dermatitis, and, to a lesser degree, asthma (Kalliomaki et al., 2001; Cordina et al., 2011; Fedorak and Demeria, 2012; Pelucchi et al., 2012).

SYNTHESIS AND CONCLUSIONS

Infectious agents, whether they are commensals or pathogens, may influence the development of autoimmune diseases in a contrasted fashion, either by stimulating, by triggering them or by slowing them down. The stimulatory effect may involve commensal bacteria, as in the example of the SFB in EAE. However, most often the stimulating effect seems rather to involve pathogens, whether bacteria or viruses. The question is more open for the protective effect, since there are strong arguments for both commensal bacteria and pathogenic infectious agents. A possible common denominator of commensal and pathogenic bacteria could be the presence of Toll-like receptor ligands in both types of agents, as indicated by the loss of the protective effect in genetically Toll-like receptor-deficient mice and by the protection afforded by synthetic Toll-like receptor agonists.

The relative loss of this protective effect in recent decades seems due for both commensal bacteria and pathogens to improved hygiene and medicine in developed countries. The fact that environmental hygiene affects both the composition of the intestinal microbiome and the rate of infections in the first years of life in humans, complicates the discussion that is the focus of this chapter, namely, the respective role of commensal bacteria and pathogens in the protective effect.

Another important issue related to the previous one is whether the protective effect operates in the first days or weeks of life or, conversely, if it can also apply later in childhood. Another central question, which concerns both commensal bacteria and pathogens, is to what extent there is a causal link between the qualitative and quantitative variations of bacterial populations and the evolution of the frequency of autoimmune diseases. In other words, do the bacteria directly influence the occurrence of autoimmune diseases or are these two correlated yet independent events, possibly under the control of a single process, most probably of immunologic nature, whose cellular and molecular mechanisms remain to be determined.

The Strength of the Protective Effect of Pathogens

A fact can be taken for granted: pathogens can induce protection *vis-à-vis* autoimmune diseases even if exposure to the pathogen in question occurs after the second or third year of life in humans, without being able to say what the age limit is beyond which the protective effect no longer occurs.

Some epidemiological evidence, particularly in multiple sclerosis, but also in allergic diseases, would tend to suggest that this age limit could be between five to fifteen years. Thus, when one follows the families of migrants from countries with a low incidence of multiple sclerosis to countries with a high incidence, the protective effect of infectious diseases that manifested itself in the country of origin no longer takes place if the migration occurs after the child reached fifteen years of age (Dean and Elian, 1997). Similar studies in allergic asthma have indicated that the age limit is about five years of age (Kuehni et al., 2007).

Importantly, the pathogens responsible for protection do not involve the intestine for some of them, as is the case in particular for mycobacteria and, more generally, for infectious agents affecting the respiratory tract. All is not as clear on this subject as we are still not able to determine among the myriad of potential pathogens, which are the protective ones and, especially, what are the mechanisms involved in their protective effect. The current state of knowledge indicates that there are several possible mechanisms and that they are likely to differ according to the pathogen or, in any case, according to the constituent of the pathogen responsible for the protection. These comments concerning the pathogens are mainly based on experimental models in which there is ample evidence that deliberate infection by a pathogen (bacteria, virus, or parasite) can completely prevent the occurrence of a spontaneous or induced autoimmune disease, even when the infection occurs in animals as adults.

We cannot exclude that commensal agents, which may act as probiotics, may also have a protective effect outside the postnatal period. Clinical trials conducted with probiotics in certain immune diseases provide some arguments in this direction. It must be recognized, however, that the therapeutic effect is modest, challenged in allergic diseases, and virtually undocumented in autoimmune diseases.

The Ambiguous Effect on Autoimmune Disease of the GF or Axenic Status

The increase in the frequency or severity of certain autoimmune diseases in GF or SPF animals compared to conventionally raised animals is, of course, very important for our present discussion. It is, however, subject to different interpretation problems. The question is not so much that of the differences that may exist between GF and SPF animals, insofar as (1) GF and SPF conditions may vary depending on the laboratory and (2) disease frequency often does not differ much in GF and SPF animals.

The main problem, in fact, at least for GF animals, is the already mentioned risk of distorting the interpretation of the results by the consequences of the GF status on the maturation of the immune system. One can indeed think that depending on the nature of the immune deficiency related to the GF status, which may relate to regulatory or effector lymphocytes, there may be a positive or negative change in the severity of the autoimmune disease. This applies to both neonatal antibiotic treatments, which are usually pursued long enough, and to GF mice derived by cesarean section. This is indeed what is seen in experimental models where one can observe in GF mice an increase (diabetes, arthritis) or a decrease (EAE) of the disease.

The Delicate Interpretation of the Reduction in the Diversity of the Intestinal Microbiome

Although the results are still limited, one cannot avoid being struck by the frequency of the reduction in the diversity of the composition of the gut microbiome in autoimmune diseases in humans. The animal data are less numerous due to the limited number of models of spontaneous autoimmune diseases.

These results are impressive, especially when they are compared with those obtained in allergic diseases (Bisgaard et al., 2011; Yap et al., 2011; Abrahamsson et al., 2012). Furthermore, experimental results have shown a clear increase of allergic reactions after neonatal treatment with some antibiotics (i.e., vancomycin but not streptomycin)

that lead to different changes in the gut microbiome composition (Russell et al., 2012).

The case of inflammatory bowel diseases is also interesting yet complicated because these appear to involve immune reactions against intestinal bacteria that cause the lesions and clinical signs observed as well as a protective effect by commensals through mechanisms mentioned above. Some studies have distinguished these two categories of bacteria without dismissing an overlap between them and without clarifying which category each bacterium belongs to (Kverka and Tlaskalova-Hogenova, 2013). A particularly good example is that of ulcerative colitis where clear anomalies in the composition of the metagenome have been observed (Dusko Ehrlich, 2010). Another interesting example is that of Crohn's disease. A study has shown that bacterium *Faecalibacterium prausnitzii* usually found in normal individuals was missing in affected patients. Interestingly, this bacterium has been shown to have an immunomodulating activity inhibiting the progression of experimental inflammatory colitis in mice (Sokol et al., 2008). However, it remains to be proven that an altered microbiome contributes to the pathophysiology of these diseases and is not rather a consequence of the disease or a concomitant characteristic of the disease state *per se* or of the individual.

Perspectives

Following these discussions, beyond the etiological, epidemiological, and pathophysiological considerations, the question arises whether we may expect some therapeutic benefits of the protective effect of commensals or infectious agents in autoimmune diseases.

With regard to commensal bacteria, we can of course discuss the possibility of administering probiotics, either mixtures of probiotics or specific bacteria. It must be recognized, however, that the results currently available, although some are encouraging, were mostly obtained in some experimental models of autoimmunity and in a few allergic diseases in man. Perhaps one could refine the use of probiotics by calibrating mixtures and especially identifying bacteria with abilities well demonstrated to slow the progression of a given autoimmune disease. Maybe we could also consider performing transplants of microbiome as it has already been done in mice presenting spontaneous autoimmune diabetes (Markle et al., 2013). The technique of transplantation of microbiome has been used in humans in cases of serious infection by *Clostridium difficile*, resistant to any treatment (Kassam et al., 2013), and could be extended to other indications, inasmuch the safety has been carefully verified. More simply one could use bacterial extracts, as we did in mice (Alyanakian et al., 2006). One may also consider using synthetic chemicals such as Toll-like receptor agonists for which we have shown a beneficial effect in autoimmune diseases and allergies in experimental models (Aumeunier et al., 2010).

In brief, a completely new, evolving, and fascinating field based on modern concepts and technologies, which may propel a conceptual revolution in our understanding of the pathophysiology, etiology, and therapeutic management of autoimmune diseases, provided more data are accumulated and validated.

ACKNOWLEDGMENTS

The work conducted in the laboratory of Prof. J.F. Bach on hygiene hypothesis and the microbiome is supported by a European Research Council Grant: Project ERC "Hygiene," 250290, ERC-2009-AgG; A.-P. is funded by Project ERC "Hygiene," 250290.

REFERENCES

Abrahamsson, T.R., Jakobsson, H.E., Anderson, A.F., Bjorksten, B., Engstrandand, L., Jenmalm, M.C., 2012. Low diversity of the gut microbiota in infants with atopic eczema. J. Allergy Clin. Immunol. 129, 434–440.

Alam, C., Bittoun, E., Bhagwat, D., Valkonen, S., Saari, A., Jaakkola, U., et al., 2011. Effects of a germ-free environment on gut immune regulation and diabetes progression in non-obese diabetic (NOD) mice. Diabetologia. 54, 1398–1406.

Allen, H.F., Klingensmith, G.J., Jensen, P., Simoes, E., Hayward, A., Chase, H.P., 1999. Effect of bacillus Calmette-Guerin vaccination on new onset type 1 diabetes. A randomized clinical study. Diabetes Care. 22, 1703–1707.

Alyanakian, M.A., Grela, F., Aumeunier, A., Chiavaroli, C., Gouarin, C., Bardel, E., et al., 2006. Transforming growth factor-beta and natural killer T-cells are involved in the protective effect of a bacterial extract on type 1 diabetes. Diabetes. 55, 179–185.

Amdekar, S., Singh, V., Singh, R., Sharma, P., Keshav, P., Kumar, A., 2011. Lactobacillus casei reduces the inflammatory joint damage associated with collagen-induced arthritis (CIA) by reducing the pro-inflammatory cytokines, Lactobacillus casei, COX-2 inhibitor. J. Clin. Immunol. 31, 147–154.

Atarashi, K., Tanoue, T., Shima, T., Imaoka, A., Kuwahara, T., Momose, Y., et al., 2011. Induction of colonic regulatory T cells by indigenous Clostridium species. Science. 331, 337–341.

Aumeunier, A., Grela, F., Ramadan, A., Pham Van, L., Bardel, E., Gomez Alcala, A., et al., 2010. Systemic toll like receptor stimulation suppresses experimental allergic asthma and autoimmune diabetes in NOD mice. PLoS One. 5, e11484.

Bach, J.F., 2002. The effect of infections on susceptibility to autoimmune and allergic diseases. N. Engl. J. Med. 347, 911–920.

Benzel, F., Erdur, H., Kohler, S., Frentsch, M., Thiel, A., Harms, L., et al., 2012. Immune monitoring of Trichuris suis egg therapy in multiple sclerosis patients. J. Helminthol. 86, 339–347.

Berer, K., Mues, M., Koutroulos, M., Rasbi, Z.A., Johner, C., Wekerle, H., et al., 2011. Commensal microbiota and myelin autoantigen cooperate to trigger autoimmune demyelination. Nature. 479, 438–541.

Bingley, P.J., Douek, F., Rogers, C.A., Gale, E.A., 2000. Influence of maternal age at delivery and birth order on risk of type 1 diabetes in childhood, prospective population based family study. Bart's Oxford Family Study Group. BMJ. 321, 420–424.

Bisgaard, H., Li, N., Bonnelykke, K., Chawes, B.L., Skov, T., Paludan-Müller, G., et al., 2011. Reduced diversity of the intestinal microbiota during infancy is associated with increased risk of allergic disease at school age. J. Allergy Clin. Immunol. 128, 646–652.

Breban, M.A., Moreau, M.C., Fournier, C., Ducluzeau, R., Kahn, M.F., 1993. Influence of the bacterial flora on collagen-induced arthritis in susceptible and resistant strains of rats. Clin. Exp. Rheumatol. 11, 61–64.

Brown, C.T., Davis-Richardson, A.G., Giongo, A., Gano, K.A., Crabb, D.B., Mukherjee, N., et al., 2011. Gut microbiome metagenomics analysis suggests a functional model for the development of autoimmunity for type 1 diabetes. PLoS One. 6, e25792.

Calcinaro, F., Dionisi, S., Marinaro, M., Candeloro, P., Bomato, V., Marzotti, S., et al., 2005. Oral probiotic administration induces interleukin-10 production and prevents spontaneous autoimmune diabetes in the non-obese diabetic mouse. Diabetologia. 48, 1565–1575.

Cardwell, C.R., Carson, D.J., Patterson, C.C., 2005. Parental age at delivery, birth order, birth weight and gestational age are associated with the risk of childhood type 1 diabetes, a UK regional retrospective cohort study. Diabet. Med. 22, 200–206.

Cardwell, C.R., Stene, L.C., Joner, G., Cinek, O., Svensson, J., Goldacre, M.J., et al., 2008. Caesarean section is associated with an increased risk of childhood-onset type 1 diabetes mellitus, a meta-analysis of observational studies. Diabetologia. 51, 726–735.

Chervonsky, A.V., 2013. Micrbiota and autoimmunity. Cold Spring Harb. Perspect. Biol.5.

Chinen, T., Volchkov, P.Y., Chervonsky, A.V., Rudensky, A.Y., 2010. A critical role for regulatory T cell-mediated control of inflammation in the absence of commensal microbiota. J. Exp. Med. 207, 2323–2330.

Cho, I., Blaser, M.J., 2012. The human microbiome, at the interface of health and disease. Nat. Rev. Genet. 13, 260–270.

Cordina, C., Shaikh, I., Shrestha, S., Camilleri-Brebnnan, J., 2011. Probiotics in the management of gastrointestinal disease, analysis of the attitudes and prescribing practices of gastroenterologists and surgeons. J. Dig. Dis. 12, 489–496.

Dean, G., Elian, M., 1997. Age at immigration to England of Asian and Caribbean immigrants and the risk of developing multiple sclerosis. J. Neurol. Neurosurg. Psychiatry. 63, 565–568.

DeFilippo, C., Cavalieri, D., Di Paola, M., Ramazzotti, M., Poullet, J.B., Massart, S., et al., 2010. Impact of diet in shaping gut microbiota revealed by a comparative study in children from Europe and rural Africa. Proc. Natl. Acad. Sci. U.S.A. 107, 14691–14696.

Dusko Ehrlich, S., 2010. Metagenomics of the intestinal microbiota, potential applications. Gastroenterol. Clin. Biol. 34 (Suppl 1), S23–S28.

Elliott, J.F., Marlin, K.L., Couch, R.M., 1998. Effect of bacilli Calmette-Guerin vaccination on C-peptide secretion in children newly diagnosed with IDDM. Diabetes Care. 21, 1691–1693.

Faustman, D.L., Wang, L., Okubo, Y., Burger, D., Ban, L., Man, G., et al., 2012. Proof of concept, randomized, controlled clinical trial of Bacillus-Calmette-Guerin for treatment of long-term type 1 diabetes. PLoS One. 7, e41756.

Fedorak, R., Demeria, D., 2012. Probiotic bacteria in the prevention and the treatment of inflammatory bowel disease. Gastroenterol. Clin. North Am. 41, 821–842.

Gaboriau-Routhiau, V., Rakotobe, S., Lécuyer, E., Mulder, I., Lan, A., Bridonneau, C., et al., 2009. The key role of segmented filamentous bacteria in the coordinated maturation of gut helper T-cell responses. Immunity. 31, 677–689.

Geddes, K., Rubino, S.J., Magalhaes, J.G., Streutker, C., Le Bourhis, L., Cho, J.H., et al., 2011. Identification of an innate T helper type 17 response to intestinal bacterial pathogens. Nat. Med. 17, 837–844.

Giongo, A., Gano, K.A., Crabb, D.B., Mukherjee, N., Novelo, L.L., Casella, G., et al., 2011. Toward defining the autoimmune microbiome for type 1 diabetes. ISME J. 5, 82–91.

deGoffau, M.C., Luopajarvi, K., Knip, M., Honen, J., Ruohtula, T., Harkonen, T., et al., 2013. Fecal microbiota composition differs between children with beta-cell autoimmunity and those without. Diabetes. 62, 1238–1244.

Goverman, J., 2009. Autoimmune T cell responses in the central nervous system. Nat. Rev. Immunol. 9, 393–407.

Hansen, C., Krych, H.L., Nielsen, D.S., Vogensen, F.K., Hansen, L.H., Sorensen, S.J., et al., 2012. Early life treatment with vancomycin propogates Akkermansia muciniphila and reduces diabetes incidence in the NOD mouse. Diabetologia. 55, 2285–2294.

Ivanov, I.I., Atarashi, K., Manel, N., Brodie, E.L., Shima, T., Karaoz, U., et al., 2009. Induction of intestinal Th17 cells by segmented filamentous bacteria. Cell. 139, 485–498.

Kalliomaki, M., Salminen, S., Arvilommi, H., Kero, P., Koskinen, P., Isolauri, E., 2001. Probiotics in primary prevention of atopic disease, a randomized placebo-controlled trial. Lancet. 357, 1076–1079.

Kassam, Z., Lee, C.H., Yaun, Y., Hunt, R.H., 2013. Fecal microbiota transplantation for clostridium difficile infection. Systemic review and meta-analysis. Am. J. Gastroenterol. 108, 500–508.

King, C., Sarvetnick, N., 2011. The incidence of type 1 diabetes in NOD mice is modulated by restricted flora not germ-free conditions. PLos One. 6, e17049.

Kohashi, O., Kuwata, J., Umehara, K., Uemura, F., Takahashi, T., Ozawa, A., 1979. Susceptibility to adjuvant-induced arthritis among germ free, specific-pathogen-free, and conventional rats. Infect. Immun. 26, 791–794.

Kondrashova, A., Reunanen, A., Romanov, A., Karvonen, A., Viskari, H., Vesikari, T., et al., 2005. A six-fold gradient in the incidence of type 1 diabetes at the eastern border of Finland. Ann. Med. 37, 67–72.

Kondrashova, A., Viskari, H., Kulmala, P., Romanov, A., Honen, J., Hyoty, H., et al., 2007. Signs of beta-cell autoimmunity in nondiabetic school children a comparison between Russian Karelia with a low incidence of type 1 diabetes and Finland with a high incidence rate. Diabetes Care. 30, 95–100.

Kriegel, M.A., Sefik, E., Hill, J.A., Wu, H.J., Benoist, C., Mathis, D., 2011. Naturally transmitted segmented filamentous bacteria segregate with diabetes protection in nonobese diabetic mice. Proc. Natl. Acad. Sci. U.S.A. 108, 11548–11553.

Kuehni, C.E., Strippoli, M.P., Low, N., Silverman, M., 2007. Asthma in young south Asian women living in the United Kingdom: the importance of early life. Clin. Exp. Allergy. 37, 47–53.

Kverka, M., Tlaskalova-Hogenova, H., 2013. Two faces of microbiota in inflammatory and autoimmune diseases, triggers and drugs. APMIS. 121, 403–421.

Lavasani, S., Dzhambazov, B., Fak, M.F., Buske, S., Molin, G., Thorlacius, H., et al., 2010. A novel probiotic mixture exerts a therapeutic effect on experimental autoimmune encephalomyelitis mediated by IL-10 producing regulatory T cells. PLoS One. 5, e9009.

Lee, Y.K., Menezes, J.S., Umesaki, Y., Mazmanian, S.K., 2011. Proinflammatory T-cell responses to gut microbiota promote experimental autoimmune encephalomyelitis. Proc. Natl. Acad. Sci. U.S. A. 108 (Suppl. 1), 4615–4622.

Li, R., Zhu, H., Ruan, J., Qian, W., Fang, X., Shi, Z., et al., 2010. De novo assembly of human genomes with massively parallel short read sequencing. Genome Res. 20, 265–272.

Liu, X., Zou, Q., Zeng, B., Fang, Y., Wei, H., 2013. Analysis of fecal lactobacillus community structure in patients with early rheumatoid arthritis. Curr. Microbiol. 67, 170–176.

Maasen, C.B., Claasen, E., 2008. Strain-dependent effects of probiotic lactobacilli on EAE autoimmunity. Vaccine. 26, 2056–2057.

Marguiles, M., Egholm, M., Altman, W.E., Attiya, S., Bader, J.S., Bemben, L.A., et al., 2005. Genome sequencing in microfabricated high-density picolitre reactors. Nature. 437, 376–380.

Markle, J.G., Frank, D.N., Mortin-Toth, S., Robertson, C.E., Feazel, L. M., Rolle-Kampczyk, U., et al., 2013. Sex differences in the gut microbiome drive hormone-dependent regulation of autoimmunity. Science. 339, 1084–1088.

Martin, R., Nauta, A.J., Ben Amor, K., Knippels, L.M., Knol, J., Garssen, J., 2010. Early life, gut microbiota and immune development in infancy. Benef. Microbes. 1, 267–382.

Mathis, D., Benoist, C., 2011. Microbiota and autoimmune disease: the hosted self. Cell Host Microbe. 10, 297–301.

Mizutani, A., Shaheen, V.M., Yoshida, H., Akaogi, J., Kuroda, Y., Nacionales, D.C., et al., 2005. Pristane-induced autoimmunity in germ free mice. Clin. Immunol. 114, 110–118.

Molloy, M.J., Bouladoux, N., Belkaid, Y., 2012. Intestinal microbiota, shaping local and systemic immune responses. Semin. Immunol. 24, 58–66.

Mulder, I.E., Schmidt, B., Stokes, C.R., Lewis, M., Bailey, M., Aminov, R.I., et al., 2009. Environmentally-acquired bacteria influence microbial diversity and natural innate immune responses at gut surfaces. BMC Biol. 7, 79.

Munn, D.H., Mellor, A.L., 2013. Indoleamine 2,3 dioxygenase and metabolic control of immune responses. Trends Immunol. 34, 137–143.

Murri, M., Leiva, I., Gomez-Zumaquero, J.M., Cardona, F., Soriguer, F., Tinahones, F.J., et al., 2013. Gut microbiota in children with type 1 diabetes differs from that in healthy children, a case control study. BMC Med. 11, 46.

Nagano, Y., Itoh, K., Honda, K., 2012. The induction of Treg cells by gut-indigenous Clostridium. Curr. Opin. Immunol. 24, 392–397.

Nowak, B., Ciszek-Lenda, M., Sróttek, M., Gamian, A., Kontny, E., Górska-Frączek, S., et al., 2012. Lactobacillus rhamnosus exopolysaccharide ameliorates arthritis induced by the systemic injection of collagen and lipopolysaccharide in DBA/1 mice. Arch. Immunol. Ther. Exp. (Warz). 60, 211–220.

Ochoa-Reparaz, J., Ivanov, I.I., Darce, J., Hattori, K., Shima, T., Umesaki, Y., et al., 2009. Role of gut commensal microflora in the development of experimental autoimmune encephalomyelitis. J. Immunol. 183, 6041–6050.

Ochoa-Repáraz, J., Mielcarz, D.W., Wang, Y., Begum-Haque, S., Dasgupta, S., Kasper, D.L., et al., 2010. A polysaccharide from the human commensal Bacteroides fragilis protects against CNS demyelinating disease. Mucosal Immunol. 3, 487–495.

Patterson, C.C., Carson, D.J., Hadden, D.R., 1996. Epidemiology of childhood IDDM in Northern Ireland 1989–1994, low incidence in areas with highest population density and most household crowding. Northern Ireland Diabetes Study Group. Diabetologia. 39, 1063–1069.

Pelucchi, C., Chatenoud, L., Turati, F., Galeone, C., Moja, L., Bach, J. F., et al., 2012. Probiotics supplementation during pregnancy or infancy for the prevention of atopic dermatitis, a meta-analysis. Epidemiology. 23, 402–414.

Pflughoeft, K.J., Versalovic, J., 2012. Human microbiome in health and disease. Annu. Rev. Pathol. 7, 99–122.

Pozzilli, P., Signore, A., Williams, A.J., Beales, P.E., 1993. NOD mouse colonies around the world—recent facts and figures. Immunol. Today. 14, 193–196.

Proal, A.D., Albert, P.J., Marshall, T., 2009. Autoimmune disease in the era of the metagenome. Autoimmun. Rev. 8, 677–681.

Qin, H.Y., Singh, B., 1997. BCG vaccination prevents insulin-dependent diabetes mellitus (IDDM) in NOD mice after disease acceleration with cyclophosphamide. J. Autoimmun. 10, 271–278.

Reid, G., Younes, J.A., Van der Mei, H.C., Gloor, G.B., Knight, R., Busscher, H.J., 2011. Microbiota restoration. Natural and supplemented recovery of human microbial communities. Nat. Rev. Microbiol. 9, 27–38.

Roesch, L.F., Lorca, G.L., Casella, G., Giongo, A., Naranjo, A., Pionzio, A. M., et al., 2009. Culture-independent identification of gut bacteria correlated with the onset of diabetes in a rat model. ISME J. 3, 536–548.

Round, J.L., Mazmanian, S.K., 2009. The gut microbiota shapes intestinal immune responses during health and disease. Nat. Rev. Immunol. 9, 313–323.

Round, J.L., Mazmanian, S.K., 2010. Inducible Fox3+ regulatory T-cell development by a commensal bacterium of the intestinal microbiota. Proc. Natl. Acad. Sci. U.S.A. 107, 12204–12209.

Russell, S.L., Gold, M.J., Hartmann, M., Willing, B.P., Thorson, L., Wlodarska, M., et al., 2012. Early life antibiotic-driven changes in microbiota enhance susceptibility to allergic asthma. EMBO Rep. 13, 440–447.

Sadelain, M., Qin, W.H.Y., Sumoski, W., Parfrey, N., Singh, B., Rabinovitch, A., 1990. Prevention of diabetes in the BB rat by early immunotherapy using Freund's adjuvant. J. Autoimmun. 3, 671–680.

Schmidt, B., Mulder, I.E., Musk, C.C., Aminov, R.I., Lewis, M., Stokes, C.R., et al., 2011. Establishemnt of normal gut microbiota is comprised under excessive hygiene conditions. PLoS One. 6, 28284.

Shanahan, F., 2013. The colonic microbiota in health and disease. Curr. Opin. Gastroenterol. 29, 49–54.

Shoda, L.K., Young, D.L., Ramanujan, S., Whiting, C.C., Atkinson, M. A., Bluestone, J.A., et al., 2005. A comprehensive review of interventions in the NOD mouse and implications for translation. Immunity. 23, 115–126.

Silva, D.G., Charlton, B., Cowden, W., Petrovsky, N., 2003. Prevention of autoimmune diabetes through immunostimulation with Q fever complement-fixing antigen. Ann. N.Y. Acad. Sci. 1005, 423–430.

Sokol, H., Pigneur, B., Watterlot, L., Lakhdari, O., Bermúdez-Humarán, L.G., Gratadoux, J.J., et al., 2008. Faecalibacterium prausnitzii is an anti-inflammatory commensal bacterium identified by gut microbiota analysis of Crohn disease patients. Proc. Natl. Acad. Sci. U.S.A. 105, 16731–16736.

Suzuki, T., Yagmado, T., Takao, T., Fujimura, T., Kawamura, E., Shimizu, M., et al., 1985. Effects of lymphocyte transfusion of the NOD or NOD nude mouse. In: Rygaard, J.B.N., Graem, N., Spang-Thomsen, M. (Eds.), Immune Deficient Animals in Biomedical Research. Karger Basel.

Takata, K., Kinoshita, M., Okuno, T., Moriya, M., Kohda, T., Honorat, J.A., et al., 2011. The lactic acid bacterium Pediococcus acidilactici suppresses autoimmune encephalomyelitis by inducing IL-10 producing regulatory T cells. PLoS One. 6, e27644.

Taniguchi, H., Makino, S., Ikegami, H., 2007. The NOD mouse and its related strains. In: Shafrir, E. (Ed.), Animal Models of Diabetes, Frontiers in Research, second ed. CRC Press. pp. 41–60.

Tlaskalova-Hogenova, H., Sterzl, J., Stepankova, R., Blabac, V., Veticka, V., Rossmann, P., et al., 1983. Development of immunological capacity under germfree and conventional conditions. Ann. N. Y. Acad. Sci. 409, 96–113.

Tlaskalova-Hogenova, H., Stepankova, R., Kozakova, H., Hudcovic, T., Vannucci, L., Tuckova, L., et al., 2011. The role of gut microbiota (commensal bacteria) and the mucosal barrier in the pathogenesis of inflammatory and autoimmune diseases and cancer, contribution of germ-free and gnotobiotic animal models of human diseases. Cell. Mol. Immunol. 8, 110–120.

Unni, K.K., Holley, K.E., McDuffie, F.C., Titus, J.L., 1975. Comparative study of NZB mice under germfree and conventional conditions. J. Rheumatol. 2, 35–44.

Vaahtovuo, J., Munukka, E., Korkeamaki, M., Luukkainen, R., Toivanen, P., 2008. Fecal microbiota in early rheumatoid arthritis. J. Rheumatol. 35, 1500–1505.

Valladares, R., Bojilova, L., Potts, A.H., Cameron, E., Gardner, C., Lorca, G., et al., 2013. Lactobacillus johnsonii inhibits indooleamine 2,3 dioxygenase and alters tryptophan metabolite levels in BioBreeding rats. FASEB J. 27, 1711–1720.

Valladares, R.D., Sankar, N., Li, E., Williams, K.K., Lai, A.S., Abdelgeliel, C.F., et al., 2010. Lactobacillus johnsonii N6.2 mitigates the development of type 1 diabetes in BB-DP rats. PLoS One. 5, c10507.

Wen, L., Ley, R.E., Volchkov, P.Y., Stranges, P.B., Avanesyan, L., Stonebaker, A.C., et al., 2008. Innate immunity and intestinal microbiota in the development of type 1 diabetes. Nature. 455, 1109–1113.

Wu, H., Ivanov II, J., Darce, J., Hattori, K., Shima, T., Umesaki, Y., et al., 2010. Gut-residing segmented filamentous bacteria drive autoimmune arthritis via T helper 17 cells. Immunity. 32, 815–827.

Yap, G.C., Chee, K.K., Hong, P.Y., Lay, C., Satria, C.D., Sumadiono, Soenarto, Y., et al., 2011. Evaluation of stool microbiota signatures in two cohorts of Asian (Singapore and Indonesia) newborns at risk of atopy. BMC Microbiol. 11, 193.

Chapter 26

Genetic Predisposition, Humans

Margaret A. Jordan[1], Judith Field[2], Helmut Butzkueven[3], and Alan G. Baxter[1]

[1]Comparative Genomics Centre, James Cook University, Townsville, Queensland, Australia, [2]Florey Institute of Neuroscience and Mental Health, Melbourne Brain Centre, The University of Melbourne, Parkville, Victoria, Australia, [3]Department of Medicine, Royal Melbourne, Parkville, Victoria, Australia

Chapter Outline

Introduction 342
Diseases of Interest 342
  Type 1 Diabetes 342
  Multiple Sclerosis 342
  Systemic Lupus Erythematosus 342
Human Leukocyte Antigen (HLA) Complex and other Candidate Genes 343
  Association of Type 1 Diabetes with HLA and other Candidate Genes 343
    INS 343
    PTPN22 344
  Association of Multiple Sclerosis with HLA and other Candidate Genes 344
  Association of Lupus with HLA and other Candidate Genes 345
    TNF 345
    C4A, C4B 345
    C2 345
    C1Q 346
    FCGR2A, FCGR3A, FCGR3B 346
    IRF5 346
  Mechanisms of Complement and Fc Associations with Autoimmunity 346
  Mechanisms of HLA Association with Autoimmunity 347
Gene Linkage Studies of Autoimmunity 347
  Linkage Studies of Type 1 Diabetes 347
    CTLA4 347
    CD25 348
    Other Loci 348
  Linkage Analyses of Combined Datasets and the Limits of Linkage Analyses 348

Linkage Studies in Multiple Sclerosis 349
Linkage Studies in Lupus 349
  TNFR1, TNFR2, LTBR 350
  STAT4 350
  Racial Heterogeneity in Systemic Lupus Erythematosus 350
Genome-Wide Association Studies of Autoimmunity 351
  Genome-Wide Association Studies of Type 1 Diabetes 351
    IFIH1 351
    IL2 352
    IL10 352
    CD69 352
  Genome-Wide Association Studies of Multiple Sclerosis 352
    CD25 352
    IL7R 352
    CD58 353
    CYP27B1 353
    CD40 353
    TNFRSF1A 353
    IRF8 353
    CD6 354
    IL12B 354
  Genome-Wide Association Studies of Systemic Lupus Erythematosus 354
    ITGAM 354
    PHRF1 355
    BLK 355
From Location to Molecular Mechanisms 355
Concluding Comments 356
Acknowledgments 356
References 356

N. Rose & I. Mackay (Eds): The Autoimmune Diseases, Fifth edition. DOI: http://dx.doi.org/10.1016/B978-0-12-384929-8.00026-5

INTRODUCTION

All common autoimmune diseases are complex genetic traits. That is, they result from a combination of many risk factors—genetic, environmental, and stochastic—each contributing a relatively small degree of risk. They are subject to genocopies (a genotype at one locus contributing to the risk of disease in a manner indistinguishable from that produced by another genotype and/or locus) and phenocopies (an environmental factor mimicking the effects of a susceptibility gene). A consequence of this is that the disease phenotype is only a weak predictor of the presence of a particular susceptibility allele. As this association underlies all current genetic approaches, the identification of susceptibility genes in complex disease traits is both practically and technologically challenging.

The main benefits of genetic studies of autoimmunity are to: (1) provide informed genetic counseling; (2) develop improved models for risk prediction; and (3) develop detailed molecular models of etiology and pathogenesis. As a generalization, the first benefit arose from work prior to the 1990s; the second has, in part, been achieved already; and the third remains a major scientific challenge.

DISEASES OF INTEREST

In any genetic study, clinical definition is critical since clinical heterogeneity associated with allelic differences weakens the statistical power. Here, we will concentrate primarily on progress in the genetics of type 1 (autoimmune) diabetes (T1D), multiple sclerosis (MS), and systemic lupus erythematosus (SLE, lupus).

Type 1 Diabetes

T1D is an endocrine disease that results from autoimmune destruction of the insulin-producing β-cells in the pancreas, leading to a loss of insulin secretion and hyperglycemia resulting in osmotic diuresis and the symptoms of polyuria, polydipsia, polyphagia, tiredness, and loss of weight. Potentially fatal complications include ketoacidosis and hyperglycaemic coma. Progression from the preclinical stage of β-cell autoimmunity (insulitis) to established diabetes can take up to a decade (Johnston et al., 1989; Bonifacio et al., 1990). Diagnostically, the major confusion is with latent autoimmune diabetes of adults (LADA), which is of later onset, and type 2 diabetes, which does not have an autoimmune origin (and therefore lacks anti-islet autoantibodies), but is common and of increasing prevalence.

Evidence for a genetic contribution to the risk of T1D includes increased prevalence of disease in first degree relatives (FDR) (2.5–6.0% risk versus 0.1–0.3% in the general population of Western countries) with a λs of

about 15 (Tillil and Köbberling, 1987; Pociot and McDermott, 2002). T1D has a high concordance in monozygotic (MZ) twins and intermediate concordance in dizygotic (DZ) twins, 27% and 3.8%, respectively (Hyttinen et al., 2003); and is associated with a lifetime risk for the twin of an affected proband of 44% and 19%, respectively (Kumar et al., 1993). The prevalence of T1D varies markedly between countries and is increasing at a rate of about 3% per year (Onkamo et al., 1999), a change that is associated with alterations in autoantibody profiles and an accelerated onset of disease from the time of identification of autoantibodies. These trends are consistent with changing environmental effects on the pathogenesis of the disease (Ziegler et al., 2011; Long et al., 2012).

Multiple Sclerosis

MS is a chronic and debilitating disease of the central nervous system (CNS) characterized by myelin loss and axonal degeneration, resulting in neurological symptoms and impairment. It primarily affects individuals of northern European descent with a prevalence of approximately 0.1–0.2 %; more females than males are affected, at a ratio of approximately 3:1. Clinically, MS can be divided into two major subtypes: relapsing-remitting MS (RRMS) and primary progressive MS (PPMS). RRMS is characterized by relapses followed by periods of remission of variable duration where there is complete or partial recovery. MS patients with RRMS may eventually progress to secondary-progressive MS (SPMS) characterized by steady decline without remit. PPMS, which affects approximately 5–15% of all individuals with MS, differs from RRMS in that there are no periods of remission. Prior to genetic studies, there was a broad acceptance that RRMS and PPMS were likely to represent pathogenetically different diseases.

Familial aggregation of MS was noted as early as the 1890s and suggested that there was a genetic influence on disease development (Eichhorst, 1896). More recently, the proportion of MS patients who have a blood relative with MS has been shown to be approximately 20% (Compston, 1991), reflecting a 3% risk in siblings of affected individuals and a λs (relative risk ratio of disease in siblings of patients) of about 25 (Robertson et al., 1996). Twin studies have demonstrated a concordance of 25–30% between MZ twin pairs, and concordance similar to that of siblings in DZ twins (Ebers et al., 1986; Sadovnick and Baird, 1988; Sadovnick et al., 1993; Robertson et al., 1996; Carton et al., 1997; Montomoli et al., 2002).

Systemic Lupus Erythematosus

Lupus is a highly variable autoimmune disease diagnosed on the basis of a combination of clinical and laboratory criteria (American College of Rheumatology Ad Hoc Committee on Systemic Lupus Erythematosus Guidelines, 1999). It may be associated with hematologic, musculo-skeletal, renal, or neuropsychiatric symptoms. It is generally characterized by the presence in plasma of antinuclear autoantibodies, primarily directed against molecules involved in transcription and translation, such as DNA, the Ul small nuclear ribonucleoprotein/Smith (Sm) complex, and the Ro/SSA and La/SSB ribonucleo-protein autoantigens. The prevalence of lupus is around 40 to 50 cases per 100,000 people, primarily affecting women (F:M ratio is 9:1); the prevalence is much higher, and the course of disease much more pernicious, in Africans and Afro-Caribbeans living in Western countries and particularly in the Aborigines of northern Australia, where the prevalence reaches >90 per 100,000 (Stoll et al., 1996; Bossingham, 2003). Lupus shows familial clustering, with approximately 1.5–3.0% of FDR affected, but the variable and often mixed racial backgrounds of patients complicates the calculation of a λs, which lies somewhere between 5.0 and 30 (Block et al., 1975; Lawrence et al., 1987; Alarcón-Segovia et al., 2005). In twin studies, 24–69% of MZ pairs and 2–3% of DZ pairs were concordant (Block et al., 1975; Deapen et al., 1992).

HUMAN LEUKOCYTE ANTIGEN (*HLA*) COMPLEX AND OTHER CANDIDATE GENES

The Major Histocompatibility Complex (MHC) was originally identified by murine allogeneic tumor transplantation (Gorer, 1937). Identification of the analogous gene complex in humans (termed the Human Leukocyte Antigen (*HLA*) Complex) was made when three groups described antibodies in sera from multitransfused patients or multiparous women that aggregated the leukocytes of many, but not all, donors (Dausset, 1958; van Rood et al., 1958; Payne and Rolfs, 1958). The collaborative dissection of the *HLA* complex is described elsewhere (Thorsby, 2009). After an association was reported between Hodgkin's disease and the 4c complex (subsequently known as *HLA-B*; Amiel, 1967), many diseases were tested for association with *HLA* alleles. The strongest *HLA* association with autoimmune disease found to date is with ankylosing spondylitis (AS); 88–96% of AS patients carry *HLA-B*27* compared with 4–8% of healthy controls (Brewerton et al., 1973; Schlosstein et al., 1973). *HLA-B*27* carries a relative risk of AS of up to 100 (Arellano et al., 1984)—the highest genetic association for any autoimmune disease. The relative risk varies between populations, and is much lower in African Americans (Khan et al., 1977).

Association of Type 1 Diabetes with HLA and other Candidate Genes

The *HLA* also shows association with T1D (locus termed *IDDM1*; Nerup et al., 1974; Bertrams, 1984; Todd, 1992; Noble et al., 1996; Cucca et al., 2001; Devendra and Eisenbarth, 2003; Kelly et al., 2003; Valdes et al., 2005) and accounts for approximately 40% of the familial aggregation of the disease; the predisposing *HLA* Class II haplotypes, *HLA-DRB1*04, DQB1*03:02* (identified by serology as DR4), and *DRB1*03:01, DQB1*02:01* (DR3) are present in 95% of affected individuals. DR3/DR4 heterozygotes carry an absolute risk of T1D of approximately 5% (compared to a cumulative incidence of $\sim$0.3% in Western communities), which rises to about 20% if a haploidentical sibling is affected (Noble et al., 1996; Valdes et al., 2001). DQ amino acid sequences directly correlate to risk of T1D and this association is largely dependent on the identity of residue 57 of the DQβ chain, Asp being protective and Ala conferring susceptibility (Todd et al., 1987), and residue 52 of the DQα chain (Arg confers susceptibility; Khalil et al., 1990). Khalil et al. (1990) reported that of 50 T1D patients, all expressed the DQα-52Arg/DQβ-57Ala susceptible heterodimer. Remarkably, the non-obese diabetic (NOD) mouse model of T1D expresses an Aβ chain homologous to DQβ with a substitution at position 57 (Todd et al., 1987).

INS

Other T1D candidate genes were examined because of their biological relevance to disease. Insulin is primarily transcribed in the beta cells of pancreatic islets, and is a major autoantigen in T1D (Kent et al., 2005). There are three common polymorphisms in strong LD in the insulin (INS) gene: −23Hph1 (an A/T polymorphism within the Hph1 restriction endonuclease site 23 bp upstream of the insulin gene transcription start site), +1140 A/C and a variable number tandem repeat (VNTR) locus. The VNTR is the best candidate because it contains binding sites for many transcription factors, including Pur1 (Kennedy et al., 1995), while there is no obvious functional role for either of the two SNPs (Barratt et al., 2004). The promoter of the INS gene on 11p15 contains the VNTR locus and the shortest alleles (class I alleles; 26–63 repeats) are associated with T1D in HLA-DR4-expressing subjects (odds ratio (OR) 1.9; *IDDM2*; Bell et al., 1984; Julier et al., 1991; Bain et al., 1992; Bennett et al., 1995). Class III alleles (the longest—209 repeats) of the VNTR are associated with marginally lower levels of insulin mRNA expression in pancreata (Bennett et al., 1995), but a two to three-fold higher expression in fetal thymus (Vafiadis et al., 1997). These data are consistent with the hypothesis that protective alleles of the INS

VNTR are responsible for increased thymic insulin expression driving more effective induction of central tolerance of insulin-reactive T cells. Although *INS* polymorphisms were associated with T1D in many Caucasian populations, the association was not seen in Chinese subjects because the frequency of the susceptible *INS* allele is approximately 95% in Chinese controls and close to 100% in Chinese T1D patients (Marron and She, unpublished data cited in Marron et al., 1997).

PTPN22

Protein tyrosine phosphatases were thought to be good candidates for autoimmunity susceptibility genes because they are involved in limiting T cell activation by dephosphorylating t cell receptor (TCR)-associated kinases and their substrates. *PTPN22*, on chromosome 1p13, encodes the lymphocyte-specific protein tyrosine phosphatase LYP, which is a negative regulator of TCR signaling via the dephosphorylation of several TCR proximal signaling molecules, including the SRC family kinases LCK and FYN, ZAP70, and TCRζ. A nonsynonymous single nucleotide polymorphism (SNP) at position 1858 of *PTPN22* was reported to be associated with T1D in many populations (OR for the homozygous TT genotype was 1.7; Bottini et al., 2004; Onengut-Gumuscu et al., 2004; Smyth et al., 2004; Zheng and She, 2005, Steck et al., 2009, reviewed in Steck and Rewers, 2011). This C1858T SNP encodes in a missense mutation that changes an arginine to a tryptophan at position 620 (R620W) causing the inability of LYP to bind its signaling molecule CSK (Vang et al., 2005), resulting in increased phosphatase activity. T cells from T1D patients and healthy subjects carrying the LYP-W620 variant show reduced production of interleukin (IL)-2 and other cytokines following TCR stimulation (Vang et al., 2005; Rieck et al., 2007). This Trp620 variant is also associated with Graves' disease (GD; autoimmune hyperthyroidism; Steck et al., 2006), rheumatoid arthritis (RA; Begovich et al., 2004), and lupus (Kyogoku et al., 2004).

TCR and immunoglobulin loci were also examined as candidates, without consistent evidence of involvement.

Association of Multiple Sclerosis with HLA and other Candidate Genes

Association of MS with the HLA Class I alleles *HLA-A*03* and *HLA-B*07* (identified by serology as A3 and B7) were reported in 1972 (Jersild et al., 1972; Jersild and Fog, 1972; Naito et al., 1972). Further studies found that both of these associations were secondary to those of the Class II alleles *HLA-DRB1*15:01* (DR2) and *HLA-DQB1*06:02* (DQ6), which can be inherited together in strong linkage disequilibrium as the HLA-DR15 haplotype

(*DRB5*01:01, DRB1*15:01, DQA1*01:02-DQB1*06:02*; Fogdell et al., 1995). This haplotype confers a relative risk of MS of between two and four (Francis et al., 1987a,b). Approximately 30% of individuals with MS carry this extended haplotype compared to 15% in the normal population; its effect is dominant and shows evidence of gene dosage (Barcellos et al., 2006). The contribution of *HLA* to total (genetic) susceptibility to MS is estimated to be between 15 and 50% (Haines et al., 1996, 1998).

There is a very strong association between Epstein−Barr virus (EBV) infection and MS: EBV is unique in being the only virus known to have infected virtually all MS patients, in contrast to healthy subjects, of whom only 85−95% are infected (Sumaya et al., 1985; Myhr et al., 1998); EBV seronegativity has an odds ratio (OR) of 0.06 (95% CI 0.03−0.13; $p < 10^{-9}$; Ascherio and Munger, 2007). *HLA-DRB1*15:01* appears to act synergistically as a risk factor with EBV exposure. The risk conferred by *HLA-DRB1*15:01* was 2.9-fold higher in patients with a history of infectious mononucleosis and the risk of MS in *HLA-DRB1*15:01* positive women increased nine-fold in those with elevated anti-EBNA-1 (EBV) antibody titers (Nielsen et al., 2009; De Jager et al., 2008). A confounding problem is the potential effects of *DRB1*15:012* on EBV susceptibility. EBV achieves penetration of the plasma membrane via the binding of its viral glycoprotein gp42 to *HLA*-DR (Li et al., 1997); the *HLA*-DR15 haplotype is associated with 15.7-, 5.2-, and 8.3-fold higher expression of DQB1, DRB5, and DRB1, respectively (Alcina et al., 2012), potentially conferring higher infection rates.

MS is also associated with childhood residence at higher geographic latitude (Acheson et al., 1960) and a significant component of this association appears to be mediated by low ultraviolet light exposure resulting in reduced 1,25(OH)2 vitamin D availability (Nieves et al., 1994; Munger et al., 2006). A functional vitamin D response element (VDRE) has been identified in the promoter region of *HLA-DRB1* and this VDRE is present on the *HLA*-DR15 haplotype (Ramagopalan et al., 2009), suggesting these genotypes may be unusual in having vitamin D-regulated MHC Class II expression.

Class I alleles also affect susceptibility to MS: The *HLA-A*03:01* allele increases the risk (OR 2.1) while *HLA-A*02:01* and *B*44* decrease it (OR 0.52 and 0.62, respectively; Fogdell-Hahn et al., 2000; Bergamaschi et al., 2010; Cree et al., 2010; Healy et al., 2010). The presence of *A*02:01* reduces the relative risk of MS conferred by the *HLA*-DR15 haplotype from 3.6 to 1.5 (Fogdell-Hahn et al., 2000).

No associations between *HLA* genotypes and specific MS subtypes have been identified (Barcellos et al., 2006), although a significant correlation between the age-of-onset of MS and a SNP tagging the HLA-DR15 haplotype has been reported (Masterman et al., 2000; International Multiple Sclerosis Genetics Consortium et al., 2011b); no associations with gender or disease severity were observed.

Other MS candidate genes that have been tested by association or transmission tests were selected largely on the basis of known or predicted roles in pathogenesis. In particular, genes encoding the TCR, IL 1 receptor (IL1R), interferons (IFN) α, β, and γ, and CTLA-4, as well as various cytokine/chemokine genes have been investigated with no consistent results.

Association of Lupus with HLA and other Candidate Genes

*HLA-DRB1*03:01* (identified by serology as DR3) is strongly associated with lupus (Freedman et al., 1993). In African American patients, *HLA-DRB1*03* was found in 62% of lupus patients, but only 20% of controls (relative risk of 6.41); in Caucasian patients, the strength of the association is a little lower: 30% vs. 13% (So et al., 1990). *DRB1*03:01* is part of the 8.1 ancestral haplotype (*HLA-A*01, C*07, B*08, DRB1*03:01, DQA1*05:01, DQB1*02:01*), so named because it includes the class I alleles *HLA-B*8* (B8) and *HLA-A*01* (A1). This haplotype therefore confers susceptibility to both lupus and T1D in Europeans, as does the $H2^{g7}$ MHC haplotype in NOD mice (Price et al., 1999; Jordan et al., 2000). It is also associated with celiac disease (Ahmed et al., 1993), myasthenia gravis (Hammarström et al., 1975), chronic active (autoimmune) hepatitis (Strettell et al., 1997), and scleroderma (Kallenberg et al., 1981).

The class II allele *HLA-DRB1*15:01* (serotype DR15, a split of DR2 and usually associated with *DQB1*06:02, DQA1*0102* (serotype DQ6, a split of DQ1)) is also associated with lupus; it was found in 41% of African American patients and 18% of controls (relative risk of 3.03). Again, in Caucasian patients, the association is a little weaker: 21% vs. 11% (So et al., 1990). The combined relative risk for lupus associated with expression of both haplotypes is 9.0 (Kachru et al., 1984).

TNF

Interest in tumor necrosis factor (*TNF*) genes in humans followed the finding of a polymorphism within the *Tnf* gene of lupus-prone (NZBxNZW)F1 hybrid mice (Jacob and McDevitt, 1988), in which decreased expression of TNF was associated with disease and TNF administration delayed nephritis. The same group applied serotyping and bioassays to determine the relevance of quantitative polymorphisms in *TNF* to lupus and lupus nephritis in patients, reporting that in lupus patients, the DR2-DQ1 serotype (inferred haplotype *DRB1*05:01, DQB1*06:02, DQA1*01:02*) was associated with low levels of induced

TNF expression and an increased incidence of nephritis. In contrast, lupus patients with the DR3 (*HLA-DRB1*03:01*) and DR4 (*HLA-DRB1*04:01*) serotypes had high TNF production and were not predisposed to nephritis (Jacob et al., 1990). One potential explanation for this association is a SNP at position −308 in the promoter of the *TNF* gene: The low expression haplotype has a G in this position, whereas the high expression haplotype has an A (Tan and Arnett, 1998; Hajeer and Hutchinson, 2001). This association with expression, as well as the SNP association with disease has been controversial, in part due to attempts to generalize the original observation to lupus (as distinct from lupus nephritis) and in part due to racial heterogeneity (Rudwaleit et al., 1996). Where an association was found, often it could not be shown to be acting independently of *HLA-DRB1* alleles (Wilson et al., 1994; Rudwaleit et al., 1996).

C4A, C4B

One of the strongest associations with lupus within the HLA is with the C4 genes in the *HLA* class III region (Christiansen et al., 1991). Both the major European DR3-associated haplotypes in lupus patients include disruption of *C4A* or *C4B*. The 8.1 ancestral haplotype common in Western and Northern Europeans contains a null allele of the gene encoding C4A (*C4A*Q0*; Fielder et al., 1983; So et al., 1990). In Caucasians, the relative risk for lupus of carrying two *C4A*Q0* alleles is 16.9 (Howard et al., 1986). Association studies of other *C4A* null alleles in African American and Asian populations, where they are present on haplotypes other than the 8.1 ancestral haplotype, indicate that *C4A* null alleles are lupus risk genes independently of *HLA-DRB1*03:01*, showing a gene dose effect and conferring a relative risk of 2.7 in African Americans (Howard et al., 1986; Yamada et al., 1990).

A null allele of the gene encoding C4B (*C4B*Q0*) is present in the other major European DR3-associated ancestral haplotype (A30::DQ2, consisting of *HLA-A*30:02, C*05:01, B*18, DRB1*03:01, DQA1*05:01, DQB1*02:01*), which occurs with frequencies around 15% in Sardinia and Basque, and between 2 and 10% in Southern Europe. The *C4B*Q0* allele is also relatively common in lupus patients (Fielder et al., 1983), and shows an association with lupus in Australian Aborigines (Christiansen et al., 1991), African Americans (relative risk 2.0; Howard et al., 1986), and Spanish populations (relative risk 6.0; Naves et al., 1998), but not other Caucasians (Howard et al., 1986).

C2

The gene encoding the C2 complement component also lies within the class III region of the HLA, between the

C4 genes and those encoding HSP70, TNF, LTα, and LTβ. Null alleles of *C2* are likewise associated with lupus and 33% of Europeans with homozygous C2 deficiency develop it (Walport, 1993). Homozygosity for null alleles is present in 0.4–2% of cases compared to 0.01% of the general population; heterozygous C2 deficiencies are present in 2.4–5.8% of cases compared to 0.7–1% of the general population (Sullivan et al., 1994; Lipsker et al., 2000). Patients with C2 deficiency tend to experience photosensitivity and other forms of skin involvement; among C2-deficient patients without lupus, benign cutaneous (discoid) lupus is also common (Agnello et al., 1972; Provost et al., 1983; Lipsker et al., 2000).

C1Q

Hereditary deficiencies of other early complement components (C1q, C1r, C1s) are powerful but rare causes of a lupus-like syndrome. For example, 90% of people with C1q deficiency develop lupus. Onset can occur in childhood (even as early as one year of age) and the disease can be associated with very severe central nervous system (CNS) and renal complications; of 30 patients, 22 died in childhood (Bowness et al., 1994).

FCGR2A, FCGR3A, FCGR3B

In the 1970s a reduction in Fc-rosette formation of red blood cells from lupus patients was identified and attributed to saturation by circulating complexes (Nakai et al., 1977). While it was known that the Fcγ receptors FcγRI (CD64), FcγRII (CD32), and FcγRIII (CD16) contribute to the clearance of IgG and IgG-containing immune complexes, they were not examined as candidates until the 1990s. A SNP in *FCGR2A* results in a His to Arg substitution at position 131 of FcγRIIa and reduces the affinity by which FcγRIIa binds IgG2 (Duits et al., 1995). This substitution also affects the clearance of IgG-coated erythrocytes and has been found to have an inconsistent association with lupus but not to nephritis (Duits et al., 1995; Salmon et al., 1996; Dijstelbloem et al., 2000).

Similarly, a SNP in *FCGR3A* results in a Val to Phe substitution at position 176 of FcγRIIIa, reducing, in 176Phe/Phe homozygotes, the binding of IgG1 and IgG3 by natural killer (NK) cells and monocytes, inhibiting NK cell activation and activation-induced cell death (Wu et al., 1997). Homozygosity for this allele is present in a significantly higher proportion of lupus patients than controls (Wu et al., 1997; Koene et al., 1998) and is associated with lupus nephritis, arthritis and serositis, or hematologic cytopenias, depending on the population (Salmon et al., 1999; Dijstelbloem et al., 2000).

Two alleles of *FCGR3B* vary in the encoded amino acid sequence of FcγRIIIb, affecting low affinity IgG binding by neutrophils. The allele associated with decreased phagocytic activity (NA2) is associated with lupus (OR 1.9; Hatta et al., 1999). *FCGR3B* also shows copy number variation and a low *FCGR3B* copy number, in particular complete FcγRIIIb deficiency is strongly associated with lupus as well as with Wegener's granulomatosis (Fanciulli et al., 2007; McKinney and Merriman, 2012).

IRF5

Increased production of type I IFNs and expression of IFN-inducible genes is commonly observed in lupus and appears to play a key role in the molecular pathogenesis of the disease (Baechler et al., 2003). Sigurdsson et al. (2005) performed linkage and association studies of 44 SNPs in 13 candidate genes involved in the type I IFN pathway on 679 Swedish, Finnish, and Icelandic patients with lupus, in 798 unaffected family members, and in 438 unrelated control individuals. Two genes were highly significantly associated with lupus: *TYK2* (19p13) and *IRF5* (7q32). Remarkably, despite the relatively low power of the study, the P value for *IRF5* reached a genome-wide level of significance. This finding was quickly and robustly replicated (Graham et al., 2006). The most highly associated SNP in the 7q32 region (*rs2004640*) lies in the splice junction of an alternate first exon. The T allele creates a 5' donor splice site allowing expression of several unique *IRF5* isoforms and is in LD with a cis-acting variant associated with elevated expression of *IRF5*. IRF5 is a transcription factor that regulates type I IFN gene expression. It is critical for the production of the proinflammatory cytokines TNF, IL-12, and IL-6 following Toll-like receptor (TLR) signaling (Takaoka et al., 2005), and it mediates type I IFN induction in response to some viruses (Barnes et al., 2001). In a genome-wide association study (GWAS) of anti-dsDNA AAb in lupus, *IRF5*, together with the *HLA*, *STAT4*, and *ITGAM*, was found to be significantly associated (Chung et al., 2011).

Mechanisms of Complement and Fc Associations with Autoimmunity

The leading hypothesis explaining the association between lupus and deficiencies in FcR and complement is that these defects impair catabolism of immune complexes by the mononuclear phagocytic system (Walport, 1993). Tracking of radio-labeled immune complexes revealed the following defects in lupus patients: (1) reduced immune complex uptake by the spleen; (2) accelerated clearance of complexes by the liver; and (3) release of those immune complexes from the liver back into circulation (Davies et al., 1992). In similar studies of a patient with C2 deficiency, splenic uptake of immune complexes was found to be entirely complement dependent, and could be restored by transfusion of fresh frozen plasma (Davies et al., 1993). As C4A binds more effectively to amino groups than C4B does, it has been proposed that it is more efficient at clearing immune complexes (Schifferli et al., 1986). This may explain the stronger association of lupus with C4A deficiencies.

Mechanisms of HLA Association with Autoimmunity

The finding of a single ancestral haplotype (8.1) associated with multiple autoimmune diseases suggests a common mechanism mediating susceptibility. The analysis of HLA recombinant patients indicates that, for many autoimmune diseases, genetic association with the HLA can be primarily attributed to associations with the genes encoding specific peptide-presenting molecules, class I or class II (Thorsby, 1997). The hypothesis arising from this observation is that disease-associated HLA class I and class II alleles permit binding of disease-inducing peptides. The question of why one particular peptide of an autoantigen should be any more disease inducing than another became the driving force behind a supplementary hypothesis: Molecular mimicry, in which it is proposed that bi-reactive TCRs permit the priming of T cells by a microbial peptide and effector activation by autoantigens. The most plausible example of putative molecular mimicry is found in AS, which on microbiologic and serologic criteria is associated with *Klebsiella* infection (Ebringer, 1992). The amino acids 72–77 of the HLA class I molecule B27 are identical to amino acids 188–193 of the nitrogenase of *Klebsiella pneumoniae* (Yu et al., 1989).

Lang et al. (2002) reported bi-reactive TCRs of MS patients that bound both DRB5*0101 presenting a peptide from the DNA polymerase of EBV as well as DRB1*1501 presenting a myelin basic protein (MBP) peptide. Crystal structure determination revealed a marked degree of structural equivalence at the surface presented for TCR recognition. In contrast, T cells from patients with lupus show no such cross-reactivity at the level of TCR/peptide/HLA. In addition to MS and lupus, *DRB1*1501* is positively associated with the autoimmune diseases Sjögren's syndrome (Guggenbuhl et al., 1998), Goodpasture syndrome (GS) (Fisher et al., 1997), and juvenile RA (JRA) (Garavito et al., 2004). Such a wide range of tissue specificities renders it most unlikely that a shared autoantigen is responsible, and there is little evidence of any etiological role for EBV in GS or JRA. The cross-reactivity identified in lupus autoantibodies can be explained by B cell polyclonal activation, support of antibody production, and inhibition of apoptosis mediated by EBV, and these activities of themselves probably provide

sufficient explanation for the association between EBV and lupus.

GENE LINKAGE STUDIES OF AUTOIMMUNITY

The availability of dense maps of polymorphic genetic markers (microsatellites and SNPs) revolutionized the localization of non-*HLA*-linked disease genes (Dietrich et al., 1992, 1996; Gyapay et al., 1994; Tsang et al., 2005). Linkage analyses rely on disproportionate transmission of alleles to affected and unaffected progeny.

Linkage Studies of Type 1 Diabetes

The first genome-wide scans for linkage to T1D were performed on large collections of T1D families with pairs of affected siblings (sibpairs) by microsatellite (variable number of tandem repeats) analysis in 1994 (Davies et al., 1994; Hashimoto et al., 1994; http://www.t1dbase.org). These studies easily confirmed linkage to the *HLA*, both by their own statistical thresholds, as well as by those of Lander and Kuglyak (1995), which are set to a 5% probability per study of a single genomic region exceeding the significance threshold by chance (i.e., a LOD score >3.6). Davies et al. (1994) calculated that the *HLA* contributes about 42% of the familial clustering of T1D. Neither group showed evidence of linkage at *INS*.

CTLA4

Owerbach and Gabbay (1995) performed a genome-wide linkage analysis in 162 type 1 diabetic families with an affected sibling pair, and subset their data by the *INS* VNTR and *HLA* haplotypes. They identified an additional susceptibility gene located on chromosome 2q31 near *HOXD8* (*IDDM7*; maximum LOD 4.8) in affected sibpairs lacking high-risk HLA-DR3/4 haplotypes and expressing homozygous high-risk class I VNTR alleles. This region is homologous to that on proximal mouse chromosome 1 where the *Idd5* T1D gene was subsequently identified in diabetes-prone NOD mice (Cornall et al., 1991) and contains the disease candidate genes *CTLA4* and *CD28*, which encode T cell receptors involved in the control of T cell activation (Walunas et al., 1994).

Candidature of *CTLA4* was also supported by a subsequent linkage analysis in 48 Italian families, transmission disequilibrium testing in 187 Italian families (138 of which had only a single affected child), and 44 Spanish families, and a population based case–control association study of 966 patients and 1058 controls from Belgium (Nisticò et al., 1996). Similar studies in British, Sardinian, and American families did not support *CTLA4* candidature (Nisticò et al., 1996). A meta-analysis of 33 independent studies showed an odds ratio of 1.45 for the G allele; with a greater effect in cases with onset <20 years of age (odds ratio 1.61; Kavvoura and Ioannidis, 2005). On the basis of *CTLA4* being 10 cM distal of the *IDDM7* linkage peak (*D2S152*), and the lack of disequilibrium between *D2S152* and *CTLA4* in the association study, the locus at 2q33 was designated *IDDM12* (Nisticò et al., 1996).

In addition to T1D, *CTLA4* is associated with GD (Yanagawa et al., 1995; Kotsa et al., 1997; Kouki et al., 2000), Hashimoto's autoimmune thyroiditis (HT) and autoimmune hypothyroidism (Kotsa et al., 1997; Donner et al., 1997), Addison's disease (Blomhoff ct al., 2004; Donner et al., 1997), MS (Harbo et al., 1999; Ligers et al., 1999), and RA (Gonzalez-Escribano et al., 1999; Gregersen et al., 2009).

Ueda et al. (2003) examined expression levels of the two major isoforms of the most disease-associated SNP (CT60): the full-length sequence, and a soluble isoform (s-CTLA-4) that lacks exon 3 (Oaks et al., 2000). The disease susceptible genotype was associated with lower expression of s-CTLA-4 in a gene dose-dependent manner. Similarly, sequence-dependent variation in *Ctla4* isoforms were identified in T1D-susceptible NOD mice, and differential expression of one appeared to mediate the allelic variation in T1D risk that maps to this chromosomal region (Oaks et al., 2000; Vijayakrishnan et al., 2004; Araki et al., 2009). CTLA-4 is expressed constitutively on regulatory T (Treg) cells and is thought, at least in part, to mediate their immunosuppressive activities (Manzotti et al., 2002) as interaction of CTLA-4 with CD80 or CD86 inhibits human T-cell activation (Vandenborre et al., 1999). Soluble CTLA-4 also has this activity (Oaks et al., 2000), and a knock-down transgene for sCTLA-4 exacerbated T1D in an NOD congenic strain that expresses the wild-type *Ctla4* allele (Gerold et al., 2011).

CD25

The 10p11-q11 region (designated *IDDM10* in unpublished data by Todd (1995); maximum LOD 2.03; Hashimoto et al. (1994)) contains the putative candidate genes *GAD2* and *CD25* (*IL2RA*). *GAD2* encodes the islet cell specific (65 kDa) form of glutamic acid decarboxylase (GAD65), a prevalent autoantigen in T1D. Association analysis of a highly polymorphic dinucleotide repeat linked to the gene did not support a significant role for GAD2 (Wapelhorst et al., 1995). In contrast, *CD25* (10p15), which encodes the IL-2 receptor α chain, was supported by a tag SNP approach and a large sample size (7457 cases and controls and 725 multiplex families; Vella et al., 2005). CD25 plays a critical role in the

development and maintenance of regulatory T cells (Treg) and may play a role in Treg expression of CD62L, which is required for their entry into lymph nodes (Malek and Bayer, 2004). In association studies, T1D was associated with two independent groups of SNPs, spanning overlapping regions of 14 and 40 kb, encompassing the first intron of *CD25* and the 5′ introgenic region (Lowe et al., 2007; Maier et al., 2009). The T1D susceptibility genotypes were also associated with lower circulating levels of soluble IL2RA (s-IL2RA; Lowe et al., 2007). Dendrou and colleagues (2009) confirmed gene–phenotype correlation at the RNA level: Individuals with one or two protective alleles (G) at *rs12722495* showed an increase in CD25 message (27%) in their CD4$^+$ memory T cells when compared to homozygous susceptible individuals (AA) or to those with protective *rs11594456* or *rs2104286* alleles. Allelic variation in *CD25* is also associated with MS (International Multiple Sclerosis Genetics Consortium et al., 2007) and Crohn's disease (Franke et al., 2010). As the most strongly associated SNP in MS is *rs2104286* (OR = 0.85; G, protective, minor allele at *rs2104286*), Dendrou et al. (2009) proposed that while the CD4$^+$ memory T cell phenotype is critical for T1D protection, naïve T cell and stimulated CD14$^+$ CD16$^+$ monocyte phenotypes are important in both diseases.

Other Loci

Other putative diabetes susceptibility loci initially identified using linkage studies were localized to chromosomes: 18q12-q21 (designated *IDDM6*; maximum LOD 3.7; Todd, 1995; Merriman et al., 1997), 6q27 (designated *IDDM8*; maximum LOD 3.4; Luo et al., 1995; Todd, 1995; Luo et al., 1996), 3q22-q25 (designated *IDDM9* (unpublished data, Todd, 1995), maximum LOD 2.4 in DR3/DR4 heterozygotes; Mein et al., 1998; Paterson et al., 1999), 14q24-q31 (designated *IDDM11*; maximum LOD 4.0, 4.6 in families without evidence of HLA linkage to T1D; Field et al., 1994), 2q34-q35 (designated *IDDM13*; maximum LOD 3.3; Morahan et al., 1996), and 6q2 (designated *IDDM15*; identified by an extension of identity-by-descent methods as adjacent to HLA, $p < 5 \times 10^{-5}$; Delépine et al., 1997). The latter locus brings to a total four putative loci on chromosome 6q: *IDDM1/HLA*, *IDDM15*, *IDDM5*, and *IDDM8*, in that order from centromere to telomere over a distance of about 100 cM.

Linkage Analyses of Combined Datasets and the Limits of Linkage Analyses

By 1998, very large collections of families were being analyzed. Mein et al. (1998) studied 356 affected sibpair families from the UK, but found significant linkage only to three regions: *IDDM1/HLA*, *IDDM10/CD25* (10p13; maximum LOD 4.7), and 16q22-24 (maximum LOD 3.4). Remarkably, most of the previously reported loci were excluded by exclusion mapping at a λs of 3 and a LOD of -2. Similarly, a two-staged analysis of 616 multiplex families from the UK and the USA identified only *IDDM1/HLA* (maximum LOD 34.2) as significant by multipoint analysis, and a single previously unreported locus on 1q of suggestive significance (LOD 3.31; Concannon et al., 1998). The data were consistent with a locus distal from the *HLA*, at *IDDM15* (6q21) with a maximum LOD 3.8, but its proximity to the *HLA* required correction for linkage disequilibrium, resulting in an adjusted LOD of 2.27. On chromosome 2q, previous studies had proposed three loci (*IDDM7*, *IDM12*, and *IDDM13*) but Concannon et al. (1998) reported a maximum LOD in this region of 1.07, and little evidence for distinct loci. By multipoint analysis, even modest contributions (λs $> = 1.5$; LOD < -2) to T1D could be excluded for *IDDM3*, *IDDM4*, *IDDM6*, *IDDM9*, and *IDDM10*. In an identity-by-descent (IBD) analysis of previously reported loci (other than *IDDM1/HLA* and *IDDM2/INS*), only *IDDM7/IDDM12/IDDM13* and *IDDM15* had LOD scores greater than 1; negligible support was found for six of the previously reported loci: *IDDM3*, *IDDM4*, *IDDM6*, *IDDM9*, *IDDM10*, and *IDDM11*.

In an attempt to further increase the power of linkage analyses, multinational consortia were formed, allowing the analysis of combined datasets. The Type 1 Diabetes Genetics Consortium (T1DGC) was established for this purpose in 2002. Concannon et al. (2005) performed, under the auspices of the T1DGC, a combined linkage analysis of four datasets, three previously published (Concannon et al., 1998; Mein et al., 1998), providing a total sample of 1435 families with 1636 affected sibpairs. By multipoint linkage analysis, only the HLA was significant (*IDDM1*; LOD 116; λs of 3.35), and four other regions showed suggestive significance (i.e., uncorrected $p < 7.4 \times 10^{-4}$): 2q31-33 (*IDDM7/IDDM12/CTLA4*; LOD3.34; λs of 1.19), 6q21 (*IDDM15*; LOD 22.39; λs of 1.56), 10p14-q11 (*IDDM10/CD25*; LOD 3.21; λs of 1.12), 16q22-24 (LOD 2.64; λs of 1.19). LOD scores above 1 were found at *IDDM2/INS*, and five other regions: 3p13-14, 9q33-34, 12q14-12, 16p12-q11, and 19p13. The 19p13 region contains the insulin receptor gene (*INSR*). In 2009, the T1DGC published a linkage analysis of 2496 multiplex families; again, only the *HLA* was significant at genome-wide significance levels (*IDDM1*; LOD 213), with significance at 6q21/*IDDM15* resulting from an effect partly due to LD with *HLA*. Suggestive linkage was found at *CTLA4* (*IDDM7/IDDM12*; LOD 3.28) and *INS* (*IDDM2*; LOD 3.16) and two regions on chromosome 19: 19p13 (*INSR*; LOD 2.84)

and 19q13 (LOD 2.54; Concannon et al., 2009). The sample size of this study provided unprecedented power to detect linkage, but provided little support for the majority of loci previously implicated in T1D.

Linkage Studies in Multiple Sclerosis

In contrast to the moderate progress in T1D, attempts to identify MS genes by linkage analysis of families such as affected sibpair analysis or patient and unaffected parent trios were relatively unsuccessful. For example, Sawcer et al. (1996) studied 282 families using a staged approach, but only obtained a maximized LOD score at the *HLA* of 2.8, compared to 8.0 for T1D (Davies et al., 1994). Only one other locus surpassed the statistical threshold for suggestive linkage, 17q22. In none of the other linkage studies did the *HLA* reach a significant maximized LOD score (Ebers et al., 1996; Haines et al., 1996; Kuokkanen et al., 1997; Broadley et al., 2001; Coraddu et al., 2001; Ban et al., 2002). Ebers et al. (1996) reported linkage to a region just outside the *HLA* (χ^2 of 10.8 by transmission disequilibrium test), Kuokkanen et al. (1997) reported linkage (maximized LOD 3.6) at 17q22-24 and the Multiple Sclerosis Genetic Group reported suggestive linkage to *HLA-DR* and 7q21-22 (Haines et al., 1996). Several groups applied a modified threshold for suggestive significance (based on reduced marker density) and identified suggestive linkage at: 1q31 (Coraddu et al., 2001), 2p13 (Ban et al., 2002), 4q26-28 (Ban et al., 2002), 6q26 (Ban et al., 2002), 10q23 (Coraddu et al., 2001), 11p15 (Coraddu et al., 2001), and Xp11 (Ban et al., 2002).

The issue of why genome-wide linkage studies were relatively successful in T1D but not MS is an important one. Where the effective strength of putative loci could be determined, they were of similar orders between the two diseases. Patient heterogeneity is also an unlikely explanation, because the consolidation of sample sets occurred later for MS than it did for T1D; as a generalization, the MS results reflected samples collected within relatively restricted geographical areas. Similarly, while the power of several of the MS studies was rather low, others used sample sizes comparable to those used in many of the T1D studies. The most likely explanation lies in the relative heritability (the proportion of variation in risk within a community attributable to genetics) of the two diseases: that of T1D is about twice that of MS (Baxter, 1997, 2007; Hawkes and MacGregor, 2009), an observation consistent with the identification of several environmental factors contributing to the risk of MS (latitude, smoking, EBV).

Linkage Studies in Lupus

Following the identification of linkage to distal chromosome 1 in the NZB/NZW and NZM mouse models of lupus, Tsao et al. (1997) examined seven markers in the syntenic region of human chromsome 1 (1q31-42) in 52 affected sibpairs and confirmed linkage to lupus.

In 1998, two major genome-wide linkage studies of lupus were published (Gaffney et al., 1998; Moser et al., 1998). Analysis of 105 families with at least two affected siblings identified just two loci surpassing the Lander and Kruglyak (1995) thresholds for significant linkage: 6p11-21 (just centromeric to the *HLA*; maximized LOD 3.9) and 16q13 (maximized LOD 3.6; Gaffney et al., 1998). Both these regions were confirmed in a subsequent reanalysis that included an additional 82 sibpair families (maximized LODs of 4.1 and 3.9, respectively; Gaffney et al., 2000). Two other regions fulfilled the criteria for suggestive linkage: 14q21-23 (maximized LOD 2.8) and 20p12 (maximized LOD 2.6). A peak, albeit nonsignificant, was consistent with linkage to 1q42, as reported in Tsao et al. (1997).

The other major analysis examined 94 African American and European American multiplex extended pedigrees identifying four regions of suggestive linkage: 1q23 (maximized LOD 3.5), 13q32 (maximized LOD 2.5), 20q13 (maximized LOD 2.5), 1q31 (maximized LOD 2.0; Moser et al., 1998). Additional suggestive loci were identified only in African American families—1q41 (maximized LOD 3.5), 11q14-23 (maximized LOD 2.1)—and only in European American families—14q11 (maximized LOD 2.2), 4p15 (maximized LOD 2.2), 11q25 (maximized LOD 2.2), 2q32 (maximized LOD 2.1), 19q13 (maximized LOD 2.1), 6q26-27 (maximized LOD 2.0), and 12p13-11 (maximized LOD 2.0). No linkage to the *HLA* (6p21) was identified, probably reflecting the reduced power of genetic studies in mixed populations. The 1q23 locus is syntenic with the major murine chromosome 1 locus (Vyse and Kotzin, 1998) and contains the lupus candidate gene *FCGR2A*, and the 1q41 linkage is consistent with that found by both Tsao et al. (1997) and Gaffney et al. (1998).

TNFR1, TNFR2, LTBR

The 12p13 locus (Moser et al., 1998) contains the genes *TNFR1* (*TNFRSF1A*) and *LTBR* (*TNFRSF3*), which encode TNF receptor 1 and the LTβ receptor, respectively. Similarly, the location of *TNFR2* (*TNFRSF1B*; encoding the TNF receptor 2) on 1p36 was sufficiently close to minor linkage peaks reported by Gaffney et al. (1998) and Shai et al. (1999) for Tsuchiya et al. (2000) to test, and confirm, association of a nonsynonymous coding SNP (587 (T→G)) with lupus in Japanese subjects. Lupus is associated with serum concentrations of soluble TNF receptor (s-TNFR; both type I and type II) sufficient to effectively inhibit the bioactivity of TNF (Aderka et al., 1993). Perhaps the clearest evidence of the

disease's heterogeneity comes from an open label trial of TNF blockade in lupus. While the majority of patients expressed increased titers of high affinity autoantibodies to dsDNA, chromatin and histones over the period of therapy, seven of nine patients with lupus nephritis experienced stabilization of serum creatinine and a reduction in proteinuria of >50%, and all five patients with lupus arthritis underwent remission lasting for weeks after treatment was halted (Aringer et al., 2009).

STAT4

A small genome-wide linkage study of RA identified a region on chromosome 2q33 with significant linkage (Amos et al., 2006). A subsequent high-resolution association study confirmed the involvement of this region in RA and implicated the gene *STAT4*, since the five most significantly associated SNPs all lay within the second intron of *STAT4* (Remmers et al., 2007). STAT4 is a cytokine-responsive transcription factor that mediates responses to IL12; it plays a critical role in the differentiation of Th1 cells. The authors also genotyped 1039 lupus patients and 1248 controls at the SNP most highly associated with RA (*rs7574865*) and found that the RA susceptibility allele (T) was also associated with lupus (Remmers et al., 2007). In lupus, this SNP was strongly associated with anti-dsDNA particularly severe nephritis, and early onset of disease (Taylor et al., 2008; Chung et al., 2011). The same risk allele confers susceptibility to primary Sjögren's syndrome (Nordmark et al., 2009).

Racial Heterogeneity in Systemic Lupus Erythematosus

Since genome-wide linkage analyses had confirmed the importance of racial heterogeneity in lupus inheritance, Shai et al. (1999) analyzed 80 families with affected sibpairs (43 Mexican American families and 37 Caucasian families) and found no significant loci and only a single suggestive locus: 1q44. An analysis of the data by race made it clear that the linkage could be attributed only to the Mexican American subgroup; there was no support for a gene in this region in the Caucasian families. Lindqvist et al. (2000) analyzed six Icelandic and 11 Swedish pedigrees with multiple affected members. The combined data set showed significant linkage to 2q37 (LOD score 4.24). This region contains the *INPP5D* gene, which encodes an SH2-containing phosphatase which is recruited through tyrosine phosphorylation of FcgRIIB, CD19, or CD22 after ligation of the B cell receptor, and is thought to be important in FcgRIIB-mediated inhibition of B cell activation. Suggestive linkage was identified at 4p15-13 and 19p13 when the Icelandic subjects were analyzed independently.

The 4p15-13 locus is syntenic with the *Lmb2* murine lupus susceptibility gene. In most cases (14/16 markers), aggregating the data from the two countries eliminated any suggestion of linkage. In many subsequent studies, particularly in the genome-wide association studies that followed, experimental power was improved by restricting racial heterogeneity—generally to populations of European descent.

GENOME-WIDE ASSOCIATION STUDIES OF AUTOIMMUNITY

Genome-wide linkage analyses were limited in resolution by the recombination frequency observable over a few generations, and in power by the relatively low number of multiplex families available. By the year 2000, a reasonable draft of the human genome sequence was completed, millions of SNPs had been deposited into public databases, and high-throughput technologies were under development for SNP genotyping. It was predicted that case–control association studies involving thousands of patients and population-based controls would provide far better resolution and power for the identification of disease-associated genes (Cardon and Bell, 2001). In contrast to linkage studies, association studies can detect alleles with much more modest effects on risk, as long as those alleles are relatively common and the sample size sufficiently large (Wang et al., 2005). In each region of the genome, pre-selected SNPs are chosen that are expected to represent the total genetic variation in linkage disequilibrium with the markers. Kruglyak (1999) estimated that in whole genome association studies, linkage disequilibrium was unlikely to extend beyond an average distance of 3 kb in the general population; this implies that a minimum of 500,000 SNPs would be required for whole genome analysis.

Genome-Wide Association Studies of Type 1 Diabetes

Smyth and colleagues (2006) performed a multi-locus case–control association study of T1D using >6500 coding, non-synonymous (ns)SNPs. Although not discussed in the paper, the rationale for studying nsSNP was the expectation that most alleles affecting common, complex diseases would alter the coding sequence, and therefore the causal variants might be among the markers selected (Weiss and Terwilliger, 2000). The study was underpowered with ~2000 cases and 1700 control samples, and, described as an "interim analysis," was not corrected for multiple hypothesis testing. The most significantly associated SNP was the previously published and confirmed C1858T SNP in *PTPN22* (Bottini et al., 2004).

IFIH1

The authors referred to the next two most significantly associated SNPs: one in *CAPSL*, which is adjacent to *IL17R*, and the other on chromosome 2q24.3 in *IFIH1* (IFN induced with helicase C domain 1; also known as *MDA5* or Helicard; risk-associated SNP *rs1990760*). The association with *rs1990760* was strengthened by genotyping an additional ~2500 cases and ~4500 controls and by examining an independent collection of parent–child trios. The IFIH1 protein functions as a pattern recognition receptor for viruses (dsRNA). The T1D-associated A allele of *rs1990760* is also associated with RA (Stahl et al., 2010) and vitiligo (Jin et al., 2010), but is a resistance allele for Crohn's disease (Barrett et al., 2008).

In 2007, the Wellcome Trust Case Control Consortium (WTCCC, 2007) published a major genetic milestone: a Genome Wide Association Study (GWAS) of seven complex diseases (bipolar disorder, coronary artery disease, Crohn's disease, hypertension, RA, T1D, and T2D) with about 2000 cases per disease, and a shared group of ~3000 controls, typed at 500,568 SNPs using the Affymetrix GeneChip500k Mapping Array Set. Prior to the genome-wide analysis of the dataset, the authors examined association at previously identified loci for confirmation by association. For T1D, they confirmed association for *HLA*, *CTLA4*, *PTPN22*, *CD25*, and *IFIH1*; *INS* could not be tested because a suitable SNP was not identified. It is sobering to note that the p-values obtained for these "proof of principle" associations only exceeded the genome-wide significance level for *HLA* and *PTPN22*. Even more concerning was the finding that even after raising the significance threshold 500-fold, the only other previously reported genetic region identified was *CD25*. The study did, however, identify three new loci significantly associated with T1D: 12q13, 12q24, and 16p13. Two other loci identified by multi-locus analysis were reported, but were unlikely to be significant after correction for the additional hypotheses tested.

In a follow-up study, the WTCCC (Todd et al., 2007) genotyped an additional 4000 cases and 5000 controls (total 6000 affected, 6200 controls) and confirmed significance for 12q24 (gene *SH2B3*), 12q13 (*ERBB3*), 16p13 (*CLEC16A*), and 18p11 (*PTPN2*). Mutations in *SH2B3* have also been associated with celiac disease (Hunt et al., 2008), MS (Alcina et al., 2010), RA (Stahl et al., 2010), and hypothyroidism (Eriksson et al., 2012); polymorphisms in *CLEC16A* are also associated with MS (International Multiple Sclerosis Genetics Consortium, 2009) and primary biliary cirrhosis (Mells et al., 2011); and the T1D-associated risk allele of *PTPN2* is also associated with celiac disease (Dubois et al., 2010).

A combined meta-analysis incorporating cases from the WTCCC studies (Todd et al., 2007) and a combined

British and US GWAS (Cooper et al., 2008) examined a total sample set of 7514 cases and 9045 reference samples (Barrett et al., 2009). At a genome-wide level of significance, they confirmed association with the previously identified regions 1p13 (gene of interest *PTPN22*), 2q24 (*IFIH1*), 2q33 (*CTLA4*), 4q27 (*IL2*), 6q15 (*BACH2*), 10p15 (*IL2RA* and *PRKCQ*), 11p15 (*INS*), 12q13 (*ERBB3*), 12q24 (*SH2B3*), 15q25 (*CTSH*), 16p13 (*CLEC16A*), 18p11 (*PTPN2*), 21p22 (*UBASH3A*), and 22q13 (*C1QTNF6*). In addition, they obtained genome-wide significance for 18 other loci, including *IL10* and *CD69*.

IL2

Within 4q27, the most significant SNP lies in the gene *KIAA1109*, which is about 200 kb 3′ of the *IL2* and *IL21* cytokine genes, and is of particular interest because it is syntenic with the NOD mouse diabetes susceptibility gene *Idd3* (Denny et al., 1997).

IL10

The most significantly associated SNP at 1q32 (*rs3024505*) is distal to the *IL10* gene. IL10 has pleiotropic effects on adaptive and innate immunity. Its ability to inhibit the production of several inflammatory cytokines and chemokines, including IL1 and TNF, contributes to its anti-inflammatory activities. It inhibits expression of MHC class II antigens, as well as the costimulators CD80 (B7) and CD86 (B7.2) on monocytes significantly affecting their T cell-activating capacity. In contrast, it enhances survival and proliferation of B cells and increases antibody production (Moore et al., 2001). While the G allele at *rs3024505* is associated with T1D, the A allele is associated with ulcerative colitis (Anderson et al., 2011) and the T allele with Crohn's disease (Franke et al., 2010). This region also contains genes encoding *IL19* and *IL20*.

CD69

CD69 is encoded at 12p13. Its expression is induced on T cell activation and mediates T cell costimulation. The most significantly associated SNP is in the first intron, which contains a cis-regulatory element (Vazquez et al., 2012). Significantly, CD69 suppresses Sphingosine 1-Phosphate Receptor-1 (S1P1) function (Bankovich et al., 2010). S1P1 plays a critical role in lymphocyte recirculation; its pharmaceutical downmodulation by the agonist Fingolimod sequesters lymphocytes in lymph nodes, inhibiting relapses of MS.

Genome-Wide Association Studies of Multiple Sclerosis

GWAS of MS soon followed those of T1D and were coordinated through the International MS Genetics Consortium (IMSGC). The first of these was performed in 2007 (International Multiple Sclerosis Genetics Consortium et al., 2007) and involved 931 trios (MS affected individual and non-affected parents) and interrogation of 334,923 SNPs. Analysis for association identified a total of 110 SNPs selected for follow-up in a replication phase consisting of 2322 MS cases, 609 parent-case trios, 789 controls, and genotyping data from two external control datasets resulting in a combined analysis of 12,360 subjects. In addition to the *HLA*, two other genes were found to be strongly associated with MS risk: *CD25* and the IL7 receptor (*IL7R*) gene.

CD25

The SNP in 10p15 most strongly associated with MS is in the first intron of *CD25*, while that associated with T1D lies about 20 kb upstream. A careful association analysis of *CD25* alleles was performed in a DNA collection of 9407 healthy controls, 2420 MS, and 6425 T1D subjects as well as 1303 MS parent−child trios. Maier et al. (2009a) observed significant complexity at this locus: one allele was associated with T1D but not MS; another was associated with susceptibility to T1D but protection from MS, and a third conferred susceptibility to both diseases. Presence of MS risk-associated variants in *CD25* correlated with increased sIL2RA expression; while sIL2RA levels were increased in very severe MS, they did not decrease with treatment (Maier et al., 2009b). In contrast the T1D-associated variants correlated with decreased sIL2RA expression (Lowe et al., 2007). Although sIL2RA inhibits IL2-mediated signaling, it promotes T cell activation and proliferation, presumably by reducing activation-induced cell death.

IL7R

IL7R on 5p13 had previously been identified in a small multi-locus case−control association study of MS as associated with the disease (Zhang et al., 2005). In the GWAS by the International Multiple Sclerosis Genetics Consortium et al., (2007) the most significantly associated SNP in the region lies within exon 6, which is alternatively spliced. This SNP has a functional effect on gene expression as it disrupts a putative exonic splicing silencer, influencing the relative proportions of soluble and membrane-bound isoforms of the protein (Gregory et al., 2007). Polymorphisms within IL7R are also associated with primary biliary cirrhosis (Mells et al., 2011).

Although not significant, moderate associations were also reported for an additional 13 SNPs, including those located within the genes *CD58* (1p13), *EVI5* (1p22), and *CLEC16A* (16p13). It was not until replication studies were performed in independent cohorts of MS cases and controls that these genes could be confirmed as MS risk-associated variants (Weber et al., 2008; Hoppenbrouwers et al., 2008; Rubio et al., 2008).

CD58

CD58 on chromosome 1p13 encodes the costimulatory molecule LFA-3. Resequencing and fine mapping of the *CD58* gene region in patients with MS and control subjects identified a *CD58* variant that provided further evidence of association with MS. The *rs2300747* SNP lies within the first intron of *CD58*. The protective (G) allele is associated with a dose-dependent increase in *CD58* mRNA expression in lymphoblastic cell lines and peripheral blood mononuclear cells from MS subjects (De Jager et al., 2009a). The possibility that increased LFA-3 expression on circulating mononuclear cells is protective is supported by the finding that *CD58* mRNA expression is increased in MS subjects during clinical remission. A potential mechanism of action is via the engagement of CD2 by LFA-3, which upregulates the expression of transcription factor FoxP3, leading to enhanced function of $CD4^+CD25^+$ Treg cells (De Jager et al., 2009b).

In 2009, an Australian study focused on an MS case versus non-affected control GWAS involving 1618 MS cases in the initial discovery phase, and replication in an independent cohort of 2256 MS cases and 2310 healthy controls (Australia and New Zealand Multiple Sclerosis Genetics Consortium, 2009). This led to the identification of two novel genetic loci, one on chromosome 12q13-14 and the other on chromosome 20q13, and replicated the association of *HLA* and *CD58* at a genome-wide level of significance (Australia and New Zealand Multiple Sclerosis Genetics Consortium, 2009).

CYP27B1

The association with the region on chromosome 12q13-14 could be due to a number of potential candidate genes, and requires further refinement due to the strong linkage disequilibrium in this region. The most strongly associated SNP lies within the 3′ untranslated region of *METTL1*, about 2 kb upstream of *CYP27B1*, which encodes the enzyme 25-hydroxy-vitamin D-1 alpha hydroxylase and is involved in vitamin D metabolism (Bailey et al., 2007). Vitamin D plays an important role in immune function, and has also been shown to regulate expression of *HLA-DR15* (Ramagopalan et al., 2009). Other genes in this region include *CDK4* also previously

shown to play a role in immune function and autoimmune disease.

CD40

The SNP most strongly associated with MS on 20q13 lies about 10 kb upstream of *CD40*. In addition to the association with MS, variants within *CD40* are also associated with RA, GD, and Crohn's disease. Of particular interest is a SNP located at −1 bp from the start of translation within the Kozak consensus sequence of the *CD40* gene (*rs1883232*), as the MS resistance allele (C) is associated with RA, GD, and Crohn's disease, and leads to increased efficiency of translation, while the MS susceptibility (T) allele leads to lower *CD40* expression (Blanco-Kelly et al., 2010).

In the same year, De Jager et al. (2009a) published a meta-analysis that combined 895 subjects from the IMSGC's original association study (International Multiple Sclerosis Genetics Consortium et al., 2007), 969 subjects from the Gene MSA consortium (Baranzini et al., 2009), and an additional unpublished set of 860 subjects, totaling 2624 cases and 7220 controls. This study confirmed, at a genome-wide level of significance, *HLA*, *CD58*, *CD25*, and *CLEC16A*. It also identified chromosomal regions at 12p13 (gene of interest *TNFRSF1A*), 16q24 (*IRF8*), and 11q12 (*CD6*) as significantly associated.

TNFRSF1A

The most significantly associated SNP at 12p13 (*rs1800693*) lies at the splice junction at the 3′ end of the sixth exon of the *TNFRSF1A* gene, which encodes TNFR1. Analysis of GWAS data in conjunction with the 1000 Genomes Project data identified this SNP as the likely causal variant in the *TNFRSF1A* region. The MS risk allele (C) generates a soluble form of TNFR1 that can block TNF signaling (Gregory et al., 2012), mimicking the effect of TNF-blocking drugs, which exacerbate MS (The Lenercept Multiple Sclerosis Study Group et al., 1999). The MS susceptibility allele at this locus also confers susceptibility to primary biliary cirrhosis (Mells et al., 2011) and this region showed mild linkage to lupus (Moser et al., 1998).

IRF8

The most significantly associated SNP at 16q24 lies ~60 kb 3′ of *IRF8*. The *IRF8* gene is a key target of vitamin D, through binding the nuclear vitamin D receptor (Ramagopalan et al., 2010). Administration of exogenous IFNγ exacerbates MS; *IRF8* is upregulated by IFNγ and cooperatively enhances IFNγ-induced apoptosis of oligodendroglial progenitor cells (Horiuchi et al., 2011).

CD6

The most significantly associated SNP in the 11q12 region (*rs17824933*) lies in the first intron of CD6. CD6 is a type 1 transmembrane glycoprotein found on T lymphocytes in association with the signaling components of the TCR. It acts as a costimulator of T cell proliferation via its interaction with the ligand, activated leukocyte cell adhesion molecule (ALCAM; Zimmerman et al., 2006). The MS susceptibility allele is associated with decreased expression of full-length *CD6* in T cells and an increase in a splice variant lacking exon 5, resulting in diminished proliferation during long-term activation of CD4$^+$ T cells (Kofler et al., 2011). Nevertheless, the role of CD6 in MS is not completely clear, as it can attenuate T cell activation, possibly via regulation of CD5 tyrosine phosphorylation (Oliveira et al., 2012), and appears to play a role in leukocyte trafficking across the blood–brain barrier and into the central nervous system via its interactions with ALCAM on the endothelium transmigratory cups (Cayrol et al., 2008).

The largest GWAS for MS to date was performed by the International MS Genetics Consortium (International Multiple Sclerosis Genetics Consortium, 2011b). This study involved approximately 10,000 MS cases and 20,000 controls collected from throughout Europe, America, and Oceania, and identified a total of 57 genetic loci associated with MS in addition to the *HLA*, of which 28 had not been previously reported (http://wattle.well.ox.ac.uk/wtccc2/external/ms/). The genes confirmed as associated with MS at a genome-wide level of significance included *HLA*, *CD58*, *CD25*, *CD6*, *TNFRSF1A*, *CYP27B1*, *CLEC16A*, and *IRF8*. New loci identified included 3p24 (gene of interest *EOMES*), 3q13 (*CD86*), and 5q33 (*IL12B*).

IL12B

The most significantly associated SNP at 5q33 is in the second exon of an uncharacterized open reading frame (ORF; *LOC285626*) about 3 kb upstream of *IL12B*, which encodes the 40 kDa subunit of IL12 and IL23. These cytokines have been strongly implicated in the pathogenesis of both MS and the mouse model of MS, experimental autoimmune encephalomyelitis (Langrish et al., 2005). The gene *IL12A* (3q25), which encodes the 35 kDa subunit of IL12, had been previously implicated as a SNP in its second intron was associated with MS by the IMSGC (International Multiple Sclerosis Genetics Consortium, 2010). IL12 is expressed by activated dendritic cells (DC), macrophages, and monocytes and plays an important role in sustaining IFNγ production and the generation and maintenance of memory/effector Th1 cells. In contrast, IL23 does not promote the development of Th1 cells, but is essential for the expansion of a pathogenic CD4 T cell population characterized by the production of IL17, IL17F, IL6, and TNF (Thakker et al., 2007). The MS-associated *IL12B* allele is also associated with psoriasis (Ellinghaus et al., 2010). Ustekinumab, a neutralizing anti-IL12 p40 mAb did not show efficacy in reducing the cumulative number of gadolinium-enhancing T1-weighted lesions in MS (Segal et al., 2008).

Once again, outside of the *HLA*, all associations showed only modest OR between 1.1 and 1.3. The majority of associated genes were located either near or within immune-system related genes, and a large proportion had previously been associated with other autoimmune diseases.

Genome-Wide Association Studies of Systemic Lupus Erythematosus

The first GWAS of lupus was performed under the auspices of the International Consortium for Systemic Lupus Erythematosus Genetics (SLEGEN) in 2007 (SLEGEN et al., 2008). It was a phased study with an initial genome-wide analysis of 720 female lupus patients of European ancestry and 2337 controls, with the most significantly associated SNPs typed in an additional 1846 patients. This study confirmed, at a genome-wide level of significance, both the *HLA* and *IRF5*. It also found significant association at four other regions: 16p11 (gene of interest *ITGAM*), 11p15.5 (*PHRF*), 3p14.3 (*PXK*), and 1q25.1.

ITGAM

The most strongly associated SNP in lupus, on 16p11.2, is in the 14th intron of *ITGAM*. This gene encodes the integrin alpha M chain, which together with the beta 2 chain (ITGB2) forms leukocyte-specific integrin CD11b (MAC1, or inactivated complement receptor 3). CD11b is important in the phagocytosis of complement coated particles as well as the adherence and emigration from the bloodstream of neutrophils and monocytes via interactions with a wide range of structurally unrelated ligands, including ICAM-1 and ICAM-2, C3bi, and fibrinogen. In a replication study, the association of lupus with *ITGAM* was confirmed. However, a SNP with stronger association was identified, *rs1143679*, which encodes a nonsynonymous polymorphism that results in an R77H substitution, so altering the conformation of the αI domain, with subsequent consequences for MAC1 ligand binding (Nath et al., 2008). In a GWAS of patients bearing anti-dsDNA autoantibodies in lupus, *ITGAM* together with the *HLA*, *STAT4*, and *IRF5* was found to be significantly associated (Chung et al., 2011).

PHRF1

The most strongly associated gene on 11p15.5 lies within the fourth intron of *PHRF1* (*KIAA1542*). The 3′ end of *PHRF1* almost immediately abuts the 3′ end of the IFN response gene *IRF7*, which is in the reverse orientation. IRF7 is a transcription factor that mediates IFNβ production in response to viral infection. Genetic variation at this locus is associated with IFNα activity in lupus and titers of anti-Sm autoantibody (Salloum et al., 2010).

Published in the same month as the SLEGEN study, Hom et al. (2008) performed a GWAS on DNA samples from 1311 patients with lupus and 1783 controls, all North Americans of European descent. Strong confirmation at a genome-wide level of significance was found for *HLA*, *IRF5*, and *STAT4*, although there was a partial overlap of subjects included in the original report of *STAT4* association (Remmers et al., 2007). In addition, two other regions of genome-wide significance were identified, 16p11 (*ITGAM*) and 8p23 (*BLK*).

BLK

The most strongly associated SNP on 8p23 is in the promoter region of *BLK*, about 3 kb upstream of the transcription initiation site. This gene encodes a Src tyrosine-kinase that has a role in B cell receptor signaling and B cell development, although *Blk*-deficient mice have no obvious phenotype (Texido et al., 2000). The lupus risk allele is associated with reduced *BLK* mRNA in transformed B cell lines (Hom et al., 2008) but in primary human B lymphocytes, cis-regulatory effects of disease-associated SNPs are restricted to naïve and transitional B cells. The allelic effect has been shown to affect protein levels (Simpfendorfer et al., 2012).

FROM LOCATION TO MOLECULAR MECHANISMS

Although a few tagging SNPs used in GWAS of autoimmune disease affect transcript splicing (Graham et al., 2006; Gregory et al., 2007; Kofler et al., 2011), in general the GWAS approach tests disease associations with individual variants that are unlikely to be causal. Many of the applications of GWAS data are dependent on identifying the functional variants, not just the tagging SNPs with which they are in LD. One approach is to examine protein-coding genes in the vicinity of risk SNPs, in order to identify overrepresented biological pathways. For example, the recent GWAS data obtained for MS were analyzed for enrichment of genes (defined as protein coding regions nearest to the lead tagging SNP) with similar function, as classified in the Gene Ontology (GO) database (Ashburner et al., 2000). The GO terms having the

most significant enrichment included genes involved in "immune system processes" ($p = 8.6 \times 10^{-11}$, OR = 9.12), particularly lymphocyte function ($p = 3.2 \times 10^{-11}$, OR = 35.96), and especially T cell activation and proliferation ($p = 1.85 \times 10^{-9}$, OR = 40.85 (International Multiple Sclerosis Genetics Consortium et al., 2011b). With this information, one can return to the genomic sequences flagging risk SNPs to identify additional putative causal variants. The sequencing of these, and their associated regulatory sequences, in patients and controls can help validate these candidates.

This approach has provided partial success, but has made it clear that few causal variants affect amino acid sequence of candidate protein coding regions. In many cases, the haplotype block in LD with tagging SNP lies within the first intron, or in regulatory sequences 5′ or 3′ of a protein-coding gene. Usually, the most important regions that regulate transcription are the promoter and the first intron, although many other regulatory elements are also required for spatiotemporally and quantitatively correct gene expression; enhancer and repressor elements frequently reside in introns up- and downstream of the transcription unit (Kleinjan and van Heyningen 2005). This finding therefore suggests that the linked causal variants in these regions are likely to be expression quantitative trait loci (eQTL), which are loci at which polymorphism affects the expression of one or more transcripts. Indeed, the data obtained on candidate genes for autoimmune diseases strongly support the hypothesis that most of the genetically encoded risk of disease is conferred by eQTL (Jacob et al., 1990; Bennett et al., 1995; Ueda et al., 2003; Graham et al., 2006; Ramagopalan et al., 2009; De Jager et al., 2009a; Maier et al., 2009b; Blanco-Kelly et al., 2010; Wang et al., 2010; Zuvich et al., 2011; Alcina et al., 2012).

The success of eQTL-based approaches is illustrated in recent studies that combine genotyping and gene expression datasets. For example, Göring et al. (2007) reported that, of around 20,000 autosomal gene transcripts, 1345 were regulated by nearby (cis) gene variants. With a false discovery rate of 5%, the median genotype-expression change was 24.6%. In a dataset combining very high density SNP genotyping and gene expression profiling of lymphoblast cell lines from 210 unrelated individuals, Veyrieras et al. (2008) found that, of 11,466 expressed genes, expression levels in 6.5% of these were highly associated with individual SNPs. The most significantly associated eQTL was an average of 7.5 kb from the transcript, and 99% of cis-eQTLs were found to lie between 110 kb upstream and 40 kb downstream of the transcription start site.

It is likely that eQTLs and splice QTLs will be cell subset specific. Dimas et al. (2009) identified eQTL in three cell types (fibroblasts, EBV-transformed B cells, and T cells) in 75 newborns enrolled in a European Gencord project. Of 1007 unique eQTLs, only 8.5% were shared among all three cell types, 12% were shared between two of three cell types and 79.5% were cell-type specific. It is therefore necessary for cell subsets to be analyzed for gene expression profiles individually. The advantages for autoimmune diseases are that so much of the disease risk appears to be conferred by genes involved in leukocyte function, and a wide range of leukocytes can be accessed via peripheral blood using commercially available kits that facilitate subset purification from whole blood or buffy coat. We are currently identifying MS-associated eQTL in five peripheral blood leukocyte subsets: CD4 T cells, CD8 T cells, B cells NK cells, and monocytes. By combining this dataset with IMSGC GWAS data (International Multiple Sclerosis Genetics Consortium et al., 2011a), we will be able to identify variants that are associated with differences in gene expression throughout the genome—whether in cis or trans. Some of these variants will also be associated with disease. These studies will dramatically increase our knowledge of each of these risk-associated haplotypes that contain eQTL: we will know what transcript it causes to be differentially expressed; we will know in what tissue that differential expression occurs; and we will know the direction of differential expression it confers, as well as the direction of change in expression that is associated with disease. With these four critical pieces of information we can generate animal models to test the validity of these candidate genes and therefore determine the molecular mechanisms of their actions.

CONCLUDING COMMENTS

In many regards, the true value of genomic studies of complex autoimmune traits are yet to be realized, and will require the identification of causal variants and their mechanisms of action. Nevertheless, work to date has strengthened our understanding of autoimmunity in many regards. We now know that some of the commonly used animal models have additional value in sharing susceptibility loci, and in some cases sharing molecular pathogenesis, with the human diseases. We now have a partial explanation for the coexistence of different autoimmune diseases within families, and in individuals, as several diseases have been found to share susceptibility alleles. And we now have a plethora or molecular clues suggesting disease aetiology, some raising intriguing questions— such as the opposite effects of many alleles on organ-specific autoimmune diseases versus the inflammatory bowel diseases. These molecular clues, and the availability of robust animal models, are likely to help dramatically improve our understanding of immune tolerance and autoimmunity over the next decade.

ACKNOWLEDGMENTS

This work was supported by the National Multiple Sclerosis Society (USA), MSRA, Lions Clubs of Australia, the Australian Research Council, and the National Health and Medical Research Council (NHMRC) of Australia. AGB is supported by an NHMRC Senior Research Fellowship; HB is supported by an NHMRC Career Development Award; MAJ is supported by an NHMRC Early Career Research Fellowship. We are greatful for discussions with our friends and colleagues, including the members of the ANZgene consortium, Jim Stankovich, Grant Morahan, and Thomas Brodnicki, and to Benjamin Crowley for assistance.

REFERENCES

Acheson, E.D., Bachrach, C.A., Wright, F.M., 1960. Some comments on the relationship of the distribution of multiple sclerosis to latitude, solar radiation, and other variables. Acta Psychiatr. Scand. Suppl. 35, 132–147.

Aderka, D., Wysenbeek, A., Engelmann, H., Cope, A.P., Brennan, F., Molad, Y., et al., 1993. Correlation between serum levels of soluble tumor necrosis factor receptor and disease activity in systemic lupus erythematosus. Arthritis Rheum. 36, 1111–1120.

Agnello, V., De Bracco, M.M., Kunkel, H.G., 1972. Hereditary C2 deficiency with some manifestations of systemic lupus erythematosus. J. Immunol. 08, 837–840.

Ahmed, A.R., Yunis, J.J., Marcus-Bagley, D., Yunis, E.J., Salazar, M., Katz, A.J., et al., 1993. Major histocompatibility complex susceptibility genes for dermatitis herpetiformis compared with those for gluten-sensitive enteropathy. J. Exp. Med. 178, 2067–2075.

Alarcón-Segovia, D., Alarcón-Riquelme, M.E., Cardiel, M.H., Caeiro, F., Massardo, L., Villa, A.R., et al., 2005. Grupo Latinoamericano de Estudio del Lupus Eritematoso (GLADEL). Familial aggregation of systemic lupus erythematosus, rheumatoid arthritis, and other autoimmune diseases in 1,177 lupus patients from the GLADEL cohort. Arthritis Rheum. 52, 1138–1147.

Alcina, A., Vandenbroeck, K., Otaegui, D., Saiz, A., Gonzalez, J.R., Fernandez, O., et al., 2010. The autoimmune disease-associated KIF5A, CD226 and SH2B3 gene variants confer susceptibility for multiple sclerosis. Genes Immun. 11, 439–445.

Alcina, A., Abad-Grau Mdel, M., Fedetz, M., Izquierdo, G., Lucas, M., Fernández, O., et al., 2012. Multiple sclerosis risk variant HLA-DRB1*1501 associates with high expression of DRB1 gene in different human populations. PLoS One. 7, e29819.

American College of Rheumatology Ad Hoc Committee on Systemic Lupus Erythematosus Guidelines, 1999. Guidelines for referral and management of systemic lupus erythematosus in adults. Arthritis Rheum. 42, 1785–1796.

Amiel, J.L., 1967. Study of the leukocyte phenotypes in Hodgkin's disease. In: Curtoni, E.S., Mattiuz, P.L., Tosi, R.M. (Eds.), Histocompatibility. Munksgaard, Copenhagen, pp. 79–81. Testing.

Amos, C.I., Chen, W.V., Lee, A., Li, W., Kern, M., Lundsten, R., et al., 2006. High-density SNP analysis of 642 Caucasian families with rheumatoid arthritis identifies two new linkage regions on 11p12 and 2q33. Genes Immun. 7, 277–286.

Anderson, C.A., Boucher, G., Lees, C.W., Franke, A., D'Amato, M., Taylor, K.D., et al., 2011. Meta-analysis identifies 29 additional ulcerative colitis risk loci, increasing the number of confirmed associations to 47. Nat. Genet. 43, 246–252.

Araki, M., Chung, D., Liu, S., Chamberlain, G., Garner, V., Hunter, K. M., et al., 2009. Genetic evidence that the differential expression of the ligand-independent isoform of CTLA-4 is the molecular basis of the Idd5.1 type 1 diabetes region in nonobese diabetic mice. J. Immunol. 183, 5146–5157.

Arellano, J., Vallejo, M., Jimenez, J., Rainbow, D.B., Chamberlain, G., Garner, V., 1984. HLA-B27 and ankylosing spondylitis in the Mexican Mestizo population. Tissue Antigens. 23, 112–116.

Aringer, M., Houssiau, F., Gordon, C., Graninger, W.B., Voll, R.E., Rath, E., et al., 2009. Adverse events and efficacy of TNF-alpha blockade with infliximab in patients with systemic lupus erythematosus, long-term follow-up of 13 patients. Rheumatology (Oxford). 48, 1451–1454.

Ascherio, A., Munger, K.L., 2007. Environmental risk factors for multiple sclerosis. Part I, the role of infection. Ann. Neurol. 61, 288–299.

Ashburner, M., Ball, C.A., Blake, J.A., Botstein, D., Butler, H., Cherry, J.M., et al., 2000. Gene ontology, tool for the unification of biology. The Gene Ontology Consortium. Nat. Genet. 25, 25–29.

Australia and New Zealand Multiple Sclerosis Genetics Consortium (ANZgene), 2009. Genome-wide association study identifies new multiple sclerosis susceptibility loci on chromosomes 12 and 20. Nat. Genet. 41, 824–828.

Baechler, E.C., Batliwalla, F.M., Karypis, G., Gaffney, P.M., Ortmann, W.A., Espe, K.J., et al., 2003. Interferon-inducible gene expression signature in peripheral blood cells of patients with severe lupus. Proc. Natl. Acad. Sci. U.S.A. 100, 2610–2615.

Bailey, R., Cooper, J.D., Zeitels, L., Smyth, D.J., Yang, J.H., Walker, N. M., et al., 2007. Association of the vitamin D metabolism gene CYP27B1 with type 1 diabetes. Diabetes. 56, 2616–2621.

Bain, S.C., Prins, J.B., Hearne, C.M., Rodrigues, N.R., Rowe, B.R., Pritchard, L.E., et al., 1992. Insulin gene region-encoded susceptibility to type 1 diabetes is not restricted to HLA-DR4-positive individuals. Nat. Genet. 2, 212–215.

Ban, M., Stewart, G.J., Bennetts, B.H., Heard, R., Simmons, R., Maranian, M., et al., 2002. A genome screen for linkage in Australian sibling-pairs with multiple sclerosis. Genes Immun. 3, 464–469.

Bankovich, A.J., Shiow, L.R., Cyster, J.G., 2010. CD69 suppresses sphingosine 1-phosophate receptor-1 (S1P1) function through inter-action with membrane helix 4. J. Biol. Chem. 285, 22328–22337.

Baranzini, S.E., Wang, J., Gibson, R.A., Galwey, N., Naegelin, Y., Barkhof, F., et al., 2009. Genome-wide association analysis of susceptibility and clinical phenotype in multiple sclerosis. Hum. Mol. Genet. 18, 767–778.

Barcellos, L.F., Sawcer, S., Ramsay, P.P., Baranzini, S.E., Thomson, G., Briggs, F., et al., 2006. Heterogeneity at the HLA-DRB1 locus and risk for multiple sclerosis. Hum. Mol. Genet. 15, 2813–2824.

Barnes, B.J., Moore, P.A., Pitha, P.M., 2001. Virus-specific activation of a novel interferon regulatory factor, IRF-5, results in the induction of distinct interferon alpha genes. J. Biol. Chem. 276, 23382–23390.

Barratt, B.J., Payne, F., Lowe, C.E., Hermann, R., Healy, B.C., Harold, D., et al., 2004. Remapping the insulin gene/IDDM2 locus in type 1 diabetes. Diabetes. 53, 1884–1889.

Barrett, J.C., Hansoul, S., Nicolae, D.L., Cho, J.H., Duerr, R.H., Rioux, J.D., et al., 2008. Genome-wide association defines more than 30 distinct susceptibility loci for Crohn's disease. Nat. Genet. 40, 955–962.

Barrett, J.C., Clayton, D.G., Concannon, P., Akolkar, B., Cooper, J.D., Erlich, H.A., et al., 2009. Genome-wide association study and meta-analysis find that over 40 loci affect risk of type 1 diabetes. Nat. Genet. 41, 703–707.

Baxter, A.G., 1997. Immunogenetics and the cause of autoimmune disease. Autoimmunity. 25, 177–189.

Baxter, A.G., 2007. The origin and application of experimental autoimmune encephalomyelitis. Nat. Rev. Immunol. 7, 904–912.

Begovich, A.B., Carlton, V.E., Honigberg, L.A., Schrodi, S.J., Chokkalingam, A.P., Alexander, H.C., et al., 2004. A missense single-nucleotide polymorphism in a gene encoding a protein tyrosine phosphatase (PTPN22) is associated with rheumatoid arthritis. Am. J. Hum. Genet. 75, 330–337.

Bell, G.I., Horita, S., Karam, J.H., 1984. A polymorphic locus near the human insulin gene is associated with insulin-dependent diabetes mellitus. Diabetes. 33, 176–183.

Bennett, S.T., Lucassen, A.M., Gough, S.C., Powell, E.E., Undlien, D. E., Pritchard, L.E., et al., 1995. Susceptibility to human type 1 diabetes at IDDM2 is determined by tandem repeat variation at the insulin gene minisatellite locus. Nat. Genet. 9, 284–292.

Bergamaschi, L., Leone, M.A., Fasano, M.E., Guerini, F.R., Ferrante, D., Bolognesi, E., et al., 2010. HLA-class I markers and multiple sclerosis susceptibility in the Italian population. Genes. Immun. 11, 173–180.

Bertrams, J., 1984. The HLA association of insulin-dependent (type I) diabetes mellitus. Behring Inst. Mitt. 75, 89–99.

Blanco-Kelly, F., Matesanz, F., Alcina, A., Teruel, M., Díaz-Gallo, L. M., Gómez-García, M., et al., 2010. CD40, novel association with Crohn's disease and replication in multiple sclerosis susceptibility. PLoS One. 5, e11520.

Block, S.R., Winfield, J.B., Lockshin, M.D., D'Angelo, W.A., Christian, C.L., 1975. Studies of twins with systemic lupus erythematosus. A review of the literature and presentation of 12 additional sets. Am. J. Med. 59, 533–552.

Blomhoff, A., Lie, B.A., Myhre, A.G., Kemp, E.H., Weetman, A.P., Akselsen, H.E., et al., 2004. Polymorphisms in the cytotoxic T lymphocyte antigen-4 gene region confer susceptibility to Addison's disease. J. Clin. Endocrinol. Metab. 89, 3474–3476.

Bonifacio, E., Bingley, P.J., Shattock, M., Dean, B.M., Dunger, D., Gale, E.A., et al., 1990. Quantification of islet-cell antibodies and prediction of insulin-dependent diabetes. Lancet. 335, 147–149.

Bossingham, D., 2003. Systemic lupus erythematosus in the far north of Queensland. Lupus. 12, 327–331.

Bottini, N., Musumeci, L., Alonso, A., Rahmouni, S., Nika, K., Rostamkhani, M., et al., 2004. A functional variant of lymphoid tyrosine phosphatase is associated with type I diabetes. Nat. Genet. 36, 337–338.

Bowness, P., Davies, K.A., Norsworthy, P.J., Athanassiou, P., Taylor-Wiedeman, J., Borysiewicz, L.K., et al., 1994. Hereditary C1q deficiency and systemic lupus erythematosus. QJM. 87, 455–464.

Brewerton, D.A., Caffrey, M., Hart, F.D., Caffrey, M., James, D.C., Sturrock, R.D., 1973. Ankylosing spondylitis and HL-A 27. Lancet. 1, 904–907.

Broadley, S., Sawcer, S., D'Alfonso, S., Hensiek, A., Coraddu, F., Gray, J., et al., 2001. A genome screen for multiple sclerosis in Italian families. Genes. Immun. 2, 205–210.

Cardon, L.R., Bell, J.I., 2001. Association study designs for complex diseases. Nat. Rev. Genet. 2, 91–99.

Carton, H., Vlietinck, R., Debruyne, J., De Keyser, J., D'Hooghe, M.B., Loos, R., et al., 1997. Risks of multiple sclerosis in relatives of patients in Flanders, Belgium. J. Neurol. Neurosurg. Psychiatr. 62, 329–333.

Cayrol, R., Wosik, K., Berard, J.L., Dodelet-Devillers, A., Ifergan, I., Kebir, H., et al., 2008. Activated leukocyte cell adhesion molecule promotes leukocyte trafficking into the central nervous system. Nat. Immunol. 9, 137–145.

Christiansen, F.T., Zhang, W.J., Griffiths, M., Mallal, S.A., Dawkins, R. L., 1991. Major histocompatibility complex (MHC) complement deficiency, ancestral haplotypes and systemic lupus erythematosus (SLE), C4 deficiency explains some but not all of the influence of the MHC. J. Rheumatol. 18, 1350–1358.

Chung, S.A., Taylor, K.E., Graham, R.R., Nititham, J., Lee, A.T., Ortmann, W.A., et al., 2011. Differential genetic associations for systemic lupus erythematosus based on anti-dsDNA autoantibody production. PLoS Genet. 7, e1001323.

Compston, A., 1991. Limiting and repairing the damage in multiple sclerosis. J. Neurol. Neurosurg. Psychiatr. 54, 945–948.

Concannon, P., Gogolin-Ewens, K.J., Hinds, D.A., Wapelhorst, B., Morrison, V.A., Stirling, B., et al., 1998. A second-generation screen of the human genome for susceptibility to insulin-dependent diabetes mellitus. Nat. Genet. 19, 292–296.

Concannon, P., Erlich, H.E., Julier, C., Morahan, G., Nerup, J., Pociot, F., et al., 2005. Type 1 diabetes, evidence for susceptibility loci from four genome-wide linkage scans in 1435 multiplex families. Diabetes. 54, 2995–3001.

Concannon, P., Chen, W.M., Julier, C., Morahan, G., Akolkar, B., Erlich, H.A., et al., 2009. Genome-wide scan for linkage to type 1 diabetes in 2,496 multiplex families from the Type 1 Diabetes Genetics Consortium. Diabetes. 58, 1018–1022.

Cooper, J.D., Smyth, D.J., Smiles, A.M., Plagnol, V., Walker, N.M., Allen, J.E., et al., 2008. Meta-analysis of genome-wide association study data identifies additional type 1 diabetes risk loci. Nat. Genet. 40, 1399–13401.

Coraddu, F., Sawcer, S., D'Alfonso, S., Plagnol, V., Walker, N.M., Allen, J.E., et al., 2001. A genome screen for multiple sclerosis in Sardinian multiplex families. Eur. J. Hum. Genet. 9, 621–626.

Cornall, R.J., Prins, J.B., Todd, J.A., Pressey, A., DeLarato, N.H., Wicker, L.S., et al., 1991. Type 1 diabetes in mice is linked to the interleukin-1 receptor and Lsh/Ity/Bcg genes on chromosome 1. Nature. 353, 262–265.

Cree, B.A., Rioux, J.D., McCauley, J.L., Gourraud, P.-A., Goyette, P., McElroy, J., et al., 2010. A major histocompatibility Class I locus contributes to multiple sclerosis susceptibility independently from HLA-DRB1*15,01. PLoS One. 5, e11296.

Cucca, F., Lampis, R., Congia, M., Angius, E., Nutland, S., Bain, S.C., et al., 2001. A correlation between the relative predisposition of MHC class II alleles to type 1 diabetes and the structure of their proteins. Hum. Mol. Genet. 10, 2025–2037.

Dausset, J., 1958. Iso-leuco-anticorps. Acta Haematol. 20, 156–166.

Davies, J.L., Kawaguchi, Y., Bennett, S.T., Copeman, J.B., Cordell, H. J., Pritchard, L.E., et al., 1994. A genome-wide search for human type 1 diabetes susceptibility genes. Nature. 371, 130–136.

Davies, K.A., Peters, A.M., Beynon, H.L., Walport, M.J., 1992. Immune complex processing in patients with systemic lupus erythematosus. In vivo imaging and clearance studies. J. Clin. Invest. 90, 2075–2083.

Davies, K.A., Erlendsson, K., Beynon, H.L., Peters, A.M., Steinsson, K., Valdimarsson, H., et al., 1993. Splenic uptake of immune complexes in man is complement-dependent. J. Immunol. 151, 3866–3873.

De Jager, P.L., Simon, K.C., Munger, K.L., Rioux, J.D., Hafler, D.A., Ascherio, A., 2008. Integrating risk factors, HLA-DRB1*1501 and Epstein-Barr virus in multiple sclerosis. Neurology. 70, 1113–1118.

De Jager, P.L., Baecher-Allan, C., Maier, L.M., Arthur, A.T., Ottoboni, L., Barcellos, L., et al., 2009a. The role of the CD58 locus in multiple sclerosis. Proc. Natl. Acad. Sci. U.S.A. 106, 5264–5269.

De Jager, P.L., Jia, X., Wang, J., de Bakker, P.I., Ottoboni, L., Aggarwal, N.T, 2009b. Meta-analysis of genome scans and replication identify CD6, IRF8 and TNFRSF1A as new multiple sclerosis susceptibility loci. Nat. Genet. 41, 776–782.

Deapen, D., Escalante, A., Weinrib, L., Horwitz, D., Bachman, B., Roy-Burman, P., et al., 1992. A revised estimate of twin concordance in systemic lupus erythematosus. Arthritis Rheum. 35, 311–318.

Delépine, M., Pociot, F., Habita, C., Hashimoto, L., Froguel, P., Rotter, J., et al., 1997. Evidence of a non-MHC susceptibility locus in type I diabetes linked to HLA on chromosome 6. Am. J. Hum. Genet. 60, 174–187.

Dendrou, C.A., Plagnol, V., Fung, E., Yang, J.H., Downes, K., Cooper, J.D., et al., 2009. Cell-specific protein phenotypes for the autoimmune locus IL2RA using a genotype-selectable human bioresource. Nat. Genet. 41, 1011–1015.

Denny, P., Lord, C.J., Hill, N.J., Goy, J.V., Levy, E.R., Podolin, P.L., et al., 1997. Mapping of the IDDM locus Idd3 to a 0.35-cM interval containing the interleukin-2 gene. Diabetes. 46, 695–700.

Devendra, D., Eisenbarth, G.S., 2003. Immunologic endocrine disorders. J. Allergy Clin. Immunol. 111, S624–S636.

Dietrich, W.F., Katz, H., Lincoln, S.E., Friedman, J., Dracopoli, N.C., Lander, E.S., 1992. A genetic map of the mouse suitable for typing intraspecific crosses. Genetics. 131, 423–447.

Dietrich, W.F., Miller, J., Steen, R., Merchant, M.A., Damron-Boles, D., Husain, Z., et al., 1996. A comprehensive genetic map of the mouse genome. Nature. 14, 149–152.

Dijstelbloem, H.M., Bijl, M., Fijnheer, R., Scheepers, R.H., Oost, W.W., Jansen, M.D., et al., 2000. Fcgamma receptor polymorphisms in systemic lupus erythematosus, association with disease and in vivo clearance of immune complexes. Arthritis Rheum. 43, 2793–2800.

Dimas, A.S., Deutsch, S., Stranger, B.E., Montgomery, S.B., Borel, C., Attar-Cohen, H., et al., 2009. Common regulatory variation impacts gene expression in a cell type-dependent manner. Science. 325, 1246–1250.

Donner, H., Braun, J., Seidl, C., Rau, H., Finke, R., Ventz, M., et al., 1997. Codon 17 polymorphism of the cytotoxic T lymphocyte antigen 4 gene in Hashimoto's thyroiditis and Addison's disease. J. Clin. Endocrinol. Metab. 82, 4130–4132.

Dubois, P.C., Trynka, G., Franke, L., Hunt, K.A., Romanos, J., Curtotti, A., et al., 2010. Multiple common variants for celiac disease influencing immune gene expression. Nat. Genet. 42, 295–302.

Duits, A.J., Bootsma, H., Derksen, R.H., Spronk, P.E., Kater, L., Kallenberg, C.G., et al., 1995. Skewed distribution of IgG Fc receptor IIa (CD32) polymorphism is associated with renal disease in systemic lupus erythematosus patients. Arthritis Rheum. 38, 1832–1836.

Ebers, G.C., Bulman, D.E., Sadovnick, A.D., Paty, D.W., Warren, S., Hader, W., et al., 1986. A population-based study of multiple sclerosis in twins. N. Engl. J. Med. 315, 1638–1642.

Ebers, G.C., Kukay, K., Bulman, D.E., Sadovnick, A.D., Rice, G., Anderson, C., et al., 1996. A full genome search in multiple sclerosis. Nat. Genet. 13, 472–476.

Ebringer, A., 1992. Ankylosing spondylitis is caused by Klebsiella. Evidence from immunogenetic, microbiologic, and serologic studies. Rheum. Dis. Clin. North Am. 18, 105–121.

Eichhorst, H., 1896. Veber infantile und hereditare multiple sclerosis. Arch. Pathol. Anat. 146, 173–192.

Ellinghaus, E., Ellinghaus, D., Stuart, P.E., Nair, R.P., Debrus, S., Raelson, J.V., et al., 2010. Genome-wide association study identifies a psoriasis susceptibility locus at TRAF3IP2. Nat. Genet. 42, 991–995.

Eriksson, N., Tung, J.Y., Kiefer, A.K., Hinds, D.A., Francke, U., Mountain, J.L., et al., 2012. Novel associations for hypothyroidism include known autoimmune risk loci. PLoS One. 7, e34442.

Fanciulli, M., Norsworthy, P.J., Petretto, E., Dong, R., Harper, L., Kamesh, L., et al., 2007. FCGR3B copy number variation is associated with susceptibility to systemic, but not organ-specific, autoimmunity. Nat. Genet. 39, 721–723.

Field, L.L., Tobias, R., Magnus, T., 1994. A locus on chromosome 15q26 (IDDM3) produces susceptibility to insulin-dependent diabetes mellitus. Nat. Genet. 8, 189–194.

Fielder, A.H., Walport, M.J., Batchelor, J.R., Rynes, R.I., Black, C.M., Dodi, I.A., et al., 1983. Family study of the major histocompatibility complex in patients with systemic lupus erythematosus, importance of null alleles of C4A and C4B in determining disease susceptibility. Br. Med. J. (Clin. Res. Ed.). 286, 425–428.

Fisher, M., Pusey, C.D., Vaughan, R.W., Rees, A.J., 1997. Susceptibility to Goodpasture's disease is strongly associated with HLA-DRB1 genes. Kidney Int. 51, 222–229.

Fogdell, A., Hillert, J., Sachs, C., Olerup, O., 1995. The multiple sclerosis- and narcolepsy-associated HLA class II haplotype includes the DRB5*0101 allele. Tissue Antigens. 46, 333–336.

Fogdell-Hahn, A., Ligers, A., Gronning, M., Olerup, O., 2000. Multiple sclerosis, a modifying influence of HLA class I genes in an HLA class II associated autoimmune disease. Tissue Antigens. 55, 140–148.

Francis, D.A., Batchelor, J.R., McDonald, W.I., Hing, S.N., Dodi, I.A., Fielder, A.H., et al., 1987a. Multiple sclerosis in north-east Scotland. An association with HLA-DQw1. Brain. 110, 181–196.

Francis, D.A., Compston, D.A., Batchelor, J.R., McDonald, W.I., 1987b. A reassessment of the risk of multiple sclerosis developing in patients with optic neuritis after extended follow-up. J. Neurol. Neurosurg. Psychiatr. 50, 758–765.

Franke, A., McGovern, D.P., Barrett, J.C., Wang, K., Radford-Smith, G.L., Ahmad, T., et al., 2010. Genome-wide meta-analysis increases to 71 the number of confirmed Crohn's disease susceptibility loci. Nat. Genet. 42, 1118–1125.

Freedman, B.I., Spray, B.J., Heise, E.R., Espeland, M.A., Canzanello, V.J., 1993. A race-controlled human leukocyte antigen frequency analysis in lupus nephritis. The South-Eastern Organ Procurement Foundation. Am. J. Kidney Dis. 21, 378–382.

Gaffney, P.M., Kearns, G.M., Shark, K.B., Ortmann, W.A., Selby, S.A., Malmgren, M.L., et al., 1998. A genome-wide search for susceptibility genes in human systemic lupus erythematosus sib-pair families. Proc. Natl. Acad. Sci. U.S.A. 95, 14875–14879.

Gaffney, P.M., Ortmann, W.A., Selby, S.A., Shark, K.B., Ockenden, T.C., Rohlf, K.E., et al., 2000. Genome screening in human systemic lupus erythematosus, results from a second Minnesota cohort and combined analyses of 187 sib-pair families. Am. J. Hum. Genet. 66, 547–556.

Garavito, G., Yunis, E.J., Egea, E., Ramirez, L.A., Malagón, C., Iglesias, A., et al., 2004. HLA-DRB1 alleles and HLA-DRB1 shared epitopes are markers for juvenile rheumatoid arthritis subgroups in Colombian mestizos. Hum. Immunol. 65, 359–365.

Gerold, K.D., Zheng, P., Rainbow, D.B., Zernecke, A., Wicker, L.S., Kissler, S., 2011. The soluble CTLA-4 splice variant protects from type 1 diabetes and potentiates regulatory T-cell function. Diabetes. 60, 1955–1963.

Gonzalez-Escribano, M.F., Rodriguez, R., Valenzuela, A., Garcia, A., Garcia-Lozano, J.R., Nuñez-Roldan, A., 1999. CTLA4 polymorphisms in Spanish patients with rheumatoid arthritis. Tissue Antigens. 53, 296–300.

Gorer, P.A., 1937. The genetic and antigenic basis of tumour transplantation. J. Pathol. Bacteriol. 44, 691–697.

Göring, H.H., Curran, J.E., Johnson, M.P., Dyer, T.D., Charlesworth, J., Cole, S.A., et al., 2007. Discovery of expression QTLs using large-scale transcriptional profiling in human lymphocytes. Nat. Genet. 39, 1208–1216.

Graham, R.R., Kozyrev, S.V., Baechler, E.C., Reddy, M.V., Plenge, R.M., Bauer, J.W., et al., 2006. A common haplotype of interferon regulatory factor 5 (IRF5) regulates splicing and expression and is associated with increased risk of systemic lupus erythematosus. Nat. Genet. 38, 550–555.

Gregersen, P.K., Amos, C.I., Lee, A.T., Lu, Y., Remmers, E.F., Kastner, D.L., et al., 2009. REL, encoding a member of the NF-kappaB family of transcription factors, is a newly defined risk locus for rheumatoid arthritis. Nat. Genet. 41, 820–823.

Gregory, A.P., Dendrou, C.A., Attfield, K.E., Haghikia, A., Xifara, D.K., Butter, F., et al., 2012. TNF receptor 1 genetic risk mirrors outcome of anti-TNF therapy in multiple sclerosis. Nature. 488, 508–511.

Gregory, S.G., Schmidt, S., Seth, P., Oksenberg, J.R., Hart, J., Prokop, A., et al., 2007. Interleukin 7 receptor alpha chain (IL7R) shows allelic and functional association with multiple sclerosis. Nat. Genet. 39, 1083–1091.

Guggenbuhl, P., Jean, S., Jego, P., Grosbois, B., Chalès, G., Semana, G., et al., 1998. Primary Sjögren's syndrome, role of the HLA-DRB1*0301-*1501 heterozygotes. J. Rheumatol. 25, 900–905.

Gyapay, G., Morissette, J., Vignal, A., Dib, C., Fizames, C., Millasseau, P., et al., 1994. The 1993–94 Genethon human genetic linkage map. Nat. Genet. 7, 246–339.

Haines, J.L., Ter-Minassian, M., Bazyk, A., Gusella, J.F., Kim, D.J., Terwedow, H., et al., 1996. A complete genomic screen for multiple sclerosis underscores a role for the major histocompatability complex. The Multiple Sclerosis Genetics Group. Nat. Genet. 13, 469–471.

Haines, J.L., Terwedow, H.A., Burgess, K., Pericak-Vance, M.A., Rimmler, J.B., Martin, E.R., et al., 1998. Linkage of the MHC to familial multiple sclerosis suggests genetic heterogeneity. The Multiple Sclerosis Genetics Group. Hum. Mol. Genet. 7, 1229–1234.

Hajeer, A.H., Hutchinson, I.V., 2001. Influence of TNFalpha gene polymorphisms on TNFalpha production and disease. Hum. Immunol. 62, 1191–1199.

Hammarström, L., Smith, E., Möller, E., Franksson, C., Matell, G., Von Reis, G., 1975. Myasthenia gravis, studies on HL-A antigens and lymphocyte subpopulations in patients with myasthenia gravis. Clin. Exp. Immunol. 21, 202−215.

Harbo, H.F., Celius, E.G., Vartdal, F., Spurkland, A., 1999. CTLA4 promoter and exon 1 dimorphisms in multiple sclerosis. Tissue Antigens. 53, 106−110.

Hashimoto, L., Habita, C., Beressi, J., Delepine, M., Besse, C., Cambon-Thomsen, A., et al., 1994. Genetic mapping of a susceptibility locus for insulin-dependent diabetes mellitus on chromosome 11q. Nature. 371, 161−164.

Hatta, Y., Tsuchiya, N., Ohashi, J., Matsushita, M., Fujiwara, K., Hagiwara, K., et al., 1999. Association of Fc gamma receptor IIIB, but not of Fc gamma receptor IIA and IIIA polymorphisms with systemic lupus erythematosus in Japanese. Genes Immun. 1, 53−60.

Hawkes, C.H., MacGregor, A.J., 2009. Twin studies and the heritability of MS, a conclusion. Mult. Scler. 15, 661−667.

Healy, B.C., Liguori, M., Tran, D., Chitnis, T., Glanz, B., Wolfish, C., et al., 2010. HLA B*44, protective effects in MS susceptibility and MRI outcome measures. Neurology. 75, 634−640.

Hom, G., Graham, R.R., Modrek, B., Taylor, K.E., Ortmann, W., Garnier, S., et al., 2008. Association of systemic lupus erythematosus with C8orf13-BLK and ITGAM-ITGAX. N. Engl. J. Med. 358, 900−909.

Hoppenbrouwers, I.A., Aulchenko, Y.S., Ebers, G.C., Ramagopalan, S. V., Oostra, B.A., van Duijn, C.M., et al., 2008. EVI5 is a risk gene for multiple sclerosis. Genes Immun. 9, 334−337.

Horiuchi, M., Itoh, A., Pleasure, D., Itoh, T., 2011. Cooperative contributions of interferon regulatory factor 1 (IRF1) and IRF8 to interferon-γ-mediated cytotoxic effects on oligodendroglial progenitor cells. J. Neuroinflammation. 8, 8.

Howard, P.F., Hochberg, M.C., Bias, W.B., Arnett Jr., F.C., McLean, R. H., 1986. Relationship between C4 null genes, HLA-D region antigens, and genetic susceptibility to systemic lupus erythematosus in Caucasian and black Americans. Am. J. Med. 81, 187−193.

Hunt, K.A., Zhernakova, A., Turner, G., Heap, G.A., Franke, L., Bruinenberg, M., et al., 2008. Newly identified genetic risk variants for celiac disease related to the immune response. Nat. Genet. 40, 395−402.

Hyttinen, V., Kaprio, J., Kinnunen, L., Koskenvuo, M., Tuomilehto, J., 2003. Genetic liability of type 1 diabetes and the onset age among 22,650 young Finnish twin pairs, a nationwide follow-up study. Diabetes. 52, 1052−1055.

International Consortium for Systemic Lupus Erythematosus Genetics (SLEGEN), Harley, J.B., Alarcón-Riquelme, M.E., Criswell, L.A., Jacob, C.O., Kimberly, R.P., et al., 2008. Genome-wide association scan in women with systemic lupus erythematosus identifies susceptibility variants in ITGAM, PXK, KIAA1542 and other loci. Nat. Genet. 40, 204−210.

International Multiple Sclerosis Genetics Consortium (IMSGC), 2009. The expanding genetic overlap between multiple sclerosis and type I diabetes. Genes Immun. 10, 11−14.

International Multiple Sclerosis Genetics Consortium (IMSGC), 2010. IL12A, MPHOSPH9/CDK2AP1 and RGS1 are novel multiple sclerosis susceptibility loci. Genes Immun. 11, 397−405.

International Multiple Sclerosis Genetics Consortium (IMSGC), 2011a. Genome-wide association study of severity in multiple sclerosis. Genes Immun. 12, 615−625.

International Multiple Sclerosis Genetics Consortium (IMSGC), Hafler, D.A., Compston, A., Sawcer, S., Lander, E.S, Daly, M.J., et al.,

2007. Risk alleles for multiple sclerosis identified by a genomewide study. N. Engl. J. Med. 357, 851−862.

International Multiple Sclerosis Genetics Consortium (IMSGC), Wellcome Trust Case Control Consortium 2, Sawcer, S., Hellenthal, G., Pirinen, M., Spencer, C.C., et al., 2011b. Genetic risk and a primary role for cell-mediated immune mechanisms in multiple sclerosis. Nature. 476, 214−219.

Jacob, C.O., McDevitt, H.O., 1988. Tumour necrosis factor-alpha in murine autoimmune "lupus" nephritis. Nature. 331, 356−358.

Jacob, C.O., Fronek, Z., Lewis, G.D., Koo, M., Hansen, J.A., McDevitt, H.O., 1990. Heritable major histocompatibility complex class II-associated differences in production of tumor necrosis factor alpha, relevance to genetic predisposition to systemic lupus erythematosus. Proc. Natl. Acad. Sci. U.S.A. 87, 1233−1237.

Jersild, C., Fog, T., 1972. Histocompatibility (HL-A) antigens associated with multiple sclerosis. Acta. Neurol. Scand.(Suppl. 51), 377.

Jersild, C., Svejgaard, A., Fog, T., 1972. HL-A antigens and multiple sclerosis. Lancet. 1, 1240−1241.

Jin, Y., Birlea, S.A., Fain, P.R., Gowan, K., Riccardi, S.L., Holland, P.J., et al., 2010. Variant of TYR and autoimmunity susceptibility loci in generalized vitiligo. N. Engl. J. Med. 362, 1686−1697.

Johnston, C., Millward, B.A., Hoskins, P., Leslie, R.D., Bottazzo, G.F., Pyke, D.A., 1989. Islet-cell antibodies as predictors of the later development of type 1 (insulin-dependent) diabetes. A study in identical twins. Diabetologia. 32, 382−386.

Jordan, M.A., Silveira, P.A., Shepherd, D.P., Chu, C., Kinder, S.J., Chen, J., et al., 2000. Linkage analysis of systemic lupus erythematosus induced in diabetes-prone nonobese diabetic mice by Mycobacterium bovis. J. Immunol. 165, 1673−1684.

Julier, C., Hyer, R.N., Daviews, J., Merlin, F., Soularue, P., Briant, L., et al., 1991. Insulin-IGF2 region on chromosome 11p encodes a gene implicated in HLA-DR4-dependent diabetes susceptibility. Nature. 354, 155−159.

Kachru, R.B., Sequeira, W., Mittal, K.K., Siegel, M.E., Telischi, M., 1984. A significant increase of HLA-DR3 and DR2 in systemic lupus erythematosus among blacks. J. Rheumatol. 11, 471−474.

Kallenberg, C.G., Van der Voort-Beelen, J.M., D'Amaro, J., The, T.H., 1981. Increased frequency of B8/DR3 in scleroderma and association of the haplotype with impaired cellular immune response. Clin. Exp. Immunol. 43, 478−485.

Kavvoura, F.K., Ioannidis, J.P., 2005. CTLA-4 gene polymorphisms and susceptibility to type 1 diabetes mellitus, a HuGE Review and meta-analysis. Am. J. Epidemiol. 162, 3−16.

Kelly, M.A., Rayner, M.L., Mijovic, C.H., Barnett, A.H., 2003. Molecular aspects of type 1 diabetes. Mol. Pathol. 56, 1−10.

Kennedy, G.C., German, M.S., Rutter, W.J., 1995. The minisatellite in the diabetes susceptibility locus IDDM2 regulates insulin transcription. Nat. Genet. 9, 293−298.

Kent, S.C., Chen, Y., Bregoli, L., Clemmings, S.M., Kenyon, N.S., Ricordi, C., et al., 2005. Expanded T cells from pancreatic lymph nodes of type 1 diabetic subjects recognize an insulin epitope. Nature. 435, 224−228.

Khalil, I., d'Auriol, L., Gobet, M., Morin, L., Lepage, V., Deschamps, I., et al., 1990. A combination of HLA-DQ beta Asp57-negative and HLA DQ alpha Arg52 confers susceptibility to insulin-dependent diabetes mellitus. J. Clin. Invest. 85, 1315−1319.

Khan, M.A., Braun, W.E., Kushner, I., Grecek, D.E., Muir, W.A., Steinberg, A.G., 1977. HLA B27 in ankylosing spondylitis, differences in frequency and relative risk in American Blacks and Caucasians. J. Rheumatol. Suppl. 3, 39–43.

Kleinjan, D.A., van Heyningen, V., 2005. Long-range control of gene expression, emerging mechanisms and disruption in disease. Am. J. Hum. Genet. 76, 8–32.

Koene, H.R., Kleijer, M., Swaak, A.J., Sullivan, K.E., Bijl, M., Petri, M. A., et al., 1998. The Fc gammaRIIIA-158F allele is a risk factor for systemic lupus erythematosus. Arthritis Rheum. 41, 1813–1818.

Kofler, D.M., Severson, C.A., Mousissian, N., De Jager, P.L., Hafler, D. A., 2011. The CD6 multiple sclerosis susceptibility allele is associated with alterations in CD4+ T cell proliferation. J. Immunol. 187, 3286–3291.

Kotsa, K., Watson, P.F., Weetman, A.P., 1997. A CTLA-4 gene polymorphism is associated with both Graves disease and autoimmune hypothyroidism. Clin. Endocrinol. (Oxf). 46, 551–554.

Kouki, T., Sawai, Y., Gardine, C.A., Fisfalen, M.E., Alegre, M.L., DeGroot, L.J., 2000. CTLA-4 gene polymorphism at position 49 in exon 1 reduces the inhibitory function of CTLA-4 and contributes to the pathogenesis of Graves' disease. J. Immunol. 165, 6606–6611.

Kruglyak, L., 1999. Prospects for whole-genome linkage disequilibrium mapping of common disease genes. Nat. Genet. 22, 139–144.

Kumar, D., Gemayel, N.S., Deapen, D., Kapadia, D., Yamashita, P.H., Lee, S., et al., 1993. North-American twins with IDDM. Genetic, etiological, and clinical significance of disease concordance according to age, zygosity, and the interval after diagnosis in first twin. Diabetes. 42, 1351–1363.

Kuokkanen, S., Gschwend, M., Rioux, J.D., Daly, M.J., Terwilliger, J. D., Tienari, P.J., et al., 1997. Genomewide scan of multiple sclerosis in Finnish multiplex families. Am. J. Hum. Genet. 61, 1379–1387.

Kyogoku, C., Langefeld, C.D., Ortmann, W.A., Lee, A., Selby, S., Carlton, V.E., et al., 2004. Genetic association of the R620W polymorphism of protein tyrosine phosphatase PTPN22 with human SLE. Am. J. Hum. Genet. 75, 504–507.

Lander, E., Kruglyak, L., 1995. Genetic dissection of complex traits, guidelines for interpreting and reporting linkage results. Nat. Genet. 11, 241–247.

Lang, H.L., Jacobsen, H., Ikemizu, S., Andersson, C., Harlos, K., Madsen, L., et al., 2002. A functional and structural basis for TCR cross-reactivity in multiple sclerosis. Nat. Immunol. 3, 940–943.

Langrish, C.L., Chen, Y., Blumenschein, W.M., Mattson, J., Basham, B., Sedgwick, J.D., et al., 2005. IL-23 drives a pathogenic T cell population that induces autoimmune inflammation. J. Exp. Med. 201, 233–240.

Lawrence, J.S., Martins, C.L., Drake, G.L., 1987. A family survey of lupus erythematosus. J. Rheumatol. 14, 913–921.

Li, Q., Spriggs, M.K., Kovats, S., Comeau, M.R., Nepom, B., Hutt-Fletcher, L.M., et al., 1997. Epstein-Barr virus uses HLA class II as a cofactor for infection of B lymphocytes. J. Virol. 71, 4657–4662.

Ligers, A., Xu, C., Saarinen, S., Hillert, J., Olerup, O., 1999. The CTLA-4 gene is associated with multiple sclerosis. J. Neuroimmunol. 97, 182–190.

Lindqvist, A.K., Steinsson, K., Johanneson, B., Kristjánsdóttir, H., Arnasson, A., Gröndal, G., et al., 2000. A susceptibility locus for human systemic lupus erythematosus (hSLE1) on chromosome 2q. J. Autoimmun. 14, 169–178.

Lipsker, D.M., Schreckenberg-Gilliot, C., Uring-Lambert, B., Meyer, A., Hartmann, D., Grosshans, E.M., et al., 2000. Lupus erythematosus associated with genetically determined deficiency of the second component of the complement. Arch. Dermatol. 136, 1508–1514.

Long, A.E., Gillespie, K.M., Rokni, S., Bingley, P.J., Williams, A.J., 2012. Rising incidence of type 1 diabetes is associated with altered immunophenotype at diagnosis. Diabetes. 61, 683–686.

Lowe, C.E., Cooper, J.D., Brusko, T., Walker, N.M., Smyth, D.J., Bailey, R., et al., 2007. Large-scale genetic fine mapping and genotype-phenotype associations implicate polymorphism in the IL2RA region in type 1 diabetes. Nat. Genet. 39, 1074–1082.

Luo, D.F., Bui, M.M., Muir, A., MacLaren, N.K., Thomson, G., She, J. X., 1995. Affected-sib-pair mapping of a novel susceptibility gene to insulin-dependent diabetes mellitus (IDDM8) on chromosome 6q25-q27. Am. J. Hum. Genet. 57, 911–919.

Luo, D.F., Buzzetti, R., Rotter, J.I., MacLaren, N.K., Raffel, L.J., Nisticò, L., et al., 1996. Confirmation of three susceptibility genes to insulin-dependent diabetes mellitus, IDDM4, IDDM5 and IDDM8. Hum. Mol. Genet. 5, 693–698.

Maier, L.M., Lowe, C.E., Cooper, J., Downes, K., Anderson, D.E., Severson, C., et al., 2009a. IL2RA genetic heterogeneity in multiple sclerosis and type 1 diabetes susceptibility and soluble interleukin-2 receptor production. PLoS Genet. 5, e1000322.

Maier, L.M., Anderson, D.E., Severson, C.A., Baecher-Allan, C., Healy, B., Liu, D.V., et al., 2009b. Soluble IL-2RA levels in multiple sclerosis subjects and the effect of soluble IL-2RA on immune responses. J. Immunol. 182, 1541–1547.

Malek, T.R., Bayer, A.L., 2004. Tolerance, not immunity, crucially depends on IL-2. Nat. Rev. Immunol. 4, 665–674.

Manzotti, C.N., Tipping, H., Perry, L.C., Mead, K.I., Blair, P.J., Zheng, Y., et al., 2002. Inhibition of human T cell proliferation by CTLA-4 utilizes CD80 and requires CD25+ regulatory T cells. Eur. J. Immunol. 32, 2888–2896.

Marron, M.P., Raffel, L.J., Garchon, H.J., Jacob, C.O., Serrano-Rios, M., Martinez Larrad, M.T., et al., 1997. Insulin-dependent diabetes mellitus (IDDM) is associated with CTLA4 polymorphisms in multiple ethnic groups. Hum. Mol. Genet. 6, 1275–1282.

Masterman, T., Ligers, A., Olsson, T., Andersson, M., Olerup, O., Hillert, J., 2000. HLA-DR15 is associated with lower age at onset in multiple sclerosis. Ann. Neurol. 48, 211–219.

McKinney, C., Merriman, T.R., 2012. Meta-analysis confirms a role for deletion in FCGR3B in autoimmune phenotypes. Hum. Mol. Genet. 21, 2370–2376.

Mein, C.A., Esposito, L., Dunn, M.G., Johnson, G.C., Timms, A.E., Goy, J.V., et al., 1998. A search for type 1 diabetes susceptibility genes in families from the United Kingdom. Nat. Genet. 19, 297–300.

Mells, G.F., Floyd, J.A., Morley, K.I., Franklin, C.S., Shin, S.Y., Heneghan, M.A., et al., 2011. Genome-wide association study identifies 12 new susceptibility loci for primary biliary cirrhosis. Nat. Genet. 43, 329–332.

Merriman, T., Twells, R., Merriman, M., Eaves, I., Cox, R., Cucca, F., et al., 1997. Evidence by allelic association-dependent methods for a type 1 diabetes polygene (IDDM6) on chromosome 18q21. Hum. Mol. Genet. 6, 1003–1010.

Montomoli, C., Prokopenko, I., Caria, A., Ferrai, R., Mander, A., Seaman, S., et al., 2002. Multiple sclerosis recurrence risk for siblings in an isolated population of Central Sardinia, Italy. Genet. Epidemiol. 22, 265–271.

Moore, K.W., de Waal Malefyt, R., Coffman, R.L., O'Garra, A., 2001. Interleukin-10 and the interleukin-10 receptor. Annu. Rev. Immunol. 19, 683–765.

Morahan, G., Huang, D., Tait, B.D., Colman, P.G., Harrison, L.C., 1996. Markers on distal chromosome 2q linked to insulin-dependent diabetes mellitus. Science. 272, 1811–1813.

Moser, K.L., Neas, B.R., Salmon, J.E., Yu, H., Gray-McGuire, C., Asundi, N., et al., 1998. Genome scan of human systemic lupus erythematosus, evidence for linkage on chromosome 1q in African-American pedigrees. Proc. Natl. Acad. Sci. U.S.A. 95, 14869–14874.

Munger, K.L., Levin, L.I., Hollis, B.W., Howard, N.S., Ascherio, A., 2006. Serum 25-hydroxyvitamin D levels and risk of multiple sclerosis. JAMA. 296, 2832–2838.

Myhr, K.M., Riise, T., Barrett-Connor, E., Myrmel, H., Vedeler, C., Grønning, M., et al., 1998. Altered antibody pattern to Epstein-Barr virus but not to other herpesviruses in multiple sclerosis, a population based case–control study from western Norway. J. Neurol. Neurosurg. Psychiatry. 64, 539–542.

Naito, S., Namerow, N., Mickey, M.R., Terasaki, P.I., 1972. Multiple sclerosis, association with HL-A3. Tissue Antigens. 2, 1–4.

Nakai, H., Morito, T., Tanimoto, K., Horiuchi, Y., 1977. Reduced Fc-receptor bearing cells in peripheral bloods of patients with systemic lupus erythematosus and in rheumatoid synovial fluids. J. Rheumatol. 4, 405–413.

Nath, S.K., Han, S., Kim-Howard, X., Viswanathan, P., Gilkeson, G.S., Chen, W., et al., 2008. A nonsynonymous functional variant in integrin-alpha(M) (encoded by ITGAM) is associated with systemic lupus erythematosus. Nat. Genet. 40, 152–154.

Naves, M., Hajeer, A.H., Teh, L.S., Davies, E.J., Ordi-Ros, J., Perez-Pemen, P., et al., 1998. Complement C4B null allele status confers risk for systemic lupus erythematosus in a Spanish population. Eur. J. Immunogenet. 25, 317–320.

Nerup, J., Platz, P., Ortved-Andersen, O., Lyngsoe, J., Poulsen, J.E., Ryder, L.P., et al., 1974. HL-A antigens and diabetes mellitus. Lancet. 2, 864–866.

Nielsen, T.R., Rostgaard, K., Askling, J., Steffensen, R., Oturai, A., Jersild, C., et al., 2009. Effects of infectious mononucleosis and HLA-DRB1*15 in multiple sclerosis. Mult. Scler. 15, 431–436.

Nieves, J.F., Cosman, J., Herbert, V., Shen, V., Lindsay, R., 1994. High prevalence of vitamin D deficiency and reduced bone mass in multiple sclerosis. Neurology. 44, 1687–1692.

Nisticò, L., Buzzetti, R., Pritchard, L.E., Van der Auwera, B., Giovannini, C., Bosi, E., et al., 1996. The CTLA-4 gene region of chromosome 2q33 is linked to, and associated with, type 1 diabetes. Hum. Mol. Genet. 5, 1075–1080.

Noble, J.A., Valdes, A.M., Cook, M., Klitz, W., Thomson, G., Erlich, H.A., 1996. The role of HLA class II genes in insulin-dependent diabetes mellitus, molecular analysis of 180 Caucasian, multiplex families. Am. J. Hum. Genet. 59, 1134–1148.

Nordmark, G., Kristjansdottir, G., Theander, E., Eriksson, P., Brun, J.G., Wang, C., et al., 2009. Additive effects of the major risk alleles of IRF5 and STAT4 in primary Sjögren's syndrome. Genes Immun. 10, 68–76.

Oaks, M.K., Hallett, K.M., Penwell, R.T., Stauber, E.C., Warren, S.J., Tector, A.J., 2000. A native soluble form of CTLA-4. Cell. Immunol. 201, 144–153.

Oliveira, M.I., Gonçalves, C.M., Pinto, M., Fabre, S., Santos, A.M., Lee, S.F., et al., 2012. CD6 attenuates early and late signaling events,

setting thresholds for T-cell activation. Eur. J. Immunol. 42, 195–205.

Onengut-Gumuscu, S., Ewens, K.G., Spielman, R.S., Concannon, P., 2004. A functional polymorphism (1858C/T) in the PTPN22 gene is linked and associated with type I diabetes in multiplex families. Genes Immun. 5, 678–680.

Onkamo, P., Väänänen, S., Karvonen, M., Tuomilehto, J., 1999. Worldwide increase in incidence of Type I diabetes—the analysis of the data on published incidence trends. Diabetologia. 42, 1395–1403, Erratum in Diabetologia 2000 43, 685.

Owerbach, D., Gabbay, K.H., 1995. The HOXD8 locus (2q31) is linked to type I diabetes. Interaction with chromosome 6 and 11 disease susceptibility genes. Diabetes. 44, 132–136.

Paterson, A.D., Rahman, P., Petronis, A., 1999. IDDM9 and a locus for rheumatoid arthritis on chromosome 3q appear to be distinct. Hum. Immunol. 60, 883–885.

Payne, R., Rolfs, M.R., 1958. Fetomaternal leukocyte incompatibility. J. Clin. Invest. 37, 1756–1762.

Pociot, F., McDermott, M.F., 2002. Genetics of type 1 diabetes mellitus (Review). Genes Immun. 3, 235–249.

Price, P., Witt, C., Allcock, R., Garlepp, M., Kok, C.C., French, M., et al., 1999. The genetic basis for the association of the 8.1 ancestral haplotype (A1, B8, DR3) with multiple immunopathological diseases. Immunol. Rev. 167, 257–274.

Provost, T.T., Arnett, F.C., Reichlin, M., 1983. Homozygous C2 deficiency, lupus erythematosus, and anti-Ro (SSA) antibodies. Arthritis Rheum. 26, 1279–1282.

Ramagopalan, S.V., Maugeri, N.J., Handunnetthi, L., Lincoln, M.R., Orton, S.M., Dyment, D.A., et al., 2009. Expression of the multiple sclerosis-associated MHC class II Allele HLA-DRB1*1501 is regulated by vitamin D. PLoS Genet. 5, e1000369.

Ramagopalan, S.V., Heger, A., Berlanga, A.J., Maugeri, N.J., Lincoln, M.R., Burrell, A., et al., 2010. A ChIP-seq defined genome-wide map of vitamin D receptor binding, associations with disease and evolution. Genome Res. 20, 1352–1360.

Remmers, E.F., Plenge, R.M., Lee, A.T., Graham, R.R., Hom, G., Behrens, T.W., et al., 2007. STAT4 and the risk of rheumatoid arthritis and systemic lupus erythematosus. N. Engl. J. Med. 357, 977–986.

Rieck, M., Arechiga, A., Onengut-Gumuscu, S., Greenbaum, C., Concannon, P., Buckner, J.H., 2007. Genetic variation in PTPN22 corresponds to altered function of T and B lymphocytes. J. Immunol. 179, 4704–4710.

Robertson, N.P., Clayton, D., Fraser, M., Deans, J., Compston, D.A., 1996. Clinical concordance in sibling pairs with multiple sclerosis. Neurology. 47, 347–352.

van Rood, J.J., Eernisse, J.G., van Leeuwen, A., 1958. Leucocyte antibodies in sera from pregnant women. Nature. 181, 1735–1736.

Rubio, J.P., Stankovich, J., Field, J., Tubridy, N., Marriott, M., Chapman, C., et al., 2008. Replication of KIAA0350, IL2RA, RPL5 and CD58 as multiple sclerosis susceptibility genes in Australians. Genes Immun. 9, 624–630.

Rudwaleit, M., Tikly, M., Khamashta, M., Gibson, K., Klinke, J., Hughes, G., et al., 1996. Interethnic differences in the association of tumor necrosis factor promoter polymorphisms with systemic lupus erythematosus. J. Rheumatol. 23, 1725–1728.

Sadovnick, A.D., Baird, P.A., 1988. The familial nature of multiple sclerosis, age-corrected empiric recurrence risks for children and siblings of patients. Neurology. 38, 990–991.

Sadovnick, A.D., Armstrong, H., Rice, G.P., Bulman, D., Hashimoto, L., Paty, D.W., et al., 1993. A population-based study of multiple sclerosis in twins, update. Ann. Neurol. 33, 281–285.

Salloum, R., Franek, B.S., Kariuki, S.N., Rhee, L., Mikolaitis, R.A., Jolly, M., et al., 2010. Genetic variation at the IRF7/PHRF1 locus is associated with autoantibody profile and serum interferon-alpha activity in lupus patients. Arthritis Rheum. 62, 553–561.

Salmon, J.E., Millard, S., Schachter, L.A., Arnett, F.C., Ginzler, E.M., Gourley, M.F., et al., 1996. Fc gamma RIIA alleles are heritable risk factors for lupus nephritis in African Americans. J. Clin. Invest. 97, 1348–1354.

Salmon, J.E., Ng, S., Yoo, D.H., Kim, T.H., Kim, S.Y., Song, G.G., 1999. Altered distribution of Fcgamma receptor IIIA alleles in a cohort of Korean patients with lupus nephritis. Arthritis Rheum. 42, 818–819.

Sawcer, S., Jones, H.B., Feakes, R., Gray, J., Smaldon, N., Chataway, J., et al., 1996. A genome screen in multiple sclerosis reveals susceptibility loci on chromosome 6p21 and 17q22. Nat. Genet. 13, 464–468.

Schifferli, J.A., Ng, Y.C., Peters, D.K., 1986. The role of complement and its receptor in the elimination of immune complexes. N. Engl. J. Med. 315, 488–495.

Schlosstein, L., Terasaki, P.I., Bluestone, R., Pearson, C.M., 1973. High association of an HL-A antigen, W27, with ankylosing spondylitis. N. Engl. J. Med. 288, 704–708.

Segal, B.M., Constantinescu, C.S., Raychaudhuri, A., Kim, L., Fidelus-Gort, R., Kasper, L.H., et al., 2008. Repeated subcutaneous injections of IL12/23 p40 neutralising antibody, ustekinumab, in patients with relapsing-remitting multiple sclerosis, a phase II, double-blind, placebo-controlled, randomised, dose-ranging study. Lancet Neurol. 7, 796–804.

Shai, R., Quismorio Jr., F.P., Li, L., Kwon, O.J., Morrison, J., Wallace, D.J., et al., 1999. Genome-wide screen for systemic lupus erythematosus susceptibility genes in multiplex families. Hum. Mol. Genet. 8, 639–644.

Sigurdsson, S., Nordmark, G., Göring, H.H., Lindroos, K., Wiman, A.C., Sturfelt, G., et al., 2005. Polymorphisms in the tyrosine kinase 2 and interferon regulatory factor 5 genes are associated with systemic lupus erythematosus. Am. J. Hum. Genet. 76, 528–537.

Simpfendorfer, K.R., Olsson, L.M., Manjarrez Orduño, N., Khalili, H., Simeone, A.M., Katz, M.S., et al., 2012. The autoimmunity-associated BLK haplotype exhibits cis-regulatory effects on mRNA and protein expression that are prominently observed in B cells early in development. Hum. Mol. Genet. 21, 3918–3925.

Smyth, D.J., Cooper, J.D., Collins, J.E., Heward, J.M., Franklyn, J.A., Howson, J.M., et al., 2004. Replication of an association between the lymphoid tyrosine phosphatase locus LYP/PTPN22 with type 1 diabetes, and evidence for its role as a general autoimmunity locus. Diabetes. 53, 3020–3023.

Smyth, D.J., Cooper, J.D., Bailey, R., Field, S., Burren, O., Smink, L.J., et al., 2006. A genome-wide association study of nonsynonymous SNPs identifies a type 1 diabetes locus in the interferon-induced helicase (IFIH1) region. Nat. Genet. 38, 617–619.

So, A.K., Fielder, A.H., Warner, C.A., Isenberg, D.A., Batchelor, J.R., Walport, M.J., 1990. DNA polymorphism of major histocompatibility complex class II and class III genes in systemic lupus erythematosus. Tissue Antigens. 35, 144–147.

Stahl, E.A., Raychaudhuri, S., Remmers, E.F., Xie, G., Eyre, S., Thomson, B.P., et al., 2010. Genome-wide association study meta-analysis identifies seven new rheumatoid arthritis risk loci. Nat. Genet. 42, 508–514.

Steck, A.K., Rewers, M.J., 2011. Genetics of type 1 diabetes. Clin. Chem. 57, 176–185.

Steck, A.K., Liu, S.Y., McFann, K., Barriga, K.J., Babu, S.R., Eisenbarth, G.S., et al., 2006. Association of the PTPN22/LYP gene with type 1 diabetes. Pediatr. Diabetes. 7, 274–278.

Steck, A.K., Baschal, E.E., Jasinski, J.M., Boehm, B.O., Bottini, N., Concannon, P., et al., 2009. rs2476601 T allele (R620W) defines high-risk PTPN22 type I diabetes-associated haplotypes with preliminary evidence for an additional protective haplotype. Genes Immun. 10, S21–S26.

Stoll, T., Seifert, B., Isenberg, D.A., 1996. SLICC/ACR Damage Index is valid, and renal and pulmonary organ scores are predictors of severe outcome in patients with systemic lupus erythematosus. Br. J. Rheumatol. 35, 248–254.

Strettell, M.D., Thomson, L.J., Donaldson, P.T., Bunce, M., O'Neill, C. M., Williams, R., 1997. HLA-C genes and susceptibility to type 1 autoimmune hepatitis. Hepatology. 26, 1023–1026.

Sullivan, K.E., Petri, M.A., Schmeckpeper, B.J., McLean, R.H., Winkelstein, J.A., 1994. Prevalence of a mutation causing C2 deficiency in systemic lupus erythematosus. J. Rheumatol. 21, 1128–1133.

Sumaya, C.V., Myers, L.W., Ellison, G.W., et al., 1985. Increased prevalence and titer of Epstein-Barr virus antibodies in patients with multiple sclerosis. Ann. Neurol. 17, 371–377.

Takaoka, A., Yanai, H., Kondo, S., Ench, Y., 2005. Integral role of IRF-5 in the gene induction programme activated by Toll-like receptors. Nature. 434, 243–249.

Tan, F.K., Arnett, F.C., 1998. The genetics of lupus. Curr. Opin. Rheumatol. 10, 399–408.

Taylor, K.E., Remmers, E.F., Lee, A.T., Ortmann, W.A., Plenge, R.M., Tian, C., et al., 2008. Specificity of the STAT4 genetic association for severe disease manifestations of systemic lupus erythematosus. PLoS Genet. 4, e1000084.

Texido, G., Su, I.H., Mecklenbräuker, I., Malek, S.N., Desiderio, S., Rajewsky, K., et al., 2000. The B-cell-specific Src-family kinase Blk is dispensable for B-cell development and activation. Mol. Cell. Biol. 20, 1227–1233.

Thakker, P., Leach, M.W., Kuang, W., Benoit, S.E., Leonard, J.P., Marusic, S., 2007. IL-23 is critical in the induction but not in the effector phase of experimental autoimmune encephalomyelitis. J. Immunol. 178, 2589–2598.

The Lenercept Multiple Sclerosis Study Group and the University of British Columbia MS/MRI Analysis Group, 1999. TNF neutralization in MS, results of a randomized, placebo-controlled multicenter study. Neurology. 53, 457–465.

Thorsby, E., 1997. Invited anniversary review, HLA associated diseases. Hum. Immunol. 53, 1–11.

Thorsby, E., 2009. A short history of HLA. Tissue Antigens. 74, 101–116.

Tillil, H., Köbberling, J., 1987. Age-corrected empirical genetic risk estimates for first-degree relatives of IDDM patients. Diabetes. 36, 93–99.

Todd, J.A., 1992. Genetic analysis of susceptibility to type 1 diabetes. Springer Semin. Immunopathol. 14, 33–58.

Todd, J.A., 1995. Genetic analysis of type 1 diabetes using whole genome approaches. Proc. Natl. Acad. Sci. U.S.A. 92, 8560–8565.

Todd, J.A., Bell, J.I., McDevitt, H.O., 1987. HLA-DQ beta gene contributes to susceptibility and resistance to insulin-dependent diabetes mellitus. Nature. 329, 599–604.

Todd, J.A., Walker, N.M., Cooper, J.D., Smyth, D.J., Downes, K., Plagnol, V., et al., 2007. Robust associations of four new chromosome regions from genome-wide analyses of type 1 diabetes. Nat. Genet. 39, 857–864.

Tsang, S., Sun, Z., Luke, B., Stewart, C., Lum, N., Gregory, M., et al., 2005. A comprehensive SNP-based genetic analysis of inbred mouse strains. Mamm. Genome. 16, 476–480.

Tsao, B.P., Cantor, R.M., Kalunian, K.C., Chen, C.J., Badsha, H., Singh, R., et al., 1997. Evidence for linkage of a candidate chromosome 1 region to human systemic lupus erythematosus. J. Clin. Invest. 99, 725–731.

Tsuchiya, N., Komata, T., Matsushita, M., Ohashi, J., Tokunaga, K., 2000. New single nucleotide polymorphisms in the coding region of human TNFR2, association with systemic lupus erythematosus. Genes Immun. 1, 501–503.

Ueda, H., Howson, J.M., Esposito, L., Heward, J., Snook, H., Chamberlain, G., et al., 2003. Association of the T-cell regulatory gene CTLA4 with susceptibility to autoimmune disease. Nature. 423, 506–511.

Vafiadis, P., Bennett, S.T., Todd, J.A., Nadeau, J., Grabs, R., Goodyer, C.G., et al., 1997. Insulin expression in human thymus is modulated by INS VNTR alleles at the IDDM2 locus. Nat. Genet. 15, 289–292.

Valdes, A.M., Noble, J.A., Genin, E., Clerget-Darpoux, F., Erlich, H.A., Thomson, G., 2001. Modeling of HLA class II susceptibility to type 1 diabetes reveals an effect associated with DPB1. Genet. Epidemiol. 21, 212–223.

Valdes, A.M., Erlich, H.A., Noble, J.A., 2005. Human leukocyte antigen class I B and C loci contribute to Type 1 Diabetes (T1D) susceptibility and age at T1D onset. Hum. Immunol. 66, 301–313.

Vandenborre, K., Van Gool, S.W., Kasran, A., Ceuppens, J.L., Boogaerts, M.A., Vandenberghe, P., 1999. Interaction of CTLA-4 (CD152) with CD80 or CD86 inhibits human T-cell activation. Immunology. 98, 413–421.

Vang, T., Congia, M., Macis, M.D., Orrú, V., Zavattari, P., Nika, K., et al., 2005. Autoimmune-associated lymphoid tyrosine phosphatase is a gain-of-function variant. Nat. Genet. 37, 1317–1319.

Vazquez, B.N., Laguna, T., Notario, L., Lauzurica, P., 2012. Evidence for an intronic cis-regulatory element within CD69 gene. Genes Immun. 13, 356–362.

Vella, A., Cooper, J.D., Lowe, C.E., Walker, N., Nutland, S., Widmer, B., et al., 2005. Localization of a type 1 diabetes locus in the IL2RA/CD25 region by use of tag single-nucleotide polymorphisms. Am. J. Hum. Genet. 76, 773–779.

Veyrieras, J.B., Kudaravalli, S., Kim, S.Y., Dermitzakis, E.T., Gilad, Y., Stephens, M., et al., 2008. High-resolution mapping of expression-QTLs yields insight into human gene regulation. PLoS Genet. 4, e1000214.

Vijayakrishnan, L., Slavik, J.M., Illés, Z., Greenwald, R.J., Rainbow, D., Greve, B., et al., 2004. An autoimmune disease-associated CTLA-4 splice variant lacking the B7 binding domain signals negatively in T cells. Immunity. 20, 563–575.

Vyse, T.J., Kotzin, B.L., 1998. Genetic susceptibility to systemic lupus erythematosus. Annu. Rev. Immunol. 16, 261–292.

Walport, M.J., 1993. The roche rheumatology prize lecture. Complement deficiency and disease. Br. J. Rheumatol. 32, 269–273.

Walunas, T.L., Lenschow, D.J., Bakker, C.Y., Linsley, P.S., Freeman, G. J., Green, J.M., et al., 1994. CTLA-4 can function as a negative regulator of T cell activation. Immunity. 1, 405–413.

Wang, H., Jin, Y., Reddy, M.V., Podolsky, R., Liu, S., Yang, P., et al., 2010. Genetically dependent ERBB3 expression modulates antigen presenting cell function and type 1 diabetes risk. PLoS One. 5, e11789.

Wang, W.Y., Barratt, B.J., Clayton, D.G., Todd, J.A., 2005. Genome-wide association studies, theoretical and practical concerns. Nat. Rev. Genet. 6, 109–118.

Wapelhorst, B., Bell, G.I., Risch, N., Spielman, R.S., Concannon, P., 1995. Linkage and association studies in insulin-dependent diabetes with a new dinucleotide repeat polymorphism at the GAD65 locus. Autoimmunity. 21, 127–130.

Weber, F., Fontaine, B., Cournu-Rebeix, I., Kroner, A., Knop, M., Lutz, S., et al., 2008. IL2RA and IL7RA genes confer susceptibility for multiple sclerosis in two independent European populations. Genes Immun. 9, 259–263.

Weiss, K.M., Terwilliger, J.D., 2000. How many diseases does it take to map a gene with SNPs? Nat. Genet. 26, 151–157.

Wellcome Trust Case Control Consortium; Australo-Anglo-American Spondylitis Consortium (TASC), Burton, P.R., et al., 2007. Association scan of 14,500 nonsynonymous SNPs in four common diseases identifies variants involved in autoimmunity. Nat. Genet. 39, 1329–1337.

Wilson, A.G., Gordon, C., di Giovine, F.S., de Vries, N., van de Putte, L.B., Emery, P., et al., 1994. A genetic association between systemic lupus erythematosus and tumor necrosis factor alpha. Eur. J. Immunol. 24, 191–195.

Wu, J., Edberg, J.C., Redecha, P.B., Bansal, V., Guyre, P.M., Coleman, K., et al., 1997. A novel polymorphism of FcgammaRIIIa (CD16) alters receptor function and predisposes to autoimmune disease. J. Clin. Invest. 100, 1059–1070.

Yamada, H., Watanabe, A., Mimori, A., Nakano, K., Takeuchi, F., Matsuta, K., et al., 1990. Lack of gene deletion for complement C4A deficiency in Japanese patients with systemic lupus erythematosus. J. Rheumatol. 17, 1054–1057.

Yanagawa, T., Hidaka, Y., Guimaraes, V., Soliman, M., DeGroot, L.J., 1995. CTLA-4 gene polymorphism associated with Graves' disease in a Caucasian population. J. Clin. Endocrinol. Metab. 80, 41–45.

Yu, D.T., Choo, S.Y., Schaack, T.M., 1989. Molecular mimicry in HLA-B27-related arthritis. Ann. Intern. Med. 111, 581–591.

Zhang, Z., Duvefelt, K., Svensson, F., Masterman, T., Jonasdottir, G., Salter, H., et al., 2005. Two genes encoding immune-regulatory molecules (LAG3 and IL7R) confer susceptibility to multiple sclerosis. Genes Immun. 6, 145–152.

Zheng, W., She, J.X., 2005. Genetic association between a lymphoid tyrosine phosphatase (PTPN22) and type 1 diabetes. Diabetes. 54, 906–908.

Ziegler, A.G., Pflueger, M., Winkler, C., Achenbach, P., Akolkar, B., Krischer, J.P., et al., 2011. Accelerated progression from islet autoimmunity to diabetes is causing the escalating incidence of type 1 diabetes in young children. J. Autoimmun. 37, 3–7.

Zimmerman, A.W., Joosten, B., Torensma, R., Parnes, J.R., van Leeuwen, F.N., Figdor, C.G., 2006. Long-term engagement of CD6 and ALCAM is essential for T-cell proliferation induced by dendritic cells. Blood. 107, 3212–3220.

Zuvich, R.L., Bush, W.S., McCauley, J.L., Beecham, A.H., De Jager, P. L.International Multiple Sclerosis Genetics Consortium et al., 2011. Interrogating the complex role of chromosome 16p13.13 in multiple sclerosis susceptibility, independent genetic signals in the CIITA-CLEC16A-SOCS1 gene complex. Hum. Mol. Genet. 20, 3517–3524.

Chapter 27

Genetic Predisposition to Autoimmune Diseases Conferred by the Major Histocompatibility Complex: Utility of Animal Models

Veena Taneja, Ashutosh Mangalam, and Chella S. David

Department of Immunology and Rheumatology, Mayo Clinic, Rochester, MN, USA

Chapter Outline

Major Histocompatibility Complex	**365**	**Post-Translational Modifications in Autoimmunity**	**371**
MHC and Autoimmunity	366	Deimination	371
The Mystery of HLA-B27 and Spondyloarthropathies	366	Deamidation	372
HLA-B27 Transgenic Mice	366	**Humanized Animal Models of Autoimmunity**	**372**
HLA-B27 and AIDS	367	Collagen-Induced Arthritis	373
HLA-B27 and Peptide Binding	367	Non-RA-Associated HLA Alleles Can Predispose to	
HLA-B27 and Natural Killer Cells	367	Autoimmunity	374
HLA-B27 and Evolution	368	HLA-DR Transgenic Mice with EAE as an Animal Model	
HLA Class II Association with Autoimmune Diseases	**368**	of MS	374
Predisposition	368	Role of DQ Molecules in Predisposition to MS	375
Onset	369	Animal Model of Celiac Disease	375
Environmental Factors	**369**	Animal Model for Type 1 Diabetes	376
Infectious Agent	369	**HLA Class II Molecules Regulate Infection Through**	
***Porphyromonas Gingivalis* and Rheumatoid Arthritis**	**370**	**Modulation of Cytokine Networks**	**376**
Smoking and Autoimmunity	370	**Concluding Remarks**	**377**
Vitamin D in Autoimmune Diseases	**370**	**References**	**377**

The biggest threat to survival of the human population is infection caused by microorganisms such as viruses, bacteria, and parasites. The major histocompatibility complex (MHC) on chromosome 6 plays a very important role in fighting these infections and comprises multiple genes encoding for molecules critical for mounting an immune response to invading pathogens. Human MHC complex is divided into three main regions, human leukocyte antigens (HLA) class I, II, and III. HLA class I and class II genes are mostly polymorphic genes in human genome. The high polymorphism in the MHC region can be attributed to strong selection pressure as the human population moved to different parts of the world, and encountered new infections leading to diversity in MHC genes through mutation, gene duplication, or gene conversion. A population with diverse HLA class I and II alleles leads to herd resistance to infection and has a survival advantage.

MAJOR HISTOCOMPATIBILITY COMPLEX

Human MHC molecules are called HLA which are homologous to the H-2 of mice. The HLA complex is located on the short arm of chromosome 6 and is 3500 kilobases long. HLA class I molecules contain one heavy chain of 44 kilodaltons (kDa) and one non-MHC encoded

N. Rose & I. Mackay (Eds): The Autoimmune Diseases, Fifth edition. DOI: http://dx.doi.org/10.1016/B978-0-12-384929-8.00027-7

non-polymorphic β2 microglobulin of 12 kDa. The heavy chain consists of three extracellular domains of 90 residues each. The polymorphic residues in class I molecules are located on α1 and α2 domains of the heavy chain. There are three class I genes designated HLA-A, HLA-B, and HLA-C which are expressed on all nucleated cells. Class I molecules can bind 8–10 amino acid-long peptides which have been processed endogenously.

HLA class II molecules are present as heterodimers on the cell surface consisting of an α chain (32–34 kDa) and a β chain (29–32 kDa), each with two extracellular domains of about 90 amino acids long (α1, α2, and β1, β2). The β chains of three class II genes, HLA-DR, DQ, and DP, are highly polymorphic while α chains are generally non-polymorphic. The class II molecules are expressed on antigen presenting cells (APCs) like B lymphocytes, macrophages, dendritic cells (DC), endothelial and other organ-specific APCs. In general, class II molecules can accommodate peptides up to 10–25 residues. In humans, DR, DQ, and DP are in linkage disequilibrium and are inherited en bloc as a haplotype. MHC genes are expressed co-dominantly in each individual. Crystal structures of the DR and DQ genes have shown that the MHC molecule has a single peptide binding cleft which can accommodate a variety of peptides which depends on the charge, stability, and binding affinity.

MHC and Autoimmunity

During evolution, HLA alleles offering an advantage during reproductive years have been selected and occur in populations with much higher frequency compared to other alleles. Abundance of HLA-DR2/DQ6, DR4/DQ8, and DR3/DQ2 haplotypes in various populations suggest the importance of these haplotypes in clearing infections and survival of the species. Although these haplotypes offered a survival advantage in terms of fighting infection, they can also generate an autoreactive response thus predisposing to a number of autoimmune diseases. Even though there are more than 450 DRB1 alleles and 75 DQB1 alleles with the possibility of generating thousands of haplotypes, only a few alleles of these three haplotypes are associated with most of the autoimmune diseases. DRB1 have the maximum allelic diversity, suggesting a rapidly evolving region due to positive or negative selective pressures. Thus nature leads to selection of alleles offering advantage over other alleles. Studies have suggested that HLA heterozygosity has an advantage over homozygosity in the generation of immune response. HLA diversity evolves via mutations, gene conversion, and genetic recombination. The most conserved haplotype, B8-DR3-DQ2, has been associated with autoimmunity, suggesting this haplotype provides an advantage over other haplotypes and is supported by a high gene frequency of HLA-DR3 in centenarians. Most of theautoimmune diseases show association with HLA class II alleles except the HLA-B27-associated spondyloarthropathies.

The Mystery of HLA-B27 and Spondyloarthropathies

Ankylosing spondylitis (AS) is a joint disease which affects the spine, the sacroiliac joints, and shoulders. In 1973, Brewerton and his colleagues showed that the MHC gene HLA-B27 is linked to susceptibility to AS (Brewerton et al., 1973). While B27 was found in 5% of the general population, 95% of AS patients were HLA-B27 positive. This was the first MHC gene found to be associated with an autoimmune-type disease. Eventually, several other closely related diseases such as psoriatic arthritis, arthritis associated with inflammatory bowel disease, and reactive arthritis were also linked to HLA-B27, although at a much lower frequency (Allen et al., 1999a). Several enterobacteria were found to be implicated in the onset of the disease (Kvien et al., 1994). These diseases are now referred to as spondyloarthropathies. In order to understand the role of HLA-B27 in these diseases, Taurog and his colleagues developed a transgenic rat expressing human HLA-B27 gene from an AS patient (Hammer et al., 1990). Transgenic rats developed spontaneous symptoms characteristic of SPA, but the disease only developed in high gene copy number rats.

HLA-B27 Transgenic Mice

Mice expressing intact HLA-B27 on the cell surface developed normally, and showed no disease symptoms. Assuming the disease may require the human β2m gene, we initiated studies to replace mouse β2m with human β2m. During this process, we noticed that mice lacking β2m altogether showed some symptoms of spondyloarthropathies (Khare et al., 1995). We found that these mice expressed about 10% of β2m free B27 heavy chains on their cell surface. Free heavy chains of class I molecules are rarely seen on the cell surface. This suggested that B27 may be a unique class I molecule capable of reaching the cell surface as free heavy chains. The frequency of symptoms increased after the mice were brought outside the pathogen-free barrier facility, suggesting environmental factors may play a role. Studies with B27⁺ CD4⁻ and CD8⁻ mice indicated that CD4 T cells were critical for the disease process. Computer simulation studies indicated that the pocket of a β2m free class I heavy chain may resemble a class II molecule with open ends which can load long exogenous peptides. Studies in Strominger's laboratory confirmed that some human B27 molecules were bound with 14–16 amino acid peptides rather than 8–9 amino acid peptides normally found in most class I molecules (Madden et al., 1991). Transporter-associated proteins (TAP) interact with a unique class I confirmation; whereas calnexin associates with multiple class I forms. Spontaneous inflammatory disease in HLA-B27 transgenic mice does not require TAP (Khare et al., 2001), and is independent of class II molecules, suggesting a direct role for B27 heavy chains and not B27-derived peptides (Khare et al., 1998).

On the basis of our studies with the HLA-B27 transgenic mice, we proposed the following hypothesis. HLA-B27 is a unique class I molecule that can be expressed on the cell surface as free heavy chains. They can load 14–16 amino acid-long exogenous bacterial peptides, and activate autoreactive CD4 T cells. Activated CD4 T cells migrate to target tissue and destroy cartilage causing various symptoms related to spondyloarthropathies.

HLA-B27 and AIDS

A major breakthrough came in the HLA-B27 field when it was identified as one of a very few HLA class I genes which protected HIV-infected individuals from progressing to full-blown disease (McMichael and Klenerman, 2002). The HLA-B27 molecules were able to bind and present multiple viral epitopes to generate a robust T cell response to clear infection (Streeck et al., 2007). The CD4 T cell level remained high and there was efficient B cell response also. Further proof came when it was shown that B27[+] individuals were also protected against hepatitis C infections and endemic malaria (Mathieu et al., 2008).

Andrew McMichael and his group at the University of Cambridge became interested in the role of HLA-B27 in clearing viral infection. They initiated in-depth studies to understand how the B27 molecule is processed and loaded with peptides in human cells. When they tried to generate B27 tetramers for their studies, they noticed that B27 heavy chains were reaching the cell surface in the absence of β2m and peptide. Further studies showed that these free chains were actually dimers of heavy chains (Allen et al., 1999b). This confirmed the findings on the HLA-B27 transgenic mice. The McMichael group expanded their studies to analyze the expression of HLA-B27 molecule in patients with spondyloarthropathies.

HLA-B27 and Peptide Binding

There are several critical residues in HLA-B27 molecules which may influence protection versus susceptibility against viral infection as well as autoimmunity. One such residue is at position 97 in the floor of the peptide binding pocket (McMichael and Jones, 2010). While most HLA class I molecules have arginine at this position, HLA-B27

has asparagine. Arginine is known to be a hindrance for peptide binding in the groove. HLA-B27 molecules in the thymus bind to multiple peptides, but there is a major difference in the affinity of the binding. While B27 bind very few peptides with high affinity, they bind many peptides with low affinity. Thus, fewer self-reactive T cells are deleted in the thymus, resulting in positive selection of autoreactive T cells. On the other hand, they may select virus specific T cells to broader fine specificity which could reduce virus options to escape by mutations, thus enhancing viral clearance.

Another key residue on the HLA-B27 molecule is at position 67 where B27 molecules have free cysteine (Bird et al., 2003). This residue enables the formation of dimers of the free heavy chains. The homodimer formation is dependent upon disulfide bonding through Cys67. Such bonding would require unwinding of the α1 helix, enabling binding of longer peptides in a class II-like groove.

The HLA-B27 molecules have several other unique characteristics. The HLA-B27 molecules continue to be associated with calnexin after making a complex with β2 microglobulin unlike other HLA molecules. However, they can be expressed on the cell surface in the absence of TAP and tapasin, which are involved in the loading of peptides into the class I molecule. We have previously shown that B27 mice in the context of the transporter-associated protein (TAP knockout) still get spontaneous disease, suggesting TAP may not be involved. Thus, HLA-B27 can be expressed on the cell surface in many different forms; as an intact molecule loaded with an endogenous peptide, or as β2m free heavy chains, homodimers, or multimers either loaded with peptide or as empty molecules. CD4 T cells have been found to recognize HLA-B27 either as homodimers or heterodimers when they are devoid of peptide (Boyle and Hill Gaston, 2003). HLA-B27 reactive CD4[+] T cells have been identified in HLA-B27[+] AS patients.

HLA-B27 and Natural Killer Cells

We had shown a potential role of natural killer (NK) cells on HLA-B27-associated arthritis (Marietta et al., 2000). Introduction into T cells of NKB1, an allelic form of KIR3DL1, produces severe arthritis in HLA-B27 transgenic mice. Thus, interaction of free MHC heavy chains with MHC receptors could play a role in the development of arthritis in our HLA-B27 transgenic mice. Killer cell immunoglobulin-like receptors (KIR family) are expressed on NK cells, T cells, and NK T cells. KIR is polymorphic and demonstrates allele-specific recognition with a cognate KIR for HLA-B27 being the 3 domain, KIR3DL1. Our work with the mice was confirmed by Kollnberger and coworkers (Kollnberger et al., 2002) who showed that HLA-B27 heavy chain homodimers and receptors for HLA-B27 homodimers are expressed on populations of peripheral blood, B and T lymphocytes, and synovial monocytes from patients with spondyloarthritis. Thus, interaction of HLA-B27 heavy chain with immunoreceptors on cells of the myelomonocytic cell lineage or lymphocytes might also be involved in the pathogenesis of spondyloarthritis.

HLA-B27 and Evolution

If HLA-B27 was a bad gene causing all of these diseases, it should have been eliminated during evolutionary time. On the contrary, HLA-B27 is one of the oldest MHC class I genes and has survived thousands of years. It is found on every continent, every geographical area, and in all ethnic and racial groups. It has one of the highest gene frequencies, and is very polymorphic with over 50 subtypes. These facts suggest that the HLA-B27 gene was positively selected during evolution and had to be a good gene.

The main function of MHC molecules is to clear infection. During thousands of years of evolution, HLA-B27 emerged as a class I molecule capable of presenting multiple epitopes of infectious agents to activate T cells to clear infection, as well as to generate cytotoxic T cells and help B cells to generate antibodies to clear infection. This could have happened by many different mechanisms. Key mutations in the peptide binding pocket could enable more promiscuous binding of multiple peptides for presentation to T cells. Mutations could have also enabled the B27 molecule to be expressed on the cell surface as free heavy chains capable of loading exogenous peptides and activating CD4 T cells. Thus, B27$^+$ individuals would have survived many infectious episodes and bottlenecks, spread all over the world, and reproduced.

Unfortunately, HLA-B27 molecules can also generate adverse effects. The free chains of HLA-B27 are also expressed in the thymus where they can bind many self-peptides with low affinity and activate autoreactive CD4 T cells. These autoreactive CD4 T cells in the periphery can be activated by various mechanisms including molecular mimicry to cause autoimmunity.

In conclusion, the many forms of HLA-B27 can activate many different T cell populations. An intact B27 molecule would activate CD8 T cells. A free heavy chain or a homodimer loaded with an exogenous peptide will activate a CD4 T cell. B27 homodimers in complex with KIR molecules can activate NK cells. Finally, the β2m free heavy chains may be able to directly interact and activate APCs such as B cells. Thus, the HLA-B27 molecule can generate a robust immune response against infectious agents to clear infections and maintain the health of the individual. On the other hand, aberrant activation of an autoreactive CD4 T cell could result in autoimmune diseases.

HLA CLASS II ASSOCIATION WITH AUTOIMMUNE DISEASES

Susceptibility to the majority of autoimmune diseases is associated with the presence of certain HLA-DR and -DQ alleles (Table 27.1). Despite the presence of a high degree of polymorphism, only a few HLA class II alleles and their linked haplotypes are associated with autoimmune diseases. Although HLA class II genes are the strongest genetic factors associated with the development of autoimmune diseases, the exact role of these molecules in disease etiology is still being deciphered.

Predisposition

In the thymus, T cells are positively selected based on their ability to bind to self-MHC molecules expressed in the thymus; T cells binding to self-peptide—MHC molecules with moderate affinity are selected, while T cells binding to self-peptide—MHC complex with strong affinity or weak affinity are deleted (von Boehmer and Kisielow, 1990; Huang et al., 2004). Although effective, there is some leakiness as some T cells binding with weak

TABLE 27.1 Association of Various Autoimmune Diseases with HLA Class II Alleles and Haplotypes.

Disease	Alleles	Haplotype
Rheumatoid arthritis	DRB1*04, DQB1*0302	DRB1*04 \DQB1*0302 DRB1*04 \DQB1*0302 DRB1*10 \DQB1*0501
Insulin dependent	DRB1*03, DRB1*04	DRB1*04 \DQB1*0302
Type 1 diabetes	DQB1*0302	DRB1*0301 \DQB1*02
Multiple sclerosis	DRB1*15	DRB1*1501 \DQB1*0602
	DRB1*0301	DRB1*0301 \DQB1*0201
Celiac disease	DRB1*0301, DRB1*0701 DQB1*0302	DRB1*0301 \DQB1*02 DRB1*0701 \DQB1*02
Graves' disease	DRB1*0301, DQB1*02	DRB1*0301, DQB1*02
Autoimmune thyroid disease	DRB1*0301	DRB1*0301, DQB1*02
Myasthenia gravis	DRB1*03	DRB1*0301, DQB1*02

affinity to the self-peptide—MHC complex escape the negative selection and circulate into the periphery. In most individuals these autoreactive T cells are kept in check through peripheral tolerance.

However, in some individuals these autoreactive T cells can be activated through an unknown mechanism and lead to the onset of autoimmune disease. Such a mechanism might explain the selection of a T cell repertoire that is protective or susceptible to autoreactivity. Elution of peptides from HLA class II molecules suggests that some of these peptides may indeed be derived from HLA molecules themselves (Chicz et al., 1994). Thus, HLA molecules not only function in the thymus by presenting other peptides but can also serve as a donor of self-peptides. This intricate relationship between MHC, self-peptides, and the T cell receptor (TCR) could determine the specificity of T cells in the periphery. Thus, the peripheral pool of T cells can recognize non-self-antigen to clear infection, recognize self-antigens to cause autoimmunity or can become tolerant/anergic. However, studies to resolve these issues in humans have been hampered by the lack of knowledge of "culprit" autoantigens as well as the difficulty in obtaining samples from affected organs. The other confounding problem has been the linkage disequilibrium of HLA class II alleles -DR and -DQ, making it difficult to interpret the association of a disease with a haplotype or specific allele. Despite this risk of autoimmunity in certain individuals, nature persisted with these HLA class II alleles due to the survival advantage associated with these genes. Thus, autoimmunity is a price we have to pay in order to control widespread infections and maintain the survival of the human population.

Onset

Among the individuals carrying the disease predisposing HLA allele/haplotype, only a small percentage develops autoimmune disease. This indicates that precipitation of disease requires a second hit in addition to genetic predisposition. Interestingly, besides genetic factors, most of the autoimmune diseases also show association with environmental factors. A number of environmental factors, both infectious as well as non-infectious, have been shown to play an important role in the onset of disease in genetically predisposed individuals (Klareskog et al., 2006). One mechanism could be molecular mimicry between infected agents and self molecules activating autoreactive T cells. Another mechanism by which pathogens can cause autoreactivity is when post-translational modification of proteins occurs to clear infections; it may inadvertently lead to the activation of self-reactive T cells.

ENVIRONMENTAL FACTORS

Infectious Agent

Among all the infectious agents associated with autoimmune diseases, such as rheumatoid arthritis (RA), multiple sclerosis (MS), and systemic lupus erythematosus (SLE), the strongest association had been reported with the presence of viruses, especially the Epstein—Barr virus (EBV) (Pender, 2003). The EBV is a ubiquitous virus found in populations all over the world. After the primary infection, the virus resides in memory B cells and secretes latent protein such as EBV nuclear antigen (EBNA). After an unknown period of latency, the virus reactivates and goes into a lytic phase infecting more cells. It has been hypothesized that EBV may cause autoimmunity by activation of autoreactive T cells either through molecular mimicry or bystander activation and the release of proinflammatory cytokines. There is strong evidence that EBV plays a central role in the etiology of autoimmune diseases including RA and MS (Alspaugh et al., 1981; Lunemann et al., 2008).

A pathophysiological link between EBV and RA was first described when 67% of patients with RA were shown to produce antibodies to EBNA (Alspaugh et al., 1981; Baboonian et al., 1989). Also, EBV-encoded protein gp110, a major replicative phase glycoprotein required for infection, shares sequence similarities with the QKRAA amino acid motif (the "shared epitope") of HLA-DRB1*0401, suggesting molecular mimicry may be one way EBV could be involved in pathogenesis of RA. In addition, the presence of HLA-DR4 is associated with 10-fold high synovial EBV DNA loads compared to controls and low T cell response in RA patients. A clonal expansion of CD8+ EBV-specific T cells that are suggested to be dysfunctional has also been observed in RA patients. Patients with RA have higher numbers of circulating EBV-reactive B cells compared to controls (Tosato et al., 1984). Thus, a combination of impaired T cell response and presence of antibodies could lead to an immune complex disease.

The mechanism linking MS and EBV is not well understood but could involve a pathological role of antibodies to EBV antigens and activation of central nervous system (CNS) myelin-specific T cells by cross-recognition of EBV-specific T cells. Patients with MS have increased antibody reactivity against several EBNA domains, of which antibodies against EBNA-1 in HLA DRB1*1501 positive individuals were associated with a 24-fold increase in risk for MS (Sundstrom et al., 2009). Further, MS patients show a selective increase of CD4+ T cell response to the EBNA1, which also cross-reacted with myelin antigens (Lunemann et al., 2008). These reports indicate that EBNA1-specific antibodies and/or myelin cross-reactive CD4+ T cells in the presence of a susceptible HLA-class II allele (HLA-DRβ1*1501) could potentially contribute to the development of MS. These reports suggest that molecular mimicry may be one way that EBV-derived protein could cause pathogenesis in autoimmune diseases.

PORPHYROMONAS GINGIVALIS AND RHEUMATOID ARTHRITIS

Porphyromonas gingivalis (*P. gingivalis*), a Gram-negative facultative anaerobe, is the major cause of an inflammatory condition of oral cavity called periodontitis (McGraw et al., 1999). Smoking has been shown to be the leading susceptibility factor for periodontitis (Klareskog et al., 2006; Lundberg et al., 2010). Further, an association between the presence of HLA-DR4 and periodontitis has been described indicating similarities with RA. *P. gingivalis* is present in more than 80% of RA patients. Recent epidemiology studies have shown an association between periodontal disease and RA (Farquharson et al., 2012). Antibodies to *P. gingivalis* are increased in RA patients and correlate with anti-citrullinated peptide antibodies (ACPAs). The potential role of *P. gingivalis* in RA pathogenesis has been suggested to be due to the presence of the bacterial peptidyl arginine deiminase (PAD) enzyme, even though there is no similarity with human PAD (Farquharson et al., 2012). These enzymes can deiminate an arginine residue to citrulline in antigens thus changing their binding affinity to HLA molecules. Further, more than 40% of RA patients are positive for antibodies to an immunodominant peptide, citrullinated alpha-enolase peptide 1, which bears sequence similarity and cross-reactivity with enolase from *P. gingivalis* (Lundberg et al., 2010). These studies suggest that molecular mimicry and immune response to a bacterial epitope may result in production of antibodies. Recent studies have shown that bacterial PAD enzyme can deiminate host fibrinogen peptides (Wegner et al., 2010), which may lead to the generation of new epitopes, so triggering an immune response in a genetically predisposed individual.

Smoking and Autoimmunity

Several retrospective and prospective studies have shown the association between cigarette smoking and susceptibility to a number of autoimmune diseases such as RA, MS, type 1 diabetes, thyroiditis, primary biliary cirrhosis, and Crohn's disease (Wingerchuk, 2012). This has led to the emergence of smoking as a risk factor linked to the onset and clinical development of these autoimmune diseases in genetically predisposed individuals. Although these studies show an association, there is no experimental proof of a direct link between smoking and autoimmune diseases, RA, and MS. Numerous studies have provided

evidence suggesting an association of smoking with development of RA. Smoking has been associated with extra-articular features of RA-like nodules and lung disease which is the third major reason for mortality in arthritis patients (Harel-Meir et al., 2007). An interaction between smoking and DRB1 alleles has been suggested to confer an increased risk of ACPA positive RA. An increase in the presence of citrulline-modified proteins observed in the lungs of smokers may be due to an increase in the PAD enzyme (Makrygiannakis et al., 2008). Although the mechanism of interaction between the RA susceptible class II alleles and environmental factors like smoking has not been elucidated, it is thought that RA onset may occur later in life (median age for RA onset is around 60 years) but the process of autoreactivity starts earlier. This is supported by the fact that autoantibodies in shared epitope positive individuals precede clinical disease, suggesting a role for smoking in triggering antibody production. A recent study using the multinational QUEST-RA database showed no significant differences in the clinical profile of RA patients who are smokers and non-smokers except for an increase in the presence of nodules in the smoker group (Naranjo et al., 2010). A study with a 3-year follow-up of patients with current smokers showed fewer swollen joints and no difference in radiologic damage, suggesting smoking may be contributing to disease by the production of autoantibodies (Harrison et al., 2001). Cigarette smoking is the most characterized environmental factor associated with pathogenesis of RA and suggests that the onset of RA may begin at a site other than joints.

Cigarette smoke can interact with other environmental factors such as EBV to increase the risk of MS, as smokers were twice as likely to have MS with high titers of anti-EBNA antibody compared to non-smokers (Simon et al., 2010). Smoking can increase risk of MS through a number of pathways such as (1) modulation of systemic immune response; (2) increasing the blood—brain barrier permeability; and (3) direct injury to CNS by neurotoxic chemicals present in smoke.

VITAMIN D IN AUTOIMMUNE DISEASES

Epidemiological studies have suggested that vitamin D deficiency is associated with a number of autoimmune diseases. Patients with autoimmune diseases such as RA, MS, T1D, as well as lupus have decreased serum levels of vitamin D3. In MS, there is both a strong north to south gradient as well as high altitude areas with low sunlight (decreased levels of vitamin D) that are associated with an increased disease incidence (Hogancamp et al., 1997; Kurtzke, 2005). African American patients are three times more likely to develop lupus as compared to Caucasian populations carrying a similar genotype. Together these studies point towards an important role of vitamin D in predisposition to autoimmune diseases. Cells involved in immune response express vitamin D receptors. Since vitamin D shows a strong immune-modulatory effect, it is hypothesized that vitamin D suppresses autoimmune disease by inhibiting disease promoting proinflammatory response and maintaining immune tolerance (Wen and Baker, 2011). Induction of regulatory T cells and suppressor macrophages by vitamin D had been suggested to play an important role in maintaining homeostasis of the immune system.

Interaction between environmental and genetic factors in the etiology of autoimmune diseases can be explained by a "Causal Pie Model" (van der Mei et al., 2011), where MHC represents the major fixed slice, while other slices represent one or another individual component (genetic or environmental) and these can interact to cause disease. To develop an autoimmune disease such as MS or RA, a person must complete the pie, though different people or groups of people might have different slices in their pie. In RA patients an inverse relationship has been described between disease activity and levels of vitamin D metabolites (Patel et al., 2007). Further, an association between a polymorphism of the vitamin D receptor and onset of RA has been observed (Gomez-Vaquero et al., 2007). Vitamin D metabolites have been shown to inhibit the production of IL-17A and stimulate IL-4 production in early RA patients (Colin et al., 2010). Thus a deficiency of vitamin D may lead to proinflammatory conditions. Patients carrying susceptible genotypes may require one or more factors, such as smoking, infection, or deficiency in vitamin D, to precipitate RA.

Similarly, in a subset of MS patients carrying the HLA-DRB1*1501 allele, immune reactivity to EBV and smoking might complete the pie, leading to clinical disease. In other individuals vitamin D and smoking or EBV and vitamin D might complete the pie and cause precipitation of disease (Ascherio and Munger, 2007). EBV may cause MS through molecular mimicry as T/B cells against the EBV antigen have been shown to cross-react with myelin antigen, leading to a break in tolerance. Smoking can also increase immune reactivity to viruses like EBV, and T cells specific to EBV antigen can further activate myelin-specific T cells through molecular mimicry (Lunemann et al., 2008). These interactions might lead to MS-related immune dysregulation that involves activation of T cells, modulation of DC function, and blood–brain barrier permeability.

POST-TRANSLATIONAL MODIFICATIONS IN AUTOIMMUNITY

Post-translational modifications of proteins occur *in vivo* frequently. In most cases, this process enables the clearance of infection and malignant cells. For example, modification of viral antigen could enable its binding to MHC molecules for activation of T cells. Similarly, malignant self-tissue could be modified to make them more antigenic. This process also occurs occasionally in normal proteins (Gyorgy et al., 2006; Greer and Shi, 2012). Unfortunately, post-translation modification of self antigen could activate autoreactive cells, for example post-translational modification of synovial or joint-related antigen could trigger an immune response which would activate autoreactive T cells in genetically predisposed individuals. There are many types of post-translational modifications (PTMs). Modifications that change an amino acid include phosphorylation, methylation, and glycosylation while enzymatic conversions include deimination and deamidation.

Deimination

The enzymatic process by which citrulline, a non-coded amino acid, is inserted in proteins is called deimination. PAD is the enzyme required for catalytic deimination of peptidyl arginine to citrulline, a process called citrullination, first described by Fearon (Fearon, 1939). Citrullination of proteins occurs under many conditions; however, an aberrant B cell response to citrullinated proteins is specific to RA. The presence of ACPAs has been shown to be specific to RA patients. RA is associated with the presence of DRB1*0401. Genome-wide association studies (GWAS) using genotyping for single nucleotide polymorphisms (SNPs) of RA patients have confirmed the association of DRB1 with RA (Wellcome Trust Case Control Consortium, 2007). Studies in some populations have shown association of RA with the PADI4 gene encoding for peptidyl arginine deiminase isotype 4 (Suzuki et al., 2003). The peptide binding region of *0401 has a positive charge, thus antigens with positive charged arginine cannot bind. Citrullination of arginine changes the charge to neutral, enabling the antigen to bind DRB1*0401 molecules for the generation of an immune response. This is supported by studies suggesting that ACPAs in RA sera strongly associate with the presence of DRB1-shared epitope alleles. In RA patients, the presence of ACPAs is used for clinical diagnosis in association with rheumatoid factor. Sera from RA patients have been shown to carry antibodies to citrullinated synovial proteins that include CII, fibrinogen, vimentin, and fibronectin. Citrullination of these proteins can potentially alter their antigenicity and function; and in genetically predisposed individuals this might lead to an autoreactive immune response.

Studies using DR4.IE transgenic mice have shown that citrullinated fibrinogen can induce arthritis although no significant difference was observed in T cell response to citrullinated and native fibrinogen. In DR4$^+$ RA patients, T cells reactive to citrullinated vimentin-derived peptides rather than native peptides have been described, suggesting a crucial role of citrullinated vimentin in RA pathogenesis. Thus post-translational conversion of peptidyl arginine to peptidyl citrulline by PAD enzymes appears to be an essential feature of many autoantigens in RA. Estrogen can increase production of the PAD enzymes required for citrullination of proteins (Senshu et al., 1989). A primary risk factor for the production of ACPAs in RA is the presence of the DRB1-shared epitope. Immunization with native CII-derived peptides that are non-responders in native form in DRB1*0401 mice followed by challenge *in vitro* with citrullinated peptide generated a higher response in female mice compared to males (Behrens et al., 2010). A higher antigen presentation has been shown by splenic cells and epithelial cells during proestrous when estrogen is high. One can speculate that the increased expression of the PAD enzyme during the estrous cycle could cause an increase in citrullination of peptides, not only in the uterus, but other tissues including synovial tissue. This could result in the citrullination of multiple synovial-specific autoantigens and their presentation by the DRB1*0401 molecule leading to activation of autoreactive CD4 T cells and autoimmunity. This could be one of the reasons for the higher incidence of autoimmune diseases in females.

Deamidation

Around 90% of proteins undergo some form of post-translational modifications, which increases the structural and functional diversity of the proteome. Post-translational modifications like deamidation have been shown to be associated with autoimmunity. Deamidation is a chemical reaction in which an amide functional group is removed from a protein leading to degradation of the protein because it damages the amide-containing side chains of the amino acids. Asparagine (Asn) and to a lesser extent glutamine (Gln) are prone to spontaneous deamidation changing them to aspartic/isoaspartic acid and glutamic acid, respectively. The rate at which Asn and Gln residues are deamidated is dependent on the neighboring residues in the peptide. The presence of glycine and serine as neighboring residues to Asn and Gln has a destabilizing effect, making them a target for deamidation.

In addition to spontaneous deamidation, enzymatic deamidation also occurs and requires transglutaminase (TG2). Transglutaminase is a calcium-dependent enzyme that is involved in deamidation of glutamine side chains. Enzymatic deamidation of glutamine converts it to glutamic acid. Tissue transglutaminase (tTg) is widely distributed and is ubiquitously present in the cytosol and the extracellular space within many connective tissues and is involved in many functions. Deamidation by tTg is dependent on the presence of either a proline residue or a hydrophobic amino acid like the Phe C terminal of the target glutamine. In celiac disease patients, an immune response to a wheat-derived protein, gliadin, can generate an autoimmune response. Celiac disease is a good example of how modified proteins induce an immune response even though the initiating antigen may not involve a self-protein. T cells of patients with celiac disease recognize peptides of gliadin that are deamidated (Glu to Gln).

Celiac disease is associated with the presence of HLA-DQ2 in the majority of patients and the remaining patients are generally positive for DQ8. Deamidation of gliadin peptides changes the charge leading to better binding of peptides to DQ2 and DQ8 and generation of an immune response. Studies in celiac disease have shown that tissue transglutaminase enzymes can deamidate peptides of gliadin which are presented by DQ8 or DQ2 leading to gluten sensitivity.

HUMANIZED ANIMAL MODELS OF AUTOIMMUNITY

The advent of transgenic mice lacking endogenous class II molecules (Aβo) but expressing human HLA-DR and HLA-DQ genes has significantly advanced the understanding of the role of individual HLA class II molecules (Mangalam et al., 2008; Taneja and David, 2010). Introduction of HLA class II transgenes in Aβo mice led to the expression of functional HLA class II molecules and reconstituted the CD4 T cell compartment, thus resulting in CD4 restricted immune response to various peptides. The HLA transgene in these mice is self and so they are tolerant to it. Experimental data from various laboratories have shown that the HLA class II molecules in these mice function in a way similar to that in humans. The first evidence came from *in vivo* and *in vitro* studies done with superantigens in HLA transgenic mice. Bacterial superantigens (SAg) have lower affinity for mouse MHC class II than for human MHC class II molecules. Because of this biological characteristic, SAg-induced toxicity is much lower in mouse models than it is in humans. When immunized with lower concentrations of SEB, HLA-DR3 transgenic mice respond vigorously, activate multiple T cells and secrete higher levels of proinflammatory cytokines than wild-type mice (DaSilva et al., 2002). The response to superantigens in transgenic mice can result in toxic shock and is dependent on the polymorphism of HLA class II alleles.

The second evidence comes from the peptide presentation by HLA class II molecules in transgenic mice. The HLA transgenic mice respond to similar epitopes as observed in humans. In a comparison study, DR3.Aβo mice recognized only one epitope comprising aa 1–20 for heat shock protein (hsp) 65 of *Mycobacterium tuberculosis* as observed with human DR3-restricted T cells (Geluk et al., 1998). The response was specific in DR3 mice as DQ8 mice did not respond to this peptide. These studies suggest that processing and presentation of the antigens in the context of class II molecules is similar in transgenic mice and humans.

The third evidence that HLA transgenes in mice function similarly to humans comes from studies with experimental autoimmune myasthenia gravis (EAMG) in DR3 transgenic mice (Infante et al., 2003). The wild-type mice show a highly conserved TCR-BV gene usage and CDR3 sequences in response to acetylcholine receptor (AChR), an autoantigen for myasthenia gravis patients. However, DR3-restricted murine hybridomas generated from DR3 mice immunized with AChR expressed a diverse set of T cell receptor β chains, similar to that observed in humans. The TCRBV sequences from human MG patients were homologous to DR3-restricted murine clones, suggesting that human and mice can recognize similar epitopes and use similar CDR3 sequences for the recognition of the same peptide–MHC complex. Thus, transgenic mice can provide an important insight into peptide presentation by different class II alleles and the resulting pathogenesis.

Collagen-Induced Arthritis

Collagen-induced arthritis has been used as a model for inflammatory arthritis where immunization of susceptible strains of mice with type II collagen leads to the development of arthritis with features similar to those of human inflammatory arthritis. The first model of autoimmunity to determine the role of human class II molecules in arthritis was established by using DQA1*0301, DQB1*0302 (DQ8) transgenic mice. DQ8 occurs in linkage disequilibrium with DR4 and has been shown to be associated with RA in certain ethnic groups (Taneja et al., 1992). Collagen-induced arthritis, an animal model for RA, was studied *in vivo* in Aβo.DQ8 mice. Immunization of Aβo.DQ8 mice with heterologous type II collagen led to a pathogenic autoimmune CD4-mediated response leading to severe arthritis and antibodies to self-type II collagen (Nabozny et al., 1996). Both CD4 T cells and B cells are required for the development of arthritis in transgenic mice (Taneja et al., 2005, 2007b). This is the first model where arthritic mice produced rheumatoid factor (RF), one of the major features in patients with RA (Taneja et al., 2002). The scenario in the development of arthritis in transgenic mice can be compared to that of RA in human. Both require presentation of an arthritogenic epitope by HLA class II molecules to CD4 T cells, leading to proliferation of autoreactive cells and production of RF

by B cells, subsequently leading to joint pathology. Further, studies using CD4-deficient and CD8-deficient mice suggested that the disease was mediated by CD4$^+$ T cells, while CD8$^+$ T cells may be the regulatory cells as CD8-deficient mice transgenic for DQ8 develop high amounts of autoantibodies including RF and anti-nuclear antibodies (ANA) (Taneja et al., 2002). A similar phenomenon can be envisaged in RA where production of autoantibodies like RF and ANAs could be related to the functional status of CD8 T cells. On the other hand, mice expressing DQA1*0103, DQB1*0601 (DQ6) were resistant to developing CIA. The double transgenic mice expressing both DQ6 and DQ8 developed moderate CIA when compared with the severe arthritis observed in DQ8 transgenic mice (Bradley et al., 1998), much like RA patients bearing both susceptible and non-susceptible HLA haplotypes. These observations contributed to the concept that polymorphism in DQ may be a major contributing factor in human RA.

Predisposition to RA has been associated with the expression of some subtypes of HLA-DR4 in most human studies ever since the first association of DW4 and RA shown by Stastny (Stastny, 1978). However, most of the studies in different ethnic groups have observed only two alleles, DRB1*0401 and *0404, which occur with increased frequency in RA patients. Thus while DRB1*0401, 0404 are associated with predisposition, DRB1*0402 is associated with resistance or protection against RA. To determine the role of DR4 molecules in RA, DRB1*0401 mice were generated in complete MHC knockout mice (AE$^{-/-}$). DRB1*0401.AE$^{-/-}$ mice develop arthritis which mimics human arthritis (Taneja et al., 2007a). AE$^{-/-}$ mice have deletion of an 80 kb region of MHC class II such that none of the classical murine class II molecules are expressed. Human T cell is unique from mice in the expression of MHC class II molecules on their cell surface. Interestingly, similar to humans, T cells from AE$^{-/-}$.DR transgenic mice express HLA-DR molecules on their cell surface and can present peptide antigen. Thus presentation of an antigen in the context of HLA by an activated T cell might also contribute towards severity.

To simulate human haplotypes, double transgenic mice expressing autoimmune associated DQ and DR alleles were generated on the AE$^{-/-}$ background. DR4\DQ8.AE$^{-/-}$ mice developed arthritis similar to DQ8 but also showed gender differences. Gender differences in CIA were not observed in DQ8 mice suggesting modulation of DQ8-restricted disease by DR4 molecules. To understand the modulation by DR polymorphism, DRB1*0402 mice were studied (Taneja et al., 2008) for their influence on CIA. DRB1*0402 mice are not susceptible to arthritis, similar to humans. Mice expressing both susceptible and resistant DR4 subtypes, 0401/0402, developed arthritis with lower incidence than *0401 mice (Taneja et al., 2003). Further, data in DR*0401/DQ8 mice suggested that APCs present DR-restricted peptides differentially, suggesting a role of hormones in influencing APCs (Behrens et al., 2010; Luckey et al., 2012). Based on the data in transgenic mice, it can be speculated that hormone-influenced PAD enzymes may lead to citrullination of antigens in females, thus enhancing presentation of certain antigens. The experimental and human data led us to hypothesize that DQ polymorphism may be responsible for susceptibility while DR may be involved in the modulation of disease. Thus both DQ and DR alleles as a haplotype influence the development of disease (Taneja et al., 1998). From the studies on DQ and DR transgenic mice, it can be extrapolated that gene complementation or interaction between DQ and DR molecules mediates susceptibility to RA in the human. Depending on the haplotypes carried by an individual, they could be susceptible to severe or mild disease. A homozygous haplotype for predisposing DQ and permissive DR will lead to severe disease. Also, heterozygous RA-susceptible haplotypes will result in very severe disease since there will be two predisposing DQ molecules. However, one predisposing and one protective haplotype should show less severity and low incidence.

Non-RA-Associated HLA Alleles Can Predispose to Autoimmunity

HLA-DQ6 alleles, DQB1*0601 and *0604, are not associated with susceptibility to develop arthritis. DQB1*0601 occurs in linkage with DQA1*0103 and DQB1*0604 with DQA1*0102. To understand if trans-heterodimers of two non-susceptible HLA alleles may have a role in rendering susceptibility to develop arthritis, we generated mice expressing DQB1*0601/DQA1*0103 (DQ6.1) and DQB1*0604/DQA1*0103 (DQ6.4). Immunization of transgenic mice leads to development of severe CIA in DQ6.4 but not DQ6.1 mice (Behrens et al., 2011). Further, data showed that DQ6.4 molecules could present CII-derived peptides similar to those presented by the CIA-susceptible DQ8 allele. These studies suggested that trans-heterodimer molecules between two DQB1 and DQA1 alleles may result in presentation of unique antigens and susceptibility to develop arthritis. Molecular modeling of the CII peptides showed that DQB1*0604/DQA1*0103 shares the p4 pocket with the arthritis-susceptible DQB1*0302 allele and further a critical role of p4 and p9 pockets is suggested with susceptibility to arthritis. This provides an explanation for the presence of non-susceptible alleles in some RA patients and a mechanism by which they can predispose to develop arthritis.

HLA-DR Transgenic Mice with EAE as an Animal Model of MS

MS, a chronic inflammatory disease of the CNS, shows strong linkage with the presence of HLA-DR2 haplotypes (DRB1*1501, DRB5*0101, DQA1*0102, and DQB1*0602) (Oksenberg et al., 1993). Besides DR2, MS has also been associated with HLA-DR3 and -DR4 haplotypes (Weinshenker et al., 1998; Coraddu et al., 2001). HLA DR3/DQ2 haplotypes have been shown to confer an increased risk for relapsing remitting MS in individuals (Weinshenker et al., 1998). The lack of a complete association to a particular HLA allele suggests that MS is a heterogeneous disease at the molecular level. MS is hypothesized to be mediated by autoreactive T cells against a variety of myelin antigens including myelin basic protein (MBP), proteolipid protein (PLP), and myelin oligodendrocytic glycoprotein (MOG).

Experimental autoimmune encephalomyelitis (EAE) has been used as an animal model of MS where immunization of susceptible strains of mice with autoantigens such as PLP, MBP, or MOG can lead to the development of inflammation and demyelination in the CNS, similar to MS pathology observed in patients (Mangalam et al., 2004; Rich et al., 2004). Induction of EAE with recombinant myelin oligodendrocyte glycoprotein (rMOG) in DR2 mice (DRB1*1501, DRB1*1502, and DRB1*1503) showed that all three strains developed EAE; however, the disease incidence and severity was higher in DRB1*1501 transgenic mice. Almost all of the T cell epitopes identified in HLA transgenic mice using overlapping epitopes of MBP, PLP, and MOG are similar to those identified among T cells isolated from peripheral blood mononuclear cells of MS patients (Kawamura et al., 2000; Khare et al., 2003). Administration of PLP91-110 peptide induced EAE in DR3 transgenic mice (Mangalam et al., 2009). Recently we have also observed that PLP178-197 peptide can induce EAE in HLA-DR4 (DRB1*0401) transgenic mice, while HLA-DR4 (DRB1*0402) transgenic mice were resistant to disease. The disease in transgenic mice was characterized by paralysis of limbs with mild demyelination while in humans demyelination is the major feature of MS. CD4$^+$ T cells have been shown to infiltrate the CNS and are responsible for inflammation and demyelination in MS. It is speculated that class II molecules on T cells may present myelin antigen in CNS and exacerbate the disease. To replicate the human disease, DR3.AEo mice were utilized for EAE with PLP peptide (Mangalam et al., 2006). The DR3.AEo transgenic mice with EAE showed severe inflammation and demyelination in the meningeal, stratum, and brain stem regions, a hallmark for human MS. HLA class II expression was detected in the CNS, especially on microglial cells. These experiments suggest that humanized HLA class II transgenic mice simulate human MS and are a good model to study the role of class II molecules in its pathogenesis.

Role of DQ Molecules in Predisposition to MS

To simulate the human haplotype, we generated double transgenic mice expressing HLA-DR2 and DQ8 (DR2/DQ8). When immunized with rMOG, 90% of mice developed disease accompanied with severe inflammatory and demyelinating lesions in the CNS as compared to DR2 single transgenic mice (Khare et al., 2005). Similarly, expression of DQ8 on disease-susceptible DR3 background (DR3/DQ8 double transgenic mice) led to the development of severe EAE upon immunization with PLP91-110 peptide (Mangalam et al., 2009). The disease in DR3/DQ8 double transgenic mice was characterized by earlier disease onset, higher clinical score, and increased inflammation and demyelination in CNS compared to single DR3 transgenic mice. Since HLA-DQ8 mice were resistant to EAE, our data suggested that DQ8 allele synergizes with disease susceptible HLA-DR allele(s) for a more severe disease phenotype suggesting its pathogenic role in disease etiology. We further determined that the increased susceptibility in DQ8/DR3 mice was due to an increased production of the proinflammatory cytokines IL-17 and GM-CSF. Higher IL-17 levels might lead to the activation and recruitment of more inflammatory cells inside the CNS, while GM-CSF has been shown to increase antigen presentation both in the periphery as well as the CNS.

In contrast HLA-DQB1*0601, observed frequently in Japanese and Asian populations, is known to be protective in MS (Amirzargar et al., 1998; Marrosu et al., 2001). DQB1*0601 transgenic mice were resistant to EAE on immunization with MOG, MBP, or PLP antigens. Expression of the HLA-DQB*0601 allele in disease susceptible HLA-DR2 or -DR3 transgenic mice led to a decrease in disease incidence and severity suggesting a protective role of the allele in disease pathogenesis. Immunization of DR2/DQB1*0601 mice with rMOG led to lower disease incidence compared to DR2 single transgenic mice. Similar findings were also observed in DR3/DQ6 mice immunized with whole myelin or human PLP91-110 (Das et al., 2000). We have further characterized that the protective effect of the DQ6 molecule is due to high levels of IFNγ produced by DQ6-restricted T cells, which suppressed proliferation of encephalitogenic DR3-restricted T cells by inducing apoptosis. Our study suggests that DQ6 modifies the PLP91-110-specific T cell response in DR3 through anti-inflammatory effects of IFNγ.

From the EAE data generated using whole myelin (CNS extract), rMOG and PLP91-110, we have observed that the presence of (1) the HLA-DR molecule is required for the development of disease; (2) HLA-DQ6 or DQ8 molecules alone are not sufficient for disease induction; (3) HLA-DQ8 on disease susceptible HLA-DR2 or HLA-DR3 transgenic mice increased the severity and incidence of disease; (4) DQ6 (DQB1*0601) molecules suppress disease incidence and severity on disease-susceptible HLA-DR2 or HLA-DR3 transgenic mice; (5) DQ6 or DQ8 on a disease-resistant background had no effect on disease induction as none of the HLA-DR2/DQ6, DR2/DQ8, or DR4/DQ8 double transgenic mice developed EAE on immunization with PLP91-110 peptide. These data would suggest that while the presence of certain DR gene(s) predisposes an individual to MS, polymorphism in DQ gene(s) might play a modulating role. This study also points out that MS is a heterogeneous disease and HLA association is specific for the various autoantigens involved.

Animal Model of Celiac Disease

We have used transgenic mice that express HLA-DQ8 to evaluate the response to gliadin (done in collaboration with Drs. Joseph Murray and Eric Marietta (Marietta et al., 2011)). Immunization of DQ8 mice with gluten led to a strong T cell response and IgG antibodies against gluten, but no enteropathy was observed. In order to introduce an autoimmune component to our mouse model of celiac disease, we back-crossed DQ8 transgenic mice to a non-obese diabetic (NOD) genetic background that was deficient in endogenous murine MHC II. This resulted in transgenic NOD mice that expressed human DQ8. With parenteral sensitization to gluten, these mice developed blistering upon the ears, reminiscent of dermatitis herpetiformis (DH), the skin manifestation that is found in 3−5% of patients with celiac disease (Marietta et al., 2004). This model had all the elements of DH, including IgA deposits at the dermal epidermal junction, infiltration of neutrophils into the dermis of the lesional tissue and, most importantly, resolution of the disease with a gluten-free diet and/or dapsone treatment. However, unlike the majority of DH patients, these mice did not develop enteropathy with gluten sensitization.

Using DQ8 mice, it was shown that T cell hybridomas generated to native peptides mounted a heteroclitic response against the deamidated peptide, suggesting a role of the class II molecule in amplifying the T cell response against dietary gluten. Thus an aberrant innate immune response to gliadin could activate tTg that would result in deamidated forms of gliadin-derived peptides. This could result in an enhanced T cell response to gliadin, causing damage and enteropathy. This heteroclitic response would also explain why most adult celiac patients have a strong T cell response against the deamidated forms of the specific gliadin-derived peptide.

Transgenic mice that express both HLA-DQ2 and DR3 (de Kauwe et al., 2009; Du Pre et al., 2011), sensitization to gliadin resulted in a strong T cell response to gliadin, but no overt enteropathy. One group went further and generated a DQ2/DR3 mouse that expressed a gliadin-specific TCR that had been identified in the gliadin-sensitization studies (de Kauwe et al., 2009). These mice responded to deamidated gliadin peptide and generated the Th1 response present in CD patients but did not develop enteropathy, suggesting a second insult to mucosa may be required for development of enteropathy in humans. Absence of pathology in the presence of antigen-specific CD4 T cells may suggest other systemic factors may be involved in disease pathogenesis.

Animal Model for Type 1 Diabetes

Type 1 diabetes shows familial clustering and is linked to the presence of HLA-DQ8/DR4 and HLA-DQ2/DR3 haplotypes. Within the HLA-DQ8/DR4 haplotype, HLA-DQ8 is believed to be the predisposing class II molecule. Most knowledge about autoimmune diabetes comes from a special strain of NOD mice which develop spontaneous diabetes. Elegant genetic studies performed in these mice have mapped the development of disease to the presence of MHC class II molecule H2-A^{g7}. Interestingly, the H2-A^{g7} molecule shows strong structural and functional homology with the human HLA-DQ8 molecule, thus strengthening the major pathogenic role of DQ8 in human T1D. Although HLA-DQ8 transgenic mice do not develop spontaneous diabetes, they lost tolerance to self-GAD65 antigen, leading to activation of autoreactive T cells in the periphery and pancreas. These transgenic mice show insulitis but do not progress to diabetes. As with DQ8 transgenic mice, the presence of a T1D predisposing MHC allele in certain individuals could result in the escape of autoreactive T cells against pancreatic antigens. However, the onset of disease might require a second hit in the pancreas. This second hit can come in the form of virus/bacterial infection, and/or overproduction of a cytokine, overexpression of an accessory molecule or other genetically-determined variations completing the causal pie and precipitation of disease in these individuals. To simulate such an insult in the pancreas, we generated HLA-DQ8 (disease-susceptible) and HLA-DQ6 (disease-resistant) transgenic mice expressing the costimulatory molecule CD80 (B7.1) in islet β cells under the rat insulin promoter (RIP) (Wen et al., 2000). HLA-DQ8/RIP/B7.1 mice developed spontaneous diabetes, while no disease was seen in DQ6/RIP/B7.1 transgenic mice. These studies further confirmed that while the HLA class II allele is the major predisposing gene for development of most if not all autoimmune diseases, other insults or signals are required for precipitation of the disease.

Further studies using double transgenic mice expressing DQ8 with HLA-DR3 or HLA-DR4 indicated that the HLA-DR molecule can modulate the diabetogenic effect of DQ8 (Rajagopalan et al., 2003), which in turn suggests that interaction between various MHC class II molecules in cis as well as trans plays an important role in predisposition, onset, as well as progression of the disease.

HLA CLASS II MOLECULES REGULATE INFECTION THROUGH MODULATION OF CYTOKINE NETWORKS

The MHC has evolved over millions of years to fight infection. Mediators such as cytokines and chemokines produced following antigen presentation play an important role in the clearance of pathogens. The association of a particular HLA class II haplotype with disease seems to depend on geographical locations as well as the ethnic composition of the populations. Evolutionarily DQ is a stable molecule with less polymorphism than observed in the DRB1 locus. The DQ8 molecule has not undergone many changes during evolution and occurs with only three known subtypes. This could be because DQ8 has the advantage of being able to bind and present multiple peptides. On the other hand, DR has many subtypes. For example, DRB1*04 has at least 50 subtypes; however, not all the subtypes are associated with susceptibility to autoimmune diseases. We speculate that DR4 polymorphism occurred to counteract the predisposition to autoimmunity imposed by the DQ8 molecule. Thus, multiple subtypes of DR4 lead to many possible DR4\DQ8 haplotypes. Only those with an advantage of presenting microbial antigens, clearing infections, and with the capacity to counter the autoimmune responses may eventually be selected. Therefore it is possible that HLA molecules were selected based on their ability to induce subsets of T cells for production of a particular cytokine that is responsible for controlling one set of microorganisms. Interferon gamma (IFNγ) is one of the signature cytokines of Th1 type of T cells and controls intracellular pathogens. At the same time interleukin (IL)-17, a signature cytokine of Th17 T cells, controls extracellular pathogens. Thus, one set of class II genes might have evolved to produce IL-17 for controlling the spread of extracellular pathogen, while others produce Th1/Th2 to control other pathogens. Using our transgenic mice we have observed that while transgenic mice expressing HLA-DQ8 induce more TH17 type of T cells, HLA-DQ6 transgenic mice induce more IFNγ producing CD4 T cells. This results in cytokine milieu that modulates disease. A scenario where interaction between HLA molecules and environmental factors leads to the onset of an autoimmune response and disease can be envisaged (Figure 27.1).

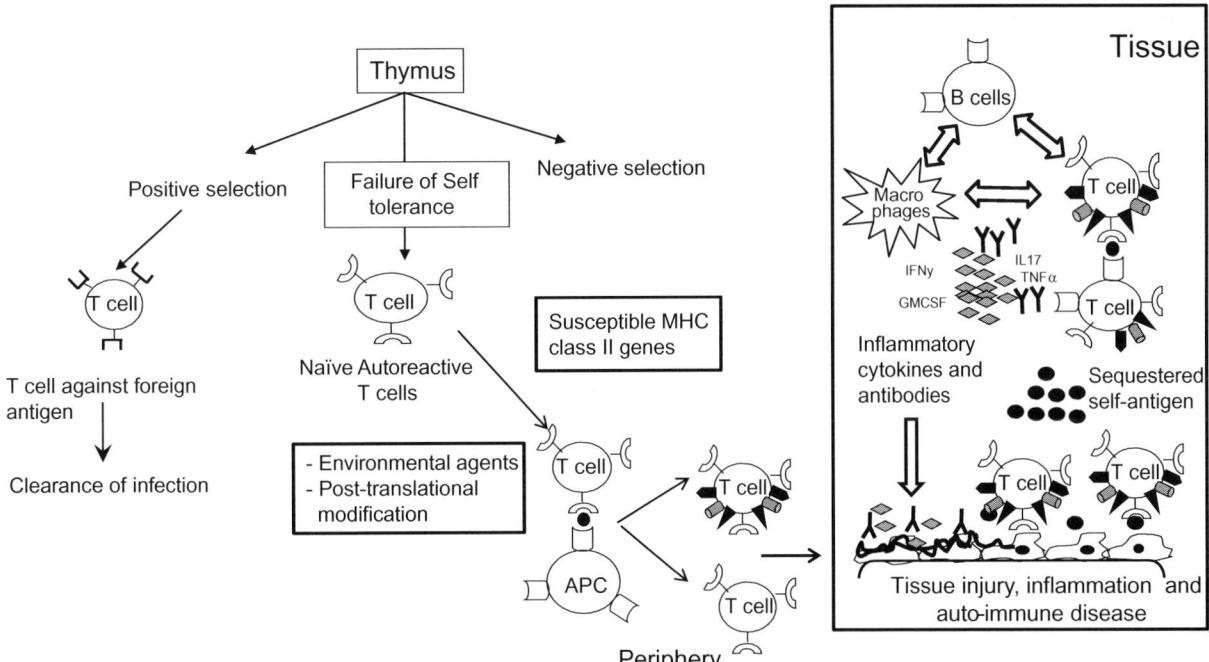

FIGURE 27.1   HLA molecules select T cell repertoire in the thymus by presenting peptides and also serving as donors of self-peptides. T cells are selected on the basis of their interaction with self-MHC molecules expressed in thymus. Thus, T cells reactive with self-peptide binding with high affinity to MHC are negatively selected in the thymus while those with weak interactions may escape negative selection. Such a mechanism may explain the selection of an autoreactive T cell repertoire. In the periphery, positively selected T cells can recognize non-self antigens and clear infection. The autoreactive T cells that have escaped can recognize viral peptide that mimic self antigen, or cryptic epitopes that are exposed during infection or post-translational modification causing activation of autoreactive T cells. These T cells can migrate to various organs, and depending on the host genotype and its interaction with the non-genetic factors, they can cause inflammation locally. The response can be exacerbated in the presence of self-peptides, that when presented by antigen presenting cells in the tissue leading to production of proinflammatory cytokines ensuing an autoimmune response.

CONCLUDING REMARKS

From various *in vivo* and *in vitro* studies, it has become clear that MHC and non-MHC genetic components are common elements for various autoimmune diseases, and in corresponding animal models. Thus polymorphism in MHC is an advantage for human survival, but autoimmunity is the price that the population must pay for combating infection effectively and for survival. In evolutionary terms, only those HLA genes which can generate strong immune responses to infections are selected. The constant mutations observed might be leading to the generation of new subtypes of an allele to circumvent autoimmunity. Haplotypes and not a single class II allele function in the selection of the T cell repertoire and susceptibility to disease.

REFERENCES

Allen, R.L., Bowness, P., McMichael, A., 1999a. The role of HLA-B27 in spondyloarthritis. Immunogenetics. 50, 220–227.

Allen, R.L., O'Callaghan, C.A., McMichael, A.J., Bowness, P., 1999b. Cutting edge: HLA-B27 can form a novel beta 2-microglobulin-free heavy chain homodimer structure. J. Immunol. 162, 5045–5048.

Alspaugh, M.A., Henle, G., Lennette, E.T., Henle, W., 1981. Elevated levels of antibodies to Epstein-Barr virus antigens in sera and synovial fluids of patients with rheumatoid arthritis. J. Clin. Invest. 67, 1134–1140.

Amirzargar, A., Mytilineos, J., Yousefipour, A., Farjadian, S., Scherer, S., Opelz, G., et al., 1998. HLA class II DRB1, DQA1 and DQB1 associated genetic susceptibility in Iranian multiple sclerosis MS patients. Eur. J. Immunogenet. 25, 297–301.

Ascherio, A., Munger, K.L., 2007. Environmental risk factors for multiple sclerosis. Part I: the role of infection. Ann. Neurol. 61, 288–299.

Baboonian, C., Halliday, D., Venables, P.J., Pawlowski, T., Millman, G., Maini, R.N., 1989. Antibodies in rheumatoid arthritis react specifically with the glycine alanine repeat sequence of Epstein-Barr nuclear antigen-1. Rheumatol. Int. 9, 161–166.

Behrens, M., Trejo, T., Luthra, H., Griffiths, M., David, C.S., Taneja, V., 2010. Mechanism by which HLA-DR4 regulates sex-bias of arthritis in humanized mice. J. Autoimmun. 35, 1–9.

Behrens, M., Papadopoulos, G.K., Moustakas, A., Smart, M., Luthra, H., David, C.S., et al., 2011. Trans heterodimer between two non-arthritis-associated HLA alleles can predispose to arthritis in humanized mice. Arthritis Rheum. 63, 1552–1561.

Bird, L.A., Peh, C.A., Kollnberger, S., Elliott, T., McMichael, A.J., Bowness, P., 2003. Lymphoblastoid cells express HLA-B27 homodimers both intracellularly and at the cell surface following endosomal recycling. Eur. J. Immunol. 33, 748–759.

von Boehmer, H., Kisielow, P., 1990. Self-nonself discrimination by T cells. Science. 248, 1369–1373.

Boyle, L.H., Hill Gaston, J.S., 2003. Breaking the rules: the unconventional recognition of HLA-B27 by CD4 + T lymphocytes as an insight into the pathogenesis of the spondyloarthropathies. Rheumatology. 42, 404–412.

Bradley, D.S., Das, P., Griffiths, M.M., Luthra, H.S., David, C.S., 1998. HLA-DQ6/8 double transgenic mice develop auricular chondritis following type II collagen immunization: a model for human relapsing polychondritis. J. Immunol. 161, 5046–5053.

Brewerton, D.A., Hart, F.D., Nicholls, A., Caffrey, M., James, D.C., Sturrock, R.D., 1973. Ankylosing spondylitis and HL-A 27. Lancet. 1, 904–907.

Chicz, R.M., Lane, W.S., Robinson, R.A., Trucco, M., Strominger, J.L., Gorga, J.C., 1994. Self-peptides bound to the type I diabetes associated class II MHC molecules HLA-DQ1 and HLA-DQ8. Int. Immunol. 6, 1639–1649.

Colin, E.M., Asmawidjaja, P.S., van Hamburg, J.P, Mus, A.M, van Driel, M, Hazes, J.M, et al., 2010. 1,25-Dihydroxyvitamin D3 modulates Th17 polarization and interleukin-22 expression by memory T cells from patients with early rheumatoid arthritis. Arthritis Rheum. 62, 132–142.

Coraddu, F., Sawcer, S., D'Alfonso, S., Lai, M., Hensiek, A., Solla, E., et al., 2001. A genome screen for multiple sclerosis in Sardinian multiplex families. Eur. J. Hum. Genet. 9, 621–626.

Das, P., Drescher, K.M., Geluk, A., Bradley, D.S., Rodriguez, M., David, C.S., 2000. Complementation between specific HLA-DR and HLA-DQ genes in transgenic mice determines susceptibility to experimental autoimmune encephalomyelitis. Hum. Immunol. 61, 279–289.

DaSilva, L., Welcher, B.C., Ulrich, R.G., Aman, M.J., David, C.S., Bavari, S., 2002. Humanlike immune response of human leukocyte antigen-DR3 transgenic mice to staphylococcal enterotoxins: a novel model for superantigen vaccines. J. Inf. Dis. 185, 1754.

Du Pre, M.F., Kozijn, A.E., van Berkel, L.A., ter Borg, M.N., Lindenbergh-Kortleve, D., Jensen, L.T., et al., 2011. Tolerance to ingested deamidated gliadin in mice is maintained by splenic, type 1 regulatory T cells. Gastroenterology. 141, 610–620.

Farquharson, D., Butcher, J.P., Culshaw, S., 2012. Periodontitis, Porphyromonas, and the pathogenesis of rheumatoid arthritis. Mucosal Immunol. 5, 112–120.

Fearon, W.R., 1939. The carbamido diacetyl reaction: a test for citrulline. Biochem. J. 33, 902–907.

Geluk, A., Taneja, V., van Meijgaarden, K.E., Zanelli, E., Abou-Zeid, C., Thole, J.E., et al., 1998. Identification of HLA class II-restricted determinants of Mycobacterium tuberculosis-derived proteins by using HLA-transgenic, class II-deficient mice. Proc. Natl. Acad. Sci. U.S.A. 95, 10797–10802.

Gomez-Vaquero, C., Fiter, J., Enjuanes, A., Nogues, X., Diez-Perez, A., Nolla, J.M., 2007. Influence of the BsmI polymorphism of the vitamin D receptor gene on rheumatoid arthritis clinical activity. J. Rheumatol. Suppl. 34, 1823.

Greer, E.L., Shi, Y., 2012. Histone methylation: a dynamic mark in health, disease and inheritance. Nat. Rev. Genet. 13, 343–357.

Gyorgy, B., Toth, E., Tarcsa, E., Falus, A., Buzas, E.I., 2006. Citrullination: a posttranslational modification in health and disease. Int. J. Biochem. Cell Biol. 38, 1662–1677.

Hammer, R.E., Maika, S.D., Richardson, J.A., Tang, J.P., Taurog, J.D., 1990. Spontaneous inflammatory disease in transgenic rats expressing HLA-B27 and human beta 2m: an animal model of HLA-B27-associated human disorders. Cell. 63, 1099–1112.

Harel-Meir, M., Sherer, Y., Shoenfeld, Y., 2007. Tobacco smoking and autoimmune rheumatic diseases. Nat. Clin. Pract. Rheumatol. 3, 707–715.

Harrison, B.J., Silman, A.J., Wiles, N.J., Scott, D.G., Symmons, D.P., 2001. The association of cigarette smoking with disease outcome in patients with early inflammatory polyarthritis. Arthritis Rheum. 44, 323–330.

Hogancamp, W.E., Rodriguez, M., Weinshenker, B.G., 1997. The epidemiology of multiple sclerosis. Mayo. Clin. Proc. 72, 871–878.

Huang, Y.H., Li, D., Winoto, A., Robey, E.A., 2004. Distinct transcriptional programs in thymocytes responding to T cell receptor, Notch, and positive selection signals. Proc. Natl. Acad. Sci. U.S.A. 101, 4936–4941.

Infante, A.J., Baillargeon, J., Kraig, E., Lott, L., Jackson, C., Hammerling, G.J., et al., 2003. Evidence of a diverse T cell receptor repertoire for acetylcholine receptor, the autoantigen of myasthenia gravis. J. Autoimmun. 21, 167–174.

de Kauwe, A.L., Chen, Z., Anderson, R.P., Keech, C.L., Price, J.D., Wijburg, O., et al., 2009. Resistance to celiac disease in humanized HLA-DR3-DQ2-transgenic mice expressing specific anti-gliadin CD4 + T cells. J. Immunol. 182, 7440–7450.

Kawamura, K., Yamamura, T., Yokoyama, K., Chui, D.H., Fukui, Y., Sasazuki, T., et al., 2000. Hla-DR2-restricted responses to proteolipid protein 95-116 peptide cause autoimmune encephalitis in transgenic mice. J. Clin. Invest. 105, 977–984.

Khare, M., Rodriguez, M., David, C.S., 2003. HLA class II transgenic mice authenticate restriction of myelin oligodendrocyte glycoprotein-specific immune response implicated in multiple sclerosis pathogenesis. Int. Immunol. 15, 535–546.

Khare, M., Mangalam, A., Rodriguez, M., David, C.S., 2005. HLA DR and DQ interaction in myelin oligodendrocyte glycoprotein-induced experimental autoimmune encephalomyelitis in HLA class II transgenic mice. J. Neuroimmunol. 169, 1–12.

Khare, S.D., Luthra, H.S., David, C.S., 1995. Spontaneous inflammatory arthritis in HLA-B27 transgenic mice lacking beta 2-microglobulin: a model of human spondyloarthropathies. J. Exp. Med. 182, 1153–1158.

Khare, S.D., Bull, M.J., Hanson, J., Luthra, H.S., David, C.S., 1998. Spontaneous inflammatory disease in HLA-B27 transgenic mice is independent of MHC class II molecules: a direct role for B27 heavy chains and not B27-derived peptides. J. Immunol. 160, 101–106.

Khare, S.D., Lee, S., Bull, M.J., Hanson, J., Luthra, H.S., David, C.S., 2001. Spontaneous inflammatory disease in HLA-B27 transgenic mice does not require transporter of antigenic peptides. Clin. Immunol. 98, 364–369.

Klareskog, L., Padyukov, L., Lorentzen, J., Alfredsson, L., 2006. Mechanisms of disease: genetic susceptibility and environmental triggers in the development of rheumatoid arthritis. Nat. Clin. Pract. Rheumatol. 2, 425–433.

Kollnberger, S., Bird, L., Sun, M.Y., Retiere, C., Braud, V.M., McMichael, A., et al., 2002. Cell-surface expression and immune receptor recognition of HLA-B27 homodimers. Arthritis Rheum. 46, 2972–2982.

Kurtzke, J.F., 2005. Epidemiology and etiology of multiple sclerosis. Phys. Med. Rehabil. Clin. N. Am. 16, 327–349.

Kvien, T.K., Glennas, A., Melby, K., Granfors, K., Andrup, O., Karstensen, B., et al., 1994. Reactive arthritis: incidence, triggering agents and clinical presentation. J. Rheumatol. 21, 115–122.

Luckey, D., Medina, K., Taneja, V., 2012. B cells as effectors and regulators of sex-biased arthritis. Autoimmunity. 45, 364–376.

Lundberg, K., Wegner, N., Yucel-Lindberg, T., Venables, P.J., 2010. Periodontitis in RA—the citrullinated enolase connection. Nat. Rev. Rheumatol. 6, 727–730.

Lunemann, J.D., Jelcic, I., Roberts, S., Lutterotti, A., Tackenberg, B., Martin, R., et al., 2008. EBNA1-specific T cells from patients with multiple sclerosis cross react with myelin antigens and co-produce IFN-gamma and IL-2. J. Exp. Med. 205, 1763–1773.

Madden, D.R., Gorga, J.C., Strominger, J.L., Wiley, D.C., 1991. The structure of HLA-B27 reveals nonamer self-peptides bound in an extended conformation. Nature. 353, 321–325.

Makrygiannakis, D., Hermansson, M., Ulfgren, A.K., Nicholas, A.P., Zendman, A.J., Eklund, A., et al., 2008. Smoking increases peptidylarginine deiminase 2 enzyme expression in human lungs and increases citrullination in BAL cells. Ann. Rheum. Dis. 67, 1488–1492.

Mangalam, A., Rodriguez, M., David, C., 2006. Role of MHC class II expressing CD4 + T cells in proteolipid protein91-110-induced EAE in HLA-DR3 transgenic mice. Eur. J. Immunol. 36, 3356–3370.

Mangalam, A., Luckey, D., Basal, E., Jackson, M., Smart, M., Rodriguez, M., et al., 2009. HLA-DQ8 DQB1*0302-restricted Th17 cells exacerbate experimental autoimmune encephalomyelitis in HLA-DR3-transgenic mice. J. Immunol. 182, 5131–5139.

Mangalam, A.K., Khare, M., Krco, C., Rodriguez, M., David, C., 2004. Identification of T cell epitopes on human proteolipid protein and induction of experimental autoimmune encephalomyelitis in HLA class II-transgenic mice. Eur. J. Immunol. 34, 280–290.

Mangalam, A.K., Rajagopalan, G., Taneja, V., David, C.S., 2008. HLA class II transgenic mice mimic human inflammatory diseases. Adv. Immunol. 97, 65–147.

Marietta, E., Trejo, T., Luthra, H., David, C., 2000. The role of natural killer NK cells on HLA-B27 associated arthritis. Arthritis Rheum. 43, S263.

Marietta, E., Black, K., Camilleri, M., Krause, P., Rogers III, R.S., David, C., et al., 2004. A new model for dermatitis herpetiformis that uses HLA-DQ8 transgenic NOD mice. J. Clin. Invest. 114, 1090–1197.

Marietta, E.V., David, C.S., Murray, J.A., 2011. Important lessons derived from animal models of celiac disease. Int. Rev. Immunol. 30, 197–206.

Marrosu, M.G., Murru, R., Murru, M.R., Costa, G., Zavattari, P., Whalen, M., et al., 2001. Dissection of the HLA association with multiple sclerosis in the founder isolated population of Sardinia. Hum. Mol. Genet. 10, 2907–2916.

Mathieu, A., Cauli, A., Fiorillo, M.T., Sorrentino, R., 2008. HLA-B27 and ankylosing spondylitis geographic distribution as the result of a genetic selection induced by malaria endemic? A review supporting the hypothesis. Autoimmun. Rev. 7, 398–403.

McGraw, W.T., Potempa, J., Farley, D., Travis, J., 1999. Purification, characterization, and sequence analysis of a potential virulence factor from Porphyromonas gingivalis, peptidylarginine deiminase. Infect. Immun. 67, 3248–3256.

McMichael, A., Klenerman, P., 2002. HIV/AIDS. HLA leaves its footprints on HIV. Science. 296, 1410–1411.

McMichael, A.J., Jones, E.Y., 2010. Genetics. First-class control of HIV-1. Science. 330, 1488–1490.

van der Mei, I.A., Simpson Jr., S., Stankovich, J., Taylor, B.V., 2011. Individual and joint action of environmental factors and risk of MS. Neurol. Clin. 29, 233–255.

Nabozny, G.H., Baisch, J.M., Cheng, S., Cosgrove, D., Griffiths, M.M., Luthra, H.S., et al., 1996. HLA-DQ8 transgenic mice are highly susceptible to collagen-induced arthritis: a novel model for human polyarthritis. J. Exp. Med. 183, 27–37.

Naranjo, A., Toloza, S., Guimaraes da Silveira, I., Lazovskis, J., Hetland, M.L., Hamoud, H., et al., 2010. Smokers and non smokers with rheumatoid arthritis have similar clinical status: data from the multinational QUEST-RA database. Clin. Exp. Rheumatol. 28, 820–827.

Oksenberg, J.R., Begovich, A.B., Erlich, H.A., Steinman, L., 1993. Genetic factors in multiple sclerosis. JAMA. 270, 2362–2369.

Patel, S., Farragher, T., Berry, J., Bunn, D., Silman, A., Symmons, D., 2007. Association between serum vitamin D metabolite levels and disease activity in patients with early inflammatory polyarthritis. Arthritis Rheum. 56, 2143–2149.

Pender, M.P., 2003. Infection of autoreactive B lymphocytes with EBV, causing chronic autoimmune diseases. Trends Immunol. 24, 584–588.

Rajagopalan, G., Kudva, Y.C., Chen, L., Wen, L., David, C.S., 2003. Autoimmune diabetes in HLA-DR3/DQ8 transgenic mice expressing the co-stimulatory molecule B7-1 in the {beta} cells of islets of Langerhans. Int. Immunol. 15, 1035–1044.

Rich, C., Link, J.M., Zamora, A., Jacobsen, H., Meza-Romero, R., Offner, H., et al., 2004. Myelin oligodendrocyte glycoprotein-35-55 peptide induces severe chronic experimental autoimmune encephalomyelitis in HLA-DR2-transgenic mice. Eur. J. Immunol. 34, 1251–1261.

Senshu, T., Akiyama, K., Nagata, S., Watanabe, K., Hikichi, K., 1989. Peptidylarginine deiminase in rat pituitary: sex difference, estrous cycle-related changes, and estrogen dependence. Endocrinology. 124, 2666–2670.

Simon, K.C., van der Mei, I.A., Munger, K.L., Ponsonby, A., Dickinson, J., Dwyer, T., et al., 2010. Combined effects of smoking, anti-EBNA antibodies, and HLA-DRB1*1501 on multiple sclerosis risk. Neurology. 74, 1365–1371.

Stastny, P., 1978. Association of the B-cell alloantigen DRw4 with rheumatoid arthritis. N. Engl. J Med. 298, 869–871.

Streeck, H., Lichterfeld, M., Alter, G., Meier, A., Teigen, N., Yassine-Diab, B., et al., 2007. Recognition of a defined region within p24 gag by CD8 + T cells during primary human immunodeficiency virus type 1 infection in individuals expressing protective HLA class I alleles. J. Virol. 81, 7725–7731.

Sundstrom, P., Nystrom, M., Ruuth, K., Lundgren, E., 2009. Antibodies to specific EBNA-1 domains and HLA DRB1*1501 interact as risk factors for multiple sclerosis. J. Neuroimmunol. 215, 102−107.

Suzuki, A., Yamada, R., Chang, X., Tokuhiro, S., Sawada, T., Suzuki, M., et al., 2003. Functional haplotypes of PADI4, encoding citrullinating enzyme peptidylarginine deiminase 4, are associated with rheumatoid arthritis. Nat. Genet. 34, 395−402.

Taneja, V., David, C.S., 2010. Role of HLA class II genes in susceptibility/resistance to inflammatory arthritis: studies with humanized mice. Immunol. Rev. 233, 62−78.

Taneja, V., Mehra, N.K., Chandershekaran, A.N., Ahuja, R.K., Singh, Y. N., Malaviya, A.N., 1992. HLA-DR4-DQw8, but not DR4-DQw7 haplotypes occur in Indian patients with rheumatoid arthritis. Rheumatol. Int. 11, 251−255.

Taneja, V., Griffiths, M.M., Luthra, H., David, C.S., 1998. Modulation of HLA-DQ-restricted collagen-induced arthritis by HLA-DRB1 polymorphism. Int. Immunol. 10, 1449−1457.

Taneja, V., Taneja, N., Paisansinsup, T., Behrens, M., Griffiths, M., Luthra, H., et al., 2002. CD4 and CD8 T cells in susceptibility/protection to collagen-induced arthritis in HLA-DQ8-transgenic mice: implications for rheumatoid arthritis. J. Immunol. 168, 5867−5875.

Taneja, V., Taneja, N., Behrens, M., Pan, S., Trejo, T., Griffiths, M., et al., 2003. HLA-DRB1*0402 DW10 transgene protects collagen-induced arthritis-susceptible H2Aq and DRB1*0401 DW4 transgenic mice from arthritis. J. Immunol. 171, 4431−4438.

Taneja, V., Taneja, N., Behrens, M., Griffiths, M.M., Luthra, H.S., David, C.S., 2005. Requirement for CD28 may not be absolute for collagen-induced arthritis: study with HLA-DQ8 transgenic mice. J. Immunol. 174, 1118−1125.

Taneja, V., Behrens, M., Mangalam, A., Griffiths, M.M., Luthra, H.S., David, C.S., 2007a. New humanized HLA-DR4-transgenic mice that mimic the sex bias of rheumatoid arthritis. Arthritis Rheum. 56, 69−78.

Taneja, V., Krco, C.J., Behrens, M.D., Luthra, H.S., Griffiths, M.M., David, C.S., 2007b. B cells are important as antigen presenting cells for induction of MHC-restricted arthritis in transgenic mice. Mol. Immunol. 44, 2988−2996.

Taneja, V., Behrens, M., Basal, E., Sparks, J., Griffiths, M.M., Luthra, H., et al., 2008. Delineating the role of the HLA-DR4 "shared epitope" in susceptibility versus resistance to develop arthritis. J. Immunol. 181, 2869−2877.

Tosato, G., Steinberg, A.D., Yarchoan, R., Heilman, C.A., Pike, S.E., De Seau, V., et al., 1984. Abnormally elevated frequency of Epstein-Barr virus-infected B cells in the blood of patients with rheumatoid arthritis. J. Clin. Invest. 73, 1789−1795.

Wegner, N., Wait, R., Sroka, A., Eick, S., Nguyen, K.A., Lundberg, K., et al., 2010. Peptidylarginine deiminase from Porphyromonas gingivalis citrullinates human fibrinogen and alpha-enolase: implications for autoimmunity in rheumatoid arthritis. Arthritis Rheum. 62, 2662−2672.

Weinshenker, B.G., Santrach, P., Bissonet, A.S., McDonnell, S.K., Schaid, D., Moore, S.B., et al., 1998. Major histocompatibility complex class II alleles and the course and outcome of MS: a population-based study. Neurology. 51, 742−747.

Wellcome Trust Case Control Consortium, 2007. Genome-wide association study of 14,000 cases of seven common diseases and 3,000 shared controls. Nature. 447, 661−678.

Wen, H., Baker, J.F., 2011. Vitamin D, immunoregulation, and rheumatoid arthritis. J. Clin. Rheumatol. 17, 102−107.

Wen, L., Wong, F.S., Tang, J., Chen, N.Y., Altieri, M., David, C., et al., 2000. In vivo evidence for the contribution of human histocompatibility leukocyte antigen HLA-DQ molecules to the development of diabetes. J. Exp. Med. 191, 97−104.

Wingerchuk, D.M., 2012. Smoking: effects on multiple sclerosis susceptibility and disease progression. Ther. Adv. Neuro.l Disord. 5, 13−22.

Chapter 28

Epigenetics and Autoimmune Diseases

Moncef Zouali

Inserm and University Paris Diderot, Sorbone Paris Cité, Paris, France

Chapter Outline

Epigenetic Modifications	**382**	Acetylation Marks	389
DNA Methylation	382	Genomic DNA Hypomethylation and the Activated	
Histone Post-Translational Modifications	382	Phenotype of RASFs	389
Acetylation and Deacetylation	383	miRNA and the Destructive Potential of RASFs	390
Histone Methylation	383	Aberrant SUMOylation	390
Arginine Methylation	383	**Systemic Sclerosis**	**390**
Ubiquitination	384	**Sjögren's Syndrome**	**390**
MicroRNAs	384	**Antineutrophil Cytoplasmic Autoantibodies-**	
Epigenetic Stability	384	**Associated Vasculitis**	**391**
Epigenetics of Immune Tolerance to Self	**384**	**Type 1 Diabetes**	**391**
Epigenetic Regulators of Tolerant T Cells	384	DNA Methylation Profiling	392
Role of CpG DNA Methylation in Treg Development and		Chromatin Remodeling and Histone Acetylation	392
Function	385	Histone Deacetylase Inhibitors in Preclinical Studies	392
Impacts of Histone Acetylation on Development and		**Multiple Sclerosis**	**393**
Function of Tregs	385	Generation of Neo-Epitopes	393
Epigenetic Modulation of Treg Stability	386	DNA Hypomethylation	393
Systemic Lupus Erythematosus	**386**	Deregulation of Acetylation Homeostasis	394
DNA Methylation	386	**Epigenetic Therapy**	**394**
DNA Methylation Control by miRNA	387	Targeting DNA Methylation	395
Histone Acetylation	388	Histone Deacetylase Inhibitors	395
Environmental Epigenetics in SLE	388	Epigenetic Generation of Tregs	396
Epigenetic Disruption of B Cell Tolerance in SLE	388	**Future Prospects**	**396**
Rheumatoid Arthritis	**389**	**References**	**396**

Alterations in genome architecture are associated with human diseases. In autoimmune diseases, however, although strong genetic bases have been found in genome-wide association studies, no unique genetic mechanism underlying immune tolerance breakdown was identified, and the significant genetic associations described are present only in a relatively small proportion of patients. As seen in other complex disorders, linkage studies and genome-wide profiling arrays have contributed to the identification of multiple genes that may exert a combinatorial effect in predisposing individuals to develop the disease (Nylander and Hafler, 2012). The largely incomplete concordance rates of autoimmune diseases in monozygotic twins strongly support other complementary mechanisms involved in gene regulation ultimately causing overt autoimmunity (Zouali, 2009). It is therefore becoming increasingly evident that gene expression based on DNA sequence alterations or mutations is not sufficient to explain the variety of manifestations observed in disease states (Feil and Fraga, 2012), and that epigenetic deregulation contributes to the severity of these diseases.

N. Rose & I. Mackay (Eds): The Autoimmune Diseases, Fifth edition. DOI: http://dx.doi.org/10.1016/B978-0-12-384929-8.00028-9

EPIGENETIC MODIFICATIONS

Epigenetics can be defined by the heritable changes that occur in gene expression caused by mechanisms other than alterations in the underlying DNA sequence. These modifications are based on a set of molecular processes that can activate, reduce, or completely disable the activity of particular genes or entire genomic regions: methylation of cytosine residues in the DNA, remodeling of chromatin structure through covalent modification of histone proteins, and recruitment of chromatin-associated small RNA molecules that provide the sequence specificity to target transcriptional silencing. The combination of these different modifications, commonly referred to as the "epigenetic code," adds a layer of complexity to the information present in the genetic code.

Several observations indicate that environmental changes can produce modifications in gene expression, suggesting that epigenetics can have a potential role in environmental/genetic interactions. First, when the diet *agouti* pregnant rodents were supplemented with foods rich in methyl donors, the offspring exhibited coat color changes, compared to mothers fed with a standard diet (Wolff et al., 1998). This observation was explained by an altered DNA methylation process that silenced the intracisternal A particle (IAP) retroviral insertional element, ultimately limiting the appearance of *agouti* alleles. A second remarkable example comes from Dutch individuals who were exposed to famine during intra-uterine life and childhood during the Second World War. Compared to non-exposed subjects, they had a well-conserved hypomethylation status of a region regulating the insulin-like growth factor 2 (IGF2) (Heijmans et al., 2008), providing an example of epigenetic imprinting.

DNA Methylation

In mammals, approximately 60% of CpG dinucleotides are methylated, and DNA methyltransferases (DNMTs) control DNA methylation of CpG residues and maintenance of methylation during cell differentiation (Bird, 2011). As a regulator of transcription, DNA methylation generally occurs on cytosines in cytosine–guanosine (CG) dinucleotides located within the promoter, most often between 1 kb and 0.8 kb upstream of the transcription start site (Figure 28.1). It consists of the addition of a methyl group to the fifth carbon of cytosine residues, converting them to 5-methylcytosines, a reaction that involves DNMT1, DNMT3a, and DNMT3b, and a methyl group donor (S-adenosylmethionine). DNA methylation can be divided into two types: *de novo* introduction of methyl group by DNMT3a and DNMT3b; and maintenance methylation associated with the replication machinery of dividing cells and involving DNMT1. However, it

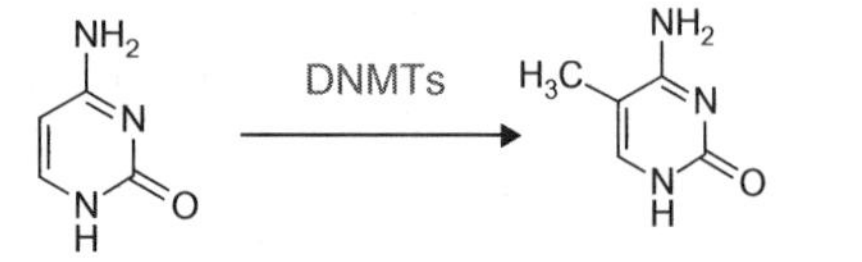

FIGURE 28.1 DNA Methylation. Methylation of DNA at 5-position of cytosine by DNA methyltransferases (DNMTs) that control DNA methylation of CpG residues and maintenance of methylation during cell differentiation.

has been reported that, in some CpG dense regions, DNMT1 is not sufficient to maintain the levels of methylated CpG during replication, and in such somatic cells, DNMT3a and DNMT3b play important roles in maintaining methylation. Altered CpG island methylation may change chromatin structure, modulating promoter–transcription factor interactions within the transcription machinery. Although DNA methylation was initially thought to be a stable modification with only passive removal of methyl groups possible, accumulating evidence suggests that DNA demethylation occurs actively, and appears to be key in a variety of cellular responses to environmental stimuli including hypoxia, hormonal signaling, and viral latency and reactivation. Furthermore, aberrant hypo- and hypermethylation may occur in specific genes within the same cell, as is the case in some neoplastic cells. Methylated CpG recruits transcriptional repressors, such as the methyl-binding proteins MBD and MeCP, and histone deacetylases (HDACs), which introduce positive charges in the histone tail, allowing tight binding to negatively charged nucleic acids and leading to the formation of closely compact nucleosomes that prevent transcription.

Histone Post-Translational Modifications

A variety of histone post-translational modifications (PTMs) that affect chromatin structure have been described, including acetylation, methylation, phosphorylation, ubiquitination, sumoylation, and adenosine diphosphate (ADP) ribosylation. They can be dynamically added or removed by a plethora of specific enzymes that can work to add or remove functional groups which are, in turn, recognized by nuclear factors. Together with the diverse nucleosome composition, these modifications can cause a change in the net charge of nucleosomes, and alter DNA–histone interactions, and affect chromatin structure. Additionally, individual histone PTMs, or specific combinations of them that form the "histone code," can provide signals to other proteins able to influence chromatin structure, thereby regulating gene expression by the formation of transcriptionally active or repressed states (Li et al., 2007a; Berger, 2007).

Histones are highly conserved proteins that reside within nuclei of eukaryotic cells. They can be categorized into two main groups: core histones (H2A, H2B, H3, and H4), and linker histones (H1, H5). Two of each of the core histones assemble to form an octameric nucleosome core particle by wrapping approximately 147 base pairs of DNA around the protein spool in a 1.7 left-handed super-helical turn (Luger et al., 1997), thus providing DNA condensation and organization in the nucleus, and modulating DNA accessibility to the transcription machinery.

Specific amino acids of histone tails are targets for several PTM, including acetylation, phosphorylation, poly-ADP ribosylation, ubiquitination, and methylation. Likewise, each histone subtype can be modified by different chemical modifications at defined amino acids, leading to transcription modulation and, therefore, cell cycle regulation, development, and differentiation. Acetylation of histones in the nucleosome increases their net negative charge, thereby interrupting their interaction with DNA and leading to open chromatin with negatively charged DNA—a structure permissive for recruitment of transcriptional machinery to initiate gene transcription and expression.

Acetylation and Deacetylation

These processes are among the most important gene expression regulatory mechanisms (Strahl and Allis, 2000). They involve the conserved ε-amino group of lysine residues at the amino terminus of nucleosomal histones (Figure 28.2). Histone acetyltransferases (HATs) decrease the overall positive charge of histones, thereby decreasing their affinity for negatively charged DNA, and

providing a platform for the binding of transcription factors to the chromatin template. Thus, transfer of acetyl groups to lysine by HATs promotes gene expression. By contrast, removal of acetyl groups by HDACs is generally associated with gene repression (Thiagalingam et al., 2003).

According to size, subcellular expression, number of enzymatic domains, and structure, HDACs are divided into four classes. Class I HDACs (HDACs 1, 2, 3, and 8) are detected in the nucleus and ubiquitously expressed in different tissues and cell lines. Class II HDACs (HDACs 4, 5, 6, 7, 9, and 10) shuttle between the nucleus and cytoplasm, and are expressed in a tissue-specific manner. For example, human HDAC4 is more abundant in skeletal muscle, brain, heart, and ovary, but not detectable in liver, lung, spleen, and placenta. HDAC5 is expressed in mouse skeletal muscle, liver, and brain, but not in spleen (Brandl et al., 2009). Class III HDACs are structurally unrelated to class I and class II HDACs, but use a unique enzymatic mechanism of action that requires the cofactor NAD^+ for their activity. Finally, HDAC1 is the only member of class IV HDACs, and its classification is still under debate.

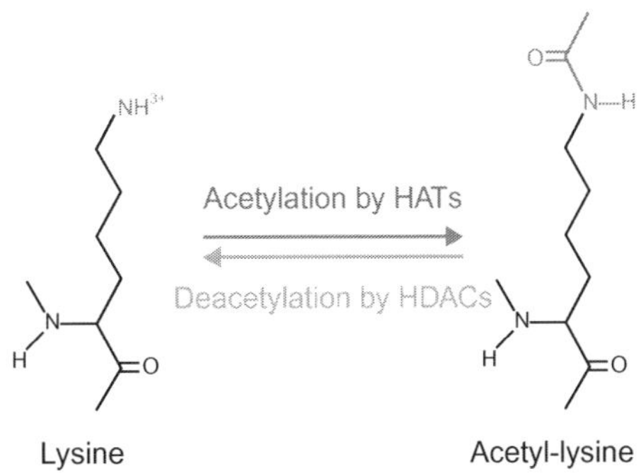

Histone Methylation

Another mechanism involves histone methylation and its effects depend on the position of the modified lysine residue within the histone tail and on the number of methyl groups added to such residues. For example, the presence of three methyl groups on lysine 4 of histone H3 (Me-H3K4) has been associated with transcriptional activation whereas the triple methylation of residues 9 or 27 determines repression (Kouzarides, 2007).

Arginine Methylation

Arginine can also be methylated/demethylated by specific enzymes (Chen et al., 1999). Methylation of arginine residue 3 on histone H4 (H4R3) and arginine 17 on histone H3 (H3R17) has been shown to induce gene activation. Remarkably, occupancy of coactivator-associated arginine methyltransferase-1 (CARM1), known to enhance transcriptional activation by nuclear receptors, together with histone H3-R17 methylation, and citrullination are regulated at the promoters of inflammatory genes in monocytes, thereby suggesting a novel role for histone arginine modifications in inflammatory diseases (Miao et al., 2006). Therefore, similar to histone lysine methylation, interest in histone arginine methylation is increasing. Based on current knowledge, the histone modification status of H3-R17 in cells can exist in at least three modes: arginine, methylated arginine, and citrullinated arginine. The biological meaning of the three modes or the "H3-R17 code" is slowly emerging, but needs more

FIGURE 28.2 **Acetylation and Deacetylation of Lysine Residues in Histone Molecules.** Histone acetylation is catalyzed by histone acetyltransferases (HATs). In general, histone acetylation is linked to transcriptional activation and associated with euchromatin. Histone deacetylases (HDACs) introduce positive charges in the histone tail, which bind tightly to negatively charged nucleic acids and lead to the formation of closely compact nucleosomes that prevent transcription.

investigation. It seems that H3-R17 methylation is associated with gene activation and that H3 arginine citrullination might be associated with repression of nuclear receptor and NF-κB-regulated genes. This could suggest additional connections between arginine epigenetic markers and human diseases.

Ubiquitination

Ubiquitin is a 76 amino acid protein involved in specific protein labeling. Ubiquitinated proteins are committed to proteosomal degradation and, thus, ubiquitination controls the stability and intracellular localization of numerous proteins. Ultimately, it influences the status of histone methylation or acetylation and modulates gene expression, as in the case of the NF-κB pathway.

MicroRNAs

Only recently has it been discovered that microRNA (miRNA) can regulate gene expression via messenger RNA (mRNA) degradation and translational repression (Bartel, 2004). miRNAs are a group of post-transcriptional regulators involved in many biological processes, including development, differentiation, proliferation, and apoptosis (Filipowicz et al., 2008). They are approximately 22-nt-long, non-coding RNAs that suppress translation by binding to complementary target mRNA species, causing the degradation of the target. miRNAs are genome-encoded and transcribed by RNA polymerase II, similar to ordinary protein-coding RNAs; and it is estimated that miRNA target <30% of the human transcriptome (Lewis et al., 2005). The role of miRNA in immunity is also beginning to be explored. For example, miR-146 was identified as a key player in innate immunity (Taganov et al., 2006), and miR-181a was found to modulate adaptive immunity, particularly T cell sensitivity and selection (Li et al., 2007c). Therefore, miRNAs are being investigated in autoimmune and chronic inflammatory conditions.

Epigenetic Stability

Maintenance of epigenetic marks during cellular division is important to maintain cell lineage commitment in progeny cells, and to shape a memory of transcriptional status. Several of the mechanisms discussed above are required for the transmission of epigenetic information through multiple cell divisions. These mechanisms also mediate the inheritance of epimutations (alterations to epigenetic marks that can be transmitted from parents to offspring via their germline), which can lead to changes in chromatin structure and transcription levels of genes in disease

conditions, such as cancer, imprinting disorders, and, potentially, autoimmune diseases.

Thus, even though DNA methylation shows dynamic changes during developmental stages, DNA methylation marks have been initially suggested to be relatively stable over time in adult individuals (Dolinoy et al., 2007). However, human and experimental studies revealed that DNA methylation can exhibit various temporal behaviors, ranging from a nearly absolute stability of the DNA sequence to the rapid variations typical of mRNA levels (Hoyo et al., 2009). Consistently, a recent study showed that DNA methylation markers in human blood DNA exhibit different degrees of short-term variability (Byun et al., 2012). Whether such variations can be extended to other cell types remains to be determined.

EPIGENETICS OF IMMUNE TOLERANCE TO SELF

In the B cell compartment, immune tolerance operates through several mechanisms (Zouali, 2007). Their epigenetic regulation has been discussed recently (see Zouali, 2013).

For T cells, central tolerance takes place in the thymus through negative selection, where developing thymocytes are deleted if they react too strongly to self-antigens presented by the major histocompatibility complex (MHC). However, since not all peripheral self-antigens are adequately presented in the thymus, central tolerance is incomplete, and self-reactive T cells escape negative selection and migrate to secondary lymphoid organs. In the periphery, autoreactive lymphocytes must be inactivated by deletion or by suppression by regulatory T cells (Tregs), and/or by cell-intrinsic programs that lead to a state of functional unresponsiveness, called anergy. Understanding the regulatory mechanisms that maintain or break T cell tolerance to self-antigens is required to prevent autoimmunity.

Epigenetic Regulators of Tolerant T Cells

Studies of histone acetylation *in vitro* and *ex vivo* suggested that immune tolerance is under epigenetic influences. A variety of HDAC inhibitors (HDACi), such as sodium butyrate or trichostatin A (TSA) and suberyolanilide hydroxamic acid (SAHA), induce anergy in Th1 cell cultures (Edens et al., 2006), as characterized by an inhibition of proliferation accompanied by a reduction of IL-2 production. The effect was attributed to chromatin remodeling at the IL-2 promoter, as well as to acetylation of transcription factors, such as NF-κB (Matsuoka et al., 2007).

To identify genes and pathways critical for maintenance of unresponsiveness, an *in vivo* mouse model was recently used to perform a microarray analysis of naïve (N), memory (M), and tolerant (T) T cells (Schietinger et al., 2012). The study revealed that T cells harbor a tolerance-specific gene signature markedly distinct from that of N and M cells, and 164 genes were identified as "tolerance-specific" gene sets representing uniquely over-expressed genes, including negative regulators of cell signaling and proliferation, transcription factors, and phosphatases. Genes modulating cell cycle, cell division, nucleosome assembly, mitosis, and DNA replication were also highly overrepresented and upregulated in T cells. Thus, T cells "remember" the tolerance program established during the initial encounter(s) with self-antigen in the periphery, raising the question of how such memory is encoded. The fact that transcripts of numerous genes regulating chromatin modification were enriched in T cells (e.g., *Jmjd3*, *Dnmt1*, *Hat1*, *Hdac2*, *Hdac3*, etc.) supports the view that epigenetic factors are involved. Consistently, genome-wide miRNA profiling revealed that N, M, and T had distinct miRNA expression patterns (Schietinger et al., 2012). Thus, these insights into the regulatory mechanisms that maintain or break self-tolerance may lead to new strategies for the treatment of autoimmunity.

Role of CpG DNA Methylation in Treg Development and Function

Foxp3 is a member of the forkhead/winged-helix family of transcription factors that acts as a "master" regulator for the development and suppressive function of Tregs. Its constitutive expression is necessary for the suppressive function of Tregs, and mutation or deficiency of *Foxp3* leads to development of autoimmune diseases. Genetic defects in *Foxp3* cause the *scurfy* phenotype in mice and IPEX syndrome (immune dysfunction, polyendocrinopathy, enteropathy, X-linked syndrome) in humans (Khattri et al., 2003). In the thymus, a subset of CD4$^+$CD25$^+$ T cells develops into Foxp3$^+$CD4$^+$ T cells, known as natural Tregs (nTregs). However, in peripheral lymphoid organs, TGF-β can induce naïve CD4$^+$CD25$^-$ T cells to develop into Foxp3$^+$CD4$^+$ T cells, known as adaptive or induced Tregs (iTregs). *In vitro* culture of peripheral naïve CD4$^+$CD25$^-$ T cells in the presence of TGF-β induces expression of Foxp3 and provides a method to generate Foxp3$^+$ Tregs *ex vivo*. Importantly, nTregs and iTregs exhibit different functional characteristics (Tran et al., 2007), and nTregs are more stable than iTregs, a feature that may be related to the epigenetic regulation of Foxp3 (Polansky et al., 2008; Lal et al., 2009).

Early studies showed that differentiation of T helper cells is under epigenetic regulation through CpG methylation (Lee et al., 2001; Wilson et al., 2009). As regards

Tregs, different regulatory *cis*-elements are present in the *Foxp3* locus, upstream of the transcriptional start site (−600 to −1 bp) at the proximal promoter where the methylation status of the CpG residues plays an essential role in Foxp3 expression. Thus, 10–45% of the CpG sites in the *Foxp3* proximal promoter (−250 to +1) are methylated in naïve CD4$^+$CD25$^-$ T cells, whereas all are demethylated in nTregs (Kim and Leonard, 2007), and TGF-β induces demethylation of CpG at this site in CD4$^+$CD25$^-$ T cells. That methylation of the proximal promoter is an important regulator of Foxp3 expression is also supported by the observation that this region is ≈70% methylated in human CD4$^+$CD25^{lo} cells compared with ≈5% in CD4$^+$CD25^{hi} T cells (Janson et al., 2008). Further support comes from the fact that CpG residues in an intronic region (+4201 to +4500) are completely methylated in naïve CD4$^+$CD25$^-$ T cells and fully demethylated in mouse (Kim and Leonard, 2007; Polansky et al., 2008) and human nTregs (Baron et al., 2007). Also, an upstream enhancer (−5786 to −5558 bp) is methylated in naive CD4$^+$CD25$^-$ T cells, activated CD4$^+$ T cells, and iFoxp3$^+$ Tregs, but is demethylated in nTregs (Lal et al., 2009). Together, these reports demonstrate that Foxp3 is regulated by complex mechanisms where many extracellular signals control transacting factors as well as chromatin remodeling through covalent modification of CpG DNA. Understanding these signals and their cumulative intracellular effect on Foxp3 *cis*-elements at different T cell developmental stages will be key for therapeutic manipulation of T cell responses.

Impacts of Histone Acetylation on Development and Function of Tregs

In addition to DNA methylation, Treg development and function are under influences of histone acetylation. For example, following T cell receptor (TCR) stimulation of murine T cells, class II HDACs are mainly expressed in Tregs (Tao et al., 2007b). On the other hand, HDACi enhance Foxp3 expression in both CD4$^+$CD25$^-$ and CD4$^+$CD25$^+$ T cells, suggesting that deacetylation directly regulates Foxp3 expression, and enhances Treg suppressive functions (Tao et al., 2007a,b; Lucas et al., 2009). Another class II histone deacetylase, HDAC9, interacts with Foxp3 and downregulates its acetylation. Treatment with the class I and II HDAC inhibitor TSA enhances Foxp3 acetylation and Treg function (Li et al., 2007b). In mice, administration of pan-HDACi increased *Foxp3* gene expression, as well as the production and suppressive function of Tregs *in vitro*. Additionally, HDAC9 proved particularly important in regulating Foxp3-dependent suppression, as demonstrated by *in vivo* data in

HDAC9 knockout mice (Tao et al., 2007a). At the molecular level, optimal functions of Treg cells required acetylation of several lysines in the forkhead domain of Foxp3 (Wang et al., 2009).

Epigenetic Modulation of Treg Stability

Several observations indicate that Foxp3$^+$CD4$^+$ Tregs encompass a heterogeneous population in mice (Komatsu et al., 2009) and humans (Miyara et al., 2009), and that their phenotype and functions are not as stable as initially thought (Zhou et al., 2009a; Lee et al., 2009). For example, a fraction of Foxp3$^+$CD4$^+$ nTregs adoptively transferred to lymphopenic mice converted into Foxp3$^-$ T cells (Komatsu et al., 2009). Under inflammatory conditions, Foxp3$^+$ Tregs lose Foxp3 expression and suppressive functions in an interleukin (IL)-6-dependent manner (Pasare and Medzhitov, 2003). The fact that different subsets of Tregs exhibit different levels of CpG DNA methylation at the Foxp3 locus suggests that Treg instability may be under epigenetic controls (Miyara et al., 2009). Thus, increased methylation of CpG at the *Foxp3* locus was linked with a lower Foxp3 expression, decreased Treg stability, and reduced suppressive Treg function (Lal et al., 2009; Miyara et al., 2009). Additionally, nTregs possess demethylated CpG at the *Foxp3* locus and show stable Foxp3 expression, whereas TGF-β-induced Tregs show methylated CpG, and do not maintain constitutive Foxp3 expression after restimulation in the absence of TGF-β. It is of further interest that HDACi can modulate Th cellular phenotypes. In one study, the HDAC inhibitor TSA could induce a profound negative effect on the emergence of IL-17-producing cells from Tregs (Koenen et al., 2008). Whereas sorted Tregs could be polarized from the Treg phenotype to Th17 cells in a defined cytokine milieu, this could be prevented by the presence of TSA (Koenen et al., 2008). Finally, while it is known that various cross-talks between (histone) methylation and acetylation exist, their impact on T cell polarization is being addressed. Investigators identified a highly conserved CpG island within a FoxP3 enhancer region that is methylated in peripheral CD4$^+$ T cells, but not in nTreg (Lal et al., 2009). This region was histone H3 acetylated and bound by Sp1 and TGF-inducible early gene-1 (TIEG1). Removing this methylation in non-Tregs resulted in an increased and stable FoxP3 expression. This effect is similar to other reported modulations of FoxP3 expression via methylation (Polansky et al., 2008).

SYSTEMIC LUPUS ERYTHEMATOSUS

In lupus, there is strong evidence that the presence of one risk allele can influence that of other risk alleles across different loci. With the recent identification of a number of gene–gene epistatic interactions (Hughes et al., 2012), it is becoming clear that epigenetic factors play a key role in systemic lupus erythematosus (SLE) pathogenesis. Likewise, interactions between environmental and genetic factors have been proposed to explain why certain individuals develop the disease while others do not, and to account for the discordance rates for the disease in monozygotic (MZ) twins (Zouali, 2005, 2011; Gourley and Miller, 2007).

DNA Methylation

This epigenetic modification has emerged as an important contributing factor in lupus. Patients exhibit global T cell hypomethylation (Richardson et al., 1990), and the changes correlate with increased disease activity (Deng et al., 2001). T cell DNA hypomethylation has been implicated in the development of drug-induced lupus by hydralazine and procainamide, and in the pathogenesis of lupus-prone MRL-*lpr* mice (Yung et al., 1997). Interruption of the extracellular signal-regulated kinase (ERK) signaling pathway in T cells and the subsequent suppression of the maintenance DNA methyltransferase DNMT1 induces anti-dsDNA antibody production and a lupus-like gene expression profile in mice (Sawalha et al., 2008).

The *CD40LG* gene, located on the X chromosome, is hypomethylated in T cells from healthy men, while healthy women have one methylated and one hypomethylated allele (Lu et al., 2007). Treatment of CD4$^+$ T cells with the DNA methylation inhibitor 5-azacytidine demethylated *CD40LG* and doubled its expression in normal healthy women, but not men (Lu et al., 2007; Zhou et al., 2009b). These findings suggest that hypomethylation of the normally inactivated and silenced X chromosome might be related to the higher prevalence of lupus in women. Indeed, men with Klinefelter's syndrome (47, XXY) have a similar risk of developing lupus as normal women (46, XX) and ~14 times higher risk to develop lupus compared to normal men (46, XY). This gene–dose effect may be achieved by hypomethylation of the X chromosome, making more than one X chromosome available for transcription (Scofield et al., 2008).

Other abnormally methylated genes include the ITGAL (CD11a), which is important for cell–cell adhesion (Lu et al., 2002), TNFSF7 (CD70), which is required for T cell proliferation, clonal expansion and promotion of effector T cell formation (Oelke et al., 2004), and CD40L, which stimulates IgG overproduction (Lu et al., 2007). Other factors, such as the gene encoding perforin 1 (PRF1) (Kaplan et al., 2004), which contributes to autoreactive killing of macrophages and release of apoptotic material, CD3 ζ chain, CTLA4, IL-2, IL-4, IL-10, and interferon (IFN)-γ (Richardson et al., 1992; Mishra et al., 2001; Lee et al., 2002; Kaplan et al., 2004; Januchowski and Jagodzinski, 2005; Lu et al., 2005; Thomas et al., 2005; Schmidl et al., 2009). In resting SLE B cells, the E1B promoter of the CD5 gene was reportedly hypomethylated (Lu et al., 2002). These data show that DNA methylation and chromatin structure can influence the expression of SLE-related genes. In mice, demethylating drugs can trigger overexpression of these same molecules and induce both autoreactive T cells and a lupus-like syndrome (Yung et al., 1997).

The observation that several susceptibility genes (*STAT4* or *MECP2*) bear connections with DNA methylation and the existence of polymorphisms in genes that can influence DNA methylation prompted further investigation of epigenetic changes in lupus. Initial candidate gene studies revealed several pathways in which aberrant gene expression due to DNA demethylation was linked with SLE development (Huck and Zouali, 1996). They have demonstrated that abnormal hypomethylation of $CD4^+$ T cell DNA can contribute to the pathogenesis of lupus-like diseases (Ballestar et al., 2006), and this phenomenon is associated with reduced expression and activity of DNMT1 in patient $CD4^+$ T cell samples (Dubroff and Reid, 1980; Deng et al., 2001; Balada et al., 2008; Lei et al., 2009). In a genome-wide DNA methylation study, 236 hypomethylated and 105 hypermethylated CG sites were identified among 27,578 CG sites located within the promoter regions of 14,495 genes in lupus $CD4^+$ T cells, as compared to normal controls (Jeffries et al., 2011). Among the hypermethylated genes identified, several genes are overrepresented in gene ontologies of metabolic pathways and responses to micronutrients, suggesting a link between environmental factors and epigenetic modifications. The data also suggest that DNA methylation changes in specific loci correlate with lupus disease activity.

Because lupus peripheral blood mononuclear cells (PBMCs) express high levels of IL-10 mRNA and protein, and since the serum levels of the potent B cell stimulator IL-10 correlate with disease activity and severity, it has been hypothesized that the Th2 cytokines IL-10 and IL-13 may be upregulated in SLE due to an aberrant DNA methylation of their promoter regions in $CD4^+$ T cells, thereby contributing to the activation of the humoral immune arm and triggering lupus disease activity. In one study, methylation of C/G pairs within the IL-10 and IL-13 promoters was found to be significantly reduced in T cells from SLE $CD4^+$ T cells, as compared with healthy control samples, and the methylation status was inversely correlated with the levels of IL-10 and IL-13 transcripts and proteins, as well as with disease severity (Zhao et al., 2010a). Furthermore, treatment of healthy $CD4^+$ T cells with the methylation inhibitor 5-azacytidine triggered IL-10 and IL-13 expression to levels similar to those observed in SLE $CD4^+$ T cells, suggesting an important role of DNA methylation in

regulating the expression of Th2 cytokines in SLE. These findings may provide a basis for the design of a new therapy aimed at reversing the epigenetic alternations of gene expression in SLE patients.

DNA Methylation Control by miRNA

In a study of 23 SLE patients and 10 healthy controls, seven miRNAs (miR-196a, miR-17-5p, miR-409-3p, miR-141, miR-383, miR-112, and miR-184) were downregulated and nine miRNAs (miR-189, miR-61, miR-78, miR-21, miR-142-3p, miR-342, miR299-3p, miR-198, and miR-298) were upregulated in patients, as compared with healthy controls (Dai et al., 2007). In further studies using pilot expression profiling, underexpression of miR146a was identified in PBMCs from SLE patients (Tang et al., 2009), and miR-146a was found to negatively regulate type I IFN induction by TLR-7 signaling. The strong association between miR-146a levels and clinical disease activity suggested that it may serve as a new disease biomarker, and that miRNA could serve as therapeutic targets for SLE treatment (Tang et al., 2009). In another study, miR-125a was found to be reduced, and the expression of its predicted target gene, KLF13 (encoding a transcription factor that regulates the expression of the chemokine (C-C motif) ligand 5 (CCL5) in T lymphocytes was increased (Zhao et al., 2010b). Additionally, miR-125a negatively regulated RANTES expression by targeting KLF13 in activated T cells.

In SLE, as well as in the anti-phospholipid syndrome (APS), there is an increased tissue factor (TF) expression in monocytes and endothelial cells. The fact that in several web databases and algorithm target predictions miR-19b and miR-20a were reported to target TF expression, led to a study that tested whether miRNA levels may influence TF levels in patients. In APS, the levels of these two miRNAs were decreased in comparison with monocytes from healthy controls. In monocytes from SLE, miR-20a levels were also lower than those from healthy subjects (Teruel et al., 2011). In addition, the reduced expression of miR-19b and miR-20a was inversely correlated with TF cell surface expression.

In line with these findings, one investigation disclosed that among the 11 microRNA that showed increased or decreased expression in SLE $CD4^+$ T cells, miR-126 was significantly overexpressed, and its upregulation was inversely correlated with DNMT1 protein levels (Zhao et al., 2011). miR-126 reportedly could directly inhibit DNMT1 translation by interacting with its 3'-UTR, leading to a significant reduction in DNMT1 protein levels. This observation suggests that overexpression of miR-126 can cause demethylation and upregulation of genes encoding LFA-1 (CD11a) and CD70, two receptors that have been linked to disease activity. Importantly, knocking down miR-126 in SLE CD4$^+$ T cells reduced their autoimmune activity and their stimulatory effect on IgG production in co-cultured B cells (Zhao et al., 2011).

Recent investigations suggest that, in SLE, miRNAs can regulate DNA methylation by targeting the DNA methylation machinery. In one study, miR-21 and miR-148a were found to be upregulated in CD4$^+$ T cells in both patients with lupus and MRL-*lpr* mice (Pan et al., 2010). Moreover, both miRNAs downregulated DNMT1 protein levels, thus resulting in hypomethylation of CD4$^+$ T cells. Whereas miR-21 indirectly downregulated DNMT1 by targeting its upstream regulator (Ras guanyl-releasing protein 1), miR-148a directly downregulated DNMT1 by targeting the protein-coding region of its transcript, leading to a derepression of autoimmune-associated methylation-sensitive genes in CD4$^+$ T cells, such as CD70 and LFA-1 (CD11a). An alleviation of hypomethylation could also be induced in CD4$^+$ T cells from lupus patients by transfection with miR-21 and miR-148a inhibitors (Pan et al., 2010).

Histone Acetylation

In addition to hypermethylation, global H3 and H4 hypoacetylation characterize CD4$^+$ T cells from SLE patients (Hu et al., 2008). Moreover, a recent study found significant clusters of aberrantly expressed genes in SLE, including those coding for chemokines, which are strongly associated with altered H4 acetylation (Zhang et al., 2010).

Environmental Epigenetics in SLE

Direct comparison of identical twins represents a unique approach to test environmental epigenetics, because DNA sequence differences, including single-nucleotide polymorphisms, which would be abundant in singleton-based studies, cannot interfere. Not surprisingly, twin studies demonstrated the existence of genome-wide epigenetic differences that potentially could explain phenotypic differences (Fraga et al., 2005; Kaminsky et al., 2009). They demonstrated how epigenetic differences between MZ twins become more pronounced with age, supporting the notion that "epigenetic drift" plays a role in divergence of MZ phenotypes (Fraga et al., 2005). More recently, a collection of identical twins discordant for SLE and two other related systemic autoimmune diseases (rheumatoid arthritis and dermatomyositis) was used to perform a high-throughput analysis of DNA methylation changes (Javierre et al., 2010). Only SLE samples exhibited significant changes in the DNA methylation status at both the global and sequence-specific levels in comparison with their healthy, discordant twins and compared with unrelated matched normal controls. Comparison of SLE twins

with their corresponding healthy twins showed a decrease in global 5-methylcytosine content and a change in DNA methylation status of the CpG-rich region of the ribosomal DNA repeat, which contains the transcribed 18S and 28S genes. The study also yielded a list of epigenetically deregulated DNA sequences in SLE. Importantly, gene ontology analysis revealed enrichment in categories associated with immune function, and individual analysis confirmed the relevance of DNA methylation changes in genes to SLE pathogenesis, supporting the notion that epigenetic alterations may be critical in the clinical manifestations (Javierre et al., 2010). The results reinforce the notion that, for a particular genetic background, environmental factors can modulate SLE onset. However, it remains unclear whether environmental factors caused the epigenetic changes observed, or whether environmental factors cause lupus by some unknown mechanisms, possibly associated with inflammatory and immune responses that give rise to epigenetic changes.

Epigenetic Disruption of B Cell Tolerance in SLE

In the B cell compartment, self-tolerance operates by several processes, including deletion, anergy, and receptor editing, a powerful mechanism that allows autoreactive B cells to revise their receptors and to escape apoptotic death (Radic and Zouali, 1996). Several studies found that receptor editing is impaired in SLE and rheumatoid arthritis, and that this abnormality could account for the ineffective silencing of B cells that have acquired autoreactive receptors (Bensimon et al., 1994; Suzuki et al., 1996; Samuels et al., 2005; Yurasov et al., 2005; Faber et al., 2006; Zouali, 2008). Further insight into the molecular basis of inefficient editing as a potential cause of autoimmunity comes from studies based on different approaches. One line of evidence comes from studies on drug-induced lupus. This autoimmune disease can be induced by more than 40 medications, such as the antihypertensive drug hydralazine (Zouali, 2011). Interestingly, aromatic amines and hydralazine derivatives can be found in a wide variety of compounds used in agriculture and industry, and commercial applications. Hydralazine itself also occurs in tobacco and tobacco smoke, and a lupus-like syndrome has been reported in individuals who have been in contact with these agents (Reidenberg et al., 1993). To test the hypothesis that drugs that alter DNA methylation and trigger a lupus-like syndrome can disrupt the mechanisms that maintain B cell tolerance, the effects of hydralazine on receptor editing were investigated in mice harboring human transgenic immunoglobulins. The studies revealed that, by disrupting the ERK signaling pathway, hydralazine reduces receptor editing in B lymphocytes and contributes to the generation of pathogenic autoreactivity (Mazari et al., 2007). The data also support the view that epigenetic alterations contribute to exacerbated activation or deregulation of the mechanisms that maintain tolerance to self-antigens in patients with lupus. Future studies will determine whether other drugs and xenobiotics that trigger autoimmunity in humans also can act through similar mechanisms.

RHEUMATOID ARTHRITIS

Like several other chronic immune-mediated diseases, the pathology of rheumatoid arthritis (RA) involves excessive production of inflammatory mediators, and large quantities of cytokines and chemokines are detectable in the synovial fluid. Another hallmark of RA is the hyperplasia of the synovium, with increased cell density and infiltration of inflammatory cells. The aggressive and invasive behavior of RA synovial fibroblasts (RASFs) and their increased resistance to apoptosis account for the fact that they are also referred to as cells with a "tumor-like phenotype" (Fassbender et al., 1992). Together with cell—cell contacts, inflammatory mediators can activate stromal fibroblast-like synoviocytes (FLS), leading to production of enzymes that degrade cartilage and bone. While there is no genetic background for these alterations, several studies suggest that epigenetic modifications could contribute to the characteristic changes of RASFs.

Acetylation Marks

Hyperacetylation and hypoacetylation are postulated to tightly regulate production of inflammatory cytokines at multiple levels, including regulation of transcription factor access to gene promoters, post-transcriptional mRNA processing, and protein secretion. In RA, analysis of human monocytes revealed that HDACi are potent anti-inflammatory agents (Leoni et al., 2002), and there are indications that decreased expression of HDACs in synovial tissue may contribute to RA pathogenesis (Huber et al., 2007a). Nuclear extracts of RA synovial tissue samples showed lower HDAC activity than those of osteoarthritis (OA) tissue samples (Huber et al., 2007a). More recently, RA PBMCs were found to exhibit increased HDAC activity compared to PBMCs from healthy individuals, and the increase was unaltered after 12 weeks of etanercept therapy (Gillespie et al., 2012).

TSA treatment of synovial macrophages reduced the level of IL-6 production and the reduction correlated with enhanced mRNA degradation in RA macrophages and RASFs (Grabiec et al., 2010). Consistently, TSA was a potent inhibitor of TNF-α and IL-6 production in both RA and healthy PBMCs (Gillespie et al., 2012). By contrast, another HDACi (MI192) inhibited TNF-α production at high concentrations and dose dependently inhibited IL-6 in RA PBMCs, but not in healthy PBMCs. More recently, HDACi were found to reduce RA FLS IL-6 production induced by cytokines and TLR ligands (Grabiec et al., 2012), providing a mechanistic evidence by which HDACi might suppress inflammatory cytokine production and supporting the view that HDACi may represent a novel therapeutic approach for RA.

In murine models of RA, nonselective HDAC inhibitors have been used with positive results, including reduced proinflammatory cytokine expression, joint destruction, and disease severity (Lin et al., 2007). However, further characterization of HDAC inhibitors is needed to better establish their role in the management of RA, and changes in RA acetylation patterns have to be firmly determined before molecular therapeutic targeting becomes feasible.

Genomic DNA Hypomethylation and the Activated Phenotype of RASFs

In RA, converging observations support the hypothesis that progressive loss of methylation marks may give rise to the activated phenotype of RASFs. For example, methylation of CpG islands in the promoter region of the Death receptor 3 (DR3) of RASFs result in a higher resistance to apoptosis (Takami et al., 2006). More recently, hypomethylated nuclei were reportedly present in the synovial tissue of RA patients, and RASFs retained their demethylation profile *in vitro* (Karouzakis et al., 2009). In further experiments, it was demonstrated that chronic treatment of normal synovial fibroblasts with the DNMT inhibitor 5-AZA (5-aza-2′-deoxycytidine) changes the cellular profile into an RASF-like phenotype.

Overall, the data support the hypothesis that genomic hypomethylation could account for the activated phenotype of RASFs, in particular with respect to their destructive potential. This hypomethylation could also explain the increased expression of multiple receptors, adhesion molecules, and matrix-degrading enzymes, which play a role in RA. It remains unclear whether the epigenetic modifications of RASFs can contribute to RA chronicity, and can be responsible, at least in part, for the fact that current therapies do not work in all patients.

Defective DNA methylation was also described in other lineages, such as lymphocytes (Schwab and Illges, 2001), potentially leading to the emergence of autoreactive T and/or B cell clones in RA, as it does in lupus. The CD21 and IL-6 promoters are also demethylated in RA PBMC and synovial fluid cells (Nile et al., 2008). However, further analysis of isolated lymphocytes is necessary to confirm whether deregulated IL-6 expression occurs in these cells as a consequence of epigenetic changes. Nevertheless, altered methylation of the IL-6 gene in RA reinforces the notion that epigenetic pathways are affected.

miRNA and the Destructive Potential of RASFs

Accumulating evidence implicates an important role of miRNAs in the regulation of immune responses and the development of autoimmunity, and recent observations suggest that altered expression and function of miRNAs may also be involved in RA pathogenesis. In one study, treatment of RASFs with TNF-α, IL-1β, lipopolysaccharide, or poly(I-C) led to an upregulation of miR-155 and miR-146, and these two miRNAs were constitutively more highly expressed in RASFs than in synovial fibroblasts of OA patients (Stanczyk et al., 2008). Peripheral blood monocytes of RA patients also displayed higher levels of miR-155. Furthermore, enforced expression of miR-155 repressed the levels of matrix metalloproteinase-3 (MMP-3), and reduced the induction of MMP-3 and MMP-1 by TLR ligands and cytokines (Stanczyk et al., 2008). The repressive effect of miR-155 on MMPs may suggest that miR-155 plays a role in the modulation of the destructive behavior of RASFs (Stanczyk et al., 2008). This conclusion is supported by another study showing an enhanced expression of miR-146 in RA synovial tissue (Nakasa et al., 2008). In that study, the expression levels of miR-146 in RASFs were increased upon stimulation with TNF-α and IL-1β. Consistently, investigation of 33 RA patients revealed that synovial fluid and peripheral blood CD4$^+$ T cells exhibit upregulation of miR-146a and downregulation of miR-363 and miR-498 (Li et al., 2010). Moreover, the levels of miR-146a expression were positively correlated with those of TNF-α. In addition, miR-146a overexpression was found to suppress T cell apoptosis, suggesting a role for miR-146a in RA pathogenesis (Li et al., 2010).

Further evidence for the involvement of miR-146a in inflammation and cytokine production comes from the observation that the expression of miR-146a was associated with that of IL-17 in the PBMC and synovium of RA patients, and that the increased expression of both molecules correlated with disease activity (Niimoto et al., 2010). A parallel survey further demonstrated that a polymorphism in the 3'-UTR of IL-1 receptor-associated kinase (IRAK1), a target gene of miR-146a, is associated with RA susceptibility (Chatzikyriakidou et al., 2010). Since overexpression of miR-146a was found to significantly deregulate the function of Th1 cells, and because miR-146a treatment *in vitro* could induce protein expression of key proinflammatory cytokines (Guo et al., 2010), the results support the hypothesis that miR-146a may be directly involved in the pathogenesis of RA and, possibly, other inflammatory diseases. Thus, in reports from different research groups, miR-146a and miR-155 have been consistently found to be upregulated in RASFs, PBMCs, synovial fluid, PBMC-derived CD4$^+$ T cells, and Th17 cells from patients with RA when compared with healthy controls or OA patients (Pauley et al., 2008; Stanczyk et al., 2008; Li et al., 2010).

Aberrant SUMOylation

In addition to DNA and histone modifications, post-translational processes can have direct or indirect effects on epigenetic events. Thus, ubiquitin and a related family of proteins, the small ubiquitin-like modifiers (SUMOs), have been shown to impact the potential of RASFs to react to Fas-induced apoptosis. In RA, SUMO is overexpressed in synovial tissue and synovial fibroblasts (Meinecke et al., 2007). However, despite the availability of chemical modulators of ubiquitination and SUMOylation, a better understanding of the molecular mechanisms that underlie these modifications must be achieved before clinical applications can be considered.

SYSTEMIC SCLEROSIS

There is increasing evidence that histone modifications of certain genes might play a role in the pathogenesis of systemic sclerosis (SSc). In one study, hypermethylation of CpG islands and deacetylation in the FLI-1 promoter region in SSc fibroblasts and skin biopsy specimens were found to be associated with the increased production of type I collagen (Wang et al., 2006). Remarkably, there was a direct influence of Dnmt3a on the degree of histone modification, and a reduced Dnmt3a expression resulted in an enhanced histone acetylation, further underlining the repressive nature of Dnmt3a on acetylation of core histones. Nevertheless, the beneficial therapeutic use of HDACi has been shown in an animal model of SSc. Knockdown of HDAC7 in skin fibroblasts and treatment of bleomycin-induced skin fibrosis in mice with TSA remarkably reduced the accumulation of extracellular matrix proteins and fibrosis (Huber et al., 2007b).

SJÖGREN'S SYNDROME

In this disease, studies have focused on analyzing DNA methylation alterations in mechanotransduction, a mechanism that allows the conversion of mechanical stimuli into chemical activity. By translating mechanical forces and deformations into biochemical signals, mechanotransduction enables cells to sense their physical three-dimensional environment. In turn, these signals can adjust cellular and extracellular structures. Experimental evidence suggests that a physical continuum directly connects the extracellular matrix (ECM) to the cellular nucleus (Herrmann et al., 2007). An example of a mechanotransduction-mediated mechanism is the production of lactotransferrin by glandular cells: high levels of lactotransferrin mRNA have been detected in a cell fraction enriched in epithelial cells from salivary glands of patients with Sjögren's syndrome (SS), together with an altered distribution of α6β4 integrin and an acinar cell shape (Perez et al., 2009). Increased transcription of the lactotransferrin gene suggests a role of mechanotransduction-signaling pathways in SS etiopathogenesis. The role of epigenetic processes in the development of glandular damage was investigated through hemidesmosome (HD) organization-mediated mechanisms. HDs are protein complexes that mediate epithelial cell adhesion to the ECM and are composed of an α6β4 integrin dimer that binds to laminin, plectin, and other proteins (bullous pemphigoid antigens BP180 and BP230). Suggestive of epigenetic control, reduced levels of BP230 mRNA were found in epithelial cells of patients with SS in comparison with controls and, in contrast, an accumulation of BP230 on the basal surface of acini was documented (Gonzalez et al., 2011). The reduced levels of BP230 mRNA could be related to an increased methylation index of CpG islands. In addition, differential methylation changes of the BP230 gene promoter may explain the up- and downregulations detected in patients with SS. It is of related interest that CD70 expression was elevated, and the changes correlated with a decrease in TNFSF7 promoter methylation in SS CD4$^+$ T cells compared to controls (Yin et al., 2010). As for SLE, demethylation of the CD70 promoter regulatory elements could contribute to CD70 overexpression in SS CD4$^+$ T cells and, thereby, to autoreactivity.

Studies of miRNAs in SS pathogenesis have centered on analyzing miRNAs from salivary exosomes. Thus, miRNA profiling of salivary glands of healthy controls and patients with SS who were classified according to a high or a low focus score revealed patterns that could distinguish control subjects and the two SS groups (Alevizos et al., 2011). In particular, expression of two miRNAs (768-3p and 574) was inversely correlated with the focus score, and downregulation of the mir-17-92 cluster was observed in half of the SS patients with a high focus score (a "focus" refers to a cluster in a labial salivary gland biopsy of at least 50 lymphocytes, based on survey of at least four lobules). Here, it is remarkable that previous studies had associated downregulation of the mir-17-92 cluster with an accumulation in pro-B cells and a marked reduction of pre-B cells, which have been associated with lymphoproliferative and autoimmune diseases (Mendell, 2008; Xiao et al., 2008). However, larger studies are required to validate the usefulness of miRNAs in salivary glands as diagnostic markers in SS.

ANTINEUTROPHIL CYTOPLASMIC AUTOANTIBODIES-ASSOCIATED VASCULITIS

Activation of neutrophils represents a hallmark of antineutrophil cytoplasmic autoantibodies (ANCA)-associated vasculitis. It results in an increased adherence and transmigration to the vascular endothelium, where neutrophils produce reactive oxygen species and release granule constituents, including proteolytic enzymes (Kallenberg et al., 2006). To account for this activation, it has been proposed that the major neutrophil granule protein ANCA autoantigens—proteinase 3 (PR3) and myeloperoxidase (MPO)—are aberrantly expressed in mature neutrophils of ANCA patients (Ohlsson et al., 2005). In contrast, silencing mechanisms would maintain normal expression of PR3 and MPO in mature neutrophils of healthy controls. Support to this view comes from recent observations showing that aberrant expression of proteolytic enzymes in ANCA disease patients could result from active gene transcription, suggesting a failure in normal gene silencing (Ciavatta et al., 2010). Specifically, at the *PR3* and *MPO* loci, levels of H3K27me3, a mark of transcriptionally silent chromatin, were reduced in neutrophils of ANCA patients relative to those of healthy controls. A potential additional silencing mechanism may be DNA methylation, because a CpG island in *MPO* was found to be unmethylated in patients, and there was a significant increase in methylated DNA at this CpG island in healthy controls (Ciavatta et al., 2010). Overall, the evidence suggests that transcriptional regulation of *PR3* and *MPO* may involve an epigenetic process in normal neutrophils that is perturbed in neutrophils of ANCA-associated patients.

TYPE 1 DIABETES

Whereas type 2 diabetes is associated with a relative lack of insulin, most commonly due to failure of the β cells to compensate for insulin resistance caused by obesity, type 1 diabetes (T1D) is associated with absolute insulin deficiency due to selective destruction of β cells. Affecting more than 30 million people worldwide, T1D is a complex autoimmune disease caused by a combination of genetic and non-genetic factors, leading to immune destruction of insulin-secreting islet cells. A role for non-genetic factors is supported by the recent rise in T1D prevalence, and by studies of twin cohorts (Leslie and Delli Castelli, 2004). Thus, even though MZ twins are genetically identical, only ~50% of twins of T1D-affected co-twins will develop the disease (Redondo et al., 2001; Hyttinen et al., 2003; Leslie and Delli Castelli, 2004). This MZ twin pair discordance for childhood-onset T1D implicates roles for genetic and non-genetic factors in the etiology of this complex auto-immune disease, including viral infections, dietary factors, or vitamin D deficiency (Knip et al., 2005).

DNA Methylation Profiling

To determine whether epigenetic variation can underlie some of the non-genetic components of T1D etiology, an epigenome-wide association study was devised (Rakyan et al., 2011). To rule out genetic differences and to establish the temporal origins of T1D-associated epigenetic variation, the study combined T1D-discordant MZ twins with longitudinally sampled pre-T1D singletons. Genome-wide DNA methylation profiling led to the identification of 132 different CpG sites at which the direction of the intra-MZ pair DNA methylation difference significantly correlated with the diabetic state, i.e., T1D-associated methylation variable positions (T1D-MVPs). Since these T1D-MVPs were found in MZ twins, they cannot be due to genetic differences. Additional experiments revealed that some of these T1D-MVPs are found in individuals before T1D diagnosis, suggesting that they arise very early in the process that leads to overt T1D and that they are not simply due to post-disease associated factors (i.e., medication or long-term metabolic changes). However, the origin of these T1D-MVPs remains unclear. First, given that stochastic epigenetic variation in humans is more common than previously appreciated, as demonstrated by genome-scale analysis of DNA methylation profiles in 114 MZ and 80 dizygotic (DZ) twins (Kaminsky et al., 2009), these T1D-MVPs could be of early life stochastic origin. Second, since disease-relevant environmental factors can operate in early life to influence disease risk (Knip et al., 2010), the T1D-MVPs could have been induced environmentally in MZ twins who were exposed to similar, but not identical, environments. Analysis of individuals before they present with autoantibodies should establish whether T1D-MVPs are valuable disease biomarkers, capable of augmenting the predictive power of autoantibodies and genetic variants.

Chromatin Remodeling and Histone Acetylation

HDAC inhibition is known to modify innate and adaptive immune responses. In monocytes isolated from patients with T1D or T2D, histone H3 was hyperacetylated in the promoters of TNF-α and the inflammatory-associated enzyme cyclooxygenase (COX)-2 (Miao et al., 2004), suggesting a potential importance of HATs and HDACs in the expression of proinflammatory genes (Miao et al., 2004).

A more recent study was based on the view that environmental factors can trigger epigenetic changes, and that variations in histone PTMs at the promoter/enhancer regions of T1D susceptible genes may be associated with T1D (Miao et al., 2012). Likewise, histone PTM variations at known T1D susceptible genes were evaluated in blood cells from T1D patients versus healthy non-diabetic controls, and key histone PTMs were profiled. Marked variations in H3K9 acetylation (H3K9Ac) levels were observed at the upstream regions of *HLA-DRB1* and *HLA-DQB1* in T1D monocytes relative to controls (Miao et al., 2012). Additional experiments demonstrated increased expression of *HLA-DRB1* and *HLA-DQB1* in response to IFN-γ and TNF-α treatment that were accompanied by changes in H3K9Ac at the same promoter regions. These results suggest that the H3K9Ac status of *HLA-DRB1* and *HLA-DQB1*, two genes highly associated with T1D, may be relevant to their regulation and transcriptional response toward external stimuli. Thus, the promoter/enhancer architecture and chromatin status of key susceptible loci could be important determinants in their functional association to T1D susceptibility. In summary, the findings point to inappropriate chromatin remodeling and histone acetylation as important pathogenetic factors in diabetes.

Histone Deacetylase Inhibitors in Preclinical Studies

In *in vitro* experiments, increased histone acetylation can be induced by high glucose concentrations and HDACi in monocytes from diabetics (Miao et al., 2004). Similarly, production of the inflammatory cytokines IL-1γ and TNF-α was induced by high glucose concentrations through activation of NF-κB (Shanmugam et al., 2003), suggesting that hyperacetylation is a consequence of hyperglycemia or other metabolic aberrancies of diabetes, rather than a cause. Such studies suggest that acetylation favors insulin expression and that HDAC activity decreases insulin expression. In support of this view, TSA and sodium butyrate (NaB) increase histone H4 acetylation and enhance insulin expression at low glucose levels (3 mmol/L), supporting a repressive role of HDACs on pre-/pro-insulin transcription (Mosley and Ozcan, 2003). Of note, TSA and NaB do not potentiate acetylation of H4 after exposure to high concentrations (30 mmol/L) of glucose (Mosley and Ozcan, 2003). A stimulatory effect of sodium valproate (VPA) on insulin release has also been reported in human islets incubated in low glucose concentrations (2.8 mmol/L). In contrast, accumulated insulin release from rat islets incubated in 11 mmol/L glucose was unaffected by SAHA and the HDAC inhibitor ITF2357, but was slightly inhibited by TSA (Lundh et al., 2010).

Overall, converging observations indicate that there is evidence of genetic association between diabetes and HDACs, and that HDACs are involved in several biological pathways relevant for the etiology and pathogenesis of T1D, but also T2D. The observations that HDACi can promote β cell development, proliferation, differentiation and function, prevent β cell inflammatory damage, improve insulin resistance, and positively affect late diabetic microvascular complications provide a strong rationale for continuing preclinical studies, with the aim of testing the clinical utility of HDACi in diabetes. On the basis of the preclinical evidence, inhibition of various HDACs represents a promising novel therapeutic principle to correct the insulin-resistant state. However, further studies are needed to clarify the differential importance of various HDAC subtypes and, thereby, different HDACi, and to optimize the concentrations of HDACi to be used. The use of more specific HDACi, along with careful titration studies, should provide even more encouraging preclinical results. Lastly, the enigma of how HDAC inhibition, an apparently nonspecific treatment, can exert therapeutic benefits in so many diverse disorders needs to be unraveled.

MULTIPLE SCLEROSIS

In this chronic, inflammatory, and demyelinating neurological disease of the central nervous system, the precise mode of inheritance is not established. Approximately 15–20% of the patients have one or more affected relatives, and first-, second- and third-degree relatives are more likely to develop the disease than the general population (Sadovnick et al., 1988). If genetic information were the sole determinant for multiple sclerosis (MS) susceptibility, one would expect that MZ twins, who are genetically identical, should display the same risk of developing the disease. By contrast, in MS the concordance rate for MZ twins is only 20–30% (Willer et al., 2003; Hansen et al., 2005), implying a multi-factorial etiology, with interactions among genetic, environmental, and stochastic factors (Dyment et al., 1997).

Generation of Neo-Epitopes

Following episodes of neuroinflammation in MS, myelin is lost in multifocal loci of demyelination, called "plaques," that are often characterized by the appearance of new myelin at the lesion edge. Pathological studies of post-mortem tissue obtained from MS brains revealed that the composition of myelin in the normal appearing white matter is different from that of non-MS brains (Moscarello et al., 1994). The coexistence of multiple cell populations in the normal appearing white matter, and the observation that HDAC is necessary for the definition of an epigenetic signature of oligodendrocytes in developing rodents (He et al., 2007), led to the proposal that, as a result of a deregulated "epigenetic identity," disease progression may result from the generation of neo-epitopes.

Further evidence that epigenetic deregulation could lead to the emergence of immunogenic forms of myelin basic protein (MBP) comes from studies of PAD2, a peptidylarginine deiminase that catalyzes the conversion of the guanidino group of arginine to citrulline in MBP. PAD2 levels are elevated in MS and in a transgenic animal model of the disease (Mastronardi et al., 2007). While in normal brains only a very small proportion of MBP is citrullinated, in chronic MS, citrullinated MBP comprises approximately 40% of the total MBP (Moscarello et al., 1994). The observation that there was over 90% citrullination of MBP in a rare acute Marburg's form of MS suggested a relationship between the amount of citrullinated MBP and MS severity. The conversion of the majority of arginines into citrullines resulted in a visible apparent mass change of MBP, and in a net reduction of its positive charge, thereby affecting the interactions of MBP with other myelin components and leading to an aberrant localization of the citrullinated form of MBP in human brain white matter biopsies (Wood et al., 1996). Altogether, citrullination of MBP caused by epigenetic deregulation of PAD2 could lead to the release of modified and/or highly immunogenic forms of MBP, which may affect disease progression (Tranquill et al., 2000; Mastronardi et al., 2007; Musse and Harauz, 2007). In one scenario, citrullination could increase the generation of immunodominant peptides, due to increased autocleavage of the protein. Alternatively, citrullination could disrupt the physico-chemical properties of MBP and thereby affect its localization within the myelin membrane. Finally, the importance of sex hormones in MS suggests that sex steroids could epigenetically modulate PAD2 gene expression by affecting chromatin components and transcriptional complexes (Kaminsky et al., 2006).

DNA Hypomethylation

DNA isolated from the white matter of MS brains contained only about one-third of the amount of methyl cytosine found in DNA from normal subjects (Mastronardi et al., 2007). This decreased methylation of cytosines in CpG islands was not the result of decreased DNMT activity, but rather the result of a two-fold higher DNMT activity (Mastronardi et al., 2007). Importantly, it was specific for MS because DNAs from the thymus of the same MS patients and patients with Alzheimer's,

Parkinson's, and Huntington's diseases were normally methylated, and the DNMT activity was unaffected (Mastronardi et al., 2007). An important target of this hypomethylation in MS brains is the activation of the PAD2 (peptidylarginine deiminase) locus. Its promoter has 74% GC content, and sequence analysis revealed that this region is hypomethylated in MS brains compared to controls (Mastronardi et al., 2007). Together with the findings of increased DNA demethylase, the data suggest that specific genes are reactivated in MS brains, due to epigenetic modulation.

Deregulation of Acetylation Homeostasis

HATs and HDACs fine-tune cellular acetylation, targeting not only histones, but also a variety of proteins with key roles in cell metabolism, signaling, and death. Several observations indicate that, within neural cells, aberrant regulation of acetylation homeostasis may represent a common pathogenetic mechanism underlying neurodegeneration in neurological diseases (Sweet et al., 2012). In an animal model of MS—experimental autoimmune encephalomyelitis (EAE) in SJL mice—the HDACi sodium phenylbutyrate (SPB) and its metabolite sodium phenylacetate (SPA) almost completely abrogated the development of adoptive transfer of EAE (Dasgupta et al., 2003). Similarly, SPA suppressed neurological impairment in MBP-primed T cell recipient mice. Both SPA pretreatment of donor EAE mice in vivo or MBP-primed T cells in vitro were able to reduce adoptive EAE symptoms and neuropathology in recipient mice (Dasgupta et al., 2003). In C57BL/6 mice immunized with the myelin oligodendrocyte glycoprotein peptide MOG35−55, injection of TSA reduced neurological impairment (Camelo et al., 2005). In that study, increased histone acetylation levels in the spinal cord of TSA-treated EAE mice correlated with reduced levels of caspase-3 and -9. In addition, TSA treatment reduced transcripts for IL-2 receptor, IL-8 receptor, IL-12, and the costimulatory molecule CD28 in the spleen of EAE mice, and proliferation to MOG35−55 as well as to nonspecific T cell activators (Camelo et al., 2005). The findings indicate that TSA treatment during EAE severely affects development of the autoimmune response.

Other studies demonstrated that immunological functions of dendritic cells (DCs), Th1, Th17, and Treg, as well as glial cells, are affected profoundly by HDACi. For example, exposure of in vitro-generated human DCs to the HDAC inhibitors valproic acid or entinostat (MS-275) impaired cell differentiation and immunogenicity (Nencioni et al., 2007). Likewise, DC production of proinflammatory cytokines (IL-6, IL-12, TNF-α) was reduced by the two HDACi. Consistently, two other HDAC inhibitors (SAHA and ITF2357) reportedly

suppressed IL-6, IL-12, and TNF-α expression by mouse bone marrow-derived DCs challenged with different activators (Reddy et al., 2008). The two HDACi also impaired costimulatory molecule expression by DCs as well as their T cell stimulatory capacity. In addition to the HDACi-dependent DC suppression, which might be relevant to MS therapy during different disease phases, different HDACi are able to impair Th1 and Th17 actions. Thus, the HDAC inhibitors TSA and SAHA could reduce the amount of IL-12 and IL-23 (two key cytokines necessary for DC-dependent polarization of T cells toward Th1 and Th17 cells) produced by human DCs in vitro or mouse DCs in vivo (Bosisio et al., 2008).

Further underscoring the therapeutic relevance of HDACi to MS therapy, several lines of evidence indicate that HDACs negatively regulate Treg generation and function. Whereas Treg transfer affords protection from EAE in rodents (Kohm et al., 2002), reduced numbers and functional deficiency of Treg have been reported in MS patients (Zhang et al., 2004). In further studies, TSA was found to assist proliferation of Treg as well as their suppressive function on effector T cells in vivo (Tao et al., 2007a). These effects are due to inhibition of HDAC9-dependent Foxp3 transcription factor deacetylation. Additional evidence indicates that the functional enhancement is also prompted in freshly isolated and expanded human Treg by several HDACi, and the promotion of Treg functions by HDACi seems to be due to increased expression of the negative immune regulator CTLA-4, also called CD152 (Akimova et al., 2010).

Overall, inhibitors of HDACs might exert protection from the autoimmune response to the nervous system via both immunosuppressive effects and promotion of neuronal survival. The preclinical evidence suggests that pharmacological inhibition of HDACs is a promising therapeutic strategy for the treatment of neurological disorders, including MS. However, based on preclinical data, the drugs also might exert detrimental effects that may contribute to MS pathogenesis. For example, HDACi can impair remyelination in cuprizone-treated mice, which may reduce the therapeutic potential of these compounds in MS in light of the emerging role of drug-induced remyelination in protection from EAE (Taveggia et al., 2010). It is also worth noting that the various HDACi used in preclinical studies are pan-HDAC inhibitors with off-target effects (Kazantsev and Thompson, 2008). It is therefore hoped that isoform-selective HDACi will be available shortly.

EPIGENETIC THERAPY

The use of drugs to correct epigenetic defects, referred to as epigenetic therapy, is a new and rapidly developing area of pharmacology. Compared to genetic defects, which are permanent, epigenetic defects are more easily reversible with pharmacological intervention. Therefore, epigenetic therapy promises to offer agents capable of controlling and, possibly, preventing various diseases (Egger et al., 2004). This offers the possibility of using epigenetic drugs to reverse patterns of epigenetic alterations and to relieve particular conditions. Epigenetic drugs can be divided into two major groups: DNMT and HDAC inhibitors.

Targeting DNA Methylation

The prototypic inhibitor 5-azacytidine was developed as a cytotoxic agent and subsequently has been discovered to possess potent DNMT inhibitor activity. Since the drug is converted into nucleotide triphosphates and is incorporated in place of cytosines into replicating DNA, it is more active in the S-phase of cells. Because it binds both RNA and DNA, it both interrupts mRNA translation and inhibits methylation by trapping DNMTs. The disadvantages of azanucleosides (instability in aqueous solutions and toxicity) might be overcome by the use of other analogues, such as zebularine, procainamide (used to treat cardiac arrhythmia), 5-fluoro-2′-deoxycytidine, and hydralazine (used to treat hypertension). Several natural products derived from tea and sponges, such as epigallocatechin-3-gallate, also show DNMT inhibitory activity (Fang et al., 2003). Clinical trials that target DNMT1 are under way in tumors (http://clinicaltrials.gov).

In autoimmune diseases, inhibiting DNA methylation would not be appropriate because the changes identified to date are hypomethylation, not hypermethylation. Furthermore, DNA demethylating agents such as hydralazine have been shown to subvert B lymphocyte tolerance and to contribute to the generation of pathogenic autoreactivity (Mazari et al., 2007). Likewise, agents should be designed to specifically increase methylation. Nevertheless gene–gene-specific hypermethylation cannot be ruled out (Ballestar et al., 2006).

Histone Deacetylase Inhibitors

HDAC and HAT enzymes play an important role in regulating gene transcription through chromatin remodeling, which comprises histone protein–DNA complexes that tightly package to form chromosomes. HATs promote the transcriptionally active "decondensed" chromatin state by catalyzing the addition of acetyl groups onto the N-terminal tails of histone lysine residues, causing spatial distortion and allowing transcription factor and RNA polymerase complex recruitment. On the other hand, HDACs catalyze the removal of acetyl groups from lysine tails and restore the transcriptionally inactive "condensed" state.

HDACi show promising anti-inflammatory properties, as demonstrated in an increasing number of animal and cellular models of inflammatory diseases (Halili et al., 2009). As indicated by their name, the molecular function of HDACs was thought to be restricted to histone deacetylation, but recent advances in phylogenetic analysis suggested that HDACs regulate the activity of a wide range of nonhistone proteins; and 3600 acetylation sites (of which only 61 were on histones) were found on 1750 proteins, including cytoplasmic proteins. Thus, the impact of acetylation in terms of post-translational regulation is comparable to that of phosphorylation. A growing number of HDACi are being developed for the treatment of an expanding range of conditions, from cancer to neurodegenerative and other inflammatory diseases.

To date, HDACi, such as SAHA and TSA, have proved to be useful for relieving lupus disease in mice (Ballestar et al., 2006). The effects of TSA on human T cells are predominantly immunosuppressive and reminiscent of the signaling aberrations that have been described in patients with SLE (Hasler and Zouali, 2001; Zouali and Sarmay, 2004). Inhibition of HDACs has also been shown to alleviate renal disease in an SLE mouse model (Mishra et al., 2003; Reilly et al., 2004). In juvenile idiopathic arthritis, HDAC inhibition provides beneficial effects (Vojinovic et al., 2011). In studies of experimental diabetes, acetylation is recognized to regulate NF-κB, the master transcription factor in inflammation, whose activation is critical in IL-1β-induced β cell death. As a result, HDAC inhibition exerts protective effects on β cells exposed to toxicity-mediating cytokines.

Studies of chemically induced experimental colitis that mimics human ulcerative colitis also show a similar trend. For example, inhibition of HDAC in trinitrobenzene- and oxazolone-induced colitis resulted in amelioration (Glauben et al., 2006, 2008). HDACi of different classes (the hydroxamic acids SAHA and ITF2357, as well as the short-chain fatty acid valproic acid) suppressed the inflammatory parameters in acute dextran sulfate sodium-induced colitis, and ameliorated weight loss, bleeding, and colon shortening (Glauben et al., 2008). These macroscopic data were paralleled by a reduction of proinflammatory cytokines at the site of inflammation in colon cultures and by a reduced histological inflammation score (Glauben et al., 2006).

However, despite encouraging preclinical observations, epigenetic therapy may have limitations. Because of lack of specificity, DNMT and HDACi may activate oncogenes, potentially resulting in accelerated tumor progression. Additionally, once corrected, epigenetic states may revert to the original state because of the reversible nature of DNA methylation patterns.

Epigenetic Generation of Tregs

Whereas a variety of methods can be used to generate Tregs, the stability of Foxp3 expression in Tregs is important for their therapeutic use (Roncarolo and Battaglia, 2007). However, the conversion of antigen-specific Tregs into effector T cells will have detrimental effects and limit clinical applicability. It is therefore possible that epigenetic regulation may be an efficient therapeutic strategy to generate stable, suppressive Tregs. *In vivo* injection of HDAC9, a member of the class II HDACi, increases Treg numbers and function in mice (Tao et al., 2007a) and rhesus monkeys (Johnson et al., 2008). Remarkably, pan-HDACi, but not class I-specific HDACi, increased the function of Foxp3$^+$ Tregs, and prevented and reduced established colitis in mice. These pan-HDACi-mediated effects were associated with increased numbers of Foxp3$^+$ Tregs within the lamina propria. As regards DNMT inhibitors, they induce strong Foxp3 expression, but are associated with cell toxicity as well as induction of Th1 and Th2 cytokines, which limits their use (Lal et al., 2009).

In humans, an epigenetic approach was followed to generate enhanced Foxp3$^+$-suppressive Tregs that could be used in cell therapy (Lal et al., 2009). Human Foxp3$^+$CD4$^+$ T cells are very heterogeneous, based on CD25, CD62L, CD45RA, HLA-DR, and ICOS expression, but can be divided into three different subsets of Foxp3$^+$CD4$^+$ T cells in the peripheral blood (Miyara et al., 2009). CD45RA$^+$Foxp3^{lo} resting Tregs and CD45RA$^-$Foxp3^{hi}-activated Tregs show completely demethylated CpG at the proximal promoter (-256 to -16 bp) and more than 85% demethylation of the intronic region promoter ($+3824$ to $+3937$ bp), and are suppressive (Miyara et al., 2009). However, CD45RA$^-$Foxp3^{lo} Tregs show less than 50% demethylation at the intronic region, secrete cytokines such as IL-2 and IFN-γ, and do not show suppressive functions (Miyara et al., 2009). These findings suggest that epigenetic mechanisms may help design better approaches to generate suppressive human Tregs.

FUTURE PROSPECTS

The above hypothesis-driven studies are being complemented by resource-generating activities. Thus, the International Human Epigenome Consortium (http://www.epigenome.org) coordinates a number of epigenomic projects in Europe, the USA, Canada, and South Korea. It aims to analyze at least 1000 epigenomes within 7 to 10 years, and at producing histone modification maps, DNA methylation maps, transcription start site maps, and catalogues of small RNAs and non-coding RNAs. The consortium also plans to compare epigenome maps of model organisms relevant to human health and disease, and to encompass a variety of human cell and tissue types from a variety of disease states, including autoimmune diseases. This could lead to the discovery and validation of epigenetic markers for diagnostic use and for the development of novel and more individualized medical treatments.

REFERENCES

Akimova, T., Ge, G., Golovina, T., Mikheeva, T., Wang, L., Riley, J.L., et al., 2010. Histone/protein deacetylase inhibitors increase suppressive functions of human FOXP3 + Tregs. Clin. Immunol. 136, 348–363.

Alevizos, I., Alexander, S., Turner, R.J., Illei, G.G., 2011. MicroRNA expression profiles as biomarkers of minor salivary gland inflammation and dysfunction in Sjogren's syndrome. Arthritis Rheum. 63, 535–544.

Balada, E., Ordi-Ros, J., Serrano-Acedo, S., Martinez-Lostao, L., Rosa-Leyva, M., Vilardell-Tarres, M., 2008. Transcript levels of DNA methyltransferases DNMT1, DNMT3A and DNMT3B in CD4 + T cells from patients with systemic lupus erythematosus. Immunology. 124, 339–347.

Ballestar, E., Esteller, M., Richardson, B.C., 2006. The epigenetic face of systemic lupus erythematosus. J. Immunol. 176, 7143–7147.

Baron, U., Floess, S., Wieczorek, G., Baumann, K., Grutzkau, A., Dong, J., et al., 2007. DNA demethylation in the human FOXP3 locus discriminates regulatory T cells from activated FOXP3(+) conventional T cells. Eur. J. Immunol. 37, 2378–2389.

Bartel, D.P., 2004. MicroRNAs: genomics, biogenesis, mechanism, and function. Cell. 116, 281–297.

Bensimon, C., Chastagner, P., Zouali, M., 1994. Human lupus anti-DNA autoantibodies undergo essentially primary V kappa gene rearrangements. Embo. J. 13, 2951–2962.

Berger, S.L., 2007. The complex language of chromatin regulation during transcription. Nature. 447, 407–412.

Bird, A., 2011. Putting the DNA back into DNA methylation. Nat. Genet. 43, 1050–1051.

Bosisio, D., Vulcano, M., DelPrete, A., Sironi, M., Salvi, V., Salogni, L., et al., 2008. Blocking TH17-polarizing cytokines by histone deacetylase inhibitors in vitro and in vivo. J. Leukoc. Biol. 84, 1540–1548.

Brandl, A., Heinzel, T., Kramer, O.H., 2009. Histone deacetylases: salesmen and customers in the post-translational modification market. Biol. Cell. 101, 193–205.

Byun, H.M., Nordio, F., Coull, B.A., Tarantini, L., Hou, L., Bonzini, M., et al., 2012. Temporal stability of epigenetic markers: sequence characteristics and predictors of short-term DNA methylation variations. PLoS One. 7, e39220.

Camelo, S., Iglesias, A.H., Hwang, D., Due, B., Ryu, H., Smith, K., et al., 2005. Transcriptional therapy with the histone deacetylase inhibitor trichostatin A ameliorates experimental autoimmune encephalomyelitis. J. Neuroimmunol. 164, 10–21.

Chatzikyriakidou, A., Voulgari, P.V., Georgiou, I., Drosos, A.A., 2010. A polymorphism in the 3'-UTR of interleukin-1 receptor-associated kinase (IRAK1), a target gene of miR-146a, is associated with rheumatoid arthritis susceptibility. Joint Bone Spine. 77, 411–413.

Chen, D., Ma, H., Hong, H., Koh, S.S., Huang, S.M., Schurter, B.T., et al., 1999. Regulation of transcription by a protein methyltransferase. Science. 284, 2174–2177.

Ciavatta, D.J., Yang, J., Preston, G.A., Badhwar, A.K., Xiao, H., Hewins, P., et al., 2010. Epigenetic basis for aberrant upregulation of autoantigen genes in humans with ANCA vasculitis. J. Clin. Invest. 120, 3209–3219.

Dai, Y., Huang, Y.S., Tang, M., Lu, T.Y., Hu, C.X., Tan, Y.H., et al., 2007. Microarray analysis of microRNA expression in peripheral blood cells of systemic lupus erythematosus patients. Lupus. 16, 939–946.

Dasgupta, S., Zhou, Y., Jana, M., Banik, N.L., Pahan, K., 2003. Sodium phenylacetate inhibits adoptive transfer of experimental allergic encephalomyelitis in SJL/J mice at multiple steps. J. Immunol. 170, 3874–3882.

Deng, C., Kaplan, M.J., Yang, J., Ray, D., Zhang, Z., Mccune, W.J., et al., 2001. Decreased Ras-mitogen-activated protein kinase signaling may cause DNA hypomethylation in T lymphocytes from lupus patients. Arthritis Rheum. 44, 397–407.

Dolinoy, D.C., Weidman, J.R., Jirtle, R.L., 2007. Epigenetic gene regulation: linking early developmental environment to adult disease. Reprod. Toxicol. 23, 297–307.

Dubroff, L.M., Reid Jr., R.J., 1980. Hydralazine-pyrimidine interactions may explain hydralazine-induced lupus erythematosus. Science. 208, 404–406.

Dyment, D.A., Sadovnick, A.D., Ebers, G.C., 1997. Genetics of multiple sclerosis. Hum. Mol. Genet. 6, 1693–1698.

Edens, R.E., Dagtas, S., Gilbert, K.M., 2006. Histone deacetylase inhibitors induce antigen specific anergy in lymphocytes: a comparative study. Int. Immunopharmacol. 6, 1673–1681.

Egger, G., Liang, G., Aparicio, A., Jones, P.A., 2004. Epigenetics in human disease and prospects for epigenetic therapy. Nature. 429, 457–463.

Faber, C., Morbach, H., Singh, S.K., Girschick, H.J., 2006. Differential expression patterns of recombination-activating genes in individual mature B cells in juvenile idiopathic arthritis. Ann. Rheum. Dis. 65, 1351–1356.

Fang, M.Z., Wang, Y., Ai, N., Hou, Z., Sun, Y., Lu, H., et al., 2003. Tea polyphenol (−)-epigallocatechin-3-gallate inhibits DNA methyltransferase and reactivates methylation-silenced genes in cancer cell lines. Cancer. Res. 63, 7563–7570.

Fassbender, H.G., Seibel, M., Hebert, T., 1992. Pathways of destruction in metacarpal and metatarsal joints of patients with rheumatoid arthritis. Scand. J. Rheumatol. 21, 10–16.

Feil, R., Fraga, M.F., 2012. Epigenetics and the environment: emerging patterns and implications. Nat. Rev. Genet. 13, 97–109.

Filipowicz, W., Bhattacharyya, S.N., Sonenberg, N., 2008. Mechanisms of post-transcriptional regulation by microRNAs: are the answers in sight?. Nat. Rev. Genet. 9, 102–114.

Fraga, M.F., Ballestar, E., Paz, M.F., Ropero, S., Setien, F., Ballestar, M. L., et al., 2005. Epigenetic differences arise during the lifetime of monozygotic twins. Proc. Natl. Acad. Sci. U.S.A. 102, 10604–10609.

Gillespie, J., Savic, S., Wong, C., Hempshall, A., Inman, M., Emery, P., et al., 2012. Histone deacetylases are dysregulated in rheumatoid arthritis and a novel histone deacetylase 3—selective inhibitor reduces interleukin-6 production by peripheral blood mononuclear cells from rheumatoid arthritis patients. Arthritis. Rheum. 64, 418–422.

Glauben, R., Batra, A., Fedke, I., Zeitz, M., Lehr, H.A., Leoni, F., et al., 2006. Histone hyperacetylation is associated with amelioration of experimental colitis in mice. J. Immunol. 176, 5015–5022.

Glauben, R., Batra, A., Stroh, T., Erben, U., Fedke, I., Lehr, H.A., et al., 2008. Histone deacetylases: novel targets for prevention of colitis-associated cancer in mice. Gut. 57, 613–622.

Gonzalez, S., Aguilera, S., Alliende, C., Urzua, U., Quest, A.F., Herrera, L., et al., 2011. Alterations in type I hemidesmosome components suggestive of epigenetic control in the salivary glands of patients with Sjogren's syndrome. Arthritis Rheum. 63, 1106–11015.

Gourley, M., Miller, F.W., 2007. Mechanisms of disease: environmental factors in the pathogenesis of rheumatic disease. Nat. Clin. Pract. Rheumatol. 3, 172–180.

Grabiec, A.M., Krausz, S., De Jager, W., Burakowski, T., Groot, D., Sanders, M.E., et al., 2010. Histone deacetylase inhibitors suppress inflammatory activation of rheumatoid arthritis patient synovial macrophages and tissue. J. Immunol. 184, 2718–2728.

Grabiec, A.M., Korchynskyi, O., Tak, P.P., Reedquist, K.A., 2012. Histone deacetylase inhibitors suppress rheumatoid arthritis fibroblast-like synoviocyte and macrophage IL-6 production by accelerating mRNA decay. Ann. Rheum. Dis. 71, 424–431.

Guo, M., Mao, X., Ji, Q., Lang, M., Li, S., Peng, Y., et al., 2010. miR-146a in PBMCs modulates Th1 function in patients with acute coronary syndrome. Immunol. Cell. Biol. 88, 555–564.

Halili, M.A., Andrews, M.R., Sweet, M.J., Fairlie, D.P., 2009. Histone deacetylase inhibitors in inflammatory disease. Curr. Top. Med. Chem. 9, 309–319.

Hansen, T., Skytthe, A., Stenager, E., Petersen, H.C., Kyvik, K.O., Bronnum-Hansen, H., 2005. Risk for multiple sclerosis in dizygotic and monozygotic twins. Mult. Scler. 11, 500–503.

Hasler, P., Zouali, M., 2001. B cell receptor signaling and autoimmunity. FASEB J. 15, 2085–2098.

He, Y., Dupree, J., Wang, J., Sandoval, J., Li, J., Liu, H., et al., 2007. The transcription factor Yin Yang 1 is essential for oligodendrocyte progenitor differentiation. Neuron. 55, 217–230.

Heijmans, B.T., Tobi, E.W., Stein, A.D., Putter, H., Blauw, G.J., Susser, E.S., et al., 2008. Persistent epigenetic differences associated with prenatal exposure to famine in humans. Proc. Natl. Acad. Sci. U.S. A. 105, 17046–17049.

Herrmann, H., Bar, H., Kreplak, L., Strelkov, S.V., Aebi, U., 2007. Intermediate filaments: from cell architecture to nanomechanics. Nat. Rev. Mol. Cell. Biol. 8, 562–573.

Hoyo, C., Murphy, S.K., Jirtle, R.L., 2009. Imprint regulatory elements as epigenetic biosensors of exposure in epidemiological studies. J. Epidemiol. Community. Health. 63, 683–684.

Hu, N., Qiu, X., Luo, Y., Yuan, J., Li, Y., Lei, W., et al., 2008. Abnormal histone modification patterns in lupus CD4 + T cells. J. Rheumatol. 35, 804–810.

Huber, L.C., Brock, M., Hemmatazad, H., Giger, O.T., Moritz, F., Trenkmann, M., et al., 2007a. Histone deacetylase/acetylase activity in total synovial tissue derived from rheumatoid arthritis and osteoarthritis patients. Arthritis Rheum. 56, 1087–1093.

Huber, L.C., Distler, J.H., Moritz, F., Hemmatazad, H., Hauser, T., Michel, B.A., et al., 2007b. Trichostatin A prevents the accumulation of extracellular matrix in a mouse model of bleomycin-induced skin fibrosis. Arthritis Rheum. 56, 2755–2764.

Huck, S., Zouali, M., 1996. DNA methylation: a potential pathway to abnormal autoreactive lupus B cells. Clin. Immunol. Immunopathol. 80, 1–8.

Hughes, T., Adler, A., Kelly, J.A., Kaufman, K.M., Williams, A.H., Langefeld, C.D., et al., 2012. Evidence for gene–gene epistatic interactions among susceptibility loci for systemic lupus erythematosus. Arthritis Rheum. 64, 485–492.

Hyttinen, V., Kaprio, J., Kinnunen, L., Koskenvuo, M., Tuomilehto, J., 2003. Genetic liability of type 1 diabetes and the onset age among 22,650 young Finnish twin pairs: a nationwide follow-up study. Diabetes. 52, 1052–1055.

Janson, P.C., Winerdal, M.E., Marits, P., Thorn, M., Ohlsson, R., Winqvist, O., 2008. FOXP3 promoter demethylation reveals the committed Treg population in humans. PLoS One. 3, e1612.

Januchowski, R., Jagodzinski, P.P., 2005. Effect of 5-azacytidine and procainamide on CD3-zeta chain expression in Jurkat T cells. Biomed. Pharmacother. 59, 122–126.

Javierre, B.M., Fernandez, A.F., Richter, J., Al-Shahrour, F., Martin-Subero, J.I., Rodriguez-Ubreva, J., et al., 2010. Changes in the pattern of DNA methylation associate with twin discordance in systemic lupus erythematosus. Genome Res. 20, 170–179.

Jeffries, M.A., Dozmorov, M., Tang, Y., Merrill, J.T., Wren, J.D., Sawalha, A.H., 2011. Genome-wide DNA methylation patterns in CD4 + T cells from patients with systemic lupus erythematosus. Epigenetics. 6, 593–601.

Johnson, J., Pahuja, A., Graham, M., Hering, B., Hancock, W.W., Bansal-Pakala, P., 2008. Effects of histone deacetylase inhibitor SAHA on effector and FOXP3 + regulatory T cells in rhesus macaques. Transplant. Proc. 40, 459–461.

Kallenberg, C.G., Heeringa, P., Stegeman, C.A., 2006. Mechanisms of disease: pathogenesis and treatment of ANCA-associated vasculitides. Nat. Clin. Pract. Rheumatol. 2, 661–670.

Kaminsky, Z., Wang, S.C., Petronis, A., 2006. Complex disease, gender and epigenetics. Ann. Med. 38, 530–544.

Kaminsky, Z.A., Tang, T., Wang, S.C., Ptak, C., Oh, G.H., Wong, A.H., et al., 2009. DNA methylation profiles in monozygotic and dizygotic twins. Nat. Genet. 41, 240–245.

Kaplan, M.J., Lu, Q., Wu, A., Attwood, J., Richardson, B., 2004. Demethylation of promoter regulatory elements contributes to perforin overexpression in CD4 + lupus T cells. J. Immunol. 172, 3652–3661.

Karouzakis, E., Gay, R.E., Michel, B.A., Gay, S., Neidhart, M., 2009. DNA hypomethylation in rheumatoid arthritis synovial fibroblasts. Arthritis. Rheum. 60, 3613–3622.

Kazantsev, A.G., Thompson, L.M., 2008. Therapeutic application of histone deacetylase inhibitors for central nervous system disorders. Nat. Rev. Drug. Discov. 7, 854–868.

Khattri, R., Cox, T., Yasayko, S.A., Ramsdell, F., 2003. An essential role for Scurfin in CD4 + CD25 + T regulatory cells. Nat. Immunol. 4, 337–342.

Kim, H.P., Leonard, W.J., 2007. CREB/ATF-dependent T cell receptor-induced FoxP3 gene expression: a role for DNA methylation. J. Exp. Med. 204, 1543–1551.

Knip, M., Veijola, R., Virtanen, S.M., Hyoty, H., Vaarala, O., Akerblom, H.K., 2005. Environmental triggers and determinants of type 1 diabetes. Diabetes. 54 (Suppl. 2), S125–S136.

Knip, M., Virtanen, S.M., Seppa, K., Ilonen, J., Savilahti, E., Vaarala, O., et al., 2010. Dietary intervention in infancy and later signs of beta-cell autoimmunity. N. Engl. J. Med. 363, 1900–1908.

Koenen, H.J., Smeets, R.L., Vink, P.M., Van Rijssen, E., Boots, A.M., Joosten, I., 2008. Human CD25highFoxp3pos regulatory T cells differentiate into IL-17-producing cells. Blood. 112, 2340–2352.

Kohm, A.P., Carpentier, P.A., Anger, H.A., Miller, S.D., 2002. Cutting edge: CD4 + CD25 + regulatory T cells suppress antigen-specific

autoreactive immune responses and central nervous system inflammation during active experimental autoimmune encephalomyelitis. J. Immunol. 169, 4712–4716.

Komatsu, N., Mariotti-Ferrandiz, M.E., Wang, Y., Malissen, B., Waldmann, H., Hori, S., 2009. Heterogeneity of natural Foxp3 + T cells: a committed regulatory T-cell lineage and an uncommitted minor population retaining plasticity. Proc. Natl. Acad. Sci. U.S.A. 106, 1903–1908.

Kouzarides, T., 2007. Chromatin modifications and their function. Cell. 128, 693–705.

Lal, G., Zhang, N., Van Der Touw, W., Ding, Y., Ju, W., Bottinger, E. P., et al., 2009. Epigenetic regulation of Foxp3 expression in regulatory T cells by DNA methylation. J. Immunol. 182, 259–273.

Lee, D.U., Agarwal, S., Rao, A., 2002. Th2 lineage commitment and efficient IL-4 production involves extended demethylation of the IL-4 gene. Immunity. 16, 649–660.

Lee, P.P., Fitzpatrick, D.R., Beard, C., Jessup, H.K., Lehar, S., Makar, K. W., et al., 2001. A critical role for Dnmt1 and DNA methylation in T cell development, function, and survival. Immunity. 15, 763–774.

Lee, Y.K., Mukasa, R., Hatton, R.D., Weaver, C.T., 2009. Developmental plasticity of Th17 and Treg cells. Curr. Opin. Immunol. 21, 274–280.

Lei, W., Luo, Y., Yan, K., Zhao, S., Li, Y., Qiu, X., et al., 2009. Abnormal DNA methylation in CD4 + T cells from patients with systemic lupus erythematosus, systemic sclerosis, and dermatomyositis. Scand. J. Rheumatol. 38, 369–374.

Leoni, F., Zaliani, A., Bertolini, G., Porro, G., Pagani, P., Pozzi, P., et al., 2002. The antitumor histone deacetylase inhibitor suberoylanilide hydroxamic acid exhibits anti-inflammatory properties via suppression of cytokines. Proc. Natl. Acad. Sci. U.S.A. 99, 2995–3000.

Leslie, R.D., Delli Castelli, M., 2004. Age-dependent influences on the origins of autoimmune diabetes: evidence and implications. Diabetes. 53, 3033–3040.

Lewis, B.P., Burge, C.B., Bartel, D.P., 2005. Conserved seed pairing, often flanked by adenosines, indicates that thousands of human genes are microRNA targets. Cell. 120, 15–20.

Li, B., Carey, M., Workman, J.L., 2007a. The role of chromatin during transcription. Cell. 128, 707–719.

Li, B., Samanta, A., Song, X., Iacono, K.T., Bembas, K., Tao, R., et al., 2007b. FOXP3 interactions with histone acetyltransferase and class II histone deacetylases are required for repression. Proc. Natl. Acad. Sci. U.S.A. 104, 4571–4576.

Li, J., Wan, Y., Guo, Q., Zou, L., Zhang, J., Fang, Y., et al., 2010. Altered microRNA expression profile with miR-146a upregulation in CD4 + T cells from patients with rheumatoid arthritis. Arthritis Res. Ther. 12, R81.

Li, Q.J., Chau, J., Ebert, P.J., Sylvester, G., Min, H., Liu, G., et al., 2007c. miR-181a is an intrinsic modulator of T cell sensitivity and selection. Cell. 129, 147–161.

Lin, H.S., Hu, C.Y., Chan, H.Y., Liew, Y.Y., Huang, H.P., Lepescheux, L., et al., 2007. Anti-rheumatic activities of histone deacetylase (HDAC) inhibitors in vivo in collagen-induced arthritis in rodents. Br. J. Pharmacol. 150, 862–872.

Lu, Q., Kaplan, M., Ray, D., Zacharek, S., Gutsch, D., Richardson, B., 2002. Demethylation of ITGAL (CD11a) regulatory sequences in systemic lupus erythematosus. Arthritis Rheum. 46, 1282–1291.

Lu, Q., Wu, A., Richardson, B.C., 2005. Demethylation of the same promoter sequence increases CD70 expression in lupus T cells and T cells treated with lupus-inducing drugs. J. Immunol. 174, 6212–6219.

Lu, Q., Wu, A., Tesmer, L., Ray, D., Yousif, N., Richardson, B., 2007. Demethylation of CD40LG on the inactive X in T cells from women with lupus. J. Immunol. 179, 6352–6358.

Lucas, J.L., Mirshahpanah, P., Haas-Stapleton, E., Asadullah, K., Zollner, T.M., Numerof, R.P., 2009. Induction of Foxp3 + regulatory T cells with histone deacetylase inhibitors. Cell. Immunol. 257, 97–104.

Luger, K., Mader, A.W., Richmond, R.K., Sargent, D.F., Richmond, T. J., 1997. Crystal structure of the nucleosome core particle at 2.8 a resolution. Nature. 389, 251–260.

Lundh, M., Christensen, D.P., Rasmussen, D.N., Mascagni, P., Dinarello, C.A., Billestrup, N., et al., 2010. Lysine deacetylases are produced in pancreatic beta cells and are differentially regulated by proinflammatory cytokines. Diabetologia. 53, 2569–2578.

Mastronardi, F.G., Noor, A., Wood, D.D., Paton, T., Moscarello, M.A., 2007. Peptidyl argininedeiminase 2 CpG island in multiple sclerosis white matter is hypomethylated. J. Neurosci. Res. 85, 2006–2016.

Matsuoka, H., Fujimura, T., Mori, H., Aramori, I., Mutoh, S., 2007. Mechanism of HDAC inhibitor FR235222-mediated IL-2 transcriptional repression in Jurkat cells. Int. Immunopharmacol. 7, 1422–1432.

Mazari, L., Ouarzane, M., Zouali, M., 2007. Subversion of B lymphocyte tolerance by hydralazine, a potential mechanism for drug-induced lupus. Proc. Natl. Acad. Sci. U.S.A. 104, 6317–6322.

Meinecke, I., Cinski, A., Baier, A., Peters, M.A., Dankbar, B., Wille, A., et al., 2007. Modification of nuclear PML protein by SUMO-1 regulates Fas-induced apoptosis in rheumatoid arthritis synovial fibroblasts. Proc. Natl. Acad. Sci. U.S.A. 104, 5073–5078.

Mendell, J.T., 2008. miRiad roles for the miR-17-92 cluster in development and disease. Cell. 133, 217–222.

Miao, F., Gonzalo, I.G., Lanting, L., Natarajan, R., 2004. In vivo chromatin remodeling events leading to inflammatory gene transcription under diabetic conditions. J. Biol. Chem. 279, 18091–18097.

Miao, F., Li, S., Chavez, V., Lanting, L., Natarajan, R., 2006. Coactivator-associated arginine methyltransferase-1 enhances nuclear factor-kappaB-mediated gene transcription through methylation of histone H3 at arginine 17. Mol. Endocrinol. 20, 1562–1573.

Miao, F., Chen, Z., Zhang, L., Liu, Z., Wu, X., Yuan, Y.C., et al., 2012. Profiles of epigenetic histone post-translational modifications at type 1 diabetes susceptible genes. J. Biol. Chem. 287, 16335–16345.

Mishra, N., Brown, D.R., Olorenshaw, I.M., Kammer, G.M., 2001. Trichostatin A reverses skewed expression of CD154, interleukin-10, and interferon-gamma gene and protein expression in lupus T cells. Proc. Natl. Acad. Sci. U.S.A. 98, 2628–2633.

Mishra, N., Reilly, C.M., Brown, D.R., Ruiz, P., Gilkeson, G.S., 2003. Histone deacetylase inhibitors modulate renal disease in the MRL-lpr/lpr mouse. J. Clin. Invest. 111, 539–552.

Miyara, M., Yoshioka, Y., Kitoh, A., Shima, T., Wing, K., Niwa, A., et al., 2009. Functional delineation and differentiation dynamics of human CD4 + T cells expressing the FoxP3 transcription factor. Immunity. 30, 899–911.

Moscarello, M.A., Wood, D.D., Ackerley, C., Boulias, C., 1994. Myelin in multiple sclerosis is developmentally immature. J. Clin. Invest. 94, 146–154.

Mosley, A.L., Ozcan, S., 2003. Glucose regulates insulin gene transcription by hyperacetylation of histone h4. J. Biol. Chem. 278, 19660–19666.

Musse, A.A., Harauz, G., 2007. Molecular "negativity" may underlie multiple sclerosis: role of the myelin basic protein family in the pathogenesis of MS. Int. Rev. Neurobiol. 79, 149–172.

Nakasa, T., Miyaki, S., Okubo, A., Hashimoto, M., Nishida, K., Ochi, M., et al., 2008. Expression of microRNA-146 in rheumatoid arthritis synovial tissue. Arthritis. Rheum. 58, 1284–1292.

Niimoto, T., Nakasa, T., Ishikawa, M., Okuhara, A., Izumi, B., Deie, M., et al., 2010. MicroRNA-146a expresses in interleukin-17 producing T cells in rheumatoid arthritis patients. BMC. Musculoskelet. Disord. 11, 209.

Nile, C.J., Read, R.C., Akil, M., Duff, G.W., Wilson, A.G., 2008. Methylation status of a single CpG site in the IL6 promoter is related to IL6 messenger RNA levels and rheumatoid arthritis. Arthritis Rheum. 58, 2686–2693.

Nylander, A., Hafler, D.A., 2012. Multiple sclerosis. J. Clin. Invest. 122, 1180–1188.

Oelke, K., Lu, Q., Richardson, D., Wu, A., Deng, C., Hanash, S., et al., 2004. Overexpression of CD70 and overstimulation of IgG synthesis by lupus T cells and T cells treated with DNA methylation inhibitors. Arthritis Rheum. 50, 1850–1860.

Ohlsson, S., Hellmark, T., Pieters, K., Sturfelt, G., Wieslander, J., Segelmark, M., 2005. Increased monocyte transcription of the proteinase 3 gene in small vessel vasculitis. Clin. Exp. Immunol. 141, 174–182.

Pan, W., Zhu, S., Yuan, M., Cui, H., Wang, L., Luo, X., et al., 2010. MicroRNA-21 and microRNA-148a contribute to DNA hypomethylation in lupus CD4 + T cells by directly and indirectly targeting DNA methyltransferase 1. J. Immunol. 184, 6773–6781.

Pasare, C., Medzhitov, R., 2003. Toll pathway-dependent blockade of CD4 + CD25 + T cell-mediated suppression by dendritic cells. Science. 299, 1033–1036.

Pauley, K.M., Satoh, M., Chan, A.L., Bubb, M.R., Reeves, W.H., Chan, E.K., 2008. Upregulated miR-146a expression in peripheral blood mononuclear cells from rheumatoid arthritis patients. Arthritis. Res. Ther. 10, R101.

Perez, P., Anaya, J.M., Aguilera, S., Urzua, U., Munroe, D., Molina, C., et al., 2009. Gene expression and chromosomal location for susceptibility to Sjogren's syndrome. J. Autoimmun. 33, 99–108.

Polansky, J.K., Kretschmer, K., Freyer, J., Floess, S., Garbe, A., Baron, U., et al., 2008. DNA methylation controls Foxp3 gene expression. Eur. J. Immunol. 38, 1654–1663.

Radic, M.Z., Zouali, M., 1996. Receptor editing, immune diversification and self-tolerance. Immunity. 5, 505–511.

Rakyan, V.K., Beyan, H., Down, T.A., Hawa, M.I., Maslau, S., Aden, D., et al., 2011. Identification of type 1 diabetes-associated DNA methylation variable positions that precede disease diagnosis. PLoS Genet. 7, e1002300.

Reddy, P., Sun, Y., Toubai, T., Duran-Struuck, R., Clouthier, S.G., Weisiger, E., et al., 2008. Histone deacetylase inhibition modulates indoleamine 2,3-dioxygenase-dependent DC functions and regulates experimental graft-versus-host disease in mice. J. Clin. Invest. 118, 2562–2573.

Redondo, M.J., Yu, L., Hawa, M., Mackenzie, T., Pyke, D.A., Eisenbarth, G.S., et al., 2001. Heterogeneity of type I diabetes:

analysis of monozygotic twins in Great Britain and the United States. Diabetologia. 44, 354–362.

Reidenberg, M.M., Drayer, D.E., Lorenzo, B., Strom, B.L., West, S.L., Snyder, E.S., et al., 1993. Acetylation phenotypes and environmental chemical exposure of people with idiopathic systemic lupus erythematosus. Arthritis Rheum. 36, 971–973.

Reilly, C.M., Mishra, N., Miller, J.M., Joshi, D., Ruiz, P., Richon, V.M., et al., 2004. Modulation of renal disease in MRL/lpr mice by suberoylanilide hydroxamic acid. J. Immunol. 173, 4171–4178.

Richardson, B., Scheinbart, L., Strahler, J., Gross, L., Hanash, S., Johnson, M., 1990. Evidence for impaired T cell DNA methylation in systemic lupus erythematosus and rheumatoid arthritis. Arthritis Rheum. 33, 1665–1673.

Richardson, B.C., Strahler, J.R., Pivirotto, T.S., Quddus, J., Bayliss, G. E., Gross, L.A., et al., 1992. Phenotypic and functional similarities between 5-azacytidine-treated T cells and a T cell subset in patients with active systemic lupus erythematosus. Arthritis Rheum. 35, 647–662.

Roncarolo, M.G., Battaglia, M., 2007. Regulatory T-cell immunotherapy for tolerance to self antigens and alloantigens in humans. Nat. Rev. Immunol. 7, 585–598.

Sadovnick, A.D., Baird, P.A., Ward, R.H., 1988. Multiple sclerosis: updated risks for relatives. Am. J. Med. Genet. 29, 533–541.

Samuels, J., Ng, Y.S., Coupillaud, C., Paget, D., Meffre, E., 2005. Impaired early B cell tolerance in patients with rheumatoid arthritis. J. Exp. Med. 201, 1659–1667.

Sawalha, A.H., Jeffries, M., Webb, R., Lu, Q., Gorelik, G., Ray, D., et al., 2008. Defective T-cell ERK signaling induces interferon-regulated gene expression and overexpression of methylation-sensitive genes similar to lupus patients. Genes Immun. 9, 368–378.

Schietinger, A., Delrow, J.J., Basom, R.S., Blattman, J.N., Greenberg, P. D., 2012. Rescued tolerant CD8 T cells are preprogrammed to reestablish the tolerant state. Science. 335, 723–727.

Schmidl, C., Klug, M., Boeld, T.J., Andreesen, R., Hoffmann, P., Edinger, M., et al., 2009. Lineage-specific DNA methylation in T cells correlates with histone methylation and enhancer activity. Genome Res. 19, 1165–1174.

Schwab, J., Illges, H., 2001. Silencing of CD21 expression in synovial lymphocytes is independent of methylation of the CD21 promoter CpG island. Rheumatol. Int. 20, 133–137.

Scofield, R.H., Bruner, G.R., Namjou, B., Kimberly, R.P., Ramsey-Goldman, R., Petri, M., et al., 2008. Klinefelter's syndrome (47, XXY) in male systemic lupus erythematosus patients: support for the notion of a gene–dose effect from the X chromosome. Arthritis Rheum. 58, 2511–2517.

Shanmugam, N., Reddy, M.A., Guha, M., Natarajan, R., 2003. High glucose-induced expression of proinflammatory cytokine and chemokine genes in monocytic cells. Diabetes. 52, 1256–1264.

Stanczyk, J., Pedrioli, D.M., Brentano, F., Sanchez-Pernaute, O., Kolling, C., Gay, R.E., et al., 2008. Altered expression of MicroRNA in synovial fibroblasts and synovial tissue in rheumatoid arthritis. Arthritis Rheum. 58, 1001–1009.

Strahl, B.D., Allis, C.D., 2000. The language of covalent histone modifications. Nature. 403, 41–45.

Suzuki, N., Harada, T., Mihara, S., Sakane, T., 1996. Characterization of a germline Vk gene encoding cationic anti-DNA antibody and role of receptor editing for development of the autoantibody in patients with systemic lupus erythematosus. J. Clin. Invest. 98, 1843–1850.

Sweet, M.J., Shakespear, M.R., Kamal, N.A., Fairlie, D.P., 2012. HDAC inhibitors: modulating leukocyte differentiation, survival, proliferation and inflammation. Immunol. Cell. Biol. 90, 14–22.

Taganov, K.D., Boldin, M.P., Chang, K.J., Baltimore, D., 2006. NF-kappaB-dependent induction of microRNA miR-146, an inhibitor targeted to signaling proteins of innate immune responses. Proc. Natl. Acad. Sci. U.S.A. 103, 12481–12486.

Takami, N., Osawa, K., Miura, Y., Komai, K., Taniguchi, M., Shiraishi, M., et al., 2006. Hypermethylated promoter region of DR3, the death receptor 3 gene, in rheumatoid arthritis synovial cells. Arthritis Rheum. 54, 779–787.

Tang, Y., Luo, X., Cui, H., Ni, X., Yuan, M., Guo, Y., et al., 2009. MicroRNA-146A contributes to abnormal activation of the type I interferon pathway in human lupus by targeting the key signaling proteins. Arthritis Rheum. 60, 1065–1075.

Tao, R., De Zoeten, E.F., Ozkaynak, E., Chen, C., Wang, L., Porrett, P. M., et al., 2007a. Deacetylase inhibition promotes the generation and function of regulatory T cells. Nat. Med. 13, 1299–1307.

Tao, R., De Zoeten, E.F., Ozkaynak, E., Wang, L., Li, B., Greene, M.I., et al., 2007b. Histone deacetylase inhibitors and transplantation. Curr. Opin. Immunol. 19, 589–595.

Taveggia, C., Feltri, M.L., Wrabetz, L., 2010. Signals to promote myelin formation and repair. Nat. Rev. Neurol. 6, 276–287.

Teruel, R., Perez-Sanchez, C., Corral, J., Herranz, M.T., Perez-Andreu, V., Saiz, E., et al., 2011. Identification of miRNAs as potential modulators of tissue factor expression in patients with systemic lupus erythematosus and antiphospholipid syndrome. J. Thromb. Haemost. 9, 1985–1992.

Thiagalingam, S., Cheng, K.H., Lee, H.J., Mineva, N., Thiagalingam, A., Ponte, J.F., 2003. Histone deacetylases: unique players in shaping the epigenetic histone code. Ann. N.Y. Acad. Sci. 983, 84–100.

Thomas, R.M., Gao, L., Wells, A.D., 2005. Signals from CD28 induce stable epigenetic modification of the IL-2 promoter. J. Immunol. 174, 4639–4646.

Tran, D.Q., Ramsey, H., Shevach, E.M., 2007. Induction of FOXP3 expression in naive human CD4 + FOXP3 T cells by T-cell receptor stimulation is transforming growth factor-beta dependent but does not confer a regulatory phenotype. Blood. 110, 2983–2990.

Tranquill, L.R., Cao, L., Ling, N.C., Kalbacher, H., Martin, R.M., Whitaker, J.N., 2000. Enhanced T cell responsiveness to citrulline-containing myelin basic protein in multiple sclerosis patients. Mult. Scler. 6, 220–225.

Vojinovic, J., Damjanov, N., D'Urzo, C., Furlan, A., Susic, G., Pasic, S., et al., 2011. Safety and efficacy of an oral histone deacetylase inhibitor in systemic-onset juvenile idiopathic arthritis. Arthritis Rheum. 63, 1452–1458.

Wang, L., Tao, R., Hancock, W.W., 2009. Using histone deacetylase inhibitors to enhance Foxp3(+) regulatory T-cell function and induce allograft tolerance. Immunol. Cell. Biol. 87, 195–202.

Wang, Y., Fan, P.S., Kahaleh, B., 2006. Association between enhanced type I collagen expression and epigenetic repression of the FLI1 gene in scleroderma fibroblasts. Arthritis Rheum. 54, 2271–2279.

Willer, C.J., Dyment, D.A., Risch, N.J., Sadovnick, A.D., Ebers, G.C., 2003. Twin concordance and sibling recurrence rates in multiple sclerosis. Proc. Natl. Acad. Sci. U.S.A. 100, 12877–12882.

Wilson, C.B., Rowell, E., Sekimata, M., 2009. Epigenetic control of T-helper-cell differentiation. Nat. Rev. Immunol. 9, 91–105.

Wolff, G.L., Kodell, R.L., Moore, S.R., Cooney, C.A., 1998. Maternal epigenetics and methyl supplements affect agouti gene expression in Avy/a mice. FASEB J. 12, 949–957.

Wood, D.D., Bilbao, J.M., O'Connors, P., Moscarello, M.A., 1996. Acute multiple sclerosis (Marburg type) is associated with developmentally immature myelin basic protein. Ann. Neurol. 40, 18–24.

Xiao, C., Srinivasan, L., Calado, D.P., Patterson, H.C., Zhang, B., Wang, J., et al., 2008. Lymphoproliferative disease and autoimmunity in mice with increased miR-17-92 expression in lymphocytes. Nat. Immunol. 9, 405–414.

Yin, H., Zhao, M., Wu, X., Gao, F., Luo, Y., Ma, L., et al., 2010. Hypomethylation and overexpression of CD70 (TNFSF7) in CD4 + T cells of patients with primary Sjogren's syndrome. J. Dermatol. Sci. 59, 198–203.

Yung, R., Chang, S., Hemati, N., Johnson, K., Richardson, B., 1997. Mechanisms of drug-induced lupus. IV. Comparison of procainamide and hydralazine with analogs in vitro and in vivo. Arthritis Rheum. 40, 1436–1443.

Yurasov, S., Wardemann, H., Hammersen, J., Tsuiji, M., Meffre, E., Pascual, V., et al., 2005. Defective B cell tolerance checkpoints in systemic lupus erythematosus. J. Exp. Med. 201, 703–711.

Zhang, X., Koldzic, D.N., Izikson, L., Reddy, J., Nazareno, R.F., Sakaguchi, S., et al., 2004. IL-10 is involved in the suppression of experimental autoimmune encephalomyelitis by CD25 + CD4 + regulatory T cells. Int. Immunol. 16, 249–256.

Zhang, Z., Maurer, K., Perin, J.C., Song, L., Sullivan, K.E., 2010. Cytokine-induced monocyte characteristics in SLE. J. Biomed. Biotechnol. 2010, 507475.

Zhao, M., Tang, J., Gao, F., Wu, X., Liang, Y., Yin, H., et al., 2010a. Hypomethylation of IL10 and IL13 promoters in CD4 + T cells of patients with systemic lupus erythematosus. J. Biomed. Biotechnol. 2010, 931018.

Zhao, S., Wang, Y., Liang, Y., Zhao, M., Long, H., Ding, S., et al., 2011. MicroRNA-126 regulates DNA methylation in CD4 + T cells and contributes to systemic lupus erythematosus by targeting DNA methyltransferase 1. Arthritis. Rheum. 63, 1376–1386.

Zhao, X., Tang, Y., Qu, B., Cui, H., Wang, S., Wang, L., et al., 2010b. MicroRNA-125a contributes to elevated inflammatory chemokine RANTES levels via targeting KLF13 in systemic lupus erythematosus. Arthritis. Rheum. 62, 3425–3435.

Zhou, X., Bailey-Bucktrout, S., Jeker, L.T., Bluestone, J.A., 2009a. Plasticity of CD4(+) FoxP3(+) T cells. Curr. Opin. Immunol. 21, 281–285.

Zhou, Y., Yuan, J., Pan, Y., Fei, Y., Qiu, X., Hu, N., et al., 2009b. T cell CD40LG gene expression and the production of IgG by autologous B cells in systemic lupus erythematosus. Clin. Immunol. 132, 362–370.

Zouali, M., 2005. Taming lupus. Sci. Am. 292, 58–65.

Zouali, M., 2008. Receptor editing and receptor revision in rheumatic autoimmune diseases. Trends. Immunol. 29, 103–109.

Zouali, M., 2011. Epigenetics in lupus. Ann. N.Y. Acad. Sci. 1217, 154–165.

Zouali, M. 2013. *Immunological Tolerance: Mechanisms*. Encyclopedia of Life Sciences. John Wiley and Sons, Ltd., in press.

Zouali, M. 2013. The epigenetic landscape of B lymphocyte tolerance to self. *FEBS Lett.* 587, 2067–73.

Zouali, M. (Ed.), 2009. The Epigenetics of Autoimmune Diseases. Wiley-Blackwell (an imprint of John Wiley and Sons Ltd.).

Zouali, M., Sarmay, G., 2004. B lymphocyte signaling pathways in systemic autoimmunity: implications for pathogenesis and treatment. Arthritis Rheum. 50, 2730–2741.

Chapter 29

Autoimmunity in Primary Immunodeficiency Disorders

Thomas A. Fleisher[1] and Arnold I. Levinson[2]

[1]Department of Laboratory Medicine, NIH Clinical Center, National Institutes of Health, Bethesda, MD, USA, [2]Perelman School of Medicine, University of Pennsylvania, Philadelphia, PA, USA

Chapter Outline

Introduction	**403**	Early Complement Component Deficiency	411
T Cell Developmental Defects	**403**	Toll-Like Receptor 3 (TLR3) Polymorphism and	
Severe Combined Immunodeficiency	403	Autoimmunity	412
Combined Immune Deficiencies	404	**Monogenic Defects Affecting Immune Homeostasis**	
DiGeorge Syndrome	405	**and/or Tolerance**	**412**
Wiskott–Aldrich Syndrome	405	Autoimmune Polyendocrinopathy, Candidiasis,	
Antibody Production Defects	**406**	Ectodermal Dystrophy	412
X-Linked Agammaglobulinemia	406	Immunodysregulation, Polyendocrinopathy, Enteropathy	
Common Variable Immunodeficiency	406	X-Linked	413
Selective IgA Deficiency	408	Autoimmune Lymphoproliferative Syndrome	414
Immunodeficiency with Hyper-IgM Syndrome	409	**Conclusion**	**414**
Innate Immune Defects	**411**	**Acknowledgment**	**416**
Chronic Granulomatous Disease	411	**References**	**416**

INTRODUCTION

It has become increasingly clear that many of the well-characterized primary immune deficiency disorders are not only associated with recurrent infections but also present with immune dysregulation that manifests as autoimmune disease. The clinical findings together with delineation of the genetic basis for many of these "experiments of nature" have led to an expanded understanding of various pathways involved in immune homeostasis and the maintenance of self tolerance. In this chapter the principal primary immune deficiency disorders associated with immune dysregulation and autoimmunity are presented, paying particular attention to the lessons provided by the etiologic genetic defects.

T CELL DEVELOPMENTAL DEFECTS

Severe Combined Immunodeficiency

Severe defects in T cell immunity can be associated with autoimmunity and an increasing appreciation for the association of T cell developmental defects producing a combination of immune deficiency and dysregulation has emerged. This has been most clearly delineated in the setting of hypomorphic mutations in genes associated with severe combined immunodeficiency (SCID). Typically in classical SCID, there is marked T cell lymphopenia with varied effects on B cells and natural killer (NK) cells depending on the genetic defect. The resulting immune deficiency is of such severity that without immune reconstitution via hematopoietic stem cell transplantation early in life, the patient has a very high likelihood of developing failure to thrive and recurrent opportunistic infections that result in death within the first 2 years of life. However, when hypomorphic mutations in *RAG1* and *RAG2* were identified in patients presenting with Omenn syndrome (OS) (Marrella et al., 2011), genes that had originally been associated with classic T-/B-/NK$^+$ SCID, it first became evident that the clinical phenotype of mutations affecting genes associated with typical SCID could vary. OS was initially recognized in the 1960s based on a presenting

N. Rose & I. Mackay (Eds): The Autoimmune Diseases, Fifth edition. DOI: http://dx.doi.org/10.1016/B978-0-12-384929-8.00029-0

clinical phenotype of susceptibility to opportunistic infections, together with generalized erythroderma involving lymphocytic infiltration, alopecia, and other forms of autoimmunity, particularly autoimmune hepatitis and other gastrointestinal tract processes. Additional findings include hepatosplenomegaly, lymphadenopathy, increased serum IgE, and eosinophilia suggesting an involvement of a Th2 polarized immune response. Unlike classical SCID, these patients also have significant numbers of circulating T cells but rather than expressing a wide array of T cell receptors, the circulating T cells are oligoclonal (evaluated by spectratyping) and highly activated based on CD45RO and HLA-DR expression. The circulating cells appear to be primarily autoreactive and prove to be incapable of providing appropriate T cell responses to microbial pathogens. Thus, hypomorphic mutations in SCID associated genes can produce a varied clinical phenotype with severe defects in host defense that require immune reconstitution similar to typical SCID but with the additional clinical findings of autoreactivity. The genetic defects associated with OS are now known to also include mutations in other SCID associated genes including genes encoding Artemis, DNA ligase IV, common gamma chain, IL-7 receptor alpha chain, adenosine deaminase, zeta-chain associated protein kinase 70 (ZAP70), and the ribonuclease mitochondrial RNA processing (RMRP) complex (Villa et al., 2008).

The association of multiple SCID genotypes with an altered clinical phenotype set the stage for investigations that have uncovered further expansion of the clinical phenotypes linked to hypomorphic ("leaky") defects in *RAG1* and *RAG2*. The range of findings appears to be linked to the level of protein function with the less severe phenotypes at the level of infectious susceptibility associated with mutations that result in residual protein activity. Autoimmunity has evolved as a major common feature in these varied clinical presentations that often includes autoimmune cytopenias. More recently there have been descriptions of later onset disease having less severe immune deficiency with autoreactive processes manifesting as granulomatous inflammation involving various organs including the skin (Niehues et al., 2010). Recently it has been recognized that some patients with hypomorphic *RAG1/RAG2* mutations can present with a mid-line granulomatous process that has many features overlapping with Wegner granulomatosis (WG) (DeRavin et al., 2010). The initial report of a WG-like presentation described a patient who first presented in adolescence with myasthenia gravis and a history of recurrent sinopulmonary infections while his older sister, who died at age 5 of sepsis, had a history of autoimmunity with cytopenias, antinuclear antibody (ANA) positive vascular disease, and symptoms consistent with myasthenia gravis.

Taken together, these findings clearly establish that genetic defects impacting T cell development not only compromise host defense but can also result in T cell dysregulation with the development of autoimmunity, albeit involving a limited range of target organs. The combination of autoimmunity and immune deficiency associated with defective T cell development may be explained by abnormalities in the thymic stroma found in experimental models of "leaky" SCID (Rucci et al., 2011). The predominant finding in these models is a reduction in the pool of medullary thymic epithelial cells (mTECs). This reduces the level of self antigen expression in the thymic medulla, which appears to diminish the effectiveness of negative selection of self reactive T cells during thympoiesis. There also appears to be a contribution of defective B cell tolerance associated with RAG gene mutations (Walter et al., 2010). In addition, findings in these models also identify a marked reduction in natural regulatory T (Treg) cells, an observation that is also likely to be contributing to the development of autoimmunity (Cassani et al., 2010). Finally, the immunological process termed homeostatic proliferation may have a role in the development of autoimmunity in congenital disorders that impact T cell development (Goyal et al., 2009). It is known that normal naïve T (and B) cells turn over slowly but in the face of significant lymphopenia undergo far more rapid cell proliferation. This process of augmented proliferation is theorized to generate an increased frequency of autoreactive T cells for reasons that have not been clarified. Thus, impaired negative thymic selection, B cell tolerance, Treg development, and/or homeostatic proliferation may largely account for the development of autoimmunity in these patients.

Combined Immune Deficiencies

Combined immune deficiencies (CID) represent T cell-based immune disorders with a somewhat less significant defect when compared to SCID. One form of CID is associated with a defect in the surface expression of class I major histocompatibility complex (MHC) proteins (often referred to as the bare lymphocyte syndrome) that presents with low levels of CD8 T cells and recurrent infections. In addition, this very rare disorder is associated with a high incidence of vasculitis-like complications including granulomatous inflammation pyoderma grangrenosa-like cutaneous manifestations, which presumably represent an autoimmune process (De la Salle et al., 1999; Villa-Forte et al., 2008). The underlying defect in this disorder is associated with mutations in genes for specific proteins (i.e., *TAP1*, *TAP2*, *TAPBP*) required for the transport of antigenic peptides to the endoplasmic reticulum necessary to assemble the MHC protein—peptide complex that is normally expressed on the cell surface.

A second CID based on a defect in the enzyme, purine nucleoside phosphorylase (PNP), a member of the purine salvage pathway, is associated with a progressive loss of T cells accompanied by an increasing risk of infection. These patients also have a high incidence of neurologic disease presumably related to the specific defect in the purine salvage pathway as well as autoimmunity typically presenting as autoimmune hemolytic anemia (AIHA) (Notarangelo, 2009). The basis of autoimmunity in patients with this enzymatic defect is not known but clearly must be linked in some fashion to the toxic metabolite's impact on T cell (and possibly B cell) function.

A more recently identified CID is associated with a defect in the stromal interaction molecule 1 (STIM1), a calcium sensing protein present in the endoplasmic reticulum that is required for the function of the calcium release activated channel (CRAC) necessary for normal T cell activation. These patients have infectious histories similar to SCID patients but also develop autoimmune cytopenias, lymphadenopathy, and hepatosplenomegaly as well as ectotermal dysplasia and congenital myopathy (Shaw and Feske, 2012). One presumed mechanism of autoimmunity in this disorder is a reduction in Treg cells based on observations in one patient as well as a murine model with T cell-specific deletion of *stim1* and *stim2* demonstrating reduced numbers and diminished function of Treg cells. In the murine model, correction of the immune dysfunction evidenced by reversal of the lymphoproliferative process is accomplished by the transfer of normal syngeneic Treg cells. However, this model does not result in the aggressive autoimmune processes seen in murine foxp3 deficiency (scurfy mouse) associated with absent Tregs, a difference presumed to be due to the defective T cell effector function associated with the abnormal calcium channel function.

A unique syndrome associated with *PLCG2* deletions was recently identified that manifests with immunodeficiency, autoimmunity, and cold urticaria (Ombrello et al., 2011). The deletions in this gene are associated with a gain of function in the signaling protein PLCγ2 causing either excessive or deficient immune functions of multiple leukocyte subsets. The autoimmunity reported includes autoimmune thyroiditis, granulomatous rash, and increased ANAs in association with a common variable-like immunodeficiency and cold urticaria. The underlying cause of autoimmunity remains to be defined in this disorder.

DiGeorge Syndrome

The DiGeorge syndrome (DGS) results from defective third and fourth pharyngeal pouch development during embryogenesis, which in many cases is associated with a chromosome 22q11.2 deletion. As a result of the developmental abnormality, patients with DGS typically have a combination of right-sided cardiac defects, defective parathyroid function often resulting in neonatal tetany, and dysmorphic facial features (e.g., low set ears, shortened philtrum, high arched or cleft palate). In addition, patients with DGS have an increased incidence of autoimmunity including cytopenias, systemic autoimmunity (particularly rheumatoid arthritis and autoimmune thyroid disease) (Zemble et al., 2010; Gennery, 2012). From an immunologic perspective, a small minority of DGS patients (1−2%) has thymic aplasia that results in marked T cell lymphopenia with increased susceptibility to opportunistic infections and among this patient group chromosomal microdeletions are only found in about 50% of patients. This group is referred to as complete DGS and among these patients is a subgroup that carries a diagnosis of complete atypical DGS with a clinical phenotype that is virtually indistinguishable from OS (Markert et al., 2004). Due to the severity of the infectious complications associated with complete (including atypical) DGS, thymic transplantation is indicated to cure the T cell deficiency. However, due to the autoreactive T cells present in the complete atypical DGS presentation, aggressive immunosuppression is required to control the autoreactive cells prior to initiating the thymus transplantation. Alternatively allogeneic bone marrow transplantation has been used and in this case reconstitution is presumably derived from long-lived donor T cells since there is no thymus present for new T cell development. Long-term follow-up studies of complete DGS (including atypical complete DGS) patients post successful thymic transplantation have demonstrated an increased incidence of autoimmune thyroid disease as well as autoimmune cytopenias. The mechanism underlying the development of autoimmunity in DGS is currently unknown but may mimic some of the immunopathogenic mechanisms thought to cause autoimmunity in "leaky" SCID.

Wiskott−Aldrich Syndrome

The Wiskott−Aldrich syndrome (WAS) is an X-linked primary immunodeficiencies (PID) that variously presents with thrombocytopenia involving small platelets, eczema, recurrent infections, autoimmunity, and malignancies (Notarangelo et al., 2008; Thrasher and Burns, 2010). Affected patients are particularly susceptible to infections with encapsulated bacteria and herpes viruses. This disorder is caused by mutations within the gene encoding the WAS protein (WASP), a critical factor in actin polymerization and skeletal remodeling initiated by cellular activation. In particular, the above-described clinical phenotype is caused by mutations that lead to abrogation of WASP expression. By contrast, hypomorphic mutations that typically affect exons 1 and 2 allow for some WASP expression and generally lead to a milder clinical phenotype characterized by X-linked thrombocytopenia (XLT). As WASP is expressed in all non-erythroid hematopoietic cells, it is not surprising that affected individuals present with a number of immunological abnormalities. These include progressive T cell lymphopenia; impaired *in vitro* T cell proliferation and IL-2 production following T cell receptor cross-linking; low serum IgM levels often associated with elevated serum IgA and IgE levels; impaired IgG antibody responses to both T-dependent and T-independent antigens; impaired migratory responses of monocytes, dendritic cells, T and B cells and neutrophils to chemokines; and impaired NK cell cytolytic activity.

Autoimmune disease affects as many as 70% of WAS patients with clinical presentation in rank order including AIHA, immune thrombocytopenia purpura (ITP), vasculitis, renal disease, Henoch–Schonlein-like purpura, and inflammatory bowel disease (Notarangelo et al., 2008; Thrasher and Burns, 2010). Autoimmunity most commonly occurs in patients with WAS but occasionally is also present in patients with XLT. Early explanations for the pathogenesis of autoimmunity referred to possible contributions of recurrent exposure to microbes and chronic inflammation as well as reduced IL-2 production and impaired clearance of apoptotic cells/bodies and debris due to the defective migration of phagocytic cells. More recently, it has become apparent that both WAS patients and WASP deficient mice are characterized by impaired natural Treg (nTreg) activity (Marangoni et al., 2007). Although the molecular basis for this abnormality remains to be established, it is tempting to speculate that impaired IL-2 secretion impacts the development and function of nTregs (Koreth et al., 2011). However, it is likely that the explanation for the development of autoimmunity extends beyond the nTreg story. A very recent report identified an intrinsic defect in WASP-deficient mouse B cells that accounted for the production of auto-antibodies, including anti-DNA antibodies following cross-linking of B cell antigen receptors or Toll-like receptors and provision of T cell-help (Becker-Herman et al., 2011). This may contribute to the findings that post hematopoietic stem cell transplantation, autoimmunity is particularly problematic in patients who remain mixed chimeras for B cells suggesting that the WASP negative B cells may be mediating autoimmunity in this situation.

As is true for many immunodeficiency disorders, the clinical phenotype of WAS does not show consistent fidelity with the genotype. This was demonstrated recently in a report of monozygotic twins, associated with WAS including autoimmune disease in one twin and a milder XLT phenotype in the other (Buchbinder et al., 2011). Interestingly, CpG methylation, diminished *WASP* gene transcripts, diminished WASP expression, and more impaired cellular function were detected in the more

symptomatic twin. These findings are consistent with the previously reported effects of epigenetic changes on the clinical expression of genetically-based autoimmune and primary immunodeficiency disorders.

ANTIBODY PRODUCTION DEFECTS

X-Linked Agammaglobulinemia

X-linked agammaglobulinemia (XLA) was the first primary antibody deficiency identified and is now known to be caused by mutations in Bruton's tyrosine kinase (*BTK*) gene necessary for B cell differentiation and signaling (Tsukada et al., 1993; Vetrie et al., 1993). Development of the B lymphocyte lineage is arrested at the pro- to pre-B cell stage of differentiation resulting in a marked deficiency of circulating B cells and panhypogammaglobulinemia but intact T cell function. Affected individuals usually present clinically by 5–6 months of age with recurrent sinopulmonary infections involving encapsulated bacteria following the loss of maternally transferred IgG antibodies.

Up to 15% of -XLA patients develop autoimmune disease including rheumatoid arthritis, inflammatory bowel disease, scleroderma, alopecia, AIHA, and type 1 diabetes (Verbruggen et al., 2005; Howard et al., 2006; Winkelstein et al., 2006). The absence of B cells and immunoglobulins in these patients suggests that, other than in autoimmune AIHA, immunoglobulin-independent, BTK-dependent processes may be involved in the pathogenesis of autoimmune disorders.

Regulatory B cells, described in mice and humans, appear to contribute to suppression of the development and expression of inflammatory reactions, particularly those mediated by T cells suggesting an important role in immune homeostasis and prevention of autoimmune and inflammatory diseases (Klinker and Lundy, 2012). In both mice and humans, B-regulatory cells comprise a small subset/s of the peripheral B cell pool and are identified by their expression of characteristic cell surface markers. In both species, regulatory B cell subsets appear to mediate immunosuppression via secretion of IL-10 and absence of these cells in XLA could also contribute to the risk of developing autoimmunity.

Common Variable Immunodeficiency

Common variable immunodeficiency (CVID) is a primary immunodeficiency that leads to a variety of clinical syndromes associated with hypogammaglobulinemia (Young et al., 2011). This is caused by a failure of terminal B cell differentiation and a decrease in the number of antibody-producing plasma cells. As a result, patients with CVID have low serum IgG and frequently low IgA and/or IgM as well as an inability to make specific antibodies to protein and carbohydrate antigens. This immunologic impairment accounts for the most characteristic clinical phenotype, namely, recurrent upper and lower respiratory tract infections caused by encapsulated bacteria. However, CVID is quite heterogeneous with regard to clinical presentation. Autoimmune disorders occur in approximately 20–40% of patients including ITP and AIHA, pernicious anemia, polyarthropathy, hypothyroidism, autoimmune hepatitis, biliary cirrhosis, and inflammatory bowel disease (Cunningham-Rundles and Bodian, 1999; Chapel et al., 2008). One of the unsolved paradoxes is how CVID patients produce IgG autoantibodies (e.g., anti-red cell) yet are unable to produce protective IgG antibodies against microbial antigens. Autoimmune disorders may appear several years prior to or after the diagnosis of CVID is made. The fact that (1) autoimmune diseases may antedate the onset of recurrent infections and (2) many CVID patients are not afflicted with autoimmune disease strongly suggests that recurrent infections are not the sole provocateurs of this complication.

In addition, upwards of 10% of patients in most series suffer from inflammatory processes including granulomatous inflammation and lymphoid hyperplasia, the latter manifested in part by lymphadenopathy and/or splenomegaly. CVID patients are at risk for non-Hodgkin lymphoma (~7%) and gastric carcinoma (~1%). Taken together, the heterogeneous clinical manifestations of CVID underscore a major role for immune dysregulation in the immunopathogenesis of this syndrome.

The most common autoimmune conditions observed in CVID are ITP and AIHA with the frequency of these disorders ranging from 5 to 8% (Cunningham-Rundles and Bodian, 1999; Chapel et al., 2008). Some patients also suffer from Evans syndrome, a concurrence of both autoimmune cytopenias. As is true for most of the autoimmune disorders, the appearance of these hematologic conditions may predate or manifest after the diagnosis of CVID. Splenomegaly is a frequent concomitant of CVID, noted at the time of diagnosis in one series in 17.5% of the cases and may not be associated with immune cytopenias.

The most common rheumatic complications include a symmetrical polyarthropathy typically involving the hands, knees, and ankles. The coexistence of systemic lupus erythematosus (SLE) and CVID is uncommon with SLE typically antedating the appearance of CVID. In many of these cases, SLE clinical activity diminished following the onset of CVID, as might be expected in an autoimmune disorder whose pathogenesis is autoantibody dependent.

Granulomatous inflammation is found in 5–10% of CVID patients. The granulomas are non-caseating involving the lungs, liver, spleen, lymph nodes, and skin. These findings mimic sarcoidosis, particularly when there are pulmonary signs and symptoms but no history of recurrent pyogenic infections. Of note, patients with sarcoidosis, unlike CVID, demonstrate polyclonal hypergammaglobulinemia at the time of presentation. The pathogenesis of CVID granulomatous disease remains a mystery without evidence for an infectious etiology and it is often associated with autoimmune disease, particularly ITP. The finding of a characteristic single-nucleotide polymorphism (SNP) in the tumor necrosis factor (TNF) α gene and elevated serum levels of TNFα in CVID patients with granulomas suggested that this cytokine may be involved in these pathologic lesions. Non-caseating lung granulomas are sometimes found along with lymphocytic interstitial infiltrates and follicular bronchitis and bronchiolitis. This pathologic picture, dubbed granulomatous interstitial lung disease (GLID), portends a poor prognosis with survival in one series reduced by 50% versus CVID patients lacking this complication.

Several autoimmune/inflammatory processes have been reported in the gastrointestinal tract of CVID patients. Inflammatory bowel disorders have been reported in 5% of patients including atrophic gastritis, nodular lymphoid hyperplasia, a gluten-insensitive enteropathy, and inflammatory bowel disease (Cunningham-Rundles and Bodian, 1999; Agarwal and Cunningham-Rundles 2009; Ahn and Cunningham-Rundles, 2009; Young et al., 2011). Putative autoimmune liver disorders include biliary cirrhosis and hepatitis (Cunningham-Rundles and Bodian, 1999; Agarwal and Cunningham-Rundles 2009; Ahn and Cunningham-Rundles, 2009; Young et al., 2011). Nodular regenerative hyperplasia (NRH) is the most common pathologic liver condition and is typically associated with cholestasis and in some series significant portal hypertension (Ward et al., 2008; Malamut et al., 2008). Histologic analysis reveals small, hyperplastic nodules in the liver parenchyma in the absence of fibrous septa around the nodules. When lymphocytic infiltrates are seen, they are predominated by CD8$^+$ T cells raising the possibility that T cell-mediated cytotoxicity somehow contributes to the pathological picture (Malamut et al., 2008). Patients with NRH were found to have a higher incidence of lymphoproliferation, granuloma, enteropathy, or cytopenias (Ward et al., 2008; Malamut et al., 2008).

Much attention has been focused on the mechanisms responsible for immune dysregulation in CVID patients. Many abnormalities in phenotype and function of B cells, T cells, and innate immunity have been reported and some track with the appearance of autoimmune disease possibly serving as biomarkers and/or pathogenic factors (Ahn and Cunningham-Rundles, 2009; Young et al., 2011; Warnatz and Voll, 2012). For example, a more pronounced defect in isotype-switched memory B cells and a decrease in naïve T cells is observed in CVID patients developing autoimmune cytopenias, lymphoid hyperplasia, splenomegaly, granulomatous disease, or chronic enteropathy (Agarwal and Cunningham-Rundles 2009; Ahn and Cunningham-Rundles, 2009). Additional studies indicate that autoimmunity and lymphoproliferation track with increased numbers of activated $CD4^+$ T cells, decreased numbers of Treg cells, and increased percentages ($>20\%$) of $CD21^{low}$ B cells (Warnatz and Voll, 2012). The majority of the latter subset appears to be comprised of mature naïve B cells. In one study, they were found to express unmutated IgM germline genes, which encode largely polyspecific autoreactivity to targets such as nuclear and cytoplasmic components, insulin, and lipopolysaccharide (Isnardi et al., 2010). However, it remains unclear whether or how the expanded $CD21^{low}$ B cell subset relates to the development of autoimmunity in CVID. They have the phenotypic and functional properties of anergic B cells and their specificities are directed at autoantigens that are not targets in patients with CVID (Isnardi et al., 2010).

Genetic defects have been demonstrated in approximately 10−15% of CVID (Young et al., 2011). These include mutations in a number of B cell signaling or survival molecules including transmembrane activator and calcium-modulating ligand interactor (TACI), the inducible costimulator (ICOS), BAFF, C19, and CD20. Those with TACI deficiency (7−10%) would appear to be particularly informative since this mutated gene is clearly associated with the development of autoimmune disease, lymphoid hyperplasia, and splenomegaly in addition to antibody deficiency and recurrent infections (Young et al., 2011). Heterozygosity for TACI C104R, one of the most common TACI mutations, appeared to show the strongest association. However, family members and rare healthy control subjects who lacked immune abnormalities shared the same heterozygous mutations (Young et al., 2011). This finding clearly suggests that other, presumably environmental and/or epigenetic, factors interact to promote the CVID clinical phenotype. Moreover, patients with homozygous TACI deficiency have less severe disease compared to patients with heterozygous TACI deficiency. This observation has spawned the hypothesis that monoallelic TACI deficiency may permit the survival of autoreactive B cell clones (Young et al., 2011). Nevertheless, homozygous TACI deficient mice develop a fulminant autoimmune syndrome, lymphadenopathy, splenomegaly, and lymphoma; findings consistent with TACI contributing to immune homeostasis. Recently, a genome-wide population-based study of CVID patients revealed an association between organ-specific autoimmunity and SNX31, a nexin possibly involved in protein sorting. Of interest SNX protein subunits are required for CD28-mediated costimulation of T cells but the biologic

significance of this association remains to be determined (Orange et al., 2011).

Another study suggested that protein tyrosine phosphatase nonreceptor type 22 (*PTPN22*) gene is linked to the development of autoimmunity in CVID (Chew et al., 2013). The *PTPN22*; R620W SNP was found with increased frequency in CVID, particularly in patients with coexistent autoimmune disease. This is of great interest since this SNP exhibits one of the strongest and most consistent associations with sporadic autoimmune diseases. Accordingly, this finding is consistent with the proposition that autoimmunity arises through a similar mechanism in patients with and without CVID. In the latter, it has been hypothesized that the associated SNP may promote the development of autoimmunity by interfering with the central deletion of autoreactive cells or the emergence of Tregs.

Two other possible mechanisms contributing to the autoimmunity seen in CVID, as yet not studied, relate to the function of B cells seen in the peripheral tissues of CVID patients. It is known that normal B cells, when activated, can secrete a myriad of cytokines including those with proinflammatory activity, e.g., IL-6 and TNFα. Thus, it is possible that B cells in CVID patients with autoimmunity and/or non-infectious inflammatory processes may contribute to the associated pathology by secreting large amounts of these molecules in the absence of sufficient counter-regulation. In addition, it is also known that a small subset/s of B cells with regulatory function contributes to immune homeostasis and suppression of inflammatory and autoimmune processes (see discussion under X-linked agammaglobulinemia). However, it is not known whether the function of these B cells is preserved in CVID patients.

Selective IgA Deficiency

Selective IgA deficiency is the most common primary immune deficiency affecting humans defined solely on the basis of serum immunoglobulin levels (Geha et al., 2007). To qualify for the diagnosis, patients must be older than 4 years and have a serum IgA of <7 mg/dl in the absence of deficits of other Ig isotypes and definable immune deficiencies. The prevalence of selective IgA deficiency varies across studied ethnic populations with a high of 1:143 on the Arabian Peninsula to a low of 1:18:500 in Japan. In the USA, the range is 1:223−1:1000 in community studies. There is considerable variability in clinical presentation with the majority of patients reported as being asymptomatic. The most common clinical manifestation occurring in the roughly 10−15% symptomatic patients is recurrent sinopulmonary infections caused by encapsulated bacteria (Geha et al., 2007). IgA deficient patients are also considered to have an increased frequency of allergic disorders and this is particularly true in younger patients (4–32 years of age) where a prevalence of 84% was reported in one study.

There is an increased prevalence of autoimmune disorders in selective IgA deficient patients with ITP occurring most commonly (Edwards et al., 2004; Jacob et al., 2008). Additional autoimmune associations include juvenile idiopathic arthritis (JIA), thyroiditis, Henoch–Schonlein purpura, type 1 diabetes mellitus, SLE, and serological positivity for a number of self-antigens including cardiolipin, Jo-1, phosphotidylserine, and collagen despite the absence of clinical pathology. First degree relatives of IgA deficient patients display an increased frequency of autoimmune disorders. In addition, patients are at risk for development of gastrointestinal complications including gluten-sensitive celiac disease caused by IgG autoantibodies specific for gliadin, tissue transglutaminase, or endomyosial proteins; lactose intolerance; nodular lymphoid hyperplasia; giardiasis; malabsorption; chronic active hepatitis; and ulcerative colitis.

The pathogenesis of IgA deficiency remains obscure in that patients have immature B cells that express surface IgA as well as IgM and IgD, but fail to differentiate into IgA secreting plasma cells (Conley and Cooper, 1981). Whereas some investigators have provided evidence of an intrinsic B cell defect, others have reported impaired IgA-specific T cell help mediated by a variety of cytokines including TGF-β, IL-4, IL-6, IL-7, IL-10, and IL-21 (Yel, 2010). These heterogeneous results create a murky picture concerning the relative importance of individual cytokines in human B cell IgA isotype switch and/or IgA secretion by IgA deficient B cells. The variation in results likely reflects differences in the *in vitro* culture techniques as well as cells studied.

No single genetic defect has been reported in IgA deficient patients although a small number of TACI deficient patients have been found with selective IgA deficiency (Castigli et al., 2005). Indeed the same TACI mutation has been found in IgA deficient patients and patients with CVID. Some patients with IgA deficiency progress to developing full-blown CVID, adding support to the contention that both disorders fall along a continuum of the same overarching PID (Aghamohammadi et al., 2008). Further support for this argument is the observation that both IgA deficiency and CVID are associated with the same common extended MHC haplotype, HLA A1, B8, DR3, and DQ2 (Mohammadi et al., 2010).

The basis of the association of this PID and autoimmunity has yet to be elucidated, although several hypotheses have been entertained. It has been posited that absent IgA results in enhanced absorption of exogenous substances at mucosal barriers, particularly in the gastrointestinal tract, that are cross-reactive with self-antigens and breach immunological tolerance to self (Cristina et al.,

2008). Such exogenous antigens may include foods and viruses. This hypothesis presupposes that additional factors must conspire to promote the development of autoimmune reactions. An alternative hypothesis relies on the knowledge that monomeric IgA, the molecular form in serum, can exert anti-inflammatory activity (Castigli et al., 2005). Once bound to Fcα receptors on phagocytic cells, IgA recruits the inhibitory tyrosine phosphatase, SHP-1, leading to a downregulation of the cellular responses mediated by activating heterologous Fcγ receptors that have been engaged by IgG-containing immune complexes. Accordingly, inflammation mediated by such heterologous activating Fc receptors would be expected to be exaggerated in IgA deficiency.

Yet another possible mechanism derives from our understanding of the important role played by TGF-β in B cell IgA isotype switch and production of IgA (Stavnezer, 1995; Cazac and Roes, 2000) and the induction and/or maintenance of immunologic tolerance (Wan and Flavell, 2008). TGF-β provides essential signals for the early induction of IgA isotype switch recombination and development of IgA secreting plasma cells in both mouse and human B cells. Interestingly, TGF-β deficient mice show a partial block in IgA production and develop a multifocal inflammatory disease with clinical autoimmune features and the production of autoantibodies. Moreover, inhibition of TGF-β expression in T cells leads to a similar but somewhat less severe autoimmune phenotype. Furthermore, mice whose TGF-β type II receptors were conditionally knocked out on their B cells developed B cell hyperplasia in Peyer's patches, elevated serum immunoglobulins, exaggerated IgG responses to a weak immunogen, anti-DNA antibodies, and an almost complete absence of serum IgA (Cazac and Roes, 2000). Finally, it is well accepted that TGF-β is a critical player in the development and maintenance of oral tolerance. Antigens delivered via the gastrointestinal tract lead to the development of CD4$^+$ Th3 regulatory cells whose suppressive activity is mediated by secreting TGF-β (Faria and Weiner, 2005). Taken together, the above findings raise the theoretical possibility that an impaired TGF-β/TGF-β type II receptor signaling apparatus might contribute to the development of not only IgA deficiency but also autoimmune complications.

Immunodeficiency with Hyper-IgM Syndrome

Immunodeficiency with hyper-IgM (HIGM) syndrome is a heterogeneous group of disorders caused by defects in genes that are critically involved in immunoglobulin B cell isotype switch recombination and somatic hypermutation (Notarangelo et al., 2006; Jesus et al., 2008). These include genes encoding CD40L and CD40, two cell surface proteins involved in cognate T cell/B cell and antigen presenting cell (APC) interactions as well as other genes that encode enzymes, which mediate the process of isotype class switch recombination and somatic hypermutation of B cells. These latter disorders are B cell-specific defects involving either activation-induced cytidine deaminase (AID) or uracil DNA glycosylase (UNG). The serological hallmark of all of these disorders is a normal to increased serum level of IgM in the face of decreased levels of IgG, IgA, and IgE.

X-linked CD40L deficiency is the most common of these disorders (65–70%) and manifests clinically with recurrent pyogenic infections as well as with an increased risk of infections with certain viruses, fungi, and parasites, most notably *Pneumocystis jiroveci* and *Cryptosporidium* species (Notarangelo et al., 2006; Jesus et al., 2008). In addition, a substantial number of patients develop autoimmune disorders (Jesus et al., 2008). In particular autoimmune neutropenia occurs in up to 50% of patients, which may be complicated by oral ulcers. Patients are also at risk for developing AIHA, severe biliary tract disease (ascending cholangitis) associated with *Cryptosporidia* infections, as well as gastrointestinal tract malignancies. The rare form of hyper-IgM associated with an autosomal recessive CD40 deficiency recapitulates the clinical phenotype of CD40L deficiency.

A review of the function of CD40L, a member of the TNF superfamily, provides a context for understanding these seemingly unrelated clinical phenotypes (Jesus et al., 2008). It is expressed transiently on activated T cells and interacts with its counter-receptor, CD40, on B cells, dendritic cells, and macrophages. The engagement on B cells is a critical proximal step in the isotype switch of naïve B cells following their encounter with T-dependent antigens. This cognate interaction initiates the activation of a number of downstream signaling molecules including TNF receptor-associated factor 2 (TRAF2), TRAF3, and TRAF6, which leads to the activation and nuclear translocation of nuclear factor-κB (NF-κB) and the expression of the genes *AID* and *UNG* triggering isotype class switch. In the absence of CD40L, patients have low serum IgA and IgG levels, normal to elevated levels of IgM, and show impaired IgG antibody responses to T-dependent antigens together with a marked reduction of circulating isotype-switched memory B cells. Lymph nodes show primary lymphoid follicles that are devoid of germinal centers. The engagement of CD40 molecules expressed on B cells, macrophages, and dendritic cells is required for the upregulation of CD80/CD86 on these populations of APCs. The interaction of these costimulatory molecules with CD28 on the collaborating T cells leads to full T cell activation and promotes their survival. Thus, it is not surprising that X-linked CD40L

deficient patients experience opportunistic infections and develop malignancies in tissues infected by the prototypical organisms.

Deficiency of UNG (5%) and AID (10%) represent autosomal forms with an infectious phenotype consisting of recurrent sinopulmonary infections with encapsulated bacteria but without opportunistic infections (Jesus et al., 2008). AID deficient patients typically present with enlarged tonsils and lymph nodes presumably related to expansion of the B cells attempting to undergo class switch as evidenced by massive germinal center expansion. Patients with UNG deficiency clinically resemble those with AID deficiency.

Two additional gene defects have more recently been associated with a hyper-IgM serological picture. Both genes are essential for activation and translocation of NF-κB to the nucleus, resulting in activation of AID and UNG. A hypomorphic mutation in one of these genes, NF-κB essential modulator (*NEMO/IKKG*), affects males who present with hypogammaglobulinemia (Jesus et al., 2008). The phenotype is varied and includes HIGM serologic findings (~25%), hypohydrotic ectodermal dysplasia (~75%), lymphedema (<5%), pyogenic infections (~85%), mycobacterial infections (~40%), and serious viral infections (~20%). These patients also develop a range of inflammatory and autoimmune conditions. This association suggests that in addition to defective host defense there is also some degree of immune dysregulation in this disorder. A defect in a second molecule, IκBα, involved in the same pathway, may also lead to the development of a HIGM phenotype (Jesus et al., 2008). Approximately 25% of patients presenting with an HIGM phenotype have no discernible genetic defects.

HIGM patients with any of the associated gene defects have a proclivity for developing autoimmune diseases (Jesus et al., 2008). This association has been best characterized in X-HIGM patients where the largest surveys have shown that substantial numbers of patients have suffered from neutropenia, ITP, AIHA, inflammatory bowel disease, and seronegative arthritis (Levy et al., 1997; Winkelstein et al., 2003). However, autoimmune disorders including ITP, AIHA, type 1 diabetes, hepatitis, seronegative polyarthritis, inflammatory bowel disease, uveitis, and the appearance of IgM autoantibodies have also been reported in 20–25% of patients with AID deficiency (Quartier et al., 2004; Durandy et al., 2005). Similarly, inflammatory and autoimmune disorders including inflammatory bowel disease, arthritis, and AIHA have been described in patients with NEMO deficiency (Orange et al., 2005).

Several mechanisms pertaining to immunologic tolerance induction and maintenance may account for autoimmune disorders in these patients (Jesus et al., 2008). The CD40L–CD40 interaction in the thymus appears to be important in the selection of the T cell repertoire as CD40L is expressed on developing thymocytes and CD40 is constitutively expressed on thymic APCs including B cells, dendritic cells, and cortical and medullary epithelial cells. Mouse models have provided evidence that the CD40L–CD40 interaction is not only important for negative selection of autoreactive T cells but also for the development of Treg1 cells and the negative selection of peripheral autoreactive B cells. Humans with CD40L deficiency appear to have intact central tolerance in the bone marrow but impaired peripheral B cell tolerance. In addition they have been reported to have a reduced frequency of $CD25^+FOXP3^+$ Treg cells compared to healthy control subjects. Finally, serum levels of BAFF, a molecule that promotes B cell survival, are increased in X-linked CD40L deficiency, offering another factor that might contribute to the expression of B cell autoimmunity.

INNATE IMMUNE DEFECTS

Chronic Granulomatous Disease

Chronic granulomatous disease (CGD) includes a group of genetic defects affecting the nicotinamide adenine dinucleotide phosphate (NADPH) oxidase system in neutrophils (and other cells) that results in recurrent bacterial and fungal infections. NADPH oxidase is the enzyme complex that produces superoxide and other reactive oxygen species upon neutrophil ingestion of microbes required for killing a variety of bacteria and fungi. This disorder is also characterized by dysregulated inflammation resulting in an inflammatory process that typically affects the gastrointestinal and genitourinary tracts often producing strictures (Rosenzweig, 2008; Kang et al., 2011). In addition, these patients may develop wound dehiscence and an inflammatory bowel disease that resembles Crohn's disease. The latter condition can be seen in upwards of 25% of CGD patients and in rare instances is the initial clinical presentation for CGD (Rosenzweig, 2008; Kang et al., 2011). The histology of the gastrointestinal (GI) lesions in CGD differs from Crohn's disease with the development of well-defined granulomata that are surrounded by dense lymphocytic infiltrates. CGD patients may also develop chorioretinal lesions that appear as asymptomatic "punch-out" retinal scars localized along retinal vessels. The mechanism underlying the increased inflammatory responses is unknown and has been observed more commonly in CGD patients with defects in the membrane bound components of NADPH oxidase (gp91phox, p22phox) that are generally associated with a greater degree of compromised NADPH oxidase function. This suggests that the oxidase pathway is not only involved in host protection but also

in controlling inflammation. However, the actual explanation for the inflammatory responses is more complicated since X-linked carriers of CGD, who show mosaicism in their neutrophils, are at increased risk for discoid lupus, oral ulcers, and other evidence of immune dysregulation, whereas the majority of carriers do not have an increased risk for infections.

Early Complement Component Deficiency

Humans with congenital deficiency of C1q, C1r/C1s, C4, or C2 are at an increased risk of developing autoimmune disease, particularly SLE (Barilla-LaBarca and Atkinson, 2003). Indeed, individuals deficient in C1q, C4, or C2 have a 90%, 75%, and 20% chance of developing SLE, respectively. Patients homozygous for C1q or C1r/s deficiency are typically younger than 20 years of age when they present predominantly with cutaneous and renal manifestations of SLE. The vast majority of patients are ANA positive with specificity for extractable nuclear antigen but anti-dsDNA antibodies are usually not detectable. Similarly, patients with homozygous C4 deficiency also present with a lupus-like disease with cutaneous manifestations and glomerulonephritis, albeit milder than in C1q deficiency. Positive ANAs are found in approximately 75% of these patients with anti-Ro and anti-La specificities being most commonly detected. Homozygous (but not heterozygous) C2 deficiency is associated in 10–20% incidence of SLE typically a milder form involving cutaneous and renal manifestations with positive ANAs associated predominantly with anti-Ro antibodies. In contrast, C3 deficiency typically manifests with recurrent bacterial infections, but there is also an increased risk of autoimmune disease including SLE-like disease and membranoproliferative glomerulonephritis. Taken together, these observations underscore the importance of the early components of the classical complement pathway in the induction and/or the maintenance of B cell tolerance or control of the inflammatory process. This relationship appeared quite paradoxical since the classical complement cascade had historically been considered to be necessary for the expression of the clinicopathologic features seen in immune complex-mediated diseases like SLE.

Transgenic mouse studies reported in the late 1990s provided a possible explanation, suggesting immature B cells encountering low levels of soluble antigen develop tolerance via anergy (Gommerman and Carroll, 2000). By contrast, immature B cells encountering membrane bound antigen were deleted. Using an adaptation of this transgenic approach, investigators discovered that the induction and maintenance of B cell anergy to a soluble selfprotein required the expression of the proteins CD21/CD35 on the surface of self-reactive B cells and the protein C4. In the mouse, one gene (*Cr2*) encodes both

CD35 (Cr1) and CD21 (Cr2), whereas in humans there are two genes: one coding for CR1 (CR1) and another for CR2 (CR2). Thus, mice deficient in CD21/CD35 would lack both Cr1, which binds C4b and C3b, and Cr2, which binds iC3b and C3d,g (Erdei et al., 2009). Furthermore, the absence of these complement receptors and the C4 protein, but not C3, in a mouse strain genetically prone to develop a lupus-like disease produced increased anti-double-stranded DNA antibodies and resulted in a more highly expressed immune complex-mediated glomerulonephritis (Gommerman and Carroll, 2000). Taken together, these results implicated CD21/CD35 and C4 in the development and the maintenance of B cell immunological tolerance to self-proteins. However, results of a later study conducted in $C1q^{-/-}$ mice provided conflicting results (Cutler et al., 2001). Thus, if the early complement components do indeed promote B cell self-tolerance, it is presumed that their silencing function is exerted when the self-reactive B cells encounter autoantigen at critical checkpoints in the bone marrow and peripheral lymphoid compartment, respectively.

A second and perhaps more compelling (but not mutually exclusive) mechanism to account for autoantibody-mediated disease relates to the role played by these molecules in the clearance of immune complexes, apoptotic bodies, and the debris released by cells undergoing apoptosis (Erdei et al., 2009). C4b and C3b are considered to be important in the uptake of immune complexes by phagocytic cells. Thus, it was reasoned that absent C1q, C4, C2, or C3 means more complexes are available to deposit in tissues where they can elicit inflammation. Currently there is more focus on the role played by these complement components, particularly C1q, in the clearance of apoptotic cells/debris. A large body of evidence indicates that such cellular rubbish must be decorated with C1q and other proteins before it can be removed by phagocytic cells like macrophages. Absent this removal, the debris, particularly nucleic acids exposing cryptic epitopes, becomes available to stimulate self-reactive B cells that have escaped self-tolerance, thereby leading to autoimmunity.

The removal of such apoptotic debris by phagocytic cells is critically important for controlling inflammation and possibly even maintaining peripheral self-tolerance. For example, studies have shown that the process of removing apoptotic neutrophils by macrophages at sites of inflammation, referred to as efferocytosis, is critical for the resolution of the inflammatory process (Bratton and Henson, 2011). A by-product of the macrophage ingestion of apoptotic neutrophils is the elaboration of a number of anti-inflammatory molecules including TGF-β, IL-10, VEGF, HGF, and PGE2. As noted above, C1q and a number of complement receptors, as well as a number of other molecules, promote tethering of apoptotic

neutrophils to their refuse collectors. The release of TGF-β by macrophages and immature dendritic cells may have yet another related effect, on orchestrating suppression of inflammatory reactions. For example, the uptake of apoptotic T cells by macrophages and immature dendritic cells was reported to lead to the production of TGF-β, which in turn induced the development of adaptive Tregs (Perruche et al., 2008). Although it remains to be determined whether early complement components are essential for the efferocytosis of apoptotic T cells or neutrophils, there is emerging evidence that complement contributes to the control of inflammation induced by self-antigens.

Toll-Like Receptor 3 (TLR3) Polymorphism and Autoimmunity

A recent report identifies that a particular variant of TLR3 (l412F) is associated with mucocutaneous candidiasis, increased susceptibility to cytomegalovirus, and autoimmunity. The autoimmune phenomena include endocrinopathies, autoimmune cytopenias, alopecia, vitiligo, arthritis, and enteritis (Nahum et al., 2012). This variant appears to diminish TLR3 mediated NF-κB activation by its natural ligand, double-stranded RNA, as well as the synthetic ligand poly I:C. The exact basis for the increase in autoimmunity is currently under investigation but is another example of specific immune dysfunction being linked to autoimmune processes.

MONOGENIC DEFECTS AFFECTING IMMUNE HOMEOSTASIS AND/OR TOLERANCE

Autoimmune Polyendocrinopathy, Candidiasis, Ectodermal Dystrophy

Autoimmune polyedocrinopathy, candidiasis, ectodermal dystrophy (APECED), also referred to as autoimmune polyendocrinopathy syndrome type 1 (APS1), is a human disorder affecting the immune system that typically presents with a triad of findings including hypoparathyroidism, adrenal insufficiency, and mucocutaneous candidiasis (CMC). Additional autoimmune features may include gonadal failure, hepatitis, type 1 diabetes, celiac disease, pernicious anemia, keratitis, vitiligo, and others. These patients also present with ectodermal dystrophy that most commonly presents as nail dystrophy.

APECED is an autosomal recessive disorder caused by mutations in the gene encoding the autoimmune regulator (AIRE) protein. There is a higher incidence of APECED in certain populations including Iranian Jews (1:9000), Sardinians (1:14,000), and Finns (1:25,000) with lower prevalence in Slovenia (1:43,000), Norway (1:80,000), and Poland (1:129,000) (Kisand and Peterson, 2011). In these settings there tend to be predominantly specific *AIRE* mutations. Importantly, the same mutation in different patients can present with varied clinical phenotypes, pointing out that additional factors impact on the clinical presentation. The AIRE protein is a transcription factor that is involved in the ectopic expression of a wide array of tissue-specific autoantigens by the medullary thymic epithelial cells (mTECs) (Rucci et al., 2011). The expression of autoantigens by the mTECs is critical in the negative selection of antigen-specific autoreactive T cells within the thymic medulla. It is now known that AIRE protein is also expressed in peripheral lymphoid tissue with the specific role played by AIRE in the periphery related to self-tolerance currently being investigated (Poliani et al., 2010). AIRE also appears to play a role in Treg cell development and studies in APECED patients have identified a decrease in forkhead box P3 protein (FOXP3) expression together with diminished *in vitro* suppressive capacity of circulating Treg cells (Laakso et al., 2010). It is clear that in APECED patients many of the autoimmune disorders are accompanied by the production of autoantibodies that in some cases may be linked to disease and in others simply serve as biomarkers of disease. Recently, the explanation for CMC in this disorder was linked to the development of high affinity, neutralizing autoantibodies to IL17A and IL-22 (Puel et al., 2010). This finding was noted in all APECED patients evaluated but was not detected in any other conditions tested. This finding fits well with prior descriptions of autoantibodies to another cytokine (α-interferon) found in the majority of these patients. The finding of the neutralizing anticytokine antibody establishes a new paradigm with an autoantibody inhibiting the activity of a critical cytokine resulting in the development of a specific host defense defect. This type of autoimmune process (i.e., anticytokine autoantibody) has also been linked to susceptibility to non-tuberculous mycobacterial infections associated with high titer, neutralizing autoantibodies to gamma interferon.

Immunodysregulation, Polyendocrinopathy, Enteropathy X-Linked

Immunodysregulation, polyendocrinopathy, enteropathy, X-linked (IPEX) syndrome is a severe disorder of immune function presenting during infancy with a clinical triad of enteritis, endocrinopathy, and dermatitis (Ochs et al., 2007; D'Hennezel et al., 2012). The GI disease produces intractable diarrhea and malabsorption causing failure to thrive. The histopathology of the enteropathy includes villous atrophy and lymphocytic infiltration of the mucosa.

The endocrinopathy typically presents as insulin-dependent type 1 diabetes mellitus and the dermatitis is a generalized eczematous-like rash. Additional autoimmune features include cytopenias, thyroid disease, renal disease, and hepatitis. Immunologic laboratory findings include eosinophilia and hypergammaglobulinemia including elevation of serum IgE, as well as the presence of a variety of autoantibodies (Tsuda et al., 2010). Early recognition of this syndrome is crucial as mortality is extremely high without therapy, which initially consists of aggressive immunosuppression to control the autoreactivity followed by hematopoietic stem cell transplantation to provide curative immune reconstitution and a source of Tregs.

The underlying genetic basis for IPEX is an X-linked recessive defect in the gene encoding FOXP3, a member of the forkhead/winged helix family of transcription factors located at Xp11.23. There have been a wide range of mutations found including single base substitutions, deletions, and splicing mutations. Defective FOXP3 expression leads to a defect in Treg cell production and this is reflected by the virtual absence of circulating CD4$^+$/CD25$^+$/FOXP3$^+$ T cells in these patients.

Confirmation that the underlying immunopathology of IPEX is related to the mutation in FOXP3 and the absence of Treg cells is supported by a murine model, the scurfy mouse. This mouse carries a mutated *foxp3 gene* and has a constellation of autoimmune disorders similar to patients with IPEX. In addition, these mice, similar to IPEX patients, demonstrate markedly impaired Treg cell development. In this model, the autoimmunity can be prevented by correcting the *foxp3* defect in the scurfy mouse using retroviral vector-based gene therapy and the same autoimmune syndrome can be created by artificially knocking down foxp3 expression in otherwise normal strains. The actual mechanism(s) mediating the immunosuppressive activity of Treg cells in humans is not fully understood although it appears to involve both inhibition by cell—cell contact and the secretion of immunomodulatory cytokines including TGF-β and IL-10. The consistently targeted organs in the IPEX syndrome suggest that Treg cell function is particularly important in developing and maintaining self-tolerance in the GI tract, (selected) endocrine organs, blood cells, and skin. However, owing to the severity of this syndrome, it is unclear if autoimmunity to other target organs could arise over time in this patient population.

There are two additional genetic defects that present with clinical findings that include significant phenotypic overlap with IPEX. The first involves an autosomal recessive defect in the gene encoding the CD25 protein, a component of the IL-2 receptor heterotrimer (IL-2 receptor alpha chain). In this disorder, patients not only have an autoimmune phenotype that resembles IPEX but also develop an SCID-like picture with early onset of opportunistic infections (Claudy et al., 2007). Findings in the murine model of CD25 deficiency suggest that Treg cell development is normal but the survival, maintenance, and competitive fitness of these cells is defective due to the absence of IL-2 signaling associated with the defective IL-2 receptor. The second overlap syndrome is an autosomal recessive disorder that involves mutations in the gene encoding STAT5B. In this disorder the patients also have an IPEX-like clinical picture together with a marked immune deficiency and growth hormone resistant dwarfism (Bernaconi et al., 2006). These patients typically present with additional distinct clinical findings including a prominent forehead, a saddle nose, and a high pitched voice. The underlying basis for this disorder is the requirement of STAT5B for effective signaling by IL-2 as well as by growth hormone. Studies in these very rare patients have demonstrated decreased numbers of circulating Treg cells that expressed diminished levels of FOXP3 and were functionally ineffective when tested *in vitro*.

Autoimmune Lymphoproliferative Syndrome

The autoimmune lymphoproliferative syndrome (ALPS) is a human disorder associated with a triad of findings that includes lymphoproliferation, increased alpha-beta TcR double negative T cells, and abnormal lymphocyte apoptosis (Oliveira et al., 2010). Clinically, ALPS patients have a high incidence of autoimmune cytopenias and a substantially increased risk for the development of non-Hodgkin and Hodgkin lymphoma. The typical course of disease in ALPS patients begins during childhood with the development of nonmalignant lymphadenopathy and splenomegaly. In many of the patients the lymphoid accumulation is followed by the development of autoimmunity that is almost exclusively immune-mediated cytopenias, most commonly AIHA and ITP. Some ALPS patients also develop neutropenia and dermatologic findings that can include an urticarial rash. Rare autoimmune findings reported in ALPS include glomerulonephritis, Guillain–Barré syndrome, autoimmune hepatitis, and polyneuropathy. A very significant problem in the most common genetic form of ALPS that is associated with a defect in the *FAS* gene linked to the increased risk for the development of Hodgkin and non-Hodgkin lymphoma (relative risk ~51- and ~14-fold, respectively).

The underlying defect in the majority of ALPS patients is an abnormality in the extrinsic apoptotic pathway linked to defective signaling via the FAS receptor (Lenardo et al., 2010). This homotrimeric receptor is a member of the TNF receptor superfamily and plays a critical role in lymphocyte homeostasis as well as in immune-mediated cytotoxicity following receptor engagement by FAS ligand (FASL). Among patients diagnosed with ALPS, ~65–70% have a heterozygous defect in the *FAS* gene that acts as a

dominant negative mutation in most patients (i.e., is autosomal dominant). These patients are now categorized as ALPS-FAS with the majority having a heterozygous germline mutation. However, more recently it has been appreciated that a significant minority of ALPS-FAS patients have a heterozygous somatic mutation affecting *FAS* (categorized as ALPS-sFAS) that can be detected primarily in the circulating alpha-beta double negative T cells. There are additional, less common genetic causes of ALPS including mutations in the genes encoding FASL (categorized as ALPS-FASL) and caspase-10 (categorized as ALPS-CASP). In addition, there remain ~20% of patients with an ALPS clinical phenotype who do not have a defined genetic defect (categorized as ALPS-U). In all ALPS cases with genetically defined mutations there is a defect in the death inducing signal mediated by FAS. This can be analyzed *in vitro* and the degree of the apoptotic defect varies based on the site of the *FAS* mutation with those affecting exons coding for the intracellular part of the protein generally conferring more severe disease with higher disease penetrance. More recently biomarkers have been identified that are strongly linked with both germline and somatic *FAS* mutations including elevation in soluble FASL, IL-10, and vitamin B12. Combining an elevation in one of these biomarkers with increased alpha-beta double negative T cells yields a greater than 95% likelihood of a *FAS* mutation (either germline or somatic).

The defect in the FAS-dependent extrinsic apoptotic pathway presumably interferes with peripheral tolerance and the normal control of specific autoreactive T cells (and possibly autoreactive B cells). Clearly, based on varied penetrance observed in extended family pedigrees, the *FAS* gene defect requires additional (currently unidentified) factors for the development of clinical disease. This situation is analogous to the murine model of autoimmunity associated with a FAS defect, the *lpr* mouse, where strain variations can significantly impact the degree of autoimmunity. As is seen in other specific genetic defects, the range of autoimmunity in ALPS is quite limited and suggests that the FAS-mediated pathway of tolerance has a more restricted role in controlling self-reactivity and the increased risk of lymphoma in ALPS patients suggests that FAS also serves as a tumor suppressor pathway.

CONCLUSION

Although at one time a perplexing paradox, coexistent autoimmunity and primary immunodeficiency now stand as two sides of the coin of immunologic dysregulation. In most of the monogenic defects that confer a primary B cell, T cell, or combined immunodeficiency, autoimmunity occurs primarily as a consequence of the impairment of one of more critical checkpoints in the development/maintenance of immunologic self-tolerance. This situation is relevant to the development of autoimmunity in certain types of SCID, STIM1 deficiency, DiGeorge syndrome, WAS, IPEX, ALPS, and immunodeficiency with hyper-IgM where various single-mutated genes lead to defects in central T cell silencing and/or peripheral T cell regulation (Table 29.1). By contrast, in APECED, the converse

TABLE 29.1 Autoimmune Manifestations of Select Primary Immunodeficiency Syndromes.

Gene	Disease	Immune Deficiency	Autoimmune/Inflammatory Manifestations	Immunological Defect[a]
T Cell Immune Defects				
RAG1	Leaky SCID	opportunistic infections	cytopenias, erythroderma, hepatitis	Tregs, homeostatic proliferation
RAG-2	Omenn			mTECs/thymic central deletion
Artemis	syndrome			
DNA-ligase4				
Common γ chain				
IL-7R				
ADA				
ZAP70				
RMP complex				
Tbx1	DiGeorge syndrome	opportunistic infections	cytopenias, RA, thyroiditis	ND
WAS	WAS	bacterial and herpes virus infections malignancy	AIHA, neutropenia, vasculitis, IBD, uveitis, type 1 diabetes mellitus	Tregs, intrinsic B cell
Antibody Production Defects				
BTK	XLA	bacterial infections	RA, IBD, scleroderma, alopecia, AIHA, type 1 diabetes	ND
TACI, ?	CVID	bacterial and opportunistic infections	ITP, AIHA, GLILD, hepatitis, biliary cirrhosis, non-gluten sensitive enteropathy, atrophic gastritis, pernicious anemia, IBD, thyroiditis, NLH	ND
?ND	Selective IgA deficiency	bacterial infections	JRA, thyroiditis, Henoch–Schonlein purpura, type 1 diabetes mellitus, SLE, gluten-sensitive enteropathy chronic active hepatitis, NLH, ulcerative colitis	? TGF-β/TGF-β receptor signaling
CD40L	X-HIgM	bacterial, viral and protozoal infections	ITP, AIHA, IBD, seronegative arthritis	? Thymic central deletion ? Peripheral B cell tolerance
Innate Immune Defects				
CYBB	CGD	bacterial and fungal infections	IBD, RA, sarcoidosis, SLE, DLE, ITP, Bechet's syndrome	?efferocytosis, ? Tregs
C1q, C2	Early		SLE, SLE-like disease	Central B cell tolerance, efferocytosis
C4	complement			
C3	component deficiency			
Monogenic Defects of Immune Dysregulation				
AIRE	APS1/APECED	CMC	hypoparathyroidism, adrenal insufficiency, gonadal failure, type 1 diabetes mellitus, hepatitis, celiac disease, pernicious anemia, vitiligo, anti-IL17 autoantibody	Thymic central deletion Tregs
FOXP3	IPEX	recurrent infections	ITP, AIHA, dermatitis, type 1 diabetes mellitus, thyroiditis, nephropathy, hepatitis	Tregs
FAS/FASL/ CASP10	ALPS	lymphadenopathy, increased risk for lymphoma	ITP, AIHA	FAS-mediated extrinsic apoptosis

[a]Immunological defect = defective immune tolerance mechanism.
Abbreviations: SCID, severe combined immunodeficiency; mTEC, medullary thymic epithelial cells; ND, not determined; WAS, Wiskott–Aldrich syndrome; RA, rheumatoid arthritis; AIHA, autoimmune hemolytic anemia; IBD, inflammatory bowel disease; ITP, immune thrombocytopenic purpura; X-HIgM, X-linked immunodeficiency with hyper-IgM; NLH, nodular lymphoid hyperplasia; JRA, juvenile rheumatoid arthritis; GLILD, granulomatous interstitial lung disease; SLE, systemic lupus erythematosus; DLE, discoid lupus erythematosus; CGD, chronic granulomatous disease; APS1, autoimmune polyendocrinopathy type 1; APECED, autoimmune polyendocrinopathy candidiasis, ectodermal dystrophy; CMC, chronic mucocutaneous candidiasis; IPEX, immunodysregulation, polyendocrinopathy, enteropathy X-linked; ALPS, autoimmune lymphoproliferative syndrome; ?, possible.

is true, i.e., autoimmunity conferred by a mutated *AIRE* gene, which impairs central T cell tolerance, leads not only to autoimmunity directed at specific end organs but also to autoimmunity that manifests as immunodeficiency presenting with chronic mucocutaneous candidiasis. Autoimmunity and inflammatory disorders arising from monogenic defects in the innate immune system that cause repeated bacterial infections, like CGD and early complement component deficiency, may be due, in part, to the failure of a principal mechanism for resolving inflammation, namely, the clearance of apoptotic debris and/or other inflammatory regulatory processes. Less clear are the reasons why autoimmunity is a fellow traveler of the two most common primary deficiencies of the adaptive immune system, whose molecular basis is less understood. Both selective IgA deficiency and CVID, which share some genetic origins, feature sizable subsets of patients who are afflicted with autoimmune disorders common to each. Although immunologic defects appear to be more expansive in CVID, immune dysregulation is a feature of both syndromes and may represent the driving force for autoimmunity.

It is important to add that the above formulation is the product of a reductionist approach. All of the primary deficiency disorders discussed are impacted by additional aberrant immune mechanisms to those summarized above. Most importantly, all of these immunodeficiency disorders, even those that are monogenic, can be quite heterogeneous with regard to their clinical phenotype whether or not they are complicated by autoimmunity. Therefore, an understanding of the molecular basis for the nexus between autoimmunity and primary immunodeficiency must await the elucidation of the matrix of factors/mechanisms, which alter gene expression in ways that influence the emergence of these respective clinical phenotypes. At the top of the list are epigenetic mechanisms including DNA methylation, histone modification, and microRNA activity through which such disease modifiers as age, gender, and environmental factors operate. Although study of these epigenetic processes in primary immunodeficiency is in its infancy, it is proceeding at a brisk pace in autoimmunity.

ACKNOWLEDGMENT

This work was supported by the Intramural Research Program of the NIH Clinical Center, National Institutes of Health.

REFERENCES

Agarwal, S., Cunningham-Rundles, C., 2009. Autoimmunity in common variable immunodeficiency. Curr. Allergy Asthma Rep. 9, 347–352.

Aghamohammadi, A., Mohammadi, J., Parvaneh, N., Rezaei, N., Moin, M., Espanol, T., et al., 2008. Progression of selective IgA deficiency to common variable immunodeficiency. Int. Arch. Allergy Immunol. 2008 (147), 87–92.

Ahn, S., Cunningham-Rundles, C., 2009. Role of B cells in common variable immune deficiency. Expert Rev. Clin. Immunol. 5, 557–564.

Barilla-LaBarca, M.L., Atkinson, J.P., 2003. Rheumatic syndromes associated with complement deficiency. Current Opin. Rheumatol. 15, 55–60.

Becker-Herman, S., Meyer-Bahlburg, A., Schwartz, M.A., Jackson, S. W., Hudkins, K.L., Liu, C., et al., 2011. WASP-deficient B cells play a critical, cell-intrinsic role in triggering autoimmunity. J. Exp. Med. 208, 2033–2042.

Bernaconi, A., Marino, R., Ribsa, A., Rossi, J., Ciaccio, M., Oleastro, M., et al., 2006. Characterization of immunodeficiency in a patient with growth hormone insensitivity secondary to a novel STAT5b gene mutation. Pediatrics. 118, 1584–1592.

Bratton, D.L., Henson, P.M., 2011. Neutrophil clearance: when the party is over, clean-up begins. Trends Immunol. 32, 350–357.

Buchbinder, D., Nadeau, K., Nugent, D., 2011. Monozygotic twin pair showing discordant phenotype for X-linked thrombocytopenia and Wiskott–Aldrich syndrome: a role for epigenetics? J. Clin. Immunol. 31, 773–777.

Cassani, B., Poliani, P.L., Moratto, D., Sobacchi, C., Marrella, V., Imperatori, L., et al., 2010. Defect in regulatory T cells in patients with Omenn syndrome. J. Allergy Clin. Immunol. 125, 209–216.

Castigli, E., Wilson, S.A., Garibyan, L., Rachid, R., Bonilla, F., Schneider, L., et al., 2005. TACI is mutant in common variable immunodeficiency and IgA deficiency. Nat. Genet. 37, 829–834.

Cazac, B.B., Roes, J., 2000. TGF-β receptor controls B cell responsiveness and induction of IgA in vivo. Immunity. 13, 443–451.

Chapel, H., Lucas, M., Lee, M., Bjorkander, J., Webster, D., Grimbacher, B., et al., 2008. Common variable immunodeficiency disorders: division into distinct clinical phenotypes. Blood. 112, 277–286.

Chew, G.Y.J., Umang, S., Gatenby, P.A., DeMalmanche, T., Adelstein, S., Garsia, R., et al., 2013. Autoimmunity in primary antibody deficiency is associated with protein tyrosine phosphatase nonreceptor type 22 (PTPN22). J. Allergy Clin. Immunol. 131, 1130–1135.

Claudy, A.A., Reddy, S.T., Chatilla, T., Atkinson, J.P., Verbsky, J.W., 2007. CD25 deficiency causes and immune dysregulation polyendocrinopathy, enteropathy, X-linked-like syndrome, and defective IL-10 expression from CD4 lymphocytes. J. Allergy Clin. Immunol. 119, 482–487.

Conley, M.E., Cooper, M.D., 1981. Immature IgA B cells in IgA-deficient patients. N. Engl. J. Med. 305, 495–497.

Cristina, M., Jacob, A., Pastorino, A.C., et al., 2008. Autoimmunity in IgA deficiency: revisiting the role of IgA as a silent housekeeper. J. Clin. Immunol. 28, 56–61.

Cunningham-Rundles, C., Bodian, C., 1999. Common variable immunodeficiency: clinical and immunological features of 248 patients. Clin. Immunol. 92, 34–48.

Cutler, A.J., Cornall, R.J., Ferry, H, Manderson, A.P., Botto, M., Walport, M.J., 2001. Intact B cell tolerance in the absence of the first component of the classical complement pathway. Eur. J. Immunol. 31, 2087–2093.

De la Salle, H., Zimmer, J., Fricker, D., Angenieux, C., Cazenave, J.P., Okubo, M., et al., 1999. HLA class I deficiencies due to mutations in subunit 1 of the peptide transporter TAP1. J. Clin. Invest. 103, R9—R13.

DeRavin, S.S., Cowen, E.W., Zarember, K.A., Whiting-Theobald, N.L., Kuhns, D.B., Sandler, N.G., et al., 2010. Hypomorphic Rag mutations can cause destructive midline granulomatous disease. Blood. 116, 1263—1271.

Durandy, A., Revy, P., Imai, K., Fischer, A., 2005. Hyper-immunoglobulin M syndromes caused by intrinsic B-lymphocyte defects. Immunol. Rev. 203, 67—79.

D'Hennezel, E., Bin Dhuban, K., Torgerson, T., Piccirillo, C., 2012. The immunogenetics of immune dysregulation, polyendocrinopathy, enteropathy, X-linked (IPEX) syndrome. J. Med. Genet. 49, 291—302.

Edwards, E., Razvi, S., Cunningham-Rundles, C., 2004. IgA deficiency: clinical correlates and responses to pneumococcal vaccine. Clin. Immunol. 111, 93—97.

Erdei, A., Isaak, A., Torok, K., Sándor, N., Kremlitzka, M., Prechl, J., et al., 2009. Expression and role of CR1 and CR2 on B and T lymphocytes under physiological and autoimmune conditions. Mol. Immunol. 46, 2767—2773.

Faria, A.M., Weiner, H.L., 2005. Oral tolerance. Immunol. Rev. 206, 232—259.

Geha, R.S., Notarangelo, L.D., Casanova, J.L., Chapel, H., Conley, M. E., Fischer, A., et al., 2007. Primary immunodeficiency diseases: an update from the International Union of Immunological Societies Primary Immunodeficiency Diseases Classification Committee. J. Allergy Clin. Immunol. 120, 776—794.

Gennery, A.R., 2012. Immunogical aspects of the 22q11.2 deletion syndrome. Cell. Mol. Life Sci. 69, 17—27.

Gommerman, J.L., Carroll, M.C., 2000. Negative selection of B lymphocytes: a novel role for innate immunity. Immunol. Rev. 173, 120—130.

Goyal, R., Bulua, A.C., Nikolov, N.P., Schwartzberg, P.L., Siegel, R.M., 2009. Rheumatologic and autoimmune manifestations of primary immunodeficiency disorders. Curr. Opin. Rheumatol. 21, 78—84.

Howard, V., Greene, J.M., Pahwa, S., Winkelstein, J.A., Boyle, J.M., Kocak, M., et al., 2006. The health status and quality of life of adults with X-linked agammaglobulinemia. Clin. Immunol. 118, 201—208.

Isnardi, I., Ng, Y.S., Menard, L., Meyers, G., Saadoun, D., Srdanovic, I., et al., 2010. Complement receptor 2/CD21 − human naïve B cells contain mostly autoreactive unresponsive clones. Blood. 115, 5026—5036.

Jacob, C.M., Pastorino, A.C., Fahl, K., Carneiro-Sampaio, M., Monteiro, R.C., 2008. Autoimmunity in IgA deficiency: revisiting the role of IgA as a silent housekeeper. J. Clin. Immunol. 28, S56—S61.

Jesus, A., Duarte, A., Oliveira, J., 2008. Autoimmunity in hyper-IgM syndrome. J. Clin. Immunol. 28, S62—S66.

Kang, E.M., Marciano, B.E., DeRavin, S., Zarember, K.A., Holland, S. M., Malech, H.L., 2011. Chronic granulomatous disease: overview and hematopoietic stem cell transplantation. J. Allergy Clin. Immunol. 127, 1319—1326.

Kisand, K., Peterson, P., 2011. Autoimmune polyendocrinopathy candidiasis ectodermal dystrophy: known and novel aspects of the syndrome. Ann. N.Y. Acad. Sci. 1246, 77—91.

Klinker, M.W., Lundy, S.K., 2012. Multiple mechanisms of immune suppression by B lymphocytes. Mol. Med. 18, 123—137.

Koreth, J., Matsuoka, K., Kim, H.T., McDonough, S.M., Bindra, B., Alyea 3rd, E.P., et al., 2011. Interleukin-2 and regulatory T cells in graft-versus-host disease. N. Engl. J. Med. 365, 2055—2066.

Laakso, S.M., Laurinolli, T.T., Rossi, L.H., Lehtoviita, A., Sairanen, H., Perheentupa, J., et al., 2010. Regulatory T cells defect in APECED patients is associated with loss of naïve FOXP3(+) precursors and impaired activated population. J. Autoimmun. 35, 351—357.

Lenardo, M.J., Oliveira, J.B., Zheng, L., Rao, V.K., 2010. ALPS—ten lessons from an international workshop on a genetic disease of apoptosis. Immunity. 26, 291—295.

Levy, J., Espanol-Boren, T., Thomas, C., Fischer, A., Tovo, P., Bordigoni, P., et al., 1997. Clinical spectrum of X-linked hyper-IgM syndrome. J. Pediatr. 131, 47—54.

Malamut, G., Ziol, M., Suarez, F., Beaugrand, M., Viallard, J.F., Lascaux, A.S., et al., 2008. Nodular regenerative hyperplasia: the main liver disease in patients with primary hypogammaglobulinemia and hepatic abnormalities. J. Hepatol. 48, 74—82.

Marangoni, F., Trifari, S., Scaramuzza, S., Panaroni, C., Martino, S., Notarangelo, L.D., et al., 2007. WASP regulates suppressor activity of human and murine CD4 + CD25 + FOXP3 + natural regulatory T cells. J. Exp. Med. 204, 369—380.

Markert, M.L., Alexieff, M.F., Li, J., Sarzotti, M., Ozaki, D.A., Devlin, B.H., et al., 2004. Complete DiGeorge syndrome: development of rash, lymphadenopathy, and oligoclonal T cells in 5 cases. J. Allergy Clin. Immunol. 113, 734—741.

Marrella, V., Maina, V., Vila, A., 2011. Omenn syndrome does not live by V(D)J recombination alone. Curr. Opin. Allergy Clin. Immunol. 11, 525—531.

Mohammadi, J., Mohammadi, J., Ramanujam, R., Rezaei, N., Aghamohammadi, A., Gregersen, P.K., et al., 2010. IgA deficiency and the MHC: assessment of relative risk and microheterogeneity within the HLA A1 B8, DR3 (8.1) haplotype. J. Clin. Immunol. 30, 138—143.

Nahum, A., Dadi, H., Bates, A., Roifman, C.M., 2012. The biological significance of TLR3 variant, L412F, in conferring susceptibility to cutaneous candidiasis, CMV and autoimmunity. Autoimmun. Rev. 11, 341—347.

Niehues, T., Perez-Becker, R., Schuetz, C., 2010. More than just SCID—the phenotypic range of combined immunodeficiencies associated with mutations in the recombinase activating genes (RAG) 1 and 2. Clin. Immunol. 135, 183—192.

Notarangelo, L.D., 2009. Primary immunodeficiencies (PIDs) presenting with cytopenias. Hematology Am. Soc. Hematol. Educ. Program.139—143.

Notarangelo, L.D., Lanzi, G., Peron, S., Durandy, A., 2006. Defects of class switch recombination. J. Allergy Clin. Immunol. 117, 855—864.

Notarangelo, L.D., Miao, C.H., Ochs, H.D., 2008. Wiskott-Aldrich syndrome. Curr. Opin. Hematol. 15, 30—36.

Ochs, H.D., Gambineri, E., Torgerson, T.R., 2007. IPEX, FOXP3 and regulatory T cells: a model for autoimmunity. Immunol. Res. 38, 112—121.

Oliveira, J.B., Bleesing, J.J., Dianzani, U., Fleisher, T.A., Jaffe, E.S., Lenardo, M.J., et al., 2010. Revised diagnostic criteria and classification for the autoimmune lymphoproliferative syndrome (ALPS): report from the 2009 NIH International Workshop. Blood. 116, e35—e40.

Ombrello, M.J., Remmers, E.F., Sun, G., Freeman, A.F., Datta, S., Torabi-Parizi, P., et al., 2011. Cold urticaria, immunodeficiency, and autoimmunity related to PLCG2 deletions. N. Engl. J. Med. 366, 330–338.

Orange, J.S., Levy, O., Geha, R.S., 2005. Human disease resulting from gene mutations that interfere with appropriate nuclear factor-kappaB activation. Immunol. Rev. 203, 21–37.

Orange, J.S., Glessner, J.T., Resnick, E., Sullivan, K.E., Lucas, M., Ferry, B., et al., 2011. Genome-wide association identifies diverse causes of common variable immunodeficiency. J. Allergy Clin. Immunol. 127, 1360–1367.

Perruche, S., Zhang, P., Liu, Y., 2008. CD3-specific antibody-induced immune tolerance involves transforming growth factor-beta from phagocytes digesting apoptotic T cells. Nat. Med. 14, 528–535.

Poliani, P.L., Kisand, K., Marrella, V., Ravanini, M., Notarangelo, L.D., Villa, A., et al., 2010. Human peripheral lymphoid tissues contain autoimmune regulator-expressing dendritic cells. Am. J. Pathol. 176, 1104–1112.

Puel, A., Doffinger, R., Natividad, A., Chrabieh, M., Barcenas-Morales, G., Picard, C., et al., 2010. Autoantibodies against IL-17A, IL17F, and IL-22 in patients with chronic mucocutaneous candidiasis and autoimmune polyendocrine syndrome type I. J. Exp. Med. 207, 291–297.

Quartier, P., Bustamante, J., Sanal, O., Plebani, A., Debré, M., Deville, A., et al., 2004. Clinical, immunologic and genetic analysis of 29 patients with autosomal recessive hyper-IgM syndrome due to activation-induced cytidine deaminase deficiency. Clin. Immunol. 110, 22–29, Erratum in: Clin. Immunol. 113, 220, 2004.

Rosenzweig, S.D., 2008. Inflammatory manifestations in chronic granulomatous disease (CGD). J. Clin. Immunol.(Suppl. 1), S67–S72.

Rucci, F., Poliani, P.L., Caraffi, S., Paganini, T., Fontana, E., Giliani, S., et al., 2011. Abnormalities of thymic stroma may contribute to immune dysregulation in murine models of leaky severe combined immunodeficiency. Front Immunol. 2, ii.

Shaw, P.J., Feske, S., 2012. Regulation of lymphocyte function by ORAI and STIM proteins in infection and autoimmunity. J. Physiol. 590, 4157–4167.

Stavnezer, J., 1995. Regulation of antibody production and class switching by TGF-β. J. Immunol. 154, 1647–1651.

Thrasher, A.J., Burns, S.O., 2010. WASP: a key immunological multitasker. Nat. Rev. Immunol. 10, 182–192.

Tsuda, M, Torgerson, T.R., Selmi, C., 2010. The spectrum of autoantibodies in IPEX syndrome is broad and includes anti-mitochondrial autoantibodies. J. Autoimmun. 35, 265–268.

Tsukada, S., Saffran, D.C., Rawlings, D.J., Parolini, O., Allen, R.C., Klisak, I., et al., 1993. Deficient expression of a B cell cytoplasmic tyrosine kinase in human X-linked agammaglobulinemia. Cell. 72, 279–290.

Verbruggen, G., De Backer., S., Deforce, D., Demetter, P., Cuvelier, C., Veys, E., et al., 2005. X linked agammaglobulinaemia and rheumatoid arthritis. Ann. Rheum. Dis. 64, 1075–1078.

Vetrie, D., Vorechovsky, I., Sideras, P., Holland, J., Davies, A., Flinter, F., et al., 1993. The gene involved in X-linked agammaglobulinaemia is a member of the src family of protein-tyrosine kinases. Nature. 361, 226–233.

Villa, A., Notarangelo, L.D., Roifman, C.M., 2008. Omenn syndrome: inflammation in leaky severe combined immunodeficiency. J. Allergy Clin. Immunol. 122, 1082–1086.

Villa-Forte, A., de la Salle, H., Fricker, D., Fricker, D., Hentges, F., Zimmer, J., 2008. HLA class I deficiency syndrome mimicking Wegener's granulomatosis. Arthritis Rheum. 58, 2579–2582.

Walter, J.E., Rucci, F., Patrizi, L., Recher, M., Regenass, S., Paganini, T., et al., 2010. Expansion of immunoglobulin-secreting cells and defects in B cell tolerance in Rag-dependent immunodeficiency. J. Exp. Med. 207, 1541–1554.

Wan, Y.Y., Flavell, R.A., 2008. TGF-β and regulatory T cell in immunity and autoimmunity. J. Clin. Immunol. 28, 647–659.

Ward, C., Lucas, M., Piris, J., Collier, J., Chapel, H., 2008. Abnormal liver function in common variable immunodeficiency disorders due to nodular regenerative hyperplasia. Clin. Exp. Immunol. 153, 331–337.

Warnatz, K., Voll, R.E., 2012. Pathogenesis of autoimmunity in common variable immunodeficiency. Front Immunol. 3, 1–6.

Winkelstein, J.A., Marino, M.C., Ochs Fuleihan, R., Scholl, P.R., Geha, R., et al., 2003. The X-linked hyper-IgM syndrome: clinical and immunologic features of 79 patients. Medicine (Baltimore). 82, 373–384.

Winkelstein, J.A., Marino, M.C., Lederman, H.M., Jones, S.M., Sullivan, K., Burks, A.W., et al., 2006. X-linked agammaglobulinemia: report on a United States registry of 201 patients. Medicine (Baltimore). 85, 193–202.

Yel, L., 2010. Selective IgA deficiency. J. Clin. Immunol. 30, 10–16.

Young, P.F.K., Thaventhiran, J.E.D., Grimbacher, B., 2011. A rose is a rose but CVID is not CVID: common variable immune deficiency (CVID). What do we know? Adv. Immunol. 11, 47–107.

Zemble, R., Luning Prak, E., McDonald, K., McDonald-McGinn, D., Zackai, E., Sullivan, K., 2010. Secondary immunologic consequences in chromosome 22q11.2 deletion syndrome (DiGeorge syndrome/velocardiofacial syndrome). Clin. Immunol. 136, 409–418.

Part 6

Experimental Models of Autoimmunity

Animal Models: Systemic Autoimmune Diseases

Masayuki Mizui and George C. Tsokos

Division of Rheumatology, Beth Israel Deaconess Medical Center, Harvard Medical School, Boston, MA, USA

Chapter Outline

Introduction   421
Spontaneous Models of Systemic Autoimmunity   421
Genetically Manipulated Models of Systemic Autoimmunity   423
    Lymphocyte Activation Molecules   423
    Ubiquitination-Protein Ligases   424
    Cytokines and their Receptors   425

Complement and Complement Receptor Proteins   426
Clearance of Dead Cells   426
    Innate Immune Cell Signaling   427
Induced Models of Systemic Autoimmunity   427
Concluding Comments   428
References   430

INTRODUCTION

Animal models have greatly facilitated the study of systemic autoimmune diseases, notably systemic lupus erythematosus (SLE) and rheumatoid arthritis (RA), and helped to develop rational new treatments. In addition, autoimmunity-prone mice have served as important tools in the study of genes involved in the expression of autoimmunity and related disease. Genes that facilitate or inhibit disease have been identified and these have in turn facilitated the study on immunogenetics and immunopathogenesis of human systemic autoimmune diseases. The etiology of both SLE (Tsokos, 2011) and RA (McInnes and Schett, 2011) is heterogeneous and complicated, but animal models bring a consistent understanding of disease pathogenesis. Mouse models of systemic autoimmune disease can be grouped into three types: spontaneous, gene manipulation derived, and induced.

SPONTANEOUS MODELS OF SYSTEMIC AUTOIMMUNITY

Commonly studied spontaneous models of lupus include the MRL-Fas$^{lpr/lpr}$ (MRL/*lpr*), (NZBxNZW)F1, and BXSB mice. These murine models that develop SLE spontaneously have generated significant information on the role of hormones (Roubinian et al., 1978; Fernandes

and Talal, 1986; Dhaher et al., 2000; Svenson et al., 2008) and the contribution of aberrant immune regulation (Handwerger et al., 1994) in the expression of the disease. Lastly, they have been used to identify loci that contribute to the genetic pool required for the development of disease (Drake et al., 1995; Reilly and Gilkeson, 2002; Kono and Theofilopoulos, 2006). Gene complementation studies have shed light on the epistatic interactions of genes (Wakeland et al., 1997; Morel and Wakeland, 1998). Candidate genes have been identified including those of the *CD2* family (Wandstrat et al., 2004), the interferon (IFN)-inducible genes (Rozzo et al., 2001), and the complement receptor gene *Cr2* (Boackle et al., 2001). Other studies have pointed to recommendations for novel treatments. For example, it has been shown that introduction of an IFN-α/β receptor null gene into New Zealand Black, H-2$_d$ (NZB) mouse results in decreased production of anti-erythrocytic antibodies (Santiago-Raber et al., 2003). Because IFN-α has been found to be increased in patients with SLE and to promote dendritic cell maturation (Blanco et al., 2001), a case can be made for the construction of biologics to limit the action of type I IFNs in systemic autoimmunity. Moreover, identification of contributing genes and loci in animal models has guided the search for orthologs in humans with systemic autoimmune diseases (Tsao et al., 1997, 2002; Gaffney et al., 1998, 2000; Harley et al., 1998; Moser et al., 1999).

N. Rose & I. Mackay (Eds): The Autoimmune Diseases, Fifth edition. DOI: http://dx.doi.org/10.1016/B978-0-12-384929-8.00030-7

The NZB mouse develops anemia due to anti-erythrocyte antibody. Hybrids with NZW (H-2^z), (NZBxNZW) F1 mice, develop systemic autoimmune disease with high titer of anti-DNA antibodies and severe glomerulonephritis (GN) that becomes apparent at 5–6 months of age. The decreased average lifespan of these mice is 8 months for females and 13 months for males (Vyse et al., 1998; Ibnou-Zekri et al., 1999). Among New Zealand Mixed (NZM) mice generated by (NZBxNZW) F1 and NZW backcross and sib mating, NZM2328 and NZM2410 were found to develop lupus-like disease. Importantly, three lupus susceptibility loci, *Sle1-3*, were identified by the lupus linkage analysis of NZM2410 mice (Morel et al., 1994). From the findings in mice, variations in many genes in these loci have been directly associated with human SLE. *Sle1b* corresponds to polymorphisms in four signaling lymphocytic activation molecule (SLAM) family member genes (Wandstrat et al., 2004), including Ly108, which was directly implicated in the regulation of B cell tolerance (Kumar et al., 2006). Variants of SLAMF3 (Ly9) and SLAMF4 (CD244) have been associated with human SLE and RA (Cunninghame Graham et al., 2008; Suzuki et al., 2008).

The MRL mouse strain was derived from several inbred lines that included LG/J (75%), AKR/J (12.6%), C3H/Dehi (12.1%), and C57BL/6 (0.3%). MRL-Fas$^{lpr/lpr}$ (MRL/lpr) mice, bearing two doses of mutation in the Fas gene, develop accelerated autoimmune disease characterized by severe lymphoadenopathy due to the accumulation of CD3$^+$CD4$^-$CD8$^-$B220$^+$ (double-negative) T cells. Disease onset with severe dermatitis and/or lymphadenopathy is seen from 10 to 12 weeks and death occurs at around 25 weeks. Disease is severe in the female and the average lifespan for female MRL/*lpr* mice is from 17 to 35 weeks depending on the environment. Mice display high concentrations of immunoglobulins including elevated levels of autoantibodies such as antinuclear antibodies (ANA), anti-ssDNA, anti-dsDNA, anti-Sm, and rheumatoid factors (Andrews et al., 1978). B cells and T cells from these mice have a defect in apoptosis due to the lack of functional Fas receptor (Reap et al., 1995). A mutation of Fas ligand gene leads to generalized lymphoproliferative disease (gld) similar to that caused by the *lpr* mutation (Takahashi et al., 1994). In humans, defective Fas signaling can lead to the development of autoimmune lymphoproliferative syndrome (ALPS) which shares many manifestations with SLE. Further study of the intense lymphoproliferation has enabled the identification of genes whose products are central to expression of systemic disease. For example, while deletion of the cyclin-dependent kinase inhibitor p21 does not lead to autoimmunity (Lawson et al., 2002, 2004), transfer of the *p21* null gene into the MRL$^{lpr/lpr}$ mouse results in reduced autoimmune disease by allowing T cell death and decreasing the accumulation of G0/G1 arrested lymphocytes cells (Lawson et al., 2004). Expression of the *lpr* mutation in non-autoimmune strains such as C3H/HeJ and C57BL/6 leads to the development of lymphoproliferation and autoantibody production but limited glomerulonephritis in female mice.

Male only BXSB mice develop severe glomerulonephritis and autoantibodies. The genetic locus responsible for the expression of the disease is located in the Y chromosome and is known as *Yaa* (Y chromosome-accelerated autoimmunity) (Izui et al., 1995). *Yaa* was first identified from a cross between a C57BL/6 female and a SB/Le male that produced the BXSB hybrid line. BXSB mice develop SLE at much higher incidence and with earlier onset in males compared to females, whereas mice from the reciprocal cross (SB/LE female and B6 male) do not show the same acceleration of disease in males. The disease is heavily dependent on the presence of the H-2b allele, because its replacement with the H-2d allele results in prolonged survival. Of interest, the (BXSBxNZW) F1 mouse develops thrombocytopenia and coronary artery disease accompanied by the presence of antiphospholipid antibodies (Kono and Theofilopoulos, 2006). Toll-like receptor 7 (TLR7), a single-stranded RNA-binding innate immune receptor, was identified as a gene responsible for the Y chromosome-linked autoimmune accelerator, as duplication of the *Tlr7* gene in *Yaa*$^+$ mice was shown to be associated with the induction of autoreactive B cells (Pisitkun et al., 2006). Moreover, deletion of the endogenous copy of *Tlr7* from X chromosome abrogates *Yaa*-induced monocytosis, lymphoid activation, splenomegaly, and glomerulonephritis, with decreased mortality (Deane et al., 2007; Santiago-Raber et al., 2008). Consistently, a human allele of the *Tlr7* gene was recently reported to be associated with increased risk for SLE development in males (Shen et al., 2010).

Palmerston North (PN) mice develop spontaneous autoimmunity manifested by the production of multiple autoantibodies, vasculitis, and glomerulonephritis. PN X NZB F1 mice develop more severe disease (Luzina et al., 1999).

Mice homozygous for the *ank* mutation, *Ank/ank* mice, develop early-onset joint ankylosis in the spine and peripheral joints resembling human spondyloarthritis (Krug et al., 1989). The Ank gene encodes a transmembrane protein expressed in joints that controls pyrophosphate levels and may be irrelevant to autoimmunity.

K/BxN T cell receptor mice, a spontaneous mouse model of autoimmune arthritis, generated fortuitously by crossing a TCR transgenic line with the non-obese diabetic (NOD) strain (Monach et al., 2004), spontaneously develop an autoimmune disease with most (although not all) of the clinical, histologic, and immunologic features of RA in humans. The murine disease is critically dependent on both T and B cells and is joint specific, but it is initiated and perpetuated by T and B cell autoreactivity to a ubiquitously expressed antigen, glucose phosphate isomerase (GPI). Transfer of serum (or purified anti-GPI immunoglobulins) from arthritic K/BxN mice into healthy animals regularly provokes arthritis within a few days, even when recipients are devoid of lymphocytes. Complement components, Fc receptors, and mast cells are important for the expression of the disease. The relevance of the K/BxN model to human RA is supported by one report showing that serum from almost two-thirds of patients with RA contain anti-GPI antibodies, which are absent from serum from normal individuals or of patients with Lyme arthritis or Sjögren's syndrome (Matsumoto et al., 2003). However, not all investigators agree. The K/BxN model has been particularly useful in illustrating the role of immune-inflammatory components in the development of arthritis and notably the characterization of the role of mast cells (Lee et al., 2002); yet, this model offers little evidence that autoantibodies are involved in the pathogenesis of RA.

SKG mice spontaneously develop T cell-mediated arthritis due to a mutation of the gene encoding a Src homology 2 (SH2) domain of ζ-associated protein of 70 kDa (ZAP-70), a key signal transduction molecule in T cells. The disturbance in the thymic T cell selection from absence of ZAP-70 results in the generation of arthritogenic T cells. Besides synovitis, SKG mice develop extra-articular lesions, including pneumonitis and vasculitis. Serologically, they develop high levels of rheumatoid factor (Marshall et al., 2003) and autoantibodies specific for type II collagen (Sakaguchi et al., 2003). A molecule termed synoviolin/Hrd1 was found to play a key role in the development of synovitis. This represents an E3 ubiquitin ligase, which, by promoting the growth of synoviovytes, facilitates the development of arthritis. Mice lacking synoviolin are resistant to arthritis (Amano et al., 2003).

Mice that develop spontaneous autoimmunity have helped our understanding of hormonal and immunoregulatory influences in autoimmunity, but obvious restraints limit direct transfer of this information to human disease. Human disease develops in individuals with a permissive genetic background in conjunction with environmental and stressful factors, possibly acting over a long period. However, these murine models allow us to analyze disease mechanisms and are very useful in testing potential therapies. Moreover, analysis of gene-manipulated mice in these genetic backgrounds enable investigators to identify a number of molecules involved in the development of disease pathogenesis. A number of cytokine/cytokine receptor signals are reported to be important for the pathogenesis of SLE, including IFN-γ/IFN-γR (Haas et al.,

1997; Balomenos et al., 1998), IL-6 (Cash et al., 2010), IFNαR (Santiago-Raber et al., 2003), IL-21/IL-21R (Bubier et al., 2009; Herber et al., 2007), and IL-23R (Zhang et al., 2009; Kyttaris et al., 2010). Intracelluar signaling molecules such as phosphoinositide 3-kinase gamma (PI3Kγ) (Barber et al., 2005), mammalian target of rapamycin (mTOR) (Lui et al., 2008), spleen tyrosin kinase (Syk) (Deng et al., 2010; Bahjat et al., 2008), and calmodulin-dependent kinase IV (CaMKIV) (Ichinose et al., 2011) were also identified to be involved in the development of lupus. These molecules could represent therapeutic targets for the treatment of human SLE and numerous clinical trials are currently in progress. What are the trials assessing?

GENETICALLY MANIPULATED MODELS OF SYSTEMIC AUTOIMMUNITY

Loss of tolerance is a fundamental immunologic abnormality in SLE. Numerous studies of mice with genetic manipulation such as gene deletions and transgenes that develop autoantibodies and other features of SLE on non-autoimmune genetic backgrounds have provided great insights into mechanisms that govern tolerance and autoimmunity and suggested novel rational treatments.

Lymphocyte Activation Molecules

Human SLE T cells are known to express less TCR-ζ chain (Liossis et al., 1998) and to use alternative signaling through the FcR-γ chain (Enyedy et al., 2001). Mice that lack the TCR-ζ chain develop autoimmune manifestation and display disturbed positive and negative thymic selection (Yamazaki et al., 1997), and the phenotype can be rescued successfully by introducing the FcR-γ chain (Shores and Love, 1997). The pathophysiology for the murine and human phenotypes may well differ and, although in mice lack of the ζ chain may lead to autoimmunity by altering early thymic events that limit the export of autoimmune T cells, in humans the rewiring of TCR with the newly upregulated FcR-γ chain will lead to increased TCR-mediated signaling processes (Tsokos et al., 2003).

The B7-CD28/CTLA-4 costimulatory pathway is pivotal for T cell activation. Signaling through this pathway is complex due to the presence of at least two B7 family members, CD80 (B7-1) and CD86 (B7-2), and two counter-receptors CD28 and CD152 (CTLA-4). CTLA-4-deficient mice rapidly develop lymphoproliferative disease with multi-organ lymphocyte proliferation and tissue destruction, with particularly severe myocarditis and pancreatitis, and die by 3—4 weeks of age (Tivol et al., 1995; Waterhouse et al., 1995). CTLA4-Ig limits effectively murine lupus (Finck et al., 1994) and the use of CTLA-4-Ig biologics has helped patients with RA (Kremer et al., 2003) and psoriatic arthritis (Abrams et al., 2000).

Programmed death-1 (PD-1) is a member of the CD28 family of receptors and its intracytoplasmic domain defines an immunoreceptor tyrosine-based inhibition motif (ITIM); engagement of PD-1 with its ligands PD-L1 and PD-L2 delivers a negative signal. Mice lacking the PD-1 gene develop either autoantibody-mediated cardiomyopathy in BALB/c (Okazaki et al., 2003) or glomerulonephritis on a C57BL/6 background (Nishimura et al., 2001). PD-1 polymorphism has been identified among SLE patients (Prokunina et al., 2002) and/or RA patients (Lin et al., 2004). PD-L1 deficient mice show accelerated autoimmune inflammation in MRL/MpJ and MRL/*lpr* mice (Lucas et al., 2008).

Src homology 2-containing phosphatase 1 (SHP1) is one of the best-characterized protein tyrosine phosphatases (PTPase). SHP inhibits cell activation through its recruitment by negative regulatory molecules containing ITIM. The homozygous loss of ITIM in mice leads to the "moth-eaten" phenotype characterized by spotty hair loss and abnormalities in the immune system that lead to systemic autoimmunity and skin inflammation (Kozlowski et al., 1993; Tsui et al., 1993; Bignon and Siminovitch, 1994). T lymphocytes from these mice are hyper-responsive to TCR stimulation (Pani et al., 1996). Since neutrophils from moth-eaten mice demonstrate increased oxidant production, surface expression of CD18, and adhesion to protein-coated plastic, the autoimmune phenotype in these mice may not directly reflect lymphocyte aberrations (Kruger et al., 2000). Furthermore, a recent report shows that only B cell specific deletion of SHP1 leads to systemic autoimmune disease (Pao et al., 2007).

Mice with beta1,6 N-acetylglucosaminyltransferase V (Mgat5) deficiency display decreased glycosylation of T cell membrane proteins, which prevents galectin binding and thereby disrupts the galectin−glycoprotein lattice leading to increased clustering of the TCR (Demetriou et al., 2001). Increased TCR clustering in these autoimmune mice provides a phenotype to some degree comparable with human SLE, involving lowered T cell activation thresholds and increased TCR signaling. In the case of T cells in human SLE, increased association of the TCR-ζ chain with lipid rafts, as well as membrane clustering, are claimed to lead to decreased tolerance and abnormal signaling (Nambiar et al., 2002; Krishnan et al., 2004). Thus, defects in the expression and function of glycosylation processes may predispose to autoimmunity and, along the same lines, glycosylation of the transcription factor Elf-1, which enables the 80-kDa form to transform to the DNA-binding 98-kDa form, is defective in human SLE T cells (Juang et al., 2002).

Other lines of evidence suggest T cells from lupus-prone mice that are transgenic for a specific receptor have decreased antigen-initiated T cell stimulation thresholds (Vratsanos et al., 2001; Bouzahzah et al., 2003). A similar concept of an "over-excitable" antigen-initiated proximal lymphocyte signaling phenotype has been proposed for human SLE (Tsokos et al., 2003).

A state of B lymphocyte hyperactivity resembling SLE is seen in mice lacking the src family kinase Lyn. Lyn is an essential inhibitory component on B cell receptor (BCR) signaling. Negative regulation of the BCR is a complex quantitative trait in which Lyn, the co-receptor CD22, and the tyrosine phosphatase SHP-1 are each limiting elements (Cornall et al., 1998). Lyn deficient mice display decreased numbers of mature peripheral B cells, greatly elevated serum IgM and IgA (Bignon and Siminovitch, 1994), and production of autoantibodies that cause autoimmune glomerulonephritis reminiscent of SLE (Chan et al., 1997). Sustained activation of Lyn *in vivo* using a targeted gain-of-function mutation (Lyn$^{up/up}$ mice) led to the development of autoantibodies and lethal autoimmune glomerulonephritis. Interestingly, B cells show a heightened calcium flux in response to BCR stimulation (Hibbs et al., 2002). These data in humans and mice suggest that mechanisms that lead to sustained BCR signaling may override control mechanisms and lead to autoimmunity.

Antigen presented in the context of immune complexes engages not only the BCR but also the FcγRIIb, which results in the phosphorylation of the ITIM defined by its intracytoplasmic domain. Recruitment of the phosphatases SHIP (Src homology 2 domain-containing inositol-5-phosphatase) and SHP1 suppresses signaling. Introduction of the FcγRIIb null phenotype into the C57BL/6 background caused production of autoantibodies and glomerulonephritis (Bolland and Ravetch, 2000) and FcγRIIb deficiency exacerbates autoimmunity in B6/lpr mice (Yajima et al., 2003). Yet the same null phenotype on the BALB/c background did not result in autoimmunity. Although SHIP is considered responsible for FcγRIIb-mediated suppression, the SHIP null phenotype does not result in autoimmunity (Helgason et al., 2000). In humans, polymorphisms of the Fc receptors have been associated with systemic autoimmunity and particularly with SLE, and granulomatous polyangiitis (formerly called Wegener's disease) (Kimberly et al., 1995).

Ubiquitination-Protein Ligases

The Cbl-b and Cbl adaptor proteins are E3 ubiquitin ligases that inhibit receptor and non-receptor tyrosine kinases by promoting ubiquitination (Bachmaier et al., 2000). Loss of Cbl-b rescues reduced calcium mobilization of anergic T cells, which was attributed to Cbl-b-mediated regulation of PLCγ-1 phosphorylation. Loss of Cbl-b in mice results in impaired induction of T cell tolerance both *in vitro* and *in vivo* and shows exacerbated autoimmunity (Jeon et al., 2004). Moreover, mice with B cell-specific deficiency of Cbl/Cbl-b exhibit impairment of anergy to self-antigen and develop lupus-like disease with anti-dsDNA, ANA, massive leukocytic infiltrates in multiple organs, and immune complex GN (Kitaura et al., 2007).

Roquin (Rc3h1), a RING-type ubiquitin ligase family member, was identified as a negative regulator of follicular helper T (Tfh) cell development. This molecule is identified by a novel forward genetic strategy: male C57BL/6 mice were treated with ethylnitrosourea (ENU), a mutagenic agent, bred the variant genome sequences to homozygosity, and progeny were screened for autoimmunity. M199R mutation within the ROQ domain of Roquin was generated by ENU mutagenesis that resulted in ANA, anti-dsDNA, glomerulonephritis, necrotizing hepatitis, anemia, and immune thrombocytopenia (Vinuesa et al., 2005). This mouse displays increased germinal center formation and expansion of memory/effector CD4$^+$ T cells, particularly Tfh cells. Tfh cells have been established as a T helper (Th) cell subset specialized for providing help to B cells in GCs (King et al., 2008). Overpresentation of Tfh cells is associated with the development of systemic autoimmunity (Linterman et al., 2009) and expansion of circulating Tfh-like cells was also detected in human SLE and associated with severe disease (Simpson et al., 2010).

Cytokines and their Receptors

Mice that are deficient in IL-2 and IL-2a have disrupted immunological homeostasis that eventually leads to fatal autoimmune manifestations (Nelson, 2002). Specifically, these mice develop autoimmune hemolytic anemia and colitis with lymphoproliferation, expansion of effector/memory phenotype T cells, polyclonal hypergammaglobulinemia, and autoantibodies. IL-2RB$^{-/-}$ mice likewise develop anemia, splenomegaly and lymphadenopathy, but not colitis. In humans, IL-2 deficiency is clinically manifested as severe combined immunodeficiency, whereas a patient lacking IL-2a was declared immunocompromised, and several organs were infiltrated with inflammatory cells (Sharfe et al., 1997). The autoimmune manifestations depend on the presence of both T and B cells and environmental antigens since, if the mice are kept under pathogen-free conditions, they do not develop autoimmunity. Activation-induced cell death (AICD) is central for the elimination of activated autoreactive cells, and this depends on IL-2 signaling. Defective AICD obviously plays a role in the development of autoimmunity. Humans with SLE have defective AICD that appears to be multifunctional: defective tumor necrosis factor (TNF)-α (Kovacs et al., 1996) and IL-2 production

(Tsokos et al., 1996). The downregulation of IL-2 production in SLE patients was found to be mediated by Ser/Thr protein phosphatase 2A (PP2A). PP2A dephosphorylates transcription factor SP-1, which results in strong binding of cyclic-AMP responsive element modulator (CREM) to the IL-2 promoter (Juang et al., 2011). T cells from patients with SLE have increased PP2A (Katsiari et al., 2005). Overexpression of PP2A in T cells in B6 mice does not lead to autoimmunity but only to granulocytosis and increased levels of IL-17 and, when challenged with an anti-glomerular basement membrane antibody, they developed exuberant glomerulonephritis (Crispin et al., 2012). Furthermore, IL-2 plays a central role in the development and maintenance of regulatory T (Treg) cells, which have been proven to be of pathogenic relevance in the development of autoimmune disease (La Cava, 2008). Low dose IL-2 treatment in patients of chronic GVHD (Koreth et al., 2011) and of hepatitis C virus-induced vasculitis (Saadoun et al., 2011) was reported to be effective with an accompanying increase of Treg cells. Vaccinia virus-mediated *in vivo* IL-2 introduction ameliorates disease progression in MRL/*lpr* mice (Gutierrez-Ramos et al., 1990). These results indicate that correction of IL-2 production could have therapeutic potential by restoring the function of T cells.

The tumor necrosis factor/receptor (TNF/TNFR) system acts on the homeostasis of the immune system in different ways. Among them, TNFSF13B (BAFF, BlyS) and TNFRSF13B (TACI) are implicated in the development of autoimmune disease. BAFF is critical for B cell survival and BAFF-transgenic or TACI-knockout mice show lupus-like disease. Moreover, serum BAFF is elevated in both BWF1 and MRL/*lpr* mice and blocking BAFF function with a soluble TACI-IgGFc protein can inhibit proteinuria and prolong survival (Gross et al., 2000). Surprisingly, T cell deficient BAFF-transgenic mice can develop lupus-like disease indistinguishable from that of BAFF-transgenic mice and the development of disease is dependent on MyD88 (Groom et al., 2007). Clinical trials using the chimeric molecule TACI-Ig (Atacicept) in SLE are now ongoing and the clinical use of anti-BAFF/BlyS (Belimumab) for active SLE patients was recently approved (Navarra et al., 2011).

The successful clinical introduction of treatment with anti-TNFα confirmed the biologic relevance of TNFα function in chronic inflammatory diseases, particularly RA and Crohn's disease. The introduction of a modified human TNF-globin hybrid transgene in mice was the first demonstration in animal models that TNF has arthritogenic properties. These mice (Tg197) spontaneously develop (with 100% penetrance and a predictable time of onset) a chronic, erosive, inflammatory polyarthritis with histologic lesions resembling human RA (Holmdahl et al., 1986; Kontoyiannis et al., 1999). Adenylate uridylate-rich elements (Holmdahl et al., 1986) are important for TNFα mRNA destabilization and translational repression in hematopoietic and stromal cells. Development of two specific pathologies in mutant mice—chronic inflammatory arthritis and colitis akin to Crohn's disease—suggests a defective function in analogous human pathologies. These mice have proven quite informative in dissecting the pleiotropic effects of TNFα on immune responses and on the expression of various forms of autoimmune pathology.

Complement and Complement Receptor Proteins

Activation of the classical pathway typically starts by interaction of C1q with immune complexes and the action of complement is the main effector mechanism of antibody-mediated immunity. The complement system also has an important role in clearing immune complexes from the circulation. It can also bind apoptotic cells and helps to eliminate these cells from tissue (Taylor et al., 2000). If the complement system fails in this function, waste material can accumulate and evoke an autoimmune response. Deficiencies of the classical pathway are associated with an increased risk of developing SLE or allied diseases in human (Manderson et al., 2004). More than 90% of individuals with C1q and C1r/C1s deficiency develop an SLE-like disorder, and 10–20% of individuals with C2 deficiency develop SLE (Truedsson et al., 2007). These phenotypes in humans do not parallel in full those in mice. Deficiency of C1q in C57BL/6 mice does not lead to the development of autoimmunity. By contrast, C1q deficient MRL/MpJ mice display accelerated disease onset and increased levels of ANA and of glomerulonephritis, particularly in females which developed severe crescentic glomerulonephritis. Moreover, C1q deficient mice on a B6x129 genetic background were shown to develop higher levels of autoantibodies compared to strain-matched controls and to develop glomerulonephritis by 8–10 months of age (Manderson et al., 2004). Thus, the expression of autoimmunity in C1q deficient mice is strongly influenced by additional background genes (Botto et al., 1998; Botto and Walport, 2002).

The B6/*lpr* mouse develops minor autoimmune features. Deficiency in this strain of the complement receptor 1 and complement receptor 2 (CR1/CR2, CD35/CD21), encoded by the Cr2 gene, permits development of intense autoimmune features (Boackle and Holers, 2003), indicating that complement receptors are important in the elimination of B cells that display reactivity with self antigens. This explanation assumes that self antigens initiate a strong B cell signal, which leads to B cell death and the absence of the CR2-mediated enhancement of the signal

permits their survival (Tsokos et al., 1990; Dempsey et al., 1996) CR1 and CR2 have been proposed to play a role in the development of SLE. Patients with SLE have around 50% lower levels of these receptors on their B cells (Levy et al., 1992; Marquart et al., 1995). MRL/*lpr* mice exhibit lower levels of these receptors on B cells prior to the onset of overt disease, suggesting that the reduction of CR1/CR2 expression may be pathogenic (Takahashi et al., 1997). Also, evidence for the involvement of Cr2 in systemic autoimmunity comes from the NZM2410 mouse. The congenic interval corresponding to *Sle1c*, one of the SLE susceptibility loci, *Sle1*, contains the Cr2 gene. NZM2410/NZW Cr2 exhibits a single nucleotide polymorphism that introduces a novel glycosylation site, resulting in higher molecular weight proteins. This polymorphism, located in the C3d binding domain, reduces ligand binding and receptor-mediated cell signaling. Molecular modeling based on the CR2 structure in complex with C3d has revealed that this glycosylation interferes with receptor dimerization (Boackle et al., 2001).

Since disruption of the C1q, C4, and CR1/CR2 leads to reduced selection against autoreactive B cells and to impaired humoral responses, C1 and C4 could act through CR1/CR2 to enhance humoral immunity and suppress autoimmunity, but each complement component appears to act independently. High titers of spontaneous ANA and SLE-like autoimmunity develop in all C4$^{-/-}$ mice and most male mice but not in Cr2$^{-/-}$ mice. The fact that the clearance of circulating immune complexes is impaired in pre-autoimmune C4$^{-/-}$ but not Cr2$^{-/-}$ mice favors the role of nuclear antigen–ANA immune complexes in the development of autoimmune disease (Chen et al., 2000).

Clearance of Dead Cells

Effective degradation of nucleotides from dead cells and digestion of cellular components by macrophages allow non-inflammatory clearance and a recycle of dead cells (Nagata et al., 2010). DNaseI is the major nuclease present in the blood, urine, and secretions. DNaseI deficiency in non-autoimmune background mice was reported to increase the incidence of SLE manifestations, including positive ANA, anti-DNA, and immune complex glomerulonephritis (Napirei et al., 2000). Reduced DNaseI activity is observed in the sera of lupus patients, which may contribute to SLE susceptibility (Tsukumo and Yasutomo, 2004). Intriguingly, an identical heterozygous nonsense mutation in DNASE1 was detected in two SLE patients (Yasutomo et al., 2001).

Deficiency in the clearance of apoptotic cells is proposed to be one of the causes of SLE. Unengulfed apoptotic cells are present in the germinal centers of the lymph nodes of some SLE patients and macrophages from these patients often show a reduced ability to engulf apoptotic cells (Gaipl et al., 2006). Milk fat globule-EGF factor 8 (MFG-E8) protein functions as a bridging protein between phosphatidylserine (PS) on apoptotic cells to avb3 or avb5 integrins on phagocytic cells (Hanayama et al., 2002). MFG-E8 is primarily expressed on CD68-positive tingible body macrophages within germinal centers. MFG-E8 deficient female mice on a B6 x129 gene background develop SLE-like autoimmune disease with anti-dsDNA, ANA, and glomerulonephritis by 40 weeks of age (Hanayama et al., 2004).

TAM family members (Tyro3, Axl, and Mer), which are tyrosine kinase receptors expressed on antigen-presenting cells (APCs), promote clearance of apoptotic cells and mice expressing a kinase-dead mutant of Mer (MerKD) develop SLE-like autoimmunity (Scott et al., 2001). TAM receptors negatively regulate the innate immune reaction and TAM-deficient dendritic cells overproduce IL-6, IFN, and TNFα, which might be responsible for the induction of autoimmunity (Lemke and Rothlin, 2008).

Innate Immune Cell Signaling

Recent studies demonstrate that DNA and RNA in apoptotic material can activate B cells and dendritic cells through TLR9, TLR7, and TLR8 (Leadbetter et al., 2002; Boule et al., 2004; Vollmer et al., 2005). As described above, overexpression of TLR7 is responsible for the development of autoimmune diseases in BXSB mice. These results indicate that TLR signaling is linked to the development of autoimmune disease and aberrant activation of innate immunity may contribute to systemic autoimmune diseases including RA and SLE (Marshak-Rothstein, 2006).

TANK (also known as I-TRAF) is a TNF receptor-associated factor (TRAF)-binding protein and binds to TRAF1, 2, 3, 5, and 6, all of which are crucial for TLR signaling. TANK is a negative regulator of proinflammatory cytokine production induced by TLR signaling and TANK deficient mice spontaneously develop lupus-like autoimmune diseases with fatal glomerulonephritis, ANA, and anti-dsDNA. Autoantibody production in TANK deficient mice is abrogated by antibiotic treatment or the absence of IL-6 or MyD88, indicating that TANK controls TLR signaling by intestinal commensal microbiota (Kawagoe et al., 2009).

Zc3h12a is an RNase activated by TLR signaling that promotes the degradation of mRNA. Zc3h12a deficient mice have early mortality associated with severe hemolytic anemia, lymphoproliferation, and ANA with an increased number of activated B cells, T cells, and plasma cells due to excessive cytokine transcription notably IL-6 and IL-12 (Matsushita et al., 2009).

INDUCED MODELS OF SYSTEMIC AUTOIMMUNITY

Information has been acquired over many years from the study of models based on induction of autoimmunity, including immunoregulatory events that lead to the expression of clinical disease and proximal events associated with triggering of autoimmune disease.

The isoprenoid alkane pristane (2, 6, 10, and 14 tetra-methylmentadecane) induces autoantibodies characteristic of SLE, including anti-Sm, anti-dsDNA, and anti-ribosomal P in BALB/c and SJL/J mice and CD1d deficiency exacerbates lupus nephritis induced by pristane (Satoh and Reeves, 1994). Pristane induces type I IFN production from Ly6C^{hi} monocyte through Toll-like receptor 7 (TLR7) and myeloid differentiation factor 88 (MyD88) pathway and triggers autoantibody production (Lee et al., 2008). Also, IL-12, IFNγ, but not IL-4, are involved in the development of pristane-induced lupus, indicating that T helper type 1 (Th1) responses are dominant. For unexplained reasons, the *lpr* and *gld* mutations protect mice from the production of antibodies routinely induced by pristane. In addition to nephritis, hemorrhagic pulmonary capillaritis and arthritis have also been observed in pristane-treated mice (Wooley et al., 1989; Chowdhary et al., 2007). The arthritis symptoms in this model include synovial hyperplasia, periostitis, and progressive marginal erosions. Pristane-induced arthritis is TNFα mediated, as treatment with neutralizing anti-TNFα antibody ameliorates the arthritis symptoms (Beech and Thompson, 1997).

Graft-versus-host-disease (GVHD)-induced models of systemic autoimmunity involve the injection of parent cells into F1 offspring and clarified early events in the induction of autoimmunity. When lymphocytes from DBA mice are transferred into (B6 X DBA) F1 mice, donor CD4$^+$ cells are stimulated by recipient major histocompatibility complex (MHC) class II cells, which presumably present a chromatin-associated nuclear antigen and produce initially IL-2 and later on IL-4 and IL-10, while the generation of CD8$^+$ CTL cells is silenced. These responses result in chronic GVHD with autoantibody and immune complex-mediated glomerulonephritis. When donor B6/H-2bm12 lymphocytes, whose MHC class II locus confers a three amino acid substitution in H-2^b, are transferred into B6 hosts, there is also development of chronic GVHD with autoantibodies and GN. This model works equally with opposite donor and recipient strains (Morris et al., 1990).

Injection of allogeneic collagen type II (CII) or certain peptides of this protein in complete or incomplete Freund's adjuvant into susceptible strains of rats or mice results in collagen-induced arthritis (CIA) resembling RA. The role of MHC in the expression of CIA is indicated, only in H-2^q mice after injection of chicken CII, whereas

H-2^r mice are susceptible to pig CII (Stuart et al., 1983; Watson et al., 1987). CD4$^+$ cells and various cytokines including IL-1 and TNF-α, as well as antibody to CII, have been shown to participate in the expression of CIA.

Immunization of BALB/c mice with partially deglycosylated human aggrecan induces chronic progressive polyarthritis and spondylitis (Glant et al., 2003). This proteoglycan (aggrecan)-induced arthritis (PGIA) resembles RA, as judged by observation, laboratory tests, radiography, and histopathology of the peripheral joints. The occurrence of PGIA depends on the development of cross-reactive T and B cell responses between the immunizing human and self (mouse) cartilage aggrecan. CIA and PGIA are two most commonly used RA models for quantitative trait locus (QTL) mapping for the identification of RA susceptibility loci.

Collagen antibody-induced arthritis (CAIA) is induced by injection of specific monoclonal CII antibodies (Holmdahl et al., 1986). The model was developed based on the findings that serum from arthritic mice or RA patients could transfer arthritis to naïve mice (Stuart and Dixon, 1983; Wooley et al., 1984). CAIA resembles CIA but is more acute and has a rapid onset, a few days after injection. Normally, the disease heals after a month and mice remain healthy. CAIA is inducible independently of MHC and T and B cell interaction (Nandakumar et al., 2004).

CONCLUDING COMMENTS

Animal models of systemic human autoimmune disease have served us well for understanding autoimmunity. Human systemic autoimmune diseases are highly

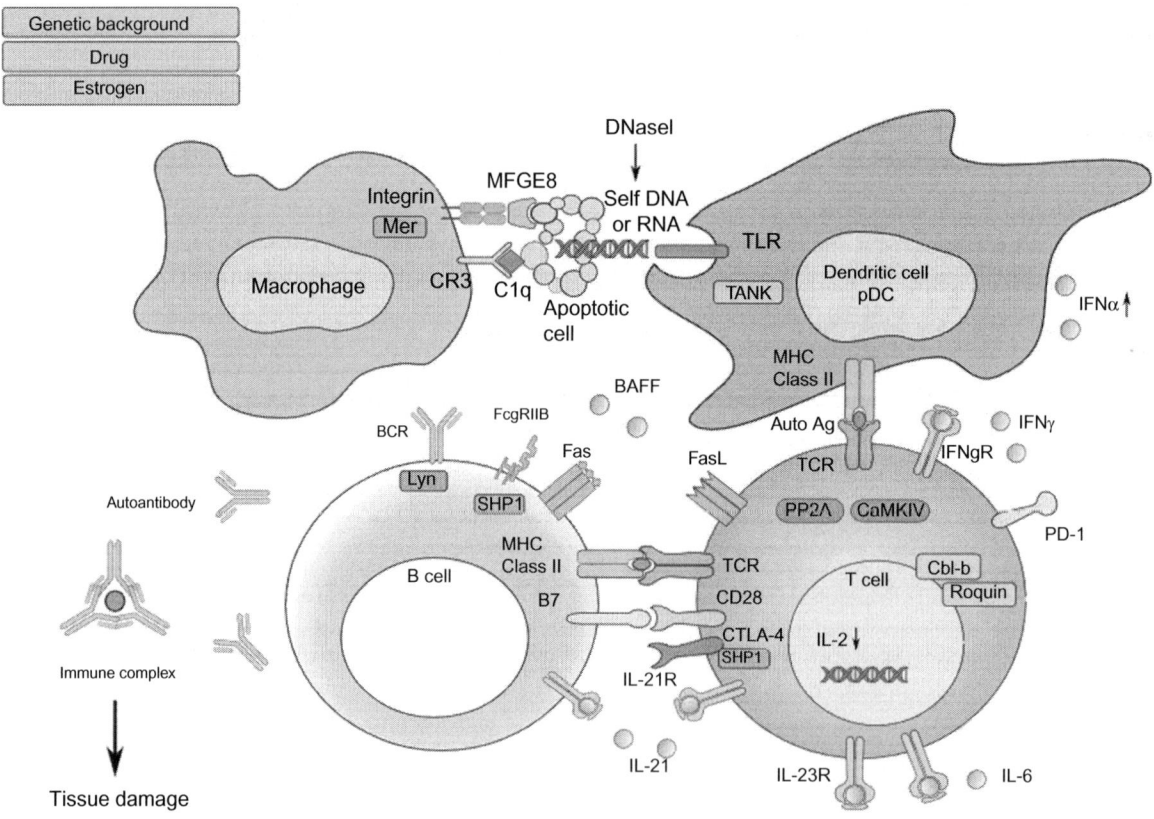

FIGURE 30.1 **Pathogenesis of systemic autoimmunity and molecules involved in the development of autoimmune disease, compiled from studies on mice and humans with systemic lupus erythematosus (SLE).** Similar to organ-specific autoimmunity, systemic autoimmunity is a function of a deleterious combination of genetic and environmental factors that lead in concert to the loss of self tolerance. T cells display numerous aberrations in the form of impaired cytokine productions, defective immunoregulatory function, and increased ability to provide help to B cells to produce autoantibodies. In systemic autoimmunity, autoantigens are frequently directed against nuclear antigens, with which they form immune complexes. Defective clearance of such immune complexes is the result of defective expression of Fc and complement receptors, and increased levels of nuclear materials may propagate the autoimmune responses. A number of cytokines including IFNα, IL-6, IL-21, IL-17, BAFF, and their receptors play critical roles for the development of lupus. IFN, interferon; IL, interleukin; MHC, major histocompatibility complex.

heterogeneous both at the clinical and pathogenic level to the point that we do not serve the field properly by lumping them along antedated criteria-counting approaches. We have presented a critical review of the animal models which have been used to understand disease processes Figure 30.1 and perform preclinical trials of putative new drugs Table 30.1 and biologics.

1. No animal model represents any systemic autoimmune disease.
2. Spontaneous models of disease can be used to obtain early insight on the consequences of lost tolerance in terms of organ damage.
3. Spontaneous models may serve preclinical testing of new rationally developed new drugs and biologics

TABLE 30.1 Representatives of Mice Models of Systemic Autoimmune Disease

Strain/Name Induction Method	Target Gene	Autoantibody Production	Arthritis	Reference(s)
Spontaneous Disease Models				
NZB		+		Ibnou-Zekri et al., 1999
NZW		+		Ibnou-Zekri et al., 1999
(NZB × NZW)F1		+		Ibnou-Zekri et al., 1999
NZM2328		+		Morel et al., 1994
NZM2410		+		Morel et al., 1994
MRL-Fas$^{lpr/lpr}$	Fas mutation	+ + +	+	Andrews et al., 1978
BXSB		+		Izui et al., 1995
Palmerston North		+		Luzina et al., 1999
K/B × N			+	Monach et al., 2004
SKG	Zap70 mutation		+	Marshall et al., 2003 Sakaguchi et al., 2003
Ank/ank	Ank mutation		+	Krug et al., 1989
Gene Manipulation-derived Models				
Lymphocyte Activation				
	PD-1 KO	+	+	Nishimura et al., 2001
	SHP-1 KO	+		Kozlowski et al., 1993 Tsui et al., 1993 Bignon and Smininovitch., 1994
	Mgat5 KO	+		Demetriou et al., 2001
	Lyn KO	+		Chan et al., 1997
	FcγRIIb KO	+		Bolland and Ravetch, 2000
Ubiquitination-protein ligases				
	Cbl-b KO	+		Bachmaier et al., 2000
	Roquin KO	+		Vinuesa et al., 2005
Cytokines and their receptors				
	L-2/IL-2R KO	+		Sharfe et al., 1997
	BAFF TG	+		Groom et al., 2007
	TNFα TG		+	Kontoyiannis et al., 1999
Complement				
	C1q KO	+		Manderson et al., 2004
	C4 KO	+		Chen et al., 2000
Molecules involved in dead cell clearance				
	DNaseIKO	+		Napirei et al., 2000
	MGF-E8 KO	+		Hanayama et al., 2002
Innate immune cell signaling molecules				
	TANK KO	+		Kawagoe et al., 2009
	Zc3h12a KO	+		Matsushita et al., 2009
Induced Models				
Pristane		+	+	Satoh and Reeves, 1994
GVHD		+		Morris et al., 1990
Collagen type II			+	Stuart et al., 1983 Watson et al., 1987
Proteoglycan			+	Glant et al., 2003
Collagen antibody			+	Holmdahl et al., 1986

although their predictive clinical value has been rather disappointing.

4. Animals which develop systemic autoimmune disease after modulation of a specific molecule known to be important in the control of maintenance of tolerance or of the immune response may only serve to address specific mechanistic questions.

5. In the study of these animals, the concepts of autoimmunity and autoimmunity-associated organ damage should be carefully considered separately.

6. Construction of animals in which modulated molecules previously identified as important in the aberrant function of SLE or RA immune cells may provide valuable information on the development of putative specific new drugs.

7. These novel animals constructed with intelligence generated from the study of human cells should provide definitive information on the relative contribution of each aberrantly expressed molecule in the expression of human systemic autoimmune disease. The B6.*CD2.PP2Ac* mouse is such an example (Crispin et al., 2012).

REFERENCES

Abrams, J.R., Kelley, S.L., Hayes, E., Kikuchi, T., Brown, M.J., Kang, S., et al., 2000. Blockade of T lymphocyte costimulation with cytotoxic T lymphocyte-associated antigen 4-immunoglobulin (CTLA4Ig) reverses the cellular pathology of psoriatic plaques, including the activation of keratinocytes, dendritic cells, and endothelial cells. J. Exp. Med. 192, 681–694.

Amano, T., Yamasaki, S., Yagishita, N., Tsuchimochi, K., Shin, H., Kawahara, K., et al., 2003. Synoviolin/Hrd1, an E3 ubiquitin ligase, as a novel pathogenic factor for arthropathy. Genes. Dev. 17, 2436–2449.

Andrews, B.S., Eisenberg, R.A., Theofilopoulos, A.N., Izui, S., Wilson, C.B., McConahey, P.J., et al., 1978. Spontaneous murine lupus like syndromes. Clinical and immunopathological manifestations in several strains. J. Exp. Med. 148, 1198–1215.

Bachmaier, K., Krawczyk, C., Kozieradzki, I., Kong, Y.Y., Sasaki, T., Oliveira-Dos-Santos, A., et al., 2000. Negative regulation of lymphocyte activation and autoimmunity by the molecular adaptor Cbl-b. Nature. 403, 211–216.

Bahjat, F.R., Pine, P.R., Reitsma, A., Cassafer, G., Baluom, M., Grillo, S., et al., 2008. An orally bioavailable spleen tyrosine kinase inhibitor delays disease progression and prolongs survival in murine lupus. Arthritis Rheum. 58, 1433–1444.

Balomenos, D., Rumold, R., Theofilopoulos, A.N., 1998. Interferon-gamma is required for lupus-like disease and lymphoaccumulation in MRL-lpr mice. J. Clin. Invest. 101, 364–371.

Barber, D.F., Bartolome, A., Hernandez, C., Flores, J.M., Redondo, C., Fernandez-Arias, C., et al., 2005. PI3Kgamma inhibition blocks glomerulonephritis and extends lifespan in a mouse model of systemic lupus. Nat. Med. 11, 933–935.

Beech, J.T., Thompson, S.J., 1997. Anti-tumour necrosis factor therapy ameliorates joint disease in a chronic model of inflammatory arthritis. Br. J. Rheumatol. 36, 1129.

Bignon, J.S., Siminovitch, K.A., 1994. Identification of PTP1C mutation as the genetic defect in motheaten and viable motheaten mice: a step toward defining the roles of protein tyrosine phosphatases in the regulation of hemopoietic cell differentiation and function. Clin. Immunol. Immunopathol. 73, 168–179.

Blanco, P., Palucka, A.K., Gill, M., Pascual, V., Banchereau, J., 2001. Induction of dendritic cell differentiation by IFN-alpha in systemic lupus erythematosus. Science. 294, 1540–1543.

Boackle, S.A., Holers, V.M., 2003. Role of complement in the development of autoimmunity. Curr. Dir. Autoimmun. 6, 154–168.

Boackle, S.A., Holers, V.M., Chen, X., Szakonyi, G., Karp, D.R., Wakeland, E.K., et al., 2001. Cr2, a candidate gene in the murine Sle1c lupus susceptibility locus, encodes a dysfunctional protein. Immunity. 15, 775–785.

Bolland, S., Ravetch, J.V., 2000. Spontaneous autoimmune disease in Fc (gamma)RIIB-deficient mice results from strain-specific epistasis. Immunity. 13, 277–285.

Botto, M., Walport, M.J., 2002. C1q, autoimmunity and apoptosis. Immunobiology. 205, 395–406.

Botto, M., Dell'agnola, C., Bygrave, A.E., Thompson, E.M., Cook, H.T., Petry, F., et al., 1998. Homozygous C1q deficiency causes glomerulonephritis associated with multiple apoptotic bodies. Nat. Genet. 19, 56–59.

Boule, M.W., Broughton, C., Mackay, F., Akira, S., Marshak-Rothstein, A., Rifkin, I.R., 2004. Toll-like receptor 9-dependent and -independent dendritic cell activation by chromatin-immunoglobulin G complexes. J. Exp. Med. 199, 1631–1640.

Bouzahzah, F., Jung, S., Craft, J., 2003. CD4 + T cells from lupus-prone mice avoid antigen-specific tolerance induction in vivo. J. Immunol. 170, 741–748.

Bubier, J.A., Sproule, T.J., Foreman, O., Spolski, R., Shaffer, D.J., Morse III, H.C., et al., 2009. A critical role for IL-21 receptor signaling in the pathogenesis of systemic lupus erythematosus in BXSB-Yaa mice. Proc. Natl. Acad. Sci. U.S.A. 106, 1518–1523.

Cash, H., Relle, M., Menke, J., Brochhausen, C., Jones, S.A., Topley, N., et al., 2010. Interleukin 6 (IL-6) deficiency delays lupus nephritis in MRL-Faslpr mice: the IL-6 pathway as a new therapeutic target in treatment of autoimmune kidney disease in systemic lupus erythematosus. J. Rheumatol. 37, 60–70.

Chan, V.W., Meng, F., Soriano, P., Defranco, A.L., Lowell, C.A., 1997. Characterization of the B lymphocyte populations in Lyn-deficient mice and the role of Lyn in signal initiation and down-regulation. Immunity. 7, 69–81.

Chen, Z., Koralov, S.B., Kelsoe, G., 2000. Complement C4 inhibits systemic autoimmunity through a mechanism independent of complement receptors CR1 and CR2. J. Exp. Med. 192, 1339–1352.

Chowdhary, V.R., Grande, J.P., Luthra, H.S., David, C.S., 2007. Characterization of haemorrhagic pulmonary capillaritis: another manifestation of Pristane-induced lupus. Rheumatology (Oxford). 46, 1405–1410.

Cornall, R.J., Cyster, J.G., Hibbs, M.L., Dunn, A.R., Otipoby, K.L., Clark, E.A., et al., 1998. Polygenic autoimmune traits: Lyn, CD22, and SHP-1 are limiting elements of a biochemical pathway regulating BCR signaling and selection. Immunity. 8, 497–508.

Crispin, J.C., Apostolidis, S.A., Rosetti, F., Keszei, M., Wang, N., Terhorst, C., et al., 2012. Cutting edge: protein phosphatase 2A confers susceptibility to autoimmune disease through an IL-17-dependent mechanism. J. Immunol. 188, 3567–3571.

Cunninghame Graham, D.S., Vyse, T.J., Fortin, P.R., Montpetit, A., Cai, Y.C., Lim, S., et al., 2008. Association of LY9 in UK and Canadian SLE families. Genes. Immun. 9, 93–102.

Deane, J.A., Pisitkun, P., Barrett, R.S., Feigenbaum, L., Town, T., Ward, J.M., et al., 2007. Control of toll-like receptor 7 expression is essential to restrict autoimmunity and dendritic cell proliferation. Immunity. 27, 801–810.

Demetriou, M., Granovsky, M., Quaggin, S., Dennis, J.W., 2001. Negative regulation of T-cell activation and autoimmunity by Mgat5 N-glycosylation. Nature. 409, 733–739.

Dempsey, P.W., Allison, M.E., Akkaraju, S., Goodnow, C.C., Fearon, D.T., 1996. C3d of complement as a molecular adjuvant: bridging innate and acquired immunity. Science. 271, 348–350.

Deng, G.M., Liu, L., Bahjat, F.R., Pine, P.R., Tsokos, G.C., 2010. Suppression of skin and kidney disease by inhibition of spleen tyrosine kinase in lupus-prone mice. Arthritis Rheum. 62, 2086–2092.

Dhaher, Y.Y., Greenstein, B., Nunn, De Fougerolles, Khamashta, E., Hughes, G.R., M., 2000. Strain differences in binding properties of estrogen receptors in immature and adult BALB/c and MRL/MP-lpr/ lpr mice, a model of systemic lupus erythematosus. Int. J. Immunopharmacol. 22, 247–254.

Drake, C.G., Rozzo, S.J., Vyse, T.J., Palmer, E., Kotzin, B.L., 1995. Genetic contributions to lupus-like disease in (NZB x NZW)F1 mice. Immunol. Rev. 144, 51–74.

Enyedy, E.J., Nambiar, M.P., Liossis, S.N., Dennis, G., Kammer, G.M., Tsokos, G.C., 2001. Fc epsilon receptor type I gamma chain replaces the deficient T cell receptor zeta chain in T cells of patients with systemic lupus erythematosus. Arthritis Rheum. 44, 1114–1121.

Fernandes, G., Talal, N., 1986. SLE: hormones and diet. Clin. Exp. Rheumatol. 4, 183–185.

Finck, B.K., Linsley, P.S., Wofsy, D., 1994. Treatment of murine lupus with CTLA4Ig. Science. 265, 1225–1227.

Gaffney, P.M., Kearns, G.M., Shark, K.B., Ortmann, W.A., Selby, S.A., Malmgren, M.L., et al., 1998. A genome-wide search for susceptibility genes in human systemic lupus erythematosus sib-pair families. Proc. Natl. Acad. Sci. U.S.A. 95, 14875–14879.

Gaffney, P.M., Ortmann, W.A., Selby, S.A., Shark, K.B., Ockenden, T.C., Rohlf, K.E., et al., 2000. Genome screening in human systemic lupus erythematosus: results from a second Minnesota cohort and combined analyses of 187 sib-pair families. Am. J. Hum Genet. 66, 547–556.

Gaipl, U.S., Kuhn, A., Sheriff, A., Munoz, L.E., Franz, S., Voll, R.E., et al., 2006. Clearance of apoptotic cells in human SLE. Curr. Dir. Autoimmun. 9, 173–187.

Glant, T.T., Finnegan, A., Mikecz, K., 2003. Proteoglycan-induced arthritis: immune regulation, cellular mechanisms, and genetics. Crit. Rev. Immunol. 23, 199–250.

Groom, J.R., Fletcher, C.A., Walters, S.N., Grey, S.T., Watt, S.V., Sweet, M.J., et al., 2007. BAFF and MyD88 signals promote a lupuslike disease independent of T cells. J. Exp. Med. 204, 1959–1971.

Gross, J.A., Johnston, J., Mudri, S., Enselman, R., Dillon, S.R., Madden, K., et al., 2000. TACI and BCMA are receptors for a TNF homologue implicated in B-cell autoimmune disease. Nature. 404, 995–999.

Gutierrez-Ramos, J.C., Andreu, J.L., Revilla, Y., Vinuela, E., Martinez, C., 1990. Recovery from autoimmunity of MRL/lpr mice after infection with an interleukin-2/vaccinia recombinant virus. Nature. 346, 271–274.

Haas, C., Ryffel, B., Le Hir, M., 1997. IFN-gamma is essential for the development of autoimmune glomerulonephritis in MRL/lpr mice. J. Immunol. 158, 5484–5491.

Hanayama, R., Tanaka, M., Miwa, K., Shinohara, A., Iwamatsu, A., Nagata, S., 2002. Identification of a factor that links apoptotic cells to phagocytes. Nature. 417, 182–187.

Hanayama, R., Tanaka, M., Miyasaka, K., Aozasa, K., Koike, M., Uchiyama, Y., et al., 2004. Autoimmune disease and impaired uptake of apoptotic cells in MFG-E8-deficient mice. Science. 304, 1147–1150.

Handwerger, B.S., Rus, V., Da Silva, L., Via, C.S., 1994. The role of cytokines in the immunopathogenesis of lupus. Springer. Semin. Immunopathol. 16, 153–180.

Harley, J.B., Moser, K.L., Gaffney, P.M., Behrens, T.W., 1998. The genetics of human systemic lupus erythematosus. Curr. Opin. Immunol. 10, 690–696.

Helgason, C.D., Kalberer, C.P., Damen, J.E., Chappel, S.M., Pineault, N., Krystal, G., et al., 2000. A dual role for Src homology 2 domain-containing inositol-5-phosphatase (SHIP) in immunity: aberrant development and enhanced function of b lymphocytes in ship$^{-/-}$ mice. J. Exp. Med. 191, 781–794.

Herber, D., Brown, T.P., Liang, S., Young, D.A., Collins, M., Dunussi-Joannopoulos, K., 2007. IL-21 has a pathogenic role in a lupus-prone mouse model and its blockade with IL-21R.Fc reduces disease progression. J. Immunol. 178, 3822–3830.

Hibbs, M.L., Harder, K.W., Armes, J., Kountouri, N., Quilici, C., Casagranda, F., et al., 2002. Sustained activation of Lyn tyrosine kinase in vivo leads to autoimmunity. J. Exp. Med. 196, 1593–1604.

Holmdahl, R., Rubin, K., Klareskog, L., Larsson, E., Wigzell, H., 1986. Characterization of the antibody response in mice with type II collagen-induced arthritis, using monoclonal anti-type II collagen antibodies. Arthritis Rheum. 29, 400–410.

Ibnou-Zekri, N., Vyse, T.J., Rozzo, S.J., Iwamoto, M., Kobayakawa, T., Kotzin, B.L., et al., 1999. MHC-linked control of murine SLE. Curr. Top. Microbiol. Immunol. 246, 275–280.

Ichinose, K., Rauen, T., Juang, Y.T., Kis-Toth, K., Mizui, M., Koga, T., et al., 2011. Cutting edge: calcium/calmodulin-dependent protein kinase type IV is essential for mesangial cell proliferation and lupus nephritis. J. Immunol. 187, 5500–5504.

Izui, S., Iwamoto, M., Fossati, L., Merino, R., Takahashi, S., Ibnou-Zekri, N., 1995. The Yaa gene model of systemic lupus erythematosus. Immunol. Rev. 144, 137–156.

Jeon, M.S., Atfield, A., Venuprasad, K., Krawczyk, C., Sarao, R., Elly, C., et al., 2004. Essential role of the E3 ubiquitin ligase Cbl-b in T cell anergy induction. Immunity. 21, 167–177.

Juang, Y.T., Solomou, E.E., Rellahan, B., Tsokos, G.C., 2002. Phosphorylation and O-linked glycosylation of Elf-1 leads to its translocation to the nucleus and binding to the promoter of the TCR zeta-chain. J. Immunol. 168, 2865–2871.

Juang, Y.T., Rauen, T., Wang, Y., Ichinose, K., Benedyk, K., Tenbrock, K., et al., 2011. Transcriptional activation of the cAMP-responsive modulator promoter in human T cells is regulated by protein phosphatase 2A-mediated dephosphorylation of SP-1 and reflects disease activity in patients with systemic lupus erythematosus. J. Biol. Chem. 286, 1795–1801.

Katsiari, C.G., Kyttaris, V.C., Juang, Y.T., Tsokos, G.C., 2005. Protein phosphatase 2A is a negative regulator of IL-2 production in patients with systemic lupus erythematosus. J. Clin. Invest. 115, 3193–3204.

Kawagoe, T., Takeuchi, O., Takabatake, Y., Kato, H., Isaka, Y., Tsujimura, T., et al., 2009. TANK is a negative regulator of Toll-like receptor signaling and is critical for the prevention of autoimmune nephritis. Nat. Immunol. 10, 965–972.

Kimberly, R.P., Salmon, J.E., Edberg, J.C., 1995. Receptors for immunoglobulin G. Molecular diversity and implications for disease. Arthritis Rheum. 38, 306–314.

King, C., Tangye, S.G., Mackay, C.R., 2008. T follicular helper (TFH) cells in normal and dysregulated immune responses. Annu. Rev. Immunol. 26, 741–766.

Kitaura, Y., Jang, I.K., Wang, Y., Han, Y.C., Inazu, T., Cadera, E.J., et al., 2007. Control of the B cell-intrinsic tolerance programs by ubiquitin ligases Cbl and Cbl-b. Immunity. 26, 567–578.

Kono, D.H., Theofilopoulos, A.N., 2006. Genetics of SLE in mice. Springer Semin. Immunopathol. 28, 83–96.

Kontoyiannis, D., Pasparakis, M., Pizarro, T.T., Cominelli, F., Kollias, G., 1999. Impaired on/off regulation of TNF biosynthesis in mice lacking TNF AU-rich elements: implications for joint and gut-associated immunopathologies. Immunity. 10, 387–398.

Koreth, J., Matsuoka, K., Kim, H.T., McDonough, S.M., Bindra, B., Alyea III, E.P., et al., 2011. Interleukin-2 and regulatory T cells in graft-versus-host disease. N. Engl. J. Med. 365, 2055–2066.

Kovacs, B., Vassilopoulos, D., Vogelgesang, S.A., Tsokos, G.C., 1996. Defective CD3-mediated cell death in activated T cells from patients with systemic lupus erythematosus: role of decreased intracellular TNF-alpha. Clin. Immunol. Immunopathol. 81, 293–302.

Kozlowski, M., Mlinaric-Rascan, I., Feng, G.S., Shen, R., Pawson, T., Siminovitch, K.A., 1993. Expression and catalytic activity of the tyrosine phosphatase PTP1C is severely impaired in motheaten and viable motheaten mice. J. Exp. Med. 178, 2157–2163.

Kremer, J.M., Westhovens, R., Leon, M., Di Giorgio, E., Alten, R., Steinfeld, S., et al., 2003. Treatment of rheumatoid arthritis by selective inhibition of T-cell activation with fusion protein CTLA4Ig. N. Engl. J. Med. 349, 1907–1915.

Krishnan, S., Nambiar, M.P., Warke, V.G., Fisher, C.U., Mitchell, J., Delaney, N., et al., 2004. Alterations in lipid raft composition and dynamics contribute to abnormal T cell responses in systemic lupus erythematosus. J. Immunol. 172, 7821–7831.

Krug, H.E., Mahowald, M.L., Clark, C., 1989. Progressive ankylosis (ank/ank) in mice: an animal model of spondyloarthropathy. III. Proliferative spleen cell response to T cell mitogens. Clin. Exp. Immunol. 78, 97–101.

Kruger, J., Butler, J.R., Cherapanov, V., Dong, Q., Ginzberg, H., Govindarajan, A., et al., 2000. Deficiency of Src homology 2-containing phosphatase 1 results in abnormalities in murine neutrophil function: studies in motheaten mice. J. Immunol. 165, 5847–5859.

Kumar, K.R., Li, L., Yan, M., Bhaskarabhatla, M., Mobley, A.B., Nguyen, C., et al., 2006. Regulation of B cell tolerance by the lupus susceptibility gene Ly108. Science. 312, 1665–1669.

Kyttaris, V.C., Zhang, Z., Kuchroo, V.K., Oukka, M., Tsokos, G.C., 2010. Cutting edge: IL-23 receptor deficiency prevents the development of lupus nephritis in C57BL/6-lpr/lpr mice. J. Immunol. 184, 4605–4609.

La Cava, A., 2008. T-regulatory cells in systemic lupus erythematosus. Lupus. 17, 421–425.

Lawson, B.R., Kono, D.H., Theofilopoulos, A.N., 2002. Deletion of p21 (WAF-1/Cip1) does not induce systemic autoimmunity in female BXSB mice. J. Immunol. 168, 5928–5932.

Lawson, B.R., Baccala, R., Song, J., Croft, M., Kono, D.H., Theofilopoulos, A.N., 2004. Deficiency of the cyclin kinase inhibitor p21(WAF-1/CIP-1) promotes apoptosis of activated/memory T

cells and inhibits spontaneous systemic autoimmunity. J. Exp. Med. 199, 547–557.

Leadbetter, E.A., Rifkin, I.R., Hohlbaum, A.M., Beaudette, B.C., Shlomchik, M.J., Marshak-Rothstein, A., 2002. Chromatin-IgG complexes activate B cells by dual engagement of IgM and Toll-like receptors. Nature. 416, 603–607.

Lee, D.M., Friend, D.S., Gurish, M.F., Benoist, C., Mathis, D., Brenner, M.B., 2002. Mast cells: a cellular link between autoantibodies and inflammatory arthritis. Science. 297, 1689–1692.

Lee, P.Y., Kumagai, Y., Li, Y., Takeuchi, O., Yoshida, H., Weinstein, J., Kellner, E.S., et al., 2008. TLR7-dependent and FcgammaR-independent production of type I interferon in experimental mouse lupus. J. Exp. Med. 205, 2995–3006.

Lemke, G., Rothlin, C.V., 2008. Immunobiology of the TAM receptors. Nat. Rev. Immunol. 8, 327–336.

Levy, E., Ambrus, J., Kahl, L., Molina, H., Tung, K., Holers, V.M., 1992. T lymphocyte expression of complement receptor 2 (CR2/CD21): a role in adhesive cell-cell interactions and dysregulation in a patient with systemic lupus erythematosus (SLE). Clin. Exp. Immunol. 90, 235–244.

Lin, S.C., Yen, J.H., Tsai, J.J., Tsai, W.C., Ou, T.T., Liu, H.W., et al., 2004. Association of a programmed death 1 gene polymorphism with the development of rheumatoid arthritis, but not systemic lupus erythematosus. Arthritis Rheum. 50, 770–775.

Linterman, M.A., Rigby, R.J., Wong, R.K., Yu, D., Brink, R., Cannons, J.L., et al., 2009. Follicular helper T cells are required for systemic autoimmunity. J. Exp. Med. 206, 561–576.

Liossis, S.N., Ding, X.Z., Dennis, G.J., Tsokos, G.C., 1998. Altered pattern of TCR/CD3-mediated protein-tyrosyl phosphorylation in T cells from patients with systemic lupus erythematosus. Deficient expression of the T cell receptor zeta chain. J. Clin. Invest. 101, 1448–1457.

Lucas, J.A., Menke, J., Rabacal, W.A., Schoen, F.J., Sharpe, A.H., Kelley, V.R., 2008. Programmed death ligand 1 regulates a critical checkpoint for autoimmune myocarditis and pneumonitis in MRL mice. J. Immunol. 181, 2513–2521.

Lui, S.L., Tsang, R., Chan, K.W., Zhang, F., Tam, S., Yung, S., et al., 2008. Rapamycin attenuates the severity of established nephritis in lupus-prone NZB/W F1 mice. Nephrol. Dial. Transplant. 23, 2768–2776.

Luzina, I.G., Knitzer, R.H., Atamas, S.P., Gause, W.C., Papadimitriou, J.C., Sztein, M.B., et al., 1999. Vasculitis in the Palmerston North mouse model of lupus: phenotype and cytokine production profile of infiltrating cells. Arthritis Rheum. 42, 561–568.

Manderson, A.P., Botto, M., Walport, M.J., 2004. The role of complement in the development of systemic lupus erythematosus. Annu. Rev. Immunol. 22, 431–456.

Marquart, H.V., Svendsen, A., Rasmussen, J.M., Nielsen, C.H., Junker, P., Svehag, S.E., et al., 1995. Complement receptor expression and activation of the complement cascade on B lymphocytes from patients with systemic lupus erythematosus (SLE). Clin. Exp. Immunol. 101, 60–65.

Marshak-Rothstein, A., 2006. Toll-like receptors in systemic autoimmune disease. Nat. Rev. Immunol. 6, 823–835.

Marshall, D., Dangerfield, J.P., Bhatia, V.K., Larbi, K.Y., Nourshargh, S., Haskard, D.O., 2003. MRL/lpr lupus-prone mice show exaggerated ICAM-1-dependent leucocyte adhesion and transendothelial migration in response to TNF-alpha. Rheumatology (Oxford). 42, 929–934.

Matsumoto, I., Lee, D.M., Goldbach-Mansky, R., Sumida, T., Hitchon, C.A., Schur, P.H., et al., 2003. Low prevalence of antibodies to glucose-6-phosphate isomerase in patients with rheumatoid arthritis and a spectrum of other chronic autoimmune disorders. Arthritis Rheum. 48, 944–954.

Matsushita, K., Takeuchi, O., Standley, D.M., Kumagai, Y., Kawagoe, T., Miyake, T., et al., 2009. Zc3h12a is an RNase essential for controlling immune responses by regulating mRNA decay. Nature. 458, 1185–1190.

McInnes, I.B., Schett, G., 2011. The pathogenesis of rheumatoid arthritis. N. Engl. J. Med. 365, 2205–2219.

Monach, P.A., Benoist, C., Mathis, D., 2004. The role of antibodies in mouse models of rheumatoid arthritis, and relevance to human disease. Adv. Immunol. 82, 217–248.

Morel, L., Wakeland, E.K., 1998. Susceptibility to lupus nephritis in the NZB/W model system. Curr. Opin. Immunol. 10, 718–725.

Morel, L., Rudofsky, U.H., Longmate, J.A., Schiffenbauer, J., Wakeland, E.K., 1994. Polygenic control of susceptibility to murine systemic lupus erythematosus. Immunity. 1, 219–229.

Morris, S.C., Cohen, P.L., Eisenberg, R.A., 1990. Experimental induction of systemic lupus erythematosus by recognition of foreign Ia. Clin. Immunol. Immunopathol. 57, 263–273.

Moser, K.L., Gray-McGuire, C., Kelly, J., Asundi, N., Yu, H., Bruner, G.R., et al., 1999. Confirmation of genetic linkage between human systemic lupus erythematosus and chromosome 1q41. Arthritis Rheum. 42, 1902–1907.

Nagata, S., Hanayama, R., Kawane, K., 2010. Autoimmunity and the clearance of dead cells. Cell. 140, 619–630.

Nambiar, M.P., Enyedy, E.J., Fisher, C.U., Krishnan, S., Warke, V.G., Gilliland, W.R., et al., 2002. Abnormal expression of various molecular forms and distribution of T cell receptor zeta chain in patients with systemic lupus erythematosus. Arthritis Rheum. 46, 163–174.

Nandakumar, K.S., Backlund, J., Vestberg, M., Holmdahl, R., 2004. Collagen type II (CII)-specific antibodies induce arthritis in the absence of T or B cells but the arthritis progression is enhanced by CII-reactive T cells. Arthritis. Res. Ther. 6, R544–R550.

Napirei, M., Karsunky, H., Zevnik, B., Stephan, H., Mannherz, H.G., Moroy, T., 2000. Features of systemic lupus erythematosus in Dnase1-deficient mice. Nat Genet. 25, 177–181.

Navarra, S.V., Guzman, R.M., Gallacher, A.E., Hall, S., Levy, R.A., Jimenez, R.E., et al., 2011. Efficacy and safety of belimumab in patients with active systemic lupus erythematosus: a randomised, placebo-controlled, phase 3 trial. Lancet. 377, 721–731.

Nelson, B.H., 2002. Interleukin-2 signaling and the maintenance of self-tolerance. Curr. Dir. Autoimmun. 5, 92–112.

Nishimura, H., Okazaki, T., Tanaka, Y., Nakatani, K., Hara, M., Matsumori, A., et al., 2001. Autoimmune dilated cardiomyopathy in PD-1 receptor-deficient mice. Science. 291, 319–322.

Okazaki, T., Tanaka, Y., Nishio, R., Mitsuiye, T., Mizoguchi, A., Wang, J., et al., 2003. Autoantibodies against cardiac troponin I are responsible for dilated cardiomyopathy in PD-1-deficient mice. Nat. Med. 9, 1477–1483.

Pani, G., Fischer, K.D., Mlinaric-Rascan, I., Siminovitch, K.A., 1996. Signaling capacity of the T cell antigen receptor is negatively regulated by the PTP1C tyrosine phosphatase. J. Exp. Med. 184, 839–852.

Pao, L.I., Lam, K.P., Henderson, J.M., Kutok, J.L., Alimzhanov, M., Nitschke, L., et al., 2007. B cell-specific deletion of protein-tyrosine phosphatase Shp1 promotes B-1a cell development and causes systemic autoimmunity. Immunity. 27, 35–48.

Pisitkun, P., Deane, J.A., Difilippantonio, M.J., Tarasenko, T., Satterthwaite, A.B., Bolland, S., 2006. Autoreactive B cell responses to RNA-related antigens due to TLR7 gene duplication. Science. 312, 1669–1672.

Prokunina, L., Castillejo-Lopez, C., Oberg, F., Gunnarsson, I., Berg, L., Magnusson, V., et al., 2002. A regulatory polymorphism in PDCD1 is associated with susceptibility to systemic lupus erythematosus in humans. Nat Genet. 32, 666–669.

Reap, E.A., Leslie, D., Abrahams, M., Eisenberg, R.A., Cohen, P.L., 1995. Apoptosis abnormalities of splenic lymphocytes in autoimmune lpr and gld mice. J. Immunol. 154, 936–943.

Reilly, C.M., Gilkeson, G.S., 2002. Use of genetic knockouts to modulate disease expression in a murine model of lupus, MRL/lpr mice. Immunol. Res. 25, 143–153.

Roubinian, J.R., Talal, N., Greenspan, J.S., Goodman, J.R., Siiteri, P.K., 1978. Effect of castration and sex hormone treatment on survival, anti-nucleic acid antibodies, and glomerulonephritis in NZB/NZW F1 mice. J. Exp. Med. 147, 1568–1583.

Rozzo, S.J., Allard, J.D., Choubey, D., Vyse, T.J., Izui, S., Peltz, G., et al., 2001. Evidence for an interferon-inducible gene, Ifi202, in the susceptibility to systemic lupus. Immunity. 15, 435–443.

Saadoun, D., Rosenzwajg, M., Joly, F., Six, A., Carrat, F., Thibault, V., et al., 2011. Regulatory T-cell responses to low-dose interleukin-2 in HCV-induced vasculitis. N. Engl. J. Med. 365, 2067–2077.

Sakaguchi, S., Takahashi, T., Hata, H., Nomura, T., Tagami, T., Yamazaki, S., et al., 2003. Altered thymic T-cell selection due to a mutation of the ZAP-70 gene causes autoimmune arthritis in mice. Nature. 426, 454–460.

Santiago-Raber, M.L., Baccala, R., Haraldsson, K.M., Choubey, D., Stewart, T.A., et al., 2003. Type-I interferon receptor deficiency reduces lupus-like disease in NZB mice. J. Exp. Med. 197, 777–788.

Santiago-Raber, M.L., Kikuchi, S., Borel, P., Uematsu, S., Akira, S., Kotzin, B.L., et al., 2008. Evidence for genes in addition to Tlr7 in the Yaa translocation linked with acceleration of systemic lupus erythematosus. J. Immunol. 181, 1556–1562.

Satoh, M., Reeves, W.H., 1994. Induction of lupus-associated autoantibodies in BALB/c mice by intraperitoneal injection of pristane. J. Exp. Med. 180, 2341–2346.

Scott, R.S., McMahon, E.J., Pop, S.M., Reap, E.A., Caricchio, R., Cohen, P.L., et al., 2001. Phagocytosis and clearance of apoptotic cells is mediated by MER. Nature. 411, 207–211.

Sharfe, N., Dadi, H.K., Shahar, M., Roifman, C.M., 1997. Human immune disorder arising from mutation of the alpha chain of the interleukin-2 receptor. Proc. Natl. Acad. Sci. U.S.A. 94, 3168–3171.

Shen, N., Fu, Q., Deng, Y., Qian, X., Zhao, J., Kaufman, K.M., et al., 2010. Sex-specific association of X-linked Toll-like receptor 7 (TLR7) with male systemic lupus erythematosus. Proc. Natl. Acad. Sci. U.S.A. 107, 15838–15843.

Shores, E.W., Love, P.E., 1997. TCR zeta chain in T cell development and selection. Curr. Opin. Immunol. 9, 380–389.

Simpson, N., Gatenby, P.A., Wilson, A., Malik, S., Fulcher, D.A., Tangye, S.G., et al., 2010. Expansion of circulating T cells resembling follicular helper T cells is a fixed phenotype that identifies a subset of severe systemic lupus erythematosus. Arthritis Rheum. 62, 234–244.

Stuart, J.M., Dixon, F.J., 1983. Serum transfer of collagen-induced arthritis in mice. J. Exp. Med. 158, 378–392.

Stuart, J.M., Tomoda, K., Yoo, T.J., Townes, A.S., Kang, A.H., 1983. Serum transfer of collagen-induced arthritis. II. Identification and localization of autoantibody to type II collagen in donor and recipient rats. Arthritis Rheum. 26, 1237–1244.

Suzuki, A., Yamada, R., Kochi, Y., Sawada, T., Okada, Y., Matsuda, K., et al., 2008. Functional SNPs in CD244 increase the risk of rheumatoid arthritis in a Japanese population. Nat. Genet. 40, 1224–1229.

Svenson, J.L., Eudaly, J., Ruiz, P., Korach, K.S., Gilkeson, G.S., 2008. Impact of estrogen receptor deficiency on disease expression in the NZM2410 lupus prone mouse. Clin. Immunol. 128, 259–268.

Takahashi, K., Kozono, Y., Waldschmidt, T.J., Berthiaume, D., Quigg, R.J., Baron, A., et al., 1997. Mouse complement receptors type 1 (CR1;CD35) and type 2 (CR2;CD21): expression on normal B cell subpopulations and decreased levels during the development of autoimmunity in MRL/lpr mice. J. Immunol. 159, 1557–1569.

Takahashi, T., Tanaka, M., Brannan, C.I., Jenkins, N.A., Copeland, N. G., Suda, T., et al., 1994. Generalized lymphoproliferative disease in mice, caused by a point mutation in the Fas ligand. Cell. 76, 969–976.

Taylor, P.R., Carugati, A., Fadok, V.A., Cook, H.T., Andrews, M., Carroll, M.C., et al., 2000. A hierarchical role for classical pathway complement proteins in the clearance of apoptotic cells in vivo. J. Exp. Med. 192, 359–366.

Tivol, E.A., Borriello, F., Schweitzer, A.N., Lynch, W.P., Bluestone, J.A., Sharpe, A.H., 1995. Loss of CTLA-4 leads to massive lymphoproliferation and fatal multiorgan tissue destruction, revealing a critical negative regulatory role of CTLA-4. Immunity. 3, 541–547.

Truedsson, L., Bengtsson, A.A., Sturfelt, G., 2007. Complement deficiencies and systemic lupus erythematosus. Autoimmunity. 40, 560–566.

Tsao, B.P., Cantor, R.M., Kalunian, K.C., Chen, C.J., Badsha, H., Singh, R., et al., 1997. Evidence for linkage of a candidate chromosome 1 region to human systemic lupus erythematosus. J Clin Invest. 99, 725–731.

Tsao, B.P., Cantor, R.M., Grossman, J.M., Kim, S.K., Strong, N., Lau, C.S., et al., 2002. Linkage and interaction of loci on 1q23 and 16q12 may contribute to susceptibility to systemic lupus erythematosus. Arthritis Rheum. 46, 2928–2936.

Tsokos, G.C., 2011. Systemic lupus erythematosus. N. Engl. J. Med. 365, 2110–2121.

Tsokos, G.C., Lambris, J.D., Finkelman, F.D., Anastassiou, E.D., June, C.H., 1990. Monovalent ligands of complement receptor 2 inhibit whereas polyvalent ligands enhance anti-Ig-induced human B cell intracytoplasmic free calcium concentration. J. Immunol. 144, 1640–1645.

Tsokos, G.C., Kovacs, B., Sfikakis, P.P., Theocharis, S., Vogelgesang, S., Via, C.S., 1996. Defective antigen-presenting cell function in patients with systemic lupus erythematosus. Arthritis Rheum. 39, 600–609.

Tsokos, G.C., Nambiar, M.P., Tenbrock, K., Juang, Y.T., 2003. Rewiring the T-cell: signaling defects and novel prospects for the treatment of SLE. Trends Immunol. 24, 259–263.

Tsui, H.W., Siminovitch, K.A., De Souza, L., Tsui, F.W., 1993. Motheaten and viable motheaten mice have mutations in the haematopoietic cell phosphatase gene. Nat. Genet. 4, 124–129.

Tsukumo, S., Yasutomo, K., 2004. DNaseI in pathogenesis of systemic lupus erythematosus. Clin. Immunol. 113, 14–18.

Vinuesa, C.G., Cook, M.C., Angelucci, C., Athanasopoulos, V., Rui, L., Hill, K.M., et al., 2005. A RING-type ubiquitin ligase family member required to repress follicular helper T cells and autoimmunity. Nature. 435, 452–458.

Vollmer, J., Tluk, S., Schmitz, C., Hamm, S., Jurk, M., Forsbach, A., et al., 2005. Immune stimulation mediated by autoantigen binding sites within small nuclear RNAs involves Toll-like receptors 7 and 8. J. Exp. Med. 202, 1575–1585.

Vratsanos, G.S., Jung, S., Park, Y.M., Craft, J., 2001. CD4(+) T cells from lupus-prone mice are hyperresponsive to T cell receptor engagement with low and high affinity peptide antigens: a model to explain spontaneous T cell activation in lupus. J. Exp. Med. 193, 329–337.

Vyse, T.J., Rozzo, S.J., Drake, C.G., Appel, V.B., Lemeur, M., Izui, S., et al., 1998. Contributions of Ea(z) and Eb(z) MHC genes to lupus susceptibility in New Zealand mice. J. Immunol. 160, 2757–2766.

Wakeland, E.K., Morel, L., Mohan, C., Yui, M., 1997. Genetic dissection of lupus nephritis in murine models of SLE. J. Clin. Immunol. 17, 272–281.

Wandstrat, A.E., Nguyen, C., Limaye, N., Chan, A.Y., Subramanian, S., Tian, X.H., et al., 2004. Association of extensive polymorphisms in the SLAM/CD2 gene cluster with murine lupus. Immunity. 21, 769–780.

Waterhouse, P., Penninger, J.M., Timms, E., Wakeham, A., Shahinian, A., Lee, K.P., et al., 1995. Lymphoproliferative disorders with early lethality in mice deficient in Ctla-4. Science. 270, 985–988.

Watson, W.C., Brown, P.S., Pitcock, J.A., Townes, A.S., 1987. Passive transfer studies with type II collagen antibody in B10.D2/old and new line and C57Bl/6 normal and beige (Chediak-Higashi) strains: evidence of important roles for C5 and multiple inflammatory cell types in the development of erosive arthritis. Arthritis Rheum. 30, 460–465.

Wooley, P.H., Luthra, H.S., Singh, S.K., Huse, A.R., Stuart, J.M., David, C.S., 1984. Passive transfer of arthritis to mice by injection of human anti-type II collagen antibody. Mayo. Clin. Proc. 59, 737–743.

Wooley, P.H., Seibold, J.R., Whalen, J.D., Chapdelaine, J.M., 1989. Pristane-induced arthritis. The immunologic and genetic features of an experimental murine model of autoimmune disease. Arthritis Rheum. 32, 1022–1030.

Yajima, K., Nakamura, A., Sugahara, A., Takai, T., 2003. FcgammaRIIB deficiency with Fas mutation is sufficient for the development of systemic autoimmune disease. Eur. J. Immunol. 33, 1020–1029.

Yamazaki, T., Arase, H., Ono, S., Ohno, H., Watanabe, H., Saito, T., 1997. A shift from negative to positive selection of autoreactive T cells by the reduced level of TCR signal in TCR-transgenic CD3 zeta-deficient mice. J. Immunol. 158, 1634–1640.

Yasutomo, K., Horiuchi, T., Kagami, S., Tsukamoto, H., Hashimura, C., Urushihara, M., et al., 2001. Mutation of DNASE1 in people with systemic lupus erythematosus. Nat. Genet. 28, 313–314.

Zhang, Z., Kyttaris, V.C., Tsokos, G.C., 2009. The role of IL-23/IL-17 axis in lupus nephritis. J. Immunol. 183, 3160–3169.

Chapter 31

Animal Models of Organ-Specific Autoimmune Disease

Ken Coppieters and Matthias von Herrath

Type 1 Diabetes Research and Development Center, Novo Nordisk, Seattle, WA, USA

Chapter Outline

What Can Animal Models Teach us about Organ-Specific
Autoimmunity? 435
  The Inciting Autoantigen 435
  Antigen-Specific Tolerization Strategies 436
  Other Immune Therapies 436
  Gene Function 436
  Understanding the Complexity of Organ-Specific
  Autoimmunity 436
Animal Models—Advantages and Disadvantages 437
Animal Models for Organ-Specific Autoimmune diseases 438
  Spontaneous Models of Organ-Specific Autoimmunity 438
    The Non-Obese Diabetic Mouse 438
  Genetically Engineered Animal Models for Organ-Specific
  Autoimmunity 439
  Induced Animal Models for Organ-Specific Autoimmune
  Diseases 439
    Breaking Tolerance is Not Easily Achieved 439
    Environmental Triggers Employed to Break Tolerance 440

    Protein/Peptide and Adjuvant 440
    Multiple Sclerosis 440
    Thyroiditis 440
    Myasthenia Gravis 441
    Autoimmune Uveitis 442
  Cell Transfer or Depletion 442
    Multiple Sclerosis 442
    Type 1 Diabetes 442
    Inflammatory Bowel Disease 442
    Autoimmune Gastritis 443
    General Conclusions from Induced Models 443
  Comparison of Organ-Specific Autoimmune Disease in
  Animal Models and Humans 444
    Type 1 Diabetes 444
    Multiple Sclerosis 444
Conclusions 444
References 444

WHAT CAN ANIMAL MODELS TEACH US ABOUT ORGAN-SPECIFIC AUTOIMMUNITY?

Without aiming to be exhaustive, we will first list some examples of scientific questions that are typically answered with the aid of animal models.

The Inciting Autoantigen

Despite intensive research over the past decades, there are some crucial elements in organ-specific autoimmunity that we do not comprehend yet. One major problem is that for many organ-specific autoimmune diseases we do not know the targets of the initial autoimmune response, while in some, such as in pemphigus vulgaris (Lin et al.,

1997), myasthenia gravis (Fambrough et al., 1973), and autoimmune gastritis (Karlsson et al., 1988), the driving autoantigen has been defined. In animal models, advantages such as homogeneous genetic background and accessibility of the target organ in theory should facilitate the search for such primary autoantigens. In the non-obese diabetic (NOD) mouse model for type 1 diabetes (T1D) it was indeed suggested that proinsulin is the primary antigenic trigger (Nakayama et al., 2005). The eventual heterogeneity in individual T and B cell repertoires, even in these inbred mice, is likely responsible for the fact that only very rarely do all individual mice exhibit the same course and severity of disease (Sercarz, 2000). In keeping with the latter theory, recent evidence from human leukocyte antigen (HLA)-A2 transgenic NOD mice reveals that individual inbred mice develop unique

N. Rose & I. Mackay (Eds): The Autoimmune Diseases, Fifth edition. DOI: http://dx.doi.org/10.1016/B978-0-12-384929-8.00031-9

patterns of CD8 T cell autoreactivity (Jarchum et al., 2007). Deciphering the underlying heterogeneity in autoreactive repertoires will be key to understanding and predicting development of autoimmune diseases. Identifying autoaggressive T-cell specificities on an individual basis is in fact emerging as an important disease biomarker (Velthuis et al., 2010).

Antigen-specific Tolerization Strategies

From a translational angle, it is still unclear whether tolerizing the "driver" T cell clones would be sufficient to reverse an ongoing autoimmune process and have therapeutic value. Some reports suggest a striking oligoclonality, which in turn indicates that deletional immunotherapy using one or a few autoantigenic determinants might be feasible (Kent et al., 2005). Animal models also suggest that T cell receptor (TCR) avidity plays a pivotal role, as it was shown that low-avidity clonotypes can act protectively (Han et al., 2005). Numerous other reports, however, suggest that low affinity clones might in fact be the driving force. Data in the rat insulin promoter (RIP)-lymphocytic choriomeningitis virus-derived proteins (LCMV) diabetes model demonstrate that, in a slow-onset variant of the model, low affinity T cells are responsible for disease induction (von Herrath et al., 1994). In human T1D, similar conclusions were drawn from studies using a preproinsulin-specific human CD8 T cell clone that is capable of inducing beta cell death (Skowera et al., 2008). Remarkably, the TCR of this clone was of extraordinarily low affinity, redefining the understanding of what constitutes a functionally relevant TCR−pMHC interaction (Bulek et al., 2012).

Animal models were used to evaluate antigen-specific therapies that are now in clinical trials, such as ECDI−peptide-coupled cell therapy in multiple sclerosis (Kennedy et al., 1990). Likewise, the NOD mouse was employed to predict responses to antigen-specific therapy based on prior antibody status (Mamchak et al., 2012). With the advent of antigen-specific therapies, mouse models will thus continue to serve as important tools for the pre-clinical validation of suitable therapeutic regimens.

Other Immune Therapies

The recent surge in clinical trials aimed at immunomodulation in large part leans on supportive data from animal models. What is remarkable is that many of the new biologicals show efficacy in multiple organ-specific autoimmune diseases. One example is the positive results that were obtained with the B cell-depleting agent infliximab in entirely distinct conditions such as T1D (Pescovitz et al., 2009) and multiple sclerosis (Hauser et al., 2008). Tumor necrosis factor (TNF) inhibition, a common

treatment for autoimmune conditions such as rheumatoid arthritis and psoriasis, was pursued in T1D (Mastrandrea et al., 2009). These results from clinical trials to some extent confirm what we had learned from their respective animal models, i.e., that disease development is characterized by overlapping immune pathways.

Can animal studies faithfully predict the success of immune intervention strategies in humans? Of course mice and men are not the same, but we conclude that data from animal models are not always fully taken into account in the clinical translation process. One example in the T1D arena is CTLA-4Ig therapy, which is able to prevent diabetes in the NOD mouse when given early but is incapable of reversing clinical disease (Lenschow et al., 1995). In a recent clinical trial, 2-year continued administration in recently diagnosed patients only showed effect in the initial few months, which to some extent only serves to confirm what was predicted by the animal data (Orban et al., 2011). Thus, choice of drug and trial design does not always seem to be rationally based upon animal research and is often more governed by the availability of certain drugs.

Gene Function

In the immunogenetic arena, animal models have provided useful insights. For diseases that are determined by one or a few genes, and where no major epigenetic factors are involved, we have learnt much from immunodeficient animals as well as humans. However, in some cases the respective human immunodeficiency will yield a different phenotype than the genetic knockout mouse, illustrating differences between men and mice that are likely linked to epigenetic and environmental factors. For example, ICOS deficiency in humans has immunologic consequences that are found in some patients with common variable immunodeficiency (Grimbacher et al., 2003). In contrast, the ICOS deficient mouse has a rather uniform phenotype involving immune deviation of T cell responses and their cytokine production, as well as effects on B cell function (Dong et al., 2001). Overall, comparison between mouse models and humans deficient in respective genes greatly contributes to our understanding of autoimmunity (e.g., AIRE, fox-P3, CD25), even if complete phenotypic homology between knockout mice and the respective human genetic deficiency is lacking.

Understanding the Complexity of Organ-Specific Autoimmunity

Animal models have helped us understand the complexity of biologic processes and be cautious in predicting the outcome of therapeutic interventions in humans (Roep et al., 2004). For example, in T1D, animal models have shown us that there are many different pathways to kill beta cells. If one of them is inactivated (i.e., perforin or interferon-gamma knockout), others will take over. The consequence is that it will be very difficult to engineer a "death-defying" beta cell that could be used for islet transplantations, since too many death pathways have to be eliminated in order to achieve resistance to immune destruction (Thomas and Kay, 2001). Present strategies therefore focus on physically shielding the transplanted islets from the immune system, an approach for which, once again, animal models have proven to be of exceptional value (Lee et al., 2009).

ANIMAL MODELS—ADVANTAGES AND DISADVANTAGES

As illustrated in Box 31.1, and as outlined above, there are several areas of investigation, where we have learned much from animal models of organ-specific autoimmunity. The first is investigation of immune responses at locations that are inaccessible in humans. Moreover, in these diseases much of what we know has often been derived from peripheral blood samples but it is unsure how this correlates to immune status at the target organ. We, for instance, were able to pioneer the *in vivo* visualization of immune responses at cellular resolution in the mouse pancreas during autoimmune diabetes development (Coppieters et al., 2012). Such information could never be gathered in human target organs with any of the technologies currently available.

Second, it is difficult to establish proof of concept in humans. Many techniques that are frequently used to unequivocally identify cellular subsets that are important in the etiology or progression of autoimmunity are impossible to implement in a clinical setting. Examples include adoptive transfers, knock-out technologies, bone marrow chimeras and many more.

Lastly, of course, the use of animal experimentation is at this point frequently indispensable to providing initial pre-clinical support for novel drugs and to defining dose ranges and regimens for immunotherapies.

How far reaching should the conclusions that we draw from observations in a given animal model be? The prevailing attitude is still that once a discovery has been made in one of the animal models thought to faithfully represent the human disease (e.g., the NOD mouse for diabetes or the experimental autoimmune encephalomyelitis (EAE) model for multiple sclerosis (MS)) there is no urgent need to look at this issue in other model systems. If the same result is found, it is considered "confirmatory," if a different result is discovered, the "secondary" model is frequently labeled as not-as-good or even flawed, for which various reasons are cited. This, we believe, can be treacherous and may hamper translation of research performed in animal models, because our pathogenetic insight into human diseases is often still rather limited due to ethical constraints. For example, only about 10% of patients with T1D exhibit the same clinical features as the NOD diabetic mouse, which is characterized by a polyglandular autoimmune syndrome affecting thyroid, salivary glands, and testes (Atkinson and Leiter, 1999; Roep et al., 2004). However, there are also striking similarities between NOD and human diabetes, for example, the occurrence of autoantibodies that precedes the development of clinical disease in NOD mice and humans (Pietropaolo and Eisenbarth, 2001).

We can now be certain that one single genetic defect or polymorphism will not be the cause for most human autoimmune disorders. We have learnt from the multitude of genome-wide association studies (GWAS) that the far more common scenario is a substantial degree of polygenic complexity. This would involve many protective and predisposing genes that act in concert, leading to disease manifestation in a fraction of their bearers. In addition to major histocompatibility complex (MHC) class II molecules that are found in association with several organ-specific autoimmune diseases such as MS and T1D, many less frequent polymorphisms in immune-related genes contribute to the expression of autoimmune disease (Bluestone et al., 2010). Immunogenetic studies in genetically identical mice can therefore not be expected to fully mimic the diverse arrays of polymorphisms that lead to disease in genetically distinct human subjects. Thus, seeking direct relevance to the human disorder becomes very important, and the assumption that there is a necessity to identify genetic defects in

---

Box 31.1 What Can Animal Models Teach Us that We Cannot Learn Otherwise?

- *In vivo* immune kinetics at *sites that are difficult to access* in humans.
- *Proof of concept* using techniques that cannot be used in humans, i.e., adoptive transfers, genetic knockouts, bone marrow chimeras, etc.
- Pre-clinical *drug validation*, large-scale assessment of *dose range, toxicity*, and immunization sites in drug and vaccine development.

Reasons to be Cautious with Animal Data.

- A single model is unlikely to cover all aspects of human pathology, concepts should therefore ideally be confirmed in multiple models.
- Genetic knockout models do not mimic the subtle and complex genetic imbalances that are thought to underlie human diseases.
- Environmental factors are usually not known and thus cannot be mimicked.

animal models in order to obtain the best pathways to cure human disease may not be correct. Indeed, in today's medicine, there is little evidence that the optimal treatment for a given disease is always the elimination of its cause. Immunogenetics in animal models might still help the adoption of novel predictive strategies and subclassifications for autoimmune diseases, which might in the future allow for more individualized treatments.

Finally, most of these genetic associations are weak enough to allow for the possibility that environmental factors in addition to genetic ones determine penetrance of disease. These factors, however, are poorly defined in most organ-specific autoimmune diseases. In the NOD mouse there appears to be a role for the gastrointestinal microbiome (Wen et al., 2008), although under normal specific pathogen-free conditions, diabetes develops without the need for an external stimulus. In human T1D, the strongest evidence for a potential trigger points toward enteroviral infection (Yeung et al., 2011). While viral infection can accelerate disease in the NOD, it is normally not required for onset. It is thus obvious that the NOD mouse does not faithfully integrate the environmental factors that seem to characterize disease in humans. Similar discordances are present in models for MS, where neuronal antigens are often injected in adjuvant to induce demyelinating disease. Such non-physiological conditions should always be kept in mind when interpreting results from animal models.

ANIMAL MODELS FOR ORGAN-SPECIFIC AUTOIMMUNE DISEASES

Again, our overview here does not intend to be complete. Instead, we will limit ourselves to a discussion of certain models that are uniquely informative on one point or another.

Spontaneous Models of Organ-Specific Autoimmunity

The Non-Obese Diabetic Mouse

The widely utilized NOD mouse expresses multiple autoimmune features in various organs—sialitis, T1D, orchitis, thyroiditis (Anderson and Bluestone, 2005)—and is prone to develop other autoimmune disorders including autoimmune cholangitis in NOD congenics (Wakabayashi et al., 2009), EAE (Winer et al., 2001), or neuritis in B7.2 deficient NOD strains (Salomon et al., 2001). The NOD strain was originally discovered in Japan and exhibits spontaneous diabetes penetrance of 20−100% depending on the environment. In addition, females develop diabetes about four times as frequently as males. In contrast to most patients with diabetes, the NOD mouse develops multiglandular and other organ-specific autoimmunity.

The immunologic causes for diabetes development are uncertain, but the genetic composition of the NOD has been studied extensively and is strikingly similar to the genetics of human T1D (Wicker et al., 2005), particularly in MHC class II molecules linked to disease expression. In addition, susceptibility loci that contain, among others, the genes for interleukin (IL)-2 and CTLA-4 have been linked to disease or protection. In the case of CTLA-4, polymorphisms have been described in the NOD mouse that might play a similar role in the human disease.

In both humans and NOD mice, environmental factors strongly influence disease expression. Monozygotic twins exhibit discordance in T1D penetrance, and NOD mice do not develop diabetes unless they are kept under specific pathogen-free (SPF) conditions. Data in the NOD mouse indicate that viral infections can have both enhancing (Serreze et al., 2000) and protective (Filippi et al., 2009) effects and an extensive meta-analysis recently confirmed the association between enteroviral infections and human T1D (Yeung et al., 2011). A growing body of evidence emphasizes the role of the intestinal microbiome in disease development in the NOD mouse (Wen et al., 2008).

Immunologically, it is still unclear to what degree NOD mice and humans with T1D are similar. The appearance of autoantibodies predicts the risk to develop islet autoimmunity and, in many cases, T1D on an individual basis; the antigens targeted, however, differ—those for NOD mice autoantibodies almost exclusively recognize insulin, whereas anti-GAD and anti-IA2 are present in humans (Eisenbarth, 2003). T lymphocytes with a Th1-like profile correlate with destructive insulitis in the NOD and also in humans (Arif et al., 2004). The Th17 immune cell subset, the discovery of which has reshaped our understanding of disease pathways in autoimmunity, was found to contribute to immunopathology in the NOD (Emamaullee et al., 2009). The question of which functional Th profile characterizes an "optimal" autoaggressive T cell is not resolved. Transfer studies in the NOD model have shown that Th1 as well as Th2 cells can cause disease in immunodeficient NOD/SCID or NOD/RAG hosts, when sufficient cell numbers are transferred (Pakala et al., 1997). In this context it should be mentioned that it appears that these Th subsets show remarkable plasticity, as was shown by Th17 cell conversion in favor of a Th1 profile in the NOD (Bending et al., 2009).

The functionality of regulatory T cells (Tregs) has been studied particularly well in the NOD mouse. Tregs are thought to control most immune responses and can be antigen induced (adaptive, i.e., peripherally generated) or "natural" (thymus derived and characterized by constitutive Foxp3 expression). In NOD mice, such cells can mediate protection from diabetes, as is the case after anti-CD3 therapy (Bresson et al., 2006). Furthermore, Tregs were shown to be involved in protection conferred by viral infection (Filippi et al., 2009). For clinical purposes, the NOD mouse has been instrumental in defining the clinical potential of future Treg cell-based immune interventions (Battaglia et al., 2006).

Finally, the predisposition to autoimmunity in the NOD mouse could also be linked to defective thymic selection and/or presentation of autoantigens in the thymus (Stratmann et al., 2003). Here, the predisposing MHC class II allele may play a role by the insufficient or inappropriate presentation of self-peptides, resulting in suboptimal elimination of a variety of autoreactive T cell specificities.

Genetically Engineered Animal Models for Organ-Specific Autoimmunity

Genetically engineered defects involving the systemic deletion or overexpression of a distinct molecule will rarely result in a disease that is limited to a single target organ. Systemic knockouts that "take the brakes off" the immune system such as foxp3 (defective Tregs), AIRE (defective thymic negative selection), or tumor growth factor (TGF)-b (defective regulation) usually result in disease affecting multiple organs and are, therefore, discussed in Chapter 30 on systemic autoimmune diseases (Shull et al., 1992; Brunkow et al., 2001; Anderson et al., 2002). There are, however, a few exceptions, one being the CD86-(B7.2) deficient NOD strain (Salomon et al., 2001). The autoimmunity that is usually directed towards the pancreatic islets in the NOD was redirected to attack peripheral nerves, resulting in neuritis. The reason may be altered local regulation of costimulatory molecules as well as defective thymic selection, resulting in higher levels of naïve T cells that can recognize neuronal antigens. One notable mouse strain with a systemic genetic defect that is commonly employed as a model for organ-specific autoimmunity, namely Crohn's disease, is the IL-10 deficient mouse (Kuhn et al., 1993). Mice are viable and develop a chronic form of enterocolitis which responds to agents such as TNF inhibitors that are clinically applied in Crohn's disease (Scheinin et al., 2003).

A more subtle variant of genetic modification includes tissue-specific gene deletion or overexpression. Here, one intends to avoid widespread autoimmunity when testing the influence of a certain gene on a specific target organ. One representative example is the series of recent papers on the *in vivo* role of the anti-inflammatory, ubiquitin-editing enzyme A20 that acts downstream of the TCR and BCR. A20 deficient mice spontaneously develop multiorgan inflammation and cachexia and die within 2 weeks of birth (Lee et al., 2000), which makes them rather irrelevant tools in the context of organ-specific autoimmunity. However, when this gene is deleted only

in specific organ systems, it is possible to mimic the development of organ-specific autoimmunity. Indeed, whereas A20 deletion in myeloid cells triggers arthritic disease (Matmati et al., 2011; a "systemic" disease), deletion in enterocytes sensitizes to organ-specific autoimmune colitis (Vereecke et al., 2010). Thus, specific gene deletion in certain tissues or organs can sometimes provoke or enhance organ-specific autoimmunity and teach us on gene function in the target organ.

An alternative approach is the introduction of a disease-provoking T cell specificity by generating TCR-transgenic animals. RIP-OVA mice express membrane-bound ovalbumin (OVA) under the control of the rat insulin promoter in the thymus and pancreas. When crossed with mice expressing an OVA-specific MHC II-restricted T cell receptor transgene (DO11.10), the double transgenic DO11.10xRIPmOVA (DORmO) mice are spontaneously diabetic, with 100% of animals becoming hyperglycemic by 20 weeks of age (Clough et al., 2008). TCR-transgenic strains that spontaneously develop EAE were also designed (Goverman et al., 1993; Pollinger et al., 2009). While these studies could yield information on some important aspects on certain driver T cells in organ-specific autoimmunity, they are clearly an oversimplification given the vast repertoire complexity in human disease.

In summary, although systemic immune defects will likely lead to more severe autoimmunity affecting multiple organs, there are exceptions to the rule. In humans, a combination of genetic factors leads to an overall predisposition state, yet not necessarily to actual clinical disease. It is thought that manifestation of organ-specific autoimmunity in most instances only occurs after a localized inflammatory insult, either a virus infection or other events that could lead to expansion of autoaggressive T cells. A thought-provoking hypothesis that was recently proposed by Wasserfall and colleagues is the "threshold hypothesis" which pictures the combined risk due to genes and environment as a continuum (Wasserfall et al., 2011). Only in extreme cases can either genes or environmental factors independently provoke autoimmunity such as is the case with Foxp3 mutations (genes only) (Brunkow et al., 2001; Bennett et al., 2001; Wildin et al., 2001) or pancreatectomy (environment only) (Lampeter et al., 1995). This theory is in agreement with the fact that in most animal models an environmental trigger is required to break tolerance, and that purely genetic models only rarely result in organ-specific autoimmunity.

Induced Animal Models for Organ-Specific Autoimmune Diseases

Breaking Tolerance is Not Easily Achieved

Provoking autoimmunity usually requires a strong artificial trigger that breaks self-tolerance. This can be achieved in susceptible mouse strains which carry a complex set of predisposing genes (e.g., SJL mice for EAE). Alternatively, many antigen-specific models for diabetes and other organ-specific autoimmune disorders are based on transgenic technology to express a defined autoantigen under the control of a tissue-specific promoter—e.g., the RIP to direct expression to beta cells or the keratin promoter to direct expression to the skin (McGargill et al., 2002). For diabetes, examples include the mouse models RIP-OVA (no spontaneous diabetes unless TCR transgenic, see above) and RIP-LCMV (Ohashi et al., 1991; Oldstone et al., 1991)). Such antigen-specific models have the advantage that the initiation of the autoaggressive response can be defined precisely, and at least the initial autoaggressive "driver" T cell is known. Notably, these mice do not develop spontaneous disease and even immunization with the protein antigen does not lead to diabetes in any of the RIP-antigen models. One could argue that according to the "threshold hypothesis" as mentioned above, these inducible models often tend to resemble the extreme end of the spectrum where genetic predisposition becomes unimportant. Despite this etiological shortcoming, inducible models are still frequently used to study effector mechanisms and test potential therapeutics. They fundamentally illustrate that breaking tolerance is generally not easy to achieve, even in the presence of a predisposing genotype.

Environmental Triggers Employed to Break Tolerance

Viral Infection

In some models, infection with a virus expressing the self-protein (transgene) or immunization in conjunction with Toll-like receptor (TLR) stimuli leads to T1D reliably (RIP-LCMV mice). These models mimic the scenario where effector T cells directly cross-react with a known autoantigen and redirect their cytotoxic action after viral clearance.

Alternatively, infection with Theile's murine encephalomyelitis virus (TMEV), which preferably replicates in neurons, results in a poliomyelitis-like syndrome reminiscent of MS (Lipton, 1975). Only certain mouse strains survive the primary infection and become persistently infected which results in a chronic progressive inflammatory demyelinating disease. The disease is initiated by virus-specific CD4 T cells while autoreactive myelin-specific CD4 T cell responses arise by epitope spreading and contribute to chronic pathology (Miller et al., 1997). Indeed, it was shown that T cell responses to the immunodominant self epitope were not a direct consequence of molecular mimicry, but rather originated from the *de novo* priming of self-reactive T cells to sequestered autoantigens released as a consequence of virus-specific T

cell-mediated demyelination. Epitope spreading is therefore considered an alternate mechanism that can link viral infection to organ-specific autoimmune diseases (Figure 31.1).

Another excellent example of a virus-triggered autoimmune disease model is the model of autoimmune myocarditis which is induced by inoculation with heart-passaged coxsackievirus B3 (Fairweather and Rose, 2007). For an in-depth discussion on this model we refer the reader to Chapter 70.

Protein/Peptide and Adjuvant

Multiple Sclerosis

The earliest evidence that encephalomyelitis could be triggered by challenging the immune system with self proteins came from side effects associated with the use of Pasteur's rabies vaccine (Mackay, 2010). The vaccine, made from the dried spinal cord from rabies-infected rabbits, in some cases led to ascending paralysis. This postvaccinal encephalomyelitis was later also shown to occur in rabbits with extracts of normal human spinal cord, or sheep brain. In the 1940s, it was more formally demonstrated that encephalomyelitis could be provoked in animals via a short course of injections of normal brain combined with Freund's complete adjuvant (FCA).

Today, the EAE model is one of the best known and most widely used examples in this category. EAE, which is primarily CD4 T cell driven, is induced in susceptible mice (SJL, PL/J) by immunization with neuronal proteins, or their respective MHC class II-restricted epitopes together with FCA and pertussis toxin (Fletcher et al., 2010). The clinical outcome is a relapsing remitting disease with severe neurologic implications. Central nervous system (CNS) histopathology shows T cell infiltration, anaphase-promoting complex (APC) and microglia activation, and disruption of the blood–brain barrier. Alternating periods of demyelination and remission characterized by remyelination occur.

Thyroiditis

Thyroid-specific autoimmunity underlies the development of Hashimoto's thyroiditis (hypothyroidism) and Graves' disease (hyperthyroidism) (Stassi and De Maria, 2002). Hashimoto's thyroiditis is the most common organ-specific autoimmune disease and is seen as a paradigm for other T cell-mediated organ-specific autoimmune diseases. Of historical interest is the series of studies by Noel Rose and Ernest Witebsky in the mid-1950s which centered on the induction of thyroid mononuclear infiltration after immunization with thyroid extracts in rabbits (Rose and Witebsky, 1956; Witebsky et al., 1957; Mackay, 2010).

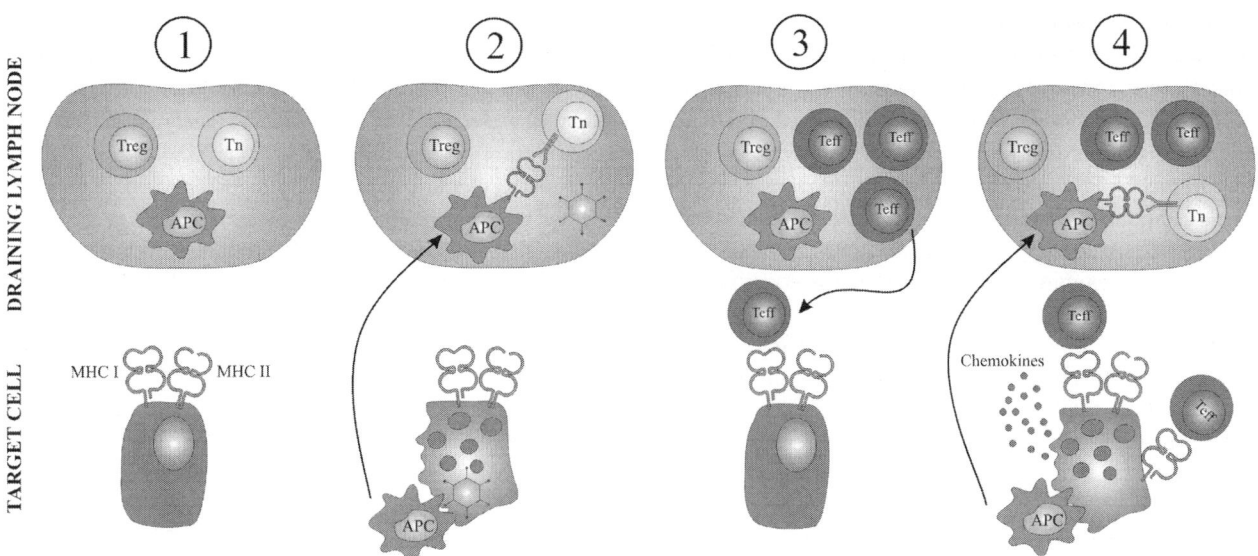

FIGURE 31.1   The development of T cell-driven organ-specific autoimmunity.   (1) While defective thymic selection may confer additional susceptibility, every individual has a certain repertoire of self-reactive cells. Under normal conditions, peripheral tolerance mechanisms governed by Treg prevent the activation of these cells. (2) When an environmental agent (here a virus) infects cells of a specific organ and causes (limited) cell death, phagocytes such as macrophages will drain self antigens to the lymph nodes. In the lymph nodes of normal individuals, Treg still maintains tolerance, whereas in susceptible individuals effector T cells are generated. Alternatively, a peripheral infection may directly activate autoreactive cells via mechanisms such as mimicry. (3) The effector T cells (here CTL) will home to their target tissue, recognize presented self antigens and initiate cellular cytoxicity. (4) Chemokine production will enhance Teff influx, leading to more cell death and antigen drainage. This, in turn, will provoke new rounds of T cell activation which expands the reactivity profile beyond the inciting antigen, a process termed "antigen spreading." As soon as a sufficient amount of target cells is killed, clinical disease typically becomes manifest.

Since the experimental outcome resembled Hashimoto's disease in humans, sera from such patients were analyzed and these, like the immunized rabbits, contained antibodies to thyroglobulin (Campbell et al., 1956).

Other experimental autoimmune thyroiditis (EAT) models have been described which rely on genetic predisposition or transfer of cells primed with thyroid antigen, collectively confirming the central role of $CD4^+$ T cells in the immunopathology (Stassi and De Maria, 2002).

In Graves' disease, $CD4^+$ T cells stimulate B cells to produce antibodies specific for the thyroid-stimulating hormone (TSH) receptor, which leads to uncontrolled thyroid hormone production. The disease can be modeled in specific mouse strains by immunization with fibroblasts that express the TSH receptor (Shimojo et al., 1996), or with an expression vector that contains the TSH receptor complementary DNA (Costagliola et al., 2000).

Myasthenia Gravis

Myasthenia gravis is an autoimmune disease where neuromuscular transmission is impaired, leading to fatigable muscle weakness in patients and, in some cases, acute respiratory failure. The cause of the disorder is the development of autoantibodies against nicotinic acetylcholine

receptors (AChR) (Spillane et al., 2012). Thus, the causal antigen is well defined.

The principal animal model of the disease, experimental autoimmune MG (EAMG), is typically induced in mice, rats, guinea pigs, or rabbits by immunization with either *Torpedo californica* or electric eel AChR in adjuvants (Lennon et al., 1975; Wu et al., 2001). In mice, strain differences greatly influence disease susceptibility, with an important role for MHC (H-2)-linked genes. In addition to current first-line therapies such as acetylcholinesterase inhibition, there is an interest in designing antigen-specific tolerization therapies such as through oral feeding of ACrR antigen (Baggi et al., 1999; Im et al., 1999) which protects from disease progression in the EAMG model.

What makes this model particularly interesting is that the pathogenesis of mouse EAMG closely resembles human myasthenia gravis. We will not elaborate on the full list of corresponding pathological features, which are reviewed in Christadoss et al. (2000). Nevertheless, it is interesting to point out the conceptual difference with other immunization-based animal models such as for instance the collagen-induced arthritis (CIA) model for rheumatoid arthritis. Both EAMG and CIA are fundamentally artificial in the sense that the underlying cause of the disease in humans is unknown and does not involve an injection of antigen in adjuvant. In rheumatoid arthritis, however, collagen-specific autoimmunity can be a contributing factor, yet collagen is not the key autoantigen that drives disease progression. In myasthenia gravis, since the key autoantigen is so well defined, immunization in the EAMG model leads not only to similar disease manifestations but arguably also a more similar underlying immunopathology. Analogous induction protocols including a combination of a defined autoantigen and adjuvant are used to induce diseases such as pemphigus vulgaris (Dsg3 immunization; Fan et al., 1999). A common shortcoming of these models is the major extent of external manipulation required to break tolerance.

Autoimmune Uveitis

Autoimmune uveitis in humans represents a heterogeneous condition with variability in both clinical presentation and disease course. The disease is typically associated with the occurrence of immune responses to retinal antigens, with retinal arrestin (S-antigen) being the most prevalent target. Notably, patients that respond to the same retinal antigen(s) do not necessarily share the same clinical symptoms (Caspi, 2011). Furthermore, it is unknown whether these uveitis-specific responses are causative or rather secondary.

In animals, different antigens were shown to result in distinct pathological outcomes (Caspi, 2006). The most widely used model is the experimental autoimmune uveitis model (EAU), which is induced by immunizing susceptible rodent strains with interphotoreceptor retinoid-binding protein (IRBP) in adjuvant (Caspi et al., 1988). Although EAU—or any other uveitis model—clearly does not reproduce the complexity of autoimmune uveitis in patients and is therefore hard to align with any clinical counterpart, the model has been informative in preclinical testing of new therapeutic concepts such as oral tolerance and more recently IL-2 receptor blockade (Caspi et al., 2008).

Chemicals

Chemical triggers usually rely on some sort of structural resemblance to non-hazardous substances that are normally taken up specifically by the target cells. The widely used model of streptozotocin (STZ)-induced diabetes is based on the structural similarity of the compound to glucose, which makes it particularly toxic to beta cells. STZ is an alkylating agent that causes DNA damage and is taken up by a glucose transporter that is specific to beta cells. While a single high dose causes non-immune beta cell deletion, a course of repeated low-dose administration mimics an autoimmune form of disease (Like and Rossini, 1976).

Another popular model is the dextran sodium sulfate (DSS) autoimmune colitis model (Okayasu et al., 1990). The exact mechanism through which DSS initiates colitis is unknown but one possible mechanism may be interference with gut permeability.

Finally, certain chemicals such as cyclophosphamide have the capacity to trigger autoimmunity, in this case diabetes, in susceptible mice (Harada and Makino, 1984). It was shown that this particular agent acts by reducing the Treg population and thus tipping the balance in favor of autoimmunity (Brode et al., 2006).

Cell Transfer or Depletion

Multiple Sclerosis

Adoptive transfer of a pathogenic "driver" T cell population is a frequently used strategy to model disease and to dissect the roles of certain functional subsets or T cell reactivities. EAE can be passively induced by adoptive transfer of T cells isolated from mice primed with myelin antigens into naïve mice (Stromnes and Goverman, 2006). This approach was instrumental in showing that myelin-specific CD8 T cells function as effector cells in MS-like pathogenesis (Huseby et al., 2001).

Type 1 Diabetes

Likewise, autoimmune diabetes can be induced by the transfer of certain diabetogenic driver clones. One approach uses the BDC2.5 CD4 T cell clone, which upon transfer rapidly triggers diabetes onset in the NOD mouse (Haskins and McDuffie, 1990). The BDC2.5 TCR is specific for a recently described pancreatic islet β-cell antigen, chromogranin A (Stadinski et al., 2010). This model offers the opportunity to study a genuine diabetogenic driver clone in the NOD and has been used for intravital imaging studies (Tang et al., 2006) or to examine functional Th plasticity (Bending et al., 2009).

Inflammatory Bowel Disease

Several key scientific breakthroughs on the role of Treg in controlling autoimmunity were based on the study of the CD45Rb transfer model for autoimmune colitis. Briefly, transfer of CD4$^+$CD45RB^{high}T cells from wild-type donor mice into immunodeficient SCID or RAG$^{-/-}$ recipients leads to wasting disease and intestinal inflammation, starting 3—5 weeks after transfer (Powrie et al., 1993). In contrast, transfer of unfractionated CD4 T cells, or transfer of the CD4$^+$CD45RB^{low}subset, does not provoke disease. When both the CD45RB^{low} and CD45RB^{high} subset are co-transferred, no disease develops, which at the time indicated that certain cells with potent regulatory function (now known as Treg) were able to control the pathogenic cells (Powrie et al., 1994).

Autoimmune Gastritis

Autoimmune gastritis is characterized by the development of a mononuclear cell infiltrate, destruction of parietal and zymogenic cells, and presence of autoantibodies specific for gastric H^+/K^+ ATPase (Field et al., 2005). Experimental autoimmune gastritis (EAG) occurs spontaneously in certain mouse strains (Alderuccio and Toh, 1998) or can be induced by a variety of methods such as immunization with gastric H^+/K^+-ATPase in FCA (Scarff et al., 1997). The latter model was instrumental in the identification of the β-subunit of the H^+/K^+ ATPase as a key autoantigen in autoimmune gastritis.

Rather than cell transfer, depletion of certain regulatory cell subsets can also lead to autoimmunity. Of major conceptual importance was the notion that neonatal thymectomy leads, in addition to a range of other autoimmune conditions, to autoimmune gastritis in 40–50% of Balb/c mice (Kojima and Prehn, 1981). Later investigations demonstrated that the early development of Treg in the thymus is essential to maintain self-tolerance later in life (Sakaguchi and Sakaguchi, 1990). This population, commonly termed "natural Treg," is now known as an essential gatekeeper against autoimmunity and in maintaining overall immune homeostasis.

General Conclusions from Induced Models

Breaking tolerance to an autoantigen is a "numbers game" and $CD8^+$ cytotoxic T lymphocytes (CTLs) can eliminate target cells such as keratinocytes or islet beta cells, when activated and able to enter the organ in sufficient numbers. Interesting differences emerge here for different target organs that express the same antigen: the pancreas and skin more readily show clinical signs of autoimmunity, but the brain appears to be capable of suppressing activated autoaggressive T cells, even after they cross the blood–brain barrier, as evidenced by mild disease in MBP-LCMV-Ag transgenic mice despite intracerebral infiltration (Evans et al., 1996). Thus, induction of organ-specific autoimmunity can be expected to follow quantitative rules and reduction of autoaggressive T cells beyond a certain threshold level will abrogate disease development.

Inflammation within any specific target organ induced by means of a local viral infection can activate macrophages and "set the stage" for further development of disease (von Herrath and Holz, 1997). Thus, breaking of tolerance might require the association with localized specific or non-specific inflammatory processes that could have, in addition to viral infections, a variety of other causes. The "fertile field" hypothesis is based on these observations and assumes that infections are required to "shape" the local target milieu and create conditions that are permissive for autoimmunity (von Herrath et al., 2003).

Regulatory cells can generally prevent autoimmune disease. Using transfer models one can clearly delineate the concept of bystander suppression, namely that a Treg with one antigenic specificity can downmodulate aggressive T cells with other antigenic specificities. This is a concept that is instrumental in the concept of antigen-specific immunotherapy. Indeed, there is a need for bystander suppression when T-cell populations with multiple autoaggressive specificities act in concert, and it might be necessary to dampen many to see an effect (Figure 31.2).

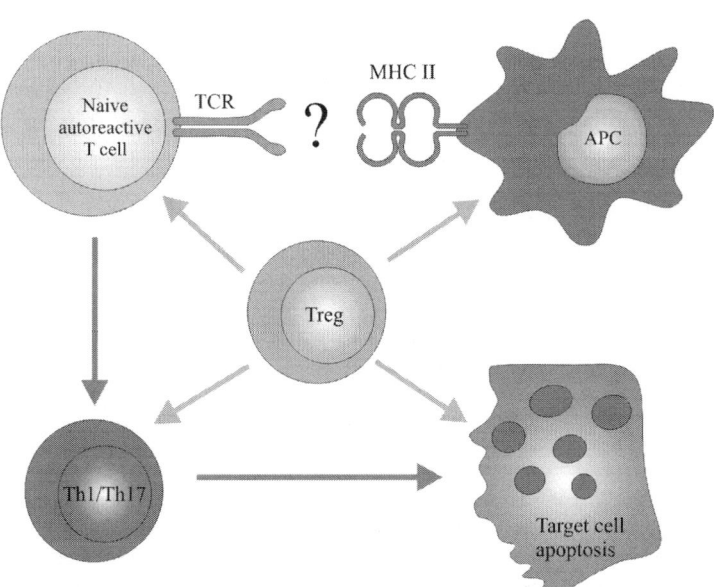

FIGURE 31.2 **The influence of Treg on autoimmunity.** In autoimmune diseases, an unknown antigen activates naïve T cells, which differentiate into pathogenic Th subsets (or CTL) and eventually kill target cells. Treg may prevent this process by direct modulation of APC function. Some studies even show Treg-mediated APC killing. Alternatively, Treg may inhibit activation or act suppressive on Th effectors. Finally, Treg can interfere with target killing and as such protect from clinical disease.

Finally, a close look at many of the induced autoimmune models suggests that the destruction of the attacked cell type or organ can occur via a variety of pathways that are not mutually exclusive. In addition, the autoaggressive response exhibits plasticity in the sense that blocking of one specific effector arm, e.g., killing of CTL by Fas or perforin or inflammatory cytokines, will result in the emergence of alternative pathways.

Comparison of Organ-Specific Autoimmune Disease in Animal Models and Humans

Every model will reflect certain aspects of the human disease and for this reason will be suited for some but not all of the scientific questions. Two examples of this are T1D and MS.

Type 1 Diabetes

The NOD model, although still considered the best model for T1D, resembles human T1D in many but not all aspects. It is evident that it lacks insufficient stringency to vigorously test preventive therapies: some 190 interventions can prevent T1D in the NOD mouse when given early enough, while many have been unsuccessful in humans (Shoda et al., 2005). Reversal of recent-onset disease, however, is much more difficult to achieve and only the most potent immune intervention regimens (e.g., anti-CD3) appear to be able to accomplish remission. Consequently, we should experimentally increase the stringency of the animal model test, and evaluate potential candidate interventions, both in NOD mice with recent-onset diabetes and in other diabetes models.

A major difference is the histopathology of the target site, the pancreatic islets. In mice, pancreatic islets are literally engulfed by a massive inflammatory infiltrate, while in humans this appears to be much more subtle. In fact, some previous studies on human cadaveric sections defined a threshold as low as five immune cells to define insulitis (Coppieters and von Herrath, 2009). Moreover, whereas prediabetic NOD mice exhibit clear signs of insulitis long before onset, studies in humans find very little evidence of ongoing pathology (In't Veld et al., 2007).

Finally, NOD mice develop antibodies to insulin, as do most patients with T1D. Some evidence was reported showing that NOD mice also develop antibody responses to GAD and IA-2. The current consensus, however, is that insulin, but not GAD and IA-2, is targeted by humoral immune response in NOD mice (Bonifacio et al., 2001). These findings indicate that there are important differences in the humoral antigenic repertoire between mouse model and human disease.

Multiple Sclerosis

In striking similarity to the NOD model for T1D, more than 90% of animal research on MS utilizes the EAE model. The model parallels MS on various levels, including genetic susceptibility in the MHC, occurrence of lesions populated by CD4 and CD8 T cells, a role for antibodies and complement, damage to the myelin sheath, and axonal degeneration.

In some instances, the EAE model shows a corresponding clinical response to treatment, as in the case of interferon (IFN)-beta therapy (Yu et al., 1996). Notable divergences, however, include TNF-alpha inhibition and IFN-gamma therapy, which are both effective in EAE but not MS (Steinman and Zamvil, 2005). Finally, in the EAE model, antibodies to myelin antigens are present in cerebrospinal fluid, while in patients these are infrequent and do not constitute the antigen specificity of the oligoclonal IgG bands that often characterize the disease (Weber et al., 2011). Whereas in animals, CNS-reactive antibodies were found to contribute in a pathogenic manner, the precise role in human disease is far from certain.

CONCLUSIONS

Today, many well-characterized models for organ-specific autoimmunity are available which together mimic a broad spectrum of human disease features. Our message is that a given animal model is only as good as the question it is used to answer, and particular models are well suited for some but not all questions. Consequently, a careful choice is needed in advance. Inbred mouse strains that are used to limit variability of *in vivo* studies will essentially tell the story of just one or a few human patients—for translating findings in animal models to human therapy, this is a particularly important realization—and a much higher degree of variation can be expected in human populations. In addition, it follows that each model will only reflect certain aspects of a given autoimmune disease accurately and, therefore, immunotherapeutic approaches should be validated in more than one model if possible. Nevertheless, the numerous animal models that are available to us are indispensable tools to study *in vivo* pathogenesis and treatments, and are a crucial step when moving from the bench to the bedside.

REFERENCES

Alderuccio, F., Toh, B.H., 1998. Spontaneous autoimmune gastritis in C3H/He mice: a new mouse model for gastric autoimmunity. Am. J. Pathol. 153, 1311–1318.

Anderson, M.S., Bluestone, J.A., 2005. The NOD mouse: a model of immune dysregulation. Annu. Rev. Immunol. 23, 447–485.

Anderson, M.S., Venanzi, E.S., Klein, L., Chen, Z., Berzins, S.P., Turley, S.J., et al., 2002. Projection of an immunological self shadow within the thymus by the aire protein. Science. 298, 1395–1401.

Arif, S., Tree, T.I., Astill, T.P., Tremble, J.M., Bishop, A.J., Dayan, C.M., et al., 2004. Autoreactive T cell responses show proinflammatory polarization in diabetes but a regulatory phenotype in health. J. Clin. Invest. 113, 451–463.

Atkinson, M.A., Leiter, E.H., 1999. The NOD mouse model of type 1 diabetes: as good as it gets? Nat. Med. 5, 601–604.

Baggi, F., Andreetta, F., Caspani, E., Milani, M., Longhi, R., Mantegazza, R., et al., 1999. Oral administration of an immunodominant T-cell epitope downregulates Th1/Th2 cytokines and prevents experimental myasthenia gravis. J. Clin. Invest. 104, 1287–1295.

Battaglia, M., Stabilini, A., Draghici, E., Migliavacca, B., Gregori, S., Bonifacio, E., et al., 2006. Induction of tolerance in type 1 diabetes via both CD4 + CD25 + T regulatory cells and T regulatory type 1 cells. Diabetes. 55, 1571–1580.

Bending, D., De La Pena, H., Veldhoen, M., Phillips, J.M., Uyttenhove, C., Stockinger, B., et al., 2009. Highly purified Th17 cells from BDC2.5NOD mice convert into Th1-like cells in NOD/SCID recipient mice. J. Clin. Invest. 119, 565–572.

Bennett, C.L., Christie, J., Ramsdell, F., Brunkow, M.E., Ferguson, P.J., Whitesell, L., et al., 2001. The immune dysregulation, polyendocrinopathy, enteropathy, X-linked syndrome (IPEX) is caused by mutations of FOXP3. Nat. Genet. 27, 20–21.

Bluestone, J.A., Herold, K., Eisenbarth, G., 2010. Genetics, pathogenesis and clinical interventions in type 1 diabetes. Nature. 464, 1293–1300.

Bonifacio, E., Atkinson, M., Eisenbarth, G., Serreze, D., Kay, T.W., Lee-Chan, E., et al., 2001. International workshop on lessons from animal models for human type 1 diabetes: identification of insulin but not glutamic acid decarboxylase or IA-2 as specific autoantigens of humoral autoimmunity in nonobese diabetic mice. Diabetes. 50, 2451–2458.

Bresson, D., Togher, L., Rodrigo, E., Chen, Y., Bluestone, J.A., Herold, K.C., et al., 2006. Anti-CD3 and nasal proinsulin combination therapy enhances remission from recent-onset autoimmune diabetes by inducing Tregs. J. Clin. Invest. 116, 1371–1381.

Brode, S., Raine, T., Zaccone, P., Cooke, A., 2006. Cyclophosphamide-induced type-1 diabetes in the NOD mouse is associated with a reduction of CD4 + CD25 + Foxp3 + regulatory T cells. J. Immunol. 177, 6603–6612.

Brunkow, M.E., Jeffery, E.W., Hjerrild, K.A., Paeper, B., Clark, L.B., Yasayko, S.A., et al., 2001. Disruption of a new forkhead/winged-helix protein, scurfin, results in the fatal lymphoproliferative disorder of the scurfy mouse. Nat. Genet. 27, 68–73.

Bulek, A.M., Cole, D.K., Skowera, A., Dolton, G., Gras, S., Madura, F., et al., 2012. Structural basis for the killing of human beta cells by CD8(+) T cells in type 1 diabetes. Nat. Immunol. 13, 283–289.

Campbell, P.N., Doniach, D., Hudson, R.V., Roitt, I.M., 1956. Autoantibodies in Hashimoto's disease (lymphadenoid goitre). Lancet. 271, 820–821.

Caspi, R.R., 2006. Ocular autoimmunity: the price of privilege? Immunol. Rev. 213, 23–35.

Caspi, R.R., 2011. Understanding autoimmune uveitis through animal models. The Friedenwald Lecture. Invest. Ophthalmol. Vis. Sci. 52, 1872–1879.

Caspi, R.R., Roberge, F.G., Chan, C.C., Wiggert, B., Chader, G.J., Rozenszajn, L.A., et al., 1988. A new model of autoimmune disease. Experimental autoimmune uveoretinitis induced in mice with two different retinal antigens. J. Immunol. 140, 1490–1495.

Caspi, R.R., Silver, P.B., Luger, D., Tang, J., Cortes, L.M., Pennesi, G., et al., 2008. Mouse models of experimental autoimmune uveitis. Ophthalmic. Res. 40, 169–174.

Christadoss, P., Poussin, M., Deng, C., 2000. Animal models of myasthenia gravis. Clin. Immunol. 94, 75–87.

Clough, L.E., Wang, C.J., Schmidt, E.M., Booth, G., Hou, T.Z., Ryan, G.A., et al., 2008. Release from regulatory T cell-mediated suppression during the onset of tissue-specific autoimmunity is associated with elevated IL-21. J. Immunol. 180, 5393–5401.

Coppieters, K., Amirian, N., Von Herrath, M., 2012. Intravital imaging of CTLs killing islet cells in diabetic mice. J. Clin. Invest. 122, 119–131.

Coppieters, K.T., Von Herrath, M.G., 2009. Histopathology of type 1 diabetes: old paradigms and new insights. Rev. Diabet Stud. 6, 85–96.

Costagliola, S., Many, M.C., Denef, J.F., Pohlenz, J., Refetoff, S., Vassart, G., 2000. Genetic immunization of outbred mice with thyrotropin receptor cDNA provides a model of Graves' disease. J. Clin. Invest. 105, 803–811.

Dong, C., Juedes, A.E., Temann, U.A., Shresta, S., Allison, J.P., Ruddle, N.H., et al., 2001. ICOS co-stimulatory receptor is essential for T-cell activation and function. Nature. 409, 97–101.

Eisenbarth, G.S., 2003. Insulin autoimmunity: immunogenetics/immunopathogenesis of type 1A diabetes. Ann. NY. Acad. Sci. 1005, 109–118.

Emamaullee, J.A., Davis, J., Merani, S., Toso, C., Elliott, J.F., Thiesen, A., et al., 2009. Inhibition of Th17 cells regulates autoimmune diabetes in NOD mice. Diabetes. 58, 1302–1311.

Evans, C.F., Horwitz, M.S., Hobbs, M.V., Oldstone, M.B., 1996. Viral infection of transgenic mice expressing a viral protein in oligodendrocytes leads to chronic central nervous system autoimmune disease. J. Exp. Med. 184, 2371–2384.

Fairweather, D., Rose, N.R., 2007. Coxsackievirus-induced myocarditis in mice: a model of autoimmune disease for studying immunotoxicity. Methods. 41, 118–122.

Fambrough, D.M., Drachman, D.B., Satyamurti, S., 1973. Neuromuscular junction in myasthenia gravis: decreased acetylcholine receptors. Science. 182, 293–295.

Fan, J.L., Memar, O., McCormick, D.J., Prabhakar, B.S., 1999. BALB/c mice produce blister-causing antibodies upon immunization with a recombinant human desmoglein 3. J. Immunol. 163, 6228–6235.

Field, J., Biondo, M.A., Murphy, K., Alderuccio, F., Toh, B.H., 2005. Experimental autoimmune gastritis: mouse models of human organ-specific autoimmune disease. Int. Rev. Immunol. 24, 93–110.

Filippi, C.M., Estes, E.A., Oldham, J.E., Von Herrath, M.G., 2009. Immunoregulatory mechanisms triggered by viral infections protect from type 1 diabetes in mice. J. Clin. Invest. 119, 1515–1523.

Fletcher, J.M., Lalor, S.J., Sweeney, C.M., Tubridy, N., Mills, K.H., 2010. T cells in multiple sclerosis and experimental autoimmune encephalomyelitis. Clin. Exp. Immunol. 162, 1–11.

Goverman, J., Woods, A., Larson, L., Weiner, L.P., Hood, L., Zaller, D.M., 1993. Transgenic mice that express a myelin basic protein-specific T cell receptor develop spontaneous autoimmunity. Cell. 72, 551–560.

Grimbacher, B., Hutloff, A., Schlesier, M., Glocker, E., Warnatz, K., Drager, R., et al., 2003. Homozygous loss of ICOS is associated with adult-onset common variable immunodeficiency. Nat. Immunol. 4, 261–268.

Han, B., Serra, P., Amrani, A., Yamanouchi, J., Maree, A.F., Edelstein-Keshet, L., et al., 2005. Prevention of diabetes by manipulation of anti-IGRP autoimmunity: high efficiency of a low-affinity peptide. Nat. Med. 11, 645–652.

Harada, M., Makino, S., 1984. Promotion of spontaneous diabetes in non-obese diabetes-prone mice by cyclophosphamide. Diabetologia. 27, 604–606.

Haskins, K., McDuffie, M., 1990. Acceleration of diabetes in young NOD mice with a CD4 + islet-specific T cell clone. Science. 249, 1433–1436.

Hauser, S.L., Waubant, E., Arnold, D.L., Vollmer, T., Antel, J., Fox, R. J., et al., 2008. B-cell depletion with rituximab in relapsing-remitting multiple sclerosis. N. Engl. J. Med. 358, 676–688.

Huseby, E.S., Liggitt, D., Brabb, T., Schnabel, B., Ohlen, C., Goverman, J., 2001. A pathogenic role for myelin-specific CD8(+) T cells in a model for multiple sclerosis. J. Exp. Med. 194, 669–676.

Im, S.H., Barchan, D., Fuchs, S., Souroujon, M.C., 1999. Suppression of ongoing experimental myasthenia by oral treatment with an acetylcholine receptor recombinant fragment. J. Clin. Invest. 104, 1723–1730.

In't Veld, P., Lievens, D., De Grijse, J., Ling, Z., Van Der Auwera, B., Pipeleers-Marichal, M., et al., 2007. Screening for insulitis in adult autoantibody-positive organ donors. Diabetes. 56, 2400–2404.

Jarchum, I., Baker, J.C., Yamada, T., Takaki, T., Marron, M.P., Serreze, D.V., et al., 2007. In vivo cytotoxicity of insulin-specific CD8 + T-cells in HLA-A*0201 transgenic NOD mice. Diabetes. 56, 2551–2560.

Karlsson, F.A., Burman, P., Loof, L., Mardh, S., 1988. Major parietal cell antigen in autoimmune gastritis with pernicious anemia is the acid-producing H + ,K + -adenosine triphosphatase of the stomach. J. Clin. Invest. 81, 475–479.

Kennedy, M.K., Tan, L.J., Dal Canto, M.C., Miller, S.D., 1990. Regulation of the effector stages of experimental autoimmune encephalomyelitis via neuroantigen-specific tolerance induction. J. Immunol. 145, 117–126.

Kent, S.C., Chen, Y., Bregoli, L., Clemmings, S.M., Kenyon, N.S., Ricordi, C., et al., 2005. Expanded T cells from pancreatic lymph nodes of type 1 diabetic subjects recognize an insulin epitope. Nature. 435, 224–228.

Kojima, A., Prehn, R.T., 1981. Genetic susceptibility to post-thymectomy autoimmune diseases in mice. Immunogenetics. 14, 15–27.

Kuhn, R., Lohler, J., Rennick, D., Rajewsky, K., Muller, W., 1993. Interleukin-10-deficient mice develop chronic enterocolitis. Cell. 75, 263–274.

Lampeter, E.F., Tubes, M., Klemens, C., Brocker, U., Friemann, J., Kolb-Bachofen, V., et al., 1995. Insulitis and islet-cell antibody formation in rats with experimentally reduced beta-cell mass. Diabetologia. 38, 1397–1404.

Lee, E.G., Boone, D.L., Chai, S., Libby, S.L., Chien, M., Lodolce, J.P., Ma, A., 2000. Failure to regulate TNF-induced NF-kappaB and cell death responses in A20-deficient mice. Science. 289, 2350–2354.

Lee, S.H., Hao, E., Savinov, A.Y., Geron, I., Strongin, A.Y., Itkin-Ansari, P., 2009. Human beta-cell precursors mature into functional insulin-producing cells in an immunoisolation device: implications for diabetes cell therapies. Transplantation. 87, 983–991.

Lennon, V.A., Lindstrom, J.M., Seybold, M.E., 1975. Experimental autoimmune myasthenia: a model of myasthenia gravis in rats and guinea pigs. J. Exp. Med. 141, 1365–1375.

Lenschow, D.J., Ho, S.C., Sattar, H., Rhee, L., Gray, G., Nabavi, N., et al., 1995. Differential effects of anti-B7-1 and anti-B7-2 monoclonal antibody treatment on the development of diabetes in the nonobese diabetic mouse. J. Exp. Med. 181, 1145–1155.

Like, A.A., Rossini, A.A., 1976. Streptozotocin-induced pancreatic insulitis: new model of diabetes mellitus. Science. 193, 415–417.

Lin, M.S., Swartz, S.J., Lopez, A., Ding, X., Fernand ez-Vina, M.A., Stastny, P., et al., 1997. Development and characterization of desmoglein-3 specific T cells from patients with pemphigus vulgaris. J. Clin. Invest. 99, 31–40.

Lipton, H.L., 1975. Theiler's virus infection in mice: an unusual biphasic disease process leading to demyelination. Infect. Immun. 11, 1147–1155.

Mackay, I.R., 2010. Travels and travails of autoimmunity: a historical journey from discovery to rediscovery. Autoimmun. Rev. 9, A251–A258.

Mamchak, A.A., Manenkova, Y., Leconet, W., Zheng, Y., Chan, J.R., Stokes, C.L., et al., 2012. Preexisting autoantibodies predict efficacy of oral insulin to cure autoimmune diabetes in combination with anti-CD3. Diabetes. 61, 1490–1499.

Mastrandrea, L., Yu, J., Behrens, T., Buchlis, J., Albini, C., Fourtner, S., et al., 2009. Etanercept treatment in children with new-onset type 1 diabetes: pilot randomized, placebo-controlled, double-blind study. Diabetes Care. 32, 1244–1249.

Matmati, M., Jacques, P., Maelfait, J., Verheugen, E., Kool, M., Sze, M., et al., 2011. A20 (TNFAIP3) deficiency in myeloid cells triggers erosive polyarthritis resembling rheumatoid arthritis. Nat. Genet. 43, 908–912.

McGargill, M.A., Mayerova, D., Stefanski, H.E., Koehn, B., Parke, E.A., Jameson, S.C., et al., 2002. A spontaneous CD8 T cell-dependent autoimmune disease to an antigen expressed under the human keratin 14 promoter. J. Immunol. 169, 2141–2147.

Miller, S.D., Vanderlugt, C.L., Begolka, W.S., Pao, W., Yauch, R.L., et al., 1997. Persistent infection with Theiler's virus leads to CNS autoimmunity via epitope spreading. Nat. Med. 3, 1133–1136.

Nakayama, M., Abiru, N., Moriyama, H., Babaya, N., Liu, E., Miao, D., et al., 2005. Prime role for an insulin epitope in the development of type 1 diabetes in NOD mice. Nature. 435, 220–223.

Ohashi, P.S., Oehen, S., Buerki, K., Pircher, H., Ohashi, C.T., Odermatt, B., et al., 1991. Ablation of "tolerance" and induction of diabetes by virus infection in viral antigen transgenic mice. Cell. 65, 305–317.

Okayasu, I., Hatakeyama, S., Yamada, M., Ohkusa, T., Inagaki, Y., Nakaya, R., 1990. A novel method in the induction of reliable experimental acute and chronic ulcerative colitis in mice. Gastroenterology. 98, 694–702.

Oldstone, M.B., Nerenberg, M., Southern, P., Price, J., Lewicki, H., 1991. Virus infection triggers insulin-dependent diabetes mellitus in a transgenic model: role of anti-self (virus) immune response. Cell. 65, 319–331.

Orban, T., Bundy, B., Becker, D.J., Dimeglio, L.A., Gitelman, S.E., Goland, R., et al., 2011. Co-stimulation modulation with abatacept in patients with recent-onset type 1 diabetes: a rand omised, double-blind, placebo-controlled trial. Lancet. 378, 412–419.

Pakala, S.V., Kurrer, M.O., Katz, J.D., 1997. T helper 2 (Th2) T cells induce acute pancreatitis and diabetes in immune-compromised non-obese diabetic (NOD) mice. J. Exp. Med. 186, 299—306.

Pescovitz, M.D., Greenbaum, C.J., Krause-Steinrauf, H., Becker, D.J., Gitelman, S.E., Goland, R., et al., 2009. Rituximab, B-lymphocyte depletion, and preservation of beta-cell function. N. Engl. J. Med. 361, 2143—2152.

Pietropaolo, M., Eisenbarth, G.S., 2001. Autoantibodies in human diabetes. Curr. Dir. Autoimmun. 4, 252—282.

Pollinger, B., Krishnamoorthy, G., Berer, K., Lassmann, H., Bosl, M.R., Dunn, R., et al., 2009. Spontaneous relapsing-remitting EAE in the SJL/J mouse: MOG-reactive transgenic T cells recruit endogenous MOG-specific B cells. J. Exp. Med. 206, 1303—1316.

Powrie, F., Leach, M.W., Mauze, S., Caddle, L.B., Coffman, R.L., 1993. Phenotypically distinct subsets of CD4 + T cells induce or protect from chronic intestinal inflammation in C.B-17 scid mice. Int. Immunol. 5, 1461—1471.

Powrie, F., Correa-Oliveira, R., Mauze, S., Coffman, R.L., 1994. Regulatory interactions between CD45RBhigh and CD45RBlow CD4 + T cells are important for the balance between protective and pathogenic cell-mediated immunity. J. Exp. Med. 179, 589—600.

Roep, B.O., Atkinson, M., Von Herrath, M., 2004. Satisfaction (not) guaranteed: re-evaluating the use of animal models of type 1 diabetes. Nat. Rev. Immunol. 4, 989—997.

Rose, N.R., Witebsky, E., 1956. Studies on organ specificity. V. Changes in the thyroid gland s of rabbits following active immunization with rabbit thyroid extracts. J. Immunol. 76, 417—427.

Sakaguchi, S., Sakaguchi, N., 1990. Thymus and autoimmunity: capacity of the normal thymus to produce pathogenic self-reactive T cells and conditions required for their induction of autoimmune disease. J. Exp. Med. 172, 537—545.

Salomon, B., Rhee, L., Bour-Jordan, H., Hsin, H., Montag, A., Soliven, B., et al., 2001. Development of spontaneous autoimmune peripheral polyneuropathy in B7-2-deficient NOD mice. J. Exp. Med. 194, 677—684.

Scarff, K.J., Pettitt, J.M., Van Driel, I.R., Gleeson, P.A., Toh, B.H., 1997. Immunization with gastric H + /K(+)-ATPase induces a reversible autoimmune gastritis. Immunology. 92, 91—98.

Scheinin, T., Butler, D.M., Salway, F., Scallon, B., Feldmann, M., 2003. Validation of the interleukin-10 knockout mouse model of colitis: antitumour necrosis factor-antibodies suppress the progression of colitis. Clin. Exp. Immunol. 133, 38—43.

Sercarz, E.E., 2000. Driver clones and determinant spreading. J. Autoimmun. 14, 275—277.

Serreze, D.V., Ottendorfer, E.W., Ellis, T.M., Gauntt, C.J., Atkinson, M.A., 2000. Acceleration of type 1 diabetes by a coxsackievirus infection requires a preexisting critical mass of autoreactive T-cells in pancreatic islets. Diabetes. 49, 708—711.

Shimojo, N., Kohno, Y., Yamaguchi, K., Kikuoka, S., Hoshioka, A., Niimi, H., et al., 1996. Induction of Graves-like disease in mice by immunization with fibroblasts transfected with the thyrotropin receptor and a class II molecule. Proc. Natl. Acad. Sci. U.S.A. 93, 11074—11079.

Shoda, L.K., Young, D.L., Ramanujan, S., Whiting, C.C., Atkinson, M.A., Bluestone, J.A., et al., 2005. A comprehensive review of interventions in the NOD mouse and implications for translation. Immunity. 23, 115—126.

Shull, M.M., Ormsby, I., Kier, A.B., Pawlowski, S., Diebold, R.J., Yin, M., et al., 1992. Targeted disruption of the mouse transforming growth factor-beta 1 gene results in multifocal inflammatory disease. Nature. 359, 693—699.

Skowera, A., Ellis, R.J., Varela-Calvino, R., Arif, S., Huang, G.C., VanKrinks, C., et al., 2008. CTLs are targeted to kill beta cells in patients with type 1 diabetes through recognition of a glucose-regulated preproinsulin epitope. J. Clin. Invest. 118, 3390—3402.

Spillane, J., Higham, E., Kullmann, D.M., 2012. Myasthenia gravis. BMJ. 345, e8497.

Stadinski, B.D., Delong, T., Reisdorph, N., Reisdorph, R., Powell, R.L., Armstrong, M., et al., 2010. Chromogranin A is an autoantigen in type 1 diabetes. Nat. Immunol. 11, 225—231.

Stassi, G., De Maria, R., 2002. Autoimmune thyroid disease: new models of cell death in autoimmunity. Nat. Rev. Immunol. 2, 195—204.

Steinman, L., Zamvil, S.S., 2005. Virtues and pitfalls of EAE for the development of therapies for multiple sclerosis. Trends Immunol. 26, 565—571.

Stratmann, T., Martin-Orozco, N., Mallet-Designe, V., Poirot, L., McGavern, D., Losyev, G., et al., 2003. Susceptible MHC alleles, not background genes, select an autoimmune T cell reactivity. J. Clin. Invest. 112, 902—914.

Stromnes, I.M., Goverman, J.M., 2006. Passive induction of experimental allergic encephalomyelitis. Nat. Protoc. 1, 1952—1960.

Tang, Q., Adams, J.Y., Tooley, A.J., Bi, M., Fife, B.T., Serra, P., et al., 2006. Visualizing regulatory T cell control of autoimmune responses in nonobese diabetic mice. Nat. Immunol. 7, 83—92.

Thomas, H.E., Kay, T.W., 2001. How beta cells die in type 1 diabetes. Curr. Dir. Autoimmun. 4, 144—170.

Velthuis, J.H., Unger, W.W., Abreu, J.R., Duinkerken, G., Franken, K., Peakman, M., et al., 2010. Simultaneous detection of circulating autoreactive CD8 + T-cells specific for different islet cell-associated epitopes using combinatorial MHC multimers. Diabetes. 59, 1721—1730.

Vereecke, L., Sze, M., McGuire, C., Rogiers, B., Chu, Y., Schmidt-Supprian, M., et al., 2010. Enterocyte-specific A20 deficiency sensitizes to tumor necrosis factor-induced toxicity and experimental colitis. J. Exp. Med. 207, 1513—1523.

Von Herrath, M., Holz, A., 1997. Pathological changes in the islet milieu precede infiltration of islets and destruction of beta-cells by autoreactive lymphocytes in a transgenic model of virus-induced IDDM. J. Autoimmun. 10, 231—238.

Von Herrath, M.G., Dockter, J., Oldstone, M.B., 1994. How virus induces a rapid or slow onset insulin-dependent diabetes mellitus in a transgenic model. Immunity. 1, 231—242.

Von Herrath, M.G., Fujinami, R.S., Whitton, J.L., 2003. Microorganisms and autoimmunity: making the barren field fertile? Nat. Rev. Microbiol. 1, 151—157.

Wakabayashi, K., Yoshida, K., Leung, P.S., Moritoki, Y., Yang, G.X., Tsuneyama, K., et al., 2009. Induction of autoimmune cholangitis in non-obese diabetic (NOD).1101 mice following a chemical xenobiotic immunization. Clin. Exp. Immunol. 155, 577—586.

Wasserfall, C., Nead, K., Mathews, C., Atkinson, M.A., 2011. The threshold hypothesis: solving the equation of nurture vs nature in type 1 diabetes. Diabetologia. 54, 2232—2236.

Weber, M.S., Hemmer, B., Cepok, S., 2011. The role of antibodies in multiple sclerosis. Biochim. Biophys. Acta. 1812, 239—245.

Wen, L., Ley, R.E., Volchkov, P.Y., Stranges, P.B., Avanesyan, L., Stonebraker, A.C., et al., 2008. Innate immunity and intestinal microbiota in the development of type 1 diabetes. Nature. 455, 1109—1113.

Wicker, L.S., Clark, J., Fraser, H.I., Garner, V.E., Gonzalez-Munoz, A., Healy, B., et al., 2005. Type 1 diabetes genes and pathways shared by humans and NOD mice. J. Autoimmun. 25 (Suppl), 29–33.

Wildin, R.S., Ramsdell, F., Peake, J., Faravelli, F., Casanova, J.L., Buist, N., et al., 2001. X-linked neonatal diabetes mellitus, enteropathy and endocrinopathy syndrome is the human equivalent of mouse scurfy. Nat. Genet. 27, 18–20.

Wincr, S., Astsaturov, I., Cheung, R., Gunaratnam, L., Kubiak, V., Cortez, M.A., et al., 2001. Type I diabetes and multiple sclerosis patients target islet plus central nervous system autoantigens; nonimmunized nonobese diabetic mice can develop autoimmune encephalitis. J. Immunol. 166, 2831–2841.

Witebsky, E., Rose, N.R., Terplan, K., Paine, J.R., Egan, R.W., 1957. Chronic thyroiditis and autoimmunization. J. Am. Med. Assoc. 164, 1439–1447.

Wu, B., Goluszko, E. and Christadoss, P. 2001. Experimental autoimmune myasthenia gravis in the mouse. Curr. Protoc. Immunol., Chapter 15, Unit 15.8.

Yeung, W.C., Rawlinson, W.D., Craig, M.E., 2011. Enterovirus infection and type 1 diabetes mellitus: systematic review and meta-analysis of observational molecular studies. BMJ. 342, d35.

Yu, M., Nishiyama, A., Trapp, B.D., Tuohy, V.K., 1996. Interferon-beta inhibits progression of relapsing-remitting experimental autoimmune encephalomyelitis. J. Neuroimmunol. 64, 91–100.

Part 7

Multisystem Autoimmune Diseases

Chapter 32

Systemic Lupus Erythematosus

Robert G. Lahita

Newark Beth Israel Medical Center, Rutgers, the New Jersey Medical School, NJ, USA

Chapter Outline

Introduction	451	Neuropsychiatric	455
Pathogenesis	451	Cardiac	456
Genetics	452	Pulmonary	457
Epidemiology	452	Hematology	457
Autoantibody	452	Dermatology	457
Clinical	453	Gastroenterological	458
Measurement of Clinical Activity	454	ENT and Eye	458
Musculoskeletal	454	Lupus Therapeutics	458
Renal	455	References	459

INTRODUCTION

Systemic lupus erythematosus (SLE), an autoimmune disease that affects many organ systems, has no known etiology and a complex pathogenesis. It is more prevalent in females, has an human leukocyte antigen (HLA)-D association and presents clinically in diverse ways. Organs and tissues commonly affected include muscle and joints, brain and peripheral nervous system, lungs, heart, kidneys, skin, serous membranes, and components of the blood. Virtually any organ can be affected. Clinical manifestations are protean, overlap with other illnesses, and are often subtle.

PATHOGENESIS

The pathogenesis of lupus is enigmatic. Although primarily immunological, the pathogenesis of the disease is influenced and modified by non-immune systems like the endocrine or clotting systems (Shapiro and Long 1999; Simantov et al., 1999). At this time, the predilection of this disease for females cannot be explained; but pathogenetic factors like sex steroids or gonadotropins play a role in the severity of disease and the different clinical presentations between the genders. Factors such as drugs, diet, and environmental toxins have been implicated in the pathogenesis of SLE through epigenetic mechanisms (Ballestar et al., 2006; Richardson, 2009) (see Chapter 28).

There are formidable roles for both T and B cells in our understanding of SLE. Patients with active SLE have lower percentages of $CD4^+CD25^+$ T cells than healthy controls and those with active disease (Zheng et al., 2004). Production of interleukin (IL)-2 and tumor growth factor (TGF)-beta is lower in SLE patients than in controls (Ohtsuka et al., 1998, 1999). In mice various methods can be used to reverse the autoimmune process by stimulating regulatory T (Treg) cell production. In murine experiments the transfer of *ex vivo*-induced Treg cells leads to tolerance with suppressive activity. This Treg population is induced with IL-2 and TGF-beta and produces enough autologous Treg cells to suppress disease activity (Baecher-Allan et al., 2002, 2003). By far the greatest progress in SLE therapy in the last few years comes from the studies of B cells (Grimaldi et al., 2005). B cells are responsible for autoantibody production and immune complex deposition that leads to tissue injury. B cells also serve as antigen presenting cells, secrete proinflammatory and immunoregulatory cytokines, IL 10, and regulate T cell activation, anergy, proliferation and the differentiation of T cells and follicular dendritic cells. The consensus of investigators was that B cells could be modulated using antigen-specific interventions or disrupting B and T cell interactions. We will discuss these pathogenetic interactions under therapy (Garaud et al., 2011; Marino and Grey, 2012).

N. Rose & I. Mackay (Eds): The Autoimmune Diseases, Fifth edition. DOI: http://dx.doi.org/10.1016/B978-0-12-384929-8.00032-0

GENETICS

Specific immune response genes in the major histocompatibility complex (MHC) class II or class III regions on chromosome 6 are associated with SLE (Johanneson and Alarcon-Riquelme, 2001). Genetic associations include other loci that are constitutive. Genetic MHC II alleles are associated with certain autoantibody groups and inherited complement deficiencies develop variants of lupus with specific clinical characteristics. There are class II antigens and HLA-D locus associations to other diseases as well. These include rheumatoid arthritis, multiple sclerosis, idiopathic thrombocytopenic purpura (ITP), and rheumatic fever; overlap syndromes such as Sjögren's, scleroderma, thyroiditis, and the inflammatory diseases of muscle. Genetic influences on the development of SLE in humans are described in Chapter 26, and in murine models in Chapter 30.

EPIDEMIOLOGY

There are several worldwide studies concerning the epidemiology of SLE. Incidence varies according to the characteristics of the population studied (age, race, gender, ethnicity, period of time considered, and diagnostic criteria used). In the USA the annual incidence of SLE is estimated as 2.2 cases per 100,000 persons per year in rural Rochester, Minnesota (Michet et al., 1985). In San Francisco, California, the incidence rises to 7.6 cases per 100,000 (Fessel, 1974). In Europe the annual incidence differs from country to country: 2.2 cases per 100,000 in Spain to 5.8 cases per 100,000 cases per year in Iceland (Hochberg, 1987). The prevalence of the disease also varies with the methods involved in case ascertainment. There are undoubtedly genetic and environmental factors that affect differences of prevalence between various locales. Even the sex distribution and age changes could affect prevalence. Hochberg reported a prevalence of 12.5 cases per 100,000 women in England and Wales and a prevalence of 17.7 cases per 100,000 among those who were 15–64 years old. In the USA the prevalence of SLE ranges from 14.6 cases per 100,000 in New York to 78.5 cases per 100,000 in Wisconsin. These variations could be explained by the variations of disease expression as well as difficulty with diagnosis of the disease.

Age is an important consideration for lupus since the incidence rates vary by age in some studies (McCarty et al., 1995). Peak rates are reported in women during the childbearing years (15–44 years). Men tend to have an onset of the disease at an older age (50–65 years). The ethnic differences in SLE are significant (Carbone and Lohr 2002; Fessler et al., 2005; Krishnan and Hubert 2006; Anderson et al., 2008; Jurencak et al., 2009). There are significant differences with regard to black versus white people with the disease. A study from the UK showed that age-adjusted incidence of SLE in Afro-Caribbean patients was 25.8 versus 4.3 cases per 100,000 persons per year. The prevalence was 112 and 21 per 100,000 cases per year for the same cohort. The incidence and prevalence rates of SLE in the Asian population of the UK were 20.7 and 46.7 cases per 100,000 persons, respectively.

AUTOANTIBODY

Although there are a few nonimmunologic laboratory characteristics of SLE, these are not specific (Aranow et al., 2011; Reeves et al., 2011). Immunological tests, which are specific to most autoimmune diseases such as lupus, include the presence of specific cytotoxic lymphocytes and a variety of autoantibodies, including a persistently positive antinuclear antibody (ANA). The diagnostic utility of test procedures for ANA is described in Chapter 77. Laboratory data in the form of an isolated false-positive syphilis test, a low platelet count, elevated partial thromboplastin time (PTT), or leukopenia may suggest many other diseases that are often considered before SLE. SLE is a clinical diagnosis that depends on a careful history and physical examination. Autoantibodies are frequently associated with no disease and occur in normal people; they alone support but are not diagnostic of the disease. A history of specific medication is particularly important, as reversible drug-induced lupus is responsible for some 10% of cases (Yung and Richardson, 2011) and is often seen in older patients, particularly males. Lupus can be related to other illnesses that can occur in the patient's family such as rheumatoid arthritis (RA), ITP, and multiple sclerosis.

Depending on the clinician, more complex immunologic laboratory tests may solidify the diagnosis when suspected clinically or contribute to the erroneous diagnosis of SLE in the absence of clinical signs.

The widespread availability of such testing, the lack of standardization, and inappropriate application of such tests may contribute to diagnostic confusion. The most useful tests for SLE are the fluorescent antinuclear antibody test, antinative DNA assay, the total hemolytic complement (CH50), and C3 and C4. All of these tests are subject to wide variation: the ANA because of substrate variability, and the tendency to use enzyme-linked immunosorbent assay (ELISA) and other nonspecific modalities; the anti-DNA because of single-stranded DNA contamination and cross-reactivity with phospholipids; and the CH50, C3, and C4 because of the temperature sensitivity of complement components (Liang et al., 1989).

One can find other reactive antibodies, such as anti-Ro, anti-La, and other ribonucleoprotein antibodies in the absence of an ANA. Antibodies to native DNA (Aranow et al., 2011) and antibodies to Smith (Sm) antigen, a nuclear ribonucleoprotein, are also quite specific for SLE. Relevant autoantibodies and their associations are given in Table 32.1 (Stahl et al., 1979).

Common laboratory assays can aid the physician in establishing the diagnosis. Most useful is the white blood cell count (WBC), which often shows leukopenia and lymphopenia (Lahita, 1992). Anemia of chronic disease or in rare instances autoimmune hemolytic anemia can be differentiated by the examination of red cell indices, a reticulocyte count, a peripheral smear, or a positive Coombs test. An abnormal urinalysis with the appearance of WBCs, red blood cells, granular casts, and proteinuria can also be helpful and raise a suspicion of lupus nephritis. While blood urea nitrogen (BUN) and creatinine levels are not usually elevated at the outset of the disease, they can be useful as baseline values in a patient who progresses to azotemia and acute renal failure. A chest X-ray and electrocardiogram should be obtained initially to rule out pulmonary pathology, to explain an enlarged cardiac silhouette, and note electrocardiographic signs of pericarditis, enlarged cardiac chambers, or signs of ischemia. This is of particular importance since accelerated atherosclerosis and early heart and vascular disease is common to this condition (Manzi, 2000) and the most common cause of death.

TABLE 32.1 Association of Specific Antibodies with Specific Clinical Findings.

Antibody	Clinical Manifestation
Anti-native DNA	Lupus nephritis, active disease
Anti-Smith (SM) and high ribonucleoprotein	SLE, scleroderma, mixed connective tissue disease
Anti-RO (SSA) and LA (SSB)	Sjögren's, SLE, neonatal lupus, subacute cutaneous lupus, C2 deficiency
Anti-ribosomal P protein	Neuropsychiatric lupus
Anti-histone	Drug-induced disease
Anti-phospholipid	Clotting, livido reticularis, false positive syphilis test

CLINICAL

The nature of the general symptoms associated with the disease includes fatigue, weight loss, and fever (Stahl et al., 1979; Robb-Nicholson et al., 1989). Often the initial complaints, they can be mistakenly attributed to causes other than lupus at first glance. Fatigue is well recognized and is the most common and often the most debilitating symptom of SLE; similar to a bout of influenza. A curious pattern of fatigue is described in SLE when compared to patients with other multisystem autoimmune diseases (Godaert et al., 2002). In SLE, fatigue decreased in the morning and increased in the evening in contrast to other conditions such as scleroderma where the opposite is true. Weight loss is common in patients with lupus and worsened when there is malabsorption due to overlapping illnesses such as CREST syndrome (calcinosis, Raynaud's, esophageal dysmotility, sclerodactyly, and telangiectasia), mixed connective tissue disease (MCTD), or scleroderma. Although anorexia is common in severely debilitated patients with associated organ disease such as renal failure, it is not an isolated finding in SLE. The fever of lupus is usually low grade and rarely exceeds 39°C (102°F), unless patients are taking immunosuppressive drugs and have a concurrent infection.

The diagnosis of SLE should be made on clinical grounds with the support of laboratory tests, not the other way around. While diagnostic criteria have been proposed for the classification of SLE (Hochberg, 1997), they are not universally applied in practice. Eleven criteria have been designated by the American College of Rheumatology (ACR) (Box 32.1) for classification. The presence of four or more criteria out of the 11 possible is mandatory for the appropriate classification of SLE. When used, these are of value in clinical practice and are 96% sensitive and specific (Parodi and Rebora, 1997). In some studies of patients with cutaneous lupus, ACR criteria showed a sensitivity of 88%, a specificity of 79%, a positive predictive value of 56%, and a negative predictive value of 96% (Asherson et al., 1991). The diagnosis of SLE is given routinely to patients in practice who fail to meet any criteria (Gilboe and Husby, 1999). Patients

Box 32.1 Classification Criteria for Systemic Lupus Erythematosus.

1. Malar rash
2. Discoid rash
3. Photosensitivity: skin rash as a result of sun exposure
4. Oral ulcers: painless
5. Arthritis (nonerosive): two or more peripheral joints with swelling and effusion
6. Serositis: pleuritis or pericarditis
7. Renal disorder: persistent proteinuria or cellular casts
8. Neurologic disorder: seizures or psychosis
9. Hematologic disorder: hemolytic anemia, leukopenia, lymphopenia, or thrombocytopenia
10. Immunologic disorders: positive antiphospholipid antibody, or anti-DNA, or anti-SM, or a false positive test for syphilis
11. Antinuclear antibody (ANA): in the absence of drugs that cause lupus

who fail to meet four of the 11 criteria have what many call lupus-like syndrome or incomplete lupus and such patients may have a related autoimmune disease. Lupus criteria can be acquired over a period. The revised ACR criteria for lupus is the standard for establishing eligibility of subjects for epidemiologic and clinical lupus studies, but exclude patients with limited disease. In 2002, the Boston weighted criteria for clinical studies were established, and these criteria were compared to the clinical rheumatologists' diagnosis of SLE. Using these criteria, the investigators were able to identify a larger number of cases with SLE. The criteria had a sensitivity of 93% and specificity of 69% compared to the ACR criteria, and 7% more patients with lupus were identified (Costenbader et al., 2002). In 2001, Wilson et al. published the criteria for antiphospholipid syndrome. These criteria, which may need revision over time, are very helpful to this important variant of SLE, which can be primary or secondary to SLE (Wilson et al., 2000).

MEASUREMENT OF CLINICAL ACTIVITY

Lupus is such a heterogeneous disease that classification of the disease and measurement of disease activity poses problems for the clinician and researcher. Over 40 instruments have been developed over many years. Recently, most observational clinical studies have used the SLEDAI and/or the BILAG in the measurement of SLE activity (Bombardier et al., 1992; Isenberg et al., 2005). These validated instruments are sensitive to change and can measure change with time. The BILAG-2004 is the latest version of this British instrument and is based on the clinician's intention to treat; there are five categories of disease severity. The SLEDAI was developed in Canada and included 37 variables for defining SLE activity. This validated measurement system was further modified during the safety of estradiol in SLE national assessment (SELENA). Descriptors were changed to insure that organ system involvement included ongoing disease activity. Additionally criteria were developed to measure flares using the BILAG 2004 index. Subsequent efforts to use the SELENA-SLEDAI index to measure flares were successful and provided a way to quantitate this aspect of the disease with particular note of specific organ involvement.

Musculoskeletal

Patients with SLE can present with isolated arthralgias, Reynaud's phenomenon, hypercoagulable states, fever of unknown origin, and respiratory symptoms such as dyspnea and pleural effusions or overt renal failure. The protean clinical manifestations of this illness can make the diagnosis difficult and if access to specialty care is unavailable the patient may elude diagnosis for many years.

The arthritis of SLE is a nonerosive, nondeforming, symmetric arthropathy. Multiple joints are involved, and 80–95% of them are tender, swollen, and effusive joints. The joints are the most frequently involved organs in SLE. The most frequently involved joints are the proximal interphalangeal, metacarpal phalangeal, wrists, and knees. The deforming arthritis of Jaccoud can occur in the lupus patient, and in such patients, swan neck deformity and profound ulnar deviation can be found. This form of joint involvement lacks erosive changes and can be differentiated from RA. The most frequent musculoskeletal X-ray changes are soft tissue swelling, acral sclerosis, and periarticular demineralization. When rare erosions of bone occur, one must consider a form of overlap syndrome (van Vugt et al., 1998). Joints such as the temporomandibular and the sacroiliac may also be involved (the latter particularly in males) in the SLE patient. Rheumatoid nodules can occur in SLE with the presence of a high rheumatoid factor (Schwartz and Grishman, 1980; Hassikou et al., 2003) but this is rare. Erosive joint changes can contribute to confusion about making a diagnosis of SLE, particularly in the elderly patient, where SLE is distinctly uncommon (Foadd et al., 1972). Avascular necrosis is a particular source of joint pain in SLE patients and should be a part of every differential diagnosis. It is a feature found in patients who are ingesting corticosteroids and those with phospholipid antibodies (Murphy Nancy et al., 1998). Avascular necrosis (AVN) is commonly found in the hips, carpal bones of the wrist, and heads of the humerus and the knees. Less commonly, the shafts of the long bones can be affected. Anywhere from 5 to 10% of patients with SLE can have AVN and these findings are not always associated with steroid use. In many cases, AVN can be asymptomatic and detected by routine X-ray evaluation. In decreasing order of sensitivity, magnetic resonance imaging (MRI), bone scan (Tc99), and plain X-ray are useful in detecting AVN; however, MRI is often positive when all other diagnostic modalities are negative. Septic arthritis must also be considered as a cause of SLE joint pain, particularly when there is swelling and intense warmth of a joint coupled with peripheral leukocytosis. An aspiration of an effusive SLE joint with subsequent culture is mandatory and can be lifesaving. Myositis is present in 3–5% of SLE patients with the creatinine phosphokinase (CPK) being greater than 1000 (Yood and Smith, 1985), but clinical features such as myalgias distinct from fibromyalgia can be found in as many as 50% of patients. The CPK is rarely elevated above 1000, but an electromyogram (EMG) can be very abnormal. Biopsy of the muscle is rarely required for a definitive diagnosis, but if the CPK is exceptionally high or there is diagnostic confusion, alternative diagnoses must be considered and anti-aldolase and anti-synthetase antibodies should be measured. The lymphocytic, monocytic, and plasma cell infiltration found in primary immune myopathies can be observed in varying degrees with SLE patients. A vacuolar myopathy is rare in SLE, but may be found in untreated patients in distal as well as proximal muscles. Myopathy in SLE can also be secondary to corticosteroid therapy, and a form of myopathy can be found in patients ingesting antimalarials (Askari et al., 1976; Posada et al., 2011).

Renal

Clinical evidence of kidney involvement is found in one-half to two-thirds of patients with SLE (Balow et al., 1999). Biopsy evidence of immune complex deposition is found in all kidneys of all patients with SLE, regardless of urine sediment. Various forms of glomerular disease listed by the World Health Organization (WHO) are helpful in establishing activity and chronicity as well as degrees of severity. Both diffuse proliferative glomerulonephritis and progressive forms of focal proliferative nephritis have poorer prognoses than membranous and mesangial forms of the disease. Each renal lesion in a lupus patient has activity and, dependent on the activity, is the need to treat the patient aggressively with large-dose steroids or immunosuppressive agents. Patients with inactive lesions (i.e., membranous nephropathy, sclerotic glomeruli, fibrous crescents, tubular atrophy, or interstitial fibrosis) may not require immunosuppressive therapy. A renal biopsy must be done to gauge the extent of disease and include two components: light microscopy and immunofluorescence. Serial renal biopsy has prognostic value and is recommended for the regulation of chemotherapy in some patients (Ginzler and Antoniadis, 1992; Yoo et al., 2000). A biopsy with immunofluorescent analysis and electron microscopy is also recommended. An adequate number of glomeruli should be obtained for verifiable diagnosis. Hypothetical problems encountered with the renal biopsy include (1) that the biopsy is static or reflective of one point in time, (2) the efficacy of the activity/chronicity index is questionable in designing treatment, and (3) no single glomerular lesion can reflect the entire renal picture.

The most serious complications of renal biopsies include pericapsular hemorrhage or clot obstruction in those patients with lupus procoagulants. In those patients with WBC, erythrocyte, hyaline, or granular casts, a BUN and creatinine are helpful in order to assess renal function. For most patients, renal function early in the course of the disease is normal despite abnormal urine sediment. If the activity of the disease progresses unchecked, these parameters change rapidly. When proteinuria is found qualitatively by urine dipstick (1 g or greater), a 24-h urine

protein and a creatinine ratio should be obtained to quantify the amounts. Urine protein is a useful measure of renal lupus activity. An incremental change of 500 mg of protein excretion is significant to predict worsening renal pathology just as a decrement can herald clinical improvement. Other reasons for decreased renal function in SLE include concomitant infections, use of aspirin, non-steroidal anti-inflammatory drugs (NSAIDs), or angiotensin-converting-enzyme (ACE) inhibitors; all affect renal circulation, as well as obstruction or thrombosis of the renal vein. Sonograms, contrast studies, or renal scans can be helpful in the evaluation of renal function when causes other than lupus nephropathy are suspected, and it is suggested that ultrasound might be of utility in the prediction of worsened renal disease (Platt et al., 1997).

Less common forms of renal involvement in SLE include interstitial nephritis, which can be the result of immune complexes (Appel et al., 2005) or the result of drug therapy. This form of renal disease may not present as a glomerulopathy but rather as a disorder of acidification and potassium transport or regulation (DeFronzo et al., 1977). Renal pathology could indicate that thrombosis of the glomerulus (Uwonkunda et al., 1998) and intraglomerular thrombi (Bhandari et al., 1998) are alternate causes of proteinuria and renal failure in SLE. Renal transplantation in lupus is as successful as that in the non-SLE population. However, renal disease can occur again in the transplanted kidneys (Amend et al., 1981). For unknown reasons, the alleviation of overall disease activity of lupus erythematosus after dialysis for chronic renal disease has been reported.

Neuropsychiatric

Neuropsychiatric manifestations can be found in as many as 66% of patients with SLE (Feinglass et al., 1976; Calabrese and Stern 1995). The pathophysiology of this clinical manifestation is not widely understood; however, thrombosis and vasculitis are not responsible for the large number of neuropsychiatric manifestations observed. It is possible that components that are both non-immunologic and immunologic might be involved, such as hormones or a direct effect of antibody. Central nervous system (CNS) manifestations include seizures, psychiatric illness, and disorders of the cranial nerves (McCune and Golbus, 1988). The frequency of organic CNS manifestations in SLE has been reported as between 35 and 75% (Jennekens and Kater, 2002a, b). The peripheral nervous system is involved in as many as 18% of patients.

Seizures are found in 15–20% of SLE patients (Johnson and Richardson, 1968). These can be the result of the disease process, such as lupus vasculitis or acute thrombosis, steroid therapy and its attendant hypertension, or a resulting metabolic problem such as uremia, seizures, or infection. Grand-mal tonic–clonic seizures are most common, although other seizures, such as Jacksonian, psychomotor, and absence attacks, have all been reported. On rare occasions, patients with SLE can present with status epilepticus. Treatment of seizures in SLE requires anticonvulsants. Corticosteroid therapy when given as pulse therapy is a cause albeit rare of status epilepticus and hence should be used with caution. Lupus can cause profound psychiatric disturbances in 50–67% of patients. Overt psychosis can occur in 12% of cases as well as a variety of organic brain syndromes. Severe depression is common to lupus patients and is thought to be a disease manifestation rather than reactive depression from chronic disease. Sleep disturbances are common in lupus and not usually related to depression. Steroid psychosis is common in lupus patients on high-dose steroids for long periods (Kohen et al., 1993).

Antiribosomal P protein antibodies are positive in over 60% of patients with SLE-related psychosis (Bonfa et al., 1987) and may help distinguish these patients from those with steroid psychosis, although there is no specific antibody associated with cerebral SLE. Ten percent of patients can have cranial nerve abnormalities, and they can be the presenting symptom in a small number. Although spinal cord involvement in SLE is rare, three types of cord involvement are seen: transverse myelitis (Lavalle et al., 1990), demyelination, and spinal cord infarction because of thrombosis (Nakano et al., 1989). These three spinal manifestations are all commonly associated with antiphospholipid antibodies. In the first 5 years of the disease, the incidence of cerebrovascular accident (CVA) is high (6.6% occurring in the first year alone) (Ginsburg et al., 1992). Patients with antiphospholipid antibodies also have an increased risk of stroke. Even though movement disorders are not common in lupus, chorea is common in children with SLE and is found in adults and children with phospholipid antibody (Lahat et al., 1989). It is virtually indistinguishable from Sydenham's chorea. Parkinsonism and cerebellar ataxia are rare. Rarer forms of CNS involvement include pseudo tumor cerebri, hypothalamic dysfunction (especially due to thalamic infarcts), aseptic meningitis (particularly related to NSAID use), myasthenia, Eaton–Lambert syndrome, a thrombotic thrombocytopenic purpura-like syndrome, and hyperprolactinemia.

Peripheral nervous system disease is found in 3–18% of patients and is largely a sensory only or combined sensorimotor neuropathy (Florica et al., 2011). Guillain–Barré syndrome, mononeuropathy, or mononeuritis multiplex has also been reported (Santos et al., 2010).

The laboratory diagnosis of central nervous system disease in SLE is difficult. Spinal fluid pleocytosis and/or high spinal fluid protein levels are the only helpful indicators that CNS disease is present. MRI and position electron tomography (PET) scanning show the most promise for diagnosing disease of the brain. Use of the newer modalities, such as Tc-99-HMAAQ brain SPECT, may have better utility in the diagnosis of CNS SLE (Colamussi et al., 1997). Infarctions and demyelinating lesions of the brain are best found with these modalities. CT scans are good for detecting focal lesions but are often unreliable. Antibodies to ribosomal P protein and anti-neuronal antibodies, as well as the finding of cytotoxic lymphocytes against myelin in blood, may eventually prove useful, but now are not very specific for cerebritis. An exciting development in the area of lupus cerebritis is the discovery of antibodies to the glutamate receptors in the brain. Originally based on a murine model of neuropsychiatric lupus and an antibody that cross-reacted with dsDNA and the N-methyl-D-aspartate (NMDA) receptors, the antibody from human SLE patients causes neuronal apoptosis when injected into mouse brains and causes significant brain pathology.

Cardiac

Cardiac involvement is very common in SLE, and some 30–50% of patients suffer from some form of heart disease (Petri, 1999; Costenbader et al., 2004). Pericarditis, the most common form of acute heart disease, occurs in 19–48% of patients. Pleural-pericardial pain can occur at any time. Echocardiography is the best diagnostic test for this manifestation. Pericarditis in SLE can be managed with NSAIDS and/or low doses of corticosteroids. Myocarditis is rare in SLE, involving only 5–10% of patients and usually presents with fever, conduction abnormalities, elevated CPK, skeletal myositis, and serositis (Lemos et al., 2008). SLE in the human results in a higher incidence of myocardial infarction because of accelerated atherosclerosis, coronary vasculitis, or coronary emboli (Manzi, 2000). Systolic cardiac murmurs are heard in up to 70% of SLE patients. These may be related to anemia, fever, or hypoxemia and are found with Libman–Sacks endocarditis, a component more frequent with antiphospholipid antibodies. The mitral and aortic valves are most commonly involved. Pulmonary arterial hypertension is common in patients with phospholipid antibodies (Bayraktar et al., 2001), and a pulmonic murmur or a loud second heart sound in the presence of an elevated PTT are clues to this diagnosis, which should be confirmed by echocardiography or cardiac angiography. Vasculitis is common in SLE and may be reflected in the presence of splinter hemorrhages, digital infarcts, or ecthymic skin lesions. Involvement of small- and medium-sized arteries may mimic polyarteritis nodosa and produce localized signs. Raynaud's phenomenon in SLE is not as common as in scleroderma or primary antiphospholipid syndrome (APLS) and is present in only 20% of patients.

The most common cause of death in SLE is early onset cardiovascular disease (CVD).

Risk factors for accelerated atherosclerotic CVD are under intense study (Svenungsson et al., 2001) (see Chapter 71). The antioxidant capacity of normal high-density lipoproteins (HDL) is lost during inflammation and the dysfunctional HDLs predispose to atherosclerosis. These dysfunctional HDLs are thought to be the single factor that increases the risk of developing subclinical atherosclerosis in SLE.

Pulmonary

The lungs are commonly affected in lupus patients (Keane and Lynch, 2000; Hughson et al., 2001a). Over 50% of SLE patients have some form of pleural disease and pleural effusions in their lifetime. These effusions are mostly exudative (>3 g protein) and less common than the pain and findings associated with simple pleuritis.

Parenchymal lung involvement can present suddenly as acute pneumonitis, dyspnea, or pleuritic pain. SLE parenchymal disease of the lung can be treated with high-dose corticosteroids, and improved pulmonary function is the desired result. Pulmonary capillaritis is also part of parenchymal disease (Franks and Koss, 2000). Hemoptysis and overt pulmonary hemorrhage are emergencies in SLE patients and are either the result of pneumonitis or pulmonary embolus, which are reversible. There is also an association of alveolar hemorrhage with renal microangiopathy (Hughson et al., 2001b).

Hematology

Sixty to 80% of lupus patients have anemia of chronic disease. Other kinds of anemia, such as autoimmune hemolytic anemia, are rare and are found in fewer than 10% of patients; however, a positive Coombs test can be found in 20–60% of patients (Simantov et al., 1999). Leukopenia can be found in over 50% of patients with SLE and is associated with either granulocytopenia or lymphopenia. Antibodies are directed to either of these cellular elements at any point in their maturation pathways. When directed against stem cells, these antibodies cause aplastic anemia. Most low cell counts in SLE can be reversed with immunosuppressive therapy. Leukopenia is often a good general sign of disease exacerbation but also occurs in response to cytotoxic agents used in lupus therapy. Platelet transfusions are contraindicated in most SLE patients except on occasions where platelets reach dangerous levels, because of the possibility that patients will be exposed to new platelet antigens that make them more refractory. Anticlotting factor antibodies have been

found in SLE and are often associated with bleeding. Antibodies are directed most commonly to factors II, VIII, IX, XI, or XII. Acquired von Willebrand syndrome is also seen. Lupus anticoagulants are found commonly in patients with SLE and are associated with mild to profoundly elevated partial thromboplastin times. This abnormality is usually associated with hypercoagulation and not with bleeding (Cockerell and Lewis, 1993). Associations have been observed, and the triad of the lupus anticoagulant, recurrent abortions, and the presence of false positive tests for syphilis is often found in patients. Patients with lupus can be hypercoagulable for a variety of reasons other than procoagulant antibodies and these include hereditary deficiencies of factors C, S, or antithrombin III. One acquired reason for hypercoagulability is the loss of antithrombin III in the urine of patients with nephrotic syndrome. If in rare instances a patient requires a splenectomy to control thrombocytopenia, laparoscopy is the best way to remove the spleen. Open laparotomy is not advisable in any except the most complicated cases.

Dermatology

Ninety percent of lupus patients have some involvement of the skin. Only 40% of patients experience sensitivity to ultraviolet (UV) light and these are mostly Caucasians (Zecevic et al., 2001). The actual percentage prevalence is 57% Caucasian vs. 11% African American. The lupus band test is the definitive test for cutaneous lupus. A biopsy shows immunoglobulin and complement deposition at the dermal/epidermal junction in nonlesional skin in greater than 60% of patients with SLE (Piette et al., 2001). However, false-positives are encountered in rosacea, RA, MCTD, renal diseases, and many other disorders. Its true value is the differentiation of discoid lupus from SLE. In discoid lupus, only lesional skin stains positive, whereas in SLE both lesional and nonlesional skin stain with immunoglobulin at the dermal epidermal junction.

Acute cutaneous lupus (30–50%) and subacute cutaneous lupus (10–15%) comprise the vast majority of patients with dermal disease. The butterfly malar rash found in 40% of patients is part of acute cutaneous lupus. Subacute cutaneous lupus (SCLE) is an annular, widespread, non-scarring, or papulosquamous/psoriasis-form lesion that is worsened by sun exposure. This form of lupus is associated with HLA-DR3, anti-Ro antibody, and high titers of ANA. SCLE has also been associated with complement component deficiencies of C2, C1q, and C1s. Chronic forms of lupus skin disease include several forms of discoid lupus and lupus profundus. These discoid lesions are usually localized to the head, scalp, and external ear, but more widespread involvement is possible. Patients with isolated discoid lupus have a 2–10% chance of developing systemic disease, whereas 10–20%

of SLE patients have discoid lesions. Discoid LE is more common in African Americans.

Alopecia can occur in all patients with SLE at some time in their disease presentation and can also be the result of therapy or hypothyroidism, which is very common in patients with SLE. Livido reticularis and livido racemosa, a more significant form of skin lesion, are found in the antiphospholipid syndrome.

Gastroenterological

The most common manifestation of gastrointestinal lupus is the occurrence of ulcers in the nose and mouth of patients. Many patients develop these ulcers at some time during the course of their disease and they indicate a flare of disease. Esophageal ulcerations and dysphagia are rarely found (Tatelman and Keech, 1966). Abdominal pain can result from a variety of causes. Pancreatitis (Baron and Brisson, 1982), ischemic bowel, perforation, or mesenteric vasculitis can suggest a surgical abdomen and mandate a laparotomy. The tumor marker CA125 can be elevated in cases of SLE-induced gastrointestinal ischemia (Koh et al., 2002). Serositis and, in some cases, vasculitis may also simulate a surgical abdomen.

Lupus peritonitis (Luman et al., 2001) is the result of small vessel involvement in the bowel serosa or retro peritoneum or the result of actual perforation of the bowel. Parenchymal liver disease as a result of lupus is uncommon and more likely represents autoimmune (chronic active) hepatitis with or without cirrhosis.

ENT and Eye

The eye is not commonly involved in SLE. Only 10% or less of patients have episcleritis or conjunctivitis. In a prospective study, retinopathy was detected in 7% of SLE patients. This retinopathy consists of microangiopathic lesions with cotton wool spots and hemorrhages that can be a significant problem in someone with a bleeding diathesis or one who is anticoagulated.

Optic neuritis, papilledema, and retinal vein occlusion are also major problems (Wong et al., 1981). Lupus retinopathy is common in patients with active SLE (88%) and in those with lupus cerebritis (73%). Patients can also have uveitis, cytoid bodies, and angle-closure glaucoma.

Less common in the patient with SLE is sicca syndrome. Patients who are older are particularly affected. Patients with lupus can have asymptomatic parotid gland enlargement with abnormal labial biopsies that suggest Sjögren's syndrome. Many of these patients have a positive anti-Ro antibody and a Sjögren's syndrome overlap. Patients with lupus may have vocal cord paralysis or present with hoarseness because of vasculitis of the recurrent laryngeal nerve. Lupus may be a cause of sensorineural learning loss. The mechanism of ear damage is not known.

LUPUS THERAPEUTICS

Besides rest and anti-inflammatory agents, the treatment of lupus involves immunosuppressants. Corticosteroids and antimalarials are the mainstay of therapy. Other drugs like mycophenolate mofetil, methotrexate, and azathioprine can be used to treat active disease. Cyclophosphamide is reserved for serious organ system involvement like renal and central nervous system disease. Standard and established therapies are described in Chapter 80.

Based upon pathogenetic mechanisms there are B cell targeted therapies that have had significant success (Furie et al., 2011). These agents include rituximab, ocrelizumab, belimumab, epratuzumab, and atacicept. Rituximab is a chimeric antiCD20 monoclonal antibody that had potential for the treatment of lupus, but did not meet its therapeutic endpoints when compared to placebo and was not approved by the Food and Drug Administration. Trial design was the likely cause of the drug's negative results. There is general agreement that the drug is a good therapeutic option. Ocrelizumab is a humanized antiCD20 antibody. The study of ocrelizumab in SLE was halted because of significant serious opportunistic infections. Belimumab is a fully humanized monoclonal antibody directed against B lymphocyte stimulating factor known as BLyS or BAFF (see Chapter 10). BLyS is part of the tumor necrosis factor (TNF) superfamily. Belimumab binds to soluble BLyS which is elevated during periods of active disease and associated with increased anti-native DNA antibody and lowered levels of complement components, both important biomarkers for disease. Belimumab was approved in 2011 by the FDA as the first biological agent approved for use in the treatment of SLE in 40 years. Epratuzumab is a humanized monoclonal antibody against CD22, an antigen involved in B cell signaling, and atacicept is another monoclonal antibody directed to a member of the TNF superfamily APRIL. Both agents are in phase II and III clinical trials as potential additions to the biological therapy of SLE. Biological therapies for SLE are further considered in Chapter 81.

The complexity of lupus along with the various instruments that have to be validated in order to ascertain clinical improvement make the evaluation of new drugs challenging. The additional need for standard therapy during clinical trials to avoid loss of patients on placebo is an additional factor for FDA consideration. Fortunately, the trial designs for the future will allow more rapid development of SLE-effective biological therapies.

REFERENCES

Amend, W.J.C., Vincenti, F., Feduska, N.J., 1981. Recurrent systemic lupus erythematosus involving renal allografts. Ann. Intern. Med. 94, 444.

Anderson, E., Nietert, P.J., Kamen, D.L., Gilkeson, G.S., 2008. Ethnic disparities among patients with systemic lupus erythematosus in South Carolina. J.Rheumatol. 35, 819–825.

Appel, G.B., Radhakrishnan, J., Ginzler, E.M., 2005. Use of mycophenolate mofetil in autoimmune and renal diseases. Transplantation. 80, S265–S271.

Aranow, C., Zhou, D., Diamond, B., et al., 2011. Anti DNA antiobdies: structure regulation and pathogenicity. In: Lahita, R.G. (Ed.), In Systemic Lupus Erythematosus., fifth ed. Academic Press, New York, pp. 235–258.

Asherson, R.A., Cervera, R., Lahita, R.G., 1991. Latent, incomplete or lupus at all? J. Rheumatol. 18, 1783–1786.

Askari, A., Vignos, P.J., Moskowitz, R.W., 1976. Steroid myopathy in connective tissue disease. Am. J. Med. 61, 485.

Baecher-Allan, C., Viglietta, V., Hafler, D.A., 2002. Inhibition of human CD4(+)CD25(+ high) regulatory T cell function. J. Immunol. 169, 6210–6217.

Baecher-Allan, C., Brown, J.A., Freeman, G.J., Hafler, D.A., 2003. CD4 + CD25 + regulatory cells from human peripheral blood express very high levels of CD25 ex vivo. Novartis. Found. Symp. 252, 67–88.

Ballestar, E., Esteller, M., Richardson, B.C., 2006. The epigenetic face of systemic lupus erythematosus. J. Immunol. 176, 7147.

Balow, J.E., Boumpas, D.T., Austin, H.A., 1999. Systemic lupus erythematosus and the kidney. In: Lahita, R.G. (Ed.), In Systemic Lupus Erythematosus, third ed. Academic Press, San Diego, pp. 657–686.

Baron, M., Brisson, M.L., 1982. Pancreatitis in systemic lupus erythematosus. Arthritis Rheum. 25, 1006.

Bayraktar, Y., Tanaci, N., Egesel, T., Gokoz, A., Balkanci, F., 2001. Antiphospholipid syndrome presenting as portopulmonary hypertension. J. Clin. Gastroenterol. 32, 359–361.

Bhandari, S., Harnden, P., Brownjohn, A.M., Turney, J.H., 1998. Association of anticardiolipin antibodies with intraglomerular thrombi and renal dysfunction in lupus nephritis. QJM. 91, 401–409.

Bombardier, C., Gladman, D.D., Urowitz, M.B., Caron, D., Chang, C.H., 1992. Derivation of the SLEDAI. A disease activity index for lupus patients. The Committee on Prognosis Studies in SLE. Arthritis Rheum. 35, 630–640.

Bonfa, E., Golombek, S.J., Kaufman, L.D., 1987. Association between lupus psychosis and anti-ribosomal P protein antibodies. N. Engl. J. Med. 317, 265–271.

Calabrese, L.V., Stern, T.A., 1995. Neuropsychiatric manifestations of systemic lupus erythematosus. Psychosomatics. 36, 344–359.

Carbone, L.D., Lohr, K.M., 2002. Ethnic differences in male lupus. J. Clin. Rheumatol. 8, 239–240.

Cockerell, C.J., Lewis, J.E., 1993. Systemic lupus erythematosus-like illness associated with syndrome of abnormally large von Willebrand's factor multimers. South. Med. J. 86, 951–953.

Colamussi, P., Trotta, F., Ricci, R., Cittanti, C., Govoni, M., Barbarella, G., et al., 1997. Brain perfusion SPET and proton magnetic resonance spectroscopy in the evaluation of two systemic lupus erythematosus patients with mild neuropsychiatric manifestations. Nucl. Med. Commun. 18, 269–273.

Costenbader, K.H., Karlson, E.W., Mandl, L.A., 2002. Defining lupus cases for clinical studies: the Boston weighted criteria for the classification of systemic lupus erythematosus. J. Rheumatol. 29, 2545–2550.

Costenbader, K.H., Wright, E., Liang, M.H., Karlson, E.W., 2004. Cardiac risk factor awareness and management in patients with systemic lupus erythematosus. Arthritis Rheum. 51, 983–988.

DeFronzo, R.A., Cooke, C.R., Goldberg, M., 1977. Impaired renal tubular potassium secretion in systemic lupus erythematosus. Ann. Intern. Med. 86, 268.

Feinglass, E.J., Arnett, F.C., Dorsch, C.A., 1976. Neuropsychiatric manifestations of systemic lupus erythematosus: diagnosis, clinical spectrum, and relationship to other features of the disease. Medicine. 55, 323.

Fessel, W.J., 1974. Systemic lupus erythematosus in the community: incidence, prevalence, outcome, and first symptoms; the high prevalence in black women. Arch. Intern. Med. 134, 1027–1035.

Fessler, B.J., Alarcon, G.S., McGwin, G., Roseman, J., Bastian, H.M., Friedmajn, A.W., et al., 2005. Systemic lupus erythematosus in three ethnic groups: XVI. Association of hydroxychloroquine use with reduced risk of damage accrual. Arthritis. Rheum. 52, 1473–1480.

Florica, B., Aghdassi, E., Su, J., Gladman, D.D., Urowitz, M.B., Fortin, P.R., 2011. Peripheral neuropathy in patients with systemic lupus erythematosus. Semin. Arthritis Rheum. 41, 203–211.

Foadd, B.S.I., Sheon, R.P., Kirsner, A.B., 1972. Systemic lupus erythematosus in the elderly. Arch. Intern. Med. 130, 743.

Franks, T.J., Koss, M.N., 2000. Pulmonary capillaritis. Curr. Opin. Pulm. Med. 6, 430–435.

Furie, R., Petri, M., Zamani, O., Cervera, R., Wallace, D.J., Tegzova, D., et al., 2011. A phase III, randomized, placebo-controlled study of belimumab, a monoclonal antibody that inhibits B lymphocyte stimulator, in patients with systemic lupus erythematosus. Arthritis Rheum. 63, 3918–3930.

Garaud, J.C., Schickel, J.N., Blaison, G., Knapp, A.M., Dembele, D., Ruer-Laventie, J., et al., 2011. B cell signature during inactive systemic lupus is heterogeneous: toward a biological dissection of lupus. PLoS One. 6, e23900.

Gilboe, I.M., Husby, G., 1999. Application of the 1982 revised criteria for the classification of systemic lupus erythematosus on a cohort of 346 Norwegian patients with connective tissue disease. Scand. J. Rheumatol. 28, 81–87.

Ginsburg, K.S., Liang, M.H., Newcomer, L., Golhaber, S.Z., Schur, P.H., Hennekens, C.H., 1992. Anticardiolipin antiobdies and the risk for ischemic stroke and venous thrombosis. Ann. Intern. Med. 117, 997–1002.

Ginzler, E.M., Antoniadis, I., 1992. Clinical manifestations of systemic lupus erythematosus, measures of disease activity, and long-term complications. Curr. Opin. Rheumatol. 4, 672–680.

Godaert, G.L., Hartkamp, A., Geenen, R., Garssen, A., Kruize, A.A., Bijlsma, J.W., et al., 2002. Fatigue in daily life in patients with primary Sjogren's syndrome and systemic lupus erythematosus. Ann. N.Y. Acad. Sci. 966, 320–326.

Grimaldi, C.M., Hicks, R., Diamond, B., 2005. B cell selection and susceptibility to autoimmunity. J. Immunol. 174, 1775–1781.

Hassikou, H., Le, G.F., Lespessailles, E., Benhamou, C.L., Martin, L., Kerdraon, R., 2003. Rheumatoid nodules in systemic lupus erythematosus: a case report. Joint Bone Spine. 70, 234–235.

Hochberg, M.C., 1987. Prevalence of systemic lupus erythematosus in England and Wales, 1981–2. Ann. Rheum. Dis. 46, 664–666.

Hochberg, M.C., 1997. Updating the American College of Rheumatology revised criteria for the classification of systemic lupus erythematosus. Arthritis Rheum. 40, 1725.

Hughson, M.D., He, Z., Henegar, J., McMurray, R., 2001. Alveolar hemorrhage and renal microangiopathy in systemic lupus erythematosus. Arch. Pathol. Lab. Med. 125, 475–483.

Isenberg, D.A., Rahman, A., Allen, E., Farewell, V., Akil, M., Bruce, I. N., et al., 2005. BILAG 2004. Development and initial validation of an updated version of the British Isles Lupus Assessment Group's disease activity index for patients with systemic lupus erythematosus. Rheumatology (Oxford). 44, 902–906.

Jennekens, F.G., Kater, L., 2002. The central nervous system in systemic lupus erythematosus. Part 2. Pathogenetic mechanisms of clinical syndromes: a literature investigation. Rheumatology (Oxford). 41, 619–630.

Johanneson, B., Alarcon-Riquelme, M.E., 2001. An update on the genetics of systemic lupus erythematosus. Isr. Med. Assoc. J. 3, 88–93.

Johnson, R.T., Richardson, D.P., 1968. The neurological manifestations of systemic lupus erythematosus. Medicine (Baltimore). 47, 337.

Jurencak, R., Fritzler, M., Tyrrell, P., Hiraki, L., Benseler, S., Silverman, E., 2009. Autoantibodies in pediatric systemic lupus erythematosus: ethnic grouping, cluster analysis, and clinical correlations. J. Rheumatol. 36, 416–421.

Keane, M.P., Lynch, J.P., 2000. Pleuropulmonary manifestations of systemic lupus erythematosus. Thorax. 55, 159–166.

Koh, M.S., Sunil, K., Howe, H.S., 2002. Late onset systemic lupus erythematosus with elevated CA125 and gastrointestinal ischaemia. Intern. Med. J. 32, 117–118.

Kohen, M., Asherson, R.A., Gharavi, A.E., Lahita, R.G., 1993. Lupus psychosis: differentiation from the steroid-induced state. Clin. Exp. Rheumatol. 11, 323–326.

Krishnan, E., Hubert, H.B., 2006. Ethnicity and mortality from systemic lupus erythematosus in the US. Ann. Rheum. Dis. 65, 1500–1505.

Lahat, E., Eshel, G., Azizi, E., 1989. Chorea associated with systemic lupus erythematosus in children: a case report. Isr. J. Med. Sci. 25, 568.

Lahita, R.G., 1992. Early diagnosis of systemic lupus erythematosus in women. J. Womens Health. 1, 117.

Lavalle, C., Pizarro, S., Drenkard, C., 1990. Transverse myelitis: a manifestation of systemic lupus erythematosus strongly associated with antiphospholipid antibodies. J. Rheumatol. 17, 34.

Lemos, J., Santos, L., Martins, I., Nunes, L., Santos, O., Henriques, P., 2008. Systemic lupus erythematosus—a diagnosis in cardiology. Rev. Port. Cardiol. 27, 841–849.

Liang, M.H., Socher, S.A., Larson, M.G., Schur, P., 1989. Reliability and validity of six systems for the clinical assessment of disease activity in systemic lupus erythematosus. Arthritis Rheum. 32, 1107–1118.

Luman, W., Chua, K.B., Cheong, W.K., Ng, H.S., 2001. Gastrointestinal manifestations of systemic lupus erythematosus. Singapore Med. J. 42, 380–384.

Manzi, S., 2000. Systemic lupus erythematosus: a model for atherogenesis? Rheumatology (Oxford). 39, 353–359.

Marino, E., Grey, S.T., 2012. B cells as effectors and regulators of autoimmunity. Autoimmunity. 45, 377–387.

McCarty, D.J., Manzi, S., Medsger, T.A., Ramsey-Goldman, R., La Porte, R.E., Kwoh, C.K., 1995. Incidence of systemic lupus erythematosus. Race and gender differences. Arthritis Rheum. 38, 1260–1270.

McCune, W.J., Golbus, J., 1988. Neuropsychiatric lupus. Rheum. Dis. Clin. North Am.(April), 149.

Michet, C.J., McKenna, C.H., Elveback, L.R., 1985. Epidemiology of systemic lupus erythematosus and other connective tissue diseases in Rochester, Minnesota 1950 through 1979. Mayo Clin. Proc. 60, 105.

Murphy, N.G., Koolvisoot, A., Schumacher, H.R., Feldt, J.M., Callegari, P.E., 1998. Musculoskeletal features in systemic lupus erythematosus and their relationship with disability [record supplied by Aries Systems]. J. Clin. Rheumatol. 4, 238–245.

Nakano, I., Mannen, T., Mizutani, T., 1989. Peripheral white matter lesions of the spinal cord with changes in small arachnoid arteries in systemic lupus erythematosus. Clin. Neuropathol. 8, 102.

Ohtsuka, K., Gray, J.D., Stimmler, M.M., Toro, B., Horwitz, D.A., 1998. Decreased production of TGF-beta by lymphocytes from patients with systemic lupus erythematosus. J. Immunol. 160, 2539–2545.

Ohtsuka, K., Gray, J.D., Stimmler, M.M., Horwitz, D.A., 1999. The relationship between defects in lymphocyte production of transforming growth factor-beta1 in systemic lupus erythematosus and disease activity or severity. Lupus. 8, 90–94.

Parodi, A., Rebora, A., 1997. ARA and EADV criteria for classification of systemic lupus erythematosus in patients with cutaneous lupus erythematosus. Dermatology. 194, 217–220.

Petri, M., 1999. Systemic lupus erythematosus and the heart. In: Lahita, R.G. (Ed.), In Systemic Lupus Erythematosus., third ed. Academic Press, San Diego, pp. 687–706.

Piette, J.C., Marinho, E., Huong, D.L., Amoura, Z., Frances, C., 2001. Lupus band test yields negative results in primary antiphospholipid syndrome. Arthritis Rheum. 44, 488–489.

Platt, J.F., Rubin, J.M., Ellis, J.H., 1997. Lupus nephritis: predictive value of conventional and Doppler US and comparison with serologic and biopsy parameters. Radiology. 203, 82–86.

Posada, C., Garcia-Cruz, A., Garcia-Doval, I., Millan, B.S., Teijeira, S., 2011. Chloroquine-induced myopathy. Lupus. 20, 773–774.

Reeves, W., Xu, Y., Zhuang, H., Li, Y.Y.L., et al., 2011. Origins of antinuclear antiobdies. In: Lahita, R.G. (Ed.), In Systemic Lupus Erythematosus, fifth ed. Academic Press, New York, pp. 213–233.

Richardson, B., 2009. Epigenetics: new insights into the pathogenesis of lupus. Transl. Res. 153, 49–50.

Robb-Nicholson, L.C., Liang, M.H., Daltroy, L., Eaton, H., Gall, V., Schwartz, J., et al., 1989. Effects of aerobic conditioning in lupus fatigue: a pilot study. J. Rheumatol. 28, 500.

Santos, M.S., De Carvalho, J.F., Brotto, M., Bonfa, E., Rocha, F.A., 2010. Peripheral neuropathy in patients with primary antiphospholipid (Hughes') syndrome.. Lupus. 19, 583–590.

Schwartz, I.S., Grishman, E., 1980. Rheumatoid nodules of the vocal cords as the initial manifestation of systemic lupus erythematosus. JAMA. 244, 2751–2752.

Shapiro, S., Long, M., 1999. Hematology: coagulation problems. In: Lahita, R.G. (Ed.), Systemic Lupus Erythematosus., third ed. Academic Press, San Diego, pp. 871–886.

Simantov, R., Laurence, J., Nachman, R., 1999. The cellular hematology of systemic lupus erythematosus. In: Lahita, R.G. (Ed.), Systemic Lupus Erythematosus., third ed. Academic Press, San Diego, pp. 765–792.

Stahl, J.I., Klippel, J.H., Decker, J.L., 1979. Fever in systemic lupus erythematosus. Am. J. Med. 67, 933.

Svenungsson, E., Jensen-Urstad, K., Heimburger, M., Silveira, A., Hamsten, A., De Faire, U., et al., 2001. Risk factors for cardiovascular disease in systemic lupus erythematosus. Circulation. 104, 1887–1893.

Tatelman, M., Keech, M.K., 1966. Esophageal motililty in systemic lupus erythematosus, rheumatoid arthritis and scleroderma. Radiology. 86, 1041.

Uwonkunda, M.R., Cosyns, J.P., Devogelaer, J.P., Houssiau, F.A., 1998. Glomerular thrombosis: an unusual cause of renal failure in systemic lupus erythematosus. Acta Clin. Belg. 53, 371–373.

van Vugt, R.M., Derksen, R.H., Kater, L., Bijlsma, J.W., 1998. Deforming arthropathy or lupus and rhupus hands in systemic lupus erythematosus. Ann. Rheum. Dis. 57 (9), 540–544.

Wilson, W.A., Gharavi, A., Koike, T., Lockshin, M.C., Branch, D.W., Piette, J.C., et al., 2000. International Consensus statement on preliminary classification criteria for definite antiphospholipid syndrome: report of an international workshop. Arthritis Rheum. 42, 1309–1311.

Wong, K., Everett, A., Verier-Jones, J., 1981. Visual loss as the initial symptom of systemic lupus erythematosus. Am. J. Opthalmol. 92, 238.

Yoo, C.W., Kim, M.K., Lee, H.S., 2000. Predictors of renal outcome in diffuse proliferative lupus nephropathy: data from repeat renal biopsy. Nephrol. Dial. Transplant. 15, 1604–1608.

Yood, R.A., Smith, T.W., 1985. Iclusion body myositis and systemic lupus erythematosus. J. Rheumatol. 12, 568.

Yung, R.L., Richardson, B., et al., 2011. Drug induced lupus. In: Lahita, R.G. (Ed.), Systemic Lupus Erythematosus, fifth ed. Academic Press, New York, pp. 385–403.

Zecevic, R.D., Vojvodic, D., Ristic, B., Pavlovic, M.D., Stefanovic, D., Karadaglic, D., 2001. Skin lesions—an indicator of disease activity in systemic lupus erythematosus? Lupus. 10, 364–367.

Zheng, S.G., Wang, J.H., Koss, M.N., Quismorio Jr., F., Gray, J.D., Horwitz, D.A., 2004. CD4 + and CD8 + regulatory T cells generated ex vivo with IL-2 and TGF-beta suppress a stimulatory graft-versus-host disease with a lupus-like syndrome. J. Immunol. 172, 1531–1539.

Chapter 33

Systemic Sclerosis, Scleroderma

Nabeel H. Borazan and Daniel E. Furst

Division of Rheumatology, University of California, Los Angeles, CA, USA

Chapter Outline

Introduction	**463**	Fra2-Transgenic Mice	469
Clinical, Pathologic, and Epidemiologic Features	**463**	TβRIIΔk Mice	469
Clinical Features	463	Wnt-10b-Transgenic Mice	469
Pathologic Features	464	**Pathogenic Mechanisms**	**469**
Epidemiologic Features	464	Vasculopathy	469
Autoimmune Features and Immunologic Markers in		Platelet Activation	469
Disease	**465**	Cytokine Abnormalities	470
Potential Pathogenetic Antibodies	465	Cellular Abnormalities	470
Diagnostic and Prognostic Antibodies	465	Immunological Abnormalities	470
Genetic Features	**466**	T Cells	470
Environmental Influences	**466**	B Cells	471
Animal Models of SSc	**467**	Antibodies	471
UCD200 Chickens	467	Cytokines	472
Tsk1 and Tsk2 Mice	468	Chemokines	472
Scl-GvHD	468	Fibrosis	472
TGF-β, CTGF, and bFGF	468	**Concluding Remarks and Future Prospects**	**473**
Bleomycin-Induced Fibrosis	468	**References**	**473**

INTRODUCTION

Scleroderma is derived from the Greek word *skleros* which means hard and *derma* which means skin. The first detailed description of scleroderma was in the early 1750s in Italy by Carlo Curzio who described the skin of these patients as dry hide and wood-like. We now know that scleroderma is a chronic, autoimmune, systemic, potentially lethal disease characterized by vasculopathy, immunological abnormalities, and excessive fibrosis that involves the skin and internal organs. The cause of scleroderma is still unclear; however, various environmental and/or genetic factors are thought to trigger complex pathogenic mechanisms that interact with each other at different levels.

CLINICAL, PATHOLOGIC, AND EPIDEMIOLOGIC FEATURES

Clinical Features

Swelling and tightening of the skin and other connective tissues is the hallmark of scleroderma, a group of related diseases (Black, 1993; Medsger, 2001). Scleroderma can be localized or systemic. Linear scleroderma and morphea are examples of the localized subtype, where the pathology is confined to the skin. Involvement of the internal organs in addition to the skin is called systemic sclerosis (SSc) (LeRoy et al., 1988; Medsger, 2004). Based solely on the extent of skin involvement, which was shown to be related to the degree of internal organ damage early in

N. Rose & I. Mackay (Eds): The Autoimmune Diseases, Fifth edition. DOI: http://dx.doi.org/10.1016/B978-0-12-384929-8.00033-2

the disease, SSc can be divided into two forms differing in the clinical course and outcome, the limited and diffuse cutaneous systemic sclerosis (lcSSc and dcSSc, respectively) (LeRoy et al., 1988; Medsger, 2004; Clements and Medsger, 2004). lcSSc is characterized by cutaneous changes affecting the extremities distal to the elbows, knees, and clavicles. CREST syndrome (calcinosis, Raynaud's phenomenon (RP), esophageal dysmotility, sclerodactyly, and telengiectasias) is an old synonym for lcSSc. The cutaneous changes in dcSSc are more proximal, and it has more severe and rapid progression than the limited subtype (LeRoy and Medsger, 2001).

Whether limited or diffuse, the early symptoms of SSc are non-specific and require a high index of suspicion to make the diagnosis. The majority of patients develop RP for variable periods of time before the appearance of skin changes. Patients may complain of fatigue, joint pain, and hand swelling early in the disease. Esophageal dysmotility, manifested as gastroesophageal reflux disease (GERD) or dysphagia, is also among the early features of SSc (LeRoy et al., 1988; Steen, 2001; Wigley, 2001).

The affected skin displays a spectrum of changes starting with edema, typically on the hands and fingers, progressing through shiny, thick, sclerotic skin that is tightly fixed to the underlying structures with loss of hair and sweat glands and ending with atrophic tethered skin. Areas of hypo- and hyperpigmentation may develop, giving a salt and pepper appearance. Telengiectasias and calcinosis may also occur (Charles et al., 2006).

Nailfold capillaroscopy can demonstrate dilated and giant capillary loops denoting impaired repair mechanisms of the injured blood vessels. Drop-out areas can also be seen classically with dcSSc. Severe vasospasm and vascular occlusive changes can lead to ulceration, infarction, and gangrene of the digits (Chandran et al., 1995). Those, as well as the gastrointestinal (GI) complications, interstitial lung disease, pulmonary hypertension, and renal involvement are responsible for the morbidity and mortality in SSc. dcSSc can display severe organ involvement that develops early in the disease. For this reason, patients should be monitored closely during the first 3–4 years of the disease for the signs and symptoms of visceral involvement (Steen and Medsger, 2000).

Pathologic Features

The pathologic picture of the involved tissues in SSc shows considerable variation depending on the stage of the disease. The understanding of these changes can help manage the patients by targeting the predominant mechanism at that particular stage.

Endothelial cell (EC) injury and apoptosis may be the earliest event in the pathogenesis of SSc (Sgonc et al., 1996). It can be detected in clinically "normal" skin.

These changes have different consequences on the integrity of the vascular and perivascular homeostasis. Perivascular edema can develop early in the disease, predisposed by increased vascular permeability.

Inflammatory cell infiltration is also among the early findings of SSc. Skin biopsies display perivascular cellular infiltration in the reticular dermis (Prescott et al., 1992). $CD4^+$ T cells and monocytes represent a major part of the cell infiltrate. Mast cells and eosinophils can also be detected but to a lesser degree (Mavilia et al., 1997). In contrast, $CD8^+$ T cells predominate in the lung tissues in addition to plasma cells, macrophages, and eosinophils (Yurovsky et al., 1996). Interestingly, the vascular pathology of the established disease is characterized as non-inflammatory obliterative vasculopathy (not vasculitis) and it shares some degree of similarity with chronic allograft arteriopathy (Furst et al., 1979; Prescott et al., 1992; Varga and Denton, 2008). Intimal thickening is caused by increased α-smooth muscle actin (α-SMA) positive myofibroblasts and upregualtion of collagen and other matrix protein synthesis. These vascular changes in the lung tissues and kidneys are behind the development of pulmonary artery hypertension (PAH) and renal crisis, respectively, in SSc (Varga and Denton, 2008; Batal et al., 2010).

Tissue fibrosis develops with further progression of the disease; dermal thickening and loss of skin appendages like hair follicles and sweat glands are caused by excessive collagen production, mainly in the deep dermal layers, followed by fat cell entrapment as a result of extension to the subcutaneous layers of skin (Varga and Denton, 2008).

Atrophy, thinning, and flattening of the rete pegs are noted in the epidermis of long-standing SSc. The dermis becomes acellular, intensely packed with dense hyalinized collagen and other extra-cellular matrix (ECM) proteins, with loss of the microvasulature, and subcutaneous fat (Davies et al., 2006).

Atrophy is more prominent than fibrosis in muscular organs like skeletal muscles and the gastrointestinal tract (GIT) (D'Angelo et al., 1969).

Epidemiologic Features

The prevalence of SSc is lower in Asia (China 10 per 100,000) (Li et al., 2012) and higher in the USA and Australia (27.6 and 23.3 per 100,000, respectively) (Roberts-Thomson et al., 2006; Helmick et al., 2008). The prevalence in Europe seems to follow a north–south gradient, with the lowest prevalence in northern European countries (Norway 9.9 vs. Italy 34.1 per 100,000) (Lo Monaco et al., 2011; Hoffmann-Vold et al., 2012). SSc shows female predominance with a female to male ratio of around 4.6:1 (Helmick et al., 2008).

A genetic influence is supported by the clustering of disease. The Choctaw Indians group in Oklahoma (66 cases per 100,000) (Arnett et al., 1996) and familial frequencies (relative risk: 15 for siblings) point towards genetic factors that increases the susceptibility for the disease (Arnett et al., 2001). African Americans may have an earlier onset and more severe disease (Helmick et al., 2008). On the other hand, case—control studies in other groups with high prevalence suggest exposure to different environmental factors including silica dust and solvents (Barnes and Mayes, 2012). These epidemiologic studies indicate a complex mix of genetics and environment which predispose to phenotypic disease.

Disease survival appears to be improving over the years, an effect that can be attributed to early detection and improved treatment (Steen and Medsger, 2007). However, other meta-analyses studies show a stable standardized mortality ratio (SMR) of 3.5 per various 10—20 year periods between 1960 and 2010 (Elhai et al., 2012). A US-wide study of the period between 1979 and 1998 showed an overall mortality rate from SSc of 3.9 per million; it is 3.5 times higher in women than men. African American women have the highest death rate from SSc (Krishnan and Furst, 2005).

Late age of onset, the diffuse cutaneous subset, anti-Scl-70 positive antibody, and cardiopulmonary involvement are associated with a poorer prognosis (Joven et al., 2010; Kim et al., 2010). Recently pulmonary fibrosis, PAH, and cardiac causes account for the majority of disease-related mortality (Steen and Medsger, 2007).

AUTOIMMUNE FEATURES AND IMMUNOLOGIC MARKERS IN DISEASE

SSc is associated with the presence of several autoantibodies, some of which may play a role in the pathogenesis of SSc and others appear to have diagnostic and prognostic value.

Potential Pathogenetic Antibodies

There are antibodies, found in SSc patients, which may play a role in SSc pathogenesis.

Tsk1 mice, an animal model of SSc, have an abnormal fibrillin-1 protein and also express *antifibrillin-1 antibodies* which might play a role in the fibrotic process of these models (Murai et al., 1998). Normal dermal fibroblasts upon exposure to these antibodies differentiate into a profibrotic phenotype. This may occur through the release of transforming growth factor beta (TGF-β) from fibrillin-1-containing microfibrils in the ECM (Zhou et al., 2005a,b). These antifibrillin-1 antibodies are of interest because a significant percent of SSc patients are positive for antifibrillin-1 antibodies and show strong

ethnic differences (100% in Choctaw American Indians, 80% in African Americans and Japanese patients, in contrast to 42% in Caucasians) (Tan et al., 2000).

Also, *antifibroblast antibodies*, which bind to antigens on the fibroblast surface, induce their activation and stimulate the production of profibrotic and angiogenic cytokines. These antibodies are more frequent in dcSSc than lcSSc (72 vs. 37%, respectively) (Chizzolini et al., 2002).

Finally, matrix metalloproteinase-1 (MMP-1)-dependent breakdown of ECM was shown to be blocked by *anti-MMP-1 IgG*, found mainly in the sera of dcSSc. The presence of the antibodies correlates with the degree of fibrosis in SSc patients (Sato et al., 2003).

Diagnostic and Prognostic Antibodies

A number of antibody tests may be useful in clinical care.

DNA topoisomerase I is an enzyme responsible for the relaxation of coiled DNA. *Anti-topoisomerase I antibodies* (also called *anti-Scl-70 antibodies*) are directed against different epitopes on this enzyme (Simon et al., 2009). Although they are considered highly specific to SSc, recent studies demonstrated the presence of these antibodies in the sera of rare healthy patients as well as patients with systemic lupus erythematosus (SLE) (up to 25%) (Spencer-Green et al., 1997; Mahler et al., 2010). Anti-Scl-70 antibodies are found in 30—40% of dcSSc (Spencer-Green et al., 1997; Derk and Jimenez, 2003) and <5% of patients with the limited disease (using highly specific assays). Seropositive patients have a higher mortality rate and are at increased risk of developing complications, including pulmonary fibrosis and cardiac involvement (Murata et al., 1998; Jacobsen et al., 2001). The level of anti-Scl-70 antibodies correlates with disease activity and skin score (Hu et al., 2003).

Anticentromere antibodies (ACA) are more specific for lcSSc and are found in up to 45—50% of these patients (Castro and Jimenez, 2010), while it can be detected in ≤5% of dcSSc (Steen et al., 1984). It recognizes different centromeric proteins (e.g., CENP-A, -B, -C) (Derk and Jimenez, 2003). Granzyme B-generated CENP-C fragments, rather than the intact CENP-C molecule, generated higher affinity antibodies in patients with ischemic digital loss (Schachna et al., 2002). This may indicate that the apoptotic process may expose hidden epitopes as targets for autoantibody production. The production of ACA is mediated by *human leukocyte antigen (HLA)-DRB1* and *HLA-DQB1* alleles (Mayes and Reveille, 2004).

Patients who are ACA positive have improved outcomes and lower mortality compared to those with anti-Scl-70 (Ho and Reveille, 2003). Moreover, ACA seropositivity was an independent protective factor for interstitial lung disease, supported by radiological and physiological studies (Kane et al., 1996; McNearney et al., 2007).

Patients who are seropositive for ACA have more recurrent and severe digital ulceration, and digital loss compared to ACA seronegative patients (Wigley et al., 1992).

Antihistone antibodies (AHA) are a heterogeneous group of antibodies directed against different histone complexes and components. IgM antibodies to H1 are related to mild clinical SSc features, while IgG antibodies to the inner core molecules of native histone, such as H2B or H2B-containing complexes, may be associated with severe pulmonary, cardiac, and renal SSc involvement (Parodi et al., 1995; Hasegawa et al., 1998).

Different studies investigated the clinical significance of antinucleolar antibodies in SSc. Antibodies directed against RNA polymerases (*anti-RNAP antibodies*) I, II, and III are highly associated with dcSSc (40%). Anti-RNAP III antibodies confer a number of risks: scleroderma renal crisis (33% are anti-RNAP III positive), systemic hypertension, synovitis, myositis, joint contracture, and malignancy within 5 years of skin manifestations (Mouthon et al., 2011; Nikpour et al., 2011).

Anti-polymyositis/scleroderma (anti-PM-Scl) antibodies are present in up to 24% of patients with polymyositis/SSc overlap syndrome. These patients tend to be younger and have pulmonary fibrosis and clacinosis as well as respond to steroids (Marguerie et al., 1992). Anti-PM-Scl positive patients follow a benign course; they have a 10-year cumulative survival rate of 91% compared to 65% of anti-PM-Scl negative patients (Koschik et al., 2012).

RNase MRP and RNase P are small nucleolar ribonucleoprotein particles (snoRNPs) that are involved in the processing of precursor ribosomal RNA (pre-rRNA) and precursor transfer RNA (pre-tRNA). Both of these snoRNPs contain Th/To antigens (Van Eenennaam et al., 2002). *Anti-Th/To antibodies* are developed against these antigens. They are associated with lcSSc and are mutually exclusive with ACA (Kuwana et al., 2002). Interestingly, anti-Th/To patients have milder skin, vascular, and esophageal involvement than lcSSc who are ACA positive. Anti-Th/To antibodies are also associated with an increased risk of developing PAH, pulmonary interstitial fibrosis, renal crisis, puffy fingers, small bowel involvement, and hypothyroidism. The survival is lower for these patients compared to ACA positive patients (Okano and Medsger, 1990; Mitri et al., 2003; Grassegger et al., 2008).

GENETIC FEATURES

In mono- and dizygotic twins the concordance rate for the molecular features of SSc is high, although it is low for clinical disease (Kuwana et al., 2001; Feghali-Bostwick et al., 2003; Zhou et al., 2005) For the last few years, genome-wide association (GWA) studies uncovered the potential relationship of some single nucleotide polymorphisms

(SNPs) that involve HLA and non-HLA loci with the development of SSc. Most of these genes are involved in the modulation of the immune system through signal transduction, cytokine production, and cell survival and proliferation. The association of *HLA-DPA1/B1, HLA-DQB1, HLADRB1, HLA-DRA* in addition to *NOTCH4*, which play a role in the TGF-β-induced pulmonary fibrosis and vascular damage, were all clearly associated with different serological and clinical subtypes of the disease (Gorlova et al., 2011). Associations of SSc with *STAT4, BLK, CD247, TNFSF4, BANK1*, and other non-HLA genes are supported by separate studies (Rueda et al., 2009, 2010; Gourh et al., 2010a,b; Radstake et al., 2010; Bossini-Castillo et al., 2011).

Some of these genes have an impact on specific serological variations and aspects of the clinical course of SSc. For instance, *SOX5* is associated with ACA positive patients, *RPL41/ESYT1* with dcSSc and *GRB10* and *IRF8* with the limited form of the disease (Gorlova et al., 2011). Separately, a certain polymorphism in the promoter region of the *IRF5* gene that downregulates *IRF5* expression is found in milder interstitial lung disease (ILD) and is associated with better long-term outcome (Sharif et al., 2012).

ENVIRONMENTAL INFLUENCES

Environmental factors can induce SSc-like syndromes by means of different mechanisms including loss of self-tolerance, direct activation of the immune system, and cytokine production or cross-reaction through molecular mimicry (Mora, 2009).

Toxic-oil syndrome traced to the consumption of colza oil (Terracini, 2004), vinyl chloride disease due to occupational exposure (Wilson et al., 1967), eosinophilia—myalgia syndrome linked to the ingestion of L-tryptophan supplements (Lindgren et al., 1991), and bleomycin-induced fibrosis are a just few examples from a long list (Adamson, 1976).

Viral triggers, like environmental effects, have been investigated. While parvovirus B19 (Ferri et al., 1999) and Epstein—Barr virus (EBV) (Arnson et al., 2009) were examined, the most interesting possibility was with cytomegalovirus (CMV). The UL94 late protein of human CMV shares some degree of similarity with an epitope on the topo-1 in patients with SSc and molecular mimicry may result in fibrogenic cytokine production (Lunardi et al., 2000).

A meta-analysis of 16 studies suggested the possibility that silica (not silicone) exposure may be a risk factor for the development of SSc, specifically in males and the male predominance may reflect an occupational bias. While interesting, the data are only associational (McCormic et al., 2010).

Recent meta-analytic studies of silicone were clear in showing no relation between silicone breast implants and SSc or other rheumatic autoimmune diseases (Janowsky et al., 2000).

Microchimerism is the presence of cells from one individual in another with each being genetically distinct. Fetomaternal microchimerism is an example of this phenomenon. It is thought that these cells might cause SSc-like disease through triggering a graft versus host (GvH)-like reaction and an increased number of michrochimeric cells are found in SSc patients, associated with increased risk of disease. This fascinating possibility requires further research (Cockrill et al., 2010).

ANIMAL MODELS OF SSc

Animal models are an important way to better understand human diseases and SSc is not an exception. There have, however, been difficulties establishing an animal model that matches the human disease with all of its phenotypic and pathological features (Table 33.1).

UCD200 Chickens

Within 1—2 weeks of hatching, UCD200 chickens spontaneously start to develop a condition somewhat similar to human SSc. They develop skin edema and Raynaud's-like features, followed by skin thickening and ischemic lesions of the toes. The disease may also involve internal organs within a few weeks. Likewise, the pathologic picture can mimic parts of SSc. Vascular obliteration, mononuclear cell infiltration, and fibroblast activation with excessive ECM production are all displayed in the lesional tissues. Furthermore, there can be detected in the serum autoantibodies including antinuclear antibodies (ANA), rheumatoid factor (RF), anticardiolipin antibodies, and anti-endothelial cell antibodies (AECA). Vascular EC apoptosis was shown to be induced by the

TABLE 33.1 Animal Models and their Similarity to Human SSc.

Models	Fibrosis	Vasculopathy	Inflammation	Autoantibodies	Principal Organs Involved	Dissimilarity to SSc
UCD200/206	++	+++	++	++	Skin, lungs, kidneys, heart, esophagus, and toes	The skin involvement is mostly confined to the comb with severe inflammation and necrosis. The skin fibrosis is not followed by sclerosis
Tsk1	+	0	0	+	Skin and heart	Hypodermal hyperplasia rather than dermal fibrosis. Unclear vascular and inflammatory changes Emphysematous lung changes rather than fibrosis
Scl-GvHD	+++	0	+++	+[a]	Skin, lungs, kidneys, liver, and parotid glands	No vascular involvement. No GI involvement
Bleomycin-induced	++	+	+	+	Skin, lungs (by endotracheal tube), esophagus, stomach	Absence of typical vascular changes. Respond to anti-inflammatory agents that are not effective in human SSc. Changes confined to the site of injection and need very high doses to see systemic involvement
TGF-β, CTGF, bFGF	+++	0	++	0	Skin	Require continuous growth factor injection. Absence of vascular and autoimmune changes. No systemic involvement
Fra2 transgenic mice	+++	+++	++	0	Skin, heart, and lungs (promising model to study PAH and different signaling pathways)	No autoimmunity. Unknown GI involvement
TβRIIΔk mice	+++	+	+	0	Skin, lungs, heart, aorta, and colon	Pathogenesis depends mainly on TGF-β. Incomplete understanding of the vascular and inflammatory changes. Absence of autoantibodies

[a]Only in modified Scl-GvHD models; +++: highly similar to human SSc; ++: moderately similar to human SSc; +: low similarity to human SSc; PAH: pulmonary artery hypertension.

AECA (Gershwin et al., 1981; Gruschwitz et al., 1993). However, this model is highly inflammatory with a combination of necrosis and widespread destruction, thus lessening its applicability to human SSc. UCD206 chickens are similar to UCD200 chickens but with more severe disease (Sgonc and Wick, 2008).

Tsk1 and Tsk2 Mice

Both tight skin mice (Tsk) type 1 and type 2 (Tsk1 and Tsk2, respectively) develop "TSK syndrome." As an autosomal dominant trait this syndrome is lethal when it is homozygotic; the homozygotes die *in utero* by 8—10 days of gestation (Green et al., 1976; Christner et al., 1995). Heterozygous mice survive and are used as an SSc model.

The mutation in Tsk1 mice was mapped on chromosome 2, and it involves the fibrillin-1 (*FBN1*) gene, resulting in an abnormally large fibrillin-1 protein that expresses more TGF-β-binding motifs (Li et al., 1993; Siracusa et al., 1996). Fibrillin-1 is a major component of the microfibrils in connective tissues and is essential for regulating the bioavailability of TGF-β (Isogai et al., 2003). In addition, Tsk1 mice produce autoantibodies to fibrillin-1 (Murai et al., 1998). Shortly after birth, heterozygous Tsk1 mice develop diffuse thickening and tethering of the skin. These changes are due to hyperplasia of the subcutaneous tissues rather than the dermis, thus not strictly mirroring human SSc. Although there is some internal organ fibrosis, the lungs develop emphysematous rather than restrictive changes (Green et al., 1976). The absence of vascular changes, the subcutaneous skin changes, and the lack of clear immune system involvement limit the usefulness of this model. The mutation in Tsk2 was mapped to chromosome 1. Tsk2 models exhibit fibrosis, inflammatory cell infiltration, and autoantibody production (Christner et al., 1995). The frequencies of ANA, anti-Scl-70, ACA, and other autoantibodies are high in this model (Gentiletti et al., 2005). However, the pathological mechanisms behind these changes are unclear.

Scl-GvHD

Manipulation of the immune system by transplantation of bone marrow (BM) or spleen from B10.D2 mice donors into intensely γ-irradiated BALB/c mice can induce a GvH reaction in Scl-GvHD models, another animal model of SSc (McCormick et al., 1999). The development of skin and lung fibrosis by the 21st day after transplantation is preceded by donor-derived monocyte and T cell infiltration with an activated phenotype. Increased TGF-β and CCL-2 are also found, promoting the production of large amounts of type I collagen mRNA and protein (Zhang

et al., 2002). Although it simulates the fibrosis and inflammation of the human disease, the absence of vascular involvement and autoimmunity, in addition to the technical difficulties of producing this model, limit the use of these models. A modified GvHD model, obtained by injection of spleen cells from B10.D2 mice into RAG-2 knockout mice, show some evidence of autoimmunity; however, lung involvement is absent in this model (Ruzek et al., 2004).

TGF-β, CTGF, and bFGF

The growth factor-induced fibrosis model of SSc is developed by subcutaneous injection of TGF-β in newborn mice which rapidly induces fibrosis that is maintained by subsequent serial application of connective tissue growth factor (CTGF) or basic fibroblast growth factor (bFGF). This demonstrates the role of TGF-β in inducing the fibrotic process and CTGF and bFGF as essential in maintaining it (Shinozaki et al., 1997; Mori et al., 1999). Transient early elevation of mast cells and constant increase in the number of macrophages was demonstrated in these models (Chujo et al., 2005).

Bleomycin-Induced Fibrosis

The murine models of bleomycin-induced fibrosis are widely used in SSc studies. Repetitive subcutaneous injection of bleomycin induces pathological changes closely similar to the human disease (Mountz et al., 1983). The skin changes are confined to the injection site and remain more than 6 weeks after the last dose of bleomycin. Various mouse strains respond differently to bleomycin, in terms of duration and intensity of fibrosis. C3H/He, DBA/2, B10.D2, and B10.A show susceptibility to bleomycin (Yamamoto et al., 2000; Oi et al., 2004). Early inflammatory cell infiltration of the dermis with T cells, monocytes/macrophages, and mast cells, followed by dermal sclerosis with accumulation of thick collagen bundles, and homogeneous materials are demonstrated in the skin. Autoantibodies can also be detected in the sera of these models (Yamamoto et al., 1999). Vascular wall thickening in the deep layers of the dermis was reported in some studies (Yamamoto and Katayama, 2011). Lung involvement with alveolar wall infiltration and thickening are among the early findings. TGF-β was shown to influence fibroblasts, myofibroblasts, and other cells to adopt a profibrotic phenotype with upregulation of collagen and other ECM materials (Yamamoto et al., 1999).

Various transgenic animal models of SSc are generated by genetic manipulation. The offspring of such models spontaneously acquire the phenotypic features of SSc.

Fra2-Transgenic Mice

Fra2 is a transcription factor that is upregulated in SSc; it acts as a downstream mediator of TGF-β and platelet-derived growth factor (PDGF) signaling (Reich et al., 2010). For the last few years, the Fra2-transgenic mouse has engendered much interest as an animal model for SSc, as it shows dermal and lung fibrosis very similar to SSc by the age of 12 weeks (Maurer et al., 2012). Joint, renal, and GI involvement have not been examined, as far as we know.

TβRIIΔk Mice

TβRIIΔk mice have fibroblast-specific and kinase-deficient TGF-β receptors II. These fibroblasts show increased proliferation, myofibroblast transdifferentiation, and expression of plasminogen activator inhibitor-1 (PAI-1), CTGF, SMAD3, SMAD4, and SMAD7 (Denton et al., 2003). By an unclear mechanism, this results in increased TGF-β signaling and leads to excessive ECM production that involves the skin, lungs, colon, heart, and aortic smooth muscles (Denton et al., 2003; Derrett-Smith et al., 2010; Thoua et al., 2012). This is an exciting model with great possibilities.

Wnt-10b-Transgenic Mice

Although thus far only under investigation, Wnt-10b-transgenic mice represent a promising animal model of skin affected by SSc. Dermal fibroblasts from this model shows persistent Wnt/β-catenin signaling with upregulation of collagen and α-SMA gene expression leading to dermal fibrosis and progressive loss of subcutaneous adipose tissue (Wei et al., 2011). The generalizability of this model and the extent to which the viscera are involved has not been published, nor have details of immune dysfunction.

PATHOGENIC MECHANISMS

Vasculopathy

RP, digital ischemia/ulcers, PAH, and renal crisis are all clear evidence of a vascular aspect to SSc and are probably among the earliest events in the disease.

SSc vasculopathy presents a wide range of changes that involve different aspects of the vascular system, including EC, capillaries, micro- and macro-vessels, and elevation of endothelium-associated adhesion molecules exemplify these effects.

For example, high intracellular adhesion molecule-1 (ICAM-1) expression and low ICAM-3 expression on the peripheral blood mononuclear cells from SSc patients suggest that adhesion molecules may be involved in some aspect of SSc (Sawaya et al., 2009). Also, endothelin-1 (ET-1), among the strongest vasoconstrictors known and with mitogenic and inflammatory effects, contributes to TGF-β-associated pulmonary fibrosis in SSc (Shi-wen et al., 2007). The use of endothelin receptor inhibitors like bosentan, ambrisentan, and sitaxentan is effective in treating SSc-PAH and this effect may be mediated through both the vasodilatory and antifibrotic effect of ET-1 (Denton et al., 2006; Shetty and Derk, 2011). The level of other adhesion molecules like thrombomodulin also correlates with the disease activity (Mercié et al., 1997).

Further, endoglin, a coreceptor for TGF-β that modulates TGF-β signaling, may well be involved in the pathogenesis of SSc (López-Casillas et al., 1991). Endoglin gene abnormalities are responsible for hereditary hemorrhagic telangiectasia which shares several features with SSc, especially the limited cutaneous subtype (McAllister et al., 1994). Studies demonstrate significantly elevated endoglin levels in limited cutaneous SSc patients compared to those seen in dcSSc, SLE, or normal controls (Fujimoto et al., 2006).

Beyond cytokines, EC abnormalities show that vasculopathy may be a central and early aspect of SSc. In a study of UCD 200/206 chickens (see above), skin EC are the first cells to undergo apoptosis, even prior to inflammation and fibrosis (Sgonc et al., 1996).

Although the mechanism of EC apoptosis is not clear, multiple pathways have been investigated as a potential cause for the EC injury, including immunological, viral, and ischemic causes (Kahaleh, 2008).

Platelet Activation

Microvascular EC injury and apoptosis can increase vascular permeability and dysregulate control of vascular tone through the release of vasoactive mediators. The edematous phase of cutaneous SSc may be a manifestation of these changes and RP is clearly a result of dysregulated vascular tone (Kahaleh and LeRoy, 1999; Generini and Matucci Cerinic, 1999). EC damage, in turn, provokes the migration of vascular smooth muscle cells and pericytes to the intimal layer of blood vessels where they transdifferentiate into collagen secreting myofibroblasts. The resulting intimal proliferation leads to intimal thickening, luminal narrowing, and blood vessel obliteration (Rajkumar et al., 1999).

Platelets are actively involved in the pathogenesis of SSc. EC injury/activation induces platelet activation, aggregation, and thrombus formation that lead to occlusion of the already narrowed blood vessels, further exacerbating tissue ischemia and necrosis (Kahaleh and LeRoy, 1999). The activated platelets also produce PDGF and TGF-β which mediate the fibrotic process and collagen synthesis (Assoian et al., 1983). On the other hand, platelets from SSc patients show increased expression of non-integrin receptors for type 1 collagen which may, in part, explain the increased platelet aggregation in SSc (Chiang et al., 2006).

Cytokine Abnormalities

Vascular endothelial growth factor (VEGF) is a potent angiogenic mediator and would be expected to be low, given the decreased angiogenesis found in SSc. Strangely, the expression of VEGF and its receptors VEGFR1 and 2 are upregulated in SSc, despite ineffective vascular repair mechanisms (Mackiewicz et al., 2002; Distler et al., 2002, 2004; Choi et al., 2003; Manetti et al., 2010). This apparent paradox was explained by recent studies which revealed the presence of VEGF isoforms with different functional properties. An angiogenic factor, VEGF165, and an angiostatic factor, VEGF165b, are the result of alternative splicing of the terminal exon of VEGF-A, premRNA. VEGF165b is significantly upregulated in SSc and is responsible for the elevation of the "total" VEGF level in SSc. Like VEGF165b, the angiogenesis inhibitor endostatin is elevated in SSc (Manetti et al., 2011).

The interaction of urokinase-type plasminogen activator (uPA) with its receptor uPAR is important in mediating the interaction of the EC with the ECM during angiogenesis. MMP-12 is responsible for cleaving domain 1 of uPAR in SSc EC, resulting in truncated and nonfunctioning receptors and thus impairing EC movement and effective new blood vessel formation (D'Alessio et al., 2004).

Cellular Abnormalities

As a physiological response to tissue ischemia, endothelial progenitor cells (EPC) can mobilize from the BM to the site of vascular lesions and differentiate into a variety of mature cells. This is a dynamic and highly complex process that requires mobilization, chemotaxis, adhesion, proliferation, and differentiation of the progenitor cells (Asahara et al., 1999). Although it is poorly understood, cytokines, tissue hypoxia, and angiogenic growth factors including granulocyte monocyte-colony stimulating factor (GM-CSF) and VEGF seem to play a major role in driving progenitor cells to the damaged tissue (Zammaretti and Zisch, 2005).

Avouac et al. (2008) demonstrated increased blood levels of EPC in SSc, supporting mobilization from the BM. Furthermore, the subset of patients with digital vascular lesions and high severity score for disease expression displayed low levels of EPC, suggesting increased homing at this stage. Other data showed a significant reduction in the number of EPC in patients with diffuse SSc when compared with healthy controls and rheumatoid arthritis patients (Kuwana et al., 2004).

Recent studies demonstrated a reduction in the differentiation capacity of EPC in SSc patients, implying impaired vasculogenesis and inadequate vascular repair mechanism (Del Papa et al., 2006).

Human mesenchymal stem cells (MSC) are multipotent cells that are present in the BM of adults and might be another source of EPC. The *in vitro* differentiation potential of MSC in patients with SSc reveals early senescence and decreased capacity to perform specific endothelial activities such as capillary morphogenesis and chemoinvasion, suggesting that endothelial repair may be impaired in SSc. Furthermore, the possibility that this impairment can be partially reversed using VEGF and stromal cell-derived factor 1 suggests that these cells might be helpful in future regenerative treatment (Cipriani et al., 2007).

Immunological Abnormalities

Activation of the immune system plays a crucial role in the vasculopathy and fibrosis of SSc (Figure 33.1).

T Cells

Macophages and activated T cells represent a large part of the cellular infiltrates in the affected tissues of SSc. The initiation of the presumed autoimmune response in SSc could be the result of interaction between the two limbs of the immune system, innate and adaptive immunity. IL-4 and IL-13 are secreted from macrophages and monocytes as part of the early activation of the innate immune system. These two cytokines are necessary for the differentiation of T helper cells Th0 into Th2 cells; the latter are predominant in SSc. Upon binding of IL-4 to its receptors on Th2, stimulation of the STAT6/GATA3 system occurs, leading to the production of IL-4, IL-5, and IL-13 with further activation of Th2 through autocrine and paracrine signaling (Higashi-Kuwata et al., 2009; O'Reilly et al., 2012). In addition, levels of regulatory T cells ($CD4^+$ $Foxp3^+$ T_{regs}), one of the major mechanisms for maintenance of self-tolerance, were low in one study (Klein et al., 2011).

The peripheral blood levels of $CD3^+$, $CD4^+$, $CD8^+$, and $CD19^+$ cells were variously low, normal, or high compared to normals, so this area remains quite controversial (Fiocco et al., 1993; Artlett et al., 2002; Ercole et al., 2003; Ingegnoli et al., 2003; Mitsuo et al., 2006; Gambichler et al., 2010).

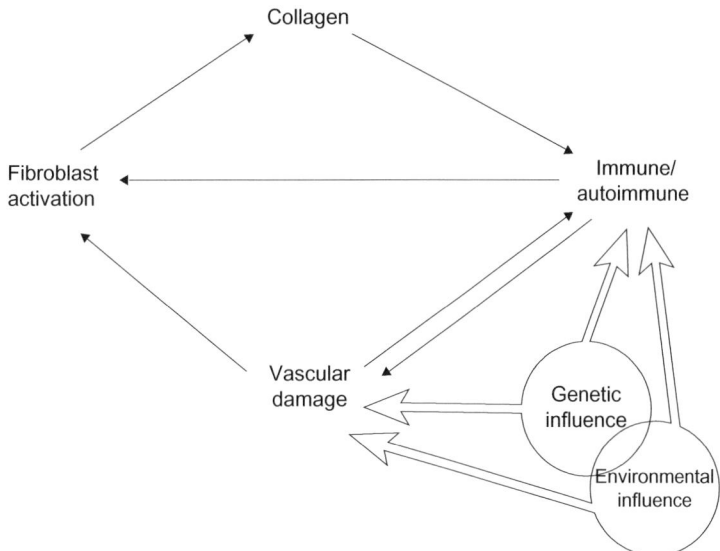

FIGURE 33.1 Relationship of potential triggering factors and the pathogenetic mechanisms involved in the development of systemic sclerosis.

B Cells

A growing body of evidence points towards the role of B cells in the initiation of the immune response in SSc. The B cell can act as an antigen presenting cell through interaction of antigen with low affinity B cell receptors (BCR) (Constant et al., 1995). CD19 is a cell surface molecule expressed on the surface of B cells that interacts with the BCR, lowering the threshold for antigen-dependent stimulation of the BCR (Carter and Fearon, 1992). The expression of CD19 was increased in SSc B cells and also in the animal models of the disease (Sato et al., 2000).

The use of rituximab (RTX) in newborn Tsk mice significantly suppresses the development of skin fibrosis, autoantibodies, and hypergammaglobulinemia, although this did not pertain when used in established disease (Hasegawa et al., 2006). In uncontrolled case reports RTX was effective in some but not all patients and a controlled trial of B cell depletion in SSc is under way (Lafyatis et al., 2009).

Antibodies

The sensitivity and specificity of different methods used in detecting autoantibodies can affect, to a certain extent, the strength and frequency of these antibodies in SSc patients (Walker and Fritzler, 2007). Indirect immunofluorescence (IIF) using rapidly dividing cell-lines is the most frequently used assay to screen for autoantibodies. Despite it being more specific, it is slower and more expensive. The use of enzyme-linked immunosorbent assay (ELISA) is becoming more popular. It is automated and also easier to use for multiple antibodies. However, it is less specific (Wiik et al., 2004).

There is a wide range of autoantibodies found in SSc and nuclear antigens represent the primary target for these antibodies. ANA are found in more than 90% of SSc patients (Medsger and Steen, 1996). Anti-Scl-70 and ACA are highly specific for SSc and support the clinical diagnosis of the disease (Reveille et al., 2003). The virtual mutually exclusive existence of these antibodies in different disease subtypes and their correlation with certain disease complications raises the likelihood that different disease processes lead to the development of these serological variations (Castro and Jimenez, 2010; Bunn and Black, 1999).

Both PDGF receptor-specific antibodies and AECA seem to be involved in SSc pathogenesis. PDGF plays an important role in the fibrotic process of SSc. Stimulatory autoantibodies against PDGF receptors were detected in SSc sera (Baroni et al., 2006); upon binding to the receptors, the RAR-ERK1/2 pathway is induced and increases the level of reactive oxygen species (ROS), and the persistence of ROS and ERK1/2 favor an increased collagen gene expression (Svegliati et al., 2005).

Although it can be detected in other diseases, AECA are present in 40−50% of SSc cases (Kahaleh, 2008) and may be linked to the development of pulmonary fibrosis in this disease (Lewandowska et al., 2013). These AECA are directed against IgG- and IgM-related antigens or CENP-B (García de la Peña-Lefebvre et al., 2004; Tamby et al., 2005; Servettaz et al., 2006). As EC apoptosis is one of the earliest events in SSc, AECA-dependent cell-mediated cytotoxicity may be an important mediator between antibodies and cellular abnormalities (Sgonc et al., 2000).

Cytokines

Various cytokines which mediate EC damage and fibrosis are elevated in SSc. Interleukin (IL)-6 receptors are expressed on the surface of monocytes, neutrophils, and B cells (Jones and Rose-John, 2002). The effect of IL-6 on EC, fibroblast, and some subsets of T cells are through a trans signaling process. This process ultimately activates STAT3 which contributes to EC injury/activation and induces the expression of adhesion molecules (Romano et al., 1997). The production of sIL-6R is mediated in part by IL-8 and leukotriene B4 (LTB4) (Marin et al., 2002). IL-6, sIL-6R, and IL-8 are elevated in SSc serum (Reitamo et al., 1993; Hasegawa et al., 1998), and LTB4 levels are elevated in the bronchoalveolar lavage (BAL) fluid of these patients (Kowal-Bielecka et al., 2005).

Like many other proinflammatory and profibrotic cytokines, the soluble receptors for IL-2 (sIL-2R), IL-6 (sIL-6R), and TNF-α (sTNF-αRI) are elevated in SSc and are linked to the activity and progression of the disease (Lis and Brzezińska-Wcisło, 2003). In all cases, however, it is not clear if these cytokines play a primary or secondary role in SSc. Further work on these proteins is necessary and is, in fact, under way.

IL-4 and IL-13 are profibrotic cytokines which mediate the production of collagen and ECM in a direct and indirect fashion via the stimulation of TGF-β. The serum levels of both IL-4 and IL-13 are elevated in SSc (Hasegawa et al., 1997).

Chemokines

Inflammatory chemokines play a major role in the pathology of SSc. They induce trafficking and accumulation of cells at the lesional sites and the expression of chemokines and their receptors are increased in SSc.

CXCR4 is expressed on the surface of multiple cell types including monocytes and fibrocytes. CXCR4 induces cell migration to lesional sites under the influence of its ligand CXCL12. Both CXCR4 and CXCL12 are elevated in the lung tissues of SSc-ILD and in the edematous skin lesions of both dcSSc and lcSSc. Fibrocytes express other receptors that respond to a wide range of chemokines and, thus, fibrocytes may play a role in the fibrotic process (Cipriani et al., 2006; Tourkina et al., 2011).

The function of chemokines goes beyond chemoattraction. CCL5 (also known as regulated upon activation, normally T cell expressed and secreted (RANTES)), for example, directly activates T cells and stimulates them to produce INF-γ (Appay et al., 2000). High levels of circulating CCL2 correlated with the modified Rodnan skin score (mRSS) (Bandinelli et al., 2012).

Fibrosis

A wide range of cells play different roles in the process of fibrosis, either directly or indirectly, through cell–cell interaction or the production of mediators. Fibroblasts act as the pivotal cells in the process of fibrous tissue production, both physiologically and pathologically, as in SSc. Proliferation of local cells and migration of others, with subsequent *in situ* differentiation to fibroblasts and myofibroblasts, tend to expand the pool of cells and upregulate ECM production (Abraham and Varga, 2005; Abraham et al., 2007). We will describe the multiple factors that affect fibrosis in SSc.

PDGF, ET-1, CTGF, and especially TGF-β, through different signaling pathways, mediate the transdifferentiation of fibrobasts and other cells into myofibroblasts, a specialized form of fibroblasts with some features of smooth muscle cell; they express α-SMA stress fibers, the ED-A variant of fibronectin, and Thy1 glycoprotein on their surface, all strongly linked to SSc. Myofibroblasts are able to contract and mechanically remodel the newly formed ECM. The persistence of active myofibroblasts is assumed to play an important part in the fibrotic process of SSc through upregulation of ECM production and increased cytokine secretion that leads to further stimulation by means of autocrine and paracrine signaling (Abraham and Varga, 2005; Abraham et al., 2007).

The ECM plays an active and complex role in influencing the survival, development, migration, proliferation, shape, and function of cells that contact it (Alberts et al., 2002). In SSc the normal equilibrium of collagen synthesis and degradation is oriented toward synthesis (Varga and Bashey, 1995).

Type I collagen is the most common collagen type and represents the major structural component of dermal ECM. It is composed of two α1 chains and one α2 chain, encoded by *COL1A1* and *COL1A2* genes, respectively (Sykes and Solomon, 1978; Huerre et al., 1982). The transcription of these genes involves the interaction of regulatory elements with transcription factors, such as specific protein 1 (Sp1), specific protein 3 (Sp3), CCAAT-binding factor (CBF), collagen-króppel box (c-Krox) and nuclear factor-$\kappa\beta$ (NF-$\kappa\beta$) (Kypriotou et al., 2007; Beachef et al., 2012).

Although human c-Krox (hc-Krox) suppresses type I collagen genes (both *COL1A1* and *COL1A2*) (Widom et al., 2001), recent data suggest that hc-Krox has a transactivating role on human *COL1A1* gene in normal and pathological dermal fibroblasts, interacting with other transcription factors to upregulate type I collagen synthesis (Kypriotou et al., 2007).

Separately, c-Krox promotes CD4$^+$ T cell lineage differentiation rather than CD8$^+$ T cells during intrathymic

T cell positive selection, indicating that c-Krox has an early role in the pathogenesis of scleroderma (Sun et al., 2005).

TGF-β plays a major role in the pathogenesis of fibrosis in SSc. TGF-β is secreted by numerous cell types including fibroblasts, immune cells, and platelets. TGF-β is a potent inducer of collagen synthesis and other ECM proteins and at the same time suppresses degradation of the matrix. TGF-β is vital in wound healing and tissue repair physiologically. However, dysregulation of TGF-β at different levels can lead to fibrosis and a wide spectrum of other diseases, including cancer and SSc (Varga and Bashey, 1995; Branton and Kopp, 1999).

The expression degree, serum/tissue levels, and activity of TGF-β is significantly altered in SSc compared to normal control groups and depends on the clinical features, stage, and type of SSc. For example, the level of TGF-β1 (one of three isoforms) is significantly elevated in the BAL fluid from patients with SSc lung disease, while the level of TGF-β2 (another isoform) is significantly less than the control group (Ludwicka et al., 1995). There were no significant differences in the levels of total serum TGF-β among dcSSc, lcSSc, and normal, but active TGF-β1 was significantly lower in dcSSc compared to the other two groups and was negatively correlated to the skin score (Dziadzio et al., 2005). This, and the evidences of increased expression of TGF-β receptors in SSc, point toward the sequestration of active TGF-β1 in affected sites (Yamane et al., 2002; Pannu et al., 2006).

TGF-β is secreted in the ECM in an inactive form and requires local activation to be biologically effective. It is frequently related to fibrotic diseases (Nakerakanti and Trojanowska, 2012). SSc patients show upregulation of thrombospondins 1 and 2 in dermal SSc fibroblasts, detailing one of the mechanisms locally activating TGF-β (Avouac et al., 2011). Other studies showed a significant elevation of other local TGF-β activators such as αvβ5 integrins (Asano et al., 2005).

Likewise, complex mechanisms have been discovered which transmit membrane ligand binding to activation of nuclear factors. SMADs 3/4 or blocking nuclear factors SMAD7 all show the degree and complexity of TGF-β regulation (Zhang et al., 1996; Nakao et al., 1997a,b; Hayashi et al., 1997).

TGF-β and other growth factors can also induce their profibrotic effects in fibroblasts via SMAD-independent pathways such as c-Abl and CTGF. c-Abl is a non-receptor tyrosine kinase which stimulates TGF-β and PDGF. c-Abl is inhibited by imatinib and its congeners; this activity seems to be part of its potential in treating SSc (Plattner et al., 1999; Daniels et al., 2004; Bhattacharyya et al., 2009).

CTGF is a matrix protein that connects the cells to the ECM. It is part of the CCN family and is induced by TGF-β, ET-1, hypoxia, shear stress, and biomechanical deformation (Gao and Brigstock, 2003; Leask and Abraham, 2006). CTGF has a clear direct profibrotic effect by inducing collagen gene expression in lung fibroblasts though a SMAD-independent pathway (Ponticos et al., 2009).

PDGF is another agent that plays a role in the pathogenicity of SSc. It is a mitoattractant factor with mitogenic and chemotactic effects on connective tissue cells (Seppä et al., 1982). PDGF is produced by smooth muscle cells, fibroblasts, EC, macrophages, in addition to platelets (Varga and Abraham, 2007). The fibroblasts from SSc skin lesions showed overexpression of PDGFR-α, leading to increased cell proliferation and transdifferentiation to myofibroblasts (Liu and Zhang, 2012).

A relatively newly described pathogenetic pathway involves the Wnt pathway and β-catenin. The Wnt family of signaling proteins regulates gene expression after cell surfacee receptor stimulation. Downstream of the Wnt signaling pathway is β-catenin which transmits the regulatory signals from the cytoplasm to the nucleus (Logan and Nusse, 2004). High β-catenin levels were found in the nucleus of SSc fibroblasts and these concentrations were directly profibrotic in SSc after exposure to increased expression of Wnt-1 and Wnt-10b (Beyer et al., 2012).

CONCLUDING REMARKS AND FUTURE PROSPECTS

Despite the number of studies on scleroderma/SSc and a great deal of progress, we are still far from a clear picture of the pathogenesis of disease. The interactions between different genetic, environmental, and molecular factors, at many levels, are behind the pathological complexity and phenotypical heterogeneity of scleroderma/SSc. Studies over many years helped uncover various mechanisms that may play a part in the development of SSc and that point to targets for new treatment strategies. This plethora of pathways and mechanisms, as their place and importance is dissected, should lead to better therapy.

Overall SSc is a combined disease which is initiated by endothelial damage and amplified by autoimmune response. One could say it is an autoimmune disease but this is just a simplification; on the other hand, one could approach treatment by considering immune suppressing medications and get a good response.

REFERENCES

Abraham, D.J., Varga, J., 2005. Scleroderma: from cell and molecular mechanisms to disease models. Trends Immunol. 26, 587–595.

Abraham, D.J., Eckes, B., Rajkumar, V., Krieg, T., 2007. New developments in fibroblast and myofibroblast biology: implications for fibrosis and scleroderma. Curr. Rheumatol. Rep. 9, 136–143.

Adamson, I.Y., 1976. Pulmonary toxicity of bleomycin. Environ Health Perspect. 16, 119–126.

Alberts, B., Johnson, A., Lewis, J., Raff, M., Roberts, K., Walter, P., 2002. Cell junctions, cell adhesion, and the extracellular matrix. In: Alberts, B., et al. (Ed.), Molecular Biology of the Cell, fourth ed. New York, NY, USA, pp. 1065–1125.

Appay, V., Dunbar, P.R., Cerundolo, V., McMichael, A., Czaplewski, L., Rowland-Jones, S., 2000. RANTES activates antigen-specific cytotoxic T lymphocytes in a mitogen-like manner through cell surface aggregation. Int. Immunol. 12, 1173–1182.

Arnett, F.C., Howard, R.F., Tan, F., Moulds, J.M., Bias, W.B., Durban, E., et al., 1996. Increased prevalence of systemic sclerosis in a Native American tribe in Oklahoma. Association with an Amerindian HLA haplotype. Arthritis Rheum. 39, 1362–1370.

Arnett, F.C., Cho, M., Chatterjee, S., Aguilar, M.B., Reveille, J.D., Mayes, M.D., 2001. Familial occurrence frequencies and relative risks for systemic sclerosis (scleroderma) in three United States cohorts. Arthritis Rheum. 44, 1359–1362.

Arnson, Y., Amital, H., Guiducci, S., Matucci-Cerinic, M., Valentini, G., Barzilai, O., et al., 2009. The role of infections in the immunopathogenesis of systemic sclerosis: evidence from serological studies. Ann. N.Y. Acad. Sci. 1173, 627–632.

Artlett, C.M., Cox, L.A., Ramos, R.C., Dennis, T.N., Fortunato, R.A., Hummers, L.K., et al., 2002. Increased microchimeric CD4 + T lymphocytes in peripheral blood from women with systemic sclerosis. Clin. Immunol. 103 (3 Pt 1), 303–308.

Asahara, T., Masuda, H., Takahashi, T., Kalka, C., Pastore, C., Silver, M., et al., 1999. Bone marrow origin of endothelial progenitor cells responsible for postnatal vasculogenesis in physiological and pathological neovascularization. Circ. Res. 85, 221–228.

Asano, Y., Ihn, H., Yamane, K., Jinnin, M., Mimura, Y., Tamaki, K., 2005. Involvement of alphavbeta5 integrin-mediated activation of latent transforming growth factor beta1 in autocrine transforming growth factor beta signaling in systemic sclerosis fibroblasts. Arthritis Rheum. 52, 2897–2905.

Assoian, R.K., Komoriya, A., Meyers, C.A., Miller, D.M., Sporn, M.B., 1983. Transforming growth factor beta in human platelets. Identification of a major storage site, purification, and characterization. J. Biol. Chem. 258, 7155–7160.

Avouac, J., Juin, F., Wipff, J., Couraud, P.O., Chiocchia, G., Kahan, A., et al., 2008. Circulating endothelial progenitor cells in systemic sclerosis: association with disease severity. Ann. Rheum. Dis. 67, 1455–1460.

Avouac, J., Clemessy, M., Distler, J.H., Gasc, J.M., Ruiz, B., Vacher-Lavenu, M.C., et al., 2011. Enhanced expression of ephrins and thrombospondins in the dermis of patients with early diffuse systemic sclerosis: potential contribution to perturbed angiogenesis and fibrosis. Rheumatology (Oxford). 50, 1494–1504.

Bandinelli, F., Del Rosso, A., Gabrielli, A., Giacomelli, R., Bartoli, F., Guiducci, S., et al., 2012. CCL2, CCL3 and CCL5 chemokines in systemic sclerosis: the correlation with SSc clinical features and the effect of prostaglandin E1 treatment. Clin. Exp. Rheumatol. 30, S44–S49.

Barnes, J., Mayes, M.D., 2012. Epidemiology of systemic sclerosis: incidence, prevalence, survival, risk factors, malignancy, and environmental triggers. Curr. Opin. Rheumatol. 24, 165–170.

Baroni, S.S., Santillo, M., Bevilacqua, F., Luchetti, M., Spadoni, T., Mancini, M., et al., 2006. Stimulatory autoantibodies to the PDGF receptor in systemic sclerosis. New Engl. J. Med. 354 (25), 2667–2676.

Batal, I., Domsic, R.T., Medsger, T.A., Bastacky, S., 2010. Scleroderma renal crisis: a pathology perspective. Int. J. Rheumatol. 2010, 543704.

Beachef, G., Bigot, N., Kypriotou, M., Renard, E., Poree, B., Widom, R., et al., 2012. The p65 subunit of NF-kB inhibits COL1A1 gene transcription in human dermal and scleroderma fibroblasts through its recruitment on promoter by protein interaction with transcriptional Activators (c-Krox, Sp1, and Sp3.). J. Biol. Chem. 287 (5), 3462–3478.

Beyer, C., Schramm, A., Akhmetshina, A., Dees, C., Kireva, T., Gelse, K., et al., 2012. β-catenin is a central mediator of pro-fibrotic Wnt signaling in systemic sclerosis. Ann. Rheum. Dis. 71, 761–767.

Bhattacharyya, S., Ishida, W., Wu, M., Wilkes, M., Mori, Y., Hinchcliff, M., et al., 2009. A non-Smad mechanism of fibroblast activation by transforming growth factor beta via c-Abl and Egr-1: selective modulation by imatinib mesylate. Oncogene. 28, 1285–1297.

Black, C.M., 1993. Scleroderma—clinical aspects. J. Intern. Med. 234, 115–118.

Bossini-Castillo, L., Broen, J.C., Simeon, C.P., Beretta, L., Vonk, M.C., Ortego-Centeno, et al., 2011. A replication study confirms the association of TNFSF4 (OX40L) polymorphisms with systemic sclerosis in a large European cohort. Ann. Rheum. Dis. 70, 638–641.

Branton, M.H., Kopp, J.B., 1999. TGF-beta and fibrosis. Microbes Infect. 1, 1349–1365.

Bunn, C.C., Black, C.M., 1999. Systemic sclerosis: an autoantibody mosaic. Clin. Exp. Immunol. 117, 207–208.

Carter, R.H., Fearon, D.T., 1992. CD19: lowering the threshold for antigen receptor stimulation of B lymphocytes. Science. 256, 105–107.

Castro, S.V., Jimenez, S.A., 2010. Biomarkers in systemic sclerosis. Biomark Med. 4, 133–147.

Chandran, G., Smith, M., Ahern, M.J., Roberts-Thomson, P.J., 1995. A study of scleroderma in South Australia: prevalence, subset characteristics and nailfold capillaroscopy. Aust. N.Z. J. Med. 25, 688–694.

Charles, C., Clements, P., Furst, D.E., 2006. Systemic sclerosis: hypothesis-driven treatment strategies. Lancet. 367, 1683–1691.

Chiang, T.M., Takayama, H., Postlethwaite, A.E., 2006. Increase in platelet non-integrin type I collagen receptor in patients with systemic sclerosis. Thromb. Res. 117, 229–306.

Chizzolini, C., Raschi, E., Rezzonico, R., Testoni, C., Mallone, R., Gabrielli, A., et al., 2002. Autoantibodies to fibroblasts induce a proadhesive and proinflammatory fibroblast phenotype in patients with systemic sclerosis. Arthritis Rheum. 46, 1602–1613.

Choi, J.J., Min, D.J., Cho, M.L., Min, S.Y., Kim, S.J., Lee, S.S., et al., 2003. Elevated vascular endothelial growth factor in systemic sclerosis. J. Rheumatol. 30, 1529–1533.

Christner, P.J., Peters, J., Hawkins, D., Siracusa, L.D., Jiménez, S.A., 1995. The tight skin 2 mouse. An animal model of scleroderma displaying cutaneous fibrosis and mononuclear cell infiltration. Arthritis Rheum. 38, 1791–1798.

Chujo, S., Shirasaki, F., Kawara, S., Inagaki, Y., Kinbara, T., Inaoki, M., et al., 2005. Connective tissue growth factor causes persistent proalpha2(I) collagen gene expression induced by transforming growth factor-beta in a mouse fibrosis model. J. Cell Physiol. 203, 447–456.

Cipriani, P., Franca Milia, A., Liakouli, V., Pacini, A., Manetti, M., Marrelli, A., et al., 2006. Differential expression of stromal cell-derived factor 1 and its receptor CXCR4 in the skin and endothelial cells of systemic sclerosis patients: pathogenetic implications. Arthritis Rheum. 54, 3022—3033.

Cipriani, P., Guiducci, S., Miniati, I., Cinelli, M., Urbani, S., Marrelli, A., et al., 2007. Impairment of endothelial cell differentiation from bone marrow-derived mesenchymal stem cells: new insight into the pathogenesis of systemic sclerosis. Arthritis Rheum. 56, 1994—2004.

Clements, P.J., Medsger Jr., T.A. 2004. Cutaneous involvement in systemic sclerosis. In: Clements, P.J., Furst, D.E. (Eds.), Systemic Sclerosis, second ed.. New York, NY, USA, pp. 129—150.

Cockrill, T., del Junco, D.J., Arnett, F.C., Assassi, S., Tan, F.K., McNearney, T., et al., 2010. Separate influences of birth order and gravidity/parity on the development of systemic sclerosis. Arthritis Care Res. (Hoboken). 62, 418—424.

Constant, S., Schweitzer, N., West, J., Ranney, P., Bottomly, K., 1995. B lymphocytes can be competent antigen-presenting cells for priming CD4 + T cells to protein antigens in vivo. J. Immunol. 155, 3734—3741.

D'Alessio, S., Fibbi, G., Cinelli, M., Guiducci, S., Del Rosso, A., Margheri, F., et al., 2004. Matrix metalloproteinase 12-dependent cleavage of urokinase receptor in systemic sclerosis microvascular endothelial cells results in impaired angiogenesis. Arthritis Rheum. 50, 3275—3285.

D'Angelo, W.A., Fries, J.F., Masi, A.T., Shulman, L.E., 1969. Pathologic observations in systemic sclerosis (scleroderma). A study of fifty-eight autopsy cases and fifty-eight matched controls. Am. J. Med. 46, 428—440.

Daniels, C.E., Wilkes, M.C., Edens, M., Kottom, T.J., Murphy, S.J., Limper, A.H., et al., 2004. Imatinib mesylate inhibits the profibrogenic activity of TGF-beta and prevents bleomycin-mediated lung fibrosis. J. Clin. Invest. 114, 1308—1316.

Davies, C.A., Jeziorska, M., Freemont, A.J., Herrick, A.L., 2006. The differential expression of VEGF, VEGFR-2, and GLUT-1 proteins in disease subtypes of systemic sclerosis. Hum. Pathol. 37, 190—197.

Del Papa, N., Quirici, N., Soligo, D., Scavullo, C., Cortiana, M., Borsotti, C., et al., 2006. Bone marrow endothelial progenitors are defective in systemic sclerosis. Arthritis Rheum. 54, 2605—2615.

Denton, C.P., Zheng, B., Evans, L.A., Shi-wen, X., Ong, V.H., Fisher, I., et al., 2003. Fibroblast-specific expression of a kinase-deficient type II transforming growth factor beta (TGFbeta) receptor leads to paradoxical activation of TGFbeta signaling pathways with fibrosis in transgenic mice. J. Biol. Chem. 278, 25109—25119.

Denton, C.P., Humbert, M., Rubin, L., Black, C.M., 2006. Bosentan treatment for pulmonary arterial hypertension related to connective tissue disease: a subgroup analysis of the pivotal clinical trials and their open-label extensions. Ann. Rheum. Dis. 65, 1336—1340.

Derk, C.T., Jimenez, S.A., 2003. Systemic sclerosis: current views of its pathogenesis. Autoimmun. Rev. 2, 181—191.

Derrett-Smith, E.C., Dooley, A., Khan, K., Shi-wen, X., Abraham, D., Denton, C.P., 2010. Systemic vasculopathy with altered vasoreactivity in a transgenic mouse model of scleroderma. Arthritis Res. Ther. 12, R69.

Distler, O., Del Rosso, A., Giacomelli, R., Cipriani, P., Conforti, M.L., Guiducci, S., et al., 2002. Angiogenic and angiostatic factors in systemic sclerosis: increased levels of vascular endothelial growth factor are a feature of the earliest disease stages and are associated with the absence of fingertip ulcers. Arthritis Res. 4, R11.

Distler, O., Distler, J.H., Scheid, A., Acker, T., Hirth, A., Rethage, J., et al., 2004. Uncontrolled expression of vascular endothelial growth factor and its receptors leads to insufficient skin angiogenesis in patients with systemic sclerosis. Circ. Res. 95, 109—116.

Dziadzio, M., Smith, R.E., Abraham, D.J., Black, C.M., Denton, C.P., 2005. Circulating levels of active transforming growth factor beta1 are reduced in diffuse cutaneous systemic sclerosis and correlate inversely with the modified Rodnan skin score. Rheumatology (Oxford). 44, 1518—1524.

Elhai, M., Meune, C., Avouac, J., Kahan, A., Allanore, Y., 2012. Trends in mortality in patients with systemic sclerosis over 40 years: a systematic review and meta-analysis of cohort studies. Rheumatology (Oxford). 51, 1017—1026.

Ercole, L.P., Malvezzi, M., Boaretti, A.C., Utiyama, S.R., Rachid, A., 2003. Analysis of lymphocyte subpopulations in systemic sclerosis. J. Investig Allergol. Clin. Immunol. 13, 87—93.

Feghali-Bostwick, C., Medsger Jr., T.A., Wright, T.M., 2003. Analysis of systemic sclerosis in twins reveals low concordance for disease and high concordance for the presence of antinuclear antibodies. Arthritis Rheum. 48, 1956—1963.

Ferri, C., Zakrzewska, K., Longombardo, G., Giuggioli, D., Storino, F. A., Pasero, G., et al., 1999. Parvovirus B19 infection of bone marrow in systemic sclerosis patients. Clin. Exp. Rheumatol. 17, 718—720.

Fiocco, U., Rosada, M., Cozzi, L., Ortolani, C., De Silvestro, G., Ruffatti, A., et al., 1993. Early phenotypic activation of circulating helper memory T cells in scleroderma: correlation with disease activity. Ann. Rheum. Dis. 52, 272—277.

Fujimoto, M., Hasegawa, M., Hamaguchi, Y., Komura, K., Matsushita, T., Yanaba, K., et al., 2006. A clue for telangiectasis in systemic sclerosis: elevated serum soluble endoglin levels in patients with the limited cutaneous form of the disease. Dermatology. 213, 88—92.

Furst, D.E., Clements, P.J., Graze, P., Gale, R., Roberts, N., 1979. A syndrome resembling progressive systemic sclerosis after bone marrow transplantation. A model for scleroderma? Arthritis Rheum. 22, 904—910.

Gambichler, T., Tigges, C., Burkert, B., Höxtermann, S., Altmeyer, P., Kreuter, A., 2010. Absolute count of T and B lymphocyte subsets is decreased in systemic sclerosis. Eur. J. Med. Res. 51, 44—46.

Gao, R., Brigstock, D.R., 2003. Low density lipoprotein receptor-related protein (LRP) is a heparin-dependent adhesion receptor for connective tissue growth factor (CTGF) in rat activated hepatic stellate cells. Hepatol. Res. 27, 214—220.

García de la Peña-Lefebvre, P., Chanseaud, Y., Tamby, M.C., Reinbolt, J., Batteux, F., Allanore, Y., et al., 2004. IgG reactivity with a 100 kDa tissue and endothelial cell antigen identified as topoisomerase 1 distinguishes between limited and diffuse systemic sclerosis patients. Clin. Immunol. 111, 241—251.

Generini, S., Matucci Cerinic, M., 1999. Raynaud's phenomenon and vascular disease in systemic sclerosis. Adv. Exp. Med. Biol. 455, 93—100.

Gentiletti, J., McCloskey, L.J., Artlett, C.M., Peters, J., Jimenez, S.A., Christner, P.J., 2005. Demonstration of autoimmunity in the tight skin-2 mouse: a model for scleroderma. J. Immunol. 175, 2418—2426.

Gershwin, M.E., Abplanalp, H., Castles, J.J., Ikeda, R.M., van der Water, J., Eklund, J., et al., 1981. Characterization of a spontaneous disease of white leghorn chickens resembling progressive systemic sclerosis (scleroderma). J. Exp. Med. 153, 1640–1659.

Gorlova, O., Martin, J.E., Rueda, B., Koeleman, B.P., Ying, J., Teruel, M., et al., 2011. Identification of novel genetic markers associated with clinical phenotypes of systemic sclerosis through a genome-wide association strategy. PLoS Genet. 7, e1002178.

Gourh, P., Agarwal, S.K., Martin, E., Divecha, D., Rueda, B., Bunting, H., et al., 2010a. Association of the C8orf13-BLK region with systemic sclerosis in North-American and European populations. J. Autoimmun. 34, 155–162.

Gourh, P., Arnett, F.C., Tan, F.K., Assassi, S., Divecha, D., Paz, G., et al., 2010b. Association of TNFSF4 (OX40L) polymorphisms with susceptibility to systemic sclerosis. Ann. Rheum. Dis. 69, 550–555.

Grassegger, A., Pohla-Gubo, G., Frauscher, M., Hintner, H., 2008. Autoantibodies in systemic sclerosis (scleroderma): clues for clinical evaluation, prognosis and pathogenesis. Wien. Med. Wochenschr. 158, 19–28.

Green, M.C., Sweet, H.O., Bunker, L.E., 1976. Tight-skin, a new mutation of the mouse causing excessive growth of connective tissue and skeleton. Am. J. Pathol. 82, 493–512.

Gruschwitz, M.S., Shoenfeld, Y., Krupp, M., Gershwin, M.E., Penner, E., Brezinschek, H.P., et al., 1993. Antinuclear antibody profile in UCD line 200 chickens: a model for progressive systemic sclerosis. Int. Arch. Allergy Immunol. 100, 307–313.

Hasegawa, M., Fujimoto, M., Kikuchi, K., Takehara, K., 1997. Elevated serum levels of interleukin 4 (IL-4), IL-10, and IL-13 in patients with systemic sclerosis. J. Rheumatol. 24, 328–332.

Hasegawa, M., Sato, S., Fujimoto, M., Ihn, H., Kikuchi, K., Takehara, K., 1998. Serum levels of interleukin 6 (IL-6), oncostatin M, soluble IL-6 receptor, and soluble gp130 in patients with systemic sclerosis. J. Rheumatol. 25, 308–313.

Hasegawa, M., Sato, S., Kikuchi, K., Takehara, K., 1998. Antigen specificity of antihistone antibodies in systemic sclerosis. Ann. Rheum. Dis. 57, 470–475.

Hasegawa, M., Hamaguchi, Y., Yanaba, K., Bouaziz, J.D., Uchida, J., Fujimoto, M., et al., 2006. B-lymphocyte depletion reduces skin fibrosis and autoimmunity in the tight-skin mouse model for systemic sclerosis. Am. J. Pathol. 169, 954–966.

Hayashi, H., Abdollah, S., Qiu, Y., Cai, J., Xu, Y.Y., Grinnell, B.W., et al., 1997. The MAD-related protein Smad7 associates with the TGF beta receptor and functions as an antagonist of TGF beta signaling. Cell. 89, 1165–1173.

Helmick, C.G., Felson, D.F., Lawrence, R.C., Gabriel, S., Hirsch, R., Kwoh, C.K., et al., 2008. Estimates of the prevalence of arthritis and other rheumatic conditions in the United States. Arthritis Rheum. 58, 15–25.

Higashi-Kuwata, N., Makino, T., Inoue, Y., Takeya, M., Ihn, H., 2009. Alternatively activated macrophages (M2 macrophages) in the skin of patient with localized scleroderma. Exp. Dermatol. 18, 727–729.

Ho, K.T., Reveille, J.D., 2003. The clinical relevance of autoantibodies in scleroderma. Arthritis Res. Ther. 5, 80–93.

Hoffmann-Vold, A.M., Midtvedt, Ø., Molberg, Ø., Garen, T., Gran, J.T., 2012. Prevalence of systemic sclerosis in south-east Norway. Rheumatology (Oxford). 51, 1600–1605.

Hu, P.Q., Fertig, N., Medsger Jr., T.A., Wright, T.M., 2003. Correlation of serum anti-DNA topoisomerase I antibody levels with disease severity and activity in systemic sclerosis. Arthritis Rheum. 48, 1363–1373.

Huerre, C., Junien, C., Weil, D., Chu, M.L., Morabito, M., Van Cong, N., et al., 1982. Human type I procollagen genes are located on different chromosomes. Proc. Natl. Acad. Sci. U.S.A. 79, 6627–6630.

Ingegnoli, F., Trabattoni, D., Saresella, M., Fantini, F., Clerici, M., 2003. Distinct immune profiles characterize patients with diffuse or limited systemic sclerosis. Clin. Immunol. 108, 21–28.

Isogai, Z., Ono, R.N., Ushiro, S., Keene, D.R., Chen, Y., Mazzieri, R., et al., 2003. Latent transforming growth factor beta-binding protein 1 interacts with fibrillin and is a microfibril-associated protein. J. Biol. Chem. 278, 2750–2757.

Jacobsen, S., Ullman, S., Shen, G.Q., Wiik, A., Halberg, P., 2001. Influence of clinical features, serum antinuclear antibodies, and lung function on survival of patients with systemic sclerosis. J. Rheumatol. 28, 2454–2459.

Janowsky, E.C., Kupper, L.L., Hulka, B.S., 2000. Meta-analysis of the relation between silicone breast implants and the risk of connective-tissue diseases. N. Engl. J. Med. 342, 781–790.

Jones, S.A., Rose-John, S., 2002. The role of soluble receptors in cytokine biology: the agonistic properties of the sIL-6R/IL-6 complex. Biochim. Biophys. Acta. 1592, 251–263.

Joven, B.E., Almodovar, R., Carmona, L., Carreira, P.E., 2010. Survival, causes of death, and risk factors associated with mortality in Spanish systemic sclerosis patients: results from a single university hospital. Semin. Arthritis Rheum. 39, 285–293.

Kahaleh, B., 2008. The microvascular endothelium in scleroderma. Rheumatology (Oxford). 47, 14–15.

Kahaleh, M.B., LeRoy, E.C., 1999. Autoimmunity and vascular involvement in systemic sclerosis (SSc). Autoimmunity. 31, 195–214.

Kane, G.C., Varga, J., Conant, E.F., Spirn, P.W., Jimenez, S., Fish, J.E., 1996. Lung involvement in systemic sclerosis (scleroderma): relation to classification based on extent of skin involvement or autoantibody status. Arthritis Rheum. 90, 223–230.

Kim, J., Park, S.K., Moon, K.W., Lee, E.Y., Lee, Y.J., Song, Y.W., et al., 2010. The prognostic factors of systemic sclerosis for survival among Koreans. Clin. Rheumatol. 29, 297–302.

Klein, S., Kretz, C.C., Ruland, V., Stumpf, C., Haust, M., Hartschuh, W., et al., 2011. Reduction of regulatory T cells in skin lesions but not in peripheral blood of patients with systemic scleroderma. Ann. Rheum. Dis. 70, 1475–1481.

Koschik III, R.W., Fertig, N., Lucas, M.R., Domsic, R.T., Medsger Jr., T.A., 2012. Anti-PM-Scl antibody in patients with systemic sclerosis. Clin. Exp. Rheumatol. 30, S12–S16.

Kowal-Bielecka, O., Kowal, K., Distler, O., Rojewska, J., Bodzenta-Lukaszyk, A., Michel, B.A., et al., 2005. Cyclooxygenase- and lipoxygenase-derived eicosanoids in bronchoalveolar lavage fluid from patients with scleroderma lung disease: an imbalance between proinflammatory and antiinflammatory lipid mediators. Arthritis Rheum. 52, 3783–3791.

Krishnan, E., Furst, D.E., 2005. Systemic sclerosis mortality in the United States: 1979–1998. Eur. J. Epidemiol. 20, 855–861.

Kuwana, M., Feghali, C.A., Medsger Jr., T.A., Wright, T.M., 2001. Autoreactive T cells to topoisomerase I in monozygotic twins discordant for systemic sclerosis. Arthritis Rheum. 44, 1654–1659.

Kuwana, M., Kimura, K., Hirakata, M., Kawakami, Y., Ikeda, Y., 2002. Differences in autoantibody response to Th/To between systemic sclerosis and other autoimmune diseases. Ann. Rheum. Dis. 61, 842—846.

Kuwana, M., Okazaki, Y., Yasuoka, H., Kawakami, Y., Ikeda, Y., 2004. Defective vasculogenesis in systemic sclerosis. Lancet. 364, 603—610.

Kypriotou, M., Beauchef, G., Chadjichristos, C., Widom, R., Renard, E., Jimenez, S.A., et al., 2007. Human collagen Krox upregulates type I collagen expression in normal and scleroderma fibroblasts through interaction with Sp1 and Sp3 transcription factors. J. Biol. Chem. 282, 32000—32014.

Lafyatis, R., Kissin, E., York, M., Farina, G., Viger, K., Fritzler, M.J., et al., 2009. B cell depletion with rituximab in patients with diffuse cutaneous systemic sclerosis. Arthritis Rheum. 60, 578—583.

LeRoy, E.C., Medsger Jr., T.A., 2001. Criteria for the classification of early systemic sclerosis. J. Rheumatol. 28, 1573—1576.

LeRoy, E.C., Black, C., Fleischmajer, R., Jablonska, S., Krieg, T., Medsger Jr., T.A., et al., 1988. Scleroderma (systemic sclerosis): classification, subsets and pathogenesis. J. Rheumatol. 15, 202—205.

Leask, A., Abraham, D.J., 2006. All in the CCN family: essential matricellular signaling modulators emerge from the bunker. J. Cell Sci. 119, 4803—4810.

Lewandowska, K., Ciurzynski, M., Gorska, E., Bienias, P., Irzyk, K., Siwicka, M., et al., 2013. Antiendothelial cells antibodies in patients with systemic sclerosis in relation to pulmonary hypertension and lung fibrosis. Adv. Exp. Med. Biol. 756, 147—153.

Li, R., Sun, J., Ren, L.M., Wang, H.Y., Liu, W.H., Zhang, X.W., et al., 2012. Epidemiology of eight common rheumatic diseases in China: a large-scale cross-sectional survey in Beijing. Rheumatology (Oxford). 51, 721—729.

Li, X., Pereira, L., Zhang, H., Sanguineti, C., Ramirez, F., Bonadio, J., et al., 1993. Fibrillin genes map to regions of conserved mouse/human synteny on mouse chromosomes 2 and 18. Genomics. 18, 667—672.

Lindgren, C.E., Walker, L.A., Bolton, P., 1991. L-tryptophan induced eosinophilia-myalgia syndrome. J. R. Soc. Health. 111, 29—30.

Lis, A.D., Brzezińska-Wcisło, L.A., 2003. [Soluble receptors of cytokines in sera of patients with systemic sclerosis: clinical correlation]. Wiad. Lek. 56, 532—536.

Liu, T., Zhang, J., 2012. Role of PDGF-A/PDGFR-α in proliferation and transdifferentiation of fibroblasts from skin lesions of patients with systemic sclerosis. Nan Fang Yi Ke Da Xue Xue Bao. 32, 496—501.

Lo Monaco, A., Bruschi, M., La Corte, R., Volpinari, S., Trotta, F., 2011. Epidemiology of systemic sclerosis in a district of northern Italy. Clin. Exp. Rheumatol. 29, S10—S14.

Logan, C.Y., Nusse, R., 2004. The Wnt signaling pathway in development and disease. Annu. Rev. Cell Dev. Biol. 20, 781—810.

López-Casillas, F., Cheifetz, S., Doody, J., Andres, J.L., Lane, W.S., Massagué, J., 1991. Structure and expression of the membrane proteoglycan betaglycan, a component of the TGF-beta receptor system. Cell. 67, 785—795.

Ludwicka, A., Ohba, T., Trojanowska, M., Yamakage, A., Strange, C., Smith, E.A., et al., 1995. Elevated levels of platelet derived growth factor and transforming growth factor beta1 in bronchoalveolar lavage fluid from patients with scleroderma. J. Rheumatol. 22, 1876—1883.

Lunardi, C., Bason, C., Navone, R., Millo, E., Damonte, G., Corrocher, R., et al., 2000. Systemic sclerosis immunoglobulin G autoantibodies bind the human cytomegalovirus late protein UL94 and induce apoptosis in human endothelial cells. Nat. Med. 6, 1183—1186.

Mackiewicz, Z., Sukura, A., Povilenaité, D., Ceponis, A., Virtanen, I., Hukkanen, M., et al., 2002. Increased but imbalanced expression of VEGF and its receptors has no positive effect on angiogenesis in systemic sclerosis skin. Clin. Exp. Rheumatol. 20, 641—646.

Mahler, M., Silverman, E.D., Schulte-Pelkum, J., Fritzler, M.J., 2010. Anti-Scl-70 (topo-I) antibodies in SLE: Myth or reality? Autoimmun. Rev. 9, 756—760.

Manetti, M., Guiducci, S., Ibba-Manneschi, L., Matucci-Cerinic, M., 2010. Mechanisms in the loss of capillaries in systemic sclerosis: angiogenesis versus vasculogenesis. J. Cell Mol. Med. 14, 1241—1254.

Manetti, M., Guiducci, S., Ibba-Manneschi, L., Matucci-Cerinic, M., 2011. Impaired angiogenesis in systemic sclerosis: the emerging role of the antiangiogenic VEGF(165)b splice variant. Trends Cardiovasc. Med. 21, 204—210.

Marguerie, C., Bunn, C.C., Copier, J., Bernstein, R.M., Gilroy, J.M., Black, C.M., et al., 1992. The clinical and immunogenetic features of patients with autoantibodies to the nucleolar antigen PM-Scl. Medicine (Baltimore). 71, 327—336.

Marin, V., Montero-Julian, F., Grès, S., Bongrand, P., Farnarier, C., Kaplanski, G., 2002. Chemotactic agents induce IL-6R alpha shedding from polymorphonuclear cells: involvement of a metalloproteinase of the TNF-alpha-converting enzyme (TACE) type. Eur. J. Immunol. 32, 2965—2970.

Maurer, B., Reich, N., Juengel, A., Kriegsmann, J., Gay, R.E., Schett, G., et al., 2012. Fra-2 transgenic mice as a novel model of pulmonary hypertension associated with systemic sclerosis. Ann. Rheum. Dis. 71, 1382—1387.

Mavilia, C., Scaletti, C., Romagnani, P., Carossino, A.M., Pignone, A., Emmi, L., et al., 1997. Type 2 helper t-cell predominance and high CD30 expression in systemic sclerosis. Am. J. Pathol. 151, 1751—1758.

Mayes, M.D. and Reveille, J.D. 2004. Epidemiology, demographics, and genetics. In: Clements, P.J., Furst, D.E. (Eds.), Systemic Sclerosis, second ed. Philadelphia, pp. 1—15.

McAllister, K.A., Grogg, K.M., Johnson, D.W., Gallione, C.J., Baldwin, M.A., Jackson, C.E., et al., 1994. Endoglin, a TGF-beta binding protein of endothelial cells, is the gene for hereditary haemorrhagic telangiectasia type 1. Nat. Genet. 8, 345—351.

McCormic, Z.D., Khuder, S.S., Aryal, B.K., Ames, A.L., Khuder, S.A., 2010. Occupational silica exposure as a risk factor for scleroderma: a meta-analysis. In. Arch. Occup. Environ. Health. 83, 763—769.

McCormick, L.L., Zhang, Y., Tootell, E., Gilliam, A.C., 1999. Anti-TGF-beta treatment prevents skin and lung fibrosis in murine sclerodermatous graft versus host disease: a model for human scleroderma. J. Immunol. 163, 5693—5699.

McNearney, T.A., Reveille, J.D., Fischbach, M., Friedman, A.W., Lisse, J.R., Goel, N., et al., 2007. Pulmonary involvement in systemic sclerosis: associations with genetic, serologic, sociodemographic, and behavioral factors. Arthritis Rheum. 57, 318—326.

Medsger Jr., T.A., 2001. Systemic sclerosis. In: Koopman, W.J. (Ed.), Arthritis and Allied Conditions, 14th ed. Philadelphia, PA, USA, pp. 1590—1624.

Medsger Jr., T.A., 2004. Classification, prognosis. In: Clements, P.J., Furst, D.E. (Eds.), Systemic Sclerosis, second ed. New York, NY, USA, pp. 129—150.

Medsger Jr., T.A., Steen, V.D. 1996. Classification, prognosis. In: Clements, P.J., Furst, D.E. (Eds.), Systemic Sclerosis, first ed. Baltimore, pp. 51—64.

Mercié, P., Seigneur, M., Constans, J., Boisseau, M., Conri, C., 1997. Assay of plasma thrombomodulin in systemic diseases. Rev. Med. Interne. 18, 126–131.

Mitri, G.M., Lucas, M., Fertig, N., Steen, V.D., Medsger Jr., T.A., 2003. A comparison between anti-Th/To- and anticentromere antibody-positive systemic sclerosis patients with limited cutaneous involvement. Arthritis Rheum. 48, 203–209.

Mitsuo, A., Morimoto, S., Nakiri, Y., Suzuki, J., Kaneko, H., Tokano, Y., et al., 2006. Decreased CD161 + CD8 + T cells in the peripheral blood of patients suffering from rheumatic diseases. Rheumatology (Oxford). 45, 1477–1484.

Mora, G.F., 2009. Systemic sclerosis: environmental factors. J. Rheumatol. 36, 2383–2396.

Mori, T., Kawara, S., Shinozaki, M., Hayashi, N., Kakinuma, T., Igarashi, A., et al., 1999. Role and interaction of connective tissue growth factor with transforming growth factor beta in persistent fibrosis: a mouse fibrosis model. J. Cell Physiol. 181, 153–159.

Mountz, J.D., Downs Minor, M.B., Turner, R., Thomas, M.B., Richards, F., Pisko, E., 1983. Bleomycin-induced cutaneous toxicity in the rat: analysis of histopathology and ultrastructure compared with progressive systemic sclerosis (scleroderma). Br. J. Dermatol. 108, 679–886.

Mouthon, L., Bérezné, A., Bussone, G., Noël, L.H., Villiger, P.M., Guillevin, L., 2011. Scleroderma renal crisis: a rare but severe complication of systemic sclerosis. Clin. Rev. Allergy Immunol. 40, 84–91.

Murai, C., Saito, S., Kasturi, K.N., Bona, C.A., 1998. Spontaneous occurrence of anti-fibrillin-1 autoantibodies in tight-skin mice. Autoimmunity. 28, 151–155.

Murata, I., Takenaka, K., Shinohara, S., Suzuki, T., Sasaki, T., Yamamoto, K., 1998. Diversity of myocardial involvement in systemic sclerosis: an 8-year study of 95 Japanese patients. Am. Heart J. 135, 960–969.

Nakao, A., Afrakhte, M., Morén, A., Nakayama, T., Christian, J.L., Heuchel, R., et al., 1997a. Identification of Smad7, a TGFbeta-inducible antagonist of TGF-beta signalling. Nature. 389 (6651), 631–635.

Nakao, A., Imamura, T., Souchelnytskyi, S., Kawabata, M., Ishisaki, A., Oeda, E., et al., 1997b. TGF-beta receptor-mediated signalling through Smad2, Smad3 and Smad4. EMBO. 16, 5353–5362.

Nakerakanti, S., Trojanowska, M., 2012. The role of TGF-β receptors in fibrosis. Open Rheumatol. J. 6, 156–162.

Nikpour, M., Hissaria, P., Byron, J., Sahhar, J., Micallef, M., Paspaliaris, W., et al., 2011. Prevalence, correlates and clinical usefulness of antibodies to RNA polymerase III in systemic sclerosis: a cross-sectional analysis of data from an Australian cohort. Arthritis Res. Ther. 13, R211.

Oi, M., Yamamoto, T., Nishioka, K., 2004. Increased expression of TGF-beta1 in the sclerotic skin in bleomycin-"susceptible"mouse strains. J. Med. Dent. Sci. 51, 7–17.

Okano, Y., Medsger Jr., T.A., 1990. Autoantibody to Th ribonucleoprotein (nucleolar 7-2 RNA protein particle) in patients with systemic sclerosis. Arthritis Rheum. 33, 1822–1828.

O'Reilly, S., Hügle, T., van Laar, J.M., 2012. T cells in systemic sclerosis: a reappraisal. Rheumatology (Oxford). 51, 1540–1549.

Pannu, J., Gardner, H., Shearstone, J.R., Smith, E., Trojanowska, M., 2006. Increased levels of transforming growth factor β receptor type I and upregulation of matrix gene program: a model of scleroderma. Arthritis Rheum. 54, 3011–3021.

Parodi, A., Drosera, M., Barbieri, L., Rebora, A., 1995. Antihistone antibodies in scleroderma. Dermatology. 191, 16–18.

Plattner, R., Kadlec, L., DeMali, K.A., Kazlauskas, A., Pendergast, A. M., 1999. c-Abl is activated by growth factors and Src family kinases and has a role in the cellular response to PDGF. Genes Dev. 13, 2400–2411.

Ponticos, M., Holmes, A.M., Shi-wen, X., Leoni, P., Khan, K., Rajkumar, V.S., et al., 2009. Pivotal role of connective tissue growth factor in lung fibrosis: MAPK-dependent transcriptional activation of type I collagen. Arthritis Rheum. 60 (7), 2142–2155.

Prescott, R.J., Freemont, A.J., Jones, C.J., Hoyland, J., Fielding, P., 1992. Sequential dermal microvascular and perivascular changes in the development of scleroderma. J. Pathol. 168, 255–263.

Radstake, T.R., Gorlova, O., Rueda, B., Martin, J.E., Alizadeh, B.Z., Palomino-Morales, R., et al., 2010. Genome-wide association study of systemic sclerosis identifies CD247 as a new susceptibility locus. Nat. Genet. 42, 426–429.

Rajkumar, V.S., Sundberg, C., Abraham, D.J., Rubin, K., Black, C.M., 1999. Activation of microvascular pericytes in autoimmune Raynaud's phenomenon and systemic sclerosis. Arthritis Rheum. 42, 930–941.

Reich, N., Maurer, B., Akhmetshina, A., Venalis, P., Dees, C., Zerr, P., et al., 2010. The transcription factor Fra-2 regulates the production of extracellular matrix in systemic sclerosis. Arthritis Rheum. 62, 280–290.

Reitamo, S., Remitz, A., Varga, J., Ceska, M., Effenberger, F., Jimenez, S., et al., 1993. Demonstration of interleukin 8 and autoantibodies to interleukin 8 in the serum of patients with systemic sclerosis and related disorders. Arch. Dermatol. 129, 189–193.

Reveille, J.D., Solomon, D.H.American College of Rheumatology Ad Hoc Committee of Immunologic Testing Guidelines, 2003. Evidence-based guidelines for the use of immunologic tests: anticentromere, Scl-70, and nucleolar antibodies. Arthritis Rheum. 49, 399–412.

Roberts-Thomson, P.J., Walker, J.G., Lu, T.Y., Esterman, A., Hakendorf, P., Smith, M.D., et al., 2006. Scleroderma in South Australia: further epidemiological observations supporting a stochastic explanation. Intern. Med. J. 36, 489–497.

Romano, M., Sironi, M., Toniatti, C., Polentarutti, N., Fruscella, P., Ghezzi, P., et al., 1997. Role of IL-6 and its soluble receptor in induction of chemokines and leukocyte recruitment. Immunity. 6, 315–325.

Rueda, B., Broen, J., Simeon, C., Hesselstrand, R., Diaz, B., Suárez, H., et al., 2009. The STAT4 gene influences the genetic predisposition to systemic sclerosis phenotype. Hum. Mol. Genet. 18, 2071–2077.

Rueda, B., Gourh, P., Broen, J., Agarwal, S.K., Simeon, C., Ortego-Centeno, N., et al., 2010. BANK1 functional variants are associated with susceptibility to diffuse systemic sclerosis in Caucasians. Ann. Rheum. Dis. 69, 700–705.

Ruzek, M.C., Jha, S., Ledbetter, S., Richards, S.M., Garman, R.D., 2004. A modified model of graft versus host-induced systemic sclerosis (scleroderma) exhibits all major aspects of the human disease. Arthritis Rheum. 50, 1319–1331.

Sato, S., Hasegawa, M., Fujimoto, M., Tedder, T.F., Takehara, K., 2000. Quantitative genetic variation in CD19 expression correlates with autoimmunity. J. Immunol. 165, 6635–6643.

Sato, S., Hayakawa, I., Hasegawa, M., Fujimoto, M., Takehara, K., 2003. Function blocking autoantibodies against matrix metalloproteinase 1 in patients with systemic sclerosis. J. Invest. Dermatol. 120, 542–547.

Sawaya, H.H., de Souza, R.B., Carrasco, S., Goldenstein-Schainberg, C., 2009. Altered adhesion molecules expression on peripheral blood mononuclear cells from patients with systemic sclerosis and clinical correlations. Clin. Rheumatol. 28, 847–851.

Schachna, L., Wigley, F.M., Morris, S., Gelber, A.C., Rosen, A., Casciola-Rosen, L., 2002. Recognition of Granzyme B-generated autoantigen fragments in scleroderma patients with ischemic digital loss. Arthritis Rheum. 46, 1873–1884.

Seppä, H., Grotendorst, G., Seppä, S., Schiffmann, E., Martin, G.R., 1982. Platelet-derived growth factor in chemotactic for fibroblasts. J. Cell Biol. 92, 584–588.

Servettaz, A., Tamby, M.C., Guilpain, P., Reinbolt, J., García de la Penã-Lefebvre, P., Allanore, Y., et al., 2006. Anti-endothelial cell antibodies from patients with limited cutaneous systemic sclerosis bind to centromeric protein B (CENP-B). Clin. Immunol. 120, 212–219.

Sgonc, R., Wick, G., 2008. Pro- and anti-fibrotic effects of TGF-beta in scleroderma. Rheumatology (Oxford). 47, 5–7.

Sgonc, R., Gruschwitz, M.S., Dietrich, H., Recheis, H., Gershwin, M.E., Wick, G., 1996. Endothelial cell apoptosis is a primary pathogenetic event underlying skin lesions in avian and human scleroderma. J. Clin. Invest. 98, 785–792.

Sgonc, R., Gruschwitz, M.S., Boeck, G., Sepp, N., Gruber, J., Wick, G., 2000. Endothelial cell apoptosis in systemic sclerosis is induced by antibody-dependent cell-mediated cytotoxicity via CD95. Arthritis Rheum. 43, 2550–2562.

Sharif, R., Mayes, M.D., Tan, F.K., Gorlova, O.Y., Hummers, L.K., Shah, A.A., et al., 2012. IRF5 polymorphism predicts prognosis in patients with systemic sclerosis. Ann. Rheum. Dis. 71, 1197–1202.

Shetty, N., Derk, C.T., 2011. Endothelin receptor antagonists as disease modifiers in systemic sclerosis. Inflamm. Allergy Drug Targets. 10, 19–26.

Shi-wen, X., Kennedy, L., Renzoni, E.A., Bou-Gharios, G., du Bois, R. M., Black, C.M., et al., 2007. Endothelin is a downstream mediator of profibrotic responses to transforming growth factor beta in human lung fibroblasts. Arthritis Rheum. 56, 4189–4194.

Shinozaki, M., Kawara, S., Hayashi, N., Kakinuma, T., Igarashi, A., Takehara, K., 1997. Induction of subcutaneous tissue fibrosis in newborn mice by transforming growth factor beta-simultaneous application with basic fibroblast growth factor causes persistent fibrosis. Biochem. Biophys. Res. Commun. 237, 292–296.

Simon, D., Czömpöly, T., Berki, T., Minir, T., Peti, A., Tóth, E., et al., 2009. Naturally occurring and disease-associated auto-antibodies against topoisomerase I: a fine epitope mapping study in systemic sclerosis and systemic lupus erythematosus. Int. Immunol. 21, 415–422.

Siracusa, L.D., McGrath, R., Ma, Q., Moskow, J.J., Manne, J., Christner, P. J., et al., 1996. A tandem duplication within the fibrillin 1 gene is associated with the mouse tight skin mutation. Genome Res. 6, 300–313.

Spencer-Green, G., Alter, D., Welch, H.G., 1997. Test performance in systemic sclerosis: anti-centromere and anti-Scl-70 antibodies. Autoimmun. Rev. 103, 242–248.

Steen, V.D., 2001. Treatment of systemic sclerosis. Am. J. Clin. Dermatol. 2, 315–325.

Steen, V.D., Medsger Jr., T.A., 2000. Severe organ involvement in systemic sclerosis with diffuse scleroderma. Arthritis Rheum. 43, 2437–2444.

Steen, V.D., Medsger, T.A., 2007. Changes in causes of death in systemic sclerosis, 1972–2002. Ann. Rheum. Dis. 66, 940–944.

Steen, V.D., Ziegler, G.L., Rodnan, G.P., Medsger Jr., T.A., 1984. Clinical and laboratory associations of anticentromere antibody in patients with progressive systemic sclerosis. Arthritis Rheum. 27, 125–131.

Sun, G., Liu, X., Mercado, P., Jenkinson, S.R., Kypriotou, M., Feigenbaum, L., et al., 2005. The zinc finger protein cKrox directs CD4 lineage differentiation during intrathymic T cell positive selection. Nat. Immunol. 6, 373–381.

Svegliati, S., Cancello, R., Sambo, P., Luchetti, M., Paroncini, P., Orlandini, G., et al., 2005. Platelet-derived growth factor and reactive oxygen species (ROS) regulate Ras protein levels in primary human fibroblasts via ERK1/2. Amplification of ROS and Ras in systemic sclerosis fibroblasts. J. Biol. Chem. 280, 36474–36482.

Sykes, B., Solomon, E., 1978. Assignment of a type I collagen structural gene to human chromosome 7. Nature. 272, 548–549.

Tamby, M.C., Chanseaud, Y., Humbert, M., Fermanian, J., Guilpain, P., García-de-la-Peña-Lefebvre, P., et al., 2005. Anti-endothelial cell antibodies in idiopathic and systemic sclerosis associated pulmonary arterial hypertension. Thorax. 60, 765–772.

Tan, F.K., Arnett, F.C., Reveille, J.D., Ahn, C., Antohi, S., Sasaki, T., et al., 2000. Autoantibodies to fibrillin 1 in systemic sclerosis: ethnic differences in antigen recognition and lack of correlation with specific clinical features or HLA alleles. Arthritis Rheum. 43, 2464–2471.

Terracini, B. 2004. Toxic Oil Syndrome: Ten Years of Progress. Europe: WHO Regional Office for Europe.

Thoua, N.M., Derrett-Smith, E.C., Khan, K., Dooley, A., Shi-Wen, X., Denton, C.P., 2012. Gut fibrosis with altered colonic contractility in a mouse model of scleroderma. Rheumatology (Oxford). 51, 1989–1998.

Tourkina, E., Bonner, M., Oates, J., Hofbauer, A., Richard, M., Znoyko, S., et al., 2011. Altered monocyte and fibrocyte phenotype and function in scleroderma interstitial lung disease: reversal by caveolin-1 scaffolding domain peptide. Fibrogenesis Tissue Repair. 4, 15.

Van Eenennaam, H., Vogelzangs, J.H., Bisschops, L., Te Boome, L.C., Seelig, H.P., Renz, M., et al., 2002. Autoantibodies against small nucleolar ribonucleoprotein complexes and their clinical associations. Clin. Exp. Immunol. 130, 532–540.

Varga, J., Abraham, D., 2007. Systemic sclerosis: a prototypic multisystem fibrotic disorder. J. Clin. Invest. 117, 557–567.

Varga, J., Bashey, R.I., 1995. Regulation of connective tissue synthesis in systemic sclerosis. Int. Rev. Immunol. 12, 187–199.

Varga, J., Denton, C.P., 2008. Systemic sclerosis and the scleroderma–spectrum disorders. In: Firestein, G.S., Budd, R.C., Harris Jr., E.D. (Eds.), Kelley's Textbook of Rheumatology, eighth ed. Philadelphia, PA, USA.

Walker, J.G., Fritzler, M.J., 2007. Update on autoantibodies in systemic sclerosis. Curr. Opin. Rheumatol. 19, 580–591.

Wei, J., Melichian, D., Komura, K., Hinchcliff, M., Lam, A.P., Lafyatis, R., et al., 2011. Canonical Wnt signaling induces skin fibrosis and subcutaneous lipoatrophy: a novel mouse model for scleroderma? Arthritis Rheum. 63, 1707–1717.

Widom, R.L., Lee, J.Y., Joseph, C., Gordon-Froome, I., Korn, J.H., 2001. The hcKrox gene family regulates multiple extracellular matrix genes. Matrix Biol. 20, 451–462.

Wigley, F.M. 2001. Systemic sclerosis: clinical features. In: Klippel, J. H. (Ed.), Primer on the Rheumatic Diseases, 12th edition. Atlanta, GA, USA.

Wigley, F.M., Wise, R.A., Miller, R., Needleman, B.W., Spence, R.J., 1992. Anticentromere antibody as a predictor of digital ischemic loss in patients with systemic sclerosis. Arthritis Rheum. 35, 688—693.

Wiik, A.S., Gordon, T.P., Kavanaugh, A.F., Lahita, R.G., Reeves, W., van Venrooij, W.J., et al., 2004. Cutting edge diagnostics in rheumatology: the role of patients, clinicians, and laboratory scientists in optimizing the use of autoimmune serology. Arthritis Rheum. 51, 291—298.

Wilson, R.H., McCormick, W.E., Tatum, C.F., Creech, J.L., 1967. Occupational acroosteolysis: report of 31 cases. JAMA. 201, 577—581.

Yamamoto, T., Katayama, I., 2011. Vascular changes in bleomycin-induced scleroderma. Int. J. Rheumatol. 2011, 270938.

Yamamoto, T., Takagawa, S., Katayama, I., Yamazaki, K., Hamazaki, Y., Shinkai, H., et al., 1999. Animal model of sclerotic skin. I: local injections of bleomycin induce sclerotic skin mimicking scleroderma. J. Invest Dermatol. 112, 456—462.

Yamamoto, T., Kuroda, M., Nishioka, K., 2000. Animal model of sclerotic skin. III: Histopathological comparison of bleomycin-induced scleroderma in various mice strains. Arch. Dermatol. Res. 292, 535—541.

Yamane, K., Ihn, H., Kubo, M., Tamaki, K., 2002. Increased transcriptional activities of transforming growth factor beta receptors in scleroderma fibroblasts. Arthritis Rheum. 46, 2421—2428.

Yurovsky, V.V., Wigley, F.M., Wise, R.A., White, B., 1996. Skewing of the CD8 + T-cell repertoire in the lungs of patients with systemic sclerosis. Hum. Immunol. 48, 84—97.

Zammaretti, P., Zisch, A.H., 2005. Adult "endothelial progenitor cells." Renewing vasculature. Int. J. Biochem. Cell Biol. 37, 493—503.

Zhang, Y., Feng, X., We, R., Derynck, R., 1996. Receptor-associated Mad homologues synergize as effectors of the TGF-beta response. Nature. 383, 168—172.

Zhang, Y., McCormick, L.L., Desai, S.R., Wu, C., Gilliam, A.C., 2002. Murine sclerodermatous graft versus host disease, a model for human scleroderma: cutaneous cytokines, chemokines, and immune cell activation. J. Immunol. 168, 3088—3098.

Zhou, X., Tan, F.K., Milewicz, D.M., Guo, X., Bona, C.A., Arnett, F.C., 2005a. Autoantibodies to fibrillin-1 activate normal human fibroblasts in culture through the TGF-beta pathway to recapitulate the "scleroderma phenotype. J. Immunol. 175, 4555—4560.

Zhou, X., Tan, F.K., Xiong, M., Arnett, F.C., Feghali-Bostwick, C.A., 2005b. Monozygotic twins clinically discordant for scleroderma show concordance for fibroblast gene expression profiles. Arthritis Rheum. 52, 3305—3314.

Chapter 34

Antiphospholipid Syndrome

Nancy Agmon-Levin[1], Angela Tincani[2], and Yehuda Shoenfeld[1,3]

[1]The Zabludowicz Center for Autoimmune Diseases, Sheba Medical Center, Tel-Hashomer, affiliated to Tel Aviv University, Israel, [2]Rheumatology and Clinical Immunology, Spedali Civili and University of Brescia, Brescia, Italy, [3]Incumbent of the Laura Schwarz-Kipp Chair for Research of Autoimmune Diseases, Sackler Faculty of Medicine, Tel Aviv University, Israel

Chapter Outline

Introduction	481	Non-Criteria aPL Antibodies	485
The Clinical Spectrum of Antiphospholipid Syndrome	482	aPL of the IGA Isotype	485
Obstetric APS	482	Low-level aPL	486
Thrombotic APS	482	The Mechanisms of aPL-Mediated Disease Expressions	486
Neurological APS	483	Thrombotic Manifestations	487
Hematologic APS	483	aPL and The Coagulation Cascade	487
Dermatologic APS	483	aPL Cellular Interactions	487
Cardiac APS	483	Obstetric Manifestations	488
Pulmonary APS	484	Neurologic Manifestations	488
Renal APS	484	The Complement System in APS	489
Catastrophic Antiphospholipid Syndrome	484	Treatment of APS	489
The Antiphospholipid Antibodies	484	Conclusions and Future Aspects	490
The b2GPI—Anti-b2GPI Complex in APS	485	References	490

INTRODUCTION

In 1983, a discrete syndrome was described by Graham Hughes in which lupus patients with antiphospholipid antibodies were prone to arterial/venous thrombosis, recurrent abortions, neurological manifestations, and occasional thrombocytopenia (Hughes, 1983). In the following years the Hughes' syndrome was delineated as a systemic disease that can affect both children and adults and can present as a primary disorder or as secondary to other autoimmune disease (Shoenfeld et al., 2009). The definition of this classical autoimmune syndrome has greatly advanced from the original reports and classification criteria for antiphospholipid syndrome (APS) formulated in Sapporo, Japan, in 1998 to the current ones published in 2006 (Miyakis et al., 2006; Cervera and Ra, 2008) (Table 34.1). For determination of APS at least one classical clinical criterion (i.e., vascular thrombosis or pregnancy morbidity) and one serological criterion (i.e., the persistence presence of anti-cardiolipin or anti-B2GPI or

lupus anticoagulant) has to be met (Giannakopoulos and Krilis 2013).

Antiphospholipid antibodies (aPL) can be detected in up to 5—6% of normal healthy subjects and in 30—40% of SLE patients (Biggioggero and Meroni, 2010). Secondary APS is estimated to appear in 10—15% of systemic lupus erythematosus (SLE) patients, and less in other autoimmune diseases, whereas the prevalence of primary APS is yet unknown (Di Prima et al., 2011).

aPL appearing in healthy subjects are usually detected transiently and at low levels. They tend to appear in older individuals and in association with infections, vaccinations, malignancies, and exposure to certain drugs. Remarkably, such aPL are frequently clinically insignificant (Shoenfeld et al., 2008a; Biggioggero and Meroni, 2010). In contrast patients with Antiphospholipid Syndrome (APS), either primary or secondary, typically present with persistent (more than 12 weeks), high-level aPL sero-positivity and significant related morbidity and mortality (Cervera et al., 2009).

N. Rose & I. Mackay (Eds): The Autoimmune Diseases, Fifth edition. DOI: http://dx.doi.org/10.1016/B978-0-12-384929-8.00034-4

TABLE 34.1 Summary of the Sydney Consensus Statement on Investigational Classification Criteria for APS[a].

Anti-phospholipids antibody syndrome is present if at least one of the clinical criteria and one of the laboratory criteria that follow are met:

Clinical criteria

1. Vascular thromboses: One or more documented episodes of arterial, venous, or small vessel thrombosis—other than superficial venous thrombosis—in any tissue or organ. Thrombosis must be confirmed by objective validated criteria. For histopathologic confirmation, thrombosis should be present without significant evidence of inflammation in the vessel wall.
2. Pregnancy morbidity:
   a. One or more unexplained deaths of a morphologically normal fetus at or beyond the 10th week of gestation, with normal fetal morphology documented by ultrasound or by direct examination of the fetus, or
   b. One or more premature births of a morphologically normal neonate before the 34th week of gestation because of: (i) eclampsia or severe pre-eclampsia defined according to standard definitions, or (ii) recognized features of placental insufficiency, or
   c. Three or more unexplained consecutive spontaneous abortions before the 10th week of gestation, with maternal anatomic or hormonal abnormalities and paternal and maternal chromosomal causes excluded.

Laboratory criteria

1. Lupus anticoagulant (LA) present in plasma, on two or more occasions at least 12 weeks apart, detected according to the guidelines of the International Society on Thrombosis and Haemostasis (Scientific Subcommittee on LAs/phospholipid-dependent antibodies).
2. Anticardiolipin antibody (aCL) of IgG and/or IgM isotype in serum or plasma, present in medium or high level (i.e., >40 GPL or MPL, or >the 99th percentile), on two or more occasions, at least 12 weeks apart, measured by a standardized ELISA.
3. Anti-b2-glycoprotein-I antibody of IgG and/or IgM isotype in serum or plasma (in level >the 99th percentile), present on two or more occasions, at least 12 weeks apart, measured by a standardized ELISA, according to recommended procedures.

[a]Miyakis et al. (2006).

In the largest survey of APS patients conducted by the Euro-Phospholipid Group (Cervera et al., 2009), 1000 APS patients, with a mean age of 42 ± 14 years at study entry were followed for a 5-year period. Among these, 20% developed recurrent thrombosis despite appropriate therapy, and 7.4% receiving oral anticoagulants presented with hemorrhage. In this cohort 5.3% of patients died within the follow-up period mostly due to bacterial infection, myocardial infarction, or stroke.

THE CLINICAL SPECTRUM OF ANTIPHOSPHOLIPID SYNDROME

APS is usually diagnosed following obstetric or thrombotic morbidity. Nonetheless the clinical spectrum of APS is considered nowadays to be wider and includes systemic and organ-specific symptoms induced by both thrombotic and immune-mediated mechanisms (Shoenfeld, 2007; Marai et al., 2004).

Obstetric APS

Obstetric complications are a hallmark of APS including mainly recurrent miscarriages and preterm deliveries. Early recurrent miscarriage (<10 weeks of gestation) occurs in about 1% of the general obstetric population of which 15% are associated with APS. Fetal loss (≥10 weeks of gestation) is less common and more strongly associated with the presence of aPL (Di Prima et al., 2011). Women with high-level aPL and a history of previous fetal loss have up to 80% risk of current pregnancy loss if not

treated (Galarza-Maldonado et al., 2012). In addition neonatal adverse outcomes as prematurity, intrauterine growth restriction, or rare fetal/neonatal thrombosis have been frequently described in patients with APS as well as maternal hypertensive disorders such as preeclampsia/eclampsia and HELLP syndrome (i.e., hemolytic anemia, elevated liver enzymes, and low platelet counts). Treatment of obstetric APS is still controversial and requires a multidisciplinary approach (Andreoli et al., 2012). The goals of such an approach are to improve maternal and fetal–neonatal outcomes by keeping to a minimum the risks recognized by both APS and its recommended therapy (Bramham et al., 2010; Galarza-Maldonado et al., 2012).

Thrombotic APS

Venous and/or arterial thrombosis are distinctive characteristic of APS (Taraborelli et al., 2012), and vessels in any site and of any size may be involved (Saponjski et al., 2011). Deep vein thromboses, pulmonary embolism, and strokes are the most commonly reported. Such thrombotic events are the main cause of morbidity and mortality in APS, and they tend to recur particularly in untreated patients (Taraborelli et al., 2012). The confirmation of thrombosis by an objective method is a requirement of the Sapporo criteria, nowadays performed by a diversity of invasive and noninvasive methods such as angiography, ultrasound, computed tomography (i.e., 64-multi-slice computed tomographic angiography), and others (Saponjski et al., 2011). Histopathology may also be utilized to confirm the diagnosis of APS-associated thrombosis once there is no evidence of inflammation in the vessel wall (Taraborelli et al., 2012).

Neurological APS

Neurological manifestations were detailed in the original description of APS and have since remained a main cause for morbidity and mortality among patients affected by this syndrome (Hughes, 1983). Central venous thrombosis, i.e., stroke and transient ischemic attack are the most common and are the only manifestations included in APS criteria (Appenzeller et al., 2012). APS-related strokes often occur in young patients and have a tendency to recur without an adequate therapy (Andreoli et al., 2012). In addition to local thrombosis mediated by aPL, vascular heart disease may become a source of emboli and related cerebrovascular events (Andreoli et al., 2012). Yet, in the last 30 years aPL positivity has been correlated with a wide variety of neurological expressions including headache, cognitive dysfunction, psychosis, depression, dementia, migraine, convulsions, chorea, transverse myelitis, Guillain–Barré syndrome and a multiple sclerosis-like illness (Shoenfeld et al., 2004; Cimaz et al., 2006; Rodrigues et al., 2010). Additionally, APS should be considered in all unexplained cases of retinal arterial and venous thromboses, as well as in cases of unusual ocular inflammations, particularly in young individuals (Arnson et al., 2010). APS-related ocular symptoms reflect both anterior and posterior pole involvement and include blurring of vision, dry eye sensation, amaurosis fugax, decreased visual acuity, diplopia, orbital and ocular pain, visual field defects, photophobia, scotoma, floaters, photopsia, and others.

Hematologic APS

Thrombocytopenia occurs in 20–40% of APS patients (Cervera et al., 2011b) and is associated with systemic involvement (Krause et al., 2005a). It is usually moderate, with platelet counts greater than 50K, rarely associated with major bleeding episodes, and does not require therapeutic intervention. Platelet reduction may be due to their destruction by autoantibodies or via their consumption following activation and aggregation (George et al., 1999). Some groups have reported anti-platelet glycoprotein antibodies which strongly correlate with thrombocytopenia whereas others observed that aPL bind directly to activated platelets via b2-glycoprotein-I thereby promoting platelet activation and aggregation (Krause et al., 2005a). Autoimmune hemolytic anemia is less frequent, reported in 6–10% of APS patients (Taraborelli et al., 2012). A significant association between the presence of aPL and a positive Coombs test as well as the co-occurrence of both autoimmune thrombocytopenia and

hemolytic anemia (named Evans syndrome) has been described (Rottem et al., 2006; Cervera et al., 2011b). Lymphopenia and neutropenia are well-recognized features of SLE, and therefore found more commonly in patients with APS associated with SLE.

Dermatologic APS

Skin manifestations are noted in 49% of APS patients and are the presenting signs in 30–40% of cases (Frances et al., 2005). The most frequent is livedo reticularis, a red or bluish alteration of the skin with a net-like pattern attributed to blood stasis in capillaries and venules (Toubi et al., 2005). The pathophysiology of livedo reticularis is not well characterized, but the relationship with arterial thrombosis such as Sneddon's syndrome suggests a possible role for an interaction of aPL with the endothelial cell or other cellular element in blood vessels (Taraborelli et al., 2012). Cutaneous necrosis is observed in 5.5% of patients with APS and the most commonly involved sites are the upper and lower extremities, helices of ears, cheeks, trunk, and forehead. These lesions may appear in the post-phlebitic state (following a thrombosis) or caused by a circumscribed skin necrosis. The latter may be confirmed by a biopsy demonstrating non-inflammatory thrombosis of dermal vessels without evidence of vasculitis. Cutaneous digital gangrene, with preceding ischemic symptoms, has also been observed in up to 7.5% of patients with APS. Many non-specific skin lesions of which some resemble vasculitis (pseudovasculitis) including red macules, purpura, cyanotic lesions on the hands and feet, ecchymoses, and painful skin nodules as well as primary anetoderma have also been reported.

Cardiac APS

The heart is one of the target organs in APS. Valve abnormalities, vegetations, and/or thickening, termed Libman–Sacks endocarditis, are the most common manifestations described in 30 to 50% of patients (Cervera et al., 2011a; Ziporen et al., 1996). Of note valve damage is more frequent in patients with secondary APS, is highly associated with the presence of aPL (Nesher et al., 1997), and coexists with neurological manifestations (Krause et al., 2005b). Myocardial infarction is diagnosed in 5.5% of patients with APS and is also significantly associated with the presence of aPL (Cervera et al., 2011a). Interestingly, in APS patients, acute myocardial infarction can occur in the absence of coronary artery lesions, especially in premenopausal women (Taraborelli et al., 2012). As a consequence of either valvular disease, myocardial infarction and secondary pulmonary hypertension, left ventricular systolic and diastolic dysfunction have both been reported. Taking it all together, echocardiographic follow-up is recommended for all APS patients (Cervera et al., 2011a).

Pulmonary APS

Pulmonary embolism and infarction constitute the most frequent pulmonary manifestation of APS. In the Europhospholipid cohort pulmonary embolism was the presenting manifestation in 9% of patients (Taraborelli et al., 2012). Leaving aside this classical thrombotic manifestation, other pulmonary expressions including pulmonary hypertension, acute respiratory distress syndrome, intra-alveolar hemorrhage, and fibrosing alveolitis have been described in the clinical spectrum of APS features (Stojanovich et al., 2012). Notably, the presence of aPL correlated with distinct pulmonary types of involvement, such as the link between aCL and pulmonary arterial thrombosis, adult respiratory distress syndrome, and fibrosing alveolitis (Stojanovich et al., 2012).

Renal APS

Anti-phospholipid-mediated thrombosis can affect different parts of the kidney depending on the type and size of the vessels. Large vessel involvement is usually in the form of thrombosis and/or stenosis that present as marked hypertension, renal dysfunction, and pain. In the case of occlusive lesions both *in situ* thrombosis and embolization from heart lesions can take place (Taraborelli et al., 2012). Involvement of smaller vessels is most commonly expressed as thrombotic microangiopathy or non-thrombotic glomerulopathies (Chaturvedi et al., 2011), clinically characterized by hypertension, renal failure, and/or proteinuria. Investigation in such cases should include a renal biopsy (Chaturvedi et al., 2011).

Catastrophic Antiphospholipid Syndrome

The term catastrophic antiphospholipid syndrome (CAPS) was first used in 1992 to define an accelerated form of APS resulting in multi-organ failure. Currently this most severe form of APS is present in less than 1% of APS patients and is defined by the clinical evidence of three or more organs affected within a short period of time. CAPS is commonly triggered by infection, trauma, surgery, pregnancy or others, and histologically multiple small vessels as well as some large vessels are concomitantly occluded (Erkan et al., 2010). In recent years following improved diagnosis and intervention, the mortality rate of CAPS decreased.

THE ANTIPHOSPHOLIPID ANTIBODIES

The aPL comprise more than 20 different autoantibodies, of which just three serve as diagnostic criteria for APS. The pathogenic effects of these antibodies are exerted through binding to various cells, including monocytes, endothelial cells, and trophoblasts, leading to the recruitment of cell surface receptors and subsequent perturbation of intracellular signaling pathways (Blank et al., 1991; Giannakopoulos and Krilis 2013). aPL target a variety of antigens including negatively charged phospholipids, phospholipid-binding proteins (particularly b2GPI and prothrombin) and factors related to hemostasis (De Groot et al., 2012). Notably, up to 5% of healthy individuals, lacking any APS features, demonstrate aPL seropositivity. In most of these cases aPL appear transiently, at low levels, following exposure to an environmental trigger, such as an infectious disease. Thus, aiming to improve the specificity of the Sapporo criteria the pathogenicity of criteria-relevant aPL was defined by three requisites (Table 34.1): (1) the detection of aPL on two or more occasions at least 12 weeks apart; (2) the presence of specific isotypes, namely IgG or IgM; and (3) the presence of aPL in medium to high levels (i.e., >40 GPL or MPL), or in levels above the 99th percentile for a specific population (Miyakis et al., 2006).

The pathogenicity of aPL is further supported by the observation that higher levels of aPL as well as the concomitant presence of the three criteria aPL (lupus anticoagulants, anti-cardiolipin, and anti-b2GPI) indicate a subgroup of high risk APS (Sciascia et al., 2011). Recently Pengo et al. (Pengo et al., 2010) analyzed data of 160 APS patients with "triple positive" sero-reactivity. At study entry, thrombosis was documented in 47%, arterial thromboembolism in 43%, pregnancy morbidity in 9.7%, and catastrophic antiphospholipid syndrome in 2.5% of patients. During 10 years of follow-up, 10 out of 160 patients died and 44.2% experienced another thrombotic event.

Another mandate of the APS criteria is the need for "standardized" laboratory assays to detect any one of the criteria-relevant aPL. The latter are detected by functional assay (lupus anticoagulant) or by solid phase immunoassay, anti-cardiolipin and anti-b2GPI (Biggioggero and Meroni, 2010). Although attempts at standardization of these tests have been conducted over the last three decades, there remain inconsistencies, inter-assay and inter-laboratory variations, as well as various issues regarding the interpretation of results. Hence, updated guidelines for lupus anticoagulants (LAC) testing (Martinuzzo et al., 2012) have been issued, followed by the formulation of a task force of scientists and pioneers in the field aiming to standardize and improve the solid phase assays (Pierangeli et al., 2011).

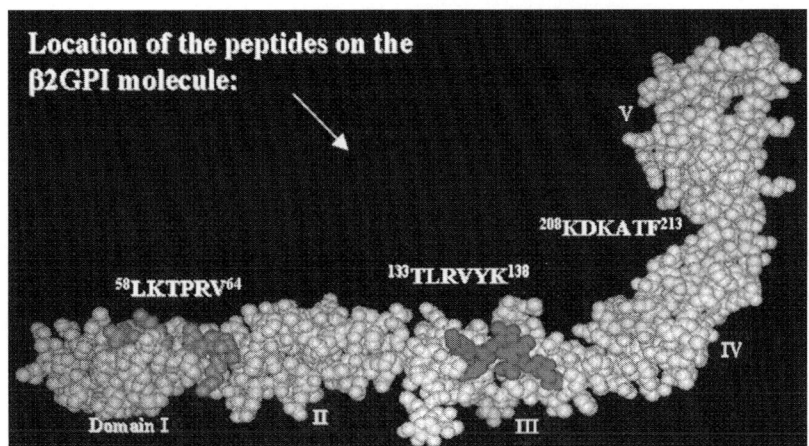

Location of the peptides on the β2GPI molecule:

V

²⁰⁸KDKATF²¹³

¹³³TLRVYK¹³⁸

⁵⁸LKTPRV⁶⁴

IV

Domain I

II

III

FIGURE 34.1 The plasma protein β(2)-glycoprotein I (b2GPI) is a phospholipid binding protein. It is constructed of five domains (I−V) that can present in a circular non-active form or in an active, open J-shaped conformation, as presented in the figure. Each of the five homologous domains of b2GPI include approximately 60 amino acids, and certain peptides in each domain have been identified as autoantigens (three of which are detailed in this figure). Anti-b2GPI antibodies can form a complex with b2GPI and activate intracellular signaling only in its open conformation while cryptic epitopes are exposed. *With acknowledgment to Prof. Miri Blank (The Zabludovicz Center for Autoimmune Diseases, Israel).*

The b2GPI−Anti-b2GPI Complex in APS

The term "antiphospholipid syndrome" is actually confusing, as most pathogenic aPL are not directed against phospholipids but towards the plasma protein β(2)-glycoprotein I (b2GPI). The latter is a phospholipid-binding protein, present either in a circulating form or bound to cells (De Groot et al., 2012). b2GPI participates in the innate immune responses (i.e., lipopolysaccharide scavenging and clearance of unwanted anionic micro-particles) and has anti-thrombotic properties. It is constructed of five domains that can present in a circular non-active form or in an open J-shaped conformation that can bind and activate intracellular signaling. The five homologous domains of b2GPI each include approximately 60 amino acids, and certain peptides in each domain have been identified as autoantigens (Figure 34.1). Domain V is located at the C terminus of the protein and contains a hydrophobic core surrounded by 14 positively charged residues that promote electrostatic interactions with negatively charged membrane components (Mahler et al., 2012). Anti-b2GPI antibodies can form a complex with b2GPI only in its open conformation (de Groot and Meijers, 2011). Moreover, this conformational change in b2GPI enables the exposure of cryptic epitopes and the formation of specific autoantibodies (de Laat et al., 2011).

The formation of b2GPI−anti-b2GPI complexes is closely linked with various manifestations of APS both in humans and in animal models of this autoimmune disease. Lately, the role of anti-b2GPI antibodies directed at different domains of b2GPI has become a focus of attention. Antibodies directed at domain I of b2GPI are associated with a higher risk of thrombosis and, to a lesser extent, pregnancy complications. In addition peptides derived from domain I of b2GPI were able to inhibit *in vivo* the pathogenicity of anti-b2GPI (Ioannou et al.,

2009; Mahler et al., 2012). Specific autoantibodies directed at other domains of b2GPI were less extensively studied. Nonetheless, the presence of an antibody directed at a peptide derived from domain III of b2GPI was found to be a significant predictor of recurrent spontaneous abortions (Shoenfeld et al., 2003). In contrast, reactivity to domains IV or V may be considered as "innocent" autoantibodies, as they were mainly identified in non-thrombotic conditions, such as healthy children born to mothers with autoimmune disease, and atopic children (Andreoli et al., 2011).

NON-CRITERIA APL ANTIBODIES

Only three aPL are considered among APS-relevant criteria, yet a number of "non-criteria" aPL have been linked with APS manifestations (Shoenfeld et al., 2008b). Likewise, in rare cases, a diagnosis of "sero-negative APS" was suggested.

aPL of the IGA Isotype

These are present in up to 40% of SLE patients with a higher rate in Afro-Caribbean individuals. Anti-cardiolipin antibodies of the IgA subtype were found to be thrombogenic in mice, whereas IgA directed at b2GPI were documented in a subgroup of sero-negative women with recurrent pregnancy losses. IgA class aPL were also an independent risk factor for cardiovascular mortality and thrombotic events in hemodialysis patients (Serrano et al., 2012) and SLE patients (Sweiss et al., 2010). Interestingly, unlike IgG directed at domains IV and V of β2GPI, IgA antibodies that bind to these domains may contribute to thrombosis atherosclerosis (Iverson et al., 2006) and early pregnancy loss (Staub et al., 2006).

Low-level aPL

Another requisite for "criteria aPL" is the presence of levels above >40 GPL or MPL, as high levels confirm both specificity and a worse outcome (Simchen et al., 2011) Even so, lower levels may still be considered if they are above the 99 percentile, an index rarely known or taken into consideration by the treating physician. Besides, aPL levels may decrease during follow-up and if determined weeks or months following a suspected event may be below the required cut-off (Faricelli et al., 2008). Moreover, technical aspects may play a role while evaluating aPL levels. Vlachoyiannopoulos et al. (Vlachoyiannopoulos et al., 1998) reported low levels of aPL in six out of 22 APS patients depending to a certain extent on the method of detection, urea resistance, and reactivity directed at a complex of cardiolipin–b2GPI rather than at the distinct antigens.

During cell apoptosis, lysophospholipids are exposed on the cell surface and can become targets for antibodies. Consequently, aPL can be directed at a heterogeneous group of non-APS criteria antigens, and antigen complexes as phosphatidylethanolamine, phosphatidylserine, vimentin, annexin A5, prothrombin, phosphatidic acid, serine proteases, and more (Alessandri et al., 2011; Pierangeli et al., 2011).

Antiphosphatidylethanolamine (aPE) were found to be associated with fetal loss and venous thrombosis (Pierangeli et al., 2011). Sugi et al. (Sugi et al., 2004) reported the prevalence of aPE in patients with unexplained recurrent early or mid-to-late pregnancy losses. In this cohort different subtypes of aPE were observed in up to 19%, suggesting an association between these antibodies and pregnancy losses. In another study Sanmarco et al. (Sanmarco et al., 2007) evaluated the role of aPE in 270 patients with APS. These antibodies were present in 15% of patients and were associated with thrombosis (odds ratio (OR) 6; $p = 0.005$) especially in the absence of criteria-type aPL.

Antiphosphatidylserine (anti-PS) positivity was documented in women with recurrent pregnancy losses who were negative for aCL (Sater et al., 2012). Additionally, anti-PS can inhibit trophoblast development and invasion, and impede syncytiotrophoblast formation further supporting their pathogenic role (Blank and Shoenfeld, 2004).

Antiprothrombin antibodies (anti-PT) similarly to anti-b2GPI are the most common aPL detected by ELISA methods, as both PT and b2GPI are phospholipid-binding proteins. The coexistence of IgG anti-PT and lupus anticoagulants was found to be an essential risk factor for venous thromboembolism in patients with SLE (Nojima et al., 2001) and to play a role in the pathogenesis of thrombosis in APS (de Groot et al., 1998; von Landenberg et al., 2003; Haj-Yahia et al., 2003). Besides, anti-PT was linked to thrombosis and disease progression

in other conditions such as acute ischemic strokes in young women (Cojocaru et al., 2008), fetal death in women with previous uneventful pregnancies and seronegative aPL (Marozio et al., 2011), and more advanced primary biliary cirrhosis (Agmon-Levin et al., 2010).

Antibodies directed at the complex phosphatidylserine/prothrombin (aPS/PT) were reported to be markers of APS with a high degree of concordance to lupus anticoagulant activity (Hoxha et al., 2012, Vlagea et al., 2013). aPS/PT correlated in a cohort of 295 individuals with particular expressions of APS, namely venous thrombosis (OR 7.44; CI 3.97–13.92) and obstetric abnormalities (OR 2.37; CI 1.04–5.43), but not with arterial thrombosis. aPS/PT were also detected at high levels in patients with cutaneous polyarteritis nodosa (Kawakami et al., 2007) and localized scleroderma, especially among patients with generalized morphea (Hasegawa et al., 2006).

The seronegative APS definition has been suggested for patients with clinical manifestations indicative of APS but with persistently negative results utilizing assays to detect criteria aPL (Rodriguez-Garcia et al., 2012). Apparently these patients exhibit similar frequencies of thrombotic events and obstetric morbidity. Transient or false-negative aPL tests may explain some of these cases, as even today anti-b2GPI is routinely tested in only a small number of laboratories, and standardization of other criteria aPL is yet to be accomplished. In addition, non-criterion aPL are currently tested in only a few research laboratories (Cervera et al., 2012). Taking it all together one may consider testing for a broad profile of aPL may enable better definition of this subgroup of patients with APS-like disease.

THE MECHANISMS OF APL-MEDIATED DISEASE EXPRESSIONS

In the last three decades much effort has been devoted to clarify the pathogenic potential of aPL (Bakimer et al., 1992). Both vascular thrombosis and pregnancy loss are the classical clinical expression of the APS, therefore aPL pathogenicity was studied focusing on these clinical aspects. Notably, aPL-related vascular thrombosis can occur both on the arterial and the venous side, making this acquired procoagulant condition very peculiar in human disease. The first evidence of the aPL-related pathogenic potential was obtained through animals that carried aPL as part of their disease (i.e., lupus-like-prone mice), or alternatively naïve mice that were infused with antibodies or stimulated to produce their own aPL (Ziporen et al., 1997; Katzav et al., 2010). In a long series of studies different polyclonal and monoclonal aPL antibodies with various specificities were utilized inducing pregnancy losses and enhancing the coagulation process. Probably in no other autoimmune disorders has there been so much evidence produced to show the pathogenicity *in vivo* of these autoantibodies. This body of evidence was pivotal in proving autoantibody-mediated damage, and at the same time prompted further *in vitro* studies aiming to define the cellular pathogenic effects of aPL. Originally both pregnancy loss and vascular occlusions were ascribed to the thrombogenic effect of aPL. Nowadays it is clear that placental thrombosis can be responsible for pregnancy failures, but at the same time it is accepted that aPL can exert a direct non-thrombotic effect on trophoblast cells (Di Simone et al., 2000) and other cells (Del Papa et al., 1995). Over the years, the concept of aPL itself has also been redefined. In fact, starting from the hypothesis that these autoantibodies were directed to phospholipids, we now know that in most cases they are directed to phospholipid-binding proteins (Giannakopoulos et al., 2011). Even if these antibodies are detected with different assays, the main target of the so-called aPL was identified as beta2-glycoprotein I (b2GPI), a phospholipid-binding protein. Almost all pathogenic effects of aPL have been shown using highly purified anti-b2GPI antibodies (Meroni et al., 2011). By reporting pathogenic effects of aPL, we will substantially refer to the effect of anti-b2GPI antibodies and anti-b2GPI–b2GPI complexes, unless otherwise specified.

Thrombotic Manifestations

aPL and The Coagulation Cascade

Several mechanisms have been described to explain the thrombophilic properties of aPL, generally related to their interaction with the coagulation and fibrinolysis systems or with cells involved in thrombus formation. These include b2GPI-anti−b2GPI complexes that were found to be localized to atherosclerotic plaques, mainly to oxidized low-density lipoprotein (LDL) (oxLDL), to induce autoimmune thombogenesis (Matsuura et al., 2003), and to amplify thrombus size (Arad et al., 2011).

Activated protein C (APC) is a natural anticoagulant that interacts with factors Va and VIIIa impairing their procoagulant activity. In the presence of b2GPI−anti-b2GPI complexes, APC cannot exert its action possibly because it is unable to bind Va/VIIIa or, alternatively, the formed APC/Va/VIIIa complex is sterically impaired in its binding to a phospholipid surface (Vlachoyiannopoulos and Routsias, 2010). Antiphospholipid antibodies can also impair the anticoagulant function of antithrombin. This can occur because some of the targets such as thrombin or activated factor IX, when bound by aPL, are no longer available for antithrombin action (Chen et al., 2010). On the other hand, aPL can interfere with the fibrinolytic cascade.

Fibrin degradation, which allows thrombus remodeling and dissolution, is mediated by the active enzyme plasmin, is derived from the conversion of plasminogen, which is mediated by its activators, tissue-type plasminogen activator (tPA) and urokinase-type plasminogen activator (uPA), of which both are controlled by specific inhibitors (plasminogen activator inhibitors PAI-1 and PAI-2). In the presence of aPL, PAI-1 activity was reported as enhanced resulting in reduction of tPA and plasminogen activation. Apparently b2GPI protects tPA from the action of PAI-1, thereby promoting fibrinolysis; if b2GPI is bound by its specific antibodies, it cannot exert its protective action with the consequent prevalent action of the inhibitory effect of PAI-1(Vlachoyiannopoulos and Routsias, 2010). Another impairment of fibrinolytic activity seems to be due to a possible direct binding of aPL to plasmin, followed by its inactivation (Yang et al., 2004). The data reported so far represent only some of the plausible mechanisms by which aPL interfere with the coagulation process, and recently another possible explanation has been formulated (Lambrianides et al., 2011). Many of the proteins involved in coagulation/fibrinolysis processes belong to the family of serine protease (SP) enzymes, such as APC, thrombin, plasmin, tPA, and others. These proteins share a high homology region at their catalytic domain. Most aPL recognize a conformational epitope that is shared by b2GPI molecule and the catalytic domain of SP. Therefore the presence of aPL can result in binding of SP molecules and impairment of their enzymatic activity, resulting in enhanced risk of thrombosis.

aPL Cellular Interactions

One of the most studied pathogenic effects of aPL deals with the interaction of antibodies with the cells involved in the coagulation process. This basically occurs through the recognition of b2GPI that has adhered to cell membranes. It is known that anti-b2GPI antibodies can upregulate adhesion molecules such as endothelial leukocyte adhesion molecule-1 (ELAM-1), vascular cell adhesion molecule-1 (VCAM-1), intracellular adhesion molecule-1 (ICAM-1), and tissue factor (TF), conditioning their expression on the cell surface.This process was described *in vitro* on monolayers of human umbilical vein endothelial cells (HUVEC) (Meroni et al., 1996) and its consequences were shown *in vivo* on CD1 mice infused with aPL: in fact in this model leukocytes were seen to adhere to vascular endothelium favoring clotting (Pierangeli et al., 1995). In the presence of aPL, HUVEC also significantly increase the production of some proinflammatory cytokines like IL-6 and IL-1β. Therefore the consequence of the aPL effect on endothelium is the shift towards a proadhesive/procoagulant as well as proinflammatory phenotype.

These profound modifications are basically due to the presence of b2GPI on the endothelial surface. A number of possible receptors for b2GPI have been described on the endothelial cell surface. Heparin sulfate, annexin2 receptor, Toll-like receptors (TLR) 2 and 4, and apolipoprotein E receptor 2 were all shown to be involved in the thrombogenic mechanisms related to aPL using *in vitro* and *in vivo* models (Poulton et al., 2012). It was also observed that animals lacking one of these receptors are only partially resistant to the pathogenic potential of aPL, suggesting that they play a similar, probably redundant, role (Meroni et al., 2011). The binding of anti-b2GPI to its antigen on the endothelial surface should produce intracellular signaling, able to upregulate the cellular expression of adhesion molecules and TF. The signal can start from the receptors that are sensitive to the clustering of b2GPI that follows their specific antibody binding. Among receptors, those having a cytoplasmic tail, TLR 2 and 4 are most likely to be the favorite candidate. Several intracellular pathways have been described as activated, including nuclear factor κB (NFκB), p-38 mitogen-activated protein kinase (MAPK), myeloid differentiation primary response protein (MyD88), and tumor necrosis factor (TNF) receptor-associated factor 6 (TRAF6). The above reported mechanisms are well defined in endothelial cells, but they are also at least partially described in monocytes, platelets, and in other cells serving as a possible target of aPL-mediated damage (Meroni et al., 2011; Poulton et al., 2012). The thrombophilic effect of aPL was also investigated at platelet level. In subjects with aPL, platelet activation was proven by the increase of thromboxane B2 and the decrease in vascular prostacyclin. Receptors of b2GPI at the platelet surface seem to be the apolipoprotein E receptor 2 and the platelet glycoprotein Ib alpha chain (Cognasse et al., 2005; Urbanus et al., 2008). *In vitro* the pathogenic effect of affinity purified anti-b2GPI antibodies was shown as an increased aggregation and intracellular signaling activation of platelets in the presence of low doses of thrombin stimulation. In this respect, a recent study (Vlachoyiannopoulos and Routsias, 2010) has underlined the importance of platelet factor 4, a protein derived from platelet alpha granules and belonging to the chemokine family. Platelet factor 4 is secreted by platelets but can also bind to the platelet surface as well as anionic molecules and b2GPI, both in solid phase and in solution. Platelet factor 4 is able to gather two b2GPI molecules, so favoring an efficient antibody binding. Complexes containing platelet factor 4, dimerized b2GPI, and anti-b2GPI antibodies can induce an activated procoagulant phenotype in platelets. Notably, platelet factor 4 is expressed in different cells such as endothelial cells, monocytes, T cells, and dendritic cells suggesting that its capacity to dimerize b2GPI could favor immune system sensitization and the production of pathogenic anti-b2GPI antibodies.

Obstetric Manifestations

Although many different obstetric expressions of APS have been described, the most typical are mid-pregnancy losses, mainly related to defective placentation and intrauterine growth restriction. Therefore the first pathogenic mechanism to be investigated was the presence of intraplacental thrombosis (Inbar et al., 1993; Levy et al., 1998). Indeed the above-described thrombophilic properties of aPL favor an increased thrombosis occurrence, particularly during pregnancy, that can work as a "second hit" since pregnancy *per se* is characterized by an increased thrombosis risk, even in the general population. A potent anticoagulant acting mainly, but not exclusively, on the trophoblast surface is annexin V that produces the so-called "protective shield," by binding negatively charged phospholipids such as phosphatidylserine. The presence of annexin V at the intervillous surface was found to be significantly reduced in patients with APS, thus confirming that b2GPI–anti b2GPI complexes are able to displace *in vivo* annexin V from the cell surface as shown *in vitro* (Hunt et al., 2011). Furthermore, it is recognized that aPL can also directly interact with trophoblast during syncytium formation (Di Simone et al., 2000) when it expresses phosphatidylserine at its outer surface. As shown by *in vitro* experiments, b2GPI can bind to negatively charged phospholipids such as phosphatidylserine on the cell surface and become a target of circulating anti-b2GPI antibodies. The antibody binding impairs the trophoblast capacity to proliferate and differentiate, and produce human chorionic gonadotropin. These changes are the final consequence of the aPL-mediated modulation of trophoblasts occurring through several intracellular biological alterations including apoptosis. This process is likely to alter the early placentation *in vivo* and can be responsible for the first trimester pregnancy failures, while late failures are probably due to uteroplacental thrombosis (De Carolis et al., 2010).

Neurologic Manifestations

Stroke was one of the historical clinical manifestations included in the APS definition supporting the neurological involvement of the disease. In fact many neurological manifestations are observed in APS patients. However, while stroke is clearly related to vascular events, this is not clear for other problems like cognitive dysfunction, mood disorder, epilepsy and others, which also occur in APS. Starting from animal models (Appenzeller et al., 2012) in which immunoglobulins from APS patients were injected into the brain of mice, it was shown that aPL can bind to neuron in the hippocampus and the cerebral cortex (Caronti et al., 1998). Importantly, the treated animals also performed poorly in a test designed to explore their cognitive capacity, proving that antibodies binding to brain cells can alter their functioning (Chapman et al., 1999). Obviously this model implies that aPL cross the blood—brain barrier, therefore requiring the coexistence of an infective-inflammatory state as a precipitating factor. However, it has been clinically observed that infective-inflammatory events can worsen the course of APS and therefore this interpretation is likely to represent a valid pathogenic mechanism. In addition, an increased prevalence of learning disabilities in children born to women with high aPL levels during pregnancy (Nacinovich et al., 2008) supports the role of aPL as mediator of brain damage. In fact, during uterine life, the absence of an effective blood—brain barrier allows maternal antibody (of the IgG isotype) to reach the fetus brain and cause impairment of its functioning as described in the animals studied.

The Complement System in APS

Complement is apparently involved in APS as antibodies cannot exert their pathogenic effect in animals that lack complement factors or receptors. This effect has been observed in both pregnancy loss (Holers et al., 2002) and in a thrombosis model (Fischetti et al., 2005). If the binding of aPL to their target cells (endothelial cells, trophoblasts) can activate complement, several activation molecules can be released. A recently described damage mechanism focused on C5a as a possible activator of neutrophils via its receptor on the cell surface (Girardi, 2010); according to this model the consequence of C5a binding to neutrophils is tissue factor production that can exert procoagulant and proinflammatory actions, and these can cause both thrombosis and fetal loss. Data observed in human disease are less clear. Decreased complement levels have been described in patients with APS (Oku et al., 2009) but are not always associated with pathological events (Reggia et al., 2012). Studying pregnancy in primary APS patients, we showed C3 and C4 levels to be significantly decreased compared with those found in the "normal" obstetrical population; however, we could not show a clearly related increased risk of pregnancy complications. Moreover, a prospective study of placentas from APS patients showed complement deposition without any relationship to pregnancy outcome or treatment (Tincani et al., 2010). Thus the role of complement activation in APS is yet to be elucidated.

TREATMENT OF APS

In contrast to the large body of evidence on the pathogenesis, mechanisms, and diagnosis of APS, there is still a gap in our knowledge on appropriate therapy for patients affected by this disease. The management of patients with APS is currently directed to antithrombotic medications. Balancing an individual's risk of thrombosis against the benefits and risks of antithrombotic therapies is crucial for optimizing management and preventing morbidity in patients with APS or aPL positive-asymptomatic ones. The international therapeutic guidelines recommend, for the secondary prevention of recurrent thrombosis, oral anticoagulation with warfarin indefinitely. However, these therapeutic guidelines lack answers for minority groups of patients such as (1) those who are appropriately anticoagulated but have recurrent thromboembolic phenomena or (2) those with prolonged clinically and serologically quiescent disease (Henriques et al., 2012). On the other hand many physicians recommend a daily low dose of aspirin for primary thrombosis prevention in asymptomatic individuals with persistent antiphospholipid antibodies. Although recent data question the effectiveness of aspirin (Puente et al., 2009) especially in patients with a high risk profile ("triple positive") (Pengo et al., 2012), the combination of aspirin and anticoagulants throughout pregnancy and the postpartum period is beneficial for the prevention of APS-associated obstetric morbidity, though the dosage and length of postpartum therapy is still an issue of debate. With proper management including low dose aspirin and/or heparin, more than 70% of pregnant women with antiphospholipid syndrome will deliver a viable infant. The role of other therapies as statins, hydroxychloroquine, steroids, and intravenous immunoglobulin (IVIG) is yet to be established (Carp et al., 2005; Blank et al., 2007; Bramham et al., 2010; Galarza-Maldonado et al., 2012).

In cases of catastrophic APS, an aggressive therapy is highly recommended using anticoagulation, glucocorticoids, and plasma exchange and/or intravenous immunoglobulins (Puente et al., 2009). This combination was retrospectively assessed and found to be advantageous (Espinosa et al., 2011), noting that APS has been revealed as a complex syndrome with multiple pathophysiological mechanisms previously unknown. In this context, new therapeutic approaches have been defended and empirically tested, with potentially promising results (Puente et al., 2009). It is well accepted that additional vascular and thrombotic risk factors such as hypertension, smoking, hyperlipidemia, and others should be actively reduced in all patients (Tuthill and Khamashta, 2009; Ruffatti et al., 2011). The potential beneficial roles of statins and hydroxychloroquine for APS-associated clinical manifestations have to be established. B cell-directed therapies have been approved for the treatment of several autoimmune diseases, and their favorable clinical and serological effects have been evident both in human and murine models of APS (Khattri et al., 2012). Vitamin D, recently defined as an immune modulator, is commonly deficient in patients with SLE and APS and deficiency was found to be associated with thrombotic manifestations and mechanisms in APS, suggesting a beneficial role for vitamin D supplementation (Agmon-Levin et al., 2011). Last but not least, though current options remain limited for the treatment of APS, the future holds much promise with the identification of multiple novel targets. These include new B cell depletion (i.e., anti-BAFF), new-generation anticoagulants, targeting components of the complement system, interfering with aPL cell-mediated activation of endothelial cells and platelets both at the cell surface level and intracellularly, and the novel concept of using a peptide-based approach to target subpopulations of aPL (Pericleous and Ioannou, 2010).

CONCLUSIONS AND FUTURE ASPECTS

APS is a systemic autoimmune disease, mediated by autoantibodies directed at phospholipids and phospholipid-binding proteins. Since its definition some 40 years ago, our understanding of the mechanisms underlining this disease has greatly improved. Nonetheless, much is yet to be accomplished regarding the definition of subgroups of APS patients, the accurate diagnosis and interpretation of criteria and non-criteria aPL, and the appropriate treatments for APS- and aPL-affected patients. These goals may be achieved by conducting well-designed, large-scale, multi-center clinical trials to explore and address the unmet needs of better, safer, and targeted management of APS.

REFERENCES

Agmon-Levin, N., Shapira, Y., Selmi, C., Barzilai, O., Ram, M., Szyper-Kravitz, M., et al., 2010. A comprehensive evaluation of serum autoantibodies in primary biliary cirrhosis. J. Autoimmun. 34, 55–58.

Agmon-Levin, N., Blank, M., Zandman-Goddard, G., Orbach, H., Meroni, P.L., Tincani, A., et al., 2011. Vitamin D: an instrumental factor in the anti-phospholipid syndrome by inhibition of tissue factor expression. Ann. Rheum. Dis. 70, 145–150.

Alessandri, C., Conti, F., Pendolino, M., Mancini, R., Valesini, G., 2011. New autoantigens in the antiphospholipid syndrome. Autoimmun. Rev. 10, 609–616.

Andreoli, L., Nalli, C., Motta, M., Norman, G.L., Shums, Z., Encabo, S., et al., 2011. Anti-beta(2)-glycoprotein I IgG antibodies from 1-year-old healthy children born to mothers with systemic autoimmune diseases preferentially target domain 4/5: might it be the reason for their "innocent" profile?. Ann. Rheum. Dis. 70, 380–383.

Andreoli, L., Fredi, M., Nalli, C., Reggia, R., Lojacono, A., Motta, M., et al., 2012. Pregnancy implications for systemic lupus erythematosus and the antiphospholipid syndrome. J. Autoimmun. 38, J197–J208.

Appenzeller, S., Lapa, A.T., Guirau, C.R., De Carvalho, J.F., Shoenfeld, Y., 2012. Cognitive impairment in antiphospholipid syndrome: evidence from animal models. Clin. Rheumatol. 31, 403–406.

Arad, A., Proulle, V., Furie, R.A., Furie, B.C., Furie, B., 2011. beta(2)-Glycoprotein-1 autoantibodies from patients with antiphospholipid syndrome are sufficient to potentiate arterial thrombus formation in a mouse model. Blood. 117, 3453–3459.

Arnson, Y., Shoenfeld, Y., Alon, E., Amital, H., 2010. The antiphospholipid syndrome as a neurological disease. Semin. Arthritis. Rheum. 40, 97–108.

Bakimer, R., Fishman, P., Blank, M., Sredni, B., Djaldetti, M., Shoenfeld, Y., 1992. Induction of primary antiphospholipid syndrome in mice by immunization with a human monoclonal anticardiolipin antibody (H-3). J. Clin. Invest. 89, 1558–1563.

Biggioggero, M., Meroni, P.L., 2010. The geoepidemiology of the antiphospholipid antibody syndrome. Autoimmun. Rev. 9, A299–A304.

Blank, M., Shoenfeld, Y., 2004. Antiphosphatidylserine antibodies and reproductive failure. Lupus. 13, 661–665.

Blank, M., Cohen, J., Toder, V., Shoenfeld, Y., 1991. Induction of antiphospholipid syndrome in naive mice with mouse lupus monoclonal and human polyclonal anti-cardiolipin antibodies. Proc. Natl. Acad. Sci. U.S.A. 88, 3069–3073.

Blank, M., Anafi, L., Zandman-Goddard, G., Krause, I., Goldman, S., Shalev, E., et al., 2007. The efficacy of specific IVIG anti-idiotypic antibodies in antiphospholipid syndrome (APS): trophoblast invasiveness and APS animal model. Int. Immunol. 19, 857–865.

Bramham, K., Hunt, B.J., Germain, S., Calatayud, I., Khamashta, M., Bewley, S., et al., 2010. Pregnancy outcome in different clinical phenotypes of antiphospholipid syndrome. Lupus. 19, 58–64.

Caronti, B., Pittoni, V., Palladini, G., Valesini, G., 1998. Anti-beta 2-glycoprotein I antibodies bind to central nervous system. J. Neurol. Sci. 156, 211–219.

Carp, H.J., Sapir, T., Shoenfeld, Y., 2005. Intravenous immunoglobulin and recurrent pregnancy loss. Clin. Rev. Allergy. Immunol. 29, 327–332.

Cervera, R, Ra, A., 2008. Antiphospholipid syndrome. Diagnostic Criteria in Autoimmune Diseases. Humana Press.

Cervera, R., Khamashta, M.A., Shoenfeld, Y., Camps, M.T., Jacobsen, S., Kiss, E., Zeher, M.M., et al., 2009. Morbidity and mortality in the antiphospholipid syndrome during a 5-year period: a multicentre prospective study of 1000 patients. Ann. Rheum. Dis. 68, 1428–1432.

Cervera, R., Tektonidou, M.G., Espinosa, G., Cabral, A.R., Gonzalez, E. B., Erkan, D., et al., 2011a. Task force on catastrophic antiphospholipid syndrome (APS) and non-criteria APS manifestations (I): catastrophic APS, APS nephropathy and heart valve lesions. Lupus. 20, 165–173.

Cervera, R., Tektonidou, M.G., Espinosa, G., Cabral, A.R., Gonzalez, E.B., Erkan, D., et al., 2011b. Task force on catastrophic antiphospholipid syndrome (APS) and non-criteria APS manifestations (II): thrombocytopenia and skin manifestations. Lupus. 20, 174–181.

Cervera, R., Conti, F., Doria, A., Iaccarino, L., Valesini, G., 2012. Does seronegative antiphospholipid syndrome really exist? Autoimmun. Rev. 11, 581–584.

Chapman, J., Cohen-Armon, M., Shoenfeld, Y., Korczyn, A.D., 1999. Antiphospholipid antibodies permeabilize and depolarize brain synaptoneurosomes. Lupus. 8, 127–133.

Chaturvedi, S., Brandao, L., Geary, D., Licht, C., 2011. Primary antiphospholipid syndrome presenting as renal vein thrombosis and membranous nephropathy. Pediatr. Nephrol. 26, 979–985.

Chen, P.P., Wu, M., Hahn, B.H., 2010. Some antiphospholipid antibodies bind to various serine proteases in hemostasis and tip the balance toward hypercoagulant states. Lupus. 19, 365–369.

Cimaz, R., Meroni, P.L., Shoenfeld, Y., 2006. Epilepsy as part of systemic lupus erythematosus and systemic antiphospholipid syndrome (Hughes syndrome. Lupus. 15, 191–197.

Cognasse, F., Hamzeh, H., Chavarin, P., Acquart, S., Genin, C., Garraud, O., 2005. Evidence of Toll-like receptor molecules on human platelets. Immunol. Cell. Biol. 83, 196–198.

Cojocaru, I.M., Cojocaru, M., Tanasescu, R., Burcin, C., Mitu, A.C., Iliescu, I., et al., 2008. Detecting anti-prothrombin antibodies in young women with acute ischemic stroke. Rom. J. Intern. Med. 46, 337–341.

De Carolis, S., Botta, A., Santucci, S., Garofalo, S., Martino, C., Perrelli, A., et al., 2010. Predictors of pregnancy outcome in antiphospholipid syndrome: a review. Clin. Rev. Allergy. Immunol. 38, 116–124.

De Groot, P.G., Meijers, J.C., 2011. beta(2)-Glycoprotein I: evolution, structure and function. J. Thromb. Haemost. 9, 1275–1284.

De Groot, P.G., Horbach, D.A., Simmelink, M.J., Van Oort, E., Derksen, R.H., 1998. Anti-prothrombin antibodies and their relation with thrombosis and lupus anticoagulant. Lupus. 7 (Suppl 2), S32–S36.

De Groot, P.G., Meijers, J.C., Urbanus, R.T., 2012. Recent developments in our understanding of the antiphospholipid syndrome. Int. J. Lab. Hematol. 34, 223–231.

De Laat, B., Van Berkel, M., Urbanus, R.T., Siregar, B., De Groot, P.G., Gebbink, M.F., Maas, C., 2011. Immune responses against domain I of beta(2)-glycoprotein I are driven by conformational changes: domain I of beta(2)-glycoprotein I harbors a cryptic immunogenic epitope. Arthritis Rheum. 63, 3960–3968.

Del Papa, N., Guidali, L., Spatola, L., Bonara, P., Borghi, M.O., Tincani, A., et al., 1995. Relationship between anti-phospholipid and anti-endothelial cell antibodies III: beta 2 glycoprotein I mediates the antibody binding to endothelial membranes and induces the expression of adhesion molecules. Clin. Exp. Rheumatol. 13, 179–185.

Di Prima, F.A., Valenti, O., Hyseni, E., Giorgio, E., Faraci, M., Renda, E., et al., 2011. Antiphospholipid syndrome during pregnancy: the state of the art. J Prenat. Med. 5, 41–53.

Di Simone, N., Meroni, P.L., De Papa, N., Raschi, E., Caliandro, D., De Carolis, C.S., et al., 2000. Antiphospholipid antibodies affect trophoblast gonadotropin secretion and invasiveness by binding directly and through adhered beta2-glycoprotein I. Arthritis Rheum. 43, 140–150.

Erkan, D., Espinosa, G., Cervera, R., 2010. Catastrophic antiphospholipid syndrome: updated diagnostic algorithms. Autoimmun. Rev. 10, 74–79.

Espinosa, G., Berman, H., Cervera, R., 2011. Management of refractory cases of catastrophic antiphospholipid syndrome. Autoimmun. Rev. 10, 664–668.

Faricelli, R., Esposito, S., Toniato, E., Flacco, M., Conti, P., Martinotti, S., et al., 2008. A new diagnostic approach to better identify antiphospholipid syndrome. Int. J. Immunopathol. Pharmacol. 21, 387–392.

Fischetti, F., Durigutto, P., Pellis, V., Debeus, A., Macor, P., Bulla, R., et al., 2005. Thrombus formation induced by antibodies to beta2-glycoprotein I is complement dependent and requires a priming factor. Blood. 106, 2340–2346.

Frances, C., Niang, S., Laffitte, E., Pelletier, F., Costedoat, N., Piette, J.C., 2005. Dermatologic manifestations of the antiphospholipid syndrome: two hundred consecutive cases. Arthritis Rheum. 52, 1785–1793.

Galarza-Maldonado, C., Kourilovitch, M.R., Perez-Fernandez, O.M., Gaybor, M., Cordero, C., Cabrera, S., et al., 2012. Obstetric antiphospholipid syndrome. Autoimmun. Rev. 11, 288–295.

George, J., Gilburd, B., Langevitz, P., Levy, Y., Nezlin, R., Harats, D., et al., 1999. Beta2 glycoprotein I containing immune-complexes in lupus patients: association with thrombocytopenia and lipoprotein (a) levels. Lupus. 8, 116–120.

Giannakopoulos, B., Krilis, S.A., 2013. The pathogenesis of the antiphospholipid syndrome. N. Engl. J. Med. 368, 1033–1044.

Giannakopoulos, B., Mirarabshahi, P., Krilis, S.A., 2011. New insights into the biology and pathobiology of beta2-glycoprotein I. Curr. Rheumatol. Rep. 13, 90–95.

Girardi, G., 2010. Role of tissue factor in the maternal immunological attack of the embryo in the antiphospholipid syndrome. Clin. Rev. Allergy. Immunol. 39, 160–165.

Haj-Yahia, S., Sherer, Y., Blank, M., Kaetsu, H., Smolinsky, A., Shoenfeld, Y., 2003. Anti-prothrombin antibodies cause thrombosis in a novel qualitative ex-vivo animal model. Lupus. 12, 364–369.

Hasegawa, M., Fujimoto, M., Hayakawa, I., Matsushita, T., Nishijima, C., Yamazaki, M., et al., 2006. Anti-phosphatidylserine-prothrombin complex antibodies in patients with localized scleroderma. Clin. Exp. Rheumatol. 24, 19–24.

Henriques, C.C., Lourenco, F., Lopez, B., Panarra, A., Riso, N., 2012. Antiphospholipid syndrome and recurrent thrombosis—limitations of current treatment strategies. BMJ Case. Rep. 2012.

Holers, V.M., Girardi, G., Mo, L., Guthridge, J.M., Molina, H., Pierangeli, S.S., et al., 2002. Complement C3 activation is required for antiphospholipid antibody-induced fetal loss. J. Exp. Med. 195, 211–220.

Hoxha, A., Ruffatti, A., Tonello, M., Bontadi, A., Salvan, E., Banzato, A., et al., 2012. Antiphosphatidylserine/prothrombin antibodies in primary antiphospholipid syndrome. Lupus. 21, 787–789.

Hughes, G.R., 1983. Thrombosis, abortion, cerebral disease, and the lupus anticoagulant. In: Clin Res (Ed.), Br. Med. J., 287. pp. 1088–1089.

Hunt, B.J., Wu, X.X., De Laat, B., Arslan, A.A., Stuart-Smith, S., Rand, J.H., 2011. Resistance to annexin A5 anticoagulant activity in women with histories for obstetric antiphospholipid syndrome. Am J Obstet Gynecol 205. 485, e17–e23.

Inbar, O., Blank, M., Faden, D., Tincani, A., Lorber, M., Shoenfeld, Y., 1993. Prevention of fetal loss in experimental antiphospholipid syndrome by low-molecular-weight heparin. Am. J. Obstet. Gynecol. 169, 423–426.

Ioannou, Y., Romay-Penabad, Z., Pericleous, C., Giles, I., Papalardo, E., Vargas, G., et al., 2009. In vivo inhibition of antiphospholipid antibody-induced pathogenicity utilizing the antigenic target peptide domain I of beta2-glycoprotein I: proof of concept. J. Thromb. Haemost. 7, 833–842.

Iverson, G.M., Von Muhlen, C.A., Staub, H.L., Lassen, A.J., Binder, W., Norman, G.L., 2006. Patients with atherosclerotic syndrome, negative in anti-cardiolipin assays, make IgA autoantibodies that preferentially target domain 4 of beta2-GPI. J. Autoimmun. 27, 266–271.

Katzav, A., Shoenfeld, Y., Chapman, J., 2010. The pathogenesis of neural injury in animal models of the antiphospholipid syndrome. Clin. Rev. Allergy. Immunol. 38, 196–200.

Kawakami, T., Yamazaki, M., Mizoguchi, M., Soma, Y., 2007. High level of anti-phosphatidylserine-prothrombin complex antibodies in patients with cutaneous polyarteritis nodosa. Arthritis Rheum. 57, 1507–1513.

Khattri, S., Zandman-Goddard, G., Peeva, E., 2012. B-cell directed therapies in antiphospholipid antibody syndrome—new directions based on murine and human data. Autoimmun. Rev. 11, 717–722.

Krause, I., Blank, M., Fraser, A., Lorber, M., Stojanovich, L., Rovensky, J., et al., 2005a. The association of thrombocytopenia with systemic manifestations in the antiphospholipid syndrome. Immunobiology. 210, 749–754.

Krause, I., Lev, S., Fraser, A., Blank, M., Lorber, M., Stojanovich, L., et al., 2005b. Close association between valvular heart disease and central nervous system manifestations in the antiphospholipid syndrome. Ann. Rheum. Dis. 64, 1490–1493.

Lambrianides, A., Turner-Stokes, T., Pericleous, C., Ehsanullah, J., Papadimitraki, E., Poulton, K., et al., 2011. Interactions of human monoclonal and polyclonal antiphospholipid antibodies with serine proteases involved in hemostasis. Arthritis Rheum. 63, 3512–3521.

Levy, R.A., Avvad, E., Oliveira, J., Porto, L.C., 1998. Placental pathology in antiphospholipid syndrome. Lupus. 7 (Suppl 2), S81–S85.

Mahler, M., Norman, G.L., Meroni, P.L., Khamashta, M., 2012. Autoantibodies to domain 1 of beta 2 glycoprotein. 1: A promising candidate biomarker for risk management in antiphospholipid syndrome. Autoimmun. Rev. 12, 313–317.

Marai, I., Zandman-Goddard, G., Shoenfeld, Y., 2004. The systemic nature of the antiphospholipid syndrome. Scand. J. Rheumatol. 33, 365–372.

Marozio, L., Curti, A., Botta, G., Canuto, E.M., Salton, L., Tavella, A.M., et al., 2011. Anti-prothrombin antibodies are associated with adverse pregnancy outcome. Am. J. Reprod. Immunol. 66, 404–409.

Martinuzzo, M.E., Cerrato, G.S., Varela, M.L., Adamczuk, Y.P., Forastiero, R.R., 2012. New guidelines for lupus anticoagulant: sensitivity and specificity of cut-off values calculated with plasmas from healthy controls in mixing and confirmatory tests. Int. J. Lab. Hematol. 34, 208–213.

Matsuura, E., Kobayashi, K., Koike, T., Shoenfeld, Y., Khamashta, M.A., Hughes, G.R., 2003. Oxidized low-density lipoprotein as a risk factor of thrombosis in antiphospholipid syndrome. Lupus. 12, 550–554.

Meroni, P.L., Papa, N.D., Beltrami, B., Tincani, A., Balestrieri, G., Krilis, S.A., 1996. Modulation of endothelial cell function by antiphospholipid antibodies. Lupus. 5, 448–450.

Meroni, P.L., Borghi, M.O., Raschi, E., Tedesco, F., 2011. Pathogenesis of antiphospholipid syndrome: understanding the antibodies. Nat. Rev. Rheumatol. 7, 330–339.

Miyakis, S., Lockshin, M.D., Atsumi, T., Branch, D.W., Brey, R.L., Cervera, R., et al., 2006. International consensus statement on an update of the classification criteria for definite antiphospholipid syndrome (APS). J. Thromb. Haemost. 4, 295–306.

Nacinovich, R., Galli, J., Bomba, M., Filippini, E., Parrinello, G., Nuzzo, M., et al., 2008. Neuropsychological development of children born to patients with antiphospholipid syndrome. Arthritis Rheum. 59, 345–351.

Nesher, G., Ilany, J., Rosenmann, D., Abraham, A.S., 1997. Valvular dysfunction in antiphospholipid syndrome: prevalence, clinical features, and treatment. Semin. Arthritis Rheum. 27, 27–35.

Nojima, J., Kuratsune, H., Suehisa, E., Futsukaichi, Y., Yamanishi, H., Machii, T., et al., 2001. Anti-prothrombin antibodies combined with lupus anti-coagulant activity is an essential risk factor for venous thromboembolism in patients with systemic lupus erythematosus. Br. J. Haematol. 114, 647–654.

Oku, K., Atsumi, T., Bohgaki, M., Amengual, O., Kataoka, H., Horita, T., et al., 2009. Complement activation in patients with primary antiphospholipid syndrome. Ann. Rheum. Dis. 68, 1030–1035.

Pengo, V., Ruffatti, A., Legnani, C., Gresele, P., Barcellona, D., Erba, N., et al., 2010. Clinical course of high-risk patients diagnosed with antiphospholipid syndrome. J. Thromb. Haemost. 8, 237–242.

Pengo, V., Ruiz-Irastorza, G., Denas, G., Andreoli, L., Khamashta, M., Tincani, A., 2012. High intensity anticoagulation in the prevention of the recurrence of arterial thrombosis in antiphospholipid syndrome: "PROS" and "CONS.". Autoimmun. Rev. 11, 577–580.

Pericleous, C., Ioannou, Y., 2010. New therapeutic targets for the antiphospholipid syndrome. Expert. Opin. Ther. Targets. 14, 1291–1299.

Pierangeli, S.S., Liu, X.W., Barker, J.H., Anderson, G., Harris, E.N., 1995. Induction of thrombosis in a mouse model by IgG, IgM and IgA immunoglobulins from patients with the antiphospholipid syndrome. Thromb. Haemost. 74, 1361–1367.

Pierangeli, S.S., De Groot, P.G., Dlott, J., Favaloro, E., Harris, E.N., Lakos, G., et al., 2011. "Criteria" aPL tests: report of a task force and preconference workshop at the 13th International Congress on Antiphospholipid Antibodies, Galveston, Texas, April 2010. Lupus. 20, 182–190.

Poulton, K., Rahman, A., Giles, I., 2012. Examining how antiphospholipid antibodies activate intracellular signaling pathways: a systematic review. Semin. Arthritis Rheum. 41, 720–736.

Puente, D., Pombo, G., Forastiero, R., 2009. Current management of antiphospholipid syndrome-related thrombosis. Expert. Rev. Cardiovasc. Ther. 7, 1551–1558.

Reggia, R., Ziglioli, T., Andreoli, L., Bellisai, F., Iuliano, A., Gerosa M., et al. 2012. Primary Antiphospholipid syndrome: any role for serum complement levels in predicting pregnancy complications? Rheumatology (Oxford). 51, 2186–2190.

Rodrigues, C.E., Carvalho, J.F., Shoenfeld, Y., 2010. Neurological manifestations of antiphospholipid syndrome. Eur. J. Clin. Invest. 40, 350–359.

Rodriguez-Garcia, J.L., Bertolaccini, M.L., Cuadrado, M.J., Sanna, G., Ateka-Barrutia, O., Khamashta, M.A., 2012. Clinical manifestations of antiphospholipid syndrome (APS) with and without antiphospholipid antibodies (the so-called "seronegative APS"). Ann. Rheum. Dis. 71, 242–244.

Rottem, M., Krause, I., Fraser, A., Stojanovich, L., Rovensky, J., Shoenfeld, Y., 2006. Autoimmune hemolytic anaemia in the antiphospholipid syndrome. Lupus. 15, 473–477.

Ruffatti, A., Del Ross, T., Ciprian, M., Bertero, M.T., Sciascia, S., Scarpato, S., et al., 2011. Risk factors for a first thrombotic event in antiphospholipid antibody carriers: a prospective multicentre follow-up study. Ann. Rheum. Dis. 70, 1083–1086.

Sanmarco, M., Gayet, S., Alessi, M.C., Audrain, M., De Maistre, E., Gris, J.C., et al., 2007. Antiphosphatidylethanolamine antibodies are associated with an increased odds ratio for thrombosis. A multicenter study with the participation of the European Forum on antiphospholipid antibodies. Thromb. Haemost. 97, 949–954.

Saponjski, J., Stojanovich, L., Djokovic, A., Petkovic, M., Mrda, D., 2011. Systemic vascular diseases in the antiphospholipid syndrome. What is the best diagnostic choice? Autoimmun. Rev. 10, 235–237.

Sater, M.S., Finan, R.R., Abu-Hijleh, F.M., Abu-Hijleh, T.M., Almawi, W.Y., 2012. Anti-phosphatidylserine, anti-cardiolipin, anti-beta2 glycoprotein I and anti-prothrombin antibodies in recurrent miscarriage at 8-12 gestational weeks. Eur J Obstet Gynecol Reprod Biol. 163, 170–174.

Sciascia, S., Cosseddu, D., Montaruli, B., Kuzenko, A., Bertero, M.T., 2011. Risk scale for the diagnosis of antiphospholipid syndrome. Ann. Rheum. Dis. 70, 1517–1518.

Serrano, A., Garcia, F., Serrano, M., Ramirez, E., Alfaro, F.J., Lora, D., et al., 2012. IgA antibodies against beta2 glycoprotein I in hemodialysis patients are an independent risk factor for mortality. Kidney. Int. 81, 1239–1244.

Shoenfeld, Y., 2007. APS—more systemic disease than SLE. Clin. Rev. Allergy. Immunol. 32, 129–130.

Shoenfeld, Y., Krause, I., Kvapil, F., Sulkes, J., Lev, S., Von Landenberg, P., et al., 2003. Prevalence and clinical correlations of antibodies against six beta2-glycoprotein-I-related peptides in the antiphospholipid syndrome. J. Clin. Immunol. 23, 377–383.

Shoenfeld, Y., Lev, S., Blatt, I., Blank, M., Font, J., Von Landenberg, P., et al., 2004. Features associated with epilepsy in the antiphospholipid syndrome. J. Rheumatol. 31, 1344–1348.

Shoenfeld, Y., Meroni, P.L., Cervera, R., 2008a. Antiphospholipid syndrome dilemmas still to be solved: 2008 status. Ann. Rheum. Dis. 67, 438–442.

Shoenfeld, Y., Twig, G., Katz, U., Sherer, Y., 2008b. Autoantibody explosion in antiphospholipid syndrome. J. Autoimmun. 30, 74–83.

Shoenfeld, Y., Meroni, P.L., Toubi, E., 2009. Antiphospholipid syndrome and systemic lupus erythematosus: are they separate entities or just clinical presentations on the same scale? Curr. Opin. Rheumatol. 21, 495–500.

Simchen, M.J., Dulitzki, M., Rofe, G., Shani, H., Langevitz, P., Schiff, E., et al., 2011. High positive antibody levels and adverse pregnancy outcome in women with antiphospholipid syndrome. Acta. Obstet. Gynecol. Scand. 90, 1428–1433.

Staub, H.L., Von Muhlen, C.A., Norman, G.L., 2006. Beta2-glycoprotein I IgA antibodies and ischaemic stroke. Rheumatology (Oxford). 45, 645–646.

Stojanovich, L., Kontic, M., Djokovic, A., Ilijevski, N., Stanisavljevic, N., Marisavljevic, D., 2012. Pulmonary events in antiphospholipid syndrome: influence of antiphospholipid antibody type and levels. Scand. J. Rheumatol. 41, 223–226.

Sugi, T., Matsubayashi, H., Inomo, A., Dan, L., Makino, T., 2004. Antiphosphatidylethanolamine antibodies in recurrent early pregnancy loss and mid-to-late pregnancy loss. J. Obstet. Gynaecol. Res. 30, 326–332.

Sweiss, N.J., Bo, R., Kapadia, R., Manst, D., Mahmood, F., Adhikari, T., et al., 2010. IgA anti-beta2-glycoprotein I autoantibodies are associated with an increased risk of thromboembolic events in patients with systemic lupus erythematosus. PLoS One. 5, e12280.

Taraborelli, M., Andreoli, L., Tincani, A., 2012. Much more than thrombosis and pregnancy loss: the antiphospholipid syndrome as a 'systemic disease'. Best. Pract. Res. Clin. Rheumatol. 26, 79–90.

Tincani, A., Cavazzana, I., Ziglioli, T., Lojacono, A., De Angelis, V., Meroni, P., 2010. Complement activation and pregnancy failure. Clin. Rev. Allergy. Immunol. 39, 153–159.

Toubi, E., Krause, I., Fraser, A., Lev, S., Stojanovich, L., Rovensky, J., et al., 2005. Livedo reticularis is a marker for predicting multisystem thrombosis in antiphospholipid syndrome. Clin. Exp. Rheumatol. 23, 499–504.

Tuthill, J.I., Khamashta, M.A., 2009. Management of antiphospholipid syndrome. J. Autoimmun. 33, 92–98.

Urbanus, R.T., Pennings, M.T., Derksen, R.H., De Groot, P.G., 2008. Platelet activation by dimeric beta2-glycoprotein I requires signaling via both glycoprotein Ibalpha and apolipoprotein E receptor 2'. J. Thromb. Haemost. 6, 1405–1412.

Vlachoyiannopoulos, P.G., Routsias, J.G., 2010. A novel mechanism of thrombosis in antiphospholipid antibody syndrome. J. Autoimmun. 35, 248–255.

Vlachoyiannopoulos, P.G., Petrovas, C., Tektonidou, M., Krilis, S., Moutsopoulos, H.M., 1998. Antibodies to beta 2-glycoprotein-I: urea resistance, binding specificity, and association with thrombosis. J. Clin. Immunol. 18, 380–391.

Vlagea, A.D., Gil, A., Cuesta, M.V., Arribas, F., Diez, J., Lavilla, P., Pascual-Salcedo, D., 2013. Antiphosphatidylserine/prothrombin. antibodies (aPS/PT) as potential markers of antiphospholipid syndrome. Clin Appl. Thromb Hemost. 19, 289–296.

Von Landenberg, P., Matthias, T., Zaech, J., Schultz, M., Lorber, M., Blank, M., et al., 2003. Antiprothrombin antibodies are associated with pregnancy loss in patients with the antiphospholipid syndrome. Am. J. Reprod. Immunol. 49, 51–56.

Yang, C.D., Hwang, K.K., Yan, W., Gallagher, K., Fitzgerald, J., Grossman, J.M., et al., 2004. Identification of anti-plasmin antibodies in the antiphospholipid syndrome that inhibit degradation of fibrin. J. Immunol. 172, 5765–5773.

Ziporen, L., Goldberg, I., Arad, M., Hojnik, M., Ordi-Ros, J., Afek, A., et al., 1996. Libman-Sacks endocarditis in the antiphospholipid syndrome: immunopathologic findings in deformed heart valves. Lupus. 5, 196–205.

Ziporen, L., Shoenfeld, Y., Levy, Y., Korczyn, A.D., 1997. Neurological dysfunction and hyperactive behavior associated with antiphospholipid antibodies. A mouse model. J. Clin. Invest. 100, 613–619.

Chapter 35

Sjögren's Syndrome

Clio P. Mavragani[1], George E. Fragoulis[2], and Haralampos M. Moutsopoulos[2]

[1]Department of Experimental Physiology, University of Athens, Athens, Greece, [2]Department of Pathophysiology, University of Athens, Athens, Greece

Chapter Outline

Introduction	495	Autoantibodies	502
Clinical Features	496	Etiopathogenesis	502
Local Manifestations (Salivary and Lachrymal Glands)	496	Genetics	502
Systemic Manifestations (Beyond Salivary and Lachrymal Glands)	496	Epigenetics	503
		Environmental Factors	503
Musculoskeletal	496	Viruses	503
Raynaud's Phenomenon	496	Stress	503
Respiratory Tract Involvement	496	Hormonal Factors	503
Gastrointestinal and Hepatobiliary Manifestations	497	Exocrine Gland Dysfunction	504
Renal Involvement	497	Apoptosis	504
Vasculitis	497	Neurotransmission	504
Neuropsychiatric Involvement	497	Aquaporins	504
Endocrine Involvement	498	Structural Abnormalities	504
Lymphoproliferative Disease	498	Tight Junctions	504
Overlapping Autoimmune Entities	498	Basal Membrane	504
Diagnosis and Differential Diagnosis	498	Therapy	504
Autoimmune Features and Pathogenic Mechanisms	498	Future Prospects	505
Immunopathology	498	References	505
Cellular Populations—Cytokine Production	498		

INTRODUCTION

Sjögren's syndrome (SjS) is a chronic, systemic autoimmune disorder, encountered in about 0.5–1% of the general population, usually in middle-aged females (female/male ratio = 9:1). It is characterized by lymphocytic infiltration of exocrine (mainly salivary and lachrymal) glands and tissue destruction. SjS has a wide spectrum of clinical features ranging from sicca symptoms (dry mouth and dry eyes) to systemic manifestations. About 5–8% of patients develop non-Hodgkin lymphoma. SjS may occur either alone as a primary process (primary SjS) or in association with other autoimmune diseases such as systemic lupus erythematosus (SLE), rheumatoid arthritis (RA), and systemic scleroderma (SScl).

B cell hyperactivity is considered as a disease hallmark as evidenced by the presence of hypergammaglobulinemia and serum autoantibodies, both specific and non-specific. These include—among others—antinuclear antibodies against ribonucleoproteinic complexes Ro/SSA and La/SSB, rheumatoid factor (RF), and cryoglobulins (Routsias and Tzioufas, 2010).

Despite the unprecedented progress, SjS etiology remains unknown. Over the last decades several studies have shed light on the underlying pathogenetic mechanisms of SjS development. According to the current belief, the interplay of environmental factors (such as viruses, stress, or hormonal factors) with the host's specific

N. Rose & I. Mackay (Eds): The Autoimmune Diseases, Fifth edition. DOI: http://dx.doi.org/10.1016/B978-0-12-384929-8.00035-6

genetic background can lead to aberrant immune responses, chronic inflammation, destruction of the affected tissue, and ensuing ocular and oral dryness. Epithelium, the principal target of SjS, has been indicated to be an active participant rather than an innocent bystander (Moutsopoulos, 2007).

CLINICAL FEATURES

While local manifestations arising from salivary and lachrymal gland involvement are considered the typical SjS-related features, virtually any other organ system can be affected in the setting of SjS giving rise to systemic manifestations. Depending on the underlying pathophysiological mechanisms, SjS-related systemic manifestations can be largely classified into those related to secretory dysfunction and to those affecting other organs beyond exocrine glands, with the latter being further segregated into non-specific, those characterized by periepithelial infiltrates in parenchymal organs (kidney, lung, liver, endocrine organs), and finally those resulting from immunocomplexes deposition as a result of B cell hyperactivity (purpura, peripheral neuropathy, glomerulonephritis) (Skopouli et al., 2000; Malladi et al., 2012). The latter connotes a disease subset associated with increased risk for lymphoma development and high mortality rates. The majority of SjS patients display an indolent benign course and in the vast majority of patients, the glandular sicca features and serologic profile remains unchanged during disease course, while lymphoma and glomerulonephritis are late events (Skopouli et al., 2000; Ioannidis et al., 2002; Voulgarelis et al., 2012).

Local Manifestations (Salivary and Lachrymal Glands)

Mouth and eye dryness are the most characteristic features of SjS, manifested as difficulty with chewing or swallowing, sore mouth, and/or a sandy feeling or itchiness of the eyes. Dry mouth is often associated with increased incidence of oral infections and development of dental caries. Fungal infections can also be observed, manifested as pseudomembranous or erythematous mucosal lesions, fissured tongue, atrophy of filiform papillae, and angular cheilitis. Salivary flow rates measured for whole saliva or for separate secretions from each major salivary gland (with or without stimulation) reveal reduced salivary flow rates. Sialography discloses various degrees of sialectasis in the majority of patients. Scintigraphy, a functional assessment of salivary glands, provides poorly specific results (Adams et al., 2003). Ultrasonography, conventional magnetic resonance imaging and magnetic resonance sialography may provide useful, non-invasive diagnostic alternatives (Milic et al., 2012). Parotid gland

enlargement (PGE) is a relatively common manifestation of SjS. It is usually bilateral, firm to palpation, asymptomatic, and is considered as an adverse prognostic factor for lymphoma development.

Diminished tear secretion leads to chronic irritation and destruction of the corneal and bulbar conjuctival epithelium [keratoconjuctivitis sicca (KCS)]. Diagnosis of ocular involvement is based on measuring tear production and tear film stability using Schirmer's test (wetting on paper strip of less than 5 mm per 5 minutes) and tear break time, respectively, and on staining of the cornea using Rose Bengal or Lissamine green staining (Vitali et al., 2002). The latter reveals punctuate or filamentary keratitis lesions, characteristics of KCS.

Systemic Manifestations (Beyond Salivary and Lachrymal Glands)

Musculoskeletal

More than half of SjS patients display musculoskeletal manifestations, the most common of which are non-erosive arthritis affecting the small joints and intermittent synovitis. Myalgias, fibromyalgia-like features, and chronic fatigue are also observed (Kassan and Moutsopoulos, 2004).

Raynaud's Phenomenon

Raynaud's phenomenon affects approximately 30–50% of primary SjS patients and often precedes sicca manifestations. The clinical picture of Raynaud's phenomenon is milder in SjS compared to other autoimmune disorders (Skopouli et al., 1990; Youinou et al., 1990; Garcia-Carrasco et al., 2002) and is associated with increased prevalence of extraglandular manifestations.

Respiratory Tract Involvement

Several manifestations of the respiratory tract have been described in the context of SjS. They are usually mild and include dry cough as a result of desiccation of tracheobronchial tree and more rarely dyspnea (xerotrachea/bronchitis sicca). A small airway obstructive pattern is usually detected by pulmonary function testing, possibly resulting from peribronchial and/or peribronchiolar mononuclear inflammation, which gives rise to a peribronchial thickening on high resolution computed tomography imaging ("dirty lung" appearance at chest X-ray). Interstitial involvement occurs less frequently and pleurisy is usually observed in SjS patients with associated lupus features (SLE-associated SjS) (Constantopoulos et al., 1984; Papiris et al., 1999, 2007; Manoussakis et al., 2004).

Gastrointestinal and Hepatobiliary Manifestations

Patients with SjS may complain of dysphagia as a result of esophageal dysmotility or of decreased saliva volume, both observed in SjS (Tsianos et al., 1985). Gastroesophageal and laryngopharyngeal reflux can also occur manifesting as unexplained hoarseness.

Primary biliary cirrhosis (PBC) is the commonest type of liver involvement occurring in SjS, in contrast to auto-immune hepatitis and primary sclerosing cholangitis, both extremely rare. Liver manifestations are usually mild and almost never the presenting manifestations of primary SjS. Liver dysfunction is evident in about 5–10% of such patients and is manifested by the elevation of cholestatic enzymes. In a substantial proportion of primary SjS patients with liver involvement, serum anti-mitochondrial (AMA) reactivity is observed (Skopouli et al., 1994). The latter antibodies are thought to be specific for the diagnosis of PBC. Pancreatic involvement has been previously described in the setting of SjS either as a result of secretory dysfunction or in the form of autoimmune pancreatitis. The latter might connote the presence of underlying IgG4-related disease and therefore should be carefully investigated, given the beneficial response to steroids (Ebert, 2012; Takahashi et al., 2012).

A recent study showed that PBC in the context of SjS remains clinically, serologically, and histologically stable, with ursodeoxycholic acid being the main therapeutic choice (Hatzis et al., 2008).

Renal Involvement

Two types of renal involvement have been described in the setting of primary SjS and include tubulointerstitial nephritis and glomerulonephritis. Interstitial nephritis is the most common renal manifestation usually encountered in young patients; it is usually subclinical and can be expressed as hypokalemia, low urine specific gravity, and alkaline urine pH (Goules et al., 2000). Distal renal tubular acidosis, which can be presented as nephrocalcinosis, can also occur (Moutsopoulos et al., 1991). An extended follow-up in a large number of SjS patients ($n = 715$) for 271.8 person-years revealed that around one-third of these patients had evidence of interstitial involvement and of those approximately two-thirds developed mild chronic renal impairment during follow-up (Goules et al., 2012).

On the other hand, glomerulonephritis is a rather rare renal SjS manifestation usually observed in the context of systemic vasculitis and often associated with hypocomplementemia and cryoglobulinemia conferring increased risk for lymphoproliferation and mortality (Goules et al., 2012). Immune deposits in renal biopsy reveal IgM and complement deposition (Moutsopoulos et al., 1978).

Vasculitis

Vasculitis is observed in about 15% of SjS patients, is usually observed many years after the diagnosis of SjS, and is associated with increased risk for lymphoma development and increased mortality. It usually affects small vessels and the skin is the most frequent site/organ affected. Skin involvement is usually manifested as palpable purpura and more rarely as urticarial lesions. Involvement of other organs, such as peripheral nerves, muscles, and kidneys, has been also described. According to histopathological findings, two types of SjS-associated vasculitis are recognized: leukocytoclastic vasculitis (infiltrates of polymorphonuclear cells) and lymphocytic vasculitis (lymphocyte and monocyte infiltrates). Cryoglobulins (type II, IgMk), high titers of rheumatoid factor, and antinuclear antibodies as well as increased levels of gammaglobulins, hypocomplementemia, and increased erythrocyte sedimentation rate are usually detected (Tsokos et al., 1987; Ramos-Casals et al., 2004).

Neuropsychiatric Involvement

The prevalence of peripheral neuropathy in SjS varies from 2 to 60% in different studies reflecting the heterogenecity of definition criteria and population characteristics. The most common types of peripheral nerve involvement in primary SjS are sensory, small fiber neuropathy (SFN), and sensorimotor neuropathy. Sensory neuropathies are expressed as distal symmetric sensory loss (glove-stocking distribution) or rarely as sensory ataxia. Small fiber neuropathy is manifested as painful and burning paresthesias and deserves particular attention since physical and electrophysiological examination are usually normal; diagnosis is undertaken by skin biopsy (Pavlakis et al., 2011, 2012). On the other hand, sensorimotor neuropathies in primary SjS patients and particularly axonal sensorimotor polyneuropathy are associated with adverse prognostic factors for lymphoma development such as hypocomplementemia, cryoglobulinemia, and vasculitic lesions. Trigeminal neuropathy, usually unilateral, as well as sensorineural hearing loss usually at high frequencies have also been said to occur in some primary SjS patients (Boki et al., 2001).

Central nervous system involvement in primary SjS remains controversial. Hemiparesis, sensory deficits, seizures, movement disorders, cerebellar defects, neurogenic bladder, transverse myelopathy, and multiple sclerosis-like picture have been described in primary SjS patients. However, other investigators using strict criteria for the classification of primary SjS have not substantiated these observations (Alexander et al., 1981; Soliotis et al., 2004).

Psychopathological features and distinct personality traits such as neuroticism, psychoticism, and obsessiveness have been also described in primary SjS patients at a higher frequency compared to healthy controls. Of interest, it has been shown that psychopathological manifestations in the setting of primary SjS are primarily dependent on premorbid personality characteristics and are associated with the presence of antibodies to specific neuropeptides (Karaiskos et al., 2010).

Endocrine Involvement

In patients with SjS, autoantibodies against organ-specific autoantigens of endocrine glands such as thyroid, adrenals, and ovaries have been previously documented at higher rates (in approximately one-fifth of patients) compared to healthy individuals. The presence of these autoantibodies indicates that the classical SjS autoimmune exocrinopathy may be associated with concomitant involvement of endocrine organs, also histopathologically characterized by the presence of lymphocytic periepithelial infiltrations and may eventually give rise to hormonal abnormalities including hypothyroidism, adrenal hyporesponsiveness, and premature ovarian failure (Euthymiopoulou et al., 2007; Mavragani et al., 2012a,b).

Lymphoproliferative Disease

Non-Hodgkin lymphoma (NHL) is encountered in about 5–8% of SjS patients and is usually of indolent course. The most common type is mucosa-associated lymphoid tissue (MALT) lymphomas followed by nodal marginal zone and diffuse large B cell lymphomas. In the majority of cases, lymphoma is located in minor and/or major salivary glands. However, other organs such as the stomach and the lungs can also be involved (Baimpa et al., 2009; Voulgarelis et al., 2012). Peripheral neuropathy, glomerulonephritis, lymphopenia, vasculitis/purpuric lesions, low C4 levels, cryoglobulinemia, and the presence of germinal centers in salivary gland biopsy are well-recognized adverse predictors for lymphoma development (Skopouli et al., 2000; Ioannidis et al., 2002; Theander et al., 2011).

Overlapping Autoimmune Entities

Given that earlier studies have shown that 5% of patients with long-standing RA present a clinically overt SjS, and subclinical sicca complaints can be affirmed by as many as 20% of such patients (Andonopoulos et al., 1987), the term "secondary SjS" has been introduced and mistakenly applied to connote sicca disorder that occurs together with any autoimmune disorder. However, this disregards the possibility for true overlapping entities. In this context, a recent study has revealed that patients with coexisting SLE and SjS appear to constitute a subgroup (9%) of SLE patients with distinct clinical, serological, pathologic, and immunogenetic features in whom SjS is expressed as an overlapping entity, which is largely similar to primary SjS

and usually precedes SLE (Manoussakis et al., 2004). Oral and/or ocular dryness are also observed in approximately 20% of patients with systemic sclerosis, often associated with fibrosis of the exocrine glands. In contrast, sicca manifestations associated with frank lymphocytic infiltrative lesions are extremely common (60%) in patients with limited systemic sclerosis (Drosos et al., 1988). Increased prevalence of autoimmune thyroid disease (ATD) and thyroid dysfunction has been previously reported in patients with primary SjS. Studies so far demonstrate rates of ATD ranging from 6 to 50% (Zeher et al., 2009; D'Arbonneau et al., 2003; Mavragani et al., 2009).

Diagnosis and Differential Diagnosis

Combined clinical, pathologic, and serologic assessment of patients can easily lead to the diagnosis. Recently, an international agreement was established for the definition of SjS, based on the "European American consensus group criteria," which requires the presence of either focal lymphocytic infiltrates in minor salivary glands with a focus score of 1 or more, or anti-SSA/SSB autoantibodies (Box 35.1) (Vitali et al., 2002). Differential diagnosis should consider various medical conditions that may cause mucosa dryness with or without salivary gland enlargement, including adverse effects of drugs, infections, tumors, metabolic disorders, and irradiation. In particular, sarcoidosis, lipoproteinemias types II, IV, and V, chronic graft-versus-host disease, lymphomas, amyloidosis, and infection by human immunodeficiency virus and hepatitis C virus might be misinterpreted as SjS (Kassan and Moutsopoulos, 2004). IgG4-related sialadenitis, formerly known as Mikulicz disease, should also be considered in SjS differential diagnosis (Nocturne et al., 2011). Clinical, pathologic, and serologic features can be helpful for the differential diagnosis. In particular, the identification of serum autoantibodies to Ro/SSA or La/SSB proteins is a strong indication for primary SjS. In elderly individuals, mucosal dryness is frequently an age-related atrophic process. In the presence of sicca symptoms together with fibromyalgia features, the diagnosis of "dry eyes and mouth syndrome" should be considered when SjS classification criteria are not fulfilled (Mariette et al., 2003).

AUTOIMMUNE FEATURES AND PATHOGENIC MECHANISMS

Immunopathology

Cellular Populations—Cytokine Production

T Lymphocytes

The classical SjS histopathological picture is characterized by the presence of periductal lymphocytic infiltrates.

Analysis of cell composition of the mononuclear infiltrates in minor salivary gland (MSG) biopsy specimens allowed the identification of histopathological patterns associating with distinct clinical and serological features.

CD4⁺T rather than CD8⁺ lymphocytes have been previously considered as the main cellular populations in the lymphoepithelial SjS lesions; however, according to recent findings, the incidence of specific immunocytes is associated with the lesion severity, with CD4⁺Th2 lymphocytes predominating in mild and B cells along with Th1 cells in more advanced lesions (Mitsias et al., 2002; Katsifis et al., 2007; Christodoulou et al., 2010). Th17 cells, a newly identified subset of CD4⁺ lymphocytes, which secrete cytokines belonging to the interleukin (IL)-17 family, are also found to contribute to the immunopathological SjS lesion (Katsifis et al., 2009). IL-22, which can exhibit a protective or inflammatory role, has also been recently shown to be produced by Th17 and natural killer (NK) cells (Ciccia et al., 2012). Th follicular cells—another CD4⁺ subset—are the main producers of IL-21 which has been shown to promote B cell differentiation in plasma cells contributing to germinal center formation. Increased IL-21 serum levels in SjS patients in association with serum IgG1 levels in conjunction with heightened expression in the lymphocytic infiltrations of SjS MSGs imply a role for this cytokine in disease pathogenesis (Kang et al., 2011; Scofield, 2011). An emerging role for IL-7 in activation of T cells at the level of SjS salivary glands was recently suggested (Bikker et al., 2012).

Regulatory T lymphocytes (Tregs), the primary suppressive component of the immune system, have recently attracted particular attention in pathogenesis of autoimmunity. In the setting of primary SjS, Tregs are possibly attracted to the site of inflammation, since an inverse correlation of Treg numbers has been observed between the affected salivary gland and the periphery. While the frequency of Tregs seems to positively correlate initially with lesion severity, the mostly advanced SjS lesions are characterized by low Treg incidence. While in early and moderate infiltrations a compensatory control of Tregs in response to Th17 expansion seems to occur, in advanced SjS lesions Tregs may fail to control the immune-mediated tissue injury (Christodoulou et al., 2008).

B Lymphocytes

B cells in the lesion contain intracytoplasmic immunoglobulins with anti-Ro(SSA) and/or anti-La(SSB) reactivity (Tengner et al., 1998). Oligoclonal B lymphocytes and germinal center formation in salivary infiltrate might represent a predisposing factor for lymphoma (Pablos et al., 1994). Comparative studies of peripheral blood and parotid glands from primary SjS patients have indicated the depletion of CD27 expressing memory B cells from

the peripheral blood and accumulation and/or retention of this antigen-experienced B cells in the inflamed salivary gland tissue (Dorner et al., 2002; Youinou et al., 2010).

Macrophages/Dendritic Cells

Increased incidence of IL-18⁺ producing macrophages (MΦ) were found in advanced histopathological lesions in association with cryoglobulinemia, low C4 levels, and salivary gland enlargement, previously regarded as adverse prognostic factors for lymphoma development (Manoussakis et al., 2007).

Dendritic cells (DCs) seem to contribute to histopathological SjS lesion, with two types of DCs being recognized; myeloid DCs (mDCs) and plasmacytoid DCs (pDCs). In early SjS lesions, reduction of blood mDCs possibly due to the preferential trafficking of mDCs into salivary glands is a common event (Ozaki et al., 2010). pDCs, the professional type I interferon (IFN) producers, have also been detected in minor salivary gland biopsies from SjS patients. They are characterized by the presence of Toll-like receptor (TLR)-7 and -9 receptors (sensed by exogenous or endogenous nucleic acids) implying the presence of a viral or viral-like trigger at the level of salivary gland tissue (Figure 35.1). In an attempt to identify possible endogenous elements that may act through TLR or other mechanisms and activate IFN-I pathways, recent work identified the transposable CpG-rich elements belonging in the long interspersed nuclear elements (LINE; L1) family as potential inducers of type I IFN activation in salivary gland tissues (Mavragani and Crow, 2010).

Despite the fact that elevated IFN levels in autoimmune disorders was first reported over 30 years ago, it was during the last few years that activation of the type I IFN system in the generation of autoimmunity attracted particular interest (Hooks et al., 1979).

In accordance with previous observations in SLE and other autoimmune disorders, activation of type I IFN in SjS was evidenced by the upregulation of IFN-related genes—the so-called interferon signature—in peripheral blood mononuclear cell (PBMC) and MSG tissues from SjS patients, heightened type I IFN levels in serum derived from SjS patients, and disease associations with genes involved in activation of type I IFN pathway. Moreover, the IFNα-producing pDCs—the professional IFNα-producing cells—were detected in the salivary glands of SjS patients, but not in controls. While the initial triggers for type I IFN production in the setting of SjS remain elusive, exogenous, such as viral agents or endogenous signals, might account for pDC activation through ligation of TLR-dependent or -independent pathways (Vakaloglou and Mavragani, 2011). Of interest, according to the findings by Ittah et al., B cell activating factor (BAFF), a member of the tumor necrosis factor (TNF) family, was shown to be overproduced by salivary gland

> **Box 35.1 European American Consensus Group Criteria**
>
> 1. Ocular symptoms (at least one present)
>   Persistent, troublesome dry eyes every day for longer than 3 months
>   Recurrent sensation of sand or gravel in the eyes
>   Use of a tear substitute more than three times a day
> 2. Oral symptoms (at least one present)
>   Feeling of dry mouth every day for at least 3 months
>   Recurrent feeling of swollen salivary glands as an adult
>   Need to drink liquids to aid in swallowing dry food
> 3. Objective evidence of dry eyes (at least one present)
>   Schirmer test ≤ 5 mm/5 mn
>   Van Bijsterveld score ≥ 4 (after lissamin test)
> 4. Objective evidence of salivary gland involvement (at least one present)
>   Salivary gland scintigraphy
>   Parotid sialography
>   Unstimulated salivary flow (≤1.5 mL per 15 min, ≤ 0.1 ml/min)
>
> 5. Histological features
>   Positive minor salivary gland biopsy sample (focus score ≥ 1: this refers to a cluster of 50 or more lymphocytes per lobule when at least four lobules are assessed)
> 6. Autoantibodies
>   Presence of antibodies to SS-A (Ro) or to SS-B (La)
>   Classification of primary Sjögren's syndrome requires:
>   - four of six criteria, including a positive minor salivary gland biopsy sample or antibody to SS-A/SS-B,
>   - or three of the four objective criteria (criteria 3 to 6)
>   Classification of secondary Sjögren's syndrome requires an established connective tissue disease and one sicca symptom (criteria 1 or 2) plus any three of the four objective criteria (items 3, 4, 5).
>
> Exclusions include previous radiotherapy to the head and neck, lymphoma, sarcoidosis, graft-versus-host disease, and infection with hepatitis C virus, or HIV, use of anticholinergic drugs.

epithelial cells (SGECs) upon stimulation with ssRNA in an IFN-I-dependent manner (Ittah et al., 2008).

The BAFF gene—located on chromosome 13q33.3—contains 6 exons and 5 introns and encodes a type II transmembrane protein of 285 amino acids in humans. A newly identified splice variant lacking the exon 4 named Δ4 BAFF has been found to act as a transcription factor for the paternal gene and to regulate innate immune and apoptosis pathways. Several single nucleotide polymorphisms of the BAFF gene have been previously described in the setting of SjS and SLE, with the rs9524828 T allele being found to associate with BAFF levels but not with disease susceptibility (Kawasaki et al., 2002; Nossent et al., 2008; Lahiri et al., 2008).

BAFF is mainly produced by cells of mononuclear lineage but also by other cell types including bone marrow cells, synoviocytes, astrocytes, and SjS salivary epithelial cells. The major receptors of BAFF include the transmembrane activator and calcium modulator ligand interactor (TACI), the B cell maturation antigen receptor (BCMA), and the BAFF receptor (BAFF-R) (Lahiri et al., 2012).

BAFF, which is crucial for the development and survival of B lymphocytes, has been found elevated in SjS serum in association with antibodies against ribonucleoproteins and B cell clonal expansion in the salivary glands and disease activity score (Nossent et al., 2008). Accordingly, BAFF-transgenic mice, which are characterized by T2 cell hyperplasia in exocrine glands and increased numbers of mature B cells, manifest an SLE-like disease, while in advanced age they develop an SjS-resembling phenotype (Mackay et al., 1999; Groom

et al., 2002; Quartuccio et al., 2012). Taken together, activation of type I IFN with subsequent BAFF induction represents a model bridging innate immune mechanisms with B cell hyperactivity, a hallmark of SjS.

Epithelial Cells

Given that the typical histopathological lesion in affected tissues (salivary, bronchial, cholangial, kidney) in the context of primary SjS is characterized by lymphocytic infiltrates that surround and sometimes invade the epithelium, the term "autoimmune epithelitis" has been proposed identifying the epithelium as an important player in the SjS pathogenesis (Moutsopoulos, 2007). Salivary gland epithelial cells exhibit a plethora of immunoreactive molecules including molecules facilitating antigen presentation (MHC-I and MHC-II), costimulation (CD40, B.7/CD80,PD-L1), cell adhesion (ICAM.1/CD54), and apoptosis-related molecules (Fas, FasL). Activated epithelia are also the source of several inflammatory cytokines (IL-1, -6, -8, TNFα, and adiponectin), chemokines, and BAFF-mediating lymphocyte recruitment and organization of germinal centers as well as activation and proliferation of B lymphocytes (Manoussakis and Kapsogeorgou, 2010; Tzioufas et al., 2012).

Additionally, recent studies demonstrated that SGECs express functional molecules of the innate immunity such as the Toll-like receptors (TLRs)-1, -2, -3, -4, -7, -9, as well as the CD91 receptor that mediates endocytosis and antigen presentation (Kawakami et al., 2007; Spachidou et al., 2007; Bourazopoulou et al., 2009). Hence, the SjS epithelial

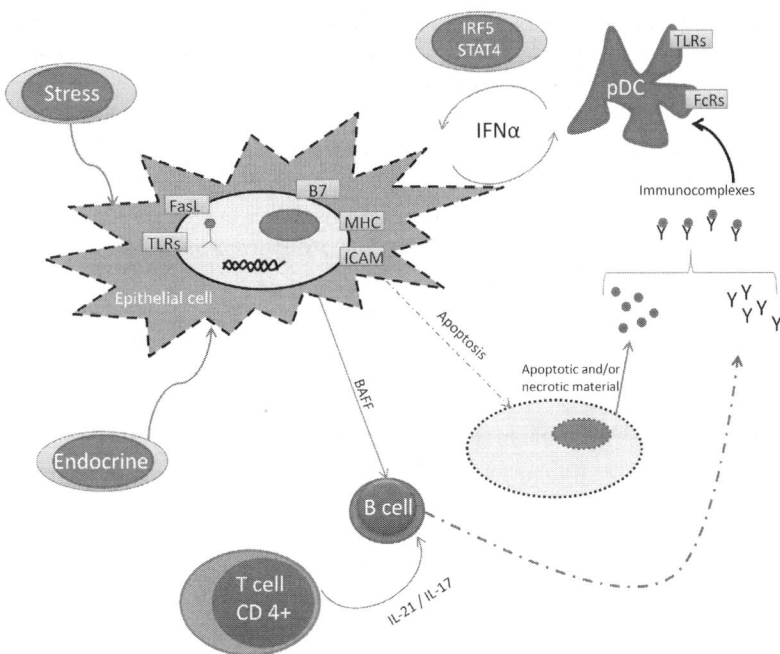

FIGURE 35.1 Epitheliotropic viruses or endogenous nucleic acids might serve as initial triggers in type I interferon (IFN) production—genetically determined by IRF-5/STAT-4 polymorphisms—by plasmacytoid dendritic cells (PDCs) through activation of Toll-like receptor (TLR)-dependent or independent pathways. Once produced, type I IFN along with environmental stressors and hormonal alterations might lead to inappropriate epithelial activation through upregulation of several immunomodulatory molecules (costimulatory, adhesion, MHC-II, etc.), BAFF production, and apoptotic events which result to exposure of autoantigens such as Ro/SSA and La/SSB and generation of disease-specific anti-Ro/SSA and La/SSB autoantibodies. The latter, in conjunction with autoantigens, would form immune complexes which in turn further promote the activation of type I IFN pathways through triggering of PDCs or other IFNα producing cells. On the other hand, the activated epithelial cell, serving as an antigen presenting cell, can activate several CD4+ T cell subtypes, which promote B cell differentiation and survival possibly through IL-17 and IL-21 secretion. IFNα perpetuates the autoimmune response through several immunomodulatory actions, including upregulation of chemotactic molecules and further recruitment of inflammatory cells, accumulation of helper and/or inducer memory T and B cells, B cell activation, autoantibody production, and ultimately tissue destruction with simultaneous B cell monoclonal expansion.

cell can act as an antigen-presenting cell to T lymphocytes since it intrinsically provides antigen-presenting and costimulatory molecules, contributes to the generation of the inflammatory microenvironment (expression of inflammatory cytokines), and can recruit, through lymphoattractant chemokines (CXCL13, CXCL21), B and T lymphocytes providing survival signals for the B lymphocytes under the effect of BAFF (Tzioufas et al., 2012) (Figure 35.1).

Proangiogenic factors shown to be produced by SGECs upon stimulation with SjS autoantibodies together with increased expression of neuropilin-1 in SjS SGECs (a co-receptor for members of the VEGF family) provide a potential mechanism for the enhanced angiogenesis shown in SjS salivary gland tissues (Sisto et al., 2012a,b). Proangiogenic factors such as VEGF and IL-8 have also been recently shown to be induced by SGECs upon stimulation of histamine receptor 4 by T cell- and dendritic cell-derived histamine at the level of salivary gland (Stegaev et al., 2012).

Apoptosis has been considered as one of the characteristic features of the SjS salivary gland epithelium. It has

been well documented that both SGECs and salivary gland tissues from SjS patients demonstrate increased *in situ* expression of pro-apoptotic molecules such as Fas, Fas-ligand, and Bax protein. The same is applied for the cultured non-neoplastic SGECs. Apoptosis mediated through Fas/FasL pathway is dependent on IFNγ which was found to reduce the survival of SGECs in a dose- and time-dependent manner (Abu-Helu et al., 2001; Manoussakis and Kapsogeorgou, 2007). The CD40 molecule, which is also upregulated by IFNγ, has been found to sensitize SGECs to apoptosis mediated by the Fas/FasL system possibly through downregulation of the anti-apoptotic protein cFLIP. The latter, and other anti-apoptotic molecules such as Bcl-2, are constitutively expressed by SGECs and are thought to act as defensive and tissue-repair mechanisms in an attempt to compensate for the increased rate of apoptosis observed in SjS (Abu-Helu et al., 2001; Dimitriou et al., 2002; Ping et al., 2005). Recent data support the role of B cells in inducing SGEC apoptosis through protein kinase C delta activation (Varin et al., 2012). Apoptosis represents a central mechanism of tolerance break through membrane expression or release of modified autoantigens (apotopes), which subsequently can trigger an inflammatory immune response at the level of SjS salivary gland tissue. Identification of apotopes, which are defined as epitopes on the surface of apoptotic cells by B cell epitope mapping techniques, appear as a promising novel diagnostic marker for both SjS and SLE. For instance, several La apotopes react with the majority of sera from mothers of infants with congenital heart block and a Ro60 apotope is specific for a subgroup of SLE patients characterized by isolated anti-Ro60 responses (Reed et al., 2007, 2008, 2010).

Another mechanism of autoantigen presentation to the immune system is mediated by small membrane vesicles (30–100 nm) of endosomal origin, the so-called exosomes. These are released by various cell types and represent a mechanism of intercellular communication and cellular material transportation. It is believed that they are able to relocate antigens to APCs or to T lymphocytes. Study from our group has shown that exosomes can be released from cultured SGECs and contain (among others) Ro, La, and Sm autoantigens, the most well-recognized antigenic targets in SjS and SLE (Kapsogeorgou et al., 2005).

Autoantibodies

From an immunological point of view, B cell activation is the hallmark of the syndrome resulting in hypergammaglobulinemia, cryoglobulinemia, and autoantibody production. The latter includes the presence of increased titers of antinuclear antibodies and rheumatoid factor as well as reactivities against the ribonucleoproteinic complexes Ro/SSA and La/SSB. Antibodies against a-fodrin—an organ-specific cytoskeletal autoantigen—initially purified by salivary glands of a murine SjS mouse model have been also detected in almost all sera from patients with primary SjS (Haneji et al., 1997; Witte et al., 2000, 2003). However, subsequent reports failed to demonstrate their superiority in terms of specificity and sensitivity in comparison to anti-Ro/SSA and anti-La/SSB testing (Ruiz-Tiscar et al., 2005; Locht et al., 2008). As a result their use in clinical practice is quite limited. Hypergammaglobulinemia has been associated with cutaneous vasculitis, articular, pulmonary or renal involvement and cryoglobulinemia with B cell lymphoma development and increased mortality rates (Skopouli et al., 2000; Ioannidis et al., 2002). Antibodies directed against Ro/SSA and La/SSB antigens are detected in approximately 60% and 30% of SjS patients, respectively, and have been previously shown to be associated with earlier disease onset, longer disease duration, parotid gland enlargement, higher frequency of extraglandular manifestations, more intense lymphocytic infiltration of the minor salivary glands, other B cell activation markers,

as well as the presence of HLADR2 and DR3. While RNA immunoprecipitation has been considered as the reference method for detection of these autoantibodies, counterimmunoelectrophoresis demonstrates increased reliability with high levels of sensitivity and specificity. Commercially available enzyme-linked immunosorbent assay (ELISA) kits are now widely used in clinical practice (Manoussakis et al., 1993; Mavragani et al., 2000; Tzioufas et al., 2002; Hernandez-Molina et al., 2011). On the other hand, anticentromere (ACA) antibodies occur in 3.7% of SjS patients designating the presence of an intermediate scleroderma-like phenotype. The ACA$^+$ SjS subgroup demonstrates a higher prevalence of Raynaud's phenomenon and dysphagia but lower rates of dry eyes, hypergammaglobulinemia, anti-Ro/SSA, and anti-La/SSB antibodies compared to ACA$^-$ SjS patients. Furthermore, compared to age–sex matched counterparts with systemic sclerosis, the ACA$^+$ SjS subset shares a less aggressive phenotype with fewer occurrences of telangiectasias, puffy fingers, sclerodactyly, Raynaud's phenomenon, digital ulcers, and gastroesophageal reflux, which rarely evolves in full blown scleroderma (Bournia et al., 2010).

Features related to the presence of peri-epithelial lesions of parenchymal organs such as the liver and the kidney have been associated with autoantibodies against mitochondrial and carbonic anhydrase, respectively (Hatzis et al., 2008; Bournia et al., 2010). The majority of AMA$^+$ primary SjS patients (5%) demonstrated lesions compatible with primary biliary cirrhosis in their liver biopsies and tended to experience slow progression in clinical, biochemical, and histological terms. Anti-carbonic anhydrase II antibody has been described in a number of patients with SjS and associated with distal renal tubular acidosis (Takemoto et al., 2005). Additionally, we have recently identified a subset of primary SjS (approximately 17% of patients) characterized by the presence of antibodies against 21-hydroxylase—a major adrenal autoantigen—which was associated with adrenal gland hyporesponsiveness and the presence of B cell activating cytokines at the level of salivary gland tissue (Mavragani et al., 2012b).

Finally, antibodies to cyclic citrullinated peptides have been previously detected in a small percentage of sera from primary SjS patients in association with the presence of synovitis, and their presence might connote progression to inflammatory arthritis (Gottenberg et al., 2005; Atzeni et al., 2008; Haga et al., 2011; Ryu et al., 2012).

ETIOPATHOGENESIS

Genetics

Multiple immunogenetic studies, familial clustering, and the increased frequency of certain major histocompatibility complex (MHC)-II alleles strongly indicate the genetic predisposition of SjS. Studies from different countries and ethnic groups have revealed an increased frequency of several HLA DR alleles. Various HLA class II alleles may have an important role in the regulation of immune responses against Ro/SSA and La/SSB ribonucleoproteins, with DR15 being associated with anti-Ro/SSA antibodies alone, and DR3 with both anti-Ro/SSA and anti-La/SSB antibodies (Mann and Moutsopoulos, 1983; Harley et al., 1986; Gottenberg et al., 2003; Cruz-Tapias et al., 2012).

Over the last years, the potential role of single nucleotide polymorphisms (SNPs) outside the HLA locus was supported by data derived from case−control association studies. Polymorphisms of the interferon regulating factor-5 (IRF5) gene, implicated in the activation of type I IFN pathway and the signal transducer and activator of transcription 4 (STAT4) gene—a transcription factor involved in Th1 and Th17 response promoting the secretion of IFNγ—seem to confer increased disease susceptibility. Of interest, the concomitant presence of IRF5 and STAT4 SNPs appears to have an additive effect in the susceptibility for SjS (Miceli-Richard et al., 2007, 2009; Nordmark et al., 2009). Polymorphisms of the genes involved in B cell differentiation and activation as well as of lymphotoxin α/lymphotoxin β/TNF locus—previously found to be upregulated in SjS salivary tissues and implicated in lymphoid tissue formation—have been also found to increase disease risk (Nordmark et al., 2011; Bolstad et al., 2012).

Epigenetics

Growing evidence is highly suggestive of the contributory role of epigenetic mechanisms such as microRNAs in pathogenesis of autoimmunity. The emerging role of these non-coding RNAs, which regulate gene expression as a potential disease biomarker, was explored in recent studies (Alevizos et al., 2011; Kapsogeorgou et al., 2011). Mir146a, previously shown to regulate innate immune responses was found to be upregulated in PBMCs from SjS patients (Kapsogeorgou et al., 2011; Pauley et al., 2011). Deep sequencing of small RNAs from SjS patients revealed the presence of previously unidentified microRNAs with high disease specificity. Further functional studies are required to delineate the role of miRNAs in the induction of autoimmune processes in the setting of SjS (Tandon et al., 2012).

Methylation mechanisms have been postulated as major epigenetic regulators with implications in the pathogenesis of autoimmunity and cancer. At the level of salivary gland biopsies, overexpression of several enzymes of the methylation machinery have been found to be strongly correlated with the mRNA expression of L1 retroelements, implying the presence of a compensatory defensive mechanism against aberrant overexpression of endogenous threats against immune homeostasis (Mavragani and

Crow, 2010). No alterations of the methylation status of the IRF5 promoter in the setting of SS have been detected (Gestermann et al., 2012).

Environmental Factors

Viruses

Viruses have been long suspected for the induction of SjS, since transient or persistent infection of epithelial cells by a putative virus may be an initiating event for autoimmune reactions. Research has been focused on various types of viruses, including cytomegalovirus, Epstein−Barr virus, human herpes virus type-6, HTLV-1, retroviruses, HCV virus, and enteroviruses; however, results have been inconclusive (Triantafyllopoulou and Moutsopoulos, 2007; Lee et al., 2012). Of interest, Epstein−Barr virus-encoded small RNA (EBER) derived from EBV infected cells in complex with the SjS-related autoantigen La/SSB can trigger type I IFN production through TL3 activation (Iwakiri et al., 2009). Endogenous viral elements have also been proposed as potential contributors in disease pathogenesis.

Stress

Stressful life events prior to disease onset in conjunction with a lack of adequate coping strategies have been previously indicated as SjS triggers (Karaiskos et al., 2009).

Hormonal Factors

Female predominance together with disease onset around menopause supports a role of hormonal factors in SjS. Estrogen deficiency in mice with a healthy background has been previously found to induce SjS-like autoimmune exocrinopathy and increased apoptosis, both resolved after estrogen administration; overexpression of the retinoblastoma-associated protein 48 (RbAp48) specific for estrogen deficiency-dependent apoptosis in the exocrine glands has been shown to account for these phenomena (Ishimaru et al., 2003, 2008). The contribution of estrogen deficiency in the generation of autoimmune responses was also shown in another mouse model lacking aromatase; deficiency of the latter which catalyzes the production of estrogens by androgens led to development of severe—SjS reminiscent—autoimmune lymphocytic exocrinopathy (Shim et al., 2004).

Estrogens have been previously shown to exert immunomodulatory actions in normal SGECs by inhibiting the IFN-γ-induced ICAM-1 expression, an adhesion molecule denoting cellular activation. Recent findings support estrogen unresponsiveness of SjS-SGECs as a potential contributor of intrinsic epithelial activation observed in SjS (Tsinti et al., 2009; Manoussakis et al., 2012).

Androgen deficiency has been additionally implicated in SjS induction. Reduced salivary gland tissue levels of dehydrotestosterone (DHT)—the active form of testosterone—were previously described in SjS patients. This might be due either to low systemic DHEA levels—the main source of DHT in females—or to defective intracrine DHT production, both observed in SjS patients. DHT has been previously suggested as an apoptosis inhibitor of salivary epithelial cells. Therefore, lack of androgen leads to unopposed induction of estrogen deficiency-dependent apoptosis in menopausal SjS patients accounting for the aberrant immune responses (Porola et al., 2008; Spaan et al., 2009; Konttinen et al., 2012).

EXOCRINE GLAND DYSFUNCTION

Despite the original belief that sicca manifestations result from exocrine gland destruction due to local lymphocytic infiltration, a growing body of evidence supports the presence of additional operative mechanisms in the alteration of glandular homeostasis (Hayashi, 2011).

Apoptosis

Several SjS animal models revealed the occurrence of hyposalivation related to apoptotic death of acinar cell events prior to lymphocytic infiltration, implying that cell death pathways might be the primary triggering events in initiation of the autoimmune process (Humphreys-Beher et al., 1998). Innate stimuli, such as TL3-ligands and IFNα itself together with other proinflammatory cytokines have been previously suggested to activate apoptotic pathways and salivary dysfunction (Deshmukh et al., 2009; Manoussakis et al., 2010).

Neurotransmission

Salivary gland secretory processes are under autonomic parasympathetic control through interaction of acetylcholine with muscarinic receptors, mainly M1 and M3 in the salivary glands. Antibodies to muscarinic receptors, proinflammatory cytokines such as TNFα, IL1α, and IL-1β, impaired neurotransmitter responsiveness, and destructions of neural innervations have been proposed as possible culprits (Pedersen et al., 2000; Gordon et al., 2001; Zoukhri and Kublin, 2002; Jin et al., 2012). Alterations of other neuropeptides, such as VIP and NPY, have been also observed in SjS (Santavirta et al., 1997).

Aquaporins

Optimal salivary secretion requires the presence of functionally adequate water channels, termed aquaporins. Abnormal distribution and expression of aquaporin 5 in SjS-SGECs has been previously proposed as a contributor in the observed hyposalivation, even in the absence of intense inflammation (Steinfeld et al., 2001).

Structural Abnormalities

Tight Junctions

Changes in tight junctions protein levels with ensuing alterations in tissue integrity at the level of salivary SjS glands, possibly under the influence of locally produced cytokines, have been previously implicated in SjS-related salivary gland dysfunction (Baker et al., 2008; Ewert et al., 2010).

Basal Membrane

Disorganization of the basal membrane in labial salivary gland acini and ducts has been attributed to altered expression of laminin/laminin receptor and collagen IV levels possibly under the effect of local cytokine milieu, allowing the invasion of T-cytotoxic lymphocytes (Defilippi et al., 1992; McArthur et al., 1993; Molina et al., 2006). Additional data support alterations in laminin levels as a result of androgen deprivation known to occur in SjS, leading to abnormal remodeling though inhibition of differentiation of intercalated duct progenitors to acinar cells (Porola et al., 2010).

THERAPY

Treatment of SjS is directed to provide symptomatic relief and to recognize and treat disease complications in a timely fashion. In particular, patients with adverse prognostic factors should be regularly followed for early identification of lymphoproliferation. For KCS, the application of eye lubricants is the mainstay of treatment. Diuretics, antidepressants, and histamines may worsen lachrymal and salivary hypofunction and should be used with caution. Patients with residual glandular function may benefit from the oral administration of the muscarinic M3 receptor agonists pilcarpine (Vivino et al., 1999) and cevimeline (Petrone et al., 2002). Corticosteroid containing ophthalmic solutions should be avoided as they may induce corneal lesions or promote infections. Dental treatment with fluoride retards damage of teeth surfaces. For tender salivary gland enlargement local application of moist heat and non-steroidal anti-inflammatory drugs may be helpful. Bacterial infection as well as lymphoma should always be considered. Vaginal lubricants may be used to treat vaginal dryness and dyspareunia. The decision for systemic therapeutic intervention remains empirical and is based on the severity of extra-glandular manifestations. Non-steroidal anti-inflammatory drugs and/or hydroxychloroquine may be administered for arthralgias/myalgias and methotrexate for persistent arthritis. Despite encouraging initial results the oral administration of natural human IFNα has shown questionable efficacy (Cummins et al., 2003). Also, studies with anti-TNF agents, infliximab and etanercept, did not show any efficacy in primary SjS possibly due to augmentation of the already activated type I interferon—BAFF pathway (Mariette et al., 2004; Mavragani et al., 2007). Patients with overt distal renal tubular acidosis may be orally treated with sodium bicarbonate to avoid nephrocalcinosis. For Raynaud's phenomenon avoidance of cold exposure, emotional stress, and smoking should be recommended. Leukocytoclastic vasculitis does not require specific therapy. Corticosteroids are mainly employed for severe extraglandular manifestations. Aggressive treatment with cytotoxic drugs carries an increased risk for lymphoma development and should be reserved for threatening systemic manifestations. The treatment of malignant lymphoma in SjS patients is based on histological type and extent. The implication of ongoing B cell activation in the pathophysiology of SjS suggests targeted anti-B cell therapies as a major therapeutic strategy (Mavragani et al., 2006; Voulgarelis et al., 2012).

Finally, the contribution of patient-based associations such as the Sjögren's Syndrome Foundation in the management of SjS is of paramount importance, through patient/family education, coping strategies enhancement, and increase of public awareness of the disease burden.

FUTURE PROSPECTS

Despite the intense research efforts worldwide, the initiating events which lead to break of tolerance and eventually to local immune injury at the level of exocrine glands remain obscure. Given the recent identification of the LINE-1 endogenous retroviral-like elements at the level of SjS salivary glands in strong correlation with local IFNα levels, elucidation of the epigenetic mechanisms underlying their inappropriate overexpression seems a logical next step. Additionally, careful characterization of various SjS clinical phenotypes and association with distinct molecular signatures would allow the designation of tailored therapies. Comorbidities in the setting of SjS have not been adequately addressed so far and would be a field of further clinical research. Finally, elucidation of underlying mechanisms of lymphomagenesis in the setting of SjS would enhance our understanding of transition between benign autoimmunity and malignant transformation eventually allowing the development of preventive strategies for high risk individuals.

REFERENCES

Abu-Helu, R.F., Dimitriou, I.D., Kapsogeorgou, E.K., Moutsopoulos, H.M., Manoussakis, M.N., 2001. Induction of salivary gland epithelial cell injury in Sjogren's syndrome: in vitro assessment of T cell-derived cytokines and Fas protein expression. J. Autoimmun. 17, 141—153.

Adams, B.K., Al Attia, H.M., Parkar, S., 2003. Salivary gland scintigraphy in Sjogren's syndrome: are quantitative indices the answer? Nucl. Med. Commun. 24, 1011—1016.

Alevizos, I., Alexander, S., Turner, R.J., Illei, G.G., 2011. MicroRNA expression profiles as biomarkers of minor salivary gland inflammation and dysfunction in Sjogren's syndrome. Arthritis Rheum. 63, 535—544.

Alexander, G.E., Provost, T.T., Stevens, M.B., Alexander, E.L., 1981. Sjogren syndrome: central nervous system manifestations. Neurology. 31, 1391—1396.

Andonopoulos, A.P., Drosos, A.A., Skopouli, F.N., Acritidis, N.C., Moutsopoulos, H.M., 1987. Secondary Sjogren's syndrome in rheumatoid arthritis. J. Rheumatol. 14, 1098—1103.

Atzeni, F., Sarzi-Puttini, P., Lama, N., Bonacci, E., Bobbio-Pallavicini, F., Montecucco, C., et al., 2008. Anti-cyclic citrullinated peptide antibodies in primary Sjogren syndrome may be associated with non-erosive synovitis. Arthritis Res. Ther. 10, R51.

Baimpa, E., Dahabreh, I.J., Voulgarelis, M., Moutsopoulos, H.M., 2009. Hematologic manifestations and predictors of lymphoma development in primary Sjogren syndrome: clinical and pathophysiologic aspects. Medicine (Baltimore). 88, 284—293.

Baker, O.J., Camden, J.M., Redman, R.S., Jones, J.E., Seye, C.I., Erb, L., et al., 2008. Proinflammatory cytokines tumor necrosis factor-alpha and interferon-gamma alter tight junction structure and function in the rat parotid gland Par-C10 cell line. Am. J. Physiol., Cell Physiol. 295, C1191—C1201.

Bikker, A., Kruize, A.A., Wenting, M., Versnel, M.A., Bijlsma, J.W., Lafeber, F.P., et al., 2012. Increased interleukin (IL-7) R alpha expression in salivary glands of patients with primary Sjogren's syndrome is restricted to T cells and correlates with IL-7 expression, lymphocyte numbers and activity. Ann. Rheum. Dis. 71, 1023—1027.

Boki, K.A., Ioannidis, J.P., Segas, J.V., Maragkoudakis, P.V., Petrou, D., Adamopoulos, G.K., et al., 2001. How significant is sensorineural hearing loss in primary Sjogren's syndrome? An individually matched case—control study. J. Rheumatol. 28, 798—801.

Bolstad, A.I., Le Hellard, S., Kristjansdottir, G., Vasaitis, L., Kvarnstrom, M., Sjowall, C., et al., 2012. Association between genetic variants in the tumour necrosis factor/lymphotoxin alpha/lymphotoxin beta locus and primary Sjogren's syndrome in Scandinavian samples. Ann. Rheum. Dis. 71, 981—988.

Bourazopoulou, E., Kapsogeorgou, E.K., Routsias, J.G., Manoussakis, M.N., Moutsopoulos, H.M., Tzioufas, A.G., 2009. Functional expression of the alpha 2-macroglobulin receptor CD91 in salivary gland epithelial cells. J. Autoimmun. 33, 141—146.

Bournia, V.K., Diamanti, K.D., Vlachoyiannopoulos, P.G., Moutsopoulos, H.M., 2010. Anticentromere antibody positive Sjogren's syndrome: a retrospective descriptive analysis. Arthritis Res. Ther. 12, R47.

Christodoulou, M.I., Kapsogeorgou, E.K., Moutsopoulos, N.M., Moutsopoulos, H.M., 2008. Foxp3 + T-regulatory cells in Sjogren's syndrome: correlation with the grade of the autoimmune lesion and certain adverse prognostic factors. Am. J. Pathol. 173, 1389—1396.

Christodoulou, M.I., Kapsogeorgou, E.K., Moutsopoulos, H.M., 2010. Characteristics of the minor salivary gland infiltrates in Sjogren's syndrome. J. Autoimmun. 34, 400—407.

Ciccia, F., Guggino, G., Rizzo, A., Ferrante, A., Raimondo, S., Giardina, A., et al., 2012. Potential involvement of IL-22 and IL-22-producing cells in the inflamed salivary glands of patients with Sjogren's syndrome. Ann. Rheum. Dis. 71, 295–301.

Constantopoulos, S.H., Drosos, A.A., Maddison, P.J., Moutsopoulos, H. M., 1984. Xerotrachea and interstitial lung disease in primary Sjogren's syndrome. Respiration. 46, 310–314.

Cruz-Tapias, P., Rojas-Villarraga, A., Maier-Moore, S., Anaya, J.M., 2012. HLA and Sjogren's syndrome susceptibility. A meta-analysis of worldwide studies. Autoimmun. Rev. 11, 7–281.

Cummins, M.J., Papas, A., Kammer, G.M., Fox, P.C., 2003. Treatment of primary Sjogren's syndrome with low-dose human interferon alfa administered by the oromucosal route: combined phase III results. Arthritis Rheum. 49, 585–593.

Defilippi, P., Silengo, L., Tarone, G., 1992. Alpha 6.beta 1 integrin (laminin receptor) is down-regulated by tumor necrosis factor alpha and interleukin-1 beta in human endothelial cells. J. Biol. Chem. 267, 18303–18307.

Deshmukh, U.S., Nandula, S.R., Thimmalapura, P.R., Scindia, Y.M., Bagavant, H., 2009. Activation of innate immune responses through Toll-like receptor 3 causes a rapid loss of salivary gland function. J. Oral Pathol. Med. 38, 42–47.

Dimitriou, I.D., Kapsogeorgou, E.K., Moutsopoulos, H.M., Manoussakis, M.N., 2002. CD40 on salivary gland epithelial cells: high constitutive expression by cultured cells from Sjogren's syndrome patients indicating their intrinsic activation. Clin. Exp. Immunol. 127, 386–392.

Dorner, T., Hansen, A., Jacobi, A., Lipsky, P.E., 2002. Immunglobulin repertoire analysis provides new insights into the immunopathogenesis of Sjogren's syndrome. Autoimmun. Rev. 1, 119–124.

Drosos, A.A., Andonopoulos, A.P., Costopoulos, J.S., Stavropoulos, E. D., Papadimitriou, C.S., Moutsopoulos, H.M., 1988. Sjogren's syndrome in progressive systemic sclerosis. J. Rheumatol. 15, 965–968.

D'Arbonneau, F., Ansart, S., Le Berre, R., Dueymes, M., Youinou, P., Pennec, Y.L., 2003. Thyroid dysfunction in primary Sjogren's syndrome: a long-term followup study. Arthritis Rheum. 49, 804–809.

Ebert, E.C., 2012. Gastrointestinal and hepatic manifestations of Sjogren syndrome. J. Clin. Gastroenterol. 46, 25–30.

Euthymiopoulou, K., Aletras, A.J., Ravazoula, P., Niarakis, A., Daoussis, D., Antonopoulos, I., et al., 2007. Antiovarian antibodies in primary Sjogren's syndrome. Rheumatol. Int. 27, 1149–1155.

Ewert, P., Aguilera, S., Alliende, C., Kwon, Y.J., Albornoz, A., Molina, C., et al., 2010. Disruption of tight junction structure in salivary glands from Sjogren's syndrome patients is linked to proinflammatory cytokine exposure. Arthritis Rheum. 62, 1280–1289.

Garcia-Carrasco, M., Siso, A., Ramos-Casals, M., Rosas, J., De La Red, G., Gil, V., et al., 2002. Raynaud's phenomenon in primary Sjogren's syndrome. Prevalence and clinical characteristics in a series of 320 patients. J. Rheumatol. 29, 726–730.

Gestermann, N., Koutero, M., Belkhir, R., Tost, J., Mariette, X., Miceli-Richard, C., 2012. Methylation profile of the promoter region of IRF5 in primary Sjogren's syndrome. Eur. Cytokine Netw. 23, 166–172.

Gordon, T.P., Bolstad, A.I., Rischmueller, M., Jonsson, R., Waterman, S.A., 2001. Autoantibodies in primary Sjogren's syndrome: new insights into mechanisms of autoantibody diversification and disease pathogenesis. Autoimmunity. 34, 123–132.

Gottenberg, J.E., Busson, M., Loiseau, P., Cohen-Solal, J., Lepage, V., Charron, D., et al., 2003. In primary Sjogren's syndrome, HLA class

II is associated exclusively with autoantibody production and spreading of the autoimmune response. Arthritis Rheum. 48, 2240–2245.

Gottenberg, J.E., Mignot, S., Nicaise-Rolland, P., Cohen-Solal, J., Aucouturier, F., Goetz, J., et al., 2005. Prevalence of anti-cyclic citrullinated peptide and anti-keratin antibodies in patients with primary Sjogren's syndrome. Ann. Rheum. Dis. 64, 114–117.

Goules, A., Masouridi, S., Tzioufas, A.G., Ioannidis, J.P., Skopouli, F. N., Moutsopoulos, H.M., 2000. Clinically significant and biopsy-documented renal involvement in primary Sjogren syndrome. Medicine (Baltimore). 79, 241–249.

Goules, A., Tatouli, I., Drosos, A., Skopouli, F., Moutsopoulos, H.M., Athanasios, G., 2012. Clinically significant and biopsy-documented renal involvement in primary Sjogren's syndrome: clinical presentation and outcome. Arthritis Rheum. 64, S510.

Groom, J., Kalled, S.L., Cutler, A.H., Olson, C., Woodcock, S.A., Schneider, P., et al., 2002. Association of BAFF/BLyS overexpression and altered B cell differentiation with Sjogren's syndrome. J. Clin. Invest. 109, 59–68.

Haga, H.J., Andersen, D.T., Peen, E., 2011. Prevalence of IgA class antibodies to cyclic citrullinated peptide (anti-CCP) in patients with primary Sjogren's syndrome, and its association to clinical manifestations. Clin. Rheumatol. 30, 369–372.

Haneji, N., Nakamura, T., Takio, K., Yanagi, K., Higashiyama, H., Saito, I., et al., 1997. Identification of alpha-fodrin as a candidate autoantigen in primary Sjogren's syndrome. Science. 276, 604–607.

Harley, J.B., Alexander, E.L., Bias, W.B., Fox, O.F., Provost, T.T., Reichlin, M., et al., 1986. Anti-Ro (SS-A) and anti-La (SS-B) in patients with Sjogren's syndrome. Arthritis Rheum. 29, 196–206.

Hatzis, G.S., Fragoulis, G.E., Karatzaferis, A., Delladetsima, I., Barbatis, C., Moutsopoulos, H.M., 2008. Prevalence and longterm course of primary biliary cirrhosis in primary Sjogren's syndrome. J. Rheumatol. 35, 2012–2016.

Hayashi, T., 2011. Dysfunction of lacrimal and salivary glands in Sjogren's syndrome: nonimmunologic injury in preinflammatory phase and mouse model. J. Biomed. Biotechnol. 2011, 407031.

Hernandez-Molina, G., Leal-Alegre, G., Michel-Peregrina, M., 2011. The meaning of anti-Ro and anti-La antibodies in primary Sjogren's syndrome. Autoimmun. Rev. 10, 123–125.

Hooks, J.J., Moutsopoulos, H.M., Geis, S.A., Stahl, N.I., Decker, J.L., Notkins, A.L., 1979. Immune interferon in the circulation of patients with autoimmune disease. N. Engl. J. Med. 301, 5–8.

Humphreys-Beher, M.G., Yamachika, S., Yamamoto, H., Maeda, N., Nakagawa, Y., Peck, A.B., et al., 1998. Salivary gland changes in the NOD mouse model for Sjogren's syndrome: is there a non-immune genetic trigger?. Eur. J. Morphol. Suppl. 247–251, 36.

Ioannidis, J.P., Vassiliou, V.A., Moutsopoulos, H.M., 2002. Long-term risk of mortality and lymphoproliferative disease and predictive classification of primary Sjogren's syndrome. Arthritis Rheum. 46, 741–747.

Ishimaru, N., Arakaki, R., Watanabe, M., Kobayashi, M., Miyazaki, K., Hayashi, Y., 2003. Development of autoimmune exocrinopathy resembling Sjogren's syndrome in estrogen-deficient mice of healthy background. Am. J. Pathol. 163, 1481–1490.

Ishimaru, N., Arakaki, R., Yoshida, S., Yamada, A., Noji, S., Hayashi, Y., 2008. Expression of the retinoblastoma protein RbAp48 in exocrine glands leads to Sjogren's syndrome-like autoimmune exocrinopathy. J. Exp. Med. 205, 2915–2927.

Ittah, M., Miceli-Richard, C., Gottenberg, J.E., Sellam, J., Eid, P., Lebon, P., et al., 2008. Viruses induce high expression of BAFF by salivary gland epithelial cells through TLR- and type-I IFN-dependent and -independent pathways. Eur. J. Immunol. 38, 1058–1064.

Iwakiri, D., Zhou, L., Samanta, M., Matsumoto, M., Ebihara, T., Seya, T., et al., 2009. Epstein-Barr virus (EBV)-encoded small RNA is released from EBV-infected cells and activates signaling from Toll-like receptor 3. J. Exp. Med. 206, 2091–2099.

Jin, M., Hwang, S.M., Davies, A.J., Shin, Y., Bae, J.S., Lee, J.H., et al., 2012. Autoantibodies in primary Sjogren's syndrome patients induce internalization of muscarinic type 3 receptors. Biochim. Biophys. Acta. 1822, 161–167.

Kang, K.Y., Kim, H.O., Kwok, S.K., Ju, J.H., Park, K.S., Sun, D.I., et al., 2011. Impact of interleukin-21 in the pathogenesis of primary Sjogren's syndrome: increased serum levels of interleukin-21 and its expression in the labial salivary glands. Arthritis Res. Ther. 13, R179.

Kapsogeorgou, E.K., Abu-Helu, R.F., Moutsopoulos, H.M., Manoussakis, M.N., 2005. Salivary gland epithelial cell exosomes: a source of autoantigenic ribonucleoproteins. Arthritis Rheum. 52, 1517–1521.

Kapsogeorgou, E.K., Gourzi, V.C., Manoussakis, M.N., Moutsopoulos, H.M., Tzioufas, A.G., 2011. Cellular microRNAs (miRNAs) and Sjogren's syndrome: candidate regulators of autoimmune response and autoantigen expression. J. Autoimmun. 37, 129–135.

Karaiskos, D., Mavragani, C.P., Makaroni, S., Zinzaras, E., Voulgarelis, M., Rabavilas, A., et al., 2009. Stress, coping strategies and social support in patients with primary Sjogren's syndrome prior to disease onset: a retrospective case-control study. Ann. Rheum. Dis. 68, 40–46.

Karaiskos, D., Mavragani, C.P., Sinno, M.H., Dechelotte, P., Zintzaras, E., Skopouli, F.N., et al., 2010. Psychopathological and personality features in primary Sjogren's syndrome—associations with autoantibodies to neuropeptides. Rheumatology (Oxford). 49, 1762–1769.

Kassan, S.S., Moutsopoulos, H.M., 2004. Clinical manifestations and early diagnosis of Sjogren syndrome. Arch. Intern. Med. 164, 1275–1284.

Katsifis, G.E., Moutsopoulos, N.M., Wahl, S.M., 2007. T lymphocytes in Sjogren's syndrome: contributors to and regulators of pathophysiology. Clin. Rev. Allergy Immunol. 32, 252–264.

Katsifis, G.E., Rekka, S., Moutsopoulos, N.M., Pillemer, S., Wahl, S.M., 2009. Systemic and local interleukin-17 and linked cytokines associated with Sjogren's syndrome immunopathogenesis. Am. J. Pathol. 175, 1167–1177.

Kawakami, A., Nakashima, K., Tamai, M., Nakamura, H., Iwanaga, N., Fujikawa, K., et al., 2007. Toll-like receptor in salivary glands from patients with Sjogren's syndrome: functional analysis by human salivary gland cell line. J. Rheumatol. 34, 1019–1026.

Kawasaki, A., Tsuchiya, N., Fukazawa, T., Hashimoto, H., Tokunaga, K., 2002. Analysis on the association of human BLYS (BAFF, TNFSF13B) polymorphisms with systemic lupus erythematosus and rheumatoid arthritis. Genes Immun. 3, 424–429.

Konttinen, Y.T., Fuellen, G., Bing, Y., Porola, P., Stegaev, V., Trokovic, N., et al., 2012. Sex steroids in Sjogren's syndrome. J. Autoimmun. 39, 49–56.

Lahiri, A., Pochard, P., Le Pottier, L., Tobon, G.J., Bendaoud, B., Youinou, P., et al., 2012. The complexity of the BAFF TNF-family members: implications for autoimmunity. J. Autoimmun. 39, 189–198.

Lahiri, D.K., Zawia, N.H., Greig, N.H., Sambamurti, K., Maloney, B., 2008. Early-life events may trigger biochemical pathways for Alzheimer's disease: the "LEARn" model. Biogerontology. 9, 375–379.

Lee, S.J., Lee, J.S., Shin, M.G., Tanaka, Y., Park, D.J., Kim, T.J., et al., 2012. Detection of HTLV-1 in the labial salivary glands of patients with Sjogren's syndrome: a distinct clinical subgroup?. J. Rheumatol. 39, 809–815.

Locht, H., Pelck, R., Manthorpe, R., 2008. Diagnostic and prognostic significance of measuring antibodies to alpha-fodrin compared to anti-Ro-52, anti-Ro-60, and anti-La in primary Sjogren's syndrome. J. Rheumatol. 35, 845–849.

Mackay, F., Woodcock, S.A., Lawton, P., Ambrose, C., Baetscher, M., Schneider, P., et al., 1999. Mice transgenic for BAFF develop lymphocytic disorders along with autoimmune manifestations. J. Exp. Med. 190, 1697–1710.

Malladi, A.S., Sack, K.E., Shiboski, S., Shiboski, C., Baer, A.N., Banushree, R., et al., 2012. Primary Sjogren's syndrome as a systemic disease: a study of participants enrolled in an international Sjogren's syndrome registry. Arthritis Care Res. (Hoboken). 64, 911–918.

Mann, D.L., Moutsopoulos, H.M., 1983. HLA DR alloantigens in different subsets of patients with Sjogren's syndrome and in family members. Ann. Rheum. Dis. 42, 533–536.

Manoussakis, M.N., Kapsogeorgou, E.K., 2007. The role of epithelial cells in the pathogenesis of Sjogren's syndrome. Clin. Rev. Allergy Immunol. 32, 225–230.

Manoussakis, M.N., Kapsogeorgou, E.K., 2010. The role of intrinsic epithelial activation in the pathogenesis of Sjogren's syndrome. J. Autoimmun. 35, 219–224.

Manoussakis, M.N., Kistis, K.G., Liu, X., Aidinis, V., Guialis, A., Moutsopoulos, H.M., 1993. Detection of anti-Ro (SSA) antibodies in autoimmune diseases: comparison of five methods. Br. J. Rheumatol. 32, 449–455.

Manoussakis, M.N., Georgopoulou, C., Zintzaras, E., Spyropoulou, M., Stavropoulou, A., Skopouli, F.N., et al., 2004. Sjogren's syndrome associated with systemic lupus erythematosus: clinical and laboratory profiles and comparison with primary Sjogren's syndrome. Arthritis Rheum. 50, 882–891.

Manoussakis, M.N., Boiu, S., Korkolopoulou, P., Kapsogeorgou, E.K., Kavantzas, N., Ziakas, P., et al., 2007. Rates of infiltration by macrophages and dendritic cells and expression of interleukin-18 and interleukin-12 in the chronic inflammatory lesions of Sjogren's syndrome: correlation with certain features of immune hyperactivity and factors associated with high risk of lymphoma development. Arthritis Rheum. 56, 3977–3988.

Manoussakis, M.N., Spachidou, M.P., Maratheftis, C.I., 2010. Salivary epithelial cells from Sjogren's syndrome patients are highly sensitive to anoikis induced by TLR-3 ligation. J. Autoimmun. 35, 212–218.

Manoussakis, M.N., Tsinti, M., Kapsogeorgou, E.K., Moutsopoulos, H. M., 2012. The salivary gland epithelial cells of patients with primary Sjogren's syndrome manifest significantly reduced responsiveness to 17beta-estradiol. J. Autoimmun. 39, 64–68.

Mariette, X., Caudmont, C., Berge, E., Desmoulins, F., Pinabel, F., 2003. Dry eyes and mouth syndrome or sicca, asthenia and polyalgia syndrome? Rheumatology (Oxford). 42, 914–915, author reply. 913–914.

Mariette, X., Ravaud, P., Steinfeld, S., Baron, G., Goetz, J., Hachulla, E., et al., 2004. Inefficacy of infliximab in primary Sjogren's syndrome: results of the randomized, controlled Trial of Remicade in Primary Sjogren's Syndrome (TRIPSS). Arthritis Rheum. 50, 1270–1276.

Mavragani, C.P., Crow, M.K., 2010. Activation of the type I interferon pathway in primary Sjogren's syndrome. J. Autoimmun. 35, 225–231.

Mavragani, C.P., Tzioufas, A.G., Moutsopoulos, H.M., 2000. Sjogren's syndrome: autoantibodies to cellular antigens. Clinical and molecular aspects. Int. Arch. Allergy Immunol. 123, 46–57.

Mavragani, C.P., Moutsopoulos, N.M., Moutsopoulos, H.M., 2006. The management of Sjogren's syndrome. Nat. Clin. Pract. Rheumatol. 2, 252–261.

Mavragani, C.P., Niewold, T.B., Moutsopoulos, N.M., Pillemer, S.R., Wahl, S.M., Crow, M.K., 2007. Augmented interferon-alpha pathway activation in patients with Sjogren's syndrome treated with etanercept. Arthritis Rheum. 56, 3995–4004.

Mavragani, C.P., Skopouli, F.N., Moutsopoulos, H.M., 2009. Increased prevalence of antibodies to thyroid peroxidase in dry eyes and mouth syndrome or sicca asthenia polyalgia syndrome. J. Rheumatol. 36, 1626–1630.

Mavragani, C.P., Fragoulis, G.E., Moutsopoulos, H.M., 2012a. Endocrine alterations in primary Sjogren's syndrome: An overview. J. Autoimmun. 39, 354–358.

Mavragani, C.P., Schini, M., Gravani, F., Kaltsas, G., Moutsopoulos, H. M., 2012b. Brief report: adrenal autoimmunity in primary Sjogren's syndrome. Arthritis Rheum. 64, 4066–4471.

McArthur, C.P., Fox, N.W., Kragel, P., 1993. Monoclonal antibody detection of laminin in minor salivary glands of patients with Sjogren's syndrome. J. Autoimmun. 6, 649–661.

Miceli-Richard, C., Comets, E., Loiseau, P., Puechal, X., Hachulla, E., Mariette, X., 2007. Association of an IRF5 gene functional polymorphism with Sjogren's syndrome. Arthritis Rheum. 56, 3989–3994.

Miceli-Richard, C., Gestermann, N., Ittah, M., Comets, E., Loiseau, P., Puechal, X., et al., 2009. The CGGGG insertion/deletion polymorphism of the IRF5 promoter is a strong risk factor for primary Sjogren's syndrome. Arthritis Rheum. 60, 1991–1997.

Milic, V., Petrovic, R., Boricic, I., Radunovic, G., Marinkovic-Eric, J., Jeremic, P, et al., 2012. Ultrasonography of major salivary glands could be an alternative tool to sialoscintigraphy in the American-European classification criteria for primary Sjogren's syndrome. Rheumatology (Oxford). 51, 1081–1085.

Mitsias, D.I., Tzioufas, A.G., Veiopoulou, C., Zintzaras, E., Tassios, I. K., Kogopoulou, O., et al., 2002. The Th1/Th2 cytokine balance changes with the progress of the immunopathological lesion of Sjogren's syndrome. Clin. Exp. Immunol. 128, 562–568.

Molina, C., Alliende, C., Aguilera, S., Kwon, Y.J., Leyton, L., Martinez, B., et al., 2006. Basal lamina disorganisation of the acini and ducts of labial salivary glands from patients with Sjogren's syndrome: association with mononuclear cell infiltration. Ann. Rheum. Dis. 65, 178–183.

Moutsopoulos, H.M., 2007. Sjogren's syndrome or autoimmune epithelitis? Clin. Rev. Allergy Immunol. 32, 199–200.

Moutsopoulos, H.M., Balow, J.E., Lawley, T.J., Stahl, N.I., Antonovych, T.T., et al., 1978. Immune complex glomerulonephritis in sicca syndrome. Am. J. Med. 64, 955–960.

Moutsopoulos, H.M., Cledes, J., Skopouli, F.N., Elisaf, M., Youinou, P., 1991. Nephrocalcinosis in Sjogren's syndrome: a late sequela of renal tubular acidosis. J. Intern. Med. 230, 187–191.

Nocturne, G., Pavy, S., Lazure, T., Taoufik, Y., Miceli, C., Mariette, X., 2011. IgG4 multiorgan lymphoproliferative syndrome as a differential diagnosis of primary Sjogren's syndrome in men? Ann. Rheum. Dis. 70, 2234–2235.

Nordmark, G., Kristjansdottir, G., Theander, E., Eriksson, P., Brun, J.G., Wang, C., et al., 2009. Additive effects of the major risk alleles of IRF5 and STAT4 in primary Sjogren's syndrome. Genes Immun. 10, 68–76.

Nordmark, G., Kristjansdottir, G., Theander, E., Appel, S., Eriksson, P., Vasaitis, L., et al., 2011. Association of EBF1, FAM167A (C8orf13)-BLK and TNFSF4 gene variants with primary Sjogren's syndrome. Genes Immun. 12, 100–109.

Nossent, J.C., Lester, S., Zahra, D., Mackay, C.R., Rischmueller, M., 2008. Polymorphism in the 5′ regulatory region of the B-lymphocyte activating factor gene is associated with the Ro/La autoantibody response and serum BAFF levels in primary Sjogren's syndrome. Rheumatology (Oxford). 47, 1311–1316.

Ozaki, Y., Ito, T., Son, Y., Amuro, H., Shimamoto, K., Sugimoto, H., et al., 2010. Decrease of blood dendritic cells and increase of tissue-infiltrating dendritic cells are involved in the induction of Sjogren's syndrome but not in the maintenance. Clin. Exp. Immunol. 159, 315–326.

Pablos, J.L., Carreira, P.E., Morillas, L., Montalvo, G., Ballestin, C., Gomez-Reino, J.J., 1994. Clonally expanded lymphocytes in the minor salivary glands of Sjogren's syndrome patients without lymphoproliferative disease. Arthritis Rheum. 37, 1441–1444.

Papiris, S.A., Maniati, M., Constantopoulos, S.H., Roussos, C., Moutsopoulos, H.M., Skopouli, F.N., 1999. Lung involvement in primary Sjogren's syndrome is mainly related to the small airway disease. Ann. Rheum. Dis. 58, 61–64.

Papiris, S.A., Tsonis, I.A., Moutsopoulos, H.M., 2007. Sjogren's syndrome. Semin. Respir. Crit. Care Med. 28, 459–471.

Pauley, K.M., Stewart, C.M., Gauna, A.E., Dupre, L.C., Kuklani, R., Chan, A.L., et al., 2011. Altered miR-146a expression in Sjogren's syndrome and its functional role in innate immunity. Eur. J. Immunol. 41, 2029–2039.

Pavlakis, P.P., Alexopoulos, H., Kosmidis, M.L., Stamboulis, E., Routsias, J.G., Tzartos, S.J., et al., 2011. Peripheral neuropathies in Sjogren syndrome: a new reappraisal. J. Neurol. Neurosurg. Psychiatr. 82, 798–802.

Pavlakis, P.P., Alexopoulos, H., Kosmidis, M.L., Mamali, I., Moutsopoulos, H.M., Tzioufas, A.G., et al., 2012. Peripheral neuropathies in Sjogren's syndrome: a critical update on clinical features and pathogenetic mechanisms. J. Autoimmun. 39, 27–33.

Pedersen, A.M., Dissing, S., Fahrenkrug, J., Hannibal, J., Reibel, J., Nauntofte, B, 2000. Innervation pattern and Ca^{2+} signalling in labial salivary glands of healthy individuals and patients with primary Sjogren's syndrome (pSS). J. Oral. Pathol. Med. 29, 97–109.

Petrone, D., Condemi, J.J., Fife, R., Gluck, O., Cohen, S., Dalgin, P., 2002. A double-blind, randomized, placebo-controlled study of cevimeline in Sjogren's syndrome patients with xerostomia and keratoconjunctivitis sicca. Arthritis Rheum. 46, 748–754.

Ping, L., Ogawa, N., Sugai, S., 2005. Novel role of CD40 in Fas-dependent apoptosis of cultured salivary epithelial cells from patients with Sjogren's syndrome. Arthritis Rheum. 52, 573–581.

Porola, P., Virkki, L., Przybyla, B.D., Laine, M., Patterson, T.A., Pihakari, A., et al., 2008. Androgen deficiency and defective intracrine processing of dehydroepiandrosterone in salivary glands in Sjogren's syndrome. J. Rheumatol. 35, 2229–2235.

Porola, P., Laine, M., Virtanen, I., Pollanen, R., Przybyla, B.D., Konttinen, Y.T., 2010. Androgens and integrins in salivary glands in Sjogren's syndrome. J. Rheumatol. 37, 1181–1187.

Quartuccio, L., Salvin, S., Fabris, M., Maset, M., Pontarini, E., Isola, M., et al., 2012. BLyS upregulation in Sjogren's syndrome associated with lymphoproliferative disorders, higher ESSDAI score and B-cell clonal expansion in the salivary glands. Rheumatology (Oxford). 52, 276–281.

Ramos-Casals, M., Anaya, J.M., Garcia-Carrasco, M., Rosas, J., Bove, A., Claver, G., et al., 2004. Cutaneous vasculitis in primary Sjogren syndrome: classification and clinical significance of 52 patients. Medicine (Baltimore). 83, 96–106.

Reed, J.H., Neufing, P.J., Jackson, M.W., Clancy, R.M., Macardle, P.J., Buyon, J.P., et al., 2007. Different temporal expression of immunodominant Ro60/60 kDa-SSA and La/SSB apotopes. Clin. Exp. Immunol. 148, 153–160.

Reed, J.H., Jackson, M.W., Gordon, T.P., 2008. B cell apotopes of the 60-kDa Ro/SSA and La/SSB autoantigens. J. Autoimmun. 31, 263–267.

Reed, J.H., Dudek, N.L., Osborne, S.E., Kaufman, K.M., Jackson, M.W., Purcell, A.W., et al., 2010. Reactivity with dichotomous determinants of Ro 60 stratifies autoantibody responses in lupus and primary Sjogren's syndrome. Arthritis Rheum. 62, 1448–1456.

Routsias, J.G., Tzioufas, A.G., 2010. Autoimmune response and target autoantigens in Sjogren's syndrome. Eur. J. Clin. Invest. 40, 1026–1036.

Ruiz-Tiscar, J.L., Lopez-Longo, F.J., Sanchez-Ramon, S., Santamaria, B., Urrea, R., Carreno, L., et al., 2005. Prevalence of IgG anti-{alpha}-fodrin antibodies in Sjogren's syndrome. Ann. N. Y. Acad. Sci. 1050, 210–216.

Ryu, Y.S., Park, S.H., Lee, J., Kwok, S.K., Ju, J.H., Kim, H.Y., et al., 2012. Follow-up of primary Sjogren's syndrome patients presenting positive anti-cyclic citrullinated peptides antibody. Rheumatol. Int. 33, 1443–1446.

Santavirta, N., Konttinen, Y.T., Tornwall, J., Segerberg, M., Santavirta, S., Matucci-Cerinic, M., et al., 1997. Neuropeptides of the autonomic nervous system in Sjogren's syndrome. Ann. Rheum. Dis. 56, 737–740.

Scofield, R.H., 2011. IL-21 and Sjogren's syndrome. Arthritis Res. Ther. 13, 137.

Shim, G.J., Warner, M., Kim, H.J., Andersson, S., Liu, L., Ekman, J., et al., 2004. Aromatase-deficient mice spontaneously develop a lymphoproliferative autoimmune disease resembling Sjogren's syndrome. Proc. Natl. Acad. Sci. U.S.A. 101, 12628–12633.

Sisto, M., Lisi, S., Lofrumento, D.D., D'Amore, M., Frassanito, M.A., Ribatti, D., 2012a. Sjogren's syndrome pathological neovascularization is regulated by VEGF-A-stimulated TACE-dependent crosstalk between VEGFR2 and NF-kappaB. Genes Immun. 13, 411–420.

Sisto, M., Lisi, S., Lofrumento, D.D., D'Amore, M., Ribatti, D., 2012b. Neuropilin-1 is upregulated in Sjogren's syndrome and contributes to pathological neovascularization. Histochem. Cell Biol. 137, 669–677.

Skopouli, F.N., Talal, A., Galanopoulou, V., Tsampoulas, C.G., Drosos, A.A., Moutsopoulos, H.M., 1990. Raynaud's phenomenon in primary Sjogren's syndrome. J. Rheumatol. 17, 618–620.

Skopouli, F.N., Barbatis, C., Moutsopoulos, H.M., 1994. Liver involvement in primary Sjogren's syndrome. Br. J. Rheumatol. 33, 745–748.

Skopouli, F.N., Dafni, U., Ioannidis, J.P., Moutsopoulos, H.M., 2000. Clinical evolution, and morbidity and mortality of primary Sjogren's syndrome. Semin. Arthritis Rheum. 29, 296–304.

Soliotis, F.C., Mavragani, C.P., Moutsopoulos, H.M., 2004. Central nervous system involvement in Sjogren's syndrome. Ann. Rheum. Dis. 63, 616–620.

Spaan, M., Porola, P., Laine, M., Rozman, B., Azuma, M., Konttinen, Y.T., 2009. Healthy human salivary glands contain a DHEA-sulphate processing intracrine machinery, which is deranged in primary Sjogren's syndrome. J. Cell. Mol. Med. 13, 1261–1270.

Spachidou, M.P., Bourazopoulou, E., Maratheftis, C.I., Kapsogeorgou, E.K., Moutsopoulos, H.M., Tzioufas, A.G., et al., 2007. Expression of functional Toll-like receptors by salivary gland epithelial cells: increased mRNA expression in cells derived from patients with primary Sjogren's syndrome. Clin. Exp. Immunol. 147, 497–503.

Stegaev, V., Sillat, T., Porola, P., Hanninen, A., Falus, A., Mieliauskaite, D., et al., 2012. First identification of the histamine 4 receptors (H(4)R) in healthy salivary glands and in focal sialadenitis in Sjogren's syndrome. Arthritis Rheum. 64, 2663–2668.

Steinfeld, S., Cogan, E., King, L.S., Agre, P., Kiss, R., Delporte, C., 2001. Abnormal distribution of aquaporin-5 water channel protein in salivary glands from Sjogren's syndrome patients. Lab. Invest. 81, 143–148.

Takahashi, H., Yamamoto, M., Tabeya, T., Suzuki, C., Naishiro, Y., Shinomura, Y., et al., 2012. The immunobiology and clinical characteristics of IgG4 related diseases. J. Autoimmun. 39, 93–96.

Takemoto, F., Hoshino, J., Sawa, N., Tamura, Y., Tagami, T., Yokota, M., et al., 2005. Autoantibodies against carbonic anhydrase II are increased in renal tubular acidosis associated with Sjogren syndrome. Am. J. Med. 118, 181–184.

Tandon, M., Gallo, A., Jang, S.I., Illei, G.G., Alevizos, I., 2012. Deep sequencing of short RNAs reveals novel microRNAs in minor salivary glands of patients with Sjogren's syndrome. Oral. Dis. 18, 127–131.

Tengner, P., Halse, A.K., Haga, H.J., Jonsson, R., Wahren-Herlenius, M., 1998. Detection of anti-Ro/SSA and anti-La/SSB autoantibody-producing cells in salivary glands from patients with Sjogren's syndrome. Arthritis Rheum. 41, 2238–2248.

Theander, E., Vasaitis, L., Baecklund, E., Nordmark, G., Warfvinge, G., Liedholm, R., et al., 2011. Lymphoid organisation in labial salivary gland biopsies is a possible predictor for the development of malignant lymphoma in primary Sjogren's syndrome. Ann. Rheum. Dis. 70, 1363–1368.

Triantafyllopoulou, A., Moutsopoulos, H., 2007. Persistent viral infection in primary Sjogren's syndrome: review and perspectives. Clin. Rev. Allergy Immunol. 32, 210–214.

Tsianos, E.B., Chiras, C.D., Drosos, A.A., Moutsopoulos, H.M., 1985. Oesophageal dysfunction in patients with primary Sjogren's syndrome. Ann. Rheum. Dis. 44, 610–613.

Tsinti, M., Kassi, E., Korkolopoulou, P., Kapsogeorgou, E., Moutsatsou, P., Patsouris, E., et al., 2009. Functional estrogen receptors alpha and beta are expressed in normal human salivary gland epithelium and apparently mediate immunomodulatory effects. Eur. J. Oral. Sci. 117, 498–505.

Tsokos, M., Lazarou, S.A., Moutsopoulos, H.M., 1987. Vasculitis in primary Sjogren's syndrome. Histologic classification and clinical presentation. Am. J. Clin. Pathol. 88, 26–31.

Tzioufas, A.G., Wassmuth, R., Dafni, U.G., Guialis, A., Haga, H.J., Isenberg, D.A., et al., 2002. Clinical, immunological, and immunogenetic aspects of autoantibody production against Ro/SSA, La/SSB and their linear epitopes in primary Sjogren's syndrome (pSS): a European multicentre study. Ann. Rheum. Dis. 61, 398–404.

Tzioufas, A.G., Kapsogeorgou, E.K., Moutsopoulos, H.M., 2012. Pathogenesis of Sjogren's syndrome: what we know and what we should learn. J Autoimmun. 39, 4–8.

Vakaloglou, K.M., Mavragani, C.P., 2011. Activation of the type I interferon pathway in primary Sjogren's syndrome: an update. Curr. Opin. Rheumatol. 23, 459–464.

Varin, M.M., Guerrier, T., Devauchelle-Pensec, V., Jamin, C., Youinou, P., Pers, J.O., 2012. In Sjogren's syndrome, B lymphocytes induce epithelial cells of salivary glands into apoptosis through protein kinase C delta activation. Autoimmun. Rev. 11, 252–258.

Vitali, C., Bombardieri, S., Jonsson, R., Moutsopoulos, H.M., Alexander, E.L., Carsons, S.E., et al., 2002. Classification criteria for Sjogren's syndrome: a revised version of the European criteria proposed by the American-European Consensus Group. Ann. Rheum. Dis. 61, 554–558.

Vivino, F.B., Al-Hashimi, I., Khan, Z., Leveque, F.G., Salisbury III, P. L., Tran-Johnson, T.K., et al., 1999. Pilocarpine tablets for the treatment of dry mouth and dry eye symptoms in patients with Sjogren syndrome: a randomized, placebo-controlled, fixed-dose, multicenter trial. P92-01 Study Group. Arch. Intern. Med. 159, 174–181.

Voulgarelis, M., Ziakas, P.D., Papageorgiou, A., Baimpa, E., Tzioufas, A.G., Moutsopoulos, H.M., 2012. Prognosis and outcome of non-Hodgkin lymphoma in primary Sjogren syndrome. Medicine (Baltimore). 91, 1–9.

Witte, T., Matthias, T., Arnett, F.C., Peter, H.H., Hartung, K., Sachse, C., et al., 2000. IgA and IgG autoantibodies against alpha-fodrin as markers for Sjogren's syndrome. Systemic lupus erythematosus. J. Rheumatol. 27, 2617–2620.

Witte, T., Matthias, T., Oppermann, M., Helmke, K., Peter, H.H., Schmidt, R.E., et al., 2003. Prevalence of antibodies against alpha-fodrin in Sjogren's syndrome: comparison of 2 sets of classification criteria. J. Rheumatol. 30, 2157–2159.

Youinou, P., Pennec, Y.L., Katsikis, P., Jouquan, J., Fauquert, P., Le Goff, P., 1990. Raynaud's phenomenon in primary Sjogren's syndrome. Br. J. Rheumatol. 29, 205–207.

Youinou, P., Devauchelle-Pensec, V., Pers, J.O., 2010. Significance of B cells and B cell clonality in Sjogren's syndrome. Arthritis Rheum. 62, 2605–2610.

Zeher, M., Horvath, I.F., Szanto, A., Szodoray, P., 2009. Autoimmune thyroid diseases in a large group of Hungarian patients with primary Sjogren's syndrome. Thyroid. 19, 39–45.

Zoukhri, D., Kublin, C.L., 2002. Impaired neurotransmission in lacrimal and salivary glands of a murine model of Sjogren's syndrome. Adv. Exp. Med. Biol. 506, 1023–1028.

Chapter 36

Rheumatoid Arthritis

Josef S. Smolen[1,2] and Kurt Redlich[1]

[1]*Division of Rheumatology, Department of Medicine 3, Medical University of Vienna, Austria,* [2]*Second Department of Medicine, Hietzing Hospital, Vienna, Austria*

Chapter Outline

Introduction	511	Pathologic Effector Mechanisms	516
Clinical, Pathologic, and Epidemiologic Features	511	Autoantibodies as Potential Immunologic Markers	517
Autoimmune Features	512	Concluding Remarks—Future Prospects	519
Genetic Features	514	Acknowledgment	519
In Vivo Models	515	References	519

INTRODUCTION

The joints are a target organ of many systemic autoimmune diseases, but in rheumatoid arthritis (RA) they are the preponderant and mostly sole evident focus of attack, with a large propensity to become destroyed. The pain and damage it elicits underlie the significant disability that can strike the patients and may lead to a wheelchair- or bed-ridden state. Thus, RA impairs all aspects of quality of life, including ability to work, and the consequences of the burden of the disease to the individual and society are enormous. For all these reasons, a better understanding of the pathogenesis of RA to develop new therapeutic agents interfering ideally with all pivotal events in all patients, or finding and abrogating the cause (or causes) of the disease, constitute a major task.

CLINICAL, PATHOLOGIC, AND EPIDEMIOLOGIC FEATURES

The *epidemiology* of RA is quite well characterized. RA is the most common chronic inflammatory joint disease, affecting 0.5−1% of the populations in the industrialized world and women more frequently than men (2−3:1) (Silman and Pearson, 2002; Helmick et al., 2008; Eriksson et al., 2013). However, in certain Native American (Eriksson et al., 2013) populations the prevalence is much higher (Helmick et al., 2008). The causes of the disease are unknown; however, several pieces of indirect evidence suggest that environmental factors play an important role: (1) RA has already at the time of its description been regarded as a disease of the poor (Landre-Beauvais, 1800) and lower levels of education and upbringing under adverse socioeconomic conditions are afflicted with a more severe course of RA and/or a higher baseline inflammatory state (Callahan and Pincus, 1997; Uhlig et al., 1999; Packard et al., 2011); (2) smoking may increase the risk and possibly also the severity of RA and is associated with increased tumor necrosis factor (TNF) and autoantibody production which in turn is related to genetic factors characteristic of RA (Silman et al., 1996; Symmons et al., 1997; Uhlig et al., 1999; Mattey et al., 2002; Glossop et al., 2006); although these associations have not been confirmed in all populations (Klareskog et al., 2011; Vesperini et al., 2013); (3) the microbiome appears to play an important role in experimental forms of arthritis (Yoshitomi et al., 2005; Abdollahi-Roodsaz et al., 2008; Wu et al., 2010) and it is conceivable that this is also the case in man, especially given the increased prevalence of periodontitis in RA and its association with particular bacteria, such as *Porphyrymonas gingivalis*, a bacterium that produces peptidyl-arginine deiminase (PADI), the enzyme responsible for citrullination (see below) (Wegner et al., 2010; Scher et al., 2012). Beyond these aspects, hormonal factors may also play a role in the development of RA (Silman and Pearson, 2002).

The main *clinical characteristics* of RA are pain and swelling of the joints. The 2010 ACR/EULAR classification

N. Rose & I. Mackay (Eds): The Autoimmune Diseases, Fifth edition. DOI: http://dx.doi.org/10.1016/B978-0-12-384929-8.00036-8

criteria (Aletaha et al., 2010), which are mainly used for clinical trial purposes but can also support the diagnostic process, require the presence of clinical synovitis (i.e., swelling due to synovial involvement) in at least one joint. The more joints that are affected (swollen or painful), the easier the patient can fulfill the criteria. Joints involved are primarily those of the wrists, fingers, toes, and knees (Smolen et al., 1995), but also many other joints can be affected, although some joints, such as the distal interphalangeal joints (DIPs), are usually spared. Affected joints are not only painful upon motion and visibly swollen (Figure 36.1A) or upon clinical examination, but also tender to mild pressure and stiff for many hours after rest, such as in the morning. RA synovitis leads to subchondral bone erosions and damage to cartilage and thus to the totality of the *pathology* of RA which can culminate in completely destroyed joints, as seen clinically (Figure 36.1A, lower photographs) and upon imaging, especially by radiography (Figure 36.1B).

AUTOIMMUNE FEATURES

The immunologic hallmark of RA is the presence of autoantibodies in the circulation (and also in the synovial fluid). Indeed, the presence of autoantibodies constitutes an important aspect of the new ACR-EULAR classification criteria of RA and contributes two points out of a maximum of 10 if detectable and even three points if at high levels (Aletaha et al., 2010).

The first autoantibody ever described in RA was *rheumatoid factor* (RF) (Waaler, 1939), subsequently recognized to be a family of autoantibodies directed against the Fc portion of immunoglobulin (Ig) G. In clinical routine, IgM-RF is most commonly determined, but RFs can be of any isotype, and next to IgM-RF, IgG-RF and IgA-RF are frequently seen. The latter has been found to be predictive for the development of RA and is associated with worse prognosis (Houssien et al., 1997; Rantapaa-Dahlqvist et al., 2003; Nell et al., 2005). Also, IgM-RF precedes the occurrence of RA and, especially at high levels ($\geq$50 IU/ml), it is associated with significant joint damage (Nielen et al., 2004; Nell et al., 2005; Aletaha et al., 2012). Moreover, the risk of developing RA for RF positive individuals in the general population may be up to 26-fold increased (Nielsen et al., 2012). This suggests an involvement of RF in the pathways to inflammation and especially joint destruction which could be a consequence of immune complex formation and subsequent Fc receptor binding, complement activation, and consequential increase in levels of inflammatory cytokines (Winchester et al., 1970; Schur et al., 1975; Mallya et al., 1982). RF are not specific for RA but can occur in other disorders, such as systemic autoimmune rheumatic diseases (SARDs) or chronic infections (Elagib et al., 1999; Bassyouni et al., 2009; Lima et al., 2013); when occurring

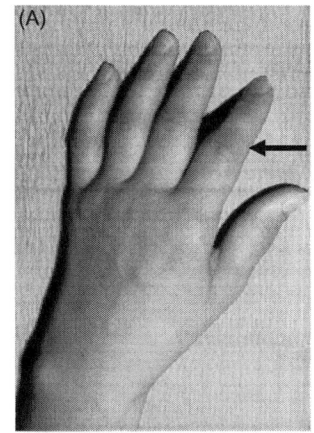
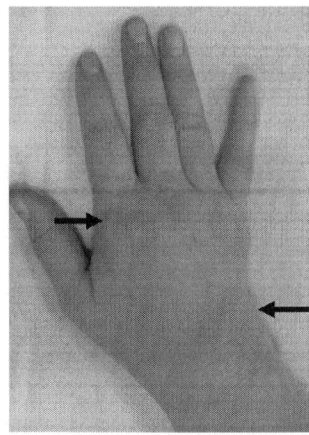
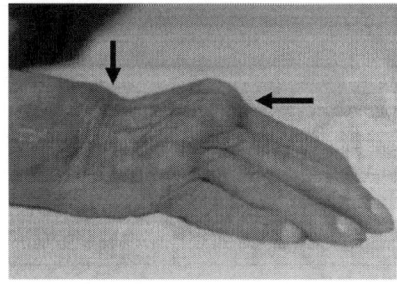
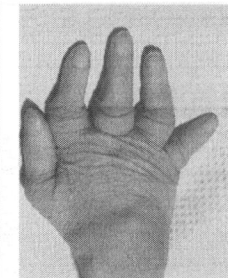
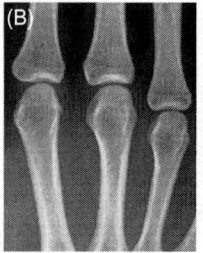
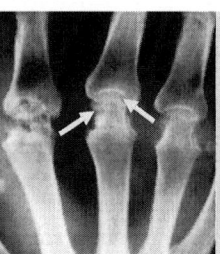
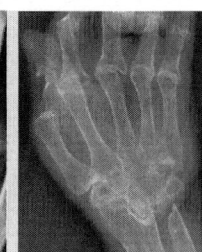

FIGURE 36.1   A. Hands of patients with RA. In the upper left image showing early RA, swelling is visible especially at the level of the proximal interphalangeal joints (arrow); in the upper right image, showing more established RA, swelling is visible at the level of the wrist, but also metacarpophalangeal joints (arrows). In the lower left image showing long-standing RA, joint damage has led to subluxation of the metacarpophalangeal joints and one can also find massive carpal joint damage (arrows). The lower right image shows a case of mutilation in virtually all joints of the hand. B. Evolution of X-ray changes from early arthritis without visible changes to severely destructive disease (bony erosions and cartilage damage seen indirectly as narrowed joint space, arrows) and ultimately mutilating disease.

in the course of acute infections, such as Epstein–Barr virus infection, they are usually of low level and transient (Halbert and Anken 1982). RF occur in up to 5% of healthy individuals, with the highest frequency in elderly people, although this has recently been disputed (Nielsen et al., 2012). The physiologic role of RFs may be to enhance immune complex clearance by amplifying complement binding and increasing immune complex size and to eliminate modified IgG (Grabar, 1975; van Snick et al., 1978). RF are found in up to 80% of RA patients and, as indicated before, a pathogenic role of RF must be assumed. RF can be produced locally by B cells infiltrating the synovial membrane (Jasin 1985; Wernick et al., 1985; Kraan et al., 1999). The observation that RF have undergone somatic mutations and isotype switching (Williams et al., 1999) suggests that RF production in RA is T cell driven. On the other hand, some RF, and especially IgM-RF, may be highly conserved and coming from a B cell population producing natural autoantibodies (Chen et al., 1986; Martin et al., 1992; Hayakawa et al., 1999), suggesting that IgM-RF may not be derived from long-lived plasma cells. In line with the latter, RF levels change quite rapidly with changes in disease activity and decrease with effective therapy (Bohler et al., 2013).

Another very important autoantibody in RA is directed against *citrullinated peptides*. Originally described as anti-keratin antibodies and anti-perinuclear factor (Nienhuis and Mandema, 1964; Young et al., 1979; Aho et al., 1993b), the autoantibody was subsequently characterized as reactive with citrullinated peptides (Schellekens et al., 1998; Girbal-Neuhauser et al., 1999). Citrulline is an amino acid derived from deimination of arginine by PADI. A large number of proteins can undergo this posttranslational modification, including fibrin, vimentin, alpha enolase, and collagen; some of these are used in ELISAs for the purposes of autoantibody testing, including a synthetic, not naturally occurring cyclic citrullinated peptide (CCP). The anti-citrullinated-protein antibodies (ACPA) have been suggested to be more predictive of RA, associated with a bad outcome and more specific for RA than RF. However, with increasing numbers of studies, an increasing number of diseases in which ACPA are present are reported, including chronic infections and other rheumatic diseases (Takasaki et al., 2004; Vossenaar ER et al., 2004; Candia et al., 2006; Bassyouni et al., 2009; Lima and Santiago 2010; Du Toit et al., 2011; Singh et al., 2011; Lima et al., 2013). Thus, while ACPA are somewhat more specific for RA than RF, they are neither pathognomonic nor of truly high specificity; this has also been accounted for in the ACR-EULAR classification criteria for RA (Aletaha et al., 2010), where both specificities are regarded as equivalent. Importantly, ACPA and RF overlap in over 90% of the patients and it has been suggested that RA is particularly severe when both specificities are present (Rantapaa-Dahlqvist et al., 2003). Interestingly, recent evidence suggests that RF and ACPA are independently associated with the progression of joint damage (De Rycke et al., 2004) and that RF may even be more strongly associated with disease activity than ACPA (Smolen et al., 2012), and it will have to be seen if this also translates into a lower effect of ACPA than RF on joint damage upon more detailed evaluation. In contrast to RF, ACPA levels do not rapidly change

with changes of disease activity or effective therapy (De Rycke et al., 2005; Bohler et al., 2013). While ACPA positivity has been reported to be associated with the shared epitope (see below) and suggested to be elicited by smoking by virtue of activation of PADI in the respiratory tract (Klareskog et al., 2006), these data stem from particular European sites and have not been uniformly confirmed in other cohorts of patients (Lee et al., 2007; Xue et al., 2008). Overall, determining ACPA is a valuable addition to the diagnostic armamentarium, but it may be sufficient to do this primarily in RF negative patients (National Collaborating Centre for Chronic Conditions, 2009). In general, autoantibody testing for RA should only be done when clinical synovitis is present in at least one joint. Interestingly, ACPA appear to precede RA for even longer periods of time than RF (Nielen et al., 2004; Brink et al., 2013); this indicates that once pre-RA becomes a recognized entity due to evidence for the efficacy of preventive therapy, ACPA testing may be an important screening method. At present, however, it appears that a significant proportion ($\sim$3%) of healthy individuals are ACPA or RF positive and, therefore, further studies to define "pre-RA" are needed (Jimenez-Boj et al., 2012).

As citrullination constitutes a post-translational protein modification, the potential autoantigenic nature of other post-translationally modified proteins was tested and, indeed, it appears that autoantibodies to carbamylated proteins also exist (anti-CarP) which are predictive of RA (Shi et al., 2013).

A variety of *other autoantibodies* can also be found in RA, confirming the broad autoimmune nature of the disease. Among these are autoantibodies to nuclear antigens, especially the heterogeneous nuclear ribonucleoprotein (hnRNP) A2 (anti-RA33) which occurs in 30–40% of RA patients, has some differential-diagnostic potential especially in RF/ACPA negative patients, and appears to be associated with a more benign form of RA (Steiner et al., 1992; Nell et al., 2003). Moreover, anti-RA33 can also precede the development of RA (Aho et al., 1993a), although this occurs closer to the time of disease onset than ACPA and RF. Anti-collagen antibodies are yet another interesting autoantibody subset, but their role appears more important in experimental models of RA (Trentham et al., 1977) than in the human disease (Steffen, 1970), although collagen might play some autoantigenic role in the context of its citrullination (Burkhardt et al., 2005).

The observation of the appearance of various autoantibodies prior to the onset of RA is similar to findings in other autoimmune diseases, such as type 1 diabetes and systemic lupus erythematosus (Arbuckle et al., 2003; Pietropaolo et al., 2012). This suggests that the activation of the autoimmune response occurs long before clinical

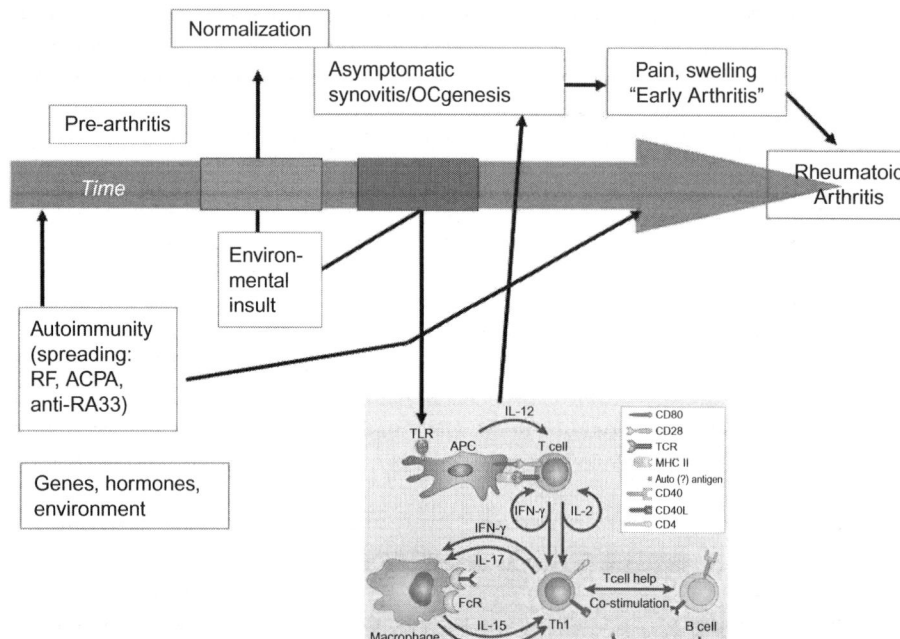

FIGURE 36.2 **A Putative Concept of Pre-arthritis and Its Evolution to Full-blown Rheumatoid Arthritis.** A host–environment interaction (with the microbiome?) could trigger the evolution of a non-pathogenic autoimmune response which, in contrast to many similar reactions, in a genetically predisposed host may persist. Another environmental insult leads to expansion (spreading) of the autoimmune response without any clinical consequence. At some point, one of such recurring environmental insults with a potentially arthrotropic agent could trigger an asymptomatic synovitis which, in the presence of autoantibodies, could ultimately become clinically manifest and due to an overwhelming cytokine response also trigger osteoclastogenesis (OCgenesis) and thus the full RA picture.

manifestations become apparent and that the evolution of disease is a multistep process which initially involves a trigger eliciting autoimmunity and a second trigger activating the disease pathology in the presence of a particular autoreactivity (Smolen et al., 2006). A depiction of a possible pathway from pre-arthritis to full-blown RA is shown in Figure 36.2.

T cell-mediated autoimmunity in RA has been described for collagen and hnRNPA2 (Trentham et al., 1978; Fritsch et al., 2002), but not for IgG-Fc or citrullinated peptides. Whether cellular immunity to autoantigens is of pathogenetic importance is hitherto unknown. Clearly, the presence of autoantibodies is the major autoimmune characteristic of RA.

GENETIC FEATURES

One of the major indications for a genetic predisposition to a disease is its increased familial occurrence. While in RA the prevalence in the general population is 0.5–1%, it rises to 2–4% in siblings and about 15% in identical twins (Silman et al., 1993; Seldin et al., 1999); however, a quantitative genetic analysis of two European populations showed a consistent heritability of RA in the order of ~60% (MacGregor et al., 2000).

The earliest observation that a particular gene may predispose to RA came from Stastny's seminal work describing the presence of human leucocyte antigen (HLA)-DRw4 in 70% of RA patients compared with 28% of controls (Stastny, 1978). The association with this major histocompatibility complex (MHC) class II

gene, located on chromosome 6p21, was subsequently numerously confirmed to constitute the most important genetic contribution to susceptibility for the disease. It was ultimately observed that in RA patients of various ethnic backgrounds the HLA-DRB1 alleles are frequently different, but each encodes a common sequence of amino acids at position 70–74 of the HLA-DRβ chain (QKRRA or similar, such as QRRAA or RRRAA) within the third hypervariable region of the HLA-DRB1 molecule (Gregersen et al., 1987), a region pivotally important for peptide binding. Thus, the risk contribution apparently comes from presentation of potentially arthritogenic antigens. The respective alleles include HLA-DRB1*0401, *0404, *0405, *0408; HLA-DRB1*0101, *0102; HLA-DRB1*1001; and HLA-DRB1*1402 which occur at different frequencies in different populations, but together are present in about 80% of RA patients. The overall odds ratio (OR) is about 3 with the biggest risk conveyed by HLA-DRB1*0401 and *0404, and especially strongly with homozygosity of the shared epitope (OR of ~30). There are also protective alleles, such as HLA-DRB1*0402. However, since HLA accounts for only about one-third of the total genetic risk in RA (Deighton et al., 1989), non-MHC genes must also contribute to susceptibility.

One of the non-MHC genes found to be associated with RA is protein tyrosine phosphatase, non-receptor type 22 (lymphoid) gene (*PTPN22*) on chromosome 1p13. A single nucleotide polymorphism (SNP) in this gene is the culprit, occurring in 14% of RA patients and 9% of controls (OR ~1.7) (Begovich et al., 2004). This phosphatase, which is expressed in hematopoietic cells, inhibits T cell receptor signal transduction and the 620W variant is associated with reduced CD4T cell activation.

SNPs in the complement component 5 (*C5*)/tumor necrosis factor receptor-associated factor 1 (*TRAF1*) region at chromosome 9q33 have likewise been found to be associated with RA (Plenge et al., 2007). Complement genes, indeed, are interesting candidates given the potential involvement of complement activation in RA pathogenesis discussed previously and below. TRAF1, on the other hand, codes for a protein which acts as a negative regulator of signaling via TNF receptors (TNFR) 1 and 2, and in light of the apparent pivotal involvement of TNF in the pathogenesis of RA (see below), there is some logic behind this association. However, it is not clear at present which of these genes is primarily associated with RA or if the association may not even be with an adjacent gene. The OR is about 1.3.

Other proteins involved in signaling are the signal transducers and activators of transcription (STATs). STATs are activated by Janus kinases (Jaks) and recently the first Jak inhibitor was approved for the treatment of RA in the USA (Burmester et al., 2013). Indeed, a variant allele of *STAT4*, located on chromosome 2q, was found associated with RA (Remmers et al., 2007). STAT4 protein mediates signaling of various cytokines, such as IL-12, IL-23, and type I interferons. The variant allele was found in 27% of patients and 22% of controls, OR ~1.3. Homozygosity of the allele was associated with a 60% increased risk of RA.

Other genetic risk factors include polymorphisms in the *CD40* and the tumor necrosis factor, alpha-induced protein 3 (*TNFAIP3*) genes (Li and Begovich, 2009).

Thus, a variety of genetic associations have been found in RA. Importantly, some of these, such as the MHC genes, are primarily related to autoantibody positive RA, indicating that immune response genes contribute their effects indeed via particular immune responses (Mattey et al., 2002; van der Helm-van Mil et al., 2006). Gene−environment interactions have been postulated in terms of genetic susceptibility in smokers to develop ACPA and RA (Klareskog et al., 2011), but have not been generally confirmed (Lee et al., 2007); thus, more information is clearly needed.

IN VIVO MODELS

Based on Koch's postulate that a causal agent must be sufficient and necessary to cause infectious disease (Koch, 1890), Witebsky et al. formulated postulates for autoimmune diseases: an autoantigen should be necessary and sufficient to cause an autoimmune disease in experimental models (Witebsky et al., 1957); in other words, the demonstration of an autoimmune nature of a disease

requires the recognition of a particular autoantigen to which antibodies or cells are autoreactive and which elicits a similar disease in an experimental model. To date, the only such autoantigen in RA is collagen, hypothesized to be the culprit several decades ago by Steffen (Steffen, 1970); collagen-specific autoantibodies and autoreactive cells exist (Menzel et al., 1975; Trentham et al., 1978; Smolen et al., 1980) and type II collagen (CII) elicits a chronic, destructive arthritis (Trentham et al., 1977). This collagen-induced arthritis (CIA) meanwhile, one of the classic RA models, depends on both the activation of T cells and the production of arthritogenic autoantibodies, but the disease itself can also only be transferred with anti-CII antibodies (Holmdahl et al., 2002). However, current views do not suggest a major role for this reactivity in eliciting human RA, and interestingly, this model responds better to IL-1- than TNF-blockade, contrasting human RA (Joosten et al., 2008). Not only CII but also other cartilage antigens, such as proteoglycan, can be used to induce experimental arthritis (Glant et al., 1987, 1998), but their role in human RA is not established.

Other autoantigens used to develop experimental models, to which autoantibodies and partly cellular immune responses exist in RA, and which are even widely used diagnostically, are immunoglobulin G (targeted by rheumatoid factors), several citrullinated proteins including fibrinogen, vimentin, alpha enolase, and collagen (targeted by ACPA), and heterogeneous nuclear ribonucleoprotein A2 (hnRNP-A2; targeted by anti-RA33 antibodies) (Steiner et al., 1992). However, none of them elicit a chronic destructive arthritis upon immunization. At most, ACPA can be detected in occasional experimental approaches, such as a study on collagen-induced arthritis (Kuhn et al., 2006), although other studies reported negative observations in this respect. Further, immunization with hnRNP-A2 can aggravate arthritis in TNF overexpressing mice (Hayer et al., 2005).

Several adjuvants can induce arthritis, in particular Freund's adjuvant ("adjuvant arthritis") and pristane, a mineral oil ("pristane-induced arthritis"); while they allow one to study certain aspects of the pathways to arthritis, they do not appear to be appropriate models for human RA (Holmdahl et al., 2001), although being free of known autoantigens, they support the involvement of environmental factors in the generation of arthritis.

That any type of immune complexes can induce arthritis has been shown by Dumonde and Glynn (Dumonde and Glynn, 1962). A particular form of an immune complex arthritis has been more recently described in the form of the KRN mouse model, originally developed to study diabetes; these mice express a transgenic T cell receptor (TCR) recognizing glucose-6-phosphoisomerase (G6PI), a ubiquitous cytoplasmic protein which is also present on the surface of articular cartilage. The ensuing autoantibodies, which by themselves can induce disease upon serum transfer, form intraarticular immune complexes followed by a severe inflammatory and destructive response, and expectedly the system is complement and mast cell dependent (Matsumoto et al., 2002). Interestingly, G6PI is not recognized as being an important autoantigen in man, but nonetheless this model confirms the role of immune complexes in chronic arthritis and especially the serum transfer model can be used to investigate the role of the innate immune system selectively. Also another model involves the TCR, namely the SKG model which is based on a spontaneous mutation of ZAP70, an important TCR signaling adaptor molecule. These mice develop a severe arthritis upon immunization with adjuvants. Of note, many of these animal models do not occur under germ-free conditions and different commensal agents can activate individual forms of experimental arthritis in hosts with particular genetic backgrounds (Wu et al., 2010), further suggesting the important involvement of the environment in the induction and maintenance of chronic arthritis (Scheinecker and Smolen, 2011; Scher and Abramson, 2011).

A number of "non-immune" models of RA also exist. The most widely used is a model in which a human TNF transgene is expressed in mice. These hTNFtg animals not only overexpress TNF but also develop a severely inflammatory and highly destructive polyarthritis (Figure 36.3A) (Keffer et al., 1991). This model has served particularly well in studies devoted to the development of bone and cartilage damage in arthritis (Redlich et al., 2002; Korb-Pap et al., 2012). Yet another example of the role of cytokine hyperactivity and consequential joint inflammation and damage is provided upon deficiency of IL-1 receptor antagonist (IL-1ra) (Horai et al., 2000), although as mentioned before IL-1 inhibition has little effect in human RA.

Thus, a variety of experimental models exist which can mimic parts of the spectrum of RA allowing studies of many aspects of pathways to arthritis and joint destruction. Some of these models even appear to fulfill Witebsky's postulate; alas, the role of the respective autoantigen(s) in human RA is not confirmed.

PATHOLOGIC EFFECTOR MECHANISMS

The detailed mechanisms leading to the expression of the disease are still insufficiently known. Figure 36.4 depicts current views on the pathways to synovitis and joint damage in RA, showing a schematic representation of the events (Smolen et al., 2007) as well as histologic and immunohistochemical characteristics of the RA synovial membrane. It is assumed that an autoantigen or hitherto unrecognized foreign antigen is taken up by antigen presenting cells (APC), prototypically dendritic cells (DCs),

leading to activation of the innate immune system (including type I interferon and IL-6 production) as well as to that of T cells (and thus also the adaptive immune response) via respective antigen presentation and costimulation. The involvement of the shared epitope (see above) suggests that either particularly arthritogenic peptides bind with high affinity to these but not other MHC molecules or that an arthritogenic T cell repertoire is selected via the shared epitope. These activated T cells, formerly thought to be Th1 (gamma interferon producing) cells, are now believed to belong mainly to the Th17 family (IL-17 producing) (Korn et al., 2009) and to be insufficiently controlled by regulatory T cells (Chavele and Ehrenstein, 2011); they in turn activate macrophages and provide B cell help. These events presumably occur partly centrally and partly within the synovial membrane into which the cells have migrated. Activated macrophages secrete proinflammatory cytokines. Activated RA B cells and their progeny produce autoantibodies which, after forming immune complexes, bind to Fc- and complement-receptors and thus increase macrophage cytokine production (Aringer and Smolen, 2012). In parallel, fibroblast-like synovial cells (FLS) become activated and also produce inflammatory mediators (Lee and Firestein 2003). Indeed, FLS may play a particularly important role, since (1) mesenchymal overexpression of TNF is sufficient to drive all aspects of destructive arthritis (Keffer et al., 1991; Bluml et al., 2010), and (2) these cells may "travel" through the bloodstream from one joint to other joints, thus spreading arthritis (Lefevre et al., 2009). Taken together, all these events lead to synovial inflammation. The inflammatory reaction is a consequence of the activation of proinflammatory cytokines (TNF, IL-6, and IL-1); based on results of clinical trials, therapies targeting TNF and IL-6 appear to play predominant roles, while that of IL-1 appears to be minor. Subsequently other mediators of inflammation, such as various chemokines, metalloproteinases, and small molecules (like prostaglandins) are induced and increase the inflammatory reaction which clinically manifests in swelling and pain as discussed above.

By whichever way the detailed events evolve (i.e., whether the innate immune reactivity, T or B cell activation are dominant), the mechanisms ultimately lead to an influx of inflammatory cells into the synovial membrane; the inflamed synovial membrane transforms into an autonomous "semimalignant" tissue (pannus) leading to destruction of bone (erosions) and cartilage. Indeed, the major feature distinguishing RA from other inflammatory joint diseases is the high propensity for joint destruction.

Cartilage damage appears to arise primarily via direct action of metalloproteinases secreted within the joint on cartilage matrix and/or via the activation of chondrocytes by cytokines and subsequent matrix degradation;

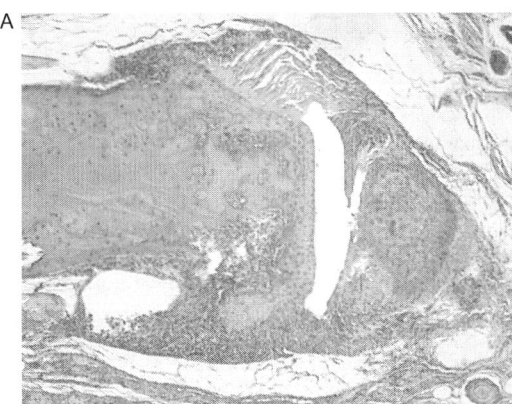

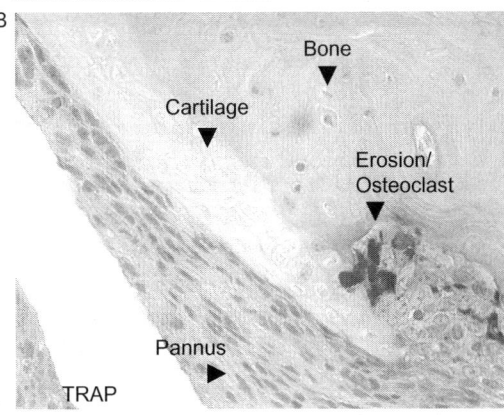

FIGURE 36.3 A. Arthritis in mice overexpressing human TNF. Note the significant inflammatory response and the dramatic destruction due to subchondral invasion of the bone by the pannus tissue. B. Bone damage is elicited by osteoclasts differentiating within the synovial membrane. The small dark blue (tartrate-resistant acid phosphatase [TRAP] positive) cells are osteoclast precursors.

attachment of the synovial membrane to cartilage appears to play an important role in these respects (Korb-Pap et al., 2012).

Bone destruction is mediated by osteoclasts activated within the synovial membrane at sites adjacent to bone (Figure 36.3B) (Gravallese et al., 1998; Redlich et al., 2002). While osteoclast differentiation and activation is pivotally dependent on receptor activator of NFκB (RANK) and its ligand (RANKL), proinflammatory cytokines enhance the generation and activity of osteoclasts (Lam et al., 2000; Teitelbaum, 2000). The much stronger destructive nature of RA compared with other inflammatory joint diseases may be explained by the higher load of cytokines like TNF and IL-6 (Partsch et al., 1997) which in turn are likely to be a consequence of the presence of autoantibodies and immune complexes in the joint (Zvaifler, 1974). Indeed, the presence of RF is related to joint damage via association with higher disease activity and also independently of disease activity (Aletaha et al., 2012).

With all due recognition of deliberations on pathogenetic pathways based on experimental models or *ex vivo* and *in vitro* studies of patient cells, tissues or body fluids, ultimately the validation of the involvement of specific pathways must come from the efficacy of therapies targeting a presumed pathogenetic principle (sort of reverse Witebsky postulate). Today, TNF and IL-6 blockade and also inhibition of T cell costimulation and B lymphocyte depletion are all approved RA therapeutics, thus validating these targets as importantly involved (although also eliciting new questions; see below). However, the fact that all these agents lead to similar clinical results, that their efficacy is not increased in patients who have failed one of the other targeted therapies, and combinations of these biological hitherto do not apparently increase efficacy although they do mostly increase serious adverse event rates, suggest that all these cells and molecules have a single major final pathway in common; this bottleneck appears to be the proinflammatory cytokine system (Smolen and Aletaha, 2013).

Still some questions arise in this respect: (1) if T cells do play a major role as suggested by the efficacy of costimulation inhibition, why is anti-CD4 therapy not effective (van der Lubbe et al., 1995)? (2) If B cells play a major role, why are several B cell directed therapies ineffective (Bluml et al., 2013)? (3) With so many similarities regarding the effects of the three major proinflammatory cytokines: TNF, IL-1, and IL-6, why is IL-1 inhibition so much less efficacious than TNF and IL-6 inhibition (Singh et al., 2009)? And, most importantly, (4) what determines the arthrotropism of the disease? Do particular antigens of the joint (cartilage components?) elicit the disease? Is it influx into the joint, with its permissive anatomical structures lacking efficient basement membranes, of non-specific bacterial products that is of decisive nature (Toivanen, 2001)? Resolving these questions will allow better insights into the pathways leading to RA, but they simply attest that proof of concept can only come from the clinic and not from theoretical considerations or experimental models.

AUTOANTIBODIES AS POTENTIAL IMMUNOLOGIC MARKERS

As discussed in the section on autoimmunity, the most important autoantibodies in RA are RF and ACPA. They are both important components in classification criteria and therefore of diagnostic help (Aletaha et al., 2010). Their sensitivity and specificity for the diagnosis of RA is similar (sensitivity about 50–60%, specificity about 85–95%) (Mjaavatten et al., 2010; Neogi et al., 2010; Nicaise-Roland et al., 2013). Both of these autoantibodies fluctuate with disease activity and effective therapy, although RF appears to do so to a much greater extent (Bohler et al., 2013); indeed, RF can become negative (seroconversion) with long-standing remission which is

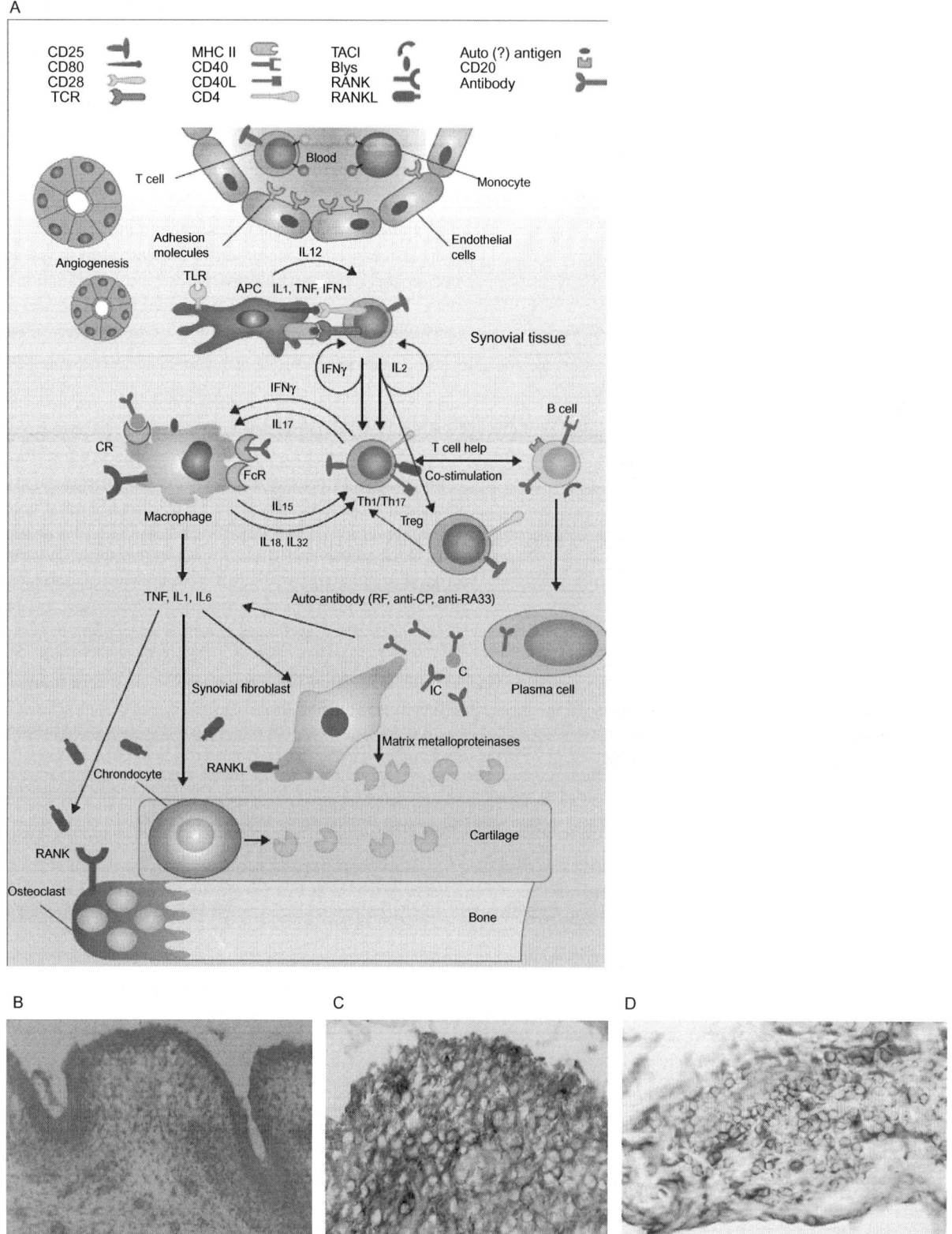

FIGURE 36.4   A. A schematic representation of the pathogenesis of RA (Smolen et al., 2007). B. Hematoxylin-eosin stain of an RA synovial membrane section showing hyperplasia of the lining layer, hypercellularity in the sublining and hypervascularity. C. TNF expression (brown) in type A (monocyte-like, blue) and type B (fibroblast-like, unstained) synovial lining cells. D. Activated T cells in synovial membrane (CD3 in brown, HLA-DR in blue).

not known for ACPA. ACPA can be tested for using several different citrullinated antigens: fibrinogen, vimentin, filaggrin, collagen type II, enolase, or a cyclic peptide. These autoantibodies differ only slightly in terms of time of appearance and frequency (Brink et al., 2013; Nicaise-Roland et al., 2013).

Another autoantibody specificity which can be of diagnostic help is anti-RA33, especially if RF and ACPA are negative (Nell et al., 2005).

All these autoantibodies can also be present in a variety of other diseases, especially other autoimmune disorders and infectious diseases, and also notably so for ACPA (Abdel Fattah et al., 2009; Bassyouni et al., 2009; Lima and Santiago 2010; Singh et al., 2011; Gokhan et al., 2013). They can also be present in healthy people and it has previously been suggested that RF positivity increases with age, but this was not seen in more recent series (Nielsen et al., 2012). Therefore, only in the right clinical setting RF and ACPA can be regarded as marker autoantibodies of the disease and as having a high weighting in the classification criteria for RA (Aletaha et al., 2010).

Of particular importance, the presence of autoantibodies can partly inform in advance on response to therapy. Thus, B cell targeted therapy with rituximab is more efficacious in RF and/or ACPA positive than negative patients (Chatzidionysiou et al., 2011). This is conceptually sound, since rituximab eliminates CD20 positive B cells and levels of these autoantibodies decrease with effective therapy. This observation appears to be specific for rituximab, since therapies targeted against cytokines or T cell costimulation do not appear to be differently effective in seropositive and seronegative patients.

CONCLUDING REMARKS—FUTURE PROSPECTS

Rheumatoid arthritis is the prototypic autoimmune joint disease. Autoreactivity, in association with a genetic predisposition, appears to play a major role in pathways to RA and the presence of autoantibodies is associated with joint damage and thus of prognostic in addition to diagnostic value. The observations that autoimmunity precedes clinical disease onset by many years and that the presence of RF in otherwise healthy individuals may increase the risk for developing RA more than 20-fold, implies that there is a pre-arthritic phase. This suggests that in the future, long before the onset of disease, preventive measures might be taken for people at risk (see Chapters 77–79). Thus, the autoimmune response may at some early point in time serve as guidance toward novel therapeutic approaches. Further, the causes of RA are still unknown: which (environmental?) provocation elicits RA? And how then does the autoimmune reaction ensue?

These questions will hopefully also find resolution over the next decade.

Finally, for patients with established disease, it is currently unknown to which therapies they will respond in the best way, ideally by attaining remission. It is conceivable that biomarkers, which may include the autoimmune reactivity pattern, will help in this regard. Thus, there is hope for the future that we may be able to predict not only people at high risk of developing RA, but also those likely to experience optimal therapeutic responsiveness.

ACKNOWLEDGMENT

The studies providing the basis for this chapter were partly supported by EU grants BT-Cure and EuroTEAM.

REFERENCES

Abdel Fattah, N.S., Hassan, H.E., Galal, Z.A., El Okda, E.S., 2009. Assessment of anti-cyclic citrullinated peptide in psoriatic arthritis. BMC Res. Notes. 2, 44.

Abdollahi-Roodsaz, S., Joosten, L.A., Koenders, M.I., Devesa, I., Roelofs, M.F., Radstake, T.R., et al., 2008. Stimulation of TLR2 and TLR4 differentially skews the balance of T cells in a mouse model of arthritis. J. Clin. Invest. 118, 205–216.

Aho, K., Steiner, G., Kurki, P., Paimela, L., Leirisalo-Repo, M., Palusuo, T., et al., 1993a. Anti-RA 33 as a marker antibody of rheumatoid arthritis in a Finnish population. Clin. Exp. Rheumatol. 11, 645–647.

Aho, K., von Essen, R., Kurki, P., Palusuo, T., Heliovaara, M., 1993b. Antikeratin antibody and antiperinuclear factor as markers for subclinical rheumatoid disease process. J. Rheumatol. 20, 1278–1281.

Aletaha, D., Neogi, T., Silman, A., Funovits, J., Felson, D., Bingham III, C.O., et al., 2010. The 2010 American College of Rheumatology/ European League Against Rheumatism Classification Criteria for Rheumatoid Arthritis. Ann. Rheum. Dis. 69, 1580–1588.

Aletaha, D., Alasti, F., Smolen, J.S., 2012. Rheumatoid factor determines structural progression of rheumatoid arthritis dependent and independent of disease activity. Ann. Rheum. Dis. 72, 875–880.

Arbuckle, M.R., McClain, M.T., Rubertone, M.V., Scofield, R.H., Dennis, G.J., James, J.A., et al., 2003. Development of autoantibodies before the clinical onset of systemic lupus erythematosus. N. Engl. J. Med. 349, 1526–1533.

Aringer, M., Smolen, J.S., 2012. Therapeutic blockade of TNF in patients with SLE-promising or crazy?. Autoimmun. Rev. 11, 321–325.

Bassyouni, I.H., Ezzat, Y., Hamdy, S., Talaat, R.M., 2009. Clinical significance of anti-cyclic citrullinated peptide antibodies in Egyptian patients with chronic hepatitis C virus genotype IV infection. Clin. Chem. Lab. Med. 47 (7), 842–847.

Begovich, A.B., Carlton, V.E., Honigberg, L.A., Schrodi, S.J., Chokkalingam, A.P., Alexander, H.C., et al., 2004. A missense single-nucleotide polymorphism in a gene encoding a protein tyrosine phosphatase (PTPN22) is associated with rheumatoid arthritis. Am. J. Hum. Genet. 75, 330–337.

Bluml, S., Binder, N.B., Niederreiter, B., Polzer, K., Hayer, S., Tauber, S., et al., 2010. Antiinflammatory effects of tumor necrosis factor on hematopoietic cells in a murine model of erosive arthritis. Arthritis Rheum. 62 (6), 1608–1619.

Bluml, S., McKeever, K., Ettinger, R., Smolen, J., Herbst, R., 2013. B-cell targeted therapeutics in clinical development. Arthritis Res. Ther. 15 (Suppl. 1), S4.

Bohler, C., Radner, H., Smolen, J.S., Aletaha, D., 2013. Serological changes in the course of traditional and biological disease modifying therapy of rheumatoid arthritis. Ann. Rheum. Dis. 72 (2), 241–244.

Brink, M., Hansson, M., Mathsson, L., Jakobsson, P.J., Holmdahl, R., Hallmans, G., et al., 2013. Multiplex analyses of antibodies against citrullinated peptides in individuals prior to development of rheumatoid arthritis. Arthritis Rheum. 65, 899–910.

Burkhardt, H.J., Sehnert, B., Bochermann, R., Engstrom, A., Kalden, J. R., Holmdahl, R., 2005. Humoral immune response to citrullinated collagen type II determinants in early rheumatoid arthritis. Europ. J. Immunol. 35, 1643–1652.

Burmester, G.R., Blanco, R., Charles-Schoeman, C., Wollenhaupt, J., Zerbini, C., Benda, B., et al., 2013. Tofacitinib (CP-690,550) in combination with methotrexate in patients with active rheumatoid arthritis with an inadequate response to tumour necrosis factor inhibitors: a randomised phase 3 trial. Lancet. 381, 1812–1813.

Callahan, L.F., Pincus, T., 1997. Education, self-care, and outcomes of rheumatic diseases: further challenges to the "biomedical model" paradigm. Arthritis Care Res. 10, 283–288.

Candia, L., Marquez, J., Gonzalez, C., Santos, A.M., Londono, J., Valle, R., et al., 2006. Low frequency of anticyclic citrullinated peptide antibodies in psoriatic arthritis but not in cutaneous psoriasis. J. Clin. Rheumatol. 12, 226–229.

Chatzidionysiou, K., Lie, E., Nasonov, E., Lukina, G., Hetland, M.L., Tarp, U., et al., 2011. Highest clinical effectiveness of rituximab in autoantibody-positive patients with rheumatoid arthritis and in those for whom no more than one previous TNF antagonist has failed: pooled data from 10 European registries. Ann. Rheum. Dis. 70, 1575–1580.

Chavele, K.M., Ehrenstein, M.R., 2011. Regulatory T-cells in systemic lupus erythematosus and rheumatoid arthritis. FEBS Lett. 585, 3603–3610.

Chen, P.P., Albrandt, K., Orida, N.K., Radoux, V., Chen, E.Y., Schrantz, R., et al., 1986. Genetic basis for the cross-reactive idiotypes on the light chains of human IgM anti-IgG autoantibodies. Proc. Natl. Acad. Sci. U.S.A. 83, 8318–8322.

De Rycke, L., Peene, I., Hoffman, I.E., Kruithof, E., Union, A., Meheus, L., et al., 2004. Rheumatoid factor and anticitrullinated protein antibodies in rheumatoid arthritis: diagnostic value, associations with radiological progression rate, and extra-articular manifestations.. Ann. Rheum. Dis. 63, 1587–1593.

De Rycke, L., Verhelst, X., Kruithof, E., van den Bosch, F., Hoffman, I. E., Veys, E.M., et al., 2005. Rheumatoid factor, but not anti-cyclic citrullinated peptide antibodies, is modulated by infliximab treatment in rheumatoid arthritis. Ann. Rheum. Dis. 64, 299–302.

Deighton, C.M., Walker, D.J., Griffiths, I.D., Roberts, D.F., 1989. The contribution of HLA to rheumatoid arthritis. Clin. Genet. 36, 178–182.

du Toit, R., Whitelaw, D., Taljaard, J.J., du Plessis, L., Esser, M., 2011. Lack of specificity of anticyclic citrullinated peptide antibodies in advanced human immunodeficiency virus infection. J. Rheumatol. 38, 1055–1060.

Dumonde, D.C., Glynn, L.E., 1962. The production of arthritis in rabbits by an immunological reaction to fibrin. Br. J. Exp. Pathol. 43, 373–383.

Elagib, K.E., Borretzen, M., Jonsson, R., Haga, H.J., Thoen, J., Thompson, K.M., et al., 1999. Rheumatoid factors in primary Sjogren's syndrome (pSS) use diverse VH region genes, the majority of which show no evidence of somatic hypermutation. Clin. Exp, Immunol. 117, 388–394.

Eriksson, J.K., Neovius, M., Ernestam, S., Lindblad, S., Simard, J.F., Askling, J., 2013. Incidence of rheumatoid arthritis in sweden: a nationwide population-based assessment of incidence, its determinants, and treatment penetration. Arthritis Care Res. (Hoboken). 65, 870–878.

Fritsch, R., Eselbock, D., Skriner, K., Jahn-Schmid, B., Scheinecker, C., Bohle, B., et al., 2002. Characterization of autoreactive T cells to the autoantigens heterogeneous nuclear ribonucleoprotein A2 (RA33) and filaggrin in patients with rheumatoid arthritis. J. Immunol. 169, 1068–1076.

Girbal-Neuhauser, E., Durieux, J.J., Arnaud, M., Dalbon, P., Sebbag, M., Vincent, C., et al., 1999. The epitopes targeted by the rheumatoid arthritis-associated antifilaggrin autoantibodies are posttranslationally generated on various sites of (pro)filaggrin by deimination of arginine residues. J. Immunol. 162, 585–594.

Glant, T.T., Mikecz, K., Arzoumanian, A., Poole, A.R., 1987. Proteoglycan-induced arthritis in BALB/c mice. Clinical features and histopathology. Arthritis Rheum. 30, 201–212.

Glant, T.T., Cs-Szabo, G., Nagase, H., Jacobs, J.J., Mikecz, K., 1998. Progressive polyarthritis induced in BALB/c mice by aggrecan from normal and osteoarthritic human cartilage. Arthritis Rheum. 41, 1007–1018.

Glossop, J.R., Dawes, P.T., Mattey, D.L., 2006. Association between cigarette smoking and release of tumour necrosis factor alpha and its soluble receptors by peripheral blood mononuclear cells in patients with rheumatoid arthritis. Rheumatology (Oxford). 45, 1223–1229.

Gokhan, A., Turkeyler, I.H., Babacan, T., Pehlivan, Y., Dag, M.S., Bosnak, V.K., et al., 2013. The antibodies cyclic citrullinated peptides (anti-CCP) positivity could be a promising marker in brucellosis patients presented with peripheric arthritis. Mod. Rheumatol.in press.

Grabar, P., 1975. The "globulines-transporteurs" theory and auto-sensitization. Med. Hypotheses. 1, 172–175.

Gravallese, E.M., Harada, Y., Wang, J.T., Gorn, A.H., Thornhill, T.S., Goldring, S.R., 1998. Identification of cell types responsiblefor bone resorption in rheumatoid arthritis and juvenile rheumatoid arthritis. Am. J. Pathol. 152, 943–951.

Gregersen, P.K., Silver, J., Winchester, R.J., 1987. The shared epitope hypothesis: an approach to understanding the molecular genetics of susceptibility to rheumatoid arthritis. Arthritis Rheum. 30, 1205–1213.

Halbert, S.P., Anken, M., 1982. Auto-antibodies in infectious mononucleosis, as determined by ELISA. Int. Arch. Allergy Appl. Immunol. 69, 257–261.

Hayakawa, K., Asano, M., Shinton, S.A., Gui, M., Allman, D., Stewart, C.L., et al., 1999. Positive selection of natural autoreactive B cells. Science. 285, 113–116.

Hayer, S., Tohidast-Akrad, M., Haralambous, S., Jahn-Schmid, B., Skriner, K., Trembleau, S., et al., 2005. Aberrant expression of the autoantigen heterogeneous nuclear ribonucleoprotein-A2 (RA33) and spontaneous formation of rheumatoid arthritis-associated anti-RA33 autoantibodies in TNF-alpha transgenic mice. J. Immunol. 175, 8327–8336.

Helmick, C.G., Felson, D.T., Lawrence, R.C., Gabriel, S., Hirsch, R., Kwoh, C.K., et al., 2008. Estimates of the prevalence of arthritis and other rheumatic conditions in the United States. Part I. Arthritis Rheum. 58, 15–25.

Holmdahl, R., Lorentzen, J.C., Lu, S., Olofsson, P., Wester, L., Holmberg, J., et al., 2001. Arthritis induced in rats with nonimmunogenic adjuvants as models for rheumatoid arthritis. Immunol. Rev. 184, 184–202.

Holmdahl, R., Bockermann, R., Backlund, J., Yamada, H., 2002. The molecular pathogenesis of collagen-induced arthritis in mice—a model for rheumatoid arthritis. Ageing Res. Rev. 1, 135–147.

Horai, R., Saijo, S., Tanioka, H., Nakae, S., Sudo, K., Okahara, A., et al., 2000. Development of chronic inflammatory arthropathy resembling rheumatoid arthritis in interleukin 1 receptor antagonist-deficient mice. J. Exp. Med. 191, 313–320.

Houssien, D.A., Jonsson, T., Davies, E., Scott, D.L., 1997. Clinical significance of IgA rheumatoid factor subclasses in rheumatoid arthritis. J. Rheumatol. 24, 2119–2122.

Jasin, H.E., 1985. Autoantibody specificities of immune complexes sequestered in articular cartilage of patients with rheumatoid arthritis and osteoarthritis. Arthritis Rheum. 28, 241–248.

Jimenez-Boj, M.E., Bauer, R., Gaertner, M., Nell-Duxneuner, V.P., Stamm, T.A., Wagner, O., et al., 2012. Prediciting rheumatoid arthritis by autoantibody testing (prera): preliminary results of a community-based investigation. Ann. Rheum. Dis. 71, 338.

Joosten, L.A., Helsen, M.M., Van De Loo, F.A., van Den Berg, W.B., 2008. Anticytokine treatment of established type II collagen-induced arthritis in DBA/1 mice: a comparative study using anti-TNFalpha, anti-IL-1alpha/beta and IL-1Ra. Arthritis Rheum. 58, S110–S122.

Keffer, J., Probert, L., Cazlaris, H., Georgopoulos, S., Kaslaris, E., Kioussis, D., et al., 1991. Transgenic mice expressing human tumour necrosis factor: a predictive genetic model of arthritis. EMBO J. 10, 4025–4031.

Klareskog, L., Malmstrom, V., Lundberg, K., Padyukov, L., Alfredsson, L., 2011. Smoking, citrullination and genetic variability in the immunopathogenesis of rheumatoid arthritis. Semin. Immunol. 23, 92–98.

Koch, R., 1890. An address on bacteriological research. Br. Med. J. 2, 380–383.

Korb-Pap, A., Stratis, A., Muhlenberg, K., Niederreiter, B., Hayer, S., Echtermeyer, F., et al., 2012. Early structural changes in cartilage and bone are required for the attachment and invasion of inflamed synovial tissue during destructive inflammatory arthritis. Ann. Rheum. Dis. 71, 1004–1011.

Korn, T., Bettelli, E., Oukka, M., Kuchroo, V.K., 2009. IL-17 and Th17 cells. Annu. Rev. Immunol. 27, 485–517.

Kraan, M.C., Haringman, J.J., Post, W.J., Versendaal, J., Breedveld, F.C., Tak, P.P., 1999. Immunohistological analysis of synovial tissue for differential diagnosis in early arthritis. Rheumatology (Oxford). 38, 1074–1080.

Kuhn, K.A., Kulik, L., Tomooka, B., Braschler, K.J., Arend, W.P., Robinson, W.H., et al., 2006. Antibodies against citrullinated proteins enhance tissue injury in experimental autoimmune arthritis. J. Clin. Invest. 116 (4), 961–973.

Lam, J., Takeshita, S., Barker, J.E., Kanagawa, O., Ross, F.P., Teitelbaum, S.L., 2000. TNF-alpha induces osteoclastogenesis by direct stimulation of macrophages exposed to permissive levels of RANK ligand. J. Clin. Invest. 106, 1481–1488.

Landre-Beauvais, A.J., 1800. Doit-on admettre une nouvelle espece de Goutte sous la denomination de Goutte Asthenique Primitive? An VIII, Paris, Brisson.

Lee, H.S., Irigoyen, P., Kern, M., Lee, A., Batliwalla, F., Khalili, H., et al., 2007. Interaction between smoking, the shared epitope, and anti-cyclic citrullinated peptide: a mixed picture in three large North American rheumatoid arthritis cohorts. Arthritis Rheum. 56, 1745–1753.

Lee, Z.H., Firestein, G.S., 2003. Fibroblasts. In: Smolen, J.S., Lipsky, P.L. (Eds.), Targeted Therapies in Rheumatology. Martin Dunitz, London–New York, pp. 133–146.

Lefevre, S., Knedla, A., Tennie, C., Kampmann, A., Wunrau, C., Dinser, R., et al., 2009. Synovial fibroblasts spread rheumatoid arthritis to unaffected joints. Nat. Med. 15, 1414–1420.

Li, Y., Begovich, A.B., 2009. Unraveling the genetics of complex diseases: susceptibility genes for rheumatoid arthritis and psoriasis. Semin. Immunol. 21, 318–327.

Lima, I., Santiago, M., 2010. Antibodies against cyclic citrullinated peptides in infectious diseases—a systematic review. Clin. Rheumatol. 29, 1345–1351.

Lima, I., Oliveira, R.C., Atta, A., Marchi, S., Barbosa, L., Reis, E., et al., 2013. Antibodies to citrullinated peptides in tuberculosis. Clin. Rheumatol.In press.

MacGregor, A.J., Snieder, H., Rigby, A.S., Koskenvuo, M., Kaprio, J., Aho, K., et al., 2000. Characterizing the quantitative genetic contribution to rheumatoid arthritis using data from twins. Arthritis Rheum. 43, 30–37.

Mallya, R.K., Vergani, D., Tee, D.E., Bevis, L., de Beer, F.C., Berry, H., et al., 1982. Correlation in rheumatoid arthritis of concentrations of plasma C3d, serum rheumatoid factor, immune complexes and C-reactive protein with each other and with clinical features of disease activity. Clin. Exp. Immunol. 48, 747–753.

Martin, T., Duffy, S.F., Carson, D.A., Kipps, T.J., 1992. Evidence for somatic selection of natural autoantibodies. J. Exp. Med. 175, 983–991.

Matsumoto, I., Maccioni, M., Lee, D.M., Maurice, M., Simmons, B., Brenner, M., et al., 2002. How antibodies to a ubiquitous cytoplasmic enzyme may provoke joint-specific autoimmune disease. Nat. Immunol. 3, 360–365.

Mattey, D.L., Dawes, P.T., Clarke, S., Fisher, J., Brownfield, A., Thomson, W., et al., 2002. Relationship among the HLA-DRB1 shared epitope smoking and rheumatoid factor production in rheumatoid arthritis. Arthritis Rheum. 47, 403–407.

Menzel, J., Steffen, C., Kolarz, G., Eberal, G., Frank, O., Thumb, N., 1975. Demonstration of antibodies to collagen and of collagen-anticollagen immune complexes in rheumatoid arthritis synovial fluids. Ann. Rheum. Dis. 35, 446–450.

Mjaavatten, M.D., van der Heijde, D., Uhlig, T., Haugen, A.J., Nygaard, H., Sidenvall, G., et al., 2010. The likelihood of persistent arthritis increases with the level of anti-citrullinated peptide antibody and immunoglobulin M rheumatoid factor: a longitudinal study of 376 patients with very early undifferentiated arthritis. Arthritis Res. Ther. 12, R76.

National Collaborating Centre for Chronic Conditions, 2009. Rheumatoid arthritis: national clinical guideline for management and treatment in adults. Royal College of Physicians, London, February 2009.

Nell, V., Machold, K.P., Stamm, T.A., Eberl, G., Heinzl, H., Uffmann, M., et al., 2005. Autoantibody profiling as early diagnostic and prognostic tool for rheumatoid arthritis. Ann. Rheum. Dis. 64, 1731–1736.

Nell, V.P.K., Machold, K.P., Eberl, G., Hiesberger, H., Hoefler, E., Smolen, J.S., et al., 2003. The diagnostic and prognostic significance of autoantibodies in patients with early arthritis. Ann. Rheum. Dis. 62, 15.

Neogi, T., Aletaha, D., Silman, A.J., Naden, R.L., Felson, D.T., Aggarwal, R., et al., 2010. The 2010 American College of Rheumatology/European League Against Rheumatism classification criteria for rheumatoid arthritis: Phase 2 methodological report. Arthritis Rheum. 62, 2582–2591.

Nicaise-Roland, P., Nogueira, I.., Demattei, C., Rincheval, N., Cornillet, M., Grootenboer-Mignot, S., et al., 2013. Autoantibodies to citrullinated fibrinogen compared with anti-MCV and anti-CCP2 antibodies in diagnosing rheumatoid arthritis at an early stage: data from the French ESPOIR cohort. Ann. Rheum. Dis. 72 (3), 357–362.

Nielen, M.M., van Schaardenburg Reesink, W.H., Van de Stadt, R.J., Van der Horst-Bruinsma, I.E., De Koning, M.G., et al., 2004. Specific autoantibodies precede the symptoms of rheumatoid arthritis: a study of serial measurements in blood donors. Arthritis Rheum. 50, 380–386.

Nielsen, S.F., Bojesen, S.E., Schnohr, P., Nordestgaard, B.G., 2012. Elevated rheumatoid factor and long term risk of rheumatoid arthritis: a prospective cohort study. BMJ. 345, e5244.

Nienhuis, R.L., Mandema, E., 1964. A new serum factor in patients with rheumatoid arthritis; the antiperinuclear factor. Ann. Rheum. Dis. 23, 302–305.

Packard, C.J., Bezlyak, V., McLean, J.S., Batty, G.D., Ford, I., Burns, H., et al., 2011. Early life socioeconomic adversity is associated in adult life with chronic inflammation, carotid atherosclerosis, poorer lung function and decreased cognitive performance: a cross-sectional, population-based study. BMC Public Health. 11, 42.

Partsch, G., Steiner, G., Leeb, B.F., Dunky, A., Broll, H., Smolen, J.S., 1997. Highly increased levels of tumor necrosis factor-alpha and other proinflammatory cytokines in psoriatic arthritis synovial fluid. J. Rheumatol. 24, 518–523.

Pietropaolo, M., Towns, R., Eisenbarth, G.S., 2012. Humoral auto-immunity in type 1 diabetes: prediction, significance, and detection of distinct disease subtypes. Cold Spring Harb. Perspect. Med. 2, 10.

Plenge, R.M., Seielstad, M., Padyukov, L., Lee, A.T., Remmers, E.F., Ding, B., et al., 2007. TRAF1-C5 as a risk locus for rheumatoid arthritis—a genomewide study. N. Engl. J. Med. 357, 1199–1209.

Rantapaa-Dahlqvist, S., De Jong, B.A., Berglin, E., Hallmans, G., Wadell, G., Stenlund, H., et al., 2003. Antibodies against cyclic citrullinated peptide and IgA rheumatoid factor predict the development of rheumatoid arthritis. Arthritis Rheum. 48, 2741–2749.

Redlich, K., Hayer, S., Ricci, R., David, J.P., Tohidast-Akrad, M., Kollias, G., et al., 2002. Osteoclasts are essential for TNF-alpha-mediated joint destruction. J. Clin. Invest. 110, 1419–1427.

Remmers, E.F., Plenge, R.M., Lee, A.T., Graham, R.R., Hom, G., Behrens, T.W., et al., 2007. STAT4 and the risk of rheumatoid arthritis and systemic lupus erythematosus. N. Engl. J. Med. 357, 977–986.

Scheinecker, C., Smolen, J.S., 2011. Rheumatoid arthritis in 2010: from the gut to the joint. Nat. Rev. Rheumatol. 7, 73–75.

Schellekens, G.A., De Jong, B.A., Van den Hoogen, F.H., Van de Putte, L.B., Van Venrooij, W.J., 1998. Citrulline is an essential constituent of antigenic determinants recognized by rheumatoid arthritis-specific autoantibodies. J. Clin. Invest. 101, 273–281.

Scher, J.U., Abramson, S.B., 2011. The microbiome and rheumatoid arthritis. Nat. Rev. Rheumatol. 7, 569–578.

Scher, J.U., Ubeda, C., Equinda, M., Khanin, R., Buischi, Y., Viale, A., et al., 2012. Periodontal disease and the oral microbiota in new-onset rheumatoid arthritis. Arthritis Rheum. 64, 3083–3094.

Schur, P.H., Britton, M.C., Franco, A.E., Corson, J.M., Sosman, J.L., Ruddy, S., 1975. Rheumatoid synovitis: complement and immune complexes. Rheumatology. 6, 34–42.

Seldin, M.F., Amos, C.I., Ward, R., Gregersen, P.K., 1999. The genetics revolution and the assault on rheumatoid arthritis. Arthritis Rheum. 42, 1071–1079.

Shi, J., Van de Stadt, L.A., Levarht, E.W., Huizinga, T.W., Toes, R.E., Trouw, L.A., et al., 2013. Anti-carbamylated protein antibodies are present in arthralgia patients and predict the development of rheumatoid arthritis. Arthritis Rheum. 65, 911–915.

Silman, A.J., Pearson, J.E., 2002. Epidemiology and genetics of rheumatoid arthritis. Arthritis Res. 4, S265–S272.

Silman, A.J., MacGregor, A.J., Thomson, W., Holligan, S., Carthy, D., Farhan, A., et al., 1993. Twin concordance rates for rheumatoid arthritis: results from a nationwide study. Br. J. Rheumatol. 32, 903–907.

Silman, A.J., Newman, J., MacGregor, A.J., 1996. Cigarette smoking increases the risk of rheumatoid arthritis. Results from a nation-wide study of disease-discordant twins. Arthritis Rheum. 39, 732–735.

Singh, J.A., Christensen, R., Wells, G.A., Suarez-Almazor, M.E., Buchbinder, R., Lopez-Olivo, M.A., et al., 2009. Biologics for rheumatoid arthritis: an overview of Cochrane reviews. Cochrane Database Syst. Rev.(4), .

Singh, U., Singh, S., Singh, N.K., Verma, P.K., Singh, S., 2011. Anticyclic citrullinated peptide autoantibodies in systemic lupus erythematosus. Rheumatol. Int. 31, 765–767.

Smolen, J.S., Aletaha, D., 2013. Forget personalised medicine and focus on abating disease activity. Ann. Rheum. Dis. 72, 3–6.

Smolen, J.S., Menzel, E.J., Scherak, O., Kojer, M., Kolarz, G., Steffen, C., et al., 1980. Lymphocyte transformation to denatured type I collagen and B lymphocyte alloantigens in rheumatoid arthritis. Arthritis Rheum. 23, 424–431.

Smolen, J.S., Breedveld, F.C., Eberl, G., Jones, I., Leeming, M., Wylie, G.L., et al., 1995. Validity and reliability of the twenty-eight-joint count for the assessment of rheumatoid arthritis activity. Arthritis Rheum. 38, 38–43.

Smolen, J.S., Aletaha, D., Machold, K., Nell, V., Redlich, K., Schett, G., et al., 2006. Pre-arthritis — a concept whose time has come. Future Rheumatol. 1, 1–4.

Smolen, J.S., Aletaha, D., Koeller, M., Weisman, M., Emery, P., 2007. New therapies for the treatment of rheumatoid arthritis. Lancet. 370, 1861–1874.

Smolen, J.S., Alasti, F., Aletaha, D., 2012. Rheumatoid factor, not antibodies to citrullinated proteins, are associated with high disease activity. Arthritis Rheum. 64, S183–S184.

van Snick, J.L., van Roost, E., Markowetz, B., Cambiaso, C.L., Masson, P.L., 1978. Enhancement by IgM rheumatoid factor of in vitro ingestion by macrophages and in vivo clearance of aggregated IgG or antigen-antibody complexes. Eur. J. Immunol. 8, 279–285.

Stastny, P., 1978. Association of the B-cell alloantigen DRw4 with rheumatoid arthritis. N. Engl. J. Med. 298, 869–871.

Steffen, C., 1970. Consideration of pathogenesis of rheumatoid arthritis as collagen autoimmunity. Z.Immunitatsforsch. Allerg. Klin. Immunol. 139, 219–227.

Steiner, G., Hartmuth, K., Skriner, K., Maurer-Fogy, I., Sinski, A., Thalmann, E., et al., 1992. Purification and partial sequencing of the nuclear autoantigen RA33 shows that it is indistinguishable from the A2 protein of the heterogeneous nuclear ribonucleoprotein complex. J. Clin. Invest. 90, 1061–1066.

Symmons, D.P., Bankhead, C.R., Harrison, B.J., Brennan, P., Barrett, E. M., Scott, D.G., et al., 1997. Blood transfusion, smoking, and obesity as risk factors for the development of rheumatoid arthritis: results from a primary care-based incident case–control study in Norfolk, England. Arthritis Rheum. 40, 1955–1961.

Takasaki, Y., Yamanaka, K., Takasaki, C., Matsushita, M., Yamada, H., Nawata, M., et al., 2004. Anticyclic citrullinated peptide antibodies in patients with mixed connective tissue disease. Mod. Rheumatol. 14, 367–375.

Teitelbaum, S.L., 2000. Bone resorption by osteoclasts. Science. 289 (5484), 1504–1508.

Toivanen, P., 2001. From reactive arthritis to rheumatoid arthritis. J. Autoimmun. 16, 369–371.

Trentham, D.E., Townes, A.S., Kang, A.H., 1977. Autoimmunity to type II collagen an experimental model of arthritis. J. Exp. Med. 146, 857–868.

Trentham, D.E., Dynesius, R.A., Rocklin, R.E., David, J.R., 1978. Cellular sensitivity to collagen in rheumatoid arthritis. N. Engl. J. Med. 299, 327–332.

Uhlig, T., Hagen, K.B., Kvien, T.K., 1999. Current tobacco smoking, formal education, and the risk of rheumatoid arthritis. J. Rheumatol. 26, 47–54.

van der Helm-van Mil, A.H., Verpoort, K.N., Breedveld, F.C., Huizinga, T.W., Toes, R.E., De Vries, R.R., 2006. The HLA-DRB1 shared epitope alleles are primarily a risk factor for anti-cyclic citrullinated peptide antibodies and are not an independent risk factor for development of rheumatoid arthritis. Arthritis Rheum. 54, 1117–1121.

van der Lubbe, PA, Dijkmans, BS, Markusse, H, Nassander, U, Breedveld, FC., 1995. A randomized, double-blind, placebo-controlled study of CD4 monoclonal antibody therapy in early rheumatoid arthritis. Arthritis Rheum. 38, 1097–1106.

Vesperini, V., Lukas, C., Fautrel, B., Le Loet, X., Rincheval, N., Combe, B., 2013. Tobacco exposure reduces radiographic progression in early rheumatoid arthritis. Results from the ESPOIR cohort. Arthritis Care Res. Jul.8. 10.1002/acr.22057.

Vossenaar, E.R., Smeets, T.J., Kraan, M.C., Raats, J.M., van Venrooij, W. J., Tak, P.P., 2004. The presence of citrullinated proteins is not specific for rheumatoid synovial tissue. Arthritis Rheum. 50, 3485–3494.

Waaler, E., 1939. On the occurrence of a factor in human serum activating the specific agglutination of sheep blood corpuscles. Acta Pathol. Microbiol. Immunol. Scand. 17, 172–182.

Wegner, N., Wait, R., Sroka, A., Eick, S., Nguyen, K.A., Lundberg, K., et al., 2010. Peptidylarginine deiminase from Porphyromonas gingivalis citrullinates human fibrinogen and alpha-enolase: implications for autoimmunity in rheumatoid arthritis. Arthritis Rheum. 62, 2662–2672.

Wernick, R.M., Lipsky, P.E., Marban-Arcos, E., Maliakkal, J.J., Edelbaum, D., Ziff, M., 1985. IgG and IgM rheumatoid factor synthesis in rheumatoid synovial membrane cell cultures. Arthritis Rheum. 28, 742–752.

Williams, D.G., Moyes, S.P., Mageed, R.A., 1999. Rheumatoid factor isotype switch and somatic mutation variants within rheumatoid arthritis synovium. Immunology. 98, 123–136.

Winchester, R.J., Agnello, V., Kunkel, H.G., 1970. Gamma globulin complexes in synovial fluids of patients with rheumatoid arthritis. Partial characterization and relationship to lowered complement levels. Clin. Exp. Immunol. 6, 689–706.

Witebsky, E., Rose, N.R., Terplan, K., Paine, J.R., Egan, R.W., 1957. Chronic thyroiditis and autoimmunization. J. Am. Med. Assoc. 164, 1439–1447.

Wu, H.J., Ivanov, I.I., Darce, J., Hattori, K., Shima, T., Umesaki, Y., et al., 2010. Gut-residing segmented filamentous bacteria drive autoimmune arthritis via T helper 17 cells. Immunity. 32, 815–827.

Xue, Y., Zhang, J., Chen, Y.M., Guan, M., Zheng, S.G., Zou, H.J., 2008. The HLA-DRB1 shared epitope is not associated with antibodies against cyclic citrullinated peptide in Chinese patients with rheumatoid arthritis. Scand. J. Rheumatol. 37, 183–187.

Yoshitomi, H., Sakaguchi, N., Kobayashi, K., Brown, G.D., Tagami, T., Sakihama, T., et al., 2005. A role for fungal {beta}-glucans and their receptor Dectin-1 in the induction of autoimmune arthritis in genetically susceptible mice. J. Exp. Med. 201 (6), 949–960.

Young, B.J., Mallya, R.K., Leslie, R.D., Clark, C.J., Hamblin, T.J., 1979. Anti-keratin antibodies in rheumatoid arthritis. Br. Med. J. 2, 97–99.

Zvaifler, N.J., 1974. Rheumatoid synovitis. An extravascular immune complex disease. Arthritis Rheum. 17, 297–305.

Chapter 37

Juvenile Idiopathic Arthritis

Clara Malattia and Alberto Martini

Pediatria II, Reumatologia, Istituto Giannina Gaslini, Genova e Dipartimento di Pediatria, Università of Genova, Genova, Italy

Chapter Outline

Epidemiology   525
Clinical Features   525
  Systemic Arthritis   525
  Rheumatoid Factor-Positive Polyarthritis   526
  Enthesitis-Related Arthritis   526
  Oligoarthritis   527
  Rheumatoid Factor-Negative Polyarthritis   527
  Psoriatic Arthritis   527
  Undifferentiated Arthritis   527
  Perspectives   527
Etiology and Pathogenesis   528

Systemic Juvenile Idiopathic Arthritis   528
  Genetics   528
  Proinflammatory Mediators   528
  Interleukin-6   528
  Interleukin-1   530
  Interleukin-18   530
  Macrophage Activation Syndrome   530
Oligoarticular Juvenile Idiopathic Arthritis   531
Treatment   532
References   533

Juvenile idiopathic arthritis (JIA) is not a disease, but an exclusion diagnosis that gathers together all forms of arthritis that begin before the age of 16 years, persist for more than 6 weeks, and are of unknown origin (Ravelli and Martini, 2007; Prakken et al., 2011) This heterogeneous group of chronic arthritides has been classified on clinical and laboratory grounds to try to identify homogeneous, mutually exclusives categories suitable for etiopathogenic studies. The more recent classification is the one proposed by the International League of Associations for Rheumatology (ILAR) (Petty et al., 2004) (Table 37.1). This classification has, however, been recently challenged and suggestions for reconsidering some aspects of classification and nomenclature, as we will discuss, have been proposed (Martini, 2003, 2012).

EPIDEMIOLOGY

JIA as a whole is the most common chronic rheumatic condition in childhood and an important cause of short- and long-term disability. Studies in Western populations have reported an incidence and a prevalence varying from 2 to 20 and from 16 to 150 per 100,000, respectively (Ravelli and Martini, 2007).

CLINICAL FEATURES

The group of diseases gathered under the umbrella term of JIA encompasses several different forms of chronic arthritis that, in the absence of etiologic clues, have been classified according to clinical criteria.

Systemic Arthritis

Systemic arthritis is considered the equivalent of "adult-onset Still's disease" and accounts for 10 to 15% of children with JIA. It is characterized by prominent systemic features, such as high spiking fever, an evanescent, non-fixed, erythematosus rash that characteristically occurs with fever peaks, hepatomegaly or splenomegaly, generalized lymphoadenopathy, and serositis. Myalgias and abdominal pain may be intense during fever peaks. Arthritis is more often symmetrical and polyarticular; it may be absent at onset and develop during disease course. Laboratory investigations show leukocytosis (with neutrophilia), thrombocytosis and very high erythrocyte sedimentation rate (ESR) and C-reactive protein concentration. A microcytic anemia is common.

About 5 to 8% of children with systemic JIA develop a life-threatening complication, named macrophage

N. Rose & I. Mackay (Eds): The Autoimmune Diseases, Fifth edition. DOI: http://dx.doi.org/10.1016/B978-0-12-384929-8.00037-X

TABLE 37.1 Frequency, Age at Onset, and Sex Distribution of the International League of Associations for Rheumatology (ILAR) Categories of Juvenile Idiopathic Arthritis. The Different Categories are Defined According to the Symptoms Presented during the First 6 Months of Disease

	Frequency[a]	Onset Age	Sex Ratio
Systemic arthritis	4–17%	Throughout childhood	F = M
Oligoarthritis	27–56%	Early childhood; peak at 2–3 years	F >>> M
Rheumatoid factor-positive polyartriris	2–7%	Late childhood or adolescence	F >> M
Rheumatoid factor-negative polyarthritis	11–28%	Biphasic distribution, early at 2–4 years and later peak at 6–12 years	F >> M
Enthesitis-related arthritis	3–11%	Late childhood or adolescence	M >> F
Psoriatic arthritis	2–11%	Biphasic distribution; early peak at 2–4 years and later peak at 9–11 years	F > M
Undiffentiated arthritis	11–21%		

[a]Percentage of all juvenile idiopathic arthritis cases.

activation syndrome (MAS) (Ravelli et al., 2012). The syndrome is a form of reactive hemophagocytic lymphohistiocytosis and is characterized by the sudden onset of sustained fever, pancytopenia, hepatosplenomegaly, liver insufficiency, coagulopathy with hemorrhagic manifestations, and neurological symptoms. Laboratory features include elevated triglycerides, low sodium levels, and markedly increased ferritin concentrations. The demonstration of active phagocytosis of hematopoietic cells by macrophage in the bone marrow is common. Early recognition and treatment of MAS before the development of severe multisystem involvement is crucial for the prognosis.

Systemic JIA (sJIA) probably does not represent a disease but rather a syndrome, the common endpoint of several different diseases all causing a marked and persistent activation of the innate immune system (Martini, 2012). The potential heterogeneity of this condition is suggested by the exquisite sensitivity to IL-1 blockade presented by a subset of patients (see below) as well as by differences in clinical course.

Indeed, in about half of patients the disease is mainly characterized by the systemic features while the arthritis usually remits when systemic features are controlled. In the other half of patients the disease follows an unremitting course; systemic symptoms may eventually resolve, leaving chronic arthritis as the major long-term problem. There are, moreover, patients who present the same systemic features observed in sJIA but never develop arthritis, and therefore cannot by definition be classified as sJIA. Currently this subgroup of patients lacks any taxonomic definition. The super-imposable systemic clinical and laboratory features suggest that they have a disease strongly related to sJIA despite the lack of arthritis. This

type of patient is indeed included in the definition of adult onset Still's disease, where the presence of arthritis is not required for diagnosis. It has been suggested to include these patients in the sJIA disease category (Martini, 2012) but, given the absence of arthritis, the term sJIA should be changed; a possible new name could be Still's disease, by analogy with the adult counterpart, adult onset Still's disease.

Rheumatoid Factor-Positive Polyarthritis

This rare (5% of patients with JIA) subgroup is the childhood equivalent of adult rheumatoid factor (RF)-positive rheumatoid arthritis; in fact, it is the only form of JIA with positive antibodies to cyclic citrullinated peptides. As in adults it is a chronic, erosive disease.

Enthesitis-Related Arthritis

This represents a form of undifferentiated spondyloarthropathy. The most common sites of enthesitis are the calcaneal insertions of the Achilles tendon and of the plantar fascia and the tarsal area. Arthritis is usually oligoarticular and affects mainly the lower limbs. Most patients are human leukocyte antigen (HLA)-B27 positive. The disease can be mild and remitting but a variable proportion of patients, who are impossible to identify at disease onset, develop the involvement of sacroiliac joints during disease course. Indeed, all the different forms of adult spondyloarthropathies can be observed in children; the major difference is the much higher proportion of undifferentiated spondyloarthropathies in childhood. The discrepancy in terminology between children and adults has been a source of confusion and it has been suggested to abandon the term enthesitis-related arthritis, which could suggest the existence of a form peculiar to childhood, and to use, with the prefix juvenile, the same terminology used to define the adult forms of spondyloarthropathies (Martini, 2012).

Oligoarthritis

Oligoarthritis is defined by the involvement of four or fewer joints during the first 6 months of disease. In Western countries the large majority of patients belongs to a quite well-defined disease entity observed only in children and characterized by an asymmetric arthritis, involving mainly large joints, an early onset (before 6 years of age), a female predilection, a high frequency of positive antinuclear antibodies (ANA), a high risk of developing chronic iridocyclitis, and consistent HLA associations. The current ILAR classification distinguishes two categories of oligoarthritis: one, often with a good long-term prognosis, in which the disease remains confined to four or fewer joints (persistent oligoarthritis) and one in which arthritis extends to more than four joints after the first 6 months of disease (extended oligoarthritis). It has, however, been shown that ANA-positive patients with persistent or with extended oligoarthritis share the same characteristics, strongly suggesting that they represent the same disease and just differ in the spread of arthritis (Ravelli et al., 2005).

A peculiar feature is a chronic, asymptomatic, nongranulomatous, anterior uveitis affecting the iris and the ciliary body (iridocyclitis) that can cause severe visual impairment and affects about 30% of patients. The onset is insidious and very often entirely asymptomatic in contrast with the painful, acute uveitis that can be observed in enthesitis-related arthritis. One or both eyes may be involved. Most children who develop uveitis do it within 5 to 7 years from the onset of arthritis. The course of uveitis may be relapsing or chronic and does not parallel the clinical course of arthritis. ANA positivity represents a strong risk factor for developing uveitis. Since uveitis is asymptomatic, children with ANA-positive JIA should be screened at least every 3 months by slit-lamp examination.

Rheumatoid Factor-Negative Polyarthritis

This is defined by the involvement of five or more joints during the first 6 months of disease and is an heterogeneous JIA category. At least two separate subsets can be identified: one, characterized by a symmetric synovitis of large and small joints, onset in school age, and negative ANA, is similar to adult-onset RF-negative rheumatoid arthritis; the other resembles oligoarthritis, except by definition for the number of joints affected in the first 6 months of disease. The similarities between this second subset and early-onset oligoarthritis led to the hypothesis

that they represent the same disease, the former representing a rapid arthritis spread in the latter (Martini, 2003). This view has been confirmed by the demonstration that those features (early age at onset, asymmetric arthritis, female predominance, ANA positivity, elevated incidence of chronic iridocyclitis) that characterize ANA-positive oligoarthritis are also present in ANA-positive, RF-negative polyarthritis, but not in ANA-negative, RF-negative polyarthritis or in ANA-negative oligoarthritis (Ravelli et al., 2005, 2011). Moreover, ANA-positive, RF-negative polyarthritis is seldom observed in those countries in which ANA-positive oligoarthritis is rare (Martini, 2003).

Of note, Barnes and co-workers (Barnes et al., 2010), studying gene expression in oligoarticular and polyarticular JIA, found that patients with early-onset arthritis (≤6 years) are characterized by a B cell signature independently from the number of joints involved; moreover, high resolution HLA class I and class II typing has also shown similarities between early-onset oligoarticular and polyarticular JIA (Hollenbach et al., 2010).

Psoriatic Arthritis

This is another inadequately defined JIA category. If Vancouver criteria (presence of arthritis and psoriasis or some psoriatic features) (Southwood et al., 1989) are used to define psoriatic arthritis two populations of patients are identified: (1) one that represents, as adult psoriatic arthritis, a form of spondyloarthropathy; (2) a second form that shares the same above-mentioned characteristics of ANA-positive, early onset oligoarthritis (Martini, 2003; Stoll et al., 2006). So the association of psoriasis with arthritis seems to lead to the identification of two different subsets of patients, one that is similar to adult psoriatic arthritis and the other that overlaps with ANA-positive, early onset oligoarthritis (Martini, 2003; Ravelli et al., 2011). The ILAR classification criteria for psoriatic arthritis, in which patients with enthesitis are by definition excluded, limit the identification of those patients that have a form of psoriatic arthritis similar to that observed in adults (Stoll et al., 2008).

Undifferentiated Arthritis

Undifferentiated arthritis does not represent a separate subset, but a category in which by definition patients that do not fulfill inclusion criteria of any of the categories, or fit criteria for more than one category, are included.

Perspectives

The ILAR classification has represented a step forward in the understanding of JIA. However, recent acquisitions call for a further refinement in order to better identify clinically homogeneous entities suitable for etiopathogenic studies.

In particular, in our opinion there is now enough evidence that some patients with ANA-positive, early-onset arthritis, a well-defined entity observed only in childhood, are in the current ILAR classification wrongly included in the RF-negative polyarthritis and in the psoriatic arthritis categories. It would be therefore advisable to group all these patients together in a new category of ANA-positive, early onset arthritis independently from the number of joints involved or the presence of psoriasis (Martini, 2012). Once these patients are removed, the RF-negative polyarthritis and the psoriatic arthritis categories would presumably mainly be represented by patients with the same clinical characteristics observed in adults.

Further advances in classification will come from immunologic, genomic, and proteomic studies in the various JIA categories as well as from differences in the response to biological agents that, by targeting specific molecules, represent a precious opportunity of "reverse translation" (from the bed to the bench side) as it has been with the inhibition of interleukin (IL)-1 in sJIA.

ETIOLOGY AND PATHOGENESIS

As discussed above, it is now clear that in children, as in adults, there are several completely different diseases which are all responsible for chronic arthritis and that are gathered under the umbrella term of JIA. With the exception of early-onset, ANA-positive arthritis, which is specific to childhood, they appear to represent the childhood counterpart of diseases also observed in adults. Therefore, in order to avoid overlaps with other chapters only those immunological aspects that belong to systemic JIA, which is far more common in children, and to early-onset ANA-positive arthritis, which occurs only in children, will be discussed in detail. For the other diseases, there are no relevant, specific immunological findings characteristic of childhood-onset forms.

Systemic Juvenile Idiopathic Arthritis

Systemic JIA (sJIA) is etiopathogenically different from all the other forms of JIA (Mellins et al., 2011). The systemic features, the marked inflammatory response, the lack of sex bias, peak age at onset, association with autoantibodies or HLA antigens are all consistent with what is observed in autoinflammatory diseases. Also, the sensitivity to treatment is different and provides evidence for a different etiopathogenesis. Indeed, methotrexate or antitumor necrosis factor (TNF) agents are less effective than in the other JIA categories, while anti-IL-6 or anti-IL-1 drugs are of impressive efficacy.

Genetics

sJIA is much more frequent in children than in adults (adult-onset Still's disease). This can suggest a role for some widely diffused infectious agents that are encountered early in life or represent the effect of a strong genetic predisposing background. The disease is considered multifactorial and multigenic although it is not known if genetic predisposition is due to the combinations of common genetic variants each providing a small contribution to inherited susceptibility or to high-penetrance rare mutations that only account for a few cases each.

Some genetic polymorphisms, particularly of cytokine genes, have been associated with sJIA (Table 37.2). A genome-wide association study is currently under way.

Consistently with the supposed autoinflammatory nature of sJIA gene expression, studies on peripheral blood mononuclear cells (PBMCs) have shown an upregulation of genes associated with the activation of monocyte/macrophage lineage and a downregulation of the gene networks involving natural killer (NK) cells, T cells, and major histocompatibility complex (MHC) antigen-related biological processes (Pascual et al., 2005; Allantaz et al., 2007; Fall et al., 2007; Ogilvie et al., 2007; Barnes et al., 2009).

Proinflammatory Mediators

Laboratory observations, as well as the therapeutic efficacy of cytokine inhibitors have provided clear evidence for a major pathogenic role of phagocyte-derived cytokines and in particular of IL-6 and IL-1.

Interleukin-6

The role of IL-6 in the pathogenesis of sJIA appears to be pivotal. Circulating levels of IL-6 are markedly elevated, increase during the peak of fever, and correlate with the extent and severity of joint involvement and with platelet counts (De Benedetti et al., 1991). Synovial fluid levels of IL-6 are also markedly increased and significantly higher than those observed in patients with polyarticular and oligoarticular JIA or in adult patients with rheumatoid arthritis (De Benedetti et al., 1997a). Moreover, in sJIA patients huge quantities of IL-6 circulate bound to the soluble receptor; this bound IL-6 seems biologically active since it correlates much better with the level of C-reactive protein than free circulating IL-6 (De Benedetti et al., 1994). At variance with findings in adult RA, anemia in sJIA is microcytic and characterized by a marked defect in iron supply for erythropoiesis, while growth of erythroid colonies is normal and erythropoietin production is appropriate (Cazzola et al., 1996). These finding are consistent with the effect of IL-6 on the bone marrow. Indeed, IL-6 stimulates both hypoxia-induced erythropoietin production and erythroid progenitor proliferation and,

TABLE 37.2 Genetic Associations with Systemic Juvenile Idiopathic Arthritis

Gene	No. of Patients	No. of Healthy Controls	Ethnicity	Genotype	Comments and Odds Ratios (OR)	Reference
5′-flanking region of the IL-6	92	383	Caucasian	-174 IL-6 CC[a]	Significant lower frequency of the CC genotype in patients with age of onset ≤ 5 yr OR 0.34, P = 0.04	Fishman et al. (1998)
5′-flanking promoter/ enhancer region of TNF-α	50	575	Japanese	-1031C -863A -857T -857T/DRB1*0405	OR 1.84, P = 0.015 OR 1.83, P = 0.022 OR 1.80, P = 0.016 OR 3.84, P = 0.0001	Date et al. (1999)
5′-flanking region of MIF	117	172	Caucasian	MIF-173*C	OR 2.3, P = 0.0005	Donn et al. (2001)
IL-18 promoter region	16 AOSD	92	Japanese	Haplotype S01 Diplotype S01/S01	OR 2.90, P = 0.0072. OR 7.81, P = 0.0005	Sugiura et al. (2002)
5′-flanking region of the MIF	136		Caucasian	MIF-173*C	Higher MIF serum and synovial fluid levels; poorer response to steroid treatment; persistence of active disease, and poor functional outcome	De Benedetti et al. (2003)
5′-flanking region of the IL-6	222 sJIA families		Caucasian	-174G IL-6	Excess transmission of the G allele to affected offspring with age at onset >5 years (P = 0.007)	Ogilvie et al. (2003)
IL-10 IL-20 (it is a member of IL-10 gene family)	172	473	Caucasian	IL-10-1082A[b] IL-20-468T IL-10-1082A/IL-20-468T haplotype	OR 1.335, P = 0.031 OR 1.507, P = 0.028 OR 2.24, P = 0.0006	Fife et al. (2006)
SLC26A2 gene for diastrophic dysplasia	133	617	Caucasian	rs1541915 rs245056 rs245055 rs245051 rs245076 rs8073	OR 2.3, P = 0.0003 OR 2.8, P = 0.00002 OR 2.5, P = 0.004 OR 2.3, P = 0.0005 OR 2.7, P = 0.0015 OR 2.3, P = 0.04	Lamb et al. (2007)
IL-1 gene family	235	335	Caucasian	IL-1 ligand cluster rs6712572 rs2071374 rs1688075 IL-1 receptor cluster rs12712122	 OR 1.32, P = 0.025 OR 1.48, P = 0.002 OR 2.04, P = 0.002 OR 1.29, P = 0.047	Stock et al. (2008)
IL-10	74	249	Caucasian	-1082A[b] -819T -592A	Increased frequency of -1082A (p < 0.001), ACC (p = 0.01) and GTC (p < 0.001) haplotypes in sJIA	Moller et al. (2010)

[a]C allele was associated with significantly lower levels of plasma-IL-6.
[b]The IL-10 promoter polymorphism -1082A was associated with low IL-10 production.
AOSD, Adult-onset Still disease.

by increasing ferritin expression and hepatic uptake of serum iron, causes a reticuloendothelial iron block. Moreover, IL-6 dramatically induces the liver production of hepcidin, a peptide that inhibits iron absorption in the small intestine and the release of recycled iron from the macrophages (Nemeth et al., 2004). This can well explain the oral iron malabsorption that has been observed in patients with sJIA (Martini et al., 1994).

Growth impairment is a well-known feature of sJIA since its first description and IL-6-transgenic mice with high circulating levels of IL-6 since birth show a decreased rate of growth, attaining 50–60% of the size of their wild-type littermates (De Benedetti et al., 1997b). Moreover, similar to patients with sJIA, IL-6-transgenic mice have normal growth hormone production but low levels of insulin-like growth factor 1 (IGF-1) and IGF binding protein 3 (IGFBP-3) (De Benedetti et al., 2001).

All these findings led to the hypothesis that sJIA is an IL-6- and not a TNF-driven disease (De Benedetti and Martini, 1998). This hypothesis was supported 10 years later by the double-blind controlled study with a withdrawal design that showed the marked efficacy of tocilizumab, a monoclonal antibody against the IL-6 soluble receptor (sIL-6R) which is essential for signal transduction (Yokota et al., 2008). These brilliant therapeutic results have been recently confirmed by a double-blind, placebo-controlled confirmatory study (De Benedetti et al., 2012).

Interleukin-1

The most compelling evidence for the important role of IL-1 in the pathogenesis of sJIA came from the quite serendipitous finding of the marked therapeutic efficacy of anakinra, an IL-1 inhibitor which is the recombinant version of the naturally occurring soluble IL-1 receptor antagonist (IL-1 Ra) (Verbsky and White, 2004; Pascual et al., 2005). The role of IL-1 is not in contrast with that of IL-6 since IL-1 is upstream to IL-6. It was also shown that serum from patients with active sJIA can induce the transcription of various IL-1-related genes (Pascual et al., 2005). However, gene expression studies mentioned above did not usually show increased expression of IL-1β. Interestingly, serum levels of myeloid-related proteins (MRPs) 8 and 14 (which are secreted by activated neutrophils and monocytes) are very high during active disease, and MRP-14 in serum of patients with sJIA has been shown to be a strong inducer of IL-1 expression in phagocytes (Frosch et al., 2009). Moreover, MRP8/14 serum concentrations have been reported to correlate closely with response to drug treatment and disease activity and might therefore also be useful in monitoring treatment of individual patients with SJIA (Holzinger et al., 2012).

Of note, it has been shown that the response to anakinra can identify two different populations of patients with sJIA (Gattorno et al., 2008). One (accounting for about 40% of patients) shows a dramatic response to IL-1 blockade (similar to that observed in cryopyrin-associated autoinflammatory syndromes) leading to complete normalization of clinical as well as laboratory features in a few days. The other is resistant to treatment or shows an intermediate response; often in this second group of patients systemic features respond well to therapy while synovitis persists although it can improve. At variance with cryopyrinopathies both groups of patients do not secrete higher amounts of IL-1 with respect to controls (Gattorno et al., 2008).

Only minor differences were observed when serum levels of 30 different cytokines and other soluble molecules were analyzed: patients with a brilliant response had higher serum levels of IL-9 and lower serum levels of granulocyte colony-stimulating factor. The main differences observed were in the number of active joints and in neutrophil count; patients with fewer joints affected or with higher neutrophil count had a higher probability of responding to anti-IL-1 therapy. Thus sJIA can be stratified in two subgroups based on responsiveness to IL-1 inhibition. The group with a bright response could represent a separate entity in which the autoinflammatory component has the leading pathogenic role and in which therefore monocytes and neutrophils, rather than lymphocytes, are the predominant effector cells. The other group, characterized by the presence of an important synovitis, seems to have, in addition, a relevant autoimmune component.

A controlled trial has also supported the efficacy of anakinra in sJIA (Quartier et al., 2011). Of interest in this trial is a "de novo" type I IFN signature (which is not a feature of untreated SJIA) which was observed in the majority of anakinra-treated patients regardless of the clinical response.

Recently, it has been suggested, in a retrospective study, that a precocious treatment with anakinra could prevent the subsequent appearance of refractory arthritis in the large majority of patients (Nigrovic et al., 2011). This hypothesis, however, needs to be confirmed in prospective randomized trials.

More recently a monoclonal antibody against IL-1β (canakinumab) has been used in the treatment of sJIA. A first dose-finding phase I/II trial has defined the correct dosage (Ruperto et al., 2012) which has been used in a subsequent phase III trial. The results have confirmed the efficacy of IL-1 inhibition in sJIA (Ruperto et al., 2012).

Interleukin-18

Systemic JIA as well as adult-onset Still's disease are characterized by very high levels of circulating IL-18 (Kawashima et al., 2001; Maeno et al., 2002). Of note, IL-18 is a member of the IL-1 cytokine superfamily, is stored as precursor protein, and, upon activation, is cleaved by caspase-1 in a manner similar to that of IL-1 to yield the active cytokine. It seems that in sJIA as well as during macrophage activation syndrome (see below) IL-18 and other proinflammatory cytokines (IFN-γ, IL-6, TNF) are mainly produced by resident macrophages (bone marrow and liver) (Maeno et al., 2004; Billiau et al., 2005). A reversible defect in phosphorylation of IL-18 receptor has been reported in patients with sJIA (de Jager et al., 2009).

Macrophage Activation Syndrome

It remains substantially a mystery why sJIA is so strongly associated with MAS. Of note MAS is seldom observed in autoinflammatory diseases. It is unclear if this complication characterizes a distinct subset of the disease. Interestingly, activated macrophages or frank hemophagocytic cells have been found in 53% of patients with sJIA who underwent bone marrow aspiration, suggesting that subclinical MAS may be present in half of the patients (Behrens et al., 2007).

As mentioned above, MAS bears a strong resemblance to a group of histiocytic disorders collectively known as hemophagocytic lymphohistiocytosis (HLH) (Janka, 2012). Two types of HLH are recognized. The primary or familial (FHLH) forms are secondary to genetic deficiency in cytolytic pathway proteins. The secondary or reactive (ReHLH) forms are associated with an identifiable infectious episode or are secondary to an autoimmune condition or to a neoplastic or a metabolic disorder.

To date, all the described genetic defects associated with HLH appear to be related to one another in the pathway of granule-mediated cytotoxicity with the lack of perforin being the most common. These genetic defects interrupt the mechanisms responsible for triggered apoptosis (mediated by cytotoxic cells on the target cell) or activation-induced apoptosis (putative suicide of activated T cell). A hallmark of HLH is therefore an impaired or absent function of NK and cytotoxic T cells. In patients with FHLH, NK cell numbers are normal and the functional defect is usually persistent; patients with ReHLH may have low NK cell numbers but NK cell number and function usually reverts to normal after treatment. Two pathogenic hypotheses have been proposed. One is an inability of cytotoxic cells to clear virally infected cells with persistent antigen stimulation, leading to activation and proliferation of T cells with escalating cytokine production and macrophage activation. The second is a failure to provide appropriate apoptotic signals for removal of APC and stimulated lymphocytes that continuously secrete IFN-γ, γ, and GM-CSF, potent activators of macrophages that secrete massive amounts of proinflammatory cytokines. HLH symptoms can be explained by the high concentration of inflammatory cytokines and by organ infiltration by lymphocytes and histiocytes. Fever is induced by IL-1 and IL-6 and pancytopenia is the consequence of high levels of TNF and interferon (IFN)-γ rather than of hemophagocytosis. TNF inhibits lipoprotein lipase leading to elevated triglycerides. Activated macrophages secrete ferritin and plasminogen activator which results in high plasmin levels and hyperfibrinolysis. Hepatosplenomegaly, increased liver enzymes, and neurological symptoms are the consequence of organ infiltration by activated lymphocytes and histiocytes. Activated lymphocytes and macrophages are respectively the source for high concentrations of circulating sIL-2 Ra and sCD163.

The best experimental model of HLH is perforin-deficient mouse in which CD 8 T cells produce large amounts of IFN-γ. The etiopathogenesis of MAS remains

unknown. Immunologic abnormalities, similar to those seen in HLH (poor NK cell cytolytic activity often associated with abnormal levels of perforin expression) but reversible have been reported (Ravelli et al., 2012). However, in many instances of sJIA/MAS, no such defects in cytotoxic cell function have been identified. This suggests that MAS represents an end-stage clinical syndrome that can be elicited by different mechanisms. In this respect other murine models of MAS have been recently reported.

It has been shown that repeated stimulation of toll-like receptor (TLR)9 produces an HLH/MAS-like syndrome on a normal genetic background, without exogenous antigen (Behrens et al., 2011). Like in perforin-deficient mice the syndrome depends on the presence of IFN-γ; however, IFN-γ is arising from different sources than CD 8 T cells, including dendritic cells and NK cells. This model shows that MAS can develop during persistent innate immune activation independently from defects in cytotoxic cell function.

Treatment of IL-6-transgenic mice with TLR ligands led to elevated levels of IL-1β, TNF, IL-6, and IL-18 and an increased fatality rate with features (high ferritin and decreased platelet and neutrophil count) similar to those observed in MAS (Strippoli et al., 2012).

Oligoarticular Juvenile Idiopathic Arthritis

As mentioned above, in Western countries most children with oligoarthritis have a definite disease, specific to childhood and characterized by an asymmetric arthritis, involving mainly large joints, an early onset (before 6 years of age), a female predilection, a high frequency of positive ANAs, and a high risk of developing chronic iridocyclitis. The homogeneity of this form of arthritis is also witnessed by consistent associations with HLA antigens. Positive associations include HLA-A2, HLA-DRB1*11 (a subtype of HLA-DR5), and HLA-DRB1*08. On the contrary, HLA-DRB1*04 and HLA-DRB1*07 have been found to be significantly decreased (Prahalad and Glass, 2008). HLA associations support an autoimmune pathogenesis and the early onset suggests that the disease could be elicited by a very common infectious agent that can be encountered early in life. In this respect evidence has been provided that T cells from patients with early-onset ANA-positive oligoarticular JIA are sensitized against epitopes that are shared between the disease-associated HLA antigens and proteins present on Epstein–Barr virus and other herpes viruses (Massa et al., 2002); herpes viruses represent a group of infectious agents to which the vast majority of children have already been exposed by 6 years of age.

ANA have been found to react against different chromatin constituents and against the DEK nuclear protein, a putative oncoprotein; however, none of these molecular targets has been found to be specific to oligoarticular JIA.

The reasons why chronic anterior uveitis is so strongly associated with the disease remain unknown.

The inflammatory synovitis observed in JIA is similar to that of adult rheumatoid arthritis. The synovium shows hyperplasia of the lining layer and infiltration of the sublining layer with mononuclear cells including T cells, B cells, macrophages, dendritic, and plasma cells. The T cell infiltrates are composed predominantly of Th-1 skewed, $CD4^+$ cells, expressing an activated memory phenotype. The inflammatory process leads to pannus formation with cartilage and bone erosions mediated by degradative enzymes such as metallo-proteinases (Ravelli and Martini, 2007).

As mentioned above, a B cell signature has been shown to characterize patients with early-onset arthritis (Barnes et al., 2010). Moreover, lymphoid aggregates and plasma cell infiltration have been found more frequently in patients with circulating ANA (Gregorio et al., 2007). These observations suggest that B cells can play a role in early-onset ANA-positive arthritis. Corcione et al. found an expansion of activated switch memory B cells and of IgG-secreting plasma blasts in the SF of oligoarticular JIA patients. Memory B cells belonged to either the $CD27^+$ or the $CD27^-$ subsets and expressed CD86, suggesting their involvement in antigen presentation to T cells (Corcione et al., 2009). Another study (Morbach et al., 2011), involving mainly patients with oligoarticular disease, has also confirmed that activated immunoglobulin class-switched $CD27^+$ and $CD27^-$ memory B cells accumulate in the joints further suggesting that B cells play an antibody-independent immunopathologic role in oligoarthritis.

Cosmi et al. (Cosmi et al., 2011) have studied Th17 cells in children with oligoarticular JIA. They showed that synovial fluid T cells could switch easily from a Th17 phenotype to a mixed Th1/Th17 phenotype, and, then, to a Th1 phenotype; the switch was linked to the presence of IL-12 in the synovial fluid. This study is in line with the findings of another study performed in JIA patients which showed that synovial fluid Th17 cells "convert" to Th17/1 in the presence of low TGFβ and high IL-12 levels, whereas Th1 cells cannot convert to Th17 (Nistala et al., 2010).

Within the joint, an inverse relationship between $IL-17^+$ T cells and $FoxP3^+$ regulatory T (Treg) cells has been found (Nistala et al., 2008). In JIA, Tregs from the peripheral blood as well as from the inflamed joints are fully functional. Nevertheless, Treg-mediated suppression of cell proliferation and cytokine production by effector cells from the site of inflammation have been shown to be severely impaired (Haufe et al., 2011; Wehrens et al., 2011). This resistance to suppression has been shown to be secondary to the activation of protein kinase B (PKB)/c-akt in inflammatory effector cells since inhibition of this kinase restores responsiveness to suppression (Wehrens et al., 2011).

The fact that in oligoarticular JIA, joint involvement can remain limited to four or fewer joints (oligoarticular persistent) or can extend to affect five or more joints after the first 6 months of disease (oligoarticular extended) provides an opportunity, in a rather homogeneous context, to study factors that are associated with disease extension.

$IL-17^+$ T cell numbers were found to be higher in patients with extended oligoarthritis as compared with patients with persistent oligoarthritis (Nistala et al., 2008). The ratio between SF regulatory and activated effector CD4 cells was found to be higher in patients with persistent oligoarticular disease with respect to those in whom the disease extended to affect five or more joints (Ruprecht et al., 2005). Hunter et al. sampled patients with recent-onset oligoarticular JIA and looked at potential differences in synovial fluid cells between patients with persistent or extended disease. Synovial CCL5 levels were higher and SF CD4:CD8 ratio was lower in children whose disease extended to a more severe phenotype. Gene expression profiling revealed increased levels of genes associated with inflammation and macrophage differentiation in patients with extended disease and of genes associated with immune regulation in patients with persistent oligoarticular disease (Hunter et al., 2010). Finnegan et al. studied the immunohistochemical features of the synovial membrane in early untreated, newly diagnosed JIA in relation with disease outcome at 2 years. CD4 expression and B cell infiltrates was significantly higher and vascularization more pronounced in patients in whom arthritis extended to involve more joints with respect to those with persistent oligoarthritis (Finnegan et al., 2011).

The fact that persistent oligoarticular JIA is self-limiting, and in about half of all cases even self-remitting, suggests an endogenous regulation. Heat shock proteins (HSPs) are endogenous proteins that are expressed upon cellular stress and are able to modulate immune responses. HSPs are highly present at sites of inflammation, like the inflamed joints of JIA patients (Boog et al., 1992). Studies have shown in JIA the presence of antigen-specific T cells against peptides derived from two types of HSPs, HSP60 and DnaJ (Kamphuis et al., 2005; Massa et al., 2007). T cell recognition of self-peptides or of peptides with a high degree of homology with self was associated with immune mechanisms with regulatory function, including the presence of T cells with the regulatory functional phenotype. These responses are significantly augmented in patients with persistent oligoarticular JIA, which again suggests a direct role in modulation of autoimmune inflammation. The identification of HSP tolerogenic peptides could have therapeutic implications in the future.

TREATMENT

The last decade has witnessed a dramatic improvement in JIA treatment. This has been due not only to the availability of the new potent biological agents but also to the implementation by the Food and Drug Administration (FDA) and the European Medicines Agency (EMA) of the so-called "pediatric rule." According to this rule, an industry that wishes to register a new treatment for a given disease in adults has to also conduct studies in children if there is a pediatric counterpart of the illness. Pediatric rheumatology was able to take a quick advantage from this rule thanks to the existence of two very large networks that have worked in a highly integrated fashion, the Pediatric Rheumatology Collaborative Study Group (PRCSG) in North America and the Paediatric Rheumatology International Trial Organization (PRINTO) in Europe and the rest of the world (Ruperto and Martini, 2004).

The widespread use of intra-articular triamcinolone hexacetonide joint injections has played an important role in preventing deformities secondary to joint contractures. Patients who do not respond to non-steroidal anti-inflammatory agents and intra-articular steroid injections are treated with methotrexate (MTX) whose maximally effective dose has been established in a randomized trial (Ruperto et al., 2004). Although a trial has shown the efficacy of leflunomide in polyarticular JIA (Silverman et al., 2005), the experience with this drug in children is still scarce.

In patients who do not respond adequately to MTX the efficacy of several anti-TNF agents (Lovell et al., 2000, 2008) as well as of abatacept (Ruperto et al., 2008) has been demonstrated in RCTs in polyarticular course JIA while a phase III controlled trial with tocilizumab has just been completed. Patients with systemic JIA are initially treated with prednisone. Systemic JIA has been shown to be less sensitive to MTX and anti-TNF agents. In those patients who are steroid dependent, anti-IL-6 and anti-IL-1 treatments, as mentioned above, have shown a dramatic efficacy. The treatment of MAS relies on high dose steroids and cyclosporine.

The safety profile of biological agents appears to be good. The initial concern raised by the FDA that treatment with anti-TNF agents could be associated with an increased rate of malignancy (Diak et al., 2010) has not been confirmed by retrospective studies that have on the contrary suggested that JIA itself and not anti-TNF therapy is associated (as adult RA) with a small increased risk of neoplasia (Beukelman et al., 2012).

In iridocyclitis, early diagnosis is very important for the success of therapy. The initial approach consists of glucocorticoid eye drops with mydriatics. In patients resistant disease systemic steroids are required. If disease remains controlled, methotrexate, cyclosporine, anti-TNF antibodies, and abatacept have been anecdotally reported to be effective.

REFERENCES

Allantaz, F., Chaussabel, D., Stichweh, D., Bennett, L., Allman, W., Mejias, A., et al., 2007. Blood leukocyte microarrays to diagnose systemic onset juvenile idiopathic arthritis and follow the response to IL-1 blockade. J. Exp. Med. 204, 2131–2144.

Barnes, M.G., Grom, A.A., Thompson, S.D., Griffin, T.A., Pavlidis, P., Itert, L., et al., 2009. Subtype-specific peripheral blood gene expression profiles in recent-onset juvenile idiopathic arthritis. Arthritis Rheum. 60, 2102–2112.

Barnes, M.G., Grom, A.A., Thompson, S.D., Griffin, T.A., Luyrink, L. K., Colbert, R.A., et al., 2010. Biologic similarities based on age at onset in oligoarticular and polyarticular subtypes of juvenile idiopathic arthritis. Arthritis Rheum. 62, 3249–3258.

Behrens, E.M., Beukelman, T., Paessler, M., Cron, R.Q., 2007. Occult macrophage activation syndrome in patients with systemic juvenile idiopathic arthritis. J. Rheumatol. 34, 1133–1138.

Behrens, E.M., Canna, S.W., Slade, K., Rao, S., Kreiger, P.A., Paessler, M., et al., 2011. Repeated TLR9 stimulation results in macrophage activation syndrome-like disease in mice. J. Clin. Invest. 121, 2264–2277.

Beukelman, T., Haynes, K., Curtis, J.R., Xie, F., Chen, L., Bemrich-Stolz, C.J., et al., 2012. Safety assessment of biological therapeutics collaboration. Rates of malignancy associated with juvenile idiopathic arthritis and its treatment. Arthritis Rheum. 64, 1263–1271.

Billiau, A.D., Roskams, T., Van Damme-Lombaerts, R., Matthys, P., Wouters, C., 2005. Macrophage activation syndrome: characteristic findings on liver biopsy illustrating the key role of activated, IFN-gamma-producing lymphocytes and IL-6- and TNF-alpha-producing macrophages. Blood. 105, 1648–1651.

Boog, C.J., de Graeff-Meeder, E.R., Lucassen, M.A., van der Zee, R., Voorhorst-Ogink, M.M., van Kooten, P.J., et al., 1992. Two monoclonal antibodies generated against human hsp60 show reactivity with synovial membranes of patients with juvenile chronic arthritis. J. Exp. Med. 175, 1805–1810.

Cazzola, M., Ponchio, L., de Benedetti, F, Ravelli, A., Rosti., V., Beguin, Y., et al., 1996. Defective iron supply for erythropoiesis and adequate endogenous erythropoietin production in the anemia associated with systemic-onset juvenile chronic arthritis. Blood. 87, 4824–4830.

Corcione, A., Ferlito, F., Gattorno, M., Gregorio, A., Pistorio, A., Gastaldi, R., et al., 2009. Phenotypic and functional characterization of switch memory B cells from patients with oligoarticular juvenile idiopathic arthritis. Arthritis Res. Ther. 11, R150.

Cosmi, L., Cimaz, R., Maggi, L., Santarlasci, V., Capone, M., Borriello, F., et al., 2011. Evidence of the transient nature of the Th17 phenotype of CD4 + CD161 + T cells in the synovial fluid of patients with juvenile idiopathic arthritis. Arthritis Rheum. 63, 2504–2515.

Date, Y., Seki, N., Kamizono, S., Higuchi, T., Hirata, T., Miyata, K., et al., 1999. Identification of a genetic risk factor for systemic juvenile rheumatoid arthritis in the 5′-flanking region of the TNFalpha gene and HLA genes. Arthritis Rheum. 42, 2577–2582.

De Benedetti, F., Martini, A., 1998. Is systemic juvenile rheumatoid arthritis an interleukin 6 mediated disease? J. Rheumatol. 25, 203–207.

De Benedetti, F., Massa, M., Robbioni, P., Ravelli, A., Burgio, G.R., Martini, A., 1991. Correlation of serum interleukin-6 levels with joint involvement and thrombocytosis in systemic juvenile rheumatoid arthritis. Arthritis Rheum. 34, 1158–1163.

De Benedetti, F., Massa, M., Pignatti, P., Albani, S., Novick, D., Martini, A., 1994. Serum soluble interleukin 6 (IL-6) receptor and

IL-6/soluble IL-6 receptor complex in systemic juvenile rheumatoid arthritis. J. Clin. Invest. 93, 2114–2119.

De Benedetti, F., Alonzi, T., Moretta, A., Lazzaro, D, Costa, P, Poli, V, et al., 1997a. Interleukin 6 causes growth impairment in transgenic mice through a decrease in insulin-like growth factor-I. A model for stunted growth in children with chronic inflammation. J. Clin. Invest. 99, 643–650.

De Benedetti, F., Pignatti, P., Gerloni, V., Massa, M., Sartirana, P., Caporali, R., et al., 1997b. Differences in synovial fluid cytokine levels between juvenile and adult rheumatoid arthritis. J. Rheumatol. 24, 1403–1409.

De Benedetti, F., Meazza, C., Oliveri, M., Pignatti, P., Vivarelli, M., Alonzi, T., et al., 2001. Effect of IL-6 on IGF binding protein-3: a study in IL-6 transgenic mice and in patients with systemic juvenile idiopathic arthritis. Endocrinology. 142, 4818–4826.

De Benedetti, F., Meazza, C., Vivarelli, M., Rossi, F., Pistorio, A., Lamb, R., et al., 2003. Functional and prognostic relevance of the -173 polymorphism of the macrophage migration inhibitory factor gene in systemic-onset juvenile idiopathic arthritis. Arthritis Rheum. 48, 1398–1407.

De Benedetti, F., Brunner, H.I., Ruperto, N., Kenwright, A., Wright, S., Calvo, I., et al., 2012. Randomized trial of tocilizumab in systemic juvenile idiopathic arthritis. N. Engl. J. Med. 367, 2385–2395.

Diak, P., Siegel, J., La Grenade, L., Choi, L., Lemery, S., McMahon, A., 2010. Tumor necrosis factor alpha blockers and malignancy in children: forty-eight cases reported to the Food and Drug Administration. Arthritis Rheum. 62, 2517–2524.

Donn, R.P., Barrett, J.H., Farhan, A., Stopford, A., Pepper, L., Shelley, E., et al., 2001. Cytokine gene polymorphisms and susceptibility to juvenile idiopathic arthritis. British Paediatric Rheumatology Study Group. Arthritis Rheum. 44, 802–810.

Fall, N., Barnes, M., Thornton, S., Luyrink, L., Olson, J., Ilowite, N.T., et al., 2007. Gene expression profiling of peripheral blood from patients with untreated new-onset systemic juvenile idiopathic arthritis reveals molecular heterogeneity that may predict macrophage activation syndrome. Arthritis Rheum. 56, 804–3793.

Fife, M.S., Gutierrez, A., Ogilvie, E.M., Stock, C.J., Samuel, J.M., Thomson, W., et al., 2006. Novel IL10 gene family associations with systemic juvenile idiopathic arthritis. Arthritis Res. Ther. 8, R148.

Finnegan, S., Clarke, S., Gibson, D., McAllister, C., Rooney, M., 2011. Synovial membrane immunohistology in early untreated juvenile idiopathic arthritis: differences between clinical subgroups. Ann. Rheum. Dis. 70, 1842–1850.

Fishman, D., Faulds, G., Jeffery, R., Mohamed-Ali, V., Yudkin, J.S., Humphries, S., et al., 1998. The effect of novel polymorphisms in the interleukin-6 (IL-6) gene on IL-6 transcription and plasma IL-6 levels, and an association with systemic-onset juvenile chronic arthritis. J. Clin. Invest. 102, 1369–1376.

Frosch, M., Ahlmann, M., Vogl, T., Wittkowski, H., Wulffraat, N., Foell, D., et al., 2009. The myeloid-related proteins 8 and 14 complex, a novel ligand of toll-like receptor 4, and interleukin-1beta form a positive feedback mechanism in systemic-onset juvenile idiopathic arthritis. Arthritis Rheum. 60, 883–891.

Gattorno, M., Piccini, A., Lasigliè, D., Tassi, S., Brisca, G., Carta, S., et al., 2008. The pattern of response to anti-interleukin-1 treatment distinguishes two subsets of patients with systemic-onset juvenile idiopathic arthritis. Arthritis Rheum. 58, 1505–1515.

Gregorio, A., Gambini, C., Gerloni, V., Parafioriti, A., Sormani, M.P., Gregorio, S., et al., 2007. Lymphoid neogenesis in juvenile idiopathic arthritis correlates with ANA positivity and plasma cells infiltration. Rheumatology (Oxford). 46, 308–313.

Haufe, S., Haug, M., Schepp, C., Kuemmerle-Deschner, J., Hansmann, S., Rieber, N., et al., 2011. Impaired suppression of synovial fluid CD4 + CD25 − T cells from patients with juvenile idiopathic arthritis by CD4 + CD25 + Treg cells. Arthritis Rheum. 63, 3153–3162.

Hollenbach, J.A., Thompson, S.D., Bugawan, T.L., Ryan, M., Sudman, M., Marion, M., et al., 2010. Juvenile idiopathic arthritis and HLA class I and class II interactions and age-at-onset effects. Arthritis Rheum. 62, 1781–1791.

Holzinger, D., Frosch, M, Kastrup, A., Prince, F.H., Otten, M.H., Van Suijlekom-Smit, L.W., et al., 2012. The Toll-like receptor 4 agonist MRP8/14 protein complex is a sensitive indicator for disease activity and predicts relapses in systemic-onset juvenile idiopathic arthritis. Ann. Rheum. Dis. 71, 974–980.

Hunter, P.J., Nistala, K., Jina, N., Eddaoudi, A., Thomson, W., Hubank, M., et al., 2010. Biologic predictors of extension of oligoarticular juvenile idiopathic arthritis as determined from synovial fluid cellular composition and gene expression. Arthritis Rheum. 62, 896–907.

Janka, G.E., 2012. Familial and acquired hemophagocytic lymphohistiocytosis. Annu. Rev. Med. 63, 233–246.

Kamphuis, S., Kuis, W., de Jager, W., Teklenburg, G., Massa, M., Gordon, G., et al., 2005. Tolerogenic immune responses to novel T-cell epitopes from heat-shock protein 60 in juvenile idiopathic arthritis. Lancet. 366, 50–56.

Kawashima, M., Yamamura, M., Taniai, M., Yamauchi, H., Tanimoto, T., Kurimoto, M., et al., 2001. Levels of interleukin-18 and its binding inhibitors in the blood circulation of patients with adult-onset Still's disease. Arthritis Rheum. 44, 550–560.

Lamb, R., Thomson, W., Ogilvie, E.M., Donn, R., 2007. British Society of Paediatric and Adolescent Rheumatology, Positive association of SLC26A2 gene polymorphisms with susceptibility to systemic-onset juvenile idiopathic arthritis. Arthritis Rheum. 56, 1286–1291.

Lovell, D.J., Giannini, E.H., Reiff, A., Cawkwell, G.D., Silverman, E.D., Nocton, J.J., et al., 2000. Etanercept in children with polyarticular juvenile rheumatoid arthritis. Pediatric Rheumatology Collaborative Study Group. N. Engl. J. Med. 342, 763–769.

Lovell, D.J., Ruperto, N., Goodman, S., Reiff, A., Jung, L., Jarosova, K., et al., 2008. Adalimumab with or without methotrexate in juvenile rheumatoid arthritis. N. Engl. J. Med. 359, 810–820.

Maeno, N., Takei, S., Nomura, Y., Imanaka, H., Hokonohara, M., Miyata, K., 2002. Highly elevated serum levels of interleukin-18 in systemic juvenile idiopathic arthritis but not in other juvenile idiopathic arthritis subtypes or in Kawasaki disease: comment on the article by Kawashima et al. Arthritis Rheum. 46, 2539–2541.

Maeno, N., Takei, S., Imanaka, H., Yamamoto, K., Kuriwaki, K., Kawano, Y., et al., 2004. Increased interleukin-18 expression in bone marrow of a patient with systemic juvenile idiopathic arthritis and unrecognized macrophage-activation syndrome. Arthritis Rheum. 50, 1935–1938.

Martini, A., 2003. Are the number of joints involved or the presence of psoriasis still useful tools to identify homogeneous disease entities in juvenile idiopathic arthritis? J.Rheumatol. 30, 1900–1903.

Martini, A., 2012. It is time to rethink juvenile idiopathic arthritis classification and nomenclature. Ann. Rheum. Dis. 71, 1437–1439.

Martini, A., Ravelli, A., Di Fuccia, G., Rosti, V., Cazzola, M., Barosi, G., 1994. Intravenous iron therapy for severe anaemia in systemic-onset juvenile chronic arthritis. Lancet. 344, 1052–1054.

Massa, M., Mazzoli, F., Pignatti, P., De Benedetti, F., Passalia, M., Viola, S., et al., 2002. Proinflammatory responses to self HLA epitopes are triggered by molecular mimicry to Epstein–Barr virus proteins in oligoarticular juvenile idiopathic arthritis. Arthritis Rheum. 46, 2721–2729.

Massa, M., Passalia, M., Manzoni, S.M., Campanelli, R., Ciardelli, L., Yung, G.P., et al., 2007. Differential recognition of heat-shock protein dnaJ-derived epitopes by effector and Treg cells leads to modulation of inflammation in juvenile idiopathic arthritis. Arthritis Rheum. 56, 1648–1657.

Mellins, E.D., Macaubas, C., Grom, A.A., 2011. Pathogenesis of systemic juvenile idiopathic arthritis: some answers, more questions. Nat. Rev. Rheumatol. 7, 416–426.

Möller, J.C., Paul, D., Ganser, G., Range, U., Gahr, M., Kelsch, R., et al., 2010. L10 promoter polymorphisms are associated with systemic onset juvenile idiopathic arthritis (SoJIA). Clin. Exp. Rheumatol. 28, 912–918.

Morbach, H., Wiegering, V., Richl, P., Schwarz, T., Suffa, N., Eichhorn, E.M., et al., 2011. Activated memory B cells may function as antigen-presenting cells in the joints of children with juvenile idiopathic arthritis. Arthritis Rheum. 63, 3458–3466.

Nemeth, E., Rivera, S., Gabayan, V., Keller, C., Taudorf, S., Pedersen, B.K., et al., 2004. IL-6 mediates hypoferremia of inflammation by inducing the synthesis of the iron regulatory hormone hepcidin. J. Clin. Invest. 113, 1271–1276.

Nigrovic, P.A., Mannion, M., Prince, F.H., Zeft, A., Rabinovich, C.E., van Rossum, M.A., et al., 2011. Anakinra as first-line disease-modifying therapy in systemic juvenile idiopathic arthritis: report of forty-six patients from an international multicenter series. Arthritis Rheum. 63, 545–555.

Nistala, K., Moncrieffe, H., Newton, K.R., Varsani, H., Hunter, P., Wedderburn, L.R., 2008. Interleukin-17-producing T cells are enriched in the joints of children with arthritis, but have a reciprocal relationship to regulatory T cell numbers. Arthritis Rheum. 58, 875–887.

Nistala, K., Adams, S., Cambrook, H., Ursu, S., Olivito, B., de Jager, W., et al., 2010. Th17 plasticity in human autoimmune arthritis is driven by the inflammatory environment. Proc. Nat. Acad. Sci. U.S.A. 107, 14751–14756.

Ogilvie, E.M., Fife, M.S., Thompson, S.D., Twine, N., Tsoras, M., Moroldo, M., et al., 2003. The -174G allele of the interleukin-6 gene confers susceptibility to systemic arthritis in children: a multicenter study using simplex and multiplex juvenile idiopathic arthritis families. Arthritis Rheum. 48, 3202–3206.

Ogilvie, E.M., Khan, A., Hubank, M., Kellam, P., Woo, P., 2007. Specific gene expression profiles in systemic juvenile idiopathic arthritis. Arthritis Rheum. 56, 1954–1965.

Pascual, V., Allantaz, F., Arce, E., Punaro, M., Banchereau, J., 2005. Role of interleukin-1 (IL-1) in the pathogenesis of systemic onset juvenile idiopathic arthritis and clinical response to IL-1 blockade. J. Exp. Med. 201, 1479–1486.

Petty, R.E., Southwood, T.R., Manners, P., Baum, J., Glass, D.N., Goldenberg, J., et al., 2004. International League of Associations for Rheumatology classification of juvenile idiopathic arthritis: second revision, Edmonton, 2001. J. Rheumatol. 31, 390–392.

Prahalad, S., Glass, D.N., 2008. A comprehensive review of the genetics of juvenile idiopathic arthritis. Pediatr. Rheumatol. Online. J. 21, 6–11.

Prakken, B., Albani, S., Martini, A., 2011. Juvenile idiopathic arthritis. Lancet. 377, 2138–2149.

Quartier, P., Allantaz, F., Cimaz, R., Pillet, P., Messiaen, C., Bardin, C., et al., 2011. A multicentre, randomised, double-blind, placebo-controlled trial with the interleukin-1 receptor antagonist anakinra in patients with systemic-onset juvenile idiopathic arthritis (ANAJIS trial). Ann. Rheum. Dis. 70, 747–754.

Ravelli, A., Martini, A., 2007. Juvenile idiopathic arthritis. Lancet. 369, 767–778.

Ravelli, A., Felici, E., Magni-Manzoni, S., Pistorio, A., Novarini, C., Bozzola, E., et al., 2005. Patients with antinuclear antibody-positive juvenile idiopathic arthritis constitute a homogeneous subgroup irrespective of the course of joint disease. Arthritis Rheum. 52, 826–832.

Ravelli, A., Varnier, G.C., Oliveira, S., Castell, E., Arguedas, O., Magnani, A., et al., 2011. Antinuclear antibody-positive patients should be grouped as a separate category in the classification of juvenile idiopathic arthritis. Arthritis Rheum. 63, 267–275.

Ravelli, A., Grom, A.A., Behrens, E.M., Cron, R.Q., 2012. Macrophage activation syndrome as part of systemic juvenile idiopathic arthritis: diagnosis, genetics, pathophysiology and treatment. Genes. Immun. 13, 289–298.

Ruperto, N., Martini, A., 2004. International research networks in pediatric rheumatology: the PRINTO perspective. Curr. Opin. Rheumatol. 16, 566–570.

Ruperto, N., Murray, K.J., Gerloni, V., Wulffraat, N., de Oliveira, S.K., Falcini, F., et al., 2004. A randomized trial of parenteral methotrexate comparing an intermediate dose with a higher dose in children with juvenile idiopathic arthritis who failed to respond to standard doses of methotrexate. Arthritis Rheum. 50, 2191–2201.

Ruperto, N., Lovell, D.J., Quartier, P., Paz, E., Rubio-Pérez, N., Silva, C.A., et al., 2008. Abatacept in children with juvenile idiopathic arthritis: a randomised, double-blind, placebo-controlled withdrawal trial. Lancet. 372, 383–391.

Ruperto, N., Quartier, P., Wulffraat, N., Woo, P., Ravelli, A., Mouy, R., et al., 2012. A phase II, multicenter, open-label study evaluating dosing and preliminary safety and efficacy of canakinumab in systemic juvenile idiopathic arthritis with active systemic features. Arthritis Rheum. 64, 557–567.

Ruperto, N., Brunner, H.I., Quartier, P., Constantin, T., Wulffraat, N., Horneff, G., et al., 2012. Two randomized trials of canakinumab in systemic juvenile idiopathic arthritis. N. Engl. J. Med. 367, 406–2396.

Ruprecht, C.R., Gattorno, M., Ferlito, F., Gregorio, A., Martini, A., Lanzavecchia, A., et al., 2005. Coexpression of CD25 and CD27 identifies FoxP3 + regulatory T cells in inflamed synovia. J. Exp. Med. 201, 1793–1803.

Silverman, E., Mouy, R., Spiegel, L., Jung, L.K., Saurenmann, R.K., Lahdenne, P., et al., 2005. Leflunomide in Juvenile Rheumatoid Arthritis (JRA) Investigator Group. Leflunomide or methotrexate for juvenile rheumatoid arthritis. N. Engl. J. Med. 352, 1655–1666.

Southwood, T.R., Petty, R.E., Malleson, P.N., Delgado, E.A., Hunt, D.W., Wood, B., et al., 1989. Psoriatic arthritis in children. Arthritis Rheum. 32, 1007–1013.

Stock, C.J., Ogilvie, E.M., Samuel, J.M., Fife, M., Lewis, C.M., Woo, P., 2008. Comprehensive association study of genetic variants in the IL-1 gene family in systemic juvenile idiopathic arthritis. Genes. Immun. 9, 349–357.

Stoll, M.L., Zurakowski, D., Nigrovic, L.E., Nichols, D.P., Sundel, R.P., Nigrovic, P.A., 2006. Patients with juvenile psoriatic arthritis comprise two distinct populations. Arthritis Rheum. 54, 3564–3572.

Stoll, M.L., Lio, P., Sundel, R.P., Nigrovic, P.A., 2008. Comparison of Vancouver and International League of Associations for rheumatology classification criteria for juvenile psoriatic arthritis. Arthritis Rheum. 59, 51–58.

Strippoli, R., Carvello, F., Scianaro, R., De Pasquale, L., Vivarelli, M., Petrini, S., et al., 2012. Amplification of the response to Toll-like receptor ligands by prolonged exposure to interleukin-6 in mice: implication for the pathogenesis of macrophage activation syndrome. Arthritis Rheum. 64, 1680–1688.

Sugiura, T., Kawaguchi, Y., Harigai, M., Terajima-Ichida, H., Kitamura, Y., Furuya, T., et al., 2002. Association between adult-onset Still's disease and interleukin-18 gene polymorphisms. Genes. Immun. 3, 394–399.

Verbsky, J.W., White, A.J., 2004. Effective use of the recombinant interleukin 1 receptor antagonist anakinra in therapy resistant systemic onset juvenile rheumatoid arthritis. J. Rheumatol. 31, 2071–2075.

Wehrens, E.J., Mijnheer, G., Duurland, C.L., Klein, M., Meerding, J., van Loosdregt, J., et al., 2011. Functional human regulatory T cells fail to control autoimmune inflammation due to PKB/c-akt hyperactivation in effector cells. Blood. 118, 3538–3548.

Yokota, S., Imagawa, T., Mori, M., Miyamae, T., Aihara, Y., Takei, S., et al., 2008. Efficacy and safety of tocilizumab in patients with systemic-onset juvenile idiopathic arthritis: a randomised, double-blind, placebo-controlled, withdrawal phase III trial. Lancet. 371, 998–1006.

de Jager, W., Vastert, S.J., Beekman, J.M., Wulffraat, N.M., Kuis, W., Coffer, P.J., et al., 2009. Defective phosphorylation of interleukin-18 receptor beta causes impaired natural killer cell function in systemic-onset juvenile idiopathic arthritis. Arthritis Rheum. 60, 2782–2793.

Chapter 38

Spondyloarthritides

Uta Syrbe and Joachim Sieper

Department of Gastroenterology, Infection Medicine and Rheumatology, Charité Campus Benjamin Franklin, Charité University Medicine Berlin, Berlin, Germany

Chapter Outline

Definition, Epidemiology, Clinical Manifestations, and Treatment	537	The Role of Non-MHC Genes in Spondyloarthritis — 540
Reactive Arthritis	538	Bacterial Trigger and Autoimmunity in the Pathogenesis of the Spondyloarthritides — 541
Arthritis with IBD	538	Cytokines in the Pathogenesis of Reactive Arthritis — 541
Psoriatic Arthritis	538	Cytokines in the Pathogenesis of Ankylosing Spondylitis — 542
The Role of HLA-B27 in the Pathogenesis of Spondyloarthritis	538	What is the Immune Target in Ankylosing Spondylitis? — 542
		Inflammation and Bone Formation — 542
Arthritogenic Peptide Hypothesis	538	Concluding Remarks—Future Prospects — 543
Misfolded HLA-B27 Hypothesis	539	References — 543

DEFINITION, EPIDEMIOLOGY, CLINICAL MANIFESTATIONS, AND TREATMENT

The spondyloarthritis (SpA) diseases comprise ankylosing spondylitis (AS), reactive arthritis (ReA), arthritis/spondylitis with inflammatory bowel disease (IBD), and arthritis/spondylitis with psoriasis. The main links between each of these is the association with human leukocyte antigen (HLA)-B27, similar clinical symptoms such as inflammatory back pain, and similar patterns of peripheral joint involvement with an asymmetric arthritis predominantly of the lower limbs, and the possible occurrence of sacroiliitis, spondylitis, enthesitis, and uveitis. Most striking is the direct relationship between the prevalence of SpA and the prevalence of HLA-B27 in the general population. This strong correlation suggests that the environmental or genetic factors that are necessary in addition to HLA-B27 to get SpA must be ubiquitous (Braun and Sieper, 2003).

Ankylosing spondylitis is regarded as the SpA with the most severe outcome. Its prevalence has been estimated to be between 0.2 and 0.9% and the disease normally starts in the second decade of life. The male-to-female ratio has more recently been estimated to be around 2:1. HLA-B27 is found to be positive in 90–95%

of patients, and IBD, psoriasis, or preceding ReA can be found in about 10% of AS patients. Back pain is the leading clinical symptom in these patients, which is characterized by morning stiffness and improvement by exercise. The disease starts in 90% or more cases with a sacroiliitis. Further in the course of the disease the whole spine can be affected with spondylitis, spondylodiscitis, and arthritis of the small intervertebral joints. As a reaction to the inflammation, ankylosis occurs, which can involve the whole spine. Relapsing uveitis, peripheral asymmetric arthritis predominantly of the lower limbs, and enthesitis are the most frequent extraspinal manifestations. Diagnosis is made by a combination of clinical symptoms (such as inflammatory back pain or limitation of spinal mobility) and the demonstration of radiologic sacroiliitis, according to the modified New York criteria (van der Linden et al., 1984). More recently, we have proposed an approach on how to make an early diagnosis before evidence of radiologic sacroiliitis by combining clinical, laboratory, and imaging parameters such as magnetic resonance imaging (MRI) (Rudwaleit et al., 2004). A new approach to an earlier diagnosis is also mandatory because of the major delay of 5–7 years between the occurrence of the first symptoms and making the diagnosis.

N. Rose & I. Mackay (Eds): The Autoimmune Diseases, Fifth edition. DOI: http://dx.doi.org/10.1016/B978-0-12-384929-8.00038-1

In the last decades, only non-steroidal anti-inflammatory drugs (NSAIDs) were used, together with physiotherapy, as an effective treatment. Rather surprisingly, disease-modifying antirheumatic drugs (DMARDs) and corticosteroids, which are highly effective in other chronic inflammatory diseases such as rheumatoid arthritis, only show an effect in patients with predominant peripheral arthritis. On this background, the finding that blockers of tumor necrosis factor (TNF) are highly effective means a breakthrough in the treatment of this disease (Braun and Sieper, 2004; van der Heijde et al., 2005; Inman et al., 2008). At least 50% of active AS patients refractory to treatment with NSAIDs show a 50% or more improvement when treated either with the monoclonal anti-TNF-α antibody infliximab (Braun and Brandt 2003; van der Heijde et al., 2005) or the soluble TNF-receptor construct etanercept (Davis et al., 2003).

Reactive Arthritis

ReA occurs after a preceding infection of the urogenital tract with *Chlamydia trachomatis* or of the gut with enterobacteriae such as *Yersinia*, *Salmonella*, *Campylobacter jejuni*, or *Shigella*, usually after a few days and up to 4−6 weeks (Sieper et al., 2000). Between 30 and 60% of patients with ReA are positive for HLA-B27; arthritis occurs in approximately 4% of the general population, but in about 25% of HLA-B27$^+$ individuals after one of these infections. The arthritis is normally an oligoarthritis, predominantly of the lower limbs, but in about 20% this will manifest as a polyarthritis. Other manifestations can be an enthesitis, conjunctivitis/uveitis, or inflammatory back pain. Usually, the patients recover in 3−6 months; however, up to 20% can run a chronic course longer than 12 months. Bacterial antigen and, in the case of *Chlamydia*, also DNA and RNA have been detected in the joint, indicating that bacterial antigens persist in the joint and drive the local immune response. For making a diagnosis of ReA, a combination of clinical manifestations (preceding infection, typical pattern of arthritis) and laboratory evidence of previous or present bacterial infection is necessary (Sieper et al., 2002). While antibiotic treatment of urogenital tract infection with antibiotics prevents the occurrence of arthritis, this is not the case for bacterial enteritis. Once an arthritis is established, long-term antimicrobial monotherapy does not seem to influence the arthritis (Sieper et al., 2000). However, as recently shown, improvement of chronic *Chlamydia*-induced arthritis can be achieved after prolonged, 6-month combination antimicrobial therapy, suggesting that antibiotic monotherapy is inefficient in eradication of ReA-inducing microbes (Carter et al., 2010).

Arthritis with IBD

In approximately 10-20% of patients with IBD, this often occurs concurrently with gut inflammation. The arthritis is often a transient peripheral arthritis of the lower limbs. About 5% of IBD patients, mostly those who are HLA-B27$^+$, will develop spondyloarthropathy. The frequency of HLA-B27 among patients with peripheral arthritis is only slightly elevated, but is present among 50−70% of patients with IBD and SpA. Treatment should primarily be directed against the gut inflammation.

Psoriatic Arthritis

Up to 50% of patients with psoriasis and arthritis show a clinical picture compatible with SpA, such as oligoarthritis of the lower limbs and/or spinal inflammation. Among these patients, HLA-B27 is positive in approximately 25% (peripheral arthritis) to 60% (spinal manifestations). Treatment is similar to that for other forms of SpA.

THE ROLE OF HLA-B27 IN THE PATHOGENESIS OF SPONDYLOARTHRITIS
Arthritogenic Peptide Hypothesis

The susceptibility to AS has been estimated to be more than 90% genetically determined, and so it has been suggested that there is a rather ubiquitous environmental factor. The most relevant genetic risk factor is HLA-B27 (Brewerton et al., 1973; Schlosstein et al., 1973). The association of HLA-B27 with SpA is the highest known major histocompatibility complex (MHC) association for human diseases (with a couple of very rare exceptions; see Chapter 75) and is the most relevant single factor for the pathogenesis of SpA. There are now considerable data from epidemiologic studies and transgenic animals to indicate a direct effect of HLA-B27, rather than that of a closely linked gene, in disease pathogenesis. It is also clear now that one copy of HLA-B27 (heterozygosity) is sufficient for the disease. Besides HLA-B27, other MHC genes such as HLA-B60 and HLA-DR1 seem to be associated, but are of minor importance. However, although MHC is the major susceptibility locus, it has been suggested that it contributes only approximately 36% to the overall genetic risk (Brown et al., 2002).

Since the main function of HLA class I molecules is to present peptide antigens to cytotoxic T cells, the antigen-presenting properties of HLA-B27 could be crucial in the pathogenesis of spondyloarthritides leading to the so-called arthritogenic peptide hypothesis (Kuon and Sieper, 2003). Thus, some HLA-B27 subtypes, due to their unique amino acid residues, can bind specific arthritogenic peptide, and so become recognized by CD8$^+$

T cells. Furthermore, in response to these bacterial peptides, autoreactive T cells recognizing antigens with sufficient structural similarity between bacteria and self might become activated by self-peptides that are present particularly in spinal joints (Figure 38.1). Major support for this hypothesis comes from studies in humans showing the differential association of some of the HLA-B27 subtypes with AS. While B*2705, B*2702, B*2704, and B*2707 are strongly associated with the disease, the HLA-B27 subtypes B*2709 in whites and B*2706 in Southeast Asians are not at all or only rarely associated. Most interestingly, B*2709 differs from the disease-associated B*2705 by only one amino acid substitution, the exchange of Asp116 to His116. B*2706 differs by only two amino acid substitutions from the disease-associated B*2704 by exchange of His114 to Asp114 and Asp116 to Tyr116 (Khan, 2000). In studies on patients, both bacteria-specific and autoreactive CD8$^+$ T cells have been demonstrated in AS and ReA. Recently, a synovial CD8$^+$ T cell response to a peptide from *Yersinia* heat shock protein 60 in patients with *Yersinia*-induced ReA and also an HLA-B27-restricted CD8$^+$ T cell response to peptides derived from several chlamydial proteins in patients with *Chlamydia*-induced ReA have been described (Kuon and Sieper, 2003). In the latter study, there was a novel approach in searching the whole chlamydial proteome to identify peptides which stimulate CD8$^+$ T cells from patients in an HLA-B27 restricted manner. Recently, there was a report of a CD8$^+$ T cell response to an Epstein–Barr virus (EBV) epitope derived from the LMP2 protein, and to a sequence-related self-peptide from the autoantigen vasoactive intestinal peptide (VIP) receptor 1

(Fiorillo et al., 2000). However, the exact identity of a potentially arthritogenic peptide has yet to be determined. An oligoclonal expansion of T cells has also been demonstrated for CD4$^+$ and CD8$^+$ T cells in AS and for CD8$^+$ T cells in ReA. Synovial T cells derived from different HLA-B27$^+$ patients suffering from ReA and triggered by different bacteria revealed an astonishingly high homology of T cell receptors (May et al., 2002). These results led to the suggestion that similar antigens are recognized by these oligoclonally expanded CD8$^+$ T cells.

Misfolded HLA-B27 Hypothesis

Beside the "classical" arthritogenic peptide theory, other hypotheses have emerged. One interesting concept, the HLA-B27 misfolding and unfolded protein response (UPR) hypothesis, states that HLA-B27 itself is directly involved in the pathologic process of SpA. That is, HLA-B27 can be misfolded, which might have implications for pathogenesis (Colbert, 2004). The misfolding is suggested to be due to a particular feature of the HLA-B27 molecule: e.g., newly synthesized HLA-B*2705 seems to fold and associate with β2-microglobulin more slowly compared with other MHC class I molecules. Allen et al. (1999) reported that as a consequence of HLA-B27 misfolding, free HLA-B27 heavy chains can form abnormal heavy-chain homodimers. This homodimer formation could be facilitated by unpaired free cysteine residues at position 67 (Cys67) of the HLA-B27 heavy chain α1 helix. Using fluorescence-tagged tetramers of HLA-B27*05 homodimers, Kollnberger et al. (2002) showed that they bind to cell surface natural killer (NK) inhibitory receptors, KIR3DL1 and KIR3DL2, and to leukocyte immunoglobulin-like receptor B2 (LILRB2) which is expressed on dendritic cells, monocytes, and macrophages. In HLA-B27$^+$ SpA patients, KIR3DL2$^+$ NK cells and CD4$^+$ T cells are expanded in peripheral blood, compared with HLA-B27$^-$ SpA, rheumatoid arthritis, and other control patients and NK cells of these patients show higher level of cytotoxicity and CD4$^+$ T cells produce IL-17 (Chan et al., 2005). It is suggested that binding of HLA-B27 heavy-chain homodimers to killer cell Ig-like receptor (KIR) and leukocyte Ig-like receptor (LILR) could promote inflammation by enhancing survival of NK and T cells and by influencing differentiation of LILR-expressing antigen-presenting cells (Kollnberger and Bowness, 2009).

Moreover, Mear et al. (1999) observed that HLA-B*2705 in cell lines showed a fraction of heavy chains undergoing degradation within the endoplasmic reticulum. These render the cells susceptible to the unfolded protein response (UPR) which is associated with the upregulation of interleukin (IL)-23, the main inducing factor for IL-17-producing T cells. The IL-23/IL-17 axis

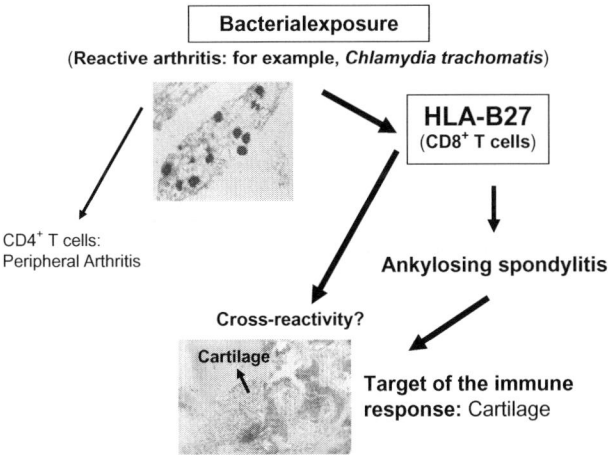

Bacterialexposure

(Reactive arthritis: for example, Chlamydia trachomatis)

HLA-B27
(CD8$^+$ T cells)

CD4$^+$ T cells:
Peripheral Arthritis

Ankylosing spondylitis

Cross-reactivity?

Cartilage

Target of the immune response: Cartilage

FIGURE 38.1 Hypothesis1 how bacterial exposure induces a peripheral arthritis, probably via a CD4$^+$ T cell response. However, axial manifestations might be mediated by CD8$^+$ T cells because of the high association with HLA-B27. The cartilage might become the primary target of the immune response through cross-reactivity with bacterial antigens.

is intriguing because IL-23 receptor polymorphisms have been shown to be associated with SpA, psoriasis, and Crohn's disease (Consortium WTC-CCaA-A-AS, 2007). Hence, the HLA-B27 misfolding and unfolded protein response hypothesis postulates a role for CD4$^+$ T and NK cells in the pathogenesis of AS and other SpA. This hypothesis is also supported by the fact that disease development and severity is unimpaired in HLA-B27 transgenic rats that lack functional CD8$^+$ T cells (Taurog et al., 2009). Similar results have been observed in cell transfer and depletion experiments (Breban et al., 1996; May et al., 2003) which challenge the arthritogenic peptide hypothesis.

THE ROLE OF NON-MHC GENES IN SPONDYLOARTHRITIS

Only a small proportion of HLA-B27 carriers develop AS (1–5% in most series) which cannot be explained by HLA-B27 subtypes. As we know from independent twin studies that the heritability of susceptibility to AS is more than 90% (Brown et al., 1997; Petersen et al., 2006), it is likely that other genes contribute to the susceptibility. Genome-wide association studies performed in recent years have identified definite associations of AS with the non-MHC genes *ERAP1* and *IL23R*, and with gene deserts 2p15 and 21q22 (Wellcome Trust Case-Control Consortium, 2007; Austrolo-Anglo-American Spondyloarthritis Consortium, 2010, 2011). Furthermore, strong evidence to support an association with AS has been demonstrated for the genes *IL-1R2*, *ANTXR2*, *TNFSF15*, *TNFR1*, *STAT3*, and a region on chromosome 16q including the gene *TRADD* (Wellcome Trust Case-Control Consortium, 2007; Austrolo-Anglo-American Spondyloarthritis Consortium 2010, 2011; Pointon et al., 2009; Zinovieva et al., 2009; Danoy et al., 2009).

The *ERAP1* gene encodes the enzyme endoplasmic reticulum aminopeptidase 1, which is involved in trimming of peptides in the endoplasmic reticulum prior to HLA class I presentation and it may be involved in trimming of cytokine receptors as well. The ERAP1 polymorphisms only affect the AS risk in HLA-B27-positive individuals suggesting that HLA-B27 operates through a mechanism involving aberrant processing of antigenic peptides (Wellcome Trust Case-Control Consortium, 2007; Austrolo-Anglo-American Spondyloarthritis Consortium, 2010, 2011).

The association of *IL-23R* with AS was confirmed in several studies and *IL-23R* was also found to be associated with IBD and psoriasis (Wellcome Trust Case-Control Consortium, 2007; Austrolo-Anglo-American Spondyloarthritis Consortium, 2010). IL-23 signals through the IL-23 receptor. IL-17-producing T cells express IL-23R, and IL-23 plays an important role in

sustaining Th17 cell responses *in vivo*. Although one study showed loss of micro-RNA-dependent regulation of one IBD-associated IL-23R variant resulting in enhanced protein production, no enhanced IL-23 levels have been found so far in AS (Zwiers et al., 2012). Thus, it is still uncertain whether the disease-associated variants of the *IL-23R* cause gain or loss of function. Also *STAT3*, which encodes a downstream signaling molecule of the IL-23 receptor, was found to be associated with Crohn's disease and also has a suggestive association with AS (Barrett et al., 2008; Danoy et al., 2009). Thus, the genetic association of *IL-23R* and *STAT3* with AS definitively suggests an impact of the IL-23/Th17 axis in pathogenesis of AS.

The association of the gene deserts 2p15 and 21q22 with AS was identified and confirmed by the TASC genome-wide association study (Austrolo-Anglo-American Spondyloarthritis Consortium, 2010). Gene deserts are lengthy regions without known genes. Therefore, these regions might contain regulatory elements, as yet unidentified genes, or regions which are involved in epigenetic gene regulation.

Apart from these confirmed genetic associations, several other genes, such as *ANTXR2*, *IL-1R2*, *TNFSF15*, *TNFR1*, and *TRADD*, show suggestive associations with AS (Pointon et al., 2009; Austrolo-Anglo-American Spondyloarthritis Consortium, 2010).

In earlier studies, two promoter polymorphisms of the TNF-α gene at positions -308 (308.1 and 308.2) and -238 (238.1 and 238.2) have been investigated in AS. The 308.2 genotype was found significantly less frequently in AS than in controls. In some studies 308.2 was associated with higher transcriptional activity (Hoehler et al., 1998). Thus, there is some evidence that TNF-α genotypes that may be associated with a low TNF-α production are present in a higher percentage in patients with ReA or AS.

Also, in earlier studies, which investigated the association of TNF-α microsatellites, an association of ReA with a TNF-α6 allele has been described; this allele has previously been associated with a low TNF-α secretion. Since, in this study from Finland, TNF-α6 was also associated with HLA-B27, the association of TNF-α6 with ReA was thought to be secondary to B27.

In another study, analyzing IL-10 gene polymorphism in ReA, a significant decrease in the promoter alleles G12 and G10 was found in the ReA group compared with HLA-B27$^+$ controls, indicating that these alleles might have a protective effect against the occurrence of ReA (Kaluza et al., 2001). Although it is not yet clear whether these alleles are associated with a higher production of IL-10, these data suggest that the relative increase of IL-10 found in ReA might be, at least partially, genetically determined.

BACTERIAL TRIGGER AND AUTOIMMUNITY IN THE PATHOGENESIS OF THE SPONDYLOARTHRITIDES

Exposure of the immune system to bacteria seems to be an important initial triggering event for AS. The best evidence for this comes from ReA, which is usually triggered by a genitourinary infection with *C. trachomatis* or an enteritis due to certain Gram-negative enterobacteria, such as *Shigella*, *Salmonella*, *Yersinia*, or *Campylobacter*. The demonstration of microbial antigens within the synovium suggests that ReA may be related to the persistence of microbial antigens at the sites of inflammatory arthritis (Granfors et al., 1989). Approximately 20–40% of HLA-B27$^+$ ReA patients develop the full clinical picture of AS after 10–20 years (Leirisalo-Repo, 1998). Although clinically diagnosed ReA arthritis precedes AS only in less than 10%, this figure may be much higher because many of the gut or urogenital infections preceding the clinical manifestation of ReA can be asymptomatic. The central role of bacteria in the pathogenesis of SpA is further supported by the relationship between Crohn's disease, HLA-B27 positivity, and the occurrence of AS: in one study, in 13 out of 24 (54%) HLA-B27$^+$ patients with Crohn's disease, AS could also be diagnosed, but only in 5 out of the 189 (2.6%) patients who were HLA-B27$^-$ (Purrmann et al., 1988). In the case of Crohn's disease, the leakage in the gut mucosa, as a consequence of the related inflammation, presumably allows an interaction of the immune system with the normal gut bacteria. It has also become clear that in about 50% of patients with so-called idiopathic AS, macroscopic or microscopic mucosal chronic lesions resembling Crohn's disease can be detected in the gut by colonoscopy (Mielants et al., 1988).

Finally, there is also evidence for the importance of B27–bacteria interaction from animal models. HLA-B27 transgenic rats develop features of ReA, including gut inflammation, peripheral arthritis, and psoriasiform skin and nail changes. The importance of environmental factors is emphasized by the observation that many of these features, including gut inflammation and arthritis, do not develop in HLA-B27 transgenic rats born and bred in a germ-free environment. Germ-free animals rapidly develop inflammatory disease on removal from the sterile environment. This can be partially prevented by treatment with antibiotics (Taurog et al., 1999).

Therefore, AS can probably be regarded as the long-term outcome for patients most of whom are HLA-B27$^+$ and who have been exposed to ReA-associated bacteria, bacteria in the gut, or other as yet unidentified bacteria.

Bacteria appear to play a crucial role as an initial event for the pathogenesis of AS; however, there is no clear evidence that they are also directly responsible for the immunopathology in AS. Although bacterial antigens are found in the joints of ReA patients, no such antigens have been found so far in sacroiliac joints (Braun et al., 1997). Therefore, AS might rather be the result of bacteria-induced autoimmunity. Particularly in the light of the strong association with MHC, research has concentrated in the past on the role of T cells in SpA. Currently, there is no evidence for any role for the humoral immune response in the pathogenesis of SpA.

CYTOKINES IN THE PATHOGENESIS OF REACTIVE ARTHRITIS

As it has been shown that bacteria persist *in vivo* in patients with ReA, most likely in the joint in the case of *Chlamydia* and in the gut mucosa or lymph nodes of the gut in the case of the enterobacteriae, the following questions arise: (1) why do these bacteria persist in some patients but not in others; and (2) why do some patients (although the minority) develop a chronic course of their arthritis. The ReA-associated bacteria are obligate (such as *Chlamydia*) or facultative intracellular bacteria. T-helper 1 (Th1) cytokines such as TNF-α and interferon-γ (IFN-γ) are crucial for an effective elimination of these bacteria, while Th2 cytokines such as IL-4 or anti-inflammatory cytokines such as IL-10 might inhibit an effective elimination. We and others showed that there is a relative deficiency of Th1 cytokines in ReA, especially of TNF-α but also of IFN-γ, both locally in synovial fluid and synovial membrane and systemically in peripheral blood (Yin et al., 1997; Braun et al., 1999). Furthermore, we could demonstrate a correlation between a low TNF-α production in peripheral blood and a longer duration of arthritic symptoms (Braun et al., 1999). Thus, a relative lack of Th1 cytokines appears to be relevant for the occurrence and persistence of ReA, probably mediated by a persistence of bacteria. IL-10 has received increasing interest recently as a potentially immunosuppressive cytokine. While upregulation of such a cytokine would be wanted in autoimmune diseases such as rheumatoid arthritis, we could show that it is relatively upregulated in ReA, and thus that it might contribute to bacterial persistence in ReA, possibly by downregulation of the Th1 cytokines, IFN-γ and TNF-α (Yin et al., 1999b). Persistence of bacterial antigens disseminated to the joints might cause aberrant inflammation at these sites which are also exposed to mechanical stress. Alternatively, persistence of antigens might cause pathological priming of T cells cross-reacting to autologous antigens.

CYTOKINES IN THE PATHOGENESIS OF ANKYLOSING SPONDYLITIS

Data are scarce on cytokines in AS. We measured by flow cytometry cytokine-positive $CD4^+$ and $CD8^+$ T cells derived from peripheral blood after mitogenic *in vitro* stimulation (Rudwaleit et al., 2001). Patients with AS had a significantly lower percentage of IFN-γ^+ or TNF-α^+ $CD4^+$ T cells compared with HLA-B27$^-$ controls, while the results for an HLA-B27$^+$ healthy control group were intermediate between the two groups. For IL-10$^+$ T cells, we found a significant increase in the $CD8^+$ T cell subpopulation from HLA-B27$^+$ AS patients compared with B27$^+$ and B27$^-$ controls, but this did not pertain for the $CD4^+$ subpopulation. This relative (small) lack of Th1 cytokines in the peripheral blood of AS patients is in contrast to the presence of abundant TNF-α in biopsies taken from the sacroiliac joint from AS patients (Braun et al., 1995) and the very strong therapeutic response to treatment with TNF blockers in AS (Braun and Sieper, 2004), suggesting that TNF-α and possibly also IFN-γ are important in the pathogenesis of AS and other SpA. This discrepancy is not easy to explain, but cytokines in peripheral blood might not accurately reflect the situation at the local site of inflammation. Furthermore, cytokines produced by innate immune cells might be of even greater impact on the pathogenesis of AS than cytokine production by adaptive immune cells. This is suggested by studies analyzing IL-17 expression within inflamed peripheral joints, where both mononuclear and polymorphonuclear synovial cell infiltrates were found to express IL-17 (Moran et al., 2011). Also in involved facet joints of AS patients increased numbers of IL-17-producing cells, primarily of myeloid origin, were found (Appel et al., 2011).

According to the misfolding hypothesis, accumulation of misfolded proteins within the endoplasmic reticulum triggers a conserved intracellular stress response that decreases protein production, enhances folding capacity of the endoplasmic reticulum, and promotes induction of gene expression. Stimulation of innate cells such as macrophages with pharmacological inducers of the unfolded protein response results in enhanced LPS-elicited production of inflammatory cytokines, in particular IFN-β and IL-23 (Smith et al., 2008). A recent study shows that peripheral blood-derived macrophages from AS patients produced strikingly higher levels of IL-23 in response to stimulation with lipopolysaccharide, even in the absence of induction by UPR (Zeng et al., 2011). This, together with the association of AS with the *IL-23R* gene, and evidence for the unrestrained signal transduction by a disease-associated variant, suggests that IL-23 production by innate immune cells might be instrumental in the pathogenesis of ankylosing spondylitis.

WHAT IS THE IMMUNE TARGET IN ANKYLOSING SPONDYLITIS?

Exposure to bacterial antigens is thought to drive AS (see above). However, since evidence for bacterial antigen in inflamed joints of the axial skeleton of AS patients is lacking, the target of the immune response in AS is still unclear. Studies using MRI have shown that the most relevant inflammatory site in SpA is an osteitis occurring at the bone/cartilage interface (McGonagle et al., 1999). This finding has been supplemented by histologic investigations in SpA from the sacroiliac joint and other structures where, especially in the early phases, mononuclear cells invade and seem to erode the cartilage at different sites (Bollow et al., 2000). Such findings have suggested that the cartilage is the primary target of the immune response in SpA (Maksymowych, 2000).

The aggrecan G1 domain has been implicated as one source of a possible T cell autoantigen in AS and similar rheumatic diseases, based both on results from animal models and on studies in patients. A specific $CD4^+$ T cell response to peptides derived from the G1 domain of aggrecan was found in animal models and also in patients with AS. Here, in 60% of patients, a $CD4^+$ response against the whole G1 protein and against a set of overlapping peptides derived from this G1 protein was evident (Zou et al., 2003).

Because of the type of tissue-specific damage in AS, other extracellular matrix proteins apart from aggrecan, derived from human cartilage and enthesis, could also be targets of an autoimmune response. Recently, a $CD8^+$ T cell response to a nonameric peptide from collagen type VI was detected in the synovial fluid from patients with AS (Atagunduz et al., 2005). Further work is in progress and will, therefore, have to focus on T cell responses against cartilage-derived antigens.

INFLAMMATION AND BONE FORMATION

A hallmark of ankylosing spondylitis is the occurrence of aberrant bone formation leading to ankylosis of joints, like the sacroiliac joints, and the formation of syndesmophytes within the spine. The factors driving this process of new bone formation in AS are not clear. Experimental models suggest that the wingless (wnt) pathway which controls osteoblastogenesis and skeletal development during embryogenesis can also control aberrant bone formation. Several members of the wnt protein family bind a receptor complex on the surface of mesenchymal cells facilitating dephosphorylation of the intracellular protein beta-catenin which then can translocate into the nucleus and bind to target genes. Activation of mesenchymal cells by wnt agonists promotes osteoblastogenesis, which is inhibited by antagonists (Miller, 2002). Inhibition of dickkopf-1 (DKK-1), which is a natural antagonist of this pathway, can reverse an erosive—destructive arthritis into a bone forming pattern of arthritis (Diarra et al., 2007). Modulation of this pathway does not change the inflammatory phenotype of arthritis suggesting that bone formation might be rather independent from inflammatory mediators. In AS, patients with progression of bone formation have reduced serum levels of wnt antagonists such as sclerostin and functional DKK-1, suggesting that the wnt pathway plays a major role in bone formation in AS (Appel et al., 2009; Heiland et al., 2012). Of note, 2-year evaluations of progression of syndesmophyte growth in patients treated with a TNF blocker did not show reduction in bone formation (van der Heijde et al., 2008a,b, 2009). This also suggests that bone formation is not controlled by Inflammatory mediators like TNF-α. Further studies are required to understand more fully the complex control of this process of aberrant bone formation in AS.

CONCLUDING REMARKS—FUTURE PROSPECTS

The spondyloarthritides, in particular ankylosing spondylitis, are among the most interesting of the rheumatic diseases. New treatment options, utilizing biologic therapy, have greatly improved the outcome of disease. However, the contribution of genes, in particular of HLA-B27, to the disease is still a matter of research. Furthermore, the interplay between immune cells and mesenchymal-derived cells facilitating bone formation is another important aspect which is just being recognized and which has a great potential for new therapeutic targets.

REFERENCES

Allen, R.L., O'Callaghan, C.A., McMichael, A.J., Bowness, P., 1999. Cutting edge: HLA-B27 can form a novel beta 2-microglobulin-free heavy chain homodimer structure. J. Immunol. 162, 5045—5048.

Appel, H., Ruiz-Heiland, G., Listing, J., Zwerina, J., Herrmann, M., Mueller, R., et al., 2009. Altered skeletal expression of sclerostin and its link to radiographic progression in ankylosing spondylitis. Arthritis Rheum. 60, 3257—3262.

Appel, H., Maier, R., Wu, P., Scheer, R., Hempfing, A., Kayser, R., et al., 2011. Analysis of IL-17(+) cells in facet joints of patients with spondyloarthritis suggests that the innate immune pathway might be of greater relevance than the Th17-mediated adaptive immune response. Arthritis Res. Ther. 20 (13), R95.

Atagunduz, P., Appel, H., Kuon, W., Wu, P., Thiel, A., Kloetzel, P.M., et al., 2005. HLA-B27 restricted CD8^{+} T cell response to cartilage-derived self-peptides in ankylosing spondylitis. Arthritis Rheum. 52, 892—901.

Austrolo-Anglo-American Spondyloarthritis Consortium (TASC), 2010. Genome-wide association study of ankylosing spondylitis identifies non-MHC susceptibility loci. Nat. Genet. 42, 123—127.

Austrolo-Anglo-American Spondyloarthritis Consortium (TASC) & Wellcome Trust Case Control Consortium 2 (WTCCC2), 2011. Interaction between ERAP1 and HLA-B27 in ankylosing spondylitis implicates peptide handling in the mechanism for HLA-B27 in disease susceptibility. Nat. Genet. 43, 761—767.

Barrett, J.C., Hansoul, S., Nicolae, D.L., et al., 2008. Genome-wide association defines more than 30 distinct susceptibility loci for Crohn's disease. Nat. Genet. 40, 955—962.

Bollow, M., Fischer, T., Reisshauer, H., Backhaus, M., Sieper, J., Hamm, B., et al., 2000. Quantitative analyses of sacroiliac biopsies in spondyloarthropathies: T cells and macro phages predominate in early and active sacroiliitis cellularity correlates with the degree of enhancement detected by magnetic resonance imaging. Ann. Rheum. Dis. 59, 135—140.

Braun, J., Sieper, J., 2003. Spondyloarthritides and related arthritides. In: Warrel, D.A., Cox, T.M., Firth, J.D., Benz, E.J. (Eds.), Oxford Textbook of Medicine, fourth ed. Oxford University Press, New York, pp. 43—53.

Braun, J., Sieper, J., 2004. Biological therapies in the spondyloarthritides— the current state. Rheumatology (Oxford). 43, 1072—1084.

Braun, J., Bollow, M., Neure, L., Seipelt, E., Seyrekbasan, F., Herbst, H., et al., 1995. Use of immunohistologic and in-situ hybridization techniques in the examination of sacroiliac joint biopsy specimens from patients with ankylosing-spondylitis. Arthritis Rheum. 38, 499—505.

Braun, J., Tuszewski, M., Ehlers, S., Haberle, J., Bollow, M., Eggens, U., et al., 1997. Nested polymerase chain reaction strategy simultaneously targeting DNA sequences of multiple bacterial species in inflammatory joint diseases. II. Examination of sacroiliac and knee joint biopsies of patients with spondyloarthropathies and other arthritides. J. Rheumatol. 24, 1101—1105.

Braun, J., Yin, Z.N., Spiller, I., Siegert, S., Rudwaleit, M., Liu, L.Z., et al., 1999. Low secretion of tumor necrosis factor alpha, but no other Th1 or Th2 cytokines, by peripheral blood mononuclear cells correlates with chronicity in reactive arthritis. Arthritis Rheum. 42, 2039—2044.

Braun, J., Brandt, J., Listing, J., Rudwaleit, M., Sieper, J., 2003. Biologic therapies in the spondyloarthritis: new opportunities, new challenges. Curr. Opin. Rheumatol. 15, 394—407.

Breban, M., Fernandez-Sueiro, J.L., Richardson, J.A, Hadavand, R.R., Maika, S.D., Hammer, R.E., et al., 1996. T cells, but not thymic exposure to HLA-B27, are required for the inflammatory disease of HLA-B27 transgenic rats. J. Immunol. 156, 794—803.

Brewerton, D.A., Hart, F.D., Nicholls, A., et al., 1973. Ankylosing spondylitis and HLA-B27. Lancet. 1, 904—907.

Brown, M.A., Kennedy, L.G., MacGregor, A.J., et al., 1997. Susceptibility to ankylosing spondylitis in twins: the role of genes, HLA, and the environment. Arthritis Rheum. 40, 1823—1828.

Brown, M.A., Wordsworth, B.P., Reveille, J.D., 2002. Genetics of ankylosing spondylitis. Clin. Exp. Rheumatol. 20, S43—S49.

Carter, J.D., Espinoza, L.R., Inman, R.D., Sneed, K.B., Ricca, L.R., Vasey, F.B., et al., 2010. Combination antibiotics as a treatment for chronic Chlamydia-induced reactive arthritis: a double-blind, placebo-controlled, prospective trial. Arthritis Rheum. 62, 1298—1307.

Chan, A.T., Kollnberger, S.D., Wedderburn, L.R., Bowness, P., 2005. Expansion and enhanced survival of natural killer cells expressing the killer immunoglobulin-like receptor KIR3DL2 in spondyloarthritis. Arthritis Rheum. 52, 3586—3595.

Colbert, R.A., 2004. The immunobiology of HLA-B27: variations on a theme. Curr. Mol. Med. 4, 21–30.

Consortium WTC-CCaA-A-AS, 2007. Association scan of 14,500 non-synonymous SNPs in four diseases identifies autoimmunity variants. Nat. Genet. 39, 1329–1337.

Danoy, P., Pryce, K., Hadler, J., et al., 2009. Evidence for genetic overlap between ankylosing spondylitis and Crohn's disease. Arthritis Rheum. 60, S249.

Davis Jr., J.C., Van Der Heijde, D., Braun, J., Dougados, M., Cush, J., Clegg, D.O., et al., 2003. Enbrel Ankylosing Spondylitis Study Group. Recombinant human tumor necrosis factor receptor (etanercept) for treating ankylosing spondylitis: a randomized, controlled trial. Arthritis Rheum. 48, 3230–3236.

Diarra, D., Stolina, M., Polzer, K., Zwerina, J., Ominsky, M.S., Dwyer, D., et al., 2007. Dickkopf-1 is a master regulator of joint remodeling. Nat. Med. 13, 156–163.

Fiorillo, M.T., Maragno, M., Butler, R., Dupuis, M.L., Sorrentino, R., 2000. CD8 + T-cell autoreactivity to an HLA-B27-restricted self-epitope correlates with ankylosing spondylitis. J. Clin. Invest. 106, 47–53.

Granfors, K., Jalkanen, S., von Essen, R., Lahesmaa-Rantala, R., Isomaki, O., Pekkola-Heino, K., et al., 1989. Yersinia antigens in synovial-fluid cells from patients with reactive arthritis. N. Engl. J. Med. 4, 216–221.

Heiland, G.R., Appel, H., Poddubnyy, D., Zwerina, J., Hueber, A., Haibel, H., et al., 2012. High level of functional dickkopf-1 predicts protection from syndesmophyte formation in patients with ankylosing spondylitis. Ann. Rheum. Dis. 71, 572–574.

Hoehler, T., Schaper, T., Schneider, P.M., zum Buschenfelde, K.H.M., Marker-Hermann, E., 1998. Association of different tumor necrosis factor alpha promoter allele frequencies with ankylosing spondylitis in HLA-B27 positive individuals. Arthritis Rheum. 41, 1489–1492.

Inman, R.D., Davis Jr., J.C., Heijde, D., Diekman, L., Sieper, J., Kim, S. I., Mack, M., et al., 2008. Efficacy and safety of golimumab in patients with ankylosing spondylitis: results of a randomized, double-blind, placebo-controlled, phase III trial. Arthritis Rheum. 58, 3402–3412.

Kaluza, W., Leirisalo-Repo, M., Marker-Hermann, E., Westman, P., Reuss, E., Hug, R., et al., 2001. IL10.G microsatellites mark promoter haplotypes associated with protection against the development of reactive arthritis in Finnish patients. Arthritis Rheum. 44, 1209–1214.

Khan, M.A., 2000. Update: the twenty subtypes of HLA-B27. Curr. Opin. Rheumatol. 12, 235–238.

Kollnberger, S., Bowness, P., 2009. The role of B27 heavy chain dimmer immune receptor interactions in spondyloarthritis. Adv. Exp. Med. 649, 277–285.

Kollnberger, S., Bird, L., Sun, M.Y., Retiere, C., Braud, V.M., McMichael, A., et al., 2002. Cell-surface expression and immune receptor recognition of HLA-B27 homodimers. Arthritis Rheum. 46, 2972–2982.

Kuon, W., Sieper, J., 2003. Identification of HLA-B27-restricted peptides in reactive arthritis and other spondyloarthropathies: computer algorithms and fluorescent activated cell sorting analysis as tools for hunting of HLA-B27-restricted chlamydial and autologous crossreactive peptides involved in reactive arthritis and ankylosing spondylitis. Rheum. Dis. Clin. N. Am. 29, 595–611.

Leirisalo-Repo, M., 1998. Prognosis, course of disease, and treatment of the spondyloarthropathies. Rheum. Dis. Clin. N. Am. 24, 737.

Maksymowych, W.P., 2000. Ankylosing spondylitis—at the interface of bone and cartilage. J. Rheumatol. 27, 2295–2301.

May, E., Dulphy, N., Frauendorf, E., Duchmann, R., Bowness, P., de Castro, J.A.L., et al., 2002. Conserved TCR beta chain usage in reactive arthritis; evidence for selection by a putative HLA-B27-associated autoantigen. Tissue Antigens. 60, 299–308.

May, E., Dorris, M.L., Satumtira, N., Iqbal, I., Rehman, M.I., Lightfoot, E., et al., 2003. CD8 alpha beta T cells are not essential to the pathogenesis of arthritis or colitis in HLA-B27 transgenic rats. J. Immunol. 170, 1099–1105.

McGonagle, D., Gibbon, W., O'Connor, P., Green, M., Pease, C., Ridgway, J., et al., 1999. An anatomical explanation for good-prognosis rheumatoid arthritis. Lancet. 353, 123–124.

Mear, J.P., Schreiber, K.L., Munz, C., Zhu, X., Stevanovic, S., Rammensee, H.G., et al., 1999. Misfolding of HLA-B27 as a result of its B pocket suggests a novel mechanism for its role in susceptibility to spondyloarthropathies. J. Immunol. 163, 6665–6670.

Mielants, H., Veys, E.M., Cuvelier, C., Devos, M., 1988. Ileocolonoscopic findings in seronegative spondylarthropathies. Br. J. Rheumatol. 27, 95–105.

Miller, J.R., 2002. The Wnts. Genome Biol. 3 (1), 3001.

Moran, E.M., Heydrich, R., Ng, C.T., Saber, T.P., McCormick, J., Sieper, J., et al., 2011. IL-17A expression is localised to both mononuclear and polymorphonuclear synovial cell infiltrates. PLoS One. 6, e24048.

Petersen, O., Svendsen, A., Ejstrup, L., et al., 2006. Heritability estimates on ankylosing spondylitis. Clin. Exp. Rheumatol. 24, 463.

Pointon, J.J., Harvey, D., Karaderi, T., et al., 2009. The chromosome 16q region associated with ankylosing spondylitis includes the candidate gene TRADD (TNF receptor type 1-associated death domain). Ann. Rheum. Dis. 69, 1243–1246.

Purrmann, J., Zeidler, H., Bertrams, J., Juli, E., Cleveland, S., Berges, W., et al., 1988. Hla antigens in ankylosing-spondylitis associated with Crohns-disease—increased frequency of the Hla phenotype B27,B44. J. Rheumatol. 15, 1658–1661.

Rudwaleit, M., Siegert, S., Yin, Z., Eick, J., Thiel, A., Radbruch, A., et al., 2001. Low T cell production of TNF alpha and IFN gamma in ankylosing spondylitis: its relation to HLA-B27 and influence of the TNF-308 gene polymorphism. Ann. Rheum. Dis. 60, 36–42.

Rudwaleit, M., van der Heijde, D., Khan, M.A., Braun, J., Sieper, J., 2004. How to diagnose axial spondyloarthritis early. Ann. Rheum. Dis. 63, 535–543.

Schlosstein, L., Teasaki, P.I., Bluestone, R., et al., 1973. High association of HL-A antigen, W27, with ankylosing spondylitis. N. Engl. J. Med. 288, 704–706.

Sieper, J., Braun, J., Kingsley, G.H., 2000. Report on the Fourth International Workshop on Reactive Arthritis. Arthritis Rheum. 43, 720–734.

Sieper, J., Rudwaleit, M., Braun, J., van der Heijde, D., 2002. Diagnosing reactive arthritis—role of clinical setting in the value of serologic and microbiologic assays. Arthritis Rheum. 46, 319–327.

Smith, J.A., Turner, M.J., DeLay, M.L., Klenk, E.I., Sowders, D.P., Colbert, R.A., 2008. Endoplasmatic reticulum stress and the unfolded protein response are linked to synergistic IFN-β induction via X-box binding protein 1. Eur. J. Immunol. 38, 1194–1203.

Taurog, J.D., Maika, S.D., Satumtira, N., Dorris, M.L., Mclean, I.L., Yanagisawa, H., et al., 1999. Inflammatory disease in HLA-B27 transgenic rats. Immunol. Rev. 169, 209–223.

Taurog, J.D., Dorris, M.L., Satumtira, N., Tran, T.M., Sharma, R., Dressel, R., 2009. Spondyloarthritis in HLA-B27/human beta 2-microglobulin-transgenic rats is not prevented by lack of CD8. Arthritis Rheum. 60, 1977–1984.

van der Heijde, D., Dijkmans, B., Geusens, P., Sieper, J., Dewoody, K., Williamson, P., et al., 2005. Efficacy and safety of infliximab in patients with ankylosing spondylitis: results of a randomized, placebo-controlled trial (ASSERT). Arthritis Rheum. 52, 582–591.

van der Heijde, D., Landewé, R., Baraliakos, X., Houben, H., van Tubergen, A., Williamson, P., et al., 2008a. Radiographic findings following two years of infliximab therapy in patients with ankylosing spondylitis. Arthritis Rheum. 58, 3063–3070.

van der Heijde, D., Landewé, R., Einstein, S., Ory, P., Vosse, D., Ni, L., et al., 2008b. Radiographic progression of ankylosing spondylitis after up to two years of treatment with etanercept. Arthritis Rheum. 58 (5), 1324–1331.

van der Heijde, D., Salonen, D., Weissman, B.N., Landewé, R., Maksymowych, W.P., Kupper, H., et al., 2009. Assessment of radiographic progression in the spines of patients with ankylosing spondylitis treated with adalimumab for up to 2 years. Arthritis Res. Ther. 11, R127.

van der Linden, S., Cats, A., Valkenburg, H.A., Khan, M.A., 1984. Evaluation of the diagnostic-criteria for ankylosing-spondylitis—a proposal for modification of the New York criteria. Br. J. Rheumatol. 23, 148–149.

Wellcome Trust Case-Control Consortium & Australo-Anglo-American Spondyloarthritis Consortium, 2007. Association scan of 14,500 nonsynonymous SNPs in four diseases identifies autoimmune variants. Nat. Genet. 39, 1329–1337.

Yin, Z., Braun, J., Grolms, M., Spiller, I., Radbruch, A., Sieper, J., 1997. IFN gamma, IL-4 and IL-10 positive cells in the CD4[+] and CD8[+] T cell population of peripheral blood in untreated patients with early rheumatoid arthritis and early reactive arthritis. Arthritis Rheum. 40, 41.

Zeng, L., Lindstrom, M.J., Smith, J.A., 2011. Ankylosing spondylitis macrophage production of higher levels of interleukin-23 in response to lipopolysaccaride without induction of a significant unfolded protein response. Arthritis Rheum. 63, 3807–3817.

Zinovieva, E., Bourgain, C., Kadi, A., et al., 2009. Comprehensive linkage and association analyses identify haplotype, near the TNFSF15 gene, significantly associated with spondyloarthritis. PLoS Genet. 5, e100528.

Zou, J., Zhang, Y., Thiel, A., Rudwaleit, M., Shi, S.L., Radbruch, A., et al., 2003. Predominant cellular immune response to the cartilage autoantigenic G1 aggrecan in ankylosing spondylitis and rheumatoid arthritis. Rheumatology. 42, 846–855.

Zwiers, A., Kraal, L., van de Pouw Kraan, T.C., Wurdinger, T., Bouma, G., Kraal, G., 2012. A variant of the IL-23R gene associated with inflammatory bowel disease induces loss of microRNA regulation and enhanced protein production. J. Immunol. 188, 1573–1577.

Chapter 39

The Autoimmune Myopathies

Livia Casciola-Rosen and Antony Rosen

Johns Hopkins University School of Medicine, Division of Rheumatology, Mason Lord Building Center Tower, Baltimore, MD, USA

Chapter Outline

Defining Autoimmune Myopathies   547
Clinical and Pathological Descriptions of Different
Phenotypes, Including IMNM   547
Characteristic Pathology, but Significant Overlap between
Phenotypes   548
Epidemiological Clues into Mechanism   548
Specific Autoantibodies are Strongly Associated with
Phenotype, Making them Useful Probes of Disease
Mechanism   549
    Myositis-Specific Autoantibodies   549
    HMG CoA Reductase Autoantibodies in Statin-Associated
    Immune-Mediated Necrotizing Myopathy   550

Mechanisms of Disease   551
    The Association of Malignancy with Myositis: Insights
    into Disease Initiation   551
    Enhanced Expression of Myositis Autoantigens in
    Regenerating Muscle Cells to Focus Propagation on
    Muscle   551
    Modification of Autoantigen Expression or Structure by
    Immune Effector Pathways to Generate a Self-Sustaining
    Phenotype   552
Therapeutic Insights   552
Concluding Remarks   553
References   553

DEFINING AUTOIMMUNE MYOPATHIES

The autoimmune myopathies are an uncommon group of disorders, unified by autoimmune damage of skeletal muscle (Mammen, 2011). The process may occur as a distinct named disease (e.g., polymyositis (PM), dermatomyositis (DM), immune-mediated necrotizing myopathy (IMNM)), or as a feature of other systemic autoimmune diseases (e.g., systemic lupus erythematosus or scleroderma). While skeletal muscle is a primary target in the autoimmune myopathies, there are frequently other tissues that may also be affected, including skin (in DM), lung, cardiac muscle, and synovial joints. Although inclusion body myositis (IBM) has features which might reflect autoimmunity (including recently described autoantibodies), the pathology of this entity and the poor response to the types of immunosuppressive therapies which characteristically are highly effective in PM and DM suggest that this entity is distinct, and we have not considered it further in this chapter.

CLINICAL AND PATHOLOGICAL DESCRIPTIONS OF DIFFERENT PHENOTYPES, INCLUDING IMNM

Like most autoimmune rheumatic diseases, the autoimmune myopathies are quite heterogeneous in their clinical presentation. These diseases are frequently characterized by the subacute onset of painless weakness, predominantly affecting proximal muscles in a symmetrical way (Robinson and Reed, 2011; Christopher-Stine et al., 2012, Miller, 2012). In some cases, there may be involvement of striated muscle of the nasopharynx and upper esophagus, with nasal regurgitation, weakness of phonation, tendency to aspiration, and difficulty swallowing. In severe cases, weakness of the respiratory muscles can occur, but this is infrequent. Muscle involvement is characterized by the leaking of various muscle enzymes, including creatine kinase (CK), and aspartyl and alaninyl transaminases (AST and ALT, which are often incorrectly interpreted as arising from liver), as well as aldolase A. Additionally, the

N. Rose & I. Mackay (Eds): The Autoimmune Diseases, Fifth edition. DOI: http://dx.doi.org/10.1016/B978-0-12-384929-8.00039-3

inflammatory myopathies are characterized by an irritable myopathy on electromyography.

Involvement of tissues other than skeletal muscle is also frequent, and may be accompanied by systemic inflammatory symptoms (malaise, fever). Skin involvement is a prominent feature in DM, with the pattern and type of skin involvement often being diagnostic features. Typical skin manifestations include (1) the characteristic heliotrope rash on the face around the eyelids; (2) Gottron's papules, inflammatory scaly papules limited to the dorsal aspect of the metacarpophalangeal and proximal interphalangeal joints; (3) a violaceous eruption involving the shawl area, the chest, the flanks, and the thighs; and (4) skin ulcers and palmar papules, which occur in a distinct subpopulation of patients with DM (Chaisson et al., 2012). Importantly, the small joints of the hands may be affected by a rheumatoid arthritis-like inflammatory synovitis; this is particularly evident in patients with the dermatopulmonary syndromes described below. Involvement of the lung is not infrequent in patients with autoimmune myopathies, with an estimated 20–65% of patients having evidence of interstitial lung disease (Labirua and Lundberg, 2010; Danoff and Casciola-Rosen, 2011).

A distinct form of IMNM associated with exposure to statins has recently been described (Christopher-Stine et al., 2010; Mammen et al., 2011). While statins are frequently associated with myalgias, which can sometimes necessitate cessation of the drug, muscle pathology is generally self-limiting, and stopping the drug results in complete resolution of the muscle process. A distinct subtype of this process presents with features of a severe autoimmune myopathy in the setting of statin exposure, where resolution does not follow cessation of statin therapy. Patients with this statin-induced IMNM have proximal muscle weakness, very high serum CK levels, irritable changes on EMG, and a prominent necrotizing myopathy on biopsy (Christopher-Stine et al., 2010; Grable-Esposito et al., 2010; Mammen et al., 2011).

CHARACTERISTIC PATHOLOGY, BUT SIGNIFICANT OVERLAP BETWEEN PHENOTYPES

Distinct pathological hallmarks of the different immune-mediated myopathies have been described. While PM is characterized by intrafascicular inflammation and regeneration (with evidence of lymphocytes surrounding morphologically normal muscle cells), the classic pattern of DM shows perifascicular atrophy and regeneration, associated with striking perivascular inflammation. In contrast, there is only a limited inflammatory infiltrate in IMNM. Although necrotic muscle cells are found in both

PM and DM, they are highly enriched in IMNM. There is an increasing appreciation that the pathological pattern in any specific patient is often less distinct, with features of the different entities present in mixed combinations (Pestronk, 2011).

It is noteworthy that biopsies reflect a single moment in time, capturing a highly dynamic and integrated homeostatic system. In the case of the autoimmune myopathies, this system includes normal, damaged, and repairing muscle cells, and various inflammatory cell subsets. Prominent among the infiltrating cells are cytotoxic lymphocytes and cells of the monocyte—macrophage and dendritic cell lineages. These different cells are not isolated, but, rather, are components of a highly interactive and reinforcing system. Indeed, the different clinical and pathological phenotypes likely represent new meta-stable states, reflecting a balance between pathways of damage and repair (see below).

EPIDEMIOLOGICAL CLUES INTO MECHANISM

The epidemiology of human disease can provide important insights into underlying mechanisms. In myositis, combining epidemiological associations with the specificity of the immunological response has been particularly instructive. For example, the recent recognition that patients with IMNM associated with statin exposure (see above) have high titer autoantibodies against HMG CoA reductase has highlighted the importance of environmental exposures in initiating autoimmunity to specific, ubiquitously expressed autoantigens, while driving injury relatively focused on skeletal muscle (Christopher-Stine et al., 2010; Mammen et al., 2011).

The association of myositis and cancer has the potential to provide similar insights into pathogenesis, but is significantly more complex for numerous reasons, including presentation of cancer either before or after myositis diagnosis, as well as effects of immunosuppressive therapy. Nevertheless, the nature of this association provides an important framework for understanding pathogenesis of spontaneous disease. The initial clinical observation that myositis and cancer are associated stimulated numerous studies over the past five decades to define the nature and kinetics of this association (Sigurgeirsson et al., 1992). Although the strength of the association of cancer with DM is higher than that with PM, there is now definitive evidence that cancer is associated with both phenotypes (Hill et al., 2001). Interestingly, the overall risk and frequency, as well as the types of cancers associated with myositis, differ between PM and DM. In one large study, cancer was found in 32% of DM patients, but in 15% of PM patients (Hill et al., 2001). Overall, the elevated risk of cancer in DM has been noted in various studies to be 3–6-fold over controls for DM, but increased only 1.3–2.0-fold in PM (Chow et al., 1995; Buchbinder et al., 2001; Hill et al., 2001; Stockton et al., 2001). In DM, the highest risk was observed for adenocarcinomas, although any tumor type could be associated (Hill et al., 2001). The most frequent cancers associated with DM include ovarian, lung, prostate, pancreatic, stomach, and colorectal cancers. Non-Hodgkin's lymphomas are also enriched in DM. PM has been associated with an increased risk of non-Hodgkin's lymphoma, and lung and bladder cancers.

Multiple studies have demonstrated a striking temporal clustering of cancer and myositis in both phenotypes, with most cancers occurring within ± 2 years of the myositis diagnosis. Indeed, standardized incidence ratios (SIRs) appear highest in the first year after diagnosis of myositis, and decrease thereafter (Stockton et al., 2001). This temporal clustering would not be expected to occur if the cancers are the result of immunosuppression, suggesting that cancer and autoimmunity might be mechanistically related (see below). Although the incidence of cancer is increased in patients with myositis, it is noteworthy that 70–85% of DM and PM patients never develop a cancer. The reason for a cancer association in only a minority of myositis patients remains unclear at this time.

SPECIFIC AUTOANTIBODIES ARE STRONGLY ASSOCIATED WITH PHENOTYPE, MAKING THEM USEFUL PROBES OF DISEASE MECHANISM

While the clinical damage in autoimmune myopathies is focused on skeletal muscle and related tissues, the described targets of the immune response in these diseases are not muscle specific (Suber et al., 2008; Casciola-Rosen and Mammen, 2012). Rather, they are expressed ubiquitously, raising important questions about the mechanisms of the tissue-specific focus of the immune response. Importantly, however, there is striking association of specific autoantibodies with distinct clinical phenotypes, suggesting that the targeting of specific molecules by the immune system might (1) participate in generating the unique phenotype or (2) that the specific immune response is stimulated by a unique series of tissue events which make that specific antigen available to drive the immune response.

A key fact remains unknown regarding the kinetics of autoimmune myopathy evolution: does the immune response to myositis-specific autoantigens precede or coincide with the onset of clinical symptoms? For most autoimmune diseases where this has been studied (e.g., systemic lupus erythematosus, rheumatoid arthritis, and type I diabetes mellitus), evidence of autoimmunity precedes clinical symptoms by several years (Baekkeskov et al., 1984; Arbuckle et al., 2003; Eisenbarth, 2003; Nielen et al., 2004; van der Helm-van Mil et al., 2005; Majka et al., 2008). For the autoimmune myopathies, no systematic data are yet available, but there have been cases where autoantibodies to histidyl tRNA synthetase preceded clinical myositis (Miller et al., 1990), suggesting that generation of the immune response may precede the establishment of the clinical phenotype.

Myositis-Specific Autoantibodies

The autoantibodies elaborated in patients with myositis recognize a family of autoantigens which have important, conserved functions in general cellular processes, and are apparently ubiquitously expressed. Prominent among these functions are protein translation (e.g., amino acyl tRNA synthetases, signal recognition particle; Mathews and Bernstein, 1983; Reeves et al., 1986), gene expression (e.g., components of the nucleosome remodeling and deacetylation complex (NuRD); Targoff and Reichlin, 1985), DNA repair machinery (e.g., double strand break and mismatch repair machinery; Casciola-Rosen et al., 1995, 2001; Suwa et al., 1996), and the exosome complex. Additionally, several autoantigens (e.g., Ro52 and MDA5) are induced by type 1 interferons (Rhodes et al., 2002; Sato et al., 2009).

Several observations about the autoantibodies in myositis are notable. With the exception of Ro52 (TRIM 21), patients generally target a single autoantigen. For example, patients with antibodies against an aminoacyl tRNA synthetase recognize only one of the multiple molecules which could be targeted in this family. Similarly, patients with antibodies against the Mi-2 component of the NuRD complex do not recognize autoantigens in the other functional families. Ro52 is an interferon-inducible antigen which is frequently targeted in myositis, and is almost always targeted in association with an autoantigen from a different protein family. For example, >50% of patients with antibodies recognizing an aminoacyl tRNA synthetase also have antibodies against Ro52. Ro52 is also frequently targeted together with antigens in other groups (Rutjes et al., 1997).

Autoantibodies in myositis have a striking association with phenotype (see Table 39.1). For example, antibodies recognizing aminoacyl tRNA synthetases are frequently associated with the "synthetase syndrome," a clinical syndrome with relatively mild myositis, Raynaud's phenomenon, inflammatory arthritis of the small joints of the hands (mechanic's hands), and interstitial lung disease of variable severity (Friedman et al., 1996). Antibodies to the signal recognition particle are associated with a particularly severe form of necrotizing myopathy, with cardiac

TABLE 39.1 Association of Myositis-specific Autoantibodies with Disease Subsets

Autoantibody	Disease subset
Anti-synthetases (anti-Jo-1, PL-7, PL-12, EJ, OJ, KS, Ha, Zo)	Anti-synthetase syndrome with polymyositis or dermatomyositis
Anti-Mi2 Anti-melanoma differentiation-associated protein (anti-MDA5, anti-CADM140) Anti-transcription intermediary factor 1γ (anti-p155) Anti-nuclear matrix protein 2 (anti-NXP2, anti-MJ) Anti-SUMO-1 activating enzyme 1 (anti-SAE1)	Dermatomyositis
Anti-signal recognition particle (SRP) Anti-3-hydroxy-3-methylglutaryl coenzyme A (anti-HMGCR)	Necrotizing myopathy

involvement. While antibodies to Mi-2 tend to be associated with the characteristic DM skin rash (including heliotrope and trunkal rash), antibodies to MDA5 have been associated with a distinct dermatopulmonary syndrome, with mild or no myositis, and mild to severe interstitial lung disease, as well as unique dermatological features (including gum pain, palmar papules, and ulceration) (Fiorentino et al., 2011; Chaisson et al., 2012). Numerous additional phenotypic features associated with the different antibodies have been described, and these are summarized in several excellent recent reviews (Mammen, 2011; Betteridge et al., 2011; Casciola-Rosen and Mammen, 2012).

An interesting feature of many of the autoantigens targeted in myositis is their striking susceptibility to cleavage by the cytotoxic lymphocyte granule protease, granzyme B (GrB) (Casciola-Rosen et al., 1999). While GrB is a fastidious protease which cleaves a minority of proteins across the proteome, it efficiently cleaves the majority of myositis autoantigens. This unusual enrichment of GrB substrates among myositis autoantigens, together with the demonstrated activity of cytotoxic cells against muscle cells in myositis patients, possibly identifies an important amplification loop in this group of diseases (see below).

New studies suggest that the autoantibodies found in myositis patients with cancer may be distinct from those found in patients where cancer does not appear. Thus, recent studies suggest that antibodies to TIF1γ (TRIM33) may be enriched in DM patients with cancer, while cancer is very uncommon in patients with Mi-2 or aminoacyl tRNA synthetases (Hoshino et al., 2010; Fujimoto et al., 2012; Trallero-Araguas et al., 2012).

Since the majority of myositis autoantigens function in pathways of general relevance to cellular function and homeostasis, it has therefore been widely assumed that these autoantigens are ubiquitously expressed. Experiments to directly address expression of autoantigens in normal and affected target tissues have only recently been attempted. These have shown that myositis autoantigens are expressed at very low levels in normal muscle, but are robustly expressed in myositis muscle, with the highest levels of autoantigen expression being found in regenerating muscle cells (Casciola-Rosen et al., 2005). This restriction of high level autoantigen expression to cells repairing muscle injury strongly suggests that normal muscle is unlikely to be the source of antigen to initiate and drive autoimmunity to these molecules in myositis, and focuses attention on other antigen sources (including cancer and repairing muscle cells) as more relevant in this regard (see model below).

Important insights have emerged from studies addressing myositis autoantigen expression in normal tissues and the relevant myositis-associated cancers. These demonstrated that myositis autoantigen expression in normal tissues is very low, but is elevated in multiple malignancies, including lung and breast (Casciola-Rosen et al., 2005). It is possible that high level autoantigen expression in the tumor can induce an immune response which cross-reacts with muscle cells. In patients with a malignancy, this reflects an effective anti-cancer response, or perhaps selection of this immune target via distinct mechanisms.

HMG CoA Reductase Autoantibodies in Statin-Associated Immune-Mediated Necrotizing Myopathy

Statin treatment is very frequent in the population, with an estimated 25 million users worldwide. Muscle-related complications related to statin therapy are widely recognized, with a spectrum from self-limited myalgias to statin-associated rhabdomyolysis (Franc et al., 2003; Graham et al., 2004; Bruckert et al., 2005). The vast majority of these cases resolve fully after stopping the statin. However, in a small group of patients, statin exposure appears to induce a self-sustaining, immune-mediated myopathy which persists despite statin discontinuation. In a recent series of studies, a novel autoantibody specificity recognizing an autoantigen migrating as a doublet of 100k/200k bands was defined in a group of immunosuppression-responsive patients with a necrotizing myopathy and very high CK levels (Christopher-Stine et al., 2010).

Interestingly, the majority of patients in that study were statin exposed. Since the target of statins is a 100 kDa protein called hydroxymethylglutaryl CoA reductase (HMGCR), the key enzyme in the *de novo* cholesterol synthesis pathway, the association with statin exposure provided an important clue for identifying the autoantigen targeted in this syndrome. While HMGCR levels are low in most cells, they are dramatically upregulated by statin exposure (Goldstein and Brown, 1990). Antibodies from INNM patients recognized higher levels of the 100k/200k antigen in statin-treated cells, leading Mammen et al. to demonstrate that the intracellular C-terminal domain containing the HMGCR active site is indeed the target of these autoantibodies (Christopher-Stine et al., 2010; Mammen et al., 2011).

As has been noted with other myositis autoantigens, high level expression of HMGCR was detected in regenerating muscle cells in biopsies of patients with HMGCR antibodies (Casciola-Rosen et al., 2005; Mammen et al., 2011). This suggests that ongoing immune effector pathways are focused onto cells attempting to repair muscle injury, thereby creating a feedforward cycle of damage and repair (Casciola-Rosen et al., 2005). The patients with HMGCR antibodies did not have the genetic polymorphism in the anion transporter frequently associated with statin myopathy, suggesting a novel mechanism underlying the targeting of this molecule in this patient subgroup. Since the majority of patients exposed to statins do not generate immune responses to HMGCR (Mammen et al., 2012b), Mammen and colleagues examined whether there might be any MHC associations with the HMGCR subgroup. Indeed, he showed a striking association of HMGCR antibodies with HLA class II DRB1*11:01 (Mammen et al., 2012a). The magnitude of this association is one of the largest described to date, suggesting that the immune response to HMGCR might be restricted by this HLA molecule, and that patients with this HLA molecule might be particularly susceptible to this syndrome.

MECHANISMS OF DISEASE

Autoimmune myopathies represent a chronic, self-sustaining process, characterized by inflammation, muscle damage, and muscle repair. While the mechanisms of disease are likely heterogeneous in different individuals, with distinct pathways playing different relative roles in different patients, recent data enable the proposal of a unifying model which incorporates the essential features

of the disease spectrum described above. This model will include the following components: (1) the important association of malignancy with myositis as a potential initiating force; (2) the enhanced expression of myositis autoantigens in regenerating muscle cells to focus propagation on muscle; and (3) the modification of autoantigen expression or structure by immune effector pathways to generate a self-sustaining phenotype. Each of these components is discussed in detail below (see Figure 39.1).

The Association of Malignancy with Myositis: Insights into Disease Initiation

In 10–20% of myositis patients who also have cancer, the two processes cluster together temporally (Chow et al., 1995; Hill et al., 2001). This kinetic clustering suggests strongly that the two processes are mechanistically related. While there are numerous potential explanations behind the connection, the observation that cancer can both precede and follow the diagnosis of myositis is important, as it reinforces that cancer is not emerging exclusively due to immunosuppressive therapy once myositis is diagnosed. The short interval separating the two diagnoses, and the occurrence of cancers in tissues often unaffected in myositis, also makes it unlikely that the inflammatory microenvironment enhances transformation and cancer growth. The available data are consistent with a mechanism in which shared antigen expression patterns in cancers and regenerating muscle cells may explain numerous features of the disease, including the kinetics noted above. In this model, natural anti-cancer immunity (including CD4 T cell and cytotoxic lymphocyte responses) develops in response to an incipient cancer.

Enhanced Expression of Myositis Autoantigens in Regenerating Muscle Cells to Focus Propagation on Muscle

The evidence showing that myositis antigens are expressed at high levels in cancers and also in myositis tissue, where robust expression is noted in regenerating muscle cells, suggests a possible mechanism whereby an initial anti-cancer immune response targeting one of the myositis autoantigens becomes secondarily focused on injured muscle, thus beginning the propagation of a self-sustaining cycle at that site (Casciola-Rosen et al., 2005). The reasons for the unusual restriction of immune responses in myositis to such a limited group of antigens remains uncertain, but may reflect the ability of only a very limited group of molecules to participate in a feedforward cycle (due to the need to both respond to and stimulate an additional immune response—see below). It is possible that anti-cancer immune responses directed even

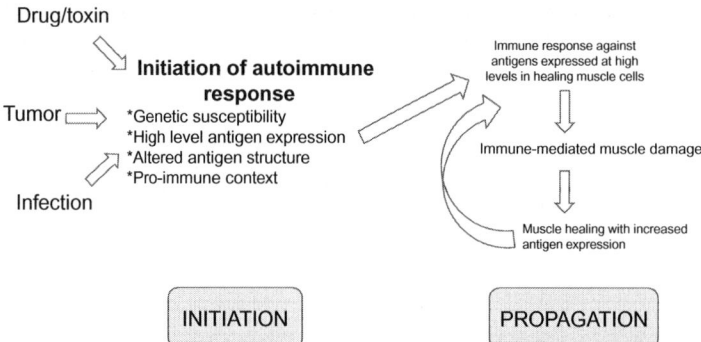

FIGURE 39.1 The Role of Autoimmunity in Myositis. Myositis arises when an immune response against myositis-specific autoantigens is initi-ated. The initiation phase may be separated spatially and temporally from propagation events, which are focused on muscle. In the absence of a stimu-lus inducing muscle injury and repair, it is possible that the autoimmune response may remain silent. In the case of cancer-associated myositis, it is possible that an unrelated muscle injury is the second hit which focuses the anti-cancer immune response onto repairing muscle, and propagates the injury there. In statin-induced necrotizing myopathy, the site of immunization with HMGCR may be muscle. The autoantigens targeted are character-ized by their shared expression patterns in immunizing tissue and regenerating muscle, and by their susceptibility to modification by immune effector pathways.

at myositis antigens might be silent, since the number of regenerating cells in unperturbed muscle is very low. Very few cells in normal muscle are therefore susceptible to immune injury focused on these "regenerating cell" antigens. In the setting of a second insult which damages muscle (strenuous exercise, drugs, viral infection), the pre-formed anti-cancer immune response could respond to antigens now expressed in regenerating muscle cells. When these cells are damaged, a self-sustaining damage-healing cycle is generated, driven by immune-mediated cytolysis and the need to continually provide additional precursors to accomplish tissue repair. This model explains several additional features of the disease, includ-ing the patchy nature of pathology, the inexact kinetic relationships between cancer and myositis, and the antigen expression patterns.

Modification of Autoantigen Expression or Structure by Immune Effector Pathways to Generate a Self-Sustaining Phenotype

A central feature of any feed-forward loop is that the activity of one component augments the amplitude of the other, which in turn augments the first. Several immune effector pathways (discussed below) are highly repre-sented in myositis muscle. These dramatically influence antigen expression and structure, and may play important roles in driving ongoing immune responses.

Several prominent myositis autoantigens (MDA5 and Ro52) are strongly interferon regulated, and interferon signatures are prominent in the muscle (PM and DM) and skin (DM) in myositis patients. Additionally, cells with the capacity to secrete large amounts of both type I (from plasmacytoid (p)DCs) and type II interferons (from

activated CD8 T cells) are enriched in DM and PM mus-cle (Goebels et al., 1996; Greenberg et al., 2005). This capacity of effector pathways to augment antigen expres-sion, and thus create additional targets for cytolytic dam-age and additional interferon secretion, may be important pathogenically, and might be particularly amenable to therapeutic manipulation.

A second potential intersection of the immune effector and antigen arms centers on the susceptibility of most myositis autoantigens to cleavage by GrB (Casciola-Rosen et al., 1999). It is noteworthy that expression of this protease is highly restricted to the cytolytic effector arm of the innate and adaptive immune systems (Darrah and Rosen, 2010). Furthermore, since GrB has a unique specificity among proteases, most antigens will not have been cleaved by GrB during development of tolerance. The potential for GrB-mediated cleavage to generate frag-ments that have not been tolerized would provide another feed-forward loop to contribute to driving myositis. In such a model, immune effector pathways generate forms of antigens not previously seen and tolerized by the immune system, thus driving the immune response, which further drives antigen generation. Multiple studies suggest that such effects are likely to be driven at the level of CD4 T cells, but this remains to be demonstrated directly.

THERAPEUTIC INSIGHTS

The therapy of myositis currently focuses entirely on mod-ification of the immune side of the pathogenic cycle. Since myositis is a rare autoimmune phenotype, there is little randomized trial-derived data about the efficacy of spe-cific agents, but clinical experience suggests efficacy with multiple immunosuppressive agents. As with all unfocused immunosuppressive strategies, the major limitations are infectious side effects. Because autoantigen expression in cells which are repairing tissue injury may be an important partner in driving the ongoing immune response and tissue damage in myositis, it is possible that focusing attention on modifying pathways of antigen expression in the target cell may be an effective strategy. If cancer is an important driver of the initial immune response, perhaps early anti-cancer treatment strategies might be of benefit.

CONCLUDING REMARKS

Although the autoimmune myopathies are uncommon, their interesting presentations and associations provide unique insights into the mechanisms of human autoimmunity, which are potentially of broad relevance, and may be of importance therapeutically. The highly focused immune response on a limited number of antigens which function in pathways of general relevance is of great interest. The association of myositis with cancer, and the shared antigen expression patterns between cancer and regenerating muscle cells, may be of importance in disease propagation. The participation of multiple interacting pathways in augmenting the amplitude of response of other partners may be critical in generating a self-sustaining feed-forward loop which characterizes these diseases, and may provide novel therapeutic opportunities. Of particular importance are the reinforcing interactions between immune effector pathways, antigen, and the target tissue.

REFERENCES

Arbuckle, M.R., McClain, M.T., Rubertone, M.V., Scofield, R.H., Dennis, G.J., James, J.A., et al., 2003. Development of autoantibodies before the clinical onset of systemic lupus erythematosus. N. Engl. J. Med. 349, 1526–1533.

Baekkeskov, S., Dyrberg, T., Lernmark, A., 1984. Autoantibodies to a 64-kilodalton islet cell protein precede the onset of spontaneous diabetes in the BB rat. Science. 224, 1348–1350.

Betteridge, Z.E., Gunawardena, H., McHugh, N.J., 2011. Novel autoantibodies and clinical phenotypes in adult and juvenile myositis. Arthritis Res. Ther. 13, 209.

Bruckert, E., Hayem, G., Dejager, S., Yau, C., Begaud, B., 2005. Mild to moderate muscular symptoms with high-dosage statin therapy in hyperlipidemic patients—the PRIMO study. Cardiovasc. Drugs Ther. 19, 403–414.

Buchbinder, R., Forbes, A., Hall, S., Dennett, X., Giles, G., 2001. Incidence of malignant disease in biopsy-proven inflammatory myopathy. A population-based cohort study. Ann. Intern. Med. 134, 1087–1095.

Casciola-Rosen, L., Mammen, A.L., 2012. Myositis autoantibodies. Curr. Opin. Rheumatol. 24, 602–608.

Casciola-Rosen, L., Andrade, F., Ulanet, D., Wong, W.B., Rosen, A., 1999. Cleavage by granzyme B is strongly predictive of autoantigen status: implications for initiation of autoimmunity. J. Exp. Med. 190, 815–826.

Casciola-Rosen, L., Nagaraju, K., Plotz, P., Wang, K., Levine, S., Gabrielson, E., et al., 2005. Enhanced autoantigen expression in regenerating muscle cells in idiopathic inflammatory myopathy. J. Exp. Med. 201, 591–601.

Casciola-Rosen, L.A., Anhalt, G.J., Rosen, A., 1995. DNA-dependent protein kinase is one of a subset of autoantigens specifically cleaved early during apoptosis. J. Exp. Med. 182, 1625–1634.

Casciola-Rosen, L.A., Pluta, A.F., Plotz, P.H., Cox, A.E., Morris, S., Wigley, F.M., et al., 2001. The DNA mismatch repair enzyme PMS1 is a myositis-specific autoantigen. Arthritis Rheum. 44, 389–396.

Chaisson, N.F., Paik, J., Orbai, A.M., Casciola-Rosen, L., Fiorentino, D., Danoff, S., et al., 2012. A novel dermato-pulmonary syndrome associated with MDA-5 antibodies: report of 2 cases and review of the literature. Medicine (Baltimore). 91, 220–228.

Chow, W.H., Gridley, G., Mellemkjaer, L., McLaughlin, J.K., Olsen, J.H., Fraumeni Jr., J.F., 1995. Cancer risk following polymyositis and dermatomyositis: a nationwide cohort study in Denmark. Cancer Causes Control. 6, 9–13.

Christopher-Stine, L., Casciola-Rosen, L.A., Hong, G., Chung, T., Corse, A.M., Mammen, A.L., 2010. A novel autoantibody recognizing 200-kd and 100-kd proteins is associated with an immune-mediated necrotizing myopathy. Arthritis Rheum. 62, 2757–2766.

Christopher-Stine, L., Robinson, D.R., Wu, C.C., Mark, E.J., 2012. Case records of the Massachusetts General Hospital. Case 37-2012. A 21-year-old man with fevers, arthralgias, and pulmonary infiltrates. N. Engl. J. Med. 367, 2134–2146.

Danoff, S.K., Casciola-Rosen, L., 2011. The lung as a possible target for the immune reaction in myositis. Arthritis Res. Ther. 13, 230.

Darrah, E., Rosen, A., 2010. Granzyme B cleavage of autoantigens in autoimmunity. Cell Death Differ. 17, 624–632.

Eisenbarth, G.S., 2003. Insulin autoimmunity: immunogenetics/immunopathogenesis of type 1A diabetes. Ann. N.Y. Acad. Sci. 1005, 109–118.

Fiorentino, D., Chung, L., Zwerner, J., Rosen, A., Casciola-Rosen, L., 2011. The mucocutaneous and systemic phenotype of dermatomyositis patients with antibodies to MDA5 (CADM-140): a retrospective study. J. Am. Acad. Dermatol. 65, 25–34.

Franc, S., Dejager, S., Bruckert, E., Chauvenet, M., Giral, P., Turpin, G., 2003. A comprehensive description of muscle symptoms associated with lipid-lowering drugs. Cardiovasc. Drugs Ther. 17, 459–465.

Friedman, A.W., Targoff, I.N., Arnett, F.C., 1996. Interstitial lung disease with autoantibodies against aminoacyl-tRNA synthetases in the absence of clinically apparent myositis. Semin. Arthritis Rheum. 26, 459–467.

Fujimoto, M., Hamaguchi, Y., Kaji, K., Matsushita, T., Ichimura, Y., Kodera, M., et al., 2012. Myositis-specific anti-155/140 autoantibodies target transcription intermediary factor 1 family proteins. Arthritis Rheum. 64, 513–522.

Goebels, N., Michaelis, D., Engelhardt, M., Huber, S., Bender, A., Pongratz, D., et al., 1996. Differential expression of perforin in muscle-infiltrating T cells in polymyositis and dermatomyositis. J. Clin. Invest. 97, 2905–2910.

Goldstein, J.L., Brown, M.S., 1990. Regulation of the mevalonate pathway. Nature. 343, 425–430.

Grable-Esposito, P., Katzberg, H.D., Greenberg, S.A., Srinivasan, J., Katz, J., Amato, A.A., 2010. Immune-mediated necrotizing myopathy associated with statins. Muscle Nerve. 41, 185–190.

Graham, D.J., Staffa, J.A., Shatin, D., Andrade, S.E., Schech, S.D., La Grenade, L., et al., 2004. Incidence of hospitalized rhabdomyolysis in patients treated with lipid-lowering drugs. JAMA. 292, 2585–2590.

Greenberg, S.A., Pinkus, J.L., Pinkus, G.S., Burleson, T., Sanoudou, D., Tawil, R., et al., 2005. Interferon-alpha/beta-mediated innate immune mechanisms in dermatomyositis. Ann. Neurol. 57, 664–678.

Hill, C.L., Zhang, Y., Sigurgeirsson, B., Pukkala, E., Mellemkjaer, L., Airio, A., et al., 2001. Frequency of specific cancer types in dermatomyositis and polymyositis: a population-based study. Lancet. 357, 96–100.

Hoshino, K., Muro, Y., Sugiura, K., Tomita, Y., Nakashima, R., Mimori, T., 2010. Anti-MDA5 and anti-TIF1-gamma antibodies have clinical significance for patients with dermatomyositis. Rheumatology (Oxford). 49, 1726–1733.

Labirua, A., Lundberg, I.E., 2010. Interstitial lung disease and idiopathic inflammatory myopathies: progress and pitfalls. Curr. Opin. Rheumatol. 22, 633–638.

Majka, D.S., Deane, K.D., Parrish, L.A., Lazar, A.A., Baron, A.E., Walker, C.W., et al., 2008. Duration of preclinical rheumatoid arthritis-related autoantibody positivity increases in subjects with older age at time of disease diagnosis. Ann. Rheum. Dis. 67, 801–807.

Mammen, A.L., 2011. Autoimmune myopathies: autoantibodies, phenotypes and pathogenesis. Nat. Rev. Neurol. 7, 343–354.

Mammen, A.L., Chung, T., Christopher-Stine, L., Rosen, P., Rosen, A., Doering, K.R., et al., 2011. Autoantibodies against 3-hydroxy-3-methylglutaryl-coenzyme A reductase in patients with statin-associated autoimmune myopathy. Arthritis Rheum. 63, 713–721.

Mammen, A.L., Gaudet, D., Brisson, D., Christopher-Stine, L., Lloyd, T.E., Leffell, M.S., et al., 2012a. Increased frequency of DRB1*11:01 in anti-hydroxymethylglutaryl-coenzyme A reductase-associated autoimmune myopathy. Arthritis Care Res. (Hoboken). 64, 1233–1237.

Mammen, A.L., Pak, K., Williams, E.K., Brisson, D., Coresh, J., Selvin, E., et al., 2012b. Rarity of anti-3-hydroxy-3-methylglutaryl-coenzyme A reductase antibodies in statin users, including those with self-limited musculoskeletal side effects. Arthritis Care Res. (Hoboken). 64, 269–272.

Mathews, M.B., Bernstein, R.M., 1983. Myositis autoantibody inhibits histidyl-tRNA synthetase: a model for autoimmunity. Nature. 304, 177–179.

Miller, F.W., 2012. New approaches to the assessment and treatment of the idiopathic inflammatory myopathies. Ann. Rheum. Dis. 71, i82–i85.

Miller, F.W., Twitty, S.A., Biswas, T., Plotz, P.H., 1990. Origin and regulation of a disease-specific autoantibody response. Antigenic epitopes, spectrotype stability, and isotype restriction of anti-Jo-1 autoantibodies. J. Clin. Invest. 85, 468–475.

Nielen, M.M., van Schaardenburg, D., Reesink, H.W., van de Stadt, R.J., van der Horst-Bruinsma, I.E., de Koning, M.H., et al., 2004.

Specific autoantibodies precede the symptoms of rheumatoid arthritis: a study of serial measurements in blood donors. Arthritis Rheum. 50, 380–386.

Pestronk, A., 2011. Acquired immune and inflammatory myopathies: pathologic classification. Curr. Opin. Rheumatol. 23, 595–604.

Reeves, W.H., Nigam, S.K., Blobel, G., 1986. Human autoantibodies reactive with the signal-recognition particle. Proc. Natl. Acad. Sci. U.S.A. 83, 9507–9511.

Rhodes, D.A., Ihrke, G., Reinicke, A.T., Malcherek, G., Towey, M., Isenberg, D.A., et al., 2002. The 52 000 MW Ro/SS-A autoantigen in Sjogren's syndrome/systemic lupus erythematosus (Ro52) is an interferon-gamma inducible tripartite motif protein associated with membrane proximal structures. Immunology. 106, 246–256.

Robinson, A.B., Reed, A.M., 2011. Clinical features, pathogenesis and treatment of juvenile and adult dermatomyositis. Nat. Rev. Rheumatol. 7, 664–675.

Rutjes, S.A., Vree Egberts, W.T., Jongen, P., Van Den Hoogen, F., Pruijn, G.J., Van Venrooij, W.J., 1997. Anti-Ro52 antibodies frequently co-occur with anti-Jo-1 antibodies in sera from patients with idiopathic inflammatory myopathy. Clin. Exp. Immunol. 109, 32–40.

Sato, S., Hoshino, K., Satoh, T., Fujita, T., Kawakami, Y., Fujita, T., et al., 2009. RNA helicase encoded by melanoma differentiation-associated gene 5 is a major autoantigen in patients with clinically amyopathic dermatomyositis: Association with rapidly progressive interstitial lung disease. Arthritis Rheum. 60, 2193–2200.

Sigurgeirsson, B., Lindelof, B., Edhag, O., Allander, E., 1992. Risk of cancer in patients with dermatomyositis or polymyositis. A population-based study. N. Engl. J. Med. 326, 363–367.

Stockton, D., Doherty, V.R., Brewster, D.H., 2001. Risk of cancer in patients with dermatomyositis or polymyositis, and follow-up implications: a Scottish population-based cohort study. Br. J. Cancer. 85, 41–45.

Suber, T.L., Casciola-Rosen, L., Rosen, A., 2008. Mechanisms of disease: autoantigens as clues to the pathogenesis of myositis. Nat. Clin. Pract. Rheumatol. 4, 201–209.

Suwa, A., Hirakata, M., Takeda, Y., Okano, Y., Mimori, T., Inada, S., et al., 1996. Autoantibodies to DNA-dependent protein kinase. Probes for the catalytic subunit. J. Clin. Invest. 97, 1417–1421.

Targoff, I.N., Reichlin, M., 1985. The association between Mi-2 antibodies and dermatomyositis. Arthritis Rheum. 28, 796–803.

Trallero-Araguas, E., Rodrigo-Pendas, J.A., Selva-O'Callaghan, A., Martinez-Gomez, X., Bosch, X., Labrador-Horrillo, M., et al., 2012. Usefulness of anti-p155 autoantibody for diagnosing cancer-associated dermatomyositis: a systematic review and meta-analysis. Arthritis Rheum. 64, 523–532.

van der Helm-van Mil, A.H., Verpoort, K.N., Breedveld, F.C., Toes, R. E., Huizinga, T.W., 2005. Antibodies to citrullinated proteins and differences in clinical progression of rheumatoid arthritis. Arthritis Res. Ther. 7, R949–R958.

Part 8

Endocrine System

Chapter 40

Thyroid Disease

Anthony P. Weetman

The Medical School, University of Sheffield, Sheffield, UK

Chapter Outline

Autoimmune Thyroiditis	557	Concluding Remarks—Future Prospects	564
Historic Background	557	**Graves' Disease**	**564**
Clinical, Pathologic, and Epidemiologic Features	557	Historic Background	564
Autoimmune Features	558	Clinical, Pathologic, and Epidemiologic	
Autoantibodies	558	Features	564
T Cell Responses	559	Autoimmune Features	565
Genetic Features	560	Autoantibodies	565
Environmental Influences	560	T Cell Responses	565
In Vivo Models	561	Genetic Features	565
Immunization-Induced Thyroiditis	561	Environmental Influences	566
Experimental Autoimmune Thyroiditis		*In Vivo* Models	566
Resulting from Immune Modulation	561	Pathologic Effector Mechanisms	567
Spontaneous Autoimmune Thyroiditis	562	Autoantibodies as Potential Immunological Markers	568
Pathologic Effector Mechanisms	562	Treatment and Outcome	568
Antibody-Mediated Injury	562	Thyroid-Associated Ophthalmopathy and Dermopathy	568
Autoantibodies as Potential Immunological Markers	563	Concluding Remarks—Future Prospects	568
Treatment and Outcome	563	**References**	**569**

AUTOIMMUNE THYROIDITIS

Historic Background

The clinical features of myxedema, the end stage of autoimmune thyroiditis (AT), defined in 1874 by Gull, and Murray, in Newcastle-upon-Tyne, was the first to give thyroid extract as treatment in 1891. The characteristic lymphocytic infiltration (struma lymphomatosa) was first noted by Hashimoto in 1912. Proof that AT was due to loss of self-tolerance came from Rose and Witebsky (1956) who showed that rabbits immunized with homologous thyroid extract and adjuvant developed a thyroid lymphocytic infiltrate and thyroglobulin (TG) antibodies. The latter were detected in Hashimoto's thyroiditis during the same year by Roitt and Doniach.

Clinical, Pathologic, and Epidemiologic Features

Several types of AT have been described (Table 40.1). Two in particular, goitrous (Hashimoto's) thyroiditis and atrophic thyroiditis (primary myxedema), result in hypothyroidism (Pearce et al., 2003). The goiter in Hashimoto's thyroiditis is usually firm and painless, with an irregular surface. Patients are often euthyroid at presentation but serum thyroid stimulating hormone (TSH) levels can be elevated even if thyroxine (T4) levels are within the reference range, representing subclinical thyroid failure. Primary myxedema is typically identified when hypothyroidism is apparent clinically and biochemically.

Autoimmunity accounts for over 90% of non-iatrogenic hypothyroidism in iodine-sufficient countries. Women are

N. Rose & I. Mackay (Eds): The Autoimmune Diseases, Fifth edition. DOI: http://dx.doi.org/10.1016/B978-0-12-384929-8.00040-X

TABLE 40.1 Types of Autoimmune Thyroiditis

Type	Course	Features
Goitrous (Hashimoto's) thyroiditis	Chronic: leads to hypothyroidism	Goiter: moderate to extensive thyroiditis lymphocytic infiltration and variable fibrosis
Atrophic thyroiditis (primary myxedema)	Chronic hypothyroidism	Atrophy: fibrosis and variable lymphocytic infiltrate
Juvenile thyroiditis	Chronic but may remit	Small goiter with moderate lymphocytic infiltrate
Postpartum thyroiditis	Transient thyrotoxicosis and/or hypothyroidism 3–6 months after delivery	Small goiter with some lymphocytic infiltrate
Silent thyroiditis	Transient thyrotoxicosis and/or hypothyroidism	Small goiter with some lymphocytic infiltrate
Focal thyroiditis	Progressive in some patients	Occurs in 20–40% thyroid specimens at autopsy: associated with thyroid carcinoma

5–10 times more likely to be affected, with a peak incidence at 50–60 years of age. The prevalence of autoimmune thyroiditis in the general Caucasian population is 0.5 per 1000 (but only half this in black people), whereas thyroid autoantibodies can be found in up to 20%, reflecting the presence of focal thyroiditis (Eaton et al., 2010).

Pathological changes in AT range from mild focal thyroiditis to extensive lymphocytic infiltration and scarring (Figure 40.1). In Hashimoto's thyroiditis there is a dense infiltration by lymphocytes, plasma cells, and macrophages, and germinal center formation. Thyroid follicles are progressively destroyed and, in the process, the cells undergo hyperplasia and oxyphil metaplasia to become Hürthle cells. In rare cases there are concurrent changes of Graves' disease, so-called hashitoxicosis. There is a variable degree of fibrosis and, when this is extensive, the picture may resemble primary myxedema, in which the gland is atrophic and there is extensive fibrosis with loss of normal lobular architecture and minimal or modest lymphocytic infiltration. Patients with high serum IgG4 levels and increased IgG4-positive plasma cells in the thyroid have more stromal fibrosis, lymphoplasmacytic infiltration, and hypothyroidism (Kakudo et al., 2011). The histology in postpartum and silent thyroiditis resembles Hashimoto's thyroiditis.

Autoimmune Features

Autoantibodies

Circulating autoantibodies against TG and thyroid peroxidase (TPO) are found, often at very high levels, in most patients with AT. These antibodies are common, albeit at low levels, in association with focal thyroiditis.

Thyroglobulin Antibodies

TG is a 660-kDa homodimeric glycoprotein secreted by thyroid follicular cells (TFC) and stored in the luminal

A
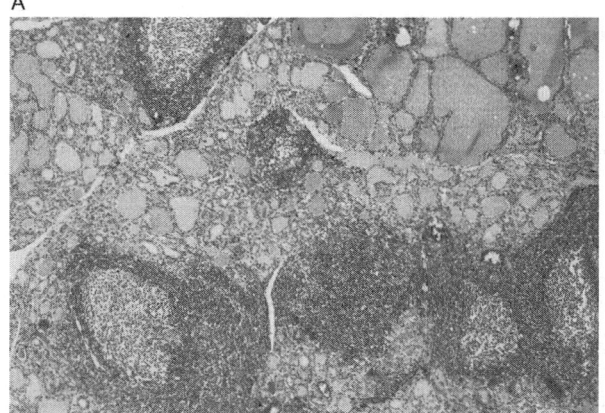

B
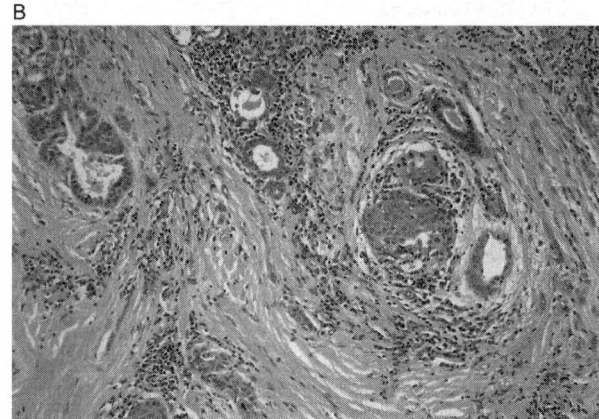

FIGURE 40.1 Pathology of Autoimmune Hypothyroidism. (A) Hashimoto's thyroiditis showing germinal center formation; (B) primary myxedema with extensive fibrosis. (Original magnification: ×100.) *Photos courtesy of Dr. Judith Channer, Northern General Hospital, Sheffield.*

colloid. At 4–8 hormonogenic sites, iodinated tyrosine residues couple to form T4 or triiodothyronine (T3). The iodination state of TG alters its immunogenicity in animals and in man (Saboori et al., 1999). There are two major and one minor antibody epitopes on each 330-kDa subunit, and the wide spacing of these prevents IgG cross-linking and therefore complement fixation. The restriction of the response to three epitopes is only relative, as TG antibodies recognize an increasing number of determinants as their titer rises and somatic hypermutation occurs (McIntosh et al., 1998). Antibody reactivity is predominantly in the IgG1 and IgG4 subclasses but not light chain restricted.

Thyroid Peroxidase Antibodies

TPO is a 100−105-kDa apical membrane protein responsible for tyrosine iodination and coupling in the formation of thyroid hormones. Molecular characterization of this autoantigen has been reviewed extensively (McLachlan and Rapoport, 2007). Antibodies to TPO have a similar IgG subclass distribution to TG, but are kappa light chain restricted (McIntosh et al., 1998). Eighty percent of TPO antibodies recognize an immunodominant region involving overlapping, conformational epitopes in two extracellular domains: specific patterns of TPO autoantibody recognition are stable in an individual and genetically transmitted in AT families (Jaume et al., 1999). In vitro, TPO can bind C4 complement component, which may contribute to the susceptibility of TFC to destruction (Blanchin et al., 2003).

Other Autoantibodies

TSH-receptor (TSH-R) blocking antibodies are found in around 20% of patients with AT (Weetman and McGregor, 1994). They contribute significantly to hypothyroidism in some patients but there is no close correlation with the presence or absence of a goiter (Feingold et al., 2009). Other thyroid-specific autoantibodies recognize a poorly characterized second (i.e., non-TG) colloid antigen, the Na^+/I^- transporter and pendrin, but any importance of these in pathogenesis is unknown (Ajjan et al., 2000; Yoshida et al., 2009). Autoantibodies against T4 and T3 occur in 15−35% of patients with autoimmune thyroiditis. AT occurs in association with many other autoimmune disorders (Boelaert et al., 2010) and the respective autoantibodies may help in diagnosing these associated conditions.

T Cell Responses

A major site of autoreactivity is within the thyroid itself, although autoimmune responses can also be detected within the draining lymph nodes and bone marrow (Weetman et al., 1984). Recruitment of lymphocytes to the thyroid requires upregulation, on endothelial cells, of various adhesion molecules and selectins, and the infiltrating lymphocytes express the reciprocal adhesion molecules, including CD11a, CD18, CD29, CD49a, and CD49e (Marazuela, 1999). The local infiltrate produces an array of chemokines

which aid homing, including CXCL12, CXCL13, and CCL22, particularly when lymphoid follicles are present, and the TFC contribute to the chemokine pool, exacerbating the autoimmune process (Liu et al., 2008). Most phenotyping and functional studies on T cells have used the readily sampled peripheral blood: this source may reflect poorly (if at all) the responses within the autoimmune target.

Studies of T Cell Phenotypes

The number of circulating human leukocyte antigen (HLA)-DR$^+$ (activated) T cells is elevated and CD8$^+$ T cells are reduced, but only in active thyroiditis (Iwatani et al., 1992). CD4$^+$ T cells predominate in the thyroid infiltrate and many of these are activated (Aichinger et al., 1985). The majority of T cells express the αβ receptor and no obvious bias in T cell receptor usage is apparent (McIntosh et al., 1997). Although a pauciclonal T cell response seems likely in early AT, by the time of clinical presentation there is spreading of the immune response to produce a polyclonal T cell response, directed against an array of autoantigens and epitopes.

Functional Studies

Weak T cell proliferative responses against TG and TPO are found in many patients and can be enhanced by interleukin (IL)-2 supplementation (Butscher et al., 2001). To identify T cell epitopes for TPO, circulating T cells from patients with autoimmune thyroiditis have been stimulated with overlapping synthetic peptides (Tandon et al., 1991). No dominant epitope has been identified; instead there is considerable heterogeneity both within and between individual patients. A T cell epitope on TG has been identified as a strong and specific binder to the micro histocompatibility complex (MHC) class II disease susceptibility HLA-DRβ1-Arg74 molecule, and this stimulates T cells from both mice and humans with AT (Menconi et al., 2010). Such an epitope could initiate an immune response that then spreads to involve other autoantigens, and fits with observations in an animal model of AT that self-tolerance may be broken first for TG and subsequently for TPO (Chen et al., 2010). Migration inhibition factor-based assays have been used in attempts to identify a defect in thyroid antigen-specific suppressor T cells in AT (Volpé, 1988; Martin and Davies, 1992) but no consistent results have been produced and there is no evidence in man yet to implicate a defect in CD4$^+$ CD25$^+$ T regulatory cells. Indeed such cells are abundant in the thyroid infiltrate and appear unable to suppress the autoimmune process (Marazuela et al., 2006).

Reverse transcription of cytokine mRNA and cDNA amplification has revealed a mixed Th1 and Th2 response in Hashimoto's thyroiditis (Ajjan et al., 1996). The demonstration of MHC class II expression on TFC in Hashimoto's thyroiditis and Graves' disease gave rise to the concept that such "aberrant" expression could initiate or perpetuate the autoimmune response by converting the TFC into antigen presenting cells (Bottazzo et al., 1983). However, class II expression is restricted to TFC adjacent to T cells producing interferon (IFN)-γ (Hamilton et al., 1991) and only this cytokine is capable of initiating class II expression *in vitro*. MHC class II expression is found on TFC in experimental autoimmune thyroiditis (EAT) induced by neonatal thymectomy (see below) but always follows the appearance of a lymphocytic infiltrate. TFC do not express costimulatory molecules even after cytokine exposure (Marelli-Berg et al., 1997). Together these results indicate that TFC are unlikely to initiate the autoimmune response.

T cell lines and clones derived from the thyroids of patients can be activated by class II-expressing TFC (Londei et al., 1985). Such T cells are likely to have been previously activated by classic antigen presenting cells and are no longer dependent on B7 costimulation (Marelli-Berg et al., 1997). Anergy can be induced in B7-dependent, naïve T cells by class II-positive TFC and this type of peripheral tolerance may be important in regulating autoreactive T cells within the normal thyroid. In established AT, however, T cells are resistant to tolerance induction (Dayan et al., 1993) and class II-expressing TFC may then help to perpetuate the autoimmune response. TFC may participate in the autoimmune process in other ways besides MHC class II expression, through the expression of other immunologically active molecules such as CD40 and CD56.

Genetic Features

The role of genetic factors in AT (Figure 40.2) is suggested by the frequent presence of thyroid autoantibodies in other family members and the association of thyroiditis with other endocrinopathies as part of the type 2 autoimmune polyglandular syndrome. Twin studies show a 0.55 concordance rate in monozygotic but not dizygotic twins, and similar findings have been reported for the aggregation of thyroid autoantibodies in euthyroid twins of individuals with AT (Brix et al., 2000, 2004).

As with most autoimmune disorders, associations with HLA alleles have been extensively investigated, producing conflicting results (Tomer and Davies, 2003). Initially it appeared that primary myxedema and Hashimoto's thyroiditis in Caucasians had distinct associations with HLA-DR3 and -DR5 respectively, but subsequent studies have shown that Hashimoto's thyroiditis is associated with HLA-DR3 and to a lesser extent -DR4. Postpartum thyroiditis has a weak association with HLA-DR5.

Polymorphisms in *CTLA-4* confer a relative risk of around 2 (Kotsa et al., 1997; Ueda et al., 2003). Genome scanning methods have suggested a number of possible susceptibility loci but these have not been reproduced in larger patient sets (Taylor et al., 2006). The existence of many genes with individual small effects, gene–gene interactions and subset effects may explain why it has been more difficult to show the effects of individual genes in patient populations than would be expected from the twin data on genetic susceptibility (Tomer, 2010). Around 45% of Turner's syndrome patients have TPO antibodies and a third become hypothyroid (Mortensen et al., 2009).

Environmental Influences

The female preponderance of AT may be due to the influence of sex steroids, although skewed X chromosome

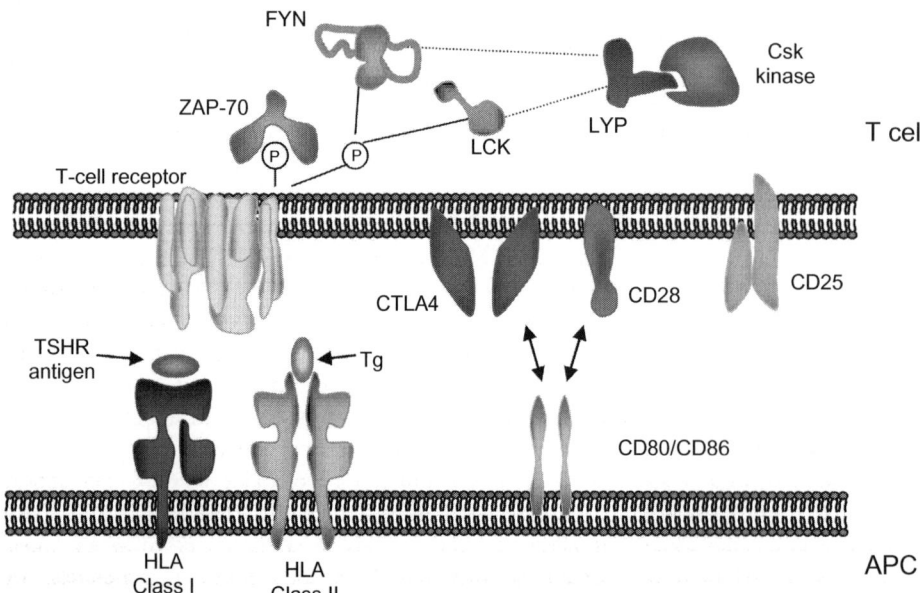

FIGURE 40.2 Genetic Associations in Autoimmune Thyroid Disease. HLA class I and II polymorphisms on the antigen presenting cell (APC) interact with presentation of the polymorphic thyroid antigens TSH-R and thyroglobulin (Tg). The binding of CTLA4 and CD28 with CD80/CD86 (B7), IL-2 signaling via CD25 and *PTPN22*-encoded LYP signaling all regulate T cell activation. *From Zeitlin et al. (2008), with permission.*

inactivation may be a further factor. Certainly in EAT, estrogens or progesterone exacerbate thyroiditis and this is reversed by testosterone (Okayasu et al., 1981; Ansar-Ahmed et al., 1983), while use of exogenous estrogens lowers the risk of developing TPO antibodies in genetically predisposed individuals (Strieder et al., 2003). Pregnancy ameliorates AT but there is an exacerbation in the year after delivery, reflected by a rise in TPO antibody levels. In some women with a previously mild thyroiditis the enhanced autoimmune response is sufficient to cause biochemical or clinical thyroid dysfunction, and this is termed postpartum thyroiditis (Muller et al., 2001). These changes may be related to the fluctuations in regulatory factors operating to maintain fetal tolerance during pregnancy (Weetman, 2010). Although usually a transient phenomenon, around a quarter of such women develop permanent hypothyroidism within 10 years, so that pregnancy is a risk factor which precipitates clinical disease in predisposed subjects. Fetal microchimerism may play a pathogenic role via intrathyroidal chimeric cells breaking immunological tolerance, and such a possibility is supported by the increase in the prevalence of high titer TPO antibodies with advancing parity (Greer et al., 2011).

A strong influence of exogenous environmental factors is suggested by epidemiological data, such as the 10-fold rise in AT prevalence over three decades in Italy (Benvenga and Trimarchi, 2008). There is no convincing evidence for a direct role of infection in etiology (Tomer and Davies, 1993) although thyroid autoantibodies can appear transiently after subacute viral thyroiditis (Iitaka et al., 1998). AT is more prevalent in areas of increased prosperity and hygiene, compatible with the "hygiene hypothesis" which suggests that exposure to microbial antigens may skew the immune response to protect against autoimmunity (Kondrashova et al., 2008). Indirect evidence for dietary iodine-induced injury is provided by studies of iodine-deficient regions, and an increase in thyroid autoantibodies and lymphocytic thyroiditis shortly after iodine supplementation has generally been reported. As well as causing thyroid injury through the generation of reactive oxygen metabolites (Bagchi et al., 1995), iodine enhances the immunogenicity of TG (Barin et al., 2005).

Anthracene derivatives and other chemicals induce EAT in the Buffalo strain rat, whereas smoking is associated with a decrease in AT (Effraimidis et al., 2009). Administration of lithium may exacerbate autoimmune thyroiditis both immunologically and biochemically, but the adverse effect of the cytokine IFN-α and other antineoplastic drugs on autoimmune thyroid dysfunction is more striking (Hamnvik et al., 2011). Radioactive fallout from the Chernobyl nuclear disaster led to an increase in the prevalence of thyroid autoantibodies in exposed children, with a small overall increase in the prevalence of AT 14–16 years later (Ostroumova et al., 2009).

In Vivo Models

AT can be induced experimentally in animals, and also occurs spontaneously, with features most closely resembling Hashimoto's thyroiditis.

Immunization-Induced Thyroiditis

In mice and rats the strength of the autoimmune response to immunization with TG in adjuvant is strain dependent. Murine EAT susceptibility (as shown by the severity of lymphocytic thyroiditis) is governed by the class II I-A subregion of the H-2 MHC (Vladutiu and Rose, 1971). H-2^{k,s} strains may even develop EAT with syngeneic TG immunization alone, demonstrating that untolerized autoreactive T cells exist in normal animals, in which they are usually under active regulation (ElRehewy et al., 1981). The influence of I-E is strain dependent, but less clear. MHC class I K and D alleles also influence susceptibility, presumably by determining the strength of effector cytotoxic T cell interaction with the thyroid cell target. Transgenic mice expressing HLA-DR3 but not HLA-DR2 develop EAT after TG immunization, confirming a role for this HLA specificity in thyroiditis (Kong et al., 1996).

Female animals have worse EAT than males and this is dependent on sex hormones, estrogen excess worsening thyroiditis, and testosterone ameliorating it (Okayasu et al., 1981). Another important influence in mice is the level of circulating TG, which can induce T regulatory cells (Kong et al., 2009). The thyroiditis after immunization consists of CD4$^+$ and CD8$^+$ T cells and macrophages, with only a small percentage of B cells. Disease can be transferred by T cells but not by TG antibodies and the critical effector cells are CD8$^+$ cytotoxic T cells which require specific CD4$^+$ T cells for their induction (Creemers et al., 1983). Immunization with the immunodominant T cell epitope of murine TPO will also induce EAT (Ng and Kung, 2006).

Experimental Autoimmune Thyroiditis Resulting from Immune Modulation

Neonatal thymectomy in certain strains of mice or rats, or thymectomy plus sublethal irradiation in certain strains of rats, results in severe EAT (Penhale et al., 1973; Kojima et al., 1976), as well as other autoimmune endocrinopathies. From these initial observations came the understanding of the crucial role of CD4$^+$, CD25$^+$ immunoregulatory T cells in preventing autoimmunity (Sakaguchi et al., 2001). Other maneuvers affecting T cells, such as treatment of neonatal mice with cyclosporin A or T cell depletion and reconstitution, can induce EAT (Sakaguchi and Sakaguchi, 1989). Depletion of CD7/CD28 in knockout mice also prevents generation of CD4$^+$, CD25$^+$ regulatory cells and results in EAT

(Sempowski et al., 2004). The induction of EAT by T cell modulation elegantly demonstrates the presence of thyroid-reactive T cells in the normal newborn repertoire. These CD4$^+$ T cells may be destined for deletion after birth but there is now strong evidence for incomplete tolerance and active suppression even later.

In addition to MHC and non-MHC genes, environmental factors play an important role in susceptibility. Rats raised under specific pathogen-free conditions until weaning are resistant to EAT following thymectomy and irradiation, but transfer of normal gut microflora results in EAT in the germ-free animals (Penhale and Young, 1988). It is unclear whether radiation-induced damage to the intestine is involved in this effect of gut microflora.

Spontaneous Autoimmune Thyroiditis

Several species develop spontaneous thyroiditis. Lymphocytic infiltration of the thyroid and TG antibodies occur in around 60% of diabetic and 10% of nondiabetic BB rats but diabetes-prone sublines have a range of prevalence, from 100% in the NB line to 5% in the BE line, suggesting that diabetes is not tightly linked genetically to EAT (Crisa et al., 1992). The Buffalo strain rat has a low spontaneous incidence of thyroiditis, reaching a maximum of 25% in old, multiparous females (Noble et al., 1976). Non-obese diabetic (NOD) mice infrequently develop thyroiditis but this trait is greatly enhanced by deficiency of the chemokine receptor CCR7, possibly related to the roles of CCR7 in negative selection of autoreactive T cells in the thymus and T regulatory cell control (Martin et al., 2009). Expression of TGFβ by thyroid cells in NOD mice inhibits the development of thyroiditis by generating an increase in thyroidal T regulatory cells (Yu et al., 2010).

Spontaneous autoimmune thyroiditis in the OS chicken is the closest animal model of Hashimoto's thyroiditis. The birds were originally bred from a White Leghorn flock of Cornell strain chickens for phenotypic features of hypothyroidism. Over time, the factors influencing disease development have changed: the importance of MHC genes and sex has diminished and the main genetic determinants in current OS chickens govern target organ susceptibility, T cell hyperreactivity, and corticosteroid responses (Wick et al., 2006). Unlike other models, OS chickens develop severe hypothyroidism as well as a lymphocytic thyroiditis and TG antibodies, and require T4 supplementation to thrive. The disease is T cell-dependent as thymectomy at birth prevents disease, although later thymectomy exacerbates thyroiditis, presumably by altering the balance of T cell-mediated regulation.

Pathologic Effector Mechanisms

Several antibody- and cell-mediated mechanisms contribute to thyroid injury in autoimmune hypothyroidism, and differences in the relative importance of each may determine some of the clinical and pathological variants described above (Figure 40.3).

Antibody-Mediated Injury

Immune complexes are deposited in the basement membrane around the thyroid follicles in Hashimoto's thyroiditis (Pfaltz and Hedinger, 1986) and terminal complement complexes are also present at this location indicating the formation of membrane attack complexes (Weetman et al., 1989). TFC are relatively resistant to lysis, through enhanced expression multiple regulators of complement activation, especially CD59, in response to cytokines derived from the infiltrating lymphocytes and macrophages (Tandon et al., 1994). After sublethal complement attack, TFC are less able to respond to TSH stimulation and also release cytokines (IL-1, IL-6), prostaglandin E_2 and reactive oxygen metabolites, which may have proinflammatory effects (Weetman et al., 1992). TPO antibodies are generally assumed to be the major mediators of complement fixation and activation within the thyroid and may also provoke damage by antibody-dependent cell-mediated cytotoxicity (Rebuffat et al., 2008). Cytokines like IL-1 may be critical in dissociating the junctional complex and thus allowing access of autoantibodies to apically-expressed TPO and other such antigens (Nilsson et al., 1998), in turn implying a secondary role for these antibodies in pathogenesis and explaining why neonates born to mothers with TPO antibodies have normal thyroid function.

Thyroid autoantibodies can also alter target cell function. TSH-R blocking antibodies have a clearly defined importance, as their placental transfer causes transient neonatal hypothyroidism (Matsuura et al., 1980). Although such antibodies have very similar characteristics to TSH-R stimulating antibodies, study of monoclonal antibodies has started to show subtle differences in binding and such approaches should allow a better understanding of their pathogenic action (Sanders et al., 2010). Although they appear to be particularly associated with atrophic thyroiditis in Asian patients (Arikawa et al., 1985), TSH-R blocking antibodies occur in both goitrous and atrophic thyroiditis in Caucasians (Kraiem et al., 1987).

T Cell-Mediated Injury

Despite the strong lead provided by studies in EAT, there is only modest direct evidence that T cell-mediated injury is important in autoimmune hypothyroidism. Two groups have derived CD8$^+$ T cell clones and lines from patients with Hashimoto's thyroiditis which lyse autologous TFC in an MHC class I-restricted fashion (MacKenzie et al., 1987; Sugihara et al., 1995). The autoantigen specificity of these T cells has not been elucidated. Indirect evidence

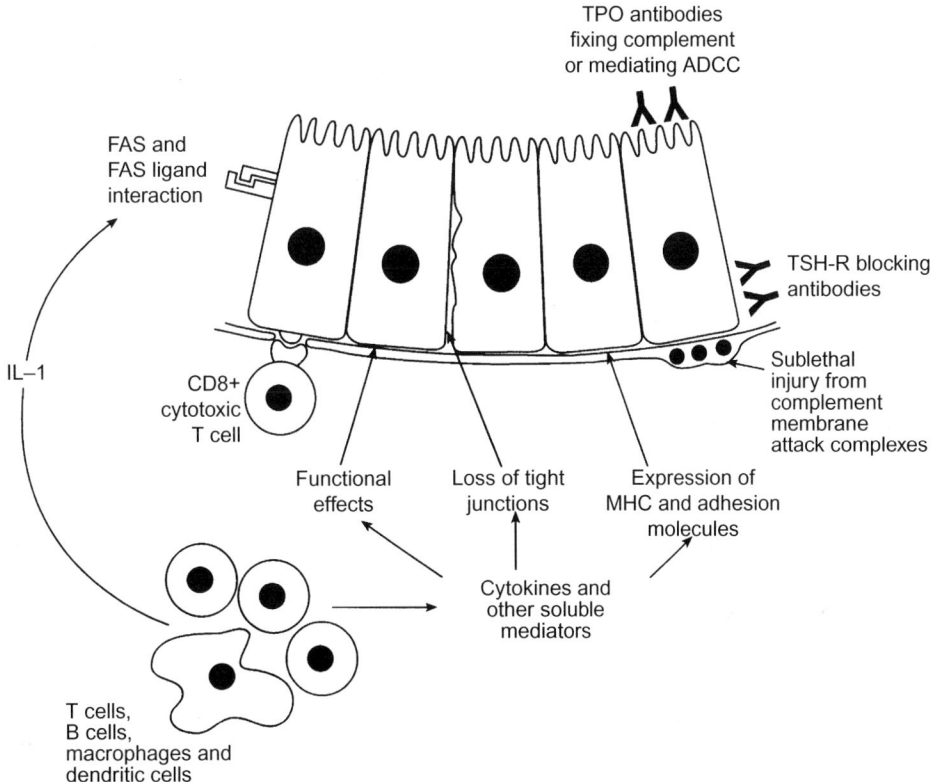

FIGURE 40.3 Mechanisms of Thyroid Destruction in Autoimmune Hypothyroidism. *From Weetman (2002), with permission.*

for the importance of cytotoxic T cells in pathogenesis is provided by the demonstration of frequent perforin-containing T cells in the intrathyroidal CD8$^+$ T cell population in Hashimoto's thyroiditis (Wu et al., 1994). In addition, TFC in Hashimoto's thyroiditis express adhesion molecules such as CD54 in response to cytokines and these increase the potential for T cell binding, thereby enhancing cytotoxicity (Weetman et al., 1990). T cells may also provoke thyroid dysfunction by the release of cytokines. There is an increase in intrathyroidal Th17 lymphocytes and enhanced synthesis of Th17 cytokines in AT, implying a role for these proinflammatory cells in pathogenesis (Figueroa-Vega et al., 2010). Hürthle cell formation results from overexpression of immunoproteasome subunits secondary to chronic inflammation (Kimura et al., 2009).

Attention has also focused on the expression of death receptor-mediated apoptosis as a major pathway for TFC destruction, based on the finding of both Fas (CD95) and Fas ligand (CD95L) on TFC in Hashimoto's thyroiditis (Giordano et al., 1997). Fas expression by TFC was upregulated by IL-1β, leading to the suggestion that cytokines could induce cytotoxicity through this pathway by suicide or fratricide as Fas interacted with FasL. Moreover, it has been proposed that FasL on TFC induces apoptosis in the infiltrating lymphocytes, suggesting that a T cell-mediated cytotoxic mechanism for thyroid destruction is less important than autocrine/paracrine Fas–FasL interaction (Stassi et al., 1999). Other interpretations have been put on the role of such apoptosis, not least because of the possible role of other decoy death receptors and regulators of apoptosis signaling and these multiple complex pathways may explain why induction of apoptosis in AT results in the destruction of thyroid cells, while apoptosis in the GD leads to damage of thyroid-infiltrating lymphocytes (Wang and Baker, 2007).

Autoantibodies as Potential Immunological Markers

The diagnosis of autoimmune hypothyroidism is usually straightforward, patients having biochemical evidence of hypothyroidism plus TG and/or TPO antibodies which can easily be measured by passive hemagglutination or immunoassays. An abnormal thyroid ultrasound pattern is also highly predictive of AT (Raber et al., 2002). Fine needle aspiration biopsy is used in difficult cases, especially to exclude an associated lymphoma.

Treatment and Outcome

It is difficult to imagine a more straightforward treatment than T4 replacement and future attempts at immunomodulation seem unlikely (Roberts and Ladenson, 2004). In around 10% of patients there may be a spontaneous remission 4–8 years after starting T4, and this is associated with the disappearance of TSH-R blocking antibodies (Takasu et al., 1992). However, the permanence of such remissions has not been established and remission in other patients has not been associated with changes in TSH-R blocking antibody levels (Cho et al., 1995).

Concluding Remarks—Future Prospects

Considerable progress in understanding the pathogenesis of AT has been made in the half century since the first demonstration of EAT and the realization that a similar process accounts for Hashimoto's thyroiditis. A major future goal is the identification of the earliest T cell responses, as these may be restricted to single T cell clones, recognizing restricted epitopes on a single inciting autoantigen, and have a particular cytokine bias. Additional work is also needed to determine the exact genetic basis for AT and to clarify the relationships between these disorders and Graves' disease, which are associated together in families and sometimes in the same individual. Finally, despite three decades of research, determining the exact role for T cell-mediated, thyroid-specific immunoregulation in preventing AT remains complex. There is no doubt that T regulatory cells are important but so far the mechanisms which control thyroid-specific T cells that have escaped central tolerance in human AT are elusive and not yet able to be exploited therapeutically.

GRAVES' DISEASE

Historic Background

Caleb Parry first described this disorder in 1825 but it was Robert Graves whose name became attached to the disease through his report of four cases published in 1835. Basedow was the first to highlight the association with exophthalmos in 1840. Originally believed to have a cardiac and then neurological origin, the role of the thyroid in Graves' disease became established in the 1890s as thyroidectomy for apparently coincidental goiter improved the other manifestations. The cause remained obscure until Adams and Purves (1956) showed that the serum from Graves' patients contained a long-acting thyroid stimulator which was distinct from TSH: working separately, Kriss and McKenzie went on to show this stimulator was an IgG.

Clinical, Pathologic, and Epidemiologic Features

Although it shares many immunological features with AT, it is the production of TSH-R stimulating antibodies which characterizes Graves' disease (Brent, 2008). It is the most common cause of hyperthyroidism, accounting for 60–80% of cases. The prevalence is around 4 per

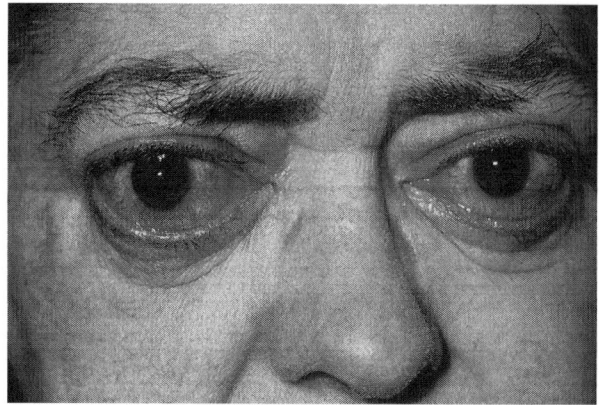

FIGURE 40.4 Eye signs in a patient with thyroid-associated ophthalmopathy showing exophthalmos, scleral injection, and periorbital edema.

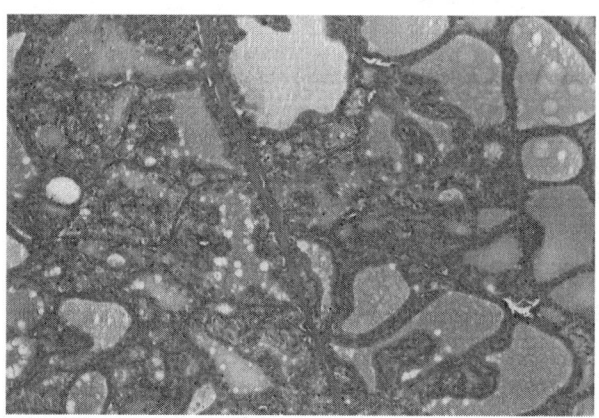

FIGURE 40.5 Pathology of Graves' disease showing columnar and folded thyroid epithelium, small new follicles, and active colloid resorption, with "scalloping" of the colloid. A lymphocytic infiltrate is not prominent in this specimen. (Original magnification: × 100.) *Photo courtesy of Dr. Judith Channer, Northern General Hospital, Sheffield.*

1000, with a 5- to 10-fold higher frequency in women (Eaton et al., 2010). Over 70% of patients with Graves' disease have thyroid-associated ophthalmopathy (TAO), which can be revealed by scanning techniques showing enlarged extraocular muscles (Bahn, 2010). Clinically obvious eye disease is apparent in around 50% of patients (Figure 40.4). TAO is not exclusive to Graves' disease, as around 5% of patients have AT and another 5% have little evidence of thyroid dysfunction. Thyroid dermopathy (or pretibial myxedema, reflecting the usual site for this complication) occurs in only 1–5% of patients, who typically also have marked TAO (Schwartz et al., 2002).

In the untreated state there is both hypertrophy and hyperplasia of the thyroid follicles; the epithelium becomes columnar and folded into the follicular lumen, new small follicles form, and there is little colloid (Figure 40.5). A variable degree of lymphocytic infiltration occurs and germinal centers may form. Antithyroid drugs diminish the lymphocytic infiltrate and the epithelium reverts to a normal appearance. Lymphoid hyperplasia may occur in the lymph nodes, thymus, and spleen, but reverses with antithyroid drugs.

Autoimmune Features

Autoantibodies

Thyroglobulin and TPO autoantibodies occur in up to 80% of patients. TSH-R stimulating antibodies (TSAb) can be detected in over 95% of patients with current assays. The TSH-R consists of a 398 amino acid extracellular domain with a series of leucine-rich repeats and a hinge region, a 266 amino acid transmembrane spanning domain with seven hydrophobic regions, and an 83 amino acid intracellular domain (Rapoport and McLachlan, 2007). The receptor undergoes complex post-translational processing at the hinge region to form two subunits linked by a disulfide bond. TFC shed the A subunit, which binds TSAb more strongly than the holoreceptor, and this may be critical in affinity maturation of the B cell autoimmune response (Mizutori et al., 2009). TSAb-induced activation of the TSH-R typically causes a rise in cAMP but TSH-R antibodies may also cause activation of other intracellular signaling pathways and these may relate to the whether such antibodies act as blockers of TSH-R activation or have no signaling (neutral) activity (Michalek et al., 2009).

The original bioassay method measured release of radioiodine from preloaded thyroid glands after injection of serum or IgG into intact animals and this activity was termed long-acting thyroid stimulator or LATS (Adams and Purves, 1956). Other early assays measured cAMP release from primary TFC cultures or thyroid cell lines (such as FRTL-5): more recently TSH-R-transfected eukaryotic cells have been utilized (Ajjan and Weetman, 2008). A separate type of assay measures displacement of TSH from solubilized or recombinant TSH-R by TSH-R antibodies in a radiolabeled or chemiluminescent format; these antibodies are called TSH-binding inhibiting immunoglobulins or TBII. Current TBII assays have a sensitivity and specificity which exceeds 95% but measure both TSAb and TSH-R blocking antibodies (which inhibit TSH-induced cAMP release). Therefore the level of TBII gives no direct information on functional activity but in practice these assays are very useful when interpreted in the clinical context (Costagliola et al., 1999). Unlike TG and TPO autoantibodies, TSAb are IgG$_1$ subclass restricted and are often λ light chain restricted (Zakarija, 1983), suggesting a pauciclonal origin for TSAb in some patients.

The majority of TSH-R B cell epitopes appear to be conformational and overlap with the binding site for TSH (Rapoport and McLachlan, 2007). Heterogeneity between patients in their antibody binding sites is apparent, for instance by using chimeric TSH/LH hormone receptors, and mutated receptors have revealed that a component of the epitope for TSH-R stimulating antibodies is on the N terminus, whereas epitopes for blocking antibodies are more diverse (Schwarz-Lauer et al., 2002). Further details on the epitope binding of TSH-R antibodies is emerging from studies of cloned monoclonal antibodies crystalized with the receptor extracellular domain, which show that a single blocking antibody binds to different regions of the leucine-rich repeat domain and more towards the N terminal than a single stimulating antibody or TSH (Sanders et al., 2011). Clearly many different monoclonal antibodies from separate patients will be required to have a more general understanding of epitope binding in relation to antibody function.

T Cell Responses

Many studies have found a reduction in circulating CD8$^+$ T cells and an increase in HLA-DR$^+$ T cells in active Graves' disease (Weetman and McGregor, 1994). Intrathyroidal T cells are CD4$^+$ and CD8$^+$ in varying proportions (Jansson et al., 1984). Similar homing mechanisms to AT account for this localization (Marazuela, 1999). Using overlapping TSH-R peptides covering the extracellular domain, a heterogeneous response was obtained using circulating or intrathyroidal T cells in proliferation assays, with multiple peptides stimulating different patients' cells (Tandon et al., 1992). There is no distinct Th1 or Th2 pattern of response by the stage of disease that specimens are available for study (Watson et al., 1994; Okumura et al., 1999). Cytokines such as IL-1, IL-6, IL-8, and IL-10 are strongly expressed, with some cytokines being in part derived from the TFC themselves. As in AT, there are plentiful T regulatory cells in the thyroid in Graves' disease, apparently without the ability to halt disease (Marazuela et al., 2006). This T regulatory cell defect may be the result of both impaired plasmacytoid dendritic cell function and elevated levels of thyroid hormone (Mao et al., 2011).

Genetic Features

Monozygotic twins are around 20–30% concordant for Graves' disease, at least 10-fold higher than for dizygotic twins (Brix et al., 1998). A consistent but weak association exists between the serologically defined specificity HLA-DR3 and Graves' disease in Caucasians, with a relative risk of around 2–3 (Tomer and Davies, 2003). The relative weakness of the contribution of HLA genes is underlined by the low concordance (7%) for Graves' disease in HLA-identical siblings (Stenszky et al., 1985). A number of candidate gene polymorphisms (encoding immune receptors, immunoglobulins, and cytokines) have been tested for associations with Graves' disease with inconsistent results

(Figure 40.2). Polymorphisms in *CTLA-4* confer a relative risk of around 2−3 (Yanagawa et al., 1995) and polymorphism in other genes affecting B and T cell responses, *PTPN22*, *CD25*, *FCRL3*, and *CD226*, have also been associated with Graves' disease (Zeitlin et al., 2008; Tomer, 2010). The sharing of these genetic associations with many other autoimmune diseases probably accounts for the frequent concurrence of other autoimmune diseases with Graves' disease and AT.

Polymorphisms in the *TSH-R* gene confers susceptibility to Graves' disease but not autoimmune hypothyroidism, and may be an important factor in determining which members of families with a predisposition to develop thyroid autoimmunity actually get Graves' disease (Brand et al., 2009). Genome scanning methods have revealed other possible loci linked to Graves' disease (Tomer and Davies, 2003) but these have not been replicated in larger studies (Taylor et al., 2006). An impressive recent genome-wide scan of thousands of Chinese individuals with Graves' disease confirmed susceptibility loci in the major histocompatibility complex, *TSHR*, *CTLA4*, and *FCRL3*, and identified two new loci; the RNASET2-FGFR1OP-CCR6 region at 6q27 and an intergenic region at 4p14 (Chu et al., 2011).

Environmental Influences

Women are predisposed to Graves' disease and, as with AT, parity increases the risk by around 10% (Jørgensen et al., 2011). Retrospective studies have shown a significantly higher number of adverse, major life events during the year preceding the recognition of Graves' disease when patients are compared to matched controls (Winsa et al., 1991; Prummel et al., 2004). Presumably this effect of stress operates through the interactions between the nervous, endocrine, and immune systems. A high iodine intake increases the risk of developing an autoimmune response against the thyroid, the type being determined by genetic factors. However, in an animal model of Graves' disease produced by immunizing NOD mice with adenovirus expressing the TSH-R A subunit, increased iodine intake increased the severity of thyroiditis but not hyperthyroidism, suggesting a dichotomy in these two autoimmune responses (McLachlan et al., 2005).

Evidence for a role of infections is circumstantial (Tomer and Davies, 1993). It remains possible that a variety of infections could precipitate Graves' disease either specifically by molecular mimicry, or modulation of TFC behavior, or non-specifically, by enhancing any ongoing immune responses. Such non-specific enhancement, presumably mediated by cytokines, would explain the association between attacks of allergic rhinitis and recurrence of Graves' disease (Hidaka et al., 1993).

Smoking is strongly associated with the development of ophthalmopathy and weakly with the development of Graves' disease, although negatively associated with the presence of TG and TPO antibodies in Graves' patients (Bartalena et al., 1995; Hou et al., 2011). Cytokine treatment is sometimes complicated by the development of Graves' disease, although this is less frequent than AT (Hamnvik et al., 2011). Perhaps the most striking example of Graves' disease caused by an obvious external agent is its appearance during the period of immune reconstitution following alemtuzumab or highly active antiretroviral treatments (Weetman, 2009). This type of response may be the result of alteration levels of T regulatory cells as the lymphocyte population is recovering.

In Vivo Models

There is still no entirely satisfactory animal model of Graves' disease. All are induced rather than spontaneous, and the likely absence of Graves' disease even in great apes suggests that there is something unique about the susceptibility factors for Graves' disease in man (Nagayama, 2007; McLachlan et al., 2011). In the first attempts to produce an animal model, immunization of BALB/c mice with the extracellular domain of TSH-R and adjuvant containing *Bordetella pertussis* induced TSH-R blocking but not stimulating antibodies and a severe thyroiditis (Costagliola et al., 1994), while genetic immunization with TSH-R cDNA produced thyroiditis but without TSAb production (Costagliola et al., 1998). Immunizing AKR/N mice with fibroblasts double transfected with human TSH-R and haploidentical MHC class II genes led to hyperthyroidism caused by TSAb, although without thyroiditis (Yamaguchi et al., 1997). A variant of this model used the hamster and Chinese hamster ovary (CHO) cells expressing TSH-R, resulting in TSAb production and a focal thyroiditis (Ando et al., 2003).

More recently, immunization experiments with adenovirus encoding the TSH-R, especially the A subunit alone, have been successful in producing a high frequency of disease in mice (Chen et al., 2004). Such immunization in transgenic mice expressing human TSH-R A subunit has provided an insight into the role for T regulatory cells in determining the disease outcome; depletion of these cells led to thyroiditis, hypothyroidism, and spreading of the autoimmune response from TSH-R to involve TPO and TG (McLachlan and Rapoport, 2007). This model has also been used to show that pre-treatment with the TSH-R A subunit can deviate the immune response from pathogenic epitopes to the production of neutral TSH-R antibodies (Misharin et al., 2009).

Reproducing ophthalmopathy has proved even more challenging. Transfer of TSH-R primed T cells appeared to offer a possible model but these results have not been replicated, possibly due to changing environmental factors (Baker et al., 2005). Recently, genetic immunization by electroporation with the TSH-R A-subunit has been shown to lead to the production of antibodies against the IGF-1 receptor, a possible autoantigen in ophthalmopathy, and orbital fibrosis, in addition to TSAb and thyroiditis (Zhao et al., 2011). This is not a consistent response in all animals but it is the closest so far to the development of a successful animal model.

Pathologic Effector Mechanisms

Clearly the main effector mechanism in Graves' disease is the production of TSAb (Figure 40.6). However, the circulating levels of TSAb do not correlate closely with the level of thyroid hormones or the clinical severity of disease because of a variable, concurrent response against other autoantigens and, in some patients, production of TSH-R blocking antibodies, which reduce the effects of TSAb. Women with the highest levels of TSAb who

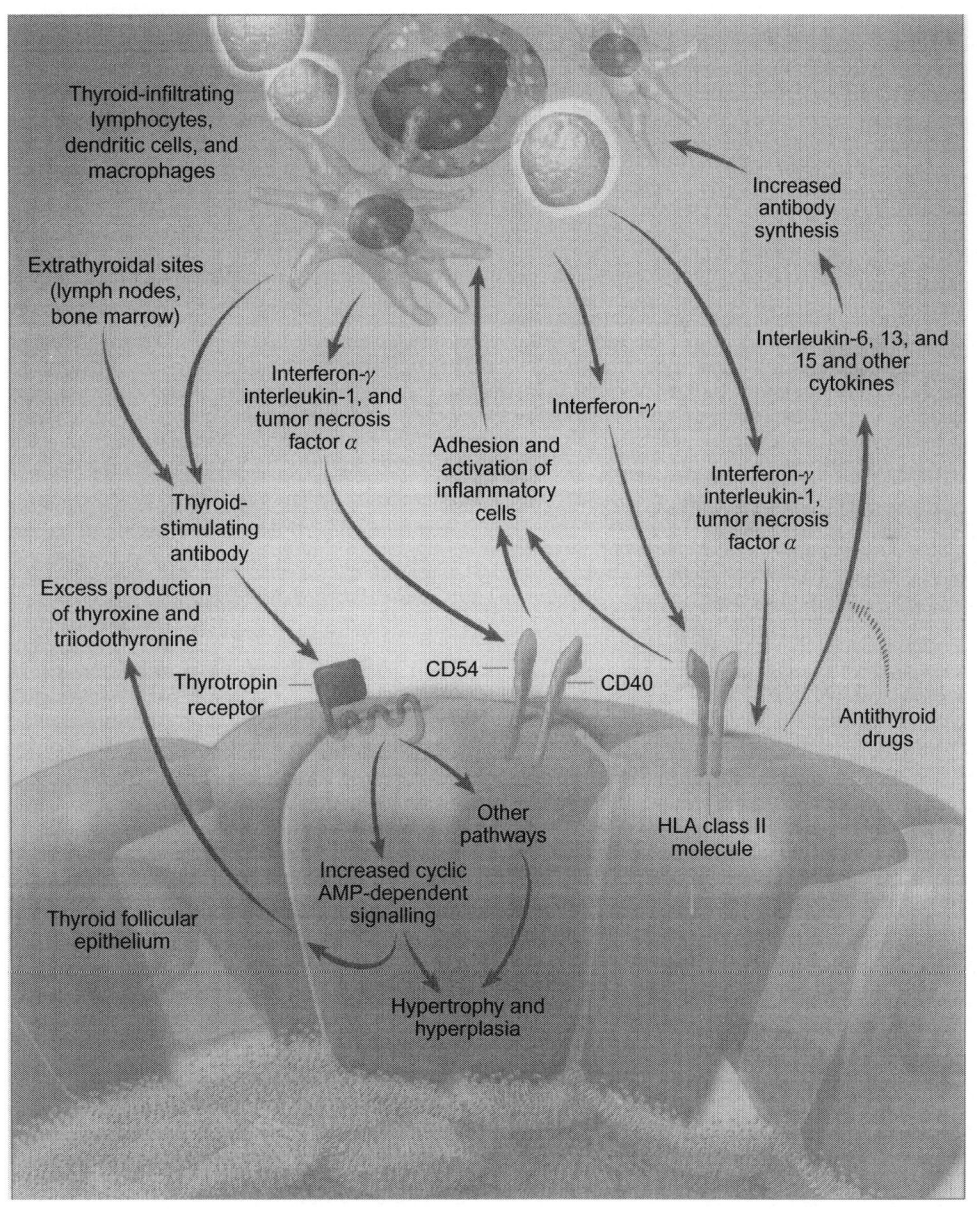

FIGURE 40.6   Pathogenesis of Graves' Disease. Hyperthyroidism is the result of TSH-R activation by thyroid stimulating antibodies. The intrathyroidal inflammatory response is enhanced by cytokines, some of which are derived from the thyroid cells themselves: antithyroid drugs interfere with this step in the pathway. Thyroid cells produce other molecules such as CD54, CD40, and HLA class II which help perpetuate the autoimmune response. *From Weetman (2000), with permission.*

become pregnant give birth to babies with transient neonatal thyrotoxicosis.

Autoantibodies as Potential Immunological Markers

TG and TPO antibodies provide readily available evidence for Graves' disease; although not specific, their presence in a patient with hyperthyroidism strongly suggests the diagnosis. These antibodies are present in 20–30% of cases 5–7 years before diagnosis (Hutfless et al., 2011). TSAb are not generally measured because present bioassays are laborious. TBII estimation is a commercially available surrogate and is useful in confirming the diagnosis of Graves' disease in the absence of clinical evidence such as ophthalmopathy. TSAb or TBII levels have been investigated as predictive markers for the success of antithyroid drug treatment in Graves' disease. Although patients with the highest levels tend to relapse the most, the results are insufficiently accurate for clinical use (Ajjan and Weetman, 2008). The most important indication for TSAb assay in Graves' disease is in women with known Graves' disease during pregnancy to predict the risk of neonatal thyrotoxicosis (Endocrine Society et al., 2007).

Treatment and Outcome

Treatment consists of antithyroid drugs (carbimazole, methimazole, or propylthiouracil), radioiodine, or thyroidectomy (Bahn et al., 2011). Around 40% of patients treated with antithyroid drugs achieve a permanent remission. These drugs ameliorate EAT and TSAb levels fall during treatment due to a decrease in the expression of proinflammatory molecules by TFC (Weetman et al., 1992). Relapse after antithyroid drugs is particularly likely in younger patients with severe hyperthyroidism or a large goiter, and those who smoke or have evidence of a strong Th2 response (Komiya et al., 2001). Radioiodine treatment is followed by a striking rise in TSH-R and other thyroid autoantibodies at 3–6 months whereas TSH-R antibody levels gradually fall in most but not all patients over the year following subtotal thyroidectomy (Laurberg et al., 2008). Complete ablation of thyroid tissue results in the disappearance of all thyroid autoantibodies, confirming the need for these autoantigens to maintain antibody production (Chiovato et al., 2003).

Thyroid-Associated Ophthalmopathy and Dermopathy

These complications of Graves' disease are most likely due to an autoimmune response which stimulates fibroblasts localized within the extraocular muscle or dermis, causing glycosaminoglycan release and edema, and accompanied by

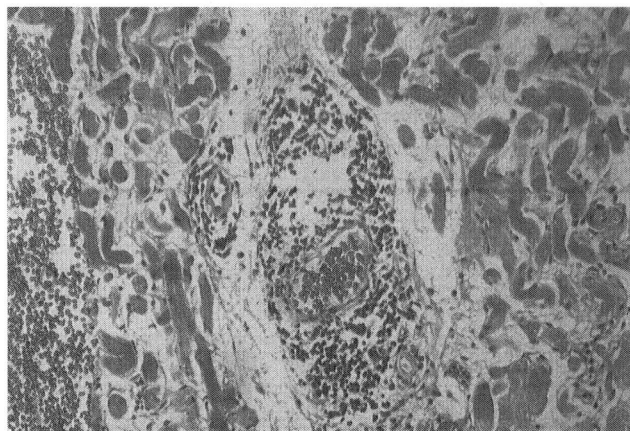

FIGURE 40.7 Photomicrograph of an extraocular muscle from a patient with thyroid-associated ophthalmopathy. There is an extensive lymphocytic infiltrate and edema: the muscle fibers are intact. (Original magnification: ×200.)

fat expansion (Naik et al., 2010). The extraocular muscles and dermis are infiltrated by activated T cells and local cytokine production (IFN-γ, IL-1, and tumor necrosis factor (TNF) can be demonstrated: these cytokines stimulate glycosaminoglycan synthesis by fibroblasts *in vitro* (Figures 40.7 and 40.8). The target of the autoimmune response appears to be the TSH-R which is expressed on a subset of fibroblasts, but the response may be enhanced by antibodies against the IGF-1 receptor (Wiersinga, 2011). Treatment of TAO usually consists of supportive measures or corticosteroids and in many the condition spontaneously becomes stable or regresses (Stiebel-Kalish et al., 2009).

Concluding Remarks—Future Prospects

Graves' disease shares many features with AT, and what determines the type of disorder is a critical issue. Apart from *TSH-R* polymorphism, genetic susceptibility factors have proven relatively non-specific, and more detailed analysis should reveal specific genotypes for Graves' disease. Future studies will clarify the relative importance of stress, iodine intake, smoking, and other environmental factors, as well as how these interact with each other and with genetic factors. It will be particularly important to study mechanisms at the earliest possible stage of disease so that an initiating rather than an enhancing role for these factors can be assessed. Experiments of nature, such as the appearance of Graves' disease after immunological treatments, may provide fresh insights into regulatory mechanisms and the early phase of disease.

The development of a robust animal model, especially one incorporating TAO, would be invaluable in clarifying the role of TSH-R as an autoantigen in TAO and its relationship to the IGF-1 receptor and other putative orbital antigens. Our current therapies for Graves' disease are

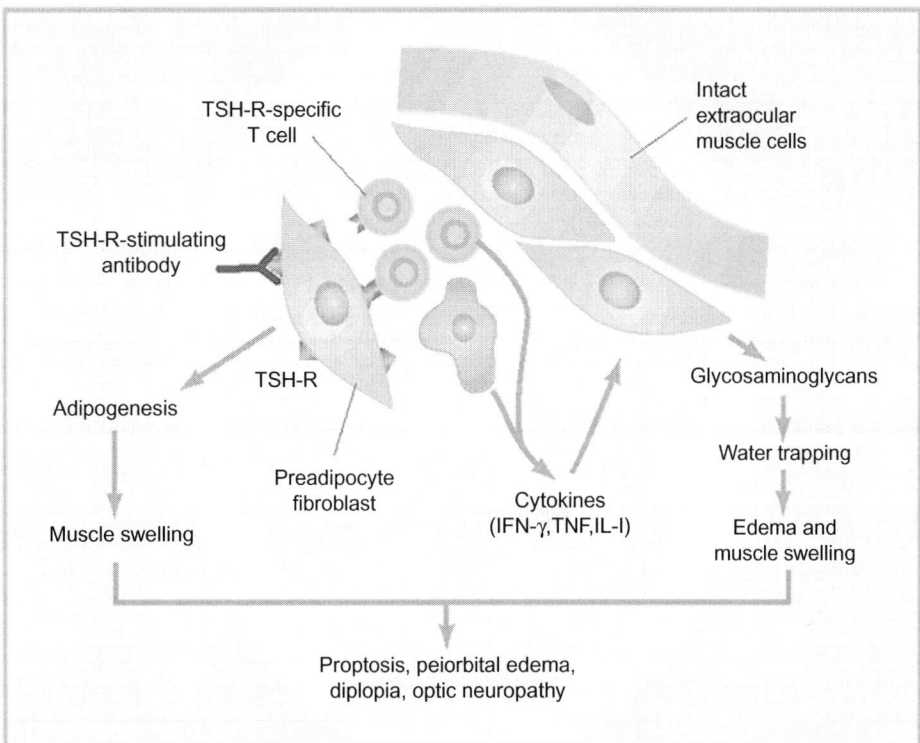

FIGURE 40.8 Pathogenic Mechanisms in Thyroid-Associated Ophthalmopathy. The inflammatory infiltrate in the orbit releases a variety of cytokines that stimulate orbital fibroblasts to secrete glycosaminoglycans (GAGs), which trap water and lead to edema; later fibroblast activation leads to fibrosis. A subset of orbital fibroblasts differentiates into adipocytes as a result of cytokine signaling, leading to fat expansion within the orbit. *From Weetman (2001), with permission.*

effective but not ideal, with many patients having recurrences or exchanging hyperthyroidism for permanent hypothyroidism. Pathogenesis-based treatment offers considerable potential advantages, but will need to be specific and innocuous: the recent description of a small molecular antagonist of TSAb suggests one possible approach (Neumann et al., 2011). An immunologically-directed strategy is even more appealing in TAO for which current treatment remains unsatisfactory.

REFERENCES

Adams, D.D., Purves, H.D., 1956. Abnormal responses in the assay of thyrotrophin. Proc. Univ. Otago Med. Sch. 34, 11–12.

Aichinger, G., Fill, H., Wick, G., 1985. In situ immune complexes, lymphocyte subpopulations, and HLA-DR-positive epithelial cells in Hashimoto thyroiditis. Lab. Invest. 52, 132–140.

Ajjan, R.A., Weetman, A.P., 2008. Techniques to quantify TSH receptor antibodies. Nat. Clin. Pract. Endocrinol. Metab. 4, 461–468.

Ajjan, R.A., Watson, P.F., McIntosh, R.S., Weetman, A.P., 1996. Intrathyroidal cytokine gene expression in Hashimoto's thyroiditis. Clin. Exp. Immunol. 105, 523–528.

Ajjan, R.A., Kemp, E.H., Waterman, E.A., Watson, P.F., Endo, T., Onaya, T., et al., 2000. Detection of binding and blocking autoantibodies to the human sodium-iodide symporter in patients with autoimmune thyroid disease. J. Clin. Endocrinol. Metab. 85, 2020–2027.

Ando, T., Imaizumi, M., Graves, P., Unger, P., Davies, T.F., 2003. Induction of thyroid-stimulating hormone receptor autoimmunity in hamsters. Endocrinology. 144, 671–680.

Ansar-Ahmed, S., Young, P.R., Penhale, W.J., 1983. The effects of female sex steroids on the development of autoimmune thyroiditis in thymectomized and irradiated rats. Clin. Exp. Immunol. 54, 351–358.

Arikawa, K., Ichikawa, Y., Yoshida, T., Shinozawa, T., Homma, M., Momotani, N., et al., 1985. Blocking type antithyrotropin receptor antibody in patients with nongoitrous hypothyroidism: its incidence and characteristics of action. J. Clin. Endocrinol. Metab. 60, 953–959.

Bagchi, N., Brown, T.R., Sundick, R.S., 1995. Thyroid cell injury is an initial event in the induction of autoimmune thyroiditis by iodine in obese strain chickens. Endocrinology. 136, 5054–5060.

Bahn, R.S., 2010. Graves' ophthalmopathy. N. Engl. J. Med. 362, 726–738.

Bahn, R.S, Burch, H.B., Cooper, D.S., Garber, J.R., Greenlee, M.C., Klein, I., et al., 2011. Hyperthyroidism and other causes of thyrotoxicosis: management guidelines of the American Thyroid Association and American Association of Clinical Endocrinologists. Endocr. Pract. 17, 456–520.

Baker, G., Mazziotti, G., von Ruhland, C., Ludgate, M., 2005. Reevaluating thyrotropin receptor-induced mouse models of Graves' disease and ophthalmopathy. Endocrinology. 146, 835–844.

Barin, J.G., Talor, M.V., Sharma, R.B., Rose, N.R., Burek, C.L., 2005. Iodination of murine thyroglobulin enhances autoimmune reactivity in the NOD.H2 mouse. Clin. Exp. Immunol. 142, 251–259.

Bartalena, L., Bogazzi, F., Tanda, M.L., Manetti, L., Dell-Unto, E., Martino, E., et al., 1995. Cigarette smoking and the thyroid. Eur. J. Endocrinol. 133, 507–512.

Benvenga, S., Trimarchi, F., 2008. Changed presentation of Hashimoto's thyroiditis in North-Eastern Sicily and Calabria (Southern Italy) based on a 31-year experience. Thyroid. 18, 429–441.

Blanchin, S., Estienne, V., Durand-Gorde, J.M., Carayon, P., Ruf, J., 2003. Complement activation by direct C4 binding to thyroperoxidase in Hashimoto's thyroiditis. Endocrinology. 144, 5422–5429.

Boelaert, K., Newby, P.R., Simmonds, M.J., Holder, R.L., Carr-Smith, J. D., Heward, J.M., et al., 2010. Prevalence and relative risk of other autoimmune diseases in subjects with autoimmune thyroid disease. Am. J. Med. 123 (183), e1–9.

Bottazzo, G.F., Pujol-Borrell, R., Hanafusa, T., Feldmann, M., 1983. Role of aberrant HLA-DR expression and antigen presentation in induction of endocrine autoimmunity. Lancet. 2, 1115–1119.

Brand, O.J., Barrett, J.C., Simmonds, M.J., Newby, P.R., McCabe, C.J., Bruce, C.K., et al., 2009. Association of the thyroid stimulating hormone receptor gene (TSHR) with Graves' disease. Hum. Mol. Genet. 18, 1704–1713.

Brent, G.A., 2008. Clinical practice. Graves' disease. N. Engl. J. Med. 358, 2594–2605.

Brix, T.H., Kyvik, K.O., Hegedüs, L., 1998. What is the evidence of genetic factors in the etiology of Graves' disease? A brief review. Thyroid. 8, 727–734.

Brix, T.H., Kyvik, K.O., Hegedüs, L., 2000. A population-based study of chronic autoimmune hypothyroidism in Danish twins. J. Clin. Endocrinol. Metab. 85, 536–539.

Brix, T.H., Hansen, P.S., Kyvik, K.O., Hegedüs, L., 2004. Aggregation of thyroid autoantibodies in first-degree relatives of patients with autoimmune thyroid disease is mainly due to genes: a twin study. Clin. Endocrinol. (Oxf.). 60, 329–334.

Butscher, W.G., Ladenson, P.W., Burek, C.L., 2001. Whole-blood proliferation assay for autoimmune thyroid disease: comparison to density-gradient separated-peripheral blood lymphocytes. Thyroid. 11, 531–537.

Chen, C.R., Pichurin, P., Chazenbalk, G.D., Aliesky, H., Nagayama, Y., McLachlan, S.M., et al., 2004. Low-dose immunization with adenovirus expressing the thyroid-stimulating hormone receptor A-subunit deviates the antibody response toward that of autoantibodies in human Graves' disease. Endocrinology. 145, 228–233.

Chen, C.R., Hamidi, S., Braley-Mullen, H., Nagayama, Y., Bresee, C., Aliesky, H.A., et al., 2010. Antibodies to thyroid peroxidase arise spontaneously with age in NOD.H-2h4 mice and appear after thyroglobulin antibodies. Endocrinology. 151, 4583–4593.

Chiovato, L., Latrofa, F., Braverman, L.E., Pacini, F., Capezzone, M., Masserini, L., et al., 2003. Disappearance of humoral thyroid autoimmunity after complete removal of thyroid antigens. Ann. Int. Med. 139, 346–351.

Cho, B.Y., Kim, W.B., Chung, J.H., Yi, K.H., Shong, Y.K., Lee, H.K., et al., 1995. High prevalence and little change in TSH receptor blocking antibody titres with thyroxine and antithyroid drug therapy in patients with non-goitrous autoimmune thyroiditis. Clin. Endocrinol. (Oxf.). 43, 465–471.

Chu, X., Pan, C.M., Zhao, S.X., Liang, J., Gao, G.Q., Zhang, X.M., et al., 2011. A genome-wide association study identifies two new risk loci for Graves' disease. Nat. Genet. 43, 897–901.

Costagliola, S., Many, M.C., Stalmans-Falys, M., Tonacchera, M., Vassart, G., Ludgate, M., et al., 1994. Recombinant thyrotropin receptor and the induction of autoimmune thyroid disease in BALB/c mice: a new animal model. Endocrinology. 135, 2150–2159.

Costagliola, S., Rodien, P., Many, M.C., Ludgate, M., Vassart, G., 1998. Genetic immunization against the human thyrotropin receptor causes thyroiditis and allows production of monoclonal antibodies recognizing the native receptor. J. Immunol. 160, 1458–1465.

Costagliola, S., Morgenthaler, N.G., Hoermann, R., Badenhoop, K., Struck, J., Freitag, D., et al., 1999. Second generation assay for thyrotropin receptor antibodies has superior diagnostic sensitivity for Graves' disease. J. Clin. Endocrinol. Metab. 84, 90–97.

Creemers, P., Rose, N.R., Kong, Y.M., 1983. Experimental autoimmune thyroiditis. In vitro cytotoxic effects of T lymphocytes on thyroid monolayers. J. Exp. Med. 157, 559–571.

Crisa, L., Mordes, J.P., Rossini, A.A., 1992. Autoimmune diabetes mellitus in the BB rat. Diab. Metab. Rev. 8, 4–37.

Dayan, C.M., Chu, N.R., Londei, M., Rapoport, B., Feldmann, M., 1993. T cells involved in human autoimmune disease are resistant to tolerance induction. J. Immunol. 151, 1606–1613.

Eaton, W.W., Pedersen, M.G., Atladóttir, H.O., Gregory, P.E., Rose, N. R., Mortensen, P.B., et al., 2010. The prevalence of 30 ICD-10 autoimmune diseases in Denmark. Immunol. Res. 47, 228–231.

Effraimidis, G., Tijssen, J.G., Wiersinga, W.M., 2009. Discontinuation of smoking increases the risk for developing thyroid peroxidase antibodies and/or thyroglobulin antibodies: a prospective study. J. Clin. Endocrinol. Metab. 94, 1324–1328.

ElRehewy, M., Kong, Y.M., Giraldo, A.A., Rose, N.R., 1981. Syngeneic thyroglobulin is immunogenic in good responder mice. Eur. J. Immunol. 11, 146–151.

Endocrine Society; American Association of Clinical Endocrinologists; Asia & Oceania Thyroid Association; American Thyroid Association; European Thyroid Association; Latin American Thyroid Association, 2007. Management of thyroid dysfunction during pregnancy and postpartum: an Endocrine Society Clinical Practice Guideline. Thyroid. 17, 1159–1167.

Feingold, S.B., Smith, J., Houtz, J., Popovsky, E., Brown, R.S., 2009. Prevalence and functional significance of thyrotropin receptor blocking antibodies in children and adolescents with chronic lymphocytic thyroiditis. J. Clin. Endocrinol. Metab. 94, 4742–4748.

Figueroa-Vega, N., Alfonso-Pérez, M., Benedicto, I., Sánchez-Madrid, F., González-Amaro, R., Marazuela, M., et al., 2010. Increased circulating pro-inflammatory cytokines and Th17 lymphocytes in Hashimoto's thyroiditis. J. Clin. Endocrinol. Metab. 95, 953–962.

Giordano, C., Stassi, G., De_Maria, R., Todaro, M., Richiusa, P., Papoff, G., et al., 1997. Potential involvement of Fas and its ligand in the pathogenesis of Hashimoto's thyroiditis. Science. 275, 960–963.

Greer, L.G., Casey, B.M., Halvorson, L.M., Spong, C.Y., McIntire, D. D., Cunningham, F.G., et al., 2011. Antithyroid antibodies and parity: further evidence for microchimerism in autoimmune thyroid disease. Am. J. Obstet. Gynecol. 205, 471.

Hamilton, F., Black, M., Farquharson, M.A., Stewart, C., Foulis, A.K., 1991. Spatial correlation between thyroid epithelial cells expressing class II MHC molecules and interferon-gamma-containing lympho-cytes in human thyroid autoimmune disease. Clin. Exp. Immunol. 83, 64–68.

Hamnvik, O.P., Larsen, P.R., Marqusee, E., 2011. Thyroid dysfunction from antineoplastic agents. J. Natl. Cancer Inst. 103, 1572–1587.

Hidaka, Y., Amino, N., Iwatani, Y., Itoh, E., Matsunaga, M., Tamaki, H., et al., 1993. Recurrence of thyrotoxicosis after attack of allergic rhinitis in patients with Graves' disease. J. Clin. Endocrinol. Metab. 77, 1667–1670.

Hou, X., Li, Y., Li, J., Wang, W., Fan, C., Wang, H., et al., 2011. Development of thyroid dysfunction and autoantibodies in Graves' multiplex families: an eight-year follow-up study in Chinese Han pedigrees. Thyroid. 21, 353–1358.

Hutfless, S., Matos, P., Talor, M.V., Caturegli, P., Rose, N.R., 2011. Significance of prediagnostic thyroid antibodies in women with autoimmune thyroid disease. J. Clin. Endocrinol. Metab. 96, E1466–E1471.

Iitaka, M., Momotani, N., Hisaoka, T., Noh, J.Y., Ishikawa, N., Ishii, J., et al., 1998. TSH receptor antoibody-associayed thyroid dysfunction following subacute thyroiditis. Clin. Endocrinol. (Oxf.). 48, 445–453.

Iwatani, Y., Amino, N., Hidaka, Y., Kaneda, T., Ichihara, K., Tamaki, H., et al., 1992. Decreases in alpha beta T cell receptor negative T cells and CD8 cells, and an increase in CD4$^+$ CD8$^+$ cells in active Hashimoto's disease and subacute thyroiditis. Clin. Exp. Immunol. 87, 444–449.

Jansson, R., Karlsson, A., Forsum, U., 1984. Intrathyroidal HLA-DR expression and T lymphocyte phenotypes in Graves' thyrotoxicosis, Hashimoto's thyroiditis and nodular colloid goitre. Clin. Exp. Immunol. 58, 264–272.

Jaume, J.C., Guo, J., Pauls, D.L., Zakarija, M., McKenzie, J.M., Egeland, J.A., et al., 1999. Evidence for genetic transmission of thyroid peroxidase autoantibody epitopic "fingerprints". J. Clin. Endocrinol. Metab. 84, 1424–1431.

Jørgensen, K.T., Pedersen, B.V., Nielsen, N.M., Jacobsen, S., Frisch, M., 2011. Childbirths and risk of female predominant and other autoimmune diseases in a population-based Danish cohort. J. Autoimmun. 38, J81–J87.

Kakudo, K., Li, Y., Hirokawa, M., Ozaki, T., 2011. Diagnosis of Hashimoto's thyroiditis and IgG4-related sclerosing disease. Pathol. Int. 61, 175–183.

Kimura, H.J., Chen, C.Y., Tzou, S.C., Rocchi, R., Landek-Salgado, M.A., Suzuki, K., et al., 2009. Immunoproteasome overexpression underlies the pathogenesis of thyroid oncocytes and primary hypothyroidism: studies in humans and mice. PLoS One. 4, e7857.

Kojima, A., Tanaka Kojima, Y., Sakakura, T., Nishizuka, Y., 1976. Spontaneous development of autoimmune thyroiditis in neonatally thymectomized mice. Lab. Invest. 34, 550–557.

Komiya, I., Yamada, T., Sato, A., Kouki, T., Nishimori, T., Takasu, N., et al., 2001. Remission and recurrence of hyperthyroid Graves' disease during and after methimazole treatment when assessed by IgE and interleukin 13. J. Clin. Endocrinol. Metab. 86, 3540–3544.

Kondrashova, A., Viskari, H., Haapala, A.M., Seiskari, T., Kulmala, P., Ilonen, J., et al., 2008. Serological evidence of thyroid autoimmunity among schoolchildren in two different socioeconomic environments. J. Clin. Endocrinol. Metab. 93, 729–734.

Kong, Y.C., Lomo, L.C., Motte, R.W., Giraldo, A.A., Baisch, J., Strauss, G., et al., 1996. HLA-DRB1 polymorphism determines susceptibility to autoimmune thyroiditis in transgenic mice: definitive association with HLA-DRB1*0301 (DR3) gene. J. Exp. Med. 184, 1167–1172.

Kong, Y.C., Morris, G.P., Brown, N.K., Yan, Y., Flynn, J.C., David, C.S., et al., 2009. Autoimmune thyroiditis: a model uniquely suited to probe regulatory T cell function. J. Autoimmun. 33, 239–246.

Kotsa, K., Watson, P.F., Weetman, A.P., 1997. A CTLA-4 gene polymorphism is associated with both Graves disease and autoimmune hypothyroidism. Clin. Endocrinol. (Oxf.). 46, 551–554.

Kraiem, Z., Lahat, N., Glaser, B., Baron, E., Sadeh, O., Sheinfeld, M., et al., 1987. Thyrotrophin receptor blocking antibodies: incidence, characterization and in-vitro synthesis. Clin. Endocrinol. (Oxf.). 27, 409–421.

Laurberg, P., Wallin, G., Tallstedt, L., Abraham-Nordling, M., Lundell, G., Tørring, O., et al., 2008. TSH-receptor autoimmunity in Graves' disease after therapy with anti-thyroid drugs, surgery, or radioiodine: a 5-year prospective randomized study. Eur. J. Endocrinol. 158, 69–75.

Liu, C., Papewalis, C., Domberg, J., Scherbaum, W.A., Schott, M., 2008. Chemokines and autoimmune thyroid diseases. Horm. Metab. Res. 40, 361–368.

Londei, M., Bottazzo, G.F., Feldmann, M., 1985. Human T-cell clones from autoimmune thyroid glands: specific recognition of autologous thyroid cells. Science. 228, 85–89.

MacKenzie, W.A., Schwartz, A.E., Friedman, E.W., Davies, T.F., 1987. Intrathyroidal T cell clones from patients with autoimmune thyroid disease. J. Clin. Endocrinol. Metab. 64, 818–824.

Mao, C., Wang, S., Xiao, Y., Xu, J., Jiang, Q., Jin, M., et al., 2011. Impairment of regulatory capacity of CD4 + CD25 + regulatory T cells mediated by dendritic cell polarization and hyperthyroidism in Graves' disease. J. Immunol. 186, 4734–4743.

Marazuela, M., 1999. Lymphocyte traffic and homing in autoimmune thyroid disorders. Eur. J. Endocrinol. 140, 287–290.

Marazuela, M., García-López, M.A., Figueroa-Vega, N., de la Fuente, H., Alvarado-Sánchez, B., Monsiváis-Urenda, A., et al., 2006. Regulatory T cells in human autoimmune thyroid disease. J. Clin. Endocrinol. Metab. 91, 3639–3646.

Marelli-Berg, F.M., Weetman, A., Frasca, L., Deacock, S.J., Imami, N., Lombardi, G., et al., 1997. Antigen presentation by epithelial cells induces anergic immunoregulatory CD45R0 + T cells and deletion of CD45RA + T cells. J. Immunol. 159, 5853–5861.

Martin, A., Davies, T.F., 1992. T cells and human autoimmune thyroid disease: emerging data show lack of need to invoke suppressor T cell problems. Thyroid. 2, 247–261.

Martin, A.P., Marinkovic, T., Canasto-Chibuque, C., Latif, R., Unkeless, J.C., Davies, T.F., et al., 2009. CCR7 deficiency in NOD mice leads to thyroiditis and primary hypothyroidism. J. Immunol. 183, 3073–3080.

Matsuura, N., Yamada, Y., Nohara, Y., Konishi, J., Kasagi, K., Endo, K., et al., 1980. Familial neonatal transient hypothyroidism due to maternal TSH-binding inhibitor immunoglobulins. N. Engl. J. Med. 303, 738–741.

McIntosh, R., Watson, P., Weetman, A., 1998. Somatic hypermutation in autoimmune thyroid disease. Immunol. Rev. 162, 219–231.

McIntosh, R.S., Watson, P.F., Weetman, A.P., 1997. Analysis of the T cell receptor V alpha repertoire in Hashimoto's thyroiditis: evidence for the restricted accumulation of CD8$^+$ T cells in the absence of CD4$^+$ T cell restriction. J. Clin. Endocrinol. Metab. 82, 1140–1146.

McLachlan, S.M., Rapoport, B., 2007. Thyroid peroxidase as an auto-antigen. Thyroid. 17, 939–948.

McLachlan, S.M., Braley-Mullen, H., Chen, C.R., Aliesky, H., Pichurin, P.N., Rapoport, B., 2005. Dissociation between iodide-induced thyroiditis and antibody-mediated hyperthyroidism in NOD.H-2h4 mice. Endocrinology. 146, 294–300.

McLachlan, S.M., Alpi, K., Rapoport, B., 2011. Review and hypothesis: does Graves' disease develop in non-human great apes? Thyroid. 21, 1359–1366.

Menconi, F., Huber, A., Osman, R., Concepcion, E., Jacobson, E.M., Stefan, M., et al., 2010. Tg.2098 is a major human thyroglobulin T-cell epitope. J. Autoimmun. 35, 45–51.

Michalek, K., Morshed, S.A., Latif, R., Davies, T.F., 2009. TSH receptor autoantibodies. Autoimmun. Rev. 9, 113–116.

Misharin, A.V., Nagayama, Y., Aliesky, H.A., Mizutori, Y., Rapoport, B., McLachlan, S.M., et al., 2009. Attenuation of induced hyperthyroidism in mice by pretreatment with thyrotropin receptor protein: deviation of thyroid-stimulating to nonfunctional antibodies. Endocrinology. 150, 3944–3952.

Mizutori, Y., Chen, C.R., Latrofa, F., McLachlan, S.M., Rapoport, B., 2009. Evidence that shed thyrotropin receptor A subunits drive affinity maturation of autoantibodies causing Graves' disease. J. Clin. Endocrinol. Metab. 94, 927–935.

Mortensen, K.H., Cleemann, L., Hjerrild, B.E., Nexo, E., Locht, H., Jeppesen, E.M., et al., 2009. Increased prevalence of autoimmunity in Turner syndrome—influence of age. Clin. Exp. Immunol. 156, 205–210.

Muller, A.F., Drexhage, H.A., Berghout, A., 2001. Postpartum thyroiditis and autoimmune thyroiditis in women of childbearing age: recent insights and consequences for antenatal and postnatal care. Endocrine Rev. 22, 605–630.

Nagayama, Y., 2007. Graves' animal models of Graves' hyperthyroidism. Thyroid. 17, 981–988.

Naik, V.M., Naik, M.N., Goldberg, R.A., Smith, T.J., Douglas, R.S., 2010. Immunopathogenesis of thyroid eye disease: emerging paradigms. Surv. Ophthalmol. 55, 215–226.

Neumann, S., Eliseeva, E., McCoy, J.G., Napolitano, G., Giuliani, C., Monaco, F., et al., 2011. A new small-molecule antagonist inhibits Graves' disease antibody activation of the TSH receptor. J. Clin. Endocrinol. Metab. 96, 548–554.

Ng, H.P., Kung, A.W., 2006. Induction of autoimmune thyroiditis and hypothyroidism by immunization of immunoactive T cell epitope of thyroid peroxidase. Endocrinology. 147, 3085–3092.

Nilsson, M., Husmark, J., Bjorkman, U., Ericson, L.E., 1998. Cytokines and thyroid epithelial integrity: interleukin-1alpha induces dissociation of the junctional complex and paracellular leakage in filter-cultured human thyrocytes. J. Clin. Endocrinol. Metab. 83, 945–952.

Noble, B., Yoshida, T., Rose, N.R., Bigazzi, P.E., 1976. Thyroid antibodies in spontaneous autoimmune thyroiditis in the Buffalo rat. J. Immunol. 117, 1447–1455.

Okayasu, I., Kong, Y.M., Rose, N.R., 1981. Effect of castration and sex hormones on experimental autoimmune thyroiditis. Clin. Immunol. Immunopathol. 20, 240–245.

Okumura, M., Hidaka, Y., Matsuzuka, F., Takeoka, K., Tada, H., Kuma, K., et al., 1999. CD30 expression and interleukin-4 and interferon-gamma production of intrathyroidal lymphocytes in Graves' disease. Thyroid. 9, 333–339.

Ostroumova, E., Brenner, A., Oliynyk, V., McConnell, R., Robbins, J., Terekhova, G., et al., 2009. Subclinical hypothyroidism after radioiodine exposure: Ukrainian-American cohort study of thyroid cancer and other thyroid diseases after the Chernobyl accident (1998–2000). Environ. Health Perspect. 117, 745–750.

Pearce, E.N., Farwell, A.P., Braverman, L.E., 2003. Thyroiditis. N. Engl. J. Med. 348, 2646–2655.

Penhale, W.J., Young, P.R., 1988. The influence of the normal microbial flora on the susceptibility of rats to experimental autoimmune thyroiditis. Clin. Exp. Immunol. 72, 288–292.

Penhale, W.J., Farmer, A., McKenna, R.P., Irvine, W.J., 1973. Spontaneous thyroiditis in thymectomized and irradiated Wistar rats. Clin. Exp. Immunol. 15, 225–236.

Pfaltz, M., Hedinger, C.E., 1986. Abnormal basement membrane structures in autoimmune thyroid disease. Lab. Invest. 55, 531–539.

Prummel, M.F., Strieder, T., Wiersinga, W.M., 2004. The environment and autoimmune thyroid diseases. Eur. J. Endocrinol. 150, 605–618.

Raber, W., Gessl, A., Nowotny, P., Vierhapper, H., 2002. Thyroid ultrasound versus antithyroid peroxidase antibody determination: a cohort study of four hundred fifty-one subjects. Thyroid. 12, 725–731.

Rapoport, B., McLachlan, S.M., 2007. The thyrotropin receptor in Graves' disease. Thyroid. 17, 911–922.

Rebuffat, S.A., Nguyen, B., Robert, B., Castex, F., Peraldi-Roux, S., 2008. Antithyroperoxidase antibody-dependent cytotoxicity in auto-immune thyroid disease. J. Clin. Endocrinol. Metab. 93, 929–934.

Roberts, C.G., Ladenson, P.W., 2004. Hypothyroidism. Lancet. 363, 793–803.

Rose, N.R., Witebsky, E., 1956. Studies in organ specificity. V. Changes in the thyroid glands of rabbits following active immunization with rabbit thyroid extracts. J. Immunol. 76, 417–427.

Saboori, A.M., Rose, N.R., Yuhasz, S.C., Amzel, L.M., Burek, C.L., 1999. Peptides of human thyroglobulin reactive with sera of patients with autoimmune thyroid disease. J. Immunol. 163, 6244–6250.

Sakaguchi, S., Sakaguchi, N., 1989. Organ-specific autoimmune disease induced in mice by elimination of T cell subsets. V. Neonatal administration of cyclosporin A causes autoimmune disease. J. Immunol. 142, 471–480.

Sakaguchi, S., Sakaguchi, N., Shimizu, J., Yamazaki, S., Sakihama, T., Itoh, M., et al., 2001. Immunologic tolerance maintained by CD25 + CD4 + regulatory T cells: their common role in controlling autoimmunity, tumor immunity, and transplantation tolerance. Immunol. Rev. 182, 18–32.

Sanders, J., Miguel, R.N., Furmaniak, J., Smith, B.R., 2010. TSH receptor monoclonal antibodies with agonist, antagonist, and inverse agonist activities. Meth. Enzymol. 485, 393–420.

Sanders, P., Young, S., Sanders, J., Kabelis, K., Baker, S., Sullivan, A., et al., 2011. Crystal structure of the TSH receptor (TSHR) bound to a blocking-type TSHR autoantibody. J. Mol. Endocrinol. 46, 81–99.

Schwartz, K.M., Fatourechi, V., Ahmed, D.D., Pond, G.R., 2002. Dermopathy of Graves' disease (pretibial myxedema): long-term outcome. J. Clin. Endocrinol. Metab. 87, 438–446.

Schwarz-Lauer, L., Chazenbalk, G.D., McLachlan, S.M., Ochi, Y., Nagayama, Y., Rapoport, B., 2002. Evidence for a simplified view of autoantibody interactions with the thyrotropin receptor. Thyroid. 12, 115–120.

Sempowski, G.D., Cross, S.J., Heinly, C.S., Scearce, R.M., Haynes, B.F., 2004. CD7 and CD28 are required for murine CD4$^+$CD25$^+$ regulatory T cell homeostasis and prevention of thyroiditis. J. Immunol. 172, 787–794.

Stassi, G., Todaro, M., Bucchieri, F., Stoppacciaro, A., Farina, F., Zummo, G., et al., 1999. Fas/Fas ligand-driven T cell apoptosis as a consequence of ineffective thyroid immunoprivilege in Hashimoto's thyroiditis. J. Immunol. 162, 263–267.

Stenszky, V., Kozma, L., Balazs, C., Rochlitz, S., Bear, J.C., Farid, N. R., et al., 1985. The genetics of Graves' disease: HLA and disease susceptibility. J. Clin. Endocrinol. Metab. 61, 735–740.

Stiebel-Kalish, H., Robenshtok, E., Hasanreisoglu, M., Ezrachi, D., Shimon, I., Leibovici, L., et al., 2009. Treatment modalities for Graves' ophthalmopathy: systematic review and metaanalysis. J. Clin. Endocrinol. Metab. 94, 2708–2716.

Strieder, T.G., Prummel, M.F., Tijssen, J.G., Endert, E., Wiersinga, W. M., 2003. Risk factors for and prevalence of thyroid disorders in a cross-sectional study among healthy female relatives of patients with autoimmune thyroid disease. Clin. Endocrinol. (Oxf.). 59, 396–401.

Sugihara, S., Fujiwara, H., Niimi, H., Shearer, G.M., 1995. Self-thyroid epithelial cell (TEC)-reactive CD8 + T cell lines/clones derived from autoimmune thyroiditis lesions. They recognize self-thyroid antigens directly on TEC to exhibit T helper cell 1-type lymphokine production and cytotoxicity against TEC. J. Immunol. 155, 1619–1628.

Takasu, N., Yamada, T., Takasu, M., Komiya, I., Nagasawa, Y., Asawa, T., et al., 1992. Disappearance of thyrotropin-blocking antibodies and spontaneous recovery from hypothyroidism in autoimmune thyroiditis. N. Engl. J. Med. 326, 513–518.

Tandon, N., Freeman, M., Weetman, A.P., 1991. T cell responses to synthetic thyroid peroxidase peptides in autoimmune thyroid disease. Clin. Exp. Immunol. 86, 56–60.

Tandon, N., Freeman, M.A., Weetman, A.P., 1992. T cell responses to synthetic TSH receptor peptides in Graves' disease. Clin. Exp. Immunol. 89, 468–473.

Tandon, N., Yan, S.L., Morgan, B.P., Weetman, A.P., 1994. Expression and function of multiple regulators of complement activation in autoimmune thyroid disease. Immunology. 81, 643–647.

Taylor, J.C., Gough, S.C., Hunt, P.J., Brix, T.H., Chatterjee, K., Connell, J.M., et al., 2006. A genome-wide screen in 1119 relative pairs with autoimmune thyroid disease. J. Clin. Endocrinol. Metab. 91, 646–653.

Tomer, Y., 2010. Genetic susceptibility to autoimmune thyroid disease: past, present, and future. Thyroid. 20, 715–725.

Tomer, Y., Davies, T.F., 1993. Infection, thyroid disease, and autoimmunity. Endocrine Rev. 14, 107–120.

Tomer, Y., Davies, T.F., 2003. Searching for the autoimmune thyroid disease susceptibility genes: from gene mapping to gene function. Endocrine Rev. 24, 694–717.

Ueda, H., Howson, J.M., Esposito, L., Heward, J., Snook, H., Chamberlain, G., et al., 2003. Association of the T-cell regulatory gene CTLA4 with susceptibility to autoimmune disease. Nature. 423, 506–511.

Vladutiu, A.O., Rose, N.R., 1971. Autoimmune murine thyroiditis relation to histocompatibility (H-2) type. Science. 174, 1137–1139.

Volpé, R., 1988. The immunoregulatory disturbance in autoimmune thyroid disease. Autoimmunity. 2, 55–72.

Wang, S.H., Baker, J.R., 2007. The role of apoptosis in thyroid autoimmunity. Thyroid. 17, 975–979.

Watson, P.F., Pickerill, A.P., Davies, R., Weetman, A.P., 1994. Analysis of cytokine gene expression in Graves' disease and multinodular goiter. J. Clin. Endocrinol. Metab. 79, 355–360.

Weetman, A.P., 2000. Graves' disease. New Engl. J. Med. 343, 1236–1248.

Weetman, A.P., 2001. Determinants of autoimmune thyroid disease. Nat. Immunol. 2, 769–770.

Weetman, A.P., 2002. Autoimmune thyroid disease. In: Wass, J.A.H., Shalet, S.M. (Eds.), Oxford Textbook of Endocrinology and Diabetes. Oxford University Press, pp. 392–408.

Weetman, A.P., 2009. Immune reconstitution syndrome and the thyroid. Best Pract. Res. Clin. Endocrinol. Metab. 23, 693–702.

Weetman, A.P., 2010. Immunity, thyroid function and pregnancy: molecular mechanisms. Nat. Rev. Endocrinol. 6, 311–318.

Weetman, A.P., McGregor, A.M., 1994. Autoimmune thyroid disease: further developments in our understanding. Endocrine Rev. 15, 788–830.

Weetman, A.P., McGregor, A.M., Wheeler, M.H., Hall, R., 1984. Extrathyroidal sites of autoantibody synthesis in Graves' disease. Clin. Exp. Immunol. 56, 330–336.

Weetman, A.P., Cohen, S.B., Oleesky, D.A., Morgan, B.P., 1989. Terminal complement complexes and C1/C1 inhibitor complexes in autoimmune thyroid disease. Clin. Exp. Immunol. 77, 25–30.

Weetman, A.P., Freeman, M., Borysiewicz, L.K., Makgoba, M.W., 1990. Functional analysis of intercellular adhesion molecule-1-expressing human thyroid cells. Eur. J. Immunol. 20, 271–275.

Weetman, A.P., Tandon, N., Morgan, B.P., 1992. Antithyroid drugs and release of inflammatory mediators by complement-attacked thyroid cells. Lancet. 340, 633–636.

Wick, G., Andersson, L., Hala, K., Gershwin, M.E., Selmi, C., Erf, G.F., et al., 2006. Avian models with spontaneous autoimmune diseases. Adv. Immunol. 92, 71–117.

Wiersinga, W.M., 2011. Autoimmunity in Graves' ophthalmopathy: the result of an unfortunate marriage between TSH receptors and IGF-1 receptors?. J. Clin. Endocrinol. Metab. 96, 2386–2394.

Winsa, B., Adami, H.O., Bergstrom, R., Gamstedt, A., Dahlberg, P.A., Adamson, U., et al., 1991. Stressful life events and Graves' disease. Lancet. 338, 1475–1479.

Wu, Z., Podack, E.R., McKenzie, J.M., Olsen, K.J., Zakarija, M., 1994. Perforin expression by thyroid-infiltrating T cells in autoimmune thyroid disease. Clin. Exp. Immunol. 98, 470–477.

Yamaguchi, K., Shimojo, N., Kikuoka, S., Hoshioka, A., Hirai, A., Tahara, K., et al., 1997. Genetic control of anti-thyrotropin receptor antibody generation in H-2K mice immunized with thyrotropin receptor-transfected fibroblasts. J. Clin. Endocrinol. Metab. 82, 4266–4269.

Yanagawa, T., Hidaka, Y., Guimaraes, V., Soliman, M., DeGroot, L. J., 1995. CTLA-4 gene polymorphism associated with Graves' disease in a Caucasian population. J. Clin. Endocrinol. Metab. 80, 41–45.

Yoshida, A., Hisatome, I., Taniguchi, S., Shirayoshi, Y., Yamamoto, Y., Miake, J, Ohkura, T., et al., 2009. Pendrin is a novel autoantigen recognized by patients with autoimmune thyroid diseases. J. Clin. Endocrinol. Metab. 94, 442–448.

Yu, S., Fang, Y., Sharp, G.C., Braley-Mullen, H., 2010. Transgenic expression of TGF-beta on thyrocytes inhibits development of spontaneous autoimmune thyroiditis and increases regulatory T cells in thyroids of NOD.H-2h4 mice. J. Immunol. 184, 5352–5359.

Zakarija, M., 1983. Immunochemical characterization of the thyroid-stimulating antibody (TSAb) of Graves' disease: evidence for restricted heterogeneity. J. Clin. Lab. Immunol. 10, 77–85.

Zeitlin, A.A., Simmonds, M.J., Gough, S.C., 2008. Genetic developments in autoimmune thyroid disease: an evolutionary process. Clin. Endocrinol. (Oxford). 68, 671–682.

Zhao, S.X., Tsui, S., Cheung, A., Douglas, R.S., Smith, T.J., Banga, J.P., et al., 2011. Orbital fibrosis in a mouse model of Graves' disease induced by genetic immunization of thyrotropin receptor cDNA. J. Endocrinol. 210, 369–377.

Chapter 41

Autoimmune (Type 1) Diabetes

Ahmed J. Delli and Åke Lernmark

Lund University, Clinical Research Center, Department of Clinical Sciences, Skåne University Hospital SUS, Malmö, Sweden

Chapter Outline

Introduction	575	Pathologic Effector Mechanisms	580
Clinical and Pathologic Features	575	Triggering Autoimmunity	580
Epidemiologic Features	577	APCs in Genetically Predisposed Subjects	581
Genetic Features	578	*In Vivo* and *In Vitro* Models	581
HLA Genetic Factors: The *DR-DQ* Alleles	578	Autoantibodies as Potential Immunologic Markers	582
Non-HLA Genetic Factors	578	Concluding Remarks—Future Prospects	582
Autoimmune Features	580	References	583

INTRODUCTION

Autoimmune (type 1) diabetes (which will be referred to in this chapter as autoimmune diabetes mellitus: AI-DM) is a disease of undetermined etiology and mode of inheritance, in which genetically predisposed individuals are exposed to a group of putative environmental exposures that trigger an aggressive and selective autoimmune response against beta cells. Our understanding of this type of diabetes has improved through years of research along with several alterations in nomenclature (Table 41.1).

AI-DM is a multi-stage disease characterized by a complex and prolonged autoimmune prodrome (pre-diabetes phase) that develops over months to years (Figure 41.1). Several autoimmune markers circulate the peripheral blood and are readily detectable during the prodrome. However, it is only near the end of stage III (Figure 41.1), when the beta cells' secretory reserves are lost, that signs of dysglycemia and eventually hyperglycemia become evident. At this point, the only possible measure to take is to restore euglycemia and its subsequent metabolic disturbance through provision of exogenous insulin. More attention and research needs to be directed to both stage II and the pre-diabetes autoimmune stage III aiming at properly identifying determinants of autoimmune response in order to improve the diagnosis and classification of autoimmune diabetes. Primary prevention should be approached in stage II. However, the only possible cure for this form of diabetes is to halt or reverse the autoimmune response through prevention or intervention measures rather than just replacing the insulin deficiency.

CLINICAL AND PATHOLOGIC FEATURES

The clinical onset of AI-DM follows after a prodromal phase of beta cell autoimmunity that is not associated with any symptoms (Figure 41.1). The diagnosis of diabetes is based on blood glucose level determinations according to combined recommendations of the World Health Organization (WHO) and the American Diabetes Association (ADA, 2013) (Table 41.2). The loss of beta cells varies with age. Young children have lost proportionally more beta cells compared to teenagers, young adults, and adults. The clinical onset is therefore not only a function of a reduced beta cell mass but also of insulin resistance. Young age at onset patients may show classic symptoms such as weight loss, thirst, frequent urination, and hunger. Adult subjects may develop diabetes symptoms that would be consistent with type 2 diabetes (T2D). It is not until beta cell autoantibodies are measured that AI-DM is properly classified. The so-called latent autoimmune diabetes in the adult (LADA) may represent 5–10% of all diabetes diagnosed above 35 years of age (Leslie et al., 2008). LADA is a useful clinical classification that requires the analysis of autoantibodies against the 65K variant of glutamic acid decarboxylase

N. Rose & I. Mackay (Eds): The Autoimmune Diseases, Fifth edition. DOI: http://dx.doi.org/10.1016/B978-0-12-384929-8.00041-1

TABLE 41.1 Variants of Diabetes Mellitus and Nomenclature Used to Describe Autoimmune (Type 1) Diabetes

Nomenclature/Acronym	Period	Basis of Classification
Juvenile diabetes	until 1970	Classification by age
Insulin-dependent diabetes (IDDM)	until 1980	Classification by treatment method
Type 1 diabetes	ongoing	Classification by clinical features
Latent autoimmune diabetes in adults (LADA)	ongoing	Classification by GAD65A positivity in adult T2DM
Latent autoimmune diabetes in the young (LADY)	ongoing	Classification by GAD65A positivity in young T2DM
Slowly progressive insulin-dependent diabetes mellitus (SPIDDM)	ongoing	Classification by clinical features
Autoimmune diabetes mellitus (AI-DM)	Proposed	Classification by immunogenetics

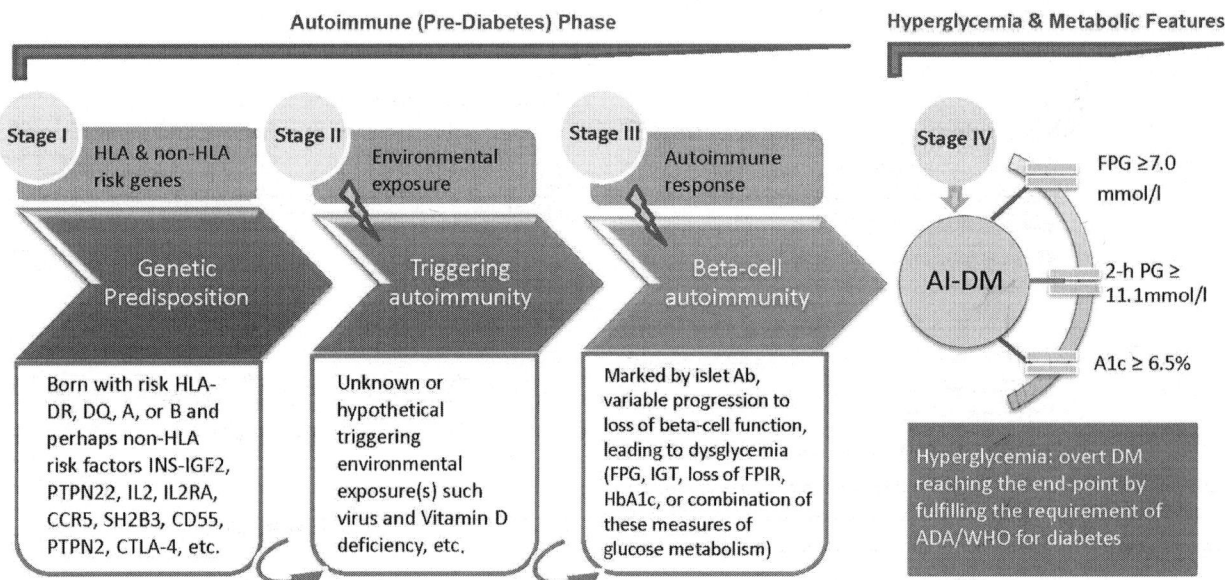

FIGURE 41.1 Stages of Autoimmune Diabetes Mellitus (AI-DM). The preclinical prodrome, which may last several months up to years, represented by three overlapping stages. Stage I represents genetic predisposition, which interacts with putative environmental factors to trigger autoimmune response in stage II. During stage III, islet autoimmunity is initiated and propagated, marked by detectable islet autoantibodies. During stages I–III, prediction, primary, and secondary prevention trials may be initiated to halt autoimmunity and progression to DM. Stage IV represents the final stage of clinical diabetes marked by metabolic consequences of insulin deficiency.

(GAD65A) as it identifies AI-DM that will require treatment with insulin within 5 years of the diagnosis of diabetes (Leslie et al., 2008). The pancreatic islet beta cells are specifically destroyed in the AI-DM. Replacement therapy with insulin is therefore introduced immediately in children and young adults diagnosed with diabetes along with symptoms of thirst, weight loss, and frequent urination. In LADA, insulin therapy will be needed after about 5 years when all other treatment approaches have failed. Insulin therapy is not a cure in AI-DM but a replacement therapy. Currently, there is no alternative to insulin replacement therapy and the many thousands of patients diagnosed each year throughout the world will all be dependent on daily insulin treatment for the rest of their lives.

Historically, the involvement of immune cells in AI-DM was described when inflammatory cell infiltrates, fibrosis, and atrophy of the islets were demonstrated in postmortem pancreatic tissues obtained from some children who died soon following diagnosis (Gepts, 1965). The pathological feature of AI-DM is the conspicuous loss of the pancreatic islet beta cells (Pipeleers et al., 2008). An infiltration of mononuclear cells in islets is often but not always observed (In't Veld, 2011). Insulitits (≥ 2 mononuclear immune cells per islets) appears as a late manifestation and is observed primarily in multiple autoantibody positive subjects prior to clinical diagnosis (In't Veld et al., 2007). Quantitative immunocytochemistry reveals a specific loss of beta cells and that the neighboring cells producing glucagon, somatostatin, pancreatic

TABLE 41.2 Basis of Diagnosis and Classification of Diabetes Mellitus (Current and Proposed)

Current criteria of diabetes diagnosis by the ADA (2013)

At least one of the following criteria is required

A1C ≥6.5% (NGSP & DCCT standardized)	Repeated in absence of unequivocal hyperglycemia
FPG ≥126 mg/dl (7.0 mmol/l)	Repeated in absence of unequivocal hyperglycemia
2-h PG ≥200 mg/dl (11.1 mmol/l) during a WHO standardized OGTT	Repeated in absence of unequivocal hyperglycemia
RPG ≥200 mg/dl (11.1 mmol/l)	In presence of hyperglycemia or hyperglycemia crisis

Criteria for increased risk of diabetes (prediabetes) by the ADA (2013)

FPG ≥100–125 mg/dl (5.6–6.9 mmol/l)	Impaired fasting glucose (IFG)
2-h PG ≥140–199 mg/dl (7.8–11.0 mmol/l)	Impaired glucose tolerance (IGT) during OGTT (WHO)
A1C ≥5.7–6.4%	

Proposed criteria for prediction and diagnosis classification of AI-DM (ongoing research)

HLA class II–DR-DQ alleles	DR4 (B1*04), DR3 (B1*03), DQ8 (B1*03:02), DQ2 (B1*05:02) (Erlich et al., 2008)
Standardized autoimmune markers	(Since 1985 through IDW, DASP and currently IASP)

Autoantigen	Marker	Abbreviation
Insulin	insulin autoantibodies	IAA
GAD65	GAD	GAD65A
Islet antigen-2	IA-2 and IA-2β	IA-2A
Zinc transporter 8 three variants	ZnT8-R (arginine), W (tryptophan) and Q (glutamine)	ZnT8-RA, ZnT8-WA, ZnT8-QA

polypeptide, or ghrelin are not affected. In subjects with insulitis, the islets of Langerhans may be infiltrated by T and B lymphocytes as well as monocytes and dendritic cells supporting a state of chronic inflammation (Eizirik et al., 2009). In some insulitis-positive islets it has been possible to demonstrate markers of inflammation along with viral antigens (Foulis et al., 1991; Foulis, 2008). The known insulitis characteristics are derived from specimens that mostly reflect an advanced stage of the disease or more extensive form of it when obtained from postmortem autopsies. Little is understood about early stages of propagation of autoimmune pathologic features in the prolonged pre-diabetes phase. T lymphocytes, especially the CD4+ and CD8+ cell subsets, dominate the insulitis (Pinkse et al., 2005), compared to B lymphocytes, and may be found in larger populations in the islets (Kent et al., 2005). Therefore, the infiltration of pancreatic islets by inflammatory cells, beta cell destruction and the resulting insulitis is a multi-step process, which may vary widely in duration and intensity before diabetes becomes clinically manifest. Furthermore, in recent-onset AI-DM, residual beta cell function was temporarily preserved through the use of monoclonal antibodies targeting CD3 on T lymphocytes (Herold et al., 2002), CD20 on B lymphocytes (Pescovitz et al., 2009), or drugs such as cyclosporine targeting monocyte/macrophage populations (Bougneres et al., 1988). These observations in addition to the significant role of cellular immunological pathway, predominantly CD8+ lymphocytes, suggest that AI-DM is primarily a cell-mediated autoimmune disease (Notkins

and Lernmark, 2001; Willcox et al., 2009). However, in the absence of specific cellular assays, stage III is defined by islet autoantibodies (Figure 41.1). The islet autoantibodies therefore represent predictive markers of an ongoing autoimmune response, yet their exact role in beta cell destruction remains to be clarified.

EPIDEMIOLOGIC FEATURES

The epidemiology of stage III AI-DM (Figure 41.1) is essentially unknown. Studies such as DIPP, BABYDIAB (Schenker et al., 1999), DAISY (Rewers et al., 1996), and DiPiS (Larsson et al., 2005) have screened newborns for AI-DM high risk human leukocyte antigen (HLA). There are four standardized tests for diabetes-relevant autoantibodies: against insulin, glutamic acid decarboxylase (GAD65), islet antigen-2 (IA-2), and the zinc transporter 8 (ZnT8) (Pietropaolo et al., 2012). All have been used to follow high HLA risk children longitudinally. Children with low risk HLA genotypes are yet to be followed. Persistent autoantibody positivity (more than 3 months) would detect AI-DM stage III. However, its epidemiology remains unknown as there is a paucity of studies screening, e.g., schoolchildren (Schlosser et al., 2002).

It is generally accepted that up to 10% of all diabetes in different age groups are classifiable as type 1 or autoimmune (ADA, 2013). In obese patients, it may sometimes be difficult to discriminate between AI-DM and T2D especially in adolescents and young adults (Pozzilli et al., 2011) and shared pathways in such patients may be present (Libman and Becker, 2003). The occurrence of AI-DM varies according to ethnic heritage and geographical locations where high-incidence regions are seen in populations of European descent especially Scandinavia (Karvonen et al., 2000). Recent estimates suggest that the annual rise in incidence of AI-DM among children under 15 years is 3% (2–5%) worldwide including low prevalence populations (IDF, 2011). AI-DM constitutes more than 85% of diabetes phenotypes in patients under 20 years in most populations (Vandewalle et al., 1997; Craig et al., 2006; Thunander et al., 2008) but it may also show a second peak between 50 and 65 years (Lorenzen et al., 1994). Nearly a quarter of patients become clinically evident during adulthood (Haller et al., 2005).

In younger patients, most AI-DM patients become clinically evident around or shortly after puberty (12–15 years in most countries), but it may be diagnosed as early as 9 months of age. This peak incidence around puberty (EURODIAB, 2000; Dabelea et al., 2007) is proposed to be related to spur of growth and upsurge metabolic demand. The highest rise in incidence was seen in younger individuals, especially preschool children indicating an increasing role of environmental factors (EURODIAB, 2000; Pundziute-Lycka et al., 2002; Berhan et al., 2011). Only 15% of newly diagnosed AI-DM patients have a first degree relative with the disease. Overall, AI-DM shows a slight male preference, which becomes evident after puberty up to 35 years (Pundziute-Lycka et al., 2002; Kyvik et al., 2004), a phenomenon that was partly linked to lack of the high risk HLA DQ2/8 genotype (Weets et al., 2004). Another significant indicator of environmental factors to the autoimmunity is the seasonal patterns of birth (Samuelsson et al., 1999; Mckinney, 2001; Willis et al., 2002; Kahn et al., 2009) and timing of diagnosis (Padaiga et al., 1999; Willis et al., 2002). The higher frequency of incident patients in colder months (Padaiga et al., 1999; Willis et al., 2002). and season of birth in spring (Mckinney, 2001) were correlated to exposure to cycles of viral infections (Knip et al., 2005) during early childhood and gestational life, respectively.

GENETIC FEATURES

AI-DM-associated genetic factors are essential yet not sufficient causal factors (Notkins and Lernmark, 2001). Among these there are more than 50 different loci on 12 chromosomes linked to AI-DM (Table 41.3). HLA class II alleles of the major histocompatibility complex (MHC) on chromosome 6p21 are the most important (Todd et al., 2007). The majority of implicated genes are essentially related to the immune response rather than predisposing to diabetes and metabolic derangements. Only few genes such as INS and ERBB3 may modulate beta cell function through affecting insulin secretion and

metabolism. Other genes such as TNFAIP3 are related to mechanisms of cell apoptosis (Todd et al., 2007; Concannon et al., 2009).

HLA Genetic Factors: The DR-DQ Alleles

The HLA-DR-DQ alleles are linked to susceptibility to AI-DM (Todd et al., 2007) and also several other autoimmune diseases such as celiac disease, multiple sclerosis, and rheumatoid arthritis, but some alleles provide protection from these diseases (Nerup et al., 1974; Owerbach et al., 1983). The AI-DM risk alleles may be found in up to 50% of the general population but only a smaller proportion develops the disease (Knip et al., 2005). The DQ8 (A1*03:01-B1*03:02) and DQ2 (A1*05:01-B1*02:01) haplotypes confer the strongest risk (Schranz and Lernmark, 1998; Erlich et al., 2008). These haplotypes share a linkage disequilibrium (LD) relationship with the DR4 (B1*04) and DR3 (B1*03), respectively (Hermann et al., 2004). Almost 90% of AI-DM patients diagnosed before 35 years of age carry one or both of these two haplotypes (Kockum et al., 1999; Komulainen et al., 1999; Graham et al., 2002). The DR3-DQ2/DR4-DQ8 genotype may be detected in 30% of patients <15 years and up to 50% of autoantibody-positive children under 5 years (AI-DM stage III) but only 2.4% of the general population (Rewers et al., 1996; Thomson et al., 2007). A sibling who is DR3-DQ2/DR4-DQ8 identical to a diabetic proband has almost 80% risk to develop islet autoantibodies and 60% for diabetes by the age of 15 years. The other main susceptibility genotypes are the homozygous DR4-DQ8/DR4-DQ8 and DR3-DQ2/DR3-DQ2 (Erlich et al., 2008).

It is frequently tested whether HLA class I genes confer risk for AI-DM independent of HLA class II (Noble et al., 2002; Aly et al., 2006; Nejentsev et al., 2007). The HLA-A*24, A*02:01, A*03:02, A*01:01, and also B*39 were associated with a lower age of onset. The A*02 allele was found to add to the class II risk haplotypes such DR4-DQ8 (Fennessy et al., 1994), while others such as the (B18 Ah 18.2) haplotype may modulate the risk of DR3-DQ2. However, as HLA class I and II genes are in strong LD, it is problematic to prove independent contributions to AI-DM risk.

Non-HLA Genetic Factors

A larger group of non-MHC genes were implicated to contribute by up to half of the AI-DM genetic risk in families with AI-DM (Risch, 1989). As indicated in Table 41.3, the majority of these genes function through regulating autoimmune responses; however, the risk of each single gene is markedly less than HLA class II (Todd et al., 2007; Todd, 2010). The genetic marker of the candidate gene/region, its chromosome location, and

TABLE 41.3 The Significant HLA and Non-HLA Genes (Confirmed Associations Loci) Associated with Autoimmune Diabetes Mellitus, Listed by Relative Risks (RR) between Homozygous

Gene/Region Chromosome Location	Marker(s)	Proposed Function	Mechanism of Action in AI-DM	Role in other AI Diseases
MHC/HLA-DRB1, DQB1, A, B. Chr.6p21	rs9268645	Expressed on surface of APCs, present antigen to T lymphocytes through interaction with TCR	Immune response	Other markers: CD, RA, MS, SLE
PTPN22 Chr.1p13	rs2476601, rs6679677	Modulates protein kinases activation through encoding protein tyrosine kinase leading to negative regulation of T cell activation	Immune response	ATD, RA, SLE, JIA, Crohn's, vitiligo
INS, INS-IGF2 Chr.11p15	rs689, rs7111341	Facilitate central tolerance through expression of insulin in the thymus	Glucose metabolism	–
IL2, IL21 Chr.4q27	rs13119723, rs13132308, rs17388568, rs2069762, rs2069763, rs4505848, rs6822844	Maintain regulatory T lymphocytes and T and B lymphocyte proliferation. Stimulate B lymphocytes and other APCs	Immune response	Celiac, RA, UC
CCR5 Chr.3p21	rs11711054, rs2097282, rs333	Chemokine receptor 5, may be important in regulating lymphocyte trafficking	Immune response	CD
SH2B3 Chr.12q24	rs3184504, rs653178, rs7137828	Encodes a negative regulator (LNK) of cell-signaling events from some receptors, including the TCR	Immune response	JIA, MS, RA
PTPN2 Chr.18p11	rs1893217, rs2847293, rs45450798, rs478582	Possible association with growth factor mediated cell signaling pathway	Immune response	CD, JIA, Crohn's, UC
IL2RA Chr.10p15	rs11594656, rs12251307, rs12722495, rs2104286, rs7090512, rs7909519	Serves as a receptor for interleukin-2, may have a significant role in proliferation of immune cells populations	Immune response	JIA, MS, RA, vitiligo
CD55, IL10 Chr.1q32	rs3024505	Causes polymorphism in the decay accelerating factor that restricts complement activation	Immune response	Crohn's, SLE, UC
CTLA-4 Chr.2q33	rs11571297, rs11571302, rs3087243	Minimize tissue damage and AI response through regulating the activation of T lymphocytes	Immune response	ATD, RA CD
IFH1 (MDA-5) Chr.2q24	rs1990760, rs2111485	When MDA5 binds to viral RNA, it may trigger production of type 1 interferon (a and b), which may enhance CD8$^+$ activity in islets.	Immune response	Graves', SLE, UC
GLIS3 Chr.9p24	rs7020673	GLIS3 transcription factor that is thought to be an autoantigen	Immune response	–
IKZF1 Chr.7p12	rs10272724	Encodes Ikaros, which is an essential regulator of lymphopoiesis and immune homeostasis	Immune response	–
UBASH3A Chr.21q22	rs11203203, rs3788013	Enhances accumulation of activated target receptors, such as TCRs, EGFR, and PDGFRB	Immune response	RA, vitiligo
BACH2 Chr.6q15	rs10806425, rs11755527	Encodes a B cell-specific transcription factor	Immune response	CD
TNFAIP3 Chr.6q23	rs10499194, rs13192841, rs17264332, rs2327832, rs6920220	May be related to mechanisms of beta cells apoptosis	Cellular apoptosis	CD, MS, RA, SLE, UC
ERBB3 Chr.12q13	rs2292239	Modulation of beta cell function and insulin secretion and metabolism	Beta cell function	–

For detailed information see http://www.t1dbase.org/.
APCs: antigen presenting cells; ATD: autoimmune thyroiditis; CD: celiac disease; JIA: juvenile idiopathic arthritis; MS: multiple sclerosis; RA: rheumatoid arthritis; SLE: systemic lupus erythematosus; UC: ulcerative colitis.
After Todd (2010).

proposed function are all summarized in Table 41.3. The possible importance of the non-HLA genetic factors in relation to AI-DM stage II (Figure 41.1) is yet to be investigated. However, it cannot be excluded that the virus-response gene *IFIH1*, also known as MDA-5 and *INS* controlling insulin gene expression in the thymus, may contribute. It will also be important to dissect to what extent the different non-HLA gene variants contribute to the variable rate of progression during AI-DM stage III.

AUTOIMMUNE FEATURES

The defining feature of AI-DM is islet (beta cell) autoimmunity (Notkins and Lernmark, 2001). The detection of islet autoantibodies in peripheral blood is currently considered as the earliest sign of AI-DM (Achenbach et al., 2005). The availability of standardized islet autoantibody tests may be used to distinguish AI-DM from other forms of diabetes (Table 41.2). Four major autoantigens have been identified in AI-DM along with a growing list of minor autoantigens (Hirai et al., 2008). Proinsulin is the exclusive beta cell-specific antigen (Pugliese et al., 2001) and insulin was described as a major target for the T lymphocyte attack especially in young children. GAD65 is specific for beta cells but is expressed in other cells as well (Karlsen et al., 1991). The IA-2 and the isoform IA-2β are important antigens especially in carriers of the HLA-DQ8 haplotype (Delli et al., 2010). The development of persistent (>3 months) single or multiple (≥2) islet autoantibodies is thought to occur shortly following killing of beta cells but this seems to occur regardless of insulitis (In't Veld et al., 2007). A larger group of minor autoantigens have also been proposed; however, the roles of T and B lymphocyte reactivity as well as autoantibodies against most of these autoantigens are not fully determined. Among these autoantigens are the secretory vesicle-associated proteins, chromogranin A, VAMP2 and NPY, HSP-60 and HSP-70, IGRP, Glima-38, and many others (for a detailed list see Wenzlau et al., 2008). It cannot be excluded that autoimmunity against these minor autoantigens reflects antigen and epitope spreading (Morran et al., 2008), meaning presentation of new antigen to inflammatory cells of the immune system leading to activation of new T lymphocytes.

The central role in autoimmune responses against islet autoantigens is related to the structural features of the HLA class II molecules and their interaction with T lymphocytes. Some of the HLA alleles coding these molecules may modify the timing, intensity, and rate of an autoimmune response and thereby affect the autoimmune feature of AI-DM. The *DQA* and *DQB* loci code for the alpha and beta subunits, the two chains of the HLA-DQ heterodimer molecules. These molecules are expressed on the cell surfaces of antigen presenting cells (APCs) and allow presentation of peptide antigens to T lymphocytes through the T lymphocyte antigen receptor (TCR). The binding of islet autoantigen peptides to HLA-DQ molecules was found to modulate the autoimmune response differentially (Eerligh et al., 2011). Binding insulin peptides to DQ8 molecules induced proinflammatory responses while binding to DQ6 molecules induced regulatory T lymphocyte responses (Eerligh et al., 2011). These differences may be related to structural differences in the DQ molecules and the affinity of these molecules to accommodate certain antigens and

thereby facilitate thymic recognition of such antigens as "self" or propagate proinflammatory response leading to activation of autoreactive T lymphocytes. Structural studies of autoantigen peptide binding to HLA-DQ2, 8, and 6.4 have suggested differences that may be related to features of AI-DM (Delli et al., 2012). It was proposed that the DQ2 heterodimer has the ability to bind multiple peptides due to a wider binding groove compared to DQ8 which is less accommodating (Lee et al., 2001; Suri et al., 2005). Structural differences between the risk-conferring alleles such as DQ8 and DQ2 and the protective allele DQ6 were suggested to modify their binding properties through modification of the volume and polarity of binding grooves (Jones et al., 2006). Similarly, HLA-DQ6.4, which is strongly associated with ZnT8 autoantibodies, showed an epitope binding pattern that would be consistent with a reduction in ZnT8 peptide presentation in the thymus. It has been speculated that a reduction in thymic presentation increases the risk for autoimmunity (Pugliese et al., 1997; Delli et al., 2012).

PATHOLOGIC EFFECTOR MECHANISMS

Triggering Autoimmunity

Normally, the HLA—autoantigen complex in the thymus presents weak and low affinity signals to T lymphocytes, which will be educated (positive selection) to identify self-antigen as "self." If these signals were deficient or were too strong, these T lymphocytes will be deleted (negative selection) as part of central tolerance induction (Ohashi, 2003). In the periphery, T regulatory (Treg) cells help to maintain normal non-responsiveness to "self" antigens through eliminating autoreactive T lymphocytes that escape negative selection in the thymus by a process called "clonal deletion," which is part of peripheral tolerance. In AI-DM, there is loss of the normal regulatory immune mechanisms, which assist in recognition of self-antigen (Morran et al., 2008). An imbalance between regulatory (Treg) and effector T lymphocytes has been described (Brusko et al., 2008), and the balance between regulatory CD4$^+$CD25$^+$ and CD4$^+$ and CD8$^+$ T lymphocytes is distorted (Brusko et al., 2008; Morran et al., 2008). The interaction between environmental and genetic factors (risk-conferring HLA alleles) may disrupt normal tolerance mechanisms and initiate or promote an aggressive autoimmune response. Many environmental factors, most importantly virus infections, have been incriminated in triggering such autoimmune response (Knip et al., 2005). It cannot be excluded that molecular mimicry may contribute. Coxsackievirus shares the sequence PEVKEK with GAD65 and it has been proposed that this type of molecular mimicry may explain the association between the virus and AI-DM (Atkinson et al., 1994). Direct viral infection of beta cells may induce local inflammatory mechanisms, secretion of proinflammatory cytokines, and involvement of APCs. This activation may elicit autoimmune response and autoreactive T lymphocytes activation; however, it has been suggested that these T lymphocytes need to be provoked by molecular mechanisms before being able to propagate autoimmunity (von Herrath et al., 2003). Other mechanisms of triggering islet autoimmunity are yet to be elucidated.

APCs in Genetically Predisposed Subjects

The cellular pathway of the immune system plays a more significant role than the humoral pathway; the CD8$^+$ autoreactive T lymphocytes are the most abundant (Pinkse et al., 2005) and the most active in beta cell destruction (Imagawa et al., 2001). It is proposed that following exposure to a putative antigen, the APCs residing in the islet process and present the autoantigen and drive CD4$^+$ T lymphocyte activation through expression of surface markers (Gepts, 1965). These APCs, including macrophages, monocytes, and dendritic cells, also express immunological abnormalities (Jansen et al., 1995; Litherland et al., 1999; Plesner et al., 2002). Antigen presentation is facilitated by the HLA class II heterodimer molecules expressed on the surfaces of these cells. The presence of risk alleles such as DQB1*03:02 or predominantly non-risk alleles such as DQ6B1*06:02 determines the magnitude and pace of beta cell killing.

CD4$^+$ cells drive and activate CD8$^+$ cells in the regional lymph nodes through formation of complexes between the autoantigen and the TCR. Once activated these autoreactive T lymphocytes will invade islets and attack and destroy beta cells (Baekkeskov et al., 1990). This is possible as antigen presentation occurs directly on the cell surface of the beta cells with the help of HLA class I molecules. CD4$^+$ may initiate direct killing of beta cells through secretion of proinflammatory mediators (Amrani et al., 2000; Plesner et al., 2002) or through inviting autoreactive CD8$^+$ T lymphocytes. Activated T lymphocytes may also secrete inflammatory mediators such as cytokines, chemokines, and perforin, which are toxic to beta cells. Simultaneously, macrophages invading the islets produce proinflammatory cytokines (such as interferon (IFN)-γ, tumor necrosis factor (TNF)-α, and interleukin (IL)-1β) and chemokines (Plesner et al., 2002) thereby recruiting additional T lymphocytes, macrophages, and dendritic cells. Cytokines are short polypeptides that serve as signaling mediators of inflammatory processes. The destruction of beta cells will expose intracellular "antigenic" component to APCs, which will further induce antigen presentation and T lymphocyte activation. This cycle of complex autoimmune interactions may be present for variable duration before the reserves of beta cells are severely diminished and hyperglycemia becomes inevitable. It is proposed

that the balance between the CD4$^+$ T-helper (Th1) and the (Th2) pathways may also be distorted by various factors including infections and stress (Ernerudh et al., 2004). Whereas the cellular mechanisms of the Th2 pathway appear to conserve beta cells, cytokines of the Th1 pathways are the likely contributors to the inflammatory process in the islets as combinations of cytokines may be toxic to beta cells and enhance the immune reactions.

B lymphocytes can also act as APCs and may present putative islet autoantigen epitopes to CD4$^+$ helper cells, which in turn invite CD8$^+$ T lymphocytes from regional lymph nodes to invade the islets. The possible role of B lymphocytes in early AI-DM stage III and late stage IV has been understudied clearly demonstrated by the ability of the CD20 monoclonal antibody rituximab that was shown to delay the loss of endogenous insulin production following the clinical onset of AI-DM (Pescovitz et al., 2009). The Rituximab-treated AI-DM patients failed to mount an immune response to neoantigens including insulin, which may temporarily have reduced disease progression.

IN VIVO AND IN VITRO MODELS

Several animal species were studied as models for AI-DM, although their diabetes phenotype was found to differ from the human type. Nevertheless, research on these animals has yielded valuable guidance to human diabetes, where ethical issues or difficulties in obtaining human pancreatic samples may limit research. AI-DM-like syndromes develop spontaneously in the BB rat (Mordes et al., 2004), the LEW.1AR1-iddm rat (Jorns et al., 2010), and the Komeda diabetes-prone (KDP) rats (Yokoi et al., 2003). All three strains of rat have features similar to human AI-DM; however, the cause (stage II, Figure 41.1) is mutations in different genes. Diabetes in all three rats is RT1.u, an ortholog of HLA-DQ2. None of the rats develop islet autoantibodies that predict AI-DM (stage III, Figure 41.1). The non-obese diabetes (NOD) mouse, which also develops diabetes with features comparable to human AI-DM, has been studied extensively (for reviews see Mathis et al., 2001; Thayer et al., 2010; Driver et al., 2011). The NOD mouse and its many congenic lines may be useful to dissect the genetic and pathogenic basis for T lymphocyte-mediated AI-DM. However, while sharing many similarities, it is becoming increasingly clear that there are not trivial but major differences in immunopathogenesis between humans and NOD mice. Combination therapy with rapamycin and IL-2 prevented NOD mouse diabetes (Rabinovitch et al., 2002) but accelerated the loss of residual beta cell function in newly diagnosed AI-DM patients (Long et al., 2012). Wild bank voles (Myodes glareolus) were reported to develop diabetes in laboratory captivity in association with autoantibodies against GAD65, IA-2, and insulin in standardized radioligand-binding assays as well as antibodies to *in vitro* transcribed and translated Ljungan virus antigens. It was speculated that bank voles may have a possible zoonotic role as a reservoir and vector for a virus that may contribute to human AI-DM (Niklasson et al., 2003).

AUTOANTIBODIES AS POTENTIAL IMMUNOLOGIC MARKERS

Islet autoantibodies are an important indicator of progression to diabetes as well as the disease outcome (Harel and Shoenfeld, 2006). The type and number of these autoantibodies signify the advancement of islet autoimmunity and therefore predict AI-DM not only in first degree relatives (FDR) (Verge et al., 1996) but also in subjects from the general population (Bingley et al., 1997). Islet cell autoantibodies have been standardized in international workshops since 1985 (Gleichmann and Bottazzo, 1987). A WHO standard assay for autoantibodies against GAD65 and IA-2 was established by the Immunology of Diabetes Workshops (IDW) (Mire-Sluis et al., 2000) and further developed by the Diabetes Autoantibody (DASP) and Islet Autoantibody Standardization Programs (IASP) (Torn et al., 2008; Schlosser et al., 2010; Lampasona et al., 2011). The inter-laboratory variation in analyzing autoantibodies to insulin, GAD65, IA-2, and ZnT8 has been reduced through the use of common standards in subsequent workshops.

Autoantibodies against all four autoantigens are used to follow children at increased genetic risk from birth to determine triggers of islet autoimmunity (stage II, Figure 41.1) (Hagopian et al., 2011; Ziegler et al., 2013), randomize subjects to secondary prevention trials (Yu et al., 2012) as well as to improve clinical classification (Delli et al., 2012). Interestingly, nearly half of all younger patients who were autoantibody negative at the time of diagnosis showed later sero-conversion (Hameed et al., 2011) indicating that islet autoantibodies may exist invariably in pre- and post- as well as at the time of diagnosis. Islet autoantibodies therefore remain robust markers of AI-DM and should prove useful to assist progress towards assays that better reflect environmental exposures (stage II, Figure 41.1) as well as sero-conversion (stage III, Figure 41.1).

The mechanisms that are responsible for the variable progression to clinical onset during stage III are poorly understood. Standardized islet autoantibody tests, primarily in first degree relatives but also in subjects from the general population, have proven useful to predict the clinical onset (Yu et al., 2012; Ziegler et al., 2013). Parallel testing for autoantibodies against GAD65 and IA-2 followed by insulin autoantibodies was found to identify 50% of patients younger than 20 years and was associated with a 71% risk within 10 years (Bingley et al., 1999). In FDR at 20−39 years of age, this strategy conferred a 51% risk. Primary screening for anti-IA-2 and anti-GAD65 autoantibodies followed by testing for insulin autoantibodies conferred a 63% risk to develop diabetes. Further studies also including subjects from the general population such as in studies of children followed since birth because of increased genetic risk for AI-DM have been reported (Hagopian et al., 2011; Ziegler et al., 2013).

CONCLUDING REMARKS—FUTURE PROSPECTS

Our understanding of the etiology and pathogenesis of AI-DM is progressing rapidly through several major efforts. First, the sequencing of the human genome has made it possible to better define the genetic contribution to the risk of islet autoimmunity and diabetes (stage I, Figure 41.1). Further studies are needed to better understand the level of genetic propensity for AI-DM when moving between countries. Second, studies from birth may uncover triggers (stage II, Figure 41.1) that launch sero-conversion. Recent data that sero-conversion tends to occur during the first 3 years of life suggest that environmental exposures in early life may have a unique impact on children with increased genetic risk for islet autoimmunity and diabetes. Third, detection, characterization, and development of standardized autoantibody assays to islet autoantigens should prove useful to uncover part of the variable progress to the clinical onset of diabetes (stage III, Figure 41.1). At present, the larger the number of islet autoantibodies, the greater the risk for clinical onset. Fourth, a current challenge is therefore to remedy the paucity of cellular studies to better uncover the series of events that contribute to islet autoimmunity. It will also be a challenge to define the APC, T and B lymphocytes during the chronic stage III of islet autoimmunity and their contribution to the variable rate of beta cell destruction. Fifth, the more than 50 non-HLA genes should be scrutinized one by one to reveal their possible contribution to the variable progression. These non-HLA genetic factors may also represent potential drug targets for secondary prevention or intervention. The limited success in secondary prevention and intervention studies with immunosuppressive agents suggest that novel approaches perhaps in combination trials with islet autoantigens will be required to successfully halt progression to clinical onset or the loss of endogenous beta cell function that invariably takes place after the clinical diagnosis.

REFERENCES

Achenbach, P., Bonifacio, E., Ziegler, A.G., 2005. Predicting type 1 diabetes. Curr. Diab. Rep. 5, 98–103.

ADA, 2013. Diagnosis and classification of diabetes mellitus. Diabetes Care. 36 (Suppl 1), S67–S74.

Aly, T.A., Ide, A., Jahromi, M.M., Barker, J.M., Fernando, M.S., Babu, S.R., et al., 2006. Extreme genetic risk for type 1A diabetes. Proc. Natl. Acad. Sci. U.S.A. 103, 14074–14079.

Amrani, A., Verdaguer, J., Thiessen, S., Bou, S., Santamaria, P., 2000. IL-1alpha, IL-1beta, and IFN-gamma mark beta cells for Fas-dependent destruction by diabetogenic CD4(+) T lymphocytes. J. Clin. Invest. 105, 459–468.

Atkinson, M.A., Bowman, M.A., Campbell, L., Darrow, B.L., Kaufman, D.L., MacLaren, N.K., 1994. Cellular immunity to a determinant common to glutamate decarboxylase and coxsackie virus in insulin-dependent diabetes. J. Clin. Invest. 94, 2125–2129.

Baekkeskov, S., Aanstoot, H.J., Christgau, S., Reetz, A., Solimena, M., Cascalho, M., et al., 1990. Identification of the 64K autoantigen in insulin-dependent diabetes as the GABA-synthesizing enzyme glutamic acid decarboxylase. Nature. 347, 151–156.

Berhan, Y., Waernbaum, I., Lind, T., Mollsten, A., Dahlquist, G., 2011. Thirty years of prospective nationwide incidence of childhood type 1 diabetes: the accelerating increase by time tends to level off in Sweden. Diabetes. 60, 577–581.

Bingley, P.J., Bonifacio, E., Williams, A.J., Genovese, S., Bottazzo, G. F., Gale, E.A., 1997. Prediction of IDDM in the general population: strategies based on combinations of autoantibody markers. Diabetes. 46, 1701–1710.

Bingley, P.J., Williams, A.J., Gale, E.A., 1999. Optimized autoantibody-based risk assessment in family members. Implications for future intervention trials. Diabetes Care. 22, 1796–1801.

Bougneres, P.F., Carel, J.C., Castano, L., Boitard, C., Gardin, J.P., Landais, P., et al., 1988. Factors associated with early remission of type I diabetes in children treated with cyclosporine. N. Engl. J. Med. 318, 663–670.

Brusko, T.M., Putnam, A.L., Bluestone, J.A., 2008. Human regulatory T cells: role in autoimmune disease and therapeutic opportunities. Immunol. Rev. 223, 371–390.

Concannon, P., Rich, S.S., Nepom, G.T., 2009. Genetics of type 1A diabetes. N. Engl. J. Med. 360, 1646–1654.

Craig, M.E., Hattersley, A., Donaghue, K., 2006. ISPAD Clinical Practice Consensus Guidelines 2006–2007. Definition, epidemiology and classification. Pediatr. Diabetes. 7, 343–351.

Dabelea, D., Bell, R.A., D'Agostino Jr., R.B., Imperatore, G., Johansen, J.M., Linder, B., et al., 2007. Incidence of diabetes in youth in the United States. JAMA. 297, 2716–2724.

Delli, A.J., Lindblad, B., Carlsson, A., Forsander, G., Ivarsson, S.A., Ludvigsson, J., et al., 2010. Type 1 diabetes patients born to immigrants to Sweden increase their native diabetes risk and differ from Swedish patients in HLA types and islet autoantibodies. Pediatr. Diabetes. 11, 513–520.

Delli, A.J., Vaziri-Sani, F., Lindblad, B., Elding-Larsson, H., Carlsson, A., Forsander, F., et al., 2012. Zinc transporter 8 autoantibodies and their association with SLC30A8 and HLA-DQ genes differ between immigrant and Swedish patients with newly diagnosed type 1 diabetes in the Better Diabetes Diagnosis study. Diabetes. 61, 2556–2564.

Driver, J.P., Serreze, D.V., Chen, Y.G., 2011. Mouse models for the study of autoimmune type 1 diabetes: a NOD to similarities and differences to human disease. Semin. Immunopathol. 33, 67–87.

Eerligh, P., Van Lummel, M., Zaldumbide, A., Moustakas, A.K., Duinkerken, G., Bondinas, G., et al., 2011. Functional consequences of HLA-DQ8 homozygosity versus heterozygosity for islet autoimmunity in type 1 diabetes. Genes Immun. 12, 415–427

Eizirik, D.L., Colli, M.L., Ortis, F., 2009. The role of inflammation in insulitis and beta-cell loss in type 1 diabetes. Nat. Rev. Endocrinol. 5, 219–226.

Erlich, H., Valdes, A.M., Noble, J., Carlson, J.A., Varney, M., Concannon, P., et al., 2008. HLA DR-DQ haplotypes and genotypes and type 1 diabetes risk: analysis of the type 1 diabetes genetics consortium families. Diabetes. 57, 1084–1092.

Ernerudh, J., Ludvigsson, J., Berlin, G., Samuelsson, U., 2004. Effect of photopheresis on lymphocyte population in children with newly diagnosed type 1 diabetes. Clin. Diagn. Lab. Immunol. 11, 856–861.

Fennessy, M., Metcalfe, K., Hitman, G.A., Niven, M., Biro, P.A., Tuomilehto, J., et al., 1994. A gene in the HLA class I region contributes to susceptibility to IDDM in the Finnish population. Childhood Diabetes in Finland (DiMe) Study Group. Diabetologia. 37, 937–944.

EURODIAB, 2000. Variation and trends in incidence of childhood diabetes in Europe. EURODIAB ACE Study Group. Lancet. 355, 873–876.

Foulis, A.K., 2008. Pancreatic pathology in type 1 diabetes in human. Novartis Found. Symp. 292, 2–13, discussion 13–18, 122–129, 202–203.

Foulis, A.K., McGill, M., Farquharson, M.A., 1991. Insulitis in type 1 (insulin-dependent) diabetes mellitus in man--macrophages, lymphocytes, and interferon-gamma containing cells. J. Pathol. 165, 97–103.

Gepts, W., 1965. Pathologic anatomy of the pancreas in juvenile diabetes mellitus. Diabetes. 14, 619–633.

Gleichmann, H., Bottazzo, G.F., 1987. Progress toward standardization of cytoplasmic islet cell-antibody assay. Diabetes. 36, 578–584.

Graham, J., Hagopian, W.A., Kockum, I., Li, L.S., Sanjeevi, C.B., Lowe, R.M., et al., 2002. Genetic effects on age-dependent onset and islet cell autoantibody markers in type 1 diabetes. Diabetes. 51, 1346–1355.

Hagopian, W.A., Erlich, H., Lernmark, A., Rewers, M., Ziegler, A.G., Simell, O., et al., 2011. The Environmental Determinants of Diabetes in the Young (TEDDY): genetic criteria and international diabetes risk screening of 421 000 infants. Pediatr. Diabetes. 12, 733–743.

Haller, M.J., Atkinson, M.A., Schatz, D., 2005. Type 1 diabetes mellitus: etiology, presentation, and management. Pediatr. Clin. North Am. 52, 1553–1578.

Hameed, S., Ellard, S., Woodhead, H.J., Neville, K.A., Walker, J.L., Craig, M.E., et al., 2011. Persistently autoantibody negative (PAN) type 1 diabetes mellitus in children. Pediatr. Diabetes. 12, 142–149.

Harel, M., Shoenfeld, Y., 2006. Predicting and preventing autoimmunity, myth or reality? Ann. N.Y. Acad. Sci. 1069, 322–345.

Hermann, R., Bartsocas, C.S., Soltesz, G., Vazeou, A., Paschou, P., Bozas, E., et al., 2004. Genetic screening for individuals at high risk for type 1 diabetes in the general population using HLA Class II alleles as disease markers. A comparison between three European populations with variable rates of disease incidence. Diabetes Metab. Res. Rev. 20, 322–329.

Herold, K.C., Hagopian, W., Auger, J.A., Poumian-Ruiz, E., Taylor, L., Donaldson, D., et al., 2002. Anti-CD3 monoclonal antibody in new-onset type 1 diabetes mellitus. N. Engl. J. Med. 346, 1692–1698.

Hirai, H., Miura, J., Hu, Y., Larsson, H., Larsson, K., Lernmark, A., et al., 2008. Selective screening of secretory vesicle-associated proteins for autoantigens in type 1 diabetes: VAMP2 and NPY are new minor autoantigens. Clin. Immunol. 127, 366–374.

Imagawa, A., Hanafusa, T., Tamura, S., Moriwaki, M., Itoh, N., Yamamoto, K., et al., 2001. Pancreatic biopsy as a procedure for detecting in situ autoimmune phenomena in type 1 diabetes: close correlation between serological markers and histological evidence of cellular autoimmunity. Diabetes. 50, 1269–1273.

International Diabetes Federation (IDF). World Atlas of Diabetes, fifth ed. 2011 [Online]. [Cited 2011 December 24.] Available from: <www.diabetesatlas.org>.

In't Veld, P., 2011. Insulitis in the human endocrine pancreas: does a viral infection lead to inflammation and beta cell replication? Diabetologia. 54, 2220–2222.

In't Veld, P., Lievens, D., De Grijse, J., Ling, Z., Van Der Auwera, B., Pipeleers-Marichal, M., et al., 2007. Screening for insulitis in adult autoantibody-positive organ donors. Diabetes. 56, 2400–2404.

Jansen, A., Van Hagen, M., Drexhage, H.A., 1995. Defective maturation and function of antigen-presenting cells in type 1 diabetes. Lancet. 345, 491–492.

Jones, E.Y., Fugger, L., Strominger, J.L., Siebold, C., 2006. MHC class II proteins and disease: a structural perspective. Nat. Rev. Immunol. 6, 271–282.

Jorns, A., Rath, K.J., Terbish, T., Arndt, T., Meyer Zu Vilsendorf, A., Wedekind, D., et al., 2010. Diabetes prevention by immunomodulatory FTY720 treatment in the LEW.1AR1-iddm rat despite immune cell activation. Endocrinology. 151, 3555–3565.

Kahn, H.S., Morgan, T.M., Case, L.D., Dabelea, D., Mayer-Davis, E.J., Lawrence, J.M., et al., 2009. Association of type 1 diabetes with month of birth among U.S. youth: The SEARCH for diabetes in youth study. Diabetes Care. 32, 2010–2015.

Karlsen, A.E., Hagopian, W.A., Grubin, C.E., Dube, S., Disteche, C.M., Adler, D.A., et al., 1991. Cloning and primary structure of a human islet isoform of glutamic acid decarboxylase from chromosome 10. Proc. Natl. Acad. Sci. U.S.A. 88, 8337–8341.

Karvonen, M., Viik-Kajander, M., Moltchanova, E., Libman, I., Laporte, R., Tuomilehto, J., 2000. Incidence of childhood type 1 diabetes worldwide. Diabetes Mondiale (DiaMond) Project Group. Diabetes Care. 23, 1516–1526.

Kent, S.C., Chen, Y., Bregoli, L., Clemmings, S.M., Kenyon, N.S., Ricordi, C., et al., 2005. Expanded T cells from pancreatic lymph nodes of type 1 diabetic subjects recognize an insulin epitope. Nature. 435, 224–228.

Knip, M., Veijola, R., Virtanen, S.M., Hyoty, H., Vaarala, O., Akerblom, H.K., 2005. Environmental triggers and determinants of type 1 diabetes. Diabetes. 54 (Suppl. 2), S125–S136.

Kockum, I., Sanjeevi, C.B., Eastman, S., Landin-Olsson, M., Dahlquist, G., Lernmark, A., 1999. Complex interaction between HLA DR and DQ in conferring risk for childhood type 1 diabetes. Eur. J. Immunogenet. 26, 361–3672.

Komulainen, J., Kulmala, P., Savola, K., Lounamaa, R., Ilonen, J., Reijonen, H., et al., 1999. Clinical, autoimmune, and genetic

characteristics of very young children with type 1 diabetes. Childhood diabetes in finland (DiMe) study group. Diabetes Care. 22, 1950–1955.

Kyvik, K.O., Nystrom, L., Gorus, F., Songini, M., Oestman, J., Castell, C., et al., 2004. The epidemiology of type 1 diabetes mellitus is not the same in young adults as in children. Diabetologia. 47, 377–384.

Lampasona, V., Schlosser, M., Mueller, P.W., Williams, A.J., Wenzlau, J.M., Hutton, J.C., et al., 2011. Diabetes antibody standardization program: first proficiency evaluation of assays for autoantibodies to zinc transporter 8. Clin. Chem. 57, 1693–1702.

Larsson, H.E., Lynch, K., Lernmark, B., Nilsson, A., Hansson, G., Almgren, P., et al., 2005. Diabetes-associated HLA genotypes affect birthweight in the general population. Diabetologia. 48, 1484–1491.

Lee, K.H., Wucherpfennig, K.W., Wiley, D.C., 2001. Structure of a human insulin peptide-HLA-DQ8 complex and susceptibility to type 1 diabetes. Nat. Immunol. 2, 501–507.

Leslie, R.D., Kolb, H., Schloot, N.C., Buzzetti, R., Mauricio, D., De Leiva, A., et al., 2008. Diabetes classification: grey zones, sound and smoke: action LADA 1. Diabetes Metab. Res. Rev. 24, 511–519.

Libman, I.M., Becker, D.J., 2003. Coexistence of type 1 and type 2 diabetes mellitus: "double" diabetes? Pediatr. Diabetes. 4, 110–113.

Litherland, S.A., Xie, X.T., Hutson, A.D., Wasserfall, C., Whittaker, D.S., She, J.X., et al., 1999. Aberrant prostaglandin synthase 2 expression defines an antigen-presenting cell defect for insulin-dependent diabetes mellitus. J. Clin. Invest. 104, 515–523.

Long, S.A., Rieck, M., Sanda, S., Bollyky, J.B., Samuels, P.L., Goland, R., et al., 2012. Rapamycin/IL-2 combination therapy in patients with type 1 diabetes augments Tregs yet transiently impairs beta-cell function. Diabetes. 61, 2340–2348.

Lorenzen, T., Pociot, F., Hougaard, P., Nerup, J., 1994. Long-term risk of IDDM in first-degree relatives of patients with IDDM. Diabetologia. 37, 321–327.

Mathis, D., Vence, L., Benoist, C., 2001. beta-Cell death during progression to diabetes. Nature. 414, 792–798.

Mckinney, P.A., 2001. Seasonality of birth in patients with childhood type I diabetes in 19 European regions. Diabetologia. 44 (Suppl 3), B67–B74.

Mire-Sluis, A.R., Gaines Das, R., Lernmark, A., 2000. The World Health Organization International Collaborative Study for islet cell antibodies. Diabetologia. 43, 1282–1292.

Mordes, J.P., Bortell, R., Blankenhorn, E.P., Rossini, A.A., Greiner, D.L., 2004. Rat models of type 1 diabetes: genetics, environment, and autoimmunity. ILAR. J. 45, 278–291.

Morran, M.P., McInerney, M.F., Pietropaolo, M., 2008. Innate and adaptive autoimmunity in type 1 diabetes. Pediatr. Diabetes. 9, 152–161.

Nejentsev, S., Howson, J.M., Walker, N.M., Szeszko, J., Field, S.F., Stevens, H.E., et al., 2007. Localization of type 1 diabetes susceptibility to the MHC class I genes HLA-B and HLA-A. Nature. 450, 887–892.

Nerup, J., Platz, P., Andersen, O.O., Christy, M., Lyngsoe, J., Poulsen, J.E., et al., 1974. HL-A antigens and diabetes mellitus. Lancet. 2, 864–866.

Niklasson, B., Hornfeldt, B., Nyholm, E., Niedrig, M., Donoso-Mantke, O., Gelderblom, H.R., et al., 2003. Type 1 diabetes in Swedish bank voles (Clethrionomys glareolus): signs of disease in both colonized and wild cyclic populations at peak density. Ann. N.Y. Acad. Sci. 1005, 170—175.

Noble, J.A., Valdes, A.M., Bugawan, T.L., Apple, R.J., Thomson, G., Erlich, H.A., 2002. The HLA class I A locus affects susceptibility to type 1 diabetes. Hum. Immunol. 63, 657—664.

Notkins, A.L., Lernmark, A., 2001. Autoimmune type 1 diabetes: resolved and unresolved issues. J. Clin. Invest. 108, 1247—1252.

Ohashi, P.S., 2003. Negative selection and autoimmunity. Curr. Opin. Immunol. 15, 668—676.

Owerbach, D., Lernmark, A., Platz, P., Ryder, L.P., Rask, L., Peterson, P.A., et al., 1983. HLA-D region beta-chain DNA endonuclease fragments differ between HLA-DR identical healthy and insulin-dependent diabetic individuals. Nature. 303, 815—817.

Padaiga, Z., Tuomilehto, J., Karvonen, M., Dahlquist, G., Podar, T., Adojaan, B., et al., 1999. Seasonal variation in the incidence of type 1 diabetes mellitus during 1983 to 1992 in the countries around the Baltic Sea. Diabet. Med. 16, 736—743.

Pescovitz, M.D., Greenbaum, C.J., Krause-Steinrauf, H., Becker, D.J., Gitelman, S.E., Goland, R., et al., 2009. Rituximab, B-lymphocyte depletion, and preservation of beta-cell function. N. Engl. J. Med. 361, 2143—2152.

Pietropaolo, M., Towns, R., Eisenbarth, G.S., 2012. Humoral autoimmunity in type 1 diabetes: prediction, significance, and detection of distinct disease subtypes. Cold Spring Harb. Perspect Med.2, a012831.

Pinkse, G.G., Tysma, O.H., Bergen, C.A., Kester, M.G., Ossendorp, F., Van Veelen, P.A., et al., 2005. Autoreactive CD8 T cells associated with beta cell destruction in type 1 diabetes. Proc. Natl. Acad. Sci. U.S.A. 102, 18425—18430.

Pipeleers, D., In't Veld, P., Pipeleers-Marichal, M., Gorus, F., 2008. The beta cell population in type 1 diabetes. Novartis Found. Symp. 292, 19—24.

Plesner, A., Greenbaum, C.J., Gaur, L.K., Ernst, R.K., Lernmark, A., 2002. Macrophages from high-risk HLA-DQB1*0201/*0302 type 1 diabetes mellitus patients are hypersensitive to lipopolysaccharide stimulation. Scand. J. Immunol. 56, 522—529.

Pozzilli, P., Guglielmi, C., Caprio, S., Buzzetti, R., 2011. Obesity, autoimmunity, and double diabetes in youth. Diabetes Care. 34 (Suppl. 2), S166—S170.

Pugliese, A., Zeller, M., Fernandez Jr., A., Zalcberg, L.J., Bartlett, R.J., Ricordi, C., et al., 1997. The insulin gene is transcribed in the human thymus and transcription levels correlated with allelic variation at the INS VNTR-IDDM2 susceptibility locus for type 1 diabetes. Nat. Genet. 15, 293—297.

Pugliese, A., Brown, D., Garza, D., Murchison, D., Zeller, M., Redondo, M.J., et al., 2001. Self-antigen-presenting cells expressing diabetes-associated autoantigens exist in both thymus and peripheral lymphoid organs. J. Clin. Invest. 107, 555—564.

Pundziute-Lycka, A., Dahlquist, G., Nystrom, L., Arnqvist, H., Bjork, E., Blohme, G., et al., 2002. The incidence of type I diabetes has not increased but shifted to a younger age at diagnosis in the 0-34 years group in Sweden 1983-1998. Diabetologia. 45, 783—791.

Rabinovitch, A., Suarez-Pinzon, W.L., Shapiro, A.M., Rajotte, R.V., Power, R., 2002. Combination therapy with sirolimus and interleukin-2 prevents spontaneous and recurrent autoimmune diabetes in NOD mice. Diabetes. 51, 638—645.

Rewers, M., Bugawan, T.L., Norris, J.M., Blair, A., Beaty, B., Hoffman, M., et al., 1996. Newborn screening for HLA markers associated with IDDM: diabetes autoimmunity study in the young (DAISY). Diabetologia. 39, 807—812.

Risch, N., 1989. Genetics of IDDM: evidence for complex inheritance with HLA. Genet. Epidemiol. 6, 143—148.

Samuelsson, U., Johansson, C., Ludvigsson, J., 1999. Month of birth and risk of developing insulin dependent diabetes in south east Sweden. Arch. Dis. Child. 81, 143—146.

Schenker, M., Hummel, M., Ferber, K., Walter, M., Keller, E., Albert, E.D., et al., 1999. Early expression and high prevalence of islet autoantibodies for DR3/4 heterozygous and DR4/4 homozygous offspring of parents with type I diabetes: the German BABYDIAB study. Diabetologia. 42, 671—677.

Schlosser, M., Strebelow, M., Wassmuth, R., Arnold, M.L., Breunig, I., Rjasanowski, I., et al., 2002. The Karlsburg type 1 diabetes risk study of a normal schoolchild population: association of beta-cell autoantibodies and human leukocyte antigen-DQB1 alleles in antibody-positive individuals. J. Clin. Endocrinol. Metab. 87, 2254—2261.

Schlosser, M., Mueller, P.W., Torn, C., Bonifacio, E., Bingley, P.J., 2010. Diabetes antibody standardization program: evaluation of assays for insulin autoantibodies. Diabetologia. 53, 2611—2620.

Schranz, D.B., Lernmark, A., 1998. Immunology in diabetes: an update. Diabetes Metab. Rev. 14, 3—29.

Suri, A., Walters, J.J., Gross, M.L., Unanue, E.R., 2005. Natural peptides selected by diabetogenic DQ8 and murine I-A(g7) molecules show common sequence specificity. J. Clin. Invest. 115, 2268—2276.

Thayer, T.C., Wilson, S.B., Mathews, C.E., 2010. Use of nonobese diabetic mice to understand human type 1 diabetes. Endocrinol. Metab. Clin. North Am. 39, 541—561.

Thomson, G., Valdes, A.M., Noble, J.A., Kockum, I., Grote, M.N., Najman, J., et al., 2007. Relative predispositional effects of HLA class II DRB1-DQB1 haplotypes and genotypes on type 1 diabetes: a meta-analysis. Tissue Antigens. 70, 110—127.

Thunander, M., Petersson, C., Jonzon, K., Fornander, J., Ossiansson, B., Torn, C., et al., 2008. Incidence of type 1 and type 2 diabetes in adults and children in Kronoberg, Sweden. Diabetes Res. Clin. Pract. 82, 247—255.

Todd, J.A., 2010. Etiology of type 1 diabetes. Immunity. 32, 457—467.

Todd, J.A., Walker, N.M., Cooper, J.D., Smyth, D.J., Downes, K., Plagnol, V., et al., 2007. Robust associations of four new chromosome regions from genome-wide analyses of type 1 diabetes. Nat. Genet. 39, 857—864.

Torn, C., Mueller, P.W., Schlosser, M., Bonifacio, E., Bingley, P.J., 2008. Diabetes Antibody Standardization Program: evaluation of assays for autoantibodies to glutamic acid decarboxylase and islet antigen-2. Diabetologia. 51, 846—852.

Vandewalle, C.L., Coeckelberghs, M.I., De Leeuw, I.H., Du Caju, M.V., Schuit, F.C., Pipeleers, D.G., et al., 1997. Epidemiology, clinical aspects, and biology of IDDM patients under age 40 years. Comparison of data from Antwerp with complete ascertainment with data from Belgium with 40% ascertainment. The Belgian Diabetes Registry. Diabetes Care. 20, 1556—1561.

Verge, C.F., Gianani, R., Kawasaki, E., Yu, L., Pietropaolo, M., Jackson, R.A., et al., 1996. Prediction of type I diabetes in first-degree relatives using a combination of insulin, GAD, and ICA512bdc/IA-2 autoantibodies. Diabetes. 45, 926—933.

Von Herrath, M.G., Fujinami, R.S., Whitton, J.L., 2003. Microorganisms and autoimmunity: making the barren field fertile? Nat. Rev. Microbiol. 1, 151–157.

Weets, I., Kaufman, L., Van Der Auwera, B., Crenier, L., Rooman, R.P., De Block, C., et al., 2004. Seasonality in clinical onset of type 1 diabetes in belgian patients above the age of 10 is restricted to HLA-DQ2/DQ8-negative males, which explains the male to female excess in incidence. Diabetologia. 47, 614–621.

Wenzlau, J.M., Hutton, J.C., Davidson, H.W., 2008. New antigenic targets in type 1 diabetes. Curr. Opin. Endocrinol. Diabetes Obes. 15, 315–320.

Willcox, A., Richardson, S.J., Bone, A.J., Foulis, A.K., Morgan, N.G., 2009. Analysis of islet inflammation in human type 1 diabetes. Clin. Exp. Immunol. 155, 173–181.

Willis, J.A., Scott, R.S., Darlow, B.A., Lewy, H., Ashkenazi, I., Laron, Z., 2002. Seasonality of birth and onset of clinical disease in children and adolescents (0–19 years) with type 1 diabetes mellitus in Canterbury, New Zealand. J. Pediatr. Endocrinol. Metab. 15, 645–647.

Yokoi, N., Namae, M., Fuse, M., Wang, H.Y., Hirata, T., Seino, S., et al., 2003. Establishment and characterization of the Komeda diabetes-prone rat as a segregating inbred strain. Exp. Anim. 52, 295–301.

Yu, L., Boulware, D.C., Beam, C.A., Hutton, J.C., Wenzlau, J.M., Greenbaum, C.J., et al., 2012. Zinc transporter-8 autoantibodies improve prediction of type 1 diabetes in relatives positive for the standard biochemical autoantibodies. Diabetes Care. 35, 1213–1218.

Ziegler, A.G., Rewers, M., Simell, O., Simell, T., Lempainen, J., Steck, A., et al., 2013. Seroconversion to multiple islet autoantibodies and risk of progression to diabetes in children. JAMA. 309, 2473–2479.

Chapter 42

Adrenalitis

Corrado Betterle and Renato Zanchetta

Endocrine Unit, Department of Medicine, University of Padova, Padova, Italy

Chapter Outline

Introduction	587	Natural History of AAD	594
Anatomy and Physiology of the Adrenals	588	Diagnosis of AAD	595
Epidemiology of Addison's Disease and Autoimmune		Clinical Manifestations	595
Adrenalitis	588	General Biochemical Indices	595
Autoimmune Addison's Disease (AAD)	589	Hormonal Tests	595
Histopathology	589	Imaging	596
Focal Lymphocytic Adrenalitis	589	Different Clinical Presentations of AAD	596
Diffuse Lymphocytic Adrenalitis	590	Association with other Autoimmune Disorders	596
Animal Models	590	Therapy	597
Induced Immunity	590	General Information	597
Spontaneous Animal Models of AD	590	Steroid Replacement during Surgery, other Illness,	
Immunologic Studies	591	Medical Procedures, Physical Activity, and	
Genetic Predisposition	591	Pregnancy	598
Cellular Immunity	591	Adrenal Crisis	598
Humoral Immunity	591	Mortality	598
Identification of 21-OH as Adrenal Antigen	592	Osteoporosis	599
Techniques for Identification of Autoantibodies to 21-		Acknowledgments	599
OH	593	References	599
Identification of other Steroidogenic Autoantigens	593		

INTRODUCTION

Bartolomeo Eustachius was the first to describe the existence of the adrenals as *"de glandulis quae renibus incumbent"* in the *Opuscola Anatomica* published in Venice on 1563. Subsequently Casserius (1561–1616) validated the discovery, depicting and naming them as *"corpuscola reni incumbentia sive renes succenturiati"* (Hiatt and Hiatt, 1997).

In 1855, Thomas Addison first proved that the adrenals were vital organs when he described the symptoms and signs of patients with "anaemia...feebleness of the heart action...a peculiar change of colour in the skin occurring in connection with a diseased condition of the suprarenal capsules."

He called this disorder "melasma suprarenale," postulating that it might be due to abnormal lesions in the adrenal glands. In this first description from the autopsies of 11 patients, he found six cases with tuberculosis, three with malignancies, one with adrenal hemorrhage, and one with adrenal fibrosis of an unknown origin. In this case Addison reported: "The two adrenals together weighed 49 grains, they appeared exceedingly small and atrophied, so that the diseased condition did not result as usual from a deposit either of a strumous or malignant character, but appears to have been occasioned by an actual inflammation, that inflammation having destroyed the integrity of the organs, which finally led to their contraction and atrophy" (Addison, 1868). Probably, this last case was the first description of an autoimmune adrenalitis. In 1856, the adrenal insufficiency was named "Addison's disease" by Trousseau.

N. Rose & I. Mackay (Eds): The Autoimmune Diseases, Fifth edition. DOI: http://dx.doi.org/10.1016/B978-0-12-384929-8.00042-3

ANATOMY AND PHYSIOLOGY OF THE ADRENALS

The adrenal glands develop from the mesenchyme—the outer part (cortex) from the mesoderm and the central part (medulla) from the neuroectoderm, which comprises part of the chromaffin system (Kannan, 1988). The cortex is divided into three layers. The *zona glomerulosa* (5–10% of the cortex) comprises discontinuous subcapsular aggregates of small cells, containing less cytoplasm than the other cortical cells; the middle zone or *fasciculata* (70% of the cortex) is formed by radial cords of large cells arranged in columns with abundant lipid-filled cytoplasm; the inner cortical zone or *zona reticularis* is composed of cells arranged in cords with compact, finely granular, eosinophilic cytoplasm (Figure 42.1A).

The adrenal cortex synthesizes three main groups of hormones (glucocorticoids, mineralocorticoids, and adrenal androgens) (Auchus and Miller, 2001). The homeostasis of glucocorticoids is regulated by a feedback mechanism through the hypothalamus by means of corticotropin-releasing hormone (CRH), the pituitary gland by ACTH, and the adrenal cortex by cortisol (Koch, 2004). The main steps in the synthesis of the adrenal cortex hormones and the enzymes involved are described in Figure 42.2.

By immunocytochemical techniques, the normal adrenal cortex shows the presence of many proteins (Thiebaut et al., 1987; Henzen-Logmans et al., 1988; Sasano et al.,

1989; Muscatelli et al., 1994; Fogt et al., 1998; Pelkey et al., 1998). Immunopositivity has been demonstrated for the class II major histocompatibility (MHC) complexes (found in 10–20% of the cortical cells) including the human antigen D-related leukocyte (HLA DR) (McNicol, 1986; Jackson et al., 1988) and interleukin-6 (Gonzalez-Hernandez et al., 1994), which is involved in the communication process between the immune and endocrine system. Using specific antibodies against the steroidogenic enzymes and cytochrome P450 (Sasano et al., 1994), it was demonstrated that cytochrome P450 is involved in the adrenal steroid biosynthesis process, while the AdBP/SF-1 transcription factor regulates the expression of the CYP genes (Orth and Kavacs, 1998).

EPIDEMIOLOGY OF ADDISON'S DISEASE AND AUTOIMMUNE ADRENALITIS

Addison's disease (AD) is a very rare disorder and formerly tuberculosis was the most frequent cause. Of the 11 cases of AD in 1855, six (55%) had tuberculosis and only one (9%) had an idiopathic fibrotic form—probably the first case of an autoimmune AD (AAD). For many years tuberculosis was the most frequent form of adrenal insufficiency. Guttman (1930) examined 566 autopsied patients with AD and found 70% with tuberculous adrenalitis. Dunlop (1963) reviewed 86 cases of AD and reported 79% with tuberculous adrenalitis. In the subsequent years the frequency of tuberculosis AD progressively decreased;

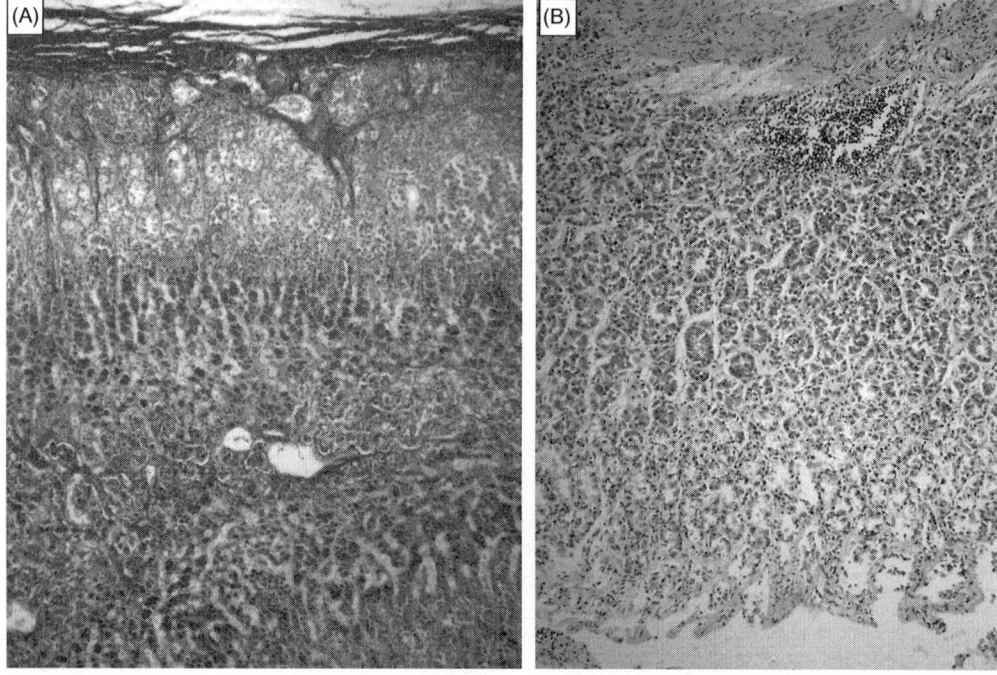

FIGURE 42.1 (A) Histopathology of the normal adrenal cortex showing the typical three layers. (B) Adrenal cortex from a patient with AAD showing atrophy of the cortex and a diffuse lymphocytic infiltration and, at top, a lymphoid follicle.

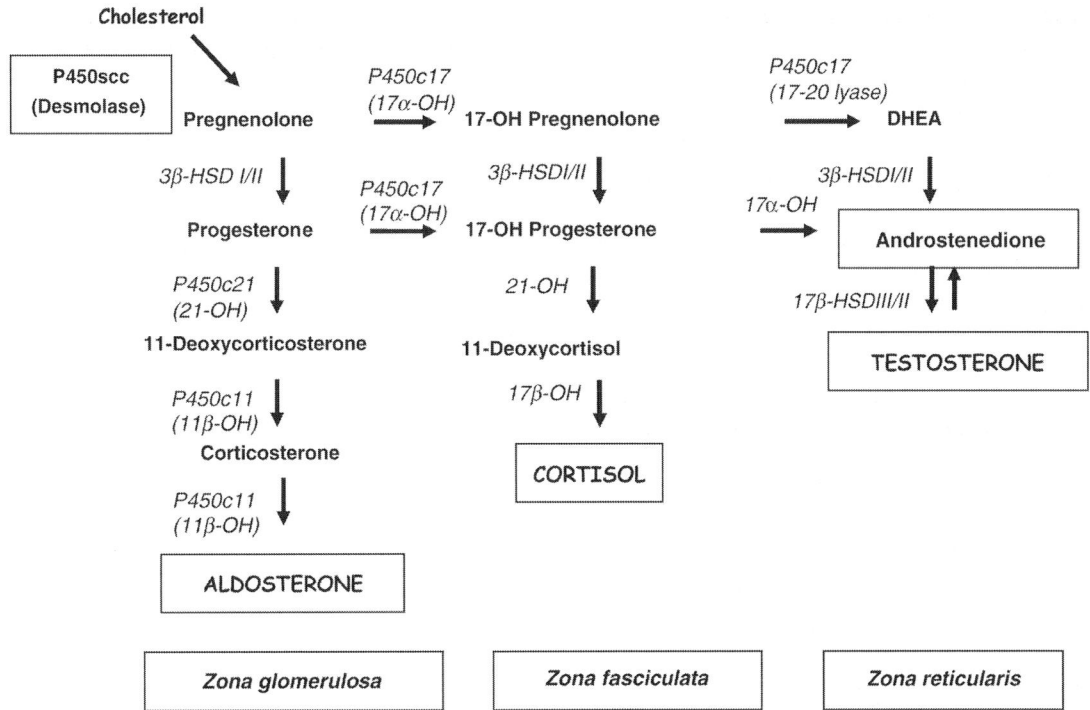

FIGURE 42.2   Main steps of the pathway of adrenal cortex hormone synthesis and the respective enzymes.

it was reported in London (Mason et al., 1968) in 31% and in Denmark (Nerup, 1974) in 17% of patients with AD. In the same years AAD progressively increased and has become the most frequent cause of AD. From 1974 to 2002, 1557 patients with AD were evaluated in various European studies, and the frequency of AAD ranged from 44.5 to 94% (Betterle et al., 2002).

In our experience, during the period 1968–2010, 633 patients with AD were collected and 524 (82.8%) were diagnosed with AAD, 57 (9.0%) with TBC-AD, 29 (4.6%) with genetic forms (G-AD), and 10 (1.6%) with adrenal cancer (C-AD); post-surgical AD (S-AD) was diagnosed in 6 (0.95%) patients, in 4 (0.63%) patients AD was caused by vascular disorders and in 3 (0.47%) AD resulted from infections affecting the adrenals, confirming that autoimmunity is by far the most frequent cause of AD in Italy (Betterle et al., 2013).

The general prevalence of AD is increasing; indeed, in London in 1968, Mason et al. found a prevalence of AD in 39 cases per million (Mason et al., 1968). In 1974 in Denmark, Nerup calculated a prevalence of 60 cases per million (Nerup, 1974), while in Coventry in 1997, Willis and Vince found a prevalence of 93 cases per million (Willis and Vince, 1997). In Nottingham in 1994, Kong and Jeffocoate reported a prevalence of 110 cases per million (Kong and jeffercoate, 1994), while in Italy Laureti et al. (1999) calculated 117 cases per million. Recently, the prevalence of AD was reported to be 144 cases per million in Norway with a calculated incidence, in the past decade, of

6.2 new cases per million per year (Erichsen et al., 2009b). The frequency of AD varies also in relation to different geographic areas: in New Zealand, Eason et al. (1982) calculated it to be 4.5 cases per million; in Japan it is five cases per million (Takayanagi et al., 2000); in the USA 50 cases per million (Jacobson et al., 1997); and in North Europe, more than 100 cases per million, as mentioned above (Kong and Jeffocoate, 1994; Laureti et al., 1999; Løvas and Husebye, 2002; Erichsen et al., 2009b). Despite the constant decrease of tuberculous forms of AD, the overall prevalence of AD has progressively increased and this may be due to the absolute increase of AAD.

AUTOIMMUNE ADDISON'S DISEASE (AAD)

AAD depends on a combination of genetic, environmental, and endogenous factors able to both induce a break of immune tolerance and initiate an autoimmune attack on the adrenal cortex, as for other autoimmune diseases (Kamradt and Mitchinson, 2001; Bratland and Husebye, 2011).

HISTOPATHOLOGY

Focal Lymphocytic Adrenalitis

In 1933 Duff and Bernstein (1933) and in 1969 Kiaer and Rytter Norgaard (1969) described a focal adrenalitis in patients without signs or symptoms of AD. Petri and Nerup (1971), studying two groups of patients (413 and

161 miscellaneous cases), reported the presence of very small numbers of lymphocytes in 15 and 18.6% of the adrenal glands, respectively. Subsequently, in up to half of the autopsied patients without AD, a focal accumulation of lymphocytes and plasma cells was demonstrated in the adrenal cortex, associated with chronic inflammatory diseases in the retroperitoneum (Fidler, 1977; Orth and Kavacs, 1998). The percentage of these infiltrates was similar to that reported in focal thyroiditis. In 1989, Hayashi et al. evaluated 174 cases at autopsy and demonstrated that mononuclear cell infiltration in the adrenal cortex increased with age, being present in about 7.4% of those aged over 49 years and 63% aged over 60 years. Immunohistochemical studies revealed that the infiltrating mononuclear cells were mainly composed of CD3[+] T cells. The major proportion of CD3[+] T cells express the CD4 phenotype, whereas CD8[+] T cells were fewer. A proportion of the CD4[+] T cells were activated (Hayashi et al., 1989). These findings indicate that the focal lymphocytic infiltration of the adrenal glands is not rare and may represent a latent adrenalitis, which, however, rarely reaches clinical expression since adrenal cortex antibodies and symptomatic AAD are extremely rare in the population.

A comprehensive investigation of the cellular and molecular components of the infiltrate has never been performed on the adrenal glands in patients with AAD so that the mechanisms by which the adrenal cortex is destroyed remain hypothetical (Bratland and Husebye, 2011).

Diffuse Lymphocytic Adrenalitis

The pathologic findings initially described by Addison (1855) as "idiopathic" are constantly present in the adrenal glands of patients affected by AAD. On macroscopic examination, both the adrenals are small (weight 1−2 g) and sometimes it is difficult to identify them in the retroperitoneal tissue. The capsule is fibrous, so that the adrenal glands are not detectable macroscopically and adrenal tissue is not detectable in multiple sections (Drury et al., 1979).

On microscopic examination, there is complete destruction of the three-layer architecture. The adrenal cortical cells are single, enlarged, or pleomorphic, with increased eosinophilia, depleted in lipids, or present as part of a cluster. Residual cortical nodules are seen as the disease progresses. The tissue is diffusely infiltrated by small lymphocytes, plasma cells, and macrophages (McNicol and Laidler, 1996). The histopathologic finding of infiltrating lymphocytes sometimes is associated with follicle formation and fibrosis (Figure 42.1B). The medulla in AAD remains normal. This pattern is present in patients with AAD, either isolated or associated in the context of autoimmune polyendocrine syndromes (McIntyre Gass, 1962; Irvine and Barnes 1975; Betterle et al., 2002).

ANIMAL MODELS

Induced Immunity

Colover and Glynn (1958) reported isoimmunization in guinea pigs by injection of adrenal antigens and complete Freund's adjuvant, with distinctive and "specific" lesions of the adrenals. Subsequently, many authors (Steiner et al., 1960; Barnett et al., 1963) reported examples of experimental autoimmune adrenalitis (EAA) in different species (rabbits, guinea pigs, rats, monkeys), including an antibody reaction in the guinea pigs and a lymphocytic infiltration in the rabbit adrenal tissue (Witebsky and Milgrom, 1962; Barnett et al., 1963). The adrenal lesions in rabbits were characterized by foci of lymphocytes and histiocytes, with a small number of plasma cells and eosinophils, and degenerative changes in adrenal cells. In 1968 Andrada et al. (1968) and in 1970 Werdelin and Witebsky (1970), EAA in a Lewis rat model was induced: adrenalitis occurred at day 7 after immunization. The histology was studied by autoradiographic tracing of H₃ thymidine and H₃ adenosine-labeled cells and demonstrated that adrenalitis was initiated with the appearance of a few specifically reactive lymphocytes, followed by an infiltration of mononuclear cells, mainly lymphocytes and plasma cells, throughout the adrenal cortex. Eosinophilia, cytoplasmic vacuolization, and a loss of nuclear definition were evident in cortical cells.

Using electron microscopy, Hoenig et al. (1970) studied the inflammatory lesions in paraffin-embedded tissues; 5 days after immunization, lymphocytes were present in sinusoids and adrenal parenchyma where damage was in the vicinity of lymphocytes, with enlargement of intercellular spaces and ischemic areas with inflammatory cells and fibrin.

It was demonstrated by Fujii et al. (1992) that in mice, repeated immunizations caused a delayed type of hypersensitivity to adrenal antigens, and that transfer of adrenalitis from an affected to a healthy animal was not possible by serum but was possible using spleen cells, confirming previous reports (Levine and Wenk, 1968; Werdelin et al., 1971) in which the disease was passively transferred by immunocytes derived from lymph nodes.

Spontaneous Animal Models of AD

Spontaneous AD occurs in dogs (Harlton, 1976; Kaufman, 1984; Little et al., 1989; Kintzer and Peterson, 1994; Sadek and Schaer, 1996; Dunn and Herrtage, 1998) and cats (Kaufman, 1984; Peterson et al., 1989; Tasker et al., 1999; Stonehewer and Tasker, 2001) with hypoadrenocorticism due to immune-mediated destruction of the adrenal glands. While biochemical laboratory data were reported, none of the authors described positivity for adrenal cortex autoantibodies, but only the presence of lymphocytic infiltration in the adrenal glands, at autopsy.

Beales et al. (2002) found the adrenal glands of a non-obese diabetic (NOD) mouse to contain a mononuclear cell infiltration in the adrenal cortex, but without signs of hypoadrenalism. Thus the NOD mouse was proposed as a spontaneous model suitable for investigating mechanisms involved in diffuse lymphocytic infiltration of the adrenal glands.

IMMUNOLOGIC STUDIES

Genetic Predisposition

As regards the genetic predisposition of AAD, it is important to remember that the majority of the studies were made in patients with isolated AAD or in the context of autoimmune polyglandular syndrome (APS) type 2. In these patients the correlation was primarily linked to class II HLA alleles in the major histocompatibility complex (MHC) (Myhre et al., 2002). Reports from several different populations have demonstrated that the risk of AAD is significantly increased in the presence of HLA-DRB1*03-DQA1*0501-DQB1*0201 (DR3/DQ2) and DRB1*0404-DQA1*0301-DQB1*0302 (DR4/4/DQ8). DRB1*0404 is much more frequent and indicates that peptides from 21-OH (21-hydroxylase) are well presented to autoreactive T lymphocytes in the presence of DR4/4. In addition to the above-mentioned alleles it has been demonstrated that HLA-B8 was significantly increased independently of DR3 (Bratland and Husebye, 2011). Furthermore, an association between AAD and the 5.1 allele of MHC class I chain-related A (MIC-A) has been demonstrated. Homozygosity for the 5.1 allele of MIC-A in the presence of high risk HLA genotype (DR3-DQ2/DR4/4-DQ8) may define subjects at very high risk of AAD. MIC-A is not involved in the antigen presentation but as a mediator of activating natural killer cells and T cytotoxic lymphocytes (Bratland and Husebye, 2011). A number of other genes outside the MHC complex have also been reported such as the cytotoxic T lymphocyte-associated protein-4 (CTLA-4), a key negative regulator in adaptive immunity, the MHC class II transactivator (MHC2TA), which regulates the expression of class II molecules, the tyrosine–protein phosphatase non-receptor type 22 (PTPN22), involved in the regulation of T cell receptor signaling, and the programmed death ligand 1 (PD-L1), an inhibitory molecule expressed on activated T cells. In addition to the above-mentioned genes AAD is associated with genes involved in the metabolism of vitamin D, with the gene encoding NACHT leucine-rich-repeat protein 1 (Bratland and Husebye, 2011).

Finally, it is important to remember that in patients with APS-1 where AAD is one of the major components, there is an association without HLA alleles but with mutations of the autoimmune regulator (AIRE) gene (Cervato et al., 2009; Bratland and Husebye, 2011). This gene is involved in the presentation of autoantigen to autoreactive T lymphocytes in order to induce tolerance, and the presence of the AIRE gene mutations with mutated proteins may inhibit the apoptosis of autoreactive T lymphocytes at the thymic level; these cells can migrate at the peripheral level where they can initiate an autoimmune aggression in a very young age in these patients.

Cellular Immunity

The early studies on AD, using the assay for migration inhibition factor, reported cell-mediated immunity in affected patients, with claims for organ-specific hypersensitivity (Nerup and Bendixen, 1969). Subsequent studies, by means of an intracutaneous test with adrenal extracts, showed a cutaneous delayed-type hypersensitivity reaction but no collateral evidence based on blast transformation experiments (Nerup et al., 1970). Other studies reported a decrease in suppressor T cell function (Verghese et al., 1980) and an increase in circulating Ia-positive T lymphocytes (Rabinowe et al., 1984), which indicated the involvement of cellular immunity. Initially, studies of cellular immunity in AAD were carried out (Freeman and Weetman, 1992) when a proliferative T cell response to an adrenal-specific protein fraction of 18–24 kDa molecular weight was described.

Recently, in order to identify the autoepitopes recognized by T lymphocytes, BALB/c and SJL inbred mouse strains were immunized with recombinant 21-OH. T lymphocytes of the immunized animals were stimulatd by a peptide 342–361 of 21-OH. This region may be involved in the pathogenesis of AAD (Husebye et al., 2006).

Subsequently, it was demonstrated that patients with AAD have circulating 21-OH-specific T cells recognizing the amino acidic fragment 342–361 of 21-OH, who constitute a disease-specific epitope presented by HLA-DRB1*0404. Furthermore, cellular proliferation and secretion of interferon-γ in response to 21-OH was significantly higher in patients with AAD respect to controls (Bratland et al., 2009).

Humoral Immunity

Anderson et al. (1957), using a complement fixation test on a homogenate of adrenal cortex tissue, demonstrated that 2/8 (25%) of patients with idiopathic AD had antibodies (adrenal cortical antibodies—ACA). From 1957 to 1970, using this technique, ACA were cumulatively reported in 57/159 (36%) patients with idiopathic AD and in 2/23 (9%) of those with the tuberculous form, reviewed

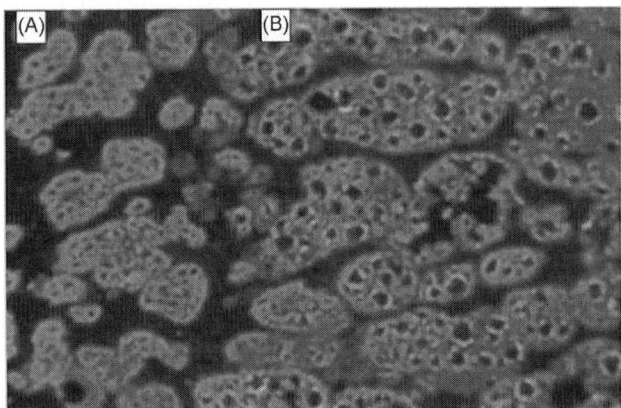

FIGURE 42.3 Immunofluorescence pattern on normal human adrenal cortex given by serum of a patient with AAD. This serum reacted with the cytoplasm of cells in all three layers of the cortex, but shown here are only glomerulosa (A) and fasciculata (B).

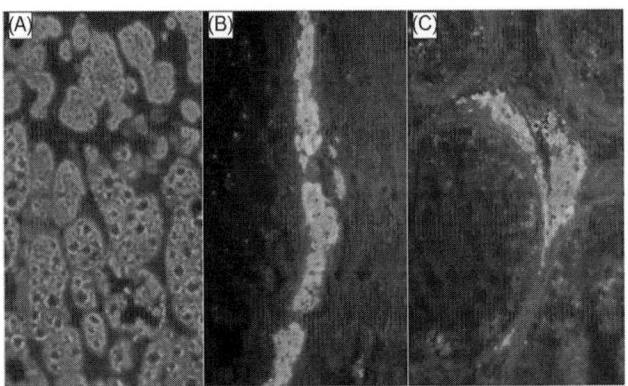

FIGURE 42.4 Immunofluorescence pattern given by serum of a patient with AAD and premature ovarian failure. This serum reacted against adrenal cortex (A), follicular theca of the ovary (B), and Leydig cells of the testis (C), and reflects autoantibodies to steroid-producing cells (StCA).

by Betterle (2004). Subsequently, Blizzard and Kyle (1963), using indirect immunofluorescence (IIF) on animal or human adrenal gland sections, demonstrated that ACA are organ-specific antibodies which react with all three layers of the adrenal cortex, producing a homogeneous cytoplasmic staining pattern (Figure 42.3). Sometimes, there is reactivity against one or two of the three layers of the cortex (Irvine and Barnes, 1975; Sotsiu et al., 1980). The autoantibodies also react with the surface of living cortical cells in culture (Khoury et al., 1981), indicating the existence of microsomal antigens on the surface of adrenal cells.

Between 1963 and 2002, IIF was used on human or animal adrenal tissues in 1637 patients with AAD and 267 with tuberculous AD, and ACA were detected in 61% and 6.7%, respectively, as reviewed by Betterle (2004).

The prevalence of ACA has varied considerably between different laboratories because of differences in the substrates used (animal or human), time of incubation, geographic or racial origins of individuals, gender, age of onset, duration of the disease, or whether other associated diseases were present (Rees Smith and Furmaniak, 1995; Betterle et al., 2002; Nigam et al., 2003). Other studies (Kendall-Taylor et al., 1988; Wulfraat et al., 1989) have reported the presence of autoantibodies blocking the ACTH receptor in 90% of patients affected by AAD, but these data could not be confirmed (Wardle et al., 1993). Finally, autoantibodies to hydrocortisone were detected in patients with an Addison-like syndrome and AIDS (Salim et al., 1988).

In 1968, steroid-producing cell antibodies (StCA) were first described (Anderson et al., 1968) in males affected by AAD without gonadal failure (Figure 42.4). Subsequently, StCA were detected in 60−80% of the

patients affected by type 1 APS, in 25−40% of those with type 2 APS, and in 18% of those with isolated AAD (Betterle et al., 2002, 2005; Betterle, 2004). The presence of these antibodies correlates with premature ovarian failure characterized by lymphocytic oophoritis (Betterle et al., 1993; Hoek et al., 1997; Betterle and Volpato, 1998).

Recent data demonstrated that in Norway 6.7% of females with AAD had premature ovarian failure (Erichsen et al., 2009b). Recent numbers from Italy confirm and extend revealing a frequency of 20% and that steroidogenic autoantibodies are not only highly correlated with the presence of premature ovarian failure, but also that there are predictive markers for future clinical manifestation (Reato et al., 2011).

Identification of 21-OH as Adrenal Antigen

With regard to the identification of adrenal autoantigens, in 1988 Furmaniak et al. described a specific 55 kDa protein in human adrenal microsomes which was reactive with the ACA (Furmaniak et al., 1988).

In 1992, two independent laboratories (Baumann-Antczak et al., 1992; Bednarek et al., 1992; Winqvist et al., 1992) demonstrated by means of purification of native 21-OH that this adrenal enzyme is a major antigen of adrenal cortical cells. Subsequently, this was confirmed in experiments with specific absorption with purified human 21-OH, using sera from six patients with different forms of AAD (Morgan et al., 2000).

21-OH is an adrenal-specific enzyme of the cytochrome P450 family and plays a key role in the synthesis of the cortical hormones (Furmaniak et al., 1999; Furmaniak and Rees Smith, 2002). 21-OH is encoded by the CYP21B gene, whereas the CYP21A gene is inactive (Wilson et al., 1995). 21-OH catalyzes the conversion of progesterone and 17-hydroxyprogesterone into 11-deoxycorticosterone and 11-deoxycortisol (see Figure 42.2). It is a 55 kDa microsomal protein containing a heme group, located in the active site of the C-terminal end of the molecule, which is important for autoantibody binding (Wedlock et al., 1993; Asawa et al., 1994) and in oxidation-reduction reactions (Picado-Leonard and Miller, 1987; Lin et al., 1994).

Analysis of autoantibody-binding sites on 21-OH indicated that the epitopes on 21-OH were conformational (Wedlock et al., 1993) and confirmed the participation of both the central and C-terminal parts of the molecule. These studies identified the presence of three different, short 5-, 6-, and 15-amino acid sequences in the C-terminal part of the 21-OH involved in the binding of antibodies to 21-OH (Chen et al., 1998). These observations are important in relation to effects of 21-OH antibodies on 21-OH enzyme activity. In fact, in studies *in vitro*, using sera positive for 21-OHAbs from patients with AAD, a dose-dependent blocking activity was identified (Furmaniak et al., 1994), although this is not usually evident *in vivo* (Boscaro et al., 1996).

Techniques for Identification of Autoantibodies to 21-OH

Following the discovery that 21-OH is the major adrenal cortex autoantigen, a specific and sensitive technique was described, by labeling the protein with ^{35}S-methionine in an *in vitro* transcription translation (TnT) system, and using a radioimmunoprecipitation assay (RIA), for the detection of antibodies (Colls et al., 1995; Falorni et al., 1995; Chen et al., 1996). Thereafter, because of certain limitations of this technique, a more convenient assay to measure 21-OHAbs was developed based on the use of ^{125}I-labeled recombinant human 21-OH and the precipitation of the immunocomplexes using solid-phase protein A (RIA) (Tanaka et al., 1997). Using these techniques, from 1995 to 2002, a group of 572 patients with AAD and 76 with tuberculosis were studied; 78% and 1.9%, respectively, were 21-OHAbs positive, reviewed by Betterle (2004).

In order to compare techniques for ACA and 21-OHAbs determinations, we studied 165 patients with AD, with different durations of disease, and found that 81% of those with AAD were positive by both techniques, whereas none with non-AAD was positive (Betterle et al., 1999). The prevalence varied in relation to both the clinical presentation (type 1 or 2 APS or isolated AAD) and the duration of the disease, being higher (100%) in patients with recent onset than in those with long-standing disease (79%) and in those with type 2 APS than in those with isolated AAD (Betterle et al., 2002). In these studies, results using IIF for ACA and RIA for 21-OHAbs were in good agreement.

Some discrepancies were reported by Falorni et al. (1997) and Betterle et al. (1999) on relationships between ACA measured using IIF and 21-OHAbs measured by RIA. For example, a few patient samples were positive for 21-OHAbs while negative for ACA and this may reflect greater sensitivity of 21-OHAbs IPA. In contrast a small number of sera were positive for ACA while negative for 21-OHAbs by RIA. This discrepancy may be related to serum reactivity with adrenal cortex antigens in the IIF that are distinct from 21-OH.

Recently, the first international standardization program for 21-OHAbs determination was carried out to compare the measurements from four different laboratories using different methods and an inter-laboratory concordance study (Falorni et al., 2011). This study has shown a very good agreement among the laboratories on reporting 21-OHAbs positive/negative samples. The sensitivity for AAD was greater than 80% in all four participating laboratories. However, the study highlighted the need to produce the international standard preparation to enable the harmonized expression of the results.

Subsequently, an International Standardization Program for 21-OHAbs measurements was organized by the EurAdrenal consortium, and 13 different laboratories across Europe and one from United States participated in this program and the results are under evaluation (Falorni et al., in preparation).

Identification of other Steroidogenic Autoantigens

With regard to steroidogenic autoantigens, in addition to 21-OH, Krohn et al. (1992) reported that screening of a human fetal adrenal cDNA expression library with sera from patients with APS type 1 identified a protein with high homology to 17α-hydroxylase (17α-OH) reacting also with a fragment of recombinant 17α-OH expressed in bacteria. 17α-OH, coded by a single gene on the human chromosome 10, showed 30% homology with 21-OH antigen.

Winqvist et al. (1992), using immunoblotting and immunoprecipitation studies, also observed a reactivity of sera from APS type 1 patients with a cytochrome P450 side chain cleavage enzyme (P450scc), a heme-binding protein coded by a single gene on human chromosome 15, that showed 20% homology with 21-OH sequence (Chung et al., 1986).

The binding sites of these two antigens and their enzyme activity have not been studied, even though Peterson and Krohn (1994) reported the presence of four distinct, reactive regions in the 17α-OH molecule and an inhibiting effect *in vivo* of the P450sccAbs in the type 1 APS serum (Winqvist et al., 1993).

The 17α-OHAbs and P450sccAbs are detectable by RIA, using recombinant human antigens, and are correlated with StCA detected by IIF (Chen et al., 1996; Reato et al., 2011).

In addition to the main antigens mentioned above, other autoantigens have also been discovered. Winqivist et al. (1996) identified an autoantibody of 51 kDa, recognizing the aromatic L-amino acid decarboxylase (AADC) involved in the generation of serotonin and dopamine. AADC was reported in the sera of patients with type 1 APS in association with chronic hepatitis, vitiligo, and type 1 diabetes mellitus (Husebye et al., 1997).

Other authors (Ekwall et al., 1998; Dal Pra et al., 2004) reported the presence of autoantibodies against a 230 kDa enzyme, tryptophan hydroxylase (TPH), involved in the synthesis of serotonin, or against histidine decarboxylase (Skoldberg ct al., 2003) in patients with type 1 APS, who have a gastrointestinal dysfunction (Scarpa et al., 2013).

Again, patients with type 1 APS and autoimmune hepatitis recognize the cytochromes P450 CYPIA2 and CYP2A6 as autoantigens (Clemente et al., 1997, 1998).

Subsequently, an autoantibody to SOX9 and SOX10 was reported in patients with type 1 APS and vitiligo (Hedstrand et al., 2001), and an antibody to tyrosine hydroxylase in those with alopecia areata (Hedstrand et al., 2000).

Some authors reported reactivities against other antigens: to 3β-hydroxysteroid dehydrogenase (Arif et al., 1996), candidal antigens, heat shock protein 90, pyruvate kinase, and alcohol dehydrogenase, and in patients with AAD and chronic mucocutaneous candidiasis (Peterson et al., 1996). Two different studies (Song et al., 1994; Peterson et al., 1997) were unable to confirm the reactivity to other enzymes (11α-hydroxylase, aromatase, adrenodoxin) in patients with AAD.

NATURAL HISTORY OF AAD

Apart from the patients with AAD, ACA can be detected in 0.2% of normal controls, in 4% of first-degree relatives of AAD patients, 4% of hospitalized patients, and 1.3% of patients with organ-specific autoimmune disease, with a much higher prevalence (2.5−20%) in premature ovarian failure or idiopathic hypoparathyroidism (Nerup, 1974; De Bellis et al., 1993; Betterle et al., 1997a,b).

AAD is a chronic disease with a long silent period marked by the presence of ACA. The natural history of the disease could entail five main phases: one potential, three subclinical, and one clinical (Betterle et al., 1988, 2002).

To recognize these different phases, it is necessary to basally measure levels of cortisol, ACTH, plasma renin activity (PRA), aldosterone, and cortisol 30 and 60 min after an intravenous injection of 250 µg of cosyntropin (α1-24-corticotropin) (ACTH test) (Stewart et al., 1988; Grinspoon and Biller, 1994).

Stage 0 is characterized by the presence of adrenal-specific autoantibodies and a normal adrenal cortical mass, in the absence of any detectable dysfunction of the adrenal glands by ACTH test, representing the "potential" phase of chronic adrenalitis. Subclinical stage 1 is characterized by an increase in PRA, together with normal/decreased levels of aldosterone (reduced production of mineralcorticoids); subclinical stage 2 by normal ACTH values with normal basal cortisol but a low cortisol peak (low reserve of glucocorticoids); subclinical stage 3 by an increase in ACTH and low level of basal cortisol, representing reduced glucocorticoid production. Stage 4, the clinical stage, is when the ACTH is significantly increased and the basal cortisol is very low (Table 42.1).

Stage 1 reveals that the *zona glomerulosa* of the adrenal glands is first affected by the autoimmune attack, or because of its greater sensitivity to diffuse lymphocyte infiltration, or because the other zones are protected by either locally produced high concentrations of corticosteroid hormones or the ability to self-regenerate (Betterle et al., 2002).

For the study of patients with ACA/21-OHAbs, it was proposed to use also an ACTH test with a low dose (1 µg) of ACTH (Laureti et al., 2000). It has been shown that this low-dose test has a diagnostic accuracy as high as that of the classical high-dose intravenous 250 µg test but it remains unclear whether "low-dose" synacthen tests have better sensitivity for detecting adrenal failure than the standard test.

From 1983 to 2000, 236 ACA-positive patients were followed in 12 studies and 28% developed AAD, but the evolution varied greatly from 0 to 90% (Betterle, 2004; Betterle et al., 2005). The highest risk was found in children with respect to adults with high antibody titers and with the presence of DR1*0404 (Betterle et al., 1997a,b; Laureti et al., 1998; Yu et al., 1999).

Subsequently, in order to estimate risk of AAD, 100 ACA-positive patients (21 children and 79 adults) with autoimmune diseases but without clinical AAD followed up for a period of 19 years were reanalyzed; 31 of the seropositive patients developed clinical AAD. The overall cumulative risk of AAD in ACA/21-OHAb-positive patients was 47.5%, with an annual incidence of 4.9%.

In order to identify the real value of the various analyzed data we assessed a multivariate analysis, including clinical (gender and age), immunologic (type of preexisting autoimmune disease, titers of autoantibodies), genetic (HLA status), and functional status (normal or subclinical adrenal cortical function). This analysis demonstrated that the occurrence of AAD was significantly correlated to gender, adrenal cortex anutoantibodies titers, adrenal cortex functional status, and type of autoimmune preexisting disease.

TABLE 42.1 ACTH Test: Stages of Adrenal Function in ACA-positive Patients

Adrenocortical Function	Stage	Autoimmune AD	ACA/ 21-OHAb	Basal PRA	Basal Aldosterone	Basal ACTH	Basal Cortisol	Cortisol Response 60 min after ACTH i.v.	Clinical Manifestations
Normal	0	Potential	+	Normal	Normal	Normal	Normal	Normal	Absent
Reduced production of mineralocorticoids	1	Subclinical	+	High	Normal or low	Normal	Normal	Normal	Absent
Reduced reserve of glucocorticoids	2	Subclinical	+	High	Low	Normal	Normal	Reduced	Absent
Reduced production of glucocorticoids	3	Subclinical	+	High	Low	High	Low	Absent	Absent
Important mineralocorticoids and glucocorticoids deficiency	4	Clinical	+	Very high	Very low	Very high	Very low	Absent	Present

On the basis of these results the probability of developing AAD can now be estimated by a mathematical model. This evaluation yielded two practical outcomes: (1) individualization of the patients with different risk grades (low, medium, or high risk) in order to monitor them at different rates (every 6, 12, or 24 months); (2) selection of patients to begin an early substitutive therapy or in future an immuno-intervention trial treatment in order to prevent the development of the clinical disease (Coco et al., 2006).

DIAGNOSIS OF AAD

Clinical Manifestations

AAD has a long pre-clinical period and clinical features do not appear until 90% or more of the adrenal cortex is destroyed. The main clinical signs at onset are general malaise, fatigue, weakness (99%), anorexia, nausea and vomiting (90%), weight loss (97%), cutaneous and mucosal hyperpigmentation (Figure 42.5) caused by the enhanced stimulation of the skin MC1-receptor by ACTH and other pro-opiomelanocortin-related peptides (98%), and severe hypotension (87%). Other signs (abdominal pain, salt craving, diarrhea, constipation, syncope) have a variable frequency (34–39%) (Williams and Dluhy, 1998). In women a loss of axillary and pubic hair, dry skin, reduced libido, and an impairment of well-being also occur.

General Biochemical Indices

In AAD at diagnosis, the serum levels of sodium, chloride, and bicarbonate are reduced, while those of potassium are elevated. The hyponatremia (in 100% of patients) is due to loss of sodium in urine and increase in

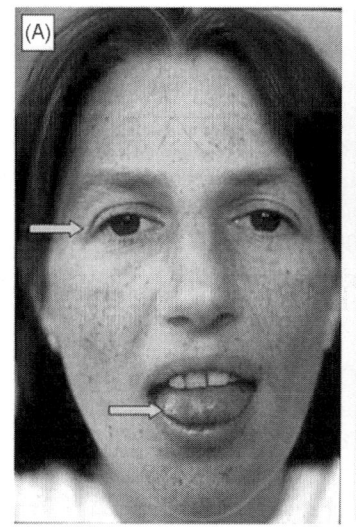
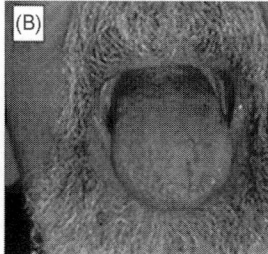
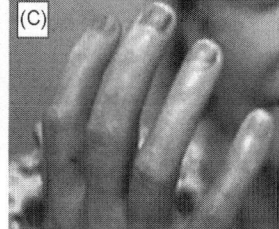

FIGURE 42.5 Clinical Manifestations of AAD at Onset. (A) Hyperpigmentation of the skin, melanosis of the tongue, and enophthalmos as a sign of dehydration. (B) Male showing a melanosis of the tongue. (C) Hyperpigmentation of the nails.

both plasma vasopressin and angiotensin II which impair free water clearance; hyperkalemia (in 50–70%) is due to aldosterone deficiency, impaired glomerular filtration, and acidosis. From 10 to 20% of patients have a mild or moderate hypercalcemia, for unknown reasons (Williams and Dluhy, 1998). Anemia is present in 40–50%, and eosinophilia and lymphocytosis in 10–15% of the cases.

Hormonal Tests

The association between a morning (8 a.m.) immunometric determination of both plasma ACTH and basal cortisol levels differentiates cases of primary adrenal failure from both a healthy status and other types of adrenal disease (Oelkers et al., 1992).

An increase in levels of ACTH (higher than 22.0 pmol/L) and decrease (below 165 nmol/L) in basal cortisol indicate primary adrenal failure. In the initial phases of AD, plasma renin activity increases above the normal range, and serum aldosterone is either subnormal or low to normal. In relation to differential diagnosis, in the case of secondary adrenal failure, levels of both ACTH and cortisol are low and, in general, aldosterone and plasma renin activity are normal. Dehydroepiandrosterone, which is the major precursor of sex steroid synthesis, is involved in the adrenal failure, causing a pronounced androgen deficiency in women, with the loss of both axillary and pubic hair, dry skin, reduced libido, and, frequently, an impairment in well-being (Arlt and Allolio, 2003).

In cases in which there are no clear clinical manifestations of AD, and/or in the presence of adrenal cortex antibodies, it may be necessary to perform an ACTH test (see above, Natural history of AAD). TSH levels are increased in 30% of patients, because of the lack of inhibiting effect of cortisol on TSH production or the presence of coexisting autoimmune hypothyroidism (Orth and Kavacs, 1998).

Recently, it has been demonstrated that the measurement of salivary and serum cortisol in the morning has a low sensitivity and specificity for detecting primary adrenal insufficiency (Raff, 2009).

Imaging

Computed tomography (CT) and nuclear magnetic resonance (NMR) show the adrenals with optimal resolution and clarity, and greatly facilitate the diagnosis and characterization of adrenal insufficiency. In patients with

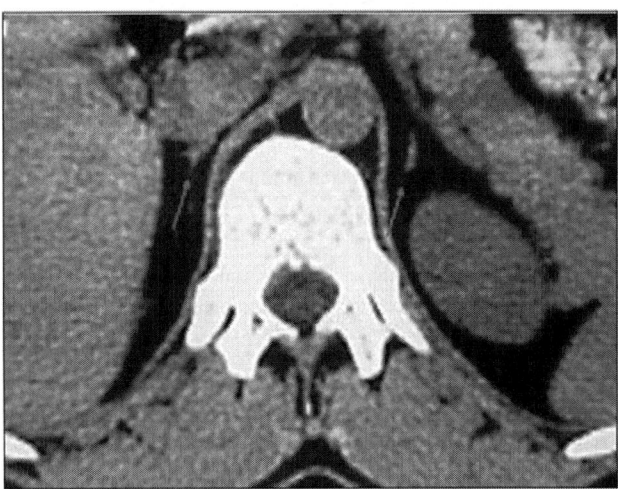

FIGURE 42.6 Adrenal Imaging. CT of the adrenal glands of a patient with autoimmune Addison's disease at diagnosis. The adrenals are small (see arrows).

AAD, either isolated or as a component of APS syndromes, the adrenal glands appear bilaterally miniscule without calcifications (Doppman, 2001) (Figure 42.6).

Recently, the imaging of the adrenal glands was performed in 250 patients with AAD. Normal adrenal glands were found in 190 patients (76%), in 59 patients (23.6%) the adrenals were reduced in size/volume or undetectable, and only in the case of one patient (0.4%) was there a modest increase in adrenal volume. None of the examined adrenal glands showed calcifications. There were no differences in the adrenal imaging between different forms of AAD in the context of the various APS/MAS (Betterle et al., 2013).

DIFFERENT CLINICAL PRESENTATIONS OF AAD

Neufeld and Blizzard (1980) proposed the classification of autoimmune syndromes into four main groups, involving different endocrine glands, and named them "autoimmune polyglandular syndromes" (APS) (see Box 42.1). According to this classification, AAD can be associated with type 1 and 2 APS.

Box 42.1 Clinical Classification of APS According to Neufeld and Blizzard (1980) (modified).

- APS-1 Chronic candidiasis, chronic hypoparathyroidism, Addison's disease (*at least two diseases must be present*)
- APS-2 Addison's disease (*always present*) + thyroid autoimmune diseases and/or type 1 diabetes mellitus
- APS-3 Thyroid autoimmune diseases + other autoimmune diseases (*excluding Addison's disease and/or hypoparathyroidism*)
- APS-4 Combinations of other autoimmune diseases not included in previous classifications

---

Betterle and Presotto (2008), in a review of multiple autoimmune syndromes (MAS), proposed the existence of three different types of APS/MAS involving AAD (type 1 when associated with chronic candidiasis and/or chronic hypoparathyroidism; type 2 when associated with autoimmune thyroid diseases and/or type 1 diabetes mellitus; and type 4 when associated with other autoimmune diseases not included in the previous list). So, AAD can present in four main clinical forms: isolated or associated with type 1, 2, or 4 APS/MAS.

Association with other Autoimmune Disorders

Every patient with a diagnosis of AAD needs to be investigated for the family and personal clinical signs or symptoms of thyroid autoimmune diseases, gastric

TABLE 42.2 Four Different Clinical Presentations of Autoimmune Adrenalitis (Number of AAD patients = 524)

Subgroups Frequency	APS-2 61.6%	APS-1 13.6%	APS-4 8%	Isolated 17.5%
F/M	2.3	2.1	1	0.6
Adults/Children	16	0.8	5,3	4
Mean age (in years) at onset of AD	34.6	15	32	32
Range	1–85	2–41	6–62	1–84
Family history for autoimmune diseases	Frequent	Frequent	Frequent	Frequent
Family history for AAD	Rare	Frequent	Rare	Rare
Genetic	HLA-DR3 and/or DR4	AIRE gene Mutations	HLA (?)	HLA(?)
Chr. candidiasis	Absent	76%	Absent	Absent
Chr. hypoparathyroidism	Absent	90%	Absent	Absent
Thyroid autoimmune dis.	93.7%	30%	Absent	Absent
Type 1 diabetes mellitus	15.5%	6%	Absent	Absent
Other autoimmune diseases (vitiligo, alopecia, autoimmune gastritis, pernicious anemia, celiac disease, myasthenia gravis, Sjögren's syndrome, Werlhof's syndrome, multiple sclerosis, etc.)	Until 43%	Until 57%	100%	Absent
Ectodermal dystrophy	Absent	Present	Absent	Absent
Cancer	5.3%	9.9%	2.6%	4.3%
ACA or	88%	91%	95%	69%
21-OHAb at onset of AD	94%	92%	100%	86%
Adrenals imaging	Normal/ atrophic	Normal/ atrophic	Normal/ atrophic	Normal/ atrophic

autoimmune diseases, gonadal failure, type 1 diabetes, chronic hypoparathyroidism, chronic candidiasis, vitiligo, alopecia, autoimmune hepatitis, and other autoimmune diseases; in the absence of the clinical manifestations of these disorders it is also important to perform an organ- and non-organ-specific autoantibody screening because a proportion of patients with apparently isolated AAD can be positive for one or more autoantibodies and this can reveal the presence of a subclinical or a potential disease with a high risk of future clinical dysfunction. In 82–87% of the patients with AAD this approach allowed the identification of one or more clinical, subclinical, or latent autoimmune diseases (Erichsen et al., 2009) which represents the autoimmune disease with the highest prevalence in relation to other autoimmune diseases in the world.

In our experience, out of 524 patients with AAD, overall 432 (82.4%) were classified to APS/MAS; in particular 323 (61.6%) had APS/MAS-2, 71 (13.6%) had APS/MAS-1, 38 (7.2%) had APS/MAS-4, and only 92 (17.6%) had an isolated AAD (Betterle et al., 2013).

Every subtype of AAD had some common features (family history for autoimmune diseases, autoantibodies to adrenal cortex, adrenal imaging of normal or atrophy) and some different features (age at onset, F/M ratio, adults/children ratio, genetic predisposition, association with the minor autoimmune diseases, association with cancer). The typical profiles of the four different forms of AAD are summarized in Table 42.2.

THERAPY

General Information

Life-saving therapy for patients with chronic adrenal insufficiency is two or three daily doses of a specific hormone replacement (Groves et al., 1988; Howlett, 1997; Williams and Dluhy, 1998; Arlt and Allolio, 2003b). Doses of 20–30 mg of hydrocortisone or 25–50 mg of cortisone acetate are required. The first dose is administered in the morning and the second in the afternoon, about 6–8 hours after the first, and the third at 6 pm or at least 4 hours before sleep. Substitutive glucocorticoid therapy is not taken with food. The dosage must be increased for obese individuals and those taking other drugs. Patients should be given relatively small doses to avert weight gain and osteoporosis.

ACTH cannot be used for the purposes of treatment surveillance, whereas a 24-hour urinary free-cortisol test has been advocated for monitoring of replacement therapy. However, urinary cortisol excretion shows considerable variability, because after oral administration and glucocorticoid absorption the cortisol-binding globulin is rapidly saturated with an increase of unutilized cortisol renal excretion (Arlt, 2009).

Some authors have proposed (Betterle et al., 2013). measurements of serum cortisol day curves to monitor replacement therapy but no agreement has been demonstrated between clinical assessment and cortisol levels (Arlt, 2009).

In order to mimic the physiological circadian biorhythm of cortisol, a once-daily dual-release hydrocortisone tablet was produced based on an immediate-release coating together with an extended-release core (Johannsson et al., 2009). The once-daily dual-release hydrocortisone tablet, compared to the conventional thrice-daily dose of conventional hydrocortisone tablets, produced a more circadian-based serum cortisol profile and reduced body weight, blood pressure, and improved glucose metabolism in patients with AD and concomitant diabetes mellitus (Johannsson et al., 2012).

Subcutaneous cortisol infusion is still an experimental treatment, but could be tested on selected patients not responding properly to regular peroral treatment (Løvås and Husebye, 2007).

Mineralocorticoid replacement is usually necessary and can be administered as a single daily dose of 0.05−0.2 mg of fludrocortisone or another aldosterone substitute. Patients should also receive an ample amount of sodium (3−4 g/daily), assessed by measurement of supine and erect blood pressure, serum electrolytes, and plasma renin activity levels (Williams and Dluhy, 1998). During the summer period, especially in Mediterranean or tropical climates, the doses of mineralocorticoids should be increased (Arlt, 2009). Complications are rare with this type of therapy. However, possible hypokalemia, hypertension, sodium retention, or heart disease should be monitored.

If essential hypertension develops in patients with mineralocorticoid replacement therapy, first, the dose may be slightly reduced; if the hypertension persists antihypertensive drugs need to be started (Arlt, 2009). DEHA (dehydroepiandrosterone) is the most important source of androgens in females; replacement therapy enhances well-being, mood, subjective health status, energy levels, and libido in women with adrenal insufficiency. For these reasons the therapy should be reserved for patients with significant impairment in well-being despite the optimized classical replacement therapy. Doses vary from 25 to 50 mg/day in a single dose in the morning (Arlt, 2009). The therapy remains optional because the drug is available only by ordering via the international pharmacy and the preparations are not pharmaceutically controlled (Arlt, 2009).

Steroid Replacement during Surgery, other Illness, Medical Procedures, Physical Activity, and Pregnancy

Patients with AD need to increase their steroid doses during surgery and medical procedures according to the stress induced.

In general, surgery, fever, gastrointestinal diseases, major dental procedures, and child delivery require parenteral hydrocortisone followed by double oral doses being tapered to replacement doses over subsequent days.

Patients undergoing regular and time-limited physical activity do not generally need to make a dose adjustment. However, in case of intense or prolonged exercise an increase in hydrocortisone and salt intake may be necessary. However, there are no systematic studies of replacement therapy during strenuous physical activity.

Pregnancy is associated with a gradual but pronounced physiological increase in corticosteroid-binding globulin (CBG) and total serum cortisol. Free cortisol levels rise during the third trimester, and some pregnant patients have a small increase in hydrocortisone requirement (by 2.5 or 5 mg daily) during the third trimester. Serum progesterone has anti-mineralocorticoid effects and hence the fludrocortisone dose may need to be increased during late pregnancy. Plasma renin activity normally increases during pregnancy. During delivery a bolus dose of 100 mg hydrocortisone should be given, and repeated if necessary. The oral dose should be doubled for 24−48 hours post-partum (Husebye et al., 2012).

In any case, patients with AD should carry a medical identification card (or a bracelet), stating the current therapy and recommendations for emergency situations such as febrile illnesses, injury, vomiting, surgical interventions, dental extractions or pregnancies, when the intake of glucocorticoids must be doubled or tripled (Oelkers, 1996).

Adrenal Crisis

The risk of adrenal crisis is a possible life-threatening event in every Addisonian patient. The crisis can be due to unnecessary reduction of the glucocorticoid therapy or to lack of stress-related glucocorticoid dose adjustment by patients or medical practitioners. Generally, oral glucocorticoid therapy should be increased or doubled during infections with fever, or during any other major stress-producing event, and, in general, needs to be orally increased but parenterally injected in case of gastrointestinal infections with diarrhea, surgical procedures, delivery, vomiting, or major traumas (Arlt, 2009).

Mortality

Three Scandinavian studies have made a contribution to the rate of mortality of AD (Bergthorsdottir et al., 2006; Bensing et al., 2008; Erichsen et al., 2009a). The two registry studies from Sweden (Bergthorsdottir et al., 2006; Bensing et al., 2008) showed that the mortality was more than double that in the control population and particularly elevated in patients with APS type 1 with an odds ratio of 4.6. The causes of death were endocrine diseases and cancer (Bensing et al., 2008). It must be said that the two Swedish registries referred exclusively to hospitalized patients, were not representative of the entire population of AD patients, and were both based on the codification of the disease without a definitive confirmation of the diagnosis. Potential assignation mistakes may have greatly influenced the outcome. More specifically, it is known that secondary adrenal insufficiency due to deficit of ACTH has an increased risk for mortality (Filipsson et al., 2006) also because of the concomitant deficit of other pituitary hormones and it is not certain that such patients have been excluded from the analysis.

A Norwegian case-control study did not report an overall increase in mortality, and also identified a subgroup of young males with doubled mortality rate, the causes of death being adrenal crisis, infections, and sudden death, while cardiovascular mortality was not increased (Erichsen et al., 2009a).

In an Italian study we examined the mortality in over 700 patients with AD followed up for a mean period of 15 years and demonstrated the existence of a normal survival rate in patients with autoimmune AD excluding those with APS type 1. Patients with APS type 1 revealed an increased mortality rate with respect to the general population matched for gender and age with the patients (Betterle et al., personal observation).

Osteoporosis

It is a constant concern that overtreatment with glucocorticoids may have negative health effects on bone mineral density. An increased incidence of osteoporosis has been reported in patients receiving daily replacement doses of 30 mg of hydrocortisone or higher, whereas replacement doses of 20–25 mg of hydrocortisone do not affect bone mineral density (Arlt, 2009).

Earlier studies have been hampered by low numbers of participants. In patients with AD a reduced bone mineral density (BMD) was reported along with polymorphisms in genes regulating steroid action influences BMD (Løvås et al., 2009). BMD revealed an inverse correlation to steroid dose, and was especially low in those taking synthetic potent glucocorticoids such as prednisolone. Despite reduced BMD, vertebral fractures were not more prevalent than in the background population. In contrast, a follow-up registry study from Sweden reported significantly increased frequencies of hip fractures in AD patients with an excess risk about 50% (Björnsdottir et al., 2011).

A recent study in 81 German patients who received low replacement doses of glucocorticoids found no reduction in BMD (Koetz et al., 2012). Thus, clinicians should aim to keep the glucocorticoid replacement dose as low as is compatible with normal well-being.

Patients with AAD should carry a medical identification card (or a bracelet), stating the current therapy; and recommendations for emergency situations such as febrile illnesses, injury, vomiting, surgical interventions, dental extractions or pregnancies, when the intake of glucocorticoids must be doubled or tripled (Oelkers, 1996).

Based on a synthesis of the EurAdrenal research, and the views and experience of the consortium's investigators, we have attempted to provide European guidelines for diagnosis, treatment, and follow-up of patients with AD (Husebye et al., 2012).

ACKNOWLEDGMENTS

We would like to thank all those who have cooperated with us over the years regarding the study of the clinical, genetic, immunologic, morphologic, and endocrine aspects of AD.

This study was supported in part by a grant from the European Union Seventh Framework Programme, the Euradrenal project: Pathophysiology and Natural Course of Autoimmune Adrenal Failure in Europe. Grant Agreement No. 2008-201167 (EURADRENAL website: www.euradrenal.org/).

REFERENCES

Addison, T., 1868. On the constitutional and local effects of disease of the suprarenal capsules. In a collection of the published writings of the late Thomas Addison MD, physician to Guy's Hospital. New Sydenham Society, London.

Anderson, J.R., Goudie, R.B., Gray, K.G., Timbury, G.C., 1957. Autoantibodies in Addison's disease. Lancet. 1, 1123–1124.

Anderson, J.U., Goudie, R.B., Gray, K., Stuart Smith, D.A., 1968. Immunological features of idiopathic Addison's disease: an antibody to cells producing steroid hormones. Clin. Exp. Immunol. 3, 107–117.

Andrada, J.A., Skelton, F.R., Andrada, E.C., Milgrom, F., Witebsky, E., 1968. Experimental autoimmune adrenalitis in rats. Lab. Invest. 19, 460–465.

Arif, S., Vallian, S., Farzaneh, F., Zanone, M.M., James, S.L., Pietropaolo, M., et al., 1996. Identification of 3-beta-hydroxysteroid dehydrogenase as a novel target of steroid cell autoantibodies: association of autoantibodies with endocrine autoimmune disease. J. Clin. Endocrinol. Metab. 81, 4439–4445.

Arlt, W., 2009. The approach to the adult with newly diagnosed adrenal insufficiency. J. Clin. Endocrinol. Metab. 94, 1059–1067.

Arlt, W., Allolio, B., 2003. Adrenal insufficiency. Lancet 361, 1881–1893.

Asawa, T., Wedlock, N., Baumann-Antczak, A., Rees Smith, B., Furmaniak, J., 1994. Naturally occurring mutations in human steroid 21-hydroxylase influence adrenal autoantibody binding. J. Clin. Endocrinol. Metab. 79, 372–376.

Auchus, R.J., Miller, W.L., 2001. The principles, pathways and enzymes of human steroidogenesis. In: fourth ed. DeGroot, L.J., Jameson, J.L. (Eds.), Endocrinology, vol. 2. W.B. Saunders.

Barnett, E.V., Dumonde, D.C., Glynn, L.E., 1963. Induction of autoimmunity to adrenal gland. Immunology 6, 382.

Baumann-Antczak, A., Wedlock, N., Bednarek, J., Kiso, Y., Krishnan, H., Fowler, S., et al., 1992. Autoimmune Addison's disease and 21-hydroxylase. Lancet. 340, 429–430.

Beales, P.E., Castri, F., Valiani, A., Rosignoli, G., Buckley, L., Pozzilli, P., 2002. Adrenalitis in the non-obese diabetic mouse. Autoimmunity. 35, 329–333.

Bednarek, J., Furmaniak, J., Wedlock, N., Kiso, Y., Baumann-Antczak, A., Fowler, S., et al., 1992. Steroid 21-hydroxylase is a major autoantigen involved in adult onset autoimmune Addison's disease. FEBS Lett. 309, 51–55.

Bensing, S., Brandt, L., Tabaroj, F., Sjöberg, O., Nilsson, B., Ekbom, A., et al., 2008. Increased death risk and altered cancer incidence pattern in patients with isolated or combined autoimmune primary adrenocortical insufficiency. Clin. Endocrinol. (Oxf). 69, 697–704.

Bergthorsdottir, R., Leonsson-Zachrisson, M., Odén, A., Johannsson, G., 2006. Premature mortality in patients with Addison's disease: a population-based study. J. Clin. Endocrinol. Metab. 91, 4849–4853.

Betterle, C., 2004. Addison's disease and autoimmune polyglandular syndromes. In: Geenen, V., Chrosus, G. (Eds.), Immunoendocrinology in Health and Disease. Dekker, New York, pp. 491–536.

Betterle, C., Presotto, F. 2008. Autoimmune polyendocrine syndromes (APS) or multiple autoimmune syndromes (MAS). In: Walker, S., Jara, L.J. (Eds.), Handbook of Systemic Autoimmune Diseases, vol. 9. Elsevier, Amsterdam, pp. 135–148.

Betterle, C., Volpato, M., 1998. Adrenal and ovarian autoimmunity. Eur. J. Endocrinol. 138, 16–25.

Betterle, C., Scalici, C., Presotto, F., Pedini, B., Moro, L., Rigon, F., et al., 1988. The natural history of adrenal function in autoimmune patients with adrenal autoantibodies. J. Endocrinol. 117, 467–475.

Betterle, C., Rossi, A., Dalla Pria, S., Artifoni, L., Pedini, B., Gavasso, S., et al., 1993. Premature ovarian failure: autoimmunity and natural history of the disease. Clin. Endocrinol. 39, 35–43.

Betterle, C., Volpato, M., Rees Smith, B., Furmaniak, J., Chen, S., Greggio, N.A., et al., 1997a. I. Adrenal cortex and steroid 21-hydroxylase autoantibodies in adult patients with organ-specific autoimmune diseases: markers of low progression to clinical Addison's disease. J. Clin. Endocrinol. Metab. 82, 932–938.

Betterle, C., Volpato, M., Rees Smith, B., Furmaniak, J., Chen, S., Zanchetta, R., et al., 1997b. II. Adrenal cortex and steroid 21-hydroxylase autoantibodies in children with organ-specific autoimmune diseases: markers of high progression to clinical Addison's disease. J. Clin. Endocrinol. Metab. 82, 939–942.

Betterle, C., Volpato, M., Pedini, B., Chen, S., Rees Smith, B., Furmaniak, J., 1999. Adrenal-cortex autoantibodies and steroid producing cells autoantibodies in patients with Addison's disease: comparison of immunofluorescence and immunoprecipitation assays. J. Clin. Endocrinol. Metab. 84, 618–622.

Betterle, C., Dal Pra, C., Mantero, F., Zanchetta, R., 2002. Autoimmune adrenal insufficiency and autoimmune polyendocrine syndromes: autoantibodies, autoantigens, and their applicability in diagnosis and disease prediction. Endocr. Rev. 23, 327–364.

Betterle, C., Coco, G., Zanchetta, R., 2005. Adrenal cortex autoantibodies in subjects with normal adrenal function. Best Pract. Res. Clin. Endocrinol. Metab. 19, 85–99.

Betterle, C., Scarpa, R., Morlin, L., Garelli, S., Lazzarotto, F., Presotto, F., et al. 2013. Addison's disease: a survey on 633 patients in Padova. Eur. J. Endocrinol Avaliable from: doi: 10.1530/EJE-13-0528.

Björnsdottir, S., Sääf, M., Bensing, S., Këmpe, O., Michaëlsson, K., Ludvigsson, J.F., 2011. Risk of hip fracture in Addison's disease: a population-based cohort study. J. Intern. Med. 270, 187–195.

Blizzard, R.M., Kyle, M., 1963. Studies on adrenal antigens and autoantibodies in Addison's disease. J. Clin. Invest. 42, 1653–1660.

Boscaro, M., Betterle, C., Volpato, M., Fallo, F., Furmaniak, J., Rees Smith, B., et al., 1996. Hormonal responses during various phases of autoimmune adrenal failure: no evidence for 21-hydroxylase enzyme activity inhibition in vivo. J. Clin. Endocrinol. Metab. 81, 2801–2804.

Bratland, E., Husebye, E.S., 2011. Cellular immunity and immunopathology in autoimmune Addison's disease. Mol. Cell. Endocrinol. 336, 180–190.

Bratland, E., Skinningsrud, B., Undlien, D.E., Mozes, E., Husebye, E.S., 2009. T cell responses to steroid cytochrome P450 21-hydroxylase in patients with autoimmune primary adrenal insufficiency. J. Clin. Endocrinol. Metab. 94, 5117–5124.

Casserius, J., Tabulae Anatomicae LXXIIX, West Germany, Druckerei Holzer, Copy 1283.

Cervato, S., Mariniello, B., Lazzarotto, F., Morlin, L., Zanchetta, R., Radetti, G., et al., 2009. Evaluation of the autoimmune regulator (AIRE) gene mutations in a cohort of Italian patients with autoimmune-polyendocrinopathy-candidiasis-ectodermal-dystrophy (APECED) and in their relatives. Clin. Endocrinol. (Oxf.). 70, 421–428.

Chen, Q.J., Lan, M.S., She, J.X., Maclaren, N.K., 1998. The gene responsible for autoimmune polyglandular syndrome type 1 maps to chromosome 21q22.3 in US patients. J. Autoimmun. 11, 117–183.

Chen, S., Sawicka, J., Betterle, C., Powell, M., Prentice, L., Volpato, M., et al., 1996. Autoantibodies to steroidogenic enzymes in autoimmune polyglandular syndrome, Addison's disease, and premature ovarian failure. J. Clin. Endocrinol. Metab. 83, 2977–2986.

Chung, B.C., Matteson, K.J., Voutilainen, R., Mohandas, T.K., Miller, W.L., 1986. Human cholesterol side-chain cleavage enzyme, P450scc: cDNA cloning, assignment of the gene to chromosome 15, and expression in the placenta. Proc. Natl. Acad. Sci. U.S.A. 83, 8962–8966

Clemente, M.G., Obermyer-Straub, P., Meloni, A., Strassburg, C.P., Arangino, V., et al., 1997. Cytochrome P450 IA2 is a hepatic autoantigen in autoimmune polyglandular syndrome type 1. J. Clin. Endocrinol. Metab. 82, 1353–1361.

Clemente, M.G., Meloni, A., Obermyer-Straub, P., Frau, F., Manns, M.P., De Virgilis, S., 1998. Two cytochrome P450 are major hepatocellular autoantigens in autoimmune polyglandular syndrome type 1. Gastroenterology. 114, 324–328.

Coco, G., Dal Pra, C., Presotto, F., Albergoni, M.P., Canova, C., Pedini, B., et al., 2006. Estimated risk for developing autoimmune Addison's disease in patients with adrenal cortex autoantibodies. J. Clin. Endocrinol. Metab. 91, 1637–1645.

Colls, J., Betterle, C., Volpato, M., Rees Smith, B., Furmaniak, J., 1995. A new immunoprecipitation assay for autoantibodies to steroid 21-hydroxylase in Addison's disease. Clin. Chem. 41, 375–380.

Colover, J., Glynn, L.E., 1958. Experimental iso-immune adrenalitis. Immunology. 2, 172–178.

Dal Pra, C., Chen, S., Betterle, C., Zanchetta, R., McGrath, V., Furmaniak, J., et al., 2004. Autoantibodies to human tryptophan hydroxylase and aromatic L-amino acid decarboxylase. Eur. J. Endocrinol. 150, 313–321.

De Bellis, A., Bizzarro, A., Rossi, R., Paglionico, V.A., Criscuolo, T., Lombardi, G., et al., 1993. Remission of subclinical adrenocortical failure in subjects with adrenal autoantibodies. J. Clin. Endocrinol. Metab. 76, 1002–1007.

Doppman, J.L. 2001. Adrenal imaging. In: DeGroot, L.J., Jameson, J.L. (Eds.), Endocrinology, vol. 2, fourth ed. W.B. Saunders Co., Philadelphia.

Drury, M.J., Keelan, D.M., Timoney, F.J., Irvine, W.J., 1979. Case report. Juvenile familial endocrinopathy. Clin. Exp. Immunol. 7, 125–132.

Duff, G.L., Bernstein, C., 1933. Five cases of Addison's disease with so-called atrophy of the adrenal cortex. Bull. Johns Hopkins Hosp. 52, 67.

Dunlop, D., 1963. Eighty-six cases of Addison's disease. Br. Med. J. 3, 887–891.

Dunn, K.J., Herrtage, M.E., 1998. Hypocortisolaemia in a Labrador retriever. J. Small Anim. Pract. 39, 90–93.

Eason, R.J., Croxon, M.S., Perry, M.C., Somerfield, S.D., 1982. Addison's disease, adrenal autoantibodies and computerized adrenal tomography. N.Z. Med. J. 95, 569–573.

Ekwall, O., Hedstrand, H., Grimelius, L., Haavik, J., Perheentupa, J., Gustafsson, J., et al., 1998. Identification of tryptophan hydroxylase as an intestinal autoantigen. Lancet. 352, 279–283.

Erichsen, M.M, Løvås, K., Fougner, K.J., Svartberg, J., Hauge, E.R., Bollerslev, J., et al., 2009a. Normal overall mortality rate in Addison's disease, but young patients are at risk of premature death. Eur. J. Endocrinol. 160, 233–237.

Erichsen, M.M., Løvås, K., Skinningsrud, B., Wolff, A.B., Undlien, D.E., Svartberg, J., et al., 2009b. Clinical, immunological, and genetic features of autoimmune primary adrenal insufficiency: observations from a Norwegian registry. J. Clin. Endocrinol. Metab. 94, 4882–4890.

Eustachius, B. 1563. Opuscula anatomica de renum structura, efficio et adminstratione. In: Luchino, V. (Ed.), Venice.

Falorni, A., Nikoshokov, A., Laureti, S., Grenbäck, E., Hulting, A.L., Casucci, G., 1995. High diagnostic accuracy for idiopathic Addison's disease with a sensitive radiobinding assay for autoantibodies against recombinant human 21-hydroxylase. J. Clin. Endocrinol. Metab. 80, 2752–2755.

Falorni, A., Laureti, S., Nikoshkov, A., et al., For the Belgian Diabetes Registry 1997. 21-Hydroxylase autoantibodies in adult patients with endocrine autoimmune diseases are highly specific for Addison's disease. Clin. Exp. Immunol. 107, 341–346.

Falorni, A., Chen, S., Zanchetta, R., Yu, L., Tiberti, C., Bacosi, M.L., et al., 2011. Measuring adrenal autoantibody response: interlaboratory concordance in the first international serum exchange for the determination of 21-hydroxylase autoantibodies. Clin. Immunol. 140, 291–299.

Fidler, W.J., 1977. Ovarian thecal metaplasma in adrenal glands. Am. J. Clin. Pathol. 67, 318–322.

Filipsson, H., Monson, J.P., Koltowska-Häggström, M., Mattsson, A., Johannsson, G., 2006. The impact of glucocorticoid replacement regimens on metabolic outcome and comorbidity in hypopituitary patients. J. Clin. Endocrinol. Metab. 92, 110–116.

Fogt, F., Vortmeyer, A.O., Poremba, C., Minda, M., Harris, C.A., Tomaszewski, J.E., 1998. Bcl2 expression in normal adrenal glands and in adrenal neoplasms. Mod. Pathol. 11, 716–720.

Freeman, M., Weetman, A.P., 1992. T and B cell reactivity to adrenal antigens in autoimmune Addison's disease. Clin. Exp. Immunol. 88, 275–279.

Fujii, Y., Kato, N., Kito, J., Asai, J., Yokochi, T., 1992. Experimental autoimmune adrenalitis: a murine model for Addison's disease. Autoimmunity. 12, 47–52.

Furmaniak, J., Rees Smith, B. 2002. Addison's disease. In: Gill, R.G. (Ed.), Immunologically Mediated Endocrine Diseases. Lippincott Williams & Williams, Philadelphia, pp. 431–451.

Furmaniak, J., Talbot, D., Reinwein, D., Benker, G., Creag, F.M., Rees Smith, B., 1988. Immunoprecipitation of human adrenal microsomal antigen. FEBS Lett. 232, 25–28.

Furmaniak, J., Kominani, S., Asawa, T., Wedlock, N., Colls, J., Rees Smith, B., 1994. Autoimmune Addison's disease. Evidence for a role of steroid 21-hydroxylase autoantibodies in adrenal insufficiency. J. Clin. Endocrinol. Metab. 79, 1517–1521.

Furmaniak, J., Sanders, J., Rees Smith, B. 1999. Autoantigens in the autoimmune endocrinopathies. In: Volpé, R. (Ed.), Contemporary Endocrinology: Autoimmune Endocrinopathies. Totowa, New York, pp. 183–216.

Gonzalez-Hernandez, J.A., Bornstein, S.R., Ehrhart-Bornstein, M., Spath-Schwalbe, E., Jirikowski, G., Scherbaum, W.A., 1994. Interleukin-6 messenger ribonucleic acid expression in human adrenal gland *in vivo*: new clue to a pancreatic or autocrine regulation of adrenal function. J. Clin. Endocrinol. Metab. 79, 1492–1497.

Grinspoon, S.K., Biller, B.M., 1994. Clinical review 62: laboratory assessment of adrenal insufficiency. J. Clin. Endocrinol. Metab. 79, 923–931.

Groves, R.W., Toms, G.C., Houghton, B.J., Monson, J.P., 1988. Corticosteroid replacement therapy: twice or thrice daily? J. R. Soc. Med. 81, 514–516.

Guttman, P.H., 1930. Addison's disease: statistical analysis of 566 cases and study of the pathology. Arch. Pathol. 10, 742–895.

Harlton, B.W., 1976. Addison's disease in a dog. Vet. Med. Small Anim. Clin. 71, 285–288.

Hayashi, Y., Hiyoshi, T., Takemura, T., Kurashima, C., Hirokawa, K., 1989. Focal lymphocytic infiltration in the adrenal cortex of the elderly: immunohistochemical analysis of infiltrating lymphocytes. Clin. Exp. Immunol. 77, 101–105.

Hedstrand, H., Ekwall, O., Haavik, J., Landgren, E., Betterle, C., Perheentupa, J., et al., 2000. Identification of tyrosine hydroxylase as an autoantigen in autoimmune polyendocrine syndrome Type 1. Biochem. Biophys. Res. Commun. 267, 456–461.

Hedstrand, H., Ekwall, O., Olsson, M.J., Landgren, E., Kemp, H.E., Weetman, A., et al., 2001. The transcription factors SOX9 and SOX10 are vitiligo autoantigens in autoimmune polyendocrine syndrome type 1. J. Biol. Chem. 276, 35390–35395.

Henzen-Logmans, S.C., Stel, H.V., Van Muijen, G.N., Mullink, H., Meijer, C.J., 1988. Expression of intermediate filament proteins in adrenal cortex and related tumors. Histopathology. 12, 359–372.

Hiatt, J.R., Hiatt, N., 1997. The conquest of Addison's disease. Am. J. Surg. 174, 280–283.

Hoek, A., Schoemaker, J., Drexhage, H.A., 1997. Premature ovarian failure and ovarian autoimmunity. Endocr. Rev. 18, 107–134.

Hoenig, E.M., Hirano, A., Levine, A., Ghatak, N.R., 1970. The early development and fine structure of allergic adrenalitis. Lab. Invest. 22, 198–205.

Howlett, T.A., 1997. An assessment of optimal hydrocortisone replacement therapy. Clin. Endocrinol. (Oxf.). 46, 263–268.

Husebye, E.S., Gebre-Medhin, G., Thuomi, T., Perheentupa, J., Landin-Olsson, M., Gustafsson, J., et al., 1997. Autoantibodies against aromatic L-amino acid decarboxylase in autoimmune polyendocrine syndrome type. I. J. Clin. Endocrinol. Metab. 82, 147–150.

Husebye, E.S., Bratland, E., Bredholt, G., Fridkin, M., Dayan, M., Mozes, E., 2006. The substrate-binding domain of 21-hydroxylase, the main autoantigen in autoimmune Addison's disease, is an immunodominant T cell epitope. Endocrinology 147, 2411–2416.

Husebye, E.S., Løvås, K., Allolio, B., Arlt, W., Badenhoop, K., Bensing, S., et al., 2012. Consensus statement on the diagnosis, treatment and follow-up of patients with primary adrenal insufficiency. JAMA, submitted.

Irvine, W.J., Barnes, E.W., 1975. Addison's disease, ovarian failure and hypoparathyroidism. Clin. Endocrinol. Metab. 4, 379–434.

Jackson, R., McNicol, A.M., Farquarson, M., Foulis, A.K., 1988. Class II MHC expression in normal adrenal cortex and cortical cell in autoimmune Addison's disease. J. Pathol. 155, 113–120.

Jacobson, D.L., Gange, S.J., Rose, N.R., Graham, N.M.H., 1997. Epidemiology and estimated population burden of selected autoimmune diseases in the United States. Clin. Immunol. Immunopathol. 84, 223–243.

Johannsson, G., Bergthorsdottir, R., Nilsson, A.G., Lennernas, H., Hedner, T., Skrtic, S., 2009. Improving glucocorticoid replacement therapy using a novel modified-release hydrocortisone tablet: a pharmacokinetic study. Eur. J. Endocrinol. 161, 119–130.

Johannsson, G., Nilsson, A.G., Bergthorsdottir, R., Burman, P., Dahlqvist, P., Ekman, B., et al., 2012. Improved cortisol exposure-time profile and outcome in patients with adrenal insufficiency: a prospective randomized trial of a novel hydrocortisone dual-release formulation. J. Clin. Endocrinol. Metab. 97, 473–481.

Kamradt, T., Mitchinson, N.A., 2001. Tolerance and autoimmunity. N. Engl. J. Med. 344, 655–664.

Kannan, C.R., 1988. Addison's disease. In: Kannan, C.R. (Ed.), The Adrenal Gland. Plenum, London, pp. 31–96.

Kaufman, J., 1984. Diseases of the adrenal cortex of dogs and cats. Mod. Vet. Pract. 65, 513–516.

Kendall-Taylor, P., Lambert, A., Mitchell, R., Robertson, W.R., 1988. Antibody that blocks stimulation of cortisol secretion by adrenocorticotrophic hormone in Addison's disease. Br. Med. J. 296, 1489–1491.

Khoury, E.L., Hammond, L., Bottazzo, G.F., Doniach, D., 1981. Surface-reactive antibodies to human adrenal cells in Addison's disease. Clin. Exp. Immunol. 45, 48–55.

Kiaer, W., Rytter Norgaard, J.O., 1969. Granulomatous hypophysitis and thyroiditis with lymphocytic adrenalitis. Acta Pathol. Microbiol. Scand. 76, 229.

Kintzer, P.P., Peterson, M.E., 1994. Diagnosis and management of primary spontaneous hypoadrenocorticism (Addison's disease) in dogs. Sem. Vet. Med. Surg. 9 (3), 148–152.

Koch, C.A. 2004. Adrenal cortex physiology. In: Martini, L. (Ed.), Encyclopedia of Endocrine Disease. Academic Press, San Diego, pp. 68–74.

Koetz, K.R., Ventz, M., Diederich, S., Quinkler, M., 2012. Bone mineral density is not significantly reduced in adult patients on low-dose glucocorticoid replacement therapy. J. Clin. Endocrinol. Metab. 97, 85–92.

Kong, M.F., Jeffcoate, W., 1994. Eighty-six cases of Addison's disease. Clin. Endocrinol. 41, 757–761.

Krohn, K., Uibo, R., Aavik, E., Peterson, P., Savilhati, K., 1992. Identification by molecular cloning of an autoantigen associated with Addison's disease as steroid 17-a-hydroxylase. Lancet 339, 770–773.

Laureti, S., De Bellis, A.M., Muccitelli, V.I., Calcinaro, F., Bizzaro, A., Rossi, R., et al., 1998. Levels of adrenocortical autoantibodies correlate with the degree of adrenal dysfunction in subjects with pre-clinical Addison's disease. J. Clin. Endocrinol. Metab. 83, 3507–3511.

Laureti, S., Vecchi, L., Santeusanio, F., Falorni, A., 1999. Is the prevalence of Addison's disease underestimated? J. Clin. Endocrinol. Metab. 84, 1762.

Laureti, S., Arvat, E., Candeloro, P., Di Vito, L., Ghigo, E., Santeusanio, F., et al., 2000. Low dose (1 g) ACTH test in the evaluation of adrenal dysfunction in pre-clinical Addison's disease. Clin. Endocrinol. 53, 107–115.

Levine, S., Wenk, E.J., 1968. The production and passive transfer of allergic adrenalitis. Am. J. Pathol. 52, 41–53.

Lin, D., Zhang, L., Chiao, E., Miller, W.L., 1994. Modeling and mutagenesis of the active site of human P450c17. Mol. Endocrinol. 8, 392–402.

Little, C., Marshall, C., Downs, J., 1989. Addison's disease in the dog. Vet. Rec. 124, 469–470.

Løvås, K., Husebye, E.S., 2002. High prevalence and increasing incidence of Addison's disease in western Norway. Clin. Endocrinol. 56, 787–791.

Løvås, K., Husebye, E.S., 2007. Continuous subcutaneous hydrocortisone infusion in Addison's disease. Eur. J. Endocrinol. 157, 109–112.

Løvås, K., Gjesdal, C.G., Christensen, M., Wolff, A.B., Almås, B., Svartberg, J., et al., 2009. Glucocorticoid replacement therapy and pharmacogenetics in Addison's disease: effects on bone. Eur. J. Endocrinol. 160, 993–1002.

Mason, A.S., Meade, T.W., Lee, J.A., Morris, J.N., 1968. Epidemiological and clinical picture of Addison's disease. Lancet 2, 744–747.

McIntyre Gass, J.D., 1962. The syndrome of keratoconjunctivitis, superficial moniliasis, idiopathic hypoparathyroidism and Addison's disease. Am. J. Ophthalmol. 54, 660–674.

McNicol, A.M., 1986. Class II MHC expression in the adrenal cortex. Lancet 2, 1282.

McNicol, A.M., Laidler, P., 1996. The adrenal gland and extra-adrenal paraganglia. In: Lewis, P.D. (Ed.), Endocrine System. Churchill Livingstone, Edinburgh.

Morgan, J., Betterle, C., Zanchetta, R., Dal Prà, C., Chen, S., Rees Smith, B., et al., 2000. Direct evidence that steroid 21-hydroxylase (21-OH) is the major antigen recognized by adrenal cortex autoantibodies (ACA). J. Endocrinol. 167, OC19.

Muscatelli, F., Strom, T.M., Walker, A.P., Zanaria., E., Recan, D., Meindl, A., et al., 1994. Mutations in the DAX-1 gene give rise to both x-linked adrenal hypoplasia congenita and hypogonadotropic hypogonadism. Nature. 372, 672–676.

Myhre, A.G., Undelien, D.A., Lovas, K., Uhlving, S., Nedrebo, B.G., Fougner, K.J., et al., 2002. Autoimmune adrenocortical failure in Norway autoantibodies and human leukocyte antigen class II association related to clinical features. J. Clin. Endocrinol. Metab. 87, 618–623.

Nerup, J., 1974. Addison's disease—clinical studies. A report of 108 cases. Acta Endocrinol. 76, 121–141.

Nerup, J., Bendixen, G., 1969. Anti-adrenal cellular hypersensitivity in Addison's disease. 2. Correlation with clinical and serological findings. Clin. Exp. Immunol. 5, 341–353.

Nerup, J., Andersen, V., Bendixen, G., 1970. Antiadrenal cellular hypersensitivity in Addison's disease. IV. *In vivo* and *in vitro* investigations of the mitochondrial fraction. Clin. Exp. Immunol. 6, 733.

Neufeld, M., Blizzard, R.M., 1980. Polyglandular autoimmune diseases. In: Pinchera, A., Doniach, D., Fenzi, G.F., Baschieri, L. (Eds.), Symposium on Autoimmune Aspects of Endocrine Disorders. Academic Press, New York, pp. 357–365.

Nigam, R., Bhatia, E., Miao, D., Brozzetti, A., Eisenbarth, G.S., Falorni, A., 2003. Prevalence of adrenal antibodies in Addison's disease among north Indian caucasians. Clin. Endocrinol. 59, 593–598.

Oelkers, W., 1996. Adrenal insufficiency. N. Engl. J. Med. 335, 1206–1212.

Oelkers, W., Diederich, S., Bahr, V., 1992. Diagnosis and therapy surveillance in Addison's disease: rapid adrenocorticotropin (ACTH) test and measurement of plasma ACTH, renin activity and aldosterone. J. Clin. Endocrinol. Metab. 75, 259–264.

Orth, D.N., Kavacs, W.J., 1998. The adrenal cortex. In: Wilson, J.D., Foster, D.W., Kronenberg, H.M., Larse, P.R. (Eds.), Williams Textbook of Endocrinology, ninth ed. W.B. Saunders, Philadelphia, pp. 517–664.

Pelkey, T.J., Frierson Jr., H.F., Mills, S.E., Stoler, M.H., 1998. The alpha subunit of inhibin in adrenal cortical neoplasia. Mod. Pathol. 11, 516–524.

Peterson, M.E., Greco, D.S., Orth, D.N., 1989. Primary hypoadrenocorticism in ten cats. J. Vet. Intern. Med. 3, 55–58.

Peterson, P., Krohn, K.J.E., 1994. Mapping of B cell epitopes on steroid 17-a-hydroxylase, an autoantigen in autoimmune polyglandular syndrome type 1. Clin. Exp. Immunol. 98, 104–109.

Peterson, P., Perheentupa, J., Krohn, K.J.E., 1996. Detection of candidal antigens in autoimmune polyglandular syndrome type I. Clin. Diagn. Lab. Immunol. 3, 290–294.

Peterson, P., Uibo, R., Peranen, J., Krohn, K.J.E., 1997. Immunoprecipitation of steroidogenic enzyme autoantigens with autoimmune polyglandular syndrome type 1 (APS I) sera; further evidence for independent humoral immunity to P450 c17 and P450c21. Clin. Exp. Immunol. 107, 335–340.

Petri, M., Nerup, J., 1971. Addison's adrenalitis. Acta Path. Microbiol. Scand. 79, 381–388.

Picado-Leonard, J., Miller, W.L., 1987. Cloning and sequence of the human gene for P450c17 (steroid 17a-hydroxylase/17,20 lyase): similarity with the gene for P450c21. DNA Cell Biol. 6, 439–448.

Rabinowe, S.L., Jackson, R.A., Dluhy, R.G., Williams, G.H., 1984. Ia-positive T lymphocytes in recently diagnosed idiopathic Addison's disease. Am. J. Med. 77, 597–601.

Raff, H., 2009. Utility of salivary cortisol measurements in Cushing's syndrome and adrenal insufficiency. J. Clin. Endocrinol. Metab. 94, 3647–3655.

Reato, G., Morlin, L., Chen, S., Furmaniak, J., Smith, B.R., Masiero., S., et al., 2011. Premature ovarian failure in patients with autoimmune Addison' disease: clinical, genetic, and immunological evaluation. J. Clin. Endocrinol. Metab. 96, E1255–E1261.

Rees Smith, B., Furmaniak, J., 1995. Editorial: adrenal and gonadal autoimmune diseases. J. Clin. Endocrinol. Metab. 80, 1502–1505.

Sadek, D., Schaer, M., 1996. Atypical Addison's disease in the dog: a retrospective survey of 14 cases. J. Am. Anim. Hosp. Assoc. 32, 159–163.

Salim, Y.S., Faber, V., Wiik, A., Andersewn, P.L., Hoier-Madsen, M., Mouritsen, S., 1988. Anti-corticosteroid antibodies in AIDS patients. Acta Pathol. Microbiol. Immunol. Scand. 96, 889–894.

Sasano, H., Nose, M., Sasano, N., 1989. Lectin histochemistry in adrenocortical hyperplasia and neoplasm with emphasis on carcinoma. Arch. Pathol. Lab. Med. 113, 68–72.

Sasano, H., Suzui, T., Shizawa, S., Kato, K., Natura, H., 1994. Transforming growth factor alpha, epidermal growth factor and epidermal growth factor receptor in normal and diseased human adrenal cortex by immunohistochemistry and in situ hybridization. Mod. Pathol. 7, 741–746.

Scarpa, R., Alaggio, R., Norberto, L., Furmaniak, J., Chen, S., Smith, B.R., et al., 2013. Tryptophan hydroxylase autoantibodies as markers of a distinct autoimmune gastrointestinal component of autoimmune polyendocrine syndrome type 1. J. Clin. Endocrinol. Metab. 98, 704–712.

Skoldberg, F., Portela-Gomes, G.M., Grimelius, L., Nilsson, G., Perheentupa, J., Betterle, C., et al., 2003. Histidine decarboxylase is a novel autoantigen of enterochromaffin-like cells in autoimmune polyendocrine syndrome type 1. J. Clin. Endocrinol. Metab. 88, 1445–1452.

Song, Y., Connor, E.L., Muir, A., She, J.X., Zorovich, B., Derovanesian, D., et al., 1994. Autoantibody epitope mapping of the 21-hydroxylase antigen in autoimmune Addison's disease. J. Clin. Endocrinol. Metab. 78, 1108–1112.

Sotsiu, F., Bottazzo, G.F., Doniach, D., 1980. Immunofluorescence studies on autoantibodies to steroid-producing cells, and to germline cells in endocrine disease and infertility. Clin. Exp. Immunol. 39, 97–111.

Steiner, J.W., Langer, B., Schatz, D.L., Volpé, R., 1960. Experimental immunologic adrenal injury: a response to injections of autologous and homologous adrenal antigens in adjuvant. J. Exp. Med. 112, 187.

Stewart, P.M., Corrie, J., Seckl, J.R., Edwards, C.R., Padfield, P.L., 1988. A rational approach for assessing the hypothalamo-pituitary-adrenal axis. Lancet 1, 1208–1210.

Stonehewer, J., Tasker, S., 2001. Hypoadrenocroticism in a cat. J. Small Anim. Pract. 42, 186–190.

Takayanagi, R., Miura, K., Nakagawa, H., Nawata, H., 2000. Epidemiological study of adrenal gland disorders in Japan. Biomed. Pharmacother. 54, 164–168.

Tanaka, H., Perez, M.S., Powell, M., Sandres, J.F., Sawicka, J., Chen, S., et al., 1997. Steroid 21-hydroxylase autoantibodies: measurements with a new immunoprecipitations assay. J. Clin. Endocrinol. Metab. 82, 1440–1446.

Tasker, S., MacKay, A.D., Sparkes, A.H., 1999. Case report. A case of feline primary hypoadrenocorticism. J. Felin. Med. Surg. 1, 257–260.

Thiebaut, F., Tsuruo, T., Hamada, H., Gottesman, M.M., Pastan, I., Willingham, M.C., 1987. Cellular localization of the multidrug resistance gene product P-glycoprotein in normal human tissues. Proc. Natl. Acad. Sci. U.S.A. 84, 7735–7738.

Trousseau, A., 1856. Bronze Addison's disease. Arch. Gen. Med. 8, 478–485.

Verghese, M.V., Ward, F.E., Eisenbarth, G.S., 1980. Decreased suppressor cell activity in patients with polyglandular failure. Clin. Res. 28, 270A.

Wardle, C.A., Weetman, A.P., Mitchell, R., Peers, N., Robertson, W.R., 1993. Adrenocorticotropic hormone receptor-blocking immunoglobulins in serum from patients with Addison's disease: a re-examination. J. Clin. Endocrinol. Metab. 77, 750–753.

Wedlock, N., Asawa, T., Baumann-Antczak, A., Rees Smith, B., Furmaniak, J., 1993. Autoimmune Addison's disease. Analysis of autoantibody sites on human steroid 21-hydroxylase. FEBS Lett. 332, 123–126.

Werdelin, O., Witebsky, E., 1970. Experimental allergic rat adrenalitis, a study on its elicitation and lymphokinetics. Lab. Invest. 23, 136–143.

Werdelin, O., Wick, G., McCluskey, R.T., 1971. The fate of newly formed lymphocytes migration from an antigen-stimulated lymph node in rats with allergic adrenalitis. Lab. Invest. 25, 279–286.

Williams, G.H., Dluhy, R.G., 1998. Disease of the adrenal cortex. In: Fauci, A.S., Braunwald, E., Isselbacher, K.J. (Eds.), Harrison's Principles of Internal Medicine, 14th ed. McGraw-Hill, New York.

Willis, A.C., Vince, F.P., 1997. The prevalence of Addison's disease in Coventry, UK. Postgrad. Med. J. 73, 286–288.

Wilson, R.C., Mercado, A.B., Cheng, K.C., New, M.I., 1995. Steroid 21-hydroxylase deficiency: genotype may not predict phenotype. J. Clin. Endocrinol. Metab. 80, 2322–3239.

Winqivist, O., Soderbergh, A., Kampe, O., 1996. The autoimmune basis of adrenal cortical destruction in Addison's disease (review). Mol. Med. Today. 2, 282–289.

Winqvist, O., Karlsson, F.A., Kampe, O., 1992. 21-hydroxylase, a major autoantigen in idiopathic Addison's disease. Lancet. 339, 1559–1562.

Winqvist, O., Gustafsson, J., Rorsman, F., Karlsson, F.A., Kampe, O., 1993. Two different cytochrome P450 enzymes are the adrenal antigens in autoimmune polyendocrine syndrome type I and Addison's disease. J. Clin. Invest. 92, 2377–2385.

Witebsky, E., Milgrom, F., 1962. Immunological studies on adrenal glands: II. Immunization with adrenals of the same species. Immunology. 5, 67–78.

Wulfraat, N.M., Drexhage, H.A., Bottazzo, G.F., Wiersinga, W.M., Jeucken, P., Van der Gaag, R., 1989. Immunoglobulins of patients with idiopathic Addison's disease block the in vitro action of adrenocotropin. J. Clin. Endocrinol. Metab. 69, 231–238.

Yu, L., Brewer, K.W., Gates, S., Wu, A., Wang, T., Babu, S.R., et al., 1999. DRB1*04 and DQ alleles: expression of 21-hydroxylase autoantibodies and risk of progression to Addison's disease. J. Clin. Endocrinol. Metab. 84, 328–335.

Chapter 43

Polyendocrine Syndromes

Pärt Peterson[1] and Eystein S. Husebye[2,3]

[1]*Molecular Pathology, University of Tartu, Tartu, Estonia,* [2]*Department of Clinical Science, University of Bergen, Bergen, Norway,* [3]*Department of Medicine, Haukeland University Hospital, Bergen, Norway*

Chapter Outline

Historical Background 605
Clinical Pathologic and Epidemiologic Features ... 606
Autoimmune Features 608
Genetic Features 608
Environmental Features 610
Animal Models 611
   AIRE-Deficient Mouse as a Model for APS-1 611
   Spontaneous Animal Models 611

Thymectomy Animal Model 611
Pathogenic Mechanisms 612
Immunologic Markers in Diagnosis 612
Treatment and Outcome 613
Concluding Remarks—Future Prospects 613
Acknowledgments 613
References 614

Autoimmune polyendocrinopathies can be divided into two distinct syndromes, autoimmune polyendocrine syndrome type 1 and type 2 (APS-1 and -2). The former is monogenic and caused by mutations in the autoimmune regulator (AIRE) gene, the latter is associated with certain major histocompatibility complex genotypes and a range of other genes. In both conditions a number of autoantibodies can be detected that correlate with clinical components. Clinically there are overlaps, but hypoparathyroidism and chronic mucocutaneous candidiasis are specific for APS-1. Recent years have provided remarkable progress in our knowledge about disease genes and immunopathology of APS, especially from studies of the AIRE-knockout mouse model. Assay of antibodies against tissue-specific enzymes, interferons, and interleukins can be used for both diagnostic purposes and to predict various disease components. However, the environmental triggers involved still remain elusive.

In this overview we summarize recent progress in the understanding of pathogenic mechanisms involved in APS-1 and APS-2, and in the corresponding animal models, and sum up similarities and differences in clinical presentation, diagnosis, and treatment.

HISTORICAL BACKGROUND

In 1855, Thomas Addison published observations linking the clinical features of "general languor and disability, feableness of the heart's action" and hyperpigmentation of the skin to disease in the suprarenal capsules (adrenals) (Addison, 1855). This disorder has since been known as Addison's disease (Wilks, 1862). Already in 1926 Schmidt (Schmidt, 1926) noticed the propensity for polyendocrinopathy by demonstrating lymphocytic infiltration in both the adrenal and thyroid glands (Schmidt syndrome, OMIM 269200); later, Carpenter (Carpenter et al., 1964) added insulin-dependent diabetes mellitus to this list. The first clinical reports on patients with Addison's disease presenting with chronic candidal infection and hypoparathyroidism appeared in the 1950s (Hetzel and Robson, 1958), although Thorpe and Hanley had already reported a case with hypoparathyroidism and candidiasis in 1929 (Thorpe and Handley, 1929). In the 1960s several reports pointed to the clinical and genetic heterogeneity among patients with Addison's disease (Blizzard and Gibbs, 1968; Spinner et al., 1968), proposing that, depending on the type of associated disorders, Addison's disease could be part of two separate and distinct clinical syndromes: autoimmune polyglandular (polyendocrine) syndromes (APS) type 1 and type 2 (Neufeld et al., 1981).

N. Rose & I. Mackay (Eds): The Autoimmune Diseases, Fifth edition. DOI: http://dx.doi.org/10.1016/B978-0-12-384929-8.00043-5

CLINICAL PATHOLOGIC AND EPIDEMIOLOGIC FEATURES

APS-1 (OMIM 240300) has a broad spectrum of clinical manifestations (Table 43.1, Figure 43.1). The disease is also referred to as autoimmune-polyendocrinopathy-candidiasis-ectodermal dystrophy (APECED) or polyglandular autoimmune syndrome (PAS) type 1. The most frequent clinical entities include chronic mucocutaneous candidiasis, hypoparathyroidism, and Addison's disease. Usually, two of the three major components need to be present in order to make the diagnosis; however, the disease variability and delay in appearance of manifestations make the diagnosis difficult in many instances. Typically, APS-1 starts in childhood with chronic candidiasis as the first manifestation followed by hypoparathyroidism and Addison's disease, but there is a wide variety of phenotypes from serious to very mild disease, even within the same family (Perheentupa, 2002, 2006).

Candida infection appears in more chronic cases as white thrush on the tongue. Candidal esophagitis is often present and the infection may spread to nails and in some cases even to skin of the hands and face. Several cases of oral carcinoma have been reported, suggesting that oral candidiasis might be carcinogenic (Perheentupa, 2002). Chronic mucocutaneous candidiasis is associated with reduced numbers of Th17 cells and presence of autoantibodies against the Th17 cell mediators IL-17F, IL-17A, and IL-22 (Kisand et al., 2010; Puel et al., 2010).

Hypoparathyroidism is the most frequent and sometimes only endocrine component in APS-1. Gonadal insufficiency is very common in females (female/male ratio, 3:1) and manifests itself in the teenage years and early twenties (Reato et al., 2011). Other endocrinopathies in falling frequencies are type 1 diabetes, autoimmune thyroid disease, and hypophysitis. Many patients suffer from gastrointestinal autoimmunity, notably enteropathy with malabsorption, hepatitis, autoimmune

TABLE 43.1   Manifestations and Organ-Specific Autoantibodies in APS-1

Main Disease Component		Autoantigen	Characteristics/Prevalence
APS-1		IFN-ω, IFN-α	Almost all patients are positive
Main triad	Hypoparathyroidism	NALP5	70–80%, childhood
	Addison's disease	P450c21	65–85%, childhood
	Candidiasis	IL-22, IL-17F, IL-17A	80–100%, childhood
Other endocrine manifestations	Ovarian failure	P450scc, P450c17, NALP5	60%
	Testicular failure	TSGA10	Adult prevalence up to 60%
	Autoimmune thyroid disease	TPO, TG	≈10%, relatively rare
	Type 1 diabetes	IA-2	0–25%
	Hypophysitis	TDRD6	Rare
Gastrointestinal	Malabsorption	TPH	Common, diarrhea, severe constipation, fatty stools
	Autoimmune gastritis		10–30%
	Autoimmune hepatitis	AADC, CYP1A2	5–20%, childhood, severe sometimes fatal
	Exocrine pancreatitis	nd	Rare
Hematological	Hypo/asplenia		10–20%, risk of septicemia
	Hypergammaglobulinemia		5%
	Pure red cell aenemia		Rare
Nephrological	Mineralocorticoid excess with hypertension		Rare
	Interstitial nephritis		Rare
Lung	Bronchiolitis obliterans	KCNRG	Rare, can be fatal
Ectodermal	Keratoconjunctivitis		Prevalence approx. 10%, may result in blindness
	Alopecia	SOX9	Common, prevalence 30–40%
	Vitiligo	TH	Prevalence ≈20%
	Periodic rash with fever		Rare
	Squamous cell carcinoma		Associated with candidosis and smoking, can be fatal
	Enamel dysplasia		Prevalence 50–70%
Muscular, neurological	Myopathy		Rare

Abbreviations: AADC, aromatic L-amino acid decarboxylase; IFN-ω, interferon-omega; IA-2, islet antigen 2; IFN-α, interferon-alpha; NALP5, NACHT-LLR-PYD-containing domain 5; KCNRG, putative potassium channel regulatory protein; SOX9, sex determining region Y-box 9; TDRD6, tudor domain-containing 6; TG, thyroglobulin; TH, tyrosine hydroxylase; TPH, tryptophan hydroxylase; TPO, thyroperoxidase; TSGA10, testis-specific gene 10 protein.

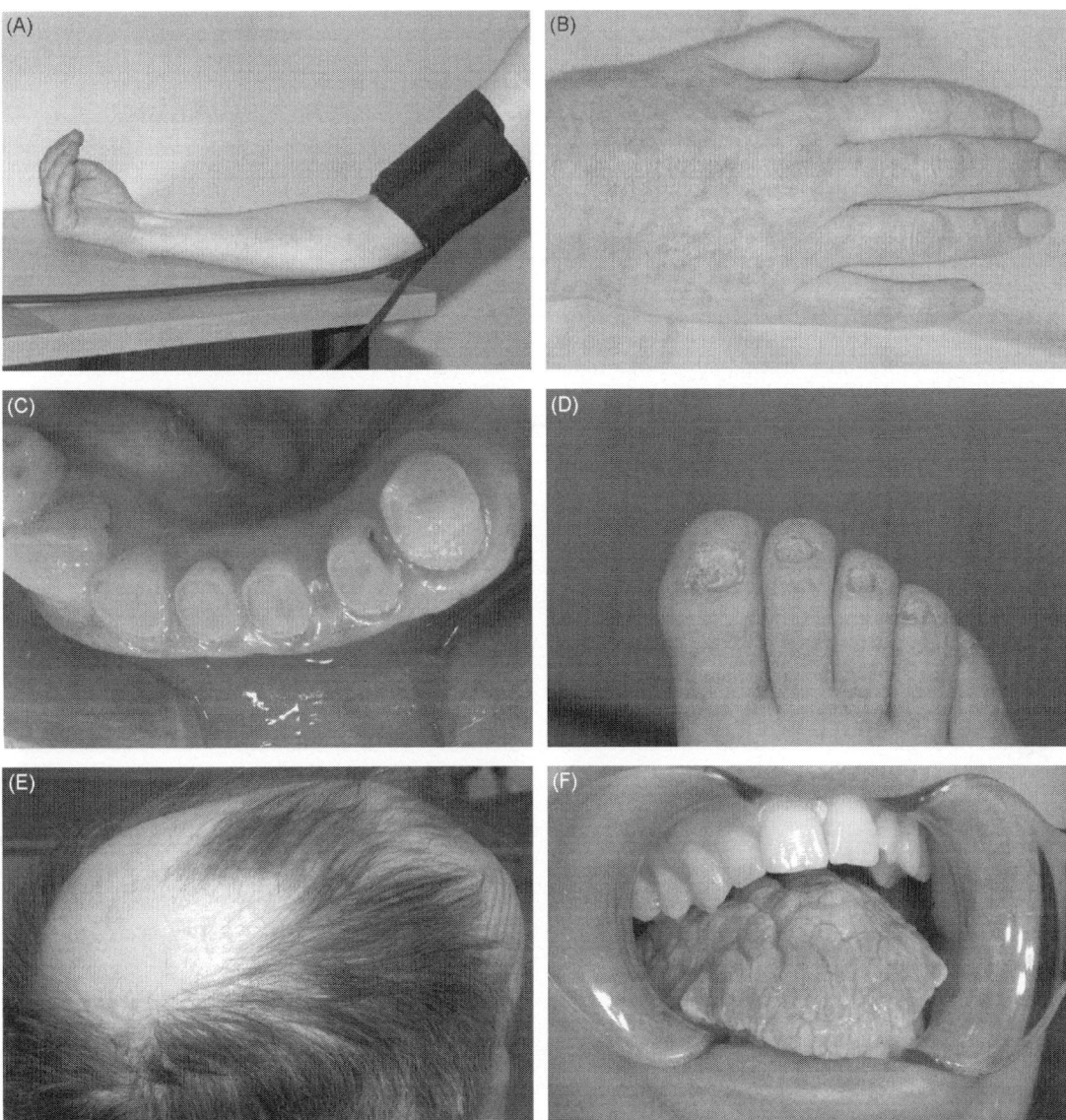

FIGURE 43.1 **Clinical manifestations of autoimmune polyendocrine syndrome type 1.**   A. Carpal spasm caused by hypocalcemia (Trousseau's sign; B. vitiligo (middle right); C. enamel hypoplasia with resultant wearing down of teeth. D. candida infection of the nail E. alopecia areata; F. candidiasis of the tongue. *Photographs courtesy Martina M. Erichsen, Haukeland University Hospital.*

gastritis with and without vitamin B12 and iron deficiencies, and exocrine pancreatitis. Many other disease associations have been reported in literature. APS-1 patients often display a number of organ-specific lesions affecting ectodermal structures, namely enamel dysplasia, vitiligo, alopecia, keratoconjuctivitis, and nail dystrophy. In addition, urticaria-like erythema and hyposplenism or splenic atrophy have been reported (Perheentupa, 2002, 2006), which render them susceptible to serious bacterial infections.

APS-2 is a genetically complex disease with a multifactorial etiology. The clinical onset usually occurs in adulthood, although it can start at any time during the lifespan. The classical definition of APS-2 (Neufeld et al.,

1981) comprises a combination of Addison's disease with autoimmune thyroid disease and/or type 1 diabetes. Probably any combinations of autoimmune disorders within the complex represent the same disorder with an inherited propensity to develop organ-specific autoimmunity (Schatz and Winter, 2002). Type 1 diabetes can develop before and after Addison's disease (Erichsen et al., 2009). In common with APS-1, manifestations such as vitiligo, alopecia, hypergonadotropic hypogonadism, and autoimmune gastritis with or without pernicious anemia are prevalent although less common and usually not present in childhood. The prevalence of APS-2 is estimated at up to 8 per 100,000 inhabitants (Erichsen et al., 2009) and first-degree relatives of patients with APS-2 are at high risk of autoimmune disorders (Michels and Eisenbarth, 2009). APS-2 affects in particular middle-aged Caucasian women with a male/female ratio of 1:2−3.

APS-3 was included in the original classification of autoimmune polyendocrine syndromes (Neufeld et al., 1981) to define the clinical entity of autoimmune thyroid disease and one or more other autoimmune diseases excluding Addison's disease. The genetic and etiological background of APS-3 is probably similar to that for APS-2. Sometimes, APS-4 is also mentioned as Addison's disease and other autoimmunity excluding autoimmune thyroid disease and type 1 diabetes. We here suggest for clarity that APS-4 is included in the group called APS-2.

AUTOIMMUNE FEATURES

Seminal evidence on the autoimmune pathogenesis in Addison's disease was provided by Anderson et al. (Anderson et al., 1957), who reported the presence of adre-nocortical cell antibodies (ACC-Ab) in patients with Addison's disease, using complement fixation. The finding of these autoantibodies was later confirmed by immunoflu-orescence (Blizzard et al., 1962) revealing 50−90% posi-tivity (Sotsiou et al., 1980; Betterle and Morlin, 2011). In addition to ACC-Ab, autoantibodies to the steroid produc-ing cells (StC-Ab) can be present reacting with the theca interna and corpus luteum of ovary, interstitial cells of tes-tis, and placental trophoblasts. These reactivities were later found to represent binding to steroidogenic P450 cyto-chrome enzymes. ACC-Ab was mainly associated with reactivity towards steroid 21-hydroxylase (P450c21 or CYP21) (Winqvist et al., 1992) expressed in the adrenal cortex, while StC-Ab was linked to reactivities against side chain cleavage enzyme (P450scc or CYP11A1) and steroid 17-alpha-hydroxylase (P450c17 or CYP17 expressed in both adrenals and gonads) (Krohn et al., 1992; Winqvist et al., 1993, 1995; Uibo et al., 1994; Brozzetti et al., 2010a; Reato et al., 2011).

Autoantibodies to several other organ-specific self antigens have been reported in APS-1 (Table 43.1). One group is decarboxylases and hydroxylases involved in neurotransmitter biosynthesis. Examples are autoantibo-dies against aromatic L-amino acid decarboxylase (AADC) correlated to type 2 autoimmune hepatitis (Husebye et al., 1997), tryptophan hydroxylase connected to autoimmune enteropathy (Ekwall et al., 1998), and tyrosine hydroxylases correlated to alopecia (Hedstrand et al., 2000). Patients also react with glutamic acid decar-boxylase 2 (GAD2/GAD65) (Skoldberg et al., 2004; Soderbergh et al., 2004) and with GAD1/GAD67 (Tuomi et al., 1996). Recently, NACHT leucine-rich-repeat pro-tein 5 (NALP5) has been identified as an autoantigen in hypoparathyroidism (Alimohammadi et al., 2008), and

potassium channel regulator KCNRG that is expressed only in the terminal bronchioli correlated with respiratory symptoms (Alimohammadi et al., 2009).

Autoantibodies to a new class of proteins were identi-fied in 2006 when type 1 interferon (IFN) antibodies were found in virtually all patients with APS-1 (Meager et al., 2006). Autoantibodies to type 1 IFN, in particular to various isoforms of IFN-α and IFN-ω, are neutralizing, occur in extremely high titers up to 1 to 10^6, are detected at very early stage of APS-1, and persist for decades. Such high frequencies of positivity renders assay of IFN-ω anti-bodies as a very useful tool to identify patients with APS-1 (Meloni et al., 2008; Oftedal et al., 2008). Finally, prevalent autoantibodies against interleukins IL-17A, IL-17F, and IL-22 were found with correlations to the pres-ence of candidiasis (Kisand et al., 2010; Puel et al., 2010).

In APS-2, most of the patients have autoantibodies to P450c21, the major autoantigen of Addison's disease (Baumann-Antczak et al., 1992; Bednarek et al., 1992; Winqvist et al., 1992; Erichsen et al., 2009). Prevalences of P450c21 antibodies in European populations are in the range of 80−90% (Falorni et al., 2011). The P450c21 auto-antibodies have been demonstrated by several methods including immunoblotting with recombinant protein expressed in bacteria, yeast, or mammalian cells or by immunoprecipitation with *in vitro* translated or luciferase-coupled protein (Burbelo et al., 2007). In approximately 15−20% of APS-2 female patients the autoantibodies to P450c17 and P450scc are detectable, which are the targets of the StC-Ab and correlate to the presence of ovarian fail-ure (Hoek et al., 1997; Betterle et al., 2002; Soderbergh et al., 2004). APS-2 patients with type 1 diabetes frequently have autoantibodies to GAD65 and/or IA-2 protein, while anti-GAD65 does not correlate to type 1 diabetes in APS-1 patients; instead an association to malabsorption was seen (Soderbergh et al., 2004). Autoantibodies to thyroid peroxi-dase are common in patients with autoimmune thyroiditis (Erichsen et al., 2009).

GENETIC FEATURES

APS-1 is inherited in an autosomal recessive manner and occurs as a defect in the autoimmune regulator (*AIRE*) gene. The prevalence worldwide is very low and population dependent. The frequency is higher among certain populations such as Finns (1/25,000) (Aaltonen et al., 1994), Iranian Jews (1/9000) (Zlotogora and Shapiro, 1992), and Sardinians (1/14,400) (Rosatelli et al., 1998). The prevalence reported from Norway at 1/80,000 (Wolff et al., 2007) probably reflects the fre-quency in most countries.

AIRE, the gene mutated in APS-1, was identified by positional cloning on chromosome 21q22.3 (Finnish-German-Consortium, 1997; Nagamine et al., 1997). To date more than 70 mutations have been found in *AIRE* gene (http://www.hgmd.cf.ac.uk/ac/gene.php?gene = AIRE). The mutations are spread throughout the coding region with two mutational hotspots. The most common mutation is amino acid arginine change to stop codon (R257X) in exon 6, which is found in 83% of the Finnish APS-1 chromosomes (Bjorses et al., 2000) but is also common in APS-1 patients of other ethnic origins (Scott et al., 1998). Another frequently occurring mutation is 967-979del13bp, which has been reported in patients from different populations (Wang et al., 1998; Pearce et al., 1998; Heino et al., 1999b; Myhre et al., 2002). Furthermore, R139X mutation is common among Sardinians (Rosatelli et al., 1998), R203X among Sicilians (Giordano et al., 2012), and Y85C among Iranian Jewish APS-1 patients (Pearce et al., 1998; Wang et al., 1998; Heino et al., 1999; Bjorses et al., 2000). Many *AIRE* mutations are nonsense mutations or deletion/insertions resulting in a truncated protein lacking SAND or PHD finger domains. Most of the missense mutations occur in the N-terminus of AIRE, a region responsible for the homodimerization and correct intracellular localization of the protein.

Despite considerable variation in the APS-1 phenotype, clear correlation of autoimmune disorders with genotype has not been found, although it is noted that among Iranian Jews the Y85C mutation has much lower frequencies of candidiasis and Addison's disease than other cohorts (Zlotogora and Shapiro, 1992). Moreover, in a study of 160 Finnish patients with the three most prevalent mutations, candidiasis was found more often in patients with homozygous R139X and R257X mutations (i.e., truncating AIRE before SAND domain) than with homozygous 967-979del13bp mutation (Kisand et al., 2010; Kisand and Peterson, 2011).

APS-1 has no clear association with the genomic region of HLA, although some components of the disease seem to correlate with certain HLA alleles or haplotypes. For example, in one study, Addison's disease was found associated with HLA DRB1*03, alopecia with DRB1*04-DQB1*0302, and type 1 diabetes correlated negatively with DRB1*15-DQB1*0602 (Halonen et al., 2002). However, another study did not find association with HLA alleles (Gylling et al., 2003).

APS-2, in contrast to APS-1, is a genetically complex disease. As for most autoimmune diseases, APS-2 is strongly associated with the HLA gene locus in chromosome 6p21 (Table 43.2). Genetic studies have demonstrated a consistent association of APS-2 with HLA DRB1*0301 (DR3), DQA1*0501, and DQB1*02 (DQ2)

TABLE 43.2 APS-2-Associated HLA Alleles and Non-HLA Genes

Genes		Details	Reference
MHC class II	DR3-DQ2 DR4 (0404)-DQ8	Antigen presentation; DR3/DR4(0404) heterozygotes have OR ≈30 for AAD	(Erichsen et al., 2009)
	DQ5	Protective; OR 0.4 for AAD	(Erichsen et al., 2009)
MHC class I	HLA-B8	Antigen presentation, DR3-B8 haplotype associated with familial AAD	(Baker et al., 2010)
	HLA-B15 (protective)	Protective for progression to overt AAD	(Baker et al., 2011)
Other genes in the MHC region	MICA5.1	Involved in NK and T cell activation, OR 18 for homozygotes with AAD	(Gambelunghe et al., 1999)
	P450c21	Steroidogenic enzyme and main autoantigen in AAD; effect could be secondary due to LD	(Peterson et al., 1995)
	Tumor necrosis factor	Inflammatory cytokine; effect could be secondary due to LD	(Partanen et al., 1994)
Non-MHC genes	CTLA4	Involved in downregulation of T cell responses; A to G SNP at position 49; 3′ untranslated region microsatellite	(Brozzetti et al., 2010b) (Blomhoff et al., 2004)
	PTPN22	Involved in T cell activation; AAD associated to the 1858 T allele and rare variants	(Skinningsrud et al., 2008a); (Roycroft et al., 2009)
	NALP1	Involved in inflammatory responses; OR 1.15 for AAD	(Magitta et al., 2009)
	CLEC16A	C-type leptin of unknown function; OR 0.76 for AAD	(Skinningsrud et al., 2008b)
	CIITA	Govern MHC class II expression; OR 1.7 for AAD	(Ghaderi et al., 2006)
	PD-LI	Downregulate cytokine production and T cell responses (CTLA4/CD28 family of costimulatory receptors); OR 1.33 for AAD	(Mitchell et al., 2009)
	CYP27B1	25-Hydroxyvitamin D3-1-alpha hydroxylase; OR 1.0−1.7 for AAD	(Lopez et al., 2004); (Jennings et al., 2005)
	FCRL3	Immune regulatory; OR 1.6 for AAD	(Owen et al., 2007)

Abbreviations: AAD, autoimmune Addison's disease; CIITA, class II, major histocompatibility complex, transactivator; CLEC16A, C-type lectin domain family 16; CTLA4, cytotoxic T lymphocyte antigen 4; CYP27B1, 25-hydroxyvitamin D3-1-alpha hydroxylase; FCRL3, Fc receptor like 3; HLA, human leukocyte antigen; MHC, major histocompatibility complex; MICA5.1, major histocompatibility complex class I chain-related MIC-A polymorphisms in exon 5; NALP1, NACHT-LRR-PYD-containing protein 1; OR, odds ratio; PTPN22, protein tyrosine phosphatase, non-receptor type 22.

alleles, which are in strong linkage equilibrium with each other (MacLaren and Riley, 1986; Partanen et al., 1994; Falorni et al., 2008). The haplotype is associated with isolated disease components of APS-2, type 1 diabetes, Graves' disease, autoimmune hypothyroidism, and Addison's disease. Most of the studies have not elucidated which of these three alleles is the primary etiological genetic factor. Another haplotype, consisting of DRB1*04 (DR4) DQA1*0301 DQB1*0302 (DQ8), was also associated with type 1 diabetes and Addison's disease (Partanen et al., 1994). The increased risk of DR4 was attributed to DRB*0404 in Addison's disease, and not DR4*0401 in variance with type 1 diabetes (Gambelunghe et al., 2005; Erichsen et al., 2009; Falorni et al., 2008). Recently, these observations were extended revealing that the association was strongest for the DRB1 locus (Skinningsrud et al., 2010). Conditioning for DRB1 indicated independent effects of HLA-B and MICA5.1 (Falorni et al., 2008; Skinningsrud et al., 2010), a positive association to HLA-B8 (Baker et al., 2010) while HLA-B15 was not protective to the formation of P450c21 antibodies, but to the progression to overt disease (Baker et al., 2011). Conversely, the haplotypes DRB1*01 (DR1) DQA1*0101 DQB1*0501 (DQ5), DRB1*1301-DQB1*0603-DQA1*0103, DRB1*1302-DQB1*0604-DQA1*0102, and DRB1*07-DQB1*0201-DQA1*0201 were protective against Addison's disease (Erichsen et al., 2009). Alleles of other genes located in HLA region, such as TNF and P450c21, have been associated with APS-2 (Partanen et al., 1994; Peterson et al., 1995; Falorni et al., 2008) but these associations could be secondary to the strong linkage disequilibrium in the HLA region.

The cytotoxic T lymphocyte-associated protein 4 (*CTLA-4*) gene on chromosome 2q33 is associated with autoimmune endocrinopathies from different populations (Brozzetti et al., 2010b). In particular, the allelic variants of an A to G single nucleotide polymorphism at position 49 and microsatellite marker in the 3' untranslated region of the *CTLA-4* gene is associated with type 1 diabetes and thyroiditis in Italian, German, and British patients (Levin and Tomer, 2003). The *CTLA-4* association with Addison's disease and APS-2 with 3' untranslated region microsatellite was significantly increased among Italian and English patients and in a meta-analysis of European studies (Kemp et al., 1998; Brozzetti et al., 2010b). Recently, autoimmune disease susceptibility was mapped to a non-coding 6.1 kb 3' region of *CTLA-4* in autoimmune thyroid disease (Ueda et al., 2003), later reproduced in Addison's disease and APS-2 (Blomhoff et al., 2004). Even if the associated allelic variation was correlated with lower messenger RNA levels of the soluble alternative splice form of *CTLA-4* (Ueda et al., 2003), the mechanism by which

CTLA-4 confers susceptibility remains incompletely understood (Scalapino and Daikh, 2008).

Additionally, a number of other susceptibility genes have been characterized in Addison's disease and APS-2 (Table 43.2). The majority of these associations are to genes involved in immunity and inflammation, and none of the associations are specific for Addison's disease or APS-2. These include PTPN22 (Skinningsrud et al., 2008a; Roycroft et al., 2009), where both association to the 1858T allele and to rare variants were found; NALP1 that could be involved in inflammation (Magitta et al., 2009); the class II, major histocompatibility complex transactivator (CIITA) (Skinningsrud et al., 2008b Ghaderi et al., 2006), the programmed death ligand 1 (PD-L1) (Mitchell et al., 2009), and the lymphocyte cell surface molecule CD226. The genetic associations have recently been reviewed (Mitchell and Pearce, 2012).

An influence of *AIRE* gene polymorphisms in APS-2 or other major autoimmune diseases is possible. The *AIRE* gene was described as a susceptible locus for the predisposition to rheumatoid arthritis in the Japanese population (Terao et al., 2011), but neither *AIRE* mutations R257X and 967-979del13bp nor SNP analyses across the AIRE gene contributed to the susceptibility to type 1 diabetes, Graves' disease, autoimmune hepatitis, or Addison's disease (Nithiyananthan et al., 2000; Vaidya et al., 2000; Boe Meyer et al., 2001; Turunen et al., 2006; Wolff et al., 2008).

ENVIRONMENTAL FEATURES

The environmental factors involved in APS are less evident than genetic factors. A recent increase in the incidence of type 1 diabetes mellitus and other autoimmune endocrine diseases in most of the developed countries points to the novel environmental influences as the genetic background has largely remained unchanged. The role of environment has been best studied in patients with type 1 diabetes (see Chapter 41) in which analysis of twins shows that the genetic background cannot be the only reason for the disease (Hyttinen et al., 2003). National prosperity and good hygiene level seem to correlate in uncertain ways with type 1 diabetes (Patterson et al., 2001). The role of viral infections in polyendocrinopathies remains unclear. Recent studies on the interaction of the intestinal microbiome with the immune system provided interesting findings. One example is that segmented filamentous bacteria seems to induce the generation of Th17 cells involved in the early phases of the immune response and linked to autoimmunity (Ivanov et al., 2009). Thus, environmental factors could mediate their effect via the intestinal microbiome (see Chapter 23).

ANIMAL MODELS

AIRE-Deficient Mouse as a Model for APS-1

AIRE-deficient mice present the autoimmune features resembling the phenotype of APS-1 patients such as multi-organ lymphocytic infiltration and circulating autoantibodies (Anderson et al., 2002; Ramsey et al., 2002). Studies on Aire mouse have been critical in elucidation of APS-1 pathogenesis and thymic tolerance (for review see Mathis and Benoist, 2009). AIRE promotes the expression of self antigens in thymic medullary epithelial cells needed for efficient negative selection of autoreactive T cells (Liston et al., 2003; Anderson et al., 2005). AIRE is also involved in the presentation of self-proteins (Kuroda et al., 2005) as it enhances the capacity of mTECs to cross-present antigen to thymic dendritic cells (Koble and Kyewski, 2009; Hubert et al., 2011) and has been implicated in the differentiation of mTECs (Nishikawa et al., 2010; Wang et al., 2012) and migration of thymocytes (Laan et al., 2009). Although AIRE deficient mice have been central to understanding AIRE-function in thymic medullary epithelial cells, the mice are also at variance with APS-1 patients in several aspects. None of the AIRE-deficient mouse models displays any of the three main components of the APS-1, although autoimmunity towards liver, gastric mucosa, and ovaries is shared. Furthermore, they do not share autoantibody targets and the reduction of Tregs seen in humans (Kekalainen et al., 2007a).

Spontaneous Animal Models

Most studied spontaneous animal models for polyendocrine autoimmunity are bio-breeding (BB) rat and non-obese diabetes (NOD) mouse. The rodent models indicate that MHC genes are major genetic factors in disease development and that other non-MHC genes are also involved. BB rat and NOD mouse also have impaired regulation of immune responses including tolerance defects and abnormal function of regulatory T cells. The BB rat develops type 1 diabetes, which is clinically similar to the diabetes seen in humans. It has have severe T cell lymphopenia which is strongly associated with diabetes development. The T cell lymphopenia is due to a single nucleotide deletion in the *Gimap5* gene (Hornum et al., 2002; MacMurray et al., 2002). The mononuclear infiltration into islets starts within first 3 weeks of age and the diabetes develops at 8–12 weeks. In addition to type 1 diabetes, BB rats frequently have lymphocytic infiltration in thyroid glands, for example in combination with distinct MHC alleles (Awata et al., 1995) or it can be potentiated by feeding rats with a high iodine diet (Allen et al., 1986). No evidence of lymphocytic infiltration to adrenal gland has been observed, but autoantibodies to gastric parietal cells and smooth muscle have been reported (Crisa et al., 1992). Recently, significant interest in the studies of spontaneous canine models of autoimmunity has been triggered by the sequencing of the dog genome (Lindblad-Toh et al., 2005). A number of breeds such as the standard poodle and Portuguese water dog are susceptible to the development of Addison's disease (Klein and Peterson, 2010) and studies are under way to use these models as a way to find human susceptibility genes.

The NOD mouse is mostly studied as a model for type 1 diabetes (see Chapter 41). In addition to pancreatic beta cell destruction, NOD mice have, although to a lesser extent, autoimmunity to submandibular and lacrimal glands. The incidence of thyroiditis is low but similarly to the BB rat, high iodine in the diet has a triggering effect on development of thyroiditis (Many et al., 1996). Lymphocytic infiltration in the adrenal and parathyroid glands has been described in NOD mice (Beales et al., 2002). Insulitis starts at an early age (4–5 weeks of age), reaching 70–90% by age of 9 weeks. Diabetes is more prevalent in females (80–90%) than in males (10–50%). The incidence of submandibular and lacrimal gland infiltration seems not to be secondary to insulitis and is more prevalent in females. In addition, many transgenic, gene-targeted, and congenic variations of NOD mice have been developed with variable effects, for example CCR7 deficiency in NOD mice leads to severe inflammation in multiple tissues including thyroid, lung, stomach, intestine, uterus, and testis (Martin et al., 2009).

Thymectomy Animal Model

A well-studied mouse model for polyendocrinopathy is thymectomy at day 3 in the Balb/C strain, which leads to multi-organ autoimmunity characterized by gastritis, thyroiditis, oophoritis, and other infiltrations. The infiltrations are T cell predominant and the mice develop autoantibodies to affected tissues. Thymectomy-induced autoimmunity depends on time of thymectomy, i.e., between the 2nd and 5th day after birth (Bonomo et al., 1995). The lack of $CD4^+CD25^+$ regulatory T cells which migrate out of the thymus in the early neonatal period was proposed to cause autoimmunity, and injection of purified regulatory T cells into the thymectomized mice was used to prevent autoimmunity (Asano et al., 1996). However, in adult age the regulatory T cell numbers in thymectomized mice are restored and even become overrepresented. More recent studies have shown that thymectomy causes lymphopenia in which development of autoimmune diabetes rather appears to be linked to effector and not to regulatory T cells (Gagnerault et al., 2009). Further implication of this model in endocrine autoimmunity was demonstrated with NALP5 (MATER), an ovarian autoantigen in APS-1, which, when transgenically expressed in MHC class II cells in thymus and secondary lymphoid system, was sufficient to mediate a significant reduction in autoimmune oophoritis after thymectomy (Otsuka et al., 2011).

PATHOGENIC MECHANISMS

The endocrine glands in APS are gradually destroyed, resulting in atrophy, or parenchymal cells are replaced by fat cells (Perheentupa, 2002). Adrenalitis in APS patients appears to be diffuse, affecting all three layers of the cortex. As an indication of T cell-mediated autoimmunity, it mainly consists of lymphocytes but macrophages and plasma cells have also been detected (Carpenter et al., 1964; Muir et al., 1993). Treatment with immunosuppressive drugs, e.g., cyclosporin A, directed against T cells, produces temporary remission of the disease in APS-2 patients (Csaszar and Patakfalvi, 1992).

It has been difficult to characterize autoreactive T cells in APS patients, partly due to the lack of specific and sensitive methods, and to the fact that T cells in contrast to autoantibodies are sequestered in the specific tissue lesions and are thus difficult to access. Recently in several reports on analysis of autoreactive T cells targeting P450c21, Bratland and co-workers showed that CD4-positive T cells in patients with autoimmune Addison's disease proliferate when exposed to recombinant P450c21 (Bratland et al., 2009). Studies of various peptides of P450c21 revealed that the main reactivity was towards a peptide close to and overlapping with the substrate binding domain. Using a slightly different experimental approach, Rottembourg and co-workers identified C-terminal immunodominant peptides and a CD8-mediated immune response in autoimmune Addison's patients (Rottembourg et al., 2010). Autoantibodies have long been regarded as merely having a bystander role, yet they still could have an important role as amplifiers of the immune response towards the adrenal cortex. Increased serum levels of proinflammatory CXCL10 chemokine have been found in patients with isolated Addison's disease, APS-2 (Rotondi et al., 2005) and APS-1 (Kisand et al., 2008). The adrenocortical cell is likely to be an active participant in the autoimmune process as it can produce CXCL10 in response to interferon gamma (Rotondi et al., 2005; Rotondi et al., 2007) (for review see Bratland and Husebye, 2011).

Studies on peripheral blood subsets in APS-1 patients have had conflicting results. CD4+ T cell numbers and a proportion of memory or activated T cells have been reported to be increased or normal (Perniola et al., 2005; Tuovinen et al., 2009). Controversial results have been found on iNKT and monocyte cell numbers (Perniola

et al., 2008; Hong et al., 2009; Lindh et al., 2010). Reports on regulatory T cells have described lower numbers, impaired function, and decreased expression of FoxP3 (Kekalainen et al., 2007b). A recent study showed the accumulation of highly differentiated and oligoclonally activated effector-like CD8+ T cells with low expression of IL7R and lack of conventional naïve CD45RA CD8+ T cells (Laakso et al., 2011).

Autoimmunity in APS-1 has been postulated, based on studies in AIRE-deficient mice, to be a consequence of defective central tolerance to the autoantigens. The lack of AIRE expression in thymus may thus lead to a defect in clonal deletion of autoreactive T cells and ultimately to autoimmunity (Liston et al., 2003; Mathis and Benoist, 2009). However, direct data are lacking on clonal deletion in human APS-1 patients. The organs targeted in APS-1 patients are limited and the syndrome typically starts with chronic mucocutaneous candidiasis, followed by hypoparathyroidism and Addison's disease indicating abovementioned phenotypic differences between human patients and AIRE mouse models. Whereas the candidiasis is associated with the early generation of anti-IL17 and IL-22 autoantibodies, the reason for the high prevalence of autoimmune hypoparathyroidism and Addison's disease remains unclear. The autoantibodies against type 1 IFN and Th17 cytokines in APS-1 have implications similar to those of thymoma patients where autoantibodies to type 1 IFN and other cytokines have also been found. An active autoimmunization process within the thymus tissue has been proposed to occur in both APS-1 and thymoma patients as both diseases are associated with thymus dysfunction (Meager et al., 2008; Kisand et al., 2011). According to this hypothesis the thymus in AIRE deficiency exports abnormal and already activated T cells capable of helping autoantibody production of B cells (Kisand and Peterson, 2011). The emerging idea of active autoimmunization in thymus, although needing validation, also points to the thymus as an important organ in protection against autoimmunity.

IMMUNOLOGIC MARKERS IN DIAGNOSIS

Autoantibodies are often diagnostic or even predictive markers for the clinical disease. The presence of high titer and persistent anti-IFN-α and IFN-ω autoantibodies in 100% of APS-1 patients provides an easier and more efficient way than AIRE mutation analysis to identify APS-1 patients. A similar test for anti-IL-17 or IL-22 autoantibodies in APS-1 could further confirm the diagnosis. These markers could be used for early detection of the disease pathogenesis as so far even samples collected before the age of 1 year appear seropositive for IFN-ω (Toth et al., 2010). In addition, autoantibodies to the steroidogenic enzymes (P450c21, P450c17, and P450scc) are significant and specific markers for onset of Addison's disease. Antibodies against at least one of the three antigens are found in 84% of the patients with Addison's disease (Soderbergh et al., 2004; Brozzetti et al., 2010a). Furthermore, hypogonadism is well associated with the presence of autoantibodies to P450scc protein. Autoantibodies to the IA-2 autoantigen, however, seem to have the strongest association with type 1 diabetes in APS-1 (Soderbergh et al., 2004). Autoantibody analyses in patients with APS-1 indicate serological markers for hepatitis (aromatic L-amino acid decarboxylase, cytochrome P450 1A2, or tryptophan hydroxylase), gastrointestinal dysfunction (tryptophan hydroxylase), and vitiligo (Hedstrand et al., 2001).

The vast majority (up to 80–90%) of patients with APS-2 have autoantibodies to P450c21 (Erichsen et al., 2009; Falorni et al., 2011). The titers of autoantibodies decrease to some extent as the disease progresses, and therefore the diagnostic value of the autoantibodies is highest at onset. The presence of anti-P450c21 antibodies in patients with autoimmune thyroid disease or type 1 diabetes, but without Addison's disease (Barker et al., 2005), would indicate risk for later development of overt Addison's disease, although the progression to overt Addison's disease may take years. Among relatives with organ-specific autoimmunity, individuals with normal adrenal function and P450c21 autoantibodies, about 15%, progressed to adrenal failure within 5 years (Coco et al., 2006).

TREATMENT AND OUTCOME

In patients with APS-1, anti-candidal drugs such as amphotericin B, ketoconazole, or fluconazole are used in the treatment of the candidiasis. Itraconazole has been reported to be effective for nail candidiasis; however, 4 to 6 months treatment is needed to eliminate the infection (Rautemaa et al., 2007, 2008a,b). Clinical follow-up of oral candidal infection is needed at least once or twice per year and, because of risk of cancer, attention should be paid to suppression of the oral infection; smokers are at particular risk. Replacement therapy with hormones has been efficiently used for Addison's disease and hypoparathyroidism. Patients with Addison's disease are treated with hydrocortisone at the smallest dose that relieves symptoms, usually $10 + 5 + 5$ mg a day (the corresponding dose of cortisone acetate is $12.5 + 6.25 + 6.25$ mg). Fludrocortisone is used to replace aldosterone. The therapy of hypoparathyroidism is aimed at maintaining normal calcium levels, and serum calcium and phosphate levels should be monitored regularly. Therapies are calciferol sterols (vitamin D hydroxylated forms, calcidiol, or calcitriol) and calcium salt preparations, preferably calcium carbonate, but these, however, do not efficiently substitute for parathyroid hormone and are difficult to regulate. As the calcium levels may vary significantly over a short time, there are significant risks for both hypo- and hypercalcemia. Recently available recombinant parathyroid hormone may improve the treatment of the hypoparathyroidism in APS-1 patients, but is still experimental (Winer et al., 2012). The patients should receive advice and written information about the symptoms, complications, and risk elements of the disease. APS-1 may cause great psychosocial burden as the persistent risk of developing new disease components can be a source of continuous distress (Perheentupa, 2006).

CONCLUDING REMARKS—FUTURE PROSPECTS

Recent years have provided remarkable progress in our knowledge about the mechanisms of autoimmune polyendocrinopathies including a clear pathogenetic distinction between APS-1 and APS-2. The autoimmune reaction destroys with high precision the endocrine organs, which often express tissue-specific proteins. The identification of the autoantibody targets in APS has revealed that the autoantigens often belong to related protein families, raising the question of exactly how the immune system selects specific targets for autoimmune reactivity. Clinically, assay of autoantibodies can be used for diagnostic purposes. Presence of antibodies against IFN-ω and IFN-α is almost diagnostic for APS-1 if myasthenia gravis and thymoma have been ruled out. The pattern of autoantibodies is an early phenomenon, which correlates with organ manifestations and could therefore predict future disease, for instance oophoritis.

Much current research effort is put into the identification of genes involved in APS-2. Clearly, MHC genes have the dominant role, but whether an Addison-specific gene association exists is not yet clear. Environmental factors in APS-2 certainly remain to be clarified and deserve more attention. Although it is a monogenic disease, APS-1 also seems to be influenced by environmental, stochastic, and/or other genetic factors to account for the variety of clinical symptoms and disease expressions. The possibility that heterozygous deficiency of *AIRE* in combination with other genetic defects might contribute to the occurrence of autoimmunity is worthy of further investigation.

ACKNOWLEDGMENTS

The authors are grateful to Dr. Kai Kisand, Prof. Kai Krohn, and Prof. Annamari Ranki for fruitful discussions.

REFERENCES

Aaltonen, J., Bjorses, P., Sandkuijl, L., Perheentupa, J., Peltonen, L., 1994. An autosomal locus causing autoimmune disease: autoimmune polyglandular disease type I assigned to chromosome 21. Nat. Genet. 8, 83–87.

Addison, T., 1855. On the Constitutional and Local Effects of Disease of the Suprarenal Capsules. New Sydenham Society 1868, London.

Alimohammadi, M., Bjorklund, P., Hallgren, A., Pontynen, N., Szinnai, G., Shikama, N., et al., 2008. Autoimmune polyendocrine syndrome type 1 and NALP5, a parathyroid autoantigen. N. Engl. J. Med. 358, 1018–1028.

Alimohammadi, M., Dubois, N., Skoldberg, F., Hallgren, A., Tardivel, I., Hedstrand, H., et al., 2009. Pulmonary autoimmunity as a feature of autoimmune polyendocrine syndrome type 1 and identification of KCNRG as a bronchial autoantigen. Proc. Natl. Acad. Sci. U.S.A. 106, 4396–4401

Allen, E.M., Appel, M.C., Braverman, L.E., 1986. The effect of iodide ingestion on the development of spontaneous lymphocytic thyroiditis in the diabetes-prone BB/W rat. Endocrinology. 118, 1977–1981.

Anderson, J.R., Goudie, R.B., Gray, K.G., Timbury, G.C., 1957. Autoantibodies in Addison's disease. Lancet. 272, 1123–1124.

Anderson, M.S., Venanzi, E.S., Klein, L., Chen, Z., Berzins, S.P., Turley, S.J., et al., 2002. Projection of an immunological self shadow within the thymus by the aire protein. Science. 298, 1395–1401.

Anderson, M.S., Venanzi, E.S., Chen, Z., Berzins, S.P., Benoist, C., Mathis, D., 2005. The cellular mechanism of Aire control of T cell tolerance. Immunity. 23, 227–239.

Asano, M., Toda, M., Sakaguchi, N., Sakaguchi, S., 1996. Autoimmune disease as a consequence of developmental abnormality of a T cell subpopulation. J. Exp. Med. 184, 387–396.

Awata, T., Guberski, D.L., Like, A.A., 1995. Genetics of the BB rat: association of autoimmune disorders (diabetes, insulitis, and thyroiditis) with lymphopenia and major histocompatibility complex class II. Endocrinology. 136, 5731–5735.

Baker, P.R., Baschal, E.E., Fain, P.R., Triolo, T.M., Nanduri, P., Siebert, J.C., et al., 2010. Haplotype analysis discriminates genetic risk for DR3-associated endocrine autoimmunity and helps define extreme risk for Addison's disease. J. Clin. Endocrinol. Metab. 95, E263–E270.

Baker, P.R., Baschal, E.E., Fain, P.R., Nanduri, P., Triolo, T.M., Siebert, J.C., et al., 2011. Dominant suppression of Addison's disease associated with HLA-B15. J. Clin. Endocrinol. Metab. 96, 2154–2162.

Barker, J.M., Yu, J., Yu, L., Wang, J., Miao, D., Bao, F., et al., 2005. Autoantibody "subspecificity" in type 1 diabetes: risk for organ-specific autoimmunity clusters in distinct groups. Diabetes Care. 28, 850–855.

Baumann-Antczak, A., Wedlock, N., Bednarek, J., Kiso, Y., Krishnan, H., Fowler, S., et al., 1992. Autoimmune Addison's disease and 21-hydroxylase. Lancet. 340, 429–430.

Beales, P.E., Castri, F., Valiant, A., Rosignoli, G., Buckley, L., Pozzilli, P., 2002. Adrenalitis in the non-obese diabetic mouse. Autoimmunity. 35, 329–333.

Bednarek, J., Furmaniak, J., Wedlock, N., Kiso, Y., Baumann-Antczak, A., Fowler, S., et al., 1992. Steroid 21-hydroxylase is a major autoantigen involved in adult onset autoimmune Addison's disease. FEBS Lett. 309, 51–55.

Betterle, C., Morlin, L., 2011. Autoimmune Addison's disease. Endocr. Dev. 20, 161–172.

Betterle, C., Dal Pra, C., Mantero, F., Zanchetta, R., 2002. Autoimmune adrenal insufficiency and autoimmune polyendocrine syndromes: autoantibodies, autoantigens, and their applicability in diagnosis and disease prediction. Endocr. Rev. 23, 327–364.

Bjorses, P., Halonen, M., Palvimo, J.J., Kolmer, M., Aaltonen, J., Ellonen, P., et al., 2000. Mutations in the AIRE gene: effects on subcellular location and transactivation function of the autoimmune polyendocrinopathy-candidiasis-ectodermal dystrophy protein. Am. J. Hum. Genet. 66, 378–392.

Blizzard, R.M., Gibbs, J.H., 1968. Candidiasis: studies pertaining to its association with endocrinopathies and pernicious anemia. Pediatrics. 42, 231–237.

Blizzard, R.M., Chandler, R.W., Kyle, M.A., Hung, W., 1962. Adrenal antibodies in Addison's disease. Lancet. 2, 901–903.

Blomhoff, A., Lie, B.A., Myhre, A.G., Kemp, E.H., Weetman, A.P., Akselsen, H.E., et al., 2004. Polymorphisms in the cytotoxic T lymphocyte antigen-4 gene region confer susceptibility to Addison's disease. J. Clin. Endocrinol. Metab. 89, 3474–3476.

Boe Wolff, A.S., Oftedal, B., Johansson, S., Bruland, O., Lovas, K., Meager, A., et al., 2008. AIRE variations in Addison's disease and autoimmune polyendocrine syndromes (APS): partial gene deletions contribute to APS, I. Genes. Immun. 9, 130–136.

Bonomo, A., Kehn, P.J., Shevach, E.M., 1995. Post-thymectomy autoimmunity: abnormal T-cell homeostasis. Immunol. Today. 16, 61–67.

Bratland, E., Husebye, E.S., 2011. Cellular immunity and immunopathology in autoimmune Addison's disease. Mol. Cell Endocrinol. 336, 180–190.

Bratland, E., Skinningsrud, B., Undlien, D.E., Mozes, E., Husebye, E.S., 2009. T cell responses to steroid cytochrome P450 21-hydroxylase in patients with autoimmune primary adrenal insufficiency. J. Clin. Endocrinol. Metab. 94, 5117–5124.

Brozzetti, A., Marzotti, S., La Torre, D., Bacosi, M.L., Morelli, S., Bini, V., et al., 2010a. Autoantibody responses in autoimmune ovarian insufficiency and in Addison's disease are IgG1 dominated and suggest a predominant, but not exclusive, Th1 type of response. Eur. J. Endocrinol. 163, 309–317.

Brozzetti, A., Marzotti, S., Tortoioli, C., Bini, V., Giordano, R., Dotta, F., et al., 2010b. Cytotoxic T lymphocyte antigen-4 Ala17 polymorphism is a genetic marker of autoimmune adrenal insufficiency: Italian association study and meta-analysis of European studies. Eur. J. Endocrinol. 162, 361–369.

Burbelo, P.D., Ching, K.H., Mattson, T.L., Light, J.S., Bishop, L.R., Kovacs, J.A., 2007. Rapid antibody quantification and generation of whole proteome antibody response profiles using LIPS (luciferase immunoprecipitation systems). Biochem. Biophys. Res. Commun. 352, 889–895.

Carpenter, C.C., Solomon, N., Silverberg, S.G., Bledsoe, T., Northcutt, R.C., Klinenberg, J.R., et al., 1964. Schmidt's syndrome (thyroid and adrenal insufficiency). A review of the literature and a report of fifteen new cases including ten instances of coexistent diabetes mellitus. Medicine (Baltimore). 43, 153–180.

Coco, G., Dal Pra, C., Presotto, F., Albergoni, M.P., Canova, C., Pedini, B., et al., 2006. Estimated risk for developing autoimmune Addison's disease in patients with adrenal cortex autoantibodies. J. Clin. Endocrinol. Metab. 91, 1637–1645.

Crisa, L., Mordes, J.P., Rossini, A.A., 1992. Autoimmune diabetes mellitus in the BB rat. Diabetes Metab. Rev. 8, 4–37.

Csaszar, T., Patakfalvi, A., 1992. Treatment of polyglandular autoimmune syndrome with cyclosporin-A. Acta Med. Hung. 49, 187–193.

Ekwall, O., Hedstrand, H., Grimelius, L., Haavik, J., Perheentupa, J., Gustafsson, J., et al., 1998. Identification of tryptophan hydroxylase as an intestinal autoantigen. Lancet. 352, 279–283.

Erichsen, M.M., Lovas, K., Skinningsrud, B., Wolff, A.B., Undlien, D.E., Svartberg, J., et al., 2009. Clinical, immunological, and genetic features of autoimmune primary adrenal insufficiency: observations from a Norwegian registry. J. Clin. Endocrinol. Metab. 94, 4882–4890.

Falorni, A., Brozzetti, A., Torre, D.L., Tortoioli, C., Gambelunghe, G., 2008. Association of genetic polymorphisms and autoimmune Addison's disease. Expert Rev. Clin. Immunol. 4, 441–456.

Falorni, A., Chen, S., Zanchetta, R., Yu, L., Tiberti, C., Bacosi, M.L., et al., 2011. Measuring adrenal autoantibody response: interlaboratory concordance in the first international serum exchange for the determination of 21-hydroxylase autoantibodies. Clin. Immunol. 140, 291–299.

Finnish-German-Consortium, 1997. An autoimmune disease, APECED, caused by mutations in a novel gene featuring two PHD-type zinc-finger domains. Nat. Genet. 17, 399–403.

Gagnerault, M.C., Lanvin, O., Pasquier, V., Garcia, C., Damotte, D., Lucas, B., et al., 2009. Autoimmunity during thymectomy-induced lymphopenia: role of thymus ablation and initial effector T cell activation timing in nonobese diabetic mice. J. Immunol. 183, 4913–4920.

Gambelunghe, G., Falorni, A., Ghaderi, M., Laureti, S., Tortoioli, C., Santeusanio, F., et al., 1999. Microsatellite polymorphism of the MHC class I chain-related (MIC-A and MIC-B. genes marks the risk for autoimmune Addison's disease. J. Clin. Endocrinol. Metab. 84, 3701–3707.

Gambelunghe, G., Kockum, I., Bini, V., De Giorgi, G., Celi, F., Betterle, C., et al., 2005. Retrovirus-like long-terminal repeat DQ-LTR13 and genetic susceptibility to type 1 diabetes and autoimmune Addison's disease. Diabetes 54, 900–905.

Ghaderi, M., Gambelunghe, G., Tortoioli, C., Brozzetti, A., Jatta, K., Gharizadeh, B., et al., 2006. MHC2TA single nucleotide polymorphism and genetic risk for autoimmune adrenal insufficiency. J. Clin. Endocrinol. Metab. 91, 4107–4111.

Giordano, C., Modica, R., Allotta, M.L., Guarnotta, V., Cervato, S., Masiero, S., et al., 2012. Autoimmune Polyendocrinopathy-Candidiasis-Ectodermal-Dystrophy (APECED) in Sicily: confirmation that R203X is the peculiar AIRE gene mutation. J. Endocrinol. Invest. 35, 384–388.

Gylling, M., Kaariainen, E., Vaisanen, R., Kerosuo, L., Solin, M.L., Halme, L., et al., 2003. The hypoparathyroidism of autoimmune polyendocrinopathy-candidiasis-ectodermal dystrophy protective effect of male sex. J. Clin. Endocrinol. Metab. 88, 4602–4608.

Halonen, M., Eskelin, P., Myhre, A.G., Perheentupa, J., Husebye, E.S., Kampe, O., et al., 2002. AIRE mutations and human leukocyte antigen genotypes as determinants of the autoimmune polyendocrinopathy-candidiasis-ectodermal dystrophy phenotype. J. Clin. Endocrinol. Metab. 87, 2568–2574.

Hedstrand, H., Ekwall, O., Haavik, J., Landgren, E., Betterle, C., Perheentupa, J., et al., 2000. Identification of tyrosine hydroxylase as an autoantigen in autoimmune polyendocrine syndrome type I. Biochem. Biophys. Res. Commun. 267, 456–461.

Hedstrand, H., Ekwall, O., Olsson, M.J., Landgren, E., Kemp, E.H., Weetman, A.P., et al., 2001. The transcription factors SOX9 and SOX10 are vitiligo autoantigens in autoimmune polyendocrine syndrome type I. J. Biol. Chem. 276, 35390–35395.

Heino, M., Peterson, P., Kudoh, J., Nagamine, K., Lagerstedt, A., Ovod, V., et al., 1999. Autoimmune regulator is expressed in the cells regulating immune tolerance in thymus medulla. Biochem. Biophys. Res. Commun. 257, 821–825.

Hetzel, B.S., Robson, H.N., 1958. The syndrome of hypoparathyroidism, Addison's disease and moniliasis. Australas. Ann. Med. 7, 27–33.

Hoek, A., Schoemaker, J., Drexhage, H.A., 1997. Premature ovarian failure and ovarian autoimmunity. Endocr. Rev. 18, 107–134.

Hong, M., Ryan, K.R., Arkwright, P.D., Gennery, A.R., Costigan, C., Dominguez, M., et al., 2009. Pattern recognition receptor expression is not impaired in patients with chronic mucocutaneous candidiasis with or without autoimmune polyendocrinopathy candidiasis ectodermal dystrophy. Clin. Exp. Immunol. 156, 40–51.

Hornum, L., Romer, J., Markholst, H., 2002. The diabetes-prone BB rat carries a frameshift mutation in Ian4, a positional candidate of Iddm1. Diabetes. 51, 1972–1979.

Hubert, F.X., Kinkel, S.A., Davey, G.M., Phipson, B., Mueller, S.N., Liston, A., et al., 2011. Aire regulates the transfer of antigen from mTECs to dendritic cells for induction of thymic tolerance. Blood. 118, 2462–2472.

Husebye, E.S., Gebre-Medhin, G., Tuomi, T., Perheentupa, J., Landin-Olsson, M., Gustafsson, J., et al., 1997. Autoantibodies against aromatic L-amino acid decarboxylase in autoimmune polyendocrine syndrome type I. J. Clin. Endocrinol. Metab. 82, 147–150.

Hyttinen, V., Kaprio, J., Kinnunen, L., Koskenvuo, M., Tuomilehto, J., 2003. Genetic liability of type 1 diabetes and the onset age among 22,650 young Finnish twin pairs: a nationwide follow-up study. Diabetes. 52, 1052–1055.

Ivanov, I.I., Atarashi, K., Manel, N., Brodie, E.L., Shima, T., Karaoz, U., et al., 2009. Induction of intestinal Th17 cells by segmented filamentous bacteria. Cell. 139, 485–498.

Jennings, C.E., Owen, C.J., Wilson, V., Pearce, S.H., 2005. A haplotype of the CYP27B1 promoter is associated with autoimmune Addison's disease but not with Graves' disease in a UK population. J. Mol. Endocrinol. 34, 859–863.

Kekalainen, E., Miettinen, A., Arstila, T.P., 2007a. Does the deficiency of Aire in mice really resemble human APECED? Nat. Rev. Immunol. 7, 1.

Kekalainen, E., Tuovinen, H., Joensuu, J., Gylling, M., Franssila, R., Pontynen, N., et al., 2007b. A defect of regulatory T cells in patients with autoimmune polyendocrinopathy-candidiasis-ectodermal dystrophy. J. Immunol. 178, 1208–1215.

Kemp, E.H., Ajjan, R.A., Husebye, E.S., Peterson, P., Uibo, R., Imrie, H., et al., 1998. A cytotoxic T lymphocyte antigen-4 (CTLA-4) gene polymorphism is associated with autoimmune Addison's disease in English patients. Clin. Endocrinol. (Oxf.). 49, 609–613.

Kisand, K., Peterson, P., 2011. Autoimmune polyendocrinopathy candidiasis ectodermal dystrophy: known and novel aspects of the syndrome. Ann. N. Y. Acad. Sci. 1246, 77–91.

Kisand, K., Link, M., Wolff, A.S., Meager, A., Tserel, L., Org, T., et al., 2008. Interferon autoantibodies associated with AIRE deficiency decrease the expression of IFN-stimulated genes. Blood. 112, 2657–2666.

Kisand, K., Boe Wolff, A.S., Podkrajsek, K.T., Tserel, L., Link, M., Kisand, K.V., et al., 2010. Chronic mucocutaneous candidiasis in APECED or thymoma patients correlates with autoimmunity to Th17-associated cytokines. J. Exp. Med. 207, 299—308.

Kisand, K., Lilic, D., Casanova, J.L., Peterson, P., Meager, A., Willcox, N., 2011. Mucocutaneous candidiasis and autoimmunity against cytokines in APECED and thymoma patients: clinical and pathogenetic implications. Eur. J. Immunol. 41, 1517—1527.

Klein, S.C., Peterson, M.E., 2010. Canine hypoadrenocorticism: part I. Can. Vet. J. 51, 63—69.

Koble, C., Kyewski, B., 2009. The thymic medulla: a unique microenvironment for intercellular self-antigen transfer. J. Exp. Med. 206, 1505—1513.

Krohn, K., Uibo, R., Aavik, E., Peterson, P., Savilahti, K., 1992. Identification by molecular cloning of an autoantigen associated with Addison's disease as steroid 17 alpha-hydroxylase. Lancet. 339, 770—773.

Kuroda, N., Mitani, T., Takeda, N., Ishimaru, N., Arakaki, R., Hayashi, Y., et al., 2005. Development of autoimmunity against transcriptionally unrepressed target antigen in the thymus of Aire-deficient mice. J. Immunol. 174, 1862—1870.

Laakso, S.M., Kekalainen, E., Rossi, L.H., Laurinolli, T.T., Mannerstrom, H., Heikkila, N., et al., 2011. IL-7 dysregulation and loss of CD8+ T cell homeostasis in the monogenic human disease autoimmune polyendocrinopathy-candidiasis-ectodermal dystrophy. J. Immunol. 187, 2023—2030.

Laan, M., Kisand, K., Kont, V., Moll, K., Tserel, L., Scott, H.S., et al., 2009. Autoimmune regulator deficiency results in decreased expression of CCR4 and CCR7 ligands and in delayed migration of CD4+ thymocytes. J. Immunol. 183, 7682—7691.

Levin, L., Tomer, Y., 2003. The etiology of autoimmune diabetes and thyroiditis: evidence for common genetic susceptibility. Autoimmun. Rev. 2, 377—386.

Lindblad-Toh, K., Wade, C.M., Mikkelsen, T.S., Karlsson, E.K., Jaffe, D.B., Kamal, M., et al., 2005. Genome sequence, comparative analysis and haplotype structure of the domestic dog. Nature. 438, 803—819.

Lindh, E., Rosmaraki, E., Berg, L., Brauner, H., Karlsson, M.C., Peltonen, L., et al., 2010. AIRE deficiency leads to impaired iNKT cell development. J. Autoimmun. 34, 66—72.

Liston, A., Lesage, S., Wilson, J., Peltonen, L., Goodnow, C.C., 2003. Aire regulates negative selection of organ-specific T cells. Nat. Immunol. 4, 350—354.

Lopez, E.R., Zwermann, O., Segni, M., Meyer, G., Reincke, M., Seissler, J., et al., 2004. A promoter polymorphism of the CYP27B1 gene is associated with Addison's disease, Hashimoto's thyroiditis, Graves' disease and type 1 diabetes mellitus in Germans. Eur. J. Endocrinol. 151, 193—197.

MacMurray, A.J., Moralejo, D.H., Kwitek, A.E., Rutledge, E.A., Van Yserloo, B., Gohlke, P., et al., 2002. Lymphopenia in the BB rat model of type 1 diabetes is due to a mutation in a novel immune-associated nucleotide (Ian)-related gene. Genome. Res. 12, 1029—1039.

Maclaren, N.K., Riley, W.J., 1986. Inherited susceptibility to autoimmune Addison's disease is linked to human leukocyte antigens-DR3 and/or DR4, except when associated with type I autoimmune polyglandular syndrome. J. Clin. Endocrinol. Metab. 62, 455—459.

Magitta, N.F., Boe Wolff, A.S., Johansson, S., Skinningsrud, B., Lie, B. A., Myhr, K.M., et al., 2009. A coding polymorphism in NALP1

confers risk for autoimmune Addison's disease and type 1 diabetes. Genes. Immun. 10, 120—124.

Many, M.C., Maniratunga, S., Denef, J.F., 1996. The non-obese diabetic (NOD) mouse: an animal model for autoimmune thyroiditis. Exp. Clin. Endocrinol. Diabetes. 104, 17—20.

Martin, A.P., Marinkovic, T., Canasto-Chibuque, C., Latif, R., Unkeless, J.C., Davies, T.F., et al., 2009. CCR7 deficiency in NOD mice leads to thyroiditis and primary hypothyroidism. J. Immunol. 183, 3073—3080.

Mathis, D., Benoist, C., 2009. Aire. Annu. Rev. Immunol. 27, 287—312.

Meager, A., Visvalingam, K., Peterson, P., Moll, K., Murumagi, A., Krohn, K., et al., 2006. Anti-interferon autoantibodies in autoimmune polyendocrinopathy syndrome type 1. PLoS Med. 3, e289.

Meager, A., Peterson, P., Willcox, N., 2008. Hypothetical review: thymic aberrations and type-I interferons; attempts to deduce autoimmunizing mechanisms from unexpected clues in monogenic and paraneoplastic syndromes. Clin. Exp. Immunol. 154, 141—151.

Meloni, A., Furcas, M., Cetani, F., Marcocci, C., Falorni, A., Perniola, R., et al., 2008. Autoantibodies against type I interferons as an additional diagnostic criterion for autoimmune polyendocrine syndrome type I. J. Clin. Endocrinol. Metab. 93, 4389—4397.

Meyer, G., Donner, H., Herwig, J., Bohles, H., Usadel, K.H., Badenhoop, K., 2001. Screening for an AIRE-1 mutation in patients with Addison's disease, type 1 diabetes, Graves' disease and Hashimoto's thyroiditis as well as in APECED syndrome. Clin. Endocrinol. (Oxf.). 54, 335—338.

Michels, A.W., Eisenbarth, G.S., 2009. Autoimmune polyendocrine syndrome type 1 (APS-1) as a model for understanding autoimmune polyendocrine syndrome type 2 (APS-2). J. Intern. Med. 265, 530—540.

Mitchell, A.L., Pearce, S.H., 2012. Autoimmune Addison disease: pathophysiology and genetic complexity. Nat. Rev. Endocrinol. 8, 306—316.

Mitchell, A.L., Cordell, H.J., Soemedi, R., Owen, K., Skinningsrud, B., Wolff, A.B., et al., 2009. Programmed death ligand 1 (PD-L1) gene variants contribute to autoimmune Addison's disease and Graves' disease susceptibility. J. Clin. Endocrinol. Metab. 94, 5139—5145.

Muir, A., Schatz, D.A., MacLaren, N.K., 1993. Autoimmune Addison's disease. Springer Semin. Immunopathol. 14, 275—284.

Myhre, A.G., Undlien, D.E., Lovas, K., Uhlving, S., Nedrebo, B.G., Fougner, K.J., et al., 2002. Autoimmune adrenocortical failure in Norway autoantibodies and human leukocyte antigen class II associations related to clinical features. J. Clin. Endocrinol. Metab. 87, 618—623.

Nagamine, K., Peterson, P., Scott, H.S., Kudoh, J., Minoshima, S., Heino, M., et al., 1997. Positional cloning of the APECED gene. Nat. Genet. 17, 393—398.

Neufeld, M., MacLaren, N.K., Blizzard, R.M., 1981. Two types of autoimmune Addison's disease associated with different polyglandular autoimmune (PGA) syndromes. Medicine (Baltimore). 60, 355—362.

Nishikawa, Y., Hirota, F., Yano, M., Kitajima, H., Miyazaki, J., Kawamoto, H., et al., 2010. Biphasic Aire expression in early embryos and in medullary thymic epithelial cells before end-stage terminal differentiation. J. Exp. Med. 207, 963—971.

Nithiyananthan, R., Heward, J.M., Allahabadia, A., Barnett, A.H., Franklyn, J.A., Gough, S.C., 2000. A heterozygous deletion of the autoimmune regulator (AIRE1) gene, autoimmune thyroid disease, and type 1 diabetes: no evidence for association. J. Clin. Endocrinol. Metab. 85, 1320–1322.

Oftedal, B.E., Wolff, A.S., Bratland, E., Kampe, O., Perheentupa, J., Myhre, A.G., et al., 2008. Radioimmunoassay for autoantibodies against interferon omega; its use in the diagnosis of autoimmune polyendocrine syndrome type, I. Clin. Immunol. 129, 163–169.

Otsuka, N., Tong, Z.B., Vanevski, K., Tu, W., Cheng, M.H., Nelson, L.M., 2011. Autoimmune oophoritis with multiple molecular targets mitigated by transgenic expression of mater. Endocrinology. 152, 2465–2473.

Owen, C., Kelly, J., Eden, H., Merriman, J.A., Pearce, M.E., Merriman, T.R., S.H., 2007. Analysis of the Fc receptor-like-3 (FCRL3) locus in Caucasians with autoimmune disorders suggests a complex pattern of disease association. J. Clin. Endocrinol. Metab. 92, 1106–1111.

Partanen, J., Peterson, P., Westman, P., Aranko, S., Krohn, K., 1994. Major histocompatibility complex class II and III in Addison's disease. MHC alleles do not predict autoantibody specificity and 21-hydroxylase gene polymorphism has no independent role in disease susceptibility. Hum. Immunol. 41, 135–140.

Patterson, C.C., Dahlquist, G., Soltesz, G., 2001. Maternal age and risk of type 1 diabetes in children. Relative risks by maternal age are biased. BMJ. 322, 1489–1490.

Pearce, S.H., Cheetham, T., Imrie, H., Vaidya, B., Barnes, N.D., Bilous, R.W., et al., 1998. A common and recurrent 13-bp deletion in the autoimmune regulator gene in British kindreds with autoimmune polyendocrinopathy type 1. Am. J. Hum. Genet. 63, 1675–1684.

Perheentupa, J., 2002. APS-I/APECED: the clinical disease and therapy. Endocrinol. Metab. Clin. North Am. 31, 295–320.

Perheentupa, J., 2006. Autoimmune polyendocrinopathy-candidiasis-ectodermal dystrophy. J. Clin. Endocrinol. Metab. 91, 2843–2850.

Perniola, R., Lobreglio, G., Rosatelli, M.C., Pitotti, E., Accogli, E., De Rinaldis, C., 2005. Immunophenotypic characterisation of peripheral blood lymphocytes in autoimmune polyglandular syndrome type 1: clinical study and review of the literature. J. Pediatr. Endocrinol. Metab. 18, 155–164.

Perniola, R., Congedo, M., Rizzo, A., Sticchi Damiani, A., Faneschi, M.L., Pizzolante, M., et al., 2008. Innate and adaptive immunity in patients with autoimmune polyendocrinopathy-candidiasis-ectodermal dystrophy. Mycoses. 51, 228–235.

Peterson, P., Partanen, J., Aavik, E., Salmi, H., Pelkonen, R., Krohn, K.J., 1995. Steroid 21-hydroxylase gene polymorphism in Addison's disease patients. Tissue Antigens. 46, 63–67.

Puel, A., Doffinger, R., Natividad, A., Chrabieh, M., Barcenas-Morales, G., Picard, C., et al., 2010. Autoantibodies against IL-17A, IL-17F, and IL-22 in patients with chronic mucocutaneous candidiasis and autoimmune polyendocrine syndrome type I. J. Exp. Med. 207, 291–297.

Ramsey, C., Winqvist, O., Puhakka, L., Halonen, M., Moro, A., Kampe, O., et al., 2002. Aire deficient mice develop multiple features of APECED phenotype and show altered immune response. Hum. Mol. Genet. 11, 397–409.

Rautemaa, R., Richardson, M., Pfaller, M., Koukila-Kahkola, P., Perheentupa, J., Saxen, H., 2007. Decreased susceptibility of Candida albicans to azole antifungals: a complication of long-term treatment in autoimmune polyendocrinopathy-candidiasis-ectodermal dystrophy (APECED) patients. J. Antimicrob. Chemother. 60, 889–892.

Rautemaa, R., Richardson, M., Pfaller, M., Perheentupa, J., Saxen, H., 2008a. Reduction of fluconazole susceptibility of Candida albicans in APECED patients due to long-term use of ketoconazole and miconazole. Scand. J. Infect. Dis. 40, 904–907.

Rautemaa, R., Richardson, M., Pfaller, M.A., Perheentupa, J., Saxen, H., 2008b. Activity of amphotericin B, anidulafungin, caspofungin, micafungin, posaconazole, and voriconazole against Candida albicans with decreased susceptibility to fluconazole from APECED patients on long-term azole treatment of chronic mucocutaneous candidiasis. Diagn. Microbiol. Infect. Dis. 62, 182–185.

Reato, G., Morlin, L., Chen, S., Furmaniak, J., Smith, B.R., Masiero, S., et al., 2011. Premature ovarian failure in patients with autoimmune Addison's disease: clinical, genetic, and immunological evaluation. J. Clin. Endocrinol. Metab. 96, E1255–E1261.

Rosatelli, M.C., Meloni, A., Meloni, A., Devoto, M., Cao, A., Scott, H.S., et al., 1998. A common mutation in Sardinian autoimmune polyendocrinopathy-candidiasis-ectodermal dystrophy patients. Hum. Genet. 103, 428–434.

Rotondi, M., Falorni, A., De Bellis, A., Laureti, S., Ferruzzi, P., Romagnani, P., et al., 2005. Elevated serum interferon-gamma-inducible chemokine-10/CXC chemokine ligand-10 in autoimmune primary adrenal insufficiency and in vitro expression in human adrenal cells primary cultures after stimulation with proinflammatory cytokines. J. Clin. Endocrinol. Metab. 90, 2357–2363.

Rotondi, M., Chiovato, L., Romagnani, S., Serio, M., Romagnani, P., 2007. Role of chemokines in endocrine autoimmune diseases. Endocr. Rev. 28, 492–520.

Rottembourg, D., Deal, C., Lambert, M., Mallone, R., Carel, J.C., Lacroix, A., et al., 2010. 21-Hydroxylase epitopes are targeted by CD8 T cells in autoimmune Addison's disease. J. Autoimmun. 35, 309–315.

Roycroft, M., Fichna, M., McDonald, D., Owen, K., Zurawek, M., Gryczynska, M., et al., 2009. The tryptophan 620 allele of the lymphoid tyrosine phosphatase (PTPN22). gene predisposes to autoimmune Addison's disease. Clin. Endocrinol. (Oxf.). 70, 358–362.

Scalapino, K.J., Daikh, D.I., 2008. CTLA-4: a key regulatory point in the control of autoimmune disease. Immunol. Rev. 223, 143–155.

Schatz, D.A., Winter, W.E., 2002. Autoimmune polyglandular syndrome. II: Clinical syndrome and treatment. Endocrinol. Metab. Clin. North Am. 31, 339–352.

Schmidt, M., 1926. Eine biglanduläre erkrankung (Nebennieren und schilddruse) bei morbus Addisonii. Verh. Dtsch. Ges. Pathol. 21, 212–221.

Scott, H.S., Heino, M., Peterson, P., Mittaz, L., Lalioti, M.D., Betterle, C., et al., 1998. Common mutations in autoimmune polyendocrinopathy-candidiasis-ectodermal dystrophy patients of different origins. Mol. Endocrinol. 12, 1112–1119.

Skinningsrud, B., Husebye, E.S., Gervin, K., Lovas, K., Blomhoff, A., Wolff, A.B., et al., 2008a. Mutation screening of PTPN22: association of the 1858T-allele with Addison's disease. Eur. J. Hum. Genet. 16, 977–982.

Skinningsrud, B., Husebye, E.S., Pearce, S.H., McDonald, D.O., Brandal, K., Wolff, A.B., et al., 2008b. Polymorphisms in CLEC16A and CIITA at 16p13 are associated with primary adrenal insufficiency. J. Clin. Endocrinol. Metab. 93, 3310–3317.

Skinningsrud, B., Lie, B.A., Lavant, E., Carlson, J.A., Erlich, H., Akselsen, H.E., et al., 2010. Multiple loci in the HLA complex are associated with Addison's disease. J. Clin. Endocrinol. Metab. 96, E1703—E1708.

Skoldberg, F., Rorsman, F., Perheentupa, J., Landin-Olsson, M., Husebye, E.S., Gustafsson, J., et al., 2004. Analysis of antibody reactivity against cysteine sulfinic acid decarboxylase, a pyridoxal phosphate-dependent enzyme, in endocrine autoimmune disease. J. Clin. Endocrinol. Metab. 89, 1636—1640.

Soderbergh, A., Myhre, A.G., Ekwall, O., Gebre-Medhin, G., Hedstrand, H., Landgren, E., et al., 2004. Prevalence and clinical associations of 10 defined autoantibodies in autoimmune polyendocrine syndrome type I. J. Clin. Endocrinol. Metab. 89, 557—562.

Sotsiou, F., Bottazzo, G.F., Doniach, D., 1980. Immunofluorescence studies on autoantibodies to steroid-producing cells, and to germline cells in endocrine disease and infertility. Clin. Exp. Immunol. 39, 97—111.

Spinner, M.W., Blizzard, R.M., Childs, B., 1968. Clinical and genetic heterogeneity in idiopathic Addison's disease and hypoparathyroidism. J. Clin. Endocrinol. Metab. 28, 795—804.

Terao, C., Yamada, R., Ohmura, K., Takahashi, M., Kawaguchi, T., Kochi, Y., et al., 2011. The human AIRE gene at chromosome 21q22 is a genetic determinant for the predisposition to rheumatoid arthritis in Japanese population. Hum. Mol. Genet. 20, 2680—2685.

Thorpe, E., Handley, H., 1929. Chronic tetany and chronic mycelial stomatitis in a child aged four and one-half years. Am. J. Dis. Child. 38, 228—238.

Toth, B., Wolff, A.S., Halasz, Z., Tar, A., Szuts, P., Ilyes, I., et al., 2010. Novel sequence variation of AIRE and detection of interferon-omega antibodies in early infancy. Clin. Endocrinol. (Oxf.). 72, 641—647.

Tuomi, T., Bjorses, P., Falorni, A., Partanen, J., Perheentupa, J., Lernmark, A., et al., 1996. Antibodies to glutamic acid decarboxylase and insulin-dependent diabetes in patients with autoimmune polyendocrine syndrome type I. J. Clin. Endocrinol. Metab. 81, 1488—1494.

Tuovinen, H., Pontynen, N., Gylling, M., Kekalainen, E., Perheentupa, J., Miettinen, A., et al., 2009. Gammadelta T cells develop independently of Aire. Cell Immunol. 257, 5—12.

Turunen, J.A., Wessman, M., Forsblom, C., Kilpikari, R., Parkkonen, M., Pontynen, N., et al., 2006. Association analysis of the AIRE and insulin genes in Finnish type 1 diabetic patients. Immunogenetics. 58, 331—338.

Ueda, H., Howson, J.M., Esposito, L., Heward, J., Snook, H., Chamberlain, G., et al., 2003. Association of the T-cell regulatory gene CTLA4 with susceptibility to autoimmune disease. Nature. 423, 506—511.

Uibo, R., Perheentupa, J., Ovod, V., Krohn, K.J., 1994. Characterization of adrenal autoantigens recognized by sera from patients with autoimmune polyglandular syndrome (APS) type I. J. Autoimmun. 7, 399—411.

Vaidya, B., Pearce, S., Kendall-Taylor, P., 2000. Recent advances in the molecular genetics of congenital and acquired primary adrenocortical failure. Clin. Endocrinol. (Oxf.). 53, 403—418.

Wang, C.Y., Davoodi-Semiromi, A., Huang, W., Connor, E., Shi, J.D., She, J.X., 1998. Characterization of mutations in patients with autoimmune polyglandular syndrome type 1 (APS1). Hum. Genet. 103, 681—685.

Wang, X., Laan, M., Bichele, R., Kisand, K., Scott, H.S., Peterson, P., 2012. Post-Aire maturation of thymic medullary epithelial cells involves selective expression of keratinocyte-specific autoantigens. Front Immunol. 3, 19.

Wilks, S., 1862. On diseases of the suprarenal capsule or morbus addisonii. Guy's Hosp. Rep. 8, 1.

Winer, K.K., Zhang, B., Shrader, J.A., Peterson, D., Smith, M., Albert, P.S., et al., 2012. Synthetic human parathyroid hormone 1-34 replacement therapy: a randomized crossover trial comparing pump versus injections in the treatment of chronic hypoparathyroidism. J. Clin. Endocrinol. Metab. 97, 391—399.

Winqvist, O., Karlsson, F.A., Kampe, O., 1992. 21-Hydroxylase, a major autoantigen in idiopathic Addison's disease. Lancet. 339, 1559—1562.

Winqvist, O., Gustafsson, J., Rorsman, F., Karlsson, F.A., Kampe, O., 1993. Two different cytochrome P450 enzymes are the adrenal antigens in autoimmune polyendocrine syndrome type I and Addison's disease. J. Clin. Invest. 92, 2377—2385.

Winqvist, O., Gebre-Medhin, G., Gustafsson, J., Ritzen, E.M., Lundkvist, O., Karlsson, F.A., et al., 1995. Identification of the main gonadal autoantigens in patients with adrenal insufficiency and associated ovarian failure. J. Clin. Endocrinol. Metab. 80, 1717—1723.

Wolff, A.S., Erichsen, M.M., Meager, A., Magitta, N.F., Myhre, A.G., Bollerslev, J., et al., 2007. Autoimmune polyendocrine syndrome type 1 in Norway: phenotypic variation, autoantibodies, and novel mutations in the autoimmune regulator gene. J. Clin. Endocrinol. Metab. 92, 595—603.

Zlotogora, J., Shapiro, M.S., 1992. Polyglandular autoimmune syndrome type I among Iranian Jews. J. Med. Genet. 29, 824—826.

Chapter 44

Autoimmune Gastritis and Pernicious Anemia

Ian R. van Driel, Eric Tu, and Paul A. Gleeson

Department of Biochemistry and Molecular Biology, Bio21 Molecular Science and Biotechnology Institute, The University of Melbourne, Parkville, Victoria, Australia

Chapter Outline

Clinical, Pathologic, and Epidemiologic Features	620	*In Vivo* and *In Vitro* Models	624
Autoimmune Features	622	Pathologic Effector Mechanisms	626
Autoantibodies	622	Autoantibodies as Potential Immunologic Markers	626
T Cell Immunity	623	Concluding Remarks—Future Prospects	626
Genetic Features	623	References	627

Pernicious anemia is the result of advanced autoimmune gastritis, which in its initial stages is an asymptomatic autoimmune disease. First reported by Addison in 1849, the link between the anemia and gastric degeneration was realized by Flint in 1860 and histologic evidence of the gastric atrophy was provided by Fenwick in 1870. In 1871, a fatal anemia was termed perniciosa by Biermer. Subacute combined degeneration was later applied to the posterolateral spinal cord lesions that can be associated with the anemia (Pearce, 2008). In 1926 Minot and Murphy discovered that feeding patients large meals of cooked liver led to a reticulocyte response and reversal of anemia, which earned them a Nobel Prize in 1934. At first, the causal connection between pernicious anemia and chronic gastritis was incomprehensible. Castle (Castle, 1953) showed that the anemia was a result of a combined deficiency of an "extrinsic factor" subsequently identified as vitamin B12 and present in the liver (Smith, 1948; Rickes et al., 1948), and an "intrinsic factor" (IF) in gastric juice (Highley et al., 1967). Oral treatment with extracts of hog stomach (Sharp, 1929; Sturgis and Isaacs, 1929; Renshaw, 1930) resulted in remission for several years (Wilkinson, 1949). However, relapses tended to occur and some cases became refractory to increasing amounts of the extract (Berlin et al., 1958a, b). This refractory state was due to a serum factor that

inhibited the effectiveness of intrinsic factor (Schwartz, 1958). Subsequently, sera from patients with pernicious anemia were shown to contain autoantibodies to intrinsic factor (Jeffries et al., 1962; Jacob and Schilling, 1966) and to gastric parietal cells (Irvine et al., 1962; Jeffries et al., 1962; Markson and Moore, 1962). However, little progress was made in understanding the pathology of the gastric lesion until a flexible biopsy tube was designed that permitted the taking of samples of the gastric mucosa for histologic examination (Wood et al., 1949).

Pernicious anemia was observed to cluster in families (McIntyre et al., 1959; Whittingham et al., 1969) and to coexist with autoimmune thyroid diseases (Tudhope and Wilson, 1960). These observations suggested a genetic component to the disorder, a suggestion further strengthened by an association with another endocrine autoimmune disease, type 1 diabetes mellitus (Ungar et al., 1968). The suggestion by Taylor (Taylor, 1959; Taylor and Morton, 1959) that the inhibitory substance to gastric intrinsic factor in the serum of patients with pernicious anemia was antibody and possibly autoantibody and the recognition that pernicious anemia fulfilled the markers of autoimmune disease put forward by Mackay and Burnet (Mackay and Burnet, 1963) led to its acceptance as an autoimmune disease of the stomach.

N. Rose & I. Mackay (Eds): The Autoimmune Diseases, Fifth edition. DOI: http://dx.doi.org/10.1016/B978-0-12-384929-8.00044-7

CLINICAL, PATHOLOGIC, AND EPIDEMIOLOGIC FEATURES

Autoimmune gastritis in the early stages is asymptomatic and demonstrable only by serologic detection of antibodies to gastric parietal cells. Pernicious anemia only manifests when stores of vitamin B12 are depleted and only 10−15% of patients with autoimmune gastritis develop pernicious anemia (Strickland and Mackay, 1973; Irvine et al., 1974) after a latent period of 20−30 years (Toh et al., 1997). Nonetheless, at an estimated prevalence of about 2% in Western adult populations at or over the age of 60 years, pernicious anemia represents the commonest cause of vitamin B12 deficiency (Carmel, 1996). Although "silent" until the end stage, the gastric lesion can be predicted years before clinical presentation by immunologic markers specific for gastric autoimmunity. Terminally, the gastritis results in deficiency of intrinsic factor, a protein that binds avidly to dietary vitamin B12 (Glass, 1963) and promotes its transport to the terminal ileum for absorption (Donaldson et al., 1967) by ileal cubulin receptors, a multifunctional endocytic receptor (Lindblom et al., 1999). Consequently, the gastritis is expressed clinically as vitamin B12 deficiency associated with megaloblastic anemia arising as a consequence of the requirement of the vitamin for DNA synthesis. The megaloblastic anemia is demonstrated by examination of blood and bone marrow (Chanarin, 1979) and is now readily controlled by vitamin B12 treatment (Carmel, 2008). Pernicious anemia usually results in low serum pepsinogen I levels and a low serum pepsinogen I/II ratio and increased serum gastrin levels which also can be diagnostically useful (Varis et al., 1979; Samloff et al., 1982; Carmel, 1988).

Pernicious anemia is uncommon before the age of 30. Reportedly more common in individuals of northern Europeans decent, the disease has been reported in blacks and in Latin Americans (Carmel and Johnson, 1978). Patients with advanced pernicious anemia are usually women of late middle age, who appear pale, tired, and depressed and may complain of a sore tongue and abdominal discomfort. Vitamin B12 deficiency can lead to neuropsychiatric syndromes such as sensory impairment, abnormal reflexes, motor impairment and spastic paraparesis, and possibly mental or psychiatric disturbances (Savage and Lindenbaum, 1995). Patients with pernicious anemia have also been reported to have a 3−5-fold higher risk of developing gastric cancer and a 13-fold increased risk of developing gastric carcinoids (Hsing et al., 1993; Fuchs and Mayer, 1995; Kokkola et al., 1998).

Strickland and Mackay (Strickland and Mackay, 1973) proposed a classification of gastritis based on histologic findings of the gastric mucosa, the presence of gastric parietal cell antibody, and serum levels of gastrin. Type A gastritis, the "pernicious anemia type," is restricted to the fundus and body of the stomach. Early lesions are characterized by chronic inflammation in the submucosa that extends into the lamina propria of the mucosa between gastric glands with accompanying loss of gastric and zymogenic cells (Figure 44.1). In advanced disease, gastric atrophy is readily recognized macroscopically and microscopically (Figures 44.2 and 44.3). The wall of the fundus and body of the stomach becomes paper thin because the gastric glands are markedly reduced or absent. In particular, parietal cells and zymogenic (chief) cells are absent from the gastric mucosa and replaced by mucus-containing cells resembling those of the intestine (intestinal metaplasia) (Figure 44.3).

Type A gastritis is characterized by circulating antibodies to gastric parietal cells (Figure 44.4) that have subsequently been shown to be directed to the gastric H^+/K^+ ATPase (Burman et al., 1989; Goldkorn et al., 1989; Toh et al., 1990, 1997), achlorhydria, and high levels of serum gastrin secreted by the intact antral glands. Strickland and Mackay observed that five out of 30 patients with type A gastritis (16%) developed overt or latent pernicious anemia during a follow-up period of 3−24 years. Type A gastritis is also the gastritis characteristic of families in

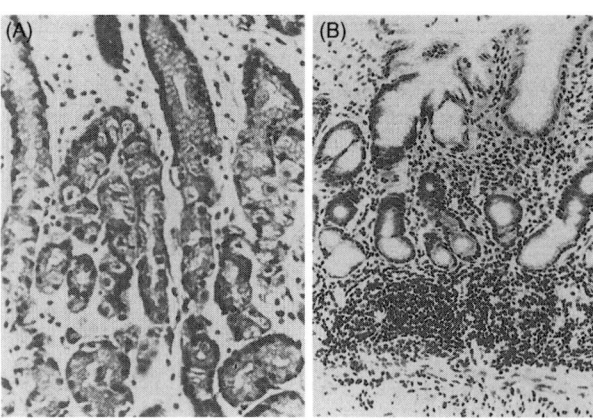

FIGURE 44.1 **The early lesion of autoimmune gastritis.** (A) The normal mucosa of the body of the stomach showing gastric glands and the absence of a chronic inflammatory infiltrate in the lamina propria. (B) An early lesion of autoimmune gastritis showing a dense chronic inflammatory infiltrate in the gastric submucosa that extends into the lamina propria with the accompanying loss of gastric parietal and zymogenic cells. ×300.

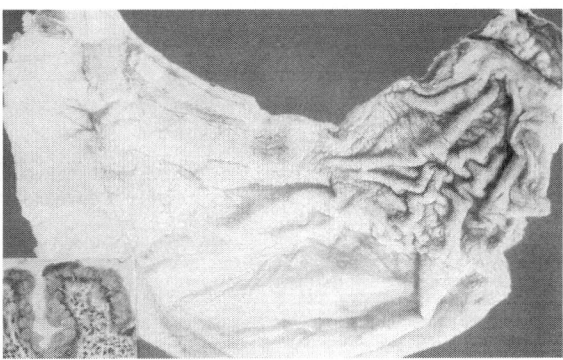

FIGURE 44.2 Macroscopic appearance of advanced autoimmune gastritis in a patient with pernicious anemia showing the extreme atrophy of the mucosa of the fundus and body of the stomach with loss of rugal folds contrasted with the healthy mucosa of the gastric antrum. Inset is the microscopic appearance of the mucosa.

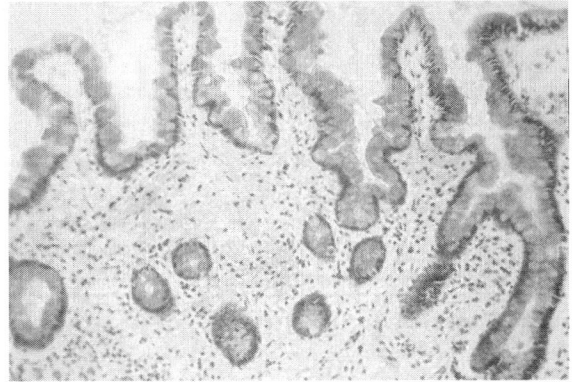

FIGURE 44.3 Microscopic appearance of the gastric mucosa of advanced autoimmune gastritis showing a chronic inflammatory infiltrate in the gastric mucosa and the loss of parietal and zymogenic cells and replacement with mucus-containing cells.

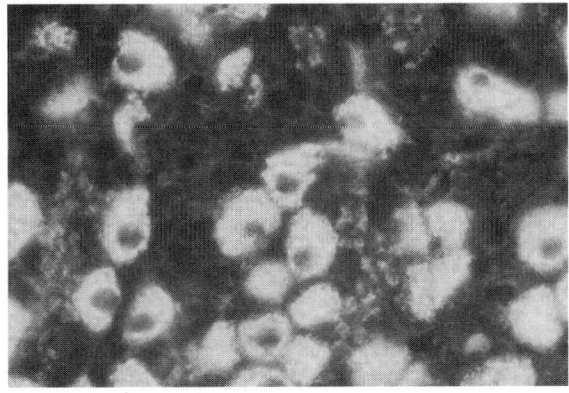

FIGURE 44.4 Indirect immunofluorescent staining of gastric parietal cells in a mouse stomach reactive with serum from a patient with autoimmune gastritis.

whom pernicious anemia predominates (Varis, 1981; Kekki et al., 1983).

Type B gastritis, the nonpernicious anemia type, involves the antrum initially but can extend to the fundus and body of the stomach and shows incomplete failure of acid secretion and low levels of serum gastrin because of the antral gastritis. Type B gastritis is usually associated with *Helicobacter pylori* infection; type A is not (Fong et al., 1991).

Pernicious anemia in patients with the common variable type of immunodeficiency associated with low levels of serum immunoglobulins can be distinguished from classic pernicious anemia on this classification. This former type of pernicious anemia usually occurs in a younger age group, is histologically type B, is associated with a negative test for antibodies to gastric parietal cells and intrinsic factor, and shows a low level of serum gastrin (Twomey et al., 1969; Hughes et al., 1972; Cowling et al., 1974). Pernicious anemia in childhood is not associated with gastritis or achlorhydria and is the result of inadequate intrinsic factor production.

The evolution of gastric atrophy in most cases of pernicious anemia probably spans 20–30 years but this is difficult to assess in individual cases. The presence of gastric parietal cell antibody in the serum is predictive of autoimmune gastritis (Irvine et al., 1965; Serafini et al., 1970). Conversely, gastric parietal cell antibody is not observed when gastritis is due to diseases affecting the body of the stomach that are not autoimmune.

There are many reports of regeneration of gastric parietal cells, improvement in gastric function, and hematologic remission after treatment with corticosteroids (Doig et al., 1957; Gordin 1959; Ardeman and Chanarin, 1965; Jeffries et al., 1966; Rodbro et al., 1967; Strickland, 1969) or azathioprine (Jorge and Sanchez, 1973). This suggests that the gastric mucosa is the direct target of an autoimmune process that can be checked by immunosuppressive drugs. The observations also suggest that precursor stem cells capable of differentiating into parietal cells and zymogenic cells are present in stomachs of patients with autoimmune gastritis and that these are responsible for the regeneration of the differentiated cells when the destructive autoimmune process is controlled. The suggestion is supported by observations in experimental models of autoimmune gastritis where there is evidence of the persistence, and even expansion, of these precursor stem cells in gastritic stomachs (see below). It is also of interest and relevance that reversal of recovery with degeneration of the gastric mucosa recurred once immunosuppressive treatment was halted (Wall et al., 1968). This highlights the persistence of autoreactive T cells that cause this disease, even in the face of immunosuppression.

Pernicious anemia associates predominantly with the autoimmune endocrinopathies and the antireceptor autoimmune diseases. The associated diseases include Hashimoto's thyroiditis, insulin-dependent type 1 diabetes mellitus, primary Addison's disease, primary ovarian failure, primary hypoparathyroidism, premature graying of the hair, vitiligo, thyrotoxicosis, myasthenia gravis, and the Lambert–Eaton syndrome. These organ-specific "thyrogastric" autoimmune diseases may occur in the same patient with pernicious anemia but aggregate in "pernicious anemia families" (Ardeman et al., 1966; Wangel et al., 1968a; Whittingham et al., 1969).

AUTOIMMUNE FEATURES

Autoantibodies

Autoimmune gastritis is associated with autoantibodies to gastric parietal cells and to their secreted product, intrinsic factor. Like most autoantibodies, these autoantibodies are polyclonal but are predominantly of the IgG isotype (Serafini et al., 1970). IgA antibodies to gastric intrinsic factor have been demonstrated in gastric juice (Goldberg and Bluestone, 1970). Autoantibodies to gastric parietal cells are routinely detected by immunofluorescence (see Figure 44.4). These autoantibodies are directed toward both the catalytic 100 kDa α subunit and the 60–90 kDa glycoprotein β-subunit of the gastric H^+/K^+ ATPase (Figure 44.5) (Karlsson et al., 1988; Burman et al., 1989; Toh et al., 1990; Callaghan et al., 1993; Ma et al., 1994). The gastric H^+/K^+ ATPase is the enzyme responsible for acidification of gastric luminal contents (Forte et al., 1989; Rabon and Reuben, 1990; Prinz et al., 1992). It belongs to a family of ion-motive P-type ATPases and is most closely related to the ubiquitous Na^+/K^+ ATPase. The gastric $H^{+/}K^+$ ATPase is located on specialized secretory membranes of gastric parietal cells (DiBona et al., 1979; Callaghan et al., 1990; Toh et al., 1990; Pettitt et al., 1995). Parietal cell antibodies have been shown to deplete H^+/K^+ ATPase activity from parietal cell membranes in vitro (Burman et al., 1989). Antibody reactivity with the α subunit of the H^+/K^+ ATPase includes an epitope on the cytosolic side of the secretory membrane (Song et al., 1994). The H^+/K^+ ATPase β subunit extracellular domain has three disulfide bonds and is highly glycosylated and these structural features are required for binding of autoantibodies (Goldkorn et al., 1989; Callaghan et al., 1993).

Human intrinsic factor is a glycoprotein with a molecular mass of 44,000. Each molecule of intrinsic factor has the capacity to bind to one molecule of vitamin B12 (Chanarin, 1979). Two distinct antibody activities are detected by radioimmunoassay; one reacts with the

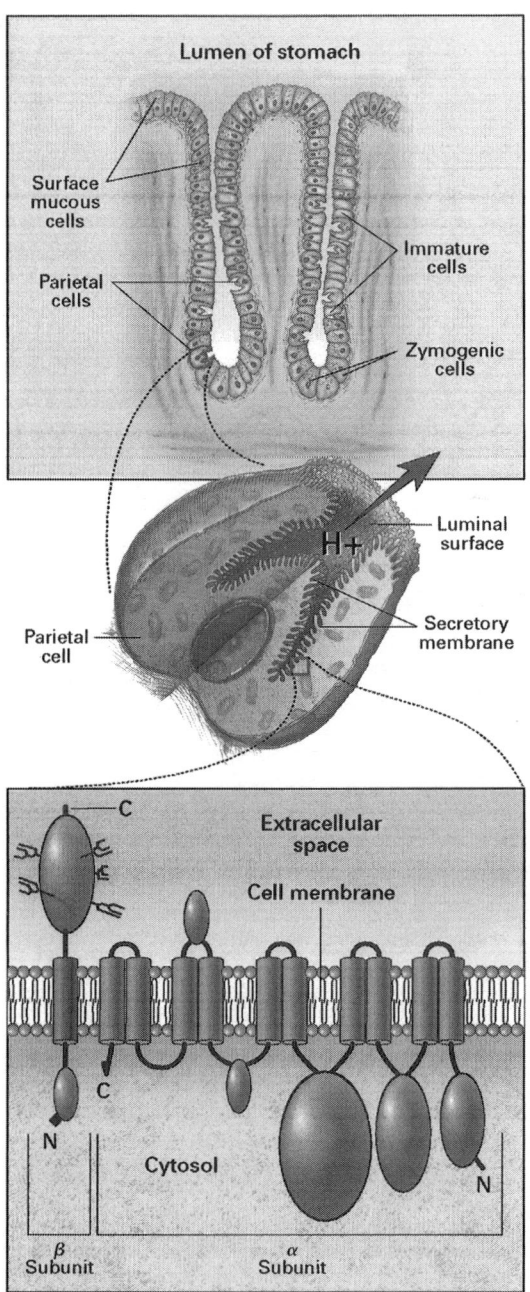

FIGURE 44.5   Gastric parietal cell H^+/K^+ ATPase as the target in autoimmune gastritis associated with pernicious anemia. Top panel represents a gastric gland showing location of parietal cells in relation to zymogenic cells, immature cells, and surface mucus cells. Middle panel represents a stimulated gastric parietal cell showing the lining membrane of the secretory canaliculus on which gastric H^+/K^+ ATPase is located. Bottom panel represents the catalytic α and the glycoprotein β subunits of the gastric H^+/K^+ ATPase showing their orientation in the membrane of the secretory canaliculus of the parietal cells. N denotes the N-terminal of protein and C the C-terminal of protein. *Reproduced with kind permission of the New England Journal of Medicine.*

binding site for vitamin B12 and blocks subsequent binding of intrinsic factor with free vitamin, and the other reacts with an antigenic determinant remote from this site (Samloff et al., 1968; Rothenberg et al., 1971).

T Cell Immunity

Studies of animal models suggest that $CD4^+$ T cells mediate the gastritic lesion (see below). In humans, a significant increase in $CD4^+$ and $CD8^+$ T cells and a sixfold increase in non-T cells (probably B cells) have been observed in the cellular infiltrate of stomachs of patients with pernicious anemia (Irvine et al., 1965; Kaye et al., 1983). Electron microscopy has shown that lymphocytes line up against the membranes of gastric parietal cells and zymogenic cells in the gastric mucosa. Phenotypic analysis of the peripheral blood T cells from patients with pernicious anemia have not shown any significant differences compared to age-matched controls (Vargas et al., 1995) although, in humans, no studies have been made on the gastric lymph nodes which are the sites appropriate for such studies.

A number of early studies suggested a T cell response to intrinsic factor and gastric extracts (Fisher et al., 1965, 1966; Tai and McGuigan, 1969; Rose et al., 1970; Fixa et al., 1972; Goldstone et al., 1973; MacCuish et al., 1974; Whittingham et al., 1975). However, the identification of the gastric H^+/K^+ ATPase as the major gastric autoantigen that was targeted by antibodies in humans and mice and T cells in mice led to the isolation of human H^+/K^+ ATPase-specific $CD4^+$ T cell clones from the gastric mucosa of patients with autoimmune gastritis. The clones were shown to recognize a number of epitopes in the H^+/K^+ ATPase α and β subunits (Bergman et al., 2003) and were biased towards the production of IFN-γ and TNF-α although some also produced IL-4 and stimulated immunoglobulin production by B cells (D'elios et al., 2001). Most clones also displayed cytotoxic activity that was either perforin or Fas dependent.

Studies in mice have shown that a T cell immune response to the gastric H^+/K^+ ATPase is essential for the initiation and development of autoimmune gastritis. These observations include the resistance to autoimmune gastritis in mice expressing the H^+/K^+ ATPase β subunit in the thymus and mice deficient in the gastric H^+/K^+ ATPase, a high incidence of disease in mice with repertoires enriched in H^+/K^+ ATPase reactive T cells, and mice immunized with purified H^+/K^+ ATPase. Initial findings suggested that the H^+/K^+ ATPase β subunit may be the primary initiating autoantigen (Alderuccio et al., 1993). However, subsequent studies indicated that both subunits are targeted in disease and that the expression of the H^+/K^+ ATPase β subunit is required for presentation of the α subunit to $CD4^+$ T cells, which explained earlier findings on antigenic hierarchy (Allen et al., 2005).

The pathways that lead to immunological tolerance to the gastric H^+/K^+ ATPase have been extensively investigated. High avidity H^+/K^+ ATPase-specific T cells exit the thymus and the H^+/K^+ ATPase-specific T cells in the periphery represent the residue of a T cell repertoire that has been subjected to partial extrathymic deletion (Read et al., 2007). This depletion occurs following antigen-specific activation of H^+/K^+ ATPase-specific $CD4^+$ T cells in the stomach-draining paragastric lymph node. Additional mechanisms of peripheral tolerance, mediated by dendritic cells and $Foxp3^+$ regulatory T cells (Treg cells), play important roles in influencing the activation of self-reactive T cells that remain after clonal deletion (Scheinecker et al., 2002; Zwar et al., 2006; Dipaolo et al., 2007; Read et al., 2007; Hogan et al., 2008; Stummvoll et al., 2008). Therefore, protection from gastritis is mediated almost exclusively by tolerogenic mechanisms in the local tissue environment.

GENETIC FEATURES

Predisposition to pernicious anemia appears to be genetically determined, at least in part. Evidence for genetic factors influencing the expression of pernicious anemia includes clustering of this disease in families and with other autoimmune diseases as well as a racial predilection for northern Europeans. Pernicious anemia is rare among southern Europeans and earlier reports suggest that it is almost nonexistent among black and Asian people (Jayaratnam et al., 1967; Irvine et al., 1969). In keeping with ethnic differences, pernicious anemia is associated with phenotypic markers that are absent or occur with low frequency in these racial groups. These markers include blue eyes, fair skin, and blood group A (Callender et al., 1957). However, a more recent study by Carmel (1992) reported a higher prevalence in black people, particularly among black women.

There have been reports of a number of Caucasian families with a high frequency of pernicious anemia over several generations (Callender et al., 1957; Callender and Denborough, 1957; McIntyre et al., 1959; Doniach et al., 1965; Ardeman et al., 1966; Wangel et al., 1968a,b; Whittingham et al., 1969). A higher but not absolute concordance of pernicious anemia has been observed in monozygotic twins (Delva et al., 1965; Balcerzak et al., 1968). While associations with susceptibility to pernicious anemia and HLA molecules have been reported (Ungar et al., 1977), such findings were not substantiated in other studies (Whittingham et al., 1991).

Studies in mice have also substantiated the role of specific genes in predisposing to autoimmune gastritis. BALB/c mouse strains are highly susceptible to autoimmune gastritis whereas C57BL/6 mice are very resistant (Kojima and Prehn, 1981; Silveira et al., 1999). To identify genes conferring susceptibility to the disease, linkage analysis was performed on (BALB/cCrSlc x C57BL/6)F2 mice. Two major genes on chromosome 4 that confer susceptibility to autoimmune gastritis, termed Gasa1 and Gasa2, were identified (Silveira et al., 1999). Further analysis found Gasa3 on chromosome 6, coincident with the MHC locus, and Gasa4 on chromosome 17 as minor gastritis susceptibility genes (Silveira et al., 2001). Experimental evidence for the Gasa1 and Gasa2 loci was obtained using congenic mouse strains that also proved that Gasa1 and Gasa2 can act independently to cause full expression of susceptibility to autoimmune disease (Ang et al., 2007).

IN VIVO AND IN VITRO MODELS

Mice can readily develop high incidence of autoimmune gastritis, either spontaneously or after manipulation. Mouse models have proven to be a very reliable and robust model of autoimmune gastritis that shares key features with human disease including antigen and epitope commonality, cytokine secretion, and pathogenic mechanisms. As a result mouse autoimmune gastritis has been used extensively to investigate basic mechanisms of immune tolerance and the cellular and molecular basis for autoimmune disease.

Spontaneous gastritis has been reported in C3H/He mice with an incidence of about 20% (Alderuccio and Toh, 1998). A variety of organ-specific autoimmune diseases can be induced by lymphopenic conditions and the particular organ affected is determined by the genetic background of the mouse strain. BALB/c mice are the most susceptible mouse strain to lymphopenia-induced autoimmune gastritis whereas C57BL/6 mice are resistant to the induction of disease (Ahmed and Penhale, 1981; Kojima and Prehn, 1981). Thymectomy-induced autoimmune gastritis is historically one of the most commonly used gastritis models. BALB/c mice thymectomized at approximately day 3 after birth develop autoimmune gastritis at ∼30–90%. Adult mice did not develop autoimmune gastritis followed by thymectomy unless the mice were treated with cyclophosphamide or irradiation (Ahmed and Penhale, 1981; Barrett et al., 1995). It was previously believed that induction of autoimmune gastritis by neonatal thymectomy was the result of a block in Treg cells being seeded into the periphery from the thymus; thus gastritogenic T cells were not suppressed (Asano et al., 1996). However, this proposal was not supported by findings that Treg cells are able to repopulate in the periphery after neonatal thymectomy and these Treg cells are fully suppressive in vivo (Asano et al., 1996; Dujardin et al., 2004; Ang et al., 2007; Samy et al., 2008).

Comparatively recently, it has been demonstrated that neonatal thymectomy results in a lymphopenic environment that promotes homeostatic proliferation of effector T cells, including expansion of gastritogenic T cell clones (Monteiro et al., 2008). Therefore, autoimmune gastritis induced by neonatal thymectomy is probably the result of a reduced Treg:effector T cell ratio that does not favor suppression by Treg cell, rather than the depletion of Treg cells per se or intrinsic defects of Treg cells.

Murine autoimmune gastritis can also be induced by immunization of adult BALB/c mice with purified gastric H^+/K^+ ATPase in complete Freund's adjuvant (Scarff et al., 1997). However, the disease induced is transient and is reversible after cessation of immunization, perhaps due to regeneration of parietal cells and zymogenic cells from the expanded stem cell population.

Autoimmune gastritis may occur as the result of the immune system being dominated by self-reactive T cells. T cell receptor (TCR) transgenic mouse lines that constitutively express H^+/K^+ ATPase-specific TCR on their T cells have been generated. A23 TCR transgenic mice contain $CD4^+$ T cells that target residues 630–641 of the H^+/K^+ ATPase α subunit and display a Th1 phenotype (McHugh et al., 2001), whereas A51 TCR transgenic mice contain $CD4^+$ T cells that target residues 889–899 of the H^+/K^+ ATPase α subunit and reveal a Th2 phenotype (Candon et al., 2004). Both A23 and A51 T cell clones were isolated from the paragastric lymph node of mice that developed autoimmune gastritis following neonatal thymectomy (Suri-Payer et al., 1999). A23 mice develop more severe autoimmune gastritis spontaneously with higher penetrance than in A51 mice due to difference in the availability of their respective autoantigenic epitopes (Levin et al., 2008). IE4 TCR transgenic mice were created using TCR genes isolated from a T cell hybridoma which was derived by immunization of a BALB/c mouse with residues 253–277 of the H^+/K^+ ATPase β subunit (Alderuccio et al., 2000; De Silva et al., 2001). Autoimmune gastritis only occurred in 20% of the mice, even though transgenic T cells in the periphery responded well to the antigenic peptide in vitro.

Constitutive expression of the cytokine granulocyte macrophage colony stimulating factor in the stomach induces autoimmune gastritis with very similar antigenic and pathological features to those of other models (Biondo et al., 2001). It is not clear which of the proinflammatory activities of granulocyte macrophage colony stimulating factor are responsible for disease initiation.

T cells from mice deficient in gastric H^+/K^+ ATPase autoantigens can induce autoimmune gastritis in sublethally irradiated mice, presumably due to the preponderance of H^+/K^+ ATPase-specific T cells that result from a lack of autoantigen-specific tolerance (Tu et al., 2011). This recent model is attractive for the study of many aspects of organ-specific autoimmunity because of a high degree of consistency of disease severity, the use of polyclonal T cells, and a specific T cell response to a bone fide autoantigen (Figure 44.6). The cardinal features of mouse autoimmune gastritis are illustrated in this disease. The gastric mucosa becomes heavily infiltrated by mononuclear cells, parietal and zymogenic cells are severely depleted, and there is overgrowth by immature cell types resulting in gastric hypertrophy visible at both microscopic and macroscopic levels (Figure 44.6A—D). The depletion of parietal cells leads to an increase in gastric pH (Figure 44.6E). High titer anti-H^+/K^+ ATPase autoantibodies develop within 4—6 weeks (Figure 44.6F, G).

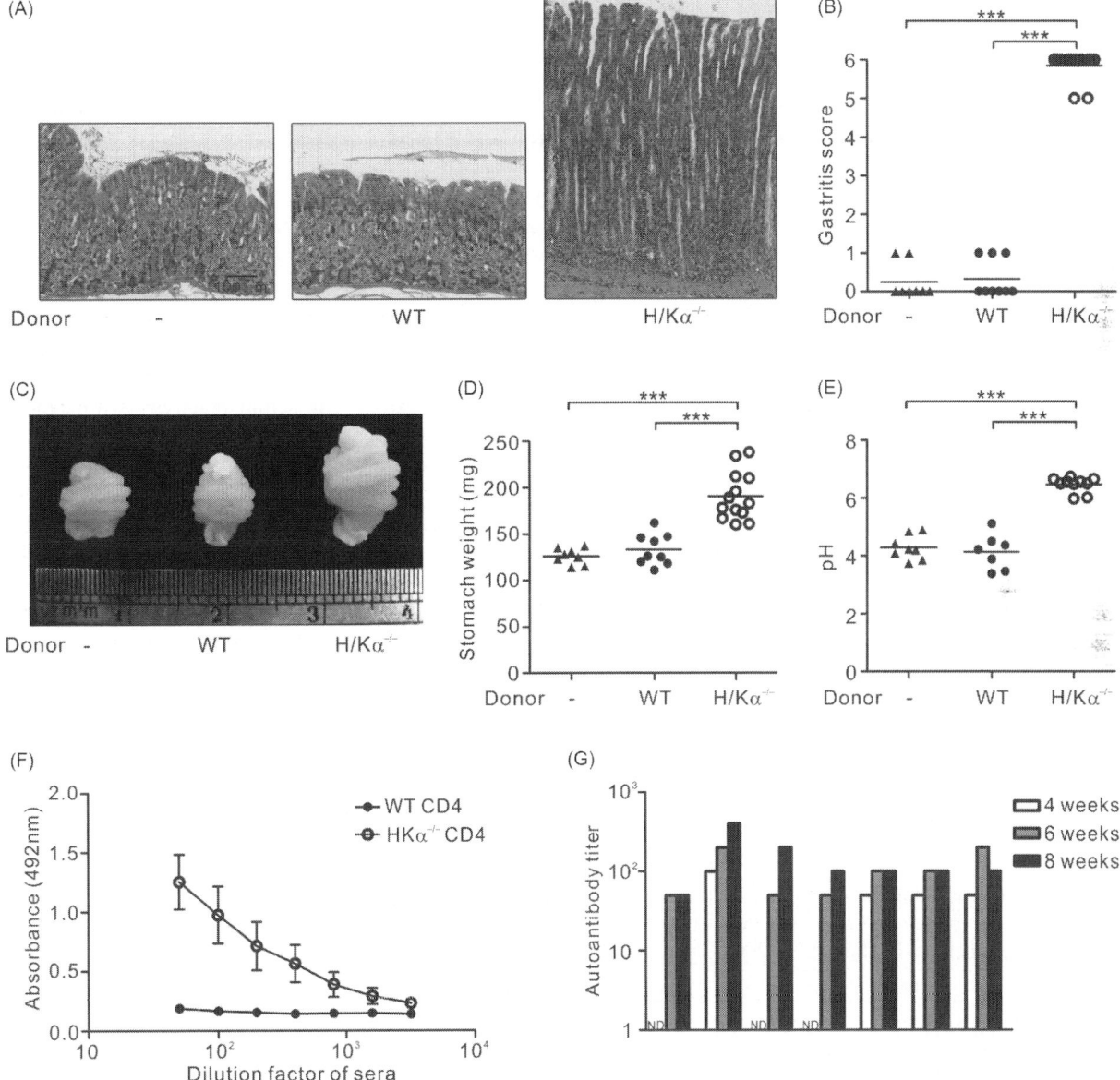

FIGURE 44.6 **A mouse model of autoimmune gastritis.** Irradiated wild-type mice that received 5×10^7 CD4$^+$ T cells from either wild-type (WT) or H^+/K^+ ATPase α subunit-deficient mice (H/K$\alpha^{-/-}$), were killed 8 weeks after transfer and compared to non-manipulated mice ($-$). (A) Hematoxylin and eosin stained sections of stomachs. (B) Gastritis scores. (C) Macroscopic views of stomachs. (D) Stomach weights after stomach contents were removed. (E) Gastric pH. Mice were starved overnight and their stomachs were rinsed in 1 ml saline which was then collected and measured by a pH meter. (F) H^+/K^+ ATPase-specific autoantibodies in serum were detected by ELISA using serial two-fold dilutions of mouse sera, with a starting dilution factor of 50. (G) Gastric H^+/K^+ ATPase autoantibody levels in mice at various times after cell transfer. Serum samples were collected at the indicated time points from each mouse after transfer of CD4$^+$ T cells from H/K$\alpha^{-/-}$ mice. Autoantibody titer was represented by the maximum dilution factor that had an absorbance reading above 50% maximum. ND = not detectable. Data pooled from four independent experiments. In (B), (D), and (E), each circle represents the data from one mouse. Mann—Whitney U test was used; bars, median and ***, $P < 0.001$.

PATHOLOGIC EFFECTOR MECHANISMS

Studies in mice have clearly indicated that autoimmune gastritis is initiated by CD4$^+$ T cells. First, gastritis can be transferred to immunocompromised hosts by CD4$^+$ T lymphocytes but not by sera from animals with autoimmune gastritis (reviewed by van Driel et al., 1984, 2005; Gleeson et al., 1996; Toh et al., 1997; van Driel and Ang, 2008). In addition, histopathologic features of gastritis occur in mice before the appearance of autoantibodies. The early gastric lesion is composed predominantly of CD4$^+$ T cells and macrophages with production of a mix of Th1- and Th2-type cytokines but not interleukin-4, suggesting a key role for these cells and their cytokines in initiation of the disease (Martinelli et al., 1996; Katakai et al., 1998). Interferon-γ, probably produced by the Th1 cells, appears to be crucial for the induction of gastritic lesion, as a single injection of antibodies to interferon-γ immediately following neonatal thymectomy prevents autoimmune gastritis (Barrett et al., 1996) and T cells from mice deficient in interferon-γ or interleukin-12 have a reduced pathogenicity in causing autoimmune gastritis (Suri-Payer and Cantor, 2001). CD8$^+$ T cells do not seem to have a role in this disease since depletion of this T cell population by treatment with anti-CD8 antibody did not reduce the capacity of the remaining T cells to transfer disease (De Silva et al., 1998). Recent data suggest that interleukin-17 may play a role in assisting the development of severe late-stage autoimmune gastritis (Tu et al., 2012). B lymphocytes tend to accumulate in gastric lesions and aggregate in follicular-like structures and it is not known if they play a functional role at these sites (Martinelli et al., 1996).

There is evidence for various mechanisms whereby T cells could cause the lesion in the gastric mucosa including direct cytotoxicity and cytokine mediated disruption of developmental pathways in the stomach (Judd et al., 1999; Marshall et al., 2002; Kang et al., 2005).

As described above, CD4$^+$ T cell clones specific for the gastric H$^+$/K$^+$ ATPase and with activities that support a pathogenic role have also been isolated from patients with pernicious anemia (D'elios et al., 2001).

AUTOANTIBODIES AS POTENTIAL IMMUNOLOGIC MARKERS

Autoimmune gastritis and pernicious anemia are typically associated with autoantibodies to parietal cells, directed to gastric H$^+$/K$^+$ ATPase and to intrinsic factor. For the diagnosis of pernicious anemia, intrinsic factor antibodies have a much higher disease specificity (>95%), albeit lower sensitivity (50–70%), than antibodies to gastric parietal cells. A recent study suggests that that assaying autoantibodies to both intrinsic factor and the H$^+$/K$^+$

ATPase results in an increased specificity and sensitivity and would aid in selection of patients for follow-up gastroscopic procedures (Lahner et al., 2009). Since the Schilling test is no longer available as a diagnostic procedure, there has been increased dependence on intrinsic factor antibodies for diagnosis. Antibodies to the vitamin B12 binding site of intrinsic factor are demonstrable in serum of $\sim$70% of patients and to a second site in $\sim$50%. These frequencies are greater if gastric juice is assayed. There may be coexisting autoantibodies specific for the various other autoimmune diseases in the thyrogastric cluster. The incidence of these antibodies rises with increasing duration of disease, almost doubling after 10 years (Ungar et al., 1967).

Parietal cell antibodies to gastric H$^+$/K$^+$ ATPase are diagnostic of the underlying pathologic lesion of autoimmune gastritis, as gastric biopsies carried out in asymptomatic patients have revealed the presence of type A gastritis (Uibo et al., 1984). These antibodies are routinely detected by indirect immunofluorescence or, to gastric H$^+$/K$^+$ ATPase, by ELISA (Chuang et al., 1992; Lahner et al., 2009). Antibodies to gastric parietal cells can be demonstrated by serum reactivity with the cytoplasm of gastric parietal cells in unfixed, air-dried, and frozen sections of mouse stomach (see Figure 44.4). Mouse stomach is preferable to rat stomach because of a lower frequency of heterophile reactions (Muller et al., 1971) that could be misinterpreted as antibody to parietal cells. The antibodies are detected by immunofluorescence in $\sim$90% of patients with pernicious anemia, with a prevalence of 2–5% in the general population, and in $\sim$30% of patients with other thyrogastric autoimmune diseases, including type 1 diabetes mellitus (De Block et al., 2000, 2001a,b). The prevalence of gastric autoantibodies increases with age and correlate with rising serum gastrin levels (Jassel et al., 1999; De Block et al., 2001a). Parietal cell mass and hence the availability of autoantigens decreases as autoimmune gastritis progresses to pernicious anemia and this may explain the observation that the prevalence of autoantibodies decreases with progression (Davidson et al., 1989) and may also explain the lower antibody prevalence in one study of pernicious anemia (Carmel, 1992).

CONCLUDING REMARKS—FUTURE PROSPECTS

As one of the most common autoimmune diseases, autoimmune gastritis has been intensively investigated and a great deal has been discovered concerning its immunological pathogenesis. The availability of excellent animal models has meant that the identity of the gastric autoantigens is well defined, and the pathway that leads to immunological tolerance in normal individuals is well understood. On the other hand, in common with most other autoimmune diseases, the reason why the immune system begins to react to gastric autoantigens to the detriment of patients is still not clear. While we know some level of detail of the genetics of autoimmune gastritis in mice, such data have not as yet been translated into the human setting. Environmental triggers for autoimmune gastritis are also unclear. While some data suggest a role for *Helicobacter* infection, this hypothesis is not supported by other epidemiological information.

From a clinical standpoint, pernicious anemia is now routinely treatable to prevent neurological complications of the disease by vitamin B12 replacement. However, this therapy does not cure the underlying cause of the disease, namely the decimation of the gastric mucosa by the autoimmune response, which increases the risk of gastric cancer. In mice, ectopic expression of the gastric autoantigen (Murphy et al., 2003) and treatment with Treg cells (Nguyen et al., 2011; Tu, Gleeson, and van Driel, unpublished) lead to long-term reversal of gastric lesions. Whether such treatments will become feasible or practical in humans remains to be seen.

REFERENCES

Ahmed, S.A., Penhale, W.J., 1981. Pathological changes in inbred strains of mice following early thymectomy and irradiation. Experientia. 37, 1341–1343.

Alderuccio, F., Toh, B.H., 1998. Spontaneous autoimmune gastritis in C3H/He mice: a new mouse model for gastric autoimmunity. Am. J. Pathol. 153, 1311–1318.

Alderuccio, F., Toh, B.H., Tan, S.S., Gleeson, P.A., van Driel, I.R., 1993. An autoimmune disease with multiple molecular targets abrogated by the transgenic expression of a single autoantigen in the thymus. J. Exp. Med. 178, 419–426.

Alderuccio, F., Cataldo, V., van Driel, I.R., Gleeson, P.A., Toh, B.H., 2000. Tolerance and autoimmunity to a gastritogenic peptide in TCR transgenic mice. Int. Immunol. 12, 343–352.

Allen, S., Read, S., DiPaolo, R., McHugh, R.S., Shevach, E.M., Gleeson, P.A., et al., 2005. Promiscuous thymic expression of an autoantigen gene does not result in negative selection of pathogenic T cells. J. Immunol. 175, 5759–5764.

Ang, D.K.Y., Brodnicki, T.C., Jordan, M.A., Wilson, W.E., Silveira, P., Gliddon, B.L., et al., 2007. Two genetic loci independently confer susceptibility to autoimmune gastritis. Int. Immunol. 19, 1135–1144.

Ardeman, S., Chanarin, I., 1965. Steroids and addisonian pernicious anemia. N. Engl. J. Med. 273, 1352–1355.

Ardeman, S., Chanarin, I., Jacobs, A., Griffiths, L., 1966. Family study in Addisonian pernicious anemia. Blood. 27, 599–610.

Asano, M., Toda, M., Sakaguchi, N., Sakaguchi, S., 1996. Autoimmune disease as a consequence of developmental abnormality of a T cell subpopulation. J. Exp. Med. 184, 387–396.

Balcerzak, S.P., Westerman, M.P., Heinle, E.W., 1968. Discordant occurrence of pernicious anemia in identical twins. Blood. 32, 701–710.

Barrett, S.P., Toh, B.H., Alderuccio, F., van Driel, I.R., Gleeson, P.A., 1995. Organ-specific autoimmunity induced by adult thymectomy and cyclophosphamide-induced lymphopenia. Eur. J. Immunol. 25, 238–244.

Barrett, S.P., Gleeson, P.A., Desilva, H., Toh, B.H., van Driel, I.R., 1996. Interferon-γ is required during the initiation of an organ-specific autoimmune disease. Eur. J. Immunol. 26, 1652–1655.

Bergman, M., Amedei, A., D'Elios, M., Azzurri, A., Benagiano, M., Tamburini, C., et al., 2003. Characterization of H+,K+ -ATPase T cell epitopes in human autoimmune gastritis. Eur. J. Immunol. 33, 539–545.

Berlin, R., Berlin, H., Brante, G., Sjoberg, S.G., 1958a. Failures in long-term oral treatment of pernicious anemia with B12-intrinsic factor preparations. Acta Med. Scand. 161, 143–150.

Berlin, R., Berlin, H., Brante, G., Sjoberg, S.G., 1958b. Refractoriness to intrinsic factor-B12 preparations abolished by massive doses of intrinsic factor; preliminary report. Acta Med. Scand. 162, 317–319.

Biondo, M., Nasa, Z., Marshall, A., Toh, B.H., Alderuccio, F., 2001. Local transgenic expression of granulocyte macrophage-colony stimulating factor initiates autoimmunity. J. Immunol. 166, 2090–2099.

Burman, P., Mardh, S., Norberg, L., Karlsson, F.A., 1989. Parietal cell antibodies in pernicious anaemia inhibit H,K-adenosine triphosphatase, the proton pump of the stomach. Gastroenterology. 96, 1434.

Callaghan, J.M., Toh, B.H., Pettitt, J.M., Humphris, D.C., Gleeson, P.A., 1990. Poly-N-acetyllactosamine-specific tomato lectin interacts with gastric parietal cells: identification of a tomato-lectin binding 60–90 × 10³ Mr membrane glycoprotein of tubulovesicles. J. Cell Sci. 95, 563–576.

Callaghan, J.M., Khan, M.A., Alderuccio, F., van Driel, I.R., Gleeson, P.A., Toh, B.H., 1993. Alpha and beta subunits of the gastric H+/K(+)-ATPase are concordantly targeted by parietal cell autoantibodies associated with autoimmune gastritis. Autoimmunity. 16, 289–295.

Callender, S.T., Denborough, M.A., 1957. A family study of pernicious anaemia. Br. J. Haematol. 3, 88–106.

Callender, S.T., Denborough, M.A., Sneath, J., 1957. Blood groups and other inherited characters in pernicious anaemia. Br. J. Haematol. 3, 107–114.

Candon, S., McHugh, R.S., Foucras, G., Natarajan, K., Shevach, E.M., Margulies, D.H., 2004. Spontaneous organ-specific Th2-mediated autoimmunity in TCR transgenic mice. J. Immunol. 172, 2917–2924.

Carmel, R., 1988. Pepsinogens and other serum markers in pernicious anemia. Am. J. Clin. Pathol. 90, 442–445.

Carmel, R., 1992. Reassessment of the relative prevalences of antibodies to gastric parietal cell and to intrinsic factor in patients with pernicious anaemia—influence of patient age and race. Clin. Exp. Immunol. 89, 74 77.

Carmel, R., 1996. Prevalence of undiagnosed pernicious anemia in the elderly. Arch Intern. Med. 156, 1097–1100.

Carmel, R., 2008. How I treat cobalamin (vitamin B12) deficiency. Blood. 112, 2214–2221.

Carmel, R., Johnson, C.S., 1978. Racial patterns in pernicious anemia. Early age at onset and increased frequency of intrinsic-factor antibody in black women. N. Engl. J. Med. 298, 647–650.

Castle, W.B., 1953. Development of knowledge concerning the gastric intrinsic factor and its relation to pernicious anemia. N. Engl. J. Med. 249, 603–614.

Chanarin, I., 1979. The Megablastic Anaemias. Blackwell, Oxford.

Chuang, J.S., Callaghan, J.M., Gleeson, P.A., Toh, B.H., 1992. Diagnostic ELISA for parietal cell autoantibody using tomato lectin-purified gastric H + /K + -ATPase (proton pump). Autoimmunity. 12, 1−7.

Cowling, D.C., Strickland, R.G., Ungar, B., Whittingham, S., Rose, W.M., 1974. Pernicious-anaemia-like syndrome with immunoglobulin deficiency. Med. J. Aust. 1, 15−17.

Davidson, R.J., Atrah, H.I., Sewell, H.F., 1989. Longitudinal study of circulating gastric antibodies in pernicious anaemia. J. Clin. Pathol. 42, 1092−1095.

De Block, C.E., De Leeuw, I.H., Decochez, K., Winnock, F., Van Autreve, J., Van Campenhout, C.M., et al., 2001a. The presence of thyrogastric antibodies in first degree relatives of type 1 diabetic patients is associated with age and proband antibody status. J. Clin. Endocrinol. Metab. 86, 4358−4363.

De Block, C.E., De Leeuw, I.H., Vertommen, J.J., Rooman, R.P., Du Caju, M.V., Van Campenhout, C.M., et al., 2001b. Beta-cell, thyroid, gastric, adrenal and coeliac autoimmunity and HLA-DQ types in type 1 diabetes. Clin. Exp. Immunol. 126, 236−241.

De Block, C.E.M., De Leeuw, I.H., Rooman, R.P.A., Winnock, F., Du Caju, M.V.L., Van Gaal, L.F., 2000. Gastric parietal cell antibodies are associated with glutamic acid decarboxylase-65 antibodies and the HLA DQA1*0501-DQB1*0301 haplotype in type 1 diabetes mellitus. Diabet. Med. 17, 618−622.

De Silva, H.D., Van Driel, I.R., La Gruta, N., Toh, B.H., Gleeson, P.A., 1998. CD4 + T cells, but not CD8 + T cells, are required for the development of experimental autoimmune gastritis. Immunology. 93, 405−408.

De Silva, H.D., Alderuccio, F., Toh, B.H., Van Driel, I.R., Gleeson, P. A., 2001. Defining T cell receptors which recognise the immunodominant epitope of the gastric autoantigen, the H/K ATPase beta-subunit. Autoimmunity. 33, 1−14.

D'elios, M.M., Bergman, M.P., Azzurri, A., Amedei, A., Benagiano, M., De Pont, J.J., et al., 2001. H + ,K + -ATPase (proton pump) is the target autoantigen of Th1-type cytotoxic T cells in autoimmune gastritis. Gastroenterology. 120 (2), 377−386.

Delva, P.L., MacDonald, J.E., Macintosh, D.C., 1965. Megaloblastic anaemia occurring simultaneously in white female monozygotic twins. Can. Med. Assoc. J. 92, 1129−1131.

DiBona, D.R., Ito, S., Berglindh, T., Sachs, G., 1979. Cellular site of gastric acid secretion. Proc. Natl. Acad. Sci. U.S.A. 76, 6689−6693.

Dipaolo, R.J., Brinster, C., Davidson, T.S., Andersson, J., Glass, D., Shevach, E.M., 2007. Autoantigen-specific TGFbeta-induced Foxp3 + regulatory T cells prevent autoimmunity by inhibiting dendritic cells from activating autoreactive T cells. J. Immunol. 179, 4685−4693.

Doig, A., Girdwood, R.H., Duthie, J.J., Knox, J.D., 1957. Response of megaloblastic anaemia of prednisolone. Lancet. 273, 966−972.

Donaldson, R.M., Mackenzie, I.L., Trier, J.S., 1967. Intrinsic factor-mediated attachment of vitamin B12 to brush borders and microvillous membranes of hamster intestine. J. Clin. Invest. 46, 1215−1228.

Doniach, D., Roitt, I.M., Taylor, K.B., 1965. Autoimmunity in pernicious anemia and thyroiditis: a family study. Ann. N. Y. Acad. Sci. 124, 605−625.

van Driel, I.R., Stearne, P.A., Grego, B., Simpson, R.J., Goding, J.W., 1984. The receptor for transferrin on murine myeloma cells: one-step

purification based on its physiology, and partial amino acid sequence. J. Immunol. 133, 3220−3224.

van Driel, I.R., Read, S., Zwar, T.D., Gleeson, P.A., 2005. Shaping the T cell repertoire to a bona fide autoantigen: lessons from autoimmune gastritis. Curr. Opin. Immunol. 17, 570−576.

Dujardin, H.C., Burlen-Defranoux, O., Boucontet, L., Vieira, P., Cumano, A., Bandeira, A., 2004. Regulatory potential and control of Foxp3 expression in newborn CD4 + T cells. Proc. Natl. Acad. Sci. U.S.A. 101, 14473−14478.

Fisher, J.M., Rees, C., Taylor, K.B., 1965. Antibodies in gastric juice. Science. 150, 1467−1469.

Fisher, J.M., Rees, C., Taylor, K.B., 1966. Intrinsic-factor antibodies in gastric juice of pernicious-anemia patients. Lancet. 2, 88−89.

Fixa, B., Thiele, H.G., Komárková, O., Nozicka, Z., 1972. Gastric auto-antibodies and cell-mediated immunity in pernicious anaemia—a comparative study. Scand. J. Gastroenterol. 7, 237−240.

Fong, T.L., Dooley, C.P., Dehesa, M., Cohen, H., Carmel, R., Fitzgibbons, P.L., et al., 1991. Helicobacter pylori infection in pernicious anemia: a prospective controlled study. Gastroenterology. 100, 328−332.

Forte, J.G., Hanzel, D.K., Urushidani, T., Wolosin, J.M., 1989. Pumps and pathways for gastric HCl secretion. Ann. N. Y. Acad. Sci. 574, 145−158.

Fuchs, C.S., Mayer, R.J., 1995. Gastric carcinoma. N. Engl. J. Med. 333, 32−41.

Glass, G.B., 1963. Gastric intrinsic factor and its function in the metabolism of vitamin B12. Physiol. Rev. 43, 529−849.

Gleeson, P.A., Toh, B.H., van Driel, I.R., 1996. Organ-specific autoimmunity induced by lymphopenia. Immunol. Rev. 149, 97−125.

Goldberg, L.S., Bluestone, R., 1970. Hidden gastric autoantibodies to intrinsic factor in pernicious anemia. J. Lab. Clin. Med. 75, 449−456.

Goldkorn, I., Gleeson, P.A., Toh, B.H., 1989. Gastric parietal cell antigens of 60−90 kDa, 92 kDa and 100−120 kDa associated with autoimmune gastritis and pernicious anaemia. Role of N-glycans in the structure and antigenicity of the 60−90 kDa component. J. Biol. Chem. 264, 18768−18774.

Goldstone, A.H., Calder, E.A., Barnes, E.W., Irvine, W.J., 1973. The effect of gastric antigens on the in vitro migration of leucocytes from patients with atrophic gastritis and pernicious anaemia. Clin. Exp. Immunol. 14, 501−508.

Gordin, R., 1959. Vitamin B12 absorption in corticosteroid-treated pernicious anaemia. Acta. Med. Scand. 164, 159−165.

Highley, D.R., Davies, M.C., Ellenbogen, L., 1967. Hog intrinsic factor. II. Some physicochemical properties of vitamin B12-binding fractions from hog pylorus. J. Biol. Chem. 242, 1010−1015.

Hogan, T.V., Ang, D.K.Y., Gleeson, P.A., van Driel, I.R., 2008. Extrathymic mechanisms of T cell tolerance: lessons from autoimmune gastritis. J. Autoimmun. 31, 268−273.

Hsing, A.W., Hansson, L.E., McLaughlin, J.K., Nyren, O., Blot, W.J., Ekbom, A., et al., 1993. Pernicious anemia and subsequent cancer—a population-based cohort study. Cancer. 71, 745−750.

Hughes, W.S., Brooks, F.P., Conn, H.O., 1972. Serum gastrin levels in primary hypogammaglobulinemia and pernicious anemia. Studies in adults. Ann. Intern. Med. 77, 746−750.

Irvine, W.J., Davies, S.H., Teitelbaum, S., Delamore, I.W., Williams, A.W., 1962. Immunological relationship between pernicious anaemia and thyroid disease. Br. Med. J. 2, 454−456.

Irvine, W.J., Davies, S.H., Teitelbaum, S., Delamore, I.W., Williams, A.W., 1965. The clinical and pathological significance of gastric parietal cell antibody. Ann. N. Y. Acad. Sci. 124, 657–691.

Irvine, W.J., McFadzean, A.J.S., Todd, D., Tso, S.C., Yeung, R.T.T., 1969. Pernicious anaemia in the chinese: a clinical and immunological study. Clin. Exp. Immunol. 4, 375–386.

Irvine, W.J., Cullen, D.R., Mawhinney, H., 1974. Natural history of autoimmune achlorhydric atrophic gastritis: a 1–15 year follow-up study. Lancet. 2, 482.

Jacob, E., Schilling, R.F., 1966. An in vitro test for the detection of serum antibody to intrinsic factor–vitamin B12 complex. J. Lab. Clin. Med. 67, 510–515.

Jassel, S.V., Ardill, J.E., Fillmore, D., Bamford, K.B., O'Connor, F.A., Buchanan, K.D., 1999. The rise in circulating gastrin with age is due to increases in gastric autoimmunity and Helicobacter pylori infection. QJM. 92, 373–377.

Jayaratnam, F.J., Seah, C.S., Da Costa, J.L., Tan, K.K., O'Brien, W., 1967. Pernicious anaemia among Asians in Singapore. Br. Med. J. 3, 18–25.

Jeffries, G.H., Hoskins, D.W., Sleisenger, M.H., 1962. Antibody to intrinsic factor in serum from patients with pernicious anemia. J. Clin. Invest. 41, 1106–1115.

Jeffries, G.H., Todd, J.E., Sleisenger, M.H., 1966. The effect of prednisolone on gastric mucosal histology, gastric secretion, and vitamin B 12 absorption in patients with pernicious anemia. J. Clin. Invest. 45, 803–812.

Jorge, A.D., Sanchez, D., 1973. The effect of azathioprine on gastric mucosal histology and acid secretion in chronic gastritis. Gut. 14, 104–106.

Judd, L.M., Gleeson, P.A., Toh, B.H., van Driel, I.R., 1999. Autoimmune gastritis results in disruption of gastric epithelial cell development. Am. J. Physiol. Gastrointest. Liver Physiol. 277, G209–G218.

Kang, W., Rathinavelu, S., Samuelson, L.C., Merchant, J.L., 2005. Interferon gamma induction of gastric mucous neck cell hypertrophy. Lab. Invest. 85, 702–715.

Karlsson, F.A., Burman, P., Loof, L., Mardh, S., 1988. Major parietal cell antigen in autoimmune gastritis with pernicious anaemia is the acid-producing H,K-adenosine triphosphatase of the stomach. J. Clin. Invest. 81, 475–479.

Katakai, T., Mori, K.J., Masuda, T., Shimizu, A., 1998. Differential localization of T(H)1 and T(H)2 cells in autoimmune gastritis. Int. Immunol. 10, 1325–1334.

Kaye, M.D., Whorwell, P.J., Wright, R., 1983. Gastric mucosal lymphocyte subpopulations in pernicious anaemia and in normal stomach. Clin. Immunol. Immunopathol. 28, 431–440.

Kekki, M., Varis, K., Pohjanpalo, H., Isokoski, M., Ihamäki, T., Siurala, M., 1983. Course of antrum and body gastritis in pernicious anemia families. Dig. Dis. Sci. 28, 698–704.

Kojima, A., Prehn, R.T., 1981. Genetic susceptibility to post-thymectomy autoimmune disease. Immunogenetics. 14, 15–27.

Kokkola, A., Sjöblom, S.M., Haapiainen, R., Sipponen, P., Puolakkainen, P., Järvinen, H., 1998. The risk of gastric carcinoma and carcinoid tumours in patients with pernicious anaemia. A prospective follow-up study. Scand. J. Gastroenterol. 33, 88–92.

Lahner, E., Norman, G.L., Severi, C., Encabo, S., Shums, Z., Vannella, L., et al., 2009. Reassessment of intrinsic factor and parietal cell autoantibodies in atrophic gastritis with respect to cobalamin deficiency. Am. J. Gastroenterol. 104, 2071–2079.

Levin, D., Dipaolo, R.J., Brinster, C., Revilleza, M.J., Boyd, L.F., Teyton, L., et al., 2008. Availability of autoantigenic epitopes controls phenotype, severity, and penetrance in TCR Tg autoimmune gastritis. Eur. J. Immunol. 38, 3339–3353.

Lindblom, A., Quadt, N., Marsh, T., Aeschlimann, D., Mörgelin, M., Mann, K., et al., 1999. The intrinsic factor-vitamin B12 receptor, cubilin, is assembled into trimers via a coiled-coil alpha-helix. J. Biol. Chem. 274, 6374–6380.

Ma, J.Y., Borch, K., Mardh, S., 1994. Human gastric H,K-adenosine triphosphatase beta-subunit is a major autoantigen in atrophic corpus gastritis—expression of the recombinant human glycoprotein in insect cells. Scand. J. Gastroenterol. 29, 790–794.

MacCuish, A.C., Urbaniak, S.J., Goldstone, A.H., Irvine, W.J., 1974. PHA responsiveness and subpopulations of circulating lymphocytes in pernicious anemia. Blood. 44, 849–855.

Mackay, I.R., Burnet, E.M., 1963. Autoimmune Diseases, Pathogenesis, Chemistry and Therapy. Charles Thomas, Springfield, IL.

Markson, J.L., Moore, J.M., 1962. Thyroid auto-antibodies in pernicious anaemia. Br. Med. J. 2, 1352–1355.

Marshall, A.C.J., Alderuccio, F., Toh, B.-H., 2002. Fas/CD95 is required for gastric mucosal damage in autoimmune gastritis. Gastroenterology. 123, 780–789.

Martinelli, T.M., van Driel, I.R., Alderuccio, F., Gleeson, P.A., Toh, B. H., 1996. Analysis of mononuclear cell infiltrate and cytokine production in murine autoimmune gastritis. Gastroenterology. 110, 1791–1802.

McHugh, R.S., Shevach, E.M., Margulies, D.H., Natarajan, K., 2001. A T cell receptor transgenic model of severe, spontaneous organ-specific autoimmunity. Eur. J. Immunol. 31, 2094–2103.

McIntyre, P.A., Hahn, R., Conley, C.L., Glass, B., 1959. Genetic factors in predisposition to pernicious anemia. Bull. Johns Hopkins Hosp. 104, 309–342.

Monteiro, J.P., Farache, J., Mercadante, A.C., Mignaco, J.A., Bonamino, M., Bonomo, A., 2008. Pathogenic effector T cell enrichment overcomes regulatory T cell control and generates autoimmune gastritis. J. Immunol. 181, 5895–5903.

Muller, H.K., McGiven, A.R., Nairn, R.C., 1971. Immunofluorescent staining of rat gastric parietal cells by human antibody unrelated to pernicious anaemia. J. Clin. Pathol. 24, 13–14.

Murphy, K., Biondo, M., Toh, B.-H., Alderuccio, F., 2003. Tolerance established in autoimmune disease by mating or bone marrow transplantation that target autoantigen to thymus. Int. Immunol. 15, 269–277.

Nguyen, T.-L.M., Sullivan, N.L., Ebel, M., Teague, R.M., Dipaolo, R.J., 2011. Antigen-specific TGF-{beta}-induced regulatory T cells secrete chemokines, regulate T cell trafficking, and suppress ongoing autoimmunity. J. Immunol. 187, 1745–1753.

Pearce, J.M.S., 2008. Subacute combined degeneration of the cord: Putnam-Dana syndrome. Eur. Neurol. 60, 53–56.

Pettitt, J.M., Humphris, D.C., Barrett, S.P., Toh, B.H., van Driel, I.R., Gleeson, P.A., 1995. Fast freeze-fixation/freeze-substitution reveals the secretory membranes of the gastric parietal cell as a network of helically coiled tubule—a new model for parietal cell transformation. J. Cell Sci. 108, 1127–1141.

Prinz, C., Kajimura, M., Scott, D., Helander, H., Shin, J.M., Besancon, M., et al., 1992. Acid secretion and the H,K-ATPase of stomach. Yale J. Biol. Med. 65, 577–596.

Rabon, E.C., Reuben, M.A., 1990. The mechanism and structure of the gastric H,K ATPase. Annu. Rev. Physiol. 52, 321–344.

Read, S., Hogan, T.V., Zwar, T.D., Gleeson, P.A., Van Driel, I.R., 2007. Prevention of autoimmune gastritis in mice requires extra-thymic T-cell deletion and suppression by regulatory T cells. Gastroenterology. 133, 547–558.

Renshaw, A., 1930. Treatment of pernicious anaemia with desiccated hog's stomach. Br. Med. J. 1, 334–335.

Rickes, E.L., Brink, N.G., Koniuszy, F.R., Wood, T.R., Folkers, K., 1948. Crystalline vitamin B12. Science. 107, 396–397.

Rodbro, P., Dige-Petersen, H., Schwartz, M., Dalgaard, O.Z., 1967. Effect of steroids on gastric mucosal structure and function in pernicious anemia. Acta. Med. Scand. 181, 445–452.

Rose, M.S., Doniach, D., Chanarin, I., Brostoff, J., Ardeman, S., 1970. Intrinsic-factor antibodies in absence of pernicious anaemia. 3–7 year follow-up. Lancet. 2, 9–12.

Rothenberg, S.P., Kantha, K.R., Ficarra, A., 1971. Autoantibodies to intrinsic factor: their determination and clinical usefulness. J. Lab. Clin. Med. 77, 476–484.

Samloff, I.M., Kleinman, M.S., Turner, M.D., Sobel, M.V., Jeffrie, G.H., 1968. Blocking and binding antibody to intrinsic factor and parietal cell antibody in pernicious anaemia. Gastroenterology. 55, 575–583.

Samloff, I.M., Varis, K., Ihamaki, T., Siurala, M., Rotter, J.I., 1982. Relationships among serum pepsinogen I, serum pepsinogen II, and gastric mucosal histology. A study in relatives of patients with pernicious anemia. Gastroenterology. 83, 204–209.

Samy, E.T., Wheeler, K.M., Roper, R.J., Teuscher, C., Tung, K.S., 2008. Cutting edge: autoimmune disease in day 3 thymectomized mice is actively controlled by endogenous disease-specific regulatory T cells. J. Immunol. 180, 4366–4370.

Savage, D.G., Lindenbaum, J., 1995. Neurological complications of acquired cobalamin deficiency: clinical aspects. Baillière's Clin. Haematol. 8, 657–678.

Scarff, K.J., Pettitt, J.M., Driel, I.R.V., Gleeson, P.A., Toh, B.H., 1997. Immunisation with gastric H/K ATPase induces reversible autoimmune gastritis. Immunology. 92, 91–98.

Scheinecker, C., McHugh, R., Shevach, E.M., Germain, R.N., 2002. Constitutive presentation of a natural tissue autoantigen exclusively by dendritic cells in the draining lymph node. J. Exp. Med. 196, 1079–1090.

Schwartz, M., 1958. Intrinsic-factor-inhibiting substance in serum of orally treated patients with pernicious anaemia. Lancet. 2, 61–62.

Serafini, U., Masala, C., Pala, A.M, 1970. Studies on gastric autoimmunity. Folia Allergol. 17, 433–434.

Sharp, E.A., 1929. An antianaemic factor in desiccated hog stomach. JAMA. 93, 749–751.

Silveira, P.A., Baxter, A.G., Cain, W.E., van Driel, I.R., 1999. A major linkage region on distal chromosome 4 confers susceptibility to mouse autoimmune gastritis. J. Immunol. 162, 5106–5111.

Silveira, P.A., Wilson, W.E., Esteban, L.M., Jordan, M.A., Hawke, C.G., van Driel, I.R., et al., 2001. Identification of the Gasa3 and Gasa4 autoimmune gastritis susceptibility genes using congenic mice and partitioned, segregative and interaction analyses. Immunogenetics. 53, 741–750.

Smith, E.L., 1948. Purification of anti-pernicious anaemia factors from liver. Nature. 161, 638–639.

Song, Y.H., Ma, J.Y., Mardh, S., Liu, T., Sjostrand, S.E., Rask, L., et al., 1994. Localization of a pernicious anaemia autoantibody epitope on the alpha-subunit of human H,K-adenosine triphosphatase. Scand. J. Gastroenterol. 29, 122–127.

Strickland, R.G., 1969. Pernicious anemia and polyendocrine deficiency. Ann. Intern. Med. 70, 1001–1005.

Strickland, R.G., Mackay, I.R., 1973. A reappraisal of the nature and significance of chronic atrophic gastritis. Am. J. Dig. Dis. 18, 426–440.

Stummvoll, G.H., DiPaolo, R.J., Huter, E.N., Davidson, T.S., Glass, D., Ward, J.M., et al., 2008. Th1, Th2, and Th17 effector T cell-induced autoimmune gastritis differs in pathological pattern and in susceptibility to suppression by regulatory T cells. J. Immunol. 181, 1908–1916.

Sturgis, C.C., Isaacs, R., 1929. Desiccated stomach in the treatment of pernicious anaemia. JAMA. 93, 747–749.

Suri-Payer, E., Cantor, H., 2001. Differential cytokine requirements for regulation of autoimmune gastritis and colitis by CD4(+)CD25(+) T cells. J. Autoimmun. 16, 115–123.

Suri-Payer, E., Amar, A.Z., McHugh, R., Natarajan, K., Margulies, D.H., Shevach, E.M., 1999. Post-thymectomy autoimmune gastritis: fine specificity and pathogenicity of anti-H/K ATPase-reactive T cells. Eur. J. Immunol. 29, 669–677.

Tai, C., McGuigan, J.E., 1969. Immunologic studies in pernicious anemia. Blood. 34, 63–71.

Taylor, K.B., 1959. Inhibition of intrinsic factor by pernicious anaemia sera. Lancet. 2, 106–108.

Taylor, K.B., Morton, J.A., 1959. An antibody to Castle's intrinsic factor. J. Pathol. Bacteriol. 77, 117–122.

Toh, B.H., Gleeson, P.A., Simpson, R.J., Moritz, R.L., Callaghan, J., Goldkorn, I., et al., 1990. The 60–90 kDa parietal cell autoantigen associated with autoimmune gastritis is a b subunit of the gastric H + K + -ATPase (proton pump). Proc. Natl. Acad. Sci. U.S.A. 87, 6418–6422.

Toh, B.H., van Driel, I.R., Gleeson, P.A., 1997. Mechanisms of disease: pernicious anemia. N. Engl. J. Med. 337, 1441–1448.

Tu, E., Ang, D.K.Y., Hogan, T.V., Read, S., Chia, C.P.Z., Gleeson, P.A., et al., 2011. A convenient model of severe, high incidence autoimmune gastritis caused by polyclonal effector T cells and without perturbation of regulatory T cells. PLoS One. 6, e27153.

Tu, E., Bourges, D., Gleeson, P.A., Ang, D.K., van Driel, I.R., 2013. Pathogenic T cells persist after reversal of autoimmune disease by immunosuppression with regulatory T cells. Eur J Immunol. 43, 1286–1296.

Tudhope, G.R., Wilson, G.M., 1960. Anaemia in hypothyroidism. Incidence, pathogenesis, and response to treatment. Q. J. Med. 29, 513–537.

Twomey, J.J., Jordan, P.H., Jarrold, T., Trubowitz, S., Ritz, N.D., Conn, H.O., 1969. The syndrome of immunoglobulin deficiency and pernicious anaemia. Am. J. Med. 47, 340–350.

Uibo, R., Krohn, K., Villako, K., Tammur, R., Tamm, A., 1984. The relationship of parietal cell, gastrin cell, and thyroid autoantibodies to the state of the gastric mucosa in a population sample. Scand. J. Gastroenterol. 19, 1075–1080.

Ungar, B., Whittingham, S., Francis, C.M., 1967. Pernicious anaemia: incidence and significance of circulating antibodies to intrinsic factor and to parietal cells. Australas. Ann. Med. 16, 226–229.

Ungar, B., Stocks, A.E., Martin, F.I., Whittingham, S., Mackay, I.R., 1968. Intrinsic-factor antibody, parietal-cell antibody, and latent pernicious anaemia in diabetes mellitus. Lancet. 2, 415–417.

Ungar, B., Mathews, J.D., Tait, B.D., Cowling, D.C., 1977. HLA patterns in pernicious anaemia. Br. Med. J. 1, 798–800.

van Driel, I.R., Ang, D.K.Y., 2008. Role of regulatory T cells in gastrointestinal inflammatory disease. J. Gastroenterol. Hepatol. 23, 171–177.

Vargas, J.A., Alvarezmon, M., Manzano, L., Albillos, A., Fernandezcorugedo, A., Albarran, F., et al., 1995. Functional defect of T cells in autoimmune gastritis. Gut. 36, 171–175.

Varis, K., 1981. Family of behaviour of chronic gastritis. Ann. Clin. Res. 13, 123–129.

Varis, K., Samloff, I.M., Ihämaki, T., Siurala, M., 1979. An appraisal of tests for severe atrophic gastritis in relatives of patients with pernicious anemia. Dig. Dis. Sci. 24, 187–191.

Wall, A.J., Whittingham, S., Mackay, I.R., Ungar, B., 1968. Prednisolone and gastric atrophy. Clin. Exp. Immunol. 3, 359–366.

Wangel, A.G., Callender, S.T., Spray, G.H., Wright, R., 1968a. A family study of pernicious anaemia. II. Intrinsic factor secretion, vitamin B12 absorption and genetic aspects of gastric autoimmunity. Br. J. Haematol. 14, 183–204.

Wangel, A.G., Callender, S.T., Spray, G.H., Wright, R., 1968b. A family study of pernicious anaemia. I. Autoantibodies, achlorhydria, serum pepsinogen and vitamin B12. Br. J. Haematol. 14, 161–181.

Whittingham, S., Ungar, B., Mackay, I.R., Mathews, J.D., 1969. The genetic factor in pernicious anaemia. A family study in patients with gastritis. Lancet. 1, 951–954.

Whittingham, S., Youngchaiyud, U., Mackay, I.R., Buckley, J.D., Morris, P.J., 1975. Thyrogastric autoimmune disease. Studies on the cell-mediated immune system and histocompatibility antigens. Clin. Exp. Immunol. 19, 289–299.

Whittingham, S., Mackay, I.R., Tait, B.D., 1991. The immunogenetics of pernicious anaemia. In: Farid, N.R (Ed.), Immunogenetics of Autoimmune Disease. CRC Press, London, pp. 215–227.

Wilkinson, J.F., 1949. Megalocytic anaemias. Lancet. 1, 249–255.

Wood, I.J., Doig, R.K., Motterham, R., Hughes, A., 1949. Gastric biopsy; report on 55 biopsies using a new flexible gastric biopsy tube. Lancet. 1, 18–21.

Zwar, T.D., Read, S., van Driel, I.R., Gleeson, P.A., 2006. CD4 + CD25 + regulatory T cells inhibit the antigen-dependent expansion of self-reactive T cells in vivo. J. Immunol. 176, 1609–1617.

Chapter 45

Autoimmune Hypophysitis

Patrizio Caturegli[1], Isabella Lupi[2], and Angelika Gutenberg[3]

[1]Department of Pathology, The Johns Hopkins University, Baltimore, MD, USA, [2]Department of Endocrinology and Metabolism, University of Pisa, Pisa, Italy, [3]Department of Neurosurgery, Medical University of Mainz, Mainz, Germany

Chapter Outline

Definition and Classification of Autoimmune Hypophysitis	633	Animal Models	640
Historical Background	633	Diagnosis	641
Epidemiology and Body of Literature	634	Treatment	641
Clinical Features	635	Outcome	642
Pathological Features	637	Hypophysitis Secondary to CTLA-4 Blockade	642
Autoimmune Features	639	Concluding Remarks—Future Perspectives	644
Genetic and Environmental Influences	640	References	644

DEFINITION AND CLASSIFICATION OF AUTOIMMUNE HYPOPHYSITIS

Autoimmune hypophysitis is a chronic inflammation of the pituitary gland that can be classified according to anatomic location, histopathology, or cause (Leporati et al., 2011).

Location distinguishes hypophysitis into adenohypophysitis, infundibulo-neurohypophysitis, or panhypophysitis depending on whether the clinical and radiological signs (and pathological findings if available) involve the anterior lobe, the posterior lobe and the stalk, or both structures.

Histopathology identifies two main forms of hypophysitis, lymphocytic and granulomatous, as well as xanthomatous, IgG4 plasmacytic, and necrotizing variants.

Etiology distinguishes primary and secondary hypophysitis. Primary hypophysitis refers to the cases that do not currently have an identifiable cause. It is the most common form of hypophysitis, has an autoimmune pathogenesis, and occurs in isolation or with other well-characterized autoimmune diseases. Secondary hypophysitis includes the cases where a clear etiological agent can be identified (for example, the administration of immunomodulatory drugs like CTLA-4 blocking antibody), the cases where the inflammation of the pituitary is considered a reaction to sellar diseases (Rathke's cleft cyst, craniopharyngioma, germinoma, and pituitary adenomas), and the cases where hypophysitis is part of a multiorgan systemic involvement (such as Wegener's granulomatosis, tuberculosis, sarcoidosis, or syphilis).

In this chapter we will discuss predominantly primary hypophysitis and dedicate a section at the end for the hypophysitis secondary to CTLA-4 blockade.

HISTORICAL BACKGROUND

Autoimmune hypophysitis of the anterior lobe (lymphocytic adenohypophysitis, LAH) was first described in 1962 by Goudie and Pinkerton in Glasgow (Goudie and Pinkerton, 1962). The authors reported a 22-year-old woman who died 14 months after her second delivery, probably because of adrenal insufficiency. Two months before admission, the patient felt increasingly tired and noticed a neck enlargement; she then developed severe lower abdominal pain, radiating to the right iliac fossa, associated with vomiting and diarrhea. She was brought to the operating room for suspected appendicitis. Surgery revealed an acutely inflamed, gangrenous appendix that, however, had not ruptured. The appendix was removed but 8 hours later the patient went into peripheral circulatory shock and died. The autopsy revealed a firm, enlarged thyroid gland, infiltrated by lymphocytes, atrophic adrenal glands, and a small pituitary. Surprisingly for that time, the adenohypophysis was extensively infiltrated by lymphocytes and a few plasma cells, aggregating in some

N. Rose & I. Mackay (Eds): The Autoimmune Diseases, Fifth edition. DOI: http://dx.doi.org/10.1016/B978-0-12-384929-8.00045-9

areas into true lymphoid follicles. The neurohypophysis was normal. Noting the presence of Hashimoto's thyroiditis, a more extensively characterized autoimmune disease, the authors concluded their discussion by writing: "It seems reasonable to assume that the coexistence of Hashimoto's disease and the mononuclear cells infiltration of the anterior pituitary is not fortuitous. Both may be explained by the onset of autoimmune reaction to thyroid and pituitary antigens released during the puerperal involution of these glands." There is no doubt that Goudie and Pinkerton were the first to postulate the autoimmune nature of this condition, at a time when the field of autoimmunity had just begun. Earlier cases, however, are probably hidden in hospital archives or published without recognition of the disease (Duff and Bernstein, 1933; Rupp and Paschkis, 1953).

Autoimmune hypophysitis of the posterior lobe and infundibulum (lymphocytic infundibulo-neurohypophysitis, LINH) was first described in 1970 by Saito et al. in Tokyo (Saito et al., 1970). The authors reported on a 66-year-old asthmatic woman with 1-month history of severe dehydration who responded strikingly to the administration of pitressin. Two months after discharge, however, she developed a severe attack of bronchial asthma and died. Autopsy revealed a marked infiltration of the neurohypophysis and the infundibular stem with lymphocytes and plasma cells, aggregating in some areas in lymphoid follicles. The adenohypophysis was normal, except for vacuolar degeneration of the basophilic cells, likely due to the prolonged use of steroids for asthma.

Autoimmune hypophysitis involving both the anterior and posterior lobe (lymphocytic panhypophysitis, LPH) was first described histologically in 1991 by Nussbaum et al. in New York (Nussbaum et al., 1991). It was a 40-year-old male with a 3-month history of headache, impotence, polyuria and polydipsia, and a sellar mass abutting the optic chiasm. Transphenoidal surgery showed that the sella turcica was filled with whitish, fibrous tissue that was almost completely removed. Histology revealed extensive infiltration of the adenohypophysis and the neurohypophysis by lymphocytes, plasma cells, and histiocytes.

Hypophysitis secondary to blockade of CTLA-4 was first reported in 2003 by Phan et al. in Bethesda. The patient was a 54-year-old male with advanced melanoma metastatic to the lungs and brain who was treated with the CTLA-4 blocking antibody ipilimumab and vaccination with melanoma peptides (Phan et al., 2003).

EPIDEMIOLOGY AND BODY OF LITERATURE

Very limited data exist to estimate the incidence of autoimmune hypophysitis. Sautner and Fehn analyzed 2500 surgical pituitary specimens collected at Hamburg, Germany, from 1970 to 1996 and found six cases (0.24%) (Sautner et al., 1995; Fehn et al., 1998). Honegger et al. analyzed 2362 specimens collected from 1982 to 1995 in Erlagen, Germany, and found seven cases (0.3%) (Honegger et al., 1997). Leung et al. reported in Charlottesville, Virginia, 13 cases of autoimmune hypophysitis among 2000 patients who underwent transphenoidal surgery for pituitary mass lesions from 1992 to 2003 (0.65%) (Leung et al., 2004). Buxton and Robertson analyzed 619 consecutive pituitary surgeries performed over 15 years at Nottingham, UK, and found five cases (0.8%) (Buxton and Robertson, 2001). Considering that their hospital served a population of approximately 3 million and that all surgery for pituitary masses was dealt with there, the yearly incidence in Nottingham can be estimated to be one case in every 10 million people. This incidence is likely an underestimate of today's incidence, also considering that some cases of autoimmune hypophysitis go undiagnosed because of their indolent, subclinical course.

At the Department of Pathology of the Johns Hopkins Hospital we maintain a database of the papers published on hypophysitis, and pituitary autoimmunity in general, as well as of clinical characteristics of the featured patients (http://pathology2.jhu.edu/hypophysitis). A total of 837 papers have been published as of March 2013, featuring 3175 different authors and 12 languages. The top three publishing authors currently are Dr. P. Caturegli (25 articles, The Johns Hopkins University, Baltimore, MD), Dr. A. De Bellis (25 articles, Federico II University of Naples, Naples, Italy), and Dr. P. Crock (16 articles, The John Hunter's Children Hospital, New South Wales, Australia). Of the languages, 682 articles (82%) were in English, 61 (7%) were in Japanese, 26 (3%) in French, and the remaining 67 articles in nine other languages. The number of papers published per year on hypophysitis has increased significantly over time, reaching a peak of 60 in 2010 (Figure 45.1). The causes underlying this increase are multifactorial: in part they relate to the widespread introduction of non-invasive imaging techniques of the sella turcica (mainly MRI); in part to the expansion of the spectrum of pituitary autoimmunity, which now includes forms of hypophysitis that were not existing a few years ago: for example, the IgG4-related form of hypophysitis and the form secondary to blockade of CTLA-4; and in part to the increased awareness of hypophysitis in the medical community.

This body of literature described a total of 857 patients, 711 with primary hypophysitis, either biopsy proven (n = 493) or clinically suspected (n = 218), and 146 with secondary hypophysitis (Table 45.1). Patients have been reported in 42 of the 193 countries in the world, but most abundantly in Japan (27% of the patients) and the USA (19%) (Figure 45.2).

LAH is more common in women (F:M ratio of 4:1), who present at a younger age (35 ± 13) than men (49 ± 16). In approximately half of the women (49%),

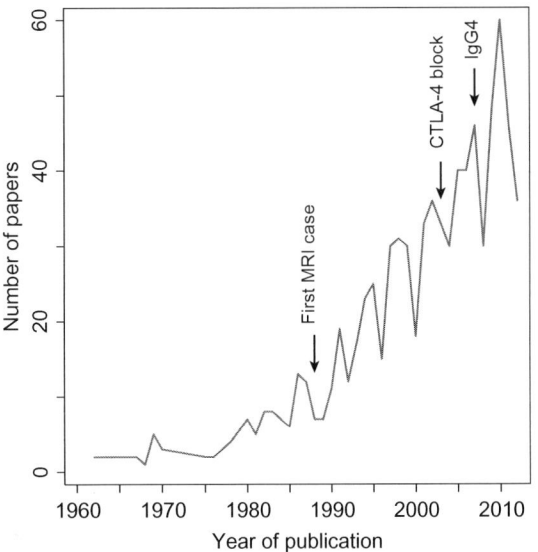

FIGURE 45.1 Yearly trend of papers published on hypophysitis and pituitary autoimmunity.

TABLE 45.1 Published Cases of Autoimmune Hypophysitis

Primary Hypophysitis (*n* = 711)	
Biopsy-proven:	
Lymphocytic	390
Granulomatous	59
Xanthomatous	17
IgG4 plasmacytic	6
Necrotizing	4
Mixed lymphocytic and granulomatous	15
Mixed xanthomatous and granulomatous	2
Clinically suspected:	218
Secondary hypophysitis (*n* = 146)	
to CTLA-4 blockade treatment:	
Individual case reports	18
In clinical trials	83
to sellar lesions:	
Rathke's cleft cyst	15
Germinoma	14
Pituitary adenoma	10
Craniopharyngioma	4
Pituitary lymphoma	2
TOTAL	857

LAH manifests during late pregnancy or early post-partum (Figure 45.3). A history of previous pregnancies does not increase the risk of developing LAH in subsequent pregnancies. This striking temporal association is one of the most interesting features of autoimmune hypophysitis, and, at the moment, remains unexplainable. LINH affects equally males and females (F:M ratio of 1:1), has a mean age at presentation of 39 ($\pm$20) years, and is not associated with pregnancy. LPH is slightly more common in women (F:M ratio of 1.9), has similar age at presentation in both sexes (43 $\pm$ 17 years), and does not show association with pregnancy. Hypophysitis secondary to CTLA-4 blockade reflects the epidemiology of the underlying oncologic populations where the treatment is used. Most commonly these are patients with metastatic melanoma, but also renal cell carcinoma, non-small-cell lung cancer, prostate cancer, and pancreatic cancer. These patients, therefore, are mainly men (90%) and of older age (55 $\pm$ 10 years) than the patients with primary hypophysitis.

CLINICAL FEATURES

The clinical presentation of autoimmune hypophysitis includes four categories of symptoms.

The most common symptoms are those originating from compression of the sellar structures and usually appear suddenly. In fact, a pituitary gland that is infiltrated by autoreactive lymphocytes initially enlarges, forming a sellar mass that expands usually upward, impinging upon the optic chiasm and the dura mater or laterally to invade the cavernous sinus. Headache is the most common presenting symptom of hypophysitis. It is severe and often generalized. Visual disturbances are the next most common symptoms. They originate from compression of the optic chiasm and typically include defects in the temporal quadrants of the visual fields and occasionally deterioration of visual acuity. Encroachment of the cavernous sinus can cause diplopia and pupillary abnormalities from compression of the third, fourth, and sixth cranial nerves. Involvement of the branches of the trigeminal nerve can result in orbital pain or facial paresthesias.

The second most common symptoms are those originating from defective production of the anterior pituitary hormones, and usually present more insidiously. These defects are considered the direct consequence of the attack of the patient's autoreactive lymphocytes onto the hormone-producing cells. The defects can be complete (panhypopituitarism) when all five adenohypophyseal axes (corticotroph, thyrotroph, gonadotroph growth hormone, and prolactin) are impaired, partial when more than one axis is involved, or isolated when only one axis is involved. The axis most commonly defective is the

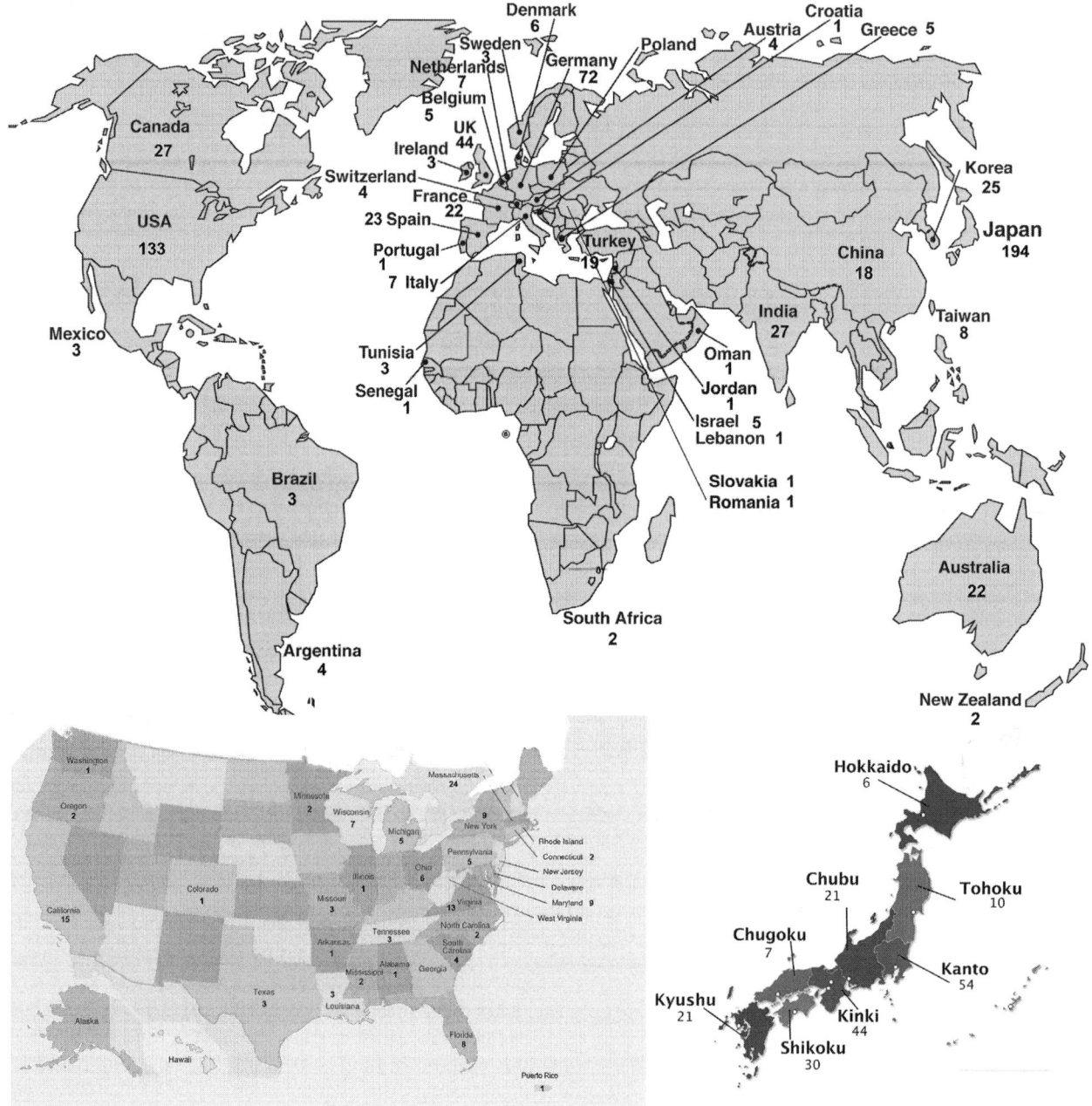

FIGURE 45.2 Geographical distribution of published patients with primary hypophysitis.

corticotroph (Table 45.2), causing symptoms like general malaise, hypotension, nausea, vomiting, dizziness, and loss of pubic and axillary hair. The resulting hypoadrenalism is often severe and can also result in acute adrenal crises that occasionally are irreversible and cause death of the patient. Next are the thyrotroph (fatigue, lethargy, cold intolerance, weight gain) and gonadotroph (decreased libido, impotence, amenorrhea) deficiencies. Prolactin deficiency, manifested in women as inability to lactate after delivery, is rare but when present should alert the astute clinician to a possible diagnosis of hypophysitis. Defects of growth hormone are considered clinically silent in adults, and consequently growth hormone is the least studied axis in this patient population. In 40% of the published patients there was no information about the growth hormone (Table 45.2), so it remains to be established whether somatotroph cells are not frequently targeted by the patient's immune system or rather their involvement has not been systematically investigated.

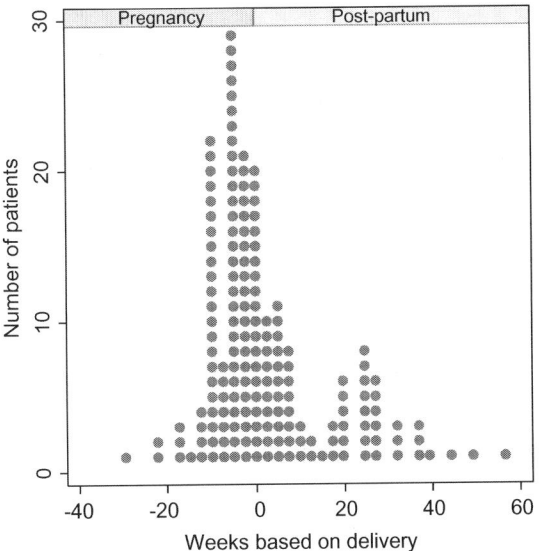

FIGURE 45.3 Distribution of symptom appearance in relation to delivery (indicated as week 0).

TABLE 45.2 Distribution of Pituitary Hormone Defects in Patients with Hypophysitis

	Secondary Decrease	Primary Decrease	Normal	Increase	Not Mentioned
Adrenal axis	53%	2%	27%	0%	18%
Thyroid axis	45%	6%	29%	2%	15%
Gonadal axis	43%	1%	30%	0%	26%
Prolactin	NA	16%	33%	27%	24%
Growth hormone	NA	23%	36%	1%	40%
Anti-diuretic hormone	NA	28%	20%	0%	25%

NA = not applicable.

The third group of symptoms are those due to deficit of the posterior pituitary (polyuria and polydipsia), which can be attributed to direct immune destruction of the neurohypophysis and infundibulum, but also compression of these structure. Diabetes insipidus is the defining symptom of LINH, but it can also be observed in about a third of the patients who have defects in the anterior pituitary axes.

Last are the signs due to hyperprolactinemia (mainly amenorrhea/oligomenorrhea and galactorrhea), which occur in about a quarter of the patients.

These clinical features of autoimmune hypophysitis are indistinguishable from those caused by other non-hormone secreting masses arising in the sella turcica (Table 45.3). Thus, although *per se* rare, hypophysitis enters in the differential diagnosis of about 30 conditions, all characterized by the presence of a sellar mass. Currently, hypophysitis can only be diagnosed with certainty by pituitary biopsy. However, a pathological specimen is not always necessary since a presumptive diagnosis of hypophysitis can often be made on the basis of a combination of clinical and radiological features. Clinical features include the association with pregnancy or post-partum, the presence of other autoimmune conditions in the same patient (co-morbidity) or family (familial aggregation), and a relatively rapid development of hypopituitarism, which is often disproportionate to the size of the pituitary mass. MRI remains the most powerful tool currently available to aid in the differential diagnosis, and will be described in detail below.

PATHOLOGICAL FEATURES

Primary hypophysitis now comprises five pathological variants: lymphocytic, granulomatous, xanthomatous, IgG4 plasmacytic, and necrotizing (Table 45.1).

Lymphocytic hypophysitis, first reported by Goudie and Pinkerton in 1962, is the most common form of hypophysitis. It is characterized by the infiltration of the pituitary gland with lymphocytes (Figure 45.4A), sometimes aggregating into lymphoid follicles with germinal centers. Immunohistochemistry reveals a mixture of T and B lymphocytes (Gutenberg et al., 2005), without a dominant subset, as is seen in other autoimmune diseases. Additional hematopoietic cell types that are found in the infiltrate include plasma cells, eosinophils, macrophages, histiocytes and neutrophils, and mast cells (Vidal et al., 2002). Fibrosis is common and often severe, explaining the toughness and adherence the surgeon finds upon entering the sella turcica. Necrosis is rare and usually of modest and focal nature. Little is known of the mechanisms by which the infiltrate causes loss of function/destruction of the endocrine cells. Staining with reticulin usually shows that the delicate connective tissue framework is conserved (Figure 45.4B), whereas in pituitary adenomas it is destroyed.

Granulomatous hypophysitis was first described in 1917 by Simmonds (Simmonds, 1917). He analyzed 2000 pituitary glands at autopsy and found four cases not related to tuberculosis or syphilis, characterized by numerous scattered collections of multinucleated giant cells, histiocytes, and occasional granulomas surrounded by lymphocytes and plasma cells. The first ante-mortem patient was reported in 1980 (Taylon and Duff, 1980). The disease is rare, affects equally males and females, and can occur together with lymphocytic hypophysitis

TABLE 45.3 Classification of Sellar Masses, with Approximate Frequency Distribution

Disease	% of all sellar masses
Hormone-secreting pituitary adenomas	**55%**
PRL-secreting adenoma	42%
ACTH-secreting adenoma	8%
GH-secreting adenoma	5%
TSH-secreting adenoma	0.25%
Non-hormone secreting sellar masses	**45%**
Developmental lesions:	
Rathke's cleft cyst	3.95%
Arachnoid cyst	0.50%
Dermoid and epidermoid cysts	0.40%
Vascular lesions:	
Pituitary apoplexy (caused by hemorrhagic necrosis)	0.08%
Intrasellar aneurysm	0.06%
Intrasellar angioma or hemangiopericytoma	0.02%
Infectious lesions:	
Tuberculosis	0.14%
Pituitary abscess	0.13%
Fungal infections	0.12%
Autoimmune and inflammatory lesions:	
Hypophysitis	0.85%
Sphenoidal sinus mucocele	0.13%
Sarcoidosis	0.12%
Wegener's granulomatosis	0.06%
Langerhans cell histiocytosis	0.06%
Benign tumors:	
Non-functioning (null cell) pituitary adenoma	32.0%
Craniopharyngioma	2.00%
Chordoma	1.30%
Meningioma	1.00%
Glioma	0.05%
Pituicytoma	0.02%
Spindle cell oncocytoma	0.02%
Malignant tumors:	
Metastasis (mainly from breast and lung cancer)	1.20%

(Continued)

TABLE 45.3 (Continued)

Disease	% of all sellar masses
Germinoma	0.24%
Lymphoma, plasmacytoma	0.12%
Astrocytoma	0.15%
Pituitary carcinoma	0.02%
Teratoma	0.02%

(McKeel, 1983; Miyamoto et al., 1988; Madsen and Karluk, 2000), and has been recently reviewed by Hunn and colleagues (Hunn et al., 2013). It is significantly more common in women (F:M ratio of 4:1) and has a mean ($\pm$ SD) age at presentation of 44 ($\pm$ 15) years.

Xanthomatous hypophysitis, originally described by Folkerth in 1998 (Folkerth et al., 1998), features an infiltration of the pituitary with foamy histiocytes and lymphocytes. The histiocytes, also called xanthoma cells, have a cytosol loaded with lipids, which confer the characteristic foamy appearance. Cystic areas can be observed in the pathological specimen and also on the MRI images. The pathogenesis of xanthomatous hypophysitis remains unknown, with autoimmune, infectious, and localized endothelial dysfunctions as postulated etiologies. Xanthomatous hypophysitis is more common in women (12 of the 17 cases reported thus far, 70%), and impairs more frequently the gonadal axis.

IgG4 plasmacytic hypophysitis is the form of most recent description. It was first reported on clinical grounds in 2004 in a 66-year-old woman with multiple pseudotumors of salivary glands, pancreas, and retroperitoneum (van der Vliet and Perenboom, 2004), and then pathologically proven in 2007 in a 77-year-old man with blurred vision, hypogonadism, and a history of autoimmune pancreatitis and sclerosing cholangitis (Wong et al., 2007). This form is more common in men (13 of the 16 reported cases are men, 81%) and in advanced ages (mean age at presentation is 69 $\pm$ 6 years). It is characterized pathologically by a mononuclear infiltrate of the pituitary gland that is rich in IgG4-producing plasma cells. We suggested a number of 10 or more IgG4 producing plasma cells in a high-power microscopic field for establishing this diagnosis (Leporati et al., 2011). Other diagnostic criteria are the increased levels of IgG4 in the serum (>140 mg/dl), and the association with IgG4-positive lesions in other organs. The disease responds extremely well to glucocorticoids and therefore a correct pre-operative diagnosis is crucial, since it can spare the patient an invasive pituitary surgery.

Necrotizing hypophysitis, first reported by Ahmed in 1993 (Ahmed et al., 1993), is the rarest form, with only five published cases, four biopsy proven (Ahmed et al., 1993; Gutenberg et al., 2012; Nater et al., 2012) and one clinically suspected (Ogawa, 1995). Patients present suddenly with severe headache and develop a long lasting hypopituitarism, features that, however, can also be seen with the other forms of hypophysitis, as well as with other non-hormone secreting sellar masses. Histologically, the pituitary appears destroyed by diffuse necrosis with surrounding lymphocytes, plasma cells, and a few eosinophils. MRI shows symmetric enlargement of the pituitary without signs of hemorrhage, and a thickened stalk, features that again are not specific enough to establish a diagnosis before surgery.

AUTOIMMUNE FEATURES

That autoimmune hypophysitis is indeed an autoimmune disease is indicated by the availability of animal models and by circumstantial evidence (Rose and Bona, 1993). The latter include the association with other diseases of known autoimmune nature, such as Hashimoto's thyroiditis (7% of the patients) and autoimmune polyglandular syndrome type 2 (2%), the improvement of symptoms upon usage of immunosuppressive drugs such as glucocorticoids, and the induction of the disease by drugs that promote immune activation like ipilimumab.

The autoantigen(s) recognized by the autoimmune attack await identification. Kobayashi's laboratory first described sera from patients with pituitary disorders that, when reacted with pituitary cytosolic extracts, recognized a 22 kDa protein (Yabe et al., 1995; Kikuchi et al., 2000), later identified by Takao et al. as growth hormone (Takao et al., 2001). Crock's laboratory subsequently reported that seven of 10 patients with biopsy-proven lymphocytic hypophysitis, and 12 of 22 patients with suspected hypophysitis, had a low titer antibody that recognized a 49 kDa cytosolic pituitary protein (Crock, 1998), later identified as alpha-enolase (O'Dwyer et al., 2002b). The authors concluded that alpha-enolase is the autoantigen targeted by the immune system in autoimmune hypophysitis and, considering its co-expression in the placenta, the basis to explain the strong association between autoimmune hypophysitis and pregnancy (O'Dwyer et al., 2002a). Antibodies recognizing alpha-enolase, however, have been reported in many other diseases, ranging from endometriosis to discoid lupus and Wegener's granulomatosis (Crock, 1998). In addition, Tanaka et al. have shown that the antibody is present in seven of 17 patients (41%) with autoimmune hypophysitis, but similarly in six of 13 (46%) patients with nonfunctioning pituitary adenoma, and in four of 17 (24%) patients with other pituitary diseases, making use of the alpha-enolase antibody inadequate as a diagnostic marker

of autoimmune hypophysitis (Tanaka et al., 2003). Finally, Nishiki et al. reported that five of 13 patients with LAH, and one of 12 patients with LINH, had antibodies that recognized 68, 49, and 43 kDa proteins in pituitary membrane extracts (Nishiki et al., 2001).

In addition to growth hormone and alpha-enolase, five candidate autoantigens have been reported in recent years: pituitary gland-specific factors 1a and 2 (Tanaka et al., 2002), secretogranin 2 (Bensing et al., 2007), chorionic somatomammotropin hormone (Lupi et al., 2008), TPIT (Smith et al., 2012), and PIT-1 (Yamamoto et al., 2011). None of them, however, has yet proven to be pathogenic in animal models, useful in clinical practice, or confirmed by independent investigators.

Antibodies to pituitary antigens have been measured occasionally in the published patients (98 of 857, 11%), mainly by indirect immunofluorescence (Bottazzo et al., 1975) or Western blotting (Crock et al., 1993). They were found positive in a minority of patients, yielding an extremely poor sensitivity (37%) (Caturegli et al., 2005). They also seem to be not specific for autoimmune hypophysitis, since they have been described in type 1 diabetes (Mirakian et al., 1982), Hashimoto's thyroiditis (Kobayashi et al., 1988), Graves' disease (Hansen et al., 1989), and normal women during postpartum (Engelberth and Jezkova, 1965). This lack of sensitivity and specificity may have several explanations. For example, patients with autoimmune hypophysitis may come to medical attention long after the onset of disease and it is known that antibodies against endocrine glands disappear over the years (Figure 45.4).

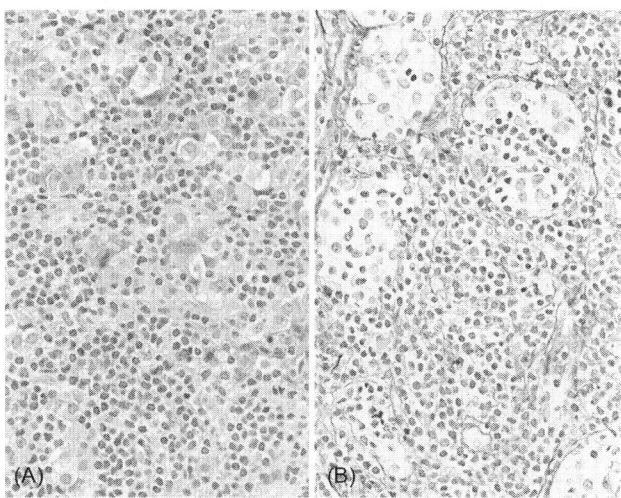

FIGURE 45.4 Histopathology of primary lymphocytic hypophysitis. (A) Hematoxylin and eosin stain showing the infiltration of lymphocytes among the endocrine cells. (B) Reticulin stain showing the conservation of the connective tissue framework.

GENETIC AND ENVIRONMENTAL INFLUENCES

Insufficient data are available to establish associations between the genes that are classically thought to influence autoimmunity, such as the MHC locus and CTLA-4, and autoimmune hypophysitis. Also no environmental agent has been involved with primary hypophysitis, with the exception of four cases presenting after a viral infection of the meningi (Vanneste and Kamphorst, 1987; Honegger et al., 1997; Sandler et al., 1998; Matta et al., 2002).

ANIMAL MODELS

The first animal model for autoimmune hypophysitis was published in 1964 by Beutner and Witesbky. The authors immunized 16 rabbits with rabbit anterior pituitary extracts, emulsified in complete Freund's adjuvant, and were able to induce specific antibody responses but no pituitary pathology (Beutner et al., 1964). In 1967 Levine immunized rats with a single intra-cutaneous injection of rat pituitary tissue, emulsified in complete Freund's adjuvant (Levine, 1967), showing that 2−3 weeks after the injection, six of the 14 rats (43%) developed infiltration of the adenohypophysis with mononuclear cells, mainly lymphocytes, monocytes, and occasional epithelioid cells. A few posterior and intermediate lobes had minimal inflammation. Disease incidence could be increased to 75% (15 out of 20 rats) by addition of a second immunologic adjuvant, pertussis toxin. He subsequently showed that pituitary extracts from guinea pig were the most potent inducer of experimental autoimmune hypophysitis (six of six rat recipients), whereas human and cow extracts were poorly effective, and dog and rabbit extracts not effective at all (Levine, 1969). In 1970 Beck and Melvin (Beck and Melvin, 1970) induced experimental autoimmune hypophysitis in one rhesus monkey by injecting her multiple times, over the course of 3 years, with human placental extracts and human chorionic gonadotropin, both emulsified with Freund's adjuvant. Histology showed infiltration of the adenohypophysis with lymphocytes and scattered plasma cells; the neurohypophysis was normal.

In 1982 Klein induced lympho-plasmacytic infiltration of the anterior pituitary by injecting 12 rabbits (seven cases and five controls) three times, at 2-week intervals, with rabbit pituitary tissue, emulsified in complete Freund's adjuvant. Eight weeks (10 rabbits) or 16 weeks (two rabbits) after the first injection, five of the seven experimental rabbits showed focal infiltration of the adenohypophysis with lymphocytes, some plasma cells, and a few eosinophils and fibrosis. None of the five controls showed histological abnormalities. In 1992, Yoon et al. immunized over 100 hamsters by injecting intra-dermally three times, at 1-week intervals, recombinant rubella virus E1 and E2 glycoproteins. Three weeks after the first injection, specific antibodies against the adenohypophysis were found in 95% of the hamsters. Eleven weeks after the first injection, a diffuse lymphocytic infiltration was found throughout the adenohypophysis. None of the hamsters that had received the control protein (nonglycosylated rubella nucleoprotein C) developed such lesions. The disease could be prevented by neonatal thymectomy, and could not be produced by passive transfer of the autoantibodies, thus indicating that T cells are critical for disease induction and that antibodies are more important as markers of disease, rather than as a pathogenic player (Yoon et al., 1992). Finally, Watanabe et al. in 2001 immunized 12 Lewis rats twice, at 1-week intervals, with rat pituitary extract emulsified in complete Freund's adjuvant. Three ($N = 6$) or 6 weeks ($N = 6$) after the first immunization, rats showed minimal lymphocytic infiltration in the adenohypophysis and developed antibodies directed against growth hormone, thyroid stimulating hormone, and luteinizing hormone (Watanabe et al., 2001). It is unclear, however, whether these hormones show that the initiating autoantigens are, rather, the natural response of the immune system to the injection of hormone-rich pituitary extracts.

A somewhat different experimental approach was taken by Stockinger's laboratory (De Jersey et al., 2002, 2004). The authors have made a transgenic mouse that expresses specifically in the anterior pituitary (as under transcriptional control of the growth hormone promoter) a nucleoprotein from the influenza virus, thus a foreign antigen. This influenza nucleoprotein contains a peptide that binds to the D^b allele of the mouse MHC locus, and is recognized by specific CD8 T cells. When the authors crossed the nucleoprotein transgenic mice to TCR transgenic mice that have CD8 T cells specific for that nucleoprotein, they observe growth hormone defect due to destruction of the growth hormone cells expressing the viral antigen. Although informative about accessibility and homing of CD8 T lymphocytes to the pituitary, this transgenic model is likely remote from the human disease where CD8 T lymphocytes are rarely seen in the infiltrate and somatotrophs are usually spared by the autoimmune attack.

In 2008 we published a comprehensive model of autoimmune hypophysitis. It is induced in SJL female mice by immunization with pituitary proteins emulsified in complete Freund's adjuvant (Tzou et al., 2008). The model mimics closely the human counterpart, featuring a female bias, a diffuse infiltration of the anterior lobe with a mixture of T and B lymphocytes, and panhypopituitarism. The model has provided useful insights into the human disease. It has shown that hypophysitis is characterized initially by an expansion of the pituitary gland but that later evolves into an atrophic structure that reflects the human empty sella condition (Lupi et al., 2011b). The model is being used to identify novel pituitary autoantigens with the intent of translating the findings to the human disease.

DIAGNOSIS

As indicated above, hypophysitis is a relatively rare condition but it enters in the differential diagnosis of other more common lesions, like the pituitary adenomas, and other masses arising in the sella turcica (classified in Table 45.3). All sellar masses share similar clinical and radiological findings, so that a diagnosis of certainty can only be achieved by examining under the microscope the pituitary tissue obtained from pituitary surgery. Clinical and immunological markers have, at the moment, low predictive values in establishing a differential diagnosis without pathology. Currently, the most powerful tool to differentiate autoimmune hypophysitis from other sellar mass is MRI. We have reviewed systematically the MRI features of the published patients with primary hypophysitis and identified a set of seven features that can orient the clinician toward a diagnosis of hypophysitis: pituitary volume, symmetry of the sellar mass, stalk diameter, status of the normal posterior pituitary bright spot, status of the mucosa lining the sphenoidal sinus, intensity of the signal after contrast, and heterogeneity of the signal after contrast (Gutenberg et al., 2009). Hypophysitis induces initially an enlargement of the pituitary gland, thus a measurable increased volume by MRI. This volume increase, however, rarely surpasses 6 mm^3, as is instead more commonly seen in non-secreting pituitary adenomas. The increase in volume is also typically symmetric in hypophysitis, with the gland assuming a sort of pear-shaped appearance, whereas in adenomas the mass typically displaces the normal (non-tumorous) pituitary tissue. The stalk (or infundibulum) is composed of the median eminence of the hypothalamus, the infundibular stem that arises from it, and the pars tuberalis of the anterior hypophysis that surrounds the stem. The normal stalk has an average antero-posterior diameter (sagittal sections) of 3.25 mm at the level of the optic chiasm and 2.32 mm at the pituitary insertion (Satogami et al., 2009). In hypophysitis the stalk thickens above 4 mm, because the inflammation either involves directly the posterior pituitary or extends to it from the involved anterior pituitary. In coronal sections the normal stalk has a transverse diameter of 3.35 mm at the optic chiasm level and 2.16 mm at the pituitary insertion, and a uniform cylindrical appearance. In hypophysitis instead the thickened stalk assumes a V shape or round appearance (Turcu et al., 2013). The stalk is of normal size and shape in pituitary adenoma. On pre-contrast images, the anterior pituitary has a signal intensity that is approximately identical to that of the gray matter whereas the stalk is hyperintense. This hyperintensity, commonly known as posterior pituitary bright spot, is believed to reflect the high phospholipid content of the ADH and oxytocin neurosecretory granules. In hypophysitis the normal posterior pituitary bright spot is lost, whereas in adenomas it is conserved. After injection of the contrast, a pituitary gland affected by hypophysitis enhances the signal strongly (similarly to the

intensity of the cavernous sinus) and homogeneously, whereas in adenomas the enhancement is less intense and more heterogeneous. Finally, the mucosa lining the sphenoidal sinus is typically normal in hypophysitis whereas it is swollen in pituitary adenomas. None of these signs is individually specific enough to diagnose with certainty hypophysitis, but in aggregate the signs classified correctly 97% of the patients, with a sensitivity of 92% and a specificity of 99% (Gutenberg et al., 2009).

More recently, Nakata and colleagues described an additional MRI feature that was considered characteristic of hypophysitis and capable of distinguishing hypophysitis from adenoma with certainty: the presence in hypophysitis of a dark signal intensity area around the pituitary and in the cavernous sinus on T2-weighted images (Nakata et al., 2010).

TREATMENT

The treatment of autoimmune hypophysitis is, at the moment, only symptomatic and aimed at reducing the size of the pituitary mass and replacing the defective hormones.

Mass reduction treatment comprises lympholytic drugs (mainly glucocorticoids), surgery, and radiotherapy. The first line of treatment is typically the use of glucocorticoids to reduce the pituitary inflammation (reviewed in Lupi et al., 2011a). They are typically given in the form of high-dose prednisone or prednisolone that are then tapered over a period of weeks to months, depending on the clinical response. Some patients, however, do not respond to glucocorticoids or experience relapses after an initial improvement. In these instances, other immunosuppressive medications such as cyclosporine (Ward et al., 1999), methotrexate (Tubridy et al., 2001), azathioprine (Lecube et al., 2003), and rituximab (Schreckinger et al., 2012) have been reported with success.

Surgery has historically been the most used way to reduce the pituitary mass in patients with primary hypophysitis. It also has the advantage of providing a tissue sample for pathological examination, which establishes a diagnosis of certainty and also expands our understanding of the disease. Nowadays surgery is recommended for patients who have significant and progressive visual loss, for those who do not respond to the various options of medical treatment outlined above, and for those with intractable symptoms. Modern pituitary surgery is typically done through the endoscopic trans-sphenoidal approach, an approach that is relatively safe and effective. The goal of the surgery is to debulk the pituitary mass to relieve the compression of the cranial nerves or relieve the pressure responsible for headache. Excision of one-third to one-half of the pituitary mass is typically sufficient, and there is no need to perform a total excision (Iuliano and Laws, 2011).

Stereotactic radiotherapy (Selch et al., 2003) and gamma knife radiosurgery (Ray et al., 2009) have been employed effectively in a few patients who failed medical and surgical treatments and experienced a disease recurrence.

Replacement of the defective pituitary hormones is the main form of long-term therapy in patients with hypophysitis. It is carried out similarly to the replacement performed for other causes of hypopituitarism. The hormones most commonly replaced are hydrocortisone for a defective corticotroph axis, thyroxine for the thyrotroph axis, desmopressin for the defective ACTH secretion, and testosterone or estradiol for a defective gonadotroph axis. The growth hormone axis, as indicated above, is not assessed systematically in patients with hypophysitis. However, a few adult patients have also had replacement recombinant growth hormone (Gachoud et al., 2002; Leung et al., 2004; Hindocha et al., 2013). Prolactin deficiency, if diagnosed and clinically significant, can be corrected with administration of recombinant prolactin (Powe et al., 2010).

OUTCOME

After a diagnosis of hypophysitis is made, either by pathology or on clinical grounds, there are five main outcomes. The majority of patients (68%) improve after the initial mass reductive treatment but the pituitary hormone deficiencies remain and require prolonged replacement. In some of these patients, a detailed imaging follow-up has shown that the pituitary gland becomes atrophic with time, yielding on the MRI the appearance of an empty sella (Karaca et al., 2009). In about a fifth of the patients (18%) the disease improves markedly after the initial mass reductive treatment and no further therapy is necessary. In a few patients (2%) the disease regresses spontaneously without any treatment. In a significant minority of patients (6%) the disease progresses and recurs despite medical and surgical attempts to contain it. In the remaining 6%, hypophysitis kills the patient, likely through the development of an irreversible adrenal insufficiency. These autopsy cases have been published sporadically but consistently throughout the years, the most recent one in 2009 (Gonzalez-Cuyar et al., 2009), reminding us that autoimmune hypophysitis can be fatal if unrecognized.

HYPOPHYSITIS SECONDARY TO CTLA-4 BLOCKADE

The introduction in the early 2000s of cancer drugs that act by blocking proteins expressed on immune cells has changed dramatically the significance of hypophysitis:

from being a rarity, it has now become a disease that most clinicians and practitioners involved in immunotherapy are familiar with. Ipilimumab (Yervory™, Medarex, and Bristol-Meyers Squibb) is one of the most used immunoregulatory drugs.

Ipilimumab is a fully human IgG1 monoclonal antibody that binds to cytotoxic T lymphocyte antigen 4 (CTLA-4). CTLA-4 is expressed on the surface of effector T cells a few hours after they become activated. It normally binds to B7 on antigen-presenting cells, initiating a negative cascade that ultimately results in T cell inhibition. Ipilimumab blocks the physiological binding of CTLA-4 to B7 and therefore prolongs T cell activation, inducing unrestrained immune responses against tumor cells but also against a variety of normal self-antigens. Ipilimumab was approved in 2011 by the FDA and the European Medicines Agency for the treatment of metastatic or unresectable melanoma, and is currently tested in several other types of cancer, including renal cell carcinoma, pancreatic cancer, prostate cancer, non-small cell lung cancer, and liver cancer. Patients undergo an induction course of ipilimumab consisting of one intravenous infusion every 3 weeks for a total of four infusions (Culver et al., 2011). The dose is usually 3 mg/kg and the price set by Bristol-Myers Squibb is $30,000 per injection, which translates to a cost of $120,000 for a course of therapy.

Patients treated with ipilimumab experience an array of autoimmune reactions collectively referred to as immune-related adverse events. As properly stated by Voskens et al., these adverse events represent "the price of tumor control" (Voskens et al., 2013). They occur in about 75% of the patients and are clinically significant (grade III or IV) in about 15% (Culver, 2011). The most common adverse events are dermatitis, enterocolitis, hepatitis, and hypophysitis, thus differing from adverse events typically reported with chemotherapy. It is unclear why hypophysitis, traditionally considered a rare autoimmune disease, is seen at increased frequency in cancer patients treated with ipilimumab. Approximately 50 clinical trials using CTLA-4 blocking antibodies have been published since 2003 (Culver, 2011). Of them, 20 reported hypophysitis as an adverse event (Table 45.4). These 20 trials included 2366 patients with advanced cancer, 83 of whom developed hypophysitis, for an average incidence of about 4%. Additional patients have been published as individual case studies.

Most patients with hypophysitis secondary to CTLA-4 blockade present with headache and symptoms from adenohypophyseal hormone deficiencies. As in primary hypophysitis, the most commonly involved axis is the corticotroph, but here the thyrotroph axis is as frequently involved as the corticotroph (almost 100% of the patients), and the gonadotroph is affected in about 85% of

TABLE 45.4 Clinical Trials using CTLA-4 Blocking Antibodies and Reporting Hypophysitis as a Side Effect

Year	First Author	Institution	CTLA-4 Blocking mAb	Cancer Type	No. of Patients	No. of AH Patients	% of AH Patients
2003	Phan	NCI	Ipilimumab	Metastatic melanoma	14	1	7.1
2005	Attia	NCI	Ipilimumab	Metastatic melanoma	56	1	1.8
2005	Blansfield	NCI	Ipilimumab	Advanced melanoma (113) and renal cell carcinoma (50)	163	8	4.9
2006	Beck	NCI	Ipilimumab	Advanced melanoma (137) and renal cell carcinoma (61)	198	13	6.6
2006	Maker	NCI	Ipilimumab	Metastatic melanoma	46	8	17.4
2007	Yang	NCI	Ipilimumab	Metastatic renal cell carcinoma	61	2	3.3
2007	Downey	NCI	Ipilimumab	Stage IV melanoma	139	13	9.4
2009	Ansell	Mayo Clinic	Ipilimumab	B cell non-Hodgkin's lymphoma	18	1	5.6
2009	Ribas	UCLA	Ipilimumab	Metastatic melanoma	16	1	6.3
2009	Fong	UCSF	Ipilimumab	Prostate cancer	24	1	4.2
2010	O'Day	MSKCC	Ipilimumab	Metastatic melanoma	155	2	1.3
2010	Wolchok	MSKCC	Ipilimumab	Metastatic melanoma	214	3	1.4
2010	Hodi	Boston	Ipilimumab	Metastatic melanoma	511	10	2.0
2010	Royal	NCI	Ipilimumab	Pancreatic cancer	27	1	3.7
2010	Ku	MSKCC	Ipilimumab	Metastatic melanoma	53	2	3.8
2011	Bronstein	Houston	Ipilimumab	Metastatic melanoma	119	2	1.7
2012	van den Eertwegh	Rotterdam	Ipilimumab	Prostate cancer	28	7	25.0
2012	Madan	NCI	Ipilimumab	Prostate cancer	30	4	13.3
2012	Lynch	Yale	Ipilimumab	Non-small-cell lung cancer	204	1	0.5
2005	Ribas	UCLA	Tremilimumab	Metastatic melanoma (34), renal cell carcinoma (4), colo-rectal cancer (1)	39	1	2.6
2010	Kirkwood	Pittsburgh	Tremilimumab	Metastatic melanoma	251	1	0.4
				TOTALS	2366	83	3.51

the male patients. As for primary hypophysitis, the growth hormone axis has not been assessed systematically. A recent case series of seven patients with metastatic melanoma treated with ipilimumab and developing secondary adrenal insufficiency, however, showed that three of five patients where the growth hormone axis was measured had low serum IGF-1. Prolactin and ADH are reported to be deficient only sporadically. In contrast to primary hypophysitis, visual disturbances are rare, likely related to the fact that the pituitary enlargement in ipilimumab patients is usually modest (Blansfield, 2005). MRI studies typically show a diffuse enlargement of the anterior pituitary, with conservation of the posterior

pituitary bright spot. All the cases reported thus far have been diagnosed on clinical and imaging grounds, therefore there is no information about the pathological lesions of hypophysitis secondary to CTLA-4 blockade.

The recommended treatment for grade 3 or 4 secondary hypophysitis is a course of high-dose glucocorticoids (like prednisone 50–60 mg/day), gradually tapered over a month to a physiological replacement dose (hydrocortisone 15–20 mg/day). It is unclear whether initial high doses are truly needed or if instead the patients could be started on physiological doses from the time of diagnosis. Thyroid hormone and sex steroids are then added as needed. No information about growth hormone replacement is available. It is now considered not necessary to discontinue ipilimumab for the treatment of CTLA4-induced hypophysitis, although initial cases did. Pituitary deficits seem to persist after treatment and long-term hormonal replacement has to be anticipated for most patients.

CONCLUDING REMARKS—FUTURE PERSPECTIVES

Autoimmune hypophysitis is a rare but increasingly recognized disease that has exploded on the medical arena due to its association with cancer immunotherapies. Its spectrum continues to expand and increase in complexity. The field will advance when a reliable serological test that identifies the autoimmune nature of hypophysitis becomes available.

ACKNOWLEDGMENTS

We dedicate this chapter to the memory of Breanna, a patient with primary autoimmune hypophysitis who, after delivery of her daughter, developed inability to lactate and adrenal insufficiency that went unrecognized. Several months later she developed an acute adrenal crisis, and died on June 18, 2010.

REFERENCES

Ahmed, S.R., Aiello, D.P., Page, R., Hopper, K., Towfighi, J., Santen, R.J., et al., 1993. Necrotizing infundibulo-hypophysitis: a unique syndrome of diabetes insipidus and hypopituitarism. J. Clin. Endocrinol. Metab. 76, 1499–1504.

Beck, J.S., Melvin, J.M., 1970. Chronic adenohypophysitis in a rhesus monkey immunised with extracts of human placenta. J. Pathol. 102, 125–129.

Bensing, S., Hulting, A.L., Hoog, A., Ericson, K., Kampe, O., 2007. Lymphocytic hypophysitis: report of two biopsy-proven cases and one suspected case with pituitary autoantibodies. J. Endocrinol. Invest. 30, 153–162.

Beutner, E.H., Djanian, A., Witebsky, E., 1964. Serological studies on rabbit antibodies to the rabbit anterior pituitary. Immunology. 7, 172–181.

Blansfield, J.A., Beck, K.E., Tran, K., Yang, J.C., Hughes, M.S., Kammula, U.S., et al., 2005. Cytotoxic T-lymphocyte-associated antigen-4 blockage can induce autoimmune hypophysitis in patients with metastatic melanoma and renal cancer. J. Immunother. 28, 593–598.

Bottazzo, G.F., Pouplard, A., Florin-Christensen, A., Doniach, D., 1975. Autoantibodies to prolactin-secreting cells of human pituitary. Lancet. 2, 97–101.

Buxton, N., Robertson, I., 2001. Lymphocytic and granulocytic hypophysitis: a single centre experience. Br. J. Neurosurg. 15, 242–245.

Caturegli, P., Newschaffer, C., Olivi, A., Pomper, M.G., Burger, P.C., Rose, N.R., et al., 2005. Autoimmune hypophysitis. Endocr. Rev. 26, 599–614.

Crock, P.A., 1998. Cytosolic autoantigens in lymphocytic hypophysitis. J. Clin. Endocrinol. Metab. 83, 609–618.

Crock, P.A., Salvi, M., Miller, A., Wall, J., Guyda, H., 1993. Detection of anti-pituitary antibodies by immunoblotting. J. Immunol. Methods. 162, 31–40.

Culver, M.E., Gatesman, M.L., Mancl, E.E., Lowe, D.K., 2011. Ipilimumab: a novel treatment for metastatic melanoma. Ann. Pharmacother. 45, 510–519.

De Jersey, J., Carmignac, D., Barthlott, T., Robinson, I., Stockinger, B., 2002. Activation of CD8 T cells by antigen expressed in the pituitary gland. J. Immunol. 169, 6753–6759.

De Jersey, J., Carmignac, D., Le Tissier, P., Barthlott, T., Robinson, I., Stockinger, B., et al., 2004. Factors affecting the susceptibility of the mouse pituitary gland to CD8 T-cell-mediated autoimmunity. Immunology. 111, 254–261.

Duff, G.L., Bernstein, C., 1933. Five cases of Addison's disease with so-called atrophy of the adrenal gland. Bull. Johns Hopkins Hosp. 52, 67–83.

Engelberth, O., Jezkova, Z., 1965. Autoantibodies in Sheehan's syndrome. Lancet. 1, 1075.

Fehn, M., Sommer, C., Ludecke, D.K., Plöckinger, U., Saeger, W., 1998. Lymphocytic Hypophysitis: light and electron microscopic findings and correlation to clinical appearance. Endocr. Pathol. 9, 71–78.

Folkerth, R.D., Price Jr., D.L., Schwartz, M., Black, P.M., De Girolami, U., 1998. Xanthomatous hypophysitis. Am. J. Surg. Pathol. 22, 736–741.

Gachoud, D., Blanc, M.H., Monnat, A., 2002. Infundibulitis, an unusual case of central diabetes insipidus. Rev. Med. Suisse. Romande. 122, 549–551.

Gonzalez-Cuyar, L.F., Tavora, F., Shaw, K., Castellani, R.J., Dejong, J. L., 2009. Sudden unexpected death in lymphocytic hypophysitis. Am. J. Forensic. Med. Pathol. 30, 61–63.

Goudie, R.B., Pinkerton, P.H., 1962. Anterior hypophysitis and Hashimoto's disease in a woman. J. Pathol. Bacteriol. 83, 584–585.

Gutenberg, A., Buslei, R., Fahlbusch, R., Buchfelder, M., Bruck, W., 2005. Immunopathology of primary hypophysitis: implications for pathogenesis. Am. J. Surg. Pathol. 29, 329–338.

Gutenberg, A., Larsen, J., Lupi, I., Rohde, V., Caturegli, P., 2009. A radiologic score to distinguish autoimmune hypophysitis from non-secreting pituitary adenoma preoperatively. AJNR Am. J. Neuroradiol. 30, 1–8.

Gutenberg, A., Caturegli, P., Metz, I., Martinez, R., Mohr, A., Bruck, W., et al., 2012. Necrotizing infundibulo-hypophysitis: an entity too rare to be true? Pituitary. 15, 202–208.

Hansen, B.L., Hegedus, L., Hansen, G.N., Hagen, C., Hansen, J.M., Hoier-Madsen, M., et al., 1989. Pituitary-cell autoantibody diversity in sera from patients with untreated Graves' disease. Autoimmunity. 5, 49–57.

Hindocha, A., Chaudhary, B.R., Kearney, T., Pal, P., Gnanalingham, K., 2013. Lymphocytic hypophysitis in males. J. Clin. Neurosci. 20, 743–745.

Honegger, J., Fahlbusch, R., Bornemann, A., Hensen, J., Buchfelder, M., Muller, M., et al., 1997. Lymphocytic and granulomatous hypophysitis: experience with nine cases. Neurosurgery. 40, 713–722.

Iuliano, S.L., Laws, E.R., 2011. The diagnosis and management of lymphocytic hypophysitis. Expert. Rev. Endocrinol. Metab. 6, 777–783.

Karaca, Z., Tanriverdi, F., Unluhizarci, K., Kelestimur, F., Donmez, H., 2009. Empty sella may be the final outcome in lymphocytic hypophysitis. Endocr. Res. 34, 10–17.

Kikuchi, T., Yabe, S., Kanda, T., Kobayashi, I., 2000. Antipituitary anti-bodies as pathogenetic factors in patients with pituitary disorders. Endocr. J. 47, 407–416.

Kobayashi, I., Inukai, T., Takahashi, M., Ishii, A., Ohshima, K., Mori, M., et al., 1988. Anterior pituitary cell antibodies detected in Hashimoto's thyroiditis and Graves' disease. Endocrinol. Jpn 35, 705–708.

Lecube, A., Francisco, G., Rodriguez, D., Ortega, A., Codina, A., Hernandez, C., et al., 2003. Lymphocytic hypophysitis successfully treated with azathioprine: first case report. J. Neurol. Neurosurg. Psychiatry. 74, 1581–1583.

Leporati, P., Landek-Salgado, M.A., Lupi, I., Chiovato, L., Caturegli, P., 2011. IgG4-related hypophysitis: a new addition to the hypo-physitis spectrum. J. Clin. Endocrinol. Metab. 96, 1971–1980.

Leung, G.K., Lopes, M.B., Thorner, M.O., Vance, M.L., Laws Jr., E.R., 2004. Primary hypophysitis: a single-center experience in 16 cases. J. Neurosurg. 101, 262–271.

Levine, S., 1967. Allergic adenophypophysitis: new experimental disease of the pituitary gland. Science. 158, 1190–1191.

Levine, S., 1969. Allergic adrenalitis and adenohypophysitis: further observations on production and passive transfer. Endocrinology. 84, 469–475.

Lupi, I., Broman, K.W., Tzou, S.C., Gutenberg, A., Martino, E., Caturegli, P., et al., 2008. Novel autoantigens in autoimmunehypo-physitis. Clin. Endocrinol. (Oxf.). 69, 269–278.

Lupi, I., Manetti, L., Raffaelli, V., Lombardi, M., Cosottini, M., Iannelli, A., et al., 2011a. Diagnosis and treatment of autoimmune hypophysitis: a short review. J. Endocrinol. Invest. 34, e245–e252.

Lupi, I., Zhang, J., Gutenberg, A., Landek-Salgado, M., Tzou, S.C., Mori, S., et al., 2011b. From pituitary expansion to empty sella: dis-ease progression in a mouse model of autoimmune hypophysitis. Endocrinology. 152, 4190–4198.

Madsen, J.R., Karluk, D., 2000. Case records of the Massachusetts General Hospital, case 34-2000: a 71-year-old woman with an enlarging pituitary mass. N. Engl. J. Med. 343, 1399–1406.

Matta, M.P., Kany, M., Delisle, M.B., Lagarrigue, J., Caron, P.H., 2002. A relapsing remitting lymphocytic hypophysitis. Pituitary. 5, 37–44.

McKeel, D.W., 1983. Common histopathologica and ultrastructural fea-tures in granulomatous and lymphoid adenohypophysitis. Endocrinology. 112 (Suppl.), 190.

Mirakian, R., Cudworth, A.G., Bottazzo, G.F., Richardson, C.A., Doniach, D., 1982. Autoimmunity to anterior pituitary cells and the pathogenesis of insulin-dependent diabetes mellitus. Lancet. 1, 755–759.

Miyamoto, M., Sugawa, H., Mori, T., Hashimoto, N., Imura, H., 1988. A case of hypopituitarism due to granulomatous and lymphocytic ade-nohypophysitis with minimal pituitary enlargement: a possible variant of lymphocytic adenohypophysitis. Endocrinol. Jpn 35, 607–616.

Nakata, Y., Sato, N., Masumoto, T., Mori, H., Akai, H., Nobusawa, H., et al., 2010. Parasellar T2 dark sign on MR imaging in patients with lymphocytic hypophysitis. AJNR Am. J. Neuroradiol. 31, 1944–1950.

Nater, A., Syro, L.V., Rotondo, F., Scheithauer, B.W., Abad, V., Jaramillo, C., et al., 2012. Necrotizing infundibuloneurohypophysi-tis: case report and literature review. Endocr. Pathol. 23, 205–211.

Nishiki, M., Murakami, Y., Ozawa, Y., Kato, Y., 2001. Serum anti-bodies to human pituitary membrane antigens in patients with autoimmune lymphocytic hypophysitis and infundibuloneurohy-pophysitis. Clin. Endocrinol. (Oxf.). 54, 327–333.

Nussbaum, C.E., Okawara, S.H., Jacobs, L.S., 1991. Lymphocytic hypo-physitis with involvement of the cavernous sinus and hypothalamus. Neurosurgery. 28, 440–444.

O'Dwyer, D.T., Clifton, V., Hall, A., Smith, R., Robinson, P.J., Crock, P.A., 2002a. Pituitary Autoantibodies in lymphocytic hypophysitis target both gamma- and alpha-enolase—a link with pregnancy? Arch. Physiol. Biochem. 110, 94–98.

O'Dwyer, D.T., Smith, A.I., Matthew, M.L., Andronicos, N.M., Ranson, M., Robinson, P.J., et al., 2002b. Identification of the 49-kDa auto-antigen associated with lymphocytic hypophysitis as alpha-enolase. J. Clin. Endocrinol. Metab. 87, 752–757.

Ogawa, R., 1995. A child with necrotizing infundibulo-neurohypophysis. Hormone to Rinsho. 43, 33–36.

Phan, G.Q., Yang, J.C., Sherry, R.M., Hwu, P., Topalian, S.L., Schwartzentruber, D.J., et al., 2003. Cancer regression and autoim-munity induced by cytotoxic T lymphocyte-associated antigen 4 blockade in patients with metastatic melanoma. Proc. Natl. Acad. Sci. USA. 100, 8372–8377.

Powe, C.E., Allen, M., Puopolo, K.M., Merewood, A., Worden, S., Johnson, L.C., et al., 2010. Recombinant human prolactin for the treat-ment of lactation insufficiency. Clin. Endocrinol. (Oxf.). 73, 645–653.

Ray, D.K., Yen, C.P., Vance, M.L., Laws, E.R., Lopes, B., Sheehan, J.P., 2010. Gamma knife surgery for lymphocytic hypophysitis. J. Neurosurg. 112, 118–121.

Rose, N.R., Bona, C., 1993. Defining criteria for autoimmune diseases (Witebsky's postulates revisited). Immunol. Today. 14, 426–430.

Rupp, J.J., Paschkis, K.E., 1953. Panhypopituitarism and hypocalcemic tet-any in a male: case presentation. Ann. Intern. Med. 39, 1103–1106.

Saito, T., Yoshida, S., Nakao, K., Takanashi, R., 1970. Chronic hyperna-tremia associated with inflammation of the neurohypophysis. J. Clin. Endocrinol. Metab. 31, 391–396.

Sandler, R., Danks, K.R., Hennigan, S.H., Hui, A.N., McElroy, K.C., 1998. The widening spectrum of lymphocytic hypophysitis. J. Ark. Med. Soc. 95, 197–200.

Satogami, N., Miki, Y., Koyama, T., Kataoka, M., Togashi, K., 2009. Normal pituitary stalk: high-resolution MR imaging at 3 T. AJNR Am. J. Neuroradiol. 31, 355–359.

Sautner, D., Saeger, W., Ludecke, D.K., Jansen, V., Puchner, M.J., 1995. Hypophysitis in surgical and autoptical specimens. Acta. Neuropathol. 90, 637–644.

Schreckinger, M., Francis, T., Rajah, G., Jagannathan, J., Guthikonda, M., Mittal, S., 2012. Novel strategy to treat a case of recurrent lym-phocytic hypophysitis using rituximab. J. Neurosurg. 116, 1318–1323.

Selch, M.T., DeSalles, A.A., Kelly, D.F., Frighetto, L., Vinters, H.V., Cabatan-Awang, C., et al., 2003. Stereotactic radiotherapy for the treatment of lymphocytic hypophysitis. Report of two cases. J. Neurosurg. 99, 591–596.

Simmonds, M., 1917. Über das Vorkommen von Riesenzelle in der Hypophyse. Virchows. Arch. 223, 281–290.

Smith, C.J., Bensing, S., Burns, C., Robinson, P.J., Kasperlik-Zaluska, A.A., Scott, R.J., et al., 2012. Identification of TPIT and other novel autoantigens in lymphocytic hypophysitis; immunoscreening of a pituitary cDNA library and development of immunoprecipitation assays. Eur. J. Endocrinol. 166, 391–398.

Takao, T., Nanamiya, W., Matsumoto, R., Asaba, K., Okabayashi, T., Hashimoto, K., 2001. Antipituitary antibodies in patients with lymphocytic hypophysitis. Horm. Res. 55, 288–292.

646

Tanaka, S., Tatsumi, K.I., Kimura, M., Takano, T., Murakami, Y., Takao, T., et al., 2002. Detection of autoantibodies against the pituitary-specific proteins in patients with lymphocytic hypophysitis. Eur. J. Endocrinol. 147, 767–775.

Tanaka, S., Tatsumi, K.I., Takano, T., Murakami, Y., Takao, T., Yamakita, N., et al., 2003. Anti-alpha-enolase antibodies in pituitary disease. Endocr. J. 50, 697–702.

Taylon, C., Duff, T.A., 1980. Giant cell granuloma involving the pituitary gland. J. Neurosurg. 52, 584–587.

Tubridy, N., Saunders, D., Thom, M., Asa, S.L., Powell, M., Plant, G.T., et al., 2001. Infundibulohypophysitis in a man presenting with diabetes insipidus and cavernous sinus involvement. J. Neurol. Neurosurg. Psychiatry. 71, 798–801.

Turcu, A.F., Erickson, B.J., Lin, E., Guadalix, S., Schwartz, K., Scheithauer, B.W., et al., 2013. Pituitary stalk lesions: the Mayo Clinic experience. J. Clin. Endocrinol. Metab. 8, 1812–1818.

Tzou, S.C., Lupi, I., Landek-Salgado, M.A., Gutenberg, A., Tzou, Y.M., Kimura, H., et al., 2008. Autoimmune hypophysitis of SJL mice: clinical insights from a new animal model. Endocrinology. 149, 3461–3469.

van der Vliet, H.J., Perenboom, R.M., 2004. Multiple pseudotumors in IgG4-associated multifocal systemic fibrosis. Ann. Intern. Med. 141, 896–897.

Vanneste, J.A., Kamphorst, W., 1987. Lymphocytic hypophysitis. Surg. Neurol. 28, 145–149.

Vidal, S., Rotondo, F., Horvath, E., Kovacs, K., Scheithauer, B.W., 2002. Immunocytochemical localization of mast cells in lymphocytic hypophysitis. Am. J. Clin. Pathol. 117, 478–483.

Voskens, C.J., Goldinger, S.M., Loquai, C., Robert, C., Kaehler, K. C., Berking, C., et al., 2013. The price of tumor control: an analysis of rare side effects of anti-CTLA-4 therapy in metastatic melanoma from the ipilimumab network. PLoS One. 8, e53745.

Ward, L., Paquette, J., Seidman, E., Huot, C., Alvarez, F., Crock, P.A., et al., 1999. Severe autoimmune polyendocrinopathy-candidiasis-ectodermal dystrophy in an adolescent girl with a novel AIRE mutation: response to immunosuppressive therapy. J. Clin. Endocrinol. Metab. 84, 844–852.

Watanabe, K., Tada, H., Shimaoka, Y., Hidaka, Y., Tatsumi, K., Izumi, Y., et al., 2001. Characteristics of experimental autoimmune hypophysitis in rats: major antigens are growth hormone, thyrotropin, and luteinizing hormone in this model. Autoimmunity. 33, 265–274.

Wong, S., Lam, W.Y., Wong, W.K., Lee, K.C., 2007. Hypophysitis presented as inflammatory pseudotumor in immunoglobulin G4-related systemic disease. Hum. Pathol. 38, 1720–1723.

Yabe, S., Murakami, M., Maruyama, K., Miwa, H., Fukumura, Y., Ishii, S., et al., 1995. Western blot analysis of rat pituitary antigens recognized by human antipituitary antibodies. Endocr. J. 42, 115–119.

Yamamoto, M., Iguchi, G., Takeno, R., Okimura, Y., Sano, T., Takahashi, M., et al., 2011. Adult combined GH, prolactin, and TSH deficiency associated with circulating PIT-1 antibody in humans. J. Clin. Invest. 121, 113–119.

Yoon, J.W., Choi, D.S., Liang, H.C., Baek, H.S., Ko, I.Y., Jun, H.S., et al., 1992. Induction of an organ-specific autoimmune disease, lymphocytic hypophysitis, in hamsters by recombinant rubella virus glycoprotein and prevention of disease by neonatal thymectomy. J. Virol. 66, 1210–1214.

Part 9

Blood Disorders

Chapter 46

Autoimmune Hemolytic Anemia

Mark A. Vickers[1] and Robert N. Barker[2]

[1]Academic Transfusion Medicine Unit, Scottish National Blood Transfusion Service, Aberdeen, UK, [2]Section of Immunology and Infection, Division of Applied Medicine, Institute of Medical Sciences, University of Aberdeen, Foresterhill, Aberdeen, UK

Chapter Outline

Historical Background	649	Etiology of AIHA and Predisposing Factors	654
Classification of AIHA	649	Genetic Predisposition	654
Animal Models of AIHA	650	Gender and Age	655
Mechanisms of RBC Destruction in AIHA	650	Infectious Agents	655
Cold Reactive Antibodies	650	Drugs	655
Warm Reactive Antibodies	651	Neoplasia	655
Pathogenicity of Warm Reactive IgG Antibodies	651	Immune Mechanisms Underlying Loss of Self Tolerance in	
Additional Mechanisms of Hemolysis by Warm		Warm AIHA	655
Antibodies	652	B Cells and Tolerance	655
RBC Autoantigens	653	T Helper (Th) Cells and Tolerance	656
Clinical Signs of AIHA	653	Concluding Remarks	657
Laboratory Diagnosis of AIHA	654	References	657
Treatment of AIHA	654		

HISTORICAL BACKGROUND

The earliest descriptions of autoimmune hemolytic anemia (AIHA) date from the 19th century, and the disease was one of the first shown to have an autoimmune pathology. Pioneering work by Donath and Landsteiner demonstrated that the destruction of red blood cells (RBC) was dependent on the absorption of hemolysins and complement from serum (Donath and Landsteiner, 1904). Further studies were impeded by the difficulty in distinguishing acquired from congenital hemolytic anemias, but an important advance was made using the antiglobulin, or Coombs', test, which detected RBC coated with autoantibodies by agglutinating them with antiserum to human globulin (Coombs et al., 1945; Boorman et al., 1946; Loutit and Mollison, 1946). Methods for measuring survival of circulating cells *in vivo* further demonstrated that RBC from patients with acquired hemolytic anemias were destroyed by a "random hemolytic process," rather than being "intrinsically defective" (Loutit and Mollison,

1946; Mollison, 1959). Together, these developments identified AIHA as a disease in which autoantibodies bind RBC and shorten their life span, affecting 1–3 per 100,000 of the population (Sokol et al., 1992; Petz and Garratty, 2004a).

CLASSIFICATION OF AIHA

AIHA can be classified both by the type of autoantibody and by the presence of underlying disease (Sokol et al., 1992; Petz and Garratty, 2004a) (Table 46.1). Pathogenic autoantibodies are divided into either cold (Petz, 2008) or warm (Packman, 2008) reactive, depending on the optimum temperature at which they bind RBC. Up to 7% of patients have "mixed" pathogenic autoantibodies of both types (Sokol et al., 1981, 1983, 1992). AIHA can also be described as primary, or idiopathic, in the absence of any associated condition, or as secondary if there is concurrent disease that may be considered causal or has shared etiology (Packman, 2008; Petz, 2008).

N. Rose & I. Mackay (Eds): The Autoimmune Diseases, Fifth edition. DOI: http://dx.doi.org/10.1016/B978-0-12-384929-8.00046-0

TABLE 46.1 Classification of AIHA by Antibody Type

Classification by Autoantibody Type

	Cold Reactive	Warm Reactive
Optimum temperature for binding RBC	4°C	37°C
Predominant autoantibody class	IgM (cold agglutinin syndrome) IgG (paroxysmal cold hematuria)	IgG
Predominant site of hemolysis	Intravascular	Extravascular (spleen, liver)
Predominant mechanism of hemolysis	Complement lysis (membrane attack complex)	Phagocytosis via macrophage IgG Fc and complement receptors

Classification by Underlying Disease

Primary (idiopathic)	Secondary
No underlying disease	Underlying disease (causal or shared etiology) Infection Other immune disease Neoplasia Drug induced

ANIMAL MODELS OF AIHA

Examples of AIHA in laboratory mice have proved valuable in understanding the pathogenesis of the disease. The New Zealand Black (NZB) mouse (Helyer and Howie, 1963; Barker et al., 1993b) develops AIHA spontaneously, and hemolysis can be recapitulated by transgenic expression of a monoclonal anti-RBC autoantibody derived from this strain (Murakami et al., 1992). AIHA is also one of the autoimmune pathologies arising in the non-obese diabetic (NOD) mouse (Baxter and Mandel, 1991), and from genetic modification to prevent expression of interleukin-2 (IL-2) (Hoyer et al., 2009). In addition to these spontaneous examples, the disease can be induced in healthy murine strains by repeated immunization with rat RBC (Playfair and Marshall-Clarke, 1973; Naysmith et al., 1981), or by infection of C3HeB/FeJ mice with the docile strain of lymphocytic choriomeningitis virus (LCMV) (Coutelier et al., 1994).

AIHA has also been described as a cause of anemia in the domestic dog (Barker et al., 1991), cat (Switzer and Jain, 1981), rabbit (Fox et al., 1971), horse (Mair et al., 1990), and ox (Dixon et al., 1978).

MECHANISMS OF RBC DESTRUCTION IN AIHA

AIHA is a classic example of type II hypersensitivity, with autoantibody-coated RBC removed from the circulation by phagocytes of the reticulo-endothelial system (RES), predominantly splenic macrophages, and/or lysis by complement fixation (Packman, 2008; Petz, 2008).

Anemia results if the hemolysis is insufficiently compensated for by increased RBC production.

Cold Reactive Antibodies

Cold reactive anti-RBC autoantibodies are responsible for 15–20% of human AIHA cases (Petz, 2008). They bind more strongly at 4°C than at higher temperatures, and the pathogenic effects of these antibodies depend more on their thermal amplitude than their titer. Cold autoagglutinins that bind RBC below 10–15°C can be demonstrated in the sera of most healthy individuals (Landsteiner and Levine, 1926). In contrast, cold autoantibodies active up to 30°C are associated with cold agglutinin syndrome (CAS) (Petz, 2008), since temperatures in the peripheral circulation can fall below this level. The antibody, usually IgM, causes intravascular hemolysis if it activates complement to form membrane attack complexes (MAC) (Engelfriet et al., 1981; Petz and Garratty, 2004b), overcoming protective regulators on the RBC such as CD35 (complement receptor 1 CR1), CD55 (decay-accelerating factor), and CD59 (protectin) (Nicholson-Weller et al., 1982; Krych-Goldberg and Atkinson, 2001; Ruiz-Argüelles and Llorente, 2007). RBC coated with C3b may also be temporarily sequestered by macrophages (Engelfriet et al., 1981). In some patients, cold IgM autoantibodies agglutinate RBC in extremities that become chilled, blocking small blood vessels and causing ischemia (Petz, 2008). CAS can be either transient, most frequently as a complication of mycoplasma infection (Costea et al., 1972), or chronic, typically associated with clonal lymphoproliferative disease (Berentsen et al., 2006).

Pathogenic cold reactive autoantibodies also include the Donath–Landsteiner (DL) hemolysins, which cause paroxysmal cold hemoglobinuria (PCH), a dramatic form of AIHA precipitated by chilling of the patient (Petz, 2008). These antibodies, which are IgG, bind RBC if the temperature falls below 37°C, then fix complement to trigger MAC formation and fulminant intravascular hemolysis when warmed again. PCH was commonly secondary to syphilis when first described in the late 19th century, but is now rare and typically follows childhood viral infections (Sokol et al., 1982, 1984, 1999).

Warm Reactive Antibodies

Warm autoantibodies are the commonest cause of AIHA and react as well, or more strongly, with RBC at 37°C than at lower temperatures (Sokol et al., 1992; Packman, 2008). Most are of the IgG class and cause extravascular hemolysis, predominantly by Fc receptor (FcγR)-mediated phagocytosis (Engelfriet et al., 1981; Petz and Garratty, 2004b; Packman, 2008). The complement regulators on the RBC membrane (Ruiz-Argüelles and Llorente, 2007) typically prevent MAC formation, but deposition of C3b and C3d is common and can strongly enhance opsonization (Kurlander et al., 1978) by interacting with specific receptors including CR1 and CR3 (Ross and Medof, 1985). Although blood monocytes and hepatic Kupffer cells also express appropriate sets of receptors, splenic macrophages are the main effectors of RBC destruction (Engelfriet et al., 1981; Petz and Garratty, 2004b; Packman, 2008). Some sensitized RBC may be only partially phagocytosed and released back into the circulation as spherocytes, which have a short half-life (Garratty, 1983).

Between 22% (Dausset and Colombani, 1959) and 81% (Pirofsky, 1976) of warm AIHA cases have been reported to be secondary, varying with different interpretations of this classification. The most common associations are with other immune-based conditions, most notably ulcerative colitis, rheumatoid arthritis, and systemic lupus erythematosus (SLE), with neoplasia, particularly chronic lymphocytic leukemia (CLL), and with a variety of infectious diseases (Sokol et al., 1992; Petz and Garratty, 2004a).

Pathogenicity of Warm Reactive IgG Antibodies

Warm reactive IgG anti-RBC autoantibodies vary in their pathogenicity, exemplified by the finding of a positive direct agglutination test (DAT) in a small proportion (1 in 7–15,000) of healthy blood donors (Hernandez-Jodra et al., 1990; Win et al., 1997; Petz and Garratty, 2004b). The ability to cause hemolysis has been attributed to multiple factors, including titer, subclass, affinity for autoantigen, patterns of heavy chain glycosylation, and also the activity of phagocytes responsible for clearance (Garratty, 1990; Sokol et al., 1992; Petz and Garratty, 2004b).

The amount of IgG blood group alloantibody coating RBC determines their rate of clearance in healthy subjects (Mollison and Hughes-Jones, 1967; Kelton et al., 1985), but it is less easy to demonstrate a similar relationship for autoantibodies in human AIHA (Rosse, 1971; Chaplin, 1990; Petz and Garratty, 2004b). Serial measurements from individual patients reveal some correlation of hemolysis with autoantibody titer, but many cross-sectional studies fail to do so, using either the DAT or more sensitive and quantitative flow cytometric or ELISA-based techniques to measure RBC-bound IgG (Van der Meulen et al., 1980; Garratty and Nance, 1990; Sokol et al., 1992; Petz and Garratty, 2004b). Autoantibody titer alone also appears to be an unreliable predictor of the severity of hemolysis in canine (Barker et al., 1992b) and murine AIHA (Naysmith et al., 1981; Shen et al., 2003).

The subclass of RBC autoantibody is a potentially important factor in its ability to cause hemolysis, by determining interactions with different types of FcγR and fixation of complement (Sokol et al., 1992; Petz and Garratty, 2004b). Comprehensive analyses of IgG subclass switch variants of monoclonal anti-RBC antibodies originally derived from NZB mice have established how differences in these Fc-associated effector functions can critically influence pathogenicity (Baudino et al., 2006), with affinity for autoantigen playing a less important role (Fossati-Jimack et al., 1999). In mice there are three activating FcγR types (FcγRI, FcγRIII, and FcγRIV), all of which are expressed on macrophages and can bind complexed IgG, while only FcγRI also has high affinity for monomeric IgG (Nimmerjahn and Ravetch, 2008). IgG$_{2a}$ and IgG$_{2b}$ autoantibody switch variants, each of which interacts efficiently with FcγRIII and activate complement, and mediate the most severe hemolysis *in vivo* (Baudino et al., 2006). FcγRIV makes an additional contribution to uptake by these isotypes, and IgG$_{2a}$ also promotes clearance via FcγRI if it coats RBC at sufficient density to compete with free monomer in serum (Baudino et al., 2008). The next most pathogenic subclass is IgG$_3$, which activates complement but does not bind any FcγR, followed by the IgG$_1$ subclass that interacts only with FcγRIII and fails to fix complement. Overall, IgG$_{2a}$ and IgG$_{2b}$ autoantibodies are 20-fold more potent in causing hemolysis than IgG$_1$ (Baudino et al., 2006). Complement fixation by the murine autoantibodies does not lead to MAC formation, but CR-mediated erythrophagocytosis can be important if there is extensive opsonization of RBC by C3 associated with binding of high affinity IgG$_{2b}$ or IgG$_3$ (da Silveira et al., 2002).

Compared with murine studies, the relationships between human RBC autoantibody subclass and hemolysis are less clear (Petz and Garratty, 2004b). Based on interactions with FcγR and complement, IgG$_3$ would be predicted to be the most pathogenic subclass, followed by IgG$_1$, with IgG$_2$ and IgG$_4$ relatively benign (Engelfriet et al., 1981; Petz and Garratty, 2004b; Sokol et al., 1992). However, in both patients with AIHA and healthy DAT-positive donors with no evidence of hemolysis, IgG$_1$ autoantibody predominates, and is the only isotype detected on RBC using agglutination-based techniques in up to 80% of each group (Garratty, 1989). Furthermore, IgG$_3$ can be detected by DAT not only in patients but also in normal blood donors, although RBC sensitization with IgG$_4$ alone may be restricted to healthy individuals (Garratty, 1989). Sensitive flow cytometric and ELISA methods (Sokol et al., 1990a; Garratty and Nance, 1990) have confirmed that increased levels of RBC-bound IgG$_3$ are not necessarily associated with disease, and suggest instead that autoantibodies of multiple IgG subclasses are common in AIHA, and that this diversity is important in promoting hemolysis via synergistic effects (Sokol et al., 1990a). The three families of human activating FcγR (FcγRI, FcγRIIa/FcγRIIc, and FcγRIIIa/FcγRIIIb) (Nimmerjahn and Ravetch, 2008) may each play a role in RBC uptake. As in mice, only FcγRI has high affinity for monomeric IgG, but may mediate erythrophagocytosis under conditions that allow RBC-bound IgG to compete with monomer in serum, particularly in the hemoconcentrated environment of the spleen (Kelton et al., 1985; Barker et al., 1992b). Although MAC formation rarely contributes to hemolysis in patients with warm antibodies, complement fixation appears to be an important determinant of disease (Petz and Garratty, 2004b). C3 can be detected by DAT in up to 50% of AIHA patients (Garratty, 1989) and is quantitatively associated with hemolysis (Freedman et al., 1982), reflecting synergy between FcγR and CR in RBC uptake (Sokol et al., 1992).

Changes in glycosylation of the CH2 domain of the IgG heavy chain may also influence interactions with FcγR and complement, with loss of either terminal sialic acid or galactose residues suggested to alter the pathogenicity of murine RBC autoantibody (Baudino et al., 2006). There is evidence in rheumatoid arthritis that IgG lacking galactose (G$_0$) can interact with mannose-binding protein, thereby fixing complement and triggering inflammation (Malhotra et al., 1995). However, in AIHA it seems likely that RBC autoantibody may be less hemolytic than G$_0$, since the loss of galactose reduces the affinity of IgG for FcγRIII (Hadley et al., 1995). Although G$_0$ RBC autoantibodies have been identified in some AIHA patients and in NZB mice, the levels can vary widely over time in individuals and show no correlation with severity of disease (Barker et al., 1999a,b).

The final, important, factor determining the hemolytic potential of warm autoantibodies is the effectiveness of the RES in clearing sensitized RBC (Sokol et al., 1992; Petz and Garratty, 2004b). The ability of macrophages to phagocytose RBC can be enhanced by infections that upregulate FcγR expression (Atkinson and Frank, 1974; Coutelier et al., 2007), or compromised by saturation with immune complexes in AIHA secondary to SLE (Frank et al., 1979). Drugs such as corticosteroids can also inhibit phagocytosis by downregulating FcγR expression (Fries et al., 1983; Kelton, 1985). The cytokine milieu is a major influence on macrophage activation state, and the severity of NZB AIHA can be ameliorated by gene therapy to increase levels of circulating IL-4 (Youssef et al., 2005).

Additional Mechanisms of Hemolysis by Warm Antibodies

Although FcγR- and CR-mediated erythrophagocytosis of IgG coated RBC is the major cause of hemolysis in warm AIHA, there is evidence for other pathogenic mechanisms (Sokol et al., 1992; Petz and Garratty, 2004b).

In rare patients with warm AIHA, the main autoantibody class may be IgM or IgA, and not IgG. If warm IgM autoantibodies predominate, they can trigger MAC formation and fulminant intravascular hemolysis (Freedman et al., 1987). IgA autoantibodies may cause hemolysis by Fc-mediated uptake and cytotoxicity (Clark et al., 1984), or hemagglutination in the spleen (Baudino et al., 2007). More sensitive techniques than the DAT detect a higher prevalence of co-sensitization of IgG with low levels of IgM and/or IgA, and such coating of RBC with multiple antibody classes is associated with severe hemolysis, suggesting the importance of synergistic effects (Sokol et al., 1990b).

Another mechanism, which may be of particular relevance in patients with very low levels of RBC-bound IgG, is that splenic macrophages are instead "armed" with the autoantibody bound to FcγRI, allowing them to capture circulating RBC (Griffiths et al., 1994). Antibody dependent cell-mediated cytotoxicity may also play a role in hemolysis (Garratty, 1983; Griffiths et al., 1994), mediated not only by macrophages but also potentially by K cells (Urbaniak and Griess, 1980) or activated neutrophils (Engelfriet et al., 1981). In some patients, there is evidence that autoantibodies can interfere with erythropoiesis (Crosby and Rappaport, 1956) or RBC egress from the bone marrow (Conley et al., 1982), as well as causing hemolysis.

RBC Autoantigens

Many of the major RBC autoantigens in AIHA have been identified (Tables 46.2 and 46.3).

Serological studies have established that cold reactive RBC autoantibodies in healthy individuals, and pathogenic species with high thermal amplitude in CAS, are most commonly directed to the Ii blood group system of carbohydrate differentiation antigens (Berentsen and Tjønnfjord, 2012). On adult RBC, the I antigen predominates, while i is expressed at low levels. Antibodies from approximately 90% of CAS patients recognize the I antigen (Jenkins et al., 1960), with anti-i (Marsh and Jenkins, 1960) accounting for most of the remainder. Other, very rare specificities for autoantibodies in CAS include Pr (Dellagi et al., 1981). In PCH, anti-P autoantibodies are detected in at least 90% of patients (Sokol et al., 1999).

The most common targets in human warm AIHA, recognized in over 70% of cases, are the Rh proteins (Weiner and Voss, 1963; Barker et al., 1992a; Leddy et al., 1993), which also express important blood groups (Avent and Reid, 2000). Autoantibodies reactive against the glycophorins, or against the RBC anion channel protein, Band 3, are produced in some patients (Victoria et al., 1990; Barker et al., 1992a; Leddy et al., 1993). The major canine RBC autoantigens are the glycophorins,

with autoantibodies from some cases specific for Band 3 (Barker et al., 1991). In mice, Band 3 is the dominant autoantigen in NZB disease (Barker et al., 1993b; de Sá Oliveira et al., 1996) and in AIHA following LCMV infection (Mazza et al., 1997), and, together with glycophorins, is also a target for autoantibodies induced by rat RBC (Barker et al., 1993a).

In addition to the autoantigens relevant to AIHA pathogenesis, RBC can also express cryptic determinants recognized by naturally occurring IgG autoantibodies. These include spectrin, the major component of the internal RBC cytoskeleton (Lutz and Wipf, 1982; Ballas, 1989; Barker et al., 1991, 1993a) and senescent red cell antigen (Alderman et al., 1981), which is exposed on Band 3 by aged RBC (Kay et al., 1990). The autoantibodies are thought to provide physiological mechanisms for disposing of damaged and effete RBC (Wiener et al., 1986; Pantaleo et al., 2008).

CLINICAL SIGNS OF AIHA

In both CAS (Petz, 2008) and warm AIHA (Packman, 2008), the predominant clinical features reflect the anemia, which most commonly causes lethargy and dyspnea. Signs include pallor and icterus, and massive hemolysis

TABLE 46.2 RBC Autoantigens in Human AIHA Caused by Cold Autoantibodies

Form of AIHA	Common Autoantibody Specificity	Rare Autoantibody Specificity
Cold agglutinin syndrome (CAS)	I (~90% patients)	i, Pr, A, B
Paroxysmal cold hematuria (PCH)	P (~90% patients)	i, p, HI, I

TABLE 46.3 RBC Autoantigens in Human and Animal AIHA Caused by Warm Autoantibodies

Species	B Cell Autoantigen (Dominant Antigen in Bold)	Th Cell Autoantigen Identified	Unprimed Autoreactive Th Cells in Health	Regulatory T Cell Response
Human AIHA	**Rh proteins (~70% patients)** Glycophorin A Band 3	Rh proteins	Yes	IL-10 response to Rh protein epitopes
Canine AIHA	**Glycophorins (~50% patients)** Band 3	Glycophorins	Yes	Not examined
Murine AIHA				
NZB mouse	**Band 3** Band 4.1 (pr) Phosphatidylcholine (pr)	Band 3	Not applicable	Weak IL-10 response to Band 3
Induced by rat RBC	**Band 3** (cr) Glycophorins (cr)	Band 3	Yes	Recovery due to suppression by CD25+ cells
Induced by LCMV	**Band 3**	Not examined	Yes	Not examined

pr = polyreactive antibody, also binds nuclear antigens, e.g. histones; cr = cross reacts with rat RBC antigen.
Modified from Barker et al. (2007).

may precipitate hemoglobinuria. In CAS there may also be cyanosis or even necrosis of the bodily extremities (Petz, 2008). AIHA due to DL antibodies is typified by recurrent bouts of anemia and hemoglobinuria precipitated by exposure to cold (Petz, 2008). In warm AIHA, splenomegaly or hepatomegaly can be associated with extravascular hemolysis (Packman, 2008). Where AIHA is secondary, the signs of the underlying disease may predominate.

LABORATORY DIAGNOSIS OF AIHA

In addition to anemia, most cases show evidence of erythroid regeneration, with a reticulocytosis (Packman, 2008; Petz, 2008). However, there can be a poor erythroid response (Liesveld et al., 1987), due to the physiological lag in increasing RBC production following acute hemolysis, or to autoimmune reactions inhibiting RBC regeneration (Conley et al., 1982), or to an underlying bone marrow disorder (Lefrere et al., 1986). Evidence of hemolysis can also be provided by increased bilirubin, aspartate transaminase, and lactate dehydrogenase levels. RBC autoagglutination or spherocytes may be seen in cold and warm AIHA, respectively.

Detection of RBC autoantibodies confirms the diagnosis of AIHA. The DAT has been the classic tool for measuring RBC-bound autoantibodies and complement (Petz and Garratty, 2004a). However, benign immunoproteins on the RBC surface can cause a positive DAT (Heddle et al., 1988; Huh et al., 1988), and the test also gives false-negative results in 3 to 11% of AIHA cases (Sokol et al., 1985, 1988; Petz and Garratty, 2004a). These limitations have led to more sensitive methods to detect RBC-bound immunoglobulins, including radioimmunoassay (Kaplan and Quimby, 1983), flow cytometry (Van der Meulen et al., 1980; Garratty and Nance, 1990), or ELISA (Sokol et al., 1985, 1988).

TREATMENT OF AIHA

Anemia in both cold and warm AIHA requires supportive care and, if life-threatening, transfusion (Packman, 2008; Petz, 2008).

Patients with pathogenic cold reactive autoantibodies should be protected from unnecessary exposure to low temperatures (Petz, 2008). Cases of secondary disease, for example CAS or PCH associated with infection, may be transient or resolve with treatment of the underlying condition. Corticosteroids or cytotoxic drugs have been used to treat CAS, but the response is frequently poor (Petz, 2008), and better results have been obtained by targeting B cells with the anti-CD20 monoclonal antibody rituximab (Berentsen et al., 2004).

Corticosteroids, such as prednisolone, are the most common therapy for warm AIHA and can be highly effective, although many patients relapse after withdrawal of these drugs (Packman, 2008). Corticosteroids can both downregulate macrophage FcγR to improve the survival of IgG-sensitized RBC (Fries et al., 1983) and reduce autoantibody production (Rosse, 1971; Sokol and Hewitt, 1985), but the rapid response they typically elicit suggests the importance of the former effect (Packman, 2008). Cytotoxic drugs such as cyclophosphamide or azathioprine may be used to suppress immune responsiveness, and splenectomy can also be considered to remove a major site of extravascular hemolysis (Packman, 2008; Crowther et al., 2011). Ablation of B cells with rituximab is now available as an effective treatment for AIHA that is refractory to conventional treatments (Zecca et al., 2003; Peñalver et al., 2010; Crowther et al., 2011).

ETIOLOGY OF AIHA AND PREDISPOSING FACTORS

It is clear that autoimmune diseases result from the interaction of multiple factors (Shoenfeld and Isenberg, 1989; Cho and Gregersen, 2011). Genetic background, gender, age, environmental factors such as infections, drugs, and neoplasia have all been implicated in the etiology of AIHA.

Genetic Predisposition

The possibility of a genetic predisposition to human AIHA was raised by rare reports of familial disease (Cordova et al., 1966; Pirofsky, 1968; Pollock et al., 1970; Lippman et al., 1982; Olanoff and Fudenberg, 1983). Particular human leucocyte antigen (HLA) haplotypes are the strongest genetic determinants of many autoimmune diseases (Shoenfeld and Schwartz, 1984; Caillat-Zucman, 2009; Cho and Gregersen, 2011; Lessard et al., 2012), and warm AIHA is positively associated with HLA-DR15, with approximately 60% of patients expressing this allele (Stott et al., 2002). Genome-wide association studies of other human autoimmune diseases reveal that large numbers of non-HLA genes further contribute to susceptibility (Cho and Gregersen, 2011; Lessard et al., 2012), and predisposition of the NZB mouse to AIHA has also been attributed to multiple loci (Chused et al., 1987; Lee et al., 2004; Scatizzi et al., 2012). The molecular bases of most such associations remain unknown. However, in common with other autoimmune-prone strains, the NZB mouse shares a promoter haplotype that is associated with reduced expression and function of the inhibitory Fc receptor FcγRIIb (Pritchard et al., 2000). The effects of the polymorphism on FcγRIIb expressed by macrophages and B cells are enhanced phagocytosis of IgG opsonized RBC, and increased antibody responsiveness (Pritchard et al., 2000; Kikuchi et al., 2006).

Gender and Age

Unlike most other human autoimmune diseases (Talal and Ahmed, 1987), the incidence of AIHA is no higher in women than in men (Pirofsky, 1976; Sokol et al., 1981, 1992). AIHA becomes progressively more common with age (Sokol et al., 1981, 1992), perhaps reflecting defects in immune regulation (Tomer and Shoenfeld, 1988; Talor and Rose, 1991; Akbar and Fletcher, 2005).

Infectious Agents

Infectious agents are commonly implicated in provoking autoimmune disease in susceptible individuals (Shoenfeld and Isenberg, 1989), with almost 10% of human AIHA patients reported to have concurrent bacterial or viral conditions (Sokol et al., 1981, 1992), and RBC autoantibodies induced in mice by LCMV (Coutelier et al., 1994). Cross-reactivity between bacterial lipopolysaccharide and the blood group antigen I has been proposed to explain the high incidence of transient CAS which follows human *Mycoplasma pneumoniae* infection (Costea et al., 1972). The potential for mimicry to induce warm AIHA is exemplified by the disease that develops in mice following repeated injections of RBC expressing cross-reactive antigens from a closely related species, the rat (Playfair and Marshall-Clarke, 1973; Barker et al., 1993a). Studies of NZB mice also suggest that cross-reactivity between a microbe and a self-epitope can focus a predisposition to autoimmunity onto a particular target, even when not a primary or sufficient cause of disease (Hall et al., 2007). A second mechanism linking infection and AIHA is the ability of innate microbial stimuli and the cytokines they induce to activate antigen-presenting cells (APC) and therefore to enhance the immunogenicity of RBC autoantigens (Elson et al., 1995; Coutelier et al., 2007). Changes to the cytokine milieu resulting from infection, particularly IFN-γ production, can also enhance RBC phagocytosis by modulating both the subclass of autoantibody and the activation of macrophages (Atkinson and Frank, 1974; Coutelier et al., 2007). Finally, particular infectious agents associated with AIHA, such as Epstein—Barr virus, may directly infect and dysregulate immune cells (Bowman et al., 1974).

Drugs

Immune-mediated hemolytic anemias are a rare side effect of many drugs, including the penicillins, but in most cases the antibodies are not strictly autoreactive and only bind RBC in the presence of the drug (Garratty, 2010). However, other examples such as α-methyldopa can induce true RBC autoantibodies that may cause AIHA (Sokol et al., 1981), by perturbing immune regulation (Kirtland et al., 1980), or altering the antigenic structure of RBC (Owens et al., 1982).

Neoplasia

Up to 22% of human AIHA cases suffer from some form of concurrent neoplastic disease (Sokol et al., 1981, 1992). Many patients with CAS have a monoclonal RBC autoantibody associated with a clonal lymphoproliferative disorder (Silberstein et al., 1986), most frequently classified as lymphoplasmacytic lymphoma (Berentsen and Tjønnfjord, 2012). Warm AIHA, and autoimmune thrombocytopenia, are both closely associated with CLL. Over 10% of AIHA cases are also diagnosed with the condition (Sokol et al., 1992), and circulating leukocytes with an abnormal CLL-like phenotype can be detected in a further 19% of patients classified with apparent primary AIHA (Mittal et al., 2008). Conversely, up to 14% of CLL patients have AIHA or elevated levels of RBC-bound autoantibody (Dearden et al., 2008). One model to explain this association is that the large numbers of the malignant CLL cells present in the spleen drive an autoimmune response to circulating cells by acting as aberrant APC (Hall et al., 2005).

IMMUNE MECHANISMS UNDERLYING LOSS OF SELF TOLERANCE IN WARM AIHA

The study of specific pathogenic responses to RBC autoantigens has enabled mechanisms underlying the loss of self tolerance in warm AIHA to be characterized.

B Cells and Tolerance

Although RBC destruction is autoantibody mediated, it is not necessary to invoke a defect in B cell repertoire selection to explain the loss of tolerance in AIHA. Central tolerance of self-reactive B cells is incomplete in healthy individuals, since anti-RBC autoantibodies with a wide range of specificities can be induced to cause AIHA in murine strains that have no predisposition to spontaneous disease (Day et al., 1989; Barker et al., 1993a). Nevertheless, one model of AIHA, created by transgenic expression of an anti-RBC monoclonal autoantibody from NZB mice, does illustrate the potential for pathology to result from failure to censor autoreactive B cells (Murakami et al., 1992). The B cells producing monoclonal antibody are sequestered in the peritoneal cavity, and survive to cause disease in only a proportion of mice, depending on whether they are deleted by contact with RBC (Murakami et al., 1992).

T Helper (Th) Cell and Tolerance

There is a long-standing belief that self tolerance in the T cell compartment is less secure than for B cells, and that, in health, antibody-mediated diseases such as AIHA are prevented due to lack of effective help (Naysmith et al., 1981; Elson and Barker, 2000). The vast majority of IgG responses are T dependent (Kelsoe, 1995), and the production of warm autoantibodies in AIHA appears to be no exception (Elson and Barker, 2000). NZB IgG autoantibody production *in vivo* is retarded by treatment with anti-CD4 monoclonal antibody (Oliveira et al., 1994), or by CD4 gene deletion (Chen et al., 1996), and splenic Th cells from NZB mice but not MHC-matched healthy strains, proliferate *in vitro* in response to the major murine RBC autoantigen, Band 3 (Perry et al., 1996; Shen et al., 1996). Furthermore, NZB disease is accelerated by immunization with an insoluble peptide bearing the dominant Th cell epitope from Band 3, and ameliorated by mucosal administration of a soluble analogue of this sequence (Shen et al., 2003). Other murine models are also Th dependent, since anti-CD4 mAb treated mice do not develop AIHA induced by LCMV (Coutelier et al., 1994), and T cell depletion prevents RBC autoantibody production in response to immunization with cross-reactive rat antigens (Naysmith et al., 1981). Findings in human AIHA are also consistent with the need for help. Rh autoantigen-specific effector Th cells that have been activated *in vivo* can be demonstrated in the peripheral blood and/or spleen from all patients with anti-Rh autoantibodies (Barker et al., 1997), but from very few healthy donors (Barker and Elson, 1994; Barker et al., 1997).

Warm AIHA in patients and NZB mice is associated with specific helper responses that are dominated by the Th1 subset, and inducing a corresponding Th2 bias can prevent or ameliorate NZB disease (Shen et al., 1996, 2003; Hall et al., 2002). Such a shift may be therapeutically beneficial partly because of the associated switch of the autoantibody to a less pathogenic isotype. Recent studies of human AIHA reveal that disease is also strongly associated with IL-17 responses to RBC, raising the possibility that Th17 cells may also provide help for autoreactive B cells to produce pathogenic IgG subclasses (Hall et al., 2012).

In common with B cells, it appears that potentially autoaggressive T cells can escape central tolerance as part of normal immune development, and that failure of peripheral mechanisms to control their activation results in AIHA. Healthy mice (Naysmith et al., 1981; Barker et al., 1993a, 2002), dogs (Corato et al., 1997), and humans (Barker and Elson, 1994) all harbor naïve Th cells that can be stimulated to proliferate *in vitro* by RBC autoantigens. Comparison with AIHA patients demonstrates they differ, not in the presence or fine specificity of circulating RBC-specific autoreactive Th cells, but in the finding that these lymphocytes are activated *in vivo* (Barker and Elson, 1994; Barker et al., 1997). One possibility is that the surviving autoreactive Th cells are specific for RBC self-epitopes that are normally inefficiently processed and presented by APC from the intact antigen (Elson et al., 1995) and therefore unavailable to induce tolerance in the thymus. This model is supported by studies of human AIHA, where activated Th cells are specific for epitopes on the Rh protein autoantigens that are "cryptic" or sub-dominant (Hall et al., 1999). Such epitopes may be more efficiently presented and drive an autoaggressive Th response if APC are activated, for example by infection (Elson et al., 1995), or by the accumulation of aberrant APC types such as CLL cells (Hall et al., 2005).

It is now recognized that CD4$^+$ regulatory T (Treg) cells are important mediators of peripheral self tolerance (Roncarolo et al., 2006; Sakaguchi et al., 2010; Shevach, 2011). AIHA induced by rat RBC immunization of mice provided an early example of such "infectious tolerance," since the autoimmune response is transient and the mice become refractory to further induction of disease, with splenocytes transferred from recovered animals providing protection to naïve recipients (Playfair and Marshall-Clarke, 1973; Naysmith et al., 1981). Both the "adaptive" IL-10$^+$ (Roncarolo et al., 2006) and "natural" CD25$^+$FoxP3$^+$ (Sakaguchi et al., 2010; Shevach, 2011) forms of Treg cell have been implicated in maintaining or restoring tolerance to RBC autoantigens. In murine AIHA induced by rat RBC, recovery is associated with protective CD25$^+$ T cells (Mqadmi et al., 2005) and the development of AIHA in gene-deleted mice that lack IL-2 has been attributed to a deficiency of the "natural" Treg population (Hoyer et al., 2009). Treg cells specific for the target Rh autoantigens can be found in the peripheral blood or spleen of patients with AIHA, and are capable of inhibiting the Th1 effector responses *in vitro* by secretion of IL-10 (Hall et al., 2002). The Rh-specific Treg cells have been cloned and shown to mediate inhibitory activity only after stimulation by cognate antigen, and not in response to polyclonal activators, illustrating the importance of specificity in their function (Ward et al., 2008). Although able to secrete the "adaptive" inhibitory cytokine IL-10, these Treg cells also express the "natural" marker FoxP3, and the Th1 transcription factor T-bet, revealing plasticity between the different regulatory forms and effector subsets (Ward et al., 2008).

CONCLUDING REMARKS

In AIHA, many of the pathogenetic mechanisms by which autoantibodies can cause disease have been defined. The identification of major human and murine RBC autoantigens has also provided unique insights into the control of specific, pathogenic immune responses in both human and experimental animal disease. This work to understand how immunological tolerance is lost and can be restored holds out the prospect of more effective, specific therapies.

REFERENCES

Akbar, A.N., Fletcher, J.M., 2005. Memory T cell homeostasis and senescence during aging. Curr. Opin. Immunol. 17, 480–485.

Alderman, E.M., Fudenberg, H.H., Lovins, R.E., 1981. Isolation and characterization of an age-related antigen present on senescent human red blood cells. Blood. 58, 341–349.

Atkinson, J.P., Frank, M.M., 1974. The effect of Bacillus Calmette-Guérin-induced macrophage activation on the *in vivo* clearance of sensitized erythrocytes. J. Clin. Invest. 53, 1742–1749.

Avent, N.D., Reid, M.E., 2000. The Rh blood group system: a review. Blood. 95, 375–387.

Ballas, S.K., 1989. Spectrin autoantibodies in normal human serum and in polyclonal blood grouping sera. Br. J. Haematol. 71, 137–139.

Barker, R.N., Elson, C.J., 1994. Multiple self-epitopes on the Rhesus polypeptides stimulate immunologically ignorant human T-cells in vitro. Eur. J. Immunol. 2, 1578–1582.

Barker, R.N., Gruffydd-Jones, T.J., Stokes, C.R., Elson, C.J., 1991. Identification of autoantigens in canine autoimmune haemolytic anaemia. Clin. Exp. Immunol. 85, 33–40.

Barker, R.N., Casswell, K.M., Reid, M.E., Sokol, R.J., Elson, C.J., 1992a. Identification of autoantigens in autoimmune haemolytic anaemia by a non-radioisotope immunoprecipitation method. Br. J. Haematol. 8, 126–132.

Barker, R.N., Gruffydd-Jones, T.J., Stokes, C.R., Elson, C.J., 1992b. Autoimmune haemolysis in the dog: relationship between anaemia and the levels of red blood cell immunoglobulins and complement measured by an enzyme-linked antiglobulin test. Vet. Immunol. Immunopathol. 3, 1–20.

Barker, R.N., Casswell, K.M., Elson, C.J., 1993a. Identification of murine erythrocyte autoantigens and cross-reactive rat antigens. Immunology. 78, 568–573.

Barker, R.N., De Sá Oliveira, G.G., Elson, C.J., Lydyard, P.M., 1993b. Pathogenic autoantibodies in the NZB mouse are specific for erythrocyte Band 3 protein. Eur. J. Immunol. 23, 1723–1726.

Barker, R.N., Hall, A.M., Standen, G.R., Jones, J., Elson, C.J., 1997. Identification of T-cell epitopes on the Rhesus polypeptides in autoimmune hemolytic anemia. Blood. 90, 2701–2715.

Barker, R.N., Leader, K.A., Elson, C.J., 1999a. Serial changes in the galactosylation of autoantibody and serum IgG in autoimmune haemolytic anaemia. Autoimmunity. 31, 103–108.

Barker, R.N., Young, R.D., Leader, K.A., Elson, C.J., 1999b. Galactosylation of serum IgG and autoantibodies in murine models of autoimmune haemolytic anaemia. Clin. Exp. Immunol. 117, 449–454.

Barker, R.N., Shen, C.-R., Elson, C.J., 2002. T-cell specificity in murine autoimmune haemolytic anaemia induced by rat red blood cells. Clin. Exp. Immunol. 129, 208–213.

Barker, R.N., Vickers, M.A., Ward, F.J., 2007. Controlling autoimmunity—lessons from the study of red blood cells as model antigens. Immunol. Lett. 108, 20–26.

Baudino, L., da Silveira, S.A., Nakata, M., Izui, S., 2006. Molecular and cellular basis for pathogenicity of autoantibodies, lessons from murine monoclonal autoantibodies. Springer Semin. Immunopathol. 28, 175–184.

Baudino, L., Fossati-Jimack, L., Chevalley, C., Martinez-Soria, E., Shulman, M.J., Izui, S., 2007. IgM and IgA anti-erythrocyte autoantibodies induce anemia in a mouse model through multivalency-dependent hemagglutination but not through complement activation. Blood. 109, 5355–5362.

Baudino, L., Nimmerjahn, F., da Silveira, S.A., Martinez-Soria, E., Saito, T., Carroll, M., et al., 2008. Differential contribution of three activating IgG Fc receptors (FcgammaRI, FcgammaRIII, and FcgammaRIV) to IgG2a- and IgG2b-induced autoimmune hemolytic anemia in mice. J. Immunol. 180, 1948–1953.

Baxter, A.G., Mandel, T.E., 1991. Hemolytic anemia in non-obese diabetic mice. Eur. J. Immunol. 21, 2051–2055.

Berentsen, S., Tjønnfjord, G.E., 2012. Diagnosis and treatment of cold agglutinin mediated autoimmune hemolytic anemia. Blood Rev. 26, 107–115.

Berentsen, S., Ulvestad, E., Gjertsen, B.T., Hjorth-Hansen, H., Langholm, R., Knutsen, H., et al., 2004. Rituximab for primary chronic cold agglutinin disease, a prospective study of 37 courses of therapy in 27 patients. Blood. 103, 2925–2928.

Berentsen, S., Ulvestad, E., Langholm, R., Beiske, K., Hjorth-Hansen, H., Ghanima, W., et al., 2006. Primary chronic cold agglutinin disease, a population based clinical study of 86 patients. Haematologica. 91, 460–466.

Boorman, K.E., Dodd, B.E., Loutit, J.F., 1946. Haemolytic icterus (acholuric jaundice), congenital and acquired. Lancet. i, 812–814.

Bowman, H.S., Marsh, W.L., Schumacher, H.R., Oyen, R., Reihart, J., 1974. Auto anti-N immunohemolytic anemia in infectious mononucleosis. Am. J. Clin. Pathol. 61, 465–472.

Caillat-Zucman, S., 2009. Molecular mechanisms of HLA association with autoimmune diseases. Tissue Antigens. 73, 1–8.

Chaplin Jr., H., 1990. Red cell-bound immunoglobulin as a predictor of severity of hemolysis in patients with autoimmune hemolytic anemia. Transfusion. 30, 576–578.

Chen, S., Takeoka, Y., Ansari, A.A., Boyd, R., Klinman, D.M., Gershwin, M.E., 1996. The natural history of disease expression in CD4 and CD8 gene-deleted New Zealand Black (NZB) Mice. J. Immunol. 157, 2676–2684.

Cho, J.H., Gregersen, P.K., 2011. Genomics and the multifactorial nature of human autoimmune disease. N. Engl. J. Med. 365, 1612–1623.

Chused, T.M., McCoy, K.L., Lal, R.B., Brown, E.M., Baker, P.J., 1987. Multigenic basis of autoimmune disease in New Zealand mice. Concepts Immunopathol. 4, 129–143.

Clark, D.A., Dessypris, E.N., Jenkins Jr., D.E., Krantz, S.B., 1984. Acquired immune hemolytic anemia associated with IgA erythrocyte coating, investigation of hemolytic mechanisms. Blood. 64, 1000–1005.

Conley, C.L., Lippman, S.M., Ness, P.M., Petz, L.D., Branch, D.R., Gallagher, M.T., 1982. Autoimmune hemolytic anemia with reticulocytopenia and erythroid marrow. N. Engl. J. Med. 306, 281–286.

Coombs, R.R.A., Mourant, A.E., Race, R.R., 1945. A new test for the detection of weak and "incomplete" Rh agglutinins. Br. J. Exp. Pathol. 26, 255–266.

Corato, A., Shen, C.-R., Mazza, G., Barker, R.N., Day, M.J., 1997. Proliferative responses of peripheral blood mononuclear cells from normal dogs and dogs with autoimmune haemolytic anaemia to red blood cell antigens. Vet. Immunol. Immunopathol. 59, 191–204.

Cordova, M.S., Baez-Villasenor, J., Mendez, J.J., Campos, E., 1966. Acquired hemolytic anemia with positive antiglobulin (Coombs') test in mother and daughter. Arch. Intern. Med. 117, 692–695.

Costea, N., Yakulis, V.J., Heller, P., 1972. Inhibition of cold agglutinins (anti-I) by *M. pneumoniae* antigens. Proc. Soc. Exp. Biol. Med. 139, 476–479.

Coutelier, J.-P., Johnston, S.J., El Idrissi, M. el-A., Pfau, C.J., 1994. Involvement of CD4 + cells in lymphocytic choriomeningitis virus-induced autoimmune anemia and hypergammaglobulinemia. J. Autoimmun. 7, 589–599.

Coutelier, J.-P., Detalle, L., Musaji, A., Meite, M., Izui, S., 2007. Two-step mechanism of virus-induced autoimmune hemolytic anemia. Ann. N.Y. Acad. Sci. 1109, 151–157.

Crosby, W.H., Rappaport, H., 1956. Reticulocytopenia in autoimmune hemolytic anemia. Blood. 11, 926–936.

Crowther, M., Chan, Y.L., Garbett, I.K., Lim, W., Vickers, M.A., Crowther, M.A., 2011. Evidence-based focused review of the treatment of idiopathic warm immune hemolytic anemia in adults. Blood. 118, 4036–4040.

da Silveira, S.A., Kikuchi, S., Fossati-Jimack, L., Moll, T., Saito, T., Verbeek, J.S., et al., 2002. Complement activation selectively potentiates the pathogenicity of the IgG2b and IgG3 isotypes of a high affinity anti-erythrocyte autoantibody. J. Exp. Med. 195, 665–672.

Dausset, J., Colombani, J., 1959. The serology and prognosis of 128 cases of autoimmune hemolytic anemia. Blood. 14, 1280–1301.

Day, M.J., Russell, J., Kitwood, A.J., Ponsford, M., Elson, C.J., 1989. Expression and regulation of erythrocyte auto-antibodies in mice following immunization with rat erythrocytes. Eur. J. Immunol. 19, 795–801.

de Sá Oliveira, G.G., Izui, S., Ravirajan, C.T., Mageed, R.A.K., Lydyard, P.M., Elson, C.J., et al., 1996. Diverse antigen specificity of erythrocyte-reactive monoclonal autoantibodies from NZB mice. Clin. Exp. Immunol. 10, 313–320.

Dearden, C., Wade, R., Else, M., Richards, S., Milligan, D., Hamblin, T., et al., 2008. The prognostic significance of a positive direct antiglobulin test in chronic lymphocytic leukemia, a beneficial effect of the combination of fludarabine and cyclophosphamide on the incidence of hemolytic anemia. Blood. 111, 1820–1826.

Dellagi, K., Brouet, J.C., Schenmetzler, C., Praloran, V., 1981. Chronic hemolytic anemia due to a monoclonal IgG cold agglutinin with anti-Pr specificity. Blood. 57, 189–191.

Dixon, P.M., Matthews, A.G., Brown, R., Millar, P.M., Ritchie, J.S.D., 1978. Bovine auto-immune haemolytic anaemia. Vet. Rec. 103, 155–157.

Donath, J., Landsteiner, K., 1904. Ueber paroxysmale Hämoglobinurie. Munch. Med. Wochenschr. 51, 1590–1593.

Elson, C.J., Barker, R.N., 2000. Helper T cells in antibody-mediated, organ specific autoimmunity. Curr. Opin. Immunol. 12, 664–669.

Elson, C.J., Barker, R.N., Thompson, S.J., Williams, N.A., 1995. Immunologically ignorant T-cells, epitope spreading and repertoire limitation. Immunol. Today. 1, 71–76.

Engelfriet, C.P., Von dem Borne, A.E.G.Kr., Beckers, D., Van der Meulen, F.W., Fleer, A., Roos, D., et al., 1981. Immune destruction of red cells. Seminar on Immune Mediated Cell Destruction. American Association of Blood Banks, Washington DC, pp. 93–130.

Fossati-Jimack, L., Reininger, L., Chicheportiche, Y., Clynes, R., Ravetch, J.V., Honjo, T., et al., 1999. High pathogenic potential of low-affinity autoantibodies in experimental autoimmune hemolytic anemia. J. Exp. Med. 190, 1689–1696.

Fox, R.R., Meier, H., Crary, D.D., Norberg, R.F., Myers, D.D., 1971. Hemolytic anemia associated with thymoma in the rabbit. Genetic studies and pathological findings. Oncology. 25, 372–382.

Frank, M.M., Hamburger, M.I., Lawley, T.J., Kimberley, R.P., Plotz, P.H., 1979. Defective reticuloendothelial system Fc-receptor function in systemic lupus erythematosus. N. Eng. J. Med. 300, 518.

Freedman, J., Ho, M., Barefoot, C., 1982. Red blood cell-bound C3d in selected hospital patients. Transfusion. 22, 515–520.

Freedman, J., Wright, J., Lim, F.C., Garvey, M.B., 1987. Hemolytic warm IgM autoagglutinins in autoimmune hemolytic anemia. Transfusion. 27, 464–467.

Fries, L.F., Brickman, C.M., Frank, M.M., 1983. Monocyte receptors for the Fc portion of IgG increase in number in autoimmune hemolytic anemia and other hemolytic states and are decreased by glucocorticoid therapy. J. Immunol. 131, 1240–1245.

Garratty, G., 1983. Mechanisms of immune red cell destruction, and red cell compatability testing. Hum. Pathol. 14, 204–212.

Garratty, G., 1989. Factors affecting the pathogenicity of red cell autoantibodies and alloantibodies. In: Nance, S.J. (Ed.), Immune Destruction of Red Blood Cells. American Association of Blood Banks, Arlington, Virginia, pp. 109–169.

Garratty, G., 1990. Predicting the clinical significance of red cell antibodies with *in vitro* cellular assays. Transfus. Med. Rev. IV, 297–312.

Garratty, G., 2010. Immune hemolytic anemia associated with drug therapy. Blood Rev. 24, 143–150.

Garratty, G., Nance, S.J., 1990. Correlation between *in vivo* hemolysis and the amount of red cell-bound IgG measured by flow cytometry. Transfusion. 30, 617–621.

Griffiths, H.L., Kumpel, B.M., Elson, C.J., Hadley, AG., 1994. The functional activity of human monocytes passively sensitized with monoclonal anti-D suggests a novel role for Fc gamma RI in the immune destruction of blood cells. Immunology. 83, 370–377.

Hadley, A.G., Zupanska, B., Kumpel, B.M., Pilkington, C., Griffiths, H.L., Leader, K.A., et al., 1995. The glycosylation of red cell autoantibodies affects their functional activity *in vitro*. Br. J. Haematol. 91, 587–594.

Hall, A.M., Stott, L.-M., Wilson, D.W.L., Urbaniak, S.J., Barker, R.N., 1999. Different epitopes are targeted by helper T-cells responding to the same human protein as an autoantigen or foreign antigen. J. Autoimmun. 27, 80.

Hall, A.M., Ward, F.J., Vickers, M.A., Stott, L-M., Urbaniak, S.J., Barker, R.N., 2002. Interleukin-10 mediated regulatory T-cell responses to epitopes on a human red blood cell autoantigen. Blood. 100, 4529–4536.

Hall, A.M., Vickers, M.A., McLeod, E., Barker, R.N., 2005. Rh autoantigen presentation to helper T cells in chronic lymphocytic leukemia by malignant B-cells. Blood. 105, 2007–2015.

Hall, A.M., Shen, C-R, Ward, F.J., Rowe, C., Bowie, L., Devine, A., et al., 2007. Deletion of the dominant autoantigen in NZB mice with autoimmune hemolytic anemia: effects on autoantibody and T-helper responses. Blood. 110, 4511–4517.

Hall, A.M., Zamzami, O.M., Whibley, N., Hampsey, D.P., Haggart, A. M., Vickers, M.A., et al., 2012. Production of the effector cytokine interleukin-17, rather than interferon-γ, is more strongly associated with autoimmune hemolytic anemia. Hematologica. Epub ahead of Print.

Heddle, N.M., Kelton, J.G., Turchyn, K.L., Ali, M.A., 1988. Hypergammaglobulinemia can be associated with a positive direct antiglobulin test, a nonreactive eluate, and no evidence of hemolysis. Transfusion. 28, 29–33.

Helyer, B.J., Howie, J.B., 1963. Spontaneous auto-immune disease in NZB/B1 mice. Br. J. Haematol. 9, 119–131.

Hernandez-Jodra, M., Hudnall, S.D., Petz, L.D., 1990. Studies of in vitro red cell autoantibody production in normal donors and in patients with autoimmune hemolytic anemia. Transfusion. 30, 411–417.

Hoyer, K.K., Kuswanto, W.F., Gallo, E., Abbas, A.K., 2009. Distinct roles of helper T-cell subsets in a systemic autoimmune disease. Blood. 113, 389–395.

Huh, Y.O., Liu, F.J., Rogge, K., Chakrabarty, L., Lichtiger, B., 1988. Positive direct antiglobulin test and high serum immunoglobulin G values. Am. J. Clin. Pathol. 90, 197–200.

Jenkins, W.J., Marsh, W.J., Noades, J., Tippett, P., Sanger, R., Race, R. R., 1960. The I antigen and antibody. Vox Sang. 5, 97–121.

Kaplan, A.V., Quimby, F.W., 1983. A radiolabelled staphylococcal protein A assay for detection of anti-erythrocyte IgG in warm agglutinin autoimmune hemolytic anemia in dogs and man. Vet. Immunol. Immunopathol. 4, 307–317.

Kay, M.M., Marchalonis, J.J., Hughes, J., Watanabe, K., Schluter, S.F., 1990. Definition of a physiologic aging autoantigen by using synthetic peptides of membrane protein band 3: localization of the active antigenic sites. Proc. Natl. Acad. Sci. U.S.A. 87, 5734–5738.

Kelsoe, G., 1995. The germinal center reaction. Immunol. Today. 16, 324–326.

Kelton, J.G., 1985. Impaired reticuloendothelial function in patients treated with methyldopa. N. Engl. J. Med. 313, 596–600.

Kelton, J.G., Singer, J., Rodger, C., Gauldie, J., Horsewood, P., Dent, P., 1985. The concentration of IgG in the serum is a major determinant of Fc-dependent reticuloendothelial function. Blood. 66, 490–495.

Kikuchi, S., Santiago-Raber, M.L., Amano, H., Amano, E., Fossati-Jimack, L., Moll, T., et al., 2006. Contribution of NZB autoimmunity 2 to Y-linked autoimmune acceleration-induced monocytosis in association with murine systemic lupus. J. Immunol. 176, 3240–3247.

Kirtland, H.H., Mohler, D.N., Horwitz, D.A., 1980. Methyldopa inhibition of suppressor-lymphocyte function. A proposed cause of autoimmune hemolytic anemia. N. Engl. J. Med. 302, 825–832.

Krych-Goldberg, M., Atkinson, J.P., 2001. Structure-function relationships of complement receptor type 1. Immunol. Rev. 180, 112–122.

Kurlander, R.J., Rosse, W.F., Logue, G.L., 1978. Quantitative influence of antibody and complement coating of red cells in monocyte-mediated cell lysis. J. Clin. Invest. 61, 1309–1319.

Landsteiner, K., Levine, P., 1926. On the cold agglutinins in human serum. J. Immunol. 12, 441–460.

Leddy, J.P., Falany, J.L., Kissel, G.E., Passador, S.T., Rosenfeld, S.I., 1993. Erythrocyte membrane proteins reactive with human (warm reacting) anti-red cell autoantibodies. J. Clin. Invest. 91, 1672–1680.

Lee, N.J., Rigby, R.J., Gill, H., Boyle, J.J., Fossati-Jimack, L., Morley, B.J., et al., 2004. Multiple loci are linked with anti-red blood cell antibody production in NZB mice—comparison with other phenotypes implies complex modes of action. Clin. Exp. Immunol. 138, 39–46.

Lefrere, J.-J., Courouce, A.-M., Bertrand, Y., Girot, R., Soulier, J.-P., 1986. Human parvovirus and aplastic crisis in chronic hemolytic anemias: a study of 24 observations. Am. J. Hematol. 23, 271–275.

Lessard, C.J., Ice, J.A., Adrianto, I., Wiley, G.B., Kelly, J.A., Gaffney, P.M., et al., 2012. The genomics of autoimmune disease in the era of genome-wide association studies and beyond. Autoimmun. Rev. 11, 267–275.

Liesveld, J.L., Rowe, J.M., Lichtman, M.A., 1987. Variability of the erythropoietic response in autoimmune hemolytic anemia. Analysis of 109 cases. Blood. 69, 820–826.

Lippman, S.M., Arnett, F.C., Conley, C.L., Ness, P.M., Meyers, D.A., Bias, W.B., 1982. Genetic factors predisposing to autoimmune diseases: autoimmune hemolytic anemia, chronic thrombocytopenic purpura and systemic lupus erythematosus. Am. J. Med. 73, 827–840.

Loutit, J.F., Mollison, P.L., 1946. Haemolytic icterus (acholuric jaundice), congenital and acquired. J. Pathol. Bacteriol. 58, 711–728.

Lutz, H.U., Wipf, G., 1982. Naturally occurring autoantibodies to skeletal proteins from human red blood cells. J. Immunol. 128, 1695–1699.

Mair, T.S., Taylor, F.G.R., Hillyer, M.H., 1990. Autoimmune haemolytic anaemia in eight horses. Vet. Rec. 126, 51–53.

Malhotra, R., Wormald, M.R., Rudd, P.M., Fischer, T.B., Dwek, R.A., Sims, R.B., 1995. Alterations in glycosylation of IgG associated with rheumatoid arthritis; activating complement via the mannose binding protein. Nat. Med. 1, 237–243.

Marsh, W.L., Jenkins, W.J., 1960. Anti-i, a new cold antibody. Nature. 188, 753.

Mazza, G., el Idrissi, M.E., Coutelier, J.P., Corato, A., Elson, C.J., Pfau, C.J., et al., 1997. Infection of C3HeB/FeJ mice with the docile strain of lymphocytic choriomeningitis virus induces autoantibodies specific for erythrocyte Band 3. Immunology. 91, 239–245.

Mittal, S., Blaylock, M., Culligan, D.J., Barker, R.N., Vickers, M.A., 2008. A high rate of "CLL phenotype" lymphocytes in autoimmune hemolytic anemia and immune thrombocytopenic purpura. Haematologica. 93, 151–152.

Mollison, P.L., 1959. Measurement of survival and destruction of red cells in haemolytic syndromes. Br. Med. Bull. 15, 59–66.

Mollison, P.L., Hughes-Jones, N.C., 1967. Clearance of Rh-positive red cells by low concentrations of Rh antibody. Immunology. 12, 63–73.

Mqadmi, A., Zheng, X., Yazdanbakhsh, K., 2005. CD4 + CD25 + regulatory T cells control induction of autoimmune hemolytic anemia. Blood. 105, 3746–3748.

Murakami, M., Tsubata, T., Okamoto, M., Shimizu, A., Kumagai, S., Imura, H., et al., 1992. Antigen-induced apoptotic death of Ly-1 B cells responsible for autoimmune disease in transgenic mice. Nature. 357, 77–80.

Naysmith, J.D., Ortega-Pierres, M.G., Elson, C.J., 1981. Rat erythrocyte-induced anti-erythrocyte autoantibody production and control in normal mice. Immunol. Rev. 55, 55–87.

Nicholson-Weller, A., Burge, J., Fearon, D.T., Weller, P.F., Austen, K. F., 1982. Isolation of a human erythrocyte membrane glycoprotein with decay accelerating activity for C_3 convertases of the human complement system. J. Immunol. 129, 184–189.

Nimmerjahn, F., Ravetch, J.V., 2008. Fcgamma receptors as regulators of immune responses. Nat. Rev. Immunol. 8, 34–47.

Olanoff, L.S., Fudenberg, H.H., 1983. Familial autoimmunity. Twenty years later. J. Clin. Lab. Immunol. 11, 105–111.

Oliveira, G.G., Hutchings, P.R., Roitt, I.M., Lydyard, P.M., 1994. Production of erythrocyte autoantibodies in NZB mice is inhibited by CD4 antibodies. Clin. Exp. Immunol. 96, 297–302.

Owens, N.A., Hui, H.L., Green, F.A., 1982. Induction of direct Coombs positivity with alpha-methyldopa in chimpanzees. J. Med. 13, 473–477.

Packman, C.H., 2008. Hemolytic anemia due to warm autoantibodies. Blood Rev. 22, 17–31.

Pantaleo, A., Giribaldi, G., Mannu, F., Arese, P., Turrini, F., 2008. Naturally occurring anti-Band 3 antibodies and red blood cell removal under physiological and pathological conditions. Autoimmun. Rev. 7, 457–462.

Peñalver, F.J., Alvarez-Larrán, A., Díez-Martin, J.L., Gallur, L., Jarque, I., Caballero, D., et al., 2010. Multi-institutional retrospective study on the use of rituximab in refractory AIHA. Rituximab is an effective and safe therapeutic alternative in adults with refractory and severe autoimmune hemolytic anemia. Ann. Hematol. 89, 1073–1080.

Perry, F.E., Barker, R.N., Mazza, G., Day, M.J., Wells, A.D., Shen, C.-R., et al., 1996. Autoreactive T-cell specificity in autoimmune hemolytic anemia of the NZB mouse. Eur. J. Immunol. 2, 136–141.

Petz, L.D., 2008. Cold antibody autoimmune hemolytic anemias. Blood Rev. 22, 1–15.

Petz, L.D., Garratty, G., 2004a. Classification and characteristics of autoimmune hemolytic anemias. In: Petz, L.D., Garratty., G. (Eds) Immune Hemolytic Anemias, second ed. Churchill Livingstone, Philadelphia, pp. 61–131.

Petz, L.D., Garratty, G. 2004b. Mechanisms of immune hemolysis. In: Petz, L.D., Garratty., G. (Eds) Immune Hemolytic Anemias, second ed. Churchill Livingstone, Philadelphia, pp. 133–165.

Pirofsky, B., 1968. Hereditary aspects of autoimmune hemolytic anemia. A retrospective analysis. Vox Sang. 14, 334–347.

Pirofsky, B., 1976. Clinical aspects of autoimmune hemolytic anemia. Semin. Hematol. 13, 251–265.

Playfair, J.H.L., Marshall-Clarke, S., 1973. Induction of red cell autoantibodies in normal mice. Nat. New Biol. 243, 213–214.

Pollock, J.G., Fenton, E., Barrett, K.E., 1970. Familial autoimmune haemolytic anaemia associated with rheumatoid arthritis and pernicious anaemia. Br. J. Haematol. 18, 171–182.

Pritchard, N.R., Cutler, A.J., Uribe, S., Chadban, S.J., Morley, B.J., Smith, K.G., 2000. Autoimmune-prone mice share a promoter haplotype associated with reduced expression and function of the Fc receptor FcgammaRII. Curr. Biol. 10, 227–230.

Roncarolo, M.G., Gregori, S., Battaglia, M., Bacchetta, R., Fleischhauer, K., Levings, M.K., 2006. Interleukin-10-secreting type 1 regulatory T cells in rodents and humans. Immunol. Rev. 212, 28–50.

Ross, G.D., Medof, M.E., 1985. Membrane complement receptors specific for bound fragments of C_3. Adv. Immunol. 37, 217–267.

Rosse, W.F., 1971. Quantitative immunology of immune hemolytic anemia. II. The relationship of cell-bound antibody to hemolysis and the effect of treatment. J. Clin. Invest. 50, 734–743.

Ruiz-Argüelles, A., Llorente, L., 2007. The role of complement regulatory proteins (CD55 and CD59) in the pathogenesis of autoimmune hemocytopenias. Autoimmun. Rev. 6, 155–161.

Sakaguchi, S., Miyara, M., Costantino, C.M., Hafler, D.A., 2010. FOXP3 + regulatory T cells in the human immune system. Nat. Rev. Immunol. 10, 490–500.

Scatizzi, J.C., Haraldsson, M.K., Pollard, K.M., Theofilopoulos, A.N., Kono, D.H., 2012. The Lbw2 locus promotes autoimmune hemolytic anemia. J. Immunol. 188, 3307–3314.

Shen, C.-R., Mazza, G., Perry, F.E., Beech, J.T., Thompson, S.J., Corato, A., et al., 1996. T-helper 1 dominated responses to erythrocyte Band 3 in NZB mice. Immunology. 8, 195–199.

Shen, C.-R., Youssef, A-R., Devine, A., Bowie, L., Hall, A.M., Wraith, D.C., et al., 2003. Peptides containing a dominant T-cell epitope from red cell Band 3 have in vivo immunomodulatory properties in NZB mice with autoimmune hemolytic anemia. Blood. 102, 3800–3806.

Shevach, E.M., 2011. Biological functions of regulatory T cells. Adv. Immunol. 112, 137–176.

Shoenfeld, Y., Isenberg, D.A., 1989. The mosaic of autoimmunity. Immunol. Today. 10, 123–126.

Shoenfeld, Y., Schwartz, R.S., 1984. Immunologic and genetic factors in autoimmune diseases. N. Engl. J. Med. 311, 1019–1029.

Silberstein, L.E., Robertson, G.A., Harris, A.C., Moreau, L., Besa, E., Nowell, P.C., 1986. Etiologic aspects of cold agglutinin disease, Evidence for cytogenetically defined clones of lymphoid cells and the demonstration that an anti-Pr cold autoantibody is derived from a chromosomally aberrant B cell clone. Blood. 67, 1705–1709.

Sokol, R.J., Hewitt, S., 1985. Autoimmune hemolysis. A critical review. CRC Crit. Rev. Oncol. Hematol. 4, 125–154.

Sokol, R.J., Hewitt, S., Stamps, B.K., 1981. Autoimmune haemolysis: an 18-year study of 865 cases referred to a regional transfusion centre. Br. Med. J. 282, 2023–2027.

Sokol, R.J., Hewitt, S., Stamps, B.K., 1982. Autoimmune haemolysis associated with Donath-Landsteiner antibodies. Acta Haemat. 68, 268–277.

Sokol, R.J., Hewitt, S., Stamps, B.K., 1983. Autoimmune haemolysis. Mixed warm and cold antibody type. Acta Haemat. 69, 266–274.

Sokol, R.J., Hewitt, S., Stamps, B.K., Hitchen, P.A., 1984. Autoimmune haemolysis in childhood and adolescence. Acta Haemat. 72, 245–257.

Sokol, R.J., Hewitt, S., Booker, D.J., Stamps, R., 1985. Enzyme linked direct antiglobulin tests in patients with autoimmune haemolysis. J. Clin. Pathol. 38, 912–914.

Sokol, R.J., Hewitt, S., Booker, D.J., Stamps, R., Booth, J.R., 1988. An enzyme-linked direct antiglobulin test for assessing erythrocyte bound immunoglobulins. J. Immunol. Meth. 106, 31–35.

Sokol, R.J., Hewitt, S., Booker, D.J., Bailey, A., 1990a. Erythrocyte autoantibodies, subclasses of IgG and autoimmune haemolysis. Autoimmunity. 6, 99–104.

Sokol, R.J., Hewitt, S., Booker, D.J., Bailey, A., 1990b. Erythrocyte autoantibodies, multiple immunoglobulin classes and autoimmune haemolysis. Transfusion. 30, 714–717.

Sokol, R.J., Booker, D.J., Stamps, R., 1992. The pathology of autoimmune haemolytic anaemia. J. Clin. Pathol. 45, 1047–1052.

Sokol, R.J., Booker, D.J., Stamps, R., 1999. Erythropoiesis: paroxysmal cold haemoglobinuria, a clinico-pathological study of patients with a positive Donath-Landsteiner test. Hematology. 4, 137–164.

Stott, L.-M., Urbaniak, S.J., Barker, R.N., 2002. Specific production of regulatory T-cell cytokines, responsiveness to the RhD blood group, and expression of HLA-DRB1*15. Immunology. 107, 6.

Switzer, J.W., Jain, N.C., 1981. Autoimmune hemolytic anemia in dogs and cats. Vet. Clin. North Am. Small Anim. Pract. 11, 405–420.

Talal, N., Ahmed, S.A., 1987. Immunomodulation by hormones—an area of growing importance. J. Rheumatol. 14, 191–193.

Talor, E., Rose, N.R., 1991. Hypothesis. The aging paradox and autoimmune disease. Autoimmunity. 8, 245–249.

Tomer, Y., Shoenfeld, Y., 1988. Ageing and autoantibodies. Autoimmunity. 1, 141–149.

Urbaniak, S.J., Griess, M.A., 1980. ADCC (K-cell) lysis of human erythrocytes sensitized with Rhesus alloantibodies. III. Comparison of IgG anti-D agglutinating and lytic (ADCC) activity and the role of IgG subclasses. Br. J. Haematol. 46, 447–453.

Van der Meulen, F.W., De Bruin, H.G., Goosen, P.C.M., Bruynes, E.C.E., Joustra-Maas, C.J., Telkamp, H.G., et al., 1980. Quantitative aspects of the destruction of red cells sensitized with IgG1 autoantibodies. An application of flow cytometry. Br. J. Haematol. 46, 47–56.

Victoria, E.J., Pierce, S.W., Branks, M.J., Masouredis, S.P., 1990. IgG red blood cell autoantibodies in autoimmune hemolytic anemia bind to epitopes on red blood cell membrane band 3 glycoprotein. J. Lab. Clin. Med. 115, 74–88.

Ward, F.J., Hall, A.M., Cairns, L.S., Leggat, A.S., Urbaniak, S.J., Vickers, M.A., et al., 2008. Clonal regulatory T cells specific for a red blood cell autoantigen in human autoimmune hemolytic anemia. Blood. 111, 680–687.

Weiner, W., Vos, G.H., 1963. Serology of acquired hemolytic anemias. Blood. 22, 606–613.

Wiener, E., Hughes-Jones, N.C., Irish, W.T., Wickramasinghe, S.N., 1986. Elution of antispectrin antibodies from red cells in homozygous β-thalassaemia. Clin. Exp. Immunol. 63, 680–686.

Win, N., Islam, S.I., Peterkin, M.A., Walker, I.D., 1997. Positive direct antiglobulin test due to antiphospholipid antibodies in normal healthy blood donors. Vox Sang. 72, 182–184.

Youssef, A.R., Shen, C-R., Lin, C.-L., Barker, R.N., Elson, C.J., 2005. IL-4 and IL-10 modulate autoimmune haemolytic anaemia in NZB mice. Clin. Exp. Immunol. 139, 84–89.

Zecca, M., Nobili, B., Ramenghi, U., Perrotta, S., Amendola, G., Rosito, P., et al., 2003. Rituximab for the treatment of refractory autoimmune hemolytic anemia in children. Blood. 101, 3857–3861.

Chapter 47

Immune Thrombocytopenia

Berengere Gruson[1] and James B. Bussel[2]

[1]Department of Hematology, Centre Hospitalier Universitaire d'Amiens, Amiens, France, [2]Departments of Pediatrics, Medicine, and Obstetrics and Gynecology, New York Presbyterian Hospital, Weill Cornell Medical Center, New York, NY, USA

Chapter Outline

Clinical, Pathologic, and Epidemiologic Features 663
General Features and Definitions 663
Diagnosis 664
Epidemiology and Clinical Presentation in Children 664
Epidemiology and Clinical Presentation in Adults 665
Autoimmune Features 665
Autoimmune Markers in Primary ITP 665
Antiphospholipid Antibodies 665
Antinuclear Antibodies 665
Antithyroid Antibodies 666
Evans Syndrome 666
ITP Secondary to Systemic Lupus Erythematosus 666
ITP Secondary to Primary Immunodeficiencies 666
Common Variable Immunodeficiency 666
Autoimmune Lymphoproliferative Syndrome 667
Wiskott–Aldrich Syndrome/X-linked
Thrombocytopenia 667
Velocardiofacial/DiGeorge Syndrome 667
Genetics Features 667

Familial ITP 667
Genetic Markers of ITP 667
In Vivo Models 668
Pathologic Effector Mechanisms 668
Increased Platelet Destruction 668
Antibody-Mediated Platelet Destruction 668
T Cell-Mediated Cytotoxicity and NK Cell Activity 669
Insufficient Platelet Production 669
Anomalies of Megakaryopoiesis 669
Serum Levels of Thrombopoietin (TPO) 669
Effect of Antiplatelet Antibodies on
Megakaryocytopoiesis 670
Infection-related Thrombocytopenia 670
Molecular Mimicry 670
Mechanisms other than Molecular Mimicry 670
Autoantibodies as Potential Immunologic Markers 670
Concluding Remarks—Future Prospects 671
References 672

CLINICAL, PATHOLOGIC, AND EPIDEMIOLOGIC FEATURES

General Features and Definitions

Immune thrombocytopenia (ITP) is an autoimmune acquired disease of adults and children characterized by transient or persistent thrombocytopenia resulting in a risk of bleeding. Antibody-mediated platelet destruction in the spleen has been the prevailing hypothesis to explain the pathogenesis of ITP; however, more and more data lend support to the notion that cell-mediated destruction of platelets as well as suppression of platelet production by autoantibodies and possibly T cells also contributes to an insufficient number of platelets (Cines et al., 2009).

Recent recommendations from an international working group defined that a platelet count less than 100 g/L is required for diagnosis and defined new categories of ITP based on disease duration. They proposed to avoid the term "acute ITP" and to use instead the term "newly diagnosed" for all patients at diagnosis, "persistent" for disease lasting between 3 and 12 months, and "chronic" if ITP lasts more than 12 months (Rodeghiero et al., 2009). ITP can be further characterized as being either primary or secondary to several associated disorders such as immunodeficiency diseases, autoimmune disorders, lymphoproliferative diseases, and certain infections. Finally, "severe" requires bleeding irrespective of the platelet count and "refractory" requires a failure to respond to splenectomy; the latter is not agreed upon for pediatric patients.

N. Rose & I. Mackay (Eds): The Autoimmune Diseases, Fifth edition. DOI: http://dx.doi.org/10.1016/B978-0-12-384929-8.00047-2

Diagnosis

Primary ITP remains a diagnosis of exclusion from both non-autoimmune causes of thrombocytopenia and secondary causes of ITP (Table 47.1). Distinguishing primary from secondary ITP and from, for example, inherited thrombocytopenia, is important because of different natural history and treatment.

TABLE 47.1 Differential Diagnosis of Primary ITP

Non-Autoimmune Causes of Thrombocytopenia	
Pseudo-Thrombocytopenia	
Decrease of platelets production	Inherited thrombocytopenia:
	Bone marrow disorders (e.g., MDS, myelofibrosis)
	Folate or vitamin B12 deficiency
	Ethanol toxicity
	Certain viral infections
Decrease of platelets survival	Thrombotic thrombocytopenic purpura
	Disseminated intravascular coagulation
	Certain drugs
	Alloimmune thrombocytopenias (e.g., post-transfusion purpura)
	Cardiopulmonary bypass
Splenic sequestration	Portal hypertension
	Infiltrative diseases of the spleen
Dilutional Thrombocytopenia	
Secondary Causes of ITP	
Viral infections	HIV, HCV, EBV
Bacterial infection	*Helicobacter pylori* infection
Autoimmune diseases including	Systemic lupus erythematosus
	Autoimmune thyroiditis
Immunodeficiency disorders	CVID
	ALPS
Lymphoproliferative disorders	CLL
	Lymphoma
Vaccination	Measles-mumps-rubella vaccine
Drugs	

MDS, myelodysplastic syndrome; CVID, common variable immunodeficiency; ALPS, autoimmune lymphoproliferative syndrome; CLL, chronic lymphocyte leukemia.

Recommendations for the diagnosis of primary ITP in children and adults include a study of familial and patient history, a physical examination that should be normal aside from bleeding manifestations, and a complete blood count that should reveal isolated thrombocytopenia with normal white and red blood cell numbers. A peripheral blood smear is also mandatory (1) to exclude schistocytes or abnormalities in blood cell morphology that may suggest an underlying bone marrow (BM) disorder such as myelodysplastic syndrome or a congenital cause of thrombocytopenia and (2) to exclude hemolysis by absence of polychromasia if a reticulocyte count is not obtained. It is generally considered that a BM examination must be performed if a patient is older than 60 years, in case a bone marrow disorder is being considered, or in patients planning to undergo splenectomy (George et al., 1996). Detection of *Helicobacter pylori* (HP) infection has been proposed in adults preferably with the urea breath test or the stool antigen test (Stasi et al., 2009). Serologic evaluation for HIV and HCV infection should be performed. Other recommended tests are quantitative immunoglobulin level testing, direct antiglobulin test (DAT), and blood group Rh(D) typing (important if anti-D immunoglobulin is being considered). Several other tests such as antiplatelet antibody assays (glycoprotein-specific antibody testing), antiphospholipid antibodies, antinuclear antibodies, antithyroid antibody, thyroid function testing or viral PCR for parvovirus, EBV, and CMV have potential utility but are not systematically required for the differential diagnosis and management of ITP (Provan et al., 2010).

Epidemiology and Clinical Presentation in Children

Recent epidemiologic studies in childhood ITP demonstrated an incidence of four to five cases per 100,000 children under 15 years of age per year with a prevalence of males (Zeller et al., 2000, 2005; Kühne et al., 2001; Watts, 2004; Segal and Powe, 2006).

The peak age of presentation of ITP in children is between 5 and 6 years, with 70% of cases presenting between ages of 1 and 10 years (Kühne et al., 2003). Approximately two-thirds of children with ITP had a preceding febrile illness due to viral infections (including rubella, varicella, mumps, and EBV) or immunizations with measles-mumps-rubella vaccine (France et al., 2008).

Affected children generally have a good prognosis and the majority of patients had no or mild mucocutaneous bleeding at diagnosis (Neunert et al., 2008). Intracranial hemorrhage is the most severe complication of childhood ITP and the primary cause of death but its incidence is very low, estimated at 0.125% to 0.5 childhood ITP (Lilleyman, 1994; Psaila et al., 2009).

Approximately 50–70% of children remit within 6 to 12 months (Kühne et al., 2003; Bennett and Tarantino, 2009), with improvement in others. Children who develop chronic ITP tend to be older, are more often female, and usually present with a higher platelet count while another predictor of chronic disease seems to be insidious onset of symptoms (Watts, 2004; Zeller et al., 2005).

Epidemiology and Clinical Presentation in Adults

Estimates of the incidence of adult ITP range from approximately 1.5 to 4 patients per 100,000 person-years depending on the threshold of platelet count used for the diagnosis. The incidence of ITP women is slightly higher compared to men, particularly in middle-aged adults. The disease incidence appears to increase with age with the absence of gender difference among older patients (Neylon et al., 2003; Schoonen et al., 2009). Mucocutaneous bleeding (petechiae, epistaxis, and gum bleeding) is the most common initial manifestation of ITP and the platelet count is predictive of more serious bleeding but not alone sufficient. Patients with platelet counts below 10×10^9/L are at risk for severe bleeding, such as intracranial hemorrhage or other internal bleeding while intracranial hemorrhage is rare in patients with platelet counts above 20×10^9/L. Bleeding risk is higher in older patients and those with a prior history of bleeding. However, propensity to bleed remains markedly heterogeneous between patients and even between different times in the same patient. The risk of bleeding and fatal hemorrhage in adults with severe chronic ITP, defined as a platelet count of 30×10^9/L at least 1 year after diagnosis, was analyzed by Cohen et al. using data from 17 adult case studies. They assessed the rate of fatal hemorrhage to be 0.0162 to 0.0389 cases per adult patient-year at risk and age-adjusted rates were 0.004, 0.012, and 0.130 cases per patient-year for age groups younger than 40, 40 to 60, and older than 60 years, respectively (Cohen et al., 2000). Michel et al. confirmed in a case–control study that ITP patients aged over 70 have an increased risk of bleeding and to a lesser extent a higher risk of some treatment-induced side effects (Michel et al., 2011). This greater risk of bleeding could be partially explained by the higher proportion of elderly patients taking anticoagulants or aspirin and also by the higher rate of comorbidities such as hypertension or renal failure. Adult patients with chronic ITP may have spontaneous, clinically significant (although not necessarily complete) remissions in 5–11% of cases (Neylon et al., 2003; Bizzoni et al., 2006).

AUTOIMMUNES FEATURES

Autoimmune Markers in Primary ITP

The 2010 international consensus report on the investigation and management of primary immune thrombocytopenia does not recommend researching systematically autoimmune markers. The panel considered that checking for the presence of antiphospholipid antibodies (aPLs), antinuclear antibodies (ANA), or antithyroid antibodies (ATA) does not belong to the basic evaluation but could be of potential utility in the management of certain ITP patients (Provan et al., 2010). We could, however, discuss the studies that support these conclusions.

Antiphospholipid Antibodies

Nearly half of ITP patients had either anticardiolipin antibodies (aCLs) and/or lupus anticoagulant (LA) at the time of diagnosis but the presence of these antibodies was not associated with sex, age, platelet count, or the severity of hemorrhages. The presence of aPLs does not appear to affect the response to ITP treatment (Stasi et al., 1994). Whether the presence of aPLs increases the incidence of thrombotic events is controversial (Diz-Kucukkaya, 2001). However, it seems that detection of LA emerged as a stronger risk factor for thrombosis than detection of aCLs (Diz-Kucukkaya, 2001). It seems reasonable to believe that patients with LA and ITP who have reached, after treatment, a normal platelet count may have a higher risk of developing thrombosis than the general population (Liebman and Stasi, 2007). The role of anti-beta2-GPI has not been well studied in ITP. One single study reported that significantly higher anti-beta2-GPI (IgG) mean concentrations occurred in chronic ITP cases compared with acute or control cases and that these increased IgG concentrations significantly correlated with steroid therapy resistance. But we do not know if anti-beta2-GPI may be a determinant cofactor for the developing risk of antiphospholipid syndrome or autoimmune diseases in ITP (El-Bostany et al., 2008).

Antinuclear Antibodies

ANA positivity is found in approximately 30% of adult and child patients with ITP but the detection of ANA positivity is insufficient to identify those patients with ITP who are at risk of developing systemic lupus erythematosus (SLE). Kurata et al. prospectively followed 66 adult patients with chronic ITP over 3 years. Twenty-nine of the 66 patients had a positive ANA, and throughout the period of follow-up none of these patients developed SLE (Kurata et al., 1994). However, ANA positivity may be an indicator of chronicity for childhood ITP as there is a statistically significant difference in terms of ANA positivity between childhood acute and chronic ITP patients (Pratt et al., 2005; Altintas et al., 2007).

Antithyroid Antibodies

About 10% of ITP patients develop clinical hyperthyroidism during the follow-up (Liebman, 2007). It may also be useful to measure ATA and thyroid-stimulating hormone (TSH) at ITP diagnosis to identify a subclinical thyroid disease (Cheung and Liebman, 2009). Isolated ATA positivity is found in about 15% of childhood ITP (Pratt et al., 2005), but this is complicated because there is a 5–10% incidence of markers of thyroid disease (primarily ATA) in otherwise healthy young women. The literature is not clear about whether screening for ATA in ITP patients would identify a patient population at greater risk of developing a thyroid disease.

Evans Syndrome

Although we can find a positive direct antiglobulin test (DAT), without hemolytic anemia, in approximately 20% of patients with ITP (Aledort et al., 2004), its clinical significance is unknown. Evans syndrome (ES) is an autoimmune disorder defined by the simultaneous or sequential development of ITP and autoimmune hemolytic anemia (AIHA) with a positive DAT and/or immune neutropenia in the absence of known underlying etiology (Evans et al., 1951). The development of the second cytopenia may occur months to years after the first immune cytopenia and may delay diagnosis of Evans syndrome (Mathew et al., 1997). Michel et al. retrospectively analyzed the data from 68 ES adults. The mean age at time of first cytopenia was 52 years with 60% of women. Both cytopenias occurred simultaneously in 54.5% of cases. ES was considered as "primary" in 50% of cases but was associated with an underlying disorder in half of the cases, including mainly SLE, lymphoproliferative disorders, and common variable immunodeficiency (Michel et al., 2009). ES is characterized by recurrent episodes of relapse and remission of both ITP and AIHA. ITP episodes seem to be more frequent and harder to control than AIHA (Mathew et al., 1997). Long-term survival data are limited. Michel et al. found a mortality rate of 24% with a follow-up of 4.8 (Michel et al., 2009). Causes of death were mainly related to hemorrhage or sepsis (Norton and Roberts, 2006), although the paucity of large patient surveys and the lack of randomized-controlled trials make it difficult to make evidence-based recommendations about the optimal management of these patients. At best, the data suggest a role for corticosteroids +/− ivIg as first-line therapy in the acute setting. Cyclosporine seems to be the best second-line option for

most patients, with mycophenolate mofetil and then multi-agent therapy or rituximab.

ITP Secondary to Systemic Lupus Erythematosus

Immune thrombocytopenia is common in SLE as it occurs in 20–30% of patients during the course of the disease and may be the initial manifestation in 5%. Conversely, SLE develops in up to 5% of adult patients with ITP (Kurata et al., 1994). The risk factors to develop SLE include being older, female, having chronic ITP, and having high ANA titers (Hazzan et al., 2006). However, the ANA titer alone was not a significant predictor for the future development of SLE (Zimmerman and Ware, 1997).

Thrombocytopenia correlates with more severe disease with higher risk of damage involving heart and kidneys (Ziakas et al., 2006) and has a negative impact on the survival of lupus patients (Zhao et al., 2010). Platelet autoantibodies to platelet membrane antigens and non-specific binding of circulating immune complexes to platelet membrane, accelerating destruction by the mononuclear phagocytic system (McMillan, 1983), or the interaction of aCLs with the platelet membrane (Harris et al., 1985) are some of the mechanisms linking ITP and SLE.

ITP Secondary to Primary Immunodeficiencies

Autoimmune manifestations have increasingly been recognized as an important component of several forms of primary immunodeficiencies. We focus on four forms of PID in which autoimmune cytopenias are particularly common and may be the first manifestation of the disease: common variable immunodeficiency (CVID), autoimmune lymphoproliferative syndrome (ALPS), Wiskott–Aldrich syndrome/X-linked thrombocytopenia (WAS/XLT), and velocardiofacial (VCF)/DiGeorge syndrome.

Common Variable Immunodeficiency

Approximately one-quarter of patients with CVID develop autoimmune diseases, autoimmune cytopenias being the most common. Since ITP may precede the diagnosis of CVID, testing for immunoglobulin levels should be performed at diagnosis of ITP. Patients with CVID in association with autoimmune cytopenias seem in certain cases to have a "particular phenotype" with lower susceptibility to infection and higher susceptibility to autoimmune manifestations (Michel et al., 2004; Notarangelo, 2009). Treatment response generally seems similar to that of ITP without CVID but physicians should be aware of the increased infection risk associated with certain treatments (e.g., splenectomy); the higher response rate to rituximab; and the occasional patient who responds completely to a short course of steroids, e.g., 1–3 months only to relapse again months to years later (Gobert et al., 2011). The recommended agents are a course of steroids (with particular attention to development of opportunistic infections which may require prophylaxis or treatment), ivIg especially at higher dose, i.e., 1 g/kg/infusion, and rituximab. After the latter and probably with steroids as well ivIg (400 mg/kg/infusion every 3–4 weeks) should be given to reduce the risk of infection.

Autoimmune Lymphoproliferative Syndrome

Autoimmune cytopenias affect over 70% of ALPS patients with a median first presentation age of 24 months. However, with increasing awareness of this condition, adults with autoimmune cytopenias are now being diagnosed more frequently (Deutsch et al., 2004) and testing for ALPS should therefore be considered in children and young adults with ES. Indeed, patients with ES frequently have other symptoms in addition to their autoimmune manifestations, which may include lymphadenopathy, hepatomegaly and splenomegaly, and these findings overlap with ALPS. Seif et al. tested 45 children with ES, measuring peripheral blood double-negative CD3+CD4−CD8− T cells (DNTs) and Fas-mediated apoptosis. ALPS was diagnosed in 47% of these patients (Seif et al., 2010). These data suggest that children with ES should be screened for ALPS. Screening is accomplished by finding an increased number of DNTs and can be confirmed functionally by *in vitro* assessment of Fas-mediated apoptosis and molecularly by finding a mutation in CD95 (Fas), which appears to be etiologic in 80–85% of patients. The pathogenesis seems to be a failure of apoptosis in autoreactive cells. Patients usually respond to immunosuppressive medications, including corticosteroids and IVIg but not as well as patients with isolated cytopenias. Splenectomy is relatively contraindicated in ALPS because of the risk of sepsis compounded, at least in children, by a lower rate of efficacy. Rituximab is highly effective but seems to create a lasting hypogammaglobulinemia for reasons not clear at this time so ideally one can avoid it in treatment. Mycophenolate mofetil may be effective in these patients as well.

Wiskott–Aldrich Syndrome/X-linked Thrombocytopenia

Wiskott–Aldrich syndrome (WAS) is an X-linked disease; affected boys exhibit microthrombocytopenia, variable degrees of eczema, combined immunodeficiency, and an increased risk for autoimmunity and lymphoid malignancies (Notarengelo et al., 2008). The disease is caused by mutations in the WAS gene, encoding the

WAS protein (WASp), a key cytoplasmic regulator of actin reorganization triggered by cell surface receptor signaling (Villa et al., 1995). The profound microthrombocytopenia seen in all individuals with WAS mutations (with the exception of a very small number of X-linked neutropenia patients) is the hallmark of the disease, and exact mechanisms underlying the thrombocytopenia of WAS/ XLT patients remain incompletely defined, although WASp-deficient platelets undergo more rapid destruction than their wild-type counterparts. WAS$^{-/-}$ mice having accelerated platelet turnover can be attributed not only to intrinsic platelet abnormalities but also in certain cases to immune-mediated mechanisms (Marathe et al., 2009).

Velocardiofacial/DiGeorge Syndrome

Velocardiofacial/DiGeorge syndrome is also known as chromosome 22q11.2 deletion syndrome, and occurs in approximately 1:4000 births. Many patients have a mild to moderate immune deficiency, and the majority of patients have a cardiac anomaly. Additional features include renal anomalies, eye anomalies, hypoparathyroidism, skeletal defects, and developmental delay (McDonald-McGinn and Sullivan, 2011). One secondary consequence of the immune deficiency is autoimmune diseases, seen in approximately 10% of patients. Juvenile idiopathic arthritis and hematologic autoimmune diseases are the most common disorders. ITP is the most common condition, occurring in 4% of patients, although platelet size and function are slightly aberrant in most patients with the deletion due to haploinsufficiency for GPIbβ (Lawrence et al., 2005).

GENETICS FEATURES

Familial ITP

Family-based linkage studies are limited since familial cases of ITP are very rare. So, familial transmission of childhood "ITP" requires consideration of other genetic disorders with thrombocytopenia- like myosin heavy chain disorders (MYH9 gene), ALPS, and Wiscott–Aldrich syndrome/X-linked thrombocytopenia. In a retrospective registry analysis, Rischewski et al. found that 2.3% of 445 patients have a positive family history with a higher likelihood of patients with familial ITP presenting at an earlier age (Rischewski et al., 2006). When familial ITP occurs, it is most commonly not in first-degree relatives.

Genetic Markers of ITP

Clinical heterogeneity in ITP course, duration, and/or in drug responsiveness may prove to have genetic bases. Single nucleotide polymorphism (SNP) chip analysis and whole genome sequencing are technically feasible but require an adequate sample size, which has been difficult to achieve in this disease. Numerous small studies have tried to demonstrate a consistent association between certain polymorphisms and ITP. Most of them, reported in the literature, affect B cell-associated genes (BAFF, Ig variable (v) gene), T cell-associated genes (CTLA4, PTPN22, SOX 13), Fcγ receptor-associated genes, cytokine-associated genes (TGF-β1, IL-4, IL-6, IL-10, TNF-α, etc.), or antigen-associated genes (HLA, HPA) (Bergmann et al., 2010). Results of these studies are often of borderline statistical significance, perhaps because of small sample size or biological heterogeneity. It is currently thought that there are genetic contributions to ITP but this is such a multifactorial heterogeneous disease that it can be very difficult to tease out the genetic factors.

IN VIVO MODELS

Passive transfer models, in which injection of platelet-specific antibodies are given to induce or maintain a state of thrombocytopenia (Nieswandt et al., 2000; Samuelsson et al., 2001; Teeling, 2001), are the most common animal models for ITP. More recently a transplantation model was developed where in splenocytes from CD61 knockout mice immunized against CD61(+) platelets were transferred into severe combined immunodeficient CD61(+) mouse recipients (Chow et al., 2010). These models will undoubtedly play a significant role in the future research of human ITP, particularly related to understanding of the pathogenesis of the disorder and the development of novel therapeutics (see the report published by Semple et al., 2010).

PATHOLOGIC EFFECTOR MECHANISMS

In the past, a shorter platelet life span was consistently seen in ITP patients compared with the 8- to 10-day platelet survival duration in healthy controls (Heyns et al., 1986). Although historically thrombocytopenia in patients with chronic ITP was caused solely by autoantibody-induced platelet destruction it has become evident that suboptimal platelet production also plays a role.

Increased Platelet Destruction

Antibody-Mediated Platelet Destruction

Antiplatelet Antibody

In the early 1950s, Harrington et al. provided first evidence that ITP is caused by a plasma antiplatelet factor by demonstrating that infusion of plasma from ITP patients induced severe thrombocytopenia that persisted several days in non-ITP controls (Harrington et al., 1953). Subsequently, the immunoglobulin (Ig)G rich serum

fraction was found to be responsible for the antiplatelet activity by Fcγ-mediated platelet destruction in the reticuloendothelial system (Shulman et al., 1965). After several studies in the 1970s reporting nonspecific elevated platelet-associated IgG in around 90% of ITP (Dixon and Rosse, 1975; McMillan, 1981), antigen-specific assays have been developed to measure autoantibodies that recognize one or more platelet surface glycoproteins (GP). The first antigen identified was the GP IIb/IIIa complex (van Leeuwen et al., 1982). Antibodies that react with GP Ib/IX or GP Ia/IIa, among others, have since been identified, and the presence of antibodies against multiple antigens is not only possible but, in patients with chronic disease, seems relatively common (Kunicki and Newman, 1992; He et al., 1994).

Antigen-Presenting Cells (APCs)

Antibody-coated platelets bind to macrophages of the reticuloendothelial system through Fcγ receptors (FcγR) and are then internalized and degraded. Gamma camera imaging of ITP patients injected with ^{111}In-labeled autologous platelets revealed that destruction occurs primarily in the spleen and liver (Stratton et al., 1989). Antigen-presenting cells not only degrade GP IIb/IIIa, thereby amplifying the initial immune response, but also may generate cryptic epitopes from other platelet glycoproteins (Cines and Blanchette, 2002). The balance between the numbers of inhibitory receptors like FcγRIIB versus activating receptors like FcγRIIA and FcγRIIIA seems to have an important role in patients with ITP, with downregulation of the inhibitory receptor FcγRIIB (Asahi et al., 2008). Moreover, studies of SNP suggest that certain polymorphisms in the FcγRIIIa gene may be overrepresented in patients with ITP (Carcao et al., 2003) and individual FcγR may correlate with response to FcγR blockade therapy (Fujimoto et al., 2001). In particular, responses to anti-D appear to depend upon FcγRIIA (Cooper et al., 2004) and rituximab upon FcγRIIIA. Complement-induced lysis following antibody binding also plays a role in this process but the response of ITP patients to a monoclonal antibody against the FcγRIIIA receptor underlines the importance of the former mechanism (Clarkson et al., 1986).

CD4[+]Th Cells

CD4[+]Th cells are also implicated in antibody production as evidenced by the fact that antibodies are usually isotype switched and harbor somatic mutations. A well-known abnormality is the oligoclonal accumulation of CD4[+]Th cells in the peripheral blood of patients with ITP (Ware and Howard, 1993). Size analysis of cDNAs for the complementarity determining region 3 (CDR3) of the T cell receptor (TCR) β-variable region genes has demonstrated the frequent use of VB3, 6, 10, and 13.1 to 14 genes (Shimomura et al., 1996). Presentation of platelet epitopes on the cell surface of activated APCs helped by costimulatory molecules (interaction between CD154 and CD40) and cytokines stimulate initiating CD4$^+$Th clones and clones with additional specificities (Cines and Blanchette, 2002). T cells autoreactive to GP IIb/IIIa have been identified in ITP patients. GP IIb/IIIa-reactive T cells respond to chemically reduced and cryptic peptides of GP IIb/IIIa but not to native GP IIb/IIIa (Kuwana et al., 1998). Moreover the Th1/Th2 balance is well known to regulate the immune system under normal conditions, and is known to be impaired in many autoimmune diseases. Several studies have found evidence supporting a Th1 polarization of the immune response in ITP (Semple et al., 1996). An increased Th1/Th2 ratio has been observed in patients with active ITP (Wang et al., 2005). An increase of the Th1 cytokines, IL-2 and IFN-γ, have been shown in patients with ITP compared with controls as well as a suppression of Th2 cytokines, IL-4 and IL-5, in patients with active disease (Panitsas et al., 2004).

In ITP patients with active disease, CD4$^+$CD25$^+$ regulatory T cells (Tregs) are both reduced in number and defective in their suppressive capacity (Liu et al., 2007; Sakakura et al., 2007; Yu et al., 2008). Impaired function of Tregs could allow activation of autoreactive Th1 cells in ITP patients and might be responsible, upon remission, for the switch to the anti-inflammatory Th2 profile (Stasi et al., 2007).

Autoreactive B Cells

Quite separately, several studies have specified B cell clonality in patients with ITP on the basis of light chain restriction in anti-platelet autoantibodies (Stockelberg et al., 1995; McMillan et al., 2001; Roark et al., 2002). However, a more recent study found no evidence of B cell receptor clonality by a more sensitive method of spectratyping analysis (Toffoletti et al., 2008). Abnormal B cells and their factors play a role in the pathogenesis of ITP. B cell activating factor (BAFF), for example, belonging to the family of tumor necrosis factor (TNF) ligands, is critical for the maintenance of normal B cell development, homeostasis, autoreactivity, and T cell costimulation (Moisini and Davidson, 2009). In addition, BAFF augments Th1-associated inflammatory responses (Sutherland et al., 2005). The levels of plasma BAFF and BAFF mRNA are elevated in active ITP patients, whereas in patients in remission, normal levels of plasma BAFF and BAFF mRNA expression were observed. The high levels of BAFF in ITP have been shown to be responsible for promoting the survival of autoreactive CD19$^+$ B cells and CD8$^+$ T cells (Zhu et al., 2009).

T Cell-Mediated Cytotoxicity and NK Cell Activity

The absence of detectable autoantibody in a subset of ITP patients as well as the failure of some patients to respond to splenectomy suggests the presence of alternative platelet destruction mechanisms. Olsson et al. were the first to demonstrate that T lymphocytes from some patients with ITP lyse human platelets and they showed increased expression of cytotoxic genes such as tumor necrosis factor α, perforin, granzyme A, and granzyme B (Olsson et al., 2003). This study was confirmed more recently in a large clinical study (Wang et al., 2005). Furthermore, a novel mouse model of ITP was recently developed that also demonstrates platelet-specific CD8$^+$ T cell immunity (Chow et al., 2010). Furthermore, genes from several members of the KIR receptor family that downregulate cytotoxic T lymphocytes were increased in patients in remission when compared with those with active ITP (Olsson et al., 2005). Similarly, an expansion of the CD56$^+$CD3$^-$ NK cell subsets has been reported in patients with active ITP (Garcia-Suarez et al., 1993).

Insufficient Platelet Production

Anomalies of Megakaryopoiesis

Autologous platelet survival studies showed that most ITP patients have normal or decreased platelet turnover, suggesting that platelet production in chronic ITP may also be impaired (Heyns et al., 1986; Ballem et al., 1987; Gernsheimer et al., 1989). Furthermore, early light microscopic observations of ITP bone marrow showed increased immature megakaryocytes with manifested degenerative changes in the nucleus and cytoplasm (Diggs and Hewlett, 1948). Various ultrastructural abnormalities of ITP megakaryocytes, including cytoplasmic vacuolization and distended demarcation membrane system, have also been described (Ridell and Branehög, 1976; Houwerzijl et al., 2004).

Serum Levels of Thrombopoietin (TPO)

TPO is a glycoprotein produced first and foremost in the liver and, to a lesser extent, in the kidney and bone marrow (Geddis et al., 2002; Kaushansky, 2005). It exerts biological effects on hematopoietic stem cells as well as megakaryocytes and platelets via its high-affinity receptors (c-Mpl) that bind and internalize the hormone receptor complex (Kuter and Rosenberg, 1995). Circulating TPO is mediated by an autoregulatory feedback loop. In thrombocytopenia, less TPO is bound to platelets and circulating levels increase, allowing binding to c-Mpl on megakaryocytes and hematopoietic stem cells, stimulating megakaryocyte development and platelet production (Li et al., 1999).

However, ITP patients demonstrate normal or only slightly increased level of TPO in contrast to the elevated levels found in patients with thrombocytopenia due to bone marrow failure (Mukai et al., 1996). This suggests that circulating TPO levels are regulated by all c-Mpl expressing cells of megakaryocyte lineage (Debili et al., 1995) and not primarily by the absolute number of circulating platelets. Because TPO could bind to the c-Mpl's increased megakaryocyte mass with subsequent internalization and degradation, the levels of TPO could be lower than expected in ITP (Kuter, 1996). This provides a rationale for the ability of supplemental TPO effect to increase platelet production.

Effect of Antiplatelet Antibodies on Megakaryocytopoiesis

As megakaryocytes also express GP IIb/III or GP Ib/IX on their surfaces during maturation (Vainchenker et al., 1982), the circulating autoantibodies could interfere with the megakaryocytes, provoke intramedullary megakaryocyte or platelet destruction, and hamper megakaryocyte maturation (McMillan et al., 1978). Chang et al. evaluated the effect of plasma from patients with childhood ITP on thrombopoietin-induced production of megakaryocytes from cord blood cells in liquid culture. They noted that plasma from ITP patients with detectable antiplatelet antibodies inhibits the *in vitro* production and maturation of megakaryocytes, whereas plasma from control subjects or ITP patients without demonstrable antibodies did not (Chang et al., 2003). These studies would imply that the number of megakaryocytes should be reduced in these patients but instead it has been repeatedly shown that the number of megakaryocytes is usually increased. This suggests that *in vivo* the megakaryocytes are made but then damaged such that they are in the marrow but relatively non-functional. T cell-mediated inhibition of megakaryocytopoiesis as well as increased apoptosis of megakaryocytes is also probably involved in the disturbance of platelet production but little studied (Figure 47.1).

Infection-related Thrombocytopenia

Mechanisms of platelet destruction in thrombocytopenia associated with lymphoproliferative disorders and collagen vascular diseases are similar to those in primary ITP, whereas infection-associated ITP occurs via various mechanisms as described below.

Molecular Mimicry

Molecular mimicry suggests that antigenic structures, such as those on infectious agents, resemble host self-antigenic structures and trigger anti-self reactivity. For example, it has been reported that HIV, HCV, and the drug quinine stimulate a particular IgG antibody that reacts with a specific amino acid domain of the platelet GP IIIa (Zhang et al., 2009; Aster, 2009). Antibodies to both HIV and HCV destroy platelets by inducing platelet-generated reactive oxygen species via NADPH oxidase activation (Zhang et al., 2009). There is also strong evidence for an association between infection with HP and ITP, which may be related to molecular mimicry (Liebman and Stasi, 2007; Stasi et al., 2009). Platelets may be activated by binding of HP antibodies to platelet FcγIIA or through an interaction between HP-bound von Willebrand factor and platelet GPIB. Activation may promote platelet clearance and antigen presentation, which augments production of antibacterial antibodies (Cines et al., 2009).

Mechanisms other than Molecular Mimicry

Other mechanisms include accelerated platelet clearance due to immune complex disease (Karpatkin et al., 1995; Samuel et al., 1999). Alternatively, chronic infection may change the cytokine milieu, encourage loss of tolerance and stimulate B cells (Yun et al., 2005). Additional evidence exists for defective platelet production and direct infection of megakaryocytes resulting in megakaryocytic apoptosis. Several studies have postulated direct HIV cytopathic infection of the megakaryocyte as a mechanism for decreased platelet production (Sato et al., 2000; Sundell and Koka, 2006), as well as the binding to and possible infection of megakaryocytes by HCV (Bordin et al., 1995). Finally, advanced hepatic fibrosis (cirrhosis) in HCV may cause altered production of TPO and also portal hypertension with enlarged spleen. The latter may play a central role in the pathogenesis of thrombocytopenia in chronic viral hepatitis of any cause (Adinolfi et al., 2001).

AUTOANTIBODIES AS POTENTIAL IMMUNOLOGIC MARKERS

Direct tests for anti-GP IIb/IIIa and/or anti-GP Ib/IX have good specificity (78–93%), but very moderate sensitivity (49–66%) in prospective studies (Warner et al., 1999; McMillan, 2003). Indirect tests were only rarely positive. This low sensitivity of platelet antibody test may have several explanations including: (1) the population's heterogeneity in the different studies, (2) the platelet autoantibodies may be missed by current monoclonal-based assays that only detect antibodies with known specificity (typically, GP IIb/IIIa and GP Ib/IX), and (3) the circulating autoantibodies may be undetectable because of their sequestration in other tissues and/or cells (particularly megakaryocytes). The diagnosis of ITP (both primary and secondary) is generally accepted to be one of exclusion.

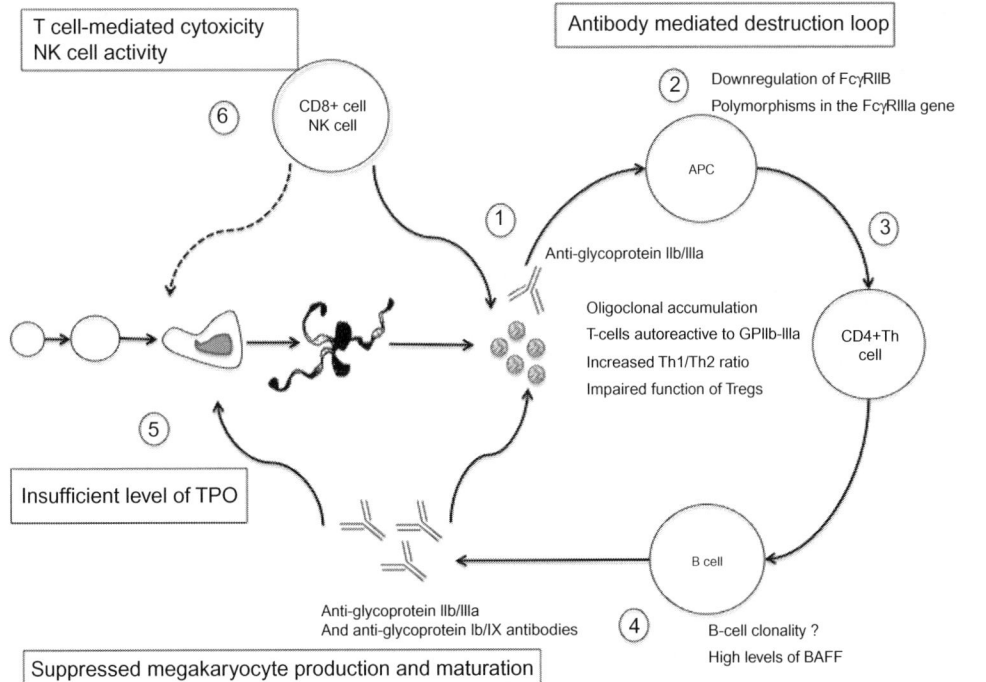

FIGURE 47.1   Central and peripheral pathogenesis of ITP.   The factors that initiate autoantibody production are unknown. Here, glycoprotein IIb/IIIa is recognized by autoantibody, whereas antibodies that recognize the glycoprotein Ib/IX complex have not been generated at this stage (1). Antibody-coated platelets bind to antigen-presenting cells (macrophages or dendritic cells) through Fcγ receptors and are then internalized and degraded (2). Antigen-presenting cells not only degrade glycoprotein IIb/IIIa thereby amplifying the initial immune response, but also may generate cryptic epitopes from other platelet glycoproteins. Activated antigen-presenting cells express these novel peptides on the cell surface along with costimulatory help and the relevant cytokines that facilitate the proliferation of the initiating CD4-positive T cell clones (3). B cell immunoglobulin receptors that recognize additional platelet antigens are thereby also induced to proliferate and synthesize anti-glycoprotein Ib/IX antibodies in addition to amplifying the production of anti-glycoprotein IIb/IIIa antibodies (4). Antiplatelet autoantibodies may also induce decreased megakaryocyte production and suppressed megakaryocyte maturation, which is compounded by an insufficient level of TPO (5). Finally, cytotoxic T cells may exert cell-mediated lysis on megakaryocytes, as well as on platelets (6).

Although three prospective studies indicate that the detection of platelet autoantibodies has a high positive diagnostic value for ITP (Brighton et al., 1996; Warner et al., 1999; McMillan et al., 2003), the utility of platelet autoantibody assays in the clinical course of ITP is still a matter of debate and is not currently recommended (Provan et al., 2010). Nevertheless, several studies highlight the prognostic value of platelet autoantibody detection (Brighton et al., 1996; Berchtold and Wenger, 1993), such as Fabris et al., who demonstrate that ITP patients with platelet autoantibodies have a worse clinical course than patients without antibodies (Fabris et al., 2004). A recent study by Zeng et al. emphasizes that steroid (and IgIV) response depends on anti-GP IIb/IIIa vs. anti-GPIbα antibodies (Zeng et al., 2012). The preliminary findings of this study suggest that the anti-GPIbα and -GP IIb/IIIa status should be assessed in future clinical trials including corticosteroids in order to test its potential relevance in deciding future treatments.

CONCLUDING REMARKS—FUTURE PROSPECTS

ITP is a heterogeneous syndrome with a complex pathogenesis. Immune platelet destruction in ITP occurs by a complex process involving multiple components of the immune system. While new insights into the complex interplay involving humoral and cellular immunity have been provided, the triggering event for ITP, for the immune dysregulation, is still unknown. The mechanism of ITP involves insufficient platelet production and autoantibody-mediated platelet destruction. Some key points of ITP pathogenesis remain unresolved, including how interruption in the normal function of the immune system occurs. The success of the TPO receptor agonists suggests a fundamental concept, namely that platelet production by megakaryocytes is often sub-optimal and increasing it might compensate for autoantibody-mediated platelet destruction.

REFERENCES

Adinolfi, L.E., Giordano, M.G., Andreana, A., Tripodi, M.F., Utili, R., Cesaro, G., et al., 2001. Hepatic fibrosis plays a central role in the pathogenesis of thrombocytopenia in patients with chronic viral hepatitis. Br. J. Haematol. 113, 590–595.

Aledort, L.M., Hayward, C.P., Chen, M.G., Nichol, J.L., Bussel, J., ITP Study Group, 2004. Prospective screening of 205 patients with ITP, including diagnosis, serological markers, and the relationship between platelet counts, endogenous thrombopoietin, and circulating antithrombopoietin antibodies. Am. J. Hematol. 76, 205–213.

Altintas, A., Ozel, A., Okur, N., Okur, N., Cil, T., Pasa, S., et al., 2007. Prevalence and clinical significance of elevated antinuclear antibody test in children and adult patients with idiopathic thrombocytopenic purpura. J. Thromb. Thrombolysis. 24, 163–168.

Asahi, A., Nishimoto, T., Okazaki, Y., Suzuki, H., Masaoka, T., Kawakami, Y., et al., 2008. Helicobacter pylori eradication shifts monocyte Fcgamma receptor balance toward inhibitory FcgammaRIIB in immune thrombocytopenic purpura patients. J. Clin. Invest. 118, 2939–2949.

Aster, R.H., 2009. Molecular mimicry and immune thrombocytopenia. Blood. 113, 3887–3888.

Ballem, P.J., Segal, G.M., Stratton, J.R., Gernsheimer, T., Adamson, J.W., Slichter, S.J., 1987. Mechanisms of thrombocytopenia in chronic autoimmune thrombocytopenic purpura. Evidence of both impaired platelet production and increased platelet clearance. J. Clin. Invest. 80, 33–40.

Bennett, C.M., Tarantino, M., 2009. Chronic immune thrombocytopenia in children: epidemiology and clinical presentation. Hematol. Oncol. Clin. North Am. 23, 1223–1238.

Berchtold, P., Wenger, M., 1993. Autoantibodies against platelet glycoproteins in autoimmune thrombocytopenic purpura: their clinical significance and response to treatment. Blood. 81, 1246–1250.

Bergmann, A.K., Grace, R.F., Neufeld, E.J., 2010. Genetic studies in pediatric ITP: outlook, feasibility, and requirements. Ann. Hematol. 89, S95–S103.

Bizzoni, L., Mazzucconi, M.G., Gentile, M., Santoro, C., Bernasconi, S., Chiarotti, F., et al., 2006. Idiopathic thrombocytopenic purpura (ITP) in the elderly: clinical course in 178 patients. Eur. J. Haematol. 76, 210–216.

Bordin, G., Ballaré, M., Zigrossi, P., Bertoncelli, M.C., Paccagnino, L., Baroli, A., et al., 1995. A laboratory and thrombokinetic study of HCV-associated thrombocytopenia: a direct role of HCV in bone marrow exhaustion?. Clin. Exp. Rheumatol. 13, S39–S43.

Brighton, T.A., Evans, S., Castaldi, P.A., Chesterman, C.N., Chong, B.H., 1996. Prospective evaluation of the clinical usefulness of an antigen-specific assay (MAIPA) in idiopathic thrombocytopenic purpura and other immune thrombocytopenias. Blood. 88, 194–201.

Carcao, M.D., Blanchette, V.S., Wakefield, C.D., Stephens, D., Ellis, J., Matheson, K., et al., 2003. Fcgamma receptor IIa and IIIa polymorphisms in childhood immune thrombocytopenic purpura. Br. J. Haematol. 120, 135–141.

Chang, M., Nakagawa, P.A., Williams, S.A., Schwartz, M.R., Imfeld, K.L., Buzby, J.S., et al., 2003. Immune thrombocytopenic purpura (ITP) plasma and purified ITP monoclonal autoantibodies inhibit megakaryocytopoiesis in vitro. Blood. 102, 887–895.

Cheung, E., Liebman, H.A., 2009. Thyroid disease in patients with immune thrombocytopenia. Hematol. Oncol. Clin. North Am. 23, 1251–1260.

Chow, L., Aslam, R., Speck, E.R., Kim, M., Cridland, N., Webster, M.L., et al., 2010. A murine model of severe immune thrombocytopenia is induced by antibody- and CD8+ T cell-mediated responses that are differentially sensitive to therapy. Blood. 115, 1247–1253.

Cines, D.B., Blanchette, V.S., 2002. Immune thrombocytopenic purpura. N. Engl. J. Med. 346, 995–1008.

Cines, D.B., Bussel, J.B., Liebman, H.A., Luning Prak, E.T., 2009. The ITP syndrome: pathogenic and clinical diversity. Blood. 113, 6511–6521.

Clarkson, S.B., Bussel, J.B., Kimberly, R.P., Valinsky, J.E., Nachman, R.L., Unkeless, J.C., 1986. Treatment of refractory immune thrombocytopenic purpura with an anti-Fc gamma-receptor antibody. N. Engl. J. Med. 314, 1236–1239.

Cohen, Y.C., Djulbegovic, B., Shamai-Lubovitz, O., Mozes, B., 2000. The bleeding risk and natural history of idiopathic thrombocytopenic purpura in patients with persistent low platelet counts. Arch Intern. Med. 160, 1630–1638.

Cooper, N., Heddle, N.M., Haas, M., Reid, M.E., Lesser, M.L., Fleit, H.B., et al., 2004. Intravenous (IV) anti-D and IV immunoglobulin achieve acute platelet increases by different mechanisms: modulation of cytokine and platelet responses to IV anti-D by FcgammaRIIa and FcgammaRIIIa polymorphisms. Br. J. Haematol. 124, 511–518.

Debili, N., Wendling, F., Katz, A., Guichard, J., Breton-Gorius, J., Hunt, P., et al., 1995. The Mpl-ligand or thrombopoietin or megakaryocyte growth and differentiative factor has both direct proliferative and differentiative activities on human megakaryocyte progenitors. Blood. 86, 2516–2525.

Deutsch, M., Tsopanou, E., Dourakis, S.P., 2004. The autoimmune lymphoproliferative syndrome (Canale-Smith) in adulthood. Clin. Rheumatol. 23, 43–44.

Diggs, L.W., Hewlett, J.S., 1948. A study of the bone marrow from 36 patients with idiopathic hemorrhagic, thrombopenic purpura. Blood. 3, 1090–1104.

Dixon, R.H., Rosse, W.F., 1975. Platelet antibody in autoimmune thrombocytopenia. Br. J. Haematol. 31, 129–134.

Diz-Kucukkaya, R., 2001. Antiphospholipid antibodies and antiphospholipid syndrome in patients presenting with immune thrombocytopenic purpura: a prospective cohort study. Blood. 98, 1760–1764.

El-Bostany, E.A., El-Ghoroury, E.A., El-Ghafar, E.A., 2008. Anti-beta2-glycoprotein I in childhood immune thrombocytopenic purpura. Blood Coagul. Fibrinolysis. 19, 26–31.

Evans, R.S., Takahashi, K., Duane, R.T., Payne, R., Liu, C., 1951. Primary thrombocytopenic purpura and acquired hemolytic anemia; evidence for a common etiology. Arch Intern. Med. 87, 48–65.

Fabris, F., Scandellari, R., Ruzzon, E., Randi, M.L., Luzzatto, G., Girolami, A., 2004. Platelet-associated autoantibodies as detected by a solid-phase modified antigen capture ELISA test (MACE) are a useful prognostic factor in idiopathic thrombocytopenic purpura. Blood. 103, 4562–4564.

France, E.K., Glanz, J., Xu, S., Hambidge, S., Yamasaki, K., Black, S.B., et al., 2008. Risk of immune thrombocytopenic purpura after measles-mumps-rubella immunization in children. Pediatrics. 121, e687–e692.

Fujimoto, T.T., Inoue, M., Shimomura, T., Fujimura, K., 2001. Involvement of Fc gamma receptor polymorphism in the therapeutic response of idiopathic thrombocytopenic purpura. Br. J. Haematol. 115, 125–130.

Garcia-Suarez, J., Prieto, A., Reyes, E., Manzano, L., Merino, J.L., Alvarez-Mon, M., 1993. Severe chronic autoimmune thrombocytopenic purpura is associated with an expansion of CD56+ CD3− natural killer cells subset. Blood. 82, 1538–1545.

Geddis, A.E., Linden, H.M., Kaushansky, K., 2002. Thrombopoietin: a pan-hematopoietic cytokine. Cytokine Growth Factor Rev. 13, 61–73.

George, J.N., Woolf, S.H., Raskob, G.E., Wasser, J.S., Aledort, L.M., Ballem, P.J., et al., 1996. Idiopathic thrombocytopenic purpura: a practice guideline developed by explicit methods for the American Society of Hematology. Blood. 88, 3–40.

Gernsheimer, T., Stratton, J., Ballem, P.J., Slichter, S.J., 1989. Mechanisms of response to treatment in autoimmune thrombocytopenic purpura. N. Engl. J. Med. 320, 974–980.

Gobert, D., Bussel, J.B., Cunningham-Rundles, C., Galicier, L., Dechartres, A., Berezne, A., et al., 2011. Efficacy and safety of rituximab in common variable immunodeficiency-associated immune cytopenias: a retrospective multicentre study on 33 patients. Br. J. Haematol. 155, 498–508.

Harrington, W.J., Sprague, C.C., Minnich, V., Moore, C.V., Aulvin, R.C., Dubach, R., 1953. Immunologic mechanisms in idiopathic and neonatal thrombocytopenic purpura. Ann. Intern. Med. 38, 433–469.

Harris, E.N., Asherson, R.A., Gharavi, A.E., Morgan, S.H., Derue, G., Hughes, G.R., 1985. Thrombocytopenia in SLE and related autoimmune disorders: association with anticardiolipin antibody. Br. J. Haematol. 59, 227–230.

Hazzan, R., Mukamel, M., Yacobovich, J., Yaniv, I., Tamary, H., 2006. Risk factors for future development of systemic lupus erythematosus in children with idiopathic thrombocytopenic purpura. Pediatr. Blood Cancer. 47, 657–659.

He, R., Reid, D.M., Jones, C.E., Shulman, N.R., 1994. Spectrum of Ig classes, specificities, and titers of serum antiglycoproteins in chronic idiopathic thrombocytopenic purpura. Blood. 83, 1024–1032.

Heyns, A.P., Badenhorst, P.N., Lötter, M.G., Pieters, H., Wessels, P., Kotzé, H.F., 1986. Platelet turnover and kinetics in immune thrombocytopenic purpura: results with autologous IIIIn-labeled platelets and homologous 51Cr-labeled platelets differ. Blood. 67, 86–92.

Houwerzijl, E.J., Blom, N.R., van der Want, J.J., Esselink, M.T., Koornstra, J.J., Smit, J.W., et al., 2004. Ultrastructural study shows morphologic features of apoptosis and para-apoptosis in megakaryocytes from patients with idiopathic thrombocytopenic purpura. Blood. 103, 500–506.

Karpatkin, S., Nardi, M.A., Hymes, K.B., 1995. Sequestration of antiplatelet GPIIIa antibody in rheumatoid factor immune complexes of human immunodeficiency virus 1 thrombocytopenic patients. Proc. Nat. Acad. Sci. USA. 92, 2263–2267.

Kaushansky, K., 2005. The molecular mechanisms that control thrombopoiesis. J. Clin. Invest. 115, 3339–3347.

Kunicki, T.J., Newman, P.J., 1992. The molecular immunology of human platelet proteins. Blood. 80, 1386–1404.

Kurata, Y., Miyagawa, S., Kosugi, S., Kashiwagi, H., Honda, S., Mizutani, H., et al., 1994. High-titer antinuclear antibodies, anti-SSA/Ro antibodies and anti-nuclear RNP antibodies in patients with idiopathic thrombocytopenic purpura. Thromb Haemost. 71, 184–187.

Kuter, D.J., 1996. The physiology of platelet production. Stem Cells. 14, 88–101.

Kuter, D.J., Rosenberg, R.D., 1995. The reciprocal relationship of thrombopoietin (c-Mpl ligand) to changes in the platelet mass during busulfan-induced thrombocytopenia in the rabbit. Blood. 85, 2720–2730.

Kuwana, M., Kaburaki, J., Ikeda, Y., 1998. Autoreactive T cells to platelet GPIIb-IIIa in immune thrombocytopenic purpura. Role in production of anti-platelet autoantibody. J. Clin. Invest. 102, 1393–1402.

Kühne, T., Imbach, P., Bolton-Maggs, P.H., Berchtold, W., Blanchette, V., Buchanan, G.R., 2001. Newly diagnosed idiopathic thrombocytopenic purpura in childhood: an observational study. Lancet. 358, 2122–2125.

Kühne, T., Buchanan, G.R., Zimmerman, S., Michaels, L.A., Kohan, R., Berchtold, W., et al., 2003. A prospective comparative study of 2540 infants and children with newly diagnosed idiopathic thrombocytopenic purpura (ITP) from the Intercontinental Childhood ITP Study Group. J. Pediatr. 143, 605–608.

Lawrence, S.E., Cummings, E.A., Gaboury, I., Daneman, D., 2005. Population-based study of incidence and risk factors for cerebral edema in pediatric diabetic ketoacidosis. J. Pediatr. 146, 688–692.

van Leeuwen, E.F., van der Ven, J.T., Engelfriet, C.P., von dem Borne, A.E., 1982. Specificity of autoantibodies in autoimmune thrombocytopenia. Blood. 59, 23–26.

Li, J., Xia, Y., Kuter, D.J., 1999. Interaction of thrombopoietin with the platelet c-mpl receptor in plasma: binding, internalization, stability and pharmacokinetics. Br. J. Haematol. 106, 345–356.

Liebman, H., 2007. Other immune thrombocytopenias. Semin. Hematol. 44, S24–S34.

Liebman, H.A., Stasi, R., 2007. Secondary immune thrombocytopenic purpura. Curr. Opin. Hematol. 14, 557–573.

Lilleyman, J.S., 1994. Intracranial haemorrhage in idiopathic thrombocytopenic purpura. Paediatric Haematology Forum of the British Society for Haematology. Arch Dis. Child. 71, 251–253.

Liu, B., Zhao, H., Poon, M.C., Han, Z., Gu, D., Xu, M., Jia, H., et al., 2007. Abnormality of CD4(+)CD25(+) regulatory T cells in idiopathic thrombocytopenic purpura. Eur. J. Haematol. 78, 139–143.

Marathe, B.M., Prislovsky, A., Astrakhan, A., Rawlings, D.J., Wan, J.Y., Strom, T.S., 2009. Antiplatelet antibodies in WASP(−) mice correlate with evidence of increased in vivo platelet consumption. Exp. Hematol. 37, 1353–1363.

Mathew, P., Chen, G., Wang, W., 1997. Evans syndrome: results of a national survey. J. Pediatr. Hematol. Oncol. 19, 433–437.

McDonald-McGinn, D.M., Sullivan, K.E., 2011. Chromosome 22q11.2 deletion syndrome (DiGeorge syndrome/velocardiofacial syndrome). Medicine (Baltimore). 90, 1–18.

McMillan, R., 1981. Chronic idiopathic thrombocytopenic purpura. N. Engl. J. Med. 304, 1135–1147.

McMillan, R., 1983. Immune thrombocytopenia. Clin. Haematol. 12, 69–88.

McMillan, R., 2003. Antiplatelet antibodies in chronic adult immune thrombocytopenic purpura: assays and epitopes. J. Pediatr. Hematol. Oncol. 25, S57–S61.

McMillan, R., Luiken, G.A., Levy, R., Yelenosky, R., Longmire, R.L., 1978. Antibody against megakaryocytes in idiopathic thrombocytopenic purpura. JAMA. 239, 2460–2462.

McMillan, R., Lopez-Dee, J., Bowditch, R., 2001. Clonal restriction of platelet-associated anti-GPIIb/IIIa autoantibodies in patients with chronic ITP. Thromb. Haemost. 85, 821–823.

McMillan, R., Wang, L., Tani, P., 2003. Prospective evaluation of the immunobead assay for the diagnosis of adult chronic immune thrombocytopenic purpura (ITP). J. Thromb. Haemost. 1, 485–491.

Michel, M., Chanet, V., Galicier, L., Ruivard, M., Levy, Y., Hermine, O., et al., 2004. Autoimmune thrombocytopenic purpura and common variable immunodeficiency. Medicine (Baltimore). 83, 254–263.

Michel, M., Chanet, V., Dechartres, A., Morin, A.S., Piette, J.C., Cirasino, L., et al., 2009. The spectrum of Evans syndrome in adults: new insight into the disease based on the analysis of 68 cases. Blood. 114, 3167–3172.

Michel, M., Rauzy, O.B., Thoraval, F.R., Languille, L., Khellaf, M., Bierling, P., et al., 2011. Characteristics and outcome of immune thrombocytopenia in elderly: results from a single center case-controlled study. Am. J. Hematol. 86, 980–984.

Moisini, I., Davidson, A., 2009. BAFF: a local and systemic target in autoimmune diseases. Clin. Exp. Immunol. 158, 155–163.

Mukai, H.Y., Kojima, H., Todokoro, K., Tahara, T., Kato, T., Hasegawa, Y., et al., 1996. Serum thrombopoietin (TPO) levels in patients with amegakaryocytic thrombocytopenia are much higher than those with immune thrombocytopenic purpura. Thromb Haemost. 76, 675–678.

Notarengelo, L.D., Miao, C.H., Ochs, H.D., 2008. Wiskott-Aldrich syndrome. Curr. Opin. Hematol. 15, 30–36.

Neunert, C.E., Buchanan, G.R., Imbach, P., Bolton-Maggs, P.H., Bennett, C.M., Neufeld, E.J., et al., 2008. Severe hemorrhage in children with newly diagnosed immune thrombocytopenic purpura. Blood. 112, 4003–4008.

Neylon, A.J., Saunders, P.W., Howard, M.R., Proctor, S.J., Taylor, P.R., Northern Region Haematology Group, 2003. Clinically significant newly presenting autoimmune thrombocytopenic purpura in adults: a prospective study of a population-based cohort of 245 patients. Br. J. Haematol. 122, 966–974.

Nieswandt, B., Bergmeier, W., Rackebrandt, K., Gessner, J.E., Zirngibl, H., 2000. Identification of critical antigen-specific mechanisms in the development of immune thrombocytopenic purpura in mice. Blood. 96, 2520–2527.

Norton, A., Roberts, I., 2006. Management of Evans syndrome. Br. J. Haematol. 132, 125–137.

Notarangelo, L.D., 2009. Primary immunodeficiencies (PIDs) presenting with cytopenias. Hematology/the Education Program of the American Society of Hematology. Hematology Am. Soc. Hematol. Educ. Program. pp. 139–143.

Olsson, B., Andersson, P.O., Jernås, M., Jacobsson, S., Carlsson, B., Carlsson, L.M., et al., 2003. T-cell-mediated cytotoxicity toward platelets in chronic idiopathic thrombocytopenic purpura. Nat. Med. 9, 1123–1124.

Olsson, B., Andersson, P.O., Jacobsson, S., Carlsson, L., Wadenvik, H., 2005. Disturbed apoptosis of T-cells in patients with active idiopathic thrombocytopenic purpura. Thromb Haemost. 93, 139–144.

Panitsas, F.P., Theodoropoulou, M., Kouraklis, A., Karakantza, M., Theodorou, G.L., Zoumbos, N.C., et al., 2004. Adult chronic idiopathic thrombocytopenic purpura (ITP) is the manifestation of a type-1 polarized immune response. Blood. 103, 2645–2647.

Pratt, E.L., Tarantino, M.D., Wagner, D., Hirsch Pescovitz, O., Bowyer, S., Shapiro, A.D., 2005. Prevalence of elevated antithyroid antibodies and antinuclear antibodies in children with immune thrombocytopenic purpura. Am. J. Hematol. 79, 175–179.

Provan, D., Stasi, R., Newland, A.C., Blanchette, V.S., Bolton-Maggs, P., Bussel, J.B., et al., 2010. International consensus report on the investigation and management of primary immune thrombocytopenia. Blood. 115, 168–186.

Psaila, B., Petrovic, A., Page, L.K., Menell, J., Schonholz, M., Bussel, J.B., 2009. Intracranial hemorrhage (ICH) in children with immune thrombocytopenia (ITP): study of 40 cases. Blood. 114, 4777–4783.

Ridell, B., Branehög, I., 1976. The ultrastructure of the megakaryocytes in idiopathic thrombocytopenic purpura (ITP) in relation to thrombokinetics. Pathol. Eur. 11, 179–187.

Rischewski, J.R., Imbach, P., Paulussen, M., Kühne, T., 2006. Idiopathic thrombocytopenic purpura (ITP): is there a genetic predisposition? Pediatr. Blood Cancer. 47, 678–680.

Roark, J.H., Bussel, J.B., Cines, D.B., Siegel, D.L., 2002. Genetic analysis of autoantibodies in idiopathic thrombocytopenic purpura reveals evidence of clonal expansion and somatic mutation. Blood. 100, 1388–1398.

Rodeghiero, F., Stasi, R., Gernsheimer, T., Michel, M., Provan, D., Arnold, D.M., et al., 2009. Standardization of terminology, definitions and outcome criteria in immune thrombocytopenic purpura of adults and children: report from an international working group. Blood. 113, 2386–2393.

Sakakura, M., Wada, H., Tawara, I., Nobori, T., Sugiyama, T., Sagawa, N., et al., 2007. Reduced Cd4 + Cd25 + T cells in patients with idiopathic thrombocytopenic purpura. Thromb Res. 120, 187–193.

Samuel, H., Nardi, M., Karpatkin, M., Hart, D., Belmont, M., Karpatkin, S., 1999. Differentiation of autoimmune thrombocytopenia from thrombocytopenia associated with immune complex disease: systemic lupus erythematosus, hepatitis-cirrhosis, and HIV-1 infection by platelet and serum immunological measurements. Br. J. Haematol. 105, 1086–1091.

Samuelsson, A., Towers, T.L., Ravetch, J.V., 2001. Anti-inflammatory activity of IVIG mediated through the inhibitory Fc receptor. Science. 291, 484–486.

Sato, T., Sekine, H., Kakuda, H., Miura, N., Sunohara, M., Fuse, A., 2000. HIV infection of megakaryocytic cell lines. Leuk. Lymphoma. 36, 397–404.

Schoonen, W.M., Kucera, G., Coalson, J., Li, L., Rutstein, M., Mowat, F., et al., 2009. Epidemiology of immune thrombocytopenic purpura in the General Practice Research Database. Br. J. Haematol. 145, 235–244.

Segal, J.B., Powe, N.R., 2006. Prevalence of immune thrombocytopenia: analyses of administrative data. J. Thromb. Haemost. 4, 2377–2383.

Seif, A.E., Manno, C.S., Sheen, C., Grupp, S.A., Teachey, D.T., 2010. Identifying autoimmune lymphoproliferative syndrome in children with Evans syndrome: a multi-institutional study. Blood. 115, 2142–2145.

Semple, J.W., 2010. Animal models of immune thrombocytopenia (ITP). Ann. Hematol. 89, S37–S44.

Semple, J.W., Milev, Y., Cosgrave, D., Mody, M., Hornstein, A., Blanchette, V., et al., 1996. Differences in serum cytokine levels in acute and chronic autoimmune thrombocytopenic purpura: relationship to platelet phenotype and antiplatelet T-cell reactivity. Blood. 87, 4245–4254.

Shimomura, T., Fujimura, K., Takafuta, T., Fujii, T., Katsutani, S., Noda, M., et al., 1996. Oligoclonal accumulation of T cells in peripheral blood from patients with idiopathic thrombocytopenic purpura. Br. J. Haematol. 95, 732–737.

Shulman, N.R., Marder, V.J., Weinrach, R.S., 1965. Similarities between known antiplatelet antibodies and the factor responsible for thrombocytopenia in idiopathic purpura. Physiologic, serologic and isotopic studies. Ann. N. Y. Acad. Sci. 124, 499–542.

Stasi, R., Stipa, E., Masi, M., Oliva, F., Sciarra, A., Perrotti, A., et al., 1994. Prevalence and clinical significance of elevated antiphospholipid antibodies in patients with idiopathic thrombocytopenic purpura. Blood. 84, 4203–4208.

Stasi, R., Del Poeta, G., Stipa, E., Evangelista, M.L., Trawinska, M.M., Cooper, N., et al., 2007. Response to B-cell depleting therapy with rituximab reverts the abnormalities of T-cell subsets in patients with idiopathic thrombocytopenic purpura. Blood. 110, 2924–2930.

Stasi, R., Sarpatwari, A., Segal, J.B., Osborn, J., Evangelista, M.L., Cooper, N., et al., 2009. Effects of eradication of Helicobacter pylori infection in patients with immune thrombocytopenic purpura: a systematic review. Blood. 113, 1231–1240.

Stockelberg, D., Hou, M., Jacobsson, S., Kutti, J., Wadenvik, H., 1995. Evidence for a light chain restriction of glycoprotein Ib/IX and IIb/IIIa reactive antibodies in chronic idiopathic thrombocytopenic purpura (ITP). Br. J. Haematol. 90, 175–179.

Stratton, J.R., Ballem, P.J., Gernsheimer, T., Cerqueira, M., Slichter, S.J., 1989. Platelet destruction in autoimmune thrombocytopenic purpura: kinetics and clearance of indium-111-labeled autologous platelets. J. Nucl. Med. 30, 629–637.

Sundell, I.B., Koka, P.S., 2006. Thrombocytopenia in HIV infection: impairment of platelet formation and loss correlates with increased c-Mpl and ligand thrombopoietin expression. Curr. HIV Res. 4, 107–116.

Sutherland, A.P., Ng, L.G., Fletcher, C.A., Shum, B., Newton, R.A., Grey, S.T., et al., 2005. BAFF augments certain Th1-associated inflammatory responses. J. Immunol. 174, 5537–5544.

Teeling, L., 2001. Therapeutic efficacy of intravenous immunoglobulin preparations depends on the immunoglobulin G dimers: studies in experimental immune thrombocytopenia. Blood. 98, 1095–1099.

Toffoletti, E., Zaja, F., Chiarvesio, A., Michelutti, A., Battista, M., Fanin, R., 2008. No evidences for B-cell clonality by spectratyping analysis in patients with idiopathic thrombocytopenic purpura undergoing rituximab therapy. Haematologica. 93, 795–796.

Vainchenker, W., Deschamps, J.F., Bastin, J.M., Guichard, J., Titeux, M., Breton-Gorius, J., et al., 1982. Two monoclonal antiplatelet antibodies as markers of human megakaryocyte maturation: immunofluorescent staining and platelet peroxidase detection in megakaryocyte colonies and in in vivo cells from normal and leukemic patients. Blood. 59, 514–521.

Villa, A., Notarangelo, L., Macchi, P., Mantuano, E., Cavagni, G., Brugnoni, D., et al., 1995. X-linked thrombocytopenia and Wiskott-Aldrich syndrome are allelic diseases with mutations in the WASP gene. Nat. Genet. 9, 414–417.

Wang, T., Zhao, H., Ren, H., Guo, J., Xu, M., Yang, R., et al., 2005. Type 1 and type 2 T-cell profiles in idiopathic thrombocytopenic purpura. Haematologica. 90, 914–923.

Ware, R.E., Howard, T.A., 1993. Phenotypic and clonal analysis of T lymphocytes in childhood immune thrombocytopenic purpura. Blood. 82, 2137–2142.

Warner, M.N., Moore, J.C., Warkentin, T.E., Santos, A.V., Kelton, J.G., 1999. A prospective study of protein-specific assays used to investigate idiopathic thrombocytopenic purpura. Br. J. Haematol. 104, 442–447.

Watts, R.G., 2004. Idiopathic thrombocytopenic purpura: a 10-year natural history study at the Childrens Hospital of Alabama. Clin. Pediatr. (Phila.). 43, 691–702.

Yu, J., Heck, S., Patel, V., Levan, J., Yu, Y., Bussel, J.B., Yazdanbakhsh, K., 2008. Defective circulating CD25 regulatory T cells in patients with chronic immune thrombocytopenic purpura. Blood. 112, 1325–1328.

Yun, C.H., Lundgren, A., Azem, J., Sjöling, A., Holmgren, J., Svennerholm, A.M., et al., 2005. Natural killer cells and Helicobacter pylori infection: bacterial antigens and interleukin-12 act synergistically to induce gamma interferon production. Infect. Immun. 73, 1482–1490.

Zeller, B., Helgestad, J., Hellebostad, M., Kolmannskog, S., Nystad, T., Stensvold, K., et al., 2000. Immune thrombocytopenic purpura in childhood in Norway: a prospective, population-based registration. Pediatr. Hematol. Oncol. 17, 551–558.

Zeller, B., Rajantie, J., Hedlund-Treutiger, I., Tedgård, U., Wesenberg, F., Jonsson, O., et al., 2005. Childhood idiopathic thrombocytopenic purpura in the Nordic countries: epidemiology and predictors of chronic disease. Acta Paediatr. 94, 178–184.

Zeng, Q., Zhu, L., Tao, L., Bao, J., Yang, M., Simpson, E.K., et al., 2012. Relative efficacy of steroid therapy in immune thrombocytopenia mediated by anti-platelet GPIIbIIIa versus GPIbα antibodies. Am. J. Hematol. 87, 206–208.

Zhang, W., Nardi, M.A., Borkowsky, W., Li, Z., Karpatkin, S., 2009. Role of molecular mimicry of hepatitis C virus protein with platelet GPIIIa in hepatitis C-related immunologic thrombocytopenia. Blood. 113, 4086–4093.

Zhao, H., Li, S., Yang, R., 2010. Thrombocytopenia in patients with systemic lupus erythematosus: significant in the clinical implication and prognosis. Platelets. 21, 380–385.

Zhu, X.J., Shi, Y., Peng, J., Guo, C.S., Shan, N.N., Qin, P., et al., 2009. The effects of BAFF and BAFF-R-Fc fusion protein in immune thrombocytopenia. Blood. 114, 5362–5367.

Ziakas, P.D., Dafni, U.G., Giannouli, S., Tzioufas, A.G., Voulgarelis, M., 2006. Thrombocytopaenia in lupus as a marker of adverse outcome—seeking Ariadne's thread. Rheumatology (Oxford). 45, 1261–1265.

Zimmerman, S.A., Ware, R.E., 1997. Clinical significance of the antinuclear antibody test in selected children with idiopathic thrombocytopenic purpura. J. Pediatr. Hematol. Oncol. 19, 297–303.

Chapter 48

Autoimmune Neutropenia

Parviz Lalezari

Montefiore Medical Center and Department of Medicine and Pathology, Albert Einstein College of Medicine, New York, NY, USA

Chapter Outline

Historical Background	677	Secondary Autoimmune Neutropenias	679
Clinical and Pathologic Features	677	Differential Diagnosis	679
Autoimmune Neutropenia of Infancy	678	Mechanisms of Cell Destruction	680
Primary Autoimmune Neutropenia in Adolescents and Adults	678	Laboratory Diagnosis	680
		Treatment	681
Neutrophil-Specific Antigens in Primary Autoimmune Neutropenias	678	Perspectives and Future Directions	681
		References	681

HISTORICAL BACKGROUND

In 1926, Charles Doan observed that sera from some patients agglutinated leukocytes from other individuals. This was the beginning of modern leukocyte immunology. The first report on autoimmune leucopenia was that of Franke (1940), who attributed the disorder to the "leukolysine" he found in a patient's serum. Later, in 1948 Hickie reported a serum inhibitor of bacterial phagocytosis in a patient who had chronic agranulocytosis. Serum of this patient also neutralized the ability of normal leukocytes to prevent growth of bacterial colonies in a culture medium. "Leukocitidin" was reported by Wiard and Robbins (1952) in the serum of a pancytopenic patient. In this patient, the widespread leukophagocytosis observed at autopsy suggested that the patient had a severe autoimmune disorder. Dausset and Nenna (1952), Moeschlin and Wagner (1952), and Goudsmit and van Loghem (1953) then established an association between leucopenia and leukoagglutinins. Steffen and Schindler (1955) introduced the antiglobulin consumption test with which "incomplete" leukocyte autoantibodies could be demonstrated in sera of some neutropenic patients. Butler (1958) showed that infusion of plasma from neutropenic patients into normal recipients could cause leukopenia. Further progress in leukocyte immunology was the discovery that leukocyte antibodies develop as a result of pregnancy (Payne and Rolfs, 1958; van Rood et al., 1959). In 1960, Lalezari and

associates demonstrated that fetal–maternal neutrophil incompatibility might cause neonatal neutropenia, a condition analogous to erythroblastosis fetalis (Lalezari et al., 1960). This led to the discovery of NA and NB neutrophil-specific antigens involved in fetal–maternal incompatibility (Lalezari and Bernard 1966; Lalezari et al., 1971). The efforts of an international cooperative research, initiated in 1964, led to the discovery of human leukocyte antigens (HLAs), the antigens that are expressed on lymphocytes and many tissues and are markers for histocompatibility (Rodney and Lalezari, 2000). The finding of neutrophil-specific antigens suggested that other nucleated cells may also express "organ-specific" antigens. Autoimmune neutropenia was then established as a definable clinical entity when neutrophil-specific antigens were demonstrated to be a target in primary autoimmune neutropenias, More recently, the structure, genetics, and functions of neutrophil-specific antigens were determined and the finding that NA is a receptor for IgG was helpful in better understanding its clinical implications. Finally, the availability of colony-stimulating factors for treatment has had a major impact on the management of all neutropenias.

CLINICAL AND PATHOLOGIC FEATURES

The levels of blood cells in circulation are determined by the rate of their production and their destruction. Neutrophil

N. Rose & I. Mackay (Eds): The Autoimmune Diseases, Fifth edition. DOI: http://dx.doi.org/10.1016/B978-0-12-384929-8.00048-4

levels are also influenced by their large marginal pool. Neutropenia is defined by reduction of absolute neutrophil and band counts forms to below 1×10^9/L in infants and to 1.5×10^9/L in adults. Autoimmune neutropenias are probably as common as the more familiar autoimmune disorders of red cells and platelets, with clinical manifestations varying from being totally asymptomatic to severe forms complicated by overwhelming sepsis. Most patients develop intermittent mucocutaneous infections. Splenomegaly is an exception. Hematologically, the patients have selective neutropenia, while monocytes, eosinophils, and basophils are either normal or increased. Lymphocyte counts are normal or occasionally reduced. Platelets are normal, and in chronic forms hypergammaglobulinemia and a mild anemia, due to persistent infections, may exist. Bone marrow shows myeloid hyperplasia with a distinctly diminished number of mature cells, resembling "maturation arrest." This is particularly relevant to cases when neutrophil-specific antigens are the targets of autoimmunity as these antigens develop after the myelocytic phase of maturation. Clinically, autoimmune neutropenia is divided into primary and secondary forms, the latter being associated with other immunological disorders. In primary forms, the diseases in children and adults are distinct.

AUTOIMMUNE NEUTROPENIA OF INFANCY

Since the first reports in which neutrophil-specific antigens were identified as the targets (Lalezari et al., 1975, 1986), many cases with similar features have been reported (McCullough et al., 1988; Bux et al., 1998). Autoimmune neutropenia of infancy (AINI) is characterized by a severe neutropenia diagnosed when infants are about 5–8 months old. Neutropenia is commonly associated with bacterial or fungal infections, and spontaneous recovery within 1–4 years is the rule. Diagnosis is made by demonstration of neutrophil-bound and circulating antineutrophil antibodies. The cause of AINI remains unclear. It was suggested that the disease represents a "physiologic state" in which strong autologous antigens provoke an immune response in infants in whom the immune regulatory system is underdeveloped (Lalezari et al., 1986). In AINI, the neutrophil counts are normal at birth probably because of immaturity of the immune system and inability to produce IgG antibodies. Later, with maturity of the immune regulatory system, autoantibody production is prevented. A long-term follow-up of AINI has confirmed that once recovered, the affected children remain immunologically normal. On rare occasions, some patients remain chronically and severely neutropenic. These patients may represent a wrong diagnosis or a subgroup of chronic autoimmune diseases seen in adults and adolescents.

PRIMARY AUTOIMMUNE NEUTROPENIA IN ADOLESCENTS AND ADULTS

Primary neutropenias in adolescents and adults are often chronic and debilitating with preponderance in females (reviewed by Shastri and Logue, 1993). Newborn infants from such mothers may develop a transient neutropenia due to transfer of the maternal autoantibodies across the placenta (Stefanini et al., 1958). Acute forms of autoimmune neutropenia are relatively rare and are self-limited. Little information is available on the specificities of the antibodies in adult forms. In a report by McCullough et al. (1988), the antibody had partial specificity for NA1. We documented NA1 specificity in a 73-year-old man who had acute neutropenia. The patient had a past history of sarcoidosis but had not received transfusion of blood or blood products. He acutely developed fever, severe pharyngitis, and gingivitis. His total leukocyte count was below 800/µl with absent neutrophils. Platelets were normal but he had a mild anemia. All other laboratory data were normal except for a positive test for antinuclear antibodies. Bone marrow was hyperplastic with absence of mature neutrophils. After 15 days of persistent severe neutropenia, treatment with prednisone was initiated and then discontinued after 3.5 months. Within 10 days after the start of treatment, the neutrophil count rose to 12,000/µl and remained normal. The blood sample obtained before prednisone treatment contained a strong agglutinating antibody that reacted with neutrophils from all 28 NA1-positive donors and none of the 12 NA1-negative donors. The blood samples obtained 3 and 6 months after recovery did not react with neutrophils from any of 30 donors tested. The patient's neutrophils, obtained after recovery, were typed as NA1/NA2 and reacted strongly with the autologous sera obtained during the neutropenic phase, but not with the recovery samples. It is of interest that the target of the autoantibody was NA1 and not NA2, suggesting that NA1 may be more immunogenic than NA2. We also diagnosed a severe autoimmune neutropenia in a 12-year-old boy who was homozygous NA2 and had a high titer anti-NA2. The patient died of overwhelming sepsis.

NEUTROPHIL-SPECIFIC ANTIGENS IN PRIMARY AUTOIMMUNE NEUTROPENIAS

NA and rarely NB neutrophil-specific antigens are often the targets of autoantibodies in primary autoimmune neutropenias in early childhood. These antigens are anchored to the outer leaflet of the lipid bilayer of neutrophils via a glycosylphosphatidylinositol structure. NA has been determined to be the low-affinity receptor for IgG (FcγRIIIb) (Ory et al., 1989) and its gene mapped to chromosome 1q22–24. The alleles of the NA are NA1,

NA2, and SH (Bux et al., 1997). Some rare individuals lack the FcγRIIIb gene and are called NA^{null} with a frequency between 0.1 and 0.8% (reviewed by Flesch et al., 1998). The NB antigen is expressed on CD177 glycoprotein (Stroncek et al., 2001) and its gene is located on chromosome 19 at 19q13.2 (Kissel et al., 2001). Recently, a glycoprotein called PRV-1 has been identified and has been shown to be overexpressed in polycythemia Vera and in some patients with essential thrombocytosis (Temerinac et al., 2000). Caruccio et al. (2004) have provided evidence that PRV-1, which belongs to the LY6/snake toxin gene and differs from NB1 in four nucleotides, is an allele of NB1, although the possibility of gene duplication has not been excluded.

The reason for involvement of neutrophil-specific antigens as the target of autoimmunity remains unclear. One possible explanation may be their strong immunogenicity. This would be similar to the strong immunogenicity of the Rh complex in the red blood cells, which are the main targets in fetal–maternal incompatibility as well as in autoimmune hemolytic anemias. An important aspect of the neutrophil-specific antigens, mainly the NA system that is most commonly targeted, is its physiological function as the IgG FcγRIIIb receptor. This receptor has a critical role in the removal and phagocytosis of opsonized bacteria, the NA2 allele being less effective that NA1 (Bredius et al., 1994). Neutrophils are crucial for host defense in the oral cavity, a reason for frequent oral infections in neutropenic patients. In studying *Porphyromonas gingivalis*, a bacterium that causes periodontitis, Kobayashi et al. (2000) and Fu et al. (2002) have demonstrated that individuals with NA2 phenotype are more susceptible to gingivitis and more resistant to treatment. These findings also suggest that in autoimmune neutropenias, patients with anti-NA1 may be more symptomatic than those with anti-NA2. Many children with AINI have been reported to have high levels of immune complexes (Lalezari et al., 1986). This may result from low absolute number of neutrophils in which the FcγII (CD32) receptors are responsible for clearance of immune complexes.

Secondary Autoimmune Neutropenias

Association of neutropenia with autoimmune hemolytic anemia or thrombocytopenia is not uncommon, as in Evans syndrome (Evans et al., 1951). A special combination, which we have designated "alternating autoimmune hemocytopenia," is characterized by being multiphasic. Initially, cytopenia is limited to thrombocytopenia, neutropenia, or hemolytic anemia, and responds to treatment. After an interval, which may last from months to years, the autoimmune process recurs, this time involving another cell type. Alternation between neutropenia, hemolytic anemia, and thrombocytopenia continues for several years, and eventually a combination prevails that is severe and resistant to treatment. Autoimmune neutropenia may be associated with hematological malignancies such as hairy cell leukemia and T-LGL (T cell large granular lymphocytic leukemia) (Loughran, 1985). T-LGL, a lymphoproliferative clonal disease of cytotoxic T cells, is associated with T cell receptor rearrangement (O'Keefe et al, 2004). Non-hematologic autoimmune disorders associated with neutropenia include systemic lupus erythematosus (SLE), Sjögren's syndrome, Graves' disease, rheumatoid arthritis, Felty's syndrome, common variable immunodeficiency, and immune complex diseases (Breedceld et al., 1986).

Little is known about the target antigens in secondary immune neutropenias. The i and I antigens, the targets of red cell cold agglutinins, are also expressed on neutrophils and platelets, and high titer cold agglutinins cause neutropenia and thrombocytopenia (Lalezari and Murphy, 1967; Markenson et al., 1975). Antineutrophil cytoplasmic antigens also have been reported to be involved in some secondary autoimmune neutropenias (Hagen et al., 1993; Coppo et al., 2004).

DIFFERENTIAL DIAGNOSIS

Diagnosis of secondary neutropenias largely depends upon recognition of the underlying disease and awareness of their potential association with neutropenia. Positive diagnosis of autoimmune neutropenia and distinction from the genetic forms in infants is an important task for physicians and a crucial issue for the anxious parents. In mild and asymptomatic patients, a form of neutropenia known as "ethnical neutropenia" should be considered before other diagnoses are made. Ethnic neutropenias occur in individuals of African descent, Sephardic Jews, and Middle Eastern Arabs. The absence of neutropenia in siblings does not exclude this diagnosis. In infants, acute neutropenia occurs in association with viral and bacterial infections because of bone marrow suppression and its limited capacity to respond to demand. In mycoplasma pneumonia and infectious mononucleosis, cold-reacting antibodies are likely to be contributing factors to neutropenia. In chronic neutropenias in infants, AINI and neonatal neutropenia due to fetal–maternal incompatibility are the most common forms. Distinction can be made between these two entities by their starting differences: in alloimmune neonatal neutropenia, infants are neutropenic at birth and the antibodies are found in both the maternal and the newborn plasma whereas in AINI, neutrophil counts are normal at birth and the infants become neutropenic after several months; antibodies are found in the infant, not the maternal, blood.

The rare genetic forms of neutropenia that must be considered after transient and immunological forms are excluded include: cyclic hematopoiesis—a dominant, genetic disorder with 21-day cycles of severe and symptomatic neutropenia at nadir and sub-normal neutrophil counts at peak; cyclic neutropenia—caused by mutations in the ELA-2 gene that encodes for neutrophil elastase (Horwitz et al., 1999); and severe congenital neutropenias (SCN), also known as Kostmann's syndrome (Kostmann, 1956)—genetically heterogeneous disorders with 35–85% ELA-2 mutations (Dale et al., 2000), characterized by severe neutropenia and maturation arrest at promyelocyte level. Most cases arise sporadically with potentially lethal autosomal dominant mutations. Ten percent develop acute myelogenous leukemia with additional mutations at the G-CSF-receptor gene, monosomy 7, trisomy 21, and ras.

Details on other congenital forms that include Schwachman–Diamond syndrome, primary congenital immunodeficiency, Barth syndrome, cartilage hair hypoplasia, and Chediak–Higashi syndrome can be found in pediatrics literature.

Mechanisms of Cell Destruction

Most information on the mechanisms of neutrophil destruction in immunologic diseases is based on laboratory observations, but relevance to *in vivo* events has not yet been established. Neutrophils usually respond to their antibodies by agglutination, a reaction which, unlike red cells, is an active process requiring living cells. Neutrophils also aggregate in the presence of activated complement and adhere to endothelial cells (Jacob et al., 1980). Some neutrophil antibodies are known to activate the complement system, and thereby initiate complement-induced neutrophil aggregation. Thus, the *in vivo* neutrophil aggregation may be a mechanism for neutrophil removal in some autoimmune neutropenias. Boxer and Stossel (1974) have shown that neutrophils coated with auto- or alloantibodies can stimulate phagocytic cells. Leukophagocytosis is seen in the spleen of some patients with autoimmune neutropenia and indicates that this organ is a location for the clearance of opsonized neutrophils. However, using [III]In-labeling techniques, McCullough et al. (1988) have shown that neutrophils are not cleared at any selective site, but are removed by phagocytic cells distributed in many tissues. Cytotoxicity, either complement mediated or cell mediated, has been shown *in vitro* by dye exclusion test or by release of [51]Cr. Inhibition of colony-forming unit (CFU)-C colonies by lymphocytes from neutropenic patients has been demonstrated in Felty's syndrome, rheumatoid disorders, and SLE. Neutrophils bind circulating immunoglobulins. This binding of immune complexes to FcγRII may not be innocuous and lead to neutropenia, by complement activation, phagocytosis, or apoptosis (Gamberle et al., 1998). Also, binding of immune complexes to neutrophils causes their activation and adherence to endothelial cells. This would change neutrophil distribution and increase the marginal pool (Breedceld et al., 1986). Many patients with known immune complex diseases, however, are not neutropenic. Neutropenia in acquired immune deficiency syndrome (AIDS) may be due to myelosuppression or to immune complexes. A positive test for a high level of neutrophil-bound immunoglobulins is a common finding in AIDS patients. Many drugs cause dose-dependent neutropenia due to myelotoxicity and interference with protein synthesis and cell replication. Some drug-induced neutropenias are not dose related and are considered to be immunologic in nature. In rare cases, the antibodies or the suppressor cells are directed against progenitor cells, causing pure white cell aplasia (Levitt et al., 1983).

Finally, autoantibodies can alter neutrophil functions. The binding of anti-NA to the Fc receptor interferes with neutrophil phagocytic functions. The report by Kramer et al. (1980) exemplifies the inhibition of neutrophil motility by an IgG autoantibody, causing a non-neutropenic clinical condition indistinguishable from chronic neutropenic states. Thus, neutrophil dysfunction may explain the severity of clinical manifestations in cases where symptoms are disproportionate to the number of neutrophils.

LABORATORY DIAGNOSIS

Techniques available for detection of neutrophil antibodies have been summarized elsewhere (McCullough et al., 1988). In autoimmune neutropenia, as in other autoimmune diseases, direct examination of the target cells should be most relevant. Because of limitations in obtaining adequate numbers of neutrophils in neutropenic patients, however, it is often necessary to use indirect techniques. One exception may be the immunofluorescence (IF) test (Verheugt et al., 1977), which requires fewer cells. In this procedure, the use of specific antiglobulin reagents and flow cytometry allows determination of the class and subclass of antibodies. In the IF test, as it is used with a microscopic aid, neutrophils should be distinguished from the frequently present monocytes that strongly react with the labeled antiglobulin reagents. In addition, neutrophils of patients who receive granulocyte-colony-stimulating factor (G-CSF) treatment overexpress Fc receptors, leading to a nonspecific positive direct IF reaction. Pre-treatment of test neutrophils for 5 minutes with 1% paraformaldehyde in phosphate buffer (Verheugt et al., 1977) significantly reduces the non-specific binding of immunoglobulins and provides reliable results.

Among the indirect tests, the neutrophil agglutination reaction can be obtained only in the presence of EDTA, which prevents spontaneous neutrophil aggregation. Antibodies may be missed if the required incubation period is shortened. In the indirect agglutination test, the probability of detecting an antibody increases if the patients' plasmas are tested against a panel of cells selected from homozygous donors for the known antigens to produce stronger reactions. Testing for cytotoxic antibodies is less useful, because sera from many non-neutropenic, normal individuals produce a positive reaction, and the results can be considered positive only if high titers are obtained. Enthusiasm for tests based on opsonization and inhibition of phagocytosis is tempered by their complexity. Moreover, in some cases of alloimmune neonatal neutropenia, strong agglutinating antibodies have failed to cause neutrophil opsonization.

Unfortunately, unlike hemoglobin in hemolytic anemia, simple and reliable markers for *in vivo* neutrophil lysis are not available. For this purpose, measurement of the released neutrophil lysozyme (Boxer et al., 1975) has had limited clinical value. In conclusion, for diagnosis of autoimmune neutropenias, especially in the primary forms, a combination of agglutination and IF tests must be used. Another consideration, especially in AINI, is the fact that the tests are positive in early phases of disease, and that in late phases and prior to recovery, antibodies become undetectable.

TREATMENT

Introduction of CSFs has changed the outcome of all neutropenias, including autoimmune forms. Many patients with primary autoimmune neutropenia, especially children, tolerate the condition well and need antibiotics and other treatments only for the management of intercurrent infections.

The effectiveness of G-CSF is due to increased neutrophil production in the bone marrow and an increase in the expression of NA antigens. G-CSF also mobilizes neutrophils from the marginal pool. These effects may result in consumption of the antibodies by mass action. Included in these effects, the possibility of suppression of the lymphoid system cannot be excluded. The dose of G-CSF must be individualized. Most patients do not require more than two to three subcutaneous injections at 2.5 ± 1 μ/kg. The treatment should be given only for control of complications and in preparation for surgical procedures. Another effective modality is intravenous administration of gammaglobulin, which temporarily reverses neutropenia (Bussel et al., 1988). Compared to hemolytic anemia and thrombocytemia, splenectomy and steroids are not as effective. These differences may reflect pathophysiologic features unique to neutrophils, particularly

the multiplicity of mechanisms involved in their destruction. Steroids cannot be fully effective when phagocytosis by macrophages plays an essential role. Neutropenic patients often have chronic infection, which causes macrophage activation. Such activated macrophages are more destructive and less susceptible to inhibition by steroids. Despite these potential shortcomings, some severe cases may be resistant to G-CSF treatment and may require treatment with steroids.

PERSPECTIVES AND FUTURE DIRECTIONS

CSFs have become the treatment of choice for neutropenias with which most patients are treated, regardless of etiology. In addition, in view of the fact that few laboratories with expertise in neutrophil antibody detection are available, an increasing number of physicians avoid laboratory work-up. Consequently, availability of laboratory material for research has noticeably diminished. In the past three decades no new neutrophil-specific antigen has been discovered and the specificities of single antibody previously reported have not been confirmed. Nevertheless, the shift of research into molecular biology has led to much progress in our understanding of the molecular genetics of neutrophil antigens and their functions. The reason for the prominence of NA as the main target for autoimmunity remains a mystery, although we have attributed it to its high antigenicity. No explanation is available, however, as to why FcγRIIa (CD32), which like FcγRIIIb (CD16) is a diallelic antigen expressed on neutrophils, is not recognized as a target for autoimmunity.

More research is needed on the effects of anti-NB1 on NB1[+] neutrophil functions, suggesting that autoantibodies may have consequences beyond obvious numerical reduction. At the clinical level, the role of regulatory T cells in the pathogenesis of autoimmune neutropenia of infancy needs to be investigated. If confirmed, this mechanism may prove to be a model for other transient autoimmune disorders in early childhood such as thrombocytopenia and hemolytic anemia. It would be most interesting to determine if similar disorders occur in non-hematological tissues. The target(s) of antibodies in secondary autoimmune neutropenias has not been fully identified, except for possible involvement of ANCAS in rare cases. To be determined also, is the possibility that neutrophil-specific antigens could be one of the targets in neutropenias associated with diseases such as SLE.

REFERENCES

Boxer, L.A., Stossel, T.P., 1974. Effects of anti-human neutrophil antibodies in vitro. Quantitative studies. J. Clin. Invest. 53, 1534–1545.

Boxer, L.A., Greenberg, M.S., Boxer, G.J., Stossel, T.P., 1975. Autoimmune neutropenia. N. Engl. J. Med. 293, 748–753.

Bredius, R.G.M., Fijen, C.A.P., de Haas, M., et al., 1994. Role of neutrophil FcγRIIa (CD32) and FcγRIIIb (CD16) polyforming forms in phagocytosis of human IgG1- and IgG3-opsonized bacteria and erythrocytes. Immunology. 83, 624–630.

Breedceld, F.C., Lafeber, G.J., de Vries, E., van Krieken, J.H., Cats, A., 1986. Immune complexes and pathogenesis of neutropenia in Felty's syndrome. Ann. Rheum. Dis. 45, 696–702.

Bussel, J.B., Lalezari, P., Fikrig, S., 1988. Intravenous treatment with gamma-globulin of autoimmune neutropenia of infancy. J. Pediatr. 112, 298–301.

Butler, J.J., 1958. Chronic idiopathic irmnune-neutropenia. Am. J. Med. 24, 145–152.

Bux, J., Stein, E.L., Bierling, P., Fromont, P., Clay, M., Stroncek, D., et al., 1997. Charactcrization of a new alloantigen (SH) on the human neutrophil Fc gamma receptor IIIb. Blood. 89, 1027–1034.

Bux, J., Bejhrens, G., Jaeger, G., Welte, K., 1998. Diagnosis and clinical course of autoimmune neutropenia of infancy: analysis of 240 cases. Blood. 91, 181–186.

Caruccio, L., Walkovich, K., Bettinetti, M., Schuller, R., Stroncek, D., 2004. CD177 polymorphisms: correlation between high-frequency single nucleotide polymorphisms and neutrophil surface protein expression. Transfusion. 44, 77–82.

Coppo, P., Ghez, D., Fuentes, V., Bengoufa, D., Oksenhendler, E., Tribout, B., et al., 2004. Antineutrophil cytoplasmic antibodies-associated neutropenia. Eur. J. Intern. Med. 7, 451–459.

Dale, D.C., Person, R.E., Bolyard, A.A., et al., 2000. Mutations in gene encoding neutrophil elastase in congenital and cyclic neutropenia. Blood. 96, 2317–2322.

Dausset, J., Nenna, A., 1952. Presence of leuko-agglutinin in the serum of a case of chronic agranulocytosis. C. R. Soc. Bioi. Fil. 146, 1539–1541.

Doan, C.A., 1926. The recognition of a biologic differentiation in the white blood cells with a specific reference to blood transfusion. JAMA. 86, 1593–1597.

Evans, R.S., Takahashi, K., Duane, R.T., Payne, R., Liu, C., 1951. Primary thrombocytopenic purpura and acquired hemolytic anemia; evidence for a common etiology. Arch. Intern. Med. 87, 48–65.

Flesch, B.K., Achtert, G., Bauer, F., Neppert, J., 1998. The NA "null" phenotype of a young man is caused by an FcγIIIRB gene deficiency while the products of the neighboring FcγRIIA and FcγIIIRA genes are present. Ann. Hematol. 76, 215–220.

Franke, E., 1940. Nachweis von Zellgiften im Blut bei Myelophthisen und deren Wirkung ouf die Hamatopoese. Klin. Wschr. 19, 1053–1058.

Fu, Y., Korostoff, J.M., Fine, D.H., Wilson, M.E., 2002. Fc gamma receptor as risk markers for localized aggressive periodontitis in African-Americans. J. Periodontol. 73, 517–523.

Gamberle, R., Giordano, M., Trevani, A.S., Andonegui, G., Geffner, J.R., 1998. Modulation of human neutrophil apoptosis by immune complexes. J. Immunol. 161, 3666–3674.

Goudsmit, R., van Loghem, J.J., 1953. Studies on the occurrence of leukocyte-antibodies. Vox Sang. 3, 58–67.

Hagen, E.C., Ballieux, B.E., van Es, L.A., Daha, M.R., van der Woude, E.J., 1993. Antineutrophil cytoplasmic autoantibodies: a review of the antigens involved, the assays, and the clinical and possible pathogenetic consequences. Blood. 80, 1996–2002.

Horwitz, M., Benson, K.F., Person, R.E., Aprikian, A.G., Dale, D.C., 1999. Mutations in ELA2, encoding neutrophil elastase, define a 21-day biological clock in cyclic hematopoiesis. Nat. Genet. 23, 433–436.

Jacob, H.S., Craddock, P.R., Hammerschmidt, D.E., Moldov, C.F., 1980. Complement-induced granulocyte aggregation: an unsuspected mechanism of disease. N. Engl. J. Med. 302, 789–794.

Kostmann, R., 1956. Infantile genetic agranulocytosis. Acta. Paediatr. 45, 1–78.

Kissel, K., Santoso, S., Hofmann, C., Stroncek, D., Bux, J., 2001. Molecular basis of the neutrophil glycoprotein NB 1 (CD 177) involved in the pathogenesis of immune neutropenias and transfusion reactions. Eur. J. Immunol. 31, 1301–1309.

Kobayashi, T., van der Pol, W.L., van der Winkel, J.G., Hara, K., et al., 2000. Relevance of IgG receptor IIIb (CD16) polymorphism to handling of Porphyromonas gingivalis: implications for the pathogenesis of adult periodontitis. J. Periodont. Res. 35, 65–73.

Kramer, N., Perez, H.D., Goldstein, L.M., 1980. An immunoglobulin (IgG) inhibitor of polymorphonuclear leukocyte motility in a patient with recurrent infection. N. Engl. J. Med. 303, 1253–1258.

Lalezari, P., Bernard, G.E., 1966. An isologous antigen-antibody reaction with human neutrophils, related to neonatal neutropenia. J. Clin. Invest. 45, 1741–1750.

Lalezari, P., Nussbaum, M.G., Gelman, S., Spaet, T.H., 1960. Neonatal neutropenia due to maternal isoimmunization. Blood. 15, 236–243.

Lalezari, P., Murphy, G.B., 1967. Cold reacting leukocyte agglutinins and their significance. In: Curtoni, E.S., Mattiuz, P.L., Tosi, R.M. (Eds.), Histocompatibility Testing. Munksgaard, Copenhagen, pp. 421–427.

Lalezari, P., Murphy, G.B., Allen, F.H., 1971. NB1, a new neutrophil antigen involved in the pathogenesis of neonatal neutropenia. J. Clin. Invest. 50, 1108–1115.

Lalezari, P., Jiang, A.P., Yegon, L., Santorineau, M., 1975. Chronic autoimmune neutropenia due to anti-NA2 antibody. N. Engl. J. Med. 293, 744–747.

Lalezari, P., Khorshidi, M., Petrosova, M., 1986. Antoimmune neutropenia of infancy. J. Pediatr. 109, 764–769.

Levitt, L., Ries, C.A., Greenberg, P.L., 1983. Pure white-cell aplasia. Antibody-mediated autoimmune inhibition of granulopoiesis. N. Engl. J. Med. 308, 1141–1146.

Loughran Jr., T.P., Kadin, M.E., Starkebaum, G., et al., 1985. Leukemia of large granular lymphocytes: association with clonal chromosomal abnormalities and autoimmune neutropenia, thrombocytopenia and hemolytic anemia. Ann. Intern. Med. 102, 169–175.

Markenson, A.L., Lalezari, P., Markenson, J.A., 1975. Proceedings of the 18th Congress of the American Society of Hematology. Grune & Stratton, Orlando, FL, USA.

McCullough, J., Clay, M.E., Press, C., Kline, W., 1988. Granulocyte Serology. A Clinical and Laboratory Guide. ASCP Press, Chicago.

Moeschlin, S., Wagner, K., 1952. Agranulocytosis due to the occurrence of leukocyte-agglutinins (pyramidon and cold agglutinins). Acta Hematol. 8, 29–41.

O'Keefe, C.L., Plasilova, M., Wlodarski, M., et al., 2004. Molecular analysis of TCR clonotypes in LGL: a clonal model for polyclonal responses. J. Immunol. 172, 1960–1969.

Ory, P.A., Clark, M.R., Kwoh, E.E., Clarkson, S.B., Goldstein, L.M., 1989. Sequences of complementary DNAs that encode the NA1 and NA2 forms of Fc receptor III on human neutrophils. J. Clin. Invest. 84, 1688–1691.

Payne, R., Rolfs, M.R., 1958. Fetomaternal leukocyte incompatibility. J. Clin. Invest. 37, 1756–1763.

Rodney, G.E., Lalezari, P., 2000. HLA and neutrophil antigen and antibody systems. In: Hoffman, R., Benz, E., Shattil, S.J. (Eds.), Hematology, Basic Principles and Practice, third ed. Churchill and Livingstone, New York, pp. 2220–2241.

Shastri, K.A., Logue, G.L., 1993. Autoimmune neutropenia. Blood. 81, 1984–1995.

Stefanini, M., Mele, R.H., Skinner, D., 1958. Transitory congenital neutropenia: a new syndrome. Am. J. Med. 25, 749–758.

Steffen, C., Schindler, H., 1955. Bericht uber die Verwendung des Antihuman Globulin-Ablenkungsversuches fur den Nachweis eines Antileukozyten-Antikorpers bei Agranulozytosen. Munch. med. Wschr. 15, 469–471.

Stroncek, D.E., Kissel, K., von dem Borne, A., Bux, J., 2001. Protein Reviews on the Web. 3, 19–24.

Temerinac, S., Klippel, S., Strunck, E.W., Lubbert, M., Lange, W., Azemar, M., et al., 2000. Cloning of PRV-I, a novel member of the uPAR receptor superfamily, which is overexpressed in polycythemia rubra vera. Blood. 95, 2569–2576.

van Rood, J.J., van Leeuwen, A., Eernisse, J.G., 1959. Leucocyte antibodies in sera of pregnant women. Vox Sang. 4, 427–444.

Verheugt, F.W.A., von dem Borne, A.E., Decary, F., Engelfriet, C.P., 1977. The detection of granulocyte alloantibodies with an indirect immunofluorescence test. Br. J. Haematol. 36, 533–544.

Wiard, B.A., Robbins, S.L., 1952. Hypersplenism. A case report with post-mortem study. Blood. 7, 631–640.

Chapter 49

Acquired Aplastic Anemia

Robert A. Brodsky and Richard J. Jones

Division of Hematology, Department of Medicine and The Sidney Kimmel Comprehensive Cancer Center at Johns Hopkins, Baltimore, MD, USA

Chapter Outline

Historical Background	685	Bone Marrow Transplantation (BMT)	688
Genetic Features	685	BMT from Unrelated Donors	688
Clinical, Pathologic, and Epidemiologic Features	685	Immunosuppressive Therapy	689
Autoimmune Features and Pathogenic Mechanisms	687	High-Dose Cyclophosphamide without BMT	689
Environmental Features	687	Aplastic Anemia and Clonality	690
Animal Models	687	Concluding Remarks—Future Prospects	691
Therapy for Aplastic Anemia	688	References	692

HISTORICAL BACKGROUND

The earliest case description of aplastic anemia in 1888 was by Dr. Paul Ehrlich (Ehrlich, 1888). He described a young woman who died following an abrupt illness characterized by severe anemia, bleeding, high fever, and a markedly hypocellular bone marrow. The term aplastic anemia was first introduced in 1904 by Chauffard. Until the early 1970s, most patients with severe aplastic anemia died within a year of diagnosis. The advent of allogeneic bone marrow transplantation (BMT) and immunosuppressive therapy markedly improved the outcome for these patients and prompted vigorous clinical and laboratory investigation. These studies have generated important insight into hematopoietic stem cell biology, immunology, and autoimmunity. Today, the majority of patients will survive this potentially fatal autoimmune disorder.

GENETIC FEATURES

Distinctive genetic abnormalities are more common with congenital bone marrow failure syndromes since most acquired aplastic anemia is autoimmune. Congenital aplastic anemia tends to present in the first decade of life and is often, but not always, associated with other physical anomalies. Fanconi anemia, the most common form of congenital bone marrow failure, predisposes to cancer and is frequently associated with other congenital abnormalities (e.g., short stature, upper-limb anomalies, hypogonadism café-au-lai spots, etc. (Bagby, 2003). Dyskeratosis congenita (DKC) is another congenital bone marrow failure disorder that can be either X-linked recessive, autosomal dominant, or autosomal recessive (Dokal and Vulliamy, 2003). The X-linked recessive form results from mutations in a gene known as *DKC1* whose gene product, dyskerin, is important for stabilizing telomerase. The resulting telomerase deficiency leads to short telomeres, bone marrow failure, and premature aging. The autosomal dominant form of DKC results from *hTERC* gene mutations, the RNA component of telomerase. This chapter will focus on the acquired form of aplastic anemia. Genetic abnormalities are less well characterized in acquired aplastic anemia; however, there appears to be an underlying genetic predisposition to acquired aplastic anemia, as evidenced by the overrepresentation of HLA DR2 subtypes (Nimer et al., 1994).

CLINICAL, PATHOLOGIC, AND EPIDEMIOLOGIC FEATURES

Aplastic anemia manifests as pancytopenia in conjunction with a hypocellular bone marrow (Brodsky and Jones, 2005). The disease may present abruptly (over days) or insidiously, over weeks to months. The most common clinical manifestations reflect the low blood counts and include dyspnea on exertion, fatigue, easy bruising,

N. Rose & I. Mackay (Eds): The Autoimmune Diseases, Fifth edition. DOI: http://dx.doi.org/10.1016/B978-0-12-384929-8.00049-6

TABLE 49.1 Aplastic anemia: diagnosis and definitions. Bone marrow cellularity must be $<25\%$ to diagnose aplastic anemia

Peripheral blood counts	Nonsevere aplastic anemia (not meeting criteria for severe disease)	Severe aplastic anemia (any 2 of 3 criteria below)	Very severe aplastic anemia (meets criteria for severe disease and absolute neutrophils <200)
Absolute neutrophils		$<500/\mu l$	$<200/\mu l$
Platelets		$<20,000/\mu l$	
Reticulocyte count		$<1.0\%$ corrected or $<60,000/\mu l$	

petechia, epistaxis, gingival bleeding, heavy menses, headaches, and fever. A complete blood count, leukocyte differential, reticulocyte count, and a bone marrow aspirate and biopsy are essential for diagnosis. Peripheral blood flow cytometry to detect GPI anchor deficient blood cells (Brodsky et al., 2000; Borowitz et al., 2010) as well as cytogenetics and fluorescent *in situ* hybridization (FISH) analysis should be performed on the bone marrow aspirate. Up to 70% of patients with acquired aplastic anemia have a detectable paroxysmal nocturnal hemoglobinuria (PNH) clone which essentially rules out inherited forms of aplastic anemia. Cytogenetic or FISH abnormalities are suggestive of a hypoplastic form of myelodysplasia. Patients under the age of 40 years should be screened for Fanconi anemia using the clastogenic agents diepoxybutane or mitomycin C (Bagby, 2003) and telomere lengths should be obtained on patients with a family history of bone marrow failure, premature graying, pulmonary fibrosis, or other stigmata of dyskeratosis congenita.

A hypocellular bone marrow is required for the diagnosis of aplastic anemia. However, some patients will have residual pockets of ongoing hematopoiesis; thus, an adequate biopsy (1–2 cm in length) is essential for establishing the diagnosis. Dyserythropoiesis is not uncommon in aplastic anemia, especially in cases with coincidental small to moderate PNH populations; however, a small percentage of myeloid blasts, or dysplastic features in the myeloid or megakaryocyte lineages, is more typical of hypoplastic myelodysplastic syndromes (MDS). CD34 is expressed on early hematopoietic progenitors and the number of CD34$^+$ cells has also been used to help discriminate between aplastic anemia and hMDS. In aplastic anemia the percentage of cells expressing CD34 is usually less than 0.1%; in hMDS the CD34 count is either normal (0.5 to 1.0%) or elevated (Matsui et al., 2006).

As with other autoimmune diseases, there is a wide spectrum of disease severity in aplastic anemia. The prognosis in aplastic anemia is proportional to degree of peripheral blood cytopenias. Accordingly, aplastic anemia is classified as non-severe, severe, and very severe based

largely upon the degree of neutropenia (Table 49.1). Severe aplastic anemia (SAA) is defined as bone marrow cellularity of less than 25% and markedly decreased values of at least two of three hematopoietic lineages (neutrophil count $<500/\mu l$, platelet count $<20,000/\mu l$, and absolute reticulocyte count of $<60,000/\mu l$). Very severe aplastic anemia satisfies the above criteria except the neutrophil count is $<200/\mu l$, while non-severe aplastic anemia is characterized by a hypocellular bone marrow but with cytopenias that do not meet the criteria for severe disease. The 2-year mortality rate with supportive care alone for patients with SAA exceeds 50% (Camitta et al., 1979), with invasive fungal infections and overwhelming bacterial sepsis being the most frequent causes of death. Non-severe aplastic anemia is seldom life threatening and in many instances requires no therapy. Although some cases of non-severe aplastic anemia will progress, many will remain stable for years, and some may spontaneously improve.

Aplastic anemia has been associated with drugs, benzene exposure, insecticides, viruses, and other agents. However, over 80% of cases are classified as idiopathic. The disease most commonly affects children and young adults but may occur at any age. Precise estimates of the incidence of aplastic anemia are difficult due to the rarity of the disease and imprecision in establishing the diagnosis. The best estimates of incidence are case–control studies that report an incidence of two cases per million inhabitants in Europe (Kaufman et al., 1991) and Israel (Modan et al., 1975), but the incidence may be two- to three-fold higher in Southeast Asia (Issaragrisil et al., 1997a; Szklo et al., 1985). A population-based case–control study of aplastic anemia in Thailand found that drugs, the most commonly implicated etiology, explain only 5% of newly diagnosed cases (Issaragrisil et al., 1997b).

An intriguing association exists between seronegative hepatitis and aplastic anemia. The hepatitis/aplastic anemia syndrome accounts for 3–5% of newly diagnosed cases of aplastic anemia. The disease predominantly affects young males, with a precipitous onset of severe pancytopenia occurring within 2 to 3 months after the onset of hepatitis (Brown et al., 1997; Locasciulli et al., 2010). Moreover, aplastic anemia has been reported to occur in up to 30% of patients following orthotopic liver transplantation for seronegative hepatitis (Tzakis et al., 1988; Cattral et al., 1994). The aplastic anemia in the hepatitis/aplastic anemia syndrome is autoimmune since most cases respond to immunosuppressive therapy (Locasciulli et al., 2010; Savage et al., 2007); however, it remains unclear whether the hepatitis results from an undiscovered virus or whether this too is autoimmune.

AUTOIMMUNE FEATURES AND PATHOGENIC MECHANISMS

Aplastic anemia was originally thought to result from a quantitative deficiency of hematopoietic stem cells precipitated by a direct toxic effect on stem cells. However, attempts to treat aplastic anemia by simple transfusion of bone marrow from an identical twin failed to reconstitute hematopoiesis in most patients. Retransplant in many of these patients following a high dose of a cyclophosphamide preparative regimen was successful, suggesting that the pathophysiology of aplastic anemia was more complicated (Champlin et al., 1984; Hinterberger et al., 1997). In the late 1960s, Mathé and colleagues were among the first to postulate an immune basis for aplastic anemia (Mathe et al., 1970). They performed BMT in patients with aplastic anemia using partially mismatched donors after administering anti-lymphocyte globulin as an immunosuppressive conditioning regimen. Although the patients failed to engraft, the investigators witnessed autologous recovery of hematopoiesis in some patients. This suggested that functional hematopoietic stem cells exist in aplastic anemia patients and that the immune system was somehow suppressing the growth and differentiation of hematopoietic stem cells. The response to immunosuppressive therapy was the first clear evidence that aplastic anemia was truly an autoimmune disease.

The first laboratory experiments implicating an autoimmune pathophysiology were co-culture experiments showing that T lymphocytes from aplastic anemia patients inhibited hematopoietic colony formation *in vitro* (Hoffman et al., 1977; Nissen et al., 1980). Since then, it has been shown that the immune destruction of hematopoietic stem cells in aplastic anemia is mediated by cytotoxic T cells and involves inhibitory Th1 cytokines and the Fas-dependent cell death pathway. The cytotoxic T cells are usually more conspicuous in the bone marrow than in the peripheral blood (Zoumbos et al., 1985; Maciejewski et al., 1994; Melenhorst et al., 1997b), and overproduce interferon-γ and tumor necrosis factor (TNF) (Nakao et al., 1992; Nistico and Young, 1994). TNF and

interferon-γ are direct inhibitors of hematopoiesis and appear to upregulate Fas expression on $CD34^+$ cells (Maciejewski et al., 1995). Immortalized $CD4^+$ and $CD8^+$ T cell clones from some aplastic anemia patients have been shown to secrete Th1 cytokines and are capable of lysing autologous CD34 cells (Nakao et al., 1997; Zeng et al., 2001). Recently, evidence for a humoral autoimmune response in aplastic anemia has also been reported (Hirano et al., 2003; Feng et al., 2004).

Studies examining T cell diversity using complementarity-determining region (CDR3) spectratyping have further implicated the role of the immune system in aplastic anemia. Several groups have now found limited heterogeneity of the T cell receptor β chain (BV) in aplastic anemia, suggesting that there is oligoclonal or even clonal expansion of T cells in response to a specific antigen (Manz et al., 1997; Melenhorst et al., 1997a; Zeng et al., 2001).

ENVIRONMENTAL FEATURES

The medical literature is replete with reports of environmental exposures, most notably benzene and radiation, causing aplastic anemia. However, rigorous epidemiologic studies supporting an association between environmental toxins and aplastic anemia are lacking. A major confounder is that benzene, radiation, and other toxins also predispose to MDS and leukemia. Older literature was unlikely to have been able to distinguish different types of marrow failure, such as aplastic anemia, MDS, and hypoplastic leukemia, leading to an overestimation of the association between benzene and aplastic anemia. While the magnitude of the risk remains uncertain, benzene is probably not a major risk factor for aplastic anemia in countries with modern standards of industrial hygiene. A large case–control study in Thailand employing modern diagnostic and epidemiologic methods found that individuals of lower economic status and younger age are at greater risk than their counterparts in other countries following exposure to solvents, glues, and hepatitis A (likely a surrogate marker). Grain farmers were also found to have a higher risk of developing aplastic anemia (relative risk = 2.7) regardless of whether they used insecticides (Issaragrisil et al., 1997a). These same investigators noted marked differences in incidence between northern and southern rural regions of Thailand and among Bangkok suburbs implicating potential environmental factors in causing the disease (Issaragrisil et al., 1999).

ANIMAL MODELS

Animal models of bone marrow failure exist, but none of these models fully replicate the human disease-acquired aplastic anemia (Chen, 2005). Busulfan, benzene, and

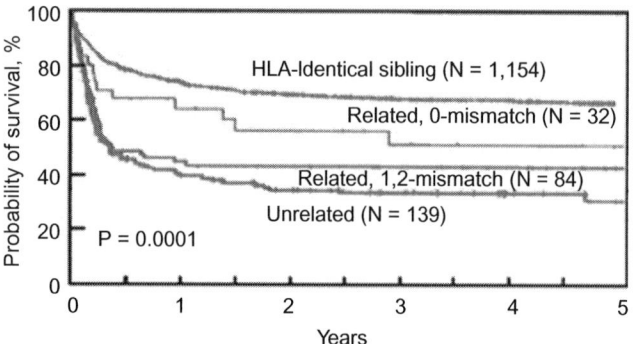

FIGURE 49.1 **Survival after allogeneic bone marrow transplantation for severe aplastic anemia.** Data for HLA-identical siblings and related matched/mismatched transplants are from the International Bone Marrow Transplant Registry (IBMTR). Data for unrelated donor transplants are from the European Bone Marrow Transplant registry (EBMT), Fred Hutchinson Cancer Research Center, IBMTR, and the IMUST study group. Survival curves are not adjusted for varying patient, disease, and transplant regimen characteristics. *Reproduced with permission from the National Bone Marrow Donor Program.*

irradiation have all been used to establish models of marrow failure. All three of these agents lead to pancytopenia and a hypocellular marrow but the marrow failure is due to stem cell injury and damage to the microenvironment rather than autoimmune-mediated suppression of hematopoiesis. More recently, infusion of lymphocytes from congenic mice was used to model immune-mediated marrow failure; this model induces a hypocellular bone marrow and severe pancytopenia, but is not truly autoimmune (Chen et al., 2004).

THERAPY FOR APLASTIC ANEMIA

Definitive therapy for aplastic anemia includes bone marrow transplantation (BMT) or immunosuppressive therapy. A variety of immunosuppressive agents have been used, but antithymocyte globulin (ATG) and cyclosporin A (CSA) are the most commonly employed. Supportive care with blood transfusions and antibiotics is commonly required. Administration of hematopoietic growth factors has not been shown to improve survival in aplastic anemia.

Bone Marrow Transplantation (BMT)

BMT is the treatment of choice for young patients who have an HLA-matched sibling donor (Figure 49.1). Cyclophosphamide (50 mg/kg/day × 4 days) with or without ATG, is most commonly used for conditioning before BMT. This regimen is non-myeloablative; however, the immunosuppression is sufficient to allow engraftment in most cases (May et al., 1993; Storb et al., 1997; Kahl et al., 2005). Alternative regimens using fludarabine, cyclophosphamide, and antithymocyte globulin are increasingly being used (Maury et al., 2009). Survival rates following matched sibling allogeneic BMT have steadily improved since the 1970s largely because of improved supportive care, improved human leukocyte antigen (HLA) typing, and better graft-versus-host-disease (GVHD) prophylaxis (Bacigalupo, 1999). Late BMT-related complications such as chronic GVHD occur

in up to one-third of patients, with many of these patients requiring long-term therapy for their GVHD (Storb et al., 2001). Patient age and the type of allograft (HLA-matched sibling, unrelated, or mismatched donors) are the most important factors influencing outcome. In patients under 30 years of age, the cure rate after HLA-matched sibling BMT ranges from 70 to 90% (Horowitz, 2000; Storb et al., 2001; Ades et al., 2004;). However, the risk of GVHD steadily increases with age, leading to reduced survival.

BMT from Unrelated Donors

BMT from HLA-matched unrelated donors (MUD) is usually reserved for patients who fail to respond to one or more courses of immunosuppressive therapy. The risk for transplant-related mortality and GVHD is almost twice that of BMT from matched sibling donors (Bacigalupo et al., 2000b). The best results have been reported in patients under 21 years of age with disease duration of less than 1 year (Margolis et al., 1996; Deeg et al., 2001, 2006). The International Bone Marrow Transplant Registry reported on the results of 318 alternative donor transplants between 1988 and 1998 (Passweg et al., 2006). Most patients in this series were young, heavily transfused, and of poor performance status. The probability of graft failure was 20% and the survival probability at 5 years was less than 40%. The Fred Hutchinson Cancer Research Center reported on the results of unrelated allogeneic bone marrow transplantation in SAA after conditioning with low-dose total body irradiation, high-dose cyclophosphamide, and ATG (Deeg et al., 2006). The median age was 19 years and with a median follow-up of 7 years. Overall survival was 61% for patients who received transplants from matched unrelated donors and 39% for patients receiving transplants from HLA mismatched unrelated donors; more than 70% of patients acquired acute GVHD and over 50% developed chronic GVHD. Nevertheless, improved typing, newer conditioning regimens, and better GVHD prophylaxis are leading to better survival, higher engraftment rates, and less GVHD. The European group for Blood and Marrow Transplanation (EBMT) has been conditioning SAA patients for BMT with fludarabine, cyclophosphamide, and antithyomcyte globulin (ATG) ± total body irradiation (TBI). The EMBT has reported survival rates as high as 75% using this conditioning regimen (Bacigalupo et al., 2010). Survival is best in children and in patients who undergo BMT within 2 years of diagnosis.

IMMUNOSUPPRESSIVE THERAPY

Antithymocyte globulin (ATG) is produced by immunizing animals (horse or rabbit) against human thymocytes and kills human T cells through its cytolytic activity. Both horse (hATG) and rabbit (rATG) are approved for use in the United States. However, difficulty in maintaining quality control has led to the withdrawal of hATG in Europe. Cyclosporine (CSA) suppresses T cell function by inhibiting the expression of nuclear regulatory proteins. Both single agent ATG and single agent CSA (Maschan et al., 1999) can induce remissions in acquired aplastic anemia; however, the combination ATG/CSA leads to a higher response rate and a greater likelihood of achieving transfusion independence (Frickhofen et al., 1991; Marsh et al., 1999). A randomized controlled trial demonstrated that hATG/CSA is superior to rATG/CSA (Scheinberg et al., 2011). The combination of ATG/CSA leads to 5-year survival rates comparable to BMT, but most of these patients are not cured of their disease (Marsh et al., 1999). Response rates to hATG/CSA range between 60 and 80%, but in contrast to BMT, most patients do not acquire normal blood counts (Frickhofen et al., 2003; Rosenfeld et al., 2003). Another limitation of this approach is that many patients relapse, become dependent on cyclosporine, or develop secondary clonal disease such as PNH or MDS (Bacigalupo et al., 2000a; Rosenfeld et al., 2003). These late events often lead to substantial morbidity and mortality. The National Institutes of Health treated 122 patients (median age, 35 years) with the combination of ATG/CSA and methylprednisolone over a period of 8 years (Rosenfeld et al., 2003). The response rate was 58% and actuarial survival at 7 years was 55%; 13% of patients died within 3 months of treatment, most from fungal infections (Figure 49.2). The relapse rate for responders was 40% and 13 patients developed MDS. In an attempt to improve response rate and survival, and to decrease the relapse rate and secondary MDS that occurs after hATG/CSA, the NIH added mycophenolate (1 gram twice daily for 18 months) to the standard hATG/CSA regimen. This three-drug regimen resulted in a 62% response rate, but 37% of the responders relapsed (most while taking mycophenolate) and 9% progressed to either MDS or leukemia; thus, the addition of mycophenolate did not improve response or survival

(Scheinberg et al., 2006). Alemtuzumab is a highly immunosuppressive monoclonal antibody that binds to cell surface CD52, which is expressed primarily on B cells, T cells, and monocytes. Alemtuzumab has activity in treating SAA, but response rates in therapy naïve patients are less than 30% (Scheinberg et al., 2012).

HIGH-DOSE CYCLOPHOSPHAMIDE WITHOUT BMT

The first successful human allogeneic BMT, reported in 1972 by Thomas et al. in a patient with aplastic anemia, employed high-dose cyclophosphamide (Thomas et al., 1972), and this remains (often in conjunction with ATG) the most commonly employed conditioning regimen for aplastic anemia (Storb et al., 2001). Complete reconstitution of autologous hematopoiesis occurs in 10–15% of patients undergoing allogeneic BMT for aplastic anemia (Thomas et al., 1976; Sensenbrenner et al., 1977; Gmur et al., 1979). The EMBT reported that 10% of SAA patients experience autologous reconstitution following BMT using a cyclophosphamide + ATG conditioning regimen. Interestingly, 10-year survival (84%) in patients with autologous recovery was better than in patients who underwent engrafting (74%) (Piccin et al., 2010).

The unique pharmacology of cyclophosphamide explains the autologous hematopoietic recovery (Emadi et al., 2009). Cyclophosphamide is a prodrug that is converted to 4-hydroxycyclophosphamide and its tautomer aldophosphamide in the liver. These compounds diffuse into the cell and are converted to the active compound phosphoramide mustard, or they are inactivated by aldehyde dehydrogenase to form the inert carboxyphosphamide. Lymphocytes have low levels of aldehyde dehydrogenase and are rapidly killed by high doses of cyclophosphamide; hematopoietic stem cells possess high levels of aldehyde dehydrogenase and are resistant to cyclophosphamide (Hilton, 1984; Jones et al., 1995). Thus, high-dose cyclophosphamide is highly immunosuppressive, but not myeloablative, allowing endogenous hematopoietic stem cells to reconstitute hematopoiesis (Figure 49.3). With this background, high-dose cyclophosphamide without BMT was used successfully in aplastic anemia patients who lacked appropriate donor (Brodsky et al., 1996, 2010; Tisdale et al., 2000; Jaime-Perez et al., 2001). The largest and most mature study with high-dose cyclophosphamide is from Johns Hopkins (Brodsky et al., 2010). These investigators treated 67 SAA patients with high-dose cyclophosphamide; 44 patients were treatment-naïve and 23 were refractory to one or more previous immunosuppressive regimens. At 10 years, the overall actuarial survival, response rate, and event-free survival was 88%, 71%, and 58%, respectively,

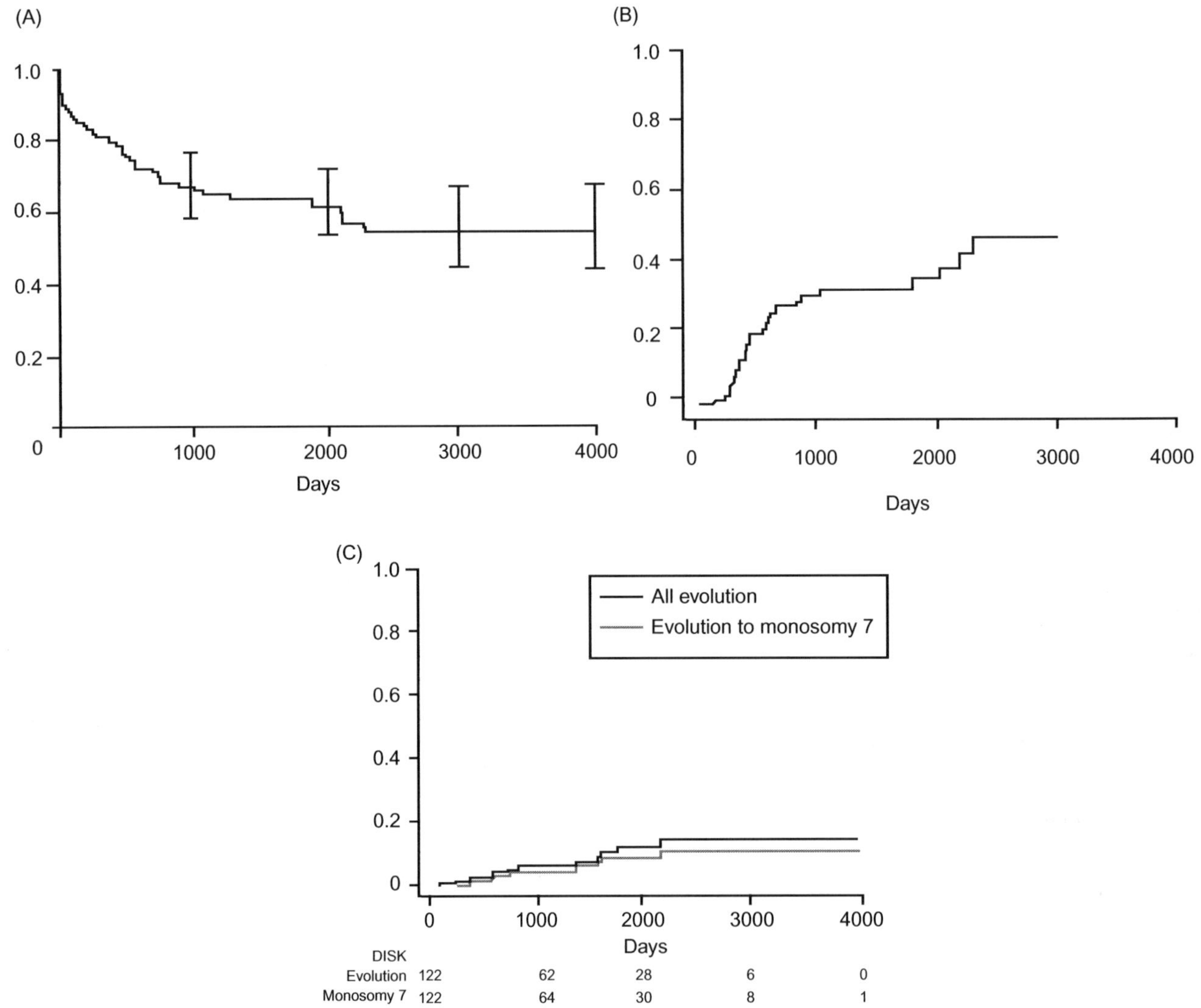

(A)

(B)

(C)

— All evolution
— Evolution to monosomy 7

DISK				
Evolution	122	62	28	6	0
Monosomy 7	122	64	30	8	1

FIGURE 49.2 (A) Survival probability for 122 patients with severe aplastic anemia following treatment with antithymocyte globulin and cyclosporine. (B) Probability of relapse in 74 patients with aplastic anemia classified as responders at 3 months after treatment with antithymocyte globulin and cyclosporine. (C) Proportion of patients experiencing clonal evolution. *Reproduced from JAMA (Rosenfeld et al., 2003) with permission.*

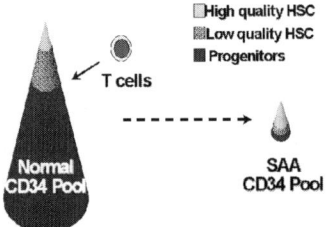

☐ High quality HSC
▨ Low quality HSC
■ Progenitors

T cells

Normal CD34 Pool

SAA CD34 Pool

FIGURE 49.3 Model depicting the pathophysiology of bone marrow failure in acquired aplastic anemia. Autoaggressive lymphocytes lyse CD34$^+$ bone marrow progenitor cells but seem to spare more immature CD34$^+$ cells known as high quality stem cells.

for the 44 treatment-naïve patients. Patients with refractory SAA fared less well; at 10 years, overall actuarial survival, response, and event-free survival rates were 62%, 48%, and 27%, respectively. For treatment-naïve patients, the median time to a neutrophil count of 0.5×10^9/L was 60 (range, 28–104) days; the median time to last platelet and red cell transfusion was 117 and 186 days, respectively. Relapse occurred in just two of the treatment-naïve patients, one of whom was retreated with high-dose cyclophosphamide into a second complete remission. Despite the high response rate and low risk of relapse and secondary clonal disease, many investigators are unwilling to accept the relatively long period of aplasia associated with this therapy (Figure 49.4).

APLASTIC ANEMIA AND CLONALITY

Survivors of aplastic anemia are at high risk of clonal progression following immunosuppressive therapy (Socie et al., 1993). PNH and MDS are the most common clonal

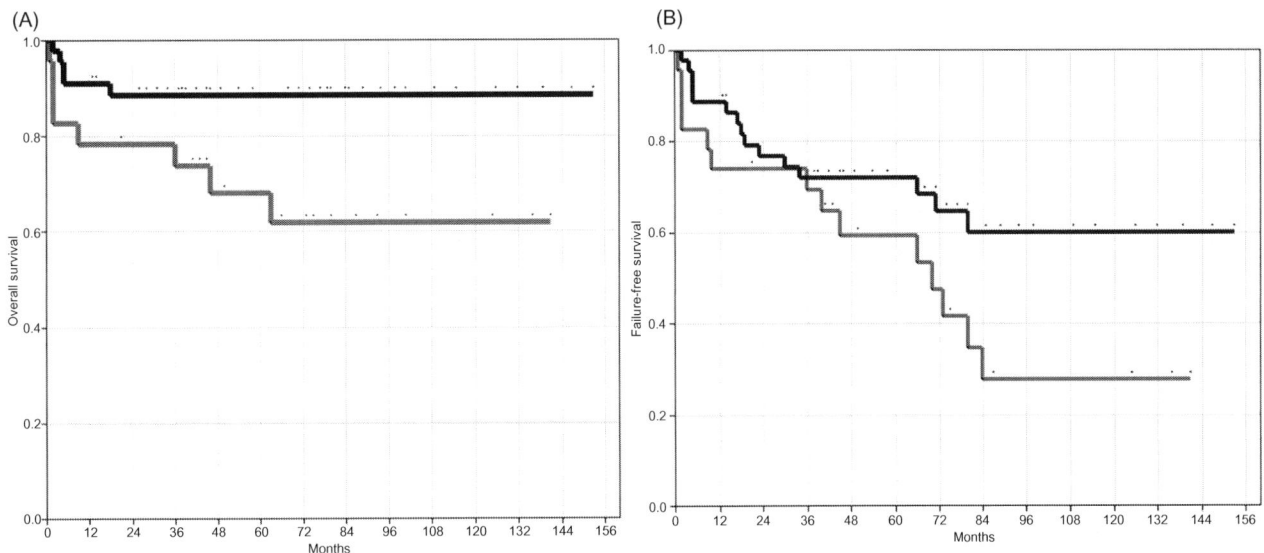

FIGURE 49.4 (A) Overall survival after high-dose cyclophosphamide therapy. Overall survival for 44 treatment-naive patients (top line) and 23 patients refractory to prior immunosuppressive therapy (bottom line). $P = .03$ (log-rank test). (B) Failure-free survival after high-dose cyclophosphamide therapy. Failure-free survival for 44 treatment-naive patients (top line) and 23 patients refractory to prior immunosuppressive therapy (bottom line). $P = .07$ (log-rank test). *Reproduced from Blood (Brodsky et al., 2010) with permission.*

disorders to evolve from aplastic anemia (Tichelli et al., 1988; de Planque et al., 1989). Even before the widespread use of immunosuppressive therapy, 5% of patients progressed to clonal hematopoiesis. This suggests that the increase in MDS and PNH following immunosuppressive therapy is not caused by the immunosuppression; rather, the increased survival following immunosuppressive therapy may allow time for these underlying clones to expand (Mukhina et al., 2001).

PNH results from the expansion of an abnormal hematopoietic stem cell that harbors a somatic mutation of the X-linked gene, termed *PIG-A* (Brodsky, 2008, 2009). The product of the *PIG-A* gene is required for glycosylphosphatidyinositol (GPI) anchor biosynthesis; consequently, PNH cells are deficient in GPI-anchored proteins. Several GPI-anchored proteins (CD59 and CD55) protect cells from complement-mediated destruction, and their absence explains the hemolytic anemia associated with PNH. It is unclear how the PNH stem cell and its progeny achieve clonal dominance in the setting of aplastic anemia, despite the fact that PNH cells are more vulnerable to complement-mediated destruction; however, it may relate to relative resistance to the autoimmune attack. Specifically, it has been suggested that PNH cells may be relatively resistant to an autoimmune attack because they are deficient in GPI-anchored ULBPs that serve as ligands for the NKG2D receptor found on natural killer cells and T cells (Hanaoka et al., 2006; Savage et al., 2009). Alternatively, it has been proposed that "second hit" mutations may also give the PNH clone a growth advantage (Inoue et al., 2006).

MDS also commonly arises in aplastic anemia patients treated with immunosuppressive therapy. In a retrospective review of children with severe aplastic anemia, 11 of 86 patients who received immunosuppressive therapy developed MDS (Ohara et al., 1997). Up to 15% of adult patients with aplastic anemia will also develop MDS following immunosuppressive therapy, with monosomy 7 being the most common chromosomal abnormality (Rosenfeld et al., 2003).

CONCLUDING REMARKS—FUTURE PROSPECTS

Aplastic anemia was originally thought to be due to a defect in hematopoietic stem cells or their microenvironment. It is now clear that most cases of acquired aplastic anemia are caused by autoreactive lymphocytes that target bone marrow stem/progenitor cells. With modern therapies, the 5-year survival rate for SAA exceeds 85%. BMT offers the best chance for cure, but its use is restricted by the relatively high morbidity and mortality in older patients and those who lack an HLA-matched sibling donor. Immunosuppressive therapy remains the standard of care for patients who are not suitable candidates for BMT. Remissions are achieved in up to 75% of patients, but the high rate of relapse and secondary clonal diseases limits the efficacy of immunosuppressive therapy. Unfortunately, the addition of newer immunosuppressive therapies (MMF, sirolimus, etc.) to ATG/CsA does not seem to improve response or decrease the risk of relapse or clonal disease. High-dose cyclophosphamide therapy seems to produce higher quality remissions with fewer relapses, but this approach has not been widely adopted due to the prolonged period of aplasia. Currently, advances in mitigating graft failure and GVHD in the setting of alternative donor BMT appear to be outpacing the development of more effective IST therapies for SAA. Over the next 5 years, there is likely to be great use of unrelated and HLA-mismatched BMT to treat SAA, especially in patients who do not respond to or relapse after immunosuppressive therapy. The development of post-transplant CY to expand the donor pool and mitigate GVHD appears promising (Brodsky et al., 2008; Dezern et al., 2011).

REFERENCES

Ades, L., Mary, J.Y., Robin, M., Ferry, C., Porcher, R., Esperou, H., et al., 2004. Long-term outcome after bone marrow transplantation for severe aplastic anemia. Blood. 103, 2490–2497.

Bacigalupo, A., 1999. Bone marrow transplantation for severe aplastic anemia from HLA identical siblings. Haematologica. 84, 2–4.

Bacigalupo, A., Bruno, B., Saracco, P., Di Bona, E., Locasciulli, A., Locatelli, F., et al., 2000a. Antilymphocyte globulin, cyclosporine, prednisolone, and granulocyte colony-stimulating factor for severe aplastic anemia: an update of the GITMO/EBMT study on 100 patients. Blood. 95, 1931–1934.

Bacigalupo, A., Oneto, R., Bruno, B., Socie, G., Passweg, J., Locasciulli, A., et al., 2000b. Current results of bone marrow transplantation in patients with acquired severe aplastic anemia. Report of the European Group for Blood and Marrow transplantation. On behalf of the Working Party on Severe Aplastic Anemia of the European Group for Blood and Marrow Transplantation. Acta Haematol. 103, 19–25.

Bacigalupo, A., Socie, G., Lanino, E., Prete, A., Locatelli, F., Locasciulli, A., et al., 2010. Fludarabine, cyclophosphamide, antithymocyte globulin, with or without low dose total body irradiation, for alternative donor transplants, in acquired severe aplastic anemia: a retrospective study from the EBMT-SAA working party. Haematologica. 95, 976–982.

Bagby Jr., G.C., 2003. Genetic basis of Fanconi anemia. Curr. Opin. Hematol. 10, 68–76.

Borowitz, M.J., Craig, F.E., DiGiuseppe, J.A., Illingworth, A.J., Rosse, W., Sutherland, D.R., et al., 2010. Guidelines for the diagnosis and monitoring of paroxysmal nocturnal hemoglobinuria and related disorders by flow cytometry. Cytometry B Clin. Cytom. 78, 211–230.

Brodsky, R.A., 2008. Narrative review: paroxysmal nocturnal hemoglobinuria: the physiology of complement-related hemolytic anemia. Ann. Intern. Med. 148, 587–595.

Brodsky, R.A., 2009. How I treat paroxysmal nocturnal hemoglobinuria. Blood. 25, 6522–6527.

Brodsky, R.A., Jones, R.J., 2005. Aplastic anaemia. Lancet. 365, 1647–1656.

Brodsky, R.A., Sensenbrenner, L.L., Jones, R.J., 1996. Complete remission in acquired severe aplastic anemia following high-dose cyclophosphamide. Blood. 87, 491–494.

Brodsky, R.A., Mukhina, G.L., Li, S., Nelson, K.L., Chiurazzi, P.L., Buckley, J.T., et al., 2000. Improved detection and characterization of paroxysmal nocturnal hemoglobinuria using fluorescent aerolysin. Am. J. Clin. Pathol. 114, 459–466.

Brodsky, R.A., Luznik, L., Bolanos-Meade, J., Leffell, M.S., Jones, R.J., Fuchs, E.J., et al., 2008. Reduced intensity HLA-haploidentical BMT with post transplantation cyclophosphamide in nonmalignant hematologic diseases. Bone Marrow Transplant. 42, 523–527.

Brodsky, R.A., Chen, A.R., Dorr, D., Fuchs, E.J., Huff, C.A., Luznik, L., et al., 2010. High-dose cyclophosphamide for severe aplastic anemia: long-term follow-up. Blood. 115, 2136–2141.

Brown, K.E., Tisdale, J., Barrett, A.J., Dunbar, C.E., Young, N.S., 1997. Hepatitis-associated aplastic anemia. N. Engl. J. Med. 336, 1059–1064.

Camitta, B.M., Thomas, E.D., Nathan, D.G., Gale, R.P., Kopecky, K.J., Rappeport, J.M., et al., 1979. A prospective study of androgens and bone marrow transplantation for treatment of severe aplastic anemia. Blood. 53, 504–514.

Cattral, M.S., Langnas, A.N., Markin, R.S., Antonson, D.L., Heffron, T.G., Fox, I.J., et al., 1994. Aplastic anemia after liver transplantation for fulminant liver failure. Hepatology. 20, 813–818.

Champlin, R.E., Feig, S.A., Sparkes, R.S., Galen, R.P., 1984. Bone marrow transplantation from identical twins in the treatment of aplastic anaemia: implication for the pathogenesis of the disease. Br. J. Haematol. 56, 455–463.

Chen, J., 2005. Animal models for acquired bone marrow failure syndromes. Clin. Med. Res. 3, 102–108.

Chen, J., Lipovsky, K., Ellison, F.M., Calado, R.T., Young, N.S., 2004. Bystander destruction of hematopoietic progenitor and stem cells in a mouse model of infusion-induced bone marrow failure. Blood. 104, 1671–1678.

de Planque, M.M., Bacigalupo, A., Wursch, A., Hows, J.M., Devergie, A., Frickhofen, N., et al., 1989. Long-term follow-up of severe aplastic anaemia patients treated with antithymocyte globulin. Br. J. Haematol. 73, 121–126.

Deeg, H.J., Amylon, I.D., Harris, R.E., Collins, R., Beatty, P.G., Feig, S., et al., 2001. Marrow transplants from unrelated donors for patients with aplastic anemia: minimum effective dose of total body irradiation. Biol. Blood Marrow Transplant. 7, 208–215.

Deeg, H.J., O'Donnell, M., Tolar, J., Agarwal, R., Harris, R.E., Feig, S.A., et al., 2006. Optimization of conditioning for marrow transplantation from unrelated donors for patients with aplastic anemia after failure of immunosuppressive therapy. Blood. 108, 1485–1491.

Dezern, A.E., Luznik, L., Fuchs, E.J., Jones, R.J., Brodsky, R.A., 2011. Post-transplantation cyclophosphamide for GVHD prophylaxis in severe aplastic anemia. Bone Marrow Transplant. 46, 1012–1013.

Dokal, I., Vulliamy, T., 2003. Dyskeratosis congenita: its link to telomerase and aplastic anaemia. Blood Rev. 17, 217–225.

Ehrlich, P., 1888. Ueber einem Fall von Anamie mit Bemer-kungen uber regenerative Veranderungen des Knochenmarks. Charite-Annalen. 13, 301–309.

Emadi, A., Jones, R.J., Brodsky, R.A., 2009. Cyclophosphamide and cancer: golden anniversary. Nat. Rev. Clin. Oncol. 6, 638–647.

Feng, X., Chuhjo, T., Sugimori, C., Kotani, T., Lu, X., Takami, A., et al., 2004. Diazepam-binding inhibitor-related protein 1: a candidate autoantigen in acquired aplastic anemia patients harboring a minor population of paroxysmal nocturnal hemoglobinuria-type cells. Blood. 104, 2425–2431.

Frickhofen, N., Kaltwasser, J.P., Schrezenmeier, H., Raghavacher, A., Vogt, H.G., Hermann, F., et al., 1991. Treatment of aplastic anemia with antilymphocyte globulin and methylprednisolone with or without cyclosporine. N. Engl. J. Med. 324, 1297–1304.

Frickhofen, N., Heimpel, H., Kaltwasser, J.P., Schrezenmeier, H., 2003. Antithymocyte globulin with or without cyclosporin A: 11-year follow-up of a randomized trial comparing treatments of aplastic anemia. Blood. 101, 1236–1242.

Gmur, J., von Felten, A., Phyner, K., Frick, P.G., 1979. Autologous hematologic recovery from aplastic anemia following high dose cyclophosphamide and HLA-matched allogeneic bone marrow transplantation. Acta Haematologica. 62, 20–24.

Hanaoka, N., Kawaguchi, T., Horikawa, K., Nagakura, S., Mitsuya, H., Nakakuma, H., et al., 2006. Immunoselection by natural killer cells of PIGA mutant cells missing stress-inducible ULBP. Blood. 107, 1184–1191.

Hilton, J., 1984. Role of aldehyde dehydrogenase in cyclophosphamide-resistant L1210 leukemia. Cancer Res. 44, 5156–5160.

Hinterberger, W., Rowlings, P.A., Hinterberger-Fischer, M., Gibson, J., Jacobsen, N, Klein, J.P., et al., 1997. Results of transplanting bone marrow from genetically identical twins into patients with aplastic anemia. Ann. Intern. Med. 126, 116–122.

Hirano, N., Butler, M.O., Bergwelt-Baildon, M.S., Maecker, B., Schultze, J.L., O'Connor, K.C., et al., 2003. Autoantibodies frequently detected in patients with aplastic anemia. Blood. 102, 4567–4575.

Hoffman, R., Zanjani, E.D., Lutton, J.D., Zalusky, R., Wasserman, L.R., 1977. Suppression of erythroid-colony formation by lymphocytes from patients with aplastic anemia. N. Engl. J. Med. 296, 10–13.

Horowitz, M.M., 2000. Current status of allogeneic bone marrow transplantation in acquired aplastic anemia. Semin. Hematol. 37, 30–42.

Inoue, N., Izui-Sarumaru, T., Murakami, Y., Endo, Y., Nishimura, J.I., Kurokawa, K., et al., 2006. Molecular basis of clonal expansion of hematopoiesis in two patients with paroxysmal nocturnal hemoglobinuria (PNH). Blood. 108, 4232–4236.

Issaragrisil, S., Chansung, K., Kaufman, D.W., Sirijirachai, J., Thamprasit, T., Young, N.S., et al., 1997a. Aplastic anemia in rural Thailand: its association with grain farming and agricultural pesticide exposure. Aplastic anemia study group. Am. J. Public Health. 87, 1551–1554.

Issaragrisil, S., Kaufman, D.W., Anderson, T., Chansung, K., Thamprasit, T., Sirijirachai, J., et al., 1997b. Low drug attributability of aplastic anemia in Thailand. Blood. 89, 4034–4039.

Issaragrisil, S., Leaverton, P.E., Chansung, K., Thamprasit, T., Porapakham, Y., Vannasaeng, S., et al., 1999. Regional patterns in the incidence of aplastic anemia in Thailand. The aplastic anemia study group. Am. J. Hematol. 61, 164–168.

Jaime-Perez, J.C., Gonzalez-Llano, O., Gomez-Almaguer, D., 2001. High-dose cyclophosphamide in the treatment of severe aplastic anemia in children. Am. J. Hematol. 66, 71.

Jones, R.J., Barber, J.P., Vala, M.S., Collector, M.I., Kaufmann, S.H., Ludeman, S.M., et al., 1995. Assessment of aldehyde dehydrogenase in viable cells. Blood. 85, 2742–2746.

Kahl, C., Leisenring, W., Deeg, H.J., Chauncey, T.R., Flowers, M.E., Martin, P.J., et al., 2005. Cyclophosphamide and antithymocyte globulin as a conditioning regimen for allogeneic marrow transplantation in patients with aplastic anaemia: a long-term follow-up. Br. J. Haematol. 130, 747–751.

Kaufman, D.W., Kelly, J.P., Levy, M., Shapiro, S., 1991. The Drug Etiology of Agranulocytosis and Aplastic Anemia. Oxford University Press, Inc., New York, 404pp.

Locasciulli, A., Bacigalupo, A., Bruno, B., Montante, B., Marsh, J., Tichelli, A., et al., 2010. Hepatitis-associated aplastic anaemia: epidemiology and treatment results obtained in Europe. A report of The EBMT aplastic anaemia working party. Br. J. Haematol. 149, 890–895.

Maciejewski, J.P., Hibbs, J.R., Anderson, S., Katevas, P., Young, N.S., 1994. Bone marrow and peripheral blood lymphocyte phenotype in patients with bone marrow failure. Exp. Hematol. 22, 1102–1110.

Maciejewski, J.P., Selleri, C., Sato, T., Anderson, S., Young, N.S., 1995. Increased expression of Fas antigen on bone marrow CD34 + cells of patients with aplastic anaemia. Br. J. Haematol. 91, 245–252.

Manz, C.Y., Dietrich, P.Y., Schnuriger, V., Nissen, C., Wodnar-Filipowicz, A., 1997. T-cell receptor beta chain variability in bone marrow and peripheral blood in severe acquired aplastic anemia. Blood Cells Mol. Dis. 23, 110–122.

Margolis, D., Camitta, B., Pietryga, D., Keever-Taylor, C., Baxter-Lowe, L.A.P.K., Kupst, M.J., et al., 1996. Unrelated donor bone marrow transplantation to treat severe aplastic anaemia in children and young adults. Br. J. Haematol. 94, 65–72.

Marsh, J., Schrezenmeier, H., Marin, P., Ilhan, O., Ljungman, P., McCann, S., et al., 1999. Prospective randomized multicenter study comparing cyclosporin alone versus the combination of antithymocyte globulin and cyclosporin for treatment of patients with nonsevere aplastic anemia: a report from the European blood and marrow transplant severe aplastic anaemia working party. Blood. 93, 2191–2195.

Maschan, A., Bogatcheva, N., Kryjanovskii, O., Shneider, M., Litvinov, D., Mitiushkina, T., et al., 1999. Results at a single centre of immunosuppression with Cyclosporine A in 66 children with aplastic anaemia. Br. J. Haematol. 106, 967–970.

Mathe, G., Amiel, J.L., Schwarzenberg, L., Choay, J., Trolard, P., Schneider, M., et al., 1970. Bone marrow graft in man after conditioning by antilymphocytic serum. Br. Med. J. 2, 131–136.

Matsui, W.H., Brodsky, R.A., Smith, B.D., Borowitz, M.J., Jones, R.J., 2006. Quantitative analysis of bone marrow CD34 cells in aplastic anemia and hypoplastic myelodysplastic syndromes. Leukemia. 20, 458–462.

Maury, S., Bacigalupo, A., Anderlini, P., Aljurf, M., Marsh, J., Socie, G., et al., 2009. Improved outcome of patients older than 30 years receiving HLA-identical sibling hematopoietic stem cell transplantation for severe acquired aplastic anemia using fludarabine-based conditioning: a comparison with conventional conditioning regimen. Haematologica. 94, 1312–1315.

May, W.S., Sensenbrenner, L.L., Burns, W.H., Ambinder, R., Carroll, M.P., Jones, R.J., et al., 1993. BMT for severe aplastic anemia using cyclosporin. Bone Marrow Transplant. 11, 459–464.

Melenhorst, J.J., Fibbe, W.E., Struyk, L., van der Elsen, P.J., Willemze, R., Landegent, J.E., et al., 1997a. Analysis of T-cell clonality in bone marrow of patients with acquired aplastic anaemia. Br. J. Haematol. 96, 85–91.

Melenhorst, J.J., van Krieken, J.H.J.M., Dreef, E., Landegent, J.E., Willemze, R., Fibbe, W.E., et al., 1997b. T cells selectively infiltrate bone marrow areas with residual haemopoiesis of patients with acquired aplastic anaemia. Br. J. Haematol. 99, 517–519.

Modan, B., Segal, S., Shani, M., Sheba, C., 1975. Aplastic anemia in Israel: evaluation of the etiological role of chloramphenicol on a community-wide basis. Am. J. Med. Sci. 270, 441–445.

Mukhina, G.L., Buckley, J.T., Barber, J.P., Jones, R.J., Brodsky, R.A., 2001. Multilineage glycosylphosphatidylinositol anchor deficient hematopoiesis in untreated aplastic anemia. Br. J. Haematol. 115, 476–482.

Nakao, S., Yamaguchi, M., Shiobara, S., Yokoi, T., Miyawaki, T., Taniguchi, T., et al., 1992. Interferon-gamma gene expression in unstimulated bone marrow mononuclear cells predicts a good response to cyclosporine therapy in aplastic anemia. Blood. 79, 2532–2535.

Nakao, S., Takami, A., Takamatsu, H., Zeng, W., Sugimori, N., Yamazaki, H., et al., 1997. Isolation of a T-cell clone showing HLA-DRBI*0405-restricted cytotoxicity for hematopoietic cells in a patient with aplastic anemia. Blood. 89, 3691–3699.

Nimer, S.D., Ireland, P., Meshkinpour, A., Frane, M., 1994. An increased HLA DR2 frequency is seen in aplastic anemia patients. Blood. 84, 923–927.

Nissen, C., Cornu, P., Gratwohl, A., Speck, B., 1980. Peripheral blood cells from patients wih aplastic anaemia in partial remission suppress growth of their own bone marrow precursors in culture. Br. J. Haematol. 45, 233–243.

Nistico, A., Young, N.S., 1994. gamma-Interferon gene expression in the bone marrow of patients with aplastic anemia. Ann. Intern. Med. 120, 463–469.

Ohara, A., Kojima, S., Hamajima, N., Tsuchida, M., Imashuku, S., Ohta, S., et al., 1997. Myelodysplastic syndrome and acute myelogenous leukemia as a late clonal complication in children with acquired aplastic anemia. Blood. 90, 1009–1013.

Passweg, J.R., Perez, W.S., Eapen, M., Camitta, B.M., Gluckman, E., Hinterberger, W., et al., 2006. Bone marrow transplants from mismatched related and unrelated donors for severe aplastic anemia. Bone Marrow Transplant. 37, 641–649.

Piccin, A., McCann, S., Socie, G., Oneto, R., Bacigalupo, A., Locasciulli, A., et al., 2010. Survival of patients with documented autologous recovery after SCT for severe aplastic anemia: a study by the WPSAA of the EBMT. Bone Marrow Transplant. 45, 1008–1013.

Rosenfeld, S., Follmann, D., Nunez, O., Young, N.S., 2003. Antithymocyte globulin and cyclosporine for severe aplastic anemia: association between hematologic response and long-term outcome. JAMA. 289, 1130–1135.

Savage, W.J., DeRusso, P.A., Resar, L.M., Chen, A.R., Higman, M.A., Loeb, D.M., et al., 2007. Treatment of hepatitis-associated aplastic anemia with high-dose cyclophosphamide. Pediatr. Blood Cancer. 49, 947–951.

Savage, W.J., Barber, J.P., Mukhina, G.L., Hu, R., Chen, G., Matsui, W., et al., 2009. Glycosylphosphatidylinositol-anchored protein deficiency confers resistance to apoptosis in PNH. Exp. Hematol. 37, 42–51.

Scheinberg, P., Nunez, O., Wu, C., Young, N.S., 2006. Treatment of severe aplastic anaemia with combined immunosuppression: antithymocyte globulin, ciclosporin and mycophenolate mofetil. Br. J. Haematol. 133, 606–611.

Scheinberg, P., Nunez, O., Weinstein, B., Scheinberg, P., Biancotto, A., Wu, C.O., et al., 2011. Horse versus rabbit antithymocyte globulin in acquired aplastic anemia. N. Engl. J. Med. 365, 430–438.

Scheinberg, P., Nunez, O., Weinstein, B., Scheinberg, P., Wu, C.O., Young, N.S., 2012. Activity of alemtuzumab monotherapy in treatment-naive, relapsed, and refractory severe acquired aplastic anemia. Blood. 119, 345–354.

Sensenbrenner, L.L., Steele, A.A., Santos, G.W., 1977. Recovery of hematologic competence without engraftment following attempted bone marrow transplantation for aplastic anemia: report of a case with diffusion chamber studies. Exp. Hematol. 77, 51–58.

Socie, G., Henry-Amar, M., Bacigalupo, A., Hows, J., Tichelli, A., Ljungman, P., et al., 1993. Malignant tumors occurring after treatment of aplastic anemia. N. Engl. J. Med. 329, 1152–1157.

Storb, R., Leisenring, W., Anasetti, C., Appelbaum, F.R., Buckner, C.D., Bensinger, W.I., et al., 1997. Long-term follow-up of allogeneic marrow transplants in patients with aplastic anemia conditioned by cyclophosphamide combined with antithymocyte globulin. Blood. 89, 3890–3891.

Storb, R., Blume, K.G., O'Donnell, M.R., Chauncey, T., Forman, S.J., Deeg, H.J., et al., 2001. Cyclophosphamide and antithymocyte globulin to condition patients with aplastic anemia for allogeneic marrow transplantations: the experience in four centers. Biol. Blood Marrow Transplant. 7, 39–44.

Szklo, M., Sensenbrenner, L., Markowitz, J., Weida, S., Warm, S., Linet, M., et al., 1985. Incidence of aplastic anemia in metropolitan Baltimore: a population-based study. Blood. 66, 115–119.

Thomas, E.D., Storb, R., Fefer, A., Slichter, S.J., Bryant, J.I., Buckner, C.D., et al., 1972. Aplastic anaemia treated by marrow transplantation. Lancet. i, 284–289.

Thomas, E.D., Storb, R., Giblett, E.R., Longpre, B., Weiden, P.L., Fefer, A., et al., 1976. Recovery from aplastic anemia following attempted marrow transplantation. Exp. Hematol. 4, 97–102.

Tichelli, A., Gratwohl, A., Wursch, A., Nissen, C., Speck, B., 1988. Late haematological complications in severe aplastic anaemia. Br. J. Haematol. 69, 413–418.

Tisdale, J.F., Dunn, D.E., Geller, N., Plante, M., Nunez, O., Dunbar, C.E., et al., 2000. High-dose cyclophosphamide in severe aplastic anaemia: a randomised trial. Lancet. 356, 1554–1559.

Tsangaris, E., Klaassen, R., Fernandez, C.V., Yanofsky, R., Shereck, E., Champagne, J., et al., 2011. Genetic analysis of inherited bone marrow failure syndromes from one prospective, comprehensive and population-based cohort and identification of novel mutations. J. Med. Genet. 48, 618–628.

Tzakis, A.G., Arditi, M., Whittington, P.F., Yanaga, K., Esquivel, C., Andrews, W.A., et al., 1988. Aplastic anemia complicating orthotopic liver transplantation for non-A, non-B hepatitis. N. Engl. J. Med. 319, 393–396.

Zeng, W., Maciejewski, J.P., Chen, G., Young, N.S., 2001. Limited heterogeneity of T cell receptor BV usage in aplastic anemia. J. Clin. Invest. 108, 765–773.

Zoumbos, N.C., Gascón, P., Djeu, J.Y., Trost, S.R., Young, N.S., 1985. Circulating activated suppressor T lymphocytes in aplastic anemia. N. Engl. J. Med. 312, 257–265.

Chapter 50

Monogenic Autoimmune Lymphoproliferative Syndromes

Joao Bosco Oliveira[1], V. Koneti Rao[2], Helen Su[3], and Michael Lenardo[4]

[1]Instituto de Medicina Integral Prof. Fernando Figueira - IMIP, Recife, PE Brazil, [2]Molecular Development Section, Laboratory of Immunology, National Institute of Allergy and Infectious Diseases, National Institutes of Health, Bethesda, MD, USA, [3]Human Immunological Diseases Unit, Laboratory of Host Defenses, National Institute of Allergy and Infectious Diseases, National Institutes of Health, Bethesda, MD, USA, [4]Molecular Development Section, Laboratory of Immunology, National Institute of Allergy and Infectious Diseases, National Institutes of Health, Bethesda, MD, USA

Chapter Outline

Introduction—Apoptosis and the Immune System 695
Clinical and Pathological Features 696
  Autoimmune Lymphoproliferative Syndrome 696
  Clinical Presentation 697
  Laboratory Evaluation 698
  Imaging Studies 699
  Treatment 699
  Prognosis 700
ALPS-Related Disorders 700
  Caspase-8 and FADD Deficiencies 700
  RAS-Associated Autoimmune Leukoproliferative Disorder (RALD) 702
  Genetic Features 702
Autoimmune Lymphoproliferative Syndrome 702
  Germline FAS Mutations 702
Somatic FAS Mutations 703
Additional Genetic Etiologies 703
RAS-Associated Autoimmune Leukoproliferative Disorder 704
  In Vivo and In Vitro Models of Disease 704
  Pathogenic Effector Mechanisms 705
    ALPS 705
    RALD 705
    CEDS 706
    BENTA Disease 706
    Disease Biomarkers 707
Conclusion 707
Acknowledgments 707
References 707

INTRODUCTION—APOPTOSIS AND THE IMMUNE SYSTEM

In the immune system, lymphocyte homeostasis is controlled by cell proliferation and cell death. Maintaining lymphocyte homeostasis is important for the normal functioning of T cells, whose numbers must rapidly expand in response to pathogens, and which subsequently contract after pathogen clearance (Lenardo et al., 1999). A key mechanism by which an organism achieves this balancing act is through a form of programmed cell death called apoptosis, which has specific morphological and biochemical hallmarks (Galluzzi et al., 2007). The hallmarks include cell shrinkage, chromatin condensation, blebbing, the formation of apoptotic bodies, and the activation of intracellular enzymes called caspases. Lymphocyte numbers can also be controlled by additional mechanisms such as programmed necrosis, which follows a set genetic pathway. In addition, stimulation of death receptors or T cell receptors can lead to a necrotic death when caspases have been inhibited and, therefore, it presumably serves as an auxiliary death mechanism for lymphocyte homeostasis (Han et al., 2011).

In lymphocytes, apoptosis can occur during the height of the immune response after cells enter late G1 or S phase of the cell cycle and become sensitive to signals generated by death receptors or after repetitive stimulation through antigenic receptors (Lenardo et al., 1999). Apoptosis also takes

N. Rose & I. Mackay (Eds): The Autoimmune Diseases, Fifth edition. DOI: http://dx.doi.org/10.1016/B978-0-12-384929-8.00050-2

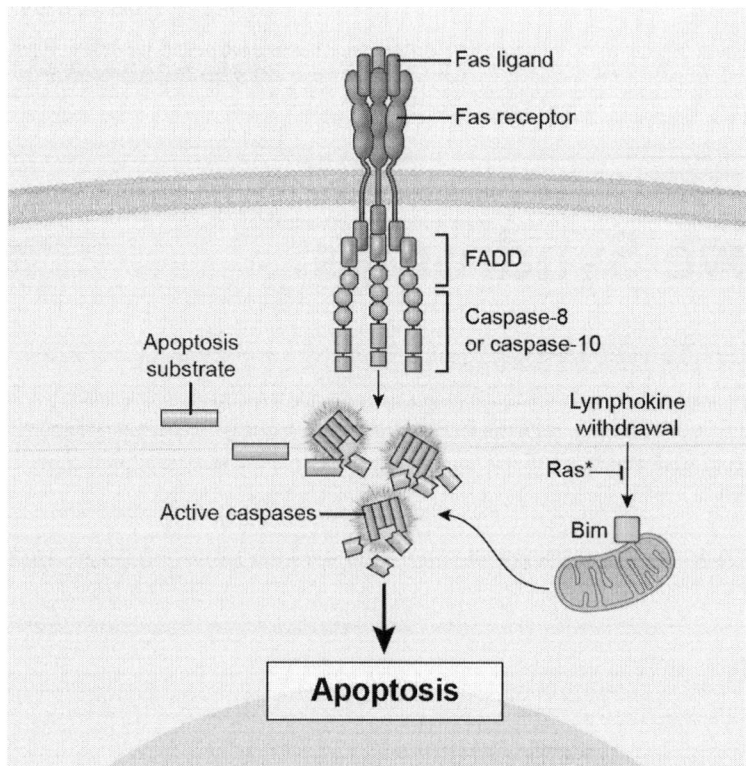

FIGURE 50.1 **Simplified scheme of immunoregulatory signaling pathways to immune cell apoptosis.** Depicted are the proteins: Fas ligand, Fas receptor, Fas-associated death domain protein (FADD), caspase-8, and caspase-10, which have been found to be mutant in ALPS and related conditions. The Fas receptor and ligand have three-fold symmetry which contributes importantly to the dominant interfering effect of heterozygous mutations. The ovals represent "death domains" in the Fas receptor and FADD, the octagons represent "death effector domains" in FADD and in caspase-8 and -10 zymogens, and the rectangles and squares represent the large and small subunits of the processed caspase proteins, respectively. The precise stoichiometry of the intracellular signaling complex is more complicated based on microscopic and crystallographic studies. Depicted on the right is the death pathway triggered through the mitochondrion by lymphokine withdrawal-induced Bim protein which also leads to caspase activation and apoptosis. The induction/stabilization of Bim is blocked by activated Ras (Ras*) in RALD leading to an apoptosis defect in response to lymphokine withdrawal.

place during the waning of an immune response after antigen clearance in response to the withdrawal of trophic factors. Together these mechanisms serve to return lymphocyte numbers almost back to their original set point at rest. Lymphocytes that escape these apoptosis mechanisms persist as memory cells with specific phenotypes and functional capabilities. The importance of these mechanisms is illustrated by inherited defects in the FAS pathway of lymphocyte apoptosis (Figure 50.1), which cause a disorder called the autoimmune lymphoproliferative syndrome (ALPS). In ALPS, the abnormal accumulation of lymphocytes leads to enlarged secondary lymphoid organs. Lymphocytes that have abnormal specificities to autoantigens, or that have acquired further mutations, also persist, leading to the development of autoimmune disease, and in some cases the malignant outgrowth of cells. This chapter will focus on ALPS and related conditions associated with defective apoptosis.

CLINICAL AND PATHOLOGICAL FEATURES

Autoimmune Lymphoproliferative Syndrome

Autoimmune lymphoproliferative syndrome is characterized by nonmalignant lymphadenopathy, splenomegaly, and multilineage cytopenias secondary to sequestration

and autoimmune peripheral destruction (Sneller et al., 1997; Bidere et al., 2006). This is the first disease known to be caused by a primary defect in programmed cell death and is the first autoimmune disease with a defined genetic basis (Fisher et al., 1995; Rieux-Laucat et al., 1995). Though others had earlier described similar manifestations of chronic lymphadenopathy simulating malignant lymphoma, a molecular basis for the disease was identified as defective lymphocyte apoptosis secondary to heterozygous mutations in the *FAS* gene in 1995 (Canale and Smith, 1967; Fisher et al., 1995; Rieux-Laucat et al., 1995). Since then, other genetic defects associated with ALPS and related disorders have been identified in both extrinsic and intrinsic apoptotic pathways (Wu et al., 1996; Wang et al., 1999; Chun et al., 2002; Holzelova et al., 2004; Del-Rey et al., 2006; Bi et al., 2007; Oliveira et al., 2007; Bolze et al., 2010; Niemela et al., 2011).

ALPS patients have mutations in the FAS pathway of apoptosis (Figure 50.1). FAS is activated upon ligation by FAS ligand (FASL), a trimeric molecule bound to the cell surface or found in soluble form. The FAS—FASL interaction triggers a conformational change in the intracellular portion of FAS, resulting in the recruitment of the adapter molecule FADD, which in turn recruits caspase-8 and -10 to the signaling complex. In close proximity, these caspases

Box 50.1 Diagnostic Criteria for ALPS Based on International ALPS Workshop 2009.

Required Criteria

1. Chronic (>6 months), nonmalignant, noninfectious lymphadenopathy and/or splenomegaly
2. Elevated CD3 + TCRαβ + CD4−CD8− DNT cells (> 1.5% of total lymphocytes or >2.5% of CD3 + lymphocytes) in the setting of normal or elevated lymphocyte counts

Additional criteria

Primary

1. Defective lymphocyte apoptosis in two separate assays
2. Somatic or germline pathogenic mutation in FAS, FASLG, or CASP10

Secondary

3. Elevated plasma sFASL levels (> 200 pg/ml), plasma IL-10 levels (>20 pg/ml), serum or plasma vitamin B12 levels (>1500 ng/L) or plasma IL-18 levels >500 pg/ml
4. Typical immunohistologic findings as reviewed by a hematopathologist
5. Autoimmune cytopenias (hemolytic anemia, thrombocytopenia, or neutropenia) with elevated IgG levels (polyclonal hypergammaglobulinemia)
6. Family history of a nonmalignant/noninfectious lymphoproliferation with or without autoimmunity

Definitive diagnosis: Both required criteria plus one primary accessory criterion.

Probable diagnosis: Both required criteria plus one secondary accessory criterion. Treat as ALPS until genetics can be done.

become activated, cleaving, in a typical signaling cascade, downstream effector caspases such as caspase-3 and -7. Upon activation, these caspases degrade several intracellular targets, leading to cell death. Mutations in all of these proteins (FAS, FASL, FADD, CASP8, and CASP10) are now known to cause ALPS or related disorders (Wu et al., 1996; Wang et al., 1999; Chun et al., 2002; Holzelova et al., 2004; Del-Rey et al., 2006; Bi et al., 2007; Oliveira et al., 2007; Bolze et al., 2010; Niemela et al., 2011). ALPS diagnostic criteria and molecular classification are shown in Box 50.1 and Table 50.1.

Clinical Presentation

ALPS usually presents in early childhood. However, this entity can be recognized in previously undiagnosed adult family members of patients following genetic counseling and testing of family members (Bidere et al., 2006; Neven et al., 2011). Most patients present with significant lymphadenopathy and splenomegaly before 3 years of age. The initial presentation of ALPS is often that of persistent lymphadenopathy and/or splenomegaly followed by an autoimmune disease such as immune thrombocytopenic purpura (ITP) or hemolytic anemia in an otherwise healthy child. Associated multilineage cytopenias due to autoantibodies and/or splenic sequestration can lead to mucocutaneous bleeding, pallor, icterus, and fatigue. Recurrent infections can also occur, mostly due to neutropenia and/or blockage of nasopharyngeal passages due to lymphadenopathy. Some patients also develop autoimmune

TABLE 50.1 ALPS Classification and Distribution of Different Categories of Patients Seen and Evaluated at National Institutes of Health Clinical Center as Part of our Current Cohort

ALPS classification	Chronic LPD/ splenomegaly	Elevated αβ DNTs	Apoptosis defect	% (no.) of ALPS cases (n = 257)
ALPS-FAS (germline mutation)	+	+	+	72 (185)
ALPS-sFAS (somatic mutation)	+	+	±	0.5 (14)
ALPS-FASLG	+	+	+	<1 (2)
ALPS-CASP10+		+	+	1.5 (4)
ALPS-U	+	+	±	20 (52)
ALPS-related apoptosis disorders				**No. of cases**
Caspase-8 deficiency state	+	±	±	4
RALD (somatic NRAS and KRAS mutations)	+	±	±	12
BENTA disease	+	−	+	2

ALPS-FAS, ALPS caused by germline FAS mutations; ALPS-sFAS, ALPS caused by somatic FAS mutations; ALPS-FASLG, ALPS caused by mutations in FAS ligand; ALPS-CASP10+, ALPS caused by caspase-10 mutations; ALPS-U, ALPS that fulfills criteria buts lacks any identifiable mutation; RALD, RAS-associated autoimmune leukoproliferative disorder.

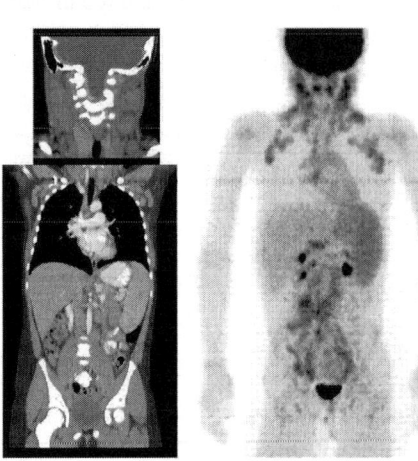
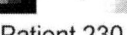

Patient 230

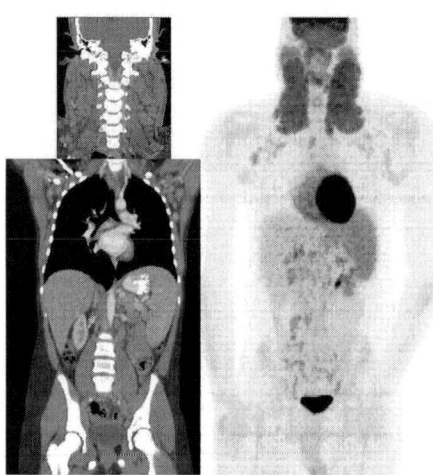

Patient 232

FIGURE 50.2 CT and FDG-PET scans featuring ALPS-FAS -associated lymphadenopathy and splenomegaly. Patient 230 is a 10-year-old girl, with asymptomatic adenopathy and splenomegaly. Patient 232 is a 22-year-old man, with asymptomatic and visible cervical and axillary lymphadenopathy and modest splenomegaly. No intervention was indicated in both patients. Note the increased uptake in the spleen as a reflection of lymphoproliferation compared with liver in both patients. *Reproduced with permission from Rao and Oliveira (2011).* © *2011 American Society of Hematology.*

Box 50.2 Differential Diagnoses of ALPS.

- Leukemia/Lymphoma
- Hemophagocytic lymphohistiocytosis (HLH)
- Mycobacterial disease
- Human immunodeficiency virus infection, acute
- Common variable immunodeficiency (CVID)
- Epstein–Barr virus infection
- Rosai–Dorfman disease
- Sarcoidosis
- Hereditary spherocytosis
- Wiskott–Aldrich syndrome
- IL-2 receptor alpha-chain deficiency
- X-lined lymphoproliferative syndrome (XLP)
- Immunodysregulation-polyendocrinopathy with enteritis, X-linked (IPEX) syndrome
- Evans syndrome
- BENTA disease

---

diseases affecting other organs such as autoimmune hepatitis, glomerulonephritis, uveitis, and encephalomyelitis (Guillain–Barré syndrome). There may also be a family history of similar disorders, usually inherited in an autosomal dominant fashion with incomplete penetrance. A thorough review of a patient's extended family for history of adenopathy, cytopenias, splenectomy, or lymphoma can provide information helpful in diagnosing ALPS.

Lymphadenopathy and hepatosplenomegaly seen in ALPS patients can often be remarkable, sometimes visibly distorting anatomic landmarks and clearly evident on CT or PET scans (Figure 50.2). Areas most commonly affected by lymphadenopathy are the neck, mediastinum, axillae, and inguinal and pelvic regions. Because of the propensity to malignant transformation of the expanded lymphocytes, ongoing lymphoma surveillance in these patients should include careful attention to the development of changes in lymph node size or appearance of new focal or generalized

lymphadenopathy and worsening splenomegaly associated with concomitant systemic symptoms such as fever, drenching night sweats, and weight loss (Rao and Oliveira, 2011).

Given that the clinical and laboratory features of ALPS can overlap with other common pediatric hematological disorders including sporadic acute ITP, Evans syndrome, and hematologic cancers, it is important for clinicians first to rule out other potentially more immediately life-threatening conditions (a short list of differential diagnose, is can be found in Box 50.2). Although rare, it is important to keep ALPS in the differential diagnosis for any child presenting with chronic non-malignant lymphadenopathy, particularly with a family history of a similar disease.

Laboratory Evaluation

Autoantibodies are frequently found in ALPS patients (Kwon et al., 2003). The most common autoantibodies occurring in ALPS patients are anti-erythrocyte antibodies detected by a Coombs direct antiglobulin test (DAT). Other common circulating autoantibodies include anti-platelet and anti-neutrophil antibodies. A complete blood count (CBC) with differential may demonstrate lymphocytosis, lymphopenia, reticulocytosis, thrombocytopenia, neutropenia, slight monocytosis, and/or eosinophilia. Polyclonal hypergammaglobulinema is also a common feature in ALPS. In addition, a polyclonal expansion in the circulation and secondary lymphoid tissue of $CD3^+TCR\alpha\beta^+$ and $CD4^-CD8^-$ lymphocytes, henceforth referred to as the double negative T (DNT) cells, is highly characteristic of ALPS (Bleesing et al., 2001a, b). Double negative gamma-delta ($CD3^+TCR\gamma\delta^+$) T cells are not characteristic of this disease. Other abnormal laboratory findings that are commonly found in patients with ALPS include elevated serum levels of vitamin B12, IL-10, soluble FAS ligand, and IL-18 (Magerus-Chatinet et al.,

2009; Caminha et al., 2010). These serve as useful bio-markers of this disease, as discussed later in this chapter.

In patients with clinical and/or laboratory features consistent with a diagnosis of ALPS, molecular genetic testing of *FAS* (*TNFRSF6*), Fas ligand (*TNFSF6*), and caspase-10 genes (*CASP10*) should be obtained. Mutations of the *FAS* gene have been identified in the majority (74%) of patients with ALPS and most of these reside in the "death domain" encoded by exon 9 (Figures 50.1 and 50.4). This includes patients with either germline *FAS* mutations or somatic *FAS* mutations limited to the DNT cell compartment. We therefore recommend first testing for *FAS* mutations, followed by analysis of the other genes only when *FAS* gene analysis fails to reveal a causative mutation (Rao and Oliveira, 2011). This testing is important for two reasons. First, it is important to provide genetic counseling to the family and invite other family members for screening evaluations if the mutation is found. Second, the location of any specific gene mutation has been shown to be important in patient prognosis as certain mutation loci are associated with a higher risk of complications including lymphoma (Straus et al., 2001; Kuehn et al., 2011). Patients with a mutation of the intracellular domain of *FAS* have been shown to have a 14-fold increased risk of non-Hodgkin lymphoma and a 51-fold increased risk of developing Hodgkin lymphoma (Straus et al., 2001).

Lymph node biopsy also reveals findings virtually pathognomonic for ALPS. These findings include follicular hyperplasia and paracortical expansion with a mixed infiltrate containing the specific DNT cells noted by immunohistochemistry for CD3, CD4, and CD8 markers (Lim et al., 1998). This specific histological pattern can help distinguish ALPS from other benign and malignant lymphoproliferative disorders. Given the chronic fluctuating nature of their lymphadenopathy, patients with ALPS may have to undergo repeated lymph node biopsies to help rule out lymphoma if they develop systemic symptoms in addition to focal change of adenopathy. Testing lymph node tissue for clonality by means of immunoglobulin and TCR gene rearrangements as well as cytogenetic analysis for chromosomal aneuploidy is also useful for evaluating the diagnosis of lymphoma in ALPS patients.

Imaging Studies

Although imaging studies are not generally used to make a diagnosis of ALPS, once the diagnosis is established, it is useful to obtain baseline and periodic computed tomography (CT) scans. CT scans of the neck, chest, abdomen, and pelvis establish the location and extent of the patient's lymphadenopathy and splenomegaly. Given the increased risk of lymphoma in patients with ALPS, surveillance with serial CT scans is an important part of the

chronic management of these patients. The degree of generalized lymphadenopathy can be documented longitudinally in a consistent fashion using the following guidelines during physical examinations: Grade: 1, few shotty nodes; 2, multiple 1–2 cm nodes; 3, multiple nodes, some >2 cm; 4, extensive visible adenopathy. Splenomegaly should also be clinically documented as a measure of its extent in the midclavicular line below the costal margin.

The use of positron emission tomography (PET) using 18-fluoro-2-deoxy-D-glucose (FDG) has become the standard in staging and follow-up evaluations of cancers including lymphomas. Whole body FDG-PET can be used to help differentiate chronic, benign lymphadenopathy in ALPS patients from ALPS-associated lymphomas, and its use decreases the number of lymph node biopsies these patients are required to endure (Rao et al., 2006). Lymph node biopsy may be indicated if sudden or dramatic change in a node is noted, particularly if these changes are associated with concerning constitutional symptoms such as weight loss, fever, or night sweats.

Treatment

Upon confirmation of a diagnosis of ALPS, patients should undergo counseling aimed at specifically addressing the risks associated with this condition. Most importantly, the increased risk of lymphomas and other malignancies should be discussed, and patients should be encouraged to seek further evaluation for any sudden fluctuations in lymph node or spleen size. In ALPS patients with intracellular *FAS* mutations, the risk of lymphoma should be particularly emphasized. Likewise, in asplenic ALPS patients, the infection risks, including opportunistic pneumococcal sepsis associated with asplenia (which may be compounded by lack of memory B cells and autoimmune neutropenia in these patients), should be stressed (Rao and Oliveira, 2011).

The massive lymphadenopathy often seen in children with ALPS may cause considerable anxiety for the patients and their families, which may lead clinicians to sympathetically treat these patients for cosmetic purposes alone. However, immunosuppressive drugs such as corticosteroids, azathioprine, cyclosporine, hydroxychloroquine, or mycophenolate mofetil do not consistently shrink lymph nodes and spleens of patients with ALPS, and treatment of these patients with such drugs for only cosmetic purposes is not indicated or desirable.

Spleen guards, made of fiberglass by an occupational therapist familiar with such devices, should be considered for ALPS patients with massive splenomegaly to help reduce the risk of traumatic splenic rupture. This is particularly important in those who are physically active (i.e., all toddlers) and/or patients involved in competitive sports. Due to their increased risk of splenic rupture, patients with splenomegaly should be discouraged from participating in contact sports such as football or ice hockey.

All ALPS patients who are asplenic should be treated with long-term antibiotic prophylaxis against pneumococcal sepsis using penicillin V. ALPS patients frequently are unable to produce or maintain protective antibodies directed against polysaccharide antigens following vaccination due to defects in memory B cell function. Nevertheless, these patients should be vaccinated against encapsulated organisms such as pneumococcus, meningococcus, and *Haemophilus influenzae* type B (HiB). Patients who have undergone surgical splenectomy are encouraged to wear medical alert bracelets, necklaces, or wallet cards warning of their risk for sepsis.

An important aspect of caring for ALPS patients is the medical treatment of the chronic and refractory autoimmune multilineage cytopenias as these frequently cause substantial morbidity including low platelet counts resulting in mucocutaneous bleeding, and even mortality. Initial management for ALPS-related autoimmune cytopenias is similar to therapies used for sporadic cytopenias in other patient populations. For autoimmune hemolytic anemia (AIHA) or ITP, this includes the use of parenteral high dose methylprednisolone (5–30 mg/kg/day for 1–2 days) followed by oral prednisone (1–2 mg/kg/day) that is tapered slowly over months. High dose intravenous immunoglobulin (1–2 g/kg) may be considered for concomitant use with pulse dose steroids for severe AIHA. Some patients with autoimmune neutropenias who experience associated infection may be treated with low dose granulocyte colony stimulating factor (G-CSF 1–2 µg/kg administered SC two to three times per week). In patients with refractory autoimmune cytopenias requiring chronic steroid therapy, mycophenolate mofetil has been shown over the last 10 years to be an effective steroid-sparing agent that maintains adequate blood cell counts and reduces the need for other immunosuppressive agents or splenectomy (Rao et al., 2005; Rao and Oliveira, 2011; Teachey, 2012).

Finally, some ALPS patients with hypersplenism and associated cytopenias have shown significant improvement following treatment with sirolimus (Teachey et al., 2009; Teachey, 2012). While these results are very encouraging in terms of avoiding splenectomy, further studies of long-term outcomes are warranted before recommendations can be made regarding which patients would benefit most from this therapy. A suggested treatment algorithm for autoimmune cytopenias associated with ALPS is included (Figure 50.3). As with many chronic diseases with an onset in childhood, adolescence and early adulthood may provide the additional treatment challenge of poor compliance with prescribed medications.

Prognosis

The overall prognosis and outcome in most patients with ALPS is good, but the mortality and morbidity varies widely in patients depending on their disease severity. Many patients are expected to live a normal lifespan with few clinical complications. Some patients, however, develop life-threatening cytopenias, requiring hospitalizations, immunosuppressive therapy, blood transfusions, or splenectomy. Patients with mutations affecting the intracellular domain of the FAS protein have more severe disease and are at increased risk for Hodgkin lymphoma and non-Hodgkin lymphoma (Jackson et al., 1999; Neven et al., 2011). A large cohort of ALPS-FAS patients showed about a 6–10% incidence of lymphoma with a median age of presentation of 17 years (Straus et al., 2001). Lymphoma can be especially difficult to discern in the setting of persistent lymphadenopathy that is commonly found even in adult ALPS patients. However, ALPS-associated lymphomas appear to be as amenable to chemotherapy as sporadic lymphomas and should be managed as such.

Lymphadenopathy and splenomegaly associated with ALPS tends to become less prominent as patients grow older. This has been observed in mice with genetic deficiencies of Fas causing lymphoproliferation. It may be due to thymic involution that begins after puberty and a decrease in input of abnormal T lymphocytes. Perhaps related to this, though the reasons remain unclear, cytopenias in most patients with ALPS also improve with age. Nevertheless, stem cell transplantation has been successful in patients with ALPS and can be considered a treatment option for those with very severe, recalcitrant disease especially when a matched donor is available. Sibling donors should be screened and demonstrated to be free of mutations in the apoptosis pathway genes. The mortality of a matched unrelated donor-derived allogenic bone marrow transplant continues to be too high to warrant the procedure in most patients with ALPS, as most of them have a near-normal life expectancy.

The major determinants of prognosis in patients diagnosed with ALPS include the severity of autoimmune disease (particularly autoimmune cytopenias) requiring chronic immunomodulatory therapy, hypersplenism, asplenia-related sepsis, and the development of lymphoma. Proper surveillance and education are vital to the prognosis of these patients.

ALPS-RELATED DISORDERS

Caspase-8 and FADD Deficiencies

Caspase-8 deficiency state (CEDS), due to an autosomal recessive mutation in the gene encoding caspase-8, was

Management Suggestions for ALPS Associated Chronic Refractory Cytopenia

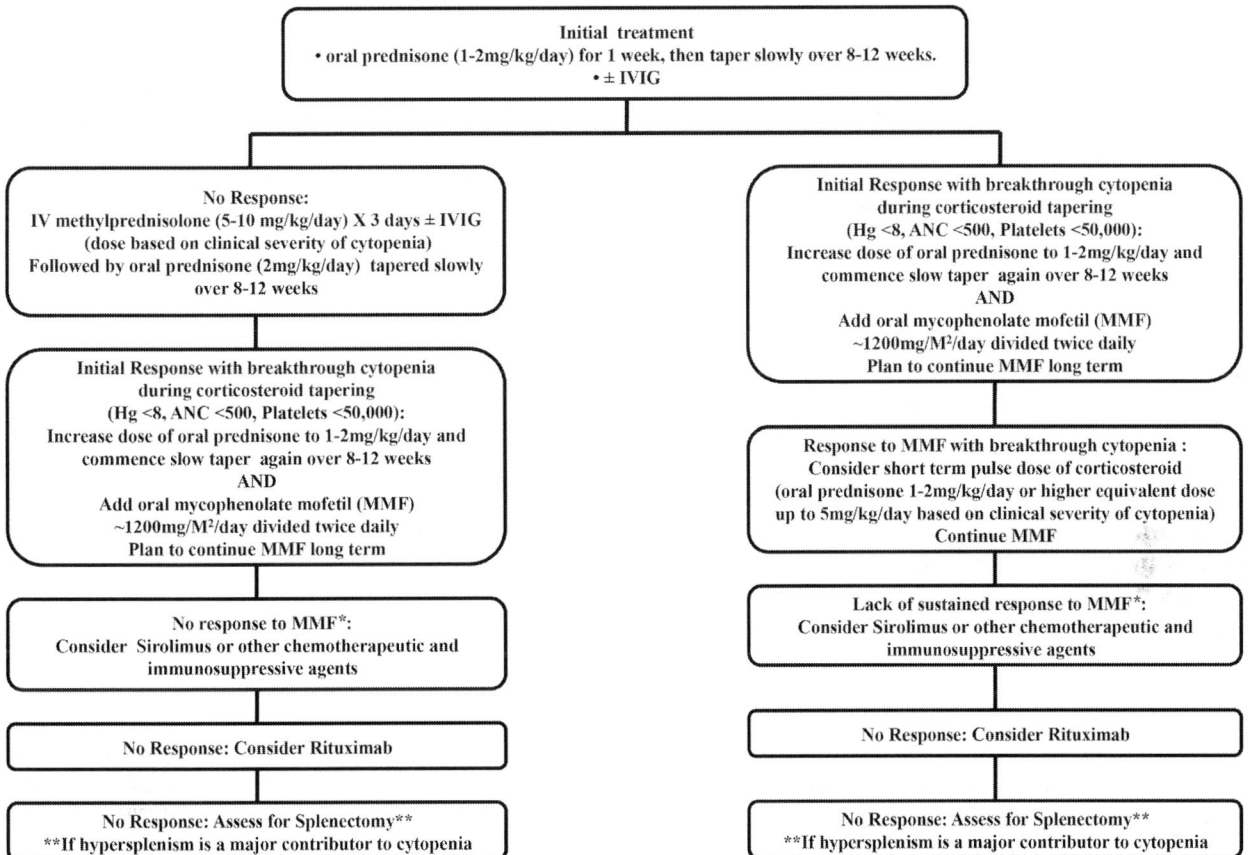

FIGURE 50.3 **Treatment algorithms for ALPS-associated cytopenias.** Note that paradigm comprises only suggested guidelines for managing ALPS patients with autoimmune multilineage cytopenias. G-CSF may be indicated for severe neutropenia associated with systemic infections. Chemotherapeutic and immunosuppressive agents including mycophenolate mofetil (MMF), sirolimus (rapamycin), vincristine, methotrexate, mercaptopurine, azathioprine, cyclosporine, and hydroxychloroquine can be considered as a steroid-sparing measure or to avoid/postpone splenectomy.

initially described in two siblings who had clinical features reminiscent of ALPS, with lymphadenopathy and splenomegaly, lymphocytosis but normal or barely elevated DNTs, defective lymphocyte apoptosis, and autoantibodies without autoimmune disease (Chun et al., 2002). However, the two patients also manifested concurrent immunodeficiency that is not typical of ALPS, with recurrent sinopulmonary and mucocutaneous herpes simplex virus infections, mild hypogammaglobulinemia, and poor pneumococcal antibodies. Recently, two more patients from the same extended family have been identified (S. Rosenzweig and J. Oliveira, unpublished results). These patients had immunodeficiency, with recurrent sinopulmonary infections, warts, molluscum contagiosum, poor pneumococcal antibodies, and normal DNTs. Besides their splenomegaly and lymphocytosis, they also had accumulation of lymphocytes in liver, lung, and brain. This is similar to the lymphocytic infiltration into parenchymal organs that develops in older mice lacking

caspase-8 within their T cells (Salmena and Hakem, 2005). Thus, CEDS in both humans and mice is characterized by a prominent combined immunodeficiency with pronounced lymphocyte accumulation and infiltration but minimal autoimmunity.

FADD assembles within the death-induced signaling complex (DISC), where it functions as an adapter molecule for apoptosis signaling. FADD can also associate with the CBM complex (but not the IKKα/β complex) upon antigen receptor stimulation, but it is also required for type I IFN antiviral immunity. Thus, FADD deficiency might be predicted to resemble CEDS. Indeed, four related patients with FADD deficiency due to autosomal recessive mutations were recently identified, who have an immunodeficiency phenotype (Bolze et al., 2010). The patients had invasive pneumococcal infections with functional hyposplenism, as well as repeated febrile episodes of encephalopathy with liver dysfunction that were associated with viral infections. However, unlike

CEDS, the viral susceptibility resulted from defective antiviral responses rather than effects on T cell proliferation. Furthermore, unlike CEDS or ALPS, none of the FADD-deficient patients had splenomegaly or lymphadenopathy. Nevertheless, one patient was demonstrated to have increased DNT cells, a lymphocyte apoptosis defect, elevated biomarkers that are usually associated with ALPS-FAS, and DAT autoantibodies without reported autoimmune disease. Taken together, FADD deficiency, like CEDS, clinically overlaps with ALPS but differs in featuring immunodeficiency prominently.

RAS-Associated Autoimmune Leukoproliferative Disorder

While studying patients with features of ALPS but without known gene mutations, in 2007 we discovered one subject with a somatic activating mutation in the gene *NRAS* (Oliveira et al., 2007). Although initially classified as ALPS, type IV, the patient had atypical features such as a history of significant leukocytosis early in life, persistent monocytosis, and a low level of αβ-DNTs, which did not infiltrate lymph nodes. Later, additional patients with an ALPS-like disease were found to have heterozygote-dominant activating mutations in *NRAS* or *KRAS* which resemble the mutations that cause activation of oncogenic RAS in a wide variety of tumors. The disease was named RAS-associated autoimmune leukoproliferative disorder (RALD) (Oliveira et al., 2007; Niemela et al., 2011; Takagi et al., 2011).

RALD patients have several clinical and laboratory features that overlap with ALPS. They were diagnosed between 1 and 47 years of life and presented with a generally mild degree of peripheral lymphadenopathy. However, they manifested significant splenomegaly and autoimmunity including AIHA, ITP, and neutropenia. In some patients, a history of recurrent mild upper and lower respiratory tract infections could be elicited (Niemela et al., 2011). Unlike ALPS patients, patients with RALD had transient or persistent elevation in granulocytes and monocytes. Some RALD patients had a clinical and laboratory phenotype very similar to juvenile myelomonocytic leukemia (JMML) early in life, with marked hepatosplenomegaly and monocytosis. However, unlike patients with JMML, the relative or absolute monocytosis tends to improve spontaneously but never disappears.

Immunophenotyping in RALD reveals mild to no elevation in DNTs and an expansion of B cells. Total lymphocyte numbers are normal to modestly decreased. In contrast, absolute or relative monocytosis is noted in all patients. Autoantibodies are typically detected, including ANA and rheumatoid factor, as well as anti-phospholipid, anti-cardiolipin, anti-platelet, anti-neutrophil, and/or anti-red cell antibodies (Oliveira et al., 2007; Niemela et al., 2011; Takagi et al., 2011). Unlike patients with ALPS, the biomarkers and *in vitro* FAS-induced apoptosis are also normal. By contrast, in RALD patients, the T cells are resistant to IL-2 withdrawal-induced cell death, pointing to a fundamentally different apoptotic defect in RALD (Oliveira et al., 2007; Niemela et al., 2011; Takagi et al., 2011). The histopathological findings include nonspecific polyclonal plasmacytosis with reactive secondary follicles, but without the typical paracortical expansion caused by DNT cells in ALPS. Given the small number of patients diagnosed to date, it is not known if these patients are at increased risk for hematological malignancy. In summary, RALD should be suspected in a patient with splenomegaly with or without lymphadenopathy, blood-cell directed autoimmunity, and relative or absolute monocytosis, in whom a malignancy or infection has been ruled out.

Genetic Features

There is marked genetic heterogeneity underlying the autoimmune lymphoproliferative syndromes. Strikingly, germline and somatic defects are seen in this patient population, complicating the molecular diagnosis in the clinical setting. We will discuss below each disorder separately.

AUTOIMMUNE LYMPHOPROLIFERATIVE SYNDROME (ALPS)

Germline *FAS* Mutations

Around 74% of ALPS patients bear heterozygous germline mutations in the *FAS* (*TNFRSF6*) gene located on chromosome 10q24.1. Mutations can be found throughout the gene, either in coding regions or in splice sites, with the majority ($\approx 2/3$) affecting the intracellular death domain (DD) encoded by exon 9 (Figure 50.4). (All mutations found to date are in the ALPS database at http://www.niaid.nih.gov/topics/ALPS/research/Pages/mutationDatabase.aspx.) Essentially all mutations are transmitted in an autosomal dominant fashion and exert a dominant-negative effect. This effect is explained by the observation that incorporation of even a single mutant Fas chain in the trimeric receptor impairs function and that very few trimers, i.e., 1/8 or 1 out of 2^3, will have exclusively wild-type subunits for heterozygous alleles encoding the trimeric receptor. Moreover, recent understanding of crystal structure of FAS protein and its oligomerization on the cell surface reveals it to be a complex structure that would make the calculations even less favorable for signaling since the mutant subunits would

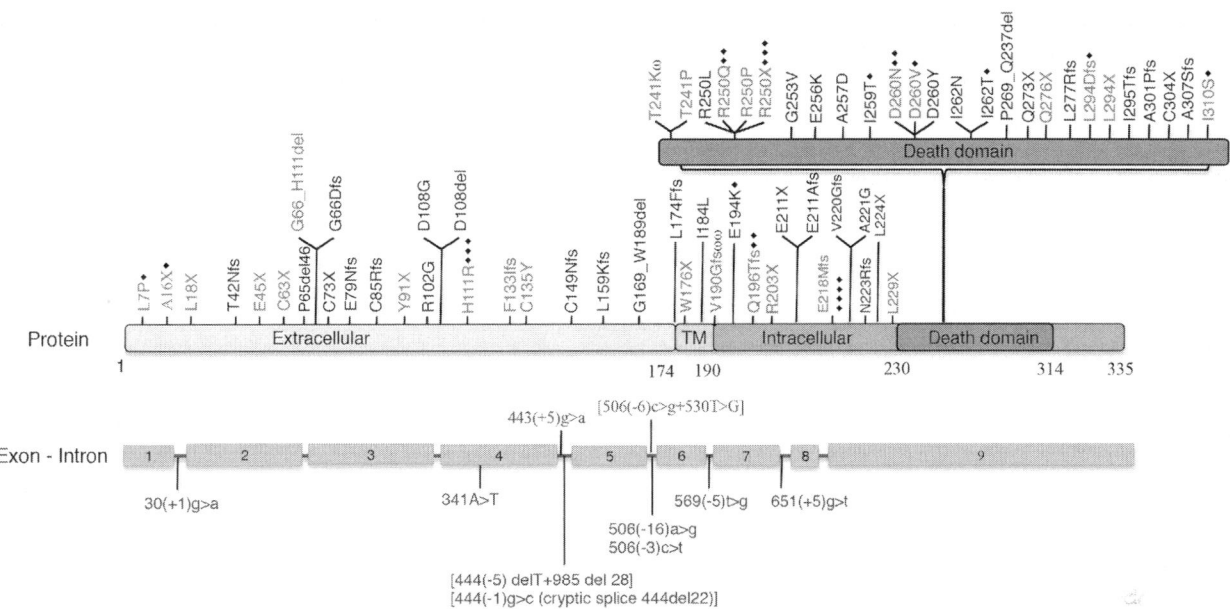

FIGURE 50.4 Schematic representation of FAS mutations in ALPS patient. Shown is the domain structure of the protein on the top (TM = transmembrane) with the amino acid position enumerated. The gene structure is shown below with the exons numbered as solid blue boxes and the introns as solid blue lines (not drawn to scale). Red text indicates mutations described in data in this chapter. Black text indicates additional known protein coding mutations. Blue text indicates complex mutations affecting the mRNA structure. Black diamonds represent the number of families with the same mutation. *From Kuehn et al. (2011).*

abrogate function of even larger superstructures of Fas receptors (Wang et al., 2010). A few ALPS cases with aggressive disease phenotype in early childhood caused by homozygous germline mutations in *FAS* have also been reported.

There are important genotype–phenotype relationships in ALPS. Disease severity and penetrance are greatest for mutations affecting the FAS intracellular DD region, which disrupt the homotypic interactions required for FADD and initiator caspase recruitment into the death-inducing signaling complex. In contrast, mutations affecting the extracellular portions of the protein are commonly associated with FAS haploinsufficiency and manifest by milder clinical disease and lower penetrance (Kuehn et al., 2011; Hsu et al., 2012). More recently, it has been described that a group of ALPS patients with extracellular mutations that develop clinically important autoimmune disease present with somatic mutation in the second allele of FAS (Magerus-Chatinet et al., 2011). This association of germline and somatic mutations in the same gene is unique and sheds light onto the genetic mechanisms underlying disease severity in ALPS.

Somatic *FAS* Mutations

Curiously, the second most common genetic cause of ALPS is somatic mutations in *FAS* (Holzelova et al., 2004; Dowdell et al., 2010). These patients present with

mutations only in blood elements, affecting most DNT cells and a small proportion of CD4, CD8, CD20, and CD34 (progenitor) cells. Notably, these patients lacked apoptosis defects *in vitro*. The somatic event is thought to happen in a hematopoietic stem cell clone that expands by survival advantage. The clinical manifestations are similar to those in patients with germline FAS mutations. These patients do share the biomarkers of patients with germline *FAS* mutations and their diagnosis can be confirmed by sequencing *FAS* in a purified DNT cell population.

Additional Genetic Etiologies

A very small proportion of ALPS patients harbor mutations in the genes encoding for caspase-10 (*CASP10*) and FAS ligand (*FASL*). *CASP10* mutations have been found in 10 patients thus far. These mutations were heterozygous and cause defective apoptosis in lymphocytes and dendritic cells (Wang et al., 1999). The clinical phenotype was indistinguishable from that of patients with *FAS* mutations. A heterozygous mutation in Fas ligand (*FASLG, TNFSF6*) was originally reported for a patient with systemic lupus erythematosus (SLE) who had lymphadenopathy, splenomegaly, and defective lymphocyte apoptosis after TCR restimulation, but no apparent DNT expansion, and in another patient with ALPS (Wu et al., 1996; Del-Rey et al., 2006). Two other ALPS

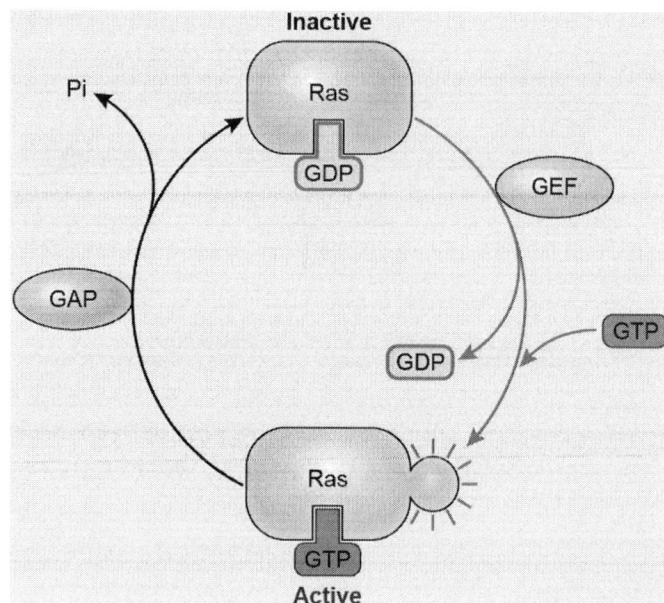

Inactive

Pi

Ras
GDP

GEF

GAP

GDP

GTP

Ras
GTP

Active

FIGURE 50.5 **RAS regulatory cycle.** RAS GTPase proteins are turned "on" by loading with a guanosine-5′-triphosphate (GTP) molecule and "off" when it is hydrolyzed to guanosine-5′-diphosphate (GDP) with the release of a phosphate group. Ras proteins carry out effector functions, such as apoptosis inhibition, in the active, GTP bound form but not in the inactive, GDP bound form. The low intrinsic GTPase activity of RAS is increased over 300-fold upon interaction with GTPase activating proteins (GAP) which turn off the Ras protein. The exchange of GTP for GDP is accelerated by GTP exchange factors (GEF), which turns on the Ras protein. Most pathogenic mutations in KRAS or NRAS disrupt the interaction of RAS with GAPs and decrease the GTPase activity thereby keeping the Ras protein in an active state. This blocks apoptosis (see Figure 50.1) and can accentuate cell proliferation.

patients were also discovered who possessed homozygous *FASLG* mutations (Del-Rey et al., 2006). Finally, a subgroup of ALPS patients fulfills diagnostic criteria including increased circulating DNT cells in peripheral blood but lacks known mutations in the FAS pathway.

RAS-ASSOCIATED AUTOIMMUNE LEUKOPROLIFERATIVE DISORDER

All 12 patients with RAS-associated autoimmune leukoproliferative disorder (RALD) described so far harbor somatic, gain-of-function mutations in *KRAS* or *NRAS*, which are present only in blood cells. Somatic activating mutations in RAS are present in up to 30% of all human cancers. Germline RAS pathway mutations have been described as causing the related Costello (*HRAS*), Noonan (*PTPN11, KRAS, SOS1, NRAS*), and cardiofaciocutaneous syndromes (*KRAS, BRAF, MEK1,* and *MEK*) (Zenker, 2011). The RAS mutations seen in RALD disrupt the interaction of RAS with the GTPase activating proteins (GAPs), significantly weakening the GTPase activity and allowing the protein to be in a permanent GTP-bound, "on" position (Figure 50.5). The consequences of this are discussed in the section below.

In Vivo and *In Vitro* Models of Disease

An important clue to the genetic etiology behind human ALPS was the unusual expansion of DNT cells which occurs in both germline and somatic Fas mutant patients (Sneller et al., 1992). Similar expansions were observed in the spontaneously arising lymphoproliferation (*lpr*) or

generalized lymphoproliferative disease (*gld*) mouse strains, which also develop lymphadenopathy, splenomegaly, hypergammaglobulinemia, autoantibodies, autoimmune disease, and lymphoma (Cohen and Eisenberg, 1991; Davidson et al., 1998). Unlike humans with ALPS who tend to have autoimmune cytopenias, autoimmune disease in their murine counterparts resembles systemic lupus erythematosus, with ANA and deposition of immune complexes leading to glomerulonephritis, arthritis, polyarteritis, sialoadenitis, and primary biliary cirrhosis. In *lpr* (and *lpr^cg*) mice, the genetic defect was mapped to the Fas gene that mediates apoptosis (Watanabe-Fukunaga et al., 1992). In the *gld* mice, the genetic defect was mapped to the Fas ligand gene that triggers apoptosis (Roths et al., 1984). In both cases, disease occurs in inbred strains of mice that are autosomal recessive for these specific loss-of-function mutations. This is consistent with a genetic "loss of function" or deficiency mechanism in the mice, which differs from the dominant interference that usually occurs in nonconsanguineous humans who have heterozygous FAS or FASL mutations. No mouse models of ALPS resulting from somatic FAS mutations have been described. Also there are no mouse models of ALPS-CASPASE-10 because caspase-10 has no ortholog in the mouse.

The availability of mouse models has been helpful in elucidating disease pathogenesis. *In vitro* apoptosis assays performed on cells from patients, or in cells transfected with mutant FAS or FAS ligand molecules, clearly demonstrate defective apoptosis whenever the mutation is present (Fisher et al., 1995). However, even though the mutation and the degree to which it interferes with apoptosis is the main factor contributing to disease, not all mutation-positive individuals exhibit disease (Sneller et al., 1997; Jackson et al., 1999). The variable penetrance argues for the additional contribution of genetic modifiers, which has been observed in mice. In *lpr* mice, the severity of autoimmune disease depends upon the inbred genetic background, with more severe disease seen in the MRL strain and less severe disease in other strains (Cohen and Eisenberg, 1991). Crosses of *lpr* mice on susceptible versus resistant backgrounds have been useful in identifying several loci that influence disease phenotype. An example of one such genetic modifier is osteopontin. Certain polymorphisms in osteopontin are associated with the development of glomerulonephritis in *lpr* mice (Miyazaki et al., 2005), or a variant of ALPS termed autoimmune lymphoproliferative disease (ALD) that lacks DNT expansion (Chiocchetti et al., 2004).

The ability to genetically manipulate mice has also facilitated other studies addressing key aspects of disease pathogenesis. For example, although DNT expansion is a defining criterion of ALPS, investigations on the provenance of these cells have been hampered by the inability to culture human or mouse DNT *in vitro*. However, mouse models suggest that DNT likely arise from senescent CD8 T cells that have lost their CD8 co-receptors (Koh et al., 1995; Merino et al., 1995). More recently, *in vivo* mouse models have also established that membrane bound but not soluble Fas ligand plays a physiological role in apoptosis induction (O'Reilly et al., 2009a), and that the normal apoptosis of antigen-presenting cells as well as T cells is crucial for establishing immune tolerance (Stranges et al., 2007). Finally, the use of mouse models has facilitated preclinical testing of potential therapies such as rapamycin that are now used to treat patients (Teachey et al., 2006, 2009). Thus, *lpr* mouse models provide a valuable complement to the clinical and laboratory investigation of ALPS.

Pathogenic Effector Mechanisms

ALPS

As described in previous sections, most ALPS patients have mutations affecting components of the FAS pathway of apoptosis. Given the crucial role of this pathway in the elimination of old, excessive, or damaged lymphocytes, the clinical consequences are predictable. The characteristic lymphadenopathy and splenomegaly are caused by local accumulation of DNT cells, which expand the paracortical areas of the lymph nodes and red pulp of the spleen. Additionally, there is marked plasmacytosis and follicular hyperplasia, also reflecting an active B cell population.

Although a hallmark of this disease, the role of the DNT cells in disease pathogenesis is important but not well understood. They seem to be derived mostly from previously activated CD8 cells, and secrete large amounts of IL-10. It has been hypothesized that the high IL-10 levels may contribute to the survival and expansion of autoreactive B cell clones, resulting in antibody-mediated blood element autoimmunity. The finding that patients with somatic *FAS* mutations, which are detected mainly in DNT cells, have essentially identical clinical manifestations to patients with germline mutations reinforces the potentially key pathogenic role of these cells. However, 10–20% of B and T cells also carry the mutation, and may also participate in disease pathogenesis. Additionally, in murine models, FAS has a role in mediating B cell selection during a germinal center reaction, and it is not known if ALPS patients have a normally selected B cell repertoire. Regarding the increased risk for lymphoma, this can be explained by the known tumor suppressor role of FAS, coupled to the chronic activation state of B cells.

Lastly, it is interesting to note the lack of T cell-mediated vasculitis in ALPS patients, despite the important role of FAS for T cell apoptosis. Also, the range of autoantibody-mediated diseases is very narrow, affecting only blood cells, with absence of organ-specific autoimmune disease such as thyroiditis, adrenalitis, or pancreatic insulitis. This points to a specific role of FAS or other as yet undefined modifier genes in controlling this specific aspect of immune tolerance.

RALD

The RAS genes (*NRAS*, *KRAS*, and *HRAS*) encode 21-kDa proteins that are members of the superfamily of small GTP-binding proteins, which have diverse intracellular signaling functions including control of cell proliferation, growth, and apoptosis. RAS activity differs when bound to GTP versus GDP (Figure 50.5). GTP-bound molecules are thought to be active signaling molecules and GDP-bound forms are thought to be inactive. The conversion from a GTP- to a GDP-bound state is catalyzed by a weak intrinsic GTPase activity, which is greatly enhanced upon interaction of RAS with GTPase activating proteins (GAPs) (de Vos et al., 1988). The *NRAS* and *KRAS* mutations seen in RALD patients are heterozygous and gain-of-function, such as p.G13D and p.G12V, similar to the ones described in tumors. These mutations disrupt the interaction of RAS with the GAPs, diminishing its GTPase activity by over 300-fold and locking the molecule in an "on" position (de Vos et al., 1988). This permanent activation state increases cell signaling through the RAS-ERK pathway, inducing the phosphorylation and destruction of the pro-apoptotic protein BIM (Ley et al., 2005; O'Reilly et al., 2009b). Consequently, the cells become resistant to certain kinds of apoptotic stimuli, such as growth-factor (IL-2)

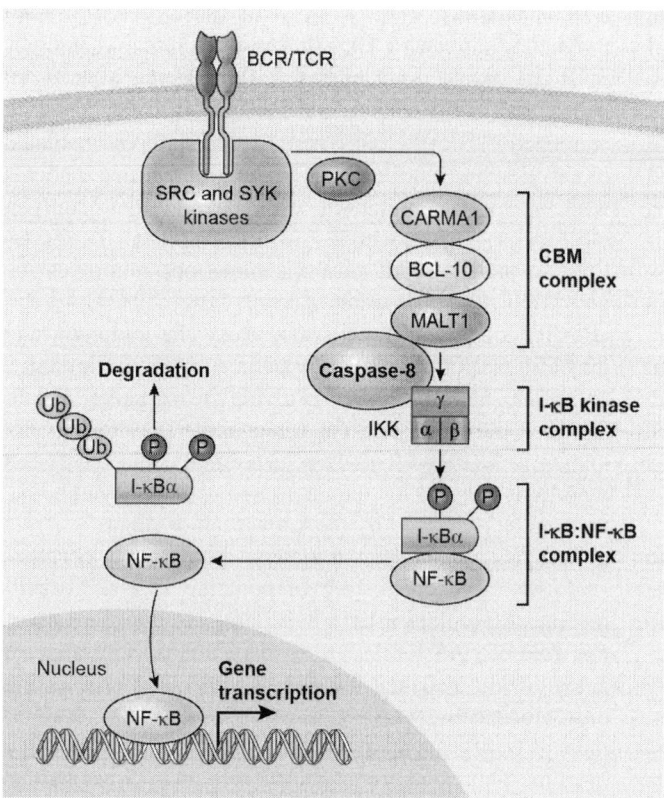

FIGURE 50.6 The role of caspase-8 in the NF-κB pathway during immune cell activation. Upon triggering of B cell, T cell, TLR, or NK receptors, a key transcriptional regulator, NF-κB, is induced which activates a large transcriptional program that coordinates the immune response. The pathway proceeds through receptor activation of Src and Syk family proximal kinases and protein kinase C isoforms (PKC) that lead to the assembly of the CARMA1-BCL10-MALT1 (CBM) complex. The CBM complex binds to and activates the I-κB kinase (IKKα/β/γ) complex using caspase-8 as a bridge (Su et al., 2005). Once recruited to the CBM complex, IKKα/β/γ phosphorylates (P) the I-κBα protein leading to its separation from NF-κB, ubiquitinylation (Ub), and degradation, while NF-κB translocates into the nucleus to activate the gene transcription program.

withdrawal, so that they can survive *in vitro* for long periods of time. Additionally, persistent ERK signaling decreases the intracellular levels of negative inhibitors of the cell cycle, namely $p27^{kip1}$, allowing for increased proliferation in the face of limiting IL-2 levels (Niemela et al., 2011). Interestingly, recent work has suggested that adequate RAS signaling is important for B cell selection, given the multiple antibody-mediated autoimmune manifestations seen in these patients with monocytosis (Limnander and Weiss, 2011; Limnander et al., 2011).

CEDS

The clinical phenotype of immunodeficiency coupled to lymphoproliferation can be explained by the dual role of caspase-8 in signaling for both apoptosis and lymphocyte activation. Upon FAS death receptor stimulation, caspase-8 is recruited into the death-inducing signaling complex (DISC) for apoptosis induction (Figure 50.1). By assembling with FAS through FADD adapter molecules, caspase-8 becomes enzymatically activated, is cleaved, and activates downstream caspases, thereby unleashing an enzymatic cascade that cleaves proteins for cell death. By contrast, upon immunoreceptor stimulation, caspase-8 assembles with the CARMA1-BCL10-MALT1 (CBM) and the IKKαβ complexes (Figure 50.6) (Su et al., 2005). Oligomerization without cleavage weakly induces

caspase-8 enzymatic activity, but not full processing of the zymogen, which is required for the holocomplex to activate the gene transcription factor NF-κB for lymphocyte activation. Thus, caspase-8 has a dual role in controlling cell activation and death.

BENTA Disease

In 1971, a form of non-malignant polyclonal B lymphocyte hyperproliferation was described in an infant that progressed in adulthood to B lymphoid chronic lymphocytic leukemia (B-CLL) (Darte et al., 1971; Snow et al., 2012). This disease, "B cell expansion with NF-κB and T cell anergy" (BENTA) has been recently attributed to germline heterozygous missense mutations in the gene encoding CARD11/CARMA1, a scaffolding protein required for antigen receptor-induced NF-κB activation in both B and T lymphocytes (Figure 50.6). Importantly, these are activating mutations that cause the CARD11 protein to spontaneously signal constitutive NF-κB activation. It is notable that similar somatic gain-of-function CARD11 mutations have been reported to cause diffuse large cell B cell lymphoma, but the germline CARD11 mutations have only been associated with a single case of B-CLL thus far. BENTA disease patients manifest B cell activation and hyperproliferation especially IgM^+ IgD^+ $CD19^+$, $CD20^+$ B cells as well as $CD10^+$ immature/transitional B cells with the relative paucity of memory (CD27$^+$) and class-switched B cells. Histological examination of spleen, lymph node, and appendix tissue showed dramatic follicular hyperplasia of B cells, containing numerous primary follicles with prominent mantles and marginal zones, but atrophic germinal centers (GCs). By contrast, the patient T cells are normal in number and distribution but markedly less functionally responsive to antigen receptor-induced activation. In apoptosis assays of T cells, Fas killing is normal, whereas RICD is mildly reduced, probably related to poor initial activation; for B cells Fas-induced apoptosis is low. B cell dysregulation in these patients can lead to autoantibodies, autoimmune cytopenias, and a positive anti-nuclear antibody. Although BENTA disease may resemble ALPS with B cell lymphoproliferation, autoantibodies, apoptosis abnormalities, mild increases in DNTs, and a propensity to lymphoid malignancy, the former can readily be distinguished by distinctive histopathology, B cell subset abnormalities, and decreased T cell function tests. Conversely, ALPS has been associated with a variety of histological types of lymphoma but not with B-CLL.

Disease Biomarkers

In recent years several biomarkers were observed to be abnormal in patients with ALPS (Magerus-Chatinet et al., 2009; Caminha et al., 2010). These include increased prototypical DNT cells, HLA-DR positive cells, and decreased memory B cells. Also, several reports described elevated serum levels of soluble FAS ligand, vitamin B12, IL-10, and IL-18. More recently, the diagnostic utility of all these markers was evaluated in a large cohort of 562 ALPS patients and their relatives, with or without FAS mutations. Although not clinically useful in isolation, the combination of these markers proved to be a powerful predictor of the presence of *FAS* mutations in patients with an ALPS clinical phenotype. Patients with a combination of DNT >4% and IL-10 >40 pg/ml or B12 >1500 ng/L or sFASL >300 pg/ml had a 97% chance of harboring a *FAS* mutation (Caminha et al., 2010). Conversely, patients with DNTs <2% and sFASL <200 pg/ml carried only a 1.7% chance of having a *FAS* mutation. These markers were also very sensitive in detecting patients with somatic *FAS* mutations (Dowdell et al., 2010). Thus, in the presence of elevated DNTs and B12 or sFASL, a negative genetic screening for germline *FAS* mutations should prompt an investigation for somatic mutations in the sorted DNT population. These biomarkers were incorporated into the recently modified ALPS diagnostic criteria (Oliveira et al., 2010).

CONCLUSION

Despite their rarity, the discovery of ALPS and related disorders and their underlying genetic defects has provided valuable lessons about the role of these molecules in human immune homeostasis, tolerance and the prevention of autoimmunity, and tumor suppression. Despite these advances, about 20% of ALPS patients have yet-to-be-discovered genetic bases. The recent developments in high throughput genomics are likely to spur a new era of discoveries at an unprecedented pace.

ACKNOWLEDGMENTS

This research was supported by the Intramural Research Program of the National Institute of Allergy and Infectious Diseases and the Clinical Center, National Institutes of Health. The authors thank the ALPS Clinical Unit personnel including Joie Davis, Susan Price, Katie Perkins, Elaine Smoot, Pat Aldridge, Janet Dale, and Stephen Straus as well as the clinical support of Clifford Lane in the NIAID Division of Clinical Research and Tom Fleisher in the Department of Laboratory Medicine, NIH Clinical Center.

REFERENCES

Bi, L.L., Pan, G., Atkinson, T.P., Zheng, L., Dale, J.K., Makris, C., et al., 2007. Dominant inhibition of Fas ligand-mediated apoptosis due to a heterozygous mutation associated with autoimmune lymphoproliferative syndrome (ALPS) type Ib. BMC Med. Genet. 8, 41.

Bidere, N., Su, H.C., Lenardo, M.J., 2006. Genetic disorders of programmed cell death in the immune system. Annu. Rev. Immunol. 24, 321–352.

Bleesing, J.J., Brown, M.R., Dale, J.K., Straus, S.E., Lenardo, M.J., Puck, J.M., et al., 2001a. TcR-alpha/beta(+) CD4(−)CD8(−) T cells in humans with the autoimmune lymphoproliferative syndrome express a novel CD45 isoform that is analogous to murine B220 and represents a marker of altered O-glycan biosynthesis. Clin. Immunol. 100, 314–324.

Bleesing, J.J., Brown, M.R., Straus, S.E., Dale, J.K., Siegel, R.M., Johnson, M., et al., 2001b. Immunophenotypic profiles in families with autoimmune lymphoproliferative syndrome. Blood. 98, 2466–2473.

Bolze, A., Byun, M., McDonald, D., Morgan, N.V., Abhyankar, A., Premkumar, L., et al., 2010. Whole-exome-sequencing-based discovery of human FADD deficiency. Am. J. Hum. Genet. 87, 873–881.

Caminha, I., Fleisher, T.A., Hornung, R.L., Dale, J.K., Niemela, J.E., Price, S., et al., 2010. Using biomarkers to predict the presence of FAS mutations in patients with features of the autoimmune lymphoproliferative syndrome. J. Allergy Clin. Immunol. 125, 946–949.

Canale, V.C., Smith, C.H., 1967. Chronic lymphadenopathy simulating malignant lymphoma. J. Pediatr. 70, 891–899.

Chiocchetti, A., Indelicato, M., Bensi, T., Mesturini, R., Giordano, M., Sametti, S., et al., 2004. High levels of osteopontin associated with polymorphisms in its gene are a risk factor for development of autoimmunity/lymphoproliferation. Blood. 103, 1376–1382.

Chun, H.J., Zheng, L., Ahmad, M., Wang, J., Speirs, C.K., Siegel, R.M., et al., 2002. Pleiotropic lymphocyte activation defects due to caspase-8 mutation cause human immunodeficiency. Nature. 419, 395–399.

Cohen, P.L., Eisenberg, R.A., 1991. Lpr and gld: single gene models of systemic autoimmunity and lymphoproliferative disease. Annu. Rev. Immunol. 9, 243–269.

Darte, J.M., McClure, P.D., Saunders, E.F., Weber, J.L., Donohue, W.L., 1971. Congenital lymphoid hyperplasia with persistent hyperlymphocytosis. N. Engl. J. Med. 284, 431−432.

Davidson, W.F., Giese, T., Fredrickson, T.N., 1998. Spontaneous development of plasmacytoid tumors in mice with defective Fas-Fas ligand interactions. J. Exp. Med. 187, 1825−1838.

De Vos, A.M., Tong, L., Milburn, M.V., Matias, P.M., Jancarik, J., Noguchi, S., et al., 1988. Three-dimensional structure of an oncogene protein: catalytic domain of human c-H-ras p21. Science. 239, 888−893.

Del-Rey, M., Ruiz-Contreras, J., Bosque, A., Calleja, S., Gomez-Rial, J., Roldan, E., et al., 2006. A homozygous Fas ligand gene mutation in a patient causes a new type of autoimmune lymphoproliferative syndrome. Blood. 108, 1306−1312.

Dowdell, K.C., Niemela, J.E., Price, S., Davis, J., Hornung, R.L., Oliveira, J.B., et al., 2010. Somatic FAS mutations are common in patients with genetically undefined autoimmune lymphoproliferative syndrome. Blood. 115, 5164−5169.

Fisher, G.H., Rosenberg, F.J., Straus, S.E., Dale, J.K., Middleton, L.A., Lin, A.Y., et al., 1995. Dominant interfering Fas gene mutations impair apoptosis in a human autoimmune lymphoproliferative syndrome. Cell. 81, 935−946.

Galluzzi, L., Maiuri, M.C., Vitale, I., Zischka, H., Castedo, M., Zitvogel, L., et al., 2007. Cell death modalities: classification and pathophysiological implications. Cell. Death Differ. 14, 1237−1243.

Han, J., Zhong, C.Q., Zhang, D.W., 2011. Programmed necrosis: backup to and competitor with apoptosis in the immune system. Nat. Immunol. 12, 1143−1149.

Holzelova, E., Vonarbourg, C., Stolzenberg, M.C., Arkwright, P.D., Selz, F., Prieur, A.M., et al., 2004. Autoimmune lymphoproliferative syndrome with somatic Fas mutations. N. Engl. J. Med. 351, 1409−1418.

Hsu, A.P., Dowdell, K.C., Davis, J., Niemela, J.E., Anderson, S.M., Shaw, P.A., et al., 2012. Autoimmune lymphoproliferative syndrome due to FAS mutations outside the signal-transducing death domain: molecular mechanisms and clinical penetrance. Genet. Med. 14, 81−89.

Jackson, C.E., Fischer, R.E., Hsu, A.P., Anderson, S.M., Choi, Y., Wang, J., et al., 1999. Autoimmune lymphoproliferative syndrome with defective Fas: genotype influences penetrance. Am. J. Hum. Genet. 64, 1002−1014.

Koh, D.R., Ho, A., Rahemtulla, A., Fung-Leung, W.P., Griesser, H., Mak, T.W., 1995. Murine lupus in MRL/lpr mice lacking CD4 or CD8 T cells. Eur. J. Immunol. 25, 2558−2562.

Kuehn, H.S., Caminha, I., Niemela, J.E., Rao, V.K., Davis, J., Fleisher, T.A., et al., 2011. FAS haploinsufficiency is a common disease mechanism in the human autoimmune lymphoproliferative syndrome. J. Immunol. 186, 6035−6043.

Kwon, S.W., Procter, J., Dale, J.K., Straus, S.E., Stroncek, D.F., 2003. Neutrophil and platelet antibodies in autoimmune lymphoproliferative syndrome. Vox Sang. 85, 307−312.

Lenardo, M., Chan, K.M., Hornung, F., McFarland, H., Siegel, R., Wang, J., et al., 1999. Mature T lymphocyte apoptosis—immune regulation in a dynamic and unpredictable antigenic environment. Annu. Rev. Immunol. 17, 221−253.

Ley, R., Ewings, K.E., Hadfield, K., Cook, S.J., 2005. Regulatory phosphorylation of Bim: sorting out the ERK from the JNK. Cell Death Differ. 12, 1008−1014.

Lim, M.S., Straus, S.E., Dale, J.K., Fleisher, T.A., Stetler-Stevenson, M., Strober, W., et al., 1998. Pathological findings in human autoimmune lymphoproliferative syndrome. Am. J. Pathol. 153, 1541−1550.

Limnander, A., Weiss, A., 2011. Ca-dependent Ras/Erk signaling mediates negative selection of autoreactive B cells. Small Gtpases. 2, 282−288.

Limnander, A., Depeille, P., Freedman, T.S., Liou, J., Leitges, M., Kurosaki, T., et al., 2011. STIM1, PKC-delta and RasGRP set a threshold for proapoptotic Erk signaling during B cell development. Nat. Immunol. 12, 425−433.

Magerus-Chatinet, A., Stolzenberg, M.C., Loffredo, M.S., Neven, B., Schaffner, C., Ducrot, N., et al., 2009. FAS-L, IL-10, and double-negative CD4 − CD8 − TCR alpha/beta + T cells are reliable markers of autoimmune lymphoproliferative syndrome (ALPS) associated with FAS loss of function. Blood. 113, 3027−3030.

Magerus-Chatinet, A., Neven, B., Stolzenberg, M.C., Daussy, C., Arkwright, P.D., Lanzarotti, N., et al., 2011. Onset of autoimmune lymphoproliferative syndrome (ALPS) in humans as a consequence of genetic defect accumulation. J. Clin. Invest. 121, 106−112.

Merino, R., Fossati, L., Iwamoto, M., Takahashi, S., Lemoine, R., Ibnou-Zekri, N., et al., 1995. Effect of long-term anti-CD4 or anti-CD8 treatment on the development of lpr CD4 − CD8 − double negative T cells and of the autoimmune syndrome in MRL-lpr/lpr mice. J. Autoimmun. 8, 33−45.

Miyazaki, T., Ono, M., Qu, W.M., Zhang, M.C., Mori, S., Nakatsuru, S., et al., 2005. Implication of allelic polymorphism of osteopontin in the development of lupus nephritis in MRL/lpr mice. Eur. J. Immunol. 35, 1510−1520.

Neven, B., Magerus-Chatinet, A., Florkin, B., Gobert, D., Lambotte, O., De Somer, L., et al., 2011. A survey of 90 patients with autoimmune lymphoproliferative syndrome related to TNFRSF6 mutation. Blood. 118, 4798−4807.

Niemela, J.E., Lu, L., Fleisher, T.A., Davis, J., Caminha, I., Natter, M., et al., 2011. Somatic KRAS mutations associated with a human non-malignant syndrome of autoimmunity and abnormal leukocyte homeostasis. Blood. 117, 2883−2886.

Oliveira, J.B., Bidere, N., Niemela, J.E., Zheng, L., Sakai, K., Nix, C.P., et al., 2007. NRAS mutation causes a human autoimmune lymphoproliferative syndrome. Proc. Natl. Acad. Sci. U.S.A. 104, 8953−8958.

Oliveira, J.B., Bleesing, J.J., Dianzani, U., Fleisher, T.A., Jaffe, E.S., Lenardo, M.J., et al., 2010. Revised diagnostic criteria and classification for the autoimmune lymphoproliferative syndrome (ALPS): report from the 2009 NIH International Workshop. Blood. 116, e35−e40.

O'Reilly, L.A., Tai, L., Lee, L., Kruse, E.A., Grabow, S., Fairlie, W.D., et al., 2009a. Membrane-bound Fas ligand only is essential for Fas-induced apoptosis. Nature. 461, 659−663.

O'Reilly, L.A., Kruse, E.A., Puthalakath, H., Kelly, P.N., Kaufmann, T., Huang, D.C., et al., 2009b. MEK/ERK-mediated phosphorylation of Bim is required to ensure survival of T and B lymphocytes during mitogenic stimulation. J. Immunol. 183, 261−269.

Rao, V.K., Oliveira, J.B., 2011. How I treat autoimmune lymphoproliferative syndrome. Blood. 118, 5741−5751.

Rao, V.K., Dugan, F., Dale, J.K., Davis, J., Tretler, J., Hurley, J.K., et al., 2005. Use of mycophenolate mofetil for chronic, refractory immune cytopenias in children with autoimmune lymphoproliferative syndrome. Br. J. Haematol. 129, 534–538.

Rao, V.K., Carrasquillo, J.A., Dale, J.K., Bacharach, S.L., Whatley, M., Dugan, F., et al., 2006. Fluorodeoxyglucose positron emission tomography (FDG-PET) for monitoring lymphadenopathy in the autoimmune lymphoproliferative syndrome (ALPS). Am. J. Hematol. 81, 81–85.

Rieux-Laucat, F., Le Deist, F., Hivroz, C., Roberts, I.A., Debatin, K.M., Fischer, A., et al., 1995. Mutations in Fas associated with human lymphoproliferative syndrome and autoimmunity. Science. 268, 1347–1349.

Roths, J.B., Murphy, E.D., Eicher, E.M., 1984. A new mutation, gld, that produces lymphoproliferation and autoimmunity in C3H/HeJ mice. J. Exp. Med. 159, 1–20.

Salmena, L., Hakem, R., 2005. Caspase-8 deficiency in T cells leads to a lethal lymphoinfiltrative immune disorder. J. Exp. Med. 202, 727–732.

Sneller, M.C., Straus, S.E., Jaffe, E.S., Jaffe, J.S., Fleisher, T.A., Stetler-Stevenson, M., et al., 1992. A novel lymphoproliferative/autoimmune syndrome resembling murine lpr/gld disease. J. Clin. Invest. 90, 334–341.

Sneller, M.C., Wang, J., Dale, J.K., Strober, W., Middelton, L.A., Choi, Y., et al., 1997. Clinical, immunologic, and genetic features of an autoimmune lymphoproliferative syndrome associated with abnormal lymphocyte apoptosis. Blood. 89, 1341–1348.

Snow, A.L., Xiao, W., Stinson, J.R., Lu, W., Chaigne-Delalande, B., Zheng, L., et al., 2012. Congenital B cell lymphocytosis explained by novel germline CARD11 mutations. J Exp Med. 209, 2247–2261.

Stranges, P.B., Watson, J., Cooper, C.J., Choisy-Rossi, C.M., Stonebraker, A.C., Beighton, R.A., et al., 2007. Elimination of antigen-presenting cells and autoreactive T cells by Fas contributes to prevention of autoimmunity. Immunity. 26, 629–641.

Straus, S.E., Jaffe, E.S., Puck, J.M., Dale, J.K., Elkon, K.B., Rosen-Wolff, A., et al., 2001. The development of lymphomas in families with autoimmune lymphoproliferative syndrome with germline Fas mutations and defective lymphocyte apoptosis. Blood. 98, 194–200.

Su, H., Bidere, N., Zheng, L., Cubre, A., Sakai, K., Dale, J., et al., 2005. Requirement for caspase-8 in NF-kappaB activation by antigen receptor. Science. 307, 1465–1468.

Takagi, M., Shinoda, K., Piao, J., Mitsuiki, N., Matsuda, K., Muramatsu, H., et al., 2011. Autoimmune lymphoproliferative syndrome-like disease with somatic KRAS mutation. Blood. 117, 2887–2890.

Teachey, D.T., 2012. New advances in the diagnosis and treatment of autoimmune lymphoproliferative syndrome. Curr. Opin. Pediatr. 24, 1–8.

Teachey, D.T., Obzut, D.A., Axsom, K., Choi, J.K., Goldsmith, K.C., Hall, J., et al., 2006. Rapamycin improves lymphoproliferative disease in murine autoimmune lymphoproliferative syndrome (ALPS). Blood. 108, 1965–1971.

Teachey, D.T., Greiner, R., Seif, A., Attiyeh, E., Bleesing, J., Choi, J., et al., 2009. Treatment with sirolimus results in complete responses in patients with autoimmune lymphoproliferative syndrome. Br. J. Haematol. 145, 101–106.

Wang, J., Zheng, L., Lobito, A., Chan, F.K., Dale, J., Sneller, M., et al., 1999. Inherited human Caspase 10 mutations underlie defective lymphocyte and dendritic cell apoptosis in autoimmune lymphoproliferative syndrome type II. Cell. 98, 47–58.

Wang, L., Yang, J.K., Kabaleeswaran, V., Rice, A.J., Cruz, A.C., Park, A.Y., et al., 2010. The Fas-FADD death domain complex structure reveals the basis of DISC assembly and disease mutations. Nat. Struct. Mol. Biol. 17, 1324–1329.

Watanabe-Fukunaga, R., Brannan, C.I., Copeland, N.G., Jenkins, N.A., Nagata, S., 1992. Lymphoproliferation disorder in mice explained by defects in Fas antigen that mediates apoptosis. Nature. 356, 314–317.

Wu, J., Wilson, J., He, J., Xiang, L., Schur, P.H., Mountz, J.D., 1996. Fas ligand mutation in a patient with systemic lupus erythematosus and lymphoproliferative disease. J. Clin. Invest. 98, 1107–1113.

Zenker, M., 2011. Clinical manifestations of mutations in RAS and related intracellular signal transduction factors. Curr. Opin. Pediatr. 23, 443–451.

Chapter 51

Autoimmune Clotting Dysfunction

Christoph Königs

J.W. Goethe University, Department of Pediatrics, Clinical and Molecular Hemostasis, Frankfurt am Main, Germany

Chapter Outline

Introduction	**711**	Characteristics and Mode of Action of Anti-FVIII	
Procoagulant Thrombotic Diseases	**712**	Antibodies	718
Autoimmune Inhibitors to ADAMTS13	713	T Cell Epitopes in aHA	719
Anticoagulant (Bleeding) Diseases	**714**	Genetic Factors in aHA	719
Autoimmune Antibody Inhibitors to Fibrinogen (Factor I)		Treatment	719
and Fibrin	714	Autoimmune Inhibitors to Factor IX	720
Autoimmune Inhibitors to Prothrombin (Factor II) and		Autoimmune Inhibitors to Factor X	720
Thrombin	714	Autoimmune Inhibitors to Factor XI	720
Autoimmune Inhibitors to Factor V	716	Autoimmune Inhibitors to Factor XII	721
Autoimmune Inhibitors to Factor VII	717	Autoimmune Inhibitors to Factor XIII	721
Autoimmune Inhibitors to Factor VIII	717	Autoimmune Inhibitors to Von Willebrand Factor	722
Properties of the Factor VIII Protein	717	Autoimmune Inhibitors to Further Proteins	722
Clinical Presentation	717	**Conclusions and Future Prospects**	**722**
Laboratory Results	718	**Acknowledgments**	**723**
		References	**723**

INTRODUCTION

Immunologically mediated dysfunction of coagulation is observed secondary to a number of different autoimmune conditions but also occurs based on an isolated, specific autoimmune response to molecules of the coagulation system. The immune response directly or indirectly leads to an imbalance of hemostasis inducing hyper- or hypocoagulability.

Autoimmunity is found in primary and secondary—also called plasmatic—hemostasis. Primary hemostasis describes the initial reaction after injury of the endothelium of the blood vessel including the contraction of the blood vessel and exposure of tissue factor followed by the activation of platelets leading to the initial closure of the injury. In parallel, secondary hemostasis is initiated transforming the initial platelet clot into a stable fibrin clot. This clot is controlled by fibrinolysis. The classical schematic presentation of the coagulation cascade and the interplay of activation and inactivation are shown in Figure 51.1 illustrating its complexity of regulation.

This chapter aims to provide a short but comprehensive overview of autoimmunity to various proteins involved in secondary hemostasis, summarizing different and independent autoimmune entities. Autoantibodies can be detected and quantified. They need to be distinguished from alloantibodies in patients with congenital bleeding disorders after substitution of plasma or plasma proteins, which are not covered in this chapter. Autoantibodies to platelets interfering with primary hemostasis are described in Chapter 47.

In general, autoimmunity to proteins of the coagulation cascade is a rare event; for some proteins, only individual cases have been described in the literature. Antibodies can be detected against such proteins and quantified. Such antibodies have been termed inhibitors historically. Therapeutic options have not yet been studied in controlled clinical trials. Thus information on therapeutic interventions provided in this chapter reflects individual reports or expert opinion based on cohort studies or case series.

N. Rose & I. Mackay (Eds): The Autoimmune Diseases, Fifth edition. DOI: http://dx.doi.org/10.1016/B978-0-12-384929-8.00051-4

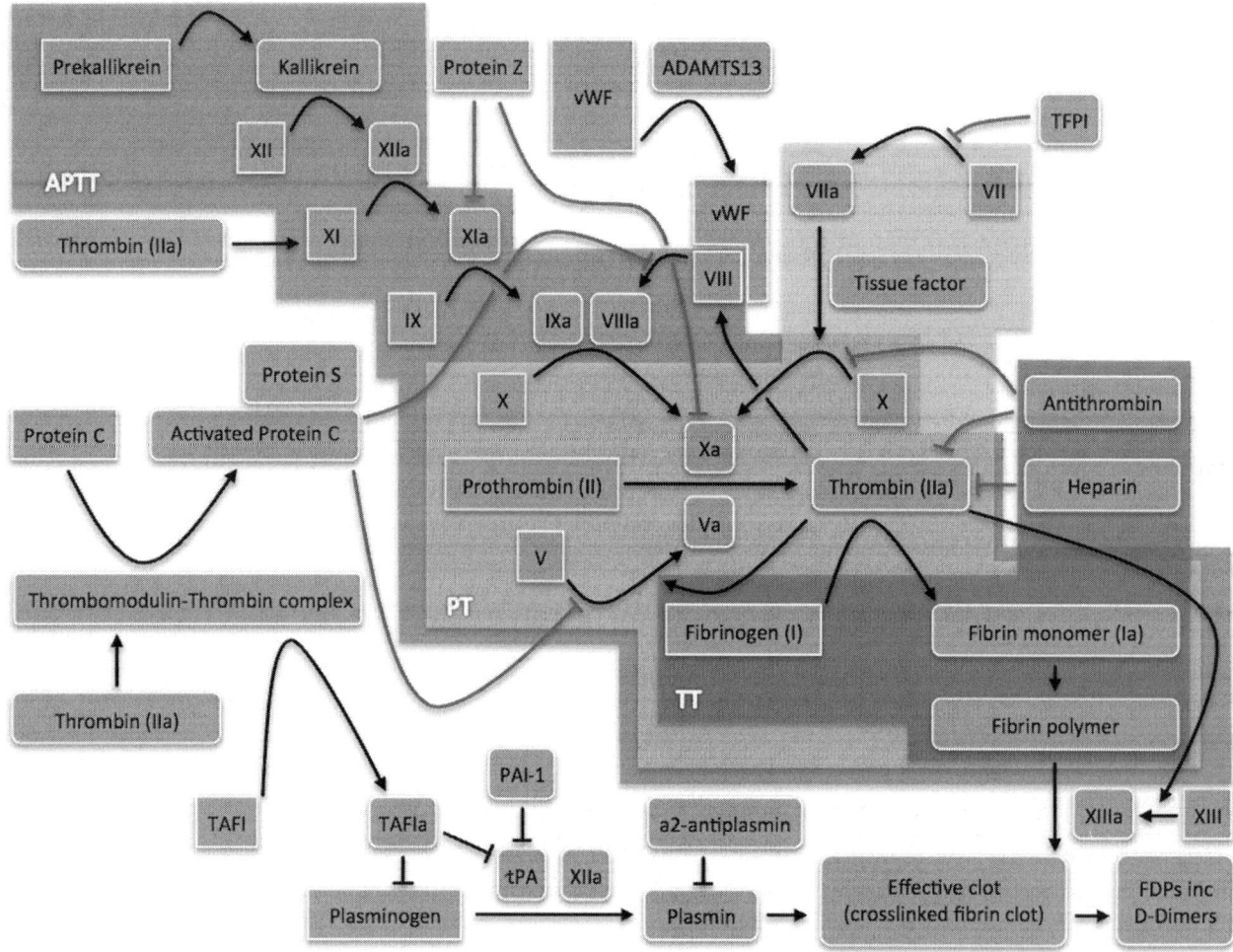

FIGURE 51.1   The coagulation cascade.   The complexity of coagulation and the interplay of the different factors with regard to inhibition and activation are illustrated in the diagram. The classical scheme has been used to demonstrate the complexity of molecules and interaction. Although extremely rare, autoimmune inhibitors have been described against most coagulation factors. The factors influencing the different global tests aPTT, PT, and TT are shaded green, gray, and red, respectively.

PROCOAGULANT THROMBOTIC DISEASES

There are several autoimmune entities known to interfere with homeostasis of the coagulation system thereby leading to a procoagulant state; in particular the antiphospolipid syndrome (APS) interferes with many components of the coagulation cascade as discussed in Chapter 34. Except for APS and antibodies to ADAMTS13 (see below) only single case reports on autoantibodies to other proteins of the coagulation cascade leading to thrombosis have been published.

Lupus anticoagulants interfere with the protein C pathway and possibly block the inactivation of FVIIIa (Urbanus and de Laat, 2010; Saenz et al., 2011). Autoantibodies to protein C and protein S have been described whereas antibodies to protein S appear to be

the more clinically relevant. Both autoantibodies were found at higher frequencies in individuals with overt thrombosis compared to healthy controls. The presence of specific IgM but not IgG autoantibodies as determined by ELISA correlated with the clinical phenotype (Rossetto et al., 2009). Also, both antibodies have been associated with fetal growth restrictions and preeclampsia (Torricelli et al., 2009). Antibodies to protein S have been detected, for example, in Behçet disease associated with thrombosis in five cases (Guermazi et al., 1997; Lechner et al., 2011). Further, they were prevalent in a number of patients with acquired protein S deficiency, and in patients with activated protein C resistance in the absence of the FV Leiden mutation with or without underlying systemic lupus erythematosus (Sorice et al., 1996; Nojima et al., 2002a, 2009). Antibodies to protein S and clinically relevant thrombosis have also been detected in children after infections, mainly varicella in several cases (Levin et al., 1995; Larakeb et al., 2009).

IgG and IgM autoantibodies to protein Z, which inactivates FXIa, have been detected in women with recurrent spontaneous miscarriages but not in healthy controls and were also associated with pregnancy complications, pre-eclampsia and fetal growth retardation (Gris et al., 2003; Erez et al., 2009; Sater et al., 2011). In a case–control study low protein Z levels and autoantibodies to protein Z were also found in patients with arterial or venous thrombosis (Pardos-Gea et al., 2008). The role of autoantibodies present in the antiphospholipid syndrome on the protein Z-mediated inactivation of FXa and on thrombosis is not clear (Forastiero et al., 2003; Sailer et al., 2008). Thrombotic complications also occur due to inhibitors to prothrombin (see below).

Autoimmune Inhibitors to ADAMTS13

Autoimmunity to ADAMTS13 (a disintegrin and metalloproteinase with a thrombospondin type 1 motif 13) causes the clinical picture of acquired thrombotic thrombocytopenic purpura (aTTP). Thrombotic events in terminal capillaries and arterioles are seen in aTTP. ADAMTS13 is a zinc protease, which cleaves the ultra large multimers of von Willebrand factor (vWF, see below) (Tsai, 1996; Furlan et al., 1997; Zheng et al., 2001; Fujikawa et al., 2001; Dong et al., 2002). Prior to the discovery of the enzyme itself the presence of ultra large multimers of vWF had already been demonstrated in aTTP patients (Moake et al., 1982). If not processed by ADAMTS13, the multimers rapidly form hyaline thrombi together with thrombocytes, mainly in the brain, kidney, adrenal gland, heart, pancreas, and spleen.

The incidence of aTTP is reported as 1.72 to 7 cases per million per year with women being affected twice as often as men. There is also a higher incidence and a more severe course seen in individuals of African descent (Torok et al., 1995; Miller et al., 2004; Terrell et al., 2005; Cataland et al., 2009). aTTP is mostly seen in adolescents and adults with a median age of 42 years (range 2–78) with a few pediatric cases being described (Scully et al., 2008; McDonald et al., 2010). aTTP can be seen in combination with underlying conditions including malignancies, drugs, infections, autoimmune diseases, primary immunodeficiency, after bone marrow transplantation, and pregnancy (Murrin and Murray, 2006; Scully et al., 2008; Yamada et al., 2011; Kawasaki et al., 2013). The combination of thrombocytopenia, hemolytic anemia, renal impairment, fever, and neurological symptoms has been described initially but the full pentad is present in fewer than half of all patients. The severe neurological symptoms are usually multifocal and often recurrent (Murrin and Murray, 2006). Typical but not pathognomonic is the paradoxical combination of thrombosis and thrombocytopenia. Additional clinical findings include petechial bleedings. The full clinical picture depends on organs affected by microthrombosis. This includes affection of the heart with pathological levels of cardiac enzymes and an abnormal ECG. Differential diagnosis includes but is not limited to hereditary TTP, hemolytic uremic syndrome, disseminated intravascular coagulation, and other microangiopathies or combinations of the above. The diagnosis may be difficult as levels of ADAMTS13 are reduced in several conditions. In suspected aTTP, diagnosis requires a blood cell count, vWF indices including multimers, ADAMTS13 activity, and levels of antigen and antibodies. Different assays to determine the enzymatic activity are available. Von Willebrand antigen and activity appear higher in TTP. In the acute phase the large vWF multimers are lacking in the plasma but reappear in remission. The extent of depleted ultra large multimers correlates with the severity of hemolysis and thrombocytopenia. Fragmented erythrocytes, an elevated LDH and creatinine, depending on kidney involvement, are observed (Whitelock et al., 2004; Wu et al., 2006; Peyvandi et al., 2010; Lotta et al., 2011).

Antibodies mainly of the isotype IgG, but also IgA and IgM, are found in almost all patients with aTTP. Most antibodies are inhibitory, but, in 10–15% of patients with ADAMTS13 deficiency, non-inhibitory antibodies are found suggesting an increased clearance of the protease (Scheiflinger et al., 2003; Tsai et al., 2006; Shelat et al., 2006; Ferrari et al., 2007; Pos et al., 2011). Antibodies isolated from peripheral B cells and class-switched memory B cells show somatic hypermutations suggestive of a role for T cells (Luken et al., 2005). IgG to ADAMTS13 is also seen in random controls but to a much lesser extent compared to aTTP patients (Tsai et al., 2006). Specific autoantibodies mainly belong to the IgG4 subclass, but also IgG1, IgG2, and IgG3 have been identified (Ferrari et al., 2009). The correlation of the type of antibodies with the outcome is still being discussed: high levels of autoantibodies and in particular high levels of IgG4 and the combination of IgG1 and IgA have been associated with an unfavorable outcome. Antibodies decrease during successful treatment (Coppo et al., 2006; Ferrari et al., 2007; Scully et al., 2007). In a different study, levels of IgA, IgG1, and IgG3 correlated with disease severity in the acute phase. Detectability of IgG in remission was also associated with a higher relapse rate (Bettoni et al., 2012). In almost all patients, antibodies against the cysteine-rich and the spacer region were identified, followed by antibodies against the metalloprotease. The cysteine-rich region is required for the cleavage of vWF. Antibodies against all other domains have been detected at lower frequencies (Soejima et al.,

2003; Klaus et al., 2004; Luken et al., 2005; Zheng et al., 2010; Yamaguchi et al., 2011).

There are indications for a genetic predisposition for the development of anti-ADAMTS13 autoantibodies: in different cohorts the MHC class II alleles DRB1*11, DQB1*0301, DQB1*02:02, and DRB3* are found more frequently in patients with aTTP, while the DRB1*04 and DRB4 alleles appear to be protective (Coppo et al., 2010; Scully et al., 2010; Pos et al., 2011; John et al., 2012).

Timely diagnosis and adequate treatment are crucial. If untreated the mortality is around 90%. Initial treatment is successful in most patients, with a relapse rate of 30–60% over 10 years (Shumak et al., 1995; Tsai, 2006; Kremer Hovinga et al., 2010). The benefit of plasmapheresis and plasma transfusions compared to transfusions alone was shown in a randomized trial (Rock et al., 1991). The combination of plasma exchange and steroids induced remission of >90% (Ferrari et al., 2007). Reported immunosuppression was mainly based on corticosteroids alone, but combinations with cyclosporine have also been successfully used (Cataland et al., 2007). Treatment with rituximab was successful and associated with a faster time to remission and fewer relapses but with the limitation of a non-stated long-term follow-up (Foley et al., 2009; Ling et al., 2009; Ojeda-Uribe et al., 2010; Scully, 2012; Tun and Villani, 2012). Successful treatment with bortezomib was reported in a patient refractory to immunosuppression including rituximab (Shortt et al., 2013). The benefit of intravenous immunoglobulin (ivIg) is doubtful; single reports discuss the benefit of defibrotide (Pogliani et al., 2000). In patients with refractory aTTP, splenectomy has been performed successfully (Kremer Hovinga et al., 2004). Thrombocyte transfusions are contraindicated, being associated with a higher mortality. Novel therapies are currently being evaluated: novel gain of function mutants resistant to autoantibodies might add to the future options in the treatment of aTTP (Jian et al., 2012). The role of recombinant ADAMTS13 in the presence of autoantibodies remains to be determined.

ANTICOAGULANT (BLEEDING) DISEASES

Autoimmune inhibitors to proteins of the coagulation cascade can cause a severe bleeding phenotype so a rapid diagnosis in these rare conditions and appropriate treatment are often crucial to the outcome for the patient. Inhibitors should be suspected in patients with hemorrhages without a personal or family bleeding history, and without trauma or use of anticoagulants. The provided algorithm describes a summary of a potential and rational approach to investigate patients with unexpected and unexplained bleeding events or abnormal coagulation tests and suspected inhibitors (Figure 51.2). For each individual protein epidemiological, clinical, and immunological aspects of inhibitors are described below.

Autoimmune Antibody Inhibitors to Fibrinogen (Factor I) and Fibrin

The fibrin clot is the final product of the coagulation cascade. Fibrin is generated from fibrinogen after thrombin cleavage. The glycoprotein fibrinogen is a heterohexamer composed respectively of two α-, β-, and γ-chains. Autoantibodies to fibrin or fibrinogen are rare. They have been described in combination with different underlying conditions, in pregnancy, or as "idiopathic." These conditions include other autoimmune disorders such as SLE or monoclonal gammopathies (Cohen et al., 1970; Coleman et al., 1972; Galanakis et al., 1978; Ruiz-Arguelles, 1988; Panzer and Thaler, 1993). Patients present with mild to severe bleeding symptoms. Antibodies to fibrin in pregnant women and newborns were not associated with a bleeding phenotype (Kondera-Anasz, 1998). More frequently cross-reactive antibodies occurred after exposure to bovine thrombin glue (see below; Chouhan et al., 1997).

Laboratory analysis reveals a prolonged TT, with both either normal or prolonged PT and aPTT. Fibrinogen levels may be normal or decreased. The TT is not corrected in mixing studies.

Antibodies against fibrinogen or fibrin usually belong to the IgG isotype; in a single report the subclasses IgG1 and IgG3 were detected (Galanakis et al., 1978). Most antibodies described interfere with the monomer formation and the release of fibrinopeptide A (Marciniak and Greenwood, 1979; Gris et al., 1992) or with the monomer polymerization (Ghosh et al., 1983). Two further cases have been described, with antibodies directed against the fibrinopeptide B also interfering with its release. These patients had no bleeding history, and a prolonged TT with a normal RT (Nawarawong et al., 1991; Llobet et al., 2007). The correlation of the clinical phenotype with the epitope location might reflect the different kinetics of thrombin cleavage for the two different fibrinopeptides and their distinct role in the three dimensional formation of the fibrin clot (Pechik et al., 2006).

The few published cases claim to show a spontaneous remission after the detection of an anti-idiotypic antibody (Ruiz-Arguelles, 1988), or report a normalization of clotting assays after treatment of the underlying disease (Panzer and Thaler, 1993). There are no treatment algorithms; an immunosuppressive or -modulatory therapy with corticosteroids or ivIg may be necessary in severe instances.

Autoimmune Inhibitors to Prothrombin (Factor II) and Thrombin

Thrombin plays a central role in coagulation by activating fibrinogen and also to some extent other proteins of the coagulation cascade. This leads to a thrombin burst by a positive feedback amplification. Thrombin also

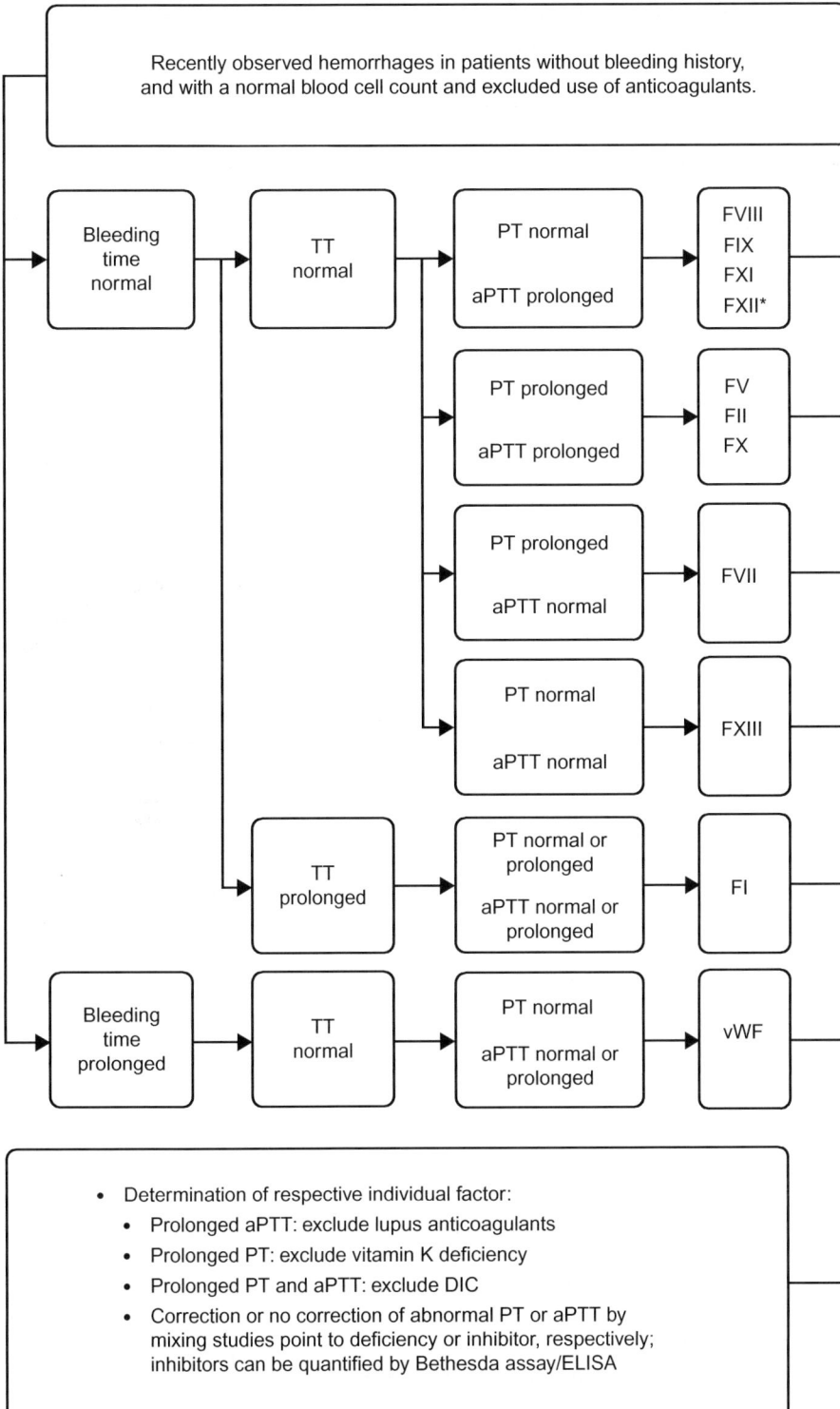

FIGURE 51.2 Possible guideline for the interpretation of coagulation tests for the diagnosis of factor inhibitors. TT: thrombin time, aPTT: activated partial thromboplastin time, PT: prothrombin time, vWF: von Willebrand factor, *: factor XII deficiency/inhibitors are not associated with a bleeding phenotype.

binds to thrombomodulin, which then activates protein C to control coagulation in a negative feedback loop. Thrombin is generated from prothombin by activated factor X and its cofactor activated factor V. Prothrombin is a glycoprotein structurally including the gamma-carboxyglutamic acid (Gla) domain, two kringle domains, and a C-terminal catalytic domain.

Antibodies to thrombin and prothrombin are rare and associated with bleeds of varying severity. Antibodies to prothrombin may also lead to a prothrombotic state

(Bertolaccini et al., 1998) as seen in patients with lupus anticoagulants (Roubey, 1998; Nojima et al., 2002b; Knobe et al., 2012; Chapter 34). Fatal cases have been described (La Spada et al., 1995). The occurrence of such antibodies has been described as "idiopathic" (La Spada et al., 1995; Knobe et al., 2012) or they may occur in association with gammopathies, liver cirrhosis, SLE, or infections including EBV (Barthels and Heimburger, 1985; Colwell et al., 1997; Bertolaccini et al., 1998; Atsumi et al., 2000).

More often antibodies to thrombin have been described during surgery after topical exposure to bovine thrombin, which is found in fibrin glues (Berruyer et al., 1993; Chouhan et al., 1997; Fastenau and Mcintyre, 2000). In some patients there is no bleeding tendency. The prolonged TT may be also an *in vitro* effect of alloantibodies to bovine thrombin, which is used in the laboratory assay; when bovine thrombin is replaced in the assay by human thrombin, the TT is normalized due to lack of cross-reactivity of the antibodies with human thrombin (Stricker et al., 1988; Flaherty et al., 1989; Lawson et al., 1990; Berruyer et al., 1993). In some patients who do develop antibodies with cross-reactivity to human thrombin, the TT does not normalize when bovine thrombin is replaced in the assay by human thrombin (Lawson et al., 1990). In a prospective trial ($n = 150$), the outcome for patients with exposure to bovine glue was less favorable (Ortel et al., 2001), but the matter is still under discussion. A possible solution is the use of human recombinant thrombin, which has been shown to be less immunogenic in clinical trials (Ballard et al., 2010).

Coagulation assays show a markedly prolonged TT and a prolonged aPTT and PT without any correction in mixing studies. RT is normal. Thrombin levels and activity are reduced (Scully et al., 1982; Gabriel et al., 1987). Antibodies can also be detected by ELISA.

Antibodies to thrombin or prothrombin may be neutralizing or non-neutralizing, increasing the clearance of prothrombin (Bajaj et al., 1985). Isotypes IgG or IgM have been identified (Bertolaccini et al., 1998). Antibody directed to the catalytic center of thrombin (Sie et al., 1991) or the exosites of thrombin blocks the corresponding functions including the cleavage of fibrinogen (Arnaud et al., 1994; La Spada et al., 1995; Mollica et al., 2006). In a single patient antibodies were described that formed a complex with prothrombin leading to an interaction with antithrombin III and a direct inactivation without the conversion to thrombin (Madoiwa et al., 2001). The affinity of anticoagulant prothrombin antibodies appeared to be lower compared to the affinity of lupus anticoagulants (Bajaj et al., 1983; Field et al., 2001).

Establishment of normal hemostasis in the presence of inhibitors to prothrombin or thrombin can be challenging. The bypassing agents, activated factor VII (FVIIa) or activated prothrombin complex concentrate (aPCC), have

been used (Giovannini et al., 2004). Other therapies including plasmapheresis, fresh frozen plasma (FFP), immunosuppressives including corticosteroids, and ivIg have been applied (Scully et al., 1982). During therapy a hypercoagulant situation may occur with the need for anticoagulation. A timely diagnosis and treatment reduces morbidity and mortality.

Autoimmune Inhibitors to Factor V

Activated factor V (FV) represents an essential cofactor of the complex converting prothrombin to thrombin. FV is structurally related to FVIII in having the A1, A2, A3, B, C1, and C2 domains. After activation by thrombin the B domain is released and an A1-A2/A3-C1-C2 heterodimer is formed (Lollar, 2005). Most FV antibodies have been described after surgical procedures especially after exposure to bovine thrombin glue, which contains traces of bovine factor V (Zehnder and Leung, 1990; Berruyer et al., 1993; Spero, 1993; Muntean and Zenz, 1994; Chouhan et al., 1997). These alloantibodies cross-react with human FV. The occurrence of "true" autoantibodies to FV has been described as idiopathic, related to the use of β lactam or aminoglycoside antibiotics (Knobl and Lechner, 1998) or to surgery (even without the use of thrombin glue), or associated with autoimmune diseases including SLE, Hashimoto thyroiditis, primary biliary cirrhosis, rheumatoid arthritis, or with malignancies or infections (Shastri et al., 1999; Takahashi et al., 2003; Ang et al., 2009; Franchini and Lippi, 2011; Franchini et al., 2012). In a recent analysis of inhibitory antibodies to FV not associated with fibrin glue, 73 cases have been described with an estimated incidence of 0.09 (Singapore) to 0.23 (Australia) cases per million person-years. About two-thirds of the patients with autoantibodies show a bleeding phenotype with hemorrhages mainly at mucosal membranes including hematuria, and gastrointestinal and gingival bleeds but also intracranial or retroperitoneal hemorrhages. Hemorrhages seem to correlate with the FV levels and with the aPTT (Favaloro et al., 2004; Ang et al., 2009).

Coagulation assays show a prolonged PT and aPTT, while the TT is normal. Again, mixing experiments fail to correct the coagulation defects, in contrast to congenital FV deficiency or due to disseminated intravascular coagulation. FV antigen and activity are reduced. FV inhibitors are also quantified by the Bethesda assay.

Inhibitors belong to the isotypes IgG and IgA (Lane et al., 1978; Ortel et al., 1992; Takahashi et al., 2003). In a single publication an FV-specific IgG4 was described (Suehisa et al., 1995). The antibodies bind to the light chain of FV (A3-C1-C2) (Ortel et al., 1992). Interestingly, antibodies from patients showing a bleeding phenotype bind to the N-terminal part of C2 and inhibit the binding of FV to phospholipids, thereby interfering with the formation of the prothrombinase complex (Ortel et al., 1998; Izumi et al., 2001). Platelet bound FV seems to be protected against most inhibitors but severe hemorrhages have been described in a patient with inhibitors against FV and platelet-associated FV (Nesheim et al., 1986; Ajzner et al., 2009). There are also non-inhibitory antibodies that increase the FV clearance. In addition to the anticoagulant nature of most FV inhibitors a single patient was identified with a FV inhibitor that mediated an activated protein C resistance and therefore led to a thrombophilic state instead of a bleeding phenotype (Kalafatis et al., 2002).

The focus of the initial therapy is the control of the acute hemorrhage. The use of platelets, fresh frozen plasma, activated prothrombin complex concentrate, and FVIIa have been described. FFP was often given prior to diagnosis and needs critical assessment due to the low content of FV. The use of aPCC and FVIIa seems more effective (Ang et al., 2009; Franchini et al., 2012). The need for eradication of FV inhibitors is discussed controversially since inhibitory antibodies can disappear spontaneously within several weeks (Knobl and Lechner, 1998). There was no statistical difference in inhibitor elimination according to whether the patients were treated or not (Ang et al., 2009). Nevertheless patients with bleeding symptoms showed benefit from eradication of the inhibitor. Several immunosuppressant approaches have been described including corticosteroids alone or in combination with immunosuppressants or rituximab. ivIg, immunoadsorption, or plasmapheresis have also been used (Jansen et al., 2001; de Raucourt et al., 2003).

Prevention seems feasible as at least half of the published cases with inhibitory antibodies to FV occurred after the use of bovine thrombin or fibrin glue and therefore appear to be preventable with using alternatives in the future (Streiff and Ness, 2002; Ballard et al., 2010).

Autoimmune Inhibitors to Factor VII

Factor VII (FVII) is a serine protease composed of a gamma-carboxyglutamic acid (Gla) domain, two epidermal growth factor (EGF) domains, and a protease domain. FVII binds to tissue factor (TF) and is activated by thrombin, FXIa, FXII, and FXa. FVIIa is a heterodimeric assembly of the light chain (Gla and EGF domain) and the heavy chain (protease domain). The complex of TF and FVIIa activates FX and FIX (Vadivel and Bajaj, 2012). Acquired FVII deficiency is mainly due to vitamin K deficiency and rarely has an autoimmune pathology. Antibody-mediated FVII deficiency has been described in only eight case reports so far and with only indirect evidence for autoimmunity. These inhibitors have been described as idiopathic or in combination with malignancies, autoimmune disorders, HIV infection or after the administration of penicillin (Campbell et al., 1980; Delmer et al., 1989; Ndimbie et al., 1989; Weisdorf et al., 1989;

Mehta et al., 1992; de Raucourt et al., 1994; Brunod et al., 1998; Okajima and Ishii, 1999; Aguilar et al., 2003). The intensity of hemorrhages varied from mild to severe and life-threatening, presenting as hematomas, ecchymosis, gastrointestinal bleeds, hematuria, and intracranial hemorrhages (Delmer et al., 1989; Okajima and Ishii, 1999). Coagulation assays show an isolated prolonged PT with normal aPTT, TT, and bleeding time. FVII antigen and activity are decreased. Mixing studies do not correct the PT. The level of inhibitors can be determined by the Bethesda assay.

FVII inhibition is mediated by an IgG autoantibody belonging to the IgG1 subclass (Campbell et al., 1980; Weisdorf et al., 1989; Brunod et al., 1998). A direct inhibition of FVIIa interaction with tissue factor or phospholipids has been proposed: an autoantibody binds to the light chain with an epitope on or near the Gla domain in a Ca^{2+}-dependent manner. In addition, there are antibodies that increase clearance of FVII without inhibition *in vitro* (Weisdorf et al., 1989; Kamikubo et al., 2000).

The initial hemorrhage is controlled by administration of FFP, FVII, or FVIIa concentrates (Delmer et al., 1989; Mullighan et al., 2004). Tranexamic acid has also been used (Aguilar et al., 2003). The use of FVII concentrate has been associated with thrombotic events in patients with FVII inhibitors and underlying disease (Brunod et al., 1998). Eradication of inhibitory antibodies has been achieved by immunosuppression with corticosteroids plus azathioprine, ivIg, or plasma exchange (Delmer et al., 1989).

Autoimmune Inhibitors to Factor VIII

Properties of the Factor VIII Protein

The factor VIII (FVIII) protein includes the domains A1, A2, A3, B, C1, C2, and acidic spacers (Toole et al., 1984; Wood et al., 1984). This domain structure is shared between FV and FVIII. FVIII is produced in several tissues; hepatocytes are the main source of the protein. During processing FVIII is cleaved to form the heavy and the light chain, which include A1-A2-B and A3-C1-C2, respectively. The heavy and light chains form a non-covalent heterodimer, which is complexed to von Willebrand factor (vWF). Upon activation by thrombin, the B domain and the acidic a3 region are cleaved off and vWF dissociates. Activated FVIII (FVIIIa) interacts with the phospholipid membrane, FIXa, and the substrate FX, which form the tenase complex and activate FX (Lenting et al., 1998; Saenko et al., 2002).

Clinical Presentation

Despite its rarity, acquired autoimmune hemophilia A (aHA) is by far the most frequent anti-coagulant autoimmune condition. A small number of studies and meta-analyses comprising 175 to 501 patients, and many case reports, have been published (Green and Lechner, 1981; Delgado et al., 2003; Collins et al., 2007). The reported incidence varies between 1.2 and 1.48 cases per million/year (Collins et al., 2004; Tay et al., 2009). Patients presenting with aHA show a biphasic age peak with postpartum women dominating in an early peak between 20 and 40 years (mean age: 33.9 years) and men dominating in the age peak above 60 years. Over all age groups, men appear to be slightly more often affected. The mean age at diagnosis is 73.9 to 78 years, depending on the cohort (Green and Lechner, 1981; Collins et al., 2007; Knoebl et al., 2012). A number of cases of aHA in children have also been described (Brodeur et al., 1980; Moraca and Ragni, 2002).

Clinically, greater than 90% of patients present with bleeds that occur spontaneously or after trauma and without a prior bleeding history. The majority of bleeds are severe, and, in contrast to congenital hemophilia A, bleeds comprise mainly large hematomas, ecchymoses, and soft tissue bleeds as well. Additionally many different clinical presentations have been reported including hematuria, gastrointestinal bleedings, intracranial hemorrhage, and hemothoraces. Around 6% of patients do not present with bleeding symptoms at the time of diagnosis. Diagnosis is often delayed and is associated with increased bleeding but without influence on the overall outcome (Micic et al., 2011; Fukushima et al., 2012; Knoebl et al., 2012; Rezaieyazdi et al., 2012; Webert, 2012). Similarly to inhibitory autoimmunity to other coagulation factors, aHA is associated with some underlying condition in about half of the cases. Among these are malignancies (11.8%) including solid tumors and hematological neoplasias, and autoimmune disorders (11.6%) including rheumatoid arthritis in one-third of the cases, and systemic lupus erythematosus. Postpartum antibody inhibitors comprised 7–15% of cases reported in cohorts (Green and Lechner, 1981; Delgado et al., 2003; Collins et al., 2007; Knoebl et al., 2012). Other conditions included exposure to certain drugs, surgery, infections, primary immunodefiency, and dermatological conditions. Disease in the remaining half of cases with no concomitant condition was termed "idiopathic aHA" (Ozgur et al., 2007; Kim et al., 2008; Shetty et al., 2011; Reitter et al., 2011; Knoebl et al., 2012). A significant number of pregnancy-associated FVIII autoantibodies are present antepartum. Hemorrhages during birth have been observed and so diagnostic evaluation of the newborn is crucial due to placental transfer of IgG (Tengborn et al., 2012).

Mortality is between 7.9 and 31%; early mortality is related to bleeding and later mortality mainly to the underlying condition or complications of immunosuppression (Green and Lechner, 1981; Lottenberg and Kentro, 1987; Morrison et al., 1993; Hay et al., 1997; Bossi et al., 1998; Collins et al., 2007). Among the largest cohort studied at the end of the follow-up period, the survival of patients with postpartum inhibitors was 100% and, in those with concomitant autoimmune disease or malignancy, was 71% and 32%, respectively, and idiopathic aHA 58% (Collins et al., 2012).

Laboratory Results

Laboratory results reveal a prolonged aPTT, low FVIII antigen levels and activity, and normal PT or TT. Mixing studies do not correct the aPTT. Antibodies can be measured by ELISA and inhibitory antibodies by the Bethesda assay (Nijmegen modification). Bethesda units or residual FVIII activity do not correlate with the bleeding phenotype (Lindgren et al., 2002; Toschi and Baudo, 2010). Inhibitors may lead to type I and type II kinetics of FVIII inactivation with the latter being the dominant one albeit not inactivating FVIII completely. There are indications that type I inhibitory antibodies block the activation of FVIII by thrombin, whereas type II inhibitors block the binding to phospholipids resulting in different clinical phenotypes (Nogami et al., 2001; Matsumoto et al., 2012). The affinity of inhibitor reactivity with FVIII might also influence the type of kinetics observed.

Characteristics and Mode of Action of Anti-FVIII Antibodies

Inhibitory antibodies are mostly of the isotype IgG and subclasses IgG4 and IgG1; IgA and IgM inhibitors have been detected at low levels (Whelan et al., 2013). The IgG population is polyclonal. Dominant IgG4 responses are associated with higher inhibitor titers (Reding et al., 2002). Antibody epitopes are mainly found on the A2 and C2 domain of FVIII; the epitope distribution differs between aHA patients and patients with congenital hemophilia A (cHA) and inhibitors (Prescott et al., 1997; Scandella, 1999; Matsumoto et al., 2001). The anti-FVIII specific IgG subclasses and the epitopes recognized differ according to different clinical conditions; a dominance of the IgG4 subclass occurs in most conditions. In postpartum aHA FVIII-specific IgG1 and IgG3 were found more frequently than in patients with other concomitant conditions. In addition, postpartum anti-FVIII antibodies more often recognized the heavy chain especially the A1a1 domain (Lapalud, 2012). Antibodies can block the interaction of FVIII with different molecules of the coagulation cascade including vWF, phospholipids, thrombin, FIX, and FX by competition or steric hindrance. Proteolytic FVIII antibodies have also been described (Wootla et al., 2008; Mahendra and Padiolleau-Lefevre, 2012). In addition, there are indications that anti-FVIII inhibitors with type II kinetics also inhibit the proteolysis of FVIIIa by activated protein C, and establish circulating immune complexes (Nogami et al., 2001). Recently the presence of hydrolyzing and activating FIX antibodies was described in aHA patients leading to thrombin generation in about a third of the patients (Wootla et al., 2011). Their clinical relevance is undetermined.

T Cell Epitopes in aHA

There are some T cell epitopes in the C2 domain of FVIII (amino acids 2291−2330) that are shared between aHA patients, cHA patients with inhibitors, and healthy individuals; there are additional epitopes including the region 2241−2290 only identified in aHA patients. In addition, distinct T cell epitopes on the A3 domain have been identified for patients with aHA that are not shared by patients with cHA and inhibitors (Reding et al., 2003, 2004).

Genetic Factors in aHA

In patients with aHA different polymorphisms in immune response genes occur more frequently than in healthy individuals: in regard to CTLA4 a higher frequency of the CTLA4 49 A/G polymorphism has been observed. Interestingly the G allele was found more frequently in patients with an underlying autoimmune disease. HLA class I haplotypes were not correlated with aHA disesase, but for HLA class II haplotypes there was a higher frequency of DRB1*16 and DQB1*0502, and a lower frequency of DRB1*15 and DQB1*0602 in affected patients. These results do not align with HLA haplotypes seen in cHA patients with inhibitors. The influence of polymorphisms in the FVIII gene itself remains to be investigated (Pavlova et al., 2008, 2010; Tiede et al., 2010).

Treatment

The treatment of patients with aHA focuses initially on reestablishing hemostasis and, later on, the induction of tolerance. Despite being the most frequent autoimmune coagulopathy, treatment recommendations are based on expert opinion due to the lack of controlled trials. With modern aHA treatment, about 70% of patients receive bypassing agents including FVIIa and aPCC to control acute bleeds. In the largest cohort studied, FVIIa was used in more than half of the bleeds and aPCC in 20%. Both agents are equally effective overall but treatment success for each differed significantly for the individual patient. The residual patients were treated with FVIII products, desmopressin, and, historically, with porcine FVIII, which is currently unavailable. Treatment with bypassing agents was more effective than treatment with FVIII or desmopressin (Morrison et al., 1993; Kessler and Ludlam,

1993; Collins et al., 2007; Baudo et al., 2012). In about 4% of patients thromboembolic events occurred during treatment with bypassing products (Knoebl et al., 2012; Sumner et al., 2007). Around one-third of patients did not require any hemostatic treatment. For AHA patients requiring surgery a successful hemostatic management with aPCC was reported for five patients (Shetty et al., 2011). In cases with antepartum inhibitors, close monitoring of the newborn is required.

Immunosuppressive therapy is necessary to induce tolerance in most aHA patients. Various regimens based on corticosteroids, cytotoxic agents, rituximab, ivIG, plasmapheresis, immune adsorption, and protocols for induction of immune tolerance from cHA patients with inhibitors using high dose FVIII have been applied (Nemes and Pitlik, 2000; Wiestner et al., 2002; Freedman et al., 2003; Stasi et al., 2004; Collins et al., 2007, 2012; Tiede et al., 2009; Muzaffar et al., 2012; Barillari and Pasca, 2013; Zanon et al., 2013). Inhibitor eradication (complete remission) was achieved in about two-thirds of the patients. In the largest cohort of patients to date (EACH2, $n = 501$) most were treated with corticosteroids either alone (43%) or in combination with cyclophosphamide (25%) or with a rituximab-based regimen (15%), achieving complete remission in 58%, 80%, or 61%, respectively. Successfully treated patients who received a combination of corticosteroids and cyclophosphamide experienced more adverse events (41%), mainly infections, compared to the group treated with steroids alone (25%). The final outcome "alive and inhibitor free at last follow-up" was achieved by 67% of patients treated with steroids alone compared to 62% of patients treated with corticosteroids and cyclophosphamide (Collins et al., 2012). The modified-Bonn−Malmö protocol combining immune adsorption, immunosuppression, FVIII administration, and FVIIa to control acute bleeds achieved remission rates of >90% for non-malignancy associated AHA (Zeitler et al., 2012, 2013).

Treatment success appears to be associated with the nature of the underlying condition, a younger age, and a lower antibody level. Spontaneous remissions have also been described. Most patients with postpartum inhibitors achieved complete remission when treated with corticosteroids (Baudo and De Cataldo, 2003). There was no improvement in survival when treatment either with corticosteroids alone or in combination with cytotoxic agents was used. Among successfully treated patients, some 20% relapsed within a median of seven months (range 1−60 weeks). When complete remission was achieved life expectancy equaled that of non-affected individuals of the same age (Collins et al., 2007).

An international expert panel recommended antihemorrhagic treatment for aHA patients using FVIIa or aPCC for first line treatment. For eradication of inhibitory antibodies a first line therapy with corticosteroids alone or in combination with cyclophosphamide is recommended. Protocols for induction of immune tolerance in cHA including immune adsorption are recommended in case of life-threatening bleedings. When hemostasis is controlled, anticoagulant prophylaxis needs to be considered (Huth-Kuhne et al., 2009). Prospective studies are currently examining treatment protocols. Also novel bypassing therapies are currently being developed such as recombinant porcine FVIII, FIX variants, and bi-specific antibodies (Kitazawa et al., 2012; Milanov et al., 2012; Kempton et al., 2012).

Autoimmune Inhibitors to Factor IX

Factor IX (FIX) is a serine protease structurally related to FVII and FX including a Gla-domain, two EGF-like domains, and a protease domain. FIX is activated by FXIa and FVIIa. FIXa forms, with FVIIIa, the tenase complex, which activates factor X (see above).

Autoimmune inhibitors of factor IX have been described only in single case reports (Roberts, 1970; Ozsoylu and Ozer, 1973; Largo et al., 1974; Reisner et al., 1977). The incidence is unknown. They have occurred mainly in elderly people, but sometimes in children (Miller et al., 1978; Mazzucconi et al., 1999; Jedidi et al., 2011). The condition was spontaneous or with various underlying diseases including hepatitis C (under therapy), autoimmune hepatitis, Sjögren syndrome, ITP, arteritis, and SLE (Castro et al., 1972; Torres et al., 1980; Carmassi et al., 2007; Campos-de-Magalhaes et al., 2011; Jedidi et al., 2011; Krishnamurthy et al., 2011). Three cases have been reported with inhibitors to both FVIII and FIX (Carmassi et al., 2007) and one with an inhibitor to FIX, FX, and prothrombin (Rochanda et al., 2012). Laboratory assessment reveals a prolonged aPTT while PT, TT, and bleeding time are normal. In mixing studies the aPTT does not correct. FIX inhibitors can be directly detected and quantified by the Bethesda assay.

With so few cases reported data are scarce on the nature of autoantibodies to FIX. Alloantibodies described in hemophilia B patients are mainly IgG and of the subclasses IgG1 and IgG4. The antibodies are mainly directed against the protease and the GLA domain, but also the EGF-like domain (Torres et al., 1980). In a single patient, in whom antibodies bound to FIX, FX, and prothrombin, the antibodies belonged to the IgG4 subclass and bound to a common motif on the Gla domain (Rochanda et al., 2012).

Acute bleeds were treated with FVIIa (Abshire and Kenet, 2008) accompanied by immunosuppression with prednisolone alone (Krishnamurthy et al., 2011), in combination with ivIg (Mazzucconi et al., 1999), or in addition with azathioprine (Carmassi et al., 2007).

Autoimmune Inhibitors to Factor X

Factor X (FX) also is a zymogen of a serine protease and is structurally related to FVII and FIX with an identical domain structure including the Gla, EGF, and protease domains. Upon activation by FVIIa and tissue factor or by the tenase complex composed of FVIIIa and FIXa, FXa cleaves prothrombin in the presence of FVa (prothrombinase complex) and phospholipids, so generating active thrombin. Antibody-mediated FX deficiency is extremely rare. Non-autoimmune acquired FX deficiency was described in the presence of amyloidosis and attributed to the adsorption of FX to amyloid fibrils (Mumford et al., 2000) and of malignancies including solid tumors and leukemias. Most cases of acquired inhibitory antibodies to FX have followed respiratory tract infections (Bayer et al., 1969; Hosker and Jewell, 1983; Currie et al., 1984; Mulhare et al., 1991); in a single childhood case the condition developed after extensive burns (Matsunaga and Shafer, 1996). Antibodies as inhibitors were identified only in recent cases. The clinical picture includes hematoma, ecchymosis, mucosal bleeds, hematuria, and also intracranial hemorrhages (Edgin et al., 1980; Lankiewicz and Bell, 1992; Smith et al., 1998; Rochanda et al., 2012). In laboratory findings PT and aPTT are prolonged while TT and bleeding time are normal. Inhibitors can be quantified by the Bethesda assay.

Anti-FX inhibitors belong to the IgG isotype. Several antibodies have been analyzed, and these bind to the light chain near or on the Gla domain. The antibody inhibited the activation of FX by the TF–FVIIa complex and by the tenase complex (Lankiewicz and Bell, 1992; Rao et al., 1994; Matsunaga and Shafer, 1996; Smith et al., 1998). Another report described an IgG4 antibody population recognizing an epitope in common with FII, FIX, and FX, and also an epitope on the Gla domain (Rochanda et al., 2012).

Treatment of acute bleeds in the presence of FX inhibitors is challenging due to the central role of FX in the coagulation cascade. The successful use of aPCC has been described, but has also been complicated by thromboembolic complications and cerebral infarctions (Henson et al., 1989; Mulhare et al., 1991; Smith et al., 1998). Transfusions of FFP have only been successful after plasma exchange followed by ivIg. Autoimmune inhibitors of FX are usually transient and treatment is not required, but corticosteroids or ivIg have been used in individual cases (Edgin et al., 1980; Matsunaga and Shafer, 1996).

Autoimmune Inhibitors to Factor XI

Factor XI (FXI) is also a zymogen of the serine protease that is activated by FXII or thrombin, or autocatalytically.

It is composed of four so-called apple domains in the heavy chain and a protease domain, and circulates as a homodimer. FXIa then activates FIX (Gailani and Smith, 2009). Autoimmune inhibitors to FXI are extremely rare and their incidence is unknown. Mostly, inhibitory antibodies to FXI have occurred with an underlying condition, including SLE, leukemias, autoimmune gastrointestinal diseases, psoriasis, or membranoproliferative glomerulonephritis (Rustgi et al., 1982; Vercellotti and Mosher, 1982; Goodrick et al., 1992; Kyriakou et al., 2002; Bortoli et al., 2009; McManus et al., 2012). Bleeding phenotypes due to FXI inhibitors differ; most are mild but a few have been life threatening (Reece et al., 1984; Bortoli et al., 2009).

In coagulation assays FXI inhibitors present with a prolongation of aPTT with a normal PT, TT, and bleeding time. Inhibitors are quantified by the Bethesda assay. The isotype of FXI inhibitors is IgG or IgM (Krieger et al., 1975). Antibodies that have developed in patients with congenital FXI deficiency are of the IgG1 or 3 subclass and are directed against the heavy chain of the molecule (De La Cadena et al., 1988). The mode of FXI inhibition has been identified as increased clearance of FXI by inhibitors or blocking of the activation of FXI (Krieger et al., 1975; Poon et al., 1984; McManus et al., 2012). No such data are available on autoimmune inhibitory antibodies to FXI.

The treatment of hemorrhages due to FXI inhibitors was based on FXI concentrate, FFP, PCC, and rFVIIa. Inhibitor eradication has been achieved either by immunosuppression with corticosteroids or by the immunosuppression used as part of the therapy of the underlying condition (Vercellotti and Mosher, 1982; Goodrick et al., 1992; Billon et al., 2001; Bern et al., 2005).

Autoimmune Inhibitors to Factor XII

Factor XII (FXII) is a monomeric zymogen of the serine protease FXIIa. FXII consists of a heavy chain including two fibronectin-type domains, two EGF-like domains, a kringle domain, and a proline-rich domain plus a light chain including the catalytic center. Polyphosphates on the surface of procoagulant thrombocytes (contact phase) pre-activate FXII, which is then activated by kallikrein. FXIIa then activates FXI and plasminogen. In addition to initiating the coagulation cascade, FXIIa starts the kallikrein–kinin system. FXII inhibitory antibodies have been described in association with particular autoimmune diseases, i.e., SLE, APS, and autoimmune hepatitis, with malignancies including lymphoma and gastric carcinoma, and with infections, particularly hepatitis B (Chalkiadakis et al., 1999; Jones et al., 2000; Davidson et al., 2005; Bertolaccini et al., 2007). The pathology of FXII inhibitors is still being discussed; they are not associated with

hemorrhages but possibly with a prothrombotic state (Aberg and Nilsson, 1972). In addition FXII inhibitors have been associated with pregnancy failure and fetal loss (Jones et al., 2001; D'Uva et al., 2005). Laboratory results show a very prolonged aPTT with a normal PT, TT, and bleeding time typically without any bleeding symptoms. Antibodies are detected by ELISA. For FXII inhibitors isotypes IgG or IgM have been identified (Jones et al., 2000; Davidson et al., 2005). In women with fetal loss most antibodies recognized the N-terminal portion of the heavy chain, which interacts with thrombocytes, whereas, in patients with APS, epitopes were identified in the catalytic domain and in the EGF-like domain (Harris et al., 2005; Inomo et al., 2008). Treatment is not required, but anticoagulation may be needed to prevent pregnancy failure.

Autoimmune Inhibitors to Factor XIII

Factor XIII (FXIII) is a tetramer composed of two A and two B domains; it is activated by thrombin and stabilizes the fibrin clot by cross-linking fibrin γ chains (Ariens et al., 2002). Autoantibodies to FXIII occur very rarely but are likely to be under-diagnosed. Some 50 individual cases have been described to date, some with underlying conditions including a monoclonal gammopathy (Luo et al., 2010) or another autoimmune disease including SLE (Ahmad et al., 1996; Lorand et al., 2002; Ajzner et al., 2009; Luo and Zhang, 2011). Antibodies to FXIII have also occurred following exposure to drugs including isoniazid (Otis et al., 1974; Shires et al., 1979; Krumdieck et al., 1991) and may develop spontaneously (Nijenhuis et al., 2004). Patients present clinically with recurrent hemorrhages of different intensity including mucosal or large soft-tissue hematomas, or with a life-threatening event such as intracranial hemorrhage (Daly et al., 1991; Lorand et al., 2002). The age of presented cases is usually between 60 and 70 years, but is wide considering all cases ranging from 10 to 87 years (Luo and Zhang, 2011). The laboratory findings reveal normal global coagulation tests like PTT, PT, bleeding time, and platelet counts. FXIII activity or levels are reduced and can be determined by chromogenic assays—ELISA for the FXIIIA or B subunits. The thromboelastogram reflects a reduced clot formation and increased fibrinolysis. Alternatively, a dissolved clot after treatment with 5M urea indicates a FXIII deficiency. Inhibitors to FXIII can be measured by mixing studies, and by ELISA to immobilized FXIII subunits. Antibodies are mainly directed against the active A domain of FXIII, and rarely against the B domain. Inhibitory antibodies block the activation by thrombin, catalysis, or the binding to fibrin or other substrates of FXIII depending on the cognate epitope (Nakamura et al., 1988; Fukue et al., 1992; Ahmad et al.,

1996; Lorand et al., 2002; Ajzner et al., 2009; Luo and Zhang, 2011).

Treatment is based on replacement therapy and immunosuppression. Despite the presence of antibodies, treatment of acute bleeds with FXIII concentrate, or with FFP (if concentrate was not available), has been successful. Treatment is mainly combined with immunosuppression with (methyl)prednisolone and/or cyclophosphamide (Tosetto et al., 1995; Ishida et al., 2010; Luo and Zhang, 2011; Hayashi et al., 2012). The use of ivIg or immune adsorption, cyclosporine, and FVIIa has also been described. Single patients have also been treated with rituximab (Gregory and Cooper, 2006; Ajzner et al., 2009).

Autoimmune Inhibitors to Von Willebrand Factor

Although von Willebrand factor (vWF) is not a classical coagulation factor, it plays a crucial role in primary as well as secondary hemostasis. This large glycoprotein includes the domains D′, D1−4, A1−3, B, and C1−2. The protein binds to FVIII prolonging its half-life prior to activation, interacts with subendothelial layers after vascular injury, and promotes thrombocyte adhesion and aggregation. The vWF monomers assemble to multimers of different sizes up to 20,000 kDa. Ultra large multimers are cleaved by ADAMTS13 (see above) (Schneppenheim and Budde, 2008).

Acquired von Willebrand disease (avWD) is a rare condition with only a few hundred patients described; one report gave an incidence of 10% in a small, preselected cohort of patients with bleeding disorders (Mohri et al., 1998). Among patients with avWD, 10−30% express an autoantibody against vWF; their overall incidence has been estimated to be 0.04% (Kumar et al., 2003). The pathophysiology of avWD in most patients is not based on autoimmune effects but rather on conditions associated with a reduced production of vWF as seen in hypothyroidism, on an increased clearance due to attachment to tumor cells or paraneoplastic products, an increased mechanical clearance, or resulting from certain drugs (Veyradier et al., 2000). Thus avWS is associated with different underlying conditions, including hypothyroidism, lympho- or myeloproliferative disorders, solid tumors including Wilms' tumor, infections, and acquired or congenital heart defects. Drugs that may cause avWD include certain antibiotics, hydroethyl starch, and valproic acid. Autoimmune avWD has been described as idiopathic or with underlying autoimmune diseases, including SLE, or monoclonal gammopathies (Federici et al., 2000; Michiels et al., 2001; Will, 2006). Patients present with a spectrum of nil to severe bleeds, mainly ecchymoses but

also epistaxis, and gastrointestinal and mucosal bleeds (Mohri et al., 1998; Collins et al., 2008). avWD patients with inhibitors show a higher bleeding tendency than patients without inhibitors. Autoantibodies bind to the large or intermediate size multimers. They have been identified as mainly of the IgG isotype, but IgA and IgM isotypes have been described, depending on the underlying condition. IgG antibodies belong to the subclasses IgG1 and IgG4. Epitopes have been mapped to the A1 and the A3 domain with inhibition of collagen binding, and display binding to GP Ib and GP IIb/IIIa (van Genderen et al., 1994; Mohri et al., 1998).

Laboratory diagnosis of avWD and differentiation from congenital vWD can be often difficult. Analysis reveals a prolonged bleeding time, with normal PT and normal or prolonged aPTT. The vWF antigen, ristocetin cofactor, or collagen binding activity is reduced. Also, FVIII activity is often reduced. Large vWF multimers are often lacking. Anti-vWF antibodies can be detected. In a Bethesda-like assay several approaches have to be considered due to the large size of vWF and different epitope-related effect of the antibodies. A pharmacokinetic analysis might be useful as non-inhibitory antibodies that enhance clearance are not detected by the Bethesda assay (Mohri et al., 1998; Luboshitz et al., 2001; Siaka et al., 2003; Tiede et al., 2008).

The treatment of avWD is based on the therapy of the underlying condition. The use of desmopressin to release vWF, and the substitution of a vWF-containing FVIII concentrate or FFP have been described to successfully treat non-autoimmune avWD and to control acute bleeds. The response to FVIII/vWF concentrates or desmopressin is usually very poor when an inhibitory antibody is present. In severe uncontrollable bleeds, FVIIa has also been used successfully. Autoimmune avWD has successfully been treated with immunomodulation including the administration of immunoglobulins and immunosuppression with corticosteroids, plasma exchange, or immune absorbtion (Collins et al., 2008; Sucker et al., 2009; Tiede et al., 2011).

Autoimmune Inhibitors to Further Proteins

In addition to autoimmune responses to proteins described above, one single case of an autoantibody to prekallikrein has been identified to date. An IgG1 and 4 polyclonal autoantibody population was detected in a single patient who presented with a prolonged aPTT without any symptoms of bleeding or thrombosis (Page et al., 1994).

CONCLUSIONS AND FUTURE PROSPECTS

Autoimmune inhibitors to coagulation factors are rare and highly diverse effectors, and remain as poorly understood

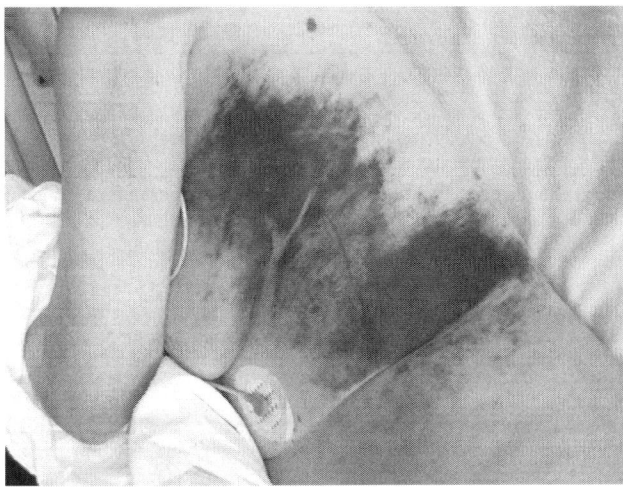

FIGURE 51.3 Severe soft tissue hemorrhage in a patient with acquired hemophilia A.

entities. Moreover, studies on the T lymphocyte component of these autoimmune reactions have been scarcely considered. In cases of bleeding in individuals without bleeding history, inhibitors to coagulation factors need to be assessed. The timely diagnosis and treatment of affected patients remains challenging. Further efforts are needed to understand the underlying pathology of autoimmunity leading to hemorrhages or thrombosis and to improve treatment outcome for affected individuals.

Understanding autoimmunity to individual proteins of the coagulation cascade may promote the understanding of autoimmunity in general. In contrast to many other autoimmune entities the autoantigens are well known and most of them well characterized. Additionally the same proteins are seen as autoantigens as well as alloantigens in patients with congenital bleeding disorders. This allows the comparison of allo- and autoimmune responses to the identical protein (Figure 51.3).

ACKNOWLEDGMENTS

The author would like to thank Stephan Schultze-Strasser, PhD and Manuela Krause, MD for assistance with or provision of figures, and Christine Heller, MD and Dirk Schwabe, MD for critical comments on the manuscript, and his family and the editors for support and patience.

REFERENCES

Aberg, H., Nilsson, I.M., 1972. Recurrent thrombosis in a young woman with a circulating anticoagulant directed against factors XI and XII. Acta. Med. Scand. 192, 419–425.

Abshire, T., Kenet, G., 2008. Safety update on the use of recombinant factor VIIa and the treatment of congenital and acquired deficiency of factor VIII or IX with inhibitors. Haemophilia. 14, 898–902.

Aguilar, C., Lucia, J.F., Hernandez, P., 2003. A case of an inhibitor autoantibody to coagulation factor VII. Haemophilia. 9, 119–120.

Ahmad, F., Solymoss, S., Poon, M.C., Berube, C., Sullivan, A.K., 1996. Characterization of an acquired IgG inhibitor of coagulation factor XIII in a patient with systemic lupus erythematosus. Br. J. Haematol. 93, 700–703.

Ajzner, E., Schlammadinger, A., Kerenyi, A., Bereczky, Z., Katona, E., Haramura, G., et al., 2009. Severe bleeding complications caused by an autoantibody against the B subunit of plasma factor XIII: a novel form of acquired factor XIII deficiency. Blood. 113, 723–725.

Ang, A.L., Kuperan, P., Ng, C.H., Ng, H.J., 2009. Acquired factor V inhibitor. A problem-based systematic review. Thromb. Haemost. 101, 852–859.

Ariens, R.A., Lai, T.S., Weisel, J.W., Greenberg, C.S., Grant, P.J., 2002. Role of factor XIII in fibrin clot formation and effects of genetic polymorphisms. Blood. 100, 743–754.

Arnaud, E., Lafay, M., Gaussem, P., Picard, V., Jandrot-Perrus, M., Aiach, M., et al., 1994. An autoantibody directed against human thrombin anion-binding exosite in a patient with arterial thrombosis: effects on platelets, endothelial cells, and protein C activation. Blood. 84, 1843–1850.

Atsumi, T., Ieko, M., Bertolaccini, M.L., Ichikawa, K., Tsutsumi, A., Matsuura, E., et al., 2000. Association of autoantibodies against the phosphatidylserine-prothrombin complex with manifestations of the antiphospholipid syndrome and with the presence of lupus anticoagulant. Arthritis Rheum. 43, 1982–1993.

Bajaj, S.P., Rapaport, S.I., Fierer, D.S., Herbst, K.D., Schwartz, D.B., 1983. A mechanism for the hypoprothrombinemia of the acquired hypoprothrombinemia-lupus anticoagulant syndrome. Blood. 61, 684–692.

Bajaj, S.P., Rapaport, S.I., Barclay, S., Herbst, K.D., 1985. Acquired hypoprothrombinemia due to non-neutralizing antibodies to prothrombin: mechanism and management. Blood. 65, 1538–1543.

Ballard, J.L., Weaver, F.A., Singla, N.K., Chapman, W.C., Alexander, W.A., 2010. Safety and immunogenicity observations pooled from eight clinical trials of recombinant human thrombin. J. Am. Coll. Surg. 210, 199–204.

Barillari, G., Pasca, S., 2013. pdFVIII/VWF may be an alternative treatment for old medical patient with acquired haemophilia A and systemic vascular disease? Transfus. Apher. Sci. 48, 59–62.

Barthels, M., Heimburger, N., 1985. Acquired thrombin inhibitor in a patient with liver cirrhosis. Haemostasis. 15, 395–401.

Baudo, F., De Cataldo, F., 2003. Acquired factor VIII inhibitors in pregnancy: data from the Italian Haemophilia Register relevant to clinical practice. BJOG. 110, 311–314.

Baudo, F., Collins, P., Huth-Kuhne, A., Levesque, H., Marco, P., Nemes, L., et al., 2012. Management of bleeding in acquired hemophilia A: results from the European Acquired Haemophilia (EACH2) Registry. Blood. 120, 39–46.

Bayer, W.L., Curiel, D., Szeto, I.L., Lewis, J.H., 1969. Acquired factor X deficiency in a Negro boy. Pediatrics. 44, 1007–1009.

Bern, M.M., Sahud, M., Zhukov, O., Qu, K., Mitchell Jr., W., 2005. Treatment of factor XI inhibitor using recombinant activated factor VIIa. Haemophilia. 11, 20–25.

Berruyer, M., Amiral, J., Ffrench, P., Belleville, J., Bastien, O., Clerc, J., et al., 1993. Immunization by bovine thrombin used with fibrin glue during cardiovascular operations. Development of thrombin and factor V inhibitors. J. Thorac. Cardiovasc. Surg. 105, 892–897.

Bertolaccini, M.L., Atsumi, T., Khamashta, M.A., Amengual, O., Hughes, G.R., 1998. Autoantibodies to human prothrombin and clinical manifestations in 207 patients with systemic lupus erythematosus. J. Rheumatol. 25, 1104–1108.

Bertolaccini, M.L., Mepani, K., Sanna, G., Hughes, G.R., Khamashta, M.A., 2007. Factor XII autoantibodies as a novel marker for thrombosis and adverse obstetric history in patients with systemic lupus erythematosus. Ann. Rheum. Dis. 66, 533–536.

Bettoni, G., Palla, R., Valsecchi, C., Consonni, D., Lotta, L.A., Trisolini, S.M., et al., 2012. ADAMTS-13 activity and autoantibodies classes and subclasses as prognostic predictors in acquired thrombotic thrombocytopenic purpura. J. Thromb. Haemost. 10, 1556–1565.

Billon, S., Le Niger, C., Escoffre-Barbe, M., Vicariot, M., Abgrall, J.F., 2001. The use of recombinant factor VIIa (NovoSeven) in a patient with a factor XI deficiency and a circulating anticoagulant. Blood Coagul. Fibrinolysis. 12, 551–553.

Bortoli, R., Monticielo, O.A., Chakr, R.M., Palominos, P.E., Rohsig, L.M., Kohem, C.L., et al., 2009. Acquired factor XI inhibitor in systemic lupus erythematosus—case report and literature review. Semin. Arthritis. Rheum. 39, 61–65.

Bossi, P., Cabane, J., Ninet, J., Dhote, R., Hanslik, T., Chosidow, O., et al., 1998. Acquired hemophilia due to factor VIII inhibitors in 34 patients. Am. J. Med. 105, 400–408.

Brodeur, G.M., O'Neill, P.J., Williams, J.A., 1980. Acquired inhibitors of coagulation in nonhemophiliac children. J. Pediatr. 96, 439–441.

Brunod, M., Chatot-Henry, C., Mehdaoui, H., Richer, C., Fonteau, C., 1998. Acquired anti-factor VII (proconvertin) inhibitor: hemorrhage and thrombosis. Thromb. Haemost. 79, 1065–1066.

Campbell, E., Sanal, S., Mattson, J., Walker, L., Estry, S., Mueller, L., et al., 1980. Factor VII inhibitor. Am. J. Med. 68, 962–964.

Campos-De-Magalhaes, M., Eduardo Brandao-Mello, C., Lucia Elias Pires, M., Cecilia Da Fonseca Salgado, M., Barcelo De Brito, S., Jose De Almeida, A., 2011. Factor VIII and IX deficiencies related to acquired inhibitors in a patient with chronic hepatitis C virus infection receiving treatment with pegylated interferon plus ribavirin. Hematology. 16, 80–85.

Carmassi, F., Giannarelli, C., De Giorgi, A., De Negri, F., 2007. Combined factor VIII and IX inhibitors in a non-haemophilic patient: successful treatment with immunosuppressive drugs. Haemophilia. 13, 106–107.

Castro, O., Farber, L.R., Clyne, L.P., 1972. Circulating anticoagulants against factors IX and XI in systemic lupus erythematosus. Ann. Intern. Med. 77, 543–548.

Cataland, S.R., Jin, M., Ferketich, A.K., Kennedy, M.S., Kraut, E.H., George, J.N., et al., 2007. An evaluation of cyclosporin and corticosteroids individually as adjuncts to plasma exchange in the treatment of thrombotic thrombocytopenic purpura. Br. J. Haematol. 136, 146–149.

Cataland, S.R., Yang, S.B., Witkoff, L., Kraut, E.H., Lin, S., George, J.N., Wu, H.M., 2009. Demographic and ADAMTS13 biomarker data as predictors of early recurrences of idiopathic thrombotic thrombocytopenic purpura. Eur. J. Haematol. 83, 559–564.

Chalkiadakis, G., Kyriakou, D., Oekonomaki, E., Tsiaoussis, J., Alexandrakis, M., Vasilakis, S., et al., 1999. Acquired inhibitors to the coagulation factor XII associated with liver disease. Am. J. Gastroenterol. 94, 2551–2553.

Chouhan, V.D., De La Cadena, R.A., Nagaswami, C., Weisel, J.W., Kajani, M., Rao, A.K., 1997. Simultaneous occurrence of human

antibodies directed against fibrinogen, thrombin, and factor V following exposure to bovine thrombin: effects on blood coagulation, protein C activation and platelet function. Thromb. Haemost. 77, 343–349.

Cohen, I., Amir, J., Ben-Shaul, Y., Pick, A., De Vries, A., 1970. Plasma cell myeloma associated with an unusual myeloma protein causing impairment of fibrin aggregation and platelet function in a patient with multiple malignancy. Am. J. Med. 48, 766–776.

Coleman, M., Vigliano, E.M., Weksler, M.E., Nachman, R.L., 1972. Inhibition of fibrin monomer polymerization by lambda myeloma globulins. Blood. 39, 210–223.

Collins, P., Macartney, N., Davies, R., Lees, S., Giddings, J., Majer, R., 2004. A population based, unselected, consecutive cohort of patients with acquired haemophilia A. Br. J. Haematol. 124, 86–90.

Collins, P., Budde, U., Rand, J.H., Federici, A.B., Kessler, C.M., 2008. Epidemiology and general guidelines of the management of acquired haemophilia and von Willebrand syndrome. Haemophilia. 14 (Suppl. 3), 49–55.

Collins, P., Baudo, F., Knoebl, P., Levesque, H., Nemes, L., Pellegrini, F., et al., 2012. Immunosuppression for acquired hemophilia A: results from the European Acquired Haemophilia Registry (EACH2). Blood. 120, 47–55.

Collins, P.W., Hirsch, S., Baglin, T.P., Dolan, G., Hanley, J., Makris, M., et al., 2007. Acquired hemophilia A in the United Kingdom: a 2-year national surveillance study by the United Kingdom Haemophilia Centre Doctors' Organisation. Blood. 109, 1870–1877.

Colwell, N.S., Tollefsen, D.M., Blinder, M.A., 1997. Identification of a monoclonal thrombin inhibitor associated with multiple myeloma and a severe bleeding disorder. Br. J. Haematol. 97, 219–226.

Coppo, P., Wolf, M., Veyradier, A., Bussel, A., Malot, S., Millot, G.A., et al., 2006. Prognostic value of inhibitory anti-ADAMTS13 antibodies in adult-acquired thrombotic thrombocytopenic purpura. Br. J. Haematol. 132, 66–74.

Coppo, P., Busson, M., Veyradier, A., Wynckel, A., Poullin, P., Azoulay, E., et al., 2010. HLA-DRB1*11: a strong risk factor for acquired severe ADAMTS13 deficiency-related idiopathic thrombotic thrombocytopenic purpura in Caucasians. J. Thromb. Haemost. 8, 856–859.

Currie, M.S., Stein, A.M., Rustagi, P.K., Behrens, A.N., Logue, G.L., 1984. Transient acquired factor X deficiency associated with pneumonia. N.Y. State. J. Med. 84, 572–573.

Daly, H.M., Carson, P.J., Smith, J.K., 1991. Intracerebral haemorrhage due to acquired factor XIII inhibitor—successful response to factor XIII concentrate. Blood Coagul. Fibrinolysis. 2, 507–514.

Davidson, S.J., Burman, J.F., Nicholson, A.G., Jones, D.W., Dusmet, M.E., 2005. Factor XII auto-antibodies present in a patient with a B-cell lymphoma. Blood Coagul. Fibrinolysis. 16, 365–367.

De La Cadena, R.A., Baglia, F.A., Johnson, C.A., Wenk, R.E., Amernick, R., Walsh, P.N., et al., 1988. Naturally occurring human antibodies against two distinct functional domains in the heavy chain of FXI/FXIa. Blood. 72, 1748–1754.

De Raucourt, E., Dumont, M.D., Tourani, J.M., Hubsch, J.P., Riquet, M., Fischer, A.M., 1994. Acquired factor VII deficiency associated with pleural liposarcoma. Blood Coagul. Fibrinolysis. 5, 833–836.

De Raucourt, E., Barbier, C., Sinda, P., Dib, M., Peltier, J.Y., Ternisien, C., 2003. High-dose intravenous immunoglobulin treatment in two patients with acquired factor V inhibitors. Am. J. Hematol. 74, 187–190.

Delgado, J., Jimenez-Yuste, V., Hernandez-Navarro, F., Villar, A., 2003. Acquired haemophilia: review and meta-analysis focused on therapy and prognostic factors. Br. J. Haematol. 121, 21–35.

Delmer, A., Horellou, M.H., Andreu, G., Lecompte, T., Rossi, F., Kazatchkine, M.D., et al., 1989. Life-threatening intracranial bleeding associated with the presence of an antifactor VII autoantibody. Blood. 74, 229–232.

Dong, J.F., Moake, J.L., Nolasco, L., Bernardo, A., Arceneaux, W., Shrimpton, C.N., et al., 2002. ADAMTS-13 rapidly cleaves newly secreted ultralarge von Willebrand factor multimers on the endothelial surface under flowing conditions. Blood. 100, 4033–4039.

D'Uva, M., Strina, I., Mollo, A., Ranieri, A., De Placido, G., Di Micco, P., 2005. Acquired factor XII deficiency in a woman with recurrent pregnancy loss: working on a differential diagnosis in a single case. J. Transl. Med. 3, 43.

Edgin, R.A., Metz, E.N., Fromkes, J.J., Beman, F.M., 1980. Acquired factor X deficiency with associated defects in platelet aggregation. A response to corticosteroid therapy. Am. J. Med. 69, 137–139.

Erez, O., Romero, R., Vaisbuch, E., Mazaki-Tovi, S., Kusanovic, J.P., Chaiworapongsa, T., et al., 2009. Maternal anti-protein Z antibodies in pregnancies complicated by pre-eclampsia, SGA and fetal death. J. Matern. Fetal. Neonatal. Med. 22, 662–671.

Fastenau, D.R., Mcintyre, J.A., 2000. Immunochemical analysis of polyspecific antibodies in patients exposed to bovine fibrin sealant. Ann. Thorac. Surg. 69, 1867–1872.

Favaloro, E.J., Posen, J., Ramakrishna, R., Soltani, S., McRae, S., Just, S., et al., 2004. Factor V inhibitors: rare or not so uncommon? A multilaboratory investigation. Blood Coagul. Fibrinolysis. 15, 637–647.

Federici, A.B., Rand, J.H., Bucciarelli, P., Budde, U., Van Genderen, P.J., Mohri, H., et al., 2000. Acquired von Willebrand syndrome: data from an international registry. Thromb. Haemost. 84, 345–349.

Ferrari, S., Scheiflinger, F., Rieger, M., Mudde, G., Wolf, M., Coppo, P., et al., 2007. Prognostic value of anti-ADAMTS 13 antibody features (Ig isotype, titer, and inhibitory effect) in a cohort of 35 adult French patients undergoing a first episode of thrombotic microangiopathy with undetectable ADAMTS 13 activity. Blood. 109, 2815–2822.

Ferrari, S., Mudde, G.C., Rieger, M., Veyradier, A., Kremer Hovinga, J.A., Scheiflinger, F., 2009. IgG subclass distribution of anti-ADAMTS13 antibodies in patients with acquired thrombotic thrombocytopenic purpura. J. Thromb. Haemost. 7, 1703–1710.

Field, S.L., Chesterman, C.N., Dai, Y.P., Hogg, P.J., 2001. Lupus antibody bivalency is required to enhance prothrombin binding to phospholipid. J. Immunol. 166, 6118–6125.

Flaherty, M.J., Henderson, R., Wener, M.H., 1989. Iatrogenic immunization with bovine thrombin: a mechanism for prolonged thrombin times after surgery. Ann. Intern. Med. 111, 631–634.

Foley, S.R., Webert, K., Arnold, D.M., Rock, G.A., Clark, W.F., Barth, D., et al., 2009. A Canadian phase II study evaluating the efficacy of rituximab in the management of patients with relapsed/refractory thrombotic thrombocytopenic purpura. Kidney Int. Suppl. 112, S55–S58.

Forastiero, R.R., Martinuzzo, M.E., Lu, L., Broze, G.J., 2003. Autoimmune antiphospholipid antibodies impair the inhibition of activated factor X by protein Z/protein Z-dependent protease inhibitor. J. Thromb. Haemost. 1, 1764–1770.

Franchini, M., Lippi, G., 2011. Acquired factor V inhibitors: a systematic review. J. Thromb. Thrombolysis. 31, 449–457.

Franchini, M., Lippi, G., Favaloro, E.J., 2012. Acquired inhibitors of coagulation factors: Part II. Semin. Thromb. Hemost. 38, 447–453.

Freedman, J., Rand, M.L., Russell, O., Davis, C., Cheatley, P.L., Blanchette, V., et al., 2003. Immunoadsorption may provide a cost-effective approach to management of patients with inhibitors to FVIII. Transfusion. 43, 1508–1513.

Fujikawa, K., Suzuki, H., McMullen, B., Chung, D., 2001. Purification of human von Willebrand factor-cleaving protease and its identification as a new member of the metalloproteinase family. Blood. 98, 1662–1666.

Fukue, H., Anderson, K., McPhedran, P., Clyne, L., McDonagh, J., 1992. A unique factor XIII inhibitor to a fibrin-binding site on factor XIIIA. Blood. 79, 65–74.

Fukushima, T., Mikane, T., Ono, D., Oku, S., Kobayashi, H., Watanabe, Y., et al., 2012. A case of acquired hemophilia A with massive hemothorax. J. Anesth. 26, 262–264.

Furlan, M., Robles, R., Solenthaler, M., Wassmer, M., Sandoz, P., Lammle, B., 1997. Deficient activity of von Willebrand factor-cleaving protease in chronic relapsing thrombotic thrombocytopenic purpura. Blood. 89, 3097–3103.

Gabriel, D.A., Carr, M.E., Cook, L., Roberts, H.R., 1987. Spontaneous antithrombin in a patient with benign paraprotein. Am. J. Hematol. 25, 85–93.

Gailani, D., Smith, S.B., 2009. Structural and functional features of factor XI. J. Thromb. Haemost. 7 (Suppl. 1), 75–78.

Galanakis, D.K., Ginzler, E.M., Fikrig, S.M., 1978. Monoclonal IgG anticoagulants delaying fibrin aggregation in two patients with systemic lupus erythematosus (SLE). Blood. 52, 1037–1046.

Ghosh, S., McEvoy, P., McVerry, B.A., 1983. Idiopathic autoantibody that inhibits fibrin monomer polymerization. Br. J. Haematol. 53, 65–72.

Giovannini, L., Appert, A., Monpoux, F., Fischer, F., Boutte, P., Sirvent, N., 2004. Successful use of recombinant factor VIIa for management of severe menorrhagia in an adolescent with an acquired inhibitor of human thrombin. Acta. Paediatr. 93, 841–843.

Goodrick, M.J., Prentice, A.G., Copplestone, J.A., Pamphilon, D.H., Boon, R.J., 1992. Acquired factor XI inhibitor in chronic lymphocytic leukaemia. J. Clin. Pathol. 45, 352–353.

Green, D., Lechner, K., 1981. A survey of 215 non-hemophilic patients with inhibitors to Factor VIII. Thromb. Haemost. 45, 200–203.

Gregory, T.F., Cooper, B., 2006. Case report of an acquired factor XIII inhibitor: diagnosis and management. Proc. (Bayl. Univ. Med. Cent.). 19, 221–223.

Gris, J.C., Schved, J.F., Branger, B., Aguilar-Martinez, P., Vecina, F., Oules, R., et al., 1992. Autoantibody to plasma fibrinopeptide A in a patient with a severe acquired haemorrhagic syndrome. Blood Coagul. Fibrinolysis. 3, 519–529.

Gris, J.C., Amadio, C., Mercier, E., Lavigne-Lissalde, G., Dechaud, H., Hoffet, M., et al., 2003. Anti-protein Z antibodies in women with pathologic pregnancies. Blood. 101, 4850–4852.

Guermazi, S., Hamza, M., Dellagi, K., 1997. Protein S deficiency and antibodies to protein S in patients with Behcet's disease. Thromb. Res. 86, 197–204.

Harris, S.L., Jones, D.W., Gallimore, M.J., Nicholls, P.J., Winter, M., 2005. The antigenic binding site(s) of antibodies to factor XII associated with the antiphospholipid syndrome. J. Thromb. Haemost. 3, 969–975.

Hay, C.R., Negrier, C., Ludlam, C.A., 1997. The treatment of bleeding in acquired haemophilia with recombinant factor VIIa: a multicentre study. Thromb. Haemost. 78, 1463–1467.

Hayashi, T., Kadohira, Y., Morishita, E., Asakura, H., Souri, M., Ichinose, A., 2012. A case of acquired FXIII deficiency with severe bleeding symptoms. Haemophilia 18, 618–620.

Henson, K., Files, J.C., Morrison, F.S., 1989. Transient acquired factor X deficiency: report of the use of activated clotting concentrate to control a life-threatening hemorrhage. Am. J. Med. 87, 583–585.

Hosker, J.P., Jewell, D.P., 1983. Transient, selective factor X deficiency and acute liver failure following chest infection treated with erythromycin BP. Postgrad. Med. J. 59, 514–515.

Huth-Kuhne, A., Baudo, F., Collins, P., Ingerslev, J., Kessler, C.M., Levesque, H., et al., 2009. International recommendations on the diagnosis and treatment of patients with acquired hemophilia A. Haematologica. 94, 566–575.

Inomo, A., Sugi, T., Fujita, Y., Matsubayashi, H., Izumi, S., Mikami, M., 2008. The antigenic binding sites of autoantibodies to factor XII in patients with recurrent pregnancy losses. Thromb. Haemost. 99, 316–323.

Ishida, F., Okubo, K., Ito, T., Okumura, N., Souri, M., Ichinose, A., 2010. Spontaneous regression of the inhibitor against the coagulation factor XIII A subunit in acquired factor XIII deficiency. Thromb. Haemost. 104, 1284–1285.

Izumi, T., Kim, S.W., Greist, A., Macedo-Ribeiro, S., Fuentes-Prior, P., Bode, W., et al., 2001. Fine mapping of inhibitory anti-factor V antibodies using factor V C2 domain mutants. Identification of two antigenic epitopes involved in phospholipid binding. Thromb. Haemost. 85, 1048–1054.

Jansen, M., Schmaldienst, S., Banyai, S., Quehenberger, P., Pabinger, I., Derfler, K., et al., 2001. Treatment of coagulation inhibitors with extracorporeal immunoadsorption (Ig-Therasorb). Br. J. Haematol. 112, 91–97.

Jedidi, I., Hdiji, S., Ajmi, N., Makni, F., Masmoudi, S., Elloumi, M., et al., 2011. [Acquired haemophilia B: a case report and literature review]. Ann. Biol. Clin. (Paris). 69, 685–688.

Jian, C., Xiao, J., Gong, L., Skipwith, C.G., Jin, S.Y., Kwaan, H.C., et al., 2012. Gain-of-function ADAMTS13 variants that are resistant to autoantibodies against ADAMTS13 in patients with acquired thrombotic thrombocytopenic purpura. Blood. 119, 3836–3843.

John, M.L., Hitzler, W., Scharrer, I., 2012. The role of human leukocyte antigens as predisposing and/or protective factors in patients with idiopathic thrombotic thrombocytopenic purpura. Ann. Hematol. 91, 507–510.

Jones, D.W., Gallimore, M.J., Mackie, I.J., Harris, S.L., Winter, M., 2000. Reduced factor XII levels in patients with the antiphospholipid syndrome are associated with antibodies to factor XII. Br. J. Haematol. 110, 721–726.

Jones, D.W., Mackie, I.J., Gallimore, M.J., Winter, M., 2001. Antibodies to factor XII and recurrent fetal loss in patients with the antiphospholipid syndrome. Br. J. Haematol. 113, 550–552.

Kalafatis, M., Simioni, P., Tormene, D., Beck, D.O., Luni, S., Girolami, A., 2002. Isolation and characterization of an antifactor V antibody causing activated protein C resistance from a patient with severe thrombotic manifestations. Blood. 99, 3985–3992.

Kamikubo, Y., Miyamoto, S., Iwasa, A., Ishii, M., Okajima, K., 2000. Purification and characterization of factor VII inhibitor found in a patient with life threatening bleeding. Thromb. Haemost. 83, 60–64.

Kawasaki, Y., Toyoda, H., Otsuki, S., Iwasa, T., Iwamoto, S., Azuma, E., et al., 2013. A novel Wiskott-Aldrich syndrome protein mutation in an infant with thrombotic thrombocytopenic purpura. Eur. J. Haematol. 90, 164–168.

Kempton, C.L., Abshire, T.C., Deveras, R.A., Hoots, W.K., Gill, J.C., Kessler, C.M., et al., 2012. Pharmacokinetics and safety of OBI-1, a recombinant B domain-deleted porcine factor VIII, in subjects with haemophilia A. Haemophilia. 18, 798–804.

Kessler, C.M., Ludlam, C.A., 1993. The treatment of acquired factor VIII inhibitors: worldwide experience with porcine factor VIII concentrate. International Acquired Hemophilia Study Group. Semin. Hematol. 30, 22–27.

Kim, M.S., Kilgore, P.E., Kang, J.S., Kim, S.Y., Lee, D.Y., Kim, J.S., et al., 2008. Transient acquired hemophilia associated with Mycoplasma pneumoniae pneumonia. J. Korean. Med. Sci. 23, 138–141.

Kitazawa, T., Igawa, T., Sampei, Z., Muto, A., Kojima, T., Soeda, T., et al., 2012. A bispecific antibody to factors IXa and X restores factor VIII hemostatic activity in a hemophilia A model. Nat. Med. 18, 1570–1574.

Klaus, C., Plaimauer, B., Studt, J.D., Dorner, F., Lammle, B., Mannucci, P.M., et al., 2004. Epitope mapping of ADAMTS13 autoantibodies in acquired thrombotic thrombocytopenic purpura. Blood. 103, 4514–4519.

Knobe, K., Tedgard, U., Ek, T., Sandstrom, P.E., Hillarp, A., 2012. Lupus anticoagulants in two children—bleeding due to nonphospholipid-dependent antiprothrombin antibodies. Eur. J. Pediatr. 171, 1383–1387.

Knobl, P., Lechner, K., 1998. Acquired factor V inhibitors. Baillieres Clin. Haematol. 11, 305–318.

Knoebl, P., Marco, P., Baudo, F., Collins, P., Huth-Kuhne, A., Nemes, L., et al., 2012. Demographic and clinical data in acquired hemophilia A: results from the European Acquired Haemophilia Registry (EACH2). J. Thromb. Haemost. 10, 622–631.

Kondera-Anasz, Z., 1998. Antibodies against fibrinogen in pregnant women, in post delivery women and in the newborns. Thromb. Haemost. 79, 963–968.

Kremer Hovinga, J.A., Studt, J.D., Demarmels Biasiutti, F., Solenthaler, M., Alberio, L., Zwicky, C., et al., 2004. Splenectomy in relapsing and plasma-refractory acquired thrombotic thrombocytopenic purpura. Haematologica. 89, 320–324.

Kremer Hovinga, J.A., Vesely, S.K., Terrell, D.R., Lammle, B., George, J.N., 2010. Survival and relapse in patients with thrombotic thrombocytopenic purpura. Blood. 115, 1500–1511, quiz 1662.

Krieger, H., Leddy, J.P., Breckenridge, R.T., 1975. Studies on a circulating anticoagulant in systemic lupus erythematosus: evidence for inhibition of the function of activated plasma thromboplastin antecedent (factor XIa). Blood. 46, 189–197.

Krishnamurthy, P., Hawche, C., Evans, G., Winter, M., 2011. A rare case of an acquired inhibitor to factor IX. Haemophilia. 17, 712–713.

Krumdieck, R., Shaw, D.R., Huang, S.T., Poon, M.C., Rustagi, P.K., 1991. Hemorrhagic disorder due to an isoniazid-associated acquired factor XIII inhibitor in a patient with Waldenstrom's macroglobulinemia. Am. J. Med. 90, 639–645.

Kumar, S., Pruthi, R.K., Nichols, W.L., 2003. Acquired von Willebrand's syndrome: a single institution experience. Am. J. Hematol. 72, 243–247.

Kyriakou, D.S., Alexandrakis, M.G., Passam, F.H., Foundouli, K., Matalliotakis, E., Koutroubakis, I.E., et al., 2002. Acquired inhibitors to coagulation factors in patients with gastrointestinal diseases. Eur. J. Gastroenterol. Hepatol. 14, 1383–1387.

La Spada, A.R., Skalhegg, B.S., Henderson, R., Schmer, G., Pierce, R., Chandler, W., 1995. Brief report: fatal hemorrhage in a patient with an acquired inhibitor of human thrombin. N. Engl. J. Med. 333, 494–497.

Lane, T.A., Shapiro, S.S., Burka, E.R., 1978. Factor V antibody and disseminated intravascular coagulation. Ann. Intern. Med. 89, 182–185.

Lankiewicz, M.W., Bell, W.R., 1992. A unique circulating inhibitor with specificity for coagulation factor X. Am. J. Med. 93, 343–346.

Lapalud, P.E.A., 2012. The IgG autoimmune response in postpartum acquired hemophilia A targets mainly the A1a1 domain of FVIII. JTH. submitted.

Larakeb, A.S., Evrard, S., Louillet, F., Kwon, T., Djaffar, H., Llanas, B., et al., 2009. Acute renal cortical necrosis due to acquired antiprotein S antibodies. Pediatr. Nephrol. 24, 207–209.

Largo, R., Sigg, P., Von Felten, A., Straub, P.W., 1974. Acquired factor-IX inhibitor in a nonhaemophilic patient with autoimmune disease. Br. J. Haematol. 26, 129–140.

Lawson, J.H., Pennell, B.J., Olson, J.D., Mann, K.G., 1990. Isolation and characterization of an acquired antithrombin antibody. Blood. 76, 2249–2257.

Lechner, K., Simonitsch, I., Haselbock, J., Jager, U., Pabinger, I., 2011. Acquired immune-mediated thrombophilia in lymphoproliferative disorders. Leuk. Lymphoma. 52, 1836–1843.

Lenting, P.J., Van Mourik, J.A., Mertens, K., 1998. The life cycle of coagulation factor VIII in view of its structure and function. Blood. 92, 3983–3996.

Levin, M., Eley, B.S., Louis, J., Cohen, H., Young, L., Heyderman, R.S., 1995. Postinfectious purpura fulminans caused by an autoantibody directed against protein S. J. Pediatr. 127, 355–363.

Lindgren, A., Wadenvik, H., Tengborn, L., 2002. Characterization of inhibitors to FVIII with an ELISA in congenital and acquired haemophilia A. Haemophilia. 8, 644–648.

Ling, H.T., Field, J.J., Blinder, M.A., 2009. Sustained response with rituximab in patients with thrombotic thrombocytopenic purpura: a report of 13 cases and review of the literature. Am. J. Hematol. 84, 418–421.

Llobet, D., Borrell, M., Vila, L., Vallve, C., Felices, R., Fontcuberta, J., 2007. An acquired inhibitor that produced a delay of fibrinopeptide B release in an asymptomatic patient. Haematologica. 92, e17–e19.

Lollar, P., 2005. Pathogenic antibodies to coagulation factors. Part II. Fibrinogen, prothrombin, thrombin, factor V, factor XI, factor XII, factor XIII, the protein C system and von Willebrand factor. J. Thromb. Haemost. 3, 1385–1391.

Lorand, L., Velasco, P.T., Hill, J.M., Hoffmeister, K.J., Kaye, F.J., 2002. Intracranial hemorrhage in systemic lupus erythematosus associated with an autoantibody against actor XIII. Thromb. Haemost. 88, 919–923.

Lotta, L.A., Lombardi, R., Mariani, M., Lancellotti, S., De Cristofaro, R., Hollestelle, M.J., et al., 2011. Platelet reactive conformation and multimeric pattern of von Willebrand factor in acquired thrombotic thrombocytopenic purpura during acute disease and remission. J. Thromb. Haemost. 9, 1744–1751.

Lottenberg, R., Kentro, T.B., Kitchens, C.S., 1987. Acquired hemophilia. A natural history study of 16 patients with factor VIII inhibitors receiving little or no therapy. Arch. Intern. Med. 147, 1077–1081.

Luboshitz, J., Lubetsky, A., Schliamser, L., Kotler, A., Tamarin, I., Inbal, A., 2001. Pharmacokinetic studies with FVIII/von Willebrand factor concentrate can be a diagnostic tool to distinguish between subgroups of patients with acquired von Willebrand syndrome. Thromb. Haemost. 85, 806–809.

Luken, B.M., Turenhout, E.A., Hulstein, J.J., Van Mourik, J.A., Fijnheer, R., Voorberg, J., 2005. The spacer domain of ADAMTS13 contains a major binding site for antibodies in patients with thrombotic thrombocytopenic purpura. Thromb. Haemost. 93, 267–274.

Luo, Y., Zhang, G., Zuo, W., Zheng, W., Dai, C., 2010. Acquired factor XIII inhibitor in monoclonal gammopathy of undetermined significance: characterization and cross-linked fibrin ultrastructure. Ann. Hematol. 89, 833–834.

Luo, Y.Y., Zhang, G.S., 2011. Acquired factor XIII inhibitor: clinical features, treatment, fibrin structure and epitope determination. Haemophilia. 17, 393–398.

Madoiwa, S., Nakamura, Y., Mimuro, J., Furusawa, S., Koyama, T., Sugo, T., et al., 2001. Autoantibody against prothrombin aberrantly alters the proenzyme to facilitate formation of a complex with its physiological inhibitor antithrombin III without thrombin conversion. Blood. 97, 3783–3789.

Mahendra, A., Padiolleau-Lefevre, S., Kaveri, S.V., Lacroix-Desmazes, S., 2012. Do proteolytic antibodies complete the panoply of the autoimmune response in acquired haemophilia A? Br. J. Haematol. 156, 3–12.

Marciniak, E., Greenwood, M.F., 1979. Acquired coagulation inhibitor delaying fibrinopeptide release. Blood. 53, 81–92.

Matsumoto, T., Shima, M., Fukuda, K., Nogami, K., Giddings, J.C., Murakami, T., et al., 2001. Immunological characterization of factor VIII autoantibodies in patients with acquired hemophilia A in the presence or absence of underlying disease. Thromb. Res. 104, 381–388.

Matsumoto, T., Nogami, K., Ogiwara, K., Shima, M., 2012. A putative inhibitory mechanism in the tenase complex responsible for loss of coagulation function in acquired haemophilia A patients with anti-C2 autoantibodies. Thromb. Haemost. 107, 288–301.

Matsunaga, A.T., Shafer, F.E., 1996. An acquired inhibitor to factor X in a pediatric patient with extensive burns. J. Pediatr. Hematol. Oncol. 18, 223–226.

Mazzucconi, M.G., Peraino, M., Bizzoni, L., Bernasconi, S., Luciani, M., Rossi, G.D., 1999. Acquired inhibitor against factor IX in a child: successful treatment with high-dose immunoglobulin and dexamethasone. Haemophilia. 5, 132–134.

Mcdonald, V., Liesner, R., Grainger, J., Gattens, M., Machin, S.J., Scully, M., 2010. Acquired, noncongenital thrombotic thrombocytopenic purpura in children and adolescents: clinical management and the use of ADAMTS 13 assays. Blood Coagul. Fibrinolysis. 21, 245–250.

Mcmanus, M.P., Frantz, C., Gailani, D., 2012. Acquired factor XI deficiency in a child with membranoproliferative glomerulonephritis. Pediatr. Blood Cancer. 59, 173–175.

Mehta, J., Singhal, S., Mehta, B.C., 1992. Factor VII inhibitor. J. Assoc. Physicians India. 40, 44.

Michiels, J.J., Budde, U., Van Der Planken, M., Van Vliet, H.H., Schroyens, W., Berneman, Z., 2001. Acquired von Willebrand syndromes: clinical features, aetiology, pathophysiology, classification and management. Best Pract. Res. Clin. Haematol. 14, 401–436.

Micic, D., Williams, E.C., Medow, J.E., 2011. Cerebellar hemorrhage as a first presentation of acquired Hemophilia A. Neurocrit. Care. 15, 170–174.

Milanov, P., Ivanciu, L., Abriss, D., Quade-Lyssy, P., Miesbach, W., Alesci, S., et al., 2012. Engineered factor IX variants bypass FVIII and correct hemophilia A phenotype in mice. Blood. 119, 602–611.

Miller, D.P., Kaye, J.A., Shea, K., Ziyadeh, N., Cali, C., Black, C., et al., 2004. Incidence of thrombotic thrombocytopenic purpura/hemolytic uremic syndrome. Epidemiology. 15, 208–215.

Miller, K., Neely, J.E., Krivit, W., Edson, J.R., 1978. Spontaneously acquired factor IX inhibitor in a nonhemophiliac child. J. Pediatr. 93, 232–234.

Moake, J.L., Rudy, C.K., Troll, J.H., Weinstein, M.J., Colannino, N.M., Azocar, J., et al., 1982. Unusually large plasma factor VIII:von Willebrand factor multimers in chronic relapsing thrombotic thrombocytopenic purpura. N. Engl. J. Med. 307, 1432–1435.

Mohri, H., Motomura, S., Kanamori, H., Matsuzaki, M., Watanabe, S., Maruta, A., et al., 1998. Clinical significance of inhibitors in acquired von Willebrand syndrome. Blood. 91, 3623–3629.

Mollica, L., Preston, R.J., Chion, A.C., Lees, S.J., Collins, P., Lewis, S., et al., 2006. Autoantibodies to thrombin directed against both of its cryptic exosites. Br. J. Haematol. 132, 487–493.

Moraca, R.J., Ragni, M.V., 2002. Acquired anti-FVIII inhibitors in children. Haemophilia. 8, 28–32.

Morrison, A.E., Ludlam, C.A., Kessler, C., 1993. Use of porcine factor VIII in the treatment of patients with acquired hemophilia. Blood. 81, 1513–1520.

Mulhare, P.E., Tracy, P.B., Golden, E.A., Branda, R.F., Bovill, E.G., 1991. A case of acquired factor X deficiency with in vivo and in vitro evidence of inhibitor activity directed against factor X. Am. J. Clin. Pathol. 96, 196–200.

Mullighan, C.G., Rischbieth, A., Duncan, E.M., Lloyd, J.V., 2004. Acquired isolated factor VII deficiency associated with severe bleeding and successful treatment with recombinant FVIIa (NovoSeven). Blood Coagul. Fibrinolysis. 15, 347–351.

Mumford, A.D., O'Donnell, J., Gillmore, J.D., Manning, R.A., Hawkins, P.N., Laffan, M., 2000. Bleeding symptoms and coagulation abnormalities in 337 patients with AL-amyloidosis. Br. J. Haematol. 110, 454–460.

Muntean, W., Zenz, W., Finding, K., Zobel, G., Beitzke, A., 1994. Inhibitor to factor V after exposure to fibrin sealant during cardiac surgery in a two-year-old child. Acta Paediatr. 83, 84–87.

Murrin, R.J., Murray, J.A., 2006. Thrombotic thrombocytopenic purpura: aetiology, pathophysiology and treatment. Blood Rev. 20, 51–60.

Muzaffar, J., Katragadda, L., Haider, S., Javed, A., Anaissie, E., Usmani, S., 2012. Rituximab and intravenous immunoglobulin (IVIG) for the management of acquired factor VIII inhibitor in multiple myeloma: case report and review of literature. Int. J. Hematol. 95, 102–106.

Nakamura, S., Kato, A., Sakata, Y., Aoki, N., 1988. Bleeding tendency caused by IgG inhibitor to factor XIII, treated successfully by cyclophosphamide. Br. J. Haematol. 68, 313–319.

Nawarawong, W., Wyshock, E., Meloni, F.J., Weitz, J., Schmaier, A.H., 1991. The rate of fibrinopeptide B release modulates the rate of clot formation: a study with an acquired inhibitor to fibrinopeptide B release. Br. J. Haematol. 79, 296–301.

Ndimbie, O.K., Raman, B.K., Saeed, S.M., 1989. Lupus anticoagulant associated with specific inhibition of factor VII in a patient with AIDS. Am. J. Clin. Pathol. 91, 491–493.

Nemes, L., Pitlik, E., 2000. New protocol for immune tolerance induction in acquired hemophilia. Haematologica. 85, 64–68.

Nesheim, M.E., Nichols, W.L., Cole, T.L., Houston, J.G., Schenk, R.B., Mann, K.G., et al., 1986. Isolation and study of an acquired inhibitor of human coagulation factor V. J. Clin. Invest. 77, 405–415.

Nijenhuis, A.V., Van Bergeijk, L., Huijgens, P.C., Zweegman, S., 2004. Acquired factor XIII deficiency due to an inhibitor: a case report and review of the literature. Haematologica. 89, ECR14.

Nogami, K., Shima, M., Giddings, J.C., Hosokawa, K., Nagata, M., Kamisue, S., et al., 2001. Circulating factor VIII immune complexes in patients with type 2 acquired hemophilia A and protection from activated protein C-mediated proteolysis. Blood. 97, 669–677.

Nojima, J., Kuratsune, H., Suehisa, E., Kawasaki, T., Machii, T., Kitani, T., et al., 2002a. Acquired activated protein C resistance associated with anti-protein S antibody as a strong risk factor for DVT in non-SLE patients. Thromb. Haemost. 88, 716–722.

Nojima, J., Kuratsune, H., Suehisa, E., Kawasaki, T., Machii, T., Kitani, T., et al., 2002b. Acquired activated protein C resistance is associated with the co-existence of anti-prothrombin antibodies and lupus anticoagulant activity in patients with systemic lupus erythematosus. Br. J. Haematol. 118, 577–583.

Nojima, J., Iwatani, Y., Ichihara, K., Tsuneoka, H., Ishikawa, T., Yanagihara, M., et al., 2009. Acquired activated protein C resistance is associated with IgG antibodies to protein S in patients with systemic lupus erythematosus. Thromb. Res. 124, 127–131.

Ojeda-Uribe, M., Federici, L., Wolf, M., Coppo, P., Veyradier, A., 2010. Successful long-term rituximab maintenance for a relapsing patient with idiopathic thrombotic thrombocytopenic purpura. Transfusion. 50, 733–735.

Okajima, K., Ishii, M., 1999. Life-threatening bleeding in a case of autoantibody-induced factor VII deficiency. Int. J. Hematol. 69, 129–132.

Ortel, T.L., Quinn-Allen, M.A., Charles, L.A., Devore-Carter, D., Kane, W.H., 1992. Characterization of an acquired inhibitor to coagulation factor V. Antibody binding to the second C-type domain of factor V inhibits the binding of factor V to phosphatidylserine and neutralizes procoagulant activity. J. Clin. Invest. 90, 2340–2347.

Ortel, T.L., Moore, K.D., Quinn-Allen, M.A., Okamura, T., Sinclair, A.J., Lazarchick, J., et al., 1998. Inhibitory anti-factor V antibodies bind to the factor V C2 domain and are associated with hemorrhagic manifestations. Blood. 91, 4188–4196.

Ortel, T.L., Mercer, M.C., Thames, E.H., Moore, K.D., Lawson, J.H., 2001. Immunologic impact and clinical outcomes after surgical exposure to bovine thrombin. Ann. Surg. 233, 88–96.

Otis, P.T., Feinstein, D.I., Rapaport, S.I., Patch, M.J., 1974. An acquired inhibitor of fibrin stabilization associated with isoniazid therapy: clinical and biochemical observations. Blood. 44, 771–781.

Ozgur, T.T., Asal, G.T., Gurgey, A., Tezcan, I., Ersoy, F., Sanal, O., 2007. Acquired factor VIII deficiency associated with a novel primary immunodeficiency suggestive of autosomal recessive hyper IgE syndrome. J. Pediatr. Hematol. Oncol. 29, 327–329.

Ozsoylu, S., Ozer, F.L., 1973. Acquired factor IX deficiency. A report of two cases. Acta Haematol. 50, 305–314.

Page, J.D., Dela Cadena, R.A., Humphries, J.E., Colman, R.W., 1994. An autoantibody to human plasma prekallikrein blocks activation of the contact system. Br. J. Haematol. 87, 81–86.

Panzer, S., Thaler, E., 1993. An acquired cryoglobulinemia which inhibits fibrin polymerization in a patient with IgG kappa myeloma. Haemostasis. 23, 69–76.

Pardos-Gea, J., Ordi-Ros, J., Serrano, S., Balada, E., Nicolau, I., Vilardell, M., 2008. Protein Z levels and anti-protein Z antibodies in patients with arterial and venous thrombosis. Thromb. Res. 121, 727–734.

Pavlova, A., Diaz-Lacava, A., Zeitler, H., Satoguina, J., Niemann, B., Krause, M., et al., 2008. Increased frequency of the CTLA-4 49 A/G polymorphism in patients with acquired haemophilia A compared to healthy controls. Haemophilia. 14, 355–360.

Pavlova, A., Zeitler, H., Scharrer, I., Brackmann, H.H., Oldenburg, J., 2010. HLA genotype in patients with acquired haemophilia A. Haemophilia. 16, 107–112.

Pechik, I., Yakovlev, S., Mosesson, M.W., Gilliland, G.L., Medved, L., 2006. Structural basis for sequential cleavage of fibrinopeptides upon fibrin assembly. Biochemistry. 45, 3588–3597.

Peyvandi, F., Palla, R., Lotta, L.A., Mackie, I., Scully, M.A., Machin, S.J., 2010. ADAMTS-13 assays in thrombotic thrombocytopenic purpura. J. Thromb. Haemost. 8, 631–640.

Pogliani, E.M., Perseghin, P., Parma, M., Pioltelli, P., Corneo, G., 2000. Defibrotide in recurrent thrombotic thrombocytopenic purpura. Clin. Appl. Thromb. Hemost. 6, 69–70.

Poon, M.C., Saito, H., Koopman, W.J., 1984. A unique precipitating autoantibody against plasma thromboplastin antecedent associated with multiple apparent plasma clotting factor deficiencies in a patient with systemic lupus erythematosus. Blood. 63, 1309–1317.

Pos, W., Luken, B.M., Sorvillo, N., Kremer Hovinga, J.A., Voorberg, J., 2011. Humoral immune response to ADAMTS13 in acquired thrombotic thrombocytopenic purpura. J. Thromb. Haemost. 9, 1285–1291.

Prescott, R., Nakai, H., Saenko, E.L., Scharrer, I., Nilsson, I.M., Humphries, J.E., et al., 1997. The inhibitor antibody response is more complex in hemophilia A patients than in most nonhemophiliacs with factor VIII autoantibodies. Recombinate and Kogenate study groups. Blood. 89, 3663–3671.

Rao, L.V., Zivelin, A., Iturbe, I., Rapaport, S.I., 1994. Antibody-induced acute factor X deficiency: clinical manifestations and properties of the antibody. Thromb. Haemost. 72, 363–371.

Reding, M.T., Lei, S., Lei, H., Green, D., Gill, J., Conti-Fine, B.M., 2002. Distribution of Th1- and Th2-induced anti-factor VIII IgG subclasses in congenital and acquired hemophilia patients. Thromb. Haemost. 88, 568–575.

Reding, M.T., Okita, D.K., Diethelm-Okita, B.M., Anderson, T.A., Conti-Fine, B.M., 2003. Human CD4 + T-cell epitope repertoire on the C2 domain of coagulation factor VIII. J. Thromb. Haemost. 1, 1777–1784.

Reding, M.T., Okita, D.K., Diethelm-Okita, B.M., Anderson, T.A., Conti-Fine, B.M., 2004. Epitope repertoire of human CD4(+) T

cells on the A3 domain of coagulation factor VIII. J. Thromb. Haemost. 2, 1385–1394.

Reece, E.A., Clyne, L.P., Romero, R., Hobbins, J.C., 1984. Spontaneous factor XI inhibitors. Seven additional cases and a review of the literature. Arch. Intern. Med. 144, 525–529.

Reisner, H.M., Roberts, H.R., Krumholz, S., Yount, W.J., 1977. Immunochemical characterization of a polyclonal human antibody to factor IX. Blood. 50, 11–19.

Reitter, S., Knoebl, P., Pabinger, I., Lechner, K., 2011. Postoperative paraneoplastic factor VIII auto-antibodies in patients with solid tumours. Haemophilia. 17, e889–e894.

Rezaieyazdi, Z., Sharifi-Doloui, D., Hashemzadeh, K., Shirdel, A., Mansouritorghabeh, H., 2012. Acquired haemophilia A in a woman with autoimmune hepatitis and systemic lupus erythematosus; review of literature. Blood Coagul. Fibrinolysis. 23, 71–74.

Roberts, H.R., 1970. Acquired inhibitors to factor IX. N. Engl. J. Med. 283, 543–544.

Rochanda, L., Del Zoppo, G.J., Feinstein, D.I., Liebman, H.A., 2012. Approach to the treatment, characterization and diagnosis of an acquired auto-antibody directed against factors prothrombin, factor X and factor IX: a case report and review of the literature. Haemophilia. 18, 102–107.

Rock, G.A., Shumak, K.H., Buskard, N.A., Blanchette, V.S., Kelton, J.G., Nair, R.C., et al., 1991. Comparison of plasma exchange with plasma infusion in the treatment of thrombotic thrombocytopenic purpura. Canadian Apheresis Study Group. N. Engl. J. Med. 325, 393–397.

Rossetto, V., Spiezia, L., Franz, F., Salmaso, L., Pozza, L.V., Gavasso, S., et al., 2009. The role of antiphospholipid antibodies toward the protein C/protein S system in venous thromboembolic disease. Am. J. Hematol. 84, 594–596.

Roubey, R.A., 1998. Mechanisms of autoantibody-mediated thrombosis. Lupus. 7 (Suppl. 2), S114–S119.

Ruiz-Arguelles, A., 1988. Spontaneous reversal of acquired autoimmune dysfibrinogenemia probably due to an antiidiotypic antibody directed to an interspecies cross-reactive idiotype expressed on antifibrinogen antibodies. J. Clin. Invest. 82, 958–963.

Rustgi, R.N., Laduca, F.M., Tourbaf, K.D., 1982. Circulating anticoagulant against factor XI in psoriasis. J. Med. 13, 289–301.

Saenko, E.L., Ananyeva, N.M., Tuddenham, E.G., Kemball-Cook, G., 2002. Factor VIII—novel insights into form and function. Br. J. Haematol. 119, 323–331.

Saenz, A.J., Johnson, N.V., Van Cott, E.M., 2011. Acquired activated protein C resistance caused by lupus anticoagulants. Am. J. Clin. Pathol. 136, 344–349.

Sailer, T., Vormittag, R., Koder, S., Quehenberger, P., Kaider, A., Pabinger, I., 2008. Clinical significance of anti-protein Z antibodies in patients with lupus anticoagulant. Thromb. Res. 122, 153–160.

Sater, M.S., Finan, R.R., Al-Hammad, S.A., Mohammed, F.A., Issa, A.A., Almawi, W.Y., 2011. High frequency of anti-protein Z IgM and IgG autoantibodies in women with idiopathic recurrent spontaneous miscarriage. Am. J. Reprod. Immunol. 65, 526–531.

Scandella, D., 1999. Epitope specificity and inactivation mechanisms of factor VIII inhibitor antibodies. Vox. Sang. 77 (Suppl. 1), S17–S20.

Scheiflinger, F., Knobl, P., Trattner, B., Plaimauer, B., Mohr, G., Dockal, M., et al., 2003. Nonneutralizing IgM and IgG antibodies to von Willebrand factor-cleaving protease (ADAMTS-13) in a patient with thrombotic thrombocytopenic purpura. Blood. 102, 3241–3243.

Schneppenheim, R., Budde, U., 2008. [Inborn and acquired von Willebrand disease]. Hamostaseologie. 28, 312–319.

Scully, M., 2012. Rituximab in the treatment of TTP. Hematology. 17 (Suppl. 1), S22–S24.

Scully, M., Cohen, H., Cavenagh, J., Benjamin, S., Starke, R., Killick, S., et al., 2007. Remission in acute refractory and relapsing thrombotic thrombocytopenic purpura following rituximab is associated with a reduction in IgG antibodies to ADAMTS-13. Br. J. Haematol. 136, 451–461.

Scully, M., Yarranton, H., Liesner, R., Cavenagh, J., Hunt, B., Benjamin, S., et al., 2008. Regional UK TTP registry: correlation with laboratory ADAMTS 13 analysis and clinical features. Br. J. Haematol. 142, 819–826.

Scully, M., Brown, J., Patel, R., McDonald, V., Brown, C.J., Machin, S., 2010. Human leukocyte antigen association in idiopathic thrombotic thrombocytopenic purpura: evidence for an immunogenetic link. J. Thromb. Haemost. 8, 257–262.

Scully, M.F., Ellis, V., Kakkar, V.V., Savidge, G.F., Williams, Y.F., Sterndale, H., 1982. An acquired coagulation inhibitor to factor II. Br. J. Haematol. 50, 655–664.

Shastri, K.A., Ho, C., Logue, G., 1999. An acquired factor V inhibitor: clinical and laboratory features. J. Med. 30, 357–366.

Shelat, S.G., Smith, P., Ai, J., Zheng, X.L., 2006. Inhibitory autoantibodies against ADAMTS-13 in patients with thrombotic thrombocytopenic purpura bind ADAMTS-13 protease and may accelerate its clearance in vivo. J. Thromb. Haemost. 4, 1707–1717.

Shetty, S., Bhave, M., Ghosh, K., 2011. Acquired hemophilia a: diagnosis, aetiology, clinical spectrum and treatment options. Autoimmun. Rev. 10, 311–316.

Shires, L., Gomperts, E.D., Bradlow, B.A., 1979. An acquired inhibitor to factor XIII: A case report. S. Afr. Med. J. 56, 70–72.

Shortt, J., Oh, D.H., Opat, S.S., 2013. ADAMTS13 antibody depletion by bortezomib in thrombotic thrombocytopenic purpura. N. Engl. J. Med. 368, 90–92.

Shumak, K.H., Rock, G.A., Nair, R.C., 1995. Late relapses in patients successfully treated for thrombotic thrombocytopenic purpura. Canadian Apheresis Group. Ann. Intern. Med. 122, 569–572.

Siaka, C., Rugeri, L., Caron, C., Goudemand, J., 2003. A new ELISA assay for diagnosis of acquired von Willebrand syndrome. Haemophilia. 9, 303–308.

Sie, P., Bezeaud, A., Dupouy, D., Archipoff, G., Freyssinet, J.M., Dugoujon, J.M., et al., 1991. An acquired antithrombin autoantibody directed toward the catalytic center of the enzyme. J. Clin. Invest. 88, 290–296.

Smith, S.V., Liles, D.K., White II, G.C., Brecher, M.E., 1998. Successful treatment of transient acquired factor X deficiency by plasmapheresis with concomitant intravenous immunoglobulin and steroid therapy. Am. J. Hematol. 57, 245–252.

Soejima, K., Matsumoto, M., Kokame, K., Yagi, H., Ishizashi, H., Maeda, H., et al., 2003. ADAMTS-13 cysteine-rich/spacer domains are functionally essential for von Willebrand factor cleavage. Blood. 102, 3232–3237.

Sorice, M., Arcieri, P., Griggi, T., Circella, A., Misasi, R., Lenti, L., et al., 1996. Inhibition of protein S by autoantibodies in patients with acquired protein S deficiency. Thromb. Haemost. 75, 555–559.

Spero, J.A., 1993. Bovine thrombin-induced inhibitor of factor V and bleeding risk in postoperative neurosurgical patients. Report of three cases. J. Neurosurg. 78, 817–820.

Stasi, R., Brunetti, M., Stipa, E., Amadori, S., 2004. Selective B-cell depletion with rituximab for the treatment of patients with acquired hemophilia. Blood. 103, 4424–4428.

Streiff, M.B., Ness, P.M., 2002. Acquired FV inhibitors: a needless iatrogenic complication of bovine thrombin exposure. Transfusion. 42, 18–26.

Stricker, R.B., Lane, P.K., Leffert, J.D., Rodgers, G.M., Shuman, M.A., Corash, L., 1988. Development of antithrombin antibodies following surgery in patients with prosthetic cardiac valves. Blood. 72, 1375–1380.

Sucker, C., Scharf, R.E., Zotz, R.B., 2009. Use of recombinant factor VIIa in inherited and acquired von Willebrand disease. Clin. Appl. Thromb. Hemost. 15, 27–31.

Suehisa, E., Toku, M., Akita, N., Fushimi, R., Takano, T., Tada, H., et al., 1995. Study on an antibody against F1F2 fragment of human factor V in a patient with Hashimoto's disease and bullous pemphigoid. Thromb. Res. 77, 63–68.

Sumner, M.J., Geldziler, B.D., Pedersen, M., Seremetis, S., 2007. Treatment of acquired haemophilia with recombinant activated FVII: a critical appraisal. Haemophilia. 13, 451–461.

Takahashi, H., Fuse, I., Abe, T., Yoshino, N., Aizawa, Y., 2003. Acquired factor V inhibitor complicated by Hashimoto's thyroiditis, primary biliary cirrhosis and membranous nephropathy. Blood Coagul. Fibrinolysis. 14, 87–93.

Tay, L., Duncan, E., Singhal, D., Al-Qunfoidi, R., Coghlan, D., Jaksic, W., et al., 2009. Twelve years of experience of acquired hemophilia A: trials and tribulations in South Australia. Semin. Thromb. Hemost. 35, 769–777.

Tengborn, L., Baudo, F., Huth-Kuhne, A., Knoebl, P., Levesque, H., Marco, P., et al., 2012. Pregnancy-associated acquired haemophilia A: results from the European Acquired Haemophilia (EACH2) registry. BJOG 119, 1529–1537.

Terrell, D.R., Williams, L.A., Vesely, S.K., Lammle, B., Hovinga, J.A., George, J.N., 2005. The incidence of thrombotic thrombocytopenic purpura-hemolytic uremic syndrome: all patients, idiopathic patients, and patients with severe ADAMTS-13 deficiency. J. Thromb. Haemost. 3, 1432–1436.

Tiede, A., Priesack, J., Werwitzke, S., Bohlmann, K., Oortwijn, B., Lenting, P., et al., 2008. Diagnostic workup of patients with acquired von Willebrand syndrome: a retrospective single-centre cohort study. J. Thromb. Haemost. 6, 569–576.

Tiede, A., Huth-Kuhne, A., Oldenburg, J., Grossmann, R., Geisen, U., Krause, M., et al., 2009. Immunosuppressive treatment for acquired haemophilia: current practice and future directions in Germany, Austria and Switzerland. Ann. Hematol. 88, 365–370.

Tiede, A., Eisert, R., Czwalinna, A., Miesbach, W., Scharrer, I., Ganser, A., 2010. Acquired haemophilia caused by non-haemophilic factor VIII gene variants. Ann. Hematol. 89, 607–612.

Tiede, A., Rand, J.H., Budde, U., Ganser, A., Federici, A.B., 2011. How I treat the acquired von Willebrand syndrome. Blood. 117, 6777–6785.

Toole, J.J., Knopf, J.L., Wozney, J.M., Sultzman, L.A., Buecker, J.L., Pittman, D.D., et al., 1984. Molecular cloning of a cDNA encoding human antihaemophilic factor. Nature. 312, 342–347.

Torok, T.J., Holman, R.C., Chorba, T.L., 1995. Increasing mortality from thrombotic thrombocytopenic purpura in the United States—analysis of national mortality data, 1968–1991. Am. J. Hematol. 50, 84–90.

Torres, A., Lucia, J.F., Oliveros, A., Vazquez, C., Torres, M., 1980. Anti-factor IX circulating anticoagulant and immune thrombocytopenia in a case of Takayasu's arteritis. Acta Haematol. 64, 338–340.

Torricelli, M., Sabatini, L., Florio, P., Scaccia, V., Voltolini, C., Biliotti, G., et al., 2009. Levels of antibodies against protein C and protein S in pregnancy and in preeclampsia. J. Matern. Fetal. Neonatal. Med. 22, 993–999.

Toschi, V., Baudo, F., 2010. Diagnosis, laboratory aspects and manage-ment of acquired hemophilia A. Intern. Emerg. Med. 5, 325–333.

Tosetto, A., Rodeghiero, F., Gatto, E., Manotti, C., Poli, T., 1995. An acquired hemorrhagic disorder of fibrin crosslinking due to IgG anti-bodies to FXIII, successfully treated with FXIII replacement and cyclophosphamide. Am. J. Hematol. 48, 34–39.

Tsai, H.M., 1996. Physiologic cleavage of von Willebrand factor by a plasma protease is dependent on its conformation and requires cal-cium ion. Blood. 87, 4235–4244.

Tsai, H.M., 2006. Current concepts in thrombotic thrombocytopenic pur-pura. Annu. Rev. Med. 57, 419–436.

Tsai, H.M., Raoufi, M., Zhou, W., Guinto, E., Grafos, N., Ranzurmal, S., et al., 2006. ADAMTS13-binding IgG are present in patients with thrombotic thrombocytopenic purpura. Thromb. Haemost. 95, 886–892.

Tun, N.M., Villani, G.M., 2012. Efficacy of rituximab in acute refractory or chronic relapsing non-familial idiopathic thrombotic thrombocy-topenic purpura: a systematic review with pooled data analysis. J. Thromb. Thrombolysis. 34, 347–359.

Urbanus, R.T., De Laat, B., 2010. Antiphospholipid antibodies and the protein C pathway. Lupus. 19, 394–399.

Vadivel, K., Bajaj, S.P., 2012. Structural biology of factor VIIa/tissue factor initiated coagulation. Front. Biosci. 17, 2476–2494.

Van Genderen, P.J., Vink, T., Michiels, J.J., Van 'T Veer, M.B., Sixma, J.J., et al., 1994. Acquired von Willebrand disease caused by an auto-antibody selectively inhibiting the binding of von Willebrand factor to collagen. Blood. 84, 3378–3384.

Vercellotti, G.M., Mosher, D.F., 1982. Acquired factor XI defi-ciency in systemic lupus erythematosus. Thromb. Haemost. 48, 250–252.

Veyradier, A., Jenkins, C.S., Fressinaud, E., Meyer, D., 2000. Acquired von Willebrand syndrome: from pathophysiology to management. Thromb. Haemost. 84, 175–182.

Webert, K.E., 2012. Acquired hemophilia A. Semin. Thromb. Hemost. 38, 735–741.

Weisdorf, D., Hasegawa, D., Fair, D.S., 1989. Acquired factor VII defi-ciency associated with aplastic anaemia: correction with bone mar-row transplantation. Br. J. Haematol. 71, 409–413.

Whelan, S.F., Hofbauer, C.J., Horling, F.M., Allacher, P., Wolfsegger, M.J., Oldenburg, J., et al., 2013. Distinct characteristics of antibody responses against factor VIII in healthy individuals and in different cohorts of hemophilia A patients. Blood. 121, 1039–1048.

Whitelock, J.L., Nolasco, L., Bernardo, A., Moake, J., Dong, J.F., Cruz, M.A., 2004. ADAMTS-13 activity in plasma is rapidly measured by a new ELISA method that uses recombinant VWF-A2 domain as substrate. J. Thromb. Haemost. 2, 485–491.

Wiestner, A., Cho, H.J., Asch, A.S., Michelis, M.A., Zeller, J.A., Peerschke, E.I., et al., 2002. Rituximab in the treatment of acquired factor VIII inhibitors. Blood. 100, 3426–3428.

Will, A., 2006. Paediatric acquired von Willebrand syndrome. Haemophilia. 12, 287–288.

Wood, W.I., Capon, D.J., Simonsen, C.C., Eaton, D.L., Gitschier, J., Keyt, B., et al., 1984. Expression of active human factor VIII from recombinant DNA clones. Nature. 312, 330–337.

Wootla, B., Dasgupta, S., Dimitrov, J.D., Bayry, J., Levesque, H., Borg, J.Y., et al., 2008. Factor VIII hydrolysis mediated by anti-factor VIII autoantibodies in acquired hemophilia. J. Immunol. 180, 7714–7720.

Wootla, B., Christophe, O.D., Mahendra, A., Dimitrov, J.D., Repesse, Y., Ollivier, V., et al., 2011. Proteolytic antibodies activate factor IX in patients with acquired hemophilia. Blood. 117, 2257–2264.

Wu, J.J., Fujikawa, K., Lian, E.C., Mcmullen, B.A., Kulman, J.D., Chung, D.W., 2006. A rapid enzyme-linked assay for ADAMTS-13. J. Thromb. Haemost. 4, 129–136.

Yamada, R., Nozawa, K., Yoshimine, T., Takasaki, Y., Ogawa, H., Takamori, K., et al., 2011. A case of thrombotic thrombocytope-nia purpura associated with systemic lupus erythematosus: Diagnostic utility of ADAMTS-13 Activity. Autoimmune Dis. 2011, 483642.

Yamaguchi, Y., Moriki, T., Igari, A., Nakagawa, T., Wada, H., Matsumoto, M., et al., 2011. Epitope analysis of autoantibodies to ADAMTS13 in patients with acquired thrombotic thrombocytopenic purpura. Thromb. Res. 128, 169–173.

Zanon, E., Milan, M., Brandolin, B., Barbar, S., Spiezia, L., Saggiorato, G., et al., 2013. High dose of human plasma-derived FVIII-VWF as first-line therapy in patients affected by acquired haemophilia A and concomitant cardiovascular disease: four case reports and a literature review. Haemophilia. 19, e50–e53.

Zehnder, J.L., Leung, L.L., 1990. Development of antibodies to throm-bin and factor V with recurrent bleeding in a patient exposed to topi-cal bovine thrombin. Blood. 76, 2011–2016.

Zeitler, H., Ulrich-Merzenich, G., Panek, D., Goldmann, G., Vidovic, N., Brackmann, H.H., et al., 2012. Extracorporeal treatment for the acute and long-term outcome of patients with life-threatening acquired hemophilia. Transfus. Med. Hemother. 39, 264–270.

Zeitler, H., Goldmann, G., Marquardt, N., Ulrich-Merzenich, G., 2013. Long term outcome of patients with acquired haemophilia—a mono-centre interim analysis of 82 patients. Atheroscler. Suppl. 14, 223–228.

Zheng, X., Chung, D., Takayama, T.K., Majerus, E.M., Sadler, J.E., Fujikawa, K., 2001. Structure of von Willebrand factor-cleaving protease (ADAMTS13), a metalloprotease involved in thrombotic thrombocytopenic purpura. J. Biol. Chem. 276, 41059–41063.

Zheng, X.L., Wu, H.M., Shang, D., Falls, E., Skipwith, C.G., Cataland, S.R., et al., 2010. Multiple domains of ADAMTS13 are targeted by autoantibodies against ADAMTS13 in patients with acquired idio-pathic thrombotic thrombocytopenic purpura. Haematologica. 95, 1555–1562.

Part 10

Central and Peripheral Nervous System

Chapter 52

Multiple Sclerosis

Amanda L. Hernandez[1], Kevin C. O'Connor[2], and David A. Hafler[3]

[1]*Department of Neurology, Interdepartmental Neuroscience Program, Yale University School of Medicine, New Haven CT, USA,* [2]*Department of Neurology, Human and Translational Immunology Program, Yale University School of Medicine, New Haven CT, USA,* [3]*Department of Neurology, Yale University School of Medicine, New Haven CT, USA*

Chapter Outline

Historical Background	735	Meningeal Ectopic B Cell Follicles	745
Clinical Features	736	**Treatment**	**745**
Imaging	737	Interferons	746
Immunological Markers in Diagnosis	738	Glatiramer Acetate (Copaxone)	747
Pathology	738	Natalizumab (Tysabri)	747
Epidemiology of MS	739	Mitoxantrone (Novantrone)	748
Genetic Factors	739	Fingolimod (Gilenya)	748
Environmental Factors	740	Teriflunomide (Aubagio)	748
Immune Pathogenesis	742	Dimethyl Fumarate, BG-12 (Tecfidera)	748
T Cell Pathogenesis	743	**Concluding Remarks**	**749**
Immune Dysregulation	744	**References**	**749**
Autoantigens	745		

HISTORICAL BACKGROUND

It is widely held that the earliest known reference of multiple sclerosis (MS) can be attributed to Scottish pathologist Robert Carswell (Murray, 2009). In his atlas, *Pathological Anatomy: Illustrations of the Elementary Forms of Disease (1838)*, Carswell described two patients affected by paralysis, both with lesions along the spinal cord and lower brain stem accompanied by atrophy. Carswell believed that the extensive paralysis the patients suffered was directly related to the impressive pathology he encountered (Behan, 1982). However compelling Carswell's account was, it was not until 30 years later that MS was named by a French neurologist, Jean Martin Charcot. Charcot first described a comprehensive account of the features of MS in 1868 by correlating the clinical and pathological features of the illness in patients he examined both while they were alive and at autopsy. He noted the accumulation of inflammatory cells in a perivascular distribution, demyelination, and axonal sparing within the lesions or "plaques" in the brain and spinal cord white matter of patients with intermittent episodes of neurologic dysfunction (Charcot, 1868a,b, 1877). This led to the term "*sclérose en plaques disseminées*," or multiple sclerosis.

Over the last 100 years there have been many important historical milestones that have led to the fundamental understanding that MS is a multifocal inflammatory disease primarily affecting central nervous system (CNS) white matter resulting in progressive neurodegeneration in genetically susceptible hosts (recently reviewed in Nylander and Hafler, 2012). The hypothesis that MS is an autoimmune disease can be attributed to observations by Thomas Rivers at the Rockefeller Institute. In 1933 Rivers demonstrated that injection of rabbit brain and spinal cord into primates resulted in a demyelinating disease in mammals (Rivers et al., 1933). This disease, known as experimental autoimmune encephalomyelitis (EAE), is the result of immunization of CNS myelin and has served as an important animal model for multiple sclerosis.

In 1965, Schumacher et al. defined clinical diagnostic criteria based on the notion that MS is a disease disseminated in time and space throughout the CNS

N. Rose & I. Mackay (Eds): The Autoimmune Diseases, Fifth edition. DOI: http://dx.doi.org/10.1016/B978-0-12-384929-8.00052-6

(Schumacker et al., 1965). Such criteria continue to be utilized and revised today. Since then, the advent of magnetic resonance imaging and FDA approval of IFN-β1b, among other therapeutic agents, have revolutionized how we examine and treat patients with MS (Young et al., 1981; Arnason, 1993). During the past 20 years, MS has evolved from a disease with no therapy to one with eight approved therapies in the USA to date. These major advances have established MS as a treatable neurological illness. Nonetheless, the development of more effective and safer treatments that can be used at the time of diagnosis for this potentially disabling illness is paramount, and predicated on a more thorough understanding of the underlying immunopathology. Advances in immunology and neurology have provided clinicians with powerful tools to better understand the underlying causes of MS, leading to new therapeutic advances. The future calls for extending the original observations of Carswell and Charcot by continuing to define the molecular pathology of MS in relation to growing knowledge surrounding immune-related pathology and DNA haplotype structure in addition to CNS and peripheral mRNA and protein expression, leading to the generation of a new series of disease-related hypotheses.

CLINICAL FEATURES

The signs and symptoms of MS are variable as the disease can affect anywhere within the CNS. Demyelinating lesions may develop at any site along myelinated CNS white matter tracts, and symptoms of MS therefore depend on the functions subserved by the pathways involved. Although the primary insult involves demyelination, edema, inflammation, gliosis, and axonal loss all contribute to the symptomatology of a lesion. The most common symptoms and signs involve alteration or loss of sensation due to involvement of spinothalamic or posterior column fibers, visual loss from optic neuritis, limb weakness and spasticity related to disruption of corticospinal tracts, tremors and incoordination of gait or limbs largely related to cerebellar or spinocerebellar fiber involvement, and abnormalities of cranial nerve function (such as double vision due to disturbance in conjugate eye movement) secondary to brainstem lesions (Noseworthy et al., 2000). Bowel, bladder, and sexual dysfunction occur in over two-thirds of patients at some time during the course of their illness (Betts et al., 1993; Mattson et al., 1995) largely due to disruption in spinal cord pathways. Fatigue, depression, and cognitive changes are common symptoms of elusive etiology that may significantly interfere with daily functioning and are now being recognized as significant contributors to disability (Whitlock and Siskind, 1980; Freal et al., 1984; Sadovnick et al., 1996). A correlation with progressive

brain atrophy, cognitive decline, and impairment on MRI has implicated axonal loss as the pathologic substrate of the cognitive deterioration in MS (Rao et al., 1989; Hohol et al., 1997; Amato et al., 2004).

While MS can have variability in clinical presentation and course of the illness, it can follow a number of rather predictable courses. MS may be divided into four clinical categories: clinically isolated syndromes (CIS), an early form of MS, relapsing—remitting multiple sclerosis (RRMS), which in a subgroup of patients becomes secondary progressive multiple sclerosis (SPMS), and primary progressive multiple sclerosis (PPMS).

CIS generally occur in young adults, and are defined by the presentation of a first episode of demyelination typically in the form of optic neuritis, cerebellar, or brainstem syndrome. During an episode, neurological symptoms develop over hours to several days, persist for days to several weeks and gradually dissipate (Miller et al., 2012). In order for such episodes of acute inflammatory CNS demyelinating events to be considered CIS, they must last for at least 24 hours with no more than 30 days between attacks (Polman et al., 2005). The resolution of symptoms appears to be due to the reduction of inflammation and edema at the site of the responsible lesion rather than to the reversal of demyelination, which may persist even in the absence of symptoms (McDonald et al., 2001). In a number of recent prospective studies, patients experiencing an initial episode suggestive of CNS demyelination and having MRI evidence indicating the presence of lesions either at the time of or within 3 months of the event is highly predictive for the development of relapses and thus clinically definite multiple sclerosis (CDMS). Without MRI lesions, the probability of developing MS is substantially less. More than half of those developing MS experienced the additional relapse within 1 year of their first episode (Achiron and Barak, 2000; Fisniku et al., 2008). Thus, it seems reasonable to label the first attack of what appears to be MS as CIS, explaining to patients that there is a high likelihood of developing multiple sclerosis (Rovira et al., 2009). This indicates to the patient there is a good understanding of the underlying problem, but the prognosis is not clear, allowing patients who never have another attack to be saved from carrying a diagnosis of MS (Miller et al., 2012).

If a patient with a CIS develops further episodes of relapses followed by a recovery with a stable course between relapses, patients are referred to as having RRMS. Early in the course of MS, patients often make complete recovery from relapses. As the disease goes on, the recovery from a relapse diminishes, which causes a patient to accrue disability. A relapsing—remitting onset is observed in 85—90% of patients, with relapses often lasting 4 weeks in duration. The outcome in patients with RRMS is variable; untreated, previous reports suggested that approximately 50% of all MS patients require the use of a walking aid by 10 years after clinical onset (Weinshenker, 1994). The consequences on prognosis of newer treatment regimens are not completely delineated; however, many studies indicate improvement of disability status following continued treatment regimens (Bates, 2011). Increased attack frequency and poor recovery from attacks in the first years of clinical disease predict a more rapid deterioration (Confavreux and Vukusic, 2006).

Ultimately, approximately 40–50% of untreated relapsing–remitting patients stop having attacks and develop what may be a neurodegenerative progressive disease secondary to the chronic CNS inflammation, known as secondary-progressive multiple sclerosis (SPMS) (Confavreux et al., 2000). The evolution to this secondary progressive form of the disease is associated with significantly fewer gadolinium-enhanced lesions and a decrease in brain parenchymal volume (Khoury et al., 1994; Filippi et al., 1995; Weiner et al., 2000). Similarly, while earlier relapsing–remitting MS is sensitive to immunosuppression (Hohol et al., 1999), as times goes on, responsiveness to immunotherapy decreases and disappears in secondary progressive disease (Rieckmann et al., 2004). Thus, rather than conceiving of MS as first a relapsing–remitting and then a secondary progressive disease, it could be hypothesized that MS is a continuum where there are acute inflammatory events early on with secondary induction of a neurodegenerative process refractory to immunologic intervention. This hypothesis awaits experimental verification.

Primary progressive MS (PPMS) occurs in close to 15% of patients, and is characterized from the onset by the absence of acute attacks and instead involves a gradual clinical decline traditionally in the form of a progressive myelopathy (Miller and Leary, 2007). Patients may also present with a progressive cerebellar syndrome in the form of ataxia. Clinically, this form of the disease is associated with a lack of response to any form of immunotherapy. Researchers had therefore posited that PPMS may in fact be a different disease than RRMS.

In the absence of a specific immune-based assay, the diagnosis of MS continues to be predicated on the clinical history and neurological exam demonstrating multiple lesions disseminated in time and space within the CNS (McDonald et al., 2001). Although using McDonald's criteria the diagnosis of MS can be made solely on the basis of history of two relapses and objective findings on exam of two lesions disseminated in the CNS (periventricular, juxtracortical, infratentorial, or spinal cord), MRI of the neuroaxis is often sought to confirm the diagnosis or to rule out other mimics of the illness. The use of the MRI and other imaging modalities has had a major impact on early diagnosis by establishing newer criteria for the diagnosis of the disease as well as a means to determine prognosis and monitor disease course and response to therapy. T1-weighted scans generally provide appreciable contrast between gray and white matter with water appearing darker and fat brighter. In T2-weighted scans fat is also differentiated from water; however, fat appears darker and water lighter in the image, making T2-weighted scans well suited for imaging edema since CSF appears lighter (Filippi and Agosta, 2009). As part of McDonald's criteria, new T1-weighted lesions or T2-weighted gadolinium enhancing lesions on follow-up MRI scans may serve as criteria for dissemination in space or time, thus allowing the diagnosis fulfilling the criteria of MS to be made with further confidence (Polman et al., 2011).

Imaging

MRI has gained a principal role in the assessment of MS because it allows clinicians to readily obtain an understanding of the pathophysiology of the lesions, CNS involvement, and ultimately the overall illness without invasive procedures. Currently, common MRI measures of disease burden include the quantification of brain lesions using T1- and T2-weighted images, gadolinium contrast, proton density, and fluid attenuated inversion recovery sequences. Each of these markers represents many possible histopathological correlates, including: demyelination, edema, axonal loss, matrix destruction, and inflammation (Filippi and Rocca, 2011). The lesions on MRI are often ovoid in shape, ranging from a few mm to more than 1 cm in size. Their location is crucial, considering that MS lesions have a high propensity to locate in the periventricular white matter, brainstem, and cerebellum. Additionally, MRI and pathological data suggest that evolution of MS lesions depends on whether they occur during early versus chronic phases of the disease course (Filippi et al., 2012).

Lesions on T2-weighted images are often clinically silent and correlate weakly with a patient's disability despite correlating well with the location on plaques in the CNS of postmortem MS patients (Newcombe et al., 1991). Hypointense lesions on T1-weighted images may be persistent or nonpersistent (Rovaris et al., 1999). Persistent hypointense T1-weighted lesions represent areas indicative of axonal loss and severe tissue destruction and correlate better than T2 lesion load with clinical severity of the disease (van Waesberghe et al., 1999). Multiple T2-weighted and/or gadolinium-enhancing lesions on initial MRI scans indicative of diffuse cortical lesions and atropy also predict a more severe subsequent course related not only to physical disability but also to diminished cognitive outcome (Calabrese et al., 2009; Deloire et al., 2011). Nonpersistent hypointense lesions on T1-weighted images represent reversible edema due to abatement of inflammation. Post-contrast gadolinium enhancement of lesions on T1-weighted images represents acute disruption of the blood–brain barrier from inflammation. On average, disruption can last 3 weeks, but may range anywhere from 2 to 6 weeks and is dependent on gadolinium dose, the characteristics and delay of image acquisition, and steroid treatment of acute attacks (Filippi, 2000).

Intermittent MRI imaging might underestimate severity of disease burden since weekly MRI scanning suggests that a significant proportion of MS lesions have very short-lived enhancement (Cotton et al., 2003). Brain and spinal cord atrophy may occur in MS and can represent loss of myelin, oligodendrocytes, and axons, in addition to contraction of astrocyte volume. Continued work in improving the use of various imaging modalities to more accurately characterize active disease is imperative in moving forward.

IMMUNOLOGICAL MARKERS IN DIAGNOSIS

CSF immunologic markers can function as adjuncts to clinical findings when considering the diagnosis of MS. The CSF of patients with MS typically shows normal glucose, a few lymphocytes (mostly T cells), normal to mildly elevated total protein, and oligoclonal immunoglobulin bands (OCBs). OCBs are uncovered when CSF from MS patients is electrophoresed. The cathode region reveals a number of discrete bands that represent excess antibody production by one or more clones of B cells. Such bands are not evident when CSF from healthy controls is electrophoresed. Often absent early in the disease, OCBs can eventually be detected in over 90% of patients with MS (Cruz et al., 1987; Mclean et al., 1990).

CSF OCBs have also been described in conditions such as subacute sclerosing panencephalomyelitis (SSPE) (Mattson et al., 1980), neurosyphilis (Pedersen et al., 1982), varicella zoster virus (VZV) infection (Vartdal et al., 1982), HIV infection (Skotzek et al., 1988), and in multisystem autoimmune diseases, cerebrovascular accidents, and up to 5% of normal individuals. Of note, OCBs are continuously present in MS regardless of disease activity, whereas they are transient in other conditions due to infection clearance (Link and Huang, 2006). Furthermore, OCBs have been reported to correlate with disease course and disability progression (Link and Huang, 2006; Mandrioli et al., 2008) and with the conversion to MS in patients with CIS and a negative MRI or an MRI with few lesions (Tintore et al., 2008). In diseases such as the viral encephalitides, OCBs commonly bind virus determinants, in contrast to MS, where the antigen against which the majority of bands are directed has not been identified to date (Olek, 2000).

Due to intrathecal synthesis from plasma cells, CSF immunoglobulin levels are also elevated in patients with MS. The immunoglobulins are mainly composed of IgG, with lesser amounts being IgM and IgA. Specifically, studies have delineated differences between IgG and IgM levels with the latter correlating more strongly with MS

disease course and IgG reflecting local B cell responses accompanying CNS inflammation. Nearly 90% of patients demonstrate elevated levels of CSF IgG production when the IgG index formula (spinal fluid IgG/spinal fluid albumin)/(serum IgG/serum albumin) is calculated. A spinal fluid IgG index greater than 0.58 implies that IgG are being synthesized in the CNS.

Apart from oligoclonal bands, numerous CSF markers have demonstrated specificity for the MS disease process. Several non-specific proteins may function as markers of disease process, including: tau protein and myelin basic protein (MBP), in addition to light and heavy neurofilament chains appearing during relapse and correlating with long-term functional outcome and the likelihood of conversion from CIS to RRMS (Graber and Dhib-Jalbut, 2011).

There are reports of serum and CSF anti-MBP, anti-MOG, and anti-PLP autoantibodies (Warren and Catz, 1994; Warren et al., 1994; Berger et al., 2003) in patients with MS. Such studies have been challenged due to the possibility of non-specific binding of low-affinity antibodies and observations that high-affinity antibodies against MOG epitopes are only present in a small proportion of patients (Menge et al., 2011). However, using sensitive solution phase assays, high-affinity autoantibodies to MBP and MOG can be detected in the serum and CSF of patients with acute disseminated encephalomyelitis and MS (O'Connor et al., 2003, 2005, 2007; Zhou et al., 2006). A recent study aiming to characterize intrathecal MOG antibodies in MS indicated that the rMOG index, a marker of intrathecal MOG antibody production, may provide complementary information to routine CSF testing in the diagnosis of MS (Klawiter et al., 2010). Moreover, anti-MOG autoantibodies can be eluted from the brain tissue of a subset of patients with MS (O'Connor et al., 2005). Such markers support the ongoing hypothesis of MS as a disease linked to immune dysfunction, ongoing inflammation, and tissue damage and repair. A serum autoantibody, neuromyelitis optica immunoglobulin (NMO-IgG), was identified in patients with neuromyelitis optica, an inflammatory demyelinating disease similar to, and considered by some to be a variant of, MS affecting the optic nerves and spinal cord, thereby highlighting the importance of the differential diagnosis between MS of NMO and NMO spectrum disorders. NMO and the associated autoantibody (NMO-IgG/anti-aquaporin 4) is discussed further in Chapter 57.

PATHOLOGY

Gross examination of MS brain tissue has largely been limited to autopsy specimens of individuals with long-standing disease. Such pathological examination reveals multiple sharply demarcated gray colored plaques in the CNS white matter with a predilection for the optic nerves and white matter tracts of the periventricular regions, brain stem, and spinal cord. The gray matter contains less myelin, and thus lesions in the gray matter are less conspicuous on gross examination (Geurts et al., 2005). When examining the histological features of an MS lesion there exist three major components: inflammation, gliosis, and demyelination. The *inflammation* in lesions is composed of lymphocytes, monocytes, and macrophages whose proportions depend on the activity and age of the lesion (Frohman et al., 2006). The second component of a lesion occurs when reactive astrocytes and fibrillary gliosis are present in the lesion.

Demyelination is an important feature of the MS lesion. Although MS is described as a disease causing a loss of myelin, the notion of axonal loss has been suggested as the major cause of irreversible disability in patients with MS. Trapp et al. first reported that substantial axonal injuries with axonal transections are also abundant throughout active MS lesions, even in patients in early stages of the disease process (Trapp et al., 1998). Axonal reduction and acute damage have previously been correlated with demyelination and meningeal inflammation (Ferguson et al., 1997). Interestingly, differences in axonal loss exist among subsets of MS, with the least axonal loss being demonstrated in PPMS and the most pronounced in SPMS (Bitsch et al., 2000). Notably, there have been case reports of early RRMS presenting with inflammatory cortical demyelination prior to the appearance of white matter lesions, indicating possible inflammation being initiated at the subpial layer (Popescu et al., 2011). Recent work aimed at elucidating the pathogenesis of axonal damage and loss has implicated several mechanisms including: inflammatory secretions, Wallerian degeneration, disruption of axonal ion concentrations, loss of myelin-derived support, damage from nitric oxide and reactive oxygen species, energy failure from mitochondrial dysfunction, and Ca^{2+} accumulation (Smith and Lassmann, 2002; Dutta and Trapp, 2007; Dziedzic et al., 2010).

MS lesions can also be classified from a pathogenesis point of view into three types based on the age of the lesion: active, chronic active, and chronic inactive (Lassmann, 1998). Macrophages are most prominent in the center of the *active plaques* and are seen to contain myelin debris, while oligodendrocyte counts are reduced and generally present in lesions demonstrating signs of remyelination. Hypertrophic astrocytes and mild astroglial scarring are also characteristic of active lesions (Frohman et al., 2006). Lymphocytes may be found in normal appearing white matter beyond the margin of active demyelination (Prineas, 1975; Booss et al., 1983). The inflammatory cell profile of active lesions is characterized by perivascular infiltration of oligoclonal T cells (Wucherpfennig et al., 1992b) consisting predominantly of clonally expanded CD8$^+$ T cells in the plaque margins and perivascular cuffs, and to a lesser extent of CD4$^+$ cells invading the normal appearing white matter around the lesion (Traugott et al., 1983; Hauser et al., 1986;

Babbe et al., 2000). The inflammatory infiltrate may also include monocytes, occasional B cells, $\gamma\delta$ T cells, and rare plasma cells (Booss et al., 1983; Wucherpfennig et al., 1992a; Babbe et al., 2000). Remarkably, demyelination in acute lesions may be related to an antimyelin antibody-mediated mechanism in which normal myelin is coated with anti-MBP immunoglobulin or anti-MOG and phagocytosed in the presence of complement by local macrophages (Genain et al., 1999). *Chronic-active lesions* are sharply demarcated with perivascular cuffs of infiltrating cells, lipid- and myelin-laden macrophages, activated microglia, and hypertrophic astrocytes. These cells disappear from the center core suggesting the presence of ongoing inflammatory activity along the lesion edge. Within the hypocellular core there are naked axons embedded within a matrix of fibrous astrocytes, lipid-laden macrophages, a few infiltrating leukocytes, and no oligodendrocytes. The *chronic-inactive plaque* does not have macrophages at the border or center of the plaque. There is vast hypocellularity and no ongoing demyelination with histology demonstrating demyelinated axons with fibrillary gliosis (Raine, 1991).

EPIDEMIOLOGY OF MS

The prevalence rates of MS in North America range between 30 and 150/100,000. Based on a weighted mean of several studies, the average annual incidence of MS in the USA is 3.2/100,000 per year. The median age of onset of symptoms is 23–24 years of age, with a peak age of onset for women in the early twenties, and for men in the late twenties (Schumacker et al., 1965; Paty et al., 1994). As in most diseases classified as autoimmune, there is a clear female predominance in MS cases, with a 3:2 female to male ratio (Olek, 2000). Studies of MS incidence rates in migrants (Dean et al., 1976) and apparent epidemics of MS at geographical locations (Kurtzke et al., 1982), also discussed below, indicate a clear role for environmental factors.

Genetic Factors

Studies in twins (Mackay and Myrianthopoulos, 1966; Williams et al., 1980; Heltberg and Holm, 1982; Ebers et al., 1986; Kinnunen et al., 1987; French Research Group on MS, 1992; Mumford et al., 1992) demonstrate shared genetic risk factors for MS. Most recently, work involving genome-wide association studies (GWAS) using single nucleotide polymorphisms (SNPs) from the haplotype map (HapMap) project have provided insights into the genetic associations involved in MS (Tishkoff and Verrelli, 2003; Frazer et al., 2007; Patsopoulos et al., 2011). While the risk of developing MS in the general population is 1/750, our early understanding of the genetic factors linked to MS has been derived from epidemiological studies and disease concordance within family members or twins. Such studies have demonstrated that approximately 15–20% of patients have a family history of MS and when both parents are affected with MS, 9% of children develop the disease (Hogancamp et al., 1997; Sadovnick et al., 1997; Sadovnick, 2006). Twin studies have indicated that the monozygotic concordance rate is 30% versus the dizygotic rate of 5% (Holmes et al., 1967; Sadovnick et al., 1993). Nevertheless, large extended pedigrees are relatively uncommon.

The sequencing of the human genome and the generation of the HapMap has finally allowed the identification of the genetic architecture underlying risk for developing MS by GWAS (Tishkoff and Verrelli, 2003). GWAS have afforded an unbiased and widespread approach in scanning the whole genome and identifying haplotypes associated with risk of developing MS. They provide an alternative approach to classic linkage analysis and have greater statistical power to detect variants conferring a modest disease risk (Risch and Merikangas, 1996; Yang et al., 2005). These studies have provided convincing evidence that MS fits into the autoimmune disease category and is caused by common allelic variants each with only subtle but important variations on function.

In 2007, the first GWAS in MS clearly identified several gene regions. Subsequent GWAS and their corresponding meta-analyses identified 14 regions with genome-wide significance, several of which have been previously identified; these regions include CD58, CD40, CD6, IL-2RA, IL-7RA, EVI5, CLEC16A, TYK2 and TNF-RSF1A, IRF8, and STAT3, all of which are of interest due to their expression on regulatory T cells, and proinflammatory Th17 cells, both $CD4^+$ subsets implicated in MS later described in detail (Wellcome Trust Case Control Consortium et al., 2007; Aulchenko et al., 2008; Comabella et al., 2008; Australia and New Zealand Multiple Sclerosis Genetics Consortium, 2009; Baranzini et al., 2009; De Jager et al., 2009b; Jakkula et al., 2010; Nischwitz et al., 2010; Sanna et al., 2010). Finally, a recent international GWAS collaboration aimed at analyzing over 9000 cases of MS succeeded in replicating many of the earlier findings in addition to highlighting 29 novel susceptibility loci, thereby identifying more than 50 regions of interest. Although each haplotype only represents a small influence on the risk of developing MS, together they account for approximately half of the genetic risk for MS (Sawcer et al., 2011) (Figure 52.1) As expected, these SNPs, upon being related to the known or likely function of nearby genes, are largely associated with lymphocyte function, providing further evidence of an immunopathogenesis of MS. A large meta-analysis with replication is now in progress.

One of the additional aims of GWAS has been to refine our understanding of the genetic risk associated with the major histocompatibility complex (MHC) through looking more closely at HLA types at six loci (A, B, C, DQA1, DQB1, and DRB1) (Sawcer et al., 2011). Prior to GWAS, our understanding of the association and linkage of MS with respect to MHC was limited to alleles and haplotypes on chromosome 6p21. Recently, studies have successfully established HLA DRB*1501 as being the allele variant involved in MS as opposed to HLA DQA1 or DQB1 (Brynedal et al., 2007; Lincoln et al., 2009). Further work has implicated HLA-A2 as being negatively associated with MS, thereby potentially serving as a protective allele with consistent effects across cohorts.

Many of the alleles identified in MS are shared not only among other autoimmune diseases but also are strongly associated with immune pathways (Torkamani et al., 2008; Xavier and Rioux, 2008; International Multiple Sclerosis Genetics Consortium, 2009; Zhernakova et al., 2009). Given these genetic commonalities, it is therefore not surprising that MS and other autoimmune diseases share related defects in immune function and regulation. Recent work aimed at uncovering the intricacies of the relationships between autoimmune diseases has confirmed commonality across seven autoimmune diseases through identifying shared genes among some but not all of the diseases (Cotsapas et al., 2011). A model addressing the overarching interconnectivity of various autoimmune disease mechanisms is likely to be elucidated in the future. As MS is a complex disease, understanding which combinations of genes within the population confer the greatest risk of developing autoimmune disease is a central goal of present genetic research efforts.

Environmental Factors

Global maps of MS prevalence rates, constructed based on multiple descriptive epidemiological studies, reveal a non-random geographical distribution of the disease. A diminishing north to south gradient of MS prevalence was described in the Northern Hemisphere (Beebe et al., 1967; Kurtzke, 1977; Kurtzke et al., 1979; Hammond et al., 1987), with an opposite trend identified in the Southern Hemisphere (Hammond et al., 1988; Hogancamp et al., 1997; Kurtzke, 2000). Notably, there is a marked absence of MS cases directly near the equator. When taking continental differences into consideration, there is increased prevalence of MS with large dispersion in Western Europe and North America, both regions being highly populated by Caucasians, whereas areas in Central and Eastern Europe, Australia, and New Zealand have lower prevalence with the lowest prevalence occurring in Asia, the Middle East, and Africa. Such variation calls into question the possibility that ethnicity might be linked to the continental differences seen (Koch-Henriksen and Sorensen, 2010).

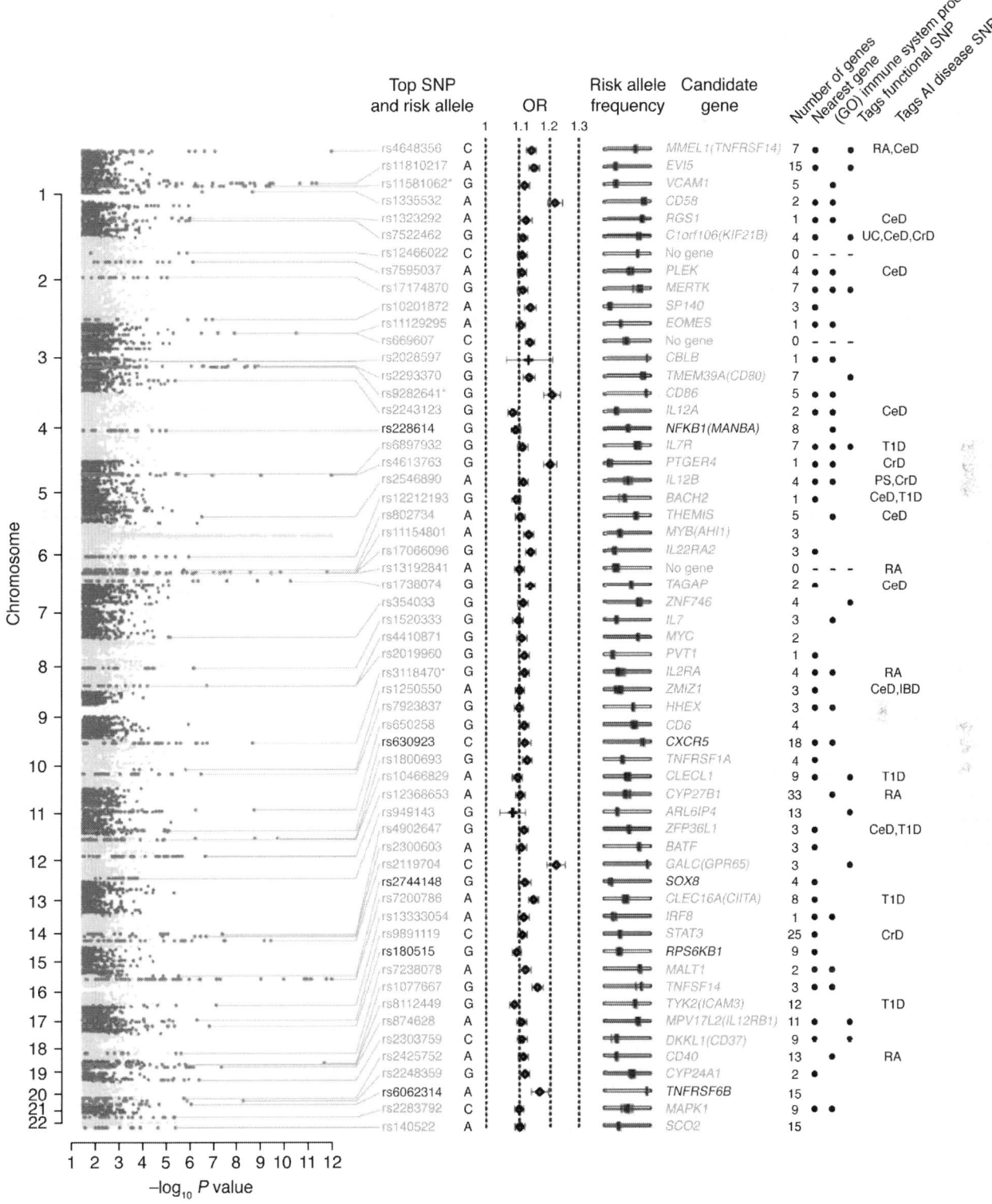

FIGURE 52.1 Regions of genome showing association to MS. Genome regions showing association with MS. Evidence for association from linear mixed model analysis of the discovery data (threshold at a −log10 P value of 12) is shown at left. Non-MHC regions containing associated SNPs are indicated in red and labeled with the rs number (green text for newly identified loci, black text for loci with strong evidence of association, and gray text for previously reported loci) and risk allele of the most significant SNP. Asterisks indicate that the locus contains a secondary SNP signal.

(Continued)

The study of latitudinal differences has demonstrated only modest effect in Europe and North America, but none within Western Europe (Lauer, 1995; Weinshenker, 1996). The only clear trend of increased incidence can be attributed to the Southern Hemisphere where the majority of studies have come from New Zealand and Australia (Skegg et al., 1987; Mcleod et al., 1994). Descendants living New Zealand and Australia have a lower risk of MS than those descendants living in the UK. These studies are rather compelling because the populations in New Zealand and Australia are relatively homogeneous due to similar British ancestry. This general distribution likely reflects a combination of genetic and environmental influences particularly with respect to exposure to sunlight (Ebers, 2008).

Relatedly, environmental deficiencies have long been associated with MS, as indicated by the inverse correlation of the world prevalence of MS and environmental supply of vitamin D. Vitamin D may be supplied from the environment via sunlight exposure or via dietary intake of vitamin D3 (Vanamerongen et al., 2004; Ascherio et al., 2010). At higher latitudes, the exposure to sunlight is insufficient to produce vitamin D given the lower exposure to the sun in winter months. Vitamin D and its immunomodulatory effect has been established both in response to sunlight and in dietary vitamin D(3) intake (Smolders et al., 2008; Kragt et al., 2009). Subtle defects in vitamin D metabolism have suggested a possible genetic origin. Identification of a highly conserved vitamin D responsive element in the promoter region of the HLA-DRB*1501 haplotype has sparked ongoing debate as to whether HLA-DRB*1501 might be involved in the response to vitamin D particularly since studies suggest that the beneficial effect of vitamin D on MS may in fact be attenuated in those with the risk allele (Ramagopalan et al., 2009; Simon et al., 2011). Nevertheless, few genetic determinants have been identified.

Epstein—Barr virus (EBV) infection has been linked to MS risk since exposure to EBV is associated with 1.5 times greater risk of developing MS. Over 99% of individuals with MS have evidence of prior infection with EBV in comparison to 90% in humans overall (Bagert, 2009). However, the role of EBV in the development of MS is not known. EBV generally infects resting B lymphocytes transforming them into memory cells that survive long-term largely undetected by the immune system (Thorley-Lawson and Gross, 2004). Interestingly, serostatus in individuals with MS has demonstrated elevated titers to EBV prior to the development of any neurologic sequelae (Thacker et al., 2006). It has been suggested that EBV may play a role in the pathogenesis of MS since postmortem analysis of brains from patients with MS have demonstrated diffuse EBV-association B cell dysregulation among the varying types of MS (Serafini et al., 2004). However, these results have been challenged due to the inability to unequivocally identify EBV infection in pathological tissues, particularly in respect to clinical scenarios unrelated to EBV-driven lymphomas or acute EBV infections. Such difficulties may be linked to differences in sensitivity and specificity of the detection methods utilized (Lassmann et al., 2011).

IMMUNE PATHOGENESIS

Until recently, there were discussions as to whether MS is a primary degenerative disease with secondary inflammation or an autoimmune disease with immune-mediated destruction of the CNS. The sharing of almost half of the allelic variants between MS and other autoimmune disorders from the GWAS has to a large extent provided convincing evidence for an autoimmune pathophysiology for the disease (Hafler, 2012). Our current understanding of MS strongly implicates involvement of the immune system and autoreactive proinflammatory T cells that are critical to the propagation of CNS tissue injury. Elucidating the mechanism of disease initiation and how it contributes to the transition from physiologic immunosurveillance to pathologic cascade continues to be an area of ongoing investigation. Our foundation is based on the understanding that peripherally activated cross-reactive T cells migrate into the CNS of genetically susceptible hosts and mount proinflammatory responses to myelin epitopes. Myelin-reactive T cells appear to be both increased in frequency and activation state in individuals with MS (Raddassi et al., 2011), suggesting a peripheral breach of tolerance to CNS antigen. However, the presence of autoreactive cells in the periphery is an insufficient explanation for the development of autoimmune disease given that myelin-reactive T cells can be found in the peripheral blood of both healthy individuals and patients with MS.

◀ Odds ratios (ORs; diamonds) and 95% confidence intervals (whiskers) are estimated from a meta-analysis of discovery and replication data (+ indicates estimates for previously known loci from discovery data only). Risk allele frequency estimates in the control populations are indicated by vertical bars (scale of 0 to 1, left to right). A candidate gene and the number of genes are reported for each region of association. Black dots indicate that the candidate gene is physically the nearest gene included in the GO immune system process term. "Tags functional SNP" indicates whether the most-significant SNP tags a SNP predicted to affect the function of the candidate gene. Where such an SNP exists, the gene is selected as the candidate gene; otherwise, the nearest gene is selected unless there are strong biological reasons for a different choice. The final column indicates whether SNPs are correlated ($r2 > 0.1$) with SNPs associated with other autoimmune diseases. CeD, celiac disease; CrD, Crohn's disease; PS, psoriasis; RA, rheumatoid arthritis; T1D, type 1 diabetes; UC, ulcerative colitis. *Reproduced with permission from Nature (Sawcer et al., 2011).*

T Cell Pathogenesis

Upon interaction of the T cell with the antigen-presenting cell (APC), the antigen-specific T cells proliferate and divide into subsets (see Figure 52.2). Of specific interest to MS are the Th1, Th2, Th17, and regulatory T cell subsets. T cells have been classified according to the cytokine profiles that they produce upon activation (Abbas et al., 1996; O'Garra, 1998; O'Shea and Paul, 2010). MHC class II restricted CD4+ T cells, producing IFN-γ, IL-2, lymphotoxin (LT), and TNF-α, have been defined as Th1 (inflammatory) cells, and have demonstrated pathogenicity in EAE models (Leonard et al., 1995; Segal et al., 1998;

Severson and Hafler, 2010). The Th1 cytokines activate macrophages for cellular immunity with the assistance of IgG1 secreted by B cells. In contrast, CD4+ T cells producing IL-4, IL-5, IL-10, or IL-13 have been termed Th2 (anti-inflammatory) cells, and have demonstrated a protective role in EAE (Khoury et al., 1992; Owens et al., 1994; Begolka et al., 1998; Antel and Owens, 1999). Th2 cytokines promote humoral immune responses alongside IgG4. Th17 cells are thought to be proinflammatory in nature and secrete the cytokines IL-17A, IL-17F, IL-21, and IL-22, which have been strongly implicated in the pathogenesis of autoimmune diseases (Harrington et al., 2005). Regulatory T cells (Tregs) are a subset of T cells that are

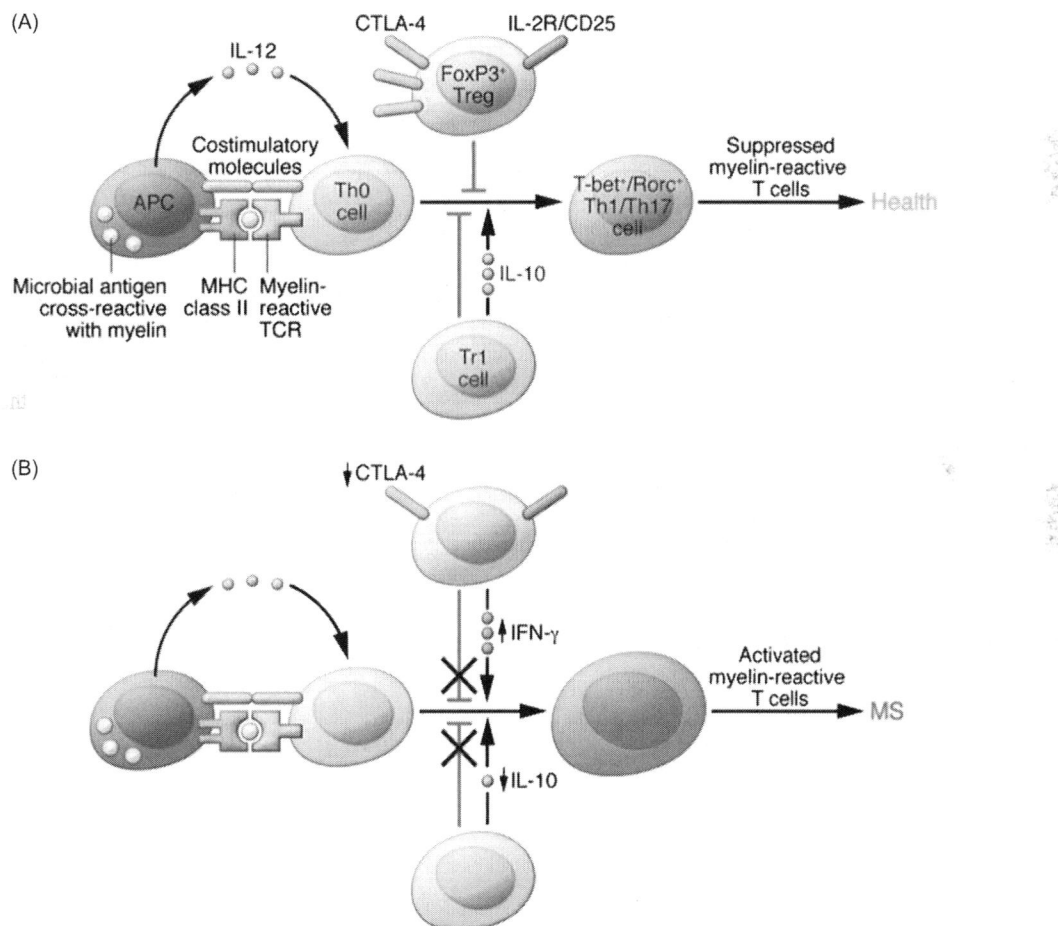

FIGURE 52.2 **Pathophysiology of MS.** Defects in peripheral immune regulation lower the activation barrier for autoreactive T cells. (A) In normal homeostasis, APCs digest microbial antigens or self proteins and present them to naïve T cells in the context of costimulatory molecules. An appropriate cytokine milieu can drive differentiation of these naïve autoreactive T cells to a Th1 or Th17 cell phenotype; however, these potentially pathogenic T cells are not activated due to the actions of peripheral regulatory immune cell populations, such as FoxP3+ Tregs and Tr1 cells. Via the actions of co-inhibitory molecules and cytokines such as IL-10 and TGF-β, autoreactive T cells become anergic and autoimmune disease is prevented. Other mechanisms, such as thymic deletion and lack of costimulatory molecules on APCs, are also involved in controlling autoreactive T cells. (B) MS patients have defects in peripheral immune regulation, including higher expression of costimulatory molecules on APCs, lower CTLA-4 levels, and lower IL-10 production. Additionally, MS patients have an increased frequency of IFN-γ-secreting Tregs relative to healthy controls. Thus, the barrier for activation of autoreactive T cells is lowered for MS patients. Activated myelin-reactive T cells can then adhere to and extravasate across the choroid plexus and BBB, where they can initiate an inflammatory milieu that gives license to further waves of inflammation and eventual epitope spreading. *Reproduced with permission from the Journal of Clinical Investigation (Nylander and Hafler, 2012).*

involved in the regulation of the immune system, maintenance of tolerance to self-antigens, and surveillance of autoimmune disease. They can secrete a variety of cytokines including, TGF-β, IL-10, and IFN-γ in addition to utilizing FoxP3 as a transcription factor (Fontenot et al., 2003; Hori et al., 2003). Current work involving Tregs has linked this subset with immune dysregulation, a concept which will be discussed later.

Several lines of evidence support the hypothesis that Th1 cells may be pathogenic in MS. Th1 and Th2 cells express distinct profiles of chemokine receptors, including CXCR3/CCR5 and CCR3/CCR4, respectively (Bonecchi et al., 2009). An increased proportion of T cells from MS patients was shown to express the characteristic Th1 chemokine receptor pattern and MS plaques were found to express increased levels of the corresponding chemokine (Siveke and Hamann, 1998; Balashov et al., 1999; Sorensen et al., 1999). Analysis of cytokine mRNA in CSF from MS patients showed a bias towards Th1 cytokines (Blain et al., 1994). Immunohistochemical studies of MS plaques *in situ* have demonstrated the presence of the proinflammatory cytokines TNF-α and IL-12 (Hofman et al., 1989; Selmaj et al., 1991; Windhagen et al., 1995). Markedly, MBP-reactive T cells derived from patients with MS secrete cytokines that are more consistent with Th1-mediated response, whereas MBP-reactive T cells from healthy individuals are more likely to produce cytokines that characterize a Th2-mediated response (Crawford et al., 2004). Interventions that shift or deviate the cytokine responses away from a Th1 and towards a Th2 profile have been deemed favorable.

Despite the prior suggestion that Th1 cells are unique in driving the inflammatory response, recent work has characterized the putative role of proinflammatory Th17 cells in establishing the MS phenotype. Studies implicate pathogenic Th17 cells in gaining early access to the CNS (Steinman, 2007; Reboldi et al., 2009). Entry to the CNS is mediated via the choroid plexus, which, in addition to producing CSF, spans the blood−CSF barrier and facilitates immune surveillance. The Th17 mechanism implicates the CCR6/CCL20 axis in disease initiation as defined in the EAE model, with Th17 cells expressing CCR6 and choroid plexus endothelial cells expressing CCL20. In applying this information to human disease, it is likely that peripherally activated Th17 cells are able to bind to adhesion molecules and chemokine receptors expressed on the choroid plexus thereby migrating across the blood − CSF barrier and gaining access to circulating CSF. Dysregulated Th17 cells are subsequently able to access perivascular tissue, initiating a cascade of proinflammatory events. Th17 cells secrete IL-23, which, in EAE models, alongside the transcription factor RORγt, promotes production of GM-CSF. This induces a positive feedback loop where further secretion of IL-23 occurs

and is implicated in the encephalogenicity and incidence of axoglial damage (Codarri et al., 2011; El-Behi et al., 2011). In relating Th17 cells to the formation of perivascular infiltrates, it is possible that their secretion of IL-17 and IL-22 may increase blood−brain barrier permeability and thus facilitate the influx of immune cells, such as autoreactive Th17 cells, Th1 (IFN-γ secreting), γδ T cells, cytotoxic CD8$^+$ cells, B cells, and immunoglobulin-secreting plasma cells (Kebir et al., 2007). This leads to the possibility of a two-step process for initiation of MS, one in which Th17 cells prime the entrance of other dysregulated immune cells and therefore creating the appropriate inflammatory environment containing infiltrates of cells that result in downstream damage of the CNS (Nylander and Hafler, 2012).

Immune Dysregulation

In elaborating on the concept of immune dysregulation, GWAS have shed light on the likely involvement of allelic variants in diseases states. A number of these variants involved genes for cytokine receptors and costimulatory molecules and have been associated with defects in Treg homeostasis. Costimulatory molecules have recently been found to function as negative regulators of the immune system. TIM-3 has been implicated in modulating Th1 and Th17 cytokine secretion and loss of TIM-3 functional T cell regulation has been established in MS patients (Koguchi et al., 2006; Yang et al., 2008; Hastings et al., 2009). GWAS studies have linked CD226 to MS risk (Hafler et al., 2009), and recent work has implicated the CD226/TIGIT axis in regulating human T cell function via a mechanism similar to that employed by CD28/CTLA4, in which binding to B7 induces coexpression of inhibitory and excitatory signals that modulate immune responses (Joller et al., 2011; Lozano et al., 2012). Costimulation between CD58/CD2 appears to be implicated in T cell receptor signaling, including activation of Tregs, and has been suggested to provide a protective effect for MS (De Jager et al., 2009a).

Recent studies have indicated that despite normal frequency of Tregs in MS patients, their suppressive ability is compromised and substantially decreased in response to autoreactive T cells in comparison to healthy individuals (Viglietta et al., 2004; Haas et al., 2005). Notably, Tregs have demonstrated great functional plasticity. Their ability to be reprogrammed suggests that Tregs may be able to function as a biomarker in MS (Nylander and Hafler, 2012). In the presence of IL-1β and IL-6, Tregs are able to produce the inflammatory cytokine IL-17, further implicating this subset in autoimmune disease (Koenen et al., 2008; Ayyoub et al., 2009; Beriou et al., 2009). Moreover, the notion of Treg reprogramming has arisen due to the observation that patients with RRMS have the ability to produce IFN-γ-secreting

Tregs, thereby characterizing a Th1-type Treg effector phenotype. This finding was observed *in vitro* under IL-12 stimulation of Tregs and recapitulated in *ex vivo* Tregs derived from patients with untreated RRMS. This role of Th1−Treg effector cells was suggested by the use of IFN-β, a first-line therapy for RRMS, which has been shown to decrease IL-12 levels and normalize the ratio of IFN-γ^+Foxp3$^+$ Tregs to that of healthy controls (Dominguez-Villar et al., 2011). Costimulatory molecules and regulatory T cell plasticity in MS undoubtedly provide fascinating clues into disease pathogenesis.

Autoantigens

Autoantigen-specific T cells have been identified both in healthy individuals and in patients with MS. Their entrance into the inflamed CNS environment is likely mediated by the immune mechanisms posited above, whereupon entering, the autoreactive T cells are able to subsequently contribute to myelin destruction and axonal damage in addition to secondary inflammation following activation by local antigen-presenting cells. Attention has been directed towards uncovering frequencies of autoantigen-specific T cell binding to myelin proteins including MOG, MBP, and proteolipid in addition to heat shock protein αB-crystallin and oligodendroglia-specific enzyme transaldolase in CD4$^+$ cells isolated from MS patients (Banki et al., 1994; Greer and Pender, 2008). Anti-MOG has previously been isolated from postmortem CNS tissue in MS patients (O'Connor et al., 2005). In an assay based on self-assembly of radiolabeled MHC tetramers, it was demonstrated that such tetramers were more sensitive for MOG autoantibody detection. Nevertheless, MOG-specific autoantibodies were found more so in patients with acute disseminated encephalomyelitis, than in adults with MS (O'Connor et al., 2007). Likewise, the ability to detect and clone autoantigen-specific T cells from blood has allowed further quantification of MOG frequencies, work which demonstrated an increase in MOG-specific T cells in MS patients in comparison to healthy individuals (Raddassi et al., 2011).

Despite the inability to identify a putative role for environmental triggers, infectious factors, or microbial antigens in establishing MS risk, studies have suggested potential cross-reactivity between epitopes with microbial antigens. Finally, regardless of what antigen event initiates the self-reactive cascade, epitope spreading is likely to contribute to an array of activated immune cells that can respond to multiple antigens. Nevertheless, no single antigen has been clearly implicated in the pathogenesis of MS.

Meningeal Ectopic B Cell Follicles

Given the marked presence of OCBs and increased levels of IgG within the CSF of individuals diagnosed with MS

in addition to the ongoing debate underlying the increased incidence of EBV and its ability to prime the immune system in individuals with MS, the notion of B cell involvement has received great attention in playing a crucial role in MS pathogenesis. There appears to be great connectivity between the cell population in the CNS and CSF since clonally expanded B cells and plasmablast clones have been associated with the observed intrathecal immunoglobulin production (Lovato et al., 2011; Obermeier et al., 2011). Recently published work indicates that related B cell clones populate the meninges, leading to the hypothesis that these aggregate structures can be related to the B cell infiltrates found in MS lesions (Lovato et al., 2011). Likewise, ectopic lymphoid follicles, strongly resembling germinal centers, have been identified in the meninges of SPMS patients (Serafini et al., 2004). These follicles contain proliferating B cells, plasma cells, T cells, and dendritic cells with the corresponding diffuse meningeal inflammation being suggested to play a role in the manifestation of cerebral cortical gray matter pathology in MS. Follicles have been located more frequently in the deep sulci of the temporal cingulate, insula, and frontal cortex (Howell et al., 2011). Apart from being associated with cortical pathology, studies have implicated that meningeal B cell follicles can be associated with early onset of disease in patients with SPMS (Magliozzi et al., 2007). Overall, such humoral activation within ectopic lymph tissue and CSF has been postulated to play an imperative role in disease progression secondary to the ongoing persistence of antigens driving a constitutive inflammatory and humoral response.

TREATMENT

Therapeutic approaches in MS may be broadly divided into treatments that are symptomatic and/or supportive in nature, and treatments that are directed at the underlying pathophysiology of the disorder. There are currently nine agents approved by the United States Food and Drug Administration (FDA) (see Table 52.1 for comparison of FDA-approved therapies) as disease-modifying therapies (DMT). They are expensive, with 10-year disease-related costs averaging US$467,712 for patients on a single disease modifying therapy (DMT) (Noyes et al., 2011). The vast majority of these DMTs have been studied in RRMS and CIS, and approved for such use, whereas the progressive forms of MS do not respond to immunotherapies. Their current use has marked a milestone for patient care. Understanding pharmacologic mechanisms of action in a number of MS DMTs has led to significant advancement in elucidating MS pathogenesis. The growing number of therapies being studied for the treatment of MS in addition to the advent of oral therapy indicates great promise for the future.

TABLE 52.1 FDA Approved Therapies for MS

	Brand name	Indications	Results	Mechanism of action
IFN-β1a (IM weekly)	Avonex®	• Treatment of RRMS	• Reduction of relapses by one-third • Reduction of new MRI T2 lesions and the volume of enlarging T2 lesions • Reduction in the number and volume of Gd-enhancing lesions • Slowing of brain atropy	• Acts on blood–brain barrier by interfering with T cell adhesion to the endothelium by binding VLA-4 on T cells or by inhibiting the T cell expression of MMP Reduction in T cell activation by interfering with HLA class II and costimulatory molecules B7/CD28 and CD40: CD40L • Immune deviation of Th2 over Th1 cytokine profile • Normalizing ratio of IFN-γ^+ Foxp3$^+$ Tregs
IFN-β1a (SC three times weekly)	Rebif®	• Treatment of RRMS	• Same as IFN-β1a	• Same as IFN-β1a
IFN-β1b (SC every other day)	Betaseron®, Extavia®	• Treatment of RRMS	• Same as IFN-β1a	• Same as IFN-β1a
Glatiramer acetate (SC daily)	Copaxone®	• Treatment of RRMS	• Reduction of relapses by one-third • Reduction of 57% in the number and volume of Gd-enhancing lesions	• Induces cytokine shift from one that is proinflammatory to one that is anti-inflammatory and regulatory in nature
Natalizumab (IV monthly infusion)	Tysabri®	• Treatment of RRMS	• Reduced rate of relapse up to 68% and the development of new MRI lesions	• Monoclonal antibody that blocks alpha 4-integrin on surface T cells preventing them from crossing the blood–brain barrier
Mitoxantrone (IV infusions every 3 months)	Novantrone®	• Worsening forms of RRMS • SPMS	• Reduction in relapses by 67% • Slowed progression on EDSS, ambulation index and MRI disease activity	• Anti-neoplastic that intercalates DNA • Suppresses cellular and humoral immune response
Fingolimod (given orally once a day)	Gilenya®	• Treatment of RRMS	• Reduction of 54% in risk of relapse • Lower risk of disability progression by 30%	• S1P agonist, causing internalization of S1P$_1$ receptors on lymph-node T cells • Subsequent decrease in migration of activation lymphocytes into circulation
Teriflunomide (given orally once a day)	Aubagio®	• Treatment of RRMS	• Reduction of 36% in risk of relapse • Lower risk of disability progression by 31%	• Inhibits *de novo* nucleotide synthesis • Decreases T cell and B cell proliferation • Interrupts T cell and APC interactions • Subsequently possesses anti-inflammatory properties
BG-12, dimethyl fumarate (given orally twice a day)	Tecfidera®	• Treatment of RRMS	• Reduction of 49% in risk of relapse • Lower risk of disability progression by 38%	• Inhibits immune cells and molecules • Decreases myelin damage in the CNS • Exhibits anti-oxidant properties that may be protective against damage to the brain and spinal cord

Interferons

Compared to placebo-treated RRMS controls, treatment with alternate-day subcutaneous injections of eight million units of IFN-β1b (Betaseron®) was shown to decrease the primary efficacy outcome measure of frequency of relapses by 34% after 2 years (The IFNB Multiple Sclerosis Study Group, 1993). A significant decrease in the accumulation of MRI lesions was observed with treatment (Paty and Li, 1993) and 5-year follow-up data reported that disease progression in the IFN-β1b treated group was 35%, compared with 46% progression in the placebo group (IFNB Multiple Sclerosis Study Group, 1995). A 30% decrease in the annual exacerbation rate in the treated group was maintained. IFN-β1a (Avonex®, weekly IM injections), a glycosylated recombinant beta-interferon, was evaluated in a 2-year study of weekly intramuscular injections of six million units (30 μg). The proportion of patients progressing by the end of the trial was 21.9% in the treated group compared to 34.9% in the placebo group. The annual exacerbation rate was decreased by 32% in the treated group versus the placebo group. Treatment was also associated with a 40% reduction in mean MRI lesion load (Jacobs et al., 1995, 1996). Clinical and MRI benefit of IFN-β1a (Rebif®, subcutaneous, three times weekly) doses for up to 4 years was demonstrated in PRISMS-4, thereby suggesting that early treatment with IFN-β1a was of increased benefit to patients with RRMS as compared with those treated later in disease course (PRISMS, 2001).

β-Interferon therapy utilizes recombinant forms of naturally occurring cytokines intrinsically possessing a wide range of properties. The mechanism of action involving β-interferons appears to be quite complex with the DMT exerting its effects on the pathophysiology of MS at several sites. Studies have suggested that β-interferons inhibit the migration of activated inflammatory cells across the blood–brain barrier (BBB) and into the CNS parenchyma through decreasing the function of the vascular cell adhesion molecule-1/very late activation antigen-4 cell adhesion axis (see Natalizumab (Tysabri®), below). IFN-β may potentially intercept inflammatory cell adhesion and subsequent migration across the BBB (Calabresi et al., 1997; Graber et al., 2005). The rapid effect of β-interferons on the gadolinium enhancing lesions of MS represents a biological marker of treatment response and establishes the BBB as an important site of action of β-inteferon therapy (Stone et al., 1997).

Studies have also suggested that the β-interferons may exert their pharmacologic effects by shifting cytokines and immune cell profiles in MS patients towards one that is anti-inflammatory and protective (Brod et al., 1996). IFN-β has also demonstrated ability to upregulate expression of costimulatory molecules needed for antigen presentation (CD80, CD86, and CD40) on monocytes, thus decreasing the generation of autoreactive T cells and limiting T cell activation. As addressed earlier, IFN-β has been implicated in normalizing the ratio of IFN-γ^+ Foxp3$^+$ Tregs to that of healthy controls and in decreasing IL-12 levels, thereby potentially restoring the ability of Tregs to regulate immune cells (Dominguez-Villar et al., 2011).

Glatiramer Acetate (Copaxone®)

Glatiramer acetate is the major noninterferon DMT used in the treatment of MS. Treatment with glatiramer acetate/copolymer 1 (Copaxone, GA, subcutaneous, daily) was associated with a 2-year relapse rate reduction of 29% compared to placebo control (Johnson et al., 1995). The clinical benefit of GA for relapse rate in comparison to placebo was sustained following an 11-month extension period utilizing the same study design (Johnson et al., 1998). Subsequent studies revealed a beneficial effect of GA in MRI with a 35% reduction in total gadolinium-enhancing lesions and 57% reduction in new gadolinium-enhancing lesions, with an overall decrease in T2 disease burden (Mancardi et al., 1998; Comi et al., 2001).

GA is a random sequence polypeptide of the four amino acids alanine (A), lysine (K), glutamate (E), and tyrosine (Y). As a sequence of amino acids, GA has been proposed to function as a T cell receptor antagonist to MBP/MHC at MBP-specific T cell receptors and operate as an altered peptide ligand to the MBP (Aharoni et al., 1999; Duda et al., 2000). Thus, research suggests that GA elicits its effect on the immune system by inducing deviation of cytokine production in response to MBP from Th1 cytokines to Th2 cytokines, a change that is characterized by increased secretion of anti-inflammatory cytokines, with prolonged GA treatment leading to a Th2 bias in MS patients (Miller et al., 1998; Duda et al., 2000; Gran et al., 2000; Neuhaus et al., 2000; Valenzuela et al., 2007;). Additionally, GA has been implicated in altering the cytokine profile to one that is more consistent with a regulatory population (Hong et al., 2005). Furthermore, increases in FoxP3$^+$ expression in Tregs have been demonstrated following GA, also supporting theories that GA facilitates a regulatory population (Hong et al., 2005).

Natalizumab (Tysabri®)

Natalizumab is a monoclonal antibody to the very late activation antigen (VLA-4), the α4β7 integrin expressed on activated T cells and monocytes, and is the ligand for vascular cell adhesion molecule (VCAM) expressed on CNS endothelial cells. Natalizumab, by preventing adhesion of activated T cells to endothelial cells, has been able to decrease influx of potentially autoreactive T cells into perivascular tissue. Natalizumab-treated patients have developed cases of progressive multifocal leukoencephalopathy, a rare and fatal disease caused by JC virus and characterized by progressive inflammatory damage of CNS white matter. This prompted both its manufacturer and the FDA to review its utility in treating MS. Regardless, its clinical benefits have been deemed to outweigh the risks involved. Its use has been restricted to individuals with highly active disease. Two trials involving RRMS patients have demonstrated interesting clinical results. The AFFIRM study compared natalizumab alone to placebo and the SENTINEL study looked at adding natalizumab to ongoing IFN-β1a therapy. The AFFIRM trial demonstrated a 42% reduced risk of sustained progression of disability, a 68% reduction in rate of clinical relapse at 1 year, and an 83% reduction in accumulation of new or enlarging hyperintense lesions over 2 years (Polman et al., 2006). Results of the SENTINEL trial were similar to those of AFFIRM with the exception of a 64% decreased risk of sustained disability progression with natalizumab (Calabresi et al., 2007; Hutchinson et al., 2009).

Mitoxantrone (Novantrone®)

Mitoxantrone, a small molecule chemotherapeutic agent able to cross the blood–brain barrier, functions as a type II topoisomerase inhibitor, which disrupts DNA synthesis and DNA repair, both events which function in an immunosuppressant capacity thereby inhibiting T cell, B cell, and macrophage proliferation. Overall, this leads to enhanced T cell suppressor function, inhibition of B cell function and antibody production, decreased secretion of proinflammatory cytokines, and inhibition of macrophage-mediated myelin degradation (Fox, 2004). Mitoxantrone, administered intravenously, has been approved by the FDA as treatment for patients with worsening forms of MS including SPMS, worsening RRMS, and PRMS. The MIMS trial indicated a 44% reduction in time to first relapse; a 24% decrease in the expanded disability status scale, however, did not demonstrate a positive impact on MRI disease burden (Hartung et al., 2002; Krapf et al., 2005). Due to concerns related to increased incidence of systolic dysfunction and therapy-related acute leukemia, its use remains relatively limited (Marriott et al., 2010).

Fingolimod (Gilenya®)

Fingolimod's pharmacologic activity is targeted towards lymphocyte migration out of lymph nodes. This action is highly dependent on the engagement of a G-protein-coupled receptor, $S1P_1$, present on the surface of the lymphocytes. Fingolimod is structurally similar to S1P and can function as an agonist by engaging four of the five known S1P receptors ($S1P_1$, $S1P_3$, $S1P_4$, $S1P_5$). This leads to a reduction in activated T cells that are able to exit the lymph node and subsequently cross the blood–brain barrier to exert their potential pathogenic effects on perivascular tissue (Schwab and Cyster, 2007; Pham et al., 2008). Studies have indicated the potential for S1P receptors to be present on other cells, including neurons, microglial cells, oligodendrocytes, and astrocytes, suggesting a putative role for fingolimod in influencing myelin repair, modulating survival of oligodendrocyte progenitor cells, and directing astrocyte migration and proliferation (Yamagata et al., 2003; Miron et al., 2008, 2010).

In September 2010 fingolimod became the first FDA-approved first-line oral agent for the treatment of MS. The FREEDOMS trial demonstrated, after 2 years, an overall 54% decreased risk of relapse in the group treated with fingolimod versus those taking placebo. The risk of disability progression was 30% lower in patients receiving the lower dose (0.5 mg) as opposed to placebo. With regard to MRI disease burden, those taking fingolimod presented with fewer new lesions and less brain tissue atrophy. The TRANSFORMS trial aimed at characterizing the efficacy of fingolimod versus intramuscular IFN-β1a (Avonex®). The group taking fingolimod had a 52% lower risk of having a relapse than those taking IFN-β1a, with 82.5% of the fingolimod group and 70% of IFN-β1a presenting with no relapses during the 1-year study period. Furthermore the group taking fingolimod had fewer signs of MRI disease burden. There was no difference among the groups in the risk of disease progression (Cohen et al., 2010). Although the arrival of fingolimod has been met with great enthusiasm, the lack of clarity surrounding long-term safety has led to caution as to its utility as a first-line agent.

Teriflunomide (Aubagio®)

Teriflunomide is the active metabolite of leflunomide, an approved therapy for rheumatoid arthritis. It inhibits *de novo* pyrimidine nucleotide synthesis and therefore potently decreases T cell and B cell proliferation (Hartung et al., 2010). Reports also indicate that teriflunomide may interrupt T cell and APC interactions in addition to possessing anti-inflammatory properties (Zeyda et al., 2005; Gold and Wolinsky, 2011). The TEMSO trial demonstrated a 31% reduction in annual relapse rate, a 21% reduction in disability progression, and a 76% reduction in number of new or enlarging T2 lesions on MRI in the higher dose cohort (O'Connor et al., 2011). Teriflunomide was approved by the FDA in September 2012 for patients with RRMS.

Dimethyl Fumarate, BG-12 (Tecfidera®)

BG-12 is an oral formulation of fumaric acid, which is metabolized to monomethyl fumarate. It was approved a second-line agent in 2013. Other oral formulations of fumaric acid have previously been used to treat psoriasis. Both dimethyl fumarate and the active metabolite induce activation of the nuclear factor E2-related factor-2 pathway, which exerts neuroprotective effects and decreases myelin damage in the CNS (Kappos et al., 2008; Fontoura and Garren, 2010; Linker et al., 2011). Anti-inflammatory mechanisms have also been attributed to dimethyl fumarate (Gold, 2011). The DEFINE trial was completed in 2011. As a randomized, double-blind, placebo-controlled phase III study, patients with RRMS were assigned to receive either oral BG-12 at a dose of 240 mg twice or thrice daily, or placebo. The primary end-point was the proportion of patients who had a relapse 2 years later in addition to disability progression and MRI disease burden. The study demonstrated positive results with a significant reduction in relapse rate (27% with BG-12 twice daily and 26% with BG-12 thrice daily vs. 46% with placebo), in the rate of disability progression, in the number of new or enlarging T2 lesions, and in new gadolinium-enhancing lesions (Gold et al., 2012). The CONFIRM trial was also completed in 2011. A phase III, randomized study, it aimed to ascertain the efficacy and safety of BG-12 at a dose of 240 twice or thrice daily in comparison to both placebo and glatiramer acetate in patients with RRMS. Similarly to the DEFINE trial, both BG-12 and glatiramer acetate significantly reduced relapse rates and MRI disease burden in relation to the placebo group (Fox et al., 2012). In early 2013, BG-12 was approved as a first-line therapy for adults with RRMS.

CONCLUDING REMARKS

Over the past decade, major strides have been made in our understanding of the immunopathogenesis underlying the development and course of MS, an autoimmune disease that predominantly impacts the CNS by way of white matter damage and demyelination of neurons thought to be primarily driven by T cell dysregulation, inflammation, and immune dysfunction. Nevertheless, our ever-growing fund of knowledge continues to inspire future directions. Novel insights are providing hints for future prospects related to early cortical demyelination, gray matter pathology, imaging, and B cell involvement in MS further establishing this disease as a multifocal entity. Overall, our increasing knowledge pertaining to MS continues to be multifactorial. The ability for clinicians and researchers to utilize our understanding of the immunopathogenesis in relation to known pharmacologic mechanisms, clinical findings, and imaging modalities will be paramount in taking the necessary steps towards eradicating MS.

REFERENCES

Abbas, A.K., Murphy, K.M., Sher, A., 1996. Functional diversity of helper T lymphocytes. Nature. 383, 787–793.

Achiron, A., Barak, Y., 2000. Multiple sclerosis-from probable to definite diagnosis: a 7-year prospective study. Arch. Neurol. 57, 974–979.

Aharoni, R., Teitelbaum, D., Arnon, R., Sela, M., 1999. Copolymer 1 acts against the immunodominant epitope 82-100 of myelin basic protein by T cell receptor antagonism in addition to major histocompatibility complex blocking. Proc. Natl. Acad. Sci. U.S.A. 96, 634–639.

Amato, M.P., Bartolozzi, M.L., Zipoli, V., Portaccio, E., Mortilla, M., Guidi, L., et al., 2004. Neocortical volume decrease in relapsing-remitting MS patients with mild cognitive impairment. Neurology. 63, 89–93.

Antel, J.P., Owens, T., 1999. Immune regulation and CNS autoimmune disease. J. Neuroimmunol. 100, 181–189.

Arnason, B.G., 1993. Interferon beta in multiple sclerosis. Neurology. 43, 641–643.

Ascherio, A., Munger, K.L., Simon, K.C., 2010. Vitamin D and multiple sclerosis. Lancet Neurol. 9, 599–612.

Aulchenko, Y.S., Hoppenbrouwers, I.A., Ramagopalan, S.V., Broer, L., Jafari, N., Hillert, J., et al., 2008. Genetic variation in the KIF1B locus influences susceptibility to multiple sclerosis. Nat. Genet. 40, 1402–1403.

Australia and New Zealand Multiple Sclerosis Genetics Consortium, 2009. Genome-wide association study identifies new multiple sclerosis susceptibility loci on chromosomes 12 and 20. Nat. Genet. 41, 824–828.

Ayyoub, M., Deknuydt, F., Raimbaud, I., Dousset, C., Leveque, L., Bioley, G., et al., 2009. Human memory FOXP3 + Tregs secrete IL-17 ex vivo and constitutively express the T(H)17 lineage-specific transcription factor RORgamma t. Proc. Natl. Acad. Sci. U.S.A. 106, 8635–8640.

Babbe, H., Roers, A., Waisman, A., Lassmann, H., Goebels, N., Hohlfeld, R., et al., 2000. Clonal expansions of CD8(+) T cells dominate the T cell infiltrate in active multiple sclerosis lesions as shown by micromanipulation and single cell polymerase chain reaction. J. Exp. Med. 192, 393–404.

Bagert, B.A., 2009. Epstein-Barr virus in multiple sclerosis. Curr. Neurol. Neurosci. Rep. 9, 405–410.

Balashov, K.E., Rottman, J.B., Weiner, H.L., Hancock, W.W., 1999. CCR5(+) and CXCR3(+) T cells are increased in multiple sclerosis and their ligands MIP-1alpha and IP-10 are expressed in demyelinating brain lesions. Proc. Natl. Acad. Sci. U.S.A. 96, 6873–6878.

Banki, K., Colombo, E., Sia, F., Halladay, D., Mattson, D.H., Tatum, A.H., et al., 1994. Oligodendrocyte-specific expression and auto-antigenicity of transaldolase in multiple sclerosis. J. Exp. Med. 180, 1649–1663.

Baranzini, S.E., Wang, J., Gibson, R.A., Galwey, N., Naegelin, Y., Barkhof, F., et al., 2009. Genome-wide association analysis of susceptibility and clinical phenotype in multiple sclerosis. Hum. Mol. Genet. 18, 767–778.

Bates, D., 2011. Treatment effects of immunomodulatory therapies at different stages of multiple sclerosis in short-term trials. Neurology. 76, S14–S25.

Beebe, G.W., Kurtzke, J.F., Kurland, L.T., Auth, T.L., Nagler, B., 1967. Studies on the natural history of multiple sclerosis. 3. Epidemiologic analysis of the army experience in World War II. Neurology. 17, 1–17.

Begolka, W.S., Vanderlugt, C.L., Rahbe, S.M., Miller, S.D., 1998. Differential expression of inflammatory cytokines parallels progression of central nervous system pathology in two clinically distinct models of multiple sclerosis. J. Immunol. 161, 4437–4446.

Behan, P.B., 1982. Sir Robert Carswell: Scotland's Pioneer Pathologist. Raven Press, New York.

Berger, T., Rubner, P., Schautzer, F., Egg, R., Ulmer, H., Mayringer, I., et al., 2003. Antimyelin antibodies as a predictor of clinically definite multiple sclerosis after a first demyelinating event. N. Engl. J. Med. 349, 139–145.

Beriou, G., Costantino, C.M., Ashley, C.W., Yang, L., Kuchroo, V.K., Baecher-Allan, C., et al., 2009. IL-17-producing human peripheral regulatory T cells retain suppressive function. Blood. 113, 4240–4249.

Betts, C.D., D'Mellow, M.T., Fowler, C.J., 1993. Urinary symptoms and the neurological features of bladder dysfunction in multiple sclerosis. J. Neurol. Neurosurg. Psychiatry. 56, 245–250.

Bitsch, A., Schuchardt, J., Bunkowski, S., Kuhlmann, T., Bruck, W., 2000. Acute axonal injury in multiple sclerosis. Correlation with demyelination and inflammation. Brain. 123 (Pt 6), 1174–1183.

Blain, M., Nalbantoglu, J., Antel, J., 1994. Interferon-gamma mRNA expression in immediately ex-vivo CSF T cells. J. Neuroimmunol. 54, 149 (abstract).

Bonecchi, R., Galliera, E., Borroni, E.M., Corsi, M.M., Locati, M., Mantovani, A., 2009. Chemokines and chemokine receptors: an overview. Front. Biosci. 14, 540–551.

Booss, J., Esiri, M.M., Tourtellotte, W.W., Mason, D.Y., 1983. Immunohistological analysis of T lymphocyte subsets in the central nervous system in chronic progressive multiple sclerosis. J. Neurol. Sci. 62, 219–232.

Brod, S.A., Marshall Jr., G.D., Henninger, E.M., Sriram, S., Khan, M., Wolinsky, J.S., 1996. Interferon-beta 1b treatment decreases tumor necrosis factor-alpha and increases interleukin-6 production in multiple sclerosis. Neurology. 46, 1633–1638.

Brynedal, B., Duvefelt, K., Jonasdottir, G., Roos, I.M., Akesson, E., Palmgren, J., et al., 2007. HLA-A confers an HLA-DRB1 independent influence on the risk of multiple sclerosis. PLoS One. 2, e664.

Calabrese, M., Agosta, F., Rinaldi, F., Mattisi, I., Grossi, P., Favaretto, A., et al., 2009. Cortical lesions and atrophy associated with cognitive impairment in relapsing-remitting multiple sclerosis. Arch. Neurol. 66, 1144–1150.

Calabresi, P.A., Giovannoni, G., Confavreux, C., Galetta, S.L., Havrdova, E., Hutchinson, M., et al., 2007. The incidence and significance of anti-natalizumab antibodies: results from AFFIRM and SENTINEL. Neurology. 69, 1391–1403.

Calabresi, P.A., Pelfrey, C.M., Tranquill, L.R., Maloni, H., Mcfarland, H.F., 1997. VLA-4 expression on peripheral blood lymphocytes is downregulated after treatment of multiple sclerosis with interferon beta. Neurology. 49, 1111–1116.

Charcot, J. 1868a. RE: Comptes rendus des seances et memoires lus a la societe de Biolgie. Mars 14.

Charcot, J., 1868b. Histologic de la sclerose en plaque. Gazette. Hopitaux. 41, 554–566.

Charcot, J., 1877. Lectures on the Diseases of the Nervous System. The New Sydenham Society, London.

Codarri, L., Gyulveszi, G., Tosevski, V., Hesske, L., Fontana, A., Magnenat, L., et al., 2011. RORgammat drives production of the cytokine GM-CSF in helper T cells, which is essential for the effector phase of autoimmune neuroinflammation. Nat. Immunol. 12, 560–567.

Cohen, J.A., Barkhof, F., Comi, G., Hartung, H.P., Khatri, B.O., Montalban, X., et al., 2010. Oral fingolimod or intramuscular interferon for relapsing multiple sclerosis. N. Engl. J. Med. 362, 402–415.

Comabella, M., Craig, D.W., Camina-Tato, M., Morcillo, C., Lopez, C., Navarro, A., et al., 2008. Identification of a novel risk locus for multiple sclerosis at 13q31.3 by a pooled genome-wide scan of 500,000 single nucleotide polymorphisms. PLoS One. 3, e3490.

Comi, G., Filippi, M., Wolinsky, J.S., 2001. European/Canadian multicenter, double-blind, randomized, placebo-controlled study of the effects of glatiramer acetate on magnetic resonance imaging—measured disease activity and burden in patients with relapsing multiple sclerosis. European/Canadian Glatiramer Acetate Study Group. Ann. Neurol. 49, 290–297.

Confavreux, C., Vukusic, S., 2006. Natural history of multiple sclerosis: a unifying concept. Brain. 129, 606–616.

Confavreux, C., Vukusic, S., Moreau, T., Adeleine, P., 2000. Relapses and progression of disability in multiple sclerosis. N. Engl. J. Med. 343, 1430–1438.

Cotsapas, C., Voight, B.F., Rossin, E., Lage, K., Neale, B.M., Wallace, C., et al., 2011. Pervasive sharing of genetic effects in autoimmune disease. PLoS Genet. 7, e1002254.

Cotton, F., Weiner, H.L., Jolesz, F.A., Guttmann, C.R., 2003. MRI contrast uptake in new lesions in relapsing-remitting MS followed at weekly intervals. Neurology. 60, 640–646.

Crawford, M.P., Yan, S.X., Ortega, S.B., Mehta, R.S., Hewitt, R.E., Price, D.A., et al., 2004. High prevalence of autoreactive, neuroantigen-specific CD8 + T cells in multiple sclerosis revealed by novel flow cytometric assay. Blood. 103, 4222–4231.

Cruz, M., Olsson, T., Ernerudh, J., Hojeberg, B., Link, H., 1987. Immunoblot detection of oligoclonal anti-myelin basic protein IgG antibodies in cerebrospinal fluid in multiple sclerosis. Neurology. 37, 1515–1519.

De Jager, P.L., Baecher-Allan, C., Maier, L.M., Arthur, A.T., Ottoboni, L., Barcellos, L., et al., 2009a. The role of the CD58 locus in multiple sclerosis. Proc. Natl. Acad. Sci. U.S.A. 106, 5264–5269.

De Jager, P.L., Jia, X., Wang, J., De Bakker, P.I., Ottoboni, L., Aggarwal, N.T., et al., 2009b. Meta-analysis of genome scans and replication identify CD6, IRF8 and TNFRSF1A as new multiple sclerosis susceptibility loci. Nat. Genet. 41, 776–782.

Dean, G., McLoughlin, H., Brady, R., Adelstein, A.M., Tallett-Williams, J., 1976. Multiple sclerosis among immigrants in Greater London. Br. Med. J. 1, 861–864.

Deloire, M.S., Ruet, A., Hamel, D., Bonnet, M., Dousset, V., Brochet, B., 2011. MRI predictors of cognitive outcome in early multiple sclerosis. Neurology. 76, 1161–1167.

Dominguez-Villar, M., Baecher-Allan, C.M., Hafler, D.A., 2011. Identification of T helper type 1-like, Foxp3 + regulatory T cells in human autoimmune disease. Nat. Med. 17, 673–675.

Duda, P.W., Schmied, M.C., Cook, S.L., Krieger, J.I., Hafler, D.A., 2000. Glatiramer acetate (Copaxone) induces degenerate, Th2-polarized immune responses in patients with multiple sclerosis. J. Clin. Invest. 105, 967–976.

Dutta, R., Trapp, B.D., 2007. Pathogenesis of axonal and neuronal damage in multiple sclerosis. Neurology. 68, S22–S31, discussion S43–S54.

Dziedzic, T., Metz, I., Dallenga, T., Konig, F.B., Muller, S., Stadelmann, C., et al., 2010. Wallerian degeneration: a major component of early axonal pathology in multiple sclerosis. Brain Pathol. 20, 976–985.

Ebers, G.C., 2008. Environmental factors and multiple sclerosis. Lancet Neurol. 7, 268–277.

Ebers, G.C., Bulman, D.E., Sadovnick, A.D., Paty, D.W., Warren, S., Hader, W., et al., 1986. A population-based study of multiple sclerosis in twins. N. Engl. J. Med. 315, 1638–1642.

El-Behi, M., Ciric, B., Dai, H., Yan, Y., Cullimore, M., Safavi, F., et al., 2011. The encephalitogenicity of T(H)17 cells is dependent on IL-1-and IL-23-induced production of the cytokine GM-CSF. Nat. Immunol. 12, 568–575.

Ferguson, B., Matyszak, M.K., Esiri, M.M., Perry, V.H., 1997. Axonal damage in acute multiple sclerosis lesions. Brain. 120 (Pt 3), 393–399.

Filippi, M., 2000. Enhanced magnetic resonance imaging in multiple sclerosis. Mult. Scler. 6, 320–326.

Filippi, M., Agosta, F., 2009. Magnetic resonance techniques to quantify tissue damage, tissue repair, and functional cortical reorganization in multiple sclerosis. Prog. Brain Res. 175, 465–482.

Filippi, M., Paty, D.W., Kappos, L., Barkhof, F., Compston, D.A., Thompson, A.J., et al., 1995. Correlations between changes in disability and T2-weighted brain MRI activity in multiple sclerosis: a follow-up study. Neurology. 45, 255–260.

Filippi, M., Rocca, M.A., 2011. MR imaging of multiple sclerosis. Radiology. 259, 659–681.

Filippi, M., Rocca, M.A., Barkhof, F., Bruck, W., Chen, J.T., Comi, G., et al., 2012. Association between pathological and MRI findings in multiple sclerosis. Lancet Neurol. 11, 349–360.

Fisniku, L.K., Brex, P.A., Altmann, D.R., Miszkiel, K.A., Benton, C.E., Lanyon, R., et al., 2008. Disability and T2 MRI lesions: a 20-year follow-up of patients with relapse onset of multiple sclerosis. Brain. 131, 808–817.

Fontenot, J.D., Gavin, M.A., Rudensky, A.Y., 2003. Foxp3 programs the development and function of CD4 + CD25 + regulatory T cells. Nat. Immunol. 4, 330–336.

Fontoura, P., Garren, H., 2010. Multiple sclerosis therapies: molecular mechanisms and future. Results Probl. Cell Differ. 51, 259–285.

Fox, E.J., 2004. Mechanism of action of mitoxantrone. Neurology. 63, S15–S18.

Fox, R.J., Miller, D.H., Phillips, J.T., Hutchinson, M., Havrdova, E., Kita, M., et al., 2012. Placebo-controlled phase 3 study of oral BG-12 or glatiramer in multiple sclerosis. N. Engl. J. Med. 367, 1087–1097.

Frazer, K.A., Ballinger, D.G., Cox, D.R., Hinds, D.A., Stuve, L.L., Gibbs, R.A., et al., 2007. A second generation human haplotype map of over 3.1 million SNPs. Nature. 449, 851–861.

Freal, J.E., Kraft, G.H., Coryell, J.K., 1984. Symptomatic fatigue in multiple sclerosis. Arch. Phys. Med. Rehabil. 65, 135–138.

French Research Group on MS, 1992. MS in 54 twinships: concordance rate is independent of zygosity. Ann. Neurol. 32, 724–727.

Frohman, E.M., Racke, M.K., Raine, C.S., 2006. Multiple sclerosis—the plaque and its pathogenesis. N. Engl. J. Med. 354, 942–955.

Genain, C.P., Cannella, B., Hauser, S.L., Raine, C.S., 1999. Identification of autoantibodies associated with myelin damage in multiple sclerosis. Nat. Med. 5, 170–175.

Geurts, J.J., Bo, L., Pouwels, P.J., Castelijns, J.A., Polman, C.H., Barkhof, F., 2005. Cortical lesions in multiple sclerosis: combined postmortem MR imaging and histopathology. AJNR Am. J. Neuroradiol. 26, 572–577.

Gold, R., 2011. Oral therapies for multiple sclerosis: a review of agents in phase III development or recently approved. CNS Drugs. 25, 37–52.

Gold, R., Kappos, L., Arnold, D.L., Bar-Or, A., Giovannoni, G., Selmaj, K., et al., 2012. Placebo-controlled phase 3 study of oral BG-12 for relapsing multiple sclerosis. N. Engl. J. Med. 367, 1098–1107.

Gold, R., Wolinsky, J.S., 2011. Pathophysiology of multiple sclerosis and the place of teriflunomide. Acta Neurol. Scand. 124, 75–84.

Graber, J., Zhan, M., Ford, D., Kursch, F., Francis, G., Bever, C., et al., 2005. Interferon-beta-1a induces increases in vascular cell adhesion molecule: implications for its mode of action in multiple sclerosis. J. Neuroimmunol. 161, 169–176.

Graber, J.J., Dhib-Jalbut, S., 2011. Biomarkers of disease activity in multiple sclerosis. J. Neurol. Sci. 305, 1–10.

Gran, B., Tranquill, L.R., Chen, M., Bielekova, B., Zhou, W., Dhib-Jalbut, S., et al., 2000. Mechanisms of immunomodulation by glatiramer acetate. Neurology. 55, 1704–1714.

Greer, J.M., Pender, M.P., 2008. Myelin proteolipid protein: an effective autoantigen and target of autoimmunity in multiple sclerosis. J. Autoimmun. 31, 281–287.

Haas, J., Hug, A., Viehover, A., Fritzsching, B., Falk, C.S., Filser, A., et al., 2005. Reduced suppressive effect of CD4 + CD25 high regulatory T cells on the T cell immune response against myelin oligodendrocyte glycoprotein in patients with multiple sclerosis. Eur. J. Immunol. 35, 3343–3352.

Hafler, D.A., 2012. Perspective: deconstructing a disease. Nature. 484, S6.

Hafler, J.P., Maier, L.M., Cooper, J.D., Plagnol, V., Hinks, A., Simmonds, M.J., et al., 2009. CD226 Gly307Ser association with multiple autoimmune diseases. Genes. Immun. 10, 5–10.

Hammond, S.R., De Wytt, C., Maxwell, I.C., Landy, P.J., English, D., Mcleod, J.G., et al., 1987. The epidemiology of multiple sclerosis in Queensland, Australia. J. Neurol. Sci. 80, 185–204.

Hammond, S.R., Mcleod, J.G., Millingen, K.S., Stewart-Wynne, E.G., English, D., Holland, J.T., et al., 1988. The epidemiology of multiple sclerosis in three Australian cities: Perth, Newcastle and Hobart. Brain. 111 (Pt 1), 1–25.

Harrington, L.E., Hatton, R.D., Mangan, P.R., Turner, H., Murphy, T.L., Murphy, K.M., et al., 2005. Interleukin 17-producing CD4 + effector T cells develop via a lineage distinct from the T helper type 1 and 2 lineages. Nat. Immunol. 6, 1123–1132.

Hartung, H.P., Aktas, O., Kieseier, B., Giancarlo Comi, G.C., 2010. Development of oral cladribine for the treatment of multiple sclerosis. J. Neurol. 257, 163–170.

Hartung, H.P., Gonsette, R., Konig, N., Kwiecinski, H., Guseo, A., Morrissey, S.P., et al., 2002. Mitoxantrone in progressive multiple sclerosis: a placebo-controlled, double-blind, randomised, multicentre trial. Lancet. 360, 2018–2025.

Hastings, W.D., Anderson, D.E., Kassam, N., Koguchi, K., Greenfield, E.A., Kent, S.C., et al., 2009. TIM-3 is expressed on activated human CD4 + T cells and regulates Th1 and Th17 cytokines. Eur. J. Immunol. 39, 2492–24501.

Hauser, S.L., Bhan, A.K., Gilles, F., Kemp, M., Kerr, C., Weiner, H.L., 1986. Immunohistochemical analysis of the cellular infiltrate in multiple sclerosis lesions. Ann. Neurol. 19, 578–587.

Heltberg, A., Holm, N., 1982. Concordance in twins and recurrence in sibships in MS. Lancet. 1, 1068.

Hofman, F.M., Hinton, D.R., Johnson, K., Merrill, J.E., 1989. Tumor necrosis factor identified in multiple sclerosis brain. J. Exp. Med. 170, 607–612.

Hogancamp, W.E., Rodriguez, M., Weinshenker, B.G., 1997. The epidemiology of multiple sclerosis. Mayo. Clin. Proc. 72, 871–878.

Hohol, M.J., Guttmann, C.R., Orav, J., Mackin, G.A., Kikinis, R., Khoury, S.J., et al., 1997. Serial neuropsychological assessment and magnetic resonance imaging analysis in multiple sclerosis. Arch. Neurol. 54, 1018–1025.

Hohol, M.J., Olek, M.J., Orav, E.J., Stazzone, L., Hafler, D.A., Khoury, S.J., et al., 1999. Treatment of progressive multiple sclerosis with pulse cyclophosphamide/methylprednisolone: response to therapy is linked to the duration of progressive disease. Mult. Scler. 5, 403–409.

Holmes, F.F., Stubbs, D.W., Larsen, W.E., 1967. Systemic lupus erythematosus and multiple sclerosis in identical twins. Arch. Intern. Med. 119, 302–304.

Hong, J., Li, N., Zhang, X., Zheng, B., Zhang, J.Z., 2005. Induction of CD4 + CD25 + regulatory T cells by copolymer-I through activation of transcription factor Foxp3. Proc. Natl. Acad. Sci. U.S. A. 102, 6449–6454.

Hori, S., Nomura, T., Sakaguchi, S., 2003. Control of regulatory T cell development by the transcription factor Foxp3. Science. 299, 1057–1061.

Howell, O.W., Reeves, C.A., Nicholas, R., Carassiti, D., Radotra, B., Gentleman, S.M., et al., 2011. Meningeal inflammation is widespread and linked to cortical pathology in multiple sclerosis. Brain. 134, 2755–2771.

Hutchinson, M., Kappos, L., Calabresi, P.A., Confavreux, C., Giovannoni, G., Galetta, S.L., et al., 2009. The efficacy of natalizumab in patients with relapsing multiple sclerosis: subgroup analyses of AFFIRM and SENTINEL. J. Neurol. 256, 405–415.

IFNB Multiple Sclerosis Study Group, The, 1993. Interferon beta-1b is effective in relapsing-remitting multiple sclerosis. I. Clinical results of a multicenter, randomized, double-blind, placebo-controlled trial. The IFNB Multiple Sclerosis Study Group. Neurology. 43, 655–661.

IFNB Multiple Sclerosis Study Group, The, 1995. Interferon beta-1b in the treatment of multiple sclerosis: final outcome of the randomized controlled trial. The IFNB Multiple Sclerosis Study Group and The University of British Columbia MS/MRI Analysis Group. Neurology. 45, 1277–1285.

International Multiple Sclerosis Genetics Consortium, 2009. The expanding genetic overlap between multiple sclerosis and type I diabetes. Genes. Immun. 110, 11–14.

Jacobs, L.D., Cookfair, D.L., Rudick, R.A., Herndon, R.M., Richert, J.R., Salazar, A.M., et al., 1996. Intramuscular interferon beta-1a for disease progression in relapsing multiple sclerosis. The Multiple Sclerosis Collaborative Research Group (MSCRG). Ann. Neurol. 39, 285–294.

Jacobs, L.D., Cookfair, D.L., Rudick, R.A., Herndon, R.M., Richert, J.R., Salazar, A.M., et al., 1995. A phase III trial of intramuscular recombinant interferon beta as treatment for exacerbating-remitting multiple sclerosis: design and conduct of study and baseline characteristics of patients. Multiple Sclerosis Collaborative Research Group (MSCRG). Mult. Scler. 1, 118–135.

Jakkula, E., Leppa, V., Sulonen, A.M., Varilo, T., Kallio, S., Kemppinen, A., et al., 2010. Genome-wide association study in a high-risk isolate for multiple sclerosis reveals associated variants in STAT3 gene. Am. J. Hum. Genet. 86, 285–291.

Johnson, K.P., Brooks, B.R., Cohen, J.A., Ford, C.C., Goldstein, J., Lisak, R.P., et al., 1995. Copolymer 1 reduces relapse rate and improves disability in relapsing-remitting multiple sclerosis: results of a phase III multicenter, double-blind placebo-controlled trial. The Copolymer 1 Multiple Sclerosis Study Group. Neurology. 45, 1268–1276.

Johnson, K.P., Brooks, B.R., Cohen, J.A., Ford, C.C., Goldstein, J., Lisak, R.P., et al., 1998. Extended use of glatiramer acetate (Copaxone) is well tolerated and maintains its clinical effect on multiple sclerosis relapse rate and degree of disability. Copolymer 1 Multiple Sclerosis Study Group. Neurology. 50, 701–708.

Joller, N., Hafler, J.P., Brynedal, B., Kassam, N., Spoerl, S., Levin, S.D., et al., 2011. Cutting edge: TIGIT has T cell-intrinsic inhibitory functions. J. Immunol. 186, 1338–1342.

Kappos, L., Gold, R., Miller, D.H., Macmanus, D.G., Havrdova, E., Limmroth, V., et al., 2008. Efficacy and safety of oral fumarate in patients with relapsing-remitting multiple sclerosis: a multicentre, randomised, double-blind, placebo-controlled phase IIb study. Lancet. 372, 1463–1472.

Kebir, H., Kreymborg, K., Ifergan, I., Dodelet-Devillers, A., Cayrol, R., Bernard, M., et al., 2007. Human TH17 lymphocytes promote blood-brain barrier disruption and central nervous system inflammation. Nat. Med. 13, 1173–1175.

Khoury, S.J., Guttmann, C.R., Orav, E.J., Hohol, M.J., Ahn, S.S., Hsu, L., et al., 1994. Longitudinal MRI imaging in multiple sclerosis: correlation between disability and lesion burden. Neurology. 44, 2120–2124.

Khoury, S.J., Hancock, W.W., Weiner, H.L., 1992. Oral tolerance to myelin basic protein and natural recovery from experimental autoimmune encephalomyelitis are associated with downregulation of inflammatory cytokines and differential upregulation of transforming growth factor beta, interleukin 4, and prostaglandin E expression in the brain. J. Exp. Med. 176, 1355–1364.

Kinnunen, E., Koskenvuo, M., Kaprio, J., Aho, K., 1987. Multiple sclerosis in a nationwide series of twins. Neurology. 37, 1627–1629.

Klawiter, E.C., Piccio, L., Lyons, J.A., Mikesell, R., O'Connor, K.C., Cross, A.H., 2010. Elevated intrathecal myelin oligodendrocyte glycoprotein antibodies in multiple sclerosis. Arch. Neurol. 67, 1102–1108.

Koch-Henriksen, N., Sorensen, P.S., 2010. The changing demographic pattern of multiple sclerosis epidemiology. Lancet Neurol. 9, 520–532.

Koenen, H.J., Smeets, R.L., Vink, P.M., Van Rijssen, E., Boots, A.M., Joosten, I., 2008. Human CD25highFoxp3pos regulatory T cells differentiate into IL-17-producing cells. Blood. 112, 2340–2352.

Koguchi, K., Anderson, D.E., Yang, L., O'Connor, K.C., Kuchroo, V.K., Hafler, D.A., 2006. Dysregulated T cell expression of TIM3 in multiple sclerosis. J. Exp. Med. 203, 1413–1418.

Kragt, J., Van Amerongen, B., Killestein, J., Dijkstra, C., Uitdehaag, B., Polman, C., et al., 2009. Higher levels of 25-hydroxyvitamin D are associated with a lower incidence of multiple sclerosis only in women. Mult. Scler. 15, 9–15.

Krapf, H., Morrissey, S.P., Zenker, O., Zwingers, T., Gonsette, R., Hartung, H.P., 2005. Effect of mitoxantrone on MRI in progressive MS: results of the MIMS trial. Neurology. 65, 690–695.

Kurtzke, J.F., 1977. Geography in multiple sclerosis. J. Neurol. 215, 1–26.

Kurtzke, J.F., 2000. Epidemiology of multiple sclerosis. Does this really point toward an etiology? Lectio Doctoralis. Neurol. Sci. 21, 383–403.

Kurtzke, J.F., Beebe, G.W., Norman Jr., J.E., 1979. Epidemiology of multiple sclerosis in U.S. veterans: 1. Race, sex, and geographic distribution. Neurology. 29, 1228–1235.

Kurtzke, J.F., Gudmundsson, K.R., Bergmann, S., 1982. MS in Iceland: 1. Evidence of a post-war epidemic. Neurology. 32, 143–150.

Lassmann, H., 1998. Neuropathology in multiple sclerosis: new concepts. Mult. Scler. 4, 93–98.

Lassmann, H., Niedobitek, G., Aloisi, F., Middeldorp, J.M., 2011. Epstein-Barr virus in the multiple sclerosis brain: a controversial issue—report on a focused workshop held in the Centre for Brain Research of the Medical University of Vienna, Austria. Brain. 134, 2772–2786.

Lauer, K., 1995. Environmental associations with the risk of multiple sclerosis: the contribution of ecological studies. Acta Neurol. Scand. Suppl. 161, 77–88.

Leonard, J.P., Waldburger, K.E., Goldman, S.J., 1995. Prevention of experimental autoimmune encephalomyelitis by antibodies against interleukin 12. J. Exp. Med. 181, 381−386.

Lincoln, M.R., Ramagopalan, S.V., Chao, M.J., Herrera, B.M., Deluca, G.C., Orton, S.M., et al., 2009. Epistasis among HLA-DRB1, HLA-DQA1, and HLA-DQB1 loci determines multiple sclerosis susceptibility. Proc. Natl. Acad. Sci. U.S.A. 106, 7542−7547.

Link, H., Huang, Y.M., 2006. Oligoclonal bands in multiple sclerosis cerebrospinal fluid: an update on methodology and clinical usefulness. J. Neuroimmunol. 180, 17−28.

Linker, R.A., Lee, D.H., Ryan, S., Van Dam, A.M., Conrad, R., Bista, P., et al., 2011. Fumaric acid esters exert neuroprotective effects in neuroinflammation via activation of the Nrf2 antioxidant pathway. Brain. 134, 678−692.

Lovato, L., Willis, S.N., Rodig, S.J., Caron, T., Almendinger, S.E., Howell, O.W., et al., 2011. Related B cell clones populate the meninges and parenchyma of patients with multiple sclerosis. Brain. 134, 534−541.

Lozano, E., Dominguez-Villar, M., Kuchroo, V., Hafler, D.A., 2012. The TIGIT/CD226 Axis Regulates Human T Cell Function. J. Immunol. 188, 3869−3875.

Mackay, R.P., Myrianthopoulos, N.C., 1966. Multiple sclerosis in twins and their relatives. Arch. Neurol. 15, 449−462.

Magliozzi, R., Howell, O., Vora, A., Serafini, B., Nicholas, R., Puopolo, M., et al., 2007. Meningeal B-cell follicles in secondary progressive multiple sclerosis associate with early onset of disease and severe cortical pathology. Brain. 130, 1089−1104.

Mancardi, G.L., Sardanelli, F., Parodi, R.C., Melani, E., Capello, E., Inglese, M., et al., 1998. Effect of copolymer-1 on serial gadolinium-enhanced MRI in relapsing remitting multiple sclerosis. Neurology. 50, 1127−1133.

Mandrioli, J., Sola, P., Bedin, R., Gambini, M., Merelli, E., 2008. A multifactorial prognostic index in multiple sclerosis. Cerebrospinal fluid IgM oligoclonal bands and clinical features to predict the evolution of the disease. J. Neurol. 255, 1023−1031.

Marriott, J.J., Miyasaki, J.M., Gronseth, G., O'Connor, P.W., 2010. Evidence report: the efficacy and safety of mitoxantrone (Novantrone) in the treatment of multiple sclerosis: Report of the Therapeutics and Technology Assessment Subcommittee of the American Academy of Neurology. Neurology. 74, 1463−1470.

Mattson, D., Petrie, M., Srivastava, D.K., Mcdermott, M., 1995. Multiple sclerosis. Sexual dysfunction and its response to medications. Arch. Neurol. 52, 862−868.

Mattson, D.H., Roos, R.P., Arnason, B.G., 1980. Isoelectric focusing of IgG eluted from multiple sclerosis and subacute sclerosing panencephalitis brains. Nature. 287, 335−337.

Mcdonald, W.I., Compston, A., Edan, G., Goodkin, D., Hartung, H.P., Lublin, F.D., et al., 2001. Recommended diagnostic criteria for multiple sclerosis: guidelines from the International Panel on the diagnosis of multiple sclerosis. Ann. Neurol. 50, 121−127.

Mclean, B.N., Luxton, R.W., Thompson, E.J., 1990. A study of immunoglobulin G in the cerebrospinal fluid of 1007 patients with suspected neurological disease using isoelectric focusing and the Log IgG-Index. A comparison and diagnostic applications. Brain. 113 (Pt 5), 1269−1289.

Mcleod, J.G., Hammond, S.R., Hallpike, J.F., 1994. Epidemiology of multiple sclerosis in Australia. With NSW and SA survey results. Med. J. Aust. 160, 117−122.

Menge, T., Lalive, P.H., Von Budingen, H.C., Genain, C.P., 2011. Conformational epitopes of myelin oligodendrocyte glycoprotein are targets of potentially pathogenic antibody responses in multiple sclerosis. J. Neuroinflammation. 8, 161.

Miller, A., Shapiro, S., Gershtein, R., Kinarty, A., Rawashdeh, H., Honigman, S., et al., 1998. Treatment of multiple sclerosis with copolymer-1 (Copaxone): implicating mechanisms of Th1 to Th2/Th3 immune-deviation. J. Neuroimmunol. 92, 113−121.

Miller, D.H., Chard, D.T., Ciccarelli, O., 2012. Clinically isolated syndromes. Lancet Neurol. 11, 157−169.

Miller, D.H., Leary, S.M., 2007. Primary-progressive multiple sclerosis. Lancet Neurol. 6, 903−912.

Miron, V.E., Jung, C.G., Kim, H.J., Kennedy, T.E., Soliven, B., Antel, J.P., 2008. FTY720 modulates human oligodendrocyte progenitor process extension and survival. Ann. Neurol. 63, 61−71.

Miron, V.E., Ludwin, S.K., Darlington, P.J., Jarjour, A.A., Soliven, B., Kennedy, T.E., et al., 2010. Fingolimod (FTY720) enhances remyelination following demyelination of organotypic cerebellar slices. Am. J. Pathol. 176, 2682−2694.

Mumford, C., Wood, N., Kellar-Wood, H., et al., 1992. The UK study of MS in twins. J. Neurol. 239, 62.

Murray, T.J., 2009. Robert Carswell: the first illustrator of MS. Int. MS J. 16, 98−101.

Neuhaus, O., Farina, C., Yassouridis, A., Wiendl, H., Then Bergh, F., Dose, T., et al., 2000. Multiple sclerosis: comparison of copolymer-1- reactive T cell lines from treated and untreated subjects reveals cytokine shift from T helper 1 to T helper 2 cells. Proc. Natl. Acad. Sci. U.S.A. 97, 7452−7457.

Newcombe, J., Hawkins, C.P., Henderson, C.L., Patel, H.A., Woodroofe, M.N., Hayes, G.M., et al., 1991. Histopathology of multiple sclerosis lesions detected by magnetic resonance imaging in unfixed postmortem central nervous system tissue. Brain. 114 (Pt 2), 1013−1023.

Nischwitz, S., Cepok, S., Kroner, A., Wolf, C., Knop, M., Muller-Sarnowski, F., et al., 2010. Evidence for VAV2 and ZNF433 as susceptibility genes for multiple sclerosis. J. Neuroimmunol. 227, 162−166.

Noseworthy, J.H., Lucchinetti, C., Rodriguez, M., Weinshenker, B.G., 2000. Multiple sclerosis. N. Engl. J. Med. 343, 938−952.

Noyes, K., Bajorska, A., Chappel, A., Schwid, S.R., Mehta, L.R., Weinstock-Guttman, B., et al., 2011. Cost-effectiveness of disease-modifying therapy for multiple sclerosis: a population-based study. Neurology. 77, 355−363.

Nylander, A., Hafler, D.A., 2012. Multiple sclerosis. J. Clin. Invest. 122, 1180−1188.

O'Connor, K.C., Appel, H., Bregoli, L., Call, M.E., Catz, I., Chan, J.A., et al., 2005. Antibodies from inflamed central nervous system tissue recognize myelin oligodendrocyte glycoprotein. J. Immunol. 175, 1974−1982.

O'Connor, K.C., Chitnis, T., Griffin, D.E., Piyasirisilp, S., Bar-Or, A., Khoury, S., et al., 2003. Myelin basic protein-reactive autoantibodies in the serum and cerebrospinal fluid of multiple sclerosis patients are characterized by low-affinity interactions. J. Neuroimmunol. 136, 140−148.

O'Connor, K.C., Mclaughlin, K.A., De Jager, P.L., Chitnis, T., Bettelli, E., Xu, C., et al., 2007. Self-antigen tetramers discriminate between myelin autoantibodies to native or denatured protein. Nat. Med. 13, 211−217.

O'Connor, P., Wolinsky, J.S., Confavreux, C., Comi, G., Kappos, L., Olsson, T.P., et al., 2011. Randomized trial of oral teriflunomide for relapsing multiple sclerosis. N. Engl. J. Med. 365, 1293–1303.

O'Garra, A., 1998. Cytokines induce the development of functionally heterogeneous T helper cell subsets. Immunity. 8, 275–283.

O'Shea, J.J., Paul, W.E., 2010. Mechanisms underlying lineage commitment and plasticity of helper CD4+ T cells. Science. 327, 1098–1102.

Obermeier, B., Lovato, L., Mentele, R., Bruck, W., Forne, I., Imhof, A., et al., 2011. Related B cell clones that populate the CSF and CNS of patients with multiple sclerosis produce CSF immunoglobulin. J. Neuroimmunol. 233, 245–248.

Olek, M.D., 2000. Multiple sclerosis and other inflammatory demyelinating diseases of the central nervous system. In: Bradley, W.D., Fenichel, G, Marsden, CD (Eds.), Neurology in Clinical Practice, third ed. Butterworth-Heinemann, Woburn.

Owens, T., Renno, T., Taupin, V., Krakowski, M., 1994. Inflammatory cytokines in the brain: does the CNS shape immune responses? Immunol. Today. 15, 566–571.

Patsopoulos, N.A., Esposito, F., Reischl, J., Lehr, S., Bauer, D., Heubach, J., et al., 2011. Genome-wide meta-analysis identifies novel multiple sclerosis susceptibility loci. Ann. Neurol. 70, 897–912.

Paty, D., Studney, D., Redekop, K., Lublin, F., 1994. MS COSTAR: a computerized patient record adapted for clinical research purposes. Ann. Neurol. 36 (Suppl), S134–S135.

Paty, D.W., Li, D.K., 1993. Interferon beta-1b is effective in relapsing-remitting multiple sclerosis. II. MRI analysis results of a multicenter, randomized, double-blind, placebo-controlled trial. UBC MS/MRI Study Group and the IFNB Multiple Sclerosis Study Group. Neurology. 43, 662–667.

Pedersen, N.S., Kam-Hansen, S., Link, H., Mavra, M., 1982. Specificity of immunoglobulins synthesized within the central nervous system in neurosyphilis. Acta Pathol. Microbiol. Immunol. Scand. C. 90, 97–104.

Pham, T.H., Okada, T., Matloubian, M., Lo, C.G., Cyster, J.G., 2008. S1P1 receptor signaling overrides retention mediated by G alpha i-coupled receptors to promote T cell egress. Immunity. 28, 122–133.

Polman, C.H., O'Connor, P.W., Havrdova, E., Hutchinson, M., Kappos, L., Miller, D.H., et al., 2006. A randomized, placebo-controlled trial of natalizumab for relapsing multiple sclerosis. N. Engl. J. Med. 354, 899–910.

Polman, C.H., Reingold, S.C., Banwell, B., Clanet, M., Cohen, J.A., Filippi, M., et al., 2011. Diagnostic criteria for multiple sclerosis: 2010 revisions to the McDonald criteria. Ann. Neurol. 69, 292–302.

Polman, C.H., Reingold, S.C., Edan, G., Filippi, M., Hartung, H.P., Kappos, L., et al., 2005. Diagnostic criteria for multiple sclerosis: 2005 revisions to the "McDonald Criteria. Ann. Neurol. 58, 840–846.

Popescu, B.F., Bunyan, R.F., Parisi, J.E., Ransohoff, R.M., Lucchinetti, C.F., 2011. A case of multiple sclerosis presenting with inflammatory cortical demyelination. Neurology. 76, 1705–1710.

Prineas, J., 1975. Pathology of the early lesion in multiple sclerosis. Hum. Pathol. 6, 531–554.

PRISMS, 2001. PRISMS-4: long-term efficacy of interferon-beta-1a in relapsing MS. Neurology. 56, 1628–1636.

Raddassi, K., Kent, S.C., Yang, J., Bourcier, K., Bradshaw, E.M., Seyfert-Margolis, V., et al., 2011. Increased frequencies of myelin oligodendrocyte glycoprotein/MHC class II-binding CD4 cells in patients with multiple sclerosis. J. Immunol. 187, 1039–1046.

Raine, C., 1991. Demyelinating diseases. In: Davis, R.L., Robertson, D.M. (Eds.), Textbook of Neuropathology, second ed. Williams and Wilkins, Baltimore.

Ramagopalan, S.V., Maugeri, N.J., Handunnetthi, L., Lincoln, M.R., Orton, S.M., Dyment, D.A., et al., 2009. Expression of the multiple sclerosis-associated MHC class II Allele HLA-DRB1*1501 is regulated by vitamin D. PLoS Genet. 5, e1000369.

Rao, S.M., Leo, G.J., Haughton, V.M., St Aubin-Faubert, P., Bernardin, L., 1989. Correlation of magnetic resonance imaging with neuropsychological testing in multiple sclerosis. Neurology. 39, 161–166.

Reboldi, A., Coisne, C., Baumjohann, D., Benvenuto, F., Bottinelli, D., Lira, S., et al., 2009. C-C chemokine receptor 6-regulated entry of TH-17 cells into the CNS through the choroid plexus is required for the initiation of EAE. Nat. Immunol. 10, 514–523.

Rieckmann, P., Toyka, K.V., Bassetti, C., Beer, K., Beer, S., Buettner, U., et al., 2004. Escalating immunotherapy of multiple sclerosis—new aspects and practical application. J. Neurol. 251, 1329–1339.

Risch, N., Merikangas, K., 1996. The future of genetic studies of complex human diseases. Science. 273, 1516–1517.

Rivers, T.M., Sprunt, D.H., Berry, G.P., 1933. Observations on attempts to produce acute disseminated encephalomyelitis in monkeys. J. Exp. Med. 58, 39–53.

Rovaris, M., Bozzali, M., Rodegher, M., Tortorella, C., Comi, G., Filippi, M., 1999. Brain MRI correlates of magnetization transfer imaging metrics in patients with multiple sclerosis. J. Neurol. Sci. 166, 58–63.

Rovira, A., Swanton, J., Tintore, M., Huerga, E., Barkhof, F., Filippi, M., et al., 2009. A single, early magnetic resonance imaging study in the diagnosis of multiple sclerosis. Arch. Neurol. 66, 587–592.

Sadovnick, A.D., 2006. The genetics and genetic epidemiology of multiple sclerosis: the "hard facts.". Adv. Neurol. 98, 17–25.

Sadovnick, A.D., Armstrong, H., Rice, G.P., Bulman, D., Hashimoto, L., Paty, D.W., et al., 1993. A population-based study of multiple sclerosis in twins: update. Ann. Neurol. 33, 281–285.

Sadovnick, A.D., Dyment, D., Ebers, G.C., 1997. Genetic epidemiology of multiple sclerosis. Epidemiol. Rev. 19, 99–106.

Sadovnick, A.D., Remick, R.A., Allen, J., Swartz, E., Yee, I.M., Eisen, K., et al., 1996. Depression and multiple sclerosis. Neurology. 46, 628–632.

Sanna, S., Pitzalis, M., Zoledziewska, M., Zara, I., Sidore, C., Murru, R., et al., 2010. Variants within the immunoregulatory CBLB gene are associated with multiple sclerosis. Nat. Genet. 42, 495–497.

Sawcer, S., Hellenthal, G., Pirinen, M., Spencer, C.C., Patsopoulos, N.A., Moutsianas, L., et al., 2011. Genetic risk and a primary role for cell-mediated immune mechanisms in multiple sclerosis. Nature. 476, 214–219.

Schumacker, G.A., Beebe, G., Kibler, R.F., Kurland, L.T., Kurtzke, J.F., Mcdowell, F., et al., 1965. Problems of Experimental trials of therapy in multiple sclerosis: report by the panel on the evaluation of experimental trials of therapy in multiple sclerosis. Ann. N. Y. Acad. Sci. 122, 552–568.

Schwab, S.R., Cyster, J.G., 2007. Finding a way out: lymphocyte egress from lymphoid organs. Nat. Immunol. 8, 1295–1301.

Segal, B.M., Dwyer, B.K., Shevach, E.M., 1998. An interleukin (IL)-10/IL-12 immunoregulatory circuit controls susceptibility to autoimmune disease. J. Exp. Med. 187, 537–546.

Selmaj, K., Raine, C.S., Cannella, B., Brosnan, C.F., 1991. Identification of lymphotoxin and tumor necrosis factor in multiple sclerosis lesions. J. Clin. Invest. 87, 949–954.

Serafini, B., Rosicarelli, B., Magliozzi, R., Stigliano, E., Aloisi, F., 2004. Detection of ectopic B-cell follicles with germinal centers in the meninges of patients with secondary progressive multiple sclerosis. Brain Pathol. 14, 164–174.

Severson, C., Hafler, D.A., 2010. T-cells in multiple sclerosis. Results Probl. Cell Differ. 51, 75–98.

Simon, K.C., Munger, K.L., Kraft, P., Hunter, D.J., De Jager, P.L., Ascherio, A., 2011. Genetic predictors of 25-hydroxyvitamin D levels and risk of multiple sclerosis. J. Neurol. 258, 1676–1682.

Siveke, J.T., Hamann, A., 1998. T helper 1 and T helper 2 cells respond differentially to chemokines. J. Immunol. 160, 550–554.

Skegg, D.C., Corwin, P.A., Craven, R.S., Malloch, J.A., Pollock, M., 1987. Occurrence of multiple sclerosis in the north and south of New Zealand. J. Neurol. Neurosurg. Psychiatry. 50, 134–139.

Skotzek, B., Sander, T., Zimmermann, J., Kolmel, H.W., 1988. Oligoclonal bands in serum and cerebrospinal fluid of patients with HIV infection. J. Neuroimmunol. 20, 151–152.

Smith, K.J., Lassmann, H., 2002. The role of nitric oxide in multiple sclerosis. Lancet Neurol. 1, 232–241.

Smolders, J., Damoiseaux, J., Menheere, P., Hupperts, R., 2008. Vitamin D as an immune modulator in multiple sclerosis, a review. J. Neuroimmunol. 194, 7–17.

Sorensen, T.L., Tani, M., Jensen, J., Pierce, V., Lucchinetti, C., Folcik, V.A., et al., 1999. Expression of specific chemokines and chemokine receptors in the central nervous system of multiple sclerosis patients. J. Clin. Invest. 103, 807–815.

Steinman, L., 2007. A brief history of T(H)17, the first major revision in the T(H)1/T(H)2 hypothesis of T cell-mediated tissue damage. Nat. Med. 13, 139–145.

Stone, L.A., Frank, J.A., Albert, P.S., Bash, C.N., Calabresi, P.A., Maloni, H., et al., 1997. Characterization of MRI response to treatment with interferon beta-1b: contrast-enhancing MRI lesion frequency as a primary outcome measure. Neurology. 49, 862–869.

Thacker, E.L., Mirzaei, F., Ascherio, A., 2006. Infectious mononucleosis and risk for multiple sclerosis: a meta-analysis. Ann. Neurol. 59, 499–503.

Thorley-Lawson, D.A., Gross, A., 2004. Persistence of the Epstein-Barr virus and the origins of associated lymphomas. N. Engl. J. Med. 350, 1328–1337.

Tintore, M., Rovira, A., Rio, J., Tur, C., Pelayo, R., Nos, C., et al., 2008. Do oligoclonal bands add information to MRI in first attacks of multiple sclerosis? Neurology. 70, 1079–1083.

Tishkoff, S.A., Verrelli, B.C., 2003. Role of evolutionary history on haplotype block structure in the human genome: implications for disease mapping. Curr. Opin. Genet. Dev. 13, 569–575.

Torkamani, A., Topol, E.J., Schork, N.J., 2008. Pathway analysis of seven common diseases assessed by genome-wide association. Genomics. 92, 265–272.

Trapp, B.D., Peterson, J., Ransohoff, R.M., Rudick, R., Mork, S., Bo, L., 1998. Axonal transection in the lesions of multiple sclerosis. N. Engl. J. Med. 338, 278–285.

Traugott, U., Reinherz, E.L., Raine, C.S., 1983. Multiple sclerosis: distribution of T cell subsets within active chronic lesions. Science. 219, 308–310.

Valenzuela, R.M., Costello, K., Chen, M., Said, A., Johnson, K.P., Dhib-Jalbut, S., 2007. Clinical response to glatiramer acetate correlates with modulation of IFN-gamma and IL-4 expression in multiple sclerosis. Mult. Scler. 13, 754–762.

Van Waesberghe, J.H., Kamphorst, W., De Groot, C.J., Van Walderveen, M.A., Castelijns, J.A., Ravid, R., et al., 1999. Axonal loss in multiple sclerosis lesions: magnetic resonance imaging insights into substrates of disability. Ann. Neurol. 46, 747–754.

Vanamerongen, B.M., Dijkstra, C.D., Lips, P., Polman, C.H., 2004. Multiple sclerosis and vitamin D: an update. Eur. J. Clin. Nutr. 58, 1095–1109.

Vartdal, F., Vandvik, B., Norrby, E., 1982. Intrathecal synthesis of virus-specific oligoclonal IgG, IgA and IgM antibodies in a case of varicella-zoster meningoencephalitis. J. Neurol. Sci. 57, 121–132.

Viglietta, V., Baecher-Allan, C., Weiner, H.L., Hafler, D.A., 2004. Loss of functional suppression by CD4 + CD25 + regulatory T cells in patients with multiple sclerosis. J. Exp. Med. 199, 971–979.

Warren, K.G., Catz, I., 1994. Relative frequency of autoantibodies to myelin basic protein and proteolipid protein in optic neuritis and multiple sclerosis cerebrospinal fluid. J. Neurol. Sci. 121, 66–73.

Warren, K.G., Catz, I., Johnson, E., Mielke, B., 1994. Anti-myelin basic protein and anti-proteolipid protein specific forms of multiple sclerosis. Ann. Neurol. 35, 280–289.

Weiner, H.L., Guttmann, C.R., Khoury, S.J., Orav, E.J., Hohol, M.J., Kikinis, R., et al., 2000. Serial magnetic resonance imaging in multiple sclerosis: correlation with attacks, disability, and disease stage. J. Neuroimmunol. 104, 164–173.

Weinshenker, B.G., 1994. Natural history of multiple sclerosis. Ann. Neurol. 36 (Suppl), S6–S11.

Weinshenker, B.G., 1996. Epidemiology of multiple sclerosis. Neurol. Clin. 14, 291–308.

Wellcome Trust Case Control Consortium, Burton, P.R., Clayton, D.G., Cardon, L.R., Craddock, N., Deloukas, P., et al., 2007. Association scan of 14,500 nonsynonymous SNPs in four diseases identifies autoimmunity variants. Nat. Genet. 39, 1329–1337.

Whitlock, F.A., Siskind, M.M., 1980. Depression as a major symptom of multiple sclerosis. J. Neurol. Neurosurg. Psychiatr. 43, 861–865.

Williams, A., Eldridge, R., McFarland, H., Houff, S., Krebs, H., McFarlin, D., 1980. Multiple sclerosis in twins. Neurology. 30, 1139–1147.

Windhagen, A., Scholz, C., Hollsberg, P., Fukaura, H., Sette, A., Hafler, D.A., 1995. Modulation of cytokine patterns of human autoreactive T cell clones by a single amino acid substitution of their peptide ligand. Immunity. 2, 373–380.

Wucherpfennig, K.W., Newcombe, J., Li, H., Keddy, C., Cuzner, M.L., Hafler, D.A., 1992a. Gamma delta T-cell receptor repertoire in acute multiple sclerosis lesions. Proc. Natl. Acad. Sci. U.S.A. 89, 4588–4592.

Wucherpfennig, K.W., Newcombe, J., Li, H., Keddy, C., Cuzner, M.L., Hafler, D.A., 1992b. T cell receptor V alpha-V beta repertoire and cytokine gene expression in active multiple sclerosis lesions. J. Exp. Med. 175, 993–1002.

Xavier, R.J., Rioux, J.D., 2008. Genome-wide association studies: a new window into immune-mediated diseases. Nat. Rev. Immunol. 8, 631–643.

Yamagata, K., Tagami, M., Torii, Y., Takenaga, F., Tsumagari, S., Itoh, S., et al., 2003. Sphingosine 1-phosphate induces the production of glial cell line-derived neurotrophic factor and cellular proliferation in astrocytes. Glia. 41, 199–206.

Yang, L., Anderson, D.E., Kuchroo, J., Hafler, D.A., 2008. Lack of TIM-3 immunoregulation in multiple sclerosis. J. Immunol. 180, 4409–4414.

Yang, Q., Khoury, M.J., Friedman, J., Little, J., Flanders, W.D., 2005. How many genes underlie the occurrence of common complex diseases in the population? Int. J. Epidemiol. 34, 1129–1137.

Young, I.R., Hall, A.S., Pallis, C.A., Legg, N.J., Bydder, G.M., Steiner, R.E., 1981. Nuclear magnetic resonance imaging of the brain in multiple sclerosis. Lancet. 2, 1063–1066.

Zeyda, M., Poglitsch, M., Geyeregger, R., Smolen, J.S., Zlabinger, G.J., Horl, W.H., et al., 2005. Disruption of the interaction of T cells with antigen-presenting cells by the active leflunomide metabolite teriflunomide: involvement of impaired integrin activation and immunologic synapse formation. Arthritis Rheum. 52, 2730–2739.

Zhernakova, A., Van Diemen, C.C., Wijmenga, C., 2009. Detecting shared pathogenesis from the shared genetics of immune-related diseases. Nat. Rev. Genet. 10, 43–55.

Zhou, D., Srivastava, R., Nessler, S., Grummel, V., Sommer, N., Bruck, W., et al., 2006. Identification of a pathogenic antibody response to native myelin oligodendrocyte glycoprotein in multiple sclerosis. Proc. Natl. Acad. Sci. U.S.A. 103, 19057–19062.

Chapter 53

Peripheral Neuropathies

Michael P.T. Lunn[1] and Kazim A. Sheikh[2]

[1]National Hospital for Neurology and Neurosurgery, Queen Square, London, UK, [2]University of Texas Medical School at Houston, TX, USA

Chapter Outline

Introduction	757
Acute Neuropathies: The Guillain–Barré Syndrome	757
Historical Background	757
Epidemiology	758
Clinical Features and Subtypes of GBS	758
Acute Inflammatory Demyelinating Polyradiculoneuropathy	758
Acute Motor Axonal Neuropathy	758
Acute Motor and Sensory Neuropathy	759
Miller Fisher Syndrome	759
Autoimmune Features	759
Molecular Mimicry	759
Anti-ganglioside Antibodies in GBS Variants	759
Gangliosides in Peripheral Nerve	761
Functional Effects of Antibodies	761
Environmental Effects	762
Animal Models of Disease	763
Cellular Mechanisms	763
Cellular and Humoral Immune Elements are Synergistic	765
Genetic Aspects of GBS	765
Treatment and Outcomes	766

Chronic Neuropathies: Chronic Inflammatory Demyelinating Polyradiculoneuropathy	766
History	766
Epidemiology and Clinical Features	766
Multifocal Motor Neuropathy with Conduction Block	766
Multifocal-acquired Demyelinating Sensory and Motor Neuropathy (MADSAM)	767
Multifocal-acquired Sensory and Motor Neuropathy (MASAM)	767
Paraproteinemic Demyelinating Peripheral Neuropathy	767
Autoimmune Features	768
Immunogenetic Features	768
Environmental Influences	768
Animal Models	768
Pathogenic Mechanisms	769
Treatment and Outcome	769
Concluding Remarks and Future Prospects	770
Acknowledgments	770
References	770

INTRODUCTION

Autoimmunity is implicated in a small but important group of peripheral nerve diseases. These include the acute inflammatory neuropathies eponymously referred to as the Guillain–Barré (GBS) and Fisher syndromes, and the chronic inflammatory demyelinating polyradiculoneuropathy (CIDP), both idiopathic and associated with a serum paraprotein. Substantial evidence exists for an autoimmune pathogenesis in GBS and its subtypes. Evidence is still gathering to support similar processes in the chronic inflammatory neuropathies including the demyelinating neuropathy associated with antibodies to myelin-associated glycoprotein (MAG). Although most current evidence supports an antibody-driven pathogenesis triggered by infection for GBS and Fisher syndrome,

T cell mechanisms predominate in CIDP and other cellular immune components are crucial effectors of disease. Experimental allergic neuritis (EAN), an inflammatory model of neuropathy, has been instructive in the detailed study of the pathogenesis of immune-mediated neuropathies and will be discussed.

ACUTE NEUROPATHIES: THE GUILLAIN–BARRÉ SYNDROME

Historical Background

Guillain, Barré, and Strohl described a rapidly evolving flaccid paralysis with areflexia and albuminocytological dissociation in the cerebrospinal fluid (CSF) in 1916

N. Rose & I. Mackay (Eds): The Autoimmune Diseases, Fifth edition. DOI: http://dx.doi.org/10.1016/B978-0-12-384929-8.00053-8

(Guillain et al., 1916). Early autopsies demonstrated both T cell inflammation and demyelination in peripheral nerves (Asbury et al., 1969; Haymaker and Kernohan, 1949) leading to the notion of GBS being a single pathophysiological entity synonymous with acute inflammatory demyelinating polyradiculoneuropathy (AIDP). AIDP is by far the most common variant of GBS in the developed world. Variants such as the Fisher syndrome (1956) (Fisher, 1956) and the axonal variants (1986) (Feasby et al., 1986), acute motor axonal neuropathy (AMAN) and acute motor and sensory axonal neuropathy (AMSAN) (Yuki et al., 1990; McKhann et al., 1991, 1993) are now part of a spectrum of disease with variable worldwide occurrence (see below and Box 53.1).

Epidemiology

Since the near eradication of poliomyelitis, GBS has become the commonest cause of acute flaccid neuromuscular paralysis in the world. The incidence of GBS is 0.81−1.89 per 100,000 (Hughes and Rees, 1997; Sejvar et al., 2011). The incidence increases steadily with advancing age (0.62 per 100,000 in 0−9 year olds and 2.99 per 100,000 in 80−89 year olds) and males are affected more than females by 1.25:1 (Hadden and Gregson, 2001; Sejvar et al., 2011). Case-control studies implicate infections as precipitating events (see later).

Severity may vary from mild with full recovery in 10% of patients only, to bedbound in 40%, to complete paralysis with ventilatory dependence in 20%. Death occurs in 3.5−12% of patients (Guillain-Barre Syndrome Study Group, 1985; Rees et al., 1998; Hughes and Cornblath, 2005).

Clinical Features and Subtypes of GBS

Acute Inflammatory Demyelinating Polyradiculoneuropathy

The diagnosis of GBS remains clinical. Electrophysiological studies patients help to subtype patients into diagnostic

> **BOX 53.1 The Diversity of Guillain–Barré Variants**
> - Acute inflammatory demyelinating polyradiculoneuropathy (AIDP)
> - Regional variants, e.g., pharyngo-cervical-brachial
> - Acute motor axonal neuropathy (AMAN)
> - Acute motor and sensory axonal neuropathy (AMSAN)
> - (Miller) Fisher syndrome (ataxia, ophthalmoplegia, and areflexia)
> - Acute panautonomic neuropathy
> - Acute pure sensory neuropathy
> - Acute motor conduction block neuropathy

categories. AIDP accounts for over 95% of patients with GBS in Europe and North America. Patients present with a rapidly evolving neuropathic (sensory-) motor paralysis, usually ascending, in two or more limbs over less than 4 weeks. The illness is monophasic. Most patients have numbness, tingling, or pain and many complain of bladder disturbance, facial weakness, or swallowing difficulty (Hughes, 1990). Autonomic disturbance is common with arrhythmia and fluctuating blood pressures. Tendon reflexes are absent or reduced. The CSF contains <50 leukocytes per μl (Asbury and Cornblath, 1990) and CSF protein is raised in 80% of cases. Antiganglioside antibodies may be detected in the serum (see below) by ELISA, often with thin layer chromatography confirmation, but novel solid phase multiplex and combinatorial ganglioside assays have emerged and are being increasingly used (Rinaldi et al., 2009). Electrophysiological studies typically show slowed motor conduction velocities, delayed F-waves, and preserved compound muscle action potential (CMAP) amplitudes consistent with demyelination, but conduction failure and axonal degeneration may complicate the picture.

Multifocal perivascular T cell infiltration with demyelination, typically patchy with involvement of proximal and terminal nerve segments, characterizes the pathology of AIDP (Asbury et al., 1969; Hall et al., 1992). Indications of blood−nerve barrier (BNB) breakdown and deposition of activated complement components can be seen in some but not all cases of AIDP (Hafer-Macko et al., 1996b). These observations raise the possibility that T cell- or antibody-mediated immune injury can predominate in an individual case, although the evidence is increasingly in favor of an antibody-driven process in humans.

Acute Motor Axonal Neuropathy

Acute motor axonal neuropathy (AMAN) is a pure motor variant of GBS seen most commonly in China, Japan, and Mexico (McKhann et al., 1991, 1993; Ogawara et al., 2000). Here it accounts for almost half of cases, but in Europe and North America it accounts for only 5−20% (Rees et al., 1995b; Visser et al., 1995), clinically probably nearer 5%. In China AMAN occurs in seasonal epidemics, affects more children (McKhann et al., 1991) and is strongly associated with *Campylobacter jejuni* infection. Sensory impairment is minimal and autonomic involvement less common. Electrophysiological studies are characterized by reduced CMAP amplitudes, absent F-waves with normal distal motor latencies and conduction velocity (Kuwabara et al., 2000) but many feel criteria of this sort misclassify AMAN as AIDP and the prevalence is higher (Uncini and Kuwabara, 2012). Sensory involvement is absent.

The pathology of axonal GBS has largely been described from AMAN cases in northern China. The pathological changes indicate an antibody-mediated immune attack directed preferentially against motor axons causing primary axonal degeneration in the absence of prominent T cell inflammation (Griffin et al., 1995, 1996a; Hafer-Macko et al., 1996a). Macrophages may be found in the periaxonal space suggesting that the antigen of interest is on the axolemma (Figure 53.1). Animal models of AMAN have disrupted nodal sodium channel clusters and detachment of paranodal myelin terminal loops. This would significantly reduce the safety factor for impulse transmission and might be responsible for the rapidly reversible conduction block frequently present in human AMAN (Yuki and Kuwabara, 2007). However, since in some patients little pathology is found (Griffin et al., 1996b) and in others recovery is too rapid for nerve fiber degeneration and regeneration (Ho et al., 1997; Kuwabara et al., 1998), axonal conduction failure and distal neuro-muscular terminal failure must also make a prominent contribution to clinical weakness in AMAN.

Acute Motor and Sensory Neuropathy

Acute motor and sensory neuropathy (AMSAN) is a more severe form of AMAN with a more severe course, sensory involvement, and delayed recovery (Feasby et al., 1986; Griffin et al., 1995). Sensory as well as motor nerve roots are involved. The pathology is similar to that of AMAN.

Miller Fisher Syndrome

The Miller Fisher or Fisher Syndrome (FS) (Fisher, 1956) accounts for approximately 5% of GBS cases and comprises ophthalmoplegia, ataxia, and areflexia without limb weakness. In common usage facial and bulbar weakness have been included as part of the syndrome. Overlapping forms with AIDP are not uncommon. This syndrome is strongly associated with preceding *C. jejuni* infection and more than 90% of patients have antibodies to the ganglioside GQ1b that are almost certainly pathogenic (see below) (Mizoguchi, 1998; O'Hanlon et al., 2001). Anti-GQ1b antibodies are also found in GBS patients with ophthalmoplegia. The pathophysiological and structural basis of the clinical manifestations in FS are still not completely resolved, although complement has been shown to be important in models of disease (Willison et al., 2008).

Autoimmune Features

Molecular Mimicry

Molecular mimicry has been invoked as a mechanism in a variety of autoimmune diseases. AMAN and FS provide some of the best available evidence to support the hypothesis of molecular mimicry as a pathogenic mechanism

underlying post-infectious autoimmune disorders. AIDP may be very similar and as more evidence of complex ganglioside antigen associations emerges AIDP may be resolved into the same pathogenic category as AMAN and FS. AMAN and FS fulfill some of the Koch−Witebsky postulates supporting autoantibody as pathogenic (Witebsky et al., 1957; Rose and Bona, 1993). Anti-ganglioside antibodies can be demonstrated in patient serum. They have cognate antigens (gangliosides) enriched in peripheral nerve. It is possible to immunize animals (see below) with ganglioside antigens either purified or as whole bacteria to produce autoantibody and disease, albeit with difficulty. Transfer of antibody from patient/model animal to a normal subject can sometimes transfer disease. Furthermore mechanisms of antibody action are now starting to be understood.

Anti-ganglioside Antibodies in GBS Variants

Antibodies to ganglioside species are found in the serum of patients with GBS (both AMAN and AIDP). They are polyclonal, predominantly IgG, and generally complement-fixing IgG1 and IgG3 (Willison and Veitch, 1994; Ogino et al., 1995; Yuki et al., 1995; Ho et al., 1999). This implies class-switching usually with T cell help, both atypical of human anti-carbohydrate responses (see below). Antibodies to single gangliosides GM1, GM1(NeuGc), GM1b, GalNAc-GM1b, GD1a, GalNAc-GD1a, GD1b, 9-0-acetyl GD1b, GD3, GT1b, GQ1b, GQ1bα, LM1, galactocerebroside, and SGPG have been reported in more than 200 papers on inflammatory neuropathies (Willison and Yuki, 2002). Clinico-serological correlations between GBS subtypes and serum antibodies to putative ganglioside antigens have been drawn (Ho et al., 1999; Ogawara et al., 2000; Rees et al., 1995a). Antibodies to gangliosides GM1 and GD1a, implicated as the major target antigens in AMAN (Hadden et al., 1998; Ho et al., 1999), can be detected in 50−60% of AMAN patients in the Far East (Ho et al., 1999; Ogawara et al., 2000). Antibodies to GalNAc-GD1a and GM1b are found in motor predominant GBS in about 10−15% of cases (Ang et al., 1999; Yuki et al., 2000). Anti-GQ1b antibodies, frequently cross-reactive with structurally related gangliosides, are present in 80−90% of patients with FS (Willison et al., 1993; Yuki et al., 1993; Carpo et al., 1998). This correlation provides the strongest association between antibodies to a specific ganglioside and a clinical phenotype.

More recently the serendipitous identification of antibodies to complex gangliosides has led to a resurgence of interest in antibodies (Kusunoki's first reference) (Greenshields et al., 2009; Kusunoki and Kaida, 2011). Antibody activity to a ganglioside species can be enhanced or entirely abrogated by the close association of a second species of ganglioside presumably making a complex epitope. Antibodies to ganglioside complexes

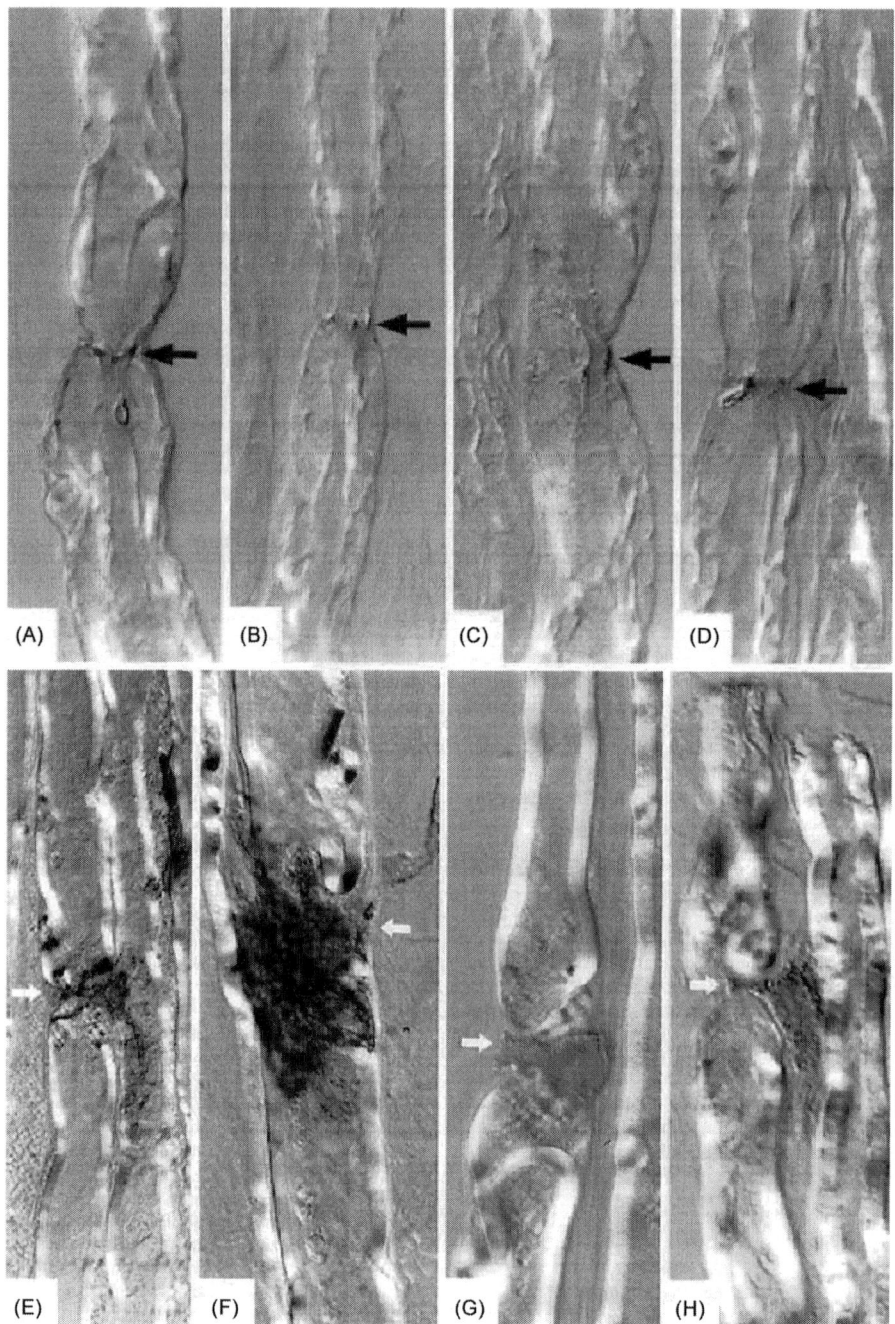

FIGURE 53.1 **Immunostained teased ventral root fibers from a case of AMAN 4 days after the onset of neurologic symptoms.** (A−D) The complement activation product C3d was localized discretely at nodes of Ranvier (black arrows) of large myelinated motor fibers. The golden-brown immunoreaction product is at the nodes. (E−H) Many motor fibers had macrophages overlying, and extending processes into, the nodes of Ranvier (white arrows designate nodes of Ranvier). (E and F were immunostained with the macrophage marker HAM-56; G and H for HLA-DR [major histocompatibility locus class II]). *Reprinted with permission of John Wiley & Sons Inc. from figure 1, p. 639 of Hafer-Macko et al. (1996a).*

may explain the lack of antibodies found in sera when only single ganglioside activities were sought, the difficulties of consistent identification of clinic-serological phenotypes, and the apparent inconsistency in spatial distribution of single gangliosides and antibody binding.

The serological studies have also identified associations of specific anti-ganglioside or -ganglioside complex antibodies with poor recovery (reviewed in Lopez et al., 2010 and Sheikh and Zhang, 2010). These association studies imply that specific anti-ganglioside antibodies can not only injure intact nerve fibers to induce neuropathy, but can also adversely affect recovery by either inducing more severe neuropathic disease or interfering with the nerve repair process required for recovery. Experimental studies with anti-ganglioside antibodies support the latter hypothesis (Lehmann et al., 2007; Lopez et al., 2010).

Gangliosides in Peripheral Nerve

Gangliosides are sialic acid containing glycolipids (see Figure 53.2), widely distributed in mammalian tissues, but enriched in the nervous system. GM1, GD1b, GD1a, and GT1b are most abundant. A simple hypothesis to explain the differences between GBS variants is based on the premise that target gangliosides have differential distribution in the PNS, but this hypothesis is being modified in response to the discovery of complex ganglioside epitopes. In relation to FS, GQ1b is relatively enriched in the oculomotor cranial nerves (Chiba et al., 1993, 1997) although anti-GQ1b antibodies may bind elsewhere (Goodyear et al., 1999). Although ganglioside immunolocalization studies are technically difficult, the AMAN-associated gangliosides GM1 and GD1a are localized at the nodes of Ranvier and in motor nerve terminals (Sheikh et al., 1999; Gong et al., 2002). Furthermore, preferential staining of motor nerve fibers has been demonstrated with monoclonal anti-GD1a antibodies in rats (Figure 53.3) and also with human anti-GD1a antibodies from a patient with AMAN (De Angelis et al., 2001). Distribution of ganglioside complexes in vivo will be even more difficult. Other factors such as variations in permeability of the blood–nerve barrier, density and accessibility of target gangliosides, and relationship to functional components of the axolemma such as ion channels, are likely to be relevant.

Functional Effects of Antibodies

Antibodies bind to nerves at nodes of Ranvier where gangliosides (especially GM1) and channels are enriched. Early studies indicated that anti-GM1 antibodies possibly blocked or altered channel function although the exact mechanism was unclear (Sheikh et al., 1999). Intraneural injection of GBS patient serum, purified immunoglobulin, or specific anti-ganglioside antibodies has produced mixed results (Saida et al., 1979; Winer et al., 1988; Sumner et al., 1992). Powerful models developed over the last 10 years have demonstrated clear binding of antibodies and complement to nodal structures, dissolution of the axonal cytoskeletal architecture, and disruption of nodal and paranodal channels (Susuki et al., 2007). The electrical effect of this is to destabilize the membrane resulting in trains of uncontrolled miniature end plate potentials identifiable in models.

An alternative site of attack is at the roots and motor nerve terminals (MNTs) where the blood–nerve barrier is

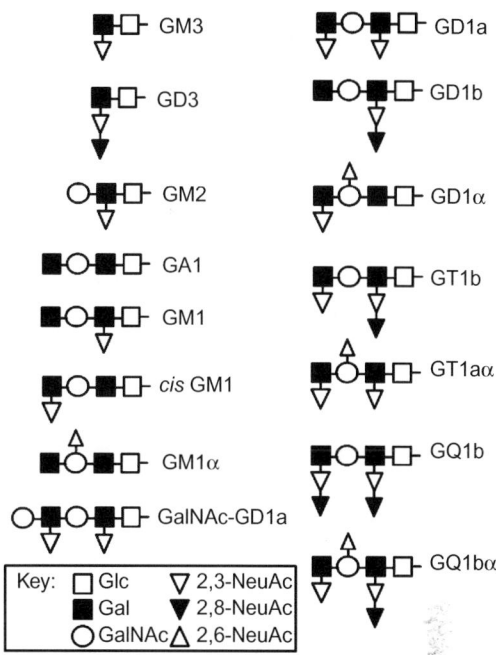

FIGURE 53.2 Some of the ganglioside species in peripheral nerve, potentially targets for neuropathy-associated antibodies. Note the similarity in structures between species, which allows for some cross-reactivity. Glc = glucose, Gal = galactose, GalNAc = N-acetylgalactosamine, NeuAc = Neuraminic (sialic) acid.

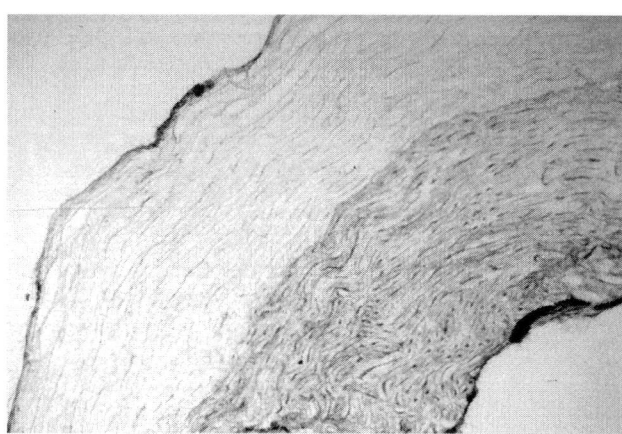

FIGURE 53.3 Unfixed fresh-frozen rat motor-sensory nerve root stained with a monospecific murine IgG anti-GD1a antibody. There is preferential strong staining of the motor axons of the ventral root (below) compared to the sensory axons of the adjacent dorsal root (above). Magnification × 320.

relatively deficient. MNTs degenerate in AMAN (Ho et al., 1997) and are disturbed electrophysiologically in FS (Uncini and Lugaresi, 1999). In an *ex vivo* phrenic nerve–diaphragm preparation, Willison et al. showed that anti-GQ1b antibodies bind to nerve terminals, cause complement-dependent quantal acetylcholine (ACh) release resulting in neuromuscular blockade and a calcium dependent disruption of the terminal bouton (Goodyear et al., 1999; Plomp et al., 1999; O'Hanlon et al., 2001). They have recently shown the same effect with anti-GD1a antibodies dependent upon GD1a antigen density (Goodfellow et al., 2005).

In a parallel series of patch-clamp experiments, IgG GQ1b, GD1a, GD1b, and GM1 antibodies have been shown to cause reversible complement independent pre- and post-synaptic blockade depending upon the antibody used (Buchwald et al., 2002).

The clinical, pathological, and electrical effects are almost entirely abrogated by the application of an inhibitor of the C5 component of complement (eculizumab) which results in failure of formation of the membrane attack complex (Halstead et al., 2008). This pathophysiological understanding and subsequent proof of concept in an animal model has led to the design of human trials.

Anti-ganglioside antibodies can inhibit neurite growth and growth cone extension in primary neuronal cultures consistent with the notion that these antibodies can adversely affect axon and nerve regeneration (Zhang et al., 2011b). Small GTPase RhoA is part of the downstream inhibitory intracellular signaling that mediates anti-ganglioside antibody-induced inhibition of axon growth (Zhang et al., 2011b). A recent study has shown that pleiotropic cytokine erythropoietin (EPO) with neurotrophic properties reverses the inhibitory effects of anti-ganglioside antibodies via EPO receptors and the Janus kinase 2/Signal transducer and activator of transcription 5 pathway (Zhang et al. 2011a).

Environmental Effects

Campylobacter jejuni is a Gram-negative, non-spore-forming enteropathogen and is one of the most common causes of bacterial gastroenteritis worldwide (Friedman et al., 2000; Oberhelman and Taylor, 2000) (see Figure 53.4). Infection with *C. jejuni* is found in 13–72% of patients with AMAN or GBS (Hughes and Rees, 1997; Hadden and Gregson, 2001) with an overall prevalence estimated around 30% (Moran et al., 2002). Only one in 1000 cases of *C. jejuni* infection is complicated by GBS. The exact characteristics of *C. jejuni that* determine whether GBS follows infection are still unclear. However, a relationship of GBS with a number of Penner serotypes is recognized (Prendergast and Moran, 2000). Penner serotyping distinguishes *C. jejuni* strains on the basis of strain-specific, heat-stable extractable capsular lipopoly- and lipooligosaccharides. Penner strains HS:19 (Rees et al., 1995b; Sheikh et al., 1998) and HS:41 (Goddard et al., 1997) are particular overrepresented in GBS and uncommon in patients with uncomplicated gastroenteritis.

The lipopolysaccharide (LPS) and lipooligosaccharide (LOS) of *C. jejuni* carry ganglioside-like moieties.

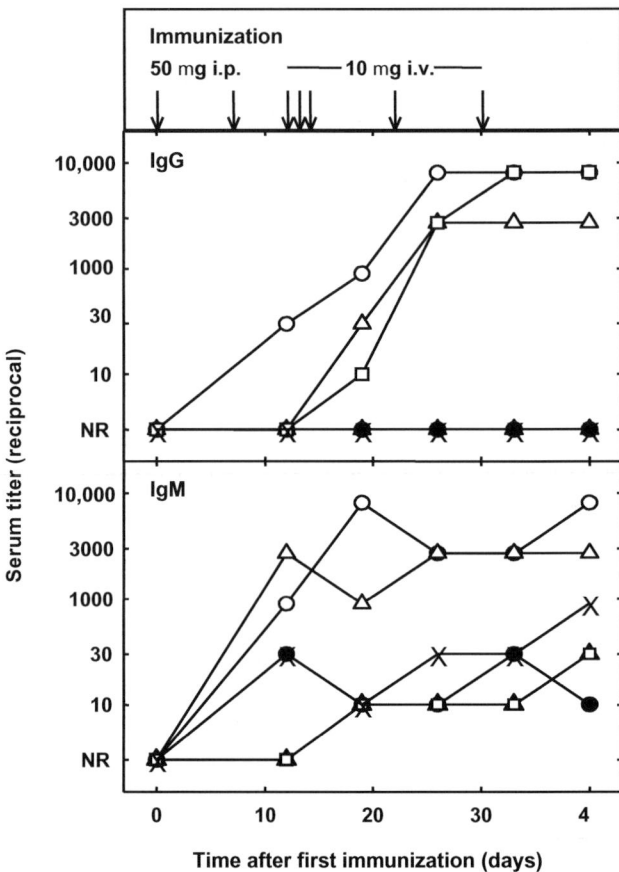

FIGURE 53.4 *Campylobacter jejuni*, a Gram-negative flagellated non-spore-forming enteropathogen, is one of the most common causes of bacterial gastroenteritis worldwide and is found in 13–72% of patients with AMAN or GBS.

Several studies have characterized these in GBS- and diarrhea-associated *C. jejuni* strains. GM1-, GD1a-, GalNAc-GD1a-, GM1b-, GT1a-, GD2-, GD3-, and GM2-like structures have all been identified (Aspinall et al., 1993; Yuki et al., 1994; Nachamkin et al., 2002). Although no GQ1b-like structure exists, antibody binding assays have shown the presence of GQ1b- and GT1a-cross-reactive moieties in *C. jejuni* LPS/LOSs (Yuki et al., 1994; Jacobs et al., 1995, 1997). It is these structures that are likely to provide the initial stimulus to auto-immune activation.

Upper respiratory tract infection or other febrile episodes caused by cytomegalovirus (CMV) (5–22%), Epstein–Barr virus (EBV) (2–10%), *Mycoplasma pneumoniae* (5%), and *Haemophilus influenzae* have all been identified as potentially causative (Hadden and Gregson, 2001). *H. influenzae* carries ganglioside-like moieties. Swine flu and rabies vaccinations have also been causatively implicated, but recent surveillance for an association with swine flu vaccination failed to demonstrate any conclusive link (Crawford et al., 2012).

Animal Models of Disease

Attempts to generate either IgG anti-ganglioside antibodies or neuropathy in animals by immunization with *C. jejuni* were for a long while either unforthcoming or not reproducible. Immunization of mice with *C. jejuni* LPSs/LOSs generates mainly low titer IgM antibodies (Wirguin et al., 1997; Goodyear et al., 1999) reflecting a high level of tolerance to self-gangliosides (Bowes et al., 2002). Tolerance to self-gangliosides can be overcome by immunization with gangliosides or *C. jejuni* LPSs conjugated to adjuvant in transgenic animals lacking complex gangliosides (Lunn et al., 2000) (see Figure 53.5). This model illustrates that where tolerance is circumvented, potentially pathogenic antibodies can be generated.

A sensory ataxic neuropathy with pathological changes in the nerve and the cord has been induced in rabbits by GD1b immunization and passive antibody transfer (Kusunoki et al., 1999). Immunization with mixed bovine brain gangliosides or GM1 alone produced an acute flaccid paralysis in rabbits reminiscent of human disease (Susuki et al., 2003). The implantation of a murine IgG antiGD1a secreting hybridoma into mice but not passive transfer of the same antibody led to an axonal neuropathy (Sheikh et al., 2004). Additional cytokine factors may be required to initiate the neuropathy.

The combined research in GBS models has clearly demonstrated that antibodies bind to ganglioside targets on the nerve, fix complement, destroy the nodal and cytoskeletal architecture through complement and calcium-dependent mechanisms, and result in electrophysiological instability and axonal dissolution (Willison et al., 2008).

A passive transfer animal model has been established to examine the effects of anti-ganglioside antibodies on peripheral nerve repair/axon regeneration (Lehmann et al., 2007). These passive transfer studies show that patient and experimental antibodies inhibit axon regeneration in a nerve crush model mimicking the regenerative response of degenerating/injured axons in GBS (Lehmann et al., 2007; Lopez et al., 2010). The impaired regenerative responses and ultrastructure of injured peripheral axons mimicked dystrophic and stalled growth cones typically seen after CNS injury. Such dystrophic/stalled growth cones can also be seen in nerve biopsy of GBS patients with poor recovery (Sheikh and Zhang, 2010). These observations support the notion that inhibition of axon regeneration is one mechanism of poor recovery in GBS patients with anti-ganglioside antibodies. Further, this antibody-induced nerve injury model was used to show beneficial proregenerative effects of EPO (Zhang et al., 2011a).

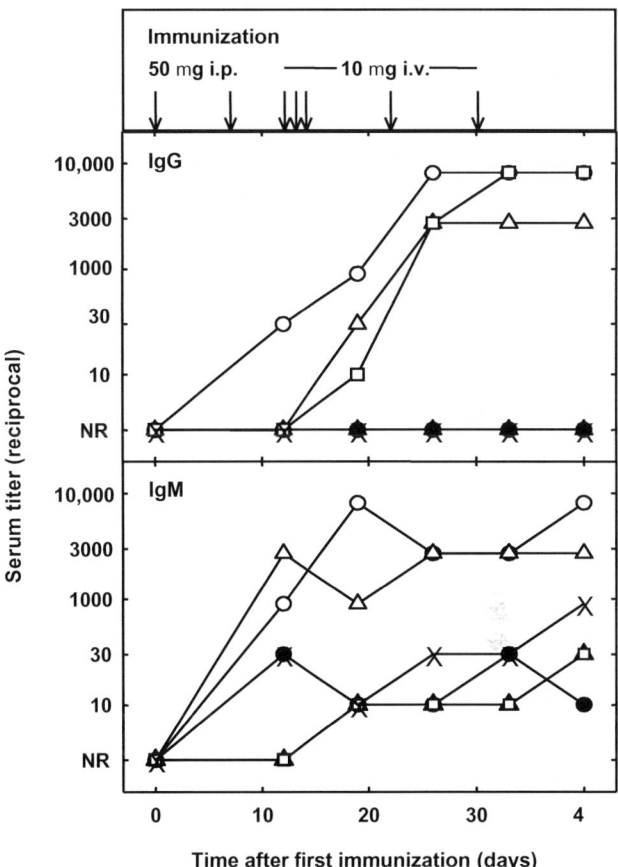

FIGURE 53.5 Mice lacking complex ganglioside species (*GalNAcT−/−*) are able to class switch to complement fixing IgG production when immunized with keyhole limpet hemocyanin (KLH)-conjugated ganglioside. Figure shows serological responses of *GalNAcT−/−* and wild-type mice immunized with GD1a-KLH or KLH alone. Sera collected at the indicated times were tested for IgG and IgM anti-GD1a antibody titers by ELISA. Open symbols, individual *GalNAcT−/−* mice immunized with GD1a-KLH; filled symbols, individual wild-type mice immunized with GD1a-KLH; X, *GalNAcT−/−* mouse immunized with unconjugated KLH. Titer values are presented as the greatest dilution resulting in a signal which exceeded 3 SD above the control mean. i.p., intraperitoneal; i.v. intravenous. *Reprinted with permission of Blackwell Publishing Ltd. from figure 2 of Lunn et al. (2000). Copyright © Blackwell Publishing Ltd. 2000.*

Cellular Mechanisms

Comprehensive evidence of T cell involvement in GBS has not been so forthcoming despite the central role of T cells in the pathogenesis of experimental allergic neuritis (EAN). Studies of animal models and predominantly human AIDP have generated a complex multi-step pathogenesis for cellular involvement in the autoimmune neuropathies (see Figure 53.6).

Multifocal lymphocytic infiltration was established as the hallmark of the pathology of GBS in early post-mortem studies (Asbury et al., 1969) but it is not always seen (Cornblath et al., 1990; Honavar et al., 1991). Circulating activated T cells are found early in the course of GBS (Taylor and

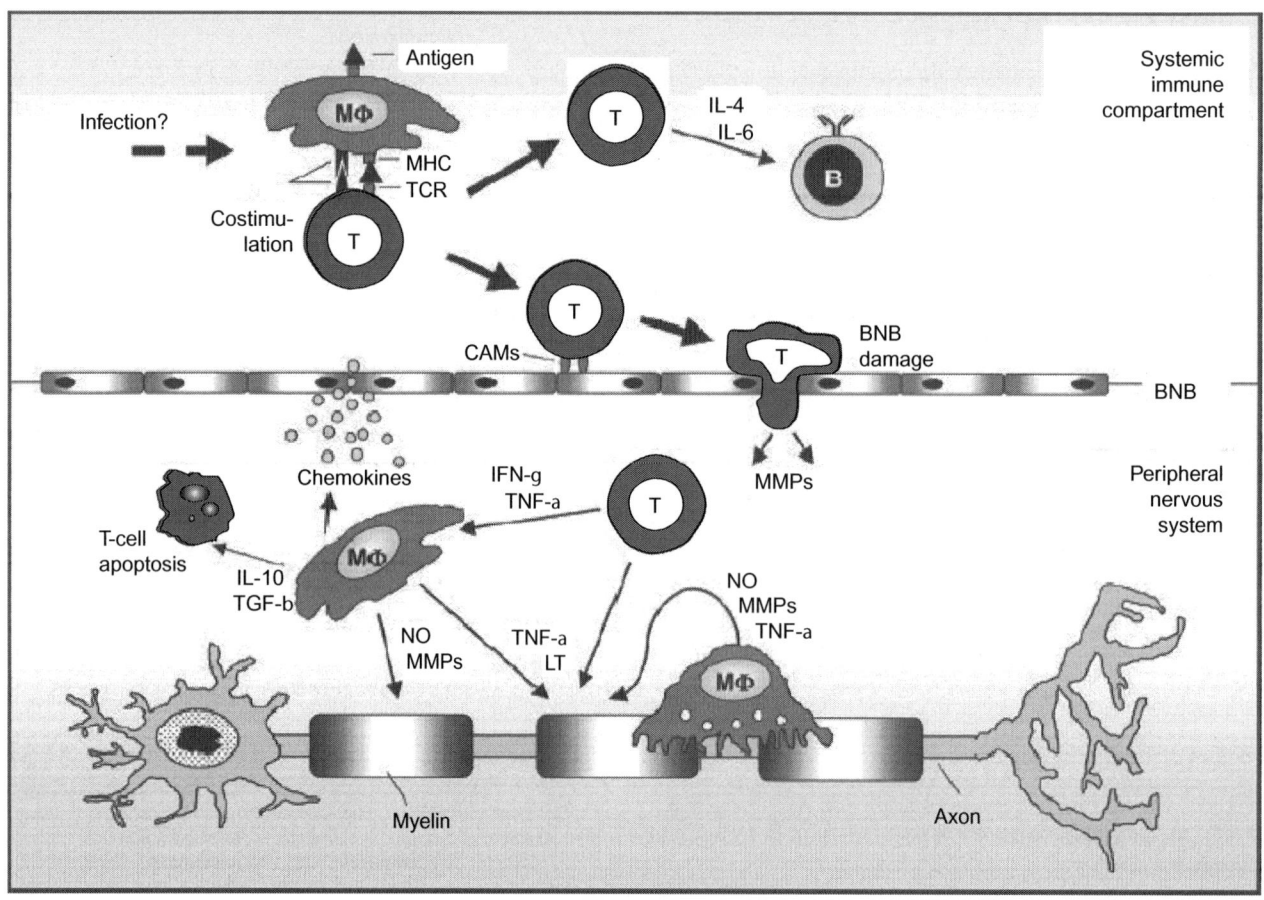

FIGURE 53.6　Schematic illustration of the immune responses in the inflamed peripheral nervous system. Basic principles of the cellular immune responses: autoreactive T cells (T) recognize a specific autoantigen presented by major histocompatibility complex (MHC) class II molecules and the simultaneous delivery of costimulatory signals on the cell surface of antigen-presenting cells, such as macrophages (MΦ), in the systemic immune compartment. Activated T lymphocytes can cross the blood–nerve barrier (BNB) in order to enter the peripheral nervous system (PNS). Within the PNS, T cells activate macrophages that enhance phagocytic activity, production of cytokines, and the release of toxic mediators, such as nitric oxide (NO), matrix metalloproteinases (MMPs), and proinflammatory cytokines, propagating demyelination and axonal loss. The termination of the inflammatory response is mediated, in part, by macrophages by the induction of T cell apoptosis and the release of anti-inflammatory Th2/Th3 cytokines, such as interleukin-10 (IL-10) and transforming growth factor-β (TGF-β). *Reprinted with permission from John Wiley & Sons Inc. from figure 1, p. 136 of Kieseier et al. (2004). Copyright © John Wiley & Sons Inc. 2004.*

Hughes, 1989; Hartung and Toyka, 1990). αβT cells with CD4 and CD8 ratios in similar proportions to peripheral blood (Cornblath et al., 1990) are the predominant cells found in nerve. Restricted usage of Vβ genes, especially Vβ15, suggests activation by a common antigen or superantigen (Khalili-Shirazi et al., 1997). Furthermore, γδT cells have also been found in, and isolated from, GBS-affected nerves (Khalili-Shirazi et al., 1998; Winer et al., 2002). γδT cells are capable of recognizing non-protein antigen and are thus candidates for responding to putative carbohydrate and ganglioside antigens (see above) (Bukowski et al., 1998). They proliferate *in vitro* in response to *C. jejuni* sonicates but require either αβT cells or IL-2/IL-15 to do so. Predominant use of Vγ8δ1 suggests activation of epithelially (possibly gut) resident γδT cells (Cooper et al., 2000). αβ and γδT cells also probably provide the necessary help to

orchestrate class-switching of anti-ganglioside antibodies to IgG1 and IgG3.

Autoantigen in the systemic compartment is processed and presented by antigen-presenting cells. EAN can be initiated with neuritogenic epitopes of peripheral nerve proteins P0, P2, and PMP22 (Hughes et al., 1999) or by adoptive transfer of sensitized T cells. Disease severity depends upon the cell or antigen dosage (Hartung et al., 1996). Disease is dependent on the presence of T cells, their normal function (Holmdahl et al., 1985; Hartung et al., 1987; Jung et al., 1992), and normal function of the costimulatory partners B7.1/CD80 or B7.2/CD86 and CTLA4/CD28 (Kiefer et al., 2000; Zhu et al., 2001; Zehntner et al., 2003).

Lymphocyte activation is revealed by greater numbers of circulating T cells bearing activation markers and increased concentrations of Th1 cytokines such as IFN-γ, IL-2, IL-2 receptor, and TNF-α (Taylor and Hughes, 1989; Hartung et al., 1991; Exley et al., 1994; Creange et al., 1996). Levels of TGF-β1 are depressed (Creange et al., 1998). In EAN levels of IFN-γ, IL-1β, IL-6, TNF-α, TNF-β, and IL-12 are raised during development of disease (Zhu et al., 1997).

Homing and migration of activated T cells to the peripheral nerve is modulated by E-selectin and mucins binding L-selectin and sialyl Lewis antigens (Hartung et al., 2002) and then VCAM-1 and ICAM-1, both upregulated early in GBS and EAN progression (Enders et al., 1998; Creange et al., 2001). Blockade of VCAM-1 or its ligand VLA-4/α4β1 integrin ameliorates EAN (Enders et al., 1998). Selectin and integrin released into the circulation may downregulate inflammation (Hartung et al., 1988). Chemokines assist in leukocyte recruitment localization and trafficking (Baggiolini, 1998; Campbell et al., 1998). The chemokine receptors CCR1, CCR2, CCR4, CCR5, and CXCR3 have been characterized in AIDP-affected nerves, differentially upregulated in infiltrating cell populations (Kieseier et al., 2002).

Diapedesis through the vascular endothelium and the basal lamina is facilitated by matrix metalloproteinases (MMPs). MMP-2, MMP-3, MMP-7, and especially MMP-9 have been implicated in the pathogenesis of EAN and GBS (Kieseier et al., 1998; Creange et al., 1999) and correlate with GBS severity.

Macrophages, both resident and recruited from the circulation (Hartung et al., 2002), remain the key component in perpetuating endoneurial inflammatory damage through the release of specific immune mediators. Under inflammatory conditions they continue to express antigen and induce Schwann cells to do so also (Gold et al., 1995). Depletion of macrophages abrogates the development of EAN, indicating their central role in the final common pathway of nerve damage. Activated macrophages target normal looking nerves and Schwann cells in EAN and AIDP (Hartung et al., 1996; Hughes et al., 1999) probably by antibody-targeted cellular cytotoxicity and complement-dependent mechanisms (Hafer-Macko et al., 1996a,b). Macrophage processes insinuate themselves between myelin lamellae and strip the myelin in AIDP (Hughes et al., 1999) or directly attack the axon in AMAN (see Figure 53.1) (Hafer-Macko et al., 1996a). In the endoneurium macrophages secrete a host of inflammatory mediators including MMPs, TNF-α, nitric oxide, eicosanoids, neutral proteases, lipases, and phospholipases, all contributing to nerve damage (Gregson and Hall, 1973; Redford et al., 1997; Smith et al., 1999).

Macrophages may also influence recovery from GBS. They direct T cell apoptosis reducing the ongoing response. During recovery, the T cell response shifts towards Th2 with rises in IL-4 in patients (Dahle et al., 1997) and

upregulation of TGF-β1, IL-10, and cytolysin in models of disease (Kiefer et al., 1996). TGF-β1 favors recovery (Vriesendorp et al., 1996; Zhu et al., 1997) and levels are correlated to severity of GBS (Creange et al., 1998).

A recent study (Mausberg et al., 2011) showed that EPO reduced disease severity and also shortened the recovery phase of EAN. The clinical improvement in this model correlated with decreased T cell inflammation within the peripheral nerve and produced less nerve fiber injury. In contrast, EPO increased the number of macrophages in the recovery phase of EAN. The beneficial effects of macrophages and the modulation of the immune system towards anti-inflammatory responses in the PNS was associated with upregulation of anti-inflammatory cytokine transforming growth factor (TGF)-beta.

Cellular and Humoral Immune Elements are Synergistic

Understanding of the pathomechanisms of the acute inflammatory neuropathies is incomplete. Neither antibodies nor T cells generate disease in isolation and immunization with any antigen induces responses in both cellular and humoral arms of the immune system. The apparent absence of T cells in some biopsies, and hence their possible non-necessity, is discussed above. Arguments against the early and significant involvement of antibodies include the absence of detectable anti-ganglioside antibodies, using current methodology, in a significant proportion of GBS (usually AIDP) cases, and the onset of adoptive transfer-EAN (AT-EAN) 4 days after transfer, before antibodies could be synthesized. However, recent advances have reduced the strength of these arguments. First, disease severity in AT-EAN is usually enhanced by co-transferring antibodies recognizing myelin or oligodendrocytes/Schwann cell epitopes (Spies et al., 1995), although this was not confirmed when pre-treatment AIDP GBS sera were co-administered to rats with mild EAN (Hadden et al., 2001). Gangliosides are not necessarily targeted by antibodies as single entities explaining why many sera were apparently negative for anti-ganglioside antibodies. Combinatorial epitopes made from adjacent but differing molecules that enhance or reduce antibody affinity in vitro and probably in vivo are recognized as targets (Kusunoki and Kaida, 2011).

Genetic Aspects of GBS

The role of host genetics in susceptibility to GBS is still in its infancy. No strong correlations have been established between disease susceptibility or GBS subtypes and host MHC class I or class II haplotypes in several studies (Magira et al., 2003; Geleijns et al., 2005a). The study of single nucleotide polymorphisms in genes for various components of the immune response has not identified any significant contributors (Geleijns et al., 2005a, b). One Dutch study identified that GBS patients homozygous for the Fcγ receptor IIa-H131 had a higher chance of developing severe disease than patients with other genotypes (van der Pol et al., 2000). Polymorphisms in CD1 molecules which present ganglioside to T cells were associated with GBS in two studies but the largest study to date failed to confirm this (Kuijf et al., 2008). Meta-analysis focusing on TNF-α, CD1, and FcγR suggests that the TNF-α 308A allele may be a moderate risk factor for GBS (Wu et al., 2012), but this awaits confirmation in directed larger studies.

Treatment and Outcomes

The effectiveness of other immunotherapies for GBS is supported by good evidence (Hughes et al., 2003). Two to five sessions of plasma exchange (PEx) hastens recovery in non-ambulant patients preferably started within 2 weeks of disease onset (Raphael et al., 2012). Intravenous immunoglobulin (ivIg) is as effective as PEx and is still probably the intervention of choice (Hughes et al., 2012). The concern about possible contamination of ivIg with prions means that written informed consent is essential before administration although advances in ivIg purification technology and prion detection may reduce this concern. The drive to search for new, more effective, and safer therapies is stronger than ever.

A large randomized controlled trial, previous smaller trials, and a Cochrane meta-analysis (Hughes and van Doorn, 2012) have shown steroids to be at best ineffective, and in some cases harmful. There is no indication for their use in GBS.

Complement inhibitors such as eculizumab are effective in other complement-mediated conditions such as paroxysmal nocturnal hemoglobinuria, and possibly effective in multifocal motor neuropathy, and clinical trials in the treatment of GBS are planned. Immunoadsorption of pathogenic anti-ganglioside antibodies has been infrequently used (Willison et al., 2004). Preclinical studies in antibody and T cell-induced models of GBS suggest that EPO neuroprotection is a viable candidate drug to develop further for neuroprotection and enhancing nerve repair in patients with GBS (Zhang et al., 2011a).

CHRONIC NEUROPATHIES: CHRONIC INFLAMMATORY DEMYELINATING POLYRADICULONEUROPATHY

Chronic inflammatory demyelinating polyradiculoneuropathy (CIDP) is an acquired peripheral nervous system disease characterized by progressive or relapsing proximal and distal weakness with or without sensory loss. There is good evidence to indicate that CIDP is autoimmune.

History

Osler recognized a chronic relapsing or progressive form of "multiple neuritis" in 1892. Austin described a slowly progressive or recurrent "steroid responsive polyneuropathy" (Austin, 1958) with histology indistinguishable from that seen in GBS. The term chronic inflammatory demyelinating polyradiculoneuropathy was coined in 1975 (Dyck et al., 1975).

Epidemiology and Clinical Features

The prevalence of CIDP is 1.25−7 per 100,000 (Lunn et al., 1998; Mygland and Monstad, 2001). Symmetrical sensory and motor deficits both proximal and distal reach their nadir over more than 8 weeks. The clinical course is commonly chronic and progressive particularly in untreated patients but some patients have a relapsing−remitting pattern of disease. Some case series have shown that up to 15% of patients with CIDP can start acutely with GBS-like onset (Dionne et al., 2010). Cranial nerve and the diaphragm are infrequently involved. CSF examination demonstrates albuminocytological dissociation with raised protein in more than 90% of cases (Bouchard et al., 1999) and the cell count is <10 mm^3 unless complicated by human immunodeficiency virus (HIV). Electrophysiology typically demonstrates multifocal motor conduction slowing, temporal dispersion, and block with delayed or absent F-waves. Half of patients require treatment at any one time and 13% require long-term aid to walk (Lunn et al., 1999). In a single study, six of 21 patients were shown to have serum antibodies to the peripheral myelin protein P0 (Yan et al., 2001) but this remains unconfirmed. Morphological examination demonstrates macrophage-associated demyelination in nerve roots, plexuses, and nerve trunks with T cells in the endoneurium. The edema, Schwann cell proliferation, and inflammatory infiltrates testify to the ongoing inflammation. Axonal degeneration occurs in severe or late cases or in distal sensory nerve biopsies (Hadden and Hughes, 2003).

As with GBS, CIDP is heterogeneous and a number of subtypes or related conditions have emerged.

Multifocal Motor Neuropathy with Conduction Block

Multifocal motor neuropathy with conduction block (MMNCB) (Pestronk et al., 1988) is a rare but treatable condition sometimes misdiagnosed as motor neurone disease. Wasting and weakness begin asymmetrically in the distribution of a motor nerve usually more distal than proximal, most commonly in the upper limb. Fasciculations and cramps occur. Males account for 70% of cases. Sensory symptoms are reported in 20% of patients. Depending upon assay methods, between 30 and 80% of patients have anti-GM1 antibodies in the serum (Sander and Latov, 2003), some as a paraprotein. Rarely anti-GD1a antibodies are described (Carpo et al., 1996). Electrophysiological studies demonstrate multifocal conduction blocks in two or more nerves with normal sensory conduction. Many studies demonstrate evidence of more widespread slowing or axonal degeneration.

The etiology of MMNCB remains unresolved, as it is seldom fatal and neuropathological material is seldom sought. Perivascular CIDP-like inflammation has been described in a motor nerve biopsy (Kaji et al., 1993), and there are minimal findings in sensory nerves (Corse et al., 1996). Inflammatory cellular infiltration and immunoglobulin deposition were described in the motor roots of an autopsy case (Oh et al., 1995). The therapeutic response to immunomodulation supports an autoimmune pathogenesis (Umapathi et al., 2005).

Multifocal-acquired Demyelinating Sensory and Motor Neuropathy (MADSAM)

Lewis and Sumner described the entity now referred to as MADSAM in 1982 (Lewis et al., 1982). Electrophysiological examination demonstrates multifocal sensory and motor involvement with conduction block.

Multifocal-acquired Sensory and Motor Neuropathy (MASAM)

This group of patients has only been recently described (Alaedini et al., 2003). Anti-ganglioside antibodies are found in the serum of 48% and there is a beneficial response to immunomodulation. The nerve conduction studies do not suggest demyelination and are more consistent with axonal degeneration. These findings require confirmation.

Paraproteinemic Demyelinating Peripheral Neuropathy

Ten percent of patients with a peripheral neuropathy will have a paraprotein in the serum. Although this should initiate a search for a malignant source, such as multiple or solitary myeloma, most are monoclonal gammopathies of undetermined significance (MGUS). A number of MGUS-neuropathy syndromes are described.

The commonest is a progressive sensory ataxic neuropathy with unsteadiness and tremor associated with an IgMκ paraprotein that reacts with the HNK-1 epitope of the peripheral nerve antigen myelin-associated

glycoprotein (MAG). Up to 80% of patients with an IgM paraprotein and a demyelinating neuropathy have anti-MAG antibodies. Nerve conduction studies reveal motor conduction slowing, particularly distally (Cocito et al., 2001). Electron microscopic examination of myelin in sural nerve biopsies reveals characteristic widening of the intraperiod line not seen in other conditions (see Figure 53.7).

Neuropathies associated with IgG or IgA paraproteins are found in a diverse group of patients with axonal and demyelinating forms of disease. No consistent pathogenesis has yet emerged. The demyelinating cases have a similar therapeutic response to CIDP (Allen et al., 2007).

Chronic ataxic neuropathy with ophthalmoplegia, M-protein, and anti-disialosyl antibodies (CANOMAD) is a rare paraproteinemic syndrome rather like a chronic Fisher syndrome. Its pathogenesis is not yet resolved.

The POEMS syndrome (polyneuropathy, organomegaly, endocrinopathy, M-protein, and skin changes) is a rare condition associated with both osteosclerotic myeloma and Castleman's disease. The paraprotein required to make the diagnosis does not seem to participate in the pathogenesis as it is often still found after successful treatment. Furthermore, cytokines (especially IL-6 and IL-1β) and vascular growth endothelial factor (VEGF) are implicated in causation (Lagueny et al., 2004; Dispenzieri, 2012).

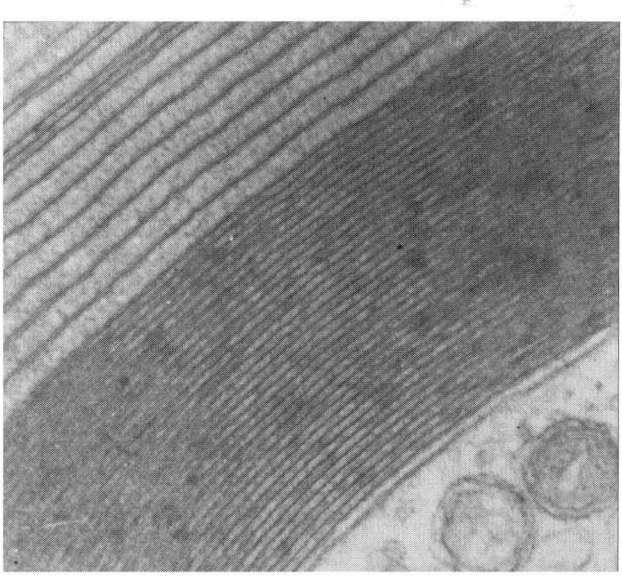

FIGURE 53.7 Widely spaced myelin. The normal myelin lamellae are tightly compacted and have a periodicity in electron microscope preparations of 12–15 nm. In the demyelinating neuropathy associated with IgM paraprotein that has activity against MAG (anti-MAG PDPN) the intraperiod line becomes split giving an overall periodicity of 30–40 nm. Note the suggestion of material within the widened spaces, possibly immunoglobulin M. Electron micrograph × 100,000.

Autoimmune Features

Many of the features of autoimmunity displayed in the acute neuropathies are also seen in CIDP. Cellular and humoral responses are both important to the pathogenesis. Raised circulating levels of IL-2 and TNF-α correlate with disease activity (Misawa et al., 2001). A TH-17 response is active with raised levels of IL-17 detectable (Chi et al., 2010), and reduced levels of CD25/CD4 and FoxP3 cells indicate reduced Treg capacity (Chi et al., 2008). T lymphocyte migration into the endoneurium is facilitated by increased levels of chemokines, cell adhesion molecules, and MMPs (Previtali et al., 2001; Kieseier et al., 2004). Expression of the blood—nerve barrier constituents claudin-5 and ZO-1 is altered in CIDP perhaps contributing to increased BNB permeability (Kanda et al., 2004). Within the endoneurium T cells secrete IFN-γ, IL-2, and TNF-α (Mathey et al., 1999) and probably others, contributing to inflammatory upregulation of effectors such as macrophages, continued recruitment, and direct nerve damage. Expression of downregulatory cytokines IL-4, IL-10, and TGF-β is also found, and in CIDP expression of NGF, GDNF, LIF, and their receptors may contribute to nerve regeneration (Yamamoto et al., 2002). Clear evidence of Fas deficiency gives support to an inability to halt the ongoing response as effectively as in a monophasic disease (Comi et al., 2009).

Macrophage and Schwann cells in the endoneurium express the costimulatory molecules CD80 (B7-1) and CD86 (B7-2) and their cognate partners CTLA-4 and CD28 are found on endoneurial T cells (Hu et al., 2007).

Antibodies to the glycopeptides P0 and P2, and glycolipids and gangliosides LM1 and GD1b, and LM1 ganglioside complexes, have been described but remain unconfirmed, or difficult to confirm, in other studies (Yan et al., 2001; Sanvito et al., 2009; Nobile-Orazio et al., 2010). The involvement of antibodies in CIDP pathogenesis remains an open question.

Unlike GBS or CIDP, in the anti-MAG paraproteinemic demyelinating peripheral neuropathy (anti-MAG PDPN) there is evidence of only antibody-mediated immunity. There is no evidence of macrophage-associated demyelination, T cell infiltration into the endoneurium or upregulation of T cell costimulatory molecules. There is quite strong evidence that anti-MAG antibodies may fulfill the Koch—Witebsky postulates. Anti-MAG antibodies can be found in the serum of patients with characteristic clinical presentation. Myelin-associated glycoprotein is expressed at the Schmidt—Lantermann incisures, the paranodes, and on the periaxonal myelin (Gabriel et al., 1998). It displays the HNK-1 carbohydrate epitope shared by several other peripheral nerve antigens. Histological studies demonstrate IgM anti-MAG deposits on Schwann cells that co-

localize with MAG (Takatsu et al., 1985). Electron-dense material seen between widened lamellae is consistent with anti-MAG IgM insinuated between the layers (Mendell et al., 1985) (see Figure 53.7). Activated complement components have been described by some researchers (Monaco et al., 1990). The disruption of MAG functions and complement-mediated damage may result in alterations in the axonal neurofilament cytoskeleton (Lunn et al., 2002) and these in turn may lead to slowing of nerve conduction and axonal degeneration.

Immunogenetic Features

Restricted usage of T cell receptor (TCR) genes has been demonstrated in CIDP. The predominant TCR in CIDP is $\alpha\beta$ but $\gamma\delta$ T cells are found in the majority of nerve biopsy specimens (Winer et al., 2002), again implying a possible non-protein immune response. No clonality has been demonstrated in isolated T cells. However, significant numbers of highly Th1 inflammatory natural killer T cells identified by expression of Vα24JαQ invariant TCR chain are found (Illes et al., 2000).

A number of putative immunogenetic modifiers have been proposed. Polymorphisms in TAG-1 are not associated with treatment response or outcome (Pang et al., 2012) and no association has been found with CD1 in small studies (Uncini et al., 2011). Recently, studies to suggest that homozygous genotype for a low number of GA repeats in SH2D2A (Uncini et al., 2011) and defective AIRE-mediated central tolerance to P0 (Su et al., 2012a) may be implicated in disease, have been presented.

Environmental Influences

A preceding illness, infection, or vaccination has been identified in patients with CIDP in 32% in the 6 months and 16% in the 6 weeks preceding their illness. Others have found no convincing evidence of vaccination being a trigger (Pritchard et al., 2002). No specific provoking environmental events have so far been recognized for CIDP or the paraproteinemic peripheral neuropathies.

Animal Models

The pathogenesis of CIDP is not completely defined. Widely accepted animal models that recapitulate all the clinical aspects of CIDP are not available. However, recently developed spontaneous autoimmune polyneuropathy (SAP) models have provided useful insights into pathogenic mechanisms involved in inflammatory demyelinating nerve injury relevant to CIDP. SAP can be seen in transgenic mice expressing the major histocompatibility complex (MHC) class II IA^b molecule. This MHC presents a single peptide, Eα52–68, in mice overexpressing interleukin (IL)-10 under the control of human *VMD2* promoter, and in non-obese diabetic (NOD) mice alongside modulations of the costimulatory molecule B7-2 (CD86) and the autoimmune regulator Aire. The subsequent pathogenic mechanisms in NOD mice are fairly well characterized. Elimination of B7-2 in NOD mice induces protection against diabetes mellitus in these animals but triggers the onset of a CIDP-like illness at 6–7 months of age that is almost 100% penetrant in female mice (Salomon et al., 2001; Ubogu et al., 2012). These mice develop a chronic progressive neuropathic disorder that has overlapping clinical, electrodiagnostic, and morphological features with CIDP (Ubogu et al., 2012). B7-2 knockout NOD mice point to the pathogenic role of costimulatory pathways such as B7-1/B7-2:CD28/CTLA-4 molecules in the development of SAP due to disruption of balance between pathogenic and regulatory T cells (Tregs) maintained by this pathway. Nerve injury in these animals is mediated by Th1 cells that are reactive against myelin P0, the most prominent PNS myelin protein (Bour-Jordan et al., 2005; Louvet et al., 2009). Sera from these animals also contain antibodies to P0, which may contribute to peripheral nerve injury (Kim et al., 2008; Su et al., 2012a).

The importance of the immunogenetic repertoire in the development of SAP is suggested by the absence of neuropathic disorder in B7-2 knockout mice on C57BL/6 or 129/Sv nonautoimmune mouse background (Salomon et al., 2001). How the immunogenetic repertoire contributes to the development of immune neuropathies was exemplified by the development of SAP in transgenic NOD mice with hypomorphic Aire gene function (NOD.Aire$^{GW/+}$ mice) (Su et al., 2012a). Aire is critical to central tolerance. Aire functions by upregulating the ectopic expression of a variety of tissue-specific self-Ags in medullary thymic epithelial cells (mTECs) (Anderson et al., 2002) and increasing the probability of negative selection of antigen-specific high affinity (developing) thymocytes (Anderson et al., 2005). Interestingly, NOD.Aire$^{GW/+}$ mice have increased immune cell and autoantibody reactivity toward P0 in the peripheral immune compartment (Su et al., 2012a). These observations support P0 being an Aire-regulated Ag in mTECs and that decreased P0 expression in mTECs is linked to the development of antigen-specific autoimmunity. Further, CD4$^+$ T cells from NOD.Aire$^{GW/+}$ mice are sufficient to transfer neuropathy and Th1 effector cells are dominant in the peripheral nerves in this model (Su et al., 2012a). The clinical relevance of these experimental findings was supported by the following observation. The patients with autoimmune polyendocrinopathy syndrome type 1 (APS1) have genetic mutations in Aire and develop multi-organ autoimmunity. Recently, a CIDP-like neuropathy was recognized as a potential novel component of APS1 in two unrelated children in whom there were confirmed Aire mutations (Valenzise et al., 2009). These patients have evidence of defective tolerance to P0 and harbor anti-P0 antibodies in their sera (Su et al., 2012a). Overall, these studies show defective tolerance to P0 and antigen-specific dysregulated cellular and humoral immune responses in both Aire-deficient mice and APS-1 patients with CIDP-like neuropathy.

The relevance of myelin P0 as a potential antigenic target in CIDP remains contentious; however, Yan et al. demonstrated that 6/21 sera (28%) from patients with CIDP responsive to plasma exchange contained IgG anti-P0 antibodies. Four of these sera containing IgG anti-P0 antibodies produced conduction block and demyelination by passive transfer when the blood–nerve barrier was breached, either by direct injection or by preceding passive T cell transfer (Yan et al., 2000).

In anti-MAG PDPN passive transfer of antibodies results in complement-mediated demyelination in cats and rabbits (Hays et al., 1987; Willison et al., 1988) although the pathological features were not similar to those seen in human disease. Widened myelin lamellae, almost pathognomonic of the condition, were demonstrated after passive transfer to chicks (Tatum, 1993). Induction of high titer IgM antibodies cross-reactive with human MAG by immunization with the peripheral nerve glycolipid sulfated glucuronyl paragloboside (SGPG) has been achieved in rats, rabbits, and cats. However, no convincing neuropathy as a result has been demonstrated.

Pathogenic Mechanisms

The final common path of macrophage-mediated demyelination in CIDP is thought to be similar to that seen in GBS (see above).

Treatment and Outcome

Steroids, ivIg, plasma exchange, and immunosuppressive drugs have all been used in the treatment of CIDP. Plasma exchange and ivIg are both very potent (Eftimov et al., 2009; Mehndiratta and Hughes, 2012). There was no statistically significant difference between steroids and ivIg in an early comparative trial (Hughes et al., 2001), and even though steroid is cheaper in the short term, ivIg was the treatment of choice. More recent evidence suggests that steroids may have a disease modifying effect, driving patients into remission more frequently and effectively than ivIg (Nobile-Orazio et al., 2012). Interferon-β1a was shown to be ineffective in otherwise treatment-resistant patients (Hadden et al., 1999). Campath-1H (alemtuzemab) and fingolimod, both designed to severely reduce circulating numbers of pathogenic T cells, are currently under trial. There is inadequate evidence to properly assess anecdotally beneficial drugs such as azathioprine, ciclosporin, and mycophenolate mofetil.

In MMNCB a dramatic therapeutic response is sometimes seen to ivIg demonstrated in controlled trials, and cyclophosphamide may have a place in primary treatment (Umapathi et al., 2012). Many other agents including interferon-β1a, rituximab, mycophenolate, azathioprine, and ciclosporin have been used with evidence for no effect for mycophenolate and only anecdotal evidence of partial benefit for the others (Umapathi et al., 2012). Plasma exchange has no effect and interestingly steroids often worsen the condition by an unknown mechanism. Predictors of favorable outcome are anti-GM1 antibodies, younger age, presence of conduction block, a normal CK, and less severe disease at outset (Hadden and Hughes, 2003). Despite treatment, conduction blocks are dynamic and weakness probably progresses slowly over time (Taylor et al., 2000).

In anti-MAG PDPN patients only need treatment for their neuropathy if it becomes severe and disabling. Randomized controlled evidence of benefit is available for ivIg in the short term (Lunn and Nobile-Orazio, 2012; Su et al., 2012a). Rituximab (an anti-CD20 monoclonal) was promising in case series but had disappointing benefit in RCTs (Lunn and Nobile-Orazio, 2012).

CONCLUDING REMARKS AND FUTURE PROSPECTS

The last decade has witnessed huge advances in the understanding of the pathogenesis of both acute and chronic inflammatory peripheral neuropathies. GBS and CIDP are heterogeneous clinical conditions in which humoral and cellular mechanisms conspire to cause disabling diseases. Although there are still innumerable advances to be made our greater understanding of pathomechanisms is inspiring trials of novel agents for treatment which will transform treatment in the next decade. Our understanding of disease with the emergence of further exciting discoveries will reduce significantly death and disability from GBS and CIDP.

ACKNOWLEDGMENTS

MPTL is supported by the Biomedical Research Centre at the National Hospital for Neurology, Queen Square, London. KAS is supported by NIH grant NS42888, NS054962, and NS070888.

REFERENCES

Alaedini, A., Sander, H.W., Hays, A.P., Latov, N., 2003. Antiganglioside antibodies in multifocal acquired sensory and motor neuropathy. Arch. Neurol. 60, 42–46.

Allen, D., Lunn, M.P., Niermeijer, J., Nobile-Orazio, E., 2007. Treatment for IgG and IgA paraproteinaemic neuropathy. Cochrane Database. Syst. Rev. 1, CD005376.

Anderson, M.S., Venanzi, E.S., Klein, L., Chen, Z., Berzins, S.P., Turley, S.J., et al., 2002. Projection of an immunological self shadow within the thymus by the aire protein. Science. 298, 1395–1401.

Anderson, M.S., Venanzi, E.S., Chen, Z., Berzins, S.P., Benoist, C., Mathis, D., 2005. The cellular mechanism of Aire control of T cell tolerance. Immunity. 23, 227–239.

Ang, C.W., Yuki, N., Jacobs, B.C., Koga, M., van Doorn, P.A., Schmitz, P.I., et al., 1999. Rapidly progressive, predominantly motor Guillain-Barre syndrome with anti-GalNAc-GD1a antibodies. Neurology. 53, 2122–2127.

Asbury, A.K., Cornblath, D.R., 1990. Current diagnostic criteria for Guillain-Barre syndrome. Ann. Neurol. 27, S22–S24.

Asbury, A.K., Arnason, B.G., Adams, R.D., 1969. The inflammatory lesion in idiopathic polyneuritis. Medicine (Baltimore). 48, 173–215.

Aspinall, G.O., McDonald, A.G., Raju, T.S., Pang, H., Moran, A.P., et al., 1993. Chemical structures of the core regions of Campylobacter jejuni serotypes O:1, O:4, O:23, and O:36 lipopolysaccharides. Eur. J. Biochem. 213, 1017–1027.

Austin, J.H., 1958. Recurrent polyneuropathies and their corticosteroid treatment. Brain. 81, 157–192.

Baggiolini, M., 1998. Chemokines and leukocyte traffic. Nature. 392, 565–568.

Bouchard, C., Lacroix, C., Plante, V., Adams, D., Chedru, F., Guglielmi, J.M., et al., 1999. Clinicopathologic findings and prognosis of chronic inflammatory demyelinating polyneuropathy. Neurology. 52, 498–503.

Bour-Jordan, H., Thompson, H.L., Bluestone, J.A., 2005. Distinct effector mechanisms in the development of autoimmune neuropathy versus diabetes in nonobese diabetic mice. J. Immunol. 175, 5649–5655.

Bowes, T., Wagner, E.R., Boffey, J., Nicholl, D., Cochrane, L., Benboubetra, M., et al., 2002. Tolerance to self gangliosides is the major factor restricting the antibody response to lipopolysaccharide core oligosaccharides in Campylobacter jejuni strains associated with Guillain-Barre syndrome. Infect. Immun. 70, 5008–5018.

Buchwald, B., Ahangari, R., Toyka, K.V., 2002. Differential blocking effects of the monoclonal anti-GQ1b IgM antibody and alpha-latrotoxin in the absence of complement at the mouse neuromuscular junction. Neurosci. Lett. 334, 25–28.

Bukowski, J.F., Morita, C.T., Band, H., Brenner, M.B., 1998. Crucial role of TCR gamma chain junctional region in prenyl pyrophosphate antigen recognition by gamma delta T cells. J. Immunol. 161, 286–293.

Campbell, J.J., Hedrick, J., Zlotnik, A., Siani, M.A., Thompson, D.A., Butcher, E.C., 1998. Chemokines and the arrest of lymphocytes rolling under flow conditions. Science. 279, 381–384.

Carpo, M., Nobile-Orazio, E., Meucci, N., Gamba, M., Barbieri, S., Allaria, S., et al., 1996. Anti-GD1a ganglioside antibodies in peripheral motor syndromes. Ann. Neurol. 39, 539–543.

Carpo, M., Pedotti, R., Lolli, F., Pitrola, A., Allaria, S., Scarlato, G., et al., 1998. Clinical correlate and fine specificity of anti-GQ1b antibodies in peripheral neuropathy. J. Neurol. Sci. 155, 186–191.

Chi, L.J., Wang, H.B., Wang, W.Z., 2008. Impairment of circulating CD4 + CD25 + regulatory T cells in patients with chronic inflammatory demyelinating polyradiculoneuropathy. J. Peripher. Nerv. Syst. 13, 54–63.

Chi, L.J., Xu, W.H., Zhang, Z.W., Huang, H.T., Zhang, L.M., Zhou, J., 2010. Distribution of Th17 cells and Th1 cells in peripheral blood and cerebrospinal fluid in chronic inflammatory demyelinating polyradiculoneuropathy. J. Peripher. Nerv. Syst. 15, 345–356.

Chiba, A., Kusunoki, S., Obata, H., Machinami, R., Kanazawa, I., 1993. Serum anti-GQ1b IgG antibody is associated with ophthalmoplegia in Miller Fisher syndrome and Guillain-Barre syndrome: clinical and immunohistochemical studies. Neurology. 43, 1911–1917.

Chiba, A., Kusunoki, S., Obata, H., Machinami, R., Kanazawa, I., 1997. Ganglioside composition of the human cranial nerves, with special reference to pathophysiology of Miller Fisher syndrome. Brain Res. 745, 32–36.

Cocito, D., Isoardo, G., Ciaramitaro, P., Migliaretti, G., Pipieri, A., Barbero, P., et al., 2001. Terminal latency index in polyneuropathy with IgM paraproteinemia and anti-MAG antibody. Muscle Nerve. 24, 1278–1282.

Comi, C., Osio, M., Ferretti, M., Mesturini, R., Cappellano, G., Chiocchetti, A., et al., 2009. Defective Fas-mediated T-cell apoptosis predicts acute onset CIDP. J. Peripher. Nerv. Syst. 14, 101–106.

Cooper, J.C., Ben Smith, A., Savage, C.O., Winer, J.B., 2000. Unusual T cell receptor phenotype V gene usage of gamma delta T cells in a line derived from the peripheral nerve of a patient with Guillain-Barre syndrome. J. Neurol. Neurosurg. Psychiatr. 69, 522–524.

Cornblath, D.R., Griffin, D.E., Welch, D., Griffin, J.W., McArthur, J.C., 1990. Quantitative analysis of endoneurial T-cells in human sural nerve biopsies. J. Neuroimmunol. 26, 113–118.

Corse, A.M., Chaudhry, V., Crawford, T.O., Cornblath, D.R., Kuncl, R.W., Griffin, J.W., 1996. Sensory nerve pathology in multifocal motor neuropathy. Ann. Neurol. 39, 319–325.

Crawford, N.W., Cheng, A., Andrews, N., Charles, P.G., Clothier, H.J., Day, B., et al., 2012. Guillain–Barré syndrome following pandemic (H1N1) 2009 influenza a immunisation in Victoria: a self-controlled case series. Med. J. Aust. 19, 574–578.

Creange, A., Belec, L., Clair, B., Raphael, J.C., Gherardi, R.K., 1996. Circulating tumor necrosis factor (TNF)-alpha and soluble TNF-alpha receptors in patients with Guillain-Barre syndrome. J. Neuroimmunol. 68, 95–99.

Creange, A., Belec, L., Clair, B., Degos, J.D., Raphael, J.C., Gherardi, R.K., 1998. Circulating transforming growth factor beta 1 (TGF-beta1) in Guillain-Barre syndrome: decreased concentrations in the early course and increase with motor function. J. Neurol. Neurosurg. Psychiatry. 64, 162–165.

Creange, A., Sharshar, T., Planchenault, T., Christov, C., Poron, F., Raphael, J.C., et al., 1999. Matrix metalloproteinase-9 is increased and correlates with severity in Guillain-Barre syndrome. Neurology. 53 (8), 1683–1691.

Creange, A., Chazaud, B., Sharshar, T., Plonquet, A., Poron, F., Eliezer, M.C., et al., 2001. Inhibition of the adhesion step of leukodiapedesis: a critical event in the recovery of Guillain-Barre syndrome associated with accumulation of proteolytically active lymphocytes in blood. J. Neuroimmunol. 114, 188–196.

Dahle, C., Ekerfelt, C., Vrethem, M., Samuelsson, M., Ernerudh, J., 1997. T helper type 2 like cytokine responses to peptides from P0

and P2 myelin proteins during the recovery phase of Guillain-Barre syndrome. J. Neurol. Sci. 153, 54–60.

De Angelis, M.V., Di Muzio, A., Lupo, S., Gambi, D., Uncini, A., Lugaresi, A., 2001. Anti-GD1a antibodies from an acute motor axonal neuropathy patient selectively bind to motor nerve fiber nodes of Ranvier. J. Neuroimmunol. 121, 79–82.

Dionne, A., Nicolle, M.W., Hahn, A.F., 2010. Clinical and electrophysiological parameters distinguishing acute-onset chronic inflammatory demyelinating polyneuropathy from acute inflammatory demyelinating polyneuropathy. Muscle Nerve. 41, 202–207.

Dispenzieri, A., 2012. How I treat POEMS syndrome. Blood. 119, 5650–5658.

Dyck, P.J., Lais, A.C., Ohta, M., Bastron, J.A., Okazaki, H., Groover, R.V., 1975. Chronic inflammatory polyradiculoneuropathy. Mayo Clin. Proc. 50, 621–637.

Eftimov, F., Winer, J.B., Vermeulen, M., de Haan, R., Van, S.I., 2009. Intravenous immunoglobulin for chronic inflammatory demyelinating polyradiculoneuropathy. Cochrane Database. Syst. Rev. 1, CD001797.

Enders, U., Lobb, R., Pepinsky, R.B., Hartung, H.P., Toyka, K.V., Gold, R., 1998. The role of the very late antigen-4 and its counterligand vascular cell adhesion molecule-1 in the pathogenesis of experimental autoimmune neuritis of the Lewis rat. Brain. 121, 1257–1266.

Exley, A.R., Smith, N., Winer, J.B., 1994. Tumour necrosis factor-alpha and other cytokines in Guillain-Barre syndrome. J. Neurol. Neurosurg. Psychiatr. 57, 1118–1120.

Feasby, T.E., Gilbert, J.J., Brown, W.F., Bolton, C.F., Hahn, A.F., Koopman, W.F., et al., 1986. An acute axonal form of Guillain-Barre polyneuropathy. Brain. 109, 1115–1126.

Fisher, M., 1956. Syndrome of ophthalmoplegia, ataxia and areflexia. N. Engl. J. Med. 255, 57–65.

Friedman, C.R., Neimann, J., Wegener, H.C., Tauxe, R.V., 2000. Epidemiology of Campylobacter jejuni infections in the United States and other industrialized nations. In: Nachamkin, I., Blaser, M. J. (Eds.), Campylobacter. American Society for Microbiology, Washington DC, pp. 121–138.

Gabriel, J.M., Erne, B., Bernasconi, L., Tosi, C., Probst, A., Landmann, L., et al., 1998. Confocal microscopic localization of anti-myelin-associated glycoprotein autoantibodies in a patient with peripheral neuropathy initially lacking a detectable IgM gammopathy. Acta Neuropathol. 95, 540–546.

Geleijns, K., Laman, J.D., van Rijs, W., Tio-Gillen, A.P., Hintzen, R.Q., van Doorn, P.A., et al., 2005a. Fas polymorphisms are associated with the presence of anti-ganglioside antibodies in Guillain-Barre syndrome. J. Neuroimmunol. 161, 183–189.

Geleijns, K., Schreuder, G.M., Jacobs, B.C., Sintnicolaas, K., van Koningsveld, R., Meulstee, J., et al., 2005b. HLA class II alleles are not a general susceptibility factor in Guillain-Barre syndrome. Neurology. 64, 44–49.

Goddard, E.A., Lastovica, A.J., Argent, A.C., 1997. Campylobacter 0:41 isolation in Guillain-Barre syndrome. Arch. Dis. Child. 76, 526–528.

Gold, R., Toyka, K.V., Hartung, H.P., 1995. Synergistic effect of IFN-gamma and TNF-alpha on expression of immune molecules and antigen presentation by Schwann cells. Cell. Immunol. 165, 65–70.

Gong, Y., Tagawa, Y., Lunn, M.P., Laroy, W., Heffer-Lauc, M., Li, C. Y., et al., 2002. Localization of major gangliosides in the PNS: implications for immune neuropathies. Brain. 125, 2491–2506.

Goodfellow, J.A., Bowes, T., Sheikh, K., Odaka, M., Halstead, S.K., Humphreys, P.D., et al., 2005. Overexpression of GD1a ganglioside sensitizes motor nerve terminals to anti-GD1a antibody-mediated injury in a model of acute motor axonal neuropathy. J. Neurosci. 25, 1620–1628.

Goodyear, C.S., O'Hanlon, G.M., Plomp, J.J., Wagner, E.R., Morrison, R., Veitch, J., et al., 1999. Monoclonal antibodies raised against Guillain-Barre syndrome-associated *Campylobacter jejuni* lipopolysaccharides react with neuronal gangliosides and paralyze muscle-nerve preparations. J. Clin. Invest. 104, 697–708.

Greenshields, K.N., Halstead, S.K., Zitman, F.M., Rinaldi, S., Brennan, K.M., O'Leary, C., et al., 2009. The neuropathic potential of anti-GM1 autoantibodies is regulated by the local glycolipid environment in mice. J. Clin. Invest. 119, 595–610.

Gregson, N.A., Hall, S.M., 1973. A quantitative analysis of the effects of the intraneural injection of lysophosphatidyl choline. J. Cell Sci. 13, 257–277.

Griffin, J.W., Li, C.Y., Ho, T.W., Xue, P., Macko, C., Gao, C.Y., et al., 1995. Guillain-Barre syndrome in northern China. The spectrum of neuropathological changes in clinically defined cases. Brain. 118, 577–595.

Griffin, J.W., Li, C.Y., Ho, T.W., Tian, M., Gao, C.Y., Xue, P., et al., 1996a. Pathology of the motor-sensory axonal Guillain-Barre syndrome. Ann. Neurol. 39, 17–28.

Griffin, J.W., Li, C.Y., Macko, C., Ho, T.W., Hsieh, S.T., Xue, P., et al., 1996b. Early nodal changes in the acute motor axonal neuropathy pattern of the Guillain-Barre syndrome. J. Neurocytol. 25, 33–51.

Guillain, G., Barré, J.A., Strohl, A., 1916. Sur un syndrome de radiculonévrite avec hyperalbuminose du liquide cephalorachidien sans réaction cellulaire. Remarques sur les caractères cliniques et graphiques des reflexes tendineux. Bull. Soc. Méd. Hôp. Paris. 40, 1462–1470.

Guillain-Barre Syndrome Study Group, 1985. Plasmapheresis and acute Guillain-Barre syndrome. Neurology. 35, 1096–1104.

Hadden, R.D., Gregson, N.A., 2001. Guillain-Barre syndrome and *Campylobacter jejuni* infection. Symp. Ser. Soc. Appl. Microbiol. 30, 145S–154S.

Hadden, R.D., Hughes, R.A., 2003. Management of inflammatory neuropathies. J. Neurol. Neurosurg. Psychiatr. 74, ii9–ii14.

Hadden, R.D., Cornblath, D.R., Hughes, R.A., Zielasek, J., Hartung, H.P., Toyka, K.V., et al., 1998. Electrophysiological classification of Guillain-Barre syndrome: clinical associations and outcome. Plasma Exchange/Sandoglobulin Guillain-Barre Syndrome Trial Group. Ann. Neurol. 44, 780–788.

Hadden, R.D., Sharrack, B., Bensa, S., Soudain, S.E., Hughes, R.A., 1999. Randomized trial of interferon beta-1a in chronic inflammatory demyelinating polyradiculoneuropathy. Neurology. 53, 57–61.

Hadden, R.D., Gregson, N.A., Gold, R., Willison, H.J., Hughes, R.A., 2001. Guillain-Barre syndrome serum and anti-Campylobacter antibody do not exacerbate experimental autoimmune neuritis. J. Neuroimmunol. 119, 306–316.

Hafer-Macko, C., Hsieh, S.T., Li, C.Y., Ho, T.W., Sheikh, K., Cornblath, D.R., et al., 1996a. Acute motor axonal neuropathy: an antibody-mediated attack on axolemma. Ann. Neurol. 40, 635–644.

Hafer-Macko, C.E., Sheikh, K.A., Li, C.Y., Ho, T.W., Cornblath, D.R., McKhann, G.M., et al., 1996b. Immune attack on the Schwann cell surface in acute inflammatory demyelinating polyneuropathy. Ann. Neurol. 39 (5), 625–635.

Hall, S.M., Hughes, R.A., Atkinson, P.F., McColl, I., Gale, A., 1992. Motor nerve biopsy in severe Guillain-Barre syndrome. Ann. Neurol. 31, 441–444.

Halstead, S.K., Zitman, F.M., Humphreys, P.D., Greenshields, K., Verschuuren, J.J., Jacobs, B.C., et al., 2008. Eculizumab prevents anti-ganglioside antibody-mediated neuropathy in a murine model. Brain. 131, 1197–1208.

Hartung, H.-P., Heininger, K., Schafer, B., Fierz, W., Toyka, K.V., 1988. Immune mechanisms in inflammatory neuropathy. Adv. Neuroimmunol. 540, 122–161.

Hartung, H.-P., Willison, H.J., Jung, S., Pette, M., Toyka, K.V., Giegerich, G., 1996. Autoimmune responses in peripheral nerve. Springer Semin. Immunopathol. 18, 97–123.

Hartung, H.P., Toyka, K.V., 1990. T-cell and macrophage activation in experimental autoimmune neuritis and Guillain-Barre syndrome. Ann. Neurol. 27, S57–S63.

Hartung, H.P., Schafer, B., Fierz, W., Heininger, K., Toyka, K.V., 1987. Ciclosporin A prevents P2 T cell line-mediated experimental autoimmune neuritis (AT-EAN) in rat. Neurosci. Lett. 83, 195–200.

Hartung, H.P., Reiners, K., Schmidt, B., Stoll, G., Toyka, K.V., 1991. Serum interleukin-2 concentrations in Guillain-Barre syndrome and chronic idiopathic demyelinating polyradiculoneuropathy: comparison with other neurological diseases of presumed immunopathogenesis. Ann. Neurol. 30, 48–53.

Hartung, H.P., Willison, H.J., Kieseier, B.C., 2002. Acute immunoinflammatory neuropathy: update on Guillain-Barre syndrome. Curr. Opin. Neurol. 15, 571–577.

Haymaker, W., Kernohan, J.W., 1949. The Landry-Guillain-Barré syndrome: a clinicopathologic report of fifty fatal cases and a critique of the literature. Medicine (Baltimore). 28, 59–141.

Hays, A.P., Latov, N., Takatsu, M., Sherman, W.H., 1987. Experimental demyelination of nerve induced by serum of patients with neuropathy and an anti-MAG IgM M-protein. Neurology. 37, 242–256.

Ho, T.W., Hsieh, S.T., Nachamkin, I., Willison, H.J., Sheikh, K., Kiehlbauch, J., et al., 1997. Motor nerve terminal degeneration provides a potential mechanism for rapid recovery in acute motor axonal neuropathy after Campylobacter infection. Neurology. 48, 717–724.

Ho, T.W., Willison, H.J., Nachamkin, I., Li, C.Y., Veitch, J., et al., 1999. Anti-GD1a antibody is associated with axonal but not demyelinating forms of Guillain-Barre syndrome. Ann. Neurol. 45, 168–173.

Holmdahl, R., Olsson, T., Moran, T., Klareskog, L., 1985. In vivo treatment of rats with monoclonal anti-T-cell antibodies. Immunohistochemical and functional analysis in normal rats and in experimental allergic neuritis. Scand. J. Immunol. 22, 157–169.

Honavar, M., Tharakan, J.K., Hughes, R.A., Leibowitz, S., Winer, J.B., 1991. A clinicopathological study of the Guillain-Barre syndrome. Nine cases and literature review. Brain. 114, 1245–1269.

Hu, W., Janke, A., Ortler, S., Hartung, H.P., Leder, C., Kieseier, B.C., et al., 2007. Expression of CD28-related costimulatory molecule and its ligand in inflammatory neuropathies. Neurology. 68, 277–282.

Hughes, R., Bensa, S., Willison, H., Van den, B.P., Comi, G., Illa, I., et al., 2001. Randomized controlled trial of intravenous immunoglobulin versus oral prednisolone in chronic inflammatory demyelinating polyradiculoneuropathy. Ann. Neurol. 50, 195–201.

Hughes, R.A., 1990. Guillain-Barré Syndrome. Springer-Verlag, London.

Hughes, R.A., Cornblath, D.R., 2005. Guillain-Barre syndrome. Lancet. 366, 1653–1666.

Hughes, R.A., Rees, J.H., 1997. Clinical and epidemiologic features of Guillain-Barre syndrome. J. Infect. Dis. 176, S92–S98.

Hughes, R.A., van Doorn, P.A., 2012. Corticosteroids for Guillain-Barre syndrome. Cochrane Database. Syst. Rev. 8, CD001446.

Hughes, R.A., Hadden, R.D., Gregson, N.A., Smith, K.J., 1999. Pathogenesis of Guillain-Barre syndrome. J. Neuroimmunol. 100, 74–97.

Hughes, R.A., Wijdicks, E.F., Barohn, R., Benson, E., Cornblath, D.R., Hahn, A.F., et al., 2003. Practice parameter: immunotherapy for Guillain-Barre syndrome: report of the Quality Standards Subcommittee of the American Academy of Neurology. Neurology. 61, 736–740.

Hughes, R.A., Swan, A.V., van Doorn, P.A., 2012. Intravenous immuno-globulin for Guillain-Barre syndrome. Cochrane Database. Syst. Rev. 7, CD002063.

Illes, Z., Kondo, T., Newcombe, J., Oka, N., Tabira, T., Yamamura, T., 2000. Differential expression of NK T cell V alpha 24J alpha Q invari-ant TCR chain in the lesions of multiple sclerosis and chronic inflam-matory demyelinating polyneuropathy. J. Immunol. 164, 4375–4381.

Jacobs, B.C., Endtz, H., van der Meche, F.G., Hazenberg, M.P., Achtereekte, H.A., van Doorn, P.A., 1995. Serum anti-GQ1b IgG antibodies recognize surface epitopes on *Campylobacter jejuni* from patients with Miller Fisher syndrome. Ann. Neurol. 37, 260–264.

Jacobs, B.C., Endtz, H.P., van der Meche, F.G., Hazenberg, M.P., De Klerk, M.A., van Doorn, P.A., 1997. Humoral immune response against *Campylobacter jejuni* lipopolysaccharides in Guillain-Barre and Miller Fisher syndrome. J. Neuroimmunol. 79, 62–68.

Jung, S., Kramer, S., Schluesener, H.J., Hunig, T., Toyka, K., Hartung, H.P., 1992. Prevention and therapy of experimental autoimmune neuritis by an antibody against T cell receptors-alpha/beta. J. Immunol. 148, 3768–3775.

Kaji, R., Oka, N., Tsuji, T., Mezaki, T., Nishio, T., Akiguchi, I., et al., 1993. Pathological findings at the site of conduction block in multi-focal motor neuropathy. Ann. Neurol. 33, 152–158.

Kanda, T., Numata, Y., Mizusawa, H., 2004. Chronic inflammatory demyelinating polyneuropathy: decreased claudin-5 and relocated ZO-1. J. Neurol. Neurosurg. Psychiatr. 75, 765–769.

Khalili-Shirazi, A., Gregson, N.A., Hall, M.A., Hughes, R.A., Lanchbury, J.S., 1997. T cell receptor V beta gene usage in Guillain-Barre syndrome. J. Neurol. Sci. 145, 169–176.

Khalili-Shirazi, A., Gregson, N.A., Londei, M., Summers, L., Hughes, R.A., 1998. The distribution of CD1 molecules in inflammatory neu-ropathy. J. Neurol. Sci. 158, 154–163.

Kiefer, R., Funa, K., Schweitzer, T., Jung, S., Bourde, O., Toyka, K.V., et al., 1996. Transforming growth factor-beta 1 in experimental autoimmune neuritis. Cellular localization and time course. Am. J. Pathol. 148, 211–223.

Kiefer, R., Dangond, F., Mueller, M., Toyka, K.V., Hafler, D.A., Hartung, H.P., 2000. Enhanced B7 costimulatory molecule expres-sion in inflammatory human sural nerve biopsies. J. Neurol. Neurosurg. Psychiatr. 69, 362–368.

Kieseier, B.C., Kiefer, R., Clements, J.M., Miller, K., Wells, G.M., Schweitzer, T., et al., 1998. Matrix metalloproteinase-9 and -7 are regulated in experimental autoimmune encephalomyelitis. Brain. 121, 159–166.

Kieseier, B.C., Dalakas, M.C., Hartung, H.P., 2002. Immune mechan-isms in chronic inflammatory demyelinating neuropathy. Neurology. 59, S7–S12.

Kieseier, B.C., Kiefer, R., Gold, R., Hemmer, B., Willison, H.J., Hartung, H.P., 2004. Advances in understanding and treatment of immune-mediated disorders of the peripheral nervous system. Muscle Nerve. 30, 131–156.

Kim, H.J., Jung, C.G., Jensen, M.A., Dukala, D., Soliven, B., 2008. Targeting of myelin protein zero in a spontaneous autoimmune poly-neuropathy. J. Immunol. 181, 8753–8760.

Kuijf, M.L., Geleijns, K., Ennaji, N., van Doorn, P.A., Jacobs, B.C., 2008. Susceptibility to Guillain-Barre syndrome is not associated with CD1A and CD1E gene polymorphisms. J. Neuroimmunol. 205, 110–112.

Kusunoki, S., Kaida, K., 2011. Antibodies against ganglioside complexes in Guillain-Barre syndrome and related disorders. J. Neurochem. 116, 828–832.

Kusunoki, S., Hitoshi, S., Kaida, K., Murayama, S., Kanazawa, I., 1999. Degeneration of rabbit sensory neurons induced by passive transfer of anti-GD1b antiserum. Neurosci. Lett. 273, 33–36.

Kuwabara, S., Yuki, N., Koga, M., Hattori, T., Matsuura, D., Miyake, M., et al., 1998. IgG anti-GM1 antibody is associated with reversible conduction failure and axonal degeneration in Guillain-Barre syn-drome. Ann. Neurol. 44, 202–208.

Kuwabara, S., Ogawara, K., Mizobuchi, K., Koga, M., Mori, M., Hattori, T., et al., 2000. Isolated absence of F waves and proximal axonal dysfunction in Guillain-Barre syndrome with antiganglioside antibodies. J. Neurol. Neurosurg. Psychiatr. 68, 191–195.

Lagueny, A., Bouillot, S., Vital, C., Ferrer, X., Larrieu, J.M., Vital, A., 2004. [POEMS syndrome (or Crow-Fukase syndrome)]. Rev. Neurol. (Paris). 160, 285–295.

Lehmann, H.C., Lopez, P.H., Zhang, G., Ngyuen, T., Zhang, J., Kieseier, B.C., et al., 2007. Passive immunization with anti-ganglioside antibodies directly inhibits axon regeneration in an ani-mal model. J. Neurosci. 27, 27–34.

Lewis, R.A., Sumner, A.J., Brown, M.J., Asbury, A.K., 1982. Multifocal demyelinating neuropathy with persistent conduction block. Neurology. 32, 958–964.

Lopez, P.H., Zhang, G., Zhang, J., Lehmann, H.C., Griffin, J.W., Schnaar, R.L., et al., 2010. Passive transfer of IgG anti-GM1 antibo-dies impairs peripheral nerve repair. J. Neurosci. 30, 9533–9541.

Louvet, C., Kabre, B.G., Davini, D.W., Martinier, N., Su, M.A., DeVoss, J.J., et al., 2009. A novel myelin P0-specific T cell receptor transgenic mouse develops a fulminant autoimmune peripheral neu-ropathy. J. Exp. Med. 206, 507–514.

Lunn, M.P., Nobile-Orazio, E., 2012. Immunotherapy for IgM anti-myelin-associated glycoprotein paraprotein-associated peripheral neuropathies. Cochrane Database Syst. Rev. 5, CD002827.

Lunn, M.P., Manji, H., Choudhary, P.P., Hughes, R.A., Thomas, P.K., 1999. Chronic inflammatory demyelinating polyradiculoneuropathy: a prevalence study in south east England. J. Neurol. Neurosurg. Psychiatr. 66, 677–680.

Lunn, M.P., Johnson, L.A., Fromholt, S.E., Itonori, S., Huang, J., Vyas, A.A., et al., 2000. High-affinity anti-ganglioside IgG anti-bodies raised in complex ganglioside knockout mice: reexamina-tion of GD1a immunolocalization. J. Neurochem. 75, 404–412.

Lunn, M.P., Crawford, T.O., Hughes, R.A., Griffin, J.W., Sheikh, K.A., 2002. Anti-myelin-associated glycoprotein antibodies alter neurofi-lament spacing. Brain. 125, 904–911.

Lunn, M.P.T., Manji, H., Choudhary, P.P., Hughes, R.A.C., Thomas, P.K., 1998. Chronic inflammatory demyelinating polyradiculoneuropathy: a prevalence study in South East England. J. Neurol. Neurosurg. Psychiatr. 66, 677–680.

Magira, E.E., Papaioakim, M., Nachamkin, I., Asbury, A.K., Li, C. Y., Ho, T.W., et al., 2003. Differential distribution of HLA-DQ beta/DR beta epitopes in the two forms of Guillain-Barre syndrome, acute motor axonal neuropathy and acute inflammatory demyelinating polyneuropathy (AIDP): identification of DQ beta epitopes associated with susceptibility to and protection from AIDP. J. Immunol. 170, 3074–3080.

Mathey, E.K., Pollard, J.D., Armati, P.J., 1999. TNF alpha, IFN gamma and IL-2 mRNA expression in CIDP sural nerve biopsies. J. Neurol. Sci. 163, 47–52.

Mausberg, A.K., Meyer zu, H.G., Dehmel, T., Stettner, M., Lehmann, H.C., Sheikh, K.A., et al., 2011. Erythropoietin ameliorates rat experimental autoimmune neuritis by inducing transforming growth factor-beta in macrophages. PLoS One. 6, e26280.

McKhann, G.M., Cornblath, D.R., Ho, T., Li, C.Y., Bai, A.Y., Wu, H.S., et al., 1991. Clinical and electrophysiological aspects of acute paralytic disease of children and young adults in northern China. Lancet. 338, 593–597.

McKhann, G.M., Cornblath, D.R., Griffin, J.W., Ho, T.W., Li, C.Y., Jiang, Z., et al., 1993. Acute motor axonal neuropathy: a frequent cause of acute flaccid paralysis in China. Ann. Neurol. 33, 333–342.

Mehndiratta, M.M., Hughes, R.A., 2012. Plasma exchange for chronic inflammatory demyelinating polyradiculoneuropathy. Cochrane Database. Syst. Rev. 9, CD003906.

Mendell, J.R., Schenk, Z., Whittaker, J.N., Trapp, B.D., Yates, A.J., Griggs, R.C., et al., 1985. Polyneuropathy and IgM monoclonal gammopathy: studies on the pathogenic role of the myelin-associated glycoprotein antibody. Ann. Neurol. 17, 243–254.

Misawa, S., Kuwabara, S., Mori, M., Kawaguchi, N., Yoshiyama, Y., Hattori, T., 2001. Serum levels of tumor necrosis factor-alpha in chronic inflammatory demyelinating polyneuropathy. Neurology. 56, 666–669.

Mizoguchi, K., 1998. Anti-GQ1b IgG antibody activities related to the severity of Miller Fisher syndrome. Neurol. Res. 20, 617–624.

Monaco, S., Bonetti, B., Ferrari, S., Moretto, G., Nardelli, E., Tedesco, F., et al., 1990. Complement-mediated demyelination in patients with IgM monoclonal gammopathy and polyneuropathy. N. Engl. J. Med. 322, 649–652.

Moran, A.P., Prendergast, M.M., Hogan, E.L., 2002. Sialosyl-galactose: a common denominator of Guillain-Barre and related disorders?. J. Neurol. Sci. 196, 1–7.

Mygland, A., Monstad, P., 2001. Chronic polyneuropathies in Vest-Agder, Norway. Eur. J. Neurol. 8, 157–165.

Nachamkin, I., Liu, J., Li, M., Ung, H., Moran, A.P., Prendergast, M.M., et al., 2002. Campylobacter jejuni from patients with Guillain-Barre syndrome preferentially expresses a GD(1a)-like epitope. Infect. Immun. 70, 5299–5303.

Nobile-Orazio, E., Giannotta, C., Briani, C., 2010. Anti-ganglioside complex IgM antibodies in multifocal motor neuropathy and chronic immune-mediated neuropathies. J. Neuroimmunol. 219, 119–122.

Nobile-Orazio, E., Cocito, D., Jann, S., Uncini, A., Beghi, E., Messina, P., et al., 2012. Intravenous immunoglobulin versus intravenous methylprednisolone for chronic inflammatory demyelinating

polyradiculoneuropathy: a randomised controlled trial. Lancet Neurol. 11, 493–502.

Oberhelman, R.A., Taylor, D.N., 2000. Campylobacter infections in developing countries. In: Nachamkin, I., Blaser, M.J. (Eds.), Campylobacter. American Society for Microbiology, Washington DC, pp. 139–153.

Ogawara, K., Kuwabara, S., Mori, M., Hattori, T., Koga, M., Yuki, N., 2000. Axonal Guillain-Barre syndrome: relation to anti-ganglioside antibodies and Campylobacter jejuni infection in Japan. Ann. Neurol. 48, 624–631.

Ogino, M., Orazio, N., Latov, N., 1995. IgG anti-GM1 antibodies from patients with acute motor neuropathy are predominantly of the IgG1 and IgG3 subclasses. J. Neuroimmunol. 58, 77–80.

Oh, S.J., Claussen, G.C., Odabasi, Z., Palmer, C.P., 1995. Multifocal demyelinating motor neuropathy: pathologic evidence of "inflammatory demyelinating polyradiculoneuropathy." Neurology. 45, 1828–1832.

O'Hanlon, G.M., Plomp, J.J., Chakrabarti, M., Morrison, I., Wagner, E. R., Goodyear, C.S., et al., 2001. Anti-GQ1b ganglioside antibodies mediate complement-dependent destruction of the motor nerve terminal. Brain. 124, 893–906.

Pang, S.Y., Chan, K.H., Mak, W.W., Kung, M.H., Lee, C.N., Tsoi, T.H., et al., 2012. Single-nucleotide polymorphism of transient axonal glycoprotein-1 and its correlation with clinical features and prognosis in chronic inflammatory demyelinating polyneuropathy. J. Peripher. Nerv. Syst. 17, 72–75.

Pestronk, A., Cornblath, D.R., Ilyas, A.A., Baba, H., Quarles, R.H., Griffin, J.W., et al., 1988. A treatable multifocal motor neuropathy with antibodies to GM1 ganglioside. Ann. Neurol. 24, 73–78.

Plomp, J.J., Molenaar, P.C., O'Hanlon, G.M., Jacobs, B.C., Veitch, J., Daha, M.R., et al., 1999. Miller Fisher anti-GQ1b antibodies: alpha-latrotoxin-like effects on motor end plates. Ann. Neurol. 45, 189–199.

Prendergast, M.M., Moran, A.P., 2000. Lipopolysaccharides in the development of the Guillain-Barre syndrome and Miller Fisher syndrome forms of acute inflammatory peripheral neuropathies. J. Endotoxin Res. 6, 341–359.

Previtali, S.C., Feltri, M.L., Archelos, J.J., Quattrini, A., Wrabetz, L., Hartung, H., 2001. Role of integrins in the peripheral nervous system. Prog. Neurobiol. 64, 35–49.

Pritchard, J., Mukherjee, R., Hughes, R.A., 2002. Risk of relapse of Guillain-Barre syndrome or chronic inflammatory demyelinating polyradiculoneuropathy following immunization. J. Neurol. Neurosurg. Psychiatr. 73, 348–349.

Raphael, J.C., Chevret, S., Hughes, R.A., Annane, D., 2012. Plasma exchange for Guillain-Barre syndrome. Cochrane Database. Syst. Rev. 7, CD001798.

Redford, E.J., Smith, K.J., Gregson, N.A., Davies, M., Hughes, P., Gearing, A.J., et al., 1997. A combined inhibitor of matrix metalloproteinase activity and tumour necrosis factor-alpha processing attenuates experimental autoimmune neuritis. Brain. 120, 1895–1905.

Rees, J.H., Gregson, N.A., Hughes, R.A., 1995a. Anti-ganglioside GM1 antibodies in Guillain-Barre syndrome and their relationship to Campylobacter jejuni infection. Ann. Neurol. 38, 809–816.

Rees, J.H., Soudain, S.E., Gregson, N.A., Hughes, R.A., 1995b. Campylobacter jejuni infection and Guillain-Barre syndrome. N. Engl. J. Med. 333, 1374–1379.

Rees, J.H., Thompson, R.D., Smeeton, N.C., Hughes, R.A., 1998. Epidemiological study of Guillain-Barre syndrome in south east England. J. Neurol. Neurosurg. Psychiatr. 64, 74–77.

Rinaldi, S., Brennan, K.M., Goodyear, C.S., O'Leary, C., Schiavo, G., Crocker, P.R., et al., 2009. Analysis of lectin binding to glycolipid complexes using combinatorial glycoarrays. Glycobiology. 19, 789–796.

Rose, N.R., Bona, C., 1993. Defining criteria for autoimmune diseases (Witebsky's postulates revisited). Immunol. Today. 14, 426–430.

Saida, K., Saida, T., Brown, M.J., Silberberg, D.H., 1979. In vivo demyelination induced by intraneural injection of anti- galactocerebroside serum: a morphologic study. Am. J. Pathol. 95, 99–116.

Salomon, B., Rhee, L., Bour-Jordan, H., Hsin, H., Montag, A., Soliven, B., et al., 2001. Development of spontaneous autoimmune peripheral polyneuropathy in B7-2-deficient NOD mice. J. Exp. Med. 194, 677–684.

Sander, H.W., Latov, N., 2003. Research criteria for defining patients with CIDP. Neurology. 60, S8–S15.

Sanvito, L., Makowska, A., Mahdi-Rogers, M., Hadden, R.D., Peakman, M., Gregson, N., et al., 2009. Humoral and cellular immune responses to myelin protein peptides in chronic inflammatory demyelinating polyradiculoneuropathy. J. Neurol. Neurosurg. Psychiatr. 80, 333–338.

Sejvar, J.J., Baughman, A.L., Wise, M., Morgan, O.W., 2011. Population incidence of Guillain-Barre syndrome: a systematic review and meta-analysis. Neuroepidemiology. 36, 123–133.

Sheikh, K.A., Zhang, G., 2010. An update on pathobiologic roles of anti-glycan antibodies in Guillain-Barre syndrome. F1000. Biol. Rep.2.

Sheikh, K.A., Nachamkin, I., Ho, T.W., Willison, H.J., Veitch, J., Ung, H., et al., 1998. Campylobacter jejuni lipopolysaccharides in Guillain-Barre syndrome: molecular mimicry and host susceptibility. Neurology. 51, 371–378.

Sheikh, K.A., Deerinck, T.J., Ellisman, M.H., Griffin, J.W., 1999. The distribution of ganglioside-like moieties in peripheral nerves. Brain. 122, 449–460.

Sheikh, K.A., Zhang, G., Gong, Y., Schnaar, R.L., Griffin, J.W., 2004. An anti-ganglioside antibody-secreting hybridoma induces neuropathy in mice. Ann. Neurol. 56, 228–239.

Smith, K.J., Kapoor, R., Felts, P.A., 1999. Demyelination: the role of reactive oxygen and nitrogen species. Brain Pathol. 9, 69–92.

Spies, J.M., Pollard, J.D., Bonner, J.G., Westland, K.W., McLeod, J.G., 1995. Synergy between antibody and P2-reactive T cells in experimental allergic neuritis. J. Neuroimmunol. 57, 77–84.

Su, M.A., Davini, D., Cheng, P., Giang, K., Fan, U., DeVoss, J.J., et al., 2012a. Defective autoimmune regulator-dependent central tolerance to myelin protein zero is linked to autoimmune peripheral neuropathy. J. Immunol. 188, 4906–4912.

Sumner, A.J., Said, G., Idy, I., Metral, S., 1992. Demyelinative conduction block produced by intraneural injection of human Guillain-Barré syndrome serum into rat sciatic nerve. Neurology. 32, A106.

Susuki, K., Nishimoto, Y., Yamada, M., Baba, M., Ueda, S., Hirata, K., et al., 2003. Acute motor axonal neuropathy rabbit model: immune attack on nerve root axons. Ann. Neurol. 54, 383–388.

Susuki, K., Rasband, M.N., Tohyama, K., Koibuchi, K., Okamoto, S., Funakoshi, K., et al., 2007. Anti-GM1 antibodies cause complement-mediated disruption of sodium channel clusters in peripheral motor nerve fibers. J. Neurosci. 27, 3956–3967.

Takatsu, M., Hays, A.P., Latov, N., Abrams, G.M., Nemni, R., Sherman, W.H., et al., 1985. Immunofluorescence study of patients with neuropathy and IgM M proteins. Ann. Neurol. 18, 173–181.

Tatum, A.H., 1993. Experimental paraprotein neuropathy, demyelination by passive transfer of human IgM anti-myelin-associated glycoprotein. Ann. Neurol. 33, 502–506.

Taylor, B.V., Wright, R.A., Harper, C.M., Dyck, P.J., 2000. Natural history of 46 patients with multifocal motor neuropathy with conduction block. Muscle Nerve. 23, 900–908.

Taylor, W.A., Hughes, R.A., 1989. T lymphocyte activation antigens in Guillain-Barre syndrome and chronic idiopathic demyelinating polyradiculoneuropathy. J. Neuroimmunol. 24, 33–39.

Ubogu, E.E., Yosef, N., Xia, R.H., Sheikh, K.A., 2012. Behavioral, electrophysiological, and histopathological characterization of a severe murine chronic demyelinating polyneuritis model. J. Peripher. Nerv. Syst. 17, 53–61.

Umapathi, T., Hughes, R.A., Nobile-Orazio, E., Leger, J.M., 2005. Immunosuppressant and immunomodulatory treatments for multifocal motor neuropathy. Cochrane Database. Syst. Rev.3.

Umapathi, T., Hughes, R.A., Nobile-Orazio, E., Leger, J.M., 2012. Immunosuppressant and immunomodulatory treatments for multifocal motor neuropathy. Cochrane Database. Syst. Rev. 4, CD003217.

Uncini, A., Kuwabara, S., 2012. Electrodiagnostic criteria for Guillain-Barre syndrome: a critical revision and the need for an update. Clin. Neurophysiol. 123, 1487–1495.

Uncini, A., Lugaresi, A., 1999. Fisher syndrome with tetraparesis and antibody to GQ1b: evidence for motor nerve terminal block. Muscle Nerve. 22, 640–644.

Uncini, A., Notturno, F., Pace, M., Caporale, C.M., 2011. Polymorphism of CD1 and SH2D2A genes in inflammatory neuropathies. J. Peripher. Nerv. Syst. 16, 48–51.

Valenzise, M., Meloni, A., Betterle, C., Giometto, B., Autunno, M., Mazzeo, A., et al., 2009. Chronic inflammatory demyelinating polyneuropathy as a possible novel component of autoimmune polyendocrine-candidiasis-ectodermal dystrophy. Eur. J. Pediatr. 168, 237–240.

van der Pol, W.L., Van den Berg, L.H., Scheepers, R.H., van der Bom, J.G., van Doorn, P.A., van Koningsveld, R., et al., 2000. IgG receptor IIa alleles determine susceptibility and severity of Guillain-Barre syndrome. Neurology. 54, 1661–1665.

Visser, L.H., van der Meche, F.G., van Doorn, P.A., Meulstee, J., Jacobs, B.C., Oomes, P.G., et al., 1995. Guillain-Barre syndrome without sensory loss (acute motor neuropathy). A subgroup with specific clinical, electrodiagnostic and laboratory features. Dutch Guillain-Barre Study Group. Brain. 118, 841–847.

Vriesendorp, F.J., Flynn, R.E., Khan, M., Pappolla, M.A., Brod, S.A., 1996. Oral administration of type I interferon modulates the course of experimental allergic neuritis. Autoimmunity. 24, 157–165.

Willison, H.J., Veitch, J., 1994. Immunoglobulin subclass distribution and binding characteristics of anti-GQ1b antibodies in Miller Fisher syndrome. J. Neuroimmunol. 50, 159–165.

Willison, H.J., Yuki, N., 2002. Peripheral neuropathies and anti-glycolipid antibodies. Brain. 125, 2591–2625.

Willison, H.J., Trapp, B.D., Bacher, J.D., Dalakas, M.C., Griffin, J.W., Quarles, R.H., 1988. Demyelination induced by intraneural injection of human antimyelin-associated glycoprotein antibodies. Muscle Nerve. 11, 1169–1176.

Willison, H.J., Veitch, J., Paterson, G., Kennedy, P.G., 1993. Miller Fisher syndrome is associated with serum antibodies to GQ1b ganglioside. J. Neurol. Neurosurg. Psychiatr. 56, 204–206.

Willison, H.J., Townson, K., Veitch, J., Boffey, J., Isaacs, N., Andersen, S.M., et al., 2004. Synthetic disialylgalactose immunoadsorbents deplete anti-GQ1b antibodies from autoimmune neuropathy sera. Brain. 127, 680–691.

Willison, H.J., Halstead, S.K., Beveridge, E., Zitman, F.M., Greenshields, K. N., Morgan, B.P., et al., 2008. The role of complement and complement regulators in mediating motor nerve terminal injury in murine models of Guillain-Barre syndrome. J. Neuroimmunol. 201–202, 172–182.

Winer, J., Hughes, S., Cooper, J., Ben Smith, A., Savage, C., 2002. Gamma delta T cells infiltrating sensory nerve biopsies from patients with inflammatory neuropathy. J. Neurol. 249, 616–621.

Winer, J.B., Gray, I.A., Gregson, N.A., Hughes, R.A., Leibowitz, S., et al., 1988. A prospective study of acute idiopathic neuropathy. III. Immunological studies. J. Neurol. Neurosurg. Psychiatr. 51, 619–625.

Wirguin, I., Briani, C., Suturkova-Milosevic, L., Fisher, T., Della-Latta, P., Chalif, P., et al., 1997. Induction of GM1 ganglioside antibodies by Campylobacter jejuni lipopolysaccharides. J. Neuroimmunol. 78, 138–142.

Witebsky, E., Rose, N.R., Terplan, K., Paine, J.R., Egan, R.W., 1957. Chronic thyroiditis and autoimmunization. J. Am. Med. Assoc. 164, 1439–1447.

Wu, L.Y., Zhou, Y., Qin, C., Hu, B.L., 2012. The effect of TNF-alpha, FcgammaR and CD1 polymorphisms on Guillain-Barre syndrome risk: evidences from a meta-analysis. J. Neuroimmunol. 243, 18–24.

Yamamoto, M., Ito, Y., Mitsuma, N., Li, M., Hattori, N., Sobue, G., 2002. Parallel expression of neurotrophic factors and their receptors in chronic inflammatory demyelinating polyneuropathy. Muscle Nerve. 25, 601–604.

Yan, W.X., Taylor, J., Andrias-Kauba, S., Pollard, J.D., 2000. Passive transfer of demyelination by serum or IgG from chronic inflammatory demyelinating polyneuropathy patients. Ann. Neurol. 47, 765–775.

Yan, W.X., Archelos, J.J., Hartung, H.P., Pollard, J.D., 2001. P0 protein is a target antigen in chronic inflammatory demyelinating polyradiculoneuropathy. Ann. Neurol. 50, 286–292.

Yuki, N., Kuwabara, S., 2007. Axonal Guillain-Barre syndrome: carbohydrate mimicry and pathophysiology. J. Peripher. Nerv. Syst. 12, 238–249.

Yuki, N., Yoshino, H., Sato, S., Miyatake, T., 1990. Acute axonal polyneuropathy associated with anti-GM1 antibodies following Campylobacter enteritis. Neurology. 40, 1900–1902.

Yuki, N., Sato, S., Tsuji, S., Ohsawa, T., Miyatake, T., 1993. Frequent presence of anti-GQ1b antibody in Fisher's syndrome. Neurology. 43, 414–417.

Yuki, N., Taki, T., Takahashi, M., Saito, K., Yoshino, H., Tai, T., et al., 1994. Molecular mimicry between GQ1b ganglioside and lipopolysaccharides of Campylobacter jejuni isolated from patients with Fisher's syndrome. Ann. Neurol. 36, 791–793.

Yuki, N., Ichihashi, Y., Taki, T., 1995. Subclass of IgG antibody to GM1 epitope-bearing lipopolysaccharide of Campylobacter jejuni in patients with Guillain-Barre syndrome. J. Neuroimmunol. 60, 161–164.

Yuki, N., Ang, C.W., Koga, M., Jacobs, B.C., van Doorn, P.A., Hirata, K., et al., 2000. Clinical features and response to treatment in Guillain-Barre syndrome associated with antibodies to GM1b ganglioside. Ann. Neurol. 47, 314–321.

Zehntner, S.P., Brisebois, M., Tran, E., Owens, T., Fournier, S., 2003. Constitutive expression of a costimulatory ligand on antigen-presenting cells in the nervous system drives demyelinating disease. FASEB J. 17, 1910–1912.

Zhang, G., Lehmann, H.C., Bogdanova, N., Gao, T., Zhang, J., Sheikh, K.A., 2011a. Erythropoietin enhances nerve repair in anti-ganglioside antibody-mediated models of immune neuropathy. PLoS One. 6, e27067.

Zhang, G., Lehmann, H.C., Manoharan, S., Hashmi, M., Shim, S., Ming, G.L., et al., 2011b. Anti-ganglioside antibody-mediated activation of RhoA induces inhibition of neurite outgrowth. J. Neurosci. 31, 1664–1675.

Zhu, J., Bai, X.F., Mix, E., Link, H., 1997. Experimental allergic neuritis: cytolysin mRNA expression is upregulated in lymph node cells during convalescence. J. Neuroimmunol. 78, 108–116.

Zhu, J., Zou, L., Zhu, S., Mix, E., Shi, F., Wang, H., et al., 2001. Cytotoxic T lymphocyte-associated antigen 4 (CTLA-4) blockade enhances incidence and severity of experimental autoimmune neuritis in resistant mice. J. Neuroimmunol. 115, 111–117.

Chapter 54

Myasthenia Gravis and Related Disorders

Stuart Viegas[1] and Angela Vincent[2]

[1]*Nuffield Department of Clinical Neurosciences, Oxford University, Oxford, UK,* [2]*Department of Neurology, St Mary's Hospital, Imperial College NHS Trust, London, UK*

Chapter Outline

Introduction	777	
The Neuromuscular Junction	777	
AChR, MuSK, and Lrp4	778	
Neuromuscular Transmission	779	
Myasthenia Gravis	779	
Epidemiology	779	
Etiology	779	
General Aspects	780	
Clinical Heterogeneity	780	
Early-onset AChR Antibody Positive MG (AChRab⁺ MG)	780	
Late-onset AChR Antibody Positive MG (AChRab⁺ MG)	781	
Thymoma-Associated MG (Thymoma MG)	781	
MuSK Antibody-Positive MG (MuSKab⁺ MG)	781	
Neonatal MG	781	
Antibodies in Myasthenia	782	
Serological Testing	782	
AChR Antibody Characteristics	782	

MuSK and Other Antibodies	783
Pathogenic Mechanisms	**783**
Evidence for Pathogenicity of AChR and MuSK Antibodies	783
AChR Antibody-Positive MG	783
MuSK Antibody-Positive MG	784
The Thymus and Cellular Immunity in MG	**784**
Role of T Lymphocytes in MG	784
The Thymus and MG	785
Lambert–Eaton Myasthenic Syndrome	**785**
Epidemiology and Etiology	786
Clinical Features	786
Investigation and Treatment	786
Pathophysiology	786
Conclusions and Future Prospects	**786**
References	**787**

INTRODUCTION

Over recent years, the recognition and ability to detect antibodies directed against receptors, ion channels, and relevant proteins within both the peripheral and the central nervous system has continued to evolve. Nevertheless, myasthenia gravis, and related autoimmune disorders of the neuromuscular junction, remains the paradigm, serving to highlight those features which help define an antibody-mediated disorder. The history of the discoveries in this archetypal autoimmune disease is summarized in Table 54.1.

The Neuromuscular Junction

The neuromuscular junction (NMJ) consists of the presynaptic motor nerve terminal and the postsynaptic motor "endplate." At the NMJ, the distal motor axon loses its myelin sheath and expands to form the boutons of the presynaptic nerve terminal. These contain mitochondria and the synaptic vesicles that store the acetylcholine (ACh). The vesicles are organized within specialized active zones, alongside voltage-gated calcium channels (VGCCs). In addition, voltage-gated potassium channels (VGKCs) are also present on the presynaptic nerve terminal (Figure 54.1).

The postsynaptic membrane is deeply infolded to create junctional folds. The crests of these, lying in close alignment to the presynaptic active zones, contain the highest density of acetylcholine receptors (AChRs). At the depths of the folds, there are relatively few AChRs, but an abundance of voltage-gated sodium channels (VGSCs). The clustering of the AChRs is critical for efficient neurotransmission. The development of the NMJ is dependent on a number of key proteins: agrin, rapsyn, muscle-specific kinase (MuSK), low density lipoprotein receptor-related protein 4 (Lrp4), and docking protein 7 (Dok-7) (Singhal and Martin, 2011) (see Figure 54.1).

N. Rose & I. Mackay (Eds): The Autoimmune Diseases, Fifth edition. DOI: http://dx.doi.org/10.1016/B978-0-12-384929-8.00054-X

TABLE 54.1 A History of Myasthenia Gravis Research

Date	Key Observation	Reference
1672	Thomas Willis publishes what is arguably the first clinical description of MG	Willis (1672)*
1895	Jolly shows that the defect is at the neuromuscular junction	Jolly (1895)*
1913 1939	Thymectomy appears to produce clinical improvement in patients with thymoma or non-thymomatous MG	Sauerbruch (1913)* Blalock (1939)*
1934	Mary Walker demonstrates the effectiveness of cholinesterase inhibitors as treatment	Walker (1934)
1960	Simpson proposes that MG is caused by antibodies to an "endplate" protein	Simpson (1960)
1962	The snake toxin α-bungarotoxin can be used as a label for acetylcholine receptors at the neuromuscular junction	Chang and Lee (1963)
1964	Elmqvist and colleagues show that the miniature endplate potentials are reduced in MG	Elmqvist et al. (1964)
1971	Several groups begin to purify AChRs from electric organs of electric rays using affinity chromatography on neurotoxin columns	
1973	Immunization against purified electric ray AChR leads to an experimental autoimmune MG (EAMG) in rabbits	Patrick and Lindstrom (1973)
1973	Acetylcholine receptors are reduced in number at neuromuscular junctions, as determined by ^{125}I-α-bungarotoxin binding	Fambrough et al. (1973)
1975	MG can be passively transferred to mice by injection of patients' IgG	Toyka et al. (1975)
1976	MG patients have acetylcholine receptor antibodies as shown by radioimmunoprecipitation of ^{125}I-α-bungarotoxin-tagged AChRs	Lindstrom et al. (1976)
1976–1978	Plasma exchange produces striking clinical improvement in MG, which correlates inversely with AChR antibody levels	Newsom-Davis et al. (1978)
1977	IgG and complement are present at the neuromuscular junctions in MG patients and in mice with EAMG	Engel et al. (1977)
1980	MG can present with different HLA, thymic pathology, age at onset, and muscle antibodies	Compston et al. (1980)
1981	The MG thymus contains plasma cells making AChR antibody	Scadding et al. (1981)
1977–present	Experimental autoimmune model used to determine pathogenic and immunological mechanisms	
1984–present	Study of T cells from MG patients and their responses to AChR epitopes	

*refer to Vincent, 2002 for further information.

The synaptic cleft between the pre- and postsynaptic membranes contains the basal lamina composed of collagen IV, heparan sulfate, and laminin. The enzyme acetylcholinesterase is anchored to the basal lamina through its collagen-like tail (ColQ).

AChR, MuSK, and Lrp4

The nicotinic AChR remains the major antigenic target in MG, followed by MuSK. Lrp4 is an antigen in rare cases of MG. The AChR is a pentameric ligand-gated ion channel that exists in adult and fetal isoforms. The adult form consists of two α-subunits and one each of the β-, δ-, and ε-subunits, with each subunit composed of a large extracellular domain, glycosylation sites, and four transmembrane domains. In the fetal form, or after denervation, the ε-subunit is replaced by a γ-subunit. The AChR subunits are organized around a central ion channel (Figure 54.1). The two ACh binding sites are between the α- and ε- or γ-subunits, and the α- and δ-subunits. Both sites need to be occupied for the ion channel to be in the open state. The main immunogenic region (MIR) is a conformation-dependent region on the extracellular component of each of the α-subunits (Lindstrom, 2000).

MuSK is a receptor tyrosine kinase. The extracellular portion consists of four immunoglobulin-like domains and a cysteine-rich domain. The intracellular portion consists of a juxtamembrane domain, followed by a tyrosine kinase catalytic domain. MuSK is critical both for the development (DeChiara et al., 1996) and ongoing maintenance (Kong

(A)   (B)

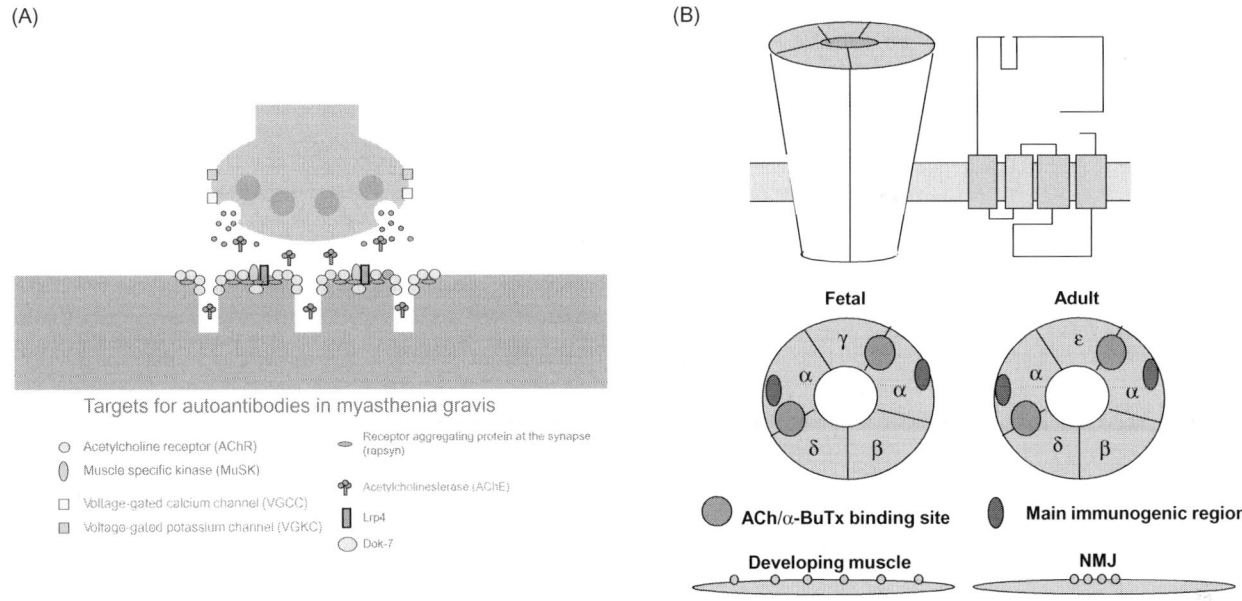

FIGURE 54.1   Ion channel targets for autoantibodies at the neuromuscular junction.   (A) Neuromuscular transmission depends on the calcium-dependent release of vesicles of acetylcholine, ACh. ACh binds to the AChRs on the postsynaptic membrane resulting in a depolarization which, if it reaches a critical threshold, initiates an action potential in the muscle leading to contraction. ACh is immediately destroyed by acetylcholinesterase. AChRs, VGCCs, and VGKCs are all targets for antibody-mediated neurological diseases. Recently, the receptor tyrosine kinase MuSK has been found to be a target for antibodies in a proportion of patients with MG without AChR antibodies. (B) The acetylcholine receptor (AChR). The acetylcholine receptor is a transmembrane protein with $(\alpha)_2,\beta,\gamma,\delta$-subunits in the fetal form and $(\alpha)_2,\beta,\delta,\varepsilon$-subunits in the adult form. A high proportion of antibodies in MG bind to the main immunogenic regions that are on both the α-subunits. In addition, many patients' antibodies bind to the fetal-specific γ-subunit. In some cases antibodies that inhibit the function of the fetal form, selectively cross the placenta causing fetal muscle paralysis with severe and often fatal deformities.

et al., 2004) of the NMJ. The activation of MuSK requires N-agrin release from the presynaptic nerve. Agrin binds to the MuSK co-receptor, Lrp4, and this binds to and activates MuSK.

released, the quantal content (QC), from these parameters (Wood and Slater, 2001). An inherent safety factor exists in normal muscle, whereby more ACh is released than is required to reach the activation threshold for the opening of the VGSCs.

Neuromuscular Transmission

Neuromuscular transmission begins with propagation of the action potential into the motor nerve terminal. This depolarization causes opening of the VGCCs and the resulting calcium influx results in the fusion and release of ACh. The release of ACh is terminated by the closing of VGCCs, and the opening of the VGKCs with subsequent repolarization of the nerve terminal. ACh binding to the AChR results in opening of the AChR central ion pore and a localized depolarization of the motor endplate. If sufficient, this will cause the opening of the VGSCs and propagation of the action potential through the muscle fiber.

The amount of ACh released by a single vesicle is termed a quantum. The spontaneous release of a single quantum is responsible for the generation of a local depolarization, termed a miniature endplate potential (MEPP); a nerve impulse releases multiple vesicles leading to a greater depolarization, termed the endplate potential (EPP). It is possible to calculate the number of quanta

MYASTHENIA GRAVIS

Epidemiology

A recent meta-analysis of 55 published studies calculated a pooled incidence rate of 5.3 per million person-years (CI 4.4–6.1) and a pooled prevalence rate of 77.7 per million (CI 64–93) (Carr et al., 2010).

Etiology

In the majority of cases no single cause is identifiable. There is genetic predisposition, which most likely reflects the contribution of polymorphic MHC class I and II loci. Other possible genetic susceptibility markers include the AChR alpha subunit (Garchon et al., 1994; Giraud et al., 2007), IgG heavy and light chains (Dondi et al., 1994), Fc gamma receptor IIa (Amdahl et al., 2007), TAP (Hjelmstrom et al., 1997), CTLA4 (Wang et al., 2008), and PTPN22 (Provenzano et al., 2012). Molecular

TABLE 54.2 MG Patients Divided on the Basis of Antibody Status, Age at Onset, Thymic Pathology and HLA Association

Subtype of MG	Age at Onset	Sex M:F	Typical Thymic Pathology	HLA Association	Associated Autoantibodies
Early onset	<41 years	1:3	Thymitis	B8, DR3	AChR. May have other tissue antibodies, e.g., thyroid
Thymoma associated	Mainly 40–60 years	1:1	Epithelial tumor containing many lymphocytes	No clear association	AChR. Titin and ryanodine receptor antibodies very common. Also cytokine antibodies
Late onset	>40 years	1.5:1	Normal or atrophied	B7, DR2 in males	AChR. Titin and ryanodine receptor antibodies common, particularly after age 60 years
AChR antibody negative MuSK antibody positive	2–70 years	1:3	Normal or atrophied in most	Not known	MuSK. No other common antibodies
AChR antibody negative MuSK antibody negative	1–80 years	2:3	Mild thymitis in some	Not known	Clustered AChR antibodies in some. Lrp4 in a small proportion.

These subgroups are not appropriate in patients with purely ocular MG, and in other ethnic populations.

mimicry between AChR subunits and microbial proteins has been proposed as a possible initiating process, with autosensitization against muscle AChR occurring as a result of determinant spreading. Certain drugs, notably penicillamine, may also trigger the development of the condition in genetically susceptible individuals (Drosos et al., 1993).

General Aspects

Myasthenia gravis (MG) is an autoimmune disorder characterized by fatigable muscle weakness. It often involves the extraocular muscles at onset, causing diplopia and/or ptosis. If it remains confined to these muscles it is termed ocular MG. If other muscle groups are involved, often facial, axial, limb, bulbar, and respiratory muscles, it is termed generalized MG. Bulbar and respiratory involvement can be life threatening.

The diagnosis rests on a compatible clinical presentation, supported by serological confirmation (see below) and/or electromyographic evidence (with repetitive nerve stimulation and/or single fiber electromyography) of a defect in neurotransmission. MG is commonly associated with thymic abnormalities, notably thymic hyperplasia and thymoma, and appropriate imaging of the thymus is therefore recommended at presentation.

Symptomatic treatment includes the use of cholinesterase inhibitors, but the majority of cases will also require immunosuppressive agents including corticosteroids and steroid sparing agents (azathioprine, mycophenolate mofetil, methotrexate, and cyclosporine). Thymectomy is a therapeutic option in younger patients with detectable AChR antibodies. Intravenous

immunoglobulin and plasma exchange may be employed in severe, life-threatening, or refractory disease. Newer biological agents, such as the monoclonal anti-CD20 agent rituximab, have shown promise in refractory cases (Maddison et al., 2011). Most of these aspects are discussed in more detail below. The treatment modalities available for MG are more fully reviewed elsewhere (Vincent and Leite, 2005; Sanders and Evoli, 2010).

CLINICAL HETEROGENEITY

MG is not a single disease entity but can be classified into different groups. Defined serologically, it is possible to delineate five main subgroups of MG (see Table 54.2) that differ also by means of age of onset, HLA association thymic pathology (Compston et al., 1980), and presence of antibodies directed against non-AChR proteins. The latter group includes MuSK, Lrp4, and the striational muscle proteins titin and ryanodine receptor (RyR).

Early-onset AChR Antibody Positive MG (AChRab⁺ MG)

These patients present before the age of the 40 years, with a female predominance and an incidence that has remained relatively stable for many years. There is an association with HLA A1, B8, DR3, DR2, and DR52 among Northern Europeans (Compston et al., 1980; Janer et al., 1999; Hill et al., 1999) and HLA DPB1, DQB1, and DR9 among the Japanese (Horiki et al., 1994). Childhood onset AChRab⁺ MG is relatively rare in Northern Europeans, but more prevalent among oriental populations (Vincent et al., 2001).

Clinically the MG often involves extra-ocular muscles at onset before generalizing, although a proportion of cases will remain purely ocular. The early response to cholinesterase inhibitors is usually good, but the majority of patients will still require some form of immunosuppressive therapy. The thymus is typically hyperplastic and thymectomy is a therapeutic option in early-onset generalized AChRab$^+$ MG, with current available evidence suggestive of benefit in over half of cases. Antibodies against titin and RyR are found in only a minority of cases.

Late-onset AChR Antibody Positive MG (AChRab$^+$ MG)

By conventional definition these patients present after 40 years of age. There is a slight male predominance. Employing a registry to identify all individuals with positive AChR antibody levels, the age-specific incidence rises between 45 and 75 years, before rapidly falling (Vincent et al., 2003). There is a weak association with HLA B7, DR2 (Compston et al., 1980) and DR4, DQw8 (Carlsson et al., 1990).

Clinically these patients have a similar phenotype to the early-onset form, although ocular MG may be more common (Zivkovic et al., 2012). The overall response to immunosuppressive treatment is similar to that with early-onset disease, but a greater proportion of patients will encounter side effects, presumably due to co-morbid disease (Sanders and Evoli, 2010). The thymus is typically atrophic. The response to thymectomy is poorer, and it is not routinely offered to patients over 60 years of age.

Over half of these late-onset cases have detectable antibodies against titin and RyR (Buckley et al., 2001) while 25% have antibodies against the cytokines, interferon-α, or interleukin-12 (Meager et al., 2003). These antibodies are more prevalent in thymoma cases and some authors have speculated that late-onset MG may represent an immune response against occult thymomas that are subsequently destroyed (Marx et al., 2010).

Thymoma-Associated MG (Thymoma MG)

Thymomas are tumors derived from thymic epithelial cells, thereby distinguishing them from lymphoma, neuroendocrine, and germ cell tumors. They are conventionally classified by means of the WHO classification (A, AB, B, and C). A coexisting thymoma is identified in 10% of MG patients. It can occur at any age, but is most common among the 40–60 age group. There is no gender difference or consistent HLA association.

Clinically the myasthenia is generalized with detectable AChR antibodies, although ocular and seronegative cases have been reported (Maggi et al., 2008). The myasthenia may be more refractory to treatment than other forms of MG (Sanders and Evoli, 2010). Following thymectomy, AChR antibody levels do not necessarily fall, without additional treatments, but in contrast to early-onset disease, the myasthenia rarely improves (Somnier, 1994).

Serum antibodies against striated muscle were recognized first in the 1960s. Their major targets are two intracellular proteins, titin and the ryanodine receptor (RyR), both of which are expressed in thymoma (Skeie et al., 1997; Mygland et al., 1995). These antibodies are typically observed in >90% of thymoma-associated MG cases, but there are no convincing data supporting their pathogenic role, and antibodies against the AChR are invariably identified. Neutralizing antibodies against interferon-α and interleukin-12 are observed in approximately 70% and 50% of cases, respectively (Buckley et al., 2001; Meager et al., 2003) (Chapter 76). These are useful markers for identification of recurrent disease.

MuSK Antibody-Positive MG (MuSKab$^+$ MG)

These patients can present at any age, with a female predominance. There is significant worldwide variation, with a correlation with geographical latitude, suggesting potential environmental influences (Vincent et al., 2008). Despite the small numbers in individual studies, a significant association with HLA DR14 and DQ5 in a Dutch cohort (Niks et al., 2006) and DRB16 and DQB5 in an Italian cohort (Bartoccioni et al., 2009) has been identified.

Clinically, the phenotype can be different from AChRab$^+$ MG with prominent ocular, bulbar, neck, and respiratory weakness (Evoli et al., 2003; Sanders et al., 2003). Muscle wasting and atrophy of the tongue and facial muscles may be evident both clinically and radiologically (Farrugia et al., 2006). The response to treatment can also differ with a comparatively poorer response (and occasionally intolerance) to cholinesterase inhibitors (Evoli et al., 2003; Pasnoor et al., 2010). A proportion can be refractory to conventional immunosuppressive treatment (Evoli et al., 2003). In such cases, plasma exchange is considered more effective than intravenous immunoglobulin (Pasnoor et al., 2010) but interestingly rituximab may be more effective in MuSK patients than in those with AChR antibodies (Maddison et al., 2011; Diaz-Manera et al., 2012). The therapeutic response to thymectomy remains uncertain (Evoli et al., 2008) and the thymus is typically normal or atrophic in direct comparison to that seen in AChRab$^+$ MG (Leite et al., 2005) (Figure 54.2). To date, there is only a single case report of MuSKab$^+$ MG associated with an underlying thymoma (Saka et al., 2005).

Neonatal MG

This is caused by passive transfer of maternal antibodies across the placenta. It may occur in up to 10% of female

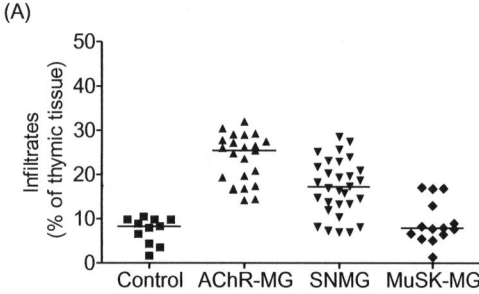
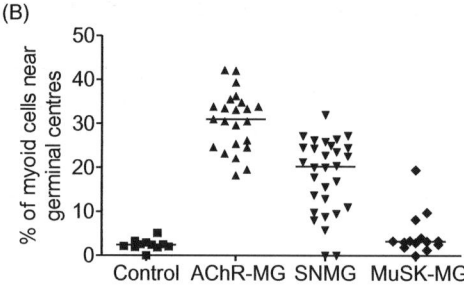

FIGURE 54.2   The thymus in different forms of myasthenia.   (A) Patients with AChR antibodies typically have hyperplastic thymuses with large lymphocytic infiltrates, whereas those with MuSK antibodies do not. Patients without either antibody (seronegative, SNMG) may have lymphocytic infiltrates and a proportion of these patients have AChR antibodies identified only by cell-based assays (Leite et al., 2008). (B) myoid cells, which express AChRs on their surface, are found close to the germinal centers or even within them, particularly in patients with AChR antibodies. *Data reproduced from Leite et al. (2007).*

patients with AChR antibodies (Vincent et al., 2001). The affected newborn babies exhibit transient symptomatic weakness, requiring the use of cholinesterase inhibitors for a few weeks. Rarely, it can occur in women who are symptom free but have AChR antibodies. Arthrogryposis multiplex congenita is a condition where the newborn have multiple joint contractures as a consequence of absent fetal movement *in utero*. It can occur if there are high levels of maternal antibodies directed against the fetal isoform of the AChR (Barnes et al., 1995). An animal model where pregnant mice are injected with maternal plasma has been described (Jacobson et al., 1999b). There are also rare case reports of neonatal MG occurring in MuSK MG, with both transient (Niks et al., 2008) and more persistent disease (Behin et al., 2008) described.

ANTIBODIES IN MYASTHENIA

Serological Testing

AChR antibodies were first detected by means of a radio-immunoprecipitation assay (RIA) employing ^{125}I α-bungarotoxin, which binds strongly to AChRs, to label AChRs in detergent extracts of human muscle (Lindstrom et al., 1976). Modern RIAs employ AChRs extracted from muscle cell lines expressing mixtures of fetal and adult AChRs (Beeson et al., 1996). Directly radiolabeled recombinant MuSK are used for detection of MuSK antibodies (Matthews et al., 2004). Enzyme-linked immunosorbent assays are not as sensitive or as specific.

Cell-based assays (CBAs) use cells transfected with DNA(s) for the antigen of interest and expressed on the cell surface. Indirect immunofluorescence can then detect binding of patients' antibodies. This method is sensitive and, importantly, measures antibodies that only bind to extracellular determinants of the antigen (Leite et al., 2010). This was demonstrated in previously seronegative cases using cells transfected with AChR subunits and

with the scaffold protein rapsyn that clusters the AChRs (Leite et al., 2008). CBAs have also been developed to detect MuSK or Lrp4 antibodies (Leite et al., 2008; Higuchi et al., 2011).

In generalized MG, 85% have AChR antibodies and 0–10% have MuSK antibodies; up to 5% may only have clustered AChR antibodies, although there are few systematic studies at present. There are rare case reports of patients with both AChR and MuSK antibodies (Saulat et al., 2007; Rajakulendran et al., 2012). Lrp4 antibodies can be found in previously seronegative patients, but a number also have MuSK antibodies (Higuchi et al., 2011).

Other antibodies that have been reported in MG include those against the striational muscle proteins actin, myosin, and titin and the ryanodine receptor (RyR) (Aarli et al., 1998). Titin is required for muscle assembly and for its ongoing ability to contract and relax, while the RyR are calcium release channels required for muscle contraction. These antibodies are typically seen in thymoma and older non-thymoma cases. Antibodies against rapsyn have also been described (Agius et al. 1998), although these are not specific for MG. All of these antigens are intracellular proteins and the antibodies are unlikely to be pathogenic.

AChR Antibody Characteristics

AChR antibodies belong to variable IgG subclasses, although IgG1 and IgG3 predominate (Rodgaard et al., 1987; Vincent et al., 1987). A significant proportion of antibodies are directed against the MIR on α-subunits, although other sites (Whiting et al., 1986) and other AChR subunits (Jacobson et al., 1999a) can also be targets. These antibodies have a high affinity (around 100 pM) and are highly specific for the intact receptor with limited binding to recombinant polypeptides or denatured AChR subunits; the antibodies bind predominantly to the extracellular portion of the receptor.

Within an individual patient, disease activity correlates well with changes in antibody level, at least in the short term. Between patients, there is variation in the antibody specificity, isoelectric heterogeneity, and avidity for the AChR, and no clear correlation with disease activity is observed (Vincent et al., 1987).

Somatic mutations of the B lymphocyte Ig genes are necessary for the synthesis of these high affinity antibodies. Lower affinity AChR antibodies have been observed in monoclonal gammopathies using ELISA, but myasthenic symptoms are rarely encountered (Eng et al., 1987).

MuSK and Other Antibodies

MuSK antibodies may also belong to variable IgG subclasses, although IgG4 predominates (McConville et al., 2004). They bind to the Ig-like domains of MuSK and have a similar affinity to that of AChR antibodies (McConville et al., 2004). No clear relationship between MuSK antibody level and disease severity is seen across the patient cohorts but for an individual patient there is a reasonable correlation in the few studies done. By contrast, Lrp4 antibodies belong predominantly to the IgG1 subclass (Higuchi et al., 2011).

PATHOGENIC MECHANISMS

Evidence for Pathogenicity of AChR and MuSK Antibodies

Both AChR and MuSK antibodies are pathogenic, satisfying the strict criteria required for establishing causation in autoimmune disease (Rose and Bona, 1993). Both are directed against autoantigens that are highly relevant to a disorder of neurotransmission, and are highly specific for MG.

The main criteria in these diseases are the passive transfer of MG from man to animal (usually mice or rats) and the response to treatments that reduce antibody levels. Passive transfer models involve injection of IgG from MG patients into animals and lead either to objective weakness or at least to neurophysiological evidence of impaired neurotransmission. Plasma exchange dramatically reduces antibody levels within a few days, and leads to striking clinical improvement even in patients with long-standing disease. In addition, maternal–fetal transfer of the disease has been reported in both serological forms of MG.

Further in vivo evidence comes from replication of the human disease in animals that have been immunized with the relevant antigen, termed experimental autoimmune myasthenia gravis (EAMG). This active immunization model has been used extensively to study the immunebiology of MG, as will be mentioned below.

AChR Antibody-Positive MG

AChR antibodies cause loss of AChRs through three principal mechanisms. These include complement-mediated destruction, cross-linking and accelerated degradation and functional blockade.

AChR antibodies belong predominantly to the complement fixing IgG1 and IgG3 subclasses (Vincent et al., 1987; Rodgaard et al., 1987). Activation of complement results in the generation of the membrane activation complex which is responsible for lysis and destruction of the postsynaptic membrane, loss of postsynaptic folding, and ultimately loss of AChR and related proteins. IgG colocalizing with activated complement is observed both in EAMG (Sahashi et al., 1978) and MG (Engel et al., 1977) muscle biopsies. The importance of complement in the pathogenesis of this form of MG comes from several lines of evidence. Depletion (Lennon et al., 1978), inhibition (Biesecker and Gomez, 1989), or blockade (Piddlesden et al., 1996) of complement all result in resistance to developing disease in EAMG. Further evidence is provided by the study of transgenic mice lacking components of the classical complement cascade (Tuzun et al., 2003) and complement regulators (Morgan et al., 2006).

AChR antibodies belonging to the IgG1, IgG2, and IgG3 subclasses are also able to divalently cross-link AChRs, increasing the rate of internalization and degradation of AChRs. This is termed antigenic modulation, and is observed in both MG (Drachman et al., 1978) and EAMG patients (Lindstrom and Einarson, 1979). It is most prominent when antibodies are directed against the MIR (Tzartos et al., 1991).

AChR antibodies have been shown to block the ACh binding sites of AChRs in cultured muscle cells (Howard et al., 1987) and even in human muscle biopsies in vitro. In EAMG they are capable of causing severe weakness, with little structural effect on the NMJ (Gomez and Richman, 1983). These blocking antibodies are often found at low levels, and while they may have a role to play in acute exacerbations, their effect is insignificant in the majority of patients.

Failure of neuromuscular transmission results from the loss of AChRs, with reduced MEPP and EPP amplitudes. The reduced EPP amplitude falls below the required threshold to initiate an action potential, leading to blocking of neurotransmission. There is partial compensation for this through an increase in the number of quanta of ACh released, which appears to be a compensatory mechanism in both MG and EAMG (Plomp et al., 1995).

MuSK Antibody-Positive MG

MuSK antibodies belong predominantly to the non-complement fixing IgG4 subclass (McConville et al., 2004). IgG4 antibodies are able to undergo Fab arm exchange to produce bispecific antibodies that do not cross-link identical antigens (van der Zee et al., 1986), and which therefore function monovalently (Schuurman et al., 1999). This suggests that the effector mechanisms are likely to be different from those in AChR-mediated disease. To date the only published human pathological study has demonstrated normal motor endplates, normal AChR numbers, and little evidence of complement deposition (Shiraishi et al., 2005). In contrast, both active immunization (Shigemoto et al., 2006; Viegas et al., 2012) and passive transfer (Cole et al., 2008; Viegas et al., 2012) models have demonstrated AChR loss in clinically affected animals, although complement deposition has not been observed and complement deficient mice remain susceptible to the disease (Mori et al., 2012). Nevertheless, both IgG4 and non-IgG4 MuSK antibodies can affect AChR clustering on myotubes in in vitro assays and the mechanisms of MuSK antibodies in general are not yet clear (Koneczny et al., 2013).

MuSK has a critical role in the ongoing maintenance of the NMJ (Kong et al., 2004; Hesser et al., 2006). Combined pre- and postsynaptic morphological changes have been observed in animal models (Cole et al., 2008; Richman et al., 2012) and may explain the severe phenotype that is observed. There is also electrophysiological evidence of both pre- and postsynaptic defects (Klooster et al., 2012; Viegas et al., 2012) with failure of the presynaptic compensatory mechanism (Plomp et al., 1995) further impacting on underlying neurotransmission.

THE THYMUS AND CELLULAR IMMUNITY IN MG

Role of T Lymphocytes in MG

High affinity AChR antibodies are thought to be dependent on CD4[+] T lymphocytes but as these are rarely observed in myasthenic muscle and almost never found at the neuromuscular junction, they are not thought to be effector cells in MG. Nevertheless their critical role in the autoimmune pathogenesis is demonstrated through several lines of evidence in both MG and EAMG. EAMG was first described following the immunization of rabbits with AChRs purified from the electric organ of *Torpedo californica* (Patrick and Lindstrom, 1973) and later reproduced in a number of other species. In the murine model there are both disease sensitive and resistant strains, related to their different H-2 alleles (Berman and Patrick, 1980).

AChR-specific CD4[+] T lymphocytes occur in both the peripheral blood and thymuses of MG patients. They may also be observed in healthy controls but the clinical improvement observed following their removal with anti-CD4 monoclonal antibodies (Ahlberg et al., 1994) and in HIV (Nath et al., 1990) supports a pathogenic role for these lymphocytes. These isolated CD4[+] T lymphocytes may respond to stimulation with the intact AChRs, recombinant subunits, or AChR peptides (Conti-Fine et al., 1998; Wang et al., 1998) and T cell lines and clones propagated from MG patients will respond more vigorously to stimulation *in vitro* than those derived from healthy controls. The epitopes are most commonly found on the α-subunit of the AChR. In EAMG a dominant epitope within the α146-162 activates MHC class II-restricted CD4[+] T lymphocytes, leading to pathogenic antibody production (Christadoss et al., 2000). A clearly immunodominant epitope has not been identified reproducibly in a high proportion of MG patients, although an epsilon subunit epitope was identified in some (Hill et al., 1999). The TCR Vβ families show preferential expansion of the Vβ 4 and 6 among MG patients (Navaneetham et al., 1998) while mice lacking Vβ 6 respond poorly to immunization with AChR (Krco et al., 1991).

Mice genetically deficient in functioning CD4[+] T lymphocytes do not develop EAMG (Kaul et al., 1994) while severe combined immunodeficiency mice will only produce AChR antibodies and develop myasthenic symptoms if the human grafted cells contain CD4[+] T lymphocytes (Wang et al., 1999).

CD4[+] T lymphocytes and the cytokines they secrete will influence the type of autoimmune response generated in both MG and EAMG. Analysis of blood from MG patients has confirmed the presence of Th1 (IFN-γ[+]), Th2 (IL-4[+]), Th17 (IL-17[+]), and Treg (Foxp[+]) cells (Li et al., 2008), but the role of these T lymphocyte subsets in the development of the disease is best examined using transgenic mice. IL-12 is essential for promoting development of Th1 cells and IL-12[-/-] mice are resistant to the development of EAMG despite a significant antibody response (Karachunski et al., 2000). The role of IFN-γ remains unclear with conflicting reports of EAMG susceptibility (Balasa et al., 1997; Wang et al., 2007). IL-4 appears to be either neutral (Balasa et al., 1998) or confer a protective effect (Karachunski et al., 1999). There is an apparent increase in Th17 and decrease in Treg cells during development of EAMG in rats (Mu et al., 2009) and administration of Treg cells to myasthenic rats inhibited progression of EAMG (Aricha et al., 2008). Initial studies identified no change in Treg cell numbers in MG subjects compared with healthy controls (Huang et al., 2004) although a specific functional impairment in those Foxp3[+] Treg cells (Balandina et al., 2005) was subsequently identified.

T cell activation requires the interaction of TCR/MHC peptide in addition to the interaction between CD28/CTLA4 on the T lymphocytes and CD80 (B7) on antigen-presenting cells (the CD28 − CD80 interaction). It also requires the cross-linking of the CD40 ligand (CD40—CD40 L interaction). Using transgenic mice it has been demonstrated that both interactions are essential for the primary immune response (Shi et al., 1998) although their contribution to the secondary response is thought to be less prominent. Here the CD278 (inducible T cell costimulator) is thought to be important for the secondary response (Scott et al., 2004).

The Thymus and MG

The thymus is an epithelial organ that can be morphologically divided into a distinct cortex, medulla, and corticomedullary zone. The cortex contains densely packed immature lymphocytes alongside a sparse population of epithelial cells and bone marrow-derived macrophages. The medulla is less cellular containing more mature T lymphocytes, more prominent epithelial cells, dendritic cells, B lymphocytes, and rare myoid cells (Pearse, 2006). The thymus has a critical role in self-tolerance with a fine balance between the generation of protective T lymphocytes and deletion of autoreactive T lymphocytes required. Relevant autoantigens including the α-subunit of the AChR are expressed on medullary thymic epithelial cells (mTECs) under the control of the autoimmune regulator gene (AIRE) (Giraud et al., 2007). Central T cell tolerance relies on the close interaction between these mTECs and nearby dendritic cells and their effect on the T lymphocyte development and subsequent differentiation.

The thymus is thought to have a critical role in the development of early-onset AChR antibody-positive MG. The cortex is typically normal but the medulla contains lymphocytic infiltrates (Figure 54.2) and germinal centers with distinct areas of B lymphocyte proliferation, differentiation, somatic hypermutation, and immunoglobulin class switching. These B lymphocytes when cultured *in vitro* are capable of secreting anti-AChR antibodies spontaneously (Vincent et al., 1978; Scadding et al., 1981). It is therefore to be expected that antibody levels fall post-thymectomy (Vincent et al., 1983) but they seldom disappear.

Whether early-onset AChR antibody-positive MG begins in the thymus, or whether these changes are a reflection of a systemic process, remains unresolved. Individual AChR subunits are expressed on mTECs (Salmon et al., 1998), presumably as part of a self-tolerance mechanism and these are targeted by both autoantibodies (Safar et al., 1991) and complement (Leite et al., 2007). Native AChR is also expressed by the muscle-like myoid cells which, while comparatively rare, are more abundant in the hyperplastic thymus (Kirchner et al., 1986). The germinal centers appear to be focused around these myoid cells (Figure 54.2). Given that they lack MHC class II or costimulatory molecules they rely on the antigen-presenting dendritic cells to prime the CD4$^+$ T lymphocytes. One proposed multi-step hypothesis is that the mTECs first present epitopes from isolated AChR subunits to CD4$^+$ T lymphocytes, evoking the production of early antibodies capable of attacking the thymic myoid cells which express the intact AChR. As the immune response continues to proliferate, germinal centers are formed which allow these antibodies to diversify allowing recognition of native AChRs (Willcox et al., 2008).

The thymus is typically involuted and atrophic in older patients. The aging thymus is gradually replaced with fat, although residual foci of mTECS may persist, and myoid cells are only rarely encountered. Histological analysis of thymus tissue from late-onset MG cases previously suggested no differences from normal controls (Myking et al., 1998). Nevertheless a more recent study looking at young and late-onset MG cases identified residual lymphocyte accumulation among the older cohort and no qualitative differences between the two groups (Ishii et al., 2007).

Thymomas are heterogeneous neoplasms of thymic epithelial cells with mixed cortical and medullary markers. They may develop from either early TEC progenitors or from more mature cortical or medullary TECs (Hasserjian et al., 2005). They are responsible for the generation of numerous maturing polyclonal T lymphocytes (thymocytes) capable of maturing into CD4$^+$ or CD8$^+$ T lymphocytes. The degree of thymopoiesis is known to vary according to the thymoma subtype (Nenninger et al., 1998). The B2 subtype is the most common type associated with MG (accounting for ≈ 50% of cases) and contains an abundance of mature CD4$^+$ T lymphocytes ready for export (Strobel et al., 2004). It should be noted that corticosteroids can deplete the immature T lymphocytes and thereby modify the histological subtype.

There are certain features in thymomas that are likely to promote inefficient self-tolerance including defective AIRE and MHC class II expression, an absence of myoid cells, and failure to generate Foxp3$^+$ Treg cells as well as defective T lymphocyte signaling (Marx et al., 2010). Antigenic targets other than AChR are also recognized which is unsurprising given the wide range of systemic, hematological, endocrine, cutaneous, gastrointestinal, and renal disorders associated with thymoma (Marx et al., 2010).

Genetic aberrations and polymorphisms may also be identified in thymoma. These include HLA genes (notably loci at 6p21) which may affect MHC class II expression and non-MHC genes (including CTLA4 and PTPN22) which influence T cell receptor signaling.

LAMBERT—EATON MYASTHENIC SYNDROME

The Lambert—Eaton myasthenic syndrome (LEMS) is clinically and electrophysiologically distinct from MG.

Approximately 50% of LEMS cases are paraneoplastic, typically associated with small cell lung carcinoma (SCLC). There are certain features that make it possible to distinguish paraneoplastic and non-paraneoplastic forms.

Epidemiology and Etiology

LEMS is less common than MG, with an annual incidence of 0.48 per million in a Dutch study (Wirtz et al., 2003). The median age of onset is 60 years in both the paraneoplastic and non-paraneoplastic forms (O'Neill et al., 1988; Titulaer et al., 2011), although there is another smaller peak at 35 years in the non-paraneoplastic forms (Titulaer et al., 2011). There is a male predominance in the paraneoplastic form, and a slight female predominance in the non-paraneoplastic form. In the latter, similarly to early onset MG there is an association with HLA B8 and DR3.

Clinical Features

The cardinal clinical features of LEMS include muscle weakness, autonomic dysfunction, and areflexia. Typical findings include proximal muscle weakness that is more marked in the lower limbs. Ocular and bulbar symptoms may occur later in the disease course. The speed of progression is often more rapid in the paraneoplastic form (Titulaer et al., 2008). Autonomic involvement is seen in over 80% of cases. Commonly encountered symptoms include dry mouth, erectile dysfunction, and constipation. Micturition difficulties and orthostatic syncope are less common. In contrast to MG, the muscle strength in LEMS will improve after a period of maximal voluntary contraction.

Investigation and Treatment

Electromyography will confirm a disorder of neurotransmission, although a significant increase in the compound muscle action potential following a period of exercise or high frequency stimulation allows electrophysiological differentiation from MG. Serological confirmation involves detection of antibodies against the P/Q type voltage-gated calcium channels which are found in approximately 90% of LEMS cases, and are invariably present in paraneoplastic SCLC cases (see below).

To detect the antibodies, the P/Q type VGCCs are extracted from mammalian brain, labeled with ^{125}I ω-conotoxin which binds specifically to these VGCCs, and used in an RIA. In addition antibodies against N type (30−40%) and L type (25%) VGCCs may be present (Johnston et al., 1994; Motomura et al., 1997). Other antibodies which have been identified include those against synaptotagmin (Takamori et al., 1995) and more recently against SOX-1 in 65% of paraneoplastic cases and around 5% of non-paraneoplastic cases (Sabater et al., 2008; Titulaer et al., 2009).

Symptomatic treatment requires 3,4-diaminopyridine. If additional treatment is required then corticosteroids and other immunosuppressive agents are used. Intravenous immunoglobulin, plasma exchange, and rituximab may be used in severe and refractory cases. Any underlying SCLC should be treated in the appropriate manner. Treatment options are reviewed in more detail in Titulaer et al. (2011).

Pathophysiology

The voltage-gated calcium channel complex contains several subunits but the α_1-subunit is primarily responsible for the biochemical and electrophysiological functions of the protein. Similarly to the MIR on the α-subunit of the AChR there may be particularly immunogenic sequences; 50% of LEMS patients have antibodies against linker domains on the α_1-subunit (Takamori et al., 1997).

Freeze fracture electron microscope studies of the presynaptic motor nerve terminal have demonstrated an ordered array of intramembranous particles. These are located close to the site of transmitter exocytosis. There is some evidence that VGCCs constitute at least some of the intramembranous particles in the active zone (Robitaille et al., 1990). LEMS patients have both a reduction in the total number of active zone particles and the number of particles per active zone (Nagel et al., 1988).

The evidence for the pathogenic nature of VGCCs comes from both clinical and experimental studies. Patients respond to plasma exchange (Newsom-Davis et al., 1982) and cases of maternal to fetal transfer of the disease have also been reported (Lecky, 2006). Passive transfer with LEMS plasma or IgG produces the same neurophysiological abnormalities in mice (Lang et al., 1983; Fukunaga et al., 1983), although no weakness was observed. Further studies confirmed the localization of IgG close to the presynaptic active zones (Fukuoka et al., 1987). Additionally, active immunization of rats with peptides from the α_1-subunit led to mild weakness and compatible neurophysiological changes (Komai et al., 1999). Finally, mice with mutations in the P/Q type VGCC (CACNA1a) share some of the electrophysiological characteristics of LEMS (Kaja et al., 2007).

CONCLUSIONS AND FUTURE PROSPECTS

Historically, the classification of MG has been based on AChR antibody status, age of onset, and thymic pathology. MuSK antibodies were first recognized over a decade ago, and while there was some initial skepticism about their relevance, it is now well established that they are pathogenic, satisfying all the necessary criteria for causation in autoimmune diseases. Defined serologically, this particular form of MG is typically more severe and more refractory to conventional immunosuppressive therapy. From an immunological perspective the predominance of the non-complement fixing IgG4 subclass contrasts with AChR antibody-mediated disease. The relative absence of complement as an effector mechanism may help explain the largely normal neuromuscular junctions that have been observed in human studies.

Over recent years further advances in serological assays for MG have been made. Alongside established radioimmunoprecipitation assays for detecting AChR and MuSK antibodies, cell-based assays have been developed that allowed us to first identify antibodies to clustered AChR, and then more recently Lrp4 antibodies. Over the next few years we need to confirm if these Lrp4 antibodies are pathogenic. Given that these antibodies are predominantly of the IgG1 subclass, we would anticipate that the role of complement may be more akin to that observed in AChR antibody-mediated MG.

Conventional treatment for MG relies on symptomatic treatment, oral immunosuppressive agents, and immuno-modulatory treatment with intravenous immunoglobulin and plasma exchange. Newer biological agents, such as rituximab, have shown promise and may benefit those with refractory disease. We should soon learn the results of the international thymectomy study. In the future, our greater understanding of the immunology of MG may allow the development of more targeted immunotherapy. Potential drugs could include those directed against the complement cascade/membrane attack complex, B lymphocyte proliferation, relevant cytokines and their receptors, and lymphocyte adhesion and migration pathways.

REFERENCES

Aarli, J.A., Skeie, G.O., Mygland, A., Gilhus, N.E., 1998. Muscle striation antibodies in myasthenia gravis. Diagnostic and functional significance. Ann. N. Y. Acad. Sci. 841, 505—515.

Agius, M.A., Zhu, S., Kirvan, C.A., Schafer, A.L., Lin, M.Y., Fairclough, R.H., et al., 1998. Rapsyn antibodies in myasthenia gravis. Ann. N. Y. Acad. Sci. 841, 516—521.

Ahlberg, R., Yi, Q., Pirskanen, R., Matell, G., Swerup, C., Rieber, E.P., et al., 1994. Treatment of myasthenia gravis with anti-CD4 antibody, improvement correlates to decreased T-cell autoreactivity. Neurology. 44, 1732—1737.

Amdahl, C., Alseth, E.H., Gilhus, N.E., Nakkestad, H.L., Skeie, G.O., 2007. Polygenic disease associations in thymomatous myasthenia gravis. Arch. Neurol. 64, 1729—1733.

Aricha, R., Feferman, T., Fuchs, S., Souroujon, M.C., 2008. Ex vivo generated regulatory T cells modulate experimental autoimmune myasthenia gravis. J. Immunol. 180, 2132—2139.

Balandina, A., Lécart, S., Dartevelle, P., Saoudi, A., Berrih-Aknin, S., 2005. Functional defect of regulatory CD4(+)CD25 + T cells in the thymus of patients with autoimmune myasthenia gravis. Blood. 105, 735—741.

Balasa, B., Deng, C., Lee, J., Bradley, L.M., Dalton, D.K., Christadoss, P., et al., 1997. Interferon gamma (IFN-gamma) is necessary for the genesis of acetylcholine receptor-induced clinical experimental autoimmune myasthenia gravis in mice. J. Exp. Med. 186, 385—391.

Balasa, B., Deng, C., Lee, J., Christadoss, P., Sarvetnick, N., 1998. The Th2 cytokine IL-4 is not required for the progression of antibody-dependent autoimmune myasthenia gravis. J. Immunol. 161, 2856—2862.

Barnes, P.R., Kanabar, D.J., Brueton, L., Newsom-Davis, J., Huson, S. M., Mann, N.P., et al., 1995. Recurrent congenital arthrogryposis leading to a diagnosis of myasthenia gravis in an initially asymptomatic mother. Neuromuscul. Disord. 5, 59—65.

Bartoccioni, E., Scuderi, F., Augugliaro, A., Chiatamone Ranieri, S., Sauchelli, D., Alboino, P., et al., 2009. HLA class II allele analysis in MuSK-positive myasthenia gravis suggests a role for DQ5. Neurology. 72, 195—197.

Beeson, D., Jacobson, L., Newsom-Davis, J., Vincent, A., 1996. A transfected human muscle cell line expressing the adult subtype of the human muscle acetylcholine receptor for diagnostic assays in myasthenia gravis. Neurology. 47, 1552—1555.

Behin, A., Mayer, M., Kassis-Makhoul, B., Jugie, M., Espil-Taris, C., Ferrer, X., et al., 2008. Severe neonatal myasthenia due to maternal anti-MuSK antibodies. Neuromuscul. Disord. 18, 443—446.

Berman, P.W., Patrick, J., 1980. Linkage between the frequency of muscular weakness and loci that regulate immune responsiveness in murine experimental myasthenia gravis. J. Exp. Med. 152, 507—520.

Biesecker, G., Gomez, C.M., 1989. Inhibition of acute passive transfer experimental autoimmune myasthenia gravis with Fab antibody to complement C6. J. Immunol. 142, 2654—2659.

Buckley, C., Newsom-Davis, J., Willcox, N., Vincent, A., 2001. Do titin and cytokine antibodies in MG patients predict thymoma or thymoma recurrence? Neurology. 57, 1579—1582.

Carlsson, B., Wallin, J., Pirskanen, R., Matell, G., Smith, C.I., 1990. Different HLA DR-DQ associations in subgroups of idiopathic myasthenia gravis. Immunogenetics. 31, 285—290.

Carr, A.S., Cardwell, C.R., McCarron, P.O., McConville, J., 2010. A systematic review of population based epidemiological studies in Myasthenia Gravis. BMC Neurol. 10, 46.

Chang, C., Lee, C., 1963. Isolation of neurotoxin from the venom of Bungarus multicinctus and their modes of neuro muscular blocking action. Arch. Int. Pharmacodyn. Ther. 144, 241—257.

Christadoss, P., Poussin, M., Deng, C., 2000. Animal models of myasthenia gravis. Clin. Immunol. 94, 75—87.

Cole, R.N., Reddel, S.W., Gervásio, O.L., Phillips, W.D., 2008. Anti-MuSK patient antibodies disrupt the mouse neuromuscular junction. Ann. Neurol. 63, 782—789.

Compston, D.A., Vincent, A., Newsom-Davis, J., Batchelor, J.R., 1980. Clinical, pathological, HLA antigen and immunological evidence for disease heterogeneity in myasthenia gravis. Brain. 103, 579—601.

Conti-Fine, B., Navaneetham, D., Karachunski, P.I., Raju, R., Diethelm-Okita, B., Okita, D., et al., 1998. T cell recognition of the acetylcholine receptor in myasthenia gravis. Ann. N. Y. Acad. Sci. 841, 283–308.

DeChiara, T.M., Bowen, D.C., Valenzuela, D.M., Simmons, M.V., Poueymirou, W.T., Thomas, S., et al., 1996. The receptor tyrosine kinase MuSK is required for neuromuscular junction formation in vivo. Cell. 85, 501–512.

Diaz-Manera, J., Martínez-Hernández, E., Querol, L., Klooster, R., Rojas-García, R., Suárez-Calvet, X., et al., 2012. Long-lasting treatment effect of rituximab in MuSK myasthenia. Neurology. 78, 189–193.

Dondi, E., Gajdos, P., Bach, J.F., Garchon, H.J., 1994. Association of Km3 allotype with increased serum levels of autoantibodies against muscle acetylcholine receptor in myasthenia gravis. J. Neuroimmunol. 51, 221–224.

Drachman, D.B., Angus, C.W., Adams, R.N., Michelson, J.D., Hoffman, G.J., 1978. Myasthenic antibodies cross-link acetylcholine receptors to accelerate degradation. N. Engl. J. Med. 298, 1116–1122.

Drosos, A.A., Christou, L., Galanopoulou, V., Tzioufas, A.G., Tsiakou, E. K., 1993. D-penicillamine induced myasthenia gravis, clinical, serological and genetic findings. Clin. Exp. Rheumatol. 11, 387–391.

Elmqvist, D., Hofmann, W.W., Kugelberg, J., Quastel, D.M., 1964. An electrophysiological investigation of neuromuscular transmission in myasthenia gravis. J. Physiol. 174, 417–434.

Eng, H., Lefvert, A.K., Mellstedt, H., Osterborg, A., 1987. Human monoclonal immunoglobulins that bind the human acetylcholine receptor. Eur. J. Immunol. 17, 1867–1869.

Engel, A.G., Lambert, E.H., Howard, F.M., 1977. Immune complexes (IgG and C3) at the motor end-plate in myasthenia gravis, ultrastructural and light microscopic localization and electrophysiologic correlations. Mayo. Clin. Proc. 52, 267–280.

Evoli, A., Tonali, P.A., Padua, L., Monaco, M.L., Scuderi, F., Batocchi, A.P., et al., 2003. Clinical correlates with anti-MuSK antibodies in generalized seronegative myasthenia gravis. Brain. 126, 2304–2311.

Evoli, A., Bianchi, M.R., Riso, R., Minicuci, G.M., Batocchi, A.P., Servidei, S., et al., 2008. Response to therapy in myasthenia gravis with anti-MuSK antibodies. Ann. N. Y. Acad. Sci. 1132, 76–83.

Fambrough, D.M., Drachman, D.B., Satyamurti, S., 1973. Neuromuscular junction in myasthenia gravis, decreased acetylcholine receptors. Science. 182, 293–295.

Farrugia, M.E., Robson, M.D., Clover, L., Anslow, P., Newsom-Davis, J., Kennett, R., et al., 2006. MRI and clinical studies of facial and bulbar muscle involvement in MuSK antibody-associated myasthenia gravis. Brain. 129, 1481–1492.

Fukunaga, H., Engel, A.G., Lang, B., Newsom-Davis, J., Vincent, A., 1983. Passive transfer of Lambert-Eaton myasthenic syndrome with IgG from man to mouse depletes the presynaptic membrane active zones. Proc. Natl. Acad. Sci. U.S.A. 80, 7636–7640.

Fukuoka, T., Engel, A.G., Lang, B., Newsom-Davis, J., Vincent, A., 1987. Lambert-Eaton myasthenic syndrome, II. Immunoelectron microscopy localization of IgG at the mouse motor end-plate. Ann. Neurol. 22, 200–211.

Garchon, H.J., Djabiri, F., Viard, J.P., Gajdos, P., Bach, J.F., 1994. Involvement of human muscle acetylcholine receptor alpha-subunit gene (CHRNA) in susceptibility to myasthenia gravis. Proc. Natl. Acad. Sci. U.S.A. 91, 4668–4672.

Giraud, M., Taubert, R., Vandiedonck, C., Ke, X., Lévi-Strauss, M., Pagani, F., et al., 2007. An IRF8-binding promoter variant and

AIRE control CHRNA1 promiscuous expression in thymus. Nature. 448, 934–937.

Gomez, C.M., Richman, D.P., 1983. Anti-acetylcholine receptor antibodies directed against the alpha-bungarotoxin binding site induce a unique form of experimental myasthenia. Proc. Natl. Acad. Sci. U.S.A. 80, 4089–4093.

Hasserjian, R.P., Ströbel, P., Marx, A., 2005. Pathology of thymic tumors. Semin. Thorac. Cardiovasc. Surg. 17, 2–11.

Hesser, B.A., Henschel, O., Witzemann, V., 2006. Synapse disassembly and formation of new synapses in postnatal muscle upon conditional inactivation of MuSK. Mol. Cell Neurosci. 31, 470–480.

Higuchi, O., Hamuro, J., Motomura, M., Yamanashi, Y., 2011. Autoantibodies to low-density lipoprotein receptor-related protein 4 in myasthenia gravis. Ann. Neurol. 69, 418–422.

Hill, M., Beeson, D., et al., 1999. Early-onset myasthenia gravis, a recurring T-cell epitope in the adult-specific acetylcholine receptor epsilon subunit presented by the susceptibility allele HLA-DR52a. Ann. Neurol. 45, 224–231.

Hjelmstrom, P., Beeson, D., Moss, P., Jacobson, L., Bond, A., Corlett, L., et al., 1997. TAP polymorphisms in Swedish myasthenia gravis patients. Tissue Antigens. 49, 176–179.

Horiki, T., Inoko, H., Moriuchi, J., Ichikawa, Y., Arimori, S., 1994. Combinations of HLA-DPB1 and HLA-DQB1 alleles determine susceptibility to early-onset myasthenia gravis in Japan. Autoimmunity. 19, 49–54.

Howard Jr., F.M., Lennon, V.A., Finley, J., Matsumoto, J., Elveback, L.R., 1987. Clinical correlations of antibodies that bind, block, or modulate human acetylcholine receptors in myasthenia gravis. Ann. N. Y. Acad. Sci. 505, 526–538.

Huang, Y.M., Pirskanen, R., Giscombe, R., Link, H., Lefvert, A.K., 2004. Circulating CD4 + CD25 + and CD4 + CD25 + T cells in myasthenia gravis and in relation to thymectomy. Scand. J. Immunol. 59, 408–414.

Ishii, W., Matsuda, M., Hanyuda, M., Momose, M., Nakayama, J., Ehara, T., et al., 2007. Comparison of the histological and immunohistochemical features of the thymus in young- and elderly-onset myasthenia gravis without thymoma. J. Clin. Neurosci. 14, 110–115.

Jacobson, L., Beeson, D., Tzartos, S., Vincent, A., 1999a. Monoclonal antibodies raised against human acetylcholine receptor bind to all five subunits of the fetal isoform. J. Neuroimmunol. 98, 112–120.

Jacobson, L., Polizzi, A., Morriss-Kay, G., Vincent, A., 1999b. Plasma from human mothers of fetuses with severe arthrogryposis multiplex congenita causes deformities in mice. J. Clin. Invest. 103, 1031–1038.

Janer, M., Cowland, A., Picard, J., Campbell, D., Pontarotti, P., Newsom-Davis, J., et al., 1999. A susceptibility region for myasthenia gravis extending into the HLA-class I sector telomeric to HLA-C. Hum. Immunol. 60, 909–917.

Johnston, I., Lang, B., Leys, K., Newsom-Davis, J., 1994. Heterogeneity of calcium channel autoantibodies detected using a small-cell lung cancer line derived from a Lambert-Eaton myasthenic syndrome patient. Neurology. 44, 334–338.

Kaja, S., van de Ven, R.C., van Dijk, J.G., Verschuuren, J.J., Arahata, K., Frants, R.R., et al., 2007. Severely impaired neuromuscular synaptic transmission causes muscle weakness in the Cacna1a-mutant mouse rolling Nagoya. Eur. J. Neurosci. 25, 2009–2020.

Karachunski, P.I., Ostlie, N.S., Okita, D.K., Conti-Fine, B.M., 1999. Interleukin-4 deficiency facilitates development of experimental myasthenia gravis and precludes its prevention by nasal administration of CD4$^+$ epitope sequences of the acetylcholine receptor. J. Neuroimmunol. 95, 73−84.

Karachunski, P.I., Ostlie, N.S., Monfardini, C., Conti-Fine, B.M., 2000. Absence of IFN-gamma or IL-12 has different effects on experimental myasthenia gravis in C57BL/6 mice. J. Immunol. 164, 5236−5244.

Kaul, R., Shenoy, M., Goluszko, E., Christadoss, P., 1994. Major histocompatibility complex class II gene disruption prevents experimental autoimmune myasthenia gravis. J. Immunol. 152, 3152−3157.

Kirchner, T., Schalke, B., Melms, A., von Kügelgen, T., Müller-Hermelink, H.K., 1986. Immunohistological patterns of nonneoplastic changes in the thymus in Myasthenia gravis. Virchows Arch., B, Cell Pathol. Incl. Mol. Pathol. 52, 237−257.

Klooster, R., Plomp, J.J., Huijbers, M.G., Niks, E.H., Straasheijm, K.R., Detmers, F.J., et al., 2012. Muscle-specific kinase myasthenia gravis IgG4 autoantibodies cause severe neuromuscular junction dysfunction in mice. Brain. 135, 1081−1101.

Komai, K., Iwasa, K., Takamori, M., 1999. Calcium channel peptide can cause an autoimmune-mediated model of Lambert-Eaton myasthenic syndrome in rats. J. Neurol. Sci. 166, 126−130.

Koneczny, I., Cossins, J., Waters, P., Beeson, D., Vincent, A., 2013. MuSK myasthenia gravis IgG4 disrupts the interaction of LRP4 with MuSK but both IgG4 and IgG1-3 can disperse preformed agrin-independent AChR clusters. PLoS one. in press.

Kong, X.C., Barzaghi, P., Ruegg, M.A., 2004. Inhibition of synapse assembly in mammalian muscle in vivo by RNA interference. EMBO Rep. 5, 183−188.

Krco, C.J., David, C.S., Lennon, V.A., 1991. Mouse T lymphocyte response to acetylcholine receptor determined by T cell receptor for antigen V beta gene products recognizing Mls-1a. J. Immunol. 147, 3303−3305.

Lang, B., Newsom-Davis, J., Prior, C., Wray, D., 1983. Antibodies to motor nerve terminals, an electrophysiological study of a human myasthenic syndrome transferred to mouse. J. Physiol. 344, 335−345.

Lecky, B.R., 2006. Transient neonatal Lambert-Eaton syndrome. J. Neurol. Neurosurg. Psychiatry. 77, 1094.

Leite, M.I., Ströbel, P., Jones, M., Micklem, K., Moritz, R., Gold, R., et al., 2005. Fewer thymic changes in MuSK antibody-positive than in MuSK antibody-negative MG. Ann. Neurol. 57, 444−448.

Leite, M.I., Jones, M., Ströbel, P., Marx, A., Gold, R., Niks, E., et al., 2007. Myasthenia gravis thymus, complement vulnerability of epithelial and myoid cells, complement attack on them, and correlations with autoantibody status. Am. J. Pathol. 171, 893−905.

Leite, M.I., Jacob, S., Viegas, S., Cossins, J., Clover, L., Morgan, B. P., et al., 2008. IgG1 antibodies to acetylcholine receptors in "seronegative" myasthenia gravis. Brain. 131, 1940−1952.

Leite, M.I., Waters, P., Vincent, A., 2010. Diagnostic use of autoantibodies in myasthenia gravis. Autoimmunity. 43, 371−379.

Lennon, V.A., Seybold, M.E., Lindstrom, J.M., Cochrane, C., Ulevitch, R., 1978. Role of complement in the pathogenesis of experimental autoimmune myasthenia gravis. J. Exp. Med. 147, 973−983.

Li, X., Xiao, B.G., Xi, J.Y., Lu, C.Z., Lu, J.H., 2008. Decrease of CD4 (+)CD25(high)Foxp3(+) regulatory T cells and elevation of CD19

(+)BAFF-R(+) B cells and soluble ICAM-1 in myasthenia gravis. Clin. Immunol. 126, 180−188.

Lindstrom, J., Einarson, B., 1979. Antigenic modulation and receptor loss in experimental autoimmune myasthenia gravis. Muscle Nerve. 2, 173−179.

Lindstrom, J.M., 2000. Acetylcholine receptors and myasthenia. Muscle Nerve. 23, 453−477.

Lindstrom, J.M., Seybold, M.E., Lennon, V.A., Whittingham, S., Duane, D.D., 1976. Antibody to acetylcholine receptor in myasthenia gravis. Prevalence, clinical correlates, and diagnostic value. Neurology. 26, 1054−1059.

Maddison, P., McConville, J., Farrugia, M.E., Davies, N., Rose, M., Norwood, F., et al., 2011. The use of rituximab in myasthenia gravis and Lambert-Eaton myasthenic syndrome. J. Neurol. Neurosurg. Psychiatry. 82, 671−673.

Maggi, L., Andreetta, F., Antozzi, C., Confalonieri, P., Cornelio, F., Scaioli, V., et al., 2008. Two cases of thymoma-associated myasthenia gravis without antibodies to the acetylcholine receptor. Neuromuscul. Disord. 18, 678−680.

Marx, A., Willcox, N., Leite, M.I., Chuang, W.Y., Schalke, B., Nix, W., et al., 2010. Thymoma and paraneoplastic myasthenia gravis. Autoimmunity. 43, 413−427.

Matthews, I., Chen, S., Hewer, R., McGrath, V., Furmaniak, J., Rees Smith, B., 2004. Muscle-specific receptor tyrosine kinase autoantibodies—a new immunoprecipitation assay. Clin. Chim. Acta. 348, 95−99.

McConville, J., Farrugia, M.E., Beeson, D., Kishore, U., Metcalfe, R., Newsom-Davis, J., et al., 2004. Detection and characterization of MuSK antibodies in seronegative myasthenia gravis. Ann. Neurol. 55, 580−584.

Meager, A., Wadhwa, M., Dilger, P., Bird, C., Thorpe, R., Newsom-Davis, J., et al., 2003. Anti-cytokine autoantibodies in autoimmunity: preponderance of neutralizing autoantibodies against interferon-alpha, interferon-omega and interleukin-12 in patients with thymoma and/or myasthenia gravis. Clin. Exp. Immunol. 132, 128−136.

Morgan, B.P., Chamberlain-Banoub, J., Neal, J.W., Song, W., Mizuno, M., Harris, C.L., 2006. The membrane attack pathway of complement drives pathology in passively induced experimental autoimmune myasthenia gravis in mice. Clin. Exp. Immunol. 146, 294−302.

Mori, S., Kubo, S., Akiyoshi, T., Yamada, S., Miyazaki, T., Hotta, H., et al., 2012. Antibodies against muscle-specific kinase impair both presynaptic and postsynaptic functions in a murine model of myasthenia gravis. Am. J. Pathol. 180, 798−810.

Motomura, M., Lang, B., Johnston, I., Palace, J., Vincent, A., Newsom-Davis, J., 1997. Incidence of serum anti-P/O-type and anti-N-type calcium channel autoantibodies in the Lambert-Eaton myasthenic syndrome. J. Neurol. Sci. 147, 35−42.

Mu, L., Sun, B., Kong, Q., Wang, J., Wang, G., Zhang, S., et al., 2009. Disequilibrium of T helper type 1, 2 and 17 cells and regulatory T cells during the development of experimental autoimmune myasthenia gravis. Immunology. 128, e826−e836.

Mygland, A., Kuwajima, G., Mikoshiba, K., Tysnes, O.B., Aarli, J. A., Gilhus, N.E., 1995. Thymomas express epitopes shared by the ryanodine receptor. J. Neuroimmunol. 62, 79−83.

Myking, A.O., Skeie, G.O., et al., 1998. The histomorphology of the thymus in late onset, non-thymoma myasthenia gravis. Eur. J. Neurol. 5, 401−405.

Nagel, A., Engel, A.G., Lang, B., Newsom-Davis, J., Fukuoka, T., 1988. Lambert-Eaton myasthenic syndrome IgG depletes presynaptic membrane active zone particles by antigenic modulation. Ann. Neurol. 24, 552–558.

Nath, A., Kerman, R.H., Novak, I.S., Wolinsky, J.S., 1990. Immune studies in human immunodeficiency virus infection with myasthenia gravis, a case report. Neurology. 40, 581–583.

Navaneetham, D., Penn, A.S., Howard Jr., J.F., Conti-Fine, B.M., 1998. TCR-Vbeta usage in the thymus and blood of myasthenia gravis patients. J. Autoimmun. 11, 621–633.

Nenninger, R., Schultz, A., Hoffacker, V., Helmreich, M., Wilisch, A., Vandekerckhove, B., et al., 1998. Abnormal thymocyte development and generation of autoreactive T cells in mixed and cortical thymomas. Lab. Invest. 78, 743–753.

Newsom-Davis, J., Vincent, A., Wilson, S.G., Ward, C.D., Pinching, A.J., Hawkey, C., 1978. Plasmapheresis for myasthenia gravis. N. Engl. J. Med. 298, 456–457.

Newsom-Davis, J., Murray, N., Wray, D., Lang, B., Prior, C., Gwilt, M., et al., 1982. Lambert-Eaton myasthenic syndrome: electrophysiological evidence for a humoral factor. Muscle Nerve. 5, S17–S20.

Niks, E.H., Kuks, J.B., Roep, B.O., Haasnoot, G.W., Verduijn, W., Ballieux, B.E., et al., 2006. Strong association of MuSK antibody-positive myasthenia gravis and HLA-DR14-DQ5. Neurology. 66, 1772–1774.

Niks, E.H., Verrips, A., Semmekrot, B.A., Prick, M.J., Vincent, A., van Tol, M.J., et al., 2008. A transient neonatal myasthenic syndrome with anti-musk antibodies. Neurology. 70, 1215–1216.

O'Neill, J.H., Murray, N.M., Newsom-Davis, J., 1988. The Lambert-Eaton myasthenic syndrome. A review of 50 cases. Brain. 111, 577–596.

Pasnoor, M., Wolfe, G.I., Nations, S., Trivedi, J., Barohn, R.J., Herbelin, L., et al., 2010. Clinical findings in MuSK-antibody positive myasthenia gravis: a U.S. experience. Muscle Nerve. 41, 370–374.

Patrick, J., Lindstrom, J., 1973. Autoimmune response to acetylcholine receptor. Science. 180, 871–872.

Pearse, G., 2006. Normal structure, function and histology of the thymus. Toxicol. Pathol. 34, 504–514.

Piddlesden, S.J., Jiang, S., Levin, J.L., Vincent, A., Morgan, B.P., 1996. Soluble complement receptor 1 (sCR1) protects against experimental autoimmune myasthenia gravis. J. Neuroimmunol. 71, 173–177.

Plomp, J.J., Van Kempen, G.T., De Baets, M.B., Graus, Y.M., Kuks, J.B., Molenaar, P.C., 1995. Acetylcholine release in myasthenia gravis: regulation at single end-plate level. Ann. Neurol. 37, 627–636.

Provenzano, C., Ricciardi, R., Scuderi, F., Maiuri, M.T., Maestri, M., La Carpia, F., et al., 2012. PTPN22 and myasthenia gravis: replication in an Italian population and meta-analysis of literature data. Neuromuscul. Disord. 22, 131–138.

Rajakulendran, S., Viegas, S., Spillane, J., Howard, R.S., 2012. Clinically biphasic myasthenia gravis with both AChR and MuSK antibodies. J. Neurol. 259, 2736–2739.

Richman, D.P., Nishi, K., Morell, S.W., Chang, J.M., Ferns, M.J., Wollmann, R.L., et al., 2012. Acute severe animal model of anti-muscle-specific kinase myasthenia: combined postsynaptic and presynaptic changes. Arch. Neurol. 69, 453–460.

Robitaille, R., Adler, E.M., Charlton, M.P., 1990. Strategic location of calcium channels at transmitter release sites of frog neuromuscular synapses. Neuron. 5, 773–779.

Rodgaard, A., Nielsen, F.C., Djurup, R., Somnier, F., Gammeltoft, S., 1987. Acetylcholine receptor antibody in myasthenia gravis: predominance of IgG subclasses 1 and 3. Clin. Exp. Immunol. 67, 82–88.

Rose, N.R., Bona, C., 1993. Defining criteria for autoimmune diseases (Witebsky's postulates revisited). Immunol. Today. 14, 426–430.

Sabater, L., Titulaer, M., Saiz, A., Verschuuren, J., Güre, A.O., Graus, F., 2008. SOX1 antibodies are markers of paraneoplastic Lambert-Eaton myasthenic syndrome. Neurology. 70, 924–928.

Safar, D., Aimé, C., Cohen-Kaminsky, S., Berrih-Aknin, S., 1991. Antibodies to thymic epithelial cells in myasthenia gravis. J. Neuroimmunol. 35, 101–110.

Sahashi, K., Engel, A.G., Linstrom, J.M., Lambert, E.H., Lennon, V.A., 1978. Ultrastructural localization of immune complexes (IgG and C3) at the end-plate in experimental autoimmune myasthenia gravis. J. Neuropathol. Exp. Neurol. 37, 212–223.

Saka, E., Topcuoglu, M.A., Akkaya, B., Galati, A., Onal, M.Z., Vincent, A., 2005. Thymus changes in anti-MuSK-positive and -negative myasthenia gravis. Neurology. 65, 782–783.

Salmon, A.M., Bruand, C., Cardona, A., Changeux, J.P., Berrih-Aknin, S., 1998. An acetylcholine receptor alpha subunit promoter confers intrathymic expression in transgenic mice. Implications for tolerance of a transgenic self-antigen and for autoreactivity in myasthenia gravis. J. Clin. Invest. 101, 2340–2350.

Sanders, D.B., Evoli, A., 2010. Immunosuppressive therapies in myasthenia gravis. Autoimmunity. 43, 428–435.

Sanders, D.B., El-Salem, K., Massey, J.M., McConville, J., Vincent, A., 2003. Clinical aspects of MuSK antibody positive seronegative MG. Neurology. 60, 1978–1980.

Saulat, B., Maertens, P., Hamilton, W.J., Bassam, B.A., 2007. Anti-musk antibody after thymectomy in a previously seropositive myasthenic child. Neurology. 69 (8), 803–804.

Scadding, G.K., Vincent, A., Newsom-Davis, J., Henry, K., 1981. Acetylcholine receptor antibody synthesis by thymic lymphocytes, correlation with thymic histology. Neurology. 31, 935–943.

Schuurman, J., Van Ree, R., Perdok, G.J., Van Doorn, H.R., Tan, K.Y., et al., 1999. Normal human immunoglobulin G4 is bispecific: it has two different antigen-combining sites. Immunology. 97, 693–698.

Scott, B.G., Yang, H., Tüzün, E., Dong, C., Flavell, R.A., Christadoss, P., 2004. ICOS is essential for the development of experimental autoimmune myasthenia gravis. J. Neuroimmunol. 153, 16–25.

Shi, F.D., He, B., Li, H., Matusevicius, D., Link, H., Ljunggren, H.G., 1998. Differential requirements for CD28 and CD40 ligand in the induction of experimental autoimmune myasthenia gravis. Eur. J. Immunol. 28, 3587–3593.

Shigemoto, K., Kubo, S., Maruyama, N., Hato, N., Yamada, H., Jie, C., et al., 2006. Induction of myasthenia by immunization against muscle-specific kinase. J. Clin. Invest. 116, 1016–1024.

Shiraishi, H., Motomura, M., Yoshimura, T., Fukudome, T., Fukuda, T., Nakao, Y., et al., 2005. Acetylcholine receptors loss and postsynaptic damage in MuSK antibody-positive myasthenia gravis. Ann. Neurol. 57, 289–293.

Simpson, J.A., 1960. Myasthenia gravis: a new hypothesis. Scot. Med. J. 5, 419–436.

Singhal, N., Martin, P.T., 2011. Role of extracellular matrix proteins and their receptors in the development of the vertebrate neuromuscular junction. Dev. Neurobiol. 71, 982–1005.

Skeie, G.O., Freiburg, A., Kolmerer, B., Labeit, S., Aarli, J.A., Appiah-Boadu, S., et al., 1997. Titin transcripts in thymomas. J. Autoimmun. 10, 551–557.

Somnier, F.E., 1994. Exacerbation of myasthenia gravis after removal of thymomas. Acta Neurol. Scand. 90, 56–66.

Strobel, P., Rosenwald, A., Beyersdorf, N., Kerkau, T., Elert, O., Murumägi, A., et al., 2004. Selective loss of regulatory T cells in thymomas. Ann. Neurol. 56, 901–904.

Takamori, M., Takahashi, M., Yasukawa, Y., Iwasa, K., Nemoto, Y., Suenaga, A., et al., 1995. Antibodies to recombinant synaptotagmin and calcium channel subtypes in Lambert-Eaton myasthenic syndrome. J. Neurol. Sci. 133, 95–101.

Takamori, M., Iwasa, K., Komai, K., 1997. Antibodies to synthetic peptides of the alpha1A subunit of the voltage-gated calcium channel in Lambert-Eaton myasthenic syndrome. Neurology. 48, 1261–1265.

Titulaer, M.J., Wirtz, P.W., Kuks, J.B., Schelhaas, H.J., van der Kooi, A. J., Faber, C.G., et al., 2008. The Lambert-Eaton myasthenic syndrome 1988–2008: a clinical picture in 97 patients. J. Neuroimmunol. 153–158, 201–202.

Titulaer, M.J., Klooster, R., Potman, M., Sabater, L., Graus, F., Hegeman, I.M., et al., 2009. SOX antibodies in small-cell lung cancer and Lambert-Eaton myasthenic syndrome: frequency and relation with survival. J. Clin. Oncol. 27, 4260–4267.

Titulaer, M.J., Lang, B., Verschuuren, J.J., 2011. Lambert-Eaton myasthenic syndrome: from clinical characteristics to therapeutic strategies. Lancet Neurol. 10, 1098–1107.

Toyka, K.V., Brachman, D.B., Pestronk, A., Kao, I., 1975. Myasthenia gravis: passive transfer from man to mouse. Science. 190, 397–399.

Tuzun, E., Scott, B.G., Goluszko, E., Higgs, S., Christadoss, P., 2003. Genetic evidence for involvement of classical complement pathway in induction of experimental autoimmune myasthenia gravis. J. Immunol. 171, 3847–3854.

Tzartos, S.J., Cung, M.T., Demange, P., Loutrari, H., Mamalaki, A., Marraud, M., et al., 1991. The main immunogenic region (MIR) of the nicotinic acetylcholine receptor and the anti-MIR antibodies. Mol. Neurobiol. 5, 1–29.

van der Zee, J.S., van Swieten, P., Aalberse, R.C., 1986. Inhibition of complement activation by IgG4 antibodies. Clin. Exp. Immunol. 64, 415–422.

Viegas, S., Jacobson, L., Waters, P., Cossins, J., Jacob, S., Leite, M.I., et al., 2012. Passive and active immunization models of MuSK-Ab positive myasthenia: electrophysiological evidence for pre and postsynaptic defects. Exp. Neurol. 234, 506–512.

Vincent, A., 2002. Unravelling the pathogenesis of myasthenia gravis. Nat. Rev. Immunol. 2, 797–804.

Vincent, A., Leite, M.I., 2005. Neuromuscular junction autoimmune disease: muscle specific kinase antibodies and treatments for myasthenia gravis. Curr. Opin. Neurol. 18, 519–525.

Vincent, A., Scadding, G.K., Thomas, H.C., Newsom-Davis, J., 1978. In-vitro synthesis of anti-acetylcholine-receptor antibody by thymic lymphocytes in myasthenia gravis. Lancet. 1, 305–307.

Vincent, A., Newsom-Davis, J., Newton, P., Beck, N., 1983. Acetylcholine receptor antibody and clinical response to thymectomy in myasthenia gravis. Neurology. 33, 1276–1282.

Vincent, A., Whiting, P.J., Schluep, M., Heidenreich, F., Lang, B., Roberts, A., et al., 1987. Antibody heterogeneity and specificity in myasthenia gravis. Ann. N. Y. Acad. Sci. 505, 106–120.

Vincent, A., Palace, J., Hilton-Jones, D., 2001. Myasthenia gravis. Lancet. 357, 2122–2128.

Vincent, A., Clover, L., Buckley, C., Grimley Evans, J., Rothwell, P.M., UK Myasthenia Gravis Survey, 2003. Evidence of underdiagnosis of myasthenia gravis in older people. J. Neurol. Neurosurg. Psychiatry. 74, 1105–1108.

Vincent, A., Leite, M.I., Farrugia, M.E., Jacob, S., Viegas, S., Shiraishi, H., et al., 2008. Myasthenia gravis seronegative for acetylcholine receptor antibodies. Ann. N. Y. Acad. Sci. 1132, 84–92.

Walker, M.B., 1934. Treatment of myasthenia gravis with physostigmine. Lancet. 1, 1200–1201.

Wang, W., Milani, M., Ostlie, N., Okita, D., Agarwal, R.K., Caspi, R.R., et al., 2007. C57BL/6 mice genetically deficient in IL-12/IL-23 and IFN-gamma are susceptible to experimental autoimmune myasthenia gravis, suggesting a pathogenic role of non-Th1 cells. J. Immunol. 178, 7072–7080.

Wang, X.B., Pirskanen, R., Giscombe, R., Lefvert, A.K., 2008. Two SNPs in the promoter region of the CTLA-4 gene affect binding of transcription factors and are associated with human myasthenia gravis. J. Intern. Med. 263, 61–69.

Wang, Z.Y., Okita, D.K., Howard Jr., J.F., Conti-Fine, B.M., 1998. CD4 + epitope spreading and differential T cell recognition of muscle acetylcholine receptor subunits in myasthenia gravis. Ann. N. Y. Acad. Sci. 841, 334–337.

Wang, Z.Y., Karachunski, P.I., Howard Jr., J.F., Conti-Fine, B.M., 1999. Myasthenia in SCID mice grafted with myasthenic patient lymphocytes: role of CD4 + and CD8 + cells. Neurology. 52, 484–497.

Whiting, P.J., Vincent, A., Newsom-Davis, J., 1986. Myasthenia gravis: monoclonal antihuman acetylcholine receptor antibodies used to analyze antibody specificities and responses to treatment. Neurology. 36, 612–617.

Willcox, N., Leite, M.I., Kadota, Y., Jones, M., Meager, A., Subrahmanyam, P., et al., 2008. Autoimmunizing mechanisms in thymoma and thymus. Ann. N. Y. Acad. Sci. 1132, 163–173.

Wirtz, P.W., Nijnuis, M.G., Sotodeh, M., Willems, L.N., Brahim, J.J., Putter, H., et al., 2003. The epidemiology of myasthenia gravis, Lambert-Eaton myasthenic syndrome and their associated tumors in the northern part of the province of South Holland. J. Neurol. 250, 698–701.

Wood, S.J., Slater, C.R., 2001. Safety factor at the neuromuscular junction. Prog. Neurobiol. 64, 393–429.

Zivkovic, S.A., Clemens, P.R., Lacomis, D., 2012. Characteristics of late-onset myasthenia gravis. J. Neurol. 259, 2167–2171.

Chapter 55

Ocular Disease

Monica D. Dalal, H. Nida Sen, and Robert B. Nussenblatt

The Laboratory of Immunology, National Eye Institute, National Institutes of Health, Bethesda, MD, USA

Chapter Outline

Historical Background	793	Pathogenic Mechanisms	798
Clinical Features	793	Ocular Immune Responses	799
Pathologic Features	795	Tissue Destruction	799
Epidemiologic Features	795	Immunologic Markers	799
Autoimmune Features	796	Treatment and Outcomes	800
Hormonal Influences	797	Concluding Remarks and Future Prospects	801
Genetic Factors	797	References	801
Animal Models	798		

HISTORICAL BACKGROUND

The concept that the eye harbors autoimmune-inducing or uveitogenic materials has been suggested by many since the beginning of the last century. It was the demonstration by Uhlenhuth (1903) of autoantibody production to the lens that pioneered investigation in this area. Several investigators used homogenates from the eye, which appeared to be capable of inducing an intraocular inflammatory response when injected into an animal eye. Noteworthy of mention are Wacker and Lipton (1968) and Faure 1980.

The presence of uveitogenic antigens in the human eye that are capable of inducing disease is a well-established concept, proposed as early as 1910 by Elschnig (Elschnig, 1910). Since then several antigens have been isolated that are capable of inducing ocular inflammatory disease similar to that seen in humans. Retinal S-antigen, or arrestin, was isolated and its immunologic properties partially characterized by Wacker et al. (1977). It is one of the most potent uveitogenic antigens defined to date. It causes an immune-mediated, bilateral inflammatory response in the eye, or experimental autoimmune uveitis (EAU), when injected in microgram quantities at a site far from the globe (Pfister et al., 1985). S-antigen and its clinical relevance in uveitis were widely studied in the 1980s by many investigators (Nussenblatt et al., 1980a,b, 1983; Graham et al., 1981; Gregerson et al., 1981, 1983; Forrester and Borthwick, 1983). Several other uveitogenic antigens have since been identified, such as interphotoreceptor retinoid-binding protein (IRBP) (Hirose et al., 1986); recoverin (Gery et al., 1994); bovine melanin protein (Chan et al., 1994); rhodopsin (Schalken et al., 1989); phosducin (Lee et al., 1990); RPE 65 (Ham et al., 2002), and tyrosinase proteins (Yamaki et al., 2000).

These studies have broadened our understanding of the ocular immune response and allowed templates to be developed with which newer approaches to immunosuppression can be tested.

CLINICAL FEATURES

The uveal tract can be divided anatomically into the iris, ciliary body, and choroid (Figure 55.1). Uveitis is usually defined as any inflammation of the uveal tract. This inflammation may be an antigen-specific, immune-mediated response, or a nonspecific response, which can be elicited by infection, trauma, or surgery. In clinical practice, any inflammatory reaction involving the structures of the eye (see Figure 55.1) is considered to be uveitis.

Episcleritis is an inflammatory disease involving the tissue that lies superficial to the sclera. Scleritis is a

N. Rose & I. Mackay (Eds): The Autoimmune Diseases, Fifth edition. DOI: http://dx.doi.org/10.1016/B978-0-12-384929-8.00055-1

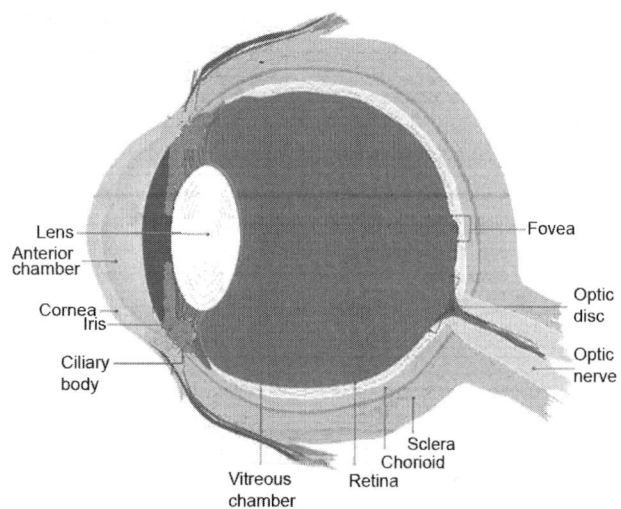

FIGURE 55.1   Key anatomic features of the eye.

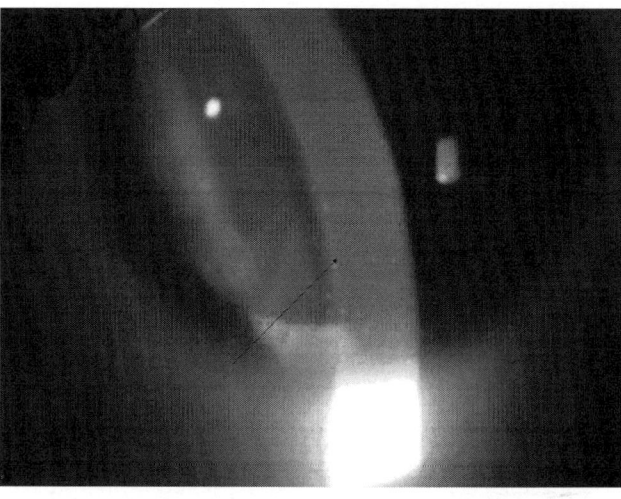

FIGURE 55.3   Slit-lamp photograph of a patient with anterior uveitis with keratic precipitates. Arrow points to corneal endothelium with keratic precipitates.

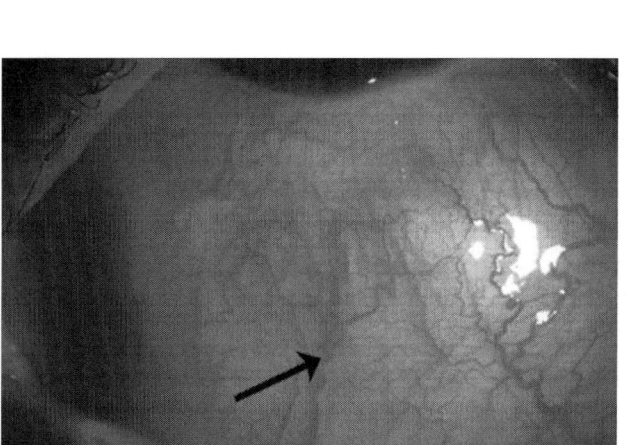

FIGURE 55.2   Slit-lamp photograph of a patient with scleritis of presumed autoimmune etiology, having ruled out infectious etiologies. Arrow indicates dilated episcleral and scleral vessels.

painful and potentially sight-threatening inflammatory disease involving the sclera. Episcleritis is typically more acute and less severe than scleritis and it is often idiopathic; however, many of the diseases associated with scleritis have also been associated with episcleritis. Clinical examination evaluates for the presence of erythema and edema of the episclera or sclera as well as injection of the deep episcleral vessels (Figure 55.2). The inflamed sclera is usually characterized by a violaceous hue which can be graded in a standardized fashion (Sen et al., 2011). Many inflammatory systemic disorders are associated with scleritis, the most common being rheumatoid arthritis. Others include juvenile idiopathic arthritis (JIA), Reiter syndrome, Crohn's disease, ankylosing

spondylitis, ulcerative colitis, polymyositis, polyarteritis nodosa, systemic lupus erythematosus (SLE), Wegener's granulomatosis, sarcoidosis, Lyme disease, and Cogan syndrome. In up to 40% of cases no associated disease can be identified (Sainz de la Maza et al., 2012).

According to standardization of uveitis nomenclature (SUN) working group criteria (Jabs et al., 2005), uveitis can be classified based on anatomic location: anterior, intermediate, posterior, and panuveitis. *Anterior uveitis* describes a disease predominantly limited to the anterior segment. In the literature it is also called iritis, iridocyclitis, and anterior cyclitis. There are many inflammatory systemic diseases associated with anterior uveitis, including juvenile idiopathic arthritis, HLA-B27-associated diseases, Behcet's disease, and sarcoidosis. The corneal examination may reveal keratic precipitates (Figure 55.3), small aggregates of inflammatory cells which can be granulomatous or non-granulomatous in nature, which accumulate on the endothelial surface of the cornea. Examination of the anterior chamber via biomicroscopy will reveal the presence of inflammatory cells and increased protein (flare), resulting from spillover of inflammation from the iris and the ciliary body, graded in a standardized fashion (Nussenblatt and Whitcup, 2004; Jabs et al., 2005). An accumulation of leukocytes associated with fibrin, layered in the lower angle of the anterior chamber, is called a hypopyon (Figure 55.4), and is commonly associated with Behcet's disease and the HLA-B27-associated uveitides. Inflammation of the iris may cause synechiae (adhesions) between the iris and the lens capsule (Figure 55.5) or the cornea. It may also develop accumulations of inflammatory cells called nodules on the papillary margin, referred to as Koeppe nodules, or on

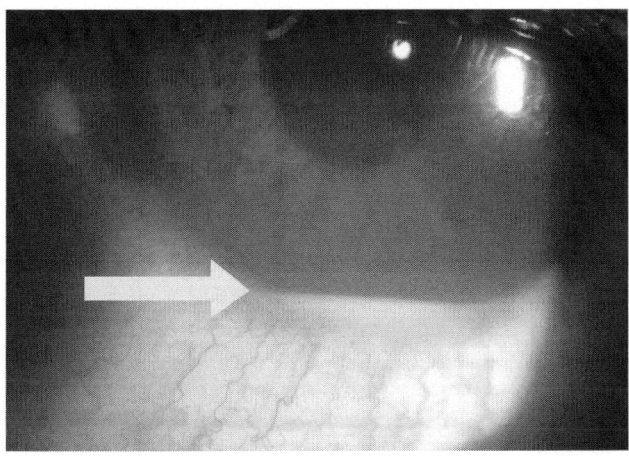

FIGURE 55.4   Slit-lamp photograph of a patient with ocular Behcet's disease and anterior uveitis, with a hypopyon. Arrow points to layer of inflammatory cells in the anterior chamber, the hypopyon.

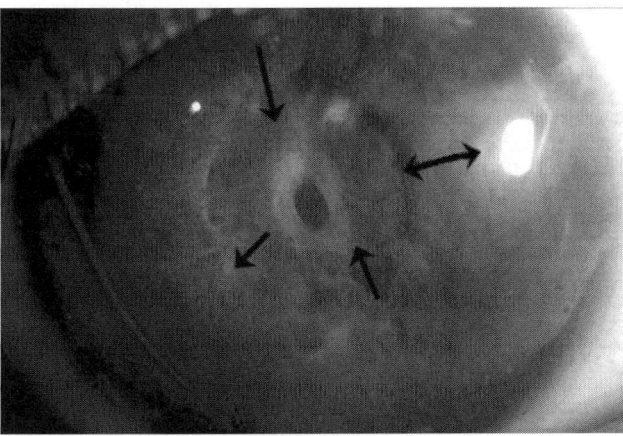

FIGURE 55.5   Slit-lamp photograph of a patient with anterior uveitis, extensive posterior synechiae, and iris adhesions to the anterior lens capsule. Arrows show the areas of adhesions.

the iris surface, known as Busacca nodules, commonly seen with sarcoidosis and other granulomatous diseases.

Intermediate uveitis refers to uveitis where the vitreous is the major site of inflammation. Inflammation in the vitreous is characterized by increased cells and protein, vitreous haze (Nussenblatt et al., 1985; Jabs et al., 2005) or pars plana exudates. Retinal inflammation may cause cystoid macular edema and retinal vasculitis. There are specific systemic autoimmune diseases associated with this type of uveitis: multiple sclerosis, sarcoidosis, and Lyme disease. A common form of intermediate uveitis is referred to as pars planitis, which is by definition idiopathic. Syphilis and tuberculosis are common infectious etiologies of intermediate uveitis.

Posterior uveitis refers to inflammation affecting the posterior segment, particularly the retina and the choroid.

There are numerous autoimmune diseases that are associated with posterior uveitis: Behcet's disease, systemic lupus erythematosus, polyarteritis nodosa, Wegener's granulomatosis, sarcoidosis, syphilis, and Vogt–Koyanagi–Harada syndrome. There are also many infectious etiologies: ocular histoplasmosis, cytomegalovirus retinitis, acute retinal necrosis (varicella zoster virus, herpes simplex virus), toxoplasmosis, and immune-mediated local ocular disorders: sympathetic ophthalmia, birdshot retinochoroidopathy, and the "white-dot syndromes," which can cause posterior uveitis. In addition, primary intraocular lymphoma can masquerade as an intermediate or posterior uveitis.

Finally, *panuveitis* is a term reserved for inflammation involving all segments of the eye and in which there is no predominant site of inflammation (Nussenblatt and Whitcup, 2004; Jabs et al., 2005). Typical systemic diseases associated with this form of uveitis are Behcet's disease, sarcoidosis, VKH syndrome, and syphilis.

PATHOLOGIC FEATURES

Uveitis can be classified as granulomatous or nongranulomatous. This is a clinical definition, based on the type of inflammatory cells infiltrating the ocular tissues, as seen by biomicroscopy. It is not based on histopathologic analysis. Biomicroscopy will reveal inflammatory precipitates throughout the eye. The most common type of corneal (keratic) precipitates is nongranulomatous, characterized by fine, white-colored lymphocytes, plasma cells, and pigment. Many etiologic factors may be responsible for this type of inflammation. Granulomatous inflammation forms large, greasy-appearing collections of lymphocytes, plasma cells, and giant cells, also called "mutton-fat" keratic precipitates. It can also cause iris nodules, vitreous inflammatory cells, called "snowballs," and retinal vascular inflammation, called "candle wax drippings." This clinical classification is an important diagnostic clue, because the etiologic agents associated with granulomatous uveitis form a fairly short list, including sarcoidosis, Vogt–Koyanagi–Harada syndrome, syphilis, tuberculosis, and toxoplasmosis.

EPIDEMIOLOGIC FEATURES

According to a study by Gritz and Wong (2004), the incidence of uveitis was 52/100,000 person-years and the period prevalence was 115/100,000 persons. It has been found that women have a higher prevalence than men, and the highest incidence and prevalence of disease are in those 65 years and older (Gritz and Wong, 2004), although the age group with the highest prevalence is still under debate. Rodriguez et al. (1996) analyzed their university/referral-based population and found 83% of cases were non-infectious in etiology. There are many demographic features that offer important clues when evaluating a patient with uveitis such as age, sex, race, ethnic heritage, and geographic residence. Specific examples include juvenile idiopathic arthritis associated with chronic anterior uveitis seen in children under age 16. One half of the JIA patients in one study reportedly had chronic uveitis by the age of 6 (Key and Kimura, 1975). It is mostly seen in young females with pauciarticular arthritis and a positive antinuclear antibody (ANA) test (Cassidy et al., 1986). The uveitis associated with ankylosing spondylitis is typically a recurrent anterior uveitis seen in young men between the ages of 20 and 30 years (Brewerton et al., 1973). Sarcoidosis affects young adults aged 20–50 years and has a slightly increased prevalence in women. It can affect all races, but African Americans are 10 times more likely to be affected compared to white persons, and with chronic sarcoidosis they are more likely to develop ocular manifestations than are white persons (Jabs and Johns, 1986). Vogt–Koyanagi–Harada syndrome is a multisystem disorder, with ocular, central nervous system, cutaneous, and vestibular-auditory manifestations; the ocular manifestation is usually a severe, bilateral, granulomatous panuveitis. It is common in Japan and certain parts of Latin America (Sugiura, 1988). We have also noted a fairly high Native American ancestry among our patients. Finally, Behcet's disease is a multisystem disorder with ocular involvement; it is especially common in the Far East and the Mediterranean basin (Ohno and Matsuda, 1986). The ocular disease may be an anterior and/or posterior uveitis, associated with retinal vasculitis (Figure 55.6).

AUTOIMMUNE FEATURES

Immunity in the eye is deviant and atypical. The eye's ability to regulate local immune responses has been attributed to several factors. First, there are several immunosuppressive substances in the aqueous humor of the eye, such as α-melanocyte-stimulating hormone (α-MSH), vasoactive intestinal peptide (VIP), transforming-growth factor-beta (TGF-β), and macrophage-migration-inhibitory factor (MIF), which act to modulate ocular immune responses. Second, there are bone marrow-derived cells in the vascularized tissues of the eye that may capture antigens and present them to immune cells. Third, surface markers, such as CD95 ligand (Griffith et al., 1996; Ferguson and Griffith, 1997), CD46 (Bora et al., 1993), and CD59 are expressed in ocular parenchymal tissues; they directly inhibit effector T cell components of complement, thus saving the eye from tissue damage. Also, inside the eye, both the retina and anterior chamber have a well-structured vascular network with blood-ocular barriers that protect the eye from intruding macromolecules.

The ability to discriminate between self and non-self is used for elimination of autoreactive cells. Because the eye is considered to be an immunologically privileged organ, it is believed that expression of ocular autoantigens occurs exclusively within the intraocular environment (Gery and Streilein, 1994). A classic example of organ-specific autoimmune disease caused by autoantigens is sympathetic ophthalmia, a rare form of intraocular inflammation in which the fellow eye develops inflammation after penetrating injury of the opposite eye. The inflammation may develop as early as several days after

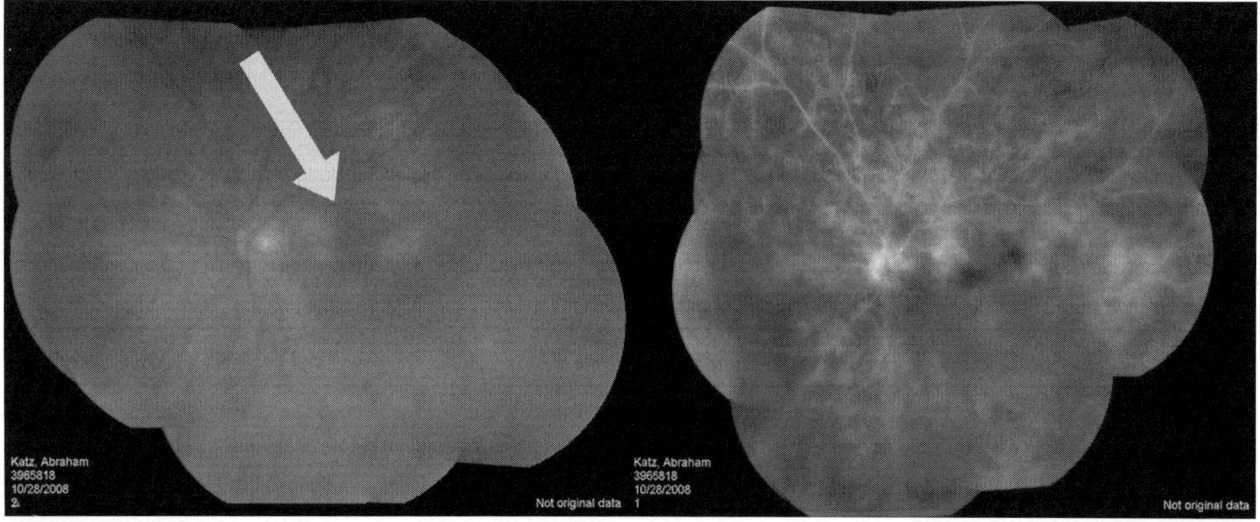

FIGURE 55.6 Fundus photograph with corresponding fluorescein angiogram of a patient with Behcet's disease and retinal vasculitis. Arrow points to areas of macular retinitis.

the penetrating insult to decades later. Typically, it occurs in the first several weeks (4–12 weeks). It is speculated that the injury causes primary immunization to self-antigens. Although the target antigen is still unknown, an experimental animal model has been developed. In this model cutaneous immunization of animals with retinal antigens (arrestin, rhodopsin, interphotoreceptor retinoid-binding protein), retinal pigment epithelial-associated antigens, and melanocyte-associated tyrosinase results in an autoimmune uveitis, with features characteristic of sympathetic ophthalmia (Rao, 1997). Substantial evidence exists that autoimmune diseases may also be initiated or aggravated by infection. This happens presumably when nonspecific polyclonal activation of the immune system, either by virus or immunostimulatory agents such as Gram-negative bacterial cell wall components, overwhelms the normal regulatory mechanisms and permits "forbidden clones" of cells to proliferate and cause tissue damage. The molecular mimicry theory states that structural similarity between invading organisms and organ tissue components may lead to persistence of the inflammatory response even after the inciting agent has been quickly cleared. This has been postulated as a mechanism for uveitis. The primary amino acid sequence of hepatitis B virus DNA polymerase shows sequence homology to the retinal S-antigen. An experimental autoimmune uveitis was induced in Lewis rats using synthetic peptides (Singh et al., 1990). Lymph nodes cells from rats immunized with this synthetic peptide or peptide M in S-antigen showed a significant degree of cross-reaction. As a clinical corollary, some types of idiopathic posterior uveitis have been reported in association with hepatitis B virus vaccine (Brezin et al., 1995; Baglivo et al., 1996). However, no definitive etiologic link has been made via histopathology or immunohistochemistry.

HORMONAL INFLUENCES

Hormones play a significant role in immunomodulation, yet the exact mechanism is not understood. Certain hormones of pregnancy, such as progesterone, α-fetoprotein, α2 pregnancy-associated globulin, and early pregnancy factor are thought to have immunomodulating properties (Anon, 1976; Chakraborty and Mandal, 1993; Harness et al., 2003). Other hormones, the levels of which increase during pregnancy, such as corticotrophin-releasing hormone, α-melanocyte stimulating hormone, estrogens, or altered estrogen/androgen ratios, are thought to be immunosuppressive (Lipton and Catania, 1997; Ilias and Mastorakos, 2003). We and other researches have reported that flares of uveitis decrease during pregnancy compared to the nonpregnant state (Rabiah and Vitale, 2003). Many women with chronic recurrent noninfectious uveitis report an association between flares and point in

the menstrual cycle. Further studies are needed to more definitively delineate hormonal influences on uveitis.

GENETIC FACTORS

Genetic factors play a significant role in the development of endogenous uveitis. The ability to respond to a specific immune stimulant is genetically determined. Genes for human leukocyte antigens (HLA) are clustered in major histocompatibility complex (MHC) proteins, located on the short arm of chromosome 6. They have been linked to various uveitic syndromes (Table 55.1).

Brewerton et al. (1973) were among the first to observe that a high percentage of white patients with ankylosing spondylitis showed HLA-B27 positivity. Khan et al. (1977) demonstrated that HLA-B7 was associated with ankylosing spondylitis in African Americans to a greater degree than HLA-B27. It is clear that HLA associations may be different for various ethnic groups. It is possible that different genes initiate responses that finally lead to a common pathway resulting in a particular disease. The reasons for association between HLA and diseases are unclear. It has been hypothesized that exogenous environmental factors may play a role in expression of a disease. For example, it has been suggested that Ia antigens are required for antigen presentation and initiation of the immune response; if Ia expression is inappropriate and other defects of immunosurveillance occur, it may result in a disease (Bottazzo et al., 1983).

Most researchers agree that mechanisms of the autoimmune disease of the eye are multifactorial, so several factors must be present to cause the disease, otherwise disease expression would be far more common. MHC plays an important role in determining disease susceptibility. Family studies in patients with uveitis show that susceptibility to particular types of idiopathic uveitis is possibly due to genetic background (Kimura and Hogan, 1963; Hogan et al., 1965; Giles and Tranton, 1980; Augsburger et al., 1981; Culbertson et al., 1983; Doft, 1983; Wetzig et al., 1988; Duinkerke-Eorela et al., 1990; Tejada et al., 1994; Lee, 1995). Genetic predisposition may determine the severity of the disease. A permissive MHC in a nonpermissive background will result in a mild disease or no disease at all (Caspi et al., 1992).

Single-nucleotide polymorphisms (SNPs) are genetic variations found normally in genes that mediate the immune response as opposed to those that control it. For example, one cytokine may have several SNP variations. Some SNPs may change the functioning of the protein. Population studies of disease groups versus controls are able to identify SNPs more commonly seen in disease groups and thus are associated with these particular autoimmune or neoplastic diseases (Shastry, 2002). A report of 102 patients with ocular Behcet's disease, who were

TABLE 55.1 Association of Selected Ocular Disease with Human Leukocyte Antigens

Human Leukocyte Antigen	Ocular Disease
HLA-A11	Sympathetic ophthalmia
HLA-A24	Tubulointerstitial nephritis–uveitis syndrome
HLA-A29	Birdshot retinochoroidopathy
HLA-B5	Adamantiades–Behcet's disease
HLA-B7	Presumed ocular histoplasmosis
	Serpiginous retinochoroidopathy
	Acute posterior multifocal placoid epitheliopathy
	Ankylosing spondylitis
HLA-B8	Acute anterior uveitis
HLA-B12	Ocular cicatricial pemphigoid
HLA-B27	Acute anterior uveitis
	Reiter syndrome
HLA-B51	Adamantiades–Behcet's disease
HLA-DQw3	Vogt–Koyanagi–Harada (VKH) syndrome
HLA-DR2	Presumed ocular histoplasmosis
HLA-DR4	Rheumatoid arthritis
	Vogt–Koyanagi–Harada (VKH) syndrome
	Relapsing polychondritis
HLA-DR6	Tubulointerstitial nephritis–uveitis syndrome
HLA-DR15	Intermediate uveitis
	Multiple sclerosis
HLA-DRB1	Sarcoidosis
HLA-DRB1*0405	Sympathetic ophthalmia
HLA-DRw53	Vogt–Koyanagi–Harada (VKH) syndrome

tested for a possible link between a specific tumor necrosis factor (TNF) SNP and the disease, found no TNF gene polymorphisms to be associated with the disease (Verity et al., 1999).

ANIMAL MODELS

Several species of mammals have been used to establish experimental autoimmune uveitis (EAU) models, including guinea pigs (Collins, 1949; Kalsow and Wacker, 1973), rabbits (Wacker and Lipton, 1968), rats (Faure 1980; de Kozak et al., 1981; Gery and Nussenblatt, 1986), mice (Caspi et al., 1988), and primates (Nussenblatt et al., 1981). Currently, mice and rats are probably the two most commonly used animals for EAU studies due to the availability of inbred and other genetically-modified strains, such as gene knockout or transgenic animals. Typically, uveitogenic antigens such as S-antigen, interphotoreceptor retinoid-binding protein (IRBP), retinal pigment epithelium-specific 65 kDa protein (RPE65), or crude extract of retina/uvea are emulsified with complete Freund's adjuvant (CFA) and injected subcutaneously into the animals ("active immunization"). Coinjection of pertussis toxin intravenously or intraperitoneally has been routinely administered to achieve maximum EAU score. EAU can also be induced by adoptively transferring primary T cells from diseased animals with active EAU or uveitogenic cell lines to syngeneic normal recipients. EAU induced by adoptive transfer typically has a shortened clinical course because of the lack of an induction phase compared to the active immunization protocol.

It is noteworthy that despite the fact that both rat and mouse EAU models have been extensively used for studying molecular mechanisms of uveitis, the clinical manifestations of the two models differ. Murine EAU seems to be less acute than rat EAU, with a later onset and longer duration. In addition, pathologic changes in murine EAU primarily involve the posterior segment with little anterior segment involvement, while rat EAU usually manifests inflammation in both anterior and posterior segments (Gery and Nussenblatt, 1986; Caspi et al., 1988). Although it was shown that passive transfer of immune serum from humans induced ocular retinitis in guinea pigs (de Kozak et al., 1976) and there is evidence of involvement of humoral immunity in EAU (Faure 1980; Gery and Nussenblatt, 1986), humoral immune response-mediated uveitis animal models have not been widely reported or used.

PATHOGENIC MECHANISMS

The establishment of extensive studies using EAU models has greatly facilitated the understanding of autoimmune uveitis. Despite some evidence of the involvement of humoral immunity (Faure 1980; Gery and Nussenblatt, 1986), cellular immunity is primarily responsible for the disease (Nussenblatt et al., 1980a,b; Gery and Nussenblatt, 1986; Caspi et al., 1986; Nussenblatt, 1987). The majority of data support the notion that helper T cells (Th) are the key players in the molecular pathogenesis of EAU models (Caspi, 1999). While the Th1 subset has been shown to play the predominant role, accumulated data also point to a role of the Th2 subset (Caspi, 2002; Kim et al., 2002). In addition, the pertussis toxin, an adjuvant routinely administered to maximize induction of

EAU, has been shown to block the induction of EAU by adoptive transfer (Su et al., 2001) underscoring a delicate balance of the immune system in this disease setting. Although limited, some data have also suggested an important role of immunosuppressive T regulatory (Tregs) and/or cytokines in EAU. Tregs were shown to be reduced in patients with active disease compared with inactive disease (Yeh et al., 2009). Coadministration of interleukin (IL)-2 could potentiate induction of oral tolerance by IRBP, accompanied by increased levels of IL-10, IL-4, and TGF-β (Rizzo et al., 1994). Induced tolerance to S-antigen after intratesticular injection of S-antigen into the Lewis rat was shown to be associated with the induction of regulatory T cells capable of secreting immunosuppressive cytokines such as IL-4, IL-10, and TGF-β (Yotsukura et al., 1997). An immunosuppressive neuropeptide believed to be associated with immune privilege of the eye, α-melanocyte-stimulating hormone, was shown to induce CD4$^+$CD25$^+$ Tregs.

Besides T cells, other immune cells have also been investigated for their roles in the pathogenesis of EAU. For example, dendritic cells and macrophages have been shown to be important in EAU induction and tissue destruction (Jiang et al., 1999). In addition, natural killer (NK) cells and natural killer T (NKT) cells have also been implied in the pathogenesis of EAU. One report suggested that NK cells might play a detrimental role in EAU (Kitaichi et al., 2002), while another study showed increased NK and NKT cells in association with interferon (IFN)-β amelioration of EAU (Suzuki et al., 2002). Nonetheless, the data point to potential roles for other cellular components of the immune system that could be critical in the pathogenesis of EAU.

Ocular Immune Responses

The ocular immune system is thought to have an innate set of mechanisms for "effector blockade" that protects the ocular tissue from the destructive effects of the secondary effector phase of the immune response arc. This blockade in the anterior chamber is known as anterior chamber-associated immune deviation (ACAID), where immunization by an anterior chamber injection in experimental animals results in an altered form of systemic immunity to that antigen (Streilein, 1993, 1997; Streilein-Stein and Streilein, 2002). The eye also has soluble and membrane-bound inhibitors, such as CD178 (FasL), which can induce apoptosis (Green and Ferguson, 2001). Additionally, the eye appears to have an immunosuppressive microenvironment of chemokines and cytokines (Granstein et al., 1990; Foxman et al., 2002). Finally, it is believed that a state of tolerance can be induced in the eye (Ferguson and Griffiths, 1997; Ferguson et al., 2002).

Tissue Destruction

During ocular inflammatory processes, there is an influx of T cells, B cells, macrophages, and polymorphonuclear leukocytes (PMNs) into the choroid, choriocapillaris, and retina. There is also local synthesis of cytokines by ocular tissue. These changes in the ocular milieu most likely contribute to the ocular tissue damage seen clinically and experimentally. The underlying pathogenesis depends on the disease process involved and thus will vary. Immunohistopathology in ocular sarcoidosis shows a predominance of lymphocytes and macrophages (Chan et al., 1987), while ocular Behcet's disease revealed predominantly lymphocytic infiltration, with some B cells and plasma cells (George et al., 1997). These reports indicate that cell-mediated immunity may play a pivotal role, while others have reported humoral-mediated immunity and also the involvement of immune complex formation (Reinsh and Moyer, 1991).

Macrophages are reported to be important effector cells for retinal tissue destruction in the animal model (Forrester et al., 1998). However, the macrophage-mediated retinal tissue destruction is probably under the control of antigen-specific T cells and the cytokines that T cells release (Jiang et al., 1999). TNF-α is a well-known cytokine capable of tissue destruction either by direct tissue damage or by induction of apoptosis (Selmaj et al., 1991; Zheng et al., 1995), but other factors such as free radicals, e.g., nitric oxide, could also contribute to inflammation-induced retinal damage (Hoey et al., 1997).

IMMUNOLOGIC MARKERS

Recent advances have demonstrated that cytokines are equally important in the pathogenesis of noninfectious uveitis. The Th1 types of cytokines, such as IFN-γ, IL-2, TNF-α, and IL-12, are considered to be the primary factors in the pathogenesis of uveitis. In humans, IFN-γ and IL-2 were found to be elevated in ocular tissues with concomitant infiltrating T cells in uveitic patients (Hooks et al., 1988). IL-6 has been shown to be elevated in the aqueous humor of patients with noninfectious uveitis (Murray et al., 1990; Franks et al., 1992). Higher levels of TNF-α and IL-1 have also been demonstrated in both peripheral sera and aqueous humor samples (Palexas et al., 1992; Sakaguchi et al., 1998). Cytokine profile analysis of peripheral T cells from uveitic patients suggested that the intracellular level of IFN-γ was increased (Frassanito et al., 2003), but similar analysis of T cells derived from aqueous humor samples showed decreased IFN-γ compared to those from peripheral blood (Hill et al., 2005). Recent interest has surrounded the role of Th17/IL-17, which is believed to play a role in chronic inflammation whereas Th1 drives the early pathogenic response (Hoyer et al., 2009).

Data derived from animal EAU studies, however, have provided more consistent insights into the molecular mechanisms of autoimmune uveitis. TNF-α was shown to be detrimental to the development of EAU (Nakamura et al., 1994; Dick et al., 1996; Robertson et al., 2003), while IL-10 and IL-12 were suggested to be protective to the development of EAU (Rizzo et al., 1998; Tarrant et al., 1999). Consistent with findings in humans, IFN-γ was also found in the ocular tissues of EAU animals, and correlated with the disease course (Charteris and Lightman, 1992). However, treatment with anti-IFN-γ antibody exacerbated EAU, while treatment with rIFN-γ ameliorated the diseases in a murine EAU model (Caspi et al., 1994), leading investigators to conclude that endogenous IFN-γ was protective for EAU. The same investigators also showed that IFN-γ gene deficient mice developed EAU similar to their wild-type littermates, suggesting that IFN-γ is not necessary for the development of EAU (Jones et al., 1997). To further complicate the issue, an independent study using IFN-γ transgenic rats showed that overexpression of IFN-γ resulted in more severe EAU (Egwuagu et al., 1999). These studies underscore the complexity of cytokine networks in the pathogenesis of EAU.

TREATMENT AND OUTCOMES

Corticosteroids have been the mainstay of therapy for ocular inflammatory disease since the early 1950s. Both systemic (oral, intravenous) and local (topical, periocular, intravitreal) formulations are available. In addition, steroid implants (fluocinolone acetonide (Retisert™) and dexamethasone (Ozurdex™)) have recently become popular choices as both adjuvant and monotherapy. They offer the benefit of sustained corticosteroid delivery to the eye while avoiding systemic complications (Larson et al., 2011).

Some diseases are steroid resistant and for others long-term steroid therapy carries the risk of developing unacceptable systemic side effects. For these patients other immunomodulatory agents need to be added as a steroid-sparing agent. Steroid-sparing agents include alkylating agents (cyclophosphamide, chlorambucil), antimetabolites (azathioprine, methotrexate, mycophenolate mofetil), cyclosporine, tacrolimus, rapamycin, antibodies, and monoclonal antibodies (daclizumab, etanercept, infliximab, adalimumab, rituximab).

Antibodies and monoclonal antibodies directed against various parts of the immune cascade represent the new era of immunomodulation through the ability to interfere with specific molecules or pathways based on our understanding of the inflammatory process (Heiligenhaus et al.,

2010; Larson et al., 2011). Daclizumab is a humanized anti-Tac monoclonal recombinant antibody. Tac is a subunit of the IL-2 receptor (IL-2R) high-affinity complex. Caspi et al. (1986) demonstrated the presence of high-affinity IL-2Rs in animal models of uveitis. It was used safely and effectively in the treatment of intermediate and posterior uveitis in adults and children, as well as active JIA-associated anterior uveitis (Yeh et al., 2008; Sen et al., 2009). However, it was pulled from the market in 2009 due to insufficient market demand (Smith et al., 2012).

TNF-α is found during the acute phase of experimental autoimmune uveoretinitis (Kim et al., 2001). Etanercept is a TNF fusion protein that binds to and inactivates TNF, while infliximab is a chimeric monoclonal antibody directed against TNF-α, and adalimumab is fully humanized monoclonal IgG1 antibody against TNF-α. Entanercept was found to be effective in some systemic diseases; however, a review of multiple case series showed new onset of uveitis in previously unaffected rheumatologic patients (Smith et al., 2012). As a result, etanercept is not used in uveitis. Infliximab has been demonstrated to be effective in several clinical studies in reducing ocular inflammation. Suhler et al. (2009) reported successful control of inflammation within 10 weeks of initiating treatment in approximately 75% of patients with refractory uveitides including idiopathic, sarcoidosis, Behcet's disease-associated uveitis, and birdshot retinochoroidopathy. Adalimumab has also been effective for the treatment of several autoimmune diseases including rheumatoid arthritis, ankylosing spondylitis, psoriatic arthritis, juvenile idiopathic arthritis, and Crohn's disease (Smith et al., 2012). Rituximab is a chimeric anti-CD20 monoclonal antibody which targets CD20, a surface antigen expressed on pre-B and mature B cells. It has demonstrated success in rheumatoid arthritis, systemic lupus erythematosus, and Wegener's-associated scleritis (Smith et al., 2012).

In our treatment approach cytotoxic agents are often used last, after corticosteroids, cyclosporine, and monoclonal antibodies, for sight-threatening intraocular inflammation. Other less widely used therapeutic modalities include intravenous immunoglobulin therapy, oral tolerance plasmapheresis, and IFN-α. In addition, nonsteroidal anti-inflammatory agents have been used for specific diseases; however, they have not been shown to be effective as a sole agent in the treatment of noninfectious uveitis.

In general, the following therapeutic guidelines can be used:

- Topical corticosteroids for anterior segment disease.
- Periocular corticosteroids for unilateral disease, the presence of intermediate or posterior complications, and in select childhood uveitis to avoid systemic complications of corticosteroids.

- Systemic immunosuppressive agents for bilateral, sight-threatening intermediate uveitis, posterior uveitis, or panuveitis. Biological immunomodulatory therapy for those who fail (or are intolerant of) standard immunosuppressive therapy.
- Consideration of corticosteroid implants for unilateral disease, contraindication or intolerance to standard agents, or multiple systemic comorbidities which limit the use of systemic immunosuppressive therapy.
- Reserving cytotoxic agents for therapeutic failures.
- For uveitis associated with infectious etiologies, specific agents are indicated, including antivirals and antitoxoplasmosis therapy.

CONCLUDING REMARKS AND FUTURE PROSPECTS

We have learned a great deal since the advent of steroids for uveitis in the early 1950s. Most therapies during the 20th century tended to be monotherapy, and combination therapy only began to be used more frequently during the 1990s. Concerns about the side effects of steroids, i.e., osteoporosis, came to the attention of treating physicians relatively early, as did the goals for therapy, including long-term approaches that reduced secondary effects. Because of this the use of local therapy, including intraocular therapy, whether by injection or a time-released device, has become more popular. So where will we be going in the 21st century? Some of the possibilities include pharmacogenetics study of variability in drug responses attributed to hereditary factors in different populations; pharmacogenomics determination and analysis of the genome and its products (RNA and proteins) as they relate to drug response; evaluation of patient genomes to identify which patients are the best candidates for a specific therapy; and finally, using cytokines or other biomarkers as a marker for inflammation, as potential therapeutic targets, and to determine the true level of immunologic quiescence in chronic uveitis.

REFERENCES

Anon, 1976. Progesterone in large amounts has immunosuppressive effect. JAMA. 236, 905–913.

Augsburger, J.J., Annesley Jr., W.H., Sergott, R.C., Fekberg, N.T., Bowman, J.H., Raymond, L.A., 1981. Familial pars planitis. Ann. Ophthalmol. 13, 553–557.

Baglivo, E., Safran, A.B., Borruat, F.X., 1996. Multiple evanescent white dot syndrome after hepatitis B vaccine. Am. J. Ophthalmol. 122, 431–432.

Bora, N.S., Gobleman, C.L., Atkinson, J.P., Pepose, J.S., Kaplan, H.J., 1993. Differential expression of the complement regulatory proteins in the human eye. Invest. Ophthalmol. Vis. Sci. 34, 3579–3584.

Bottazzo, G.F., Pujol-Borrel, R., Hanafusa, T., Feldmann, M., 1983. Role of aberrant HLA-Dr expression and antigen presentation in induction of endocrine autoimmunity. Lancet. 2, 1115–1119.

Brewerton, D.A., Hart, F.D., Nicholls, A., Cafferey, M., James, D.C., Sturrock, R.D., 1973. Ankylosing spondylitis and HLA-B27. Lancet. 1, 904–907.

Brezin, A.P., Massin-Korobelnik, P., Boudin, M., Gauric, A., Le Hoang, P., 1995. Acute posterior multifocal placoid pigment epitheliopathy after hepatitis B vaccine. Arch. Ophthalmol. 113, 297–300.

Caspi, R.R., 1999. Immune mechanisms in uveitis. Springer Semin. Immunopathol. 21, 113–124.

Caspi, R.R., 2002. Th1 and Th2 responses in pathogenesis and regulation of experimental autoimmune uveoretinitis. Int. Rev. Immunol. 21, 197–208.

Caspi, R.R., Chan, C.C., Grubbs, B.G., Silver, P.B., Wiggert, B., Parsa, C.F., et al., 1994. Endogenous systemic IFN-gamma has a protective role against ocular autoimmunity in mice. J. Immunol. 152, 890–899.

Caspi, R.R., Grubbs, B.G., Chan, C.C., Chader, G.J., Wiggert, B., 1992. Genetic control of susceptibility to experimental autoimmune uveoretinitis in the mouse model: concomitant regulation by MHC and non-MHC genes. J. Immunol. 148, 2384–2389.

Caspi, R.R., Roberge, F.G., Chan, C.C., Wiggert, B., Chadar, G.J., Rozenszajn, L.A., et al., 1988. A new model of autoimmune disease. Experimental autoimmune uveoretinitis induced in mice with two different retinal antigens. J. Immunol. 140, 1490–1495.

Caspi, R.R., Roberge, F.G., McAllister, C.G., el-Saied, M., Kuwabara, T., Gery, I., et al., 1986. T cell lines mediating experimental autoimmune uveoretinitis (EAU) in the rat. J. Immunol. 136, 928–933.

Cassidy, J.T., Levinson, J.E., Bass, J.C., Baum, J., Brewer Jr., E.J., Fink, C.W., et al., 1986. A study of classification criteria for a diagnosis of juvenile rheumatoid arthritis. Arthritis Rheum. 29, 274–281.

Chakraborty, M., Mandal, C., 1993. Immunosuppresive effect of human alpha-fetoprotein: a cross species study. Immunol. Invest. 22, 329–339.

Chan, C.C., Hikita, N., Dastgheib, J., Dastgheib, K., Whitcup, S.M., Gery, I., et al., 1994. Experimental melaninprotein-induced uveitis in the Lewis rat immunopathologic processes. Ophthalmology. 101, 1275–1280.

Chan, C.C., Wetzig, R.P., Palestine, A.G., Kuwabara, T., Nusenblatt, R.B., 1987. Immunohistopathology of ocular sarcoidosis: report of a case and discussion of immunopathogenesis. Arch. Ophthalmol. 105, 1398–1402.

Charteris, D.G., Lightman, S.L., 1992. Interferon-gamma (IFNgamma) production in vivo in experimental autoimmune uveoretinitis. Immunology. 75, 463–467.

Collins, R.C., 1949. Experimental studies on sympathetic ophthalmia. Am. J. Ophthalmol. 32, 1687–1699.

Culbertson, W.W., Giles, C.L., West, C., Stafford, T., 1983. Familial pars planitis. Retina. 3, 179–181.

de Kozak, Y., Sakai, J., Thillaye, B., Faure, J.P., 1981. S antigen induced experimental autoimmune uveo-retinitis in rats. Curr. Eye Res. 1, 327–337.

de Kozak, Y., Youn, W.S., Bogossian, M., Faure, J.P., 1976. Humoral and cellular immunity to retinal antigens in guinea pigs. Mod. Probl. Ophthalmol. 16, 51–58.

Dick, A.D., McMenamin, P.G., Korner, H., Scallon, B.J., Ghrayeb, J., Forrester, J.V., et al., 1996. Inhibition of tumor necrosis factor activity minimizes target organ damage in experimental autoimmune uveoretinitis despite quantitatively normal activated T cell traffic to the retina. Eur. J. Immunol. 26, 1018–1025.

Doft, B.H., 1983. Pars planitis in identical twins. Retina. 3, 32–33.

Duinkerke-Eorela, K.U., Pinkers, A., Cruysberg, J.R.M., 1990. Pars planitis in father and son. Ophthal. Pediatr. Genet. 11, 305–308.

Egwuagu, C.E., Szetein, J., Mandi, R.M., Li, W., Chao-Chan, C., Smith, J.A., et al., 1999. IFNgamma increases the severity and accelerates the onset of experimental autoimmune uveitis in transgenic rats. J. Immunol. 162, 510–517.

Elschnig, A., 1910. Studien zur sympathischen ophthalmic:die antigen wirkung des augenpigmentes. Albrecht von Graefes Arch. Ophthalmol. 76, 509–546.

Faure, J.P., 1980. Autoimmunity and the retina. Curr. Top Eye Res. 2, 215–302.

Ferguson, T.A., Griffith, T.S., 1997. A vision of cell death: insights into immune privilege. Immunol. Rev. 156, 167–184.

Ferguson, T.A., Green, D.R., Griffith, T.S., 2002. Cell death and immune privilege. Int. Rev. Immunol. 21, 153–172.

Forrester, J.V., Borthwick, G.M., 1983. Clinical relevance of S-antigen induced experimental uveoretinitis. Trans. Ophthalmol. Soc. U.K. 103, 497–502.

Forrester, J.V., Huitinga, I., Lumsden, L., Dijkstra, C.D., 1998. Marrow-derived activated macrophages are required during the effector phase of experimental autoimmune uveoretinitis in rats. Curr. Eye Res. 17, 426–437.

Foxman, E.F., Zhang, M., Hurst, S.D., Muchamuel, T., Shen, D., Wawrousek, E.F., et al., 2002. Inflammatory mediators in uveitis: differential induction of cytokines and chemokines in Th 1 versus Th2 mediated ocular inflammation. J. Immunol. 168, 2483–2492.

Franks, W.A., Limb, G.A., Stanford, M.R., Ogilvie, J., Wolstencroft, R. A., Crignell, A.H., et al., 1992. Cytokines in human intraocular inflammation. Curr. Eye. Res. 11 (Suppl.), 187–191.

Frassanito, M.A., Dammacco, R., Fusaro, T., Cusmai, A., Guerriero, S., Sborgia, C., 2003. Combined cyclosporin-A /prednisone therapy of patients with active uveitis suppresses IFN-gamma production and the function of dendritic cells. Clin. Exp. Immunol. 133, 233–239.

George, R.K., Chan, C.C., Whitcup, S.M., Nussenblatt, R.B., 1997. Ocular immunopathology of Behcet's disease. Surv. Ophthalmol. 42, 157–162.

Gery, I., Streilen, J.W., 1994. Autoimmunity in the eye and its regulation. Curr. Opin. Immunol. 6, 938–945.

Gery, I., Chanaud III, N.P., Anglade, E., 1994. Recoverin is highly uveitogenic in Lewis rats. Invest. Ophthalmol. Vis. Sci. 35, 3342–3345.

Gery, I.M., Nussenblatt, R.B., 1986. Retinal specific antigens and immunopathologic processes they provoke. Prog. Ret. Res. 5, 75–109.

Giles, C.L., Tranton, J.H., 1980. Peripheral uveitis in three children of one family. J. Pediatr. Ophthalmol. Strabismus. 17, 297–299.

Graham, E., Spalton, D.J., Sanders, M.D., 1981. Immunological investigations in retinal vasculitis. Trans. Ophthalmol. Soc. U.K. 101, 12–16.

Granstein, R., Satszewski, R., Knisely, T., Zeira, E., Nazareno, R., Latina, M., et al., 1990. Aqueous humor contains transforming growth factor beta and a small (<3500 daltons) inhibitor of thymocyte proliferation. J. Immunol. 144, 3021–3027.

Green, D.R., Ferguson, T.A., 2001. The role of FAS ligand in immune privilege. Nat. Rev. Mol. Cell Biol. 2, 917–924.

Gregerson, D.S., Abrahams, I.W., 1983. Immunologic and biochemical properties of several retinal proteins bound by antibodies in sera from animals with experimental autoimmune uveitis and uveitis patients. J. Immunol. 131, 259–264.

Gregerson, D.S., Abrahams, I.W., Thirkill, C.E., 1981. Serum antibody levels of uveitis patients to bovine retinal antigens. Invest. Ophthalmol. Vis. Sci. 21, 669–680.

Griffith, T.S., Yu, X., Herndon, J.M., Green, D.R., Ferguson, T.A., 1996. CD95-induced apoptosis of lymphocytes in an immune privileged site induces immunological tolerance. Immunity. 5, 7–16.

Gritz, D.C., Wong, I.G., 2004. Incidence and prevalence of uveitis in Northern California; the Northern California epidemiology of uveitis study. Ophthalmology. 111, 491–500.

Ham, D.I., Gentleman, S., Chan, C.C., McDowell, J.H., Redmond, T.M., Gery, I., 2002. RPE65 is highly uveitogenic in rats. Invest. Ophthalmology. Vis. Sci. 43, 2258–2263.

Harness, J., Cavanagh, A., Morton, H., McCombe, P., 2003. A protective effect of early pregnancy factor on experimental autoimmune encephalomyelitis induced in Lewis rats by inoculation with myelin basic protein. J. Neurol. Sci. 216, 33–41.

Heiligenhaus, A., Thurau, S., Hennig, M., Grajewski, R.S., Wildner, G., 2010. Anti-inflammatory treatment uveitis with biologicals: new treatment options that reflect pathogenetic knowledge of the disease. Graefes Arch. Clin. Exp. Ophthalmol. 248, 1531–1551.

Hill, T., Galatowicz, F., Akerele, T., Lau, C.H., Calder, V., Lightman, S., 2005. Intracellular T lymphocyte cytokine profiles in the aqueous humour of patients with uveitis and correlation with clinical phenotype. Clin. Exp. Immunol. 139, 132–137.

Hirose, S., Kuwabara, T., Nussenblatt, R.B., Wiggert, B., Redmond, T.M., Gery, I., 1986. Uveitis induced in primates by interphotoreceptor retinoid-binding protein. Arch. Ophthalmol. 104, 1698–1702.

Hoey, S., Grabowski, P.S., Ralston, S.H., Forrester, J.V., Liversidge, J., 1997. Nitric oxide accelerates the onset and increases the severity of experimental autoimmune uveoretinitis through an IFN-gamma dependent mechanism. J. Immunol. 159, 5132–5142.

Hogan, M.J., Kimura, S.J., O'Connor, G.R., 1965. Peripheral retinitis and chronic cyclitis in children. Trans. Ophthalmol. Soc. U.K. 85, 39–51.

Hooks, J.J., Chan, C.C., Detrick, B., 1988. Identification of the lymphokines, interferon-gamma and interleukin-2, in inflammatory eye diseases. Invest. Ophthalmol. Vis. Sci. 29, 1444–1451.

Hoyer, K.K., Kuswanto, W.F., Gallo, E., Abbas, A.K., 2009. Distinct roles of helper T-cell subsets in a systemic autoimmune disease. Blood. 113, 389–395.

Ilias, I., Mastorakos, G., 2003. The emerging role of peripheral corticotrophin-releasing hormone. J. Endocrinol. Invest. 26, 364–371.

Jabs, D.A., Johns, C.J., 1986. Ocular involvement in chronic sarcoidosis. Am. J. Ophthalmol. 102, 297–301.

Jabs, D.A., Nussenblatt, R.B., Rosenbaum, J.T., 2005. Standardization of uveitis nomenclature for reporting clinical data. Results of the first international workshop. Am. J. Ophthalmol. 140, 509–516.

Jiang, H.R., Lumsden, L., Forrester, J.V., 1999. Macrophages and dendritic cells in IRBP-induced experimental autoimmune uveoretinitis in B10RIII mice. Invest. Ophthalmol. Vis. Sci. 40, 3177–3185.

Jones, L.S., Rizzo, L.V., Agarwal, R.K., Tarrant, T.K., Chan, C.C., Wiggert, B., Caspi, R.R., 1997. IFN-gamma-deficient mice develop experimental autoimmune uveitis in the context of a deviant effector response. J. Immunol. 158, 5997–6005.

Kalsow, C.M., Wacker, W.B., 1973. Localization of a uveitogenic soluble retinal antigen in the normal guinea pig eye by an indirect fluorescent antibody technique. Int. Arch. Allergy Appl. Immunol. 44, 11–20.

Key III, S.W., Kimura, S.J., 1975. Iridocyclitis associated with juvenile rheumatoid arthritis. Am. J. Ophthalmol. 80, 425–429.

Khan, M.A., Kushner, I., Braun, W.E., Zachary, A.A., Steinberg, A.G., 1977. HLA-B7 and ankylosing spondylitis in American blacks. N. Engl. J. Med. 297, 513.

Kim, H.S., Yoon, S.K., Joo, C., 2001. The expression of multiple cytokines and inducible nitric oxide synthase in experimental melanin protein induced uveitis. Ophthal. Res. 33, 329–355.

Kim, S.J., Zhang, M., Vistica, B.P., Chan, C.C., Shen, D.F., Wawrousek, E.F., Gery, I., 2002. Induction of ocular inflammation by T-helper lymphocytes type 2. Invest. Ophthamol. Vis. Sci. 43, 758–765.

Kimura, S.J., Hogan, M.J., 1963. Chronic cyclitis. Trans. Am. Ophthalmol. Soc. 61, 397–413.

Kitaichi, N., Kotake, S., Morohashi, T., Onoe, K., Ohno, S., Taylor, A.W., 2002. Diminution of experimental autoimmune uveoretinitis (EAU) in mice depleted of NK cells. J. Leukoc. Biol. 72, 1117–1121.

Larson, T., Nussenblatt, R.B., Sen, H.N., 2011. Emerging drugs for uveitis. Expert Opin. Emerg. Drugs. 16, 309–322.

Lee, A.G., 1995. Fam pars planitis. Ophthalmol. Genet. 16, 17–19.

Lee, R.H., Fowler, A., McGinnis, J.F., Lolley, R.N., Craft, C.M., 1990. Amino acid cDNA sequence of bovine phosducin, a soluble phosphoprotein from photoreceptor cells. J. Biol. Chem. 265, 15867–15873.

Lipton, J.M., Catania, A., 1997. An anti-inflammatory action of the neuromodulator a-MSH. Immunol. Today. 18, 140–145.

Murray, P.I., Hoekzema, R., van Haren, M.A., de Hon, F.D., Kijlstra, A., 1990. Aqueous humor interleukin-6 levels in uveitis. Invest. Ophthalmol. Vis. Sci. 31, 917–920.

Nakamura, S., Yamakawa, T., Sugita, M., Kijima, M., Ishioka, M., Tanake, S., et al., 1994. The role of tumor necrosis factor-alpha in the induction of experimental autoimmune uveoretinitis in mice. Invest. Ophthalmol. Vis. Sci. 35, 3884–3889.

Nussenblatt, R.B., 1987. Basic and clinical immunology in uveitis. Jpn. J. Ophthalmol. 31, 368–374.

Nussenblatt, R.B., Whitcup, S.M., 2004. Uveitis: Fundamentals and Clinical Practice. third ed. Mosby, Philadelphia.

Nussenblatt, R.B., Gery, I., Wacker, W.B., 1980a. Experimental autoimmune uveitis: cellular immune responsiveness. Invest. Ophthalmol. Vis. Sci. 19, 686–690.

Nussenblatt, R.B., Gery, I., Ballintine, E.J., Wacker, W.B., 1980b. Cellular immune responsiveness of uveitis patients to retinal S-antigen. Am. J. Ophthalmol. 89, 173–179.

Nussenblatt, R.B., Kuwabara, T., de Monasterio, F.M., Wacker, W.B., 1981. S-antigen uveitis in primates. A new model for human disease. Arch. Ophthalmol. 99, 1090–1092.

Nussenblatt, R.B., Palestine, A.G., Chan, C.C., Roberge, F., 1985. Standardization of vitreal inflammatory activity in intermediate and posterior uveitis. Ophthalmology. 92, 467–471.

Nussenblatt, R.B., Salinas-Carmona, M., Leake, W., Scher, I., 1983. T lymphocyte subsets in uveitis. Am. J. Ophthalmol. 95, 614–621.

Ohno, S., Matsuda, H., 1986. Studies of HLA antigens in Behçet's disease in Japan. In: Lehner, T., Barnes, C. (Eds.), Recent Advances in Behçet's Disease. Royal Society of Medicine Press, London, pp. 11–16.

Palexas, G.N., Sussman, G., Welsh, N.H., 1992. Ocular and systemic determination of IL-1 beta and tumour necrosis factor in a patient with ocular inflammation. Scand. J. Immunol. 11 (Suppl.), 173–175.

Pfister, C., Chabre, M., Plouet, J., Tuyen, V.V., de Kozak, Y., Faure, J.P., et al., 1985. Retinal S antigen identified as the 48K protein regulating light-dependent phosphodiesterase in rods. Science. 228, 891–893.

Rabiah, P.K., Vitale, A.T., 2003. Non-infectious uveitis and pregnancy. Am. J. Ophthalmol. 136, 91–98.

Rao, N.A., 1997. Mechanisms of inflammatory response in sympathetic ophthalmia and VKH syndrome. Eye. 11, 213–216.

Reinsh, C.L., Moyer, C.F., 1991. Animal models of vasculitis. In: Churg, A., Churg, J. (Eds.), Systemic Vasculitis, the Biologic Basis. Igaku-Shoin, New York, pp. 31–40.

Rizzo, L.V., Miller-Rivero, N.E., Chan, C.C., Wiggert, B., Nussenblatt, R.B., Caspi, R.R., 1994. Interleukin-2 treatment potentiates induction of oral tolerance in a murine model of autoimmunity. J. Clin. Invest. 94, 1668–1672.

Rizzo, L.V., Xu, H., Chan, C.C., Wiggert, B., Caspi, R.R., 1998. IL-10 has a protective role in experimental autoimmune uveoretinitis. Int. Immunol. 10, 807–814.

Robertson, M., Liversidge, J., Forrester, J.V., Dick, A.D., 2003. Neutralizing tumor necrosis factor-alpha activity suppresses activation of infiltrating macrophages in experimental autoimmune uveoretinitis. Invest. Ophthalmol. Vis. Sci. 44, 3034–3041.

Rodriguez, A., Calonge, M., Pedroza-Seres, M., Akova, Y.A., Messmer, E.M., D'Amico, D.J., et al., 1996. Referral patterns of uveitis in a tertiary eye care center. Arch. Ophthalmol. 114, 593–599.

Sainz de la Maza, M., Molina, N., Gonzalez-Gonzalez, L.A., Doctor, P.P., Tauber, J., Foster, C.S., 2012. Clinical characteristics of a large cohort of patients with scleritis and episcleritis. Ophthalmol. 119, 43–50.

Sakaguchi, M., Sugita, S., Sagawa, K., Itoh, K., Machizuki, M., 1998. Cytokine production by T cells infiltrating in the eye of uveitis patients. Jpn J. Ophthalmol. 42, 262–268.

Schalken, J.J., Winkens, H.J., van Vugt, A.H.M., De Grip, W.J., Broekhuyse, R.M., 1989. Rhodopsin induced experimental autoimmune uveoretinitis in monkey. Br. J. Ophthalmol. 73, 168–172.

Selmaj, K., Raime, C.S., Farooq, M., Norton, W.T., Brosnan, C.F., 1991. Cytokine cytotoxicity against oligodendrocytes. Apoptosis induced by lymphotoxin. J. Immunol. 147, 1522–1529.

Sen, H.N., Levy-Clarke, G., Faia, L.J., Li, Z., Yeh, S., Barron, K.S., et al., 2009. High-dose daclizumab for the treatment of juvenile idiopathic arthritis-associated active anterior uveitis. Am. J. Ophthalmol. 148, 696–703.

Sen, H.N., Sangave, A.A., Goldstein, D.A., Suhler, E.B., Cunningham, D., Vitale, S., et al., 2011. A standardized grading system for scleritis. Ophthalmology. 118, 768–771.

Shastry, B.S., 2002. SNP alleles in human disease and evolution. J. Hum. Genet. 47, 561–566.

Singh, V.K., Kalra, H.K., Yamaki, K., Abe, T., Donoso, L.A., Shinohara, T., 1990. Molecular mimcry between a uveitopathogenic site of S antigen and viral peptides. Induction of experimental autoimmune uveitis in Lewis rats. J. Immunol. 144, 1282–1287.

Smith, W.M., Sen, H.N., Nussenblatt, R.B., 2012. Noncorticosteroid immune therapy for ocular inflammation. In: Tasman, W., Jaeger, E. A., (Eds.), Duane's Ophthalmology. Lippincott Williams & Wilkins, Philadelphia, Chapter 31.

Streilein, J.W., 1993. Immune privilege as the result of local tissue barriers and immunosuppressive microenvironments. Curr. Opin. Immunol. 5, 428–432.

Streilein-Stein, J., Streilein, J.W., 2002. Anterior chamber associated immune deviation (ACAID): regulation, biological relevance, and implications for therapy. Int. Rev. Immunol. 21, 123–152.

Streiline, J.W., 1997. Molecular basis of ACAID. Ocul. Immunol. Inflamm. 5, 217–218.

Su, S.B., Silver, P.B., Zhang, M., Chan, C.C., Caspi, R.R., 2001. Pertussis toxin inhibits induction of tissue-specific autoimmune disease by disrupting G protein-coupled signals. J. Immunol. 167, 250–256.

Sugiura, S., 1988. Vogt-Koyanagi-Harada disease. Jpn J. Ophthalmol. 32, 334–343.

Suhler, E.B., Smith, J.R., Giles, T.R., Lauer, A.K., Wertheim, M.S., Kurz, D.E., et al., 2009. Infliximab therapy for refractory uveitis: 2-year results of a prospective trial. Arch. Ophthalmol. 127, 819–822.

Suzuki, J., Sakai, J., Okada, A.A., Takeda, E., Usui, M., Mizuguchi, J., 2002. Oral administration of interferon-beta suppresses experimental autoimmune uveoretinitis. Graefes Arch. Clin. Exp. Ophthalmol. 240, 314–321.

Tarrant, T.K., Silver, P.B., Wahlsten, J.L., Rizzo, L.V., Chan, C.C., Wiggert, B., et al., 1999. Interleukin 12 protects from a T helper type 1-mediated autoimmune disease, experimental autoimmune uveitis, through a mechanism involving interferon gamma, nitric oxide, and apoptosis. J. Exp. Med. 189, 219–230.

Tejada, P., Sanz, A., Criado, D., 1994. Pars planitis in a family. Int. Ophthalmol. 18, 111–113.

Uhlenhuth, P., 1903. Zur lehre von der unterscheidung verscheidener eiweissarten mit hilfe spezifischer sera. Fetschrift zum 60 Geburtstag von Robert Koch. Fischer, Jena (pp. 49–74).

Verity, D.H., Wallace, G.R., Vaughan, R.W., Kondeati, E., Madanat, W., Zureitkat, H., et al., 1999. HLA and tumor necrosis factor (TNF) polymorphism in ocular Behçet's disease. Tissue Antigen. 54, 264–272.

Wacker, W.B., Lipton, M.M., 1968. Experimental allergic uveitis. I. Production in the guinea pig and rabbit by immunization with retina in adjuvant. J. Immunol. 101, 151–156.

Wacker, W.B., Donoso, L.A., Kalsow, C.M., Yankeelov Jr., J.A., Organisciak, D.T., 1977. Experimental allergic uveitis: isolation characterization, localization of a soluble uveitopathogenic antigen from bovine retina. J. Immunol. 119, 1949–1958.

Wetzig, R.P., Chan, C.C., Nussenblatt, R.B., Palestine, A.G., Mazur, D. O., Mittal, K.K., 1988. Clinical and immunopathological studies of pars planitis in a family. Br. J. Ophthalmol. 72, 5–10.

Yamaki, K., Kondo, I., Nakamura, H., Miyano, M., Konno, S., Sakuragi, S., 2000. Ocular and extraocular inflammation induced by immunization of tyrosinase related protein 1 and 2 in Lewis rats. Exp. Eye Res. 71, 361–369.

Yeh, S., Li, Z., Forooghian, F., Hwang, F.S., Cunningham, M.A., Pantanelli, S., et al., 2009. CD4 + Foxp3 + T-regulatory cells in noninfectious uveitis. Arch. Ophthalmol. 127, 407–413.

Yeh, S., Wroblewski, K., Buggage, R., Li, Z., Kurup, S.K., Sen, H.N., et al., 2008. High dose humanized anti-IL-2 receptor alpha antibody (daclizumab) for the treatment of active, non-infectious uveitis. J. Autoimmun. 31, 91–97.

Yotsukura, J., Huang, H., Singh, A.K., Shichi, H., 1997. Regulatory cells generated by testicular tolerization to retinal S-antigen: possible involvement of IL-4, IL-10, and TGF-beta in the suppression of experimental autoimmune uveoretinitis. Cell. Immunol. 182, 89–98.

Zheng, L., Fisher, G., Miller, R.E., Peschon, J., Lynch, D.H., Lenardo, M.J., 1995. Induction of apoptosis in mature T cells by tumour necrosis factor. Nature. 377, 348–351.

Chapter 56

Immune-Mediated Inner Ear Disease

Claudio Lunardi[1] and Antonio Puccetti[2]

[1]Department of Medicine, University Hospital, Verona, Italy, [2]Institute Giannina Gaslini and Department of Experimental Medicine, University of Genova, Genova, Italy

Chapter Outline

Introduction	805	Genetic Susceptibility	810
Clinical Features	805	Animal Models	810
IMIED Associated with Systemic Autoimmune Diseases	806	Treatment	811
IMIED Associated with Primary Vasculitides	807	Concluding Remarks and Future Perspectives	812
Cogan's Syndrome	807	Acknowledgments	812
Evidence of Autoimmunity	808	References	812

INTRODUCTION

The hypothesis that a syndrome of sensorineural hearing loss (SNHL) often accompanied by vestibular symptoms might be of autoimmune origin was first proposed by McCabe (1979), who based his findings on clinical features, presence of abnormal immunological tests, and a positive response to immunosuppressive therapy. Since then, a number of syndromes characterized by SNHL with overlapping clinical features have been described and termed in different ways: autoimmune SNHL, immune-mediated inner ear disease (IMIED), idiopathic progressive bilateral SNHL, sudden SNHL, idiopathic SNHL, bilateral immune-mediated Ménière's disease, and autoimmune vestibulo-cochlear disorders (Rahman et al., 2001a), generating a great confusion in the identification of patients and in the evaluation of different studies. SNHL in adult patients remains idiopathic in the vast majority of cases (71%); known causes are viral infections (12.8%), inner ear abnormality (4.7%), trauma (4.2%), vascular or hematologic (2.8%), neoplastic (2.3%), and CNS abnormality (Chau et al., 2010). In a series of children with idiopathic SNHL, Berti et al. confirmed an autoimmune origin in the majority of the cases included in the study (manuscript submitted).

It is still debated whether we can define "autoimmune" in the majority of cases of SNHL without any apparent cause (Greco et al., 2011). Although most of the authors in the field refer to these cases as "autoimmune inner ear disease (AIED)" or "autoimmune sensorineural hearing loss (ASHL)" (Solares et al., 2003; Mathews and Kumar, 2003), we and others (Stone and Francis, 2000; Garcìa-Berrocal et al., 2003) still prefer the definition of IMIED, since an autoimmune process cannot always be identified. Immune-mediated inner ear disease may be a process confined to the inner ear, and antibodies against a vast array of different molecular weight inner ear antigens may be found in a percentage of these patients; in this case the process can be identified as an organ-specific autoimmune disease. In other cases, IMIED is a feature of a systemic disorder such as primary vasculitides or of systemic autoimmune diseases. Indeed a systemic autoimmune disorder can be present in one-third of the patients with IMIED.

CLINICAL FEATURES

Immune-mediated inner ear disease is characterized by the presence of rapidly progressive, often bilateral SNHL, and frequently by vertigo, tinnitus, and a sense of aural fullness, sometimes indistinguishable from Ménière's disease at the beginning. Immune-mediated inner ear disease usually leads to irreversibile damage within hours or days from the onset and involves both ears often asynchronously. Sometimes the disease shows an initial fluctuating

N. Rose & I. Mackay (Eds): The Autoimmune Diseases, Fifth edition. DOI: http://dx.doi.org/10.1016/B978-0-12-384929-8.00056-3

course of remissions and relapses typical of an autoimmune disease. Since the devastating sequelae of IMIED may be avoided with the early institution of aggressive immunosuppression, a prompt diagnosis represents a major goal for the clinician. Indeed the clinical manifestations are shared with entities of different etiologies such as vascular, toxic, metabolic, genetic, traumatic, and infective (Beyea et al., 2012; Massimo et al., 2012; Yariz et al., 2012; Abdelfatah et al., 2013; Gao et al., 2013; Lin et al., 2013). Therefore all the possible non-immune-mediated causes of SNHL need to be excluded. Overall, the incidence of SNHL has been estimated to range from five to 20 per 100,000 subjects per year (Chau et al., 2010).

Ménière's syndrome, characterized by hearing loss and episodes of vertigo, tinnitus, and aural fullness, may accompany several causes of inner ear inflammation, including IMIED. In the absence of an identifiable cause, usually viral, this syndrome is termed Ménière's disease, considered of autoimmune origin at least in 30–40% of the cases although the immunological mechanisms involved are not clear (Riente et al., 2004; Greco et al., 2012). Time course is the most important criterion to differentiate IMIED from Ménière's disease where hearing loss occurs over a long period of time, sometimes several years. Moreover, Ménière's disease is usually limited to one ear in the majority of the cases.

Due to the many different etiologies which can lead to SNHL and to the absence of specific diagnostic markers, Garcìa-Berrocal and Ramìrez-Camacho (2002a) proposed the following criteria to correctly assess IMIED as a distinct entity:

1. Major criteria: bilateral involvement, presence of systemic autoimmune disease, positive antinuclear antibodies (ANA), reduced number of naïve T cells (CD4RA) and recovery of hearing >80%.
2. Minor criteria: unilateral involvement, young/middle-aged patient, often female, presence of antibodies against heat shock protein70 (HSP70) and good response to steroid therapy.

The suspicion of IMIED would be supported by the presence of three major criteria or two major and more than two minor criteria. The same authors (in 2003) used these criteria to characterize and evaluate the response to therapy of 69 patients with recent onset SNHL of different origin such as viral, vascular, immune mediated, and idiopathic. Patients with IMIED had the best and the earliest recovery rate of hearing after therapy, but also a higher rate of recurrence, typical of an autoimmune disorder. However, profound hearing loss (>90 dB) presents a low percentage of recoveries, regardless of the etiology. The criteria proposed by Garcìa-Berrocal et al. still need to be validated by different groups in a greater number of patients. In particular, we think that the presence not only

of ANA but also of other autoantibodies such as anticardiolipin antibodies, antithyroid antibodies, rheumatoid factor, or myeloperoxidase-antineutrophil cytoplasmic antibodies (Takagi et al., 2004; Toubi et al., 2004; Bachor et al., 2005) may suggest the presence of an autoimmune aggression of the inner ear. Moreover we believe that a positive therapeutic response to corticosteroid administration should be considered a major criterion for the diagnosis of IMIED (Ruckenstein, 2004; Gallo et al., 2013).

Due to the lack of a reliable diagnostic tests (Bovo et al., 2009), MRI–PET of the inner ear, in association with anti-HSP70 antibody determination, had been proposed as a useful technique for assessing IMIED (Mazlumzadeh et al., 2003).

However, the utility of the determination of anti-HSP70 antibodies is still unclear and they are no more frequent in Ménière's disease compared to healthy controls; moreover, the presence of such autoantibodies was not correlated with bilateral disease, activity, or stage of the disease (Hornibrook et al., 2011).

IMIED Associated with Systemic Autoimmune Diseases

Hearing loss, both sensorineural and conductive, has been reported in patients with rheumatoid arthritis (Raut et al., 2001; Ozcan et al., 2002; Salvinelli et al., 2004), with psoriatic arthritis (Giani et al., 2006), and with primary Sjögren's syndrome (Boki et al., 2001). Anticardiolipin antibodies have been found associated with the presence of SNHL in patients with Sjögren's syndrome (Tumiati et al., 1997; Tucci et al., 2005) and with systemic lupus erythematosus (SLE) (Naarendorp and Spiera, 1998; Green and Miller, 2001; Kastanioudakis et al., 2002; Batueca-Caletrio et al., 2013). Moreover SNHL can be present in patients with primary antiphospholipid syndrome (Vyse et al., 1994; Chapman et al., 2003). The histopathologic features of temporal bone described in subjects affected by SLE showed various degrees of hair cell loss and atrophy of the organ of Corti, marked cochlear inflammatory infiltrate or formation of fibrous tissue and new bone throughout the cochlea, and degeneration of the spiral ligament, findings very similar to the known features of IMIED (Sone et al., 1999).

Similarly, the histopathology in four patients with Sjögren's syndrome showed severe loss of intermediate cells of stria vascularis and immunoglobulin G deposition on the basement membrane of stria vascularis blood vessels. These pathologic changes are very similar to the inner ear histology found in a mouse model of Sjögren's syndrome (Calzada et al., 2012a).

Sensorineural hearing loss has also been reported in progressive systemic sclerosis (Kastanioudakis et al.,

2001) and in ulcerative colitis (Kumar et al., 2000). Granulomatous inner ear disease has been described in Crohn's disease (Dettmer et al., 2011).

Finally, Ménière's disease displays an elevated prevalence of systemic autoimmune diseases such as RA, SLE, and ankylosis spondylitis (Gazquez et al., 2011).

In conclusion, the presence of a systemic autoimmune disease needs always to be ruled out in SNHL (Mijovic et al., 2013).

IMIED Associated with Primary Vasculitides

Sensorineural hearing loss is often an early symptom of primary vasculitides, which usually affect both the middle and the inner ear. The best example is granulomatosis with polyangitis, previously known as Wegener's granulomatosis (Kempf et al., 1989; Takagi et al., 2002), characterized by chronic otitis media leading to conductive hearing loss; SNHL is often associated and is related to vasculitis of the inner ear. Similar findings may be present in patients with relapsing polychondritis (Malard et al., 2002), characterized by vasculitis of the labyrinthine artery and inflammation of the cartilage within the inner ear. Sensorineural hearing loss has been described in polyarteritis nodosa (Tsunoda et al., 2001), microscopic polyangiitis (Koseki et al., 1997), Behcet's disease (Adler et al., 2002), and Kawasaki disease (Silva et al., 2002).

Cogan's Syndrome

Cogan's syndrome is a rare chronic inflammatory disease characterized by three main clinical features: vestibulo-auditory dysfunction, interstitial keratitis, and vasculitis (St. Clair and McCallum, 1999; Greco et al., 2013). It occurs primarily in children and young adults and was first described by Cogan in 1945. Systemic manifestations occur in approximately half of the cases (Van Doornum et al., 2001); fever and weight loss are associated with active vasculitis which can involve the aorta, aortic arch vessels, or medium vessels (Vollersten, 1990; Weissen-Plenz et al., 2010; Branislava et al., 2011)). Central and peripheral nervous system abnormalities may be present in up to 50% of the subjects (Bicknell and Holland, 1978; Albayram et al., 2001).

Morbidity in Cogan's syndrome results from permanent hearing loss and from cardiovascular disease.

Inner ear pathology reveals endolymphatic hydrops, infiltration of the spiral ligament with lymphocytes and plasma cells, degeneration of the sensory receptors and supporting structures of the cochlea and vestibular apparatus, and demyelinization and atrophy of the vestibular and cochlear branches of the eighth cranial nerve. In some cases extensive new bone formation can be observed.

The cause of the disease is unknown; upper respiratory tract infections may precede the onset of the disease, suggesting an infectious origin (Vollertsen et al., 1986). Autoimmunity has been implicated because of the presence of serum antibodies to a mixture of corneal antigens and inner ear extracts (Disher et al., 1997; Helmchen et al., 1999). In a few cases, anti-neutrophil cytoplasmic autoantibodies (ANCA) have been reported.

We have demonstrated that Cogan's syndrome is an autoimmune disease and that DEP1/CD148 is the pathogenetically relevant autoantigen (Lunardi et al., 2002). Using the peptide library approach (Puccetti and Lunardi, 2010), already applied to the study of systemic sclerosis (Lunardi et al., 2000), we identified a peptide recognized by the sera of all the patients. The peptide shares homology with autoantigens and with the major core protein lambda 1 (Bartlett and Joklik, 1988) of reovirus type III, which causes mild rhinitis and pharyngitis. Peptide-specific IgG antibodies isolated from patients' sera recognized the viral protein, suggesting a viral involvement in the pathogenesis of the disease, possibly through a molecular mimicry mechanism (Zhao et al., 1998).

The peptide showed homology with the high cell density enhanced protein tyrosine phosphatase-1 (DEP-1/CD148), which is highly expressed on both endothelial cells (Takahashi et al., 1999) and supporting cells of the inner ear (Kruger et al., 1999) and with connexin-26, a gap-junction protein expressed in the inner ear (Kikuchi et al., 2000). Affinity-purified antibodies against the peptide obtained from the patients recognized CD148 and connexin-26 in human cochlear extracts. DEP1/CD148 is a widespread cell-surface antigen and its distribution explains the clinical spectrum of Cogan's syndrome. Connexin-26 represents a major system of intercellular communication and its loss results in local intoxication of the Corti organ, leading to hearing loss; moreover mutations at the connexin-26 gene are responsible for the majority of congenital deafness. Connexin-26 shows homology with connexin-43 and connexin-50, gap-junction proteins present in corneal fibroblasts and epithelium and this homology may explain the eye involvement in the disease. Peptide-specific antibodies bind human cochlea by immunohistochemistry (Figure 56.1A, B).

To prove that these autoantibodies are pathogenic and that the identified autoantigen is relevant to Cogan's syndrome we induced the clinical features of the disease in animals (Balb/c mice and rabbits NZW) following either passive transfer of peptide-specific autoantibodies or active immunization with autoantigen peptides. The animal developed hearing loss as assessed by auditory brainstem responses evaluation (Figure 56.2).

We have so far tested many patients with Cogan's syndrome and with idiopathic SNHL for the presence of antibodies directed against the Cogan peptide, DEP-1/CD148,

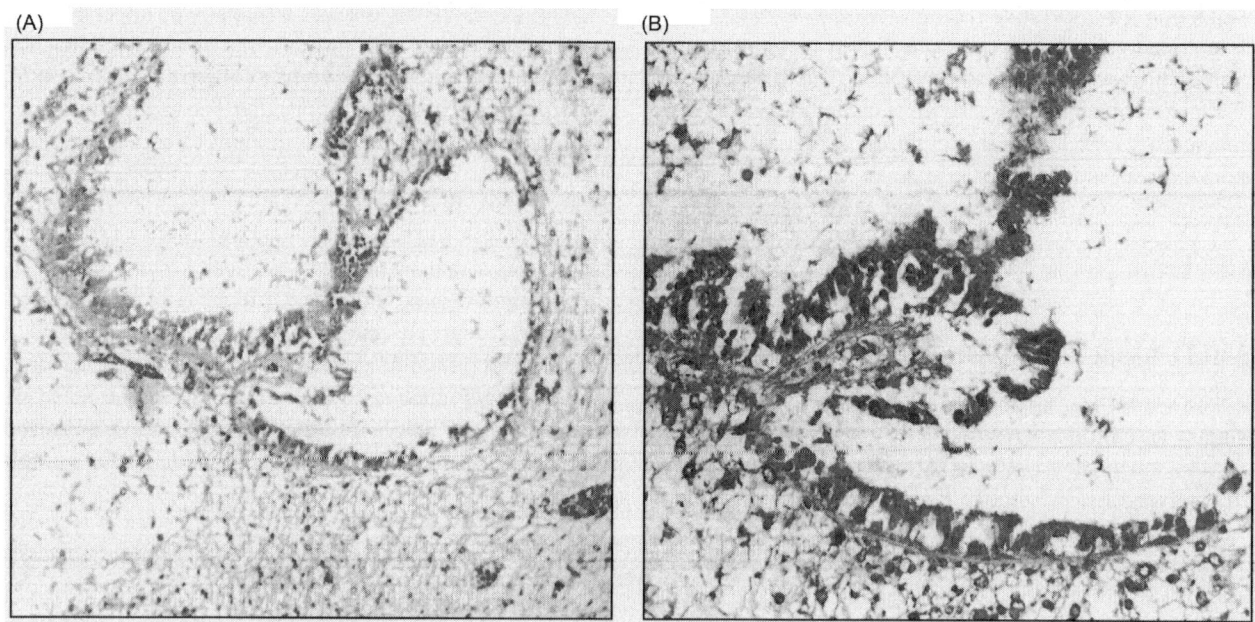

FIGURE 56.1 Antibodies against the Cogan peptide bind human cochlea. Human cochlea immunostained with antibodies purified against an irrelevant peptide (negative control (A)) and with antibodies purified against the Cogan peptide (higher magnitude, (B)). *Reprinted with permission from Elsevier; The Lancet, 2002, 360, 915–921.*

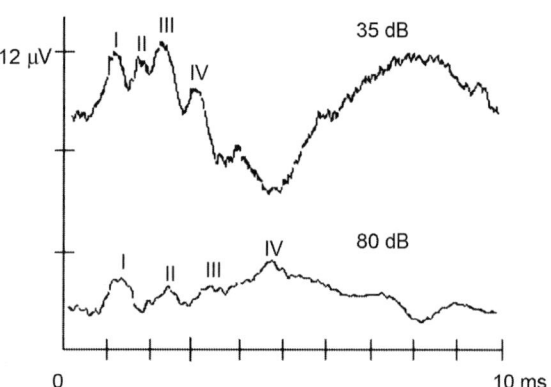

FIGURE 56.2 Grand average of auditory brainstem responses (ABRs) obtained from the same six mice before (upper trace) and 1 week after (lower trace) the third injection of purified antibodies directed against the Cogan peptide. A higher stimulus intensity (80 versus 35 dB) was needed to obtain much smaller and delayed responses (lower trace), consistent with hearing loss. The traces shown were obtained with above-threshold stimuli in order to clearly identify the single components. The delay of waves II, III, and IV suggests an impaired transmission along the auditory pathway from the acoustic nerve to the midbrain. Data represent amplitude of the response in microvolts (μV) (vertical axis); time elapsed from stimulus in milliseconds (horizontal axis). The time of stimulus delivery (click) is coincident with the 0 of the horizontal axis; no pre-stimulus baseline is shown. *Reprinted with permission from Elsevier; The Lancet, 2002, 360, 915–921.*

reovirus, and connexin-26 peptides in order to define the specificity and the sensitivity of the test. We consider positive those patients who have at least two antibodies directed against the four peptides, and one of the two positivities needs to be either anti-Cogan peptide or anti-DEP1/CD148 antibodies. Interestingly, antibodies against Cogan peptide and DEP1/CD148 have been found also in patients diagnosed as affected by autoimmune SNHL.

EVIDENCE OF AUTOIMMUNITY

Autoantibodies and autoreactive T cells have been implicated in the etiopathogenesis of idiopathic SNHL (Yehudai et al., 2006). Different antibodies directed either against inner ear-specific or widely distributed autoantigens have been described in patients with SNHL of unknown origin. Antibodies against type II and type IX collagens as well as against other autoantigens in patients with Ménière's disease and with IMIED have been reported (Yoo et al., 2002). The Kresge Hearing Research Institute-3 (KHRI-3) antibody binds to guinea pig inner ear supporting cell antigen which has been found to be homologous to the human choline transporter-like protein 2, expressed in the inner ear, making this protein a possible target for autoimmune aggression in IMIED (Nair et al., 2004). Anti-endothelial cell autoantibodies have been reported in some patients with SNHL and may represent a marker of vasculitis or vascular damage of inner ear which leads to leukocyte infiltration and local immunoglobulin production (Cadoni et al., 2002; Mathews and Kumar, 2003). The detection of antibodies against the myelin protein P0 (30 kDa) has given conflicting results (Passali et al., 2004; Pham et al., 2007). Besides

TABLE 56.1 Putative Autoantigen Targets in IMIED and Cogan's Syndrome

	Molecular Weight	Ref.	Induces Hearing Loss in Animals	Ref.
IMIED				
Collagen type II		Yoo et al. (2002)	No	Harris et al. (1986)
Collagen type IX		Yoo et al. (2002)	?	–
Myelin protein P0	30 kDa	Boulassel et al. (2001a)	No	Boulassel et al. (2001a)
Beta actin	42 kDa	Boulassel et al. (2001a)	?	–
HSP-70	68 kDa	Billings et al. (1995)	No	Billings et al. (1998)
		Bloch et al. (1999)		
Cochlin	58 kDa	Boulassel et al. (2001b)	Yes	Solares et al. (2004)
Beta tectorin	43 kDa	Boulassel et al. (2001b)	Yes	Solares et al. (2004)
Beta tubulin	55 kDa	Zhou et al. (2011a)	Yes	Zhou et al. (2011a)
CTL2	68–72 kDa	Kommareddi et al. (2009)	?	–
Cogan's syndrome				
DEP1/CD148	200 kDa	Lunardi et al. (2002)	Yes	Lunardi et al. (2002)
Connexin 26	26 kDa	Lunardi et al. (2002)	Yes	Lunardi et al. (2002)

antibodies against the 30 kDa protein, Boulassel et al. (2001a) reported also the presence of antibodies against a 42 kDa protein identified as beta-actin and against a 68 kDa protein identified as HSP70 by some authors (Billings et al., 1998; Bloch et al., 1999) but not by others (Yeom et al., 2003). The Western blot test for HSP70 has a very low sensitivity (Garcìa-Berrocal et al., 2002b); however, its positivity seems to correlate with steroid responsiveness in subjects with IMIED (Hirose et al., 1999). The 58 kDa inner ear protein recognized by the sera of some patients with SNHL has been identified as cochlin, a molecule highly expressed in the cochlea (Boulassel et al., 2001b). Mutation at the "coagulation factor C homology gene" (COCH gene) encoding for cochlin causes progressive DFNA9 hearing loss and vestibular disorder (Roberston et al., 2006). Increased expression of cochlin and decreased expression of its associated basement membrane proteins have been found also in Ménière's disease (Calzada et al., 2012b).

Another protein, highly expressed in the inner ear tissues, such as hair cells, supporting cells, and spiral ligament of stria vascularis, is beta-tubulin. Antibodies against the 55 kDa protein beta-tubulin have been identified in 59% of patients with autoimmune SNHL and Ménière's disese (Zhou et al., 2011a).

Cochlin, β-tectorin, and β-tubulin have been used to induce SNHL in animal models (see below). A 68–72 kDa inner ear membrane glycoprotein called choline transporter-like protein 2 (CTL2) has been identified as a target of autoantibodies in patients with autoimmune hearing loss. Moreover, the presence of these antibodies seems to be correlated with response to corticosteroids (Kommareddi et al., 2009). Table 56.1 summarizes the putative autoantigens believed or proved to be involved in the pathogenesis of IMIED.

We can conclude that sera of patients with SNHL recognize a large array of proteins of variable molecular weight, only a few of which have been identified so far. However, there is no direct proof that any of the antibodies directed against such autoantigens may be immunopathogenic and cochleopathic in IMIED. Indeed the majority of them could not induce SNHL in immunized animals (see below).

The first evidence for an implication of autoreactive T cells was reported by McCabe and McCormick (1984), who observed leukocyte migration inhibition by T cells exposed to inner ear extracts. Lorenz et al. (2002) reported an increased number of inner ear-specific IFN-γ producing T cells in the peripheral blood of patients with SNHL believed to be of autoimmune origin. This finding indicated that proinflammatory T cells specific for as yet unknown inner ear antigens may play a role in the development and progression of inner ear autoimmunity.

GENETIC SUSCEPTIBILITY

As IMIED and Ménière's disease can be of autoimmune origin, interactions between genetic factors and environmental factors play a pivotal role in the pathogenesis of the disease.

Variability in acute immune response genes could determine susceptibility and prognosis of SNHL.

Functional allelic variants of genes encoding for the proinflammatory cytokines tumor necrosis factor alpha (TNF-alpha), interferon gamma, and macrophage migration inhibitory factor have not been found associated with disease susceptibility or hearing loss progression in patients with Ménière's disease (Gásquez et al., 2012).

Since increased permeability of blood vessels, as shown by MRI, suggests inflammation of the inner ear, different genes involved in inflammatory pathways have been analyzed; polymorphisms of the gene encoding for IL-6 (Hiramatsu et al., 2012) and for IL-1β (Um et al., 2013) have been found associated with risk of sudden SNHL. Moreover, IL-1β seems to be overexpressed and aberrantly regulated in patients with autoimmune inner ear disease who are non-responders to steroid therapy (Pathak et al., 2011). Finally, SNHL has been observed in autoinflammatory syndromes such as Muckle–Wells syndrome, whose hallmark is IL-1β dysregulation (Kuemmerle-Deschmer et al., 2013). Therefore IL-1β blockade may be an alternative method to restore hearing in patients who do not respond to steroid therapy.

Oxidative stress seems to be related to the pathology of inner ear; however, polymorphisms of genes involved in oxidative stress have not been found associated with the risk of SNHL or Ménière's disease (Teranishi et al., 2012).

Aquaporins are water channel proteins that play a pivotal role in the regulation of perilymph and endolymph volume; two of the eight aquaporin subtypes seems to be involved in impaired fluid regulation present in Ménière's disease and in Sjögren's syndrome (Eckhard et al., 2012).

Finally, the study of coagulation has identified risk factors such as hyperhomocysteinemia and polymorphism of the MTHFR gene associated with SNHL (Massimo et al., 2012), whereas decrease of plasminogen activator inhibitor-1 (PAI-1) levels due to gene polymorphism may be associated with reduced risk of sudden SNHL in the Italian population (Cho et al., 2012).

ANIMAL MODELS

A major barrier in understanding the pathophysiology of IMIED derives from the paucity of available inner ear tissue. This problem underlines the importance of animal models of this disorder, which may provide insights into pathogenesis, diagnosis, and treatment of IMIED.

A recent animal model of autoimmune inner ear disease has been obtained in Sprague-Dawley rats by combination with a high dose of pertuxis toxin: cellular infiltration, missing hair cells, degeneration of the spiral ganglion cells, endolymphatic hydrops, and autoantibodies directed to inner ear-specific antigens were all noted after immunization (Kong et al., 2011).

Immunization with the better characterized putative autoantigens, such as collagen type II, HSP70, and myelin P0, has failed to elicit hearing loss (Harris et al., 1986; Billings et al., 1998; Boulassel et al., 2001c). Attempts to develop animal models of IMIED have been made by immunizing guinea pigs with either isologous or bovine inner ear homogenates (Harris, 1987; Gong et al., 2002); this model was hampered by the vast array of immunologically active components involved, making it impossible to identify the specific self-antigens involved in disease initiation and progression. The use of fractions of inner ear proteins has partially addressed this problem (Tomiyama, 2002), which will be solved by the availability of recombinant antigens (Billings, 2004). Gloddek et al. (1999) induced SNHL in naïve Lewis rats following passive transfer of activated T cells specific for bovine inner ear extract, demonstrating the role of T cells in the initiation and pathogenesis of SNHL. A confirmation of the importance of T cells was recently provided by Solares et al. (2004), who showed that SWXJ mice immunized with peptides derived from two proteins of the inner ear, cochlin and β-tectorin, had significant hearing loss. Two selected peptides elicited a CD4$^+$ T cell response of the Th1-like phenotype. Moreover the passive transfer of peptide-activated CD4$^+$ T cells into naïve SWXJ recipient induced leukocytic infiltration of inner ear and hearing loss. However, it is not clear whether cochlin and β-tectorin are implicated in IMIED in humans and how accurately this model reflects events occurring in the spontaneous disease (Billings, 2004). Zhou et al. (2011a) have shown that immunization of Balb/c mice with β-tubulin is able to cause lesions in the cochlear hair cells and cochlear damage of the spiral ganglion, mediated by CD4$^+$ T cells producing IFN-γ. Hearing loss was induced by the passive transfer of CD4$^+$ T cells specific for β-tubulin to naïve mice and this is accompanied by a decreased frequency and impaired suppressive function of regulatory T cells. In this murine model of autoimmune hearing loss, systemic infusion of adipose tissue-derived mesenchymal stem cells significantly improved hearing function and protected hair cells by decreasing proliferation of antigen-specific Th1/Th17 cells and by inducing generation of antigen-specific Treg cells (Zhou et al., 2011b). Moreover, the severity of β-tubulin-induced experimental autoimmune hearing loss is exacerbated by IL-10 deficiency (Zhou et al., 2012).

Interestingly, oral administration of β-tubulin in female C57BL/6 mice induced decreased hearing loss and inner ear damage through induction of oral tolerance by increasing Th2-type cytokines (Cai et al., 2009).

The administration of monoclonal antibodies directed either against the guinea pig inner ear supporting cell antigen (KHRI-3 antibody) (Nair et al., 1995) or against type II collagen fragment CB11 peptide-induced SNHL with loss of hair cells, inflammatory cell migration, and endolymphatic hydrops (Matsuoka et al., 2002) suggests that antibodies also play a critical role in autoimmunity of the inner ear.

IL-1β has been observed highly expressed in an animal model of autoimmune inner ear disease; in this model, LPS was required in addition to Ag re-exposure to initiate cochlear IL-1β expression, leukocyte ingress into the cochlea, and hearing loss (Pathak et al., 2011).

TREATMENT

Since IMIED may result in severe deafness and vestibular dysfunction, patients must be treated aggressively and immediately after the onset of the symptoms. The mainstay of therapy is high-dose corticosteroids (1 mg/kg/day) (Chen et al., 2003) continued for at least 2 weeks and then for another 2 weeks in the case of improvement. The steroid is then tapered in a period variable between 2 and 3 months and in some cases maintained at low dosage for a long period (e.g., methylprednisolone 4 mg/day). Different steroid administration schemes, including intratympanic dexamethasone and 6-methylprednisolone injections, have been used with good results (Garcia-Berrocal et al., 2006; Alexander et al., 2009; Lim et al., 2012; Gallo et al., 2013). In the case of deterioration of symptoms or of a not significant improvement during the first 2 weeks of treatment, other immunosuppressive agents (Buniel et al., 2009) are added such as cyclophosphamide (CYP), 2 mg/kg/day, or methotrexate (MTX), 7.5−20 mg/wk. Because of the well-known side effects of CYP, clinicians prefer the use of MTX; however, despite the preliminarily favorable responses (Kilpatrick et al., 2000; Matteson et al., 2001; Rahman et al., 2001; Matteson et al., 2003), the unique controlled trial published so far does not support the efficacy of long-term MTX in maintaining the improvement achieved with glucocorticoid therapy (Harris et al., 2003). Since MTX is slow acting, its effect may start too late in a disease that rapidly leads to hearing loss. In 1989 McCabe reported the promising results obtained with the CYP−prednisolone combination therapy. We have used oral methylprednisolone and CYP pulse therapy in two particularly rapid and severe cases; this therapy blocked and reversed the hearing loss.

The results obtained with steroids and aggressive immunosuppression are variable (Broughton et al., 2004; Loveman et al., 2004; Ruckenstein, 2004) depending on the characteristics of the patients included, on the severity of the hearing loss at the beginning of the treatment, and on how early the therapy is started. Also proinflammatory cytokines and cytokines receptors polymorphisms may affect the steroid responsiveness (Vambutas et al., 2009).

Biological agents can play a role in the management of patients with IMIED (reviewed by Lobo et al., 2012): most studies achieved a hearing improvement or stabilization in more than 70% of patients treated. The biological agents used include anti-TNF-alpha inhibitors (etanercept, infliximab, adalimumab), anti-IL-1 antagonist (anakinra), and anti-CD20 surface antigen (rituximab). Infliximab has been also delivered locally through transtympanic administration (Van Wijk et al., 2006) and has been used in the treatment of Cogan's syndrome (Beccastrini et al., 2010).

There are reports on the utility of plasmapheresis (Luetje and Berliner, 1997), therapeutic apheresis of LDL (Bosch, 2003), and fibrinogen (Suzuki et al., 2003). Suckfull and the Hearing Loss Study Group (2002) reported the beneficial effects of a single fibrinogen/LDL apheresis compared to conventional infusion treatment and prednisolone for 10 days. In controlled studies the use of antiviral therapy with valacyclovir (Tucci et al., 2002) and acyclovir (Uri et al., 2003; Westerlaken et al., 2003) in addition to steroids was no more beneficial than steroids alone. Finally, there are recent reports on the utility of low molecular weight heparins (Yue et al., 2003; Mora et al., 2004) and antioxidants (Joachims et al., 2003) in addition to the usual therapy and the efficacy of intravenous infusion of tissue plasminogen activator (Mora et al., 2003) alone.

In the case of permanent severe bilateral hearing loss, auditory function may be partially replaced with a cochlear implant, an electrical prosthesis with electrodes inserted into the cochlea through mastoidectomy (Cohen et al., 1993). Cochlear implantation has been successfully used in patients with SNHL (Gaylor et al., 2013), with IMIED, and with Cogan's syndrome (Aftab et al., 2010; Wang et al., 2010; Malik et al., 2012). Of the 17 patients with Cogan's syndrome we are following at the moment, nine (age 7−30) have undergone multichannel cochlear implant, resulting in a great improvement to their quality of life, without any complication.

Cochlear implantation has been applied with benefit in children 12 months of age or younger (Holman et al., 2013). Bilateral cochlear implantation seems to be more beneficial than unilateral implantation (van Schoonhoven et al., 2013).

Hematopoietic stem cell transplantation led to improvement in sensorineural hearing in patients with mucopolysaccharidosis (Da Costa et al., 2012). The recent emergence of stem cell technology has the potential to open new approaches for hair cell regeneration (Okano and Kelley, 2012).

CONCLUDING REMARKS AND FUTURE PERSPECTIVES

It is now evident that the inner ear is not an "immunologically privileged" site and may mount an immune response against both foreign and self-antigens. The association of IMIED with systemic autoimmune diseases provides evidence that autoimmunity can damage the inner ear, but it does not address organ-specific disease (Mijovic et al., 2013). Antibodies directed against different inner ear antigens have been identified in some patients; however, they are neither diagnostic nor correlate with disease state. In the future the major goals for research in this field will be: (1) the identification of pathogenetically relevant autoantigen(s); (2) the development of a highly specific diagnostic test; and (3) gaining better knowledge of the immunopathological mechanisms in an organ as inaccessible as the inner ear and allied to the above, defining the best timing and treatment for the disease.

ACKNOWLEDGMENTS

We are grateful to Dr. C. Bason.

REFERENCES

Abdelfatah, N., McComiskey, D.A., Doucette, L., Griffin, A., Moore, S. J., Negrijn, C., et al., 2013. Identification of a novel in-frame deletion in KCNQ4 (DFNA2A) and evidence of multiple phenocopies of unknown origin in a family with ADSNHL. Eur. J. Hum. Genet. Feb 27 [Epub ahead of print].

Adler, Y.D., Jovanovic, S., Jivanjee, A., Krause, L., Zouboulis, C.C., 2002. Adamantiades-Behcet's disease with inner ear involvement. Clin. Exp. Rheumatol. 20, S40–S42.

Aftab, S., Semaan, M.T, Murray, G.S., Megerian, C.A., 2010. Cochlear implantation outcomes in patients with autoimmune and immune-mediated inner ear disease. Otol. Neurotol. 31, 1337–1342.

Albayram, M.S., Wityk, R., Yousem, D.M., Zinreich, S.J., 2001. The cerebral angiographic findings in Cogan syndrome. Am. J. Neuroradiol. 22, 751–754.

Alexander, T.H., Weisman, M.H., Derebery, J.M., Espeland, M.A., Gantz, B.J., Gulya, A.J., et al., 2009. Safety of high-dose corticosteroids for the treatment of autoimmune inner ear disease. Otol. Neurotol. 30, 443–448.

Bachor, E., Kremmer, S., Kreuzfelder, E., Jahnke, K., Seidahmadi, S., 2005. Antiphospholipid antibodies in patients with sensorineural hearing loss. Eur. Arch. Otorhinolaryngol. 262, 622–626.

Bartlett, J.A., Joklik, W.K., 1988. The sequence of the reovirus serotype 3 L3 genome segment which encodes the major core protein lambda 1. Virology. 167, 31–37.

Batueca-Caletrio, A., Del Pin-Montes, J., Cordero-Civantos, C., Calle-Cabanillas, M., Lopez-Escamez, J., 2013. Hearing and vestibular disorders in patients with systemic lupus erythematosus. Lupus. Feb 19 (Epub ahead of print).

Beccastrini, E., Emmi, G., Squatrito, D., Vannucchi, P., Emmi, L., 2010. Infliximab and Cogan's syndrome. Clin. Otolaryngol. 35, 439–450.

Beyea, J.A., Agrawal, S.K., Parnes, L.S., 2012. Recent advances in viral inner ear disorders. Curr. Opin. Otolaryngol. Head Neck Surg. 20, 404–408.

Bicknell, J.M., Holland, J.V., 1978. Neurologic manifestations of Cogan's syndrome. Neurology. 28, 278–288.

Billings, P., 2004. Experimental autoimmune hearing loss. J. Clin. Invest. 113, 1114–1117.

Billings, P.B., Keithley, E.M., Harris, J.P., 1995. Evidence linking the 68 kilodalton antigen identified in progressive sensorineural hearing loss patient sera with heat shock protein 70. Ann Otol Rhinol Laryngol. 104, 181–188.

Billings, P., Shin, S.O., Harris, J.P., 1998. Assessing the role of anti-hsp70 in cochlear function. Hear. Res. 126, 210–212.

Bloch, D.B., Gutierrez, J.A., Guerriero Jr., V., Rauch, S.D., Bloch, K.J., 1999. Recognition of a dominant epitope in bovine heat-shock protein 70 in inner ear disease. Laryngoscope. 109, 621–625.

Boki, K.A., Ioannidis, J.P., Segas, J.V., Maragkoudakis, P.V., Petrou, D., Adamopoulos, G.K., et al., 2001. How significant is sensorineural hearing loss in primary Sjogren's syndrome? An individually matched case-control study. J. Rheumatol. 28, 798–801.

Bosch, T., 2003. Recent advances in therapeutic apheresis. J. Artif. Organs. 6, 1–8.

Boulassel, M.R., Deggouj, N., Tomasi, J.P., Gersdorff, M., 2001a. Inner ear autoantibodies and their targets in patients with autoimmune inner ear diseases. Acta Otolaryngol. 121, 28–34.

Boulassel, M.R., Tomasi, J.P., Deggouj, N., Gersdorff, M., 2001b. COCH5B2 is a target antigen of anti-inner ear antibodies in autoimmune inner ear diseases. Otol. Neurotol. 22, 614–618.

Boulassel, M.R., Guerit, J.M., Denison, S., de Tourtchaninoff, M., Wenderickx, L., Botterman, N., et al., 2001c. No evidence of auditory dysfunction in guinea pigs immunized with myelin P0 protein. Hear. Res. 152, 10–16.

Bovo, R., Ciorba, A., Martini, A., 2009. The diagnosis of autoimmune inner ear disease: evidence and critical pitfalls. Eur. Arch. Otorhinolaryngol. 266, 37–40.

Branislava, I., Marijana, T., Nemanja, D., Dragan, S., Maja, Z., 2011. Atypical Cogan's syndrome associated with coronary disease. Chin. Med. J. 124, 3192–3194.

Broughton, S.S., Meyerhoff, W.E., Cohen, S.B., 2004. Immune-mediated inner ear disease: 10-year experience. Semin. Arthritis Rheum. 34, 544–548.

Buniel, M.C., Geelan-Hansen, K., Weber, P.C., Tuohy, V.K., 2009. Immunosuppressive therapy for autoimmune inner ear disease. Immunotherapy. 1, 425–434.

Cadoni, G., Fetoni, A.R., Agostino, S., DeSantis, A., Manna, R., Ottaviani, F, et al., 2002. Autoimmunity in sudden sensorineural hearing loss: possible role of anti-endothelial cell autoantibodies. Acta Otolaryngol. Suppl. 548, 30–33.

Cai, Q., Du, X., Zhou, B., Cai, C., Kermany, M.H., Yoo, T., 2009. Induction of tolerance by oral administration of beta-tubulin in an animal model of autoimmune inner ear disease. ORL. 71, 135–141.

Calzada, A.P., Balaker, A.E., Ishiyama, G., Lopez, I.A., Ishiyama, A., 2012a. Temporal bone histopathology and immunoglobulin deposition in Sjögren's syndrome. Otol. Neurotol. 33, 258–266.

Calzada, A.P., Lopez, I.A., Parrazal, L.B., Ishiyama, A., Ishiyama, G., 2012b. Cochlin expression in vestibular endorgans obtained from patients with Meniere's disease. Cell Tissue Res. 350, 373–384.

Chapman, J., Rand, J.H., Brey, R.L., Levine, S.R., Blatt, I., Khamashta, M.A., et al., 2003. Non-stroke neurological syndromes associated with antiphospholipid antibodies: evaluation of clinical and experimental studies. Lupus. 12, 514–517.

Chau, J.K., Lin, J.R.J., Atashband, S., Irvine, R.A., Westerberg, B.D., 2010. Systematic review of the evidence for the etiology of adult sudden sensorineural hearing loss. Laryngoscope. 120, 1011–1021.

Chen, C.Y., Halpin, C., Rauch, S.D., 2003. Oral steroid treatment of sudden sensorineural hearing loss: a ten year retrospective analysis. Otol. Neurotol. 24, 728–733.

Cho, S.H., Chen, H., Kim, I.S., Yokose, C., Kang, J., Cho, D., et al., 2012. Association of the 4 g/5 g polymorphism of plasminogen activator inhibitor-1 gene with sudden sensorineural hearing loss. A case control study. BMC Ear Nose Throat Disord. 6, 12–15.

Cogan, D., 1945. Syndrome of nonsyphilitic interstitial keratitis and vestibuloauditory symptoms. Arch Ophthalmol. 33, 144–149.

Cohen, N.L., Waltzman, S.B., Fisher, S.G., the Department of Veterans Affair Cochlear Implant Study Group, 1993. A prospective, randomized study of cochlear implants. N. Engl. J. Med. 328, 233–237.

Da Costa, V., O'Grady, G., Jackson, L., Kaylie, D., Raynor, E., 2012. Improvements in sensorineural hearing loss after cord blood transplant in patients with mucopolysaccharidosis. Arch. Otolaryngol. Head Neck Surg. 138, 1071–1076.

Dettmer, M., Hegemann, I., Hegemann, S.C., 2011. Extraintestinal Crohn's disease mimicking autoimmune inner ear disease: a histopathological approach. Audiol. Neurootol. 16, 36–40.

Disher, M.J., Ramakrishnan, A., Nair, T.S., Miller, J.M., Telian, S.A., Arts, H.A., et al., 1997. Human autoantibodies and monoclonal antibody KHRI-3 bind to a phylogenetically conserved inner-ear supporting cell antigen. Ann. N.Y. Acad. Sci. 830, 253–267.

Eckhard, A., Gleiser, C., Arnold, H., Rask-Andersen, H., Kumagami, H., Müller, M., et al., 2012. Water channel proteins in the inner ear and their link to hearing impairment and deafness. Mol. Aspects Med. 33, 612–637.

Gallo, E., Khojasteh, E., Gloor, M., Hegemann, S.C., 2013. Effectiveness of systemic high-dose dexamethasone therapy for idiopathic sudden sensorineural hearing loss. Audiol. Neurootol. 18, 161–170.

Gao, Y., Yechikov, S., Vazquez, A.E., Chen, D., Nie, L., 2013. Distinct roles of molecular chaperones HSP90α and HSP90β in the biogenesis of KCNQ4 channels. PloS One. 8, e57282.

Garcìa-Berrocal, J.R., Ramìrez-Camacho, R., 2002a. Sudden sensorineural hearing loss: supporting the immunologic theory. Ann. Otol. Rhinol. Laryngol. 111, 989–997.

Garcìa-Berrocal, J.R., Ramìrez-Camacho, R., Arellano, B., Vargas, J.A., 2002b. Validity of the Western blot immunoassay for heat shock protein-70 in associated and isolated immunorelated inner ear disease. Laryngoscope. 112, 304–309.

Garcìa-Berrocal, J.R., Ramìrez-Camacho, R., Millàn, I., Gorriz, C., Trinidad, A., Arellano, B., et al., 2003. Sudden presentation of immune-mediated inner ear disease: characterization and acceptance of a cochleovestibular dysfunction. J. Laryngol. Otol. 117, 775–779.

Garcia-Berrocal, J.R., Ibañez, A., Rodrìguez, A., Gonzàlez-Garcìa, J.A., Verdaguer, J.M., Trinidad, A., et al., 2006. Alternatives to systemic steroid therapy for refractory immune-mediated inner ear disease: a physiopathologic approach. Eur. Arch. Otorhinolaryngol. 263, 977–982.

Gásquez, I., Moreno, A., Requena, T., Ohmen, J., Santos-Perez, S., Aran, I., et al., 2012. Functional variants of MIF, INFG and TFNA genes are not associated with disease susceptibility or hearing loss progression in patients with Ménière's disease. Eur. Arch. Otorhinolaryngol. Nov. 21. [Epub ahead of print].

Gaylor, J.M., Raman, G., Chung, M., Lee, J., Rao, M., Lau, J., et al., 2013. Cochlear implantation in adults: a systematic review and meta-analysis. JAMA Otolaryngol. Head Neck Surg. 21, 1–8.

Gazquez, I., Soto-Varela, A., Aran, I., Santos, S., Batuecas, A., Trinidad, G., et al., 2011. High prevalence of systemic autoimmune diseases in patients with Menière's disease. PloS One. 6, 1–7.

Giani, T., Simonini, G., Lunardi, C., Puccetti, A., De Martino, M., Falcini, F., 2006. Juvenile psoriatic arthritis and acquired sensorineural hearing loss in a teenager: is there an association? Clin. Exp. Rheumatol. 24, 344–346.

Gloddek, B., Gloddek, J., Arnold, W., 1999. A rat T cell line that mediates autoimmune disease of the inner ear in the Lewis rat. ORL. J. Otorhinolaryngol. Relat. Spec. 61, 181–187.

Gong, S.S., Yu, D.Z., Wang, J.B., 2002. Relationship between three inner ear antigens with different molecular weights and autoimmune inner ear disease. Acta. Otolaryngol. 122, 5–9.

Greco, A., Fusconi, M., Gallo, A., Marinelli, C., Macri, G.F., De Vincentiis, M., 2011. Sudden sensorineural hearing loss: an autoimmune disease? Autoimmun. Rev. 10, 756–761.

Greco, A., Gallo, A., Fusconi, M., Marinelli, C., Macri, G.F., De Vincentiis, M., 2012. Meniere's disease might be an autoimmune condition? Autoimmun. Rev. 11, 731–738.

Greco, A., Gallo, A., Fusconi, M., Magliulo, G., Turchetta, R., Marinelli, C., et al., 2013. Cogan's syndrome: an autoimmune inner ear disease. Autoimmun. Rev. 12, 396–400.

Green, L., Miller, E.B., 2001. Sudden sensorineural hearing loss as a first manifestation of systemic lupus erythematosus: association with anticardiolipin antibodies. Clin. Rheumatol. 20, 220–222.

Harris, J.P., 1987. Experimental autoimmune sensorineural hearing loss. Laryngoscope. 97, 63–76.

Harris, J.P., Sharp, P., 1990. Inner ear autoantibodies in patients with rapidly progressive sensorineural hearing loss. Laryngoscope. 100, 516–524.

Harris, J.P., Woolf, N.K., Ryan, A.F., 1986. A re-examination of experimental type II collagen autoimmunity: middle and inner ear morphology and function. Ann. Otol. Rhinol. Laryngol. 95, 176–180.

Harris, J.P., Weisman, M.H., Derebery, J.M., Espeland, M.A., Gantz, B. J., Gulya, A.J., et al., 2003. Treatment of corticosteroid-responsive autoimmune inner ear disease with methotrexate: a randomized controlled trial. JAMA. 290, 1875–1883.

Helmchen, C., Arbusow, V., Jager, L., Strupp, M., Stocker, W., Schulz, P., 1999. Cogan's syndrome: clinical significance of antibodies against inner ear and cornea. Acta Otolaryngol. 119, 528–536.

Hiramatsu, M., Teranishi, M., Uchida, Y., Nishio, N., Suzuki, H., Kato, K., et al., 2012. Polymorphisms in genes involved in inflammatory pathways in patients with sudden sensorineural hearing loss. J. Neurogenet. 26, 387–396.

Hirose, K., Wener, M.H., Duckert, L.G., 1999. Utility of laboratory testing in autoimmune inner ear disease. Laryngoscope. 109, 1749–1754.

Holman, M.A., Carison, M.L., Driscoll, C.L., Grim, K.J., Petersson, R. S., Sladen, D.P., et al., 2013. Cochlear implantation in children 12 months of age and younger. Otol. Neurotol. 34, 251–258.

Hornibrook, J., George, P., Spellerberg, M., Gourley, J., 2011. HSP70 antibodies in 80 patients with "clinically certain" Meniere's disease. Ann. Otol. Rhinol. Laryngol. 120, 651–655.

Joachims, H.Z., Segal, J., Golz, A., Netzer, A., Goldenberg, D., 2003. Antioxidants in treatment of idiopathic sudden hearing loss. Otol. Neurotol. 24, 572–575.

Kastanioudakis, I., Ziavra, N., Politi, E.N., Exarchakos, G., Drosos, A.A., Skevas, A., 2001. Hearing loss in progressive systemic sclerosis patients: a comparative study. Otolaryngol. Head Neck Surg. 124, 522–525.

Kastanioudakis, I., Ziavra, N., Voulgari, P.V., Exarchakos, G., Skevas, A., Drosos, A.A., 2002. Ear involvement in systemic lupus erythematosus patients: a comparative study. J. Laryngol. Otol. 116, 103–107.

Kempf, H.G., 1989. Ear involvement in Wegener's granulomatosis. Clin. Otorhinolaryngol. 14, 451–456.

Kikuchi, T., Kimura, R.S., Paul, D.L., Takasaka, T., Adams, J.C., 2000. Gap junction systems in the mammalian cochlea. Brain Res. Rev. 32, 163–166.

Kilpatrick, J.K., Sismanis, A., Spencer, R.F., Wise, C.M., 2000. Low dose oral methotrexate management of patients with bilateral Meniere's disease. Ear Nose Throat J. 79, 82–83, 86–88, 91–92.

Kommareddi, P.K., Nair, T.S., Vallurupalli, M., Telian, S.A., Arts, H.A., El-Kshlan, H.K., et al., 2009. Autoantibodies to recombinant human CTL2 in autoimmune hearing loss. Laryngoscope. 119, 924–932.

Kong, W.J., Wang, D.Y., Huang, X., Ding, G.F., 2011. High dose combination pertussis toxin induces autoimmune inner ear disease in Sprague-Dawley rats. Acta Otolaryngol. 131, 692–700.

Koseki, Y., Suwa, A., Nojima, T., Ishijama, K., Nakajima, A., Tanabe, M., et al., 1997. A case of microscopic polyangiitis accompanied by hearing loss as the initial sign of the disease. Ryumachi. 37, 804–809.

Kruger, R.P., Goodyear, R.J., Legan, P.K., Warchol, M.E., Raphael, Y., Cotanche, D.A., et al., 1999. The supporting-cell antigen: a receptor-like protein tyrosine phosphatase expressed in the sensory epithelia of the avian inner ear. J. Neurosci. 19, 4815–4827.

Kuemmerle-Deschner, J.B., Koitschev, A., Ummenhofer, K., Hansmann, S., Plontke, S.K., Koitschev, C., et al., 2013. Hearing loss in Muckle-Wells syndrome. Arthritis Rheum. 65, 824–831.

Kumar, B.N., Smith, M.S.H., Walsh, R.M., 2000. Sensorineural hearing loss in ulcerative colitis. Clin. Otolaryngol. 25, 143–145.

Lim, H.J., Kim, Y.T., Choi, S.J., Lee, J.B., Park, K., Choung, Y.H., 2012. Efficacy of 3 different steroid treatments for sudden sensorineural hearing loss: a prospective, randomized trial. Otolaryngol. Head Neck Surg. Oct. 16. [Epub ahead of print].

Lin, C., Lin, S.W., Weng, S.F., Lin, Y.S., 2013. Increased risk of sudden sensorineural hearing loss in patients with human immunodeficiency virus aged 18 to 35 years: a population-based cohort study. JAMA Otolaryngol. Head Neck Surg. 21, 1–5. [Epub ahead of print].

Lobo, D., Garcia-Berrocal, JR., Trinidad, A., Verdaguer, J.M., Ramirez-Camacho, R., 2012. Review of the biologic agents used for immune-mediated inner ear disease. Acta Otorrinolaringol. Esp. Jul 4. [Epub ahead of print].

Lorenz, R.R., Solares, C.A., Williams, P., Sikora, J., Pelfrey, C.M., Hughes, G.B., et al., 2002. Interferon-gamma production to inner ear antigens by T cells from patients with autoimmune sensorineural hearing loss. J. Neuroimmunol. 130, 173–178.

Loveman, D.M., de Comarmond, C., Cepero, R., Baldwin, D.M., 2004. Autoimmune sensorineural hearing loss: clinical course and treatment outcome. Semin. Arthritis Rheum. 34, 538–543.

Luetje, C.M., Berliner, K.I., 1997. Plasmapheresis in autoimmune inner ear disease: long-term follow-up. Am. J. Otol. 18, 572–576.

Lunardi, C., Bason, C., Navone, R., Millo, E., Damonte, G., Corrocher, R., et al., 2000. Systemic sclerosis immunoglobulin G autoantibodies bind the human cytomegalovirus late protein UL94 and induce apoptosis in human endothelial cells. Nat. Med. 6, 1183–1186.

Lunardi, C., Bason, C., Leandri, M., Navone, R., Lestani, M., Millo, E., et al., 2002. Autoantibodies to inner ear and endothelial antigens in Cogan's syndrome. Lancet. 360, 915–921.

Malard, O., Hamidou, M., Toquet, C., Bailleul, S., Bordure, P., Beauvillain De Montreuil, C., 2002. Relapsing polychondritis revealed by ENT symptoms: clinical characteristics in three patients. Ann. Otolarynol. Chir. Cervicofac. 119, 202–208.

Malik, M.U., Pandian, V., Masood, H., Diaz, D.A., Varela, V., Dávalos-Balderas, A.J., et al., 2012. Spectrum of immune-mediated inner ear disease and cochlear implant results. Laryngoscope. 122, 2557–2562.

Massimo, F., Antonio, C., Armand de, V., Antonio, G., Fulvio, M., Rosaria, T., et al., 2012. Sudden sensorineural hearing loss: a vascular cause? Analysis of prothrombic risk factors in head and neck. Int. J. Audiol. 51, 800–805.

Mathews, J., Kumar, B.N., 2003. Autoimmune sensorineural hearing loss. Clin. Otolaryngol. 28, 479–488.

Matsuoka, H., Kwon, S.S., Yazawa, Y., Barbieri, M., Yoo, T.J., 2002. Induction of endolymphatic hydrops by directly infused monoclonal antibody against type II collagen CB11 peptide. Ann. Otol. Rhinol. Laryngol. 111, 587–592.

Matteson, E.L., Fabry, D.A., Facer, G.W., Beatty, W., Driscoll, C.L., Strome, S.E., et al., 2001. Open trial of methotrexate as treatment for autoimmune hearing loss. Arthritis Rheum. 45, 146–150.

Matteson, E.L., Fabry, D.A., Strome, S.E., Driscoll, C.L., Beatty, C.W., McDonald, T.J., 2003. Autoimmune inner ear disease: diagnostic and therapeutic approaches in a multidisciplinary setting. J. Am. Acad. Audiol. 14, 225–230.

Mazlumzadeh, M., Lowe, V.J., Mullan, B.P., Fabry, D.A., McDonald, T.J., Matteson, E.L., 2003. The utility of positron emission tomography in the evaluation of autoimmune hearing loss. Otol. Neurotol. 24, 201–204.

McCabe, B.F., 1979. Autoimmune sensorineural earing loss. Ann. Otol. Rhinol. Laryngol. 88, 585–589.

McCabe, B.F., 1989. Autoimmune inner ear disease: therapy. Am. J. Otol. 10, 196–197.

McCabe, B.F., McCormick, K.J., 1984. Tests for autoimmune disease in otology. Am. J. Otol. 5, 447–449.

Mijovic, T., Zeitouni, A., Colmegna, I., 2013. Autoimmune sensorineural hearing loss: the otology-rheumathology interface. Rheumatology. Feb. 21. [Epub ahead of print].

Mora, R., Barbieri, M., Mora, F., Mora, M., Yoo, T.J., 2003. Intravenous infusion of recombinant tissue plasminogen activator for treatment of patients with sudden and/or chronic hearing loss. Ann. Otol. Rhinol. Laryngol. 112, 665–670.

Mora, R., Mora, F., Passali, F.M., Cordone, M.P., Crippa, B., Barbieri, M., 2004. Restoration of immune-mediated sensorineural hearing loss with sodium enoxaparin: a case report. Acta Otolaryngol. Suppl. 552, 25–28.

Naarendorp, M., Spiera, H., 1998. Sudden sensorineural hearing loss in patients with systemic lupus erythematosus or lupus-like syndromes and antiphospholipid antibodies. J. Rheumatol. 25, 589–592.

Nair, T.S., Raphael, Y., Dolan, D.F., Parrett, T.J., Perlman, L.S., Brahmbhatt, V.R., et al., 1995. Monoclonal antibody induced hearing loss. Hear. Res. 83, 101–113.

Nair, T.S., Kozma, K.E., Hoefling, N.L., Kommareddi, P.K., Ueda, Y., Gong, T.W., et al., 2004. Identification and characterization of choline transporter-like protein 2, an inner ear glycoprotein of 68 and 72 kDa that is the target of antibody-induced hearing loss. J. Neurosci. 24, 1772–1779.

Okano, T., Kelley, M.W., 2012. Stem cell therapy for the inner ear: recent advances and future directions. Trends Amplif. 16, 4–18.

Ozcan, M., Karakus, M.F., Gunduz, O.H., Tuncel, U., Sahin, H., 2002. Hearing loss and middle ear involvement in rheumatoid arthritis. Rheumatol. Int. 22, 16–19.

Passali, D., Damiani, V., Mora, R., Passali, F.M., Pssali, G.C., Bellussi, L., 2004. P0 antigen detection in sudden hearing loss and Meniere's disease: a new diagnostic marker? Acta Otolaryngol. 124, 1145–1148.

Pathak, S., Goldofsky, E., Vivas, E.X., Bonagura, V.R., Vambutas, A., 2011. Il-1β is overexpressed and aberrantly regulated in corticosteroid nonresponders with autoimmune inner ear disease. J. Immunol. 186, 1870–1879.

Pham, B.-N., Rudic, M., Bouccara, D., Sterkers, O., Belmatoug, N., Bébéar, J.-P., et al., 2007. Antibodies to myelin protein zero (P0) protein as markers of auto-immune inner ear diseases. Autoimmunity. 40, 202–207.

Puccetti, A., Lunardi, C., 2010. The role of peptide libraries in the identification of novel autoantigen targets in autoimmune diseases. Discov. Med. 9, 224–228.

Rahman, M.U., Poe, D.S., Choi, H.K., 2001. Autoimmune vestibulo-cochlear disorders. Curr. Opin. Rheumatol. 13, 184–189.

Raut, V.V., Cullen, J., Cathers, G., 2001. Hearing loss in rheumatoid arthritis. J. Otolaryngol. 30, 289–294.

Riente, L., Bongiorni, F., Nacci, A., Migliorini, P., Segnini, G., Delle Sedie, A., et al., 2004. Antibodies to inner ear antigens in Meniere's disease. Clin. Exp. Immunol. 135, 159–163.

Roberston, N.G., Cremers, C.W.R.J., Huygen, P.L.M., Ikezono, T., Krastins, B., Kremer, H., et al., 2006. Cochlin immunostaining of inner ear pathologic deposits and proteomic analysis in DFNA9 deafness and vestibular dysfunction. H. Mol. Genetics. 15, 1071–1085.

Ruckenstein, M.J., 2004. Autoimmune inner ear disease. Curr. Opin. Otolaryngol. Head Neck Surg. 12, 426–430.

Salvinelli, F., Cancilleri, F., Casale, M., Luccarelli, V., Di Peco, V., D'Ascanio, L., et al., 2004. Hearing thresholds in patients affected by rheumatoid arthritis. Clin. Otolaryngol. 29, 75–79.

Silva, C.H., Roscoe, I.C., Fernandes, K.P., Novaes, R.M., Lazari, C.S., 2002. Sensorineural hearing loss associated to Kawasaki disease. J. Pediatr. 78, 71–74.

Solares, C.A., Hughes, G.B., Tuohy, V.K., 2003. Autoimmune sensorineural hearing loss: an immunologic perspective. J. Neuroimmunol. 138, 1–7.

Solares, C.A., Edling, A.E., Johnson, J.M., Baek, M., Hirose, K., Hughes, G.B., et al., 2004. Murine autoimmune hearing loss mediated by CD4+ T cells specific for inner ear peptides. J. Clin. Invest. 113, 1210–1217.

Sone, M., Schachern, P.A., Paparella, M.M., Morizono, N., 1999. Study of systemic lupus erythematosus in temporal bones. Ann. Otol. Rhinol. Laryngol. 108, 338–344.

St. Clair, E.W., McCallum, R.M., 1999. Cogan's syndrome. Curr. Opin. Rheumatol. 11, 47–52.

Stone, J.H., Francis, H.W., 2000. Immune-mediated inner ear disease. Curr. Opin. Rheumatol. 12, 32–40.

Suckfull, M., the Hearing Loss Study Group, 2002. Fibrinogen and LDL apheresis in treatment of sudden hearing loss: a randomized multicentre trial. Lancet. 360, 1811–1817.

Suzuki, H., Furukawa, M., Kumagai, M., Takahashi, E., Matsuura, K., Katori, Y., et al., 2003. Defibrinogenation therapy for idiopathic sudden sensorineural hearing loss in comparison with high-dose steroid therapy. Acta Otolaryngol. 123, 46–50.

Takagi, D., Nakamaru, Y., Maguchi, S., Furuta, Y., Fukuda, S., 2002. Otologic manifestations of Wegener's granulomatosis. Laryngoscope. 112, 1684–1690.

Takagi, D., Nakamaru, Y., Maguchi, S., Furuta, Y., Fukuda, S., 2004. Clinical features of bilateral progressive hearing loss associated with myeloperoxidase-antineutrophil cytoplasmic antibody. Ann. Otol. Rhinol. Laryngol. 113, 388–393.

Takahashi, T., Takahashi, K., Mernaugh, R., Drozdoff, V., Sipe, C., Schoecklmann, H., et al., 1999. Endothelial localization of receptor tyrosine phosphatase, ECRTP/DEP1, in developing and mature renal vasculature. J. Am. Soc. Nephrol. 10, 2135–2145.

Teranishi, M., Uchida, Y., Nishio, N., Kato, K., Otake, H., Yoshida, T., et al., 2012. Polymorphisms in genes involved in oxidative stress response in patients with sudden sensorineural hearing loss and Ménière's disease in a Japanese population. DNA Cell Biol. 31, 1555–1562.

Tomiyama, S., 2002. Experimental autoimmune labyrinthitis: assessment of molecular size of autoantigens in fractions of inner ear proteins eluted on the Mini Whole Gel Eluter. Acta Otolaryngol. 122, 692–697.

Toubi, E., Ben-David, J., Kessel, A., Hals, K., Sabo, E., Luntz, M., 2004. Immune-mediated disorders associated with idiopathic sudden sensorineural hearing loss. Ann. Otol. Rhinol. Laryngol. 113, 445–449.

Tsunoda, K., Akaogi, J., Ohya, N., Murofushi, T., 2001. Sensorineural hearing loss as the initial manifestation of polyateritis nodosa. J. Laryngol. Otol. 115, 311–312.

Tucci, D.L., Farmer Jr., J.C., Kitch, R.D., Witsell, D.L., 2002. Treatment of sudden sensorineural hearing loss with systemic steroids and valacyclovir. Otol. Neurotol. 23, 301–308.

Tucci, M., Quatraro, C., Silvestris, F., 2005. Sjögren's syndrome: an autoimmune disorder with otolaryngological involvement. Acta Otorhinolaryngol. Ital. 25, 139–144.

Tumiati, B., Casoli, P., Parmeggiani, A., 1997. Hearing loss in Sjogren's syndrome. Ann. Intern. Med. 126, 450–453.

Um, J.Y., Jang, C.H., Kim, H.L., Cho, Y.B., Park, J., Lee, S.J., et al., 2013. Proinflammatory cytokine IL-1β polymorphisms in sudden sensorineural hearing loss. Immunopharmacol. Immunotoxicol. 35, 52–56.

Uri, N., Doweck, I., Cohen-Kerem, R., Greenberg, E., 2003. Acyclovir in the treatment of idiopathic sudden sensorineural hearing loss. Otolaryngol. Head Neck Surg. 128, 544–549.

Vambutas, A., DeVoti, J., Goldofsky, E., Gordon, M., Lesser, M., Bonagura, V., 2009. Alternate splicing of interleukin-1 receptor type II (IL1R2) in vitro correlates with clinical glucocorticoid responsiveness in patients with AIED. PloS One. 4, 1–9.

Van Doornum, S., McColl, G., Walter, M., Jennens, I., Bhathal, P., Wicks, I.P., 2001. Prolonged prodrome, systemic vasculitis, and deafness in Cogan's syndrome. Ann. Rheum. Dis. 60, 69–71.

Van Schoonhoven, J., Sparreboom, M., van Zanten, B.G., Scholten, R.J., Mylanus, E.A., Dreschler, W.A., et al., 2013. The effectiveness of bilateral cochlear implants for severe-to-profound deafness in adults: a systemic review. Otol. Neurotol. 34, 190–198.

Van Wijk, F., Staecker, H., Keithley, E., Lefebvre, P.P., 2006. Local perfusion of the tumor necrosis factor alpha blocker infliximab to the inner ear improves autoimmune neurosensory hearing loss. Audiol. Neurootol. 11, 357–365.

Vollersten, R., 1990. Vasculitis and Cogan's syndrome. Rheum. Dis. Clin. North Am. 16, 433–438.

Vollertsen, R.S., McDonald, T.J., Younge, B.R., Banks, P.M., Stanson, A.W., Ilstrup, D.M., 1986. Cogan's syndrome: 18 cases and a review of the literature. Mayo Clin. Proc. 61, 344–361.

Vyse, T., Luxon, L.M., Walport, M.J., 1994. Audiovestibular manifestations of the antiphospholipid syndrome. J. Laryngol. Otol. 108, 57–59.

Wang, J.R., Yuen, H.W., Shipp, D.B., Stewart, S., Lin, V.Y.W., Chen, J. M., et al., 2010. Cochlear implantation in patients with autoimmune inner ear disease including Cogan syndrome: a comparison with age- and sex-matched controls. Laryngoscope. 120, 2478–2483.

Weissen-Plenz, G., Sezer, Ö., Vahlhaus, C., Robenek, H., Hoffmeier, A., Tjan, T.D.T., et al., 2010. Aortic dissection associated with Cogan's syndrome: deleterious loss of vascular structural integrity is associated with GM-CSF overstimulation in macrophages and smooth muscle cells. J. Cardiothorac. Surg. 5, 66–70.

Westerlaken, B.O., Stokroos, T.J., Dhooge, I.J., Wit, H.P., Albers, F.W., 2003. Treatment of idiopathic sudden sensorineural hearing loss with antiviral therapy: a prospective, randomised, double-blind clinical trial. Ann. Otol. Rhinol. Laryngol. 112, 993–1000.

Yariz, K.O., Duman, D., Seco, C.Z., Dallman, J., Huang, M., Peters, T. A., et al., 2012. Mutations in OTOGL, encoding the inner ear protein otogelin-like, cause moderate sensorineural hearing loss. Am. J. Hum. Genet. 91, 872–882.

Yehudai, D., Shoenfeld, Y., Toubi, E., 2006. The autoimmune characteristics of progressive or sudden sensorineural hearing loss. Autoimmunity. 39, 153–158.

Yeom, K., Gray, J., Nair, T.S., Arts, H.A., Telian, S.A., Disher, M.J., et al., 2003. Antibodies to HSP-70 in normal donors and autoimmune hearing loss patients. Laryngoscope. 113, 1770–1776.

Yoo, T.J., Du, X., Known, S.S., 2002. Molecular mechanism of autoimmune hearing loss. Acta Otolaryngol. (Suppl. 548), 3–9.

Yue, W.L., Li, P.Y., Qi, P.Y., Li, H.J., Zhou, H., 2003. Role for low-molecular-weight heparins in the treatment of sudden hearing loss. Am. J. Otol. 24, 328–333.

Zhao, Z.S., Granucci, F., Yeh, L., Schaffer, P.A., Cantor, H., 1998. Molecular mimicry by herpes simplex virus-type 1: autoimmune disease after viral infection. Science. 279, 1344–1347.

Zhou, B., Kermany, M.H., Glickstein, J., Cai, Q., Cai, C., Zhou, Y., et al., 2011a. Murine autoimmune hearing loss mediated by CD4 + T cells specific for β-tubulin. Clin. Immunol. 138, 222–230.

Zhou, Y., Yuan, J., Zhou, B., Lee, A.J, Lee, A.J, Ghawji Jr., M., et al., 2011b. The therapeutic efficacy of human adipose tissue-derived mesenchymal stem cells on experimental autoimmune hearing loss in mice. Immunology. 133, 133–140.

Zhou, B., Kermany, M.H., Cai, C., Zhou, Y., Nair, U., Liu, W., et al., 2012. Experimental autoimmune hearing loss is exacerbated in IL-10-deficient mice and reversed by IL-10 gene transfer. Gene. Ther. 19, 228–235.

Chapter 57

Encephalomyelopathies

Eric Lancaster

Department of Neurology, University of Pennsylvania, Philadelphia, PA, USA

Chapter Outline

Introduction	817	Glycine Receptor (GlyR)	822
Neurological Syndromes of Autoimmune Causation	818	Voltage-Gated Potassium Channel Complex (VGKC)	823
Cerebral Syndromes	818	LGI1	823
Ataxia	818	Caspr2	824
Spinal Myelitis	818	PCA-Tr	824
Stiff Person Syndrome	818	CNS Diseases with Autoantibodies to Intracellular Antigens	824
Systemic Immunopathic Disorders with Encephalitis and Myelitis	818	GAD65	824
Systemic Lupus Erythematosus	818	Amphiphysin I	824
Sarcoidosis	819	Neuronal Nuclear Antigens (NNA)	825
Sjögren's Syndrome	819	ANNA-1/anti-Hu	825
Behçet's Disease	820	ANNA-2 (anti-Ri)	825
Diseases with Autoantibodies to Cell-surface Channels, Receptors	820	ANNA-3	825
Neuromyelitis Optica (NMO; Devic's disease)	820	Ma1/Ma2 (Ma and Ta)	825
Encephalitis with Antibodies to N-methyl-d-aspartate Receptor (NMDAR)	821	Purkinje Cell Antigen-1 (PCA-1; Yo)	826
Anti-AMPAR	822	PCA-2	826
Anti-GABA-B-R	822	Conclusions and Future Prospects	826
Group 1 Metabotropic Glutamate Receptors (mGluR1, mGluR5)	822	Acknowledgments	827
		Abbreviations	827
		References	827

INTRODUCTION

A new understanding of neuronal autoimmunity has evolved rapidly over the last few decades. Historically, multisystem autoimmune disorders, notably systemic lupus erythematosus (SLE, lupus) and sarcoidosis, have been long recognized to affect the central nervous system (CNS). Autoimmunity to specific neuronal antigens was the first-described involvement of the peripheral nervous system (PNS) with the recognition in myasthenia gravis of pathogenic autoantibodies to the acetylcholine receptor (AChR). Subsequently numerous autoantibodies to intracellular CNS and PNS antigens, starting with ANNA-1 (Hu), were associated with neurological syndromes, often in the setting of an extraneural malignancy. These "paraneoplastic" syndromes can affect the brain, brainstem, spinal cord, cerebellum, nerve roots, and peripheral nerves. Although the syndromes appear to reflect damage to neurons expressing the antigens, the symptoms bear little relationship to the actual functions of these antigens. It was proposed initially that these "onconeuronal" antibodies were directly pathogenic, but more likely they mark a cell-lethal T cell response. Next, and starting with autoantibodies to the voltage-gated potassium channel (VGKC) complex, a series of antibodies to various neurotransmitter receptors, synaptic proteins, and cell adhesion molecules were described. Here, the autoantibodies likely do have direct effects on the target antigens, and the symptoms so induced resemble those caused by genetic or pharmacologic disruption of the cognate receptor. Notably, the discovery of aquaporin-4 (AQP4) antibodies has provided a plausible mechanism for neuromyelitis optica (NMO) and

N. Rose & I. Mackay (Eds): The Autoimmune Diseases, Fifth edition. DOI: http://dx.doi.org/10.1016/B978-0-12-384929-8.00057-5

related disorders. The particular focus of this chapter is on autoimmune disorders associated with encephalitis or myelitis, subdivided into three groups: (1) systemic diseases with CNS manifestations, (2) CNS diseases with antibodies to synaptic and cell-surface proteins, and (3) CNS diseases with antibodies to intracellular antigens.

NEUROLOGICAL SYNDROMES OF AUTOIMMUNE CAUSATION

Autoimmunity affecting the CNS may result in diverse clinical syndromes, including encephalitis, psychiatric symptoms, acquired epilepsy, cerebellitis, stiff person syndrome, and myelitis. Before surveying the implicated disorders, these clinical presentations should be considered.

The diagnosis of autoimmune CNS disorders requires clinical history and neurological examination to define the syndrome, neuro-imaging and laboratory testing to exclude other causes, and specific serological testing to confirm an autoimmune basis. Since these autoimmune syndromes are often treatable, their recognition is important. We can list the clinical presentations as follows.

Cerebral Syndromes

Autoimmune encephalitis which most often develops sub-acutely, over weeks or months, with memory loss, confusion, unusual behaviors including hallucinations or delusions, and fluctuating levels of consciousness.

Psychiatric disorders which may be prominent early, as in encephalitis with disruption of critical receptors, NMDAR and AMPAR, thus resembling schizophrenia or new onset psychosis.

Epilepsy wherein onset of seizures or unusual movements or features of autonomic disorder should prompt consideration of autoimmune encephalitis.

Ataxia

Ataxia due to cerebellitis which may occur as an isolated syndrome or as part of a more general encephalitis wherein patients typically have ataxia of limb, trunk, and/or ocular movements with nystagmus, diplopia, vertigo, and nausea.

In these presentations, an infectious cause such as herpes simplex virus encephalitis will be suspected and excluded after CSF analysis and other specific testing. Also, patients will be assessed for inflammatory/autoimmune conditions (SLE, sarcoidosis), fulminant multiple sclerosis and paraneoplastic causes, including cancer screening and testing for paraneoplastic autoantibodies. While many cases of encephalitis lack any specific clues to an autoimmune etiology, there are findings that do suggest a specific diagnosis. Thus, NMDA receptor autoantibodies are associated with a distinct clinical syndrome described

below, and autoantibodies to the VGKC complex mark patients with coexisting neuromyotonia, thymoma, and/or myasthenia gravis. Autoantibodies to Tr (or more precisely DNER) or rarely to mGluR1 are found in some patients with cerebellitis in the setting of Hodgkin's lymphoma. If specific clues are lacking, testing for autoantibodies to a panel of candidate antigens is appropriate.

Spinal Myelitis

Spinal myelitis affects the long tracts of the spinal cord resulting in numbness and weakness of the extremities. Damage to spinal cord gray matter also results in flaccid paralysis and/or depressed tendon reflexes at affected levels. Due to the longer fiber tracts between brain and lower spinal cord, symptoms affecting the lower extremities, bowel, and bladder are the most prominent. Sensory loss is characterized by a spinal sensory level, or differential effects on the sensory pathways for pain/temperature and vibration/proprioception, which may run along different sides of the cord and be unequally disrupted. Rapidly progressive disorders may initially present as "spinal shock" with suppressed reflexes, whereas in sub-acutely progressive cases, or the chronic state, hyper-reflexia and upper motor neuron signs become prominent.

Stiff Person Syndrome

Stiff person syndrome presents as stiffness of the limbs and/or trunk. Patients lack sensory deficits, abnormal reflexes, or upper motor neuron signs, so that Parkinson's disease or a related disorder is suspected. An autoimmune basis is confirmed by positive serological tests and/or improvement with immunotherapy. While a specific autoantibody syndrome cannot be distinguished with certainty, particular findings suggest specific diagnoses. Thus, stiffness with acquired hyperekplexia (an extremely exaggerated startle response) has been associated with autoantibodies to the glycine receptor, and stiff person syndrome in the setting of gynecologic cancers with autoantibodies to amphiphysin.

SYSTEMIC IMMUNOPATHIC DISORDERS WITH ENCEPHALITIS AND MYELITIS

Various of the multisystem/vasculitic diseases have a well-described involvement of the CNS but, striking as the features may be, there is no consistently demonstrable CNS-specific mechanism of neuronal damage.

Systemic Lupus Erythematosus

SLE may have diverse neuropsychiatric expressions, including cerebrovascular events, stroke, transient ischemic attack

(TIA), encephalitis, movement disorders most commonly chorea, headache, seizures, anxiety, and/or psychosis (see Chapter 32). The American College of Rheumatology (1999) proposed criteria for 19 distinct neuropsychiatric symptoms associated with SLE with 12 involving the CNS. The large retrospective analysis of Chiewthanakul et al. (2012) showed that 13% of patients with SLE were affected by these CNS disorders, most often seizures, vascular events, and/or psychosis: their mortality rate was 18.8%. In patients with neuropsychiatric features attributed to SLE, these were the presenting signs in some 40% (Padovan et al., 2012). A standardized set of measurements for neuropsychiatric impairment associated with SLE has been proposed for clinical trials (Mikdashi et al., 2007). In SLE, many of the neurological syndromes have a high frequency in the general population (e.g., headache) or have other risk factors (e.g., hypertension for stroke), making it unclear whether or not SLE is causally involved. However, several studies have associated antiphospholipid antibodies with neurovascular complications (Sanna et al., 2003; Mikdashi and Handwerger, 2004; Govoni et al., 2012).

Some 1–2% of patients with SLE are affected by transverse myelitis (Provenzale et al., 1994); these were more likely to be African American, and to have an elevated CSF IgG index and erythrocyte sedimentation rate (Schulz et al., 2011). Birnbaum and colleagues distinguished two subgroups with myelitis: those with primarily long-tract signs (spasticity, hyper-reflexia) and those with flaccid paralysis (indicating gray matter damage) (Birnbaum et al., 2009). The former group was more likely to meet criteria for neuromyelitis optica, and the second group had a worse outcome (Birnbaum et al., 2009). Episodes of transverse myelitis are accompanied by other signs of active SLE in only half of the cases, and in 25% of patients with SLE-associated myelitis there were no prior systemic signs of SLE (Espinosa et al., 2010). Patients typically have sensory, motor, and urinary dysfunction (Espinosa et al., 2010). MR imaging shows T2 hyperintense lesions of the cervical or mid-lower thoracic spinal cord in some patients with less extensive disease and in almost all with lesions involving more than four cord segments (Kovacs et al., 2000; Espinosa et al., 2010). Therapy with steroids, cyclophosphamide, rituximab, mycophenolate mofetil and other agents has given mixed results (Mok et al., 1998, 2006; Kovacs et al., 2000; Birnbaum et al., 2009). Two case series showed statistically non-significant associations between early immunotherapy and better outcomes (Harisdangkul et al., 1995; Lu et al., 2008). A minority of patients recover completely. Recurrences are common (Provenzale et al., 1994).

Several immune mechanisms have been proposed to cause CNS disorders associated with lupus. Thrombosis and infarction, such as may be associated with the prothrombotic state (e.g., aPL antibodies), may result in stroke or venous sinus thrombosis (Sanna et al., 2003; Mikdashi and Handwerger, 2004; Govoni et al., 2012). More rarely, vasculitis may be implicated. Inflammatory cytokines have been proposed to affect cognition and injure neurons. Antineuronal antibodies are more common in SLE patients with CNS disease than those without CNS manifestations (Kang et al., 2008; Cojocaru et al., 2010). Specific antibodies to several different neuronal antigens have also been reported (Iizuka et al., 2010). However, it has not been established whether any of these antibodies are pathogenic. Antibodies whose pathogenesis is more likely (e.g., NMDAR or AMPAR) may also be found in lupus patients

Sarcoidosis

Sarcoidosis is not formally enumerable as an autoimmune disease, although this possibility has been raised from time to time. Neural tissues are affected in 5–13% of patients, including peripheral nerves, cranial nerves, meninges, brain (including hypothalamus), and/or spinal cord (Lacomis, 2011). In about half of the cases, the neurological symptoms were the initial presentation (Chapelon et al., 1990; Zajicek et al., 1999; Joseph and Scolding, 2009). Cranial nerve involvement of the optic, facial, or multiple cranial nerves was the most common manifestation (Zajicek et al., 1999; Joseph and Scolding, 2009; Pawate et al., 2009). Meningitis particularly affecting the basilar meninges may occur with or without associated cranial neuropathies (Gullapalli and Phillips, 2002). The definitive demonstration of non-caseating granulomas in the affected areas of the nervous system is available only in a minority of cases. More often, a diagnosis of probable neurosarcoidosis is made based upon accessory evidence (Zajicek et al., 1999). Treatment with corticosteroids is usual and some patients do improve (Lower et al., 1997; Joseph and Scolding, 2009; Lacomis, 2011). Patients refractory to initial therapy have received numerous other immunosuppressive medications, including azathioprine, cyclophosphamide, and methotrexate (Lower et al., 1997; Scott et al., 2007), or even cranial irradiation (Chapelon et al., 1990; Agbogu et al., 1995) but optimal regimens are not yet established. The actual immunological nature of the sarcoid process remains obscure.

Sjögren's Syndrome

Sjögren's syndrome is an autoimmune inflammatory disease affecting salivary and lacrimal glands. Approximately 25% of patients have features of PNS or CNS involvement, most typically sensory neuropathy, sensory neuronopathy, or mononeuritis multiplex (Sene et al., 2011). However, the true percentage of neurologically affected patients is controversial, in part due to the wide diversity of manifestations (Soliotis et al., 2004) such as encephalitis, cerebellitis, aseptic meningitis, brainstem syndromes, migraines, seizures, and psychiatric symptoms. Alexander et al. (Alexander, 1993; Alexander et al., 1986, 1994) demonstrated intrathecal antibody synthesis in patients with encephalopathic Sjögren's syndrome and suggested vasculopathy as a pathogenic mechanism, and reported an association between the presence in serum of anti-Ro (SS-A) and more severe CNS disease. More recently, Estiasari et al. found that one-third of patients with Sjögren's syndrome, particularly those with spinal cord lesions or optic neuritis, had antibodies to AQP4 (Estiasari et al., 2012). Given the important prognostic therapeutic and mechanistic implications of these antibodies (see following section on NMO), a patient with Sjögren's syndrome and CNS symptoms should be tested for anti-AQP4. The pathophysiology of anti-AQP4-negative patients with Sjögren's syndrome and CNS symptoms is unclear and may involve other as yet undiscovered autoimmune reactivities.

Behçet's Disease

Behçet's disease is a multisystem inflammatory vasculitic disorder characterized by oral aphthae, genital ulcerations, and uveitis. The typical patient is male, aged 30–40 years, with recurrent attacks of inflammation affecting the eye, oral and genital mucosa, the gastrointestinal (GI) tract, large vessels, or CNS (Sakane et al., 1999). The disease is most common in a region extending from Turkey to East Asia (Nishiyama et al., 1999; Siva and Saip, 2009). Some 50% of patients experience neurological disorder, almost always involving the CNS (Akman-Demir et al., 1999; Borhani Haghighi et al., 2005). Involvement of pyramidal motor pathways is common, particularly in the brainstem, and other presentations included sensory deficits, cerebellar ataxia, and/or cranial nerve or brainstem abnormalities. Most patients have discrete attacks, most commonly including hemiparesis, and a half have behavioral changes. Inirect effects on the CNS from venous sinus thrombosis or the superior vena cava syndrome may occur (Siva and Saip, 2009), possibly as part of a thrombophilia affecting other tissues (Yazici et al., 2007). Pathological studies have revealed perivascular lymphocytic infiltrates, especially in the basal ganglia, midbrain, and thalamus (Borhani Haghighi et al., 2007), whereas others report perivascular neutrophilic infiltrates (Arai et al., 2006). Brain perfusion MRI showed prolonged mean transit time for cerebral blood flow and decreased relative cerebral blood flow in patients with neuro-Behçet's disease and Behçet's disease without neurological symptoms (Alkan et al., 2012), suggesting that sub-clinical CNS involvement may be common,

and that distinction between patients with and without CNS symptoms is simply a matter of degree.

DISEASES WITH AUTOANTIBODIES TO CELL-SURFACE CHANNELS, RECEPTORS

Neuromyelitis Optica (NMO; Devic's disease)

NMO has been the subject of the transformative discovery of autoimmunity affecting a water channel, aquaporin-4 (AQP4). Long considered a variant of multiple sclerosis, NMO is characterized by episodes of often bilateral optic neuritis, spinal cord lesions often longitudinally extensive and very disabling, and a relative paucity of brain lesions. The identification in NMO of an initially characteristic pattern for an autoantibody response, subsequently defined as specific anti-AQP4 antibodies, has revolutionized our understanding of this disorder (Lennon et al., 2004): as many as 77% of patients with a clinical diagnosis of NMO have AQP4 antibodies (Waters et al., 2012). In addition to lesions of the optic nerves and spinal cord, half of the patients show brain lesions on MRI (Nagaishi et al., 2011) particularly frequently in children (Pena et al., 2011), and such may be the presenting feature in children or adults (Kim et al., 2011).

Detection of AQP4 antibodies has important clinical implications including presence during an initial clinical event suggesting a risk of further attacks (Weinshenker et al., 2006). The severe disability caused by NMO should prompt potent therapies immediately upon diagnosis (Sato et al., 2012). Notably, interferon-β therapy, successfully used to treat MS, appears to worsen rather than benefit NMO (Kim et al., 2012); also, in a single case report, there was worsening in a patient given the drug fingolimod used orally in MS (Min et al., 2012). But other "suppressive" therapies such as the anti-IL-6 monoclonal antibody tocilizumab (Araki et al., 2013) and azathioprine (Costanzi et al., 2011) do appear to be effective in NMO. Finally, studies on anti-idiotypic antibodies directed against patients' AQP4 antibodies might provide a highly specific therapy for NMO (Tradtrantip et al., 2012). A recent open-label study of eculizumab, a monoclonal antibody that inhibits the complement protein C5, showed promising results for stopping attacks and improving disability in patients with active NMO (Pittock et al., 2013).

AQP4 proteins are water channels expressed in astrocytes and other cells, and organize into large molecular aggregates called orthogonal arrays of particles (Jung et al., 1994; Rossi et al., 2012). AQP4 channels are important for regulating brain water balance, astrocyte migration, glial scar formation, and responses to brain edema and injury (Verkman et al., 2006). AQP4 antibodies target extracellular (surface) epitopes, predominantly in the C-loop, and these surface epitopes may be formed by the interactions of APQ4 subunits in functional tetramers (Iorio and Lennon, 2012). AQP4 antibodies are thought to cause internalization of AQP4 channels, along with the closely associated glutamate transporter EAAT2, disrupting both water and glutamate homeostasis for astrocytes (Hinson et al., 2008). AQP4 exists as two major isoforms, M23 and M1, that have identical extracellular domains but are affected differently by patients' antibodies (Crane et al., 2009; Hinson et al., 2012). The M1 isoform is internalized but the M23 isoform is found in the large orthogonal arrays that resist internalization, and more effectively activate complement. Antibodies disrupt the ability of both types of channel to conduct water, but complement fixation may be important for determining the severity of clinical attacks; sera from patients experiencing severe attacks is more effective at fixing complement on AQP4-expressing cells than sera from patients with milder attacks and a similar anti-AQP4 level (Hinson et al., 2009). The strongest evidence that AQP4 antibodies are directly pathogenic comes from animal experiments in which IgG from affected humans is directly injected into the brain of rodents. The IgG, particularly along with complement, reproduced the characteristic pathology of neuromyelitis optica (Bradl et al., 2009; Saadoun et al., 2010) and this pathology was abrogated in aquaporin-4-null mice, confirming that AQP4-specific antibodies are critical for the disease. The promising effects of the C5 complement inhibitor eculizumab on patients' attacks provides a powerful argument that complement activation is important for pathogenesis in humans (Pittock et al., 2013).

It is unknown what triggers development of AQP4 antibodies and NMO. Patients generally do not have unusual mutations or polymorphisms of AQP4 (Matiello et al., 2011). Some with NMO have coexisting myasthenia gravis (Jarius et al., 2012; Leite et al., 2012) and, in one series, 19% had co-morbid Sjögren's syndrome and 13% co-morbid thyroid disease, suggesting predisposition in NMO to form multiple autoantibodies (Nagaishi et al., 2011). Reported pedigrees of multiple affected family members suggest a complex genetic susceptibility to formation of AQP4 antibodies (Matiello et al., 2010).

Testing for NMO antibody reactivity initially involved indirect immunofluorescence against a composite substrate of mouse tissues, specifically at the blood–brain barrier, to detect a characteristic pattern of reactivity (Lennon et al., 2004). A recent study comparing the multiple methods available now found ELISA and detecting IgG binding to transfected cells (by flow cytometry or visual observation with fluorescent antibodies) to be most sensitive and specific (Waters et al., 2012). The recent identification of antibodies to the Kir4.1 inwardly-rectifying potassium channel in a subset of patients with

MS hints that other specific autoantibody-associated syndromes might account for other subsets currently diagnosed with MS (Srivastava et al., 2012).

Encephalitis with Antibodies to N-methyl-d-aspartate Receptor (NMDAR)

NMDAR targets an ionotropic, excitatory glutamate receptor that has a relatively high permeability to calcium, and hence is important for triggering calcium-dependent synaptic plasticity. NMDARs are structurally and functionally diverse tetramers comprised of many combinations of the eight GluN1 isoforms, the four GluN2 isoforms, and the two GluN3 isoforms (Paoletti, 2011). Antibodies to the GluN1 (NR1) subunit were initially reported in young women with encephalitis and ovarian teratoma, some of whom responded to tumor therapy and/or immunotherapy (Dalmau et al., 2007). Subsequently, hundreds of cases have been reported, so expanding and further clarifying the associated disorder (Dalmau et al., 2011). Some patients have an initial prodrome resembling a viral illness, and the onset of disease, whether behavioral or psychiatric, includes hallucinations, delusions, agitation, inappropriate (violent or hypersexual) behaviors, and/or decreased speech. Memory loss is nearly universal, although often overlooked in the setting of dramatic psychotic features resembling those seen initially in schizophrenia. Patients then develop seizures, decreased responsiveness, and/or autonomic instability. Writhing movements of the face, tongue, and extremities may occur. A catatonic or comatose state develops, and central respiratory failure may require mechanical ventilation. With treatment, patients usually become more responsive, but may pass through the "psychotic" stage of the illness again before recovering more fully. The resemblance of symptoms to effects of pharmacologic NMDAR blockade has been noted (Dalmau et al., 2011). Anti-NMDAR encephalitis affects children, and symptoms may differ from those in adults: behavioral change is a common presenting sign and language disruption, sleep disruption, seizures, and abnormal movements are common at diagnosis (Florance et al., 2009).

Based on the rapid accrual of cases, anti-NMDAR is probably the most common type of CNS synaptic autoantibody (Dalmau et al., 2011). Some 80% of patients are female and 59% have ovarian teratomas (Dalmau et al., 2008). Neuronal tissues within these teratomas express NMDAR, and patients' antibodies are found bound to these receptors, indicating that the teratomas trigger the immune response; in patients without teratomas the source of the response is unknown, but some of the patients appear predisposed to forming autoantibodies. While peak age incidence appears to be between 13 and 30, all ages may be affected, including infants and the elderly (Dalmau et al., 2011). Although clinical trials to define the optimal treatment have not been done, treatment of the tumor and/or with immunotherapy is associated with better outcomes. Treatment with corticosteroids and IVIg is usually followed, failing a good response, by second line treatment with cyclophosphamide and/or rituximab. Approximately 75% of patients have a substantial recovery (Dalmau et al., 2011).

NMDAR antibodies appear to be directly pathogenic. IgG from patients causes cross-linking and internalization of synaptic NMDARs, resulting in decreased NMDAR-mediated synaptic currents (Dalmau et al., 2008; Hughes et al., 2010). This rapid functional disruption of NMDAR-mediated neurotransmission would account for patients' symptoms by disruption of NMDAR-dependent synaptic circuits (Moscato et al., 2010). Notably, affected neurons are able to restore their synapses and function after removal of the antibodies. Consistent with this, autopsy studies have shown widespread antibody binding to CNS neurons but not significant neuronal death (Tuzun et al., 2009).

Testing for anti-NMDAR consists in screening with indirect immunofluorescence for IgG reactivity to cultured cells expressing the NR1 subunit of the receptor.

Anti-AMPAR

The extracellular domains of the GluR1 and GluR2 subunits of the 2-amino-3-(5-methyl-3-oxo-1,2-oxazol-4-yl) propanoic acid receptor, (AMPAR) is the reactant for autoantibodies (anti-AMPAR) that have been reported in patients with encephalitis (Lai et al., 2009). AMPAR is the other main ionotropic glutamate receptor, along with NMDAR, used in the human brain for rapid excitatory synaptic transmission; it is critical for learning and memory (Lee and Kirkwood, 2011). Patients with anti-AMPAR may present with either encephalitis or psychiatric symptoms, and the patients may have tumors of the lung, breast, or thymus (Bataller et al., 2010; Graus et al., 2010). Anti-AMPAR antibodies have effects similar to those of anti-NMDAR in causing antibody-mediated capping and internalization of the receptor, and disruption of AMPAR-mediated synaptic transmission (Lai et al., 2009).

Testing for anti-AMPAR is by screening with indirect immunofluorescence for IgG reactivity to cultured cells expressing the GluR1 and GluR2 subunits of the receptor.

Anti-GABA-B-R

The γ-amino-butyric acid receptor B is a metabotropic GABA receptor that can exert both pre- and post-synaptic inhibitory effects. In particular, autoantibodies to the extracellular domain of the B1 subunit are found in patients with encephalitis, especially encephalitis with severe seizures or status epilepticus (Lancaster et al., 2010). The receptors consist of two subunits, a B1 subunit

important for GABA binding, and a B2 subunit important for effecting inhibition (Bettler et al., 2004). Small cell lung cancer is found in about half of the patients; in fact, GABA-B-R may be the most common type of synaptic autoantibody in patients with this tumor type (Boronat et al., 2011). The clinical improvement of some patients with tumor- and/or immune-therapy supports a functional effect of the antibodies.

Testing for anti-GABA-B-R is carried out by screening with indirect immunofluorescence for IgG reactivity to cultured cells expressing the GABA-B1 subunit of the receptor.

Group 1 Metabotropic Glutamate Receptors (mGluR1, mGluR5)

These receptors are closely homologous (85% by amino acid structure) but serve distinct functions: mGluR1 is critical for rapid synaptic transmission in the cerebellum, whereas mGluR5 is more important for synaptic plasticity in the hippocampus, for learning, and for memory (Ichise et al., 2000; Faas et al., 2002). Autoantibodies to mGluR1 have been reported in four patients with cerebellitis, two having Hodgkin's lymphoma (HL) (Sillevis Smitt et al., 2000; Coesmans et al., 2003; Marignier et al., 2010; Lancaster et al., 2011a). These antibodies have demonstratively functional effects on neurons. Interestingly, neoplastic HL cells are not thought to express mGluR1, but may rather trigger the disease by causing dysregulation of the immune system. mGluR1 antibodies may be directly pathogenic, since injection of mGluR1 antibodies near the cerebellum of rodents induces reversible ataxia, and mGluR1 antibodies partially attenuated long-term depression (LTD) in cerebellar slices (Coesmans et al., 2003).

Antibodies to mGluR5 have been found in two patients with Ophelia syndrome, a form of encephalitis associated with Hodgkin's lymphoma that improves rapidly with tumor treatment (Lancaster et al., 2011a). Despite the close homology between these two antigens, the autoimmune syndromes are clinically and immunologically distinct—and the antibodies do not cross-react. These two rare disorders raise the distinct possibility that there are other synaptic proteins and receptors that are autoantigenic causes of presently uncharacterized syndromes.

Testing for mGluR1 and mGluR5 antibodies is done by screening with indirect immunofluorescence for IgG reactivity to cultured cells expressing the respective receptors.

Glycine Receptor (GlyR)

GlyR is the major inhibitory ionotropic receptor in the brainstem and spinal cord, and consists of five units (α1–4, β) (Hernandes and Troncone, 2009). Pharmacologic inhibition of the GlyR with strychnine results in painful and debilitating muscle spasms, and pathologically exaggerated startle responses, but preserved consciousness. Genetic mutations of GlyR are found in patients with hereditary hyperekplexia (human startle disease) (Harvey et al., 2008). Autoantibodies to the α1 subunit of the GlyR were first reported in a patient with progressive encephalitis with myoclonus and rigidity (PERM), a disorder characterized by muscle spasms, stiffness, and exaggerated startle responses (Hutchinson et al., 2008); subsequently, similar patients were identified (Mas et al., 2011; Piotrowicz et al., 2011). Thereafter a series of patients with stiff person syndrome and its variants associated with anti-GlyR antibodies, to the α1 subunit and other subunits as well, has been reported (McKeon, 2012). This disorder is not known to be cancer associated, and sometimes responds to immunotherapy. The resemblance of the autoimmune syndrome to effects of pharmacological and genetic disruption of the receptor suggests a functional effect of the antibodies. Testing for these glycine receptor antibodies is performed by screening with indirect immunofluorescence for IgG reactivity to cultured cells expressing the receptor subunits.

Voltage-Gated Potassium Channel Complex (VGKC)

The VGKC contained Kv1.1/Kv1.2, "Kv1," and regulates, voltage-gated potassium channels, and thus the excitability of neurons, shaping action potential discharge and synaptic transmission, and controlling axonal excitability (Robbins and Tempel, 2012). Kv1 channels are homo- or hetero meric tetramers of α subunits, along with four associated β subunits, allowing for functional diversity. Antibodies to the VGKC complex were first detected in patients with Isaacs' syndrome, an autoimmune disorder of acquired peripheral nerve hyperexcitability (Hart et al., 1997). Patients with Isaacs' syndrome have the subacute onset of muscle twitching, cramps, and stiffness, sometimes accompanied by hyperhidrosis, and electrodiagnostic testing showed abnormal spontaneous action potential discharges originating from peripheral nerve axons (Isaacs, 1961, 1967). Some patients were found to have thymomas and some responded to plasmapheresis, suggesting an antibody-mediated pathogenesis (Sinha et al., 1991; Shillito et al., 1995). Due to the resemblance of Isaacs' syndrome to poisoning with the Kv1 toxin α-dendrotoxin, it seemed plausible that patients might have autoantibodies to the VGKC complex. A test for VGKC complex antibodies was therefore designed based on the ability of patients' IgG to immunoprecipitate Kv1 channels labeled with ^{125}I-α-dendrotoxin. Over the last 15 years hundreds of patients have been reported with these antibodies (Apiwattanakul et al., 2010; Irani et al., 2010). These patients may have peripheral nerve

hyperexcitability, encephalitis, or both encephalitis and peripheral nerve hyperexcitability (Morvan's syndrome) (Tan et al., 2008). Several other less common clinical accompaniments, such as unexplained epilepsy and pain syndromes, have also been reported.

While the autoantibodies were initially thought to directly target Kv1 subunits (Kleopa et al., 2006), recent work has shown that other members of the VGKC complex are actually the primary autoantigens, such as leucine-rich gliomainactivated 1 (LGI1) and contactin-associated protein-like 2 (Caspr2) (Irani et al., 2010; Lai et al., 2010). A small fraction of those with anti-VGKC may have autoantibodies that directly target Kv1 subunits. Another small group of patients have antibodies reactive with contactin-2 but, since many also have antibodies to LGI or Caspr2, the clinical significance of this finding is uncertain (Irani et al., 2010). It should be noted that in a considerable fraction of cases with antibodies to the VGKC complex, particularly those with solely peripheral nervous system manifestations, the target autoantigens are unknown. Since the ^{125}I-α-dendrotoxin assay detects most, but not all, patients with LGI1 and Caspr2 antibodies, it is often used as a screening test. Specific detection of LGI1 or Caspr2 antibodies is done with indirect immunofluorescence of sera or CSF against cells transfected to express the proteins.

LGI1

This is a secreted protein that binds to pre- and post-synaptic proteins at CNS synapses (Fukata et al., 2010). LGI1 interacts with presynaptic Kv1 channels via the transmembrane protein ADAM23, and also with post-synaptic AMPA receptors via the transmembrane protein ADAM22 (Fukata et al., 2006; Sagane et al., 2008). Genetic mutations of LGI1 in humans account for a relatively common form of inherited epilepsy known as autosomal dominant lateral temporal lobe epilepsy or autosomal dominant partial epilepsy with auditory features (Gu et al., 2002; Kalachikov et al., 2002; Morante-Redolat et al., 2002). Animals with genetic deletion of LGI1 die of intractable seizures about 10–14 days after birth (Yu et al., 2010). Patients with anti-LGI1 have encephalitis without peripheral nerve manifestations, consistent with the CNS expression pattern of LGI1 (Irani et al., 2010; Lai et al., 2010). Some patients may have prominent myoclonus and cognitive impairment, and there may be an initial clinical suspicion of Creutzfeld–Jakob disease (Geschwind et al., 2008). Most patients improve with treatment and outcomes are relatively good. There are no strong associations with cancer in these patients. It is unknown how antibodies to LGI1 cause disease. LGI1 associates with Kv1 channels, explaining the positive ^{125}I-α-dendrotoxin assay results, but it also associates with other synaptic proteins such as

AMPA receptors. Therefore, while anti-LGI1 may well disrupt the VGKC complex, other equally plausible mechanisms are proposed (Lancaster and Dalmau, 2012).

Caspr2

Caspr2 is a transmembrane protein expressed on CNS and PNS axons (Poliak et al., 1999). Caspr2 is critical for concentrating Kv1 potassium channels at the juxtapara-nodes of myelinated axons, although the precise mechanism by which this is accomplished is unknown (Traka et al., 2003; Horresh et al., 2010). Genetic mutations in the human gene encoding Caspr2, *CNTNAP2*, have been associated with epilepsy, autism and other intellectual disabilities, and defective neuronal migration (Verkerk et al., 2003; Arking et al., 2008; Gregor et al., 2011; Penagarikano et al., 2011; Whalley et al., 2011). Patients with anti-Caspr2 may have encephalitis or peripheral nerve hyperexcitability or both (Irani et al., 2010; Lancaster et al., 2011b). The symptoms may occur in either order, potentially months or years apart. Some patients with anti-Caspr2 have thymoma and/or myasthenia gravis, but most do not have any tumor. Outcomes are relatively good; most patients improve with immunotherapy although relapses occur.

PCA-Tr

Autoantibodies to PCA-Tr (Tr antibodies) are associated with paraneoplastic cerebellar degeneration (PCD) in the setting of Hodgkin's lymphoma (HL), or more rarely non-Hodgkin's lymphoma (Bernal et al., 2003). Anti-PCA-Tr are probably rarer than either Yo or Hu antibodies among patients with PCD (see below), but are more common than mGluR1 antibodies (Shams'ili et al., 2003). Anti-PCD-Tr react with cerebellar Purkinje cells, and were initially defined by their fine granular staining of these neurons (Graus et al., 1997). Recent work has shown the Delta/notch-like epidermal growth factor-related receptor (DNER) to be the actual autoantigen (de Graaff et al., 2012), but the precise mechanisms of pathogenesis are unknown. Since the antibodies react with surface epitopes of the DNER on living neurons, an antibody-mediated mechanism is possible. However, pathological studies from these patients typically show a permanent loss of cerebellar neurons and patients often respond poorly to immunotherapy (Bernal et al., 2003). These findings suggest cytotoxic effects of either the antibodies or a coexisting T cell-mediated response.

While testing for anti-Tr initially involved recognizing a pattern of reactivity with cerebellar neurons, screening with indirect immunofluorescence for IgG reactivity to cultured cells expressing the DNER is more specific for this disorder.

CNS DISEASES WITH AUTOANTIBODIES TO INTRACELLULAR ANTIGENS

GAD65

The 65 kd isoform of glutamic carboxylase (GAD) is the autoantigen for prevalent autoantibodies associated with stiff person syndrome (SPS) and cerebellar ataxia, and, more rarely, other syndromes such as encephalitis and epilepsy (Meinck et al., 2001; Pittock et al., 2006). Anti-GAD65 is characteristically associated with type 1 diabetes (Baekkeskov et al., 1990). Along with the GAD67 isoform (which is not intrinsically autoantigenic), GAD65 is one of two enzyme isoforms of the GAD enzyme that neurons use to synthesize GABA. GAD65 is concentrated in presynaptic terminals and is important for maintaining GABA-ergic transmissions during sustained neuronal activity (Soghomonian and Martin, 1998; Tian et al., 1999; Fenalti et al., 2007). Anti-GAD65 B cell and T cell immune responses predominantly target the COOH terminal of the enzyme (Fenalti et al., 2008), and the target epitopes differ in patients with SPS from those in patients with type 1 diabetes (Ali et al., 2011).

Anti-GAD65 are very weakly associated with thymoma, but most patients do not have any malignancy (Vernino and Lennon, 2004; McKeon et al., 2012, 2013) and anti-GAD65 are frequently found in patients with other neuronal autoantibodies, perhaps explaining some of the diversity of symptoms in these patients (Pittock et al., 2005; Lai et al., 2009; Lancaster et al., 2010). Anti-GAD65 interfere with GABA synthesis in tissue extracts and affect GABA-ergic transmission when applied to tissue slices (Dinkel et al., 1998; Ishida et al., 1999, 2008), and also are reported to cause abnormal spontaneous electrical discharges in spinal motor neurons (Manto et al., 2007, 2011). It is not clear whether these antibody-mediated effects *in vitro* are relevant *in vivo*.

The presence of anti-GAD65 may signify a T cell-mediated pathophysiological mechanism. Immunization of mice with GAD65 produced T cells that react to GAD65 (Burton et al., 2008, 2010), and such mice developed encephalomyelitis; retrogenic transfer of these T cells to naïve mice also produced encephalomyelitis. Transfer to mice that lacked B cells produced identical findings, substantiating a T cell-mediated effect. While mice with intact B cells developed anti-GAD65, these did not influence the encephalomyelitis.

Amphiphysin I

Amphiphysin I is a reactant for autoantibodies found in patients with stiff-person syndrome, encephalitis and certain other syndromes. Some 90% of patients with anti-amphiphysin I have breast cancer, although adenocarcinoma has also been reported (Dropcho, 1996). Compared to patients with stiff person syndrome and anti-GAD65 antibodies, those with anti-amphiphysin I tend to be older and female, have prominent cervical stiffness, are responsive to benzodiazepine therapy, and show abnormal spontaneous activity on EMG (Murinson and Guarnaccia, 2008). Amphiphysins are proteins of the BAR superfamily required for regulating membrane curvature, particularly of clathrin-coated synaptic vesicles (Zhang and Zelhof, 2002; Wu et al., 2009). Amphiphysin I is strongly expressed in brain, and genetic deletion of amphiphysin I in mice results in seizures and cognitive deficits, findings that may be influenced by indirect effects on amphiphysin II in this animal model (Di Paolo et al., 2002). Anti-amphiphysin I are reported to cause direct effects on neurons. Transferred patient antibodies, or selectively purified patient-derived antibodies to amphiphysin I, cause stiffness in mice (Sommer et al., 2005; Geis et al., 2009, 2010), but these studies were from samples from only two patients and, in the case of non-purified antibodies, could be confounded by other coexisting autoantibodies. A postmortem study of a patient who died of brainstem encephalitis associated with anti-amphiphysin I showed an intense CD8$^+$ predominant T lymphocytic infiltrate, along with neuronal loss, and perivascular lymphocytic cuffs in affected brainstem areas (Wessig et al., 2003). Pathological studies of another patient also showed CD8$^+$ T cell infiltrates in the brainstem, spinal cord, and dorsal root ganglia (Pittock et al., 2005). Thus a T cell-dependent disease process is likely.

Neuronal Nuclear Antigens (NNA)

Autoantibodies to NNA (ANNA 1-3) have acquired a dual terminology. In the earlier days of autoimmunity, antigens for newly discovered autoantibodies were identified by the initial letters of the donor patient's surname (e.g., Sm for the lupus autoantigen from patient Smith), and hence the derivation of the neuronal nuclear antigens *Hu* and *Ri*. Autoantibodies to neuronal nuclear antigens ANNA-1 and ANNA-2 correspond to anti-Hu and anti-Ri, respectively. These autoantibody reactivities are observed mostly in paraneoplastic diseases.

ANNA-1/anti-Hu

These are associated with subacute neuropathy, cerebellitis, encephalitis, and autonomic dysfunction (Dalmau et al., 1992; Lucchinetti et al., 1998; Graus et al., 2001), with many of the patients having small-cell lung cancer. Mortality is high (20% three-year survival) due to the serious underlying malignancy and poor responses of the neurological symptoms to treatment. react with HuD (embryonic lethal abnormal vision-like 4, ELAVL4) and

three related RNA-binding proteins, HuC, Hel-N1, and Hel-N2 (Dalmau et al., 1990; Szabo et al., 1991; King and Dropcho, 1996). HuD is expressed in neurons and neuroendocrine tumor cells, and is important for cell-cycle regulation and neuronal development (Okano and Darnell, 1997; Hubers et al., 2011). Several lines of evidence suggest that ANNA-1/anti-Hu are not directly pathogenic, being found in many patients with malignancy but without neurological symptoms (Darnell and Posner, 2003), failing when injected into animals to recapitulate neurological symptoms (Sillevis Smitt et al., 1995), and failing to induce any CNS disorder using antibodies to Hu raised by immunization of rodents (Sillevis Smitt et al., 1996; Carpentier et al., 1998). Pathological studies point more to T cell responses to neurons as the disease mechanism (Wanschitz et al., 1997; Plonquet et al., 2002; Rousseau et al., 2005).

ANNA-2 (anti-Ri)

These are associated with cerebellar degeneration, opsoclonus—myoclonus, encephalitis, myelitis, or other CNS disorders. Patients have small-cell lung cancer or breast cancer (Pittock et al., 2003; Shams'ili et al., 2003) and ANNA-2, like ANNA-1, may be found in cancer patients without neurological symptoms (Drlicek et al., 1997). ANNA-2/anti-Ri react with Nova-1, an RNA-binding protein expressed by various subcortical neurons (Buckanovich et al., 1993). While ANNA-2 block the binding of Nova-1 to RNA *in vitro*, it is unknown how relevant this might be *in vivo* (Buckanovich and Darnell, 1997).

ANNA-3

These are associated with diverse neurological phenotypes including neuropathy, myelopathy, ataxia, and brain stem and limbic encephalopathy, and are detected in patients with lung cancer (Chan et al., 2001). The autoantigen is an unidentified and functionally unknown 170 kDa protein expressed by nuclei of Purkinje and granular neurons, enteric neurons, and small-cell lung cancer cells.

Ma1/Ma2 (Ma and Ta)

These autoantigens are reactants for the closely related Ma and Ta antibodies; Ma antibodies target the onconeural proteins PNMA-1 (paraneoplastic Ma antigen-1; the Ma1 response) and PNMA-2 (paraneoplastic Ma antigen-2; the Ma2 response); also, anti-Ta react with PNMA-2 (Graus et al., 2004). Patients with anti-Ma most often have limbic encephalitis, but cerebellitis, brainstem encephalitis, and polyneuropathy have also been described (Rosenfeld et al., 2001; Hoffmann et al., 2008). Anti-Ma1 are strongly associated with cancer, but many different tumor types have been reported, and response to therapy is poor. Anti-Ma2 are usually detected in young men with germ cell tumors, among whom outcome is more favorable (Dalmau et al., 2004).

There are four known PNMA proteins and these are expressed by brain, testes, and other tissues (Schuller et al., 2005). PNMA-1 is a pro-apoptotic protein in developing brain, and increased PNMA-1 expression has been proposed to contribute to neurodegenerative diseases (Chen and D'Mello, 2010). In a rat model of PNMA-1 immunity, immunization with PNMA-1 elicited specific $CD4^+$ T cells and an antibody response to PNMA-1, and transfer of T cells to naïve rats resulted in a CNS inflammatory response but no neurological symptoms (Pellkofer et al., 2004); thus a PNMA-1 antibody response was generated but not associated with neurological findings. These studies suggest that a T cell rather than a direct antibody response may be more relevant, and that a strong immune tolerance to PNMA proteins must be overcome for disease to occur.

Purkinje Cell Antigen-1 (PCA-1; Yo)

This is the reactant for anti-Purkinje cell antibodies (APSA, anti-Yo) that are associated with paraneoplastic cerebellar degeneration (PCD) in women. Patients typically have limb and truncal ataxia, nystagmus, and dysarthria, resulting in significant disability within a few months of diagnosis. Less often they have rigidity, spasticity, cognitive impairment, or emotional dysregulation. Almost all patients are eventually diagnosed with breast or gynecological cancer (Peterson et al., 1992). These tumors often respond to treatment, but the neurological symptoms less so (Rojas et al., 2000).

Anti-PCA-1 were initially defined by their reactivity with the cytoplasm of Purkinje cells (Greenlee and Brashear, 1983). The minor and major target antigens are two unrelated proteins of 34 kDa and 62 kDa, cerebellar degeneration related-34 (CDR34; CDR1; OMIM 302650), and cerebellar degeneration related-62 (CDR62; CDR2; OMIM 117340), respectively (Fathallah-Shaykh et al., 1991; Dropcho, 1996). CDR1 is a neuroectodermal protein, strongly expressed in Purkinje cells, with a unique tandem hexapeptide repeat structure and unknown function (Furneaux et al., 1989; Chen et al., 1990). CDR2 has a leucine zipper motif and may be involved in cell-cycle regulation, mitosis, and transcriptional regulation (Okano et al., 1999; O'Donovan et al., 2010). Tumor tissues express the target antigens (Peterson et al., 1992), and CDR2-selective T cells kill tumor cells *in vitro* (Santomasso et al., 2007), but the immune response seems ineffective for control of tumors *in vivo* (Rojas et al., 2000; Mathew et al., 2006). CDR2 is expressed in all ovarian tumors and normal ovary, with no apparent differences in expression of CDR2 in cancer patients with or without anti-PCA-1 (Totland et al., 2011). Post-mortem studies have

shown T cell infiltration of the cerebellum with extensive loss of Purkinje cells, but no deposits of IgG or complement, or B cell infiltrates (Giometto et al., 1997; Storstein et al., 2009). Despite the lack of B cell infiltrates, there is evidence of intrathecal antibody synthesis, which is important for establishing CNS antibody titers (Peterson et al., 1992; Stich and Rauer, 2007). T cell infiltrates have also been described in tumors of patients with anti-PCA-1. Interestingly, patients with PCA-1 antibodies and related disorders may have lower levels of regulatory T lymphocytes, suggestive of T cell dysregulation (Tani et al., 2008). Two reports have described cytotoxic T cell responses to CDR2 in patients with anti-PCA-1 (Albert et al., 1998, 2000), but others find that most patients do not have such cytotoxic T lymphocyte responses (Sutton et al., 2004), leaving it unclear what antigen in brain is actually targeted. When DNA immunization was used to induce CDR2 reactive T cells and antibodies in mice, the T cells killed antigen-expressing cells *in vitro*, but the animals remained asymptomatic (Sakai et al., 2001). A direct toxic effect of the antibodies has been proposed. Anti-PCA-1 are taken up by cerebellar neurons in slice culture and induce cell death, in contrast to normal IgG which does enter the Purkinje cell cytoplasm but is cleared without toxicity (Greenlee et al., 2010). Similarly, anti-PCA-1 injected into guinea pigs intraventricularly, or intraperitoneally with blood—brain barrier disruption into rats, are taken up by Purkinje cells, but have not been shown to cause neuronal death *in vivo* (Graus et al., 1991; Greenlee et al., 1995).

PCA-2

PCA-2 is an antigen for autoantibodies that are strongly associated with lung cancer, and with neurological presentations that include encephalitis, cerebellitis, neuropathy, and Lambert—Eaton myasthenic syndrome (Vernino and Lennon, 2000). Anti-PCA-2 are defined by a characteristic pattern of Purkinje cell staining, involving the soma and dendrites. The antigen is an unidentified 280 kDa protein. Anti-PCA-2 are frequently encountered together with other co-morbid antibodies, and it is unknown how the antibodies relate to the pathophysiology of the disorders (Lennon et al., 2004).

CONCLUSIONS AND FUTURE PROSPECTS

The field of autoimmune CNS disorders is rapidly evolving and touches on many aspects of neurology and neuroscience. The autoimmune disorders targeting synaptic proteins provide interesting insights into the effects of disrupting key neurotransmitter receptors in the adult nervous system. Vague descriptive diagnoses of unclear pathophysiology, such as encephalitis lethargica, are gradually being replaced by disorders defined by specific autoantibodies, such as anti-NMDAR encephalitis. Recognition of these disorders may lead to the search for specific tumors, and should prompt tumor and/or immunotherapy since, with appropriate treatment, even profoundly ill patients can recover. With some of these disorders, the autoantibodies are directly pathogenic and in others they mark a specific T cell response. The antibody tests are generally very helpful for confirming a specific diagnosis, but in some patients with multiple autoantibodies, it can be difficult to determine which immune response is causing disease. Thus, future research should focus not just on detection of the various autoantibodies, but also on the pathophysiology of the accompanying disorders, and on mechanisms for clearly differentiating incidental findings from pathological responses. This should lead to more informative diagnostic testing, precisely targeted therapies, and better outcomes. For immunology in general, it seems not too much to expect that insights from these strange paraneoplastic disorders will enlighten us on maintenance of self-tolerance and evasion of autoimmunity.

ACKNOWLEDGMENTS

I would like to thank my mentors, Dr. Josep Dalmau, Dr. Steven S. Scherer, and Dr. Rita Balice-Gordon. I am grateful to Dr. Vanda Lennon, who suggested I write this chapter. I also thank the National Institutes of Health (NIH), National Organization for Rare Disorders (NORD), and the Dana Foundation for their generous support.

ABBREVIATIONS

AMPAR	2-amino-3-(5-methyl-3-oxo-1,2-oxazol-4-yl) propanoic acid receptor
ANNA-1 (-2, -3)	autoantibodies to neuronal nuclear antigens -1 (-2, -3)
AQP4	aquaporin-4
Caspr2	contactin-associated protein-like 2
DNER	delta/notch-like epidermal growth factor-related receptor
GABA-B-R	γ-amino-butyric acid receptor B
Kv1	voltage-gated potassium channels containing Kv1.1 and/or Kv1.2 subunits
LGI1	leucine-rich, glioma inactivated 1
NMDAR	N-methyl-d-aspartate receptor
PCA	Purkinje cell antibodies
SPS	stiff person syndrome
VGCC	voltage-gated calcium channel
VGKC	voltage-gated potassium channel

REFERENCES

Agbogu, B.N., Stern, B.J., Sewell, C., Yang, G., 1995. Therapeutic considerations in patients with refractory neurosarcoidosis. Arch. Neurol. 52, 875–879.

Akman-Demir, G., Serdaroglu, P., Tasci, B., 1999. Clinical patterns of neurological involvement in Behcet's disease, evaluation of 200 patients. The Neuro-Behcet Study Group. Brain. 122 (11), 2171–2182.

Albert, M.L., Austin, L.M., Darnell, R.B., 2000. Detection and treatment of activated T cells in the cerebrospinal fluid of patients with paraneoplastic cerebellar degeneration. Ann. Neurol. 47, 9–17.

Albert, M.L., Darnell, J.C., Bender, A., Francisco, L.M., Bhardwaj, N., Darnell, R.B., 1998. Tumor-specific killer cells in paraneoplastic cerebellar degeneration. Nat. Med. 4, 1321–1324.

Alexander, E.L., 1993. Neurologic disease in Sjögren's syndrome: mononuclear inflammatory vasculopathy affecting central/peripheral nervous system and muscle. A clinical review and update of immunopathogenesis. Rheum.Dis. Clin North. Am. 19, 869–908.

Alexander, E.L., Lijewski, J.E., Jerdan, M.S., Alexander, G.E., 1986. Evidence of an immunopathogenic basis for central nervous system disease in primary Sjögren's syndrome. Arthritis. Rheum. 29, 1223–1231.

Alexander, E.L., Ranzenbach, M.R., Kumar, A.J., Kozachuk, W.E., Rosenbaum, A.E., Patronas, N., et al., 1994. Anti-Ro (SS-A) autoantibodies in central nervous system disease associated with Sjögren's syndrome (CNS-SS): clinical, neuroimaging, and angiographic correlates. Neurology. 44, 899–908.

Ali, F., Rowley, M., Jayakrishnan, B., Teuber, S., Gershwin, M.E., Mackay, I.R., 2011. Stiff-person syndrome (SPS) and anti-GAD-related CNS degenerations, protean additions to the autoimmune central neuropathies. J. Autoimmun. 37, 79–87.

Alkan, A., Goktan, A., Karincaoglu, Y., Kamisli, S., Dogan, M., Oztanir, N., et al., 2012. Brain perfusion MRI findings in patients with Behcet's disease. Sci. World J. 2012, 261502.

Apiwattanakul, M., McKeon, A., Pittock, S.J., Kryzer, T.J., Lennon, V.A., 2010. Eliminating false-positive results in serum tests for neuromuscular autoimmunity. Muscle Nerve. 41, 702–704.

Arai, Y., Kohno, S., Takahashi, Y., Miyajima, Y., Tsutusi, Y., 2006. Autopsy case of neuro-Behcet's disease with multifocal neutrophilic perivascular inflammation. Neuropathology. 26, 579–585.

Araki, M., Aranami, T., Matsuoka, T., Nakamura, M., Miyake, S., Yamamura, T., 2013. Clinical improvement in a patient with neuromyelitis optica following therapy with the anti-IL-6 receptor monoclonal antibody tocilizumab. Mod. Rheumatol. 23, 827–831.

Arking, D.E., Cutler, D.J., Brune, C.W., Teslovich, T.M., West, K., Ikeda, M., et al., 2008. A common genetic variant in the neurexin superfamily member CNTNAP2 increases familial risk of autism. Am. J. Hum. Genet. 82, 160–164.

Baekkeskov, S., Aanstoot, H.J., Christgau, S., Reetz, A., Solimena, M., Cascalho, M., et al., 1990. Identification of the 64 K autoantigen in insulin-dependent diabetes as the GABA-synthesizing enzyme glutamic acid decarboxylase. Nature. 347, 151–156.

Bataller, L., Galiano, R., Garcia-Escrig, M., Martinez, B., Sevilla, T., Blasco, R., et al., 2010. Reversible paraneoplastic limbic encephalitis associated with antibodies to the AMPA receptor. Neurology. 74, 265–267.

Bernal, F., Shams'ili, S., Rojas, I., Sanchez-Valle, R., Saiz, A., Dalmau, J., et al., 2003. Anti-Tr antibodies as markers of paraneoplastic cerebellar degeneration and Hodgkin's disease. Neurology. 60, 230–234.

Bettler, B., Kaupmann, K., Mosbacher, J., Gassmann, M., 2004. Molecular structure and physiological functions of GABA(B) receptors. Physiol. Rev. 84, 835–867.

Birnbaum, J., Petri, M., Thompson, R., Izbudak, I., Kerr, D., 2009. Distinct subtypes of myelitis in systemic lupus erythematosus. Arthritis. Rheum. 60, 3378–3387.

Borhani Haghighi, A., Pourmand, R., Nikseresht, A.R., 2005. Neuro-Behcet disease. A review. Neurologist. 11, 80–89.

Borhani Haghighi, A., Sharifzad, H.R., Matin, S., Rezaee, S., 2007. The pathological presentations of neuro-Behcet disease, a case report and review of the literature. Neurologist. 13, 209–214.

Boronat, A., Sabater, L., Saiz, A., Dalmau, J., Graus, F., 2011. GABA (B) receptor antibodies in limbic encephalitis and anti-GAD-associated neurologic disorders. Neurology. 76, 795–800.

Bradl, M., Misu, T., Takahashi, T., Watanabe, M., Mader, S., Reindl, M., et al., 2009. Neuromyelitis optica, pathogenicity of patient immunoglobulin in vivo. Ann. Neurol. 66, 630–643.

Buckanovich, R.J., Darnell, R.B., 1997. The neuronal RNA binding protein Nova-1 recognizes specific RNA targets in vitro and in vivo. Mol. Cell. Biol. 17, 3194–3201.

Buckanovich, R.J., Posner, J.B., Darnell, R.B., 1993. Nova, the paraneoplastic Ri antigen, is homologous to an RNA-binding protein and is specifically expressed in the developing motor system. Neuron. 11, 657–672.

Burton, A.R., Baquet, Z., Eisenbarth, G.S., Tisch, R., Smeyne, R., Workman, C.J., et al., 2010. Central nervous system destruction mediated by glutamic acid decarboxylase-specific CD4 + T cells. J. Immunol. 184, 4863–4870.

Burton, A.R., Vincent, E., Arnold, P.Y., Lennon, G.P., Smeltzer, M., Li, C.S., et al., 2008. On the pathogenicity of autoantigen-specific T-cell receptors. Diabetes. 57, 1321–1330.

Carpentier, A.F., Rosenfeld, M.R., Delattre, J.Y., Whalen, R.G., Posner, J.B., Dalmau, J., 1998. DNA vaccination with HuD inhibits growth of a neuroblastoma in mice. Clin. Cancer Res. 4, 2819–2824.

Chan, K.H., Vernino, S., Lennon, V.A., 2001. ANNA-3 anti-neuronal nuclear antibody, marker of lung cancer-related autoimmunity. Ann. Neurol. 50, 301–311.

Chapelon, C., Ziza, J.M., Piette, J.C., Levy, Y., Raguin, G., Wechsler, B., et al., 1990. Neurosarcoidosis, signs, course and treatment in 35 confirmed cases. Medicine. 69, 261–276.

Chen, H.L., D'Mello, S.R., 2010. Induction of neuronal cell death by paraneoplastic Ma1 antigen. J. Neurosci. Res. 88, 3508–3519.

Chen, Y.T., Rettig, W.J., Yenamandra, A.K., Kozak, C.A., Chaganti, R.S., Posner, J.B., et al., 1990. Cerebellar degeneration-related antigen, a highly conserved neuroectodermal marker mapped to chromosomes X in human and mouse. Proc. Nat. Acad. Sci. U.S.A. 87, 3077–3081.

Chiewthanakul, P., Sawanyawisuth, K., Foocharoen, C., Tiamkao, S., 2012. Clinical features and predictive factors in neuropsychiatric lupus. Asian. Pac. J. Allergy. Immunol. 30, 55–60.

Coesmans, M., Smitt, P.A., Linden, D.J., Shigemoto, R., Hirano, T., Yamakawa, Y., et al., 2003. Mechanisms underlying cerebellar motor deficits due to mGluR1-autoantibodies. Ann. Neurol. 53, 325–336.

Cojocaru, I.M., Cojocaru, M., Botnaru, L., Miu, G., Sapira, V., Tanasescu, R., 2010. Detection of serum of IgG anti-neuronal antibodies in systemic lupus erythematosus patients with central nervous system manifestations. Rom. J. Intern. Med. 48, 267–269.

Costanzi, C., Matiello, M., Lucchinetti, C.F., Weinshenker, B.G., Pittock, S.J., Mandrekar, J., et al., 2011. Azathioprine, tolerability, efficacy, and predictors of benefit in neuromyelitis optica. Neurology. 77, 659–666.

Crane, J.M., Bennett, J.L., Verkman, A.S., 2009. Live cell analysis of aquaporin-4 m1/m23 interactions and regulated orthogonal array assembly in glial cells. J. Biol. Chem. 284, 35850–35860.

Dalmau, J., Graus, F., Rosenblum, M.K., Posner, J.B., 1992. Anti-Hu-associated paraneoplastic encephalomyelitis/sensory neuronopathy. A clinical study of 71 patients. Medicine. 71, 59–72.

Dalmau, J., Furneaux, H.M., Gralla, R.J., Kris, M.G., Posner, J.B., 1990. Detection of the anti-Hu antibody in the serum of patients with small cell lung cancer—a quantitative western blot analysis. Ann. Neurol. 27, 544–552.

Dalmau, J., Lancaster, E., Martinez-Hernandez, E., Rosenfeld, M.R., Balice-Gordon, R., 2011. Clinical experience and laboratory investigations in patients with anti-NMDAR encephalitis. Lancet Neurol. 10, 63–74.

Dalmau, J., Graus, F., Villarejo, A., Posner, J.B., Blumenthal, D., Thiessen, B., et al., 2004. Clinical analysis of anti-Ma2-associated encephalitis. Brain. 127, 1831–1844.

Dalmau, J., Gleichman, A.J., Hughes, E.G., Rossi, J.E., Peng, X., et al., 2008. Anti-NMDA-receptor encephalitis, case series and analysis of the effects of antibodies. Lancet Neurol. 7, 1091–1098.

Dalmau, J., Tuzun, E., Wu, H.Y., Masjuan, J., Rossi, J.E., Voloschin, A., et al., 2007. Paraneoplastic anti-N-methyl-D-aspartate receptor encephalitis associated with ovarian teratoma. Ann. Neurol. 61, 25–36.

Darnell, R.B., Posner, J.B., 2003. Paraneoplastic syndromes involving the nervous system. N. Engl. J. Med. 349, 1543–1554.

de Graaff, E., Maat, P., Hulsenboom, E., van den Berg, R., van den Bent, M., Demmers, J., et al., 2012. Identification of delta/notch-like epidermal growth factor-related receptor as the Tr antigen in paraneoplastic cerebellar degeneration. Ann. Neurol. 71, 815–824.

Di Paolo, G., Sankaranarayanan, S., Wenk, M.R., Daniell, L., Perucco, E., Caldarone, B.J., et al., 2002. Decreased synaptic vesicle recycling efficiency and cognitive deficits in amphiphysin 1 knockout mice. Neuron. 33, 789–804.

Dinkel, K., Meinck, H.M., Jury, K.M., Karges, W., Richter, W., 1998. Inhibition of gamma-aminobutyric acid synthesis by glutamic acid decarboxylase autoantibodies in stiff-man syndrome. Ann. Neurol. 44, 194–201.

Drlicek, M., Bianchi, G., Bogliun, G., Casati, B., Grisold, W., Kolig, C., et al., 1997. Antibodies of the anti-Yo and anti-Ri type in the absence of paraneoplastic neurological syndromes, a long-term survey of ovarian cancer patients. J. Neurol. 244, 85–89.

Dropcho, E.J., 1996. Antiamphiphysin antibodies with small-cell lung carcinoma and paraneoplastic encephalomyelitis. Ann. Neurol. 39, 659–667.

Espinosa, G., Mendizabal, A., Minguez, S., Ramo-Tello, C., Capellades, J., Olive, A., et al., 2010. Transverse myelitis affecting more than 4 spinal segments associated with systemic lupus erythematosus, clinical, immunological, and radiological characteristics of 22 patients. Semin. Arthritis Rheum. 39, 246–256.

Estiasari, R., Matsushita, T., Masaki, K., Akiyama, T., Yonekawa, T., Isobe, N., et al., 2012. Comparison of clinical, immunological and neuroimaging features between anti-aquaporin-4 antibody-positive and antibody-negative Sjogren's syndrome patients with central nervous system manifestations. Mult. Scler. 18, 807–816.

Faas, G.C., Adwanikar, H., Gereau, R., Saggau, P., 2002. Modulation of presynaptic calcium transients by metabotropic glutamate receptor activation, a differential role in acute depression of synaptic transmission and long-term depression. J. Neurosci. 22, 6885–6890.

Fathallah-Shaykh, H., Wolf, S., Wong, E., Posner, J.B., Furneaux, H.M., 1991. Cloning of a leucine-zipper protein recognized by the sera of patients with antibody-associated paraneoplastic cerebellar degeneration. Proc. Nat. Acad. Sci. U.S.A. 88, 3451–3454.

Fenalti, G., Hampe, C.S., O'Connor, K., Banga, J.P., Mackay, I.R., Rowley, M.J., et al., 2007. Molecular characterization of a disease associated conformational epitope on GAD65 recognised by a human monoclonal antibody b96.11. Mol. Immunol. 44, 1178–1189.

Fenalti, G., Hampe, C.S., Arafat, Y., Law, R.H., Banga, J.P., Mackay, I.R., et al., 2008. COOH-terminal clustering of autoantibody and T-cell determinants on the structure of GAD65 provide insights into the molecular basis of autoreactivity. Diabetes. 57, 1293–1301.

Florance, N.R., Davis, R.L., Lam, C., Szperka, C., Zhou, L., Ahmad, S., et al., 2009. Anti-N-methyl-D-aspartate receptor (NMDAR) encephalitis in children and adolescents. Ann. Neurol. 66, 11–18.

Fukata, Y., Adesnik, H., Iwanaga, T., Bredt, D.S., Nicoll, R.A., Fukata, M., 2006. Epilepsy-related ligand/receptor complex LGI1 and ADAM22 regulate synaptic transmission. Science. 313, 1792–1795.

Fukata, Y., Lovero, K.L., Iwanaga, T., Watanabe, A., Yokoi, N., Tabuchi, K., et al., 2010. Disruption of LGI1-linked synaptic complex causes abnormal synaptic transmission and epilepsy. Proc. Nat. Acad. Sci. U.S.A. 107, 3799–3804.

Furneaux, H.M., Dropcho, E.J., Barbut, D., Chen, Y.T., Rosenblum, M.K., Old, L.J., et al., 1989. Characterization of a cDNA encoding a 34-kDa Purkinje neuron protein recognized by sera from patients with paraneoplastic cerebellar degeneration. Proc. Nat. Acad. Sci. U.S.A. 86, 2873–2877.

Geis, C., Beck, M., Jablonka, S., Weishaupt, A., Toyka, K.V., Sendtner, M., et al., 2009. Stiff person syndrome associated anti-amphiphysin antibodies reduce GABA associated [Ca(2 +)]i rise in embryonic motoneurons. Neurobiol. Dis. 36, 191–199.

Geis, C., Weishaupt, A., Hallermann, S., Grunewald, B., Wessig, C., Wultsch, T., et al., 2010. Stiff person syndrome-associated autoantibodies to amphiphysin mediate reduced GABAergic inhibition. Brain. 133, 3166–3180.

Geschwind, M.D., Tan, K.M., Lennon, V.A., Barajas Jr., R.F., Haman, A., Klein, C.J., et al., 2008. Voltage-gated potassium channel autoimmunity mimicking Creutzfeldt-Jakob disease. Arch. Neurol. 65, 1341–1346.

Giometto, B., Marchiori, G.C., Nicolao, P., Scaravilli, T., Lion, A., Bardin, P.G., et al., 1997. Sub-acute cerebellar degeneration with anti-Yo autoantibodies, immunohistochemical analysis of the immune reaction in the central nervous system. Neuropathol. Appl. Neurobiol. 23, 468–474.

Govoni, M., Bombardieri, S., Bortoluzzi, A., Caniatti, L., Casu, C., Conti, F., et al., 2012. Factors and comorbidities associated with first neuropsychiatric event in systemic lupus erythematosus, does a risk profile exist? A large multicentre retrospective cross-sectional study on 959 Italian patients. Rheumatology (Oxford). 51, 157–168.

Graus, F., Illa, I., Agusti, M., Ribalta, T., Cruz-Sanchez, F., et al., 1991. Effect of intraventricular injection of an anti-Purkinje cell antibody (anti-Yo) in a guinea pig model. J. Neurol. Sci. 106, 82–87.

Graus, F., Keime-Guibert, F., Rene, R., Benyahia, B., Ribalta, T., Ascaso, C., et al., 2001. Anti-Hu-associated paraneoplastic encephalomyelitis, analysis of 200 patients. Brain. 124, 1138–1148.

Graus, F., Dalmau, J., Valldeoriola, F., Ferrer, I., Rene, R., Marin, C., et al., 1997. Immunological characterization of a neuronal antibody (anti-Tr) associated with paraneoplastic cerebellar degeneration and Hodgkin's disease. J. Neuroimmunol. 74, 55–61.

Graus, F., Boronat, A., Xifro, X., Boix, M., Svigelj, V., Garcia, A., et al., 2010. The expanding clinical profile of anti-AMPA receptor encephalitis. Neurology. 74, 857–859.

Graus, F., Delattre, J.Y., Antoine, J.C., Dalmau, J., Giometto, B., Grisold, W., et al., 2004. Recommended diagnostic criteria for paraneoplastic neurological syndromes. J. Neurol. Neurosurg. Psychiatry. 75, 1135–1140.

Greenlee, J.E., Brashear, H.R., 1983. Antibodies to cerebellar Purkinje cells in patients with paraneoplastic cerebellar degeneration and ovarian carcinoma. Ann. Neurol. 14, 609–613.

Greenlee, J.E., Burns, J.B., Rose, J.W., Jaeckle, K.A., Clawson, S., 1995. Uptake of systemically administered human anticerebellar antibody by rat Purkinje cells following blood–brain barrier disruption. Acta. Neuropathol. 89, 341–345.

Greenlee, J.E., Clawson, S.A., Hill, K.E., Wood, B.L., Tsunoda, I., Carlson, N.G., 2010. Purkinje cell death after uptake of anti-Yo antibodies in cerebellar slice cultures. J. Neuropathol. Exp. Neurol. 69, 997–1007.

Gregor, A., Albrecht, B., Bader, I., Bijlsma, E.K., Ekici, A.B., Engels, H., et al., 2011. Expanding the clinical spectrum associated with defects in CNTNAP2 and NRXN1. BMC Med. Genet. 12, 106.

Gu, W., Brodtkorb, E., Steinlein, O.K., 2002. LGI1 is mutated in familial temporal lobe epilepsy characterized by aphasic seizures. Ann. Neurol. 52, 364–367.

Gullapalli, D., Phillips II, L.H., 2002. Neurologic manifestations of sarcoidosis. Neurol. Clin. 20, 59–83, vi.

Harisdangkul, V., Doorenbos, D., Subramony, S.H., 1995. Lupus transverse myelopathy, better outcome with early recognition and aggressive high-dose intravenous corticosteroid pulse treatment. J. Neurol. 242, 326–331.

Hart, I.K., Waters, C., Vincent, A., Newland, C., Beeson, D., Pongs, O., et al., 1997. Autoantibodies detected to expressed K + channels are implicated in neuromyotonia. Ann. Neurol. 41, 238–246.

Harvey, R.J., Topf, M., Harvey, K., Rees, M.I., 2008. The genetics of hyperekplexia: more than startle! Trends Genet. 24, 439–447.

Hernandes, M.S., Troncone, L.R., 2009. Glycine as a neurotransmitter in the forebrain, a short review. J. Neural. Transm. 116, 1551–1560.

Hinson, S.R., McKeon, A., Fryer, J.P., Apiwattanakul, M., Lennon, V.A., Pittock, S.J., 2009. Prediction of neuromyelitis optica attack severity by quantitation of complement-mediated injury to aquaporin-4-expressing cells. Arch. Neurol. 66, 1164–1167.

Hinson, S.R., Roemer, S.F., Lucchinetti, C.F., Fryer, J.P., Kryzer, T.J., Chamberlain, J.L., et al., 2008. Aquaporin-4-binding autoantibodies in patients with neuromyelitis optica impair glutamate transport by down-regulating EAAT2. J. Exp. Med. 205, 2473–2481.

Hinson, S.R., Romero, M.F., Popescu, B.F., Lucchinetti, C.F., Fryer, J.P., Wolburg, H., et al., 2012. Molecular outcomes of neuromyelitis optica (NMO)-IgG binding to aquaporin-4 in astrocytes. Proc. Nat. Acad. Sci. U.S.A. 109, 1245–1250.

Hoffmann, L.A., Jarius, S., Pellkofer, H.L., Schueller, M., Krumbholz, M., Koenig, F., et al., 2008. Anti-Ma and anti-Ta associated paraneoplastic neurological syndromes: 22 newly diagnosed patients and review of previous cases. J. Neurol. Neurosurg. Psychiatry. 79, 767–773.

Horresh, I., Bar, V., Kissil, J.L., Peles, E., 2010. Organization of myelinated axons by Caspr and Caspr2 requires the cytoskeletal adapter protein 4.1B. J. Neurosci. 30, 2480–2489.

Hubers, L., Valderrama-Carvajal, H., Laframboise, J., Timbers, J., Sanchez, G., Cote, J., 2011. HuD interacts with survival motor neuron protein and can rescue spinal muscular atrophy-like neuronal defects. Hum. Mol. Genet. 20, 553–579.

Hughes, E.G., Peng, X., Gleichman, A.J., Lai, M., Zhou, L., Tsou, R., et al., 2010. Cellular and synaptic mechanisms of anti-NMDA receptor encephalitis. J. Neurosci. 30, 5866–5875.

Hutchinson, M., Waters, P., McHugh, J., Gorman, G., O'Riordan, S., Connolly, S., et al., 2008. Progressive encephalomyelitis, rigidity, and myoclonus, a novel glycine receptor antibody. Neurology. 71, 1291–1292.

Ichise, T., Kano, M., Hashimoto, K., Yanagihara, D., Nakao, K., Shigemoto, R., et al., 2000. mGluR1 in cerebellar Purkinje cells essential for long-term depression, synapse elimination, and motor coordination. Science. 288, 1832–1835.

Iizuka, N., Okamoto, K., Matsushita, R., Kimura, M., Nagai, K., Arito, M., et al., 2010. Identification of autoantigens specific for systemic lupus erythematosus with central nervous system involvement. Lupus. 19, 717–726.

Iorio, R., Lennon, V.A., 2012. Neural antigen-specific autoimmune disorders. Immunol. Rev. 248, 104–121.

Irani, S.R., Alexander, S., Waters, P., Kleopa, K.A., Pettingill, P., Zuliani, L., et al., 2010. Antibodies to Kv1 potassium channel-complex proteins leucine-rich, glioma inactivated 1 protein and contactin-associated protein-2 in limbic encephalitis, Morvan's syndrome and acquired neuromyotonia. Brain. 133, 2734–2748.

Isaacs, H., 1961. A syndrome of continuous muscle-fibre activity. J. Neurol. Neurosurg. Psychiatry. 24, 319–325.

Isaacs, H., 1967. Continuous muscle fibre activity in an Indian male with additional evidence of terminal motor fibre abnormality. J. Neurol. Neurosurg. Psychiatry. 30, 126–133.

Ishida, K., Mitoma, H., Mizusawa, H., 2008. Reversibility of cerebellar GABAergic synapse impairment induced by anti-glutamic acid decarboxylase autoantibodies. J. Neurol. Sci. 271, 186–190.

Ishida, K., Mitoma, H., Song, S.Y., Uchihara, T., Inaba, A., Eguchi, S., et al., 1999. Selective suppression of cerebellar GABAergic transmission by an autoantibody to glutamic acid decarboxylase. Ann. Neurol. 46, 263–267.

Jarius, S., Paul, F., Franciotta, D., de Seze, J., Munch, C., Salvetti, M., et al., 2012. Neuromyelitis optica spectrum disorders in patients with myasthenia gravis: ten new aquaporin-4 antibody positive cases and a review of the literature. Mult. Scler. 18, 1135–1143.

Joseph, F.G., Scolding, N.J., 2009. Neurosarcoidosis: a study of 30 new cases. J. Neurol. Neurosurg. Psychiatry. 80, 297–304.

Jung, J.S., Bhat, R.V., Preston, G.M., Guggino, W.B., Baraban, J.M., Agre, P., 1994. Molecular characterization of an aquaporin cDNA from brain: candidate osmoreceptor and regulator of water balance. Proc. Nat. Acad. Sci. U.S.A. 91, 13052–13056.

Kalachikov, S., Evgrafov, O., Ross, B., Winawer, M., Barker-Cummings, C., Martinelli Boneschi, F., et al., 2002. Mutations in LGI1 cause autosomal-dominant partial epilepsy with auditory features. Nat. Genet. 30, 335–341.

Kang, E.H., Shen, G.Q., Morris, R., Metzger, A., Lee, E.Y., Lee, Y.J., et al., 2008. Flow cytometric assessment of anti-neuronal antibodies in central nervous system involvement of systemic lupus erythematosus and other autoimmune diseases. Lupus. 17, 21–25.

Kim, S.H., Kim, W., Li, X.F., Jung, I.J., Kim, H.J., 2012. Does interferon beta treatment exacerbate neuromyelitis optica spectrum disorder?. Mult. Scler. 18 , 1480–1483.

Kim, W., Kim, S.H., Lee, S.H., Li, X.F., Kim, H.J., 2011. Brain abnormalities as an initial manifestation of neuromyelitis optica spectrum disorder. Mult. Scler. 17, 1107–1112.

King, P.H., Dropcho, E.J., 1996. Expression of Hel-N1 and Hel-N2 in small-cell lung carcinoma. Ann. Neurol. 39, 679–681.

Kleopa, K.A., Elman, L.B., Lang, B., Vincent, A., Scherer, S.S., 2006. Neuromyotonia and limbic encephalitis sera target mature Shaker-type K+ channels: subunit specificity correlates with clinical manifestations. Brain. 129, 1570–1584.

Kovacs, B., Lafferty, T.L., Brent, L.H., DeHoratius, R.J., 2000. Transverse myelopathy in systemic lupus erythematosus, an analysis of 14 cases and review of the literature. Ann. Rheum. Dis. 59, 120–124.

Lacomis, D., 2011. Neurosarcoidosis. Curr. Neuropharmacol. 9, 429–436.

Lai, M., Huijbers, M.G., Lancaster, E., Graus, F., Bataller, L., Balice-Gordon, R., et al., 2010. Investigation of LGI1 as the antigen in limbic encephalitis previously attributed to potassium channels, a case series. Lancet Neurol. 9, 776–785.

Lai, M., Hughes, E.G., Peng, X., Zhou, L., Gleichman, A.J., Shu, H., et al., 2009. AMPA receptor antibodies in limbic encephalitis alter synaptic receptor location. Ann. Neurol. 65, 424–434.

Lancaster, E., Dalmau, J., 2012. Neuronal autoantigens-pathogenesis, associated disorders and antibody testing. Nat. Rev. Neurol. 8, 380–390.

Lancaster, E., Martinez-Hernandez, E., Titulaer, M.J., Boulos, M., Weaver, S., Antoine, J.C., et al., 2011a. Antibodies to metabotropic glutamate receptor 5 in the Ophelia syndrome. Neurology. 77, 1698–1701.

Lancaster, E., Huijbers, M.G., Bar, V., Boronat, A., Wong, A., Martinez-Hernandez, E., et al., 2011b. Investigations of caspr2, an autoantigen of encephalitis and neuromyotonia. Ann. Neurol. 69, 303–311.

Lancaster, E., Lai, M., Peng, X., Hughes, E., Constantinescu, R., Raizer, J., et al., 2010. Antibodies to the GABA(B) receptor in limbic encephalitis with seizures, case series and characterisation of the antigen. Lancet Neurol. 9, 67–76.

Lee, H.K., Kirkwood, A., 2011. AMPA receptor regulation during synaptic plasticity in hippocampus and neocortex. Semin. Cell Dev. Biol. 22, 514–520.

Leite, M.I., Coutinho, E., Lana-Peixoto, M., Apostolos, S., Waters, P., Sato, D., et al., 2012. Myasthenia gravis and neuromyelitis optica spectrum disorder, a multicenter study of 16 patients. Neurology. 78, 1601–1607.

Lennon, V.A., Wingerchuk, D.M., Kryzer, T.J., Pittock, S.J., Lucchinetti, C.F., Fujihara, K., et al., 2004. A serum autoantibody marker of neuromyelitis optica, distinction from multiple sclerosis. Lancet. 364, 2106–2112.

Lower, E.E., Broderick, J.P., Brott, T.G., Baughman, R.P., 1997. Diagnosis and management of neurological sarcoidosis. Arch. Intern. Med. 157, 1864–1868.

Lu, X., Gu, Y., Wang, Y., Chen, S., Ye, S., 2008. Prognostic factors of lupus myelopathy. Lupus. 17, 323–328.

Lucchinetti, C.F., Kimmel, D.W., Lennon, V.A., 1998. Paraneoplastic and oncologic profiles of patients seropositive for type 1 antineuronal nuclear autoantibodies. Neurology. 50, 652–657.

Manto, M.U., Hampe, C.S., Rogemond, V., Honnorat, J., 2011. Respective implications of glutamate decarboxylase antibodies in stiff person syndrome and cerebellar ataxia. Orphanet. J. Rare Dis. 6, 3.

Manto, M.U., Laute, M.A., Aguera, M., Rogemond, V., Pandolfo, M., Honnorat, J., 2007. Effects of anti-glutamic acid decarboxylase antibodies associated with neurological diseases. Ann. Neurol. 61, 544–551.

Marignier, R., Chenevier, F., Rogemond, V., Sillevis Smitt, P., Renoux, C., Cavillon, G., et al., 2010. Metabotropic glutamate receptor type 1 autoantibody-associated cerebellitis: a primary autoimmune disease? Arch. Neurol. 67, 627–630.

Mas, N., Saiz, A., Leite, M.I., Waters, P., Baron, M., Castano, D., et al., 2011. Antiglycine-receptor encephalomyelitis with rigidity. J. Neurol. Neurosurg. Psychiatry. 82, 1399–1401.

Mathew, R.M., Cohen, A.B., Galetta, S.L., Alavi, A., Dalmau, J., 2006. Paraneoplastic cerebellar degeneration, Yo-expressing tumor revealed after a 5-year follow-up with FDG-PET. J. Neurol. Sci. 250, 153–155.

Matiello, M., Schaefer-Klein, J.L., Hebrink, D.D., Kingsbury, D.J., Atkinson, E.J., Weinshenker, B.G., 2011. Genetic analysis of aquaporin-4 in neuromyelitis optica. Neurology. 77, 1149 1155.

Matiello, M., Kim, H.J., Kim, W., Brum, D.G., Barreira, A.A., Kingsbury, D.J., et al., 2010. Familial neuromyelitis optica. Neurology. 75, 310–315.

McKeon, A., Robinson, M.T., McEvoy, K.M., Matsumoto, J.Y., Lennon, V.A., Ahlskog, J.E., et al., 2012. Stiff-man syndrome and variants: clinical course, treatments, and outcomes. Arch. Neurol. 69, 230–238.

McKeon, A., Martinez–Hernandez, E., Lancaster, E., Matsumoto, J.Y., Harvey, R.J., McEvoy, K.M., et al., 2013. Glycine receptor autoimmune spectrum with stiff-man syndrome phenotype. Neurology. 70, 44–50.

Meinck, H.M., Faber, L., Morgenthaler, N., Seissler, J., Maile, S., Butler, M., et al., 2001. Antibodies against glutamic acid decarboxylase: prevalence in neurological diseases. J. Neurol. Neurosurg. Psychiatry. 71, 100–103.

Mikdashi, J., Handwerger, B., 2004. Predictors of neuropsychiatric damage in systemic lupus erythematosus: data from the Maryland lupus cohort. Rheumatology (Oxford). 43, 1555–1560.

Mikdashi, J.A., Esdaile, J.M., Alarcon, G.S., Crofford, L., Fessler, B.J., Shanberg, L., et al., 2007. Proposed response criteria for neurocognitive impairment in systemic lupus erythematosus clinical trials. Lupus. 16, 418–425.

Min, J.H., Kim, B.J., Lee, K.H., 2012. Development of extensive brain lesions following fingolimod (FTY720) treatment in a patient with neuromyelitis optica spectrum disorder. Mult. Scler. 18, 113–115.

Mok, C.C., Mak, A., To, C.H., 2006. Mycophenolate mofetil for lupus related myelopathy. Ann. Rheum. Dis. 65, 971–973.

Mok, C.C., Lau, C.S., Chan, E.Y., Wong, R.W., 1998. Acute transverse myelopathy in systemic lupus erythematosus, clinical presentation, treatment, and outcome. J. Rheumatol. 25, 467–473.

Morante-Redolat, J.M., Gorostidi-Pagola, A., Piquer-Sirerol, S., Sáenz, A., Poza, J.J., Galán, J., et al., 2002. Mutations in the LGI1/Epitempin gene on 10q24 cause autosomal dominant lateral temporal epilepsy. Hum. Mol. Genet. 11, 1119–1128.

Moscato, E.H., Jain, A., Peng, X., Hughes, E.G., Dalmau, J., Balice-Gordon, R.J., 2010. Mechanisms underlying autoimmune synaptic encephalitis leading to disorders of memory, behavior and cognition: insights from molecular, cellular and synaptic studies. Eur. J. Neurosci. 32, 298–309.

Murinson, B.B., Guarnaccia, J.B., 2008. Stiff-person syndrome with amphiphysin antibodies: distinctive features of a rare disease. Neurology. 71, 1955–1958.

Nagaishi, A., Takagi, M., Umemura, A., Tanaka, M., Kitagawa, Y., Matsui, M., et al., 2011. Clinical features of neuromyelitis optica in a large Japanese cohort: comparison between phenotypes. J. Neurol. Neurosurg. Psychiatry. 82, 1360–1364.

Nishiyama, M., Nakae, K., Yukawa, S., Hashimoto, T., Inaba, G., Mochizuki, M., et al., 1999. A study of comparison between the nationwide epidemiological survey in 1991 and previous surveys on Behcet's disease in Japan. Environ. Health Prev. Med. 4, 130–134.

O'Donovan, K.J., Diedler, J., Couture, G.C., Fak, J.J., Darnell, R.B., 2010. The onconeural antigen cdr2 is a novel APC/C target that acts in mitosis to regulate c-myc target genes in mammalian tumor cells. PloS One. 5, e10045.

Okano, H.J., Darnell, R.B., 1997. A hierarchy of Hu RNA binding proteins in developing and adult neurons. J. Neurosci. 17, 3024–3037.

Okano, H.J., Park, W.Y., Corradi, J.P., Darnell, R.B., 1999. The cytoplasmic Purkinje onconeural antigen cdr2 down-regulates c-Myc function: implications for neuronal and tumor cell survival. Genes Dev. 13, 2087–2097.

Padovan, M., Castellino, G., Bortoluzzi, A., Caniatti, L., Trotta, F., Govoni, M., 2012. Factors and comorbidities associated with central nervous system involvement in systemic lupus erythematosus: a retrospective cross-sectional case-control study from a single center. Rheumatol. Int. 32, 129–135.

Paoletti, P., 2011. Molecular basis of NMDA receptor functional diversity. Eur. J. Neurosci. 33, 1351–1365.

Pawate, S., Moses, H., Sriram, S., 2009. Presentations and outcomes of neurosarcoidosis: a study of 54 cases. QJM. 102, 449–460.

Pellkofer, H., Schubart, A.S., Hoftberger, R., Schutze, N., Pagany, M., Schuller, M., et al., 2004. Modelling paraneoplastic CNS disease: T-cells specific for the onconeuronal antigen PNMA1 mediate autoimmune encephalomyelitis in the rat. Brain. 127, 1822–1830.

Pena, J.A., Ravelo, M.E., Mora-La Cruz, E., Montiel-Nava, C., 2011. NMO in pediatric patients: brain involvement and clinical expression. Arq. Neuropsiquiatr. 69, 34–38.

Penagarikano, O., Abrahams, B.S., Herman, E.I., Winden, K.D., Gdalyahu, A., Dong, H., et al., 2011. Absence of CNTNAP2 leads to epilepsy, neuronal migration abnormalities, and core autism-related deficits. Cell. 147, 235–246.

Peterson, K., Rosenblum, M.K., Kotanides, H., Posner, J.B., 1992. Paraneoplastic cerebellar degeneration. I. A clinical analysis of 55 anti-Yo antibody-positive patients. Neurology. 42, 1931–1937.

Piotrowicz, A., Thumen, A., Leite, M.I., Vincent, A., Moser, A., 2011. A case of glycine-receptor antibody-associated encephalomyelitis with rigidity and myoclonus (PERM): clinical course, treatment and CSF findings. J. Neurol. 258, 2268–2270.

Pittock, S.J., Lucchinetti, C.F., Lennon, V.A., 2003. Anti-neuronal nuclear autoantibody type 2: paraneoplastic accompaniments. Ann. Neurol. 53, 580–587.

Pittock, S.J., Yoshikawa, H., Ahlskog, J.E., Tisch, S.H., Benarroch, E.E., Kryzer, T.J., et al., 2006. Glutamic acid decarboxylase autoimmunity with brainstem, extrapyramidal, and spinal cord dysfunction. Mayo Clin. Proc. 81, 1207–1214.

Pittock, S.J., Lennon, V.A., McKeon, A., Mandrekar, J., Weinshenker, B.G., Lucchinetti, C.F., et al., 2013. Eculizumab in AQP4-IgG-positive relapsing neuromyelitis optica spectrum disorders: an open-label pilot study. Lancet Neurol. 12, 554–562.

Pittock, S.J., Lucchinetti, C.F., Parisi, J.E., Benarroch, E.E., Mokri, B., Stephan, C.L., et al., 2005. Amphiphysin autoimmunity: paraneoplastic accompaniments. Ann. Neurol. 58, 96–107.

Plonquet, A., Gherardi, R.K., Creange, A., Antoine, J.C., Benyahia, B., Grisold, W., et al., 2002. Oligoclonal T-cells in blood and target tissues of patients with anti-Hu syndrome. J. Neuroimmunol. 122, 100–105.

Poliak, S., Gollan, L., Martinez, R., Custer, A., Einheber, S., Salzer, J.L., et al., 1999. Caspr2, a new member of the neurexin superfamily, is localized at the juxtaparanodes of myelinated axons and associates with K + channels. Neuron. 24, 1037–1047.

Provenzale, J.M., Barboriak, D.P., Gaensler, E.H., Robertson, R.L., Mercer, B., 1994. Lupus-related myelitis: serial MR findings. AJNR Am. J. Neuroradiol. 15, 1911–1917.

Robbins, C.A., Tempel, B.L., 2012. Kv1.1 and Kv1.2: similar channels, different seizure models. Epilepsia. 53 (Suppl. 1), 134–141.

Rojas, I., Graus, F., Keime-Guibert, F., Rene, R., Delattre, J.Y., Ramon, J.M., et al., 2000. Long-term clinical outcome of paraneoplastic cerebellar degeneration and anti-Yo antibodies. Neurology. 55, 713–715.

Rosenfeld, M.R., Eichen, J.G., Wade, D.F., Posner, J.B., Dalmau, J., 2001. Molecular and clinical diversity in paraneoplastic immunity to Ma proteins. Ann. Neurol. 50, 339–348.

Rossi, A., Moritz, T.J., Ratelade, J., Verkman, A.S., 2012. Super-resolution imaging of aquaporin-4 orthogonal arrays of particles in cell membranes. J. Cell Sci. 125, 4405–4412.

Rousseau, A., Benyahia, B., Dalmau, J., Connan, F., Guillet, J.G., Delattre, J.Y., et al., 2005. T cell response to Hu-D peptides in patients with anti-Hu syndrome. J. Neurooncol. 71, 231–236.

Saadoun, S., Waters, P., Bell, B.A., Vincent, A., Verkman, A.S., Papadopoulos, M.C., 2010. Intra-cerebral injection of neuromyelitis optica immunoglobulin G and human complement produces neuromyelitis optica lesions in mice. Brain. 133, 349–361.

Sagane, K., Ishihama, Y., Sugimoto, H., 2008. LGI1 and LGI4 bind to ADAM22, ADAM23 and ADAM11. Int. J. Biol. Sci. 4, 387–396.

Sakai, K., Shirakawa, T., Kitagawa, Y., Li, Y., Hirose, G., 2001. Induction of cytotoxic T lymphocytes specific for paraneoplastic cerebellar degeneration-associated antigen in vivo by DNA immunization. J. Autoimmun. 17, 297–302.

Sakane, T., Takeno, M., Suzuki, N., Inaba, G., 1999. Behcet's disease. N. Engl. J. Med. 341, 1284–1291.

Sanna, G., Bertolaccini, M.L., Cuadrado, M.J., Laing, H., Khamashta, M.A., Mathieu, A., et al., 2003. Neuropsychiatric manifestations in systemic lupus erythematosus: prevalence and association with antiphospholipid antibodies. J. Rheumatol. 30, 985–992.

Santomasso, B.D., Roberts, W.K., Thomas, A., Williams, T., Blachere, N.E., Dudley, M.E., et al., 2007. A T cell receptor associated with naturally occurring human tumor immunity. Proc. Nat. Acad. Sci. U.S.A. 104, 19073–19078.

Sato, D., Callegaro, D., Lana-Peixoto, M.A., Fujihara, K., 2012. Treatment of neuromyelitis optica: an evidence based review. Arq. Neuropsiquiatr. 70, 59–66.

Schuller, M., Jenne, D., Voltz, R., 2005. The human PNMA family: novel neuronal proteins implicated in paraneoplastic neurological disease. J. Neuroimmunol. 169, 172–176.

Schulz, S.W., Shenin, M., Mehta, A., Kebede, A., Fluerant, M., Derk, C.T., 2012. Initial presentation of acute transverse myelitis in systemic lupus erythematosus: demographics: diagnosis, management and comparison to idiopathic cases. Rheumatol. Int. 32, 2623–2627.

Scott, T.F., Yandora, K., Valeri, A., Chieffe, C., Schramke, C., 2007. Aggressive therapy for neurosarcoidosis: long-term follow-up of 48 treated patients. Arch. Neurol. 64, 691–696.

Sene, D., Jallouli, M., Lefaucheur, J.P., Saadoun, D., Costedoat-Chalumeau, N., Maisonobe, T., et al., 2011. Peripheral neuropathies associated with primary Sjogren syndrome: immunologic profiles of nonataxic sensory neuropathy and sensorimotor neuropathy. Medicine. 90, 133–138.

Shams'ili, S., Grefkens, J., de Leeuw, B., van den Bent, M., Hooijkaas, H., van der Holt, B., et al., 2003. Paraneoplastic cerebellar degeneration associated with antineuronal antibodies: analysis of 50 patients. Brain. 126, 1409–1418.

Shillito, P., Molenaar, P.C., Vincent, A., Leys, K., Zheng, W., van den Berg, R.J., et al., 1995. Acquired neuromyotonia: evidence for autoantibodies directed against K + channels of peripheral nerves. Ann. Neurol. 38, 714–722.

Sillevis Smitt, P., Manley, G., Dalmau, J., Posner, J., 1996. The HuD paraneoplastic protein shares immunogenic regions between PEM/PSN patients and several strains and species of experimental animals. J. Neuroimmunol. 71, 199–206.

Sillevis Smitt, P., Kinoshita, A., De Leeuw, B., Moll, W., Coesmans, M., Jaarsma, D., et al., 2000. Paraneoplastic cerebellar ataxia due to autoantibodies against a glutamate receptor. N. Engl. J. Med. 342, 21–27.

Sillevis Smitt, P.A., Manley, G.T., Posner, J.B., 1995. Immunization with the paraneoplastic encephalomyelitis antigen HuD does not cause neurologic disease in mice. Neurology. 45, 1873–1878.

Sinha, S., Newsom-Davis, J., Mills, K., Byrne, N., Lang, B., Vincent, A., 1991. Autoimmune aetiology for acquired neuromyotonia (Isaacs' syndrome). Lancet. 338, 75–77.

Siva, A., Saip, S., 2009. The spectrum of nervous system involvement in Behcet's syndrome and its differential diagnosis. J. Neurol. 256, 513–529.

Soghomonian, J.J., Martin, D.L., 1998. Two isoforms of glutamate decarboxylase: why? Trends Pharmacol. Sci. 19, 500–505.

Soliotis, F.C., Mavragani, C.P., Moutsopoulos, H.M., 2004. Central nervous system involvement in Sjogren's syndrome. Ann. Rheum. Dis. 63, 616–620.

Sommer, C., Weishaupt, A., Brinkhoff, J., Biko, L., Wessig, C., Gold, R., et al., 2005. Paraneoplastic stiff-person syndrome: passive transfer to rats by means of IgG antibodies to amphiphysin. Lancet. 365, 1406–1411.

Srivastava, R., Aslam, M., Kalluri, S.R., Schirmer, L., Buck, D., Tackenberg, B., et al., 2012. Potassium channel KIR4.1 as an immune target in multiple sclerosis. N. Engl. J. Med. 367, 115–123.

Stich, O., Rauer, S., 2007. Antigen-specific oligoclonal bands in cerebrospinal fluid and serum from patients with anti-amphiphysin- and anti-CV2/CRMP5 associated paraneoplastic neurological syndromes. Eur. J. Neurol. 14, 650–653.

Storstein, A., Krossnes, B.K., Vedeler, C.A., 2009. Morphological and immunohistochemical characterization of paraneoplastic cerebellar degeneration associated with Yo antibodies. Acta. Neurol. Scand. 120, 64–67.

Sutton, I.J., Steele, J., Savage, C.O., Winer, J.B., Young, L.S., 2004. An interferon-gamma ELISPOT and immunohistochemical investigation of cytotoxic T lymphocyte-mediated tumour immunity in patients with paraneoplastic cerebellar degeneration and anti-Yo antibodies. J. Neuroimmunol. 150, 98–106.

Szabo, A., Dalmau, J., Manley, G., Rosenfeld, M., Wong, E., Henson, J., et al., 1991. HuD, a paraneoplastic encephalomyelitis antigen, contains RNA-binding domains and is homologous to Elav and Sex-lethal. Cell. 67, 325–333.

Tan, K.M., Lennon, V.A., Klein, C.J., Boeve, B.F., Pittock, S.J., 2008. Clinical spectrum of voltage-gated potassium channel autoimmunity. Neurology. 70, 1883–1890.

Tani, T., Tanaka, K., Idezuka, J., Nishizawa, M., 2008. Regulatory T cells in paraneoplastic neurological syndromes. J. Neuroimmunol. 196, 166–169.

Tian, N., Petersen, C., Kash, S., Baekkeskov, S., Copenhagen, D., Nicoll, R., 1999. The role of the synthetic enzyme GAD65 in the control of neuronal gamma-aminobutyric acid release. Proc. Natl. Acad. Sci. U.S.A. 96, 12911–12916.

Totland, C., Aarskog, N.K., Eichler, T.W., Haugen, M., Nostbakken, J.K., Monstad, S.E., et al., 2011. CDR2 antigen and Yo antibodies. Cancer Immunol. Immunother. 60, 283–289.

Tradtrantip, L., Zhang, H., Saadoun, S., Phuan, P.W., Lam, C., Papadopoulos, M.C., et al., 2012. Anti-aquaporin-4 monoclonal antibody blocker therapy for neuromyelitis optica. Ann. Neurol. 71, 314–322.

Traka, M., Goutebroze, L., Denisenko, N., Bessa, M., Nifli, A., Havaki, S., et al., 2003. Association of TAG-1 with Caspr2 is essential for the molecular organization of juxtaparanodal regions of myelinated fibers. J. Cell Biol. 162, 1161–1172.

Tuzun, E., Zhou, L., Baehring, J.M., Bannykh, S., Rosenfeld, M.R., Dalmau, J., 2009. Evidence for antibody-mediated pathogenesis in anti-NMDAR encephalitis associated with ovarian teratoma. Acta. Neuropathol. 118, 737–743.

Verkerk, A.J., Mathews, C.A., Joosse, M., Eussen, B.H., Heutink, P., Oostra, B.A., 2003. CNTNAP2 is disrupted in a family with Gilles de la Tourette syndrome and obsessive compulsive disorder. Genomics. 82, 1–9.

Verkman, A.S., Binder, D.K., Bloch, O., Auguste, K., Papadopoulos, M.C., 2006. Three distinct roles of aquaporin-4 in brain function revealed by knockout mice. Biochim. Biophys. Acta. 1758, 1085–1093.

Vernino, S., Lennon, V.A., 2000. New Purkinje cell antibody (PCA-2): marker of lung cancer-related neurological autoimmunity. Ann. Neurol. 47, 297–305.

Vernino, S., Lennon, V.A., 2004. Autoantibody profiles and neurological correlations of thymoma. Clin. Cancer Res. 10, 7270–7275.

Wanschitz, J., Hainfellner, J.A., Kristoferitsch, W., Drlicek, M., Budka, H., 1997. Ganglionitis in paraneoplastic subacute sensory neuronopathy: a morphologic study. Neurology. 49, 1156–1159.

Waters, P.J., McKeon, A., Leite, M.I., Rajasekharan, S., Lennon, V.A., Villalobos, A., et al., 2012. Serologic diagnosis of NMO, a multicenter comparison of aquaporin-4-IgG assays. Neurology. 78, 665–671.

Weinshenker, B.G., Wingerchuk, D.M., Vukusic, S., Linbo, L., Pittock, S.J., Lucchinetti, C.F., et al., 2006. Neuromyelitis optica IgG predicts relapse after longitudinally extensive transverse myelitis. Ann. Neurol. 59, 566–569.

Wessig, C., Klein, R., Schneider, M.F., Toyka, K.V., Naumann, M., Sommer, C., 2003. Neuropathology and binding studies in anti-amphiphysin-associated stiff-person syndrome. Neurology. 61, 195–198.

Whalley, H.C., O'Connell, G., Sussmann, J.E., Peel, A., Stanfield, A.C., Hayiou-Thomas, M.E., et al., 2011. Genetic variation in CNTNAP2 alters brain function during linguistic processing in healthy individuals. Am. J. Med. Genet. B Neuropsychiatr. Genet. 156B, 941–948.

Wu, Y., Matsui, H., Tomizawa, K., 2009. Amphiphysin I and regulation of synaptic vesicle endocytosis. Acta. Med. Okayama. 63, 305–323.

Yazici, H., Fresko, I., Yurdakul, S., 2007. Behcet's syndrome: disease manifestations, management, and advances in treatment. Nat. Clin. Pract. Rheumatol. 3, 148–155.

Yu, Y.E., Wen, L., Silva, J., Li, Z., Head, K., Sossey-Alaoui, K., et al., 2010. Lgi1 null mutant mice exhibit myoclonic seizures and CA1 neuronal hyperexcitability. Hum. Mol. Genet. 19, 1702–1711.

Zajicek, J.P., Scolding, N.J., Foster, O., Rovaris, M., Evanson, J., Moseley, I.F., et al., 1999. Central nervous system sarcoidosis—diagnosis and management. QJM, Monthly Journal of the Association of Physicians. 92, 103–117.

Zhang, B., Zelhof, A.C., 2002. Amphiphysins, raising the BAR for synaptic vesicle recycling and membrane dynamics. Bin-Amphiphysin-Rvsp. Traffic. 3, 452–460.

Chapter 58

Paraneoplastic Neurologic Syndromes

Paula K. Rauschkolb and Jerome B. Posner

Department of Neurology, Memorial Sloan-Kettering Cancer Center, New York, NY, USA

Chapter Outline

Introduction	835	Anti-Ganglionic Neuronal Acetylcholine Receptor	843
Pathogenesis	836	Anti-Voltage-Gated Potassium Channel	844
Diagnosis	837	Treatment	844
Antibodies	838	Clinical Syndromes	844
Nuclear/Nucleolar Antibodies	838	Paraneoplastic Cerebellar Degeneration	844
Anti-Hu (ANNA1)	838	Paraneoplastic Encephalomyelitis	845
Anti-Ri (ANNA2)	840	Paraneoplastic Limbic Encephalitis	845
Anti-Ma	841	Brainstem Encephalitis	846
Cytoplasmic Antibodies	841	Myelitis	846
Anti-Yo (PCA1)	841	Subacute Sensory Neuronopathy	846
Anti-Tr	842	Autonomic Neuropathy	846
Anti-CRMP5 (Anti-CV2)	842	Vision Loss	847
Synaptic/Cell Surface Antibodies	842	Retinopathy	847
Anti-Amphiphysin	842	Optic Neuropathy	847
Anti-Glutamic Acid Decarboxylase	843	Stiff Person Syndrome	847
Anti-N-Methyl-D-Aspartate Receptor	843	Lambert–Eaton Myasthenic Syndrome	847
Ion Channel Antibodies	843	References	848

INTRODUCTION

The term paraneoplastic describes syndromes caused by cancer, but not as a direct result of invasion or infiltration of the target organ or tissue by the primary tumor or its metastases. Paraneoplastic syndromes have several different causes, only some of which are fully understood (Table 58.1). An autoimmune reaction to the tumor that secondarily affects the nervous system is one mechanism, and that is the focus of this chapter. A more comprehensive review can be found in a recently published monograph (Darnell and Posner, 2011).

Paraneoplastic disorders can affect any part of the nervous system (Box 58.1). The syndrome may cause destruction of a single cell type, such as the Purkinje cell of the cerebellum (paraneoplastic cerebellar degeneration, PCD), a single area of the nervous system such as the medial temporal lobes (limbic encephalopathy, LE), or multiple areas of the nervous system simultaneously (carcinomatous encephalomyeloradiculopathy). In some instances, the disorder targets a specific receptor such as the NMDA receptor on the cell surface of hippocampal neurons causing limbic encephalitis, or the presynaptic voltage-gated calcium channel causing the Lambert–Eaton myasthenic syndrome (LEMS).

Paraneoplastic neurologic syndromes can be categorized as classical or non-classical (Box 58.1). Classical syndromes are those so commonly associated with cancer that they demand a rigorous evaluation for an underlying neoplasm. Non-classical syndromes can also be associated with malignancy, but are more likely to occur in patients without cancer. Despite this distinction, classical paraneoplastic syndromes are sometimes found in patients without cancer. In a

N. Rose & I. Mackay (Eds): The Autoimmune Diseases, Fifth edition. DOI: http://dx.doi.org/10.1016/B978-0-12-384929-8.00058-7

TABLE 58.1 Pathogenesis of Paraneoplastic Syndromes

Pathogenesis	Example(s)	Neurologic Symptoms
Ectopic secretion of ectopic substance(s) by the tumor	ACTH ADH	Cushing syndrome (myopathy, psychosis) SIADH (seizures)
Destruction of non-nervous system organs	Liver Bone (hypercalcemia)	Hepatic encephalopathy Muscle weakness, delirium
Immunosuppression	Sepsis, meningitis	Seizures, headache
?Exosome secretion	Hypercoagulability	Stroke
Anorexia	Vitamin deficiency	Wernicke encephalopathy
Cytokine secretion	?Interleukin-6	Cachexia, weakness
Immune response to tumor	PCD, LE	Refer to text below

ACTH, adrenocorticotropic hormone; ADH, antidiuretic hormone; SIADH, syndrome of inappropriate antidiuretic hormone secretion; PCD, paraneoplastic cerebellar degeneration; LE, limbic encephalopathy.

Box 58.1 Paraneoplastic Nervous System Syndromes
- Brain (supratentorial)
  - Encephalomyelitis*
  - Limbic encephalitis*
  - Demyelinating encephalopathy
  - Chorea
  - Parkinsonism
- Brainstem and cerebellum
  - Brainstem encephalitis
  - Cerebellar degeneration*
  - Opsoclonus–myoclonus*
- Cranial nerves
  - Cancer-associated retinopathy (CAR)*
  - Melanoma-associated retinopathy (MAR)*
  - Optic neuropathy
  - Bilateral diffuse uveal melanocytic proliferation (BDUMP)
- Spinal cord
  - Necrotizing myelopathy/neuromyelitis optica
  - Inflammatory myelitis
  - Motor neuron disease (ALS)
  - Subacute motor neuronopathy*
  - Stiff person syndrome
- Dorsal root ganglia and peripheral nerves
  - Sensory neuronopathy*
  - Autonomic neuropathy
  - Chronic gastrointestinal pseudo-obstruction*
  - Acute sensorimotor neuropathy
  - Polyradiculopathy (Guillain–Barré)
  - Brachial neuropathy
  - Chronic sensorimotor neuropathy
  - Polyneuropathy, organomegaly, endocrinopathy, monoclonal protein, skin changes (POEMS)*
  - Vasculitic neuropathy
  - Neuromyotonia

(Continued)

Box 58.1 (Continued)
- Neuromuscular junction and muscle
  - Lambert–Eaton myasthenic syndrome*
  - Myasthenia gravis
  - Dermatomyositis*
  - Polymyositis
  - Inclusion body myositis
  - Necrotizing myopathy
  - Myotonia

*Classical paraneoplastic syndromes (see text).

few instances, an identifiable cancer has regressed or even disappeared with the emergence of a paraneoplastic syndrome (Byrne et al., 1997).

PATHOGENESIS

Although the syndromes discussed in this chapter are considered to be the result of an immune response to a cancer, the exact pathogenesis is not yet fully understood. The most straightforward explanation is that an antigen normally restricted to the nervous system (or sometimes the testes, also an immunologically privileged site) is ectopically expressed in a tumor. The antigen present in the tumor is structurally identical to that found in the nervous system, but is recognized by the immune system as "foreign" (Schreiber and Rowley, 2008). The antigen expressed by the tumor triggers an immune response and the result is two-fold. Structures in the nervous system containing the antigen are damaged or destroyed causing neurological signs and symptoms. The same immune response may slow the growth of the tumor or sometimes even cause regression. For this reason, in up to three-quarters of patients, the

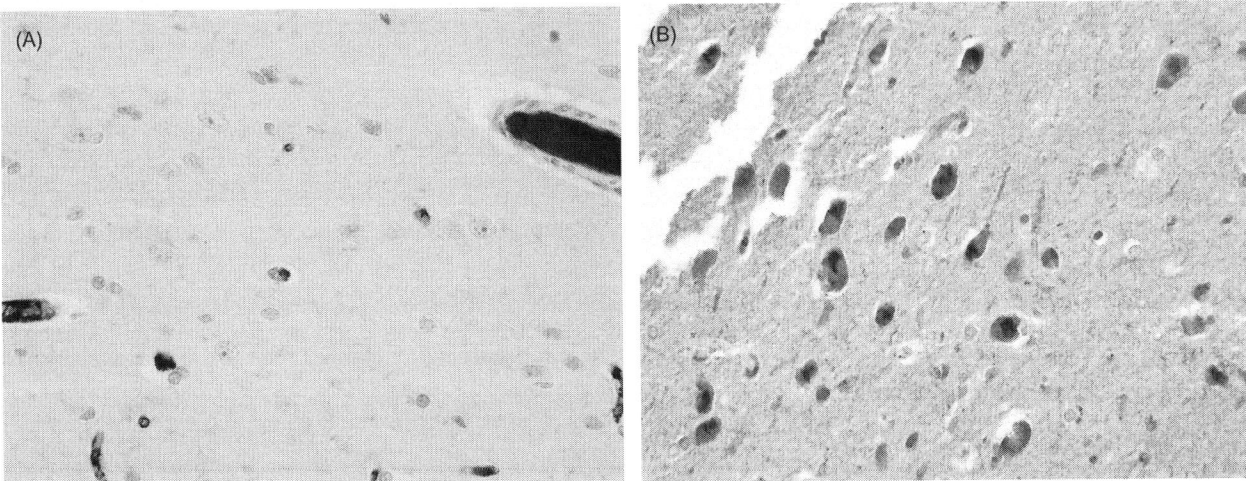

FIGURE 58.1   Five years after he developed an anti-Hu limbic encephalitis, this man underwent a temporal lobe resection for the treatment of intractable seizures. The surgery was successful. The surgical material was as assayed for the presence of IgG within the brain. (A) Section of the lateral temporal cortex. There is no evidence of IgG within the brain, but there is ample staining within small blood vessels. (B) Section of the parahippocampus. IgG is seen decorating the brain parenchyma as well as most neurons, sparing the glia. The neurons do not appear to be degenerating. *Photos courtesy of Dr. Mark Rosenblum.*

neurologic signs appear when the tumor is small or even undetectable.

In a few paraneoplastic syndromes such as LEMS, well-characterized animal models implicate B cells (antibodies) as the major culprit. The same is probably true for anti-NMDA receptor encephalopathy (Dalmau et al., 2011) and stiff person syndrome, for which there is also an animal model (Hansen et al., 2013). However, the underlying mechanism for most syndromes, particularly those involving the brain, remains to be elucidated. The primary question is whether those syndromes are mediated by T cells (the majority opinion), B cells, or both. T cells are thought to play a major role when the antigen triggering the paraneoplastic syndrome is intracellular, whereas B cells may be more important when the antigen is on the surface and accessible to antibodies. In some reports, IgG has been detected in the brains and even within the affected neurons of patients with paraneoplastic syndromes (Graus et al., 2004) (Figure 58.1). However, others have been skeptical.

DIAGNOSIS

The diagnosis of a paraneoplastic syndrome can only be unequivocally established if an antibody is detected in the serum of a patient, and it is then found to react with both the affected portion of the nervous system and the cells of a neoplasm identified in the same patient. In the absence of this type of clear-cut evidence, one may refer to a set of diagnostic criteria that has been established to assist the clinician (Graus et al., 2004) (Box 58.2).

Box 58.2 Diagnostic Criteria for Paraneoplastic Neurologic Syndromes

Definite paraneoplastic neurologic syndromes

1. A classical syndrome and cancer that develops within 5 years of the diagnosis of the neurological disorder
2. A nonclassical syndrome that resolves or significantly improves after cancer treatment without concomitant immunotherapy, provided that the syndrome is not susceptible to spontaneous remission
3. A nonclassical syndrome with onconeural antibodies (well characterized or not) and cancer that develops within 5 years of diagnosis of the neurological disorder
4. A neurological syndrome (classical or not) with well-characterized onconeural antibodies (anti-Hu, Yo, CV2, Ri, Ma-2, or amphiphysin), and no cancer

Possible paraneoplastic neurologic syndromes

1. A classical syndrome, no onconeural antibodies, no cancer but at high risk to have an underlying cancer
2. A neurologic syndrome (classical or not) with partially characterized onconeural antibodies and no cancer
3. A nonclassical syndrome, no onconeural antibodies, and cancer present within 2 years of diagnosis

From Graus et al. (2004), with permission.

Characteristics which should lead the clinician to suspect a paraneoplastic syndrome in a patient with neurologic signs and symptoms include the following:

1. Most paraneoplastic syndromes begin quickly and follow a subacute course, progressing over several days to weeks or months and then stabilizing. Occasionally a

patient develops a severe neurologic disability overnight.

2. Most paraneoplastic syndromes cause severe neurologic disability. Mild sensory symptoms and nonspecific imbalance are likely due to other causes. Many cancer patients present with minor neurologic symptomatology which may or may not be paraneoplastic (Erlington et al., 1991).

3. In patients with a paraneoplastic syndrome involving the central nervous system (CNS), cerebrospinal fluid (CSF) often reveals a lymphocytic pleocytosis (typically 20–100). Protein concentration may be increased, with elevated gamma globulin and oligoclonal bands. The latter may represent paraneoplastic antibody IgG (Stich and Rauer, 2007). The inflammatory infiltrate, if present, typically disappears after several weeks.

4. As indicated in Box 58.1, almost any constellation of neurologic symptoms can occur in patients with a paraneoplastic syndrome. However, one should be most suspicious in patients who present with a clinical syndrome affecting a specific portion of the nervous system such as the cerebellar Purkinje cell, the dorsal root ganglion, or the cholinergic synapse. Widespread nervous system damage, e.g., encephalomyelitis, is less specific.

5. A physical examination with careful attention to lymph nodes, breasts, prostate, and testes may reveal signs of an underlying malignancy that was previously unsuspected.

ANTIBODIES

Measurement of paraneoplastic antibodies in the serum is the most important diagnostic test. In addition to its value in establishing the diagnosis of a paraneoplastic syndrome, the antibody identified may reveal the likely underlying tumor. However, it is important to remember that not all paraneoplastic syndromes are antibody positive. For example, opsoclonus–myoclonus syndrome associated with neuroblastoma is clearly the result of an autoimmune process, yet a specific antibody has never been identified in the serum of affected children (Bolognani et al., 2007). Conversely, not all patients with serum antibodies have a paraneoplastic syndrome. This is illustrated by LEMS and myasthenia gravis in which the same antibodies (voltage-gated calcium channel and acetylcholine receptor, respectively) are found in patients with and without an underlying malignancy. In addition, low titers of paraneoplastic antibodies may be found in patients with cancer but without neurological symptoms (Tanner et al., 2008). Table 58.2 lists many of the serum antibodies found in paraneoplastic syndromes and the

malignancies with which they are typically associated. More common syndromes are discussed in the text that follows.

It is usually not necessary to measure paraneoplastic antibodies in the CSF. However, there are instances in which CSF testing is positive while serum levels are very low or undetectable (Tora et al., 1997; Graus et al., 2001; Fornaro et al., 2007). Higher activity of antibody in the CSF relative to serum indicates intrathecal antibody synthesis (Graus et al., 1997; Lucchinetti et al., 1998; Jarius et al., 2008a,b).

Paraneoplastic antibodies can be divided into two large groups (Stich et al., 2009). Group 1 consists of intracellular antigens, either cytoplasmic or nuclear, while Group 2 is composed of antibodies directed against antigens on the surface of the neuron or at it synapses. This classification also effectively divides the antibodies based upon likelihood of treatment response and probable pathogenesis. In Group 2, the antibodies are probably causal and these disorders typically respond to treatment. For disorders resulting from Group 1 antibodies, in which pathogenesis may be T cell mediated, treatment response is usually poor.

Some have further subdivided these broad groups (Budde-Steffen et al., 1988). Group 1A consists of antigens that are usually paraneoplastic; Group 1B consists of intracellular antigens that are cancer specific, but not specific to a paraneoplastic syndrome; Group 1C is composed of intracellular antigens associated with autoimmune disorders of the nervous system that are only sometimes paraneoplastic. Group 2A consists of surface antigens associated with autoimmune CNS syndromes which are only sometimes paraneoplastic and Group 2B is composed of surface antigens associated with paraneoplastic disorders.

Of note, the nomenclature of paraneoplastic antibodies has varied over time. Prior to formal identification, the Memorial Sloan-Kettering group named the antibodies after the first two letters of the last name of the index patient (e.g., Anti-Yo). However, the Mayo Clinic group named the same antibodies after the clinical syndrome (e.g., PCD1—anti-paraneoplastic cerebellar degeneration 1). Once characterized, the name changed to that of the antigen (e.g., VGCC—anti-voltage-gated calcium channel).

Nuclear/Nucleolar Antibodies

Anti-Hu (ANNA1)

The anti-Hu antibody reacts with the nuclei and, to a lesser extent, the cytoplasm of all neurons in both the central and peripheral nervous systems (Figure 58.2A). This antibody identifies a family of proteins of approximately 37 kDa, of

TABLE 58.2 Selected Paraneoplastic Antibodies and the Cancers and Neurologic Syndromes with which they are Associated

Antibody	Cancer	Neurologic disorder
Anti-Hu (-1*)	SCLC, neuroblastoma, prostate	PEM, PSN, autonomic dysfunction
Anti-Yo (PCA-1*)	Ovary, breast, lung	PCD
Anti-Ri (ANNA-2*)	Breast, gynecologic, lung, bladder	Ataxia/opsoclonus, brainstem encephalitis
Anti-CRMP5 (anti-CV2*)	SCLC, thymoma	PEM, PCD, chorea, optic/sensory neuropathy
Anti-Ma2	Testis	Limbic, brainstem (diencephalic) encephalitis
Anti-amphiphysin	Breast, SCLC	SPS
Anti-Sox (AGNA-1*)	SCLC	LEMS
Anti-Tr (PCA-Tr*)	Hodgkin	PCD
Anti-recoverin	SCLC	CAR
Anti-alpha-enolase	SCLC	CAR
Anti-bipolar	Melanoma	MAR
Anti-titin	Thymoma	MG
Anti-AChR	Thymoma	MG
Anti-ryanodine receptor	Thymoma	MG (severe form)
Anti-VGCC	SCLC	LEMS
Anti-NMDAR	Ovarian teratoma	PEM
Anti-AMPAR	Thymoma, breast, lung	LE
Anti-nAChR	SCLC, thymoma	Autonomic neuropathy
Anti-VGKC (LGI1/CASPR2)	Thymoma	LE, peripheral nerve hyperexcitability
Anti-GAD	Several (renal, Hodgkin, SCLC)	SPS, cerebellar ataxia
Anti-glycine receptor	Lung cancer	PERM
Anti-GABA-AR	??	SPS
Anti-GABA-BR	SCLC	LE
Anti-MuSK	Thymoma	MG

*Nomenclature used at the Mayo Clinic laboratory (based upon immunohistochemistry staining patterns).
CAR, cancer-associated retinopathy; LE, limbic encephalopathy; LEMS, Lambert–Eaton myasthenic syndrome; MAR, melanoma-associated retinopathy; MG, myasthenia gravis; PCD, paraneoplastic cerebellar degeneration; PEM, paraneoplastic encephalomyelitis; PERM, progressive encephalomyelitis, rigidity and myoclonus; PSN, paraneoplastic sensory neuropathy; SPS, stiff person syndrome.

which the most relevant in paraneoplastic syndromes is a neuron-specific protein designated HuD. The exact function of the Hu protein has not been definitively established. They bind to AU-rich elements of several different mRNAs *in vitro* and are believed to be important in the development and maintenance of neurons (Bolognani et al., 2007; Tanner et al., 2008; Perrone-Bizzozero and Bird, 2013). Electron microscopic studies have identified the protein at the site of nuclear pores, within layers of the Golgi apparatus and within the mitochondria (Fornaro et al., 2007). The antigen also has been reported to be expressed on the surface

membranes of small cell lung cancer (SCLC) and neuroblastoma cells in tissue culture (Tora et al., 1997).

Although the antibody is associated with a wide variety of neurological symptoms (Lucchinetti et al., 1998; Graus et al., 2001), the two most common findings are subacute sensory neuronopathy and limbic encephalitis. The most frequently associated malignancy is SCLC. The antigen is expressed in all SCLC tumors and in many other neuroendocrine tumors. Once the symptoms have become relatively severe, the prognosis for neurologic recovery is poor despite treatment. However, low titer antibodies are

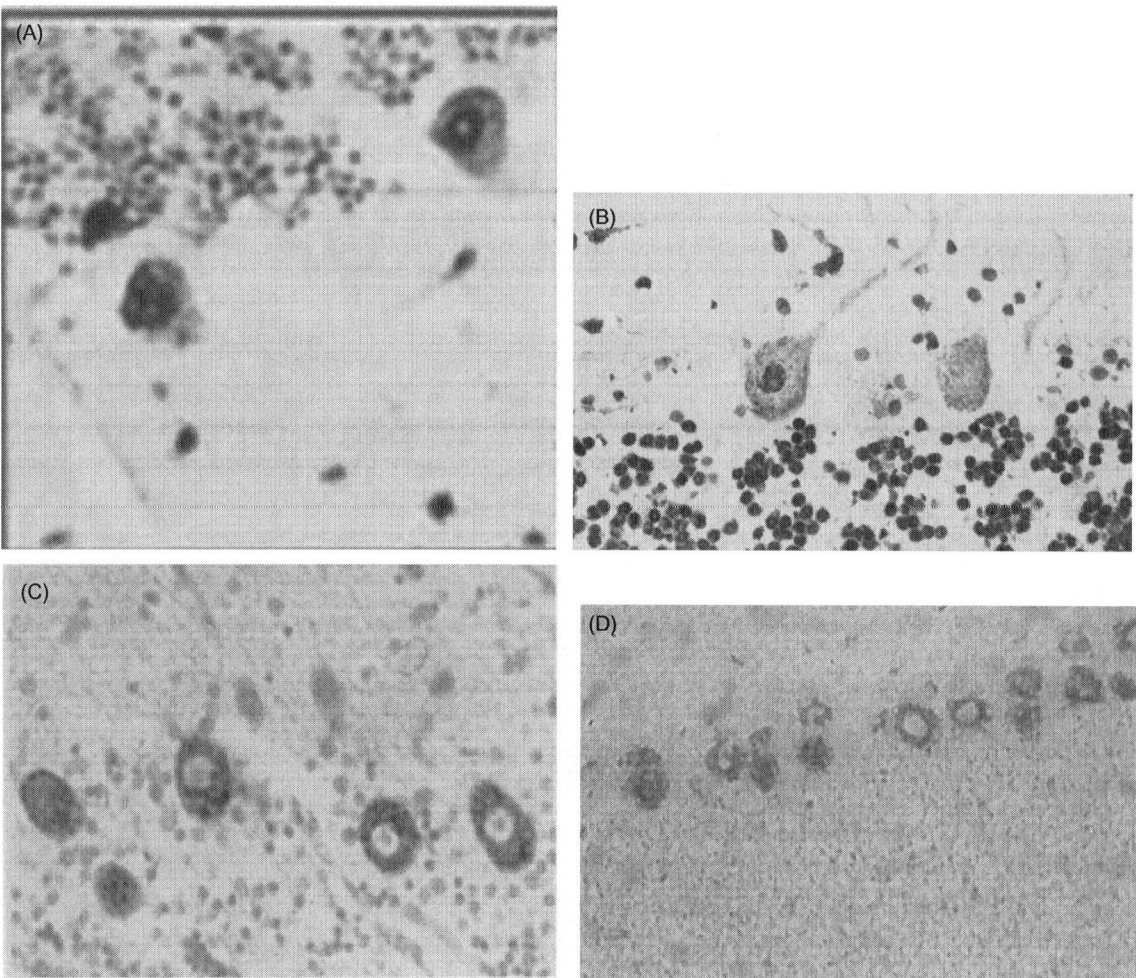

FIGURE 58.2   Several paraneoplastic antibodies reacted with sections of cerebellum.   (A) Anti-Hu antibody. There is intense staining of the nuclei of all of the cells in the Purkinje, molecular and granule cell layer. All neurons in both central and peripheral nervous system react the same. (B) Anti-Ri antibody. The reaction predominantly with the nuclei of neurons is the same as with anti-Hu. The difference is that the anti-Ri antibody does not react with neurons in the peripheral nervous system. (C) Anti-Yo antibody. The reaction is with the cytoplasmic Purkinje cells. Other cells in the cerebellum are spared. (D) Anti-Tr antibody. The Purkinje cell reaction is similar but reaction product is also seen in the molecular layer, presumably in Purkinje cell dendrites.

identified in approximately 20% of SCLC patients without a paraneoplastic syndrome, and when present suggest a better prognosis for the tumor (Graus et al., 1997a).

Anti-Ri (ANNA2)

The anti-Ri antibody is structurally similar to the anti-Hu antibody and reacts with the nuclei of all neurons in the CNS; however, unlike anti-Hu, it does not affect neurons in the peripheral nervous system (Figure 58.2B). The antibody is detectable in both serum and CSF, with higher titers in the CSF (Jarius et al., 2008a,b). In one patient, an increase in the antibody level preceded relapse of the underlying malignancy (Stich et al., 2009), suggesting that quantification of antibody levels may be useful in predicting relapse of cancer.

Western blot against cortical neurons identifies bands at 55 and 80 kDa (Budde-Steffen et al., 1988). The Ri antigens are RNA-binding proteins (Lewis et al., 1999) that identify two genes, Nova-1 and Nova-2 (neuro-onco-logical ventral antigen). The Nova-1 protein is highly expressed in the ventral portion of the brainstem and spinal cord, while Nova-2 is expressed predominantly in the neocortex. Both genes regulate alternative splicing of RNAs encoding synaptic proteins (Licatalosi et al., 2008) and appear to be particularly involved in regulating synaptic proteins, including the regulation of splicing of the inhibitory glycine receptor (Ratti et al., 2008); such inhibition could lead to uncontrollable eye movements.

In one patient, autopsy revealed deposits of IgG in the cytoplasm and the nuclei of neurons throughout the brain, most impressively in the brainstem. Likewise, Western blot

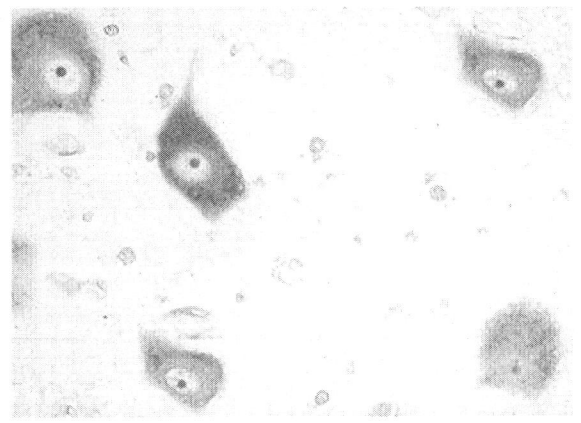

FIGURE 58.3 **Anti-Ma 2 antibody.** The primary reaction is in nucleoli of neurons. The remainder of the nucleus is spared.

analysis revealed the presence of anti-Ri IgG in the brain, with its distribution most prominent in the brainstem. There was little in the cerebellum, perhaps because there were no detectable Purkinje cells (Hormigo et al., 1994).

The characteristic findings of the anti-Ri syndrome are opsoclonus–myoclonus and truncal ataxia (Hormigo et al., 1994). Other manifestations of brainstem encephalitis, including dystonia and laryngospasm (Pittock et al., 2010), may also occur. The antibody is associated with a variety of cancers, of which breast cancer and SCLC are the most common (Pittock et al., 2010). Opsoclonus–myoclonus often responds to immunosuppressive treatment or may resolve spontaneously (Pittock et al., 2003). Other neurologic symptoms, including cognitive difficulties, have been less responsive.

Anti-Ma

Anti-Ma antibodies react with all neurons of the central and peripheral nervous system, including sympathetic and dorsal root ganglia and the myenteric plexus. They react mainly with the nuclei and nucleoli of neurons, predominantly the nucleoli, and to a lesser degree with the cytoplasm (Figure 58.3). The antibodies do not react with other tissues with the notable exception of testicular germ cells, especially spermatocytes and early spermatids which react with Ma1 but not Ma2.

Western blot using either nervous system or testicular tissue identifies an antigen of approximately 40 kDa (Rosenfeld et al., 2001). The Ma proteins are a family of highly homologous proteins that contain several potential phosphorylation sites for protein kinase C, casein kinase II, and cyclic AMP-dependent protein kinase. The first three genes are the most important in paraneoplastic Ma2 encephalitis (Rosenfeld et al., 2001; Schuller et al., 2005).

The typical anti-Ma2 (anti-Ta) patient is a young man not known to have cancer who develops limbic encephalopathy, diencephalic symptoms, brainstem encephalitis, or a combination of these. A report of 38 patients identified 34 with isolated or combined limbic, diencephalic, or brainstem dysfunction (Dalmau et al., 2004). Other neurologic findings in this or other reports include narcolepsy with low hypocretin1 CSF levels (Overeem et al., 2004), gaze palsy (Compta et al., 2007), and parkinsonism (Adams et al., 2011).

Anti-Ma2 is typically associated with testicular cancer, but occurs in other tumors including lymphoma (Kraemer and Berlit, 2007). The tumor may be occult; in some cases, despite a complete clinical work-up, pathology following orchiectomy will reveal microscopic tumor (Landolfi, 2003).

Treatment of neurological symptoms appears to be effective in some anti-Ma2-positive patients. Of 33 patients in one series, 11 improved following treatment of the underlying tumor, immunotherapy (usually intravenous immunoglobulin, IVIg), or both (Dalmau et al., 2004). Seven others stabilized, while nine deteriorated despite treatment. Six patients received neither tumor nor immunological therapy and all deteriorated.

Cytoplasmic Antibodies

Anti-Yo (PCA1)

The anti-Yo antibody reacts predominantly with Purkinje cells of the cerebellum (Figure 58.2C) and with some neurons in the deep cerebellar nuclei. The reaction is cytoplasmic, sparing the nucleus. On immunoelectron microscopy, the antibodies are found to bind clusters of ribosomes, granular endoplasmic reticulum, and the *trans* face of the vesicles of the Golgi complex in Purkinje cells, suggesting that at least one of the autoantigens may be a glycoprotein specific to cerebellar tissue (Rodriguez et al., 1988).

On Western blot against extracts of Purkinje cells, the antibody identifies two groups of antigens, the first 62 kDa and the second 34 kDa (Cunningham et al., 1986). The major antigen, CDR2, encodes a leucine zipper motif, suggesting that the protein might interact with other proteins that also express that motif (Sakai et al., 2002). Serum from patients blocks the interaction between c-Myc and CDR2 *in vitro* (Okano et al., 1999), effectively preventing downregulation of c-Myc activity by CDR2. The failure of downregulation may allow c-Myc transport to the nucleus promoting dysregulated cell signaling and apoptosis.

Although CDR2 mRNA is expressed in all tissues, significant amounts of the protein are detectable only in the brain and testes (Corradi et al., 1997). In brain tissue, the mRNA is confined primarily to neurons in the cerebellum and brainstem, and in the retina and olfactory bulb. However, the protein is widely expressed in gynecologic tumors, most of which do not elicit an immune response (Darnell et al., 2000).

Most patients with paraneoplastic syndromes resulting from anti-Yo antibodies have ovarian or gynecologic cancers and the most common manifestation is paraneoplastic cerebellar degeneration (see below). The neurologic symptoms only occasionally respond to treatment (Keime-Guibert et al., 2000; Phuphanich and Brock, 2007).

Anti-Tr

The anti-Tr antibody reacts exclusively with cytoplasm of Purkinje cells, in a pattern less granular than that of the anti-Yo antibody. It further differs from anti-Yo in that it diffusely stains the molecular layer of the cerebellum in a manner that originally suggested reaction with dendritic spines of Purkinje cells (Graus et al., 1997b, 1998) (Figure 58.2D). A recent report has identified the antigen as a delta/notch-like epidermal growth factor-related receptor (de Graaf et al., 2012). The antigen may mediate neuron−glia interactions through notch signaling. Experimental animals lacking the antigen exhibit motor incoordination.

The anti-Tr antibody is almost always associated with paraneoplastic cerebellar degeneration. It is typically associated with Hodgkin disease or other lymphomas. Anti-Tr-positive patients have been reported to improve after successful treatment of the underlying tumor (Geromin et al., 2006) and/or immunosuppressive treatment (Taniguchi et al., 2006).

Anti-CRMP5 (Anti-CV2)

This antibody, originally named anti-CV2, was later found by Yu and colleagues from Dr. Lennon's laboratory (Yu et al., 2001) to react with a protein which is a member of the collapsing response mediator family and was thus renamed anti-CRMP5. It reacts with the cytoplasm of glial cells and, to a lesser extent, with neurons in cerebral cortex, cerebellum, and optic nerve. A staining pattern resembling amphiphysin (see below) is found in the cerebellar cortex (Yu et al., 2001). The antibody also reacts with enteric neurons, but not with Purkinje cell cytoplasm, smooth muscle, kidney, or gut (Yu et al., 2001). Oligoclonal bands in the CSF are specific for the CRMP5 antigen (Stich and Rauer, 2007).

Immunofluorescence and Western blotting techniques identify the antibody less frequently than does immunoprecipitation (only one of 10 SCLC patients positive by competitive radioimmunoassay and five of nine thymoma patients). The titer is generally lower than in those patients with paraneoplastic syndromes (Monstad et al., 2008).

Collapsin response mediator protein 5 is a member of a family of five developmentally regulated neuronal phosphoproteins that are highly expressed during brain development. The protein is located predominantly in the dendrites of neurons, including cortical pyramidal neurons, hippocampal CA1 pyramidal cells and Purkinje cells. In tissue culture, the protein is equally distributed throughout cell bodies, axons, and dendrites. Oligodendroglia also express the protein in cell bodies and processes in both adult brain and primary cultures (Bretin et al., 2005). The CRMP proteins are involved in apoptosis and proliferation, as well as migration and differentiation in the developing brain (Charrier et al., 2003). Their function in the adult brain is less clear.

The antibody may be associated with a wide variety of neurologic disorders affecting cranial nerves and both the central and peripheral (Antoine et al., 2001) nervous system. Findings that strongly suggest the presence of the anti-CRMP5 antibody include optic neuropathy with or without uveitis (Antoine et al., 1993; Vernino et al., 2002), chorea (Vernino et al., 2002), and sometimes an associated obsessive compulsive behavioral disorder (Muehlschlegel et al., 2005). SCLC and thymoma are the most common tumors (Yu et al., 2001). Treatment of the underlying tumor and/or immunosuppressive therapy leads to resolution of the neurologic disorder in some cases.

Synaptic/Cell Surface Antibodies

Anti-Amphiphysin

Serum and CSF of patients with anti-amphiphysin antibodies react with the neuropil of brain (Folli et al., 1993) and spinal cord, and also react diffusely with the cytoplasm of large hippocampal neurons (Dropcho, 1996). There is somewhat less intense staining of Purkinje cell cytoplasm, often concentrated at the periphery of the perikarya, suggesting reaction with synaptic terminals.

Western blot against brain extracts or breast cancer tissue of patients harboring the antibody identified bands at 128 kDa (De Camilli et al., 1993) and 108 kDa (Floyd et al., 1998). One laboratory reported that, in 38% of patients, the antibody coexists with other paraneoplastic antibodies, particularly CRMP-5 and voltage-gated calcium channel antibodies (Pittock et al., 2004).

The antigen identified in the serum of patients with anti-amphiphysin antibodies is amphiphysin I, a 128 kDa protein highly concentrated in nerve terminals where it appears to be involved in synaptic vesicle recycling (Murthy and De, 2003; Dawson et al., 2006; Nguyen-Huu et al., 2006).

The paraneoplastic syndrome most strongly associated with antibodies against amphiphysin is the stiff person syndrome, and it is usually found in patients with breast cancer

(Nguyen-Huu et al., 2006). Immunotherapy with IVIg or rituximab is sometimes effective (Baker et al., 2005) in treating the neurological disorder. Baclofen, administered orally or intrathecally, or propofol may be effective in relieving some of the stiffness (Hattan et al., 2008).

Anti-Glutamic Acid Decarboxylase

The anti-glutamic acid decarboxylase (anti-GAD65) antibody recognizes cerebellar neurons, reacting with the cytoplasm of Purkinje cells and nerve terminals in both molecular and granular cell layers (Solimena et al., 1990). The antibody also reacts with nerve terminals throughout the neuraxis, but when applied to hippocampal neurons, appears to have a different labeling pattern depending on the underlying neurologic disease (Vianello et al., 2006). Although antibodies are present in most patients with type 1 diabetes (Taplin and Barker, 2008), titers are considerably higher in patients with antibody-associated neurologic disorders (Honnorat et al., 2001).

On Western blot, the antibody usually recognizes the 65 kDa isoform of GAD, the enzyme that catalyzes the conversion of glutamic acid to gamma-aminobutyric acid, but not the similar 67 isoform (Fenalti and Rowley, 2008). A radioimmunoassay is sensitive and specific (Vianello et al., 2005). In patients with antibody-associated CNS disorders, the specific activity of antibody is higher in the CSF than in the serum, indicating intrathecal synthesis (Rakocevic et al., 2004).

SPS associated with anti-GAD antibodies is found primarily in patients without cancer, and in many with diabetes. It is also reported in association with several neurologic disorders, either alone or in combination, most of which are non-paraneoplastic (Saiz et al., 2008).

In cases of paraneoplastic SPS, the patient may also present with myasthenia gravis or encephalomyelitis (Saiz et al., 2008). Several tumors have been associated with SPS, including Hodgkin disease, renal cell carcinoma, multiple myeloma, and colon cancer. The disorder often responds to immunosuppression, as does its non-neoplastic counterpart.

Anti-N-Methyl-D-Aspartate Receptor

The anti-N-methyl-D-aspartate receptor (anti-NMDAR) antibody is present on the surface of hippocampal neurons and their processes (Florance et al., 2009). It specifically reacts with the NR1 subunit of the NMDA receptor. The antibody is present at relatively higher titer in the CSF than in the serum indicating intrathecal synthesis, and there appears to be a correlation between the CSF titer and the severity of clinical symptomatology (Dalmau et al., 2008). The NMDA receptor is one of three ion channel glutamate receptors at the post-synaptic excitatory synapse. The other two NMDA receptors are the AMPA receptor (alpha-amino-3-hydroxy-5-methylisoxazole-4-propionic acid) and the kainite receptor (Kalia et al., 2008).

The paraneoplastic syndrome is typically characterized by an encephalitis with clinical abnormalities referable to the medial temporal lobe (limbic encephalitis), the hypothalamus (sleepiness, weight gain), and the brainstem (respiratory failure), and may progress to coma (Dalmau et al., 2008). A neoplasm is not always present, but when identified is most often an ovarian teratoma. Many patients recover after treatment of the underlying tumor and with immunosuppressive therapy (Dalmau et al., 2008).

Ion Channel Antibodies

Several ion channel antibodies have been associated with autoimmune disorders, only some of which are paraneoplastic (Vincent, 2010). These antibodies include anti-acetylcholine receptor (anti-AChR) and muscle-specific kinase (anti-MuSK) antibodies in myasthenia gravis, P/Q type voltage-gated calcium channel (anti-VGCC) antibodies in LEMS and paraneoplastic cerebellar degeneration, α3 nicotinic muscle-specific kinase acetylcholine receptor (anti-α 3AChR) antibodies in autonomic neuropathy, and voltage-gated potassium channel (anti-VGKC) antibodies in limbic encephalitis and myotonia. Only the last two are discussed here.

Anti-Ganglionic Neuronal Acetylcholine Receptor

Nicotinic acetylcholine receptors are ligand-gated cation channels that are present throughout the nervous system (Vernino et al., 2008). Immunizations with the antigen can induce the clinical syndrome in experimental animals (Lennon et al., 2003).

The primary clinical manifestation in patients with antibodies to this ligand-gated channel is a subacutely-developing autonomic neuropathy (Altermatt et al., 1991; Wang et al., 2007; Vernino et al., 2008). Neurologic abnormalities may also include peripheral neuropathy, myasthenia gravis, and CNS dysfunction. Those with high titers were more likely to have dysautonomia (McKeon et al., 2009).

The disorder is not paraneoplastic in all cases of antibody-positive autonomic neuropathy (Vincent et al., 2006). In a recent study of 155 patients, 30 of 78 tested for cancer were found have a malignancy. Neoplasm was more likely in those with high or medium titers versus low but positive titers (McKeon et al., 2009). The most commonly associated cancers are SCLC or thymoma.

Anti-Voltage-Gated Potassium Channel

Although the term voltage-gated potassium channel antibodies is now entrenched in the literature, the measurements actually encompass at least two different antibodies linked to the potassium channel. These antibodies, called LGI1 and CASPR2, are associated with limbic encephalitis and neuromyotonia, respectively (Vincent, 2009). LGI1 is not actually an ion channel protein, but instead is a secreted protein.

Most patients with the antibody do not have cancer, but, when it is present, SCLC and thymoma are the most commonly found types. A report of positive voltage-gated potassium channel antibodies should prompt additional analysis to differentiate between LGI1 and CASPR2. The former is associated with limbic encephalitis and the latter with neuromyotonia or Morvan syndrome (Abou-Zeid et al., 2012). Patients often respond to immunotherapy (Buckley et al., 2001).

TREATMENT

There are two components to the treatment of a paraneoplastic syndrome. The first and foremost is to identify and treat an underlying malignancy. Effective treatment of the tumor often prevents progression of the neurologic syndrome and sometimes reverses it, probably by removing the inciting antigen. It is important to note that suppression of the immune response does not appear to worsen the outcome of the tumor (Keime-Guibert et al., 1999).

The second approach is immunosuppression, which may include plasmapheresis, IVIg, immunosuppressive drugs such as corticosteroids, cyclophosphamide, cyclosporin or tacrolimus, or immunosuppressive antibodies, e.g., rituximab (Table 58.3) (Viaccoz and Honnarat, 2013).

Because many chemotherapeutic agents are also immunosuppressive, treatment of the tumor may achieve both effects. However, several of the neurologic syndromes are so devastating that concomitant immunosuppression and tumor treatment is warranted. Table 58.3 summarizes treatment recommendations and the likelihood of success for various clinical syndromes. The earlier tumor treatment and/or immunosuppressive therapy is begun, the more likely the patient is to stabilize or improve (Sillevis et al., 2002).

CLINICAL SYNDROMES

The list of paraneoplastic syndromes is provided in Box 58.1. Following are brief descriptions of some key clinical syndromes. References to less common neurologic disorders are not described due to space limitations but can be found in a recently published monograph (Darnell and Posner, 2011).

Paraneoplastic Cerebellar Degeneration

Paraneoplastic cerebellar degeneration (PCD) is the most common paraneoplastic disorder of the CNS. In the Euronetwork database (Giometto et al., 2010), PCD represented one-quarter of all paraneoplastic disorders and one-half of all CNS paraneoplastic syndromes. PCD usually occurs in isolation but may also occur as one manifestation of paraneoplastic encephalomyelitis (see below).

The clinical syndrome is so distinct that one must always search for an underlying malignancy when it is encountered. Patients with PCD present with relatively rapid onset (sometimes overnight) of signs of cerebellar dysfunction and including nausea and vomiting, vertigo, diplopia, incoordination, imbalance, and dysarthria. A viral-like syndrome with dizziness, nausea, and vomiting precedes cerebellar signs by a few days in some cases. Symptoms typically worsen progressively over the course of days to weeks only to stabilize in several weeks to a few months, often (but not always) with severe disability. Extra-cerebellar neurologic symptoms including cognitive dysfunction and extensor plantar responses, and evidence of peripheral neuropathy is present in some patients but it is usually mild (Peterson et al., 1992).

Imaging is typically normal at onset, although a rare patient will show evidence of inflammation (contrast enhancement) in cerebellar folia. With time, cerebellar atrophy becomes apparent. CSF usually shows a lymphocytic pleocytosis (10–50 cells) early in the illness, with elevated protein and immunoglobulin concentration and oligoclonal bands. Lymphocytes generally normalize over time but protein abnormalities remain.

The three most common antibodies are anti-Yo (gynecologic and breast cancers), anti-Hu (SCLC), and anti-Tr (Hodgkin disease). CSF antibody titers are usually higher than in serum, and in anti-Tr may be detectable only in the CSF (Bernal et al., 2003). Mimics of PCD are few, and include post-infectious cerebellitis, Miller–Fischer syndrome, and HIV infection. Other disorders, including alcoholism, vitamin deficiency, metastases, celiac disease, and spongiform encephalopathy, are rarely so abrupt in onset or involve so much of the cerebellum simultaneously.

The pathogenesis of the Purkinje cell destruction is not established. Cerebellar slice cultures bind the antibody and cause Purkinje cell death (Greenlee et al., 2010).

It is essential that treatment begin as early as possible in an effort to avoid further destruction of remaining Purkinje cells (Greenlee, 2013). Treatment usually will not reverse the illness, but may help to stabilize it. A few case reports describe a favorable response to immunosuppressive therapy (Counsell et al., 1994; Esposito et al., 2008).

TABLE 58.3 Approach to Treatment of Neurologic Paraneoplastic Syndromes

Syndrome	Treatment
Syndromes that usually respond to treatment*	
Lambert–Eaton myasthenic syndrome	IVIg, plasma exchange, 2,3-diaminopyridine, immunosuppression**
Myasthenia gravis	IVIg, plasma exchange, immunosuppression, acetylcholinesterase inhibitors
Dermatomyositis	IVIg, immunosuppression
Opsoclonus–myoclonus (pediatric)	IVIg, corticosteroids, ACTH, rituximab
Neuropathy associated with osteosclerotic myeloma	Radiation, chemotherapy
Anti-NMDAR encephalitis	First line: corticosteroids, IVIg, plasma exchange
	Second line: cyclophosphamide, rituximab
Anti-LGI1 encephalitis	Corticosteroids, IVIg, plasma exchange
Anti-cell surface antigens other than NMDAR and LGI1 (AMPA receptor, GABA(B) receptor, CASPR2)	Corticosteroids, IVIg, plasma exchange, cyclophosphamide
Syndromes that may respond to treatment	
Stiff person syndrome	IVIg, steroids, diazepam, baclofen
Neuromyotonia	IVIg, plasma exchange, phenytoin, carbamazepine
Guillain–Barré (in Hodgkin lymphoma)	IVIg, plasma exchange
Vasculitis of nerve and muscle	Corticosteroids, cyclophosphamide
Limbic encephalitis	IVIg, corticosteroids
Opsoclonus–myoclonus (adults)	Corticoteroids, cyclophosphamide, protein A column, clonazepam, thiamine
Anti-MAG-associated peripheral neuropathy (Waldenstrom macroglobulinemia)	IVIg, plasma exchange, chlorambucil, cyclophosphamide, fludarabine, rituximab
Acute necrotizing myopathy	Immunosuppression
Syndromes that usually do not respond to treatment	
Encephalomyelitis	
Sensory neuronopathy	
Autonomic dysfunction	
Cerebellar degeneration	
Cancer- and melanoma-associated retinopathy	

*In all cases, initial treatment should focus on identifying and treating the underlying tumor.
**Immunosuppression includes corticosteroids, azathioprine.
IVIg = intravenous immunoglobulin.
Modified from Dalmau and Posner (1998), with permission.

Paraneoplastic Encephalomyelitis

Paraneoplastic encephalomyelitis (PEM) is an inflammatory disorder that includes limbic encephalitis, brainstem encephalitis, myelitis, dorsal root ganglionitis (sensory neuronopathy), and autonomic neuropathy. One or all of these areas may be involved. The disorder was diagnosed in 5.6% of 979 patients in the Euronetwork database (Giometto et al., 2010). The full-blown syndrome is usually caused by SCLC associated with the anti-Hu antibody.

Paraneoplastic Limbic Encephalitis

Paraneoplastic limbic encephalitis (LE) is the most common paraneoplastic syndrome affecting the cerebral hemispheres. It was identified in 10% of patients in the

Euronetwork database (Giometto et al., 2010). Patients with LE typically present with short-term memory loss, behavioral changes, and/or seizures. Symptoms may begin with changes in mood and personality over days to weeks, progressing relatively rapidly, with development of potentially severe memory deficits. In some cases, patients present with short-term memory loss but otherwise preserved cognitive function, the so-called Ophelia syndrome (Carr, 1982). When the disorder is associated with anti-NMDAR antibodies, florid psychiatric symptoms are especially common at onset. When associated with other antibodies, LE more commonly presents with short-term memory loss and otherwise normal cognitive function, with or without complex partial seizures.

Although LE can be associated with a variety of antibodies (Table 58.2), the most prominent are anti-Hu, anti-LGI1 (previously anti-VGKC), and anti-NMDAR. Almost all anti-Hu patients have SCLC and respond relatively poorly to treatment. In contrast, only about 15% of patients with anti-LGI1-associated LE have cancer. Many of these patients respond to immunosuppressive treatment regardless of etiology.

Many patients with anti-NMDAR antibodies demonstrate a characteristic EEG pattern called extreme delta brush (Rosenfeld et al., 2012). There is also a fronto-temporo-parieto-occipital gradient of glucose metabolism that correlates with disease activity (Rosenfeld et al., 2012). These patients may also develop brainstem encephalitis with respiratory dysfunction and coma. Anti-NMDAR antibody patients are typically young women with ovarian teratomas (non-malignant). Most of these patients respond to treatment, sometimes even after weeks of coma.

Brainstem Encephalitis

Brainstem encephalitis can cause a multitude of symptoms and signs including movement disorders, deafness, gaze palsies, respiratory dysfunction, and even coma. The only relatively common symptom of brainstem dysfunction that occurs in isolation is opsoclonus, with or without myoclonus and with or without ataxia. Opsoclonus is characterized by involuntary, arrhythmic, multidirectional, high amplitude conjugate saccades occurring in all directions and without an inter-saccadic interval. Myoclonus and/or ataxia may also be present.

When opsoclonus occurs in children, approximately 40% of cases are paraneoplastic, usually caused by neuroblastoma (Singhi et al., 2013). However, only about 3% of patients with neuroblastoma have opsoclonus. When the syndrome occurs, it usually portends a good prognosis with regard to the neuroblastoma. While neurologic symptoms do respond to immunosuppression, patients are often left with other evidence of brain damage (Gorman, 2010).

A number of antibodies have been identified in the childhood syndrome but none, with the possible exception of a recently described cell surface antibody (Blaes et al., 2008), appears to be clearly related to the paraneoplastic disorder. In adults, the paraneoplastic disorder, which represents about 20% of adult cases of opsoclonus, is associated with a number of well-characterized paraneoplastic antibodies including anti-Hu and anti-Ri. Causal tumors include SCLC as well as breast and gynecological cancers.

The symptoms sometimes resolve spontaneously and have been reported to respond to immunosuppression including removal of antibodies via protein A column (Cher et al., 1995). Although included here as a brainstem symptom, the actual site of pathology is unknown. Pathologic study of the brainstem in affected patients failed to show specific abnormalities.

Myelitis

Acute or subacute inflammatory transverse myelitis may occur in isolation or be associated with the encephalomyelitis syndrome. In the vast majority of patients, transverse myelitis is not paraneoplastic. When it is, it is usually associated with the anti-Hu syndrome. Clinical findings that mimic amyotrophic lateral sclerosis may be the presenting symptom, followed by signs of more widespread encephalomyelitis. Other transverse myelopathies that are sometimes paraneoplastic include necrotizing myelopathy, demyelinating myelopathy, and neuromyelitis optica, the last disorder only rarely associated with cancer.

Subacute Sensory Neuronopathy

This disorder is as common as PCD, having been identified in 24% of 979 patients with paraneoplastic syndromes in the Euronetwork database (Giometto et al., 2010). Unlike most other sensory neuropathies, it has a rapid onset and is characterized by sensory loss and paresthesias. While symptoms can begin distally in all four extremities (as is typical of many neuropathies), in subacute sensory neuronopathy patients may present with symptoms beginning in other areas such as the trunk or the neck, or sensory changes may occur in the hands before the feet. Symptoms are often, but not always, asymmetric. Sensation to all modalities is affected—e.g., pain, temperature, vibration, proprioception—and most patients become very ataxic as a result of the proprioceptive deficit. Deep tendon reflexes are usually lost. Motor function is generally spared.

The most common cancer is SCLC and the most common antibody is anti-Hu. Treatment may stabilize or improve symptoms; patients usually do not fully recover and many progress despite treatment.

Autonomic Neuropathy

Autonomic neuropathy may present as a prominent or a minor deficit in patients with encephalomyelitis. It may also occur in isolation. A variety of symptoms of autonomic dysfunction may occur, including orthostatic hypotension, impotence, incontinence, pupillary abnormalities, anhydrosis, xerostomia, or xerophthalmia; however, the most significant distressing symptom is constipation/pseudoobstruction, which may be the presenting or sole complaint in patients with SCLC and anti-Hu antibody syndrome. Autonomic neuropathy is also associated with the anti-ganglionic neuronal acetylcholine receptor antibody (Vernino et al., 1998), which is only sometimes paraneoplastic.

Vision Loss

Paraneoplastic syndromes can cause vision loss by affecting either the retina or the optic nerve or both (Cornblath, 2004; Thirkill, 2005; Shildkrot et al., 2011; Braithwaite et al., 2012). The retinal disorder can affect photoreceptors—rods, cones or both—or can cause retinal vasculitis. Paraneoplastic visual disorders may occur as an isolated phenomenon or as part of a widespread encephalomyelopathy.

Retinopathy

Paraneoplastic photoreceptor degeneration has two causes: cancer-associated retinopathy (CAR), which usually occurs in association with SCLC and gynecological tumors, and melanoma-associated retinopathy (MAR). Visual symptoms—which include episodic visual obscurations, night blindness, light-induced glare, photosensitivity, and impaired color vision—precede the diagnosis of cancer (Shildkrot et al., 2011). Symptoms progress to painless vision loss. Visual testing demonstrates peripheral and ring scotomata, and loss of acuity. Fundoscopic examination may reveal arteriolar narrowing and abnormal mottling of the retinal pigment epithelium. The electroretinogram is abnormal. CSF is typically normal, although elevated immunoglobulin levels have been reported. Inflammatory cells are sometimes seen in the vitreous by slit-lamp examination.

Pathologically, a loss of photoreceptors and ganglion cells with inflammatory infiltrates and macrophages is usually noted. MAR is usually less severe than CAR, typically occurs in patients already known to have melanoma, and is generally associated with better vision. Symptoms include night blindness, photopsias, and visual glare (Dhingra et al., 2011).

Several autoantibodies have been identified in patients with CAR. The most common is recoverin (Shildkrot et al., 2011), a 23 kDa protein that modulates dark and light adaptation through calcium-dependent regulation of rhodopsin phosphorylation in photoreceptor cells. Recoverin antibodies can cross the blood–brain barrier gaining access to photoreceptor cells within the aqueous humor (Ohguro et al., 2002). Similar to CAR, a number of antibodies have been detected in the serum of patients with MAR (Lu et al., 2009) and, as in CAR, treatment is usually ineffective.

Optic Neuropathy

Paraneoplastic optic neuropathy occurring in the absence of other neurological symptoms is extremely uncommon (Ko et al., 2008). Cross and colleagues described 16 patients with optic neuritis (five of whom also had retinitis), all of whom harbored antibodies to CRMP5 (Cross et al., 2003). The patients had subacute vision loss. Optic discs were swollen and visual field defects were present. All patients had other neurological symptoms including cognitive changes, ataxia, sensory neuropathy, and myelopathy. Some patients had symptoms resembling those of neuromyelitis optica (Cree, 2008). SCLC was the most commonly associated malignancy.

Stiff Person Syndrome

Originally termed the stiff man syndrome, this disorder affects more women than men. It is characterized by muscle stiffness and rigidity that is usually painful (Rakocevic and Floeter, 2012; Ciccoto et al., 2013). The paraspinal and abdominal muscles are almost always involved, and those of the lower extremity are usually affected as well.

Sustained muscle contraction results in abnormal posture, such as an exaggerated lumbar lordosis. In addition to chronic contractions, severe muscle spasms may be precipitated by voluntary movements, unexpected environmental stimuli, and emotional upset. Muscles are firm on palpation and may be difficult to move passively. The EMG is characterized by sustained continuous motor unit activity that disappears during sleep and general anesthesia.

The non-paraneoplastic disorder is associated with diabetes and anti-GAD65 antibodies (Pittock et al., 2006). Paraneoplastic SPS is associated with antibodies against amphiphysin (Pittock et al., 2005), anti-GAD antibodies, anti-Ri antibodies, gephyrin, and glycine receptor alpha-1 subunit antibody (McKeon et al., 2013). GABA$_A$ receptor has also been reported in isolated cases. The common tumors include breast cancer, SCLC, Hodgkin disease, and colon cancer. Although the pathogenesis of the disorder is not fully understood (Rakocevic and Floeter, 2012), the disorder may be antibody mediated; injection of either anti-GAD65 (Hansen et al., 2013) or anti-amphiphysin antibodies (Geis et al., 2009) into experimental animals reproduces the syndrome.

Benzodiazepines and baclofen may relieve symptoms. Treatment of the underlying tumor and immunosuppression with corticosteroids, IVIg, or repeated plasmapheresis (Casa-Fages et al., 2012) are sometimes effective.

Lambert–Eaton Myasthenic Syndrome

Lambert–Eaton myasthenic syndrome (LEMS) is the most common of the classical paraneoplastic syndromes. The likelihood of cancer (usually SCLC) in the presence of LEMS is relatively high, at approximately 40–60%. However, the chance that a patient with SCLC will develop LEMS remains low, at less than 6% (Seute et al., 2004).

Patients typically present with progressive proximal weakness and fatigue (Wirtz et al., 2002). Early in the disease course they may complain of difficulty in walking up stairs, in rising from a chair without using hands to push off, or in opening windows. Weakness may fluctuate, which can lead to an inconsistent and confusing clinical presentation. Patients may complain of cramping with exercise. Cranial nerve involvement is less common than in myasthenia gravis, especially at onset of the condition. Autonomic symptoms are common early in the course and may include erectile dysfunction in men or xerostomia and/or metallic taste in either sex. Orthostatic hypotension is less common but may also occur.

Exam typically reveals proximal weakness (hip and shoulder girdles) and diminished or absent deep tendon reflexes. In some patients, strength and reflexes will transiently improve after brief exercise, followed shortly thereafter by increased weakness and recurrence of hyporeflexia or areflexia. All patients, whether paraneoplastic or not, harbor serum anti-VGCC antibodies.

The most important initial step is treatment of the underlying malignancy (usually SCLC), which may ameliorate symptoms from LEMS as well. However, if symptoms are severe one can administer concomitant immunosuppressive therapy such as plasma exchange, IVIg, oral agents (e.g., corticosteroids, azathioprine), or possibly rituximab. For patients who remain symptomatic, consideration may be given to medications that increase the availability of acetylcholine at the neuromuscular junction.

REFERENCES

Abou-Zeid, E., Boursoulian, L.J., Metzer, W.S., Gundogdu, B., 2012. Morvan syndrome, a case report and review of the literature. J. Clin. Neuromuscul. Dis. 13, 214−227.

Adams, C., McKeon, A., Silber, M.H., Kumar, R., 2011. REM sleep behavior disorder, and supranuclear gaze palsy associated with Ma1 and MAa2 antibodies and tonsillar carcinoma. Arch. Neurol. 68, 521−524.

Altermatt, H.J., Rodriguez, M., Scheithauer, B.W., Lennon, V.A., 1991. Paraneoplastic anti-Purkinje and type I anti-neuronal nuclear autoantibodies bind selectively to central, peripheral, and autonomic nervous system cells. Lab. Invest. 65, 412−420.

Antoine, J.C., Honnorat, J., Vocanson, C., Koenig, F., Aguera, M., Belin, M.F., et al., 1993. Posterior uveitis, paraneoplastic encephalomyelitis and autoantibodies reacting with developmental protein of brain and retina. J. Neurol. Sci. 117, 215−223.

Antoine, J.C., Honnorat, J., Camdessanché, J.P., Magistris, M., Absi, L., Mosnier, J.F., et al., 2001. Paraneoplastic anti-CV2 antibodies react with peripheral nerve and are associated with a mixed axonal and demyelinating peripheral neuropathy. Ann. Neurol. 49, 214−221.

Baker, M.R., Das, M., Isaacs, J., Fawcett, P.R., Bates, D., 2005. Treatment of stiff person syndrome with rituximab. J. Neurol. Neurosurg. Psychiatry. 76, 999−1001.

Bernal, F., Shams'ili, S., Rojas, I., Sanchez-Valle, R., Saiz, A., Dalmau, J., et al., 2003. Anti-Tr antibodies as markers of paraneoplastic cerebellar degeneration and Hodgkin's disease. Neurology. 60, 230−234.

Blaes, F., Pike, M.G., Lang, B., 2008. Autoantibodies in childhood opsoclonus-myoclonus syndrome. J. Neuroimmunol. 201−202, 221−226.

Bolognani, F., Qiu, S., Tanner, D.C., Paik, J., Perrone-Bizzozero, N.I., Weeber, E.J., 2007. Associative and spatial learning and memory deficits in transgenic mice overexpressing the RNA-binding protein HuD. Neurobiol. Learn. Mem. 87, 635−643.

Braithwaite, T., Vugler, A., Tufail, A., 2012. Autoimmune retinopathy. Ophthalmologica. 228, 131−142.

Bretin, S., Reibel, S., Charrier, E., Maus-Moatti, M., Auvergnon, N., Thevenoux, A., et al., 2005. Differential expression of CRMP1, CRMP2A, CRMP2B, and CRMP5 in axons or dendrites of distinct neurons in the mouse brain. J. Comp. Neurol. 486, 1−17.

Buckley, C., Oger, J., Clover, L., Tüzün, E., Carpenter, K., Jackson, M., et al., 2001. Potassium channel antibodies in two patients with reversible limbic encephalitis. Ann. Neurol. 50, 73−78.

Budde-Steffen, C., Anderson, N.E., Rosenblum, M.K., Graus, F., Ford, D., Synek, B.J., et al., 1988. An anti-neuronal autoantibody in paraneoplastic opsoclonus. Ann. Neurol. 23, 528−531.

Byrne, T., Mason, W.P., Posner, J.B., Dalmau, J., 1997. Spontaneous neurological improvement in anti-Hu associated encephalomyelitis. J. Neurol. Neurosurg. Psychiatry. 62, 276−278.

Carr, I., 1982. The Ophelia syndrome: memory loss in Hodgkin's disease. Lancet. 1, 844−845.

Casa-Fages, B., Anaya, F., Gabriel-Ortemberg, M., Grandas, F., 2012. Treatment of stiff-person syndrome with chronic plasmapheresis. Mov. Disord. 28, 396−397.

Charrier, E., Reibel, S., Rogemond, V., Aguera, M., Thomasset, N., Honnorat, J., 2003. Collapsin response mediator proteins (CRMPs): involvement in nervous system development and adult neurodegenerative disorders. Mol. Neurobiol. 28, 51−64.

Cher, L.M., Hochberg, F.H., Teruya, J., Nitschke, M., Valenzuela, R.F., Schmahmann, J.D., et al., 1995. Therapy for paraneoplastic neurologic syndromes in six patients with protein A column immunoadsorption. Cancer. 75, 1678−1683.

Ciccoto, G., Blaya, M., Kelley, R.E., 2013. Stiff person syndrome. Neurol. Clin. 31, 319−328.

Corradi, J.P., Yang, C.W., Darnell, J.C., Dalmau, J., Darnell, R.B., 1997. A post-transcriptional regulatory mechanism restricts expression of the paraneoplastic cerebellar degeneration antigen cdr2 to immune privileged tissues. J. Neurosci. 17, 1406−1415.

Compta, Y., Iranzo, A., Santamaria, J., Casamitjana, R., Graus, F., 2007. REM sleep behavior disorder and narcoleptic features in anti-Ma2-associated encephalitis. Sleep. 30, 767−769.

Cornblath, W.T., 2004. Paraneoplastic disorders of ophthalmic interest. Ophthalmol. Clin. North Am. 17, 447−454.

Counsell, C.E., McLeod, M., Grant, R., 1994. Reversal of subacute paraneoplastic cerebellar syndrome with intravenous immunoglobulin. Neurology. 44, 1184−1185.

Cree, B., 2008. Neuromyelitis optica: diagnosis, pathogenesis, and treatment. Curr. Neurol. Neurosci. Rep. 8, 427−433.

Cross, S.A., Salomao, D.R., Parisi, J.E., Kryzer, T.J., Bradley, E.A., Mines, J.A., et al., 2003. Paraneoplastic autoimmune optic neuritis with retinitis defined by CRMP-5-IgG. Ann. Neurol. 54, 38−50.

Cunningham, J., Graus, F., Anderson, N., Posner, J.B., 1986. Partial characterization of the Purkinje cell antigens in paraneoplastic cerebellar degeneration. Neurology. 36, 1163–1168.

Dalmau, J., Graus, F., Villarejo, A., Posner, J.B., Blumenthal, D., Thiessen, B., et al., 2004. Clinical analysis of anti-Ma2-associated encephalitis. Brain. 127, 1831–1844.

Dalmau, J., Gleichman, A.J., Hughes, E.G., Rossi, J.E., Peng, X., Lai, M., et al., 2008. Anti-NMDA-receptor encephalitis, case series and analysis of the effects of antibodies. Lancet Neurol. 7, 1091–1098.

Dalmau, J., Lancaster, E., Martinez-Hernandez, E., Rosenfeld, M.R., Balice-Gordon, R., 2011. Clinical experience and laboratory investigations in patients with anti-NMDAR encephalitis. Lancet Neurol. 10, 63–74.

Darnell, J.C., Albert, M.L., Darnell, R.B., 2000. Cdr2, a target antigen of naturally occurring human tumor immunity, is widely expressed in gynecological tumors. Cancer Res. 15 (60), 2136–2139.

Darnell, R.B., Posner, J.B., 2011. Paraneoplastic Syndromes. Oxford University Press, New York.

David, C., McPherson, P.S., Mundigl, O., De Camilli, P., 1996. A role of amphiphysin in synaptic vesicle endocytosis suggested by its binding to dynamin in nerve terminals. Proc. Natl. Acad. Sci. U.S.A. 93, 331–335.

Dawson, J.C., Legg, J.A., Machesky, L.M., 2006. Bar domain proteins, a role in tubulation, scission and actin assembly in clathrin-mediated endocytosis. Trends Cell Biol. 16, 493–498.

De Camilli, P., Thomas, A., Cofiell, R., Folli, F., Lichte, B., Piccolo, G., et al., 1993. The synaptic vesicle-associated protein amphiphysin is the 128-kD autoantigen of stiff-man syndrome with breast cancer. J. Exp. Med. 178, 2219–2223.

de Graaf, E., Maat, P., Hulsenboom, E., van den Berg, R., van den Bent, M., Demmers, J., et al., 2012. Identification of delta/notch-like epidermal growth factor-related receptor as the Tr antigen in paraneoplastic cerebellar degeneration. Ann. Neurol. 71, 815–824.

Dhingra, A., Fina, M.E., Neinstein, A., Ramsey, D.J., Xu, Y., Fishman, G.A., et al., 2011. Autoantibodies in melanoma-associated retinopathy target TRPM1 cation channels of retinal ON bipolar cells. J. Neurosci. 31, 3962–3967.

Dropcho, E.J., 1996. Antiamphiphysin antibodies with small-cell lung carcinoma and paraneoplastic encephalomyelitis. Ann. Neurol. 39, 659–667.

Erlington, G.M., Murray, N.M., Spiro, S.G., Newsom-Davis, J., 1991. Neurological paraneoplastic syndromes in patients with small cell lung cancer. A prospective survey of 150 patients. J. Neurol. Neurosurg. Psychiatry. 54, 764–767.

Esposito, M., Penza, P., Orefice, G., Pagano, A., Parente, E., Abbadessa, A., et al., 2008. Successful treatment of paraneoplastic cerebellar degeneration with rituximab. J. Neurooncol. 86, 363–364.

Fenalti, G., Rowley, M.J., 2008. GAD65 as a prototypic autoantigen. J Autoimmun. 31, 228–232.

Florance, N.R., Davis, R.L., Lam, C., Szperka, C., Zhou, L., Ahmad, S., et al., 2009. Anti-N-methyl-D-aspartate receptor (NMDAR) encephalitis in children and adolescents. Ann Neurol. 66, 11–18.

Floyd, S., Butler, M.H., Cremona, O., David, C., Freyberg, Z., Zhang, X., et al., 1998. Expression of amphiphysin I, an autoantigen of paraneoplastic neurological syndromes, in breast cancer. Mol. Med. 4, 29–39.

Folli, F., Solimena, M., Cofiell, R., Austoni, M., Tallini, G., Fassetta, G., et al., 1993. Autoantibodies to a 128-kd synaptic protein in three women with the stiff-man syndrome and breast cancer. N. Engl. J. Med. 328, 546–551.

Fornaro, M., Raimondo, S., Lee, J.M., Giacobini-Robecchi, M.G., 2007. Neuron-specific Hu proteins sub-cellular localization in primary sensory neurons. Ann. Anat. 189, 223–228.

Geis, C., Beck, M., Jablonka, S., Weishaupt, A., Toyka, K.V., Sendtner, M., et al., 2009. Stiff person syndrome associated anti-amphiphysin antibodies reduce GABA associated $[Ca^{2+}]$i rise in embryonic motoneurons. Neurobiol. Dis. 36, 191–199.

Geromin, A., Candoni, A., Marcon, G., Ferrari, S., Sperotto, A., De Luca, S., et al., 2006. Paraneoplastic cerebellar degeneration associated with anti-neuronal anti-Tr antibodies in a patient with Hodgkin's disease. Leuk. Lymphoma. 47, 1960–1963.

Giometto, B., Grisold, W., Vitaliani, R., Graus, F., Honnorat, J., Bertolini, G., 2010. Paraneoplastic neurologic syndrome in the PNS Euronetwork database, a European Study from 20 centers. Arch. Neurol. 67, 330–335.

Gorman, M.P., 2010. Update on diagnosis, treatment, and prognosis in opsoclonus-myoclonus-ataxia syndrome. Curr. Opin. Pediatr. 22, 745–750.

Graus, F., Dalmau, J., René, R., Tora, M., Malats, N., Verschuuren, J.J., et al., 1997a. Anti-Hu antibodies in patients with small-cell lung cancer. Association with complete response to therapy and improved survival. J. Clin. Oncol. 15, 2866–2872.

Graus, F., Dalmau, J., Valldeoriola, F., Ferrer, I., Reñe, R., Marin, C., et al., 1997b. Immunological characterization of a neuronal antibody (anti-Tr) associated with paraneoplastic cerebellar degeneration and Hodgkin's disease. J. Neuroimmunol. 74, 55–61.

Graus, F., Delattre, J.Y., Antoine, J.C., Dalmau, J., Giometto, B., Grisold, W., et al., 2004. Recommended diagnostic criteria for paraneoplastic neurological syndromes. J. Neurol. Neurosurg. Psychiatry. 75, 1135–1140.

Graus, F., Gultekin, S.H., Ferrer, I., Reiriz, J., Alberch, J., Dalmau, J., 1998. Localization of the neuronal antigen recognized by anti-Tr antibodies from patients with paraneoplastic cerebellar degeneration and Hodgkin's disease in the rat nervous system. Acta Neuropathol. (Berl.). 96, 1–7.

Graus, F., Keime-Guibert, F., Reñe, R., Benyahia, B., Ribalta, T., Ascaso, C., et al., 2001. Anti-Hu-associated paraneoplastic encephalomyelitis: analysis of 200 patients. Brain. 124, 1138–1148.

Greenlee, J.E., 2013. Treatment of paraneoplastic cerebellar degeneration. Curr. Treat Options Neurol. 15, 185–200.

Greenlee, J.E., Clawson, S.A., Hill, K.E., Wood, B.L., Tsunoda, I., Carlson, N.G., 2010. Purkinje cell death after uptake of anti-yo antibodies in cerebellar slice cultures. J. Neuropathol. Exp. Neurol. 69, 997–1007.

Hansen, N., Grunewald, B., Weishaupt, A., Colaço, M.N., Toyka, K.V., Sommer, C., et al., 2013. Human stiff person syndrome IgG-containing high-titer anti-GAD65 autoantibodies induce motor dysfunction in rats. Exp. Neurol. 239, 202–209.

Hattan, E., Angle, M.R., Chalk, C., 2008. Unexpected benefit of propofol in stiff-person syndrome. Neurology. 70, 1641–1642.

Honnorat, J., Saiz, A., Giometto, B., Vincent, A., Brieva, L., de Andres, C., et al., 2001. Cerebellar ataxia with anti-glutamic acid decarboxylase antibodies. Study of 14 patients. Arch. Neurol. 58, 225–230.

Hormigo, A., Dalmau, J., Rosenblum, M.K., River, M.E., Posner, J.B., 1994. Immunological and pathological study of anti-Ri-associated encephalopathy. Ann. Neurol. 36, 896–902.

Jarius, S., Stich, O., Rasiah, C., Voltz, R., Rauer, S., 2008a. Qualitative evidence of Ri specific IgG-synthesis in the cerebrospinal fluid from patients with paraneoplastic neurological syndromes. J. Neurol. Sci. 268, 65–68.

Jarius, S., Wandinger, K.P., Borowski, K., Stoecker, W., Wildemann, B., 2008b. Antibodies to CV2/CRMP5 in neuromyelitis optica-like disease, case report and review of the literature. Clin. Neurol. Neurosurg. 114, 331–335.

Kalia, L.V., Kalia, S.K., Salter, M.W., 2008. NMDA receptors in clinical neurology, excitatory times ahead. Lancet Neurol. 7, 742–755.

Keime-Guibert, F., Graus, F., Broet, P., René, R., Molinuevo, J.L., Ascaso, C., et al., 1999. Clinical outcome of patients with anti-Hu-associated encephalomyelitis after treatment of the tumor. Neurology. 53, 1719–1723.

Keime-Guibert, F., Graus, F., Fleury, A., René, R., Honnorat, J., Broet, P., et al., 2000. Treatment of paraneoplastic neurological syndromes with antineuronal antibodies (Anti-Hu, Anti-Yo) with a combination of immunoglobulins, cyclophosphamide, and methylprednisolone. J. Neurol. Neurosurg. Psychiatry. 68, 479–482.

Ko, M.W., Dalmau, J., Galetta, S.L., 2008. Neuro-ophthalmologic manifestations of paraneoplastic syndromes. J. Neuroophthalmol. 28, 58–68.

Kraemer, M., Berlit, P., 2007. Anti-Ma2 antibodies in B-cell primary CNS lymphoma. J. Neurol. 254, 1286–1287.

Landolfi, J.C., 2003. Paraneoplastic limbic encephalitis and possible narcolepsy in a patient with testicular cancer, case study. Neuro-Oncology. 5, 214–216.

Lennon, V.A., Ermilov, L.G., Szurszewski, J.H., Vernino, S., 2003. Immunization with neuronal nicotinic acetylcholine receptor induces neurological autoimmune disease. J. Clin. Invest. 111, 907–913.

Lewis, H.A., Chen, H., Edo, C., Buckanovich, R.J., Yang, Y.Y., Musunuru, K., et al., 1999. Crystal structures of Nova-1 and Nova-2 K-homology RNA-binding domains. Structure Fold Des. 7, 191–203.

Licatalosi, D.D., Mele, A., Fak, J.J., Ule, J., Kayikci, M., Chi, S.W., et al., 2008. HITS-CLIP yields genome-wide insights into brain alternative RNA processing. Nature. 456, 464–469.

Lu, Y., Jia, L., He, S., Leys, M.J., Jayasundera, T., Heckenlively, J.R., 2009. Melanoma-associated retinopathy, a paraneoplastic autoimmune complication. Arch. Ophthalmol. 127, 1572–1580.

Lucchinetti, C.F., Kimmel, D.W., Lennon, V.A., 1998. Paraneoplastic and oncologic profiles of patients seropositive for type 1 antineuronal nuclear autoantibodies. Neurology. 50, 652–657.

McKeon, A., Lennon, V.A., Lachance, D.H., Fealey, R.D., Pittock, S.J., 2009. Ganglionic acetylcholine receptor autoantibody, oncological, neurological, and serological accompaniments. Arch. Neurol. 66, 735–741.

McKeon, A., Martinez-Hernandez, E., Lancaster, E., Matsumoto, J.Y., Harvey, R.J., McEvoy, K.M., et al., 2013. Glycine receptor autoimmune spectrum with stiff-man syndrome phenotype. JAMA Neurol. 70, 44–50.

Monstad, S.E., Drivsholm, L., Skeie, G.O., Aarseth, J.H., Vedeler, C.A., 2008. CRMP5 antibodies in patients with small-cell lung cancer or thymoma. Cancer Immunol. Immunother. 57, 227–232.

Muehlschlegel, S., Okun, M.S., Foote, K.D., Coco, D., Yachnis, A.T., Fernandez, H.H., 2005. Paraneoplastic chorea with leukoencephalopathy presenting with obsessive-compulsive and behavioral disorder. Mov. Disord. 20, 1523–1527.

Murthy, V.N., De, C.P., 2003. Cell biology of the presynaptic terminal. Annu. Rev. Neurosci. 26, 701–728.

Nguyen-Huu, B.K., Urban, P.P., Schreckenberger, M., Dieterich, M., Werhahn, K.J., 2006. Antiamphiphysin-positive stiff-person syndrome associated with small cell lung cancer. Mov. Disord. 21, 1285–1287.

Ohguro, H., Maruyama, I., Nakazawa, M., Oohira, A., 2002. Antirecoverin antibody in the aqueous humor of a patient with cancer-associated retinopathy. Am. J. Ophthalmol. 134, 605–607.

Okano, H.J., Park, W.Y., Corradi, J.P., Darnell, R.B., 1999. The cytoplasmic Purkinje onconeural antigen CDR2 down-regulates c-Myc function: implications for neuronal and tumor cell survival. Genes Dev. 13, 2087–2097.

Overeem, S., Dalmau, J., Bataller, L., Nishino, S., Mignot, E., Verschuuren, J., et al., 2004. Hypocretin-1 CSF levels in anti-Ma2 associated encephalitis. Neurology. 62, 138–140.

Perrone-Bizzozero, N., Bird, C.W., 2013. Role of HuD in nervous system function and pathology. In: Schol (Ed.), Front Biosci., 5. pp. 554–563.

Peterson, K., Rosenblum, M.K., Kotanides, H., Posner, J.B., 1992. Paraneoplastic cerebellar degeneration. I. A clinical analysis of 55 anti-Yo antibody positive patients. Neurology. 42, 1931–1937.

Phuphanich, S., Brock, C., 2007. Neurologic improvement after high-dose intravenous immunoglobulin therapy in patients with paraneoplastic cerebellar degeneration associated with anti-Purkinje cell antibody. J. Neurooncol. 81, 67–69.

Pittock, S.J., Lucchinetti, C.F., Lennon, V.A., 2003. Anti-neuronal nuclear autoantibody type 2, paraneoplastic accompaniments. Ann. Neurol. 53, 580–587.

Pittock, S.J., Kryzer, T.J., Lennon, V.A., 2004. Paraneoplastic antibodies coexist and predict cancer, not neurological syndrome. Ann. Neurol. 56, 715–719.

Pittock, S.J., Lucchinetti, C.F., Parisi, J.E., Benarroch, E.E., Mokri, B., Stephan, C.L., et al., 2005. Amphiphysin autoimmunity: paraneoplastic accompaniments. Ann. Neurol. 58, 96–107.

Pittock, S.J., Yoshikawa, H., Ahlskog, J.E., Tisch, S.H., Benarroch, E.E., Kryzer, T.J., et al., 2006. Glutamic acid decarboxylase autoimmunity with brainstem, extrapyramidal, and spinal cord dysfunction. Mayo Clin. Proc. 81, 1207–1214.

Pittock, S.J., Parisi, J.E., McKeon, A., Roemer, S.F., Lucchinetti, C.F., Tan, K.M., et al., 2010. Paraneoplastic jaw dystonia and laryngospasm with antineuronal nuclear autoantibody type 2 (anti-ri). Arch. Neurol. 67, 1109–1115.

Rakocevic, G., Floeter, M.K., 2012. Autoimmune stiff person syndrome and related myelopathies: understanding of electrophysiological and immunological processes. Muscle Nerve. 45, 623–634.

Rakocevic, G., Raju, R., Dalakas, M.C., 2004. Anti-glutamic acid decarboxylase antibodies in the serum and cerebrospinal fluid of patients with Stiff-Person syndrome correlation with clinical severity. Arch. Neurol. 61, 902–904.

Ratti, A., Fallini, C., Colombrita, C., Pascale, A., Laforenza, U., Quattrone, A., et al., 2008. Post-transcriptional regulation of neuro-oncological ventral antigen 1 by the neuronal RNA-binding proteins ELAV. J. Biol. Chem. 283, 7531–7541.

Rodriguez, M., Truh, L.I., O'Neill, B.P., Lennon, V.A., 1988. Autoimune paraneoplastic cerebellar degeneration, ultrastructural localization of antibody-binding sites in Purkinje cells. Neurology. 38, 1380–1386.

Rosenfeld, M.R., Eichen, J.G., Wade, D.F., Posner, J.B., Dalmau, J., 2001. Molecular and clinical diversity in paraneoplastic immunity to Ma proteins. Ann. Neurol. 50, 339–348.

Rosenfeld, M.R., Titulaer, M.J., Dalmau, J., 2012. Paraneoplastic syndromes and autoimmune encephalitis. Five new things. Neurol. Clin. Pract. 2, 215–223.

Saiz, A., Blanco, Y., Sabater, L., González, F., Bataller, L., Casamitjana, R., et al., 2008. Spectrum of neurological syndromes associated with glutamic acid decarboxylase antibodies: diagnostic clues for this association. Brain. 131, 2553–2563.

Sakai, K., Shirakawa, T., Li, Y.Y., Kitagawa, Y., Hirose, G., 2002. Interaction of a paraneoplastic cerebellar degeneration-associated neuronal protein with the nuclear helix-loop-helix leucine zipper protein MRG X. Mol. Cell Neurosci. 19, 477–484.

Schreiber, H., Rowley, D.A., 2008. Cancer. Quo vadis, specificity? Science. 319, 164–165.

Schuller, M., Jenne, D., Voltz, R., 2005. The human PNMA family, novel neuronal proteins implicated in paraneoplastic neurological disease. J. Neuroimmunol. 169, 172–176.

Seute, T., Leffers, P., Ten Velde, G.P., Twijnstra, A., 2004. Neurologic disorders in 432 consecutive patients with small cell lung carcinoma. Cancer. 100, 801–806.

Shildkrot, Y., Sobrin, L., Gragoudas, E.S., 2011. Cancer-associated retinopathy, update on pathogenesis and therapy. Semin. Ophthalmol. 26, 321–328.

Sillevis, S.P., Grefkens, J., De Leeuw, B., van den Bent, M., van Putten, W., Hooijkaas, H., et al., 2002. Survival and outcome in 73 anti-Hu positive patients with paraneoplastic encephalomyelitis/sensory neuronopathy. J. Neurol. 249, 745–753.

Singhi, P., Sahu, J.K., Sarkar, J., Bansal, D., 2013. Clinical profile and outcome of children with opsoclonus-myoclonus syndrome. J. Child. Neurol. Epub ahead of print.

Solimena, M., Folli, F., Aparisi, R., Pozza, G., De Camilli, P., 1990. Autoantibodies to GABA-ergic neurons and pancreatic beta cells in stiff-man syndrome. N. Engl. J. Med. 322, 1555–1560.

Stich, O., Rauer, S., 2007. Antigen-specific oligoclonal bands in cerebrospinal fluid and serum from patients with anti-amphiphysin- and anti-CV2/CRMP5-associated paraneoplastic neurological syndromes. Eur. J. Neurol. 14, 650–653.

Stich, O., Rasiah, C., Rauer, S., 2009. Paraneoplastic antibody during follow-up of a patient with anti-Ri-associated paraneoplastic neurological syndrome. Acta Neurol. Scand. 119, 338–340.

Taniguchi, Y., Tanji, C., Kawai, T., Saito, H., Marubayashi, S., Yorioka, N., 2006. A case report of plasmapheresis in paraneoplastic cerebellar ataxia associated with anti-Tr antibody. Ther. Apher. Dial. 10, 90–93.

Tanner, D.C., Qiu, S., Bolognani, F., Partridge, L.D., Weeber, E.J., Perrone-Bizzozero, N.I., 2008. Alterations in mossy fiber physiology and GAP-43 expression and function in transgenic mice overexpressing HuD. Hippocampus. 18, 814–823.

Taplin, C.E., Barker, J.M., 2008. Autoantibodies in type 1 diabetes. Autoimmunity. 41, 11–18.

Thirkill, C.E., 2005. Cancer-induced, immune-mediated ocular degenerations. Ocul. Immunol. Inflamm. 13, 119–131.

Tora, M., Graus, F., De Bolòs, C., Real, F.X., 1997. Cell surface expression of paraneoplastic encephalomyelitis/sensory neuronopathy-associated Hu antigens in small-cell lung cancers and neuroblastomas. Neurology. 48, 735–741.

Vernino, S., Adamski, J., Kryzer, T.J., Fealey, R.D., Lennon, V.A., 1998. Neuronal nicotinic ACh receptor antibody in subacute autonomic neuropathy and cancer-related syndromes. Neurology. 50, 1806–1813.

Vernino, S., Tuite, P., Adler, C.H., Meschia, J.F., Boeve, B.F., Boasberg, P., et al., 2002. Paraneoplastic chorea associated with CRMP-5 neuronal antibody and lung carcinoma. Ann. Neurol. 51, 625–630.

Vernino, S., Sandroni, P., Singer, W., Low, P.A., 2008. Autonomic ganglia, target and novel therapeutic tool. Neurology. 70, 1926–1932.

Viaccoz, A., Honnorat, J., 2013. Paraneoplastic neurological syndromes, general treatment overview. Curr. Treat Options Neurol. 15, 150–168.

Vianello, M., Keir, G., Giometto, B., Betterle, C., Tavolato, B., Thompson, E.J., 2005. Antigenic differences between neurological and diabetic patients with anti-glutamic acid decarboxylase antibodies. Eur. J. Neurol. 12, 294–299.

Vianello, M., Giometto, B., Vassanelli, S., Canato, M., Betterle, C., Mucignat, C., 2006. Peculiar labeling of cultured hippocampal neurons by different sera harboring anti-glutamic acid decarboxylase autoantibodies (GAD-Ab). Exp. Neurol. 202, 514–518.

Vincent, A., 2009. Antibodies to contractin-associated protein 2 (CASPR2). Ann. Neurol. 66, T72.

Vincent, A., 2010. Autoimmune channelopathies: well-established and emerging immunotherapy-responsive diseases of peripheral and central nervous systems. J. Clin. Immunol. Supp. 1, s97–s102.

Vincent, A., Lang, B., Kleopa, K.A., 2006. Autoimmune channelopathies and related neurological disorders. Neuron. 52, 123–138.

Wang, Z., Low, P.A., Jordan, J., Freeman, R., Gibbons, C.H., Schroeder, C., et al., 2007. Autoimmune autonomic ganglionopathy: IgG effects on ganglionic acetylcholine receptor current. Neurology. 68, 1917–1921.

Wirtz, P.W., Smallegange, T.M., Wintzen, A.R., Verschuuren, J.J., 2002. Differences in clinical features between the Lambert-Eaton myasthenic syndrome with and without cancer, an analysis of 227 published cases. Clin. Neurol. Neurosurg. 104, 359–363.

Yu, Z., Kryzer, T.J., Griesmann, G.E., Kim, K., Benarroch, E.E., Lennon, V.A., 2001. CRMP-5 neuronal autoantibody, marker of lung cancer and thymoma-related autoimmunity. Ann. Neurol. 49, 146–154.

Part 11

Gastrointestinal System

Chapter 59

Celiac Disease

Ludvig M. Sollid[1] and Knut E.A. Lundin[1,2]

[1]Centre for Immune Regulation and Department of Immunology, University of Oslo and Oslo University Hospital – Rikshospitalet, Oslo, Norway,
[2]Department of Gastroenterology, Oslo University Hospital – Rikshospitalet, Oslo, Norway

Chapter Outline

Clinical, Pathologic and Epidemiologic Features	855	**Pathogenic Mechanisms**	861
Clinical Features and Associated Disorders	855	Gluten-reactive CD4+ T Cells	861
Pathology of the Intestinal Lesion	856	Role of Transglutaminase 2	861
Epidemiology	856	Gluten Antigen Presentation by Disease-associated DQ	
Autoimmune Features	857	Molecules	862
Autoantibodies	857	Mucosal Antigen-presenting Cells	864
Autoreactive Intraepithelial Lymphocytes (IELs)	859	Effector Mechanisms Leading to Mucosal Alterations	864
Genetic Features	859	**Autoantibodies as Potential Immunologic Markers**	864
HLA Genes	859	Serology	864
Non-HLA Genes	859	Staining of Immune Complexes	865
Environmental Influences	860	**Treatment and Outcome**	865
Gluten Proteins	860	Current Treatment and Outcome	865
Other Environmental Factors	860	Novel Therapeutic Options	865
***In Vivo* and *In Vitro* Models**	861	**Concluding Remarks—Future Prospects**	866
Animal Models	861	**Acknowledgments**	866
Organ Culture Assays	861	**References**	866

Celiac disease (also termed gluten sensitive enteropathy) has autoimmune features of which the highly disease-specific antibodies to the enzyme transglutaminase 2 (TG2), a.k.a. tissue transglutaminase, are particularly striking. The disease is precipitated in genetically susceptible individuals by the ingestion of cereal gluten proteins of wheat, barley, and rye. Some historical findings which have lead to our current understanding of the pathogenesis of celiac disease are listed in Box 59.1. If the critical role of gluten was not known in celiac disease, this disorder would not have been related to food hypersensitivity, but rather been considerered a bona fide autoimmune disease with tissue-specific destruction of enterocytes in the small bowel—not very different from the destruction of islet cells in the pancreas in type 1 diabetes. The combinantion of the knowledge of the disease-driving antigen, the easy access to the target organ by gastroduodeno-scopy, and an unusually clear HLA association has led to a detailed understanding of pathogenic mechanisms.

Thus, among the chronic inflammatory disorders with autoimmune components, celiac disease stands out as a particularly good model. Insight into the pathogenesis of this disorder is relevant for diseases for which the genetic and environmental components are poorly characterized.

CLINICAL, PATHOLOGIC AND EPIDEMIOLOGIC FEATURES

Clinical Features and Associated Disorders

Celiac disease may present in early childhood soon after the introduction of gluten-containing food. A dramatic and even fatal clinical picture with diarrhea, anorexia, failure to thrive, abdominal distension, and growth retardation was once regarded as typical. This is now rare, and most children and adults present with a milder, pauci- or mono-symptomatic disease (Mäki et al., 1988). Many of the symptoms associated with the milder disease form, like chronic

N. Rose & I. Mackay (Eds): The Autoimmune Diseases, Fifth edition. DOI: http://dx.doi.org/10.1016/B978-0-12-384929-8.00059-9

fatigue, joint pain, and neuropsychological problems, do not directly point to a small intestinal disorder (Murray, 1999; Fasano and Catassi, 2001; Farrell and Kelly, 2002). Neither do complications like osteoporosis, reduced fertility, peripheral neuropathy, epilepsy with cerebral calcifications or dermatitis herpetiformis (Ciacci et al., 1995; Collin and Reunala, 2003; Hadjivassiliou et al., 2003; Sanders et al., 2003). The coexistence of autoimmune diseases is striking; in particular there is an overrepresentation of type 1 diabetes (Green et al., 1962; Koletzko et al., 1988; Cronin et al., 1997), Sjögren's syndrome (Collin et al., 1994), autoimmune thyroid disorders (Collin et al., 1994; Counsell et al., 1994), connective tissue disease (Collin et al., 1994), and IgA deficiency (Mawhinney and Tomkin, 1971; Cataldo et al., 1997; Wang et al., 2011). Like many autoimmune disorders, pediatric and adult celiac disease show a gender bias with a female to male ratio of approximately 2:1 (Ciacci et al., 1995; Ivarsson et al., 2003b).

Recently there has been much interest in the clinical entity of "non-celiac gluten sensitivity." Such patients may have symptoms resembling celiac disease, but the enteropathy, serology, and HLA association typical of celiac disease are lacking as are clear diagnostic criteria (Ludvigsson et al., 2012).

Pathology of the Intestinal Lesion

The intestinal lesion in celiac disease can be classified into three dynamically connected stages as suggested by Marsh; the infiltrative, the hyperplastic, and the destructive lesion (Marsh, 1992) (Figure 59.1). In the infiltrative lesion (Marsh 1) the mucosal architecture is normal, but there is an increased infiltration of intraepithelial lymphocytes (IEL) in the villous epithelium. The hyperplastic lesion (Marsh 2) is similar to the infiltrate lesion, but in addition has enlarged hyperplastic crypts. The last stage is the destructive lesion which can be subgrouped into partial, subtotal, or total villous atrophy (Marsh 3 A–C) (Oberhuber et al., 1999). The latter corresponds to the classic flat lesion, which in addition to the increased IEL, is characterized by swelling and infiltration of plasma cells, CD4$^+$ αβ T cells, macrophages/dendritic cells, mast cells, and neutrophils in the lamina propria (Figure 59.2).

Epidemiology

Celiac disease has a world wide distribution, but is primarily a disease of Caucasians. The prevalence in Europe and USA is around 1:130–1:300 (Catassi et al., 1996; Fasano et al., 2003). There are unexplained differences in prevalence between European countries with adult prevalence figures ranging from 2.4% in Finland to 0.3% in Germany (Mustalahti et al., 2010). More than half the cases are now diagnosed in adult life, and the disease can be diagnosed even after the age of 60 years. Many patients may have had undetected celiac disease in childhood, whereas in others, the disease has started later. The natural history and the timing for conversion to seropositivity and/or mucosal inflammation are not fully understood. Studies from Finland suggest that some children may have transient positive serology that normalizes without dietary manipulation (Mäki et al., 2003; Simell et al., 2007). These rare events suggest that at least some aspects of celiac disease may be transient.

Between 1985 and 1995 there was an epidemic of celiac disease in Sweden among children below 2 years with a three-fold increase in incidence (Ivarsson et al., 2000). The sharp rise and subsequent abrupt decrease in incidence was likely related to changes in infant feeding habits, including the amount of gluten given, the age at introduction of gluten to the diet, and whether

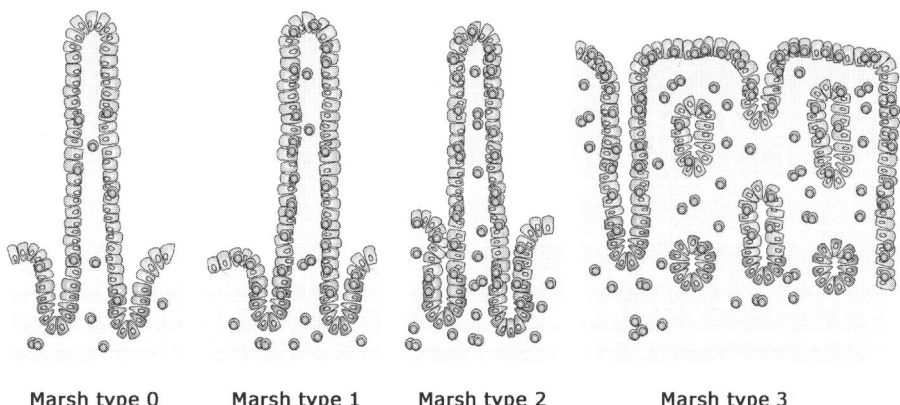

Marsh type 0   Marsh type 1   Marsh type 2   Marsh type 3

FIGURE 59.1   Schematic representation of the stages of the intestinal lesion in celiac disease according to Marsh.   The stages are dynamically related. The normal stage is Marsh type 0. In Marsh type 1 there are increased numbers of intraepithelial lymphocytes (IELs). Marsh type 2 has increased numbers of IELs and enlarged, hyperplastic crypts. Marsh type 3 has, in addition to increased numbers of IELs and crypt hyperplasia, also partial to complete blunting of the villous structures. The numbers of leukocytes in the lamina propria, such as plasma cells and T cells, are increased in the full blown celiac disease lesion, but their presence is not included as parameters for the Marsh staging. *Courtesy of A.-C.R. Beitnes and Jorunn Stamnaes.*

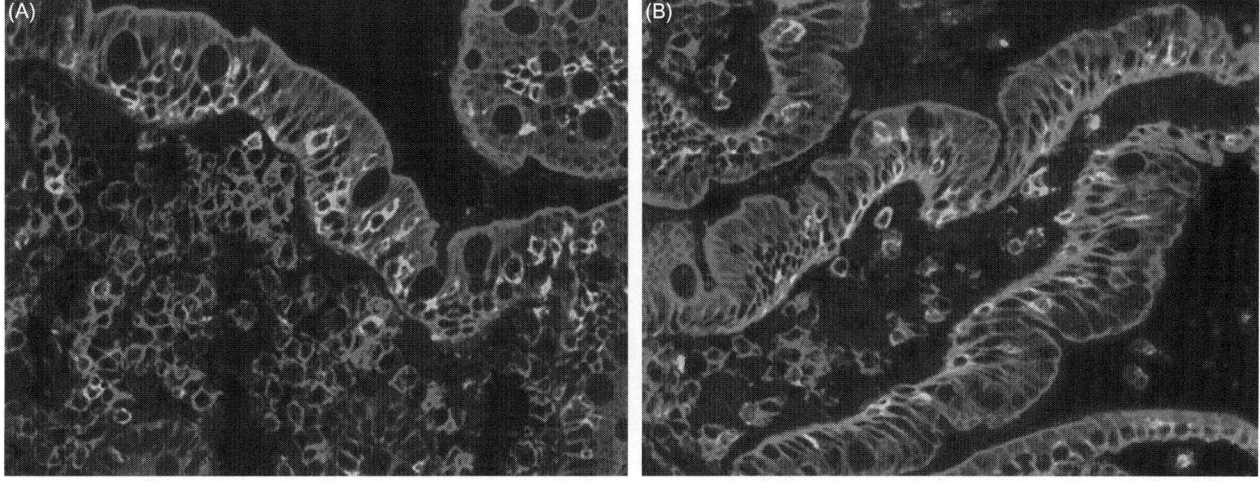

FIGURE 59.2   The celiac lesion is characterized by increased infiltration of T cells and plasma cells.   Immunohistochemical staining of T cells (CD3, green), plasma cells (CD138, red) and epithelial cells (cytokeratin, blue) in biopsy sections of (A) a patient with untreated celiac disease and (B) a normal subject. *Courtesy of A.-C.R. Beitnes.*

breastfeeding was ongoing or not when gluten was introduced. Notably, breastfeeding reduced the risk of early celiac disease (Ivarsson et al., 2002). Later follow-up at the age of 12 years has shown an astonishingly high prevalence of 3% for celiac disease in these children (Myleus et al., 2009). The increase is not, however, confined to these high-risk cohorts and celiac disease has become far more prevalent in Sweden.

AUTOIMMUNE FEATURES

Autoantibodies

Untreated celiac disease patients (on a regular diet) usually have increased levels of antibodies against gluten, other food antigens, and autoantigens. Initially, autoantibodies in celiac disease were detected as anti-reticulin antibodies by staining of various rat tissue (Alp and Wright, 1971; Seah et al., 1971). Later IgA anti-endomysium antibodies (EMA) either as detected by staining of monkey esophagus (Chorzelski et al., 1984) or human umbilical cord (Ladinser et al., 1994) were recognized. The main antigen recognized by anti-reticulin antibodies and EMA was identified as the enzyme transglutaminse 2 (TG2) (Dieterich et al., 1997), although antibodies to calreticulin and actin are also found (Clemente et al., 2000; Sanchez et al., 2000). The antibodies to TG2 are both of the IgA and IgG isotypes, but the IgA antibodies are most closely linked with celiac disease (Rostom et al., 2005).

Anti-TG2 antibodies only occur in individuals who are HLA-DQ2 or HLA-DQ8 (Bjorck et al., 2010). Moreover, the production of the IgA anti-TG2 antibodies is entirely dependent on dietary gluten exposure (Dieterich et al., 1998; Sulkanen et al., 1998). These two observations indicate that gluten-reactive T cells are implicated in the generation of these antibodies. A model has been proposed where gluten-reactive T cells provide help to TG2-specific B cells by means of hapten carrier-like gluten–TG2 complexes (Sollid et al., 1997) (Figure 59.3c). This model can explain why the serum TG2 antibodies in celiac disease disappear when the patients are put on a gluten-free diet. When the gluten goes, so does the T cell help needed for the B cells to switch isotype and differentiate to plasma cells (Sollid et al., 1997).

Production of anti-TG2 antibodies is vigorous in the active celiac lesion, and on average 10% of the plasma cells in the lesion produce anti-TG2 antibodies (Di Niro et al., 2012). IgA is the dominating isotype, and such cells

are absent in celiac patients on a gluten-free diet (Di Niro et al., 2012). The TG2 antibodies have a unique repertoire with overusage of VH5-51 (Marzari et al., 2001; Di Niro et al., 2012), and they have few mutations despite being part of a chronic inflammatory response (Di Niro et al., 2012). The somatic mutations, though they are modest, speak of T cell involvement in the antibody response as the displacement mutations dominate silent mutations (Di Niro et al., 2012; Marzari et al., 2001) and as reversion of some selected antibodies to germline sequence lead to reduction in antibody affinity (Di Niro et al., 2012).

It is uncertain whether autoantibodies play a role in the pathogenesis. High incidence of celiac disease in IgA deficiency (Wang et al., 2011) argues that IgA antibodies *per se* play a minor pathogenic role. The involvement of the humoral immune system does not need to be at the level of soluble antibodies, but could at the level of B cells. If TG2-specific B cells are indeed able to present gluten peptides to gluten-specific T cells, this would be an extremely effective amplification step in the anti-gluten T cell response.

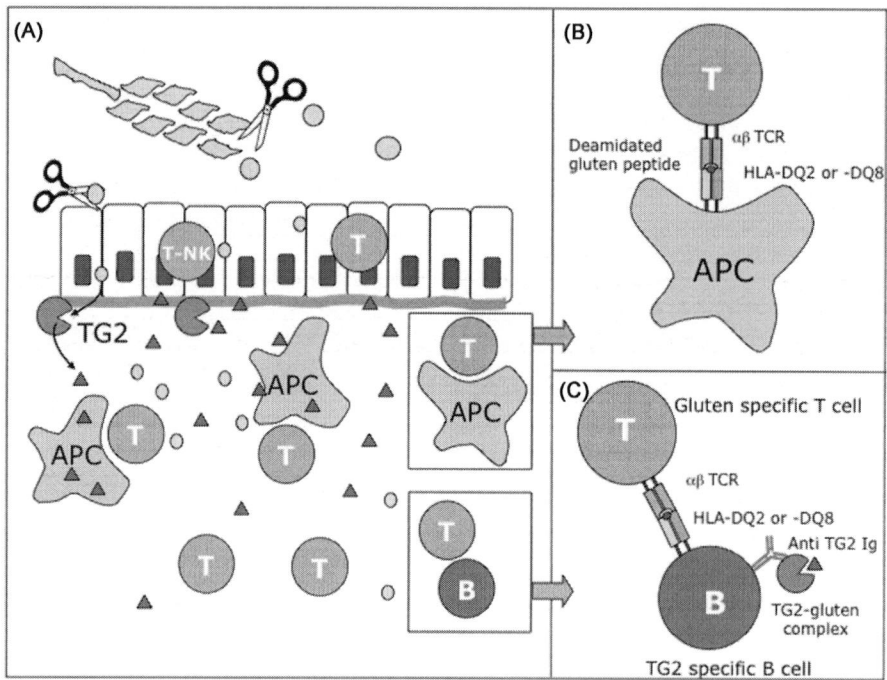

FIGURE 59.3 The celiac small intestinal lesion. (A) Depiction of the intestinal mucosa with emphasis on the factors taking part in the development and control of celiac disease. The parts of the gluten proteins that are resistant to processing by luminal and brush border enzymes will survive digestion, and can be transported across the epithelial barrier as polypeptides. Gluten peptides are deamidated by transglutaminase 2 (TG2), which, in the intestinal mucosa, is mainly located extracellularly in the subepithelial region, but is also found in the brush border. TG2 may also be expressed by antigen-presenting cells (APCs [l.c.]) like macrophages and dendritic cells. CD4+ T cells in the lamina propria recognize predominantly deamidated gluten peptides, presented by HLA-DQ2 or -DQ8 molecules on the cell surface of the APC. (B) HLA-DQ2 and -DQ8 molecules have preference for binding peptides with negatively charged amino acids (DQ2 in positions P4, P6, and P7; DQ8 in positions P1 and P9) and thereby bind gluten peptides deamidated by TG2 with increased affinities. (C) Model of how gluten-reactive T cells control the formation of antibodies to TG2 by intramolecular help. TG2 and gluten can form complexes. Such complexes of gluten and TG2 bound by surface immunoglobulin of TG2-specific B cells (anti TG2 Ig) will be endocytosed, and deamidated gluten peptides can be released for binding to DQ2 or DQ8 molecules. After transport to the cell surface of the HLA molecules with bound peptides, gluten-reactive T cells can recognize the deamidated gluten peptides and thereby provide T cell help to the TG2-specific B cells.

Involvement of TG2-specific B cells in the pathogenesis of celiac disease could then explain why anti-TG2-specific antibodies are such precise predictors of disease.

The autoantibodies may well be implicated in the extraintestinal manifestations of celiac disease. In dermatitis herpetiformis, which could be considered as celiac disease with additional skin lesions, IgA autoantibodies are prime suspects. These patients, in addition to anti-TG2 antibodies, have antibodies that target transglutaminase 3 (TG3), and the IgA anti-TG3 antibodies are more closely associated with the disease than the IgA anti-TG2 antibodies (Sardy et al., 2002). TG3 is closely related to TG2 and is also able to modify gluten peptides, but is paradoxically not expressed in the dermal papillae where the granular IgA deposits in dermatitis herpetiformis are located.

Autoreactive Intraepithelial Lymphocytes (IELs)

Untreated celiac disease is characterized by an increased density of proliferating $TCR\alpha\beta^+$ $CD8^+CD4^-$ and $TCR\gamma\delta^+$ $CD8^-CD4^-$ cells in the villous epithelium. In contrast to the $TCR\alpha\beta + CD8^+$ IELs that return to normal when gluten is removed from the diet, the $TCR\gamma\delta^+$ IELs remain at an elevated level (Kutlu et al., 1993). This may suggest that these two types of T cells play different roles in the pathogenesis process. Many of the IELs co-express innate (NK cell) receptors recognizing non-classical HLA molecules like MIC molecules and HLA-E. In celiac disease there is a decrease in IELs expressing the inhibitory receptor CD94-NKG2A (Meresse et al., 2006) and an increase of IELs expressing the activating receptors NKG2D (Hüe et al., 2004; Meresse et al., 2004) and CD94/NKG2C (Meresse et al., 2006) (Figure 59.3A). These activated IELs can kill enterocytes by use of the NK cell receptors possibly without involvement of the T cell receptor (Hüe et al., 2004; Meresse et al., 2004).

GENETIC FEATURES

A high prevalence (10%) among first-degree relatives of celiac disease patients indicates that susceptibility to develop celiac disease is strongly influenced by inherited factors (Ellis, 1981). Familial clustering is stronger in celiac disease than in most other chronic inflammatory diseases with a multifactorial etiology (Risch, 1987). The strong genetic influence in celiac disease is further supported by a high concordance rate ($\sim 75\%$) in monozygotic twins (Greco et al., 2002). Both HLA and non-HLA genes contribute to the genetic predisposition.

HLA Genes

The strongest HLA association in celiac disease is the presence of a variant of HLA-DQ2 which is often termed HLA-DQ2.5 (Figure 59.4). Usually 90% or more of the celiac disease patients carry this HLA molecule. The DQ2.5 molecule is found in individuals who carry the DR3-DQ2 haplotype encoded by DQA1 and DQB1 alleles (DQA1*05:01 and DQB1*02:01) which are located on the same chromosome (cis position). Alternatively it can be expressed by indiduals who are DQ5DQ7/ /DR7DQ2 heterozygous and then the alleles (DQA1*05:05 and DQB1*02:02) are located on opposite chromosomes (trans position). About half of the remaining celiac patients carry HLA-DQ8 encoded by the DQA1*03 and DQB1*03:02 alleles. The rest of the patients are DQ2.2 or DQ7.5 (Karell et al., 2003); thus they carry either the α-chain or the β-chain of the DQ2.5 molecule. DQ2.5 and DQ8 have population frequencies each around 20–25% in most Caucasian populations so the majority of the individuals with these HLA types do not develop celiac disease. Because of the strong HLA association in celiac disease, HLA can be considered a necessary but not sufficient genetic factor for disease development.

Non-HLA Genes

Genome-wide association studies (GWAS) have greatly advanced the knowledge of non-HLA genes in celiac disease. So far 39 loci outside of HLA have been identified to harbor one or more genes predisposing to or protecting against celiac disease (Trynka et al., 2011). Individually, these non-HLA genes contribute little to genetic risk. It has been estimated that with a population prevalence of 1% and a heritability of 50%, the 39 non-HLA loci account for 14% of the genetic variance whereas HLA in comparison accounts for 40% (Trynka et al., 2011). Evidence suggests the existence of many additional non-HLA genes with even smaller effect than those identified to date. However, these genes would make little contribution to the overall genetic risk, and it is unclear what should account for the remaining half of the heritability. Unprecise heritability estimates and complex gene–gene interactions have been suggested to be relevant factors.

Most of the 39 non-HLA loci contain genes with immunological functioning. Many of these genes are associated with the functioning of T cells. Thus the pathogenesis model established by studies of immune cells of celiac disease patients is confirmed by the findings of the GWAS. Most celiac disease-associated risk variants in the 39 non-HLA loci are not located in protein coding regions but rather in regions implicated in gene regulation. This suggests that differences in gene expression play an important factor in the pathogensis of celiac disease. Finally, celiac

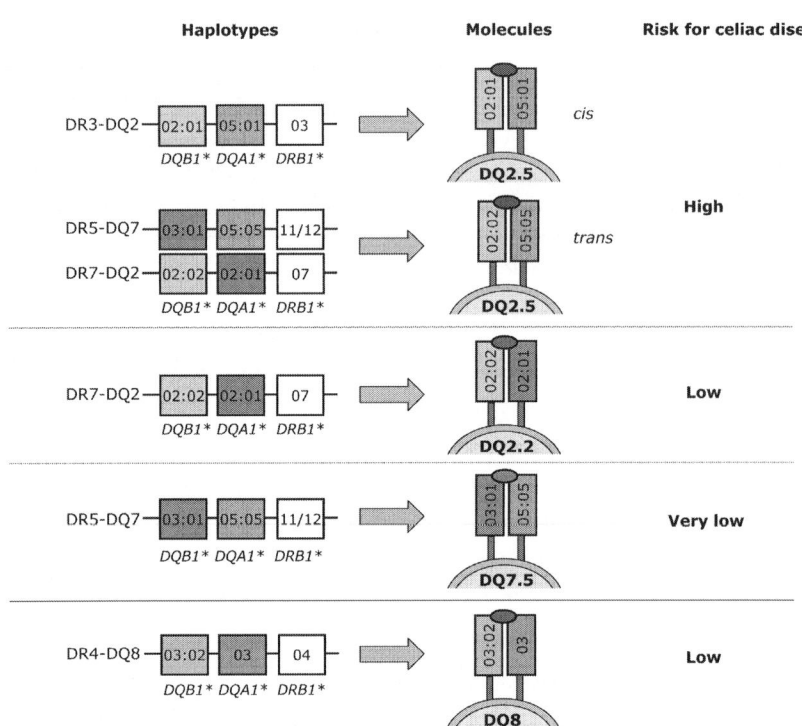

FIGURE 59.4 HLA association in celiac disease. The majority of celiac disease patients carry the HLA-DQ2.5 molecule, which can be encoded in *cis* or in *trans* positions. Most of the remaining patients express HLA-DQ8 whereas the rest of the celiac disease patients express HLA-DQ2.2 or HLA-DQ7.5. The polypeptides encoded by DQA1*05:01 and DQA1*05:05 differ by one residue in the leader peptide, whereas those encoded by DQB1*02:01 and DQB1*02:02 differ by one residue in the membrane proximal domain. It is unlikely that these substitutions have functional consequences.

disease and other immune-mediated dieases, in particular type 1 diabetes (Smyth et al., 2008), share risk gene variants speaking of sharing of critical pathways in the development of the various diseases. New therapeutics for treatment of autoimmune diseases, including biologicals, may thus find a rational basis for testing in celiac disease as well.

ENVIRONMENTAL INFLUENCES

Gluten Proteins

Gluten is the cohesive mass that remains when dough is washed to remove starch. Gluten was originally used to denote wheat proteins only, but is now increasingly used as a term for proline- and glutamine-rich proteins of wheat, barley, rye, and also oat. In wheat, gluten consists of the gliadin and glutenin subcomponents. The gliadin proteins can be subdivided into α-, γ-, and ω-gliadins, while the glutenin proteins can be subdivided into high molecular weight (HMW) and low molecular weight (LMW) subunits (Shewry et al., 2003). The number of unique gluten proteins in common bread wheat is huge due to a hexaploid genome, multiple encoding loci, and allelic variation. Thus, in a single wheat variety there are several hundred different gluten proteins, many of which only differ by a few amino acids. The high content of proline residues makes the gluten proteins particularly resistant to gastrointestinal digestion (Shan et al., 2002). This has important implications for their immunogenicity for T cells.

The gluten proteins of barley are termed hordeins, those of rye, secalins, and those of oat, avenins. Clinical observations suggest that the gluten proteins of barley and rye are also toxic for celiac disease patients (Farrell and Kelly, 2002), and T cell epitopes of barley and rye have been defined (see below). In general, feeding studies have indicated that oat is safe for celiac disease patients (Janatuinen et al., 1995, 2002; Hoffenberg et al., 2000). Rare cases of oat-intolerant celiac patients exist (Lundin et al., 2003; Arentz-Hansen et al., 2004). The lesions of these rare patients harbor T cells specific for oat avenin peptides that closely resemble gliadin T cell epitopes, but which are present in low amounts (Arentz-Hansen et al., 2004).

Other Environmental Factors

Infections may play a role in the development of celiac disease. Some of the best evidence comes from studies in Sweden. In children below the age of 2 years, a positive correlation was found between celiac disease risk and being born during the summer, and children born in the summer are first exposed to dietary gluten during the winter when infections are more prevalent (Ivarsson et al., 2003a). Moreover, in the same population case−control studies indicated that celiac subjects experience three or more infection episodes, more frequently than referents.

IN VIVO AND *IN VITRO* MODELS

Animal Models

With the possible exception of gluten-sensitivite conditions in macaques (Bethune et al., 2008) and in horses (van der Kolk et al., 2012), there exists no good animal model for celiac disease. Several attempts have been made to establish a mouse model, so far with limited success. Gluten-sensitive enteropathy could not be induced in mice made transgenic for HLA-DQ2.5 (Chen et al., 2002, 2003) or HLA-DQ8 (Black et al., 2002). Not even HLA-DQ2.5 transgenic mice made trangenic also for T cell receptors specific for celiac disease-relevant gluten epitopes developed enteropathy (de Kauwe et al., 2009; Du Pre et al., 2011). Notably, dermatitis herpetiformis like skin lesions occurred in a fraction of HLA-DQ8 transgenic mice on a NOD background after systemic immunization with gluten, but without enteropathy (Marietta et al., 2004). Oral tolerance to dietary antigens is strong in rodents, and this could be one of the reasons why gluten-sensitive enteropathy does not develop in these models. Studying immune responses to dietary antigens, it was demonstrated that mice made transgenic for IL-15 and given retinoic acid lost oral tolerance to gliadin and developed gliadin-specific T cells producing IFN-γ (DePaolo et al., 2011). However, also these mice lacked enteropathy suggesting yet other factors are required for the formation of full blown celiac disease.

Organ Culture Assays

Culturing of small intestinal biopsies *ex vivo* has frequently been used to dissect pathogenic events in celiac disease. This assay for instance has been used to examine innate effects of gluten (Maiuri et al., 2003), and to show that gluten challenge induces a stress response with upregulation of IL-15, MICA, and heat shock proteins (Hüe et al., 2004). Although the *ex vivo* culture system has been very important in clarifying the pathogenic mechanisms of celiac disease (Lindfors et al., 2012), the result should be carefully interpreted. One of the problems with the *ex vivo* organ culture system may relate to uneven distribution of inflammatory cells in the mucosa (our unpublished results).

PATHOGENIC MECHANISMS

The strong HLA association in celiac disease and the overrepresentation of non-HLA susceptibility genes related to T cell function strongly suggests that T cells are important in the pathogenesis of celiac disease.

Gluten-reactive CD4[+] T Cells

CD4[+] T cells specific for gluten proteins can be isolated from the small intestinal biopsies of the majority of celiac disease patients (Lundin et al., 1993; van de Wal et al., 1998b), but not from biopsies obtained from disease controls (Molberg et al., 1997). In contrast, patients and many control subjects have gliadin-reactive T cells in their peripheral blood. These T cells use many different HLA molecules for presentation (DR, DQ, and DP) (Gjertsen et al., 1994), and their reactivity is not enhanced by deamidation of the gliadin (Molberg et al., 1998). This implies that many individuals can be immunologically sensitized to gluten without having small intestinal pathology. The gluten-specific T cells derived from the intestinal celiac lesions display a remarkable feature as they are invariably restricted by the disease-associated HLA-DQ molecules (Lundin et al., 1993, 1994) (Figure 59.3B). Most gluten proteins appear to be recognized by such DQ2.5 and DQ8 restricted T cells, although with variable frequency (Lundin et al., 1997; Sjöström et al., 1998; van de Wal et al., 1999; Anderson et al., 2000; Arentz-Hansen et al., 2000, 2002; Vader et al., 2002b; Molberg et al., 2003). The intestinal T cell responses to gluten are thus characterized by heterogeneity and many T cell epitopes exist (Sollid et al., 2012) (Figure 59.5). T cells responsive to the same epitopes are usually not detectable in the peripheral blood, but they can be detected in this compartment in patients in remission after a short-term oral gluten challenge either by ELISPOT (Anderson et al., 2000) or by HLA tetramer staining (Ráki et al., 2007; Brottveit et al., 2011). DQ2 tetramers are recombinantly made DQ2.5 molecules with tethered gluten epitopes that are multimerized (Quarsten et al., 2001), and which hence have sufficient avidity to stain antigen-specific T cells. Also celiac patients who are DQ2.2 but not DQ2.5 or DQ8 have gluten-reactive T cells in the intestinal lesions (Bodd et al., 2012).

Role of Transglutaminase 2

The role of the TG2 enzyme in the pathogenesis of celiac disease is not completely understood, but it clearly encompasses more than simply being the target of the autoantibodies in the disease. There are elevated levels of active TG2 in tissue homogenates made from biopsies of untreated celiac disease patients (Bruce et al., 1985) and the gluten proteins are excellent substrates for TG2. Most importantly, however, the T cells within the celiac lesions predominantly recognize gluten peptides modified by TG2 (Molberg et al., 1998; van de Wal et al., 1998a).

TG2 catalyzes a post-translational transamidation or deamidation of specific glutamine residues within its substrate proteins (Folk, 1983; Lorand and Graham, 2003).

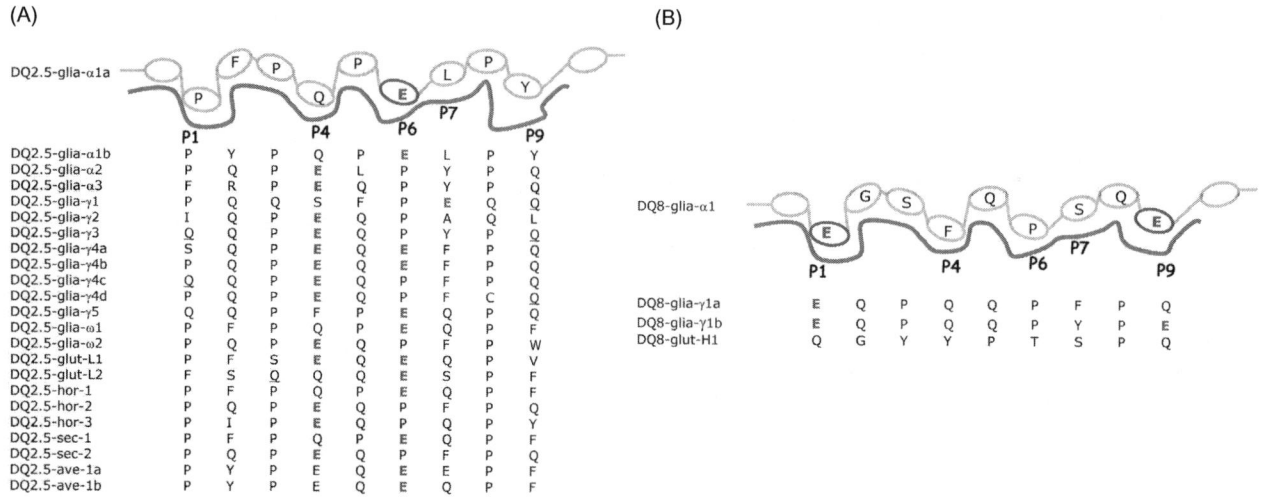

FIGURE 59.5　T cell epitopes of gluten recognized by CD4⁺ T cells of celiac disease patients.　Epitopes presented by HLA-DQ2.5 are shown in (A) and epitopes presented by HLA-DQ8 are shown in (B). The 9-mer core regions of the epitopes are given with one letter amino acid codes in the register with which they bind to the HLA molecules. T cell receptors recognizing the epitopes often are sensitive to residues outside the 9-mer core region. Glutamate residues (E) formed by TG2-mediated deamidation, which are important for recognition by T cells, are shown in red. Additional glutamine residues (Q) also targeted by TG2 are underlined. Of note is the abundance of proline (P) residues within the epitopes. Further information about epitopes and epitope nomenclature can be found in. *Sollid et al. (2012).*

In the transamidation reaction, the glutamine becomes cross-linked to a protein-bound lysine or a polyamine, whereas the deamidation reaction results in conversion of the glutamine to glutamic acid. The enzyme displays regional selectivity for glutamine residues in gliadin peptides, and QXP is a particularly good target sequence (Fleckenstein et al., 2002; Piper et al., 2002; Vader et al., 2002a). There is now strong evidence that the enzyme is involved in the selection of DQ2.5 restricted T cell epitopes (see later).

Gluten Antigen Presentation by Disease-associated DQ Molecules

HLA class II molecules bind antigenic peptides in a groove in their membrane distal part. In this groove there are pockets which accommodate side chains of amino acids of the peptide, so-called anchor residues. In HLA class II peptides anchor residues are found at positions P1, P4, P6, P7, and P9. Both DQ2.5 and DQ8, which are associated with celiac disease, have a fairly unique preference for binding peptides with multiple negatively charged residues. DQ2.5 has a preference for negatively charged anchor residues at positions P4, P6, and P7 (Kim et al., 2004; Tollefsen et al., 2006), whereas DQ8 has preference for negatively charged anchor residues at positions P1 and P9 (Tollefsen et al., 2006; Henderson et al., 2007) (Figure 59.6). The HLA association in celiac disease can thus be explained by a superior ability of the disease-associated HLA-DQ molecules to bind the biased repertoire of proline-rich gluten peptides that have

survived gastrointestinal digestion and which have been deamidated by TG2.

There is a hierachy among the gluten T cell epitopes both in terms of how many T cells of a single patient respond to each, and in terms of the responder frequency among different patients (Marti et al., 2005; Tye-Din et al., 2010). The same epitopes dominate in each of these settings, likely reflecting variation in immunogenicity between the epitopes. In α-gliadin of wheat there are two immunodominant epitopes (i.e., DQ2.5-glia-α1a/b and DQ2.5-gli-α2) (Arentz-Hansen et al., 2000). In some α-gliadin proteins these epitopes are expressed in, altogether, six copies within a 33-mer fragment. This potent antigen is resistant to degradation by gastric, pancreatic, and intestinal brush border membrane proteases (Shan et al., 2002). Other immunodominant epitopes are the DQ2.5-glia-ω2 which comes from ω-gliadin of wheat, and a shared 9 amino acid sequence found in wheat, rye, and barley (termed DQ2.5.glia-ω1, DQ2.5-hor-1, and DQ2-sec-1) (Tye-Din et al., 2010). A similar hierarcy probably exists for HLA-DQ8 restricted epitopes. Celiac disease patients who express DQ2.2 but not DQ2.5 or DQ8, do not have T cells that respond to the common DQ2.5 restricted epitopes but often respond to an immunodominant DQ2.2 restricted epitope (DQ2.2-glut-L1) (Bodd et al., 2012). The common DQ2.5 restricted epitopes bind stably to DQ2.5 but unstably to DQ2.2 (Fallang et al., 2009), and interestingly the immunodominant DQ2.2 epitope binds stably to DQ2.2 (Bodd et al., 2012).

Stable binding of a gluten peptide to the HLA molecule thus seems to be important for a successful T cell

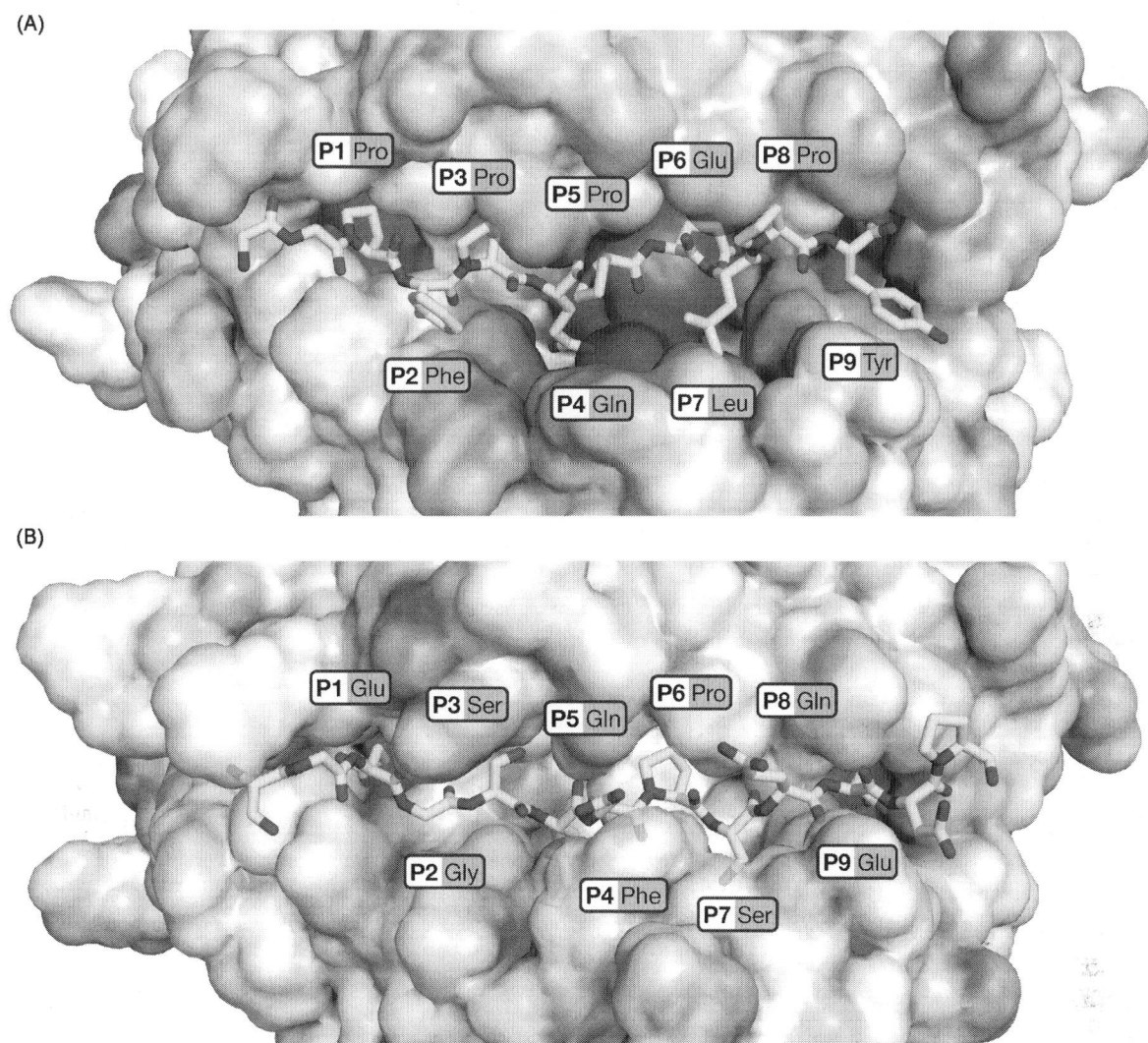

FIGURE 59.6   Three-dimensional structures of the binding sites of HLA-DQ2.5 in (A) and HLA-DQ8 (B) complexed with deamidated gliadin peptide epitopes (carbon = yellow, nitrogen = blue, oxygen = red; amino acid residues in positions P1 to P9 are labeled).The electrostatic potential surface of the HLA molecules is shown as red (=negative) and blue (=positive). HLA-DQ2.5 (PDB 1S9V) (Kim et al., 2004) is complexed with the DQ2.5-glia-α1a epitope, and HLA-DQ8 (PDB 2NNA) (Henderson et al., 2007) is complexed with the DQ8-glia-α1 epitope. *Courtesy of K. Hotta.*

priming, possibly because the peptide in complex with the HLA molecule has to be transported on the surface of antigen-presenting cells from the mucosa to the mesenteric lymph node where the priming most likely takes place (Fallang et al., 2009). Notably, deamidation of gluten peptides decreases the off-rate for binding to DQ2.5 (Xia et al., 2005), and one effect of demidation could be that more gluten−DQ complexes reach the lymph node resulting in productive priming.

Only few sequences in the huge gluten proteome give rise to T cell epitopes. This suggests that there are strong guidance factors in the selection of T cell epitopes. Three factors have been identified as being particularly important: protease resistance, MHC binding, and TG2

efficiency. The clustering of epitopes to regions of gluten proteins which have a high content of proline residues and which are protelytically stable is evidence that proteolytic stability is important. Antigen concentration is important for T cell stimulation, and fragments that are resistant to breakdown will survive at higher concentrations. The selection by MHC would relate to selection of peptides with the correct binding motif as well as selection of peptides that form stable HLA complexes. The observation that HLA-DQ2.5 and HLA-DQ8 in general select discrete epitopes in gluten epitopes underscores the effect of the former factor (Tollefsen et al., 2006). Finally, TG2 specificity appears to be important. There is a correlation between how frequently T cell epitopes are recognized by celiac disease patients and their propensity to be targeted as substrates for TG2 (Dorum et al., 2009). Moreover, using TG2 to select its best substrates from a proteolytic digest of gluten consisting of several thousand different peptides, the majority of about 30 peptides selected contained celiac disease-related T cell epitopes (Dorum et al., 2010). This suggests that TG2 specificity is a major force in T cell epitope selection.

Mucosal Antigen-presenting Cells

Several types of HLA-DQ positive cells can serve as antigen presenting cells in the small intestinal mucosa (Raki et al., 2006; Beitnes et al., 2011). There are $CD163^+CD11c^-$ macrophages and $CD11c^+$ dendritic cells which express either CD163 or CD103 and CD1c. The $CD163^+CD11c^+$ dendritic cells likely derive from circulating monocytes as they co-express CD14 and CCR2. The $CD11c^+$ dendritic cells expressing $CD103^+$ or $CD1c^+$ do not express CD163 or CD14, suggesting the existence of separate functional lineages. In the active celic disease lesion there is an increase of $CD163^+CD11c^+$ dendritic cells, whereas $CD163^+CD11c^-$ macrophages and $CD103^+$ and $CD1c^+$ dendritic cells are all decreased (Beitnes et al., 2011). Based on studies in mice (Schulz et al., 2009) it is tempting to speculate that the $CD11c^+CD103^+$ dendritic cells function to transport antigen to mesenteric lymph nodes for presentation to naïve or central memory cells T cells whereas the $CD163^+CD11c^-$ macrophages and $CD163^+CD11c^+$ dendritic cells serve to present antigen locally to effector T cells.

Effector Mechanisms Leading to Mucosal Alterations

Despite the lack of detailed knowledge of effector mechanisms involved in creation of the celiac lesion, evidence suggests that inflammatory cytokines, particularly interferon-γ, are involved. Messenger RNA for IFN-γ is abundant in biopsies taken from untreated patients and is rapidly induced when biopsies from treated patients are challenged *ex vivo* with gluten (Nilsen et al., 1998). IFN-γ is also produced by the intestinal, gluten-specific $CD4^+$ T cells (Nilsen et al., 1995), and by IELs (Forsberg et al., 2002; Olaussen et al., 2002).

IL-15 is another important cytokine in celiac disease. In active celiac disease there is increased expression of IL-15, both in the lamina propria (Maiuri et al., 2000) and in the epithelium (Mention et al., 2003). Enterocyte bound IL-15 can activate and expand IELs (Mention et al., 2003), and can induce epithelial Fas expression promoting apoptosis of epithelial cells (Maiuri et al., 2000). The expression of IL-15 increases following *in vitro* gluten challenge of celiac biopsies, and certain gluten peptides appear to cause innate immune activation and IL-15 production (Maiuri et al.,

2003). IL-15 is a key factor for reprogramming IELs in celiac disease, where the IELs downregulate inhibitory and upregulate activating NK cell receptors (Meresse et al., 2006) (Figure 59.3A). Activated IELs can kill stressed enterocytes, and this seems to be a crucial step in creating the celiac lesion (Jabri and Sollid, 2009).

Taken together, currently available data places the activation of $CD4^+$ T cells recognizing gluten peptides presented by HLA-DQ2 or HLA-DQ8 molecules as the central key gateway for the control of celiac disease development. The activation of naïve T cells probably takes place in mesenteric lymph nodes, and effector cells then seed to the lamina propria in the small intestine where they are reactivated upon challenge with gluten. This model would explain the dominant genetic role of HLA. The products of the other predisposing genes likely feed into the processes that lead to T cell activation or tissue destruction, but as the non-HLA susceptibility genes each has small effects this indicates a lack of critical checkpoints or redundancy in pathways.

AUTOANTIBODIES AS POTENTIAL IMMUNOLOGIC MARKERS

The diagnosis of celiac disease in adults requires demonstration of enteropathy corresponding to Marsh 3 (Kagnoff, 2006; Ludvigsson et al., 2012). Serology is supportive of the diagnosis. Moreover, it is clear that even less pronounced enteropathy can be compatible with celiac disease, and there is a need for both a combined approach and revision of guidelines (Kurppa et al., 2009). New European guidelines for children were recently published (Husby et al., 2012), but are not yet generally implemented. These guidelines state that the diagnosis in some cases can be made without assessment of intestinal histology by using a combination of strongly positive serology, HLA typing, and clinical criteria.

Serology

More than 95% of untreated celiac disease patients (at least in selected patient cohorts) have high titers of serum IgA antibodies reactive with TG2 (Dieterich et al., 1998; Sulkanen et al., 1998). Most tests are ELISA based with human recombinant TG2 as antigen. In the recent European guidelines for pediatric celiac disease (Husby et al., 2012), the EMA test is included in the diagnostic algorithm as this test was judged to outperform the anti-TG2 ELISA for prediction of celiac disease (Giersiepen et al., 2012). This may relate to the fact that the celiac anti-TG2 antibodies are reactive with conformational epitopes and that the TG2 antigen in some commercial kits is suboptimally folded. If so, one may expect that anti-TG2 ELISA kits will replace the EMA test when the TG2 antigen is produced carefully and the test is performed in an optimal way. IgG anti-TG2 antibodies can be useful for evaluation in patients with selective IgA deficiency, but should otherwise not be tested for (Collin, 1999; Murray, 1999).

Patients with untreated celiac disease also have increased levels of IgA and IgG anti-gluten antibodies. Monitoring of such antibodies, in particular anti-gliadin antibodies, was for many years used in the clinical workup of celiac disease. However, the IgA EMA and anti-TG2 tests gradually took over in clinical practice due to better performance. Some of the anti-gluten antibodies are directed against deamidated epitopes (Osman et al., 2000), and tests based on reactivity to deamidated gliadin peptides perform at the level of anti-TG2 tests (Lewis and Scott, 2010). A problem is that the performance of serological tests is less impressive in clinical practice, at least for adults, when the tests are used in unselected, "everyday" patients as compared to the majority of publications where the proportion of serology-positive celiac disease has been high (Leffler and Schuppan, 2010).

Some celiac disease patients present with negative serology (Dahele et al., 2001; Kaukinen et al., 2002), and an intestinal biopsy should therefore always be taken when there is high clinical suspicion of celiac disease (Farrell and Kelly, 2002). Notably, false-positive anti-TG2 tests do also occur, particularly in patients with inflammatory bowel disease (Dahele et al., 2001; Carroccio et al., 2002).

Staining of Immune Complexes

In patients with active celiac disease there are deposits of IgA in the small intestine corresponding to the distribution of fibronectin bound extracellular TG2, typically as a band beneath the epithelium (Korponay-Szabo et al., 2004). Such deposits of specific IgA complexed with TG2 can be found in the intestinal mucosa even in those patients where serum autoantibodies are undetectable (Salmi et al., 2006b). In IgA deficient patients, these deposits are made up of IgM (Borrelli et al., 2010). Case reports have described autoantibody deposits years before any intestinal damage was observed, and the production of TG2-specific autoantibodies is therefore considered an early marker for developing celiac disease (Salmi et al., 2006a). Because detection of IgA deposits can only be done with frozen tissue sections, this method has not reached widespread usage.

TREATMENT AND OUTCOME

Current Treatment and Outcome

The current treatment of celiac disease is a life-long gluten exclusion diet. The disease is largely a benign disorder, and particularly so in patients detected by screening

(West et al., 2003). Although celiac patients overall have an increased relative risk for non-Hodgkin's lymphoma of the gastrointestinal tract, the absolute risk is low and lower than previously anticipated (Askling et al., 2002; Catassi et al., 2002). In an Italian study it was found that the overall mortality rate in celiac disease was two times greater than in the controls (Corrao et al., 2001). This increased mortality was accounted for by increased death rates in the first 3 years after diagnosis. The gluten-free diet has been considered to be protective against development of malignancy, but this notion was not supported by a study from the United States (Green et al., 2003). Persistent mucosal inflammation (compatible with either lack of compliance or other autoimmune phenomena) is of particular concern (Ludvigsson et al., 2009).

The most frequent reason for absent or incomplete clinical improvement is poor diet compliance (Ciacci et al., 2002), but it is clear that some patients have refractory disease that does not respond to an adequate diet. A majority of the patients with refractory celiac disease have monoclonal expansions of intraepithelial lymphocytes that can progress to become overt enteropathy-associated T cell lymphoma (Cellier et al., 2000). The management of severe complications in this condition is difficult and has yet to be based on recommendations obtained by multi-center trials (Rubio-Tapia and Murray, 2010).

Novel Therapeutic Options

Many patients cope with the gluten-free diet easily. Others find that the dietary restrictions are laborious and negatively impact their quality of life. Better alternatives are thus called for. It is hence promising that the insight into the molecular mechanisms involved in the intestinal T cell reactivity to gluten has uncovered novel targets for therapy. Several avenues are being pursued for the development of new therapies. One possibility, which is basically an extension of today's treatment with a gluten-free diet, is to produce cereals with bread-making properties that are devoid of T cell epitopes, either by breeding programs or transgenic technology (Gil-Humanes et al., 2010). Another possibility is enzyme supplementation with the aim either to destroy T cell epitopes directly or to facilitate their gastrointestinal proteolysis (Hausch et al., 2002; Gass et al., 2007; Mitea et al., 2008). Prolyl endopeptidases are particularly attractive enzymes as they will target the proline-rich regions of gluten that harbor the T cell epitopes. TG2 is a target for intervention because of the critical role it plays in generating gluten T cell epitopes, and a series of TG2 inhibitors have been developed (Badarau et al., 2011) that potentially may be useful in therapy of celiac disease. A potential problem with this approach may be that TG2 inhibitors can have unacceptable side effects, as TG2 is involved in many different physiological processes (Lorand and Graham, 2003). TG2 inhibitors may also not be specific for TG2, but may affect the function of other transglutaminases. Another strategy would be to aim directly at the gluten-reactive T cells. This can possibly be achieved by peptide vaccination or by deletion of antigen-specific T cells. Yet another possible target would be to block presentation of gluten peptides by DQ2 and DQ8, and thereby activation of gluten-reactive T cells. The challenge with this approach will be to find an efficient way to target and block the binding sites of DQ molecules, which are continuously synthesized by antigen-presenting cells. Whatever new therapeutic modality is introduced in celiac disease, it will have to prove as good as or better than the current gluten-free diet regime, with regard to its long-term safety and outcome. This fact must be taken into consideration when devising new treatments.

CONCLUDING REMARKS—FUTURE PROSPECTS

Considerable progress has been made in recent years on the understanding of the molecular basis for celiac disease, but several new questions have emerged. Many of these relate to the autoimmune aspects of the disease. Is celiac disease an autoimmune disorder? To what extent are the autoimmune components of celiac disease involved in disease development? What is the key event transforming the mucosal immune system from gluten tolerant to gluten intolerant? How relevant are the findings of T cell recognition of post-translationally modified peptides and autoantibody formation driven by an exogenous food antigen for other autoimmune disorders? Can it be that other autoimmune disorders are driven by immune responses to foreign, not yet identified, antigens? Finally, in the coming years it will be interesting to see if any of the novel therapies being developed become real alternatives to the gluten-free diet.

ACKNOWLEDGMENTS

Studies in the author's laboratory are funded by grants from the Research Council of Norway, the European Commission (BMH4-CT98-3087, QLRT-1999-00037, QLRT-2000-00657), the European Research Council, the South-Eastern Norway Regional Health Authority, and the Jahre Foundation, and by EXTRA funds from the Norwegian Foundation for Health and Rehabilitation. We thank Ann-Christin R. Beitnes, Jorunn Stamnaes, and Kinya Hotta for help in preparation of figures.

REFERENCES

Alp, M.H., Wright, R., 1971. Autoantibodies to reticulin in patients with idiopathic steatorrhoea, coeliac disease, and Crohn's disease, and their relation to immunoglobulins and dietary antibodies. Lancet. 2, 682—685.

Anderson, R.P., Degano, P., Godkin, A.J., Jewell, D.P., Hill, A.V., 2000. In vivo antigen challenge in celiac disease identifies a single transglutaminase-modified peptide as the dominant A-gliadin T-cell epitope. Nat. Med. 6, 337—342.

Arentz-Hansen, H., Körner, R., Molberg, Ø., Quarsten, H., Vader, W., Kooy, Y.M., et al., 2000. The intestinal T cell response to α-gliadin in adult celiac disease is focused on a single deamidated glutamine targeted by tissue transglutaminase. J. Exp. Med. 191, 603—612.

Arentz-Hansen, H., McAdam, S.N., Molberg, Ø., Fleckenstein, B., Lundin, K.E., Jorgensen, T.J., et al., 2002. Celiac lesion T cells recognize epitopes that cluster in regions of gliadins rich in proline residues. Gastroenterology. 123, 803—809.

Arentz-Hansen, H., Fleckenstein, B., Molberg, Ø., Scott, H., Koning, F., Jung, G., et al., 2004. The molecular basis for oat intolerance in patients with celiac disease. PLoS Med. 1, e1.

Askling, J., Linet, M., Gridley, G., Halstensen, T.S., Ekstrom, K., Ekbom, A., 2002. Cancer incidence in a population-based cohort of individuals hospitalized with celiac disease or dermatitis herpetiformis. Gastroenterology. 123, 1428—1435.

Badarau, E., Collighan, R.J., Griffin, M., 2013. Recent advances in the development of tissue transglutaminase (TG2) inhibitors. Amino Acids. 44,119—127.

Beitnes, A.C., Raki, M., Lundin, K.E., Jahnsen, J., Sollid, L.M., et al., 2011. Density of CD163 + CD11c + dendritic cells increases and CD103 + dendritic cells decreases in the coeliac lesion. Scand. J. Immunol. 74, 186—194.

Bethune, M.T., Borda, J.T., Ribka, E., Liu, M.X., Phillippi-Falkenstein, K., Jandacek, R.J., et al., 2008. A non-human primate model for gluten sensitivity. PLoS One. 3, e1614.

Bjorck, S., Brundin, C., Lorinc, E., Lynch, K.F., Agardh, D., 2010. Screening detects a high proportion of celiac disease in young HLA-genotyped children. J. Pediatr. Gastroenterol. Nutr. 50, 49—53.

Black, K.E., Murray, J.A., David, C.S., 2002. HLA-DQ determines the response to exogenous wheat proteins: a model of gluten sensitivity in transgenic knockout mice. J. Immunol. 169, 5595—5600.

Bodd, M., Kim, C.Y., Lundin, K.E., Sollid, L.M., 2012. T-cell response to gluten in patients with HLA-DQ2.2 reveals requirement of peptide-MHC stability in celiac disease. Gastroenterology. 142, 552—561.

Borrelli, M., Maglio, M., Agnese, M., Paparo, F., Gentile, S., Colicchio, B., et al., 2010. High density of intraepithelial gammadelta lymphocytes and deposits of immunoglobulin (Ig)M anti-tissue transglutaminase antibodies in the jejunum of coeliac patients with IgA deficiency. Clin. Exp. Immunol. 160, 199—206.

Brottveit, M., Raki, M., Bergseng, E., Fallang, L.E., Simonsen, B., Lovik, A., et al., 2011. Assessing possible celiac disease by an HLA-DQ2-gliadin tetramer test. Am. J. Gastroenterol. 106, 1318—1324.

Bruce, S.E., Bjarnason, I., Peters, T.J., 1985. Human jejunal transglutaminase: demonstration of activity, enzyme kinetics and substrate specificity with special relation to gliadin and coeliac disease. Clin. Sci. 68, 573—579.

Carroccio, A., Vitale, G., Di, P.L., Chifari, N., Napoli, S., La, R.C., et al., 2002. Comparison of anti-transglutaminase ELISAs and an anti-endomysial antibody assay in the diagnosis of celiac disease: a prospective study. Clin. Chem. 48, 1546–1550.

Cataldo, F., Marino, V., Bottaro, G., Greco, P., Ventura, A., 1997. Celiac disease and selective immunoglobulin A deficiency. J. Pediatr. 131, 306–308.

Catassi, C., Fabiani, E., Ratsch, I.M., Coppa, G.V., Giorgi, P.L., Pierdomenico, R., et al., 1996. The coeliac iceberg in Italy. A multicentre antigliadin antibodies screening for coeliac disease in school-age subjects. Acta Paediatr. (Suppl. 412), 29–35.

Catassi, C., Fabiani, E., Corrao, G., Barbato, M., De, R.A., Carella, A. M., et al., 2002. Risk of non-Hodgkin lymphoma in celiac disease. JAMA. 287, 1413–1419.

Cellier, C., Delabesse, E., Helmer, C., Patey, N., Matuchansky, C., Jabri, B., et al., 2000. Refractory sprue, coeliac disease, and enteropathy-associated T-cell lymphoma. Lancet. 356, 203–208.

Chen, D., Ueda, R., Harding, F., Patil, N., Mao, Y., Kurahara, C., et al., 2003. Characterization of HLA DR3/DQ2 transgenic mice: a potential humanized animal model for autoimmune disease studies. Eur. J. Immunol. 33, 172–182.

Chen, Z., Dudek, N., Wijburg, O., Strugnell, R., Brown, L., Deliyannis, G., et al., 2002. A 320-kilobase artificial chromosome encoding the human HLA DR3-DQ2 MHC haplotype confers HLA restriction in transgenic mice. J. Immunol. 168, 3050–3056.

Chorzelski, T.P., Beutner, E.H., Sulej, J., Tchorzewska, H., Jablonska, S., et al., 1984. IgA anti-endomysium antibody. A new immunological marker of dermatitis herpetiformis and coeliac disease. Br. J. Dermatol. 111, 395–402.

Ciacci, C., Cirillo, M., Sollazzo, R., Savino, G., Sabbatini, F., Mazzacca, G., 1995. Gender and clinical presentation in adult celiac disease. Scand. J. Gastroenterol. 30, 1077–1081.

Ciacci, C., Cirillo, M., Cavallaro, R., Mazzacca, G., 2002. Long-term follow-up of celiac adults on gluten-free diet: prevalence and correlates of intestinal damage. Digestion. 66, 178–185.

Clemente, M.G., Musu, M.P., Frau, F., Brusco, G., Sole, G., Corazza, G. R., et al., 2000. Immune reaction against the cytoskeleton in coeliac disease. Gut. 47, 520–526.

Collin, P., 1999. New diagnostic findings in coeliac disease. Ann. Med. 31, 399–405.

Collin, P., Reunala, T., 2003. Recognition and management of the cutaneous manifestations of celiac disease: a guide for dermatologists. Am. J. Clin. Dermatol. 4, 13–20.

Collin, P., Reunala, T., Pukkala, E., Laippala, P., Keyrilainen, O., Pasternack, A., 1994. Coeliac disease—associated disorders and survival. Gut. 35, 1215–1218.

Corrao, G., Corazza, G.R., Bagnardi, V., Brusco, G., Ciacci, C., Cottone, M., et al., 2001. Mortality in patients with coeliac disease and their relatives: a cohort study. Lancet. 358, 356–361.

Counsell, C.E., Taha, A., Ruddell, W.S., 1994. Coeliac disease and autoimmune thyroid disease. Gut. 35, 844–846.

Cronin, C.C., Feighery, A., Ferriss, J.B., Liddy, C., Shanahan, F., Feighery, C., 1997. High prevalence of celiac disease among patients with insulin-dependent (type I) diabetes mellitus. Am. J. Gastroenterol. 92, 2210–2212.

Dahele, A.V., Aldhous, M.C., Humphreys, K., Ghosh, S., 2001. Serum IgA tissue transglutaminase antibodies in coeliac disease and other gastrointestinal diseases. QJM. 94, 195–205.

de Kauwe, A.L., Chen, Z., Anderson, R.P., Keech, C.L., Price, J.D., Wijburg, O., et al., 2009. Resistance to celiac disease in humanized HLA-DR3-DQ2-transgenic mice expressing specific antigliadin CD4 + T cells. J. Immunol. 182, 7440–7450.

DePaolo, R.W., Abadie, V., Tang, F., Fehlner-Peach, H., Hall, J.A., Wang, W., et al., 2011. Co-adjuvant effects of retinoic acid and IL-15 induce inflammatory immunity to dietary antigens. Nature. 471, 220–224.

Di Niro, R., Mesin, L., Zheng, N.Y., Stamnaes, J., Morrissey, M., Lee, J. H., et al., 2012. High abundance of plasma cells secreting transglutaminase 2-specific IgA autoantibodies with limited somatic hypermutation in celiac disease intestinal lesions. Nat. Med. 18, 441–445.

Dicke, W.K., 1950. Coeliac disease. Investigations of the harmful effects of certain types of cereal on patients suffering from coeliac disease: Thesis. University of Utrecht.

Dieterich, W., Ehnis, T., Bauer, M., Donner, P., Volta, U., Riecken, E. O., et al., 1997. Identification of tissue transglutaminase as the autoantigen of celiac disease. Nat. Med. 3, 797–801.

Dieterich, W., Laag, E., Schopper, H., Volta, U., Ferguson, A., Gillett, H., et al., 1998. Autoantibodies to tissue transglutaminase as predictors of celiac disease. Gastroenterology. 115, 1317–1321.

Dorum, S., Qiao, S.W., Sollid, L.M., Fleckenstein, B., 2009. A quantitative analysis of transglutaminase 2-mediated deamidation of gluten peptides: implications for the T-cell response in celiac disease. J. Proteome. Res. 8, 1748–1755.

Dorum, S., Arntzen, M.O., Qiao, S.W., Holm, A., Koehler, C.J., Thiede, B., et al., 2010. The preferred substrates for transglutaminase 2 in a complex wheat gluten digest are peptide fragments harboring celiac disease T-cell epitopes. PLoS One. 5, e14056.

Du Pre, M.F., Kozijn, A.E., van Berkel, L.A., ter Borg, M.N., Lindenbergh-Kortleve, D., Jensen, L.T., et al., 2011. Tolerance to ingested deamidated gliadin in mice is maintained by splenic, type 1 regulatory T cells. Gastroenterology. 141, 610–620.

Ellis, A., 1981. Coeliac disease: previous family studies. In: McConnell, R.B. (Ed.), The Genetics of Coeliac Disease. MTP Press, Lancaster, pp. 197–200.

Falchuk, Z.M., Rogentine, G.N., Strober, W., 1972. Predominance of histocompatibility antigen HL-A8 in patients with gluten-sensitive enteropathy. J. Clin. Invest. 51, 1602–1605.

Fallang, L.E., Bergseng, E., Hotta, K., Berg-Larsen, A., Kim, C.Y., Sollid, L.M., 2009. Differences in the risk of celiac disease associated with HLA-DQ2.5 or HLA-DQ2.2 are related to sustained gluten antigen presentation. Nat. Immunol. 10, 1096–1101.

Farrell, R.J., Kelly, C.P., 2002. Celiac sprue. N. Engl. J. Med. 346, 180–188.

Fasano, A., Catassi, C., 2001. Current approaches to diagnosis and treatment of celiac disease: an evolving spectrum. Gastroenterology. 120, 636–651.

Fasano, A., Berti, I., Gerarduzzi, T., Not, T., Colletti, R.B., Drago, S., et al., 2003. Prevalence of celiac disease in at-risk and not-at-risk groups in the United States: a large multicenter study. Arch. Intern. Med. 163, 286–292.

Ferguson, A., MacDonald, T.T., McClure, J.P., Holden, R.J., 1975. Cell-mediated immunity to gliadin within the small-intestinal mucosa in coeliac disease. Lancet. 1, 895–897.

Fleckenstein, B., Molberg, Ø., Qiao, S.W., Schmid, D.G., Von Der, M.F., Elgstoen, K., et al., 2002. Gliadin T cell epitope selection by tissue transglutaminase in celiac disease. Role of enzyme specificity and pH influence on the transamidation versus deamidation process. J. Biol. Chem. 277, 34109–34116.

Folk, J.E., 1983. Mechanism and basis for specificity of transglutaminase-catalyzed ε-(γ-glutamyl) lysine bond formation. Adv. Enzymol. Relat. Areas. Mol. Biol. 54, 1–56.

Forsberg, G., Hernell, O., Melgar, S., Israelsson, A., Hammarstrom, S., Hammarstrom, M.L., 2002. Paradoxical coexpression of proinflammatory and down-regulatory cytokines in intestinal T cells in childhood celiac disease. Gastroenterology. 123, 667–678.

Gass, J., Bethune, M.T., Siegel, M., Spencer, A., Khosla, C., 2007. Combination enzyme therapy for gastric digestion of dietary gluten in patients with celiac sprue. Gastroenterology. 133, 472–480.

Gee, S.J., 1888. On the coeliac affection. St. Bartholomew's Hosp. Res. 24, 17–20.

Giersiepen, K., Lelgemann, M., Stuhldreher, N., Ronfani, L., Husby, S., Koletzko, S., et al., 2012. Accuracy of diagnostic antibody tests for coeliac disease in children: Summary of an evidence report. J. Pediatr. Gastroenterol. Nutr. 54, 229–241.

Gil-Humanes, J., Piston, F., Tollefsen, S., Sollid, L.M., Barro, F., 2010. Effective shutdown in the expression of celiac disease-related wheat gliadin T-cell epitopes by RNA interference. Proc. Natl. Acad. Sci. U.S.A. 107, 17023–17028.

Gjertsen, H.A., Sollid, L.M., Ek, J., Thorsby, E., Lundin, K.E.A., 1994. T cells from the peripheral blood of coeliac disease patients recognize gluten antigens when presented by HLA-DR, -DQ, or -DP molecules. Scand. J. Immunol. 39, 567–574.

Greco, L., Romino, R., Coto, I., Di, C.N., Percopo, S., Maglio, M., et al., 2002. The first large population based twin study of coeliac disease. Gut. 50, 624–628.

Green, P.A., Wollaeger, E.E., Sprague, R.G., Brown, A.L., 1962. Diabetes mellitus associated with tropical sprue. Diabetes. 18, 388–392.

Green, P.H., Fleischauer, A.T., Bhagat, G., Goyal, R., Jabri, B., Neugut, A.I., 2003. Risk of malignancy in patients with celiac disease. Am. J. Med. 115, 191–195.

Haas, S.V., 1932. Celiac disease, its specific treatment and cure without nutritional relapse. JAMA. 99, 448–452.

Hadjivassiliou, M., Grunewald, R., Sharrack, B., Sanders, D., Lobo, A., Williamson, C., et al., 2003. Gluten ataxia in perspective: epidemiology, genetic susceptibility and clinical characteristics. Brain. 126, 685–691.

Hausch, F., Shan, L., Santiago, N.A., Gray, G.M., Khosla, C., 2002. Intestinal digestive resistance of immunodominant gliadin peptides. Am. J. Physiol. Gastrointest. Liver Physiol. 283, G996–G1003.

Henderson, K.N., Tye-Din, J.A., Reid, H.H., Chen, Z., Borg, N.A., Beissbarth, T., et al., 2007. A structural and immunological basis for the role of human leukocyte antigen DQ8 in celiac disease. Immunity. 27, 23–34.

Hoffenberg, E.J., Haas, J., Drescher, A., Barnhurst, R., Osberg, I., Bao, F., et al., 2000. A trial of oats in children with newly diagnosed celiac disease. J. Pediatr. 137, 361–366.

Husby, S., Koletzko, S., Korponay-Szabo, I.R., Mearin, M.L., Phillips, A., Shamir, R., et al., 2012. European Society for Pediatric Gastroenterology, Hepatology, and Nutrition guidelines for the diagnosis of coeliac disease. J. Pediatr. Gastroenterol. Nutr. 54, 136–160.

Hüe, S., Mention, J.J., Monteiro, R.C., Zhang, S., Cellier, C., Schmitz, J., et al., 2004. A direct role for NKG2D/MICA interaction in villous atrophy during celiac disease. Immunity. 21, 367–377.

Ivarsson, A., Persson, L.A., Nystrom, L., Ascher, H., Cavell, B., Danielsson, L., et al., 2000. Epidemic of coeliac disease in Swedish children. Acta Paediatr. 89, 165–171.

Ivarsson, A., Hernell, O., Stenlund, H., Persson, L.A., 2002. Breastfeeding protects against celiac disease. Am. J Clin. Nutr. 75, 914–921.

Ivarsson, A., Hernell, O., Nystrom, L., Persson, L.A., 2003a. Children born in the summer have increased risk for coeliac disease. J. Epidemiol. Community Health. 57, 36–39.

Ivarsson, A., Persson, L.A., Nystrom, L., Hernell, O., 2003b. The Swedish coeliac disease epidemic with a prevailing twofold higher risk in girls compared to boys may reflect gender specific risk factors. Eur. J. Epidemiol. 18, 677–684.

Jabri, B., Sollid, L.M., 2009. Tissue-specific immune responses tissue-mediated control of immunopathology in coeliac disease. Nat. Rev. Immunol. 9, 858–870.

Janatuinen, E.K., Pikkarainen, P.H., Kemppainen, T.A., Kosma, V.M., Jarvinen, R.M., Uusitupa, M.I., et al., 1995. A comparison of diets with and without oats in adults with celiac disease. N. Engl. J. Med. 333, 1033–1037.

Janatuinen, E.K., Kemppainen, T.A., Julkunen, R.J., Kosma, V.M., Maki, M., Heikkinen, M., et al., 2002. No harm from five year ingestion of oats in coeliac disease. Gut. 50, 332–335.

Kagnoff, M.F., 2006. AGA Institute medical position statement on the diagnosis and management of celiac disease. Gastroenterology. 131, 1977–1980.

Karell, K., Louka, A.S., Moodie, S.J., Ascher, H., Clot, F., Greco, L., et al., 2003. HLA types in celiac disease patients not carrying the DQA1*05-DQB1*02 (DQ2) heterodimer: results from the European Genetics Cluster on Celiac Disease. Hum. Immunol. 64, 469–477.

Kaukinen, K., Sulkanen, S., Maki, M., Collin, P., 2002. IgA-class transglutaminase antibodies in evaluating the efficacy of gluten-free diet in coeliac disease. Eur. J. Gastroenterol. Hepatol. 14, 311–315.

Kim, C.Y., Quarsten, H., Bergseng, E., Khosla, C., Sollid, L.M., 2004. Structural basis for HLA-DQ2-mediated presentation of gluten epitopes in celiac disease. Proc. Natl. Acad. Sci. U.S.A. 101, 4175–4179.

Koletzko, S., Burgin-Wolff, A., Koletzko, B., Knapp, M., Burger, W., Gruneklee, D., et al., 1988. Prevalence of coeliac disease in diabetic children and adolescents. A multicentre study. Eur. J. Pediatr. 148, 113–117.

Korponay-Szabo, I.R., Halttunen, T., Szalai, Z., Laurila, K., Kiraly, R., Kovacs, J.B., et al., 2004. In vivo targeting of intestinal and extraintestinal transglutaminase 2 by coeliac autoantibodies. Gut. 53, 641–648.

Kurppa, K., Collin, P., Viljamaa, M., Haimila, K., Saavalainen, P., Partanen, J., et al., 2009. Diagnosing mild enteropathy celiac disease: a randomized, controlled clinical study. Gastroenterology. 136, 816–823.

Kutlu, T., Brousse, N., Rambaud, C., Le Deist, F., Schmitz, J., Cerf-Bensussan, N., 1993. Numbers of T cell receptor (TCR) αβ + but not of TcR γδ + intraepithelial lymphocytes correlate with the grade of villous atrophy in coeliac patients on a long term normal diet. Gut. 34, 208–214.

Ladinser, B., Rossipal, E., Pittschieler, K., 1994. Endomysium antibodies in coeliac disease: an improved method. Gut. 35, 776–778.

Leffler, D.A., Schuppan, D., 2010. Update on serologic testing in celiac disease. Am. J. Gastroenterol. 105, 2520–2524.

Lewis, N.R., Scott, B.B., 2010. Meta-analysis: deamidated gliadin peptide antibody and tissue transglutaminase antibody compared as screening tests for coeliac disease. Aliment. Pharmacol. Ther. 31, 73–81.

Lindfors, K., Rauhavirta, T., Stenman, S., Maki, M., Kaukinen, K., 2012. In vitro models for gluten toxicity: relevance for celiac disease pathogenesis and development of novel treatment options. Exp. Biol. Med. 237, 119–125.

Lorand, L., Graham, R.M., 2003. Transglutaminases: crosslinking enzymes with pleiotropic functions. Nat. Rev. Mol. Cell Biol. 4, 140–156.

Ludvigsson, J.F., Montgomery, S.M., Ekbom, A., Brandt, L., Granath, F., 2009. Small-intestinal histopathology and mortality risk in celiac disease. JAMA. 302, 1171–1178.

Ludvigsson, J.F., Leffler, D.A., Bai, J.C., Biagi, F., Fasano, A., Green, P.H., et al., 2013. The Oslo definitions for coeliac disease and related terms. Gut. 62, 43–52.

Lundin, K.E.A., Scott, H., Hansen, T., Paulsen, G., Halstensen, T.S., Fausa, O., et al., 1993. Gliadin-specific, HLA-DQ(α1*0501,β1*0201) restricted T cells isolated from the small intestinal mucosa of celiac disease patients. J. Exp. Med. 178, 187–196.

Lundin, K.E.A., Scott, H., Fausa, O., Thorsby, E., Sollid, L.M., 1994. T cells from the small intestinal mucosa of a DR4, DQ7/DR4, DQ8 celiac disease patient preferentially recognize gliadin when presented by DQ8. Hum. Immunol. 41, 285–291.

Lundin, K.E.A., Sollid, L.M., Norén, O., Anthonsen, D., Molberg, Ø., Thorsby, E., et al., 1997. Heterogenous reactivity patterns of HLA-DQ-restricted small intestinal T-cell clones from patients with celiac disease. Gastroenterology. 112, 752–759.

Lundin, K.E.A., Nilsen, E.M., Scott, H.G., Løberg, E.M., Gjøen, A., Bratlie, J., et al., 2003. Oats induced villous atrophy in coeliac disease. Gut. 52, 1149–1152.

MacDonald, W.C., Dobbins, I.W.O., Rubin, C.E., 1965. Studies of the familial nature of celiac sprue using biopsy of the small intestine. N. Engl. J. Med. 272, 448–456.

Maiuri, L., Ciacci, C., Auricchio, S., Brown, V., Quaratino, S., Londei, M., 2000. Interleukin 15 mediates epithelial changes in celiac disease. Gastroenterology. 119, 996–1006.

Maiuri, L., Ciacci, C., Ricciardelli, I., Vacca, L., Raia, V., Auricchio, S., et al., 2003. Association between innate response to gliadin and activation of pathogenic T cells in coeliac disease. Lancet. 362, 30–37.

Mäki, M., Kallonen, K., Lähdeaho, M.L., Visakorpi, J.K., 1988. Changing pattern of childhood coeliac disease in Finland. Acta. Paediatr. Scand. 77, 408–412.

Mäki, M., Mustalahti, K., Kokkonen, J., Kulmala, P., Haapalahti, M., Karttunen, T., et al., 2003. Prevalence of celiac disease among children in Finland. N. Engl. J. Med. 348, 2517–2524.

Marietta, E., Black, K., Camilleri, M., Krause, P., Rogers, R.S., David, C., et al., 2004. A new model for dermatitis herpetiformis that uses HLA-DQ8 transgenic NOD mice. J. Clin. Invest. 114, 1090–1097.

Marsh, M.N., 1992. Mucosal pathology in gluten sensitivity. In: Marsh, M.N. (Ed.), In Coeliac Disease. Blackwell Scientific Publications, Oxford, pp. 136–191.

Marti, T., Molberg, Ø., Li, Q., Gray, G.M., Khosla, C., Sollid, L.M., 2005. Prolyl endopeptidase-mediated destruction of T cell epitopes in whole gluten: chemical and immunological characterization. J. Pharmacol. Exp. Ther. 312, 19–26.

Marzari, R., Sblattero, D., Florian, F., Tongiorgi, E., Not, T., Tommasini, A., et al., 2001. Molecular dissection of the tissue transglutaminase autoantibody response in celiac disease. J. Immunol. 166, 4170–4176.

Mawhinney, H., Tomkin, G.H., 1971. Gluten enteropathy associated with selective IgA deficiency. Lancet. 2, 121–124.

Meeuwisse, G.W., 1970. European Society for Paediatric Gastroenterology Meeting in Interlaken September 18, 1969. Acta Paediat. Scand. 59, 461–463.

Mention, J.J., Ben Ahmed, M., Begue, B., Barbe, U., Verkarre, V., et al., 2003. Interleukin 15: a key to disrupted intraepithelial lymphocyte homeostasis and lymphomagenesis in celiac disease. Gastroenterology. 125, 730–745.

Meresse, B., Chen, Z., Ciszewski, C., Tretiakova, M., Bhagat, G., Krausz, T.N., et al., 2004. Coordinated induction by IL15 of a TCR-independent NKG2D signaling pathway converts CTL into lymphokine-activated killer cells in celiac disease. Immunity. 21, 357–366.

Meresse, B., Curran, S.A., Ciszewski, C., Orbelyan, G., Setty, M., Bhagat, G., et al., 2006. Reprogramming of CTLs into natural killer-like cells in celiac disease. J. Exp. Med. 203, 1343–1355.

Mitea, C., Havenaar, R., Drijfhout, J.W., Edens, L., Dekking, L., Koning, F., 2008. Efficient degradation of gluten by a prolyl endoprotease in a gastrointestinal model: implications for celiac disease. Gut. 57, 25–32.

Molberg, Ø., Kett, K., Scott, H., Thorsby, E., Sollid, L.M., Lundin, K.E.A., 1997. Gliadin specific, HLA DQ2-restricted T cells are commonly found in small intestinal biopsies from coeliac disease patients, but not from controls. Scand. J. Immunol. 46, 103–109.

Molberg, Ø., McAdam, S.N., Kärner, R., Quarsten, H., Kristiansen, C., Madsen, L., et al., 1998. Tissue transglutaminase selectively modifies gliadin peptides that are recognized by gut-derived T cells. Nat. Med. 4, 713–717.

Molberg, Ø., Solheim, F.N., Jensen, T., Lundin, K.E., Arentz-Hansen, H., Anderson, O.D., et al., 2003. Intestinal T-cell responses to high-molecular-weight glutenins in celiac disease. Gastroenterology. 125, 337–344.

Murray, J.A., 1999. The widening spectrum of celiac disease. Am. J. Clin. Nutr. 69, 354–365.

Mustalahti, K., Catassi, C., Reunanen, A., Fabiani, E., Heier, M., McMillan, S., et al., 2010. The prevalence of celiac disease in Europe: results of a centralized, international mass screening project. Ann. Med. 42, 587–595.

Myleus, A., Ivarsson, A., Webb, C., Danielsson, L., Hernell, O., Hogberg, L., et al., 2009. Celiac disease revealed in 3% of Swedish 12-year-olds born during an epidemic. J. Pediatr. Gastroenterol. Nutr. 49, 170–176.

Nilsen, E.M., Lundin, K.E.A., Krajci, P., Scott, H., Sollid, L.M., Brandtzaeg, P., 1995. Gluten specific, HLA-DQ restricted T cells from coeliac mucosal produce cytokines with Th1 or Th0 profile dominated by interferon [gamma]. Gut. 37, 766–776.

Nilsen, E.M., Jahnsen, F.L., Lundin, K.E.A., Johansen, F.E., Fausa, O., Sollid, L.M., et al., 1998. Gluten induces an intestinal cytokine response strongly dominated by interferon gamma in patients with celiac disease. Gastroenterology. 115, 551–563.

Oberhuber, G., Granditsch, G., Vogelsang, H., 1999. The histopathology of coeliac disease: time for a standardized report scheme for pathologists. Eur. J. Gastroenterol. Hepatol. 11, 1185–1194.

Olaussen, R.W., Johansen, F.E., Lundin, K.E., Jahnsen, J., Brandtzaeg, P., Farstad, I.N., 2002. Interferon-gamma-secreting T cells localize to the epithelium in coeliac disease. Scand. J. Immunol. 56, 652–664.

Osman, A.A., Gunnel, T., Dietl, A., Uhlig, H.H., Amin, M., Fleckenstein, B., et al., 2000. B cell epitopes of gliadin. Clin. Exp. Immunol. 121, 248–254.

Paulley, J.W., 1954. Observations on the aetiology of idiopathic steatorrhoea—jejunal and lymph-node biopsies. Br. Med. J. 2, 1318–1321.

Piper, J.L., Gray, G.M., Khosla, C., 2002. High selectivity of human tissue transglutaminase for immunoactive gliadin peptides: implications for celiac sprue. Biochemistry. 41, 386–393.

Quarsten, H., McAdam, S.N., Jensen, T., Arentz-Hansen, H., Molberg, O., Lundin, K.E., et al., 2001. Staining of celiac disease-relevant T cells by peptide-DQ2 multimers. J. Immunol. 167, 4861–4868.

Raki, M., Tollefsen, S., Molberg, O., Lundin, K.E., Sollid, L.M., Jahnsen, F.L., 2006. A unique dendritic cell subset accumulates in the celiac lesion and efficiently activates gluten-reactive T cells. Gastroenterology. 131, 428–438.

Ráki, M., Fallang, L.E., Brottveit, M., Bergseng, E., Quarsten, H., Lundin, K.E., et al., 2007. Tetramer visualization of gut-homing gluten-specific T cells in the peripheral blood of celiac disease patients. Proc. Natl. Acad. Sci. U.S.A. 104, 2831–2836.

Risch, N., 1987. Assessing the role of HLA-linked and unlinked determinants of disease. Am. J. Hum. Genet. 40, 1–14.

Rostom, A., Dube, C., Cranney, A., Saloojee, N., Sy, R., Garritty, C., et al., 2005. The diagnostic accuracy of serologic tests for celiac disease: a systematic review. Gastroenterology. 128, S38–S46.

Rubin, C.E., Brandborg, L.L., Phelps, P.C., Taylor, H.C., 1960. Studies of celiac disease. I. Apparent identical and specific nature of the duodenal and proximal jejunal lesion in celiac disease and idiopathic sprue. Gastroenterology. 38, 28–49.

Rubio-Tapia, A., Murray, J.A., 2010. Classification and management of refractory coeliac disease. Gut. 59, 547–557.

Salmi, T.T., Collin, P., Jarvinen, O., Haimila, K., Partanen, J., Laurila, K., et al., 2006a. Immunoglobulin A autoantibodies against transglutaminase 2 in the small intestinal mucosa predict forthcoming coeliac disease. Aliment. Pharmacol. Ther. 24, 541–552.

Salmi, T.T., Collin, P., Korponay-Szabo, I.R., Laurila, K., Partanen, J., Huhtala, H., et al., 2006b. Endomysial antibody-negative coeliac disease: clinical characteristics and intestinal autoantibody deposits. Gut. 55, 1746–1753.

Sanchez, D., Tuckova, L., Sebo, P., Michalak, M., Whelan, A., Sterzl, I., et al., 2000. Occurrence of IgA and IgG autoantibodies to calreticulin in coeliac disease and various autoimmune diseases. J. Autoimmun. 15, 441–449.

Sanders, D.S., Patel, D., Stephenson, T.J., Ward, A.M., McCloskey, E.V., Hadjivassiliou, M., et al., 2003. A primary care cross-sectional study of undiagnosed adult coeliac disease. Eur. J. Gastroenterol. Hepatol. 15, 407–413.

Sardy, M., Karpati, S., Merkl, B., Paulsson, M., Smyth, N., 2002. Epidermal transglutaminase (TGase 3) is the autoantigen of dermatitis herpetiformis. J. Exp. Med. 195, 747–757.

Schulz, O., Jaensson, E., Persson, E.K., Liu, X., Worbs, T., Agace, W.W., et al., 2009. Intestinal CD103 + , but not CX3CR1 + , antigen

sampling cells migrate in lymph and serve classical dendritic cell functions. J. Exp. Med. 206, 3101–3114.

Seah, P.P., Fry, L., Rossiter, M.A., Hoffbrand, A.V., Holborow, E.J., 1971. Anti-reticulin antibodies in childhood coeliac disease. Lancet. 2, 681–682.

Shan, L., Molberg, Ø., Parrot, I., Hausch, F., Filiz, F., Gray, G.M., et al., 2002. Structural basis for gluten intolerance in celiac sprue. Science. 297, 2275–2279.

Shewry, P.R., Halford, N., Lafiandra, D., 2003. Genetics of wheat gluten proteins. Adv. Genet. 49, 111–184.

Simell, S., Hoppu, S., Hekkala, A., Simell, T., Stahlberg, M.R., Viander, M., et al., 2007. Fate of five celiac disease-associated antibodies during normal diet in genetically at-risk children observed from birth in a natural history study. Am. J. Gastroenterol. 102, 2026–2035.

Sjöström, H., Lundin, K.E.A., Molberg, Ø., Körner, R., McAdam, S.N., Anthonsen, D., et al., 1998. Identification of a gliadin T-cell epitope in coeliac disease: general importance of gliadin deamidation for intestinal T-cell recognition. Scand. J. Immunol. 48, 111–115.

Smyth, D.J., Plagnol, V., Walker, N.M., Cooper, J.D., Downes, K., Yang, J.H., et al., 2008. Shared and distinct genetic variants in type 1 diabetes and celiac disease. N. Engl. J. Med. 359, 2767–2777.

Sollid, L.M., Markussen, G., Ek, J., Gjerde, H., Vartdal, F., Thorsby, E., 1989. Evidence for a primary association of celiac disease to a particular HLA-DQ αβ heterodimer. J. Exp. Med. 169, 345–350.

Sollid, L.M., Molberg, Ø., McAdam, S., Lundin, K.E., 1997. Autoantibodies in coeliac disease: tissue transglutaminase—guilt by association? Gut. 41, 851–852.

Sollid, L.M., Qiao, S.W., Anderson, R.P., Gianfrani, C., Koning, F., 2012. Nomenclature and listing of celiac disease relevant gluten T-cell epitopes restricted by HLA-DQ molecules. Immunogenetics. 64, 455–460

Stokes, P.L., Asquith, P., Holmes, G.K., Mackintosh, P., Cooke, W.T., 1972. Histocompatibility antigens associated with adult coeliac disease. Lancet. 2, 162–164.

Sulkanen, S., Halttunen, T., Laurila, K., Kolho, K.L., Korponay-Szabo, I.R., Sarnesto, A., et al., 1998. Tissue transglutaminase autoantibody enzyme-linked immunosorbent assay in detecting celiac disease. Gastroenterology. 115, 1322–1328.

Tollefsen, S., Arentz-Hansen, H., Fleckenstein, B., Molberg, Ø., Raki, M., Kwok, W.W., et al., 2006. HLA-DQ2 and -DQ8 signatures of gluten T cell epitopes in celiac disease. J. Clin. Invest. 116, 2226–2236.

Trynka, G., Hunt, K.A., Bockett, N.A., Romanos, J., Mistry, V., Szperl, A., et al., 2011. Dense genotyping identifies and localizes multiple common and rare variant association signals in celiac disease. Nat. Genet. 43, 1193–1201.

Tye-Din, J.A., Stewart, J.A., Dromey, J.A., Beissbarth, T., van Heel, D.A., Tatham, A., et al., 2010. Comprehensive, quantitative mapping of T cell epitopes in gluten in celiac disease. Sci. Transl. Med. 2, 41ra51.

Vader, L.W., de Ru, A., van Der, W.Y., Kooy, Y.M., Benckhuijsen, W., Mearin, M.L., et al., 2002a. Specificity of tissue transglutaminase explains cereal toxicity in celiac disease. J. Exp. Med. 195, 643–649.

Vader, W., Kooy, Y., van Veelen, P., de Ru, A., Harris, D., Benckhuijsen, W., et al., 2002b. The gluten response in children with celiac disease is directed toward multiple gliadin and glutenin peptides. Gastroenterology. 122, 1729—1737.

van de Wal, Y., Kooy, Y., van Veelen, P., Peña, S., Mearin, L., Papadopoulos, G., et al., 1998a. Selective deamidation by tissue transglutaminase strongly enhances gliadin-specific T cell reactivity. J. Immunol. 161, 1585—1588.

van de Wal, Y., Kooy, Y.M., van Veelen, P.A., Peña, S.A., Mearin, L.M., Molberg, Ø., et al., 1998b. Small intestinal T cells of celiac disease patients recognize a natural pepsin fragment of gliadin. Proc. Natl. Acad. Sci. U.S.A. 95, 10050—10054.

van de Wal, Y., Kooy, Y.M., van Veelen, P., Vader, W., August, S.A., Drijfhout, J.W., et al., 1999. Glutenin is involved in the gluten-driven mucosal T cell response. Eur. J. Immunol. 29, 3133—3139.

van der Kolk, J.H., van Putten, L.A., Mulder, C.A., Grinwis, G.C.M., Reijm, M., Butler, C.M., 2012. Gluten-dependent antibodies in horses with inflammatory small bowel disease (ISBD). Vet. Q. First. 1—9.

Wang, N., Shen, N., Vyse, T.J., Anand, V., Gunnarson, I., Sturfelt, G., et al., 2011. Selective IgA deficiency in autoimmune diseases. Mol. Med. 17, 1383—1396.

West, J., Logan, R.F., Hill, P.G., Lloyd, A., Lewis, S., Hubbard, R., et al., 2003. Seroprevalence, correlates, and characteristics of undetected coeliac disease in England. Gut. 52, 960—965.

Xia, J., Sollid, L.M., Khosla, C., 2005. Equilibrium and kinetic analysis of the unusual binding behavior of a highly immunogenic gluten peptide to HLA-DQ2. Biochemistry. 44, 4442—4449.

Chapter 60

Inflammatory Bowel Diseases

Vera Kandror Denmark[1] and Lloyd Mayer[2,†]

[1]*Newton Wellesley Hospital, Newton, MA*, [2]*Immunology Institute, Mount Sinai School of Medicine, New York, NY, USA*

Chapter Outline

Introduction	873	Serologic Markers	879
History	873	**Treatment**	**879**
Epidemiology and Environmental Factors	874	Medical	879
Clinical and Pathologic Features	874	Aminosalicylates	879
Disease Presentation	874	Glucocorticoids	879
Crohn's Disease	874	Thiopurines	880
Ulcerative Colitis	875	Cyclosporine	880
Pathology	875	Methotrexate	880
Genetics	875	Anti-TNF Antibody Therapies	880
Immunopathogenesis	876	Inhibitors of Leukocyte Infiltration	881
Epithelial Barrier and Innate Immunity	877	New Biologic Therapies	881
Adaptive Immunity	877	Surgical	881
Host–Microbial Interactions	878	**Future Prospects**	**882**
Biomarkers	878	**References**	**882**
Fecal Markers	878		

INTRODUCTION

Inflammatory bowel disease (IBD) is divided into two distinct but related entities: Crohn's disease (CD) and ulcerative colitis (UC). While the two diseases share some features, there are important clinical differences between them and thus they will be presented separately for part of this discussion. It should also be noted that the etiology and pathophysiology of IBD is not yet clearly established; furthermore, the degree to which these diseases are truly autoimmune in nature is unclear.

HISTORY

Numerous case reports exist from the 19th century describing inflammatory diseases of the small and large intestine that may have represented CD (Baron, 2000). Ileocecal inflammation as seen in CD is also characteristic of intestinal tuberculosis, which was the most commonly recognized disease of the small intestine at that time. As microscopy evolved, case series have emerged of patients with inflammation and strictures of the ileocecal region that were determined to be neither tuberculous nor malignant. These strongly suggest that CD, as we presently know it, existed at least as far back as the 19th century.

The seminal work describing CD was a paper from the Mount Sinai Hospital in New York by Burrill B. Crohn, Leon Ginzburg, and Gordon D. Oppenheimer (1932) entitled "Regional Ileitis: A Pathologic and Clinical Entity." The authors described a series of 14 patients operated upon by Dr. A.A. Berg with granulomatous inflammation of the terminal ileum. The title of the paper reflected Crohn's belief that the disease affected only the ileum (Wells, 1952) despite evidence presented by Ginzburg and Oppenheimer (1932) and others of cases affecting the small and large intestine. Interestingly, the

---

† With their deepest regret, the Editors note the death of Dr Lloyd Mayer during the composition of this text. The Editors' Preface contains a tribute to his many valued achievements and contributions. The corresponding author is Vera Denmark.

disease came to be known as Crohn's only because the authors agreed to list their names alphabetically and because the surgeon Berg humbly declined to be included as an author (Baron, 2000).

Early work on UC was also complicated by difficulty in distinguishing it from infectious colitides such as bacillary dysentery. Credit for the discovery of UC as a distinct entity has been given to Samuel Wilks (1859) who termed it "idiopathic colitis." The term "ulcerative colitis" was first used by Hale-White (1888), although in retrospect these patients may not have had UC but rather irritable bowel syndrome (Baron, 2000). Further work was facilitated by the introduction of the electric sigmoidoscope; studies by Sir William Hurst (1909) and also Lockhart-Mummery (1907) helped to clarify the appearance of the colon in UC.

EPIDEMIOLOGY AND ENVIRONMENTAL FACTORS

The highest of rates of IBD are found in northern Europe, the United Kingdom, and North America (Loftus, 2004). However, it is increasingly recognized that IBD can occur in persons from other areas such as Africa, Latin America, and Asia. Extrapolation of incidence and prevalence rates for North America as presented by Loftus (2004) and suggests the following: approximately 780,000 persons in the USA and Canada have UC and 630,000 have CD. Between 7000 and 46,000 new diagnoses of UC are made yearly and between 10,000 and 47,000 new diagnoses of CD are made. Similarly to multiple sclerosis, IBD does appear to be more frequently found in the northern latitudes (Blanchard et al., 2001; Sonnenberg et al., 1991).

IBD may present at any age; however, it is most commonly diagnosed in the second or third decade of life. There does not seem to be a major gender preference in IBD. Other than genetic risk factors, which will be addressed in a separate section, several environmental risk factors have been hypothesized to predict the development or course of IBD. Cigarette smoking is an important risk factor with divergent effects on CD and UC. Numerous studies have confirmed that smoking is associated with a higher risk of developing CD (Calkins, 1989), an earlier need for surgery for CD (Sands et al., 2003), and earlier relapse after surgery (Timmer et al., 1998). Conversely, cigarette smokers are less likely to develop UC (Calkins, 1989) or to require colectomy for UC (Boyko et al., 1988). In numerous case–control studies as well as a meta-analysis by Koutroubakis et al. (2002), appendectomy for appendicitis has been shown to protect against a subsequent diagnosis of UC. The pathophysiologic effects of smoking and appendectomy are as of yet unclear. Numerous other environmental factors have been studied,

TABLE 60.1 Major Categories in the Differential Diagnosis of IBD

Category	Examples
Infectious	Bacterial (*Salmonella, Shigella, E. coli, Yersinia, Clostridium difficile, Campylobacter*)
	Viral (*Cytomegalovirus*)
	Mycobacterial (*M. tuberculosis, M. avium-intracellulare*)
	Parasitic (*Entamoeba histiolytica, Strongyloides, Giardia*)
Vascular	Vasculitis (polyarteritis nodosa, Henoch–Schönlein purpura)
	Radiation-induced enteritis
	Ischemia
Oncologic	Lymphoma, adenocarcinoma, carcinoid, metastatic disease
Inflammatory	Microscopic colitis, diverticular colitis, diversion colitis, celiac disease
Functional	Irritable bowel syndrome
Drug-induced	Non-steroidal anti-inflammatory drugs

including breast feeding, diet, measles vaccination, oral contraceptives, and various infectious agents. However, none of these has been conclusively shown to affect the development or course of IBD (see Table 60.1).

CLINICAL AND PATHOLOGIC FEATURES

Disease Presentation

Crohn's Disease

A hallmark of CD is its ability to involve any part of the gastrointestinal tract from mouth to anus. Multiple sites of disease can be affected in the same individual. The inflammation in CD, as distinct from UC, is discontinuous; diseased bowel is separated by areas of healthy bowel (so-called "skip lesions"). The location of CD in the bowel usually falls into one of three patterns: isolated small bowel disease, combined small and large bowel disease, and isolated colitis. The most commonly affected segment of bowel is the terminal ileum, which is diseased in two-thirds of patients (Munkholm and Binder, 2004). Colonic involvement in CD typically does not involve the rectum, which is always involved in UC. A small percentage of patients have disease of the jejunum or esophagus only.

CD can also be divided into three types of disease behavior: pure inflammatory, stricturing, or fistulizing. These behavior types are not mutually exclusive; however, the combination of disease behavior and location can nonetheless often dictate clinical presentation. For example, a common presentation of CD is inflammatory disease of the terminal ileum with symptoms of pain, diarrhea, and weight loss. When inflammatory disease involves the colon, a more UC-type syndrome ensues with diarrhea and occasional rectal bleeding. Stricturing disease can be more subtle in development, with a long time course of relatively normal bowel function before symptoms of pain, bloating, and eventually obstruction ensue.

The ability of CD to cause fistulae reflects its transmural nature. UC involves only the mucosal layer of the GI tract while CD can involve all layers from mucosa to serosa. When inflammation is severe enough to extend from mucosa to serosa, fistulae result such that the contents of the intestinal tract spill out into an adjacent space. The perianal region is the most common site of fistula development in CD. About 20% of patients with CD will have perianal fistulas (Schwartz et al., 2002) which present clinically with perianal abscesses that may spontaneously drain. Fistulas can also arise in the bowel and invade other parts of bowel, bladder, vagina, or psoas muscles causing abscesses or frank drainage of stool.

Ulcerative Colitis

UC affects only the colon. As a result, its presentation is more consistent than that of CD. UC usually presents with symptoms of diarrhea and rectal bleeding. Abdominal pain and constitutional symptoms (fever, weight loss) are less frequent than in CD, except in severe UC flares. The amount of colon that is involved in UC can vary from the entire colon (pan-colitis) to just the most distal part (left-sided colitis or proctitis). As a rule, the more proximal colon will only be affected when the more distal area is as well. Thus the endoscopic findings of isolated right-sided colitis (in combination with other features such as rectal sparing) argue strongly for a diagnosis of CD as opposed to UC. Isolated proctitis can present as tenesmus or rectal bleeding in the absence of diarrhea given the normal proximal colon. Infrequently, pan-colitis can progress to toxic megacolon, a massively dilated colon with accompanying fever and tachycardia; immediate surgery is indicated for this condition.

Pathology

Microscopy of specimens from endoscopic mucosal biopsies or surgical resections can help ascertain the diagnosis of IBD and frequently distinguish between UC and CD. Common features of IBD include ulceration, acute and chronic inflammatory infiltrate, crypt abscesses, and crypt distortion. Though suggestive of IBD, these changes can sometimes be seen in other conditions such as infectious colitis. The findings of transmural inflammation (usually possible only in surgical specimens) or of non-caseating granulomas suggest a diagnosis of CD as opposed to UC. Unfortunately, granulomas may be identified in as few as 15% of endoscopic biopsies (Okada et al., 1991) and thus the absence of granulomas does not rule out CD. The cellular infiltrate in the Crohn's mucosa is one of activated lymphocytes (mostly T cells) and macrophages. In UC, neutrophils and mast cells predominate although activated lymphocytes and macrophages are present as well.

GENETICS

Several factors point to a genetic contribution to the etiology of IBD. Rates of IBD are considerably higher in certain ethnic groups such as Ashkenazi Jews as compared with others living in the same geographic area. Relatives of patients with IBD also have a higher rate of developing the disease. For monozygotic twins, the concordance rate is about 40–60% for CD and about 5–20% for UC (Subhani et al., 1998; Orholm et al., 2000; Halfvarson et al., 2003). This suggests that CD may have more of a genetic basis, but clearly since both rates are much less than 100% the environment and possibly the microbiome must play a role as well. Five to 15% of patients with IBD will have an affected first-degree relative, and the subtype (CD vs. UC) will be the same in 75–80% of cases (Binder, 1998). This corresponds to about a 15-fold increased risk of disease if one has a first-degree relative with IBD (Satsangi et al., 1994; Peeters et al., 1996).

Genome-wide association studies have identified 99 non-overlapping susceptibility loci for CD, including 28 that are shared between CD and UC (Anderson et al., 2011). Approximately 50% of IBD susceptibility loci have also been associated with other autoimmune diseases. Analysis of genetic loci implicated in IBD underscore the importance of several pathways that are involved in the maintenance of gut homeostasis: epithelial restitution and barrier function, regulation of innate and adaptive immunity, microbial defense, and autophagy. Each of these pathways will be discussed in the subsequent section. A few of the major IBD susceptibility loci will be reviewed here.

NOD2 (*CARD15*) (see Table 60.2) was the first CD susceptibility gene identified, emphasizing the importance of defects in innate immunity in the pathogenesis of CD (Hugot et al., 2001; Ogura et al., 2001a; Hampe et al., 2001). It is present in 8–25% of CD patients and is encountered in the greatest percentage of the patients as compared to other mutations. *NOD2* is an intracellular receptor for muramyl dipeptide, a motif present in bacterial cell walls. It appears to modulate signaling through Toll-like receptor pathways, thereby activating NF-κB. *NOD2* may also trigger autophagy after detecting

TABLE 60.2 Genomic Regions Associated with Inflammatory Bowel Disease in Genome-wide Association Studies of Patients of European Descent

Predominantly Associated with CD	Predominantly Associated with UC	Significant Associations with CD and UC
NOD2 (16q12)	MHC region (6p21)	Factors in IL-23 pathway (12q13, 5q33, 19p13
ATG16L1 (2q37)	FCGR2A (1q23, Fc fragment receptor)	1q32 (region includes IL-10)
IRGM (5q33.1)	Loci that affect epithelial defenses (7q22)	Gene deserts (5p13, 9q32)
5q31	12q14	9q34 (region includes CARD9)
9q32	20q13	Transcription factors (10q22, 10q24, 15q22)
10q21		
18p11		
22q13		
12q12		

Adapted from Cho and Brant (2011). Gastro enterology 140, 1704–1712.

intracellular bacteria (Zaki et al., 2010). Interestingly, *NOD2* variants associated with CD result in loss of function of the *NOD2* protein. This is puzzling as increased, rather than reduced, inflammatory activity is observed in CD patients. This loss of function of a key component of innate immunity may be overcompensated for by the adaptive immunity arm, which may drive the inappropriate inflammatory response observed in CD patients. This theory remains to be proven, however.

CARD9 is an IBD-implicated adaptor protein which integrates signals from many innate immune receptors that recognize microbial motifs (Ogura et al., 2001b). *CARD9* is required for the development of an appropriate intestinal immune response in the steady state and in the colitis setting. *CARD9* knockout (KO) mice exhibit defective expression of IL-17A and IL-22 in the recovery phase following DSS-induced injury (Sokol et al., 2006). In addition, KO mice show a decrease proportion of Th1, Th17, and innate lymphoid cells (ILCs). Thus, *CARD9* is notably involved in Th17 and IL-22 responses that are required to eradicate some intestinal pathogens and to recover after intestinal inflammation.

The IL-23/IL-12 pathway has been extensively studied in respect of IBD as it determines differentiation of naïve T cells into effector Th1 cells (driven by IL-12) or Th17 cells (driven by IL-23). Variants in the IL-23 receptor gene (IL-23R) on chromosome 1p31 were found to be associated with CD susceptibility (Duerr et al., 2006). This association was also confirmed in UC (Tremelling et al., 2007). Other components of the Th17 pathway have been associated with CD, including signal transducers STAT2 and JAK3, the chemokine receptor CCR6 and costimulatory molecule ICOS-L, highlighting the

important role the Th17 pathway plays in the pathogenesis of CD (Barrett et al., 2008). Interestingly, *NOD2* and *IL-23R* were not found to be associated with IBD in Japan (Yamazaki et al., 2007).

Genetic analyses have revealed a role for autophagy in innate immunity and IBD, implicating two genes, *ATG16L1* and *IRGM*, in IBD pathogenesis (Hampe et al., 2007; McCarroll et al., 2008). Autophagy is involved in the degradation and recycling of cytosolic contents and organelles, as well as in the removal of intracellular microbes. *ATG16L1* is essential for all forms of autophagy and the coding mutation T300A is associated with increased risk of CD. Epithelial cells and dendritic cells containing CD-associated *ATG16L1* and *NOD2* variants show defects in antibacterial autophagy (Cooney et al., 2010; Travassos et al., 2010). These results suggest that genetic polymorphisms may affect both pathways concomitantly and underscore a close relationship between *NOD2*, *ATG16L1*, and autophagy.

IBD represents a complex genetic disorder in which each gene mutation contributes to the disease. However, other than NOD2, the other 98 genes identified in the genome-wide association studies contribute only 1% or less to the risk of developing IBD. Many healthy controls carry the same genetic mutations but do not have the disease. Thus, predicting the development of IBD remains a challenge.

IMMUNOPATHOGENESIS

Inflammatory bowel disease (IBD) is a chronic disease of the intestinal tract, which results from a complex interplay between genetic factors and environmental triggers.

It is believed that aberrant innate immune responses to commensal flora play an important role in IBD pathogenesis. Patients with IBD develop strong immune responses to common bacterial antigens that do not trigger an immune response in a normal host (Dahan et al., 2007). Controlling inflammatory responses to commonly encountered antigens presents a challenge to the mucosal immune system of patients with IBD. The basal state of mucosal immune suppression observed in healthy people is important to prevent a pathologic response to the constant presence of commensal flora and dietary antigens. While the immunologic tone of a mucosa-associated lymphoid tissue (MALT) in a normal host is that of hyporesponsiveness or suppression, the immunologic tone of the MALT in an IBD patient is that of activation. The mechanisms responsible for the healthy tone of hyporesponsiveness in a normal host involve complex interactions between the intestinal epithelial cell (IEC) of the GI tract and the underlying T lymphocyte in the lamina propria. We will discuss each of the three major players in the pathogenesis of IBD (the epithelial barrier, the innate and adaptive immune responses, and the host–microbial interactions) separately.

Epithelial Barrier and Innate Immunity

The first line of defense against luminal pathogens is a layer of mucus produced by specialized cells within the epithelial lining called goblet cells. Mice deficient in the main component of goblet cell mucus, Muc2, develop spontaneous colitis (Heazlewood et al., 2008). Patients with IBD frequently have a compromised mucus layer and increased mucolytic bacteria. In addition to the mucus layer, another layer of protection is provided by Paneth cells that are located in the crypts of the small intestine. Paneth cells are the primary source of antimicrobial peptides. Interestingly, patients with CD carrying the *ATG16L1* (T300A) mutation have Paneth cell granule abnormalities (Cadwell et al., 2008). This defect in Paneth cell biology may define a subset of patients with CD.

Intestinal epithelial cells (IECs) perform both barrier and signal-transduction functions. The structure of tight junctions is crucial for the integrity of the epithelial layer. Genetic studies have shown that truncated forms of the adherens junction protein E-cadherin (encoded by *CDH1*, a CD susceptibility gene) are associated with CD. Intestinal biopsies from patients with these CD alleles show inappropriate protein localization and cytosolic accumulation.

We now know that the epithelial cell not only serves as a physical barrier between the intestinal lumen and the underlying lymphoid tissue, but is also involved in the regulation of innate and adaptive immune responses (Dahan et al., 2007). IECs produce intestinal alkaline phosphatase, which can mediate lipopolysaccharide detoxification. IECs can also attenuate neutrophil transmigration by generating resolving-E1 through the action of cyclooxygenase-2 (Campbell et al., 2010). IECs can also modulate adaptive immune responses by functioning as nonprofessional antigen-presenting cells to the T lymphocytes in the lamina propria (Campbell et al., 2002). Epithelial antigen processing occurs in a highly polarized fashion, with apical antigens being sorted and presented exclusively basolaterally. Studies from the Mayer lab have identified a regulatory/suppressor CD8$^+$ T cell population, CD8$^+$CD28$^-$CD103$^+$, which undergoes oligoclonal expansion in the lamina propria of the gut after interacting with an MHC class I-like complex on the basolateral surface of an epithelial cell (Allez et al., 2002). This suppressor T cell population is absent or markedly reduced in the lamina propria of IBD patients (Brimnes et al., 2005). A lack of activation of this regulatory lymphocyte population may contribute to the uncontrolled inflammation seen in IBD.

Adaptive Immunity

Professional and nonprofessional antigen-presenting cells (APCs), such as dendritic cells, macrophages, and intestinal epithelial cells, communicate with lamina propria lymphocytes through a broad array of cytokines. Cytokines have been demonstrated to play a central role in fostering gut inflammation in CD. Inflammatory responses in UC are driven by a complex of activated T cells, while inflammation in CD is driven by an interplay between Th1 and Th17 responses, creating a constantly evolving cytokine milieu (Kamada et al., 2010; Strober et al., 2010). The conventional Th1 response is characterized by an increased production of IL-12 and IFN-γ. This response is followed by a Th17 response, characterized by an increase in IL-23 and IL-17. Indeed, increased IL-17 production occurs in the lamina propria of CD patients and IFN-γ levels correlate with disease severity (Strober et al., 2010). In addition, CD patients harbor increased numbers of circulating IL-17 and IFN-γ producing memory cells. IL-17 and IFN-γ, the major players in the CD inflammatory response, induce production of "downstream" cytokines, such as TNF-α, IL-6 and IL-1β that play important roles in the mediation of inflammation and tissue destruction. A unique IL-17$^+$ FoxP3$^+$ T cell population has recently been identified in the lamina propria of CD patients but not in patients with UC or healthy controls (Hovhannisyan et al., 2011). This CD4$^+$ population shares phenotypic characteristics of both Th17 and Treg cells and shows potent suppressor activity *in vitro*. Thus, the specific microenvironmental cues likely determine cellular commitment to either lineage and affect the balance between regulation and inflammation.

Another example of the diverse effects environmental cues have on cellular/cytokine behavior is illustrated by a newly discovered cytokine IL-22, a member of the IL-10 family. IL-22 has recently been found to be upregulated in the inflamed mucosa of CD patients (Brand et al., 2006). Although IL-22 has been shown to promote epithelial barrier function by inducing epithelial cell differentiation, co-secretion of IL-22 with proinflammatory cytokines such as TNF-α, IFN-γ, and IL-17 results in a dramatic increase in an inflammatory immune reaction (Eyerich et al., 2010). Thus, IL-22 can be a pro- as well as an anti-inflammatory cytokine depending on the microenvironment.

Host—Microbial Interactions

Accumulating evidence suggests that luminal flora is a requisite factor in the development of IBD. The animal models have served to underscore the role of the luminal flora, In virtually every model identified to date (over 50 described), the animals fail to develop disease when reared in a germ-free environment (Podolsky, 1997) (see Table 60.3). When normal flora is added, disease ensues rapidly. Microbial signals also shape innate and adaptive immune responses. Germ-free animals have underdeveloped Peyer's patches, as well as fewer lamina propria CD4$^+$ cells, underscoring the role microbiota plays in generating mature adaptive immune responses.

Studies of luminal bacterial composition in patients with IBD have revealed a decrease in beneficial bacteria such as the bifidobacteria *Lactobacilli* and *Firmicutes* and an increase in putative pathogenic bacteria such as *Bacteroides* and *E. coli* (Swidsinski et al., 2002; Sokol et al., 2006). This dysbiosis may promote inflammation by altering the balance between protective and harmful intestinal bacteria. Recently, adherent-invasive *E. coli* (AIEC) has been shown to adhere to IECs in the ileal mucosa in CD patients but not to ileal mucosa of normal controls, implicating AIEC as a potential inflammatory trigger in CD patients (Barnich et al., 2007). It is still unclear, however, whether the abundance of AIEC in the terminal ileum of CD patients is the cause of inflammation or a consequence of the disease. CEACAM6, a surface epithelial glycoprotein, has been shown to be the receptor for AIEC. CEACAM6 is expressed to a greater extent in ileal IECs of CD patients as compared to normal controls. Therefore, it is unclear whether the presence of AIEC in the terminal ileum of CD patients stimulates CEACAM6 expression and facilitates its own cell adhesion or whether the abnormal ileal expression of CEACAM6 during inflammation in CD mediates binding of pathogenic *E. coli*.

In summary, IBD appears to occur in the setting of host genetic susceptibility due to impaired function in host defense against intestinal bacteria, induced by polymorphisms in innate effector systems, such as NOD2 and autophagy pathways.

BIOMARKERS

Numerous fecal and serological biomarkers have been proposed to be used for the purpose of identifying patients with IBD, differentiating between active and quiescent disease, predicting disease course and monitoring response to therapy. Here we will briefly describe the major biomarkers used in clinical practice.

Fecal Markers

The two fecal markers most commonly utilized are calprotectin and lactoferrin. Calprotectin is a calcium- and zinc-binding protein that represents 60% of cytosolic proteins in granulocytes. Lactoferrin is an iron-binding protein found in neutrophil granules and is secreted by mucosal membranes. Both markers are indirect measures of the neutrophil infiltrate in the bowel mucosa (Kane et al., 2003; Vermeire et al., 2006). Based on a recent meta-analysis, the estimate sensitivity and specificity values for the two fecal markers for the identification of patients with IBD, compared to those without, are 82—89% and 81%, respectively ((Lewis, 2011). Concentrations of fecal calprotectin and lactoferrin have

TABLE 60.3 Prevalence of pANCA and ASCA Positivity in Controls and Patients with CD or UD

Reference	UC		CD		Controls	
	pANCA+	ASCA+	pANCA+	ASCA+	pANCA+	ASCA+
Peeters et al. (1996)	50%	14%	6%	60%	3—8%	3—11%
Quinton et al. (1998)	65%	12%	15%	61%	1%	1%
Ruemmele et al. (1998)	57%[a]	6%[b]	13%[a]	55%[b]	0%[a]	5%[b]

[a]Indirect immunofluorescence after DNase.
[b]IgG or IgA ASCA.

respectively been correlated with histologic and endo-scopic disease activity in patients with UC and CD. Fecal markers correlated better with colonic than with ileal disease (Sipponen et al., 2008). The sensitivities of these tests to detect any active mucosal disease ranged from 70 to 100%, while specificities ranged from 44 to 100%, depending on the cut-off points used (Lewis, 2011). Despite the high predictive value of fecal tests, a combination of clinical symptoms and elevated serum CRP values was superior to fecal tests in predicting endoscopic disease activity (Solem et al., 2005). Of note, fecal calprotectin is increased in other infectious and inflammatory conditions, such as infectious and ischemic colitis and non-IBD inflammatory disorders.

Serologic Markers

C-reactive protein (CRP) is one of many acute phase reactants that increase in the serum of patients with active IBD. CRP is elevated in close to 100% of patients with active CD and only in about 50% of patients with active UC (Poullis et al., 2002). Erythrocyte sedimentation rate (ESR) has also been found in some studies to correlate with CD activity but it is used less widely than CRP in CD because ESR levels do not change as quickly with disease activity. However, in UC the ESR is more of a reliable marker.

A number of circulating antibodies directed against self-antigens as well as microbial components have been found in sera of IBD patients. These biomarkers have been used in attempts to help differentiate between CD and UC in 10% of patients with IBD-type unclassified, in whom the exact diagnosis is difficult to make. Antibodies associated with CD are anti-*Saccharomyces cerevisiae* antibodies (ASCA), anti-*Escherichia coli* outer membrane porin (OmpC), anti-*Pseudomonas fluorescens*-associated sequence (I2), and anti-flagellin (CBir1). On the other hand, patients with UC have higher titers of perinuclear antineutrophil cytoplasmic antibodies (pANCA) than CD patients. These tests are specific but not sensitive in identifying patients with IBD; thus, close to 50% of patients with IBD may have normal titers of these circulating antibodies (Reese et al., 2006). Additional anti-microbial antibodies have been described (such as anti-glycan antibodies) and these appear to be directed towards fungi.

In addition to being used for diagnostic purposes, combinations of seromarkers have been used to predict disease behavior over time, such as the development of fistulizing and penetrating complications and the need for surgery. Studies by Mow et al. and Dubinsky et al. have demonstrated that ASCA, OmpC, and I2 were each associated with features of complicated disease and that the number of positive tests for antibodies and the concentrations of antibodies were associated with complications

such as stenosis, penetrating disease, and the need for small bowel surgery (Mow et al., 2004; Dubinsky et al., 2006, 2008). It is still unclear, however, whether early aggressive intervention in patients with markers of a worse prognosis will change long-term outcomes.

TREATMENT

Medical

The medical treatment of IBD involves a growing armamentarium of medications, as a fundamental knowledge of disease pathogenesis expands. Many of these drugs are used for both UC and CD. Clinical trials are hampered by a consistent finding of placebo response rates of about 30%. The various classes of medications will be presented here, with specific mention of their use in CD and UC.

Aminosalicylates

The first aminosalicylate used in IBD was sulfasalazine, which consists of 5-aminosalicylic acid (5-ASA) bound to the antibiotic sulfapyridine via an azo-bond. This bond is split by enzymes present in colonic bacteria. It is the free 5-ASA that is released into the colon to exert the therapeutic effect. 5-ASA has multiple anti-inflammatory properties including inhibition of production of IL-1 (Mahida et al., 1991), interference with binding of TNF (Shanahan et al., 1990), and as a free radical scavenger (Ahnfelt-Ronne et al., 1990). These effects appear to be mediated in part by inhibition of activation of NF-κB (Bantel et al., 2000). The most commonly used aminosalicyate in the treatment of IBD today is mesalamine. Various mesalamine preparations exist including coated drugs designed to delay release until the terminal ileum or colon is reached, and topical enemas or suppositories for treatment of the distal colon and rectum.

The aminosalicylates are effective first-line agents in the induction and the maintenance of remission in moderately active ulcerative colitis. There is no convincing evidence of the superiority of any one preparation over another (Mahadevan and Sandborn, 2004). Evidence for the effectiveness of aminosalicylates in the treatment of active CD is not as strong as for UC. Sulfasalazine may be effective in the treatment of active colonic disease whereas controlled-release mesalamine is preferred for treatment of ileal disease. Studies of mesalamine for maintenance of remission show little if any benefit (Sandborn, 2004).

Glucocorticoids

Corticosteroids are used extensively in the treatment of IBD. Glucocorticoids are steroid hormones that bind to cytosolic receptors and are then translocated to the nucleus where they affect transcription of various genes. This leads to inhibition of various proinflammatory mediators such as cytokines, leukotrienes, adhesion molecules, and nitric oxide synthase (Sands, 2002). Most patients with active UC or CD will respond to a course of oral glucocorticoids, although occasionally the intravenous route is required for severe disease. In many patients, however, tapering the drug will lead to a flare; this phenomenon is termed steroid dependence. The well-known side effects of chronic steroid use are common and troublesome; these include diabetes, bone loss, acne, moon facies, and adrenal suppression. Attempts to limit these side effects have resulted in other formulations such as topical foam and enemas which can be effective for left-sided colonic disease. Budesonide is an oral glucocorticoid that undergoes extensive first-pass metabolism in the liver. As a result, high topical levels are achieved in the GI tract with only about 10% systemic absorption and thus fewer steroid side effects (Edsbacker et al. 1999). Budesonide has been shown to have some efficacy as a treatment for mild to moderately active CD (Greenberg et al., 1994; Tremaine et al., 2002).

Thiopurines

The thiopurines include azathioprine and 6-mercaptopurine (6-MP). Azathioprine is metabolized to 6-MP, which can eventually be converted into a number of metabolites including 6-thioguanine nucleotides (6-TG). The exact mechanism of action of the thiopurines is unknown, but studies have shown that their therapeutic effect is either due to blocking of the TcR signaling pathway, which leads to T cell apoptosis, or 6-TG inhibition of purine synthesis. The beneficial effect of thiopurines is generally not seen until 3−6 months of use. The ideal use of thiopurines is as a so-called "steroid-sparing" agent: to allow for the discontinuation of steroids in the patient who requires chronic or frequent use. Clinical studies have confirmed the utility of thiopurines as steroid-sparing agents effective in inducing and maintaining remission in CD and UC (Present et al., 1980; George et al., 1996). The side effects of thiopurines are far less than those of glucorticoids but include leukopenia, pancreatitis, and hepatitis. The leucopenia is a result of 6-MP metabolism to 6-TG, whereas the hepatitis is associated with the accumulation of the 6-MMP metabolite. Interestingly, genetic variations in the enzyme thiopurine methyltransferase increase the risk of leukopenia by increasing 6-TG levels.

Cyclosporine

Cyclosporine is a fungal product that functions as an inhibitor of calcineurin, a cytoplasmic enzyme required for activation of T cells (Mahadevan and Sandborn, 2004).

Intravenous cyclosporine is an effective treatment for severe steroid-refractory UC (Lichtiger et al., 1994). The utility of cyclosporine is limited by significant side effects including hypertension, seizures, and nephrotoxicity.

Methotrexate

Methotrexate is a folate analogue that inhibits dihydrofolate reductase. Its anti-inflammatory effect is due to a reduction in various proinflammatory cytokines, an induction of lymphocyte apoptosis, and perhaps an increase in extracellular adenosine (Mahadevan and Sandborn, 2004). Intramuscular methotrexate is effective in inducing and maintaining remission in patients with CD (Feagan et al., 1995; Arora et al., 1999). Side effects of methotrexate at doses used for CD include rare hepatotoxicity, pneumonitis, and rash.

Anti-TNF Antibody Therapies

Infliximab (Remicade) was the first anti-TNF agent to be approved for use in IBD. It is a chimeric monoclonal antibody against TNF-α administered as an i.v. infusion. Neutralization of soluble TNF seems not to be the primary mechanism since the soluble TNF-receptor etanercept is not effective in CD (Sandborn et al., 2001). It appears that binding of infliximab to membrane-bound TNF on inflammatory cells leads to T cell apoptosis, thereby reducing the effector cell pool (Lugering et al., 2001; Van den Brande et al., 2003).

Infliximab has initially been shown to induce and maintain remission in patients with moderate to severe luminal (non-fistulizing) CD (Targan et al., 1997). Since the initial studies showing efficacy of infliximab in luminal CD, it has also been found to be effective for healing of perianal fistulas due to CD (Present et al., 1999), as well as for the induction and maintenance of remission in fistulizing CD (Sands et al., 2004). Subsequent studies have demonstrated efficacy of infliximab as induction and maintenance therapy in UC (Rutgeerts et al., 2005). Antibodies to infliximab (ATIs) are of concern in that they appear to increase the risk of infusion reactions and limit effectiveness (Baert et al., 2003). Increasing the dose given at each infusion, shortening the interval between infusions, and dosing infliximab based on trough levels are strategies that are currently being explored in patients who lose response to infliximab over time.

Adalimumab (Humira), a fully human anti-TNF monoclonal antibody administered subcutaneously, has also been shown to induce and maintain remission in patients with moderate to severe CD (Colombel et al., 2007). In addition, adalimumab demonstrated fistula healing and improved quality of life in patients with CD who failed prior infliximab therapy (Lichtiger et al., 2010).

Certolizumab pegol (Cimzia), a polyethylene glycolated Fab′ fragment of humanized anti-TNF monoclonal antibody administered subcutaneously, has been found to be effective in inducing and maintaining remission in CD patients who have lost response to infliximab (Sandborn et al., 2010). However, in patients with moderate to severe CD who were naïve to anti-TNF agents certolizumab pegol was not found to be effective at inducing remission (Sandborn et al., 2011). In a subgroup analysis, CD patients with elevated CRP levels (>5 mg/L at entry) had remission rates at week 6 that were significantly higher than placebo.

Inhibitors of Leukocyte Infiltration

A new approach to biologic therapy has been the development of inhibitors of various elements in the leukocyte infiltration process. The main targets of these new agents are the integrins α4β1 and α4β7, which interact with VCAM-1 and MAdCAM-1, respectively, to mediate interactions between leukocytes and endothelial cells. Here we will focus on the monoclonal antibodies natalizumab and MLN0002, which target α4 and α4β, respectively.

Natalizumab (Tysabri) is a humanized monoclonal antibody against α4 integrin. Natalizumab has recently been approved for use in CD after being found to be superior to placebo in inducing remission in patients with elevated CRP levels (Targan et al., 2007). The limiting factor in the use of this agent is a high rate of JC virus reactivation, which results in progressive multifocal leukoencephalopathy (PML). It is estimated that one in 1000 patients treated with natalizumab will develop PML (Yousry et al., 2006). It is recommended that patients be tested for JC virus seropositivity prior to undergoing therapy with natalizumab, as it is the seropositive patients that develop JC virus reactivation in the setting of immune suppression.

Another antibody against α4β7 integrin, MLN0002, demonstrated a dose-dependent beneficial effect on clinical remission in patients with active CD in a phase 2 randomized, double-blind, placebo-controlled trial (Feagan et al., 2008). In addition, MLN0002 was demonstrated to be more efficacious than placebo in inducing clinical and endoscopic remission at 6 weeks in patients with active UC (Feagan et al., 2005). More studies are needed to examine long-term efficacy of anti-α4β7 integrin in patients with CD and UC.

New Biologic Therapies

New biologic therapies aim to reduce pathogenic T cell activation and its effects by inhibiting the actions of proinflammatory cytokines, blocking T cell co-stimulation and inducing T cell apoptosis. Monoclonal antibodies

against the following proinflammatory cytokine targets have been developed: α-chain (CD25) of the IL-2 receptor, IFN-γ, IL-6, IL-6 receptor, IL-13, IL-17, IL-18, and IL-22. Unfortunately, antibodies against both IL-2R and IFN-γ failed to show benefit over placebo in inducing remission in patients with UC and CD, respectively (Van Assche et al., 2006;Reinisch et al., 2010). Of interest, the monoclonal antibody against IL-17 was tested in a phase II trial in CD patients. Not only did the patients not respond to anti-IL-17 but their condition worsened. The other monoclonal antibodies against proinflammatory cytokines are entering phase I trials.

Visilizumab is a monoclonal antibody against the CD3 chain of the T cell antigen receptor. CD3 is expressed on all T cells and its blockade leads to T cell apoptosis. Visilizumab was tested in severe, steroid-resistant UC in phase I/II trials. All patients reported significant adverse events, such as abdominal abscesses, atrial fibrillation, cytokine release syndrome, CMV, and herpes zoster reactivation (Baumgart et al., 2010). Visilizumab was not shown to be efficacious in the management of IBD in larger trials.

Stimulators of the innate immune system have been tested in CD. Granulocyte−monocyte colony-stimulating factor (GM-CSF), sargramostim, underwent an open-label trial and was found to produce a clinical response in patients with moderate to severe CD (Dieckgraefe and Korzenik, 2002). However, follow-up trials did not meet their primary therapeutic end points (Egea et al., 2010).

Surgical

Around 70−80% of CD patients and 30−40% of UC patients will require surgery at some point in their lives (Larson and Pemberton, 2004). Indications for surgery in UC include toxic megacolon, severe disease not responding to maximal medical therapy, medication side effects, dysplasia or cancer, severe hemorrhage, and intractable extraintestinal manifestations. In almost all cases, complete removal of the entire colon and rectum (total proctocolectomy) is required to eliminate the risk of recurrent or residual disease as well as subsequent cancer.

Indications for surgery in CD are similar to those for UC but include the complications of stricturing or fistulizing disease such as obstruction and abscess. The most common operation performed for ileal disease is the ileocolic resection, in which the terminal ileum and cecum are resected and an anastomosis is performed between ileum and ascending colon. For the treatment of strictures in patients with multiple prior resections or with multiple skip lesions, a stricturoplasty can be performed in which the stricture is widened without resection. For colitis, in which the rectum is usually spared, a subtotal colectomy with ileorectal or ileosigmoid anastomosis can usually be performed with good functional results. If there is rectal involvement or perianal disease, a total proctocolectomy with permanent ileostomy is usually required.

FUTURE PROSPECTS

During the last 15 years there have been great advances in the understanding of processes involved in the pathogenesis of both types of IBD, Crohn's disease and ulcerative colitis. These were earlier thought to be based on adaptive autoimmune responses but newer concepts have arisen. These recently elucidated pathways have in turn led to the development of new therapies for IBD. A major challenge now is to determine which inflammatory pathways predominate in which subgroups of patients. Studies are needed to determine how the products of the numerous IBD susceptibility genes modify immune responses and, ultimately, responses to different therapeutic agents. Combined analysis of clinical phenotypes, genotypes and peripheral and mucosal cytokine profiles will be called for, to predict responses to different therapies including biological agents. Current studies indicate that starting biologic therapy early in the course of the disease, and targeting patients with the more aggressive disease phenotype, improves long-term disease control. However, better pathogenesis-driven markers are needed for risk-stratification of patients into aggressive and non-aggressive phenotypes. Studies on families with multiple affected family members may help identify genetic loci predisposing to aggressive disease type. The identification of the dominant inflammatory pathway(s) prior to, or at the time of, diagnosis would allow for individualized tailoring of therapeutic options. In addition, new serologic and mucosal markers likely will identify post-operative patients (especially with CD) at a high risk for disease recurrence, sparing low-risk patients of exposure to biologic therapies and affording high-risk patients the best available post-operative prophylaxis. Better understanding of the genetics and immune pathways involved in the pathogenesis of the IBDs will move clinical practice closer towards individualized therapy.

REFERENCES

Ahmad, T., Armuzzi, A., Bunce, M., Mulcahy-Hawes, K., Marshall, S. E., Orchard, T.R., et al., 2002. The molecular classification of the clinical manifestations of Crohn's disease. Gastroenterology. 122, 854–866.

Ahmad, T., Tamboli, C.P., Jewell, D., Colombel, J.F., 2004. Clinical relevance of advances in genetics and pharmacogenetics of IBD. Gastroenterology. 126, 1533–1549.

Ahnfelt-Ronne, I., Nielsen, O.H., Christensen, A., Langholz, E., Binder, V., Riis, P., 1990. Clinical evidence supporting the radical scavenger mechanism of 5-aminosalicylic acid. Gastroenterology. 98, 1162–1169.

Allez, M., Brimnes, J., Dotan, I., Mayer, L., 2002. Expansion of CD8 + T cells with regulatory function after interaction with intestinal epithelial cells. Gastroenterology. 123, 1516–1526.

Anderson, C.A, Boucher, G., Lees, C.W., Franke, A., D'Amato, M., et al., 2011. Meta-analysis identifies 29 additional ulcerative colitis risk loci, increasing the number of confirmed associations to 47. Nat. Genet. 43, 246–252.

Arora, S., Katkov, W., Cooley, J., Kemp, J.A., Johnston, D.E., Schapiro, R. H., et al., 1999. Methotrexate in Crohn's disease: results of a randomized, double-blind, placebo-controlled trial. Hepatogastroenterology. 46, 1724–1729.

Axelsson, L.G., Landstrom, E., Goldschmidt, T.J., Gronberg, A., Bylund-Fellenius, A.C., 1996. Dextran sulfate sodium (DSS) induced experimental colitis in immunodeficient mice: effects in CD4(+)-cell depleted, athymic and NK-cell depleted SCID mice. Inflamm. Res. 45, 181–191.

Baert, F., Noman, M., Vermeire, S., Van Assche, G., D'Haens, G., Carbonez, A., et al., 2003. Influence of immunogenicity on the long-term efficacy of infliximab in Crohn's disease. N. Engl. Med. 348, 601–608.

Bantel, H., Berg, C., Vieth, M., Stolte, M., Kruis, W., Schulze-Osthoff, K., 2000. Mesalazine inhibits activation of transcription factor NF-κB in inflamed mucosa of patients with ulcerative colitis. Am. J. Gastroenterol. 95, 3452–3457.

Barnich, N., Carvalho, F.A., Glasser, A.L., Darcha, C., Jantscheff, P., Allez, M., et al., 2007. CEACAM6 acts as a receptor for adherent-invasive E. coli, supporting ileal mucosa colonization in Crohn disease. J. Clin. Invest. 117, 1566–1574.

Baron, J.H., 2000. Inflammatory bowel disease up to 1932. Mt. Sinai J. Med. 67 (3), 174–189.

Barrett, J.C., Hansoul, S., Nicolae, D.L., Cho, J.H., Duerr, R.H., Rioux, J. D., et al., 2008. Genome-wide association defines more than 30 distinct susceptibility loci for Crohn's disease. Nat. Genet. 40, 955–962.

Baumgart, D.C., Lowder, J.N., Targan, S.R., Sandborn, W.J., Frankel, M.B., 2009. Transient cytokine-induced liver injury following administration of the humanized anti-CD3 antibody visilizumab (HuM291) in Crohn's disease. Am. J. Gastroenterol. 104, 868–876.

Baumgart, D.C., Targan, S.R., Dignass, A.U., Mayer, L., van Assche, G., Hommes, D.W., et al., 2010. Prospective randomized open-label multicenter phase I/II dose escalation trial of visilizumab (HuM291) in severe steroid-refractory ulcerative colitis. Inflamm. Bowel Dis. 16, 620–629.

Berg, D.J., Zhang, J., Weinstock, J.V., Ismail, H.F., Earle, K.A., Alila, H., et al., 2002. Rapid development of colitis in NSAID-treated IL-10-deficient mice. Gastroenterology. 123, 1527–1542.

Binder, V., 1998. Genetic epidemiology in inflammatory bowel disease. Dig. Dis. 16, 351–355.

Blanchard, J.F., Bernstein, C.N., Wajda, A., Rawsthorne, P., 2001. Small-area variations and sociodemographic correlates for the incidence of Crohn's disease and ulcerative colitis. Am. J. Epidemiol. 154, 328–335.

Boirivant, M., Marini, M., Di Felice, G., Pronio, A.M., Montesani, C., Tersigni, R., et al., 1999. Lamina propria T cells in Crohn's disease and other gastrointestinal inflammation show defective CD2 pathway-induced apoptosis. Gastroenterology. 116, 557–565.

Bonen, D.K., Nicolae, D.L., Moran, T., Turkyilmaz, M.A., Ramos, R., Karaliukas, R., et al., 2002. Racial differences in Nod2 variation: characterization of Nod2 in African-Americans with Crohn's disease. Gastroenterology. 122, A29.

Boyko, E.J., Perera, D.R., Keopsell, T.D., Keane, E.M., Inui, T.S., 1988. Effect of cigarette smoking on the clinical course of ulcerative colitis. Scand. J. Gastroenterol. 23, 1147–1152.

Brand, S., Beigel, F., Olszak, T., Zitmann, K., Eichhorst, S.T., Otte, J. M., et al., 2006. IL-22 is increased in active Crohn's disease and promotes proinflammatory gene expression and intestinal epithelial cell mirgration. Am. J. Physiol. Gastrointest. Liver Physiol. 290 (4), G827–G838.

Brimnes, J., Allez, M., Dotan, I., Shao, L., Nakazawa, A., Mayer, L., 2005. Defects in CD8 + regulatory T cells in the lamina propria of patients with inflammatory bowel disease. J. Immunol. 174 (9), 5814–5822.

Cadwell, K., Liu, J.Y., Brown, S.L., Miyoshi, H., Loh, J., Lennerz, J.K., et al., 2008. A key role for autophagy and the autophagy gene Atg16l1 in mouse and human intestinal Paneth cells. Nature. 456, 259–263.

Cadwell, K., Patel, K.K., Maloney, N.S., Liu, T.C., Ng, A.C., Storer, C. E., et al., 2010. Virus-plus-susceptibility gene interaction determines Crohn's disease gene Atg16L1 phenotypes in intestine. Cell. 141, 1135–1145.

Calkins, B.M., 1989. A meta-analysis of the role of smoking in inflammatory bowel disease. Dig. Dis. Sci. 34, 1841–1854.

Campbell, E.L., MacManus, C.F., Kominsky, D.J., Keely, S., Glover, L.E., Bowers, B.E., et al., 2010. Resolvin E1-induced intestinal alkaline phosphatase promotes resolution of inflammation through LPS detoxification. Proc. Natl. Acad. Sci. U.S.A. 107, 14289–14303.

Campbell, N.A., Kim, H.S., Blumberg, R.S., Mayer, L., 1999. The non-classical class I molecule CD1d associates with the novel CD8 ligand gp180 on intestinal epithelial cells. J. Biol. Chem. 274, 26259–26265.

Campbell, N.A., Park, M.S., Toy, L.S., Yio, X.Y., Devine, L., Kavathas, P., et al., 2002. A non-class I MHC intestinal epithelial surface glycoprotein, gp180, binds to CD8. Clin. Immunol. 102 (3), 267–274.

Chalifoux, L.V., Bronson, R.T., 1981. Colonic adenocarcinoma associated with chronic colitis in cotton top marmosets, Saguinus oedipus. Gastroenterology. 80, 942–946.

Chamaillard, M., Girardin, S.E., Viala, J., Philpott, D., 2003. Nods, Nalps and Naip: intracellular regulators of bacterial-induced inflammation. Cell. Microbiol. 5, 581–592.

Colombel, J.F., Sandborn, W.J., Rutgeerts, P., Enns, R., Hanauer, S.B., Panaccione, R., et al., 2007. Adalimumab for maintenance of clinical response and remission in patients with Crohn's disease: the CHARM trial. Gastroenterology. 132, 52–65.

Colpaert, S., Vastraelen, K., Liu, Z., Maerten, P., Shen, C., Penninckx, F., et al., 2002. In vitro analysis of interferon gamma (IFN-gamma) and interleukin-12 (IL-12) production and their effects in ileal Crohn's disease. Eur. Cytokine Netw. 13, 431–437.

Cooney, R., Baker, J., Brain, O., Danis, B., Pichulik, T., Allan, P., et al., 2010. NOD2 stimulation induces autophagy in dendritic cells influencing bacterial handling and antigen presentation. Nat. Med. 16, 90–97.

Cooper, H.S., Murthy, S.N., Shah, R.S., Sedergran, D.J., 1993. Clinicopathologic study of dextran sulfate sodium experimental murine colitis. Lab. Invest. 69, 238–249.

Dahan, S., Roth-Walter, F., Arnaboldi, P., Agarwal, S., Mayer, L., 2007. Immunol. Rev. 215, 243–253.

Danese, S., 2012. New therapies for inflammatory bowel disease: from the bench to the bedside. Gut. 61, 918–932.

Davidson, N.J., Hudak, S.A., Lesley, R.E., Menon, S., Leach, M.W., Rennick, D.M., 1998. IL-12, but not IFN-gamma, plays a major role in sustaining the chronic phase of colitis in IL-10-deficient mice. J. Immunol. 161, 3143–3149.

Dieckgraefe, B.K., Korzenik, J.R., 2002. Treatment of active Crohn's disease with recombinant human granulocyte-macrophage colony-stimulating factor. Lancet. 360, 1478–1480.

Dubinsky, M.C., Lin, Y.C., Dutridge, D., Picornell, Y., Landers, C.J., Farrior, S., et al., 2006. Serum immune responses predict rapid disease progression among children with Crohn's disease: immune responses predict disease progression. Am. J. Gastroenterol. 101, 360–3607.

Dubinsky, M.C., Kugathasan, S., Mei, L., Picornell, Y., Nebel, J., Wrobel, I., et al., 2008. Increased immune reactivity predicts aggressive complicating Crohn's disease in children. Clin. Gastroenterol. Hepatol. 6, 1105–1111.

Duchmann, R., Kaiser, I., Hermann, E., Mayet, W., Ewe, K., Meyer zum Buschenfelde, K.H., 1995. Tolerance exists towards resident intestinal flora but is broken in active inflammatory bowel disease (IBD). Clin. Exp. Immunol. 102, 448–455.

Duerr, R.H., Taylor, K.D., Brant, S.R., Rioux, J.D., Silverberg, M.S., Daly, M.J., et al., 2006. A genome-wide association study identifies IL23R as an inflammatory bowel disease gene. Science. 314, 1461–1463.

Eaden, J., Abrams, K.R., Mayberry, J.F., 2001. The risk of colorectal cancer in ulcerative colitis: a meta-analysis. Gut. 48, 526–535.

Edsbacker, S., 2000. Budesonide capsules: scientific basis. Drugs Today. 38, 9–23.

Ehrhardt, R.O., Ludviksson, B.R., Gray, B., Neurath, M., Strober, W., 1997. Induction and prevention of colonic inflammation in IL-2-deficient mice. J. Immunol. 158, 566–573.

Eyerich, S., Eyerich, K., Pennino, D., Carbone, T., Nasorri, F., Pallotta, S., et al., 2010. IL-17 and IL-22: siblings, not twins. Trends Immunol. 31 (9), 354–361.

Egea, L., Hirata, Y., Kagnoff, M., 2010. GM:CSF: a role in immune and inflammatory reactions in the intestine. Expert Reviews Gastroenterology and Hepatology. 4, 723–731.

Feagan, B.G., Rochon, J., Fedorak, R.N., Irvine, E.J., Wild, G., Sutherland, L., et al., 1995. Methotrexate for the treatment of Crohn's disease. The North American Crohn's Study Group Investigators. N. Engl. J. Med. 332, 292–297.

Feagan, B.G., Greenberg, G.R., Wild, G., Fedorak, R.N., Paré, P., McDonald, J.W., et al., 2005. Treatment of ulcerative colitis with a humanized antibody to the alpha4beta7 integrin. N. Engl. J. Med. 352, 2499–2507.

Feagan, B.G., Greenberg, G.R., Wild, G., Fedorak, R.N., Paré, P., McDonald, J.W., et al., 2008. Treatment of active Crohn's disease with MLN0002, a humanized antibody to the alpha4beta7 integrin. Clin. Gastroenterol. Hepatol. 6, 1370–1377.

Feagan, B.G., Sandborn, W.J., Wolf, D.C., Coteur, G., Purcaru, O., Brabant, Y., et al., 2011. Randomised clinical trial: improvement in health outcomes with certolizumab pegol in patients with active Crohn's disease with prior loss of response to infliximab. Aliment. Pharmacol. Ther. 33, 541–550.

Fleshner, P.R., Vasiliauskas, E.A., Kam, L.Y., Fleshner, N.E., Gaiennie, J., Abreu-Martin, M.T., et al., 2001. High level perinuclear antineutrophil cytoplasmic antibody (pANCA) in ulcerative colitis patients before colectomy predicts the development of chronic pouchitis after ileal pouch-anal anastomosis. Gut. 49, 671–677.

George, J., Present, D.H., Pou, R., Bodian, C., Rubin, P.H., 1996. The long-term outcome of ulcerative colitis treated with 6-mercaptopurine. Am. J. Gastroenterol. 91, 1711–1714.

Ghosh, S., Goldin, E., Gordon, F.H., Malchow, H.A., Rask-Madsen, J., Rutgeerts, P., et al., 2003. Natalizumab for active Crohn's disease. N. Engl. J. Med. 348, 24–32.

Ginzburg, L., Oppenheimer, G.D., 1932. Non-specific granulomata of the intestines (inflammatory tumors and strictures of the bowel). Trans. Am. Gastro-Enterol. Assoc. 35, 241–283.

Gionchetti, P., Rizzello, F., Venturi, A., Brigidi, P., Matteuzzi, D., Bazzocchi, G., et al., 2000. Oral bacteriotherapy as maintenance treatment in patients with chronic pouchitis: a double-blind, placebo-controlled trial. Gastroenterology. 119, 305–309.

Girardin, S.E., Boneca, I.G., Viala, J., Chamaillard, M., Labigne, A., Thomas, G., et al., 2003. Nod2 is a general sensor of peptidoglycan through muramyl dipeptide (MDP) detection. J. Biol. Chem. 278, 8869–8872.

Greenberg, G.R., Feagan, B.G., Martin, F., Sutherland, L.R., Thomson, A.B., Williams, C.N., et al., 1994. Oral budesonide for active Crohn's disease. Canadian Inflammatory Bowel Disease Study Group. N. Engl. J. Med. 331, 836–841.

Greenstein, A., Janowitz, H.D., Sachar, D.B., 1976. The extra-intestinal complications of Crohn's disease and ulcerative colitis. Medicine. 55, 401–412.

Hale-White, W., 1888. On simple ulcerative colitis and other rare intestinal ulcers. Guys. Hosp. Rep. 30, 131–162, 3rd series.

Halfvarson, J., Bodin, L., Tysk, C., Lindberg, E., Jarnerot, G., 2003. Inflammatory bowel disease in a Swedish twin cohort: a long-term follow-up of concordance and clinical characteristics. Gastroenterology. 124, 1767–1773.

Hampe, J., Cuthbert, A., Croucher, P.J., Mirza, M.M., Mascheretti, S., Fisher, S., et al., 2001. Association between insertion mutation in NOD2 gene and Crohn's disease in German and British populations. Lancet. 357, 1925–1928.

Hampe, J., Franke, A., Rosenstiel, P., Till, A., Teuber, M., Huse, K., et al., 2007. A genome-wide association scan of nonsynonymous SNPs identifies a susceptibility variant for Crohn disease in ATG16L1. Nat. Genet. 39, 207–211.

Hanai, H., Watanabe, F., Yamada, M., Sato, Y., Takeuchi, K., Iida, T., et al., 2004. Adsorptive granulocyte and monocyte apheresis versus prednisolone in patients with corticosteroid-dependent moderately severe ulcerative colitis. Digestion. 70, 36–44.

Hanauer, S.B., Feagan, B.G., Lichtenstein, G.R., Mayer, L.F., Schreiber, S., Colombel, J.F., et al., 2002. Maintenance infliximab for Crohn's disease: the ACCENT I randomised trial. Lancet. 359, 1541–1549.

Hanauer, S.B., Panes, J., Colombel, JF., Bloomfield, R., Schreiber, S., Sandborn, W.J., 2010. Clinical trial: impact of prior infliximab therapy on the clinical response to certolizumab pegol maintenance therapy for Crohn's disease. Aliment. Pharmacol. Ther. 32, 384–393.

Heazlewood, C.K., Cook, M.C., Eri, R., Price, G.R., Tauro, S.B., Taupin, D., et al., 2008. Aberrant mucin assembly in mice causes endoplasmic reticulum stress and spontaneous inflammation resembling ulcerative colitis. PloS Med. 5, e54.

Heller, F., Fuss, I.J., Nieuwenhuis, E.E., Blumberg, R.S., Strober, W., 2002. Oxazolone colitis, a Th2 colitis model resembling ulcerative colitis, is mediated by IL-13-producing NK-T cells. Immunity. 17, 629–638.

Hisamatsu, T., Suzuki, M., Reinecker, H.C., Nadeau, W.J., McCormick, B. A., Podolsky, D.K., 2003. CARD15/NOD2 functions as an antibacterial factor in human intestinal epithelial cells. Gastroenterology. 124, 993–1000.

Hovhannisyan, Z., Treatman, J., Littman, D.R., Mayer, L., 2011. Characterization of interleukin-17-producing regulatory T cells in inflamed intestinal mucosa from patients with inflammatory bowel disease. Gastroenterology. 140 (3), 957–965.

Hugot, J.P., Chamaillard, M., Zouali, H., Lesage, S., Cezard, J.P., Belaiche, J., et al., 2001. Association of NOD2 leucine-rich repeat variants with susceptibility to Crohn's disease. Nature. 411, 599–603.

Hurst, A.F., 1909. Ulcerative colitis. Guy's Hosp. Rep. 71, 26.

Inoue, N., Tamura, K., Kinouchi, Y., Fukuda, Y., Takahashi, S., Ogura, Y., et al., 2002. Lack of common Nod2 variants in Japanese patients with Crohn's disease. Gastroenterology. 123, 86–91.

Itzkowitz, S.H., 2004. Colorectal cancer in inflammatory bowel disease: molecular considerations. In: Sartor, R.B., Sandborn, W.J. (Eds.), Kirsner's Inflammatory Bowel Diseases. Saunders, New York, USA, pp. 230–242.

Joossens, S., Reinisch, W., Vermeire, S., Sendid, B., Poulain, D., Peeters, M., et al., 2002. The value of serologic markers in indeterminate colitis: a prospective follow-up study. Gastroenterology. 122, 1242–1247.

Jung, H.C., Eckmann, L., Yang, S.K., Panja, A., Fierer, J., Morzycka-Wroblewska, E., et al., 1995. A distinct array of proinflammatory cytokines is expressed in human colon epithelial cells in response to bacterial invasion. J. Clin. Invest. 95, 55–65.

Kaiserlian, D., Vidal, K., Revillard, J.P., 1989. Murine enterocytes can present soluble antigen to specific class II-restricted CD4 + T cells. Eur. J. Immunol. 19, 1513–1516.

Kamada, N., Hisamatsu, T., Honda, H., Kobayashi, T., Chinene, H., Takayama, T., Kitazume, M.T., et al., 2010. TL1A produced by lamina propria macrophages induces Th1and Th17 immune responses in cooperation with IL-23 in patients with Crohn's disease. Inflamm. Bowel Dis. 16 (4), 568–575.

Kamm, M.A., Hanauer, S.B., Panaccione, R., Colombel, J.F., Sandborn, W.J., Pollack, P.F., et al., 2011. Adalimumab sustains steroid-free remission after 3 years of therapy for Crohn's disease. Aliment. Pharmacol. Ther. 34, 306–317.

Kane, S.V., Sandborn, W.J., Rufo, P.A., Zholudev, A., Boone, J., Lyerly, D., et al., 2003. Fecal lactoferrin is a sensitive and specific marker in identifying intestinal inflammation. Am. J. Gastroenterol. 98, 1309–1314.

Kitajima, S., Morimoto, M., Sagara, E., Shimizu, C., Ikeda, Y., 2001. Dextran sodium sulfate-induced colitis in germ-free IQI/Jic mice. Exp. Anim. 50, 387–395.

Kneitz, B., Herrmann, T., Yonehara, S., Schimpl, A., 1995. Normal clonal expansion but impaired Fas-mediated cell death and anergy induction in interleukin-2-deficient mice. Eur. J. Immunol. 25, 2572–2577.

Koutroubakis, I.E., Vlachonikolis, I.G., Kouroumalis, E.A., 2002. Role of appendicitis and appendectomy in the pathogenesis of ulcerative colitis: a critical review. Inflamm. Bowel Dis. 8, 277–286.

Kraus, T.A., Toy, L., Chan, L., Childs, J., Mayer, L., 2004. Failure to induce oral tolerance to a soluble protein in patients with inflammatory bowel disease. Gastroenterology. 126, 1771–1778.

Kuhn, R., Lohler, J., Rennick, D., Rajewsky, K., Muller, W., 1993. Interleukin-10-deficient mice develop chronic enterocolitis. Cell. 75, 263–274.

Landers, C.J., Cohavy, O., Misra, R., Yang, H., Lin, Y.C., Braun, J., et al., 2002. Selected loss of tolerance evidenced by Crohn's disease-associated immune responses to auto- and microbial antigens. Gastroenterology. 123, 689–699.

Larson, D.W., Pemberton, J.H., 2004. Current concepts and controversies in surgery for IBD. Gastroenterology. 126, 1611–1619.

Lennard, L., 1992. The clinical pharmacology of 6-mercaptopurine. Eur. J. Clin. Pharmacol. 43, 329–339.

Lesage, S., Zouali, H., Cezard, J.P., Colombel, J.F., Belaiche, J., et al., 2002. CARD15/NOD2 mutational analysis and genotype-phenotype correlation in 612 patients with inflammatory bowel disease. Am. J. Hum. Genet. 70, 845–857.

Lewis, J.D., 2011. The utility of biomarkers in the diagnosis and therapy of inflammatory bowel disease. Gastroenterology. 140 (6), 1817–1826.

Lichtiger, S., Present, D.H., Kornbluth, A., Gelernt, I., Bauer, J., Galler, G., et al., 1994. Cyclosporine in severe ulcerative colitis refractory to steroid therapy. N. Engl. J. Med. 330, 1841–1845.

Lichtiger, S., Binion, D.G., Wolf, D.C., Present, D.H., Bensimon, A.G., Wu, E., et al., 2010. The CHOICE trial: adalimumab demonstrates safety, fistula healing, improved quality of life and increased work productivity in patients with Crohn's disease who failed prior infliximab therapy. Aliment. Pharmacol. Ther. 32, 1228–1239.

Lindsay, J.O., Hodgson, H.J., 2001. Review article: the immunoregulatory cytokine interleukin-10—a therapy for Crohn's disease? Aliment. Pharmacol. Ther. 15, 1709–1716.

Loftus, E.V., 2004. Clinical epidemiology of inflammatory bowel disease. Gastroenterology. 126, 1504–1517.

Lugering, A., Schmidt, M., Lugering, N., Pauels, H.G., Domschke, W., Kucharzik, T., 2001. Infliximab induces apoptosis in monocytes from patients with chronic active Crohn's disease by using a caspase-dependent pathway. Gastroenterology. 121, 1145–1157.

Madsen, K.L., Doyle, J.S., Tavernini, M.M., Jewell, L.D., Rennie, R.P., Fedorak, R.N., 2000. Antibiotic therapy attenuates colitis in interleukin 10 gene-deficient mice. Gastroenterology. 118, 1094–1105.

Mahadevan, U., Sandborn, W.J., 2004. Clinical pharmacology of inflammatory bowel disease therapy. In: Sartor, R.B., Sandborn, W.J. (Eds.), Kirsner's Inflammatory Bowel Diseases. Saunders, New York, USA, pp. 484–502.

Mahida, Y.R., Lamming, C.E., Gallagher, A., Hawthorne, A.B., Hawkey, C.J., 1991. 5-Aminosalicylic acid is a potent inhibitor of interleukin 1 beta production in organ culture of colonic biopsy specimens from patients with inflammatory bowel disease. Gut. 32, 50–54.

Mannon, P.J., Fuss, I.J., Mayer, L., Elson, C.O., Sandborn, W.J., Present, D., et al., 2004. Anti-IL-12 Crohn's Disease Study Group. Anti-interleukin-12 antibody for active Crohn's disease. N. Engl. J. Med. 351, 2069–2079.

Matsumoto, S., Okabe, Y., Setoyama, H., Takayama, K., Ohtsuka, J., Funahashi, H., et al., 1998. Inflammatory bowel disease-like enteritis and caecitis in a senescence accelerated mouse P1/Yit strain. Gut. 43, 71–78.

Mayer, L., Eisenhardt, D., 1990. Lack of induction of suppressor T cells by intestinal epithelial cells from patients with inflammatory bowel disease. J. Clin. Invest. 86, 1255–1260.

Mayer, L., Shlien, R., 1987. Evidence for function of Ia molecules on gut epithelial cells in man. J. Exp. Med. 166, 1471–1483.

McCarroll, S.A., Huett, A., Kuballa, P., Chilewski, S.D., Landry, A., Goyette, P., et al., 2008. Deletion polymorphism upstream of IRGM associated with altered IRGM expression and Crohn's disease. Nat. Genet. 40, 1107–1112.

McLeod, R.S., 2004. Surgery for Crohn's disease. In: Sartor, R.B., Sandborn, W.J. (Eds.), Kirsner's Inflammatory Bowel Diseases. Saunders, New York, USA, pp. 614–630.

Meddings, J.B., 1997. Review article: intestinal permeability in Crohn's disease. Aliment. Pharmacol. Ther. 11 (Suppl 3), 47–53.

Mombaerts, P., Mizoguchi, E., Grusby, M.J., Glimcher, L.H., Bhan, A.K., Tonegawa, S., 1993. Spontaneous development of inflammatory bowel disease in T cell receptor mutant mice. Cell. 75, 274–282.

Monteleone, G., Biancone, L., Marasco, R., Morrone, G., Marasco, O., Luzza, F., et al., 1997. Interleukin 12 is expressed and actively released by Crohn's disease intestinal lamina propria mononuclear cells. Gastroenterology. 112, 1169–1178.

Morrissey, P.J., Charrier, K., Braddy, S., Liggitt, D., Watson, J.D., 1993. CD4 + T cells that express high levels of CD45RB induce wasting disease when transferred into congenic severe combined immunodeficient mice. Disease development is prevented by cotransfer of purified CD4 + T cells. J. Exp. Med. 178, 237–244.

Mostov, K.E., 1994. Transepithelial transport of immunoglobulins. Annu. Rev. Immunol. 12, 63–84.

Mow, W.S., Vasiliauskas, E.A., Lin, Y.C., Fleshner, P.R., Papadakis, K.A., Taylor, K.D., et al., 2004. Association of antibody responses to microbial antigens and complications of small bowel Crohn's disease. Gastroenterology. 126, 414–424.

Muise, A.M., Walters, T.D., Glowacka, W.K., Griffiths, A.M., Ngan, B.Y., Lan, H., et al., 2001. Polymorphisms in E-cadherin (CDH1) result in a mis-localised cytoplasmic protein that is associated with Crohn's disease. Gut. 58 (8), 1121–1127.

Mummery, L.P., 1907. The causes of colitis with special reference to its surgical treatment. With an account of 36 cases. Lancet. 1, 1638–1643.

Munkholm, P., Binder, V., 2004. Clinical features and natural history of Crohn's disease. In: Sartor, R.B., Sandborn, W.J. (Eds.), Kirsner's Inflammatory Bowel Diseases. Saunders, New York, USA, pp. 289–300.

Neurath, M., Fuss, I., Strober, W., 2000. TNBS-colitis. Int. Rev. Immunol. 19, 51–62.

Ogura, Y., Bonen, D.K., Inohara, N., Nicolae, D.L., Chen, F.F., Ramos, R., et al., 2001a. A frameshift mutation in NOD2 associated with susceptibility to Crohn's disease. Nature. 411, 603–606.

Ogura, Y., Inohara, N., Benito, A., Chen, F.F., Yamaoka, S., Nunez, G., 2001b. Nod2, a Nod1/Apaf-1 family member that is restricted to monocytes and activates NF-κB. J. Biol. Chem. 276, 4812–4818.

Okada, M., Maeda, K., Yao, T., Iwashita, A., Nomiyama, Y., Kitahara, K., 1991. Minute lesions of the rectum and sigmoid colon in patients with Crohn's disease. Gastrointest. Endosc. 37, 319–324.

Orchard, T.R., Jewell, D.P., 2004. Extraintestinal manifestations: skin, joints, and mucocutaneous manifestations. In: Sartor, R.B., Sandborn, W.J. (Eds.), Kirsner's Inflammatory Bowel Diseases. Saunders, New York, USA, pp. 658–672.

Orholm, M., Binder, V., Sorensen, T.I., Rasmussen, L.P., Kyvik, K.O., 2000. Concordance of inflammatory bowel disease among Danish twins. Results of a nationwide study. Scand. J. Gastroenterol. 35, 1075–1081.

Pallone, F., Fais, S., Squarcia, O., Biancone, L., Pozzilli, P., Boirivant, M., 1987. Activation of peripheral blood and intestinal lamina propria lymphocytes in Crohn's disease. In vivo state of activation and in vitro response to stimulation as defined by the expression of early activation antigens. Gut. 28, 745–753.

Papadakis, K.A., Shaye, O.A., Vasiliauskas, E.A., Ippoliti, A., Dubinsky, M.C., Birt, J., et al., 2005. Safety and efficacy of adalimumab (D2E7) in Crohn's disease patients with an attenuated response to infliximab. Am. J. Gastroenterol. 100, 75–79.

Peeters, M., Nevens, H., Baert, F., Hiele, M., de Meyer, A.M., Vlietinck, R., et al., 1996. Familial aggregation in Crohn's disease: increased age-adjusted risk and concordance in clinical characteristics. Gastroenterology. 111, 597–603.

Peltekova, V.D., Wintle, R.F., Rubin, L.A., Amos, C.I., Huang, Q., Gu, X., et al., 2004. Functional variants of OCTN cation transporter genes are associated with Crohn disease. Nat. Genet. 36, 471–475.

Podolsky, D.K., 1997. Lessons from genetic models of inflammatory bowel disease. Acta Gastroenterol. Belg. 60, 163–165.

Poullis, A.P., Zar, S., Sundaram, K.K., Moodie, S.J., Risley, P., Theodossi, A., et al., 2002. A new, highly sensitive assay for C-reactive protein can aid the differentiation of inflammatory bowel disorders from constipation- and diarrhoea-predominant functional bowel disorders. European Journal of Gastroenterology and Hepatology. 14, 409–412.

Powrie, F., 1995. T cells in inflammatory bowel disease: protective and pathogenic roles. Immunity. 3, 171–174.

Present, D.H., Korelitz, B.I., Wisch, N., Glass, J.L., Sachar, D.B., Pasternack, B.S., 1980. Treatment of Crohn's disease with 6-mercaptopurine. A long-term, randomized, double-blind study. N. Engl. J. Med. 302, 981–987.

Present, D.H., Rutgeerts, P., Targan, S., Hanauer, S.B., Mayer, L., van Hogezand, R.A., et al., 1999. Infliximab for the treatment of fistulas in patients with Crohn's disease. N Engl J Med. 340, 1398–1405.

Quinton, J.F., Sendid, B., Reumaux, D., Duthilleul, P., Cortot, A., Grandbastien, B., et al., 1998. Anti-Saccharomyces cerevisiae mannan antibodies combined with antineutrophil cytoplasmic autoantibodies in inflammatory bowel disease: prevalence and diagnostic role. Gut. 42, 788–791.

Rath, H.C., Schultz, M., Freitag, R., Dieleman, L.A., Li, F., Linde, H.J., et al., 2001. Different subsets of enteric bacteria induce and perpetuate experimental colitis in rats and mice. Infect. Immun. 69, 2277–2285.

Reese, G.E., Constantinides, V.A., Simillis, C., Darzi, A.W., Orchard, T.R., Fazio, V.W., et al., 2006. Diagnostic precision of anti-Saccharomyces cerevisiae antibodies and perinuclear antineutrophil cytoplasmic antibodies in inflammatory bowel disease. Am. J. Gastroenterol. 101, 2410–2422.

Reinisch, W., Nahavandi, H., Santella, R., Zhang, Y., Gasche, C., Moser, G., et al., 2001. Extracorporeal photochemotherapy in patients with steroid-dependent Crohn's disease: a prospective pilot study. Aliment. Pharmacol. Ther. 15, 1313–1322.

Reinisch, W., de Villiers, W., Bene, L., Simon, L., Rácz, I., Katz, S., et al., 2010. Fontolizumab in moderate to severe Crohn's disease: a phase 2, randomized, double-blind, placebo-controlled, multiple-dose study. Inflamm. Bowel Dis. 16, 233–242.

Reinisch, W., Sandborn, W.J., Hommes, D.W., D'Haens, G., Hanauer, S., Schreiber, S., et al., 2011. Adalimumab for induction of clinical remission in moderately to severely active ulcerative colitis: results of a randomised controlled trial. Gut. 60, 780–787.

Rioux, J.D., Xavier, R.J., Taylor, K.D., Silverberg, M.S., Goyette, P., Huett, A., et al., 2007. Genome-wide association study identifies new susceptibility loci for Crohn disease and implicates autophagy in disease pathogenesis. Nat. Genet. 39, 596–604.

Ruemmele, F.M., Targan, S.R., Levy, G., Dubinsky, M., Braun, J., Seidman, E.G., 1998. Diagnostic accuracy of serological assays in pediatric inflammatory bowel disease. Gastroenterology. 115, 822–829.

Rutgeerts, P., Sandborn, W.J., Feagan, B.G., Reinisch, W., Olson, A., Johanns, J., et al., 2005. Infliximab for induction and maintenance therapy for ulcerative colitis. N. Engl. J. Med. 353, 2462–2476.

Sachar, D.B., 1994. Cancer in Crohn's disease: dispelling the myths. Gut. 35, 1507–1508.

Sadlack, B., Merz, H., Schorle, H., Schimpl, A., Feller, A.C., Horak, I., 1993. Ulcerative colitis-like disease in mice with a disrupted interleukin-2 gene. Cell. 75, 253–261.

Sandborn, W.J., 2004. Medical therapy for Crohn's disease. In: Sartor, R.B., Sandborn, W.J. (Eds.), Kirsner's Inflammatory Bowel Diseases. Saunders, New York, USA, pp. 531–554.

Sandborn, W.J., Hanauer, S.B., Katz, S., Safdi, M., Wolf, D.G., Baerg, R.D., et al., 2001. Etanercept for active Crohn's disease: a randomized, double-blind, placebo-controlled trial. Gastroenterology. 121, 1088–1094.

Sandborn, W.J., Feagan, B.G., Radford-Smith, G., Kovacs, A., Enns, R., Innes, A., et al., 2004. CDP571, a humanised monoclonal antibody to tumour necrosis factor alpha, for moderate to severe Crohn's disease: a randomised, double blind, placebo controlled trial. Gut. 53, 1485–1493.

Sandborn, W.J., Abreu, M.T., D'Haens, G., Colombel, J.F., Vermeire, S., Mitchev, K., et al., 2010. Certolizumab pegol in patients with moderate to severe Crohn's disease and secondary failure to infliximab. Clin. Gastroenterol. Hepatol. 8, 688–695.

Sandborn, W.J., Schreiber, S., Feagan, B.G., Rutgeerts, P., Younes, Z.H., Bloomfield, R., et al., 2011. Certolizumab pegol for active Crohn's disease: a placebo-controlled, randomized trial. Clin. Gastroenterol. Hepatol. 9, 670–678.

Sands, B., 2002. Crohn's disease. In: Feldman, M, Friedman, L.S., Tschumy, W.O., Sleisenger, M.H. (Eds.), Sleisenger and Fordtran's Principles of Gastrointestinal Disease. Saunders, New York, USA, pp. 2005–2038.

Sands, B.E., Arsenault, J.E., Rosen, M.J., Alsahli, M., Bailen, L., Banks, P., et al., 2003. Risk of early surgery for Crohn's disease: implications for early treatment strategies. Am. J. Gastroenterol. 98, 2712–2718.

Sands, B.E., Anderson, F.H., Bernstein, C.N., Chey, W.Y., Feagan, B. G., Fedorak, R.N., et al., 2004. Infliximab maintenance therapy for fistulizing Crohn's disease. N. Engl. J. Med. 350, 876–885.

Sartor, R.B., 2004. Animal models of intestinal inflammation. In: Sartor, R.B., Sandborn, W.J. (Eds.), Kirsner's Inflammatory Bowel Diseases. Saunders, New York, USA, pp. 120–137.

Satsangi, J., Jewell, D.P., Rosenberg, W.M., Bell, J.I., 1994. Genetics of inflammatory bowel disease. Gut. 35, 696–700.

Schultz, M., Clarke, S.H., Arnold, L.W., Sartor, R.B., Tonkonogy, S.L., 2001. Disrupted B-lymphocyte development and survival in interleukin-2-deficient mice. Immunology. 104, 127–134.

Schwartz, D.A., Loftus Jr., E.V., Tremaine, W.J., Panaccione, R., Harmsen, W.S., Zinsmeister, A.R., et al., 2002. The natural history of fistulizing in Crohn's Disease in Olmstead County, Minnesota. Gastroenterology. 122, 875–880.

Sellon, R.K., Tonkonogy, S., Schultz, M., Dieleman, L.A., Grenther, W., Balish, E., et al., 1998. Resident enteric bacteria are necessary for development of spontaneous colitis and immune system activation in interleukin-10-deficient mice. Infect. Immun. 66, 5224–5231.

Sendid, B., Colombel, J.F., Jacquinot, P.M., Faille, C., Fruit, J., Cortot, A., et al., 1996. Specific antibody response to oligomannosidic epitopes in Crohn's disease. Clin. Diag. Lab. Immunol. 3, 219–226.

Shanahan, F., Niederlehner, A., Carramanzana, N., Anton, P., 1990. Sulfasalazine inhibits the binding of TNF alpha to its receptor. Immunopharmacology. 20, 217–224.

Sipponen, T., Savilahti, E., Kolho, K.L., Nuutinen, H., Turunen, U., Färkkilä, M., 2008. Crohn's disease activity assessed by fecal calprotectin and lactoferrin: correlation with Crohn's disease activity index and endoscopic findings. Inflamm. Bowel Dis. 14, 40–46.

Sokol, H., Seksik, P., Rigottier-Gois, L., Lay, C., Lepage, P., Podglajen, I., et al., 2006. Specificities of the fecal microbiota in inflammatory bowel disease. Inflamm. Bowel Dis. 12, 106–111.

Solem, C.A., Loftus Jr., E.V., Tremaine, W.J., Harmsen, W.S., Zinsmeister, A.R., Sandborn, W.J., 2005. Correlation of C-reactive protein with clinical, endoscopic, histologic, and radiographic activity in inflammatory bowel disease. Inflamm. Bowel Dis. 11, 707–712.

Sonnenberg, A., McCarty, D.J., Jacobsen, S.J., 1991. Geographic variation of inflammatory bowel disease within the United States. Gastroenterology. 100, 143–149.

Stokkers, P.C., Reitsma, P.H., Tytgat, G.N., van Deventer, S.J., 1999. Inflammatory bowel disease and the genes for the natural resistance-associated macrophage protein-1 and the interferon-gamma receptor 1. Int. J. Colorectal. Dis. 14, 13–17.

Stoll, M., Corneliussen, B., Costello, C.M., Waetzig, G.H., Mellgard, B., Koch, W.A., et al., 2004. Genetic variation in DLG5 is associated with inflammatory bowel disease. Nat. Genet. 36, 476–480.

Strober, W., Zhang, F., Kinati, A., Fuss, I., Fitchner-Feigl, S., 2010. Proinflammatory cytokines underlying the inflammation of Crohn's disease. Curr. Opin. Gastroenterol. 26 (4), 310–317.

Subhani, J., Montgomery, S., Pounder, R., Wakefield, A., 1998. Concordance rates of twins and siblings in inflammatory bowel diseases. Gut. 42, A40.

Sundberg, J.P., Elson, C.O., Bedigian, H., Birkenmeier, E.H., 1994. Spontaneous, heritable colitis in a new substrain of C3H/HeJ mice. Gastroenterology. 107, 1726–1735.

Swidsinski, A., Ladhoff, A., Pernthaler, A., Swidsinski, S., Loening-Baucke, V., Ortner, M., et al., 2002. Mucosal flora in inflammatory bowel disease. Gastroenterology. 122, 44–54.

Targan, S.R., Karp, L.C., 2004. Serology and laboratory markers of disease activity. In: Sartor, R.B., Sandborn, W.J. (Eds.), Kirsner's Inflammatory Bowel Diseases. Saunders, New York, USA, pp. 442–450.

Targan, S.R., Hanauer, S.B., van Deventer, S.J., Mayer, L., Present, D.H., Braakman, T., et al., 1997. A short-term study of chimeric monoclonal antibody cA2 to tumor necrosis factor alpha for Crohn's disease. Crohn's Disease cA2 Study Group. N. Engl. J. Med. 337, 1029–1035.

Targan, S.R., Feagan, B.G., Fedorak, R.N., Lashner, B.A., Panaccione, R., Present, D.H., et al., 2007. Natalizumab for the treatment of active Crohn's disease: results of the ENCORE Trial. Gastroenterology. 132, 1672–1683.

Taylor, K.D., Plevy, S.E., Yang, H., Landers, C.J., Barry, M.J., Rotter, J.I., et al., 2001. ANCA pattern and LTA haplotype relationship to clinical responses to anti-TNF antibody treatment in Crohn's disease. Gastroenterology. 120, 1347–1355.

Timmer, A., Sutherland, L.R., Martin, F., 1998. Oral contraceptive use and smoking are risk factors for relapse in Crohn's disease. Gastroenterology. 114, 1115–1143.

Travassos, L.H., Carneiro, L.A., Ramjeet, M., Hussey, S., Kim, Y.G., Magalhães, J.G., et al., 2010. Nod1 and Nod2 direct autophagy by recruiting ATG16L1 to the plasma membrane at the site of bacterial entry. Nat. Immunol. 11, 55–62.

Tremaine, W.J., 2004. Pouchitis. In: Sartor, R.B., Sandborn, W.J. (Eds.), Kirsner's Inflammatory Bowel Diseases. Saunders, New York, USA, pp. 673–681.

Tremaine, W.J., Hanauer, S.B., Katz, S., Winston, B.D., Levine, J.G., Persson, T., et al., 2002. Budesonide CIR capsules (once or twice daily divided-dose) in active Crohn's disease: a randomized placebo-controlled study in the United States. Am. J. Gastroenterol. 97, 1748–1754.

Tremelling, M., Cummings, F., Fisher, S.A., Mansfield, J., Gwilliam, R., Keniry, A., et al., 2007. IL23R variation determines susceptibility but not disease phenotype in inflammatory bowel disease. Gastroenterology. 132, 1657–1664.

Van Assche, G., Sandborn, W.J., Feagan, B.G., Salzberg, B.A., Silvers, D., Monroe, P.S., et al., 2006. Daclizumab, a humanised monoclonal antibody to the interleukin 2 receptor (CD25), for the treatment of moderately to severely active ulcerative colitis: a randomised, double blind, placebo controlled, dose ranging trial. Gut. 55, 1568–1574.

Van den Brande, J.M., Braat, H., van den Brink, G.R., Versteeg, H.H., Bauer, C.A., Hoedemaeker, I., et al., 2003. Infliximab but not etanercept induces apoptosis in lamina propria T-lymphocytes from patients with Crohn's disease. Gastroenterology. 124, 1774–1785.

Vasiliauskas, E.A., Plevy, S.E., Landers, C.J., Binder, S.W., Ferguson, D.M., Yang, H., et al., 1996. Perinuclear anti-neutrophil cytoplasmic antibodies in patients with Crohn's disease define a clinical subgroup. Gastroenterology. 110, 1810–1819.

Vermeire, S., Van Assche, G., Rutgeerts, P., 2006. Laboratory markers in IBD: useful, magic, or unnecessary toys? Gut. 55, 426–431.

Watanabe, T., Kitani, A., Murray, P.J., Strober, W., 2004. NOD2 is a negative regulator of Toll-like receptor 2-mediated T helper type 1 responses. Nat. Immunol. 5, 800–808.

Wells, C., 1952. Ulcerative colitis and Crohn's disease. Ann. R. Surg. Engl. 11, 105–120.

Welte, T., Zhang, S.S., Wang, T., Zhang, Z., Hesslein, D.G., Yin, Z., et al., 2003. STAT3 deletion during hematopoiesis causes Crohn's disease-like pathogenesis and lethality: a critical role of STAT3 in innate immunity. Proc. Natl. Acad. Sci. U.S.A. 100, 1879–1884.

Wilks, S., 1859. Lectures on Pathological Anatomy. third ed. Longmans, London, UK.

Winter, T.A., Wright, J., Ghosh, S., Jahnsen, J., Innes, A., Round, P., 2004. Intravenous CDP870, a PEGylated Fab′ fragment of a humanized antitumour necrosis factor antibody, in patients with moderate-to-severe Crohn's disease: an exploratory study. Aliment. Pharmacol. Ther. 20, 1337–1346.

Yamamoto, T., Umegae, S., Kitagawa, T., Yasuda, Y., Yamada, Y., Takahashi, D., et al., 2004. Granulocyte and monocyte adsorptive apheresis in the treatment of active distal ulcerative colitis: a prospective, pilot study. Aliment. Pharmacol. Ther. 20, 783–792.

Yamazaki, K., Onouchi, Y., Takazoe, M., Kubo, M., Nakamura, Y., Hata, A., 2007. Association analysis of genetic variants in IL23R, ATG16L1 and 5p13.1 loci with Crohn's disease in Japanese patients. J. Hum. Genet. 52, 575–583.

Yousry, T.A., Major, E.O., Ryschkewitsch, C., Fahle, G., Fischer, S., Hou, J., et al., 2006. Evaluation of patients treated with natalizumab for progressive multifocal leukoencephalopathy. N. Engl. J. Med. 354, 924–933.

Zaki, M.H., Boyd, K.L., Vogel, P., Kastan, M.B., Lamkanfi, M., Kanneganti, T.D., 2010. The NLRP3 inflammasome protects against loss of epithelial integrity and mortality during experimental colitis. Immunity. 32, 379–391.

Chapter 61

Hepatitis

Diego Vergani[1], Ian R. Mackay[2], and Giorgina Mieli-Vergani[3]

[1]Institute of Liver Studies, King's College London School of Medicine at King's College Hospital, London, UK, [2]Department of Biochemistry and Molecular Biology, Monash University, Clayton, Victoria, Australia, [3]Paediatric Liver, GI & Nutrition Centre, King's College London School of Medicine at King's College Hospital, London, UK

Chapter Outline

Clinical, Pathologic, and Epidemiologic Features	890	Treatment and Outcome	900
Clinical Features	890	Standard Treatment	900
Pathologic Features	891	Alternative Treatments	901
Epidemiologic Features	892	Duration of Treatment	902
Autoimmune Features	892	Liver Transplantation	902
Autoantibodies as Potential Immunologic Markers	893	Future Treatment Approaches	902
Genetic Features	896	Concluding Remarks—Future Prospects	903
Animal Models	897	References	903
Pathologic Effector Mechanisms	898		

Autoimmune hepatitis (AIH) is an inflammatory liver disease, affecting mainly females, characterized by elevated transaminase and immunoglobulin G (IgG) levels, interface hepatitis on histology, and positive autoantibodies, whose profile allows its distinction into two types. The etiology of AIH is said to be unknown but, as for complex diseases in general, it results from interplay of multiple predisposing causes, genetic and environmental. The outcome is immune reactivity against host liver antigens. AIH responds to immunosuppressive treatment, which should be instituted as soon as the diagnosis is made, as untreated disease progresses to liver failure.

Historically, a chronic hepatitis with a female preponderance associated with high serum proteins was noted as early as the 1940s (Meyer zum Büschenfelde, 2003). A fuller description of AIH was given by the Swedish physician Jan Gösta Waldeström at the German Society for Digestive and Metabolic Disorders meeting in September 1950 (Waldenstrom, 1950). He described six patients, five female, with "hepatitis sui generis," characterized by a marked elevation of gamma globulins, in whom administration of ACTH to investigate the nature of amenorrhea resulted in a striking subjective improvement and a dramatic fall in the erythrocyte sedimentation rate.

Waldeström concluded that these "patients may benefit from ACTH treatment." This early report defines key characteristics of AIH: female preponderance, hyperglobulinemia, and response to corticosteroid drugs. It was suspected that a persisting virus in the liver was to blame. In 1951, confirming Waldeström's observation, Henry George Kunkel in New York noted that some patients had additional clinical features such as fever and joint involvement (Kunkel et al., 1951). In 1954 the Italian physician Leoni reported the lupus erythematosus (LE) cell phenomenon ("fenomeno LE") in the ascites fluid of a patient with cirrhosis (Leoni, 1954), and in 1955 Joske and King (Joske and King, 1955) in Melbourne, Australia, described LE cells in the blood of two patients with hypergammaglobulinemic active chronic hepatitis. In a landmark article in 1956 (Mackay et al., 1956), Mackay and co-workers reported five additional hypergammaglobulinemic chronic hepatitis patients recruited in the same unit, and, in view of the presence of LE cells, proposed the term of "lupoid hepatitis" to define this condition. A decade later, when it became clear that liver disease is rare in typical systemic lupus erythematosus (SLE) and that LE cells reflect the presence of anti-nuclear antibody, Mackay suggested the alternative name of "autoimmune hepatitis" (Mackay

N. Rose & I. Mackay (Eds): The Autoimmune Diseases, Fifth edition. DOI: http://dx.doi.org/10.1016/B978-0-12-384929-8.00061-7

et al., 1965). This term, however, was universally accepted only in the 1990s, after several different labels (mostly "chronic active hepatitis") had been given to this condition over the years. In addition to seropositivity for anti-nuclear antibodies (ANA), reports from the early 1960s showed that anti-smooth muscle antibodies (SMA) are also markers of what is known today as AIH type 1 (Meyer zum Büschenfelde, 2003). Thirty years after the first description of "lupoid hepatitis," AIH type 2, characterized by the presence in the serum of anti-liver kidney microsomal type 1 and/or anti-liver cytosol type 1 antibodies, was described (Homberg et al., 1987; Martini et al., 1988).

Awareness over the years that the clinical and pathological picture of chronic hepatitis may be due to causes other than AIH, such as persistent infection with the hepatotropic viruses B and C, alcohol abuse, and non-alcoholic steatohepatitis, prompted the establishment in the 1990s of an expert panel with the brief of defining criteria for the diagnosis of AIH (International Autoimmune Hepatitis Group, IAIHG (Johnson and McFarlane, 1993)).

CLINICAL, PATHOLOGIC, AND EPIDEMIOLOGIC FEATURES

Clinical Features

The diagnosis of AIH is based on a combination of clinical, biochemical, immunological, and histological features and the exclusion of other known causes of liver disease. Liver biopsy is needed to confirm the diagnosis and to evaluate the severity of liver damage (Krawitt, 2006; Manns et al., 2010a), as transaminase and IgG levels do not reflect the degree of tissue inflammatory changes or indicate the presence or absence of cirrhosis. Conditions that may share serological and histological features with AIH, such as viral hepatitis B and C, Wilson disease, non-alcoholic steatohepatitis, and drug-induced liver disease, must be excluded by accurate clinical history and appropriate investigations.

Three-quarters of patients with AIH are female. AIH type 1 affects all ages with two peaks, one in childhood/adolescence, and the other in adulthood around the age of 40 years. Only 20% of patients are diagnosed after the age of 60 years (Krawitt, 2006; Manns et al., 2010a). AIH type 2 affects mainly children and young adults, being rare, though not absent, in older individuals. In pediatrics, AIH type 2 represents one-third of all cases and has a clinical course similar to AIH type 1, though anti-LKM1-positive children present at a younger age, more often with an acute onset, including fulminant hepatitis, and have associated IgA deficiency (Gregorio et al., 1997; Oettinger et al., 2005).

Forty to 60% of adult patients with AIH type 1 have a chronic disease course with non-specific symptoms such as fatigue, nausea, abdominal pain, and arthralgia (Czaja et al., 1983; Al-Chalabi et al., 2008). AIH may be diagnosed after the incidental finding of abnormal liver function tests during routine investigations.

About one-third of adult patients present acutely with jaundice, arthralgia, anorexia, and fatigue, symptoms indistinguishable from those of an acute hepatitis due to other causes (Crapper et al., 1986; Amontree et al., 1989). Acute hepatitic episodes alternating with spontaneous clinical and biochemical improvement are not uncommon, being a relapsing pattern that often leads to a dangerous delay in diagnosis and treatment. Occasionally the first symptoms of AIH are complications of portal hypertension, e.g., gastrointestinal bleeding or hypersplenism, without previous knowledge of liver disease. The acute presentation is more commonly observed in children and young adults than in older patients. At times AIH, particularly AIH type 2, presents as fulminant hepatic failure (Gregorio et al., 1997). Because of the variability of its presenting features, AIH should be suspected and excluded in all patients with symptoms and signs of prolonged, relapsing, or severe liver disease, so that the appropriate treatment can be instituted promptly.

At least one-third of patients with AIH already have cirrhosis at the time of diagnosis, irrespective of the mode of presentation (Roberts et al., 1996; Gregorio et al., 1997), indicating that the disease process is longstanding. Also patients presenting acutely have often advanced fibrosis or cirrhosis on liver biopsy.

About 40% of patients with AIH have a family history of autoimmune disorders, and associated autoimmune features (e.g., thyroiditis, inflammatory bowel disease, type 1 diabetes, arthritis, hemocytopenias, vitiligo) are present at diagnosis or develop during follow-up in some 20% of patients (Gregorio et al., 1997; Mieli-Vergani and Vergani, 2011).

In children and young adults, a form of sclerosing cholangitis, known as autoimmune sclerosing cholangitis (ASC), and characterized by ANA and SMA positivity, high levels of IgG, and interface hepatitis, is as prevalent as AIH type 1 (Gregorio et al., 2001). Alkaline phosphatase and gamma glutamyl transpeptidase levels, which are usually elevated in cholestatic disease, are often normal or only mildly increased in the early disease stages of ASC and a cholangiography is needed to make the diagnosis. In the absence of bile duct imaging, these patients are diagnosed and treated as AIH type 1. The presence of sclerosing cholangitis may be discovered during follow-up, after the appearance of an overt cholestatic biochemical profile. In childhood, ASC affects equally males and females (Gregorio et al., 2001). If treatment is started early, the parenchymal liver damage in ASC responds well to the same immunosuppressive treatment used for AIH, with good medium- to long-term survival. However,

TABLE 61.1 International Autoimmune Hepatitis Group Revised Diagnostic Scoring System

Parameter	Feature	Score
Sex	Female	+2
ALP: AST (or ALT) ratio	>3	−2
	1.5–3	0
	<1.5	+2
Serum globulins or IgG	>2.0	+3
(times above normal)	1.5–2.0	+2
	1.0–1.5	+1
	<1.0	0
ANA, SMA or anti-LKM1	>1:80	+3
titers	1:80	+2
	1:40	+1
	<1:40	0
AMA	Positive	−4
Viral markers of active	Positive	−3
infection	Negative	+3
Hepatotoxic drug history	Yes	−4
	No	+2
Average alcohol	<25 g/day	+2
	>60 g/day	−2
Histological features	Interface hepatitis	+3
	Plasma cells	+1
	Rosettes	+1
	None of the above	−5
	Biliary changes[a]	−3
	Atypical changes[b]	−3
Immune diseases	Thyroiditis, colitis, other	+2
HLA	DR3 or DR4	+1
Seropositivity for other	Anti-SLA/LP, actin,	+2
autoantibodies	ASGPR, pANNA	
Response to therapy	Remission	+2
	Relapse	+3

[a]Including granulomatous cholangitis, concentric periductal fibrosis, ductopenia, marginal bile duct proliferation and cholangiolitis.
[b]Any other prominent feature suggesting a different etiology.
Pre-treatment score >15: definite AIH; 10–15: probable AIH.
Post-treatment score >17: definite AIH; 12–17: probable AIH.
ALP, alkaline phosphatase; AST, aspartate aminotransferase; ALT, alanine aminotransferase; IgG, immunoglobulin G; ANA, anti-nuclear antibody; SMA, anti-smooth muscle antibody; anti-LKM1, anti-liver kidney microsomal type 1 antibodies; AMA, anti-mitochondrial antibodies; SLA/LP, soluble liver antigen/liver pancreas; ASGPR, asialoglycoprotein receptor; pANNA, peripheral anti-nuclear neutrophil antibody; HLA, human leukocyte antigen.
Adapted from Alvarez et al. (1999a).

TABLE 61.2 Simplified Criteria for the Diagnosis of Autoimmune Hepatitis

Variable	Cut-off	Points
ANA or SMA	≥1:40	1
ANA or SMA	≥1:80	2[a]
or anti-LKM1	≥1:40	
or SLA	Positive	
IgG	>upper limit of normal	1
	>1.10 times upper limit of normal	2
Liver histology	Compatible with AIH	1
	Typical of AIH	2
Absence of viral hepatitis	Yes	2

[a]Additional points for all autoantibodies cannot exceed a maximum of 2.
Score ≥6: probable AIH; ≥7: definite AIH.
ANA, anti-nuclear antibody; SMA, anti-smooth muscle antibody; anti-LKM1, anti-liver kidney microsomal antibody type 1; SLA, soluble liver antigen; IgG, immunoglobulin G; AIH, autoimmune hepatitis.
Adapted from Hennes et al. (2008b).

form of the disease, in which diagnostically relevant auto-antibodies often have titers lower than the cut-off value considered positive in adults. In addition, neither system can distinguish between AIH and ASC.

Pathologic Features

The typical histological feature of AIH is interface hepatitis, which is, however, not exclusive to this condition (Czaja and Carpenter, 1997). Interface hepatitis is characterized by a dense inflammatory infiltrate composed of lymphocytes and plasma cells, which crosses the limiting plate and invades the surrounding parenchyma (Figure 61.1). Hepatocytes surrounded by inflammatory cells become swollen and undergo pyknotic necrosis, representing apoptosis (Searle et al., 1987). We emphasize this feature because not only was the liver the site wherein apoptosis was first recognized nearly a century ago but also, in some other autoimmune diseases, disordered apoptosis can yield potently immunogenic particles—apoptopes (Lleo et al., 2009). Though plasma cells are characteristically abundant at the interface and within the lobule, their presence in low number does not exclude the diagnosis of AIH. When AIH presents acutely, and during episodes of relapse, a common histological finding is panlobular hepatitis with bridging necrosis and, if the disease takes a fulminant course, massive necrosis and multilobular collapse.

Though sampling variation may occur in needle biopsy specimens, particularly in cirrhotic livers, the severity of the histological appearance is usually of prognostic value. Inflammatory changes surrounding the bile ducts are present in a small proportion of adult patients with AIH, but

the bile duct disease progresses in about 50% of patients despite treatment (Gregorio et al., 2001).

In the absence of a single diagnostic test for AIH, the IAIHG has devised a diagnostic system for comparative and research purposes, which includes several positive and negative scores, the sum of which gives a value indicative of probable or definite AIH (Johnson and McFarlane, 1993; Alvarez et al., 1999a) (Table 61.1). A simplified IAIHG scoring system published more recently is better suited to clinical application (Hennes et al., 2008b) (Table 61.2). However, neither the original nor the simplified scoring system is perfect, particularly for the juvenile

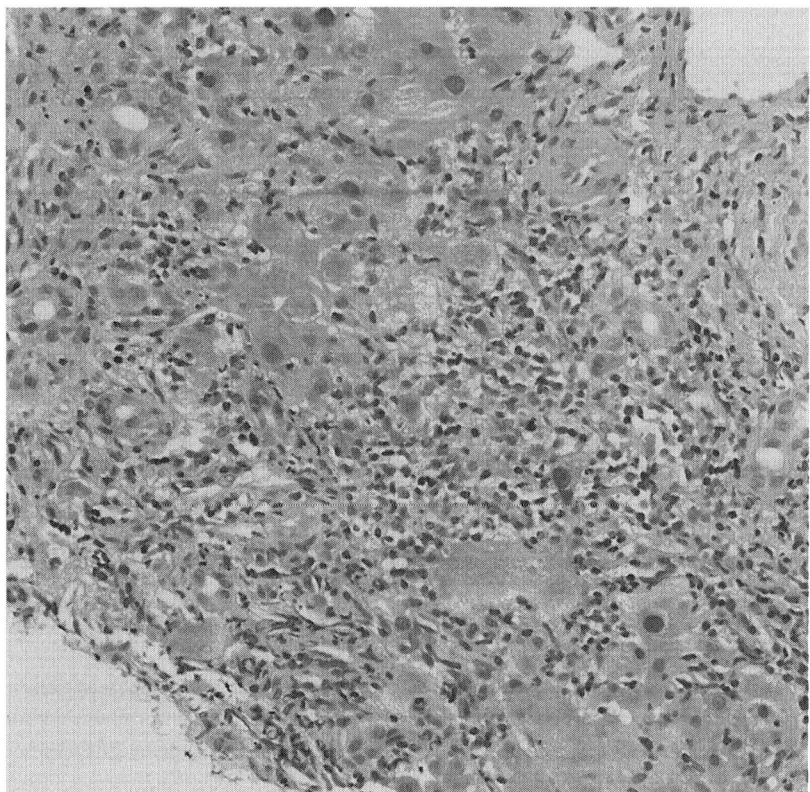

FIGURE 61.1 **Interface hepatitis.** Interface hepatitis is the typical histological feature of AIH and is characterized by a dense portal and peri-portal lymphocyte and plasma cell infiltrate that disrupts the parenchymal limiting plate. Hematoxylin and eosin staining. Original magnification × 40. *Courtesy of Dr. Alberto Quaglia.*

when conspicuous they suggest an overlap with sclerosing cholangitis (Gregorio et al., 2001).

Epidemiologic Features

AIH occurs worldwide, but its prevalence remains to be established. Most information on prevalence had been obtained for AIH type 1 before the introduction of the IAIHG diagnostic scoring system (Johnson and McFarlane, 1993; Alvarez et al., 1999a), therefore without standard criteria for patient inclusion. Prevalences reported in early papers range from 1.9 cases/100,000 in Norway (Boberg et al., 1998) and 1/200,000 in the US general population (Manns et al., 1998), to 20/100,000 in females over 14 years of age referred to a tertiary center in Spain (Primo et al., 2004). A more recent study from a UK secondary referral center reported an AIH annual incidence of 3.5/100,000 (Whalley et al., 2007). Two studies using standardized criteria for the diagnosis of AIH published in 2002 and 2010 report a point prevalence of 24.5/100,000 in New Zealand (Ngu et al., 2010) and of 34.5/100,000 in Alaskan natives (Hurlburt et al., 2002). In Asia, AIH was widely considered less frequent than in Western countries, with a reported incidence in Japan ranging between 0.08 and 0.15 cases/100,000/year (Nishioka and McFarlane, 1998). A better awareness of its clinical characteristics has led to an increased frequency in the diagnosis of AIH in China, where this condition was hitherto considered very rare (Qiu et al., 2011). It is likely, however, that all these

epidemiological figures are underestimates, since AIH may remain undiagnosed for several years and present eventually with decompensated liver disease attributed to "cryptogenic" cirrhosis.

The prevalence of AIH type 2, which affects mainly children and young adults, is unknown, also because the diagnosis is often overlooked. Intriguingly AIH type 2 has been reported more frequently in Europe that in the USA (Czaja and Freese, 2002), possibly because of the lack of testing for anti-LKM1 antibodies in the latter, due to the unsubstantiated belief that AIH type 2 is rare and therefore that testing for anti-LKM1 antibodies is not cost-effective (Duchini et al., 2000).

At the King's College Hospital tertiary pediatric hepatology referral center there has been a seven-fold increase in incidence of AIH over the last decade, perhaps a result in part of increased awareness of the disease. AIH represents approximately 10% of some 500 new referrals per year, two-thirds of the cases being AIH type 1 and one-third AIH type 2.

AUTOIMMUNE FEATURES

AIH has several characteristics of an organ-specific autoimmune disease: it affects mainly females, it is accompanied by serological features of autoimmunity (organ and non-organ-specific autoantibodies; high levels of IgG), it is associated with human leukocyte antigen (HLA) allotypes predisposing to autoimmunity, it has a strong connectivity with other autoimmune disorders, and it responds satisfactorily to immunosuppressive treatment.

AUTOANTIBODIES AS POTENTIAL IMMUNOLOGIC MARKERS

Key to the diagnosis of AIH is positivity for circulating autoantibodies (Johnson and McFarlane, 1993; Alvarez et al., 1999a; Vergani et al., 2004; Hennes et al., 2008b). Their detection by indirect immunofluorescence (Figures 61.2–61.5) on a rodent substrate not only assists in the diagnosis but also allows differentiation into two forms of AIH. ANA and SMA characterize AIH type 1, while anti-LKM1 and anti-LC1 define AIH type 2. The two autoantibody profiles rarely occur simultaneously (Vergani et al., 2004). As interpretation of the immuno-fluorescence patterns can be difficult, guidelines have been provided by the IAIHG regarding methodology and interpretation of liver autoimmune serology (Vergani et al., 2004). A major advantage of testing for autoantibodies by indirect immunofluorescence on a freshly prepared rodent substrate that includes kidney, liver, and stomach is that it allows the concurrent detection of several autoreactivities relevant to AIH. These include ANA, SMA, anti-LKM1, and anti-LC1, as well as anti-mitochondrial antibody (AMA), the serological hallmark of primary biliary cirrhosis (PBC), the presence of which weighs against the diagnosis of AIH (Johnson and McFarlane, 1993; Alvarez

et al., 1999a; Vergani et al., 2004; Hennes et al., 2008b). Autoantibodies are considered positive when present at a dilution of 1:40 or more in adults, while in children, who are rarely positive for autoantibodies in health, positivity at a dilution ≥1:20 for ANA and SMA or ≥1:10 for anti-LKM1 is clinically significant (Mieli-Vergani et al., 2009). Both in adults and in children autoantibodies may be present at a low titer or even be negative at disease onset, to become detectable during follow-up (Gregorio et al., 2001). If AIH is suspected, it is advisable to repeat autoantibody testing and to ask the laboratory to report any level of positivity.

ANA is detectable on all rodent tissues and in AIH usually has a homogeneous pattern (Figure 61.2). For a clearer and easier definition of the pattern, HEp2 cells that have prominent nuclei are used (Figure 61.2), though these cells, derived from a laryngeal carcinoma, should be used with caution for screening purposes, because of a high proportion of low titer positivity within the normal population (Tan et al., 1997). There are no ANA molecular targets specific for AIH. A varied profile of ANA reactivities reminiscent of that found in SLE (e.g., to nuclear chromatin, histones, centromere, double-stranded DNA and single-stranded DNA, and ribonucleoproteins) (Peakman et al., 1989; Burlingame et al., 1993; Czaja et al., 1994; Strassburg et al., 1996a; Bogdanos et al., 2008, 2009) has been reported in AIH, but at least a third of AIH patients positive for ANA do not react with known nuclear targets (Bogdanos et al., 2008, 2009).

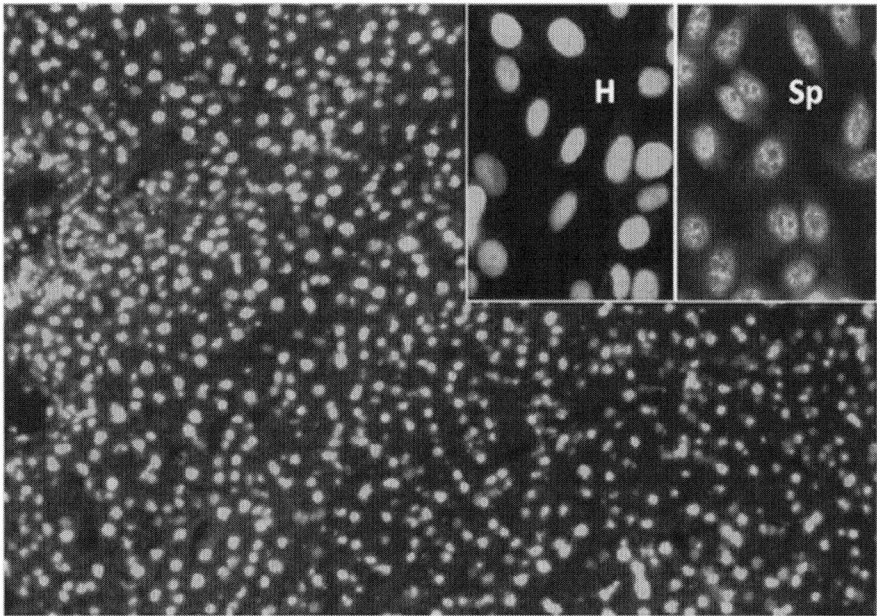

FIGURE 61.2 Antinuclear antibodies. Immunofluorescence pattern of antinuclear autoantibodies on rodent liver (main image) and HEp2 cells (inset), which, because of their large nuclei, allow pattern recognition. The homogeneous pattern (inset left) is the most common in autoimmune hepatitis; the speckled pattern (inset right) is much rarer. HEp2 cells should not be used for sample screening because of a high frequency of false-positive results. H = homogeneous; Sp = speckled.

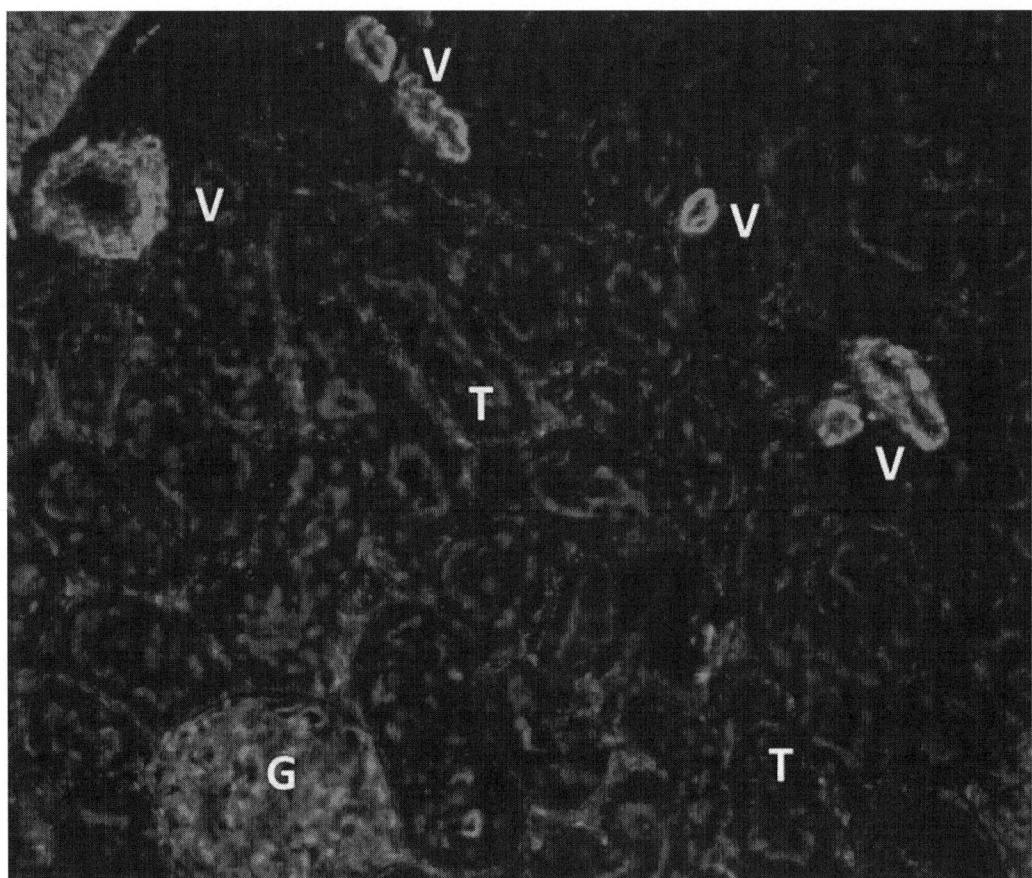

FIGURE 61.3   Anti-smooth muscle antibodies. Immunofluorescence pattern of smooth muscle autoantibodies (SMA) on rodent kidney. SMA stains the smooth muscle of arterial vessels (V), glomeruli (G), and tubules (T). *Courtesy of Dr. Luigi Muratori.*

Immunofluorescence remains therefore the gold standard for ANA testing, as recently surmised by the American College of Rheumatology ANA Task Force (Meroni and Schur, 2010), but is not universally practiced. There is an impression, albeit poorly documented, that higher levels of autoantibody and/or multiple autoantibodies are a pointer to a diagnosis of AIH, as pertains in type 1 diabetes.

The immunofluorescent staining of SMA is detected in the arterial walls of rodent kidney, liver, and stomach. In the kidney, SMA can have three patterns: V (vessels), G (glomeruli), and T (tubules) (Bottazzo et al., 1976) (Figure 61.3). The V pattern is present also in non-autoimmune inflammatory liver disease, in autoimmune diseases not affecting the liver, and in viral infections, but the VG and VGT patterns are indicative of AIH. The VGT pattern corresponds to the "F actin" or microfilament (MF) pattern observed using cultured fibroblasts as substrate. Neither the VGT nor the anti-MF patterns are, however, entirely specific for the diagnosis of AIH type 1. The molecular target of the microfilament reactivity observed in AIH type 1 remains to be identified. Though "anti-actin" reactivity is strongly associated with AIH type 1,

some 20% of SMA-positive AIH type 1 patients do not have the F-actin/VGT pattern. The absence, therefore, of anti-actin SMA does not exclude the diagnosis of AIH (Muratori et al., 2002).

The anti-LKM1 pattern is characterized by bright staining of the hepatocyte cytoplasm and of the P3 portion of the renal tubules (Figure 61.4). Anti-LKM1 is frequently confused with AMA, as both autoantibodies stain liver and kidney, though AMA, in contrast to anti-LKM1, also stains gastric parietal cells. The identification of the molecular targets of anti-LKM1, cytochrome P4502D6 (CYP2D6), and of AMA, enzymes of the 2-oxo-acid dehydrogenase complexes, has allowed the establishment of immuno-assays using recombinant or purified antigens (Vergani et al., 2004), which can be used to resolve doubtful cases. In the context of AIH, there can be positivity for AMA in a small subset of patients (3–5%) in whom there are overlapping features with PBC (Montano-Loza et al., 2008; O'Brien et al., 2008). Additional LKM reactivities have been described. Anti-LKM2 antibodies, which target cytochrome P4502C9, are of historical interest only because of their association

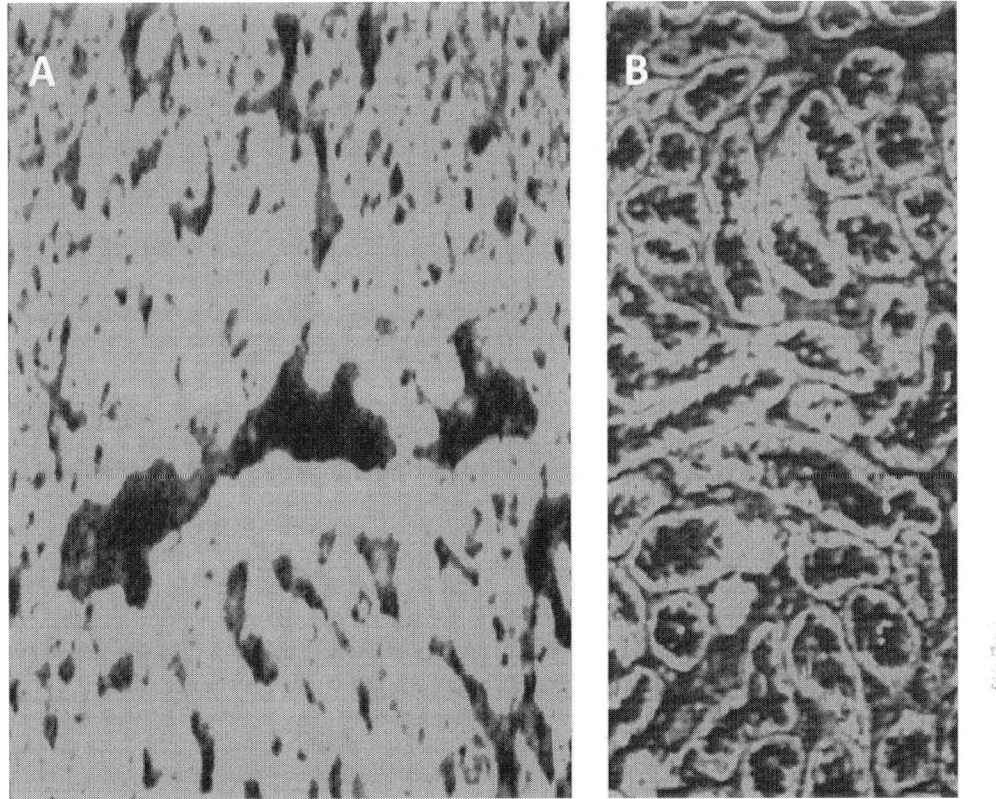

FIGURE 61.4 **Anti-liver kidney microsomal type 1 antibodies.** Immunofluorescence pattern of anti-liver kidney microsomal type 1 (LKM1) autoantibodies on liver (A) and kidney (B) rodent sections; anti-LKM1 stains the cytoplasm of hepatocytes and proximal renal tubules.

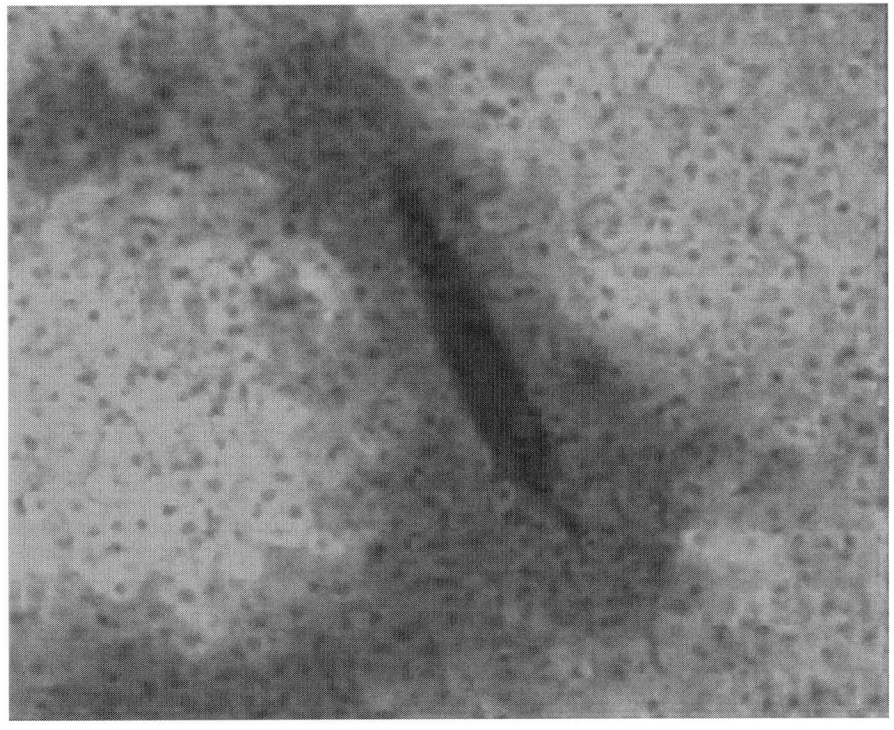

FIGURE 61.5 **Anti-liver cytosol type 1 antibodies.** Immunofluorescence pattern of anti-liver cytosol type 1 (anti-LC1) antibodies on a rodent liver section: they stain the cytoplasm of hepatocytes with a weakening of the staining around the central vein.

with ticrynafen-induced hepatitis, a uricosuric diuretic withdrawn from clinical use in 1980 because of its severe hepatotoxicity. Anti-LKM3 antibodies are specific for members of the uridine glucuronosyltransferase (UGT) family 1 and give an immunofluorescence pattern similar to anti-LKM1. Although anti-LKM3 are most commonly detected in patients with hepatitis delta, they have also been reported in approximately 10% of patients with AIH type 2 (Strassburg et al., 1996b).

Anti-LC1 (Figure 61.5), which is an additional marker for AIH type 2, can be present on its own, but frequently occurs in association with anti-LKM1, and targets formimino-transferase cyclodeaminase (FTCD) (Lapierre et al., 1999). Anti-FTCD antibody can be detected by commercial ELISA (Vergani et al., 2004).

Other autoantibodies less commonly tested, but of diagnostic importance, include anti-soluble liver antigen (anti-SLA) and anti-perinuclear neutrophil cytoplasm (pANCA) antibodies.

Anti-SLA is highly specific for the diagnosis of AIH, usually type 1 (Baeres et al., 2002). Its presence identifies patients with more severe disease and worse outcome (Czaja et al., 2002; Ma et al., 2002). Anti-SLA was thought to identify a third type of AIH in which tests for conventional autoantibodies were negative (Manns et al., 1987). However, early reports predated the publication of the IAIHG recommendations and used a cut-off point for conventional autoantibody levels higher than that currently used for the diagnosis of AIH. Several patients considered to have AIH type 3 were positive for conventional autoantibodies. At variance with standard diagnostic autoantibodies, anti-SLA is not detectable by immunofluorescence. The molecular target of anti-SLA is Sep (O-phosphoserine) tRNA:Sec (selenocysteine) tRNA synthase (SEPSECS) (Costa et al., 2000; Wies et al., 2000; Palioura et al., 2009). Cloning of this reactant has led to the availability of molecularly-based diagnostic assays for anti-SLA, but their full evaluation is still under way.

In AIH type 1, akin to primary sclerosing cholangitis and inflammatory bowel disease, pANCA are frequently detected, but they are atypical, since they react with peripheral nuclear membrane components (perinuclear anti-nuclear neutrophil antibodies, pANNA) (Bogdanos et al., 2009). In curious contrast to AIH type 1, pANNA are virtually absent in AIH type 2 (Vergani et al., 2004).

Anti-asialoglycoprotein receptor antibodies (ASGPR) were identified in 1984 during an attempt to detect putative autoantigenic targets located on the hepatocyte membrane. ASGPR is the main constituent of the crude liver cell extract known as liver-specific protein (LSP) and is the only liver-specific autoantigen discovered so far (Bogdanos et al., 2009). Some 50–90% of patients with AIH type 1 or 2 are anti-ASGPR/anti-LSP seropositive (Gregorio et al., 2001); anti-ASGPR is found in combination with ANA, SMA, and anti-LKM1 and its level correlates with disease activity. However, the detection of anti-ASGPR requires either purified or recombinant antigen, and the development of reliable molecular assays has been difficult; therefore their applicability to clinical practice is limited. Moreover, since these autoantibodies have also been detected in patients with viral hepatitis, drug-induced hepatitis, and PBC, they are not disease specific (Bogdanos et al., 2009).

GENETIC FEATURES

AIH is a "complex trait" disease, i.e., a condition not inherited in a Mendelian autosomal dominant, autosomal recessive, or sex-linked fashion (Donaldson, 2002, 2004). The mode of inheritance of a complex trait disorder involves one or more genes, operating alone or in concert, to increase or reduce the risk of the trait, and interacting with environmental factors.

Several genes have been reported to confer susceptibility to AIH, and influence clinical manifestations, response to treatment, and prognosis. Most are located within the human leukocyte antigen (HLA) region (the human major histocompatibility complex [MHC]), the gene products of which are involved in the presentation of antigenic peptides to T cells and the initiation of adaptive immune responses. The strongest associations lie within the HLA-DRB1 locus, with alleles encoding the HLA-DR3 (*DRB1*0301*) and DR4 (*DRB1*0401*) molecules conferring susceptibility to AIH type 1 in European and North American populations (Donaldson, 2002, 2004). These associations are sufficiently strong to score positively for the diagnosis of AIH according to the revised diagnostic IAIHG system (Hennes et al., 2008b). Links have been reported between possession of these alleles and clinical manifestations, response to treatment, and prognosis. Thus, among white Northern Europeans, *DRB1*0301* is more common in patients who deteriorate despite corticosteroid treatment (Donaldson, 2002, 2004). The residues within the cleft of the HLA class II molecules specifically linked to the pathogenesis of AIH reported from various countries differ, suggesting that the antigenic peptides recognized by T cell-mediated immune responses in AIH may derive from different exogenous triggers and that they are embraced by geographically/ethnically distinct HLA molecules (Donaldson, 2002, 2004). These HLA associations may be the molecular footprints of the prevailing triggers that precipitate AIH in different environments. In this context, it is of interest that in South America possession of the HLA *DRB1*1301* allele, which predisposes to pediatric AIH type 1 in that population, is also associated with persistent infection with the endemic hepatitis A virus (Fainboim et al., 2001).

Susceptibility to, and severity of, AIH type 2 has been linked to alleles encoding the DRB1*0301 and

DRB1*0701 molecules in the United Kingdom and Brazil. Allelic variation within HLA-DRB1 has been linked to differences in the autoantibody seropositivity profiles of AIH type 2 patients (Djilali-Saiah et al., 2006).

There are also reports of susceptibility to AIH linked to polymorphisms in genes located outside the MHC; the cytotoxic T lymphocyte antigen-4 (CTLA-4) (Agarwal et al., 2000), the tumor necrosis factor alpha (TNF-α) gene promoter (Cookson et al., 1999), and Fas (Agarwal et al., 2007) are notable examples.

A form of AIH serologically resembling AIH type 2 affects some 20% of patients with autoimmune polyendocrinopathy-candidiasis-ectodermal dystrophy (APECED) (see Chapter 43). APECED is a monogenic autosomal recessive disorder caused by homozygous mutations in the *AIRE1* gene and characterized by a variety of organ-specific autoimmune diseases, the most common of which are hypoparathyroidism and primary adrenocortical failure, accompanied by chronic mucocutaneous candidiasis (Simmonds and Gough, 2004; Liston et al., 2005). Interestingly there are neutralizing autoantibodies to type 1 interferons, perhaps accounting for the associated immune deficiencies (see Chapter 76). APECED has a high level of variability in symptoms, especially between populations. Carriers of a single *AIRE1* mutation (heterozygotes) do not develop APECED. However, although the inheritance pattern of APECED indicates a strictly recessive disorder, there are anecdotal data of mutations in a single copy of *AIRE1* being associated with human autoimmunity of a less severe form than classically defined APECED (Simmonds and Gough, 2004; Liston et al., 2005).

The role of the *AIRE1* heterozygote state in the development of type 2 AIH remains to be established, though heterozygous *AIRE1* mutations have been reported in three children with severe AIH type 2 and extrahepatic autoimmune manifestations (Lankisch et al., 2005).

ANIMAL MODELS

Research on the pathogenesis of AIH has been hampered by the lack of animal models reproducing faithfully the human condition. Findings in animal models of AIH have been recently reviewed by Hardtke-Wolenski et al. (2012). Most animal models of AIH, though informative regarding single steps leading to liver inflammation and damage, do not mimic the chronic relapsing course of the human disease. In fact, they demonstrate the difficulty in breaking tolerance towards liver antigens, and the involvement of regulatory mechanisms in maintaining it.

A widely studied model of experimental hepatitis is that induced by concanavalin A (Tiegs et al., 1992). Though this model does not reflect accurately the pathological entity of AIH in humans, it has provided evidence that liver damage mainly occurs within a Th1 scenario, with the involvement of activated CD4 T cells and release of the proinflammatory cytokines interferon gamma and tumor necrosis factor alpha against a specific genetic background. Interleukin-4, a cytokine with mainly regulatory activity, is also required for the establishment of concanavalin A-induced hepatitis. This finding and those of Takeda and collaborators, who have shown that NKT cells, which secrete both interleukin-4 (IL-4) and interferon gamma, are critical to the development of concanavalin A-induced hepatitis in C57/B6 mice, suggest that both adaptive and innate immunity are involved (Takeda et al., 2000).

The ideal model for AIH should have a well-defined initiating event followed by chronic inflammation leading to fibrosis. More recently, researchers have focused on animal models of AIH type 2, since in this condition the autoantigens are well defined. The model produced by the group of Alvarez (Lapierre et al., 2004) is based on immunizing every 2 weeks for three times C57BL/6 female mice with a plasmid containing the antigenic region of human CYP2D6, the target of anti-LKM1, and FTCD, the target of anti-LC1, together with the murine end terminal region of cytotoxic T lymphocyte antigen 4 (CTLA-4). The latter was added to facilitate antigen uptake by antigen-presenting cells. In a parallel set of experiments a plasmid containing the DNA encoding IL-12, a Th1 skewing proinflammatory cytokine, was also used. When autoantigens and IL-12 were used to break tolerance, antigen-specific autoantibodies were produced, a relatively modest elevation of transaminase levels at 4 and 7 months was observed, and a portal and periportal inflammatory infiltrate composed of CD4 and CD8 T cells and, to a lesser extent, B cells was demonstrated 8–10 months after the third immunization. When the same immunization protocol was used in different mouse strains, either a mild hepatitis or no inflammatory changes were observed, indicating the importance of a specific genetic background. Recently, these authors have shown, in the same animal model, that adoptive transfer of *ex vivo* expanded Tregs expressing the chemokine receptor CXCR3 targets efficiently the inflamed liver, restores peripheral tolerance to FTCD, and induces disease remission (Lapierre et al., 2013). Using FTDC as immunogen in an adenovirus shuttle vector, Hartke-Wolenski et al. have described a model of AIH evolving to portal and lobular fibrosis, in which the genetic predisposition afforded by the NOD background was key to the development of the disease (Hardtke-Wolenski et al., 2013).

Another model of AIH type 2 uses CYP2D6 transgenic mice and aims at breaking tolerance with an adenovirus-CYP2D6 vector (Holdener et al., 2008). While focal hepatocyte necrosis was seen both in mice treated with the Adenovirus-CYP2D6 vector and in control mice treated with Adenovirus alone, only the former developed chronic histological changes, including fibrosis, reminiscent of AIH. The hepatic lesion was associated with a specific immune response to an immunodominant region of CYP2D6 and a cytotoxic T cell response to Adenovirus-CYP2D6 vector-infected target cells.

A complex and somewhat artificial strategy, involving neonatal thymectomy to prevent Treg development and egress from the thymus, was used in PD-1 deficient mice to produce a fulminant hepatitis characterized by spontaneous and severe CD4 and CD8 T cell liver infiltration, lobular necrosis, and elevated titers of ANA. Also in this model, adoptive transfer of Tregs was able to reverse progression to fatal hepatitis, providing support for a protective role of this cell population in AIH (Kido et al., 2008).

Though these experimental approaches provide useful information on some of the possible pathogenic mechanisms leading to AIH type 2, a model more closely representative of type 1 AIH in humans is still missing.

PATHOLOGIC EFFECTOR MECHANISMS

In patients with increased genetic susceptibility to AIH, immune responses to liver autoantigens could be triggered by molecular mimicry. Cross-reactivity is an inherent property of the cells of the adaptive immune system (Vergani et al., 2002), derived from the need of T and B lymphocytes to recognize a potentially infinite number of non-self antigens without any prior information as to their structure. This implies that these cells, rather than responding to single antigen specificities, are able to cross-reactively respond to a number of antigens, thus expanding the antigenic specificities of the immune system to a level that reflects the antigenic diversity of the external environment.

This inherent potential for cross-reactivity, while allowing efficient responses to a vast array of pathogens, also provides the immune system with the potential to cross-react with self, leading to autoimmunity. This concept has been termed "molecular mimicry," where immune responses to external pathogens become directed towards structurally similar self components.

The strongest support to this model is in the context of AIH type 2, where T lymphocytes that target a key epitope of CYP2D6 also react with self-mimicking exogenous sequences present on the hepatitis C virus and members of the herpes virus family, cytomegalovirus, Epstein–Barr virus, and herpes simplex virus (Vergani et al., 2002). It is conceivable that, in genetically predisposed individuals, T cells targeting the self-epitope may be primed and expanded through exposure to the self-mimicking exogenous sequences with consequent initiation and perpetuation of liver autoimmunity.

This potential scenario is supported by a case report describing a 10-year-old girl who acquired HCV infection following a liver transplant for end-stage liver disease caused by alpha1-anti-trypsin deficiency. Two weeks after HCV infection, IgM anti-LKM1 autoantibodies appeared, followed by IgG anti-LKM1 antibodies, suggestive of HCV as the initiator of a primary anti-LKM1/anti-CYP2D6 autoimmune response (Mackie et al., 1994); 10 years later, the patient developed florid AIH type 2, which responded satisfactorily to immunosuppressive treatment, but by this time there was no trace of the previous HCV infection (Bogdanos et al., 2004).

Putative mechanisms of autoimmune liver damage are depicted in Figure 61.6. The immune response in AIH is believed to be initiated by the presentation of self-antigenic peptides (as yet unknown) to the T cell receptor (TCR) of uncommitted naïve CD4$^+$ T-helper (Th0) lymphocytes. Self-antigenic peptides are processed and presented by professional antigen-presenting cells (APCs), including dendritic cells (DCs), macrophages, and B lymphocytes. The liver is home to several specialized APC populations, including liver sinusoidal endothelial cells (LSECs), Kupffer cells, and DCs, where antigen presentation to both CD4 and CD8 effector T cells can occur *in situ*, perhaps averting the need for trafficking to the regional lymphoid tissues (Crispe, 2011; Ebrahimkhani et al., 2011).

During antigen presentation, in the presence of appropriate costimulatory signals, CD4$^+$ Th0 cells become activated and undergo differentiation into distinct T-helper cell subsets, depending on the cytokine milieu to which they are exposed. In the presence of IL-12 or IL-4, Th0 lymphocytes differentiate into Th1 or Th2 cells respectively, while predominance of IL-1beta and IL-6 favors differentiation into Th17 cells. Differentiation into Th1 cells leads to the production of IL-2 and IFN-gamma and the concomitant activation of CD8 T lymphocytes that produce IFN-gamma and TNF-alpha and exert cytotoxicity upon recognition of an antigen/MHC class I complex (Ichiki et al., 2005). Exposure of hepatocytes to IFN-gamma results in the upregulation of MHC class I and in the aberrant expression of MHC class II molecules, which leads to further T cell activation and to the perpetuation of liver damage (Lobo-Yeo et al., 1990; Senaldi et al., 1991). IFN-gamma also favors monocyte differentiation, promotes macrophage and immature DC activation (Delneste et al., 2003), and contributes to enhanced natural killer (NK) cell killing (Schroder et al., 2004).

Differentiation of Th0 into Th2 cells leads to the secretion of IL-10, IL-4, and IL-13, cytokines essential for B cell maturation into plasma cells and consequently to the production of autoantibodies, which can participate in mechanisms of damage such as antibody-mediated cellular cytotoxicity and complement activation (Longhi et al., 2010). Of note,

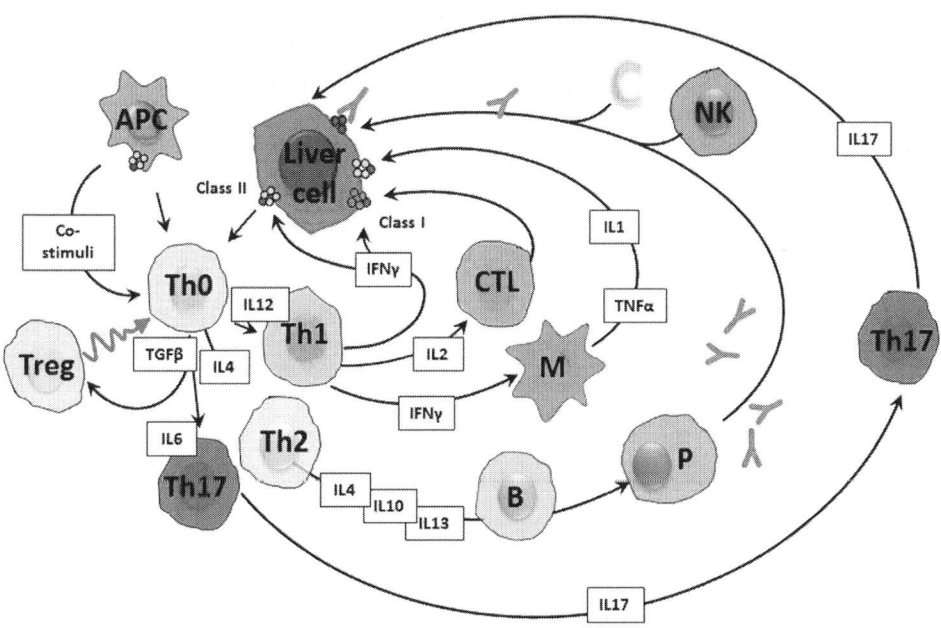

FIGURE 61.6 Autoimmune attack to the hepatocyte. An autoantigen is presented to uncommitted T-helper (Th0) lymphocytes within the HLA class II molecule of an antigen-presenting cell (APC) either in the regional lymph nodes or within the liver itself. Activated Th0 cells differentiate into Th1 or Th2 cells in the presence of interleukin (IL)-2 or IL-4, respectively, and according to the nature of the antigen. This triggers a series of immune reactions determined by the cytokines they produce. Th1 cells secrete IL-2 and interferon (IFN)-γ, which are cytokines that stimulate cytotoxic T lymphocytes (CTL), enhance expression of class I HLA molecules, induce expression of class II HLA molecules on the liver cells, and activate macrophages. Macrophages (M) release IL-1 and tumor necrosis factor (TNF). TH2 cells secrete mainly IL-4, IL-10, and IL-13, and stimulate autoantibody production by B lymphocytes. Regulatory T cells (Tregs) are derived from Th0 in the presence of transforming growth factor (TGF)-β. In the presence of defective Treg, hepatocyte destruction ensues from the engagement of damaging effector mechanisms, including CTL, cytokines released by Th1 and by activated macrophages, complement activation, or adhesion of natural killer (NK) cells to autoantibody-coated hepatocytes through their Fc receptors. Th17 cells produce the inflammatory cytokine IL-17 and derive from Th0 cells in the presence of TGF-β and IL-6. They are the focus of current investigations.

the titers of several autoantibodies, including anti-liver-specific protein and its components, correlate with indices of disease severity (Jensen et al., 1978; McFarlane et al., 1986). Moreover, in AIH type 2, the target of the disease-defining antibody anti-LKM1, CYP2D6 is present not only in the endoplasmic reticulum, but also is expressed on the membrane of hepatocytes and therefore readily accessible to the immune attack (Muratori et al., 2000).

Th17 cells contribute to autoimmunity by producing the proinflammatory cytokines IL-17, IL-22, and TNF-alpha, and inducing hepatocytes to secrete IL-6 (Zhao et al., 2011a), which further enhances Th17 activation. The role of Th17 cells, which has been documented in PBC (Harada et al., 2009), is currently under investigation in AIH, where an elevated level of Th17 cells has been reported in both blood and liver (Zhao et al., 2011a).

Gamma/delta T cells, which account for a low proportion of circulating lymphocytes, are relatively abundant in the liver (Wen et al., 1992) and might contribute to the pathogenesis of AIH, as they are elevated during active disease phases. Moreover, in AIH, gamma/delta T cells produce high levels of granzyme B and IFN-gamma the expression of which correlates with

biochemical indices of liver damage, suggesting a direct involvement of this cell population in hepatic injury (Ferri et al., 2010).

A deficiency of immunoregulation, enabling the auto-immune response to develop, has been repeatedly reported in AIH. Thus, earlier, patients with AIH had low levels of circulating CD8[+] T cells and impaired T cell suppressor function which segregated with disease-predisposing HLA alleles B8/DR3 and was correctable by therapeutic doses of corticosteroids (Nouri-Aria et al., 1982). Furthermore, there was a defect in a subpopulation of T cells controlling the immune response to liver-specific membrane antigens (Vento et al., 1984). More recent evidence based on the now "genuine" Treg cells confirms an impairment of immunoregulatory function in AIH. Among recently defined T cell subsets with potential immunosuppressive function, CD4 cells constitutively expressing the IL-2 receptor alpha chain (CD25) (T-regulatory cells, Tregs) have emerged as the dominant subset. These cells, representing 5–10% of all peripheral CD4 cells in health, control innate and adaptive immune responses by limiting the proliferation and effector function of autoreactive T cells (Sakaguchi, 2000). Their mechanism of action involves mainly a direct contact with the target cells, and to a lesser extent the release of immunoregulatory cytokines, such as IL-10 and tissue growth factor beta 1.

In addition to CD25, which is also present on T cells undergoing activation, Tregs express a number of additional markers such as the glucocorticoid-induced tumor necrosis factor receptor, CD62L, CTLA4, and the fork-head/winged helix transcription factor FOXP3, whose expression has been associated with the acquisition of regulatory properties. Treg impairment is linked with various human autoimmune diseases including AIH (Sakaguchi et al., 2010). In patients with AIH type 1 and type 2, Tregs are defective in number compared to normal controls and this reduction is disease stage related, being more evident at diagnosis and during relapses than during drug-induced remission (Longhi et al., 2005; Longhi et al. 2010; Ferri et al., 2010). The percentage of Tregs inversely correlated with markers of disease severity, such as anti-SLA and anti-LKM1 autoantibody titers, suggesting that reductions in regulatory T cells favor manifestations of autoimmune liver disease. Moreover, Tregs from AIH patients at diagnosis are impaired in their ability to control the proliferation of CD4 and CD8 effector cells compared to Tregs isolated from AIH patients at remission or from healthy subjects (Longhi et al., 2005; Ferri et al., 2010). Though most published literature indicates a numerical and functional Treg defect in AIH, these findings were disputed in a recent paper which used a different methodological approach (Peiseler et al., 2012; reply Longhi et al., 2012).

The immunoregulatory defects described above have been complemented recently by findings that effector CD4 T cells in AIH are less susceptible to restraints exerted by Tregs. This defect is linked to reduced expression of the receptor molecule Tim-3 (inhibitory receptor T-cell-immunoglobulin-and-mucindomain-containing-molecule-3, which upon ligation of galectin-9 expressed by Tregs, induces effector cell death) (Liberal et al., 2012a). Thus data so far point to failure in homeostatic mechanisms in which Th17 cells override Tregs.

If loss of immunoregulation were central to the pathogenesis of autoimmune liver disease, treatment should concentrate on restoring the ability of Tregs to expand, with consequent increase in their number and function. However, we must be mindful that further confirmatory data are needed, and that the studies in AIH type 1 are being performed in the "vacuum" of lack of any knowledge of the provocative liver autoantigen.

TREATMENT AND OUTCOME

The aim of treatment in AIH is to attain an early complete remission to prevent disease progression and to maintain the remission long term using the lowest possible dose of medication. In all types of presentation apart from a fulminant onset with encephalopathy, AIH responds well to immunosuppressive treatment whatever the degree of liver impairment with a reported remission rate of ≈80% (Krawitt, 2006).

Standard Treatment

Since the late 1960s a combination of predniso(lo)ne and azathioprine has remained the basis of treatment for AIH (Mackay, 1968; Cook et al., 1971; Soloway et al., 1972; Murray-Lyon et al., 1973). The earlier unfounded suggestion of waiting for 6 months before starting immunosuppression has long been abandoned, since it is now clear that treatment should be started as soon as possible to avoid disease progression (Manns et al., 2010a).

The American Association for the Study of Liver Diseases (AASLD) practice guidelines, published in 2010, recommend for adult patients either an initial dose of 30 mg predniso(lo)ne combined with 1–2 mg of azathioprine daily, or monotherapy with prednis(lo)ne at a starting dose of 40–60 mg daily (Manns et al., 2010a). For children, a dose of 1–2 mg/kg predniso(lo)ne up to a daily dose of 60 mg is recommended in combination with azathioprine (1–2 mg/kg) or its parent drug 6-mercaptopurine (6MP) (1.5 mg/kg) (Mieli-Vergani et al., 2009). As azathioprine can be hepatotoxic, particularly in the presence of frank icterus, jaundiced patients should be treated with high-dose prednisolone first and azathioprine should be added later when partial disease control is achieved and jaundice has subsided.

The most common corticosteroid side effect affecting most patients after prolonged administration is Cushingoid changes, and recurrent cutaneous warts are also frequent. Less common but severe side effects include osteoporosis, vertebral collapse, diabetes, cataract, hypertension, and psychosis. But only ≈13% of treated patients develop side effects that necessitate dose reduction or premature drug withdrawal, this being usually for cosmetic changes or obesity, osteopenia with vertebral collapse, and brittle diabetes (Czaja and Freese, 2002). Indeed the impression exists that corticosteroids are tolerated relatively well in AIH. Adverse effects of azathioprine (cholestatic hepatitis, veno-occlusive disease, pancreatitis, nausea and vomiting, rash, bone marrow suppression) affect less than 10% of patients and usually subside upon drug withdrawal (Manns et al., 2010a). Determination of thiopurine methyltransferase activity is only warranted when there is pre-treatment or intra-treatment cytopenia, or the need for higher than conventional doses of azathioprine to maintain remission (Czaja, 2008), as only patients with near-zero erythrocyte concentrations of the enzyme are at risk of developing myelosuppression during treatment (Lennard et al., 1989; Ben Ari et al., 1995).

Criteria for complete remission are the disappearance of clinical symptoms, normalization of transaminase and IgG levels in adults and children, and, in addition, abrogation or reduction to a very low titer of the autoantibodies in children (Mieli-Vergani et al., 2009). Histological resolution of inflammation lags well behind biochemical improvement (Sogo et al., 2006; Ustundag et al., 2008; Manns et al., 2010a). Response to immunosuppressive treatment in AIH is usually so swift that a lack of response should prompt investigation of other causes of liver disease.

Relapse is characterized by an increased level in serum of transaminase enzymes, and is common, occurring in 40–80% of patients usually during attempts to withdraw treatment or because of non-adherence, and requires a temporary increase in the steroid dose (Gregorio et al., 1997; Czaja and Freese, 2002; Krawitt, 2006; Manns et al., 2010a). Non-adherence is particularly common in young adults and adolescents (Kerkar et al., 2006) and should not be mistaken for inefficacy of the drugs. Most patients, including those with cirrhosis (Manns et al., 2010a), attain complete remission on the above treatment schedules. In the presence of severe steroid side effects, remission can be maintained with azathioprine alone at a dose of up to 2 mg/kg daily (Johnson et al., 1995; Czaja, 2008). Treatment with both steroids and azathioprine can be safely continued during pregnancy (Heneghan et al., 2001; Candia et al., 2005; Terrabuio et al., 2009). Though azathioprine is classified as a category D drug by the FDA, it has no reported teratogenic effects in humans. If concerns remain about its use, women can be switched to steroid monotherapy.

For adult patients who are asymptomatic, paucisymptomatic, or are identified incidentally, the benefit of therapy should be weighed against the adverse effects of corticosteroids, particularly in postmenopausal women or elderly patients, with the histological severity of inflammation and liver damage being the best guide. In contrast, children, despite being rarely symptomatic, should start treatment promptly, even if the diagnosis is made incidentally, as they have a more aggressive and rapidly progressive disease (Czaja et al., 2005).

Long-term immunosuppressive treatment could be associated with the development of malignancies since extrahepatic cancers, including non-Hodgkin lymphoma and skin cancer, are reported to be more frequent in patients with AIH than in age-matched and sex-matched normal populations (Wang et al., 1989; Werner et al., 2009). The risk of developing primary hepatocellular carcinoma (HCC) in AIH is associated with the presence of cirrhosis, akin to other chronic liver diseases (Yeoman et al., 2008; Wong et al., 2011); hence the AASLD

Autoimmune Hepatitis Guidelines recommend active surveillance for HCC (Manns et al., 2010a).

Alternative Treatments

Cyclosporine and tacrolimus, calcineurin inhibitors, have been used as steroid-sparing agents in an attempt to induce remission while avoiding high-dose steroid adverse effects (Van Thiel et al., 1995; Alvarez et al., 1999b; Debray et al., 1999; Cuarterolo et al., 2006), but whether the use of these toxic and expensive drugs confers any advantage over standard treatment remains to be evaluated in controlled studies.

A large European trial investigating the effect of a combination of budesonide and azathioprine in AIH reported remission in a higher proportion of non-cirrhotic patients with less adverse effects than medium-dose standard prednisone and azathioprine (Manns et al., 2010b). This study compared the effect of budesonide at a dose of 3 mg three times daily, decreased upon response, with prednisone 40 mg once daily reduced per protocol, irrespective of response. Six months after starting treatment, remission was observed in 60% of the budesonide group but in only 39% of the prednisone group. When pediatric patients were considered separately, no difference in response was observed between the budesonide and prednisone groups at 6 months (16% versus 15%) and 12 months (50% versus 42%) (Woynarowski et al., 2013). Of note, the remission rate in the prednisone arm of this study is considerably less than that reported both in adults and children ($\approx$80%) when a higher starting dose of predniso(lo)ne is used and tapered according to biochemical response (Kanzler et al., 2001; Gregorio et al., 1997). A limitation of budesonide, moreover, is that it is ineffective in patients with cirrhosis, who represent at least one-third of all AIH cases (Roberts et al., 1996; Gregorio et al., 1997). Despite limitations, this trial does show budesonide to be a valid alternative in patients at selected risk of adverse effects from prednisolone.

Difficult-to-treat cases are reported to respond to mycophenolate mofetil at a dose of 20 mg/kg twice daily in association with prednisone (Richardson et al., 2000; Devlin et al., 2004; Aw et al., 2009) although this experience is not unanimous (Hennes et al., 2008a). In adults, mycophenolate mofetil appears to be effective in patients intolerant of, but not in those unresponsive to, azathioprine (Hennes et al., 2008a). For patients who do not respond to, or are intolerant to, mycophenolate mofetil (headache, diarrhea, nausea, dizziness, hair loss, and neutropenia), a calcineurin inhibitor in combination with prednisone is suggested (Manns et al., 2010a). In patients particularly difficult to treat, the use of rituximab (Barth and Clawson, 2010) and infliximab (Weiler-Normann et al., 2009; Weiler-Normann et al., 2013) has been recently reported, but with variable outcomes. An important risk of these biological treatments is the occurrence of severe infections.

Duration of Treatment

No optimal length of treatment has been established. Most authors recommend at least 3 years of continuous therapy (Manns et al., 2010a). Treatment should cease only when a follow-up liver biopsy shows resolution of inflammation. Cessation should proceed with caution during or immediately before puberty, when relapses are more frequent, possibly because of poor adherence to treatment during adolescence (Kerkar et al., 2006).

During withdrawal close monitoring is needed as relapse may be severe and even fatal. Successful stopping of immunosuppression should be followed up long term, as relapses can occur even several years later (Manns et al., 2010a). Some 20% of patients with juvenile type 1 AIH can stop treatment successfully and permanently, but treatment cessation is achieved only rarely for patients with type 2 AIH (Gregorio et al., 1997). Levels of autoantibody and IgG (Gregorio et al., 2002; Luth et al., 2008) are important markers of disease activity and are useful to monitor response to treatment. Most AIH patients who respond to immunosuppressive treatment have an excellent outcome and lead a normal life on low-dose medication.

Liver Transplantation

Liver transplantation is the treatment of choice for patients who present with fulminant hepatic failure (grade II–IV encephalopathy), or who progress to end-stage liver disease despite immunosuppression ($\approx$10–20% of patients). Recurrence of AIH, characterized by high transaminase levels, positive autoantibodies, interface hepatitis, and/or steroid dependence, occurs in $\approx$20% of patients receiving transplant (Milkiewicz et al., 1999; Duclos-Vallee et al., 2003) and can happen even years after transplantation. Prednisolone treatment long term and at a dose higher than that generally used after liver transplantation for other conditions is recommended to avoid recurrence. Besides recurrent AIH, there is a form of graft dysfunction characterized by chronic liver damage with interface hepatitis, high transaminase and IgG levels, and positive tests for autoantibodies that occurs in $\approx$6–10% of patients receiving transplants for non-autoimmune disorders. It has been named "de novo AIH" (Kerkar et al., 1998; Liberal et al., 2012b). This condition does not respond satisfactorily to anti-rejection regimens but only to the addition of standard treatment for AIH (Liberal et al., 2012b) or, in resistant cases, rapamycin (Kerkar et al., 2005); an early diagnosis is needed to avoid graft loss.

Future Treatment Approaches

As loss of immunoregulation appears central to the pathogenesis of AIH, so treatment should concentrate on restoring the ability of Tregs to expand in number, with consequent increase in their function. The immunotherapeutic use of autologous $CD4^+CD25^+$ Tregs derived from patients, however, is hindered by their limited ability to proliferate and by their propensity to apoptosis (Akbar et al., 2003), which usually precludes cell numbers adequate for treatment. The partial Treg restoration in patients during remission (Longhi et al., 2004, 2005) indicates that Tregs in AIH, although impaired, can expand and regain function. Following *in vitro* exposure to polyclonal T cell stimulation, Tregs can be expanded not only in healthy individuals, but also in patients with AIH (Longhi et al., 2008). While maintaining the phenotypic features of original $CD4^+CD25^+$ T cells, expanded Tregs express increased FOXP3 and display augmented suppressor function.

Studies in mice show that Tregs with autoantigen specificity suppress immune effectors more efficiently than do their non-antigen-specific counterparts (Tarbell et al., 2004; Albert et al., 2005). In this regard, type 2 AIH is an excellent model for specific reconstitution of self-tolerance since not only is the key autoantigen, CYP2D6, known, but also the specific autoepitope regions ($CYP2D6_{217-260}$ and $CYP2D6_{305-348}$), targeted by B cells, CD4 cells, and CD8 T cells (Kerkar et al., 2003; Ma et al., 2006; Longhi et al., 2007). Antigen-specific Tregs have been obtained from patients with type 2 AIH and exert a more powerful immunosuppressive effect than polyclonally expanded Tregs (Longhi et al., 2011). The most efficient suppression of autoreactive T cells was achieved after Tregs were exposed to CYP2D6 peptides co-cultured with semi-mature dendritic cells loaded with the same peptide. Thus adoptive transfer of autologous CYP2D6-specific Tregs could become an effective and even curative therapy for type 2 AIH, as suggested also in an animal model of type 2 AIH (Lapierre et al., 2013). In type 1 AIH, immune intervention based on SLA might be a possibility, since at least 50% of patients have autoantibodies to this autoantigen. An even higher proportion of patients with type 1 AIH have cellular immune reactivity to HLA DRB1*0301 (Meda et al., 2007) or HLA DRB1*0401 (Zhao et al., 2011b)-restricted SLA epitopes. SLA-specific Tregs could, therefore, be considered for antigen-specific immune intervention in type 1 AIH as well.

Another possible therapeutic approach is exploitation of the Treg response to low doses of IL-2, since Saadoun et al. (2011) report encouraging results in the treatment of hepatitis C virus-associated vasculitis that was refractory to conventional antiviral therapy and anti-CD20 monoclonal antibody, using repeated courses of low-dose IL-2, which led to an increase in Treg numbers and also clinical improvement.

CONCLUDING REMARKS—FUTURE PROSPECTS

AIH requires consideration in the differential diagnosis of any instance in serum of increase in liver enzyme levels. Several pathogenic aspects of AIH have been elucidated, including predisposing genetic factors and (to a degree) disease-specific humoral and cellular immune responses. Prompt immunosuppressive treatment provides a good outcome with a mostly symptom-free long-term survival.

Even so, type 1 (but not type 2) AIH is one of those autoimmune diseases for which clear knowledge on initiation, immunopathogenic mechanisms, and effector processes remains quite lacking. The necessary better understanding of each of these aspects could facilitate our tasks for the future which include establishment of novel treatments aimed specifically at arresting liver autoaggression or, ideally, at reinstating failed tolerance to liver autoantigens, thereby abrogating our hitherto long reliance on non-specific immunosuppression with all of its discomforts and hazards.

REFERENCES

Agarwal, K., Czaja, A.J., Jones, D.E., Donaldson, P.T., 2000. Cytotoxic T lymphocyte antigen-4 (CTLA-4) gene polymorphisms and susceptibility to type 1 autoimmune hepatitis. Hepatology. 31, 49–53.

Agarwal, K., Czaja, A.J., Donaldson, P.T., 2007. A functional Fas promoter polymorphism is associated with a severe phenotype in type 1 autoimmune hepatitis characterized by early development of cirrhosis. Tissue Antigens. 69, 227–235.

Akbar, A.N., Taams, L.S., Salmon, M., Vukmanovic-Stejic, M., 2003. The peripheral generation of CD4+ CD25+ regulatory T cells. Immunology. 109, 319–325.

Al-Chalabi, T., Underhill, J.A., Portmann, B.C., McFarlane, I.G., Heneghan, M.A., 2008. Impact of gender on the long-term outcome and survival of patients with autoimmune hepatitis. J. Hepatol. 48, 140–147.

Albert, M.H., Liu, Y., Anasetti, C., Yu, X.Z., 2005. Antigen-dependent suppression of alloresponses by Foxp3-induced regulatory T cells in transplantation. Eur. J. Immunol. 35, 2598–2607.

Alvarez, F., Berg, P.A., Bianchi, F.B., Bianchi, L., Burroughs, A.K., Cancado, E.L., et al., 1999a. International Autoimmune Hepatitis Group Report: review of criteria for diagnosis of autoimmune hepatitis. J. Hepatol. 31, 929–938.

Alvarez, F., Ciocca, M., Canero-Velasco, C., Ramonet, M., de Davila, M.T.G., Cuarterolo, M., et al., 1999b. Short-term cyclosporine induces a remission of autoimmune hepatitis in children. J. Hepatol. 30, 222–227.

Amontree, J.S., Stuart, T.D., Bredfeldt, J.E., 1989. Autoimmune chronic active hepatitis masquerading as acute hepatitis. J. Clin. Gastroenterol. 11, 303–307.

Aw, M.M., Dhawan, A., Samyn, M., Bargiota, A., Mieli-Vergani, G., 2009. Mycophenolate mofetil as rescue treatment for autoimmune liver disease in children: a 5-year follow-up. J. Hepatol. 51, 156–160.

Baeres, M., Herkel, J., Czaja, A.J., Wies, I., Kanzler, S., Cancado, E.L., et al., 2002. Establishment of standardised SLA/LP immunoassays: specificity for autoimmune hepatitis, worldwide occurrence, and clinical characteristics. Gut. 51, 259–264.

Barth, E., Clawson, J., 2010. A case of autoimmune hepatitis treated with rituximab. Case Rep. Gastroenterol. 4, 502–509.

Ben Ari, Z., Mehta, A., Lennard, L., Burroughs, A.K., 1995. Azathioprine-induced myelosuppression due to thiopurine methyltransferase deficiency in a patient with autoimmune hepatitis. J. Hepatol. 23, 351–354.

Boberg, K.M., Aadland, E., Jahnsen, J., Raknerud, N., Stiris, M., Bell, H., 1998. Incidence and prevalence of primary biliary cirrhosis, primary sclerosing cholangitis, and autoimmune hepatitis in a Norwegian population. Scand. J. Gastroenterol. 33, 99–103.

Bogdanos, D., Ma, Y., Hadzic, N., Portmann, B., Mieli-Vergani, G., Vergani, D., 2004. Virus-self crossreactivity inducing de novo autoimmune hepatitis eight-years after liver transplantation. J. Pediatr. Gastroenterol. Nutr. 39, s169.

Bogdanos, D.P., Invernizzi, P, Mackay, I.R., Vergani, D., 2008. Autoimmune liver serology: current diagnostic and clinical challenges. World J. Gastroenterol. 14, 3374–3387.

Bogdanos, D.P., Mieli-Vergani, G., Vergani, D., 2009. Autoantibodies and their antigens in autoimmune hepatitis. Semin. Liver Dis. 29, 241–253.

Bottazzo, G.F., Florin-Christensen, A., Fairfax, A., Swana, G., Doniach, D., Groeschel-Stewart, U., 1976. Classification of smooth muscle autoantibodies detected by immunofluorescence. J. Clin. Pathol. 29, 403–410.

Burlingame, R.W., Rubin, R.L., Rosenberg, A.M., 1993. Autoantibodies to chromatin components in juvenile rheumatoid arthritis. Arthritis Rheum. 36, 836–841.

Candia, L., Marquez, J., Espinoza, L.R., 2005. Autoimmune hepatitis and pregnancy: a rheumatologist's dilemma. Semin Arthritis Rheum. 35, 49–56.

Cook, G., Mulligan, R., Sherlock, S., 1971. Controlled prospective trial of corticosteroid therapy in active chronic hepatitis. Q. J. Med. 40, 159–185.

Cookson, S., Constantini, P.K., Clare, M., Underhill, J.A., Bernal, W., Czaja, A.J., et al., 1999. Frequency and nature of cytokine gene polymorphisms in type 1 autoimmune hepatitis. Hepatology. 30, 851–856.

Costa, M., Rodriguez-Sanchez, J.L., Czaja, A.J., Gelpi, C., 2000. Isolation and characterization of cDNA encoding the antigenic protein of the human tRNP(Ser)Sec complex recognized by autoantibodies from patients with type-1 autoimmune hepatitis. Clin. Exp. Immunol. 121, 364–374.

Crapper, R.M., Bhathal, P.S., Mackay, I.R., Frazer, I.H., 1986. "Acute" autoimmune hepatitis. Digestion. 34, 216–225.

Crispe, I.N., 2011. Liver antigen-presenting cells. J. Hepatol. 54, 357–365.

Cuarterolo, M., Ciocca, M., Velasco, C.C., Ramonet, M., Gonzalez, T., Lopez, S., et al., 2006. Follow-up of children with autoimmune hepatitis treated with cyclosporine. J. Pediatr. Gastroenterol. Nutr. 43, 635–639.

Czaja, A.J., 2008. Safety issues in the management of autoimmune hepatitis. Expert Opin. Drug Saf. 7, 319–333.

Czaja, A.J., Carpenter, H.A., 1997. Histological findings in chronic hepatitis C with autoimmune features. Hepatology. 26, 459–466.

Czaja, A.J., Freese, D.K., 2002. Diagnosis and treatment of autoimmune hepatitis. Hepatology. 36, 479–497.

Czaja, A.J., Davis, G.L., Ludwig, J., Baggenstoss, A.H., Taswell, H.F., 1983. Autoimmune features as determinants of prognosis in steroid-treated chronic active hepatitis of uncertain etiology. Gastroenterology. 85, 713–717.

Czaja, A.J., Nishioka, M., Morshed, S.A., Hachiya, T., 1994. Patterns of nuclear immunofluorescence and reactivities to recombinant nuclear antigens in autoimmune hepatitis. Gastroenterology. 107, 200–207.

Czaja, A.J., Donaldson, P.T., Lohse, A.W., 2002. Antibodies to soluble liver antigen/liver pancreas and HLA risk factors for type 1 autoimmune hepatitis. Am. J. Gastroenterol. 97, 413–419.

Czaja, A.J., Bianchi, F.B., Carpenter, H.A., Krawitt, E.L., Lohse, A.W., Manns, M.P., et al., 2005. Treatment challenges and investigational opportunities in autoimmune hepatitis. Hepatology. 41, 207–215.

Debray, D., Maggiore, G., Giradet, J.P., Mallet, E., Bernard, O., 1999. Efficacy of cyclosporin A in children with type 2 autoimmune hepatitis. J. Pediatr. 135, 111–114.

Delneste, Y., Charbonnier, P., Herbault, N., Magistrelli, G., Caron, G., Bonnefoy, J.Y., et al., 2003. Interferon-gamma switches monocyte differentiation from dendritic cells to macrophages. Blood. 101, 143–150.

Devlin, S.M., Swain, M.G., Urbanski, S.J., Burak, K.W., 2004. Mycophenolate mofetil for the treatment of autoimmune hepatitis in patients refractory to standard therapy. Can. J. Gastroenterol. 18, 321–326.

Djilali-Saiah, I., Fakhfakh, A., Louafi, H., Caillat-Zucman, S., Debray, D., Alvarez, F., 2006. HLA class II influences humoral autoimmunity in patients with type 2 autoimmune hepatitis. J. Hepatol. 45, 844–848.

Donaldson, P., 2002. Genetics in autoimmune hepatitis. Semin. Liver Dis. 22, 353–364.

Donaldson, P.T., 2004. Genetics of liver disease: immunogenetics and disease pathogenesis. Gut. 53, 599–608.

Duchini, A., McHutchison, J.G., Pockros, P.J., 2000. LKM-positive autoimmune hepatitis in the western United States: a case series. Am. J. Gastroenterol. 95, 3238–3241.

Duclos-Vallee, J.C., Sebagh, M., Rifai, K., Johanet, C., Ballot, E., Guettier, C., et al., 2003. A 10 year follow up study of patients transplanted for autoimmune hepatitis: histological recurrence precedes clinical and biochemical recurrence. Gut. 52, 893–897.

Ebrahimkhani, M.R., Mohar, I., Crispe, I.N., 2011. Cross-presentation of antigen by diverse subsets of murine liver cells. Hepatology. 54, 1379–1387.

Fainboim, L., Canero Velasco, M.C., Marcos, C.Y., Ciocca, M., Roy, A., Theiler, G., et al., 2001. Protracted, but not acute, hepatitis A virus infection is strongly associated with HLA-DRB*1301, a marker for pediatric autoimmune hepatitis. Hepatology. 33, 1512–1517.

Ferri, S., Longhi, M.S., De Molo, C., Lalanne, C., Muratori, P., Granito, A., et al., 2010. A multifaceted imbalance of T cells with regulatory function characterizes type 1 autoimmune hepatitis. Hepatology. 52, 999–1007.

Gregorio, G.V., Portman, B., Reid, F., Donaldson, P.T., Doherty, D.G., McCartney, M., et al., 1997. Autoimmune hepatitis in childhood: a 20-year experience. Hepatology. 25, 541–547.

Gregorio, G.V., Portmann, B., Karani, J., Harrison, P., Donaldson, P.T., Vergani, D., et al., 2001. Autoimmune hepatitis/sclerosing cholangitis overlap syndrome in childhood: a 16-year prospective study. Hepatology. 33, 544–553.

Gregorio, G.V., Mcfarlane, B., Bracken, P., Vergani, D., Mieli-Vergani, G., 2002. Organ and non-organ specific autoantibody titres and IgG levels as markers of disease activity: a longitudinal study in childhood autoimmune liver disease. Autoimmunity. 35, 515–519.

Harada, K., Shimoda, S., Sato, Y., Isse, K., Ikeda, H., Nakanuma, Y., 2009. Periductal interleukin-17 production in association with biliary innate immunity contributes to the pathogenesis of cholangiopathy in primary biliary cirrhosis. Clin. Exp. Immunol. 157, 261–270.

Hardtke-Wolenski, M., Taubert, R., Jaeckel, E., 2012. Animal models for autoimmune liver disease—what is relevant for immune-mediated liver disease. Dig. Dis. 30, S1–S20.

Hardtke-Wolenski, M., Fischer, K., Noyan, F., Schlue, J., Falk, C., Stahlhut, M., et al., 2013. Genetic predisposition and environmental danger signals initiate chronic autoimmune hepatitis driven by CD4+ T cells. Hepatology. 58, 718–728.

Heneghan, M.A., Norris, S.M., O'Grady, J.G., Harrison, P.M., McFarlane, I.G., 2001. Management and outcome of pregnancy in autoimmune hepatitis. Gut. 48, 97–102.

Hennes, E.M., Oo, Y.H., Schramm, C., Denzer, U., Buggisch, P., Wiegard, C., et al., 2008a. Mycophenolate mofetil as second line therapy in autoimmune hepatitis? Am. J. Gastroenterol. 103, 3063–3070.

Hennes, E.M., Zeniya, M., Czaja, A.J., Pares, A., Dalekos, G.N., Krawitt, E.L., et al., 2008b. Simplified criteria for the diagnosis of autoimmune hepatitis. Hepatology. 48, 169–176.

Holdener, M., Hintermann, E., Bayer, M., Rhode, A., Rodrigo, E., Hintereder, G., et al., 2008. Breaking tolerance to the natural human liver autoantigen cytochrome P450 2D6 by virus infection. J. Exp. Med. 205, 1409–1422.

Homberg, J.C., Abuaf, N., Bernard, O., Islam, S., Alvarez, F., Khalil, S.H., et al., 1987. Chronic active hepatitis associated with antiliver/kidney microsome antibody type 1: a second type of autoimmune hepatitis. Hepatology. 7, 1333–1339.

Hurlburt, K.J., McMahon, B.J., Deubner, H., Hsu-Trawinski, B., Williams, J.L., Kowdley, K.V., 2002. Prevalence of autoimmune liver disease in Alaska Natives. Am. J. Gastroenterol. 97, 2402–2407.

Ichiki, Y., Aoki, C.A., Bowlus, C.L., Shimoda, S., Ishibashi, H., Gershwin, M.E., 2005. T cell immunity in autoimmune hepatitis. Autoimmun. Rev. 4, 315–321.

Jensen, D.M., McFarlane, I.G., Portmann, B.S., Eddleston, A.L., Williams, R., 1978. Detection of antibodies directed against a liver-specific membrane lipoprotein in patients with acute and chronic active hepatitis. N. Engl. J. Med. 299, 1–7.

Johnson, P.J., McFarlane, I.G., 1993. Meeting report: International Autoimmune Hepatitis Group. Hepatology. 18, 998–1005.

Johnson, P.J., McFarlane, I.G., Williams, R., 1995. Azathioprine for long-term maintenance of remission in autoimmune hepatitis. N. Engl. J. Med. 333, 958–963.

Joske, R.A., King, W.E., 1955. The L.E.-cell phenomenon in active chronic viral hepatitis. Lancet. 269, 477–480.

Kanzler, S., Lohr, H., Gerken, G., Galle, P.R., Lohse, A.W., 2001. Long-term management and prognosis of autoimmune hepatitis (AIH): a single center experience. Z. Gastroenterol. 39, 339–341.

Kerkar, N., Hadzic, N., Davies, E.T., Portmann, B., Donaldson, P.T., Rela, M., et al., 1998. De-novo autoimmune hepatitis after liver transplantation. Lancet. 351, 409–413.

Kerkar, N., Choudhuri, K., Ma, Y., Mahmoud, A., Bogdanos, D.P., Muratori, L., et al., 2003. Cytochrome P4502D6(193–212): a new immunodominant epitope and target of virus/self cross-reactivity in liver kidney microsomal autoantibody type 1-positive liver disease. J. Immunol. 170, 1481–1489.

Kerkar, N., Dugan, C., Rumbo, C., Morotti, R.A., Gondolesi, G., Shneider, B.L., et al., 2005. Rapamycin successfully treats post-transplant autoimmune hepatitis. Am. J. Transplant. 5, 1085–1089.

Kerkar, N., Annunziato, R.A., Foley, L., Schmeidler, J., Rumbo, C., Emre, S., et al., 2006. Prospective analysis of nonadherence in autoimmune hepatitis: a common problem. J. Pediatr. Gastroenterol. Nutr. 43, 629–634.

Kido, M., Watanabe, N., Okazaki, T., Akamatsu, T., Tanaka, J., Saga, K., et al., 2008. Fatal autoimmune hepatitis induced by concurrent loss of naturally arising regulatory T cells and PD-1-mediated signaling. Gastroenterology. 135, 1333–1343.

Krawitt, E.L., 2006. Autoimmune hepatitis. N. Engl. J. Med. 354, 54–66.

Kunkel, H.G., Ahrens Jr., E.H., Eigenmernger, W.J., Bongiovanni, A.M., Slater, R.J., 1951. Extreme hypergammaglobulinemia in young women with liver disease of unknown etiology [abstract]. J. Clin. Invest. 30, 654.

Lankisch, T.O., Strassburg, C.P., Debray, D., Manns, M.P., Jacquemin, E., 2005. Detection of autoimmune regulator gene mutations in children with type 2 autoimmune hepatitis and extrahepatic immune-mediated diseases. J. Pediatr. 146, 839–842.

Lapierre, P., Hajoui, O., Homberg, J.C., Alvarez, F., 1999. Formiminotransferase cyclodeaminase is an organ-specific autoantigen recognized by sera of patients with autoimmune hepatitis. Gastroenterology. 116, 643–649.

Lapierre, P., Djilali-Saiah, I., Vitozzi, S., Alvarez, F., 2004. A murine model of type 2 autoimmune hepatitis: xenoimmunization with human antigens. Hepatology. 39, 1066–1074.

Lapierre, P., Beland, K., Yang, R., Alvarez, F., 2013. Adoptive transfer of ex vivo expanded regulatory T cells in an autoimmune hepatitis murine model restores peripheral tolerance. Hepatology. 57, 217–227.

Lennard, L., Van Loon, J.A., Weinshilboum, R.M., 1989. Pharmacogenetics of acute azathioprine toxicity: relationship to thiopurine methyltransferase genetic polymorphism. Clin. Pharmacol. Ther. 46, 149–154.

Leoni, A., 1954. The specificity of L.E. phenomenon. Minerva Med. 45, 1022–1027.

Liberal, R., Grant, C.R., Holder, B.S., Ma, Y., Mieli-Vergani, G., Vergani, D., et al., 2012a. The impaired immune regulation of autoimmune hepatitis is linked to a defective galectin-9/tim-3 pathway. Hepatology. 56, 677–686.

Liberal, R., Longhi, M.S., Grant, C.R., Mieli-Vergani, G., Vergani, D., 2012b. Autoimmune hepatitis after liver transplantation. Clin. Gastroenterol. Hepatol. 10, 346–353.

Liston, A., Lesage, S., Gray, D.H., Boyd, R.L., Goodnow, C.C., 2005. Genetic lesions in T-cell tolerance and thresholds for autoimmunity. Immunol. Rev. 204, 87–101.

Lleo, A., Selmi, C., Invernizzi, P., Podda, M., Coppel, R.L., Mackay, I.R., et al., 2009. Apotopes and the biliary specificity of primary biliary cirrhosis. Hepatology. 49, 871–879.

Lobo-Yeo, A., Senaldi, G., Portmann, B., Mowat, A.P., Mieli-Vergani, G., Vergani, D., 1990. Class I and class II major histocompatibility complex antigen expression on hepatocytes: a study in children with liver disease. Hepatology. 12, 224–232.

Longhi, M.S., Ma, Y., Bogdanos, D.P., Cheeseman, P., Mieli-Vergani, G., Vergani, D., 2004. Impairment of CD4(+)CD25(+) regulatory T-cells in autoimmune liver disease. J. Hepatol. 41, 31–37.

Longhi, M.S., Ma, Y., Mitry, R.R., Bogdanos, D.P., Heneghan, M., Cheeseman, P., et al., 2005. Effect of CD4+ CD25+ regulatory T-cells on CD8 T-cell function in patients with autoimmune hepatitis. J. Autoimmun. 25, 63–71.

Longhi, M.S., Hussain, M.J., Bogdanos, D.P., Quaglia, A., Mieli-Vergani, G., Ma, Y., et al., 2007. Cytochrome P450IID6-specific CD8 T cell immune responses mirror disease activity in autoimmune hepatitis type 2. Hepatology. 46, 472–484.

Longhi, M.S., Meda, F., Wang, P., Samyn, M., Mieli-Vergani, G., Vergani, D., et al., 2008. Expansion and de novo generation of potentially therapeutic regulatory T cells in patients with autoimmune hepatitis. Hepatology. 47, 581–591.

Longhi, M.S., Ma, Y., Mieli-Vergani, G., Vergani, D., 2010. Aetiopathogenesis of autoimmune hepatitis. J. Autoimmun. 34, 7–14.

Longhi, M.S., Hussain, M.J., Kwok, W.W., Mieli-Vergani, G., Ma, Y., Vergani, D., 2011. Autoantigen-specific regulatory T cells, a potential tool for immune-tolerance reconstitution in type-2 autoimmune hepatitis. Hepatology. 53, 536–547.

Longhi, M.S., Ma, Y., Mieli-Vergani, G., Vergani, D., 2012. Regulatory T cells in autoimmune hepatitis. J. Hepatol. 57, 932–933.

Luth, S., Herkel, J., Kanzler, S., Frenzel, C., Galle, P.R., Dienes, H.P., et al., 2008. Serologic markers compared with liver biopsy for monitoring disease activity in autoimmune hepatitis. J. Clin. Gastroenterol. 42, 926–930.

Ma, Y., Okamoto, M., Thomas, M.G., Bogdanos, D.P., Lopes, A.R., Portmann, B., et al., 2002. Antibodies to conformational epitopes of soluble liver antigen define a severe form of autoimmune liver disease. Hepatology. 35, 658–664.

Ma, Y., Bogdanos, D.P., Hussain, M.J., Underhill, J., Bansal, S., Longhi, M.S., et al., 2006. Polyclonal T-cell responses to cytochrome P450IID6 are associated with disease activity in autoimmune hepatitis type 2. Gastroenterology. 130, 868–882.

Mackay, I.R., 1968. Chronic hepatitis: effect of prolonged suppressive treatment and comparison of azthioprine with prednisolone. Quart. J. Med. 37, 379–392.

Mackay, I.R., Taft, L.I., Cowling, D.C., 1956. Lupoid hepatitis. Lancet. ii, 1323–1326.

Mackay, I.R., Weiden, S., Hasker, J., 1965. Autoimmune hepatitis. Ann. N.Y. Acad. Sci. 124, 767–780.

Mackie, F.D., Peakman, M., Yun, M., Sallie, R., Smith, H., Davies, E.T., et al., 1994. Primary and secondary liver/kidney microsomal autoantibody response following infection with hepatitis C virus. Gastroenterology. 106, 1672–1675.

Manns, M., Gerken, G., Kyriatsoulis, A., Staritz, M., Meyer Zum Büschenfelde, K.H., 1987. Characterisation of a new subgroup of autoimmune chronic active hepatitis by autoantibodies against a soluble liver antigen. Lancet. 1, 292–294.

Manns, M.P., Luttig, B., Obermayer-Straub, P., 1998. Autoimmune hepatitis. In: Rose, N.R., Mackay, I.R. (Eds.), The Autoimmune Diseases, third ed. Academic Press.

Manns, M.P., Czaja, A.J., Gorham, J.D., Krawitt, E.L., Mieli-Vergani, G., Vergani, D., et al., 2010a. Diagnosis and management of autoimmune hepatitis. Hepatology. 51, 2193–2213.

Manns, M.P., Woynarowski, M., Kreisel, W., Lurie, Y., Rust, C., Zuckerman, E., et al., 2010b. Budesonide induces remission more effectively than prednisone in a controlled trial of patients with autoimmune hepatitis. Gastroenterology. 139, 1198–1206.

Martini, E., Abuaf, N., Cavalli, F., Durand, V., Johanet, C., Homberg, J.C., 1988. Antibody to liver cytosol (anti-LC1) in patients with autoimmune chronic active hepatitis type 2. Hepatology. 8, 1662–1666.

Mcfarlane, B.M., McSorley, C.G., Vergani, D., McFarlane, I.G., Williams, R., 1986. Serum autoantibodies reacting with the hepatic asialoglycoprotein receptor protein (hepatic lectin) in acute and chronic liver disorders. J. Hepatol. 3, 196–205.

Meda, F., Wang, P., Longhi, M.S., Bogdanos, D., Mieli-Vergani, G., Vergani, D., et al., 2007. Identification of HLA-DR3 restricted CD4 T-cell epitopes on soluble liver antigen in autoimmune hepatitis type 1. J. Hepatol. 46, S13.

Meroni, P.L., Schur, P.H., 2010. ANA screening: an old test with new recommendations. Ann. Rheum. Dis. 69, 1420–1422.

Meyer Zum Büschenfelde, K.H., 2003. Autoimmune hepatitis: "Hepatitis sui generis". J. Hepatol. 38, 130–135.

Mieli-Vergani, G., Vergani, D., 2011. Autoimmune hepatitis. Nat. Rev. Gastroenterol. Hepatol. 8, 320–329.

Mieli-Vergani, G., Heller, S., Jara, P., Vergani, D., Chang, M.H., Fujisawa, T., et al., 2009. Autoimmune hepatitis. J. Pediatr. Gastroenterol. Nutr. 49, 158–164.

Milkiewicz, P., Hubscher, S.G., Skiba, G., Hathaway, M., Elias, E., 1999. Recurrence of autoimmune hepatitis after liver transplantation. Transplantation. 68, 253–256.

Montano-Loza, A.J., Carpenter, H.A., Czaja, A.J., 2008. Frequency, behavior, and prognostic implications of antimitochondrial antibodies in type 1 autoimmune hepatitis. J. Clin. Gastroenterol. 42, 1047–1053.

Muratori, L., Parola, M., Ripalti, A., Robino, G., Muratori, P., Bellomo, G., et al., 2000. Liver/kidney microsomal antibody type 1 targets CYP2D6 on hepatocyte plasma membrane. Gut. 46, 553–561.

Muratori, P., Muratori, L., Agostinelli, D., Pappas, G., Veronesi, L., Granito, A., et al., 2002. Smooth muscle antibodies and type 1 autoimmune hepatitis. Autoimmunity. 35, 497–500.

Murray-Lyon, I.M., Stern, R.B., Williams, R., 1973. Controlled trial of prednisone and azathioprine in active chronic hepatitis. Lancet. 1, 735–737.

Ngu, J.H., Bechly, K., Chapman, B.A., Burt, M.J., Barclay, M.L., Gearry, R.B., et al., 2010. Population-based epidemiology study of autoimmune hepatitis: a disease of older women? J. Gastroenterol. Hepatol. 25, 1681–1686.

Nishioka, M., McFarlane, I.G., 1998. Geographical variation in the frequency and characteristics of autoimmune liver diseases. In: Krawitt, E.L., Nishioka, M. (Eds.), Autoimmune Liver Diseases. Elsevier, Amsterdam.

Nouri-Aria, K.T., Hegarty, J.E., Alexander, G.J., Eddleston, A.L., Williams, R., 1982. Effect of corticosteroids on suppressor-cell activity in autoimmune and viral chronic active hepatitis. N. Engl. J. Med. 307, 1301–1304.

O'Brien, C., Joshi, S., Feld, J.J., Guindi, M., Dienes, H.P., Heathcote, E.J., 2008. Long-term follow-up of antimitochondrial antibody-positive autoimmune hepatitis. Hepatology. 48, 550–556.

Oettinger, R., Brunnberg, A., Gerner, P., Wintermeyer, P., Jenke, A., Wirth, S., 2005. Clinical features and biochemical data of Caucasian children at diagnosis of autoimmune hepatitis. J. Autoimmun. 24, 79–84.

Palioura, S., Sherrer, R.L., Steitz, T.A., Soll, D., Simonovic, M., 2009. The human SepSecS-tRNASec complex reveals the mechanism of selenocysteine formation. Science. 325, 321–325.

Peakman, M., Bevis, L., Mieli-Vergani, G., Mowat, A.P., Vergani, D., 1989. Double stranded DNA binding in autoimmune chronic active hepatitis and primary sclerosing cholangitis starting in childhood. Autoimmunity. 3, 271–280.

Peiseler, M., Sebode, M., Franke, B., Wortmann, F., Schwinge, D., Quaas, A., et al., 2012. FOXP3 + regulatory T cells in autoimmune hepatitis are fully functional and not reduced in frequency. J. Hepatol. 57, 125–132.

Primo, J., Merino, C., Fernandez, J., Moles, J.R., Llorca, P., Hinojosa, J., 2004. [Incidence and prevalence of autoimmune hepatitis in the area of the Hospital de Sagunto (Spain)]. Gastroenterol. Hepatol. 27, 239–243.

Qiu, D., Wang, Q., Wang, H., Xie, Q., Zang, G., Jiang, H., et al., 2011. Validation of the simplified criteria for diagnosis of autoimmune hepatitis in Chinese patients. J. Hepatol. 54, 340–347.

Richardson, P.D., James, P.D., Ryder, S.D., 2000. Mycophenolate mofetil for maintenance of remission in autoimmune hepatitis in patients resistant to or intolerant of azathioprine. J. Hepatol. 33, 371–375.

Roberts, S.K., Therneau, T.M., Czaja, A.J., 1996. Prognosis of histological cirrhosis in type 1 autoimmune hepatitis. Gastroenterology. 110, 848–857.

Saadoun, D., Rosenzwajg, M., Joly, F., Six, A., Carrat, F., Thibault, V., et al., 2011. Regulatory T-cell responses to low-dose interleukin-2 in HCV-induced vasculitis. N. Engl. J. Med. 365, 2067–2077.

Sakaguchi, S., 2000. Regulatory T cells: key controllers of immunologic self-tolerance. Cell. 101, 455–458.

Sakaguchi, S., Miyara, M., Costantino, C.M., Hafler, D.A., 2010. FOXP3+ regulatory T cells in the human immune system. Nat. Rev. Immunol. 10, 490–500.

Schroder, K., Hertzog, P.J., Ravasi, T., Hume, D.A., 2004. Interferon-gamma: an overview of signals, mechanisms and functions. J. Leukoc. Biol. 75, 163–189.

Searle, J., Harmon, B.V., Bishop, C.S., Kerr, J.F.R., 1987. The significance of cell death by apoptosis in hepatobiliary disease. J. Gastroenterol. Hepatol. 2, 77–96.

Senaldi, G., Lobo-Yeo, A., Mowat, A.P., Mieli-Vergani, G., Vergani, D., 1991. Class I and class II major histocompatibility complex antigens on hepatocytes: importance of the method of detection and expression in histologically normal and diseased livers. J. Clin. Pathol. 44, 107–114.

Simmonds, M.J., Gough, S.C., 2004. Genetic insights into disease mechanisms of autoimmunity. Br. Med. Bull. 71, 93–113.

Sogo, T., Fujisawa, T., Inui, A., Komatsu, H., Etani, Y., Tajiri, H., et al., 2006. Intravenous methylprednisolone pulse therapy for children with autoimmune hepatitis. Hepatol. Res. 34, 187–192.

Soloway, R.D., Summerskill, W.H., Baggenstoss, A.H., Geall, M.G., Gitnick, G.L., Elveback, I.R., et al., 1972. Clinical, biochemical, and histological remission of severe chronic active liver disease: a controlled study of treatments and early prognosis. Gastroenterology. 63, 820–833.

Strassburg, C.P., Obermayer-Straub, P., Alex, B., Durazzo, M., Rizzetto, M., Tukey, R.H., et al., 1996a. Autoantibodies against glucuronosyltransferases differ between viral hepatitis and autoimmune hepatitis. Gastroenterology. 111, 1576–1586.

Strassburg, C.P., Alex, B., Zindy, F., Gerken, G., Luttig, B., Meyer Zum Büschenfelde, K.H., et al., 1996b. Identification of cyclin A as a molecular target of antinuclear antibodies (ANA) in hepatic and non-hepatic autoimmune diseases. J. Hepatol. 25, 859–866.

Takeda, K., Hayakawa, Y., Van Kaer, L., Matsuda, H., Yagita, H., Okumura, K., 2000. Critical contribution of liver natural killer T cells to a murine model of hepatitis. Proc. Natl. Acad. Sci. USA. 97, 5498–5503.

Tan, E.M., Feltkamp, T.E., Smolen, J.S., Butcher, B., Dawkins, R., Fritzler, M.J., et al., 1997. Range of antinuclear antibodies in "healthy" individuals. Arthritis Rheum. 40, 1601–1611.

Tarbell, K.V., Yamazaki, S., Olson, K., Toy, P., Steinman, R.M., 2004. CD25+ CD4+ T cells, expanded with dendritic cells presenting a single autoantigenic peptide, suppress autoimmune diabetes. J. Exp. Med. 199, 1467–1477.

Terrabuio, D.R., Abrantes-Lemos, C.P., Carrilho, F.J., Cancado, E.L., 2009. Follow-up of pregnant women with autoimmune hepatitis: the disease behavior along with maternal and fetal outcomes. J. Clin. Gastroenterol. 43, 350–356.

Tiegs, G., Hentschel, J., Wendel, A., 1992. A T cell-dependent experimental liver injury in mice inducible by concanavalin A. J. Clin. Invest. 90, 196–203.

Ustundag, G., Kuloglu, Z., Kirsaclioglu, C.T., Kansu, A., Erden, E., Girgin, N., 2008. Complete regression of cirrhosis after immunosuppressive treatment in autoimmune hepatitis. Pediatr. Int. 50, 711–713.

Van Thiel, D.H., Wright, H., Carroll, P., Abu-Elmagd, K., Rodriguez-Rilo, H., McMichael, J., et al., 1995. Tacrolimus: a potential new treatment for autoimmune chronic active hepatitis: results of an open-label preliminary trial. Am. J. Gastroenterol. 90, 771–776.

Vento, S., Hegarty, J.E., Bottazzo, G., Macchia, E., Williams, R., Eddleston, A.L., 1984. Antigen specific suppressor cell function in autoimmune chronic active hepatitis. Lancet. 1, 1200–1204.

Vergani, D., Choudhuri, K., Bogdanos, D.P., Mieli-Vergani, G., 2002. Pathogenesis of autoimmune hepatitis. Clin. Liver Dis. 6, 439–449.

Vergani, D., Alvarez, F., Bianchi, F.B., Cancado, E.L., Mackay, I.R., Manns, M.P., et al., 2004. Liver autoimmune serology: a consensus statement from the committee for autoimmune serology of the International Autoimmune Hepatitis Group. J. Hepatol. 41, 677–683.

Waldenstrom, J., 1950. Leber, Blutproteine und Nahrungseiweiss. Dtsch. Z. Verdau. Staffwechselkr. 15, 113–119.

Wang, K.K., Czaja, A.J., Beaver, S.J., Go, V.L., 1989. Extrahepatic malignancy following long-term immunosuppressive therapy of severe hepatitis B surface antigen-negative chronic active hepatitis. Hepatology. 10, 39–43.

Weiler-Normann, C., Wiegard, C., Schramm, C., Lohse, A.W., 2009. A case of difficult-to-treat autoimmune hepatitis successfully managed by TNF-alpha blockade. Am. J. Gastroenterol. 104, 2877–2878.

Weiler-Normann, C., Schramm, C., Quaas, A., Wiegard, C., Glaubke, C., Pannicke, N., et al., 2013. Infliximab as a rescue treatment in difficult-to-treat autoimmune hepatitis. J. Hepatol. 58, 529–534.

Wen, L., Peakman, M., Mieli-Vergani, G., Vergani, D., 1992. Elevation of activated gamma delta T cell receptor bearing T lymphocytes in patients with autoimmune chronic liver disease. Clin. Exp. Immunol. 89, 78–82.

Werner, M., Almer, S., Prytz, H., Lindgren, S., Wallerstedt, S., Bjornsson, E., et al., 2009. Hepatic and extrahepatic malignancies in autoimmune hepatitis. A long-term follow-up in 473 Swedish patients. J. Hepatol. 50, 388–393.

Whalley, S., Puvanachandra, P., Desai, A., Kennedy, H., 2007. Hepatology outpatient service provision in secondary care: a study of liver disease incidence and resource costs. Clin. Med. 7, 119–124.

Wies, I., Brunner, S., Henninger, J., Herkel, J., Kanzler, S., Meyer Zum Büschenfelde, K.H., et al., 2000. Identification of target antigen for SLA/LP autoantibodies in autoimmune hepatitis. Lancet. 355, 1510–1515.

Wong, R.J., Gish, R., Frederick, T., Bzowej, N., Frenette, C., 2011. Development of hepatocellular carcinoma in autoimmune hepatitis patients: a case series. Dig. Dis. Sci. 56, 578–585.

Woynarowski, M., Nemeth, A., Baruch,Y., Koletzko, S., Melter, M., Rodeck, B., et al. 2013. Budesonide vs. prednisone with azathioprine for the treatment of autoimmune hepatitis in children and adolescents. J. Pediatr. doi: 10.1016/j.jpeds.2013.05.042.

Yeoman, A.D., Al-Chalabi, A.T., Karani, J.B., Quaglia, A., Devlin, J., Mieli-Vergani, G., et al., 2008. Evaluation of risk factors in the development of HCC in AIH: Implications for follow-up and screening. Hepatology. 48, 863–870.

Zhao, L., Tang, Y., You, Z., Wang, Q., Liang, S., Han, X., et al., 2011a. Interleukin-17 contributes to the pathogenesis of autoimmune hepatitis through inducing hepatic interleukin-6 expression. PLoS One. 6, e18909.

Zhao, Y., Zhang, Y., Liu, Y.M., Liu, Y., Feng, X., Liao, H.Y., et al., 2011b. Identification of T cell epitopes on soluble liver antigen in Chinese patients with auto-immune hepatitis. Liver Int. 31, 721–729.

Chapter 62

Primary Biliary Cirrhosis

Carlo Selmi[1,2], Ian R. Mackay[3], and M. Eric Gershwin[1]

[1]*Division of Rheumatology, Allergy, and Clinical Immunology, University of California at Davis, Davis, CA, USA,* [2]*Division of Rheumatology and Clinical Immunology, Humanitas Clinical and Research Center, University of Milan, Italy,* [3]*Department of Biochemistry and Molecular Biology, Monash University, Clayton, Victoria, Australia*

Chapter Outline

Clinical, Pathologic, and Epidemiologic Features	**909**		Epigenetic Effects	915
History	909		Fetal Microchimerism	916
Diagnosis	909		Genes on the X Chromosome	916
Pathology	910		**Environmental Provocation of PBC**	**916**
Clinical Features	910		Infections	916
Epidemiology and Natural History	910		Xenobiotics	916
Treatment	913		**Experimental Animal Models**	**916**
Autoimmune Features	**913**		**Pathologic Effector Mechanisms**	**917**
Genetic Features	**914**		**Autoantibodies as Potential Immunologic Markers**	**918**
Familial PBC: Twins and Relatives	914		**Concluding Remarks—Future Prospects**	**919**
HLA Association	915		**References**	**920**
Genome-wide Association Studies (GWAS)	915			

CLINICAL, PATHOLOGIC, AND EPIDEMIOLOGIC FEATURES

History

Biliary cirrhosis, although possibly secondary, was first reported in the work of the Italian pathologist Giovanni Battista Morgagni in 1761. The first report of non-obstructive biliary cirrhosis was by Addison and Gull in 1851. The term primary biliary cirrhosis (PBC) became accepted in medical literature following the report of Ahrens et al. (Ahrens et al., 1950). The first long-term study of PBC cases observed that the patients presented with pruritus as well as jaundice and features of end-stage liver disease (Sherlock, 1959), but there have been significant changes in the clinical presentation at diagnosis since then. In 1965 was recognized the association between serum antimitochondrial antibody (AMA) and PBC from the immunofluorescence pattern given by serum with reactivity against antigens present in cytoplasmic organelles: such reactivity was found almost exclusively in affected individuals (Walker et al., 1965). Some 20 years later gene cloning revealed the identity of the autoantigen as an enzyme of the pyruvate dehydrogenase complex (PDC) located on the inner mitochondrial membrane (Gershwin et al., 1987). This led to more sensitive assays for AMA testing, although indirect immunofluorescence remains the method of routine testing in most clinical centers.

Diagnosis

The diagnosis of PBC is based on three criteria: increased serum alkaline phosphatase levels indicating cholestasis for longer than 6 months, a positive test for AMA in serum by indirect immunofluorescence (IIF) at a titer of or >1:40, and a compatible liver histology (Selmi et al., 2011). Patients who lack AMA presence but otherwise present signs of PBC are specified as "AMA-negative PBC" as they follow a natural history similar to AMA-positive patients (Selmi et al., 2008a).

N. Rose & I. Mackay (Eds): The Autoimmune Diseases, Fifth edition. DOI: http://dx.doi.org/10.1016/B978-0-12-384929-8.00062-9

Pathology

Liver biopsy remains critical for histological staging, but it is currently uncertain whether it is still needed for the diagnosis of PBC when the other two diagnostic criteria are met. It should be done when the diagnosis is suspected but AMA testing is negative and/or alkaline phosphatase levels are normal, and when it is required to stage the disease, both at presentation and in the follow-up (Heathcote, 2000). Sampling error should always be considered and if one biopsy appears to have variable staging the highest stage should be accepted (Ludwig, 2000). Histological classification (Ludwig et al., 1978) identifies four stages of PBC. Stage I shows portal-tract inflammation with predominantly lymphoplasmacytic infiltrates, loss of septal and interlobular bile ducts (diameter <100 μm), and non-caseating granulomas in absence of features of sarcoidosis or tuberculosis. Stage II shows a periportal inflammatory infiltrate, cholangitis, granulomas, and proliferation of ductules. Stage III shows septal or bridging fibrosis, ductopenia (over half of the interlobular bile ducts have vanished) and copper deposition in periportal and paraseptal hepatocytes. Stage IV is frank cirrhosis. The non-caseating epithelioid granulomas in PBC, as seen too in sarcoidosis, remain a mysterious feature since these are not a histological characteristic of any other autoimmune disease. Granulomas encountered in unselected liver biopsies are mostly attributable to PBC, but their pathogenic significance (if any) remains unknown (You et al., 2012).

Clinical Features

Unlike in the past, in the majority of cases (20–60%) the diagnosis of PBC is now made in the absence of symptoms that indicate a liver condition or cholestasis. This is due to the increased awareness of the disease and the availability of more sensitive and non-invasive tests, such as those for AMA detection. Interestingly, however, symptomless patients are commonly older than the symptomatic ones, possibly indicating a difference in the progression of PBC in these two groups (Howel et al., 2000). During extended clinical follow-up, most apparently normal AMA-positive patients will eventually develop PBC (Metcalf et al., 1997). In the last cirrhotic stage of PBC features of advanced liver disease, such as portal hypertension, jaundice, ascites, porto-systemic encephalopathy, and upper digestive bleeding, are predominant as with liver cirrhosis from any cause.

Fatigue is the most common symptom, affecting 70% of patients, but prevalence rates vary across cohorts. The fatigue is sufficient to cause severe distress and disability. The severity of fatigue is independent of the severity of liver disease or other symptoms and of psychiatric factors. The cause of fatigue is unknown, and numerous pathological and neurophysiological mechanisms have been unconvincingly proposed including daytime somnolence, autonomic dysfunction, and cognitive impairment (Hollingsworth et al., 2008, 2009; Newton et al., 2011; Pearce et al., 2011; Hale et al., 2012). Pruritus is the second most common symptom of PBC; long-term observations showed that most patients experience pruritus, especially at advanced stages. It can anticipate jaundice by months or years. Pruritus is usually diffuse, typically worsens at night and following contact with certain fabrics (wool), or in a warm climate. Recent studies point towards lysophosphatidic acid (LPA), a potent neuronal activator, as a pruritogen in cholestasis pruritus (Kremer et al., 2011). Specific treatments are awaited. Cholestyramine (4 g before and after the first meal) improves pruritus. The only other pharmaceutical therapies are short cycles of rifampin or opiate antagonists. Intractable pruritus can require liver transplantation. Portal hypertension develops in over 50% of untreated patients over a 4-year follow-up and may manifest at upper digestive endoscopy before other signs of liver cirrhosis appear.

Metabolic bone disease in PBC is secondary to reduced bone deposition. Therapy includes oral calcium supplementation, weight-bearing activity, and vitamin D replacement if a deficiency is present; bisphosphonates appear to be safe but benefits are inconclusive (Rudic et al., 2011). Dyslipidemia is present in up to 85% of patients with PBC and may precede the diagnosis with elevations of both serum cholesterol and serum triglyceride levels but these do not correlate with the risk of cardiovascular events or atherosclerosis as measured by intima-media thickness of carotid arteries (Longo et al., 2002).

Coexistence with other autoimmune diseases occurs with PBC in 70% of patients (Table 62.1) with co-morbidities including keratoconjunctivitis sicca, Raynaud's phenomenon, and limited cutaneous systemic sclerosis (lcSS). Systemic lupus erythematosus (lupus) was highlighted as a frequently self-reported coexistence in one large cohort of patients with PBC but this was unconfirmed in other studies and could be an overestimation attributable to autoantibody misinterpretation.

Hepatocellular carcinoma (HCC) is a risk in PBC as for other chronic cirrhotic liver conditions, and should be monitored for using ultrasonography (and CT in selected cases), particularly when orthotopic liver transplantation (OLT) is being considered (Cavazza et al., 2009). There is no association with cholangiocarcinoma in contrast to primary sclerosing cholangitis (PSC) (see Chapter 63) or with breast carcinoma as previously suspected.

Epidemiology and Natural History

PBC epidemiology is mainly descriptive. Published studies have major methodological flaws such as non-uniform

TABLE 62.1 Prevalence of Disorders Associated with PBC Derived from Clinical Studies. Other associations Suggested by Limited Case Reports are Not Indicated Herein

	Prevalence in PBC	Reference
Keratoconjunctivitis sicca	75%	Tsianos et al. (1990)
Renal tubular acidosis[a]	50%	Pares et al. (1981)
Reduced alveolar diffusion capacity[a]	39%	Costa et al. (1995)
Raynaud's phenomenon	32%	Marasini et al. (2001)
Hashimoto's disease	11%	Elta et al. (1983)
Celiac disease	6%	Kingham and Parker (1998)
Systemic sclerosis	12%	Marasini et al. (2001)

[a]Usually of limited clinical significance.

case definition; even so in most cases such definition is more solid compared to other similar autoimmune or chronic inflammatory diseases, notably PSC. Indeed, ideal population-based studies have not been performed to establish the true prevalence of PBC, as a noninvasive highly sensitive marker is not currently available. The most specific candidate marker is AMA, but this is negative in 5–10% of patients as discussed below, and the absence of disease registers precludes the recognition of all cases. Tables 62.2 and 62.3 cite PBC and AMA epidemiology in available studies. PBC is considered to be most prevalent among northern European and northern American populations, as shown in Table 62.2. The highest prevalence rate reported is 402 cases/million, but a true prevalence is undetermined as case finding methods overlook asymptomatic subjects marked only by abnormal tests of liver function and a positive test for AMA and, moreover, depend on physician awareness. Further, incidence rates appear to be increasing over time, perhaps real or secondary to more sensitive AMA laboratory tests and availability of better administrative datasets. Evidence suggests an unexplained seasonal and time clustering of newly diagnosed cases (McNally et al., 2009, 2011). There is a striking female predominance, about 10:1 (Table 62.2); yet, notably, the sex ratio among all AMA-positive samples in large serum collections is significantly lower, only 2–3:1. This suggests that a discrimination bias may apply also in this case, similar to what has been proposed for disease prevalence (Podda et al., 2013) (Table 62.3), or that "femaleness" may continue to influence progression after initial seroconversion. The characteristic female predominance in PBC could result from sex hormones acting on the immune system, the number of pregnancies, or sex chromosome abnormalities, as explained later.

Risk factors for PBC have been hypothesized from both epidemiological studies and a susceptible genetic background. In epidemiological surveys, history of recurrent urinary tract infections, co-morbidity like other autoimmune diseases, and lifestyle factors, such as smoking and a high-fat diet, are the most consistent findings, while less notable associations were reported for frequent use of hair dye or nail polish, and a higher family income (Prince et al., 2010) (Box 62.1). This latter factor is of interest as PBC is mainly asymptomatic and a higher social status may lead to better healthcare and an earlier recognition of the disease, and in women a more frequent use of cosmetics.

PBC progresses at a variable pace over time. One final note is related to the proposed ethnic and racial factors that may contribute to the cause of PBC. There is a variable prevalence, with subjects of African American descent being underrepresented among collected cases when compared to other chronic liver diseases or to the general population, and these show a more aggressive disease progression (Peters et al., 2007). Whether this could be related to genetics or to environmental factors, possibly insufficient vitamin D, remains to be determined.

Some patients have a stable disease without symptoms for decades and others rapidly advance towards end-stage liver disease. We can identify three periods: (1) an asymptomatic stage lasting even for decades in which the diagnosis is usually incidental; (2) a phase with non-specific symptoms and mild jaundice, with a shorter duration; and (3) a rapidly progressing pre-terminal stage with frank jaundice and complications of liver cirrhosis. The presence of symptoms at the time of diagnosis constitutes a major factor limiting survival (Pares and Rodes, 2003). Nevertheless, a shorter survival of presymptomatic patients was reported possibly secondary to a higher prevalence of non-hepatic causes

TABLE 62.2 Synopsis of Population-based Epidemiological Studies of PBC, with Further Details given by Boonstra et al. (2012)

Location	No. of Cases	Yearly Incidence	Prevalence	Sex Ratio (M/F)
Sheffield, UK	34	5.8	54	1:16
Dundee, UK	21	10.6	40.2	1:9.5
Newcastle, UK	117	10	37–144	1:14
Malmo, Sweden	33	4–24	28–92	1:3
Western Europe	569	4	23 (5–75)	1:10
Orebro, Sweden	18	14	128	1:3.5
Glasgow, UK	373	11–15	70–93	–
Umea, Sweden	111	13.3	151	1:6
Ontario, Canada	225	3.26	22.4	1:13
Northern England	347	19	129–154	1:9
Victoria, Australia	84	–	19.1	1:11
Estonia	69	2.27	26.9	1:22
Newcastle, UK	160	14–32	240	1:10
Olmsted County, MN (USA)	46	27	402	1:8
Sabadell, Spain	87	17	195	1:30
Alberta, Canada	137	30	227	1:5
Southern Israel	138	20	238	1:19
Iceland	168	22.5	383	1:4

Data are given per million and were obtained from multiple studies (Triger, 1980; Eriksson and Lindgren, 1984; Lofgren et al., 1985; Danielsson et al., 1990; James and Myszor, 1990; Myszor and James, 1990; Remmel et al., 1995; Metcalf et al., 1997; Berdal et al., 1998; Boberg et al., 1998; James et al., 1999; Kim et al., 2000; Pla et al., 2007; Rautiainen et al., 2007; Myers et al., 2009; Baldursdottir et al., 2012; Delgado et al., 2012).

TABLE 62.3 Synopsis of Population-Based Epidemiological Studies of Serum AMA Positivity

Reference	Region	No. of Subjects	AMA$^+$	Males (%)
Turchany et al. (1997)	Estonia	1565	14 (0.89%)	21
Mattalia et al. (1998)	Northern Italy	1530	9 (0.59%)	44
Shibata et al. (2004)	Japan	1714	11 (0.64%)	27
Lazaridis et al. (2007)	USA	196	2 (1.00%)	0
Liu X. et al. (2010)	Southern China	8126	35 (0.43%)	43

of death compared to deaths related to PBC (Prince et al., 2004). Multivariate analysis among symptomatic patients has indicated several factors that can negatively influence the outcome in PBC including clinical features (older age, ascites, edema, hepatic encephalopathy), analytical features (hyperbilirubinemia, hypoalbuminemia), and histological features (fibrosis or cirrhosis) (Pares and Rodes, 2003). The prognostic model based on the Mayo risk score is widely used for survival estimations (Grambsch et al., 1989) while PBC-specific ANA may also identify patients with a worse outcome, as discussed later.

Significant Associations

- Female sex
- Family history for PBC
- Non-PBC autoimmune disease (particularly autoimmune thyroiditis, Sjögren's syndrome, lupus)
- Pregnancies
- Former smoking habit
- History of recurrent vaginal of urinary tract infection
- Previous tonsillectomy
- Frequent use of hair dye
- Frequent use of nail polish
- Unlikely associations
- Previous surgery (particularly appendectomy, uterine surgery)
- Previous hepatitis A infection
- Use of contraceptive pill

No Association

- Dietary fat intake
- Childhood diseases
- Breast cancer

Treatment

Ursodeoxycholic acid (UDCA) is the only therapy that has received US Food and Drug Administration approval (Serfaty and Poupon, 2012). UDCA accounts for 4% of the bile acid pool in human bile and is more hydrophilic compared to other bile acids. UDCA action depends on (1) modification of the bile-acid pool, (2) reduction in proinflammatory cytokines, and (3) decreases in degrees of apoptosis and levels of vasoactive mediators (Poupon, 2012). Doses ranging from 13 to 20 mg/kg of UDCA lead to optimum bile enrichment, and long-term survival with UDCA therapy is higher than predictions based on mathematical models of survival for PBC. However, a meta-analysis of published trials indicated that UDCA influences biochemical factors and histology without improving survival, at least according to the Cochrane data base (Rudic et al., 2012). But, notably, a complete biochemical response to UDCA with normalization of serum liver tests in the absence of cirrhosis was achieved in some 40% of treated patients (Leuschner et al., 2000), and recent data suggested that a response at 12 months does predict a different outcome in patients receiving an adequate UDCA dose (Zhang et al., 2013).

The use of immunosuppressive/immunomodulatory drugs including azathioprine, cyclosporine, penicillamine, and colchicine is not recommended unless combined with UDCA in the autoimmune hepatitis–PBC overlap syndromes, while methotrexate with UDCA may prove beneficial in a subgroup of patients despite some safety concerns (Leung et al., 2011). Data on the effects of corticosteroids and fibrates in PBC are inconclusive particularly at early stages and their long-term use is not recommended pending longer clinical trials (Poupon, 2011) or unless autoimmune hepatitis features coexist (Tanaka et al., 2011a). Recent data on the use of B cell depletion for PBC suggest that this approach may help in UDCA non-responders (Tsuda et al., 2012), thus raising interesting questions on the role of B cells in PBC pathogenesis.

OLT is considered the *extrema ratio* treatment for end-stage PBC: interestingly, the effects of UDCA are making it less frequently needed (Singal et al., 2013). Post-OLT survival rates are excellent with either living or cadaver donors (Kashyap et al., 2010; Kaneko et al., 2012). A re-transplantation is needed in fewer than 10% of patients despite high recurrence rates of disease, possibly influenced by the use of specific immunosuppressive post-OLT regimens (Ilyas et al., 2011). The use of UDCA in patients receiving transplans is safe and needed when disease recurs since one would expect a similar natural history with AMA appearance and subsequent histological stages. PBC frequently recurs after OLT and data suggest incidence rates of 21–37% and 43% at 10 and 15 years, respectively, when histology is assessed (Carbone and Neuberger, 2011).

AUTOIMMUNE FEATURES

An autoimmune pathogenesis for PBC appears indisputable according to different lines of evidence, notably high levels/counts of serum autoantibodies and autoreactive T cells directed at overlapping epitopes on the mitochondrial constituent pyruvate dehydrogenase complex (Folci et al., 2012), and/or reactivity to nuclear autoantigens (ANA) of very particular specificities. Detectable AMA in serum exist in some 90% of affected individuals, but AMA negative cases are clinically similar, and AMA titers do not correlate with disease staging or grading (Selmi et al., 2008b). If ANA positivity were taken into account, then nearly all cases of PBC could show seropositivity. Autoreactive T cells were equally detectable in the peripheral blood of AMA positive and negative PBC cases and virtually all patients with PBC, and recognize the same overlapping epitopes within the PDC-E2 autoantigens as do AMA (Selmi et al., 2011b). There is no direct proof for a pathogenic role of serum AMA in the bile duct injury observed in PBC but, as is well known, this applies to many other of the disease-specific autoantibodies with the exception of damaging anti-double-stranded DNA (dsDNA) antibody in lupus nephritis. Finally there is no established benefit from immunosuppressants in PBC but we should also note that long-term treatment is required and thus adequate clinical trials are poorly feasible.

AMA are directed against components of the 2-oxoacid dehydrogenase complexes (2-OADCs), a family of functionally related enzymes within the mitochondrial respiratory chain. Recognized autoantigens include particularly the E2 subunit of the pyruvate dehydrogenase complex (PDC), the E3 binding protein (E3BP) of PDC, and the E2 subunit of the 2-oxoglutarate dehydrogenase complex (OGDC-E2) and the branched-chain 2-oxo acid dehydrogenase complex (BCOADC-E2). In particular, these autoantigens include closely-related conformational epitopes, notably the inner lipoylated domains of all three complexes. The lipoic acid cofactor has been suggested as contributing to epitope recognition (Bruggraber et al., 2003), but results on this have been conflicting.

Antinuclear antibodies (ANA) are detectable in PBC sera by indirect immunofluorescence (IIF), and three patterns are described, i.e., "nuclear rim," "multiple nuclear dots" (MND), and anti-centromere. The nuclear rim pattern depends on the recognition of proteins gp210 and nucleoporin 62 within the nuclear pore complex and on the MND pattern on the Sp100 and promyelocytic leukemia (PML) proteins, and the anti-centromere pattern is seen in cases of lcSS. Interestingly, the presence of serum reactivity against proteins from the nuclear pore complex (gp210, p62) in PBC was found to be associated with a more severe disease in longitudinal studies (Wesierska-Gadek et al., 2006; Nakamura et al., 2007). The nuclear body protein Sp100 and PML, giving the MND pattern, have been shown to be complexed with small ubiquitin-like molecules (SUMO) for cell transport regulation, and SUMO are in turn independent antigens specific for ANA-positive PBC (Janka et al., 2005). The anti-centromere antibodies (ACA) in patients with PBC and limited cutaneous systemic sclerosis possibly signify a more benign PBC phenotype (Rigamonti et al., 2006).

Cumulatively, serum ANAs are detected in 30−50% of patients with PBC but, as for AMA, their pathogenic role is undetermined. The IIF staining patterns of these PBC-related ANAs do not in any way point to a coexisting SLE. The T cell response in PBC is characterized by a multilineage reactivity to PDC-E2 epitopes with participation of Th1 CD4$^+$ T cells and CD8$^+$ T cells: the latter are considered as the true effectors by reason of their prevalence at sites of bile duct injury (Shimoda et al., 2008b) and capacity to transfer biliary disease in animal models (Yang et al., 2008; Kawata et al., 2013). Most recently, a detailed phenotype of the CD8$^+$ T cell subpopulations in PBC was derived using peripheral blood, demonstrating a higher frequency of effector memory CD8 T cells (CD45RO^{high} CD57$^+$ CD8^{high}) and the gut homing integrin $\alpha 4\beta 7$ (Tsuda et al., 2011). Such CD8^{high} effector memory T cells accumulate within the portal

areas of PBC liver samples, respond to the peptide epitope of PDC-E2 associated with HLA class I, and thus contribute to the destruction of intrahepatic bile ducts; this in turn may further costimulate an overall T cell response (Kamihira et al., 2005). Likely participants are also autoreactive CD4$^+$ T cells of phenotype Th1 that respond to PDC-E2 163-176 in a "universal" fashion, regardless of serum AMA positivity (Shimoda et al., 2008a). These results can be aligned with the striking observation in PBC of a 100−150-fold increase in the precursor frequency of PDC-E2-specific T cells in the hilar lymph nodes and liver compared with counts in peripheral blood (Shimoda et al., 1998). The Th17 and T regulatory profiles also have been investigated in PBC, as in other autoimmune conditions. There is an elevation of levels in blood of Th17-related cytokines and the number of Th17 cells in peripheral blood of patients with PBC (Rong et al., 2009), and in liver of PBC animal models (Lan et al., 2009), and numbers of T regulatory cells (FoxP3 expression) are significantly reduced in PBC (Rong et al., 2009). This is similar to autoimmune hepatitis where Tregs are quantitatively reduced (Longhi et al., 2012) and possibly functionally impaired, although the latter observation has not been confirmed and its relevance needs to be determined (Fenoglio et al., 2012).

GENETIC FEATURES
Familial PBC: Twins and Relatives

The concordance for PBC among monozygotic (MZ) twins is 63%, among the highest reported among autoimmune diseases (Bogdanos et al., 2012), and significantly higher than concordance for dizygotic twins (Selmi et al., 2004). Nevertheless, phenotype differences are found also in twin pairs concordant for PBC including significant differences in disease progression and severity. Further, the frequency of PBC is higher among relatives of affected individuals and the term "familial PBC" has been coined to indicate families that have more than one case. Variable rates of familial PBC are seen in different geographical areas, possibly due to different methods of case ascertainment but also perhaps to differences in local environmental provocation. As with disease prevalence estimates, family studies have significant limits, since the reported methodology was substantially based on case-note review, with criteria for case ascertainment neither uniform nor clearly illustrated, no attempt made to calculate the size of the patient pedigree, and no control group available for comparison of the population prevalence rate. In general, data indicate that 1−6% of PBC cases have at least one other family member with the disease (Table 62.4), and a higher prevalence is ascertained for serum AMA (Lazaridis et al., 2007). Of note, serum AMA in first-

TABLE 62.4 Prevalence of Familial Cases of PBC

Affected Families	First-Degree Relatives	Author, Year
17 (4.3%)	–	Bach and Schaffner (1994)
6 (3.8%)	8 (1.1%)	Brind et al. (1995)
10 (6.4%)	5 (3.2%)	Floreani et al. (1997)
8 (5.1%)	8 (5.0%)	Jones et al. (1999)
8 (3.6%)	8 (5.1 %)	Tsuji et al. (1999)
17 (4.3%)	57 (5.5%)	
57 (5.5%)	8 (3.6%)	Corpechot et al. (2010)

degree relatives supports the role of genetic factors in loss of tolerance towards mitochondrial antigens. Earlier studies based on indirect immunofluorescence for AMA reported familial prevalence rates for AMA between 4.9 and 7.4% (Feizi et al., 1972; Galbraith et al., 1974), but recent data for first-degree relatives using recombinant mitochondrial autoantigens gave an overall 13.1% prevalence, with higher rates, as expected, in siblings (Lazaridis et al., 2007) that had been largely excluded from previous studies. In conclusion, the occurrence of PBC among first-degree relatives of patients—"familial PBC"—is common and these have a 50–100-fold higher risk to develop PBC (Selmi et al., 2008a), particularly so for mothers, sisters, and daughters (Lazaridis et al., 2007). Cumulatively, the sibling relative risk, that is the risk for having PBC of a subject with a sibling affected by the disease, is 10.5, among the highest for autoimmune diseases.

HLA Association

An HLA association with one or another class 2 DR alleles is such a characteristic of human autoimmune diseases that we are surprised by the weakness and regionality of such an association for PBC; this has not been satisfactorily explained (Invernizzi, 2011). The susceptibility (DR8) and protective (DR11) associations have now been confirmed in different populations and fine mapping has most recently proposed a better definition of the associated loci (Invernizzi et al., 2012), following GWAS data (Hirschfeld and Invernizzi, 2011) and pathway-based analyses (Kar et al., 2013).

Genome-wide Association Studies (GWAS)

GWAS studies can provide substantial information about gene polymorphisms and disease association provided that adequately large and well-characterized samples of patients and, more importantly, controls are included (see Chapter 26). Recent studies have disclosed consistent

associations but the candidate polymorphisms were found only in a fraction of patients, thus limiting the clinical use of the data. Patients from Canada and the USA (Hirschfeld et al., 2009) or Italy (Liu X et al., 2010) were included in the earlier studies that reported associations with the gene loci for IL12A, IL12RB2, and STAT4 while a combined analysis of both cohorts confirmed these associations and identified new susceptibility loci at SPIB, IRF5-TNPO3, and a chromosome 17 region containing IKZF3-ZPBP2-GSDMB-ORMDL3 with unclear functional significance (Hirschfeld and Invernizzi, 2011). A GWAS on patients from Japan disclosed similar associations (Tanaka et al., 2011b). Among candidate genes, IL12A and IL12RB2 are pivotal in the immune responses against certain infectious diseases (Filipe-Santos et al., 2006), so that the PBC genetic association discerned by GWAS could be responsible of an impaired response to infection and determine an augmented risk to generate autoimmune responses (Selmi and Gershwin, 2009) and ultimately indicate new biotherapeutic approaches (Yeilding et al., 2011). Further studies have identified additional linked loci (Mells et al., 2011; Hirschfeld et al., 2012), and a pathway analysis supports an association with the tumor necrosis factor/stress-related signaling system (Kar et al., 2013). We may expect that next generation sequencing will provide new clues to genetic susceptibility to PBC.

Epigenetic Effects

Epigenetic effects are emerging as a promising field of research for autoimmune disease pathogenesis (see Chapter 28) but so far data for PBC are limited to just one study in monozygotic twins supporting the role of X chromosome gene methylation (Mitchell et al., 2011). We foresee that the genome-wide approach on specific cell subpopulations will in the coming years provide new data on the methylome and histone code associated with PBC, particularly in the unique model of monozygotic twin pairs.

Fetal Microchimerism

Similarly to other autoimmune diseases that are prevalent in women following their reproductive years (Selmi et al., 2012a,b,c), an effect of fetal microchimerism has been a suggested contributor to PBC, according to small amounts of fetal (paternal) DNA being found in the maternal liver (Stevens et al., 2004). This is an intriguing hypothesis wherein microchimerism due to replicating fetus-derived lymphocytes induces a condition analogous to chronic graft-versus-host disease (Nelson, 2003). However, the data are cumulatively unconvincing (Tanaka et al., 1999).

Genes on the X Chromosome

There are genes on the X chromosome, including but not limited to the gene for FoxP3, that are critical to the maintenance of physiological sex hormone levels and, more importantly, of immune responsiveness (see Chapter 24, Selmi, 2012b). This is well represented in clinical practice by autoimmune features in women with a constitutional X monosomy, i.e., Turner syndrome (Lleo et al., 2012a). An age-dependent enhanced monosomy X in peripheral blood leukocytes of women with PBC was reported (Invernizzi et al., 2004) indicative of a polygenic model for PBC with an X-linked major locus of susceptibility in which genes escaping inactivation are major candidates (Mitchell et al., 2011). These data, of note, have been recapitulated in other autoimmune diseases with an advanced age onset, such as systemic sclerosis (scleroderma) and autoimmune thyroid disease (Invernizzi et al., 2005), but not in younger women with systemic lupus erythematosus (Invernizzi et al., 2007). Finally, one fascinating observation is the enhanced loss of the Y chromosome in men with PBC (Lleo et al., 2013).

ENVIRONMENTAL PROVOCATION OF PBC

The paucity in PBC of strong genetic associations and the less than complete concordance in MZ twins suggest that environmental influences must contribute to autoimmunity in PBC (Liang et al., 2011). As other evidence there is a latitudinal gradient for PBC prevalence, coined geoepidemiology, quite similar to that pertaining for other autoimmune diseases. The epidemiology data report the highest incidence of PBC in northern European countries, namely northern England and Scandinavia, and northern American regions, i.e., in one Minnesota county. However, these data may be biased by different and usually better methodologies for diagnosis (Selmi, 2012a,c).

Infections

The ability of infectious agents, particularly bacteria, to induce autoimmune responses in the human setting is well accepted, noting the association between streptococcal infections and rheumatic carditis. Molecular mimicry is the most widely studied explanation. In the case of PBC, evidence points to *Escherichia coli* according to reports of an increased prevalence of urinary tract infections, *Chlamydia pneumoniae* infections despite some conflicting results, and occurrence of *Novosphingobium aromaticivorans* infection (Selmi et al., 2003). Whether the proposed associations are based merely on cross-reactivity noting the high similarity of PDC-E2 across species (yeast and some bacteria) remains to be determined (Ortega-Hernandez et al., 2010). In the case of *N. aromaticivorans*, data from infected mice support a more direct pathogenic role (Mattner et al., 2008).

Xenobiotics

These are foreign (non-self) compounds that may either alter or form complexes with defined self proteins, so inducing a change in the molecular structure of the native protein sufficient to induce an immune response to the complexed self protein (Selmi et al., 2010). Such an immune response may then result in the cross-recognition of the self form, thereby perpetuating the immune response and leading on to chronic autoimmunity (Selmi et al., 2011b). Results from experiments in animals and serological data in humans support this hypothesis as a cause of PBC (Leung et al., 2012), and data include the induction of PBC-like liver lesions in experimental models and the study in humans of serum reactivity against specific compounds included in cosmetic products (Leung et al., 2007; Wakabayashi et al., 2009; Chen et al., 2013). This latter association appears fascinating in the context of the female predisposition to PBC and the role of other PBC risk factors. A provocative effect for a number of specific environmental compounds has been proposed for various other autoimmune conditions (see Chapter 21), and are shown in Table 62.5. Whatever the case, it is difficult to escape the conclusion that the "etiology" of PBC (and most other autoimmune diseases) depends on unfortunate combinations of multiple genetic and environmental risk factors each individually conferring a relatively low risk but cumulatively "spilling over" to create an autoimmune phenotype.

EXPERIMENTAL ANIMAL MODELS

Obviously the availability of a valid animal model would be extremely helpful in elucidating the multi-factorial causation and relentless progression of human PBC. Several models,

TABLE 62.5 The Role of Xenobiotics in Autoimmune Disease

Compound	Associated Autoimmune Condition
Mercury	Immune complex formation
	Glomerulonephritis
Iodine	Autoimmune thyroiditis
Vinyl chloride	Scleroderma-like disease
Contaminated L-tryptophan	Eosinophilia myalgia syndrome
Toxic oil	Scleroderma-like disease
Silica	Rheumatoid arthritis
	Systemic lupus erythematosus (SLE)
	Scleroderma
Halothane	Autoimmune hepatitis
Canavanine	SLE-like syndromes
6-Bromohexanoate	PBC

For a complete discussion please refer to the recent NIEHS workshop results (Germolec et al., 2012; Selmi et al., 2012a,b,c).

mostly murine, were proposed in earlier years, albeit with some limitations. However, from 2006, novel and informative experimental models of PBC have been developed. These are subdivisible into spontaneously occurring models based on germline genetic modifications, and induced models based on immunization with xenobiotics structurally similar to PDC-E2 (Tsuneyama et al., 2012). These models are listed and compared in Table 62.6. The spontaneous models include (1) NOD.c3c4 congenic mice, (2) dominant negative TGF-β receptor II mice, (3) IL-2a (CD25)$^{-/-}$ mice, (4) Ae2$_{a,b}$$^{-/-}$ mice, and (5) scurfy mice. The induced xenobiotic-immunized models are represented by (1) 6-bromohexanoate-immunized guinea pigs, and (2) 2-octanoic acid-immunized mice. Of note, all models share the occurrence of high-titer serum AMA (and sometimes other autoantibodies as well) and exhibit hepatocellular and cholangiocellular injury inflicted by the infiltrating lymphocytes, and express a similar proinflammatory cytokine profile. Some of these models have already been used to investigate the impact of pathway-specific treatments, as in the case of B cell depletion (Dhirapong et al., 2011) or IL-12 (Lleo et al., 2012b). In this case, the deletion of the gene encoding for one IL-12 subunit led to an amelioration of the PBC-like pathology in the TGF-βRII model (Yoshida et al., 2009). Nevertheless, the nature of the liver pathology is frequently unclear as some models manifest features uncommon in human PBC, i.e., peritonitis in the 2-octanoic acid-induced model or inflammatory bowel disease in the

CD25$^{-/-}$ model; also the models fail to recapitulate the female sex imbalance characteristic of human PBC.

Several obstacles still militate against the development of a consistent and reliable animal model for PBC, one being a long latency between the appearance of AMA and the occurrence of liver pathology as pertains also in humans, and may well be reflective of autoimmune disease in general. However, it is a drawback given the short life expectancy of the experimental mice. On the positive side the models developed so far have provided very useful lessons in (1) showing the tightness of the nexus between AMA reactivity and biliary epithelial cell pathology, (2) indicating that deficiency in the Treg compartment is highly complicit in the genesis of human PBC, (3) identifying target-specific pathways that might be utilized to modulate the disease, and (4) maintaining confidence in the participation of environment (xenobiotic agents) in pathogenesis.

PATHOLOGIC EFFECTOR MECHANISMS

The striking tissue specificity of the pathology observed in PBC has been the focus of different lines of research. An earlier thesis was that anti-PDC-E2 antisera reacted not only with PDC-E2 in mitochondria but additionally with material located at the apical end of the biliary epithelial cell (BEC) in close apposition to the cell surface (Van de Water et al., 1993). Similarly postulated was an

TABLE 62.6 PBC Animal Models Proposed since 2006

	NOD.c3c4 mice (Irie et al., 2006)	dnTGF-βRII mice (Oertelt et al., 2006)	IL-2 Rα$^{-/-}$ mice (Wakabayashi et al., 2006)	Scurfy mice (Zhang et al., 2009)	Ae2$_{a,b}$$^{-/-}$ mice (Salas et al., 2008)	6-BH- immunized guinea pigs (Leung et al., 2007)	2-OA- immunized mice (Wakabayashi et al., 2008)
AMA	50–6%	100%	100%	10%	40–80%	100%	100%
Biliary damage	+	+	+	+	+	+	+
Granuloma	+	+	+/−	−		+	+
Proinflammatory cytokines	+	+	+	+	+	+	+
Collateral observations	Biliary dilatation	Moderate colitis	Severe colitis Severe hemolytic anemia	Short lifespan	Late onset	Late onset	peritonitis

In all cases the main AMA target is PDC-E2.
Modified from Tsuneyama et al. (2012).

aberrant expression in PBC of a molecule that shared epitopes with PDC-E2 and was located exclusively in the BECs targeted by the immune system (Joplin et al., 1997). If this material were to be derived from PDC-E2, there could be sequence variants common in PBC patients that lead to an altered turnover of the molecule, and high accumulation of PDC-E2 specifically in BECs. Moreover, chemicals (xenobiotics) metabolized by the liver could significantly modify PDC-E2, so leading to the production of such variants (Leung et al., 2012). It is noteworthy that the material is found in association with IgA and the polymeric Ig receptor (Migliaccio et al., 1998; Fukushima et al., 2002) on the cell membranes of cholangiocytes. However, interest in this line of research has waned.

A more contemporary theory seeks to explain PBC tissue specificity by unique features of apoptosis affecting the cholangiocyte. Thus during apoptosis PDC-E2 remains intact and maintains its immunogenicity, due to a cell-specific lack of glutathionylation within BECs, and the postulate is that intact PDC-E2 in apoptotic fragments could be taken up by local antigen-presenting cells and transferred to regional (portal) lymph nodes for priming of cognate T cells, thus initiating the PBC cascade (Lleo and Invernizzi, 2013). As direct evidence of this, Lleo and colleagues demonstrated that PDC-E2 is found in the blebs of human intrahepatic bile duct cells undergoing apoptosis and this effect was not observed in other epithelial cell lines (Lleo et al., 2009). Although the biliary epithelium represents only a small proportion of all liver cells, these cells contribute to the induction of immune activity against microbes and foreign antigens as they express HLA and adhesion molecules. Thus cholangiocytes may be implicated in the failure of immune tolerance by impairment of a correct clearance process of apoptotic cells by specific local phagocytes, and cell lysates can release intracellular molecules initiating the autoimmune reaction when taken up by local macrophages. Similar ideas have been invoked by others in different contexts, with the immunogenic apoptosis-derived material being specified as an "apotope" (Lleo et al., 2008; Reed et al., 2008; Rudic et al., 2011). Additional items, as recently suggested (Rong et al., 2009; Fenoglio et al., 2012), include alterations in the balance of Th17 cells and Tregs (Fenoglio et al., 2012), and activity of NK and NKT cells (Shimoda et al., 2012). B cell/antibody effects have received relatively little attention as pathogenic effectors, but we draw attention to the sometimes prominent presence of plasma cells among the periductular lymphoid infiltrates in human PBC, and the ameliorative effects in PBC of the anti-CD20 monoclonal rituximab (Tsuda et al., 2012). All in all, PBC well illustrates the multiplicity of contributors to the autoimmune-orchestrated response against intrahepatic cholangiocytes.

AUTOANTIBODIES AS POTENTIAL IMMUNOLOGIC MARKERS

The significance of serum autoantibodies in PBC pathogenesis was the subject of a previous paragraph but we discuss here the appropriate clinical use of the available diagnostic tests. Serum AMA remains the most widely utilized test when PBC is suspected and indirect immunofluorescence is the routine test for their detection. Notably, there is significantly lower operator variability than for serum ANA patterns. However, increasingly, less labor-intensive methods such as commercially available ELISAs and immunoblots are being used, at least for preliminary screens, and comparative tests are becoming available (Liu X et al., 2010; Bizzaro et al., 2012). Although "traditionalists" prefer to use indirect immunofluorescence primarily, they would call on second-level tests (Western blot and ELISA) to confirm the immunofluorescence results, and particularly to detect AMA in a suspected case of PBC with a negative test by IIF. Because of the higher sensitivity of the ELISA test, the number of AMA-negative PBC patients has been decreasing (Liu X et al., 2010; Bizzaro et al., 2012). On the contrary, Western blot (which detects autoantibodies to the E2 subunit of all three of the 2-OADC enzymes) represents the most specific method for AMA detection. The introduction of a triple hybrid recombinant mitochondrial preparation for Western blot and ELISA has increased the sensitivity and the specificity of the diagnostic tests with reduction in the proportion of AMA-negative PBC (Moteki et al., 1996). The presence of AMA in as many as 73% of IIF-negative patients was identified using a recombinant mitochondrial preparation in an ELISA format (Miyakawa et al., 2001), and the use of a multiplex platform further increased the sensitivity of detection methods (Oertelt et al., 2007). However, and of particular note, head-to-head comparisons of the available tests have not been performed in a rigorous fashion using histology as the gold standard, meaning that we do not really know the rate of "falsely positive" tests for PBC by any test format. Some may hold that a positive test always heralds "incipient" PBC but we cannot be sure of this.

As previously discussed, 30–50% of PBC sera are also ANA positive, and possibly even more among those AMA negative by IIF. It is a pity that the historically embedded term "ANA" has been retained for these because this term is so tightly linked in practitioners' minds with lupus. In fact PBC-associated ANA has nothing to do with lupus, particularly since the homogeneous pattern characteristic of lupus is virtually absent in PBC, while one or another of the other three "PBC-related" ANA patterns by IIF are common. One of these, anti-centromere, specifies the unique syndrome of mixed PBC-limited cutaneous systemic sclerosis. Other PBC-specific ANA antigens include those that give by IIF the multiple nuclear dot pattern (Sp100/PML), or rim pattern (gp210/p62) for which serological kits are commercially available and their detection may prove helpful in AMA-negative cases suspect for PBC (Liu X et al., 2010). Among less specific serum markers, variable proportions of PBC sera manifest positivity for rheumatoid factor, smooth muscle antibody, anti-thyroglobulin antibody, and anti-ribonucleoprotein antibody, but definitive data on the significance of these other autoantibodies in PBC are not available despite observations that anti-RNP antibody-positive subjects frequently manifest PBC (Takada et al., 2008). One serum antibody that warrants further investigation is that directed at Ro52/TRIM21 which is observed, albeit not specifically, in a proportion of PBC cases (Chou et al., 1995; Takada et al., 2007). So, in conclusion, it is not too much to say that with the present availability of serological tests for ANA and AMA based on recombinant antigens, PBC is the most amenable among all of autoimmune diseases to expect an accurate laboratory serological diagnosis.

CONCLUDING REMARKS—FUTURE PROSPECTS

PBC is indeed a characteristic disease within the ambit of autoimmunity and amply fulfills the defining features for autoimmune disorders, including the association with highly epitope-specific autoantibodies and autoreactive T cells. Yet there are some unusual features, notably (1) the insensitivity of PBC to conventional immunosuppressive drugs but responsiveness to UDCA which is not a first-line therapy for any other autoimmune disease, (2) the relative weakness of the genetic associations, including HLA, and (3) the histological non-caseating granulomas among the cellular infiltrates in the liver. However, regarding genetics, informative immune models in animals, mainly inbred mice, indicate that genetically-based immune derangements are critical to pathogenesis, notwithstanding disappointing data from GWAS so far. The extreme female predisposition to the disease is puzzling but may be just the top end of the general female predisposition to autoimmunity. Also, the pathogenetic pathways to the characteristic terminal cholangiolitic damage are not clear, although immunohistological evidence in human PBC points to CD8$^+$ T cell cytotoxicity. From where might come the solution to the riddle of autoimmunity in PBC? One opinion is that this might come from the study of very large numbers of PBC cases and their families, and more searching GWAS with even larger cohorts of cases categorized according to location and disease features, along with the implementation of next generation deep sequencing that could at least unravel the complex genetic basis of PBC. Or it could come from the development in the laboratory of novel experimental models that are more directly representative than those hitherto of human PBC. Or it could even come from some serendipitous result obtained by an astute researcher whose primary investigational enquiries bore no direct relationship to PBC.

REFERENCES

Ahrens Jr., E.H., Payne, M.A., Kunkel, H.G., Eisenmenger, W.J., Blondheim, S.H., 1950. Primary biliary cirrhosis. Medicine (Baltimore). 29, 299–364.

Bach, N., Schaffner, F., 1994. Familial primary biliary cirrhosis. J. Hepatol. 20, 698–701.

Baldursdottir, T.R., Bergmann, O.M., Jonasson, J.G., Ludviksson, B.R., Axelsson, T.A., Björnsson, E.S., 2012. The epidemiology and natural history of primary biliary cirrhosis, a nationwide population-based study. Eur. J. Gastroenterol. Hepatol. 24, 824–830.

Berdal, J.E., Ebbesen, J., Rydning, A., 1998. [Incidence and prevalence of autoimmune liver diseases]. Tidsskr. Nor. Laegeforen. 118, 4517–4519.

Bizzaro, N., Covini, G., Rosina, F., Muratori, P., Tonutti, E., Villalta, D., et al., 2012. Overcoming a probable diagnosis in antimitochondrial antibody negative primary biliary cirrhosis, study of 100 sera and review of the literature. Clin. Rev. Allergy Immunol. 42, 288–297.

Boberg, K., Aadland, E., Jahnsen, J., Raknerud, N., Stiris, M., Bell, H., 1998. Incidence and prevalence of primary biliary cirrhosis, primary sclerosing cholangitis, and autoimmune hepatitis in a Norwegian population. Scand. J. Gastroenterol. 33, 99–103.

Bogdanos, D.P., Smyk, D.S., Rigopoulou, E.I., Mytilinaiou, M.G., Heneghan, M.A., Selmi, C., et al., 2012. Twin studies in autoimmune disease: genetics, gender and environment. J. Autoimmun. 38, J156–J169.

Boonstra, K., Beuers, U., Ponsioen, C.Y., 2012. Epidemiology of primary sclerosing cholangitis and primary biliary cirrhosis: a systematic review. J. Hepatol. 56, 1181–1188.

Brind, A.M., Bray, G.P., Portmann, B.C., Williams, R., 1995. Prevalence and pattern of familial disease in primary biliary cirrhosis. Gut. 36, 615–617.

Bruggraber, S.F., Leung, P.S., Amano, K., Quan, C., Kurth, M.J., Nantz, M.H., et al., 2003. Autoreactivity to lipoate and a conjugated form of lipoate in primary biliary cirrhosis. Gastroenterology. 125, 1705–1713.

Carbone, M., Neuberger, J., 2011. Liver transplantation in PBC and PSC: indications and disease recurrence. Clin. Res. Hepatol. Gastroenterol. 35, 446–454.

Cavazza, A., et al., 2009. Incidence, risk factors, and survival of hepatocellular carcinoma in primary biliary cirrhosis: comparative analysis from two centers. Hepatology. 50, 1162–1168.

Chen, R.C., Caballería, L., Floreani, A., Farinati, F., Bruguera, M., Caroli, D., et al., 2013. Antimitochondrial antibody heterogeneity and the xenobiotic etiology of primary biliary cirrhosis. Hepatology. 57, 1498–1508.

Chou, M.J., Lee, S.L., Chen, T.Y., Tsay, G.J., 1995. Specificity of antinuclear antibodies in primary biliary cirrhosis. Ann. Rheum. Dis. 54, 148–151.

Corpechot, C., Chrétien, Y., Chazouillères, O., Poupon, R., 2010. Demographic, lifestyle, medical and familial factors associated with primary biliary cirrhosis. J. Hepatol. 53, 162–169.

Costa, C., Sambataro, A., Baldi, S., Modena, V., Todros, L., Libertucci, D., et al., 1995. Primary biliary cirrhosis: lung involvement. Liver. 15, 196–201.

Danielsson, A., Boqvist, L., Uddenfeldt, P., 1990. Epidemiology of primary biliary cirrhosis in a defined rural population in the northern part of Sweden. Hepatology. 11, 458–464.

Delgado, J.S., Vodonos, A., Delgado, B., Jotkowitz, A., Rosenthal, A., Fich, A., et al., 2012. Primary biliary cirrhosis in Southern Israel: a 20 year follow up study. Eur. J. Intern. Med. 23, e193–e198.

Dhirapong, A., Lleo, A., Yang, G.X., Tsuneyama, K., Dunn, R., Kehry, M., et al., 2011. B cell depletion therapy exacerbates murine primary biliary cirrhosis. Hepatology. 53, 527–535.

Elta, G.H., Sepersky, R.A., Goldberg, M.J., Connors, C.M., Miller, K.B., Kaplan, M.M., 1983. Increased incidence of hypothyroidism in primary biliary cirrhosis. Dig. Dis. Sci. 28, 971–975.

Eriksson, S., Lindgren, S., 1984. The prevalence and clinical spectrum of primary biliary cirrhosis in a defined population. Scand. J. Gastroenterol. 19, 971–976.

Feizi, T., Naccarato, R., Sherlock, S., Doniach, D., 1972. Mitochondrial and other tissue antibodies in relatives of patients with primary biliary cirrhosis. Clin. Exp. Immunol. 10, 609–622.

Fenoglio, D., Bernuzzi, F., Battaglia, F., Parodi, A., Kalli, F., Negrini, S., et al., 2012. Th17 and regulatory T lymphocytes in primary biliary cirrhosis and systemic sclerosis as models of autoimmune fibrotic diseases. Autoimmun. Rev. 12, 300–304.

Filipe-Santos, O., Bustamante, J., Chapgier, A., Vogt, G., de Beaucoudrey, L., Feinberg, J., et al., 2006. Inborn errors of IL-12/23- and IFN-gamma-mediated immunity: molecular, cellular, and clinical features. Semin. Immunol. 18, 347–361.

Floreani, A., Naccarato, R., Chiaramonte, M., 1997. Prevalence of familial disease in primary biliary cirrhosis in Italy. J. Hepatol. 26, 737–738.

Folci, M., Meda, F., Gershwin, M.E., Selmi, C., 2012. Cutting-edge issues in primary biliary cirrhosis. Clin. Rev. Allergy. Immunol. 42, 342–354.

Fukushima, N., Nalbandian, G., Van De Water, J., White, K., Ansari, A. A., Leung, P., et al., 2002. Characterization of recombinant monoclonal IgA anti-PDC-E2 autoantibodies derived from patients with PBC. Hepatology. 36, 1383–1392.

Galbraith, R.M., et al., 1974. High prevalence of seroimmunologic abnormalities in relatives of patients with active chronic hepatitis or primary biliary cirrhosis. N. Engl. J. Med. 290 (2), 63–69.

Germolec, D., Smith, M., Mackenzie, R.M., Tee, D.E., Doniach, D., Williams, R., 2012. Animal models used to examine the role of the environment in the development of autoimmune disease: findings from an NIEHS Expert Panel Workshop. J. Autoimmun. 39, 285–293.

Gershwin, M.E., Mackay, I.R., Sturgess, A., Coppel, R.L., 1987. Identification and specificity of a cDNA encoding the 70 kD mitochondrial antigen recognized in primary biliary cirrhosis. J. Immunol. 138, 3525–3531.

Grambsch, P.M., Dickson, E.R., Kaplan, M., LeSage, G., Fleming, T.R., Langworthy, A.L., 1989. Extramural cross-validation of the Mayo primary biliary cirrhosis survival model establishes its generalizability. Hepatology. 10, 846–850.

Hale, M., Newton, J.L., Jones, D.E., 2012. Fatigue in primary biliary cirrhosis. BMJ. 345, e7004.

Heathcote, E.J., 2000. Management of primary biliary cirrhosis. The American Association for the Study of Liver Diseases practice guidelines. Hepatology. 31, 1005–1013.

Hirschfield, G.M., Invernizzi, P., 2011. Progress in the genetics of primary biliary cirrhosis. Semin. Liver Dis. 31, 147–156.

Hirschfield, G.M., Liu, X., Xu, C., Lu, Y., Xie, G., Lu, Y., et al., 2009. Primary biliary cirrhosis associated with HLA, IL12A, and IL12RB2 variants. N. Engl. J. Med. 360, 2544–2555.

Hirschfield, G.M., Xie, G., Lu, E., Sun, Y., Juran, B.D., Chellappa, V., et al., 2012. Association of primary biliary cirrhosis with variants in the CLEC16A, SOCS1, SPIB and SIAE immunomodulatory genes. Genes. Immun. 13, 328–335.

Hollingsworth, K.G., Newton, J.L., Taylor, R., McDonald, C., Palmer, J.M., Blamire, A.M., et al., 2008. Pilot study of peripheral muscle function in primary biliary cirrhosis, potential implications for fatigue pathogenesis. Clin. Gastroenterol. Hepatol. 6, 1041–1048.

Hollingsworth, K.G., Jones, D.E., Aribisala, B.S., Thelwall, P.E., Taylor, R., Newton, J.L., et al., 2009. Globus pallidus magnetization transfer ratio, T(1) and T(2) in primary biliary cirrhosis: relationship with disease stage and age. J. Magn. Reson. Imaging. 29, 780–784.

Howel, D., Fischbacher, C.M., Bhopal, R.S., Gray, J., Metcalf, J.V., James, O.F., 2000. An exploratory population-based case-control study of primary biliary cirrhosis. Hepatology. 31, 1055–1060.

Ilyas, J.A., O'Mahony, C.A., Vierling, J.M., 2011. Liver transplantation in autoimmune liver diseases. Best. Pract. Res. Clin. Gastroenterol. 25, 765–782.

Invernizzi, P., 2011. Human leukocyte antigen in primary biliary cirrhosis: an old story now reviving. Hepatology. 54, 714–723.

Invernizzi, P., Miozzo, M., Battezzati, P.M., Bianchi, I., Grati, F.R., Simoni, G., et al., 2004. Frequency of monosomy X in women with primary biliary cirrhosis. Lancet. 363, 533–535.

Invernizzi, P., Miozzo, M., Selmi, C., Persani, L., Battezzati, P.M., Zuin, M., et al., 2005. X chromosome monosomy, a common mechanism for autoimmune diseases. J. Immunol. 175, 575–578.

Invernizzi, P., Miozzo, M., Oertelt-Prigione, S., Meroni, P.L., Persani, L., Selmi, C., et al., 2007. X monosomy in female systemic lupus erythematosus. Ann. N.Y. Acad. Sci. 1110, 84–91.

Invernizzi, P., Ransom, M., Raychaudhuri, S., Kosoy, R., Lleo, A., Shigeta, R., et al., 2012. Classical HLA-DRB1 and DPB1 alleles account for HLA associations with primary biliary cirrhosis. Genes Immun. 13, 461–468.

Irie, J., Wu, Y., Wicker, L.S., Rainbow, D., Nalesnik, M.A., Hirsch, R., et al., 2006. NOD.c3c4 congenic mice develop autoimmune biliary disease that serologically and pathogenetically models human primary biliary cirrhosis. J. Exp. Med. 203, 1209–1219.

James, O.F., Myszor, M., 1990. Epidemiology and genetics of primary biliary cirrhosis. Prog. Liver Dis. 9, 523–536.

James, O.F., Bhopal, R., Howel, D., Gray, J., Burt, A.D., Metcalf, J.V., 1999. Primary biliary cirrhosis once rare, now common in the United Kingdom? Hepatology. 30, 390–394.

Janka, C., Selmi, C., Gershwin, M.E., Will, H., Sternsdorf, T., 2005. Small ubiquitin-related modifiers, a novel and independent class of autoantigens in primary biliary cirrhosis. Hepatology. 41, 609–616.

Jones, D.E., Watt, F.E., Metcalf, J.V., Bassendine, M.F., James, O.F., 1999. Familial primary biliary cirrhosis reassessed: a geographically-based population study. J. Hepatol. 30, 402–407.

Joplin, R.E., Wallace, L.L., Lindsay, J.G., Palmer, J.M., Yeaman, S.J., Neuberger, J.M., 1997. The human biliary epithelial cell plasma membrane antigen in primary biliary cirrhosis: pyruvate dehydrogenase X? Gastroenterology. 113, 1727–1733.

Kamihira, T., Shimoda, S., Nakamura, M., Yokoyama, T., Takii, Y., Kawano, A., et al., 2005. Biliary epithelial cells regulate autoreactive T cells: implications for biliary-specific diseases. Hepatology. 41, 151–159.

Kaneko, J., Sugawara, Y., Tamura, S., Aoki, T., Hasegawa, K., Yamashiki, N., et al., 2012. Long-term outcome of living donor liver transplantation for primary biliary cirrhosis. Transpl. Int. 25, 7–12.

Kar, S.P., Seldin, M.F., Chen, W., Lu, E., Hirschfield, G.M., Invernizzi, P., et al., 2013. Pathway-based analysis of primary biliary cirrhosis genome-wide association studies. Genes Immun. 14, 179–186.

Kashyap, R., Safadjou, S., Chen, R., Mantry, P., Sharma, R., Patil, V., et al., 2010. Living donor and deceased donor liver transplantation for autoimmune and cholestatic liver diseases—an analysis of the UNOS database. J. Gastrointest. Surg. 14, 1362–1369.

Kawata, K., et al., 2013. Clonality, activated antigen specific CD8 T cells and development of autoimmune cholangitis in dnTGFbetaRII mice. Hepatology. 10.1002/hep.26418.

Kim, W.R., Lindor, K.D., Locke III, G.R., Therneau, T.M., Homburger, H.A., Batts, K.P., et al., 2000. Epidemiology and natural history of primary biliary cirrhosis in a US community. Gastroenterology. 119, 1631–1636.

Kingham, J.G., Parker, D.R., 1998. The association between primary biliary cirrhosis and coeliac disease: a study of relative prevalences. Gut. 42, 120–122.

Kremer, A.E., Oude Elferink, R.P., Beuers, U., 2011. Pathophysiology and current management of pruritus in liver disease. Clin. Res. Hepatol. Gastroenterol. 35, 89–97.

Lan, R.Y., Salunga, T.L., Tsuneyama, K., Lian, Z.X., Yang, G.X., Hsu, W., et al., 2009. Hepatic IL-17 responses in human and murine primary biliary cirrhosis. J. Autoimmun. 32, 43–51.

Lazaridis, K.N., Juran, B.D., Boe, G.M., Slusser, J.P., de Andrade, M., Homburger, H.A., et al., 2007. Increased prevalence of antimitochondrial antibodies in first-degree relatives of patients with primary biliary cirrhosis. Hepatology. 46, 785–792.

Leung, J., Bonis, P.A., Kaplan, M.M., 2011. Colchicine or methotrexate, with ursodiol, are effective after 20 years in a subset of patients with primary biliary cirrhosis. Clin. Gastroenterol. Hepatol. 9, 776–780.

Leung, P.S., Park, O., Tsuneyama, K., Kurth, M.J., Lam, K.S., Ansari, A., et al., 2007. Induction of primary biliary cirrhosis in guinea pigs following chemical xenobiotic immunization. J. Immunol. 179, 2651–2657.

Leung, P.S., Lam, K., Kurth, M.J., Coppel, R.L., Gershwin, M.E., 2012. Xenobiotics and autoimmunity: does acetaminophen cause primary biliary cirrhosis? Trends Mol. Med. 18, 577–582.

Leuschner, M., Dietrich, C.F., You, T., Seidl, C., Raedle, J., Herrmann, G., et al., 2000. Characterisation of patients with primary biliary cirrhosis responding to long term ursodeoxycholic acid treatment. Gut. 46, 121–126.

Liang, Y., Yang, Z., Zhong, R., 2011. Smoking, family history and urinary tract infection are associated with primary biliary cirrhosis: A meta-analysis. Hepatol. Res. 41, 572–578.

Liu, H., Liu, Y., Wang, L., Xu, D., Lin, B., Zhong, R., et al., 2010a. Prevalence of primary biliary cirrhosis in adults referring hospital for annual health check-up in Southern China. BMC Gastroenterol. 10, 100.

Liu, H., Norman, G.L., Shums, Z., Worman, H.J., Krawitt, E.L., Bizzaro, N., et al., 2010b. PBC screen, an IgG/IgA dual isotype ELISA detecting multiple mitochondrial and nuclear autoantibodies specific for primary biliary cirrhosis. J. Autoimmun. 35, 436–442.

Liu, X., Invernizzi, P., Lu, Y., Kosoy, R., Lu, Y., Bianchi, I., et al., 2010. Genome-wide meta-analyses identify three loci associated with primary biliary cirrhosis. Nat. Genet. 42, 658–660.

Lleo, A., Invernizzi, P., 2013. Apotopes and innate immune system. Novel players in the primary biliary cirrhosis scenario. Dig. Liver Dis. 45, 630–636.

Lleo, A., Selmi, C., Invernizzi, P., Podda, M., Gershwin, M.E., 2008. The consequences of apoptosis in autoimmunity. J. Autoimmun. 31, 257–262.

Lleo, A., Selmi, C., Invernizzi, P., Podda, M., Coppel, R.L., Mackay, I. R., et al., 2009. Apotopes and the biliary specificity of primary biliary cirrhosis. Hepatology. 49, 871–879.

Lleo, A., Gershwin, M.E., Mantovani, A., Invernizzi, P., 2012a. Towards common denominators in primary biliary cirrhosis: the role of IL-12. J. Hepatol. 56, 731–733.

Lleo, A., Moroni, L., Caliari, L., Invernizzi, P., 2012b. Autoimmunity and Turner's syndrome. Autoimmun. Rev. 11, A538–A543.

Lleo, A., Oertelt-Prigione, S., Bianchi, I., Caliari, L., Finelli, P., Miozzo, M., et al., 2013. Y chromosome loss in male patients with primary biliary cirrhosis. J. Autoimmun. 41, 87–91.

Lofgren, J., Järnerot, G., Danielsson, D., Hemdal, I., 1985. Incidence and prevalence of primary biliary cirrhosis in a defined population in Sweden. Scand. J. Gastroenterol. 20, 647–650.

Longhi, M.S., Ma, Y., Mieli-Vergani, G., Vergani, D., 2012. Regulatory T cells in autoimmune hepatitis. J. Hepatol. 57, 932–933.

Longo, M., Crosignani, A., Battezzati, P.M., Squarcia Giussani, C., Invernizzi, P., Zuin, M., et al., 2002. Hyperlipidaemic state and cardiovascular risk in primary biliary cirrhosis. Gut. 51, 265–269.

Ludwig, J., 2000. The pathology of primary biliary cirrhosis and autoimmune cholangitis. Baillieres Best Pract. Res. Clin. Gastroenterol. 14, 601–613.

Ludwig, J., Dickson, E.R., McDonald, G.S., 1978. Staging of chronic nonsuppurative destructive cholangitis (syndrome of primary biliary cirrhosis). Virchows. Arch. A. Pathol. Anat. Histol. 379, 103–112.

Marasini, B., Gagetta, M., Rossi, V., Ferrari, P., 2001. Rheumatic disorders and primary biliary cirrhosis: an appraisal of 170 Italian patients. Ann. Rheum. Dis. 60, 1046–1049.

Mattalia, A., Quaranta, S., Leung, P.S., Bauducci, M., Van de Water, J., Calvo, P.L., et al., 1998. Characterization of antimitochondrial antibodies in health adults. Hepatology. 27, 656–661.

Mattner, J., Savage, P.B., Leung, P., Oertelt, S.S., Wang, V., Trivedi, O., et al., 2008. Liver autoimmunity triggered by microbial activation of natural killer T cells. Cell Host. Microbe. 3, 304–315.

McNally, R.J., Ducker, S., James, O.F., 2009. Are transient environmental agents involved in the cause of primary biliary cirrhosis? Evidence from space-time clustering analysis. Hepatology. 50, 1169–1174.

McNally, R.J., James, P.W., Ducker, S., James, O.F., 2011. Seasonal variation in the patient diagnosis of primary biliary cirrhosis: further evidence for an environmental component to etiology. Hepatology. 54, 2099–2103.

Mells, G.F., Floyd, J.A., Morley, K.I., Cordell, H.J., Franklin, C.S., Shin, S.Y., et al., 2011. Genome-wide association study identifies 12 new susceptibility loci for primary biliary cirrhosis. Nat. Genet. 43, 329–332.

Metcalf, J.V., Bhopal, R.S., Gray, J., Howel, D., James, O.F., 1997. Incidence and prevalence of primary biliary cirrhosis in the city of Newcastle upon Tyne, England. Int. J. Epidemiol. 26, 830–836.

Migliaccio, C., Nishio, A., Van de Water, J., Ansari, A.A., Leung, P.S., Nakanuma, Y., et al., 1998. Monoclonal antibodies to mitochondrial E2 components define autoepitopes in primary biliary cirrhosis. J. Immunol. 161, 5157–5163.

Mitchell, M.M., Lleo, A., Zammataro, L., Mayo, M.J., Invernizzi, P., Bach, N., et al., 2011. Epigenetic investigation of variably X chromosome inactivated genes in monozygotic female twins discordant for primary biliary cirrhosis. Epigenetics. 6, 95–102.

Miyakawa, H., Tanaka, A., Kikuchi, K., Matsushita, M., Kitazawa, E., Kawaguchi, N., et al., 2001. Detection of antimitochondrial autoantibodies in immunofluorescent AMA-negative patients with primary biliary cirrhosis using recombinant autoantigens. Hepatology. 34, 243–248.

Moteki, S., Leung, P.S., Coppel, R.L., Dickson, E.R., Kaplan, M.M., Munoz, S., et al., 1996. Use of a designer triple expression hybrid clone for three different lipoyl domain for the detection of antimitochondrial autoantibodies. Hepatology. 24, 97–103.

Myers, R.P., Shaheen, A.A., Fong, A., Burak, K.W., Wan, A., Swain, M. G., et al., 2009. Epidemiology and natural history of primary biliary cirrhosis in a Canadian health region: a population-based study. Hepatology. 50, 1884–1892.

Myszor, M., James, O.F., 1990. The epidemiology of primary biliary cirrhosis in north-east England: an increasingly common disease?. Q. J. Med. 75, 377–385.

Nakamura, M., Kondo, H., Mori, T., Komori, A., Matsuyama, M., Ito, M., et al., 2007. Anti-gp210 and anti-centromere antibodies are different risk factors for the progression of primary biliary cirrhosis. Hepatology. 45, 118–127.

Nelson, J.L., 2003. Microchimerism in human health and disease. Autoimmunity. 36, 5–9.

Newton, J.L., Elliott, C., Frith, J., Ghazala, C., Pairman, J., Jones, D.E., 2011. Functional capacity is significantly impaired in primary biliary cirrhosis and is related to orthostatic symptoms. Eur. J. Gastroenterol. Hepatol. 23, 566–572.

Oertelt, S., Lian, Z.X., Cheng, C.M., Chuang, Y.H., Padgett, K.A., He, XS., et al., 2006. Anti-mitochondrial antibodies and primary biliary cirrhosis in TGF-beta receptor II dominant-negative mice. J. Immunol. 177, 1655–1660.

Oertelt, S., Rieger, R., Selmi, C., Invernizzi, P., Ansari, A.A., Coppel, R. L., et al., 2007. A sensitive bead assay for antimitochondrial antibodies. Chipping away at AMA-negative primary biliary cirrhosis. Hepatology. 45, 659–665.

Ortega-Hernandez, O.D., Levin, N.A., Altman, A., Shoenfeld, Y., 2010. Infectious agents in the pathogenesis of primary biliary cirrhosis. Dis. Markers. 29, 277–286.

Pares, A., Rodes, J., 2003. Natural history of primary biliary cirrhosis. Clin. Liver. Dis. 7, 779–794.

Pares, A., Rimola, A., Bruguera, M., Mas, E., Rodés, J., 1981. Renal tubular acidosis in primary biliary cirrhosis. Gastroenterology. 80, 681–686.

Pearce, R.M., Jones, D.E., Newton, J.L., 2011. Development of an evidence-based patient information medium, empowering newly diagnosed patients with primary biliary cirrhosis. J. Vis. Commun. Med. 34, 4–13.

Peters, M.G., Di Bisceglie, A.M., Kowdley, K.V., Flye, N.L., Luketic, V.A., Munoz, S.J., et al., 2007. Differences between Caucasian, African American, and Hispanic patients with primary biliary cirrhosis in the United States. Hepatology. 46, 769–775.

Pla, X., Vergara, M., Gil, M., Dalmau, B., Cisteró, B., Bella, R.M., et al., 2007. Incidence, prevalence and clinical course of primary biliary cirrhosis in a Spanish community. Eur. J. Gastroenterol. Hepatol. 19, 859–864.

Podda, M., Selmi, C., Lleo, A., et al., 2013. The limitations and hidden gems in the epidemiology of primary biliary cirrhosis. J. Autoimmun. 46, 81–87.

Poupon, R., 2011. Treatment of primary biliary cirrhosis with urso-deoxycholic acid, budesonide and fibrates. Dig. Dis. 29, 85–88.

Poupon, R., 2012. Ursodeoxycholic acid and bile-acid mimetics as thera-peutic agents for cholestatic liver diseases, an overview of their mechanisms of action. Clin. Res. Hepatol. Gastroenterol. 36, S3–12.

Prince, M.I., Chetwynd, A., Craig, W.L., Metcalf, J.V., James, O.F., 2004. Asymptomatic primary biliary cirrhosis, clinical features, prognosis, and symptom progression in a large population based cohort. Gut. 53, 865–870.

Prince, M.I., Ducker, S.J., James, O.F., 2010. Case-control studies of risk factors for primary biliary cirrhosis in two United Kingdom populations. Gut. 59, 508–512.

Rautiainen, H., Salomaa, V., Niemelä, S., Karvonen, A.L., Nurmi, H., Isoniemi, H., et al., 2007. Prevalence and incidence of primary bili-ary cirrhosis are increasing in Finland. Scand. J. Gastroenterol. 42, 1347–1353.

Reed, J.H., Jackson, M.W., Gordon, T.P., 2008. A B cell apotope of Ro 60 in systemic lupus erythematosus. Arthritis. Rheum. 58, 1125–1129.

Remmel, T., Remmel, H., Uibo, R., Salupere, V., 1995. Primary biliary cirrhosis in Estonia. With special reference to incidence, prevalence, clinical features, and outcome. Scand. J. Gastroenterol. 30, 367–371.

Rigamonti, C., Shand, L.M., Feudjo, M., Bunn, C.C., Black, C.M., Denton, C.P., et al., 2006. Clinical features and prognosis of primary biliary cirrhosis associated with systemic sclerosis. Gut. 55, 388–394.

Rong, G., Zhou, Y., Xiong, Y., Zhou, L., Geng, H., Jiang, T., et al., 2009. Imbalance between T helper type 17 and T regulatory cells in patients with primary biliary cirrhosis, the serum cytokine profile and peripheral cell population. Clin. Exp. Immunol. 156, 217–225.

Rudic, J.S., Giljaca, V., Krstic, M.N., Bjelakovic, G., Gluud, C., 2011. Bisphosphonates for osteoporosis in primary biliary cirrhosis. Cochrane Database Syst. Rev. 7,CD009144.

Rudic, J.S., Poropat, G., Krstic, M.N., Bjelakovic, G., Gluud, C., 2012. Ursodeoxycholic acid for primary biliary cirrhosis. Cochrane. Database. Syst. Rev. 12, CD000551.

Salas, J.T., Banales, J.M., Sarvide, S., Recalde, S., Ferrer, A., Uriarte, I., et al., 2008. Ae2a,b-deficient mice develop antimitochondrial anti-bodies and other features resembling primary biliary cirrhosis. Gastroenterology. 134, 1482–1493.

Selmi, C., Gershwin, M.E., 2009. The role of environmental factors in primary biliary cirrhosis. Trends Immunol. 30, 415–420.

Selmi, C., Balkwill, D.L., Invernizzi, P., Ansari, A.A., Coppel, R.L., Podda, M., et al., 2003. Patients with primary biliary cirrhosis react against a ubiquitous xenobiotic-metabolizing bacterium. Hepatology. 38, 1250–1257.

Selmi, C., Invernizzi, P., Keeffe, E.B., Coppel, R.L., Podda, M., Rossaro, L., et al., 2004. Epidemiology and pathogenesis of primary biliary cirrhosis. J. Clin. Gastroenterol. 38, 264–271.

Selmi, C., Zuin, M., Bowlus, C.L., Gershwin, M.E., 2008a. Anti-mitochondrial antibody-negative primary biliary cirrhosis. Clin. Liver. Dis. 12, 173–185.

Selmi, C., Zuin, M., Gershwin, M.E., 2008b. The unfinished business of primary biliary cirrhosis. J. Hepatol. 49, 451–460.

Selmi, C., Affronti, A., Ferrari, L., Invernizzi, P., 2010. Immune-mediated bile duct injury. The case of primary biliary cirrhosis. World J. Gastrointest. Pathophysiol. 1, 118–128.

Selmi, C., Bowlus, C.L., Gershwin, M.E., Coppel, R., 2011a. Primary biliary cirrhosis. Lancet. 377, 1600–1609.

Selmi, C., Mackay, I.R., Gershwin, M.E., 2011b. The autoimmunity of primary biliary cirrhosis and the clonal selection theory. Immunol. Cell. Biol. 89, 70–80.

Selmi, C., Maria Papini, A., Pugliese, P., Claudia Alcaro, M., Gershwin, M.E., 2011c. Environmental pathways to autoimmune diseases: the cases of primary biliary cirrhosis and multiple sclerosis. Arch. Med. Sci. 7, 368–380.

Selmi, C., Lu, Q., Humble, M.C., 2012a. Heritability versus the role of the environment in autoimmunity. J. Autoimmun. 39, 249–252.

Selmi, C., Brunetta, E., Raimondo, M.G., Meroni, P.L., 2012b. The X chromosome and the sex ratio of autoimmunity. Autoimmun. Rev. 11, A531–A537.

Selmi, C., Leung, P.S., Sherr, D.H., Diaz, M., Nyland, J.F., Monestier, M., et al., 2012c. Mechanisms of environmental influence on human autoimmunity: a National Institute of Environmental Health Sciences expert panel workshop. J. Autoimmun. 39, 272–284.

Serfaty, L., Poupon, R., 2012. Therapeutic approaches for hepatobiliary disorders with ursodeoxycholic acid and bile-acid derivatives. Clin. Res. Hepatol. Gastroenterol. 36, S1.

Sherlock, S., 1959. Primary biliary cirrhosis (chronic intrahepatic obstructive jaundice). Gastroenterology. 37, 574–586.

Shibata, M., Onozuka, Y., Morizane, T., Koizumi, H., Kawaguchi, N., Miyakawa, H., et al., 2004. Prevalence of antimitochondrial antibody in Japanese corporate workers in Kanagawa prefecture. J. Gastroenterol. 39, 255–259.

Shimoda, S., Van de Water, J., Ansari, A., Nakamura, M., Ishibashi, Coppel, R.L., et al., 1998. Identification and precursor frequency analysis of a common T cell epitope motif in mitochondrial auto-antigens in primary biliary cirrhosis. J. Clin. Invest. 102, 1831–1840.

Shimoda, S., Miyakawa, H., Nakamura, M., Ishibashi, H., Kikuchi, K., Kita, H., et al., 2008a. CD4 T-cell autoreactivity to the mitochon-drial autoantigen PDC-E2 in AMA-negative primary biliary cirrho-sis. J. Autoimmun. 31, 110–115.

Shimoda, S., Harada, K., Niiro, H., Yoshizumi, T., Soejima, Y., Taketomi, A., et al., 2008b. Biliary epithelial cells and primary bili-ary cirrhosis: the role of liver-infiltrating mononuclear cells. Hepatology. 47, 958–965.

Shimoda, S., Tsuneyama, K., Kikuchi, K., Harada, K., Nakanuma, Y., Nakamura, M., et al., 2012. The role of natural killer (NK) and NK T cells in the loss of tolerance in murine primary biliary cirrhosis. Clin. Exp. Immunol. 168, 279–284.

Singal, A.K., Guturu, P., Hmoud, B., Kuo, Y.F., Salameh, H., Wiesner, R.H., 2013. Evolving frequency and outcomes of liver transplanta-tion based on etiology of liver disease. Transplantation. 95, 755–760.

Stevens, A.M., McDonnell, W.M., Mullarkey, M.E., Pang, J.M., Leisenring, W., Nelson, J.L., 2004. Liver biopsies from human females contain male hepatocytes in the absence of transplantation. Lab. Invest. 84, 1603–1609.

Takada, K., Suzuki, K., Matsumoto, M., Okada, M., Nakanishi, T., Horikoshi, H., et al., 2007. Primary biliary cirrhosis in female subjects with sicca-associated antibodies. Mod. Rheumatol. 17, 486–491.

Takada, K., Suzuki, K., Matsumoto, M., Okada, M., Nakanishi, T., Horikoshi, H., et al., 2008. Clinical characteristics of patients with both anti-U1RNP and anti-centromere antibodies. Scand. J. Rheumatol. 37, 360–364.

Tanaka, A., Lindor, K., Gish, R., Batts, K., Shiratori, Y., Omata, M., et al., 1999. Fetal microchimerism alone does not contribute to the induction of primary biliary cirrhosis. Hepatology. 30, 833–838.

Tanaka, A., Invernizzi, P., Ohira, H., Kikuchi, K., Nezu, S., Kosoy, R., et al., 2011a. Replicated association of 17q12-21 with susceptibility of primary biliary cirrhosis in a Japanese cohort. Tissue Antigens. 78, 65–68.

Tanaka, A., Harada, K., Ebinuma, H., Komori, A., Yokokawa, J., Yoshizawa, K., et al., 2011b. Primary biliary cirrhosis–autoimmune hepatitis overlap syndrome: a rationale for corticosteroids use based on a nation-wide retrospective study in Japan. Hepatol. Res. 41, 877–886.

Triger, D.R., 1980. Primary biliary cirrhosis, an epidemiological study. Br. Med. J. 281, 772–775.

Tsianos, E.V., Hoofnagle, J.H., Fox, P.C., Alspaugh, M., Jones, E.A., Schafer, D.F., et al., 1990. Sjogren's syndrome in patients with primary biliary cirrhosis. Hepatology. 11, 730–734.

Tsuda, M., Ambrosini, Y.M., Zhang, W., Yang, G.X., Ando, Y., Rong, G., et al., 2011. Fine phenotypic and functional characterization of effector cluster of differentiation 8 positive T cells in human patients with primary biliary cirrhosis. Hepatology. 54, 1293–1302.

Tsuda, M., Moritoki, Y., Lian, Z.X., Zhang, W., Yoshida, K., Wakabayashi, K., et al., 2012. Biochemical and immunologic effects of rituximab in patients with primary biliary cirrhosis and an incomplete response to ursodeoxycholic acid. Hepatology. 55, 512–521.

Tsuji, K., Watanabe, Y., Van De Water, J., Nakanishi, T., Kajiyama, G., Parikh-Patel, A., et al., 1999. Familial primary biliary cirrhosis in Hiroshima. J. Autoimmun. 13, 171–178.

Tsuneyama, K., Moritoki, Y., Kikuchi, K., Nakanuma, Y., 2012. Pathological features of new animal models for primary biliary cirrhosis. Int. J. Hepatol. 2012, 403954.

Turchany, J.M., Uibo, R., Kivik, T., Van de Water, J., Prindiville, T., Coppel, R.L., et al., 1997. A study of antimitochondrial antibodies in a random population in Estonia. Am. J. Gastroenterol. 92, 124–126.

Van de Water, J., Turchany, J., Leung, P.S., Lake, J., Munoz, S., Surh, C.D., et al., 1993. Molecular mimicry in primary biliary cirrhosis.

Evidence for biliary epithelial expression of a molecule cross-reactive with pyruvate dehydrogenase complex-E2. J. Clin. Invest. 91, 2653–2664.

Wakabayashi, K., Lian, Z.X., Moritoki, Y., Lan, R.Y., Tsuneyama, K., Chuang, Y.H., et al., 2006. IL-2 receptor alpha(−/−) mice and the development of primary biliary cirrhosis. Hepatology. 44, 1240–1249.

Wakabayashi, K., Lian, Z.X., Leung, P.S., Moritoki, Y., Tsuneyama, K., Kurth, M.J., et al., 2008. Loss of tolerance in C57BL/6 mice to the autoantigen E2 subunit of pyruvate dehydrogenase by a xenobiotic with ensuing biliary ductular disease. Hepatology. 48, 531–540.

Wakabayashi, K., Yoshida, K., Leung, P.S., Moritoki, Y., Yang, G.X., Tsuneyama, K., et al., 2009. Induction of autoimmune cholangitis in non-obese diabetic (NOD)1101 mice following a chemical xenobiotic immunization. Clin. Exp. Immunol. 155, 577–586.

Walker, J.G., Doniach, D., Roitt, I.M., Sherlock, S., 1965. Serological tests in diagnosis of primary biliary cirrhosis. Lancet. 1, 827–831.

Wesierska-Gadek, J., Penner, E., Battezzati, P.M., Selmi, C., Zuin, M., Hitchman, E., et al., 2006. Correlation of initial autoantibody profile and clinical outcome in primary biliary cirrhosis. Hepatology. 43, 1135–1144.

Yang, G.X., Lian, Z.X., Chuang, Y.H., Moritoki, Y., Lan, R.Y., Wakabayashi, K., et al., 2008. Adoptive transfer of CD8(+) T cells from transforming growth factor beta receptor type II (dominant negative form) induces autoimmune cholangitis in mice. Hepatology. 47, 1974–1982.

Yeilding, N., Szapary, P., Brodmerkel, C., Benson, J., Plotnick, M., Zhou, H., et al., 2011. Development of the IL-12/23 antagonist ustekinumab in psoriasis, past, present, and future perspectives. Ann. N. Y. Acad. Sci. 1222, 30–39.

Yoshida, K., Yang, G.X., Zhang, W., Tsuda, M., Tsuneyama, K., Moritoki, Y., et al., 2009. Deletion of interleukin-12p40 suppresses autoimmune cholangitis in dominant negative transforming growth factor beta receptor type II mice. Hepatology. 50, 1494–1500.

You, Z., Wang, Q., Bian, Z., Liu, Y., Han, X., Peng, Y., et al., 2012. The immunopathology of liver granulomas in primary biliary cirrhosis. J. Autoimmun. 39, 216–221.

Zhang, L.N., Shi, T.Y., Shi, X.H., Wang, L., Yang, Y.J., Liu, B., et al., 2013. Early biochemical response to ursodeoxycholic acid and long-term prognosis of primary biliary cirrhosis. Results of a 14-year cohort study. Hepatology. 58, 264–272.

Zhang, W., Sharma, R., Ju, S.T., He, X.S., Tao, Y., Tsuneyama, K., et al., 2009. Deficiency in regulatory T cells results in development of antimitochondrial antibodies and autoimmune cholangitis. Hepatology. 49, 545–552.

Chapter 63

Primary Sclerosing Cholangitis

John E. Eaton[1], Jayant A. Talwalkar[1], and Keith D. Lindor[2]

[1]Mayo Clinic, Rochester, MN, USA, [2]Arizona State University, Phoenix, AZ, USA

Chapter Outline

Epidemiology and Risk Factors	925
Epidemiologic Features	925
Risk Factors	925
Natural History, Clinical Features, and PSC-IBD	926
Natural History and Clinical Features	926
PSC-IBD	926
Diagnosis	926
Biochemical Features	926
Cholangiography	927
Histology	927
PSC Subtypes and Pediatric PSC	927
Small Duct PSC	927
PSC-AIH	928
Pediatric PSC	928
PSC-Associated Malignancies	929
Colorectal Neoplasia	929
Cholangiocarcinoma (CCA)	929
Gallbladder Neoplasia	929
Hepatocellular Carcinoma	929
Genetics	929
Animal Models	930
Overview	930
Summary of PSC Models	930
Potential Pathogenic Mechanisms	930
Overview	930
Bacterial Translocation, Pathogen-associated Molecular Patterns, and Innate Immune Response	930
Adhesion Molecules, Lymphocyte Homing, and the Liver–Gut Axis	931
Antibodies, Memory, and Regulatory T cells	931
Transporter Defects and Bile Acids	931
Autoimmune Features	932
Treatment	932
Medical Therapy	932
Therapeutic Endoscopy	932
Liver Transplantation	932
Concluding Remarks	933
References	933

EPIDEMIOLOGY AND RISK FACTORS

Epidemiologic Features

Adult primary sclerosing cholangitis (PSC) affects mainly patients in their third to fourth decade of life with a male-to-female ratio of 2:1 (Lee and Kaplan, 1995). Although an uncommon disease, the diagnosis of PSC is increasing over time (Molodecky et al., 2011). Population-based cohorts suggest the incidence rate of PSC in North American populations is 1 per 100,000 inhabitants (Bambha et al., 2003; Kaplan et al., 2007). The prevalence of PSC in North America and Europe is reported to be between six and 16 cases per 100,000 individuals (Bambha et al., 2003; Berdal et al., 1998; Lindkvist et al., 2010). Contemporary data suggests PSC is less common in Southern Europe and Asian populations (Escorsell et al., 1994; Ang et al., 2002).

Risk Factors

Risk factors for PSC are poorly understood. Inflammatory bowel disease (IBD) is the primary risk factor and condition associated with PSC. Among patients with PSC, up to 86% will have concurrent IBD, typically ulcerative colitis (UC) (Chapman et al., 2010). In contrast only 4% of patients with UC will have PSC (Olsson et al., 1991; Chapman et al., 2010). Even after controlling for UC, smoking may be protective of PSC whereas male gender and a family history of PSC appear to be associated with the disease (Mitchell et al., 2002; Bergquist et al., 2005; Molodecky et al., 2011).

N. Rose & I. Mackay (Eds): The Autoimmune Diseases, Fifth edition. DOI: http://dx.doi.org/10.1016/B978-0-12-384929-8.00063-0

NATURAL HISTORY, CLINICAL FEATURES, AND PSC-IBD

Natural History and Clinical Features

Classic PSC is associated with progressive stricturing and dilation of the extra and/or intrahepatic bile ducts. Approximately 50% of patients with PSC are asymptomatic at the time of diagnosis and the condition is detected based on the presence of abnormal liver tests (Broome et al., 1996). Following a diagnosis of asymptomatic PSC, nearly 25% will develop clinical symptoms after 5 years and the majority of patients will have some clinical or objective evidence of progression 6 years after the diagnosis (Porayko et al., 1990; Broome et al., 1996). Patients who present with asymptomatic disease have a better long-term prognosis compared to those who are symptomatic at the time of diagnosis (Broome et al., 1996). However, asymptomatic patients have a worse survival compared to the general population (Porayko et al., 1990).

Over time biliary strictures can lead to the development of symptoms, progressive cholestasis, and cirrhosis. When symptoms do develop, patients may present with fatigue, abdominal pain, jaundice, or fever. It is unusual for decompensated liver failure to be the initial manifestation (Broome et al., 1996). Refractory pruritus, metabolic bone disease, IBD, complications from portal hypertension and cholangitis (occurring in 10–45% of patients) add to the morbidity and can impact the quality of life of affected individuals (Chapman et al., 1980; Lee and Kaplan, 2002). Dominant strictures (stenosis ≤1.5 mm in common bile duct or ≤1.0 mm in hepatic duct) have been reported in up to 50% of PSC patients (Stiehl et al., 2002; Chapman et al., 2010). Among those with a dominant stricture 10–30% will be symptomatic (Kaya et al., 2001; Stiehl et al., 2002). It is important to note that both colorectal cancer and cholangiocarcinoma (CCA) can be present at the time of diagnosis in many patients regardless of the presence of symptoms (see below) (Razumilava et al., 2011).

Various studies have reported median a time of 9–18 years to the development of death or liver transplantation (LT) for all patients with PSC (Broome et al., 1996; Porayko et al., 1990; Ponsioen et al., 2002). Among population-based studies, the survival for PSC patients is estimated to be 65% after 10 years (Bambha et al., 2003). Prognostic models such as the revised Mayo PSC Risk score are not recommended for routine use in individual patients (Chapman et al., 2010).

PSC-IBD

The most common co-morbid condition associated with PSC is IBD, particularly UC. IBD can be diagnosed at any point in the disease course, even after LT (Verdonk et al., 2006). Similarly, PSC can develop after a colectomy for UC (Chapman et al., 1980). Approximately 86% will have features consistent with UC whereas 13% of PSC patients have features more typical of Crohn's disease (Chapman et al., 2010). PSC-IBD may represent a unique phenotype. For example, the colonic involvement with PSC-IBD is more extensive, yet with minimal endoscopic inflammation despite a greater degree of histologic inflammation (Loftus et al., 2005; Jorgensen et al., 2012a). Some have reported an increased presence of backwash ileitis and rectal sparing compared to UC alone (Loftus et al., 2005). PSC-IBD patients are associated with an increased risk of colorectal neoplasia compared to those with IBD alone (Soetikno et al., 2002). Following proctocolectomy, PSC-IBD patients are at an increased risk of pouchitis and parastomal varices (Penna et al., 1996; Soetikno et al., 2002). Interestingly, recent studies have suggested patients with more severe colitis tend to have less severe liver disease, and vice versa (Marelli et al., 2011; Navaneethan et al., 2012). Because of the prevalence of IBD in PSC, patients with a new diagnosis of PSC should immediately undergo a colonoscopy with surveillance biopsies to screen for IBD and malignancy, regardless of symptoms (Chapman et al., 2010).

DIAGNOSIS

Biochemical Features

For many patients, an elevated alkaline phosphatase level may be the only laboratory abnormality. Fluctuations in alkaline phosphatase can occur throughout the disease course and improvement in alkaline phosphatase has been associated with improved outcomes (Stanich et al., 2011). Elevations in aminotransaminases less than 3–4 times the upper limit of normal can also be observed. Bilirubin can be increased particularly in the presence of a severe stricturing disease. Abnormalities in hepatic synthetic function are rare unless cirrhosis is present (Chapman et al., 2010). Liver enzyme abnormalities such as an isolated alkaline phosphatase in someone with IBD should immediately raise the suspicion for PSC.

A variety of autoantibodies can be detected in the sera of patients with PSC (see below) (Chapman et al., 2010). However, autoantibodies are non-specific and do not play a role in the diagnostic evaluation of patients with typical PSC. In retrospective studies, elevated IgG4 levels have been described in 9–12% of patients with a previous diagnosis of PSC. The distinction of IgG4-associated cholangitis and PSC with elevated IgG4 levels can be challenging (Mendes et al., 2006; Bjornsson et al., 2011). In contrast to classic PSC, IgG4-associated cholangitis is associated with steroid responsive biliary strictures and a lymphoplasmacytic infiltrate on biopsy. Because a subset of patients with biochemical and cholangiographic features of PSC may have IgG4, it is recommended that a serum IgG4 be measured in all cases of suspected PSC (Chapman et al., 2010). Importantly, CCA in PSC patients can be associated with an elevated IgG4. Although an elevated IgG4 greater than four times the upper limit of normal has been reported to have a high specificity for IgG4-associated cholangitis, it is still important to carefully exclude malignancy in patients with elevations in IgG4 (Oseini et al., 2011).

Cholangiography

Cholangiography plays a central role in the diagnosis and management of patients with PSC. After laboratory testing raises the possibility of PSC, cholangiography can help secure the diagnosis without the need for additional testing. Cholangiography can reveal typical multifocal strictures with dilatations in the intrahepatic and or extrahepatic bile ducts in patients with typical PSC (Figure 63.1). Compared to endoscopic retrograde cholangiography (ERC), magnetic resonance cholangiography (MRC) is less invasive, avoids radiation, and is a cost -effective method to diagnosis PSC (Talwalkar et al., 2004; Kaltenthaler et al., 2004). ERC is an essential therapeutic tool for the management of biliary strictures and for characterizing biliary lesions suspicious for CCA.

Histology

The histologic findings in classic PSC are often nonspecific. Rarely are the pathognomonic "onion skin" lesions present (Figure 63.2). The Batts–Ludwig grading system has historically divided the pathologic features of classic PSC based on the presence or absence of bile ducts and degree of fibrosis into four stages (Ludwig et al., 1986). A liver biopsy is rarely needed and should be reserved for suspected small duct PSC, or primary sclerosing cholangitis–autoimmune hepatitis (PSC-AIH) overlap.

PSC SUBTYPES AND PEDIATRIC PSC

There are several key PSC subtypes which appear to have different features compared to classic large duct PSC. Recognition of these phenotypic differences is important as these subtypes often have an improved prognosis and the treatment may differ when compared to large duct PSC.

Small Duct PSC

Small duct PSC should be suspected among individuals with elevations in alkaline phosphatase and a normal

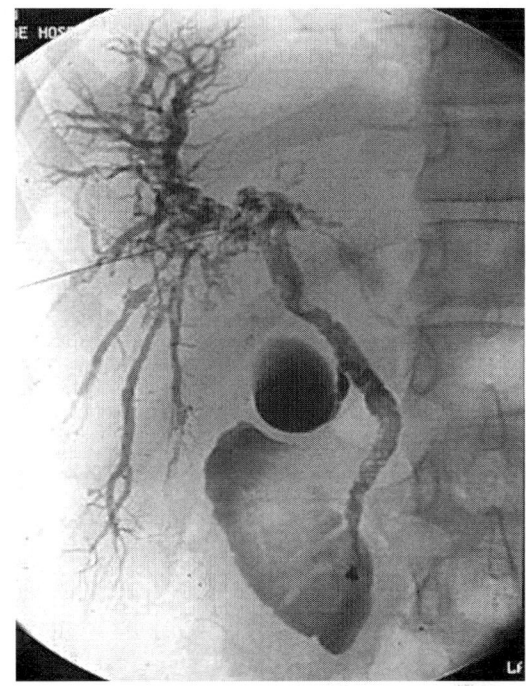

FIGURE 63.1   Cholangiogram of an adult patient with primary sclerosing cholangitis showing severe widespread strictures and dilatations of the intra- and extrahepatic bile ducts.

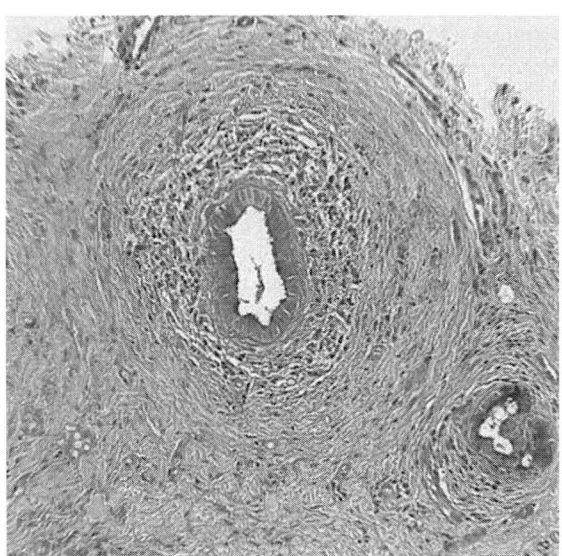

FIGURE 63.2   "Onionskin" fibrosis around a damaged bile duct. This is the characteristic lesion of sclerosing cholangitis, but is rarely seen in percutaneous liver biopsies.

cholangiogram. A liver biopsy is required to secure the diagnosis and the histologic features are similar to classic PSC. Among IBD patients with evidence of chronic cholestasis despite a normal cholangiogram, nearly 6%

will have small duct PSC (Angulo et al., 2002). The prevalence of IBD in small duct PSC is similar to typical large duct PSC (Bjornsson et al., 2008). Classic features of large duct PSC will eventually develop in 12–23% of patients with small duct PSC over 7–10 years (Bjornsson et al., 2002, 2008). Therefore, it is unclear if some small duct PSC patients represent an early form of classic PSC. Although both small duct and classic PSC can have similar symptoms, patients with small duct PSC rarely develop CCA and have an improved prognosis compared to those with classic PSC (Bjornsson et al., 2008).

PSC-AIH

PSC-AIH overlap syndrome is characterized by cholangiographic features of typical PSC with histologic and laboratory evidence suggestive of AIH. The frequency of PSC-AIH is unclear, but has been reported to occur in 1–17% of patients with PSC (Chapman et al., 2010). This wide variability may be related to differences in case ascertainment, varying diagnostic criteria, and center location. PSC-AIH tends to be diagnosed in younger patients compared to classic PSC but the coexistence of IBD is comparable between the two disorders (Abdalian et al., 2008; Trivedi and Hirschfield, 2012). Patients with PSC-AIH have a worse prognosis compared to those with AIH alone or other overlap syndromes yet their survival is improved compared to patients with classic PSC (Floreani et al., 2005; Al-Chalabi et al., 2008).

There are no standard diagnostic criteria for PSC-AIH. It should be suspected in patients diagnosed with AIH who have concurrent IBD, or are refractory to immunosuppression. Conversely, PSC-AIH should be suspected among those diagnosed with PSC if serum transaminases are elevated (particularly if greater than five times the upper limit of normal). High titers of antinuclear antibody (ANA), antismooth muscle antibodies (ASMA), or IgG may also raise the suspicion of concurrent AIH, but such tests are not diagnostic since these antibodies can be found in those with PSC alone (Trivedi and Hirschfield, 2012). Although the simplified international autoimmune hepatitis group criteria can aid in the diagnosis of AIH, it is not recommended this be applied to diagnose subgroups. Instead, individual patients should be categorized based on the dominant disease entity. Supportive histologic findings include lymphoplasmacytic portal-based infiltrates and interface hepatitis (Trivedi and Hirschfield, 2012). Unlike classic PSC, immunosuppression may have a role in the treatment of patients with PSC-AIH (Chapman et al., 2010).

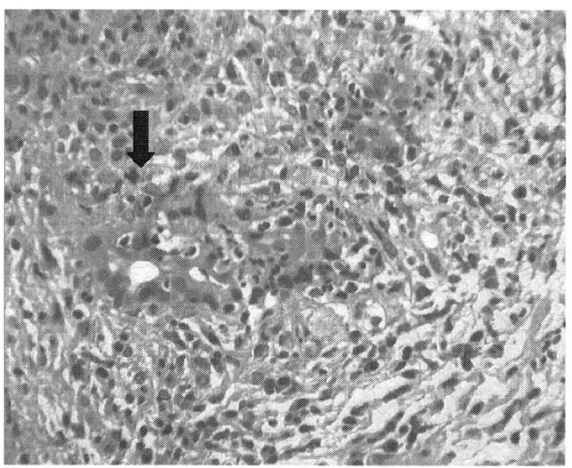

FIGURE 63.3 Portal tract inflammatory cell infiltrate in a case of juvenile sclerosing cholangitis positive for anti-nuclear and anti-smooth muscle antibodies. Plasma cells and lymphocytes cross the limiting plate invading the parenchyma (interface hepatitis). The arrow points to a damaged bile duct.

Pediatric PSC

Pediatric PSC is less common than classic adult PSC with an incidence rate of 0.2 per 100,000 person-years (Ghazale et al., 2008). Most cases occur in pre-teen years. However, it should be noted that inherited conditions such as cystic fibrosis and immunologic defects may present in a manner similar to PSC in childhood.

It is unresolved whether pediatric PSC represents a distinct pathologic entity or an earlier form of classic PSC. However, adult and pediatric PSC share several features. For example, both are often associated with IBD, are more common in males, and have similar cholangiographic features (Ibrahim and Lindor, 2011). Similarly to adults, the median transplant-free survival in children is 13 years and pediatric PSC is associated with a worse survival compared to age and gender-matched controls in the general population (Feldstein et al., 2003). In contrast to adult PSC, pediatric patients with PSC are more likely to be symptomatic upon presentation (81% in one retrospective study) and have higher elevations in serum aminotransferases and gamma glutamyltranspeptidase levels (Floreani et al., 1999; Miloh et al., 2009). Furthermore, pediatric PSC patients are more likely to have AIH overlap features which include elevated ANA, SMA, and IgG titers along with interface hepatitis (Figure 63.3). In one center the frequency of pediatric PSC-AIH was 25% and small duct PSC occurred in 34% of pediatric patients (Miloh et al., 2009). Therefore, histology may play a more important role in the diagnostic evaluation in pediatric patients. Finally, dominant strictures and malignancy such as CCA are rare in childhood PSC (Chapman et al., 2010).

PSC-ASSOCIATED MALIGNANCIES

Colorectal Neoplasia

Patients with PSC-UC are four times more likely to develop colorectal neoplasia than patients with UC alone (Soetikno et al., 2002). The risk is also elevated in PSC patients with concurrent Crohn's disease (Lindstrom et al., 2011). Colorectal neoplasia is often present shortly after the conditions are diagnosed (Thackeray et al., 2011). Consequently once PSC-IBD is diagnosed, a colonoscopy with surveillance biopsies for flat neoplasia should be undertaken to evaluate for cancer or dysplasia. Surveillance colonoscopy with biopsies should continue annually. The risk of colorectal neoplasia does not dissipate after LT and surveillance should be continued in post-transplant patients (Chapman et al., 2010). Indications for colectomy include cancer, high grade dysplasia, and unresectable low grade dysplasia that have been confirmed by two expert pathologists. Several studies have suggested that ursodeoxycholic acid (UDCA) may reduce the risk of colorectal neoplasia in PSC-IBD patients (Tung et al., 2001; Pardi et al., 2003). However, studies have been inconsistent and some studies suggest UDCA may increase the risk of colorectal neoplasia (Wolf et al., 2005; Eaton et al., 2011; Jorgensen et al., 2012b; Lindstrom et al., 2012). Therefore, routine use of UDCA to prevent colorectal neoplasia is not recommended at this time (Chapman et al., 2010).

Cholangiocarcinoma (CCA)

CCA is one of the most feared complications related to PSC. The lifetime risk is up to 10% with an annual risk of 1−2% (Bergquist et al., 2002). Similar to colorectal neoplasia, CCA is frequently detected within the first 3 years after the diagnosis of PSC (Bergquist et al., 2002). The diagnosis is often challenging. The development of CCA should be suspected with worsening cholestasis or the development of dominant strictures. Distinguishing between dominant strictures and CCA is difficult, in part because CCA is a desmoplastic malignancy making tissue sampling challenging. Consequently, traditional cytology has a low sensitivity. Fluorescence *in situ* hybridization (FISH) utilizes centromeric probes against specific chromosomes and is able to detect the abnormal loss or gain of chromosomes. Polysomy in PSC patients is 46% sensitive and 88% specific for CCA and patients with recurrent polysomy are more likely to develop CCA compared to those without recurrent polysomy (75% versus 18% after 3 years) (Bangarulingam et al., 2010; Barr Fritcher et al., 2011). Therefore, patients with polysomy who otherwise do not have CCA should be monitored closely.

Treatment options for CCA are limited and the 5-year survival rates remain 10% or less (Rosen and Nagorney, 1991). In a highly selective group of patients with unresectable hilar CCA less than 3 cm may be candidates for an intensive multimodal approach that culminates with an LT. There appear to be good long-term outcomes following LT for this indication (Darwish Murad et al., 2012).

Gallbladder Neoplasia

PSC patients commonly have cholelithiasis and are at a higher risk for gallbladder neoplasia. Although the exact prevalence of gallbladder neoplasia in PSC is unclear, when gallbladder polyps are detected (particularly if greater than 8 mm) they are often malignant. For example, in one series 14% of PSC patients had gallbladder lesions detected and 57% were malignant (Buckles et al., 2002). Current guidelines suggest an annual ultrasound to detect gallbladder lesions in PSC patients and if a gallbladder polyp is detected they should undergo a cholecystectomy (Chapman et al., 2010). However, the natural history of gallbladder polyps less than 8 mm is less clear and the risks and benefits of undergoing a cholecystectomy for small polyps should be discussed with each patient (Eaton et al., 2012).

Hepatocellular Carcinoma

Cirrhosis is an important risk factor for hepatocellular carcinoma and the prevalence of this malignancy in PSC associated with cirrhosis is 2% (Harnois et al., 1997). Therefore, screening every 6 months with an ultrasound is recommended once cirrhosis is detected (Bruix and Sherman, 2011).

GENETICS

Patients with a first degree relative with PSC are at a higher risk for developing the condition, which suggests a genetic predisposition for the development of the disease. The strongest genetic risk factors to date have been localized to the human leukocyte antigen (HLA) complex. Haplotypes that have been associated with PSC include HLA-DRB1*1501-DQB1*0602, HLA-DRB1*1301-DQB1* 0603, and HLA-A1-B8-DRB1*0301-DQB1*0201 (Farrant et al., 1992; Mehal et al., 1994; Olerup et al., 1995; Spurkland et al., 1999). Genome-wide association studies have also revealed strong associations with PSC near HLA-B at chromosome 6p21 (Karlsen et al., 2010). HLA DR4 may be a marker for rapid disease progression (Mehal et al., 1994). In contrast, DRB1*04, DQB1*302, DRB1*0701 DQB10303, and MICA*002 have been shown to be protective from PSC (Norris et al., 2001; Donaldson and Norris, 2002).

Genome-wide association studies have also revealed potential non-HLA associations. To date, many of the non-HLA associations appear to play an immunoregulatory role. Examples include GPC5/GPC6 region on chromosome 13q21 (function unknown but may regulate inflammatory cytokines in cholangiocytes), GPBAR1 on chromosome 2q35 (may represent a bile acid suppressor), MST1 on chromosome 3p21 (encodes a protein that inhibits lipopolysaccharide induced nuclear factor $\kappa\beta$ signaling), and BCL2L11 (encodes Bcl-2 interacting protein which maintains tolerance through induction of apoptosis of autoreactive T cells) (Karlsen et al., 2010; Melum et al., 2011).

ANIMAL MODELS

Overview

Currently, there is no single animal model for PSC. This may be related to the uncertainty regarding the pathophysiology of PSC and the multifactorial processes that are involved in the development of this condition. Consequently, multiple models may be necessary to study the various facets of PSC.

Summary of PSC Models

Key models for PSC currently fall into the following broad categories: (1) creation of cholangitis secondary to infectious organisms (example, *Cryptosporidium parvum*); (2) creation of cholangitis via chemicals (example, lithocholic acid); (3) bacteria or cell wall components inducing hepatobiliary injury (example, small intestinal bacterial overgrowth); (4) apoptosis in cholestatic liver disease (example, death receptor 5 and TNF-related apoptosis inducing ligand deficient mice); (5) knockout mice (example, Mdr2$^{-/-}$); (6) experimental biliary obstruction (example, bile duct ligation in mice); and (7) models of biliary and endothelial cell injury (example, graft versus host disease models in mice) (Takeda et al., 2008; Pollheimer et al., 2011).

POTENTIAL PATHOGENIC MECHANISMS

Overview

The inciting etiology of PSC and the precise pathogenic mechanism remain elusive. Several hypotheses and indirect lines of evidence are outlined below. It likely involves one or more environmental triggers in a genetically susceptible individual which probably leads to a series of events resulting in the activation of the innate immune system, lymphocyte homing, cholangiocyte immune-mediated damage, and progressive fibrosis.

Bacterial Translocation, Pathogen-associated Molecular Patterns, and Innate Immune Response

Translocation of bacteria across a permeable, inflamed bowel with subsequent immune activation which leads to biliary inflammation has been suggested as a potential mechanism. Although bacterial overgrowth and introducing bacterial antigens into the portal circulation have been shown to result in cholangitis in animal models, it appears that in humans portal venous bacteremia in UC patients is uncommon (Palmer et al., 1980; Lichtman and Sartor, 1991; Yamada et al., 1994; O'mahony and Vierling 2006; Pollheimer et al., 2011). Intestinal flora express the protein FtsZ, which is cross-reactive with p-ANCA (Terjung et al., 2010). This raises the possibility of an inappropriate immune response towards intestinal bacteria (Terjung and Spengler, 2009). The role of the microbiome in the development and progression of PSC is unknown and further studies are needed.

Biliary epithelial cells are normally exposed to pathogen-associated molecular patterns such as lipopolysaccharides. Lipopolysaccharide exposure to colonic and biliary epithelial cells has been shown to disrupt tight junctions through a Toll-like receptor 4 (TLR-4)-dependent mechanism (Sheth et al., 2007; Guo et al., 2013). Disruption of critical paracellular barriers could expose cholangiocytes to a variety of factors, such as bile acids (see below) that could promote injury. Indeed animal models suggest that disruption in bile duct tight junctions is a key step in the development of sclerosing cholangitis (Fickert et al., 2004). Despite this exposure, the innate immune system appears relatively downregulated in normal individuals (Medvedev et al., 2006; Mueller et al., 2011). In contrast, PSC patients exhibit features of innate system upregulation when exposed to such endotoxins. Interferon-γ (IFN-γ) and tumor necrosis factor-α (TNF-α) likely mediate a TLR4-mediated endotoxin incorporation in biliary cells and a diminished ability to deactivate the TLR4 signaling cascade. TNF-α inhibition partly restored the protective innate immune tolerance in one *in vitro* study (Mueller et al., 2011). Cholangiocytes from PSC liver explants have an increased expression of TLRs, nucleotide-binding domains, MyD88/IRAK complex formation, TNF-α, IFN-γ, and interleukin-8 (IL-8). Upregulation of TLR, IL-8, and TNF-α is more pronounced in late stage PSC (Mueller et al., 2011). Therefore, based on this observation, the innate immune system hyperresponsiveness observed in *in vitro* studies may bolster the inflammatory response as the disease progresses rather than act as an inciting event. In contrast, others have suggested that the innate immune system could play a key early role in the development of PSC. This hypothesis involves pathogen-associated molecular patterns activating macrophages, NK cells, and dendritic cells through pattern recognition receptors including TLRs which ultimately leads to NK and lymphocyte activation (Aron and Bowlus, 2009).

Adhesion Molecules, Lymphocyte Homing, and the Liver–Gut Axis

A variety of adhesion molecules such as intercellular adhesion molecules (ICAM), mucosal addressin cellular adhesion molecule 1 (MAdCAM-1), and vascular adhesion molecule-1 (VCAM-1) are upregulated in PSC patients. Increased expression of chemokines such as CCL25, CCL28, CXCL12, and CXCL16 has been described in PSC. Activation of $\alpha 4\beta 7$ integrins is achieved through this increase in CCL25 and CCL28 which enables lymphocytes to bind to MAdCAM-1 (located in gut and liver). CCL28 also activates $\alpha 4\beta 1$ integrins to enhance adhesion to VCAM-1 (primarily expressed in the portal and sinusoidal endothelial cells of the liver). It has been postulated that once lymphocytes enter the portal tract, CXCL12 and CXCL16 aid in lymphocyte binding to the bile duct epithelium (Borchers et al., 2009).

Some have proposed that lymphocyte homing between the so-called liver–gut axis may play an important role in the pathogenesis of PSC (Grant et al., 2002). Chemokines and specific adhesion molecules, particularly those shared by the gut and liver, may mediate immune cell trafficking and binding. For example, vascular adhesion protein 1 (VAP-1) is found in liver endothelial cells and in mucosal vessels. The chronic inflammation observed in patients with IBD upregulates VAP-1 in the gut venules. This activation of VAP-1 has been shown to increase the expression of MAdCAM-1—primarily expressed in the gut—in hepatic vessels. This may result in the recruitment of effector lymphocytes to the liver (Liaskou et al., 2011). In addition, $\alpha 4\beta 7^+CCR9^+CD8^+$ T cells found in the liver in PSC are primed by dendritic cells in the gut rather than antigen-presenting cells in the liver (Eksteen et al., 2009). Subclinical inflammation in patients without a diagnosis of IBD being sufficient to trigger cross-talk between immune cells from liver and the gastrointestinal tract as a potential explanation why a subset of PSC patients do not have IBD, is unclear. Nonetheless the above observations suggest a possible role for lymphocyte trafficking along the liver–gut axis in PSC patients.

Antibodies, Memory, and Regulatory T cells

PSC patients have a variety of nonspecific autoantibodies. In addition to atypical p-ANCA which cross-reacts with a ubiquitous protein in intestinal bacteria (see above), nearly two-thirds of PSC patients have autoantibodies against cholangiocytes (Xu et al., 2002). These autoantibodies may cause cholangiocytes to express CD44 and

increase IL-6 production which could potentially lead to the recruitment of memory T cells via CD44 and upregulation of the innate immune system via ERK1/2 transcription factor signaling and upregulation of TLRS (Xu et al., 2002; Karrar et al., 2007). T cells in the liver and bile ducts of PSC patients may have oligoclonal restriction (Broome et al., 1997; Probert et al., 1997). Furthermore, the proportion of $\gamma\delta^+$ T cells in the liver and peripheral circulation is increased in PSC patients. The peripheral $\gamma\delta^+$ T cells co-express CD45RO and IL-2 receptors which suggests they have an activated memory phenotype (Wen et al., 1992; Martins et al., 1996). $CD4^+CD25^+$ T regulatory cells are believed to play an important role in autoimmune diseases. Indeed, patients with PSC-UC appear to have a higher peripheral proportion of $CD4^+CD25^+$ T cells when compared to UC patients without PSC (Kekilli et al., 2013). The significance of this observation remains unclear but warrants further study.

Transporter Defects and Bile Acids

Normally, bile acids and biliary phospholipids are transported into bile via the canalicular phospholipid flippase (multidrug resistance gene 2 [Mdr2]/Abcb4) and the bile salt export pump (Bsep/Abcb11) to form mixed micelles which protect cholangiocytes from bile acid toxicity (Trauner and Boyer, 2003). Disruption of the Mdr2 gene in mice results in an impairment of biliary phospholipid secretion and an increased concentration of bile acids that ultimately cause bile duct injury (Fickert et al., 2004; Lammert et al., 2004). In addition, the human MDR3 (analogue to rodent Mdr2) has been associated with a variety of cholestatic syndromes (Trauner et al., 2007). For example, MDR3 mutations have been associated with pediatric small duct PSC (Jacquemin et al., 2001; Chapman et al., 2010). Patients with cystic fibrosis can have cholangiographic features similar to those seen in PSC patients. Indeed, there have been mutations in the cystic fibrosis transmembrane conductance regulator (CFTR) gene described in PSC patients (Sheth et al., 2003). The precise role of MDR3 and CFTR is unclear but a central role in the pathophysiology of PSC in the majority of patients seems unlikely.

Lithocholic acid (LCA) is a hydrophobic secondary bile acid that is primarily formed in the intestine by bacterial metabolism of chenodeoxycholic acid. LCA-fed mice developed bile duct crystals with bile infarcts and a destructive cholangitis that was followed by myofibroblast proliferation. One of the proposed mechanisms behind these findings involved alteration of cholangiocyte tight junctions leading to permeable bile ducts (Fickert et al., 2006). In another animal model, bile was able to reflux into the portal tracts in the presence of altered bile duct tight junctions and basal membrane integrity. This resulted in an inflammatory response with an influx of CD4 and CD8-positive T cells and overexpression of TNF-α, IL-1β, IL-6, and transforming growth factor β1 (TGF-β1). This proinflammatory infiltrate resulted in activation of myofibroblasts, which lead to periductal fibrosis (Fickert et al., 2004).

Autoimmune Features

A variety of other autoantibodies have been described in PSC patients including ANA, SMA, antimitochondrial antibodies, and antineutrophil cytoplasmic antibodies (Hov et al., 2008). Sera from nearly two-thirds of patients with PSC have circulating autoantibodies against amino acid sequences shared in common by colon and biliary epithelial cells (Mandal et al., 1994) and anti-biliary epithelial cell antibodies (Xu et al., 2002). The significance of this observation on the pathogenesis of PSC and the relationship between PSC and IBD is unclear. Other autoantibodies include anti-endothelial cell antibody (35%) (Gur et al., 1995), anticardiolipin antibody (4–66%) (Angulo et al., 2000), antithyroperoxidase (7–16%) (Angulo et al., 2000), antithyroglobulin (4%) (Gur et al., 1995), and rheumatoid factor (15%) (Angulo et al., 2000). An increased level of circulating immune complexes and activation of the classical complement pathway has been described (Bodenheimer et al., 1983; Senaldi et al., 1989). No autoantibody to date is specific enough to play a role in the diagnosis of classic PSC. Nonetheless the presence of autoantibodies coupled with the genetic association with HLA haplotypes, influx of lymphocytes, particularly T lymphocytes with an increase in circulating memory T cells plus the strong association with PSC and other immune-mediated conditions, are several of the key indirect lines of evidence that suggest PSC is mediated by an autoimmune phenomenon. In contrast, the lack of a proven response to immunosuppression and male predominance are features which suggest PSC is not a classic autoimmune disorder.

TREATMENT

Medical Therapy

To date, there are no proven effective therapies for PSC. The use of immunosuppressive agents has not demonstrated benefit for the treatment of classic PSC. Of the numerous agents examined, UDCA has been investigated the most extensively. One of the first randomized studies utilizing UDCA showed improvement in liver biochemistries and histology (Beuers et al., 1992). Subsequent studies did not show differences in liver-related endpoints between the placebo and UDCA treatment group. Another study which utilized 17–23 mg/kg/day of UDCA was not associated with improved survival; however, it may have been underpowered (Olsson et al., 2005). A North American randomized control trial found high-dose UDCA (28–30 mg/kg/day) was associated with worse outcomes and another study showed an increased risk of colorectal neoplasia in the high-dose group (Lindor et al., 2009; Eaton et al., 2011). The American Association for the Study of Liver Disease advises against the use of UDCA for PSC while the European Association for the Study of Liver Disease neither approves nor advises against the use of UDCA (Chapman et al., 2009, 2010). Treatment for patients with PSC-AIH, as for patients with AIH alone, can be initiated using corticosteroids and other immunosuppressive agents (Chapman et al., 2010).

Therapeutic Endoscopy

New or worsening symptoms of cholestasis in PSC patients should alert the clinician to the possible development of a dominant stricture or CCA. Cholangitis may also be a manifestation of progressive disease. Endoscopic therapy, either dilation or stenting, via ERC plays a key role in the management of symptomatic biliary strictures and can provide patients with long-term symptomatic relief. Retrospective data suggest expansion of strictures with dilation (compared to dilation plus stenting) is associated with fewer complications (Kaya et al., 2001). However, biliary stent placement may be necessary in cases where dilation is unable to maintain patency of the bile duct lumen. Upper endoscopy plays a key role in the surveillance, diagnosis, and treatment of gastroesophageal varices in patients with cirrhosis.

Liver Transplantation

Currently, liver transplantation (LT) is the most effective therapy for PSC. Indications for deceased donor transplant are similar to other LT indications and priority is determined based on the model for end stage liver disease (MELD) score. As mentioned above, a select group of patients with CCA and PSC may be eligible for LT. Patients with other disease-related complications of PSC such as recurrent cholangitis and intractable pruritus may be eligible to undergo living related donor LT despite a low MELD score. Outcomes following LT for PSC are excellent with reported 5-year survival rates exceeding 80% (Graziadei et al., 1999).

Recurrent PSC can develop in 25% of cases following a LT (Chapman et al., 2010). The diagnosis is typically established based on elevated liver tests and classic features on cholangiography. A liver biopsy can provide a supportive role in the diagnosis. Other conditions that can mimic recurrent PSC such as hepatic artery thrombosis, CMV infection, non-anastomotic biliary strictures, and

ABO incompatible mismatch LT should be excluded (Fosby et al., 2012). There is no effective therapy for recurrent PSC and some patients may undergo a repeat LT.

CONCLUDING REMARKS

PSC remains a rare but important cause of cholestatic liver disease. Although the pathophysiology is poorly understood, there are key direct and indirect lines of evidence which suggest PSC is an immune-mediated disorder that develops in susceptible individuals. Clarifying the pathophysiology through a variety of methods such as genome-wide association studies should help shed light on the underlying pathophysiology, important PSC disease modifiers, and open the door to novel therapeutic targets. Contemporary management of PSC depends on establishing the diagnosis, early recognition, and treatment of PSC-associated malignancies and other co-morbid conditions, and transplantation for select individuals. Future therapies may employ novel bile acids or target lymphocyte migration and adhesion, or progression of fibrosis.

REFERENCES

Abdalian, R., Dhar, P., Jhaveri, K., Haider, M., Guindi, M., Heathcote, E.J., 2008. Prevalence of sclerosing cholangitis in adults with autoimmune hepatitis: evaluating the role of routine magnetic resonance imaging. Hepatology. 47, 949–957.

Al-Chalabi, T., Portmann, B.C., Bernal, W., Mcfarlane, I.G., Heneghan, M.A., 2008. Autoimmune hepatitis overlap syndromes: an evaluation of treatment response, long-term outcome and survival. Aliment. Pharmacol. Ther. 28, 209–220.

Ang, T.L., Fock, K.M., Ng, T.M., Teo, E.K., Chua, T.S., Tan, J.Y., 2002. Clinical profile of primary sclerosing cholangitis in Singapore. J. Gastroenterol. Hepatol. 17, 908–913.

Angulo, P., Peter, J.B., Gershwin, M.E., Desotel, C.K., Shoenfeld, Y., Ahmed, A.E., et al., 2000. Serum autoantibodies in patients with primary sclerosing cholangitis. J. Hepatol. 32, 182–187.

Angulo, P., Maor-Kendler, Y., Lindor, K.D., 2002. Small-duct primary sclerosing cholangitis: a long-term follow-up study. Hepatology. 35, 1494–1500.

Aron, J.H., Bowlus, C.L., 2009. The immunobiology of primary sclerosing cholangitis. Semin. Immunopathol. 31, 383–397.

Bambha, K., Kim, W.R., Talwalkar, J., Torgerson, H., Benson, J.T., Therneau, T.M., et al., 2003. Incidence, clinical spectrum, and outcomes of primary sclerosing cholangitis in a United States community. Gastroenterology. 125, 1364–1369.

Bangarulingam, S.Y., Bjornsson, E., Enders, F., Barr Fritcher, E.G., Gores, G., Halling, K.C., et al., 2010. Long-term outcomes of positive fluorescence in situ hybridization tests in primary sclerosing cholangitis. Hepatology. 51, 174–180.

Barr Fritcher, E.G., Kipp, B.R., Voss, J.S., Clayton, A.C., Lindor, K.D., Halling, K.C., et al., 2011. Primary sclerosing cholangitis patients with serial polysomy fluorescence in situ hybridization results are at increased risk of cholangiocarcinoma. Am. J. Gastroenterol. 106, 2023–2028.

Berdal, J.E., Ebbesen, J., Rydning, A., 1998. Incidence and prevalence of autoimmune liver diseases. Tidsskr. Nor. laegeforen. 118, 4517–4519.

Bergquist, A., Ekbom, A., Olsson, R., Kornfeldt, D., Loof, L., Danielsson, A., et al., 2002. Hepatic and extrahepatic malignancies in primary sclerosing cholangitis. J. Hepatol. 36, 321–327.

Bergquist, A., Lindberg, G., Saarinen, S., Broome, U., 2005. Increased prevalence of primary sclerosing cholangitis among first-degree relatives. J. Hepatol. 42, 252–256.

Beuers, U., Spengler, U., Kruis, W., Aydemir, U., Wiebecke, B., Heldwein, W., et al., 1992. Ursodeoxycholic acid for treatment of primary sclerosing cholangitis: a placebo-controlled trial. Hepatology. 16, 707–714.

Bjornsson, E., Boberg, K.M., Cullen, S., Fleming, K., Clausen, O.P., Fausa, O., et al., 2002. Patients with small duct primary sclerosing cholangitis have a favourable long term prognosis. Gut. 51, 731–735.

Bjornsson, E., Olsson, R., Bergquist, A., Lindgren, S., Braden, B., Chapman, R.W., et al., 2008. The natural history of small-duct primary sclerosing cholangitis. Gastroenterology. 134, 975–980.

Bjornsson, E., Chari, S., Silveira, M., Gossard, A., Takahashi, N., Smyrk, T., et al., 2011. Primary sclerosing cholangitis associated with elevated immunoglobulin G4: clinical characteristics and response to therapy. Am. J. Ther. 18, 198–205.

Bodenheimer Jr., H.C., Larusso, N.F., Thayer Jr., W.R., Charland, C., Staples, P.J., Ludwig, J., 1983. Elevated circulating immune complexes in primary sclerosing cholangitis. Hepatology. 3, 150–154.

Borchers, A.T., Shimoda, S., Bowlus, C., Keen, C.L., Gershwin, M.E., 2009. Lymphocyte recruitment and homing to the liver in primary biliary cirrhosis and primary sclerosing cholangitis. Semin. Immun. 31, 309–322.

Broome, U., Olsson, R., Loof, L., Bodemar, G., Hultcrantz, R., Danielsson, A., et al., 1996. Natural history and prognostic factors in 305 Swedish patients with primary sclerosing cholangitis. Gut. 38, 610–615.

Broome, U., Grunewald, J., Scheynius, A., Olerup, O., Hultcrantz, R., 1997. Preferential V beta3 usage by hepatic T lymphocytes in patients with primary sclerosing cholangitis. J. Hepatol. 26, 527–534.

Bruix, J., Sherman, M., 2011. Management of hepatocellular carcinoma: an update. Hepatology. 53, 1020–1022.

Buckles, D.C., Lindor, K.D., Larusso, N.F., Petrovic, L.M., Gores, G.J., 2002. In primary sclerosing cholangitis, gallbladder polyps are frequently malignant. Am. J. Gastroenterol. 97, 1138–1142.

Chapman, R., Fevery, J., Kalloo, A., et al., 2010. Diagnosis and management of primary sclerosing cholangitis. Hepatology. 51, 660–678.

Chapman, R.W., Arborgh, B.A., Rhodes, J.M., Summerfield, J.A., Dick, R., Scheuer, P.J., et al., 1980. Primary sclerosing cholangitis: a review of its clinical features, cholangiography, and hepatic histology. Gut. 21, 870–877.

Darwish Murad, S., Kim, W.R., Harnois, D.M., Douglas, D.D., Burton, J., Kulik, L.M., et al., 2012. Efficacy of neoadjuvant chemoradiation, followed by liver transplantation, for perihilar cholangiocarcinoma at 12 US centers. Gastroenterology. 143, 88–98.

Donaldson, P.T., Norris, S., 2002. Evaluation of the role of MHC class II alleles, haplotypes and selected amino acid sequences in primary sclerosing cholangitis. Autoimmunity. 35, 555–564.

EASL Clinical Practice Guidelines: Management of Cholestatic Liver Diseases, 2009. J. Hepatol. 51, 237–267.

Eaton, J.E., Silveira, M.G., Pardi, D.S., Sinakos, E., Kowdley, K.V., Luketic, V.A., et al., 2011. High-dose ursodeoxycholic acid is associated with the development of colorectal neoplasia in patients with ulcerative colitis and primary sclerosing cholangitis. Am. J. Gastroenterol. 106, 1638–1645.

Eaton, J.E., Thackeray, E.W., Lindor, K.D., 2012. Likelihood of malignancy in gallbladder polyps and outcomes following cholecystectomy in primary sclerosing cholangitis. Am. J. Gastroenterol. 107, 431–439.

Eksteen, B., Mora, J.R., Haughton, E.L., Henderson, N.C., Lee-Turner, L., Villablanca, E.J., et al., 2009. Gut homing receptors on CD8 T cells are retinoic acid dependent and not maintained by liver dendritic or stellate cells. Gastroenterology. 137, 320–329.

Escorsell, A., Pares, A., Rodes, J., Solis-Herruzo, J.A., Miras, M., De La Morena, E., 1994. Epidemiology of primary sclerosing cholangitis in Spain. Spanish Association for the Study of the Liver. J. Hepatol. 21, 787–791.

Farrant, J.M., Doherty, D.G., Donaldson, P.T., Vaughan, R.W., Hayllar, K.M., Welsh, K.I., et al., 1992. Amino acid substitutions at position 38 of the DR beta polypeptide confer susceptibility to and protection from primary sclerosing cholangitis. Hepatology. 16, 390–395.

Feldstein, A.E., Perrault, J., El-Youssif, M., Lindor, K.D., Freese, D.K., Angulo, P., 2003. Primary sclerosing cholangitis in children: a long-term follow-up study. Hepatology. 38, 210–217.

Fickert, P., Fuchsbichler, A., Wagner, M., Zollner, G., Kaser, A., Tilg, H., et al., 2004. Regurgitation of bile acids from leaky bile ducts causes sclerosing cholangitis in Mdr2 (Abcb4) knockout mice. Gastroenterology. 127, 261–274.

Fickert, P., Fuchsbichler, A., Marschall, H.U., Wagner, M., Zollner, G., Krause, R., et al., 2006. Lithocholic acid feeding induces segmental bile duct obstruction and destructive cholangitis in mice. Am. J. Path. 168, 410–422.

Floreani, A., Zancan, L., Melis, A., Baragiotta, A., Chiaramonte, M., 1999. Primary sclerosing cholangitis (PSC): clinical, laboratory and survival analysis in children and adults. Liver. 19, 228–233.

Floreani, A., Rizzotto, E.R., Ferrara, F., Carderi, I., Caroli, D., Blasone, L., et al., 2005. Clinical course and outcome of autoimmune hepatitis/primary sclerosing cholangitis overlap syndrome. Am. J. Gastroenterol. 100, 1516–1522.

Fosby, B., Karlsen, T.H., Melum, E., 2012. Recurrence and rejection in liver transplantation for primary sclerosing cholangitis. World J. Gastroenterol. 18, 1–15.

Ghazale, A., Chari, S.T., Zhang, L., Smyrk, T.C., Takahashi, N., Levy, M.J., et al., 2008. Immunoglobulin G4-associated cholangitis: clinical profile and response to therapy. Gastroenterology. 134, 706–715.

Grant, A.J., Lalor, P.F., Salmi, M., Jalkanen, S., Adams, D.H., 2002. Homing of mucosal lymphocytes to the liver in the pathogenesis of hepatic complications of inflammatory bowel disease. Lancet. 359, 150–157.

Graziadei, I.W., Wiesner, R.H., Marotta, P.J., Porayko, M.K., Hay, J.E., Charlton, M.R., et al., 1999. Long-term results of patients undergoing liver transplantation for primary sclerosing cholangitis. Hepatology. 30, 1121–1127.

Guo, S., Al-Sadi, R., Said, H.M., Ma, T.Y., 2013. Lipopolysaccharide causes an increase in intestinal tight junction permeability in vitro and in vivo by inducing enterocyte membrane expression and localization of TLR-4 and CD14. Am. J. Path. 182, 375–387.

Gur, H., Shen, G., Sutjita, M., Terrberry, J., Alosachie, I., Barka, N., et al., 1995. Autoantibody profile of primary sclerosing cholangitis. Pathobiology. 63, 76–82.

Harnois, D.M., Gores, G.J., Ludwig, J., Steers, J.L., Larusso, N.F., Wiesner, R.H., 1997. Are patients with cirrhotic stage primary sclerosing cholangitis at risk for the development of hepatocellular cancer? J. Hepatol. 27, 512–516.

Hov, J.R., Boberg, K.M., Karlsen, T.H., 2008. Autoantibodies in primary sclerosing cholangitis. World J. Gastroenterol. 14, 3781–3791.

Ibrahim, S.H., Lindor, K.D., 2011. Current management of primary sclerosing cholangitis in pediatric patients. Paediatr. Drugs. 13, 87–95.

Jacquemin, E., De Vree, J.M., Cresteil, D., Sokal, E.M., Sturm, E., Dumont, M., et al., 2001. The wide spectrum of multidrug resistance 3 deficiency: from neonatal cholestasis to cirrhosis of adulthood. Gastroenterology. 120, 1448–1458.

Jorgensen, K.K., Grzyb, K., Lundin, K.E., Clausen, O.P., Aamodt, G., Schrumpf, E., et al., 2012a. Inflammatory bowel disease in patients with primary sclerosing cholangitis: clinical characterization in liver transplanted and nontransplanted patients. Inflamm. Bowel Dis. 18, 536–545.

Jorgensen, K.K., Lindstrom, L., Cvancarova, M., Castedal, M., Friman, S., Schrumpf, E., et al., 2012b. Colorectal neoplasia in patients with primary sclerosing cholangitis undergoing liver transplantation: a Nordic multicenter study. Scand. J. Gastroenterol. 8–9, 1021–1029.

Kaltenthaler, E., Vergel, Y.B., Chilcott, J., Thomas, S., Blakeborough, T., Walters, S.J., et al., 2004. A systematic review and economic evaluation of magnetic resonance cholangiopancreatography compared with diagnostic endoscopic retrograde cholangiopancreatography. Health Technol. Assess. 8 (iii), 1–89.

Kaplan, G.G., Laupland, K.B., Butzner, D., Urbanski, S.J., Lee, S.S., 2007. The burden of large and small duct primary sclerosing cholangitis in adults and children: a population-based analysis. Am. J. Gastroenterol. 102, 1042–1049.

Karlsen, T.H., Franke, A., Melum, E., Kaser, A., Hov, J.R., Balschun, T., et al., 2010. Genome-wide association analysis in primary sclerosing cholangitis. Gastroenterology. 138, 1102–1111.

Karrar, A., Broome, U., Sodergren, T., Jaksch, M., Bergquist, A., Bjornstedt, M., et al., 2007. Biliary epithelial cell antibodies link adaptive and innate immune responses in primary sclerosing cholangitis. Gastroenterology. 132, 1504–1514.

Kaya, M., Petersen, B.T., Angulo, P., Baron, T.H., Andrews, J.C., Gostout, C.J., et al., 2001. Balloon dilation compared to stenting of dominant strictures in primary sclerosing cholangitis. Am. J. Gastroenterol. 96, 1059–1066.

Kekilli, M., Tunc, B., Beyazit, Y., Kurt, M., Onal, I.K., Ulker, A., et al., 2013. Circulating CD4+ CD25+ regulatory T cells in the pathobiology of ulcerative colitis and concurrent primary sclerosing cholangitis. Dig. Dis. Sci. 58, 1250–1255.

Lammert, F., Wang, D.Q., Hillebrandt, S., Geier, A., Fickert, P., Trauner, M., et al., 2004. Spontaneous cholecysto- and hepatolithiasis in Mdr2 −/− mice: a model for low phospholipid-associated cholelithiasis. Hepatology. 39, 117–128.

Lee, Y.M., Kaplan, M.M., 1995. Primary sclerosing cholangitis. N. Engl. J. Med. 332, 924–933.

Lee, Y.M., Kaplan, M.M., 2002. Management of primary sclerosing cholangitis. Am. J. Gastroenterol. 97, 528–534.

Liaskou, E., Karikoski, M., Reynolds, G.M., Lalor, P.F., Weston, C.J., Pullen, N., et al., 2011. Regulation of mucosal addressin cell adhesion molecule 1 expression in human and mice by vascular adhesion protein 1 amine oxidase activity. Hepatology. 53, 661—672.

Lichtman, S.N., Sartor, R.B., 1991. Hepatobiliary injury associated with experimental small-bowel bacterial overgrowth in rats. Immunol. Res. 10, 528—531.

Lindkvist, B., Valle, Benito De, Gullberg, M., Bjornsson, E., B., 2010. Incidence and prevalence of primary sclerosing cholangitis in a defined adult population in Sweden. Hepatology. 52, 571—577.

Lindor, K.D., Kowdley, K.V., Luketic, V.A., Harrison, M.E., Mccashland, T., Befeler, A.S., et al., 2009. High-dose ursodeoxycholic acid for the treatment of primary sclerosing cholangitis. Hepatology. 50, 808—814.

Lindstrom, L., Lapidus, A., Ost, A., Bergquist, A., 2011. Increased risk of colorectal cancer and dysplasia in patients with Crohn's colitis and primary sclerosing cholangitis. Dis. Colon Rectum. 54, 1392—1397.

Lindstrom, L., Boberg, K.M., Wikman, O., Friis-Liby, I., Hultcrantz, R., Prytz, H., et al., 2012. High dose ursodeoxycholic acid in primary sclerosing cholangitis does not prevent colorectal neoplasia. Aliment. Pharmacol. Ther. 35, 451—457.

Loftus Jr., E.V., Harewood, G.C., Loftus, C.G., Tremaine, W.J., Harmsen, W.S., Zinsmeister, A.R., et al., 2005. PSC-IBD: a unique form of inflammatory bowel disease associated with primary sclerosing cholangitis. Gut. 54, 91—96.

Ludwig, J., La Russo, N., Wiesner, R.H., 1986. Primary sclerosing cholangitis. In: Peters, R.L., Craig, J.R. (Eds.), Contemporary Issues in Surgical Pathology: Liver Pathology, vol. 8. Churchill Livingstone, New York, pp. 193—213.

Mandal, A., Dasgupta, A., Jeffers, L., Squillante, L., Hyder, S., Reddy, R., et al., 1994. Autoantibodies in sclerosing cholangitis against a shared peptide in biliary and colon epithelium. Gastroenterology. 106, 185—192.

Marelli, L., Xirouchakis, E., Kalambokis, G., Cholongitas, E., Hamilton, M.I., Burroughs, A.K., 2011. Does the severity of primary sclerosing cholangitis influence the clinical course of associated ulcerative colitis? Gut. 60, 1224—1228.

Martins, E.B., Graham, A.K., Chapman, R.W., Fleming, K.A., 1996. Elevation of gamma delta T lymphocytes in peripheral blood and livers of patients with primary sclerosing cholangitis and other autoimmune liver diseases. Hepatology. 23, 988—993.

Medvedev, A.E., Sabroe, I., Hasday, J.D., Vogel, S.N., 2006. Tolerance to microbial TLR ligands: molecular mechanisms and relevance to disease. J. Endotoxin. Res. 12, 133—150.

Mehal, W.Z., Lo, Y.M., Wordsworth, B.P., Neuberger, J.M., Hubscher, S.C., Fleming, K.A., et al., 1994. HLA DR4 is a marker for rapid disease progression in primary sclerosing cholangitis. Gastroenterology. 106, 160—167.

Melum, E., Franke, A., Schramm, C., Weismuller, T.J., Gotthardt, D.N., Offner, F.A., et al., 2011. Genome-wide association analysis in primary sclerosing cholangitis identifies two non-HLA susceptibility loci. Nat. Genet. 43, 17—19.

Mendes, F.D., Jorgensen, R., Keach, J., Katzmann, J.A., Smyrk, T., Donlinger, J., et al., 2006. Elevated serum IgG4 concentration in patients with primary sclerosing cholangitis. Am. J. Gastroenterol. 101, 2070—2075.

Miloh, T., Arnon, R., Shneider, B., Suchy, F., Kerkar, N., 2009. A retrospective single-center review of primary sclerosing cholangitis in children. Clin. Gastroenterol. Hepatol. 7, 239—245.

Mitchell, S.A., Thyssen, M., Orchard, T.R., Jewell, D.P., Fleming, K.A., Chapman, R.W., 2002. Cigarette smoking, appendectomy, and tonsillectomy as risk factors for the development of primary sclerosing cholangitis: a case control study. Gut. 51, 567—573.

Molodecky, N.A., Kareemi, H., Parab, R., Barkema, H.W., Quan, H., Myers, R.P., et al., 2011. Incidence of primary sclerosing cholangitis: a systematic review and meta-analysis. Hepatology. 53, 1590—1599.

Mueller, T., Beutler, C., Pico, A.H., Shibolet, O., Pratt, D.S., Pascher, A., et al., 2011. Enhanced innate immune responsiveness and intolerance to intestinal endotoxins in human biliary epithelial cells contributes to chronic cholangitis. Liver Int. 31, 1574—1588.

Navaneethan, U., Venkatesh, P.G., Mukewar, S., Lashner, B.A., Remzi, F.H., Mccullough, A.J., et al., 2012. Progressive primary sclerosing cholangitis requiring liver transplantation is associated with reduced need for colectomy in patients with ulcerative colitis. Clin. Gastroenterol. Hepatol. 10, 540—546.

Norris, S., Kondeatis, E., Collins, R., Satsangi, J., Clare, M., Chapman, R., et al., 2001. Mapping MHC-encoded susceptibility and resistance in primary sclerosing cholangitis: the role of MICA polymorphism. Gastroenterology. 120, 1475—1482.

O'mahony, C.A., Vierling, J.M., 2006. Etiopathogenesis of primary sclerosing cholangitis. Semin. Liver Dis. 26, 3—21.

Olerup, O., Olsson, R., Hultcrantz, R., Broome, U., 1995. HLA-DR and HLA-DQ are not markers for rapid disease progression in primary sclerosing cholangitis. Gastroenterology. 108, 870—878.

Olsson, R., Danielsson, A., Jarnerot, G., Lindstrom, E., Loof, L., Rolny, P., et al., 1991. Prevalence of primary sclerosing cholangitis in patients with ulcerative colitis. Gastroenterology. 100, 1319—1323.

Olsson, R., Boberg, K.M., De Muckadell, O.S., Lindgren, S., Hultcrantz, R., Folvik, G., et al., 2005. High-dose ursodeoxycholic acid in primary sclerosing cholangitis: a 5-year multicenter, randomized, controlled study. Gastroenterology. 129, 1464—1472.

Oseini, A.M., Chaiteerakij, R., Shire, A.M., Ghazale, A., Kaiya, J., Moser, C.D., et al., 2011. Utility of serum immunoglobulin G4 in distinguishing immunoglobulin G4-associated cholangitis from cholangiocarcinoma. Hepatology. 54, 940—948.

Palmer, K.R., Duerden, B.I., Holdsworth, C.D., 1980. Bacteriological and endotoxin studies in cases of ulcerative colitis submitted to surgery. Gut. 21, 851—854.

Pardi, D.S., Loftus Jr., E.V., Kremers, W.K., Keach, J., Lindor, K.D., 2003. Ursodeoxycholic acid as a chemopreventive agent in patients with ulcerative colitis and primary sclerosing cholangitis. Gastroenterology. 124, 889—893.

Penna, C., Dozois, R., Tremaine, W., Sandborn, W., Larusso, N., Schleck, C., et al., 1996. Pouchitis after ileal pouch-anal anastomosis for ulcerative colitis occurs with increased frequency in patients with associated primary sclerosing cholangitis. Gut. 38, 234—239.

Pollheimer, M.J., Trauner, M., Fickert, P., 2011. Will we ever model PSC?—"it's hard to be a PSC model!". Clin. Res. Hepatol. Gastroenterol. 35, 792—804.

Ponsioen, C.Y., Vrouenraets, S.M., Prawirodirdjo, W., Rajaram, R., Rauws, E.A., Mulder, C.J., et al., 2002. Natural history of primary sclerosing cholangitis and prognostic value of cholangiography in a Dutch population. Gut. 51, 562—566.

Porayko, M.K., Wiesner, R.H., Larusso, N.F., Ludwig, J., Maccarty, R.L., Steiner, B.L., et al., 1990. Patients with asymptomatic primary sclerosing cholangitis frequently have progressive disease. Gastroenterology. 98, 1594–1602.

Probert, C.S., Christ, A.D., Saubermann, L.J., Turner, J.R., Chott, A., Carr-Locke, D., et al., 1997. Analysis of human common bile duct-associated T cells: evidence for oligoclonality, T cell clonal persistence, and epithelial cell recognition. J. Immunol. 158, 1941–1948.

Razumilava, N., Gores, G.J., Lindor, K.D., 2011. Cancer surveillance in patients with primary sclerosing cholangitis. Hepatology. 54, 1842–1852.

Rosen, C.B., Nagorney, D.M., 1991. Cholangiocarcinoma complicating primary sclerosing cholangitis. Semin. Liver Dis. 11, 26–30.

Senaldi, G., Donaldson, P.T., Magrin, S., Farrant, J.M., Alexander, G.J., Vergani, D., et al., 1989. Activation of the complement system in primary sclerosing cholangitis. Gastroenterology. 97, 1430–1434.

Sheth, P., Delos Santos, N., Seth, A., Larusso, N.F., Rao, R.K., 2007. Lipopolysaccharide disrupts tight junctions in cholangiocyte monolayers by a c-Src-, TLR4-, and LBP-dependent mechanism. Am. J. Physiol. Gastrointest. Liver Physiol. 293, G308–G318.

Sheth, S., Shea, J.C., Bishop, M.D., Chopra, S., Regan, M.M., Malmberg, E., et al., 2003. Increased prevalence of CFTR mutations and variants and decreased chloride secretion in primary sclerosing cholangitis. Hum. Genet. 113, 286–292.

Soetikno, R.M., Lin, O.S., Heidenreich, P.A., Young, H.S., Blackstone, M.O., 2002. Increased risk of colorectal neoplasia in patients with primary sclerosing cholangitis and ulcerative colitis: a meta-analysis. Gastrointest. Endosc. 56, 48–54.

Spurkland, A., Saarinen, S., Boberg, K.M., Mitchell, S., Broome, U., Caballeria, L., et al., 1999. HLA class II haplotypes in primary sclerosing cholangitis patients from five European populations. Tissue Antigens. 53, 459–469.

Stanich, P.P., Bjornsson, E., Gossard, A.A., Enders, F., Jorgensen, R., Lindor, K.D., 2011. Alkaline phosphatase normalization is associated with better prognosis in primary sclerosing cholangitis. Dig. Liv. Dis. 43, 309–313.

Stiehl, A., Rudolph, G., Kloters-Plachky, P., Sauer, P., Walker, S., 2002. Development of dominant bile duct stenoses in patients with primary sclerosing cholangitis treated with ursodeoxycholic acid: outcome after endoscopic treatment. J. Hepatol. 36, 151–156.

Takeda, K., Kojima, Y., Ikejima, K., Harada, K., Yamashina, S., Okumura, K., et al., 2008. Death receptor 5 mediated-apoptosis contributes to cholestatic liver disease. Proc. Natl. Acad. Sci. USA. 105, 10895–10900.

Talwalkar, J.A., Angulo, P., Johnson, C.D., Petersen, B.T., Lindor, K.D., 2004. Cost-minimization analysis of MRC versus ERCP for the diagnosis of primary sclerosing cholangitis. Hepatology. 40, 39–45.

Terjung, B., Spengler, U., 2009. Atypical p-ANCA in PSC and AIH: a hint toward a "leaky gut"?. Clin. Rev. Allergy Immunol. 36, 40–51.

Terjung, B., Sohne, J., Lechtenberg, B., Gottwein, J., Muennich, M., Herzog, V., et al., 2010. p-ANCAs in autoimmune liver disorders recognise human beta-tubulin isotype 5 and cross-react with microbial protein FtsZ. Gut. 59, 808–816.

Thackeray, E.W., Charatcharoenwitthaya, P., Elfaki, D., Sinakos, E., Lindor, K.D., 2011. Colon neoplasms develop early in the course of inflammatory bowel disease and primary sclerosing cholangitis. Clin. Gastroenterol. Hepatol. 9, 52–56.

Trauner, M., Boyer, J.L., 2003. Bile salt transporters: molecular characterization, function, and regulation. Physiol. Rev. 83, 633–671.

Trauner, M., Fickert, P., Wagner, M., 2007. MDR3 (ABCB4) defects: a paradigm for the genetics of adult cholestatic syndromes. Semin. Liver Dis. 27, 77–98.

Trivedi, P.J., Hirschfield, G.M., 2012. Review article: overlap syndromes and autoimmune liver disease. Aliment. Pharmacol. Ther. 36, 517–533.

Tung, B.Y., Emond, M.J., Haggitt, R.C., Bronner, M.P., Kimmey, M.B., Kowdley, K.V., et al., 2001. Ursodiol use is associated with lower prevalence of colonic neoplasia in patients with ulcerative colitis and primary sclerosing cholangitis. Ann. Intern. Med. 134, 89–95.

Verdonk, R.C., Dijkstra, G., Haagsma, E.B., Shostrom, V.K., Van Den Berg, A.P., Kleibeuker, J.H., et al., 2006. Inflammatory bowel disease after liver transplantation: risk factors for recurrence and de novo disease. Am. J. Transplant. 6, 1422–1429.

Wen, L., Peakman, M., Mieli-Vergani, G., Vergani, D., 1992. Elevation of activated gamma delta T cell receptor bearing T lymphocytes in patients with autoimmune chronic liver disease. Clin. Exp. Immunol. 89, 78–82.

Wolf, J.M., Rybicki, L.A., Lashner, B.A., 2005. The impact of ursodeoxycholic acid on cancer, dysplasia and mortality in ulcerative colitis patients with primary sclerosing cholangitis. Aliment. Pharmacol. Ther. 22, 783–788.

Xu, B., Broome, U., Ericzon, B.G., Sumitran-Holgersson, S., 2002. High frequency of autoantibodies in patients with primary sclerosing cholangitis that bind biliary epithelial cells and induce expression of CD44 and production of interleukin 6. Gut. 51, 120–127.

Yamada, S., Ishii, M., Liang, L.S., Yamamoto, T., Toyota, T., 1994. Small duct cholangitis induced by N-formyl L-methionine L-leucine L-tyrosine in rats. J. Gastroenterol. 29, 631–636.

Chapter 64

Autoimmune Pancreatitis and IgG4-related Disease

Shigeyuki Kawa[1], Hideaki Hamano[2], and Kendo Kiyosawa[3]

[1]Center for Health, Safety and Environmental Management, Shinshu University, Matsumoto, Japan, [2]Department of Medical Information, Shinshu University School of Medicine, Matsumoto, Japan, [3]Department of Medicine, Nagano Red Cross Hospital, Nagano, Japan

Chapter Outline

Historical Background · 937
Autoimmune Pancreatitis – Clinical, Pathologic, and Epidemiological Features · 938
 Clinical Features · 938
  Symptoms · 938
  Laboratory Tests · 938
  Ultrasound and Radioimage Findings · 938
  Misdiagnosis of Pancreatic Cancer · 938
 Extra-pancreatic Lesions · 939
 Pathological Features · 939
 Epidemiologic Features · 940
 Autoimmune Features · 940
 Genetic Features · 941
Animal Models · 942
Pathological Mechanisms · 942
Immunological Markers in Diagnosis · 944
Treatment and Outcome · 944
IgG4-related Disease · 944
 Definition · 944
 Historical Background · 945
 Epidemiology · 945

Clinical Features of IgG4-related Disease · 945
Definite IgG4-related Diseases · 945
 IgG4-related Lacrimal and Salivary Gland Lesions · 945
 IgG4-related Lung Disease · 945
 IgG4-related Sclerosing Cholangitis · 946
 IgG4-related Liver Disease · 946
 IgG4-related Kidney Disease · 946
 IgG4-related Retroperitoneal Fibrosis · 946
Possible IgG4-related Diseases · 946
 IgG4-related Hypophysitis · 946
 IgG4-related Hypertrophic Pachymeningitis · 946
 IgG4-related Thyroid Disease · 946
 Gastrointestinal Disease · 947
 Prostate Disease · 947
Pathological Features · 947
Autoimmune Features, Genetic Features, Animal Models, and Pathological Mechanisms · 947
Diagnosis · 947
Treatment · 947
Concluding Remarks: Future Prospects · 948
References · 948

HISTORICAL BACKGROUND

In 1961, Sarles et al. first reported a specific type of pancreatitis as chronic inflammatory sclerosis of the pancreas that showed hyperglobulinemia and histologically marked lymphocytic infiltration (Sarles et al., 1961). In 1978, Nakano et al. reported the first case that had been successfully treated with corticosteroids (Nakano et al., 1978). In 1991, Kawaguchi designated this condition as a lymphoplasmacytic sclerosing pancreatitis (LPSP) based on a detailed pathological study (Kawaguchi et al., 1991). In 1992, Toki et al. reported chronic pancreatitis showing diffuse irregular narrowing of the entire main pancreatic duct (Toki et al., 1992). Yoshida and Toki et al. summarized the clinical features and designated this condition as autoimmune pancreatitis based on clinical findings of hypergammaglobulinemia, positive tests for autoantibodies and lymphoplasmacytic infiltration in the pancreas, and a favorable response to corticosteroid treatment (Yoshida et al., 1995). Since then, many patients have been diagnosed based on these characteristic clinical findings, and a number of reports on single cases or small series of cases have been published. In 2001, Hamano et al. reported that patients with autoimmune pancreatitis

N. Rose & I. Mackay (Eds): The Autoimmune Diseases, Fifth edition. DOI: http://dx.doi.org/10.1016/B978-0-12-384929-8.00064-2

frequently and specifically have high serum IgG4 concentrations that correlate well with disease activity, suggesting that this disease is a discrete clinical entity different from ordinary chronic pancreatitis (Hamano et al., 2001). In 2002, Hamano et al. first reported abundant IgG4-bearing plasma cell infiltration in the pancreas and extra-pancreatic sites of disease, and this remains as a histological hallmark of autoimmune pancreatitis and IgG4-related disease (Hamano et al., 2002). In 2002 and 2006, the Japanese Pancreas Society and the Research Committee of Intractable Diseases of the Pancreas proposed Japanese diagnostic criteria for autoimmune pancreatitis (Steinberg et al., 2003; Okazaki et al., 2006). Subsequently, diagnostic criteria for autoimmune pancreatitis were proposed in other countries, and the International Consensus Diagnostic Criteria (ICDC) for Autoimmune Pancreatitis was published in 2011 (Shimosegawa et al., 2011). The ICDC allow diagnosis of autoimmune pancreatitis based on the international standards and differentiate this condition from pancreatic cancer and other types of pancreatitis.

Notably, there has been reported another type of autoimmune pancreatitis that is based pathologically on granulocyte infiltration into the pancreatic duct epithelium. These pathological findings were termed "idiopathic duct-centric chronic pancreatitis" (IDCP) (Notohara et al., 2003) or "autoimmune pancreatitis with granulocytic epithelial lesions" (AIP with GEL) (Zamboni et al., 2004). Recently, the LPSP form of autoimmune pancreatitis which was closely associated with IgG4 was designated as type 1 autoimmune pancreatitis, whereas the IDCP/AIP with GEL form was designated as type 2 (Sugumar et al., 2009). Although the IDCP/AIP with GEL form of autoimmune pancreatitis seems to be prevalent in Western countries, the clinical features, including the autoimmune nature, remain obscure. Accordingly, this article focuses on the LPSP form of autoimmune pancreatitis.

AUTOIMMUNE PANCREATITIS – CLINICAL, PATHOLOGIC, AND EPIDEMIOLOGICAL FEATURES

Clinical Features

Symptoms

We analyzed the clinical findings in 98 patients with autoimmune pancreatitis that fulfilled the diagnostic criteria proposed by the ICDC. The summarized clinical features based on our results and published reports are as follows. The male-to-female ratio was 75:23 (male 77%), and the median age of occurrence was 63 years (range 38–85), suggesting that this disease shows an elderly male preponderance. Few patients complained of severe attacks of pancreatitis, but many (80%) had mild to moderate epigastralgia or discomfort, thus different from those of classical acute pancreatitis. A striking feature was obstructive jaundice in 70%, caused by the stenosis or obstruction of the intra-pancreatic common bile duct (Yoshida et al., 1995; Horiuchi et al., 1998, 2001; Kawa et al., 2011a). Diabetes mellitus (DM) was often observed, and the majority were thought to have type 2 DM. Some patients improved after steroid therapy (Tanaka et al., 2000).

Laboratory Tests

Laboratory tests showed several abnormal findings related to the obstructive jaundice such as elevated serum levels of bilirubin, biliary enzymes, and transaminases in 70–80% of patients. The tumor-associated antigen, CA19-9, showed elevated levels in 50% of patients, probably due to cholestasis rather than a malignant process. Serum elevations of pancreatic enzyme were mild or moderate, and were found in 60% of patients. Serum elevations of γ-globulin and IgG were found in 60% and 70%, respectively. Positive rates for antinuclear antibody were 40%, and those of other antibodies were 10–30%. Decreased exocrine and endocrine function by the bentiromide test and HbA1c were found in 66% and 51%, respectively (Horiuchi et al., 1998, 2001; Kawa et al., 2011a).

Ultrasound and Radioimage Findings

Abdominal ultrasonography (US) showed characteristic sonolucent swelling, a so-called sausage-like appearance, and dilatation of the common bile duct. Computed tomography (CT) with contrast material revealed swelling and delayed enhancement of parenchyma, resulting in a peripheral low-density area and a capsule-like rim (Figure 64.1). Endoscopic retrograde cholangiopancreatography (ERCP) showed a characteristic pancreatogram of diffuse but irregular narrowing (Figure 64.2). Cholangiography showed severe narrowing of the lower bile duct, which was caused by swelling of the head of the pancreas. However, intraductal ultrasonography (IDUS) showed that thickening of the bile duct wall also contributed to narrowing of the bile duct. In some cases, bile duct changes extended to extrapancreatic regions such as the intrahepatic bile duct system and resembled primary sclerosing cholangitis (PSC) (Figure 64.3). Gallium-67 scintigraphy and fluorine-18 fluorodeoxyglucose positron emission tomography (FDG-PET) showed characteristic pancreatic and extra-pancreatic accumulation during the active stage of the disease (Saegusa et al., 2003; Ozaki et al., 2007).

Misdiagnosis of Pancreatic Cancer

Patients with autoimmune pancreatitis sometimes receive the erroneous diagnosis of pancreatic cancer because of the preponderance of the disease in the elderly together with

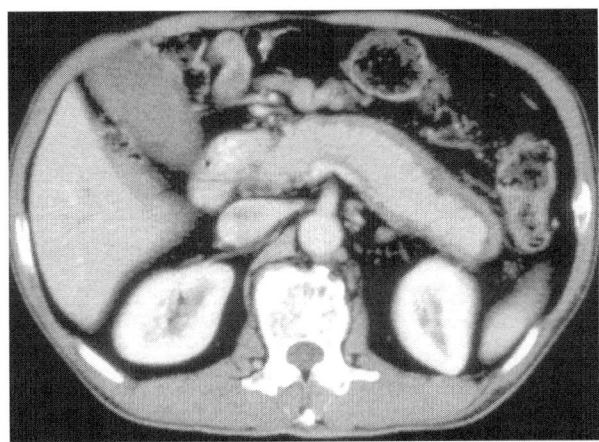

FIGURE 64.1 Contrast-enhanced computed tomography (CT) image of autoimmune pancreatitis, showing swelling and delayed enhancement of parenchymal tissue. The result is a peripheral low-density area and a capsule-like rim.

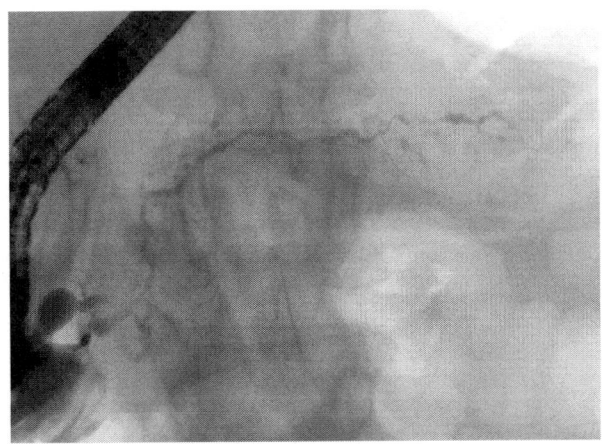

FIGURE 64.2 Endoscopic retrograde cholangiopancreatography (ERCP) showing the characteristic pancreatogram of diffuse irregular narrowing seen in autoimmune pancreatitis.

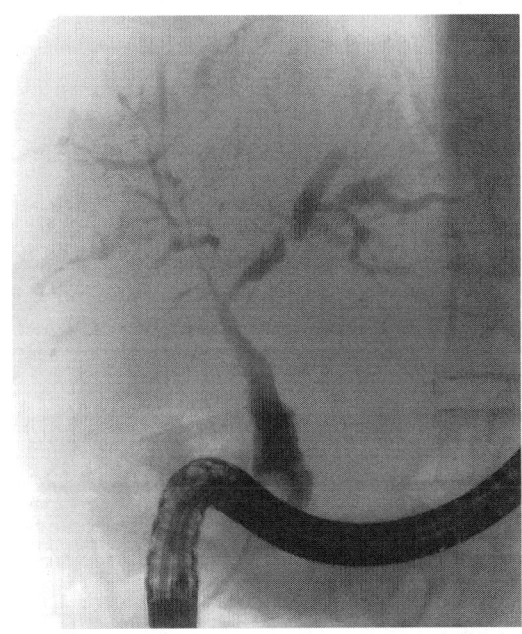

FIGURE 64.3 Endoscopic retrograde cholangiopancreatography (ERCP) showing the characteristic intrahepatic bile duct changes in autoimmune pancreatitis that are similar to those in primary sclerosing cholangitis (PSC).

obstructive jaundice, serum elevations of CA19-9, and irregular narrowing or obstruction of the pancreatic duct. Pathological analysis after pancreaticoduodenectomy (Whipple resection), performed because of a diagnosis of pancreatic cancer, disclosed results representative of autoimmune pancreatitis (lymphoplasmacytic sclerosing pancreatitis: LPSP) in 2.2% of patients (Hardacre et al., 2003). Because of similar pathological findings, this disease has also been diagnosed as pancreatic lymphoma (Horiuchi et al., 1996).

Extra-pancreatic Lesions

Autoimmune pancreatitis is characterized by extra-pancreatic lesions (Figure 64.4) (Hamano et al., 2006; Fujinaga et al.,

2009) such as swelling of the lacrimal and salivary glands (Figure 64.5) (Kamisawa et al., 2003a; Yamamoto et al., 2005a), sclerosing cholangitis (Figure 64.3) (Erkelens et al., 1999; Nakazawa et al., 2001; Horiuchi et al., 2001), retroperitoneal fibrosis (Hamano et al., 2002), interstitial lung disease (Taniguchi et al., 2004), hilar lymphadenopathy (Saegusa et al., 2003), lung nodules (Zen et al., 2005), tubulointerstitial nephritis (Takeda et al., 2004; Saeki et al., 2010), liver disease or IgG4-hepatopathy (Umemura et al., 2007a), hypophysitis (van der Vliet et al., 2004), gastric ulcer (Shinji et al., 2004), hypothyroidism (Komatsu et al., 2005), and prostatitis (Yoshimura et al., 2006). These extra-pancreatic lesions share common clinical and pathological features, i.e., favorable response to corticosteroid therapy and IgG4-bearing plasma cell infiltration, suggesting the presence of systemic disease, i.e., IgG4-related disease (Kamisawa et al., 2003b; Kawa and Sugai, 2011b; Umehara et al., 2012a,b). Autoimmune pancreatitis is now recognized as the pancreatic manifestation of IgG4-related disease.

Pathological Features

On gross examination, the involved pancreas appears glistening white, is firm or hard, and may be enlarged or show mass lesions. The lesion may be limited to one portion of the pancreas, most often the head, or may involve the body, tail, or entire organ. Lymphoplasmacytic infiltration and fibrosis are characteristic microscopic features of the pancreatic lesions, and in some cases result in the formation of

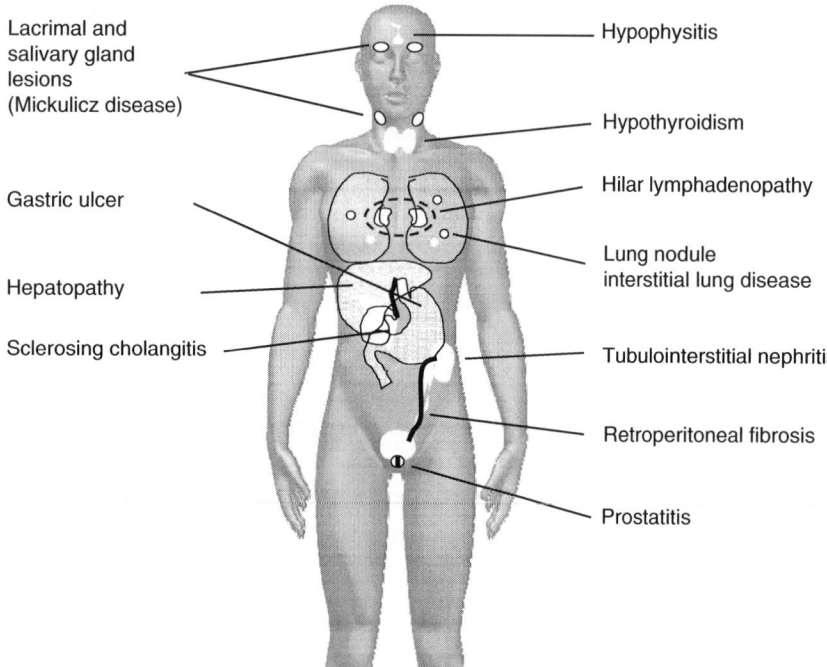

FIGURE 64.4 Extra-pancreatic lesions associated with autoimmune pancreatitis. These lesions are comprehensively termed IgG4-related disease.

Lacrimal and salivary gland lesions (Mickulicz disease)

Gastric ulcer

Hepatopathy

Sclerosing cholangitis

Hypophysitis

Hypothyroidism

Hilar lymphadenopathy

Lung nodule interstitial lung disease

Tubulointerstitial nephritis

Retroperitoneal fibrosis

Prostatitis

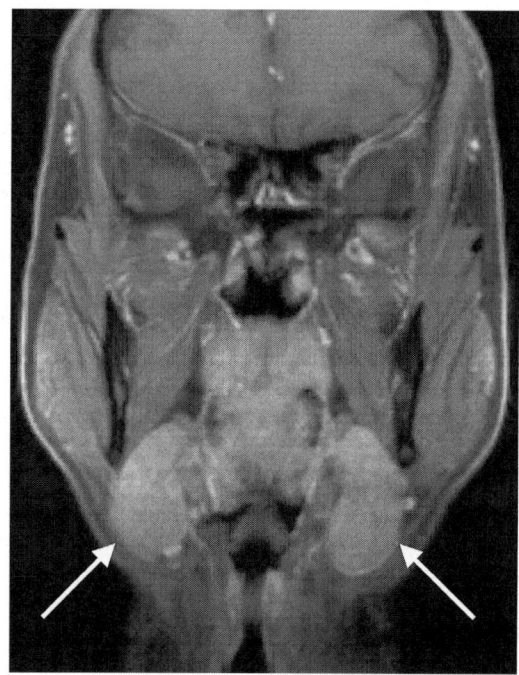

FIGURE 64.5 Magnetic resonance imaging (MRI) showing swelling of salivary glands (arrows) complicated with autoimmune pancreatitis.

resulting in stenosis or obstruction of the duct, stasis of the pancreatic secretions, and damage to the pancreatic lobules. Obliterating phlebitis is another characteristic feature, which shows a marked cellular infiltration of the venous wall and venous thrombosis (Kawaguchi et al., 1991). The histological features observed in the extra-pancreatic lesions such as in the salivary glands (Kamisawa et al., 2003a) or retroperitoneal fibrosis (Hamano et al., 2002) resemble those seen in the pancreas.

Epidemiologic Features

A nationwide survey in Japan by the Research Committee of Intractable Diseases of the Pancreas showed a prevalence of 0.82/100,000 inhabitants, corresponding roughly to 2% of all patients with chronic pancreatitis (Nishimori et al., 2007; Shimosegawa and Kanno, 2009). Due to diagnostic criteria proposals, the number of patients in Japan and other countries has increased (Hart et al., 2012). However, autoimmune pancreatitis is a relatively rare disorder, and its exact prevalence remains unknown.

Autoimmune Features

Positive rates for antinuclear antibody were 40%, and those of other antibodies were 10–30%. We found no patients with positive test for SS-A/Ro or SS-B/La antibodies, or anti-mitochondrial antibodies that represent disease-specific antibodies for the diagnosis of Sjögren's syndrome or primary biliary cirrhosis (PBC), respectively. These findings suggest that the autoantibodies found in

lymphoid follicles. Immunostaining has demonstrated that T cells predominate over B cells among the infiltrating lymphocytes. The infiltrating plasma cells characteristically bear IgG4 (Hamano et al., 2002) (Figure 64.6). The cell infiltration is prominent around the pancreatic duct,

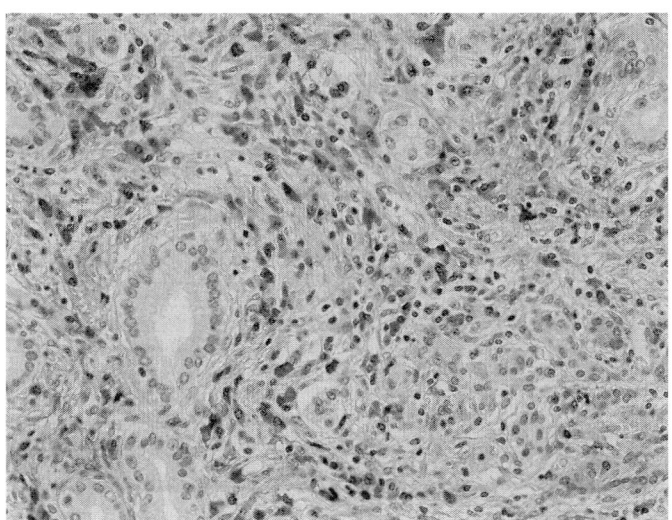

FIGURE 64.6 IgG4 immunostaining of pancreatic tissue with autoimmune pancreatitis, showing abundant infiltration of IgG4-bearing plasma cells.

this disease are not pathogenic, and that patients have a tendency to produce various autoantibodies that are neither disease specific nor of primary relevance. However, the occasional coexistence of pancreatitis with salivary gland lesions and cholangitis suggests shared target antigens. Carbonic anhydrase II (CA II) and lactoferrin are distributed in the cells of several exocrine organs, including the pancreas, salivary glands, and biliary duct. In this context, CA II or lactoferrin have been proposed as a candidate target antigen, but the presence of autoantibodies for these antigens is not sufficiently specific or sensitive (Kino-Ohsaki et al., 1996).

Protein electrophoresis of patients' sera showed a polyclonal band in the rapidly migrating fraction of γ-globulins. Later, immunoelectrophoresis confirmed that this polyclonal band was caused by a high serum concentration of IgG4. We confirmed that serum IgG4 elevation could be found in 90% of patients with autoimmune pancreatitis, but in very few patients with other conditions including pancreatic cancer, chronic pancreatitis, and Sjögren's syndrome, suggesting that IgG4 is a sensitive and specific marker for this disease. In addition, levels of IgG4 correlate well with disease activity (Hamano et al., 2001).

Genetic Features

Autoimmune diseases are multifactorial, and pathogenesis involves a complex interplay of multiple genetic and environmental factors. Several genes, including human leukocyte antigen (HLA), Fc receptor-like 3 (FCRL3), and cytotoxic T lymphocyte antigen (CTLA4), contribute to autoimmune diseases. HLA serotypes DR4 and DQ4 are the markers most frequently associated with autoimmune pancreatitis among the major histocompatibility complex

(MHC) class I and class II molecules. Among the DR4 and DQ4 subtypes, the frequencies of DRB1*0405 and DQB1*0401 are significantly higher in autoimmune pancreatitis patients than in normal subjects or in patients with chronic pancreatitis. In the Japanese population, DRB1*0405 is known to be in strong linkage disequilibrium with DQB1*0401, resulting in the DRB1*0405-DQB1*0401 haplotype. This haplotype is specifically associated with susceptibility to autoimmune pancreatitis and may play a functional role in antigen presentation and induction of an autoimmune response (Kawa et al., 2002). HLA-DR*0405 transgenic mice experience a high prevalence of autoimmune pancreatitis after sublethal irradiation and adoptive transfer of CD90[+] T cells. HLA-DR*0405 transgenic mice can also develop unprovoked autoimmune pancreatitis, whereas HLA-DR*0401, HLA-DQ8, and HLA-DR*0405/DQ8 transgenic controls all remained normal, even after irradiation and adoptive transfer of CD90[+] T cells. Since HLA-DR*0405 expression fails to protect mice from autoimmune pancreatitis, this allele appears to be an important risk factor for autoimmune pancreatitis in the HLA-DRB1*0405/DQB1*0401 haplotype (Freitag et al., 2010). In a case-control study using microsatellite markers distributed throughout the HLA region, we mapped autoimmune pancreatitis susceptibility to two regions of the telomeric region of HLA adjacent to the C3-2-11 marker and to HLA DRB1-DQB1. The region adjacent to C3-2-11 contains the ATP-binding cassette sub-family F (ABCF1) gene, which is regulated by TNF-α, a major cytokine that participates in inflammatory and autoimmune reactions (Ota et al., 2007).

Although autoimmune pancreatitis responds well to corticosteroid therapy, relapse is not uncommon during maintenance therapy or after the cessation of corticosteroids. A previous study found that DQβ1 mutations with substitutions in aspartic acid at residue 57 were significantly associated with relapses of autoimmune pancreatitis (Park do et al., 2008).

Polymorphisms in the *FCRL* genes alter the binding affinity of nuclear factor κB and regulate *FCRL3* expression. An analysis of genotype frequencies for *FCRL3-110* polymorphisms revealed a significant association between the −110A/A genotype and autoimmune pancreatitis, and serum IgG4 concentrations were significantly and positively correlated with the number of susceptibility alleles (Umemura et al., 2006).

The *CTLA4* (or *CD152*) gene product is an inhibitory receptor expressed on the surface of activated memory T cells and CD4$^+$CD25$^+$ regulatory T cells (Tregs); this receptor largely acts as a negative regulator of T cell responses. The *CTLA4* +49A/G single nucleotide polymorphism (SNP) has been associated with susceptibility to autoimmune diseases. We found that the frequency of the +6230G/G genotype was significantly higher in Japanese patients with autoimmune pancreatitis than in those without the disease, and that the +49A/A and +6230A/A genotypes were associated with an enhanced risk of autoimmune pancreatitis relapse (Umemura et al., 2008). The *CTLA-4* 49A polymorphism and the −318C/+49A/CT60G haplotype have also been associated with autoimmune pancreatitis in a Chinese population (Chang et al., 2007).

An association analysis involving 400 microsatellite markers with an average spacing of 10.8 cM in the genome revealed the association of autoimmune pancreatitis with seven SNPs within the 20-kb region around the potassium voltage-gated channel, shaker-related subfamily, member 3 gene (*KCNA3*). Further analysis of *KCNA3* by SNP genotyping revealed four SNPs that were significantly associated with autoimmune pancreatitis susceptibility (Ota et al., 2011). Notably, *KCNA3* is involved in immunomodulation of autoreactive effector T cell- and memory T cell-mediated autoimmune diseases.

ANIMAL MODELS

Putative animal models of autoimmune pancreatitis have been developed by immunizing thymectomized neonatal mice with carbonic anhydrase (CA II) and lactoferrin and transferring immunized spleen cells to nude mice (Uchida et al., 2002). In that study, inflammation was present in the pancreas of the immunized thymectomized neonatal mice and in all mice that received whole spleen cells or CD4$^+$ cells. CA II- or lactoferrin-immunized mice develop apoptotic duct cells or acinar cells, respectively. Taken together, these observations suggest that an immunological response to CA II or lactoferrin is involved in pathogenesis of these pancreatitis models in which the effector cells are Th1-type CD4$^+$ T cells. Adoptive transfer of amylase-

specific CD4$^+$ T cells in rats also results in pancreatitis characterized by mononuclear cell infiltrates and destruction of lobular tissue (Davidson et al., 2005). Another animal model for autoimmune pancreatitis was developed by exposing C57BL/6 mice to heat-killed *Escherichia coli*, which results in marked cellular infiltration with fibrosis in the exocrine pancreas and salivary gland. Antibodies for CA II and lactoferrin, as well as antinuclear antibody, occur in the sera of mice inoculated with heat-killed *E. coli* (Haruta et al., 2010). These findings suggest that silently infiltrating microorganisms such as avirulent bacteria can engage pathogen-associated molecular patterns (PAMPs) and thereby activate the innate immune systems so as to elicit a host immune response to the target antigen by molecular mimicry, and at the same time result in the establishment of autoimmune pancreatitis (Oldstone, 1998; Haruta et al., 2010).

PATHOLOGICAL MECHANISMS

An aberrant immune response to microbial antigens may underlie the immunopathogenesis of autoimmune pancreatitis. Antigens derived from intestinal microflora may activate the host's innate immune system via pattern recognition receptors such as the Toll-like receptors (TLRs) and nucleotide-binding oligomerization (NOD)-like receptors (NLRs). Peripheral blood mononuclear cells, presumably B cells, from patients with autoimmune pancreatitis show enhanced production of IgG4 upon stimulation with NLR and TLR ligands, which is associated with release of B cell-activating factor (BAFF) (Yamanishi et al., 2011; Watanabe et al., 2011). Since the systemic IgG4 response is one of the most important immunological features of autoimmune pancreatitis, abnormal innate immune responses via NLRs and TLRs may underlie the immunopathogenesis of IgG4-related autoimmune pancreatitis (Watanabe et al., 2011).

Helicobactor pylori infection may also trigger autoimmune pancreatitis, possibly as a result of molecular mimicry. There is substantial homology between human CA II and *H. pylori* alpha-carbonic anhydrase; the homologous segments contain the binding motif of the HLA molecule *DRB1*04:05*, which is closely associated with autoimmune pancreatitis (Kawa et al., 2002). These data led to the hypothesis that the *DRB1*0405*-restricted peptide of CA II is presented in genetically predisposed subjects, and reactive T cells injure pancreatic tissue via interaction with the CA II of pancreatic ductal cells (Guarneri et al., 2005). To identify pathogenetically relevant autoantigen targets, a random peptide library derived from pooled IgGs obtained from patients with autoimmune pancreatitis was screened. Selected peptides exhibited homology with an amino acid sequence from the plasminogen-binding protein (PBP) of *H. pylori* and with ubiquitin-protein ligase E3 component n-recognin 2 (UBR2), an enzyme that is highly expressed in acinar cells of the pancreas. Antibodies against the PBP peptide were detected at high levels in patients with autoimmune pancreatitis but were barely detectable in patients with pancreatic cancer. It seems likely that UBR2 from pancreatic acinar cells may be targeted by an autoantibody against PBP of *H. pylori* in patients with autoimmune pancreatitis (Frulloni et al., 2009).

Since the serum IgG4 and IgG4-type immune complexes are closely associated with disease activity, they may play a major role in the pathogenesis of autoimmune pancreatitis. However, the exact role(s) of IgG4 remains unclear, and may be either beneficial or harmful. To date, the pathological effects of IgG4 and IgG4-type immune complexes have been reported in limited settings, such as in groups of patients with pemphigus or idiopathic membranous nephropathy. Pemphigus vulgaris and pemphigus foliaceus are autoimmune skin diseases that are characterized by the presence of IgG4-type autoantibodies against the cell adhesion molecules desmoglein-3 and desmoglein-1 (see Chapter 65). The IgG4-type anti-desmoglein antibodies may cause the skin lesions characteristic of acantholysis. Idiopathic membranous nephropathy has been characterized by IgG4-subclass glomerular deposits, and IgG4-type antibodies against phospholipase A_2 receptor (PLA$_2$R) were found in a majority of patients. PLA$_2$R is present in podocytes in normal human glomeruli and in immune deposits in these patients, indicating that PLA$_2$R is a major target antigen in this disease (Beck et al., 2009). In autoimmune pancreatitis, IgG4-type autoantibodies may elicit an inflammatory response after interacting with an undefined target antigen.

Recent studies have shown that IgG4 has two outstanding characteristics: Fab-arm exchange (van der Neut Kolfschoten et al., 2007) and rheumatoid factor-like activity (Figure 64.7) (Kawa et al., 2008). These properties may enable IgG4 to contribute to the defense against disease progression. Specifically, dynamic Fab-arm exchange in the IgG4 molecule results in bispecific activity, loss of monospecific cross-linking activity, and loss of the ability to form immune complexes, resulting in anti-inflammatory effects (van der Neut Kolfschoten et al., 2007). IgG4 has also been reported to bind IgG or exert rheumatoid factor activity; however, IgG4 Fc, but not IgG4 Fab, binds to IgG Fc, indicating that IgG4 binding to IgG Fc occurs via an Fc–Fc interaction, not via rheumatoid activity *per se* (Figure 64.7). The role of the IgG4 Fc–IgG Fc interaction is unclear, but its rheumatoid factor-like activity may promote the formation of large circulating immune complexes that are easily eliminated from the circulation (Kawa et al., 2008).

Previous investigations have addressed the effector cells in autoimmune pancreatitis (Okazaki et al., 2011;

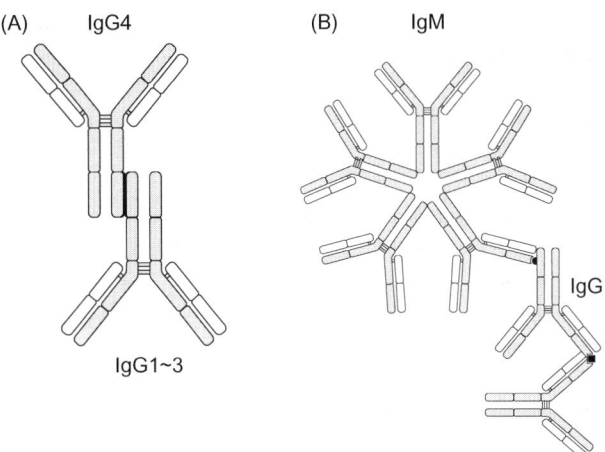

FIGURE 64.7 Rheumatoid factor-like activity of IgG4. IgG4 Fc, but not IgG4 Fab, binds to IgG Fc, indicating that IgG4 binding to IgG Fc is via an Fc–Fc interaction (A), not via rheumatoid activity *per se* (B) (Kawa et al., 2008).

Zen et al., 2011). In peripheral blood or pancreatic tissue, activated CD4$^+$ or CD8$^+$ T cells bearing HLA-DR molecules are aggregated mainly around the pancreatic duct, which expresses HLA-DR molecules (Okazaki et al., 2000). CD4$^+$ T cells are subdivided into Th1 and Th2 cells based on cytokine production profiles (see Chapter 6). In some cases, CD4$^+$ Th1 cells predominate over Th2 cells, suggesting that Th1 cytokines are essential for the induction and maintenance of autoimmune pancreatitis, with Th2 cytokines involved in disease progression (Okazaki and Chiba, 2002). However, there is evidence that a Th2-predominant immune response is predominant in autoimmune pancreatitis (Zen et al., 2007). Thus an immunopathological study using histological specimens to assess cytokine production *in situ* revealed higher expression levels of Th2 cytokines such as IL-4, IL-5, and IL-13, and quantitative real-time PCR revealed significantly higher ratios of IL-4/IFN-γ, IL-5/IFN-γ, and IL-13/IFN-γ (Zen et al., 2007).

TGF-β secreted from naïve Th0 cells can induce CD4$^+$ CD25$^+$ Tregs, which have potent inhibitory function via the transcription factor forkhead box P3 (Foxp3). In peripheral blood, numbers of Tregs were significantly increased in patients with autoimmune pancreatitis, and this increase was correlated with increased serum concentrations of IgG4. In contrast, naïve Tregs are significantly decreased in patients with autoimmune pancreatitis. These observations suggest that increased numbers of Tregs may influence IgG4 production and reflect disease progression, whereas decreased numbers of naïve Tregs may be involved in the pathogenesis of autoimmune pancreatitis (Miyoshi et al., 2008). The ratio of Foxp3-positive cells to infiltrated mononuclear cells (Foxp3/Mono) in patients with autoimmune pancreatitis is significantly higher than in patients with alcoholic chronic pancreatitis, and the Foxp3/Mono and IgG4/Mono ratios have a positive correlation with each other (Kusuda et al., 2011). In the periphery, two functionally different subsets of effector Tregs, inducible costimulatory molecule (ICOS)$^+$ or ICOS$^-$ effector Tregs, actively produce the suppressive cytokines IL-10 and TGF-β, respectively. Levels of ICOS$^+$ Tregs and IL-10$^+$ Tregs are significantly higher in patients with autoimmune pancreatitis, suggesting that ICOS$^+$ Tregs may influence IgG4 production via IL-10 in this disease (Kusuda et al., 2011). Further, fibrosis may be regulated by TGF-β, which is secreted by ICOS$^-$ Tregs.

Taking these observations into account, the following pathogenesis pathway was proposed for autoimmune pancreatitis. An initial response to self-antigens, such as lactoferrin, CA II, or the PBP peptide of *H. pylori*, may be induced by decreased levels of naïve Tregs and followed by a Th1-type immune response that releases proinflammatory cytokines (IFN-γ, IL-1β, IL-2, TNF-α). Next, Th2-type immune responses that produce IgG, IgG4, and autoantibodies are involved in the pathophysiology of progression. IgG4 and fibrosis may be regulated by increased levels of IL-10 and TGF-β, respectively, which are secreted from inducible memory Tregs (Okazaki et al., 2011).

IMMUNOLOGICAL MARKERS IN DIAGNOSIS

In patients with autoimmune pancreatitis, the positive rates for various immunological markers are as follows: increased γ-globulin, 60%; increased IgG, 70%; any of the autoantibodies noted above, 80%; and increased IgG4, 90%. Serum IgG4 elevation is seldom observed in patients who have conditions other than autoimmune pancreatitis, suggesting that IgG4 is the most sensitive and specific immunological marker for diagnosis (Hamano et al., 2001). Interestingly, decreased IgA and IgM concentrations were detected in patients with increased IgG4 levels (Taguchi et al., 2009). Serum concentrations of the complement proteins C3 and C4 were reduced in 36% of patients, suggesting that the complement activation system may contribute to the pathogenesis of autoimmune pancreatitis (Muraki et al., 2006). The serum immune complex value, as determined by the monoclonal rheumatoid factor method, also reflects disease activity (Kawa et al., 2009). Although autoantibodies to CA II and lactoferrin have been reported to be useful markers, their diagnostic value for autoimmune pancreatitis has not been fully accepted due to insufficient sensitivity and specificity (Kino-Ohsaki et al., 1996; Okazaki and Chiba, 2002).

TREATMENT AND OUTCOME

Steroid treatment should be standard therapy for patients with autoimmune pancreatitis (Ito et al., 2007; Okazaki et al., 2009). Pancreatic tissue obtained by needle biopsy after corticosteroid therapy showed marked histological improvements (Song et al., 2005; Ko et al., 2010). Most patients with obstructive jaundice, diffuse enlargement of the pancreas, associated extra-pancreatic involvement, and abdominal pain are good candidates for steroid therapy, although spontaneous remission has been observed in patients with low disease activity (Kamisawa et al., 2009). In general, patients are started on 30–40 mg, or 0.6 mg/kg, per day of prednisolone for 2–4 weeks with careful assessment of clinical findings and laboratory and imaging results. Thereafter, the dosage is reduced and maintained (Ito et al., 2007; Kamisawa et al., 2009; Okazaki et al., 2009). Some patients with high disease activity may thus continue maintenance therapy for 3 years. Studies of long-term outcomes of autoimmune pancreatitis show recurrence and pancreatic stone formation, indicating that autoimmune pancreatitis has the potential to be a progressive disease with pancreatic lithiasis (Takayama et al., 2004; Kawa et al., 2009). Narrowing of the pancreatic ducts was a risk factor for pancreatic stone formation; this presumably leads to pancreatic juice stasis and stone development (Maruyama et al., 2012), and possibly transforms this condition into classical chronic pancreatitis (Maruyama et al., 2013).

IgG4-related DISEASE

Definition

IgG4-related disease includes systemic syndromes characterized by tumefactive lesions, a high serum IgG4 concentration, abundant lymphoplasmacytic infiltration with a large number of IgG4-positive plasma cells, a favorable response to corticosteroid treatment, and various associated diseases. The major characteristic is autoimmune pancreatitis. The concept of IgG4-related disease was developed for disorders that include extra-pancreatic lesions related to autoimmune pancreatitis and have the common features of lymphoplasmacytic infiltration with IgG4-bearing plasma cells and a favorable response to corticosteroids (Kawa et al., 2011a; Zen et al., 2011). In IgG4-related disease, lesions may exist in almost any organ including the central nervous system, eye and salivary glands, respiratory system, hepato-biliary-pancreatic system, retroperitoneum, aorta, renal system, genitourinary system, and endocrine system (Figure 64.4). In addition, other previously recognized conditions are now considered as IgG4-related disease, including multifocal idiopathic fibrosclerosis, Mikulicz's disease, Küttner's tumor, Ormond's disease, and idiopathic hypertrophic pachymeningitis (Stone et al., 2012).

Historical Background

In 1967, Comings reported on multifocal idiopathic fibrosclerosis (MIF), a systemic disease with retroperitoneal fibrosis, mediastinal fibrosis, sclerosing cholangitis, Riedel's thyroiditis, and sicca complex (Comings et al., 1967). Later, pancreatic lesions were added as a component of MIF by Clark and Levy (Clark et al., 1988; Levey and Mathai, 1998). In 1991, Kawaguchi described the histology of autoimmune pancreatitis as lymphoplasmacytic sclerosing pancreatitis (LPSP), and suggested that LPSP be categorized with MIF (Kawaguchi et al., 1991). The disease distribution of MIF seemed similar to that of the extra-pancreatic lesions of autoimmune pancreatitis (Kamisawa et al., 2003a) or IgG4-related disease; as a result, MIF is now considered under the IgG4-related disease category. In 2001, Hamano reported the close association between autoimmune pancreatitis and a high serum IgG4 concentration (Hamano et al., 2001). In 2002, Hamano also reported IgG4-bearing plasma cell infiltration as a histological hallmark of autoimmune pancreatitis and extra-pancreatic lesions (Hamano et al., 2002). Various styles of nomenclature associated with IgG4 were then proposed, including: IgG4-related autoimmune disease (Kamisawa et al., 2003b), IgG4-related plasmacytic disease (Yamamoto et al., 2006), hyper-IgG4 disease (Neild et al., 2006), and IgG4-positive multi-organ lymphoproliferative syndrome (Masaki et al., 2008). In 2010, Japanese researchers agreed on the nomenclature of "IgG4-related disease" (Umehara et al., 2012a,b), which was accepted worldwide at the first international symposium for IgG4-related disease (Stone et al., 2012).

Epidemiology

The prevalence and distribution of the disorders included within the IgG4-related disease category are unclear because most are recognized as complications of autoimmune pancreatitis (Figure 64.4) or Mikulicz's disease. Based on images, a radiologist reported the following prevalence of extra-pancreatic lesions in autoimmune pancreatitis: lacrimal and salivary gland lesions, 48%; lung lesions, 54%; biliary tract lesions, 78%; renal lesions, 14%; retroperitoneal fibrosis, 20%; and prostate lesions, 10% (Fujinaga et al., 2009). Correspondingly a gastroenterologist showed the prevalence based on clinical findings was: lacrimal and salivary gland lesions, 39%; thyroid lesions, 22%; hilar lymphadenopathy, 80%; biliary tract lesions, 74%; and retroperitoneal fibrosis, 13% (Hamano et al., 2006). Finally, based on pathological findings, the prevalence of the location of IgG4-related disease was reported as: head and neck, 20%; thoracic, 14%; hepatic and pancreatobiliary (HPB), 24%; retroperitoneal, 11%; and systemic, 31% (Zen et al., 2010).

Clinical Features of IgG4-related Disease

IgG4-related disease appears as single or multiple organ lesions. In multiple organ lesions, each lesion appears simultaneously or metachronously with the other lesions. In general, multiple organ lesions represent a highly active state with a high serum IgG4 concentration (Hamano et al., 2006). Disease activity may differ in each IgG4-related disease: for example, lacrimal and salivary gland lesions usually represent a higher state of activity, whereas retroperitoneal fibrosis represents a lower state (Hamano et al., 2006). IgG4-related disease can be erroneously diagnosed as an inherent disease of the affected organ, especially when autoimmune pancreatitis or Mikulicz's disease is not present. Intensive differentiation with histological evidence is needed, especially when IgG4-related disease mimics malignant conditions. IgG4-related disease may be divided into definite and probable entities, with the latter lacking supporting evidence such as characteristic histological findings or sufficient case numbers.

Definite IgG4-related Diseases

IgG4-related Lacrimal and Salivary Gland Lesions

IgG4-related lacrimal and salivary gland lesions include Mikulicz's disease or Küttner's tumor and show symmetrical swelling of lacrimal and salivary glands (Figure 64.5). These lesions have been observed in ≈14−39% of patients with autoimmune pancreatitis and were sometimes misdiagnosed as Sjögren's syndrome (Kamisawa et al., 2003a; Yamamoto et al., 2005a, b, 2006). Compared with Sjögren's syndrome, IgG4-related lacrimal and salivary gland lesions show milder exocrine dysfunction, are negative for anti-SS-A/Ro and SS-B/La autoantibodies, and have an excess of submandibular gland lesions (Yamamoto et al., 2005b).

IgG4-related Lung Disease

There are a variety of IgG4-related respiratory lesions, which may result in interstitial pneumonia (Taniguchi et al., 2004), inflammatory pseudotumor (Zen et al., 2005), hilar or mediastinal lymphadenopathy (Saegusa et al., 2003), and bronchial wall thickening (Ito et al., 2009). Interstitial pneumonia has been observed in ≈8−13% of patients with autoimmune pancreatitis. Clinical findings include dry cough, high serum Krebs von den Lungen-6 (KL-6) concentrations, and a ground glass appearance in the middle and lower lung fields and honeycombing in the lower lung field in CT imaging (Kobayashi et al., 2007). An inflammatory pseudotumor presents as nodular lesions in a chest X-ray or CT, which correspond to a plasma cell granuloma, and this is frequently misdiagnosed as a lung tumor (Zen et al., 2005). CT, gallium scintigraphy, and FDG-PET revealed hilar and mediastinal lymphadenopathy in ≈60−70% of patients with autoimmune pancreatitis (Saegusa et al., 2003). CT showed bronchial wall thickening, which results in central airway stenosis. Central airway stenosis and hilar lymphadenopathy should be differentiated from sarcoidosis, and the absence of raised serum levels of angiotensin-converting enzyme (ACE) and histological examination may help differentiate between these conditions (Ito et al., 2009).

IgG4-related Sclerosing Cholangitis

IgG4-related sclerosing cholangitis has been observed in ≈60−70% of patients with autoimmune pancreatitis, and is found in any part of the biliary system (Erkelens et al., 1999; Horiuchi et al., 2001; Nakazawa et al., 2001). Lower bile duct lesions should be differentiated from pancreatic cancer, and intrahepatic or hilar lesions from primary sclerosing cholangitis (PSC) and biliary malignancies (Figure 64.3). PSC is usually observed in young and middle-aged patients and may accompany inflammatory bowel disease (Nakazawa et al., 2005). On cholangiography, the characteristics of PSC include a band-like stricture, beaded or pruned tree appearance, and diverticulum-like outpouchings. In contrast, cholangiography of IgG4-related sclerosing cholangitis showed evidence of lower bile duct stenosis and relatively long strictures from the hilar to intrahepatic biliary systems with distal duct dilatation (Figure 64.3) (Nakazawa et al., 2004).

IgG4-related Liver Disease

IgG4-related liver disease consists of a variety of histological changes, including portal inflammation, interface hepatitis, large bile-duct obstructive features, portal sclerosis, lobular hepatitis, and canalicular cholestasis, which are collectively designated as IgG4 hepatopathy (Umemura et al., 2007a). Some of these lesions mimic those observed in autoimmune hepatitis (AIH) and have a similar clinical presentation; therefore, they fulfill the diagnostic criteria of AIH (Umemura et al., 2007b).

IgG4-related Kidney Disease

Most IgG4-related kidney disease involves the uriniferous tubules, with few being glomerular; in addition, there is tubulointerstitial nephritis with hypocomplementemia and deposits of immune complexes and C3 in tubular basement membranes (Takeda et al., 2004; Saeki et al., 2010). CT shows renal cortical lesions with decreased enhancement that appear as small peripheral cortical nodules and round or wedge-shaped lesions (Takahashi et al., 2007; Fujinaga et al., 2009).

IgG4-related Retroperitoneal Fibrosis

Retroperitoneal fibrosis, observed in about 10−20% of patients with autoimmune pancreatitis, may affect the urinary system or aorta (Hamano et al., 2002; Fujinaga et al., 2009). CT or MRI shows soft tissue density or masses around the aorta and ureters (Fujinaga et al., 2009). Patients with peri-ureteral lesions sometimes complain of lumbago or back pain due to hydronephrosis, which may result in renal atrophy and renal failure (Hamano et al., 2002). Thickening of the aortic wall or aneurysms are sometimes observed, which gave rise to the concept of IgG4-related periaortitis (Ito et al., 2008).

Possible IgG4-related Diseases

IgG4-related Hypophysitis

IgG4-related hypophysitis presents with compressive optic neuropathy, panhypopituitarism, pituitary hypothyroidism, adrenocortical insufficiency, and syndrome of inappropriate secretion of antidiuretic hormone (SIADH) (van der Vliet and Perenboom, 2004; Taniguchi et al., 2006; Tanabe et al., 2006; Shimatsu et al., 2009). MRI analysis revealed pituitary gland and pituitary stalk swelling that produced a high signal on T1-weighted images and early enhancement on dynamic studies, findings which disappeared after corticosteroid treatment (Taniguchi et al., 2006; Tanabe et al., 2006; Shimatsu et al., 2009).

IgG4-related Hypertrophic Pachymeningitis

Hypertrophic pachymeningitis is a rare fibroinflammatory lesion, which causes thickening of the dura in the cranium and/or spinal canal and presents as radiculomyelopathy, headache, or cranial nerve palsies depending on the site of involvement. Hypertrophic pachymeningitis was considered a member of MIF and histological findings showed IgG4-positive plasma cell infiltration in the dura, suggesting a close association with IgG4-related disease (Chan et al., 2009; Riku et al., 2009).

IgG4-related Thyroid Disease

Hypothyroidism has been reported as a complication of autoimmune pancreatitis (Komatsu et al., 2005). Patients with Hashimoto's thyroiditis were classified as having

TABLE 64.1 Comprehensive Clinical Diagnostic Criteria for IgG4-related Disease, 2011

1. Clinical examination showing characteristic diffuse/localized swelling or masses in single or multiple organs.
2. Hematological examination shows elevated serum IgG4 concentrations (135 mg/dl).
3. Histopathologic examination shows:
   a. Marked lymphocyte and plasmacyte infiltration and fibrosis.
   b. Infiltration of IgG4$^+$ plasma cells: ratio of IgG4$^+$/IgG$^+$ cells >40% and >10 IgG4$^+$ plasma cells/HPF.

Definite: (1) + (2) + (3); Probable: (1) + (3); Possible: (1) + (2)

However, it is important to differentiate IgG4-RD from malignant tumors of each organ (e.g., cancer, lymphoma) and similar diseases (e.g., Sjögren's syndrome, primary sclerosing cholangitis, Castleman's disease, secondary retroperitoneal fibrosis, Wegener's granulomatosis, sarcoidosis, Churg–Strauss syndrome) by additional histopathological examination.

Even when patients cannot be diagnosed using the CCD criteria, they may be diagnosed using organ-specific diagnostic criteria for IgG4-RD.

IgG4 thyroiditis and non-IgG4 thyroiditis, based on immunostaining of IgG4 (Li et al., 2009). IgG4-related disease is also significantly associated with hypothyroidism that favorably responds to corticosteroid therapy, suggesting the existence of an IgG4-related thyroid disease or an IgG4-related thyroiditis (Watanabe et al., 2013).

Gastrointestinal Disease

Gastric ulcers may be associated with autoimmune pancreatitis and they occur independently from NSAID medication or *Helicobacter pylori* infection (Shinji et al., 2004). Swelling of the main duodenal papilla is observed in ≈40–65% of patients with autoimmune pancreatitis that responds well to corticosteroid therapy (Unno et al., 2002; Kubota et al., 2007). Similarly to pancreatic lesions, significant numbers of IgG4-positive plasma cells have been detected in these lesions, suggesting that tissue assays may provide an alternative to pancreatic tissue biopsy (Kubota et al., 2007).

Prostate Disease

Some patients with autoimmune pancreatitis have experienced an improvement in symptoms associated with prostatitis, polyuria, dysuria, and nocturia, after corticosteroid therapy, suggesting the existence of an IgG4-related prostatitis (Yoshimura et al., 2006). Patients present with a symmetrical, non-tender, swollen prostate, and imaging has shown severe inflammatory lesions, mainly in the central and transition zones (Uehara et al., 2008).

Pathological Features

The pathological findings of each type of IgG4-related disease share common features that are also seen in autoimmune pancreatitis; however, there are subtle variations among some organs or organ-specific features (Zen et al., 2010). Unique pathological features include dense fibrosis in lacrimal gland lesions, numerous lymph follicles in

lacrimal and salivary gland lesions, and obliterative arteritis in lung lesions (Zen et al., 2010). Obliterative phlebitis is scarcely found in lacrimal gland lesions. Semiquantitative analysis of IgG4-bearing plasma cells may help to distinguish IgG4-related disease from other conditions (Deshpande et al., 2006; Dhall et al., 2010). The ratio of IgG4-bearing plasma cells to IgG-bearing plasma cells further assists in confirming the diagnosis of IgG4-related disease, with a ratio higher than 50% being very suggestive of this diagnosis. The closest histopathological mimics of IgG4-related disease are lymphomas, and clonality studies are necessary to differentiate these two conditions (Stone et al., 2012).

Autoimmune Features, Genetic Features, Animal Models, and Pathological Mechanisms

These are as described in the section on autoimmune pancreatitis.

Diagnosis

Diagnostic criteria have been proposed for some of the IgG4-related diseases, such as autoimmune pancreatitis (Kawa et al., 2011a; Shimosegawa et al., 2011), Mikulicz's disease (Masaki et al., 2010), and IgG4-related kidney disease (Kawano et al., 2011). Japanese researchers proposed comprehensive diagnostic criteria for IgG4-related disease in 2011, based on morphological, serological, and pathological findings (Table 64.1) (Umehara et al., 2012b).

Treatment

When vital organs are involved and serious organ dysfunction or failure may occur, aggressive treatment is needed. However, not all forms of IgG4-related disease require immediate treatment and simple observation is justified in some cases. The correlation between the extent of disease and the need for treatment is imperfect, and the establishment of guidelines for the treatment of each IgG4-related disease is desirable (Stone et al., 2012). Glucocorticoids are typically the first line treatment as described in the autoimmune pancreatitis section.

CONCLUDING REMARKS: FUTURE PROSPECTS

Autoimmune pancreatitis and IgG4-related diseases provide a new disease concept which consists of a distinctive disease profile characterized by high serum IgG4 concentrations and IgG4-bearing plasma cell infiltration. In the future, researchers need to clarify the following: (1) the pathogenesis and role of elevated serum IgG4; (2) the detailed characteristics and the global prevalence of IgG4-related disease; and (3) the long-term outcome with respect to structure and function and predisposition to malignancy.

Autoimmune pancreatitis has received particular attention in Japan, from where the early reports on this disease were mainly published. However, there are now reports from Europe, the United States, and East Asia (Hart et al., 2012). Affected patients in other countries may have been overlooked, or categorized as having other diseases (Kim et al., 2004). The use of the ICDC criteria will enable the correct diagnosis based on internationally recognized standards. A growing awareness of autoimmune pancreatitis and IgG4-related disease will result in an increase in diagnoses as well as more international studies in the future.

REFERENCES

Beck Jr., L.H., Bonegio, R.G., Lambeau, G., Beck, D.M., Powell, D.W., Cummins, T.D., et al., 2009. M-type phospholipase A2 receptor as target antigen in idiopathic membranous nephropathy. N. Engl. J. Med. 361, 11–21.

Chan, S.K., Cheuk, W., Chan, K.T., Chan, J.K., 2009. IgG4-related sclerosing pachymeningitis: a previously unrecognized form of central nervous system involvement in IgG4-related sclerosing disease. Am. J. Surg. Pathol. 33, 1249–1252.

Chang, M.C., Chang, Y.T., Tien, Y.W., Liang, P.C., Jan, I.S., Wei, S.C., et al., 2007. T-cell regulatory gene CTLA-4 polymorphism/haplotype association with autoimmune pancreatitis. Clin. Chem. 53, 1700–1705.

Clark, A., Zeman, R.K., Choyke, P.L., White, E.M., Burrell, M.I., Grant, E.G., et al., 1988. Pancreatic pseudotumors associated with multifocal idiopathic fibrosclerosis. Gastrointest. Radiol. 13, 30–32.

Comings, D.E., Skubi, K.B., Van Eyes, J., Motulsky, A.G., 1967. Familial multifocal fibrosclerosis. Findings suggesting that retroperitoneal fibrosis, mediastinal fibrosis, sclerosing cholangitis, Riedel's thyroiditis, and pseudotumor of the orbit may be different manifestations of a single disease. Ann. Intern. Med. 66, 884–892.

Davidson, T.S., Longnecker, D.S., Hickey, W.F., 2005. An experimental model of autoimmune pancreatitis in the rat. Am. J. Pathol. 166, 729–736.

Deshpande, V., Chicano, S., Finkelberg, D., Selig, M.K., Mino-Kenudson, M., Brugge, W.R., et al., 2006. Autoimmune pancreatitis: a systemic immune complex mediated disease. Am. J. Surg. Pathol. 30, 1537–1545.

Dhall, D., Suriawinata, A.A., Tang, L.H., Shia, J., Klimstra, D.S., 2010. Use of immunohisto-chemistry for IgG4 in the distinction of autoimmune pancreatitis from peritumoral pancreatitis. Hum. Pathol. 41, 643–652.

Erkelens, G.W., Vleggaar, F.P., Lesterhuis, W., van Buuren, H.R., van der Werf, S.D., 1999. Sclerosing pancreato-cholangitis responsive to steroid therapy. Lancet. 354, 43–44.

Freitag, T.L., Cham, C., Sung, H.H., Beilhack, G.F., Durinovic-Belló, I., Patel, S.D., et al., 2010. Human risk allele HLA-DRB1*0405 predisposes class II transgenic Ab0 NOD mice to autoimmune pancreatitis. Gastroenterology. 139, 281–291.

Frulloni, L., Lunardi, C., Simone, R., Dolcino, M., Scattolini, C., Falconi, M., et al., 2009. Identification of a novel antibody associated with autoimmune pancreatitis. N. Engl. J. Med. 361, 2135–2142.

Fujinaga, Y., Kadoya, M., Kawa, S., Hamano, H., Ueda, K., Momose, M., et al., 2009. Characteristic findings in images of extra-pancreatic lesions associated with autoimmune pancreatitis. Eur. J. Radiol. 76, 228–238.

Guarneri, F., Guarneri, C., Benvenga, S., 2005. Helicobacter pylori and autoimmune pancreatitis: role of carbonic anhydrase via molecular mimicry? J. Cell. Mol. Med. 9, 741–744.

Hamano, H., Kawa, S., Horiuchi, A., Unno, H., Furuya, N., Akamatsu, T., et al., 2001. High serum IgG4 concentrations in patients with sclerosing pancreatitis. N. Engl. J. Med. 344, 732–738.

Hamano, H., Kawa, S., Ochi, Y., Unno, H., Shiba, N., Wajiki, M., et al., 2002. Hydronephrosiis associated with retroperitoneal fibrosis and sclerosing pancreatitis. Lancet. 359, 1403–1404.

Hamano, H., Arakura, N., Muraki, T., Ozaki, Y., Kiyosawa, K., Kawa, S., 2006. Prevalence and distribution of extrapancreatic lesions complicating autoimmune pancreatitis. J. Gastroenterol. 41, 1197–1205.

Hardacre, J.M., Lacobuzio-Donahue, C.A., Sohn, T.A., Abraham, S.C., Yeo, C.J., Lillemoe, K.D., et al., 2003. Results of pancreaticoduodenectomy for lymphoplasmacytic sclerosing pancreatitis. Ann. Surg. 237, 853–859.

Hart, P.A., Kamisawa, T., Brugge, W.R., Chung, J.B., Culver, E.L., Czakó, L., et al., 2012. Long-term outcomes of autoimmune pancreatitis: a multicentre, international analysis. Gut. [Epub ahead of print].

Haruta, I., Yanagisawa, N., Kawamura, S., Furukawa, T., Shimizu, K., Kato, H., et al., 2010. A mouse model of autoimmune pancreatitis with salivary gland involvement triggered by innate immunity via persistent exposure to avirulent bacteria. Lab. Invest. 90, 1757–1769.

Horiuchi, A., Kaneko, T., Yamamura, S., Nagata, A., Nakamura, T., Akamatsu, T., et al., 1996. Autoimmune chronic pancreatitis simulating pancreatic lymphoma. Am. J. Gastroenterol. 91, 2607–2609.

Horiuchi, A., Kawa, S., Aoli, Y., Mukawa, K., Furuya, N., Ochi, Y., et al., 1998. Characteristic pancreatic duct appearance in autoimmune chronic pancreatitis: a case report and review of the Japanese literature. Am. J. Gastroenterol. 93, 260–263.

Horiuchi, A., Kawa, S., Hamano, H., Ochi, Y., Kiyosawa, K., 2001. Sclerosing pancreato- cholangitis responsive to corticosteroid therapy: report of 2 case reports and review. Gastrointest. Endosc. 53, 518—522.

Ito, T., Nishimori, I., Inoue, N., Kawabe, K., Gibo, J., Arita, Y., et al., 2007. Treatment for autoimmune pancreatitis: consensus on the treatment for patients with autoimmune pancreatitis in Japan. J. Gastroenterol. 42 (Suppl. 18), 50—58.

Ito, H., Kaizaki, Y., Noda, Y., Fujii, S., Yamamoto, S., 2008. IgG4-related inflammatory abdominal aortic aneurysm associated with autoimmune pancreatitis. Pathol. Int. 58, 421—426.

Ito, M., Yasuo, M., Yamamoto, H., Tsushima, K., Tanabe, T., Yokoyama, T., et al., 2009. Central airway stenosis in a patient with autoimmune pancreatitis. Eur. Respir. J. 33, 680—683.

Kamisawa, T., Funata, N., Hayashi, Y., Tsuruta, K., Okamoto, A., Amemiya, K., et al., 2003a. Close relationship between autoimmune pancreatitis and multifocal fibrosclerosis. Gut. 52, 683—687.

Kamisawa, T., Funata, N., Hayashi, Y., et al., 2003b. A new clinico-pathological entity of IgG4-related autoimmune disease. J. Gastroenterol. 38, 982—984.

Kamisawa, T., Shimosegawa, T., Okazaki, K., Nishino, T., Watanabe, H., Kanno, A., et al., 2009. Standard steroid treatment for autoimmune pancreatitis. Gut. 58, 1504—1507.

Kawa, S., Ota, M., Yoshizawa, K., Horiuchi, A., Hamano, H., Ochi, Y., et al., 2002. HLA DRB1*0405- DQB1*0401 haplotype is associated with autoimmune pancreatitis in the Japanese population. Gastroenterology. 122, 1264—1269.

Kawa, S., Kitahara, K., Hamano, H., Ozaki, Y., Arakura, N., Yoshizawa, K., et al., 2008. A novel immunoglobulin—immunoglobulin interaction in autoimmunity. PLoS One. 3, e1637

Kawa, S., Hamano, H., Ozaki, Y., Ito, T., Kodama, R., Chou, Y., et al., 2009. Long-term follow-up of autoimmune pancreatitis: characteristics of chronic disease and recurrence. Clin. Gastroenterol. Hepatol. 7, S18—S22.

Kawa, S., Fujinaga, Y., Ota, M., Hamano, H., Bahram, S., 2011a. Autoimmune pancreatitis and diagnostic criteria. Curr. Immunol. Rev. 7, 144—161.

Kawa, S., Sugai, S., 2011b. History of autoimmune pancreatitis and Mikulicz's disease. Curr. Immunol. Rev. 7, 137—143.

Kawaguchi, K., Koike, M., Tsuruta, K., Okamoto, A., Tobata, I., Fujita, N., 1991. Lymphoplasmacytic sclerosing pancreatitis with cholangitis: a variant of primary sclerosing cholangitis extensively involving pancreas. Hum. Pathol. 22, 387—395.

Kawano, M., Saeki, T., Nakashima, H., Nishi, S., Yamaguchi, Y., Hisano, S., et al., 2011. Proposal for diagnostic criteria for IgG4-related kidney disease. Clin. Exp. Nephrol. 15, 615—626.

Kim, K.P., Kim, M.H., Song, M.H., Lee, S.S., Seo, D.W., Lee, S.K., 2004. Autoimmune chronic pancreatitis. Am. J. Gastroenterol. 99, 1605—1616.

Kino-Ohsaki, J., Nishimori, I., Morita, M., Okazaki, K., Yamamoto, Y., Onishi, S., et al., 1996. Serum antibodies to carbonic anhydrase I and II in patients with idiopathic pancreatitis and SjS. Gastroenterology. 110, 1579—1586.

Ko, S.B., Mizuno, N., Yatabe, Y., Yoshikawa, T., Ishiguro, H., Yamamoto, A., et al., 2010. Corticosteroids correct aberrant cystic fibrosis transmembrane conductance regulator localization in the duct and regenerate acinar cells in autoimmune pancreatitis. Gastroenterology. 138, 1988—1996.

Kobayashi, H., Shimokawaji, T., Kanoh, S., Motoyoshi, K., Aida, S., 2007. IgG4-positive pulmonary disease. J. Thorac. Imaging. 22, 360—362.

Komatsu, K., Hamano, H., Ochi, Y., Takayama, M., Muraki, T., Yoshizawa, K., et al., 2005. High prevalence of hypothyroidism in patients with autoimmune pancreatitis. Dig. Dis. Sci. 50, 1052—1057.

Kubota, K., Iida, H., Fujisawa, T., Ogawa, M., Inamori, M., Saito, S., et al., 2007. Clinical significance of swollen duodenal papilla in autoimmune pancreatitis. Pancreas. 35, e51—e60.

Kusuda, T., Uchida, K., Miyoshi, H., Koyabu, M., Satoi, S., Takaoka, M., et al., 2011. Involvement of inducible costimulator- and interleukin 10-positive regulatory T cells in the development of igG4-related autoimmune pancreatitis. Pancreas. 40, 1120—1130.

Levey, J.M., Mathai, J., 1998. Diffuse pancreatic fibrosis: an uncommon feature of multifocal idiopathic fibrosclerosis. Am. J. Gastroenterol. 93, 640—642.

Li, Y., Bai, Y., Liu, Z., Ozaki, T., Taniguchi, E., Mori, I., et al., 2009. Immunohistochemistry of IgG4 can help subclassify Hashimoto's autoimmune thyroiditis. Pathol. Int. 59, 636—641.

Masaki, Y., Dong, L., Kurose, N., et al., 2008. Proposal for a new clinical entity, IgG4-positive multi-organ lymphoproliferative syndrome: Analysis of 64 cases of IgG4-related disorders. Ann. Rheum. Dis. 68, 1310—1315.

Maruyama, M., Arakura, N., Ozaki, Y., Watanabe, T., Ito, T., Yoneda, S., et al., 2012. Risk factors for pancreatic stone formation in autoimmune pancreatitis over a long-term course. J. Gastroenterol. 47, 553—560.

Maruyama, M., Arakura, N., Ozaki, Y., Watanabe, T., Ito, T., Yoneda, S., et al., 2013. Type 1 autoimmune pancreatitis can transform into chronic pancreatitis: a long-term follow-up study of 73 Japanese patients. Int. J. Rheumatol. submitted.

Masaki, Y., Sugai, S., Umehara, H., 2010. IgG4-related diseases including Mikulicz's disease and sclerosing pancreatitis: diagnostic insights. J. Rheum. 37, 1380—1385.

Miyoshi, H., Uchida, K., Taniguchi, T., Yazumi, S., Matsushita, M., Takaoka, M., et al., 2008. Circulating naïve and CD4+ CD25 high regulatory T cells in patients with autoimmune pancreatitis. Pancreas. 36, 133—140.

Muraki, T., Hamano, H., Ochi, Y., Komatsu, K., Komiyama, Y., Arakura, N., et al., 2006. Autoimmune pancreatitis and complement activation system. Pancreas. 32, 16—21.

Nakano, S., Takeda, I., Kitamura, K., 1978. Vanishing tumor of the abdomen in patients with Sjogren's syndrome. Dig. Dis. Sci. 23, 75—79.

Nakazawa, T., Ohara, H., Yamada, T., Ando, H., Sano, H., Kajino, S., et al., 2001. Atypical primary sclerosing cholangitis cases associated with unusual pancreatitis. Hepatogastroenterology. 48, 625—630.

Nakazawa, T., Ohara, H., Sano, H., Aoki, S., Kobayashi, S., Okamoto, T., et al., 2004. Cholangiography can discriminate sclerosing cholangitis with autoimmune pancreatitis from primary sclerosing cholangitis. Gastrointest. Endosc. 60, 937—944.

Nakazawa, T., Ohara, H., Sano, H., Ando, T., Aoki, S., Kobayashi, S., et al., 2005. Clinical differences between primary sclerosing cholangitis and sclerosing cholangitis with autoimmune pancreatitis. Pancreas. 30, 20—25.

Neild, G.H., Rodriguez-Justo, M., Wall, C., Connolly, J.O. 2006. Hyper-IgG4 disease: report and characterisation of a new disease. BMC Med. 4, 23.

Nishimori, I., Tamakoshi, A., Otsuki, M., 2007. Prevalence of autoimmune pancreatitis in Japan from a nationwide survey in 2002. J. Gastroenterol. 42 (Suppl. 18), 6–8.

Notohara, K., Burgart, L.J., Yadav, D., Chari, S., Smyrk, TC., 2003. Idiopathic chronic pancreatitis with periductal lymphoplasmacytic infiltration: clinicopathologic features of 35 cases. Am. J. Surg. Pathol. 27, 1119–1127.

Okazaki, K., Uchida, K., Ohana, M., Nakase, H., Uose, S., Inai, M., et al., 2000. Autoimmune-related pancreatitis is associated with auto antibodies and Th1/Th2-type cellular immune response. Gastroenterology. 118, 573–581.

Okazaki, K., Chiba, T., 2002. Autoimmune related pancreatitis. Gut. 51, 1–4.

Okazaki, K., Kawa, S., Kamisawa, T., Naruse, S., Tanaka, S., Nishimori, I., et al., 2006. Clinical diagnostic criteria of autoimmune pancreatitis: revised proposal. J. Gastroenterol. 41, 626–631.

Okazaki, K., Kawa, S., Kamisawa, T., Ito, T., Inui, K., Irie, H., et al., 2009. Japanese clinical guidelines for autoimmune pancreatitis. Pancreas. 38, 849–866.

Okazaki, K., Uchida, K., Koyabu, M., Miyoshi, H., Takaoka, M., 2011. Recent advances in the concept and diagnosis of autoimmune pancreatitis and IgG4-related disease. J. Gastroenterol. 46, 277–288.

Oldstone, M.B.A., 1998. Molecular mimicry and immune-mediated diseases. FASEB J. 12, 1255–1265.

Ota, M., Katsuyama, Y., Hamano, H., Umemura, T., Kimura, A., Yoshizawa, K., et al., 2007. Two critical genes (HLA-DRB1 and ABCF1) in the HLA region are associated with the susceptibility to autoimmune pancreatitis. Immunogenetics. 59, 45–52.

Ota, M., Ito, T., Umemura, T., Katsuyama, Y., Yoshizawa, K., Hamano, H., et al., 2011. Polymorphism in the KCNA3 gene is associated with susceptibility to autoimmune pancreatitis in the Japanese population. Dis. Markers. 31, 223–229.

Ozaki, Y., Oguchi, K., Hamano, H., Arakura, N., Muraki, T., Kiyosawa, K., et al., 2007. Differentiation of autoimmune pancreatitis from suspected pancreatic cancer by fluorine-18 fluorodeoxyglucose positron emission tomography. J Gastroenterol. 43, 144–151.

Park do, H., Kim, M.H., Oh, H.B., Kwon, O.J., Choi, Y.J., Lee, S.S., et al., 2008. Substitution of aspartic acid at position 57 of the DQbeta1 affects relapse of autoimmune pancreatitis. Gastroenterology. 134, 440–446.

Riku, S., Hashizume, Y., Yoshida, M., Riku, Y., 2009. Is hypertrophic pachymeningitis a dural lesion of IgG4-related systemic disease? Rinsho Shinkeigaku. 49, 594–596.

Saegusa, H., Momose, M., Kawa, S., Hamano, H., Ochi, Y., Takayama, M., et al., 2003. Hilar and pancreatic gallium-67 accumulation is characteristic feature of autoimmune pancreatitis. Pancreas. 27, 20–25.

Saeki, T., Nishi, S., Imai, N., Ito, T., Yamazaki, H., Kawano, M., et al., 2010. Clinicopathological characteristics of patients with IgG4-related tubulointerstitial nephritis. Kidney Int. 78, 1016–1023.

Sarles, H., Sarles, J.C., Muratore, R., Gulen, C., 1961. Chronic inflammatory sclerosis of the pancreas—an autonomous pancreatitis disease? Am. J. Dig. Dis. 6, 688–698.

Shimatsu, A., Oki, Y., Fujisawa, I., Sano, T., 2009. Pituitary and stalk lesions (infundibulo-hypophysitis) associated with immunoglobulin G4-related systemic disease: an emerging clinical entity. Endocr. J. 56, 1033–1041.

Shimosegawa, T., Kanno, A., 2009. Autoimmune pancreatitis in Japan: overview and perspective. J. Gastroenterol. 44, 503–517.

Shimosegawa, T., Chari, ST., Frulloni, L., Kamisawa, T., Kawa, S., Mino-Kenudson, M., et al., 2011. International Consensus Diagnostic Criteria for Autoimmune Pancreatitis: Guidelines of the International Association of Pancreatology. Pancreas. 40, 352–358.

Shinji, A., Sano, K., Hamano, H., Unno, H., Fukushima, M., Nakamura, N., et al., 2004. Autoimmune pancreatitis is closely associated with gastric ulcer presenting with abundant IgG4-bearing plasma cell infiltration. Gastroint. Endoscop. 59, 506–511.

Song, M.H., Kim, M.H., Lee, S.K., Seo, D.W., Lee, S.S., Han, J., et al., 2005. Regression of pancreatic fibrosis after steroid therapy in patients with autoimmune chronic pancreatitis. Pancreas. 30, 83–86.

Steinberg, W.M., Barkin, J.S., Bradley 3rd, E.L., DiMagno, E., Layer, P., 2003. Controversies in clinical pancreatology: autoimmune pancreatitis: does it exist? Pancreas. 27, 1–13.

Stone, J.H., Zen, Y., Deshpande, V., 2012. IgG4-related disease. N. Engl. J. Med. 366, 539–551.

Sugumar, A., Kloppel, G., Chari, S.T., 2009. Autoimmune pancreatitis: pathologic subtypes and their implications for its diagnosis. Am. J. Gastroenterol. 104, 2308–2310.

Taguchi, M., Kihara, Y., Nagashio, Y., Yamamoto, M., Otsuki, M., Harada, M., 2009. Decreased production of immunoglobulin M and A in autoimmune pancreatitis. J. Gastroenterol. 44, 1133–1139.

Takahashi, N., Kawashima, A., Fletcher, J.G., Chari, S.T., 2007. Renal involvement in patients with autoimmune pancreatitis: CT and MR imaging findings. Radiology. 242, 791–801.

Takayama, M., Hamano, H., Ochi, Y., Saegusa, H., Komatsu, K., Muraki, T., et al., 2004. Recurrent attacks of autoimmune pancreatitis result in pancreatic stone formation. Am. J. Gastroenterol. 99, 932–937.

Tanaka, S., Kobayashi, T., Nakanishi, K., Okubo, M., Murase, T., Hashimoto, M., et al., 2000. Corticosteroid-responsive diabetes mellitus associated with autoimmune pancreatitis. Lancet. 356, 910–911.

Takeda, S., Haratake, J., Kasai, T., Takaeda, C., Takazakura, E., 2004. IgG4-associated idiopathic tubulointerstitial nephritis complicating autoimmune pancreatitis. Nephrol. Dial. Transplant. 19, 474–476.

Tanabe, T., Tsushima, K., Yasuo, M., Urushihata, K., Hanaoka, M., Koizumi, T., et al., 2006. IgG4-associated multifocal systemic fibrosis complicating sclerosing sialadenitis, hypophysitis, and retroperitoneal fibrosis, but lacking pancreatic involvement. Intern. Med. 45, 1243–1247.

Taniguchi, T., Ko, M., Seko, S., Nishida, O., Inoue, F., Kobayashi, H., et al., 2004. Interstitial pneumonia associated with autoimmune pancreatitis. Gut. 53, 770–771.

Taniguchi, T., Hamasaki, A., Okamoto, M., 2006. A case of suspected lymphocytic hypophysitis and organizing pneumonia during maintenance therapy for autoimmune pancreatitis associated with autoimmune thrombocytopenia. Endocr. J. 53, 563–566.

Toki, F., Kozu, T., Oi, I., 1992. An unusual type of chronic pancreatitis showing diffuse irregular narrowing of the entire main pancreatic duct on ERCP—a report of four cases. Endoscopy. 24, 640.

Uchida, K., Okazaki, K., Nishi, T., Uose, S., Nakase, H., Ohana, M., et al., 2002. Experimental immune-mediated pancreatitis in neonatally thymectomized mice immunized with carbonic anhydrase II and lactoferrin. Lab. Invest. 82, 411–424.

Uehara, T., Hamano, H., Kawakami, M., Koyama, M., Kawa, S., Sano, K., et al., 2008. Autoimmune pancreatitis-associated prostatitis: distinct clinicopathological entity. Pathol. Int. 58, 118–125.

Umehara, H., Okazaki, K., Masaki, Y., Kawano, M., Yamamoto, M., Saeki, T., et al., 2012a. A novel clinical entity, IgG4-related disease (IgG4RD): general concept and details. Mod. Rheumatol. 22, 1−14.

Umehara, H., Okazaki, K., Masaki, Y., Kawano, M., Yamamoto, M., Saeki, T., et al., 2012b. Comprehensive diagnostic criteria for IgG4-related disease (IgG4-RD). Mod. Rheumatol. 22, 21−30.

Umemura, T., Ota, M., Hamano, H., Katsuyama, Y., Kiyosawa, K., Kawa, S., 2006. Genetic association of Fc receptor-like 3 polymorphisms with autoimmune pancreatitis in Japanese patients. Gut. 55, 1367−1368.

Umemura, T., Zen, Y., Hamano, H., Kawa, S., Nakanuma, Y., Kiyosawa, K., 2007a. Immunoglobin G4-hepatopathy: association of immunoglobin G4-bearing plasma cells in liver with autoimmune pancreatitis. Hepatology. 46, 463−471.

Umemura, T., Zen, Y., Hamano, H., Ichijo, T., Kawa, S., Nakanuma, Y., et al., 2007b. IgG4 associated autoimmune hepatitis: a differential diagnosis for classical autoimmune hepatitis. Gut. 56, 1471−1472.

Umemura, T., Ota, M., Hamano, H., Katsuyama, Y., Muraki, T., Arakura, N., et al., 2008. Association of autoimmune pancreatitis with cytotoxic T-lymphocyte antigen 4 gene polymorphisms in Japanese patients. Am. J. Gastroenterol. 103, 588−594.

Unno, H., Saegusa, H., Fukushima, M., Hamano, H., 2002. Usefulness of endoscopic observation of the main duodenal papilla in the diagnosis of sclerosing pancreatitis. Gastrointest. Endosc. 56, 880−884.

van der Neut Kolfschoten, M., Schuurman, J., Losen, M., Bleeker, W.K., Martinez-Martinez, P., Vermeulen, E., et al., 2007. Anti-inflammatory activity of human IgG4 antibodies by dynamic Fab arm exchange. Science. 317, 1554−1557.

van der Vliet, H.J., Perenboom, R.M., 2004. Multiple pseudotumors in IgG4-associated multifocal systemic fibrosis. Ann. Intern. Med. 141, 896−897.

Watanabe, T., Yamashita, K., Fujikawa, S., Sakurai, T., Kudo, M., Shiokawa, M., et al., 2011. Involvement of activation of toll-like receptors and nucleotide-binding oligomerization domain-like receptors in enhanced IgG4 responses in autoimmune pancreatitis. Arthritis Rheum. 64, 914−924.

Watanabe, T., Maruyama, M., Ito, T., Fujinaga, Y., Ozaki, Y., Maruyama, M., et al., 2013. Clinical features of a new disease concept, IgG4-related thyroiditis. Scand. J. Rheumatol. 42, 325−330.

Yamamoto, M., Harada, S., Ohara, M., Suzuki, C., Naishiro, Y., Yamamoto, H., et al., 2005a. Clinical and pathological differences between Mikulicz's disease and Sjogren's syndrome. Rheumatology. (Oxford). 44, 227−234.

Yamamoto, M., Takahashi, H., Sugai, S., Imai, K., 2005b. Clinical and pathological characteristics of Mikulicz's disease (IgG4-related plasmacytic exocrinopathy). Autoimmun. Rev. 4, 195−200.

Yamamoto, M., Takahashi, H., Ohara, M., Suzuki, C., Naishiro, Y., Yamamoto, H., et al., 2006. A new conceptualization for Mikulicz's disease as an IgG4-related plasmacytic disease. Mod. Rheumatol. 16, 335−340.

Yamanishi, H., Kumagi, T., Yokota, T., Azemoto, N., Koizumi, M., Kobayashi, Y., et al., 2011. Clinical significance of B cell-activating factor in autoimmune pancreatitis. Pancreas. 40, 840−845.

Yoshida, K., Toki, F., Takeuchi, T., Watanabe, S., Shiratori, K., Hayashi, N., 1995. Chronic pancreatitis caused by an autoimmune abnormality. Proposal of the concept of autoimmune pancreatitis. Dig. Dis. Sci. 40, 1561−1568.

Yoshimura, Y., Takeda, S., Ieki, Y., Takazakura, E., Koizumi, H., Takagawa, K., 2006. IgG4-associated prostatitis complicating autoimmune pancreatitis. Intern. Med. 45, 897−901.

Zamboni, G., Luttges, J., Capelli, P., Frulloni, L., Cavallini, G., Pederzoli, P., et al., 2004. Histopathological features of diagnostic and clinical relevance in autoimmune pancreatitis: a study on 53 resection specimens and 9 biopsy specimens. Virchows. Arch. 445, 552−563.

Zen, Y., Kitagawa, S., Minato, H., Kurumaya, H., Katayanagi, K., Masuda, S., et al., 2005. IgG4-positive plasma cells in inflammatory pseudotumor (plasma cell granuloma) of the lung. Hum. Pathol. 36, 710−717.

Zen, Y., Fujii, T., Harada, K., Kawano, M., Yamada, K., Takahira, M., et al., 2007. Th2 and regulatory immune reactions are increased in immunoglobin G4-related sclerosing pancreatitis and cholangitis. Hepatology. 45, 1538−1546.

Zen, Y., Nakanuma, Y., 2010. IgG4-related disease: a cross-sectional study of 114 cases. Am. J. Surg. Pathol. 34, 1812−1819.

Zen, Y., Bogdanos, D.P., Kawa, S., 2011. Type 1 autoimmune pancreatitis. Orphanet. J. Rare Dis. 7, 82.

Part 12

Skin Diseases

Chapter 65

Autoimmune Bullous Skin Diseases—Pemphigus and Pemphigoid

Donna A. Culton, Zhi Liu, and Luis A. Diaz

Department of Dermatology, University of North Carolina at Chapel Hill, Chapel Hill, NC, USA

Chapter Outline

Introduction	955	Other Types of Pemphigus	962
Pemphigus Vulgaris	956	Paraneoplastic Pemphigus	962
Clinical, Pathologic, and Epidemiologic Features	956	Drug-induced Pemphigus	962
Autoimmune Features	956	IgA Pemphigus	962
Autoantibodies	956	Bullous Pemphigoid	963
T Cell Activation	958	Clinical, Pathologic, and Epidemiologic Features	963
Genetic Features	959	Autoimmune Features	963
In Vivo and in Vitro Models	959	Autoantibodies	963
Autoantibody Passive Transfer Model	959	T Cell Activation	963
Active Immunization Model	959	Genetic Features	963
Pathologic Effector Mechanisms	959	In Vivo and In Vitro Models	963
Pathogenic Role of Autoantibodies	959	Pathologic Effector Mechanisms	964
Autoantibodies as Potential Immunologic Markers	960	Autoantibodies as Potential Immunologic Markers	964
Pemphigus Foliaceus	960	Other Subepidermal Bullous Diseases	964
Clinical, Pathologic, and Epidemiologic Features	960	Herpes Gestationis (Pemphigoid Gestationis)	964
Autoimmune Features	960	Cicatricial Pemphigoid	964
Autoantibodies	960	Linear IgA Disease	965
T Cell Activation	961	Epidermolysis Bullosa Acquisita	965
Genetic Features	961	Dermatitis Herpetiformis	965
In Vivo and In Vitro Models	961	Treatment of Autoimmune Bullous Diseases	965
Pathologic Effector Mechanisms	961	Concluding Remarks	966
Autoantibodies as Potential Immunologic Markers	961	References	966
Environmental Factors involved in Fogo Selvagem	961		

INTRODUCTION

Autoimmune bullous diseases are rare disorders affecting skin and mucous membranes. These diseases are mediated by pathogenic autoantibodies against keratinocyte adhesion molecules (Diaz and Giudice, 2000). In the epidermis, neighboring keratinocytes adhere to each other through organelles known as desmosomes, whereas dermal–epidermal junction adhesion is mediated by hemidesmosomes. The majority of antigens recognized by these autoantibodies are desmosomal and hemidesmosomal transmembrane glycoproteins involved in epidermal cell–cell and epidermal–dermal adherence.

The desmosome contains two parallel intracellular plaques, which are located just beneath the cell membranes of neighboring cells (Figure 65.1). Transmembrane glycoproteins emerge from the desmosomal plaques and meet in the narrow extracellular space shared by the two cells, constituting the desmosomal core. The desmosomal plaques are composed of plakin family proteins and serve as insertion sites of intracellular keratins, whereas the core is composed of transmembrane calcium-dependent cell

N. Rose & I. Mackay (Eds): The Autoimmune Diseases, Fifth edition. DOI: http://dx.doi.org/10.1016/B978-0-12-384929-8.00065-4

adhesion molecules known as desmosomal cadherins. The desmosomal cadherins include desmogleins (Dsg1−4) and desmocollins (Dsc1−3) (Getsios et al., 2004), the isoforms of which vary in expression throughout the epidermis and in different squamous epithelial tissues. For example, in the skin Dsg1 is expressed throughout the epidermis with predominance in the upper layers of this tissue, whereas Dsg3 is expressed mainly in the suprabasal layers of the epidermis.

The hemidesmosomes, located on the dermal pole of the epidermal basal cells, also contain an intracellular plaque and a core structure (Figure 65.1). The extracellular space, termed the lamina lucida (corresponding to the desmosomal core), separates these cells from the underlying lamina densa (composed of collagen IV) (Diaz and Giudice, 2000). The sub-lamina densa region contains other matrix molecules and the anchoring fibrils (collagen VII). The hemidesmosomal plaque, linked to the keratin network, contains the intracellular proteins BP230 and plectin. The lamina lucida contains the ectodomains of transmembrane proteins BP180, $\alpha6\beta4$ integrin, and laminin 5.

The pemphigus group includes diseases that are characterized by autoantibodies against desmosomal cadherins (Dsg and Dsc) (Beutner and Jordon, 1964; Anhalt and Diaz, 2001), and intraepidermal cell−cell detachment known as acantholysis (Civatte, 1943). This group comprises the two classical forms of pemphigus: pemphigus vulgaris (PV) and pemphigus foliaceus (PF). PV is characterized by suprabasilar acantholysis and anti-Dsg3 IgG autoantibodies, whereas PF is characterized by subcorneal acantholysis and anti-Dsg1 IgG autoantibodies. Other infrequent forms of pemphigus include paraneoplastic pemphigus (PNP), drug-induced pemphigus, and IgA pemphigus (Table 65.1).

The pemphigoid group and other rare subepidermal autoimmune blistering diseases (Table 65.1) are characterized by separation of the epidermis from the dermis. Bullous pemphigoid (BP), the most common autoimmune bullous disease seen in the elderly (Lever, 1965), is characterized by subepidermal blisters and autoantibodies against the hemidesmosomal BP180 and BP230 antigens (Stanley et al., 1981; Mutasim et al., 1985; Labib et al., 1986). Other subepidermal blistering diseases such as cicatricial pemphigoid (CP), herpes gestationis (HG), and linear IgA dermatosis (LAD) exhibit distinctive clinical, histological, and immunologic features, yet share a humoral autoimmune response to BP180 and occasionally other antigens. The remainder of the acquired subepidermal blistering diseases show autoantibody responses to structural molecules of the dermal extracellular matrix. They include epidermolysis bullosa acquisita (EBA) with a target antigen of collagen VII and dermatitis herpetiformis (DH) with a target antigen of epidermal transglutaminase.

While the autoantibody response in most of these autoimmune skin diseases belongs to the IgG class, there are exceptions (IgE and IgM in endemic PF, IgE in BP, and IgA in IgA pemphigus, LAD, and DH).

In this chapter we shall review the current clinical, histological, and immunological features of the most common forms of autoimmune bullous diseases (PV, PF, and BP) (Figure 65.2), and briefly discuss other infrequent forms of pemphigus and other subepidermal autoimmune bullous diseases.

PEMPHIGUS VULGARIS

Clinical, Pathologic, and Epidemiologic Features

Pemphigus vulgaris (PV) is the most severe and common form of pemphigus (Lever, 1965). The disease usually begins with painful ulcerations or erosions of the oral mucosa (mucosal PV), which may last for several months. This process is gradually followed by involvement of the skin (mucocutaneous PV) where the disease produces flaccid blisters and erosions. Other squamous epithelial tissues (e.g., nasal, esophageal, larynx, pharynx, conjunctival, vaginal, and rectal) may also be involved.

Histologically, the lesions of PV show intra-epidermal separation just above the basal cell layer of the epidermis with acantholysis, or rounding up of individual cells (Figure 65.2, left panel). The basal cells remain attached to the dermis but laterally detached from each other producing the histological sign known as "row of tombstones" (Civatte, 1943). Inflammatory infiltration is usually mild and composed of lymphocytes and eosinophils in the superficial dermis.

The incidence of PV ranges from one to five new cases per million persons per year, with a mean age of onset of 50 to 60 years of age (Chams-Davatchi et al., 2005). Although found in all ethnic and racial groups, the disease is more prevalent in patients harboring certain HLA class II alleles (see Genetic Features, below).

Autoimmune Features

Autoantibodies

The serum of PV patients contains IgG autoantibodies that stain the epidermal intercellular spaces (ICS) by indirect immunofluorescence (IF) producing titers that roughly correlate with disease activity (Beutner and Jordon, 1964). Direct IF of perilesional skin reveals IgG bound to keratinocyte cell surfaces. These autoantibodies are predominantly of the IgG4 subclass (Jones et al., 1988). Noteworthy, non-pathogenic anti-Dsg3 autoantibodies have been detected in first-degree relatives of PV

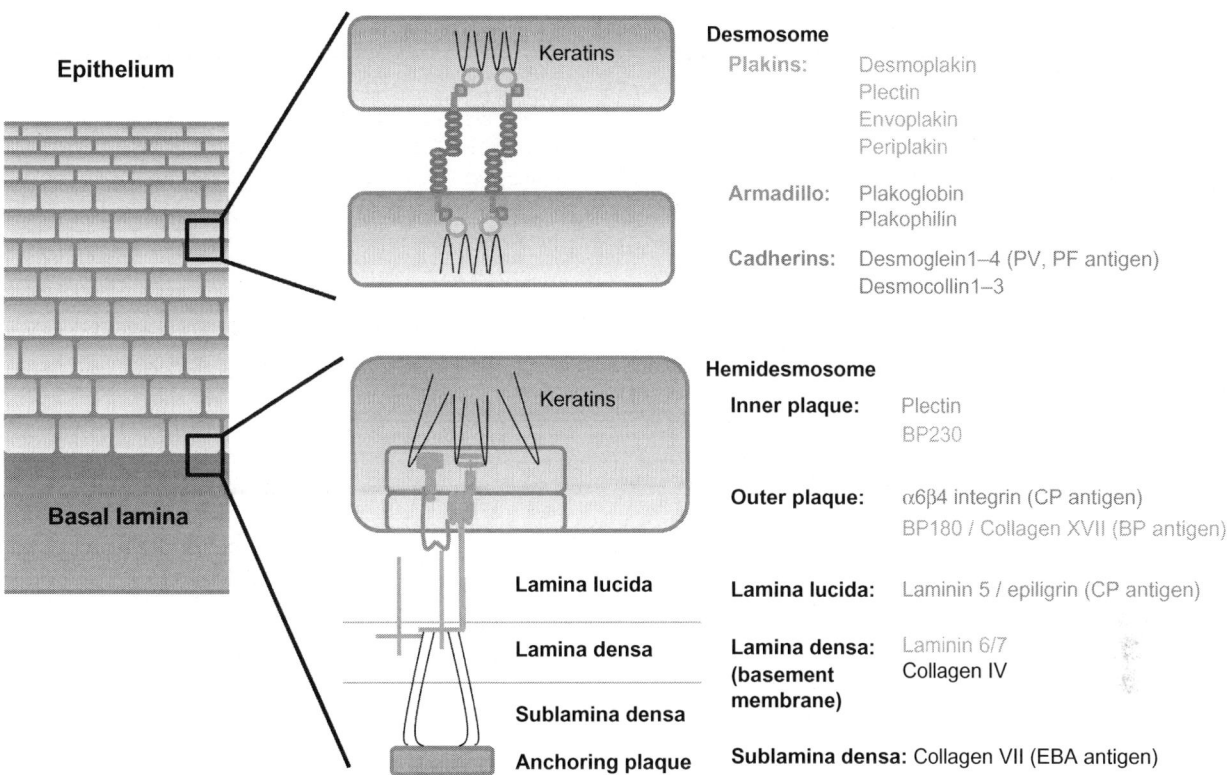

FIGURE 65.1   Diagrammatic representation of the desmosome and the hemidesmosome.

TABLE 65.1 Autoimmune Blistering Diseases of the Skin

Diseases	Cleavage Site	Skin Organelle	Autoantigens	Pathogenic Autoantibodies
Pemphigus vulgaris	Suprabasilar acantholysis	Desmosome	Desmoglein 3	Passive transfer
Pemphigus foliaceus	Subcorneal acantholysis	Desmosome	Desmoglein 1	Passive transfer
Paraneoplastic pemphigus	Suprabasilar acantholysis	Desmosome, hemidesmosome	Desmoglein 3, desmoglein 1 and plakin family	Passive transfer (Dsg3)
Drug-induced pemphigus	Subcorneal acantholysis (commonly)	Desmosome	Desmoglein 1	?
IgA pemphigus	Subcorneal/intraepidermal pustules	Desmosome	Desmocollin 1	?
Bullous pemphigoid	Subepidermal	Hemidesmosome	BP180 and BP230	Passive transfer (BP180)
Herpes gestationis	Subepidermal	Hemidesmosome	BP180	Passive transfer
Cicatricial pemphigoid	Subepidermal	Hemidesmosome	BP180, laminin 5, α6β4 integrin	Passive transfer (laminin 5)
Linear IgA dermatosis	Subepidermal	Hemidesmosome	BP180 fragments	?
Epidermolysis bullosa acquisita	Subepidermal	Anchoring fibrils	Type VII collagen	Passive transfer

patients, which are mainly IgG1 subclass (Bhol et al., 1995; Kricheli et al., 2000).

The target antigen recognized by PV autoantibodies is desmoglein 3 (Dsg3), a 130-kDa desmosomal core glycoprotein (Amagai et al., 1991). While patients with limited mucosal lesions have autoantibodies to Dsg3 exclusively, patients who develop skin lesions may possess autoantibodies against Dsg1 as well (Ding et al., 1997). It is

PV   PF   BP

(A)

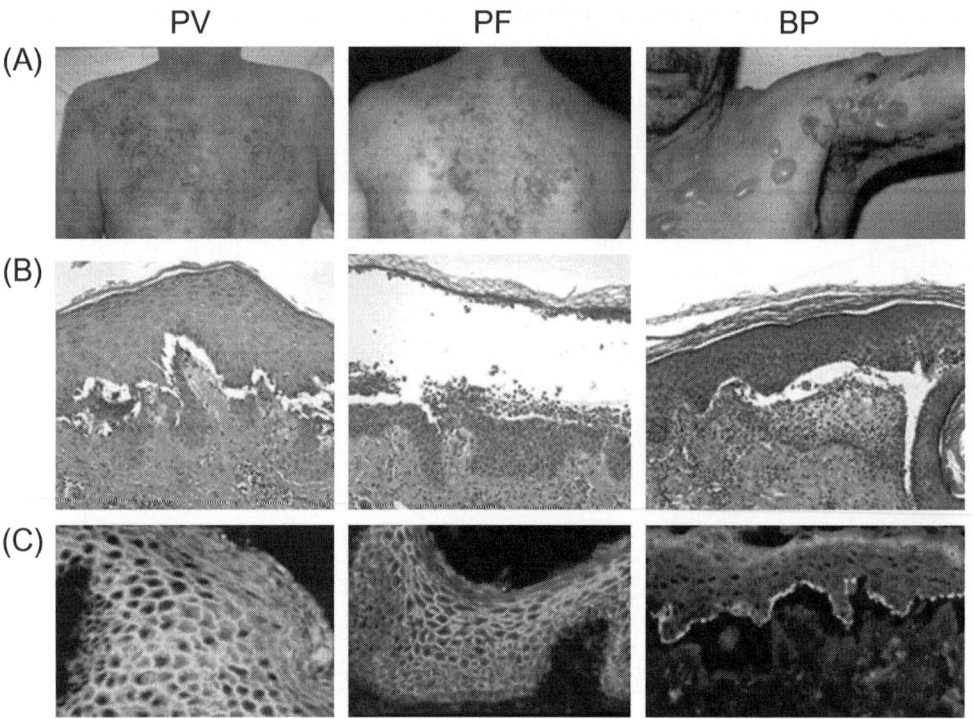

(B)

(C)

FIGURE 65.2   Clinical, histologic, and immunofluorescent features of pemphigus vulgaris, pemphigus foliaceus, and bullous pemphigoid human disease. The clinical (A), histological (B), and immunofluorescent (C) features of pemphigus vulgaris (PV, left panel), pemphigus foliaceus (PF, middle panel), and bullous pemphigoid (BP, right panel) are shown.

well established that about 50% of PV patients show auto-antibodies against Dgs3 and Dsg1.

Dsg1 and Dsg3 belong to the cadherin superfamily of calcium-dependent cell adhesion molecules and share high sequence homology (Getsios et al., 2004). The ectodomain of these glycoproteins is composed of four cadherin repeats (EC1−4) and a variable extracellular anchor (EC5). The six putative calcium-binding motifs of the ectodomain are believed to be involved in maintaining the conformation and adhesive function of Dsg3. A putative adhesion site (RAL) is located on the EC1 domain. The ectodomain of Dsg3 has been expressed in the baculovirus system and employed to adsorb pathogenic auto-antibodies from PV serum. The Dsg3 affinity-purified autoantibodies are sufficient to induce suprabasilar acantholysis when passively transferred to neonatal mice (Amagai et al., 1992; Ding et al., 1999). These pathogenic autoantibodies recognize conformational and calcium-dependent epitopes located on the EC1 domain of Dsg3 (Sekiguchi et al., 2001), which is believed to be involved in the adhesion function of the molecule.

T Cell Activation

Like most other antibodies, induction of anti-Dsg3 auto-antibodies is T cell dependent. Indeed, *in vitro* anti-Dsg3

antibody production by autoreactive B cells is abolished upon depletion of CD4$^+$ T cells (Nishifuji et al., 2000). Other investigators have successfully derived T cell clones from PV patients that proliferated when stimulated with various Dsg3 peptides (Wucherpfennig et al., 1995; Lin et al., 1997; Veldman et al., 2004). Most of the T cell epitopes identified are located in the first three ectodomains of Dsg3. The HLA restrictions and cytokine profiles of the T cell clones have been characterized. The reactivity of one of these T cell clones with the Dsg3 peptide (residues190−204) is restricted to PV-associated DRB1*0402 allele and associated with high levels of Th2 cytokines (Wucherpfennig et al., 1995). Similarly, CD4$^+$ T cells from PV patients responsive to three polypeptides (residues 145−192, 240−303, and 570−614) were also restricted to HLA-DR and exhibit a Th2-like cytokine profile (Lin et al., 1997). These studies suggest that Th2 cells are relevant in the induction of Dsg3-specific auto-antibodies. Not only autoreactive Th2 cells, but also Th1 cells are found in PV patients (Veldman et al., 2004). Both Th1 and Th2 cells may be involved in the production of PV autoantibodies, since the ratio of Dsg3-specific Th1/Th2 cells in PV patients correlated well with the serum autoantibody titers of the patients. In addition, recent studies have shown that an imbalance of Dsg3-specific type 1 regulatory T cells and Th2 cells may be critical for the loss of tolerance against Dsg3 in PV (Veldman et al., 2009).

Interestingly, Dsg3-specific T cells are not only detected in PV patients, but are also detected in healthy individuals who carry PV susceptible HLA alleles (Veldman et al., 2004). However, in contrast to PV patients, Dsg3-responsive T cell clones from the healthy donors exhibit exclusively Th1 (IFN-1) cytokine profiles.

Recent studies have shown that Dsg3-specific CD4$^+$ T cells can induce pemphigus vulgaris in mice, further underscoring the importance of T cells in initiation of disease (Takahashi et al., 2011).

Genetic Features

IILA alleles may play important roles in the development and progression of PV (Sinha et al., 1988; Delgado et al., 1997). Two haplotypes, HLA-DR4 and HLA-DR6, are strongly associated with PV in different ethnic groups (Todd et al., 1988). In the non-Jewish population, DRB1*0402 and DQB1*0503 are the two candidate alleles most likely associated with disease susceptibility, whereas in the Ashkenazi Jewish population DRB1*0402 seems to be singularly associated with PV (Lee et al., 2006).

In Vivo and *in Vitro* Models

Autoantibody Passive Transfer Model

As described in previous sections, neonatal mice have been used as targets for passive transfer experiments of PV IgG (Anhalt et al., 1982). The small size of the animals and the lack of hair allow the use of smaller amounts of IgG and the lesions are easily visible on the hairless skin. PV IgG transferred to neonatal mice reproduces the clinical, histological, and immunological features of human disease within the first 24 hours post injection (Figure 65.3, left panel). The disease induced in these animals is dose dependent and also correlates with the titers of PV autoantibodies detected in the sera of the injected mice.

Active Immunization Model

The efforts to induce PV phenotype in adult mice by conventional active immunization with human Dsg3 have been largely unsuccessful. While the immunized animals produce anti-Dsg3 antibodies that were able to induce skin blisters when passively transferred into neonatal mice, the animals themselves do not develop disease (Fan et al., 1999). Amagai et al. have developed an active mouse model of PV using a novel strategy to overcome the barrier of self-tolerance (Amagai et al., 2000). They immunized Dsg3 knockout mice (Koch et al., 1997) with human Dsg3, and adoptively transferred the splenocytes from these immunized animals to immunodeficient

Rag-2$^{-/-}$ mice which express Dsg3 in their epidermis. The recipient mice producedanti-Dsg3 antibodies and show suprabasilar acantholysis histologically. Some of the animals developed spontaneous crusted erosions on the skin around the snout.

Pathologic Effector Mechanisms

Pathogenic Role of Autoantibodies

Several studies have demonstrated the correlation of PV autoantibody titers and disease extent and activity. *In vitro* studies also showed that PV IgG can induce acantholysis in skin organ cultures and cell detachment in primary epidermal cell cultures. The *in vivo* passive transfer studies demonstrating that PV IgG is able to faithfully reproduce the disease in neonatal mice finally attributed a pathogenic role for PV autoantibodies (Figure 65.3, left panel) (Anhalt et al., 1982). These pioneer studies were extended to demonstrate that PV autoantibodies are able to induce disease by passive transfer in a process that is independent of activation of complement or plasminogen activator (Anhalt et al., 1986; Mascaro et al., 1997; Mahoney et al., 1999).

Another area of intensive research is addressing the molecular mechanisms of acantholysis, i.e., how PV autoantibodies trigger cell detachment. Recent studies have shown that PV autoantibodies bind Dsg3 on the keratinocyte cell surfaces forming clusters that are internalized and fused with lysosomes (Calkins et al., 2006). It has been proposed that PV IgG may alter the assembly/disassembly of desmosomes by impairing the dynamics of the soluble and insoluble pools of Dsg3, which in turn may lead to acantholysis (Jennings et al., 2011). The epidermis of mice passively transferred with PV IgG shows binding of these autoantibodies to the epidermal ICS, and initiation of the cell detachment process begins in the space between desmosomes. This process was followed by desmosome splitting and complete cell detachment (Takahashi et al., 1985). Similar findings were reported in an active mouse model for PV (Shimizu et al., 2004), and thus lead to the appealing hypothesis that autoantibodies to non-desmosomal cadherins, i.e., E-cadherin, may play a role in pemphigus acantholysis.

A longstanding theory for autoantibody-mediated pathogenesis is the steric hindrance theory, in which binding of the autoantibodies to Dsg3 directly impairs the adhesive ability of the molecules thereby causing cell separation (Diaz and Marcelo, 1978). However, substantial evidence is accumulating in support of a complementary hypothesis in which binding of PV autoantibodies to Dsg3 leads to activation of intracellular signaling pathways that ultimately lead to acantholysis. Several signaling pathways have been shown to be activated upon

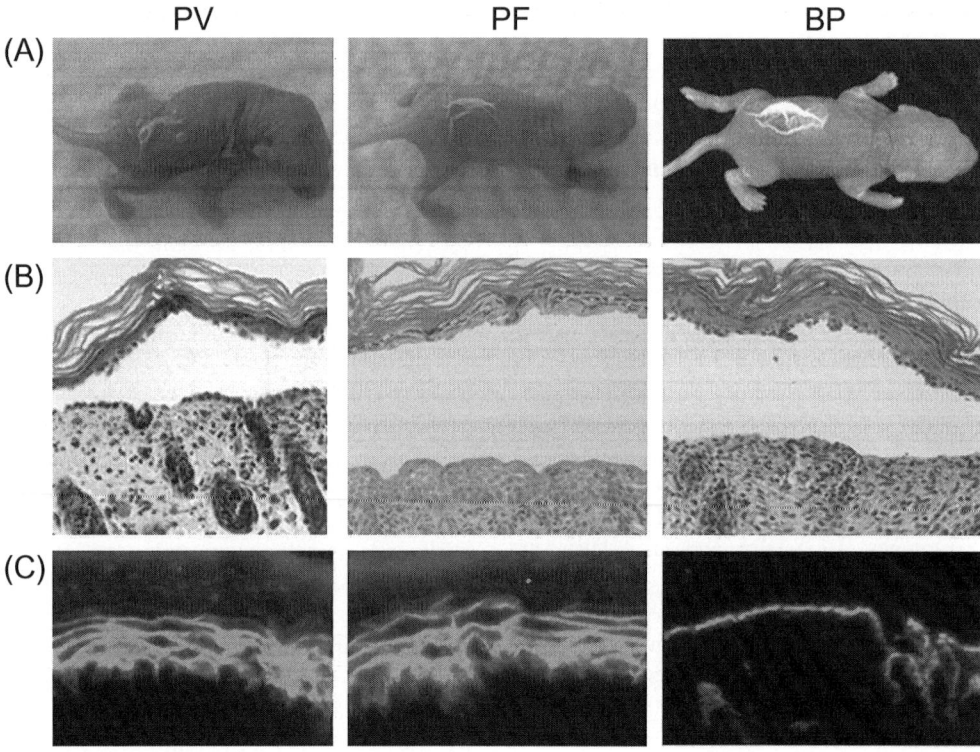

FIGURE 65.3 Clinical, histologic, and immunofluorescent features of the murine models of pemphigus vulgaris, pemphigus foliaceus, and bullous pemphigoid. The clinical (A), histological (B), and immunofluorescent (C) features of pemphigus vulgaris (PV, left panel), pemphigus foliaceus (PF, middle panel), and bullous pemphigoid (BP, right panel) murine models are shown. The animals passively transferred with human IgG (and IgG4) develop skin lesions (A), which histologically (B) are similar to the human disease. The human autoantibodies are detected bound to lesional skin (C) and circulating in the mouse serum.

autoantibody binding to Dsg3 including p38MAPK/ HSP27, Rho family GTPase, c-myc, protein kinase C, and phospholipase C (Caldelari et al., 2001; Kitajima, 2003; Sharma et al., 2007; Berkowitz et al., 2008). Furthermore, modulation of these pathways can prevent autoantibody-induced acantholysis.

Autoantibodies as Potential Immunologic Markers

As PV autoantibodies are the direct effectors of keratinocyte dissociation and blister formation, anti-Dsg3 and anti-Dsg1 autoantibodies are not merely immunologic markers of PV, but are critical for the diagnosis.

PEMPHIGUS FOLIACEUS

Clinical, Pathologic, and Epidemiologic Features

Unlike PV, PF affects skin only and the disease is manifested by superficial blisters and erosions which may lead to crusting and formation of keratotic plaques (Figure 65.2, middle panel). The skin lesions initially involve the central areas of the face, scalp, the mid chest, and the upper back. From these areas the disease may spread to involve the entire body, producing an exfoliative erythroderma. Histological examination of these lesions reveals subcorneal vesicles and acantholysis, predominantly in the upper layers of the stratum spinosum (Lever, 1965).

The classic form of PF is non-endemic and seen sporadically in different parts of the world with an incidence of less than one case per million persons per year. A second form of PF is endemic and was originally described in certain states of Brazil with the name of fogo selvagem (FS) and with a prevalence of 1−3% (Diaz et al., 1989). Endemic forms of PF have also been reported in Colombia and Tunisia. Epidemiological studies suggest environmental triggers for FS development (Aoki et al., 2004).

Autoimmune Features

Autoantibodies

Similarly to PV, PF patients are characterized by anti-epidermal ICS autoantibodies, predominantly of the IgG4 subclass (Rock et al., 1989). These autoantibodies are detected bound to diseased epidermis and circulating in the serum of the patients, with titers that roughly correlate with disease extent and activity.

Dsg1, expressed mostly in the superficial layers of the epidermis, is the target antigen of PF autoantibodies. Affinity-purified anti-Dsg1 antibodies from PF serum are able to induce disease in neonatal mice (Amagai et al., 1995). The majority of PF autoantibodies recognize conformational and calcium-dependent epitopes residing in the NH_2-terminal amino acid 1-161 of Dsg1 (Sekiguchi et al., 2001). In the pre-clinical stage of FS, during disease remission, and in some normal individuals exhibiting no skin disease, the anti-Dsg1 autoantibodies recognize the EC5 domain only. On the contrary, FS anti-Dsg1 autoantibodies from patients showing active disease or during disease relapses recognize the EC1/EC2 domains (Li et al., 2003). Although the majority of PF/FS autoantibodies are of IgG4 subclass, it appears that epitope specificity, rather than the subclass of IgG, is the driver of the pathogenicity of the autoantibodies (Li et al., 2002). Considering these findings we hypothesize that an environmental agent(s) cross-reacts with the EC5 domain of Dsg1 and triggers an initial nonpathogenic anti-EC5 autoimmune response (Diaz et al., 2004). In genetically predisposed individuals, the autoimmune response may undergo intramolecular epitope spreading toward pathogenic epitopes on the EC1/EC2 domains of Dsg1, which leads to disease onset.

T Cell Activation

It has been demonstrated that $CD4^+$ T cell lines and clones derived from peripheral blood of FS patients show a proliferative response when incubated with the Dsg1 ectodomain (Lin et al., 2000a). The stimulation of these $CD4^+$ T cells is HLA-DR restricted. Moreover, these cells secrete Th2-like cytokines.

Genetic Features

HLA alleles strongly associated with FS are DRB1*0404, *1406, *1402 (relative risk = 14) and *0102 (relative risk = 7.3) (Moraes et al., 1997). A common epitope of LLEQRRAA, the residues 67–74 of the third hypervariable region of the DRB1 molecule, is shared by these susceptibility alleles. Similarly, a strong association of DRB1*0102 and DRB1*0404 is also found in non-endemic PF patients in France (Loiseau et al., 2000). Interestingly, two susceptible alleles in PV, DRB1*1401 and DQB1*0503, have been also reported with high frequencies in Italian and Japanese PF patients (Lombardi et al., 1999; Miyagawa et al., 1999).

In Vivo and *In Vitro* Models

The classic animal model of PF was developed by passively transferring IgG from patients into neonatal mice (Roscoe et al., 1985). The animals develop skin blisters, which show the typical histological features of the human disease, i.e., subcorneal vesicles (Figure 65.3, middle panel). The extent of the disease correlates well with the indirect IF titers of human autoantibodies detected in the mouse. These animals develop classic ultrastructural subcorneal acantholysis (Futamura et al., 1989). The disease is induced as a complement-independent process and by monovalent PF IgG fragments as well (Espana et al., 1997). Despite the availability of recombinant human and murine Dsg1, the studies on inducing disease by active immunization have been unsuccessful.

Pathologic Effector Mechanisms

The IgG4 autoantibodies are pathogenic as demonstrated by passive transfer studies (Figure 65.3, middle panel) (Rock et al., 1989). Activation of the complement cascade and plasminogen activator is not required for the induction of acantholysis by these autoantibodies in the mouse model (Espana et al., 1997; Mahoney et al., 1999).

Autoantibodies as Potential Immunologic Markers

The importance of anti-Dsg1 autoantibodies as markers of disease has been illustrated in the FS population, where IgG4 anti-Dsg1 autoantibodies serve as a novel classifier/predictor that identifies FS patients with high sensitivity and specificity (92% and 97%, respectively). In an FS prone population with an incidence of 3%, detection of IgG4 anti-Dsg1 autoantibodies has a positive predictive value of 49% and a negative predictive value of 99.7% (Qaqish et al., 2009).

Environmental Factors involved in Fogo Selvagem

A remarkable characteristic of FS is its epidemiology. Several independent lines of evidence indicate that FS is precipitated by exposure to an environmental factor(s) (Aoki et al., 2004). Anti-Dsg1 autoantibodies are detected in 55% of normal individuals living in an area exhibiting a high prevalence (3.4%) of FS (Warren et al., 2000). Remarkably, anti-Dsg1 autoantibodies are also detected in FS patients from one to several years before the clinical onset of disease (Qaqish et al., 2009). These antibodies are a mixture of IgG1 and IgG4 subclasses and recognize the EC5 domain of Dsg1 (Li et al., 2003; Warren et al., 2003).

A case–control epidemiological study points to hematophagous insects as a prime etiological agent of FS (Aoki et al., 2004). For example, anti-Dsg1 EC5 antibodies have been detected in the sera of patients with onchocerciasis, leishmaniasis, and Chagas disease, though the patients exhibit no skin lesions of FS (Diaz et al., 2004). It is known that hematophagous vectors (black flies, sand flies, and kissing bugs, respectively) are involved in the transmission of the respective tropical diseases. It is postulated that the saliva of these vectors may contain proteins that contain specific epitopes that cross-react with Dsg1, thus inducing a non-pathogenic anti-EC5 domain autoantibody response. Detection of anti-Dsg1 autoantibodies of the IgM and IgE classes provides further support of an environmental trigger (Diaz et al., 2008; Qian et al., 2011).

OTHER TYPES OF PEMPHIGUS

Paraneoplastic Pemphigus

Paraneoplastic pemphigus (PNP) is a severe mucocutaneous disease that runs a usually lethal course in patients with underlying lymphoproliferative malignancy, i.e., non-Hodgkin's lymphoma, chronic lymphocytic leukemia, and Castleman's diseases (Anhalt et al., 1990, 2004). Patients exhibit severe stomatitis and skin lesions that may be vesiculobullous in some patients or show erythema multiforme or lichen planus features in other patients. In approximately 30% of the patients there is a bronchiolitis obliterans syndrome with severe respiratory insufficiency.

Histological examination of the skin lesions reveals keratinocyte necrosis, basal cell vacuolization, and suprabasilar acantholysis. Direct IF shows deposition of IgG and C3 in the epidermal intercellular spaces (as in pemphigus) and along the basement membrane zone (BMZ). The unique and characteristic immunological finding in PNP patients is the polyclonal autoantibody response against structural antigens of the desmosome and hemidesmosome. The antigens that have been characterized besides Dsg3 and Dsg1 are members of the plakin family of proteins that includes desmoplakin I and II, BP230, envoplakin, periplakin, and plectin. Removal of anti-Dsg3 autoantibodies from PNP sera abrogates the pathogenicity of the IgG fraction (Amagai et al., 1998). Affinity-purified anti-Dsg3 antibodies and monoclonal anti-Dsg3 antibodies derived from PNP patients (Saleh et al., 2012) are able to induce skin lesions in neonatal mice. Autoantibody-mediated disease may explain only part of the complex epithelial injury found in these patients. Other mechanisms of tissue injury that have been proposed are those of T cell-mediated cytotoxicity.

It has been proposed that the autoantibody response in PNP is primarily directed against tumor antigens that cross-react with epithelial structural proteins. Additionally the tumor may produce cytokines that modulate the autoimmune response. Interestingly, Wang et al. (2004) have demonstrated that tumor B cells are able to produce anti-epidermal antibodies. In those patients that receive rituximab, the B cell-mediated aspect of the disease, and, therefore, autoantibody detection, wanes. In these cases, the T cell-mediated aspect predominates and the disease takes on a distinct lichenoid pattern with absent or low PNP autoantibodies (Cummins et al., 2007).

The diagnosis of PNP is made clinically, histologically, and immunologically. By indirect IF, the serum of PNP patients typically stains rat bladder epithelium, which produces negative results when stained with the serum of PV or PF. Immunoprecipitation techniques using radiolabeled keratinocyte extracts reveal reactivity with the plakin proteins.

Drug-induced Pemphigus

Certain drugs, particularly thiol-containing drugs, such as penicillamine and captopril, may induce clinical and histological features of PF, and less commonly PV. The majority of drug-induced pemphigus patients exhibit circulating autoantibodies to the epidermal ICS and epidermal-bound IgG. In cases of drug-induced PF, the autoantibodies recognize Dsg1. Some of these drugs have been shown to cause acantholysis *in vitro* directly. Drug-induced pemphigus may be transient and usually resolves upon withdrawal of the medication, although in rare cases the disease may run a chronic course. The mechanisms involved in the induction of the autoimmune response by drugs in pemphigus remain obscure (Brenner and Goldberg, 2011).

IgA Pemphigus

This variant of pemphigus is unique because of its clinical and histological phenotype. Clinically, the patients show superficial clusters of small vesicles and pustules, in some cases producing annular patterns. The Nikolsky sign is positive and the great majority of patients show no mucosal lesions. The histological features show, in addition to the acantholysis, an intense neutrophilic infiltrate in the epidermis. This infiltrate may be subcorneal (subcorneal pustular dermatosis type or SPD type) or located in the mid-epidermis (intraepidermal neutrophilic type or IEN type). The immunological hallmark of this form of pemphigus is the presence of IgA class autoantibodies directed to the epidermal ICS (like PV or PF). The antigen recognized in the SPD type has been shown to be another desmosomal cadherin, desmocollin 1, whereas for the IEN type, the target antigen appears to be a non-desmosomal cell surface protein (Hashimoto, 2001). The pathogenic role of these IgA autoantibodies has not been demonstrated. Further, the intense neutrophilic infiltrate of the epidermis and a rapid response of the disease to dapsone (a neutrophilic-targeted drug) might indicate a unique IgA-mediated pathway of tissue damage (Tsuruta et al., 2011).

BULLOUS PEMPHIGOID

Clinical, Pathologic, and Epidemiologic Features

Bullous pemphigoid (BP) is the most common autoimmune bullous disease affecting the skin primarily (Lever, 1965). The incidence of disease is 7–14 cases per million per year in France, Germany, and Scotland (Bernard et al., 1995; Zillikens et al., 1995; Gudi et al., 2005). Recent studies suggest that the incidence may be as high as 43 cases per million per year in the United Kingdom (Langan et al., 2008). BP occurs most frequently in the elderly (60 to 80 years of age) and affects men and women equally. The skin lesions usually begin as urticarial plaques or erythematous papules, which evolve into large, tense bullae filled with clear fluid (Figure 65.2, right panel). Histological examination of these lesions shows detachment of the epidermis from the dermis, producing subepidermal blisters. The upper dermis exhibits an inflammatory infiltrate including eosinophils, neutrophils, lymphocytes, and monocytes/macrophages. The predominant inflammatory cells in early lesions are usually eosinophils and eosinophilic spongiosis may be present. Histological evidence of mast cell degranulation has also been reported.

Autoimmune Features

Autoantibodies

BP patients have circulating and tissue-bound IgG autoantibodies described by Jordon et al. (Jordon et al., 1967), which are directed against two hemidesmosomal proteins (Mutasim et al., 1985) known as the BP230 (BPAG1) and the BP180 (BPAG2, type XVII collagen) antigens (Jordon et al., 1967; Stanley et al., 1981; Labib et al., 1986). The autoantibodies in BP sera are predominantly of IgG1 and IgG4 subclasses (Laffitte et al., 2001). In addition to IgG autoantibodies, IgE autoantibodies to BP180 are found in the majority of untreated BP patients (Dimson et al., 2003). Only antibodies to BP180 have been demonstrated to be pathogenic in neonatal mice (Figure 65.3, right panel) (Liu et al., 1993).

The BP230 antigen is an intracellular hemidesmosomal plaque protein belonging to the plakin family (Tanaka et al., 1991), whereas the BP180 antigen is a hemidesmosomal transmembrane protein belonging to the collagen family (Giudice et al., 1992). The BP180 protein shows a type II orientation, with its amino-terminal region toward the intracellular hemidesmosomal plaque and its carboxy-terminal half projecting into the extracellular milieu of the BMZ. The anti-BP180 autoantibodies from BP patients recognize multiple epitopes that cluster within the noncollagen 16A (NC16A) domain of the BP180 ectodomain (Giudice et al., 1993). It has been reported recently that the serum levels of autoantibodies to BP180 NC16A in patients are directly correlated to disease severity (Haase et al., 1998; Tsuji-Abe et al., 2005).

Intra- and intermolecular epitope spreading has also been reported in BP and may shape the course of individual disease (Di Zenzo et al., 2011).

T Cell Activation

It has been recently reported that BP180-specific autoreactive T cells recognize epitopes located predominantly on the NC16A domain of the molecule (Budinger et al., 1998; Lin et al., 2000b). These T lymphocytes express CD4 memory T cell surface markers and exhibit a Th1/Th2 mixed cytokine profile.

Genetic Features

Earlier HLA studies involving American, Japanese, and British BP patients showed no significant association between the disease and HLA-A, B, C, and DR loci, while a marked increase in the HLA-DR5 allele was found in BP patients from France. Recent studies have demonstrated that HLA-DQB1*0301 is associated with Caucasian BP (Delgado et al., 1996), whereas DRB1*0403, 0406 or DRB1*1101 has high frequency in Japanese BP (Okazaki et al., 2000).

In Vivo and *In Vitro* Models

Early studies on passive transfer of human BP IgG containing anti-BP180 and anti-BP230 autoantibodies to neonatal mice were unsuccessful. It was found later that the murine BP180 protein did not react with human anti-BP180 antibodies largely due to differences at the amino acid level of the NC16A domain of the molecule. This problem was overcome by raising rabbit antibodies against a segment of murine BP180 homologous to the human epitope. It was demonstrated that these anti-BP180 antibodies were pathogenic if passively transferred into neonatal mice. The animals recapitulate the key clinical and histological features of the human disease (Figure 65.3, right panel) (Liu et al., 1993).

In contrast to PV and PF mouse models, the subepidermal blistering in mice induced by anti-BP180 antibodies depends on complement activation and a subsequent cascade of inflammatory events including mast cell degranulation and neutrophil infiltration. Proteolytic enzymes released from recruited neutrophils are the final effector molecules that cause the epidermal–dermal separation seen in skin lesions (Liu, 2004).

To directly test the pathogenicity of anti-BP180 IgG autoantibodies from BP patients, humanized BP180 mice were generated which harbor the human BP180 or NC16A domain in place of the murine protein (Nishie et al., 2007; Liu et al., 2008). Injection of anti-BP180 IgG into these humanized mice leads to subepidermal blister formation in a process dependent on complement, mast cells, and neutrophils (Nishie et al., 2007; Liu et al., 2008).

IgE purified from BP patient sera was also shown to be pathogenic upon passive transfer into athymic nude mice with human skin grafts. The human skin grafts developed urticarial plaques and subepidermal splitting at higher doses (Fairley et al., 2007).

Pathologic Effector Mechanisms

As opposed to the pemphigus group where the autoantibodies directly induce blister formation, bullous pemphigoid is the result of autoantibody deposition leading to a complex inflammatory cascade. In addition to autoantibody deposition at the basement membrane zone, inflammatory cells are present in the upper dermis and bullous cavity, including both intact and degranulating eosinophils, neutrophils, and mast cells (Wintroub et al., 1978; Dvorak et al., 1982; Czech et al., 1993; Borrego et al., 1996). Proteinases including plasmin, MMP-9, collagenase, and elastase are present in blister fluid and lead to blister formation by their ability to degrade BP180 and other extracellular matrix proteins (Ujiie et al., 2011).

Autoantibodies as Potential Immunologic Markers

Detection of anti-BP180 autoantibodies by DIF, indirect IF, and/or ELISA is critical for the diagnosis of BP. However, a recent study of 337 patients with various non-BP dermatologic disorders suggests that 4% of individuals without BP show a low positive level of anti-BP180 by ELISA. The relevance of anti-BP180 autoantibodies in these patients is unclear (Wieland et al., 2010).

OTHER SUBEPIDERMAL BULLOUS DISEASES

Herpes Gestationis (Pemphigoid Gestationis)

Herpes gestationis (HG), also known as pemphigoid gestationis (PG), is a variant of BP affecting pregnant women primarily. The incidence is about one in 50,000 pregnancies. The disease usually develops during the second or third trimester of pregnancy or in the immediate postpartum period. HG has rarely been associated with underlying trophoblastic tumors. Similarly to BP, HG patients develop subepidermal blisters and linear deposition of C3 at the BMZ (Provost and Tomasi, 1973). The sera of these patients are usually negative by conventional indirect IF assays but become positive when complement fixation to the skin is assayed (HG factor) (Provost and Tomasi, 1973). The HG factor was found to be a complement fixing autoantibody against the BP180 antigen (Jordon et al., 1976; Katz et al., 1976; Morrison et al., 1988; Giudice et al., 1993). This autoantibody is predominantly IgG1 and recognizes the same epitope (within the BP180 NC16A domain) as do BP autoantibodies. BP180-specific T cells also recognize the BP180 NC16A and express a $CD4^+$ Th1 memory phenotype (Lin et al., 1999). Like BP, HG is also associated with DQB1*0301. The mechanism of autoimmunity in HG and the role of pregnancy are not fully understood.

Cicatricial Pemphigoid

Cicatricial pemphigoid (CP), also known as mucous membrane pemphigoid, is a group of heterogeneous diseases characterized by subepithelial blistering involving mucous membranes exclusively (Korman and Cooper, 2000). The oral and ocular surfaces are most commonly involved, while skin lesions occur only in one-third of CP patients. A striking clinical feature of CP is that healing of the lesions leads to scarring and dysfunction of the affected organs. For example, ocular involvement may cause blindness due to corneal scarring and fibrosis. Direct IF reveals linear deposition of IgG, IgA, or C3 along the epithelial BMZ (Egan et al., 2003). CP is also associated with DQB1*0301 (Delgado et al., 1996).

The majority of CP patients show circulating IgG autoantibodies against BP180 antigen (Balding et al., 1996). Some of these CP autoantibodies recognize the C-terminal domain of BP180, which is different from BP. A subset of CP patients exhibits circulating autoantibodies against laminin 5 (epiligrin), also known as epiligrin (Domloge-Hultsch et al., 1994; Egan et al., 1999). Experimentally, it was shown that anti-laminin 5 antibodies are able to induce subepidermal blisters in neonatal mice (Lazarova et al., 1996). There appears to be a relationship of anti-laminin 5 with underlying malignancy (Egan et al., 2003). Many patients with ocular involvement have autoantibodies against α6β4 integrin (Tyagi et al., 1996). The pathogenic role of the various autoantibodies found in CP and their link to scarring remain to be elucidated.

Linear IgA Disease

Linear IgA disease (LAD) is a subepidermal blistering disorder characterized by pruritic lesions and linear deposition of IgA autoantibodies at the BMZ (Nemzer et al., 2000). Mucosal membrane involvement is common (60–80%). LAD can be subdivided into adult-onset, childhood-onset, and drug-induced LAD (Zone et al., 2004). The histology of lesional and perilesional skin reveals subepidermal vesicles with neutrophilic infiltration along the BMZ and in the superficial dermis.

IgA autoantibodies in LAD serum react with multiple antigenic peptides derived from the BP180 ectodomain. The most common antigenic peptides for the major type of LAD (lamina lucida type), detected by immunoblotting using epidermal extracts, are the 97-kDa protein (LABD97) and the 120-kDa antigens (LAD-1), which are considered to be the proteolytic fragments of the BP180 polypeptide (Zone et al., 2004). These findings suggest that the majority of LAD autoantibodies recognize epitopes on LABD97 and LAD-1, which are different from those bound by BP autoantibodies on the intact BP180 molecule.

Epidermolysis Bullosa Acquisita

Epidermolysis bullosa acquisita (EBA) is an acquired subepithelial blistering disease of the skin and mucous membranes mediated by IgG autoantibodies against type VII collagen (O'Toole and Woodley, 2000). Lesions occur predominantly on areas of trauma and often heal with scarring, like CP. Subepidermal blisters are formed as a result of detachment of the epidermis at the level of the sublamina densa area as demonstrated by ultrastructural studies (Figure 65.1). EBA is associated with HLA-DR2 (Gammon et al., 1988).

The target antigen of EBA is type VII collagen (C-VII), which is confined to anchoring fibrils of the sublamina densa region of the skin. EBA autoantibodies react with four major epitopes within the amino-terminal non-collagenous NC1 domain of C-VII. It is hypothesized that binding of these autoantibodies may interfere with dimer formation of the C-VII molecule or may impair the association of C-VII with its ligands, laminin 5 and fibronectin. It has also been suggested that complement activation by the autoantibodies induces inflammation and blistering. Rabbit anti-human type VII collagen NC1 domain IgG induced EBA-like lesions in adult hairless mice and nude mice bearing human skin grafts (Chen et al., (2004)). Furthermore, rabbit antibodies specific to a murine portion of type VII collagen induced subepidermal blistering when passively transferred into adult mice, thereby reproducing the clinical, histological, and immunopathological features of human disease in a complement-dependent fashion (Sitaru et al., 2005).

Dermatitis Herpetiformis

Dermatitis herpetiformis (DH) is an IgA-mediated skin blistering disease characterized by intensive pruritic erythematous papules and vesicles symmetrically distributed over extensor surfaces (Bagheri and Hall, 2000). The skin rash is gluten dependent and responsive to gluten-free diet. Skin biopsies from DH lesions show a characteristic neutrophilic infiltration in the upper dermis involving the dermal papillae. Perilesional and normal skin in DH show a granular deposition of IgA along the BMZ. Recently it has been shown that DH patients possess in their sera IgA autoantibodies that recognize epidermal transglutaminase (Sardy et al., 2002). It is unknown if these anti-transglutaminase autoantibodies are pathogenic or an epiphenomenon, but the autoantibodies can be used as a sensitive serologic marker for DH. A remarkable feature of DH is its high association with celiac disease (CD), another IgA-mediated gluten-sensitive (GSE) disorder involving the small intestine. Patients with DH and GSE share an increased expression of the HLA-A1, HLA-B8, HLA-DR3, and HLA-DQA1*0505 and DQB1*02 genes (Sollid, 2000) and a humoral response to transglutaminases. Both diseases are exacerbated by the intake of gluten-containing food. The mechanisms of gluten-induced autoimmunity and the relationship of the IgA autoantibody response to transglutaminase in DH remain unclear.

TREATMENT OF AUTOIMMUNE BULLOUS DISEASES

The aim of the therapy in all autoimmune blistering diseases of the skin is to abrogate the pathogenic autoantibodies and to decrease the tissue inflammatory response triggered by some of these antibodies. Elimination of pathogenic autoantibodies from the patient is accomplished by immunosuppression or plasmapheresis. The inflammatory response in the skin may be modulated by using topical or systemic steroids or drugs that are known to impair the effector function of neutrophils such as dapsone. It is understood that systemic steroids may modulate the production of antibody and also benefit the local inflammatory response in the skin.

Systemic corticosteroids are the first line of therapy for patients with all clinical forms of pemphigus and pemphigoid. Doses of prednisone in the range of 1.0 mg/kg q.a.m. are used initially. If patients continue to develop new lesions, the dose of prednisone can be increased incrementally to 2.0 mg/kg; however, in our practice we rarely exceed a total prednisone dose of 100 mg q.d. The use of azathioprine, cyclophosphamide, methotrexate, or mycophenolate mofetil, as adjunctive therapy, is beneficial in controlling the disease of these patients. The use of these drugs enhances the chances of inducing a prolonged remission of the disease. They are excellent steroid sparing agents. The patients must be fully evaluated clinically and tested to reveal hematological, renal, and liver function parameters. The doses and side effects for any of these drugs are described in detail in dermatological textbooks. The mortality rate for patients with pemphigus has been reduced to less than 10%; however, these patients are prone to develop severe complications of the therapy, e.g., osteoporosis, diabetes, hypertension, and obesity.

It is well documented that some patients are "resistant" to all these therapeutic modalities. These rare patients may benefit from the use of plasmapheresis or parenteral infusions of human immunoglobulin. Recently, therapy with anti-CD20 humanized monoclonal antibodies has been shown to induce clinical and serological remissions in severe cases of pemphigus.

Dapsone is the drug of choice in dermatitis herpetiformis (DH); it exerts its anti-inflammatory effects by direct action on the neutrophil by interfering with the myeloperoxidase–hydrogen peroxide–halide-mediated cytotoxic system in neutrophils. Dapsone can cause hemolysis and methemoglobinemia; therefore, it is mandatory to assay the levels of the enzyme glucose 6-phosphate dehydrogenase (G6PD) prior to beginning dapsone as G6PD deficient patients may experience severe hemolysis. There are other side effects of dapsone such as hepatitis and thrombocytopenia that may need to be monitored. Not only patients with DH, but also those with LAD, IgA pemphigus show a remarkable clinical response to dapsone. These diseases may be kept in remission with small doses of dapsone. Additionally, CP and certain cases of BP might respond favorably to dapsone as well.

The therapy for patients with EBA is limited since most of the drugs used to control other autoimmune blistering diseases do not change the course of the disease in most patients. The use of systemic steroids, immunosuppressive drugs, or dapsone may be individualized in each patient. Removal of underlying malignancy, steroids, immunosuppressive drugs, and supportive therapy has

been attempted in PNP patients. The prognosis of these patients, however, is poor.

CONCLUDING REMARKS

The autoimmune blistering disorders represent classic antibody-mediated organ-specific autoimmune diseases that can serve as models for understanding the development and pathogenesis of antibody-mediated autoimmune disease in general. New treatments continue to emerge based on our current understanding of disease pathogenesis. Furthermore, unique disease responses to some of these treatments have led investigators back to the bench to further explore the immunologic aberrations present in these patients.

REFERENCES

Amagai, M., Klaus-Kovtun, V., Stanley, J., 1991. Autoantibodies against a novel epithelial cadherin in pemphigus vulgaris, a disease of cell adhesion. Cell. 67, 869–877.

Amagai, M., Karpati, S., Prussick, R., Klaus-Kovtun, V., Stanley, J., 1992. Autoantibodies against the amino-terminal cadherin-like binding domain of pemphigus vulgaris antigen are pathogenic. J. Clin. Invest. 90, 919–926.

Amagai, M., Hashimoto, T., Green, K., Shimizu, N., Nishikawa, T., 1995. Antigen-specific immunoadsorption of pathogenic autoantibodies in pemphigus foliaceus. J. Invest. Dermatol. 104, 895–901.

Amagai, M., Nishikawa, T., Nousari, H., Anhalt, G., Hashimoto, T., 1998. Antibodies against desmoglein 3 (pemphigus vulgaris antigen) are present in sera from patients with paraneoplastic pemphigus and cause acantholysis in vivo in neonatal mice. J. Clin. Invest. 102, 775–782.

Amagai, M., Tsunoda, K., Suzuki, H., Nishifuji, K., Koyasu, S., Nishikawa, T., 2000. Use of autoantigen-knockout mice in developing an active autoimmune disease model for pemphigus. J. Clin. Invest. 105, 625–631.

Anhalt, G., 2004. Paraneoplastic pemphigus. J. Investig. Dermatol. Symp. Proc. 9, 29–33.

Anhalt, G., Diaz, L., 2001. Prospects for autoimmune disease: research advances in pemphigus. JAMA. 285, 652–654.

Anhalt, G., Labib, R., Voorhees, J., Beals, T., Diaz, L., 1982. Induction of pemphigus in neonatal mice by passive transfer of IgG from patients with the disease. N. Engl. J. Med. 306, 1189–1196.

Anhalt, G., Till, G., Diaz, L., Labib, R., Patel, H., Eaglstein, N., 1986. Defining the role of complement in experimental pemphigus vulgaris in mice. J. Immunol. 137, 2835–2840.

Anhalt, G., Kim, S., Stanley, J., Korman, N., Jabs, D., Kory, M., et al., 1990. Paraneoplastic pemphigus. An autoimmune mucocutaneous disease associated with neoplasia. N. Engl. J. Med. 323, 1729–1735.

Aoki, V., Millikan, R., Rivitti, E., Hans-Filho, G., Eaton, D., Warren, S., et al., 2004. Environmental risk factors in endemic pemphigus foliaceus (fogo selvagem). J. Investig. Dermatol. Symp. Proc. 9, 34–40.

Bagheri, B., Hall, R., III, 2000. Dermatitis herpetiformis. In: Jordon, R. (Ed.), Atlas of Bullous Disease. Churchill Livingstone, New York.

Balding, S., Prost, C., Diaz, L., Bernard, P., Bedane, C., Aberdam, D., et al., 1996. Cicatricial pemphigoid autoantibodies react with multiple sites on the BP180 extracellular domain. J. Invest. Dermatol. 106, 141–146.

Berkowitz, P., Diaz, L., Hall, R., Rubenstein, D., 2008. Induction of p38MAPK and HSP27 phosphorylation in pemphigus patient skin. J. Invest. Dermatol. 128, 738–740.

Bernard, P., Vaillant, L., Labeille, B., Bedane, C., Arbeille, B., Denoeux, J., et al., 1995. Incidence and distribution of subepidermal autoimmune bullous skin diseases in three French regions. Bullous Diseases French Study Group. Arch Dermatol. 131, 48–52.

Beutner, E., Jordon, R., 1964. Demonstration of skin antibodies in sera of pemphigus vulgaris patients by indirect immunofluorescent staining. Proc. Soc. Exp. Biol. Med. 117, 505–510.

Bhol, K., Natarajan, K., Nagarwalla, N., Mohimen, A., Aoki, V., Ahmed, A., 1995. Correlation of peptide specificity and IgG subclass with pathogenic and nonpathogenic autoantibodies in pemphigus vulgaris: a model for autoimmunity. Proc. Natl. Acad. Sci. USA. 92, 5239–5243.

Borrego, L., Maynard, B., Peterson, E., George, T., Iglesias, L., Peters, M., et al., 1996. Deposition of eosinophil granule proteins precedes blister formation in bullous pemphigoid. Comparison with neutrophil and mast cell granule proteins. Am. J. Pathol. 148, 897–909.

Brenner, S., Goldberg, I., 2011. Drug-induced pemphigus. Clin. Dermatol. 29, 455–457.

Budinger, L., Borradori, L., Yee, C., Eming, R., Ferencik, S., Grosse-Wilde, H., et al., 1998. Identification and characterization of autoreactive T cell responses to bullous pemphigoid antigen 2 in patients and healthy controls. J. Clin. Invest. 102, 2082–2089.

Caldelari, R., De Bruin, A., Baumann, D., Suter, M., Bierkamp, C., Balmer, V., et al., 2001. A central role for the armadillo protein plakoglobin in the autoimmune disease pemphigus vulgaris. J. Cell Biol. 153, 823–834.

Calkins, C., Setzer, S., Jennings, J., Summers, S., Tsunoda, K., Amagai, M., et al., 2006. Desmoglein endocytosis and desmosome disassembly are coordinated responses to pemphigus autoantibodies. J. Biol. Chem. 281, 7623–7634.

Chams-Davatchi, C., Valikhani, M., Daneshpazhooh, M., Esmaili, N., Balighi, K., Hallaji, Z., et al., 2005. Pemphigus: analysis of 1209 cases. Int. J. Dermatol. 44, 470–476.

Chen, M., Saadat, P., Atha, T., Lipman, K., Ram, R., Woodley, D.T., 2004. A passive transfer model of epidermolysis bullosa acquisita using antibodies generated against the noncollagenous (NC1) domain of human type VII collagen on human skin grafted onto mice. J. Invest. Dermatol. 122, A11.

Civatte, A., 1943. Diagnostic histopathologique de la dermatite polymorphe douloureseou maladie de During-Brocq. Ann. Dermatol. Syph. 3, 1–30.

Cummins, D., Mimouni, D., Tzu, J., Owens, N., Anhalt, G., Meyerle, J., 2007. Lichenoid paraneoplastic pemphigus in the absence of detectable antibodies. J. Am. Acad. Dermatol. 56, 153–159.

Czech, W., Schaller, J., Schopf, E., Kapp, A., 1993. Granulocyte activation in bullous diseases: release of granular proteins in bullous pemphigoid and pemphigus vulgaris. J. Am. Acad. Dermatol. 29, 210–215.

Delgado, J., Turbay, D., Yunis, E., Yunis, J., Morton, E., Bhol, K., et al., 1996. A common major histocompatibility complex class II allele HLA-DQB1* 0301 is present in clinical variants of pemphigoid. Proc. Natl. Acad. Sci. USA. 93, 8569–8571.

Delgado, J., Hameed, A., Yunis, J., Bhol, K., Rojas, A., Rehman, S., et al., 1997. Pemphigus vulgaris autoantibody response is linked to HLA-DQB1*0503 in Pakistani patients. Hum. Immunol. 57, 110–119.

Di Zenzo, G., Thoma-Uszynski, S., Calabresi, V., Fontao, L., Hofmann, S., Lacour, J., et al., 2011. Demonstration of epitope-spreading phenomena in bullous pemphigoid: results of a prospective multicenter study. J. Invest. Dermatol. 131, 2271–2280.

Diaz, L., Giudice, G., 2000. End of the century overview of skin blisters. Arch. Dermatol. 136, 106–112.

Diaz, L., Marcelo, C., 1978. Pemphigoid and pemphigus antigens in cultured epidermal cells. Br. J. Dermatol. 98, 631–637.

Diaz, L., Sampaio, S., Rivitti, E., Martins, C., Cunha, P., Lombardi, C., et al., 1989. Endemic pemphigus foliaceus (fogo selvagem): II. Current and historic epidemiologic studies. J. Invest. Dermatol. 92, 4–12.

Diaz, L., Arteaga, L., Hilario-Vargas, J., Valenzuela, J., Li, N., Warren, S., et al., 2004. Anti-desmoglein-1 antibodies in onchocerciasis, leishmaniasis and Chagas disease suggest a possible etiological link to Fogo selvagem. J. Invest. Dermatol. 123, 1045–1051.

Diaz, L., Prisayanh, P., Dasher, D., Li, N., Evangelista, F., Aoki, V., et al., 2008. The IgM anti-desmoglein 1 response distinguishes Brazilian pemphigus foliaceus (fogo selvagem) from other forms of pemphigus. J. Invest. Dermatol. 128, 667–675.

Dimson, O., Giudice, G., Fu, C., Van Den Bergh, F., Warren, S., Janson, M., et al., 2003. Identification of a potential effector function for IgE autoantibodies in the organ-specific autoimmune disease bullous pemphigoid. J. Invest. Dermatol. 120, 784–788.

Ding, X., Aoki, V., Mascaro Jr., J., Lopez-Swiderski, A., Diaz, L., Fairley, J., 1997. Mucosal and mucocutaneous (generalized) pemphigus vulgaris show distinct autoantibody profiles. J. Invest. Dermatol. 109, 592–596.

Ding, X., Diaz, L., Fairley, J., Giudice, G., Liu, Z., 1999. The anti-desmoglein 1 autoantibodies in pemphigus vulgaris sera are pathogenic. J. Invest. Dermatol. 112, 739–743.

Domloge-Hultsch, N., Anhalt, G., Gammon, W., Lazarova, Z., Briggaman, R., Welch, M., et al., 1994. Antiepiligrin cicatricial pemphigoid. A subepithelial bullous disorder. Arch Dermatol. 130, 1521–1529.

Dvorak, A., Mihm Jr., M., Osage, J., Kwan, T., Austen, K., Wintroub, B., 1982. Bullous pemphigoid, an ultrastructural study of the inflammatory response: eosinophil, basophil and mast cell granule changes in multiple biopsies from one patient. J. Invest. Dermatol. 78, 91–101.

Egan, C., Hanif, N., Taylor, T., Meyer, L., Petersen, M., Zone, J., 1999. Characterization of the antibody response in oesophageal cicatricial pemphigoid. Br. J. Dermatol. 140, 859–864.

Egan, C., Lazarova, Z., Darling, T., Yee, C., Yancey, K., 2003. Anti-epiligrin cicatricial pemphigoid: clinical findings, immunopathogenesis, and significant associations. Medicine (Baltimore). 82, 177–186.

Espana, A., Diaz, L., Mascaro Jr., J., Giudice, G., Fairley, J., Till, G., et al., 1997. Mechanisms of acantholysis in pemphigus foliaceus. Clin. Immunol. Immunopathol. 85, 83–89.

Fairley, J., Burnett, C., Fu, C., Larson, D., Fleming, M., Giudice, G., 2007. A pathogenic role for IgE in autoimmunity: bullous pemphigoid IgE reproduces the early phase of lesion development in human skin grafted to nu/nu mice. J. Invest. Dermatol. 127, 2605–2611.

Fan, J., Memar, O., McCormick, D., Prabhakar, B., 1999. BALB/c mice produce blister-causing antibodies upon immunization with a recombinant human desmoglein 3. J. Immunol. 163, 6228–6235.

Futamura, S., Martins, C., Rivitti, E., Labib, R., Diaz, L., Anhalt, G., 1989. Ultrastructural studies of acantholysis induced in vivo by passive transfer of IgG from endemic pemphigus foliaceus (fogo selvagem). J. Invest. Dermatol. 93, 480–485.

Gammon, W., Heise, E., Burke, W., Fine, J., Woodley, D., Briggaman, R., 1988. Increased frequency of HLA-DR2 in patients with autoantibodies to epidermolysis bullosa acquisita antigen: evidence that the expression of autoimmunity to type VII collagen is HLA class II allele associated. J. Invest. Dermatol. 91, 228–232.

Getsios, S., Huen, A., Green, K., 2004. Working out the strength and flexibility of desmosomes. Nat. Rev. Mol. Cell Biol. 5, 271–281.

Giudice, G., Emery, D., Diaz, L., 1992. Cloning and primary structural analysis of the bullous pemphigoid autoantigen BP180. J. Invest. Dermatol. 99, 243–250.

Giudice, G., Emery, D., Zelickson, B., Anhalt, G., Liu, Z., Diaz, L., 1993. Bullous pemphigoid and herpes gestationis autoantibodies recognize a common non-collagenous site on the BP180 ectodomain. J. Immunol. 151, 5742–5750.

Gudi, V., White, M., Cruickshank, N., Herriot, R., Edwards, S., Nimmo, F., et al., 2005. Annual incidence and mortality of bullous pemphigoid in the Grampian region of north-east Scotland. Br. J. Dermatol. 153, 424–427.

Haase, C., Budinger, L., Borradori, L., Yee, C., Merk, H., Yancey, K., et al., 1998. Detection of IgG autoantibodies in the sera of patients with bullous and gestational pemphigoid: ELISA studies utilizing a baculovirus-encoded form of bullous pemphigoid antigen 2. J. Invest. Dermatol. 110, 282–286.

Hashimoto, T., 2001. Immunopathology of IgA pemphigus. Clin. Dermatol. 19, 683–689.

Jennings, J., Tucker, D., Kottke, M., Saito, M., Delva, E., Hanakawa, Y., et al., 2011. Desmosome disassembly in response to pemphigus vulgaris IgG occurs in distinct phases and can be reversed by expression of exogenous Dsg3. J. Invest. Dermatol. 131, 706–718.

Jones, C., Hamilton, R., Jordon, R., 1988. Subclass distribution of human IgG autoantibodies in pemphigus. J. Clin. Immunol. 8, 43–49.

Jordon, R., Beutner, E., Witebsky, E., Blumental, G., Hale, W., Lever, W., 1967. Basement zone antibodies in bullous pemphigoid. JAMA. 200, 751–756.

Jordon, R., Heine, K., Tappeiner, G., Bushkell, L., Provost, T., 1976. The immunopathology of herpes gestationis. Immunofluorescence studies and characterization of "HG factor". J. Clin. Invest. 57, 1426–1431.

Katz, S., Hertz, K., Yaoita, H., 1976. Herpes gestationis. Immunopathology and characterization of the HG factor. J. Clin. Invest. 57, 1434–1441.

Kitajima, Y., 2003. Current and prospective understanding of clinical classification, pathomechanisms and therapy in pemphigus. Arch. Dermatol. Res. 295 (Suppl. 1), S17–S23.

Koch, P., Mahoney, M., Ishikawa, H., Pulkkinen, L., Uitto, J., Shultz, L., et al., 1997. Targeted disruption of the pemphigus vulgaris antigen (desmoglein 3) gene in mice causes loss of keratinocyte cell adhesion with a phenotype similar to pemphigus vulgaris. J. Cell Biol. 137, 1091–1102.

Korman, N., Cooper, K., 2000. Cicatricial pemphigoid. In: Jordon, R. (Ed.), Atlas of Bullous Disease. Churchill Livingstone, New York.

Kricheli, D., David, M., Frusic-Zlotkin, M., Goldsmith, D., Rabinov, M., Sulkes, J., et al., 2000. The distribution of pemphigus vulgaris-IgG subclasses and their reactivity with desmoglein 3 and 1 in pemphigus patients and their first-degree relatives. Br. J. Dermatol. 143, 337–342.

Labib, R., Anhalt, G., Patel, H., Mutasim, D., Diaz, L., 1986. Molecular heterogeneity of the bullous pemphigoid antigens as detected by immunoblotting. J. Immunol. 136, 1231–1235.

Laffitte, E., Skaria, M., Jaunin, F., Tamm, K., Saurat, J., Favre, B., et al., 2001. Autoantibodies to the extracellular and intracellular domain of bullous pemphigoid 180, the putative key autoantigen in bullous pemphigoid, belong predominantly to the IgG1 and IgG4 subclasses. Br. J. Dermatol. 144, 760–768.

Langan, S., Smeeth, L., Hubbard, R., Fleming, K., Smith, C., West, J., 2008. Bullous pemphigoid and pemphigus vulgaris—incidence and mortality in the UK: population based cohort study. BMJ. 337, a180.

Lazarova, Z., Yee, C., Darling, T., Briggaman, R., Yancey, K., 1996. Passive transfer of anti-laminin 5 antibodies induces subepidermal blisters in neonatal mice. J. Clin. Invest. 98, 1509–1518.

Lee, E., Lendas, K., Chow, S., Pirani, Y., Gordon, D., Dionisio, R., et al., 2006. Disease relevant HLA class II alleles isolated by genotypic, haplotypic, and sequence analysis in North American Caucasians with pemphigus vulgaris. Hum. Immunol. 67, 125–139.

Lever, W., 1965. Pemphigus and Pemphigoid. Charles C. Thomas Publisher, Springfield IL, USA.

Li, N., Liu, Z., Diaz, L.A., 2002. Pemphigus foliaceus autoantibodies recognize two dominant pathogenic epitopes located in EC1 and EC2 domains of desmoglein-1. J. Invest. Dermatol. 119, A305.

Li, N., Aoki, V., Hans-Filho, G., Rivitti, E., Diaz, L., 2003. The role of intramolecular epitope spreading in the pathogenesis of endemic pemphigus foliaceus (fogo selvagem). J. Exp. Med. 197, 1501–1510.

Lin, M., Swartz, S., Lopez, A., Ding, X., Fernandez-Vina, M., Stastny, P., et al., 1997. Development and characterization of desmoglein-3 specific T cells from patients with pemphigus vulgaris. J. Clin. Invest. 99, 31–40.

Lin, M., Gharia, M., Swartz, S., Diaz, L., Giudice, G., 1999. Identification and characterization of epitopes recognized by T lymphocytes and autoantibodies from patients with herpes gestationis. J. Immunol. 162, 4991–4997.

Lin, M., Fu, C., Aoki, V., Hans-Filho, G., Rivitti, E., Moraes, J., et al., 2000a. Desmoglein-1-specific T lymphocytes from patients with endemic pemphigus foliaceus (fogo selvagem). J. Clin. Invest. 105, 207–213.

Lin, M., Fu, C., Giudice, G., Olague-Marchan, M., Lazaro, A., Stastny, P., et al., 2000b. Epitopes targeted by bullous pemphigoid T lymphocytes and autoantibodies map to the same sites on the bullous pemphigoid 180 ectodomain. J. Invest. Dermatol. 115, 955–961.

Liu, Z., 2004. Bullous pemphigoid: using animal models to study the immunopathology. J. Investig. Dermatol. Symp. Proc. 9, 41–46.

Liu, Z., Diaz, L., Troy, J., Taylor, A., Emery, D., Fairley, J., et al., 1993. A passive transfer model of the organ-specific autoimmune disease, bullous pemphigoid, using antibodies generated against the hemidesmosomal antigen, BP180. J. Clin. Invest. 92, 2480–2488.

Liu, Z., Sui, W., Zhao, M., Li, Z., Li, N., Thresher, R., et al., 2008. Subepidermal blistering induced by human autoantibodies to BP180 requires innate immune players in a humanized bullous pemphigoid mouse model. J. Autoimmun. 31, 331–338.

Loiseau, P., Lecleach, L., Prost, C., Lepage, V., Busson, M., Bastuji-Garin, S., et al., 2000. HLA class II polymorphism contributes to specify desmoglein derived peptides in pemphigus vulgaris and pemphigus foliaceus. J. Autoimmun. 15, 67–73.

Lombardi, M., Mercuro, O., Ruocco, V., Lo Schiavo, A., Lombari, V., Guerrera, V., et al., 1999. Common human leukocyte antigen alleles in pemphigus vulgaris and pemphigus foliaceus Italian patients. J. Invest. Dermatol. 113, 107–110.

Mahoney, M., Wang, Z., Stanley, J., 1999. Pemphigus vulgaris and pemphigus foliaceus antibodies are pathogenic in plasminogen activator knockout mice. J. Invest. Dermatol. 113, 22–25.

Mascaro Jr., J., Espana, A., Liu, Z., Ding, X., Swartz, S., Fairley, J., et al., 1997. Mechanisms of acantholysis in pemphigus vulgaris: role of IgG valence. Clin. Immunol. Immunopathol. 85, 90–96.

Miyagawa, S., Amagai, M., Niizeki, H., Yamashina, Y., Kaneshige, T., Nishikawa, T., et al., 1999. HLA-DRB1 polymorphisms and autoimmune responses to desmogleins in Japanese patients with pemphigus. Tissue Antigens. 54, 333–340.

Moraes, M., Fernandez-Vina, M., Lazaro, A., Diaz, L., Filho, G., Friedman, H., et al., 1997. An epitope in the third hypervariable region of the DRB1 gene is involved in the susceptibility to endemic pemphigus foliaceus (fogo selvagem) in three different Brazilian populations. Tissue Antigens. 49, 35–40.

Morrison, L., Labib, R., Zone, J., Diaz, L., Anhalt, G., 1988. Herpes gestationis autoantibodies recognize a 180-kD human epidermal antigen. J. Clin. Invest. 81, 2023–2026.

Mutasim, D., Takahashi, Y., Labib, R., Anhalt, G., Patel, H., Diaz, L., 1985. A pool of bullous pemphigoid antigen(s) is intracellular and associated with the basal cell cytoskeleton-hemidesmosome complex. J. Invest. Dermatol. 84, 47–53.

Nemzer, P., Egan, C., Zone, J., 2000. Linear IgA bullous dermatosis. In: Jordon, R. (Ed.), Atlas of Bullous Disease. Churchill Livingstone, New York.

Nishie, W., Sawamura, D., Goto, M., Ito, K., Shibaki, A., McMillan, J., et al., 2007. Humanization of autoantigen. Nat. Med. 13, 378–383.

Nishifuji, K., Amagai, M., Kuwana, M., Iwasaki, T., Nishikawa, T., 2000. Detection of antigen-specific B cells in patients with pemphigus vulgaris by enzyme-linked immunospot assay: requirement of T cell collaboration for autoantibody production. J. Invest. Dermatol. 114, 88–94.

Okazaki, A., Miyagawa, S., Yamashina, Y., Kitamura, W., Shirai, T., 2000. Polymorphisms of HLA-DR and -DQ genes in Japanese patients with bullous pemphigoid. J. Dermatol. 27, 149–156.

O'Toole, E., Woodley, D., 2000. Epidermolysis bullosa acquisita. In: Jordon, R. (Ed.), Atlas of Bullous Disease. Churchill Livingstone, New York.

Provost, T., Tomasi Jr., T., 1973. Evidence for complement activation via the alternate pathway in skin diseases, I. Herpes gestationis, systemic lupus erythematosus, and bullous pemphigoid. J. Clin. Invest. 52, 1779–1787.

Qaqish, B., Prisayanh, P., Qian, Y., Andraca, E., Li, N., Aoki, V., et al., 2009. Development of an IgG4-based predictor of endemic pemphigus foliaceus (fogo selvagem). J. Invest. Dermatol. 129, 110–118.

Qian, Y., Prisayanh, P., Andraca, E., Qaqish, B., Aoki, V., Hans-Filhio, G., et al., 2011. IgE, IgM, and IgG4 anti-desmoglein 1 autoantibody profile in endemic pemphigus foliaceus (fogo selvagem). J. Invest. Dermatol. 131, 985–987.

Rock, B., Martins, C., Theofilopoulos, A., Balderas, R., Anhalt, G., Labib, R., et al., 1989. The pathogenic effect of IgG4 autoantibodies in endemic pemphigus foliaceus (fogo selvagem). N. Engl. J. Med. 320, 1463–1469.

Roscoe, J., Diaz, L., Sampaio, S., Castro, R., Labib, R., Takahashi, Y., et al., 1985. Brazilian pemphigus foliaceus autoantibodies are pathogenic to BALB/c mice by passive transfer. J. Invest. Dermatol. 85, 538–541.

Saleh, M., Ishii, K., Yamagami, J., Shirakata, Y., Hashimoto, K., Amagai, M., 2012. Pathogenic anti-desmoglein 3 mAbs cloned from a paraneoplastic pemphigus patient by phage display. J. Invest. Dermatol. 132, 1141–1148.

Sardy, M., Karpati, S., Merkl, B., Paulsson, M., Smyth, N., 2002. Epidermal transglutaminase (TGase 3) is the autoantigen of dermatitis herpetiformis. J. Exp. Med. 195, 747–757.

Sekiguchi, M., Futei, Y., Fujii, Y., Iwasaki, T., Nishikawa, T., Amagai, M., 2001. Dominant autoimmune epitopes recognized by pemphigus antibodies map to the N-terminal adhesive region of desmogleins. J. Immunol. 167, 5439–5448.

Sharma, P., Mao, X., Payne, A., 2007. Beyond steric hindrance: the role of adhesion signaling pathways in the pathogenesis of pemphigus. J. Dermatol. Sci. 48, 1–14.

Shimizu, A., Ishiko, A., Ota, T., Tsunoda, K., Amagai, M., Nishikawa, T., 2004. IgG binds to desmoglein 3 in desmosomes and causes a desmosomal split without keratin retraction in a pemphigus mouse model. J. Invest. Dermatol. 122, 1145–1153.

Sinha, A., Brautbar, C., Szafer, F., Friedmann, A., Tzfoni, E., Todd, J., et al., 1988. A newly characterized HLA DQ beta allele associated with pemphigus vulgaris. Science. 239, 1026–1029.

Sitaru, C., Mihai, S., Otto, C., Chiriac, M., Hausser, I., Dotterweich, B., et al., 2005. Induction of dermal-epidermal separation in mice by passive transfer of antibodies specific to type VII collagen. J. Clin. Invest. 115, 870–878.

Sollid, L., 2000. Molecular basis of celiac disease. Annu. Rev. Immunol. 18, 53–81.

Stanley, J., Hawley-Nelson, P., Yuspa, S., Shevach, E., Katz, S., 1981. Characterization of bullous pemphigoid antigen: a unique basement membrane protein of stratified squamous epithelia. Cell. 24, 897–903.

Takahashi, H., Kouno, M., Nagao, K., Wada, N., Hata, T., Nishimoto, S., et al., 2011. Desmoglein 3-specific CD4 + T cells induce pemphigus vulgaris and interface dermatitis in mice. J. Clin. Invest. 121, 3677–3688.

Takahashi, Y., Patel, H., Labib, R., Diaz, L., Anhalt, G., 1985. Experimentally induced pemphigus vulgaris in neonatal BALB/c mice: a time-course study of clinical, immunologic, ultrastructural, and cytochemical changes. J. Invest. Dermatol. 84, 41–46.

Tanaka, T., Parry, D., Klaus-Kovtun, V., Steinert, P., Stanley, J., 1991. Comparison of molecularly cloned bullous pemphigoid antigen to desmoplakin I confirms that they define a new family of cell adhesion junction plaque proteins. J. Biol. Chem. 266, 12555–12559.

Todd, J., Acha-Orbea, H., Bell, J., Chao, N., Fronek, Z., Jacob, C., et al., 1988. A molecular basis for MHC class II-associated autoimmunity. Science. 240, 1003–1009.

Tsuji-Abe, Y., Akiyama, M., Yamanaka, Y., Kikuchi, T., Sato-Matsumura, K., Shimizu, H., 2005. Correlation of clinical severity and ELISA indices for the NC16A domain of BP180 measured using BP180 ELISA kit in bullous pemphigoid. J. Dermatol. Sci. 37, 145–149.

Tsuruta, D., Ishii, N., Hamada, T., Ohyama, B., Fukuda, S., Koga, H., et al., 2011. IgA pemphigus. Clin. Dermatol. 29, 437–442.

Tyagi, S., Bhol, K., Natarajan, K., Livir-Rallatos, C., Foster, C., Ahmed, A., 1996. Ocular cicatricial pemphigoid antigen: partial sequence and biochemical characterization. Proc. Natl. Acad. Sci. USA. 93, 14714–14719.

Ujiie, H., Nishie, W., Shimizu, H., 2011. Pathogenesis of bullous pemphigoid. Dermatol. Clin. 29, 439–446, ix.

Veldman, C., Gebhard, K., Uter, W., Wassmuth, R., Grotzinger, J., Schultz, E., et al., 2004. T cell recognition of desmoglein 3 peptides in patients with pemphigus vulgaris and healthy individuals. J. Immunol. 172, 3883–3892.

Veldman, C., Pahl, A., Hertl, M., 2009. Desmoglein 3-specific T regulatory 1 cells consist of two subpopulations with differential expression of the transcription factor Foxp3. Immunology. 127, 40–49.

Wang, L., Bu, D., Yang, Y., Chen, X., Zhu, X., 2004. Castleman's tumours and production of autoantibody in paraneoplastic pemphigus. Lancet. 363, 525–531.

Warren, S., Lin, M., Giudice, G., Hoffmann, R., Hans-Filho, G., Aoki, V., et al., 2000. The prevalence of antibodies against desmoglein 1 in endemic pemphigus foliaceus in Brazil. Cooperative Group on Fogo Selvagem Research. N. Engl. J. Med. 343, 23–30.

Warren, S., Arteaga, L., Rivitti, E., Aoki, V., Hans-Filho, G., Qaqish, B., et al., 2003. The role of subclass switching in the pathogenesis of endemic pemphigus foliaceus. J. Invest. Dermatol. 120, 104–108.

Wieland, C., Comfere, N., Gibson, L., Weaver, A., Krause, P., Murray, J., 2010. Anti-bullous pemphigoid 180 and 230 antibodies in a sample of unaffected subjects. Arch. Dermatol. 146, 21–25.

Wintroub, B., Mihm Jr., M., Goetzl, E., Soter, N., Austen, K., 1978. Morphologic and functional evidence for release of mast-cell products in bullous pemphigoid. N. Engl. J. Med. 298, 417–421.

Wucherpfennig, K., Yu, B., Bhol, K., Monos, D., Argyris, E., Karr, R., et al., 1995. Structural basis for major histocompatibility complex (MHC)-linked susceptibility to autoimmunity: charged residues of a single MHC binding pocket confer selective presentation of self-peptides in pemphigus vulgaris. Proc. Natl. Acad. Sci. USA. 92, 11935–11939.

Zillikens, D., Wever, S., Roth, A., Weidenthaler-Barth, B., Hashimoto, T., Brocker, E., 1995. Incidence of autoimmune subepidermal blistering dermatoses in a region of central Germany. Arch. Dermatol. 131, 957–958.

Zone, J., Egan, C., Taylor, T., Meyer, L., 2004. IgA autoimmune disorders: development of a passive transfer mouse model. J. Investig. Dermatol. Symp. Proc. 9, 47–51.

Chapter 66

Non-bullous Skin Diseases: Alopecia Areata, Vitiligo, Psoriasis, and Urticaria

Stanca A. Birlea, Marc Serota, and David A. Norris

Department of Dermatology, University of Colorado School of Medicine, Anschutz Medical Campus, University of Colorado Denver, CO, USA

Chapter Outline

Alopecia Areata	**971**
Clinical, Pathologic, and Epidemiologic Features	971
Autoimmune Features	972
Genetic Features	973
In Vivo and *In Vitro* Models	973
Pathologic Effector Mechanisms	973
Autoantibodies as Potential Immunologic Markers	974
Concluding Remarks—Future Prospects	974
Vitiligo	**974**
Clinical, Pathologic, and Epidemiologic Features	974
Autoimmune Features	975
Genetic Features	976
In Vivo and *In Vitro* Models	976
Pathogenetic Mechanism	977
Autoantibodies as Potential Immunologic Markers	977
Concluding Remarks—Future Prospects	978
Psoriasis	**978**
Clinical, Pathologic, and Epidemiologic Features	978

Autoimmune Features	978
Genetic Features	980
In Vivo and *In Vitro* Models	980
In Vivo Models	980
In Vitro Models	981
Pathogenic Mechanism	981
Autoantibodies as Potential Immunologic Markers	981
Concluding Remarks—Future Prospects	982
Chronic Urticaria	**982**
Clinical, Pathologic, and Epidemiologic Features	982
Autoimmune Features	982
Genetic Features	983
In Vivo and *In Vitro* Models	983
Pathologic Effector Mechanisms	983
Autoantibodies as Potential Immunologic Markers	984
Concluding Remarks—Future Prospects	984
References	**984**

ALOPECIA AREATA

Clinical, Pathologic, and Epidemiologic Features

Alopecia areata (AA) is perhaps the most common autoimmune disease, affecting 5.3 million Americans including males and females across all ethnic groups (Petukhova et al., 2011), with a lifetime risk of 1.7% (Safavi et al., 1995). The most common presentation of AA is reversible loss of one or a few patches of hair called transient alopecia areata (TAA). More extensive persistent hair loss is classified as patchy persistent alopecia areata (PPAA) (Figure 66.1). Loss of all hair of the scalp is called alopecia totalis (AT), and loss of all scalp and body hair is termed alopecia universalis

(AU). Loss of hair localized to the retroauricular area and occipital areas is called ophiasis, and has a poor prognosis. Onset early in life, severe and long-lasting course (Chu et al., 2011), extensive disease, and associated nail dystrophy (pits, ridges, or trachonychia), also indicate poor prognosis.

In AA a mononuclear cell inflammatory infiltrate attacks the hair follicle (HF) bulb, the factory which produces the hair shaft. T cell cytokines and cytotoxic T cells produce cytotoxic damage (Whiting, 2003) and disrupt the normal function of the HF. This leads to production of thin, fragile hairs, which easily break off or detach from the follicle and fall out. Since the hairs which fall out in AA are in actively growing anagen follicles, AA is classified as a form of anagen effluvium.

N. Rose & I. Mackay (Eds): The Autoimmune Diseases, Fifth edition. DOI: http://dx.doi.org/10.1016/B978-0-12-384929-8.00066-6

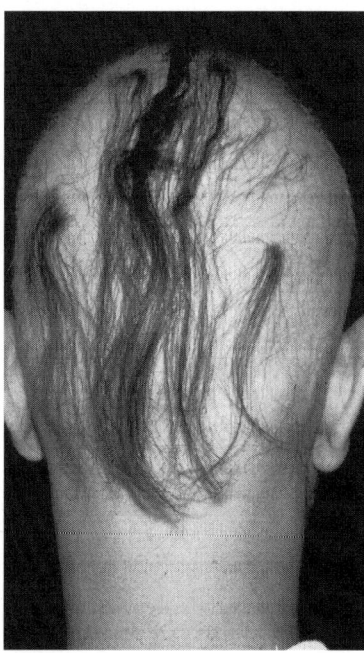

FIGURE 66.1 Patchy persistent, extensive alopecia areata.

Alopecia areata is commonly associated with atopy, especially in severe forms, where the incidence of atopy may be 50% or more (Barahmani et al., 2009). AA is highly associated with other autoimmune diseases, the most common being hypothyroidism, especially autoimmune thyroiditis (Goh et al., 2006). Because the immune damage is localized to the hair bulb, the stem cell populations are preserved and normal cycling HF can be regenerated, and regrowth of the hair can occur even years after total hair loss.

Autoimmune Features

There are multiple observations supporting the concept that AA is an autoimmune disease:

1. AA HFs are surrounded by an immune infiltrate of activated T helper(h) cells, cytotoxic T cells and natural killer (NK) cells, and a Th1-type cytokine profile (Petukhova et al., 2011).
2. The target of the immune response in AA appears to be the pigmented anagen HF. Anagen is the growing phase of the hair cycle. Neither resting HFs (telogen phase) nor white hair-containing follicles are affected in AA.
3. Autoantibodies are common both in human AA and in the C3H/HeJ mouse model of AA, and their specificities are quite different from the antibody specificities in human vitiligo (Cui et al., 1992; Tobin et al., 1997) where melanocytes are the targets. Antibodies in the C3H/HeJ mouse and in human AA appear to react to

proteins of 40−46 kDa, possibly HF-specific keratins (Tobin et al., 1997). Other candidate targets are trichohyalin, an HF keratin-associated protein, and keratin 16 (Tobin, 2003; Leung et al., 2010). Attempts to identify antibodies specific for HF melanocytes have not been successful.

4. Autoreactive T cells and NK cells are necessary for hair loss in AA, as demonstrated in a xenograft model in which hair-bearing skin from AA patients is grafted onto the severe combined immunodeficiency (SCID) mouse. This is followed by injection into the graft of leukocytes from the AA patient stimulated *in vitro* with various melanocyte antigens (Gilhar et al., 1998). In this model CD4$^+$ and CD8$^+$ T lymphocytes transferred the disease after they were primed *in vitro* by the melanocyte antigens gp100, MART-1, or tyrosinase (Gilhar et al., 2001). In a recent update of this model, leukocytes from AA patients are first stimulated with IL-2 (not melanocyte antigens), producing hair loss dependent on NK cells, CD8$^+$NG2D$^+$, and CD8$^+$CD56$^+$ cells (Gilhar et al., 2012, 2013).
5. CD8$^+$ T cells are necessary for local HF cytotoxicity, while CD4$^+$CD25$^+$ T cells can transfer the disease systemically in the C3H/HeJ mouse (McElwee et al., 2005).
6. The adhesion pair Cadm-1/CRTAM-1 appears to be necessary to mediate CD8$^+$ T cell cytotoxicity in AA. Cadm-1 is expressed by epidermal cells and mediates heterotypic adhesion to lymphocytes expressing the class 1-restricted T cell-associated molecule (CRTAM). Overexpression of Cadm-1 in a mouse model of alopecia

increased the progression of alopecia (Giangreco et al., 2012).

7. It has been hypothesized that low expression of class I and II MHC molecules in the HF, together with local expression of potent immunosuppressants, maintains a state of immune privilege of HF, in which the cytotoxic immune attack on the HF is suppressed (Ito et al., 2008). Several reports indicated that AA occurs because of the breakdown in this immune privilege in the follicle (Paus et al., 2003; Ito et al., 2008; Kang et al., 2010). According to this hypothesis, proinflammatory signals such as interferon (IFN)-γ and substance P cause upregulation of class I MHC molecules and allow the presentation of previously sequestered HF antigens to preexisting autoreactive CD8$^+$ T cells. Costimulatory signals from CD4$^+$ T cells and mast cells also facilitate the attack of lymphocytic infiltrates on the HF (Gilhar et al., 2012).

Genetic Features

As the approaches to studying the genetics of AA have broadened from observed heritability in first-degree relatives, twin studies, and family-based linkage studies (Martinez-Mir et al., 2007), to genome-wide association studies or deep sequencing of key areas of the genome, it has been increasingly clear that genetic control of innate and acquired immunity is the most powerful factor in determining the susceptibility to all variants of AA, from patchy disease to alopecia universalis. The two GWAS studies performed in AA to date (Petukhova et al., 2010; Jagielska et al., 2012) provided compelling evidence for the implication of numerous individual genes, most of them with immune function, and have established the major determinants of autoimmunity in AA (Table 66.1) (Petukhova et al., 2010).

In Vivo and In Vitro Models

Since AA is a complex immune process attacking the human anagen HF, and since the exact targets of autoimmune damage are not known, in vitro experiments based on single cell populations have not been very useful. However, both naturally occurring and engineered animal models have been extremely useful in defining disease mechanisms in AA, in identifying potential drug targets, and more recently, in testing new drugs for future use in human experimentation.

The C3H/HeJ mouse has been an indispensable tool in defining the immunoregulatory AA genes (Sundberg et al., 2004). As in humans, the alopecia developed in these mice is strongly IFN-γ and IL-2 dependent (Freyschmidt-Paul et al., 2005) and is characterized by a diffuse inflammatory hair loss, which closely mimics in terms of histology, gene

TABLE 66.1 Alopecia Areata Major Susceptibility Genes with Role in Innate or Acquired Immunity

Mechanism	Genes
Innate Immunity	
NK cell activation	NKG2D ligands: *ULBP6, ULBP3, MICA*
Cytokine	*IL-2, IL-21, IL2RA*
Acquired Immunity	
Antigen presentation	*HLA-DRA, HLA-DQA1, HLA-DQA2, HLA-DQB2, HLA-DOB9*
T cell proliferation	*CTLA4, ICOS, IL-21, IL-2, IL2RA, IKZF4, BTNL2*
T cell differentiation	*NOTCH4*
Tregs	*CTLA4, IKZF4, IL-2, IL2RA*
B cell proliferation	*IL13*
End Organ	
Anti-oxidant	*PRDX5*
Premature graying	*STX17*
With supposed immune function	*KIAA0350/CLEC16A*

expression, and response to treatment, the human disease AA. The AA phenotype could be adoptively transferred to a whole colony of other syngeneic C3H/HeJ mice by transplanting involved alopecic skin, providing the ability to synchronize AA development in large cohorts of mice, and an exciting basic and clinical research platform (Sun et al., 2008). Newer engineered mouse models promise to validate T cell and NK cell roles in AA pathogenesis (Alli et al., 2012; Gilhar et al., 2012).

The xenograft mouse model using hairy skin from AA patients and autologous PBMC sensitized in vitro has already been described in a review by Gilhar et al. (Gilhar et al., 1998). This model has been instrumental in showing that melanocyte-specific CD4$^+$, CD8$^+$, and NK cells are effectors of hair loss in AA.

Pathologic Effector Mechanisms

At the recent AA Research Summit "From Basepairs to Bedside: Innovations in the Immunology and Clinical Science of Alopecia Areata," Raphael Clynes and Angela Christiano presented their recent investigations on the inflammatory cascade in AA. As summarized in Table 66.2, the effector cascade in AA encompasses danger signals, NK/innate immune first responders, APC/Sentinel presentation of HF antigens and adaptive responses dependent on the interplay of multiple T and B cell populations, and a complex cytokine network (Petukhova et al., 2011). Their studies on gene expression in AA lesions show that 16 of the top 20 signals are IFN-γ response genes.

TABLE 66.2 Inflammatory Response Underlying Alopecia Areata

Type of Response	Cells and Signaling Molecules
Innate/NKG2D response	Alarms: hair follicle TNF-α, IL-15, IFN-γ, MICA, UBLP-3, UBLP-6, Rae-1 First responders: DETC, NK, NKT, γ/8T
APC/Sentinel	Cellular sentinels: Langerhans cells, dermal dendritic cells, dermal macrophage, mast cells Determinants: HLA, TAP, IFN-γ
Adaptive immunity	Immune cells: CD4⁺ T cells, CD8⁺ T cells, Tregs, B cells, CTLA4, iCOS, IL-2, IL-2R, IL-21 Cytokine network: IL-2, IL-6, IL-17, IL-21, IFN-γ, IFN-α Downstream signaling pathways: Jak 1/2, Syk

Autoantibodies as Potential Immunologic Markers

To date, no widely accepted or validated antibody markers in AA have been identified. Research is under way to use validated techniques to identify and quantitate autoantibodies in AA.

Concluding Remarks— Future Prospects

It is widely accepted that current treatments for AA are inadequate. As stated in a recent Cochrane review, "There is no good trial evidence that any treatments provide long-term benefit to patients with alopecia areata, Totalis and universalis" (Delamere et al., 2008). Initial studies of biologics that are highly effective in psoriasis were stunningly unsuccessful in AA. The National Alopecia Areata Foundation (NAAF) has organized a program to develop and test new treatments in AA. This includes an intensive effort to design and validate a uniform clinical research platform for testing effectiveness of new treatments. Multiple new approaches using drugs effective in other

autoimmune diseases are being developed: anti-CTLA4, anti-Jak {1/2}, anti-Syk, anti-IL-15, anti-NKG2D (Colonna et al., 2010; Petukhova et al., 2011).

It is unknown whether it is necessary to purposefully reactivate affected HF in AA.

Future research programs will determine the effectiveness of direct HF stimuli to reactivate hair growth in AA.

VITILIGO

Clinical, Pathologic, and Epidemiologic Features

Vitiligo is the most common acquired type of leukoderma, causing significant social and psychological difficulties in people with darker skin phototypes. The hallmark of the disease is the white patch with well-defined borders, affecting the skin and mucous membranes (Birlea et al., 2012). Based on the lesions' distribution, extension and number, the disease is divided into non-segmental vitiligo (NSV), segmental vitiligo (SV), mixed, and unclassified (Taieb et al., 2013) (Table 66.3). In general,

TABLE 66.3 Classification of Vitiligo

Types and Subtypes of Disease	Features
1. Non-segmental vitiligo (NSV)	
1.1. Generalized/vulgaris	Presents as multiple scattered lesions over the body
1.2. Acrofacial	Begins typically on the fingers and feet and around facial orifices
1.3. Universalis	Depigmentation over the whole body
2. Segmental vitiligo (SV)	
2.1. Uni/pluri-segmental	Follows a dermatomal distribution; stops at the midline; most common type in childhood
2.2. Focal	
2.3. Mucosal	One/few macules in one site. Lesions on multiple sites
3. Mixed	NSV + SV
4. Unclassified	
4.1. Focal	At onset; an earlier stage of generalized type
4.2. Multifocal asymmetrical NSV	Becomes generalized/mixed over time
4.3. Mucosal	Lesions on one site

Modified from Taieb et al., 2012

NSV is characterized by symmetrical depigmentation (Figure 66.2) with earlier onset and progression over time. SV is characterized by a unilateral distribution that may be dermatomal, rapid in onset, and with involvement of both epidermal and hair follicle (HF) melanocytes (Taieb et al., 2013). Vitiligo often occurs in a photodistribution, and commonly affects body folds and periorificial areas. The most common triggers include sunburn, physical trauma, repeated rubbing of the skin (so-called Koebner phenomenon), psychological stress, and pregnancy. The clinical course of vitiligo is unpredictable; in general, NSV is gradually progressive, while most SV cases rapidly stabilize.

In atypical cases of vitiligo, pathologic exam of lesional skin is necessary to confirm the diagnosis. It shows an epidermal basal layer completely devoid of melanocytes in the center of the lesions (Le Poole et al., 1993a); cells expressing melanocyte markers are sometimes observed at the margins of lesions. In early vitiligo or in episodes of progression, the dermis at the margin of lesions may contain sparse perivascular and perifollicular infiltrates, consistent with cell-mediated immune processes destroying melanocytes *in situ* (Kim et al., 2008).

Vitiligo affects all races and geographic areas with a frequency of 0.3–0.5% (Birlea et al., 2012). Generalized vitiligo (GV), the most common subtype, occurs with equal frequency in males and females and may manifest at any time in life, with the average age of onset of 24 years (Spritz, 2010).

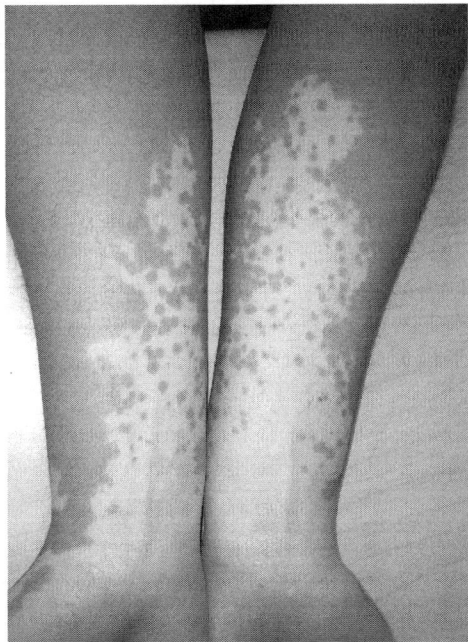

FIGURE 66.2 Generalized symmetric vitiligo of the anterior forearms with perifollicular repigmentation process (brown dots).

Autoimmune Features

Several clinical and experimental observations support the autoimmune basis of vitiligo:

1. In GV subjects of white European ancestry there is a 15–25% incidence of at least one additional concomitant autoimmune disease, particularly autoimmune thyroid disease, pernicious anemia, rheumatoid arthritis, psoriasis, type 1 diabetes, Addison's disease, or systemic lupus erythematosus. These diseases also occur at increased frequencies in first-degree relatives of patients with GV (Spritz, 2010), indicating a heritable autoimmune diathesis in vitiligo. In contrast with GV, in SV the occurrence of other autoimmune diseases is uncommon (el-Mofty and el-Mofty, 1980; Koga and Tango, 1988; Park et al., 1988).

2. Circulating anti-melanocyte antibodies (anti-tyrosinase, anti-tyrosinase-related protein-1, anti-dopachrome tautomerase) have been described in GV. Vitiligo antibodies were initially described by immunoprecipitation studies using melanoma cell extracts; they were most commonly directed against antigens with molecular weights of 35, 40–45, 75, 90, and 150 kDa; the antigens of 35 and 90 kDa were preferentially expressed on melanocytes (Cui et al., 1992). Antigens of 45, 65, and 110 kDa have been identified in immunoblotting studies with melanocyte extracts (Hann et al., 1996b; Park et al., 1996), while vitiligo-associated antibodies have been demonstrated to recognize melanoma cell proteins of 68, 70, 88, 90, 110, and 165 kDa (Hann et al., 1996a; Rocha et al., 2002). Other vitiligo-associated antibody targets have been reported (lamin A, MCHR-1, PM-17, SOX-9, SOX-10, tyrosine hydroxylase).

3. The presence of circulating skin-homing cytotoxic T cells (Tc) (Ogg et al., 1998) and infiltrates containing activated cytotoxic T cells and macrophages was described at the margins of active vitiligo lesions (Gross et al., 1987; Badri et al., 1993a, Le Poole et al., 1993b, 1996). The Tc were shown to target melanocyte-specific antigens [including Melan-A (MART-1), gp100 (Pmel17) and tyrosinase] (Ogg et al., 1998; Lang et al., 2001; Palermo et al., 2001) and to express high levels of the skin-homing receptor cutaneous lymphocyte-associated antigen (CLA). The frequency of Tc correlated with both the extent and activity of the disease (Lang et al., 2001). In progressive disease, the CD4/CD8 ratio was reported decreased among skin-infiltrating T cells, which exhibited a predominant Th1 cytokine secretion profile (Wankowicz-Kalinska et al., 2003). It is accepted that skin-homing, autoreactive, melanocyte-specific T cells cause melanocyte destruction in vitiligo, and that regulatory cells ineffectively restrain autoreactive T cells in GV (Klarquist et al., 2010).

4. Recent evidence suggests that immune responses may also contribute to the pathogenesis of SV, in which the melanocyte loss, which remains more localized, seems to be related to a lymphocytic infiltrate of interferon-γ-producing CD8$^+$ and of some CD4$^+$ T cells found at the lesional margin of early stages, similar to those observed in GV (van Geel et al., 2011).

5. An immune mechanism in vitiligo was also implied by experimental observations in occupational vitiligo (Manga et al., 2006). So-called chemical leukoderma can initially occur on upper extremities of subjects coming in contact with cleaning solutions containing phenolic compounds (like 4-tertiary butyl phenol). It was hypothesized that these agents are directly toxic to melanocytes, in the context of a possible genetic susceptibility of patients' melanocytes to chemical injuries, which can lead to melanocyte death, release of intracellular proteins, and subsequent autoimmunity.

6. Vitiligo-like depigmentation occurring during interleukin-2 immunotherapy for malignant melanoma was proposed to follow an autoimmune mechanism. Since some melanoma-associated antigens (such as MART-1, gp100, and tyrosinase) are shared by normal melanocytes and melanoma, the onset of vitiligo suggests that the cytotoxic T cells activated by IL-2 (Feliciani et al., 1996; Verheyen et al., 2001) can also attack normal tissue (Phan et al., 2001), producing vitiligo-like depigmentation.

7. Lymphocyte-mediated destruction of melanocytes can occur in other non-vitiligo scenarios: (a) intratumor depigmentation during melanoma regression; (b) leukoderma acquisitum centrifugum around melanoma and nevi (the latter defining the "halo nevi" phenomenon), and (c) vitiligo-like depigmentation, observed at distant sites from primary melanoma (Birlea et al., 2012).

8. Immunosuppressive drugs may induce repigmentation in vitiligo. As such, topical calcineurin inhibitors (tacrolimus or pimecrolimus) are first-line therapy in vitiligo and exert an immunosuppressive effect on T cells, by blocking the action of the cytokine gene-activating cofactor calcineurin (Homey et al., 1998; Boone et al., 2007; Hartmann et al., 2008; Kemp et al., 2011). Topical corticosteroids have anti-inflammatory and immunosuppressive effects and are recommended typically in children and adults with SV or NSV of recent onset (Abu Tahir et al., 2010; Gawkrodger et al., 2010). Systemic corticosteroids, which represent a second-line alternative, can halt the progression of the rapid-spreading vitiligo. Unfortunately, well-established depigmented vitiligo lesions often do not repigment in response to immunosuppressives or corticosteroids. In these circumstances, was ultraviolet light-based therapies are necessary to trigger repigmentation (Figure 66.2), through a regenerative process involving hair follicle melanocyte precursors (Birlea et al., 2012).

Genetic Features

Epidemiologic studies showed that 15−20% of vitiligo patients have one or more affected first-degree relatives, although most vitiligo cases occur sporadically. A single-locus Mendelian pattern of transmission was not supported for vitiligo. Most reports favored a polygenic, multifactorial model involving multiple genes and also environmental risk factors, features that define a "complex trait" (Spritz, 2011). In addition to the genetic factors, a considerable effect of non-genetic, environmental triggers has been implicated by the observation of a low concordance rate of 23% in monozygotic twins (Alkhateeb et al., 2003). Different earlier approaches, like candidate gene association studies (Birlea et al., 2011) or genome-wide linkage studies (Spritz, 2011), tested the involvement of susceptibility genes in vitiligo pathogenesis, some of which could not be confirmed to date. More successful in gene identification were the genome-wide association studies applied more recently; they have produced a rich yield of validated GV susceptibility genes that encode components of biological pathways reaching from immune cells to the melanocyte (Birlea et al., 2010, 2013; Jin et al., 2010a,b, 2012a; Quan et al., 2010). Among the most informative signals in Caucasians (Jin et al., 2010a) were those within MHC class I single nucleotide polymorphisms (SNP) rs12206499 which tags the HLA-A*02a marker that was associated with a favorable response to melanoma therapy. Also significant, and within the *TYR* gene locus, was the R402Q polymorphism which is associated with susceptibility to malignant melanoma (Spritz, 2011). Currently, the corresponding underlying causal variants for the two above-mentioned signals have already been identified by next generation resequencing (Jin et al., 2012b).

In Vivo and *In Vitro* Models

Several animal models of naturally occurring vitiligo (the Smyth line chicken, the gray horse, the vitiligo mouse, and the Sinclair pig) were identified and described (Boissy and Lamoreux, 1988). Of these, the Smyth line chicken continues to be studied extensively because it recapitulates the entire spectrum of clinical and biological manifestations of the human disease (mainly an inherent defect in the melanocytes in feathers and ocular tissue, and an associated autoimmune response that eliminates pigment cells). Recently, a new spontaneous mouse model for autoimmune vitiligo was created by introducing a human T cell receptor to human tyrosinase (h3T) into mice, combined with transgenic expression of the associated human HLA-A*0201 molecule (Mehrotra et al., 2012; Mosenson et al., 2013). The ensuing h3TA2 mice develop rapid, symmetrical, and progressive depigmentation of the pelage during adolescence.

Research in vitiligo using *in vitro* models has greatly advanced over the past two decades, providing a range of methodological options to study discrete mechanistic questions, as cited by Dell'anna et al. (2012):

1. Histological, immunofluorescence, and molecular techniques to test the destruction of melanocyte in vitiligo, and the migration of melanocytes to the interfolliclular epidermis during vitiligo repigmentation.
2. Monolayer cell culture studies from vitiligo skin to characterize the response of vitiligo melanocytes to various pharmacological agents, and to study melanocyte differential susceptibility to noxious stimuli (UVB, cumene, hydroperoxide, and tert-butyl-phenol).
3. Three-dimensional skin models, like reconstructed epidermis with keratinocytes and melanocytes on dead de-epidermized dermis (DDD) offer the possibility of reproducing the epidermal melanin unit.
4. Analysis of peripheral blood mononuclear cells (PBMC) in vitiligo consists in characterization of the immunological status of such cells, their ability to recognize specific melanocyte antigens, their cytotoxic effects to melanocytes or melanoma cell lines, and their redox status and responses to DNA damage.
5. Computer simulation models where structural and functional features can be reproduced to define better the sequence of events that possibly lead to functional defects.
6. Fluorescence-based assays, like microscopy and flow cytometry, represent easy methods to study some functional parameters and cell morphology.

Pathogenetic Mechanism

One of the most important factors in vitiligo pathogenesis is the unique nature of the human melanocyte as a target of cytotoxic damage. Melanocytes are factories for melanin, a heterogeneous protein product that absorbs light over a broad range of wavelengths. The melanization apparatus is enclosed in the melanosome, an organelle that separates the toxic intermediates of melanization from the cytoplasm of melanocytes. These melanocytes are transferred to surrounding keratinocytes to produce an intact pigment network. Melanocytes are terminally differentiated cells of neuroendocrine lineage. They have limited regenerative capacity and are highly resistant to

apoptotic cell death because of high expression of Bcl-2, Bcl-X, and Mcl-1 (Bowen et al., 2003). As discussed in the "Autoimmune features" section, melanocyte-specific Tc can cause the progressive depigmentation seen in vitiligo (van den Boorn et al., 2009). Moreover, vitiligo-associated antibodies are able to destroy melanocytes and melanoma cells *in vitro* and *in vivo* by complement-mediated damage and antibody-dependent cellular cytotoxicity (Fishman et al., 1993; Gilhar et al., 1995; Norris et al., 1998a; Gottumukkala et al., 2006). However, the current opinion is that these autoantibodies reflect a humoral response secondary to melanocyte destruction, rather than a primary cause of GV (Kemp, 2007). There is also extensive evidence that other mechanisms participate in the development and progression of disease, and in the induction of autoimmunity (Le Poole et al., 1993a; Norris et al., 1994). *In vitro* studies have connected cellular oxidative stress (Schallreuter et al., 1991, 2001, 2005; Dell'anna and Picardo, 2006) with the immune response in vitiligo: stressed melanocytes were found to mediate dendritic cell activation with the consequent dendritic cell effector functions playing a role in the destruction of melanocytes (Kroll et al., 2005). These experimental observations suggest that, like other autoimmune diseases, intrinsic damage to melanocytes could be the initiating event in vitiligo, followed by a secondary immune response by Tc lymphocytes which exacerbates the destruction of melanocytes (Le Poole and Luiten, 2008; Hariharan et al., 2010; van den Boorn et al., 2011).

The observation that depigmented lesions develop at a site previously exposed to a physical trauma (Le Poole and Luiten, 2008) suggests that immune response follows melanocyte damage. Cryptic epitopes of several vitiligo-associated intracellular melanocyte autoantigens such as tyrosinase and gp100 could be released during apoptosis and lead to T cell activation (Namazi, 2007; Westerhof and d'Ischia, 2007; Kemp et al., 2011). Antibodies could then be produced following the stimulation of B lymphocytes by activated helper T cells (Namazi, 2007); activated Tc could directly attack melanocytes that express antigenic peptides on their surface in the context of MHC class I molecules (Le Poole et al., 1993b; Hedley et al., 1998; Kemp et al., 2011). The selective destruction of melanocytes in vitiligo might occur because they are intrinsically more sensitive to immune-mediated injury than other skin cells (Norris et al., 1988b).

Autoantibodies as Potential Immunologic Markers

The use of melanocyte antibodies as markers of vitiligo activity is a controversial subject. While a recent study reported no correlation between the presence of antibodies and recent disease activity or different clinical parameters (e.g., age, gender, extension, and duration of vitiligo) (Kroon et al., 2012), other reports found the incidence and/or level of melanocyte antibodies linked to the activity and extent of vitiligo (Naughton et al., 1986; Aronson and Hashimoto, 1987; Harning et al., 1991; Yu et al., 1993; Kemp et al., 2011).

Following treatment with systemic steroids, a reduction in anti-melanocyte antibody levels and in antibody-mediated anti-melanocyte cytotoxicity has been reported (Hann et al., 1993; Takei et al., 1984). After therapy with psoralen and ultraviolet radiation (PUVA), decreased expression of vitiligo-associated melanocyte antigens was noted, leading to a blocking of antibody-dependent cell-mediated cytotoxicity against melanocytes (Kao and Yu, 1992; Viac et al., 1997). The presence or levels of anti-melanocyte antibodies have not yet been effectively developed as diagnostic tools or markers of disease activity.

Concluding Remarks—Future Prospects

Vitiligo has been observed and treated since antiquity, but it still remains an enigmatic disorder in which combined genetic and non-genetic factors can cause the autoimmune-mediated destruction of melanocytes from epidermis, but often sparing HF melanocytes. Treatment in vitiligo must consider two distinct aspects: (1) limitation of the immune process which halts the progression of depigmentation and (2) stimulation of repigmentation of vitiligo lesions by mobilizing the stem cell populations to proliferate, migrate, and differentiate to regenerate the interfollicular melanocytes. Effective treatment of vitiligo involves topical medications and phototherapy to both suppress the immune response and to activate melanocyte regeneration from HF reservoirs of pluripotent stem cells (Birlea et al., 2012). New research initiatives are focusing on the repopulation of affected interfollicular epidermis with melanocyte precursors from the bulge region of the HF. This process is a classic example of regenerative medicine, based on stem cell activation. The key to improving therapeutic approaches for vitiligo is targeted stimulation of the principal repigmentation genes/proteins or designing new compounds which are potent and selective inducers of melanocyte activation, migration, and differentiation.

PSORIASIS

Clinical, Pathologic, and Epidemiologic Features

Psoriasis is a common, chronic, immune-mediated inflammatory skin disease with polygenic inheritance, characterized by erythematous scaly plaques that can range from a few scattered lesions to involvement of the entire body surface. Psoriasis may progressively worsen with age, or wax and wane in severity (Stern et al., 2004; Gelfand et al., 2005; Kurd and Gelfand, 2009; Parisi et al., 2013). The disease prevalence is 2–4% of the population in Western countries (Parisi et al., 2013), ranging from 0.91% (United States) (Robinson et al., 2006) to 8.5% (Norway) (Bø et al., 2008). Psoriasis can present at any age (see Table 66.4); type I psoriasis presents in younger patients and has a poor prognosis, while type II psoriasis presents in elderly patients and is easier to control. When psoriasis has extensive distribution, especially involving the groin and hands or feet, it produces significant morbidity and a decrease in the quality of life (Nestle et al., 2009). The prototypic lesion is plaque psoriasis, characterized by raised, well-demarcated, erythematous, oval plaques with adherent silvery-white, dry scales (Figure 66.3). The histopathology of psoriasis characteristically shows a thickened epidermis with an expanded proliferative compartment, premature maturation of keratinocytes and incomplete cornification with retention of nuclei in the stratum corneum (parakeratosis) (Nestle et al., 2009). The dermal inflammatory infiltrate consists mainly of dendritic cells, macrophages, and T cells, while the epidermis contains neutrophils and some T cells. Erythema in lesions is due to increased numbers of tortuous capillaries in the rete ridges, covered by a very thin epidermis (Nestle et al., 2009). Psoriasis may be triggered by trauma or injury (Koebner's phenomenon), infections (Leung et al., 1995, 1998), xerosis, and reactions to various drugs (Gudjonsson and Elder, 2008). Psoriatic arthritis presents as distal interphalangeal disease, axial arthritis, or symmetrical arthritis (Winchester, 2008) (see Chapter 38). Nail involvement may be present, particularly associated with arthritis. The various types and presentations of psoriasis are outlined in Table 66.4 (Langley et al., 2005) and guttate and pustular psoriasis are presented in Figures 66.4 and 66.5.

Autoimmune Features

It is now generally accepted that psoriatic lesions are caused by abnormal reactivity of specific T cells in the skin. It is also accepted that alterations in the epidermal barrier, in innate immune defenses, and in processing of inflammatory signals may all contribute to the triggering of nonspecific innate immune mechanisms. The effector mechanisms in the epidermis include increased production of IL-23 and Th1- and Th17-type cytokines (Gudjonsson and Johnston, 2009).

The concept of an autoimmune basis for psoriasis notwithstanding the presence of a dysregulated immune

TABLE 66.4 Classification of Psoriasis

Types and Subtypes of Disease	Features
1. Plaque psoriasis/vulgaris type	— sharply circumscribed, round-oval, or nummular (coin-sized) plaques — plaques occur on elbows, knee, trunk, back — most common type, occurring in 85–90% of patients
2. Guttate psoriasis	— small, 2–10 mm diameter; acute onset, centripetal distribution — lesions occur shortly after an acute streptococcal infection of the pharynx or tonsils — common in children; occasionally in adults
3. Flexural (inverse) psoriasis	— affects the flexures (inframammary, perineal, and axillary) — lesions devoid of scale appear as red, shiny, well demarcated plaques — differential diagnosis: candidal intertrigo, dermatophyte infections

4. Erythroderma
  a. chronic plaque psoriasis
  b. unstable psoriasis
	— total or subtotal involvement of the body skin
	— may impair the thermoregulatory capacity of the skin, leading to hypothermia, high output cardiac failure, and metabolic changes
	  a. lesions gradually progress as plaques and become confluent and extensive
	  b. precipitated by infection, tar, drugs, withdrawal of corticosteroids; becomes rapidly extensive

5. Generalized pustular psoriasis (von Zumbusch)	— monomorphic, sterile pustules, which may coalesce to form sheets — active, unstable disease; sometimes requires hospital admission — precipitated by withdrawal of systemic or potent topical corticosteroids and by infections
6. Palmoplantar pustulosis	— sterile, yellow pustules on erythemato-squamous background — frequently with nail involvement — prevalent in women, in the 4th–6th decade, and in smokers
7. Psoriatic nail disease	— small pits, onycholysis, "oil spots" thickening, dystrophy, discoloration, subungual hyperkeratosis

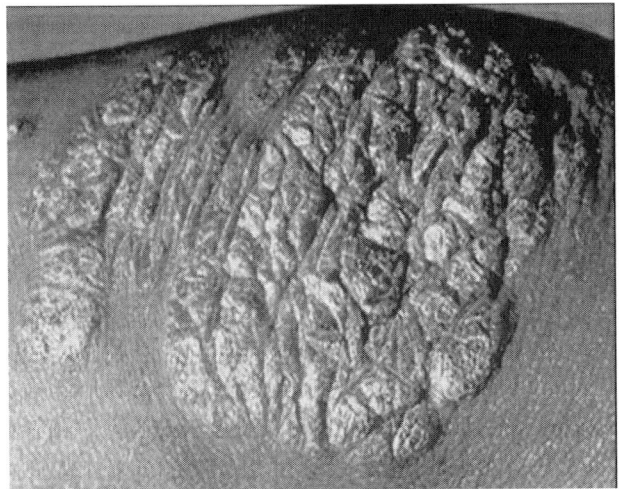

FIGURE 66.3 Typical plaque of psoriasis.

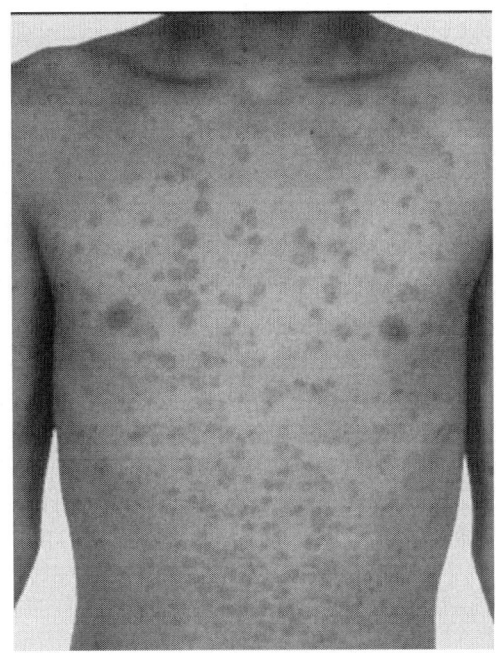

FIGURE 66.4 Guttate psoriasis of the trunk.

system (Nestle et al., 2009) is supported by the following:

1. Increased numbers of immune cells (mainly dendritic and T cells) within the lesions, and the appearance of oligoclonal T cells in lesions over time.
2. Oligoclonal T cell activation in psoriatic lesions (Lin et al., 2001).
3. Efficacy of T cell-targeted treatments (cyclosporine, efalizumab, alefacept) (Lowes et al., 2007), drugs that inhibit Th1 and Th17 cells and their cytokines

(ustekinumab), or therapies that are thought to target the adaptive immune system rather than modify keratinocyte function (corticosteroids, UVB) (Schwarz, 2008; Bergboer et al., 2012).

4. Genetic associations that are largely immunologic (discussed below).
5. Xenograft animal models (Bergboer et al., 2012) that have focused on the functional role of T cells and cytokines (Nestle et al., 2009).
6. The observation that bone marrow transplantation into psoriasis patients may cure the disease, and that psoriasis can be transferred from a psoriatic transplant donor to the recipient (Nestle et al., 2009).

However, as yet there is no convincing evidence identifying the specificity of autoreactive T cell clones in psoriasis. Although it has been proposed that CD4$^+$ T cell activation initiates psoriasis and CD8$^+$ intraepidermal T cells cause lesion persistence, there is no evidence that these cells are activated by self-antigens (Lin et al., 2001). Many of the triggers for psoriasis are not antigen specific (Leung et al., 1993, 1998), and several of the most effective treatments such as anti-tumor necrosis factor (TNF) biologics may affect both innate and acquired immunity as well as inflammation in general.

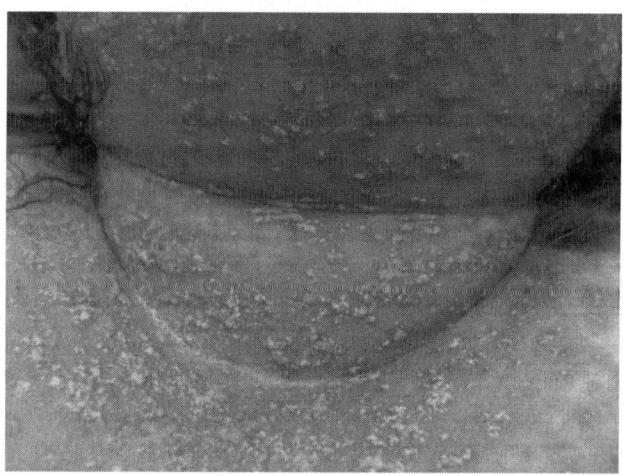

FIGURE 66.5   Pustular psoriasis of the neck and upper chest.

Genetic Features

The importance of a hereditary component in the pathogenesis of psoriasis has been established through population-based studies (Gudjonsson and Elder, 2008). They indicate that the incidence of psoriasis is greater among first-degree and second-degree relatives of patients than among the general population (Nestle et al., 2009). Twin studies showed a concordance rate of 35–72% in monozygotic twins and 12–23% in dizygotic twins (Bowcock and Krueger, 2005). About 71% of the patients with childhood psoriasis report a positive family history (Morris et al., 2001). In the past decades, several linkage studies and genome-wide association studies (Bergboer et al., 2012) identified susceptibility loci for psoriasis. Genome-wide linkage analysis has identified at least nine chromosomal loci with statistically significant linkage to psoriasis (called PSORS1 through PSORS9) (Nestle et al., 2009). Genomic signatures in psoriatic lesions point to dendritic cells as a key cell type, and IFN-γ and TNF-α as key cytokines; this reinforces the concept that cells and mediators of the immune system have essential roles in susceptibility to and maintenance of psoriasis (Nestle et al., 2009). The psoriasis genome-wide association signals confirmed (Bergboer et al., 2012) are listed in Table 66.5.

In Vivo and *In Vitro* Models

In Vivo *Models*

Spontaneous Mouse Models

A number of spontaneous mouse mutations give rise to psoriasiform inflammatory and scaly phenotypes (Sundberg and King, 1996; Raychaudhuri et al., 2001), which usually represent only a limited set of psoriatic features (Gudjonsson et al., 2007; Nestle et al., 2009).

Genetically Engineered Mouse Models

Transgenic mice have been generated that overexpress adhesion molecules, cytokines, transcription factors, and inflammatory mediators in both keratinocytes and immunocytes to define the important cell types in psoriasis disease initiation. Epidermal overexpression of molecules

TABLE 66.5 Top Psoriasis Signals with Immune Function

Putative Biological Pathway	Gene/Locus
Adaptive immunity	IL23R, ERAP1, IL-12B, TNF, TRAG3IP2, IL-4, IL-13, IL-23A, ZNF313/RNF114, HLA-C
Barrier skin function	LCERB, LCE3C, CDSN, DEFB, GJB2
Innate immunity	IF1H1, REL, TNIP1, TNFAIP3, IL-28RA, NFKBIA, FBXL19, NOS2, TYK2

under the control of promoters in the epidermis (e.g., keratin (K)5, K14, and K10, or involucrin) induce the development of a psoriasis-like disease in several mouse models. The K5-STAT3C mouse develops a psoriasis-like disease, with keratinocyte hyperplasia, loss of stratum granulosum, and parakeratosis.

Knockout or hypomorphic mice, in which the genetic element has been removed or attenuated, respectively, have also been used to study a given mediator in psoriasis. Mice develop a condition that resembles psoriatic skin disease after *ITGB2*, *ITGAE*, *IL1RN*, and *IRF2* genes are knocked out (Wagner et al., 2010).

Transplantation Models (Nestle et al., 2009; Gudjonsson et al., 2007)

Psoriasis-like findings were observed in Prkdc^scid mice receiving CD4$^+$-CD45-RBhi T cells from donors who were MHC matched, but mismatched for minor histocompatibility antigens (Schön et al., 1997). Humanized xenotransplantation models most closely resemble psoriasis. Their advantage is that both human skin and immune cell infiltrate are transplanted and can be studied directly.

In Vitro *Models*

Because of the complex nature of psoriasis, *in vivo* models are the preferred platform for investigation of most aspects of disease. However, *in vitro* studies have been useful in isolating infiltrating lymphocytes from lesional areas, in studying selected functions in psoriatic keratinocytes, and showing the effects of de-epidermized psoriatic dermis on the disease process.

Pathogenic Mechanism

The mechanism of evolution of a psoriatic lesion from initiation to persistence of disease has been thoroughly studied (Nestle et al., 2009).

1. Initial triggers (e.g., physical trauma or bacterial products) start a cascade of events that include the formation of DNA–LL-37 complexes, activation of plasmacytoid dendritic cells, and secretion of the cytokine IFN-α (both found increased in early psoriatic lesions). Clinical observation points to an important role of IFN-α as an inducer of psoriasis (Funk et al., 1991).

2. Psoriatic keratinocytes are a rich source of antimicrobial peptides, including LL-37, β-defensins, and psoriasin. In addition, keratinocytes are responsive to key dendritic cell-derived and T cell-derived cytokines, including interferons, TNF, IL-17, and IL-20, and in turn will produce proinflammatory cytokines including IL-1, IL-6, and TNF-α.

3. Myeloid dermal dendritic cells are increased in psoriatic lesions and induce proliferation of T cells and production of Th1 cytokines. Activated myeloid dendritic cells migrate into draining lymph nodes and stimulate differentiation of naïve T cells into effector cells, Th17 or type 17 cytotoxic T cells (Tc)17, Th1 or Tc1 (Nestle et al., 1994). They have proinflammatory effects, producing TNF-α and nitric oxide synthase (NOS) (Lowes et al., 2005).

4. Effector cells recirculate and slow down in skin capillaries in the presence of selectin- and integrin-guided receptor–ligand interactions. Immune cells expressing the chemokine receptors CCR6, CCR4, and CXCR3 emigrate into skin tissue along these chemokine gradients. Key processes during disease maintenance are the presentation of putative autoantigens to T cells and the release of IL-23 by dermal dendritic cells, the production of proinflammatory mediators such as TNF-α and nitric oxide (NO) by TNF-α and inducible NOS-producing dendritic cells, and the production of IL-17 and IL-22 by Th17 and Tc17 cells, and of IFN-γ and TNF-α by Th1 and Tc1 cells. These mediators act on keratinocytes, leading to the activation, proliferation, and production of antimicrobial peptides (e.g., LL-37, cathelicidin, and β-defensins), chemokines (e.g., CXCL1, CXCL9 through CXCL11, and CCL20), and S100 proteins by keratinocytes. Dendritic and T cells form perivascular clusters in the presence of CCL19 produced by macrophages. An essential event is the migration of T cells from the dermis into the epidermis, controlled through the interaction of $\alpha1\beta1$ integrin (very late antigen 1 [VLA-1]) on T cells with collagen IV at the basement membrane.

5. Natural killer (NK) T cells contribute to the disease process.

6. Feedback loops involving keratinocytes, fibroblasts, and endothelial cells contribute to tissue reorganization with endothelial cell activation and proliferation and deposition of extracellular matrix. Neutrophils in the epidermis are attracted by chemokines, including CXCL8 and CXCL1.

7. Studies have indicated a defect in the overall suppressive activity of T regulatory (Treg) cells (Sugiyama et al., 2005), with decreased contra-regulation of the proinflammatory state (Nestle et al., 2009).

Autoantibodies as Potential Immunologic Markers

Autoantibodies to keratin-associated intermediate filaments (Shigenobu et al., 1989), to U1 and U2 small nuclear ribonucleoproteins (Reeves et al., 1986), to cal-pastatin (Matsushita et al., 2005), and to other epidermal proteins have been described in psoriasis, but none has proven reliable as a biomarker of disease activity, or has been accepted as a participant in disease pathogenesis.

Concluding Remarks—Future Prospects

Psoriasis is a common inflammatory skin disease of undetermined etiology in which an autoimmune basis is suspected, but is far from established. There is no cure, although multiple treatments can produce worthwhile disease remissions (UV light phototherapy, methotrexate, biologicals); all of the treatments that induce remissions decrease the population of activated T cells within the lesions. This heterogeneous, cutaneous, inflammatory disorder is histopathologically characterized by prominent epidermal hyperplasia and a distinct inflammatory infiltrate. Crosstalk between immunocytes and keratino-cytes, which results in the production of cytokines, chemokines, and growth factors, is thought to mediate the disease. Given that psoriasis is only observed in humans, numerous genetic approaches to model psoriasis in mice have been undertaken (Wagner et al., 2010). Existing and new mouse models are needed in order to dissect this complex disease and to provide novel insights into the molecular mechanisms and pathways that incite the disease initiating events, and also those which are responsible for recurrences following success-ful treatment. Biological therapies are already giving promising results but, owing to the heterogeneity of psoriasis, optimal treatments are unlikely to be restricted to individual targets. Combination treatments intended to reduce the immune activation and angiogenesis and to restore differentiation of keratinocytes in a disease stage-dependent manner will be beneficial.

CHRONIC URTICARIA

Clinical, Pathologic, and Epidemiologic Features

Chronic urticaria (CU) is a relatively common type of urticaria, defined as hives lasting longer than 6 weeks (Kaplan, 2004). It affects around 0.1% of the population including both adults and children (Schocket, 2006), with a higher predilection in women than in men (2:1), and with significant adverse effects on quality of life (Schocket, 2006). CU is currently divided into three sub-categories (Greaves and Tan, 2007): (1) urticarial vasculi-tis (leukocytoclastic vasculitis of the small vessels with hives duration of more than 24 hours which can accom-pany autoimmune rheumatic diseases, inflammatory bowel disease, viral hepatitis, and paraproteinemia); (2)

physical urticarias (with several subtypes, e.g., solar, cold, aquagenic, delayed pressure, vibratory, cholinergic, and dermographism); and (3) chronic autoimmune urti-caria (which is caused by anti-FCεRI antibodies, and less often by anti-IgE antibodies).

Chronic spontaneous urticaria (with more than 6 weeks' duration of symptoms) is a subtype of urticaria in which there is no identifiable cause (Zuberbier, 2012).

The characteristic clinical lesion of both acute urti-caria and CU is the hive; hives present as pruritic, ery-thematous, blanching, circumscribed macular or raised lesions, involving the superficial layers of the skin (Joint Task Force on Practice, 2000). Up to 40% of CU patients have associated angioedema (swelling of the deeper struc-tures) (Kaplan, 2004). Generally an individual CU lesion does not persist in the same location for greater than 24 hours (Joint Task Force on Practice, 2000). Untreated CU should virtually always be associated with pruritus. In the absence of pruritus the clinician should consider alterna-tive diagnoses. A thorough history is critical to identify-ing known causes of urticaria.

CU is diagnosed clinically. The patient history is criti-cal in making the diagnosis, identifying a potential trig-ger, and ruling out other diseases. For both acute and chronic urticaria, important specific points of history include physical triggers, recent changes in medications, recent travel, infections (including parasitic), history of atopy, and a complete review of systems. Additional der-matologic conditions should be considered in the differen-tial diagnosis: erythema annulare centrifugum, erythema chronicum migrans, and erythema multiforme.

The principal histologic finding in CU is dermal edema. There is variable cellular infiltrate around vessels, with predominance of neutrophils and eosinophils in early lesions and of lymphocytes accompanied by neutrophils and eosinophils in advanced lesions (Lee et al., 2002).

Autoimmune Features

The presence of autoimmunity in a significant proportion of CU patients was initially suggested by demonstration of skin reactivity to the injection of the patient's own serum, the so-called autologous serum skin test (ASST) (Grattan et al., 1986, 1990). Later, it was shown that the serum and purified IgG of a subset of patients with chronic idiopathic urticaria releases histamine from baso-phils and dermal mast cells when incubated with leuko-cytes prepared from peripheral blood from two healthy human donors. This release could be inhibited by preincu-bation with recombinant FcεR1α, the α-chain of the high-affinity IgE receptor. In a small proportion of patients (5%), the histamine-releasing factor was inhibited not by the α-chain of FcεR1 but by IgE itself (Hide et al., 1993; Niimi et al., 1996).

CU has been shown to be associated with an autoimmune mechanism in 30–50% of idiopathic urticaria cases. In addition, other concomitant autoimmune disorders including autoimmune thyroid disorders, rheumatoid arthritis, type 1 diabetes mellitus, celiac disease, Sjögren's syndrome, and systemic lupus erythematosus were significantly more prevalent in patients with CU when compared to the general population (Confino-Cohen et al., 2012). Moreover, in the same population, CU patients showed a higher prevalence of other serologic markers of autoimmunity, notably rheumatoid factor and antinuclear antibodies, as compared with non-CU controls (Confino-Cohen et al., 2012). The association of CU with thyroid autoimmunity was described earlier (Leznoff et al., 1983), followed by the observation that suppression of thyroid activity results in CU remission (Schocket, 2006).

The presence of an inflammatory perivascular infiltrate in many CU patients also supports the immune basis of this disease. This infiltrate is predominantly composed of T lymphocytes, specifically CD4$^+$, T helper cells, and a small number of CD8$^+$ cytotoxic T cells (Mekori et al., 1983).

Genetic Features

Autoimmune CU is a complex multifactorial disease with probably genetic and environmental components. CU clusters in families, being more frequent among the first-degree relatives of affected individuals than in the general population (Asero, 2002). There is a paucity of literature on proposed genetic susceptibilities, mainly consisting of small candidate genes studies, of which results are still unconfirmed. These studies targeted protein tyrosine phosphatase-22 (*PTPN22*) (Brzoza et al., 2012), formyl peptide receptor like 1 (*FPRL1*) (Yang et al., 2010), HLA-DRB1, and HLA-DQB1 (Chen et al., 2005).

In Vivo and *In Vitro* Models

While it is understood that autoimmune mechanisms are responsible for a subset of CU, no single test is diagnostic, and therefore all require clinical correlation. Biopsy and histologic evaluation is only valuable to confirm features consistent with urticaria when the diagnosis is in doubt, or when alternative diagnoses are being strongly considered. While there is evidence suggesting the presence of IgG directed against both the IgE receptor α subunit and the Fc region of IgE (Sabroe and Greaves, 2006), there remains significant debate as to the clinical utility of the available testing modalities. One of the earliest tests performed on patients with CU is the ASST. This involves intradermal injection of autologous serum on the volar surface of an unaffected arm along with positive and negative controls (typically saline and histamine).

The test is read 30 minutes later and is considered positive if the wheal at the serum site is 1.5 mm greater than that of the wheal at the negative control. The sensitivity was calculated at 65–81% and specificity 71–78% (Sabroe et al., 1999). Other authors have shown unacceptably high false-positive reactions in healthy controls with the autologous serum skin test as high as 56% (Taskapan et al., 2008).

Other testing modalities including basophil activation and commercial assays for detecting anti-FcεR1α antibodies (sometimes referred to as the CU index) are available although there remains much debate regarding their clinical utility. More recently an assay focusing on a unique connective tissue mast cell line has been proposed (Posthumus et al., 2012).

Animal models for contact urticaria were previously described; however, a suitable model for CU has not been reported so far.

Pathologic Effector Mechanisms

Histamine-releasing IgG autoantibodies directed against both the IgE receptor α subunit and the Fc region of IgE remain the basis of the autoimmune subset within CU (Hide et al., 1993; Niimi et al., 1996; Kaplan 2004; Mlynek et al., 2008). It was also suggested that the sera from patients with CU containing FcεRIα antibody release mediators and tumor necrosis factor (TNF)-α by activating human foreskin mast cells (Lee et al., 2002). Mast cells are considered to be the primary effector cells in CU, by releasing a variety of inflammatory mediators such as leukotrienes, tryptase, prostaglandins, histamine, interleukin (IL)-1, IL-6, IL-8, and TNF-α (Lee et al., 2002), which regulate the emigration of leukocytes; these mediators induce a sequential upregulation of endothelial adhesion molecules [P-selectin, E-selectin, intercellular adhesion molecules 1 (ICAM-1)], and vascular cell adhesion molecule-1 (VCAM-1) (Lee et al., 2002), which facilitate the binding of the activated leukocytes to endothelial cells, and then transmigrate into tissues. Recent literature has suggested alternative mast cell activating factors relate to the coagulation cascade. Activation of the classical complement pathway and formation of C5a are important for dermal mast cell activation and for neutrophil and eosinophil chemoattraction (Greaves and Tan, 2007). Autologous sera from some patients with CU retain the ability to induce a wheal-and-flare reaction when injected intracutaneously even after depletion of IgG (Mlynek et al., 2008). Other studies have demonstrated that thrombin causes edema development by both direct endothelial and indirect inflammatory mediator mechanisms (Asero et al., 2006, 2007a,b). This effect is reduced by antihistamines and completely absent if mast cell granules are eliminated. One recent study showed high serum levels of the Th17 cell profile of cytokines including IL-17, IL-23, and TNF-α among chronic spontaneous urticaria patients (Atwa et al., 2013). Other recent work has focused on a possible hormonal component given that CU is twice as prevalent in women. To date there is no evidence to suggest a hormonal mechanism.

Autoantibodies as Potential Immunologic Markers

Numerous attempts to develop immunoassays that measure serum levels of IgG and anti-FcϵR1 or anti-IgE antibodies in urticaria, although successful, have shown low specificity and poor correlation with *in vitro* serum histamine release and disease activity (Greaves and Tan, 2007).

Concluding Remarks—Future Prospects

Regardless of the mechanism, first-line treatment for CU remains H1 antihistamines. Second-line treatments include addition of an H2 antihistamine, or of a leukotriene modifier (Tilles, 2005). Using oral glucocorticoids is a common practice for refractory symptoms. In light of the likely adverse effects with long-term use, most clinicians recommend using them for short periods (usually 3−7 days) at the minimally effective dose to control symptoms. Third-line treatments include immunomodulators, but evidence for efficacy with these agents is largely based on clinical experience and small-scale studies. Management guidelines also recommend dapsone as the next line of therapy. In patients with anemia, sulfasalazine is used as an alternative. In patients with only modest impairment in quality of life, use of hydroxychloroquine was suggested given its slow onset of action (Reeves, 2004). Alternative immunomodulators used for refractory cases include other calcineurin inhibitors (Trojan and Khan, 2012), mycophenolate mofetil (Zimmerman et al., 2012), immunglobulin (Asero, 2000), TNF inhibitors, colchicine (Pho et al., 2011), methotrexate (Gach et al., 2001; Perez et al., 2010; Sagi et al., 2011), and cyclophosphamide (Bernstein et al., 2002; Asero, 2005). Phototherapy has also been shown to be effective and is a treatment option for patients desiring to avoid systemic medications (Berroeta et al., 2004; Engin et al., 2008; Aydogan et al., 2012). More recently, omalizumab, a human monoclonal antibody against the high-affinity IgE receptor FcϵRI, has been shown to be effective, although cost remains a limiting factor (Maurer et al., 2013).

Although CU is a relatively common condition, identifying the precise trigger in individual patients is usually not possible. Better testing for antigen specificities is a high priority to correct this important issue and is essential for the best treatment outcomes. Blocking mast cell degranulation or blocking the effects of released mast cell mediators is often an inadequate approach to treatment.

The addition of immunosuppressive drugs and specific anti-IgE biologics has enhanced the effectiveness of treatment for recalcitrant CU patients. Nevertheless, better tools for immunologic characterization of the autoimmune mechanism in individual patients, better drugs for mast cell stabilization, and better drugs to block the autoimmune mechanisms of CU are all important to enhance the effectiveness of treating these patients.

REFERENCES

Abu Tahir, M., Pramod, K., Ansari, S.H., Ali, J., 2010. Current remedies for vitiligo. Autoimmun. Rev. 9, 516−520.

Alkhateeb, A., Fain, P.R., Thody, A., Bennett, D.C., Spritz, R.A., 2003. Epidemiology of vitiligo and associated autoimmune diseases in Caucasian probands and their relatives. Pigment Cell Res. 16, 208−214.

Alli, R., Nguyen, P., Boyd, K., Sundberg, J.P., Geiger, T.L., 2012. A mouse model of clonal CD8+ T lymphocyte-mediated alopecia areata progressing to alopecia universalis. J. Immunol. 188, 477−486.

Aronson, P.J., Hashimoto, K., 1987. Association of IgA anti-melanoma antibodies in the sera of vitiligo patients with active disease. J. Invest. Dermatol. 88, 475.

Asero, R., 2000. Are IVIG for chronic unremitting urticaria effective? Allergy 55, 1099−1101.

Asero, R., 2002. Chronic idiopathic urticaria: a family study. Ann. Allergy Asthma Immunol. 89, 195−196.

Asero, R., 2005. Oral cyclophosphamide in a case of cyclosporin and steroid-resistant chronic urticaria showing autoreactivity on autologous serum skin testing. Clin. Exp. Dermatol. 30, 582−583.

Asero, R., Riboldi, P., Tedeschi, A., Cugno, M., Meroni, P., 2007a. Chronic urticaria: a disease at a crossroad between autoimmunity and coagulation. Autoimmun. Rev. 7, 71−76.

Asero, R., Tedeschi, A., Coppola, R., Griffini, S., Paparella, P., Riboldi, P., et al., 2007b. Activation of the tissue factor pathway of blood coagulation in patients with chronic urticaria. J. Allergy Clin. Immunol. 119, 705−710.

Asero, R., Tedeschi, A., Riboldi, P., Cugno, M., 2006. Plasma of patients with chronic urticaria shows signs of thrombin generation, and its intradermal injection causes wheal-and-flare reactions much more frequently than autologous serum. J. Allergy Clin. Immunol. 117, 1113−1117.

Atwa, M.A., Emara, A.S., Youssef, N., Bayoumy, N.M., 2013. Serum concentration of IL-17, IL-23 and TNF-alpha among patients with chronic spontaneous urticaria: association with disease activity and autologous serum skin test. J. Eur. Acad. Dermatol. Venereol. Epub ahead of print.

Aydogan, K., Karadogan, S.K., Tunali, S., Saricaoglu, H., 2012. Narrowband ultraviolet B (311 nm, TL01) phototherapy in chronic ordinary urticaria. Int. J. Dermatol. 51, 98−103.

Badri, A.M., Todd, P.M., Garioch, J.J., Gudgeon, J.E., Stewart, D.G., Goudie, R.B., 1993. An immunohistological study of cutaneous lymphocytes in vitiligo. J. Pathol. 170, 149−155.

Barahmani, N., Schabath, M.B., Duvic, M., National Alopecia Areata Registry, 2009. History of atopy or autoimmunity increases risk of alopecia areata. J. Am. Acad. Dermatol. 61, 581−591.

Bergboer, J.G., Zeeuwen, P.L., Schalkwijk, J., 2012. Genetics of psoriasis: evidence for epistatic interaction between skin barrier abnormalities and immune deviation. J. Invest. Dermatol. 132, 2320–2321.

Bernstein, J.A., Garramone, S.M., Lower, E.G., 2002. Successful treatment of autoimmune chronic idiopathic urticaria with intravenous cyclophosphamide. Ann. Allergy Asthma Immunol. 89, 212–214.

Berroeta, L., Clark, C., Ibbotson, S.H., Ferguson, J., Dawe, R.S., 2004. Narrow-band (TL-01) ultraviolet B phototherapy for chronic urticaria. Clin. Exp. Dermatol. 29, 97–98.

Birlea, S.A., Ahmad, F.J., Uddin, R.M., Ahmad, S., Pal, S.S., Begum, R., et al., 2013. Association of generalized vitiligo with MHC Class II Loci in patients from the Indian subcontinent. J. Invest. Dermatol. 133, 1369–1372.

Birlea, S.A., Gowan, K., Fain, P.R., Spritz, R.A., 2010. Genome-wide association study of generalized vitiligo in an isolated European founder population identifies SMOC2, in close proximity to IDDM8. J. Invest. Dermatol. 130, 798–803.

Birlea, S.A., Jin, Y., Bennett, D.C., Herbstman, D.M., Wallace, M.R., McCormack, W.T., et al., 2011. Comprehensive association analysis of candidate genes for generalized vitiligo supports XBP1, FOXP1, and TSLP. J. Invest. Dermatol. 131, 371–381.

Birlea, S.A., Spritz, R.A., Norris, D.A., 2012. Vitiligo. In: Wolff, K., Goldsmith, L.A., Katz, S.I., Gilchrest, B.A., Paller, A.S., Leffell, D.J. (Eds.), Fitzpatrick's Dermatology in General Medicine, eighth ed. McGraw-Hill, New York, pp. 792–803.

Bø, K., Thoresen, M., Dalgard, F., 2008. Smokers report more psoriasis, but not atopic dermatitis or hand eczema: results from a Norwegian population survey among adults. Dermatology. 216, 40–45.

Boissy, R.E., Lamoreux, M.L., 1988. Animal models of an acquired pigmentary disorder: vitiligo. In: J. Bagnara, J. (Ed.), Advances in Pigment Cell Research. Alan R. Liss Inc., New York, USA, pp. 207–218.

Boone, B., Ongenae, K., Van Geel, N., Vernijns, S., De Keyser, S., Naeyaert, J.M., 2007. Topical pimecrolimus in the treatment of vitiligo. Eur. J. Dermatol. 17, 55–61.

Bowcock, A.M., Krueger, J.G., 2005. Getting under the skin: the immunogenetics of psoriasis. Nat. Rev. Immunol. 5, 699–711.

Bowen, A.R., Hanks, A.N., Allen, S.M., Alexander, A., Diedrich, M.J., Grossman, D., 2003. Apoptosis regulators and responses in human melanocytic and keratinocytic cells. J. Invest. Dermatol. 120, 48–55.

Brzoza, Z., Grzeszczak, W., Rogala, B., Trautsolt, W., Moczulski, D., 2012. PTPN22 polymorphism presumably plays a role in the genetic background of chronic spontaneous autoreactive urticaria. Dermatology. 224, 340–345.

Chen, J., Tan, Z., Li, J., Xiong, P., 2005. Association of HLA-DRB1, DQB1 alleles with chronic urticaria. J. Huazhong Univ. Sci. Technol. Med. Sci. 25, 354–356.

Chu, S.Y., Chen, Y.J., Tseng, W.C., et al., 2011. Comorbidity profiles among patients with alopecia areata: the importance of onset age, a nationwide population-based study. J. Am. Acad. Dermatol. 65, 949–956.

Colonna, L., Catalano, G., Chew, C., et al., 2010. Therapeutic targeting of Syk in autoimmune diabetes. J. Immunol. 185, 1532–1543.

Confino-Cohen, R., Chodick, G., Shalev, V., Leshno, M., Kimhi, O., Goldberg, A., 2012. Chronic urticaria and autoimmunity: associations found in a large population study. J. Allergy Clin. Immunol. 129, 1307–1313.

Cui, J., Harning, R., Henn, M., Bystryn, J.C., 1992. Identification of pigment cell antigens defined by vitiligo antibodies. J. Invest. Dermatol. 98, 162–165.

Delamere, F.M., Sladden, M.M., Dobbins, H.M., Leonardi-Bee, J., 2008. Interventions for alopecia areata. Cochrane Database Syst. Rev. 16, CD004413.

Dell'anna, M.L., Cario-André, M., Bellei, B., Taieb, A., Picardo, M., 2012. In vitro research on vitiligo: strategies, principles, methodological options and common pitfalls. Exp. Dermatol. 21, 490–496.

Dell'anna, M.L., Picardo, M., 2006. A review and a new hypothesis for non-immunological pathogenetic mechanisms in vitiligo. Pigment Cell Res. 19, 406–411.

el-Mofty, A.M., el-Mofty, M., 1980. Vitiligo. A symptom complex. Int. J. Dermatol. 19, 237–244.

Engin, B., Ozdemir, M., Balevi, A., Mevlitoglu, I., 2008. Treatment of chronic urticaria with narrowband ultraviolet B phototherapy: a randomized controlled trial. Acta Derm. Venereol. 88, 247–251.

Feliciani, C., Gupta, A.K., Sauder, D.N., 1996. Keratinocytes and cytokine/growth factors. Crit. Rev. Oral Biol. Med. 7, 300–318.

Fishman, P., Azizi, E., Shoenfeld, Y., Sredni, B., Yecheskel, G., Ferrone, S., et al., 1993. Vitiligo autoantibodies are effective against melanoma. Cancer. 72, 2365–2369.

Freyschmidt-Paul, P.M., Zoller, K.J., McElwee, J., et al., 2005. The functional relevance of the type 1 cytokines IFN-gamma and IL-2 in alopecia areata of C3H/HeJ mice. J. Investig. Dermatol. Symp. Proc. 10, 282–283.

Funk, J., Langeland, T., Schrumpf, E., Hanssen, L.E., 1991. Psoriasis induced by interferon-alpha. Br. J. Dermatol. 125, 463–465.

Gach, J.E., Sabroe, R.A., Greaves, M.W., Black, A.K., 2001. Methotrexate-responsive chronic idiopathic urticaria: a report of two cases. Br. J. Dermatol. 145, 340–343.

Gawkrodger, D.J., Ormerod, A.D., Shaw, L., Mauri-Sole, I., Whitton, M.E., Watts, M.J., et al., 2010. Vitiligo: concise evidence based guidelines on diagnosis and management. Postgrad. Med. J. 86, 466–471.

Gelfand, J.M., Weinstein, R., Porter, S.B., Neimann, A.L., Berlin, J.A., Margolis, D.J., 2005. Prevalence and treatment of psoriasis in the United Kingdom: a population-based study. Arch Dermatol. 141, 1537–1541.

Giangreco, A., Hoste, E., Takai, Y., Rosewell, I., Watt, F.M., 2012. Epidermal Cadm1 expression promotes autoimmune alopecia via enhanced T cell adhesion and cytotoxicity. J. Immunol. 188, 1514–1522.

Gilhar, A., Ftzion, A.I., Paus, R., 2012. Alopecia Areata. N. Engl. J. Med. 366, 1515–1525.

Gilhar, A., Keren, A., Shemer, A., d'Ovidio, R., Ullmann, Y., Paus, R., 2013. Autoimmune disease induction in a healthy human organ: a humanized mouse model of alopecia areata. J. Invest. Dermatol. 133, 844–847.

Gilhar, A., Landau, M., Assy, B., Shalaginov, R., Serafimovich, S., Kalish, R.S., 2001. Mediation of alopecia areata by cooperation between CD4+ and CD8+ T lymphocytes: transfer to human scalp explants on Prkdc (scid) mice. J. Invest. Dermatol. 117, 1357–1362.

Gilhar, A., Ullmann, Y., Berkutzki, T., Assy, B., Kalish, R.S., 1998. Autoimmune hair loss alopecia areata transferred by T lymphocytes to human scalp explants on SCID mice. J. Clin. Invest. 101, 62–67.

Gilhar, A., Zelickson, B., Ulman, Y., Etzioni, A., 1995. In vivo destruction of melanocytes by the IgG fraction of serum from patients with vitiligo. J. Invest. Dermatol. 105, 683–686.

Goh, C., Finkel, M., Christos, P.J., Sinha, A.A., 2006. Profile of 513 patients with alopecia areata: associations of disease subtypes with atopy, autoimmune disease and positive family history. J. Eur. Acad. Dermatol. Venereol. 20, 1055–1060.

Gottumukkala, R.V.S.R.K., Gavalas, N.G., Akhtar, S., Metcalfe, R.A., Gawkrodger, D.J., Haycock, J.W., et al., 2006. Function blocking autoantibodies to the melanin-concentrating hormone receptor in Vitiligo patients. Lab. Invest. 86, 781–789.

Grattan, C.E., Boon, A.P., Eady, R.A., Winkelmann, R.K., 1990. The pathology of the autologous serum skin test response in chronic urticaria resembles IgE-mediated late-phase reactions. Int. Arch. Allergy Appl. Immunol. 93, 198–204.

Grattan, C.E., Wallington, T.B., Warin, R.P., Kennedy, C.T., Bradfield, J.W., 1986. A serological mediator in chronic idiopathic urticaria—a clinical, immunological and histological evaluation. Br. J. Dermatol. 114, 583–590.

Greaves, M.W., Tan, K.T., 2007. Chronic urticaria: recent advances. Clin. Rev. Allergy Immunol. 33, 134–143.

Gross, A., Tapia, F.J., Mosca, W., Perez, R.M., Briceño, L., Henriquez, J.J., et al., 1987. Mononuclear cell subpopulations and infiltrating lymphocytes in erythema dyschromicum perstans and vitiligo. Histol. Histopathol. 2, 277–283.

Gudjonsson, J.E., Elder, J.T., 2008. Psoriasis. In: Wolff, K., et al., (Eds.), Fitzpatrick's Dermatology in General Medicine, seventh ed. McGraw-Hill, New York, pp. 169–193.

Gudjonsson, J.E., Johnston, A., 2009. Current understanding of the genetic basis of psoriasis. Expert Rev. Clin. Immunol. 5, 433–443.

Gudjonsson, J.E., Johnston, A., Dyson, M., Valdimarsson, H., Elder, J.T., 2007. Mouse models of psoriasis. J. Invest. Dermatol. 127, 1292–1308.

Hann, S.K., Kim, H.I., Im, S., Park, Y.K., Cui, J., Bystryn, J.C., 1993. The change of melanocyte cytotoxicity after systemic steroid treatment in vitiligo patients. J. Dermatol. Sci. 6, 201–205.

Hann, S.K., Koo, S.W., Kim, J.B., Park, Y.K., 1996a. Detection of antibodies to human melanoma cells in vitiligo and alopecia areata by Western blot analysis. J. Dermatol. 23, 100–103.

Hann, S.K., Shin, H.K., Park, S.H., Reynolds, S.R., Bystryn, J.C., 1996b. Detection of antibodies to melanocytes in vitiligo by western immunoblotting. Yonsei Med. J. 37, 365–370.

Hariharan, V., Klarquist, J., Reust, M.J., Koshoffer, A., McKee, M.D., Boissy, R.E., et al., 2010. Monobenzyl ether of hydroquinone and 4-tertiary butyl phenol activate markedly different physiological responses in melanocytes: relevance to skin depigmentation. J. Invest. Dermatol. 130, 211–220.

Harning, R., Cui, J., Bystryn, J.C., 1991. Relation between the incidence and level of pigment cell antibodies and disease activity in vitiligo. J. Invest. Dermatol. 97, 1078–1080.

Hartmann, A., Brocker, E.B., Hamm, H., 2008. Occlusive treatment enhances efficacy of tacrolimus 0.1% ointment in adult patients with vitiligo: results of a placebo controlled 12-month prospective study. Acta Derm. Venereol. 88, 474–479.

Hedley, S.J., Metcalfe, R., Gawkrodger, D.J., Weetman, A.P., MacNeil, S., 1998. Vitiligo melanocytes in long-term culture show normal constitutive and cytokine-induced expression of intercellular adhesion molecule-1 and major histocompatibility complex class I and class II molecules. Br. J. Dermatol. 139, 965–973.

Hide, M., Francis, D.M., Grattan, C.E., Hakimi, J., Kochan, J.P., Greaves, M.W., 1993. Autoantibodies against the high-affinity IgE receptor as a cause of histamine release in chronic urticaria. N. Engl. J. Med. 328, 1599–1604.

Homey, B., Assmann, T., Vohr, H.W., Ulrich, P., Lauerma, A.I., Ruzicka, T., et al., 1998. Topical FK506 suppresses cytokine and costimulatory molecule expression in epidermal and local draining lymph node cells during primary skin immune responses. J. Immunol. 160, 5331–5340.

Ito, T., Ito, N., Saatoff, M., Hashizume, H., Fukamizu, H., Nickoloff, B.J., et al., 2008. Maintenance of hair follicle immune privilege is linked to prevention of NK cell attack. J. Invest. Dermatol. 128, 1196–1206.

Jagielska, D., Redler, S., Brockschmidt, F.F., Herold, C., Pasternack, S.M., Garcia Bartels, N., 2012. Follow-up study of the first genome-wide association scan in alopecia areata: IL13 and KIAA0350 as susceptibility loci supported with genome-wide significance. J. Invest. Dermatol. 132, 2192–2197.

Jin, Y., Birlea, S.A., Fain, P.R., Ferrara, T.M., Ben, S., Riccardi, S.L., et al., 2012a. Genome-wide association analyses identify 13 new susceptibility loci for generalized vitiligo. Nat. Genet. 44, 676–680.

Jin, Y., Birlea, S.A., Fain, P.R., Gowan, K., Riccardi, S.L., Holland, P.J., et al., 2010a. Variant of TYR and autoimmunity susceptibility loci in generalized vitiligo. N. Engl. J. Med. 362, 1686–1697.

Jin, Y., Birlea, S.A., Fain, P.R., Mailloux, C.M., Riccardi, S.L., Gowan, K., et al., 2010b. Common variants in FOXP1 are associated with generalized vitiligo. Nat. Genet. 42, 576–578.

Jin, Y., Ferrara, T., Gowan, K., Holcomb, C., Rastrou, M., Erlich, H.A., et al., 2012b. Next-generation DNA re-sequencing identifies common variants of TYR and HLA-A that modulate the risk of generalized vitiligo via antigen presentation. J. Invest. Dermatol. 132, 1730–1733.

Joint Task Force on Practice Parameters, 2000. The diagnosis and management of urticaria: a practice parameter part I: acute urticaria/angioedema part II: chronic urticaria/angioedema. Ann. Allergy Asthma Immunol. 85, 521–544.

Kang, H., Wu, W.Y., Lo, B.K.K., Yu, M., Leung, G., Shapiro, J. and et al. 2010. Hair follicles from alopecia areata patients exhibit alterations in immune privilege-associated gene expression in advance of hair loss. 130, 2677–2680.

Kaplan, A.P., 2004. Chronic urticaria: pathogenesis and treatment. J. Allergy. Clin. Immunol. 114, 465–474.

Kao, C.H., Yu, H.S., 1992. Comparison of the effect of 8-methoxypsoralen (8-MOP) plus UVA (PUVA) on human melanocytes in vitiligo vulgaris and in vitro. J. Invest. Dermatol. 98, 734–740.

Kemp E.H., Gavalsa N.G., Gawkrodger D.J., Weetman A.P., 2007. Autoantibody responses to melanocytes in the depigmented skin disease vitiligo. Autoimmun Rev. 6, 138–142.

Kim, Y.C., Kim, Y.J., Kang, H.Y., Sohn, S., Lee, E.S., 2008. Histopathologic features in vitiligo. Am. J. Dermatopathol. 30, 112–116.

Klarquist, J., Denman, C.J., Hernandez, C., Wainwright, D.A., Strickland, F.M., Overbeck, A., et al., 2010. Reduced skin homing by functional Treg in vitiligo. Pigment Cell Melanoma Res. 23, 276–286.

Koga, M., Tango, T., 1988. Clinical features and course of type A and type B vitiligo. Br. J. Dermatol. 118, 223–228.

Kroll, T.M., Bommiasamy, H., Boissy, R.E., Hernandez, C., Nickoloff, B.J., Mestril, R., et al., 2005. 4-tertiary butyl phenol exposure sensitizes human melanocytes to dendritic cell-mediated killing: relevance to vitiligo. J. Invest. Dermatol. 124, 798–806.

Kroon, M.W., Kemp, E.H., Wind, B.S., Krebbers, G., Bos, J.D., Gawkrodger, D.J., et al., 2012. Melanocyte antigen-specific antibodies cannot be used as markers for recent disease activity in patients with vitiligo. J. Eur. Acad. Dermatol. Venereol. 27, 1172–1175.

Kurd, S.K., Gelfand, J.M., 2009. The prevalence of previously diagnosed and undiagnosed psoriasis in US adults: results from NHANES 2003–2004. J. Am. Acad. Dermatol. 60, 218–224.

Lang, K.S., Caroli, C.C., Muhm, D., Wernet, D., Moris, A., Schittek, B., et al., 2001. HLA-A2 restricted, melanocyte-specific CD8 + T lymphocytes detected in vitiligo patients are related to disease activity and are predominantly directed against MelanA/MART1. J. Invest. Dermatol. 116, 891–897.

Langley, R.G., Krueger, G.G., Griffiths, C.E., 2005. Psoriasis: epidemiology, clinical features, and quality of life. Ann. Rheum. Dis. 64, 18–23.

Lee, K.H., Kim, J.Y., Kang, D.S., Choi, Y.J., Lee, W.J., Ro, J.Y., 2002. Increased expression of endothelial cell adhesion molecules due to mediator release from human foreskin mast cells stimulated by autoantibodies in chronic urticaria sera. J. Invest. Dermatol. 118, 658–663.

Le Poole, I.C., Luiten, R.M., 2008. Autoimmune etiology of generalized vitiligo. Curr. Dir. Autoimmun. 10, 227–243.

Le Poole, I.C., van den Wijngaard, R.M., Westerhof, W., Dutrieux, R.P., Das, P.K., 1993a. Presence or absence of melanocytes in vitiligo lesions: an immunohistochemical investigation. J. Invest. Dermatol. 100, 816–822.

Le Poole, I.C., Das, P.K., van den Wijngaard, R.M., Bos, J.D., Westerhof, W., 1993b. Review of the etiopathomechanism of vitiligo: a convergence theory. Exp. Dermatol. 2, 145–153.

Le Poole, I.C., van den Wijngaard, R.M., Westerhof, W., Das, P.K., 1996. Presence of T cells and macrophages in inflammatory vitiligo skin parallels melanocyte disappearance. Am. J. Pathol. 148, 1219–1228.

Leung, D.Y., Hauk, P., Strickland, I., Travers, J.B., Norris, D.A., 1998. The role of superantigens in human diseases: therapeutic implications for the treatment of skin diseases. Br. J. Dermatol. 139 (53), 17–29.

Leung, D.Y.M., Travers, J.B., Giorno, R., Norris, D.A., Skinner, R., Aelion, J., et al., 1995. Evidence for a streptococcal superantigen-driven process in acute guttate psoriasis. J. Clin. Invest. 96, 2106–2112.

Leung, M.C., Sutton, C.W., Fenton, D.A., Tobin, D.J., 2010. Trichohyalin is a potential major autoantigen in human alopecia areata. J. Proteome Res. 9, 5153–5163.

Leznoff, A., Josse, R.G., Denburg, J., Dolovich, J., 1983. Association of chronic urticaria and angioedema with thyroid autoimmunity. Arch. Dermatol. 119, 636–640.

Lin, W.J., Norris, D.A., Achziger, M., Kotzin, B.L., Tomkinson, B., 2001. Oligoclonal expansion of intraepidermal T cells in psoriasis lesions. J. Invest. Dermatol. 117, 1546–1553.

Lowes, M.A., Bowcock, A.M., Krueger, J.G., 2007. Pathogenesis and therapy of psoriasis. Nature. 445, 866–873.

Lowes, M.A., Chamian, F., Abello, M.V., Fuentes-Duculan, J., Lin, S.L., Nussbaum, R., et al., 2005. Increase in TNF-alpha and inducible nitric oxide synthase-expressing dendritic cells in psoriasis and reduction with efalizumab (anti-CD11a). Proc. Natl. Acad. Sci. USA. 102, 19057–19062.

Manga, P., Sheyn, D., Yang, F., Sarangarajan, R., Boissy, R.E., 2006. A role for tyrosinase-related protein 1 in 4-tert-butylphenol-induced toxicity in melanocytes: Implications for vitiligo. Am. J. Pathol. 169, 1652–1662.

Martinez-Mir, A., Zlotogorski, A., Gordon, D., et al., 2007. Genomewide scan for linkage reveals evidence of several susceptibility loci for alopecia areata. Am. J. Hum. Genet. 80, 316–328.

Matsushita, Y., Shimada, Y., Kawara, S., Takehara, K., Sato, S., 2005. Autoantibodies directed against the protease inhibitor calpastatin in psoriasis. Clin. Exp. Immunol. 139, 355–362.

Maurer, M., Rosen, K., Hsieh, H.J., Saini, S., Grattan, C., Gimenez-Arnau, A., et al., 2013. Omalizumab for the treatment of chronic idiopathic or spontaneous urticaria. N. Engl. J. Med. 368, 924–935.

McElwee, K.J., Freyschmidt-Paul, P., Hoffmann, R., Kissling, S., Hummel, S., Vitacolonna, M., et al., 2005. Transfer of CD8(+) cells induces localized hair loss whereas CD4(+)/CD25(−) cells promote systemic alopecia areata and CD4(+)/CD25(+) cells blockade disease onset in the C3H/HeJ mouse model. J. Invest. Dermatol. 124, 947–957.

Mehrotra, S., Al-Khami, A.A., Klarquist, J., Husain, S., Naga, O., Eby, J.M., et al., 2012. A coreceptor-independent transgenic human TCR mediates anti-tumor and anti-self immunity in mice. J. Immunol. 189, 1627–1638.

Mekori, Y.A., Giorno, R.C., Anderson, P., Kohler, P.F., 1983. Lymphocyte subpopulations in the skin of patients with chronic urticaria. J. Allergy Clin. Immunol. 72, 681–684.

Mlynek, A., Maurer, M., Zalewska, A., 2008. Update on chronic urticaria: focusing on mechanisms. Curr. Opin. Allergy Clin. Immunol. 8, 433–437.

Morris, A., Rogers, M., Fischer, G., Williams, K., 2001. Childhood psoriasis: a clinical review of 1262 cases. Pediatr. Dermatol. 18, 188–198.

Mosenson, J.A., Zloza, A., Nieland, J.D., Garrett-Mayer, E., Eby, J.M., Huelsmann, E.J., et al., 2013. Mutant HSP70 reverses autoimmune depigmentation in vitiligo. Sci. Transl. Med. 5, 174.

Namazi, M.R., 2007. Neurogenic dysregulation, oxidative stress, and melanocytorrhagy in vitiligo: can they be interconnected? Pigment Cell Res. 20, 360–363.

Naughton, G.K., Reggiardo, M.D., Bystryn, J.C., 1986. Correlation between vitiligo antibodies and extent of depigmentation in vitiligo. J. Am. Acad. Dermatol. 15, 978–981.

Nestle, F.O., Kaplan, D.H., Barker, J., 2009. Psoriasis. N. Engl. J. Med. 361, 496–509.

Nestle, F.O., Turka, L.A., Nickoloff, B.J., 1994. Characterization of dermal dendritic cells in psoriasis: autostimulation of T lymphocytes and induction of Th1 type cytokines. J. Clin. Invest. 94, 202–209.

Niimi, N., Francis, D.M., Kermani, F., O'Donnell, B.F., Hide, M., Kobza-Black, A., et al., 1996. Dermal mast cell activation by autoantibodies against the high affinity IgE receptor in chronic urticaria. J. Invest. Dermatol. 106, 1001–1006.

Norris, D.A., Capin, L., Muglia, J.J., Osborn, R.L., Zerbe, G.O., Bystryn, J.C., et al., 1988b. Enhanced susceptibility of melanocytes to different immunologic effector mechanisms in vitro: potential mechanisms for post-inflammatory hypopigmentation and vitiligo. Pigment Cell Res. 1, 113–123.

Norris, D.A., Horikawa, T., Morelli, J.G., 1994. Melanocyte destruction and repopulation in vitiligo. Pigment Cell Res. 7, 193–203.

Norris, D.A., Kissinger, R.M., Naughton, G.M., Bystryn, J.C., 1988a. Evidence for immunologic mechanisms in human vitiligo: patients' sera induce damage to human melanocytes in vitro by complement-mediated damage and antibodydependent cellular cytotoxicity. J. Invest. Dermatol. 90, 783–789.

Ogg, G.S., Dunbar, P.R., Romero, P., Chen, J.L., Cerundolo, V., 1998. High frequency of skin-homing melanocyte-specific cytotoxic T lymphocytes in autoimmune vitiligo. J. Exp. Med. 188, 1203–1208.

Palermo, B., Campanelli, R., Garbelli, S., Mantovani, S., Lantelme, E., Brazzelli, V., et al., 2001. Specific cytotoxic T lymphocyte responses against Melan-A/MART1, tyrosinase and gp100 in vitiligo by the use of major histocompatibility complex/peptide tetramers: the role of cellular immunity in the etiopathogenesis of vitiligo. J. Invest. Dermatol. 117, 326–332.

Parisi, R., Symmons, D.P., Griffiths, C.E., Ashcroft, D.M., 2013. Identification and Management of Psoriasis and Associated Comorbidity (IMPACT) project team, Global epidemiology of psoriasis: a systematic review of incidence and prevalence. J. Invest. Dermatol. 133, 377–385.

Park, K.C., Youn, J.I., Lee, Y.S., 1988. Clinical study of 326 cases of vitiligo. Korean J. Dermatol. 26, 200–205.

Park, Y.K., Kim, N.S., Hann, S.K., Im, S.J., 1996. Identification of auto-antibody to melanocytes and characterization of vitiligo antigen in vitiligo patients. Dermatol. Sci. 11, 111–120.

Paus, R., Ito, N., Takigawa, M., Ito, T., 2003. The hair follicle and immune privilege. J. Investig. Dermatol. Symp. Proc. 8, 188–194.

Perez, A., Woods, A., Grattan, C.E., 2010. Methotrexate: a useful steroid-sparing agent in recalcitrant chronic urticaria. Br. J. Dermatol. 162, 191–194.

Petukhova, L., Cabral, R.M., Mackay-Wiggan, J., Clynes, R., Christiano, A.M., 2011. The genetics of alopecia areata: what's new and how will it help our patients? Dermatol. Ther. 24, 326–336.

Petukhova, L., Duvic, M., Hordinsky, M., Norris, D., Price, V., Shimomura, Y., et al., 2010. Genome-wide association study in alopecia areata implicates both innate and adaptive immunity. Nature. 466, 113–117.

Phan, G.Q., Attia, P., Steinberg, S.M., White, D.E., Rosenberg, S.A., 2001. Factors associated with response to high-dose interleukin-2 in patients with metastatic melanoma. J. Clin. Oncol. 19, 3477–3482.

Pho, L.N., Eliason, M.J., Regruto, M., Hull, C.M., Powell, D.L., 2011. Treatment of chronic urticaria with colchicine. J. Drugs Dermatol. 10, 1423–1428.

Posthumus, J., Tinana, A., Mozena, J.D., Steinke, J.W., Borish, L., 2012. Autoimmune mechanisms in chronic idiopathic urticaria. J. Allergy Clin. Immunol. 130, 814–816.

Quan, C., Ren, Y.Q., Xiang, L.H., Sun, L.D., Xu, A.E., Gao, X.H., et al., 2010. Genome-wide association study for vitiligo identifies susceptibility loci at 6q27 and the MHC. Nat. Genet. 42, 614–618.

Raychaudhuri, S.P., Dutt, S., Raychaudhuri, S.K., Sanyal, M., Farber, E.M., 2001. Severe combined immunodeficiency mouse-human skin chimeras: a unique animal model for the study of psoriasis and cutaneous inflammation. Br. J. Dermatol. 144, 931–939.

Reeves G.E., Boyle M.J., Bonfield J., Dobson P., Loewenthal M., 2004. Impact of hydroxychloroquine therapy on chronic urticaria: chronic autoimmune urticaria study and evaluation. Intern Med J. 34:182–186.

Reeves, W.H., Fisher, D., Wisniewolski, R., Gottlieb, A.B., Chiorazzi, N., 1986. Psoriasis Raynaud's phenomenon associated with

autoantibodies to U1 and U2 small nuclear ribonucleoproteins. N. Engl. J. Med. 315, 105–111.

Robinson Jr., D., Hackett, M., Wong, J., Kimball, A.B., Cohen, R., Bala, M., et al., 2006. Co-occurrence and comorbidities in patients with immune-mediated inflammatory disorders: an exploration using US healthcare claims data, 2001–2002. Curr. Med. Res. Opin. 22, 989–1000.

Rocha, I.M., Oliveira, L.J., De Castro, L.C., De Araujo Pereira, L.I., Chaul, A., Guerra, J.G., et al., 2002. Recognition of melanoma cell antigens with antibodies present from patients with vitiligo. Int. J. Dermatol. 39, 840–843.

Sabroe, R.A., Grattan, C.E., Francis, D.M., Barr, R.M., Kobza Black, A., Greaves, M.W., 1999. The autologous serum skin test: a screening test for autoantibodies in chronic idiopathic urticaria. Br. J. Dermatol. 140, 446–452.

Sabroe, R.A., Greaves, M.W., 2006. Chronic idiopathic urticaria with functional autoantibodies: 12 years on. Br. J. Dermatol. 154, 813–819.

Safavi, K.H., Muller, S.A., Suman, V.J., Moshell, A.N., Melton III, L.J., 1995. Incidence of alopecia areata in Olmsted County, Minnesota, 1975 through 1989. Mayo Clin. Proc. 70, 628–633.

Sagi, L., Solomon, M., Baum, S., Lyakhovitsky, A., Trau, H., Barzilai, A., 2011. Evidence for methotrexate as a useful treatment for steroid-dependent chronic urticaria. Acta Derm. Venereol. 91, 303–306.

Schallreuter, K.U., Chavan, B., Rokos, H., Hibberts, N., Panske, A., Wood, J.M., 2005. Decreased phenylalanine uptake and turnover in patients with vitiligo. Mol. Genet. Metabol. 86, S27–S33.

Schallreuter, K.U., Moore, J., Wood, J.M., Beazley, W.D., Peters, E.M. J., Marles, L.K., et al., 2001. Epidermal H$_2$O$_2$ accumulation alters tetrahydrobiopterin (6BH4) recycling in vitiligo: identification of a general mechanism in regulation of all 6BH4-dependent processes? J. Invest. Dermatol. 116, 167–174.

Schallreuter, K.U., Wood, J.M., Berger, J., 1991. Low catalase levels in the epidermis of patients with vitiligo. J. Invest. Dermatol. 97, 1081–1085.

Schocket, A.L., 2006. Chronic urticaria: pathophysiology and etiology, or the what and why. Allergy Asthma Proc. 27, 90–95.

Schön, M.P., Detmar, M., Parker, C.M., 1997. Murine psoriasis-like disorder induced by naive CD4+ T cells. Nat. Med. 3, 183–188.

Schwarz, T., 2008. 25 years of UV-induced immunosuppression mediated by T cells—from disregarded T suppressor cells to highly respected regulatory T cells. Photochem. Photobiol. 84, 10–18.

Shigenobu, A., Yaoita, H., Kitajima, Y., 1989. An elevated level of auto-antibodies against 48- to 50-kd keratins in the serum of patients with psoriasis. J. Invest. Dermatol. 92, 179–183.

Spritz, R.A., 2010. The genetics of generalized vitiligo: autoimmune pathways and an inverse relationship with malignant melanoma. Genome Med. 2, 78.

Spritz, R.A., 2011. Recent progress in the genetics of generalized vitiligo. J. Genet. Genomics. 38, 271–278.

Stern, R.S., Nijsten, T., Feldman, S.R., Margolis, D.J., Rolstad, T., 2004. Psoriasis is common, carries a substantial burden even when not extensive, and is associated with widespread treatment dissatisfaction. J. Investig. Dermatol. Symp. Proc. 9, 136–139.

Sugiyama, H., Gyulai, R., Toichi, E., Garaczi, E., Shimada, S., Stevens, S.R., et al., 2005. Dysfunctional blood and target tissue CD4+CD25 high regulatory T cells in psoriasis: mechanism underlying unrestrained pathogenic effector T cell proliferation. J. Immunol. 174, 164–173.

Sun, J., Silva, K.A., McElwee, K.J., King Jr., L.E., Sundberg, J.P., 2008. The C3H/HeJ mouse and DEBR rat models for alopecia areata: review of preclinical drug screening approaches and results. Exp. Dermatol. 17, 793–805.

Sundberg, J.P., King Jr., L.E., 1996. Mouse mutations as animal models and biomedical tools for dermatological research. J. Invest. Dermatol. 106, 368–376.

Sundberg, J.P., Silva, K.A., Li, R., Cox, G.A., King, L.E., 2004. Adult-onset alopecia areata is a complex polygenic trait in the C3H/HeJ mouse model. J. Invest. Dermatol. 123, 294–297.

Taieb, A., Alomar, A., Böhm, M., Dell'anna, M.L., De Pase, A., Eleftheriadou, V., et al., 2013. Guidelines for the management of vitiligo: the European Dermatology Forum consensus, in: Vitiligo European Task Force (VETF); European Academy of Dermatology and Venereology (EADV); Union Europenne des Medecins Specialistes (UEMS). Br. J. Dermatol. 168, 5–19.

Takei, M., Mishima, Y., Uda, H., 1984. Immunopathology of vitiligo vulgaris, Sutton's leukoderma and melanoma-associated vitiligo in relation to steroid effects. I. Circulating antibodies for cultured melanoma cells. J. Cutan. Pathol. 11, 107–113.

Taskapan, O., Kutlu, A., Karabudak, O., 2008. Evaluation of autologous serum skin test results in patients with chronic idiopathic urticaria, allergic/non-allergic asthma or rhinitis and healthy people. Clin. Exp. Dermatol. 33, 754–758.

Tilles, S.A., 2005. Approach to therapy in chronic urticaria: when benadryl is not enough. Allergy Asthma Proc. 26, 9–12.

Tobin, D.J., Sundberg, J.P., King Jr., L.E., Boggess, D., Bystryn, J.C., 1997. Autoantibodies to hair follicles in C3H/HeJ mice with alopecia areata-like hair loss. J. Invest. Dermatol. 109, 329–333.

Tobin, D.J., 2003. Characterization of hair follicle antigens targeted by the anti-hair follicle response. J. Investig. Dermatol. Symp. Proc. 8, 176–181.

Trojan, T.D., Khan, D.A., 2012. Calcineurin inhibitors in chronic urticaria. Curr. Opin. Allergy Clin. Immunol. 12, 412–420.

van den Boorn, J.G., Konijnenberg, D., Dellemijn, T.A., van der Veen, J.P., Bos, J.D., Melief, C.J., et al., 2009. Autoimmune destruction of skin melanocytes by perilesional T cells from vitiligo patients. J. Invest. Dermatol. 129, 2220–2232.

van den Boorn, J.G., Picavet, D.I., van Swieten, P.F., van Veen, H.A., Konijnenberg, D., van Veelen, et al., 2011. Skin-depigmenting agent monobenzone induces potent T-cell autoimmunity toward pigmented cells by tyrosinase haptenation and melanosome autophagy. J. Invest. Dermatol. 131, 1240–1251.

van Geel, N., De Lille, S., Vandenhaute, S., Gauthier, Y., Mollet, I., Brochez, L., et al., 2011. Different phenotypes of segmental vitiligo based on a clinical observational study. J. Eur. Acad Dermatol. Venereol. 25, 673–678.

Verheyen, J., Bonig, H., Banning, U., Shin, D.I., Mauz-Körholz, C., Körholz, D., 2001. Co-operation of IL-1 and IL-2 on T-cell activation in mononuclear cell cultures. Immunol. Invest. 30, 289–302.

Viac, J., Groujon, C., Misery, L., Staniek, V., Faure, M., Schmitt, D., et al., 1997. Effect of UVB 311 mm irradiation on normal human skin. Photodermatol. Photoimmunol. Photomed. 13, 103–108.

Wagner, E.F., Schonthaler, H.B., Guinea-Viniegra, J., Tschachler, E., 2010. Psoriasis: what we have learned from mouse models. Nat. Rev. Rheumatol. 6, 704–714.

Wankowicz-Kalinska, A., van den Wijngaard, R.M., Tigges, B.J., Westerhof, W., Ogg, G.S., Cerundolo, V., et al., 2003. Immunopolarization of CD4+ and CD8+ T cell to type-1-like is associated with melanocyte loss in human vitiligo. Lab. Invest. 83, 683–695.

Westerhof, W., d'Ischia, M., 2007. Vitiligo puzzle: the pieces fall in place. Pigment Cell Res. 20, 345–359.

Whiting, D.A., 2003. Histopathologic features of alopecia areata: a new look. Arch Dermatol. 139, 1555–1559.

Winchester, R., 2008. In: Wolff, K., et al., (Eds.), Psoriatic arthritis. Fitzpatrick's Dermatology in General Medicine, seventh ed. McGraw-Hill, New York, pp. 194–207.

Yang, E.M., Kim, S.H., Kim, N.H., Park, H.S., 2010. The genetic association of the FPRL1 promoter polymorphism with chronic urticaria in a Korean population. Ann. Allergy Asthma Immunol. 105, 96–97.

Yu, H.S., Kao, C.H., Yu, C.L., 1993. Coexistence and relationship of antikeratinocyte and antimelanocyte antibodies in patients with nonsegmental-type vitiligo. J. Invest. Dermatol. 100, 823–828.

Zimmerman, A.B., Berger, E.M., Elmariah, S.B., Soter, N.A., 2012. The use of mycophenolate mofetil for the treatment of autoimmune and chronic idiopathic urticaria: experience in 19 patients. J. Am. Acad. Dermatol. 66, 767–770.

Zuberbier, T., 2012. Chronic urticaria. Curr. Allergy. Asthma Rep. 12, 267–272.

Part 13

Nephropathies and Reproductive System

Autoimmune Disease in the Kidney

Gloria A. Preston and Ronald J. Falk

UNC Kidney Center, Division of Nephrology and Hypertension, Department of Medicine, University of North Carolina at Chapel Hill, Chapel Hill, NC, USA

Chapter Outline

Introduction	993	Hyperactivity of Fc–FcR Pathway	997
Are there Hallmarks of Autoimmune Disease?	993	Antigenic Alterations of "Self" Proteins	997
Autoantibodies and Their Antigens	993	Susceptibility to Environmental Impacts	999
Hallmarks of Autoimmune Diseases of the Kidney	994	Microbial Infections	999
Autoreactive T and B Cells Evade Deletion	994	Summary	1001
Pre-existence of Asymptomatic "Normal"		Future Directions	1001
Autoantibodies	996	References	1001

INTRODUCTION

Autoimmune diseases as a whole are a diverse class of over 80 diseases that affect different organs and tissue types. Because of this diversity, we tend to study them as individual diseases rather than as a whole. This is comparable to cancer, which is also a diverse group of diseases that are studied individually such a colon or lung cancer. This view was changed quite radically by Hanahan and Weinberg in their proposed Hallmarks of Cancer (Hanahan and Weinberg, 2000). They proposed that all cancer types (organ, species) could be characterized by a small number of acquired characteristics. This approach might also be applied to autoimmune diseases, leading to a "small number of underlying principles."

ARE THERE HALLMARKS OF AUTOIMMUNE DISEASE?

By definition, a *hallmark* is a distinguishing characteristic, trait, or feature. What are the enabling characteristics or hallmarks that drive the inception of autoimmune disease? In this chapter, we propose a holistic view of common traits among autoimmune diseases of the kidney. Diseases considered in this discussion include anti-glomerular basement membrane (anti-GBM) disease, systemic lupus erythematosus (SLE) nephritis,

and anti-neutrophil-cytoplasmic-autoantibody (ANCA) pauci-immune small vessel vasculitis. IgA nephropathy will not be included, although it is now considered to be immune mediated, as the diseases listed above provide ample support for the point of discussion in this chapter. A brief description of the three diseases discussed is given in the following section.

Autoantibodies and Their Antigens

Anti-GBM disease is the only kidney disease in which it is definitely known that antibodies develop against a native renal antigen, the $\alpha 3$ helix of collagen IV. Rapidly progressive glomerulonephritis in GBM disease is mediated by autoantibodies binding to the non-collagenous NC1 domain of $\alpha 3$(IV) collagen in the glomerular basement membrane (Borza and Hudson, 2003). The epitope is made up of nine discontinuous amino acids in the C-terminal non-collagenous domain of the $\alpha 3$ helix (abbreviated $\alpha 3$(IV)NC1) (Hellmark et al., 1999; Gunnarsson et al., 2000). Anti-GBM antibodies bind to the renal and alveolar basement membranes, inducing complement fixation and leukocyte recruitment and activation. Anti-IgG stains show intense diffuse linear staining of the glomerular basement membrane in all patients.

Numerous human and animal studies support the hypothesis that lupus nephritis is an immune complex

N. Rose & I. Mackay (Eds): The Autoimmune Diseases, Fifth edition. DOI: http://dx.doi.org/10.1016/B978-0-12-384929-8.00067-8

disease. The diversity of the autoantibody repertoire associated with SLE is well recognized. Lupus nephritis can occur in any SLE patient with any autoantibody profile; however, specific antibodies or antibody repertoires are associated with a higher incidence of kidney disease (Lefkowith and Gilkeson, 1996; Lefkowith et al., 1996). The strongest association identified thus far is with circulating antibodies directed against RNA complexes or anti-Sm antibodies with or without concurrent anti-U_1RNP, which predicts development of nephritis in approximately 50% of SLE patients. Other circulating antibodies associated with nephritis include anti-C1q-CLR, anti-heparan sulfate, and anti-endothelial cell antibodies (D'Cruz et al., 1991; Coremans et al., 1995; Ravirajan et al., 2001). Autoantibodies frequently found deposited within kidneys of lupus patients include anti-C1q-CLR, anti-SSA, anti-Sm, anti-SSB, antihistone, and antichromatin antibodies (Mannik et al., 2003). Immunoglobulin deposition can occur in subepithelial or subendothelial spaces and typically contains predominantly IgG and complement with variable levels of IgM and IgA (reviewed in Couser, 1990). For example, anti-dsDNA and anti-histone antibodies in particular are thought to be more nephritogenic than other autoantibodies due to overall charge and due to their potential to cross-react with native GBM antigens (Foster et al., 1993; Xie et al., 2003; Cortes-Hernandez et al., 2004). Although serum autoantibody titers generally correlate with presence and severity of nephritis, some patients with high titers do not develop kidney disease while others with low titers may have severe nephritis (Chien et al., 2001; Horvath et al., 2001; Reveille, 2004; Linnik et al., 2005). This inconsistency is reflected in findings that, in some cases, the antigen specificity of antibodies eluted from a lupus nephritis kidney are different from those detected in the serum (Mannik et al., 2003), alluding to the importance of the properties of the immune complexes, such as antigen specificity and charge, for binding within the kidney (Vogt et al., 1990; Suenaga and Abdou, 1993; Woitas and Morioka, 1996).

ANCAs occur in more than 80% of patients with pauci-immune small vessel vasculitis. These antibodies are specific for neutrophil and monocyte granule proteins, with a given patient typically having antibody reactivity to a single antigen (Charles et al., 1992). The major neutrophil granule protein targets of ANCAs are proteinase-3 (PR3, a serine protease) and myeloperoxidase (MPO, a lysosomal enzyme that produces hypochlorous acid). Indirect immunofluorescence staining of neutrophils using sera from ANCA patients results in cytoplasmic fluorescence. PR3-ANCAs produce a cytoplasmic staining pattern (C-ANCA pattern), whereas MPO-ANCAs produce a perinuclear cytoplasmic staining pattern (P-ANCA) (Jennette and Falk, 1990).

ANCAs are IgG, mostly of the IgG1 subclass, with lesser amounts of IgG3 and IgG4 (Segelmark and Wieslander, 1993). There is no single epitope on either PR3 or MPO that is uniformly recognized by ANCAs from different patients; additionally a single ANCA patient can have antibodies against multiple epitopes of a single protein target (Bini et al., 1992; Russell et al., 2001; Rarok et al., 2003; Pfister et al., 2004; Selga et al., 2004; Farrag et al., 2007). ANCA binding to their specific antigens in combination with Fc region binding to an Fc receptor results in neutrophil and monocyte activation with induction of the respiratory burst, degranulation, and release of cellular inflammatory products into the microenvironment (Falk et al., 1990b; Keogan et al., 1992; Savage et al., 1992; Mulder et al., 1994; Porges et al., 1994; Johnson et al., 1997). Interaction of these leukocytes and their products with the endothelium causes inflammatory injury and vasculitis (Falk and Jennette, 1988; Gross et al., 1993; De'Oliviera et al., 1995). Rapidly progressive glomerulonephritis secondary to vasculitis is one of the most common clinical manifestations (Castillo et al., 1993). Renal involvement is found in approximately 90% of patients with microscopic polyangiitis (MPA), 80% of patients with granulomatous polyangiitis (GPA), 45% of patients with the Churg–Strauss syndrome and, by definition, 100% of patients with renal-limited small vessel ANCA vasculitis (Falk and Jennette, 1988; Jennette and Falk, 1997a,b).

HALLMARKS OF AUTOIMMUNE DISEASES OF THE KIDNEY

Not everyone who develops self-reactive autoantibodies develops autoimmune disease. Autoimmune disease is a multistep process with a succession of genetic and epigenetic changes, culminating in susceptibility to disease. Collectively, these changes dictate physiologic changes whereby novel capabilities are acquired. How many traits must an individual acquire before onset of disease? Moreover, what are these traits or hallmarks leading to disease? The following sections address these questions. After review of existing information, we propose six traits or hallmarks that are highly likely to be common to, and contribute to, disease onset (Figure 67.1).

Autoreactive T and B Cells Evade Deletion

Both basic and translational research efforts are expanding our understanding of how humeral immune cell regulation may be subverted or disrupted to such an extent so as to trigger and perpetuate autoimmune disease. For example, anti-GBM disease is devastating if unrecognized or when treatment is delayed, typically resulting

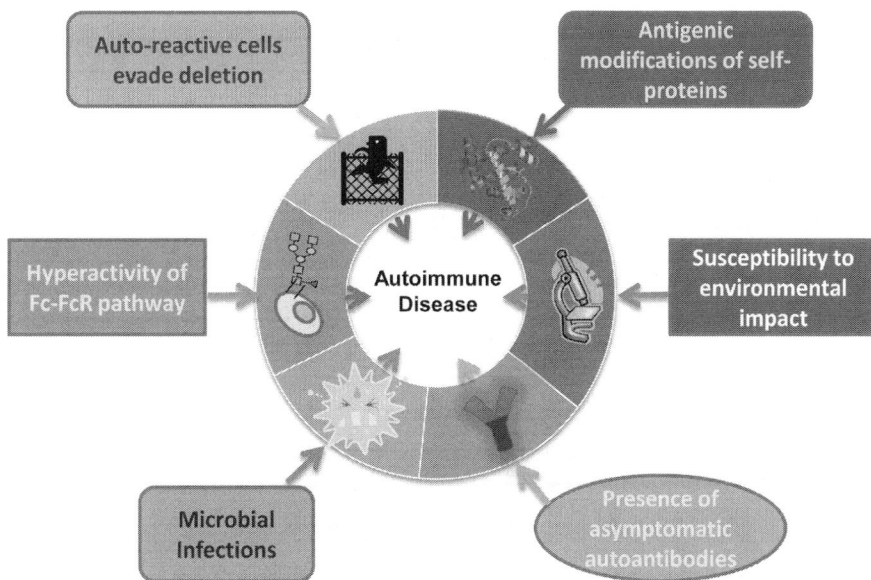

FIGURE 67.1   Hallmarks of autoimmune diseases of the kidney.

in irreversible renal failure and the risk of pulmonary hemorrhage but, unlike ANCA vasculitis and lupus nephritis, the risk of relapse following treatment for anti-GBM disease is generally very low (Savige et al., 1991). Recent evidence indicates that this is attributable to the development of protective regulatory T cell subsets (adaptive Tregs) (Ooi et al., 2011; Peto and Salama, 2011). The opposite appears to occur in relapsing diseases SLE and ANCA vasculitis, where regulatory T cells not only fail to develop but may be dysfunctional at the onset (Marinaki et al., 2005; Yoshimura et al., 2010). Tregs are central to maintaining order in the immune system. Without regulation, "effector T cells are free to cause destruction," leading to injury for the host (Walters et al., 2009). In autoimmune disease, an acquired trait common among diseases is an increased level of effector T cells that are resistant to Treg suppression. The phenomenon of repression-resistant effector T cells has "prompted a shift in focus from how Tregs rule to how their jurisdiction can be overturned" (Walker, 2009). For example, a deficiency in α3(IV) NC1-specific $CD4^+CD25^+$ Tregs in anti-GBM disease is attributed to unrestrained expansion of autoreactive T lymphocytes that cause disease (Salama et al., 2003; Robertson et al., 2005). Similarly, persistent or aberrant T cell activation was identified as an initiating defect in SLE; abnormal CD40L expression on lymphocytes and decreased $CD4^+CD25^+$ Treg activity have both been implicated (Desai-Mehta et al., 1996; Powrie and Maloy, 2003). In ANCA disease effector T cells appeared to be activated above normal levels, with exaggerated skewing of cytokine profiles in response to

antigenic stimulation (Gross et al., 1998). In addition, a newly described $CD4^+CD25^{intermediate}$ effector cell population is linked with ANCA disease and lupus nephritis (Free et al., 2013). This unusual effector T cell subset (1) comprises the majority of the peripheral $CD4^+$ T population, (2) is antigen-experience, (3) produces proinflammatory cytokines, and (4) is resistant to Treg suppression (Figure 67.2) (Free et al., 2013). In these same individuals, Treg frequency was increased not decreased, counterintuitive in light of the expanded effector cell population. Functionality studies showed that the suppressive capability of Tregs was disrupted due to expression of a FoxP3 splice variant in which exon 2, an essential domain for Treg function, was spliced out (Figure 67.3). A hint that this phenotype may be an acquired trait of susceptibility lies in the fact that patients in disease remission continue to express the splice variant, raising the question of its existence before disease onset. Investigations in other autoimmune diseases may prove expression of the FoxP3 splice variant to be a predisposing trait, or hallmark, of autoimmune diseases.

If the amalgamation of experimental data and clinical observations persuades us of the central importance of autoantibodies in the pathogenesis of glomerular injury for anti-GBM, lupus nephritis, and ANCA-vasculitis, then it also signals a fundamental need to unravel the identity of the key autoreactive B cells. Perturbations of B cell populations exist in the peripheral blood of patients with SLE and ANCA vasculitis, in particular a subset of $CD19^{HI}CD27^+$ memory B cells that may be linked to autoantibody production (Culton et al., 2007).

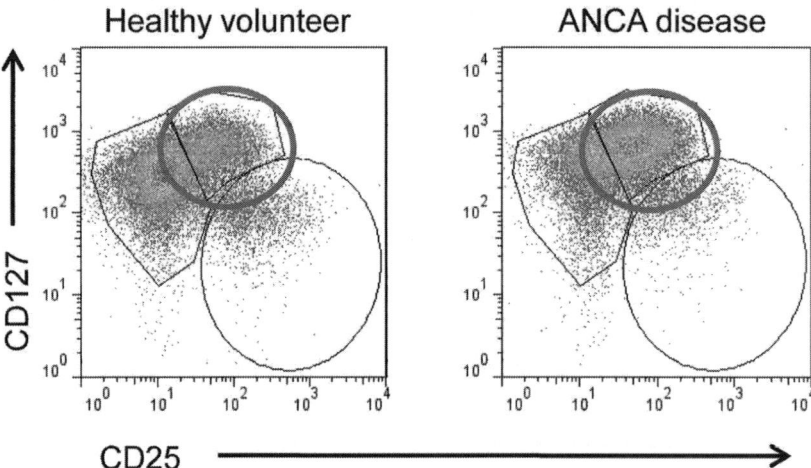

FIGURE 67.2 Altered effector T cell dynamics in disease. Representative flow cytometric analysis of CD3⁺ CD4⁺ lymphocytes, when stratified by CD127 versus CD25 reactivity, identified a CD25int T cell population.

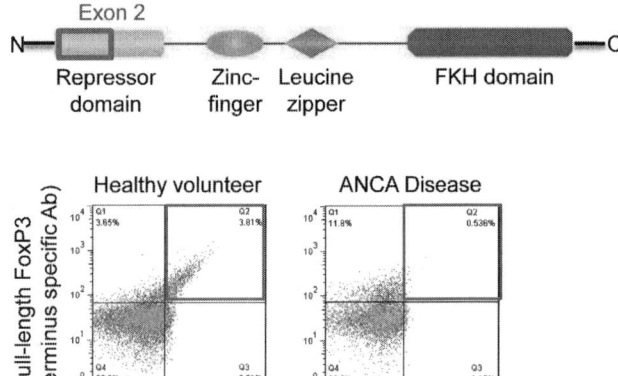

FIGURE 67.3 Regulatory CD4⁺ T cells are dysfunctional due to FoxP3 splice variant. Exon 2-deficient FoxP3 splice variant predominates in AAV. Schematic highlights the repressor domain of FoxP3 protein coded by exon 2. Representative flow cytometric analysis of CD4⁺ T cells plotting reactivity to antibody recognizing exon 2 on the X-axis versus reactivity to an antibody reactivity to the full-length N-terminus of FoxP3. Dual positive cells were detected in healthy individuals but were absent in patients.

CD19 is a B cell receptor (BCR) co-receptor that enhances BCR signal transduction to activate CD21 binding, the receptor for complement component C3d(g) (Walters et al., 2009). Complexes of antigen and C3d(g) are 10,000 times more potent in B cell activation than antigen alone (Lee et al., 2005b). Concomitant with CD19ʰⁱ B cells is a decrease in CD5 expression, which functions as a negative regulator of the B cell receptor (Bunch et al., 2013).

Pre-existence of Asymptomatic "Normal" Autoantibodies

Does pre-existence of self-reactive autoantibodies predispose an individual to autoimmune disease? Are they a hallmark of autoimmune disease? Anti-GBM autoantibodies were detected in sera of ostensibly healthy individuals months to years before onset of anti-GBM disease (Olson et al., 2011). Similarly, circulating autoantibodies were found in healthy individuals who eventually develop SLE (Arbuckle et al., 2003), and natural autoantibodies against MPO and PR3 were detected in healthy individuals (Cui et al., 2010). The presence of serologically-detectable autoantibodies years prior to disease onset compels one to consider whether the presence of these autoantibodies predispose individuals to develop disease. The clinical utility of testing for autoantibodies is apparent but even robust associations between specific immunoglobulins and particular autoimmune diseases or patterns of organ involvement do not guarantee a causal link. An epitope specificity study of "normal" autoantibodies provides a, somewhat incriminating, clue (Roth et al., 2013). The study aims were to (1) determine if differences in ANCA epitope specificity would explain why, in some cases, conventional serologic assays do not correlate well with disease activity, especially in MPO-ANCA, (2) explore why naturally occurring anti-MPO autoantibodies can exist in disease-free individuals, and (3) address the question of why ANCAs are not detected in patients with ANCA-negative disease. Using a highly sensitive excision/mass spectrometry approach, data indicated that autoantibodies from healthy individuals had different epitopes than

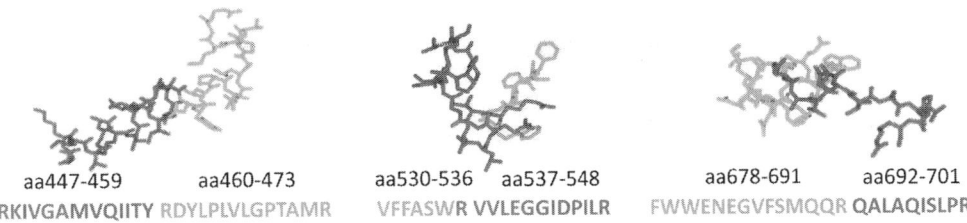

FIGURE 67.4   Visualization of anti-MPO autoantibodies binding sites on the crystal structure of MPO showed epitopes of asymptomatic or "natural" autoantibodies (green) are spatially adjacent to epitopes exclusive to active disease (blue). Amino acids predicted to be required for autoantibody binding are highlighted in red.

autoantibodies from diseased patients. However, visualization of amino acid sequences of epitopes on the three-dimensional crystal structure of MPO (pdb 3f9) revealed an interesting adjacency of "natural" epitopes to epitopes exclusive to active disease (Figure 67.4). This suggests the possibility that an asymptomatic or "natural" autoantibody response to MPO may precede the onset of autoimmune disease, and that epitope spreading to epitopes exclusive to active disease may be one step of a cascade that initiates disease onset. Epitope spreading has been hypothesized to drive the pathogenesis of autoimmune diseases, where autoreactive lymphocytes react with determinants distinct from the initial, disease-inducing epitope as a result of chronic tissue damage (Vanderlugt and Miller, 1996). Lastly, another consideration would be that antigen binding by asymptomatic autoantibodies may structurally distort the conformation of the antigen exposing cryptic epitopes leading to production of pathogenic autoantibodies.

MPO-ANCA, reactive with a sole linear sequence on MPO, are now known to be present in sera from patients with what has been historically labeled, "ANCA-negative disease" (Figure 67.5) (Roth et al., 2013). Why had these autoantibodies gone undetected by routine clinical tests? Detection required prior purification of IgG from sera (Roth et al., 2013). When screening for autoantibodies specific for this epitope, it was found that assays using sera were negative due to the presence of a proteolytic fragment of an abundant protein in sera, a fragment of ceruloplasmin, which obscured antibody binding. The broader issue raised by these data is that management of many autoantibody-mediated diseases relies on tests that explore antibody reactivity to the whole molecule rather than target epitopes, and utilize sera where critical epitope recognition is marked and correlates well with disease activity.

Hyperactivity of Fc–FcR Pathway

All antibodies are glycosylated at conserved positions in their constant regions. At least 36 structurally unique oligosaccharide chains may be attached at each Asn-297

residue in both of the C_H2 domains of the Fc region. More than 50% of Fc oligosaccharides are accounted for by three main glycans: G0, G1, and G2 (designated according to the numbers of terminal Gal) (Figure 67.6). Reduction in galactosylation is routinely measured by comparing the relative abundances of glycoforms G0, G1, and G2 using mass spectrometry. The structure of the attached carbohydrates can affect antibody activity. Hyposialylation and hypoglycosylation of total IgG-Fc from serum was reported for PR3-ANCA disease, as indicated by elevated levels of G0 truncated N-glycans lacking the terminal galactose (Holland et al., 2002, 2006). This deficit results in a positive amplification of the Fc/cReceptor signaling and has been linked with active PR3-ANCA disease (Espy et al., 2011). Further, IgG glycan hydrolysis attenuates ANCA-mediated glomerulonephritis (van Timmeren et al., (2010)). Changes in the glycan structures of some glycoproteins have been observed in SLE and rheumatoid arthritis (Tomana et al., 1988). A deficiency of α-mannosidase II, which is associated with branching in N-glycans, has been found to induce SLE-like glomerular nephritis in a mouse model (Hashii et al., 2009).

Effects of altered glycoforms of the Fc are intertwined with Fc receptor polymorphisms, which are also known to contribute to autoimmune disease (reviewed in Bournazos et al., 2009). The genes with the strongest association with development of lupus nephritis are Fc receptor polymorphisms thought to increase susceptibility and affect its rate of progression by altering or inhibiting clearance of immune complexes, or by inappropriately activating leukocytes, which bind deposited complexes (Salmon and Roman, 2001; Yun et al., 2001; Zuniga et al., 2001).

Antigenic Alterations of "Self" Proteins

What causes the autoimmune response to begin and what causes it to worsen into autoimmune disease? In the case of anti-GBM disease, mounting evidence indicates it is initiated by exposure of epitopes normally sequestered or buried, as conceptualized in the Cryptic Epitope Theory

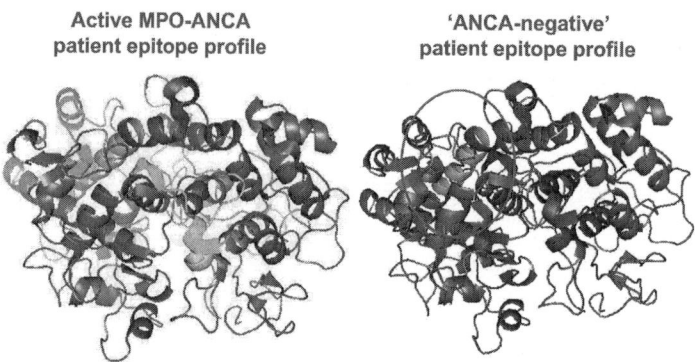

Active MPO-ANCA patient epitope profile

'ANCA-negative' patient epitope profile

FIGURE 67.5   ANCA-negative small vessel vasculitis develops a restricted autoantibody response against a linear epitope on MPO (aa447-459), shown in red.

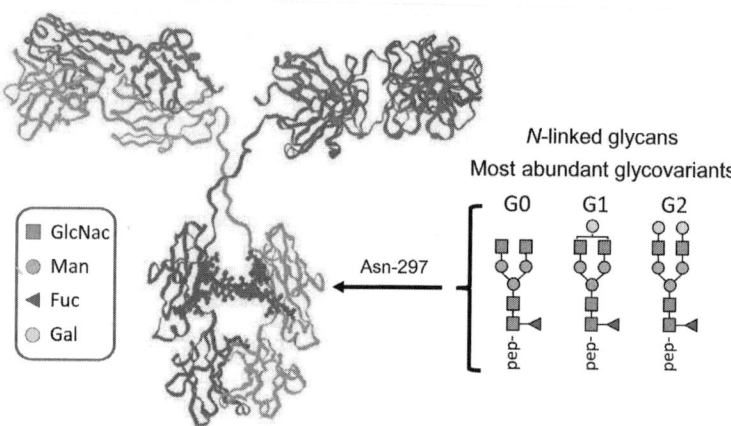

N-linked glycans

Most abundant glycovariants

G0   G1   G2

GlcNac   Man   Fuc   Gal

Asn-297

FIGURE 67.6   Antibody glycosylation deficit autoimmune diseases.   At least 36 structurally unique oligosaccharide chains may be attached at each Asn-297 residue in both of the C_H2 domains of the Fc region. More than 50% of Fc oligosaccharides are accounted for by three main glycans: G0, G1, and G2 (designated according to the numbers of terminal Gal). The sugar moiety functions as a molecular switch to enhance either the proinflammatory or anti-inflammatory activity of IgG.

(Lanzavecchia, 1995). Epitopes reactive with anti-GBM autoantibodies are cryptic (sequestered) within the NC1 hexamers of the alpha3alpha4alpha5(IV) collagen network. Disruption in the hexamer structure, through some unknown mechanism, causes disassociation of the endogenous hexamer structure of the α-3 chain of type IV collagen and exposure of a pathogenic epitope (Borza et al., 2005). A pathogenic autoantibody may be available for months to years prior to disease but the target epitope had been concealed. Do naturally occurring autoantibodies contribute to disruption, or is it due to post-translational changes, proteolytic cleavage by exogenous environmental factors, or is it a combination of events? As discussed above, it is conceivable that asymptomatic autoantibodies reactive to one part of a target antigen could pry open or disrupt autoantigen conformation.

Apoptosis has been implicated in the onset of autoimmune disease whereby an accumulation of autoantigens on the surface of apoptotic cells coupled with a defect in clearance of apoptotic material helps to drive systemic autoimmune diseases (Rosen and Casciola-Rosen, 1999). Proximal defects in the classical complement pathway, leading to aberrant clearance of apoptotic cells, are well understood as potential initiators of autoimmune disease, in particular SLE (Prokunina et al., 2002). The autoantigens of SLE are exposed on dead and dying cells and released from injured tissues. Large quantities of antigen become available, so large numbers of small immune complexes are produced continuously and are deposited in the walls of small blood vessels in the renal glomerulus, in glomerular basement membrane in joints, and in other organs. Inefficient clearance of apoptotic cells may also have a role in ANCA vasculitis; macrophages that have engulfed apoptotic neutrophils appear to be diverted away from a non-phlogistic phenotype and this may contribute to the failure of effective healing (Ohlsson et al., 2012).

Additionally, the presence of ANCA accelerates neutrophil apoptosis without promoting concomitant externalization of phosphatidylserine which likely impairs neutrophil clearance and promotes secondary necrosis, amplifying tissue damage.

Proteins processed with modifications in glycosylation, phosphorylation, or proteolysis, etc., have differences in structure resulting in new epitopes or "neoantigenic determinants." New antigenic determinants may give rise to specific autoantibodies and/or autoreactive T cells that now attack cells/tissues that bear the self-antigen. ANCA disease research suggests that the molecular architecture of PR3 and MPO, which are aberrantly transcribed in mature neutrophils, may be compromised producing neoantigenic determinants (Yang et al., 2004). How do cells transport these proteins? Are they secreted, or does the cell see them as misfolded proteins and shuttle them to lysosomes? Neutrophils have the ability to function as antigen-presenting cells (Cao et al., 2011). Peripheral neutrophils from patients homozygous for *DRB1*1501* expressed surface of DRB1*15 protein, in response to TNF-α exposure, that bound amino acids sequences of sense-PR3, purportedly an antigenic epitope in an experimental setting. Neutrophils expressing modified proteins in the periphery of patients could deliver proteins for MHC class II presentation through the process of autophagy. Autophagy is now emerging as a spotlight in trafficking events that activate adaptive immunity due, in part, to promoting MHC class II presentation of peptides from intracellular source proteins (Dengjel et al., 2005). This may explain why HLA genes are highly linked with susceptible genetic background for autoimmune diseases (Lyons et al., 2012). Analysis of the MHC class II ligandome shows that 20 to 30% of self-class II epitopes are derived from cytosolic and nuclear proteins (Dengjel et al., 2005; Fissolo et al., 2009; Nedjic et al., 2009). The *HLA-DB1*15* alleles were identified as a risk factor for PR3-ANCA disease in African Americans with an odds ratio of 73.3 ($p = 2.3 \times 10^{-9}$) (Cao et al., 2011). Patients with anti-GBM disease carry the HLA-DRB1*1501 or HLA-DRB1*04 alleles in approximately 80% of cases, as compared to only 20% of people in the general population (Phelps and Rees, 1999).

Susceptibility to Environmental Impacts

There are numerous articles implicating aging, chronic stress, hormones, even sunlight as "triggers" for the development of autoimmune disease. Epigenetics is receiving unprecedented attention as evidence mounts that autoimmune diseases arise from a combination of genetic susceptibility and environmental factors. Epigenetic mechanisms link external stimuli and gene expression. Perturbation of epigenetic regulation of gene transcription was discovered as a manifestation of ANCA disease (Ciavatta et al., 2010).

The result was increased expression of the known autoantigens PR3 and MPO, raising questions of increased antigen availability as a pathogenic factor (Yang et al., 2004; Ciavatta et al., 2010). These observations, among others, depict the neutrophil, not as a terminally differentiated, transcriptionally silent cell, but as a cell poised to respond to external stimuli. Probing deeper, it was found that silencing was deficient in patients due, at least in part, to inadequate levels of RUNX3, a transcriptional repressor with binding sites within both the PR3 and MPO genes. An article by Ben Harden in *Science News* reads, "All Roads Lead to RUNX: Several Autoimmune Diseases Share One Bad Actor." A central role for RUNX proteins in the development of autoimmunity was first described in 2003 (Alarcon-Riquelme, 2003). Normally, RUNX3 mediates histone methylation by carrying the H3K27 methyltransferase, EXH2, to the RUNX3-specific DNA binding sites.

Another "sensor" and "transmitter" of environmental signals, protein tyrosine phosphatase-N22 (PTPN22), is linked to increased susceptibility to autoimmune disease (Bottini et al., 2004; Begovich et al., 2004, 2005; Kyogoku et al., 2004; Behrens et al., 2005; Canton et al., 2005; Carlton et al., 2005; Criswell et al., 2005; Jagiello et al., 2005; Ladner et al., 2005; Lee et al., 2005a; Burkhardt et al., 2006; Carr et al., 2009; Fiorillo et al., 2010; Martorana et al., 2012). In this case the genetic polymorphism responsible conferred a gain-of-function phenotype. This gain-of-function allele strongly correlates with numerous autoimmune diseases including SLE and ANCA disease.

Environmental factors known to impact ANCA and SLE diseases, at both disease onset and relapse, include aging (Hogan et al., 2005, 2007), seasonal changes (Falk et al., 1990a), and silica exposure (Hogan et al., 2001). The Mitochondrial−Lysosomal Axis Theory suggests that oxidized proteins, generated by reactive oxygen species (ROS), coupled with their inefficient breakdown by lysosomes, leads to generation of antigenic protein−protein cross-links (Kannan, 2005). Hydrocarbon and cigarette smoke exposures have been associated with anti-GBM disease, particularly in patients with significant pulmonary hemorrhage (Stevenson et al., 1995). Similarly, lithotripsy, MPO-ANCA, and other causes of "renal trauma" have occasionally been reported to be associated with development of anti-GBM disease (Xenocostas et al., 1999).

Microbial Infections

Scientific evidence has linked autoimmune disorders with infection for well over a century. What is the connection? Epidemiologic studies and case reports have suggested an association between anti-GBM disease and microbial infections. The first description of two patients with influenza-like clinical signs, and sporadic reports of an association between these two diseases, can still be found (Salama et al., 2001). One study raised the possibility that a single T cell epitope mimicry by microbial Ag may be sufficient to induce the anti-GBM disease (Arends et al., 2006). The fact that 20 to 60% of patients report a pro-dromal upper respiratory tract infection increases suspicion of involvement of infection or toxin-triggered events (Perez et al., 1974). The most consistent microbial trigger in ANCA disease appears to be *Staphylococcus aureus*, which produces a superantigen response that may play a role in some patients (Stegeman et al., 1994; Mayet et al., 1999; Hellmich et al., 2001; Tadema et al., 2011).

Microbes carry proteins molecularly similar to "host" proteins. The Theory of Molecular Mimicry posits that a bacterial or viral protein is sufficiently similar, in either sequence and/or structure, to a host protein to cause a breakdown of immune tolerance to the host protein (Albert and Inman, 1999). Sequence similarities between foreign and self-peptides are sufficient to result in the cross-activation of autoreactive T or B cells by pathogen-derived proteins (Fujinami et al., 1983; Levin et al., 2002; Kohm et al., 2003). For example, GBM disease was induced in a rat model with microbial peptides that mimicked a previously identified T cell epitope that could induce the disease (Arends et al., 2006). Molecular mimicry has been implicated as a mechanism for initiation of ANCA by a group who found that patients had anti-LAMP-2 autoantibodies that cross-reacted with Fim-H, a bacterial adhesion protein (Kain et al., 2008).

Generally listed alongside molecular mimicry as a possible mechanism of autoimmunity caused by viral infection is the Direct Bystander Effect Theory which posits that an infection leading to inflammatory tissue damage and necrosis of cells uncovers epitopes of autoantigens that reactivate resting autoreactive T cells (Horwitz et al., 1998). This leads to the discussion of the recently discovered neutrophil extracellular traps (NETs), also called TRAPS. NETS are thought to be formed through a novel cell death program. Upon activation, neutrophils release granule proteins and chromatin that together form extracellular fibers that bind Gram-positive and -negative bacteria. Thus, NETs appear to be a form of innate response that binds microorganisms, prevents them from spreading, and ensures a high local concentration of anti-microbial agents to degrade virulence factors and kill bacteria. PR3 was shown to be present in these NETS (Brinkmann et al., 2004; Fuchs et al., 2007; Bosch, 2009).

While these examples of molecular mimicry in auto-immune disease are compelling, they do not satisfy the question of why there aren't more examples given the plethora of microbial and viral sequences similar to human proteins. Alternative ideas for how infectious agents induce autoimmune disease continue to build on the Theory of Autoantigen Complementarity (Pendergraft et al., 2004). This theory is in line with a hypothesis published in 1983 of how a viral infection leads to autoimmune disease (Figure 67.7) (Plotz, 1983). The host-cell receptor is envisioned as an internal image of the virus. The variable region of the primary antibody against the viral protein is similar in shape to the host receptor. The anti-idiotypic antibody against the variable region of the primary antibody consequently has a shape similar to the viral protein thus producing an internal image cascade. The anti-idiotypic antibody which now carries the internal image of the viral protein can bind to the host receptor and act as an autoantibody. The process of internal image binding to a protein opposite in shape is termed "complementarity." Proteins complementary to the auto-antigen PR3 are carried by many different microbes and viruses. Among these microbes are Ross River virus, *Staphylococcus aureus*, and *Entamoeba histolytica*, all of which have been previously linked with ANCA disease (Davies et al., 1982; Pudifin et al., 1994; Stegeman et al., 1994). Pertinent to this finding, the onset of ANCA disease is commonly associated with a flu-like illness (Falk et al., 1990a). Alternatively patients may be producing complementary PR3 protein themselves. Investigations of ANCA patients' leukocytes reveal the presence of PR3 antisense RNA in approximately one-half of the patients tested (Pendergraft et al., 2004). The question remains whether these antisense transcripts are, or can be translated into, a protein product to produce the complementary protein. Translation of an antisense transcript has been reported (Van Den Eynde et al., 1999). It may be that aberrantly expressed antisense transcripts are a component of a range of human diseases (Lavorgna et al., 2004).

In support, it has been suggested that molecular complementarity contributes to the pathogenesis of other, non-renal autoimmune diseases as well. Evidence already exists for molecular complementarity in patients with Sjögren's syndrome and SLE (Papamattheou et al., 2004). Anti-idiotypic antibodies were detected in patients' sera using peptides complementary to the autoantigen B cell epitopes, and mice immunized with either the B cell epitope peptide or its complement developed antibodies against both immunogens (Routsias et al., 2003; Papamattheou et al., 2004).

In conclusion, after producing over 20,000 papers on autoimmune disease of the kidney, we are yet to understand when and how autoimmune disease develops. These hallmarks of the disease provide a comprehensive and cohesive foundation for the field that will influence bio-medical researchers in their quest for new treatments. We suggest that a holistic approach may provide clarity of mechanism and help to understand how and what treatments would be efficacious for treatment of disease.

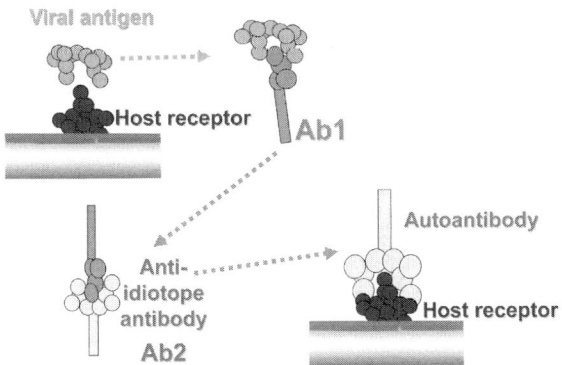

FIGURE 67.7 Hypothesis of how a viral infection leads to autoimmune disease. The host-cell receptor is envisioned as an internal image of the virus. The inciting antigen is not the autoantigen, but a viral protein complementary in shape to the host's cell surface protein. This complementary protein elicits an antibody response, which in turn elicits an anti-antibody, referred to as an anti-idiotypic response. The anti-antibody then reacts with the host's cell surface protein, now becoming an autoantigen. This process relies upon the activation of the immune system's idiotypic network.

SUMMARY

This chapter enumerates six tentative hallmarks that represent common denominators of autoantibody-mediated autoimmune disease of the kidney. These hallmarks are autoreactive cells to achieve the capability to evade deletion, the presence of asymptomatic autoantibodies, hyperactivity of the Fc—FcR pathway, enhanced susceptibility to environmental factors, antigenic modifications of self-proteins, and microbial infections.

FUTURE DIRECTIONS

A major challenge is to dissect the interconnectedness between the candidate hallmarks and their relative contributions to disease with the final goal of identifying pharmaceutical targets to develop new treatment approaches with minimal side effects.

REFERENCES

Alarcon-Riquelme, M., 2003. A RUNX trio with a taste for autoimmunity. Nat. Genet. 35, 299—300.

Albert, L., Inman, R., 1999. Molecular mimicry and autoimmunity. N. Engl. J. Med. 341, 2068—2074.

Arbuckle, M., McClain, M., Rubertone, M., Scofield, R., Dennis, G., James, J., et al., 2003. Development of autoantibodies before the clinical onset of systemic lupus erythematosus. N. Engl. J. Med. 349, 1526—1533.

Arends, J., Wu, J., Borillo, J., Troung, L., Zhou, C., Vigneswaran, N., et al., 2006. T cell epitope mimicry in antiglomerular basement membrane disease. J. Immunol. 176, 1252—1258.

Begovich, A., Carlton, V., Honigberg, L., Schrodi, S., Chokkalingam, A., Alexander, H., et al., 2004. A missense single-nucleotide polymorphism in a gene encoding a protein tyrosine phosphatase (PTPN22) is associated with rheumatoid arthritis. Am. J. Hum. Genet. 75, 330—337.

Begovich, A., Caillier, S., Alexander, H., Penko, J., Hauser, S., Barcellos, L., et al., 2005. The R620W polymorphism of the protein tyrosine phosphatase PTPN22 is not associated with multiple sclerosis. Am. J. Hum. Genet. 76, 184—187.

Behrens, T., Graham, R., Kyogoku, C., Baechler, E., Ramos, P., Gillett, C., et al., 2005. Progress towards understanding the genetic pathogenesis of systemic lupus erythematosus. Novartis Found Symp. 267, 145—160, discussion 160—164.

Bini, P., Gabay, J., Teitel, A., Melchior, M., Zhou, J., Elkon, K., 1992. Antineutrophil cytoplasmic autoantibodies in Wegener's granulomatosis recognize conformational epitope(s) on proteinase 3. J. Immunol. 149, 1409—1415.

Borza, D., Hudson, B., 2003. Molecular characterization of the target antigens of anti-glomerular basement membrane antibody disease. Springer Semin. Immunopathol. 24, 345—361.

Borza, D., Bondar, O., Colon, S., Todd, P., Sado, Y., Neilson, E., et al., 2005. Goodpasture autoantibodies unmask cryptic epitopes by selectively dissociating autoantigen complexes lacking structural reinforcement: novel mechanisms for immune privilege and autoimmune pathogenesis. J. Biol. Chem. 280, 27147—27154.

Bosch, X., 2009. LAMPs and NETs in the pathogenesis of ANCA vasculitis. J. Am. Soc. Nephrol. 20, 1654—1656.

Bottini, N., Musumeci, L., Alonso, A., Rahmouni, S., Nika, K., Rostamkhani, M., et al., 2004. A functional variant of lymphoid tyrosine phosphatase is associated with type I diabetes. Nat. Genet. 36, 337—338.

Bournazos, S., Woof, J., Hart, S., Dransfield, I., 2009. Functional and clinical consequences of Fc receptor polymorphic and copy number variants. Clin. Exp. Immunol. 157, 244—254.

Brinkmann, V., Reichard, U., Goosmann, C., Fauler, B., Uhlemann, Y., Weiss, D., et al., 2004. Neutrophil extracellular traps kill bacteria. Science. 303, 1532—1535

Bunch, D., McGregor, J., Khandoobhai, N., Aybar, L., Burkart, M., Hu, Y., et al., 2013. Decreased CD5 + B cells in active ANCA vasculitis and relapse after rituximab. Clin. J. Am. Soc. Nephrol 8, 382—391.

Burkhardt, H., Huffmeier, U., Spriewald, B., Bohm, B., Rau, R., Kallert, S., et al., 2006. Association between protein tyrosine phosphatase 22 variant R620W in conjunction with the HLA-DRB1 shared epitope and humoral autoimmunity to an immunodominant epitope of cartilage-specific type II collagen in early rheumatoid arthritis. Arthritis Rheum. 54, 82—89.

Canton, I., Akhtar, S., Gavalas, N., Gawkrodger, D., Blomhoff, A., Watson, P., et al., 2005. A single-nucleotide polymorphism in the gene encoding lymphoid protein tyrosine phosphatase (PTPN22) confers susceptibility to generalised vitiligo. Genes. Immun. 6, 584—587.

Cao, Y., Schmitz, J., Yang, J., Hogan, S., Bunch, D., Hu, Y., et al., 2011. DRB1*15 allele is a risk factor for PR3-ANCA disease in African Americans. J. Am. Soc. Nephrol. 22, 1161—1167.

Carlton, V., Hu, X., Chokkalingam, A., Schrodi, S., Brandon, R., Alexander, H., et al., 2005. PTPN22 genetic variation: evidence for multiple variants associated with rheumatoid arthritis. Am. J. Hum. Genet. 77, 567—581.

Carr, E., Niederer, H., Williams, J., Harper, L., Watts, R., Lyons, P., et al., 2009. Confirmation of the genetic association of CTLA4 and PTPN22 with ANCA-associated vasculitis. BMC Med. Genet. 10, 121.

Castillo, A., Valderrama, G., Ardiles, L., Caorsi, I., Mezzano, S., 1993. [Rapidly progressive glomerulonephritis without immune deposits: detection of neutrophil anticytoplasmic antibodies]. Rev. Med. Chil. 121, 260–264.

Charles, L., Falk, R., Jennette, J., 1992. Reactivity of antineutrophil cytoplasmic autoantibodies with mononuclear phagocytes. J. Leukoc. Biol. 51, 65–68.

Chien, J., Lin, C., Yang, L., 2001. Correlation between anti-Ro/La titers and clinical findings of patients with systemic lupus erythematosus. Zhonghua Yi Xue Za Zhi (Taipei). 64, 283–291.

Ciavatta, D., Yang, J., Preston, G., Badhwar, A., Xiao, H., Hewins, P., et al., 2010. Epigenetic basis for aberrant upregulation of autoantigen genes in humans with ANCA vasculitis. J. Clin. Invest. 120, 3209–3219.

Coremans, I., Spronk, P., Bootsma, H., Daha, M., Van Der Voort, E., Kater, L., et al., 1995. Changes in antibodies to C1q predict renal relapses in systemic lupus erythematosus. Am. J. Kidney Dis. 26, 595–601.

Cortes-Hernandez, J., Ordi-Ros, J., Labrador, M., Bujan, S., Balada, E., Segarra, A., et al., 2004. Antihistone and anti-double-stranded deoxyribonucleic acid antibodies are associated with renal disease in systemic lupus erythematosus. Am. J. Med. 116, 165–173.

Couser, W., 1990. Mediation of immune glomerular injury. J. Am. Soc. Nephrol. 1, 13–29.

Criswell, L., Pfeiffer, K., Lum, R., Gonzales, B., Novitzke, J., Kern, M., et al., 2005. Analysis of families in the multiple autoimmune disease genetics consortium (MADGC) collection: the PTPN22 620 W allele associates with multiple autoimmune phenotypes. Am. J. Hum. Genet. 76, 561–571.

Cui, Z., Zhao, M., Segelmark, M., Hellmark, T., 2010. Natural autoantibodies to myeloperoxidase, proteinase 3, and the glomerular basement membrane are present in normal individuals. Kidney Int. 78, 590–597.

Culton, D., Nicholas, M., Bunch, D., Zhen, Q., Kepler, T., Dooley, M., et al., 2007. Similar CD19 dysregulation in two autoantibody-associated autoimmune diseases suggests a shared mechanism of B-cell tolerance loss. J. Clin. Immunol. 27, 53–68.

Davies, D., Moran, J.E., Niall, J.F., Ryan, G.B., 1982. Segmental necrotising glomerulonephritis with antineutrophil antibody: possible arbovirus aetiology? Br. Med. J. (Clin. Res. Ed.). 285, 606–610.

Dengjel, J., Schoor, O., Fischer, R., Reich, M., Kraus, M., Muller, M., et al., 2005. Autophagy promotes MHC class II presentation of peptides from intracellular source proteins. Proc. Natl. Acad. Sci. USA. 102, 7922–7927

Desai-Mehta, A., Lu, L., Ramsey-Goldman, R., Datta, S., 1996. Hyperexpression of CD40 ligand by B and T cells in human lupus and its role in pathogenic autoantibody production. J. Clin. Invest. 97, 2063–2073.

De'Oliviera, J., Gaskin, G., Dash, A., Rees, A., Pusey, C., 1995. Relationship between disease activity and anti-neutrophil cytoplasmic antibody concentration in long-term management of systemic vasculitis. Am. J. Kidney Dis. 25, 380–389.

D'Cruz, D., Houssiau, F., Ramirez, G., Baguley, E., McCutcheon, J., Vianna, J., et al., 1991. Antibodies to endothelial cells in systemic lupus erythematosus: a potential marker for nephritis and vasculitis. Clin. Exp. Immunol. 85, 254–261.

Espy, C., Morelle, W., Kavian, N., Grange, P., Goulvestre, C., Viallon, V., et al., 2011. Sialylation levels of anti-proteinase 3 antibodies are associated with the activity of granulomatosis with polyangiitis (Wegener's). Arthritis Rheum. 63, 2105–2115.

Falk, R., Jennette, J., 1988. Anti-neutrophil cytoplasmic autoantibodies with specificity for myeloperoxidase in patients with systemic vasculitis and idiopathic necrotizing and crescentic glomerulonephritis. N. Engl. J. Med. 318, 1651–1657.

Falk, R., Hogan, S., Carey, T., Jennette, J., 1990a. Clinical course of anti-neutrophil cytoplasmic autoantibody-associated glomerulonephritis and systemic vasculitis. The Glomerular Disease Collaborative Network [see comments]. Ann. Intern. Med. 113, 656–663.

Falk, R., Terrell, R., Charles, L., Jennette, J., 1990b. Anti-neutrophil cytoplasmic autoantibodies induce neutrophils to degranulate and produce oxygen radicals in vitro. Proc. Natl. Acad. Sci. USA. 87, 4115–4119

Farrag, L., Pendergraft III, W., Yang, J., Jennette, J., Falk, R., Preston, G., 2007. A study of conformational restraints on reactivity of human PR3-specific autoantibodies (ANCA) facilitated through protein folding manipulations of a new recombinant proteinase 3 protein. Autoimmunity. 40, 503–511.

Fiorillo, E., Orru, V., Stanford, S., Liu, Y., Salek, M., Rapini, N., et al., 2010. Autoimmune-associated PTPN22 R620 W variation reduces phosphorylation of lymphoid phosphatase on an inhibitory tyrosine residue. J. Biol. Chem. 285, 26506–26518.

Fissolo, N., Haag, S., De Graaf, K., Drews, O., Stevanovic, S., Rammensee, H., et al., 2009. Naturally presented peptides on major histocompatibility complex I and II molecules eluted from central nervous system of multiple sclerosis patients. Mol. Cell Proteomics. 8, 2090–2101

Foster, M., Sabbaga, J., Line, S., Thompson, K., Barrett, K., Madaio, M., 1993. Molecular analysis of spontaneous nephrotropic anti-laminin antibodies in an autoimmune MRL-lpr/lpr mouse. J. Immunol. 151, 814–824.

Free, M., Bunch, D., McGregor, J., Poulton, C.E., Jones, B., Berg, E., et al., 2013. Patients with antineutrophil cytoplasmic antibody-associated vasculitis have defective Treg cell function exacerbated by the presence of a suppression-resistant effector cell population. Arthritis Rheum. 65, 1922–1923.

Fuchs, T., Abed, U., Goosmann, C., Hurwitz, R., Schulze, I., Wahn, V., et al., 2007. Novel cell death program leads to neutrophil extracellular traps. J. Cell Biol. 176, 231–241.

Fujinami, R., Oldstone, M., Wroblewska, Z., Frankel, M., Koprowski, H., 1983. Molecular mimicry in virus infection: crossreaction of measles virus phosphoprotein or of herpes simplex virus protein with human intermediate filaments. Proc. Natl. Acad. Sci. USA. 80, 2346–2350.

Gross, W., Schmitt, W., Csernok, E., 1993. ANCA and associated diseases: immunodiagnostic and pathogenetic aspects. Clin. Exp. Immunol. 91, 1–12.

Gross, W., Trabandt, A., Csernok, E., 1998. Pathogenesis of Wegener's granulomatosis. Ann. Med. Interne. (Paris). 149, 280–286.

Gunnarsson, A., Hellmark, T., Wieslander, J., 2000. Molecular properties of the Goodpasture epitope. J. Biol. Chem. 275, 30844–30848.

Hanahan, D., Weinberg, R., 2000. The hallmarks of cancer. Cell. 100, 57–70.

Hashii, N., Kawasaki, N., Itoh, S., Nakajima, Y., Kawanishi, T., Yamaguchi, T., 2009. Alteration of N-glycosylation in the kidney in a mouse model of systemic lupus erythematosus: relative quantification of N-glycans using an isotope-tagging method. Immunology. 126, 336—345

Hellmark, T., Burkhardt, H., Wieslander, J., 1999. Goodpasture disease. Characterization of a single conformational epitope as the target of pathogenic autoantibodies. J. Biol. Chem. 274, 25862—25868.

Hellmich, B., Ehren, M., Lindstaedt, M., Meyer, M., Pfohl, M., Schatz, H., 2001. Anti-MPO-ANCA-positive microscopic polyangiitis following subacute bacterial endocarditis. Clin. Rheumatol. 20, 441—443.

Hogan, S., Satterly, K., Dooley, M., Nachman, P., Jennette, J., Falk, R., 2001. Silica exposure in anti-neutrophil cytoplasmic autoantibody-associated glomerulonephritis and lupus nephritis. J. Am. Soc. Nephrol. 12, 134—142.

Hogan, S., Falk, R., Chin, H., Cai, J., Jennette, C., Jennette, J., et al., 2005. Predictors of relapse and treatment resistance in antineutrophil cytoplasmic antibody-associated small-vessel vasculitis. Ann. Intern. Med. 143, 621—631.

Hogan, S., Cooper, G., Savitz, D., Nylander-French, L., Parks, C., Chin, H., et al., 2007. Association of silica exposure with anti-neutrophil cytoplasmic autoantibody small-vessel vasculitis: a population-based, case-control study. Clin. J. Am. Soc. Nephrol. 2, 290—299.

Holland, M., Takada, K., Okumoto, T., Takahashi, N., Kato, K., Adu, D., et al., 2002. Hypogalactosylation of serum IgG in patients with ANCA-associated systemic vasculitis. Clin. Exp. Immunol. 129, 183—190.

Holland, M., Yagi, H., Takahashi, N., Kato, K., Savage, C., Goodall, D., et al., 2006. Differential glycosylation of polyclonal IgG, IgG-Fc and IgG-Fab isolated from the sera of patients with ANCA-associated systemic vasculitis. Biochim. Biophys. Acta. 1760, 669—677.

Horvath, L., Czirjak, L., Fekete, B., Jakab, L., Pozsonyi, T., Kalabay, L., et al., 2001. High levels of antibodies against Clq are associated with disease activity and nephritis but not with other organ manifestations in SLE patients. Clin. Exp. Rheumatol. 19, 667—672.

Horwitz, M., Bradley, L., Harbertson, J., Krahl, T., Lee, J., Sarvetnick, N., 1998. Diabetes induced by Coxsackie virus: initiation by bystander damage and not molecular mimicry. Nat. Med. 4, 781—785.

Jagiello, P., Aries, P., Arning, L., Wagenleiter, S., Csernok, E., Hellmich, B., et al., 2005. The PTPN22 620W allele is a risk factor for Wegener's granulomatosis. Arthritis Rheum. 52, 4039—4043.

Jennette, J., Falk, R., 1990. Antineutrophil cytoplasmic autoantibodies and associated diseases: a review. Am. J. Kidney Dis. 15, 517—529.

Jennette, J., Falk, R., 1997a. Diagnosis and management of glomerular diseases. Med. Clin. North Am. 81, 653—677.

Jennette, J., Falk, R., 1997b. Small-vessel vasculitis. N. Engl. J. Med. 337, 1512—1523.

Johnson, P., Alexander, H., Mcmillan, S., Maxwell, A., 1997. Upregulation of the granulocyte adhesion molecule Mac-1 by autoantibodies in autoimmune vasculitis. Clin. Exp. Immunol. 107, 513—519.

Kain, R., Exner, M., Brandes, R., Ziebermayr, R., Cunningham, D., Alderson, C., et al., 2008. Molecular mimicry in pauci-immune focal necrotizing glomerulonephritis. Nat. Med. 14, 1088—1096.

Kannan, S., 2005. Molecular mechanism of chemotherapeutic drug(s)-induced autoimmunity: a mitochondrial-lysosomal axis theory. Med. Hypotheses. 64, 1068.

Keogan, M., Esnault, V., Green, A., Lockwood, C., Brown, D., 1992. Activation of normal neutrophils by anti-neutrophil cytoplasm antibodies. Clin. Exp. Immunol. 90, 228—234.

Kohm, A., Fuller, K., Miller, S., 2003. Mimicking the way to autoimmunity: an evolving theory of sequence and structural homology. Trends Microbiol. 11, 101—105.

Kyogoku, C., Langefeld, C., Ortmann, W., Lee, A., Selby, S., Carlton, V., et al., 2004. Genetic association of the R620W polymorphism of protein tyrosine phosphatase PTPN22 with human SLE. Am. J. Hum. Genet. 75, 504—507.

Ladner, M., Bottini, N., Valdes, A., Noble, J., 2005. Association of the single nucleotide polymorphism C1858T of the PTPN22 gene with type 1 diabetes. Hum. Immunol. 66, 60—64.

Lanzavecchia, A., 1995. How can cryptic epitopes trigger autoimmunity? J. Exp. Med. 181, 1945—1948.

Lavorgna, G., Dahary, D., Lehner, B., Sorek, R., Sanderson, C., Casari, G., 2004. In search of antisense. Trends Biochem. Sci. 29, 88—94.

Lee, A., Li, W., Liew, A., Bombardier, C., Weisman, M., Massarotti, E., et al., 2005a. The PTPN22 R620W polymorphism associates with RF positive rheumatoid arthritis in a dose-dependent manner but not with HLA-SE status. Genes Immun. 6, 129—133.

Lee, Y., Haas, K., Gor, D., Ding, X., Karp, D., Greenspan, N., et al., 2005b. Complement component C3d-antigen complexes can either augment or inhibit B lymphocyte activation and humoral immunity in mice depending on the degree of CD21/CD19 complex engagement. J. Immunol. 175, 8011—8023.

Lefkowith, J., Gilkeson, G., 1996. Nephritogenic autoantibodies in lupus: current concepts and continuing controversies. Arthritis Rheum. 39, 894—903.

Lefkowith, J., Kiehl, M., Rubenstein, J., Divalerio, R., Bernstein, K., Kahl, L., et al., 1996. Heterogeneity and clinical significance of glomerular-binding antibodies in systemic lupus erythematosus. J. Clin. Invest. 98, 1373—1380.

Levin, M., Lee, S., Kalume, F., Morcos, Y., Dohan Jr., F., Hasty, K., et al., 2002. Autoimmunity due to molecular mimicry as a cause of neurological disease. Nat. Med. 8, 509—513.

Linnik, M., Hu, J., Heilbrunn, K., Strand, V., Hurley, F., Joh, T., 2005. Relationship between anti-double-stranded DNA antibodies and exacerbation of renal disease in patients with systemic lupus erythematosus. Arthritis Rheum. 52, 1129—1137.

Lyons, P., Rayner, T., Trivedi, S., Holle, J., Watts, R., Jayne, D., et al., 2012. Genetically distinct subsets within ANCA-associated vasculitis. N. Engl. J. Med. 367, 214—223.

Mannik, M., Merrill, C., Stamps, L., Wener, M., 2003. Multiple autoantibodies form the glomerular immune deposits in patients with systemic lupus erythematosus. J. Rheumatol. 30, 1495—1504.

Marinaki, S., Neumann, I., Kalsch, A., Grimminger, P., Breedijk, A., Birck, R., et al., 2005. Abnormalities of CD4 T cell subpopulations in ANCA-associated vasculitis. Clin. Exp. Immunol. 140, 181—191.

Martorana, D., Maritati, F., Malerba, G., Bonatti, F., Alberici, F., Oliva, E., et al., 2012. PTPN22 R620W polymorphism in the ANCA-associated vasculitides. Rheumatology (Oxford) 51, 805—812.

Mayet, W., Marker-Hermann, E., Schlaak, J., Meyer Zum Buschenfelde, K., 1999. Irregular cytokine pattern of CD4 + T lymphocytes in response to Staphylococcus aureus in patients with Wegener's granulomatosis. Scand. J. Immunol. 49, 585–594.

Mulder, A., Heeringa, P., Brouwer, E., Limburg, P., Kallenberg, C., 1994. Activation of granulocytes by anti-neutrophil cytoplasmic antibodies (ANCA): a Fc gamma RII-dependent process. Clin. Exp. Immunol. 98, 270–278.

Nedjic, J., Aichinger, M., Mizushima, N., Klein, L., 2009. Macroautophagy, endogenous MHC II loading and T cell selection: the benefits of breaking the rules. Curr. Opin. Immunol. 21, 92–97.

Ohlsson, S., Pettersson, A., Ohlsson, S., Selga, D., Bengtsson, A., Segelmark, M., et al., 2012. Phagocytosis of apoptotic cells by macrophages in anti-neutrophil cytoplasmic antibody-associated systemic vasculitis. Clin. Exp. Immunol. 170, 47–56.

Olson, S., Arbogast, C., Baker, T., Owshalimpur, D., Oliver, D., Abbott, K., et al., 2011. Asymptomatic autoantibodies associate with future anti-glomerular basement membrane disease. J. Am. Soc. Nephrol. 22, 1946–1952.

Ooi, J., Snelgrove, S., Engel, D., Hochheiser, K., Ludwig-Portugall, I., Nozaki, Y., et al., 2011. Endogenous foxp3(+) T-regulatory cells suppress anti-glomerular basement membrane nephritis. Kidney Int. 79, 977–986.

Papamattheou, M., Routsias, J., Karagouni, E., Sakarellos, C., Sakarellos-Daitsiotis, M., Moutsopoulos, H., et al., 2004. T cell help is required to induce idiotypic-anti-idiotypic autoantibody network after immunization with complementary epitope 289-308aa of La/SSB autoantigen in non-autoimmune mice. Clin. Exp. Immunol. 135, 416–426.

Pendergraft III, W., Preston, G., Shah, R., Tropsha, A., Carter Jr., C., Jennette, J., et al., 2004. Autoimmunity is triggered by cPR-3(105-201), a protein complementary to human autoantigen proteinase-3. Nat. Med. 10, 72–79.

Perez, G., Bjornsson, S., Ross, A., Aamato, J., Rothfield, N., 1974. A mini-epidemic of Goodpasture's syndrome clinical and immunological studies. Nephron. 13, 161–173.

Peto, P., Salama, A., 2011. Update on antiglomerular basement membrane disease. Curr. Opin. Rheumatol. 23, 32–37.

Pfister, H., Ollert, M., Froehlich, L., Quintanilla-Martinez, L., Colby, T., Specks, U., et al., 2004. Anti-neutrophil cytoplasmic autoantibodies (ANCA) against the murine homolog of proteinase 3 (Wegener's autoantigen) are pathogenic in vivo. Blood. 104, 1411–1418.

Phelps, R., Rees, A., 1999. The HLA complex in Goodpasture's disease: a model for analyzing susceptibility to autoimmunity. Kidney Int. 56, 1638–1653.

Plotz, P., 1983. Autoantibodies are anti-idiotype antibodies to antiviral antibodies. Lancet. 2, 824–826.

Porges, A., Redecha, P., Kimberly, W., Csernok, E., Gross, W., Kimberly, R., 1994. Anti-neutrophil cytoplasmic antibodies engage and activate human neutrophils via Fc gamma RIIa. J. Immunol. 153, 1271–1280.

Powrie, F., Maloy, K., 2003. Immunology. Regulating the regulators. Science. 299, 1030–1031.

Prokunina, L., Castillejo-Lopez, C., Oberg, F., Gunnarsson, I., Berg, L., Magnusson, V., et al., 2002. A regulatory polymorphism in PDCD1 is associated with susceptibility to systemic lupus erythematosus in humans. Nat. Genet. 32, 666–669.

Pudifin, D., Duursma, J., Gathiram, V., Jackson, T., 1994. Invasive amoebiasis is associated with the development of anti-neutrophil cytoplasmic antibody. Clin. Exp. Immunol. 97, 48–51.

Rarok, A., Van Der Geld, Y., Stegeman, C., Limburg, P., Kallenberg, C., 2003. Diversity of PR3-ANCA epitope specificity in Wegener's granulomatosis. Analysis using the biosensor technology. J. Clin. Immunol. 23, 460–468.

Ravirajan, C., Rowse, L., Macgowan, J., Isenberg, D., 2001. An analysis of clinical disease activity and nephritis-associated serum autoantibody profiles in patients with systemic lupus erythematosus: a cross-sectional study. Rheumatology (Oxford). 40, 1405–1412.

Reveille, J., 2004. Predictive value of autoantibodies for activity of systemic lupus erythematosus. Lupus. 13, 290–297

Robertson, J., Wu, J., Arends, J., Glass II, W., Southwood, S., Sette, A., et al., 2005. Characterization of the T-cell epitope that causes anti-GBM glomerulonephritis. Kidney Int. 68, 1061–1070.

Rosen, A., Casciola-Rosen, L., 1999. Autoantigens as substrates for apoptotic proteases: implications for the pathogenesis of systemic autoimmune disease. Cell Death Differ. 6, 6–12.

Roth, A., Ooi, J., Hess, J.J., Van Timmeren, M., Berg, E., Jennette, C., et al., 2013. Epitope specificity determines pathogenicity and detectability in ANCA-associated vasculitis. Clin. Invest. 123, 1773–1783.

Routsias, J., Dotsika, E., Touloupi, E., Papamattheou, M., Sakarellos, C., Sakarellos-Daitsiotis, M., et al., 2003. Idiotype-anti-idiotype circuit in non-autoimmune mice after immunization with the epitope and complementary epitope 289-308aa of La/SSB: implications for the maintenance and perpetuation of the anti-La/SSB response. J. Autoimmun. 21, 17–26.

Russell, K., Fass, D., Specks, U., 2001. Antineutrophil cytoplasmic antibodies reacting with the pro form of proteinase 3 and disease activity in patients with Wegener's granulomatosis and microscopic polyangiitis. Arthritis. Rheum. 44, 463–468.

Salama, A., Levy, J., Lightstone, L., Pusey, C., 2001. Goodpasture's disease. Lancet. 358, 917–920

Salama, A., Chaudhry, A., Holthaus, K., Mosley, K., Kalluri, R., Sayegh, M., et al., 2003. Regulation by CD25+ lymphocytes of autoantigen-specific T-cell responses in Goodpasture's (anti-GBM) disease. Kidney Int. 64, 1685–1694.

Salmon, J., Roman, M., 2001. Accelerated atherosclerosis in systemic lupus erythematosus: implications for patient management. Curr. Opin. Rheumatol. 13, 341–344.

Savage, C., Pottinger, B., Gaskin, G., Pusey, C., Pearson, J., 1992. Autoantibodies developing to myeloperoxidase and proteinase 3 in systemic vasculitis stimulate neutrophil cytotoxicity toward cultured endothelial cells. Am. J. Pathol. 141, 335–342.

Savige, J., Gallicchio, M., Chang, L., Parkin, J., 1991. Autoantibodies in systemic vasculitis. Aust. N.Z. J. Med. 21, 433–437.

Segelmark, M., Wieslander, J., 1993. IgG subclasses of antineutrophil cytoplasm autoantibodies (ANCA). Nephrol. Dial. Transplant. 8, 696–702.

Selga, D., Segelmark, M., Wieslander, J., Gunnarsson, L., Hellmark, T., 2004. Epitope mapping of anti-PR3 antibodies using chimeric human/mouse PR3 recombinant proteins. Clin. Exp. Immunol. 135, 164–172.

Stegeman, C., Tervaert, J., Sluiter, W., Manson, W., De Jong, P., Kallenberg, C., 1994. Association of chronic nasal carriage of Staphylococcus aureus and higher relapse rates in Wegener granulomatosis. Ann. Intern. Med. 120, 12–17.

Stevenson, A., Yaqoob, M., Mason, H., Pai, P., Bell, G., 1995. Biochemical markers of basement membrane disturbances and occupational exposure to hydrocarbons and mixed solvents. QJM. 88, 23–28.

Suenaga, R., Abdou, N., 1993. Cationic and high affinity serum IgG anti-dsDNA antibodies in active lupus nephritis. Clin. Exp. Immunol. 94, 418–422.

Tadema, H., Abdulahad, W., Lepse, N., Stegeman, C., Kallenberg, C., Heeringa, P., 2011. Bacterial DNA motifs trigger ANCA production in ANCA-associated vasculitis in remission. Rheumatology. (Oxford). 50, 689–696.

Tomana, M., Schrohenloher, R., Koopman, W., Alarcon, G., Paul, W., 1988. Abnormal glycosylation of serum IgG from patients with chronic inflammatory diseases. Arthritis Rheum. 31, 333–338.

Van Den Eynde, B., Gaugler, B., Probst-Kepper, M., Michaux, L., Devuyst, O., Lorge, F., et al., 1999. A new antigen recognized by cytolytic T lymphocytes on a human kidney tumor results from reverse strand transcription. J. Exp. Med. 190, 1793–1800.

Van Timmeren, M., Van Der Veen, B., Stegeman, C., Petersen, A., Hellmark, T., Collin, M., et al., 2010. IgG glycan hydrolysis attenuates ANCA-mediated glomerulonephritis. J. Am. Soc. Nephrol. 21, 1103–1114.

Vanderlugt, C., Miller, S., 1996. Epitope spreading. Curr. Opin. Immunol. 8, 831–836.

Vogt, A., Schmiedeke, T., Stockl, F., Sugisaki, Y., Mertz, A., Batsford, S., 1990. The role of cationic proteins in the pathogenesis of immune complex glomerulonephritis. Nephrol. Dial. Transplant. 5 (Suppl. 1), 6–9.

Walker, L., 2009. Regulatory T cells overturned: the effectors fight back. Immunology. 126, 466–474

Walters, S., Webster, K., Sutherland, A., Gardam, S., Groom, J., Liuwantara, D., et al., 2009. Increased CD4+ Foxp3+ T cells in BAFF-transgenic mice suppress T cell effector responses. J. Immunol. 182, 793–801.

Woitas, R., Morioka, T., 1996. Influence of isoelectric point on glomerular deposition of antibodies and immune complexes. Nephron. 74, 713–719.

Xenocostas, A., Jothy, S., Collins, B., Loertscher, R., Levy, M., 1999. Anti-glomerular basement membrane glomerulonephritis after extracorporeal shock wave lithotripsy. Am. J. Kidney Dis. 33, 128–132.

Xie, C., Liang, Z., Chang, S., Mohan, C., 2003. Use of a novel elution regimen reveals the dominance of polyreactive antinuclear autoantibodies in lupus kidneys. Arthritis Rheum. 48, 2343–2352.

Yang, J., Pendergraft, W., Alcorta, D., Nachman, P., Hogan, S., Thomas, R., et al., 2004. Circumvention of normal constraints on granule protein gene expression in peripheral blood neutrophils and monocytes of patients with antineutrophil cytoplasmic autoantibody-associated glomerulonephritis. J. Am. Soc. Nephrol. 15, 2103–2114.

Yoshimura, J., Fukami, K., Koike, K., Nagano, M., Matsumoto, T., Iwatani, R., et al., 2010. Interstitial Foxp3-positive T cells may predict renal survival in patients with myeroperoxidase anti-neutrophil cytoplasmic antibody-associated glomerulonephritis. Clin. Exp. Pharmacol. Physiol. 37, 879–883.

Yun, H., Koh, H., Kim, S., Chung, W., Kim, D., Hong, K., et al., 2001. FcgammaRIIa/IIIa polymorphism and its association with clinical manifestations in Korean lupus patients. Lupus. 10, 466–472

Zuniga, R., Ng, S., Peterson, M., Reveille, J., Baethge, B., Alarcon, G., et al., 2001. Low-binding alleles of Fcgamma receptor types IIA and IIIA are inherited independently and are associated with systemic lupus erythematosus in Hispanic patients. Arthritis Rheum. 44, 361–367.

Chapter 68

Autoimmune Orchitis and Autoimmune Oophoritis

Livia Lustig[1], Claudia Rival[2], and Kenneth S.K. Tung[2]

[1]Instituto de Investigaciones Biomédicas, Facultad de Medicina, Universidad de Buenos Aires, Paraguay, Argentina, [2]Beirne Carter Center for Immunology Research and Department of Pathology, University of Virginia, Charlottesville, VA, USA

Chapter Outline

Introduction 1007
Experimental Autoimmune Disease of the Testis 1008
  Autoimmune Orchitis in the Dark Mink 1008
  Autoimmune Orchitis in Rats Expressing Transgenic Human HLA B27 and Human β2 Microglobulin 1008
  Post-vasectomy Autoimmune Orchitis in Mice with Treg Depletion and Post-vasectomy Tolerance to Testis Antigens 1008
  Autoimmune Orchitis Associated with Viral Infection 1009
  Autoimmune Orchitis in Day 3 Thymectomized (d3tx) Mice 1009
  Classical Experimental Autoimmune Orchitis Induced by Immunization with Testis Antigen in Adjuvant 1009
    Historical Aspect 1009
    Testicular Immunoprivilege (Local Regulation) 1009
    Testicular Antigens 1010
    Mechanisms of Disease Initiation 1010
Clinical Autoimmune Disease of the Testis 1011
  Idiopathic Male Infertility 1011
  Infertility and ASA Coexist with Other Autoimmune Diseases 1012
  Vasectomy, Sperm Granuloma, and Cystic Fibrosis 1012
  Orchitis Associated with Virus Infections 1012
Experimental Autoimmune Disease of the Ovary 1013
  Spontaneous Autoimmune Ovarian Disease (AOD) in AIRE Null Mice 1013
  AOD in Day 3 Thymectomized (d3tx) Mice 1013
  AOD in Neonatal Mice by Maternal Antibody to Murine ZP3 1014
  Classical Experimental Autoimmune Oophoritis 1014
Clinical Autoimmune Disease of the Ovary 1015
Concluding Remarks 1016
Acknowledgments 1016
References 1016

INTRODUCTION

Experimental studies predict a frequent occurrence of human gonadal autoimmunity. In spontaneous autoimmune model targeting multiple organs, the testis and ovary are the dominant targets. Sperm autoimmunity commonly occurs after vasectomy, and autoimmune orchitis can be induced by testis antigens without adjuvant; thus male meiotic germ cell antigens are highly immunogenic to the autologous host. Autoimmune disease of the testis (orchitis) occurs spontaneously in essentially all animal species examined. Despite these observations, human gonadal disease with proven autoimmune etiology has yet to be identified and characterized. The slow progress in clinical research is in part explained by the success of assisted reproduction techniques that

partly overcome the adverse effects of antisperm antibodies. Nonetheless, the experimental studies have yielded exceptional information on the fundamental mechanisms of tolerance and autoimmunity. They include: the discovery and functional analysis of the CD4$^+$CD25$^+$ Foxp3$^+$ regulatory T cells (Treg) and of the autoimmune response (AIRE) gene, molecular mimicry as a basis of autoreactive T cell response, and the epitope spreading phenomenon in autoantibody production. In addition, they provide guidelines for translational research into human gonadal autoimmunity, and for better understanding of chronic inflammatory conditions of the gonads associated with subfertility and infertility. In this chapter, we will present the experimental autoimmune models, followed by a description of existing data supporting an autoimmune basis in human testicular and ovarian diseases.

N. Rose & I. Mackay (Eds): The Autoimmune Diseases, Fifth edition. DOI: http://dx.doi.org/10.1016/B978-0-12-384929-8.00068-X

EXPERIMENTAL AUTOIMMUNE DISEASE OF THE TESTIS

Classical experimental autoimmune orchitis (EAO) is induced by immunization with testis antigen in adjuvant. In addition, autoimmune orchitis occurs spontaneously after manipulation of the immune system or following vasectomy, without Ag immunization. Studies on the spontaneous orchitis models have addressed the genetic and cellular mechanisms that terminate tolerance, leading to spontaneous autoimmune disease. Studies on the classical EAO model clarified the local immune mechanisms by which the protection of the testis is compromised, leading to autoimmune tissue injury.

Autoimmune Orchitis in the Dark Mink

Inbreeding of mink for a dark fur, co-selected male infertility in this seasonal breeder (Tung et al., 1981), but also affects mink with other fur colors (Pelletier, 1986). There are two histopathologic patterns: one has massive granulomatous inflammation, and the other extensive germ cell loss with little inflammation. In the latter, antibodies to sperm acrosome form an immune complex, with IgG and complement C3 depositing in the basement membrane outside the Sertoli cell barrier (SCB). Interestingly, there is an association of autoimmune orchitis with abnormal hypothalamic-pituitary-testicular function since correction of the hormonal defect prevented testis pathology (Tung et al., 1984). A study by Pelletier et al. (2009) has critically analyzed the spermatogenic cycle in this seasonal breeder and provided evidence that defects in the regulatory clearance mechanisms favor the breakdown of self-tolerance during spontaneous autoimmune orchitis in mink.

Autoimmune Orchitis in Rats Expressing Transgenic Human HLA B27 and Human β2 Microglobulin

Lewis rats with transgenic human HLA B27/β2m spontaneously develop spondyloarthritis and rheumatoid arthritis that mimic human disease (Taurog, 2009). Unexpectedly, severe autoimmune orchitis occurs in the transgenic rats several months before the onset of joint disease (Taurog et al., 2012). Inflammation first appears in the ductus efferentes at 3 weeks when the first wave of apoptotic testicular germ cells begins to transit the ductus efferentes to reach the epididymis. B27/β2m transgene expression somehow reduces male germ cell specific tolerance. When autoreactive T cells respond to their cognate peptides in this vulnerable region of male reproductive tract, they trigger persistent granulomatous inflammation. Interestingly, it takes another 3 months before the inflammation shifts to the testis and ultimately eliminates sperm production. Importantly, bilateral surgical excision of the orchitic testes prevents arthritis development and documents for the first time a causal link between two organ-specific autoimmune diseases (Taurog et al., 2012). The new model will provide an excellent opportunity to investigate molecular mimicry, and the finding supports the hypothesis of persistent innate cell activation as a factor in rheumatoid arthritis (Noss and Brenner, 2008). Although autoimmune orchitis has not been reported in men with spondyloarthritis, recent study detected sperm abnormalities in these patients (Villiger et al., 2010). Notably, lower urinary tract infections may be associated with this male-dominant human spondyloarthritis.

Post-vasectomy Autoimmune Orchitis in Mice with Treg Depletion and Post-vasectomy Tolerance to Testis Antigens

Vasectomy is a major global contraceptive method adopted by over 0.5 million men in the USA alone. Autoimmune orchitis with immune complex deposition occurs in vasectomized rabbits, guinea pigs, monkeys, and others (Bigazzi, 1981). Although vasectomized men develop sperm antibody, well-characterized autoimmune orchitis has not been documented. A recent study on the early autoimmune response to vasectomy discovered that the Treg response critically controls the response to sperm antigens that influence long-term outcome. Post-vasectomy autoimmune orchitis does not occur in the susceptible A/J or (B6xA/J) F1 mice unless Treg are partially (60%) depleted, whereas in the genetically resistant C57BL/6 mice, 98% Treg depletion is required. Unexpectedly, vasectomy alone does not lead to autoimmune orchitis at least within 10 weeks. Instead, sperm antigen-specific tolerance is the outcome. When subsequently immunized with tissue antigens in adjuvant, the vasectomized mice resist experimental autoimmune orchitis but not experimental autoimmune encephalomyelitis induction, indicating that vasectomized mice developed sperm-specific tolerance (Wheeler et al., 2011). Thus, sperm antigens released from the post-vasectomy epididymal granuloma induce tolerance or autoimmunity depending on the balance of effector Treg and effector T cell responses. The long-term immune sequel of vasectomy is likely determined by the genetic control of this dual response, including the individual's Treg capacity.

Autoimmune Orchitis Associated with Viral Infection

Infection may be followed by an autoimmune response that prolongs inflammation and tissue damage. Orchitis occurs in rabbits with infection of myxoma virus (Fountain et al., 1997) and Sendai virus closely related to mumps virus (Melaine et al., 2003). In mice unilaterally infected with *Listeria monocytogenes*, the contralateral testis develops orchitis without detectable microorganisms, providing evidence for an autoimmune component of infectious orchitis (Mukasa et al., 1995). Indeed, CD4$^+$ T cells from infected donors transfer orchitis to uninfected recipients. In this study, $\gamma\delta$ T cells are found to regulate $\alpha\beta$ pathogenic T cells by cytokines, notably IL-10 and TGF-β (Mukasa et al., 1998).

Autoimmune Orchitis in Day 3 Thymectomized (d3tx) Mice

D3tx B6AF1 mice produce sperm-specific and oocyte-specific autoantibodies (autoAb). The testis and epididymis, and the ovary, are three of the five organs that develop autoimmune disease. A more detailed description of the d3tx autoimmune model is presented in the section on autoimmune oophoritis.

Classical Experimental Autoimmune Orchitis Induced by Immunization with Testis Antigen in Adjuvant

Historical Aspect

EAO, the first "tissue antigen/adjuvant" autoimmune model, was described by Voisin et al. (1951) and by Freund et al. (1953). Attempts to transfer disease by serum antibody to normal guinea pig failed but the study clarified regional differences in different spermatogenic compartments, and supported the physiological findings in the normal testis (Tung et al., 1971a; Johnson, 1973). Lymphocytes retrieved from immunized guinea pig induced EAO when they were injected directly into the testis, but not intravenously (Tung et al., 1971b). The finding supports the notion that normal recipients are resistant to Ab transfer of autoimmune disease, and T cells need to express tissue homing receptor to enter target organs. Further progress in the EAO mechanism has come from mouse and rat models. In general, EAO induction requires co-injection of testis antigen in complete Freund's adjuvant (CFA) and/or pertussis toxin (Kohno et al., 1983; Doncel et al., 1989); however, murine EAO can also be induced by subcutaneous injections of viable testicular cells without adjuvant (Sakamoto et al., 1985; Itoh et al., 1991, 2005). A detailed description of the

protocols for testicular autoimmune disease was described by Tung et al. (1994).

Testicular Immunoprivilege (Local Regulation)

Head et al. (1983) discovered the prolonged survival of an allogeneic organ engrafted in the testicular interstitium, and called attention to the testis as an immunoprivileged organ (reviewed by Fijak et al., 2011a and Li et al., 2012). Since then, many soluble and cell-based immunosuppressive factors have been discovered in the testis interstitium, largely based on *in vitro* studies. The testis resident macrophages, peritubular cells, Leydig cells, and Sertoli cells have documented immunoregulatory properties (Meinhardt and Hedger, 2011). Testosterone has an immunosuppressive role and may directly enhance Treg function (Fijak et al., 2011b). These interstitial regulatory mechanisms can reduce local inflammation and prevent the efferent arm of immune response to self or microbial antigens, and are likely to operate in an antigen-independent manner. Recent *in vivo* studies emphasize the critical regulatory functions of the Sertoli cells. Co-implantation with Sertoli cells led to prolonged survival of functioning allogeneic pancreatic islets in diabetic mice (Selawry and Cameron, 1993; Mital et al., 2010). Mechanistically, the Sertoli cell expresses the Tyro-3 family receptors (Tyro 3, Axl, and Mer) (Lu et al., 1999) that normally regulate the innate cellular response to Toll-like receptor stimulation (Rothlin et al., 2007). Major defect in spermatogenesis occurs in mice with triple genetic deletion of the TAM receptors (Lu et al., 1999). The Sertoli cells produce TGF-β; and through a cell-to-cell immunomodulatory action, they can inhibit CD8$^+$ T cell proliferation via B7-H1, and increase Tregs (Dal Secco et al., 2008). In addition, Sertoli cell-specific androgen receptor deletion led to breakdown of the SCB, which normally separates the antigenic and immunogenic meiotic germ cells from the interstitial space. There is reduced expression of claudin 3, a component of the SCB, and the emergence of interstitial inflammation and sperm antibody response (Meng et al., 2011).

Immature or tolerogenic testis dendritic cells (DCs) or macrophages in the testis may also control the inductive phase of an autoimmune response to meiotic germ cell antigens. But the current dogma, that these antigens are completely sequestered by the SCB, would deem this scenario unlikely. However, it should be emphasized that the truism of the dogma has never been tested experimentally. In addition, study on vasectomy and spontaneous orchitis models support Treg-dependent systemic tolerance to testis antigen, and this would require continuous priming of Tregs by germ cell antigens (Setiady et al., 2006). It is therefore very likely that at least some of the meiotic germ cell antigens are not sequestered.

Testicular Antigens

Orchitogenic antigens are localized in male meiotic germ cells including the spermatozoa. Their identity and immunogenicity are only partially known (reviewed by Frayne and Hall, 1999 and Tung et al., 2000). Some orchitogenic antigens are not testis specific, and they react with sera from rats with EAO, and their identity is revealed by a proteomics approach. These include heat shock protein 70, disulfide isomerase ER-60 and heterogeneous nuclear ribonucleoprotein H1 (Fijak et al., 2005). Recently, a murine orchitogenic antigen has been identified as the glycosylated murine zonadhesin (Wheeler et al., 2011). Zonadhesin is expressed on the outer acrosomal membrane of spermatids and sperm. It binds to the zona pellucida and prevents interspecies sperm—oocyte interaction (Hardy and Garbers, 1994; Tardif et al., 2010).

Mechanisms of Disease Initiation

T Cell and Autoantibody

CD4$^+$ T cells are pivotal in EAO pathogenesis. Polyclonal or monoclonal murine CD4$^+$ T cells adoptively transfer severe EAO (Tung et al., 1987; Yule and Tung, 1993). In rat EAO, an increase in the testicular IL-17 and IL-23 was detected, suggesting the involvement of Th17 subsets (Jacobo et al., 2011a). Variations in the number and cytokine profile (Th1 and Th17) of CD8$^+$ T cells are also identified in EAO testis, in the chronic stage of the disease (Jacobo et al., 2009, 2011a). Tregs are distributed as clusters in subcapsular seminiferous tubules of rats with classical EAO (Jacobo et al., 2009). Tregs isolated from regional lymph nodes (LN) are more potent suppressors of polyclonal T cell response than the Tregs from other LN *in vitro* (Jacobo et al., 2010). However, Tregs fail to effectively suppress ongoing inflammation *in vivo*. This may be caused by T cell imbalance induced by cytokines in the inflamed testis, leading to effector T cell resistance to suppression or to reduction of the Treg suppressive function (Jacobo et al., 2011b).

Autoantibody participation in EAO is supported by immune complex detection in the tubular basement membrane in murine EAO and in the spontaneous autoimmune orchitis. Immune complexes are characterized by granular deposition of immunoglobulin (Ig) G and complement C3 (Figure 68.1D). Although antibody *per se* does not transfer EAO to normal recipients, antibody can synergize with effector T cells to induce severe EAO (Wheeler et al., 2011). The detection of immune complexes in frozen sections of human testis biopsies would provide more definitive evidences for an ongoing autoimmune process. See the oophoritis section for further discussion on autoantibody action.

Mechanism of Testis Inflammation

When orchitogenic T cells are adoptively transferred to normal recipients, they initially target the straight tubules and the ductus efferentes, and subsequently spread to the seminiferous tubules (Tung et al., 1987). In contrast, EAO induced by active immunization is initiated equally between the region of the rete testis and seminiferous tubules. After migration from blood vessels into testis interstitium, the macrophages, DCs, and T cells form multiple cell clusters around the seminiferous tubule. In many species, with the exception of rat EAO, the cells invade the SCB and enter the seminiferous tubules. It is important to understand how T cells enter the testis, damage the SCB, and injure the seminiferous tubules. Recent studies in the rat support the following scenario in active EAO induction. Chemokines and cytokines upregulate adhesion molecules on the endothelial cell (EC), and support T cell attachment to EC, and extravasation into the interstitial space. Contact between the activated form of CD44 on lymphocytes and its major ligand hyaluronic acid expressed on EC is required (Guazzone et al., 2005). Chemokines (which include CCL2/MCP-1, CCL3/MIP-1α, and CCL4/MIP-1β) expressed by testicular cells convert the leukocyte rolling into cell arrest. In addition, the higher percentage of leukocytes expressing CD49d integrin and the increased expression of CD106/VCAM ligand in endothelial cells mediate the step of firm adhesion. Finally, inflammatory cell transmigration occurs via the interaction of CD106 and CD31/PECAM-1 (Guazzone et al., 2009, 2012).

Interstitial macrophages and DCs play a critical role in testis inflammation. They express high levels of MHC class II, CD80, and CD86 and increase in number in the testicular interstitium of rats with EAO (Rival et al., 2008). They produce proinflammatory cytokines (mainly TNF-α, IL-6, and IFN-γ) (Suescun et al., 2003; Rival et al., 2006) and nitric oxide (Jarazo-Dietrich et al., 2012). In EAO of the B27/β2m transgenic rats, there is distinct distribution between the testis M1 and M2 macrophages; and the M1 macrophages dominantly target the seminiferous tubules (Taurog et al., 2012). Importantly, *in vivo* depletion of macrophages and DCs in rat EAO by clodronate-containing liposomes significantly reduces EAO incidence and severity suggesting that they are derived from circulating monocytes (Rival et al., 2008). Proinflammatory cytokines and nitric oxide alter the integrity and function of Sertoli adherens and tight junctions facilitating germ cell sloughing (Lee and Cheng, 2003; Pérez et al., 2011, 2012). Finally, germ cell apoptosis involves the TNF-α/TNFR1, IL-6/IL-6R, and FasL/Fas systems (Suescun et al., 2003; Theas et al., 2003, 2008; Rival et al., 2006). Death receptor and mitochondrial apoptotic pathways are involved

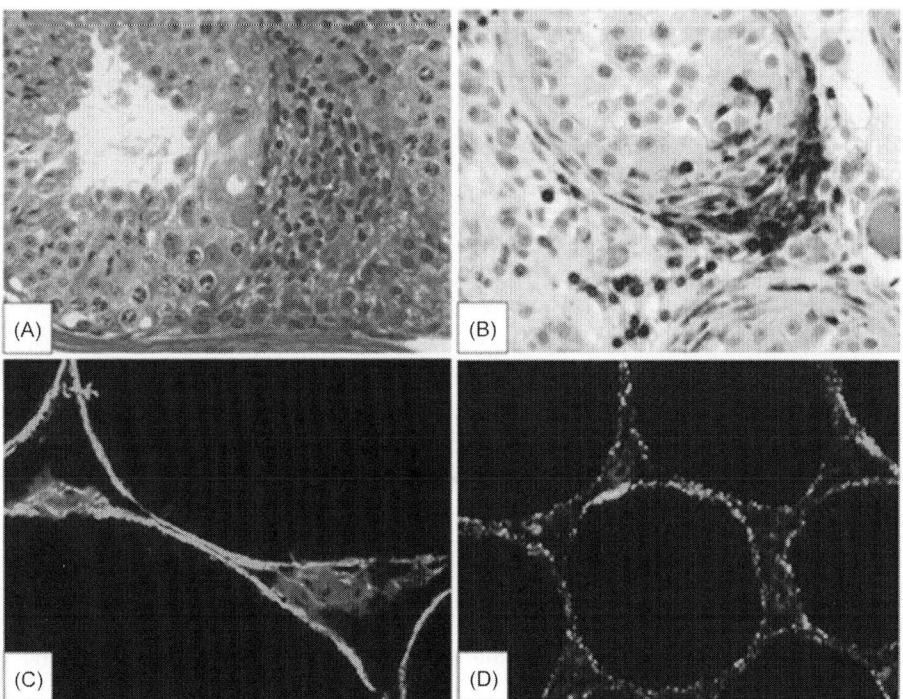

FIGURE 68.1   Comparing the immunopathology shared between autoimmune orchitis in mice and human orchitis with unexplained infertility.   Frames A, C, and D illustrate immunopathology of autoimmune orchitis in mice. (A) A typical monocytic inflammatory cell cluster that "cups" the perimeter of seminiferous tubule. Although the inflammatory cells remain external to the SCB, the adjacent Sertoli cells and germ cells inside the tubule have disappeared ($\times 100$, hematoxylin and eosin). (C) Dendritic cells in the cell cluster (red fluorescence: CD11c) detected by immunofluorescence on frozen section, adjacent to a split myoid cell layer (green fluorescence: alpha actin) ($\times 400$). Not shown are co-localized T cells and macrophages in the cell cluster. (D) Direct immunofluorescence detection of testicular immune complexes on a frozen section of mouse testis with EAO. Immune complexes appear as peri-tubular IgG granules (green fluorescence). Frame B represents an immunoperoxidase study of the testis biopsy from a patient with unexplained infertility. CD3$^+$ T cells form a peritubular "cup" that resembles the murine EAO shown in frame A. Note some T cells are inside the hypospermatogenic seminiferous tubule in B ($\times 400$, anti-CD3). *Tung, K., Meinhardt, A., Schuppe, H.C., Bergmann, M. and Kliesch, S., personal observation.*

(Theas et al., 2006). Excessive male germ cell antigens released into the interstitium during EAO further stimulate T cell response in the testicular draining LN (TLN). The TLN-specific DCs from these rats are more mature and express more IL-12p35 mRNA than do DCs from non-draining LN (Guazzone et al., 2011). Loss of SCB integrity is important in EAO pathogenesis, as documented by the finding in Sertoli cell-specific deletion of androgen receptor, reported by Meng et al. (2011).

CLINICAL AUTOIMMUNE DISEASE OF THE TESTIS

Idiopathic Male Infertility

The advent of the immunobead assay allows for objective semi-quantitation of anti-sperm antibody (ASA) of different Ig classes against antigens present in different surface domains of viable spermatozoa (Marshburn and Kutteh, 1994). ASA are found in 3−12% of men with

infertility, compared to 0−2% of the general male population (reviewed by Turek and Lipshultz, 1994). In principle, ASA may cause infertility by interfering with sperm transport and other fertilization events. ASA from infertile patients and animals can affect many steps of fertilization *in vitro*, such as sperm motility, cervical mucus penetration, acrosome reaction, zona binding, zona penetration, oolema binding, and pronucleus formation in the fertilized oocyte (reviewed by Tung et al., 2002). The detection of ASA of IgA and IgG isotypes to sperm head in the local genital secretion is strongly associated with male infertility (reviewed by Marshburrn and Kutteh, 1994). Deciphering the nature of the cognate sperm antigens will add insight into ASA-mediated human infertility (Frayne and Hall, 1999) because ASA is also a component of autoimmune response that causes autoimmune orchitis and gonadal failure.

The diagnosis of human autoimmune orchitis depends on immunopathologic evaluation of testis biopsies; however, testis biopsy is rarely performed. The common finding of reduction in spermatogenesis is not diagnostic of an autoimmune process. More important are the findings of orchitis and immune complexes. Two types of human orchitis with possible autoimmune basis are reported. The first is granulomatous orchitis of non-infectious origin. Clinically, patients present mild scrotal pain or swelling, or a hard scrotal mass. Histologically, the seminiferous tubules are replaced by granulomatous inflammation consisting of T cells, macrophages, and multinucleated giant cells (Figure 68.2). These findings mimic the changes in rat EAO (Doncel et al., 1989; Taurog et al., 2012). The second and more common type of orchitis contains multiple foci of monocytic inflammation (Suominen and Söderström 1982; Chan and Schlegel, 2002a,b) (Figure 68.1B), and resembles the finding in early lesions found in EAO of mice and guinea pig. T cell and macrophage clusters are located at the boundary of seminiferous tubules and penetrate them through disrupted SCB (Figure 68.1A, C) (Kohno et al., 1983; Schuppe et al., 2008). A recent study detected IL-17, IL-21, and IL-23 among the inflammatory cells, and suggests involvement of the proinflammatory Th17 pathway in human orchitis (Duan et al., 2011). Finally, in addition to chronic inflammation of unknown etiology associated with infertility, infectious orchitis can mimic autoimmune orchitis, and similar lymphocyte infiltrations are found in testicular biopsies in patients with other diseases including cryptorchic testes and testicular cancer *in situ* (Nistal et al., 2002; Jahnukainen et al., 1995).

Even more helpful in autoimmune orchitis diagnosis is the detection of testis immune complexes. Technically, the most accurate and convincing method of tissue immune complex detection is immunofluorescence on frozen testis sections. They are readily detected by this approach in many types of experimental autoimmune orchitis (Tung, 1978; Tung et al., 1981; Bigazzi, 1981; Lustig et al., 1987, 2000). Surprisingly, a systematic study of human testis biopsy with this approach has not been reported. However, earlier light and electron microscope studies show deposits or electron dense material in the tubular basement membrane that reacts with antibody to human IgG and complement C3 (Salomon et al., 1982; Lehmann et al., 1987).

Infertility and ASA Coexist with Other Autoimmune Diseases

The major evidence for an autoimmune basis of human autoimmune orchitis comes from patients with the autoimmune polyglandular syndrome (APS) (see Chapter 43 for details). APS-1 is a rare autosomal recessive disease caused by AIRE gene mutation (Kisand and Peterson,

2011). About 30% of male patients develop testis failure with autoantibody to steroidogenic enzymes and other antigens expressed in the Leydig cells (Maclaren et al., 2001).

Vasectomy, Sperm Granuloma, and Cystic Fibrosis

Patients with vasectomy commonly produce ASA, detectable several months after surgery. Post-vasectomy ASA may be a cause of infertility in men with vasovasostomy and adequate sperm count (Lee et al., 2009). Focal orchitis has also been reported in the testes of vasectomized men (McDonald, 1997), and by epidemiological analysis (Goldacre et al., 2007). However, a systematic immunopathologic analysis of the human testes and epididymis in vasectomized subjects is still lacking. Epididymal sperm granuloma commonly occurs in vasectomized mice (>80%), and also occurs in men, but the incidence in human is unknown without histopathologic data. Finally, ASA response also occurs in patients with congenital absence of the vas deferens and seminal vesicles associated with cystic fibrosis (D'Cruz et al., 1991).

Orchitis Associated with Virus Infections

Virus infection of the testis may cause orchitis by disrupting local immune privilege besides a direct viral cytopathological effect. The best-known orchitogenic viruses are mumps virus and HIV. The symptoms of mumps in prepubertal boys are limited to parotitis; however, 5–37% of male adults with mumps infection also develop orchitis (Erpenbach, 1991). Lymphocytic infiltration followed by oligozoospermia with tubular atrophy and fibrosis contribute to transient or permanent subfertility or infertility. Mumps virus does not appear to induce germ cell transformation, and may not be directly spermatogenotoxic. However, mumps virus replicates in Leydig cells *in vitro*, inhibits testosterone secretion and induces production of the chemokine CXCL10 that recruits leukocytes to the testis (Le Goffic et al., 2002; Mouchel et al., 2002). ASA is reported in AIDS patients who develop orchitis, hypogonadism, oligozoospermia, or azoospermia. The reduced testosterone levels in AIDS may result from a reduction of Leydig cell number or function. Proinflammatory cytokines may also alter the hypothalamic-pituitary-gonadal regulation of Leydig cell function (reviewed by Dejucq and Jégou, 2001), and affect SCB integrity (Xia et al., 2009). Sexual transmission of acquired immunodeficiency disease by HIV-infected macrophages from inflamed testis has been proposed but not further investigated.

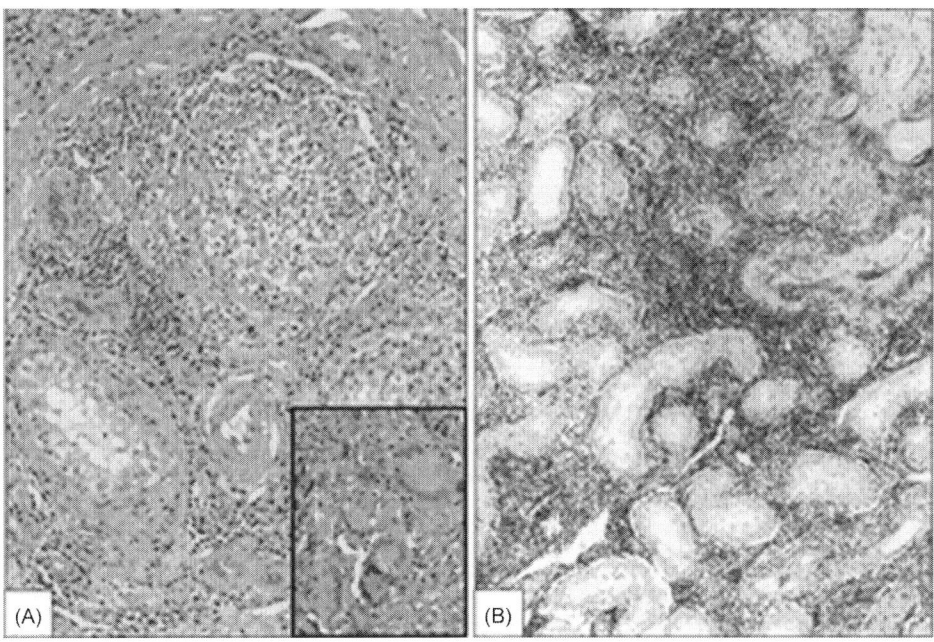

FIGURE 68.2   Immunopathology of human granulomatous orchitis.   (A) Seminiferous tubules, devoid of germ cells, are filled with monocytic inflammatory cells with associated peritubular and interstitial fibrosis ($\times 200$), and multi-nucleated giant cells ($\times 400$, insert) (hematoxylin and eosin). (B) Immunoperoxidase stain showing massive infiltration of CD3$^+$ T cells in the interstitial space and inside the seminiferous tubular lumen devoid of germ cells ($\times 100$, CD3 stain). *Tung, K., Meinhardt, A., Schuppe, H.C., Bergmann, M. and Kliesch, S., personal observation.*

EXPERIMENTAL AUTOIMMUNE DISEASE OF THE OVARY

Spontaneous Autoimmune Ovarian Disease (AOD) in AIRE Null Mice

Mice with AIRE deficiency resemble humans with the APS1 syndrome including a high incidence of spontaneous AOD (Kuroda et al., 2005; Cheng et al., 2007). AIRE regulates the transcription of many tissue-specific antigens that are ectopically expressed in thymic medullary epithelial cells. These antigens, presented by epithelial cells or DC, participate in central tolerance by either deleting autoreactive effector T cells, or by promoting development of antigen-specific natural Treg (Anderson et al., 2002; Derbinski et al., 2005). In AIRE null mice, the lack of thymic expression of ovarian antigens allows the emergence of pathogenic effector T and B cell responses against the autoantigens and AOD development. The ovarian disease in AIRE null mice is associated with lymphocytic infiltration in both ovarian follicles and the interstitial space. Severe AOD causes loss of oocytes and ovarian atrophy. The autoantibody in AIRE null mice in the AOD background reacts with the oocyte antigen NALP5/MATER (Cheng and Nelson, 2011). The similarity between AIRE null mice and the d3tx mice raises the intriguing possibility that the two diseases share common mechanisms.

AOD in Day 3 Thymectomized (d3tx) Mice

Autoimmune disease in d3tx B6AF1 mice most commonly targets the ovary (Figure 68.3), lacrimal gland, prostate, and epididymis (Nishizuka and Sakakura, 1969). The d3tx disease was once thought to be due to depletion of Tregs of late ontogeny. However, this notion has been challenged by several independent studies (Dujardin et al., 2004; Ang et al., 2007; Samy et al., 2008). Notably, normal day 3-old mice were found to have functional Tregs; and their depletion greatly enhanced disease frequency and severity. Monteiro et al. (2008) further reported enhanced effector T cells in alymphopenic environment due to imbalance in Tregs and effectors, possible modified thymic T cell repertoire, and lymphopenia. Although the d3tx disease is not due entirely to Treg depletion, the process is effectively inhibited by early infusion of exogenous CD4 Tregs from normal donors (Nishizuka and Sakakura, 1969). Indeed, this is the key experiment that ultimately led to the discovery of CD25$^+$ Foxp3$^+$ Tregs (Sakaguchi et al., 1995; Fontenot et al., 2003; Hori et al., 2003). In d3tx mice, effector T cells spontaneously respond to endogenous ovarian antigens in the ovarian draining LN (Alard et al., 2001). Disease suppression achieved by exogenous Tregs occurs in the ovarian draining LN where abundant antigen-specific donor Tregs accumulate (Samy et al., 2005). Subsequently, antigen-specific polyclonal Tregs in normal mice were also found

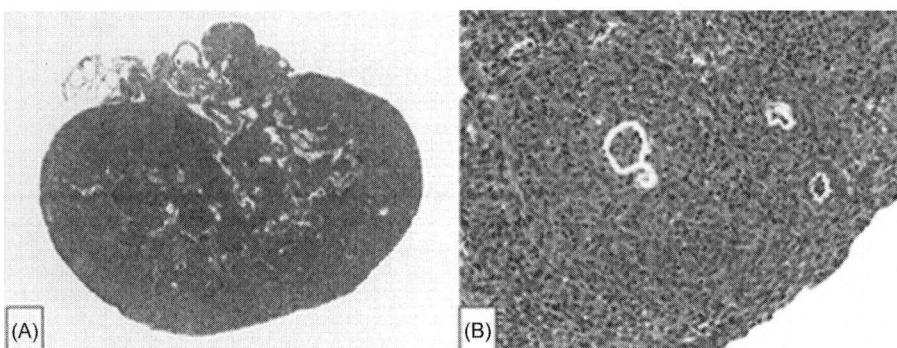

FIGURE 68.3 Immunopathology of autoimmune oophoritis in d3tx mice. (A) Atrophic ovary with absence of ovarian follicles and minimal oophoritis in severe and late AOD (× 50, hematoxylin and eoxin). (B) Inflammatory mononuclear cells surrounding and infiltrating ovarian follicles and surrounding interstitial atretic follicle; note leukocytes inside the oocyte space (× 200). *Wheeler, K. and Tung, K., personal observation.*

to accumulate in regional LN of the internal organs; and they exert Ag-specific and Ag-dependent protection of the antigens in the draining organs (Samy et al., 2005, 2006, 2008; Setiady et al., 2006; Wheeler et al., 2009). Importantly, the repertoires of Treg antigen receptors present in individual LN are unique (Hsieh et al., 2012).

AOD in Neonatal Mice by Maternal Antibody to Murine ZP3

AOD is induced in neonatal mice (neonatal AOD or nAOD) by passive transfer of maternal antibody specific for a ZP3 B cell epitope 335-342 (Setiady et al., 2003, 2004). Although ZP3 antibody readily forms immune complex in the zona pellucida of both neonatal and adult ovaries, AOD occurs only in the neonatal but not adult mice. The immune complexes are targeted by activated FcγRIII$^+$ NK cells, which are critical for nAOD induction. The increased susceptibility of newborns to nAOD is not explained by ovarian ontogenetic differences (Setiady et al., 2003). In fact, the activating FcγRIII-positive antigen-presenting cells located in both neonatal and adult ovaries can process ZP3 antigens, and stimulate a *de novo* pathogenic T cell response that can adoptively transfer nAOD to naïve recipients. The unique neonatal NK cells are required for both induction and effector functions of the autoreactive T cell response in adoptive transfer of nAOD (Setiady et al., 2003, 2004).

Classical Experimental Autoimmune Oophoritis

AOD was first induced in rabbit by immunization with pig zona pellucida in complete Freund adjuvant (CFA)

(Wood et al., 1981), and this was soon confirmed by AOD induction in dogs (Mahi-Brown et al., 1982). Extensive mechanistic study of AOD began after the disease was induced in mice immunized with a 13-mer murine ZP3 peptide (pZP3) (Rhim et al., 1992). The pZP3 contains both T cell and a native B cell epitopes. AOD can be induced by immunization with microbial and tissue peptides that mimic the pZP3. This T cell epitope molecular mimicry depends on very limited partial sharing of residues critical for induction of the ZP3 specific T cell response (Luo et al., 1993; Garza and Tung, 1995). Th1 subset is the major pathogenic T cell, and AOD is dependent on both CD28 and CD40 costimulatory pathways (Griggs et al., 1996). pZP3-specific Th2 cells also elicit AOD with dominant eosinophilic inflammation, and this can be transferred by T cell clones that produce IL-4 and IL-5 but not IFN-γ (Lou et al., 2000; Agersborg et al., 2001). While most human ovarian autoimmune inflammation is monocytic, some are dominantly eosinophilic (Lewis, 1993). The enteric nematode (the rodent pinworm) strongly promotes a Th2 autoimmune response to pZP3, particularly in the neonatal period. Without adjuvant, pZP3 plus pinworm infection elicits strong Th2 response and eosinophilic AOD in neonatal mice. Moreover, this imprints long-term Th2 memory for pZP3, and mice develop rapid and intense Th2-mediated autoimmune response upon secondary challenge (Agersborg et al., 2001).

The pZP3-AOD model revealed unexpected mechanisms of autoAb induction and autoAb actions in tissue inflammation. Surprisingly, mice with ongoing pZP3-specific T cell response rapidly developed antibodies to antigenic determinants outside the pZP3 (Lou et al., 1996; Bagavant et al., 1999). Thus, when immunized with a truncated pZP3 lacking its native B cell epitope, mice develop ZP3 antibodies that recognize distant native B cell epitopes of ZP3, and the antibodies do not cross-react with the truncated pZP3. This amplified antibody response is driven by endogenous ovarian antigen as it is abrogated in mice with ovarian ablation. Thus autoreactive B cells to ovarian antigens are not tolerized but are normally "primed" by endogenous antigens. This discovery preceded the study on diversification of lupus autoantibody, and provided the first definitive evidence that endogenous antigens can drive diversified autoantibody response (Lou and Tung, 1993). Second, although ZP antibodies do not cause adult AOD, they influence the distribution of AOD induced by CD4$^+$ T cells. Atretic follicles in the ovarian interstitial space are the prime targets for pathogenic T cells, and T cell-mediated interstitial oophoritis is compatible with normal ovarian function (Bagavant et al., 1999). However, in the presence of ZP antibody, which binds to the oocytes in normal follicles, the T cell-mediated inflammation is "retargeted" to those ovarian follicles, leading to ovarian atrophy and infertility (Lou et al., 2000). The results from the experimental testis and ovarian models have provided insight into the pathogenetic role of autoAb in organ-specific autoimmunity. Although autoAb do not induce autoimmune disease when transferred to normal mice, they do so in "modified" recipients. This includes: (1) neonatal mice with unusual NK cell function and (2) recipients with ongoing T cell response, either by redirecting the T cells to new a new target within the organ, or by enhancing T cell mediated injury as in postvasectomy orchitis.

CLINICAL AUTOIMMUNE DISEASE OF THE OVARY

Premature ovarian insufficiency (POI) occurs in 1% of women before the age of 40 years, with amenorrhea, sex steroid deficiency, and elevated levels of gonadotropins (Conway, 2002; Rees and Purdie, 2006; Rebar, 2006; La Marca et al., 2010). POI has known genetic, developmental and environmental causes, but many POI cases are idiopathic. Kim et al. (1995) and Hoek et al. (1997) summarized the arguments for autoimmunity as a basis for idiopathic POI: circulating autoantibodies against ovarian targets, association with other autoimmune diseases, ovarian function recovery after immunosuppressive therapy, and ovarian lymphocytic infiltration.

Human autoimmune ovarian disease is best documented in POI patients with adrenal autoimmunity; they, in fact, produce antibody to antigens shared by the two organs (Hoek et al., 1997; Bakalov et al., 2005). Two to 10% of the POI cases show this association (LaBarbera et al., 1988; Betterle et al., 1993; Kim et al., 1997; Bakalov et al., 2002), which can manifest as part of the autoimmune polyglandular syndrome type 1

(APS-1) or type 2 (APS-2). APS-1 of early childhood is characterized by mucocutaneous candidiasis, hypoparathyroidism, and adrenal insufficiency, and the incidence of POI is found in 60% of APS-1 patients. APS-1 patients have mutations in the AIRE gene on chromosome 21 (Nagamine et al., 1997; The Finnish-German APECED Consortium, 1997). Although the prevalent paradigm that explains autoimmunity in APS patients is the incomplete deletion of autoreactive T cells, Kriegel et al. (2004) demonstrated that patients with this disease exhibit a defective Treg function. Antibodies against antigenic enzymes common to ovary and adrenal gland include: cytochrome P450 side-chain cleavage enzyme (P450SCC), 17-α hydroxylase/17, 20-lyase (CYP17A1), and 21-hydroxylase (CYP21). Indirect immunofluorescence on frozen adrenal gland sections, and CYP21 antibody detection by radioimmunoassays are sensitive diagnostic tests (Falorni et al., 2002a,b; Dal Pra et al., 2003). The theca cells of preantral and antral follicles are the main targets in some POI cases.

POI also occurs as an independent autoimmune ovarian disease, which can result in unsuccessful IVF–embryo transfer therapy. Recent studies have identified cognate antigenic peptides recognized by the serum antibodies from POI patients, including alpha actinin 4, heat shock 70 protein 5, and actin beta (Mande et al., 2011). Although they are not ovary specific, mice immunized with the peptides develop loss of ovarian structure and partial fertility reduction (Mande et al., 2012). In general, POI patients have a higher risk in autoimmune disease (Hoek et al., 1997); and some POI patients produce autoAb to antigens other than those of the steroidogenic cells (Hoek et al., 1997). The most common association is thyroid autoimmunity at 20% (Hoek et al., 1997; Kim et al., 1997); less common are autoimmune gastritis with parietal cell antibodies (4%), myasthenia gravis with acetylcholine receptor antibodies (2%), and/or insulin-dependent diabetes (2%) (Hoek et al., 1997; Kim et al., 1997).

Histopathologically, the ovaries from POI patients may show complete or partial loss of ovarian follicles (Hoek et al., 1997). Oophoritis is represented by infiltration of monocytes, lymphocytes (mainly effector CD4$^+$ T cells), macrophages, and plasma cells in the theca layer of large, antral follicles, while earlier stage follicles are consistently free of lymphocytic infiltration (Bakalov et al., 2005; La Marca et al., 2010). There is upregulation of class II MHC antigen expression in granulosa cells and an increase in the number of CD8$^+$ T cells and NK cells (Hill et al., 1990; Giglio et al., 1994; Wu et al., 2004). Because the primordial follicles are unaffected in POI, fertility may be partially conserved in autoimmune oophoritis, but may progress to severe POI and infertility (Gloor and Hurlimann, 1984; Bannatyne et al., 1990).

CONCLUDING REMARKS

EAO and AOD research has provided new approaches to investigate human gonadal autoimmunity and chronic inflammation of the gonads associated with subfertility and infertility. We have described the experimental autoimmune diseases that occur in animals with perturbed immune regulation, in this chapter. They include: d3tx, Treg depletion/vasectomy, AIRE deficiency, and transgenic HLA B27/β2m expression. In all instances, the testis and the ovary are among the few organs affected. Moreover, the major regulatory elements that have been perturbed are Treg and AIRE. We propose that the gonads, and their unique functions, demand exceptional protection from autoimmune destruction, and this requires the Treg. We also hypothesize that a unique Treg function may in fact be the protection of the continuum of physiological events in reproduction, which include gamete production, gamete transfer, embryo implantation, and maintenance of the pregnancy itself (Trowsdale and Betz, 2006; Mold et al., 2008; Guerin et al., 2009; Kahn and Baltimore, 2010; Samstein et al., 2012), to assure successful procreation.

ACKNOWLEDGMENTS

We wish to thank the following graduate students and postdoctoral fellows for their contribution to the chapter: Sallie Agersborg, Harini Bagavant, Kristina Garza, Vanesa Guazzone, Patricia Jacobo, Sabrina Jarazo-Dietrich, Yahuan Lou, Cecilia Pérez, Claudia Rival, Eileen Samy, Yulius Setiady, Hedy Smith, Cristian Sobarzo, María Theas, Karen Wheeler, and Terecita Yule.

REFERENCES

Agersborg, S.S., Garza, K.M., Tung, K.S., 2001. Intestinal parasitism terminates self tolerance and enhances neonatal induction of autoimmune disease and memory. Eur. J. Immunol. 31, 851–859.

Alard, P., Thompson, C., Agersborg, S.S., Thatte, J., Setiady, Y., Samy, E., et al., 2001. Endogenous oocyte antigens are required for rapid induction and progression of autoimmune ovarian disease following day-3 thymectomy. J. Immunol. 166, 4363–4369.

Anderson, M.S., Venanzi, E.S., Klein, L., Chen, Z., Berzins, S.P., Turley, S.J, et al., 2002. Projection of an immunological self shadow within the thymus by the aire protein. Science. 298, 1395–1401.

Ang, D.K., Brodnicki, T.C., Jordan, M.A., Wilson, W.E., Silveira, P., Gliddon, B.L., et al., 2007. Two genetic loci independently confer susceptibility to autoimmune gastritis. Int. Immunol. 19, 1135–1144.

Bagavant, H., Adams, S., Terranova, P., Chang, A., Kraemer, F.W., Lou, Y., et al., 1999. Autoimmune ovarian inflammation triggered by proinflammatory (Th1) T cells is compatible with normal ovarian function in mice. Biol. Reprod. 61, 635–642.

Bakalov, V.K., Vanderhoof, V.H., Bondy, C.A., Nelson, L.M., 2002. Adrenal antibodies detect asymptomatic auto-immune adrenal insufficiency in young women with spontaneous premature ovarian failure. Hum. Reprod. 17, 2096–2100.

Bakalov, V.K., Anasti, J.N., Calis, K.A., Vanderhoof, V.H., Premkumar, A., Chen, S., et al., 2005. Autoimmune oophoritis as a mechanism of follicular dysfunction in women with 46,XX spontaneous premature ovarian failure. Fertil. Steril. 84, 958–965.

Bannatyne, P., Russell, P., Shearman, R.P., 1990. Autoimmune oophoritis: a clinicopathologic assessment of 12 cases. Int. J. Gynecol. Pathol. 9, 191–207.

Betterle, C., Rossi, A., Dalla, P.S., Artifoni, A., Pedini, B., Gavasso, S., 1993. Premature ovarian failure: autoimmunity and natural history. Clin. Endocrinol. 39, 35–43.

Bigazzi, P., 1981. Immunologic effects of vasectomy in men and experimental animals. Prog. Clin. Biol. Res. 70, 461–476.

Chan, P.T., Schlegel, P.N., 2002a. Inflammatory conditions of the male excurrent ductal system.Part I. J. Androl. 23, 453–460.

Chan, P.T., Schlegel, P.N., 2002b. Inflammatory conditions of the male excurrent ductal system. Part II. J. Androl. 23, 461–469.

Cheng, M.H., Nelson, L.M., 2011. Mechanisms and models of immune tolerance breakdown in the ovary. Semin. Reprod. Med. 29, 308–316.

Cheng, M.H., Shum, A.K., Anderson, M.S., 2007. What's new in the Aire. Trends Immunol. 28, 321–327.

Conway, S., 2002. Primary ovarian failure. In: Wass, A.H., Shalet, S.M. (Eds.), Endocrinology and Diabetes. Oxford University Press, Oxford, UK, pp. 1107–1113.

Dal Pra, C., Chen, S., Furmaniak, J., Smith, B.R., Pedini, B., Moscon, A., et al., 2003. Autoantibodies to steroidogenic enzymes in patients with premature ovarian failure with and without Addison's disease. Eur. J. Endocrinol. 148, 565–570.

Dal Secco, V., Riccioli, A., Padula, F., Ziparo, E., Filippini, A., 2008. Mouse Sertoli cells display phenotypical and functional traits of antigen-presenting cells in response to interferon gamma. Biol. Reprod. 7, 234–242.

Dejucq, N., Jégou, B., 2001. Viruses in the mammalian male genital tract and their effects on the reproductive system. Microb. Mol. Biol. Rev. 65, 208–231.

Derbinski, J., Gabler, J., Brors, B., Tierling, S., Jonnakuty, S., Hergenhahn, M., et al., 2005. Promiscuous gene expression in thymic epithelial cells is regulated at multiple levels. J. Exp. Med. 202, 33–45.

Doncel, G.F., Di Paola, J.A., Lustig, L., 1989. Sequential study of the histopathology and cellular and humoral immune response during the development of an autoimmune orchitis in Wistar rats. Am. J. Reprod. Immunol. 20, 44–51.

Duan, Y.G., Yu, C.F., Novak, N., Bieber, T., Zhu, C.H., Schuppe, H.C., et al., 2011. Immunodeviation towards a Th17 immune response associated with testicular damage in azoospermic men. Int. J. Androl. 34, 536–545.

Dujardin, H.C., Burlen-Defranoux, O., Boucontet, L., Vieira, P., Cumano, A., Bandeira, A., 2004. Regulatory potential and control of Foxp3 expression in newborn CD4 + T cells. Proc. Natl. Acad. Sci. U.S.A. 101, 14473–14478.

D'Cruz, O.J., Haas, G.G., de La Rocha, R., Lambert, H., 1991. Ocurrence of serum antisperm antibodies in patients with cystic fibrosis. Fertil. Steril. 56, 519–527.

Erpenbach, K.H., 1991. Systemic treatment with interferon-alpha 2B: an effective method to prevent sterility after bilateral mumps orchitis. J. Urol. 146, 54–56.

Falorni, A., Laureti, S., Santeusanio, F., 2002a. Autoantibodies in autoimmune polyendocrine syndrome type II. Endocrinol. Metab. Clin. North Am. 31, 369–389.

Falorni, A., Laureti, S., Candeloro, P., Perrino, S., Coronella, C., Bizzarro, A., et al., 2002b. Steroid-cell auto-antibodies are preferentially expressed in women with premature ovarian failure who have adrenal autoimmunity. Fertil. Steril. 78, 270–279.

Fijak, M., Iosub, R., Schneider, E., Linder, M., Respondek, K., Klug, J., et al., 2005. Identification of immunodominant autoantigens in rat autoimmune orchitis. J. Pathol. 207, 127–138.

Fijak, M., Bhushan, S., Meinhardt, A., 2011a. Immunoprivileged sites: the testis. Methods Mol. Biol. 67, 459–470.

Fijak, M., Schneider, E., Klug, J., Bhushan, S., Hackstein, H., Schuler, G., et al., 2011b. Testosterone replacement effectively inhibits the development of experimental autoimmune orchitis in rats: evidence for a direct role of testosterone on regulatory T cell expansion. J. Immunol. 186, 5162–5172.

Finnish-German APECED Consortium, The, 1997. An autoimmune disease, APECED, caused by mutations in a novel gene featuring two PHD-type zinc-finger domains. Nat. Genet. 17, 393–398.

Fontenot, J.D., Gavin, M.A., Rudensky, A.Y., 2003. Foxp3 programs the development and function of CD4 + CD25 + regulatory T cells. Nat. Immunol. 4, 330–336.

Fountain, S., Holland, M.K., Hinds, L.A., Janssens, P.A., Kerr, P, 1997. Interstitial orchitis with impaired steroidogenesis and spermatogenesis in the testes of rabbits infected with an attenuated strain of myxoma virus. J. Reprod. Fertil. 110, 161–169.

Frayne, J., Hall, L., 1999. The potential use of sperm antigens as targets for immunocontraception: past, present and future. J. Reprod. Immunol. 43, 1–33.

Freund, J., Lipton, M.M., Thompson, G.E., 1953. Aspermatogenesis in guinea pig induced by testicular tissue and adjuvant. J. Exp. Med. 97, 711–725.

Garza, K.M., Tung, K.S., 1995. Frequency of molecular mimicry among T cell peptides as the basis for autoimmune disease and autoantibody induction. J. Immunol. 155, 5444–5448.

Giglio, T., Imro, M.A., Filaci, G., Scudeletti, M., Puppo, F., De Cecco, L., et al., 1994. Immune cell circulating subsets are affected by gonadal function. Life Sci. 54, 1305–1312.

Gloor, E., Hurlimann, J., 1984. Autoimmune oophoritis. Am. J. Clin. Pathol. 81, 105–109.

Goldacre, M.J., Wotton, C.J., Seagroatt, V., Yeates, D., 2007. Immune-related disease before and after vasectomy: an epidemiological database study. Hum. Reprod. 22, 1273–1278.

Griggs, N.D., Agersborg, S.S., Noelle, R.J., Ledbetter, J.A., Linsley, P. S., Tung, K.S., 1996. The relative contribution of the CD28 and gp39 costimulatory pathways in the clonal expansion and pathogenic acquisition of self-reactive T cells. J. Exp. Med. 1183, 801–810.

Guazzone, V., Denduchis, B., Lustig, L., 2005. Involvement of CD44 in testicular leukocyte recruitment in experimental autoimmune orchitis. Reproduction. 129, 603–609.

Guazzone, V.A., Jacobo, P., Theas, M.S., Lustig, L., 2009. Cytokines and chemokines in testicular inflammation: a brief review. Microsc. Res. Tech. 72, 620–628.

Guazzone, V.A., Hollwegs, S., Mardirosian, M., Jacobo, P., Hackstein, H., Wygrecka, M., et al., 2011. Characterization of dendritic cells in testicular draining lymph nodes in a rat model of experimental autoimmune orchitis. Int. J. Androl. 34, 276–289.

Guazzone, V.A., Jacobo, P., Denduchis, B., Lustig, L., 2012. Expression of cell adhesion molecules, chemokines and chemokine receptors involved in leukocyte traffic in rats undergoing autoimmune orchitis. Reproduction. 143, 651–662.

Guerin, L.R., Prins, J.R., Robertson, S.A., 2009. Regulatory T-cells and immune tolerance in pregnancy: a new target for infertility treatment? Hum. Reprod. Update. 15, 517–535.

Hardy, D.M., Garbers, D.L., 1994. Species-specific binding of sperm proteins to the extracellular matrix (zona pellucida) of the egg. J. Biol. Chem. 269, 19000–19004.

Head, J.R., Neaves, W.B., Billingham, R.E., 1983. Immune privilege in the testis. I. Basic parameters of allograft survival. Transplantation. 36, 423–431.

Hill, J.A., Welch, W.R., Faris, H.M., Anderson, D.J., 1990. Induction of class II major histocompatibility complex antigen expression in human granulosa cells by interferon gamma: a potential mechanism contributing to autoimmune ovarian failure. Am. J. Obstet. Gynaecol. 162, 534–540.

Hoek, A., Schoemaker, J., Drexhage, H.A., 1997. Premature ovarian failure and ovarian autoimmunity. Endocr. Rev. 18, 107–134.

Hori, S., Nomura, T., Sakaguchi, S., 2003. Control of regulatory T cell development by the transcription factor Foxp3. Science. 299, 1057–1061.

Hsieh, C.S., Lee, H.M., Lio, C.W., 2012. Selection of regulatory T cells in the thymus. Nat. Rev. Immunol. 12, 157–167.

Itoh, M., Hiramine, C., Hojo, K., 1991. A new murine model of autoimmune orchitis induced by immunization with viable syngeneic testicular germ cells alone. I. Immunological and histological studies. Clin. Exp. Immunol. 83, 137–142.

Itoh, M., Terayama, H., Naito, M., Ogawa, Y., Tainosho, S., 2005. Tissue microcircumstances for leukocytic infiltration into the testis and epididymis in mice. J. Reprod. Immunol. 67, 57–67.

Jacobo, P., Guazzone, V.A., Jarazo-Dietrich, S., Theas, M.S., Lustig, L., 2009. Differential changes in CD4 + and CD8 + effector and regulatory T lymphocyte subsets in the testis of rats undergoing autoimmune orchitis. J. Reprod. Immunol. 81, 44–54.

Jacobo, P., Guazzone, V.A., Pérez, C., Jarazo-Dietrich, S., Theas, M.S., Lustig, L., 2010. Functional studies of Foxp3 + regulatory T cells in autoimmune orchitis. Translational Biomed. 1 (3), 4 (Abstract).

Jacobo, P., Guazzone, V.A., Theas, M.S., Lustig, L., 2011b. Testicular autoimmunity. Autoimmun. Rev. 10, 201–204.

Jacobo, P.V., Pérez, C.V., Theas, M.S., Guazzone, V.A., Lustig, L., 2011a. CD4 + and CD8 + T cells producing Th1 and Th17 cytokines are involved in the pathogenesis of autoimmune orchitis. Reproduction. 141, 249–258.

Jahnukainen, K., Jorgensen, N., Pöllänen, P., Giwercman, A., Skakkebaek, N.E., 1995. Incidence of testicular mononuclear cell infiltrates in normal human males and in patients with germ cell neoplasia. Int. J. Androl. 18, 313–320.

Jarazo-Dietrich, S., Jacobo, P., Pérez, CV., Guazzone, V.A, Lustig, L., Theas, M.S., 2012. Up regulation of nitric oxide synthase–nitric oxide system in the testis of rats undergoing autoimmune orchitis. Immunobiology. 217, 778–787.

Johnson, M.H., 1973. Physiological mechanisms for the immunological isolation of spermatozoa. Adv. Reprod. Physiol. 6, 297–324.

Kahn, D.A., Baltimore, D., 2010. Pregnancy induces a fetal antigen-specific maternal T regulatory cell response that contributes to tolerance. Proc. Natl. Acad. Sci. USA. 107, 9299–9304.

Kim, J.G., Moon, S.Y., Chang, Y.S., Lee, J.Y., 1995. Autoimmune premature ovarian failure. J. Obstet. Gynaecol. 21, 59–66.

Kim, T.J., Anasti, J.N., Flack, M.R., Kimzey, L.M., Defensor, R.A., Nelson, L.M., 1997. Routine endocrine screening for patients with karyotypically normal spontaneous premature ovarian failure. Obstet. Gynecol. 89, 777–779.

Kisand, K., Peterson, P., 2011. Autoimmune polyendocrinopathy candidiasis ectodermal dystrophy: known and novel aspects of the syndrome. Ann. N.Y. Acad. Sci. 1246, 77–91.

Kohno, S., Munoz, J.A., Williams, T.M., Teuscher, C., Bernard, C.C.A., Tung, K.S.K., 1983. Immunopathology of murine experimental allergic orchitis. J. Immunol. 130, 2675–2682.

Kriegel, M.A., Lohmann, T., Gabler, C., Blank, N., Kalden, J.R., Lorenz, H.M., 2004. Defective suppressor function of human CD4 + CD25 + regulatory T cells in autoimmune polyglandular syndrome Type II. J. Exp. Med. 199, 1285–1291.

Kuroda, N., Mitani, T., Takeda, N., Ishimaru, N., Arakaki, R., Hayashi, Y., et al., 2005. Development of autoimmunity against transcriptionally unrepressed target antigen in the thymus of AIRE-deficient mice. J. Immunol. 174, 1862–1870.

La Marca, A., Brozzetti, A., Sighinolfi, G., Marzotti, S., Volpea, A., Falorni, A., 2010. Primary ovarian insufficiency: autoimmune causes. Curr. Opin. Obst. Gynecol. 22, 277–282.

LaBarbera, A.R., Miller, M.M., Ober, C., Rebar, R.W., 1988. Autoimmune etiology in premature ovarian failure. Am. J. Reprod. Immunol. Microbiol. 16, 115–122.

Le Goffic, R., Mouchel, T., Aubry, F., Patard, J.J., Ruffault, A., Jégou, B., et al., 2002. Production of the chemokines monocyte chemotactic protein-1, regulated on activation normal T cell expressed and secreted protein, growth-related oncogene, and interferon-γ-inducible protein-10 is induced by the Sendai virus in human and rat testicular cells. Endocrinology. 143, 1434–1440.

Lee, N.P., Cheng, C.Y., 2003. Regulation of Sertoli cell tight junction dynamics in the rat testis via the nitric oxide synthase/soluble guanylate cyclase/3′,5′-cyclic guanosine monophosphate/protein kinase G signaling pathway: an in vitro study. Endocrinology. 144, 3114–3129.

Lee, R., Goldstein, M., Ullery, B.W., Ehrlich, J., Soares, M., Razzano, R.A., et al., 2009. Value of serum antisperm antibodies in diagnosing obstructive azoospermia. J. Urol. 181, 264–269.

Lehmann, D., Temminch, D., Da Rugna, D., Leibundgut, B., Sulmoni, A., Muller, H.J., 1987. Role of immunological factors in male infertility: Immunohistochemical and serological evidence. Lab. Invest. 57, 21–28.

Lewis, J., 1993. Eosinophilic perifolliculitis: a variant of autoimmune oophoritis? Int. J. Gynecol. Pathol. 12, 360–364.

Li, N., Wang, T., Han, D., 2012. Structural, cellular and molecular aspects of immune privilege in the testis. Front. Immunol. 3, 152.

Lou, Y.H., Tung, K.S.K., 1993. T cell peptide of a self protein elicits autoantibody to the protein antigen: Implications for specificity and pathogenetic role of antibody in autoimmunity. J. Immunol. 151, 5790–5799.

Lou, Y.H., McElveen, M.F., Garza, K.M., Tung, K.S., 1996. Rapid induction of autoantibodies by endogenous ovarian antigens and activated T cells: implication in autoimmune disease pathogenesis and B cell tolerance. J. Immunol. 156, 3535–3540.

Lou, Y.H., Park, K.K., Agersborg, S., Alard, P., Tung, K.S., 2000. Retargeting T cell-mediated inflammation: a new perspective on autoantibody action. J. Immunol. 2164, 5251–5257.

Lu, Q., Gore, M., Zhang, Q., Camenisch, T., Boast, S., Casagranda, F., et al., 1999. Tyro-3 family receptors are essential regulators of mammalian spermatogenesis. Nature. 398, 723–728.

Luo, A.M., Garza, K.M., Hunt, D., Tung, K.S., 1993. Antigen mimicry in autoimmune disease sharing of amino acid residues critical for pathogenic T cell activation. J. Clin Invest. 92, 2117–2123.

Lustig, L., Doncel, G.F., Berensztein, E., Denduchis, B., 1987. Testis lesions, cell and humoral immune response induced in rats by immunization with laminin. Am. J. Reprod. Inmunol. Microbiol. 14, 123–128.

Lustig, L., Denduchis, B., Ponzio, R., Lauzon, M., Pelletier, R.M., 2000. Passive immunization with anti-laminin immunoglobulin G modifies the integrity of the seminiferous epithelium and induces arrest of spermatogenesis in the guinea pig. Biol. Reprod. 62, 1505–1514.

Maclaren, N., Chen, Q.Y., Kukreja, A., Marker, J., Zhang, C.H., Sun, Z.S., 2001. Autoimmune hypogonadism as part of an autoimmune polyglandular syndrome. J. Soc. Gynecol. Investig. 8 (1 Suppl Proceedings), S52–S54.

Mahi-Brown, C.A., Huang Jr., T.T., Yanagimachi, R., 1982. Infertility in bitches induced by active immunization with porcine zonae pellucidae. J. Exp. Zool. 222, 89–95.

Mande, P.V., Parikh, F.R., Hinduja, I., Zaveri, K., Vaidya, R., Gajbhiye, R., et al., 2011. Identification and validation of candidate biomarkers involved in human ovarian autoimmunity. Reprod. Biomed. 23, 471–483.

Mande, P.V., Thomas, S., Khan, S., Jadhav, S., Khole, V.V., 2012. Immunization with ovarian autoantigens leads to reduced fertility in mice following follicular dysfunction. Reproduction. 143, 309–323.

Marshburn, P.B., Kutteh, W.H., 1994. The role of antisperm antibody in infertility. Fertil. Steril. 5, 799–811.

McDonald, S.W., 1997. Is vasectomy harmful to health? Br. J. Gen. Pract. 47, 381–386.

Meinhardt, A., Hedger, M.P., 2011. Immunological, paracrine and endocrine aspects of testicular immune privilege. Mol. Cell. Endocrinol. 335, 60–68.

Melaine, N., Ruffault, A., Dejucq-Rainsford, N., Jégou, B., 2003. Experimental inoculation of the adult rat testis with Sendai virus: effect on testicular morphology and leukocyte population. Human Reprod. 18, 1574–1579.

Meng, J., Greenlee, A.R., Taub, C.J., Braun, R.E., 2011. Sertoli cell-specific deletion of the androgen receptor compromises testicular immune privilege in mice. Biol. Reprod. 85, 254–260.

Mital, P., Kaur, G., Dufour, J.M., 2010. Immunoprotective Sertoli cells: making allogeneic and xenogeneic transplantation feasible. Reproduction. 139, 485–504.

Mold, J.E., Michaëlsson, J., Burt, T.D., Muench, M.O., Beckerman, K.P., Busch, M.P., et al., 2008. Maternal alloantigens promote the development of tolerogenic fetal regulatory T cells in utero. Science. 322, 1562–1565.

Monteiro, J.P., Farache, J., Mercadante, A.C., Mignaco, J.A., Bonamino, M., Bonomo, A., 2008. Pathogenic effector T cell enrichment overcomes regulatory T cell control and generates autoimmune gastritis. J. Immunol. 181, 5895–5903.

Mouchel, T., Le Goffic, R., Patard, J.J., Samson, M., 2002. Le virus ourlien et l'orchite: vers une approche physiopathologique. Progr. Urol. 12, 124–128.

Mukasa, A., Hiromatsu, K., Matsuzaki, G., O'Brien, R., Born, W., Nomoto, K., 1995. Bacterial infection of the testis leading to autoaggressive immunity triggers apparently opposed responses of αβ and γδ T cells. J. Immunol. 155, 2047–2056.

Mukasa, A., Yoshida, H., Kobayashi, N., Matsuzaki, G., Nomoto, K., 1998. γδ T cells in infection-induced and autoimmune-induced testicular inflammation. Immunology. 95, 395–401.

Nagamine, K., Peterson, P., Scott, H., 1997. Positional cloning of the APECED gene. Nat. Genet. 17, 393–397.

Nishizuka, Y., Sakakura, T., 1969. Thymus and reproduction: sex-linked dysgenesia of the gonad after neonatal thymectomy in mice. Science. 166, 753–755.

Nistal, M., Riestra, M.L., Paniagua, R., 2002. Focal orchitis in undescended testes. Arch. Pathol. Lab. Med. 126, 64–69.

Noss, E.H., Brenner, M.B., 2008. The role and therapeutic implications of fibroblast-like synoviocytes in inflammation and cartilage erosion in rheumatoid arthritis. Immunol. Rev. 223, 252–270.

Pelletier, R.M., 1986. Cyclic formation and decay of the blood-testis barrier in the mink (Mustela vison), a seasonal breeder. Am. J. Anat. 175, 91–117.

Pelletier, R.M., Yoon, S.R., Akpovi, C.D., Silvas, E., Vitale, M.L., 2009. Defects in the regulatory clearance mechanisms favor the breakdown of self-tolerance during spontaneous autoimmune orchitis. Am. J. Physiol. Regul. Integr. Comp. Physiol. 296, 743–762.

Pérez, C.V., Sobarzo, C., Jacobo, P., Jarazo-Dietrich, S., Theas, M., Denduchis, B., et al., 2011. Impaired expression and distribution of adherens and gap junction proteins in the seminiferous tubules of rats undergoing autoimmune orchitis. Int. J. Androl. 34, e566–e577.

Pérez, C.V., Sobarzo, C.M., Jacobo, P.V., Pellizzari, E.H., Cigorraga, S. B., Denduchis, B., et al., 2012. Loss of occludin expression and impairment of blood-testis barrier permeability in rats with autoimmune orchitis: effect of interleukin 6 on Sertoli cell tight junctions. Biol Reprod. 87, 122.

Rebar, R.W., 2006. Premature ovarian failure. Obstet. Gynecol. 113, 1355–1363.

Rees, M., Purdie, D., 2006. Premature menopause. In: Management of the Menopause: The Handbook, fourth ed. Royal Society of Medicine Press Ltd., London, pp. 142–149.

Rhim, S.H., Millar, S.E., Robey, F., Luo, A.M., Lou, Y.H., Yule, T., et al., 1992. Autoimmune disease of the ovary induced by a ZP3 peptide from the mouse zona pellucida. J. Clin. Invest. 89, 28–35.

Rival, C., Theas, M.S., Guazzone, V.A., Lustig, L., 2006. Interleukin-6 and IL-6 receptor cell expression in testis of rats with autoimmune orchitis. J. Reprod. Immunol. 70, 43–54.

Rival, C., Theas, M.S., Suescun, M.O., Jacobo, P., Guazzone, V.A., van Rooijen, N., et al., 2008. Functional and phenotypic characteristics of testicular macrophages in experimental autoimmune orchitis. J. Pathol. 215, 108–117.

Rothlin, C.V., Ghosh, S., Zuniga, EI., Oldstone, M.B., Lemke, G., 2007. TAM receptors are pleiotropic inhibitors of the innate immune response. Cell. 131, 1124–1136.

Sakaguchi, S., Sakaguchi, N., Asano, M., Itoh, M., Toda, M., 1995. Immunologic self-tolerance maintained by activated T cells expressing IL-2 receptor alpha-chains (CD25). Breakdown of a single mechanism of self-tolerance causes various autoimmune diseases. J. Immunol. 155, 1151–1164.

Sakamoto, H., Himeno, K., Sanui, H., Yoshida, S., Nomoto, K., 1985. Experimental allergic orchitis in mice. I. A new model induced by immunization without adjuvants. Clin. Immunol. Immunopathol. 37, 360–368.

Salomon, F., Saremaslani, P.P., Jakob, M., Hedinger, C.F., 1982. Immune complex orchitis in infertile men. Lab. Invest. 47, 555–567.

Samstein, R.M., Josefowicz, S.Z., Arvey, A., Treuting, P.M., Rudensky, A.Y., 2012. Extrathymic generation of regulatory T cells in placental mammals mitigates maternal-fetal conflict. Cell. 150, 29–38.

Samy, E.T., Parker, L.A., Sharp, C.P., Tung, K.S., 2005. Continuous control of autoimmune disease by antigen-dependent polyclonal CD4 + CD25 + regulatory T cells in the regional lymph node. J. Exp. Med. 202, 771–781.

Samy, E.T, Setiady, Y.Y., Ohno, K., Pramoonjago, P., Sharp, C., Tung, K.S., 2006. The role of physiological self-antigen in the acquisition and maintenance of regulatory T-cell function. Immunol. Rev. 212, 170–184.

Samy, E.T., Wheeler, K.M., Roper, R.J., Teuscher, C., Tung, K.S.K., 2008. Cutting edge: autoimmune disease in day 3 thymectomized mice is actively controlled by endogenous disease-specific regulatory T cells. J. Immunol. 180, 4366–4370.

Schuppe, H.C., Meinhardt, A., Allam, J.P., Bergmann, M., Weidner, W., Haidl, G., 2008. Chronic orchitis: a neglected cause of male infertility? Andrologia. 40, 84–91.

Selawry, H.P., Cameron, D.F., 1993. Sertoli cell-enriched fractions in successful islet cell transplantation. Cell Transplant. 2, 123–129.

Setiady, Y., Pramoonjago, P., Tung, K.S., 2004. Requirements of NK cells and proinflammatory cytokines in T cell-dependent neonatal autoimmune ovarian disease triggered by immune complex. J. Immunol. 173, 1051–1058.

Setiady, Y.Y., Samy, E.T., Tung, K.S., 2003. Maternal autoantibody triggers de novo T cell-mediated neonatal autoimmune disease. J. Immunol. 170, 4656–4664.

Setiady, Y.Y., Ohno, K., Samy, E.T., Bagavant, H., Qiao, H., Sharp, C., et al., 2006. Physiologic self antigens rapidly capacitate autoimmune disease-specific polyclonal CD4 + CD25 + regulatory T cells. Blood. 107, 1056–1062.

Suescun, M.O., Rival, C., Theas, M.S., Calandra, R.S., Lustig, L., 2003. Involvement of tumor necrosis factor-alpha in the pathogenesis of autoimmune orchitis in rats. Biol. Reprod. 68, 2114–2121.

Suominen, J., Söderström, K.O., 1982. Lymphocyte infiltration in human testicular biopsies. Int. J. Androl. 5, 461–466.

Tardif, S., Wilson, M.D., Wagner, R., Hunt, P., Gertsenstein, M., Nagy, A., et al., 2010. Zonadhesin is essential for species specificity of sperm adhesion to the egg zona pellucida. J. Biol. Chem. 285, 24863–24870.

Taurog, J.D., 2009. Animal models of spondyloarthritis. Adv. Exp. Med. Biol. 649, 245–254.

Taurog, J.D., Rival, C., van Duivenvoorde, L.M., Satumtira, N., Dorris, M. L., Sun, M., et al., 2012. Autoimmune epididymo-orchitis is essential to the pathogenesis of male-specific spondyloarthritis in HLA-B27 transgenic rats. Arthritis Rheum. 64, 2518–2528.

Theas, M.S., Rival, C., Lustig, L., 2003. Germ cell apoptosis in autoimmune orchitis: involvement of the Fas-Fas L system. Am. J. Reprod. Immunol. 50, 166–176.

Theas, M.S., Rival, C., Jarazo-Dietrich, S., Guazzone, V.A., Lustig, L., 2006. Death receptor and mitochondrial pathways are involved in germ cell apoptosis in an experimental model of autoimmune orchitis. Hum. Reprod. 21, 1734–1742.

Theas, M.S., Rival, C., Jarazo-Dietrich, S., Jacobo, P., Guazzone, V.A., Lustig, L., 2008. Tumour necrosis factor-alpha released by testicular macrophages induces apoptosis of germ cells in autoimmune orchitis. Hum. Reprod. 23, 1865–1872.

Trowsdale, J., Betz, A.G., 2006. Mother's little helpers: mechanisms of maternal—fetal tolerance. Nat. Immunol. 7, 241—246.

Tung, K.S., 1978. Autoimmunity to sperm. Andrologia. 10, 247—249.

Tung, K.S., Ellis, L.E., Childs, G.V., Dufau, M., 1984. The dark mink: a model of male infertility. Endocrinology. 114, 922—929.

Tung, K.S.K, Unanue, E.R., Dixon, F.J., 1971a. Pathogenesis of experimental allergic orchitis. I. Transfer with immune lymph node cells. J. Immunol. 106, 1453—1462.

Tung, K.S.K., Unanue, E.R., Dixon, F.J., 1971b. Pathogenesis of experimental allergic orchitis. II. The role of antibody. J. Immunol. 106, 1463—1472.

Tung, K.S.K., Ellis, L., Teuscher, C., Meng, A., Blaustein, J.C., Kohno, S., et al., 1981. The black mink (Mustela vison): a natural model of immunologic male infertility. J. Exp. Med. 154, 1016—1032.

Tung, K.S.K., Yule, T.D., Mahi-Brown, C.A., Listrom, M.B., 1987. Distribution of histopathology and Ia positive cells in actively-induced and adoptively-transferred experimental autoimmune orchitis. J. Immunol. 138, 752—759.

Tung, K.S.K., Fusi, F., Teuscher, C., 2002. Autoimmune disease of the spermatozoa, ovary and testis. In: Theofilopoulos, A.N., Bona, C.A. (Eds.), The Molecular Pathology of Autoimmune Diseases. Taylor & Francis, New York, pp. 1031—1045.

Turek, P.J., Lipshultz, L.I., 1994. Immunologic infertility. Urol. Clin. North Am. 21, 447—468.

Villiger, P.M., Caliezi, G., Cottin, V., Forger, F., Senn, A., Ostensen, M., 2010. Effects of TNF antagonists on sperm characteristics in patients with spondyloarthritis. Ann. Rheum. Dis. 69, 1842—1844.

Voisin, G.A., Delauney, A., Barber, M., 1951. Sur les lesions tésticulaires provoqueés chez les cobayes par iso- et autosensibilisation. Ann. Inst. Pasteur. (Paris). 81, 48—63.

Wheeler, K.M., Samy, E.T., Tung, K.S., 2009. Cutting edge: normal regional lymph node enrichment of antigen-specific regulatory T cells with autoimmune disease-suppressive capacity. J. Immunol. 183, 7635—7638.

Wheeler, K.M., Tardif, S., Rival, C., Luu, B., Bui, E., Del Rio, R., et al., 2011. Regulatory T cells control tolerogenic versus autoimmune response to sperm in vasectomy. Proc. Natl. Acad. Sci. USA. 108, 7511—7516.

Wood, D.M., Liu, C., Dunbar, B.S., 1981. Effect of alloimmunization and heteroimmunization with zonae pellucidae on fertility in rabbits. Biol. Reprod. 25, 439—450.

Wu, R., Van der Hoek, K.H., Ryan, N.K., Norman, R.J., Robker, R.L., 2004. Macrophage contributions to ovarian function. Hum. Reprod. Update. 10, 119—133.

Xia, W., Wong, E.W., Mruk, D.D., Cheng, C.Y., 2009. TGF-beta 3 and TNF-alpha perturb blood—testis barrier (BTB) dynamics by accelerating the clathrin-mediated endocytosis of integral membrane proteins: a new concept of BTB regulation during spermatogenesis. Dev. Biol. 327, 48—61.

Yule, T.D., Tung, K.S.K., 1993. Experimental autoimmune orchitis induced by testis and sperm antigen-specific T cell clones: an important pathogenic cytokine is tumor necrosis factor. Endocrinology. 133, 1098—1107.

Part 14

Cardiovascular System and Lungs

Rheumatic Fever and Rheumatic Heart Disease

L. Guilherme[1,3] and J. Kalil[1,2,3]

[1]Heart Institute (InCor), School of Medicine, University of São Paulo, São Paulo, Brazil, [2]Clinical Immunology and Allergy Division, School of Medicine, University of São Paulo, São Paulo, Brazil, [3]Immunology Investigation Institute, National Institute for Science and Technology, University of São Paulo, São Paulo, Brazil

Chapter Outline

Clinical, Pathological, and Epidemiologic Features	**1023**		*CTLA4* Gene	1027
Autoimmune Features	**1024**		Both Innate and Adaptive Immune Response	1027
Genetic Features	**1024**		***In Vivo* and *In Vitro* Models**	**1027**
Innate Immune Response	1024		*In Vivo* Model of Myocarditis and Valvulitis	1027
MBL2 Gene	1024		*In Vitro* Model of Rheumatic Heart Disease Autoimmune	
TLR-2 Gene	1025		Reactions	1028
Ficolin Gene	1025		**Pathologic Effector Mechanisms**	**1028**
FcγRIIA Gene	1025		**Autoantibodies as Potential Immunologic Markers**	**1029**
Adaptive Immune Response	1025		**Concluding Remarks—Future Prospects**	**1030**
Major Histocompatibility Complex (MHC): *DRB1*,			**References**	**1030**
DRB3, DQB1, DQA1 Genes	1027			

CLINICAL, PATHOLOGICAL, AND EPIDEMIOLOGIC FEATURES

The clinical profile of rheumatic fever (RF) was first described by Cheadle in 1889 and the manifestation of the disease follows defined criteria established by Jones in 1944, which were updated in 1992 and remain useful today (Dajani et al., 1993). Briefly, the disease follows an untreated *S. pyogenes* infection in children and teenagers that present some genetic factors that predispose to the diverse clinical manifestations. The diagnosis is made on a clinical basis. The major manifestations include polyarthritis, carditis, chorea, subcutaneous nodules, and erythema marginatum. The minor manifestations are fever, arthralgia (clinical) and prolonged PR interval, increased erythrocyte sedimentation rate, and presence of C-reactive protein.

Polyarthritis and carditis are the most frequent manifestations of the disease and occur in around 70% of children. Arthritis is one of the earliest and most common

features of the disease, present in 60–80% of patients. It usually affects the peripheral large joints; small joints and the axial skeleton are rarely involved. Knees, ankles, elbows, and wrists are most frequently affected. The arthritis is usually migratory and very painful. Carditis is the most serious manifestation of the disease, occurring a few weeks after the infection, and usually present as a pancarditis. Endocarditis is the most severe sequel and frequently leads to chronic rheumathic heart disease (RHD). Mitral and aortic regurgitation are the most common events caused by valvulitis. Sydenham's chorea is less common (30–40%), characterized by involuntary movements, especially of the face and limbs, muscular weakness, and disturbances of speech, gait, and voluntary movements. It is usually a delayed manifestation, and often the sole manifestation of acute rheumatic fever. Other manifestations such as subcutaneous nodules and erythema marginatum can also occur during RF episodes and are characterized by nodules on the surface of joints and skin lesions, respectively (Mota et al., 2009).

N. Rose & I. Mackay (Eds): The Autoimmune Diseases, Fifth edition. DOI: http://dx.doi.org/10.1016/B978-0-12-384929-8.00069-1

Streptococcus pyogenes, or group A streptococcus, was identified in 1941 by Rebecca Lancefield through serology based on its cell wall polysaccharide that is composed of carbohydrates such as N-acetyl β-D-glucosamine linked to a polymeric rhamnose backbone. Group A streptococci contain M, T, and R surface proteins and lipoteichoic acid (LTA), involved in bacterial adherence to throat epithelial cells. The M protein, which extends from the cell wall, is composed of two polypeptide chains with approximately 450 amino acid residues, in an alpha-helical coiled-coil configuration. The amino-terminal (N-terminal) portion is composed of two regions, A and B, which present variable numbers of amino acid residues. The A region shows high polymorphism and defines the different M types, currently more than 225 according to CDC (Centers for Disease Control and Prevention, http://www.cdc.gov/ncidod/biotech/strep/strepblast.htm). The C-terminal portion (regions C and D) is highly conserved (Smeesters et al., 2010).

The incidence of ARF in some developing countries exceeds 50 per 100,000 children. The worldwide incidence of RHD is of at least 15.6 million cases and the major cause of around 233,000 deaths/year. However, since these estimates are based on conservative assumptions, the actual disease burden is probably substantially higher. The incidence of ARF can vary from 0.7 to 508 per 100,000 children per year in different populations from several countries (Carapetis et al., 2005). In Brazil, according to the WHO epidemiological model and data from IBGE (Brazilian Institute of Geography and Statistics), the number of streptococcal pharyngitis infections is around 10 million cases, which could lead to 30,000 new cases of RF, of which around 15,000 could develop to cardiac lesions (Barbosa et al., 2009).

AUTOIMMUNE FEATURES

RHD is the most serious complication of RF and depends on several host factors that mediate a heart tissue-driven autoimmune response triggered by a defensive immune response against *S. pyogenes*.

Genetic predisposition is one of the leading factors contributing to the development of autoimmunity. In the last 5 years, using molecular biology tools, several new single nucleotide polymorphisms of genes involved with the activation of both innate and adaptive immune responses were associated with the development of RF/RHD (see Genetic Features).

The first genetic associations described in the 1980s focused on HLA class II alleles coded by HLA-DRB1 and DQB1 genes. The HLA class II molecules are expressed in the surface of antigen-presenting cells (APCs), e.g., macrophages, dendritic cells, and B lymphocytes, and trigger

activation of the immune system. In the case of RF/RHD, T cell populations activated upon specific self antigen stimulation will trigger autoimmune reactions. The production of several inflammatory cytokines will perpetuate the heart-tissue damage. These observations are corroborated by the fact that during the acute phase of disease, Aschoff bodies, a granulomatous lesion containing macrophages, Anitschkow cells, multinucleated cells, and polymorphonuclear leukocytes develop in the myocardium and/or endocardium of RHD patients. Inflammatory cytokines such as IL-1, TNF-alpha, and IL-2 have been found, depending on the developmental phase of the Aschoff bodies (Fraser et al., 1997) and as mentioned above, probably initiate the inflammatory process leading to heart tissue rheumatic lesions.

More recently, other molecules were described involved with the inflammatory process like integrins and chemokines and cytokines such as IFN-gamma, IL-23, and IL-17 that play a role in the recruitment of both T and B lymphocytes leading to the autoimmune reactions observed in rheumatic heart lesions (reviewed by Guilherme et al., 2011). T and B lymphocytes react against self antigens through molecular mimicry, first in the periphery and later in the heart tissue. The mechanisms of T cell receptor degeneracy and epitope spreading amplifies the autoimmune reactions (see Pathologic Effector Mechanisms). All these steps are represented in Figure 69.1.

GENETIC FEATURES

RF and RHD occur in 1 to 5% of untreated children with genetic predisposition. The disease is associated with several genes, some of which are related to the innate or adaptive immune response or both (Table 69.1).

In order to facilitate the comprehension of the role of implicated genes known up to now, we describe the associated genes/alleles based on their role.

Innate Immune Response

MBL2 Gene

MBL (mannan-binding lectin) is an acute phase inflammatory protein and functions as a soluble pathogen recognition receptor. It binds to a wide variety of sugars on the surface of pathogens and plays a major role in innate immunity due to its ability to opsonize pathogens, enhancing their phagocytosis and activating the complement cascade via the lectin pathway (Jack et al., 2001). Different variants of the promoter and exon 1 regions of the *MBL2* gene, which encodes mannan-binding lectin, have been reported in patients with RF/RHD. Interestingly, the A allele that codes for high production of MBL was associated with development of mitral

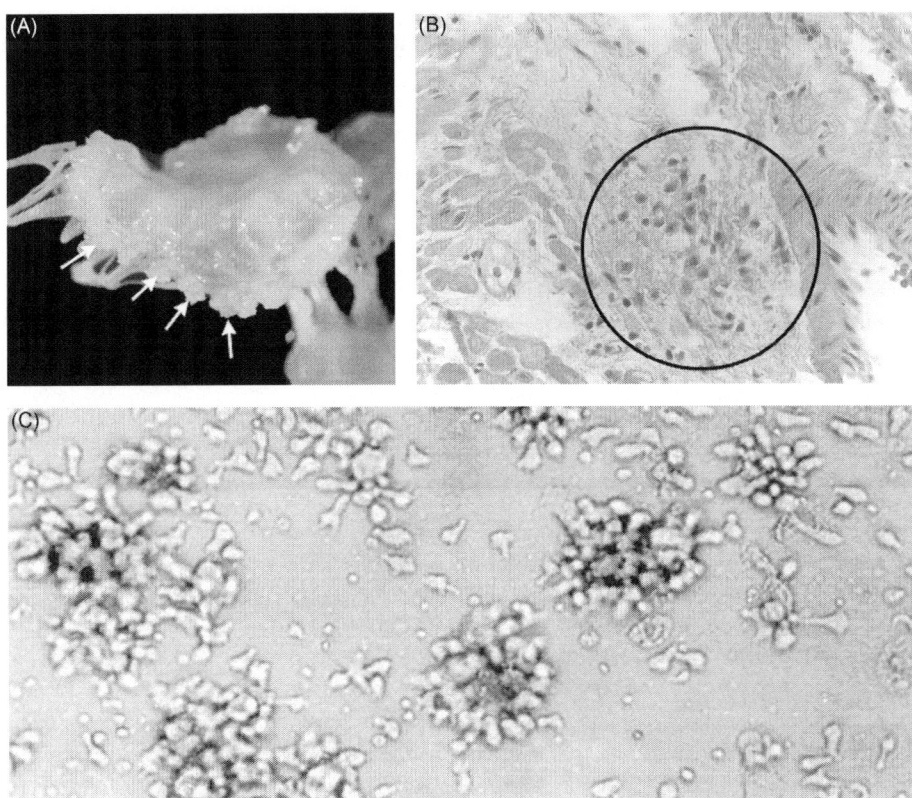

FIGURE 69.1   Acute phase rheumatic lesions (A and B) and cultured intralesional T lymphocytes (C).

stenosis (MS) and most of these patients presented high serum levels of MBL (Messias-Reason et al., 2006). In contrast, RHD patients with aortic regurgitation (AR) presented the O allele that codes for low production of MBL, and the patients presented low serum levels of MBL (Ramasawmy et al., 2008).

TLR-2 Gene

Toll-like receptors (TLRs) are sensors of foreign microbial products, which initiate host defense responses in multicellular organisms. A polymorphism of TLR-2 at codon 753 generally leads to the replacement of arginine with glutamine. The genotype 753Arg/Gln was more frequent in a Turkish ARF cohort when compared to controls (Berdeli et al., 2005).

Ficolin Gene

Ficolins trigger the innate immune response by either binding collectin cellular receptors or initiating the complement lectin pathway (Meassias-Reason et al., 2009). In Brazilian chronic RHD patients, with prolonged time of infection or repeated streptococcal infections, the haplotype G/G/A (-986/-602/-4) was found to be more frequent

than in controls, and was also correlated with low expression levels of this protein.

FcγRIIA Gene

This protein plays a role in the clearance of immune complexes by macrophages, neutrophils, and platelets (Hirsch et al., 1996). ARF patients presented histidine (H) in the codon 131, which typically encodes for argenin (A); consequently RF/RHD patients present a protein with low binding capacity to the immune complex, favoring the inflammatory response.

Adaptive Immune Response

The HLA (human leukocytes antigens) system is located in the short arm of the human chromosome 6 and codes for diverse proteins; it is considered the most polymorphic system, composed of several genes with several alleles. The class I proteins are present in all nucleated cells; however, the class II are expressed only in specialized cells of the immune system (B lymphocytes, activated T lymphocytes, monocytes/macrophages, and dendritic cells). These proteins are involved with antigen recognition and presentation of self and foreign (microbes) antigens.

TABLE 69.1　Genetic Polymorphism Associated with Development of RF/RHD

Immune response	Gene	Chromosome localization	Polymorphism	Allele/Genotype/Haplotype associated with disease	Clinical picture	Population studied	References
INNATE	MBL-2	10q11.2-q21	−221 X,YA (52C, 54G, 57G), O (52T, 54A, 57A)	YA/YA, YA/XA	RHD-MS	Brazilian	Messias-Reason et al. (2006)
			A (52C, 54G, 57G), O (52T, 54A, 57A)	O, O/O	RHD-AR	Brazilian	Ramasawmy et al. (2008)
	TLR-2	4q32	2258A/G (753 Arg/Gln)	753Gln, Arg753Gln	ARF	Turkish	Berdeli et al. (2005)
	FCN-2	9q34	−986G/A, −602G/A, −4G/A	G/G/A	RHD	Brazilian	Messias-Reason et al. (2009)
	FCγRIIA	1q21-q23	494A/G (131H/R)	131R, R/R (high risk), R/H (intermediate risk)	ARF	Turkish	Hirsch et al. (1996)
ADAPTIVE	MHC	6p21.31	DRB1, DRB3, DQB1, DQA1	Several alleles	RF/RHD	Several	Guilherme et al. (2011) (review)
	CTLA-4	2q33.2	+49A/G	G/G	RHD	Turkish	Düzgün et al. (2009)
BOTH INNATE and ADAPTIVE	TNF-α	6p21.3	−308G/A	A	RHD	Mexican	Hernandez-Pacheco et al. (2003a)
				A/A, G/G	RHD- MVL, MVD	Egyptian	Sallakci et al. (2005)
				A	ARF/RHD	Brazilian	Ramasawmy et al. (2007)
				A	ARF/RHD	Turkish	Berdeli et al. (2006)
			−238G/A	G, G/G	RHD	Mexican	Hernandez-Pacheco et al. (2003b)
				A	ARF/RHD	Brazilian	Ramasawmy et al. (2007)
	IL-1RA	2q14.2	A1, A2, A3, A4	A1/A1	RHD	Egyptian	Settin et al. (2007)
				A1, A1/A1	RHD	Brazilian	Azevedo et al. (2010)
	TGF-β1	19q13.1	−509C/T	T, T/T	RHD	Egyptian	Kamal et al. (2010)
			869T/C	C/C	RHD	Egyptian	Chou et al. (2004)
	IL-10	1q31-q32	−1082G/A	G/G	RHD-MVD	Egyptian	Settin et al. (2007)
				A/A	RHD-MVL	Egyptian	Settin et al. (2007)

MHC: major histocompatibility complex; TNF-α: tumor necrosis factor alpha; TGF-β: transforming growth factor beta; IL-1RA: IL-1 receptor antagonist; MBL: mannan binding lectin; TLR-2: Toll-like receptor 2; FCN-2: ficolin 2; FCγRIIA: IgG Fc receptor; CTLA-4: cytotoxic T cell lymphocyte antigen 4; ARF: acute rheumatic fever; RHD: rheumatic heart disease; AR: aortic regurgitation; MS: mitral stenosis; MVD: mitral valve disease; MVL: multivalvular lesions.

Major Histocompatibility Complex (MHC): *DRB1, DRB3, DQB1, DQA1* Genes

Several HLA class II alleles have been described in association with RF/RHD. Patarroyo et al. (1979) described an alloantigen on the surface of B cells, designated 883, probably related to the HLA class II molecules, which was present in a high frequency in RF patients. Later, a monoclonal antibody (D8/17 MoAb) was produced against B cells from RF patients bearing the 883 alloantigen. Studies performed by Zabriskie et al. (1985) showed an increased frequency of this alloantigen in RF patients.

The susceptibility of developing RF/RHD was first associated with alleles of HLA class II genes (*DRB1, DRB3, DQB, and DQA*), which are located on human chromosome 6 (Table 69.1). Briefly, HLA-DR7 was the allele most consistently associated with RF (Guilherme et al., 1991; Ozkan et al., 1993; Weidebach et al., 1994, Guedez et al., 1999; Visanteiner et al., 2000; Stanevicha et al., 2003). In addition, the association of DR7 with different DQ-B or DQ-A alleles seems to be related to the development of multiple valvular lesions (MVL) or mitral valve regurgitation (MVR) in RHD patients (Guedez et al., 1999; Stanevicha et al., 2003). HLA-DR53 coded by the *DRB3* gene is another HLA class II molecule in linkage disequilibrium with HLA-DR4, DR7, and DR9. This allele was strongly associated with RF/RHD in two studies with Mulatto Brazilian patients (Guilherme et al., 1991; Weidebach et al., 1994), but not in Brazilian Caucasian patients (Visanteiner et al., 2000). Although DR53 has not been described in previous studies, DR4 and DR9 were associated with RF in American Caucasian and Arabian patients (Ayoub, 1984; Rajapkase et al., 1987), whereas in Egyptian and Latvian patients, DR7 was associated with the disease (Guedez et al., 1999; Stanevicha et al., 2003) (Table 69.1). In Japanese RHD patients, susceptibility to mitral stenosis seems to be in part controlled by the HLA-DQA gene or by genes in close disequilibrium linkage with HLA-DQA*0104 and DQB1*05031 (Koyanagi et al., 1996). HLA-DQA*0501 DQB*0301 with DRB1*1601 (DR2) were associated with RHD in a Mexican Mestizo population (Hernandez-Pacheco et al., 2003a).

The molecular mechanism by which MHC class II molecules confer susceptibility to autoimmune diseases is not clear. However, since the role of HLA molecules is to present antigens to the T cell receptor, it is probable that the associated alleles facilitate the presentation of some streptococcal peptides that will later trigger autoimmune reactions mediated by molecular mimicry mechanisms.

CTLA-4 Gene

This gene is an essential inhibitor of T cell responses. It is a strong candidate susceptibility gene in autoimmunity and several studies suggest disease-associated polymorphisms (reviewed by Gough et al., 2005).

Both Innate and Adaptive Immune Response

More recently, with new technologies that have allowed the description of gene variability by single nucleotide polymorphisms (SNPs), other associations have been established that could clarify some reactions related to both the innate and the adaptive immune response leading the autoimmune reactions in RF/RHD.

- *TNF-α* gene, also located in the chromosome 6, between HLA class I and II genes, codes for a proinflammatory cytokine that plays a role during the *S. pyogenes* infection and later in the inflammatory process in the valves. Polymorphisms at -308 G/A and -238 G/A were associated with the susceptibility of RHD patients from several countries (Hernandez-Pacheco et al., 2003b; Sallakci et al., 2005; Berdeli et al., 2006; Ramasawmy et al., 2007).

- *IL-10* gene is responsible for the production of IL-10, an anti-inflammatory cytokine. The genotype -1082 G/A, misrepresented in RHD patients, is apparently associated with the development of multivalvular lesions (MVL) and with the severity of RHD (Settin et al., 2007).

- *TGF-B1* is a gene that controls the proliferation and differentiation of cells. The polymorphisms of both the SNPs 869 T and -509 T alleles were considered as possible risk factors for the development of valvular RHD lesions in Egyptian and Taiwanese RHD patients (Chou et al., 2004; Kamal et al., 2010).

- *IL-1Ra* gene, for which the most frequent alleles are 1 and 2, encodes the antagonist of IL-1α and IL-1β, which are inflammatory cytokines. Two studies in Brazilian and Egyptian RHD patients with severe carditis showed low frequencies of allele 1, suggesting lack of inflammatory control (Settin et al., 2007; Azevedo et al., 2010).

IN VIVO AND *IN VITRO* MODELS

In Vivo Model of Myocarditis and Valvulitis

Humans are unique hosts for *S. pyogenes* infections. However, several studies have been performed to determine a suitable animal model and numerous different species (mice, rats, hamsters, rabbits, and primates) have been tested for the development of autoimmune reactions that resemble those observed in RF/RHD patients (Unny and Middlebrooks, 1983), all with little success.

In the last decade, a model that appears to be useful for the study of RF/RHD has been developed with Lewis rats. These rats have already been used to induce experimental autoimmune myocarditis and to study the pathogenesis of RF/RHD (Li et al., 2004)

Immunization of Lewis rats with recombinant M6 protein induced focal myocarditis, myocyte necrosis, and valvular heart lesions in three out of six animals. The disease in these animals included verruca-like nodules and the presence of Anitschkow cells, which are large macrophages (also known as caterpillar cells), in mitral valves. Lymph node cells from these animals showed a proliferative response against cardiac myosin, but not skeletal myosin or actin. A CD4$^+$ T cell line responsive to both the M protein and cardiac myosin was also obtained. Taken together, these results confirmed the cross-reactivity between the M protein and cardiac myosin triggered by molecular mimicry, as observed in humans, possibly causing a break in tolerance and consequently leading to autoimmunity (Quin et al., 2001).

In another study done by the same group, Lewis rats were immunized with a pool of synthetic peptides from the conserved region of the M5 protein. Mononuclear spleen cells from these animals were able to proliferate in response to peptides from both the C-terminal region of M5 protein and the N-terminal region of a heterologous protein (M1) and myosin. These rats developed focal infiltration of mononuclear cells predominantly in the aortic valve, although no evidence of Aschoff bodies, the hallmark of RF lesions, or Anitschkow cells was observed (Lymbury et al., 2003).

Another study immunized Lewis rats with recombinant M5 or synthetic peptides from the B- and C-regions of GAS M5 (Gorton et al., 2009). Sera and T cells from these animals recognized a peptide (M5-B.6) from the B-repeat of the N-terminal portion of M5 protein and induced heart lesions (Gorton et al., 2010), confirming the previous results. The immunized rats (five out of seven) developed mononuclear cell infiltration in the myocardial or valvular tissue. Histopathological analysis of valve lesions showed the presence of both CD4$^+$ T cells and CD68$^+$ macrophages (Gorton et al., 2010), consistent with human studies (Guilherme et al., 1995).

Altogether, these studies indicated that the Lewis rats could be a model of autoimmune valvulitis.

In Vitro Model of Rheumatic Heart Disease Autoimmune Reactions

The major sequels of rheumatic fever are heart tissue lesions that lead to chronic rheumatic heart disease, which is characterized by permanent valvular lesions. The heart disease starts by pericarditis, followed by myocarditis episodes in which the healing process results in varied degrees of valvular damage (Mota et al., 2009).

By isolating infiltrating T lymphocytes from damaged valvular tissue, we could establish the mechanism by which the immune response in the heart leads to autoimmune reactions (Guilherme et al., 1995). Figure 69.1 shows a damaged mitral valve in which verrucae lesions are observed, indicative of an acute rheumatic fever episode. Furthermore, the presence of Aschoff bodies in the myocardium tissue allowed for histological diagnosis of an active episode of rheumatic disease. *In vitro* tissue culture of small pieces of the surgical fragment allowed the isolation of infiltrating T cells.

The *in vitro* analysis of these tissue infiltrating T cells showed their ability to recognize several streptococcal-M protein peptides and self antigens by molecular mimicry mechanisms. We identified some mitral valve-derived proteins such as vimentin, PDIA3 (protein disulfide isomerase ER-60 precursor), and HSPA5 (78 kDa glucose-regulated protein precursor) that were recognized by both peripheral and intralesional T cell clones (Faé et al., 2008).

The identification of heart-M protein cross-reactive T cell clones directly from rheumatic valvular lesions established their involvement in the pathogenesis of the disease.

PATHOLOGIC EFFECTOR MECHANISMS

The term "molecular mimicry" was introduced in 1964 by Damian to define the mechanism by which self antigens are recognized after an infection by cross-reactivity (Damian, 1964).

Pathogen and self antigens can be recognized by T lymphocytes and antibodies through molecular mimicry by four different mechanisms. They can recognize (1) identical amino acid sequences, (2) homologous but non-identical sequences, (3) common or similar amino acid sequences of different molecules (proteins, carbohydrates), and (4) structural similarities between the microbe or environmental agent and its host (Peterson and Fujinami, 2007).

RF/RHD is the most convincing example of molecular mimicry in human pathological autoimmunity, in light of the cross-reactions between streptococcal antigens and human tissue proteins, mainly heart tissue proteins, that follow throat infection by *S. pyogenes* in susceptible individuals.

The inflammatory process that follows an *S. pyogenes* throat infection in individuals with genetic predisposition leads to intense cytokine production by monocytes and macrophages that trigger the activation of B and T lymphocytes.

Several heart-reactive antibodies described from 1945 until nowadays (reviewed by Cunningham, 2000 and Guilherme et al., 2011) also play role in the development of the disease.

Streptococcal and heart tissue cross-reactive antibodies activate the heart tissue valvular endothelial cells, increasing the expression of adhesion molecules such as VCAM1, which facilitates cellular infiltration by neutrophils, monocytes, B and T cells (Yegin et al., 1997) The "rolling" of leukocytes through vessels is triggered by chemokines expressed by activated endothelial cells that induce the expression of integrins, selectins, and subsequent trans-endothelial migration. Recently we identified increased expression of ICAM, another adhesion molecule, and a few chemokines (CCL-1, CCL-3, and CCL9), as well as some integrins (P- and E-selectins) in the myocardium and valvular tissue of RHD patients (Guilherme, L. in preparation). All of these molecules are involved with the inflammatory process and T and B lymphocyte infiltration leading to rheumatic valvular tissue damage.

CD4$^+$ infiltrating T cells are predominant in heart rheumatic lesions (Raizada et al., 1983; Kemeny et al., 1989), and the first evidence of the molecular mimicry between streptococcus and heart tissue was obtained through an analysis of these heart tissue-infiltrating T cells. Three immunodominant regions of the M5 protein (residues 1−25, 81−103, and 163−177), heart tissue proteins (myocardium and valve-derived proteins, as well as vimentin), and synthetic peptides of the beta chain of cardiac myosin-light meromyosin region (LMM) were recognized by cross-reactivity by intralesional T cell clones (Guilherme et al., 1995, 2001; Ellis et al., 2005; Faé et al., 2006). Peripheral T cell clones also recognized human purified myosin, tropomyosin, laminin, and cardiac myosin-derived peptides from LMM and S2 regions (Guilherme et al., 1995).

Employing a proteomics approach, we characterized a number of mitral valve proteins identified by molecular weight (MW) and isoelectric point (pI). Four valve-derived proteins with molecular masses ranging between 52 and 79 kDa and different pI cross-reacted with the M5 immunodominant peptides, and were recognized in proliferation assays by intralesional T cell clones from patients with severe RHD. Vimentin was one of the identified proteins, a result that reinforces the role of this protein as a putative autoantigen involved in the rheumatic lesions. Novel heart tissue proteins were also identified, including disulfide isomerase ER-60 precursor (PDIA3) protein and a 78-kDa glucose-regulated protein precursor (HSPA5). The role of PDIA3 in RHD pathogenesis and other autoimmune diseases is not clear (Table 69.2) (Faé et al., 2008).

The analysis of the T cell receptors (TCRs) of autoreactive T lymphocytes that infiltrate both myocardium and valves allowed us to evaluate the Vβ chains usage of TCR and the degree of clonality of heart tissue infiltrating T cells (Guilherme et al., 2000). In the heart tissue (myocardium and valves) of both chronic and acute RHD patients, several expanded T cell populations with an oligoclonal profile were found. Such oligoclonal expansions were identified by T cell receptor (TCR) analyses (Guilherme et al., 2000). The finding of oligoclonal T cell populations is in contrast with the peripheral blood scenario, which contains polyclonal TCR-BV families. The fact that a high number of T cell oligoclonal expansions could be found in the valvular tissue indicates that specific and cross-reactive T cells migrate to the valves (Guilherme et al., 2000) and proliferate upon specific cytokine stimulation at the site of the lesions.

Cytokines are important secondary signals following an infection because they trigger effective immune responses in most individuals and probably deleterious responses in patients with autoimmune diseases. Three subsets of T helper cytokines are currently described. Antigen-activated CD4$^+$ T cells polarize to the Th1, Th2, or Th17 subsets, depending on the cytokine secreted. Th1 is involved with the cellular immune response and produces IL-2, IFN-γ, and TNF-α. Th2 cells mediate humoral and allergic immune responses and produce IL-4, IL-5, and IL-13.

Another lineage of CD4$^+$ T cells, namely Th17 cells, have been more recently described and produce a complex set of cytokines initially identified as IL-17, TGF-β, IL-6, and IL-23. This subset of cells has been described in and associated with several autoimmune diseases (reviewed by Volin and Shahrara, 2011).

In RHD in both myocardium and valvular tissue, we found large numbers of infiltrating mononuclear cells secreting the inflammatory cytokines IFN-γ and TNF-α. However, mononuclear cells secreting IL-10 and IL-4, which are regulatory cytokines, were also found in the myocardium tissue; nonetheless, in the valvular tissue, only a few cells secrete IL-4, suggesting that low numbers of IL4-producing cells may contribute to the progression of valvular RHD lesions (Guilherme et al., 2004).

Recently, using immunohistochemistry, we identified IL-17$^+$ and IL-23$^+$ infiltrating cells in both myocardium and valvular tissue. The expression of these cytokines was also observed in the valvular endothelium (manuscript in preparation), confirming that Th17 cells also play an important role in the inflammatory process in RHD heart lesions.

AUTOANTIBODIES AS POTENTIAL IMMUNOLOGIC MARKERS

Several streptococcal and human cross-reactive antibodies have been found in the sera of RF patients and immunized rabbits and mice over the last 50 years and have been recently reviewed (Cunningham, 2000; Guilherme

TABLE 69.2 Mitral Valve Proteins Identified by 2D Gel Electrophoresis and Mass Spectrometry Analysis Recognized by Peripheral and Intralesional T Cells

Protein	Accession number	Coverage (%)	Masses matched/total	MW/pI
Vimentin	P08670	34	20/23	53.0/5.4 53.7/5.1
Vimentin	P08670	49	23/87	51.0/5.9
PDIA3 Protein disulfide isomerase	P30101	45	19/92	56.0/6.7
ER-60 precursor				56.0/6.0
HSPA5 78 kDa glucose-regulated protein precursor	P11021	43	27/69	68.0/5.9

MW: molecular weight; pI: isoelectrical point; coverage (%): percentage of matched peptides identification in terms of amino acid residues.
Adapted from Faé et al., 2008.

et al., 2004). N-acetyl β-D-glucosamine, which is present in both the streptococcal cell wall and heart valvular tissue, is one of the major targets of the humoral response in RF/RHD, and antibodies against this polysaccharide displayed cross-reactivity with laminin, an extracellular matrix alpha-helical coiled-coil protein that surrounds heart cells and is also present in the valves (Cunningham et al., 1989; Cunningham, 2000).

Cardiac myosin is the most important protein in the myocardium and by using affinity purified anti-myosin antibodies, Cunningham's group identified a five amino acid residue (Gln-Lys-Ser-Lys-Gln) epitope of the N-terminal M5 and M6 proteins as being cross-reactive with cardiac myosin (Cunningham et al., 1989).

The permanent rheumatic lesions that damage the valves and antibodies against vimentin, an abundant protein in the valvular tissue, probably play a role in the valvular lesions (Cunningham, 2000).

In conclusion, antibodies against N-acetyl β-D-glucosamine, some epitopes of cardiac myosin, and vimentin can be considered as immunological markers of the disease.

CONCLUDING REMARKS—FUTURE PROSPECTS

RF/RHD is the most convincing example of molecular mimicry in which the response against *S. pyogenes* triggers autoimmune reactions with human tissues. RF/RHD lesions result from a complex network of several genes that control both innate and adaptive immune responses after an *S. pyogenes* throat infection. An inflammatory process permeates the development of heart lesions, in which adhesion molecules and specific chemokines facilitate the valvular tissue infiltration by B and T cells. CD4⁺ T lymphocytes are the prime effectors of heart lesions. Several self antigens such as vimentin, myosin, and other mitral valve-derived proteins are recognized by molecular mimicry of streptococcal immunodominant peptides, particularly in individuals with genetic predisposition. Production of inflammatory cytokines (IFN-γ, TNF-α, IL-17, and IL-23), and low numbers of IL-4 producing cells, a regulatory cytokine, lead to local inflammation.

All this information creates a new scenario for the development of RHD, opening new possibilities for immunotherapy. Molecular knowledge of the autoimmune reactions mediated by intralesional T cells will certainly assist in the choice of streptococcal protective epitopes for the construction of an effective and safe vaccine.

REFERENCES

Ayoub, E.M., 1984. The search for host determinants of susceptibility to rheumatic fever: the missing link. T. Duckett Jones Memorial Lecture. Circulation. 69, 197–201.

Azevedo, P.M., Bauer, R., de Caparbo, V.F., Silva, C.A., Bonfá, E., Pereira, R.M., 2010. Interleukin-1 receptor antagonist gene (IL1RN) polymorphism possibly associated to severity of rheumatic carditis in a Brazilian cohort. Cytokine. 49, 109–113.

Barbosa, P.J.B., Muller, R.E., Latado, A., Achutti, A.C., Ramos, A.I.O., Weksler, C., et al., 2009. Brazilian guidelines for diagnostis, treatment and prevention of rheumatic fever. Arq. Bras. Cardiol. 93, 1–18.

Berdeli, A., Celik, H.A., Ozyürek, R., Dogrusoz, B., Aydin, H.H., 2005. TLR-2 gene Arg753Gln polymorphism is strongly associated with acute rheumatic fever in children. J. Mol. Med. 83, 535–541.

Berdeli, A., Tabel, Y., Celik, H.A., Ozyurek, R., Dogrusoz, B., Aydin, H.H., et al., 2006. Lack of association between TNFalpha gene polymorphism at position −308 and risk of acute rheumatic fever in Turkish patients. Scand. J. Rheumatol. 35, 44–47.

Carapetis, J.R., Steer, A.C., Mulholland, E.K., Weber, M., 2005. The global burden of group A streptococcal disease. Lancet Infect. Dis. 5, 685–694.

Chou, H.T., Chen, C.H., Tsai, C.H., Tsai, F.J., 2004. Association between transforming growth factor-beta1 gene C-509T and T869C polymorphisms and rheumatic heart disease. Am. Heart J. 148, 181–186.

Cunningham, M.W., 2000. Pathogenesis of group A streptococcal infections. Clin. Microbiol. Rev. 13, 470–511.

Cunningham, M.W.., McCormack, J.M., Fenderson, P.G., Ho, M.K., Beachey, E.H., Dale, J.B., 1989. Human and murine antibodies cross-reactive with streptococcal M protein and myosin recognize the sequence GLN-LYS-SER-LYS-GLN in M protein. J Immunol. 143, 2677–2683.

Dajani, A.A., Ayoub, E.M., Bierman, F.Z., Bisno, A.L., Deny, F.W., et al., 1993. Guidelines for the diagnosis of rheumatic fever: Jones criteria, update 1992. Circulation. 87, 302–307.

Damian, R.T., 1964. Molecular mimicry. Antigen sharing by parasite and host and its consequences. Am. Naturalist. 98, 129–149.

Düzgün, N., Duman, T., Haydardedeoðlu, F.E., Tutkak, H., 2009. Cytotoxic T lymphocyte-associated antigen-4 polymorphism in patients with rheumatic heart disease. Tissue Antigens. 74, 539–542.

Ellis, N.M., Li, Y., Hildebrand, W., Fischetti, V.A., Cunningham, M. W., 2005. T cell mimicry and epitope specificity of cross-reactive T cell clones from rheumatic heart disease. J. Immunol. 175, 5448–5456.

Fae, K.C., Silva, D.D., Oshiro, S.E., Tanaka, A.C., Pomerantzeff, P.M., Douay, C., et al., 2006. Mimicry in recognition of cardiac myosin peptides by heart-intralesional T cell clones from rheumatic heart disease. J. Immunol. 176, 5662–5670.

Faé, K.C., Diefenbach da Silva, D., Bilate, A.M., Tanaka, A.C., Pomerantzeff, P.M., Kiss, M.H., et al., 2008. PDIA3, HSPA5 and vimentin, proteins identified by 2-DE in the valvular tissue, are the target antigens of peripheral and heart infiltrating T cells from chronic rheumatic heart disease patients. J. Autoimmun. 31, 136–141.

Fraser, W.J., Haffejee, Z., Jankelow, D., Wadee, A., Cooper, K., 1997. Rheumatic Aschoff nodules revisited. II. Cytokine expression corroborates recently proposed sequential stages. Histopathology. 31, 460–464.

Gorton, D., Govan, B., Olive, C., Ketheesan, N., 2009. B- and T-cell responses in group A Streptococcus M-protein- or peptide-induced experimental carditis. Infect. Immun. 77, 2177–2183.

Gorton, D., Blyth, S., Gorton, J.G., Govan, B., Ketheesan, N., 2010. An alternative technique for the induction of autoimmune valvulitis in a rat model of rheumatic heart disease. J. Immunol. Meth. 355, 80–85.

Gough, S.C., Walker, L.S., Sansom, D.M., 2005. CTLA4 gene polymorphism and autoimmunity. Immunol. Rev. 204, 102–115.

Guedez, Y., Kotby, A., El-Demellawy, M., Galal, A., Thomson, G., Zaher, S., et al., 1999. HLA class II associations with rheumatic heart disease are more evident and consistent among clinically homogeneous patients. Circulation. 99, 2784–2790.

Guilherme, L., Weidebach, W., Kiss, M.H., Snitcowsky, R., Kalil, J., 1991. Association of human leukocyte class II antigens with rheumatic fever or rheumatic heart disease in a Brazilian population. Circulation. 83, 1995–1998.

Guilherme, L., Cunha-Neto, E., Coelho, V., Snitcowsky, R., Pomerantzeff, P.M., Assis, R.V., et al., 1995. Human heart-infiltrating T-cell clones from rheumatic heart disease patients recognized both streptococcal and cardiac proteins. Circulation. 92, 415–420.

Guilherme, L., Dulphy, N., Douay, C., Coelho, V., Cunha-Neto, E., Oshiro, S.E., et al., 2000. Molecular evidence for antigen-driven immune responses in cardiac lesions of rheumatic heart disease patients. Int. Immunol. 12, 1063–1074.

Guilherme, L., Oshiro, S.E., Fae, K.C., Cunha-Neto, E., Renesto, G., Goldberg, A.C., et al., 2001. T cell reactivity against streptococcal antigens in the periphery mirrors reactivity of heart infiltrating T lymphocytes in rheumatic heart disease patients. Infect. Immun. 69, 5345–5535.

Guilherme, L., Cury, P., Demarchi, L.M., Coelho, V., Abel, L., Lopez, A.P., et al., 2004. Rheumatic heart disease, proinflammatory cytokines play a role in the progression and maintenance of valvular lesions. Am. J. Pathol. 165, 1583–1591.

Guilherme, L., Köhler, K.F., Kalil, J., 2011. Rheumatic heart disease: mediation by complex immune events. Adv. Clin. Chem. 53, 31–50.

Hernandez-Pacheco, G., Aguilar-Garcia, J., Flores-Dominguez, C., Rodríguez-Pérez, J.M., Pérez-Hernández, N., Alvarez-Leon, E., et al., 2003a. MHC class II alleles in Mexican patients with rheumatic heart disease. Int. J. Cardiol. 92, 49–54.

Hernandez-Pacheco, G., Flores-Domínguez, C., Rodríguez-Pérez, J.M., Pérez-Hernández, N., Fragoso, J.M., Saul, A., Alvarez-León, E., et al., 2003b. Tumor necrosis factor-alpha promoter polymorphisms in Mexican patients with rheumatic heart disease. J. Autoimmun. 21, 59–63.

Hirsch, E., Irikura, V.M., Paul, S.M., Hirsh, D., 1996. Functions of interleukin 1 receptor antagonist in gene knockout and overproducing mice. Proc. Natl. Acad. Sci. USA. 93, 11008–11013.

Jack, D.L., Klein, N.J., Turner, M.W., 2001. Mannose-binding lectin targeting the microbial world for complement attack and opsonophagocytosis. Immunol. Rev. 180, 86–89.

Kamal, H., Hussein, G., Hassoba, H., Mosaad, N., Gad, A., Ismail, M., et al., 2010. Transforming growth factor-beta1 gene C-509T and T869C polymorphisms as possible risk factors in rheumatic heart disease in Egypt. Acta Cardiol. 65, 177–183.

Kemeny, E., Grieve, T., Marcus, R., Sareli, P., Zabriskie, J.B., 1989. Identification of mononuclear cells and T cell subsets in rheumatic valvulitis. Clin. Immunol. Immunopathol. 52, 225–237.

Kodama, M., Matsumoto, Y., Fujiwara, M., Masani, F., Izumi, T., Shibata, A., et al., 1990. A novel experimental model of giant cell myocarditis induced in rats by immunization with cardiac myosin fraction. Clin. Immunol. Immunopathol. 57, 250–262.

Koyanagi, T., Koga, Y., Nishi, H., Toshima, H., Sasazuki, T., Imaizumi, T., et al., 1996. DNA typing of HLA class II genes in Japanese patients with rheumatic heart disease. J. Mol. Cell Cardiol. 28, 1349–1353.

Li, Y., Heuser, J.S., Kosanke, S.D., Hemric, M., Cunningham, M.W., 2004. Cryptic epitope identified in rat and human cardiac myosin S2 region induces myocarditis in the Lewis rat. J. Immunol. 172, 3225–3234.

Lymbury, R.S., Olive, C.O., Powell, K.A., Good, M.F., Hirst, R.G., Labrooy, J.T, et al., 2003. Induction of autoimmune valvulitis in lewis rats following immunization with peptides from the conserved region of group A streptococcal M protein. J. Autoimmun. 20, 211–217.

Messias-Reason, I.J., Schafranski, M.D., Jensenius, J.C., Steffensen, R., 2006. The association between mannose-binding lectin gene polymorphism and rheumatic heart disease. Hum. Immunol. 67, 991–998.

Messias-Reason, I.J., de, Schafranski, M.D., Kremsner, P.G., Kun, J.F., 2009. Ficolin 2 (FCN2) functional polymorphisms and the risk of rheumatic fever and rheumatic heart disease. Clin. Exp. Immunol. 157, 395–399.

Mota, C.C., Aiello, D.V., Anderson, R.H., 2009. Chronic rheumatic heart disease. In: Anderson, R.H., Baker, E.J., Penny, D.J. (Eds.), Pediactric Cardiology, third ed. Churchill Livingstone/Elsevier, Philadelphia, pp. 1091–1133.

Ozkan, M., Carin, M., Sonmez, G., Senocak, M., Ozdemir, M., Yakut, C., et al., 1993. HLA antigens in Turkish race with rheumatic heart disease. Circulation. 87, 1974–1978.

Patarroyo, M.E., Winchester, R.J., Vejerano, A., Gibofsky, A., Chalem, F., Zabriskie, J.B., et al., 1979. Association of a B-cell alloantigen with susceptibility to rheumatic fever. Nature. 278, 173–174.

Peterson, L.K., Fujinami, R.S., 2007. Molecular mimicry. In: Shoenfeld, Y., Gershwin, M.E., Meroni, P.L. (Eds.), Autoantibodies, second ed. Elsevier, Burlington, pp. 13–19.

Quinn, A., Kosanke, S., Fischetti, V.A., Factor, S.M., Cunningham, M.W., 2001. Induction of autoimmune valvular heart disease by recombinant streptococcal M protein. Infect. Immun. 69, 4072–4078.

Raizada, V., Williams Jr., R.C., Chopra, P., et al., 1983. Tissue distribution of lymphocytes in rheumatic heart valves as defined by monoclonal anti-T cells antibodies. Am. J. Med. 74, 225–237.

Rajapakse, C.N., Halim, K., Al-Orainey, I., Al-Nozha, M., Al-Aska, A.K., 1987. A genetic marker for rheumatic heart disease. Br. Heart J. 58, 659–662.

Ramasawmy, R., Fae, K.C., Spina, G., Victora, G.D., Tanaka, A.C., Palácios, S.A., et al., 2007. Association of polymorphisms within the promoter region of the tumor necrosis factor alpha with clinical outcomes of rheumatic fever. Mol. Immunol. 44, 1873–1878.

Ramasawmy, R., Spina, G., Fae, K.C., Pereira, A.C., Nisihara, R., Messias Reason, I.J., et al., 2008. Association of mannose-binding lectin gene polymorphism but not of mannose-binding serine protease 2 with chronic severe aortic regurgitation of rheumatic etiology. Clin. Vaccine Immunol. 15, 932–936.

Sallakci, N., Akcurin, G., Köksoy, S., Kardelen, F., Uguz, A., Coskun, M., et al., 2005. TNF-alpha G-308A polymorphism is associated with rheumatic fever and correlates with increased TNF-alpha production. J. Autoimmun. 25, 150–154.

Settin, A., Abdel-Hady, H., El-Baz, R., Saber, I., 2007. Gene polymorphisms of TNF-alpha(-308), IL-10(-1082), IL-6(-174), and IL-1Ra (VNTR) related to susceptibility and severity of rheumatic heart disease. Pediatr. Cardiol. 28, 363–371.

Smeesters, P.R., McMillan, D., Sriprakash, K.S., 2010. The streptococcal M protein, a highly versatile molecule. Trends Microbiol. 18, 275–282.

Stanevicha, V., Eglite, J., Sochnevs, A., Gardovska, D., Zavadska, D., Shantere, R., et al., 2003. HLA class II associations with rheumatic heart disease among clinically homogeneous patients in children in Latvia. Arthritis Res. Ther. 5, 340–346.

Unny, S.K., Middlebrooks, B.L., 1983. Streptococcal rheumatic carditis. Microbiol. Rev. 47, 97–120.

Visentainer, J.E., Pereira, F.C., Dalalio, M.M., Tsuneto, L.T., Donadio, P.R., Moliterno, R.A., et al., 2000. Association of HLA-DR7 with rheumatic fever in the Brazilian population. J. Rheumatol. 27, 1518–1520.

Volin, M.V., Shahrara, S., 2011. Role of Th17 cells in rheumatic and other autoimmune diseases. Rheumatology. 1, 2169.

Weidebach, W., Goldberg, A.C., Chiarella, J.M., Guilherme, L., Snitcowsky, R., Pileggi, F., et al., 1994. HLA class II antigens in rheumatic fever. Analysis of the DR locus by restriction fragment-length polymorphism and oligotyping. Hum. Immunol. 40, 253–258.

Yegin, O., Coskun, M., Ertug, H., 1997. Cytokines in acute rheumatic fever. Eur. J. Pediatr. 156, 25–29.

Zabriskie, J.B., Lavenchy, D., Williams Jr., R.C., Fu, S.M., Yeadon, C.A., Fotino, M., et al., 1985. Rheumatic fever-associated B cell alloantigens as identified by monoclonal antibodies. Arthritis Rheum. 28, 1047–1051.

Chapter 70

Myocarditis and Dilated Cardiomyopathy

Noel R. Rose[1] and Ziya Kaya[2]

[1]*Department of Pathology and W. Harry Feinstone Department of Molecular Microbiology and Immunology, The Johns Hopkins University Medical Institutions, Baltimore, MD, USA,* [2]*Department of Cardiology, University of Heidelberg, Heidelberg, Germany*

Chapter Outline

Historical Background   1033
Clinical, Pathologic, and Epidemiologic Features   1033
  Myocarditis   1033
  Dilated Cardiomyopathy   1035
Autoimmune Features and Immunologic Markers   1037
  Circulating Antibodies   1037
  Immunofluorescence   1037
  Western Immunoblot   1038
  Immunoassay with Defined Antigens   1038

Immunologic Assessment of Biopsies   1038
Genetic Features   1039
Environmental Features   1039
Animal Models and Pathogenic Mechanisms   1040
Treatment and Outcome   1043
Personal Thoughts   1044
Acknowledgments   1044
References   1044

HISTORICAL BACKGROUND

The role of autoimmunity in cardiovascular disease has long been a topic of investigation in the clinic and the laboratory. Years of research effort were devoted to establishing a link between streptococcal infection and rheumatic heart disease on the basis of an autoimmune response (see Chapter 69). Chagas' disease is still believed to be based on a cross-reaction of antibodies to *Trypanosoma cruzi* with myocardial or cardiac conductive tissue (Coura and Borges-Pereira, 2012). Finally, post-pericardiotomy syndrome and post-myocardial infarction syndrome are sometimes cited as instances of an autoimmune response instigated by damaged or necrotic tissue (Maisch et al., 1979). This chapter reviews the evidence linking autoimmunity with two important forms of heart disease, myocarditis and dilated cardiomyopathy (DCM). It must be stated, *ab initio*, that immunologic testing has so far not been effective in allowing a clear distinction between autoimmune and other etiologies of these diseases.

The classic description of myocarditis was given by Corvisart in 1812 (referenced in Gravanis and Sternby, 1991), but for many years progress in studying the disease was impeded by the uncertainties of clinical diagnosis. Definitive diagnosis was dependent upon autopsy examination. Interest in the disease increased in recent years because of the availability of better antemortem diagnostic tools, especially the endomyocardial biopsy, greater understanding of the role of cardiotropic viruses, and the potential of new modalities of therapy.

CLINICAL, PATHOLOGIC, AND EPIDEMIOLOGIC FEATURES

Myocarditis

While myocarditis may be asymptomatic, the major features include arrhythmias (palpitations, dizziness, syncope, or sudden cardiac death), embolic events, congestive heart failure, or cardiogenic shock. These clinical findings can be supported by electrocardiographic changes, such as nonspecific ST-T wave abnormalities and atrial or ventricular arrhythmias. Two-dimensional echocardiography, a noninvasive way of evaluating heart size and function, may show normal ventricular size with thick walls and decreased contractility early in the illness or progressive heart enlargement with thinning of the muscle in chronic cases. Biventricular enlargement is seen in chronic cases. A pericardial rub may be detected, indicating pericardial irritation with or without a pericardial effusion. As the disease progresses, gallop rhythms and signs of congestive

N. Rose & I. Mackay (Eds): The Autoimmune Diseases, Fifth edition. DOI: http://dx.doi.org/10.1016/B978-0-12-384929-8.00070-8

heart failure appear. The patient may recall a recent viral illness with symptoms of malaise, chills and fever, upper respiratory or gastrointestinal symptoms, myalgia, and chest pain. The majority of cases, however, cannot be traced back to an obvious preceding illness. Most patients with myocarditis present with either left ventricular failure or arrhythmias as their only clinical signs.

Studies of the occurrence of myocarditis in North America, Europe, and Japan have suggested that the incidence varies widely in different areas (Jacobson et al., 1997). Prevalence figures of 1.06, 3.5, 5.4, and as high as 10 have been reported in different series (Gravanis and Sternby, 1991). The reasons for these wide differences are not known, but may be related to the differing diagnostic criteria used or may reflect exposures to different types and strains of cardiotropic viruses, as well as genetic differences in the host populations. The 5-year survival of biopsy-proven acute or chronic myocarditis in adults is only 56% (Grogan et al., 1995). In pediatric populations, the prevalence and mortality are even higher. Noren et al. (1976) described histologic evidence of latent myocarditis in 4.2% of accidental deaths of children and 16.7% of unexplained, unexpected deaths, suggesting that unsuspected myocarditis may be a significant cause of unexpected death in children (Liberthson, 1996). Fabre et al. describe myocarditis in up to 12% of cases of sudden death in young adults (Fabre and Sheppard, 2006). Prospective studies have also revealed a grave prognosis for myocarditis patients, with a 5- to 10-year survival rate of 25–46%, mostly due to manifestations of DCM and sudden cardiac death (Dec et al., 1985; McCarthy et al., 2000; Magnani et al., 2006; Caforio et al., 2007).

The clinical diagnosis of myocarditis remains a challenge (Schultheiss and Kuhl, 2011). Myocarditis can be classified by etiology, histology, immunohistology, clinical pathologic, or clinical criteria (Table 70.1). Felker et al. (2000) and McCarthy et al. (2000) have demonstrated that the prognosis of cardiomyopathy in patients with myocarditis is dependent on the clinical pathologic classification of their initial disorder. Patients with fulminant myocarditis, who do not die within the first 2 weeks, have a survival rate which is virtually identical to that of age-matched controls. Patients with subacute myocarditis who develop persistent left ventricular dysfunction have an outcome that is virtually identical to that of patients with idiopathic DCM. Patients with chronic persistent myocarditis, while they continue to have myocardial inflammation, have no deterioration in ventricular function and usually have a normal survival. Patients with chronic active myocarditis and who have ongoing inflammation and fibrosis develop a restrictive cardiomyopathy severe enough to require transplantation within

TABLE 70.1 An Exemplary Classification Scheme for Myocarditis (Modified from Sagar et al., 2011)

Etiologic	Histologic	Clinicopathologic
Viral, such as enteroviruses (e.g., Coxsackie B),	Eosinophilic	Fulminant
Erythroviruses (eg, Parvovirus B19), adenoviruses, and Herpes viruses	Giant cell	Acute
Bacterial, such as Corynebacterium diphtheria, Staphylococcus aureus, Borrelia burgdorferi, and Ehrlichia species	Granulomatous	Chronic active
Protozoal, such as Babesia Trypanosomal, such as Trypanosoma cruzi	Lymphocytic	Chronic persistent
Toxic: alcohol, radiation, chemicals (hydrocarbons and Arsenic), and drugs, including doxorubicin		
Hypersensitivity: sulfonamides and penicillins		

2–3 years (Lieberman et al., 1991). Patients with giant cell or necrotizing eosinophilic myocarditis (Sagar et al., 2012) develop rapidly progressive mildly dilated but severely hypofunctional cardiomyopathy and have a life expectancy, without vigorous treatment, that is measured in months.

The so-called Dallas criteria, the consensus of a group of cardiovascular pathologists, led to better standardization of the histopathologic examination (Aretz et al., 1986). Active myocarditis requires the presence of mononuclear inflammation associated with adjacent myocyte damage (Figure 70.1). Myocyte damage can take the form of necrosis or myocyte vacuolization. The term borderline myocarditis is applied when an unequivocal diagnosis of myocarditis cannot be made either because the inflammatory infiltrate is too sparse or because the damage to the myocyte is not clearly demonstrable (Figure 70.2). The terminology used for subsequent biopsies is ongoing, resolving, or resolved myocarditis. Ongoing myocarditis indicates persistent myocardial inflammation associated with myocyte damage. Resolving myocarditis resembles borderline myocarditis, but reparative fibrosis is evident. Resolved or healed myocarditis is diagnosed if no inflammatory infiltrate is seen. The Dallas criteria also require that myocarditis be distinguished from the histologic pattern of myocardial injury evident in ischemic heart disease. The inflammatory infiltrate in myocarditis is composed primarily of mononuclear cells, although in the

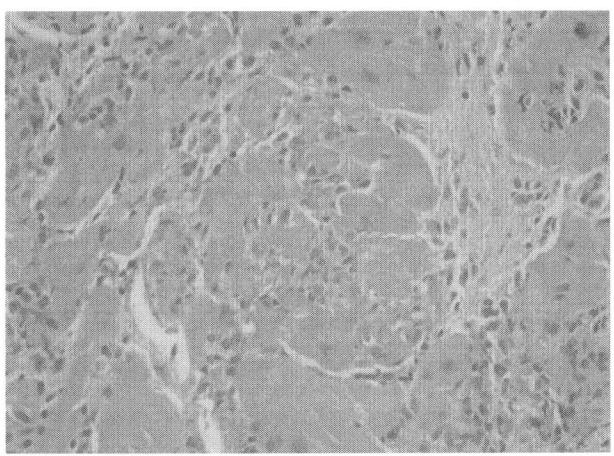

FIGURE 70.1 **Lymphocytic myocarditis.**   There is a heavy infiltrate of large activated lymphocytes throughout the myocardium. Myocyte necrosis is noted in the middle of this image. Fibrosis is present on the right side of the image. (H&E 400×)

more acute phases polymorphonuclear cell infiltration is common. Giant cells and prominent eosinophilia are seen in some cases of myocarditis and often indicate a dire outcome.

The Dallas criteria, which have been used extensively for clinical trials, may be too insensitive to diagnose many patients with inflammatory heart disease. In one trial, only 9.6% of 2233 patients with a clinical diagnosis of myocarditis were positive by the rigid Dallas criteria (Mason and O'Connell, 1989). Utilizing the Dallas criteria even in patients who have died of myocarditis, and with five tissue samples, it is only possible to establish a histologic diagnosis of myocarditis in 54% of patients (Chow et al., 1989; Hauck et al., 1989). Additionally, in Towbin et al.'s (1994) study of children with suspected clinical myocarditis (67% of these patients had adenoviral infection), 13 of the 26 patients positive for viral nucleic acid by the polymerase chain reaction (PCR) did not display the histopathologic features that would allow the diagnosis of myocarditis to be established. The standard Dallas criteria are further limited by variability in interpretation as well as low sensitivity. These limitations have led to alternative pathological classifications. Wojnicz et al. (2001) and Frustaci et al. (2003), utilizing upregulation of HLA by endomyocardial biopsy or the presence of antiheart antibodies as markers of an autoimmune response, identified patients with suspected myocarditis who appeared to respond to immunosuppressive therapy.

Additional criteria rely on cell-specific immunoperoxidase stains for surface antigens, such as anti-CD3, anti-CD4, anti-CD20, anti-CD68, and anti-human leukocyte antigen (HLA) (Herskowitz et al., 1990; Maisch et al., 2000). Criteria that are based on immunoperoxidase staining have greater sensitivity and may have prognostic value.

Nevertheless there is the diagnostic lack due to sampling error. Noninvasive cardiac magnetic resonance imaging (MRI) may provide additional diagnostic value (Jesirich et al., 2010). With the unique potential for tissue characterization using T1- and T2-weighted images, cardiac MRI can evaluate three important markers of tissue injury: (1) intracellular and interstitial edema; (2) hyperemia and capillary leakage; and (3) necrosis and fibrosis (Mahrholdt et al., 2004; Abdel-Aty et al., 2005; Gutberlet et al., 2008; Friedrich et al., 2009). In practice, although the number of medical centers performing endomyocardial biopsy has been increased, it is still not routinely performed in all patients and all centers.

There are several distinct histologic forms of myocarditis (Basso et al., 2012). Drug- or allergy-mediated myocarditis is characterized by an eosinophilic infiltrate. Fulminant myocarditis demonstrates intense infiltration in virtually all sections with marked myocyte necrosis (Figure 70.3). Chronic active myocarditis reveals ongoing myocardial inflammation associated with fibrosis and occasional giant cells (Lieberman et al., 1993). Giant-cell myocarditis is a rare but frequently fatal form of myocarditis (Figure 70.4) (Elamm, et al., 2012). The victims are primarily young, healthy adults who die suddenly of heart failure or ventricular arrhythmia. Although cardiac transplantation may be curative, several instances of recurrent disease in the transplanted heart have been reported. Histologic findings in giant-cell myocarditis are diffuse myocardial necrosis with numerous multinucleated giant cells and a mixed inflammatory infiltrate of lymphocytes and macrophages. Collections of eosinophils are seen in some of these patients.

Dilated Cardiomyopathy

Dilated cardiomyopathy (DCM) is a chronic form of heart disease characterized by left and right ventricular dilatation and impaired contraction (Gravanis and Ansari, 1987). The clinical spectrum is broad, ranging from individuals with asymptomatic cardiomegaly to patients who present with severe congestive heart failure. Patients may also display symptoms or signs of arrhythmia or systemic embolization with or without congestive heart failure. Other signs include systemic or pulmonary venous congestion, cardiomegaly, gallop rhythms, and mitral or tricuspid regurgitation. The diagnosis requires exclusion of heart failure due to other causes, such as coronary artery disease, toxic exposure, drug allergy, medication (adriamycin) effect, or physical agent injury. Once heart failure is established in a patient with DCM, the expected outcome is poor, with a 5-year mortality of 46% (Grogan et al., 1995). D'Ambrosio et al. describe in long-term follow-up studies in patients with acute myocarditis the development of DCM in 21% of patients over a mean follow-up period of 3 years (D'Ambrosio et al., 2001).

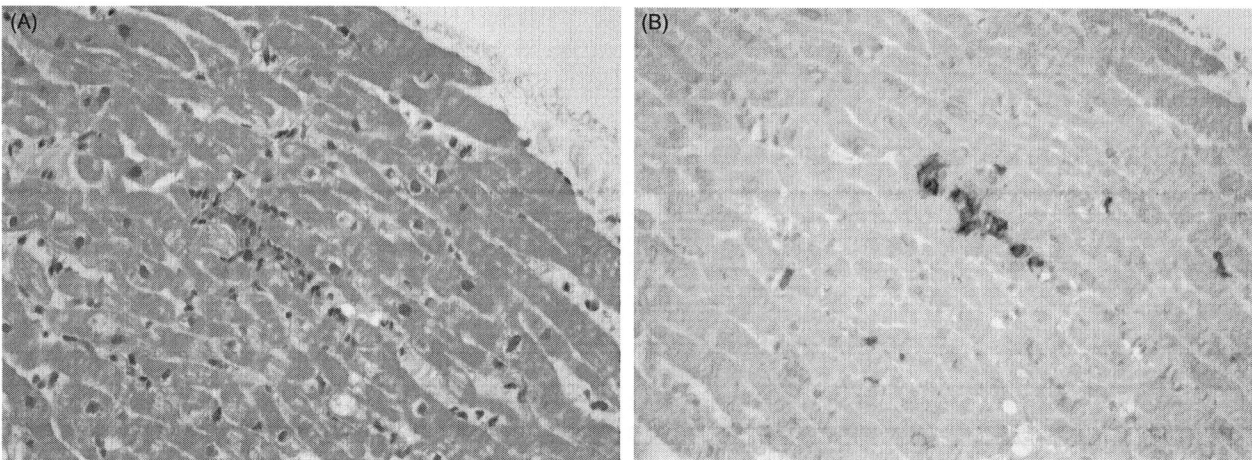

FIGURE 70.2 **Borderline myocarditis.** (A) A single cluster of perivascular lymphocytes is present. No myocardial damage is identified. (H&E 400×). (B) A CD8 immunohistochemical stain highlights the infiltrating T lymphocytes. (H&E 400×)

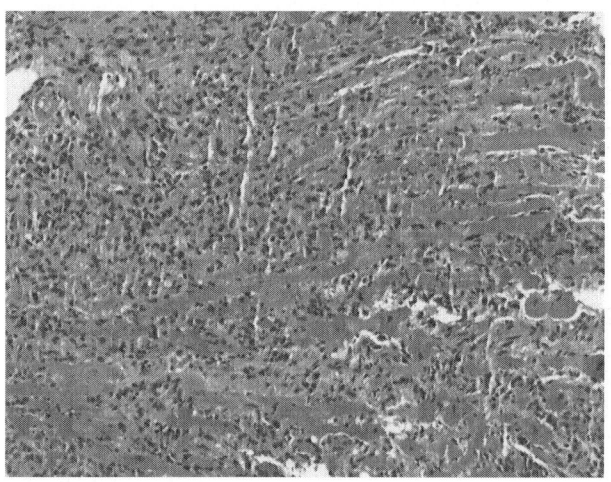

FIGURE 70.3 **Fulminant myocarditis.** The myocardium is replaced by a marked polymorphous inflammatory infiltrate composed predominantly of lymphocytes and macrophages with rarer eosinophils and neutrophils. Global myocyte injury and loss is noted. No giant cells are present. (H&E 100×)

Several studies have investigated the frequency of familial dilated cardiomyopathy. Petretta et al. report in their meta-analysis an estimated clinically confirmed FDC of 23% (95% confidence interval 0.17 to 0.31) was found (Petretta et al., 2011). Furthermore, a large number of other etiologic agents have been associated with DCM (Felker et al., 2000), including infections and metabolic, endocrinologic, and nutritional disturbances, as well as toxins and drugs. However, in approximately 50% of patients, no specific etiology can be identified. The same pathologic process probably results from a number of different etiologies.

Evidence for pathophysiologic relevance of autoimmunity in DCM has substantially increased over the past years. Several circulating autoantibodies, some of them heart specific, have been described in animal experiments and first clinical pilot studies suggest that antibodies, including antibodies to the β1-adrenoceptor, play a crucial role in the induction and progression of heart failure. But the precise mechanisms on how these autoantibodies perpetuate or even induce an organ-specific autoimmune response are not yet fully understood (Leuschner et al., 2008; Deubner et al., 2010; Kaya et al., 2010, 2012). Clinical observations on prognostic relevance of autoantibodies have the prompted therapeutic trials focused on nonspecific removal of autoantibodies from the circulation via immunoadsorption. There are early reports on a beneficial outcome in patients treated by immunoadsorption (Felix and Staudt, 2006).

To address cardiac autoimmunity the prospective Etiology, Titer-Course, and effect on Survival (ETiCS) of cardiac autoantibodies has been initiated. It is the largest European clinical diagnostic study initiated so far in the field of cardiac autoimmunity. ETiCS will enhance current knowledge on autoimmunity in human heart disease and promote endeavors to develop novel therapies targeting cardiac autoantibodies (Deubner et al., 2010).

In 1985, the prevalence of DCM in Olmsted County, Minnesota, was 36.5 in 100,000. African American race and male gender were associated with increased risk (Cetta and Michels, 1995). The incidence of DCM in Malmö, Sweden, was reported to be 10 in 100,000 per year (Torp, 1981), and estimated in Great Britain at 0.7—7.5 in 100,000 per year, with a prevalence in 1985 of 8.3 cases in 100,000 (Williams and Olsen, 1985). In a nationwide study in Finland, the incidence of DCM among children and adolescents was 0.34 in 100,000 per

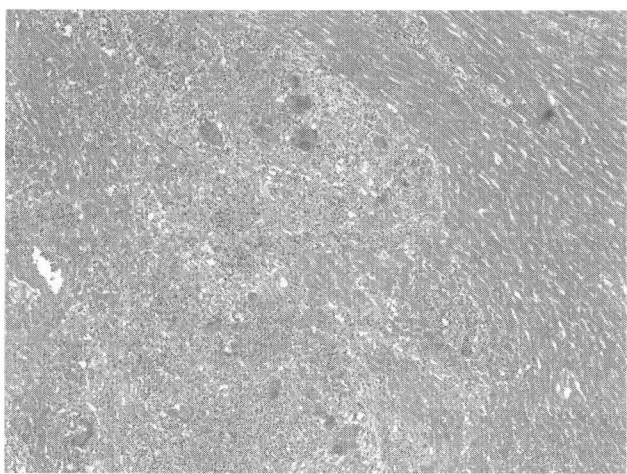

FIGURE 70.4 Giant cell myocarditis. The myocardium is infiltrated by a patchy and diffuse inflammatory infiltrate composed primarily of lymphocytes and macrophages. Multiple collections of giant cells are seen within the infiltrate along with eosinophils. There is significant injury and loss of myocytes in areas of inflammation, while adjacent myocardium is relatively uninvolved. (H&E 50×).

year, with a prevalence in 1991 of 2.6 in 100,000. In children, the incidence is higher in boys than girls, and higher in babies younger than 1 year than in older children (Jefferies and Towbin, 2010). Although the male predominance in this disease is not great, it stands in contrast to most autoimmune disorders that occur more frequently in females. The basis of the male predominance is still not clearly understood, but appears to be related to sex-based differences in cytokine formation. The number of new cases increased each year over the 10-year study period (Arola et al., 1997). Since a number of these patients utilize significant medical resources in their care or eventually require cardiac transplantation, there is a great need for early and definitive diagnosis.

Cases representing progression from myocarditis to DCM can be termed inflammatory DCM (Maisch et al., 2000); Kline and Saphir (1960) documented progressive myocardial failure and death in a series of patients within months to years after acute myocarditis. Miklozek et al. (1986) found that 12 of 16 patients diagnosed as having viral myocarditis had continued cardiac functional abnormalities. Abelmann (1984) reported that half of 16 patients had cardiac symptoms or physical evidence of persistent cardiac dysfunction after recovery from acute myocarditis. Most symptomatic relatives of DCM patients with left ventricular dysfunction have evidence of myocardial inflammation consistent with early or mild myocarditis (Mahon et al., 2002).

Like myocarditis, DCM may be associated with Coxsackievirus infection. In 50 infants and children with DCM, Ayuthya et al. (1974) found significantly increased titers of neutralizing antibody to Coxsackieviruses B3.

Initially, Bowles et al. (1986) and Kandolf et al. (1987) demonstrated Coxsackievirus B-specific nucleic acid sequences in heart tissue of a small number of patients with DCM. Since then molecular testing has become increasingly sophisticated. Towbin et al. (1994) demonstrated that children with suspected myocarditis were PCR positive for viral etiologies on endomyocardial biopsy (26 of 38 samples from 34 patients). Additionally, the viral sequences demonstrated were more frequently adenoviral (15) than enteroviral (8).

In cases of DCM, the heart assumes a globular shape due to enlargement of all of the chambers, especially the left ventricle (Gravanis and Ansari, 1987). The histologic findings are generally nonspecific, and include myocardial cell hypertrophy and an increase in interstitial fibrous connective tissue. In areas of degeneration of the myocardial fibers, small clusters of lymphocytes may be seen. This finding may blur the distinction of DCM from myocarditis.

AUTOIMMUNE FEATURES AND IMMUNOLOGIC MARKERS

Circulating Antibodies

The ambiguities in diagnosing inflammatory disease of the heart muscle are evident. Although the availability of endomyocardial biopsy has helped to clarify the situation, many cases are still inconclusive. There is, at present, a need for noninvasive, inexpensive diagnostic procedures to distinguish autoimmune from other forms of inflammatory heart disease. Much evidence points to a significant role of autoimmunity in some animal models of heart muscle disease. It is logical, therefore, to propose that serologic tests, based on the demonstration of circulating autoantibodies to cardiac antigens, might be useful in the identification of autoimmune forms of myocarditis and DCM in humans. The literature has been reviewed by Caforio et al. (2002), Cihakova and Rose (2008), and, most recently, Kaya et al. (2012).

Immunofluorescence

Immunofluorescence tests utilize cardiac tissue of rat or human origin. Both frozen sections and isolated myocytes have been employed. Antibody generally localizes at the surface of the myocyte, giving a sarcolemmal or myolemmal pattern, or on the striations, producing a fibrillar pattern. Whether these two immunofluorescent patterns represent antibodies of different specificities is unclear, because both patterns can be seen in sera from mice immunized with purified cardiac myosin. A major problem in the interpretation of indirect immunofluorescence is the high prevalence of reactions obtained with sera from healthy control subjects. Maisch (1987) found that 91% of patients with myocarditis gave positive reactions with human or rat cardiocytes, but 31–35% of healthy controls showed similar reactions, although generally at lower levels. Neumann et al. (1990) used more conservative criteria, 59% of patients with biopsy-proven myocarditis being positive, as were 20% of patients with DCM. In contrast, none of the healthy controls and only 4% of patients with ischemic heart disease were positive in this test under the conditions used.

Western Immunoblot

The Western immunoblot is potentially more sensitive than immunofluorescence and is capable of identifying particular antigens recognized by heart-reactive antibodics. Ncumann et al. (1990) detected heart-reactive antibodies in 48 of 103 samples from biopsy-proven myocarditis or DCM patients by immunofluorescence, whereas 97 of the 103 samples exhibited reactivity by Western immunoblotting. No single pattern of antigen reactivity was unique to patients with myocarditis or DCM, but myocarditis sera showed an elevated prevalence of antibody against myosin heavy chain, whereas cardiomyopathy sera exhibited a greater prevalence of reactivity against cardiac muscle actin. Many normal sera reacted with the same antigen, but generally in lower titers. A quantitative immunoassay, such as an enzyme-linked immunosorbent assay (ELISA) using purified human cardiac myosin heavy chain, therefore, is needed for clinical evaluation of these antibodies.

Immunoassay with Defined Antigens

Among the well-characterized antigens used for the study by immunoassay of antibodies in sera of patients with myocarditis and DCM are myosin (Neumann et al., 1990; Caforio et al., 1992), laminin (Wolff et al., 1989), β1-adrenergic receptors (Limas et al., 1989), and the mitochondrial components, adenine nucleotide translocator (ANT) protein (Schultheiss et al., 1986) and branched-chain ketodehydrogenase (BCKD) (Ansari et al., 1988).

These results show that many patients with myocarditis and DCM develop autoantibodies to a number of cardiac constituents. Large-scale evaluation is necessary before it can be concluded that detection of any single antibody, or group of antibodies, is sufficiently sensitive and specific to replace the endomyocardial biopsy as a primary diagnostic tool. It does seem, even at this early stage of investigation, that a decline in some antibody titers during treatment may predict a favorable therapeutic response (Müller et al., 2000).

None of these antibodies to cardiac antigens is known to play a direct pathogenic role in the disease. However,

the presence of antibodies to β1-adrenergic receptors in DCM is highly suggestive of a direct pathogenic effect, since the antigen is accessible on the surface of the myocardiocyte. β1-Adrenergic receptor antibodies can induce apoptosis in isolated adult cardiomyocytes (Staudt et al., 2003) and antibodies activating the receptors are associated with reduced cardiac function in chronic heart failure (Jahns et al., 2010).

While the pathogenic importance of antibodies is still controversial, the finding that reduction of immunoglobulins in plasma by an immunoadsorption column benefits cardiomyopathy patients provides strong evidence of their involvement (Winters, 2012). Although immunoadsorption does not establish the specificity of the autoantibodies that are depleted, reduction of certain immunoglobulin subclasses (IgG3) may be especially beneficial (Nagatomo et al., 2011). In a preliminary study, absorption columns using β1-adrenergic receptors benefited patients with the corresponding antibody (Dandel et al., 2012).

Although the role of T cells in the pathogenesis of myocarditis has been difficult to study in humans, animal models have proved to be invaluable in discovering their pathogenic mechanisms. Findings in mice indicate that they play a key role in inducing myocarditis (Smith and Allen, 1991).

Immunologic Assessment of Biopsies

In addition to studies of circulating antibody, immunologic methods can contribute to the diagnosis of heart disease by the identification of immunoglobulin and complement in biopsy specimens. Hammond et al. (1988) found that 55% of patients with active myocarditis had deposits of IgG and complement component C3 in their biopsies. Thirty-nine percent of borderline myocarditis (inflammation without myocyte necrosis) cases and 6% of DCM cases were also positive. Patients with other autoimmune diseases, such as systemic lupus erythematosus and scleroderma, sometimes showed deposits of IgG and C3 in their heart tissue, but these usually were coarse, granular deposits in the interstitial spaces of the myocardium or endocardium, probably representing immune complexes.

Immunofluorescence with defined antisera has been used to identify infiltrating cells in cardiac biopsies. Luppi et al. (2003) found that the myocardium of myocarditis and DCM patients was infiltrated by macrophages and CD4[+] and CD8[+] T lymphocytes. In the majority of patients, the T cell receptor (TCR) repertoire was restricted with a polyclonal expansion of the Vb7 gene family. Evidence of Coxsackievirus infection was also found.

The expression of MHC class I and class II antigens in biopsy specimens was evaluated by Herskowitz et al.

(1990). In control samples, only low levels of MHC class I molecules were expressed on interstitial cells and vascular epithelium, while MHC class II could not be demonstrated immunohistologically. Increased myocardial expression of MHC class I and *de novo* expression of class II antigens were found in 85% of the myocarditis patients and 33% of the DCM patients.

GENETIC FEATURES

Because of the possible autoimmune origin of myocarditis and DCM in humans, and the well-documented association of experimental myocarditis with the major histocompatibility complex (MHC) in mice (Rose et al., 1988), a number of studies to determine the relationship with the human MHC (HLA) have been carried out. Anderson et al. (1984) reported that DCM patients had an increased frequency of HLA-DR4 and a decreased frequency of HLA-DR6. These findings were corroborated by Limas et al. (1990), who also demonstrated an increased frequency of HLA-DR4 in DCM patients. A genetic predisposition toward cardiac autoimmunity was demonstrated, in that 72% of HLA-DR4$^+$ patients had anti-β1-adrenergic receptor antibodies compared with 21% of HLA-DR4$^-$ patients. In the largest study to date, Carlquist et al. (1991) reconfirmed these findings and also found that the DR4-DQw4 haplotype conferred heightened risk of disease. In a meta-analysis of five studies, they confirmed that the DR4 association with myocarditis was sustained among different patient populations. No differences in disease phenotypes have been reported.

A predominance of myocarditis in males has been reported in a number of studies. The proportion of male patients is about 60% (Lieberman et al., 1991; et al., 1995). In this respect, myocarditis differs from most autoimmune diseases, which predominantly affect females.

ENVIRONMENTAL FEATURES

Myocarditis has both infectious and noninfectious causes. As noninfectious agents of myocarditis, a number of drugs have been implicated, acting either directly as toxic agents or as triggers of an allergic response. This section deals with infectious myocarditis; there is less information on cardiac autoimmunity in other forms (see Table 70.1).

Acute myocarditis is associated with infections of many types, including bacterial, rickettsial, viral, mycotic, protozoan, and helminthic. Several viruses have been implicated in this disease and, in some cases, multiple viruses may be detected in the heart. In Europe and North America, among the most common agents are the enteroviruses and the adenoviruses. Grist and Bell (1974)

reported that Coxsackievirus group B infections were associated with at least half of the acute cases of myocarditis. By immunofluorescence, Burch et al. (1968) found Coxsackievirus B antigen in the myocardium of 30.9% of routine autopsy specimens of myocarditis. Serotype B3 is identified most frequently. Other studies have suggested that adenoviruses are more prevalent in pediatric patients (Bowles et al., 2003).

By using molecular genetic methods, enteroviral and adenoviral genomes were detected in 10–35% of endomyocardial biopsies from patients with myocarditis or DCM (Baboonian and McKenna, 2003; Pauschinger et al., 2004). In a study in Europe, 32.6% of biopsies in the study group contained enteroviral RNA, 8.1% adenovirus DNA, 36.6% parvovirus B19 DNA, and 10.5% human herpesvirus type 6 DNA. In 12.2% of the samples, dual infection with PVB19 and herpesvirus was present (Kuhl et al., 2003). A study carried out in the United States identified parvovirus DNA in 12% of samples, but its presence did not correlate with clinical presentation (Stewart et al., 2011).

Like other enteroviruses, Coxsackieviruses enter the alimentary tract and are acid stable. They multiply in the small intestine. Following replication, viremia develops, seeding the infectious agents in selected tissues. As an obligatory intracellular parasite, the virus must enter a cell through receptor-mediated endocytosis. The virus receptor determines the tropism of the virus. Cardiotropic CB3 employs myocyte surface molecules as receptors, whereas hepatotropic or diabetogenic virus strains utilize receptors on hepatocytes or pancreatic islet cells, respectively. The infection may cause cell death directly, or act indirectly to stimulate an immunopathic host response (Huber, 1997). Coxsackievirus B3 RNA can persist in the myocardium for many days after infectious virus is no longer demonstrable (Klingel et al., 1992) and may, even without the ability to multiply, cause ventricular compromise in the face of a stimulated immune system (Wessely et al., 1998; Esfandiarei and McManus, 2008).

The CB3 genome is a single molecule of positive-sense RNA of approximately 7400 nucleotides in length. The genome codes for four capsid proteins as well as for the nonstructural proteins necessary for viral replication. A comparison of cloned cDNA from cardiovirulent and noncardiovirulent strains showed that sites within a nontranslated region and in the capsid protein affect virulence (Tracy et al., 1996).

Nutrition also plays a role in determining susceptibility to viral myocarditis. Beck et al. (1995) demonstrated that mice fed a diet deficient in selenium and infected with a noncardiovirulent strain of CB3 developed severe myocardial damage. Virus isolated from the hearts was fully virulent; six point mutations distinguished the virulent strains. The accumulation of these multiple mutations may be the result of greater viral replication in the hearts of selenium-deficient mice and may be attributable to decreased immune responses compared to selenium-adequate mice (Levander and Beck, 1997). These results may shed light on the etiology of an endemic form of cardiomyopathy known as Keshan disease, seen primarily in selenium-deficient regions of China (Abelmann, 1984).

Chagas' disease is a major cause of heart muscle disease in Latin America, responsible for 8 to 9 million cases annually (Hashimoto and Yoshioka, 2012). It is caused by the hemoflagellate *Trypanosoma cruzi*, which is transmitted to humans via the bite of the reduviid triatomine bug. Most patients initially have only mild, influenza-like symptoms, but 10−30% of infected individuals develop fulminant myocarditis. Chronic Chagas' disease may present with arrhythmias, thromboembolic events, and congestive heart failure. It represents a particularly lethal form of cardiomyopathy, as survival after presentation is two- to four-fold shorter than that of patients with other forms of DCM (Cunha-Neto et al., 2004).

Antibodies to a number of cardiac antigens, including fibronectin, laminin, and myosin, are found in many patients with chronic Chagas' disease, as well as with other forms of DCM (Ballinas-Vedugo et al., 2003). Molecular mimicry between *T. cruzi* and heart disease has been cited as a mechanism to explain the production of autoantibodies during infection (Kalil and Cunha-Neto, 1996). A number of candidate antigens have been described, including a heart-specific epitope of cardiac myosin heavy chain and a 12-amino acid peptide of Fl160, a 160-kDa protein on the surface of *T. cruzi* that mimics a similar protein found on mammalian axonal and myenteric plexus cells (Van Voorhis et al., 1991). The latter antibody is of special interest because of the occurrence of megacolon, megaesophagus, and other neuropathies during chronic Chagas' disease. Among the other antigens described as possible initiators of cross-reactive responses are a peptide of the second extracellular loop of the β1-adrenergic receptor (Ferrari et al., 1995), a *T. cruzi* ribosomal protein R13 (Motran et al., 2000), a ribosomal P protein (Kaplan et al., 1997), and Cha. The latter antigen is recognized by T cells of patients as well as antibodies (Girones et al., 2001). An early decision about the course of immunity is made during the early innate response determined by activation of Toll-like receptors and macrophage development. The subsequent adaptive immunity may be protective or pathogenic (Pellegrini et al 2012).

Kawasaki syndrome is an acute febrile disease of infants and young children that is often associated with myocarditis (see Chapter 72). In addition to prolonged fever lasting more than 5 days, the principal signs are diffuse mucosal inflammation, bilateral nonpurulent conjunctivitis, dysmorphic skin rashes, indurative angioedema of hands and feet, and cervical lymphadenopathy (Kuo et al., 2012). Although the etiology is uncertain, available evidence implicates bacterial infection. Cunningham et al. (1999) showed that sera from five of 13 patients with Kawasaki syndrome recognized peptides from the light meromysin region of human cardiac myosin and had a different pattern of reactivity from acute rheumatic fever sera.

ANIMAL MODELS AND PATHOGENIC MECHANISMS

Since enteroviruses are most often implicated in human myocarditis and DCM, these agents have been widely used to investigate the pathogenic mechanisms of these diseases. Although infections by CB3 are relatively common, the development of clinically significant, ongoing myocardial disease in humans is relatively uncommon, suggesting that differences in host response play a critical role in disease susceptibility. These differences are likely to be genetically determined and may relate to the expression of virus-specific receptor on heart tissue or to the immune response of the host. Because it is difficult to examine the role that genetic polymorphisms play in humans, investigators have developed models of Coxsackievirus-induced myocarditis in mice, for which a large number of genetically different, inbred strains are available.

A model of the timecourse of viral myocarditis is illustrated in Figure 70.5. All strains of mice tested developed acute myocarditis starting 2 or 3 days after CB3 infection. The disease reached its peak on day 7 and gradually resolved so that by day 21 the heart was histologically normal. No infectious virus was found after day 9. In a few strains of mice, however, the myocarditis persisted (Rose et al., 1987; Cihakova and Rose, 2008), but the histologic picture shifted. The first phase was characterized by focal necrosis of myocytes and accompanying a focal acute inflammatory response with a mixed cell infiltrate consisting of polymorphonuclear and mononuclear cells. In those mice that developed the second phase of disease, the inflammatory process was diffuse rather than focal and consisted mainly of mononuclear interstitial infiltrates, including both T and B lymphocytes and little or no myocyte necrosis. In the mice that developed the second phase of disease, heart-reactive autoantibodies were present and shown to be specific for the cardiac isoform of myosin (Neu et al., 1987a). This finding suggested that the second phase represented an autoimmune response initiated by the viral infection. Direct evidence to support this hypothesis was produced by immunizing the susceptible strains of mice with purified cardiac myosin and showing that they developed a very similar histologic picture of myocarditis (Neu et al., 1987b). No heart disease was found in animals

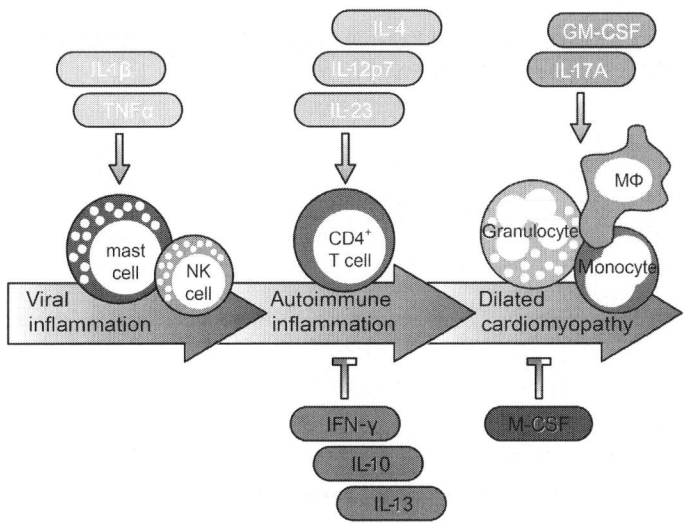

FIGURE 70.5 Schematic of the pathogenesis of viral myocarditis.

that received skeletal myosin and none appeared in the strains of mice that were not genetically susceptible to the second phase. They found evidence that this form of inflammatory heart disease was due to an immune response to cardiac myosin, assembled by inducing specific tolerance to cardiac myosin (Wang et al., 2000; Fousteri et al., 2011). This finding suggested that the second phase represents an autoimmune response initiated by molecular mimicry between the virus and heart antigens (Cunningham, 2004). On the other hand, available evidence suggests that the autoimmune response depends upon virus-induced damage to the heart since Horwitz et al. (2000) found that transgenic mice expressing interferon gamma (IFN-γ) in their pancreatic cells failed to produce CB3-induced myocarditis, even though the virus proliferated great in other sites. These findings suggest that the virus infection may serve as an adjuvant for cardiac antigens that have been expressed or liberated during the viral infection of the heart (Rose, 2000). Of importance is the finding that a number of other viruses unrelated to Coxsackieviruses such as cytomegalovirus produce a similar autoimmune myocarditis following infection. The experiments showing that myocarditis can be produced by immunization with cardiac myosin in animals that have not undergone viral infection demonstrate that the disease does not depend upon persisting virus even though it is possible to demonstrate traces of viral RNA in the heart of Coxsackievirus B3 infected animals.

Unless subjected to exercise stress, most mice survived the autoimmune phase of myocarditis whether induced by viruses, infection, or by immunization with cardiac myosin. Gradually the disease waned in severity (Rose and Hill, 1996; Cihakova and Rose, 2008). Under some conditions, however, the histologic picture changed again to

produce a mainly fibrotic disease. As the process continued, there was a thinning of the ventricular cell walls and a large increase in size of the left ventricle. By day 35, after infection or immunization there were definite signs of cardiac insufficiency and by day 60, most of the animals with these changes died of heart failure. This form of the disease, whether induced by viral infection or myosin autoimmunity, replicated the major characteristics of dilated cardiomyopathy, suggesting that DCM can represent an end stage of autoimmune myocarditis in some instances.

The striking finding from the investigations described above was that strains of mice highly susceptible to the autoimmune myocarditis following viral infection were also the strains most susceptible to the myosin-induced disease. On the other hand, other strains were relatively resistant to both forms of myocarditis. These observations indicated that the disease susceptibility was under a large measure of genetic control. As in most autoimmune diseases, genes of the major histocompatibility complex have an important influence on the development and course of autoimmune disease (Li et al., 2008a). Thus, in both the viral and myosin-induced models, the H-2^s, H-2^a, and H-2^b alleles were associated with increased morbidity of autoimmune myocarditis, whereas the H-2^b allele is associated with a relatively low susceptibility. These MHC polymorphisms were further reflected in the prevalence and titer of cardiac-specific autoantibodies. The genetic findings in the mouse can be related to human myocarditis through experiments by Hayward et al. (2006) and Taneja and David (2009), who demonstrated a spontaneous myocarditis model in NOD mice carrying the transgenically introduced human HLA-DQ8 allele associated with greater susceptibility to human

DCM. Like many autoimmune diseases in animals and humans, non-MHC genes play a determining role in susceptibility to myocarditis. To determine the non-MHC genes that affect susceptibility to myosin-induced myocarditis, genome-wide linkage analysis was carried out and revealed at least two prominent loci that had significant effects on susceptibility to autoimmune myocarditis. A putative susceptibility gene, *eam1*, was located on the proximal end of chromosome 1 and *eam2* on the distal region of chromosome 6. Both of these chromosomal segments bore genes determining susceptibility to a number of other autoimmune diseases such as autoimmune encephalomyelitis and autoimmune arthritis as well as spontaneous diabetes.

In addition to lending themselves to genetic studies, the experimental models of autoimmune myocarditis provide the opportunity of following the inflammatory process from the beginning to the end (Rose, 2011). The first major question to be considered was the basis of the susceptibility to autoimmune myocarditis following the virus infection. Studies show that two critical cytokines, IL-1β and TNF-α, were both necessary and sufficient for the progression from viral myocarditis to autoimmune myocarditis. Blocking either one of these two cytokines prevented the transition from viral to autoimmune myocarditis even in the most highly susceptible strains. Even more important was the demonstration that providing either of these two cytokines in recombinant form allowed normally resistant mice to develop the autoimmune form of myocarditis just like their genetically susceptible counterparts. The earlier signs of susceptibility to autoimmune myocarditis become evident very early in the course of viral infection. In fact, significant elevations of IL-1β were found as early as 8 hours after viral infection (Fairweather et al., 2004a,b). Thus, the innate immune response to the virus is the determining factor in later susceptibility to autoimmune disease. Some evidence points to the mast cell as particularly important in producing the mediators that determine the course of innate immunity to the virus. In addition, NK cells which are also activated during the innate immune response are responsible for downregulating susceptibility to the autoimmune response.

An important lesson to be learned from these experiments is that the early steps in innate immunity determine the later course of adaptive autoimmune diseases. Adoptive transfer experiments using myosin or myosin peptide-induced disease have shown that the induction of autoimmune myocarditis depends upon myosin-specific CD4 T cells (Smith and Allen, 1991; Li et al., 2008b; Chen et al., 2012). The course of the inflammation during autoimmune myocarditis can be traced to the relative proportions of certain key cytokines. Severe forms of autoimmune myocarditis are associated with greater production of IL-12 P40 (a Th1 signal), IL-4 (a Th2 signal), and IL-23 (a signal of the Th17 response) (Rose, 2011). On the other hand, IFN-γ, a signature of Th1 responses, definitely retards the development of autoimmune myocarditis as do two cytokines associated with Th2 responses, IL-10 and IL-13. These findings are striking examples of the cytokine "interactome"; they further suggest a balance of cytokines affects not only the severity, but the profile of inflammation. For example, IL-4 promotes a particularly severe form of eosinophilic giant-cell myocarditis in A/J mice. IL-17A, a cytokine associated with neutrophilic inflammation in some other autoimmune conditions, has little impact on the severity of inflammation in the myosin-induced autoimmune disease. It is, however, critical for the later progression to dilated cardiomyopathy; animals deprived of IL-17A fail to develop the subsequent fibrotic disease. The disease can actually be prevented by administering antibody to IL-17A earlier in the course of inflammation. This key role of IL-17 may be related to its established ability to increase granulocyte proliferation as well as to activate macrophages. A cytokine acting with IL-17, i-GM-CSF, stimulates both granulocytes and monocytes. On the other hand, M-CSF, which acts only to increase monocytes, retards the development of dilated cardiomyopathy.

An issue critical to understanding the pathogenesis of autoimmune myocarditis is the dynamic balance of mediators tending to favor inflammation and cardiomyocyte injury with mediators that reduce or retard inflammation. In contrast to some other experimental models of autoimmune disease, IFN-γ is downregulatory in myocarditis and its deficiency produces a particularly severe form of the disease. IL-10 and IL-13 are also downregulatory whereas IL-4 and IL-5 contribute to severity of the disease. In fact, elevated IL-5 production induces a disease with a Th2 phenotype and extensive infiltration by eosinophils, like the disease in humans, eosinophilic myocarditis in mice tends to be rapidly fatal.

As mentioned previously, other cardiac-specific antigens can induce autoimmune myocarditis. Goser et al. (2006) demonstrated the provocation of an autoimmune response to cardiac troponin I, which induces severe inflammation in the myocardium of mice followed by fibrosis and heart failure, with marked mortality. These investigators identified two sequence motifs of cardiac troponin I that induced inflammation and fibrosis in the myocardium (Kaya et al., 2008). Interestingly, these same animals eventually developed immunity to cardiac myosin following at least 90 days of inflammation. Thus, autoimmune myocarditis, like most autoimmune diseases, is characterized by the production of multiple organ-specific autoantibodies.

TREATMENT AND OUTCOME

Until recently, the only treatment for myocarditis and DCM was supportive therapies, such as bedrest and treatment of heart failure, arrhythmias, and embolic events if present. In many centers, cardiac transplantation has become the eventual treatment of choice in patients with refractory heart failure. In patients whose condition deteriorates despite optimal medical management, mechanical circulatory support, such as ventricular assist devices or extracorporeal membrane oxygenation, serve as a bridge to transplantation or recovery.

The role of immunosuppressive therapy in myocarditis remains controversial (Maisch et al., 2004). Numerous reported studies on relatively small numbers of patients have generally found that, while some individuals respond well to immunosuppression (prednisone and cyclosporine), others fail to respond or even have serious adverse reactions that preclude continued treatment. The major problem at present is surely the difficulty in distinguishing immune-mediated cardiac disease from infectious, genetic, or toxic forms of the disease. Obviously, until there are reliable biomarkers to distinguish autoimmune myocarditis/DCM, treatment cannot be rational or capable of statistical evaluation.

A placebo-controlled study of the treatment of idiopathic DCM was performed by Parrillo et al. (1989). The study demonstrated that unselected patients with DCM overall did not benefit substantially from immunosuppressive therapy, but a small, if transient, benefit was demonstrated in patients who had histologic evidence of active inflammation by biopsy.

Mason et al. (1995) assigned a series of patients with a histopathologic diagnosis of myocarditis (based on the Dallas criteria) and a low left ventricular ejection fraction to receive conventional therapy, with or without a 24-week course of prednisone plus cyclosporine or azathioprine. The outcome assessed was improvement in the left ventricular ejection fraction at 28 weeks compared with a placebo control group. No significant functional improvement was seen with immunosuppressive therapy. It should be noted, however, that during the establishment of the trial as many as 2233 patients with a clinical and pathologic diagnosis of myocarditis were presented for entry by their cardiologists, but only 111 met the strict Dallas criteria; i.e., some 95% of patients with a preliminary diagnosis of myocarditis failed to fulfill the Dallas criteria. The patients who would be expected to benefit most from immunosuppressive treatment are those with primarily autoimmune rather than viral myocarditis.

This interpretation is favored by the report of Kühl and Schultheiss (1995), who selected 48 patients presenting with mild-to-severe heart failure and immunohistologic evidence of an active immunologic process on biopsy.

After a 6-month treatment with 6-methylprednisolone, 23 experienced objective improvement in cardiac function. The suggestion of this study is that in a subgroup of patients with an active immunopathologic process immunosuppressive treatment will confer clinical benefit.

Wojnicz et al. (2001) evaluated 202 patients with idiopathic DCM by endomyocardial biopsy. Eighty-four of these 202 on biopsy had expression of HLA class II molecules. Those patients were randomized to immunosuppressive therapy or placebo. While the major outcome of the trial (death, transplantation, or hospitalization) was unchanged by treatment, the ejection fraction in the treated population rose from 24 to 36%, while it was virtually unchanged in the placebo group (25 to 27%). In addition, subjective parameters of improvement were noted at 3 months in 72% of the immunosuppressive therapy patients compared with only 21% of the control group. Frustaci et al. (2003) identified 112 of 652 patients with new-onset left ventricular compromise who had a presentation compatible with myocarditis. Forty-one of the 112 had progressive heart failure despite standard heart failure management. This patient population was treated with prednisone and azathioprine. Twenty of the 41 patients responded while 21 did not. The investigators determined retrospectively that those who responded had antiheart antibodies by immunofluorescence, and those who failed to respond had persistent virus demonstrated by PCR analysis of the endomyocardial biopsy. Additionally, Jones et al. (1991) demonstrated that in 20 patients with Dallas criteria-positive myocarditis, those with borderline myocarditis had a greater improvement in their ejection fraction by echocardiography and stroke work index from right heart catheterization than those with frank myocarditis. These studies suggest that there soon may be more sensitive and specific biomarkers for immune-mediated heart disease than are currently available by the Dallas criteria.

Different myocarditis populations may respond differently. Patients with fulminant myocarditis usually resolve spontaneously and there is suggestive evidence that immunosuppressive therapy may worsen the outcome. In contrast, the treatment of giant-cell myocarditis with immunosuppression may improve the prognosis by slowing progression of the disease (Cooper, 2002), suggesting that this form of the disease is an autoimmune variant.

Other therapeutic approaches have been based on the possible pathogenic role of humoral antibodies. As described above, several investigators reduced the level of circulating immunoglobulin by means of an immunoabsorption column, and showed improvement in cardiac function. McNamara et al. (2001) demonstrated in a trial of 72 patients with new onset cardiomyopathy that 2 g/kg of intravenous immunoglobulin failed to improve ejection fraction or survival when compared with placebo-treated patients. Early trials have shown promising results using extra corporeal immunoadsorption of antibodies to the p1-adrenoreceptor in the IgG3 subclass (Staudt et al., 2002, 2003; Winters, 2012).

On the premise that many patients with myocarditis or idiopathic DCM have an undisclosed persistent viral infection, Miric et al. (1994) treated a series of 180 patients with IFN-α or thymomodulin. Left ventricular function, exercise tolerance, and survival rate were significantly improved in patients given the immunomodulatory therapy. Kühl et al. (2003) treated 22 patients with proven viral myocarditis with IFN-β. The treatment was well tolerated. All patients cleared the viral genome and showed improved left ventricular function.

The above studies make it obvious that treatment of myocarditis and DCM is still problematic. As more is learned about the pathogenic mechanisms in these diseases, treatments can be individualized.

PERSONAL THOUGHTS

The diseases described in this chapter exemplify the broad range of cardiovascular disorders with which autoimmune responses have been implicated. Until very recently the role of autoimmunity in cardiovascular diseases had been rather neglected. Yet, before the early 1960s, rheumatic fever was a major topic of investigation. Although the decline of rheumatic fever in the 1960s accounted for a loss of interest in this topic, it must be recognized that the studies of rheumatic fever were the stimulus for many current concepts of autoimmunity and autoimmune disease. A renaissance in cardiovascular immunology followed efforts to define the role of autoimmunity in myocarditis and DCM. There is now a substantial challenge in developing reliable and robust *in vitro* assays that define autoimmune heart disorders with the same sensitivity and specificity now available in autoimmune disorders affecting other major organs. These studies will also serve as the impetus to delineate the contribution of autoimmunity to other enigmatic cardiovascular diseases such as atherosclerosis (see Chapter 71). Further, they provide as a general model for studying the steps relating infection to the onset of autoimmune disease (see Chapter 19).

ACKNOWLEDGMENTS

The figures were prepared by Dr. Marc Halushka and Dr. Jobert Barin, Department of Pathology, Johns Hopkins School of Medicine. The authors dedicate this chapter to their late colleague, Kenneth Baughman, a co-author of the original chapter.

REFERENCES

Abdel-Aty, H., Boye, P., Zagrosek, A., Wassmuth, R., Kumar, A., Messroghli, D., et al., 2005. Diagnostic performance of cardiovascular magnetic resonance in patients with suspected acute myocarditis: comparison of different approaches. J. Am. Coll. Cardiol. 45, 1815–1822.

Abelmann, W.H., 1984. Classification and natural history of primary myocardial disease. Prog. Cardiovasc. Dis. 27, 73–94.

Anderson, J.L., Carlquist, J.F., Lutz, J.R., DeWitt, C.W., Hammond, E. H., 1984. HLA A, B and DR typing in idiopathic dilated cardiomyopathy: a search for immune response factors. Am. J. Cardiol. 53, 473–487.

Ansari, A.A., Herskowitz, A., Danner, D.J., Neckelmann, N., Gershwin, M.E., Gravanis, M.B., et al., 1988. Identification of mitochondrial proteins that serve as targets for autoimmunity in human dilated cardiomyopathy. Circulation. 78, 457.

Aretz, H.T., Billingham, M.E., Edwards, W.D., Factor, S.M., Fallon, J.T., Fenoglio Jr., J.J., et al., 1986. Myocarditis. A histopathologic definition and classification. Am. J. Cardiovasc. Pathol. 1, 3–14.

Arola, A., Jokinen, E., Ruuskanen, O., Saraste, M., Pesonen, E., Kuusela, A.L., et al., 1997. Epidemiology of idiopathic cardiomyopathies in children and adolescents. A nationwide study in Finland. Am. J. Epidemiol. 146, 385–393.

Ayuthya, P.S.N., Jayavasu, J., Pongpanich, B., 1974. Coxsackie group B virus and primary myocardial disease in infants and children. Am. Heart J. 88, 311–314.

Baboonian, C., McKenna, W., 2003. Eradication of viral myocarditis. Is there hope? J. Am. Coll. Cardiol. 42, 473–476.

Ballinas-Vedugo, M.A., Alejandre-Aguilar, R., Aranda-Fraustro, A., Reyes, P., Monteon, M., 2003. Anti-myosin autoantibodies are more frequent in non-Chagas cardiomyopathy than in Chagasic cardiomyopathy patients. Int. J. Cardiol. 92, 101–102.

Basso, C., Calabrese, F., Angelini, A., Carturan, E., Thiene, G., 2012. Classification and histological, immunohistochemical, and molecular diagnosis of inflammatory myocardial disease. Heart Fail. Rev. 10.1007/s10741-012-9355-6.

Beck, M.A., Shi, Q., Morris, V.C., Levander, O.A., 1995. Rapid genomic evolution of a non-virulent Coxsackievirus B3 in selenium-deficient mice results in selection of identical virulent isolates. Nat. Med. 1, 433–436.

Bowles, N.E., Richardson, P.J., Olsen, E.G.J., Archard, L.C., 1986. Detection of Coxsackie-B-virus-specific RNA sequences in myocardial biopsy samples from patients with myocarditis and dilated cardiomyopathy. Lancet. i.1120–1122.

Bowles, N.E., Ni, J., Kearney, D.L., Pauschinger, M., Schultheiss, H.-P., McCarthy, R., et al., 2003. Detection of viruses in myocardial tissues by polymerase chain reaction; evidence of adenovirus as a common cause of myocarditis in children and adults. J. Am. Coll. Cardiol. 42, 466–472.

Burch, G.E., Sun, S.C., Chu, K.C., Sohal, R.S., Colcolough, H.L., 1968. Interstitial and Coxsackievirus B myocarditis in infants and children. A comparative histologic and immunofluorescent study of 50 autopsied hearts. J. Am. Med. Assoc. 203, 55–62.

Caforio, A.L., Calabrese, F., Angelini, A., Tona, F., Vinci, A., Bottaro, S., et al., 2007. A prospective study of biopsy-proven myocarditis: prognostic relevance of clinical and aetiopathogenetic features at diagnosis. Eur. Heart J. 28, 1326–1333.

Caforio, A.L.P., Grazzini, M., Mann, J.M., Keeling, P.J., Bottazzo, G.F., McKenna, W.J., et al., 1992. Identification of a- and b-cardiac myosin heavy chain isoforms as major autoantigens in dilated cardiomyopathy. Circulation. 85, 1734–1742.

Caforio, A.L.P., Mahon, N.J., Tona, F., McKenna, W.J., 2002. Circulating cardiac autoantibodies in dilated cardiomyopathy and myocarditis: pathogenetic and clinical significance. Eur. J. Heart Failure. 4, 411–417.

Carlquist, J.F., Menlove, R.L., Murray, M.B., O'Connell, J.B., Anderson, J.L., 1991. HLA class II (DR and DQ) antigen associations in idiopathic dilated cardiomyopathy. Circulation. 83, 515–522.

Cetta, F., Michels, V.V., 1995. The autoimmune basis of dilated cardiomyopathy. Ann. Med. 27, 169–173.

Chen, P., Baldeviano, G.C., Ligons, D.L., Talor, M.V., Barin, J.G., Rose, N.R., et al., 2012. Susceptibility to autoimmune myocarditis is associated with intrinsic differences in CD4(+) T cells. Clin. Exp. Immunol. 169, 79–88.

Chow, L.H., Radio, S.J., Sears, T.D., McManus, G.M., 1989. Insensitivity of right ventricular endomyocardial biopsy in the diagnosis of myocarditis. J. Am. Coll. Cardiol. 14, 915–920.

Cihakova, D., Rose, N.R., 2008. Pathogenesis of myocarditis and dilated cardiomyopathy. Adv. Immunol. 99, 95–114.

Cooper, L.T., 2002. Idiopathic giant cell myocarditis. In: Cooper, L.T. (Ed.), Myocarditis from Bench to Bedside. Humana Press, Totowa, NJ, pp. 405–420.

Coura, J.R., Borges-Pereira, J., 2012. Chagas disease: what is known and what should be improved: a systemic review. Rev. Soc. Bras. Med. Trop. 45, 286–296.

Cunha-Neto, E., Iwai, L.K., Morand, B., Bilate, A., Goncalves-Fonseca, S., Kalil, J., 2004. Autoimmunity in Chagas' Disease. In: Shoenfeld, Y., Rose, N.R. (Eds.), Infection and Autoimmunity. Elsevier, Amsterdam, pp. 449–466.

Cunningham, M.W., 2004. T cell mimicry in inflammatory heart disease. Mol. Immunol. 40, 1121–1127.

Cunningham, M.W., Meissner, H.C., Heuser, J.S., Pietra, B.A., Kurahara, D.K., Leung, D.Y.M., 1999. Anti-human cardiac myosin autoantibodies in Kawasaki syndrome. J. Immunol. 163, 1060–1065.

Dandel, M., Wallukat, G., Potapov, E., Hetzer, R., 2012. Role of beta (1)-adrenoceptor autoantibodies in the pathogenesis of dilated cardiomyopathy. Immunobiology. 217, 511–520.

Dec Jr., G.W., Palacios, I.F., Fallon, J.T., Aretz, H.T., Mills, J., Lee, D.C., et al., 1985. Active myocarditis in the spectrum of acute dilated cardiomyopathies. Clinical features, histologic correlates, and clinical outcome. N. Engl. J. Med. 312, 885–890.

Deubner, N., Berliner, D., Schlipp, A., Gelbrich, G., Caforio, A.L., Felix, S.B., et al., 2010. Cardiac beta1-adrenoceptor autoantibodies in human heart disease: rationale and design of the Etiology, Titre-Course, and Survival (ETiCS) Study. Eur. J. Heart Fail. 12, 753–762.

D'Ambrosio, A., Patti, G., Manzoli, A., Sinagra, G., Di Lenarda, A., Silvestri, F., et al., 2001. The fate of acute myocarditis between spontaneous improvement and evolution to dilated cardiomyopathy: a review. Heart. 85, 499–504.

Elamm, C., Fairweather, D., Cooper, L.T., 2012. Pathogenesis and diagnosis of myocarditis. Heart. 98 (11), 835–840.

Esfandiarei, M., McManus, B.M., 2008. Molecular biology and pathogenesis of viral myocarditis. Annu. Rev. Pathol. 3, 127–155.

Fabre, A., Sheppard, M.N., 2006. Sudden adult death syndrome and other non-ischaemic causes of sudden cardiac death. Heart. 92, 316–320.

Fairweather, D., Frisancho-Kiss, S., Gatewood, S., Njoku, D., Steele, R., Barrett, M., et al., 2004a. Mast cells and innate cytokines are associated with susceptibility to autoimmune heart disease following Coxsackievirus B3 infection. Autoimmunity. 37, 131–145.

Fairweather, D., Afanasyeva, M., Rose, N.R., 2004b. Cellular immunity: a role for cytokines. In: Doria, A., Pauletto, P. (Eds.), Handbook of Systemic Autoimmune Diseases, Vol. 1: The Heart in Systemic Autoimmune Diseases. Elsevier, Amsterdam, pp. 3–17.

Felix, S.B., Staudt, A., 2006. Non-specific immunoadsorption in patients with dilated cardiomyopathy: mechanisms and clinical effects. Int. J. Cardiol. 112, 30–33.

Felker, G.M., Thompson, R.E., Hare, J.M., Hurban, R.H., Clemetson, D.E., Howard, D.L., et al., 2000. Underlying causes and long-term survival in patients with initially unexplained cardiomyopathy. N. Engl. J. Med. 342, 1077–1084.

Ferrari, I., Levin, M.J., Wallukat, G., Elies, R., Lebesgue, D., Chiale, P., et al., 1995. Molecular mimicry between the immunodominant ribosomal protein P0 of Trypanosoma cruzi and a functional epitope on the human beta1-adrenergic receptor. J. Exp. Med. 182, 59–65.

Fousteri, G., Dave, A., Morin, B., Omid, S., Croft, M., von Herrath, M.G., 2011. Nasal cardiac myosin peptide treatment and OX40 blockade protect mice from acute and chronic virally-induced myocarditis. J. Autoimmun. 36, 210–220.

Friedrich, M.G., Sechtem, U., Schulz-Menger, J., Holmvang, G., Alakija, P., Cooper, L.T., et al., 2009. Cardiovascular magnetic resonance in myocarditis: a JACC White Paper. J. Am. Coll. Cardiol. 53, 1475–1487.

Frustaci, A., Chimenti, C., Calabrese, F., Pieroni, M., Thiene, G., Maseri, A., 2003. Immunosuppressive therapy for active lymphocytic myocarditis. Virological and immunologic profile of responders versus nonresponders. Circulation. 107, 857–863.

Girones, N., Rodriguez, C.I., Carrasco-Marin, E., Hernaez, R.F., de Rego, J.L., Fresno, M., 2001. Dominant T- and B-cell epitopes in an autoantigen linked to Chagas' disease. J. Clin. Invest. 107, 985–993.

Goser, S., Andrassy, M., Buss, S.J., Leuschner, F., Volz, C.H., Ottl, R., et al., 2006. Cardiac troponin I but not cardiac troponin T induces severe autoimmune inflammation in the myocardium. Circulation. 114, 1693–1702.

Gravanis, M.B., Ansari, A.A., 1987. Idiopathic cardiomyopathies. A review of pathologic studies and mechanisms of pathogenesis. Arch. Pathol. Lab. Med. 111, 915–929.

Gravanis, M.B., Sternby, N.H., 1991. Incidence of myocarditis: a 10-year autopsy study from Malmö, Sweden. Arch. Pathol. Lab. Med. 115, 390–392.

Grist, N.R., Bell, E.J., 1974. A six-year study of coxsackievirus B infections in heart disease. J. Hygiene. 73, 165–172.

Grogan, M., Redfield, M.M., Bailey, K.R., Reeder, G.S., Gersh, B.J., Edwards, W.D., et al., 1995. Long-term outcome of patients with biopsy-proved myocarditis: comparison with idiopathic dilated cardiomyopathy. J. Am. Coll. Cardiol. 26, 80–84.

Gutberlet, M., Spors, B., Thoma, T., Bertram, H., Denecke, T., Felix, R., et al., 2008. Suspected chronic myocarditis at cardiac MR: diagnostic accuracy and association with immunohistologically detected inflammation and viral persistence. Radiology. 246, 401–409.

Hammond, E.H., Menlove, R.L., Anderson, J.L., 1988. Immunofluorescence microscopy in the diagnosis and follow-up of myocarditis. A critical review. In: Schultheiss, H.-P. (Ed.), New Concepts in Viral Heart Disease. Springer-Verlag, Berlin, pp. 303–311.

Hashimoto, K., Yoshioka, K., 2012. Review: surveillance of Chagas disease. Adv. Parasitol. 79, 375–428.

Hauck, A.J., Kearney, D.L., Edwards, W.D., 1989. Evaluation of postmortem endomyocardial biopsy specimens from 38 patients with lymphocytic myocarditis: implications for role of sampling error. Mayo Clinic. Proc. 64, 1235–1245.

Hayward, S.L., Bautista-Lopez, N., Suzuki, K., Atrazhev, A., Dickie, P., Elliott, J.F., 2006. CD4 T cells play major effector role and CD8 T cells initiating role in spontaneous autoimmune myocarditis of HLA-DQ8 transgenic IAb knockout nonobese diabetic mice. J. Immunol. 176, 7715–7725.

Herskowitz, A., Ahmed-Ansari, A., Neumann, D.A., Beschorner, W.E., Rose, N.R., Soule, L.M., et al., 1990. Induction of major histocompatibility complex antigens within the myocardium of patients with active myocarditis: a nonhistologic marker of myocarditis. J. Am. Coll. Cardiol. 15, 624–632.

Horwitz, M.S., La Cava, A., Fine, C., Rodriguez, E., Ilic, A., Sarvetnick, N., 2000. Pancreatic expression of interferon-gamma protects mice from lethal coxsackievirus B3 infection and subsequent myocarditis. Nat. Med. 6, 693–697.

Huber, S.A., 1997. Animal models of human disease. Autoimmunity in myocarditis: relevance of animal models. Clin. Immunol. Immunopathol. 83, 93–102.

Jacobson, D.L., Gange, S.J., Rose, N.R., Graham, N.M.H., 1997. Epidemiology and estimated population burden of selected autoimmune diseases in the United States. Clin. Immunol. Immunopathol. 84, 223–243.

Jahns, R., Schlipp, A., Boivin, V., Lohse, M.J., 2010. Targeting receptor antibodies in immune cardiomyopathy. Semin. Thromb. Hemost. 36, 212–218.

Jefferies, J.L., Towbin, J.A., 2010. Dilated cardiomyopathy. Lancet. 375, 752–762.

Jeserich, M., Konstantinides, S., Olschewski, M., Pavlik, G., Bode, C., Geibel, A., 2010. Diagnosis of early myocarditis after respiratory or gastrointestinal tract viral infection: insights from cardiovascular magnetic resonance. Clin. Res. Cardiol. 99, 707–714.

Jones, S.R., Herskowitz, H.M., Hutchins, H.M., Baughman, K.L., 1991. Effects of immunosuppressive therapy in biopsy-proved myocarditis and borderline myocarditis on left ventricular function. Am. J. Cardiol. 68, 370–376.

Kalil, J., Cunha-Neto, E., 1996. Autoimmunity in Chagas' disease cardiomyopathy: fulfilling the criteria at last? Parasitol. Today. 12, 396–399.

Kandolf, R., Ameis, D., Kirschner, P., Canue, A., Hofschneider, P.H., 1987. In situ detection of enteroviral genomes in myocardital cells by nucleic acid hybridization: an approach to the diagnosis of viral heart disease. Proc. Natl. Acad. Sci. USA. 84, 6272–6276.

Kaplan, D., Ferrari, I., Bergami, P.L., Mahler, E., Levitus, G., Chiale, P., et al., 1997. Antibodies to ribosomal P proteins of Trypanosoma cruzi in Chagas' disease possess functional autoreactivity with heart tissue and differ from anti-P autoantibodies in lupus. Proc. Natl. Acad. Sci. USA. 94, 10301–10306.

Kaya, Z., Goser, S., Buss, S.J., Leuschner, F., Ottl, R., Li, J., et al., 2008. Identification of cardiac troponin I sequence motifs leading to heart failure by induction of myocardial inflammation and fibrosis. Circulation. 118, 2063–2072.

Kaya, Z., Katus, H.A., Rose, N.R., 2010. Cardiac troponins and autoimmunity: their role in the pathogenesis of myocarditis and of heart failure. Clin. Immunol. 134, 80–88.

Kaya, Z., Leib, C., Katus, H.A., 2012. Autoantibodies in heart failure and cardiac dysfunction. Circ. Res. 110, 145–158.

Kline, I.K., Saphir, O., 1960. Chronic pernicious myocarditis. Am. Heart J. 59, 681–697.

Klingel, K.C., Hohenadl, A., Canu, M., Albrecht, M., Seemann, M., Mall, G., et al., 1992. Ongoing enterovirus-induced myocarditis is associated with persistent heart muscle infection: quantitative analysis of virus replication, tissue damage, and inflammation. Proc. Natl. Acad. Sci. USA. 89, 314–318.

Kuo, H.C., Yang, K.D., Chang, W.C., Ger, L.P., Hsieh, K.S., 2012. Kawasaki disease: an update on diagnosis and treatment. Pediatr. Neonatol. 53, 4–11.

Kühl, U., Schultheiss, H.-P., 1995. Treatment of chronic myocarditis with corticosteroids. Eur. Heart J. 16, 168–172.

Kühl, U., Pauschinger, M., Schwimmbeck, P.L., Seeberg, B., Lober, C., Noutsias, M., et al., 2003. Interferon-b treatment eliminates cardiotropic viruses and improves left ventricular function in patients with myocardial persistence of viral genomes and left ventricular dysfunction. Circulation. 107, 2793–2798.

Leuschner, F., Li, J., Goser, S., Reinhardt, L., Ottl, R., Bride, P., et al., 2008. Absence of auto-antibodies against cardiac troponin I predicts improvement of left ventricular function after acute myocardial infarction. Eur. Heart. 29, 1949–1955.

Levander, O.A., Beck, M.A., 1997. Interacting nutritional and infectious etiologies of Keshan disease. Insights from Coxsackie virus B-induced myocarditis in mice deficient in selenium or vitamin E. Biol. Trace. Elem. Res. 56, 1–16.

Li, H.S., Ligons, D.L., Rose, N.R., 2008a. Genetic complexity of autoimmune myocarditis. Autoimmun. Rev. 7, 168–173.

Li, H.S., Ligons, D.L., Rose, N.R., Guler, M.L., 2008b. Genetic differences in bone marrow-derived lymphoid lineages control susceptibility to experimental autoimmune myocarditis. J. Immunol. 180, 7480–7484.

Liberthson, R.R., 1996. Sudden death from cardiac causes in children and young adults. N. Engl. J. Med. 334, 1039–1044.

Lieberman, E.B., Hutchins, G.M., Herskowitz, A., Rose, N.R., Baughman, K.L., 1991. Clinicopathologic description of myocarditis. J. Am. Coll. Cardiol. 18, 1617–1626.

Lieberman, E.B., Herskowitz, A., Rose, N.R., Baughman, K.L., 1993. A clinicopathologic description of myocarditis. Clin. Immunol. Immunopathol. 68, 191–196.

Limas, C.J., Goldenberg, I.F., Limas, C., 1989. Autoantibodies against beta-adrenoreceptors in human idiopathic dilated cardiomyopathy. Circ. Res. 64, 97–103.

Limas, C.J., Limas, C., Kubo, S.H., Olivari, M.T., 1990. Anti-beta receptor antibodies in human dilated cardiomyopathy and correlation with HLA-DR antigens. Am. J. Cardiol. 65, 483–487.

Luppi, P., Rudert, W., Licata, A., Riboni, S., Betters, D., Cotrufo, M., et al., 2003. Expansion of specific αβ+ T-cell subsets in the myocardium of patients with myocarditis and idiopathic dilated cardiomyopathy associated with Coxsackievirus B infection. Hum. Immunol. 64, 194–210.

Magnani, J.W., Danik, H.J., Dec Jr., G.W., DiSalvo, T.G., 2006. Survival in biopsy-proven myocarditis: a long-term retrospective analysis of the histopathologic, clinical, and hemodynamic predictors. Am. Heart J. 151, 463–470.

Mahon, N.G., Madden, B.P., Caforio, A.L.P., Elliott, P.M., Haven, A.J., Keogh, B.E., et al., 2002. Immunohistologic evidence of myocardial disease in apparently healthy relatives of patients with dilated cardiomyopathy. J. Am. Coll. Cardiol. 39, 455–462.

Mahrholdt, H., Goedecke, C., Wagner, A., Meinhardt, G., Athanasiadis, A., Vogelsberg, H., et al., 2004. Cardiovascular magnetic resonance assessment of human myocarditis: a comparison to histology and molecular pathology. Circulation. 109, 1250–1258.

Maisch, B., 1987. Immune regulation, humoral and cell-mediated immune reactions in myocarditis and dilated cardiomyopathy. In: Kawai, C., Abelmann, W.H. (Eds.), Pathogenesis of Myocarditis and Cardiomyopathy. University of Tokyo Press, Tokyo, pp. 245–267.

Maisch, B., Berg, P.A., Kochsiek, K., 1979. Clinical significance of immunopathological findings in patients with post-periocardiotomy syndrome. I. Relevance of antibody pattern. Clin. Exp. Immunol. 38, 189–197.

Maisch, B., Portig, I., Ristic, A., Hufnagel, G., Pankuweit, S., 2000. Definition of inflammatory cardiomyopathy (myocarditis): on the way to consensus. A status report. Herz. 25, 200–209.

Maisch, B., Hufnagel, G., Kolsch, S., Funck, R., Richter, A., Rupp, H., et al., 2004. Treatment of inflammatory dilated cardiomyopathy and (Peri)myocarditis with immunosuppression and i.v. immunoglobulins. Herz. 29, 624–636.

Mason, J.W., O'Connell, J.B., 1989. Clinical merit of endomyocardial biopsy. Circulation. 79, 971–979.

Mason, J.W., O'Connell, J.B., Herskowitz, A., Rose, N.R., McManus, B. M., Billingham, M.E., et al., 1995. A clinical trial of immunosuppressive therapy for myocarditis. N. Engl. J. Med. 333, 269–275.

McCarthy III, R.M., Boehmer, J.P., Hruban, R.H., Hutchins, G.M., Kasper, E.K., Hare, J.M., et al., 2000. Long-term outcome of fulminant myocarditis as compared with acute (nonfulminant) myocarditis. N. Engl. J. Med. 342, 690–695.

McNamara, D.M., Holubko, V.R., Starling, R.C., Dee, G.W., Loh, E., Tirre-Amione, G., et al., 2001. Controlled trial of intravenous immunoglobulin in recent onset dilated cardiomyopathy. Circulation. 103, 2254–2259.

Miklozek, C.L., Kingsley, E.M., Crumpaker, C.S., Modlin, J.F., Royal Henry, D., Come, P.C., et al., 1986. Serial cardiac function tests in myocarditis. Postgrad. Med. J. 62, 577–579.

Miric, M., Miskovic, A., Brkic, S., Vasiljevic, J., Keserovic, N., Pesic, M., 1994. Long-term follow-up of patients with myocarditis and idiopathic dilated cardiomyopathy after immunomodulatory therapy. FEMS Immunol. Med. Microbiol. 10, 65–74.

Motran, C.C., Fretes, R.E., Cerban, F.M., Rivarola, H.W., Bottero de Cima, E., 2000. Immunization with the C-terminal region of Trypanosoma cruzi ribosomal P1 and P2 proteins induces long-term duration cross-reactive antibodies with heart functional and structural alterations in young and aged mice. Clin. Immunol. 97, 89–94.

Müller, J., Wallukat, G., Dandel, M., Bieda, H., Brandes, K., Spiegelsberger, S., et al., 2000. Immunoglobulin adsorption in patients with idiopathic dilated cardiomyopathy. Circulation. 101, 385–401.

Nagatomo, Y., Baba, A., Ito, H., Naito, K., Yoshizawa, A., Kurita, Y., et al., 2011. Specific immunoadsorption therapy using a tryptophan column in patients with refractory heart failure due to dilated cardiomyopathy. J. Clin. Apher. 26, 1–8.

Neu, N., Beisel, K.W., Traystman, M.D., Rose, N.R., Craig, S.W., 1987a. Autoantibodies specific for the cardiac myosin isoform are found in mice susceptible to Coxsackievirus B3-induced myocarditis. J. Immunol. 138, 2488–2492.

Neu, N., Rose, N.R., Beisel, K.W., Herskowitz, A., Gurri-Glass, G., Craig, S.W., 1987b. Cardiac myosin induces myocarditis in genetically predisposed mice. J. Immunol. 139, 3630–3636.

Neumann, D.A., Burek, C.L., Baughman, K.L., Rose, N.R., Herskowitz, A., 1990. Circulating heart-reactive antibodies in patients with myocarditis or cardiomyopathy. J. Am. Coll. Cardiol. 16, 839–846.

Noren, G.R., Staley, N.A., Bandt, C.M., Kaplan, E.L., 1976. Occurrence of myocarditis in sudden death in children. J. Forensic Sci. 22, 188–196.

Parrillo, J.E., Cunnion, R.E., Epstein, S.E., Parker, M.M., Suffredini, A. F., Brenner, M., et al., 1989. A prospective, randomized, controlled trial of prednisone for dilated cardiomyopathy. N. Engl. J. Med. 321, 1061–1068.

Pauschinger, M., Chandrasekharan, K., Noutsias, M., Kühl, U., Schwimmbeck, L.P., Schultheiss, H.-P., 2004. Viral heart disease: molecular diagnosis, clinical prognosis, and treatment strategies. Med. Microbiol. Immunol. (Berl.). 193, 65–69.

Pellegrini, A., Guinazu, N., Giordanengo, L., Cano, R.C., Gea, S., 2012. The role of Toll-like receptors and adaptive immunity in the development of protective or pathological immune response triggered by the Trypanosoma cruzi protozoan. Future Microbiol. 6, 1521–1533.

Petretta, M., Pirozzi, F., Sasso, L., Paglia, A., Bonaduce, D., 2011. Review and metaanalysis of the frequency of familial dilated cardiomyopathy. Am. J. Cardiol. 108, 1171–1176.

Rose, N.R., 2000. Viral damage or "molecular mimicry": placing the blame in myocarditis. Nat. Med. 6, 5–6.

Rose, N.R., 2011. Critical cytokine pathways to cardiac inflammation. J. Interferon Cytokine Res. 31 (10), 705–710.

Rose, N.R., Hill, S.L., 1996. The pathogenesis of postinfectious myocarditis. Clin. Immunol. Immunopathol. 80, S92–S99.

Rose, N.R., Beisel, K.W., Herskowitz, A., Neu, N., Wolfgram, L.J., Alvarez, F.L., et al., 1987. Cardiac myosin and autoimmune myocarditis. In: Evered, D., Whelan, J. (Eds.), Ciba Symposium 129. John Wiley & Sons, Chichester, pp. 3–24.

Rose, N.R., Neumann, D.A., Herskowitz, A., Traystman, M., Beisel, K.W., 1988. Genetics of susceptibility to viral myocarditis in mice. Pathol. Immunopathol. Res. 7, 266–278.

Sagar, S., Liu, P.P., Cooper Jr., J.T., 2012. Myocarditis. Lancet. 379, 738–747.

Schultheiss, H.-P., Schulze, K., Kühl, U., Ulrich, G., Klingenberg, M., 1986. The ADP/ATP carrier as a mitochondrial auto-antigen—facts and perspectives. Ann. N.Y. Acad. Sci. 488, 44–64.

Schultheiss, H.P., Kuhl, U., 2011. Why is diagnosis of infectious myocarditis such a challenge? Expert Rev. Anti. Infect. Ther. 9, 1093–1095.

Smith, S.C., Allen, P.M., 1991. Myosin-induced acute myocarditis is a T cell-mediated disease. J. Immunol. 147, 2141–2147.

Staudt, A., Böhm, M., Knebel, F., Grosse, Y., Bischoff, C., Hummel, A., et al., 2002. Potential role of autoantibodies belonging to the immunoglobulin G-3 subclass in cardiac dysfunction among patients with dilated cardiomyopathy. Circulation. 106, 2448–2453.

Staudt, Y., Mobini, R., Fu, M., Felix, S.B., Kuhn, J.P., Staudt, A., 2003. Beta1-adrenoceptor antibodies induce apoptosis in adult isolated cardiomyocytes. Eur. J. Pharmacol. 466, 1–6.

Stewart, G.C., Lopez-Molina, J., Gottumukkala, R.V., Rosner, G.F., Anello, M.S., Hecht, J.L., et al., 2011. Myocardial parvovirus B19 persistence: lack of association with clinicopathologic phenotype in adults with heart failure. Circ. Heart Fail. 4, 71–78.

Taneja, V., David, C.S., 2009. Spontaneous autoimmune myocarditis and cardiomyopathy in HLA-DQ8.NODAbo transgenic mice. J. Autoimmun. 33, 260–269.

Torp, A., 1981. Incidence of congestive cardiomyopathy. In: Goodwin, J.F., Hjalmarson, A., Olsen, E.G.J. (Eds.), Congestive Cardiomyopathy. A.B. Hässle, Molndal, pp. 18–22.

Towbin, J.A., Li, H., Taggart, R.T., Lehman, M.H., Schwartz, P.J., Satler, C.A., et al., 1994. Molecular and cellular cardiovascular medicine: evidence of genetic heterogeneity in Romano-Ward long QT syndrome: analysis of 23 families. Circulation. 90, 2635–2644.

Tracy, S., Chapman, N.M., Romero, J., Ramsingh, A.I., 1996. Genetics of coxsackievirus B cardiovirulence and inflammatory heart muscle disease. Trends Microbiol. 4, 175–179.

Van Voorhis, W.C., Schlekewy, L., Trong, H.L., 1991. Molecular mimicry by Tryponosoma cruzi: the Fl-160 epitope that mimics mammalian nerve can be mapped to a 12-amino acid peptide. Proc. Natl. Acad. Sci. USA. 88, 5993–5997.

Wang, Y., Afanasyeva, M., Hill, S.L., Kaya, A., Rose, N.R., 2000. Nasal administration of cardiac myosin suppresses autoimmune myocarditis in mice. J. Am. Coll. Cardiol. 36, 1992–1999.

Wessely, R., Henke, A., Zell, R., Kandolf, R., Knowlton, K.U., 1998. Low-level expression of a mutant coxsackieviral cDNA induces a myocytopathic effect in culture: an approach to the study of enteroviral persistence in cardiac myocytes. Circulation. 98, 450–457.

Williams, D.G., Olsen, E.G.L., 1985. Prevalence of overt dilated cardiomyopathy in two regions of England. Br. Heart J. 54, 153–155.

Winters, J.L., 2012. Apheresis in the treatment of idiopathic dilated cardiomyopathy. J. Clin. Apher. 27, 312–319.

Wojnicz, R., Nawalany-Kozielska, E., Wojciechowska, C., Glanowska, G., Wilczewski, P., Niklewski, T., et al., 2001. Randomized, placebo-controlled study for immunosuppressive treatment of inflammatory dilated cardiomyopathy: two-year follow-up results. Circulation. 104, 39–45.

Wolff, P., Kühl, U., Schultheiss, H.-P., 1989. Laminin distribution and autoantibodies in idiopathic dilated cardiomyopathy and myocarditis. Am. Heart J. 117, 1303–1309.

Chapter 71

Atherosclerosis

Ban-Hock Toh[1], Tin Kyaw[1], Peter Tipping[2], and Alex Bobik[3]

[1]Centre for Inflammatory Diseases, Department of Medicine, Southern Clinical School, Faculty of Medicine, Nursing and Health Sciences, Monash University, Victoria, Australia, [2]Prince Henry's Institute of Medical Research, Clayton, Victoria, Australia, [3]Vascular Biology and Atherosclerosis Laboratory, Baker IDI Heart and Diabetes Institute, Victoria, Australia

Chapter Outline

Introduction	**1049**	CD8 T Cells	1055
Development of Atherosclerotic Lesions	**1050**	Conventional B2 Cells	1055
Mouse Models of Atherosclerosis	**1050**	Innate-like B1a Cells	1056
Culprit Autoantigens	**1050**	Other Key Cellular Players	1056
Oxidized Low-density Lipoprotein (oxLDL)	1050	Smooth Muscle Cells (SMCs)	1056
Heat Shock Protein 60 (HSP60)	1050	Endothelial Cells	1056
β2 Glycoprotein 1 (β2-GP1)	1050	Immune System Activation	1056
Immune Responses in Atherosclerosis	**1051**	Activation Sites	1056
Innate Immunity in Atherosclerosis	1051	Dendritic Cells	1057
Macrophages	1051	TLR	1057
NKT Cells	1053	Costimulatory Molecules	1057
NK Cells	1053	Leukocyte Recruitment: Adhesion Molecules	1057
Neutrophils	1053	Monocyte Homing	1058
Mast Cells	1054	T Cell Homing	1059
Adaptive Immunity in Atherosclerosis	1054	B Cell Homing	1059
Th1 CD4 T Cells	1054	Experimental Therapeutics: A Protective "Vaccine" for Atherosclerosis	1059
Th2 CD4+ T Cells	1054	Implications for Clinical Translation	1060
Th17 CD4+ T Cells	1054	**References**	**1061**
Foxp3 Regulatory CD4+ T Cells	1055		

INTRODUCTION

Atherosclerosis is a chronic inflammatory disease of large and medium sized arteries initiated by entry of low density lipoprotein (LDL) into the arterial intima. Atherosclerotic lesions are characterized by progressive accumulation of chronic inflammatory cells in the intima leading to development of vulnerable plaques characterized by large necrotic cores and thin fibrous caps (Tabas, 2011; Yla-Herttuala et al., 2011). Rupture of vulnerable plaques initiates thrombotic occlusion, end-organ infarction, heart attacks, and strokes—leading causes of death in our community.

An *autoimmune basis* for development of inflammatory lesions in atherosclerosis is supported by the presence of cognate immune cells, demonstration of autoimmunity to antigens localized within atherosclerotic plaques, attenuated atherosclerosis with establishment of tolerance to putative autoantigens, a family history, association with DRB1 (Gonzalez-Gay et al., 2007) and aggravated lesions in systemic lupus erythematosus (Asanuma et al., 2003; Roman et al., 2003), and rheumatoid arthritis (Shoenfeld et al., 2005; Steen et al., 2009).

Using mouse models, a reductionist approach has identified culprit autoantigens and roles of atherogenic and atheroprotective cells of the innate and adaptive immune system in atherogenesis.

N. Rose & I. Mackay (Eds): The Autoimmune Diseases, Fifth edition. DOI: http://dx.doi.org/10.1016/B978-0-12-384929-8.00071-X

DEVELOPMENT OF ATHEROSCLEROTIC LESIONS

Atherosclerotic lesions develop early intimal thickening due to proliferation of intimal smooth muscle cells (Ross and Glomset, 1973) thus forming the "soil" in which atherosclerotic lesions develop. Initial steps in atherosclerotic lesion formation involve lipid accumulation within the intima together with activation of the endothelium. P-selectin and vascular cell adhesion molecule-1 (VCAM-1) are focally expressed by endothelial cells at sites of lesion development in hypercholesterolemic rabbits before intimal accumulation of macrophages and T cells (Sakai et al., 1997). Fatty streaks, the initial stages of atherosclerosis, involve accumulation of macrophages and T cells with macrophages accumulating lipids to form foam cells. Subsequently, multiple types of immune cells accumulate driving these early lipid-rich lesions to develop into atheromas containing necrotic cores and subsequently to more complex lesions that may be either stable fibrous plaques or unstable, rupture-prone, soft-centered lipid laden lesions with thin collagen and vascular smooth muscle cell caps (Figure 71.1) (Davies, 1996; Yla-Herttuala et al., 2011).

MOUSE MODELS OF ATHEROSCLEROSIS

Murine models have proved powerful tools in identification of the roles of immunocytes and potential autoantigens in atherogenesis. Although wild-type strains of mice are relatively resistant to atherosclerosis development even on high-fat diets, gene knockout approaches have given two useful models. The apolipoprotein E knockout (ApoE$^{-/-}$) mouse, generated in 1992, develops atherosclerotic lesions on standard chow diet, which is greatly accelerated by a high-fat "Western" diet and the LDL receptor (LDLR) deficient mouse develop small lesions on standard chow diet and robust lesions on high-fat diet. ApoE$^{-/-}$ mouse lesions have been most thoroughly characterized. These lesions develop fibrofatty plaques with characteristics similar to those of human plaques but rarely rupture (Jawien et al., 2004). Many variants of ApoE$^{-/-}$ and LDLR$^{-/-}$ mice have been studied (Kleemann et al., 2008), generated by cross-breeding with different knockout and transgenic mice. One mouse model, ApoE$^{-/-}$SR-B1$^{-/-}$, deficient in HDL receptor scavenger receptor class B and on a mixed C57Bl/6 × 129 background, develops exceptional severe occlusive coronary artery atherosclerosis, and exhibits spontaneous myocardial infarctions, severe cardiac dysfunction, and premature death (Braun et al., 2002). The mechanisms leading to myocardial infarction in these mice are yet to be elucidated.

CULPRIT AUTOANTIGENS

Three autoantigens have been identified. Whether immune activation by these antigens occurs concurrently or sequentially following intermolecular spreading is unknown. The epitopes that drive the autoimmune response are also unknown.

Oxidized Low-density Lipoprotein (oxLDL)

oxLDL is a major component of atherosclerotic lesions, and T lymphocytes reactive to oxLDL have been recovered from human atherosclerotic plaques (Stemme et al., 1995). It seems likely that the oxidation of oxLDL renders the molecule non-self, thus initiating an autoimmune response. In LDLR-deficient mice, oral feeding of oxLDL induced oxLDL-specific TGF-β, producing Foxp3 regulatory T cells and attenuated development of atherosclerosis, strongly suggesting that oxLDL is an autoantigen in this model (van Puijvelde et al., 2006).

Heat Shock Protein 60 (HSP60)

HSP60 has generated much interest as an autoantigen with potential to drive inflammatory processes in atherosclerosis (Wick et al., 2004; Grundtman and Wick, 2011; Grundtman et al., 2011). Mixed CD4$^+$ and CD8$^+$ T cells isolated from human carotid endarterectomy specimens show an oligoclonal TCR repertoire and enhanced proliferation to human HSP60 (Rossmann et al., 2008). HSP60 is co-expressed with ICAM-1, VCAM-1, and ELAM-1 in human endothelial cells in response to stimulation by cytokines and oxLDL (Amberger et al., 1997). Atherosclerosis risk factors may act as endothelial stressors to provoke expression of HSP60 that acts as a "danger signal" (Grundtman et al., 2011). Studies in LDLR$^{-/-}$ mice provide evidence that immune responses to HSP60 are atherogenic. Oral feeding of HSP60 (or HSP60 peptides) attenuated atherosclerosis in LDLR$^{-/-}$ mice that correlated with increased Foxp3 regulatory T cells, increased expression of Foxp3, CD25, and CTLA-4 in lesions, and IL-10 and TGF-β production by lymph node cells (van Puijvelde et al., 2007).

β2 Glycoprotein 1 (β2-GP1)

β2-GP1 is a recognized autoantigen associated with antiphospholipid syndrome in humans. It has also been proposed as a potential autoantigen in atherosclerosis, either on its own or complexed with oxLDL (Matsuura et al., 2009; Shen et al., 2011). Human β2-GP1, co-localizing with CD4 T cells, is expressed in human lesions (George et al., 1999). Oral feeding of human or bovine β2-GP1 attenuated atherosclerosis in LDLR$^{-/-}$ mice, inhibited

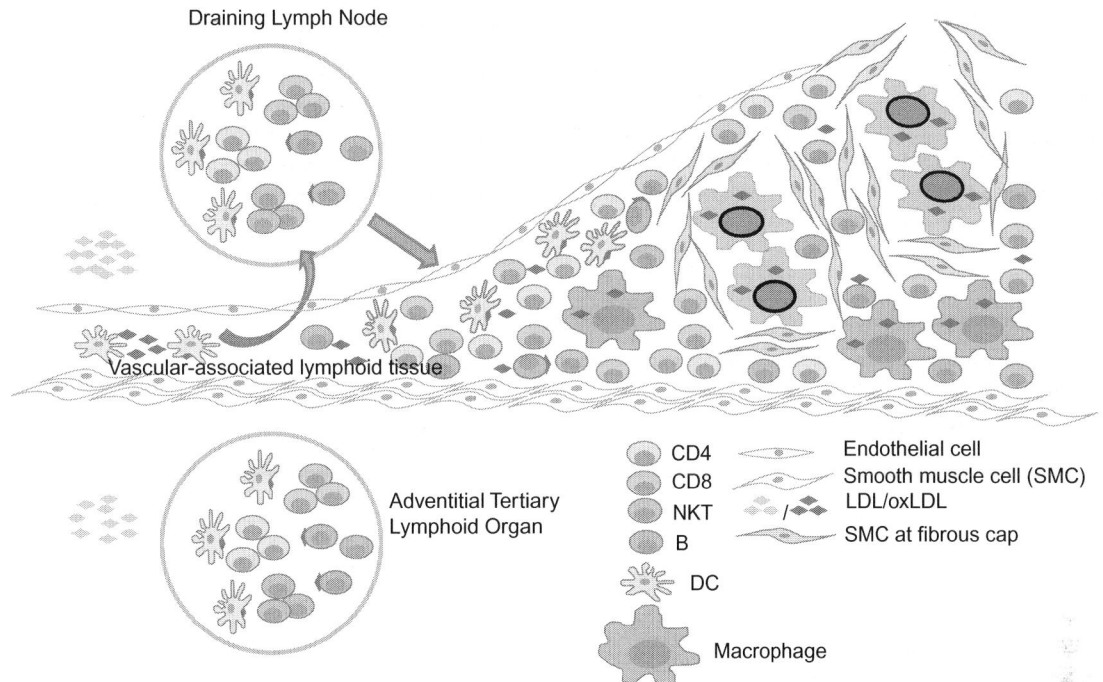

Draining Lymph Node

Vascular-associated lymphoid tissue

Adventitial Tertiary
Lymphoid Organ

CD4
CD8
NKT
B
DC

Macrophage

Endothelial cell
Smooth muscle cell (SMC)
LDL/oxLDL
SMC at fibrous cap

FIGURE 71.1 **Immune cells in adaptive immune response of atherosclerosis.** Low density lipoprotein (LDL) entry into the intima through dysfunctional endothelial cells initiates atherosclerosis. After modification to oxidized LDL (oxLDL), it is captured and processed by tissue dendritic cells. Dendritic cells (DCs) with captured antigen activate resident naïve T cells and NKT cells *in situ* in "vascular-associated lymphoid tissue" and/or migrate to draining lymph nodes to activate these circulating lymphocytes. Activated lymphocytes in draining lymph nodes return to the intima to promote inflammation by secreting proinflammatory cytokines and cytotoxins. B cells can also capture antigen to activate immune responses. As local inflammation increases, more immune cells are recruited into lesion areas, and apoptotic cells and necrotic core areas appear and are contained by smooth muscle and collagen caps. Cap disruption initiates thrombotic arterial occlusion leading to heart attacks and strokes. Concomitantly, adventitial DCs and B cells activate an immune response to generate adventitial tertiary lymphoid organs (ATLO).

lymph node cell reactivity to β2-GP1 and oxLDL, and upregulated IL-4 and IL-10 production, indicating tolerance induced by this antigen is atheroprotective (George et al., 2004), but not antigen specific.

IMMUNE RESPONSES IN ATHEROSCLEROSIS

The role of innate and adaptive immunity in atherosclerosis is summarized in Table 71.1.

Innate Immunity in Atherosclerosis

Macrophages

Macrophages are the major leukocyte subset in human and mouse lesions (Woollard and Geissmann, 2010). Several lines of evidence indicate a key role for macrophages in atherogenesis. Treatment of hypercholesterolemic rabbits with clodronate-containing liposomes, which depletes macrophages, markedly reduced atherosclerosis (Oksala et al., 1994). Administering diphtheria toxin to transgenic mice expressing diphtheria toxin receptor regulated by the

macrophage-specific promoter CD11b attenuated early lesions (Stoneman et al., 2007). Inhibiting macrophage apoptosis augments lesion development (Gautier et al., 2009a) while induction of macrophage apoptosis in advanced lesions elevates chemokine expression to further increase monocyte accumulation and lesion size (Gautier et al., 2009a). Monocytes accumulate continuously during atheroma development and this is further increased with hypercholesterolemia (Swirski et al., 2006). In human lesions, macrophages contain PPARγ that may regulate expression of MMP-9 implicated in plaque rupture (Marx et al., 1998). In mice, atherosclerosis drives rapid influx of inflammatory Ly-6C(+) and patrolling Ly-6C(−) monocytes. Recruited Ly-6C(+) monocytes differentiate to inflammatory macrophages and dendritic cells (Ley et al., 2007). Resident macrophages also probably participate in atherogenesis. LDL entry into the intima is a key event in recruiting macrophages. oxLDL generated by oxidation of LDL is taken up by macrophages via scavenger receptors to form foam cells that accumulate in the intima and are responsible for fatty streaks.

Macrophages produce proinflammatory cytokines including TNF-α, IL-1α and -β, IL-18, IL-6, IL-12, and

TABLE 71.1 Cellular Components Involved in Pathogenesis of Atherosclerosis

Innate Immune Cells	Role in Atherosclerosis	Reference
Macrophages	*Atherogenic* Inflammatory cytokines	Gown et al. (1986); Marx et al. (1998); George et al. (1999, 2004); Swirski et al. (2006); Gautier et al. (2009a); Kamari et al. (2011)
NK cells	*? Atherogenic*	Nakai et al. (2004); Tupin et al. (2004)
Neutrophils	*Atherogenic*	Naruko et al. (2002); van Leeuwen et al. (2008); Drechsler et al. (2010)
Mast cells	*Atherogenic* Inflammatory cytokines Cell proliferation initiator	Brawand et al. (2000); Lappalainen et al. (2004)
B1a cells	*Atheroprotective* Low-affinity natural IgM antibody	Wardemann et al. (2002); Kyaw et al. (2011a); Kyaw et al. (2012)

Adaptive Immune Cells		
Th1 CD4$^+$ T cells	*Atherogenic* IFN-γ IL-12	Hansson et al. (1989); Emeson et al. (1996); Whitman et al. (2002); Schieffer et al. (2004); Sun et al. (2007)
TH2 CD4$^+$ T cells	*Mixed* IL-4 (yet to be defined) IL-5 (*atherogenic*) IL-10 (*anti-atherogenic*)	Zhou et al. (2000); Whitman et al. (2002) Zhou et al. (2006) Gupta et al. (1997)
Th17 CD4$^+$ T cells	?	Eid et al. (2009); Taleb et al. (2010); Kurowska-Stolarska et al. (2011)
CD8$^+$ T cells	?	Roselaar et al. (1996); Weber et al. (2008)
NKT cells	*Atherogenic* Inflammatory cytokines	Geng and Libby (1995); Bobryshev and Lord (2005); Rogers et al. (2008); To et al. (2009); Iyer et al. (2009); Kyriakakis et al. (2010); Hansson and Klareskog (2011)
Conventional B2 B cells	*Atherogenic*	Yla-Herttuala et al. (1994); Ludewig et al., (2000); Houtkamp et al. (2001a)
Regulatory CD4$^+$ Foxp3$^+$ T cells	*Atheroprotective*	Taleb et al. (2009); Danzaki et al. (2011)

Non-immune Cells		
Smooth muscle cells	*Atherogenic* Adhesion molecules Inflammatory cytokines	Binder et al. (2005); Lewis et al. (2009); O'Garra et al. (1992)
Endothelial cells	*Atherogenic* Adhesion molecules Inflammatory cytokines	Inaba et al. (1992); Schecter et al. (2003); Swirski et al. (2006); Butoi et al. (2011)

IL-15 (Osterud and Bjorklid, 2003; Tedgui and Mallat, 2006; Ait-Oufella et al., 2011). Macrophages from human plaques produce TNF-α and IL-1 (Tipping and Hancock, 1993). TNF-α-deficient ApoE$^{-/-}$ mice, chimeric ApoE$^{-/-}$ mice transplanted with bone marrow from TNF-α-deficient ApoE$^{-/-}$ mice, or ApoE$^{-/-}$ mice treated with soluble TNF receptor 1 pellets attenuate atherosclerosis (Branen et al., 2004) associated with decreased ICAM-1, VCAM-1, and MCP-1 expression (Ohta et al., 2005). Atherosclerosis is attenuated in IL-1β-deficient ApoE$^{-/-}$ mice associated with decreased mRNA levels of VCAM-1 and MCP-1

(Kirii et al., 2003). IL-1α deficiency in ApoE$^{-/-}$ mice also attenuated atherosclerosis (Kamari et al., 2011). IL-18 augments atherosclerosis by secreting IFN-γ (Whitman et al., 2002) while its deficiency in ApoE$^{-/-}$ mice attenuated atherosclerosis (Elhage et al., 2003). Lesions are enhanced lesions in IL-6-deficient ApoE$^{-/-}$ mice (Schieffer et al., 2004). IL-12 has been localized to macrophages of atherosclerotic lesions and daily IL-12 administration increased serum oxLDL antibodies and accelerated atherosclerosis in young ApoE$^{-/-}$ mice (Lee et al., 1999). IL-12 appears atherogenic in early disease in ApoE$^{-/-}$ mice (Davenport and

Tipping, 2003) and selective IL-12 synthesis defect in 12/15-lipoxygenase-deficient macrophages reduced atherosclerosis (Zhao et al., 2002). IL-12 was induced in monocytes *in vitro* in response to oxLDL (Uyemura et al., 1996). IL-15 is associated with oxLDL-positive macrophages and co-localizes with CD40L-positive T cells (Houtkamp et al., 2001a); its deficiency reduced atherosclerosis in LDLR$^{-/-}$ mice (van Es et al., 2011).

Inflammatory macrophages have a short half-life. After undergoing apoptosis, they may be phagocytosed by surrounding macrophages or, if phagocytosis is overwhelmed, can undergo secondary necrosis, forming necrotic cores (Silva, 2010; Ley et al., 2011; Moore and Tabas, 2011; Thorp et al., 2011). In humans, apoptosis in macrophages has been reported in advanced lesions and may contribute to plaque rupture (Geng and Libby, 1995; Bjorkerud and Bjorkerud, 1996). Necrotic cells can further aggravate inflammation through Nlrp3 inflammasome activation (Iyer et al., 2009; Hansson and Klareskog, 2011).

NKT Cells

Given the role of lipid in atherogenesis and in NKT cell activation, these cells are candidates for linking innate with adaptive immunity. Indeed, invariant NKT (iNKT) cells from human plaques produce inflammatory cytokines when stimulated by CD1d expressing antigen-present cells presenting α-gal-cer (Kyriakakis et al., 2010). NKT cells recognize lipid antigens presented by the major histocompatibility complex (MHC) class 1-like molecule CD1d, producing copious amounts of IFN-γ and IL-4 when activated. In human lesions they accumulate within rupture-prone regions where they co-localize with dendritic cells (Bobryshev and Lord, 2005). NKT cell depletion by neonatal thymectomy ameliorated atherosclerosis while their adoptive transfer to thymectomized mice aggravated atherosclerosis (To et al., 2009). Similarly, Jα18 gene deletion which depletes Vα14 NKT cells also decreased atherosclerosis (Rogers et al., 2008) while adoptive transfer of NKT cells from Jα18Vα14 transgenic mice aggravated atherosclerosis (VanderLaan et al., 2007). Also, CD1d deficiency decreased atherosclerosis whereas NKT cell activation by α-gal-cer aggravated atherosclerosis (Major et al., 2004; Nakai et al., 2004; Tupin et al., 2004). Atherogenic NKT cells have been identified as belonging to the CD4$^+$ and not the double negative (DN) subset because adoptive transfer of CD4$^+$ NKT cells and not the DN subset to NKT cell-deficient thymectomized mice augmented atherosclerotic lesions (To et al., 2009). The differential effects were not attributable to differences in homing to developing atherosclerotic lesions. DN NKT cells expressed at least three-fold higher levels of inhibitory Ly49 receptors (Ly49A, Ly49C/I, and Ly49G2) than CD4$^+$ NKT cells,

and lesions expressed large amounts of their MHC class I ligand. *In vitro* these inhibitory receptors initiated greater effects in DN NKT cells. Culture of each NKT cell subset with TAP-deficient (MHC class I-deficient) dendritic cells and α-gal-cer led to secretion of similar amounts of proatherogenic cytokines IL-2, IFN-γ, and TNF but, when cultured with MHC class I-positive dendritic cells, CD4$^+$ NKT cells secreted more of these cytokines.

NK Cells

NK cells secrete proinflammatory cytokines, in particular IFN-γ as well as cytoxins such as perforin and granzyme B. The LILB1 receptor expressed by human NK cells is associated with human atherosclerotic disease (Romo et al., 2011). The lack of a mouse model with specific genetic deletion of NK cells has made it difficult to define the precise role of these cells in atherosclerosis, although a proatherogenic role might be envisaged. NK cell function is reduced in mice having a beige mutation (Roder and Duwe, 1979). LDLR-deficient mice with a beige mutation exhibit a modest increase in atherosclerotic lesion size suggesting a protective role (Schiller et al., 2002). In contrast, mice deficient in functional NK cells through expression of a transgene encoding Ly49A under a granzyme A promoter exhibit reduced atherosclerosis, suggesting a proatherogenic role (Whitman et al., 2004). However, this transgenic construct also induces overexpression of Ly49A in CD8$^+$ T cells, which attenuates their antigen-specific responses (Brawand et al., 2000).

Neutrophils

In humans, neutrophil infiltration in plaques is associated with acute coronary events, with particularly high neutrophil numbers demonstrated in ruptured plaques (Naruko et al., 2002). Neutrophil infiltration is also a feature of culprit lesions in acute coronary syndromes in humans (Naruko et al., 2002); both eroded and ruptured human lesions frequently contained neutral endopeptide expressing neutrophils while they are low in number or largely absent in stable plaques. Hyperlipidemia generated by feeding ApoE-deficient mice a high-fat diet promoted neutrophilia associated with neutrophil infiltration during early stages of atherosclerosis (Drechsler et al., 2010). Neutrophil accumulation peaked at 4 weeks after starting a high-fat diet and declined thereafter and neutropenia reduced early plaque development but not the later stages of atherosclerosis. In LDLR-deficient mice, introduction of a high-fat diet was associated with elevated circulating levels of myeloperoxidase. Neutrophils expressing myeloperoxidase were observed to be attached to atherosclerotic caps and in the adventitial regions of lesions (van Leeuwen et al., 2008). The precise role of neutrophils in plaque rupture is yet to be defined.

Mast Cells

Mast cells accumulate in all stages of human atherosclerotic lesion development and at sites of coronary lesion rupture, erosion, and neovascularization. In human lesions mast cells produce FGF-2, which promotes vascularization and contributes to lesion progression (Lappalainen et al., 2004). Mast cells in human lesions (Atkinson et al., 1994; Jeziorska et al., 1997) are a common feature of advanced plaques complicated by fissure, hemorrhage, and thrombosis. The chemokines responsible for attracting mast cells to developing lesions are largely unknown. Mast cells have a unique expression of CCR3 which is mainly located intracellularly. Upon activation, CCR3 is relocated to the cell surface enabling them to respond to chemokines such as eotaxin which is produced by macrophages in lesions (Haley et al., 2000; Juremalm and Nilsson, 2005). Mast cells also contribute to lesion development. Mast cell-deficient Ldlr$^{-/-}$ Kit$^{W-sh/W-sh}$ mice have decreased lesions. Transfer of wild-type or TNF-α-deficient but not IL-6- or IFN-γ-deficient mast cells restored atherogenesis to Ldlr$^{-/-}$ Kit$^{W-sh/W-sh}$ mice, implying that mast cell-derived IL-6 and IFN-γ promote atherogenesis (Sun et al., 2007),

Adaptive Immunity in Atherosclerosis

Th1 CD4 T Cells

Activated oxLDL-reactive T cells have been recovered from human atherosclerotic lesions (Hansson et al., 1989; Stemme et al., 1995). In human lesions, mRNA for the key inducer of Th1 cytokines, IL12p40, and p70 are abundant (Uyemura et al., 1996). In mice, a number of experimental approaches have demonstrated the proatherogenic role of T cells. CD4 lymphocyte depletion using a monoclonal antibody reduced lesion size (Emeson et al., 1996). T cell-deficient nude (nu/nu) mice develop smaller lesions than do their heterozygote litter mates. ApoE$^{-/-}$ mice crossed with immunodeficient scid/scid mice had reduced fatty streaks while transfer of CD4 T cells increased lesions associated with infiltration of transferred T cells into lesions (Zhou et al., 2000). Transfer of CD4 T cells from oxLDL-immunized mice had substantially larger lesions. The increase in serum IFN-γ levels was proportional to the accelerated atherosclerosis (Zhou et al., 2006), consistent with involvement of a Th1 cell subset. Indeed, IFN-γ co-localizes with CD4 T cells in atherosclerotic lesions and IFN-γ-deficient ApoE$^{-/-}$ mice had markedly attenuated atherosclerosis, reduced lesion cellularity, and increased lesion collagen (Gupta et al., 1997), while exogenous IFN-γ augmented atherosclerotic lesions (Whitman et al., 2000).

ApoE$^{-/-}$ mice deficient in IL-12 also displayed reduced atherosclerosis (Davenport and Tipping, 2003).

Th2 CD4$^+$ T Cells

There are mixed reports of the role of the Th2 cytokine IL-4, with reduced atherosclerosis in mice deficient in IL-4 (King et al., 2002; Davenport and Tipping, 2003) but aggravated atherosclerosis in mice deficient in the Th2 cytokine IL-5 (Binder et al., 2004). IL-10-deficient C57Bl/6 mice fed an atherogenic diet increased lesion size associated with T cell infiltration, IFN-γ expression, and decreased collagen content. Transfer of murine IL-10 reduced lesion size (Mallat et al., 1999). Treatment with IL-33, a novel IL-1-like cytokine that signals via ST2, reduced lesions in ApoE$^{-/-}$ mice associated with elevated oxLDL antibody and a Th1–Th2 switch supported by increased levels of IL-4, -5, and -13, but decreased levels of IFN-γ in serum and lymph node cells (Miller et al., 2008). Conversely, mice treated with soluble ST2, a decoy receptor that neutralizes IL-33, developed larger plaques in the aortic sinus of ApoE$^{-/-}$ mice. Furthermore, co-administration of an anti-IL-5 mAb with IL-33 prevented reduction in plaque size; IL-33 and ST2 are present in normal and atherosclerotic vasculature of mice and humans. The IL-33 receptor, consisting of ST2 and IL-1 receptor accessory protein, is widely expressed, particularly in Th2 cells and mast cells (Liew et al., 2010). IL-33 can act both as a nuclear factor and as a soluble mediator; however, the precise role of IL-33 within the nucleus is not clear. As a cytokine, IL-33 is suggested to function as an alarmin that is released upon endothelial or epithelial cell damage (Kurowska-Stolarska et al., 2011).

Th17 CD4$^+$ T Cells

There are contradictory reports of the role of Th17 in atherosclerosis (Taleb et al., 2010).

An atherogenic role is supported by the report that IL-17 produced concomitantly with IFN-γ by human coronary artery-infiltrating T cells, act synergistically to induce proinflammatory responses in vascular smooth muscle cells (Eid et al., 2009). Patients with acute coronary syndrome show increased peripheral Th17 numbers, Th17-related cytokines (IL-17, IL-6, and IL-23), and transcription factor (RORγt) levels and decreased Treg number, Treg-related cytokines (IL-10 and TGF-β1), and transcription factor (Foxp3) levels (Cheng et al., 2008). In ApoE$^{-/-}$ mice, an increased proportion of Th17 cells and higher expression in plaques of IL-17, retinoic acid-related orphan receptor (ROR)γt, and IL-17A-expressing T cells have been reported. Treatment with neutralizing anti-IL-17 antibody or with adenovirus-produced IL-17 receptor inhibited atherosclerosis development while rIL-17 augmented lesions (Gao et al., 2010; Smith et al., 2010). However, an atheroprotective role for IL-17A is supported by the report that IL-17A-deficient ApoE$^{-/-}$ mice accelerated unstable atherosclerotic plaque formation after 8 weeks on high-fat diet (Danzaki et al., 2011). An atheroprotective role is also suggested by attenuated atherosclerosis arising from increased IL-17 and IL-10 production with loss of SOCS3 in T cells (Taleb et al., 2009). On the other hand, transplantation of IL-17R bone marrow into LDLR$^{-/-}$ mice attenuated atherosclerosis accompanied by reduced IL-6 but increased IL-10 production (van Es et al., 2009). Attenuated atherosclerosis in Fcγ-chain-deficient ApoE$^{-/-}$ mice is associated with decreased Th17 cells, decreased IL-17 secretion by activated CD4 T cells, decreased IL-6 release by APC, and STAT-3 phosphorylation essential for Th17 cell genesis while regulatory T cells, TGF-β, and IL-10 were increased (Ng et al., 2011).

Foxp3 Regulatory CD4$^+$ T Cells

Regulatory T cells and their adoptive transfer suppress atherosclerosis in several mouse models (Ait-Oufella et al., 2006; Mor et al., 2007). TGF-β is implicated in suppression because partial depletion of regulatory T cells ameliorated atherosclerosis in ApoE$^{-/-}$ mice but not in ApoE$^{-/-}$ mice expressing dominant negative TGR-β type 2 receptor under control of the CD4 promoter. Various experimental manipulations modulate atherosclerosis through regulatory T cells. For instance, local delivery of IL-12 attenuated atherosclerosis by expanding regulatory T cells (Dietrich et al., 2011) and CCL17-expressing dendritic cells restrain regulatory T cell homeostasis in ApoE$^{-/-}$ mice (Weber et al., 2011). Caveolin-1 deficiency in ApoE$^{-/-}$ mice attenuated atherosclerosis by hampering leukocyte influx into the arterial wall and generating a regulatory T cell response (Engel et al., 2011). The findings are consistent with a role for caveolin-1 in LDL transcytosis and on inflammation. Amygdalin (vitamin B17) derived from the seeds of a variety of plants reduced atherosclerosis in ApoE$^{-/-}$ mice and increased regulatory T cells and expression of IL-10 and TGF-β (Jiagang et al., 2011). Oral administration of an active form of vitamin D3 (calcitriol) decreased atherosclerosis in ApoE$^{-/-}$ mice and reduced macrophage and CD4 T cell accumulation by increasing Foxp3 regulatory T cells and immature dendritic cells with tolerogenic functions; mRNA for IL-10 was increased while IL-12 was reduced (Takeda et al., 2010). Treatment of ApoE$^{-/-}$ mice with ApoB100 peptides reduced development and progression of established atherosclerosis and increased collagen content indicative of plaque stabilization (Herbin et al., 2012). Conversely, ICOS-deficient LDR$^{-/-}$-chimeric mice displayed augmented atherosclerotic lesions accompanied by decreased numbers of Foxp3 regulatory T cells, impaired their suppressive function, and increased CD4 T cells, macrophages, smooth muscle

cells, and collagen content. CD4 T cells from ICOS-deficient chimeras proliferated more and secreted more interferon-γ and tumor necrosis factor-α (Gotsman et al., 2006).

CD8 T Cells

In human lesions, CD8 T lymphocytes are the dominant leukocyte infiltrate, representing up to 50% in advanced plaques (van der Wal et al., 1989; Gewaltig et al., 2008; Rossmann et al., 2008). In mouse lesions, CD8 T cells predominate early (Kolbus et al., 2010) and accumulate throughout lesion development (Roselaar et al., 1996). A role for CD8 T cells remains unresolved (Weber et al., 2008; Galkina and Ley, 2009; Hansson and Hermansson, 2011). Previous studies have given contradictory results. MHC class I-deficient β2 microglobulin (β2 m) knockout had increased atherosclerosis, suggesting that CD8 T cells are atheroprotective. However, β2 m gene disruption affects development of CD8α/α but not Kb and Db-dependent CD8α/β CD8 T cells, and CD8$^+$ CTL clones have been reported in β2m-deficient mice (Cook et al., 1995). In ApoE$^{-/-}$ mice rendered CD8 T cell deficient by CD8 gene targeting, no change in lesions was reported (Elhage et al., 2004). Indirect evidence for a damaging role is suggested by increased CD8 T cells in lesions aggravated by treatment with CD137 agonist (Olofsson et al., 2008), PDL1/L2 deficiency (Gotsman et al., 2007), and infection with microbes (Krebs et al., 2007), and in a transgenic mouse model of arterial inflammation and hypercholesterolemia (Ludewig et al., 2000).

Conventional B2 Cells

B lymphocytes accumulate in lesions in humans and mice (Yla-Herttuala et al., 1994; Zhou and Hansson, 1999; Houtkamp et al., 2001b). An atherogenic role for B cells is supported by the observation that their depletion by monoclonal antibody to CD20 ameliorates atherosclerosis (Ait-Oufella et al., 2010; Kyaw et al., 2010). The atherogenic B subset responsible was identified as conventional B2 cells by their adoptive transfer to lymphocyte-deficient or to μMT B cell-deficient ApoE$^{-/-}$ mice (Kyaw et al., 2010). Augmented atherosclerosis following B2 cell transfer to lymphocyte-deficient mice indicates that B2 cells can potently promote atherosclerosis development entirely on their own in the total absence of all other lymphocyte populations. Additionally, these B2 cells can also significantly augment atherosclerosis development in the presence of T cells and all other lymphocyte populations because the lesions in mice deficient only in B cells only had a four-fold increase in lesion size compared to transfer to lymphocyte-deficient mice. Attenuated atherosclerosis was also observed in BAFF receptor-deficient ApoE$^{-/-}$

mice (Kyaw et al., 2012) consistent with the dependence of B2 cells on BAFF for their development and survival (Mackay et al., 2010). Aortic atherosclerotic lesions were decreased and B cells were absent in atherosclerotic lesions of BAFF receptor-deficient ApoE$^{-/-}$ mice as were IgG1 and IgG2a immunoglobulins produced by B2 cells, despite low but measurable numbers of B2 cells and IgG1 and IgG2a immunoglobulin concentrations in plasma. Plasma IgM and IgM deposits in atherosclerotic lesions were also reduced. BAFF-R deficiency in ApoE2/2 mice also potently reduced arterial inflammation as reflected by reduced expression of VCAM-1 and fewer macrophages, dendritic cells, CD4$^+$ and CD8$^+$ T cell infiltrates and PCNA$^+$ cells in lesions, and reduced expression of proinflammatory cytokines, TNF-α, IL-1β, and proinflammatory chemokine MCP-1.

Innate-like B1a Cells

Transfer of unfractionated spleen B cells to splenectomized mice with aggravated atherosclerosis suggested B cells are atheroprotective but the protective B cell subset was not identified (Caligiuri et al., 2002). The protective B cell subset was identified as peritoneal B1a cells as these cells are specifically depleted in splenectomized mice (Wardemann et al., 2002) and their adoptive transfer to splenectomized mice ameliorated atherosclerosis (Kyaw et al., 2011a). These B1a lymphocytes likely belong to a population designated as regulatory B cells (Fillatreau et al., 2008; Kyaw et al., 2011b). Protection is mediated by IgM secreted by B1a cells because the adoptive transfer of IgM-deficient B1a cells failed to confer atheroprotection. Transfer of IgM-sufficient B1a cells restored plasma total and oxLDL IgM levels and lesion IgM deposits; and potently attenuated atherosclerotic lesions, with reduced lesion necrotic cores, oxidized low-density lipoprotein, and apoptotic cells. The findings are consistent with an atheroprotective role for IgM (Lewis et al., 2009) and for IgM secreted by B1a cells to confer protection by providing a scavenger role in removing apoptotic cells and oxLDL (Binder et al., 2005; Ehrenstein and Notley, 2010). As B1a cells are also major B cell producers of the immunosuppressive cytokine IL-10 (O'Garra et al., 1992) it is possible that IL-10 may also have a suppressive role in atherosclerosis.

Other Key Cellular Players

Smooth Muscle Cells (SMCs)

Although the majority of SMCs in the vessel wall of humans are contained within the medial layer, a significant number exist within the intima in "intimal thickenings" (Doran et al., 2008). Intimal SMCs differ from medial SMCs in being predominantly synthetic rather than contractile and are major producers of extracellular matrix including collagen. Like macrophages, SMCs have receptors for lipid uptake and can form foam-like cells (Inaba et al., 1992), thereby participating in early accumulation of plaque lipid. Intimal and media SMC express MCSF (CSF1) receptor and proliferate following stimulation with MCSF. Like endothelial cells, SMCs can express adhesion molecules such as VCAM-1 and ICAM-1 to which monocytes and lymphocytes can adhere and migrate into the vessel wall. Through these adhesion molecules, SMCs can also stabilize macrophages and T cells against apoptosis. SMCs also possess functional chemokine receptors, including CCR5, CXCR4, and a receptor for MCP-1 (Schecter et al., 2003) and produce many cytokines such as PDGF, TGF-β, IFN-γ, IL-1, IL-18, MIF, and MCP-1(CCL2), which contribute to the inflammatory response to lipid (Doran et al., 2008). Cross-talk between SMC and monocytes augments the inflammatory response in both cell types as revealed by increased expression of TNF-α, IL-1β, IL-6, CX3CR1, and MMPs. Upregulation of TNF-α, CX3CR1, and MMP-9 is further increased upon interaction of SMC with activated monocytes and is dependent on the fractalkine/CXRCR1 pair (Butoi et al., 2011).

Endothelial Cells

Nitric oxide inhibits oxidation of low-density lipoprotein. A defect in production or activity of nitric oxide leads to endothelial dysfunction, an early marker for atherosclerosis, and is detected before structural changes to the vessel wall are apparent on angiography or ultrasound. Many of the risk factors that predispose to atherosclerosis can also cause endothelial dysfunction, and the presence of multiple risk factors predicts endothelial dysfunction (Davignon and Ganz, 2004). Endothelial cells express the adhesion molecules VCAM-1, ICAM-1, E-selectin, and P-selectin for leukocyte adhesion and a variety of cytokines such as IL-1, IL-6, and IL-8 (Ait-Oufella et al., 2011). IL-1 induces IL-6 expression by human endothelial cells (Sironi et al., 1989) while IL-17F produced by activated T cells induced endothelial cells to produce IL-2, TGF-β, and MCP-1 (CCL2) (Starnes et al., 2001). RANTES (CCL5) can be induced in human endothelial cells by combined TNF-α and IFN-γ stimulation and is inhibited by IL-4 and IL-13 (Marfaing-Koka et al., 1995).

Immune System Activation

Activation Sites

As draining lymph nodes are sites of immune activation in response to infectious microorganisms, the para-aortic lymph nodes draining the aorta are possible sites of auto-immune activation. Activation at these sites would require antigen-presenting cells in arteries, such as dendritic cells, to capture cognate antigen that then migrate to the draining lymph nodes to activate circulating lymphocytes as they transit through the lymph node. Following activation, the lymphocytes would be required to acquire homing receptors to return to the artery. However, activation at draining para-aortic sites has not thus far been investigated or demonstrated.

The observation that mononuclear cells pre-exist in the intima at bifurcation sites of normal arteries has led to designation of these aggregates as "vascular-associated lymphatic tissue" akin to "mucosa-associated lymphatic tissue." According to this hypothesis, the vasculature is an integral component of the lymphoid system and activation of the immune system occurs *in situ* in the vessel wall. B and T lymphocytes and some macrophages and dendritic cells are already present in the adventitia of normal/noninflamed mouse aortas and adoptively transfer lymphocytes constitutively homed to the aorta (Galkina et al., 2006) presumably transiting through vasa vasorum.

Whether activation occurs in para-aortic lymph nodes or in vascular-associated lymphoid tissue, concurrently or sequentially, is not known.

Dendritic Cells

Dendritic cells (DCs) in human atherosclerotic intima (Bobryshev and Lord, 1995) probably participate in all phases of atherosclerosis, from early fatty streaks to mature lesions. Small numbers of DCs in healthy arteries dramatically increase with atherosclerosis development. During plaque growth, new DCs are recruited, and egress from vessels is dampened. DCs are also present in adventitial tertiary lymphoid aggregates (Figure 71.1) (Koltsova and Ley, 2011). Given their key role as peripheral sentinels of the immune system, DCs likely play a key role in antigen presentation and activation of the immune system in atherosclerosis (Figure 71.2). In addition, dendritic cells appear to have a role in cholesterol homeostasis in atherosclerosis. Whereas DC expansion decreased plasma cholesterol levels, DC depletion raised these levels (Gautier et al., 2009b). Resident dendritic cells, like their macrophage counterparts, also accumulate lipid and contribute to initiation of the atherosclerotic process (Paulson et al., 2010).

TLR

In human lesions, TLR1, 2, and 4 expression is markedly enhanced (Edfeldt et al., 2002). Atherosclerosis is reduced in mice lacking MyD88 (Bjorkbacka et al., 2004). TLR4 deficiency reduced atherosclerosis with reduced circulating levels of IL-12 and MCP 1, plaque lipid, macrophages,

and cyclooxygenase 2. Endothelial-leukocyte adhesion in response to minimally modified LDL was also reduced in aortic endothelial cells from MyD88-deficient mice (Michelsen et al., 2004). TLR2 deficiency reduced atherosclerosis but loss of TLR2 expression from BM-derived cells had no effect. However, BM-derived cells deficient in TLR2 protected against atherosclerosis aggravated by Pam3CSK4, a TLR2 agonist (Mullick et al., 2005). Increased endothelial TLR2 expression at sites of disturbed blood flow exacerbated early atherosclerosis (Mullick et al., 2008). TLR 3 is atheroprotective as its deficiency augmented atherosclerosis (Cole et al., 2011).

Costimulatory Molecules

B7/CD28 Family

Costimulatory B7.1 and B7.2 are found in human plaques (de Boer et al., 1997). Mice deficient in B7.1 and B7.2 have reduced early lesions and CD4$^+$ T cells from these mice secreted lower amounts of IFN-γ in response to mouse HSP60 (Buono et al., 2004). ICOS-deficient mice had augmented lesions displaying increased CD4 T cells, and CD4 T cells from ICOS-deficient chimeras proliferated more and secreted more interferon-γ and TNF-α. FoxP3 regulatory T cells constitutively express high ICOS levels and ICOS-deficient mice had decreased numbers of FoxP3 regulatory T cells and impaired *in vitro* suppressive function (Gotsman et al., 2006). PD-L1/2 deficiency augmented lesions, increased numbers of lesional CD4$^+$ and CD8$^+$ T cells, activated CD4$^+$ T cells, and had higher serum TNF-α levels. PD-L1/2-deficient APCs were more effective in activating CD4$^+$ T cells *in vitro* (Gotsman et al., 2007).

TNF/TNF Receptor Family

CD40L is expressed on human macrophages, smooth muscle cells, and endothelial cells (Mach et al., 1997). An atherogenic role for CD40 is indicated by attenuated lesions, fewer lesional macrophages and T lymphocytes, and decreased VCAM-1 expression following treatment with antibody against mouse CD40L (Mach et al., 1998). Targeted mutation of OX40L decreased lesions (Wang et al., 2005), as did treatment with anti-OX40L antibody, whereas overexpression of OX40L increased lesions. CD137 is present on T cells and endothelial cells in human atherosclerotic lesions. Treatment of mice with a CD137 agonist augmented lesions and promoted T cell infiltration (mainly CD8 T cells) and proinflammatory cytokine expression (Olofsson et al., 2008).

Leukocyte Recruitment: Adhesion Molecules

In human atherosclerotic plaques, P-selectin is highly expressed by the endothelium overlying active but not

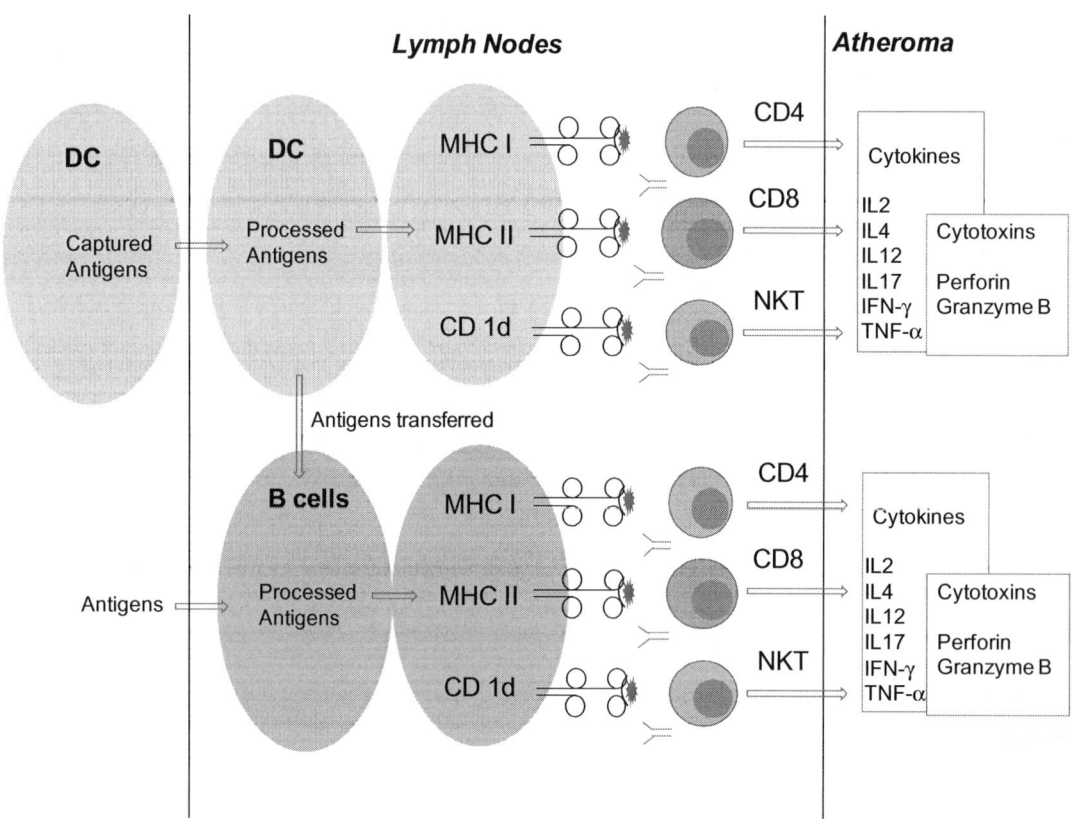

FIGURE 71.2   Activation of naïve T and NKT cells in adaptive immunity.   Dendritic cells in the intima and adventitia capture and process modified LDL that are presented to naïve T and NKT cells in draining lymph nodes and adventitia leading to formation of adventitial tertiary lymphoid organ formation. Activated T and NKT cells in draining lymph nodes home to the intima where they produce inflammatory and cytotoxic mediators. B cells are shown as functional antigen-presenting cells.

inactive atherosclerotic plaques; its expression correlates with ICAM-1 expression (Bourdillon et al., 2006). In ApoE$^{-/-}$ mice, P-selectin deficiency attenuated atherosclerosis in mice fed a chow but not a high-fat diet (Bourdillon et al., 2006), while lymphocyte traffic into lesions is partially L-selectin dependent. In LDLR$^{-/-}$ mice, VCAM-1 and ICAM-1 are expressed in atherosclerotic lesions but VCAM-1 appears to have the dominant role in leukocyte recruitment because VCAM-1 but not ICAM-1 deficiency in LDLR$^{-/-}$ mice attenuated atherosclerosis

Monocyte Homing

Monocytes utilize CCR2, CCR5, CXCR2, and CX3CR1 chemokine receptors, and CXCR4 as non-cognate ligands of MIF and receptors for MCSF(CSF1) for homing to arteries.

CCL2(MCP-1) and its receptor (CCR2) are critical for macrophage recruitment into lesions as their deficiency in LDLR$^{-/-}$ and in ApoE$^{-/-}$ mice attenuated atherosclerosis accompanied by reduced macrophage accumulation. CCL5 (RANTES) and its receptor CCR5 but not CCR1 is

also implicated in atherosclerosis because CCR5 but not CCR1 deficiency attenuated atherosclerosis. CXCL1, CXCL8 (IL-8), and their receptor CXCR2 are expressed on macrophages, and CXCR2 deficiency in LDLR$^{-/-}$ mice reduced macrophage accumulation and attenuated atherosclerosis. Deficiency of macrophage migration inhibitory factor in LDLR$^{-/-}$ mice also attenuated atherosclerosis. CX3CL1/CX3CR1 is essential for macrophage recruitment with reduced atherosclerotic lesion formation in CX3CR1-deficient ApoE$^{-/-}$ mice, while combined inhibition of CX3CR1, CCL2, and CCR5 abrogates Ly6C(hi) and Ly6C(lo) monocytosis and almost abolishes atherosclerosis in hypercholesterolemic mice. Two monocyte subsets are differentiated by different chemokine receptor patterns: CCR2(+)CX3CR1(+)Ly-6C (hi) and CCR2(−)CX3CR1(++)Ly-6C(lo). Blood monocyte counts elevated in ApoE$^{-/-}$ mice were skewed toward an increased frequency of CCR2(+)Ly-6C(hi) monocytes in ApoE$^{-/-}$ mice fed a high-fat diet. CCR2 (+)Ly-6C(hi) monocytes efficiently accumulated in plaques, whereas CCR2(−)Ly-6C(lo) monocytes entered less frequently but were more prone to develop into plaque cells expressing the dendritic cell-associated marker

CD11c, indicating that phagocyte heterogeneity in plaques is linked to distinct types of entering monocytes. CCR2(−) monocytes did not rely on CX3CR1 to enter plaques but were partially dependent upon CCR5, which they selectively upregulated, whereas CCR2(+)Ly-6C(hi) monocytes required CX3CR1 in addition to CCR2 and CCR5 to accumulate within plaques

CXCR2 and CXCR4 were identified as functional receptors for MIF (macrophage migration inhibitory factor). MIF triggered G(alpha)- and integrin-dependent arrest and chemotaxis of monocytes and T cells, rapid integrin activation, and calcium influx through CXCR2 or CXCR4. MIF competed with cognate ligands for CXCR4 and CXCR2 binding, and directly bound to CXCR2. CXCR2 and CD74 formed a receptor complex, and monocyte arrest elicited by MIF in inflamed or atherosclerotic arteries involved both CXCR2 and CD74. *In vivo*, MIF deficiency impaired monocyte adhesion to the arterial wall in atherosclerosis-prone mice, and MIF-induced leukocyte recruitment required Il8rb (which encodes Cxcr2). Blockade of MIF but not of canonical ligands of Cxcr2 or Cxcr4 in mice with advanced atherosclerosis led to plaque regression and reduced monocyte and T cell content in plaques.

A role for MCSF for monocyte homing is supported by the report of attenuated atherosclerosis in MCSF-deficient ApoE$^{-/-}$ mice (Smith et al., 1995). With GMCSF, there are conflicting reports. On the one hand, GMCSF deficiency in ApoE$^{-/-}$ mice aggravated atherosclerosis by reducing cholesterol efflux through reduction of macrophage PPARγ and ABCA1. On the other hand, systemic injection of GM-CSF into LDLR$^{-/-}$ mice markedly increased cell proliferation in early lesions, whereas function-blocking anti-GM-CSF antibody inhibited proliferation (Zhu et al., 2009).

T Cell Homing

T cells utilize CCR7, CXCR3, and CXCR6 chemokine receptors as well as CXCR2 and CXCR4 as non-cognate ligands of MIF for homing to arteries.

CCR7 deficiency resulted in reduced atherosclerotic plaque development. CCR7-deficient T cells showed impaired entry and exit behavior from atherosclerotic lesions. Adoptive transfer of C57BL/6 wild-type T cells but not CCR7-deficient T cells primed with oxLDL-pulsed dendritic cells reconstituted atherogenesis in CCR7-deficient LDLR$^{-/-}$ mice. These results demonstrate that both CCR7-dependent T cell priming in secondary lymphoid organs and CCR7-dependent recirculation of T cells between secondary lymphoid organs and inflamed tissue are crucially involved.

CXCR3, a common receptor for CXCL9, CXCL10, and CXCL11, is expressed on activated T cells. CXCR3-

deficient ApoE$^{-/-}$ mice displayed significantly reduced atherosclerotic lesion development within abdominal aortas that correlated with upregulation of anti-inflammatory molecules IL-10, IL-18BP, and endothelial nitric oxide synthase and with an increased number of regulatory T lymphocytes within atherosclerotic lesions. Similarly, LDLR$^{-/-}$ mice treated with a specific CXCR3 antagonist displayed attenuated atherosclerotic lesions, and lymph nodes draining the aortic arch were significantly smaller and enriched in regulatory T cells and contained fewer activated T cells, whereas markers for regulatory T cells within the lesion were enhanced. CXCL10-deficient ApoE$^{-/-}$ mice showed reduced atherosclerotic lesions, a decreased accumulation of CD4$^+$ T cells, and CXCR3 expression, but Foxp3 regulatory T cell numbers and activity were enhanced as well as increases in Treg-associated cytokines IL-10 and TGF-β.

CXCR6 expressed on a subset of CD4 T cells. CXCR6-deficient ApoE$^{-/-}$ mice displayed attenuated atherosclerosis accompanied by reduced CXCR6$^+$ T cells in the aorta, reduced macrophage accumulation, and reduced IFN-γ in atherosclerotic lesions. Short-term homing experiments demonstrated that CXCR6 is involved in the recruitment of CXCR6$^+$ leukocytes into the atherosclerosis-prone aortic wall.

B Cell Homing

Loss of Id3 in ApoE$^{-/-}$ mice resulted in early and increased atherosclerosis with reduced B cells in the aorta but not the spleen, lymph nodes, and circulation. Similarly, B cells transferred from Id3(−/−) ApoE$^{-/-}$ mice into B cell-deficient mice reconstituted spleen, lymph node, and blood, but aortic reconstitution and B cell-mediated inhibition of diet-induced atherosclerosis was significantly impaired. In addition to retarding initiation of atherosclerosis, B cells homed to regions of existing atherosclerosis reduced macrophage content in plaque, and attenuated disease progression. The chemokine receptor CCR6 was identified as an important Id3 target mediating aortic homing and atheroprotection (Doran et al., 2012).

Figure 71.3 sums key events in the immunopathogenesis of atherosclerosis.

Experimental Therapeutics: A Protective "Vaccine" for Atherosclerosis

Vaccination strategies using antigens based on LDL have been explored to expand immunosuppressive populations of regulatory T and B cells to attenuate atherosclerosis. For instance, immunization of ApoE$^{-/-}$ mice with an LDL-associated apolipoprotein B peptide vaccine aBp210 based on amino acids 3136 to 3155 of apoB-100 (p210) is

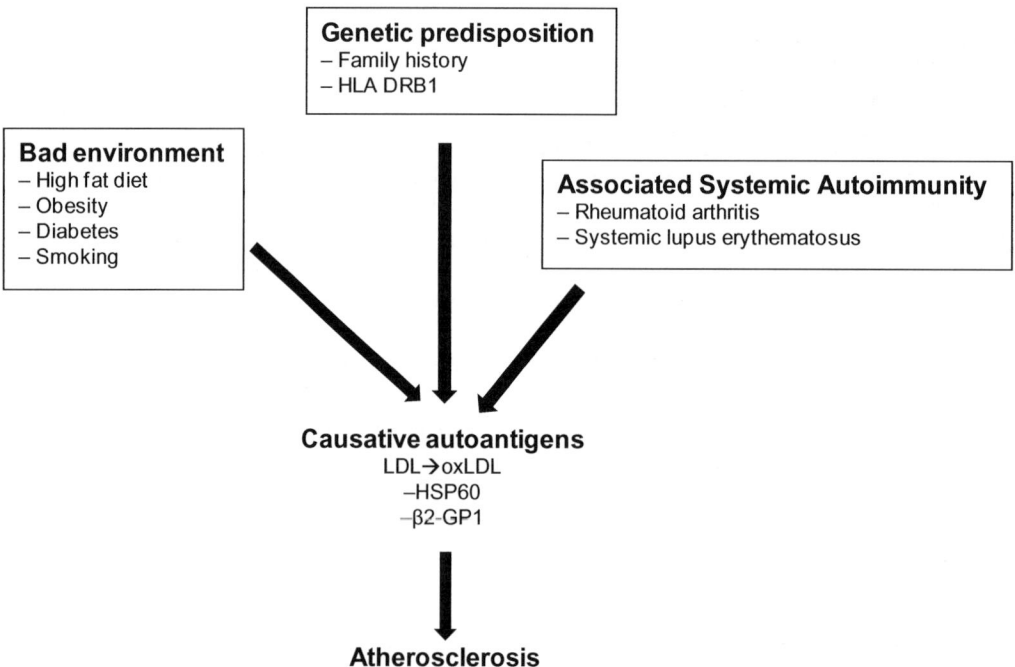

FIGURE 71.3 Immunopathogenesis of atherosclerosis. Interplay of genetic predisposition, bad environment, and systemic autoimmune diseases in initiating an immune response driven by causative autoantigens to generate atherosclerotic lesions.

associated with activation of Tregs. The atheroprotective effect of the vaccine was blocked by administration of antibodies against CD25 that depleted Tregs. These peptide-based vaccines are based on the earlier observation that active immunization with native or modified LDL reduced atherosclerosis in hypercholesterolemic rabbits and mice. As an example of harnessing the immunosuppressive properties of B1a-derived IgM, active immunization in LDLR knockout mice with *Streptococcus pneumoniae* resulted in induction of high levels of oxidized LDL-specific IgM and a modest reduction of atherosclerosis (Binder et al., 2003).

Implications for Clinical Translation

Despite lipid-lowering statins, atherosclerosis-based heart attacks and strokes remain leading causes of deaths; statins reduce cardiovascular risk by around 30%. Recognition of the role of inflammation in atherosclerosis based on studies in genetically modified mice has raised prospects of anti-inflammatory therapy to improve clinical outcomes. Recent clinical trials with statins have also provided evidence for inflammation associated with human atherosclerosis and inflammation associated with myocardial infarction even when cholesterol is "normal." The importance of inflammation is highlighted by the report that patients with low levels of the inflammatory biomarker C-reactive protein (CRP) after statin therapy have better clinical outcomes than those with higher CRP levels, regardless of the resultant level of LDL cholesterol.

The finding is further reinforced by the report that with apparently healthy persons without hyperlipidemia but with elevated high-sensitivity C-reactive protein levels, rosuvastatin significantly reduced the incidence of major cardiovascular events. Immunopathic cell types in mice are found in human lesions, suggesting that they play similar pathological roles. Nonetheless caution has been expressed in translating mouse studies to humans (Libby et al., 2011). A prospective study in patients treated with methotrexate indicated that methotrexate may provide substantial survival benefit by reducing cardiovascular mortality (Choi et al., 2002). A review of low dose methotrexate in chronic inflammation showed that its use is associated with a lower cardiovascular risk (Micha et al., 2011). To test the hypothesis that anti-inflammatory treatment may reduce cardiovascular risk and open novel therapeutic approaches, the cardiovascular inflammation reduction trial (CIRT) proposed to allocate stable coronary artery disease patients with persistently elevated hsCRP to placebo or very low dose methotrexate (10 mg weekly), a proven anti-inflammatory regimen that reduces TNF-α, IL-6, and CRP levels (Ridker, 2009). Another trial proposed to evaluate whether selective inhibition by IL-1β by canakinumab, a human monoclonal antibody, can reduce recurrent myocardial infarction, stroke, and cardiovascular death among stable patients with coronary artery disease who remain at high vascular risk due to persistently elevated hsCRP despite contemporary secondary prevention strategies (Ridker et al., 2011). Future potential strategies include those with demonstrated efficacy in mouse models. These include the deletion of pathogenic inflammatory clones or expansion of regulatory clones (Kyaw et al., 2011b). Potential deletion therapies include B cell (Kyaw et al., 2010; Ait-Oufella et al., 2010) or specific B2 cell deletion. As B2 cells are BAFF dependent, BAFF receptor knockout mice have attenuated atherosclerosis. As BAFF blocking reagents are currently in clinical trials to treat human autoimmune diseases (Moisini and Davidson, 2009). BAFF blockers could be considered as ancillary strategies to treat atherosclerotic-based vascular lesions.

REFERENCES

Ait-Oufella, H., Salomon, B.L., Potteaux, S., Robertson, A.K., Gourdy, P., Zoll, J., et al., 2006. Natural regulatory T cells control the development of atherosclerosis in mice. Nat. Med. 12, 178–180.

Ait-Oufella, H., Herbin, O., Bouaziz, J.D., Binder, C.J., Uyttenhove, C., Laurans, L., et al., 2010. B cell depletion reduces the development of atherosclerosis in mice. J. Exp. Med. 207, 1579–1587.

Ait-Oufella, H., Taleb, S., Mallat, Z., Tedgui, A., 2011. Recent advances on the role of cytokines in atherosclerosis. Arterioscler. Thromb. Vasc. Biol. 31, 969–979.

Amberger, A., Maczek, C., Jürgens, G., Michaelis, D., Schett, G., Trieb, K., et al., 1997. Co-expression of ICAM-1, VCAM-1, ELAM-1 and Hsp60 in human arterial and venous endothelial cells in response to cytokines and oxidized low-density lipoproteins. Cell Stress Chaperones. 2, 94–103.

Asanuma, Y., Oeser, A., Shintani, A.K., Turner, E., Olsen, N., Fazio, S., et al., 2003. Premature coronary-artery atherosclerosis in systemic lupus erythematosus. N. Eng. J. Med. 349, 2407–2415.

Atkinson, J.B., Harlan, C.W., Harlan, G.C., Virmani, R., 1994. The association of mast cells and atherosclerosis: a morphologic study of early atherosclerotic lesions in young people. Hum. Pathol. 25, 154–159.

Binder, C.J., Hörkkö, S., Dewan, A., Chang, M.K., Kieu, E.P., Goodyear, C.S., et al., 2003. Pneumococcal vaccination decreases atherosclerotic lesion formation: molecular mimicry between Streptococcus pneumoniae and oxidized LDL. Nat. Med. 9, 736–743.

Binder, C.J., Hartvigsen, K., Chang, M.K., Miller, M., Broide, D., Palinski, W., et al., 2004. IL-5 links adaptive and natural immunity specific for epitopes of oxidized LDL and protects from atherosclerosis. J. Clin. Invest. 114, 427–437.

Binder, C.J., Shaw, P.X., Chang, M.K., Boullier, A., Hartvigsen, K., Hörkkö, S., et al., 2005. The role of natural antibodies in atherogenesis. J. Lipid Res. 46, 1353–1363.

Bjorkbacka, H., Kunjathoor, V.V., Moore, K.J., Koehn, S., Ordija, C.M., Lee, M.A., et al., 2004. Reduced atherosclerosis in MyD88-null mice links elevated serum cholesterol levels to activation of innate immunity signaling pathways. Nat. Med. 10, 416–421.

Bjorkerud, S., Bjorkud, B., 1996. Apoptosis is abundant in human atherosclerotic lesions, especially in inflammatory cells (macrophages and T cells), and may contribute to the accumulation of gruel and plaque instability. Am. J. Pathol. 149, 367–380.

Bobryshev, Y.V., Lord, R.S., 1995. Ultrastructural recognition of cells with dendritic cell morphology in human aortic intima. Contacting interactions of vascular dendritic cells in athero-resistant and athero-prone areas of the normal aorta. Arch. Histol. Cytol. 58, 307–322.

Bobryshev, Y.V., Lord, R.S., 2005. Co-accumulation of dendritic cells and natural killer T cells within rupture-prone regions in human atherosclerotic plaques. J. Histochem. Cytochem. 53, 781–785.

Bourdillon, M.C., Randon, J., Barek, L., Zibara, K., Covacho, C., Poston, R.N., et al., 2006. Reduced atherosclerotic lesion size in P-selectin deficient apolipoprotein E-knockout mice fed a chow but not a fat diet. J. Biomed. Biotechnol. 2006, 49193.

Branen, L., Hovgaard, L., Nitulescu, M., Bengtsson, E., Nilsson, J., Jovinge, S., 2004. Inhibition of tumor necrosis factor-alpha reduces atherosclerosis in apolipoprotein E knockout mice. Arterioscler. Thromb. Vasc. Biol. 24, 2137–2142.

Braun, A., Trigatti, B.L., Post, M.J., Sato, K., Simons, M., Edelberg, J.M., et al., 2002. Loss of SR-BI expression leads to the early onset of occlusive atherosclerotic coronary artery disease, spontaneous myocardial infarctions, severe cardiac dysfunction, and premature death in apolipoprotein E-deficient mice. Circ. Res. 90, 270–276.

Brawand, P., Lemonnier, F.A., MacDonald, H.R., Cerottini, J.C., Held, W., 2000. Transgenic expression of Ly49A on T cells impairs a specific antitumor response. J. Immunol. 165, 1871–1876.

Buono, C., Pang, H., Uchida, Y., Libby, P., Sharpe, A.H., Lichtman, A.H., 2004. B7-1/B7-2 costimulation regulates plaque antigen-specific T-cell responses and atherogenesis in low-density lipoprotein receptor-deficient mice. Circulation. 109, 2009–2015.

Butoi, E.D., Gan, A.M., Manduteanu, I., Stan, D., Calin, M., Pirvulescu, M., et al., 2011. Cross talk between smooth muscle cells and monocytes/activated monocytes via CX3CL1/CX3CR1 axis augments expression of pro-atherogenic molecules. Biochim. Biophys. Acta. 1813, 2026–2035.

Caligiuri, G., Nicoletti, A., Poirier, B., Hansson, G.K., 2002. Protective immunity against atherosclerosis carried by B cells of hypercholesterolemic mice. J. Clini. Invest. 109, 745–753.

Cheng, X., Yu, X., Ding, Y.J., Fu, Q.Q., Xie, J.J., Tang, T.T., et al., 2008. The Th17/Treg imbalance in patients with acute coronary syndrome. Clini. Immunol. 127, 89–97.

Choi, H.K., Hernán, M.A., Seeger, J.D., Robins, J.M., Wolfe, F., 2002. Methotrexate and mortality in patients with rheumatoid arthritis: a prospective study. Lancet. 359, 1173–1177.

Cole, J.E., Navin, T.J., Cross, A.J., Goddard, M.E., Alexopoulou, L., Mitra, A.T., et al., 2011. Unexpected protective role for Toll-like receptor 3 in the arterial wall. Proc. Nat. Acad. Sci. U.S.A. 108, 2372–2377.

Cook, J.R., Solheim, J.C., Connolly, J.M., Hansen, T.H., 1995. Induction of peptide-specific CD8 + CTL clones in beta 2-microglobulin-deficient mice. J. Immunol. 154, 47–57.

Danzaki, K., Matsui, Y., Ikesue, M., Ohta, D., Ito, K., Kanayama, M., et al., 2011. Interleukin-17A deficiency accelerates unstable atherosclerotic plaque formation in apolipoprotein E-deficient mice. Arterioscler. Thromb. Vasc. Biol. 32, 273–280.

Davenport, P., Tipping, P.G., 2003. The role of interleukin-4 and interleukin-12 in the progression of atherosclerosis in apolipoprotein E-deficient mice. Am. J. Pathol. 163, 1117–1125.

Davies, M.J., 1996. Stability and instability: two faces of coronary atherosclerosis. The Paul Dudley White Lecture 1995. Circulation. 94, 2013–2020.

Davignon, J., Ganz, P., 2004. Role of endothelial dysfunction in athero-sclerosis. Circulation. 109, III27–III32.

de Boer, O.J., Hirsch, F., van der Wal, A.C., van der Loos, C.M., Das, P.K., Becker, A.E., 1997. Costimulatory molecules in human athero-sclerotic plaques: an indication of antigen specific T lymphocyte activation. Atherosclerosis. 133, 227–234.

Dietrich, T., Hucko, T., Schneemann, C., Neumann, M., Menrad, A., Willuda, J., et al., 2011. Local delivery of IL-2 reduces atherosclerosis via expansion of regulatory T cells. Atherosclerosis. 220, 329–336.

Doran, A.C., Meller, N., McNamara, C.A., 2008. Role of smooth muscle cells in the initiation and early progression of atherosclerosis. Arterioscler. Thromb. Vasc. Biol. 28, 812–819.

Doran, A.C., Lipinski, M.J., Oldham, S.N., Garmey, J.C., Campbell, K.A., Skaflen, M.D., et al., 2012. B-cell aortic homing and atheroprotection depend on id3. Circ. Res. 110, e1–e12.

Drechsler, M., Megens, R.T., van Zandvoort, M., Weber, C., Soehnlein, O., 2010. Hyperlipidemia-triggered neutrophilia promotes early atheroscle-rosis. Circulation. 122, 1837–1845.

Edfeldt, K., Swedenborg, J., Hansson, G.K., Yan, Z.Q., 2002. Expression of toll-like receptors in human atherosclerotic lesions: a possible pathway for plaque activation. Circulation. 105, 1158–1161.

Ehrenstein, M.R., Notley, C.A., 2010. The importance of natural IgM: scavenger, protector and regulator. Nat. Rev. Immunol. 10, 778–786.

Eid, R.E., Rao, D.A., Zhou, J., Lo, S.F., Ranjbaran, H., Gallo, A., et al., 2009. Interleukin-17 and interferon-gamma are produced concomi-tantly by human coronary artery-infiltrating T cells and act synergis-tically on vascular smooth muscle cells. Circulation. 119, 1424–1432.

Elhage, R., Jawien, J., Rudling, M., Ljunggren, H.G., Takeda, K., Akira, S., et al., 2003. Reduced atherosclerosis in interleukin-18 deficient apoli-poprotein E-knockout mice. Cardiovasc. Res. 59, 234–240.

Elhage, R., Gourdy, P., Brouchet, L., Jawien, J., Fouque, M.J., Fiévet, C., et al., 2004. Deleting TCR alpha beta + or CD4 + T lymphocytes leads to opposite effects on site-specific atherosclerosis in female apo-lipoprotein E-deficient mice. Am. J. Pathol. 165, 2013–2018.

Emeson, E.E., Shen, M.L., Bell, C.G., Qureshi, A., 1996. Inhibition of atherosclerosis in CD4 T-cell-ablated and nude (nu/nu), C57BL/6 hyperlipidemic mice. Am. J. Pathol. 149, 675–685.

Engel, D., Beckers, L., Wijnands, E., Seijkens, T., Lievens, D., Drechsler, M., et al., 2011. Caveolin-1 deficiency decreases ath-erosclerosis by hampering leukocyte influx into the arterial wall and generating a regulatory T-cell response. FASEB J. 25, 3838–3848.

Fillatreau, S., Gray, D., Anderton, S.M., 2008. Not always the bad guys: B cells as regulators of autoimmune pathology. Nat. Rev. Immunol. 8, 391–397.

Galkina, E., Ley, K., 2009. Immune and inflammatory mechanisms of atherosclerosis. Annu. Rev. Immunol. 27, 165–197.

Galkina, E., Kadl, A., Sanders, J., Varughese, D., Sarembock, I.J., Ley, K., 2006. Lymphocyte recruitment into the aortic wall before and during development of atherosclerosis is partially L-selectin dependent. J. Exp. Med. 203, 1273–1282.

Gao, Q., Jiang, Y., Ma, T., Zhu, F., Gao, F., Zhang, P., et al., 2010. A critical function of Th17 proinflammatory cells in the development of atherosclerotic plaque in mice. J. Immunol. 185, 5820–5827.

Gautier, E.L., Huby, T., Saint-Charles, F., Ouzilleau, B., Pirault, J., Deswaerte, V., et al., 2009a. Conventional dendritic cells at the

crossroads between immunity and cholesterol homeostasis in athero-sclerosis. Circulation. 119, 2367–2375.

Gautier, E.L., Huby, T., Witztum, J.L., Ouzilleau, B., Miller, E.R., Saint-Charles, F., et al., 2009b. Macrophage apoptosis exerts diver-gent effects on atherogenesis as a function of lesion stage. Circulation. 119, 1795–1804.

Geng, Y.J., Libby, P., 1995. Evidence for apoptosis in advanced human atheroma. Colocalization with interleukin-1 beta-converting enzyme. Am. J. Pathol. 147, 251–266.

George, J., Harats, D., Gilburd, B., Afek, A., Levy, Y., Schneiderman, J., et al., 1999. Immunolocalization of beta2-glycoprotein I (apolipopro-tein H), to human atherosclerotic plaques: potential implications for lesion progression. Circulation. 99, 2227–2230.

George, J., Yacov, N., Breitbart, E., Bangio, L., Shaish, A., Gilburd, B., et al., 2004. Suppression of early atherosclerosis in LDL-receptor deficient mice by oral tolerance with beta 2-glycoprotein I. Cardiovasc. Res. 62, 603–609.

Gewaltig, J., Kummer, M., Koella, C., Cathomas, G., Biedermann, B.C., 2008. Requirements for CD8 T-cell migration into the human arte-rial wall. Hum. Pathol. 39, 1756–1762.

Gonzalez-Gay, M.A., Gonzalez-Juanatey, C., Lopez-Diaz, M.J., Piñeiro, A., Garcia-Porrua, C., Miranda-Filloy, J.A., et al., 2007. HLA-DRB1 and persistent chronic inflammation contribute to cardiovascular events and cardiovascular mortality in patients with rheumatoid arthritis. Arthritis Rheum. 57, 125–132.

Gotsman, I., Grabie, N., Gupta, R., Dacosta, R., MacConmara, M., Lederer, J., et al., 2006. Impaired regulatory T-cell response and enhanced atherosclerosis in the absence of inducible costimulatory molecule. Circulation. 114, 2047–2055.

Gotsman, I., Grabie, N., Dacosta, R., Sukhova, G., Sharpe, A., Lichtman, A.H., 2007. Proatherogenic immune responses are regu-lated by the PD-1/PD-L pathway in mice. J. Clin. Invest. 117, 2974–2982.

Gown, A.M., Tsukada, T., Ross, R., 1986. Human atherosclerosis. II. Immunocytochemical analysis of the cellular composition of human atherosclerotic lesions. Am. J. Pathol. 125, 191–207.

Grundtman, C., Wick, G., 2011. The autoimmune concept of atheroscle-rosis. Curr. Opin. Lipidol. 22, 327–334.

Grundtman, C., Kreutmayer, S.B., Almanzar, G., Wick, M.C., Wick, G., 2011. Heat shock protein 60 and immune inflammatory responses in atherosclerosis. Arterioscler. Thromb. Vasc. Biol. 31, 960–968.

Gupta, S., Pablo, A.M., Jiang, X.C., Wang, N., Tall, A.R., Schindler, C., 1997. IFN-gamma potentiates atherosclerosis in ApoE knock-out mice. J. Clin. Invest. 99, 2752–2761.

Haley, K.J., Lilly, C.M., Yang, J.H., Feng, Y., Kennedy, S.P., Turi, T.G., et al., 2000. Overexpression of eotaxin and the CCR3 receptor in human atherosclerosis: using genomic technology to identify a poten-tial novel pathway of vascular inflammation. Circulation. 102, 2185–2189.

Hansson, G.K., Hermansson, A., 2011. The immune system in athero-sclerosis. Nat. Immunol. 12, 204–212.

Hansson, G.K., Klareskog, L., 2011. Pulling down the plug on athero-sclerosis: cooling down the inflammasome. Nat. Med. 17, 790–791.

Hansson, G.K., Holm, J., Jonasson, L., 1989. Detection of activated T lymphocytes in the human atherosclerotic plaque. Am. J. Pathol. 135, 169–175.

Herbin, O., Ait-Oufella, H., Yu, W., Fredrikson, G.N., Aubier, B., Perez, N., et al., 2012. Regulatory T-cell response to apolipoprotein B100-derived peptides reduces the development and progression of atherosclerosis in mice. Arterioscler. Thromb. Vasc. Biol. 32, 605–612.

Houtkamp, M.A., de Boer, O.J., van der Loos, C.M., van der Wal, A. C., Becker, A.E., 2001a. Adventitial infiltrates associated with advanced atherosclerotic plaques: structural organization suggests generation of local humoral immune responses. J. Pathol. 193, 263–269.

Houtkamp, M.A., van Der Wal, A.C., de Boer, O.J., van Der Loos, C.M., de Boer, P.A., Moorman, A.F., et al., 2001b. Interleukin-15 expression in atherosclerotic plaques: an alternative pathway for T-cell activation in atherosclerosis?. Arterioscler. Thromb. Vasc. Biol. 21, 1208–1213.

Inaba, T., Yamada, N., Gotoda, T., Shimano, H., Shimada, M., Momomura, K., et al., 1992. Expression of M-CSF receptor encoded by c-fms on smooth muscle cells derived from arteriosclerotic lesion. J. Biol. Chem. 267, 5693–5699.

Iyer, S.S., Pulskens, W.P., Sadler, J.J., Butter, L.M., Teske, G.J., Ulland, T. K., et al., 2009. Necrotic cells trigger a sterile inflammatory response through the Nlrp3 inflammasome. Proc. Natl. Acad. Sci. U.S.A. 106, 20388–20393.

Jawien, J., Nastalek, P., Korbut, R., 2004. Mouse models of experimental atherosclerosis. J. Physiol. Pharmacol. 55, 503–517.

Jeziorska, M., McCollum, C., Woolley, D.E., 1997. Mast cell distribution, activation, and phenotype in atherosclerotic lesions of human carotid arteries. J. Pathol. 182, 115–122.

Jiagang, D., Li, C., Wang, H., Hao, E., Du, Z., Bao, C., et al., 2011. Amygdalin mediates relieved atherosclerosis in apolipoprotein E deficient mice through the induction of regulatory T cells. Biochem. Biophys. Res. Commun. 411, 523–529.

Juremalm, M., Nilsson, G., 2005. Chemokine receptor expression by mast cells. Chem. Immunol. Allergy. 87, 130–144.

Kamari, Y., Shaish, A., Shemesh, S., Vax, E., Grosskopf, I., Dotan, S., et al., 2011. Reduced atherosclerosis and inflammatory cytokines in apolipoprotein-E-deficient mice lacking bone marrow-derived interleukin-1alpha. Biochem. Biophys. Res. Commun. 405, 197–203.

King, V.L., Szilvassy, S.J., Daugherty, A., 2002. Interleukin-4 deficiency decreases atherosclerotic lesion formation in a site-specific manner in female LDL receptor −/− mice. Arterioscler. Thromb. Vasc. Biol. 22, 456–461.

Kirii, H., Niwa, T., Yamada, Y., Wada, H., Saito, K., Iwakura, Y., et al., 2003. Lack of interleukin-1beta decreases the severity of atherosclerosis in ApoE-deficient mice. Arterioscler. Thromb. Vasc. Biol. 23, 656–660.

Kleemann, R., Zadelaar, S., Kooistra, T., 2008. Cytokines and atherosclerosis: a comprehensive review of studies in mice. Cardiovasc. Res. 79, 360–376.

Kolbus, D., Ramos, O.H., Berg, K.E., Persson, J., Wigren, M., Bjorkbacka, H., 2010. CD8 + T cell activation predominate early immune responses to hypercholesterolemia in Apoe(/) mice. BMC Immunol. 11, 58.

Koltsova, E.K., Ley, K., 2011. How dendritic cells shape atherosclerosis. Trends Immunol. 32, 540–547.

Krebs, P., Scandella, E., Bolinger, B., Engeler, D., Miller, S., Ludewig, B., 2007. Chronic immune reactivity against persisting microbial antigen in the vasculature exacerbates atherosclerotic lesion formation. Arterioscler. Thromb. Vasc. Biol. 27, 2206–2213.

Kurowska-Stolarska, M., Hueber, A., Stolarski, B., McInnes, I.B., 2011. Interleukin-33: a novel mediator with a role in distinct disease pathologies. J. Intern. Med. 269, 29–35.

Kyaw, T., Tay, C., Khan, A., Dumouchel, V., Cao, A., To, K., et al., 2010. Conventional B2 B cell depletion ameliorates whereas its adoptive transfer aggravates atherosclerosis. J. Immunol. 185, 4410–4419.

Kyaw, T., Tay, C., Krishnamurthi, S., Kanellakis, P., Agrotis, A., Tipping, P., et al., 2011a. B1a B lymphocytes are atheroprotective by secreting natural IgM that increases IgM deposits and reduces necrotic cores in atherosclerotic lesions. Circ. Res. 109, 830–840.

Kyaw, T., Tipping, P., Toh, B.H., Bobik, A., 2011b. Current understanding of the role of B cell subsets and intimal and adventitial B cells in atherosclerosis. Curr. Opin. Lipidol. 22, 373–379.

Kyaw, T., Tay, C., Hosseini, H., Kanellakis, P., Gadowski, T., MacKay, F., et al., 2012. Depletion of B2 but not B1a B cells in BAFF receptor-deficient ApoE mice attenuates atherosclerosis by potently ameliorating arterial inflammation. PLoS One. 7, e29371.

Kyriakakis, E., Cavallari, M., Andert, J., Philippova, M., Koella, C., Bochkov, V., et al., 2010. Invariant natural killer T cells: linking inflammation and neovascularization in human atherosclerosis. Eur. J. Immunol. 40, 3268–3279.

Lappalainen, H., Laine, P., Pentikäinen, M.O., Sajantila, A., Kovanen, P.T., 2004. Mast cells in neovascularized human coronary plaques store and secrete basic fibroblast growth factor, a potent angiogenic mediator. Arterioscler. Thromb. Vasc. Biol. 24, 1880–1885.

Lee, T.S., Yen, H.C., Pan, C.C., Chau, L.Y., 1999. The role of interleukin 12 in the development of atherosclerosis in ApoE-deficient mice. Arterioscler. Thromb. Vasc. Biol. 19, 734–742.

Lewis, M.J., Malik, T.H., Ehrenstein, M.R., Boyle, J.J., Botto, M., Haskard, D.O., 2009. Immunoglobulin M is required for protection against atherosclerosis in low-density lipoprotein receptor-deficient mice. Circulation. 120, 417–426.

Ley, K., Miller, Y.I., Hedrick, C.C., 2011. Monocyte and macrophage dynamics during atherogenesis. Arterioscler. Thromb. Vasc. Biol. 31, 1506–1516.

Libby, P., Ridker, P.M., Hansson, G.K., 2011. Progress and challenges in translating the biology of atherosclerosis. Nature. 473, 317–325.

Liew, F.Y., Pitman, N.I., McInnes, I.B., 2010. Disease-associated functions of IL-33: the new kid in the IL-1 family. Nat. Rev. Immunol. 10, 103–110.

Ludewig, B., Freigang, S., Jäggi, M., Kurrer, M.O., Pei, Y.C., Vlk, L., et al., 2000. Linking immune-mediated arterial inflammation and cholesterol-induced atherosclerosis in a transgenic mouse model. Proc. Natl. Acad. Sci. U.S.A. 97, 12752–12757.

Mach, F., Schönbeck, U., Sukhova, G.K., Bourcier, T., Bonnefoy, J.Y., Pober, J.S., et al., 1997. Functional CD40 ligand is expressed on human vascular endothelial cells, smooth muscle cells, and macrophages: implications for CD40-CD40 ligand signaling in atherosclerosis. Proc. Natl. Acad. Sci. U.S.A. 94, 1931–1936.

Mach, F., Schönbeck, U., Sukhova, G.K., Atkinson, E., Libby, P., 1998. Reduction of atherosclerosis in mice by inhibition of CD40 signalling. Nature. 394, 200–203.

Mackay, F., Figgett, W.A., Saulep, D., Lepage, M., Hibbs, M.L., 2010. B-cell stage and context-dependent requirements for survival signals from BAFF and the B-cell receptor. Immunol. Rev. 237, 205–225.

Major, A.S., Wilson, M.T., McCaleb, J.L., Ru, Su, Y., Stanic, A.K., Joyce, S., et al., 2004. Quantitative and qualitative differences in proatherogenic NKT cells in apolipoprotein E-deficient mice. Arterioscler. Thromb. Vasc. Biol. 24, 2351–2357.

Mallat, Z., Besnard, S., Duriez, M., Deleuze, V., Emmanuel, F., Bureau, M.F., et al., 1999. Protective role of interleukin-10 in atherosclerosis. Circ. Res. 85, e17–e24.

Marfaing-Koka, A., Devergne, O., Gorgone, G., Portier, A., Schall, T.J., Galanaud, P., et al., 1995. Regulation of the production of the RANTES chemokine by endothelial cells. Synergistic induction by IFN-gamma plus TNF-alpha and inhibition by IL-4 and IL-13. J. Immunol. 154, 1870–1878.

Marx, N., Sukhova, G., Murphy, C., Libby, P., Plutzky, J., 1998. Macrophages in human atheroma contain PPARgamma: differentiation-dependent peroxisomal proliferator-activated receptor gamma (PPARgamma) expression and reduction of MMP-9 activity through PPARgamma activation in mononuclear phagocytes in vitro. Am. J. Pathol. 153, 17–23.

Matsuura, E., Kobayashi, K., Matsunami, Y., Shen, L., Quan, N., Makarova, M., et al., 2009. Autoimmunity, infectious immunity, and atherosclerosis. J. Clin. Immunol. 29, 714–721.

Micha, R., Imamura, F., Wyler von Ballmoos, M., Solomon, D.H., Hernán, M.A., Ridker, P.M., et al., 2011. Systematic review and meta-analysis of methotrexate use and risk of cardiovascular disease. Am. J. Cardiol. 108, 1362–1370.

Michelsen, K.S., Wong, M.H., Shah, P.K., Zhang, W., Yano, J., Doherty, T.M., et al., 2004. Lack of toll-like receptor 4 or myeloid differentiation factor 88 reduces atherosclerosis and alters plaque phenotype in mice deficient in apolipoprotein E. Proc. Natl. Acad. Sci. U.S.A. 101, 10679–10684.

Miller, A.M., Xu, D., Asquith, D.L., Denby, L., Li, Y., Sattar, N., et al., 2008. IL-33 reduces the development of atherosclerosis. J. Exp. Med. 205, 339–346.

Moisini, I., Davidson, A., 2009. BAFF: a local and systemic target in autoimmune diseases. Clin Exp Immunol. 158, 155–163.

Moore, K.J., Tabas, I., 2011. Macrophages in the pathogenesis of atherosclerosis. Cell. 145, 341–355.

Mor, A., Planer, D., Luboshits, G., Afek, A., Metzger, S., Chajek-Shaul, T., et al., 2007. Role of naturally occurring CD4 + CD25 + regulatory T cells in experimental atherosclerosis. Arterioscler. Thromb. Vasc. Biol. 27, 893–900.

Mullick, A.E., Tobias, P.S., Curtiss, L.K., 2005. Modulation of atherosclerosis in mice by Toll-like receptor 2. J. Clin. Invest. 115, 3149–3156.

Mullick, A.E., Soldau, K., Kiosses, W.B., Bell III, T.A., Tobias, P.S., Curtiss, L.K., 2008. Increased endothelial expression of Toll-like receptor 2 at sites of disturbed blood flow exacerbates early atherogenic events. J. Exp. Med. 205, 373–383.

Nakai, Y., Iwabuchi, K., Fujii, S., Ishimori, N., Dashtsoodol, N., Watano, K., et al., 2004. Natural killer T cells accelerate atherogenesis in mice. Blood. 104, 2051–2059.

Naruko, T., Ueda, M., Haze, K., van der Wal, A.C., van der Loos, C.M., Itoh, A., et al., 2002. Neutrophil infiltration of culprit lesions in acute coronary syndromes. Circulation. 106, 2894–2900.

Ng, H.P., Burris, R.L., Nagarajan, S., 2011. Attenuated atherosclerotic lesions in apoE-Fcgamma-chain-deficient hyperlipidemic mouse model is associated with inhibition of Th17 cells and promotion of regulatory T cells. J. Immunol. 187, 6082–6093.

Ohta, H., Wada, H., Niwa, T., Kirii, H., Iwamoto, N., Fujii, H., et al., 2005. Disruption of tumor necrosis factor-alpha gene diminishes the development of atherosclerosis in ApoE-deficient mice. Atherosclerosis. 180, 11–17.

Oksala, O., Ylä-Herttuala, S., Ylitalo, P., 1994. Effects of clodronate (dichloromethylene bisphosphonate) on the development of experimental atherosclerosis in rabbits. J. Lab. Clin. Med. 123, 769–776.

Olofsson, P.S., Söderström, L.A., Wågsäter, D., Sheikine, Y., Ocaya, P., Lang, F., et al., 2008. CD137 is expressed in human atherosclerosis and promotes development of plaque inflammation in hypercholesterolemic mice. Circulation. 117, 1292–1301.

Osterud, B., Bjorklid, E., 2003. Role of monocytes in atherogenesis. Physiol. Rev. 83, 1069–1112.

O'Garra, A., Chang, R., Go, N., Hastings, R., Haughton, G., Howard, M., 1992. Ly-1 B (B-1) cells are the main source of B cell-derived interleukin 10. Eur. J. Immunol. 22, 711–717.

Paulson, K.E., Zhu, S.N., Chen, M., Nurmohamed, S., Jongstra-Bilen, J., Cybulsky, M.I., 2010. Resident intimal dendritic cells accumulate lipid and contribute to the initiation of atherosclerosis. Circ. Res. 106, 383–390.

Ridker, P.M., 2009. Testing the inflammatory hypothesis of atherothrombosis: scientific rationale for the cardiovascular inflammation reduction trial (CIRT). J. Thromb. Haemost. 7, 1332–1339.

Ridker, P.M., Thuren, T., Zalewski, A., Libby, P., 2011. Interleukin-1 inhibition and the prevention of recurrent cardiovascular events: rationale and design of the Canakinumab Anti-inflammatory Thrombosis Outcomes Study (CANTOS). Am. Heart J. 162, 597–605.

Roder, J., Duwe, A., 1979. The beige mutation in the mouse selectively impairs natural killer cell function. Nature. 278, 451–453.

Rogers, L., Burchat, S., Gage, J., Hasu, M., Thabet, M., Willcox, L., et al., 2008. Deficiency of invariant V alpha 14 natural killer T cells decreases atherosclerosis in LDL receptor null mice. Cardiovasc. Res. 78, 167–174.

Roman, M.J., Shanker, B.A., Davis, A., Lockshin, M.D., Sammaritano, L., Simantov, R., et al., 2003. Prevalence and correlates of accelerated atherosclerosis in systemic lupus erythematosus. N. Engl. J. Med. 349, 2399–2406.

Romo, N., Fitó, M., Gumá, M., Sala, J., García, C., Ramos, R., et al., 2011. Association of atherosclerosis with expression of the LILRB1 receptor by human NK and T-cells supports the infectious burden hypothesis. Arterioscler. Thromb. Vasc. Biol. 31, 2314–2321.

Roselaar, S.E., Kakkanathu, P.X., Daugherty, A., 1996. Lymphocyte populations in atherosclerotic lesions of apoE−/− and LDL receptor−/− mice. Decreasing density with disease progression. Arterioscler. Thromb. Vasc. Biol. 16, 1013–1018.

Ross, R., Glomset, J.A., 1973. Atherosclerosis and the arterial smooth muscle cell: proliferation of smooth muscle is a key event in the genesis of the lesions of atherosclerosis. Science. 180, 1332–1339.

Rossmann, A., Henderson, B., Heidecker, B., Seiler, R., Fraedrich, G., Singh, M., et al., 2008. T-cells from advanced atherosclerotic lesions recognize hHSP60 and have a restricted T-cell receptor repertoire. Exp. Gerontol. 43, 229–237.

Sakai, A., Kume, N., Nishi, E., Tanoue, K., Miyasaka, M., Kita, T., 1997. P-selectin and vascular cell adhesion molecule-1 are focally expressed in aortas of hypercholesterolemic rabbits before intimal accumulation of macrophages and T lymphocytes. Arterioscler. Thromb. Vasc. Biol. 17, 310–316.

Schecter, A.D., Berman, A.B., Taubman, M.B., 2003. Chemokine receptors in vascular smooth muscle. Microcirculation. 10, 265–272.

Schieffer, B., Selle, T., Hilfiker, A., Hilfiker-Kleiner, D., Grote, K., Tietge, U.J., et al., 2004. Impact of interleukin-6 on plaque development and morphology in experimental atherosclerosis. Circulation. 110, 3493–3500.

Schiller, N.K., Boisvert, W.A., Curtiss, L.K., 2002. Inflammation in atherosclerosis: lesion formation in LDL receptor-deficient mice with perforin and Lyst (beige) mutations. Arterioscler. Thromb. Vasc. Biol. 22, 1341–1346.

Shen, L., Matsunami, Y., Quan, N., Kobayashi, K., Matsuura, E., Oguma, K., 2011. In vivo oxidation, platelet activation and simultaneous occurrence of natural immunity in atherosclerosis-prone mice. Isr. Med. Assoc. J. 13, 278–283.

Shoenfeld, Y., Gerli, R., Doria, A., Matsuura, E., Cerinic, M.M., Ronda, N., et al., 2005. Accelerated atherosclerosis in autoimmune rheumatic diseases. Circulation. 112, 3337–3347.

Silva, M.T., 2010. Secondary necrosis: the natural outcome of the complete apoptotic program. FEBS Letters. 584, 4491–4499.

Sironi, M., Breviario, F., Proserpio, P., Biondi, A., Vecchi, A., Van Damme, J., et al., 1989. IL-1 stimulates IL-6 production in endothelial cells. J. Immunol. 142, 549–553.

Smith, J.D., Trogan, E., Ginsberg, M., Grigaux, C., Tian, J., Miyata, M., et al., 1995. Decreased atherosclerosis in mice deficient in both macrophage colonystimulating factor (op) and apolipoprotein E. Proc. Natl. Acad. Sci. U.S.A. 92, 8264–8268.

Smith, E., Prasad, K.M., Butcher, M., Dobrian, A., Kolls, J.K., Ley, K., et al., 2010. Blockade of interleukin-17A results in reduced atherosclerosis in apolipoprotein E-deficient mice. Circulation. 121, 1746–1755.

Starnes, T., Robertson, M.J., Sledge, G., Kelich, S., Nakshatri, H., Broxmeyer, H.E., et al., 2001. Cutting edge: IL-17F, a novel cytokine selectively expressed in activated T cells and monocytes, regulates angiogenesis and endothelial cell cytokine production. J. Immunol. 167, 4137–4140.

Steen, K.S., Lems, W.F., Visman, I.M., Heierman, M., Dijkmans, B.A., Twisk, J.W., et al., 2009. High incidence of cardiovascular events in patients with rheumatoid arthritis. Ann. Rheu. Dis. 68, 1509–1510.

Stemme, S., Faber, B., Holm, J., Wiklund, O., Witztum, J.L., Hansson, G.K., 1995. T lymphocytes from human atherosclerotic plaques recognize oxidized low density lipoprotein. Proc. Natl. Acad. Sci. U.S.A. 92, 3893–3897.

Stoneman, V., Braganza, D., Figg, N., Mercer, J., Lang, R., Goddard, M., et al., 2007. Monocyte/macrophage suppression in CD11b diphtheria toxin receptor transgenic mice differentially affects atherogenesis and established plaques. Circ. Res. 100, 884–893.

Sun, J., Sukhova, G.K., Wolters, P.J., Yang, M., Kitamoto, S., Libby, P., et al., 2007. Mast cells promote atherosclerosis by releasing proinflammatory cytokines. Nat. Med. 13, 719–724.

Swirski, F.K., Pittet, M.J., Kircher, M.F., Aikawa, E., Jaffer, F.A., Libby, P., et al., 2006. Monocyte accumulation in mouse atherogenesis is progressive and proportional to extent of disease. Proc. Natl. Acad. Sci. U.S.A. 103, 10340–10345.

Tabas, I., 2011. Pulling down the plug on atherosclerosis: finding the culprit in your heart. Nat. Med. 17, 791–793.

Takeda, M., Yamashita, T., Sasaki, N., Nakajima, K., Kita, T., Shinohara, M., et al., 2010. Oral administration of an active form of vitamin D3 (calcitriol), decreases atherosclerosis in mice by inducing regulatory T cells and immature dendritic cells with tolerogenic functions. Arterioscler. Thromb. Vasc. Biol. 30, 2495–2503.

Taleb, S., Romain, M., Ramkhelawon, B., Uyttenhove, C., Pasterkamp, G., Herbin, O., et al., 2009. Loss of SOCS3 expression in T cells reveals a regulatory role for interleukin-17 in atherosclerosis. J. Exp. Med. 206, 2067–2077.

Taleb, S., Tedgui, A., Mallat, Z., 2010. Interleukin-17: friend or foe in atherosclerosis? Curr. Opin. Lipidol. 21, 404–408.

Tedgui, A., Mallat, Z., 2006. Cytokines in atherosclerosis: pathogenic and regulatory pathways. Physiol. Rev. 86, 515–581.

Thorp, E., Subramanian, M., Tabas, I., 2011. The role of macrophages and dendritic cells in the clearance of apoptotic cells in advanced atherosclerosis. Eur. J. Immunol. 41, 2515–2518.

Tipping, P.G., Hancock, W.W., 1993. Production of tumor necrosis factor and interleukin-1 by macrophages from human atheromatous plaques. Am. J. Pathol. 142, 1721–1728.

To, K., Agrotis, A., Besra, G., Bobik, A., Toh, 2009. NKT cell subsets mediate differential proatherogenic effects in ApoE − / − mice. Arterioscler. Thromb. Vasc. Biol. 29, 671–677.

Tupin, E., Nicoletti, A., Elhage, R., Rudling, M., Ljunggren, H.G., Hansson, G.K., et al., 2004. CD1d-dependent activation of NKT cells aggravates atherosclerosis. J. Exp. Med. 199, 417–422.

Uyemura, K., Demer, L.L., Castle, S.C., Jullien, D., Berliner, J.A., Gately, M.K., et al., 1996. Cross-regulatory roles of interleukin IL-12 and IL-10 in atherosclerosis. J. Clin. Invest. 97, 2130–2138.

van der Wal, A.C., Das, P.K., Bentz van de Berg, D., van der Loos, C.M., Becker, A.E., 1989. Atherosclerotic lesions in humans. In situ immunophenotypic analysis suggesting an immune mediated response. Lab. Invest. 61, 166–170.

van Es, T., van Puijvelde, G.H., Ramos, O.H., Segers, F.M., Joosten, L.A., van den Berg, W.B., et al., 2009. Attenuated atherosclerosis upon IL-17R signaling disruption in LDLr deficient mice. Biochem. Biophys. Res. Commun. 388, 261–265.

van Es, T., van Puijvelde, G.H., Michon, I.N., van Wanrooij, E.J., de Vos, P., et al., 2011. IL-15 aggravates atherosclerotic lesion development in LDL receptor deficient mice. Vaccine. 29, 976–983.

van Leeuwen, M., Gijbels, M.J., Duijvestijn, A., Smook, M., van de Gaar, M.J., Heeringa, P., et al., 2008. Accumulation of myeloperoxidase-positive neutrophils in atherosclerotic lesions in LDLR−/− mice. Arterioscler. Thromb. Vasc. Biol. 28, 84–89.

van Puijvelde, G.H., Hauer, A.D., de Vos, P., van den Heuvel, R., van Herwijnen, M.J., van der Zee, R., et al., 2006. Induction of oral tolerance to oxidized low-density lipoprotein ameliorates atherosclerosis. Circulation. 114, 1968–1976.

van Puijvelde, G.H., van Es, T., van Wanrooij, E.J., Habets, K.L., de Vos, P., van der Zee, R., et al., 2007. Induction of oral tolerance to HSP60 or an HSP60-peptide activates T cell regulation and reduces atherosclerosis. Arterioscler. Thromb. Vasc. Biol. 27, 2677–2683.

VanderLaan, P.A., Reardon, C.A., Sagiv, Y., Blachowicz, L., Lukens, J., Nissenbaum, M., et al., 2007. Characterization of the natural killer T-cell response in an adoptive transfer model of atherosclerosis. Am. J. Pathol. 170, 1100–1107.

Wang, X., Ria, M., Kelmenson, P.M., Eriksson, P., Higgins, D.C., Samnegård, A., et al., 2005. Positional identification of TNFSF4, encoding OX40 ligand, as a gene that influences atherosclerosis susceptibility. Nat. Genet. 37, 365–372.

Wardemann, H., Boehm, T., Dear, N., Carsetti, R., 2002. B-1a B cells that link the innate and adaptive immune responses are lacking in the absence of the spleen. J. Exp. Med. 195, 771–780.

Weber, C., Zernecke, A., Libby, P., 2008. The multifaceted contributions of leukocyte subsets to atherosclerosis: lessons from mouse models. Nat. Rev. Immunol. 8, 802–815.

Weber, C., Meiler, S., Döring, Y., Koch, M., Drechsler, M., Megens, R.T., et al., 2011. CCL17-expressing dendritic cells drive atherosclerosis by restraining regulatory T cell homeostasis in mice. J. Clin. Invest. 121, 2898–2910.

Whitman, S.C., Ravisankar, P., Elam, H., Daugherty, A., 2000. Exogenous interferon-gamma enhances atherosclerosis in apolipoprotein E−/− mice. Am. J. Pathol. 157, 1819–1824.

Whitman, S.C., Ravisankar, P., Daugherty, A., 2002. Interleukin-18 enhances atherosclerosis in apolipoprotein E(−/−) mice through release of interferon-gamma. Circ. Res. 90, E34–E38.

Whitman, S.C., Rateri, D.L., Szilvassy, S.J., Yokoyama, W., Daugherty, A., 2004. Depletion of natural killer cell function decreases atherosclerosis in low-density lipoprotein receptor null mice. Arterioscler. Thromb. Vasc. Biol. 24, 1049–1054.

Wick, G., Knoflach, M., Xu, Q., 2004. Autoimmune and inflammatory mechanisms in atherosclerosis. Annu. Rev. Immunol. 22, 361–403.

Woollard, K.J., Geissmann, F., 2010. Monocytes in atherosclerosis: subsets and functions. Nature Reviews. Cardiology. 7, 77–86.

Yla-Herttuala, S., Palinski, W., Butler, S.W., Picard, S., Steinberg, D., Witztum, J.L., 1994. Rabbit and human atherosclerotic lesions contain IgG that recognizes epitopes of oxidized LDL. Arterioscler. Thromb. 14, 32–40.

Yla-Herttuala, S., Bentzon, J.F., Daemen, M., Falk, E., Garcia-Garcia, H.M., Herrmann, J., et al., 2011. Stabilisation of atherosclerotic plaques. Position paper of the European Society of Cardiology (ESC). Working Group on Atherosclerosis and Vascular Biology. Thromb. Haemost. 106, 1–19.

Zhao, L., Cuff, C.A., Moss, E., Wille, U., Cyrus, T., Klein, E.A., et al., 2002. Selective interleukin-12 synthesis defect in 12/15-lipoxygenase-deficient macrophages associated with reduced atherosclerosis in a mouse model of familial hypercholesterolemia. J. Biol. Chem. 277, 35350–35356.

Zhou, X., Hansson, G.K., 1999. Detection of B cells and proinflammatory cytokines in atherosclerotic plaques of hypercholesterolaemic apolipoprotein E knockout mice. Scand. J. Immunol. 50, 25–30.

Zhou, X., Nicoletti, A., Elhage, R., Hansson, G.K., 2000. Transfer of CD4(+) T cells aggravates atherosclerosis in immunodeficient apolipoprotein E knockout mice. Circulation. 102, 2919–2922.

Zhou, X., Robertson, A.K., Hjerpe, C., Hansson, G.K., 2006. Adoptive transfer of CD4 + T cells reactive to modified low-density lipoprotein aggravates atherosclerosis. Arterioscler. Thromb. Vasc. Biol. 26, 864–870.

Zhu, S.N., Chen, M., Jongstra-Bilen, J., Cybulsky, M.I., 2009. GM-CSF regulates intimal cell proliferation in nascent atherosclerotic lesions. J. Exp. Med. 206, 2141–2149.

Chapter 72

Necrotizing Arteritis and Small Vessel Vasculitis

J. Charles Jennette[1] and Ronald J. Falk[2]

[1]*Department of Pathology and Laboratory Medicine, University of North Carolina, Chapel Hill, NC, USA,* [2]*Department of Medicine, University of North Carolina, Chapel Hill, NC, USA*

Chapter Outline

Historical Background	**1067**	Environmental Influences	1075
Necrotizing Arteritis	1067	*In Vivo* Models	1076
Purpura and Small Vessel Vasculitis	1069	Pathologic Effector Mechanisms	1076
Polyarteritis Nodosa	**1070**	Autoantibodies as Immunologic Markers	1077
Clinical, Epidemiologic, and Pathologic Features	1070	**Cryoglobulinemic Vasculitis**	**1079**
Autoimmune Features	1070	Clinical, Pathologic, and Epidemiologic Features	1079
Genetic Features and Environmental Influences	1070	Autoimmune Features	1079
In Vivo Models	1071	Genetic Features and Environmental Influences	1079
Pathologic Effector Mechanisms	1071	*In Vivo* Models	1080
Autoantibodies as Potential Immunologic Markers	1071	Pathologic Effector Mechanisms	1080
Kawasaki's Disease	**1071**	Autoantibodies as Immunologic Markers	1080
Clinical, Pathologic, and Epidemiologic Features	1071	**IgA Vasculitis (Henoch–Schönlein Purpura)**	**1080**
Autoimmune Features	1072	Clinical, Pathologic, and Epidemiologic Features	1080
Genetic Features and Environmental Influences	1072	Autoimmune Features	1081
In Vivo Models	1072	Genetic Features and Environmental Influences	1081
Pathologic Effector Mechanisms	1072	*In Vivo* Models	1081
Autoantibodies as Potential Immunologic Markers	1073	Pathologic Effector Mechanisms	1081
ANCA-associated Vasculitis (AAV)	**1073**	Autoantibodies as Potential Immunologic Markers	1081
Clinical, Pathologic, and Epidemiologic Features	1073	**Concluding Remarks—Future Prospects**	**1082**
Autoimmune Features	1074	**References**	**1082**
Genetic Features	1075		

HISTORICAL BACKGROUND

The three major categories of systemic vasculitis are large vessel vasculitis (chronic granulomatous arteritis), medium vessel vasculitis (necrotizing arteritis), and small vessel vasculitis (necrotizing polyangiitis) (Figure 72.1, Box 72.1). A subsequent chapter will review large vessel vasculitis. Necrotizing arteritis was first recognized because of the grossly discernible segmental inflammatory nodular lesions that occur along major arteries (Kussmaul and Maier, 1866). Small vessel vasculitis (SVV) was first recognized

because of the palpable purpura that is caused by inflammation of dermal venules (Willan, 1808).

Necrotizing Arteritis

Kussmaul and Maier (1866) gave the first detailed pathologic and clinical description of systemic necrotizing arteritis. They reported a patient with fever, anorexia, muscle weakness, paresthesias, myalgias, abdominal pain, and oliguria, who was found to have inflammatory

N. Rose & I. Mackay (Eds): The Autoimmune Diseases, Fifth edition. DOI: http://dx.doi.org/10.1016/B978-0-12-384929-8.00072-1

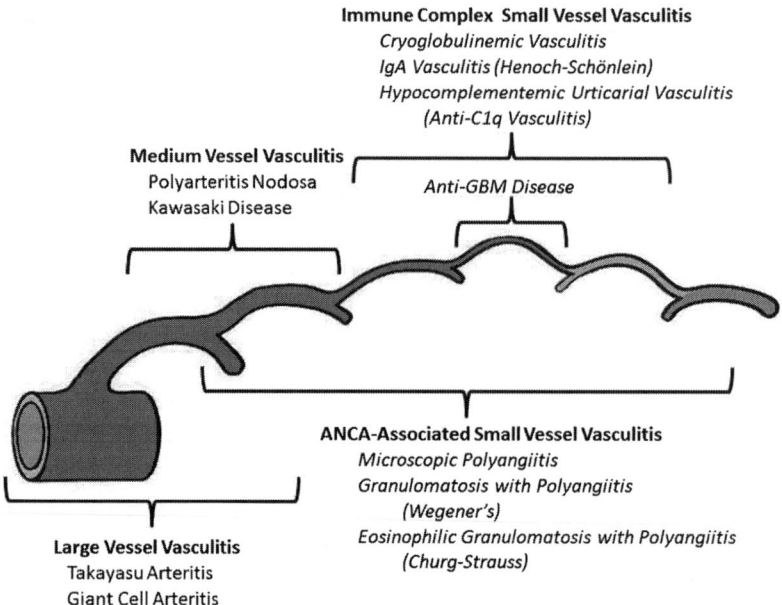

FIGURE 72.1   Overlapping predominant vascular distributions (brackets) of large vessel vasculitis, medium vessel vasculitis, and small vessel vasculitis. *Reproduced with permission from Jennette et al. (2013a).*

Box 72.1 Names for Vasculitides Proposed by the 2012 International Chapel Hill Consensus Conference on the Nomenclature of Vasculitides

- Large vessel vasculitis (LVV)
  - Takayasu arteritis (TAK)
  - Giant cell arteritis (GCA)
- Medium vessel vasculitis (MVV)
  - Polyarteritis nodosa (PAN)
  - Kawasaki's disease (KD)
- Small vessel vasculitis (SVV)
- Antineutrophil cytoplasmic antibody (ANCA)-associated vasculitis (AAV)
  - Microscopic polyangiitis (MPA)
  - Granulomatosis with polyangiitis (Wegener's) (GPA)
  - Eosinophilic granulomatosis with polyangiitis (Churg–Strauss) (EGPA)
- Immune complex SVV
  - Anti-glomerular basement membrane (anti-GBM) disease
  - Cryoglobulinemic vasculitis (CV)

- IgA vasculitis (Henoch-Schönlein) (IgAV)
- Hypocomplementemic urticarial vasculitis (HUV) (anti-C1q vasculitis)
- Variable vessel vasculitis (VVV)
  - Behçet's disease (BD)
  - Cogan's syndrome (CS)
- Single-organ vasculitis (SOV)
- Vasculitis associated with systemic disease
  - Lupus vasculitis
  - Rheumatoid vasculitis
  - Others
- Vasculitis associated with probable etiology
  - Hepatitis C virus-associated cryoglobulinemic vasculitis
  - Hepatitis B virus-associated vasculitis
  - Drug-associated immune complex vasculitis
  - Drug-associated ANCA-associated vasculitis
  - Cancer-associated vasculitis
  - Others

Jennette et al., 2013a.

---

nodules scattered over medium-sized and small arteries in many organs. They coined the term "periarteritis nodosa" for this process, which, over the following decades, evolved into "polyarteritis nodosa" as it became clear that the inflammation arose in the walls of arteries rather than in the perivascular tissue.

Soon after the recognition of polyarteritis nodosa (PAN), a number of investigators noted that some patients with necrotizing arteritis also had vasculitis affecting arteries that could be seen only by microscopy, and that some patients also had vasculitis affecting glomerular capillaries (glomerulonephritis) and pulmonary capillaries (alveolar capillaritis) (Arkin, 1930; Davson et al., 1948; Zeek et al., 1948; Zeek, 1952; Godman and Churg, 1954). Davson, and Godman and Churg, called this the "microscopic form of periarteritis," and Zeek called it "hypersensitivity angiitis." Today, this form of vasculitis usually is designated microscopic polyangiitis (Jennette et al., 2013a,b).

By the 1950s, Wegener's granulomatosis and Churg–Strauss syndrome had been recognized as variants of vasculitis that could have necrotizing arteritis combined with granulomatous inflammation and vasculitis in small vessels (Klinger, 1931; Wegener, 1939; Churg and Strauss, 1951; Godman and Churg, 1954). In their landmark publication in 1954, Godman and Churg concluded that the "microscopic form or periarteritis," Wegener's granulomatosis, and Churg–Strauss syndrome are pathologically and clinically distinct from PAN, and probably have a related etiology and pathogenesis. This concept has been borne out by the discovery that microscopic polyangiitis, Wegener's granulomatosis, and Churg–Strauss syndrome are associated with, and are probably caused by, antineutrophil cytoplasmic autoantibodies (ANCAs), whereas PAN is not (Jennette and Falk, 1997; Jennette et al., 2013a). These forms of ANCA-associated vasculitis (AAV) now are designated microscopic polyangiitis (MPA), granulomatosis with polyangiitis (GPA), and eosinophilic granulomatosis with polyangiitis (EGPA).

An additional form of necrotizing arteritis was discovered that is associated with the mucocutaneous lymph node syndrome (Kawasaki, 1967; Tanaka et al., 1971). This disease has been called "infantile polyarteritis nodosa" because it almost always occurs in young children (Magilavy et al., 1977); however, the clinical, pathologic, and pathogenetic features of Kawasaki's disease are clearly distinct from those of PAN (Jennette et al., 2013a).

Purpura and Small Vessel Vasculitis

The evaluation of patients with cutaneous palpable purpura revealed vasculitis involving predominantly small vessels. Although purpura had been described in medical writings at least since the time of Hippocrates, Willan (1808) was one of the first to separate purpura caused by febrile infectious disease from noninfectious purpura. The occurrence of purpura in children with arthralgias and arthritis was reported (Schönlein, 1837). Later, Henoch (1868, 1882) described the association of purpura with abdominal pain, nephritis, small visceral hemorrhages, and pathologic changes in small vessels in the skin and internal organs. These pediatric patients probably had what today would be called Henoch–Schönlein purpura.

At the turn of the 20th century, William Osler (1895, 1914) reported numerous adult patients with a more aggressive form of SVV most consistent with what today would be called microscopic polyangiitis. These patients had a broad spectrum of SVV manifestations, including purpura, arthritis, peripheral neuropathy, abdominal pain, pulmonary hemorrhage, epistaxis, iritis, and nephritis, including rapidly progressive renal disease with death from uremia in several months and the autopsy finding of glomeruli with "every tuft compressed by a crescentic mass."

The pathologic findings in SVV of extensive acute inflammation with numerous neutrophils and conspicuous leukocytoclasia that resembled the Arthus reaction suggested a possible "hypersensitivity" pathogenesis (Winklemann, 1958). A hypersensitivity or allergic cause also was supported by the association of SVV with exposure to certain drugs and with serum sickness (Clark and Kaplan, 1937; Zeek et al., 1948; Winklemann, 1958; Alarcon Segovia and Brown, 1964). In the 1960s, the widespread application of immunofluorescence microscopy revealed that certain forms of SVV had substantial vascular localization of immunoglobulins and complement, suggesting an immune complex pathogenesis. Some patients with pulmonary–renal syndrome had linear deposits of immunoglobulin along glomerular and pulmonary capillary basement membranes (Sturgill and Westervelt, 1965), which were shown to be pathogenic autoantibodies directed against basement membrane collagen (Lerner et al., 1967). Patients with circulating cryoglobulins associated with signs and symptoms of SVV, such as purpura and glomerulonephritis, were found to have granular deposits of IgM, IgG, and complement in vessels walls (Meltzer et al., 1966), indicating an immune complex pathogenesis. This concept of immune complex-mediated SVV was further supported by the detection of hepatitis B antigens and antibodies in the walls of vessels in patients with SVV associated with hepatitis B virus (HBV) infection (Gower et al., 1978). Children with Henoch–Schönlein purpura were found to have deposits of IgA and C3 in dermal venules and glomerular capillaries supporting a distinct type of immune complex pathogenesis (Baart de la Faille-Kuyber et al., 1973). Neutrophilic SVV with extensive leukocytoclastic angiitis also was identified in the acute phase of Behçet's disease (Jorizzo et al., 1985).

By the end of the 1970s, there was a widespread belief that most if not all SVV was mediated by immune complexes (Fauci et al., 1978). However, not all immunohistologic studies of vasculitis showed evidence for substantial vessel wall deposition of immunoglobulins or complement. This was especially true in some of the most common forms of SVV in adults, including Wegener's granulomatosis (GPA) (Ronco et al., 1983; Weiss and Crissman, 1984). Davies et al., (1982) reported a new type of autoantibody that reacted with neutrophil cytoplasm in patients with SVV who did not have deposits of immunoglobulin or complement in inflamed glomeruli. Three years later, van der Woude et al. (1985) identified these autoantibodies in patients with GPA. Numerous subsequent studies have documented the association of these ANCAs with several clinicopathologic expressions of SVV (MPA, GPA, and EGPA) that are characterized by the absence or paucity of immunoglobulin and complement deposits in the vessel walls, which suggests a pathogenesis that does not involve extensive vascular deposition of immune complexes (Jennette and Falk, 1997; Jennette et al., 2013a). In fact, there is strong evidence that ANCA-associated pauci-immune SVV is caused by direct activation of neutrophils by autoantibodies directed against granule proteins (Jennette et al., 2013b).

POLYARTERITIS NODOSA

Clinical, Epidemiologic, and Pathologic Features

The hallmark of PAN is necrotizing inflammation of medium-sized or small arteries. The prevalence is somewhere between 10 and 30 cases per million population (Mahr et al., 2004; Watts and Scott, 2004). The vascular inflammation initially contains predominantly neutrophils, but within a few days the infiltrates contain predominantly mononuclear leukocytes. Segmental inflammation and necrosis may produce pseudoaneurysms by eroding through the vessel wall into the surrounding tissue. Thrombosis can cause acute ischemia, including infarction. Rupture of pseudoaneurysms results in hemorrhage, which may be severe and life-threatening.

PAN is an acute disease that typically has one major episode with only rare recurrences if remission is attained (Guillevin, 1999). Clinical manifestations include cutaneous erythematous nodules and ulcers caused by dermal and subcutaneous arteritis; peripheral neuropathy (e.g., mononeuritis multiplex) caused by arteritis in epineural arteries; myalgias and elevated circulating muscle enzymes caused by arteritis in skeletal muscle; and pain and dysfunction in virtually any viscera caused by arteritis in the parenchyma. Involvement of the skin and gut is common, whereas involvement of the lungs is rare (Agard et al., 2003). Imaging studies may reveal arterial aneurysms (pseudoaneurysms), visceral infarcts, or gut perforation. Diagnosis of PAN in a patient with necrotizing arteritis requires the exclusion of other diseases that also cause arteritis, including Kawasaki's disease, MPA, GPA, and EGPA (Agard et al., 2003; Mahr et al., 2004; Jennette et al., 2013a). Glomerulonephritis or alveolar capillaritis rule out a diagnosis of PAN and indicate some form of SVV, such as microscopic polyangiitis (Agard et al., 2003; Jennette et al., 2013a). Renal involvement can result in renal insufficiency, hematuria, and low-level proteinuria, but this is the result of infarction and hemorrhage rather than glomerulonephritis. Myocardial infarction caused by coronary artery involvement is a rare complication.

Corticosteroids and cytotoxic drugs have been the most frequently used therapy for PAN and many other forms of noninfectious vasculitis. Guillevin (1999) advocates the use of corticosteroids alone for patients with PAN who lack all of the following five factors that indicate a worse prognosis: renal insufficiency, proteinuria >1 g/day, cardiac involvement, central nervous system (CNS) involvement, or gastrointestinal involvement. If one or more of these five factors are present, treatment should include combined steroids and cyclophosphamide. If one of these five factors is identified, the 5-year mortality is 25%; if two are identified it is 46%; and if none is identified it is 12%.

The optimal treatment of HBV-associated PAN includes a combination of antiviral and immunosuppressive therapies (Guillevin, 1999; Han, 2004; Janssen et al., 2004). In fact, control of HBV replication may be the most important factor in the resolution of HBV-associated PAN (Janssen et al., 2004). Guillevin (1999) advocates an initial short regimen of corticosteroids to subdue the arteritis, which is most intense during the first weeks of disease. Steroids are then stopped. Continued treatment of the putative immune complex mechanism can be pursued with plasmapheresis if manifestations of arteritis persist. Antiviral therapy also should be instituted, e.g., with interferon (IFN)-α or lamivudine.

Autoimmune Features

Most patients with PAN do not have recognized evidence for an autoimmune pathogenesis. Exceptions are the few patients with systemic lupus erythematosus who have a vasculitis that is pathologically similar to idiopathic PAN (lupus arteritis) (Korbet et al., 1984). PAN is not associated with ANCAs (Jennette et al., 2013a). As noted later, the serologic detection of ANCAs in a patient who is suspected of having PAN should raise the possibility of pauci-immune SVV instead (Guillevin et al., 1995; Jennette et al., 2013a).

Genetic Features and Environmental Influences

There is no evidence that genetic factors play a substantial role in the development of PAN. Familial occurrences of PAN are rare and may be related to hepatitis B virus (HBV) infection (Reveille et al., 1989; Mason et al., 1994). No genetic features of HBV have been identified that correlate with the induction of PAN (Janssen et al., 2004).

The most commonly recognized environmental factor is infection by HBV (Guillevin, 1999; Janssen et al., 2004). There are anecdotal reports of PAN associated with other infections, such as hepatitis C virus (HCV), human immunodeficiency virus (HIV), and parvovirus B19, but a statistically significant relationship has been established only for HBV infection.

In Vivo Models

Rich (1942) proposed that PAN was mediated by immunologic mechanisms because he observed arteritis in patients who had serum sickness or had been treated with antibiotics. He acquired support for this hypothesis by inducing necrotizing arteritis in rabbits after injection of horse serum (Rich and Gregory, 1943). However, serum sickness in animals actually is a better model for SVV than for PAN because glomerulonephritis is a very frequent component (Germuth, 1953; Dixon et al., 1958). Interestingly, Pearl Zeek, who was one of the pioneers in delineating the clinical and pathologic features of PAN, studied an animal model of systemic arteritis that resembled PAN and that was induced by implanting pieces of silk in the perirenal tissue of rats (Zeek et al., 1948).

Pathologic Effector Mechanisms

As noted above, at least some examples of PAN are thought to be mediated by immune complex deposition in vessel walls (Figure 72.2). HBV infection may be the source of pathogenic antigens in patients with PAN (Han, 2004; Janssen et al., 2004); however, the vasculitis that is associated with HBV infection often has more features of SVV than necrotizing arteritis alone.

When arterial wall immune complexes are present, they cause inflammation by activating the many interconnected humoral and cellular inflammatory mediator systems; e.g., the complement, kinin, plasmin, and coagulation humoral systems, and the neutrophil, mononuclear phagocyte, lymphocyte, and platelet cellular systems. Endothelial cells and mural smooth muscle cells are capable of modulating vascular inflammation, e.g., by producing lipid metabolites with cytokine activity, and, in the case of endothelial cells, by secreting cytokines, upregulating leukocyte adhesion molecules, and altering surface thrombogenicity (Pober, 1988). This complex interplay of humoral and cellular events results in the influx of inflammatory cells (especially neutrophils), necrosis, and sometimes thrombosis.

Autoantibodies as Potential Immunologic Markers

Serologic testing for ANCA helps distinguish between PAN and AAV (MPA, GPA, EGPA) in a patient with arteritis because <5% of patients with PAN have a positive ANCA (Agard et al., 2003) compared to >80% of

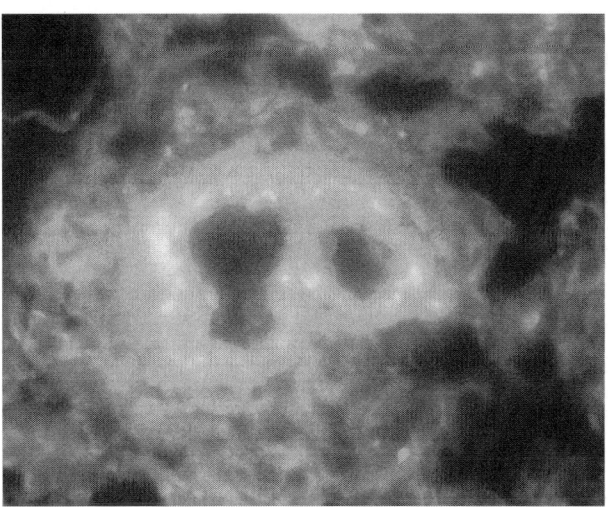

FIGURE 72.2 Direct immunofluorescence photomicrograph demonstrating granular IgG deposits in an artery from the subcutaneous tissue of a patient with hepatitis B-associated polyarteritis nodosa, showing granular vessel wall staining for C3.

patients with pauci-immune SVV. For example, if a patient with mononeuritis multiplex and a peripheral nerve biopsy showing arteritis is ANCA-positive, pauci-immune SVV (e.g., microscopic polyangiitis) is a more likely possibility than PAN. Serologic identification of HBV infection by detection of antigens or antibodies supports a diagnosis of PAN because of the strong association between PAN and hepatitis B (Agard et al., 2003; Janssen et al., 2004) and the rare occurrence of hepatitis B in other forms of vasculitis (Guillevin, 1999).

KAWASAKI'S DISEASE

Clinical, Pathologic, and Epidemiologic Features

Kawasaki's disease is a self-limited febrile illness with systemic necrotizing arteritis that affects predominantly children, usually under 2 years of age (Yim et al., 2013). It was first described in Japan (Kawasaki, 1967), but occurs worldwide. The incidence of Kawasaki's disease in children under 5 years of age ranges from roughly 100 in 100,000 in Japan to 15 in 100,000 in the USA to 10 in 100,000 in Europe (Watts and Scott, 2004).

The clinical hallmark of Kawasaki's disease is the mucocutaneous lymph node syndrome, which is characterized by oral mucosal changes, e.g., erythema of the oropharynx; "strawberry tongue," and dryness, redness or fissuring of the lips; skin lesions, e.g., erythema, indurative edema, or desquamation of the distal extremities, or polymorphous macular exanthema on the trunk; bilateral conjunctivitis; and lymphadenopathy (Kawasaki, 1967; Rauch and Hurwitz, 1985; Newburger and Fulton, 2004).

The vasculitis of Kawasaki's disease involves medium-sized and small arteries, most notably the coronary arteries. The lesions are characterized histologically by segmental mural necrosis with infiltration by predominantly mononuclear leukocytes with less conspicuous neutrophils (Jennette, 2002). Necrosis occurs but typically has less fibrinoid material, more edema, and more macrophages than seen with PAN. Mural thickening, especially from intimal inflammation, may result in narrowing of the lumen and ischemia. Pseudoaneurysms are most common in the proximal coronary arteries and may be occluded by thrombus, resulting in myocardial infarction. Kawasaki's disease is the major cause of myocardial infarction in young children. Kawasaki's disease has surpassed acute rheumatic fever as the leading cause of acquired heart disease in children in the USA (Newburger and Fulton, 2004).

The conventional therapy for Kawasaki's disease is aspirin and intravenous gamma-globulin (Furusho et al., 1984; Nagashima et al., 1987; Rowley et al., 1988; Newburger and Fulton, 2004). If the interaction of anti-endothelial cell antibodies (AECAs) with cytokine-activated endothelial cells is the major pathogenic mechanism in Kawasaki's disease, intravenous gamma-globulin could be acting by reducing, e.g., through negative feedback control, or neutralizing, e.g., by anti-idiotypic binding, AECAs, or preventing cytokine stimulation of endothelial cells. Leung et al. (1989) have studied these possibilities, and have concluded that the beneficial effects of intravenous gamma-globulin result from reduced circulating cytokines and reduced endothelial cell activation, and not from reduced anti-endothelial cell antibodies (AECA) activity. Interestingly, intravenous gamma-globulin therapy but not aspirin is effective in reducing the severity and complications of the coronary arteritis (Newburger and Fulton, 2004), which indirectly supports the role of antibodies in the pathogenesis of the arteritis.

Autoimmune Features

Some investigators have reported evidence that patients with Kawasaki's disease have circulating autoantibodies that react with activated endothelial cells (Leung et al., 1986a,b, 1989; Grunebaum et al., 2002; Kaneko et al., 2004). Kaneko et al. (2004) identified a number of candidate target antigens using a cDNA expression library derived from tumor necrosis factor (TNF)-α-stimulated human umbilical vein endothelial cells. Tropomyosin was the most likely autoantigen recognized by anti-endothelial cell autoantibodies. Mor et al. (2002) have identified autoantibodies to tropomyosin in another form of vasculitis, Behçet's disease.

Cunningham et al. (1999) have reported IgM autoantibodies to cardiac myosin in Kawasaki's disease. These autoantibodies differ from the antimyosin antibodies of patients with acute rheumatic fever.

Genetic Features and Environmental Influences

A role for genetic factors in the pathogenesis of Kawasaki's disease is supported by the observation that children of parents who had Kawasaki's disease in childhood are at greater risk for developing the disease (Uehara et al., 2003). In addition, a child is at 10-fold greater risk of developing the disease within 1 year of onset of the disease in a sibling (Fujita et al., 1989). However, the genetic basis for this familial susceptibility has not been defined. No definite HLA genotype associations have been detected.

The clinical and epidemiologic features of Kawasaki's disease, especially the temporal clustering and seasonality, suggest an infectious or environmental etiology. However, in spite of extensive efforts over many decades, no specific infectious agent or environmental factor has been identified (Newburger and Fulton, 2004; Burns et al., 2005).

In Vivo Models

Takahashi et al. (2004) have developed an animal model of vasculitis that has a remarkable pathologic similarity to the arteritis of Kawasaki's disease. They injected a *Candida albicans* extract intraperitoneally for 5 consecutive days into a variety of mouse strains. Arteritis developed in 66% of CD-1 mice and most often affected the coronary arteries and aortic root close to the orifice of coronary arteries. The gross distribution and histologic pattern of injury closely mimics coronary arteritis in patients with Kawasaki's disease. Not all strains of mice developed disease, indicating a genetic susceptibility in certain strains.

Duong et al. (2003) have described a similar model of coronary arteritis induced by injection of *Lactobacillus casei* cell wall extract into mice. They hypothesized that the pathogenicity of *L. casei* cell wall extract may derive from its ability to function as a superantigen.

Pathologic Effector Mechanisms

Although not fully verified, AECAs have been incriminated in the pathogenesis of vascular injury in patients with Kawasaki's disease by Leung et al. (1986a,b). They observed that patients with Kawasaki's disease have IgG and IgM AECAs that cause complement-mediated lysis of human umbilical and saphenous vein endothelial cells that had been pretreated with IFN-γ, interleukin (IL)-1, or TNF. From these observations, they hypothesized that the pathogenesis of vasculitis in Kawasaki's disease entails two events: production of AECAs (possibly related to the polyclonal B cell activation that occurs in Kawasaki's disease) and increased cytokine production (possibly related to the increased activity of CD4 T lymphocytes and monocytes that also occurs in Kawasaki's disease). The AECAs would bind to upregulated endothelial antigens, and cause endothelial death and vascular inflammation.

A role for bacterial superantigen has been postulated because of selective expansion of T cell receptor (TCR) Vβ families in some patients with Kawasaki's disease (Newburger and Fulton, 2004; Yim et al., 2013). As noted earlier, observations in animal models also support this possibility.

Autoantibodies as Potential Immunologic Markers

No autoantibodies have been recognized that can be used for routine diagnosis of Kawasaki's disease (Newburger and Fulton, 2004). Erythrocyte sedimentation rate and C-reactive protein are consistently elevated but are completely nonspecific.

ANCA-ASSOCIATED VASCULITIS (AAV)

Clinical, Pathologic, and Epidemiologic Features

ANCA-associated vasculitis (AAV) has three major clinicopathologic expressions: microscopic polyangiitis (MPA), granulomatosis with polyangiitis (GPA), and eosinophilic granulomatosis with polyangiitis (EGPA) (Falk and Jennette, 2010; Jennette et al., 2013a) (see Box 72.1). GPA was formerly called Wegener's granulomatosis and EGPA, Churg–Strauss syndrome (Jennette et al., 2013a). All three are characterized by a pauci-immune SVV (i.e., with little or no immunoglobulin in the walls of involved vessels). GPA has necrotizing granulomatous inflammation superimposed on the vasculitis. EGPA has asthma, eosinophilia, and granulomatous inflammation in addition to the vasculitis. MPA has only the vasculitis, without granulomatous inflammation, asthma, or eosinophilia. As the term AAV implies, AAV is associated with circulating ANCAs; however, it is important to realize that not all patients with these clinicopathologic expressions of vasculitis are positive in current clinical assays for ANCA.

Patients with all clinicopathologic expressions of AAV share a common pathologic manifestation of small vessel inflammation (Jennette, 1991, 2002; Jennette and Falk, 1998). This lesion is characterized by mural fibrinoid necrosis with karyorrhexis and infiltrating leukocytes (Figure 72.3). Neutrophils predominate in early lesions but are replaced by mononuclear leukocytes as soon as 48 h after the onset of acute lesions.

The clinical manifestations are protean and can affect many different organs individually or in combination. For example, vasculitis affecting dermal venules causes palpable purpura in skin; inflammation of glomerular capillaries causes glomerulonephritis (see Figure 72.3); pulmonary capillaritis causes pulmonary hemorrhage; vasculitis of small vessels in the upper respiratory tract mucosa causes sinusitis and otitis; vasculitis of the small vessels in the uvea (vascular tunic) of the eye causes uveitis; vasculitis affecting small epineural arteries and arterioles causes peripheral neuropathy (usually mononeuritis multiplex); vasculitis in small

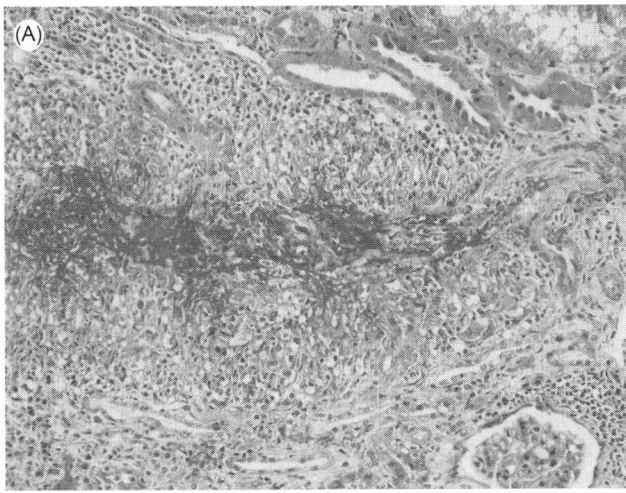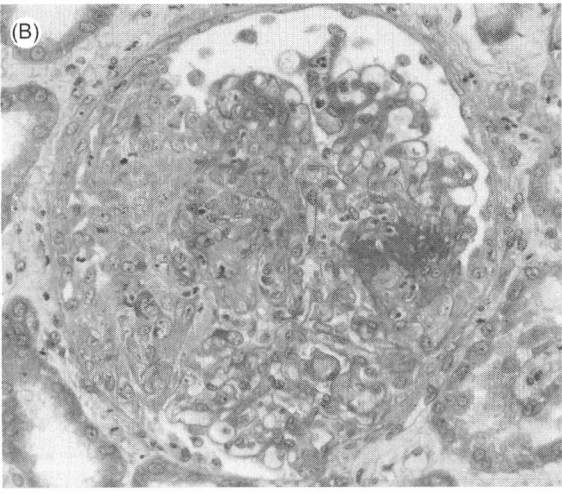

FIGURE 72.3 (A) Necrotizing arteritis in a small artery and (B) necrotizing glomerulonephritis in a patient with microscopic polyangiitis. The artery and glomerulus have bright red staining for fibrinoid necrosis in this Masson trichrome stain. The artery and adjacent tissue are infiltrated by neutrophils and mononuclear leukocytes. The glomerulus has a cellular crescent.

TABLE 72.1 Approximate Frequency of Organ System Manifestations in Several Forms of Small Vessel Vasculitis

Organ system	MPA (%)	GPA (%)	EGPA IgA (%)	Vasculitis (%)	Cryoglobulinemic vasculitis (%)
Renal	90	80	45	50	55
Cutaneous	40	40	60	90	90
Pulmonary	50	90	70	<5	<5
Ear, nose, and throat	35	90	50	<5	<5
Musculoskeletal	60	60	50	75	70
Neurologic	30	50	70	10	40
Gastrointestinal	50	50	50	60	30

Jennette and Falk, 1997

vessels in the gastrointestinal mucosa and submucosa causes abdominal pain and blood in the stool; and vasculitis affecting small visceral arteries, e.g., in the liver and pancreas, causes pain, dysfunction, and release of intracellular enzymes into the blood. The different clinicopathologic categories of AAV have overlapping clinical features with each other and with other forms of SVV (Table 72.1). Patients with GPA may have clinical manifestations of the necrotizing granulomatous inflammation, such as pulmonary nodules and cavities, perforation of the nasal septum, or collapse of the nasal septum causing saddle nose deformity.

In a review of multiple studies, Watts and Scott (2004) reported that the prevalence of GPA ranged from 24 to 157 in 1,000,000, adults that of microscopic polyangiitis from 9 to 66, and that of Churg–Strauss syndrome from 2 to 38. In accord with this, Mahr et al. (2004) determined that the prevalence of pauci-immune SVV in 1,000,000 adults in France was 25 for microscopic polyangiitis, 24 for GPA, and 11 for Churg–Strauss syndrome. The incidence in 1,000,000 adults ranged from 5 to 11 for GPA, from 3 to 12 for microscopic polyangiitis, and from 1 to 3 for Churg–Strauss syndrome (Watts and Scott, 2004).

ANCA vasculitis is usually a very aggressive disease that often will be complicated by end-stage renal disease or life-threatening pulmonary hemorrhage if not treated with high-dose corticosteroids and cytotoxic drugs, especially cyclophosphamide (Nachman et al., 1996; Jayne, 2003; Little and Pusey, 2004; Falk and Jennette, 2010). Although there is general agreement about the use of corticosteroid and cytotoxic therapy for the induction of remission in patients with pauci-immune SVV, there is controversy over the dose, method of administration, and duration of treatment. Approximately 80% of ANCA SVV patients will enter remission with aggressive immunosuppressive therapy. However, up to 40% will have a relapse within 2 years. There is controversy over how best to treat relapses. A repeat course of corticosteroids

and cyclophosphamide often is used for relapses, but less toxic alternatives are azathioprine or mycophenolate mofetil (Little and Pusey, 2004).

Intravenous gamma-globulin and plasma exchange may have a beneficial effect on ANCA SVV, especially in patients with aggressive or persistent disease that does not respond well to conventional therapy (Jordan, 1995; Jayne et al., 2000; Little and Pusey, 2004). Anti-idiotypic antibodies that inhibit ANCA *in vitro* are present in pooled human gamma-globulin preparations, but whether or not an anti-idiotypic effect is the basis for the therapeutic benefits has not been determined. Plasma exchange reduces circulating ANCA levels, which is potentially beneficial if these autoantibodies are in fact pathogenic.

Autoimmune Features

Over 80% of patients with acute untreated pauci-immune SVV have circulating ANCAs (Jennette and Falk, 1997; Falk and Jennette, 2010). ANCAs are specific for proteins in the cytoplasm of neutrophils and monocytes. When detected by indirect immunofluorescence microscopy using alcohol-fixed neutrophils as substrate, the two major antigen specificities cause two different staining patterns: cytoplasmic (C-ANCA) and perinuclear (P-ANCA) (Figure 72.4). The perinuclear pattern is an artifact of substrate preparation caused by diffusion of antigens from the cytoplasm to the nucleus (Charles et al., 1989). When analyzed by specific immunoassays, the most frequent C-ANCA antigen specificity is for proteinase 3 (PR3-ANCA) (Goldschmeding et al., 1989; Niles et al., 1989; Jennette et al., 1990; Ludemann et al., 1990) and the most frequent P-ANCA specificity is for myeloperoxidase (MPO-ANCA) (Falk and Jennette, 1988).

T cells with specificity for ANCA antigens are present in patients with ANCA vasculitis (Griffith et al., 1996; Clayton and Savage, 2000). T cells are probably involved

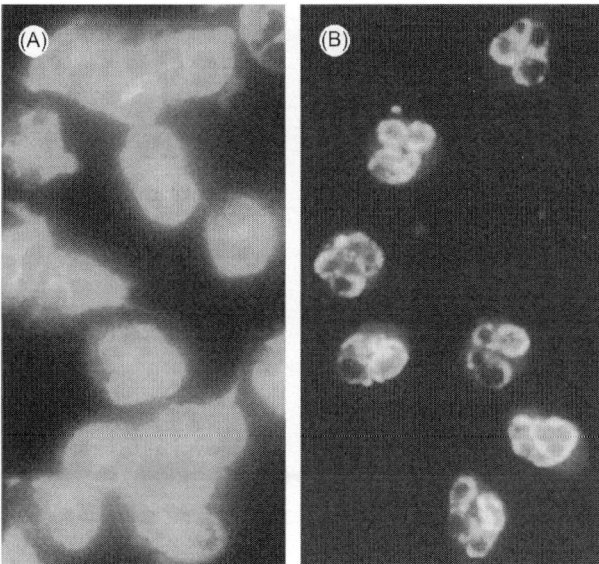

FIGURE 72.4 Indirect immunofluorescence microscopy photomicrograph of (A) C-ANCA- and (B) P-ANCA-staining patterns on alcohol-fixed human neutrophils.

in the immunogenesis of the autoimmune response, but their role in the pathogenesis of injury is unknown.

Some patients with GPA and MPA have circulating AECAs, often concurrent with ANCA (Chan et al., 1993; Del Papa et al., 1996; Holmen et al., 2004). There is controversy over the diagnostic utility and pathogenic significance of AECAs in pauci-immune SVV.

Genetic Features

A gene-wide association study (GWAS) has revealed a genetic influence on AAV that correlated best with MPO-ANCA and PR3-ANCA autoantigen specificity rather than clinicopathologic phenotype (Lyons at al., 2012). PR3-ANCA was associated with HLA-DP and genes encoding α1-antitrypsin (SERPINA1) and proteinase 3 (PRTN3). MPO-ANCA was associated with HLA-DQ. These HLA associations suggest that antigen specificity of antigen binding sites on HLA molecules influences the initiation of the autoimmune response.

The predilection for the disease in white persons and the low prevalence in African Americans suggests that a genetic background contributes to disease induction. In accord with a role for MHC antigen specificity in the immunogenesis of ANCA, Cao et al. (2011) found that African Americans with PR3-ANCA AAV had 73.3-fold higher odds of having HLA-DRB1*15 alleles than healthy controls. Further, DRB1*1501 protein binds with high affinity to amino acid sequences of both sense-PR3 and antisense (complementary) PR3, suggesting that the MHC antigen binding site is important in disease induction.

Esnault et al. (1993) and Elzouki et al. (1994) reported the association of α1-antitrypsin-deficiency phenotypes with PR3-ANCA-positive SVV. The fact that α1-antitrypsin is the major inhibitor in the blood of PR3 is intriguing, but the relevance of this to the relationship between α1-antitrypsin deficiency and PR3-ANCA is unknown.

Gencik et al. (2000) identified an association between GPA and a polymorphism in the PR3 promotor affecting a possible transcription factor binding site. In addition, Borgmann and Haubitz (2004) concluded that the neutrophil expression of PR3 is genetically regulated and correlates with onset and relapse of PR3-ANCA-associated SVV.

Environmental Influences

Drug exposure can induce ANCA formation and SVV. For example, a minority of patients who receive propylthiouracil develop ANCAs concurrent with the onset of pauci-immune SVV and glomerulonephritis (Choi et al., 2000). Minocycline and hydralazine also have been associated with the development of ANCA disease (Elkayam et al., 1996; Choi et al., 2000). Cocaine contaminated with levamisole also can cause AAV (McGrath, 2011).

Silica exposure and farming are risk factors for the development of ANCA SVV (Gregorini et al., 1993; Hogan et al., 2001; Lane et al., 2003), possibly by having an adjuvant effect on macrophages in the respiratory tract. For example, Hogan et al. noted that silica dust exposure was reported by 46% of patients with ANCA SVV, compared with 20% of control subjects ($P = 0.001$). The odds ratio of exposure to silica dust was 4.4 times greater for patients with ANCA SVV compared with control subjects ($P = 0.013$) (Hogan et al., 2001).

Approximately two-thirds of patients with GPA are chronic nasal carriers of *Staphylococcus aureus*. This is a risk factor for relapse, and prophylactic treatment with antibiotics that eliminate staphylococcal nasal carriage reduces relapse frequency (Stegman et al., 1996). The mechanistic relationship between staphylococcal infection and ANCA disease onset or exacerbation is not clear. However, observations by Pendergraft et al. (2004, 2005) raise the possibility that exposure to certain pathogens can result in the induction of the autoimmune ANCA response (see Chapter 60). They propose that pathogens can initiate an autoantibody response through induction of an appropriate antibody response to microbial proteins that have an amino acid sequence that mimics the antisense sequence (complementary sequence) of the autoantigen. These antibodies to the complementary peptide in turn induce anti-idiotypic antibodies that cross-react with the autoantigen (i.e., are autoantibodies). In support of this theory, patients with PR3-ANCA disease have circulating antibodies that react with peptides that have an amino acid sequence that is complementary to PR3, and these antibodies react with anti-PR3 antibodies as an anti-idiotypic pair. Further, immunization of mice with a complementary PR3 peptide induces not only an antibody response to the complementary PR3 peptide but also to native PR3. Interestingly, *Staph. aureus*, which is associated with PR3-ANCA disease, contains a protein that has a sequence that mimics the antisense sequence of PR3. According to the theory of autoantigen complementarity, an antibody response to the *Staph. aureus* peptide that mimics a complementary PR3 peptide results in an anti-idiotypic immune response that targets PR3, resulting in PR3-ANCA production. Also in support of this concept is the association between PR3-ANCA and infection with Ross River virus and *Entamoeba histolytica*, both of which contain proteins with amino acid sequences that mimic complementary peptides of PR3 (Pendergraft et al., 2004).

In Vivo Models

Multiple animal models of MPO-ANCA SVV have been developed, but no widely accepted model of PR3-ANCA SVV has been reported (Jennette et al., 2011). The first convincing animal model of ANCA-induced SVV was described by Xiao et al. (2002). MPO knockout mice were immunized with murine MPO and produced anti-MPO antibodies. Splenocytes (including T and B cells) or isolated antibodies were then transferred from MPO$^{-/-}$ mice that had been immunized with MPO to Rag2$^{-/-}$ mice (lacking functional T and B cells), resulting in the development of necrotizing and crescentic glomerulonephritis in all mice and varying degrees of extrarenal SVV in many mice, including pulmonary capillaritis or necrotizing granulomatous inflammation, leukocytoclastic angiitis in the skin, and necrotizing arteritis in multiple viscera (Figure 72.5). The disease in the mice that received splenocytes is complicated by a background of immune complex localization in glomeruli; however, the Rag2$^{-/-}$ mice or wild-type mice that receive anti-MPO IgG alone develop a pauci-immune glomerulonephritis and vasculitis that is pathologically identical to human ANCA-associated pauci-immune disease. Because this disease can be induced in mice with no functional T cells, T cells are not required for pathogenesis. However, neutrophils are required because elimination of circulating neutrophils with a cytotoxic rat antibody completely abrogates disease induction by anti-MPO IgG (Xiao et al., 2005). Activation of the alternative complement pathway also is required (Xiao et al., 2007).

Pathologic Effector Mechanisms

By definition, pauci-immune SVV has little or no localization of immunoglobulin in vessel walls and thus

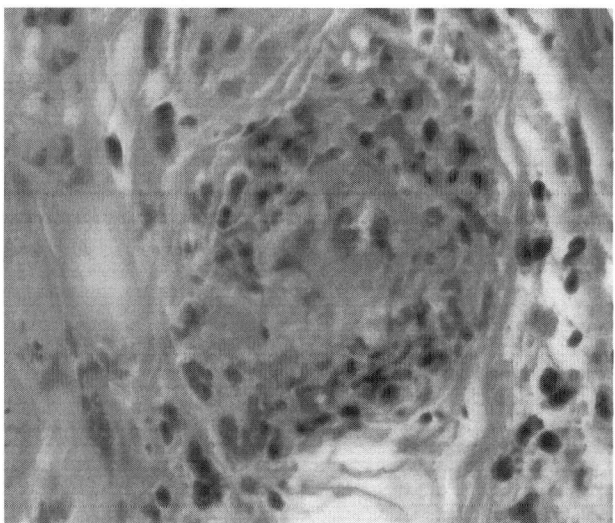

FIGURE 72.5   Necrotizing arteritis in a small artery in the dermis of a mouse 6 days after intravenous injection of mouse antimyeloperoxidase IgG. There is a central area of deeply eosinophilic fibrinoid necrosis surrounded by leukocytes with leukocytoclasia (H&E stain).

appears to have a pathogenic mechanism that differs from classical immune complex-mediated vasculitis. The presence of ANCA in the circulation and the correlation of ANCA titers with disease activity raise the possibility that ANCAs have a pathogenic role (Kallenberg et al., 1994; Han et al., 2003; Falk and Jennette, 2010). But not all patients have ANCA detectable by current clinical serologic methods, and disease activity does not correlate very well with the titers obtained with these assays. This may change with the development of more sensitive and activity-specific assays (Roth et al., 2013). Using an epitope-specific assay, Roth et al. (2013) were able to detect three categories of MPO-ANCA epitope specificity: (1) epitope specificity confined to AAV patients with active disease, (2) epitope specificity detected in patients with active disease and in remission, and (3) epitope specificity that was seen is patients as well as in very low titer in healthy controls (natural ANCA). Further, they also were able to detect MPO-ANCA with very restricted epitope specificity in many patients who were ANCA-negative by conventional clinical assays.

The induction of ANCA and pauci-immune SVV by drug exposure, discussed above, is strong clinical evidence for the pathogenic importance of ANCA. The report of a neonate who developed pulmonary hemorrhage and nephritis following transplacental transfer of maternal MPO-ANCA IgG supports a pathogenic role for ANCA (Bansal and Tobin, 2004), but this phenomenon has not been observed in other patients.

In addition to the animal models described earlier, there are numerous *in vitro* observations that support the pathogenic potential of ANCA IgG (Jennette and Falk, 1998; Rarok et al., 2003; Williams et al., 2005). Incubation of ANCA IgG with primed neutrophils induces the release of toxic reactive oxygen species and lytic granule enzymes (Falk et al., 1990a). Neutrophil priming, as occurs with exposure to certain cytokines, results in the expression of small amounts of ANCA antigens at the surface of neutrophils where they can interact with ANCA. The resultant activation of neutrophils is mediated by a combination of Fc receptor-dependent events (Porges et al., 1994; Mulder et al., 1994), as well as F(ab')2-mediated events (Kettritz et al., 1997; Williams and Savage, 2005).

In vitro, ANCA-activated neutrophils kill primed endothelial cells (Ewert et al., 1992a; Savage et al., 1992). This process requires adhesion of the neutrophils to endothelial cells via b2 integrins (Ewert et al., 1992b). Further, Radford et al. (2000) have shown that exposure to ANCA IgG causes rolling neutrophils to adhere to endothelial cells in culture through integrin-mediated adhesion.

Instead of, or in addition to, reacting with antigens expressed on the surface of neutrophils and monocytes, ANCAs might react with antigens (e.g., MPO and PR3) that have become planted in vessel walls. Vargunam et al. (1992) have shown that MPO binds to cultured endothelial cells by a charge-dependent mechanism and can subsequently react with ANCA to form immune complexes *in situ*. If this occurs *in vivo*, the magnitude of vessel wall immune complex formation must be substantially less than in conventional immune complex disease because of the absence or paucity of staining for immunoglobulin in vessel walls in ANCA SVV.

An inflammatory process, such as a viral respiratory tract infection, may cause increased levels of circulating cytokines, which in turn prime neutrophils to interact with circulating ANCAs to induce vasculitis (Jennette and Falk, 1998). With respect to this hypothesis, it is interesting to note that approximately 90% of patients report a "flu-like illness" shortly before the onset of the signs and symptoms of ANCA vasculitis (Falk et al., 1990b). Experimental support for this hypothesis is provided by the observation that injection of bacterial lipopolysaccharide into mice prior to induction of glomerulonephritis with anti-MPO IgG causes more severe injury (Huugen et al., 2005).

In summary, the *in vitro* observations support the hypothesis that antigens (PR3 and MPO) that are expressed at the surface of cytokine-primed neutrophils react with ANCA, causing neutrophil activation through both Fc receptor engagement and F(ab')2 attachment to antigens, and activation of the alternative complement pathway, resulting in the attachment to and injury of vascular endothelial cells (Figure 72.6) (Jennette et al., 2013b).

AECAs have been detected in some patients with pauci-immune SVV. Del Papa et al. (1996) observed that AECAs from patients with GPA are not toxic to endothelial cells but cause these cells to upregulate adhesion molecules and to release proinflammatory cytokines. Holmen et al. (2004) reported that patients with GPA have noncytotoxic AECAs that selectively bind surface antigens on unstimulated nasal, kidney, and lung endothelial cells, and that serum from patients with GPA caused agglutination of cytokine-stimulated nasal endothelial cells. AECA could synergize with ANCA to cause disease; however, the pathogenic importance of AECA in pauci-immune SVV has not been clearly delineated.

Autoantibodies as Immunologic Markers

In a patient with signs and symptoms of SVV, serology and/or immunohistology may demonstrate diagnostic immunologic markers that distinguish between vasculitides that have very different prognoses and treatments (Table 72.2). For example, in a patient with purpura, arthralgias, hematuria, and proteinuria, IgA-dominant immune deposits in dermal vessels support a diagnosis of IgA vasculitis (Henoch–Schönlein purpura); serum cryoglobulins and antihepatitis C antibodies support cryoglobulinemic vasculitis; serum anti-DNA and hypocomplementemia support lupus vasculitis; and serum ANCAs support one of the categories of pauci-immune SVV. Similarly, in a patient with hemoptysis and rapidly progressive glomerulonephritis (i.e., pulmonary–renal vasculitic syndrome), serum antiglomerular basement membrane (GBM) antibodies indicate anti-GBM disease, whereas ANCAs indicate one of the ANCA-associated vasculitides.

ANCA testing should include a specific immunochemical method [e.g., enzyme-linked immunosorbent assay (ELISA)] that will detect MPO-ANCA and PR3-ANCA, not merely an indirect immunofluorescence assay for C-ANCA and P-ANCA (Lim et al., 1999; Savige et al., 1999). This improves diagnostic specificity without a significant drop in sensitivity. As mentioned earlier, the studies by Roth et al. (2013) suggest that epitope-specific assays may be more useful for the diagnosis and follow-up of AAV than assays with the whole molecules as substrate.

An added complexity of serologic testing for ANCA disease and anti-GBM disease is the increased frequency of anti-GBM antibodies in patients with ANCA and *vice versa* (Saxena et al., 1991; Jennette, 2003; Levy et al., 2004). Patients with both autoantibodies have a worse prognosis than patients with ANCA alone. When both autoantibodies are present, a patient is at risk for manifesting vasculitic features of ANCA-associated disease that do not occur with anti-GBM disease alone, such as cutaneous, skeletal muscle, or gut

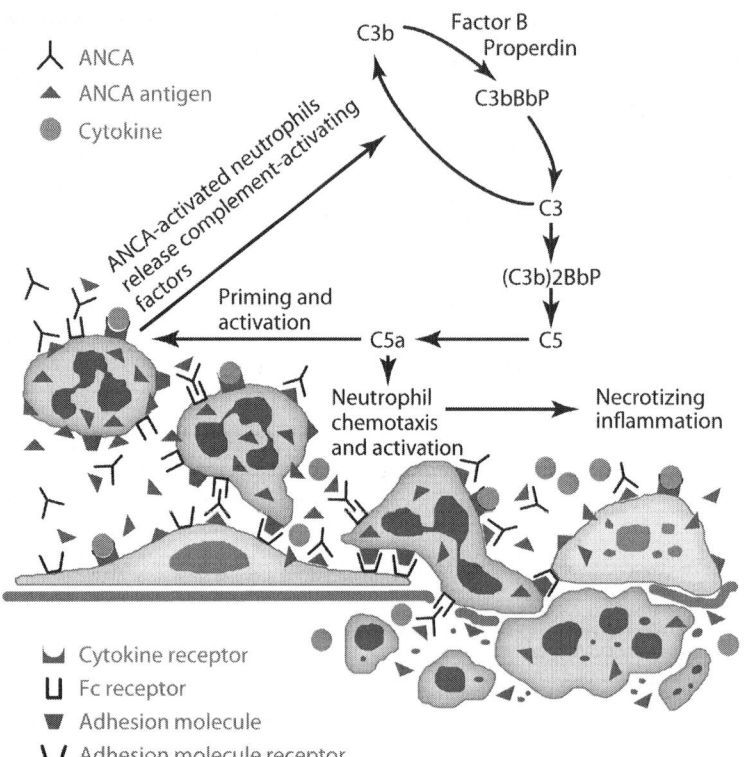

FIGURE 72.6 Putative pathogenic mechanisms for antineutrophil cytoplasmic autoantibody (ANCA)-induced vasculitis. ANCA antigens (granule proteins) that are normally within the cytoplasm of neutrophils are transferred to the surface by cytokine priming, where they can interact with ANCAs. Some antigens also are released and can bind to endothelial cells. These free and bound antigens can also react with ANCAs. The interaction of neutrophils with ANCAs induces full activation with respiratory burst and degranulation, which releases factors that activate the alternative pathway of complement activation. The resultant inflammation causes vascular injury (vasculitis). *Reproduced with permission from Jennette et al. (2013b).*

TABLE 72.2 Differential Diagnostic Features of Several Forms of Small Vessel Vasculitis (SVV)

Diagnostic feature	MPA	GPA	EGPA	IgA vasculitis	Cryoglobulinemic vasculitis
SVV signs and symptoms*	+	+	+	+	+
IgA-dominant deposits	−	−	−	+	−
Cryoglobulins	−	−	−	−	+
ANCAs in blood	+	+	+	−	−
Necrotizing granulomas	−	+	+	−	−
Asthma and eosinophilia	−	−	+	−	−

*All of these SVVs can manifest any or all of the shared features of SVV, such as purpura, nephritis, abdominal pain, peripheral neuropathy, myalgias, and arthralgias. Each is distinguished by the presence and, just as importantly, the absence of certain specific features.
ANCAs, antineutrophil cytoplasmic autoantibodies.
Jennette and Falk, 1997

vasculitis. In some patients, the anti-GBM component of their autoimmune disease resolves, leaving more persistent ANCA disease.

Serology alone cannot make the distinction between MPA, GPA, EGPA, or isolated pauci-immune crescentic glomerulonephritis because each syndrome can be associated with either C-ANCA (PR3-ANCA) or P-ANCA (MPO-ANCA). However, the relative frequencies of ANCA specificities vary among the disease variants. For example, most patients with GPA have C-ANCA (PR3-ANCA) and most patients with renal-limited disease have

P-ANCA (MPO-ANCA) (Jennette et al., 2013b) (Table 72.3).

Diseases other than pauci-immune SVV can be associated with ANCAs, especially with ANCAs that are not specific for MPO or PR3. P-ANCAs that do not have specificity for MPO are associated with a number of nonvasculitic inflammatory diseases, such as ulcerative colitis, sclerosing cholangiitis, autoimmune hepatitis, and Felty syndrome (Jennette and Falk, 1993; Bartunkova et al., 2002). C-ANCAs that are not associated with SVV occur in patients with cystic fibrosis (Bartunkova et al., 2002).

TABLE 72.3 Approximate Frequency of PR3-ANCA and MPO-ANCA in Patients with Pauci-immune Small Vessel Vasculitis

	GPA	MPA	EGPA[a]	Renal-limited AAV
PR3-ANCA	75	40	5	20
MPO-ANCA	20	50	40	70
Negative	5	10	55	10

[a]EGPA with glomerulonephritis is >75% ANCA-positive.

CRYOGLOBULINEMIC VASCULITIS

Clinical, Pathologic, and Epidemiologic Features

Cryoglobulinemic vasculitis is characterized pathologically by inflammation in small vessels (Figure 72.7) that is associated with deposits of cryoglobulins and complement in vessel lumens and walls. Skin, joints, gut, and glomeruli often are involved (see Table 72.1). Cryoglobulinemic vasculitis affects vessels of many types, including postcapillary venules (e.g., in the dermis), capillaries (e.g., glomerular and rarely pulmonary alveolar capillaries), arterioles, and rarely small arteries (Ferri et al., 2004). Immunofluorescence microscopy reveals granular deposits of immunoglobulins and complement in vessel walls, and sometimes lumenal aggregates of cryoglobulins and complement. The clinical and pathologic manifestations of cryoglobulinemic vasculitis overlap with those of other systemic vasculitides, including purpura with leukocytoclastic angiitis, proliferative and membranoproliferative glomerulonephritis, and, in rare severe cases, pulmonary hemorrhage with alveolar capillaritis. As with many systemic vasculitides, arthralgias and arthritis caused by synovitis are common features.

The prevalence of cryoglobulinemic vasculitis is not well defined, but it is more common in southern Europe than in northern Europe or North America (Ferri et al., 2004). There is a close association between HCV infection and cryoglobulinemia (D'Amico and Fornasieri, 1995; Ferri et al., 2004).

If there are circulating pathogenic autoantibodies or immune complexes in patients with vasculitis, theoretically, plasmapheresis combined with immunosuppression would be beneficial. Plasmapheresis has been used in severe cryoglobulinemia (D'Amico and Fornasieri, 1995). Plasmapheresis is combined with corticosteroid and cytotoxic therapy, which makes it difficult to determine what effect plasmapheresis alone is having on the disease. Therapy with IFN-α, in addition to the immunosuppressive drugs, has also been advocated in patients with cryoglobulinemic vasculitis secondary to HCV infection (D'Amico and Fornasieri, 1995).

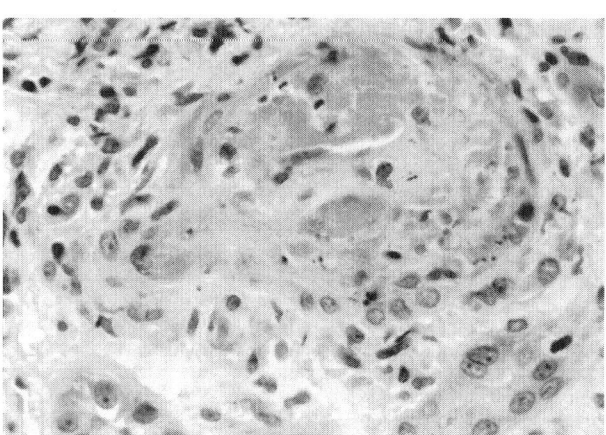

FIGURE 72.7 Cryoglobulinemic vasculitis affecting a small artery in the kidney. The deeply acidophilic material in the vessel probably is a mixture of thrombus, fibrinoid necrosis, and aggregated cryoglobulins. The vessel wall and adjacent tissue are infiltrated by leukocytes with leukocytoclasia.

Autoimmune Features

Most cryoglobulins that cause vasculitis contain autoantibodies directed against immunoglobulins, i.e., rheumatoid factors (Ferri et al., 2004; Sansonno and Dammacco, 2005). Cryoglobulins are divided into three major types: monoclonal (type I), mixed monoclonal–polyclonal (type II), and polyclonal (type III). Mixed cryoglobulins are more pathogenic than monoclonal or polyclonal cryoglobulins. Monoclonal cryoglobulins usually occur in patients with plasma cell dyscrasias or B cell lymphomas, and cause morbidity primarily by precipitating within vessels and producing occlusion. Monoclonal cryoglobulins are not effective activators of inflammatory mediator systems, and therefore rarely cause overt vasculitis. Mixed cryoglobulins, however, are immune complexes that are capable of activating inflammatory mediators, including the complement system, and therefore characteristically cause systemic vasculitis.

The mechanism of cryoglobulin induction by HCV is not fully elucidated. HCV may initially induce production of polyclonal IgM lacking rheumatoid factor activity that evolves through somatic mutations to monoclonal IgM with anti-IgG reactivity (Sansonno and Dammacco, 2005).

Genetic Features and Environmental Influences

Not all patients with HCV infection develop cryoglobulinemia. The likelihood of developing cryoglobulinemia is not determined by serum HCV RNA titer or HCV genotype; thus, host factors, including genetic susceptibility, are incriminated as risk factors for this complication. In studies of relatively small numbers of patients,

Amoroso et al. (1998) reported an increased frequency of DRB1*11 (DR5) (36% vs. 20%, $P = 0.0035$), Congia et al. (1996) an increased frequency of DRB1*1101−4 (DR5), DQB1*0301, DRB1*0301 (DR3), and DQB1*0201, and Lenzi et al. (1998) an increased frequency of HLA-B8 and HLA-DR3 in patients with cryoglobulinemia compared to healthy controls or patients with hepatitis C but no cryoglobulinemia.

There is a strong association between cryoglobulinemic vasculitis and HCV infection (D'Amico and Fornasieri, 1995; Ferri et al., 2004; Sansonno and Dammacco, 2005). HCV antibodies and RNA are detected in the serum of 75−95% of patients with vasculitis and glomerulonephritis caused by mixed cryoglobulins. The HCV is both hepatotropic and lymphotropic. One hypothesis proposes that infection of B cells by HCV triggers the production of polyclonal and monoclonal rheumatoid factors that participate in cryoglobulin formation (D'Amico and Fornasieri, 1995). Another proposes that HCV lipoprotein induces an IgM response that is initially reactive with a virus−self complex but subsequently mutates to have rheumatoid factor activity (Agnello, 1995).

In Vivo Models

Gyotoku et al. (1987) have described an experimental animal model of cryoglobulinemic vasculitis. They established monoclonal IgG rheumatoid factor-secreting hybridomas from MRL/lpr mice. These monoclonal rheumatoid factor antibodies were capable of forming cryoglobulins, and, when injected into normal mice, caused peripheral vasculitis and glomerulonephritis resembling that seen in patients with mixed cryoglobulinemia. Kikuchi et al. (2002) implanted mice with a hybridoma that secreted an IgG3 anti-IgG2a rheumatoid factor. The mice developed circulating cryoglobulins, acute glomerulonephritis, and cutaneous leukocytoclastic vasculitis.

Pathologic Effector Mechanisms

Cryoglobulinemic vasculitis is mediated by the deposition of mixed cryoglobulins in small vessels. These immune complexes composed of mixed cryoglobulins activate complement and initiate acute inflammation through mechanisms that were discussed above in the section on PAN. In patients with HCV-associated cryoglobulinemic vasculitis, immune complexes contain nonenveloped nucleocapsid proteins and whole HCV virions (Sansonno et al., 2005).

Autoantibodies as Immunologic Markers

The laboratory hallmark of cryoglobulinemic vasculitis is the detection of cryoglobulins in the circulation (see Table 72.2). The most common types of cryoglobulin contain monoclonal (type II) or polyclonal (type III) autoantibodies (rheumatoid factors) that bind to other immunoglobulin molecules to form large immune complexes that precipitate from serum upon cooling. Type I cryoglobulins are composed of monoclonal IgM. Testing for cryoglobulins requires that the blood be kept warm prior to testing. In a proper clinical setting, hypocomplementemia, positive rheumatoid factor assay, and positive serology for HCV infection support a diagnosis of cryoglobulinemia. The hypocomplementemia characteristically has low C4 but normal or near normal C3, supporting predominantly classical/lectin complement pathway activation rather than alternative pathway activation.

IgA VASCULITIS (HENOCH−SCHÖNLEIN PURPURA)

Clinical, Pathologic, and Epidemiologic Features

IgA vasculitis was previously called Henoch−Schönlein purpura, but the name was changed to reflect the pathogenic role of IgA1 vessel wall deposits in the disease, and to emphasize that the resultant clinical syndrome (e.g., purpura, arthralgias, nephritis, abdominal pain) can be caused by many different forms of SVV (e.g., AAV) (Jennette et al., 2013a).

IgA vasculitis is the most common form of vasculitis in children with an incidence of approximately 20 in 100,000 children, with the highest frequency between 4 and 6 years old (Gardner-Medwin et al., 2002), although it can occur at any age. IgA vasculitis is SVV with IgA-dominant immune deposits affecting small vessels, i.e., capillaries, venules, or arterioles (Jennette et al., 2013a). It typically involves skin, gut, and glomeruli, and is associated with arthralgias or arthritis (Ting and Hashkes, 2004). The purpura typically affects the buttocks and lower extremities. Table 72.1 provides estimates of involvement of different organs, although this differs among cohorts. Immunofluorescence microscopy of dermal venules and renal glomeruli reveals granular vessel wall deposits of predominantly IgA1 and C3, supporting a pathogenic mechanism that involves IgA-dominant immune deposits (Mestecky et al., 2013).

IgA vasculitis usually is a mild, self-limited, vasculitis that does not warrant corticosteroid or cytotoxic therapy (Robson and Leung, 1994; Mestecky et al., 2013). Less than 5% of patients have serious complications, usually progressive renal failure. Patients with rapidly progressive glomerulonephritis or severe CNS disease benefit from immunosuppressive therapy, e.g., with high-dose corticosteroids, cytotoxic drugs, or plasmapheresis (Gedalia, 2004; Ting and Hashkes, 2004). The overall prognosis is excellent even though one-third to one-half of patients will have one or more recurrences of symptoms, usually within 6 weeks, but rarely years later (Gedalia, 2004).

Autoimmune Features

Davin et al. (1987) detected IgA anti-α-galactosyl antibodies in the serum of children with active IgA vasculitis nephritis and IgA nephropathy. This finding is intriguing because of the known association between IgA vasculitis and infection with pathogens that have α-galactosyl residues on their surfaces, but the relevance of these antibodies to the pathogenesis of IgA vasculitis is uncertain. More recently, incriminating evidence for a role for antibodies directed against abnormally glycosylated IgA1 has emerged in the pathogenesis of IgA nephropathy and IgA vasculitis (Mestecky et al., 2013).

Genetic Features and Environmental Influences

There is evidence from family studies that there may be a genetic predisposition for having circulating potentially pathogenic abnormally glycosylated IgA1 (Boyd and Barratt, 2011; Kiryluk et al., 2011).

No HLA-A, HLA-B, or HLA-C associations were observed in 26 patients with IgA vasculitis (Ostergaard et al., 1990). Amoli et al. (2002a,b) reported an increased prevalence of HLA-DRB101 and a decreased prevalence of HLA-DRB107 among IgA vasculitis patients. They also observed an increased prevalence of HLA-B35 and IL-1 allele polymorphism in IgA vasculitis patients with glomerulonephritis (Amoli et al., 2004). The severity of nephritis and renal outcome were influenced by the IL-1 gene polymorphism.

Approximately 40% of children have an upper respiratory tract infection near the time of onset of IgA vasculitis, most commonly with group A *Streptococcus* (Masuda et al., 2003; Gonzalez-Gay et al., 2004; Ting and Hashkes, 2004). The pathogenic relationship between the infection and the onset of disease is unclear. Theoretically, this association could be because of a specific acquired immune response that is initiated by the infection, or because of a nonspecific amplification of immune activation that augments an underlying pathogenic mechanism, such as production of aberrantly glycosylated IgA (Allen et al., 1998).

In Vivo Models

There is no good animal model for IgA vasculitis. There are a few animal models of IgA nephropathy, which is the glomerular lesion of IgA vasculitis. Many of these involve oral or nasal immunization with dietary or infectious antigens (Amore et al., 2004). Uteroglobin gene knockout and uteroglobin antisense transgenic mice develop pathologic features of human IgA nephropathy (Zheng et al., 1999), but the relevance of this to human disease is unclear because reduced uteroglobin has not been observed in patients with IgA nephropathy (Coppo et al., 2002). Okazaki et al. (2012) use ddY mice as a model of spontaneously developing IgA nephropathy and have shown that aberrant IgA glycosylation influences progression of this murine IgAN.

Pathologic Effector Mechanisms

A leading hypothesis is that IgA vasculitis is an immune complex vasculitis resulting from a dysregulated mucosal immune response to environmental or infectious antigens in a genetically predisposed individual. IgA-dominant immune complex deposits in vessel walls are the putative mediators of the inflammation. The predominant subclass is IgA1. The major antigen in the complexes, if any, is unknown. Because of the association with infections, an antigen derived from a pathogen has been sought. Masuda et al. (2003) reported the discovery of streptococcal antigens in the glomeruli of patients with IgA vasculitis glomerulonephritis, but this has not been independently confirmed. The IgA1 deposits may contain predominantly self-aggregated IgA1 or IgA1 complexed with anti-IgA1 autoantibodies, without a contribution by a specific exogenous antigen (Mestecky et al., 2013).

Human IgA1 has an O-glycosylated hinge region not present in other immunoglobulin classes, and this hinge region has reduced galactosyl residues in patients with IgA nephropathy and IgA vasculitis (Allen et al., 1998; Lau et al., 2007; Mestecky et al., 2013; Suzuki et al., 2009). This reduced galactosylation may be due to a functional defect in plasma cell β-1,3-galactosyltransferase. The abnormal glycosylation alters IgA1 structure and function, resulting in IgA1 aggregation, greater affinity for matrix proteins in vessel walls (including glomerular mesangium), and greater complement activation, which could result in localization of pathogenic IgA1-dominant deposits in vessel walls with resultant complement activation and vasculitis.

Vessel wall immune deposits contain not only IgA1 but also C3, C3c, C3d, and variable amounts of IgG and IgM, but little or no C1q or C4. The complement profile suggests predominantly alternative pathway activation.

Autoantibodies as Potential Immunologic Markers

The immunohistologic identification of IgA-dominant immune deposits in vessels is currently the only accepted diagnostic marker for IgA nephropathy, and is a defining feature of IgA vasculitis (Jennette et al., 2013a). However, the amount of circulating abnormally glycosylated IgA1 or IgG autoantibodies specific for abnormally glycosylated IgA1 may become a useful diagnostic marker in the future (Mestecky et al., 2013).

CONCLUDING REMARKS—FUTURE PROSPECTS

A variety of pathogenic immunologic mechanisms, including autoimmune processes, mediate necrotizing arteritis and SVV. Clinically, and even pathologically, identical disease can be produced by distinctly different mechanisms; and a given pathogenic mechanism can produce more than one clinical and pathologic pattern of vasculitis. Because different organs can be affected in different patients, the clinical manifestations of even relatively specific types of vasculitis are extremely variable among patients. Therefore, the diagnosis of systemic vasculitis, including autoimmune vasculitis, is difficult, and requires skillful integration of clinical, pathologic, and laboratory data. Although difficult, precise diagnosis is essential for proper management, because the prognosis and appropriate treatment vary substantially among different categories of vasculitis. As knowledge of pathogenic immunologic mechanisms and inflammatory mediator systems increases, more effective treatments for autoimmune-mediated vasculitis will emerge, which will make precise diagnosis even more important.

REFERENCES

Agard, C., Mouthon, L., Mahr, A., Guillevin, L., 2003. Microscopic polyangiitis and polyarteritis nodosa: how and when do they start? Arthritis Rheum. 49, 709–715.

Agnello, V., 1995. The aetiology of mixed cryoglobulinaemia associated with hepatitis C virus infection. Scand. J. Immunol. 42, 179–184.

Alarcon Segovia, D., Brown Jr, A.L., 1964. Classification and etiologic aspects of necrotizing angiitides: an analytic approach to a confused subject with a critical review of the evidence for hypersensitivity in polyarteritis nodosa. Mayo Clin. Proc. 39, 205–222.

Allen, A.C., Willis, F.R., Beattie, T.J., Feehally, J., 1998. Abnormal IgA glycosylation in Henoch-Schönlein purpura restricted to patients with clinical nephritis. Nephrol. Dial. Transplant. 13, 930–934.

Amoli, M.M., Alansari, A., El Magadmi, M., Thomson, W., Hajeer, A.H., Calvino, M.C., et al., 2002a. Lack of association between A561C E-selectin polymorphism and large and small-sized blood vessel vasculitides. Clin. Exp. Rheumatol. 20, 575–576.

Amoli, M.M., Thomson, W., Hajeer, A.H., Calvino, M.C., Garcia-Porrua, C., Ollier, W.E., et al., 2002b. Interleukin 1 receptor antagonist gene polymorphism is associated with severe renal involvement and renal sequelae in Henoch-Schönlein purpura. J. Rheumatol. 29, 1404–1407.

Amoli, M.M., Calvino, M.C., Garcia-Porrua, C., Llorca, J., Ollier, W.E., Gonzalez-Gay, M.A., 2004. Interleukin 1beta gene polymorphism association with severe renal manifestations and renal sequelae in Henoch-Schönlein purpura. J. Rheumatol. 31, 295–298.

Amore, A., Coppo, R., Nedrud, J.G., Sigmund, N., Lamm, M.E., Emancipator, S.N., 2004. The role of nasal tolerance in a model of IgA nephropathy induced in mice by Sendai virus. Clin. Immunol. 113, 101–108.

Amoroso, A., Berrino, M., Canale, L., Cornaglia, M., Guarrera, S., Mazzola, G., et al., 1998. Are HLA class II and immunoglobulin constant region genes involved in the pathogenesis of mixed cryo-globulinemia type II after hepatitis C virus infection? J. Hepatol. 29, 36–44.

Arkin, A., 1930. A clinical and pathological study of periarteritis nodosa. A report of five cases, one histologically healed. Am. J. Pathol. 6, 401–426.

Bansal, P.J., Tobin, M.C., 2004. Neonatal microscopic polyangiitis secondary to transfer of maternal myeloperoxidase-antineutrophil cytoplasmic antibody resulting in neonatal pulmonary hemorrhage and renal involvement. Ann. Allergy. Asthma Immunol. 93, 398–401.

Baart de la Faille-Kuypen, E.H., Kater, L., Kuijten, R.H., et al., 1976. Occurrence of vascular IgA deposits in clinically normal skin of patients with renal disease. Kidney. Int. 9, 424–429.

Bartunkova, J., Kolarova, I., Sediva, A., Holzelova, E., 2002. Antineutrophil cytoplasmic antibodies, anti-Saccharomyces cerevi-siae antibodies, and specific IgE to food allergens in children with inflammatory bowel diseases. Clin. Immunol. 102, 162–168.

Borgmann, S., Haubitz, M., 2004. Genetic impact of pathogenesis and prognosis of ANCA-associated vasculitides. Clin. Exp. Rheumatol. 22 (Suppl. 36), S79–S86.

Boyd, J.K., Barratt, J., 2011. Inherited IgA glycosylation pattern in IgA nephropathy and HSP nephritis: where do we go next? Kidney. Int. 80, 8–10.

Burns, J.C., Cayan, D.R., Tong, G., Bainto, E.V., Turner, C.L., Shike, H., et al., 2005. Seasonality and temporal clustering of Kawasaki syndrome. Epidemiology. 16, 220–225.

Cao, A.Y., Schmitz, J., Yang, J.J., Hogan, S.L., Bunch, D.O., Jennette, C.E., et al., 2011. DRB1*15 Allele is a risk factor for PR-3 ANCA disease in African Americans. J. Am. Soc. Nephrol. 22, 1161–1167.

Chan, T.M., Frampton, G., Jayne, D.R., Perry, G.J., Lockwood, C.M., Cameron, J.S., 1993. Clinical significance of anti-endothelial cell antibodies in systemic vasculitis: a longitudinal study comparing anti-endothelial cell antibodies and anti-neutrophil cytoplasm antibodies. Am. J. Kidney Dis. 22, 387–392.

Charles, L.A., Falk, R.J., Jennette, J.C., 1989. Reactivity of antineutrophil cytoplasmic autoantibodies with HL-60 cells. Clin. Immunol. Immunopathol. 53, 243–253.

Choi, H.K., Merkel, P.A., Walker, A.M., Niles, J.L., 2000. Drug-associated antineutrophil cytoplasmic antibody-positive vasculitis: prevalence among patients with high titers of antimyeloperoxidase antibodies. Arthritis Rheum. 43, 405–413.

Churg, J., Strauss, L., 1951. Allergic granulomatosis, allergic angiitis and periarteritis nodosa. Am. J. Pathol. 27, 277–301.

Clark, E., Kaplan, B., 1937. Endocardial, arterial and other mesenchymal alterations associated with serum disease in man. Arch. Pathol. 24, 458–475.

Clayton, A.R., Savage, C.O., 2000. What you should know about PR3-ANCA. Evidence for the role of T cells in the pathogenesis of systemic vasculitis. Arthritis Res. 2, 260–262.

Congia, M., Clemente, M.G., Dessi, C., Cucca, F., Mazzoleni, A.P., Frau, F., et al., 1996. HLA class II genes in chronic hepatitis

C virus-infection and associated immunological disorders. Hepatology. 24, 1338–1341.

Coppo, R., Chiesa, M., Cirina, P., Peruzzi, L., Amore, A., 2002. In human IgA nephropathy uteroglobin does not play the role inferred from transgenic mice. Am. J. Kidney Dis. 40, 495–503.

Cunningham, M.W., Meissner, H.C., Heuser, J.S., Pietra, B.A., Kurahara, D.K., Leung, D.Y., 1999. Anti-human cardiac myosin autoantibodies in Kawasaki syndrome. J. Immunol. 163, 1060–1065.

D'Amico, G., Fornasieri, A., 1995. Cryoglobulinemic glomerulonephritis: a membranoproliferative glomerulonephritis induced by hepatitis C virus. Am. J. Kidney Dis. 25, 361–369.

Davies, D.J., Moran, J.E., Niall, J.F., Ryan, G.B., 1982. Segmental necrotising glomerulonephritis with antineutrophil antibody: possible arbovirus aetiology? BMJ Clin. Res. Ed. 285, 606.

Davin, J.C., Malaise, M., Foidart, J., Mahieu, P., 1987. Antialphagalactosyl antibodies and immune complexes in children with Henoch-Schönlein purpura or IgA nephropathy. Kidney Int. 31, 1132–1139.

Davson, J., Ball, J., Platt, R., 1948. The kidney in periarteritis nodosa. Q. J. Med. 17, 75–202.

Del Papa, N., Guidali, L., Sironi, M., Shoenfeld, Y., Mantovani, A., Tincani, A., et al., 1996. Anti-endothelial cell IgG antibodies from patients with Wegener's granulomatosis bind to human endothelial cells in vitro and induce adhesion molecule expression and cytokine secretion. Arthritis Rheum. 39, 758–766.

Dixon, F.J., Wazuez, J.J., Weigle, W.O., 1958. Pathogenesis of serum sickness. Arch. Pathol. 65, 18–28.

Duong, T.T., Silverman, E.D., Bissessar, M.V., Yeung, R.S., 2003. Superantigenic activity is responsible for induction of coronary arteritis in mice: an animal model of Kawasaki disease. Int. Immunol. 15, 79–89.

Elkayam, O., Yaron, M., Caspi, D., 1996. Minocycline induced arthritis associated with fever, livedo reticularis, and pANCA. Ann. Rheum. Dis. 55, 769–771.

Elzouki, A.N., Segelmark, M., Wieslander, J., Eriksson, S., 1994. Strong link between the alpha 1-antitrypsin PiZ allele and Wegener's granulomatosis. J. Intern. Med. 236, 543–548.

Esnault, V.L., Testa, A., Audrain, M., Roge, C., Hamidou, M., Barrier, J.H., et al., 1993. Alpha 1-antitrypsin genetic polymorphism in ANCA-positive systemic vasculitis. Kidney Int. 43, 1329–1332.

Ewert, B.H., Jennette, J.C., Falk, R.J., 1992a. Anti-myeloperoxidase antibodies stimulate neutrophils to damage human endothelial cells. Kidney Int. 41, 375–383.

Ewert, B.H., Becker, M., Jennette, J.C., Falk, R.J., 1992b. Anti-myeloperoxidase antibodies stimulate neutrophils to adhere to cultured human endothelial cells utilizing the beta-2 integrin CD 11/18. J. Am. Soc. Nephrol. 3, 585.

Falk, R.J., Jennette, J.C., 1988. Anti-neutrophil cytoplasmic autoantibodies with specificity for myeloperoxidase in patients with systemic vasculitis and idiopathic necrotizing and crescentic glomerulonephritis. N. Engl. J. Med. 318, 1651–1657.

Falk, R.J., Hogan, S., Carey, T.S., Jennette, J.C., 1990a. Clinical course of anti-neutrophil cytoplasmic autoantibody-associated glomerulonephritis and systemic vasculitis. The Glomerular Disease Collaborative Network. Ann. Intern. Med. 113, 656–663.

Falk, R.J., Terrell, R.S., Charles, L.A., Jennette, J.C., 1990b. Anti-neutrophil cytoplasmic autoantibodies induce neutrophils to degranulate and produce oxygen radicals in vitro. Proc. Natl. Acad. Sci. USA. 87, 4115–4119.

Falk, R.J., Jennette, J.C., 2010. ANCA disease: where is this field going? J. Am. Soc. Nephrol. 21, 745–752.

Fauci, A.S., Haynes, B., Katz, P., 1978. The spectrum of vasculitis: clinical, pathologic, immunologic and therapeutic considerations. Ann. Intern. Med. 89, 660–676.

Ferri, C., Sebastiani, M., Giuggioli, D., Cazzato, M., Longombardo, G., Antonelli, A., et al., 2004. Mixed cryoglobulinemia: demographic, clinical, and serologic features and survival in 231 patients. Semin. Arthritis Rheum. 33, 355–374.

Fujita, Y., Nakamura, Y., Sakata, K., Hara, N., Kobayashi, M., Nagai, M., et al., 1989. Kawasaki disease in families. Pediatrics. 84, 666–669.

Furusho, K., Kamiya, T., Nakano, H., Kiyosawa, N., Shinomiya, K., Hayashidera, T., et al., 1984. High-dose intravenous gammaglobulin for Kawasaki disease. Lancet. 2, 1055–1058.

Gardner-Medwin, J.M., Dolezalova, P., Cummins, C., Southwood, T.R., 2002. Incidence of Henoch-Schönlein purpura, Kawasaki disease, and rare vasculitides in children of different ethnic origins. Lancet. 360, 1197–1202.

Gedalia, A., 2004. Henoch-Schönlein purpura. Curr. Rheumatol. Rep. 6, 195–202.

Gencik, M., Meller, S., Borgmann, S., Fricke, H., 2000. Proteinase 3 gene polymorphisms and Wegener's granulomatosis. Kidney Int. 58, 2473–2477.

Germuth Jr., F.G., 1953. A comparative histologic and immunologic study in rabbits of induced hypersensitivity of the serum sickness type. J. Exp. Med. 97, 257–282.

Godman, G.C., Churg, J., 1954. Wegener's granulomatosis. Pathology and review of the literature. Arch. Pathol. Lab. Med. 58, 533–553.

Goldschmeding, R., van der Schoot, C.E., ten Bokkel Huinink, D., Hack, C.E., van den Ende, M.E., Kallenberg, C.G., et al., 1989. Wegener's granulomatosis autoantibodies identify a novel diisopropylfluorophosphate-binding protein in the lysosomes of normal human neutrophils. J. Clin. Invest. 84, 1577–1587.

Gonzalez-Gay, M.A., Calvino, M.C., Vazquez-Lopez, M.E., Garcia-Porrua, C., Fernandez-Iglesias, J.L., Dierssen, T., et al., 2004. Implications of upper respiratory tract infections and drugs in the clinical spectrum of Henoch-Schönlein purpura in children. Clin. Exp. Rheumatol. 22, 781–784.

Gower, R.G., Sausker, W.F., Kohler, P.F., Thorne, G.E., McIntosh, R.M., 1978. Small vessel vasculitis caused by hepatitis B virus immune complexes. Small vessel vasculitis and HBsAG. J. Allergy Clin. Immunol. 62, 222–228.

Gregorini, G., Ferioli, A., Donato, F., Tira, P., Morassi, L., Tardanico, R., et al., 1993. Association between silica exposure and necrotizing crescentic glomerulonephritis with p-ANCA and anti-MPO antibodies: a hospital-based case-control study. Adv. Exp. Med. Biol. 336, 435–440.

Griffith, M.E., Coulthart, A., Pusey, C.D., 1996. T cell responses to myeloperoxidase (MPO) and proteinase 3 (PR3) in patients with systemic vasculitis. Clin. Exp. Immunol. 103, 253–258.

Grunebaum, E., Blank, M., Cohen, S., Afek, A., Kapolovic, J., Meroni, P.L., et al., 2002. The role of anti-endothelial cell antibodies in Kawasaki disease—in vitro and in vivo studies. Clin. Exp. Immunol. 130, 233–240.

Guillevin, L., 1999. Treatment of classic polyarteritis nodosa in 1999. Nephrol. Dial. Transplant. 14, 2077–2079.

Guillevin, L., Lhote, F., Brauner, M., Casassus, P., 1995. Antineutrophil cytoplasmic antibodies (ANCA) and abnormal angiograms in polyarteritis nodosa and Churg-Strauss syndrome: indications for the diagnosis of microscopic polyangiitis. Ann. Med. Interne (Paris). 146, 548–550.

Gyotoku, Y., Abdelmoula, M., Spertini, F., Izui, S., Lambert, P.H., 1987. Cryoglobulinemia induced by monoclonal immunoglobulin G rheumatoid factors derived from autoimmune MRL/MpJ-lpr/lpr mice. J. Immunol. 138, 3785–3792.

Han, S.H., 2004. Extrahepatic manifestations of chronic hepatitis B. Clin. Liver Dis. 8, 403–418.

Han, W.K., Choi, H.K., Roth, R.M., McCluskey, R.T., Niles, J.L., 2003. Serial ANCA titers: useful tool for prevention of relapses in ANCA-associated vasculitis. Kidney Int. 63, 1079–1085.

Henoch, E., 1868. Uber den zusammenhang von purpura und intestinalstoerungen. Berl. Klin. Wochenschur. 5, 517–519.

Henoch, E., 1882. Lectures on Diseases of Children: A Handbook for Physicians and Students. W. Wood & Co, New York.

Hogan, S.L., Satterly, K.K., Dooley, M.A., Nachman, P.H., Jennette, J.C., Falk, R.J., 2001. Silica exposure in anti-neutrophil cytoplasmic autoantibody-associated glomerulonephritis and lupus nephritis. J. Am. Soc. Nephrol. 12, 134–142.

Holmen, C., Christensson, M., Pettersson, E., Bratt, J., Stjarne, P., Karrar, A., et al., 2004. Wegener's granulomatosis is associated with organ-specific antiendothelial cell antibodies. Kidney Int. 66, 1049–1060.

Huugen, D., Xiao, H., van Esch, A., Falk, R.J., Peutz-Kootstra, C.J., Buurman, W.A., et al., 2005. Aggravation of anti-myeloperoxidase antibody induced glomerulonephritis by bacterial lipopolysaccharide: role of tumor necrosis factor alpha. Am. J. Pathol. 167, 47–58.

Janssen, H.L., van Zonneveld, M., van Nunen, A.B., Niesters, H.G., Schalm, S.W., de Man, R.A., 2004. Polyarteritis nodosa associated with hepatitis B virus infection. The role of antiviral treatment and mutations in the hepatitis B virus genome. Eur. J. Gastroenterol. Hepatol. 16, 801–807.

Jayne, D., 2003. Current attitudes to the therapy of vasculitis. Kidney Blood Press. Res. 26, 231–239.

Jayne, D.R., Chapel, H., Adu, D., Misbah, S., O'Donoghue, D., Scott, D., et al., 2000. Intravenous immunoglobulin for ANCA-associated systemic vasculitis with persistent disease activity. Q. J. Med. 93, 433–439.

Jennette, J.C., 1991. Antineutrophil cytoplasmic autoantibody-associated diseases: a pathologist's perspective. Am. J. Kidney Dis. 18, 164–170.

Jennette, J.C., 2002. Implications for pathogenesis of patterns of injury in small- and medium-sized-vessel vasculitis. Cleve. Clin. J. Med. 69, SII33–SII38.

Jennette, J.C., 2003. Rapidly progressive crescentic glomerulonephritis. Kidney Int. 63, 1164–1177.

Jennette, J.C., Falk, R.J., 1993. Antineutrophil cytoplasmic autoantibodies in inflammatory bowel disease. Am. J. Clin. Pathol. 99, 221–223.

Jennette, J.C., Falk, R.J., 1997. Small-vessel vasculitis. N. Engl. J. Med. 337, 1512–1523.

Jennette, J.C., Falk, R.J., 1998. Pathogenesis of the vascular and glomerular damage in ANCA-positive vasculitis. Nephrol. Dial. Transplant. 13, 16–20.

Jennette, J.C., Hoidal, J.R., Falk, R.J., 1990. Specificity of anti-neutrophil cytoplasmic autoantibodies for proteinase 3. Blood. 75, 2263–2264.

Jennette, J.C., Xiao, H., Falk, R., Gasim, A.M., 2011. Experimental models of vasculitis and glomerulonephritis induced by antineutrophil cytoplasmic autoantibodies. Contrib. Nephrol. 169, 211–220.

Jennette, J.C., Falk, R.J., Bacon, P.A., Basu, N., Cid, M.C., Ferrario, F., et al., 2013a. 2012 Revised International Chapel Hill Consensus Conference nomenclature of vasculitides. Arthritis Rheum. 65, 1–11.

Jennette, J.C., Falk, R.J., Hu, P., Xiao, H., 2013b. Pathogenesis of anti-neutrophil cytoplasmic autoantibody associated small vessel vasculitis. Annu. Rev. Pathol. Mech. Dis. 8, 139–160.

Jordan, S.C., 1995. Treatment of systemic and renal-limited vasculitic disorders with pooled human intravenous immune globulin. J. Clin. Immunol. 15, 76S–85S.

Jorizzo, J.L., Solomon, A.R., Cavallo, T., 1985. Behçet's syndrome. Immunopathologic and histopathologic assessment of pathergy lesions is useful in diagnosis and follow-up. Arch. Pathol. Lab. Med. 109, 747–751.

Kallenberg, C.G., Brouwer, E., Weening, J.J., Tervaert, J.W., 1994. Anti-neutrophil cytoplasmic antibodies: current diagnostic and pathophysiological potential. Kidney Int. 46, 1–15.

Kaneko, M., Ono, T., Matsubara, T., Yamamoto, Y., Ikeda, H., Yoshiki, T., et al., 2004. Serological identification of endothelial antigens predominantly recognized in Kawasaki disease patients by recombinant expression cloning. Microbiol. Immunol. 48, 703–711.

Kawasaki, T., 1967. Acute febrile mucocutaneous syndrome with lymphoid involvement with specific desquamation of the fingers and toes in children. Arerugi Jpn J. Allergol. 16, 178–222.

Kettritz, R., Jennette, J.C., Falk, R.J., 1997. Crosslinking of ANCA-antigens stimulates superoxide release by human neutrophils. J. Am. Soc. Nephrol. 8, 386–394.

Kikuchi, S., Pastore, Y., Fossati-Jimack, L., Kuroki, A., Yoshida, H., Fulpius, T., et al., 2002. A transgenic mouse model of autoimmune glomerulonephritis and necrotizing arteritis associated with cryoglobulinemia. J. Immunol. 169, 4644–4650.

Kiryluk, K., Moldoveanu, Z., Sanders, J.T., Eison, T.M., Suzuki, H., Julian, B.A., et al., 2011. Aberrant glycosylation of IgA1 is inherited in both pediatric IgA nephropathy and Henoch-Schönlein purpura nephritis. Kidney Int. 80, 79–87.

Klinger, H., 1931. Grenzformen der Periarteritis nodosa. Frankf. Ztschr. Pathol. 42, 455–480.

Korbet, S.M., Schwartz, M.M., Lewis, E.J., 1984. Immune complex deposition and coronary vasculitis in systemic lupus erythematosus. Report of two cases. Am. J. Med. 77, 141–146.

Kussmaul, A., Maier, R., 1866. Uber eine bisher nicht besch-reibene eigenthumliche Arterienerkrankung (Periarteritis nodosa), die mit Morbus Brightii und rapid fortschreitender allgemeiner Muskellahmung einhergeht. Dtsch. Arch. Klin. Med. 1, 484–518.

Lane, S.E., Watts, R.A., Bentham, G., Innes, N.J., Scott, D.G., 2003. Are environmental factors important in primary systemic vasculitis? A case-control study. Arthritis Rheum. 48, 814–823.

Lau, K.K., Wyatt, R.J., Moldoveanu, Z., Tomana, M., Julian, B.A., Hogg, R.J., et al., 2007. Serum levels of galactose-deficient IgA in children with IgA nephropathy and Henoch-Schönlein purpura. Pediatr. Nephrol. 22, 2067–2072.

Lenzi, M., Frisoni, M., Mantovani, V., Ricci, P., Muratori, L., Francesconi, R., et al., 1998. Haplotype HLA-B8-DR3 confers susceptibility to hepatitis C virus-related mixed cryoglobulinemia. Blood. 91, 2062−2066.

Lerner, R.A., Glassock, R.J., Dixon, F.J., 1967. The role of anti-glomerular basement membrane antibody in the pathogenesis of human glomerulonephritis. J. Exp. Med. 126, 989−1004.

Leung, D.Y., Collins, T., Lapierre, L.A., Geha, R.S., Pober, J.S., 1986a. Immunoglobulin M antibodies present in the acute phase of Kawasaki syndrome lyse cultured vascular endothelial cells stimulated by gamma interferon. J. Clin. Invest. 77, 1428−1435.

Leung, D.Y., Geha, R.S., Newburger, J.W., Burns, J.C., Fiers, W., Lapierre, L.A., et al., 1986b. Two monokines, interleukin 1 and tumor necrosis factor, render cultured vascular endothelial cells susceptible to lysis by antibodies circulating during Kawasaki syndrome. J. Exp. Med. 164, 1958−1972.

Leung, D.Y., Cotran, R.S., Kurt-Jones, E., Burns, J.C., Newburger, J.W., Pober, J.S., 1989. Endothelial cell activation and high interleukin-1 secretion in the pathogenesis of acute Kawasaki disease. Lancet. 2, 1298−1302.

Levy, J.B., Hammad, T., Coulthart, A., Dougan, T., Pusey, C.D., 2004. Clinical features and outcome of patients with both ANCA and anti-GBM antibodies. Kidney Int. 66, 1535−1540.

Lim, L.C., Taylor III, J.G., Schmitz, J.L., Folds, J.D., Wilkman, A.S., Falk, R.J., et al., 1999. Diagnostic usefulness of antineutrophil cytoplasmic autoantibody serology. Comparative evaluation of commercial indirect fluorescent antibody kits and enzyme immunoassay kits. Am. J. Clin. Pathol. 111, 363−369.

Little, M.A., Pusey, C.D., 2004. Rapidly progressive glomerulonephritis: current and evolving treatment strategies. J. Nephrol. 17, S10−S19.

Ludemann, J., Utecht, B., Gross, W.L., 1990. Anti-neutrophil cytoplasm antibodies in Wegener's granulomatosis recognize an elastinolytic enzyme. J. Exp. Med. 171, 357−362.

Lyons, P.A., Rayner, T.F., Trivedi, S., Holle, J.U., Watts, R.A., Jayne, D.R., et al., 2012. Genetically distinct subsets within ANCA-associated vasculitis. N. Engl. J. Med. 367, 214−223.

Magilavy, D.B., Petty, R.E., Cassidy, J.T., Sullivan, D.B., 1977. A syndrome of childhood polyarteritis. J. Pediatr. 91, 25−30.

Mahr, A., Guillevin, L., Poissonnet, M., Ayme, S., 2004. Prevalences of polyarteritis nodosa, microscopic polyangiitis, Wegener's granulomatosis, and Churg−Strauss syndrome in a French urban multiethnic population in 2000: a capture-recapture estimate. Arthritis Rheum. 51, 92−99.

Mason, J.C., Cowie, M.R., Davies, K.A., Schofield, J.B., Cambridge, J., Jackson, J., et al., 1994. Familial polyarteritis nodosa. Arthritis Rheum. 37, 1249−1253.

Masuda, M., Nakanishi, K., Yoshizawa, N., Iijima, K., Yoshikawa, N., 2003. Group A streptococcal antigen in the glomeruli of children with Henoch-Schönlein nephritis. Am. J. Kidney Dis. 41, 366−370.

McGrath, M.M., Isakova, T., Rennke, H.G., Mottola, A.M., Laliberte, K.A., Niles, J.L., 2011. Contaminated cocaine and antineutrophil cytoplasmic antibody-associated disease. Clin. J. Am. Soc. Nephrol. 6, 2799−2805.

Meltzer, M., Franklin, E.C., Elias, K., McCluskey, R.T., Cooper, N., 1966. Cryoglobulinemia—a clinical and laboratory study. II. Cryoglobulins with rheumatoid factor activity. Am. J. Med. 40, 837−856.

Mestecky, J., Raska, M., Julian, B.A., Gharavi, A.G., Renfrow, M.B., Moldoveanu, Z., et al., 2013. IgA nephropathy: molecular mechanisms of the disease. Annu. Rev. Pathol. 24, 217−240.

Mor, F., Weinberger, A., Cohen, I.R., 2002. Identification of alpha-tropomyosin as a target self-antigen in Behçet's syndrome. Eur J Immunol. 32, 356−365.

Mulder, A.H., Herringa, P., Brouwer, E., Limburg, P.C., Kallenberg, C.G., 1994. Activation of granulocytes by anti-neutrophil cytoplasmic antibodies (ANCA): a Fc gamma RII-dependent process. Clin. Exp. Immunol. 98, 270−278.

Nachman, P.H., Hogan, S.L., Jennette, J.C., Falk, R.J., 1996. Treatment response and relapse in antineutrophil cytoplasmic autoantibody-associated microscopic polyangiitis and glomerulonephritis. J. Am. Soc. Nephrol. 7, 33−39.

Nagashima, M., Matsushima, M., Matsuoka, H., Ogawa, A., Okumura, N., 1987. High-dose gammaglobulin therapy for Kawasaki disease. J. Pediatr. 110, 710−712.

Newburger, J.W., Fulton, D.R., 2004. Kawasaki disease. Curr. Opin. Pediatr. 16, 508−514.

Niles, J.L., McCluskey, R.T., Ahmad, M.F., Arnaout, M.A., 1989. Wegener's granulomatosis autoantigen is a novel neutrophil serine proteinase. Blood. 74, 1888−1893.

Okazaki, K., Suzuki, Y., Otsuji, M., Suzuki, H., Kihara, M., Kajiyama, T., et al., 2012. Development of a model of early-onset IgA nephropathy. J. Am. Soc. Nephrol. 23, 1364−1374.

Osler, W., 1895. On the visceral complications of erythema eudativum multiforme. Am. J. Med. Sci. 2, 629−647.

Osler, W., 1914. The visceral lesions of purpura and allied conditions. BMJ. 1, 517−525.

Ostergaard, J.R., Storm, K., Lamm, L.U., 1990. Lack of association between HLA and Schoenlein-Henoch purpura. Tissue Antigens. 35, 234−235.

Pendergraft III, W.F., Preston, G.A., Shah, R.R., Tropsha, A., Carter Jr., C.W., Jennette, J.C., et al., 2004. Autoimmunity is triggered by cPR-3(105−201), a protein complementary to human autoantigen proteinase-3. Nat. Med. 10, 72−79.

Pendergraft III, W.F., Pressler, B.M., Jennette, J.C., Falk, R.J., Preston, G.A., 2005. Autoantigen complementarity: a new theory implicating complementary proteins as initiators of autoimmune disease. J. Mol. Med. 83, 12−25.

Pober, J.S., 1988. Warner-Lambert/Parke-Davis award lecture. Cytokine-mediated activation of vascular endothelium. Physiology and pathology. Am. J. Pathol. 133, 426−433.

Porges, A.J., Redecha, P.B., Kimberly, W.T., Csernok, E., Gross, W.L., Kimberly, R.P., 1994. Anti-neutrophil cytoplasmic antibodies engage and activate human neutrophils via Fc gamma RIIa. J. Immunol. 153, 1271−1280.

Radford, D.J., Savage, C.O., Nash, G.B., 2000. Treatment of rolling neutrophils with antineutrophil cytoplasmic antibodies causes conversion to firm integrin-mediated adhesion. Arthritis Rheum. 43, 1337−1345.

Rarok, A.A., Limburg, P.C., Kallenberg, C.G., 2003. Neutrophil-activating potential of antineutrophil cytoplasm autoantibodies. J. Leukoc. Biol. 74, 3−15.

Rauch, A.M., Hurwitz, E.S., 1985. Centers for Disease Control (CDC) case definition for Kawasaki syndrome. Pediatr. Infect. Dis. J. 4, 702−703.

Reveille, J.D., Goodman, R.E., Barger, B.O., Acton, R.T., 1989. Familial polyarteritis nodosa: a serologic and immunogenetic analysis. J. Rheumatol. 16, 181–185.

Rich, A.R., 1942. The role of hypersensitivity in periarteritis nodosa. As indicated by seven cases developing during serum sickness and sulfonamide therapy. Bull. Johns Hopkins Hosp. 71, 123–140.

Rich, A.R., Gregory, J.E., 1943. The experimental demonstration that periarteritis nodosa is a manifestation of hypersensitivity. Bull. Johns Hopkins Hosp. 72, 65–88.

Robson, W.L., Leung, A.K., 1994. Henoch-Schönlein purpura. Adv. Pediatr. 41, 163–194.

Ronco, P., Verroust, P., Mignon, F., Kourilsky, O., Vanhille, P., Meyrier, A., et al., 1983. Immunopathological studies of polyarteritis nodosa and Wegener's granulomatosis: a report of 43 patients with 51 renal biopsies. Q. J. Med. 52, 212–223.

Roth, A.J., Ooi, J., Hess, J.J., van Timmeren, M.M., Berg, E.A., Jennette, C.E., et al., 2013. ANCA epitope specificity determines pathogenicity, detectability and clinical predictive value. J. Clin. Invest. 123, 1773–1783.

Rowley, A.H., Duffy, C.E., Shulman, S.T., 1988. Prevention of giant coronary artery aneurysms in Kawasaki disease by intravenous gamma globulin therapy. J. Pediatr. 113, 290–294.

Sansonno, D., Dammacco, F., 2005. Hepatitis C virus, cryoglobulinaemia, and vasculitis: immune complex relations. Lancet Infect Dis. 5, 227–236.

Savage, C.O., Pottinger, B.E., Gaskin, G., Pusey, C.D., Pearson, J.D., 1992. Autoantibodies developing to myeloperoxidase and proteinase 3 in systemic vasculitis stimulate neutrophil cytotoxicity toward cultured endothelial cells. Am. J. Pathol. 141, 335–342.

Savige, J., Gillis, D., Benson, E., Davies, D., Esnault, V., Falk, R.J., et al., 1999. International consensus statement on testing and reporting of antineutrophil cytoplasmic antibodies (ANCA). Am. J. Clin. Pathol. 111, 507–513.

Saxena, R., Bygren, P., Rasmussen, N., Wieslander, J., 1991. Circulating autoantibodies in patients with extracapillary glomerulonephritis. Nephrol. Dialysis Transpl. 6, 389–397.

Schönlein, J.L., 1837. Allgemeine und specielle Pathologie und Therapie. third ed. Literatur-Comptoir, Herisau.

Stegeman, C.A., Tervaert, J.W., de Jong, P.E., Kallenberg, C.G., 1996. Trimethoprim-sulfamethoxazole (co-trimoxazole) for the prevention of relapses of Wegener's granulomatosis. Dutch Co-Trimoxazole Wegener Study Group. N. Engl. J. Med. 335, 16–20.

Sturgill, B.C., Westervelt, F.B., 1965. Immunofluorescence studies in a case of Goodpasture's syndrome. JAMA. 194, 914–916.

Suzuki, H., Fan, R., Zhang, Z., Brown, R., Hall, S., Julian, B.A., et al., 2009. Aberrantly glycosylated IgA1 in IgA nephropathy patients is recognized by IgG antibodies with restricted heterogeneity. J. Clin. Invest. 119, 1668–1677.

Takahashi, K., Oharaseki, T., Wakayama, M., Yokouchi, Y., Naoe, S., Murata, H., 2004. Histopathological features of murine systemic vasculitis caused by Candida albicans extract—an animal model of Kawasaki disease. Inflamm. Res. 53, 72–77.

Tanaka, N., Naoe, S., Kawasaki, T., 1971. Pathological study on autopsy cases of mucocutaneous lymph node syndrome. J. Jpn Red Cross Cent. Hosp. 2, 85–94.

Ting, T.V., Hashkes, P.J., 2004. Update on childhood vasculitides. Curr. Opin. Rheumatol. 16, 560–565.

Uehara, R., Yashiro, M., Nakamura, Y., Yanagawa, H., 2003. Kawasaki disease in parents and children. Acta Paediatr. 92, 694–697.

van der Woude, F.J., Rasmussen, N., Lobatto, S., Wiik, A., Permin, H., van Es, L.A., et al., 1985. Autoantibodies against neutrophils and monocytes: tool for diagnosis and marker of disease activity in Wegener's granulomatosis. Lancet. 1, 425–429.

Vargunam, M., Adu, D., Taylor, C.M., Michael, J., Richards, N., Neuberger, J., Thompson, R.A., 1992. Endothelium myeloperoxidase–antimyeloperoxidase interaction in vasculitis. Nephrol. Dialysis Transpl. 7, 1077–1081.

Watts, R.A., Scott, D.G., 2004. Epidemiology of the vasculitides. Semin. Respir. Crit. Care Med. 25, 455–464.

Wegener, F., 1939. Uber eine eigenartige rhinogene Granulomatose mit besonderer Beteiligung des Arteriensystems under der Nieren. Beitrage Zur Pathologieschen Anatomie. 102, 36–68.

Weiss, M.A., Crissman, J.D., 1984. Renal biopsy findings in Wegener's granulomatosis: segmental necrotizing glomerulonephritis with glomerular thrombosis. Hum. Pathol. 15, 943–956.

Willan, R., 1808. On Cutaneous Diseases. Kimber & Conrad, pp. 452–471.

Williams, J.M., Savage, C.O., 2005. Characterization of the regulation and functional consequences of p21ras activation in neutrophils by antineutrophil cytoplasm antibodies. J. Am. Soc. Nephrol. 16, 90–96.

Williams, J.M., Kamesh, L., Savage, C.O., 2005. Translating basic science into patient therapy for ANCA-associated small vessel vasculitis. Clin. Sci. (Lond.). 108, 101–112.

Winkelman, R.K., 1958. Clinical and pathologic findings in the skin in anaphylactoid purpura (allergic purpura). Proc. Mayo Clin. 33, 277–288.

Xiao, H., Heeringa, P., Hu, P., Liu, Z., Zhao, M., Aratani, Y., et al., 2002. Antineutrophil cytoplasmic autoantibodies specific for myeloperoxidase cause glomerulonephritis and vasculitis in mice. J. Clin. Invest. 110, 955–963.

Xiao, H., Heeringa, P., Liu, Z., Huugen, D., Hu, P., Falk, R.J., et al., 2005. The role for neutrophils in the induction of glomerulonephritis by anti-myeloperoxidase antibody. Am. J. Pathol. 167, 39–45.

Xiao, H., Schreiber, A., Heeringa, P., Falk, R.J., Jennette, J.C., 2007. Alternative complement pathway in the pathogenesis of disease mediated by anti-neutrophil cytoplasmic autoantibodies. Am. J. Pathol. 170, 52–56.

Yim, D., Curtis, N., Cheung, M., Burgner, D., 2013. Update on Kawasaki disease: epidemiology, aetiology and pathogenesis. J. Paediatr. Child Health. 49, 704–708.

Zeek, P.M., 1952. Periarteritis nodosa: a critical review. Am. J. Clin. Pathol. 22, 777–790.

Zeek, P.M., Smith, C.C., Weeter, J.C., 1948. Studies on periarteritis nodosa. III. The differentiation between the vascular lesions of periarteritis nodosa and of hypersensitivity. Am. J. Pathol. 24, 889–917.

Zheng, F., Kundu, G.C., Zhang, Z., Ward, J., DeMayo, F., Mukherjee, A.B., 1999. Uteroglobin is essential in preventing immunoglobulin A nephropathy in mice. Nat. Med. 5, 1018–1025.

Chapter 73

Large and Medium Vessel Vasculitides

Cornelia M. Weyand and Jörg J. Goronzy

Department of Medicine, Division of Immunology and Rheumatology, Stanford University School of Medicine, Stanford, CA, USA

Chapter Outline

Vasculitides of Large and Medium-sized Blood Vessels   **1087**
Giant Cell Arteritis   **1087**
    Historical Background   1088
    Clinical, Pathologic, and Epidemiologic Features   1089
    The Vascular Lesion   1091
    Epidemiology   1091
    Genetic Features   1091
    Pathogenic Mechanisms   1091
    T Cells and Antigen-Presenting Cells in Giant Cell Arteritis   1092
    Macrophages in Giant Cell Arteritis   1093
    Intimal Hyperplasia   1094

    Immuno-stromal Interactions Promoting Vasculitis   1094
    The Systemic Inflammatory Syndrome   1094
    Treatment, Monitoring, and Outcome   1095
Takayasu's Arteritis   **1096**
    Historical Background   1096
    Clinical, Pathologic, and Epidemiologic Features   1096
    Genetic Features   1098
    Pathogenic Mechanisms   1098
    Treatment and Outcome   1098
Concluding Remarks—Future Perspectives   **1099**
Acknowledgment   **1100**
References   **1100**

VASCULITIDES OF LARGE AND MEDIUM-SIZED BLOOD VESSELS

Among the immune-mediated diseases vasculitides stand out for their potential to rapidly progress to serious, and at times life-threatening, complications. Inflammation in the wall of medium-sized and large blood vessels is considered a medical emergency that requires prompt diagnosis and therapeutic management. Arteritides threaten the host through two different mechanisms (Weyand and Goronzy, 2003b). Destruction of the vessel wall leads to dissection, aneurysm formation, rupture, and hemorrhage. Alternatively, arteritis initiates luminal stenosis with subsequent occlusion, tissue ischemia, and infarct.

Inflammation in venous vessels is rare, whereas the layered wall structure of large arteries appears to be a preferred site for granulomatous vasculitis, such as giant cell arteritis (GCA) and Takayasu's arteritis (TA) (Table 73.1). Both target the aorta and its major branches. However, the overlap in affected vascular territories is only partial, and each entity also manifests in unique arterial beds. Aortitides can be associated with other syndromes, such as relapsing polyarthritis, sarcoidosis, inflammatory bowel disease, and infections; however, GCA and TA are the most frequent causes of aortic wall inflammation (Rojo-Leyva et al., 2000). Notably, host age is a strong risk factor for each for these vasculitides with the old susceptible to GCA and the young susceptible to TA. The pathologic and radiographic features can be indistinguishable, and clinical information is necessary to allow for proper diagnosis and classification (Gravanis, 2000).

The etiology of vasculitis in the aorta and its major branches remains unresolved. Both the innate and the adaptive immune system contribute to pathogenesis. Some aspects of the abnormal immunity resemble an autoimmune reaction, but classical autoantigens have not been identified. An emerging concept proposes that vasculitides are one side of the spectrum of vascular inflammation that also includes atherosclerosis (see Chapter 71), with overlap in pathogenic mechanisms but differences in the intensity of inflammation.

GIANT CELL ARTERITIS

Giant cell arteritis is also known as temporal arteritis, cranial arteritis, granulomatous arteritis, polymyalgia arteritis, and Horton's disease. Typically, granulomatous lesions are formed in the wall of medium-sized arteries,

N. Rose & I. Mackay (Eds): The Autoimmune Diseases, Fifth edition. DOI: http://dx.doi.org/10.1016/B978-0-12-384929-8.00073-3

TABLE 73.1 Principal Features of Giant Cell Arteritis and Takayasu's Arteritis

	Giant cell arteritis	Takayasu's arteritis
Clinical	Subacute disease onset Restricted to individuals older than 50 years Highest incidence in individuals with Northern European ancestry Often combined with polymyalgia rheumatica	Subacute disease onset 90% of patients are female Highest risk in Asian and South American populations Systemic inflammatory syndrome with malaise, fever, arthralgias, and chest pain
Preferred vascular territories	Extracranial branches of the carotid artery Subclavian—axillary junction Aorta	Aorta Innominate, carotid, subclavian, mesenteric, renal arteries
Severe complications	Blindness Stroke Aortic aneurysm Wasting	Stroke Pulselessness Visual impairment Aortic regurgitation Hypertension
Pathogenesis	Key cellular elements in vasculitic lesions: arterial wall dendritic cells, IFN-γ-producing CD4$^+$ T cells, IL-17-producing CD4$^+$ T cells, tissue-injurious macrophages Trigger of immune-mediated vascular inflammation unknown Intense systemic inflammation with highly elevated IL-6 and hepatic acute phase reactants	Key cellular elements in the vascular lesions: perforin-producing T cells and natural killer cells Instigator of vessel wall inflammation unknown Systemic inflammatory syndrome

particularly in the upper extremity and cranial branches of the aorta. CD4$^+$. T cells are recruited to the adventitia of affected blood vessels where they interact with tissue-residing dendritic cells (DCs) and undergo *in situ* activation. At least two distinct lineages of CD4 T cells, Th1 cells and Th17 cells, participate in the intramural inflammation. Activated T cells regulate the differentiation of macrophages into tissue-injurious effector cells and orchestrate the production of growth factors intimately involved in the process of intimal hyperplasia. Vessel stenosis/occlusion leads to ischemia, and blindness-inducing ischemic optic neuropathy is one of the most feared clinical manifestations. Variations exist in the vascular inflammation, which translate into differences of the clinical disease profile. The diagnosis can be made by biopsy of the temporal artery. Almost all patients are older than 50 years of age, and the highest incidence has been reported in persons of northern European ancestry. If diagnosed early and treated appropriately, the clinical outcome is excellent (Weyand and Goronzy, 2003a,b). However, recent data strongly suggest that GCA is not a self-limiting disease. The early phase of vasculitis, mediated by Th1 and Th17 cells, partially responds to corticosteroid therapy. The late phase, a Th1-dependent disease process, appears relatively steroid resistant and manifests as a smoldering arteritis.

Historical Background

In 1932, Bayard Horton and colleagues (Horton et al., 1932) reported on two patients admitted to the Mayo Clinic with "fever, weakness, anorexia, weight loss, anemia and painful, tender areas over the scalp and along the temporal vessels." Histomorphology of the removed temporal artery described periarteritis and arteritis with granulation tissue in the adventitia. Horton recognized that this type of arteritis was distinct from all other vasculitic syndromes and named it "temporal arteritis." Prior descriptions of temporal artery disease suggest that GCA may be a very old disease. In 1890, the English surgeon Jonathan Hutchinson described a patient with a red and swollen temporal artery who had difficulties wearing his hat (Hutchinson, 1890). In the grave of Pa-Aton-Ern-Hebs, built during the Amarna period (around AD 1350), a blind harpist was shown with nodularity and swelling of the temporal artery. And Ali Ibn Isa (940—1010 BC), an ophthalmologist in Baghdad, recommended removal of the temporal artery not only to treat headaches, but also inflammation of the scalp muscles associated with blindness (Henriet et al., 1989).

Horton deserves credit for recognizing the connection between the constitutional symptoms and the arteritis of the temporal vessels and for introducing temporal artery biopsy as a diagnostic test.

TABLE 73.2 The Clinical Profile in Giant Cell Arteritis

Sign/Symptom	Frequency (%)	Pathology
Headaches	80	Vascular stenosis
Scalp tenderness	70	
Jaw claudication	30	
Ocular symptoms (blindness, amaurosis, fugax, motor deficit)	<20	
Painful dysphagia	<10	
Cough	<10	
Limb claudication	10	
Absent pulses	<10	
Asymmetrical blood pressure readings	<10	
CNS ischemia	<5	
Peripheral neuropathy	<5	
Aortic regurgitation	<5	Vascular dilatation
Intense acute phase response (elevated ESR, CRP, IL-6)	90	Systemic inflammation
Anemia	70	
Polymyalgia rheumatica	40	
Wasting syndrome	30	
Synovitis	<5	

CRP, C-reactive protein; ESR, erythrocyte sedimentation rate; IL-6, interleukin 6.

Clinical, Pathologic, and Epidemiologic Features

The clinical manifestations of GCA are characterized by two major dimensions: (1) arterial stenosis and occlusion of arteries causing impaired blood flow, ischemia, and tissue infarction; and (2) systemic inflammation leading to a massive increase in acute phase proteins, liver abnormalities, anemia, weight loss, malaise, and fever (Table 73.2) (Evans and Hunder, 2000; Weyand and Goronzy, 2003a). Evidence suggests that the systemic inflammatory syndrome precedes rather than follows vascular inflammation, responds promptly to corticosteroid immunosuppression, and is mediated by a distinct immune abnormality: the excessive production of IL-6 and related cytokines. Clinical symptoms vary depending on the nature of the vascular lesions and the vascular bed is preferentially affected. For clinical purposes it is helpful to subdivide the GCA syndrome into different subtypes, including cranial GCA, nonstenosing GCA, large vessel GCA, and polymyalgia rheumatica (PMR).

In cranial GCA, the major focus of the vasculopathy lies in the branches of the aorta that supply the head and the neck. Most often affected are the superficial temporal artery, the vertebral artery, the ophthalmic and posterior ciliary arteries, and, less frequently, the internal and external carotid artery. Clinical consequences of vascular insufficiency include headaches, scalp tenderness, claudication of the masseter muscles, and vision loss due to ischemia in the visual pathway. The headaches are often intense, throbbing and sharp in character, and can be combined with temporal tenderness. On physical examination, the temporal vessels are thickened, with nodules and absence of pulses. Other arteries of the scalp can be involved. Vision loss is one of the reasons that GCA is considered a prime ophthalmic emergency. Occlusion in branches of the ophthalmic artery results in ischemic optic neuropathy that causes sudden and pain-free blindness. Amaurosis fugax can precede complete vision loss. Patients with blindness in one eye are at high risk to suffer additional visual loss in the other eye. Vascular insufficiency of arteries supplying the orbita can cause a wide spectrum of ophthalmic complications, but ischemic optic neuropathy remains the most frequent ophthalmic manifestation (Chan et al., 2005). Intermittent claudication of the masseter and temporal muscles is a relatively disease-specific symptom but only affects a fraction of patients (Smetana and Shmerling, 2002). Usually, jaw claudication is induced by chewing or prolonged talking.

Claudication of the tongue and painful dysphagia can occur. Impaired blood flow in the vertebrobasilar and carotid arteries causes ischemia of the central nervous system, e.g., transient ischemic attacks or stroke. Chronic nonproductive cough has been attributed to vasculitis of pulmonary artery branches.

In a subset of patients, the primary targets of vasculitis are the subclavian, axillary, and carotid arteries, and the aorta itself (Brack et al., 1999; Salvarani, 2003). Presenting symptoms of upper extremity vasculitis are claudication of the arms, loss of pulses, paresthesisas, and, only rarely, frank gangrene. Temporal artery biopsies are often negative, and, in the majority of patients, symptoms indicative of cranial ischemia are lacking (Brack et al., 1999). Aortitis can coexist with cranial arteritis or large vessel involvement and predominantly manifests in the thoracic aorta. Silent aneurysm, aortic dissection, or rupture is a consequence of destruction of the elastic membranes (Evans et al., 1994; Lie, 1995). Not unusually, histomorphologic evidence of vasculitis is found during surgical repair of aortic aneurysm. Aortic involvement is typically seen in patients many years after the initial diagnosis of GCA, suggesting a smoldering disease process and is associated with increased mortality (Kermani et al., 2012).

Inflammation of medium-sized arteries in GCA does not necessarily lead to vascular stenosis but may manifest as nonstenosing vasculitis. Only in recent years has it become clear that patients with nonstenosing GCA present with a different clinical profile than those who have lumenal occlusion (Weyand et al., 1997). In nonstenosing GCA, the dominant features are those of intense systemic inflammation, often manifesting as fever and wasting. Frequently such patients seek medical attention because of nonspecific symptoms such as malaise, depression, anorexia, and weight loss and are subjected to a work-up for underlying malignancy. Lack of cranial symptoms, such as headaches, scalp tenderness, and abnormal temporal artery, can generate a challenging clinical scenario in which only the experienced clinician will search actively for vasculitis. Temporal artery biopsy is the diagnostic procedure of choice.

The vasculitic component of GCA may remain subclinical with the systemic inflammatory syndrome appearing in isolation (Weyand and Goronzy, 2003a). Signs and symptoms of impaired blood flow are missing, and clinical findings are dominated by myalgias, stiffness, and laboratory signs of heightened acute phase response. This subtype of GCA is best known as PMR, a clinical syndrome that is about two- to three-fold more frequent in incidence than GCA (Doran et al., 2002; Kermani and Warrington, 2013). Polymyalgia rheumatica and GCA are closely related entities, affecting the same patient population. They can occur together, and PMR can precede or follow GCA. Histologic examination of arterial biopsies is unrevealing, but molecular analysis of arterial tissues demonstrates the activation of immune responses in the vessel wall (Weyand et al., 1994a). Lead symptoms are those of shoulder girdle and pelvic girdle pain and stiffness. Synovitis of hip and shoulder joints has been described in some patients with PMR and recent provisional classification criteria have been expanded to include cases with bursitis and synovitis (Dasgupta et al., 2012). The diagnosis of PMR remains founded on nonspecific findings, such as pain and elevated acute phase proteins, and, in some cases, inflammation of joint-related structures. Further widening of the diagnostic category of PMR is suggested by recent reports that the diffuse myalgias associated with statin therapy may also fulfill the criteria for PMR (de Jong et al., 2012). Urgent need exists to replace the non-specific clinical classification criteria with objective, histological, and molecularly based criteria. Until that goal is reached, PMR remains a diagnosis of exclusion and includes an assortment of conditions.

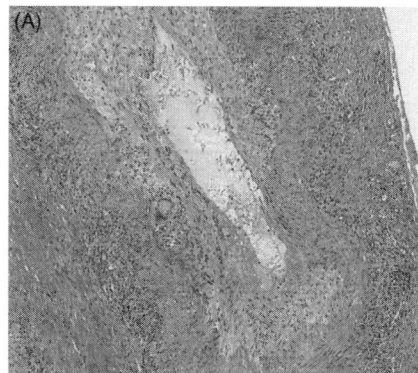 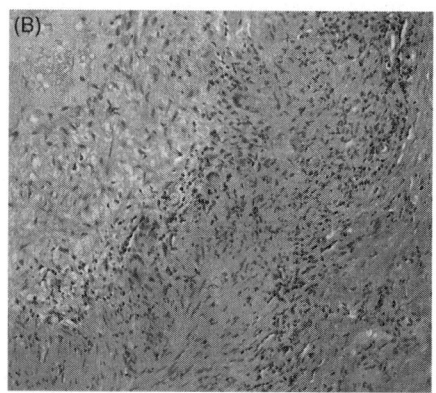

FIGURE 73.1   Giant cell arteritis.   Cross-section of the temporal artery from a 78-year-old patient. (A) Transmural inflammation with granuloma formation in the inner media and along the intimal–medial junction. Partial occlusion of the lumen by thickened intima. (B) Detailed view of several multinucleated giant cells, close to the fragmented internal elastic lamina. *Reproduced with permission from Weyand and Goronzy (2003b).*

The Vascular Lesion

In its typical form, GCA is a panarteritis with T lymphocytes and macrophages infiltrating into all layers of the vessel wall (Figure 73.1) (Gravanis, 2000). In about half of the cases, granulomatous formations are seen. Giant cells, which give the name to the syndrome, are not necessarily present. They have a tendency to accumulate at the media-intima border, often closely related to the fragmented internal elastic lamina. Inflammatory infiltrates are usually segmental but can be circumferential. Most typical is the focal placement of lesions producing the so-called "skip" pattern of vasculitis. In some patients, the infiltrates are predominantly composed of lymphocytes without granuloma formation. The intima is hyperplastic, obstructing the lumen. Frequently, the adventitia is infiltrated by T cells and macrophages. Clusters of lymphocytes and macrophages in the adventitia, at times arranged as cuffs around vasa vasorum, should be considered sufficient to establish the diagnosis of GCA (Bjornsson, 2002). In some cases, the small vessels in the adventitia are the primary target for the inflammatory infiltrates, leaving the main temporal artery unaffected (Chatelain et al., 2008).

Epidemiology

Among the vasculitic syndromes, GCA is the most frequent in the Western world. Age is the most significant risk factor; the disease almost exclusively occurs in individuals older than 50 years of age, and susceptibility increases as individuals get older (Machado et al., 1988; Salvarani et al., 2004). The female-to-male ratio of patients is 3:1. A characteristic feature of GCA is pronounced geographical variations in prevalence. The range of incidence rates spans between 1 and 25 cases per 100,000 persons aged 50 years and older. Highest incidence rates have been reported in northern Europe, including Iceland, Denmark, and Sweden (Baldursson et al., 1994; Nordborg et al., 2003), as well as in areas of North America settled by populations of Scandinavian origin (Machado et al., 1988), such as Minnesota. Conversely, blacks and Hispanics are infrequently affected (Smith et al., 1983; Gonzalez et al., 1989).

Genetic Features

Giant cell arteritis is an HLA class II-associated disease (Weyand et al., 1992, 1994b). HLA-DR4 confers the highest risk to develop arteritis. Several allelic variants of HLA DR B1*04 are overrepresented among affected individuals. Sharing of sequence polymorphisms in the antigen-binding groove of HLA-DR molecules has been cited as evidence for a role of antigenic peptides in disease initiation. HLA class II polymorphisms seem not to influence the patterning or severity of the disease. Minor effects of polymorphisms in multiple non-HLA genes, such as corticotrophin-releasing hormone, CCL5 (RANTES), intracellular adhesion molecule 1 (ICAM-1), and interleukin 6 (IL-6), have been reported and larger studies are awaited to confirm or refute such associations (Alvarez-Rodriguez et al., 2011; Rodriguez-Rodriguez et al., 2011a,b). It is possible that the marked geographical variations in disease susceptibility are related to differences in population genetics, for example, the representation of HLA class II haplotypes.

Pathogenic Mechanisms

Progress has been made in deciphering the pathogenic mechanisms relevant for the inflammatory injury of the vessel wall (Weyand, 2000; Weyand and Goronzy, 2003b; Weyand et al., 2012). Data on the systemic component with the massive upregulation of acute phase responses are more limited. A comprehensive pathogenic model would have to explain why individuals of Scandinavian origin develop granulomatous lesions in the walls of selected medium-sized arteries when they reach the seventh to eighth decades of their lives; how panarteritis translates into occlusive vasculopathy; and how vascular insufficiency is related to the clinical profile of the syndrome. Over the last decade, much progress has been made in understanding the pathways of immunostimulation in the artery and how the immune system regulates vessel stenosis/occlusion (Figure 73.2). A concept explaining the target tissue susceptibility of selected arterial territories is emerging.

Principally, GCA is a chronic inflammatory disease in which $CD4^+$ T lymphocytes establish stable lymphoid microstructures in the arterial wall and orchestrate the differentiation of tissue-injurious macrophages (Figure 73.2) (see also Chapter 11). The response-to-injury program of the vessel is maladaptive and leads to overshooting proliferation of the intimal layer resulting in luminal occlusion, ischemia, and infarct of dependent organ structures. Age-related changes in the immune system as well as in the arterial system represent risk factors for the development of this granulomatous arteritis (Mohan et al., 2011). Dysfunctional immunity is only one aspect of the pathogenic process; the blood vessel participates as an equal partner in destabilizing the immune protection ordinarily guarding blood vessel walls from inflammation. Vascular cells actively interact with immune cells to break tissue tolerance and provide signals that amplify tissue-destructive feed-forward circuits sustaining vasculitis (Weyand and Goronzy, 2013). Specifically, wall-resident cells, such as endothelial cells and vascular smooth muscle cells, may provide activation and survival signals for

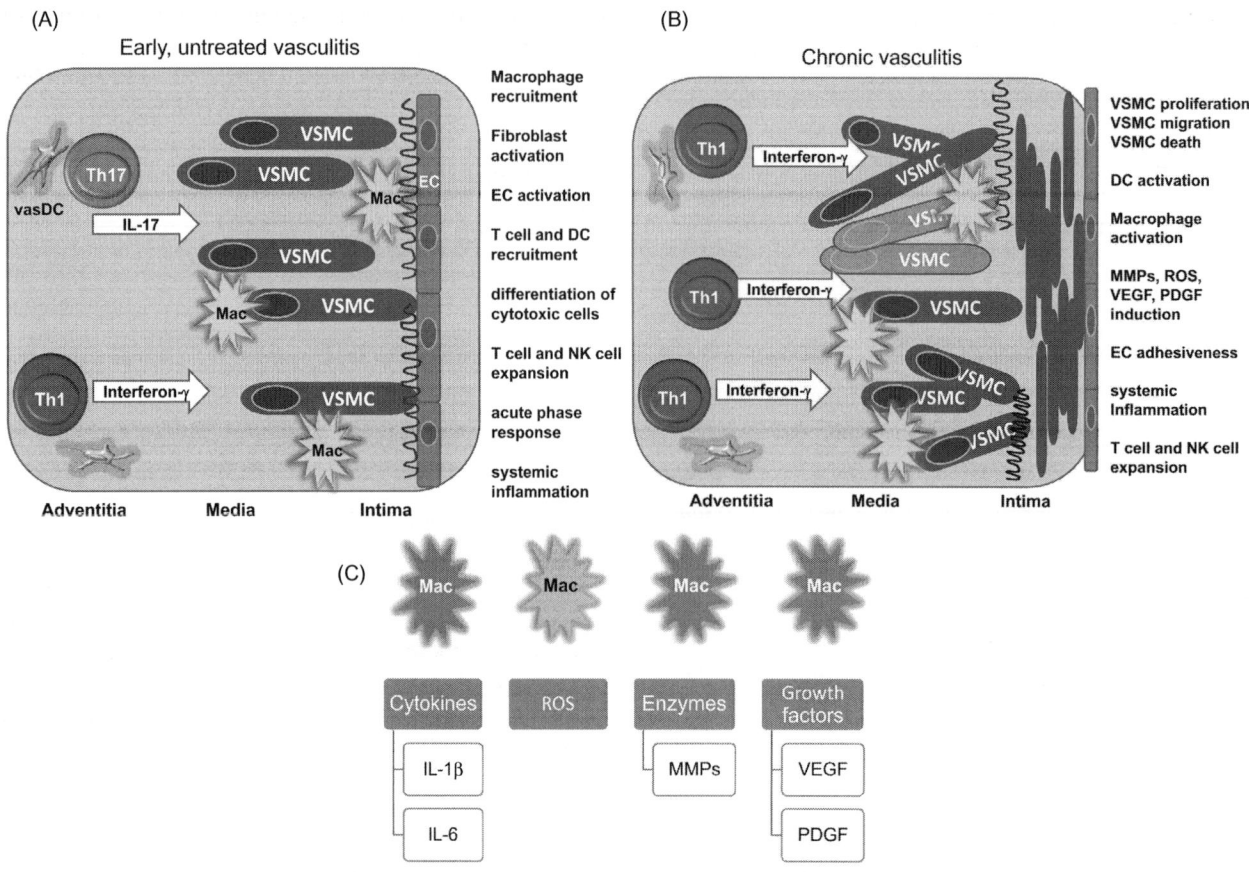

FIGURE 73.2 (A) Medium-sized human arteries host a population of dendritic cells (vasDC) positioned in the adventitia. When stimulated, such vasDC begin to recruit and activate CD4 T cells. In early vasculitis, both IFN-γ-producing Th1 cells and IL-17-producing Th17 cells are represented in the infiltrate. Release of IFN-γ and IL-17 recruits and stimulates macrophages and targets vessel-wall cells (VSMC and EC). The misplaced T cell response amplifies inflammation, creates a permissive microenvironment and organizes the infiltrating immune cells in granulomatous arrangements. (B) Chronic giant cell arteritis. In temporal arteries of corticosteroid-treated patients Th17 cells are rare but Th1 cells dominate the infiltrates. Secretion of IFN-γ into the tissue niche activates macrophages and directs their differentiation into a multitude of proinflammatory and tissue-damaging populations (see Figure 73.3). VSMC respond to IFN-γ stimulation with proliferation, migration, and secretory differentiation. Activated myofibroblasts form hyperplastic intima, which obstructs the lumen. IFN-γ can also cause VSMC death and thinning of the media. (C) Macrophages in giant cell arteritis. Directed by tissue-infiltrating T cells, macrophages differentiate into several distinct populations, which specialize in different aspects of tissue damage. IL-1β and IL-6 production supports proinflammatory feed-forward circuits. ROS release damages vessel-wall structures. Enzyme production sustains digestion of elastic membes. Growth factors promote growth and activity of myofibroblasts and enable neo-angiogenesis through the release of VEGF.

infiltrating immune cells that allow them to be retained in the tissue niche and undergo chronic activation.

T Cells and Antigen-Presenting Cells in Giant Cell Arteritis

The vast majority of T cells in the lesions are CD4[+] T cells of the memory phenotype (Andersson et al., 1987). CD4[+] T cells enter the vessel wall through the vasa vasorum and infiltrate into the adventitia recruited by chemokines that derive from DCs positioned at the adventitia–media border (Krupa et al., 2002) (Figure 73.2). Adventitial DCs are an indigenous cell

population that was only recently described (Ma-Krupa et al., 2004). They form a circumferential ring along the lamina elastica externa. They express typical DC markers, such as CD11c, fascin, and S-100 but lack CD1a and thus are distinct from Langerhans cells in the skin. Functional profiling has demonstrated that they possess Toll-like receptors (TLRs) and respond to pathogen-associated molecular patterns (Pryshchep et al., 2008).

Toll-like receptors are characteristically found on cells of the innate immune system and typical ligands are lipo-polysaccharides, flagellin, viral RNA, bacterial DNA, and also heat-shock proteins (see Chapter 12). The triggering of TLRs, together with additional signals, initiates the maturation of immature DCs. Upon maturation, such DCs switch their chemokine receptor profile, become migratory, and travel via lymphatic vessels to secondary lymphoid tissues, such as lymph nodes. There they home to the T cell zones, become stationary, start producing T cell-attracting chemokines, and upregulate the expression of antigen-presenting HLA molecules and costimulatory molecules.

It is not known what the physiological role of adventitial DCs is and what they are checking for. Experiments that utilized the implantation of human temporal arteries into immunodeficient mice have revealed that such adventitial DCs respond to LPS and undergo rapid activation when triggered by blood-borne mediators (Ma-Krupa et al., 2004). In GCA, almost all DCs in the arterial wall are highly activated and have adopted a functional profile reminiscent of that in lymph node-positioned DCs (Krupa et al., 2002). They produce high amounts of chemokines, are no longer migratory, and can present antigen to T cells. It has been proposed that one of the pathomechanisms in GCA is the trapping of arterial wall DCs in the tissue instead of allowing them to migrate to lymph nodes, which leads to a misplaced immune response.

Experiments in patients with PMR who lack T cell infiltrates in the temporal artery have supported the concept that DC activation is a very early step in the disease process (Krupa et al., 2002). In fact, DCs in PMR arteries have already acquired the capability to produce T cell-attracting chemokines. If appropriate T cells are made available, they will initiate T cell recruitment and *in situ* activation. How patients with PMR are protected from accumulating T cells in the artery, although tissue-residing DCs have already matured, is not understood.

Once CD4$^+$ T cells have made their entrance into the adventitial layer of medium-sized arteries, they undergo local activation (Weyand et al., 1994c; Brack et al., 1997). Studies in right-sided and left-sided temporal artery specimens from the same patient have shown that identical T cell clonotypes emerge in physically separated lesions (Weyand et al., 1994c), providing strong support for antigen-driven selection (Weyand and Goronzy, 1995). Recent studies have emphasized that several functional T cell lineages participate in the vasculitic lesions. A major subset of tissue-infiltrating CD4 T cells produce interferon-γ (IFN-γ) and represent Th1 cells (Wagner et al., 1996; Deng et al., 2010; Samson et al., 2012; Terrier et al., 2012). However, GCA is not a "pure" Th1 disease. Rather, also present in the lesions are Th17 cells (Deng et al., 2010; Samson et al., 2012). Evidence for nonoverlapping actions of both T cell lineages comes from the analysis of consecutive temporal artery biopsies in untreated and treated patients (Deng et al., 2010). Corticosteroids essentially eliminate Th17 cells but leave Th1 cells unaffected. The emerging pathogenic concept distinguishes between early untreated GCA, a Th1—Th17-driven process and chronic-persistent GCA, a Th1-dependent pathology (Weyand et al., 2011).

CD4$^+$ T cells undergo clonal expansion and regulate macrophage recruitment (Figure 73.2). The intensity of IFN-γ production, which could be viewed as a measure of T cell activation in the vasculitic lesions, has been correlated with the clinical manifestations of this disease. Patients with high production of IFN-γ in the artery have more intense intimal hyperplasia, more visual symptoms, and cranial ischemia. Patients with distinctly low production of IFN-γ in the temporal artery sample often lack vessel occlusion and tend to present with fever of unknown origin or other constitutional symptoms (Weyand et al., 1997).

Depletion experiments have indicated that CD83$^+$ DCs are the critical antigen-presenting cells and thus have gatekeeper function in the disease (Ma-Krupa et al., 2004). Since DCs sit in a unique position in the artery (outside of the lamina elastica externa), their absence or presence may dictate whether a particular artery is susceptible to be targeted by GCA. Indeed, different arterial beds in the human body carry vascular DC with distinct profiles of pattern recognition receptors (Pryshchep et al., 2008), providing a molecular basis for variations in the target tissues and a possible mechanism for the unusual patterning of temporal arteritis.

Macrophages in Giant Cell Arteritis

There are no data to suggest that T lymphocytes accumulating in the vasculitic infiltrates have direct involvement in wall injury (Weyand and Goronzy, 1999). Rather, multiple pathways have been identified through which macrophages mediate tissue damage (Figure 73.2). Macrophage function is closely related to the positioning in the wall, suggesting a tight interaction between infiltrating macrophages and the cellular and matrix components of the particular microenvironment (Weyand et al., 1996).

Adventitial macrophages focus on the production of proinflammatory cytokines, such as IL-1β and IL-6. Tumor necrosis factor-α (TNF-α) has been reported to be present in inflamed arteries with the staining pattern suggesting production in the media (Hernandez-Rodriguez et al., 2004). Macrophages in the media specialize in generating reactive oxygen intermediates (Rittner et al., 1999b). Toxic aldehydes, products of lipid peroxidation, have been detected in the medial smooth muscle cell layer (Rittner et al., 1999b). The formation of nitrotyrosine, a marker of nitrosative stress, has also been localized to the media (Borkowski et al., 2002). Interestingly, only endothelial cells of medial neovessels are affected by nitrotyrosine formation. These studies have pinpointed tissue injury pathways, identified the cellular players, and at least partially described target structures incurring damage.

A noteworthy aspect of the presence of oxidative stress in the media is the induction of protective mechanisms, such as the induction of aldose reductase, a ketoreductase with a role in metabolizing toxic aldehydes (Rittner et al., 1999a). Blocking aldose reductase in GCA lesions increased apoptosis rates of smooth muscle cells, demonstrating a protective role of the enzyme. There is no information about whether patients actually vary in the induction of such protective mechanisms, making them more or less susceptible to oxidative damage.

Other functional properties of media-located macrophages include the secretion of matrix metalloproteinases (MMPs) (Sorbi et al., 1996; Tomita and Imakawa, 1998). CD68-expressing macrophages in the vicinity of the lamina elastica interna are prone to produce MMP-2 as well as MMP-9. Such metalloproteinases almost certainly are the mechanisms underlying the typical fragmentation of the elastic membranes. So far, macrophages captured in the intima have not been assigned to particular injury pathways (Weyand et al., 1996). They have been described as staining positive for NOS-2, but downstream effects of nitrosative stress have not been detected in the intima itself.

Progress in macrophage biology has led to the identification of functionally different macrophage populations, including proinflammatory M1 macrophages and reparative M2 macrophages. IL-33, a cytokine associated with M2 polarization, has been localized in temporal artery biopsies (Ciccia et al., 2013). Why tissue-damaging macrophages functions dominate the vasculitic lesions remains unexplored.

Intimal Hyperplasia

Blockage of the vascular lumen by hyperplastic intima is the mechanism through which GCA causes vascular insufficiency and tissue ischemia (Figure 73.2). Myofibroblasts in the intima proliferate and deposit matrix. They have migrated to the intima from deeper wall layers, either the media or the adventitia. Factors regulating myofibroblast migration and differentiation thus have gatekeeper function in the disease process.

Inflamed temporal artery walls produce platelet-derived growth factor (PDGF), which derives from at least two cell types, CD68^{+} macrophages and resident wall cells (Kaiser et al., 1999). Numerically, the most important sources are macrophages in the media, often close to the lamina elastica interna. Multinucleated giant cells can also produce this growth factor. Fibroblast growth factor has been described to be present in vasculitic lesions; its function is unexplored.

The outgrowth of the expanding intimal layer needs to be supported by the formation of new blood vessels (Kaiser et al., 1998; Cid, 2002). Neoangiogenesis typically affects the media and the hyperplastic intima. Newly formed blood vessels are highly organized. Multinucleated giant cells have been found to secrete vascular endothelial growth factor (VEGF) (Kaiser et al., 1998). In essence, tissue-infiltrating macrophages appear to have a critical role in regulating the process of intimal proliferation and neoangiogenesis. Interestingly, VEGF production is correlated with IFN-γ production, thereby connecting the wall remodeling in the intima and media with the adaptive immune responses in the adventitia.

Immuno-stromal Interactions Promoting Vasculitis

While the immune system participates in vasculitic responses through a multitude of mechanisms, the blood vessel wall is not just an innocent bystander. Vascular cells, including vascular smooth muscle cells (VSMC) and endothelial cells, contribute to the intramural inflammation. Specifically, expression of receptors and ligands of the NOTCH family of molecules enables VSMC to directly communicate with infiltrating T cells and regulate their activity. The majority of CD4 T cells in GCA patients are spontaneously positive for NOTCH1, a receptor that binds to VSMC-expressed ligands in the lesions (Piggott et al., 2011). Blockade of the NOTCH signaling pathway has profound immunosuppressive effects, emphasizing the relevance of T cell–VSMC communications in GCA.

The Systemic Inflammatory Syndrome

Mechanisms driving the systemic inflammatory component of GCA are less well understood. Patients with PMR in whom vascular inflammatory infiltrates are undetectable by standard histology are equally affected by systemic inflammation as GCA patients with full-fledged vasculitis (Wagner et al., 1994; Weyand et al., 1999). This clinical constellation has supported the concept that systemic inflammation is not a "spillover" from the vasculitis.

Typical findings include a massive acute phase response with manifestations in multiple organ systems (Weyand and Goronzy, 2003a). Patients show signs of abnormalities in hematopoiesis, such as anemia and thrombocytosis. Liver function is often abnormal and shows elevation of alkaline phosphatase levels. By affecting the central nervous system, the acute phase response causes fever, malaise, and depression. Profound elevation of the erythrocyte sedimentation rate (ESR), a typical laboratory marker of GCA, is also a consequence of excessive production of acute phase proteins.

The only known pathomechanism related to the systemic inflammatory syndrome is the production of high amounts of IL-6 (Roche et al., 1993; Wagner et al., 1994; Weyand et al., 2000), a cytokine that has been implicated in inducing acute phase proteins in hepatocytes. In patients with GCA, as well as those with PMR, circulating monocytes are found to be spontaneously activated and produce IL-6 (Wagner et al., 1994). These data suggest initiator function of an activated innate immune system in the syndrome.

Elegant studies in interstitial fluids collected from PMR-affected muscles have shown local enrichment of proinflammatory cytokines and pain-inducing substances, such as glutamate and PGE(2), strongly supporting a pathogenic role of intramuscular abnormalities as a local manifestation of a systemic process (Kreiner et al., 2010; Kreiner and Galbo, 2011).

Treatment, Monitoring, and Outcome

The gold standard for treatment of GCA is the use of corticosteroids. Patients respond explicitly well, with prompt and substantial improvement of symptoms within 24—48 hours. Initial doses of 60 mg of prednisone (or approx. 1 mg per kg body weight) have been found to be effective in almost all patients. Indeed, current discussions center on the question of whether at least some patients could be successfully treated with lower doses (Chevalet et al., 2000).

Once patients are stabilized on high doses of corticosteroids, daily prednisolone doses should be tapered. A reduction of 10—20% every 2 weeks has proven to be a clinically useful guidance. Both clinical symptoms and laboratory markers of inflammation are monitored to guide the tapering process. There is preliminary evidence that IL-6 is a more sensitive marker of disease activity than ESR, but properly designed clinical trials have not been performed (Weyand et al., 2000). A frequent clinical dilemma is a discrepancy between clinical and laboratory findings. To avoid overutilization of corticosteroids, it has been recommended that treatment decisions should not be solely based on laboratory results.

Many patients develop signs of flaring disease when corticosteroids are reduced. Fortunately, severe manifestations, such as sight-threatening ischemic complications, appear to be rare (Weyand et al., 2000; Martinez-Lado et al., 2011). Instead, most disease flares present as PMR or constitutional symptoms. Dose adjustments of corticosteroids can effectively recapture disease control.

Corticosteroids can be discontinued in many patients after about 2 years of therapy. There is evidence that the disease process does not enter remission but continues

with smoldering activity (Uddhammar, 2000; Weyand et al., 2000, 2012). Whether that chronic state of inflammation requires continued immunosuppression or can be managed by watchful monitoring remains a matter of discussion.

One of the serious long-term consequences of GCA is the development of aortic aneurysm (Evans et al., 1994; Kermani et al., 2012). Patients need to be informed about this complication, and monitoring for aortic wall thickness and aortic dimension has been recommended (Mackie et al., 2012). However, population-based data estimating the risk for aortic aneurysm development are lacking and it is unknown whether continuous immunosuppression can prevent aortic wall damage.

With an average age of almost 75 years at disease onset and the duration of therapy for several years, patients are prone to show steroid side effects (Proven et al., 2003). Monitoring of blood glucose and blood pressure is obvious. Also, bone sparing therapy with calcium, vitamin D substitution, bisphosphonates, etc. should be a fixed component of management.

Given the high rate of steroid side effects, efforts have been made to identify steroid-sparing therapies. In an experimental model of GCA with human temporal arteries implanted into immunodeficient mice, aspirin effectively suppressed IFN-γ production and augmented the anti-inflammatory effects of corticosteroids (Weyand et al., 2002). In contrast to other chronic inflammatory diseases, patients with GCA seem not to benefit from methotrexate as an immunosuppressant. Although results of clinical trials have been controversial, a well-designed clinical study with a large cohort of patients could not demonstrate any advantage for methotrexate/corticosteroid combination therapy compared to corticosteroids alone (Jover et al., 2001; Spiera et al., 2001; Hoffman et al., 2002). A meta-analysis has suggested a mild steroid-sparing effect of MTX after 48 weeks of combination therapy for female but not for male patients (Mahr et al., 2007). Similar modest effects have been reported for azathioprine as a steroid-sparing agent (De Silva and Hazleman, 1986). While anti-TNF biologics provide powerful immunosuppression in patients with rheumatoid arthritis, clinical trials testing the use of a combination therapy with corticosteroids plus infliximab compared to corticosteroids alone have been disappointing (Hoffman et al., 2007; Salvarani et al., 2007) and TNF-α blockade is not considered a first-line therapy in this vasculitis. Considering the role of IL-6 as an inducer of the acute phase response, blocking IL-6 has been pursued as a means of treating GCA and encouraging results have been reported for seven patients with large-vessel GCA (Seitz et al., 2011). In more recent reports, results were much less impressive with sustained aortic wall inflammation in patients with

Takayasu's arteritis (Xenitidis et al., 2013). Whether these differences reflect differential response patterns of GCA and TA needs to be addressed in appropriately designed clinical trials. Predictions based on recent progress in understanding the immunopathogenesis of GCA would point towards the importance of IL-6 independent disease mechanisms which cannot be controlled by IL-6 blockade.

Overall, the outcome of GCA is good. No shortening of life expectancy has been reported, emphasizing that highly aggressive therapies may have to be used with caution (Matteson et al., 1996; Gran et al., 2001).

TAKAYASU'S ARTERITIS

Takayasu's arteritis (TA) is a systemic arteritis that predominantly manifests in the aorta and its major branches. It is also known as pulseless disease or occlusive thromboaortopathy. The typical patient is a female of Asian or South American origin presenting with vascular insufficiency and generalized inflammation in the second or third decades of life. But care has to be taken not to miss the diagnosis in males and middle-aged individuals. Inflammatory infiltrates in the wall of large elastic arteries induce thickening of the adventitia, destruction of the media, and hyperplasia of the intima (Figure 73.3) (Gravanis, 2000). Recently, diagnosis and management of TA have benefited from advances in noninvasive imaging methods and more aggressive use of surgical procedures (Luqmani, 2012). Over the last decade, the prognosis of TA has continued to improve with more rapid diagnosis, more aggressive immunosuppression, and fewer vaso-occlusive complications (Ohigashi et al., 2012).

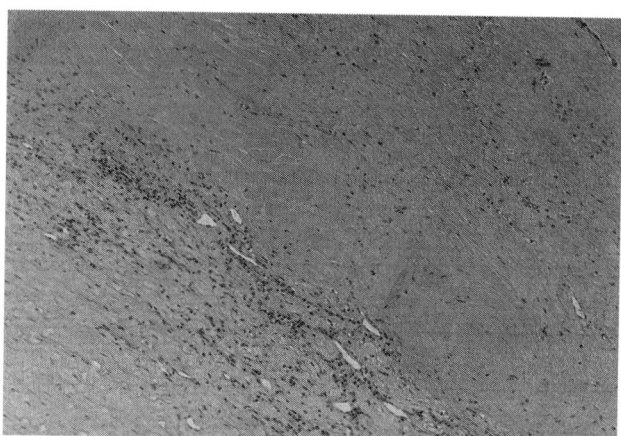

FIGURE 73.3 Takayasu's arteritis. Cross-section of an innominate artery. Note transmural round cell infiltration with dominance of inflammation along the media—adventitia border. Extensive neovascularization has occurred in the media. The adventitia slows fibrotic expansion.

Historical Background

In 1830, Rokushu Yamamoto reported the first case of TA. In 1905, Mikito Takayasu was the first to describe peculiar optic fundus abnormalities with coronal anastomosis (Takayasu, 1908), which 40 years later were interpreted as neovascularization and anastomosis secondary to ischemia caused by the occlusion of cervical vessels. In 1951, Shimizu and Sano described a cohort of 31 cases and made the connection between pulselessness, coronal anastomosis of retinal vessels, and carotid abnormalities and called it pulseless disease (Shimizu and Sano, 1951).

Clinical, Pathologic, and Epidemiologic Features

Takayasu's arteritis is a rare disease with incidence rates of 1—2 cases in 1 million individuals per year (Watts et al., 2009). The most significant risk factors are female sex, age less than 40 years, and selected ethnic origin. The highest prevalence rates have been reported for Asian countries, including Japan, Korea, China, India, Thailand, and Turkey (Koide, 1992). South American countries, such as Mexico, Brazil, Columbia and Peru, are now also considered higher incidence areas (Dabague and Reyes, 1996). The disease does occur in whites, can affect males, and needs to be kept in mind as a differential diagnosis in older individuals with aortitis or large vessel vasculitis.

Prominent histomorphologic findings include the thickening of the aortic wall which may involve all three layers (see Figure 73.3) but often is most significant in the adventitia (Gravanis, 2000; Bjornsson, 2002). Extensions of inflammatory infiltrates and fibrosis into the periaortic tissues are not unusual. Most often, the aortic lumen is compromised, but stenotic lesions can alternate with aneurysmal dilatation giving rise to fusiform or saccular aneurysms. Also characteristic are "skipped" areas with normal vessel wall next to densely inflamed regions. Besides the aorta and its primary branches, coronary and pulmonary arteries can be involved.

Microscopic examination shows inflammatory infiltrates composed of lymphocytes and plasma cells primarily around the vasa vasorum, causing vasa vasoritis with lumenal stenosis. Lymphocytes, plasma cells, and occasional giant cells accumulate in the media, sometimes complicating the distinction between GCA and TA (Gravanis, 2000). Patches of medial necrosis can occur, and destruction of elastic membranes is typical. Growth of fibroblasts and smooth muscle cells and deposition of acid mucopolysaccharides result in widening of the intimal layer, similar to that found in fibromuscular hyperplasia. Vascular insufficiency in the aortic branches is related to ostial stenosis or more extended involvement.

TABLE 73.3 The Clinical Spectrum in Takayasu's Arteritis

Organ system	Sign/Symptom	Frequency (%)
Vascular	Bruit	70
	Claudication	70
	Reduced/absent pulses	60
	Asymmetrical blood pressure	50
CNS	Dizziness	40
	Visual abnormalities	30
	Stroke/TIA	10
Constitutional	Malaise	70
	Fever	30
	Weight loss	20
Cardiac	Aortic regurgitation	20
	Angina	10
	Congestive heart failure	<5

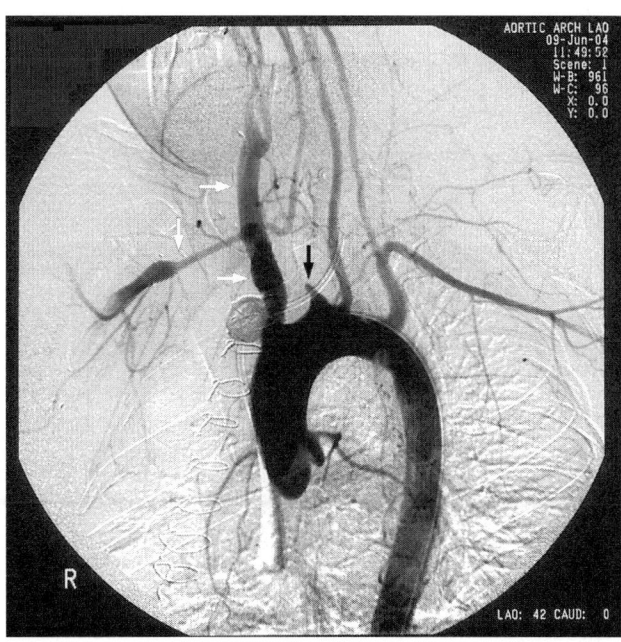

FIGURE 73.4 **Takayasu's arteritis. Angiography of the aortic arch and the cervical vessels.** The native brachiocephalic artery (black arrow) is occluded just distal to its origin. A graft has been placed (white arrows) from the ascending aorta to the right common carotid artery with a separate limb connecting to the right subclavian artery. The left carotid artery and both vertebral arteries are normal.

Available data suggest that the clinical spectrum of TA is different in distinct geographic areas (Numano, 1997). Japanese, Korean, and North American patients are more likely to present with impairment of cervical, cerebral, and upper extremity blood flow and aortic regurgitation, due to involvement of the ascending aorta and the primary aortic arch branches. Conversely, in Indian patients, the abdominal aorta, including the renal arteries, appears to be the preferred target resulting in renovascular hypertension. Overall, blindness and severe retinal ischemia are less common now than they used to be (Numano, 2002).

Initial presentation may be dominated by a generalized inflammatory syndrome with fever, night sweats, weakness, arthralgias, and chest pain (Kerr et al., 1994). Direct complications of vessel wall inflammation include headaches, syncope, visual disturbances, and face and neck pain from insufficient blood flow in the cervical vessels (see Table 73.3). Stenotic lesions in the brachiocephalic and subclavian arteries lead to arm claudication, pulselessness, and discrepant blood pressure measurements (Figure 73.4). Ischemic heart disease is a result of reduction in coronary blood flow. A feared complication of TA is aortic regurgitation caused by dilatation of the ascending aorta. Congestive heart failure is not unusual (Endo et al., 2003).

Marked progress has been made in imaging modalities, compensating at least partially for the difficulties in accessing tissue to establish the diagnosis of TA and follow its course for patients receiving therapy. Besides conventional angiography, which has been the standard imaging tool for diagnosing and evaluating patients with

TA (see Figure 73.4), a number of alternatives have emerged, including magnetic resonance (MR) imaging and MR angiography, computed tomography (CT), Doppler ultrasound, and metabolic imaging with positron emission tomography (PET) (Kissin and Merkel, 2004; Litmanovich et al., 2012; Tezuka et al., 2012; Cheng et al., 2013;). Ultrasound is particularly useful in evaluating the carotid arteries, with high sensitivity for submillimeter changes in wall thickness. The diffuse circumferential thickening (halo) of the carotid artery wall in TA has been named the "macaroni sign" (Keo et al., 2013). CT and MR imaging provide excellent visualization of vessels and their relationship to neighboring structures and demonstrate both lumenal and mural abnormalities. Contrast enhancement is necessary for the CT to depict the vessel lumen, but it can provide fast information about the aorta and its wall; MR imaging has inherent multiplanar imaging capabilities, can be used with or without contrast enhancement, and lends itself to the evaluation of the aorta and its major branches (Matsunaga et al., 2003; Nastri et al., 2004). With the potential to assess mural edema and vascularity, it has been hoped that it would be an ideal instrument to monitor disease activity and progress in patients on immunosuppression. However, a recent study has cast doubt on the utility of edema-weighted MR as a sole means to estimate disease activity (Tso et al., 2002). A role for PET, which detects areas of active glucose metabolism in the vascular wall in identifying early disease, has been suggested (Webb et al., 2004), but no large-scale controlled studies are available. A recent study has reported only moderate sensitivity of 18FDG-PET in estimating disease activity in TA (Cheng et al., 2013), whereas a study of 39 Japanese patients with TA suggested superiority of FDG-PET/CT over use of ESR and CRP values in detecting active disease (Tezuka et al., 2012).

Genetic Features

Like GCA, TA is an HLA-associated disease (Kerr et al., 1994; Salazar et al., 2000). More than half of the Japanese patients carry the HLA A24-B52-DR2 haplotype (Kimura et al., 1996). Nonpolymorphic HLA molecules, specifically MICA, have also been reported to be enriched among patients (Kimura et al., 1998).

Pathogenic Mechanisms

Despite considerable overlap in the histomorphology and clinical presentation of GCA and TA, evidence suggests that pathogenic mechanisms are distinct (Seko, 2002) (Figure 73.5). Whereas CD4$^+$ T cells producing IFN-γ have been identified as key regulators in the vascular

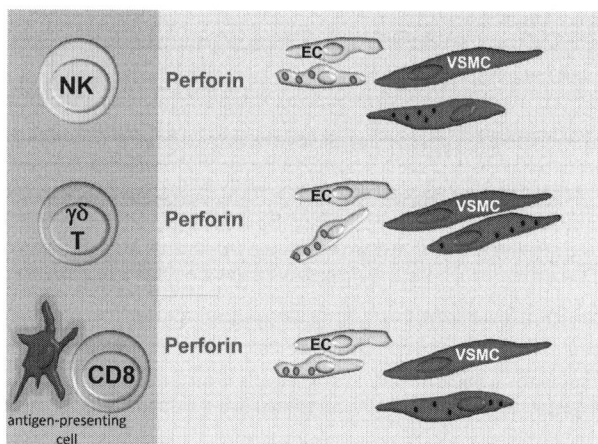

FIGURE 73.5 Immune-mediated tissue damage in Takayasu's arteritis. Multiple damage pathways in the wall of the inflamed aorta have been identified in Takayasu's arteritis. A common denominator is the production of the cytolytic mediator perforin, which allows for cell-mediated cytotoxicity. Damage of VSMC leads to loss of the tunica media. Injury of endothelial cells may cause local ischemia and tissue necrosis. The triggers of perforin release by NK cells and $\gamma\delta$ T cells is not known. Perforin release by CD8 T cells involves recognition of HLA class I molecules and antigen on the surface of antigen-presenting cells (APC).

lesions of GCA, they appear to be less important in TA. In the vascular infiltrates of TA, $\gamma\delta$ T cells account for 31% of the cells, natural killer cells for 20%, and CD8$^+$ cytotoxic T cells for 15% (Seko, 2000). CD4$^+$ T cells, macrophages, and B cells were less frequent. In support for the concept that cytotoxic cells directly damage resident cells in the aorta, Seko et al. (1994) have shown cellular expression of perforin and deposition of perforin directly onto wall resident cells. Heat shock proteins, in particular HSP65, have been proposed as the antigen stimulating cytotoxic lymphocytes (Seko et al., 2000). Restricted usage of T cell receptor AV and BV genes in tissue infiltrating T cells also supports the concept of selective expansion of antigen-reactive T cells in the vessel wall infiltrates (Seko et al., 1996). Dense expression of costimulatory molecules is in line with a role for adaptive immune responses driving the disease process. Data suggesting a possible role of metalloproteinases as biomarkers of disease activities refocuses interest on macrophage-dependent disease mechanisms (Matsuyama et al., 2003). Destruction of elastic membranes points towards release of elastolytic enzymes, likely derived from tissue-infiltrating macrophages.

Much less is known about the pathomechanism of the systemic inflammatory syndrome. Cytokine levels of IL-6 and RANTES have been reported to be elevated and to correlate with clinical activity (Noris et al., 1999). Serum IL-18 levels have been correlated with disease activity (Park et al., 2006). IL-18 is a Th1 immunity promoting cytokine, suggesting a role for IFN-γ-producing T cells in this vasculitis. Possible, not yet validated biomarkers of disease activity include pentraxin-3 and MMP-9.

Treatment and Outcome

Immunosuppressive therapy remains the mainstay of treatment for this arteritis, but, in contrast to GCA, surgical procedures are gaining in importance for managing patients with TA (Perrotta et al., 2012). While endovascular treatment of TA has been associated with poor outcomes with respect to patency, more recent experience with newer endovascular techniques appears to be associated with better results (Qureshi et al., 2011).

As with most rare diseases, randomized controlled treatment trials are explicitly difficult to perform, are missing, or are based on small patient numbers. The immunosuppressants of choice are corticosteroids, which are started at a dose of 40−60 mg/day prednisone. Clinicians in Japan have advocated doses of only 20−30 mg/day (Numano, 2002). Once acute disease activity is controlled, an effort needs to be made to reduce corticosteroids. Tapering by 5 mg/day every 2−3 weeks has been adopted as a useful guideline. However, there has been agreement that a target maintenance dose of

5–10 mg/day should be kept stable over a prolonged period to avoid exacerbation of vascular and generalized inflammation. Although not formally tested, most patients receive aspirin or an alternative agent to reduce platelet aggregation and thrombus formation.

About 50% of patients may be considered to be insufficiently treated with corticosteroid monotherapy (Kerr et al., 1994). Some of these patients may benefit from methotrexate as a steroid-sparing agent (Hoffman et al., 1994). Mycophenolate mofetil has been reported to show clinical efficiency in a small patient cohort (Daina et al., 1999). TNF-α blocking agents have been reported to induce sustained remission in a subset of patients, but about 50% of patients fail treatment with anti-TNF-α (Schmidt et al., 2012). Given the role of IL-6 in driving inflammation in TA, rescue therapy with anti-IL-6 blocking antibodies has been reported for selected cases (Salvarani et al., 2012). More recent reports of persistent aortic wall inflammation despite IL-6-blocking therapy have raised concerns that this therapeutic approach may be less effective than expected (Xenitidis et al., 2013).

Monitoring for and managing hypertension is prudent in patients with TA. There is an ongoing discussion about whether vascular inflammation predisposes for the accelerated development and progression of atherosclerosis, although it may be difficult to separate these disease processes (Numano et al., 2000). Accelerated atherosclerosis demands appropriate monitoring for risk factors and treatment of dyslipidemia.

Critical renal artery stenosis, limiting claudication of extremities, cerebrovascular ischemia, coronary ischemia, and aortic regurgitation may represent indications for surgical intervention. If clinically possible, quiescence of vascular inflammation should be aimed for prior to surgery. Prevention of stroke may be possible if critical stenosis of cervical vessels is bypassed with grafts originating from the ascending aorta. Percutaneous transluminal angioplasty has emerged as an alternative to bypass surgery, specifically for renal artery stenosis (Weaver et al., 2004), and may be useful for preserving the competence of vessels in other territories.

The best outcome data for TA are available from Japan where all patients with TA are registered by the government. Analysis of 897 patients through 1998 showed that more than 70% of patients had well-controlled disease, enjoying almost normal lives. Twenty-five percent of patients had severe complications. Cardiac manifestations have become the most common cause of death among TA patients (Numano, 2002). Modern imaging techniques are enabling close monitoring of vessel wall inflammation. The time between disease onset and diagnosis is shortening (Isobe, 2013) and the overall prognosis is improving.

CONCLUDING REMARKS—FUTURE PERSPECTIVES

Vasculitides are infrequent yet clinically challenging diseases because they threaten blood supply to vital organs. Damage to large and medium-sized arteries immediately puts the host at risk for severe clinical consequences, as compensatory mechanisms for losing the function of the aorta and its major branches are very limited. In contrast to noninflammatory vasculopathies, arteritides are characterized by a combination of ischemic tissue damage and a syndrome of generalized inflammation. Pathogenic mechanisms relevant for these two dimensions of disease may be distinct and respond differentially to therapy. Systemic inflammation is caused by the excessive production of cytokines. In the cases of GCA and TA, induction of an abrupt and massive acute phase response is typical. As part of the acute phase response, patients produce hepatic acute phase proteins that give rise to diagnostically important laboratory abnormalities, such as increases in ESR and C-reactive protein (CRP).

In both GCA and TA, T lymphocytes are the key regulators of tissue injury in the blood vessel wall. They either mediate direct cellular damage, as in the case of TA, or orchestrate the functional activity of tissue-injurious macrophages, as in GCA. Arterial wall injury causes hyperproliferation of myofibroblasts and results in thickening of the intima, the underlying mechanism of vessel stenosis/occlusion. In GCA, tissue-resident dendritic cells have been implicated in initiating T cell activation, possibly after being triggered by blood-borne stimuli (Weyand et al., 2011). There is no evidence that autoantibodies or other B cell-dependent functions contribute to large vessel vasculitis (Martinez-Taboada et al., 1996).

Giant cell arteritis and TA are unique among the chronic inflammatory diseases in that they respond very well to corticosteroids. However, even prolonged therapy can usually not induce complete remission, and side effects are common. So far, alternative immunosuppressive agents have been amazingly ineffective in treating GCA but may have a role in TA. Major progress could be made by targeting disease pathways, such as the oxidative damage of vessel wall resident cells, and the process of intimal hyperplasia (Weyand and Goronzy, 2003a).

Despite advances in noninvasive imaging methods, monitoring patients for disease activity still remains a challenge. Cytokines may be useful biomarkers in assessing the "burden of disease," at least as far as the systemic inflammatory syndrome is concerned. Well-designed clinical trials are necessary to validate the use of cytokine levels, particularly for IL-6, as a marker of disease in patients.

The ultimate challenge in understanding GCA and TA remains the identification of the initial triggers of the disease process. Although infections have been suspected, scientific evidence for their role in starting arteritis is lacking (Regan et al., 2002; Nordborg and Nordborg, 2003). Local factors intrinsic to the artery itself, such as dendritic cells positioned in the adventitia of medium-sized and large arteries, may be instrumental in breaking tolerance and giving rise to misplaced immune responses (Ma-Krupa et al., 2004; Pryshchep et al., 2008). Also, age is a major risk factor in GCA and TA, suggesting that age-related changes in T cell function may be critical determinants of disease susceptibility (Miller, 1990; Weyand and Goronzy, 2003a; Goronzy and Weyand, 2013).

ACKNOWLEDGMENT

Supported in part by grants from the National Institutes of Health (AR42527, AI44142, AI57266, and EY11916).

REFERENCES

Alvarez-Rodriguez, L., Munoz Cacho, P., Lopez-Hoyos, M., Beares, I., Mata, C., Calvo-Alen, J., et al., 2011. Toll-like receptor 4 gene polymorphism and giant cell arteritis susceptibility: a cumulative meta-analysis. Autoimmun. Rev. 10, 790−792.

Andersson, R., Jonsson, R., Tarkowski, A., Bengtsson, B.A., Malmvall, B.E., 1987. T cell subsets and expression of immunological activation markers in the arterial walls of patients with giant cell arteritis. Ann. Rheum. Dis. 46, 915−923.

Baldursson, O., Steinsson, K., Bjornsson, J., Lie, J.T., 1994. Giant cell arteritis in Iceland. An epidemiologic and histopathologic analysis. Arthritis. Rheum. 37, 1007−1012.

Bjornsson, J., 2002. Histopathology of primary vasculitis disorders. In: Hoffman, G.S., Weyand, C.M. (Eds.), Inflammatory Diseases of Blood Vessels. Marcel Dekker, Inc., New York, pp. 255−265.

Borkowski, A., Younge, B.R., Szweda, L., Mock, B., Bjornsson, J., Moeller, K., et al., 2002. Reactive nitrogen intermediates in giant cell arteritis: selective nitration of neocapillaries. Am. J. Pathol. 161, 115−123.

Brack, A., Geisler, A., Martinez-Taboada, V.M., Younge, B.R., Goronzy, J.J., Weyand, C.M., 1997. Giant cell vasculitis is a T cell-dependent disease. Mol. Med. 3, 530−543.

Brack, A., Martinez-Taboada, V., Stanson, A., Goronzy, J.J., Weyand, C.M., 1999. Disease pattern in cranial and large-vessel giant cell arteritis. Arthritis Rheum. 42, 311−317.

Chan, C.C., Paine, M., O'Day, J., 2005. Predictors of recurrent ischemic optic neuropathy in giant cell arteritis. J. Neuroophthalmol. 25, 14−17.

Chatelain, D., Duhaut, P., Loire, R., Bosshard, S., Pellet, H., Piette, J.C., et al., 2008. Small-vessel vasculitis surrounding an uninflamed temporal artery: a new diagnostic criterion for polymyalgia rheumatica? Arthritis Rheum. 58, 2565−2573.

Cheng, Y., Lv, N., Wang, Z., Chen, B., Dang, A., 2013. 18FDG-PET in assessing disease activity in Takayasu arteritis: a meta-analysis. Clin. Exp. Rheumatol. 31 (1 Suppl 75), S22−S27.

Chevalet, P., Barrier, J.H., Pottier, P., Magadur-Joly, G., Pottier, M.A., Hamidou, M., et al., 2000. A randomized, multicenter, controlled trial using intravenous pulses of methylprednisolone in the initial treatment of simple forms of giant cell arteritis: a one year followup study of 164 patients. J. Rheumatol. 27, 1484−1491.

Ciccia, F., Alessandro, R., Rizzo, A., Raimondo, S., Giardina, A., Raiata, F., et al., 2013. IL-33 is overexpressed in the inflamed arteries of patients with giant cell arteritis. Ann. Rheum. Dis. 72, 258−264.

Cid, M.C., 2002. Endothelial cell biology, perivascular inflammation, and vasculitis. Cleve. Clin. J. Med. 69 (Suppl 2), SII45−SII49.

Dabague, J., Reyes, P.A., 1996. Takayasu arteritis in Mexico: a 38-year clinical perspective through literature review. Int. J. Cardiol. 54 (Suppl), S103−S109.

Daina, E., Schieppati, A., Remuzzi, G., 1999. Mycophenolate mofetil for the treatment of Takayasu arteritis: report of three cases. Ann. Intern. Med. 130, 422−426.

Dasgupta, B., Cimmino, M.A., Kremers, H.M., Schmidt, W.A., Schirmer, M., Salvarani, C., et al., 2012. 2012 Provisional classification criteria for polymyalgia rheumatica: a European League Against Rheumatism/American College of Rheumatology collaborative initiative. Arthritis Rheum. 64, 943−954.

de Jong, H.J., Saldi, S.R., Klungel, O.H., Vandebriel, R.J., Souverein, P. C., Meyboom, R.H., et al., 2012. Statin-associated polymyalgia rheumatica. An analysis using WHO global individual case safety database: a case/non-case approach. PLoS One. 7, e41289.

De Silva, M., Hazleman, B.L., 1986. Azathioprine in giant cell arteritis/polymyalgia rheumatica: a double-blind study. Ann. Rheum. Dis. 45, 136−138.

Deng, J., Younge, B.R., Olshen, R.A., Goronzy, J.J., Weyand, C.M., 2010. Th17 and Th1 T-cell responses in giant cell arteritis. Circulation. 121, 906−915.

Doran, M.F., Crowson, C.S., O'Fallon, W.M., Hunder, G.G., Gabriel, S.E., 2002. Trends in the incidence of polymyalgia rheumatica over a 30 year period in Olmsted County, Minnesota, USA. J. Rheumatol. 29, 1694−1697.

Endo, M., Tomizawa, Y., Nishida, H., Aomi, S., Nakazawa, M., Tsurumi, Y., et al., 2003. Angiographic findings and surgical treatments of coronary artery involvement in Takayasu arteritis. J. Thorac. Cardiovasc. Surg. 125, 570−577.

Evans, J.M., Hunder, G.G., 2000. Polymyalgia rheumatica and giant cell arteritis. Rheum. Dis. Clin. North Am. 26, 493−515.

Evans, J.M., Bowles, C.A., Bjornsson, J., Mullany, C.J., Hunder, G.G., 1994. Thoracic aortic aneurysm and rupture in giant cell arteritis. A descriptive study of 41 cases. Arthritis Rheum. 37, 1539−1547.

Gonzalez, E.B., Varner, W.T., Lisse, J.R., Daniels, J.C., Hokanson, J.A., 1989. Giant-cell arteritis in the southern United States. An 11-year retrospective study from the Texas Gulf Coast. Arch. Intern. Med. 149, 1561−1565.

Goronzy, J.J., Weyand, C.M., 2013. Understanding immunosenescence to improve responses to vaccines. Nat. Immunol. 14, 428−436.

Gran, J.T., Myklebust, G., Wilsgaard, T., Jacobsen, B.K., 2001. Survival in polymyalgia rheumatica and temporal arteritis: a study of 398 cases and matched population controls. Rheumatology (Oxford). 40,

1238—1242.

Gravanis, M.B., 2000. Giant cell arteritis and Takayasu aortitis: morphologic, pathogenetic and etiologic factors. Int. J. Cardiol. 75 (Suppl 1), S21—S33, discussion S35—S36.

Henriet, J.P., Marin, J., Gosselin, J., Hamel-Desnos, C., Ducrocq, M., Brard, G., et al., 1989. The history of Horton's disease or…10 centuries of a fascinating adventure. J. Mal. Vasc. 14 (Suppl C), 93—97.

Hernandez-Rodriguez, J., Segarra, M., Vilardell, C., Sanchez, M., Garcia-Martinez, A., Esteban, M.J., et al., 2004. Tissue production of pro-inflammatory cytokines (IL-1beta, TNFalpha and IL-6) correlates with the intensity of the systemic inflammatory response and with corticosteroid requirements in giant-cell arteritis. Rheumatology (Oxford). 43, 294—301.

Hoffman, G.S., Leavitt, R.Y., Kerr, G.S., Rottem, M., Sneller, M.C., Fauci, A.S., 1994. Treatment of glucocorticoid-resistant or relapsing Takayasu arteritis with methotrexate. Arthritis Rheum. 37, 578—582.

Hoffman, G.S., Cid, M.C., Hellmann, D.B., Guillevin, L., Stone, J.H., Schousboe, J., et al., 2002. A multicenter, randomized, double-blind, placebo-controlled trial of adjuvant methotrexate treatment for giant cell arteritis. Arthritis Rheum. 46, 1309—1318.

Hoffman, G.S., Cid, M.C., Rendt-Zagar, K.E., Merkel, P.A., Weyand, C.M., Stone, J.H., et al., 2007. Infliximab for maintenance of glucocorticosteroid-induced remission of giant cell arteritis: a randomized trial. Ann. Intern. Med. 146, 621—630.

Horton, B.T., Magath, T.B., Brown, G.E., 1932. An undescribed form of arteritis of the temporal vessels. P. Staff M. Mayo Clin. 7, 700—701.

Hutchinson, J., 1890. Diseases of the arteries. On a peculiar form of thrombolic arteritis of the aged which is sometimes productive of gangrene. Arch. Surg. 1, 323—329.

Isobe, M., 2013. Takayasu arteritis revisited: current diagnosis and treatment. Int. J. Cardiol. 168, 3—10.

Jover, J.A., Hernandez-Garcia, C., Morado, I.C., Vargas, E., Banares, A., Fernandez-Gutierrez, B., 2001. Combined treatment of giant-cell arteritis with methotrexate and prednisone. a randomized, double-blind, placebo-controlled trial. Ann. Intern. Med. 134, 106—114.

Kaiser, M., Weyand, C.M., Bjornsson, J., Goronzy, J.J., 1998. Platelet-derived growth factor, intimal hyperplasia, and ischemic complications in giant cell arteritis. Arthritis Rheum. 41, 623—633.

Kaiser, M., Younge, B., Bjornsson, J., Goronzy, J.J., Weyand, C.M., 1999. Formation of new vasa vasorum in vasculitis. Production of angiogenic cytokines by multinucleated giant cells. Am. J. Pathol. 155, 765—774.

Keo, H.H., Caliezi, G., Baumgartner, I., Diehm, N., Willenberg, T., 2013. Increasing echogenicity of diffuse circumferential thickening ("macaroni sign") of the carotid artery wall with decreasing inflammatory activity of Takayasu arteritis. J. Clin. Ultrasound. 41, 59—62.

Kermani, T.A., Warrington, K.J., 2013. Polymyalgia rheumatica. Lancet. 381, 63—72.

Kermani, T.A., Warrington, K.J., Crowson, C.S., Ytterberg, S.R., Hunder, G.G., Gabriel, S.E., et al., 2012. Large-vessel involvement in giant cell arteritis: a population-based cohort study of the incidence-trends and prognosis. Ann. Rheum. Dis. doi:10.1136/annrheumdis-2012-202408.

Kerr, G.S., Hallahan, C.W., Giordano, J., Leavitt, R.Y., Fauci, A.S., Rottem, M., et al., 1994. Takayasu arteritis. Ann. Intern. Med. 120, 919—929.

Kimura, A., Kitamura, H., Date, Y., Numano, F., 1996. Comprehensive analysis of HLA genes in Takayasu arteritis in Japan. Int. J. Cardiol. 54 (Suppl), S61—S69.

Kimura, A., Kobayashi, Y., Takahashi, M., Ohbuchi, N., Kitamura, H., Nakamura, T., et al., 1998. MICA gene polymorphism in Takayasu's arteritis and Buerger's disease. Int. J. Cardiol. 66 (Suppl 1), S107—S113, discussion S115.

Kissin, E.Y., Merkel, P.A., 2004. Diagnostic imaging in Takayasu arteritis. Curr. Opin. Rheumatol. 16, 31—37.

Koide, K., 1992. Takayasu arteritis in Japan. Heart Vessels Suppl. 7, 48—54.

Kreiner, F., Galbo, H., 2011. Elevated muscle interstitial levels of pain-inducing substances in symptomatic muscles in patients with polymyalgia rheumatica. Pain. 152, 1127—1132.

Kreiner, F., Langberg, H., Galbo, H., 2010. Increased muscle interstitial levels of inflammatory cytokines in polymyalgia rheumatica. Arthritis Rheum. 62, 3768—3775.

Krupa, W.M., Dewan, M., Jeon, M.S., Kurtin, P.J., Younge, B.R., Goronzy, J.J., et al., 2002. Trapping of misdirected dendritic cells in the granulomatous lesions of giant cell arteritis. Am. J. Pathol. 161, 1815—1823.

Lie, J.T., 1995. Aortic and extracranial large vessel giant cell arteritis: a review of 72 cases with histopathologic documentation. Semin. Arthritis Rheum. 24, 422—431.

Litmanovich, D.E., Yildirim, A., Bankier, A.A., 2012. Insights into imaging of aortitis. Insights Imaging. 3, 545—560.

Luqmani, R., 2012. Large vessel vasculitides: update for the cardiologist. Curr. Opin. Cardiol. 27, 578—584.

Ma-Krupa, W., Jeon, M.S., Spoerl, S., Tedder, T.F., Goronzy, J.J., Weyand, C.M., 2004. Activation of arterial wall dendritic cells and breakdown of self-tolerance in giant cell arteritis. J. Exp. Med. 199, 173—183.

Machado, E.B., Michet, C.J., Ballard, D.J., Hunder, G.G., Beard, C.M., Chu, C.P., et al., 1988. Trends in incidence and clinical presentation of temporal arteritis in Olmsted County, Minnesota, 1950—1985. Arthritis Rheum. 31, 745—749.

Mackie, S.L., Hensor, E.M., Morgan, A.W., Pease, C.T., 2012. Should I send my patient with previous giant cell arteritis for imaging of the thoracic aorta? A systematic literature review and meta-analysis. Ann. Rheum. Dis. doi:10.1136/annrheumdis-2012-202145.

Mahr, A.D., Jover, J.A., Spiera, R.F., Hernandez-Garcia, C., Fernandez-Gutierrez, B., Lavalley, M.P., et al., 2007. Adjunctive methotrexate for treatment of giant cell arteritis: an individual patient data meta-analysis. Arthritis Rheum. 56, 2789—2797.

Martinez-Lado, L., Calvino-Diaz, C., Pineiro, A., Dierssen, T., Vazquez-Rodriguez, T.R., Miranda-Filloy, J.A., et al., 2011. Relapses and recurrences in giant cell arteritis: a population-based study of patients with biopsy-proven disease from northwestern Spain. Medicine (Baltimore). 90, 186—193.

Martinez-Taboada, V., Brack, A., Hunder, G.G., Goronzy, J.J., Weyand, C.M., 1996. The inflammatory infiltrate in giant cell arteritis selects against B lymphocytes. J. Rheumatol. 23, 1011—1014.

Matsunaga, N., Hayashi, K., Okada, M., Sakamoto, I., 2003. Magnetic resonance imaging features of aortic diseases. Top. Magn. Reson. Imaging. 14, 253—266.

Matsuyama, A., Sakai, N., Ishigami, M., Hiraoka, H., Kashine, S., Hirata, A., et al., 2003. Matrix metalloproteinases as novel disease markers in Takayasu arteritis. Circulation. 108, 1469—1473.

Matteson, E.L., Gold, K.N., Bloch, D.A., Hunder, G.G., 1996. Long-term survival of patients with Wegener's granulomatosis from the American College of Rheumatology Wegener's Granulomatosis Classification Criteria Cohort. Am. J. Med. 101, 129–134.

Miller, J.D., 1990. Fiberoptic pressure monitors. J. Neurosurg. 73, 642.

Mohan, S.V., Liao, Y.J., Kim, J.W., Goronzy, J.J., Weyand, C.M., 2011. Giant cell arteritis: immune and vascular aging as disease risk factors. Arthritis Res. Ther. 13, 231.

Nastri, M.V., Baptista, L.P., Baroni, R.H., Blasbalg, R., de Avila, L.F., Leite, C.C., et al., 2004. Gadolinium-enhanced three-dimensional MR angiography of Takayasu arteritis. Radiographics. 24, 773–786.

Nordborg, C., Johansson, H., Petursdottir, V., Nordborg, E., 2003. The epidemiology of biopsy-positive giant cell arteritis: special reference to changes in the age of the population. Rheumatology (Oxford). 42, 549–552.

Nordborg, E., Nordborg, C., 2003. Giant cell arteritis: epidemiological clues to its pathogenesis and an update on its treatment. Rheumatology (Oxford). 42, 413–421.

Noris, M., Daina, E., Gamba, S., Bonazzola, S., Remuzzi, G., 1999. Interleukin-6 and RANTES in Takayasu arteritis: a guide for therapeutic decisions? Circulation. 100, 55–60.

Numano, F., 1997. Differences in clinical presentation and outcome in different countries for Takayasu's arteritis. Curr. Opin. Rheumatol. 9, 12–15.

Numano, F., Kishi, Y., Tanaka, A., Ohkawara, M., Kakuta, T., Kobayashi, Y., 2000. Inflammation and atherosclerosis. Atherosclerotic lesions in Takayasu arteritis. Ann. N.Y. Acad. Sci. 902, 65–76.

Numano, F. (Ed.), 2002. Takayasu's Arteritis: Clinical Aspects. Marcel Dekker, Inc., New York.

Ohigashi, H., Haraguchi, G., Konishi, M., Tezuka, D., Kamiishi, T., Ishihara, T., et al., 2012. Improved prognosis of Takayasu arteritis over the past decade—comprehensive analysis of 106 patients. Circ. J. 76, 1004–1011.

Park, M.C., Lee, S.W., Park, Y.B., Lee, S.K., 2006. Serum cytokine profiles and their correlations with disease activity in Takayasu's arteritis. Rheumatology (Oxford). 45, 545–548.

Perrotta, S., Radberg, G., Perrotta, A., Lentini, S., 2012. Aneurysmatic disease in patients with Takayasu disease: a case review. Herz. 37, 347–353.

Piggott, K., Deng, J., Warrington, K., Younge, B., Kubo, J.T., Desai, M., et al., 2011. Blocking the NOTCH pathway inhibits vascular inflammation in large-vessel vasculitis. Circulation. 123, 309–318.

Proven, A., Gabriel, S.E., Orces, C., O'Fallon, W.M., Hunder, G.G., 2003. Glucocorticoid therapy in giant cell arteritis: duration and adverse outcomes. Arthritis Rheum. 49, 703–708.

Pryshchep, O., Ma-Krupa, W., Younge, B.R., Goronzy, J.J., Weyand, C.M., 2008. Vessel-specific Toll-like receptor profiles in human medium and large arteries. Circulation. 118, 1276–1284.

Qureshi, M.A., Martin, Z., Greenberg, R.K., 2011. Endovascular management of patients with Takayasu arteritis: stents versus stent grafts. Semin. Vasc. Surg. 24, 44–52.

Regan, M.J., Wood, B.J., Hsieh, Y.H., Theodore, M.L., Quinn, T.C., Hellmann, D.B., et al., 2002. Temporal arteritis and Chlamydia pneumoniae: failure to detect the organism by polymerase chain reaction in ninety cases and ninety controls. Arthritis Rheum. 46, 1056–1060.

Rittner, H.L., Hafner, V., Klimiuk, P.A., Szweda, L.I., Goronzy, J.J., Weyand, C.M., 1999a. Aldose reductase functions as a detoxification system for lipid peroxidation products in vasculitis. J. Clin. Invest. 103, 1007–1013.

Rittner, H.L., Kaiser, M., Brack, A., Szweda, L.I., Goronzy, J.J., Weyand, C.M., 1999b. Tissue-destructive macrophages in giant cell arteritis. Circ. Res. 84, 1050–1058.

Roche, N.E., Fulbright, J.W., Wagner, A.D., Hunder, G.G., Goronzy, J.J., Weyand, C.M., 1993. Correlation of interleukin-6 production and disease activity in polymyalgia rheumatica and giant cell arteritis. Arthritis Rheum. 36, 1286–1294.

Rodriguez-Rodriguez, L., Carmona, F.D., Castaneda, S., Miranda-Filloy, J.A., Morado, I.C., Narvaez, J., et al., 2011a. Role of rs1343151 IL23R and rs3790567 IL12RB2 polymorphisms in biopsy-proven giant cell arteritis. J. Rheumatol. 38, 889–892.

Rodriguez-Rodriguez, L., Castaneda, S., Vazquez-Rodriguez, T.R., Morado, I.C., Gomez-Vaquero, C., Mari-Alfonso, B., et al., 2011b. Role of the rs6822844 gene polymorphism at the IL2-IL21 region in biopsy-proven giant cell arteritis. Clin. Exp. Rheumatol. 29, S12–S16.

Rojo-Leyva, F., Ratliff, N.B., Cosgrove III, D.M., Hoffman, G.S., 2000. Study of 52 patients with idiopathic aortitis from a cohort of 1,204 surgical cases. Arthritis Rheum. 43, 901–907.

Salazar, M., Varela, A., Ramirez, L.A., Uribe, O., Vasquez, G., Egea, E., et al., 2000. Association of HLA-DRB1*1602 and DRB1*1001 with Takayasu arteritis in Colombian mestizos as markers of Amerindian ancestry. Int. J. Cardiol. 75 (Suppl 1), S113–S116.

Salvarani, C., 2003. Large vessel vasculitis. Clin. Exp. Rheumatol. 21, S133–S134.

Salvarani, C., Crowson, C.S., O'Fallon, W.M., Hunder, G.G., Gabriel, S.E., 2004. Reappraisal of the epidemiology of giant cell arteritis in Olmsted County, Minnesota, over a fifty-year period. Arthritis Rheum. 51, 264–268.

Salvarani, C., Macchioni, P., Manzini, C., Paolazzi, G., Trotta, A., Manganelli, P., et al., 2007. Infliximab plus prednisone or placebo plus prednisone for the initial treatment of polymyalgia rheumatica: a randomized trial. Ann. Intern. Med. 146, 631–639.

Salvarani, C., Magnani, L., Catanoso, M.G., Pipitone, N., Versari, A., Dardani, L., et al., 2012. Rescue treatment with tocilizumab for Takayasu arteritis resistant to TNF-alpha blockers. Clin. Exp. Rheumatol. 30, S90–S93.

Samson, M., Audia, S., Fraszczak, J., Trad, M., Ornetti, P., Lakomy, D., et al., 2012. Th1 and Th17 lymphocytes expressing CD161 are implicated in giant cell arteritis and polymyalgia rheumatica pathogenesis. Arthritis Rheum. 64, 3788–3798.

Schmidt, J., Kermani, T.A., Bacani, A.K., Crowson, C.S., Matteson, E.L., Warrington, K.J., 2012. Tumor necrosis factor inhibitors in patients with Takayasu arteritis: experience from a referral center with long-term followup. Arthritis Care Res. (Hoboken). 64, 1079–1083.

Seitz, M., Reichenbach, S., Bonel, H.M., Adler, S., Wermelinger, F., Villiger, P.M., 2011. Rapid induction of remission in large vessel vasculitis by IL-6 blockade. A case series. Swiss. Med. Wkly. 141, w13156.

Seko, Y., 2000. Takayasu arteritis: insights into immunopathology. Jpn Heart J. 41, 15–26.

Seko, Y., 2002. Takayasu's arteritis: pathogenesis. In: Hoffman, G.S. (Ed.), Inflammatory Diseases of Blood Vessels. Marcel Dekker, New York, pp. 443–453.

Seko, Y., Minota, S., Kawasaki, A., Shinkai, Y., Maeda, K., Yagita, H., et al., 1994. Perforin-secreting killer cell infiltration and expression of a 65-kD heat-shock protein in aortic tissue of patients with Takayasu's arteritis. J. Clin. Invest. 93, 750–758.

Seko, Y., Sato, O., Takagi, A., Tada, Y., Matsuo, H., Yagita, H., et al., 1996. Restricted usage of T-cell receptor Valpha-Vbeta genes in infiltrating cells in aortic tissue of patients with Takayasu's arteritis. Circulation. 93, 1788–1790.

Seko, Y., Takahashi, N., Tada, Y., Yagita, H., Okumura, K., Nagai, R., 2000. Restricted usage of T-cell receptor Vgamma-Vdelta genes and expression of costimulatory molecules in Takayasu's arteritis. Int. J. Cardiol. 75 (Suppl 1), S77–S83, discussion S85–S87.

Shimizu, K., Sano, K., 1951. Pulseless disease. J. Neuropath. Clin. Neuro. 1, 37–47.

Smetana, G.W., Shmerling, R.H., 2002. Does this patient have temporal arteritis? JAMA. 287, 92–101.

Smith, C.A., Fidler, W.J., Pinals, R.S., 1983. The epidemiology of giant cell arteritis. Report of a ten-year study in Shelby County, Tennessee. Arthritis Rheum. 26, 1214–1219.

Sorbi, D., French, D.L., Nuovo, G.J., Kew, R.R., Arbeit, L.A., Gruber, B.L., 1996. Elevated levels of 92-kd type IV collagenase (matrix metalloproteinase 9) in giant cell arteritis. Arthritis Rheum. 39, 1747–1753.

Spiera, R.F., Mitnick, H.J., Kupersmith, M., Richmond, M., Spiera, H., Peterson, M.G., et al., 2001. A prospective, double-blind, randomized, placebo controlled trial of methotrexate in the treatment of giant cell arteritis (GCA). Clin. Exp. Rheumatol. 19, 495–501.

Takayasu, M., 1908. A case with peculiar changes of the central retinal vessels. Acta. Soc. Ophthal. Japan. 12, 554–555.

Terrier, B., Geri, G., Chaara, W., Allenbach, Y., Rosenzwajg, M., Costedoat-Chalumeau, N., et al., 2012. Interleukin-21 modulates Th1 and Th17 responses in giant cell arteritis. Arthritis Rheum. 64, 2001–2011.

Tezuka, D., Haraguchi, G., Ishihara, T., Ohigashi, H., Inagaki, H., Suzuki, J., et al., 2012. Role of FDG PET-CT in Takayasu arteritis: sensitive detection of recurrences. JACC Cardiovasc. Imaging. 5, 422–429.

Tomita, T., Imakawa, K., 1998. Matrix metalloproteinases and tissue inhibitors of metalloproteinases in giant cell arteritis: an immunocytochemical study. Pathology. 30, 40–50.

Tso, E., Flamm, S.D., White, R.D., Schvartzman, P.R., Mascha, E., Hoffman, G.S., 2002. Takayasu arteritis: utility and limitations of magnetic resonance imaging in diagnosis and treatment. Arthritis Rheum. 46, 1634–1642.

Uddhammar, A.C., 2000. Von Willebrand factor in polymyalgia rheumatica and giant cell arteritis. Clin. Exp. Rheumatol. 18, S32–S33.

Wagner, A.D., Goronzy, J.J., Weyand, C.M., 1994. Functional profile of tissue-infiltrating and circulating CD68 + cells in giant cell arteritis. Evidence for two components of the disease. J. Clin. Invest. 94, 1134–1140.

Wagner, A.D., Bjornsson, J., Bartley, G.B., Goronzy, J.J., Weyand, C.M., 1996. Interferon-gamma-producing T cells in giant cell vasculitis represent a minority of tissue-infiltrating cells and are located distant from the site of pathology. Am. J. Pathol. 148, 1925–1933.

Watts, R., Al-Taiar, A., Mooney, J., Scott, D., MacGregor, A., 2009. The epidemiology of Takayasu arteritis in the UK. Rheumatology (Oxford). 48, 1008–1011.

Weaver, F.A., Kumar, S.R., Yellin, A.E., Anderson, S., Hood, D.B., Rowe, V.L., et al., 2004. Renal revascularization in Takayasu arteritis-induced renal artery stenosis. J. Vasc. Surg. 39, 749–757.

Webb, M., Chambers, A., Mason, J.C., Maudlin, L., Rahman, L., Frank, J., 2004. The role of 18F-FDG PET in characterising disease activity in Takayasu arteritis. Eur. J. Nucl. Med. Mol. Imaging. 31, 627–634.

Weyand, C.M., 2000. The Dunlop-Dottridge Lecture: the pathogenesis of giant cell arteritis. J. Rheumatol. 27, 517–522.

Weyand, C.M., Goronzy, J.J., 1995. Giant cell arteritis as an antigen-driven disease. Rheum. Dis. Clin. North. Am. 21, 1027–1039.

Weyand, C.M., Goronzy, J.J., 1999. Arterial wall injury in giant cell arteritis. Arthritis Rheum. 42, 844–853.

Weyand, C.M., Goronzy, J.J., 2003a. Giant-cell arteritis and polymyalgia rheumatica. Ann. Intern. Med. 139, 505–515.

Weyand, C.M., Goronzy, J.J., 2003b. Medium- and large-vessel vasculitis. N. Engl. J. Med. 349, 160–169.

Weyand, C.M., Goronzy, J.J., 2013. Immune mechanisms in medium and large vessel vasculitis. Nat. Rev. Rheumatol. In press.

Weyand, C.M., Hicok, K.C., Hunder, G.G., Goronzy, J.J., 1992. The HLA-DRB1 locus as a genetic component in giant cell arteritis. Mapping of a disease-linked sequence motif to the antigen binding site of the HLA-DR molecule. J. Clin. Invest. 90, 2355–2361.

Weyand, C.M., Hicok, K.C., Hunder, G.G., Goronzy, J.J., 1994a. Tissue cytokine patterns in patients with polymyalgia rheumatica and giant cell arteritis. Ann. Intern. Med. 121, 484–491.

Weyand, C.M., Hunder, N.N., Hicok, K.C., Hunder, G.G., Goronzy, J.J., 1994b. HLA-DRB1 alleles in polymyalgia rheumatica, giant cell arteritis, and rheumatoid arthritis. Arthritis Rheum. 37, 514–520.

Weyand, C.M., Schonberger, J., Oppitz, U., Hunder, N.N., Hicok, K.C., Goronzy, J.J., 1994c. Distinct vascular lesions in giant cell arteritis share identical T cell clonotypes. J. Exp. Med. 179, 951–960.

Weyand, C.M., Wagner, A.D., Bjornsson, J., Goronzy, J.J., 1996. Correlation of the topographical arrangement and the functional pattern of tissue-infiltrating macrophages in giant cell arteritis. J. Clin. Invest. 98, 1642–1649.

Weyand, C.M., Tetzlaff, N., Bjornsson, J., Brack, A., Younge, B., Goronzy, J.J., 1997. Disease patterns and tissue cytokine profiles in giant cell arteritis. Arthritis Rheum. 40, 19–26.

Weyand, C.M., Fulbright, J.W., Evans, J.M., Hunder, G.G., Goronzy, J.J., 1999. Corticosteroid requirements in polymyalgia rheumatica. Arch. Intern. Med. 159, 577–584.

Weyand, C.M., Fulbright, J.W., Hunder, G.G., Evans, J.M., Goronzy, J.J., 2000. Treatment of giant cell arteritis: interleukin-6 as a biologic marker of disease activity. Arthritis Rheum. 43, 1041–1048.

Weyand, C.M., Kaiser, M., Yang, H., Younge, B., Goronzy, J.J., 2002. Therapeutic effects of acetylsalicylic acid in giant cell arteritis. Arthritis Rheum. 46, 457–466.

Weyand, C.M., Younge, B.R., Goronzy, J.J., 2011. IFN-gamma and IL-17: the two faces of T-cell pathology in giant cell arteritis. Curr. Opin. Rheumatol. 23, 43–49.

Weyand, C.M., Liao, Y.J., Goronzy, J.J., 2012. The immunopathology of giant cell arteritis: diagnostic and therapeutic implications. J. Neuroophthalmol. 32, 259–265.

Xenitidis, T., Horger, M., Zeh, G., Kanz, L., Henes, J.C., 2013. Sustained inflammation of the aortic wall despite tocilizumab treatment in two cases of Takayasu arteritis. Rheumatology (Oxford). 52, 1729–1731.

Chapter 74

Idiopathic and Autoimmune Interstitial Lung Disease

Brian Gelbman[1] and Ronald G. Crystal[1,2]

[1]*Division of Pulmonary and Critical Care Medicine, Weill Medical College of Cornell University, New York, NY, USA,* [2]*Department of Genetic Medicine, Weill Medical College of Cornell University, New York, NY, USA*

Chapter Outline

Introduction	1105	Cryptogenic Organizing Pneumonia	1113
History	1105	Idiopathic Pulmonary Fibrosis	1113
Cryptogenic Organizing Pneumonia	1105	Pathologic Effector Mechanisms	1113
Idiopathic Pulmonary Fibrosis	1106	Cryptogenic Organizing Pneumonia	1113
Clinical, Pathological, and Epidemiological Features	1106	Idiopathic Pulmonary Fibrosis	1114
Cryptogenic Organizing Pneumonia	1106	Treatment and Outcome	1116
Idiopathic Pulmonary Fibrosis	1107	Cryptogenic Organizing Pneumonia	1116
Autoimmune Features	1109	Idiopathic Pulmonary Fibrosis	1116
Cryptogenic Organizing Pneumonia	1109	Corticosteroids	1116
Idiopathic Pulmonary Fibrosis	1110	Cytotoxic Agents	1116
Genetic Features	1112	Anti-fibrotic Agents	1117
Cryptogenic Organizing Pneumonia	1112	Conclusions	1117
Idiopathic Pulmonary Fibrosis	1112	Acknowledgments	1118
In Vivo and *In Vitro* Models	1113	References	1118

INTRODUCTION

Interstitial lung disease is a broad category of heterogeneous diseases which share the common feature of inflammatory and fibrotic changes that primarily affect the alveoli and small airways. The two most common manifestations are idiopathic pulmonary fibrosis (IPF) and cryptogenic organizing pneumonia (COP), both of which can occur as "idiopathic" conditions or in association with several autoimmune diseases. Although both are classified as "lung disorders of unknown etiology," there are multiple clues suggesting that autoimmune mechanisms play a role in the pathogenesis of both disorders. The focus of this chapter is to explore the link between autoimmune mechanisms underlying COP and IPF as models for autoimmune disorders of the lung. To do so, we will first discuss the history and the clinical features of COP and IPF, followed by a summary of the autoimmune, genetic, environmental features, current concepts of pathogenesis, and the therapies currently available and under investigation for both disorders.

HISTORY

Although both COP and IFP are inflammatory/fibrotic disorders, because they are centered on the bronchioles and alveoli, respectively, and have different clinical, radiologic, and pathologic features, they have always been considered to be different disorders.

Cryptogenic Organizing Pneumonia

The term "bronchiolitis obliterans" was first used by Lange in 1901 (Lange, 1901), when he described two patients in whom the bronchioles were blocked by plugs of granulation tissue, though those patients likely had what is now known as "cryptogenic organizing

N. Rose & I. Mackay (Eds): The Autoimmune Diseases, Fifth edition. DOI: http://dx.doi.org/10.1016/B978-0-12-384929-8.00074-5

pneumonia." In 1966, Baar et al. (Baar and Galindo, 1966) used the term "bronchiolitis fibrosa obliterans" to describe concentric rings of fibrotic tissue in the wall of the airways. In 1973, Gosink et al. (Gosink et al., 1973) employed "bronchiolitis obliterans" to describe a group of patients that had submucosal and peribronchiolar infiltrate of granulation tissue resulting in extrinsic narrowing of the bronchiolar lumen. During the 1970s, several rheumatological conditions, particularly rheumatoid arthritis, were recognized to be associated with bronchiolitis obliterans, as were adverse reactions to therapies used for rheumatoid arthritis such as gold and penicillamine (Geddes et al., 1977).

In 1983, Davison et al. (Davison et al., 1983) first used the term "cryptogenic organizing pneumonitis" to describe eight patients that had pulmonary infiltrates and histology similar to bronchopneumonia, yet no organism was identified and they responded to steroids. In 1985, Epler et al. (Epler et al., 1985), similarly described 50 patients with bronchiolitis obliterans, but also with granulation tissue in airways, airway ducts, and alveoli, and coined the term bronchiolitis obliterans organizing pneumonia (BOOP). COP and BOOP are now believed to represent the same disease and COP is the preferred term. Current usage of the term "bronchiolitis obliterans" is reserved primarily for transplant-related lung injury that occurs almost exclusively at the bronchiole.

Idiopathic Pulmonary Fibrosis

The first recognition of the broad category of idiopathic interstitial lung diseases, which includes idiopathic pulmonary fibrosis, is credited to William Osler in 1892, when he described a chronic fibrinoid change occurring between the alveolus and the blood vessels (Osler, 1892). Osler demonstrated great foresight by also noting that there were diverse patterns of the disease that made classification difficult.

Idiopathic pulmonary fibrosis, also referred to as "cryptogenic fibrosing alveolitis," "idiopathic interstitial pneumonitis," "usual interstitial pneumonitis," and "idiopathic interstitial pneumonia," was first described by the Czech pathologist Sandoz in 1907, but went largely unnoticed (Sandoz, 1907). Hamman and Rich are frequently credited with the first description of IPF in 1935 (Hamman and Rich, 1935), despite the fact that their initial cases were more acute in presentation, unlike classic IPF, and may have been descriptions of acute respiratory distress syndrome. In 1964, Scadding coined the term "cryptogenic fibrosing alveolitis" to describe IPF as a diffuse inflammatory and fibrotic lung disease affecting primarily the alveoli (Scadding, 1964). Scadding advanced the concept that IPF was a slow, progressive disease that

was distinctly different from the relatively acute process described by Hamman and Rich.

IPF was further defined by Liebow and Carrington in the 1960s using histologic criteria. These investigators separated IPF into two morphologic patterns, which they referred to as "usual interstitial pneumonia" (UIP, now often referred to as "usual interstitial pneumonitis") and desquamative interstitial pneumonia (DIP) (Liebow and Carrington, 1969). The inflammatory component of IPF was characterized by our group using bronchoalveolar lavage to distinguish IPF from other interstitial lung disorders (Crystal et al., 1976; Reynolds et al., 1977). The pathological pattern of UIP was furthered refined over the next several decades, including the description of nonspecific interstitial pneumonia (NSIP) by Katzenstein and Fiorelli in 1994 as a distinct entity (Katzenstein and Fiorelli, 1994). The classification system developed by the American Thoracic Society and European Respiratory Society in 2001 separates IPF from NSIP and DIP based primarily on pathologic findings (2002).

CLINICAL, PATHOLOGICAL, AND EPIDEMIOLOGICAL FEATURES

Cryptogenic Organizing Pneumonia

Cryptogenic organizing pneumonia is identified pathologically by a proliferation of granulation resulting in near obstruction of the small airways and can extend into the alveoli with a surrounding interstitial lymphoplasmacyctic infiltrate (Murray and Nadel, 2000). Overall, there is preservation of the underlying lung architecture and apparent temporal homogeneity, with very little fibrotic changes present. These findings may also be present during the "organizing" phase of a bacterial or viral pneumonia, but when they occur in the absence of an infectious disease, the term used is "cryptogenic organizing pneumonia." Thus, the definition relies on both pathologic and clinical features.

Individuals with COP usually present with persistent cough and worsening dyspnea on exertion, which can mimic bronchopneumonia. The physical exam is notable for crackles in the affected lobe. Most patients will have a mild obstructive pattern on pulmonary function testing, although the disease can present with normal, restrictive or mixed pattern (King and Mortenson, 1992). Routine chest radiographs may reveal bilateral air-space opacities, peripherally located, which can be migratory. High resolution computed tomography (HRCT) reveals patchy air-space consolidations or ground glass opacities that can be indistinguishable from bacterial pneumonia or eosinophilic pneumonia. Fibrosis or honeycombing is rarely seen. The areas affected by COP are scattered and patchy in distribution. For this reason, transbronchial lung biopsy is insensitive as a diagnostic tool, as it often misses the involved area, and thus a surgical lung biopsy is often necessary to make the diagnosis.

There have been no epidemiological studies performed to quantify the overall prevalence of COP, although one study found a yearly cumulative incidence of six to seven cases per 100,000 hospital admissions (Alasaly et al., 1995). It is generally considered a rare disease, although it is likely that COP is underdiagnosed and may account for a small percentage of cases misdiagnosed as bacterial or viral pneumonia.

Idiopathic Pulmonary Fibrosis

Idiopathic pulmonary fibrosis (sometimes referred to as "cryptogenic fibrosing alveolitis" in Europe) refers to a distinctive type of chronic inflammatory/fibrotic interstitial lung disorder of unknown cause that is limited to the lungs and associated with a histologic pattern of usual interstitial pneumonia (UIP) (American Thoracic Society, 2002) (see Figure 74.1). The pattern of UIP on surgical lung biopsy is also seen in patients with multisystem autoimmune disease who present with similar pulmonary-related clinical features to those of IPF (Harrison et al., 1991).

Individuals with IPF typically present with the gradual onset of symptoms, most commonly dyspnea on exertion and non-productive cough. Most will have had at least 6 months of symptoms before presentation, with an average duration of 24 months (ATS, 2002). The clinical course typically involves gradual deterioration, occasionally punctuated by periods of rapid decline, although some of the disease stabilizes in some individuals. The best

estimates for life expectancy from time of diagnosis to death are derived from case–control cohort studies, because they are not biased like prevalence studies, which tend to be overrepresented by survivors. According to two such studies, the average survival from the time of diagnosis to death is 3 to 4 years (Hubbard et al., 1998; Mapel et al., 1998).

On physical exam, patients with IPF may have digital clubbing (25 to 50%) and fine, inspiratory, Velcro-like crackles confined to the bases of the lungs. As there is progressive loss of alveoli, and the diffusing capacity drops below 50% predicted, pulmonary hypertension develops, first with exercise, and later at rest (Crystal et al., 1976; McLees et al., 1979). Once established at rest, the pulmonary hypertension is associated with an increased pulmonary component of the S2 on cardiac exam, and eventual fixed split of the second sound. In the late stages of the disease there can be signs of right heart failure, such as peripheral edema.

Pulmonary function testing usually shows a restrictive pattern of ventilatory defects and a decrease in diffusing capacity, although in early stages of the disease, these tests can be normal (Fulmer et al., 1979; Keogh and Crystal, 1980; Cherniack et al., 1995). Individuals with IPF typically have mild to moderate hypoxemia with concomitant low resting oxygen saturation that falls with exercise (Keogh and Crystal, 1980).

Chest radiographs of individuals with IPF are routinely abnormal, with a reticular pattern seen at the periphery and in the bases. Later in the disease there is honeycombing and volume loss in the lower lobes (Staples et al., 1987). In early stages of the disease, chest

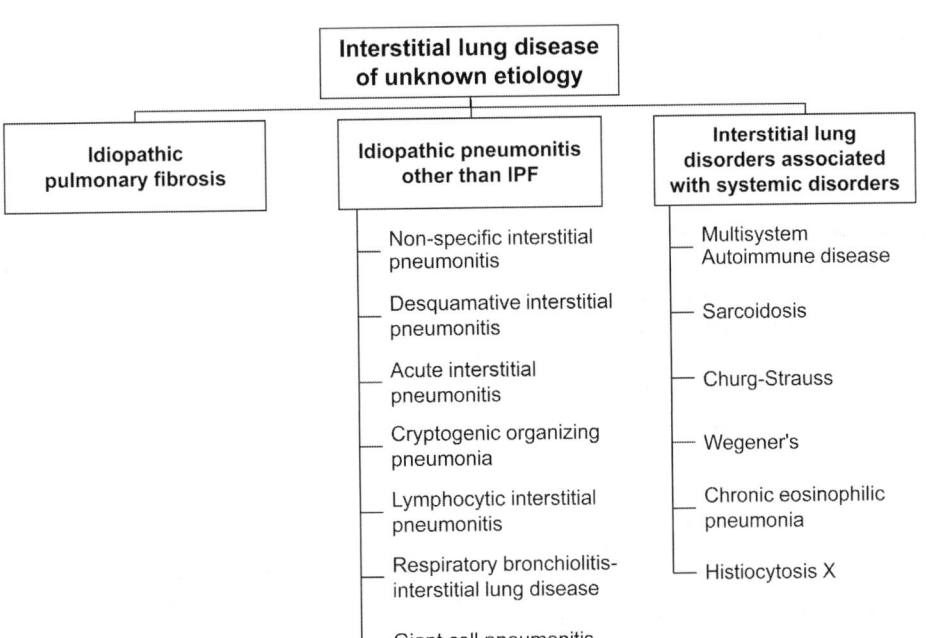

FIGURE 74.1 Relationship of idiopathic pulmonary fibrosis to other idiopathic interstitial disorders. Some of the rare disorders have been left off the lists. *see American Thoracic Society, 2002; Crystal, 1984; Schoenberger and Crystal, 1983 for further details.*

radiographs may be normal. HRCT is more sensitive and is the preferred imaging modality. The typical HRCT findings are reticular–nodular opacities (Figure 74.2). Later in the disease, traction bronchiectasis is commonly seen in the peripheral and basal segments of the lower lobes. Volume loss and ground glass opacities are frequently present. As the disease progresses, honeycomb cysts develop and enlarge over time (Staples et al., 1987). The chest X-ray and HRCT appearance of IPF is nearly identical to that seen in pulmonary fibrosis associated with the rheumatic disorders, with the lone exception of possibly more basal involvement seen on HRCT in IPF (Chan et al., 1997).

Transbronchial biopsies are insufficient to diagnose IPF because the biopsy specimen is too small and does not preserve the architecture of the lung. However, transbronchial biopsies may be useful to rule out other conditions, such as sarcoidosis, that can mimic IPF. A surgical

lung biopsy has been required in the past to firmly establish the diagnosis. However, the consensus statement by the American Thoracic Society (ATS) and European Respiratory Society (ERS) permits the diagnosis of IPF when there are typical clinical and HRCT findings of IPF (Hunninghake et al., 2001, ATS, 2002; Raghu et al., 2011). Surgical lung biopsies are still recommended whenever there are atypical clinical or HRCT features.

The histological pattern characteristic for IPF is referred to as usual interstitial pneumonia (UIP) (Figure 74.3). This pattern is distinct from the other forms of idiopathic interstitial lung disorders such as desquamative interstitial pneumonia, lymphocytic interstitial pneumonia, cryptogenic organizing pneumonia, non-specific interstitial pneumonia, and acute interstitial pneumonia (Liebow and Carrington, 1969; Katzenstein and Fiorelli, 1994, ATS, 2002). There is typically a heterogeneous distribution of interstitial fibrosis interspersed within areas

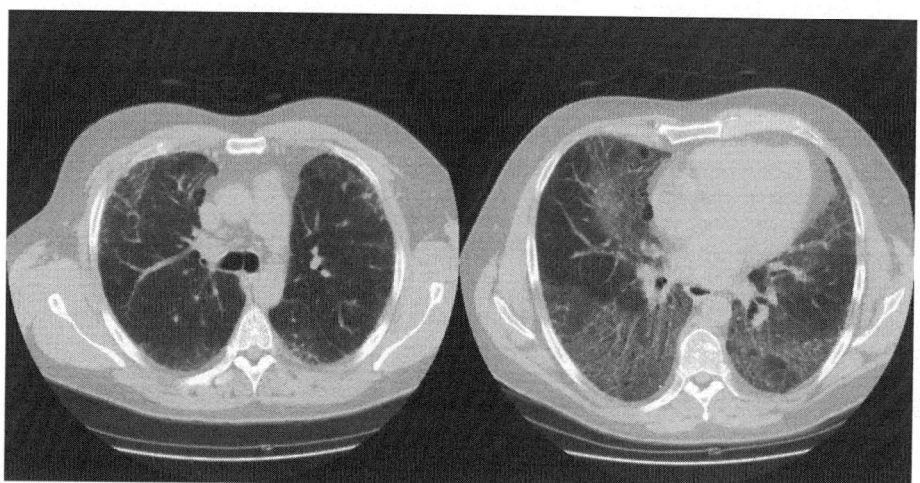

FIGURE 74.2 Diffuse reticular–nodular pattern on high resolution chest tomography commonly observed in idiopathic pulmonary fibrosis. Note areas of honeycombing.

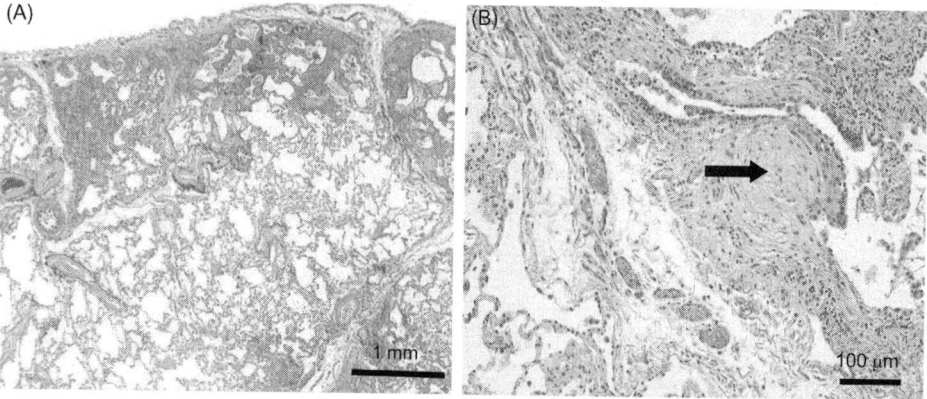

FIGURE 74.3 **Histologic pattern of idiopathic pulmonary fibrosis.** The patterns are often referred to as "usual interstitial pneumonitis." (A) Subpleural, paraseptal, and interstitial collagen deposition together with areas of mildly abnormal alveolar parenchyma (hematoxylin and eosin, bar = 1 mm). (B) Thickened interstitium with collagen deposition, mild to moderate alveolar septal mononuclear cell infiltrates, mainly lymphocytes, cuboidalization of the epithelium and a large fibroblastic foci (thick arrow). The fibroblastic foci are composed of spindled mesenchymal cells and are thought to represent the "leading edge" of the progressive fibroinflammatory process (hematoxylin and eosin; bar = 100 Φm).

of normal lung, suggesting different temporal stages of involvement. There is patchy inflammation, dominated by alveolar macrophages, and to a lesser extent lymphocytes, neutrophils, and sometimes eosinophils. The alveolar epithelium undergoes marked changes, referred to as "cuboidalization," with a loss of type I epithelial cells, and their replacement with cuboidal cells, both alveolar type II epithelial cells and bronchiolar epithelium. One hallmark finding in IPF is the subepithelial "fibroblastic focus," which is a nodule of spindle-shaped, mesenchymal cells that produce an abundant deposition of extracellular matrix. These "foci" are believed to be the "leading edge" of the fibrotic process. Occasionally, the interstitial fibrosis extends through breaks in the epithelium into the alveolar space to form intra-alveolar fibrosis (Basset et al., 1986). Later in the disease there is architectural destruction and fibrosis with honeycombing. Frequently, the subpleural parenchyma is the most severely involved region. When a biopsy shows areas of both UIP and non-specific interstitial pneumonitis, the default pathologic diagnosis becomes the clinical diagnosis IPF, as these patients have been shown to have behavior similar to that seen in IPF with UIP-only pattern (Flaherty et al., 2001; Raghu et al., 2011).

The histological features of pulmonary fibrosis associated with multisystem autoimmune disease can be classified into the same pathological descriptions of idiopathic interstitial pneumonias put forth by the American Thoracic Society and European Respiratory Society, including usual interstitial pneumonia (UIP), non-specific interstitial pneumonitis (NSIP), desquamative interstitial pneumonia (DIP), and cryptogenic organizing pneumonia (COP) (Figure 74.1). The UIP pattern that is seen with multisystem autoimmune diseases is essentially identical to the pattern seen in the IPF. In polymyositis, dermatomyositis, and scleroderma, NSIP is the most frequently seen histologic pattern followed by UIP (Douglas et al., 2001; Bouros et al., 2002). The prevalence of the different histologic subtypes of idiopathic interstitial pneumonias has not been well characterized in the other multisystem autoimmune diseases.

The estimated annual incidence of idiopathic pulmonary fibrosis is 7 per 100,000 for women and 10 per 100,000 for men. Most patients present between 50 and 70 years of age; however, the incidence, prevalence, and death rate rise with age (Coultas et al., 1994).

Several studies have tried to establish the prevalence of pulmonary fibrosis in patients with the multisystem autoimmune diseases, but the results have varied depending on the method by which patients are screened for pulmonary involvement. Studies that utilize autopsy or lung biopsy data are subject to overdiagnosis, since they have been shown to detect subclinical disease that can fail to progress (Cervantes-Perez et al., 1980). Likewise, HRCT

screening studies may also overestimate the prevalence of disease by detecting parenchymal changes that may not be clinically significant. In rheumatoid arthritis, cross-sectional studies using chest radiographs estimate the prevalence to be less than 5% of patients (Hyland et al., 1983). When HRCT is used to screen patients, the prevalence appears to be between 20 and 50%, although these studies are limited by selection bias (Remy-Jardin et al., 1994; Gabbay et al., 1997). Pulmonary fibrosis is most prevalent in scleroderma, where autopsy series have shown it to be present in 70% of cases and chest radiograph series estimate the prevalence between 25 and 65% (Wiedemann and Matthay, 1989; Minai et al., 1998). The prevalence of clinically overt pulmonary fibrosis is 30% in polymyositis and dermatomyositis, 5% in systemic lupus erythematosus, and 10% in Sjögren's syndrome (Eisenberg et al., 1973; Gardiner, 1993; Schwarz, 1998).

AUTOIMMUNE FEATURES

Cryptogenic Organizing Pneumonia

Cryptogenic organizing pneumonia has been reported in association with many different types of autoimmune disorders, including rheumatoid arthritis (RA), lupus erythematosus, ankylosing spondylitis, Sjögren's syndrome, and scleroderma (Colby, 1998; Ryu et al., 2003). COP is most frequently seen with rheumatoid arthritis, and in one case series of 40 RA patients undergoing open lung biopsy, COP was the second most common diagnosis behind rheumatoid nodules of the lung (Yousem et al., 1985). In rheumatoid arthritis, bronchiolar involvement typically presents in the fifth and sixth decades of life and is more frequently seen in women (Geddes et al., 1977; Epler et al., 1979; Herzog et al., 1981). Most patients with COP in association with RA have long-standing symptoms of arthritis, though occasionally the pulmonary involvement predates the rheumatologic disease. Occasionally, COP will appear at the same time as a flare in arthritic symptoms and there is a case report of it occurring simultaneously with the onset of pernicious anemia, an autoimmune disease. Further support for the autoimmune basis is the fact that most cases of COP in RA will have a positive rheumatoid factor (85%) and usually have very high titers (Mori et al., 2008). Immunofluorescence stains in affected regions of the lung of patients with RA show IgM and IgG depositions in the alveolar septum (Begin et al., 1982; Yousem et al., 1985), and many cells are positive for S-100 protein (Yoshinouchi et al., 1999).

The bronchoalveolar lavage (BAL) fluid from patients with COP is notable for a marked activation of macrophages and lymphocytes, and an overall Th1 helper response (Cordier, 2006). BAL obtained from patients with COP has elevated levels of tryptase, mast cells, and interleukins-10, -12, and -18 (Pesci et al., 1996; Forlani et al., 2002). Platelet-derived growth factor and interleukin-8 also appear to play a role in the pathogenesis of COP (Carre et al., 1994; Aubert et al., 1997).

Indirect evidence for autoimmune mechanisms in COP comes from the bronchiolitis obliterans syndrome associated with both lung and allogeneic stem cell transplants. These cases, which can be viewed as *in vivo* human models of bronchiolar disease, have been more extensively studied than COP or rheumatic disease-associated COP. The bronchiolitis obliterans syndrome in association with lung transplantation is the main cause of morbidity and mortality (Arcasoy and Kotloff, 1999). It is a form of chronic lung rejection that is mediated by B cell and T cell activation against mismatched HLA class I and II antigens (Kelly and Hertz, 1997). Bronchiolitis obliterans associated with allogeneic bone marrow transplants is also thought to represent graft versus host disease. The disease progresses from inflammatory changes around the bronchioles to fibrosis and scarring (Ratanatharathorn et al., 2001). It is interesting to note that in bronchiolitis obliterans syndrome associated with lung transplant or with bone marrow transplant, the bronchioles are the more frequent site for chronic rejection, not the lung parenchyma.

Idiopathic Pulmonary Fibrosis

Although the etiology of IPF remains unknown, it has been hypothesized for 30 years that autoimmune mechanisms to external stimuli are the driving force for repeated injury and inflammation that ultimately lead to fibrosis (Crystal et al., 1976, 1981, 1984). Although no clear infectious or environmental agent has been found as the etiology of IPF (Gross and Hunninghake, 2001), there are extensive data regarding autoimmune cellular and humoral processes ongoing in this disorder.

Initial studies in IPF relevant to autoimmunity focused on identifying autoantibodies that target the pulmonary parenchyma. Turner-Warwick demonstrated that 40% of patients with IPF had circulating, non-specific autoantibodies such as anti-nuclear antibodies (ANA) and rheumatoid factor (Turner-Warwick and Doniach, 1965). Increases in circulating ANA and rheumatoid factor were observed in 30% of our patients (Crystal et al., 1976). Similar studies which evaluated the presence of autoantibodies to nuclear antigens, DNA topoisomerase, and cytokeratin detected the antibodies in some patients (Table 74.1). More recent studies have focused on antibodies that are specific to lung proteins, although these studies have also shown variable expression of autoantibodies (Wallace et al., 1994; Robinson et al., 2001). These results raise the possibility that autoantibodies are a secondary consequence of the ongoing immune activation in

the setting of inflammation and tissue damage, rather than the causative mechanism.

Similarly, investigations have evaluated the role that immune complex deposition plays in the pathogenesis of inflammation and fibrosis in IPF. Early studies observed elevated levels of circulating immune complexes in certain subsets of patients with IPF; however, these were performed prior to the current classification system and included patients with other forms of interstitial lung disease (Dreisin et al., 1978; Haslam et al., 1979). Hunninghake et al. (Hunninghake et al., 1981) demonstrated a correlation between the level of immune complexes in bronchoalveolar lavage fluid and the levels of neutrophil chemotactic factor released by alveolar macrophages in patients with IPF. Other studies have also seen elevated levels of immune complex in lavage fluid, but the levels are variable and do not correlate with disease activity.

More recently, attention has turned to immune-based microvascular injury as the ongoing trigger for pulmonary fibrosis. In scleroderma-associated pulmonary fibrosis, studies have shown complement and immunoglobulin deposition in the microvasculature. Some have hypothesized that perhaps anti-endothelial cell antibodies, which are present in the circulation in several autoimmune conditions, may be responsible for the injury. Several studies have correlated the presence of anti-endothelial cell antibodies with the development and severity of IPF (Magro et al., 2007).

The lack of clear evidence for a humoral mechanism as the primary cause for IPF shifted the focus towards cellular immunity. One popular theory is that an unknown stimulus triggers a dysregulated activation of cell-mediated immune response that results in the fibrotic process analogous to that observed in abnormal wound healing. This theory rests on the belief that a normal cell-mediated defense to a pulmonary insult would be a Th1 response, as seen in most infections and in hypersensitivity pneumonitis (Wallace et al., 1995; Lukacs et al., 2001; Kunkel, 2004). The Th1 response is characterized by the release of interferon-γ and the activation of neutrophils and macrophages for efficient clearing of the antigen, as well as suppression of fibroblast activation and collagen deposition. Cytokine profiles in IPF are closer to Th2 response which are typified by elevated IL-4, IL-5, and IL-13 levels, and result in fibroblast activation (Hancock et al., 1998; Wallace and Howie, 1999). Early evidence for this T cell-mediated mechanism in IPF was demonstrated by Kravis et al. (Kravis et al., 1976), who discovered that circulating lymphocytes from patients with IPF would release migration inhibitor factor after exposure to collagen and would lyse collagen-coated sheep red blood cells.

One experimental model used to demonstrate a cell-mediated autoimmune mechanism is the adoptive transfer, hapten immune pulmonary interstitial fibrosis model (Stein-Streilein et al., 1987). In this model, donor mice are

TABLE 74.1 Autoantibodies Associated with Idiopathic Pulmonary Fibrosis[1]

Antigens	Number of patients	Result	Reference
Fresh unfixed lung tissue, rheumatoid factor, nuclear, thyroglobulin, gastric parietal cells	48 IPF	Sensitivity: Positive titers for: RF 49%, ANA 28%, rat liver homogenate 19%, gastric cells 0%; no autoantibodies specific to lung were detected by immunofluorescence	Turner-Warwick and Doniach (1965)
Nuclear[2] ANA, nRNP, ds-DNA, Sm, SS-A and SS-B	68 IPF 54 PF-AID 47 controls	Sensitivity: ANA present in 21% of IPF and 46% of PF-AID. Anti-nRNP present in 15% of IPF and PF-AID. Other antibodies were not significantly different from control group Specificity: ANA 94%, anti-nRNP 98%	Chapman et al. (1984)
Nuclear ANA, ds-DNA, ss-DNA, RF[3]	53 IPF 33 SLE[4] 50 controls	Sensitivity: IPF patients had 42% ANA (titer >1/10), 25% anti-dsDNA, and 100% anti-ssDNA titers that were two standard deviations above the normal range; levels did not correlate with disease activity	Holgate et al. (1983)
Histidyl-tRNA synthetase (Jo-1 antigen)	62 IPF 19 PF-AID (myositis) 53 myositis alone	Sensitivity: Antibody present in 68% of PF-AID (myositis) patients compared to 3% IPF alone and 7.5% myositis alone Specificity: >99% normal and 98% autoimmune controls	Bernstein et al. (1984)
Topoisomerase II	41 IPF	Sensitivity: 44% positive. Remained elevated in 17 of 19 follow-up patients. Did not correlate with disease activity	Meliconi et al. (1993)
Collagen types I, II, III, IV	16 IPF 29 controls	Sensitivity: 75% of IPF patients had antibody titers to at least one type of collagen >1:16. Specificity: 83% using cut-off titer 1:16. Negative correlation between antibody level and duration of disease	Nakos et al. (1993)
Lung proteins derived from IPF, sarcoid, and normal lung	17 IPF 17 controls	Sensitivity: 71% of IPF patients had IgG that reacted to lung proteins in the 70–90 kDa range by Western blot; IgG reacted to alveolar lining cells Specificity: 82%	Wallace et al. (1994)
Cytokeratin 19	26 IPF 11 PF-AID 52 controls	Significantly higher mean serum levels in IPF compared to control. No cut-off value determined by ELISA because of overlap between groups	Fujita et al. (1999)
Expressed cDNA library from lung cancer cell line	11 IPF	Serum from index patient used to probe expressed cDNA library. Antigens recognized were unique to index patient (including anti-alanyl-tRNA synthetase), but not shared with sera from other 10 patients	Robinson et al. (2001)
Endothelial cell protein extract	45 PF-AID (scleroderma) 16 controls	Sensitivity: 93% PF-AID had positive staining using an indirect immunofluorescent assay against rodent lung tissue Specificity: 88%	Wusirika et al. (2003)

[1] Summary of autoantibody studies in patients with idiopathic pulmonary fibrosis (IPF). PF-AID, pulmonary fibrosis associated with autoimmune disease.
[2] Nuclear antigens: ANA, anti-nuclear antibodies; nRNP, nuclear ribonucleoprotein, Sm, Smith antigen, SS-A and SS-B, Sjögren's syndrome A and B antigens.
[3] RF, rheumatoid factor.
[4] SLE, systemic lupus erythematosus.

sensitized by a hapten, and then lymph nodes and spleen are transferred to recipient mice. When the recipient mice are then challenged with intratracheal administration of the hapten, they develop pulmonary fibrosis in 7 to 14 days. Interestingly, when the adoptive transfer with Th1 cells was used, an alveolitis developed, but not fibrosis, thus supporting the Th2 theory regarding the pathogenesis of the fibrotic component of IPF (Irifune et al., 2003).

In pulmonary fibrosis associated with the multisystem autoimmune disease, several serological and genetic markers are linked to the development of lung disease. For instance, patients with rheumatoid arthritis that have high levels of rheumatoid factor and prominent rheumatoid nodules are at increased risk for developing pulmonary fibrosis (Hyland et al., 1983). In systemic sclerosis, the presence of anti-topoisomerase antibodies and diffuse cutaneous involvement are associated with pulmonary fibrosis (Fanning et al., 1998).

Perhaps the best evidence for associating autoantibodies to pulmonary fibrosis is in patients with polymyositis and dermatomyositis, in which antibodies (Targoff, 1993) against the aminoacyl-tRNA synthetases have been shown to be highly correlated with pulmonary fibrosis (Bernstein et al., 1984; Targoff, 1993). At least five known forms of the autoantibodies have been identified, which include anti-alanyl-tRNA synthetase (PL), anti-histidyl-tRNA synthetase (Jo-1), anti-isoleucyl-tRNA synthetase (OJ), anti-glycyl tRNA synthetase, and anti-threonyl tRNA synthetase. The strongest correlation appears to be with anti-Jo-1 antibodies, which have been reported to have a frequency of interstitial lung disease between 50% (Hochberg et al., 1984) and 100% (Yoshida et al., 1983). Patients with polymyositis or dermatomyositis can frequently present with the "antisynthetase syndrome" characterized by pulmonary fibrosis in 50–75% of patients, arthritis, Raynaud's phenomenon, and fevers. Occasionally, the antisynthetase syndrome can occur in the absence of clinical myositis (Marguerie et al., 1990). There are also several case series of patients with isolated pulmonary fibrosis occurring in association with aminoacyl-tRNA synthetase antibodies (Friedman et al., 1996; Sauty et al., 1997). These patients have been shown to have a CD8 lymphocyte predominant bronchoalveolar lavage and non-specific interstitial pneumonitis pattern on lung biopsy. Most of the patients described in these case series have been more responsive to therapy with cyclosporine and azathioprine than patients with IPF.

GENETIC FEATURES

Cryptogenic Organizing Pneumonia

Given the rarity of COP, there are no studies that demonstrate a genetic predisposition to this condition. The same is true for the autoimmune-associated forms of COP.

Idiopathic Pulmonary Fibrosis

Up to 3% of cases of IPF occur in clusters of families, suggesting that a genetic predisposition may be responsible for susceptibility to disease (Hodgson et al., 2002). A simple pattern of Mendelian inheritance has not been observed. Familial cases appear to be inherited in an autosomal dominant pattern, although the penetrance is variable. In familial cases of IPF, children of individuals with fibrotic lung disease can have evidence of inflammatory alveolitis in bronchial lavage fluid, without having clinical evidence of disease (Bitterman et al., 1986). There have been several reports of pulmonary fibrosis occurring in separately raised monozygotic twins, underscoring the role of genetic factors (Javaheri et al., 1980; Peabody et al., 1950). Using a candidate gene approach in one large family kindred with IPF, Thomas and colleagues (Thomas et al., 2002) identified a mutation in the highly conserved coding region of surfactant protein C, resulting in aberrant cellular distribution of SP-C in the lung tissue of affected individuals.

In addition to the familial form of the disease, there is evidence for a genetic basis for the more common, sporadic form of the disease. A study from Finland demonstrated a clustering of sporadic cases of IPF in areas where familial cases were found, suggesting a founder's effect (Hodgson et al., 2002). One prevailing hypothesis is that susceptibility does not lie in one gene locus, but, rather, within multiple genes that interact through inflammatory and fibrotic mechanisms, creating a background genotype of fibrotic potential, yet still requiring an insult to create the profibrotic phenotype. This theory would explain why the familial form of the disease has an earlier age of onset (55 vs. 67), yet still presents relatively later in life, implying that a reduced threshold for the development of fibrosis exists in familial types (Marshall et al., 2000). This theory is also supported by the fact that only a small proportion of individuals who receive drugs known to cause pulmonary fibrosis (such as bleomycin or amiodarone) actually develop the disease (Tisdale et al., 1995).

One major limitation in the search for genetic sources for susceptibility is that the sizes of the association studies are limited because of the rarity of the disease. Polymorphisms in several genes have been explored as potential causes for the inherited susceptibility to IPF; however, these studies utilized a traditional candidate gene approach which is limited by our current understanding of the disease and may lead to false-positive associations. These studies are typically focused on genes involved in the inflammatory pathways, such as interleukin-1α and tumor necrosis factor-α, and have shown conflicting results (Whyte et al., 2000; Pantelidis et al., 2001). Xaubet et al. (2003) recently demonstrated that transforming growth factor-β polymorphisms were related to disease progression, but they found no association with susceptibility to IPF.

Given recent advances in genomics, microarray analysis, and proteomics, there is an excellent opportunity to perform genome-wide searches for linkage in patients with IPF to identify novel genes that are involved in pathogenesis and may represent therapeutic targets. Many of these genetic approaches are simply hypothesis generators; however, this may be a necessary first step to decipher the complex interactions of multiple loci. Additionally, microarray technology can be used for "molecular fingerprinting" to identify subclassifications within the general category of IPF.

IN VIVO AND *IN VITRO* MODELS

Animal models of the classical human Mendelian genetic diseases are relatively easy to produce because the genotype typically involves one affected gene, and knockout models of that gene, in mice for instance, can usually approximate the phenotype. Generating an animal model of a complex polygenic disease poses far more challenges because it involves multiple genes, each exerting a relatively small effect.

Cryptogenic Organizing Pneumonia

The best animal model for COP involves inoculating CBA/J mice with reovirus serotype 1 via intranasal route (Bellum et al., 1997). These CBA/J mice develop intraluminal fibrosis and lymphocytic, peribronchial infiltrates that are identical to the pathologic findings of COP in human disease. Interestingly, the COP pathological changes appear when titers of 10^6 are used; however, when 10^7 titers of the same virus are used, the CBA/J mice develop diffuse alveolar damage, the pathological finding of acute respiratory distress syndrome (ARDS). This suggests that the tendency towards COP vs. ARDS may be due to severity of the initial insult (London et al., 2002a,b).

Other animal models for COP are designed to mimic bronchiolitis obliterans, the transplant-associated form of the disease. One model frequently used is the heterotopic murine tracheal transplant, whereby grafts of trachea and main bronchi are placed subcutaneously into allogeneic mismatched recipients (Hertz et al., 1993). By 21 days, grafts demonstrate fibroproliferation in the airway lumen, a characteristic for the human chronic rejection process. Subsequent studies on this model have shown that this is mediated by cellular and humoral immunity (Kelly and Hertz, 1997). Although this model can successfully mimic the phenotypic changes of IBO, it has limited applicability to understand IBO because the entire graft tracheo-bronchial graft is an immunogenic stimulus, which is not likely the case in the idiopathic or autoimmune-associated forms of the disease.

Idiopathic Pulmonary Fibrosis

There is no animal model for IPF that clearly represents human IPF. However, there are several animal models for

susceptibility to developing experimental pulmonary fibrosis. The susceptibility to bleomycin-induced interstitial lung disease has been correlated with both immune-related (TH2 type) and non-immune-related genes in different strains of mice (Rossi et al., 1987). Transforming growth factor-β has been shown to induce pulmonary fibrotic changes when overexpressed via intratracheal administration of an adenoviral vector (Liu et al., 2001). Likewise, when mice are treated with an adenoviral vector expressing SMAD-7, an inhibitory regulator of TGF-β production, they appear to be protected against bleomycin-induced lung injury (Nakao et al., 1999).

Many different transgenic and knockout mice have also been developed to investigate the molecular pathways that lead to pulmonary fibrosis. One example is mice that overexpress TNF-α and that develop pulmonary fibrosis, and have some of the features of human IPF (Miyazaki et al., 1995). Knockout mice with targeted deletions of genes necessary for fibrosis (e.g., adhesion molecules, ICAM-1, and L-selectin, which facilitate the accumulation of leukocytes) show significantly decreased fibrosis in response to bleomycin (Hamaguchi et al., 2002).

Many of these models are focused on only a select number of candidate genes, which may or may not have relevance to human disease. While these studies have been useful to identify genes that may play a role in susceptibility, the actual human form of the disease is likely far more complex and polygenic, which may prohibit creating a comprehensive animal model that reflects the underlying pathogenesis.

PATHOLOGIC EFFECTOR MECHANISMS

Cryptogenic Organizing Pneumonia

The sequence of events that ultimately leads to organizing pneumonia has been established in multiple studies. The common initial event is airway epithelial injury, with necrosis and denudation of the pneumocytes, but preservation of basal laminae and endothelial cells. This is distinctly different from ARDS, where there is believed to be a breakdown in the basal membrane leading to hyaline membrane formation. The first alveolar changes involve formation of inflammatory cell clusters (macrophages, lymphocytes, and neutrophils) bound together by fibrin. The next stage involves migration of fibroblasts through the basal lamina and proliferation of fibrotic and inflammatory "buds" in the airway. The final stage is when these buds progress to a mature stage and there is less inflammatory component and the alveolar space begins to clear of fibrin (Peyrol et al., 1990; Kuhn and McDonald, 1991; Myers and Colby, 1993). Vascular endothelial growth factor and basic fibroblast growth factor are highly expressed in COP and this results in a proliferation of capillary tissue as is normally seen in response to wound healing (Lappi-Blanco et al., 2002).

Environmental factors are clearly linked to the development of cryptogenic organizing pneumonia in general, although specific causative environmental factors for COP are difficult to identify. Perhaps the best documented environmental cases of COP occurred after exposure to aerosolized textile dye acramin FWN (Moya et al., 1994; Sole et al., 1996; Camus and Nemery, 1998; Romero et al., 1998).

In addition, inhalational injuries can progress into bronchiolitis obliterans, which is similar pathologically to COP, except the injury is predominantly bronchiolar in location, without necessarily an inflammatory alveolar infiltrate. The mechanism is believed to be due to inflammation caused by the irritant in the bronchioles that progresses into irreversible fibrosis and airway obstruction. Frequently, this occurs after exposure to water-insoluble gases (such as oxides of nitrogen in the case of silo-filler's lung) and organic dusts or fumes, which are not rapidly absorbed in the mucous membranes of the upper airways (Ramirez and Dowell, 1971; Fleming et al., 1979). Nitrous fumes are a significant industrial hazard and can be found in the agriculture, fire-fighting, and chemical industries. The timing of the injury can be delayed from the exposure because the gases are slowly hydrolyzed into acids that act as powerful oxidants which eventually penetrate the small airways and cause severe tissue injury. Clinical symptoms may present as acute, subacute, or chronic. The chronic form usually presents as a new clinical illness, weeks to months after recovery from the initial acute illness (King, 2003).

There have been many case reports of industrial exposures followed by the development of bronchiolitis obliterans in unrelated industries such as battery workers, food flavoring workers, and nylon flock workers (Konichezky et al., 1993; Eschenbacher et al., 1999; Kreiss et al., 2002). It is difficult to prove causation when only a few workers are affected. Kreiss and colleagues (Kreiss et al., 2002) reported a high incidence of bronchiolitis obliterans in 7% (8 out of 117) of workers at a microwave popcorn plant, which was attributed to inhalation of the volatile agent diacetyl in the butter flavoring. This observation was supported by toxicity studies of diacetyl inhalation in rats (Hubbs et al., 2002). Bronchiolitis obliterans has also been described in a truck driver who inhaled fly ash, as well as in a young man with smoke inhalation from a fire (Boswell and McCunney, 1995; Tasaka et al., 1995). Both cases recovered from the acute illness only to have their symptoms recur and progress weeks to months later.

Organizing pneumonia can also occur as a sequela from prior pulmonary infections, most commonly seen with adenovirus, but also associated with other viruses (RSV, influenza) and mycoplasma (Wright et al., 1992; Penn and Liu, 1993; Chan et al., 1997). When an organizing pneumonia pattern is observed after an infection, it is referred to as "secondary organizing pneumonia." COP has been reported to occur in the contralateral lung in women undergoing breast radiation for breast cancer (Stover et al., 2001). Some medications have been implicated as etiological agents in the development of COP, including amiodarone, amphotericin, bleomycin, mesalazine, methotrexate, phenytoin, and sirolimus (Cordier, 2006). Both gold and penicillamine have been suspected; however, it is difficult to determine if the COP results from the medication or the underlying disease (Geddes et al., 1977).

Idiopathic Pulmonary Fibrosis

The original theory for the pathogenesis of IPF rested on the premise that inflammation of the alveoli was followed by fibrosis (Crystal et al., 1976, 1981, 1984; Hunninghake et al., 1979). There are many observations that support this hypothesis. Early studies that used bronchial lavage demonstrated increased numbers of alveolar macrophages, neutrophils, eosinophils, and lymphocytes (Crystal et al., 1976; Reynolds et al., 1977; Weinberger et al., 1978). Gallium scans, which are non-specific markers of inflammation with macrophages and neutrophils, are positive in about 70% of all patients with IPF (Crystal et al., 1976; Line et al., 1978). Biopsies that are performed in early stages of the disease reveal large amounts of inflammation and alveolar wall derangement compared to biopsies taken in the later stages of disease when fibrosis predominates (Carrington et al., 1978). Alveolar macrophages are believed to play a central role in the inflammatory process through the release of cytokines that affect other cells. Alveolar macrophages from patients with IPF have been shown to secrete neutrophil chemotactic factor, which does not occur in normal non-activated alveolar macrophages (Hunninghake et al., 1980, 1981). Animal models have shown the presence of inflammation preceding fibrosis, and the suppression of the inflammatory response attenuates the progression to fibrosis (Snider, 1986).

More recently, there has been a focus on the fibrotic aspect of the disease as also playing an important role. These theories about the pathogenesis of IPF involve the idea of recurrent, ongoing stimulus and injury to the lung, with abnormal wound healing. The abnormal wound healing is believed to result from a complex interplay of the genetic background of the individual, the predominant inflammatory phenotype (Th1 or Th2), and the environmental triggers. The stimulus that acts as the driving force remains a mystery, as does the mechanism that promotes a pathological fibrotic response instead of the normal reparative response.

The lung parenchyma regulates its immune and fibrotic processes through cytokine signaling between the cells of the interstitium, including epithelial cells, endothelial cells, fibroblasts, and macrophages, and it is likely that these cells contribute to the pathogenesis of IPF (Martinet et al., 1987; Standiford et al., 1991; Selman et al., 2001). Although the exact sequence of chemokine signaling that leads to the progression of fibrosis is not understood, it has been shown that cytokines are responsible for the cell-to-cell communication and fibroblast activation, proliferation, and collagen production.

One theory is that an imbalance in inflammatory phenotype, shifted towards a Th2 response, is responsible for the fibrotic phenotype. Support for this theory comes from the observation that IL-4 and IL-13, major Th2-type cytokines, have been shown to be major stimuli for fibroblast derived extracellular matrix deposition (Furuie et al., 1997; Hancock et al., 1998). Interferon-γ, one of the major Th1-type cytokines, has been shown to suppress the production of collagen and fibronectin by fibroblasts (Goldring et al., 1986). The increased presence of eosinophils, which have been associated with Th2 cytokine expression in asthma and parasitic infections, in association with fibrotic changes in IPF, is consistent with the concepts of the Th2 paradigm of abnormal healing. Davis et al. (Davis et al., 1984) demonstrated that eosinophils represented greater than 5% of the cells in the lavage fluid of 20% of patients with IPF compared to less than 1% of the normal controls. These eosinophils were shown to have collagenase activity and have the capacity to injure lung parenchymal cells.

The pathogenetic mechanisms that lead to the development of pulmonary fibrosis associated with rheumatic diseases have been most extensively studied in scleroderma. The most common theory, which may or may not be applicable to the idiopathic form, is that an initial environmental injury triggers an ongoing, amplified immune response in the lung. TNF-α and TGF-β have both been shown to be upregulated early in the course of the disease (Corrin et al., 1994; Bolster et al., 1997) and there is a cytokine shift from Th1 to Th2 in helper T cells (Bolster et al., 1997). Bronchoalveolar lavage fluid from patients with scleroderma has increased levels of several inflammatory cytokines such as IL-8, TNF-α, and macrophage inflammatory protein (Southcott et al., 1995). The lavage is also believed to have prognostic value in patients with systemic sclerosis. Scleroderma patients with a neutrophil and eosinophil predominant bronchoalveolar lavage have been associated with more extensive pulmonary fibrosis seen on CT and more rapid clinical deterioration (Rossi et al., 1987; Silver et al., 1990; Behr et al., 1996; Friedman et al., 1996; Witt et al., 1999).

The stimulus that leads to the inflammatory response in the lungs of patients with scleroderma is also unknown, but one hypothesis suggests that aspiration of refluxed esophageal and gastric contents may be the cause. The premise behind this theory arises from the fact that many patients with systemic sclerosis have both esophageal dysmotility and pulmonary fibrosis. This association was initially observed in a relatively small cohort of 12 patients (Johnson et al., 1989a). Subsequent studies have found conflicting results when trying to correlate pulmonary function parameters meant to be a surrogate marker of pulmonary fibrosis (such as total lung capacity and diffusion capacity) with esophageal manometry (Troshinsky et al., 1994; Lock et al., 1998). These studies are limited by confounding factors because both esophageal dysmotility and pulmonary fibrosis may be independent markers of scleroderma disease severity, without having a causal link.

Several environmental factors have been investigated for an etiological role in IPF. The premise of an environmental stimulus that leads to repeated lung injury followed by abnormal wound healing fits nicely into one theory of the pathogenesis of IPF (see below). The search for these stimuli is challenging because the offending agent may be different between individuals based on individual differences in genetic susceptibility. Nevertheless, epidemiological studies have identified links between occupational exposures, medications and infectious agents, and IPF.

Four separate case-control studies have looked at the association between occupational exposure and IPF. Although these studies are limited because of recall bias, there were some consistent observations. Metal dust exposure was significantly associated with IPF in every study and in a dose–response relationship (Iwai et al., 1994; Hubbard et al., 1996; Baumgartner et al., 1997, 2000). Two studies showed a significant association with livestock exposure, farming, and agricultural exposure (Iwai et al., 1994; Baumgartner et al., 2000). Paraquat, a herbicide used in agriculture, has been found to cause fatal pulmonary fibrosis in humans and experimental animals after oral, inhalational, or cutaneous exposure (Schoenberger et al., 1984). Anecdotal case reports have linked cases of IPF with occupations that result in toxic dust or fume exposure such as diamond polishing, dairy work, welding, gold extraction, and dental work (Baumgartner et al., 1997).

Pulmonary fibrosis is a well-known side effect of several medications, most notably bleomycin, amiodarone, methotrexate, and nitrofurantoin (Holmberg and Boman, 1981; Schoenberger and Crystal, 1983; Martin and Rosenow, 1988; Israel-Biet et al., 1991; Sleijfer, 2001). It has also been found as a rare complication of more commonly used medications such as beta blockers, antidepressants, anti-convulsants, and non-steroidal anti-inflammatory drugs. However, these associations have been difficult to prove given the ubiquity of these medications and the relative rarity of IPF (Coultas et al., 1994).

The effect of smoking on the natural history of IPF is controversial, but of four case–control studies examining the association of smoking with pulmonary fibrosis, three show a significant link between smoking and the development of IPF (Iwai et al., 1994; Hubbard et al., 1996; Baumgartner et al., 1997, 2000). Some studies have shown improved survival in smokers with IPF compared to non-smokers (Cherniack et al., 1995; King et al., 2001). However, this observation may be due to lead time bias in the smoking group, and simply reflect a greater severity of disease in the non-smoking groups.

TREATMENT AND OUTCOME

Cryptogenic Organizing Pneumonia

One of the defining features of COP is that it usually has an excellent response to corticosteroids. Although there have not been any randomized clinical trials to prove their efficacy, there is widespread consensus based on individual experience that corticosteroids are highly efficacious. When patients respond, there is typically complete radiographic and clinical resolution of the organizing pneumonia. There is no consensus on duration of treatment, with some authorities suggesting 6 to 8 weeks, while others advocate 1 year. Spontaneous remissions are unusual, except when a precipitating factor is identified and withdrawn, e.g., new medication. Second line agents, e.g., cytotoxic agents or macrolid antibiotics, can be used when steroids are contraindicated, but high quality data for these are lacking.

Idiopathic Pulmonary Fibrosis

IPF usually portends a poor prognosis and is typically poorly responsive to therapy. Early diagnosis and treatment have traditionally been advocated so that therapy can be initiated and hopefully prevent irreversible fibrosis. Therefore, the typical medications used to treat IPF work through anti-inflammatory and immunosuppressant mechanisms. However, these traditional approaches have failed to show that the inflammatory or fibrotic process can be altered or reversed. As the understanding of the pathogenesis of the disease improves, newer agents are being developed based on cellular mechanisms to inhibit fibrogenesis. No therapy for IPF has been shown in a prospective, randomized, double-blind, placebo-controlled trial to improve survival.

Prior studies have suggested that the prognosis may be favorable for patients with pulmonary fibrosis associated with systemic sclerosis (Wells et al., 1994). However, Hubbard and Venn (Hubbard and Venn, 2002) demonstrated with actuarial data that the mortality rates for patients with pulmonary fibrosis associated with all rheumatic disorders, predominantly rheumatoid arthritis in their study, are remarkably similar to those that are idiopathic in origin.

Corticosteroids

The most common medications used to treat IPF are corticosteroids, despite the fact that they have not been properly evaluated in a large clinical trial. Early studies showed that 10 to 30% of patients with IPF appear to improve or survive longer when treated with corticosteroids (Stack et al., 1972; Turner-Warwick et al., 1980). Unfortunately, these studies likely included other forms of idiopathic interstitial pneumonia, such as non-specific interstitial pneumonia or cryptogenic organizing pneumonia, which tend to have a more favorable prognosis than IPF. When histopathological criteria are used for the diagnosis of IPF, the clinical response (0–16%) and survival rates are much worse than for the other pathological patterns (Daniil et al., 1999; Ziesche et al., 1999; Nicholson et al., 2000). Despite the lack of evidence for a beneficial role of corticosteroids, many pulmonologists use a 3- to 6-month trial of corticosteroids with close monitoring for radiographic or physiologic improvement. Patients who improve with corticosteroids or who remain stable are then kept on a maintenance dose of 10 to 20 mg of prednisone per day (ATS, 2002). Intravenous pulse corticosteroids for 3 to 5 days are generally recommended for an acute exacerbation of IPF, as Keogh and colleagues (Keogh et al., 1983) have shown that higher doses of corticosteroids can significantly reduce the neutrophil accumulation during an active alveolitis of IPF.

Cytotoxic Agents

Other anti-inflammatory and cytotoxic agents have been investigated for a beneficial role in IPF. Cyclophosphamide, when used in combination with corticosteroids, had promising results towards a survival advantage compared to corticosteroids alone in an early randomized control trial (Johnson et al., 1989b; Baughman and Lower, 1992). Cyclophosphamide has been shown to reduce the neutrophil component of the active alveolitis after 3 and 6 months of therapy (O'Donnell et al., 1987). However, subsequent studies have shown cyclophosphamide to have limited efficacy and a high frequency of side effects when used to treat patients with IPF who failed to respond to corticosteroid therapy (Zisman et al., 2000). Cyclophosphamide may be particularly effective in patients with scleroderma-associated pulmonary fibrosis, as it was shown to improve pulmonary function testing in this population. Scleroderma patients with a neutrophil predominant bronchoalveolar lavage seemed to have the best outcomes, although these studies were limited by either small sample size, lack of a control group, or selection bias from retrospective review (Silver et al., 1990; Schnabel et al., 1998; White et al., 2000). It is currently considered as a second line drug for patients with progressive IPF. Side effects include leukopenia, thrombocytopenia, and hemorrhagic cystitis.

Azathioprine has been shown to have some efficacy in the treatment for IPF in small prospective case series (Winterbauer et al., 1978; Raghu et al., 1991). Azathioprine exerts cytotoxic effects on lymphocytes and also suppresses the activity of natural killer cells and antibody production. It is also considered a second line therapy for patients who fail corticosteroids, or may be given in conjunction with corticosteroids.

A randomized control trial comparing acetylcysteine vs. placebo in patients with IPF who were also receiving prednisone and azathioprine demonstrated significantly slower declines in both vital capacity and diffusing capacity in the acetylcysteine group. However, there were no improvements in mortality, quality of life, or radiography (Hunninghake, 2005). One possible explanation is that the addition of acetylcysteine simply attenuates the harmful effects of cytotoxic therapy. More studies of this combination therapy are needed before this can be determined.

Anti-fibrotic Agents

Colchicine has been postulated to have a role in the treatment of IPF because it inhibits collagen formation *in vitro* and suppresses the release of alveolar macrophage-derived growth factor (Rennard et al., 1988). Colchicine has been suggested in small randomized control trials to be as effective as corticosteroids in treatment of IPF, but has not been followed up with large, controlled studies (Peters et al., 1993; Douglas et al., 1998).

Interferon γ-1b was used by Ziesche and colleagues (Ziesche et al., 1999) in a 1-year study of 18 patients with IPF randomized to receive interferon γ-1b and prednisolone, compared to prednisolone alone. Interferon γ-1b has been shown to downregulate the expression of TGF-α1 and inhibit the proliferation of fibroblasts, both of which are considered important roles in the pathogenesis of pulmonary fibrosis (Clark et al., 1989; Narayanan et al., 1992). Ziesche's study (Ziesche et al., 1999) suggested a significant improvement in total lung capacity and partial pressure of arterial oxygen, and a decrease in the level of transcription of TGF-α1 and connective-tissue growth factor in the individuals who received interferon γ-1b.

This led to a multi-center, double-blind, placebo-controlled trial of interferon γ-1b in patients with IPF who failed to respond to corticosteroids. Interferon γ-1b did not improve any of the main outcomes: progression-free survival, pulmonary function, or quality of life (Raghu et al., 2004). Additionally, there were more adverse side effects in the group that received interferon γ-1b. There was a trend towards increased survival in the group that received interferon γ-1b (16 out of 162 patients in the interferon γ-1b group died compared with 28 out of 168 patients in the placebo group, an absolute reduction of 7%). However, the relatively short follow up of 1 year, coupled with the fact that this was not a primary endpoint of the trial, raises the concern that this trend may be misleading. At this time, interferon γ-1b should not be considered as a proven therapy for IPF, unless used as part of a clinical trial.

Many other novel strategies have been investigated in the treatment of IPF, including cyclosporin A, pirfenidone, bosentan, and etanercept (Raghu et al., 2011). These therapies focus on different aspects of the pathogenesis of the disease, such as anti-oxidants, inhibitors of cytokines, proteases, and fibroblast growth factors. However, all of these agents have failed to demonstrate clinically meaningful responses and therefore the joint statement by the American Thoracic Society and European Respiratory Society strongly recommended against using corticosteroids, colchicine, interferon γ-1b, cyclosporine, pirfenidone, bosentan, or etanercept for treatment of IPF (Raghu et al., 2011).

Lung transplantation should be considered for individuals who progress despite optimized medical management. Patients should be referred to a transplant center relatively early in their course, since wait times on the list can exceed 2 years due to limited donor availability. Those who receive a successful transplant can experience significant improvement in arterial oxygenation, pulmonary hypertension, and right ventricular dysfunction. Unfortunately, the 5-year survival rates for lung transplant are only about 60%, with death frequently due to graft failure, infection, or bronchiolitis obliterans (Lu and Bhorade, 2004).

CONCLUSIONS

The autoimmune disorders of the lung, notably cryptogenic organizing pneumonia and idiopathic pulmonary fibrosis, have long been recognized as inflammatory and fibrotic processes that are associated with variable prognosis, whether idiopathic in nature or in association with the multisystem autoimmune diseases. Both diseases appear to be mediated through repetitive cell-mediated injury directed at the bronchioles and alveoli/interstitium, followed by wound healing. Recent advances in the classification and diagnostic testing for these diseases have improved our ability to study their incidence, prognosis, and response to therapy. While much progress has been made, the search for antigenic stimuli and genetic polymorphisms that are responsible for disease pathogenesis continues. Only through a better understanding of the disease process will we be able to offer new therapies for these diseases.

ACKNOWLEDGMENTS

We thank J. Kaplan and N. Mohamed for help in preparing this manuscript.

REFERENCES

American Thoracic Society/European Respiratory Society International Multidisciplinary Consensus Classification of the Idiopathic Interstitial Pneumonias 2002 Am. J. Respir. Crit. Care Med. 165, 277–304.

Alasaly, K., Muller, N., Ostrow, D.N., Champion, P., FitzGerald, J.M., 1995. Cryptogenic organizing pneumonia. A report of 25 cases and a review of the literature. Medicine (Baltimore). 74, 201–211.

Arcasoy, S.M., Kotloff, R.M., 1999. Lung transplantation. N. Engl. J. Med. 340, 1081–1091.

Aubert, J.D., Pare, P.D., Hogg, J.C., Hayashi, S., 1997. Platelet-derived growth factor in bronchiolitis obliterans-organizing pneumonia. Am. J. Respir. Crit. Care Med. 155, 676–681.

Baar, H.S., Galindo, J., 1966. Bronchiolitis fibrosa obliterans. Thorax. 21, 209–214.

Basset, F., Ferrans, V.J., Soler, P., Takemura, T., Fukuda, Y., Crystal, R.G., 1986. Intraluminal fibrosis in interstitial lung disorders. Am. J. Pathol. 122, 443–461.

Baughman, R.P., Lower, E.E., 1992. Use of intermittent, intravenous cyclophosphamide for idiopathic pulmonary fibrosis. Chest. 102, 1090–1094.

Baumgartner, K.B., Samet, J.M., Coultas, D.B., Stidley, C.A., Hunt, W.C., Colby, T.V., et al., 2000. Occupational and environmental risk factors for idiopathic pulmonary fibrosis: a multicenter case–control study. Collaborating Centers. Am. J. Epidemiol. 152, 307–315.

Baumgartner, K.B., Samet, J.M., Stidley, C.A., Colby, T.V., Waldron, J.A., 1997. Cigarette smoking: a risk factor for idiopathic pulmonary fibrosis. Am. J. Respir. Crit. Care Med. 155, 242–248.

Begin, R., Masse, S., Cantin, A., Ménard, H.A., Bureau, M.A., 1982. Airway disease in a subset of nonsmoking rheumatoid patients. Characterization of the disease and evidence for an autoimmune pathogenesis. Am. J. Med. 72, 743–750.

Behr, J., Vogelmeier, C., Beinert, T., Meurer, M., Krombach, F., König, G., et al., 1996. Bronchoalveolar lavage for evaluation and management of scleroderma disease of the lung. Am. J. Respir. Crit. Care Med. 154, 400–406.

Bellum, S.C., Dove, D., Harley, R.A., Greene, W.B., Judson, M.A., London, L., et al., 1997. Respiratory reovirus 1/L induction of intraluminal fibrosis. A model for the study of bronchiolitis obliterans organizing pneumonia. Am. J. Pathol. 150, 2243–2254.

Bernstein, R.M., Morgan, S.H., Chapman, J., Bunn, C.C., Mathews, M.B., Turner-Warwick, M., et al., 1984. Anti-Jo-1 antibody: a marker for myositis with interstitial lung disease. Br. Med. J. (Clin. Res. Ed.). 289, 151–152.

Bitterman, P.B., Rennard, S.I., Keogh, B.A., Wewers, M.D., Adelberg, S., Crystal, R.G., 1986. Familial idiopathic pulmonary fibrosis. Evidence of lung inflammation in unaffected family members. N. Engl. J. Med. 314, 1343–1347.

Bolster, M.B., Ludwicka, A., Sutherland, S.E., Strange, C., Silver, R. M., 1997. Cytokine concentrations in bronchoalveolar lavage fluid of patients with systemic sclerosis. Arthritis Rheum. 40, 743–751.

Boswell, R.T., McCunney, R.J., 1995. Bronchiolitis obliterans from exposure to incinerator fly ash. J. Occup. Environ. Med. 37, 850–855.

Bouros, D., Wells, A.U., Nicholson, A.G., Colby, T.V., Polychronopoulos, V., Pantelidis, P., et al., 2002. Histopathologic subsets of fibrosing alveolitis in patients with systemic sclerosis and their relationship to outcome. Am. J. Respir. Crit. Care Med. 165, 1581–1586.

Camus, P., Nemery, B., 1998. A novel cause for bronchiolitis obliterans organizing pneumonia: exposure to paint aerosols in textile workshops. Eur. Respir. J. 11, 259–262.

Carre, P.C., King Jr., T.E., Mortensen, R., Riches, D.W., 1994. Cryptogenic organizing pneumonia: increased expression of interleukin-8 and fibronectin genes by alveolar macrophages. Am. J. Respir. Cell Mol. Biol. 10, 100–105.

Carrington, C.B., Gaensler, E.A., Coutu, R.E., FitzGerald, M.X., Gupta, R.G., 1978. Natural history and treated course of usual and desquamative interstitial pneumonia. N. Engl. J. Med. 298, 801–809.

Cervantes-Perez, P., Toro-Perez, A.H., Rodriguez-Jurado, P., 1980. Pulmonary involvement in rheumatoid arthritis. JAMA. 243, 1715–1719.

Chan, T.Y., Hansell, D.M., Rubens, M.B., du Bois, R.M., Wells, A.U., 1997. Cryptogenic fibrosing alveolitis and the fibrosing alveolitis of systemic sclerosis: morphological differences on computed tomographic scans. Thorax. 52, 265–270.

Chapman, J.R., Charles, P.J., Venables, P.J., Thompson, P.J., Haslam, P.L., Maini, R.N., et al., 1984. Definition and clinical relevance of antibodies to nuclear ribonucleoprotein and other nuclear antigens in patients with cryptogenic fibrosing alveolitis. Am. Rev. Respir. Dis. 130, 439–443.

Cherniack, R.M., Colby, T.V., Flint, A., Thurlbeck, W.M., Waldron Jr., J.A., Ackerson, L., et al., 1995. Correlation of structure and function in idiopathic pulmonary fibrosis. Am. J. Respir. Crit. Care Med. 151, 1180–1188.

Clark, J.G., Dedon, T.F., Wayner, E.A., Carter, W.G., 1989. Effects of interferon-gamma on expression of cell surface receptors for collagen and deposition of newly synthesized collagen by cultured human lung fibroblasts. J. Clin. Invest. 83, 1505–1511.

Colby, T.V., 1998. Bronchiolitis. Pathologic considerations. Am. J. Clin. Pathol. 109, 101–109.

Cordier, J.F., 2006. Cryptogenic organising pneumonia. Eur. Respir. J. 28, 422–446.

Corrin, B., Butcher, D., McAnulty, B.J., Dubois, R.M., Black, C.M., Laurent, G.J., et al., 1994. Immunohistochemical localization of transforming growth factor-beta 1 in the lungs of patients with systemic sclerosis, cryptogenic fibrosing alveolitis and other lung disorders. Histopathology. 24, 145–150.

Coultas, D.B., Zumwalt, R.E., Black, W.C., Sobonya, R.E., 1994. The epidemiology of interstitial lung diseases. Am. J. Respir. Crit. Care Med. 150, 967–972.

Crystal, R.G., Bitterman, P.B., Rennard, S.I., Hance, A.J., Keogh, B.A., 1984. Interstitial lung diseases of unknown cause. Disorders characterized by chronic inflammation of the lower respiratory tract. N. Engl. J. Med. 310, 235–244.

Crystal, R.G., Fulmer, J.D., Roberts, W.C., Moss, M.L., Line, B.R., Reynolds, H.Y., 1976. Idiopathic pulmonary fibrosis. Clinical, histologic, radiographic, physiologic, scintigraphic, cytologic, and biochemical aspects. Ann. Intern. Med. 85, 769–788.

Crystal, R.G., Gadek, J.E., Ferrans, V.J., Fulmer, J.D., Line, B.R., Hunninghake, G.W., 1981. Interstitial lung disease: current concepts of pathogenesis, staging and therapy. Am. J. Med. 70, 542–568.

Daniil, Z.D., Gilchrist, F.C., Nicholson, A.G., Hansell, D.M., Harris, J., Colby, T.V., et al., 1999. A histologic pattern of nonspecific interstitial pneumonia is associated with a better prognosis than usual interstitial pneumonia in patients with cryptogenic fibrosing alveolitis. Am. J. Respir. Crit. Care Med. 160, 899–905.

Davis, W.B., Fells, G.A., Sun, X.H., Gadek, J.E., Venet, A., Crystal, R.G., 1984. Eosinophil-mediated injury to lung parenchymal cells and interstitial matrix. A possible role for eosinophils in chronic inflammatory disorders of the lower respiratory tract. J. Clin. Invest. 74, 269–278.

Davison, A.G., Heard, B.E., McAllister, W.A., Turner-Warwick, M.E., 1983. Cryptogenic organizing pneumonitis. Q. J. Med. 52, 382–394.

Douglas, W.W., Ryu, J.H., Swensen, S.J., Offord, K.P., Schroeder, D.R., Caron, G.M., et al., 1998. Colchicine versus prednisone in the treatment of idiopathic pulmonary fibrosis. A randomized prospective study. Members of the Lung Study Group. Am. J. Respir. Crit. Care Med. 158, 220–225.

Douglas, W.W., Tazelaar, H.D., Hartman, T.E., Hartman, R.P., Decker, P.A., Schroeder, D.R., et al., 2001. Polymyositis-dermatomyositis-associated interstitial lung disease. Am. J. Respir. Crit. Care Med. 164, 1182–1185.

Dreisin, R.B., Schwarz, M.I., Theofilopoulos, A.N., Stanford, R.E., 1978. Circulating immune complexes in the idiopathic interstitial pneumonias. N. Engl. J. Med. 298, 353–357.

Eisenberg, H., Dubois, E.L., Sherwin, R.P., Balchum, O.J., 1973. Diffuse interstitial lung disease in systemic lupus erythematosus. Ann. Intern. Med. 79, 37–45.

Epler, G.R., Colby, T.V., McLoud, T.C., Carrington, C.B., Gaensler, E.A., 1985. Bronchiolitis obliterans organizing pneumonia. N. Engl. J. Med. 312, 152–158.

Epler, G.R., Snider, G.L., Gaensler, E.A., Cathcart, E.S., FitzGerald, M.X., Carrington, C.B., 1979. Bronchiolitis and bronchitis in connective tissue disease A possible relationship to the use of penicillamine. JAMA. 242, 528–532.

Eschenbacher, W.L., Kreiss, K., Lougheed, M.D., Pransky, G.S., Day, B., Castellan, R.M., 1999. Nylon flock-associated interstitial lung disease. Am. J. Respir. Crit. Care Med. 159, 2003–2008.

Fanning, G.C., Welsh, K.I., Bunn, C., Du Bois, R., Black, C.M., 1998. HLA associations in three mutually exclusive autoantibody subgroups in UK systemic sclerosis patients. Br. J. Rheumatol. 37, 201–207.

Flaherty, K.R., Travis, W.D., Colby, T.V., Toews, G.B., Kazerooni, E.A., Gross, B.H., et al., 2001. Histopathologic variability in usual and non-specific interstitial pneumonias. Am. J. Respir. Crit. Care Med. 164, 1722–1727.

Fleming, G.M., Chester, E.H., Montenegro, H.D., 1979. Dysfunction of small airways following pulmonary injury due to nitrogen dioxide. Chest. 75, 720–721.

Forlani, S., Ratta, L., Bulgheroni, A., Cascina, A., Paschetto, E., Cervio, G., et al., 2002. Cytokine profile of broncho-alveolar lavage in BOOP and UIP. Sarcoidosis Vasc. Diffuse Lung Dis. 19, 47–53.

Friedman, A.W., Targoff, I.N., Arnett, F.C., 1996. Interstitial lung disease with autoantibodies against aminoacyl-tRNA synthetases in the absence of clinically apparent myositis. Semin. Arthritis Rheum. 26, 459–467.

Fujita, J., Dobashi, N., Ohtsuki, Y., Yamadori, I., Yoshinouchi, T., Kamei, T., et al., 1999. Elevation of anti-cytokeratin 19 antibody in sera of the patients with idiopathic pulmonary fibrosis and pulmonary fibrosis associated with collagen vascular disorders. Lung. 177, 311–319.

Fulmer, J.D., Roberts, W.C., von Gal, E.R., Crystal, R.G., 1979. Morphologic-physiologic correlates of the severity of fibrosis and degree of cellularity in idiopathic pulmonary fibrosis. J. Clin. Invest. 63, 665–676.

Furuie, H., Yamasaki, H., Suga, M., Ando, M., 1997. Altered accessory cell function of alveolar macrophages: a possible mechanism for induction of Th2 secretory profile in idiopathic pulmonary fibrosis. Eur. Respir. J. 10, 787–794.

Gabbay, E., Tarala, R., Will, R., Carroll, G., Adler, B., Cameron, D., et al., 1997. Interstitial lung disease in recent onset rheumatoid arthritis. Am. J. Respir. Crit. Care Med. 156, 528–535.

Gardiner, P., 1993. Primary Sjogren's syndrome. Baillieres Clin. Rheumatol. 7, 59–77.

Geddes, D.M., Corrin, B., Brewerton, D.A., Davies, R.J., Turner-Warwick, M., 1977. Progressive airway obliteration in adults and its association with rheumatoid disease. Q. J. Med. 46, 427–444.

Goldring, M.B., Sandell, L.J., Stephenson, M.L., Krane, S.M., 1986. Immune interferon suppresses levels of procollagen mRNA and type II collagen synthesis in cultured human articular and costal chondrocytes. J. Biol. Chem. 261, 9049–9055.

Gosink, B.B., Friedman, P.J., Liebow, A.A., 1973. Bronchiolitis obliterans. Roentgenologic-pathologic correlation. Am. J. Roentgenol. Radium. Ther. Nucl. Med. 117, 816–832.

Gross, T.J., Hunninghake, G.W., 2001. Idiopathic pulmonary fibrosis. N. Engl. J. Med. 345, 517–525.

Hamaguchi, Y., Nishizawa, Y., Yasui, M., Hasegawa, M., Kaburagi, Y., Komura, K., et al., 2002. Intercellular adhesion molecule-1 and L-selectin regulate bleomycin-induced lung fibrosis. Am. J. Pathol. 161, 1607–1618.

Hamman, L., Rich, A.R., 1935. Fulminating diffuse interstitial fibrosis of the lungs. Trans. Am. Clin. Climatol. Assoc. 51, 154–163.

Hancock, A., Armstrong, L., Gama, R., Millar, A., 1998. Production of interleukin 13 by alveolar macrophages from normal and fibrotic lung. Am. J. Respir. Cell Mol. Biol. 18, 60–65.

Harrison, N.K., Myers, A.R., Corrin, B., Soosay, G., Dewar, A., Black, C.M., et al., 1991. Structural features of interstitial lung disease in systemic sclerosis. Am. Rev. Respir. Dis. 144, 706–713.

Haslam, P.L., Thompson, B., Mohammed, I., Townsend, P.J., Hodson, M.E., Holborow, E.J., et al., 1979. Circulating immune complexes in patients with cryptogenic fibrosing alveolitis. Clin. Exp. Immunol. 37, 381–390.

Hertz, M.I., Jessurun, J., King, M.B., Savik, S.K., Murray, J.J., 1993. Reproduction of the obliterative bronchiolitis lesion after heterotopic transplantation of mouse airways. Am. J. Pathol. 142, 1945–1951.

Herzog, C.A., Miller, R.R., Hoidal, J.R., 1981. Bronchiolitis and rheumatoid arthritis. Am. Rev. Respir. Dis. 124, 636–639.

Hochberg, M.C., Feldman, D., Stevens, M.B., Arnett, F.C., Reichlin, M., 1984. Antibody to Jo-1 in polymyositis/dermatomyositis: association with interstitial pulmonary disease. J. Rheumatol. 11, 663–665.

Hodgson, U., Laitinen, T., Tukiainen, P., 2002. Nationwide prevalence of sporadic and familial idiopathic pulmonary fibrosis: evidence of founder effect among multiplex families in Finland. Thorax. 57, 338–342.

Holgate, S.T., Haslam, P., Turner-Warwick, M., 1983. The significance of antinuclear and DNA antibodies in cryptogenic fibrosing alveolitis. Thorax. 38, 67–70.

Holmberg, L., Boman, G., 1981. Pulmonary reactions to nitrofurantoin. 447 cases reported to the Swedish Adverse Drug Reaction Committee 1966–1976. Eur. J. Respir. Dis. 62, 180–189.

Hubbard, R., Johnston, I., Britton, J., 1998. Survival in patients with cryptogenic fibrosing alveolitis: a population-based cohort study. Chest. 113, 396–400.

Hubbard, R., Lewis, S., Richards, K., Johnston, I., Britton, J., 1996. Occupational exposure to metal or wood dust and aetiology of cryptogenic fibrosing alveolitis. Lancet. 347, 284–289.

Hubbard, R., Venn, A., 2002. The impact of coexisting connective tissue disease on survival in patients with fibrosing alveolitis. Rheumatology (Oxford). 41, 676–679.

Hubbs, A.F., Battelli, L.A., Goldsmith, W.T., Porter, D.W., Frazer, D., Friend, S., et al., 2002. Necrosis of nasal and airway epithelium in rats inhaling vapors of artificial butter flavoring. Toxicol. Appl. Pharmacol. 185, 128–135.

Hunninghake, G.W., 2005. Antioxidant therapy for idiopathic pulmonary fibrosis. N. Engl. J. Med. 353, 2285–2287.

Hunninghake, G.W., Gadek, J.E., Fales, H.M., Crystal, R.G., 1980. Human alveolar macrophage-derived chemotactic factor for neutrophils: stimuli and partial characterization. J. Clin. Invest. 66, 473–483.

Hunninghake, G.W., Gadek, J.E., Kawanami, O., Ferrans, V.J., Crystal, R.G., 1979. Inflammatory and immune processes in the human lung in health and disease: evaluation by bronchoalveolar lavage. Am. J. Pathol. 97, 149–206.

Hunninghake, G.W., Gadek, J.E., Lawley, T.J., Crystal, R.G., 1981. Mechanisms of neutrophil accumulation in the lungs of patients with idiopathic pulmonary fibrosis. J. Clin. Invest. 68, 259–269.

Hunninghake, G.W., Zimmerman, M.B., Schwartz, D.A., King Jr., T.E., Lynch, J., Hegele, R., et al., 2001. Utility of a lung biopsy for the diagnosis of idiopathic pulmonary fibrosis. Am. J. Respir. Crit. Care Med. 164, 193–196.

Hyland, R.H., Gordon, D.A., Broder, I., Davies, G.M., Russell, M.L., Hutcheon, M.A., et al., 1983. A systematic controlled study of pulmonary abnormalities in rheumatoid arthritis. J. Rheumatol. 10, 395–405.

Irifune, K., Yokoyama, A., Kohno, N., Sakai, K., Hiwada, K., 2003. T-helper 1 cells induce alveolitis but do not lead to pulmonary fibrosis in mice. Eur. Respir. J. 21, 11–18.

Israel-Biet, D., Labrune, S., Huchon, G.J., 1991. Drug-induced lung disease: 1990 review. Eur. Respir. J. 4, 465–478.

Iwai, K., Mori, T., Yamada, N., Yamaguchi, M., Hosoda, Y., 1994. Idiopathic pulmonary fibrosis. Epidemiologic approaches to occupational exposure. Am. J. Respir. Crit. Care Med. 150, 670–675.

Javaheri, S., Lederer, D.H., Pella, J.A., Mark, G.J., Levine, B.W., 1980. Idiopathic pulmonary fibrosis in monozygotic twins. The importance of genetic predisposition. Chest. 78, 591–594.

Johnson, D.A., Drane, W.E., Curran, J., Cattau Jr., E.L., Ciarleglio, C., Khan, A., et al., 1989a. Pulmonary disease in progressive systemic sclerosis. A complication of gastroesophageal reflux and occult aspiration? Arch. Intern. Med. 149, 589–593.

Johnson, M.A., Kwan, S., Snell, N.J., Nunn, A.J., Darbyshire, J.H., Turner-Warwick, M., 1989b. Randomised controlled trial comparing prednisolone alone with cyclophosphamide and low dose prednisolone in combination in cryptogenic fibrosing alveolitis. Thorax. 44, 280–288.

Katzenstein, A.L., Fiorelli, R.F., 1994. Nonspecific interstitial pneumonia/fibrosis. Histologic features and clinical significance. Am. J. Surg. Pathol. 18, 136–147.

Kelly, K., Hertz, M.I., 1997. Obliterative bronchiolitis. Clin. Chest Med. 18, 319–338.

Keogh, B.A., Bernardo, J., Hunninghake, G.W., Line, B.R., Price, D.L., Crystal, R.G., 1983. Effect of intermittent high dose parenteral corticosteroids on the alveolitis of idiopathic pulmonary fibrosis. Am. Rev. Respir. Dis. 127, 18–22.

Keogh, B.A., Crystal, R.G., 1980. Clinical significance of pulmonary function tests. Pulmonary function testing in interstitial pulmonary disease. What does it tell us? Chest. 78, 856–865.

King Jr., T.E., 2003. Bronchiolitis. In: Schwarz, M.I, King Jr., T.E (Eds.), Interstitial lung Disease. BD Decker Inc, London, pp. 787–824.

King Jr., T.E., Mortenson, R.L., 1992. Cryptogenic organizing pneumonitis. The North American experience. Chest. 102, 8S–13S.

King Jr., T.E., Tooze, J.A., Schwarz, M.I., Brown, K.R., Cherniack, R.M., 2001. Predicting survival in idiopathic pulmonary fibrosis: scoring system and survival model. Am. J. Respir. Crit. Care Med. 164, 1171–1181.

Konichezky, S., Schattner, A., Ezri, T., Bokenboim, P., Geva, D., 1993. Thionyl-chloride-induced lung injury and bronchiolitis obliterans. Chest. 104, 971–973.

Kravis, T.C., Ahmed, A., Brown, T.E., Fulmer, J.D., Crystal, R.G., 1976. Pathogenic mechanisms in pulmonary fibrosis: collagen-induced migration inhibition factor production and cytotoxicity mediated by lymphocytes. J. Clin. Invest. 58, 1223–1232.

Kreiss, K., Gomaa, A., Kullman, G., Fedan, K., Simoes, E.J., Enright, P.L., 2002. Clinical bronchiolitis obliterans in workers at a microwave-popcorn plant. N. Engl. J. Med. 347, 330–338.

Kuhn, C., McDonald, J.A., 1991. The roles of the myofibroblast in idiopathic pulmonary fibrosis. Ultrastructural and immunohistochemical features of sites of active extracellular matrix synthesis. Am. J. Pathol. 138, 1257–1265.

Kunkel, S.L., 2004. Cytokine phenotypes and the progression of chronic pulmonary fibrosis. In: Lenfant, C. (Ed.), Idiopathic Pulmonary Fibrosis. Marcel Decker, Inc., New York, pp. 303–320.

Lange, W., 1901. Uber eine eigentumliche Erkrankung der kleinen Bronchien obliterans. Dtsch. Arch. Klin. Med. 70, 342–364.

Lappi-Blanco, E., Soini, Y., Kinnula, V., et al., 2002. VEGF and bFGF are highly expressed in intraluminal fibromyxoid lesions in bronchiolitis obliterans organizing pneumonia. J. Pathol. 196, 220–227.

Liebow, A.A., Carrington, D., 1969. The interstitial pneumonias. In: Simon, M., Potchen, E., LeMay, M. (Eds.), Frontiers of Pulmonary Radiology. Grune & Stratton, New York, pp. 102–141.

Line, B.R., Fulmer, J.D., Reynolds, H.Y., Roberts, W.C., Jones, A.E., Harris, E.K., et al., 1978. Gallium-67 citrate scanning in the staging of idiopathic pulmonary fibrosis: correlation and physiologic and morphologic features and bronchoalveolar lavage. Am. Rev. Respir. Dis. 118, 355–365.

Liu, J.Y., Sime, P.J., Wu, T., Warshamana, G.S., Pociask, D., Tsai, S.Y., et al., 2001. Transforming growth factor-beta(1) overexpression in tumor necrosis factor-alpha receptor knockout mice induces fibroproliferative lung disease. Am. J. Respir. Cell Mol. Biol. 25, 3–7.

Lock, G., Pfeifer, M., Straub, R.H., Zeuner, M., Lang, B., Schölmerich, J., et al., 1998. Association of esophageal dysfunction and pulmonary function impairment in systemic sclerosis. Am. J. Gastroenterol. 93, 341–345.

London, L., Majeski, E.I., Paintlia, M.K., Harley, R.A., London, S.D., 2002a. Respiratory reovirus 1/L induction of diffuse alveolar damage: a model of acute respiratory distress syndrome. Exp. Mol. Pathol. 72, 24–36.

London, L., Majeski, E.I., tman-Hamamdzic, S., Enockson, C., Paintlia, M.K., Harley, R.A., et al., 2002b. Respiratory reovirus 1/L induction of diffuse alveolar damage: pulmonary fibrosis is not modulated by corticosteroids in acute respiratory distress syndrome in mice. Clin. Immunol. 103, 284–295.

Lu, B.S., Bhorade, S.M., 2004. Lung transplantation for interstitial lung disease. Clin. Chest Med. 25, 773–782.

Lukacs, N.W., Hogaboam, C., Chensue, S.W., Blease, K., Kunkel, S.L., 2001. Type 1/type 2 cytokine paradigm and the progression of pulmonary fibrosis. Chest. 120, 5S–8S.

Magro, C.M., Ross, P., Marsh, C.B., Allen, J.N., Liff, D., Knight, D.A., et al., 2007. The role of anti-endothelial cell antibody-mediated microvascular injury in the evolution of pulmonary fibrosis in the setting of collagen vascular disease. Am. J. Clin. Pathol. 127, 237–247.

Mapel, D.W., Hunt, W.C., Utton, R., Baumgartner, K.B., Samet, J.M., Coultas, D.B., 1998. Idiopathic pulmonary fibrosis: survival in population based and hospital based cohorts. Thorax. 53, 469–476.

Marguerie, C., Bunn, C.C., Beynon, H.L., Bernstein, R.M., Hughes, J.M., So, A.K., et al., 1990. Polymyositis, pulmonary fibrosis and autoantibodies to aminoacyl-tRNA synthetase enzymes. Q. J. Med. 77, 1019–1038.

Marshall, R.P., Puddicombe, A., Cookson, W.O., Laurent, G.J., 2000. Adult familial cryptogenic fibrosing alveolitis in the United Kingdom. Thorax. 55, 143–146.

Martin, W.J., Rosenow III, E.C., 1988. Amiodarone pulmonary toxicity. Recognition and pathogenesis (Part I). Chest. 93, 1067–1075.

Martinet, Y., Rom, W.N., Grotendorst, G.R., Martin, G.R., Crystal, R.G., 1987. Exaggerated spontaneous release of platelet-derived growth factor by alveolar macrophages from patients with idiopathic pulmonary fibrosis. N. Engl. J. Med. 317, 202–209.

McLees, B.D., Adair, N., Moss, J., Fulmer, J.D., Keogh, B., Crystal, R.G., 1979. Patterns of pulmonary hemodynamic dysfunction: similarities between idiopathic pulmonary fibrosis and panacinar emphysema. Am. Rev. Respir. Dis. 119, 380.

Meliconi, R., Negri, C., Borzi, R.M., Facchini, A., Sturani, C., Fasano, L., et al., 1993. Antibodies to topoisomerase II in idiopathic pulmonary fibrosis. Clin. Rheumatol. 12, 311–315.

Minai, O.A., Dweik, R.A., Arroliga, A.C., 1998. Manifestations of scleroderma pulmonary disease. Clin. Chest Med. 19, 713–732.

Miyazaki, Y., Araki, K., Vesin, C., Garcia, I., Kapanci, Y., Whitsett, J.A., et al., 1995. Expression of a tumor necrosis factor-alpha transgene in murine lung causes lymphocytic and fibrosing alveolitis. A mouse

model of progressive pulmonary fibrosis. J. Clin. Invest. 96, 250–259.

Mori, S., Cho, I., Koga, Y., Sugimoto, M., 2008. A simultaneous onset of organizing pneumonia and rheumatoid arthritis, along with a review of the literature. Mod. Rheumatol. 18, 60–66.

Moya, C., Anto, J.M., Taylor, A.J., 1994. Outbreak of organising pneumonia in textile printing sprayers. Collaborative Group for the Study of Toxicity in Textile Aerographic Factories. Lancet. 344, 498–502.

Murray, J.F., Nadel, J.A., 2000. Idiopathic interstitial pneumonias. In: Murray, J.F., Nadel, J.A. (Eds.), Murray and Nadel's Textbook of Respiratory Medicine. Saunders, Philadelphia PA, pp. 1686–1687.

Myers, J.L., Colby, T.V., 1993. Pathologic manifestations of bronchiolitis, constrictive bronchiolitis, cryptogenic organizing pneumonia, and diffuse panbronchiolitis. Clin. Chest Med. 14, 611–622.

Nakao, A., Fujii, M., Matsumura, R., Kumano, K., Saito, Y., Miyazono, K., et al., 1999. Transient gene transfer and expression of Smad7 prevents bleomycin-induced lung fibrosis in mice. J. Clin. Invest. 104, 5–11.

Nakos, G., Adams, A., Andriopoulos, N., 1993. Antibodies to collagen in patients with idiopathic pulmonary fibrosis. Chest. 103, 1051–1058.

Narayanan, A.S., Whithey, J., Souza, A., Raghu, G., 1992. Effect of gamma-interferon on collagen synthesis by normal and fibrotic human lung fibroblasts. Chest. 101, 1326–1331.

Nicholson, A.G., Colby, T.V., du Bois, R.M., Hansell, D.M., Wells, A.U., 2000. The prognostic significance of the histologic pattern of interstitial pneumonia in patients presenting with the clinical entity of cryptogenic fibrosing alveolitis. Am. J. Respir. Crit. Care Med. 162, 2213–2217.

O'Donnell, K., Keogh, B., Cantin, A., Crystal, R.G., 1987. Pharmacologic suppression of the neutrophil component of the alveolitis in idiopathic pulmonary fibrosis. Am. Rev. Respir. Dis. 136, 288–292.

Osler, W., 1892. The Principles and Practice of Medicine. Appleton, New York.

Pantelidis, P., Fanning, G.C., Wells, A.U., Welsh, K.I., Du Bois, R.M., 2001. Analysis of tumor necrosis factor-alpha, lymphotoxin-alpha, tumor necrosis factor receptor II, and interleukin-6 polymorphisms in patients with idiopathic pulmonary fibrosis. Am. J. Respir. Crit Care. Med. 163, 1432–1436.

Peabody, J.W., Peabody Jr., J.W., Hayes, E.W., Hayes Jr., E.W., 1950. Idiopathic pulmonary fibrosis; its occurrence in identical twin sisters. Dis. Chest. 18, 330–344.

Penn, C.C., Liu, C., 1993. Bronchiolitis following infection in adults and children. Clin. Chest Med. 14, 645–654.

Pesci, A., Majori, M., Piccoli, M.L., Casalini, A., Curti, A., Franchini, D., et al., 1996. Mast cells in bronchiolitis obliterans organizing pneumonia. Mast cell hyperplasia and evidence for extracellular release of tryptase. Chest. 110, 383–391.

Peters, S.G., McDougall, J.C., Douglas, W.W., Coles, D.T., DeRemee, R.A., 1993. Colchicine in the treatment of pulmonary fibrosis. Chest. 103, 101–104.

Peyrol, S., Cordier, J.F., Grimaud, J.A., 1990. Intra-alveolar fibrosis of idiopathic bronchiolitis obliterans-organizing pneumonia. Cell-matrix patterns. Am. J. Pathol. 137, 155–170.

Raghu, G., Brown, K.K., Bradford, W.Z., Starko, K., Noble, P.W., Schwartz, D.A., et al., 2004. A placebo-controlled trial of interferon gamma-1b in patients with idiopathic pulmonary fibrosis. N. Engl. J. Med. 350, 125–133.

Raghu, G., Collard, H.R., Egan, J.J., Martinez, F.J., Behr, J., Brown, K.K., et al., 2011. An official ATS/ERS/JRS/ALAT statement: idiopathic pulmonary fibrosis: evidence-based guidelines for diagnosis and management. Am. J. Respir. Crit. Care Med. 183, 788–824.

Raghu, G., Depaso, W.J., Cain, K., Hammar, S.P., Wetzel, C.E., Dreis, D.F., et al., 1991. Azathioprine combined with prednisone in the treatment of idiopathic pulmonary fibrosis: a prospective double-blind, randomized, placebo-controlled clinical trial. Am. Rev. Respir. Dis. 144, 291–296.

Ramirez, J., Dowell, A.R., 1971. Silo-filler's disease: nitrogen dioxide-induced lung injury. Long-term follow-up and review of the literature. Ann. Intern. Med. 74, 569–576.

Ratanatharathorn, V., Ayash, L., Lazarus, H.M., Fu, J., Uberti, J.P., 2001. Chronic graft-versus-host disease: clinical manifestation and therapy. Bone Marrow Transplant. 28, 121–129.

Remy-Jardin, M., Remy, J., Cortet, B., Mauri, F., Delcambre, B., 1994. Lung changes in rheumatoid arthritis: CT findings. Radiology. 193, 375–382.

Rennard, S.I., Bitterman, P.B., Ozaki, T., Rom, W.N., Crystal, R.G., 1988. Colchicine suppresses the release of fibroblast growth factors from alveolar macrophages in vitro. The basis of a possible therapeutic approach to the fibrotic disorders. Am. Rev. Respir. Dis. 137, 181–185.

Reynolds, H.Y., Fulmer, J.D., Kazmierowski, J.A., Roberts, W.C., Frank, M.M., Crystal, R.G., 1977. Analysis of cellular and protein content of broncho-alveolar lavage fluid from patients with idiopathic pulmonary fibrosis and chronic hypersensitivity pneumonitis. J. Clin. Invest. 59, 165–175.

Robinson, C., Callow, M., Stevenson, S., Robinson, B.W., Lake, R.A., 2001. Private specificities can dominate the humoral response to self-antigens in patients with cryptogenic fibrosing alveolitis. Respir. Res. 2, 119–124.

Romero, S., Hernandez, L., Gil, J., Aranda, I., Martín, C., Sanchez-Payá, J., 1998. Organizing pneumonia in textile printing workers: a clinical description. Eur. Respir. J. 11, 265–271.

Rossi, G.A., Szapiel, S., Ferrans, V.J., Crystal, R.G., 1987. Susceptibility to experimental interstitial lung disease is modified by immune- and non-immune-related disease. Am. Rev. Respir. Dis. 135, 448–455.

Ryu, J.H., Myers, J.L., Swensen, S.J., 2003. Bronchiolar disorders. Am. J. Respir. Crit. Care Med. 168, 1277–1292.

Sandoz, E., 1907. Über zwei Falle von "Fotaler Bronchektasie". Beitr. Pathol. Anat. 41, 495–516.

Sauty, A., Rochat, T., Schoch, O.D., Hamacher, J., Kurt, A.M., Dayer, J.M., et al., 1997. Pulmonary fibrosis with predominant CD8 lymphocytic alveolitis and anti-Jo-1 antibodies. Eur. Respir. J. 10, 2907–2912.

Scadding, J.G., 1964. Fibrosing alveolitis. Br. Med. J. 5410, 686.

Schnabel, A., Reuter, M., Gross, W.L., 1998. Intravenous pulse cyclophosphamide in the treatment of interstitial lung disease due to collagen vascular diseases. Arthritis Rheum. 41, 1215–1220.

Schoenberger, C.I., Crystal, R.G., 1983. Drug induced lung disease. In: Isselbacher, K.J., Adams, R.D., Braunwald, E.M.J.B., Petersdorf, R.G., Wilson, J.D. (Eds.), Harrison's Principles of Internal Medicine Update IV. McGraw-Hill, New York, pp. 49–74.

Schoenberger, C.I., Rennard, S.I., Bitterman, P.B., Fukuda, Y., Ferrans, V.J., Crystal, R.G., 1984. Paraquat-induced pulmonary fibrosis. Role of the alveolitis in modulating the development of fibrosis. Am. Rev. Respir. Dis. 129, 168–173.

Schwarz, M.I., 1998. The lung in polymyositis. Clin. Chest Med. 19, 701–712.

Selman, M., King, T.E., Pardo, A., 2001. Idiopathic pulmonary fibrosis: prevailing and evolving hypotheses about its pathogenesis and implications for therapy. Ann. Intern. Med. 134, 136–151.

Silver, R.M., Miller, K.S., Kinsella, M.B., Smith, E.A., Schabel, S.I., 1990. Evaluation and management of scleroderma lung disease using bronchoalveolar lavage. Am. J. Med. 88, 470–476.

Sleijfer, S., 2001. Bleomycin-induced pneumonitis. Chest. 120, 617–624.

Snider, G.L., 1986. Interstitial pulmonary fibrosis. Chest. 89, 115S–121S.

Sole, A., Cordero, P.J., Morales, P., Martínez, M.E., Vera, F., Moya, C., 1996. Epidemic outbreak of interstitial lung disease in aerographics textile workers—the "Ardystil syndrome": a first year follow up. Thorax. 51, 94–95.

Southcott, A.M., Jones, K.P., Li, D., Majumdar, S., Cambrey, A.D., Pantelidis, P., et al., 1995. Interleukin-8. Differential expression in lone fibrosing alveolitis and systemic sclerosis. Am. J. Respir. Crit. Care Med. 151, 1604–1612.

Stack, B.H., Choo-Kang, Y.F., Heard, B.E., 1972. The prognosis of cryptogenic fibrosing alveolitis. Thorax. 27, 535–542.

Standiford, T.J., Kunkel, S.L., Phan, S.H., Rollins, B.J., Strieter, R.M., 1991. Alveolar macrophage-derived cytokines induce monocyte chemoattractant protein-1 expression from human pulmonary type II-like epithelial cells. J. Biol. Chem. 266, 9912–9918.

Staples, C.A., Muller, N.L., Vedal, S., Abboud, R., Ostrow, D., Miller, R.R., 1987. Usual interstitial pneumonia: correlation of CT with clinical, functional, and radiologic findings. Radiology. 162, 377–381.

Stein-Streilein, J., Lipscomb, M.F., Fisch, H., Whitney, P.L., 1987. Pulmonary interstitial fibrosis induced in hapten-immune hamsters. Am. Rev. Respir. Dis. 136, 119–123.

Stover, D.E., Milite, F., Zakowski, M., 2001. A newly recognized syndrome—radiation-related bronchiolitis obliterans and organizing pneumonia. A case report and literature review. Respiration. 68, 540–544.

Targoff, I.N., 1993. Humoral immunity in polymyositis/dermatomyositis. J. Invest. Dermatol. 100, 116S–123S.

Tasaka, S., Kanazawa, M., Mori, M., Fujishima, S., Ishizaka, A., Yamasawa, F., et al., 1995. Long-term course of bronchiectasis and bronchiolitis obliterans as late complication of smoke inhalation. Respiration. 62, 40–42.

Thomas, A.Q., Lane, K., Phillips III, J., Prince, M., Markin, C., Speer, M., et al., 2002. Heterozygosity for a surfactant protein C gene mutation associated with usual interstitial pneumonitis and cellular nonspecific interstitial pneumonitis in one kindred. Am. J. Respir. Crit. Care Med. 165, 1322–1328.

Tisdale, J.E., Follin, S.L., Ordelova, A., Webb, C.R., 1995. Risk factors for the development of specific noncardiovascular adverse effects associated with amiodarone. J. Clin. Pharmacol. 35, 351–356.

Troshinsky, M.B., Kane, G.C., Varga, J., Cater, J.R., Fish, J.E., Jimenez, S.A., et al., 1994. Pulmonary function and gastroesophageal reflux in systemic sclerosis. Ann. Intern. Med. 121, 6–10.

Turner-Warwick, M., Burrows, B., Johnson, A., 1980. Cryptogenic fibrosing alveolitis: clinical features and their influence on survival. Thorax. 35, 171–180.

Turner-Warwick, M., Doniach, D., 1965. Auto-antibodies studies in interstitial pulmonary fibrosis. Br. Med. J. 5439, 886–891.

Wallace, W.A., Howie, S.E., 1999. Immunoreactive interleukin 4 and interferon-gamma expression by type II alveolar epithelial cells in interstitial lung disease. J. Pathol. 187, 475–480.

Wallace, W.A., Ramage, E.A., Lamb, D., Howie, S.E., 1995. A type 2 (Th2-like) pattern of immune response predominates in the pulmonary interstitium of patients with cryptogenic fibrosing alveolitis (CFA). Clin. Exp. Immunol. 101, 436–441.

Wallace, W.A., Schofield, J.A., Lamb, D., Howie, S.E., 1994. Localisation of a pulmonary autoantigen in cryptogenic fibrosing alveolitis. Thorax. 49, 1139–1145.

Weinberger, S.E., Kelman, J.A., Elson, N.A., Young Jr, R.C., Reynolds, H.Y., Fulmer, J.D., et al., 1978. Bronchoalveolar lavage in interstitial lung disease. Ann. Intern. Med. 89, 459–466.

Wells, A.U., Cullinan, P., Hansell, D.M., Rubens, M.B., Black, C.M., Newman-Taylor, A.J., et al., 1994. Fibrosing alveolitis associated with systemic sclerosis has a better prognosis than lone cryptogenic fibrosing alveolitis. Am. J. Respir. Crit. Care Med. 149, 1583–1590.

White, B., Moore, W.C., Wigley, F.M., Xiao, H.Q., Wise, R.A., 2000. Cyclophosphamide is associated with pulmonary function and survival benefit in patients with scleroderma and alveolitis. Ann. Intern. Med. 132, 947–954.

Whyte, M., Hubbard, R., Meliconi, R., Whidborne, M., Eaton, V., Bingle, C., et al., 2000. Increased risk of fibrosing alveolitis associated with interleukin-1 receptor antagonist and tumor necrosis factor-alpha gene polymorphisms. Am. J. Respir. Crit. Care Med. 162, 755–758.

Wiedemann, H.P., Matthay, R.A., 1989. Pulmonary manifestations of the collagen vascular diseases. Clin. Chest Med. 10, 677–722.

Winterbauer, R.H., Hammar, S.P., Hallman, K.O., Hays, J.E., Pardee, N.E., Morgan, E.H., et al., 1978. Diffuse interstitial pneumonitis. Clinicopathologic correlations in 20 patients treated with prednisone/azathioprine. Am. J. Med. 65, 661–672.

Witt, C., Borges, A.C., John, M., Fietze, I., Baumann, G., Krause, A., 1999. Pulmonary involvement in diffuse cutaneous systemic sclerosis: bronchoalveolar fluid granulocytosis predicts progression of fibrosing alveolitis. Ann. Rheum. Dis. 58, 635–640.

Wright, J.L., Cagle, P., Churg, A., Colby, T.V., Myers, J., 1992. Diseases of the small airways. Am. Rev. Respir. Dis. 146, 240–262.

Wusirika, R., Ferri, C., Marin, M., Knight, D.A., Waldman, W.J., Ross Jr., P., et al., 2003. The assessment of anti-endothelial cell antibodies in scleroderma-associated pulmonary fibrosis. A study of indirect immunofluorescent and western blot analysis in 49 patients with scleroderma. Am. J. Clin. Pathol. 120, 596–606.

Xaubet, A., Marin-Arguedas, A., Lario, S., Ancochea, J., Morell, F., Ruiz-Manzano, J., et al., 2003. Transforming growth factor-beta1 gene polymorphisms are associated with disease progression in idiopathic pulmonary fibrosis. Am. J. Respir. Crit. Care Med. 168, 431–435.

Yoshida, S., Akizuki, M., Mimori, T., Yamagata, H., Inada, S., Homma, M., 1983. The precipitating antibody to an acidic nuclear protein antigen, the Jo-1, in connective tissue diseases. A marker for a subset of polymyositis with interstitial pulmonary fibrosis. Arthritis Rheum. 26, 604–611.

Yoshinouchi, T., Ohtsuki, Y., Ueda, R., Sato, S., Ueda, N., 1999. Myofibroblasts and S-100 protein positive cells in idiopathic pulmonary fibrosis and rheumatoid arthritis-associated interstitial pneumonia. Eur. Respir. J. 14, 579–584.

Yousem, S.A., Colby, T.V., Carrington, C.B., 1985. Follicular bronchitis/bronchiolitis. Hum. Pathol. 16, 700–706.

Ziesche, R., Hofbauer, E., Wittmann, K., Petkov, V., Block, L.H., 1999. A preliminary study of long-term treatment with interferon gamma-1b and low-dose prednisolone in patients with idiopathic pulmonary fibrosis. N. Engl. J. Med. 341, 1264–1269.

Zisman, D.A., Lynch III, J.P., Toews, G.B., Kazerooni, E.A., Flint, A., Martinez, F.J., 2000. Cyclophosphamide in the treatment of idiopathic pulmonary fibrosis: a prospective study in patients who failed to respond to corticosteroids. Chest. 117, 1619–1626.

Part 15

Unclassified Expressions of Autoimmunity

Cameos: Candidates and Curiosities

Ian R. Mackay

Department of Biochemistry and Molecular Biology, Monash University, Clayton, Victoria, Australia

Chapter Outline

Introduction   1127
Autoimmune/Inflammatory Syndrome Induced by
Adjuvants   1127
Autonomic Neuropathy   1128
Birdshot Retinopathy   1129
Cystitis, Interstitial   1129
Endometriosis   1130
Epilepsy   1131
Fatigue Syndrome   1131
Folate Deficiency   1132
Lichen Sclerosus   1132

Lymphocytic Mastitis   1133
Metabolic–Genetic Storage Diseases   1133
Movement Disorders   1133
Narcolepsy   1134
Osteoarthritis   1134
Parathyroid Disease   1135
Polychondritis, Relapsing   1136
Prostatitis   1136
Sarcoidosis   1137
References   1137

INTRODUCTION

Previous editions (3rd, 1998, Chapter 37 and 4th, 2006, Chapter 71) described various candidate autoimmune diseases or rare ill-defined conditions with autoimmune features—cameos. Several have been developed as full chapters in the 4th or this present 5th edition. Others together with some new entities are retained as cameos because of their rarity, controversial evidence for an autoimmune causation, or autoimmunity being just one of several contributing elements to pathogenesis.

AUTOIMMUNE/INFLAMMATORY SYNDROME INDUCED BY ADJUVANTS

The "autoimmune/inflammatory syndrome induced by adjuvants" (ASIA) (Shoenfeld and Agmon-Levin, 2011) merits serious attention since the strongly suspected environmental contributors to the occurrence of autoimmunity are proving so hard to identify. The concept of ASIA was derived from a composite of features of four conditions interconnected by their occurrence on a background of medicinally introduced chemical agents, prototypically aluminum hydroxide (alum), used in vaccines as an adjuvant with the capacity to enhance immunizing potency.

Thus the specifications for ASIA were derived from (1) undefined syndromes that can occur after routine vaccinations with preparations that contain aluminum hydroxide (alum); (2) the macrophage myofasciitis syndrome (MMF); (3) the Gulf War syndrome (GWS); and (4) siliconosis in women after rupture/leakage of cosmetic breast implants.

1. Vaccination against infectious diseases is practiced worldwide and, expectedly, miscellaneous adverse effects do ensue. However, the last widespread illness was in the 1970s when vaccination (against swine flu) was associated with polyneuropathy attributed to adjuvant used in the vaccine. Nowadays vaccines are so well linked to the components of vaccine preparations that adjuvants as a cause *per se* of adverse effects are minimized (see Chapter 20).
2. The post-vaccination myalgia-fatigue (MMF) syndrome, reported particularly from France and investigated by Gherardi and colleagues (Gherardi et al., 1998, 2001), could be adjuvant related and associated with the practice of intramuscular (deltoid muscle) injection of vaccines that contain alum. Histological and ultrastructural studies on deltoid muscle biopsies showed osmiophilic deposits together with inflammatory changes and

N. Rose & I. Mackay (Eds): The Autoimmune Diseases, Fifth edition. DOI: http://dx.doi.org/10.1016/B978-0-12-384929-8.00075-7

macrophage activation; these deposits were membrane bound and had a finely spicular appearance, with potential capacity for inflammasome activation.

3. Those affected by Gulf War syndrome, which is marked by fatigue and fibromyalgia and afflicts veterans of the first Iraq–Persian Gulf conflict in 1991, had received intensive vaccinations. These included six shots of anthrax vaccine with adjuvants that included alum and squalene, which is usually derived from shark liver oil and botanic sources; however, it is synthesized also by animals and humans and thus could be regarded as an autoantigen. It was claimed that vaccine recipients versus non-recipients had serum antibodies to squalene but, in a brief and rather skeptical literature review, squalene was described as a poor immunogen, and antibodies to it were non-discriminatory for disease (Lippi et al., 2010).

4. Silicone is another chemical agent with potential adjuvant activities, and thus discussed in the context of ASIA. Exposure to silicone in humans can occur by rupture/leakage of cosmetic breast implants with a presumed ensuing syndrome of "connective tissue disease"—siliconosis. Silicone-gel prosthetic devices came into use in the 1960s, and were chosen by over one million women in the United States (Gabriel et al., 1994). Some women who experienced illness after cosmetic injection with silicone or paraffin were thought to have "human adjuvant disease" (HAD) (Miyoshi et al., 1964), perhaps akin to the classical adjuvant arthritis model developed in Lewis rats by Pearson and Wood (1959). The features of claimed HAD seemed to resemble those associated with multisystem autoimmune diseases including scleroderma but large surveys of women with breast implants in the United States failed to show any clear association with autoimmune diseases. For example, in a retrospective study by Hennekens et al. (1996) comprising 395,543 female health professionals between 1962 and 1991 there were 10,830 who had had an implant, and 11,805 who reported some form of "connective tissue disease": the (small) relative risk conferred by a breast implant for "connective tissue disease" was 1.24 (95% CI 1.08–1.41, $p = 0.0015$), but the authors acknowledged possible selection bias in the self-reported nature of the data. Various ideas emerged. First, the silicone-containing breast implant itself might have adjuvant properties sufficient to initiate a multisystem autoimmune disease; second, there existed a "breast implant syndrome" comprising diffuse muscle pains, intermittent fever, fatigue, and other symptoms attributable to the inflammatory potential of silicone leaking from the implant; third, the breast implant and any concurrent diseases were coincidental. Whatever the case, the substantial litigation that followed led to an embargo in 1992 in the United States on silicone breast implants

(Angell, 1996). One point to consider is the overall latency between an inductive stimulus and any ensuing autoimmune disease—in the case of breast implants it could take quite some years before leakage from an implant, then more time for an immune/inflammatory response to be generated, and still more time for occurrence of overt disease. But, whatever the case, several influential academic and governmental agencies refuted the possibility that silicone breast implants confer risk for autoimmune disease (Rosenbaum, 1997), as further established by a meta-analysis of many published studies (Janowski et al., 2000). Whether or not breast implants provoke an autoantibody reaction also has been investigated. Of 24 patients with silicone exposure and rheumatic symptoms, 11 had some defined rheumatic syndrome and 13 did not, and the frequencies of ANA were 10 of 11 and 7 of 13 for the two groups (Press et al., 1992); the ANA specificities in group II were not typical of those seen in any recognized autoimmune disease. The frequency of ANA reactivity in women with breast implants was higher than in controls according to Bridges (1994) and Bar-Meir et al. (1995), but not according to Gabriel et al. (1994). Antibodies to native or denatured collagen types I and II was assessed in our laboratory by Western blot in 70 women with a breast implant, 94 with rheumatoid arthritis, and 133 healthy controls: the frequency in the three groups of antibodies to type I collagen was 26, 23, and 3%, and to type II collagen 23, 36, and 4% (Rowley et al., 1996). So, in brief, large epidemiological studies, albeit with relatively short surveillance periods, appear to exonerate silicone in breast implants as a cause of either recognized multisystem autoimmune diseases, or undifferentiated connective tissue disease but consider in some instances that they may provoke an autoimmune response to tissue constituents including collagen perhaps secondarily to an inflammatory response to the implant.

In conclusion, there does exist persuasive evidence for ASIA including the well-confirmed adjuvant arthritis model inducible in rats by injection of Freund's complete adjuvant and, given this, the syndrome could be reflective of "human adjuvant disease." Thus a return to the rat model of adjuvant disease could well be justified.

AUTONOMIC NEUROPATHY

Unmyelinated autonomic nerve fibers that innervate cardiovascular, gastrointestinal, urogenital, thermoregulatory, sudomotor, and pupillary structures are subject to neuropathies of disparate cause affecting nerve fibers or ganglionic structures, resulting in autonomic failure (dysautonomia). It is well recognized that paraneoplastic dysautonomia occurs usually in association with other paraneoplastic expressions (Freeman, 2005). The accompanying autoantibody is usually to nicotinic acetyl choline receptors (AChR) in autonomic ganglia (Vernino et al., 2000) or to the Hu family autoantigen (ANNA-1) or peripherin, or less often to presynaptic voltage-gated calcium channels (Iorio and Lennon, 2012). Alternatively, an autoimmune autonomic neuropathy occurs spontaneously independently of neoplasia (Vernino et al., 2000). Some 50% of patients with autoimmune gangliopathy are reactive with autonomic ganglia that are similar structurally to AChR pentamers at the neuromuscular junction and, among the spontaneous cases, one or another clinical expression of dysautonomia may be the more prominent, often intestinal hypomotility causing gastric stasis or constipation. In a reported case of neuropathic gastric stasis with type 1 diabetes (T1D), histological examination revealed a complete and presumably autoimmune depletion of interstitial cells of Cajal of the myenteric plexus (He et al., 2001). Experimentally, rabbits immunized with the a3 subunit of the AChR developed an autonomic neuropathy (Lennon et al., 2003) that was passively transferable to mice with IgG from serum of affected rabbits and, from limited data, with sera from diseased humans (Vernino et al., 2004).

BIRDSHOT RETINOPATHY

The slender reasons, additional to the piquancy of the title, for considering this rare ocular disease among the cameos is the presumed dependency for pathogenesis on the retinal S antigen and the remarkably high disease association with the class 1 MHC molecule, HLA A29. Autoimmune inflammatory eye diseases (see Chapter 55) comprise responses to antigens in uvea or retina but serological responses to a putative characterized autoantigenic molecule are not readily demonstrable as in other autoimmune diseases. Birdshot retinopathy affects predominantly individuals of northern European background and occurs usually in mid-adult life, and there is a slight female excess. It is rare, accounting for only about 1% of all cases presenting clinically as "uveitis." Birdshot retinopathy is seen at retinoscopy as multiple separate cream-colored spots on the post-equatorial fundus. Opportunity for pathologic examination is most infrequent; the retina is predominantly affected, and microscopy reveals a T lymphocytic and granulomatous infiltrate (Gasch et al., 1999). A claimed serologic reactivity *in vitro* to retinal S antigen is not well documented. The risk conferred by the class I MHC allele HLA A29 (50- to 224-fold) is higher than that for any other disease, and is greater for the A29.1 than the A29.2 subtype of HLA29. There are only a few other human diseases wherein a demonstrable HLA association is with a class I rather than a class II HLA molecule, including

spondyloarthropathies (B27, Chapter 38) and psoriasis (Cw6, Tillikainen et al., 1980). Birdshot retinopathy is attributed to specific reactivity of CD8[+] cytotoxic T cells against the retinal S antigen. The provocation for this disease is unknown.

CYSTITIS, INTERSTITIAL

Hunner's report (1914) of chronic recurrent edematous ulceration of the bladder in eight young women is taken to be the first on putative autoimmune cystitis; *interstitial* was subsequently added to accommodate the accompanying diffuse fibrosis of the bladder wall. Hand (1949) described a larger case series, 204 women and 19 men, representing almost 5% of urologically investigated patients in his clinic. Oravisto et al. (1970) reported on 54 cases from a urology clinic over a 10-year period, all female aged 16−80 years, mean 59, with symptoms of urinary frequency and urgency, suprapubic pain, and hematuria; cystoscopic appearances were included comprising a greatly reduced bladder capacity and a bladder wall with stellate scars, clusters of granulations, and punctuate hemorrhages likened to an "angry scratch." Microscopically, the bladder wall reveals mucosal ulcerations, edema, lymphoid-plasma cell infiltrates and prominence of mast cells (Sant and Theoharides, 1994) and, in longstanding cases, fibrosis. The best evidence for autoimmunity in interstitial cystitis is the disease association with SLE (Fister, 1938; Shipton, 1965; Boye et al., 1979), Sjögren's syndrome, and autoimmune thyroiditis (Oravisto, 1980). In 129 cases, Peeker et al. (2003) supplemented these associations with cases of "hypersensitivity/allergic disorders," rheumatoid arthritis, and inflammatory bowel diseases. The high population frequency of interstitial cystitis (1−2 per 1000, overall, predominantly among women, ≈90%), has led in the USA to a patient support group being founded (Interstitial Cystitis Association). Subtypes of interstitial cystitis are sometimes cited for case classification into ulcerative (typical) or non-ulcerative types, and into primary (sole disorder) or secondary (associated with SLE or other immune-mediated disease) (de la Serna and Alarcon-Segovia, 1981; Alarcon-Segovia et al., 1984). Biomarkers are needed to assess accuracy of diagnosis and efficacy of treatment, with formal criteria for diagnosis being specified by the National Institute of Diabetes and Digestive and Kidney Diseases of the NIH (USA).

Serologic studies have not been helpful. Bladder-specific autoantibodies were reported by Silk (1970), but have not been confirmed. Frequencies of ANA were raised according to Oravisto et al. (1970) and Jokinen et al. (1972). However, in a more contemporary study Ochs et al. (1994) assembled 96 patients whose sera were tested for ANA by immunofluorescence on tissue sections and on HEp-2 cells, and additionally a cultured bladder epithelial cell line was used for Western blotting. Autoantibodies specific to bladder cells were not demonstrable, but there was an increased frequency, 36% versus 8% in female controls, of non-tissue-specific autoantibodies (cut-off titer 1:40); the reactivities were mostly ANA with staining patterns usually speckled or nucleolar, unlike what pertains in SLE, and tests for AMA were positive in three cases. The findings of Ochs et al. (1994) were not seen as indicative of a primary autoimmune attack on the bladder wall but rather as a consequence of an undefined chronic inflammatory process, with autoantibodies secondarily augmenting this process.

Experimental models of autoimmune cystitis have been attempted in mice and rats, first by direct immunization with bladder wall extracts (Bullock et al., 1992), and later by introduction of transgenically encoded protein antigen (Liu et al., 2007). Immunization of Balb/c AN mice with bladder extract induced cystitis shown histologically by edema, fibrosis, and lymphocytic and mast cell infiltrations; specific reactivities of serum antibodies or T cells were not described, but disease was transferable adoptively by lymphoid cells from affected mice. Cystitis was similarly inducible in Lewis rats, and was adoptively transferable with splenocytes (Luber-Narod et al., 1996). More recently Liu et al. (2007) developed mice that transgenically expressed on bladder epithelial cells the model "self" antigen ovalbumin (URO-OVA). Such mice are unresponsive to OVA stimulation. Adoptive transfer studies were performed wherein naïve OVA-specific T cells showed proliferation and infiltration into the bladder mucosa but no cystitis, whereas transfer of activated OVA-specific T cells did induce an inflammatory cystitis. Their model was further developed to demonstrate that bladder epithelium was capable of presenting a self antigen in association with MHC class I, that activation of T cells occurred in bladder regional lymph nodes, and that features of the ensuing cystitis simulated those of the human counterpart.

In conclusion, human interstitial cystitis remains on the fringe of autoimmunity, since neither pathogenic nor disease-specific marker autoantibodies are regularly demonstrable, immune-mediated mechanisms of bladder wall damage in humans remain obscure, and lacking are genetic analyses and well-controlled studies of efficacy of corticosteroid or immunosuppressive drugs—yet the experimental transgenic models are persuasive. Perhaps there exist as yet undefined co-contributory mechanisms of pathogenesis such as a harmful constituent of urine to which the bladder wall could be persistently exposed.

ENDOMETRIOSIS

Endometriosis was so named to convey the idea that fragments of sloughed uterine endometrium become distributed in the pelvic peritoneum and sites further afield (Sampson, 1921; Ridley, 1968; Giudice and Koo, 2004). The estimated frequency of this disease is 1–2% of all women and one of five women of reproductive age. Clinical expressions include (1) gynecologic symptoms, pelvic pain, menorrhagia, dysmenorrhea, and dyspareunia, (2) dysfunction of the pelvic colon or bladder, (3) infertility, and (4) repeated pregnancy loss. Definitive diagnosis requires laparoscopic surgery. Unsurprisingly, dysfunctions of the immune system are implicated in pathogenesis at various levels (Giudice and Koo, 2004) and include compromised natural killer cell (NK) activity resulting in decreased surveillance/removal of ectopic tissue (Wilson et al., 1994), activation of peritoneal macrophages and upregulation of proinflammatory cytokines, and there are various pointers to autoimmune reactivity. Thus Weed and Arquembourg (1980) surmised that "non-self" ectopic endometrial implants in the pelvis generated endometrial tissue-specific antibodies, with ensuing infertility. In general, autoimmunity has not been held to explain the actual occurrence of displaced endometrium in the pelvis, but rather particular consequences of this displacement. Yet despite considerable immunological investigation in the 1980s, results were relatively unimpressive (Dmowski, 1987). Even so, impetus was given to the autoimmune concept by Grimes et al. (1985), whose case-control study showed that endometriosis was associated with a two-fold (but non-significantly) increased risk for developing SLE, and by increased frequencies of non-tissue-specific autoantibodies, Gleicher et al. (1987) found that among 59 cases 28.5% gave a positive test for ANA and 45.5% for lupus anticoagulant, and Taylor et al. (1991) compared 71 age-matched cases with 109 control women and reported that there was a very significantly increased frequency of autoantibodies to nuclei, ribonucleoproteins (Ro and La), to smooth muscle antigens, and to anticardiolipin and lupus anticoagulant. While Gleicher et al. (1987) asserted that endometriosis "fulfills all the classic characteristics of an autoimmune disease," Taylor et al. (1991) took a more reserved interpretation of the reported autoantibody responses. A serological study on 12 patients and various controls, based on immunofluorescence on endometrial tissues sections, and Western blotting on extracts of endometrial tissue, failed to show any disease-specific autoimmune serological reactivity (Switchenko et al., 1991). However, Fernández Shaw Hicks et al. (1993) reported, and convincingly illustrated, results from an improved immunohistochemical procedure by which sera of women with endometriosis specifically reacted with the cytoplasm of endometrial glands whereas all control sera were negative, concluding that the demonstrable anti-endometrial antibodies could be reactive *in vivo* and impair fertility. Mathur et al. (1995) reinvestigated the question of endometrial autoantigens using Western blotting and found that sera did react with endometrial tissue extracts from affected individuals, observing five reactive components with molecular weights of 34, 46/48, 64, 94, and 120 kDa that were not seen with control sera; moreover sera of rabbits immunized with endometrial extracts, or reactive proteins eluted after electrophoretic separation, bound to the same components as did the patients' sera. Finally, Walter et al. (1995) characterized by Western blotting a 48 kDa molecule from a human endometrial adenocarcinoma cell preparation that was sequenced as *alpha-enolase*, and a recombinant enzyme protein was derived for use in a diagnostic assay (although the utility of this has not been established); also two linear autoepitopes reactive with endometriosis sera were mapped and characterized. However, in the event, interest in endometrium-specific autoimmune reactants over the last decade has faded. The most recent information on the immunopathology of endometriosis, obtained using a gene array procedure, is that of Hever et al. (2007). These authors compared endometriosis tissue with normal endometrium and found that the former was enriched in plasma cells and activated macrophages; the gene arrays did not point to the presence of mature B or T cells, but did show that there was activation of genes for the B cell activating cytokine BAFF/BLyS. The BAFF-driven plasma cells were likely of the marginal zone B-1 type, and the likely source of the various non-tissue-specific autoantibodies described in endometriosis.

In conclusion, endometriosis perhaps has less relevance to autoimmunity than to physiological immunology by indicating that autoantibodies may in fact serve to remove unwanted/ectopic tissue (Grabar, 1975), in this case displaced uterine endometrium.

EPILEPSY

Autoimmunity became implicated from the early 1990s in seizure disorders when a severe form of childhood encephalitis with seizures (Rasmussen disease, RD) was linked with antibodies to excitatory glutamate receptors in the CNS. Rabbits immunized simply to raise antibodies to glutamate receptor subunit 3 (GluR3) developed seizures and histological encephalitis, and this led to a search for autoantibodies to glutamate receptors in RD in children (Rogers et al., 1994). This is reminiscent of the discovery of the causation of myasthenia gravis by autoantibody to the nicotinic acetylcholine receptor (AChR) after the unexpected occurrence of myasthenia in rabbits immunized merely to raise an antiserum to AChR (Patrick and Lindstrom, 1973). However, at present, anti-GluR3 figures much less prominently in autoimmune epilepsy in adults than do autoantibodies to various other neuronal antigens such as glutamic acid decarboxylase of 65 kDa (GAD65). Importantly, recognition in blood or cerebrospinal fluid of such autoantibodies is a distinct directive to immunotherapy.

It was the description of epilepsy-relevant autoantibodies during the 1990s that eventually led to the nomination in 2000 of certain epilepsies—particularly refractory and localization-related types—as "autoimmune" (Palace and Lang, 2000; Peltola et al., 2000), after which there have been various corroborative reports specifying associated autoimmune reactants notably anti-GAD65 (Saiz et al., 2008) (and others) in the context of the stiff person syndrome (Ali et al., 2011), voltage-gated potassium channels (VGKC) (Irani et al., 2011; Iorio and Lennon, 2012; Quek et al., 2012) in the context of chronic encephalitis syndromes, or N-methyl-D-aspartate receptor (NMDA-R) implicated mostly in neuropsychiatric dysfunctions other than epilepsy (Diamond et al., 2009; Dalmau et al., 2011). Quek et al. (2012) described 32 patients with an "exclusive or predominant seizure presentation" and suspected neuronal autoimmunity; among these were autoantibodies to VGKC complexes in 56%, GAD65 in 22%, collapsin response-mediator protein in 6%, and NMDA-R in just 3% (one case). "VGKC complexes" is used advisedly as this is a broad term that covers macromolecular assemblies that contain various potentially antigenic constituents (Iorio and Lennon, 2012). A further neuronal antibody species, often paraneoplastic, was characterized in cases of limbic encephalitis with early and prominent seizures being directed to the B1 subunit of the GABAB receptor; the assay used was a cell line transfected with rodent GABA receptor (Lancaster et al., 2010).

The two important points are, first, that "autoimmune epilepsy" should now be regarded as a definitive neurological entity for which there are valid serological diagnostic assays, and second, that immunotherapies can provide substantial relief from seizures in cases in which conventional anti-epilepsy drugs have failed.

FATIGUE SYNDROME

The "fatigue syndrome" was derived in 1955 from an outbreak of an unexplainable illness at the Royal Free Hospital in London that affected 292 staff members (Medical Staff of the Royal Free Hospital, 1957). The features were severe fatigue, loss of energy, poor exercise tolerance, muscle discomfort, fibromyalgia, and other nonspecific symptoms including malaise, neck stiffness, lymphadenopathy, and fever. A preceding viral illness was often implicated. The name "myalgic encephalomyelitis" (ME) was proposed by "an unusually uncritical Lancet editorialist" (Byrne, 1988). "Myalgic encephalomyelitis" faded from use, but the fatigue syndrome attracted ongoing attention from patient support groups and various medical specialties: some argued for a functional basis and others for an unknown organic basis. By the 1980s, the syndrome had become accepted as an entity, and in 1987 was formally designated as chronic fatigue syndrome (CFS), with recommended diagnostic criteria from the Centers for Disease Control (CDC) in Atlanta, GA (Holmes et al., 1988). The two major criteria for diagnosis were (1) a new onset of fatigue lasting 6 months and reducing activity to less than 50%, and (2) exclusion of any other condition usually producing fatigue, and 11 minor criteria (of which eight should be fulfilled) including eight symptomatic and three physical features, these being mild fever, nonexudative pharyngitis, and palpable cervical or axillary lymph nodes up to 2 cm in diameter. High among claimed causes of CFS are chronic viral infections, notably Epstein–Barr virus; the case for a murine retrovirus, XMRV, has been convincingly refuted. Other candidates are allergies, autoimmunity, hyper-reactive responses to unusual environmental exposures, and psychosomatic disorder. Despite evidence in CFS for immune activation and/or impaired indices of cell-mediated immunity (Lloyd et al., 1989, 1990; Buchwald and Komaroff, 1991), data from the conventional indications of inflammatory activity or tissue destruction (ESR, C-reactive protein) are non-supportive. Benefit from immunomodulatory treatment with intravenous immunoglobulin, of known efficacy in some well-defined antibody-mediated autoimmune diseases, is controversial, either endorsed (Lloyd et al., 1990) or refuted (Peterson et al., 1990).

Analysis of an autoimmune component in CFS encounters issues such as specification of a clear associated diagnosis and a scarcity of affirmative evidence, perhaps indicative of unpublished negative studies, opposed to which is the known occurrence of fatigue in certain well-accepted autoimmune disorders. The major question then is whether, among cases fulfilling CDC criteria for CFS, there can be regularly identified a highly raised level of any autoantibody specificity, particularly antinuclear autoantibody (ANA). Positive studies include that of Behan et al. (1985) (50 cases) and another group (60 cases) (Konstantinov et al., 1996; von Mikecz et al., 1997) which cited a frequency of autoantibodies of 83% versus 17% in a control group, predominantly of ANA specificity, and directed particularly to nuclear envelope proteins, together with cytoplasmic staining patterns of intermediate filament-vimentin type thought to be indicative of viral infection. On the other hand, there are negative results for ANA in CFS (Skowera et al., 2002), or only modestly positive results (Vernon and Reeves, 2005).

It is not the purpose here to review all the varied suppositions on the basis of CFS because none is sufficiently convincing. It can be said that autoimmunity does not provide an explanation for all cases of CFS, that autoantibodies when present might reflect some other as yet unidentified cause, and that autoimmunity likely is but one among a conglomerate of causes for CFS.

FOLATE DEFICIENCY

Maldevelopment of the embryonic neural tube resulting in spina bifida, anencephaly, or other defects occurs in infants at a prevalence of about one in 1000. It has been widely ascertained that periconceptual folic acid supplements to mothers strikingly alleviate this, even though the mothers usually do not have evident folate deficiency (Rothenberg et al., 2004). The observation was made that antiserum to folate receptors in pregnant rats resulted in embryonic mal-development, and this prompted the search for autoantibodies to folate receptors in women in whom a pregnancy had resulted in an infant affected with a neural tube defect (Rothenberg et al., 2004). The procedure used was the specific blocking of (^{3}H) folic acid to folate receptors on placental membranes and to indicator cell lines. The results were that nine of 12 women (versus two of 20 controls) with affected children had a receptor blocking antibody. The same authors (Ramaekers et al., 2005) in a further study investigated infantile-onset cerebral folate deficiency that develops 4–6 months after birth and is expressed as mental and psychomotor retardation, cerebellar ataxia, dyskinesis, seizures, visual disorder, and autism. There were low levels of 5-methyl tetrahydrofolate (5-MTHF) in the cerebrospinal fluid but normal levels in serum, and lack of evidence of extracerebral folate deficiency. Serum from 25 of 28 affected children, versus none of 28 controls, contained high-affinity blocking autoantibodies against membrane-bound folate receptors on the choroid plexus, indicating impediment to the passage of folic acid from serum to brain. This could be normalized by oral calcium folinate that led to clinical improvement. Notably, none of five tested mothers had autoantibodies. Perhaps the induction of the anti-folate receptor antibodies in these affected children was due to soluble folate-binding proteins in milk, or to other unknown antigens (Ramaekers et al., 2005). This story is indeed a legitimate "cameo" in the world of autoimmunity, since anti-folate receptor autoantibody could be generated either in the pregnant mother or the newborn child, causing neural developmental disorders. Indeed Schwartz (2005) was prompted to comment that "autoimmunization lurks behind every pillar." And there is the added point that the catastrophic consequences in this particular example are remediable by a very simple therapy, folic acid.

LICHEN SCLEROSUS

"Lichen," a compound plant (fungi in symbiotic union with algae) that spreads on rocks and trees, gives its name to chronic skin diseases seen mostly as thickened but sometimes atrophic inflammatory patches on skin or mucus membranes with, histologically, damage and cellular infiltration between the epidermis and dermis. There are many variants described of mucocutaneous lichenoid eruptions according to their location and visual appearances. The prototype is lichen planus for which no single specific cause has been identified, although one interesting association is infection with hepatitis C virus (Le Cleach et al., 2010). The lichenoid eruption described as lichen sclerosus is, however, consistently linked to autoimmunity. Lichen sclerosus particularly affects the anogenital skin, and the vulval mucosa in women. The population prevalence is at least ≈ 1 per 1000 with a female:male ratio of at least 6:1; histologically, there is hydropic degeneration of basal keratinocytes with inflammatory changes (Dalziel and Shaw, 2010). The evidence for autoimmunity specified by Oyama et al. (2003) includes familial occurrence, association with the class II HLA allele DQ7 as seen in other mucus membrane/pemphigoid diseases, and co-occurrence with other autoimmune diseases and/or autoantibodies, mainly of the "thyrogastric" cluster, i.e., thyroiditis, pernicious anemia, diabetes, vitiligo, and others, but better immunological data on these disease associations are called for.

Previous findings of "pemphigoid" autoantibodies in skin diseases with basement membrane pathology (see Chapter 65) led a search for analogous autoantibodies to extracellular matrix protein 1 (ECM1) in lichen sclerosus (Oyama et al., 2003). The autoantigen ECM1 was chosen based on the observation that loss-of-function mutations of the gene encoding ECM1 result in a lichen sclerosus-like pathology (lipoid proteinosis, LP). The sera studied were from 86 patients with lichen sclerosus, 85 healthy controls, and 107 "other disease" contrast cases, and the technical procedures included Western immunoblotting (WB) on extracts from normal skin and LP skin that lacks ECM1, and indirect immunofluorescence (IIF) microscopy using affinity purified IgG. In brief, there was a specific signal for anti-ECM1 from lichen sclerosus sera by WB (to the low titer of 1:20), absence of signal using extracts from LP skin lacking ECM1, and specific reactivity by IIF of affinity-purified serum IgG with the basal keratinocyte layer of normal skin. Passive transfer of lichen sclerosus lesions to mice by serum or IgG was a contemplated next step.

LYMPHOCYTIC MASTITIS

The female breast is subject to a non-neoplastic multinodular fibrosing disease expressed clinically by recurrent mastalgia, and histologically by periductular lymphocytic infiltrations. An early report described the case of a woman with a multisystem-like disease in whom there were dense collections of lymphoid cells within diseased breast tissue, with underlying autoimmunity thus implicated (Shelley and Hurley, 1960), but the idea of an "autoimmune mastitis" was not picked up. The disease (or diseases) characterized by lymphocytic mastitis has acquired several descriptors, granulomatous mastitis—although giant multinuclear cells are actually inconspicuous (Donn et al., 1994), diabetic mastopathy by reason of a frequent association with clinical diabetes (Tomaszewski et al, 1992; Camuto et al., 2000), fibrocystic mastitis, and some cases classed as IgG4 mastitis (Ogura et al., 2010). Lymphocytic mastitis may represent an immunological response to extruded breast milk, or to acinar or ductular breast tissue, but immunocytological examination of the characteristic lymphocytic infiltrates has received rather little attention, so the condition remains "idiopathic."

METABOLIC–GENETIC STORAGE DISEASES

Batten disease is a rare, recessively inherited, and fatal neurodegenerative disease of children due to a mutation in both copies of a gene *CLN3*, so leading to accumulation of ceroid lipofuscin in neurons. A gene-disruption model in mice revealed altered expression of enzymes required for the synthesis of the neurotransmitter glutamate, and circulating antibodies to brain proteins including GAD65. This prompted a search for anti-GAD65 in human Batten disease, with positive results (Chattopadhyay et al., 2002). As yet, the role (if any) of anti-GAD in the overall pathogenesis of Batten disease is uncertain.

Sandhoff disease is another metabolic autoimmune curiosity. It is a recessively inherited lysosomal storage disease of infancy in which neuronal cell death results from an enzyme deficiency that causes accumulation of gm2 gangliosides in lysosomes of brain cells. A murine equivalent has been created by knockout of the *hexb* gene that encodes the hexosamidase enzyme. It is claimed that antiganglioside antibodies in Sandhoff disease accelerate premature neuronal death, perhaps via complexes of antibody and ganglioside that cause inflammatory activation of microglial cells. Similar events are postulated for the human counterpart (Yamaguchi et al., 2004).

MOVEMENT DISORDERS

A miscellaneous group of movement disorders, observed particularly in children, and sharing the features of an antecedent streptococcal infection, are claimed to have in common the expression of autoantibodies to neurons of basal ganglia in the brain. Prototypic among these is Sydenham's chorea, marked by frequent unintended jerky movements, and long known to occur occasionally in association with streptococcal-related rheumatic carditis. Others include the Tourette syndrome of motor and vocal tics, and a pediatric autoimmune neuropsychiatric disorder associated with streptococcal infections (PANDAS) (Shulman, 1999). Speculative extensions have brought in other entities including obsessive–compulsive and attention-deficit disorders. Autoimmunity has been implicated, but on rather slender evidence: (1) the claimed antecedent streptococcal infections that provide a reasoning for the occurrence of autoimmunity similar to that proposed for the onset of rheumatic carditis (see Chapter 69), (2) positive tests for antineuronal autoantibodies particularly to autoantigens of basal ganglia neurons, and (3) a claimed capacity of patients' sera to transfer disease passively after direct injection into the striatum of rats. However, the autoantibody studies are in earlier literature and have not been convincingly confirmed (reviewed by Dale, 2005), and the validity of the data on passive transfer to animals by serum is likewise questionable (Giovannoni, 2005).

NARCOLEPSY

Narcolepsy is a sleep–wake disorder with onset during adolescence in which there is irresistible daytime sleepiness. It is now confidently attributed to deficient neurotransmission dependent on a neurotransmitter that sustains wakefulness, known according to the discoverers as either hypocretin or orexin. Deficiency of this transmitter, synthesized by neurons in the hypothalamus, is the underlying fault—in canines with narcolepsy there is a profound loss of hypocretin-secreting neurons in the hypothalamus. *Prima facie*, narcolepsy would seem hardly likely as an autoimmune disease, yet there is a long-known extreme and puzzling co-association with the class II MHC allele, HLA DQB1*0602. Inconveniently for theorists, an autoantibody relevant to narcolepsy against hypocretin/orexin, or the cognate receptor, has not been demonstrated by conventional assays. However, some evidence for a serum factor was obtained by a bioassay based on passive transfer to mice of IgG from narcolepsy patients, by a readout of increased contractile responses of detrusor muscle strips (Smith et al., 2004); but these preliminary bioassay data would seem to require further work. There is a published personal account of a narcolepsy sufferer annotating the curious symptoms, together with comments on the occurrence of narcolepsy in inbred Doberman Pinscher dogs (although this is attributed to a genetically faulty cell receptor, see below), the extreme immunogenetic HLA D locus bias (DQ6// DQB1*0602 &/or DR2/DRB11501) and seasonal (springtime) peak incidences suggesting an antecedent infection (Nicholls, 2012). Suspected infections include either H1N1 influenza, or streptococcal throat infection substantiated by raised levels in childhood narcolepsy of antistreptolysin O, as implicated also in movement disorders of childhood described above.

A possible disease pathway can now be specified based on the interaction of hypocretin/orexin and the cognate receptor. The first hints in the 1990s came from the identification of hitherto unknown hormone-like agents in the brain of rats and mice, hypocretins/orexins, and one group further identified the structure of the orexin receptors (Sarkurai et al., 1998), although these authors directed their attention to the role of the orexin system in energy balance and eating behavior rather than sleep patterns. However, it was evident from other investigations that the hypothalamic cells that secrete hypocretin/orexin hormones provide also send "stay awake" messages to other cells in the CNS via the orexin-receptor pathway. Reliable detection of antibody or T cell reactivity to hypocretin/orexin or to the cognate receptor is still awaited. Meanwhile further immunogenetic and immunological anomalies have come to light (reviewed by Faraco and Mignot, 2011) and include polymorphism of the alpha chain of the T cell antigen receptor (Hallmayer et al., 2009), with three single nucleotide polymorphisms within the TCRA locus showing significant association with narcolepsy syndromes across various ethnic groups; another susceptibility locus is the gene for the P2RY11 purinergic receptor. There is an autoantibody association too, depending on the tribbles2 homolog protein (trib2), in 14–26% of DQB1 (cataplexy-associated) cases, but trib2 is a ubiquitously expressed protein, and there are no indications that antibodies to it are related to narcolepsy. One wonders how the story will eventually pan out!

OSTEOARTHRITIS

Osteoarthritis (OA) is prototypically a "degenerative" articular disease with usually a late-in-life onset and a relationship to articular stresses and previous trauma, but there can be an early inflammatory phase with an obviously acute onset. In tests for specificity of serological reactants used for the diagnosis of rheumatic diseases, i.e., autoantibodies to citrullinated peptides or native collagen type II (nCII), a degree of reactivity is usually observed. In regard to anti-nCII, Xiang et al. (2004) reported that sera from patients with osteoarthritis reacted more with denatured than with native CII, and Burkhardt et al. (2002) found that OA sera were reactive but, in contrast to rheumatoid arthritis (RA), sera engaged different antibody epitopes of nCII, notably CII-F4 located at the C-terminal region of nCII, rather than the characteristic RA-related epitopes, CII-Cl and CII-M2139. Interestingly, a murine anti-CII-F4 monoclonal antibody (mAb), in contrast to other mAbs reactive with specific epitopes of nCII, is not pathogenic on passive transfer in mice but actually inhibits the adverse effects (matrix disruption) of mAbs that do react with nCII epitopes other than F4 (Burkhardt et al., 2002). Xiang et al. (2004)

further found that those OA sera, as well as reacting with CII-F4, reacted with an antigen of different provenance, triose phosphate isomerase. In regard to pathogenicity, the capacity of autoantibodies to nCII to perpetrate articular damage remains an open question.

T lymphocytes have not been neglected in OA, according to a recent review by Sakkas and Platsoukas (2007). T cell infiltrates are demonstrable in the affected articular cartilage, and particularly in the synovial membrane, appearing as nodular aggregates suggestive of an antigen-driven process, although a provocative cartilagenous autoantigen has not so far been identified, despite much search and speculation. Curiously, erosive effects of cartilage/synovial inflammation associated with activated T lymphocytes infiltrating subchondral bone, as seen in rheumatoid arthritis, are not evident in OA. The T cells demonstrable in synovial membrane in OA are of the Th1 subtype and their activated phenotype is revealed by transcripts for cytokines such as IL-12, detectable in synovial fluid. Sakkas and Platsoukas (2007) discuss the utility of future procedures to assess the degree of clonality of T cell infiltrates in joints in OA.

However, while few of the conventional markers (particularly reactivity with an "accepted" autoantigenic structure) are fulfilled, it remains difficult to ascribe OA to an adaptive autoimmune response. In addition, results of a large (and latest) GWAS that included stratified cases of OA defined some eight candidate loci for association with OA, although none could be aligned with those often associated with autoimmune disease (arcOGEN Consortium and arcOGEN Collaborators, 2012).

Hence it is of interest to consider a new slant on the immunological contribution to OA, namely an inflammatory association with an anomaly of the complement cascade. Wang et al. (2011) found in mice that injury to articular cartilage in the setting of dysregulation of complement gene expression in joint tissues led to formation of the membrane attack complex (MAC) on chondrocytes, with either killing or production of matrix degrading enzymes, so linking OA to such age-related diseases as macular degeneration and Alzheimer's disease. Possible applications of this concept to define subsets of human OA are awaited. This theme was developed in a recent review in which various components of innate immunity were implicated, without recourse to an adaptive response (Haseeb and Haqqi, 2013). So perhaps OA may be better placed in the category of autoinflammatory diseases (see Chapter 4).

PARATHYROID DISEASE

An autoimmune basis for hypoparathyroidism was proposed by Solomon and Blizzard (1963), and then by Seemann (1967), whose histological study revealed lymphocyte–plasma cell infiltrates—hence "lymphocytic

parathyroiditis." In our first edition of this text, Maclaren and Blizzard (1985) described autoimmune polyendocrine syndrome (APS) types 1 and 2. For type 1 the three major components appeared usually in a uniform sequential order: candidiasis, hypoparathyroidism, and Addison's disease. Autoimmune hypoparathyroidism, despite being a characteristic feature of APS type 1, did not occur in any of 224 cases of APS type 2. However, serological reactivity with parathyroid tissue was insufficiently convincing to generate clinical laboratory assays, although accompanying autoantibodies were reported to bind to the cell surface of human parathyroid cells and to inhibit parathyroid cell secretion. Perhaps these autoantibodies were related to those revealed by a monoclonal antibody raised by immunizing mice with parathyroid tissue and shown to react with a parathyroid cell surface antigen called PTA (Cance et al., 1986). An autoimmune basis was strengthened when Li et al. (1996) demonstrated, in both APS1-associated and sporadic cases of hypothyroidism, serological reactivity with the ubiquitous calcium-sensing receptor (Ca-SR) on the parathyroid cell surface; an immunoprecipitation assay showed that the extracellular domain of the Ca-SR contained the reactive epitopes. This autoimmune reactivity, anti-Ca-SR, was demonstrable in 56% of 25 cases and was far more frequent among females than males. Also, cases were recognized wherein antibodies to the parathyroid Ca-SR had an inactivating effect, so rendering the glands insensitive to ambient calcium, such that the ensuing oversecretion of parathyroid hormone had effects like those seen with parathyroid adenomas, causing hypocalciuric hypercalcemia (Pallais et al., 2004). These antibodies were functionally active but nondestructive, were of the IgG4 subclass, and in one case were associated with autoimmune pancreatitis, perhaps illustrating another facet of "IgG4 disease" (see Chapter 64). Thus the clinical expressions of autoimmune parathyroiditis with anti-Ca-SR reactivity may be either hypoparathyroidism if the antibodies are non-blocking as pertains when the glands are subject to lymphocytic-mediated destruction, or hyperparathyroidism if the antibodies are blocking and the glands retain functional activity.

In 2008 a novel autoimmune reactant was discovered by screening a cDNA expression library with serum samples from cases of APS type 1, identified as the NACHT leucine-rich-repeat protein 5 (NALP5) (Alimohammadi et al., 2008). These authors, in their Introduction, negated the role of other described autoantigens in parathyroiditis, although anti-Ca-SR reactivity in parathyroiditis had been well established in earlier studies (see Gavalas et al., 2007). The authors of the NALP5 study decisively showed that autoantibody was limited to cases of APS type 1 hypoparathyroidism with AIRE mutations, was not demonstrable in "isolated" (sporadic) hypoparathyroidism, and was detectable as a subcellular autoantigen only in the chief and not the oxyphilic cells of the parathyroid gland. Still to come are studies on patterns of T cell reactivity to NALP5, and the relative contributions of defective thymic deletional tolerance versus Treg-mediated suppressive tolerance to this putative parathyroid autoantigen.

POLYCHONDRITIS, RELAPSING

Relapsing polychondritis (RP) was so named by Pearson et al. (1960) to designate recurring inflammatory damage to, and degradation of, (mainly) type II collagenous cartilage throughout the body (Michet et al., 1986). More particularly vulnerable is cartilage of nasal, auricular, tracheobronchial, and audiovestibular sites than is articular cartilage. However, there is a very wide distribution of lesions to non-cartilaginous sites, such as ocular sclera, heart valves, skin, and others, and therefore RP is called "an autoimmune disease with many faces" (Lahmer et al., 2010). There is clustering in some 30% of cases with one or another systemic autoimmune rheumatic disease, notably rheumatoid arthritis and SLE. Lymphoid cell accumulation is prominent at affected sites. There is a weak association with the MHC class II allele HLA DR4, and clear benefit accrues from prednisolone (McAdam et al., 1976). Thus polychondritis has most of the hallmarks of an autoimmune process.

Specific antibodies to cartilage were detected using IIF and cartilage substrate from mouse leg, or from human costochondral and tracheal cartilage, after preincubation with hyaluronidase to remove masking proteoglycan (Dolan et al., 1976; Foidart et al., 1978). Autoantibodies were more readily detected in the acute stages, were of IgG class and non-complement-binding, and levels correlated with disease severity. Absorption exclusively with type II collagen removed reactivity with cartilage from serum. Using a direct immunofluorescence procedure, and serum from in a single case, Bergfeld (1978) detected deposits *in vivo* of IgG, IgA, and C3 in affected cartilage. In a subsequent study, positive results were reported in six of nine patients for antibodies to cartilage, and there was association with organ (thyroid)-specific autoantibodies as well (Ebringer et al., 1981). Assays for T cell-mediated immune responses to cartilage proved indecisive (Foidart et al., 1978; Ebringer et al., 1981).

Reactivity of serum with type II collagen (CII) has been investigated in polychondritis. This was rather low by ELISA among Japanese patients, 202 with rheumatoid arthritis, 26 with polychondritis, and 92 with other rheumatic diseases, positivity being only 42%, 11%, and 0.3%, respectively (Terato et al., 1990). In tests using peptides derived by cyanogen bromide (CB) digestion of CII, polychondritis sera reacted preferentially with the CB 9.7 kDa peptide, unlike the anti-CII reactivity of sera

from other diseases, and the species of anti-CII antibody detectable in polychondritis lacked the epitope specificity of sera from patients with erosive articular inflammation (Burkhardt et al., 2002). However, subsequent studies have indicated that the primary reactant in polychondritis might not be CII, since reactivity of serum antibodies and T cells was greater with collagens IX and XII (Yang et al., 1993). Moreover, in NOD mice carrying a human HLA DQ1 transgene and immunized with CII, there developed an auricular chondritis that simulated the abnormality seen in human polychondritis, and sera reacted to CIX as well as CII (Taneja et al., 2003). Perhaps, then, in polychondritis, anti-CII occurs secondarily by epitope spreading.

The cartilage protein matrilin is another suggested autoantigen in polychondritis (Hansson et al., 2004). Matrilin is a cartilage-specific protein abundant at sites affected in polychondritis (trachea, ears) but sparse in sites that are spared (joints). A model of polychondritis induced in mice by active immunization with matrilin I showed that functional B cells and complement factor V were required for disease expression, and that passive transfer could be accomplished by a mAb to matrilin I suggesting that polychondritis, in this model at least, is essentially an antibody-mediated autoimmune disease (Hansson et al., 2004).

The disease itself, and in particular expressions of it, limit survival, e.g., after 10 years to 55%. Therapists have relied mainly upon corticosteroid drugs that are of variable efficacy, supplemented with the conventional immunosuppressives. Successful use of TNF antagonists is reported but in very limited case studies (Lahmer et al., 2010) and a recent review on the utility of biological therapies identified some benefits with the authors deploring the limitations of the data available (Kempta Lekpa et al., 2012).

PROSTATITIS

Aging men become afflicted by the urinary obstructive effects of benign prostatic hyperplasia due to prostatic cell proliferation. Often a component of inflammation is demonstrable histologically despite no evident infection. The question thus has arisen whether BPH is an "immune inflammatory disease" (Kremer et al., 2007), or even whether autoimmunity is implicated. From the earlier days, prostate-specific autoantigens were demonstrable by immunization of rabbits with a saline extract of prostate tissue that provoked an autoantibody response (Shulman et al., 1965) but histological data were not provided.

However, interest waned, as judged by a lapse in citations on inflammatory prostatitis until the post-2000 era, according to Penna et al. (2009). These authors implicated stromal cells in the prostate as having the properties of immune accessory cells, i.e., antigen-presenting cells, that induced expression of MHC class II molecules, costimulatory molecules and demonstrability of high levels of the two inter-related cytokines, IL-12p75 and IL-23p40, as well as other cytokines and chemokines characteristic of immunoinflammatory reactivity (see Chapter 22). Penna et al. (2009) also cited publications on the detection in semen from cases of chronic prostatitis of proinflammatory cytokines IL-6, IL-8, IL-1beta, and TNF-alpha, together with other data suggesting that products of immunoreactive cells in the prostate foster chronic inflammation and prostate cell growth. A credible sequence for an autoimmune prostatitis would require a candidate prostate-specific autoantigen; among those cited is the controversial cancer marker, prostate-specific antigen (PSA). There is clearly more work needed, but considerations such as the high frequency of prostatitis among aging males and its dependency on hormonal influences leave open the idea of an autoimmune component to prostate disease in men.

SARCOIDOSIS

An early suspicion that sarcoidosis could have an autoimmune connection (Mackay and Burnet, 1963) proved not sustainable, although few other more credible pathogeneses have emerged. Epidemiological data implicate an environmental influence, with possible person-to-person transmission, or a shared response to a provocative transmissible agent (Newman et al., 1997).

The disease expressions depend on non-caseating granulomatous lesions in multiple sites—skin, lymph nodes, lung, liver or CNS, and pathogenicity depends either on inflammatory fibrosis as in the lungs, or pressure effects of lesions as in the CNS. The immune system is clearly implicated as judged by the Th1-directed granulomatous histopathology. Also, there is solid evidence from a comparative population study in Italy of co-association with other autoimmune diseases, notably autoimmune thyroiditis, although the strength of this association is questionable (Antonelli et al., 2006).

Ho et al. (2005) drew on the known Th1-biased CD4$^+$ T cell response in sarcoidosis, together with possible involvement of the natural killer T (NKT) cell system. NKT cells are activated by glycolipid antigens presented by CD1 molecules on antigen-presenting cells (APCs) (Chapter 8). There is a particular class of CD1 (CD1d) that, after interaction with NKT cells with an invariant receptor (Va24/JaQ, paired with Vb11), can exert regulatory effects. Also, in mice at least, the CD1-restricted repertoire includes autoreactive T cells (Park et al., 2001). Ho et al. (2005) ascertained in sarcoidosis a deficiency (for unknown reasons) of Va24 NKT cells, with ensuing loss of their normal regulatory effect on CD1d-dependent reactivity. However, for sarcoidosis to be confidently ascribed to autoimmunity, depletion of Va24 NKT cells would need to be associated with persistent stimulation of the Th1 T cell pathway by some endogenous autoantigen, for which the evidence is meager, at best.

REFERENCES

Alarcon-Segovia, D., Abud-Mendoza, C., Reyes-Gutierrez, E., Iglesias-Gammara, A., Diaz-Jovanen, E., 1984. Involvement of the urinary bladder in systemic lupus erythematosus: a pathologic study. J. Rheum. 111, 208—210.

Ali, F., Rowley, M.J., Jayakrishnan, B., Teuber, S., Gershwin, M.E., Mackay, I.R., 2011. Stiff-person syndrome (SPS) and anti-GAD-related CNS degenerations: protean additions to the autoimmune central neuropathies. J. Autoimmunity. 37, 79—87.

Alimohammadi, M., Bjorklund, P., Hallgren, A., Pontynen, N., Szinnai, G., Shikama, N., et al., 2008. Autoimmune polyendocrine syndrome type 1 and NALP5, a parathyroid autoantigen. N. Engl. J. Med. 358, 1018—1028.

Angell, M., 1996. Shattuck lecture—Evaluatng the health risks of breast implants: the interplay of medical science, the law and public opinion. New Engl J Med. 34, 1513—1518.

Antonelli, A., Fazzi, P., Fallah, P., Ferrani, S.M., Ferannini, E., 2006. Prevalence of hypothyroidism and Graves' disease in sarcoidosis. Chest. 130, 526—532.

arcOGEN Consortium and arcOGEN Collaborators, 2012. Identification of new susceptibility loci for osteoarthritis: a genome wide association study. Lancet. 380, 815—823.

Bar-Meir, E., Teuber, S.S., Lin, H.C., Alosacie, I., Goddard, G., Terybery, J., et al., 1995. Multiple autoantibodies in patients with silicone breast implants. J. Autoimmunity. 8, 267—277.

Behan, P.O., Behan, W.M., Bell, E.J., 1985. The post-viral fatigue syndrome—an analysis of the findings in 50 cases. J. Infect. 10, 211—222.

Bergfeld, W.F., 1978. Relapsing polychondritis with positive direct immunofluorescence (letter). Arch. Dermatol. 114, 127.

Boye, E., Morse, M., Huttner, M., Erlanger, I., MacKinnon, K.J., Klassen, J., 1979. Immune complex-mediated interstitial cystitis as a major manifestation of systemic lupus erythematosus. Clin. Immunol. Immunopathol. 13, 67—76.

Bridges, A.J., 1994. Autoantibodies in patients with silicone breast implants. Semin. Arthritis Rheum. 23 (4 (Suppl.)), 24—60.

Buchwald, D., Komaroff, A.L., 1991. Review of laboratory findings for patients with chronic fatigue syndrome. Rev. Infect. Dis. 13, 512—518.

Bullock, A.D., Becich, M.J., Klutke, C.G., Ratliff, T.L., 1992. Experimental autoimmune cystitis: a potential murine model for ulcerative interstitial cystitis. J. Urol. 148, 1951—1956.

Burkhardt, H., Koller, T., Engstrom, A., Nandakumar, S.K., Turnay, J., Kraetsch, H.G., et al., 2002. Epitope-specific recognition of type II collagen by rheumatoid arthritis antibodies is shared with recognition by antibodies that are arthritogenic in collagen-induced arthritis in the mouse. Arthritis Rheum. 46, 2339—2348.

Byrne, E., 1988. Idiopathic chronic fatigue and myalgia syndrome myalgic encephalomyelitis. Some thoughts on nomenclature and aetiology. Med. J. Aust. 148, 80—82.

Camuto, P.M., Zetrenne, E., Ponn, T., 2000. Diabetic mastopathy. A report of 5 cases and a review of the literature. Arch. Surg. 135, 1190—1193.

Cance, W.G., Wells Jr., S.A., Dilley, W.G., Welch, M.J., Otsuka, F.L., Davie, J.M., 1986. Human parathyroid antigen, characterization and localization with monoclonal antibodies. Proc. Nat. Acad. Sci. U.S.A. 83, 6112–6116.

Chattopadhyay, S., Ito, M., Cooper, J.D., Brocks, A.L., Curran, T.M., Powers, J.M., et al., 2002. An autoantibody inhibitory to glutamic acid decarboxylase in the neurodegenerative disorder Batten disease. Hum. Mol. Genet. 11, 1421–1431.

Dale, R.C., 2005. Post-streptococcal autoimmune disorders of the central nervous system. Dev. Med. Child Neurol. 47, 785–791.

Dalmau, J., Lancaster, E., Martinez-Hernandez, E., Rosenfeld, M.R., Balice-Gordon, R., 2011. Clinical experience and laboratory investigations in patients with anti-NMDAR encephalitis. Lancet Neurol. 10, 63–74.

Dalziel, K., Shaw, S., 2010. Lichen sclerosus. BMJ. 340, 757–761.

de la Serna, A.R., Alarcon-Segovia, D., 1981. Chronic interstitial cystitis as an initial major manifestation of systemic lupus erythematosus. J. Rheumatol. 8, 808–810.

Diamond, B., Huerta, P.T., Mina-Osorio, P., Kowal, C., Volpe, B.T., 2009. Losing your nerves? Maybe it's the antibodies. Nat. Rev. Immunol. 9, 449–456.

Dmowski, W.P., 1987. Immunologic aspects of endometriosis. Contrib. Gynecol. Obstet. 16, 48–55.

Dolan, D.L., Lemmon, G.B., Teitelbaum, S.L., 1976. Relapsing polychondritis. Analytical literature review and studies on pathogenesis. Am. J. Med. 41, 285–297.

Donn, W., Rebbeck, P., Wilson, C., Gilks, C.B., 1994. Idiopathic granulomatous mastitis. Arch. Path. Lab. Med. 118, 822–825.

Ebringer, R., Rook, G., Swana, G.T., Bottazzo, G.F., Donaich, D., 1981. Autoantibodies to cartilage and type II collagen in relapsing polychondritis and other rheumatic diseases. Ann. Rheum. Dis. 40, 473–479.

Faraco, J., Mignot, E., 2011. Immunological and genetic aspects of narcolepsy. Sleep Med. Res. 2, 1–9.

Fernandez-Shaw, S., Hicks, B.R., Yudkin, P.L., Kennedy, S., Barlow, D.H., Starkey, P.M., 1993. Anti-endometrial and anti-endothelial autoantibodies in women with endometriosis. Hum. Reprod. 8, 310–315.

Fister, G.M., 1938. Similarity of interstitial cystitis (Hunner's ulcus) to lupus erythematosus. J. Urol. 40, 37–51.

Foidart, J.-M., Abe, S., Martin, G.R., Zizic, T.M., Barnett, E.V., Lawley, T.J., et al., 1978. Antibodies to type II collagen in relapsing polychondritis. N. Engl. J. Med. 299, 1203–1207.

Freeman, R., 2005. Autonomic peripheral neuropathy. Lancet. 365, 1259–1270.

Gabriel, S.E., O'Fallon, W.M., Kurland, L.T., Beard, C.M., Woods, J.E., Melton 3rd, L.J., 1994. Risk of connective-tissue diseases and other disorders after breast implantation. N. Eng. J. Med. 330, 1697–1702.

Gasch, A.T., Smith, J.A., Whitcup, S.M., 1999. Birdshot retinochoroidopathy. Br. J. Ophthalmol. 83, 241–249.

Gavalas, N.G., Kemp, E.H., Krohn, K.J., Brown, E.M., Watson, P.F., Weetman, A.P., 2007. The calcium-sensing receptor is a target of autoantibodies in patients with autoimmune polyendocrine syndrome type 1. J. Clin. Endocrinol. Metab. 92, 2107–2114.

Gherardi, R.K., Coquet, M., Cherin, P., Authier, F.J., Laforet, P., Belec, L., et al., 1998. Macrophagic myofasciitis, an emerging entity. Lancet. 352, 347–352.

Gherardi, R.K., Couquet, M., Cherin, P., Belec, L., Moretto, P.A., 2001. Macrophagic myofasciitis lesions assess long-term persistence of vaccine-derived aluminium hydroxide in muscle.. Brain. 124, 1821–1831.

Giovannoni, G., 2005. Anti-neruronal antibodies and movement disorders. J. Neuroimmunol. 163, 5–7.

Giudice, L.C., Koo, L., 2004. Endometriosis. Lancet. 364, 1789–1793.

Gleicher, N., el-Roeiy, A., Confino, E., Friberg, J., 1987. Is endometriosis an autoimmune disease? Obstet. Gynecol. 70, 115–122.

Grabar, P., 1975. Hypothesis. Autoantibodies and immunological theories. An analytic review. Clin. Immunol. Immunopathol. 4, 453–466.

Grimes, D.A., Lebolt, S.C., Grimes, K.R., Wingo, P.A., 1985. Systemic lupus erythematosus and reproductive function. A case-control study. Am J Obstet Gynecol. 153, 179–186.

Hallmayer, J., Faraco, J., Lin, L., Hesselson, S., Winkelmann, J., Kawashima, M., et al., 2009. Narcolepsy is strongly associated with the T-cell receptor alpha locus. Nat. Genet. 41, 708–711.

Hand, J.R., 1949. Interstitial cystitis: report of 223 cases 204 women and 19 men. J. Urol. 61, 291–310.

Hansson, A.-S., Johanneson, M., Svensson, L., Nandakumar, K.S., Heinegad, D., Holmdahl, R., 2004. Relapsing polychondritis, induced in mice with Matrilin 1, is an antibody and complement-dependent disease. Am. J. Pathol. 164, 959–966.

Haseeb, A., Haqqi, T.M., 2013. Immunopathogenesis of osteoarthritis. J. Clin. Immunol. 146, 185–196.

He, C., Soffer, E.E., Ferris, C.D., Walsh, R.M., Szurszewski, J.H., Farrugia, G., 2001. Loss of interstitial cells of Cajal and inhibitory innervation in insulin-dependent diabetes. Gastroenterology. 121, 427–434.

Hennekens, C.H., Lee, I.M., Cook, N.R., Hebert, P.R., Karlson, E.W., LaMotte, F., et al., 1996. Self-reported breast implants and connective-tissue diseases in female health professionals. A retrospective cohort study. JAMA. 275, 616–621.

Hever, A., Roth, R.B., Hevezi, P., Marin, M.E., Acosta, J.A., Acosta, H., et al., 2007. Human endometriosis is associated with plasma cells and overexpression of B lymphocyte stimulator. Proc. Natl. Acad. Sci. 104, 12451–12456.

Ho, L.-P., Urban, B.C., Thickett, D.R., Davis, R.J.O., McMichael, A.J., 2005. Deficiency of a subset of T cells with immunoregulatory properties in sarcoidosis. Lancet. 365, 1062–1072.

Holmes, G.P., Kaplan, J.E., Gantz, N.M., Komaroff, A.L., Schonberger, L.B., Straus, S.E., et al., 1988. Chronic fatigue syndrome. A working case definition. Ann. Intern. Med. 108, 387–389.

Hunner, G.L., 1914. A rare type of bladder ulcer in women. Trans. South Surg. Gynec. Assoc. 27, 247–292.

Iorio, R., Lennon, V.A., 2012. Neural antigen-specific autoimmune disorders. Immunol. Rev. 248, 104–121.

Irani, S.R., Bien, C.G., Lang, B., 2011. Autoimmune epilepsies. Curr. Opin. Neurol. 24, 146–153.

Janowski, E.C., Kuppe, L.L., Hulka, B.S., 2000. Meta-Analysis of the relation between silicone breast implants and the risk of connective-tissue diseases. New Engl J Med. 342, 781–790.

Jokinen, E.J., Alfthan, O.S., Oravisto, K.J., 1972. Anti-tissue antibodies in interstitial cystitis. Clin. Exp. Immunol. 11, 333–339.

Kempta Lekpa, F., Kraus, V.B., Chevalier, X., 2012. Biologics in relapsing polychondritis; a literature review. Sem. Arthritis Rheum. 41, 712–719.

Konstantinov, K., von Mikecz, A., Buchwald, D., Jones, J., Gerace, L., Tan, E.M., 1996. Autoantibodics to nuclear envelope antigens in chronic fatigue syndrome. J. Clin. Invest. 98, 1888–1996.

Kremer, G.D., Mitteregger, D., Marberger, M., 2007. Is Benign Prostatic Hyperplasia (BPH) an immune inflammatory disease? Eur. Urol. 51, 1202–1216.

Lahmer, T., Treiber, M., von Verder, A., Foeger, F., von Knopf, A., Heemann, U., et al., 2010. Relapsing polychondritis: an autoimmune disease with many faces. Autoimmunity Rev. 9, 540–546.

Lancaster, E., Lai, M., Peng, X., Hughes, E., Constantinescu, R., Raizer, J., et al., 2010. Antibodies to the GABA(B) receptor in limbic encephalitis with seizures, case series and characterization of the antigen. Lancet Neurol. 9, 67–76.

Le Cleach, L., Chosidow, O., 2012. Lichen planus. New Engl J Med. 366, 723–732.

Lennon, V.A., Ermilov, L.G., Szurzewski, J.H., Vernino, S., 2003. Immunization with neuronal nicotinic acetylcholine receptor induces neurological autoimmune disease. J. Clin. Invest. 111, 907–913.

Li, Y., Song, Y.-H., Rais, N., Connor, E., Schatz, D., Muir, A., et al., 1996. Autoantibodies to the extracellular domain of the calcium sensing receptor in patients with acquired hypoparathyroidism. J. Clin. Invest. 97, 910–914.

Lippi, G., Targher, G., Franchini, M., 2010. Vaccination, squalene and anti-squalene antibodies, facts or fiction? Eur. J. Intern. Med. 21, 70–73.

Liu, W., Evanoff, D.P., Chen, X., Luo, Y., 2007. Urinary bladder epithelium antigen induces CD8 + T cell tolerance, activation, and autoimmune response. J. Immunol. 178, 539–546.

Lloyd, A.R, Wakefield, D., Boughton, CR., Dwyer, J.M., 1989. Immunological abnormalities in the chronic fatigue syndrome. Med. J. Aust. 151, 122–124.

Lloyd, A., Hickie, I., Wakefield, D., Boughton, C., Dwyer, J., 1990. A double-blind placebo-controlled trial of intravenous immunoglobulin therapy in patients with chronic fatigue syndrome. Am. J. Med. 89, 561–568.

Luber-Narod, J., Austin-Ritchie, T., Banner, B., Hollins, C., Maramag, C., Price, H., et al., 1996. Experimental autoimmune cystitis in the Lewis rat, a potential animal model for interstitial cystitis. Urol. Res. 24, 367–373.

Mackay, I.R., Burnet, F.M., 1963. The Autoimmune Diseases: Pathogenesis, Chemistry and Therapy. Charles C Thomas, Springfield IL, pp. 242–243.

Maclaren, N.K., Blizzard, R.N., 1985. Adrenal autoimmunity and autoimmune polyglandular syndromes. In: Rose, N.R., Mackay, I.R. (Eds.), The Autoimmune Diseases. Academic Press, Orlando, pp. 201–225.

Mathur, S., Butler, W.J., Chihal, H.J., Isaacson, K.B., Gleicher, N., 1995. Target antigen(s) in endometrial autoimmunity of endometriosis. Autoimmunity. 20, 211–222.

McAdam, L.P., O'Hanlan, M.A., Bluestone, R., Pearson, C.M., 1976. Relapsing polychondritis. Prospective study of 23 patients and a review of the literature. Medicine (Baltimore). 55, 193–215.

Medical Staff of the Royal Free Hospital, 1957. An outbreak of encephalomyelitis in the Royal Free Hospital Group, London, in 1955. Br. Med. J. 2, 1436–1437.

Michet Jr, C.J., McKenna, C.H., Luthra, H.S., O'Fallon, W.M., 1986. Relapsing polychondritis. Survival and predictive role of early disease manifestations. Ann. Intern. Med. 104, 74–78.

Miyoshi, K., Miyaoka, T., Kobayashi, Y., Itakura, T., Nishijo, K., Higashibara, N., et al., 1964. Hypergammaglobulinemia by prolonged adjuvanticity in man. Disorders developed after augmentation mammoplasty. Ijishimpo. 2122, 9–14.

Newman, L.S., Rose, C.S., Maier, L.A., 1997. Sarcoidosis. N. Engl. J. Med. 336, 1224–1234.

Nicholls, H., 2012. Eyes wide shut. New Sci. 24 (March), 48–51.

Ochs, R.L., Stein Jr., T.W., Peebles, C.L., Gittes, R.F., Tan, E., 1994. Autoantibodies in interstitial cystitis. J. Urol. 151, 587–592.

Ogura, K., Matsumoto, T., Aoki, Y., Kitabatake, T., Fujisawa, M., Kojima, K., 2010. IgG4-related tumour-forming mastitis with histological appearances of granulomatous lobular mastitis, comparison with other types of tumour-forming mastitis. Histopathology. 57, 39–45.

Oravisto, K.J., 1980. Interstitial cystitis as an autoimmune disease. A review. Eur. Urol. 6, 10–13.

Oravisto, K.J., Alftahn, O.S., Jokinen, E.J., 1970. Interstitial cystitis: clinical and immunological findings. Scand. J. Urol. Nephrol. 4, 37–42.

Oyama, N., Chan, I., Neill, S.M., Hamada, T., South, A.P., Wessagowit, V., et al., 2003. Autoantibodies to extracellular matrix protein 1 in lichen sclerosus. Lancet. 362, 118–123.

Palace, J., Lang, B., 2000. Epilepsy, an autoimmune disease. J. Neurol. Neurosurg. Psychiatr. 69, 711–714.

Pallais, J.C., Kifor, O., Chen, Y.-B., Slovik, D., Brown, E.M., 2004. Acquired hypocalciuric hypercalemia due to autoantibodies against the calcium-sensing receptor. N. Engl. J. Med. 351, 362–364.

Park, S.-H., Weiss, A., Benlagha, K., Kyin, T., Teyton, L., Bendelac, A., 2001. The mouse CD1d-restricted repertoire is dominated by a few autoreactive T-cell families. J. Exp. Med. 193, 893–904.

Patrick, J., Lindstrom, J., 1973. Autoimmune response to acetyl choline receptor. Science. 180, 871–872.

Pearson, C.M., Wood, F.D., 1959. Studies of polyarthritis and other lesions induced in rats by injection of mycobacterial adjuvant. General clinical and pathologic characteristics and some modifying factors. Arthritis Rheum. 2, 440–459.

Pearson, C.M., Kline, H.M., Newcomer, V.D., 1960. Relapsing polychondritis. N. Engl. J. Med. 263, 51–58.

Peeker, R., Atanasiu, L., Logadottir, Y., 2003. Intercurrent autoimmune conditions in classic and non-ulcer interstitial cystitis. Scand. J. Urol. Nephrol. 37, 60–63.

Peltola, J., Kulmala, P., Isojärvi, J., Saiz, A., Latvala, K., Palmio, J., et al., 2000. Antibodies to glutamic acid decarboxylase in patients with therapy resistant epilepsy. Neurology. 55, 46–50.

Penna, G., Fibbi, B., Amuchastegui, S., Cossetti, C., Aquilano, F., Laverny, G., et al., 2009. Human benign prostatic hyperplasia stromal cells as inducers and targets of chronic immuno-mediated inflammation. J. Immunol. 182, 4056–4064.

Peterson, P.K., Shepard, J., Macres, M., Schenck, C., Crosson, J., Rechtman, D., et al., 1990. A controlled trial of intravenous immunoglobulin G in chronic fatigue syndrome. Am. J. Med. 89, 554–560.

Press, R.L., Peebles, C.L., Kumagai, Y., Ochs, R.L., Tan, E.M., 1992. Anti-nuclear autoantibodies in women with silicone breast implants. Lancet. 340, 1304–1307.

Quek, A.M.L., Britton, J.W., McKeon, A., So, A., Lennon, V.A., Shin, C., et al., 2012. Autoimmune epilepsy. Clinical characteristics and response to immunotherapy. Arch. Neurol. 69, 582–593.

Ramaekers, V.T., Rothenberg, S.P., Sequeira, J.M., Opladen, T., Blau, N., et al., 2005. Autoantibodies to folate receptors in the cerebral folate deficiency syndrome. N. Engl. J. Med. 352, 1985–1991.

Ridley, J.H., 1968. The histogenesis of endometriosis: a review of facts and fancies. Obstet. Gynecol. Surv. 23, 1–35.

Rogers, S.W., Andrews, P.I., Gahring, L.C., Whisenand, T., Cauley, K., Crain, B., et al., 1994. Autoantibodies to glutamate receptor GluR3 in Rasmussen's encephalitis. Science. 265, 648–651.

Rosenbaum, J.T., 1997. Lessons from litigation over silicone breast implants, a call for activism by scientists. Science. 276, 1524–1525.

Rothenberg, S.P., da Costa, M.P., Sequeira, J.M., Cracco, J., Roberts, J.L., Weedon, J., et al., 2004. Autoantibodies against folate receptors in women with a pregnancy complicated by neural-tube defect. N. Engl. J. Med. 350, 134–142.

Rowley, M.J., Cook, A.D., Mackay, I.R., Teuber, S.S., Gershwin, M.E., 1996. Comparative epitope mapping of antibodies to collagen in women with silicone breast implants, systemic lupus erythematosus and rheumatoid arthritis. In: Immunology of Silicones. Potter, M., Rose, N.R. (Eds.), Current Topics in Microbiology and Immunology. Springer Verlag, Berlin, 210, 307–316.

Saiz, A., Blanco, Y., Sabater, L., Gonzalez, F., Bataller, L., Casamitjana, R., et al., 2008. Spectrum of neurological syndromes associated with glutamic acid decarboxylase antibodies, diagnostic clues for this association. Brain. 13, 2553–2563.

Sakkas, L.T., Platsoukas, C.D., 2007. The role of T cells in the pathogenesis of osteoarthritis. Arthritis Rheum. 56, 409–424.

Sampson, J.A., 1921. Perforating hemorrhagic (chocolate) cysts of the ovary: their importance and especially their relation to pelvic Adenomas of the endometrial type ("adenomyoma" of the uterus, rectovaginal septum, sigmoid etc.). Arch. Surg. 3, 245–323.

Sant, G.R., Theoharides, T.C., 1994. The role of the mast cell in interstitial cystitis. Urol. Clin. N. Am. 21, 41–53.

Sarkurai, T., Amemiya, A., Ishii, M., Matzusaki, I., Chemelli, R.M., et al., 1998. Orexin and orexin receptors, a family of hypothalamic neuropeptides and G protein-coupled receptors that regulate feeding behavior. Cell. 92, 573–585.

Schwartz, R.S., 2005. Autoimmune folate deficiency and the rise and fall of "horror autotoxicus" [d.q.]. N. Engl. J. Med. 352, 1948–1950.

Seemann, N., 1967. Untersuchungen zur Häufigkeit der lymphozytären Parathyreoiditis. Dtsch. Med. Wschr. 92, 106–108.

Shelley, W.B., Hurley, H.J., 1960. An unusual autoimmune syndrome. Erythema annulare centrifugum, generalized pigmentation and breast hypertrophy. Arch. Dermat. 81, 889–897.

Shipton, E.A., 1965. Hunner's ulcus (chronic interstitial cystitis). A manifestation of collagen disease. Br. J. Urol. 37, 443–449.

Shoenfeld, Y., Agmon-Levin, N., 2011. Autoimmune/inflammatory syndrome induced by adjuvants. J. Autoimmun. 36, 4–8.

Shulman, S., Yantorno, C., Barnes, G.W., Gonder, M.J., Soanes, W.A., Witebsky, E., 1965. Studies on autosensitization to prostatic tissue and related tissues. Ann. N.Y. Acad. Sci. 124, 279–291.

Shulman, S.T., 1999. Pediatric autoimmune neuropsychiatric disorders associated with streptococci (PANDAS). Pediatr. Infect. Dis. J. 18, 281–282.

Silk, M.R., 1970. Bladder antibodies in interstitial cystitis. J. Urol. 103, 307–309.

Skowera, A., Stewart, E., Davis, E.T., Cleare, A.J., Unwin, C., Hull, L., et al., 2002. Antinuclear autoantibodies in Gulf War-related illness and chronic fatigue syndrome patients. Clin. Exp. Immunol. 129, 354–358.

Smith, A.J., Jackson, M.W., Neufing, P., McEvoy, R.D., Gordon, T.P., 2004. A functional autoantibody in narcolepsy. Lancet. 364, 2122–21224.

Solomon, I.L., Blizzard, R.M., 1963. Autoimmune disorders of the endocrine glands. J. Pediatr. 63, 1021–1033.

Switchenko, A.C., Kauffman, R.S., Becker, M., 1991. Are there antiendometrial antibodies in sera of women with endometriosis? Fertil. Steril. 56, 235–241.

Taneja, V., Griffiths, M., Behrens, M., Luthra, H.S., David, C.S., 2003. Auricular chondritis in NOD.DQ8.Aβo (Ag7 − / −) transgenic mice resembles human relapsing polychondritis. J. Clin. Invest. 112, 1843–1850.

Taylor, P.V., Maloney, M.D., Campbell, J.M., Skerrow, S.M., Nip, M.M.C., Parmar, A., Tate, G., 1991. Autoreactivity in women with endometriosis. Br J Obstet Gynecol. 98, 680–684.

Terato, K., Shimozuru, Y., Katayama, K., Takemitsu, Y., Yamashita, I., Miyatsu, M., et al., 1990. Specificity of antibodies to type II collagen in rheumatoid arthritis. Arthritis Rheum. 33, 1493–1500.

Tillikainen, A., Lassus, A., Karvonen, J., Vartiainen, P., Julin, M., 1980. Psoriasis and HLA-Cw6. B J Dermatol. 102, 179–184.

Tomaszewski, J.E., Brooks, J.S., Hicks, D., Livolsi, V.A., 1992. Diabetic mastopathy: a distinctive clinicopathologic entity. Hum. Pathol. 23, 780–786.

Vernino, S., Low, P.A., Fealey, R.D., Stewart, J.D., Farrugia, G., Lennon, V.A., 2000. Autoantibodies to ganglionic acetylcholine receptors in autoimmune autonomic neuropathies. N. Engl. J. Med. 343, 847–855.

Vernino, S., Ermilov, L.G., Sha, L., Szurszewski, J.H., Low, P.A., Lennon, V., 2004. Passive transfer of autoimmune autonomic neuropathy to mice. J. Neurosci. 24, 7037–7042.

Vernon, S.D., Reeves, W.C., 2005. Evaluation of autoantibodies to common and neuronal cell antigens in chronic fatigue syndrome. J. Autoimmune Dis. 2, 5.

von Mikecz, H., Konstantinov, K., Buchwald, D.S., Gerace, I., Tan, E.M., 1997. High frequency of autoantibodies to insoluble cellular antigens in patients with chronic fatigue syndrome. Arthritis Rheum. 40, 295–305.

Walter, M., Berg, H., Leidenberger, F.A., Schweppe, K.W., Northemann, W., 1995. Autoreactive epitopes within the human alpha-enolase and their recognition by sera from patients with endometriosis. J. Autoimmun. 8, 931–945.

Wang, Q., Rozelle, A.L., Lepus, C.M., Scanzello, C.R., Song, S.S., Larsen, D.M., et al., 2011. Identification of a central role for complement in osteoarthritis. Nature Med. 17, 1674–1679.

Weed, J.C., Arquembourg, P.C., 1980. Endometriosis: can it produce an autoimmune response resulting in infertility? Clin. Obstet. Gynecol. 23, 885–893.

Wilson, T.J., Hertzog, P.J., Angus, D., Munnery, L., Wood, E.C., Kola, I., 1994. Decreased natural killer cell activity in endometriosis patients: relationship to disease pathogenesis. Fertil. Steril. 62, 1086–1088.

Xiang, Y., Sekine, T., Nakamura, H., Imajoh-Ohmi, S., Fukuda, H., Nishioka, K., et al., 2004. Proteomic surveillance of autoimmunity in osteoarthritis: identification of triosephosphate isomerase as an autoantigen in patients with osteoarthritis. Arthritis Rheum. 50, 1511–1521.

Yamaguchi, A., Katsuyama, K., Nagahama, K., Takai, T., Aoki, I., Yamanaka, S., 2004. Possible role of autoantibodies in the pathophysiology of GM2 gangliosides. J. Clin. Invest. 113, 200–208.

Yang, C.L., Brinkmann, J., Rui, H.F., Vehring, K.H., Lehmann, H., Kakow, J., et al., 1993. Autoantibodies to cartilage collagens in relapsing polychondritis. Arch. Dermatol. Res. 285, 245–249.

Chapter 76

Autoantibodies Against Cytokines

John W. Schrader[1] and James W. Goding[2]

[1]The Biomedical Research Centre, University of British Columbia, Vancouver, Canada, [2]Department of Physiology, Monash University, Victoria, Australia

Chapter Outline

Introduction   1142
Autoantibodies Against Cytokines in Humans   1142
   Autoantibodies Against Type I and Type II Interferon   1142
   Autoantibodies Against IL-1α   1142
   Autoantibodies Against Tumor Necrosis Factor (TNF)   1142
   Autoantibodies Against IL-6   1142
   Autoantibodies against Granulocyte-Macrophage Colony-Stimulating Factor   1143
Pathogenicity of Autoantibodies Against Cytokines—General Comments   1143
   Autoantibodies Against GM-CSF Cause Idiopathic Pulmonary Alveolar Proteinosis   1143
   Autoantibodies Against Erythropoietin Cause Pure Red Cell Aplasia   1144
   Autoantibodies Against IFN-γ Cause Mycobacteria Infections   1144
   Autoantibodies Against IL-17A, IL-17F, and IL-22 Correlate with Mucocutaneous Candidiasis in Autoimmune-Polyendocrinopathy-Candidiasis-Ectodermal Dystrophy   1144
   Opportunistic Infections in Patients with a Thymoma   1144
   Autoantibodies Against the Bioactivity of Osteoprotegerin   1144
   Autoantibodies Against IL-8   1145
   Autoantibodies Against IL-1α   1145
   Autoantibodies Against IL-6   1145
   What Is the Therapeutic Benefit of Autoantibodies against Cytokines from Pharmaceutically Prepared Immunoglobulin?   1145
Are Anti-Cytokine Autoantibodies Against a Range of Cytokines in all Healthy Humans?   1145
Analysis of a Panel of Neutralizing Monoclonal Antibodies to GM-CSF   1146
   The Advantage of Studying Monoclonal Autoantibodies with Natural and Authentic H and L Chain Pairing   1146

The Autoantibodies Against GM-CSF Were all Polyclonal, Excluding a "Forbidden B Cell Clone"   1146
No Preferred V-gene Usage in Autoantibodies to GM-CSF   1147
Multiple Epitopes Recognized by Pathogenic Monoclonal Autoantibodies to GM-CSF   1147
Mechanism of Pathogenicity of Monoclonal Autoantibodies to GM-CSF   1147
Inhibitory Activity Is Strengthened by Formation of Stable High-avidity Complexes Comprising Multiple Antibodies Binding to Multiple Epitopes   1147
Somatic Mutation of Autoantibodies to GM-CSF   1148
Is Antibody Autoreactivity a Consequence of Somatic Mutation?   1148
Could Autoantibodies Arise in Response to a B Cell Epitope on a Pathogen Antigen that Mimics a Self-antigen GM-CSF?   1148
Autoantibodies to GM-CSF: Implications for B Cell Tolerance to Cytokines   1149
   General B Cell Tolerance   1149
   Antibodies Binding to Multiple Epitopes on GM-CSF Suggest that B Cells Lack Tolerance to Cytokines   1149
Role of T Cells and the Thymus in Pathogenesis of Autoantibodies to Cytokines   1150
   General T Cell Tolerance   1150
   Role of the AIRE Gene in T Cell Tolerance   1150
   T Cell Tolerance to Cytokines   1150
   T Cell Tolerance Is Incomplete and Breakable   1150
   Autoantibodies against Cytokines in APECED   1151
   Autoantibodies against Cytokines in Patients with Thymoma   1152
Induction of Autoantibodies as a Consequence of Therapy with Recombinant Cytokines   1152
Conclusions and Future Prospects   1153
References   1154

N. Rose & I. Mackay (Eds): The Autoimmune Diseases, Fifth edition. DOI: http://dx.doi.org/10.1016/B978-0-12-384929-8.00076-9

INTRODUCTION

Research on purified cytokines started in the late 1970s following the development of technologies for analyzing minute amounts of proteins and producing recombinant cytokines, and was soon followed by reports of human autoantibodies against human cytokines in infections, cancer, and autoimmune diseases. Shortly thereafter, autoantibodies against the specific cytokines, IFN-α, IL-1α, and IL-6 were reported in healthy normal humans, in various frequencies, probably reflecting differences in affinity and the sensitivity of the assay (Bendtzen et al., 2000). Neutralizing autoantibodies against a cytokine would be expected to be pathogenic by reducing the development of mature, differentiated cells or reducing activation of effector cells dependent on it, and if resistance to a certain pathogen is dependent on that cytokine, such autoantibodies might make the patient unusually susceptible.

Antibodies against cytokines that neutralize the bioactivity of the cytokine *in vitro* can block the biological action of the cytokine *in vivo* when present in high concentrations (Finkelman et al., 1993; Kawade et al., 2003). On the other hand, antibodies against cytokines in low concentrations can sometimes prolong their half-lives, which are typically short, by acting as carrier-proteins in the plasma and extracellular fluid. This may occur whether they neutralize the bioactivity of the cytokine (Finkelman et al., 1993; Boyman et al., 2006) or not (Rosenblum et al., 1985; Jones and Ziltener, 1993). Following the discovery of autoantibodies against cytokines in healthy humans, it was proposed that they might act as physiological regulators of cytokine action (Jeffes et al., 1989; Bendtzen et al., 1990; Ross et al., 1990; Hansen et al., 1995; van der Meide and Schellekens, 1997), but this notion is unproven.

The mechanisms that result in the formation of autoantibodies against cytokines are still poorly understood, and it is conceivable that autoantibodies against specific cytokines may have different etiologies and different biological consequences. We will explore some examples in the following section.

AUTOANTIBODIES AGAINST CYTOKINES IN HUMANS

Autoantibodies Against Type I and Type II Interferon

The first report of natural autoantibodies against cytokines was in 1981, when an aged woman with a varicella zoster infection was found to have autoantibodies against the type 1 interferon interferon-alpha (IFN-α) (Mogensen et al., 1981). A year later, neutralizing autoantibody against IFN-α was found in one out of six female patients with systemic lupus erythematosus (Panem et al., 1982),

and the following year it was noted that two cancer patients had natural autoantibodies against IFN-α (Trown et al., 1983). One report examined 200 sera from normal humans and all contained autoantibodies that neutralized the antiviral bioactivity against type I IFN (IFN-α and IFN-β) and type II IFN (IFN-γ) (Ross et al., 1990). The autoantibodies were also detectable in immunoglobulin pools. Autoantibodies against IFN-γ have been shown to be increased in viral infection but these did not neutralize the antiviral activity of IFN-γ (Caruso et al., 1990). Autoantibodies against IFN-α were found at high levels in 12/15 preparations of pharmaceutically prepared pooled IgG (Ross et al., 1995). The autoantibodies neutralized IFN-α and to a less extent IFN-β, but not IFN-γ.

Autoantibodies Against IL-1α

Autoantibodies against another cytokine, IL-1α, were found in the sera of 10% of healthy humans (Svenson et al., 1989) and 75% of people with autoimmune diseases (Hansen et al., 1991a). These autoantibodies against IL-1α increased with age (Ohmoto et al., 1997). High affinity autoantibodies against IL-1α that neutralized the bioactivity of IL-1α were also found in pharmaceutically prepared immunoglobulin pools (Svenson et al., 1993).

The first human monoclonal autoantibody against a cytokine was immortalized with Epstein—Barr virus from a human who had high levels of autoantibodies against IL-1α (Garrone et al., 1996). This monoclonal autoantibody specifically recognized and neutralized the bioactivity of IL-1α but did not recognize IL-1β or IL-1 receptor antagonist (IL-1RA). It was found to be somatically mutated and bound with high affinity ($K_d = 1.2 \times 10^{-10}$ M).

Autoantibodies Against Tumor Necrosis Factor (TNF)

Autoantibodies against TNF and against lymphotoxin have been found in healthy humans and it was speculated that these autoantibodies might be therapeutic in certain diseases (Jeffes et al., 1989). Autoantibodies against TNF that were affinity purified from a patient with rheumatoid arthritis neutralized the bioactivity of TNF in a tumor cell killing assay (Sioud et al., 1994). However, no high-affinity, neutralizing autoantibodies against TNF were observed in batches of pharmaceutically prepared immunoglobulin prepared from normal healthy humans (Svenson et al., 1993; Wadhwa et al., 2000).

Autoantibodies Against IL-6

Hansen et al. (Hansen et al., 1991b) found autoantibodies against IL-6 in about 10% of healthy humans. The autoantibodies were polyclonal, and two IgG molecules could bind to one IL-6 molecule. In another study, autoantibodies against IL-6 were found in 9/52 patients with systemic sclerosis, whereas ≈ 2% of normal people or 0–5% of people with rheumatoid disease exhibited autoantibodies against IL-6 (Takemura et al., 1992). The difference in incidence in normal people between these two studies (10% versus 2%) presumably reflects differences in sensitivity of the assays used. Autoantibodies against IL-6 that inhibited the bioactivity of IL-6 and bound to IL-6 with high affinity have been found in pharmaceutical human immunoglobulin preparations (Svenson et al., 1993).

Autoantibodies against Granulocyte-Macrophage Colony-Stimulating Factor

Autoantibodies against granulocyte-macrophage colony-stimulating factor (GM-CSF) were found in 5 of 300 normal humans (Ragnhammar et al., 1994). Later, autoantibodies against GM-CSF were found in pharmaceutically prepared pooled immunoglobulin (Svenson et al., 1998). All batches of pharmaceutically prepared pooled immunoglobulin contained detectable autoantibodies against GM-CSF, but when 1258 single plasma samples were tested only four were positive. The fact that the antibodies were detectable when diluted by a factor of about 300 (1258/4) suggests that the titer in the four positive samples must have been quite high. The authors also demonstrated that circulating autoantibodies against GM-CSF were detectable in the patients treated with a batch of immunoglobulin. Another group has also demonstrated that autoantibodies against GM-CSF in pharmaceutically prepared pooled immunoglobulin neutralized the bioactivity of GM-CSF (Wadhwa et al., 2000).

The largest panel of pathogenic human monoclonal autoantibodies against cytokines so far described is that cited in our recent publication which documented 19 monoclonal autoantibodies against GM-CSF from six patients with idiopathic pulmonary alveolar proteinosis (IPAP) (Wang et al., 2013). The monoclonal autoantibodies against GM-CSF were genetically unrelated, with multiple clonotypes in individual patients. The characteristics of these antibodies will be discussed later in this chapter.

PATHOGENICITY OF AUTOANTIBODIES AGAINST CYTOKINES—GENERAL COMMENTS

Formal evidence that autoantibodies against cytokines are pathogenic (Sakagami et al., 2009) exists only for the rare autoimmune disease IPAP (Kitamura et al., 1999; Trapnell et al., 2009), although there is also strong evidence that autoantibodies against erythropoietin can cause pure red aplasia (Casadevall et al., 1996). There is

suggestive evidence that autoantibodies to various cytokines are pathogenic in specific infectious diseases (Browne and Holland, 2010a,b; Burbelo et al., 2010; Kisand et al., 2010; Puel et al., 2010; Kampitak et al., 2011; Browne et al., 2012a).

Most pathogenic autoantibodies against cytokines occur against a single cytokine, such as autoantibodies against GM-CSF in IPAP (Kitamura et al., 1999), or against erythropoietin in pure red aplasia (Casadevall et al., 1996), or autoantibodies against IFN-γ (Browne and Holland, 2010a). In patients with IPAP, there are autoantibodies against GM-CSF but not autoantibodies against IFN-α or against IFN-γ (Burbelo et al., 2010). There are reports of autoantibodies against IFN-γ in humans with non-tuberculous mycobacterial infections, but those patients exhibited no autoantibodies against IFN-α (Burbelo et al., 2010).

However, autoantibodies against clusters of cytokines have been documented. Patients with APECED/APS-1 had autoantibodies against IFN-α, IL-17A, IL-17F, and IL-22 but not against other cytokines like IL-10, IL-18, or transforming growth factor beta (TGF-β) (Kisand et al., 2010; Puel et al., 2010). A patient with a thymoma and chronic mucocutaneous candidiasis had similar findings (Kisand et al., 2010). A second report described patients with thymoma who had autoantibodies against IFN-α but no autoantibodies against IFN-γ or GM-CSF (Burbelo et al., 2010).

Autoantibodies Against GM-CSF Cause Idiopathic Pulmonary Alveolar Proteinosis

Idiopathic pulmonary alveolar proteinosis (IPAP) is a lung disease caused by the accumulation of surfactant protein in the alveoli leading to severe respiratory distress (Trapnell et al., 2009). The role of GM-CSF in the syndrome was first documented in mice in which the GM-CSF gene had been disrupted (Dranoff et al., 1994; Stanley et al., 1994), but in humans this is caused by autoantibodies that neutralize the bioactivity of the GM-CSF (Kitamura et al., 1999; Tanaka et al., 1999; Uchida et al., 2003), although congenital cases of pulmonary alveolar proteinosis are caused by mutations in the GM-CSF receptor (Trapnell et al., 2009).

The bioactivity of GM-CSF is necessary for the proper maturation of alveolar macrophages, which normally catabolize surplus surfactant in the alveoli (Stanley et al., 1994; Nishinakamura et al., 1995). Formal proof of the role of autoantibodies to GM-CSF was obtained by transfer of affinity-purified autoantibodies to GM-CSF from patients suffering from IPAP into non-human primates, which caused the development of the characteristic features of IPAP, including milky bronchoalveolar lavage

(BAL) fluid, increased concentration of surfactants in BAL fluid and serum, and increased pulmonary leukocytosis (Sakagami et al., 2009).

Additional evidence that the IPAP is caused by a deficiency in the bioactivity of GM-CSF is amelioration of IPAP by GM-CSF nebulized into the lungs or delivered systemically (Bonfield et al., 2002; Seymour et al., 2003). The disease is also ameliorated by reducing the concentration of autoantibodies against GM-CSF by plasmapheresis (Luisetti et al., 2009) or the anti-CD20 monoclonal antibody rituximab (Borie et al., 2011).

Autoantibodies against GM-CSF have also been implicated in Crohn's disease (Han et al., 2009) but in contrast, antibodies against GM-CSF were found to ameliorate a mouse model of colitis (Griseri et al., 2012). Autoantibodies against GM-CSF have also been implicated in opportunistic infection in IPAP (Browne and Holland, 2010a).

Autoantibodies Against Erythropoietin Cause Pure Red Cell Aplasia

Pure red cell aplasia is often associated with thymomas, and is cured in a quarter of cases by thymectomy (Jacobs et al., 1959). The reason remained obscure until 1967, when an inhibitor of erythropoiesis was discovered in the plasma of patients with pure red aplasia (Krantz and Kao, 1967). It is now clear that the inhibitor consisted of autoantibodies to erythropoietin (Casadevall et al., 1996).

Very rarely, patients treated with human recombinant erythropoietin make antibodies against both human recombinant erythropoietin and endogenous erythropoietin, producing pure red aplasia (Casadevall et al., 2002). Supporting evidence that autoantibodies against erythropoietin cause pure red cell aplasia comes from reports that rituximab, which depletes B lymphocytes, ameliorates pure red cell aplasia (Behler et al., 2009).

Autoantibodies Against IFN-γ Cause Mycobacteria Infections

There is suggestive evidence that autoantibodies to IFN-γ are pathogenic. Patients who had autoantibodies to IFN-γ were susceptible to disseminated *Mycobacterium tuberculosis* and *Mycobacterium chelonae* infections (Madariaga et al., 1998; Doffinger et al., 2004). Autoantibodies to IFN-γ were also associated with severe infections with *Burkholderia cocovenenans* and *Mycobacterium chelonae* (Hoflich et al., 2004). Patients with autoantibodies to IFN-γ who had infections with non-tuberculous mycobacteria and who were treated with rituximab resolved their infections and inflammation in parallel with reduction in autoantibodies to IFN-γ (Browne et al., 2012b).

Chi et al. found that patients with autoantibodies against IFN-γ had a higher frequency of the HLA alleles DRB1*16:02 and DQB1*05:02 (Chi et al., 2013), and suggested that these MHC class II polymorphisms permitted the formation of T cell epitopes that cross-reacted between the peptide of a hypothetical pathogen antigen and peptides from IFN-γ.

Autoantibodies Against IL-17A, IL-17F, and IL-22 Correlate with Mucocutaneous Candidiasis in Autoimmune-Polyendocrinopathy-Candidiasis-Ectodermal Dystrophy

Many subjects with autoimmune-polyendocrinopathy-candidiasis-ectodermal dystrophy (APECED) suffer from chronic mucocutaneous candidiasis. Th17 cells produce IL-17 family members, IL-22, GM-CSF, and TNF and can damage or protect in autoimmune disease (Gaffen, 2011; Iwakura et al., 2011; Marwaha et al., 2012). In APECED, autoantibodies against IL-17A, IL-17F, and IL-22 strongly correlated with candidiasis (Kisand et al., 2010; Puel et al., 2010). Kisand et al. (2010) reported that there were reduced numbers of cells that synthesized IL-22 and IL-17F in APECED patients with chronic mucocutaneous candidiasis. They speculated that cell-mediated attack on Th17 subsets, perhaps by antibody-dependent cellular cytotoxicity reactions or by T cells, could produce a deficiency of IL-22 and IL-17F.

Opportunistic Infections in Patients with a Thymoma

Patients with opportunistic infections with a thymoma were found to have autoantibodies against 16 of 39 cytokines tested (Burbelo et al., 2010). The autoantibodies blocked *in vitro* the bioactivity of IFN-α, IFN-β, IL-1α, IL-12p35, IL-12p40, and IL-17A. Kisand et al. (Kisand et al., 2010) found autoantibodies against IL-17 and IL-22 in two patients with thymoma that had chronic mucocutaneous candidiasis, but they did not find autoantibodies against IL-17 and IL-22 in 33 patients with a thymoma without chronic mucocutaneous candidiasis. This is suggestive evidence that autoantibodies against IL-17 and IL-22 patients with a thymoma cause chronic mucocutaneous candidiasis.

Autoantibodies Against the Bioactivity of Osteoprotegerin

Osteoprotegerin is a member of the TNF receptor family but it is secreted and acts like a cytokine. Osteoprotegerin is the decoy receptor which binds and thereby opposes RANK ligand, another cytokine which activates osteoclasts and causes bone resorption (Riches et al., 2009). One report contains suggestive evidence of pathogenic autoantibodies against osteoprotegerin that cause osteoporosis (Riches et al., 2009). The patient was found to have neutralizing autoantibodies against the bioactivity of osteoprotegerin (Riches et al., 2009). A further 3/15 patients with celiac disease had autoantibodies against osteoprotegerin but none of the healthy controls had autoantibodies against osteoprotegerin (Riches et al., 2009).

Autoantibodies Against IL-8

Autoantibodies against IL-8, a chemokine, were reported in BAL fluid in adult respiratory distress syndrome (Kurdowska et al., 1996). The autoantibodies against IL-8 were high affinity and blocked IL-8 binding to its receptor. Autoantibodies against IL-8 have also been reported in heparin-associated thrombocytopenia (Amiral et al., 1996) and in association with ovarian cancer (Lokshin et al., 2006).

Autoantibodies Against IL-1α

Autoantibodies that neutralized the bioactivity of IL-1α have been believed to ameliorate disease in rheumatoid arthritis (Graudal et al., 2002; Miossec, 2002) and chronic polyarthritis (Jouvenne et al., 1997), but the entire role of IL-1α in arthritis is still unknown.

Autoantibodies Against IL-6

It has been suggested that patients with alcoholic cirrhosis had more infections and a higher risk of death if they had autoantibodies against IL-6 (Homann et al., 1996). A child with staphylococcal cellulitis and abscesses was found to have high titers of autoantibodies that neutralized the bioactivity of IL-6 (Puel et al., 2008).

What Is the Therapeutic Benefit of Autoantibodies against Cytokines from Pharmaceutically Prepared Immunoglobulin?

Most batches of pharmaceutically prepared immunoglobulin had detectable amounts of antibodies against GM-CSF (Svenson et al., 1998), IL-1α (Svenson et al., 1993), IL-6 (Svenson et al., 1993), IFN-α (Ross et al., 1990, 1995), IFN-γ (Ross et al., 1990), and IL-10 (Svenson et al., 1998). High-affinity, neutralizing autoantibodies against cytokines were found in pharmaceutically prepared IgG against IL-1α, IFN-α, IL-6 (Svenson et al., 1993), and against GM-CSF (Svenson et al., 1998), but no high-affinity, neutralizing autoantibodies against IL-1β or TNF were observed (Svenson et al., 1993). Wadhwa et al. (2000) also demonstrated that batches of immunoglobulin neutralized the bioactivity of IL-1α and IFN-α,

IFN-β, and IFN-ω. They found no neutralizing autoantibodies to granulocyte colony-stimulating factor (G-CSF), macrophage colony-stimulating factor (M-CSF), stem cell factor (SCF), IL-1β, IL-2, IL-3, IL-4, IL-6, IL-9, IL-10, IL-12, TNF, oncostatin M, or IFN-γ (Wadhwa et al., 2000).

Svenson et al. (1998) also tested pharmaceutically prepared immunoglobulin for other autoantibodies against other cytokines, including G-CSF, IL-1RA, IL-2, IL-3, IL-4, IL-5, and IL-10. Only one batch tested positive for high-avidity autoantibodies against IL-5 and 13/15 batches bound weakly to IL-10, agreeing with Menetrier-Caux et al. that there exist rare autoantibodies to IL-10 (Menetrier-Caux et al., 1996).

In the light of all these observations, the suggestion was made that some of the therapeutic benefit of treating humans with pharmaceutically prepared immunoglobulin (intravenous immunoglobulin: ivIg) could be due to autoantibodies against certain cytokines (Svenson et al., 1993; see also Bendtzen et al., 2000). Patients with autoimmune diseases treated with human IgG preparations had higher titers of autoantibodies against IFN-α, IL-1α, IL-6 (Ross et al., 1997), and GM-CSF (Svenson et al., 1998). It is unclear whether these antibodies had any effect on the disease. It seems unlikely that they were present in sufficient amounts to give therapeutic effects, and the question addressed by Svenson et al. (1993) is probably answered in the negative.

ARE ANTI-CYTOKINE AUTOANTIBODIES AGAINST A RANGE OF CYTOKINES IN ALL HEALTHY HUMANS?

Early studies reported that significant numbers of healthy humans have autoantibodies against against IL-1α (10%) (Svenson et al., 1989), IFN-α, IFN-β, and IFN-γ (100%) (Ross et al., 1990), IL-6 (10%) (Hansen et al., 1991b), and GM-CSF (0.3–1.7%) (Ragnhammar et al., 1994; Svenson et al., 1998). Neutralizing autoantibodies against cytokines were also found in pharmaceutically prepared immunoglobulin pools, IFN-α, IFN-β, and IFN-γ (Ross et al., 1990), IL-1α (Svenson et al., 1993), IL-6 (Svenson et al., 1993), and GM-CSF (Svenson et al., 1998; Wadhwa et al., 2000).

More recently, it was reported that all of 15 healthy humans had autoantibodies against IL-2, IL-8, TNF, vascular endothelial growth factor (VEGF), and G-CSF (Watanabe et al., 2007). These authors dissociated autoantibody complexes with cytokine by treating the sera with low pH buffer (pH 2.7), separated the cytokines from autoantibodies by size, and measured the separated autoantibodies by ELISA (Watanabe et al., 2007).

Autoantibodies against IL-4, IL-6, IL-10, and IFN-γ were at a lower frequency and there were no autoantibodies against IL-3, osteopontin, and macrophage-colony stimulating factor (CSF-1) (Watanabe et al., 2007).

The same group also reported a surprisingly high incidence and concentration of autoantibodies against GM-CSF in 72/72 healthy humans, once again using the technique of acid treatment (Uchida et al., 2009). They also found extremely high concentrations of the total GM-CSF concentration in normal plasma, 99.9% of which was bound by neutralizing autoantibodies against GM-CSF, and concluded that autoantibodies against GM-CSF can scavenge free GM-CSF and thereby block myeloid functions. They calculated the levels of autoantibodies against GM-CSF that correlated with pathogenesis and the onset of IPAP, and concluded that the difference between healthy individuals and IPAP patients was a pathogenic increase in levels of autoantibodies against GM-CSF rather than a novel autoantibody response.

For many reasons, we believe that these results should be regarded with caution. The concentration of GM-CSF complexed with autoantibodies claimed in normal plasma in these studies was surprisingly high, but paradoxically its free concentration was so low that it would be totally inactive. Moreover, protocols in which serum is treated with acid and neutralized have received substantial criticism on many grounds (Bazin et al., 2010; Meager et al., 2010; see also response by Uchida et al., 2010). In particular, acid treatment has been well documented to cause partial degradation of specificity, presumably due to incomplete refolding or chemical modification. It is also well known that treatment of antibodies by acid and subsequent neutralization results in the formation of aggregates (Goding, 1996) which can cause substantial errors in ELISA and other assays.

If Watanabe and his colleagues are correct that there are autoantibodies against all of these cytokines, GM-CSF, IL-2, IL-8, TNF, VEGF, and G-CSF in healthy humans, then these could be assayed by different techniques, rather than using low pH buffer to separate the autoantibodies/cytokine complexes. An alternative assay is to measure the frequency of memory B autoantibodies specific for these cytokines when memory B cells from peripheral blood are polyclonally activated (Wen et al., 1987; Pinna et al., 2009) at limit dilution. Autoantibodies against each cytokine could be measured by ELISA and the frequency calculated by Poisson's distribution. If there is an ongoing autoantibody response, the high-affinity memory B cells specific for these cytokines will be in the lymph nodes and not in the peripheral blood. Another assay would be to test the plasmablasts in the blood (Odendahl et al., 2005) or bone marrow plasma cells that are secreting autoantibodies against cytokines by an Elispot assay.

ANALYSIS OF A PANEL OF NEUTRALIZING MONOCLONAL ANTIBODIES TO GM-CSF

The Advantage of Studying Monoclonal Autoantibodies with Natural and Authentic H and L Chain Pairing

It is generally accepted that at least for B cells, most autoimmune reactions are polyclonal. Accordingly, the analysis of autoantibodies from serum is fraught with the difficulties of dealing with a poorly defined chemical mixture. Moreover, the assessment of the nature, origin, and importance of serum autoantibodies to cytokines depends greatly on the sensitivity and specificity of the assays used, and published results have shown marked variation between investigators. Phage-display monoclonal antibodies have been generated from peripheral blood mononuclear cells with H and L chain genes from many autoimmune diseases. However, the data are compromised because random pairs of H and L chain genes have been selected with autoantigens. Multiple monoclonal antibodies with authentic H and L chains that bind to autoantigens would have many advantages. Monoclonal antibodies that have authentic H and L chain pairs are pure, chemically defined entities and their V genes can be sequenced and somatic mutations identified with ease. If they use multiple V genes rather than preferred V genes and consist of multiple clonotypes, epitope mapping can determine whether they bind to multiple non-overlapping epitopes.

Pathogenic monoclonal autoantibodies should take the analysis of autoimmunity to a higher level of precision and may shed light on some central questions. Does B cell tolerance to cytokines exist? Are autoantibodies driven by antigen? If so, are they driven by their self-antigen or the cytokine, or are they initiated and perpetuated by a cross-reacting exogenous antigen? And what can monoclonal antibodies tell us about the role of helper T cells in autoantibody generation?

We have generated a panel of 19 anti-GM-CSF-secreting cell lines from six patients with IPAP and have used them to conduct a detailed characterization of clones secreting autoantibodies to GM-CSF (Wang et al., 2013). Our results may help in the understanding of the origin of pathogenic autoantibodies in general.

The Autoantibodies Against GM-CSF were all Polyclonal, Excluding a "Forbidden B Cell Clone"

The monoclonal autoantibodies against GM-CSF were polyclonal and genetically unrelated. Multiple clonotypes against GM-CSF existed in different patients with IPAP, excluding a single "forbidden" clone for pathogenic auto-antibodies in one patient (Burnet, 1972; Mackay, 2008).

No Preferred V-gene Usage in Autoantibodies to GM-CSF

There is no suggestion of preferred V-gene usage in auto-antibodies to GM-CSF (Wang et al., 2013). Monoclonal pathogenic autoantibodies with authentic H and L chains that bind to desmoglein-3 and cause pemphigus vulgaris also had no preferred V-gene usage (Di Zenzo et al., 2012). In contrast, monoclonal autoantibodies against transglutaminase-2 that are diagnostic for celiac disease use preferred V genes (Di Niro et al., 2012).

Multiple Epitopes Recognized by Pathogenic Monoclonal Autoantibodies to GM-CSF

The pathogenic monoclonal autoantibodies against GM-CSF bound to four non-overlapping, conformational epitopes on GM-CSF and one that overlapped two of the non-overlapping epitopes (Wang et al., 2013). There were at least three non-overlapping epitopes in two patients with IPAP.

All 19 monoclonal autoantibodies against GM-CSF from IPAP patients were conformational and dependent on the native structure. None of the autoantibodies against GM-CSF bound to reduced, boiled GM-CSF on an immuno-blot (Wang et al., 2013), and all neutralized the bioac-tivity of GM-CSF (Wang et al., 2013).

B cell epitopes are conformational and depend on the three-dimensional structure of the protein. The area bur-ied in a protein—antibody complex is 600—935 square Å (Laver et al., 1990), and although it can only be deter-mined through direct crystallography (Laver et al., 1990), a great deal of useful information can be obtained by combining molecular modeling based on known struc-tures with site-directed mutagenesis and physico-chemical analysis.

Mechanism of Pathogenicity of Monoclonal Autoantibodies to GM-CSF

All autoantibodies to GM-CSF neutralized the bioactivity of GM-CSF (Wang et al., 2013) but they bound to five epitopes. How did each monoclonal autoantibody to GM-CSF block the signaling of GM-CSF? The signaling com-plex of the GM-CSF:GM-CSF receptor is a dodecamer and contains four GM-CSF molecules, four GMRα and four βc subunits (Hansen et al., 2008). The fraction of the total surface area of GM-CSF buried by the GMRα is 19%. The one molecule of the GM-CSF in the signaling complex interacts with two βc subunits, domain 1 of βc

and domain 4 of a different βc monomer. The total surface area of GM-CSF buried by domain 1 of βc is 4% and the total surface area of GM-CSF buried by domain 4 of a dif-ferent βc is 7% (Wang et al., 2013). The total surface area of GM-CSF buried by the ternary complex is ≈ 30 %.

In view of their neutralizing activity, we hypothesized that these autoantibodies against GM-CSF bound to the surfaces of GM-CSF that bind to the GM-CSF receptor subunits, the GM-CSF receptor alpha (GMRα) and two binding sites on different beta common (βc) subunits. Using site-directed mutagenesis of GM-CSF, we were able to map two non-overlapping receptor-binding epi-topes, one that interacted with the α subunit of the GM receptor, and the second that interacted with the βc sub-unit. The potential for steric hindrance by autoantibodies binding GM-CSF is great because the signaling GM-CSF: GM-CSF receptor complex contains 12 proteins, four GM-CSF molecules, four GMRα molecules, and four GMRβc molecules.

There was an overall correlation between affinity/off-rate and the potency of neutralizing the bioactivity of GM-CSF, but the highest-affinity autoantibody against GM-CSF was not the most potent at neutralizing the bio-activity of GM-CSF (Wang et al., 2013). The autoanti-body against GM-CSF that was most potent at neutralizing the bioactivity of GM-CSF bound to an over-lapping epitope that spanned the two non-overlapping epi-topes (Wang et al., 2013).

Inhibitory Activity Is Strengthened by Formation of Stable High-avidity Complexes Comprising Multiple Antibodies Binding to Multiple Epitopes

Although GM-CSF is a monomer, IgG is bivalent, and it has been shown that two different IgG molecules can bind to distinct epitopes on two cytokine molecules to form a circular complex, with each cytokine bound by two non-overlapping epitopes (Moyle et al., 1983). If one antigen-binding site of the IgG dissociates from the cytokine and the other arm of IgG is still bound to the same epitope on another cytokine of the circular autoantibody—cytokine complex, the antigen-binding site of the IgG will be in high molar local concentration and will therefore probably reassociate. Thus, if autoantibodies against cytokines bind to multiple epitopes, multiple molecules of the cytokine and autoantibodies are likely to form high-avidity com-plexes (Moyle et al., 1983). Hansen et al. (Hansen et al., 1991b) found that in healthy humans, two IgG autoanti-bodies against IL-6 could bind to one IL-6 molecule.

We have shown that three individual IgG molecules could bind a single molecule of GM-CSF (Wang et al., 2013), and the probability of cytokine bound by three immunoglobulin molecules dissociating will be small; accordingly the free cytokine concentration will be low.

Somatic Mutation of Autoantibodies to GM-CSF

Affinity maturation of IgG antibodies in secondary responses requires T cell help, and is mediated by passage through germinal centers, somatic hypermutation, and Darwinian selection based on competition for antigen on follicular dendritic cells (Nossal, 1992). A high-affinity human monoclonal autoantibody against IL-1α in a healthy human showed evidence of somatic mutations (Garrone et al., 1996).

All the autoantibodies against GM-CSF exhibited high levels of somatic mutation (Wang et al., 2013), indicating T cell help and passage through germinal centers. We observed a high number of somatic mutations in the *IGHV* gene and the *IGKV* and *IGLV* genes (Wang et al., 2013). The median rate of somatic mutations in *IGHV* was 30, compared with typical observed rates for memory B cells and germinal center B cells of 13.6 ± 4.8 (Wrammert et al., 2008). The highest number of somatic mutations in *IGHV* of all of the autoantibodies against GM-CSF was 52 and correlated with the highest affinity antibody, which had a K_d of 3.7×10^{-11} (Wang et al., 2013), indicating that memory B cells had probably re-entered the germinal center many times. This is confirmed by the high levels of somatic mutations found in monoclonal pathogenic autoantibodies with authentic H and L chains that bind to desmoglein-3 in pemphigus vulgaris (Di Zenzo et al., 2012). It may be concluded that these two pathogenic classes of monoclonal autoantibodies need the help of follicular helper T cells.

Is Antibody Autoreactivity a Consequence of Somatic Mutation?

It seems virtually inevitable that some somatic mutations that increase affinity for exogenous antigens will by chance react with self-antigens, but the crystallographic studies of somatically mutated antibodies show that affinity-matured antibodies are very different from germline antibodies. In a germline antibody the CDR loops are flexible and the antigen-binding site or paratope has a diversity of conformations, and the single paratope is to a degree polyspecific, binding many antigens (Manivel et al., 2000). Since only one of these conformations is likely to bind to a single antigen, the association rate of a germline antibody to bind to a single antigen is low. If a germline antibody binds to a single antigen and the paratope is thereby locked in a single conformation, there is a big entropy reduction because there is a loss of freedom

for the CDR loops (Manivel et al., 2000). In contrast, in an affinity-matured antibody, the CDR loops are less flexible, supported by somatic mutations, the antigen-binding site is more rigid, and the association rate may be higher—the affinity-matured antibody interaction with antigen is like a lock and key rather than a handshake. In addition, of course, affinity-matured antibodies show greatly decreased dissociation rates.

Conformational freedom of germline CDRs is likely to account for the observation that 55–75% of the expressed recombinant antibodies from early immature B cells bind to self-antigens (Wardemann et al., 2003). Many of the early immature B cells that are self-reactive are purged and only a small fraction of the expressed recombinant antibodies from mature naïve B cells bind to intracellular self-antigens in human Hep-2 cells, although about 47% of expressed recombinant somatically mutated antibodies from IgG memory B cells from healthy humans showed low levels of self-reactivity with intracellular antigens of HEp-2 cells (Tiller et al., 2007). It is concluded that affinity-matured antibodies that react with intra-cellular self-antigens are low affinity and non-pathogenic. The same group subsequently showed that there is a reduced frequency of plasma cells in the bone marrow that make antibodies that react with HEp-2 cells, although plasma cells had higher somatic mutation rates than IgG memory B cells (Scheid et al., 2011).

Di Zenzo et al. proposed that the pathogenic autoantibodies that bind to desmoglein-3 and cause pemphigus vulgaris were initiated by an unrelated exogenous antigen that started the affinity-maturation process, and fortuitous somatic mutations made the antigen-binding site react with desmoglein-3 (Di Zenzo et al., 2012). However, the authors observed that the autoantibodies bound to at least three to four non-overlapping, conformational epitopes on desmoglein-3 (Di Zenzo et al., 2012). The probability that chance somatic mutations against an unrelated exogenous antigen would create multiple unrelated clonotypes binding to multiple conformational epitopes seems vanishingly small. Two crystallographic studies (Thomson et al., 2008; Schmidt et al., 2013) showed that the antigen-binding site of germline antibodies and affinity-matured antibodies has the same general conformation and it is unlikely that fortuitous somatic mutations of an affinity-maturation process initiated by a single antigen could change the general conformation of the antigen-binding site.

Could Autoantibodies Arise in Response to a B Cell Epitope on a Pathogen Antigen that Mimics a Self-antigen GM-CSF?

It has been suggested that autoantibodies might arise in response to a B cell epitope on a pathogen-associated antigen that mimics a self-antigen (Rowley and Jenkin, 1962). This scenario might envisage a pathogen antigen that cross-reacts with GM-CSF initiating an antibody response which is followed by GM-CSF-driven affinity-maturation via somatic mutations. However, crystallography has demonstrated that a low-affinity, unmutated antigen-binding site has the same general conformation as the high-affinity somatically mutated antibody and has similar antigen contacts (Thomson et al., 2008; Schmidt et al., 2013). Accordingly, the B cell epitope of the pathogen antigen cross-reacting with GM-CSF must overlap the original epitope of the pathogen antigen, but our monoclonal autoantibodies against GM-CSF bound to four non-overlapping, conformational epitopes on GM-CSF, with at least three non-overlapping epitopes in two patients with IPAP. It would therefore seem very improbable that antigens from a pathogen could mimic three to four non-overlapping, conformational B cell epitopes on GM-CSF.

AUTOANTIBODIES TO GM-CSF: IMPLICATIONS FOR B CELL TOLERANCE TO CYTOKINES

General B Cell Tolerance

Contact with self-antigens early in B cell development leads to cell death (Hartley et al., 1993), anergy (Glynne et al., 2000; Zikherman et al., 2012), or receptor editing (Nemazee and Hogquist, 2003). Presumably because signaling via membrane immunoglobulin requires cross-linking, tolerance is most easily induced in B cells by membrane-associated antigens which are by their very nature presented in a multivalent form (Hartley et al., 1993; but see Akkaraju et al., 1997). In contrast, most cytokines are soluble and monomeric, and tolerance to monomeric and monovalent soluble antigens is much less robust (Adelstein et al., 1991). There are several known and perhaps many as yet unknown checkpoints for self-reactive B cells which may allow some self-reactive B lymphocytes to be functional in protecting against pathogens without harming the host (Goodnow, 2007).

In humans, 55–75% of early immature B cells make antibodies that bind to self-antigens and about 50% of these early immature B cells are deleted (Wardemann et al., 2003), leaving 5–25% of the naïve B cell repertoire reactive with self-antigens. If a V gene facilitates protective antibodies against important pathogens, there will be evolutionary pressure on retaining that V gene even if it reacts with a self-antigen (Wardemann et al., 2003). It may be hypothesized that low-affinity self-reactive B cells may do no harm, and their complete deletion may leave the species vulnerable to infectious pathogens. For example, we have reported that the germline ancestor

of a hypermutated protective human mAb that neutralized human cytomegalovirus (HCMV) was autoreactive (McLean et al., 2006). On the other hand, there may be a counter-evolutionary pressure for pathogen antigens to resemble human self-antigens so that their hosts are tolerant to the self-antigens and cannot respond (Rowley and Jenkin, 1962).

Antibodies Binding to Multiple Epitopes on GM-CSF Suggest that B Cells Lack Tolerance to Cytokines

A critical question concerns the lower limit of concentration below which a protein antigen is simply not seen by B cells, and therefore for which there can be no B cell tolerance. There is experimental evidence for B cell anergy for soluble protein antigens at serum concentrations greater than 100 pM (Adelstein et al., 1991), but since most soluble cytokines are present at very low or sub-picomolar levels in normal plasma they are unlikely to produce B cell tolerance or anergy. Indeed, there is no experimental evidence for induction of B cell tolerance or anergy to cytokines, and thus we assume that there is no B cell anergy or no B cell tolerance for these self-antigens.

If there is no B cell tolerance to cytokines, we would anticipate the entire surface of each cytokine to be potentially immunogenic, and we would expect to find antibodies that bind to multiple epitopes on the cytokine, and this is what is observed. In healthy humans who had autoantibodies against IL-6, autoantibodies bound to two non-overlapping epitopes on IL-6 (Hansen et al., 1991b). Uchida et al. (2003) observed that autoantibodies against GM-CSF in IPAP patients bound to multiple epitopes. In our panel of 19 human monoclonal autoantibodies against GM-CSF cloned from six IPAP patients we observed three monoclonal autoantibodies against GM-CSF that bound to three non-overlapping epitopes, and three monoclonal autoantibodies were able to bind simultaneously to a single monomer of GM-CSF (Wang et al., 2013). The formation of stable, high-avidity, multi-molecular complexes formed by autoantibodies against GM-CSF is entirely compatible with the idea that B cells show no tolerance to this cytokine and, by inference, no B cell tolerance to any cytokine.

The production of B cell memory and high-affinity IgG production requires T cell help, and as long as the corresponding T cells are tolerant, there would seem to be no compelling reason why B cell tolerance to all self-cytokines would be a biological necessity. Without T cell help, the worst that might happen might be transient IgM responses which may do little if any harm. On the other hand, lack of tolerance to a particular self-cytokine in B cells leaves the body open to the possibility of autoimmunity if for any reason a T cell of the appropriate specificity becomes activated. Indeed, such a scenario may explain many aspects of autoantibody production against cytokines, as will be discussed in the next section.

ROLE OF T CELLS AND THE THYMUS IN PATHOGENESIS OF AUTOANTIBODIES TO CYTOKINES

We have already discussed the evidence that production of high-affinity IgG autoantibodies to cytokines requires T cell help (see above).

General T Cell Tolerance

The thymus plays a major but incomplete role in the establishment of self-tolerance via a sequence of positive and negative selection steps in which the T cell receptor (TCR) for antigen recognizes linear peptides in the groove of MHC proteins on the surface of specialized thymic epithelial cells. Because the thymus is largely isolated from the exterior of the body, the overwhelming probability is that these peptides will be "self." The first step involves positive selection for T cells that are capable of at least weak interaction with MHC−peptide complexes. T cells that are incapable of this interaction die by apoptosis. A second step involves apoptotic deletion of potentially harmful T cells with strong reactivity to these MHC−self-peptide complexes.

If every protein that the body is capable of making were expressed in the thymus, such a mechanism would have the potential to generate a set of mature T cells capable of defending the body against any intruder, while avoiding attack against the body. However, if any proteins synthesized elsewhere in the body are not expressed in the thymus, mature T cells reactive to these proteins could emerge, and they would have the potential to cause autoimmunity. Cytokines may represent a case in point.

Most cytokines are tissue-restricted self-antigens that might not be expressed in the thymus. Many are synthesized only in emergencies such as infection or trauma, while some are synthesized continuously at local sites such as skin and mucous membranes which bacteria colonize, for example IFN-α in the gut (Abt et al., 2012; Ganal et al., 2012).

Role of the AIRE Gene in T Cell Tolerance

A unique mechanism exists to deal with this problem. An unusual transcription factor with very broad activity on many promoters is present in thymic medullary epithelial cells and acts as an autoimmune regulator (AIRE) by causing transcription of many genes that would otherwise not be expressed in the thymus, allowing deletion of T cells that would otherwise have the potential to cause autoimmunity in tissues or organs where there are tissue-restricted antigens.

The AIRE gene was discovered by mapping and cloning the mutant gene causing autoimmune-polyendocrinopathy-candidiasis-ectodermal dystrophy (APECED), also known as autoimmune polyglandular syndrome 1 (APS-1) (Nagamine et al., 1997) (see Chapter 43). It was found that AIRE is expressed in medullary thymic epithelial cells (Zuklys et al., 2000), where it would be ideally situated to mediate negative selection of self-reactive T cells.

A mouse with a deletion of the AIRE gene developed APECED-like multi-organ autoimmune disease (Anderson et al., 2002), but the mechanism by which AIRE controls promiscuous expression of tissue-restricted self-antigens in medullary thymic epithelial cells and in the secondary lymphoid organs is still under investigation (Akirav et al., 2011).

T Cell Tolerance to Cytokines

AIRE has the potential to facilitate induction of tolerance to any cytokines that are not expressed in the thymus. However, its role in tolerance to cytokines is still unclear, and Meager and colleagues (Kisand et al., 2010) comment that functional AIRE is not necessary to produce T cell tolerance against IFN-α or IL-17. They point out that IFN-α is made by macrophages and dendritic cells in the thymus (Meager et al., 2006) and that IL-17 is made by thymocytes (Marks et al., 2009). Other cytokines are made in the thymus without the need for tolerogenic AIRE, including IL-7 and chemokines such as CCL25, CXCL12, CCL19, CCL21, CCL17, and CCL22 that direct thymocyte migration to different parts of the thymus to make mature T cells. We will return to speculate on the possible role of AIRE later in this chapter.

T Cell Tolerance is Incomplete and Breakable

Notwithstanding the expression of ubiquitous proteins and many more tissue-restricted proteins in the thymus via AIRE, deletion of self-reactive T cells in the thymus is incomplete, as is the case for B cell tolerance in the bone marrow or spleen (Akkaraju et al., 1997; Wardemann et al., 2003). And even if intrathymic purging of these dangerous T cells is complete, the process could be reversed by a rare event such as a somatic mutation in a mature T cell that alters its specificity or activation threshold, or an encounter with a rare pathogen.

Perhaps for this reason, a further layer of protection against autoimmunity is provided by the so-called regulatory T cells (Tregs). Tregs are characterized by high levels of expression of CD25 and the transcription factor *Foxp3*. Kim et al. constructed a mouse in which the 3′ untranslated region of the mRNA for *Foxp3* contained a gene for the receptor for diphtheria toxin driven by an internal ribosome entry site (IRES), so that cells expressing *Foxp3* could be killed by administration of diphtheria toxin, to which mice are normally resistant. Interestingly, when Tregs were eliminated in this way, mice were found to die from autoimmunity with splenomegaly and lymphadenopathy within 10–21 days (Kim et al., 2007), indicating/suggesting that potentially pathogenic autoreactive T cells do indeed escape the thymus but are normally kept in check by Tregs.

Yet, in spite of all the mechanisms in place to prevent or control autoimmunity, "the best-laid schemes o' mice an' men gang aft a-gley." There is a chance that a pathogen might be able to stimulate a T cell that cross-reacts with a peptide on a self-antigen, especially if the pathogen antigen comes with danger-associated molecular patterns that stimulate a Toll-ligand receptor or an inflammasome that "licensed" antigen-presenting cells (Heath and Carbone, 2001). The self-cytokine T cell epitope need not correspond to the amino acid sequence of the T cell epitope in the pathogen, because the T cell antigen receptor (TCR) is polyreactive and multiple peptides of different sequences on the MHC class II can be recognized by the same TCR (Felix et al., 2007).

If AIRE were to control T cell tolerance to most cytokines, how could autoantibodies be made without T cell help? The probable answer is that T cell deletion is incomplete, and low-avidity T cells reactive with self-peptides from cytokines do escape from the thymus. All that is needed is an infection in a local site with a pathogen that stimulates cytokine production in the local site and that has pathogen-associated molecular patterns. This stimulates an antigen-presenting cell and if it has receptors for the cytokine, the antigen-presenting cell endocytoses the cytokine, proteolyses it, and presents a T cell cytokine epitope to activate low-avidity T cells. Antigen-presenting cells have receptors for IFN-α, IFN-β, IL-1α, IL-6, and GM-CSF, and a percentage of healthy humans have autoantibodies against these cytokines (see above). If there is no B cell tolerance to most cytokines, the B cells specific for the cytokine will endocytose the cytokine and present a/the peptide of the cytokine bound to MHC class II to the activated T cells.

An alternative scenario is that a pathogen antigen has a higher-avidity T cell epitope that cross-reacts with a low-avidity T cell epitope of a cytokine and activates T cells. B cells that make antibodies that bind to the cytokine will endocytose the cytokine and present the low-avidity, cross-reactive T cell epitope of the cytokine to get help from those T cells activated by higher-avidity T cell epitopes of the pathogen antigen.

To take an example, healthy humans very frequently produce autoantibodies against IFN-α. The microbiome in the gut normally stimulates the gut to produce IFN-α (Abt et al., 2012; Ganal et al., 2012), and if local antigen-presenting cells exhibit receptors for IFN-α and if they are stimulated by pathogen-associated molecular patterns, they will present a T cell epitope from the IFN-α to activate low-avidity T cells that have escaped from tolerance mechanisms in the thymus.

We speculate that in the case of IPAP a pathogen cross-reactive with a T cell epitope in GM-CSF will present pathogen-associated molecular patterns to antigen-presenting cells and activate T cells. If the pathogen stimulates the release of GM-CSF from macrophages and nearby GM-CSF-specific B cells endocytose GM-CSF, they will present the low-avidity GM-CSF peptide–MHC complex to the T cells activated by the pathogen high-avidity T epitope. The frequency of IPAP is increased in smokers. Cigarette smoke is an irritant causing chronic inflammation and recurrent infection in the lung, and is also a potent source of mutagens that cause cancer in the lung and elsewhere. The putative pathogen does not have to be in the lung. It could be in the gut or the skin where perhaps an unusual bacterium colonizes. Even if there is no pathogen antigen cross-reactive with a T cell epitope in GM-CSF, a pathogen with a pathogen-associated molecular pattern may activate the antigen-presenting cell, which has receptors for GM-CSF and can present a low-avidity T cell epitope of GM-CSF to a low-avidity T cell that has not been tolerized in the thymus.

Autoantibodies against Cytokines in APECED

APECED is caused by mutations in AIRE, although the onset of the disease expression is highly variable (Perheentupa, 2006). Among the many autoantibodies seen in this syndrome, Meager et al. found high titers of neutralizing autoantibodies against IFN-α or IFN-ω (Meager et al., 2006). On the other hand, autoantibodies against IFN-γ, IL-10, and IL-12 were rarer and did not neutralize.

The pathogenesis of chronic mucocutaneous candidiasis has been associated with defects in the so-called Th17 cytokine family IL-17A, IL-17F, and IL-22. It is therefore of interest that neutralizing autoantibodies to these cytokines are particularly prevalent in APECED patients, particularly those with chronic mucocutaneous candidiasis (Kisand et al., 2010; Puel et al., 2010).

It has been suggested that the AIRE mutation in APECED may have caused a loss of T cell tolerance for IL-17A, IL-17F, and IL-22 (Puel et al., 2010). If there is no B cell tolerance to those cytokines, a lack of T cell tolerance could explain how the autoantibodies against IL-17A, IL-17F, and IL-22 were generated. However, the selective incidence of autoantibodies against Th17 cytokines is difficult to understand given that mutations in AIRE do not seem to result in a global loss of tolerance to cytokines. Autoantibodies were only weakly present in low titers against IL-6, IL-9, IL-12, IL-21, IL-23, IL-26, IL- 29, or RANTES and no autoantibodies were found in APECED patients against IL-1, IL-2, IL-4, IL-8, IL-10, IL-18, TGF-β, or TNF (Kisand et al., 2010). Similarly, Puel et al. (2010) found no autoantibodies against GM-CSF, IFN-γ, IL-6, IL-1β, IL-10, IL-12, IL-18, IL-21, IL-23, IL-26, IFN-β, TNF, or TGF-β in APECED patients. Control experiments found no autoantibodies against IL-17A, IL-17F, and IL-22 in plasma from the control group of 37 healthy individuals or 103 patients with various other autoimmune conditions (Puel et al., 2010).

Autoantibodies against Cytokines in Patients with Thymoma

Thymomas are tumors of thymic epithelial cells. They rarely metastasize and generally behave in a relatively non-malignant fashion, although in advanced cases they may show local invasion. They are frequently associated with autoimmunity, most commonly with myasthenia gravis and related disorders, but also with a variety of other autoimmune paraneoplastic syndromes (Marx et al., 2010) (see Chapters 54, 57, and 58). These associations are particularly remarkable given that the thymus is the classical site of tolerance induction (Marx et al., 2010). The clue seems to be that thymomas are often capable of supporting thymopoiesis of T cells, but in a disorganized environment (Buckley et al., 2001; Marx et al., 2010). It may be significant that they do not seem to support the production of Tregs (Strobel et al., 2004). In addition, thymomas are almost devoid of AIRE expression (Offerhaus et al., 2007; Scarpino et al., 2007; Strobel et al., 2007). Thymomas usually have low or absent MHC class II expression, and frequently there is loss of heterozygosity at the MHC region which would be expected to limit their ability to present self-peptides (Marx et al., 2010).

Patients with thymoma and autoimmune disease have been found to have neutralizing antibodies against numerous cytokines including IL-12 (Shiono et al., 2003) and all 12 types of IFN-α and IFN-ω, which has 60% amino acid identity (Meager et al., 1997; Shiono et al., 2003; Marx et al., 2010).

Neutralizing autoantibodies to Th17 cytokines are also very prevalent in patients with thymoma, especially those with chronic mucocutaneous candidiasis, reminiscent of

similar findings in patients with mutant AIRE-associated APECED (Kisand et al., 2010; Browne and Holland, 2010b; see earlier). Autoantibodies that bind GM-CSF were occasionally associated with thymoma and autoimmune disease but only a small fraction neutralized the bioactivity of GM-CSF (Meager et al., 1999).

Marx et al. (2010) commented that the neutralizing ability of autoantibodies to cytokines in thymoma strongly implies autoimmunization by the cells expressing the native molecules (Marx et al., 2010); the finding that the titers increased markedly when the thymomas recurred in 12 of the 13 cases studied supports this concept (Buckley et al., 2001; Marx et al., 2010). They speculated that disorganized thymopoiesis in thymoma may have resulted in immunization of T cells rather than tolerance induction.

Alternatively, we speculate that in thymoma, thymocytes may not be completely deleted of thymocytes reactive with tissue-restricted self-cytokines. If there are self-reactive T cells against cytokines, the cytokine-specific T cells may be activated if a pathogen stimulates dendritic cells. If there is no B cell tolerance to cytokines, they will endocytose the cytokines and present cytokine peptides to cytokine-specific T cells.

INDUCTION OF AUTOANTIBODIES AS A CONSEQUENCE OF THERAPY WITH RECOMBINANT CYTOKINES

According to Rossert et al. (2004), "There is probably not a single recombinant molecule used in clinical medicine that has not been found to induce antibody formation in at least some cases" (see also Macdougall et al., 2012). This situation might be seen as a loss of self-tolerance rather than a classical immune response to a foreign entity, and is a puzzle for immunologists and a serious concern for physicians and patients. Humans treated with human recombinant IFN-α made antibodies against human recombinant IFN-α that affected therapy (von Wussow et al., 1987; Antonelli et al., 1996). Patients who were injected with recombinant cytokines in some cases made antibodies against the recombinant cytokines and the natural cytokine.

If there is no B cell tolerance to cytokines and deletion of self-reactive T cells in the thymus is incomplete, potentially self-reactive helper T cells specific for cytokines could emerge from the thymus. Even if the self-reactive T cells are normally kept in check by regulatory T cells, it is not inconceivable that this "fail safe" mechanism could break down.

All cytokines are glycosylated *in vivo*, but the great majority of therapeutic recombinant cytokines are synthesized in *E. coli* and therefore non-glycosylated. When non-glycosylated human recombinant GM-CSF produced in *E. coli* was injected into non-immunocompromised patients, 95% of the patients developed antibodies that bound to GM-CSF (Ragnhammar et al., 1994). The presence of antibodies against GM-CSF significantly reduced the GM-CSF-induced increase of neutrophils, the therapeutic effect the clinicians were aiming for (Ragnhammar et al., 1994).

A native glycosylation site on a naturally produced cytokine could prevent T cell tolerance to a T cell epitope in many different ways. The native glycosylation site could: (1) prevent access to the TCR to the peptide in the groove on the MHC; (2) prevent binding of the T cell epitope to the MHC; and (3) interfere with proteolysis of a cytokine to make a short linear T cell epitope. If any of these things happen with the endogenous cytokine, the T cell epitope might be invisible to thymocytes and hence the T cells would not be tolerant of that particular T cell epitope. If a recombinant human cytokine is produced in *E. coli* or a mammalian cell-line with a different size of glycan chain and if the recombinant cytokine produces a new T cell epitope, it would be regarded as clearly nonself. If there were no B cell tolerance to the cytokine, the T cell activated by this epitope could provide help for B cells for the formation of autoantibodies against both the recombinant and endogenous forms. If this scenario is correct, cessation of therapy with the recombinant cytokine might result in gradual waning of the antibodies.

Rarely, humans treated with human recombinant erythropoietin (EPO) have been found to make antibodies against human recombinant erythropoietin and endogenous erythropoietin, producing severe anemia and pure red aplasia (Casadevall et al., 2002). Many possibilities have been considered, but this apparent loss of tolerance to an endogenous protein is still not well understood. Differences in glycosylation of recombinant EPO have been considered but have not been incriminated. The formation of aggregates has been frequently raised as a possible means by which immunogenicity could be increased, although this would only apply to B cells; but since the relevant form seen by T cells is a short linear peptide in the MHC groove, it is hard to see how the presence of aggregates in the therapeutic preparation could circumvent T cell tolerance.

The route of immunization has been raised as a possible association with the formation of autoantibodies to EPO; autoantibody formation seems to have been more common after subcutaneous administration as compared to intravenous administration, but the data are not clear-cut. Extraneous material in recombinant EPO has included human serum albumin, polysorbate 80 and "lee-chates" from rubber stoppers (Macdougall et al., 2012). None of these has been definitively implicated. Leechates from the stoppers have been shown to have adjuvant activity when tested with mice immunized with ovalbumin, but have not been shown to be involved in loss of tolerance to EPO.

The ingredient with the greatest index of suspicion is tungsten in trace amounts resulting from the way that the syringes are manufactured. Evidently tungsten can promote protein denaturation and the formation of disulfide-bonded aggregates which might be seen as foreign to T cells, but at present there is no definitive answer (Macdougall et al., 2012).

The fact that instances of autoantibodies against endogenous EPO as a result of therapy are so rare means that the search for a universal external cause may be futile, and we may need to consider host factors. In a few cases in Thailand, certain HLA alleles have been found to be overrepresented, but this finding is not general (Macdougall et al., 2012). A somatic mutation in a mature T cell would have a great deal of explanatory power, and its relative rarity would also fit the observed rarity of this perplexing condition.

CONCLUSIONS AND FUTURE PROSPECTS

The concept of a cross-reacting environmental antigen seems to be contradicted by the emerging evidence that autoantibodies against cytokines involve multiple conformational epitopes, which would be extremely unlikely. Another concept of the generation of autoantibodies is that an unrelated, exogenous antigen initiated the immune response and started the affinity maturation process and that, by chance, somatic mutations change the conformations of the antigen-binding site so it binds to multiple, conformational B cell epitopes on a cytokine. Given that the two crystallographic analyses of antigen-binding sites of germline antibody and somatically mutated antibody derived from the same germline antibody have the same general conformation, this concept is very improbable. We have concluded from the literature that there is no B cell tolerance to cytokines but definitive experiments need to be undertaken in the future. If the production of a particular cytokine is constant, there will be a continuing source of antigen and the process of antigen-driven autoantibody production will be ongoing. There is abundant evidence that the process of autoantibody formation against cytokines is antigen driven, and shows all the features of a typical secondary immune response with passage through germinal centers, somatic mutations, and affinity maturation, all of which require T cell help. When the autoantibodies are associated with thymoma, removal of the thymoma often results in a decline in the autoantibody titer, and the titer may rise again if the thymoma recurs. In the case of type 1 diabetes mellitus, when the pancreatic islets are destroyed, the autoantibodies against insulin fade away to undetectability, as might be expected for an antigen-driven process.

We conclude from the literature that T cell tolerance in the thymus is leaky and that T cells with specificity for low-avidity T cell epitopes of self-cytokines exist. What initiates the autoimmune process? It has been suggested that the simultaneous exposure to a cross-reacting exogenous antigen and the adjuvant effects of "danger signals" from a rare pathogen might break self-tolerance at the T cell level for a cytokine, but this remains a theoretical possibility for which there is no direct experimental evidence. Inflammation may be essential for normal immunity, and does not usually lead to autoantibodies. Autoantibodies provoked by the injection of a recombinant cytokine that cross-reacts with the natural cytokine might be explained by the fact that native cytokines are glycosylated while recombinant cytokines are generally not. This could lead to a lack of T cell tolerance for recombinant cytokines. However, there are no hard data.

In the future there will many more studies of pathogenic or non-pathogenic monoclonal autoantibodies against cytokines with authentic H and L chain pairs, including attempts to map the T cell epitopes in cytokines. It remains a mystery why APECED patients that lack functional AIRE show production of autoantibodies against certain cytokines but not against others. Perhaps autoantibodies against cytokines in healthy humans will inform us of how these processes are initiated.

REFERENCES

Abt, M.C., Osborne, L.C., Monticelli, L.A., Doering, T.A., Alenghat, T., Sonnenberg, G.F., et al., 2012. Commensal bacteria calibrate the activation threshold of innate antiviral immunity. Immunity. 37, 158–170.

Adelstein, S., Pritchard-Briscoe, H., Anderson, T.A., Crosbie, J., Gammon, G., Loblay, R.H., et al., 1991. Induction of self-tolerance in T cells but not B cells of transgenic mice expressing little self antigen. Science. 251, 1223–1225.

Akirav, E.M., Ruddle, N.H., Herold, K.C, 2011. The role of AIRE in human autoimmune disease. Nat. Rev. Endocrinol. 7, 25–33.

Akkaraju, S., Canaan, K., Goodnow, C.C., 1997. Self-reactive B cells are not eliminated or inactivated by autoantigen expressed on thyroid epithelial cells. J. Exp. Med. 186, 2005–2012.

Amiral, J., Marfaing-Koka, A., Wolf, M., Alessi, M.C., Tardy, B., Boyer-Neumann, C., et al., 1996. Presence of autoantibodies to interleukin-8 or neutrophil-activating peptide-2 in patients with heparin-associated thrombocytopenia. Blood. 88, 410–416.

Anderson, M.S., Venanzi, E.S., Klein, L., Chen, Z., Berzins, S.P., Turley, S.J., et al., 2002. Projection of an immunological self shadow within the thymus by the aire protein. Science. 298, 1395–1401.

Antonelli, G., Giannelli, G., Currenti, M., Simeoni, E., Del Vecchio, S., Maggi, F., et al., 1996. Antibodies to interferon (IFN) in hepatitis C patients relapsing while continuing recombinant IFN-alpha2 therapy. Clin. Exp. Immunol. 104, 384–387.

Bazin, R., St-Amour, I., Laroche, A., Lemieux, R., 2010. Activated cryptic granulocyte-macrophage colony-stimulating factor autoantibodies in intravenous immunoglobulin preparations. Blood. 115, 431.

Behler, C.M., Terrault, N.A., Etzell, J.E., Damon, L.E., 2009. Rituximab therapy for pure red cell aplasia due to anti-epoetin antibodies in a woman treated with epoetin-alfa: a case report. J. Med. Case. Rep. 3, 7335.

Bendtzen, K., Svenson, M., Jonsson, V., Hippe, E., 1990. Autoantibodies to cytokines—friends or foes? Immunol. Today. 11, 167–169.

Bendtzen, K., Hansen, M.B., Ross, C., Svenson, M., 2000. Detection of autoantibodies to cytokines. Mol. Biotechnol. 14, 251–261.

Bonfield, T.L., Kavuru, M.S., Thomassen, M.J., 2002. Anti-GM-CSF titer predicts response to GM-CSF therapy in pulmonary alveolar proteinosis. Clin. Immunol. 105, 342–350.

Borie, R., Danel, C., Debray, M.P., Taille, C., Dombret, M.C., Aubier, M., et al., 2011. Pulmonary alveolar proteinosis. Eur. Respir. Review. 20, 98–107.

Boyman, O., Kovar, M., Rubinstein, M.P., Surh, C.D., Sprent, J., 2006. Selective stimulation of T cell subsets with antibody-cytokine immune complexes. Science. 311, 1924–1927.

Browne, S.K., Holland, S.M., 2010a. Anticytokine autoantibodies in infectious diseases, pathogenesis and mechanisms. Lancet Infect. Dis. 10, 875–885.

Browne, S.K., Holland, S.M., 2010b. Immunodeficiency secondary to anticytokine autoantibodies. Curr. Opin. Allergy Clin. Immunol. 10, 534–541.

Browne, S.K., Burbelo, P.D., Chetchotisakd, P., Suputtamongkol, Y., Kiertiburanakul, S., Shaw, P.A., et al., 2012a. Adult-onset immunodeficiency in Thailand and Taiwan. N. Engl. J. Med. 367, 725–734.

Browne, S.K., Zaman, R., Sampaio, E.P., Jutivorakool, K., Rosen, L.B., Ding, L., et al., 2012b. Anti-CD20 (rituximab) therapy for anti-IFN-gamma autoantibody-associated nontuberculous mycobacterial infection. Blood. 119, 3933–3939.

Browne, S.K., Zaman, R., Sampaio, E.P., Jutivorakool, K., Rosen, L.B., Ding, L., et al., 2012c. Anti-CD20 (rituximab) therapy for anti-IFN-gamma autoantibody-associated nontuberculous mycobacterial infection. Blood. 119, 3933–3939.

Buckley, C., Douek, D., Newsom-Davis, J., Vincent, A., Willcox, N., 2001. Mature, long-lived CD4 + and CD8 + T cells are generated by the thymoma in myasthenia gravis. Ann. Neurol. 50, 64–72.

Burbelo, P.D., Browne, S.K., Sampaio, E.P., Giaccone, G., Zaman, R., Kristosturyan, E., et al., 2010. Anti-cytokine autoantibodies are associated with opportunistic infection in patients with thymic neoplasia. Blood. 116, 4848–4858.

Burnet, F.M., 1972. A reassessment of the forbidden clone hypothesis of autoimmune disease. Aust. J. Exp. Biol. Med. Sci. 50, 1–9.

Caruso, A., Bonfanti, C., Colombrita, D., De Francesco, M., De Rango, C., Foresti, I., et al., 1990. Natural antibodies to IFN-gamma in man and their increase during viral infection. J. Immunol. 144, 685–690.

Casadevall, N., Dupuy, E., Molho-Sabatier, P., Tobelem, G., Varet, B., Mayeux, P., 1996. Autoantibodies against erythropoietin in a patient with pure red-cell aplasia. N. Engl. J. Med. 334, 630–633.

Casadevall, N., Nataf, J., Viron, B., Kolta, A., Kiladjian, J.J., Martin-Dupont, P., et al., 2002. Pure red-cell aplasia and antierythropoietin antibodies in patients treated with recombinant erythropoietin. N. Engl. J. Med. 346, 469–475.

Chi, C.Y., Chu, C.C., Liu, J.P., Lin, C.H., Ho, M.W., Lo, W.J., et al., 2013. Anti-IFN-gamma autoantibodies in adults with disseminated nontuberculous mycobacterial infections are associated with HLA-DRB1*16, 02 and HLA-DQB1*05, 02 and the reactivation of latent varicella-zoster virus infection. Blood. 121, 1357–1366.

Di Niro, R., Mesin, L., Zheng, N.Y., Stamnaes, J., Morrissey, M., Lee, J.H., et al., 2012. High abundance of plasma cells secreting transglutaminase 2-specific IgA autoantibodies with limited somatic hypermutation in celiac disease intestinal lesions. Nat. Med. 18, 441–445.

Di Zenzo, G., Di Lullo, G., Corti, D., Calabresi, V., Sinistro, A., Vanzetta, F., et al., 2012. Pemphigus autoantibodies generated through somatic mutations target the desmoglein-3 cis-interface. J. Clin. Invest. 122, 3781–3790.

Doffinger, R., Helbert, M.R., Barcenas-Morales, G., Yang, K., Dupuis, S., Ceron-Gutierrez, L., et al., 2004. Autoantibodies to interferon-gamma in a patient with selective susceptibility to mycobacterial infection and organ-specific autoimmunity. Clin. Infect. Dis. 38, e10–14.

Dranoff, G., Crawford, A.D., Sadelain, M., Ream, B., Rashid, A., Bronson, R.T., et al., 1994. Involvement of granulocyte-macrophage colony-stimulating factor in pulmonary homeostasis. Science. 264, 713–716.

Felix, N.J., Donermeyer, D.L., Horvath, S., Walters, J.J., Gross, M.L., Suri, A., et al., 2007. Alloreactive T cells respond specifically to multiple distinct peptide-MHC complexes. Nat. Immunol. 8, 388–397.

Finkelman, F.D., Madden, K.B., Morris, S.C., Holmes, J.M., Boiani, N., Katona, I.M., et al., 1993. Anti-cytokine antibodies as carrier proteins. Prolongation of in vivo effects of exogenous cytokines by injection of cytokine-anti-cytokine antibody complexes. J. Immunol. 151, 1235–1244.

Gaffen, S.L., 2011. Recent advances in the IL-17 cytokine family. Curr. Opin. Immunol. 23, 613–619.

Ganal, S.C., Sanos, S.L., Kallfass, C., Oberle, K., Johner, C., Kirschning, C., et al., 2012. Priming of natural killer cells by non-mucosal mononuclear phagocytes requires instructive signals from commensal microbiota. Immunity. 37, 171–186.

Garrone, P., Djossou, O., Fossiez, F., Reyes, J., Ait-Yahia, S., Maat, C., et al., 1996. Generation and characterization of a human monoclonal autoantibody that acts as a high affinity interleukin-1 alpha specific inhibitor. Mol. Immunol. 33, 649–658.

Glynne, R., Akkaraju, S., Healy, J.I., Rayner, J., Goodnow, C.C., Mack, D.H., 2000. How self-tolerance and the immunosuppressive drug FK506 prevent B-cell mitogenesis. Nature. 403, 672–676.

Goding, J.W., 1996. Monoclonal Antibodies, Principles and Practice. third ed. Academic Press, London.

Goodnow, C.C., 2007. Multistep pathogenesis of autoimmune disease. Cell. 130, 25–35.

Graudal, N.A., Svenson, M., Tarp, U., Garred, P., Jurik, A.G., Bendtzen, K., 2002. Autoantibodies against interleukin 1alpha in rheumatoid arthritis, association with long term radiographic outcome. Ann. Rheum. Dis. 61, 598–602.

Griseri, T., McKenzie, B.S., Schiering, C., Powrie, F., 2012. Dysregulated hematopoietic stem and progenitor cell activity promotes interleukin-23-driven chronic intestinal inflammation. Immunity. 37, 1116–1129.

Han, X., Uchida, K., Jurickova, I., Koch, D., Willson, T., Samson, C., et al., 2009. Granulocyte-macrophage colony-stimulating factor autoantibodies in murine ileitis and progressive ileal Crohn's disease. Gastroenterology. 136 (1261–1271), e1261–e1263.

Hansen, G., Hercus, T.R., McClure, B.J., Stomski, F.C., Dottore, M., Powell, J., et al., 2008. The structure of the GM-CSF receptor complex reveals a distinct mode of cytokine receptor activation. Cell. 134, 496–507.

Hansen, M.B., Svenson, M., Bendtzen, K., 1991a. Human anti-interleukin 1 alpha antibodies. Immunol. Lett. 30, 133–139.

Hansen, M.B., Svenson, M., Diamant, M., Bendtzen, K., 1991b. Anti-interleukin-6 antibodies in normal human serum. Scand. J. Immunol. 33, 777–781.

Hansen, M.B., Svenson, M., Diamant, M., Abell, K., Bendtzen, K., 1995. Interleukin-6 autoantibodies: possible biological and clinical significance. Leukemia. 9, 1113–1115.

Hartley, S.B., Cooke, M.P., Fulcher, D.A., Harris, A.W., Cory, S., Basten, A., et al., 1993. Elimination of self-reactive B lymphocytes proceeds in two stages: arrested development and cell death. Cell. 72, 325–335.

Heath, W.R., Carbone, F.R., 2001. Cross-presentation in viral immunity and self-tolerance. Nat. Rev. Immunol. 1, 126–134.

Hoflich, C., Sabat, R., Rosseau, S., Temmesfeld, B., Slevogt, H., Docke, W.D., et al., 2004. Naturally occurring anti-IFN-gamma autoantibody and severe infections with Mycobacterium chelonae and Burkholderia cocovenenans. Blood. 103, 673–675.

Homann, C., Hansen, M.B., Graudal, N., Hasselqvist, P., Svenson, M., Bendtzen, K., et al., 1996. Anti-interleukin-6 autoantibodies in plasma are associated with an increased frequency of infections and increased mortality of patients with alcoholic cirrhosis. Scand. J. Immunol. 44, 623–629.

Iwakura, Y., Ishigame, H., Saijo, S., Nakae, S., 2011. Functional specialization of interleukin-17 family members. Immunity. 34, 149–162.

Jacobs, E.M., Hutter, R.V., Pool, J.L., Ley, A.B., 1959. Benign thymoma and selective erythroid aplasia of the bone marrow. Cancer. 12, 47–57.

Jeffes III, E.W., Ininns, E.K., Schmitz, K.L., Yamamoto, R.S., Dett, C.A., Granger, G.A., 1989. The presence of antibodies to lymphotoxin and tumor necrosis factor in normal serum. Arthritis. Rheum. 32, 1148–1152.

Jones, A.T., Ziltener, H.J., 1993. Enhancement of the biologic effects of interleukin-3 in vivo by anti-interleukin-3 antibodies. Blood. 82, 1133–1141.

Jouvenne, P., Fossiez, F., Banchereau, J., Miossec, P., 1997. High levels of neutralizing autoantibodies against IL-1 alpha are associated with a better prognosis in chronic polyarthritis, a follow-up study. Scand. J. Immunol. 46, 413–418.

Kampitak, T., Suwanpimolkul, G., Browne, S., Suankratay, C., 2011. Anti-interferon-gamma autoantibody and opportunistic infections, case series and review of the literature. Infection. 39, 65–71.

Kawade, Y., Finter, N., Grossberg, S.E., 2003. Neutralization of the biological activity of cytokines and other protein effectors by antibody, theoretical formulation of antibody titration curves in relation to antibody affinity. J. Immunol. Methods. 278, 127–144.

Kim, J.M., Rasmussen, J.P., Rudensky, A.Y., 2007. Regulatory T cells prevent catastrophic autoimmunity throughout the lifespan of mice. Nat. Immunol. 8, 191–197.

Kisand, K., Boe Wolff, A.S., Podkrajsek, K.T., Tserel, L., Link, M., Kisand, K.V., et al., 2010. Chronic mucocutaneous candidiasis in APECED or thymoma patients correlates with autoimmunity to Th17-associated cytokines. J. Exp. Med. 207, 299–308.

Kitamura, T., Tanaka, N., Watanabe, J., Uchida, Kanegasaki, S., Yamada, Y., et al., 1999. Idiopathic pulmonary alveolar proteinosis as an autoimmune disease with neutralizing antibody against granulocyte/macrophage colony-stimulating factor. J. Exp. Med. 190, 875–880.

Krantz, S.B., Kao, V., 1967. Studies on red cell aplasia. I. Demonstration of a plasma inhibitor to heme synthesis and an antibody to erythroblast nuclei. Proc. Natl. Acad. Sci. U.S.A. 58, 493–500.

Kurdowska, A., Miller, E.J., Noble, J.M., Baughman, R.P., Matthay, M.A., Brelsford, W.G., et al., 1996. Anti-IL-8 autoantibodies in alveolar fluid from patients with the adult respiratory distress syndrome. J. Immunol. 157, 2699–2706.

Laver, W.G., Air, G.M., Webster, R.G., Smith-Gill, S.J., 1990. Epitopes on protein antigens, misconceptions and realities. Cell. 61, 553–556.

Lokshin, A.E., Winans, M., Landsittel, D., Marrangoni, A.M., Velikokhatnaya, L., Modugno, F., et al., 2006. Circulating IL-8 and anti-IL-8 autoantibody in patients with ovarian cancer. Gynecol. Oncol. 102, 244–251.

Luisetti, M., Rodi, G., Perotti, C., Campo, I., Mariani, F., Pozzi, E., et al., 2009. Plasmapheresis for treatment of pulmonary alveolar proteinosis. Eur. Respir. J. 33, 1220–1222.

Macdougall, I.C., Roger, S.D., de Francisco, A., Goldsmith, D.J., Schellekens, H., Ebbers, H., et al., 2012. Antibody-mediated pure red cell aplasia in chronic kidney disease patients receiving erythropoiesis-stimulating agents, new insights. Kidney. Int. 81, 727–732.

Mackay, I.R., 2008. Autoimmunity since the 1957 clonal selection theory: a little acorn to a large oak. Immunol. Cell. Biol. 86, 67–71.

Madariaga, L., Amurrio, C., Martin, G., Garcia-Cebrian, F., Bicandi, J., Lardelli, P., et al., 1998. Detection of anti-interferon-gamma autoantibodies in subjects infected by Mycobacterium tuberculosis. Int. J. Tuberc. Lung Dis. 2, 62–68.

Manivel, V., Sahoo, N.C., Salunke, D.M., Rao, K.V., 2000. Maturation of an antibody response is governed by modulations in flexibility of the antigen-combining site. Immunity. 13, 611–620.

Marks, B.R., Nowyhed, H.N., Choi, J.Y., Poholek, A.C., Odegard, J.M., Flavell, R.A., et al., 2009. Thymic self-reactivity selects natural interleukin 17-producing T cells that can regulate peripheral inflammation. Nat. Immunol. 10, 1125–1132.

Marwaha, A.K., Leung, N.J., McMurchy, A.N., Levings, M.K., 2012. TH17 Cells in autoimmunity and immunodeficiency, protective or pathogenic? Front. Immunol. 3, 129.

Marx, A., Willcox, N., Leite, M.I., Chuang, W.Y., Schalke, B., Nix, W., et al., 2010. Thymoma and paraneoplastic myasthenia gravis. Autoimmunity. 43, 413–427.

McLean, G.R., Cho, C.W., Schrader, J.W., 2006. Autoreactivity of primary human immunoglobulins ancestral to hypermutated human antibodies that neutralize HCMV. Mol. Immunol. 43, 2012–2022.

Meager, A., Vincent, A., Newsom-Davis, J., Willcox, N., 1997. Spontaneous neutralising antibodies to interferon-alpha and interleukin-12 in thymoma-associated autoimmune disease. Lancet. 350, 1596–1597.

Meager, A., Wadhwa, M., Bird, C., Dilger, P., Thorpe, R., Newsom-Davis, J., et al., 1999. Spontaneously occurring neutralizing antibodies against granulocyte-macrophage colony-stimulating factor in patients with autoimmune disease. Immunology. 97, 526–532.

Meager, A., Visvalingam, K., Peterson, P., Moll, K., Murumagi, A., Krohn, K., et al., 2006. Anti-interferon autoantibodies in autoimmune polyendocrinopathy syndrome type 1. PLoS Med. 3, e289.

Meager, A., Cludts, I., Thorpe, R., Wadhwa, M., 2010. Are neutralizing anti-GM-CSF autoantibodies present in all healthy persons? Blood. 115, 433–434.

Menetrier-Caux, C., Briere, F., Jouvenne, P., Peyron, E., Peyron, F., Banchereau, J., 1996. Identification of human IgG autoantibodies specific for IL-10. Clin. Exp. Immunol. 104, 173–179.

Miossec, P., 2002. Anti-interleukin 1alpha autoantibodies. Ann. Rheum. Dis. 61, 577–579.

Mogensen, K.E., Daubas, P., Gresser, I., Sereni, D., Varet, B., 1981. Patient with circulating antibodies to alpha-interferon. Lancet. 2, 1227–1228.

Moyle, W.R., Anderson, D.M., Ehrlich, P.H., 1983. A circular antibody-antigen complex is responsible for increased affinity shown by mixtures of monoclonal antibodies to human chorionic gonadotropin. J. Immunol. 131, 1900 1905.

Nagamine, K., Peterson, P., Scott, H.S., Kudoh, J., Minoshima, S., Heino, M., et al., 1997. Positional cloning of the APECED gene. Nat. Genet. 17, 393–398.

Nemazee, D., Hogquist, K.A., 2003. Antigen receptor selection by editing or downregulation of V(D)J recombination. Curr. Opin. Immunol. 15, 182–189.

Nishinakamura, R., Nakayama, N., Hirabayashi, Y., Inoue, T., Aud, D., et al., 1995. Mice deficient for the IL-3/GM-CSF/IL-5 beta c receptor exhibit lung pathology and impaired immune response, while beta IL3 receptor-deficient mice are normal. Immunity. 2, 211–222.

Nossal, G.J., 1992. The molecular and cellular basis of affinity maturation in the antibody response. Cell. 68, 1–2.

Odendahl, M., Mei, H., Hoyer, B.F., Jacobi, A.M., Hansen, A., Muehlinghaus, G., et al., 2005. Generation of migratory antigen-specific plasma blasts and mobilization of resident plasma cells in a secondary immune response. Blood. 105, 1614–1621.

Offerhaus, G.J., Schipper, M.E., Lazenby, A.J., Montgomery, E., Morsink, F.H., Bende, R.J., et al., 2007. Graft-versus-host-like disease complicating thymoma, lack of AIRE expression as a cause of non-hereditary autoimmunity? Immunol. Lett. 114, 31–37.

Ohmoto, Y., Ogushi, F., Muraguchi, M., Yamakawa, M., Sone, S., 1997. Age-related increase of autoantibodies to interleukin 1 alpha in healthy Japanese blood donors. JMI. 44, 89–94.

Panem, S., Check, I.J., Henriksen, D., Vilcek, J., 1982. Antibodies to alpha-interferon in a patient with systemic lupus erythematosus. J. Immunol. 129, 1–3.

Perheentupa, J., 2006. Autoimmune polyendocrinopathy-candidiasis-ectodermal-dystrophy. J. Clin. Endocrinol. Metab. 91, 2843–2850.

Pinna, D., Corti, D., Jarrossay, D., Sallusto, F., Lanzavecchia, A., 2009. Clonal dissection of the human memory B-cell repertoire following infection and vaccination. Eur. J. Immunol. 39, 1260–1270.

Puel, A., Picard, C., Cypowyj, S., Lilic, D., Abel, L., Casanova, J.-L. Inborn errors of mucocutaneous immunity to Candida albicans in humans, a role for IL-17 cytokines? Curr. Opin. Immunol. 22, 467–474.

Puel, A., Picard, C., Lorrot, M., Pons, C., Chrabieh, M., Lorenzo, L., et al., 2008. Recurrent staphylococcal cellulitis and subcutaneous abscesses in a child with autoantibodies against IL-6. J. Immunol. 180, 647–654.

Puel, A., Doffinger, R., Natividad, A., Chrabieh, M., Barcenas-Morales, G., Picard, C., et al., 2010. Autoantibodies against IL-17A, IL-17F, and IL-22 in patients with chronic mucocutaneous candidiasis and autoimmune polyendocrine syndrome type I. J. Exp. Med. 207, 291—297.

Ragnhammar, P., Friesen, H.J., Frodin, J.E., Lefvert, A.K., Hassan, M., Osterborg, A., et al., 1994. Induction of anti-recombinant human granulocyte-macrophage colony-stimulating factor (Escherichia coli-derived) antibodies and clinical effects in nonimmunocompromised patients. Blood. 84, 4078—4087.

Riches, P.L., McRorie, E., Fraser, W.D., Determann, C., van't Hof, R., Ralston, S.H., 2009. Osteoporosis associated with neutralizing auto-antibodies against osteoprotegerin. N. Engl. J. Med. 361, 1459—1465.

Rosenblum, M.G., Unger, B.W., Gutterman, J.U., Hersh, E.M., David, G.S., Frincke, J.M., 1985. Modification of human leukocyte interferon pharmacology with a monoclonal antibody. Cancer. Res. 45, 2421—2424.

Ross, C., Hansen, M.B., Schyberg, T., Berg, K., 1990. Autoantibodies to crude human leucocyte interferon (IFN), native human IFN, recombinant human IFN-alpha 2b and human IFN-gamma in healthy blood donors. Clin. Exp. Immunol. 82, 57—62.

Ross, C., Svenson, M., Hansen, M.B., Vejlsgaard, G.L., Bendtzen, K., 1995. High avidity IFN-neutralizing antibodies in pharmaceutically prepared human IgG. J. Clin. Invest. 95, 1974—1978.

Ross, C., Svenson, M., Nielsen, H., Lundsgaard, C., Hansen, M.B., Bendtzen, K., 1997. Increased in vivo antibody activity against interferon alpha, interleukin-1alpha, and interleukin-6 after high-dose Ig therapy. Blood. 90, 2376—2380.

Rossert, J., Casadevall, N., Eckardt, K.U., 2004. Anti-erythropoietin antibodies and pure red cell aplasia. J. Am. Soc. Nephrol. 15, 398—406.

Rowley, D., Jenkin, C.R., 1962. Antigenic cross-reaction between host and parasite as a possible cause of pathogenicity. Nature. 193, 151—154.

Sakagami, T., Uchida, K., Suzuki, T., Carey, B.C., Wood, R.E., Wert, S.E., et al., 2009. Human GM-CSF autoantibodies and reproduction of pulmonary alveolar proteinosis. N. Engl. J. Med. 361, 2679—2681.

Scarpino, S., Di Napoli, A., Stoppacciaro, A., Antonelli, M., Pilozzi, E., Chiarle, R., et al., 2007. Expression of autoimmune regulator gene (AIRE) and T regulatory cells in human thymomas. Clin. Exp. Immunol. 149, 504—512.

Scheid, J.F., Mouquet, H., Kofer, J., Yurasov, S., Nussenzweig, M.C., Wardemann, H., 2011. Differential regulation of self-reactivity discriminates between IgG + human circulating memory B cells and bone marrow plasma cells. Proc. Natl. Acad. Sci. U.S.A. 108, 18044—18048.

Schmidt, A.G., Xu, H., Khan, A.R., O'Donnell, T., Khurana, S., King, L.R., et al., 2013. Preconfiguration of the antigen-binding site during affinity maturation of a broadly neutralizing influenza virus antibody. Proc. Natl. Acad. Sci. U.S.A. 110, 264—269.

Seymour, J.F., Doyle, I.R., Nakata, K., Presneill, J.J., Schoch, O.D., Hamano, E., et al., 2003. Relationship of anti-GM-CSF antibody concentration, surfactant protein A and B levels, and serum LDH to pulmonary parameters and response to GM-CSF therapy in patients with idiopathic alveolar proteinosis. Thorax. 58, 252—257.

Shiono, H., Wong, Y.L., Matthews, I., Liu, J.L., Zhang, W., Sims, G., et al., 2003. Spontaneous production of anti-IFN-alpha and anti-IL-12 autoantibodies by thymoma cells from myasthenia gravis patients suggests autoimmunization in the tumor. Int. Immunol. 15, 903—913.

Sioud, M., Dybwad, A., Jespersen, L., Suleyman, S., Natvig, J.B., Farre, O., 1994. Characterization of naturally occurring autoantibodies against tumour necrosis factor-alpha (TNF-alpha), in vitro function and precise epitope mapping by phage epitope library. Clin. Exp. Immunol. 98, 520—525.

Stanley, E., Lieschke, G.J., Grail, D., Metcalf, D., Hodgson, G., Gall, J.A., et al., 1994. Granulocyte/macrophage colony-stimulating factor-deficient mice show no major perturbation of hematopoiesis but develop a characteristic pulmonary pathology. Proc. Natl. Acad. Sci. U.S.A. 91, 5592—5596.

Strobel, P., Rosenwald, A., Beyersdorf, N., Kerkau, T., Elert, O., Murumagi, A., et al., 2004. Selective loss of regulatory T cells in thymomas. Ann. Neurol. 56, 901—904.

Svenson, M., Poulsen, L.K., Fomsgaard, A., Bendtzen, K., 1989. IgG autoantibodies against interleukin 1 alpha in sera of normal individuals. Scand. J. Immunol. 29, 489—492.

Strobel, P., Murumagi, A., Klein, R., Luster, M., Lahti, M., Krohn, K., et al., 2007. Deficiency of the autoimmune regulator AIRE in thymomas is insufficient to elicit autoimmune polyendocrinopathy syndrome type 1 (APS-1). J. Pathol. 211, 563—571.

Svenson, M., Hansen, M.B., Ross, C., Diamant, M., Rieneck, K., Nielsen, H., et al., 1998. Antibody to granulocyte-macrophage colony-stimulating factor is a dominant anti-cytokine activity in human IgG preparations. Blood. 91, 2054—2061.

Svenson, M., Hansen, M.B., Bendtzen, K., 1993. Binding of cytokines to pharmaceutically prepared human immunoglobulin. J. Clin. Invest. 92, 2533—2539.

Takemura, H., Suzuki, H., Yoshizaki, K., Ogata, A., Yuhara, T., Akama, T., et al., 1992. Anti-interleukin-6 autoantibodies in rheumatic diseases. Increased frequency in the sera of patients with systemic sclerosis. Arthritis. Rheum. 35, 940—943.

Tanaka, N., Watanabe, J., Kitamura, T., Yamada, Y., Kanegasaki, S., Nakata, K., 1999. Lungs of patients with idiopathic pulmonary alveolar proteinosis express a factor which neutralizes granulocyte-macrophage colony stimulating factor. FEBS Lett. 442, 246—250.

Thomson, C.A., Bryson, S., McLean, G.R., Creagh, A.L., Pai, E.F., Schrader, J.W., 2008. Germline V-genes sculpt the binding site of a family of antibodies neutralizing human cytomegalovirus. EMBO J. 27, 2592—2602.

Tiller, T., Tsuiji, M., Yurasov, S., Velinzon, K., Nussenzweig, M.C., Wardemann, H., 2007. Autoreactivity in human IgG + memory B cells. Immunity. 26, 205—213.

Trapnell, B.C., Carey, B.C., Uchida, K., Suzuki, T., 2009. Pulmonary alveolar proteinosis, a primary immunodeficiency of impaired GM-CSF stimulation of macrophages. Curr. Opin. Immunol. 21, 514—521.

Trown, P.W., Kramer, M.J., Dennin Jr., R.A., Connell, E.V., Palleroni, A.V., Quesada, J., et al., 1983. Antibodies to human leucocyte interferons in cancer patients. Lancet. 1, 81—84.

Uchida, K., Nakata, K., Trapnell, B.C., Terakawa, T., Hamano, E., Mikami, A., et al., 2003. High affinity autoantibodies specifically eliminate granulocyte-macrophage colony-stimulating factor activity in the lungs of patients with idiopathic pulmonary alveolar proteinosis. Blood. 103, 1089—1098.

Uchida, K., Nakata, K., Suzuki, T., Luisetti, M., Watanabe, M., Koch, D.E., et al., 2009. Granulocyte/macrophage-colony-stimulating factor autoantibodies and myeloid cell immune functions in healthy subjects. Blood. 113, 2547—2556.

Uchida, K., Carey, B., Suzuki, T., Nakata, K., Trapnell, B., 2010. Response: Granulocyte/macrophage colony-stimulating factor autoantibodies and myeloid cell immune functions in healthy persons. Blood. 115, 431–433.

van der Meide, P.H., Schellekens, H., 1997. Anti-cytokine autoantibodies, epiphenomenon or critical modulators of cytokine action. Biotherapy. 10, 39–48.

von Wussow, P., Freund, M., Block, B., Diedrich, H., Poliwoda, H., Deicher, H., 1987. Clinical significance of anti-IFN-alpha antibody titres during interferon therapy. Lancet. 2, 635–636.

Wadhwa, M., Meager, A., Dilger, P., Bird, C., Dolman, C., Das, R.G., et al., 2000. Neutralizing antibodies to granulocyte-macrophage colony-stimulating factor, interleukin-1alpha and interferon-alpha but not other cytokines in human immunoglobulin preparations. Immunology. 99, 113–123.

Wang, Y., Thomson, C.A., Allan, L.L., Jackson, L.M., Olson, M., Hercus, T.R., et al., 2013. Characterization of pathogenic human monoclonal autoantibodies against GM-CSF. Proc. Natl. Acad. Sci. U.S.A. 110, 7832–7837.

Watanabe, M., Uchida, K., Nakagaki, K., Kanazawa, H., Trapnell, B.C., Hoshino, Y., et al., 2007. Anti-cytokine autoantibodies are ubiquitous in healthy individuals. FEBS Lett. 581, 2017–2021.

Wardemann, H., Yurasov, S., Schaefer, A., Young, J.W., Meffre, E., Nussenzweig, M.C., 2003. Predominant autoantibody production by early human B cell precursors. Science. 301, 1374–1377.

Wen, L., Hanvanich, M., Werner-Favre, C., Brouwers, N., Perrin, L.H., Zubler, R.H., 1987. Limiting dilution assay for human B cells based on their activation by mutant EL4 thymoma cells, total and antimalaria responder B cell frequencies. Eur. J. Immunol. 17, 887–892.

Wrammert, J., Smith, K., Miller, J., Langley, W.A., Kokko, K., Larsen, C., et al., 2008. Rapid cloning of high-affinity human monoclonal antibodies against influenza virus. Nature. 453, 667–671.

Zikherman, J., Parameswaran, R., Weiss, A., 2012. Endogenous antigen tunes the responsiveness of naive B cells but not T cells. Nature. 489, 160–164.

Zuklys, S., Balciunaite, G., Agarwal, A., Fasler-Kan, E., Palmer, E., Hollander, G.A., 2000. Normal thymic architecture and negative selection are associated with Aire expression, the gene defective in the autoimmune-polyendocrinopathy-candidiasis-ectodermal dystrophy (APECED). J. Immunol. 165, 1976–1983.

Part 16

Diagnosis, Prevention, and Therapy

Autoantibody Assays: Performance, Interpretation, and Standardization

Marvin J. Fritzler

Faculty of Medicine, University of Calgary, Calgary, Canada

Chapter Outline

Introduction 1161
Spectrum of Autoantibodies 1163
Assays and Technologies for Autoantibody Testing 1165
Clinical Interpretation and Application of Autoantibody Testing 1166
Clinical Practice Guidelines 1167
Laboratory Reports, Electronic Medical Records, and Cost Analysis 1167
Standardization and Quality Assurance 1170
Conclusions and Future Prospects 1170
References 1170

INTRODUCTION

The history of autoantibodies (aab) dates back more than a century to Ehrlich's description of "horror autotoxicus" (Ehrlich, 1900) and the development of Wasserman test for syphilis that was initially based on agglutination and complement fixation (Wassermann et al., 1906). Despite this long history, the detection of aab lagged from about 1900 to 1950 and was largely relegated to organ-specific autoimmune diseases (reviewed in Conrad et al., 2011). However, in the following 50 years (1950–2000) autoantibodies achieved prominence in the laboratory and clinical settings.

The more recent advances in aab testing dates to the seminal observation of the lupus erythematosus (LE) cell phenomenon in 1948 (Hargraves et al., 1948) and then the advent of the LE cell test (Conn, 1994). In the ensuing 20 years, a number of techniques such as indirect immunofluorescence (IIF), immunodiffusion (ID), hemagglutination, and complement fixation were developed and refined (reviewed in Fritzler, 1986). IIF was described by Coons, Kaplan and Weller in the early 1950s (Warde, 2011) and this assay stands out as one of the few techniques that is still widely used today in clinical diagnostic laboratories, particularly as a screening test in the diagnosis of systemic autoimmune rheumatic disease (SARD) (reviewed in Fritzler and Wiik, 2006).

In the 60 years following the inception of IIF, a variety of substrates were utilized, but cryopreserved sections of rodent organs became the mainstay for the first 25 years (Holborow et al., 1957; Beck, 1961; Hijmans et al., 1964; Kunkel and Tan, 1964). In the mid-1970s it was discovered that human tissue culture cells such as HeLa and HEp-2 were superior to organ sections in the identification of aab in SARD primarily because they had larger nuclei, they expressed target antigens in various stages of the cell cycle, and kits using these substrates were relatively economical to manufacture (Nakamura et al., 1984; Nakamura and Tan, 1977). The adoption of tissue culture cells (e.g., almost exclusively HEp-2 cells) as the substrate of choice for IIF led to what some regard as the "golden age" of aab detection (Fritzler, 2012).

The increased sensitivity of the IIF techniques using tissue culture cells became an issue of concern that led to a study by the Serology Subcommittee of the International Union of Immunology Societies/World Health Organization/Arthritis Foundation (IUIS/WHO/AF) who recommended that sera should be screened at dilutions of 1/40 and 1/160 but that a cut-off of 1/160 was the most appropriate to achieve a balance of sensitivity and specificity for the diagnosis of adult SARD (Tan et al., 1997). This advice achieved limited acceptance because many laboratories preferred to screen at serum dilutions that provided the

N. Rose & I. Mackay (Eds): The Autoimmune Diseases, Fifth edition. DOI: http://dx.doi.org/10.1016/B978-0-12-384929-8.00077-0

appropriate balance of sensitivity and specificity in their clinical environment.

An unanticipated advantage of using HEp-2 cell substrates was the identification of novel aab targets that were weakly expressed, selectively expressed, or not expressed in highly differentiated tissues. This led to the identification of novel aab targets and also provided cell and molecular biologists with valuable probes for studies of novel cell structures and macromolecules (Tan, 1991; Luqmani et al., 2011). These included anti-proliferating cell nuclear antigen (PCNA) and other cell cycle-related targets (Mahler et al., 2010), anti-centromere (Fritzler et al., 2010), and a number of targets in nucleoli (Reimer et al., 1987; Welting et al., 2003), nuclear envelope (Enarson et al., 2004), and cytoplasm (Stinton et al., 2004; Fritzler et al., 2007). The identification of these novel targets occurred in parallel with the emergence of new assays, such as immunoblotting (IB), expression cloning, and rapid and economical DNA sequencing.

The remarkable advances in identifying and cataloguing the molecular targets bound by aab led to the next generation of diagnostic technologies that included antigen-specific immunoassays using novel platforms including enzyme linked immunoassays (ELISA) (Halbert et al., 1981; Reichlin and Harley, 1986; Tonuttia et al., 2004), dot blots (Stott, 1989; Nezlin and Mozes 1995), line immunoassays (LIA) (Pottel et al., 2004; Damoiseaux et al., 2005), and multiplexed immunoassays such as addressable laser bead immunoassays (ALBIA) (Fritzler 2006; Fritzler and Fritzler, 2009) and chemiluminescence (CLA) (Mahler et al., 2011b) (Table 77.1). Other emerging technologies include lateral flow (Renger et al., 2010), antigen arrays on planar surfaces (Baker et al., 2004; Balboni et al., 2008; Chandra et al., 2011), and nanobarcodes (Freeman et al., 2005). Such advances are progressively being adopted by modern diagnostic laboratories because they are automated and contribute to high throughput and shortened turnaround times resulting in considerable laboratory cost savings. In addition, some of these platforms, such as lateral flow, have applications in point of care diagnostics.

The continued use of IIF has many advantages, but the limitations of this technology in the context of ever-changing clinical algorithms should not be overlooked. Numerous studies have pointed to deficiencies of IIF assays (reviewed in Fritzler, 2011a,c, 2012). In the context of new and emerging technologies and the background of the more familiar IIF, it has become clear that, depending on the assay used, the results from any one immunoassay can be at considerable variance with other assays. This has prompted concerns about the relative value of old and new diagnostic platforms where the implications of false-negative and false-positive test results are being debated (reviewed in Fritzler, 2011c). Many clinicians prefer to adhere to assay results that are easily understood, fit within existing diagnostic paradigms, and

are clinically relevant. Hence, for the present time, some prefer test results derived from IIF on specified substrates (i.e., HEp-2 and certain tissue sections) and regard them as the "gold standard" for aab testing (Satoh et al., 2009; Meroni and Schur, 2010).

One of the arguments supporting continued use of IIF on HEp-2 substrates is that this substrate contains more than 100 different target antigens, whereas newer screening technologies such as ELISA, LIA, or ALBIA are currently limited to less than 20 (American College of Rheumatology, 2011). However, it is obvious that IIF does not detect all aab in a given human sera even when they are directed to an autoantigen that is highly expressed in HEp-2 cells. For example, a significant proportion of sera that have aab directed to Jo-1 (histdyl tRNA synthase), ribosomal P proteins (Mahler et al., 2004, 2008), PCNA (Mahler et al., 2010), GWB (Stinton et al., 2010), and PM/Scl (Mahler and Fritzler, 2009) (to name a few) are scored as negative in IIF test results derived from HEp-2 substrates. It has been suggested that these "false-negative" IIF results are likely attributable to low aab titers, hidden or cryptic epitopes, secondary antibodies, and/or characteristics of the substrate (i.e., cell density, growth media, fixation protocols). However, the evidence to support these contentions is not well documented. In addition, even when IIF results are read and interpreted by the same cadre of technologists on different manufacturer substrates and using a characterized set of SARD sera, the agreement of five assays from different manufacturers was only 78% (Copple et al., 2012). And within the specific groups of serum samples, agreement ranged from only 44% for SSc samples to 72% agreement for the SLE sera but, reassuringly, 93% for healthy control sera. In this particular study, variations in slide and substrate quality (i.e., clarity, consistency of fluorescence, cell size, number and quality of mitotic cells) from different manufacturers were also noted. Therefore, along with problems of subjective interpretation, IIF on HEp-2 substrates are subject to problematic standardization issues that are akin to other methods for ANA screening (Copple et al., 2007).

It is interesting that some of the issues plaguing IIF assays, particularly subjective reader bias, are being addressed through the development of technology platforms that provide automated, digital reading of IIF slides (Hiemann et al., 2009; Egerer et al., 2010). This technology has advantages of machine learning algorithms and being able to archive digital images of the IIF result for subsequent review. However, disadvantages of current iterations of this technology include limited throughput capacity (fewer than 10 slides loaded per run) and difficulty distinguishing IIF patterns in sera where multiple or less common aab are present.

Taken together, the rapid proliferation of aab specificities and the emergence and adoption of novel technologies has created a dilemma for standardization of aab testing

TABLE 77.1 Contemporary and Emerging Technologies Used to Detect Autoantibodies in Human Sera

Assay	Essential technology	Applications
Indirect immunofluorescence (IIF)	• Tissue or cell substrates • Fluorochrome-labeled secondary antibodies • Microscope fitted with UV source and optics	Screening test Specific aab detection by staining pattern
Line immunoassays (LIA)	• Native or recombinant antigens on solid phase substrate • Enzyme-labeled secondary antibodies • Densitometry/Scanner	Test aab reactivity to specific targets Arrays typically based on disease groups
Addressable laser bead immunoassays (ALBIA)	• Antigen of interest bound to addressable microbeads • Dual laser flow (Luminex)	Test aab reactivity to specific targets Arrays based on disease groups
Cell-based assays (CBA)	• Cell lines transfected with and express cDNA encoding antigen of interest • IIF protocols	Detect aab directed to antigens of low expression Detect aab directed to highly conformational epitopes
Chemiluminescence (CLA)	• Antigen of interest bound to addressable microbeads • Fluorochrome-labeled secondary antibodies • Chemiluminescence • Laser flow technology • (Bio Flash)	Test aab reactivity to specific targets Arrays based on disease groups
Lateral flow assays	• Similar to LIA but two or three step protocol • Line array enclosed in a portable cassette • Small hand-held densitometer	Point of care diagnostics
*Antigen arrays on planar surfaces	• High density autoantigen arrays printed on glass or other matrices	Personalized medicine
*Microfluidics or "lab on a chip"	• Portable microdevices with all components embedded	Point of care diagnostics
*Electrochemiluminescence arrays	• Antigen arrays on solid phase • Specialized detection system (mesoscale discovery)	Personalized medicine
*Nanotechnology	• High density autoantigen arrays ("nanobarcodes") printed or absorbed to nanoscale devices	Personalized medicine Point of care diagnostics
*Mass and NMR spectroscopy	• Early development depends on decreasing footprint and cost of technology	Personalized medicine High throughput diagnostics

*Not in wide use; in developmental stage.
Abbreviations: aab, autoantibodies; IIF, indirect immunofluorescence; LIA, line immunoassay; NMR, nuclear magnetic resonance.

protocols and the results that are communicated to clinicians (Fritzler et al., 2003a; Wiik et al., 2004). Rapid advances in diagnostic technologies have made it difficult for even the most modern laboratory to keep abreast of the changes, not to mention clinicians who are hard pressed to keep abreast of new diagnostic paradigms that follow the adoption of the newer technologies.

SPECTRUM OF AUTOANTIBODIES

In a single chapter, it is virtually impossible to cover the spectrum of aab that are now in wide use as diagnostic and prognostic biomarkers, although many of the clinically relevant aab are covered in earlier chapters of this book or summarized in other publications (Conrad et al., 2007, 2011). Given the variation of observations with the same technology or between different technologies, the spectrum of aab and their associated sensitivity or specificity is much wider than can be summarized in Table 77.2. Such information needs to be interpreted in the context of the reader's own clinical and laboratory setting. As an example of the complexity of data sets, there are now over 10 different diagnostics platforms (Table 77.1) and in autoimmune conditions such as systemic lupus erythematosus (SLE) there are now

TABLE 77.2 Autoantibodies Used in Diagnosis of Autoimmune Diseases

Autoantibody	Disease	Sensitivity/Specificity	Assay
dsDNA	SLE DIL[a]	45–60/80–90	IIF, ELISA, IP
Sm (U2–U4-6 RNP)	SLE	10–20/95	ELISA, ID, IP, ALBIA, LIA, CLA
U1RNP	MCTD SLE	90/90–95 40/30	ELISA, ID, IP, ALBIA, LIA, CLA
SS-A/Ro 60	SjS SLE	50–70/80 45/25	ELISA, ID, IP, ALBIA, LIA, CLA
SS-B/La	SjS SLE	40/70–90 15/10	ELISA, ID, IP, ALBIA, LIA, CLA
Ro52/TRIM21	SARD	Varies from disease to disease	ELISA, LIA, ALBIA, CLA
Histone/chromatin	SLE DIL	70/20 80/20	ELISA, IB, ALBIA, LIA, CLA
Topoisomerase I/Scl-70	SSc	20/90	ELISA, IB, IP, ALBIA, LIA, CLA
U3 RNP/Fibrillarin	SSc	15/95	IIF, IP, LIA
Centromere	SSc	50–60/90	IIF, ELISA, IB, ALBIA, LIA, CLA
Jo-1/histidyl tRNA synthetase	PM/DM	20–30/90–95	ELISA, IB, IP, ALBIA, LIA, CLA
Citrullinated peptides and proteins	RA	65–85/85–95	ELISA
Proteinase 3	GPA	60–70/90–95	ELISA, IB, LIA, CLA
Myeloperoxidase	MPA	65/80	ELISA, IIF, CLA (pANCA)
Pyruvate dehydrogenase complex (M2)	PBC	75–80/85	IIF, IB, ELISA, IP, LIA, CLA
Smooth muscle F-actin	Chronic active hepatitis	70/25	IIF, ELISA
Intrinsic factor	Pernicious anemia	90/70	IIF, ELISA
Human tissue transglutaminase	Celiac disease	85/90	IIF, ELISA
Cardiolipin complex	APS	80/50	ELISA
β2-glycoprotein I	APS	80/90	ELISA
Basement membrane (α4 domain of type IV collagen)	Anti-GBM disease (Goodpasture's syndrome)	80/80	IIF, ELISA
Acetylcholine receptor	Myasthenia gravis	80/90	ELISA, IB
Thyroid microsomes (thyroid peroxidase)	Hashimoto's thyroiditis	90/75	IIF, ELISA
Cadherins	Pemphigus vulgaris	90/90	ELISA
Skin basement membrane zone	Bullous pemphigoid	80/80	ELISA
Yo/Purkinje cell	PCD	70/95	IIF, IB, LIA
Hu	PEM	70/90	IIF, IB, IP, LIA
Aquaporin 4	NMO/Devic's disease	75/85	CBA, ELISA
NMDA/NR1 receptor	Autoimmune encephalitis	MSR	CBA, ELISA
PLA2R	Membranous glomerulonephritis	MSR	CBA, ELISA, ALBIA

[a]Some patients treated with anti-TNF and other biological therapeutics develop features of drug-induced lupus and anti-dsDNA and other aab.
Abbreviations: ALBIA, addressable laser bead immunoassay; APS, anti-phospholipid syndrome; CBA, cell-based assay; CLA, chemiluminescence assay; DIL, drug-induced lupus; ELISA, enzyme linked immunoassay; GBM, glomerular basement membrane; GPA, granulomatosis with polyangiitis—formerly Wegener's syndrome; IB, immunoblotting; IIF, indirect immunofluorescence; IP, immunoprecipitation; LIA, line immunoassay; MCTD, mixed connective tissue disease; MPA, microscopic polyangiitis; MSR, more studies required; NMDAR, N-methyl-D-aspartate (glutamate) receptor; NMO, neuromyelitis optica; NPSLE, neuropsychiatric systemic lupus erythematosus; PBC, primary biliary cirrhosis; PCD, paraneoplastic cerebellar degeneration, PEM, paraneoplastic encephalomyelitis; PLA2R, phospholipase A2 receptor; PM, polymyositis; RNP, ribonucleoprotein; SARD, systemic autoimmune rheumatic diseases; SjS, Sjögren's syndrome; SLE, systemic lupus erythematosus; SSc, systemic sclerosis; TRIM, tripartite motif.

over 150 autoantibodies catalogued (Sherer et al., 2004; Sherer and Shoenfeld, 2007) and over 30 in scleroderma (Ho and Reveille, 2003; Walker and Fritzler, 2007; Mehra et al., 2013), with not infrequent overlaps between these two and other SARD. In most organ-localized diseases, the autoantibodies tend to be directed to only one or a few antigens that tend to be harbored in the affected organ (Conrad et al., 2011).

One of the relatively new arrivals on the aab scene are a class of autoimmune diseases referred to as IgG4-related disease (IgG4-RD) that encompasses a variety of clinical entities once regarded as being separate diseases (Khosroshahi et al., 2011; Nirula et al., 2011; Carruthers et al., 2012; Stone et al., 2012) (see Chapter 64). Clinical manifestations of IgG4-RD have been reported in virtually all organ systems where they display consistent histopathological similarities: diffuse lymphoplasmacytic infiltrates, abundant IgG(4)-positive plasma cells, modest tissue eosinophilia, and extensive fibrosis (Khosroshahi et al., 2011). Polyclonal elevations of serum IgG4 are found in approximately 70% of patients and in some cases IgG4 aab directed to specific targets are found (Bruschi et al., 2011; Debiec and Ronco, 2011; Hofstra et al., 2011; Klooster et al., 2012).

ASSAYS AND TECHNOLOGIES FOR AUTOANTIBODY TESTING

As mentioned above, the IIF technique using HEp-2 or other cellular substrates continues to be the preferred screening immunoassay to detect aab in SARD. However, as also referenced above, it is important to appreciate that a negative IIF screen does not necessarily exclude the presence of a wide spectrum of autoantibodies (reviewed in Fritzler, 2012). Therefore, in the setting of high clinical suspicion of a SARD or another autoimmune disease and a negative IIF test, the identification of aab should include a more specific and sensitive assay that includes an array of relevant autoantigens. Such tests could be reflexed to newer technologies as described in more detail below (Fritzler and Fritzler 2006, 2009; Mahler et al., 2011a). The strength of aab associations with autoimmune disease subgroups can vary according to the diagnostic techniques being used but also depends on demographic and genetic factors (Fritzler, 2006; Fritzler and Fritzler, 2009). With the emergence of more sensitive immunoassays, care must be taken to ensure that cutoffs are based on appropriate local normal and comparative disease controls (Fritzler et al., 2003a; Shoenfeld et al., 2007; Bossuyt et al., 2008). Also the source and characteristics (i.e., recombinant vs. native, peptide vs. full length) of the autoantigen used in newer assays can affect the results. Despite years of attempts, standardization of aab assays continues to be a

major challenge (Kessenbrock et al., 2007; Satoh et al., 2009; Mahler and Fritzler, 2010; Mahler et al., 2011a). Because the evolution of clinically recognizable SARD and other autoimmune conditions can span decades before a full clinical picture is evident or a diagnosis is firmly established, long-term longitudinal studies are ideally required to reach definitive conclusions about aab specificities.

Many laboratories rely on ccommercial aab assay kits that employ a variety of technologies such as IIF, ID, IP, IB, LIA, ELISA, and more recently ALBIA, CLA (Mahler et al., 2011b) and antigen arrays (Fritzler, 2002; Robinson et al., 2002; Sokolove et al., 2012). The use and application of these diagnostic platforms has been attended by certain considerations that are not always apparent to the clinician (Box 77.1). One of the more popular assay platforms is based on the ELISA because it offers high sensitivity, efficient throughput and relatively low cost while requiring only modest equipment to perform the assay. Unfortunately, little has been done to standardize these kits (Feltkamp, 1996; Tan et al., 1999; Fritzler et al., 2003b) and postmarketing surveillance and quality assurance is largely left to the manufacturers (Fritzler et al., 2003a). Although the ELISA kits are constantly being improved, some high titer aab to a variety of autoantigens (i.e., fibrillarin, PM/Scl, centromere, nuclear envelope) are often not detected. Hence, a report that indicates a

> **Box 77.1 Considerations Regarding the Clinical Interpretation of Autoantibody Testing**
>
> - Sera from first degree relatives, infectious diseases, malignancies, and normal individuals contain autoantibodies
> - Disease-specific autoantibodies can antedate diagnosis
> - Definition of a positive autoantibody test is based on an empirically defined threshold
> - Some assays such as IIF are based on subjective interpretation
> - While IIF is a good screening test for some autoantibodies, it is less sensitive for others
> - There is a lack of standardized antibodies and reagents
> - There is a growing variety of immunoassays and diagnostic assay platforms
> - High throughput assays are often adopted before validation of local performance
> - The advent of electronic medical records is enhancing the autoantibody reporting system
> - Short-term cost and budget restraints on autoantibody testing have an impact
> - Long-term impact of autoantibody testing on total health care costs and quality adjusted life years are mostly unknown

"negative ELISA" screen should not be interpreted as "negative for all relevant autoantibodies," because they might otherwise be detected by IIF and/or other diagnostic technologies.

While the experience with ALBIA is not nearly as extensive as ELISA, there is evidence indicating that these assays are far from perfect (Shovman et al., 2005a; Fritzler and Fritzler, 2009; Hanly et al., 2010), especially when comparing the results for specific analytes such as anti-dsDNA although they have generally good agreement with other platforms (Shovman et al., 2005b; Avaniss-Aghajani et al., 2007; Caramaschi et al., 2007; Bardin et al., 2009; Albon et al., 2011) There is general consensus that because there is considerable variation in the sensitivity of the various commercial diagnostic kits, the identity of the particular assay used to generate the test result should be made available to the clinician (Meroni and Schur, 2010; American College of Rheumatology, 2011). In addition, because of the growing trend to use automated immunoassay systems that provide quantitative results, these laboratories should follow standards of chemistry instrumentation including a requirement to demonstrate analytical measured ranges and periodic calibrations. Clinical laboratories that adopt multiplexed assays (i.e., ALBIA) must establish reference ranges and cutoff values for each analyte, and the sensitivity and specificity must be established with care as the laboratory findings may present a difficult problem for the clinician who has to interpret the results.

CLINICAL INTERPRETATION AND APPLICATION OF AUTOANTIBODY TESTING

As referred to earlier, it is important to appreciate some considerations and certain limitations that impact on the interpretation and clinical application of aab tests (Box 77.1). Many of these issues are due to a lack of thorough knowledge of autoimmunity, such as the perpetuation and perturbations of aab production, and the continuum of B cell responses that span innate to acquired immunity (Fritzler, 2012). It is firmly established that any human serum contains a wide range of aab of varying concentrations (Rose, 1996). It is also important to understand that the measurement and assignment of an abnormal or elevated aab test requires an empirically defined threshold that is dependent on numerous factors such as the equipment used to generate the assays, secondary antibodies, and adherence to manufacturer's protocols (Fritzler et al., 2003a; Wiik et al., 2004). Of significant clinical relevance, some disease-specific autoantibodies can antedate and predict overt disease by many years (reviewed in Bizzaro et al., 2007; Rose, 2007; Fritzler, 2008, 2011a;

Meroni and Shoenfeld, 2008; Kallenberg, 2011). For example, antibodies to centromere proteins (CENPs) may antedate the clinical diagnosis of SSc by many years (Kallenberg et al., 1988; Wigley et al., 1992) and antibodies to Scl-70 (topoisomerase I) have been linked to the development of pulmonary fibrosis and higher mortality (Kuwana et al., 1994; Scussel-Lonzetti et al., 2002). These and numerous other examples in the literature should certainly give pause to clincians before labeling an aab test result as a "false-positive" test. The performance characteristics of each test must be known to avoid misinterpretation, incorrect diagnosis, and potentially harmful treatment, a feature that is commonly reflected in so-called "false-positive" tests. It is equally important to consider the impact of "false-negative" tests that can lead to delayed diagnoses and unnecessary morbidity (Fritzler, 2011c). Therefore, to achieve significant clinical utility, it is important to perform aab tests that discriminate between disease and the absence of disease, between emerging or subclinical disease, or between disease and confounding clinical conditions (Conrad et al., 2012).

As very few prospective, unbiased, and multicenter studies have been published, the clinical accuracy of many aab tests is still uncertain. Studies based on literature review and meta-analysis have been published as "evidence-based guidelines" (Kavanaugh and Solomon, 2002; Solomon et al., 2002; Reveille et al., 2003) but the translation of this information is limited because of the wide variety of newer assays and assay parameters that have come into wide use since these studies and recommendations were published.

Decades of clinical experience and research have led to the development of classification and diagnostic criteria to support a diagnosis of a number of autoimmune diseases, many of which include aab biomarkers (Masi et al., 1980; Kasukawa, 1987; Alarcon-Segovia and Cardiel, 1989; Cassidy et al., 1989; Leavitt et al., 1990; Jennette et al., 1994; Savige et al., 1999; Wilson et al., 1999; Petri et al., 2013). Since SARD are characterized by multiple organ system involvement, separate sets of criteria are required to support accurate classification. As a consequence, it is rare that a single pathognomonic criterion can be translated into certainty that a given diagnosis is correct. To ensure that results from the immunology laboratory gain maximum utility for clinicians, it is important to study the performance of each aab assay as an aid to diagnostics in early disease because that is the time at which a serologic result would impact prognostic and diagnostic considerations the most (Fenger et al., 2004; Conrad et al., 2012). Since the clinical diagnosis often may be established only after months or years of clinical follow-up, the more knowledgeable the clinician is with regard to the clinical and laboratory characteristics of diseases, the greater the chance that a correct diagnosis will be made.

Many of the diseases listed in Table 77.2 have clinical subgroups with somewhat dissimilar manifestations and, hence, prognosis. Of relevance to this discussion, these subgroups are often associated with different aab profiles and specificities (Permin et al., 1978; Cervera et al., 1993, 2002; Kuwana et al., 1994; Mustila et al., 2000; Wiik, 2001; Scussel-Lonzetti et al., 2002; Targoff, 2002). Therefore, certain aab are valuable biomarkers of a disease subgroup with markedly different clinical features, end organ involvement, and prognosis. Accordingly, the information imparted by aab profiles, in combination with other biomarkers, is likely to be valuable in the future as an approach to tailoring therapeutic strategies (i.e., personalized or prescriptive medicine) (Franssen et al., 1998; Andrade, 2009; Fritzler, 2011b; Plenge and Bridges, 2011; Tak, 2012).

In the entire spectrum of aab described to date, those with high disease specificity, regarded as disease-specific markers, tend to be rare (von Muhlen and Tan, 1995). This is especially true today when newer diagnostic platforms (ELISA, ALBIA, CLA) have achieved higher sensitivity than older immunoassays. Thus, with the introduction and adoption of newer diagnostic technology platforms, aab that were thought to be specific for one disease based on older or even outdated technologies, may subsequently turn out to be associated with a variety of autoimmune diseases (van Eenennaam et al., 2002). The appreciation that multiple disease-related aab occur in a single serum and that aab expression may change over time in individual patients (von Muhlen and Tan, 1995; Blass et al., 1999; Vasiliauskiene et al., 2001; Visser et al., 2002) holds potential that aab serology in combination with other biomarkers (i.e., genomics, cytokines, metabolomics, transcriptomics) may lead to an earlier and more accurate diagnosis, and, by extension, more effective therapeutic interventions (Fritzler, 2011b; Plenge and Bridges, 2011). While some evidence indicates that certain aab are stable over the disease course (Ippolito et al., 2011), other evidence indicates that aab profiles as determined by array technologies will likely change over time (reviewed in Fritzler, 2012). Evidence supporting this notion includes observations that aab to RNA helicase occur only early in the course of SLE (Yamasaki et al., 2007), and only clinically distinct neuropsychiatric events attributed to SLE that occurred around the time of diagnosis were found to be associated with anti-P antibodies and the lupus anticoagulant (anti-phospholipid, anti-cardiolipin) (Hanly et al., 2008). Hence, multiplexed and autoantigen array technologies that are now emerging provide more extensive aab profiles in a given patient (Kessenbrock et al., 2007; Mahler and Fritzler, 2010) are altering approaches to diagnostics and therapeutics (Fritzler, 2002; Robinson et al., 2002; Schachna et al., 2002).

CLINICAL PRACTICE GUIDELINES

Because of the complexity of modern autoimmune serology, there continues to be a pressing need for clinical practice guidelines (CPG) that outline the appropriate and economic use of serologic testing. If a limited number of clinicians are involved in ordering diagnostic testing, it is easier to achieve a consensus on testing strategies. However, there is a growing trend toward amalgamated regional and national laboratories that provide service to a widening spectrum of health care providers. Thus, clearly articulated CPG are required to lay out criteria for aab screening and an evidence-based testing algorithm that limits unnecessary testing (Wiik et al., 2004). A related strategy is to develop aab order forms in such a way that the doctor chooses between tentative diagnoses, after which only evidence-based tests are done. It is important to realize that the pre-test probability to detect a useful diagnostic laboratory result increases dramatically when each clinical feature or diagnostic criterion has been incorporated into the tentative diagnosis (Keren and Nakamura, 1997).

LABORATORY REPORTS, ELECTRONIC MEDICAL RECORDS, AND COST ANALYSIS

Many laboratories use an aab testing algorithm that includes a rapid and inexpensive screening test (i.e., IIF) followed by more specific tests (i.e., LIA, ALBIA, ELISA) as an approach to evidence-based screening for serum aab. For example, the IIF test or whole cell lysate ELISAs are often used to detect autoantibodies in SARD and other diseases (reviewed in Stinton and Fritzler, 2007; Fritzler, 2011c, 2012). This serves two purposes: first, as an approach to triage for further reflex testing; second, if the IIF or screening ELISA test is negative, unless there is a compelling clinical evidence to do so, no further testing is required and the result is reported accordingly. However, as discussed earlier there is a caveat inasmuch as the sensitivity of IIF testing is not as high as some presume and is attended by significant "false-negative" results (Fritzler, 2011c). Third, many autoantibodies can be quite accurately identified solely by an IIF screening approach (Table 77.3).

It is very important that aab test results should be validated and, in this context, borderline (low positive) results can be especially troublesome. It is recommended that borderline positive results must be confirmed or refuted by use of a second well-established independent technique to ensure that only certified positive results are reported to the physician or clinic. If controversy about the result persists, the laboratory should add a note of caution to the clinician that the result may have little significance in supporting a diagnosis and/or may

TABLE 77.3 Autoantibodies Determined by IIF Patterns that may be Useful in Clinical Diagnostics

Cellular structure/IIF staining pattern	Molecular targets	Disease associations
Coiled bodies	p80 coilin	Localized SSc, Raynaud's syndrome
Golgi complex	Golgins, giantin	SLE, SjS, RA overlap syndromes, malignancy, viral infection
Mitotic spindle apparatus – Centrioles – NuMa pattern – Spindle microtubules	enolase, pericentrin, ninein NuMa 235 HsEg5	SSc, SjS, post-viral syndromes, *Mycoplasma* infection SLE, SjS SjS, SLE
Multiple nuclear dots	Sp-100	Primary biliary cirrhosis
Nuclear envelope	Lamins A/C, B1, B2, LAP1/2	SLE, SjS, CAH, APS, SNP
Nuclear pore complex	p62, gp210, Tpr	PBC, SjS
GW bodies	GW182, hAgo2, Ge-1/Hedls, RAP55	SjS, sensory/motor neuropathy, SLE, PBC
Dense fine speckles	DFS70/LEDGF	Rare in SARD, in isolation, may rule out diagnosis of SARD

Abbreviations: APS, anti-phospholipid antibody syndrome; CAH, chronic active hepatitis; DFS, dense fine speckles; LEDGF; lens epithelium derived growth factor; NuMA, nuclear mitotic apparatus; PBC, primary biliary cirrhosis; RA, rheumatoid arthritis; SARD, systemic autoimmune rheumatic diseases; SjS, Sjögren's syndrome; SLE, systemic lupus erythematosus; SNP, seronegative polyarthritis; SSc, systemic sclerosis; Tpr, translocated promoter region.

recommend retesting a new serum sample in 1 to 3 months. Some regulatory agencies mandate that borderline positive tests should be reported as positive until proven otherwise after repeat or follow-up testing at appropriate intervals. High and intermediate positive results of a single credible technique can be reported without independent confirmation by a second technique. To aid in the interpretation of laboratory results the chosen limit for positivity should be stated in the report along with ranges of low, intermediate, and strong positivity.

A problem is that easy-to-perform and high throughput techniques are often adopted by clinical laboratories without proper clinical validation. Screening for aab by ELISA that have adsorbed complex mixtures of native and/or recombinant autoantigens or nuclear extracts is now used by many laboratories instead of IIF ANA screening (Meroni and Schur, 2010; Fritzler, 2011a,c). This practice continues despite data showing that many patients with Sjögren's syndrome (SjS), systemic sclerosis (SSc), autoimmune myopathies, and juvenile idiopathic arthritis (JIA) score negative for ANA using such composite ELISA screening techniques (Keren and Nakamura, 1997; Fawcett et al., 1999). While the technology has remarkably improved in the last few years, HEp-2-IIF screening of these "false-negative" sera reveals that many of these sera contain aab to nucleoli, nuclear matrix, nuclear envelope, nuclear pores, coiled bodies, promyelocyte leukemia (PML) domains, cell cycle-specific antigens such as proliferating cell nuclear antigen (PCNA) and mitotic spindle apparatus components, or other cytoplasmic organelles and structures such as mitochondria, Golgi apparatus, signal recognition particles or ribosomal proteins (Bayer et al., 1999; Wiik, 2003a,b; Stinton et al., 2004) (Tables 77.2 and 77.3).

Studies using older screening ELISAs have shown that some of these aab are readily recognized by experienced technicians (Wiik and Lam, 2001) but are missed by ELISAs for ANA screening (Bayer et al., 1999). Some of these aab have defined clinical associations and should be identified as such (Table 77.3). It needs to be emphasized that newer technologies and wider testing have not supported clinical associations of some aab. For example, anti-PCNA aab once thought to be highly specific for SLE, have recently been shown to lack specific disease associations (Vermeersch et al., 2009; Mahler et al., 2012b). Aab that lack proven clinical value should be reported but it must be clearly stated that neither their diagnostic specificity nor their value has been clearly established.

It is important to point out that not all aab are diagnostic of or associated with clinically apparent autoimmune diseases. This goes beyond established evidence that disease-specific aab can be detected in first-degree relatives of autoimmune diseases patients, in a variety of bacterial and viral infections, or in apparently unrelated conditions and normal individuals. Several lines of evidence indicate that approximately 20% of serum samples from healthy individuals have a positive ANA test, the majority of which produce an IIF pattern known as dense fine speckles (DFS) (Mahler et al., 2012a). The typical IIF DFS staining pattern is typically observed as small

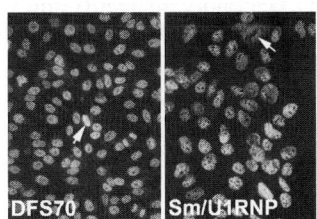

FIGURE 77.1   IIF pattern of dense fine speckles (DFS) on HEp-2 cell substrate.   Anti-DFS antibodies (left panel) typically stain the nucleus and metaphase chromatin (arrow) as compared to antibodies to Sm/U1RNP (right panel) which also stain the nucleoplasm but do not stain the metaphase chromatin (arrow). It is important to appreciate that consistent staining characteristics of anti-DFS sera can vary from manufacturer to manufacturer of HEP-2 substrates. ImmunoConcepts HEp-2000 substrate; original magnification 250 ×.

Box 77.2 Advantages and Disadvantages of the EMR

Advantages

- Improved turnaround time and accessibility to laboratory results
- Eliminating part of "paper trail": improved accuracy of reporting
- Increased knowledge of the patient's disease status
- Improved interaction of patient with health care providers
- Increased patient safety
- More knowledgeable patients involved in self-management
- Enhanced communication with health care team
- Elimination of lower security multiple paper records and mailed/faxed paper reports
- Higher security of health information

Disadvantages

- Challenges interpreting reports and data
- Additional security protocols and standard operating procedures add extra workload
- Consultation content changed
- Altered face-to-face patient–provider interactions

---

speckles that are somewhat uniformly distributed throughout the nucleus and on metaphase chromatin (Figure 77.1). Of note, the DFS staining pattern has been reported in 33% of ANA-positive healthy individuals, but not in ANA positive SARD sera (Mariz et al., 2011). Since their first description, anti-DFS70 antibodies have been found in the sera of patients with a variety of chronic inflammatory conditions, such as interstitial cystitis and atopic dermatitis, as well as in cancer patients and in healthy individuals (reviewed in Mahler et al., 2012a). The target autoantigen is a 70-kDa protein. This autoantigen was initially termed DFS70, but the primary autoantigen

was eventually identified as the lens epithelium-derived growth factor (LEDGF) (reviewed in Ganapathy and Casiano, 2004). As the intended use of the ANA HEp-2 test is to primarily serve as a screening test to aid in the diagnosis of SARD, the reporting of anti-DFS70 antibodies as a positive test significantly reduces the specificity and the positive likelihood of the ANA IIF test. This has important implications for ANA test algorithms because if these results are widely validated, it suggests that aab associated with DFS70/LEDGF can be used to rule out the diagnosis of SARD (Mahler et al., 2012a).

When aab are detected, the positive result is usually communicated in a printed report that is sent directly to the requesting physician or the referring laboratory. Unfortunately, in some jurisdictions, regulatory constraints (i.e., Health Protection Act and Freedom of Information Protection Act) prohibit the transmission of a digital report directly to the referring physician's computer or other digital devices. Nevertheless, there is a trend in many jurisdictions to rapidly adopt electronic medical records (EMR) that will accommodate uploading encrypted or otherwise secure data files directly to online or "cloud" storage of patient medical records. For many laboratories, this has added another layer of protocols and standard operating procedures that are intended to protect patient confidentiality. Efforts to develop consensus on the format and structure of the EMR, along with consensus terminology and content of aab results, would be an important step forward in standardizing the aab testing system (Vogt et al., 2004; Pincus et al., 2009; Malaviya and Gogia, 2010; Wiik et al., 2010). A number of advantages and disadvantages of the EMR have been identified (Liao et al., 2010; van der Vaart et al., 2012) (Box 77.2). At the present time, the question regarding unlimited access of patients to their EMR is unsettled (van der Vaart et al., 2012). While information on diagnosis, treatment plan, and consultations might be released for patient access, more complex data, such as physical examinations, laboratory results, and radiographic images, are more controversial. There is some thought that providing patients random access to their EMR might be an important step to empowering and enhancing patient service, provided that clinical and personal data and information security is optimal, and content and presentation of data are constructed so that they are clearly understood by patient and physician alike. A description of the most common diagnostic associations related to an aab found in diagnostic testing should be included with the result. Also, the level (titer) of the aab or the strength of expression should be mentioned together with how these relate to cut-off values and how they were established (i.e., disease controls, normal controls, and the range of credible measurements).

There is a serious deficiency in our knowledge of the actual costs incurred through inappropriate laboratory testing, although the actual costs of laboratory diagnostic testing can readily be calculated. In Scandinavia, the estimated cost of all types of *in vitro* diagnostic testing in laboratories is between 2 and 3% of the total budget for health care. The prospects for health care financing are intimately linked to the three overarching tenets of clinical medicine: (1) disease prevention is of utmost importance, (2) an early and accurate diagnosis is the next most important, and (3) appropriate, effective treatment follows the first two. Many health care providers and payers jump from (1) to (3) without much consideration of (2). An estimation of long-term costs related to early accurate diagnosis and therapeutic intervention compared to a missed or a wrong diagnosis, with or without treatment, needs to be performed to highlight the value of high quality laboratory diagnostics.

STANDARDIZATION AND QUALITY ASSURANCE

A number of jurisdictions have recognized the importance of standardizing aab testing (Wiik et al., 2006; Shoenfeld et al., 2007) and a set of standardized sera provided by the IUIS/AF/WHO/CDC Serology Committee (www.autoab. org) have been made available through the CDC in Atlanta (Chan et al., 2007). The reference sera available through this program are continually monitored and more recent additions to the reference sera available include those with defined aab directed to cardiolipin/β2-glycoprotein I, RNA polymerase I/III, ribosomal P proteins, proteinase 3, and myeloperoxidase (c- and p-ANCA, respectively). Sera used as standards for a particular methodology or technology platform need to be reviewed from time to time as exemplified by the re-evaluation of AF/CDC reference sera by a variety of contemporary techniques (Smolen et al., 1997; Copple et al., 2012). Although it would likely decrease inter-laboratory variation in performance, standardized secondary antibodies are not widely available.

All clinical laboratories should participate in quality assurance and quality improvement programs such as the one administered by the College of American Pathologists (www.cap.org). The Clinical Laboratory Improvement Amendments of 1988 set standards for all laboratories engaged in clinical testing. These standards include requirements for trained and competent supervisory and testing personnel, record keeping and instrument maintenance, daily quality control practices, result reporting, and laboratory inspection and maintenance. It is not clear that these standards are being met in routine practice. In Europe the most widely used quality assurance and management program (DS/EN ISO/IEC 17025:2000)

additionally sets laboratory standards aimed to prove that an assay actually gives results that are useful for clinical diagnostics.

CONCLUSIONS AND FUTURE PROSPECTS

The detection of aab can serve as biomarkers that focus the clinician's attention to involved tissues or organs using classical diagnostic tools such as histopathology, imaging techniques, and organ function testing. Clinical practice guidelines to facilitate the communication between clinicians and laboratories need to be formulated, along with mutually accepted algorithms for test ordering and interpretation. The emergence of the EMR is a significant step forward but is attended by some challenges.

In contemporary medical practice, changes in laboratory diagnostics and new technologies to detect aab are being introduced at a rapid pace. This is attended by concerns that certain key matters, such as clinical utility, are not thoroughly addressed. In many cases, the manufacturer has often been assumed to be the root cause for shortcomings in aab testing; however, the use of commercial kits and their appropriate application in a clinical setting involves a rather complex set of contingencies (Fritzler et al., 2003a; Fritzler, 2012). It has been suggested that a higher level of commitment and partnership between all of the participants is required to achieve the goal of improving the quality of patient care through the use of aab testing and analysis (Wiik et al., 2004).

REFERENCES

Alarcon-Segovia, D., Cardiel, M.H., 1989. Comparison between 3 diagnostic criteria for mixed connective tissue disease: study of 539 patients. J. Rheumatol. 16, 328–334.

Albon, S., Bunn, C., Swana, G., Karim, Y., 2011. Performance of a multiplex assay compared to enzyme and precipitation methods for anti-ENA testing in systemic lupus and systemic sclerosis. J. Immunol. Methods. 365, 126–131.

American College of Rheumatology, 2011. Position paper: methodology of testing for antinuclear antibodies. Available at: <http://www.rheumatology.org/practice/ana_position_stmt.pdf>.

Andrade, L.E., 2009. Future perspective for diagnosis in autoimmune diseases. An. Acad. Bras. Cienc. 81, 367–380.

Avaniss-Aghajani, E., Berzon, S., Sarkissian, A., 2007. Clinical value of multiplexed bead based immunoassays for detection of autoantibodies to nuclear antigens. Clin. Vaccine Immunol. 14, 505–509.

Baker, C.A., Lu, Z.Y., Manuelidis, L., 2004. Early induction of interferon-responsive mRNAs in Creutzfeldt-Jakob disease. J. Neurovirol. 10, 29–40.

Balboni, I., Limb, C., Tenenbaum, J.D., Utz, P.J., 2008. Evaluation of microarray surfaces and arraying parameters for autoantibody profiling. Proteomics. 8, 3443–3449.

Bardin, N., Desplat-Jego, S., Daniel, L., Jourde, C.N., Sanmarco, M., 2009. BioPlex 2200 multiplexed system: simultaneous detection of anti-dsDNA and anti-chromatin antibodies in patients with systemic lupus erythematosus. Autoimmunity. 42, 63–68.

Bayer, P.M., Bauerfeind, S., Bienvenu, J., Fabien, N., Frei, P.C., Gilburd, B., et al., 1999. Multicenter evaluation study on a new HEp2 ANA screening enzyme immune assay. J. Autoimmun. 13, 89–93.

Beck, J.S., 1961. Variations in the morphological patterns of "autoimmune" nuclear fluorescence. Lancet. 1, 1203–1207.

Bizzaro, N., Tozzoli, R., Shoenfeld, Y., 2007. Are we at a stage to predict autoimmune rheumatic diseases? Arthritis Rheum. 56, 1736–1744.

Blass, S., Engel, J.-M., Burmester, G.R., 1999. The immunologic homunculus in rheumatoid arthritis. Arthritis Rheum. 42, 2499–2506.

Bossuyt, X., Louche, C., Wiik, A., 2008. Standardisation in clinical laboratory medicine: an ethical reflection. Ann. Rheum. Dis. 67, 1061–1063.

Bruschi, M., Carnevali, M.L., Murtas, C., Candiano, G., Petretto, A., Prunotto, M., et al., 2011. Direct characterization of target podocyte antigens and auto-antibodies in human membranous glomerulonephritis: Alfa-enolase and borderline antigens. J. Proteomics. 74, 2008–2017.

Caramaschi, P., Ruzzenente, O., Pieropan, S., Volpe, A., Carletto, A., Bambara, L.M., et al., 2007. Determination of ANA specificity using multiplexed fluorescent microsphere immunoassay in patients with ANA positivity at high titres after infliximab treatment: preliminary results. Rheumatol. Int. 27, 649–654.

Carruthers, M.N., Stone, J.H., Khosroshahi, A., 2012. The latest on IgG4-RD: a rapidly emerging disease. Curr. Opin. Rheumatol. 24, 60–69.

Cassidy, J.T., Levinson, J.E., Brewer, E.J., 1989. The development of classification criteria for children with juvenile rheumatoid arthritis. Bull. Rheum. Dis. 38, 1–7.

Cervera, R., Khamashta, M.A., Font, J., Sebastiani, G.D., Gil, A., Lavilla, P., et al., 1993. Systemic lupus erythematosus: Clinical and immunologic patterns of disease expression in a cohort of 1,000 patients. Medicine (Baltimore). 72, 113–124.

Cervera, R., Piette, J.C., Font, J., Khamashta, M.A., Cervera, R., Piette, J.C., et al., 2002. Antiphospholipid syndrome—clinical and immunologic manifestations and patterns of disease expression in a cohort of 1,000 patients. Arthritis Rheum. 46, 1019–1027.

Chan, E.K.L., Fritzler, M.J., Wiik, A., Andrade, L.E., Reeves, W.H., Tincani, A., et al., 2007. AutoAbSC.Org—Autoantibody Standardization Committee in 2006. Autoimmun. Rev. 6, 577–580.

Chandra, P.E., Sokolove, J., Hipp, B.G., Lindstrom, T.M., Elder, J.T., Reveille, J.D., et al., 2011. Novel multiplex technology for diagnostic characterization of rheumatoid arthritis. Arthritis Res. Ther. 13, R102.

Conn, R.B., 1994. Practice parameter—the lupus erythematosus cell test. Am. J. Clin. Pathol. 101, 65–66.

Conrad, K., Schlosser, W., Hiepe, F., Fritzler, M.J., 2007. Autoantibodies in Systemic Autoimmune Diseases: A Diagnostic Reference, second ed. Pabst Scientific Publishers, Lengerich.

Conrad, K., Schlosser, W, Hiepe, F., Fritzler, M.J., 2011. Autoantibodies in Organ Specific Autoimmune Diseases: A Diagnostic Reference, third ed. Pabst Science Publishers, Lengerich.

Conrad, K., Roggenbuck, D., Reinhold, D., Sack, U., 2012. Autoantibody diagnostics in clinical practice. Autoimmun. Rev. 11, 207–211.

Copple, S.S., Martins, T.B., Masterson, C., Joly, E., Hill, H.R., 2007. Comparison of three multiplex immunoassays for detection of antibodies to extractable nuclear antibodies using clinically defined sera. Ann. N.Y. Acad. Sci. 1109, 464–472.

Copple, S.S., Giles, S.R., Jaskowski, T.D., Gardiner, A.E., Wilson, A.M., Hill, H.R., 2012. Screening for IgG antinuclear autoantibodies by HEp-2 indirect fluorescent antibody assays and the need for standardization. Am. J. Clin. Pathol. 137, 825–830.

Damoiseaux, J., Boesten, K., Giesen, J., Austen, J., Tervaert, J.W., 2005. Evaluation of a novel line-blot immunoassay for the detection of antibodies to extractable nuclear antigens. Ann. N.Y. Acad. Sci. 1050, 340–347.

Debiec, H., Ronco, P., 2011. PLA2R autoantibodies and PLA2R glomerular deposits in membranous nephropathy. N. Engl. J. Med. 364, 689–690.

Egerer, K., Roggenbuck, D., Hiemann, R., Weyer, M.G., Buettner, T., Radau, B., et al., 2010. Automated evaluation of autoantibodies on human epithelial-2 cells as an approach to standardize cell-based immunofluorescence tests. Arthritis Res. Ther. 12, R40.

Ehrlich, P., 1900. On immunity with special reference to cell life. Proc. R. Soc. Lond. 66, 424–448.

Enarson, P., Rattner, J.B., Ou, Y., Miyachi, K., Horigome, T., Fritzler, M.J., 2004. Autoantigens of the nuclear pore complex. J. Mol. Med. 82, 423–433.

Fawcett, P.T., Rose, C.D., Gibney, K.M., Emerich, M.J., Athreya, B.H., Doughty, R.A., 1999. Use of ELISA to measure antinuclear antibodies in children with juvenile rheumatoid arthritis. J. Rheumatol. 26, 1822–1826.

Feltkamp, T.E.W., 1996. Antinuclear antibody determination in a routine laboratory. Ann. Rheum. Dis. 55, 723–727.

Fenger, M., Wiik, A., Hoier-Madsen, M., Lykkegaard, J.J., Rozenfeld, T., Hansen, M.S., et al., 2004. Detection of antinuclear antibodies by solid-phase immunoassays and immunofluorescence analysis. Clin. Chem. 50, 2141–2147.

Franssen, C., Gans, R., Kallenberg, C., Hageluken, C., Hoorntje, S., 1998. Disease spectrum of patients with antineutrophil cytoplasmic autoantibodies of defined specificity: distinct differences between patients with anti-proteinase 3 and anti-myeloperoxidase autoantibodies. J. Intern. Med. 244, 209–216.

Freeman, R.G., Raju, P.A., Norton, S.M., Walton, I.D., Smith, P.C., He, L., et al., 2005. Use of nanobarcodes particles in bioassays. Methods Mol. Biol. 303, 73–83.

Fritzler, M.J., 1986. Autoantibody testing: procedures and significance in systemic rheumatic diseases. Meth. Achiev. Exp. Pathol. 12, 224–260.

Fritzler, M.J., 2002. New technologies in the detection of autoantibodies. In: Conrad, K., Fritzler, M.J., Meuer, M., Sack, U., Shoenfeld, Y. (Eds.), Autoantigens, Autoantibodies, Autoimmunity, third ed. Pabst Scientific Publishers, Lengerich, pp. 50–63.

Fritzler, M.J., 2006. Advances and applications of multiplexed diagnostic technologies in autoimmune diseases. Lupus. 15, 422–427.

Fritzler, M.J., 2008. Challenges to the use of autoantibodies as predictors of disease onset, diagnosis and outcomes. Autoimmun. Rev. 7, 616–620.

Fritzler, M.J., 2011a. Autoantibody testing: current challenges and future opportunities. In: Conrad, K., Chan, E.K.L., Fritzler, M.J., Humbel, R.L., Meroni, P.L., Shoenfeld, Y. (Eds.), From Prediction to Prevention of Autoimmune Diseases, vol. 7. Pabst Science Publishers, Berlin, pp. 584–596.

Fritzler, M.J., 2011b. Personalized medicine approaches in rheumatoid arthritis and other systemic autoimmune rheumatic diseases. In: Conrad, K., Chan, E.K.L., Fritzler, M.J., Humbel, R.L., Meroni, P.L., Shoenfeld, Y. (Eds.), From Prediction to Prevention of Autoimmune Diseases, vol. 7. Pabst Science Publishers, Berlin, pp. 127–137.

Fritzler, M.J., 2011c. The antinuclear antibody (ANA) test: last or lasting gasp? Arthritis Rheum. 16, 19–22.

Fritzler, M.J., 2012. Toward a new autoantibody diagnostic orthodoxy: understanding the bad, good and indifferent. Autoimmun. Highlights. 10.1007/s13317-012-0030-7.

Fritzler, M.J., Fritzler, M.L., 2006. The emergence of multiplexed technologies as diagnostic platforms in systemic autoimmune diseases. Curr. Med. Chem. 13, 2503–2512.

Fritzler, M.J., Fritzler, M.L., 2009. Microbead-based technologies in diagnostic autoantibody detection. Expert Opin. Med. Diag. 3, 81–89.

Fritzler, M.J., Wiik, A., 2006. Autoantibody assays, testing, and standardization. In: Rose, N.R., Mackay, I.R. (Eds.), The Autoimmune Diseases, fourth ed. Elsevier Academic Press, pp. 1011–1022.

Fritzler, M.J., Wiik, A., Fritzler, M.L., Barr, S.G., 2003a. The use and abuse of commercial kits used to detect autoantibodies. Arthritis Res. Ther. 5, 192–201.

Fritzler, M.J., Wiik, A., Tan, E.M., Smolen, J.S., McDougal, J.S., Chan, E.K.L., et al., 2003b. A critical evaluation of enzyme immunoassay kits for detection of antinuclear antibodies of defined specificities. III. Comparative performance characteristics of academic and manufacturers' laboratories. J. Rheumatol. 30, 2374–2381.

Fritzler, M.J., Stinton, L.M., Chan, E.K.L., 2007. Autoantibodies to cytoplasmic autoantigens in endosomes, exosomes and the Golgi complex. In: Conrad, K., Chan, E.K.L., Fritzler, M.J., Sack, U., Shoenfeld, Y., Wiik, A. (Eds.), From Etiopathogenesis to the Prediction of Autoimmune Diseases: Relevance of Autoantibodies, fifth ed. Pabst Science Publishers, Lengerich, Germany, pp. 194–209.

Fritzler, M.J., Rattner, J.B., Luft, L.M., Edworthy, S.M., Casiano, C.A., Peebles, C., et al., 2010. Historical perspectives on the discovery and elucidation of autoantibodies to centromere proteins (CENP) and the emerging importance of antibodies to CENP-F. Autoimmun. Rev. 10, 194–200.

Ganapathy, V., Casiano, C.A., 2004. Autoimmunity to the nuclear autoantigen DFS70 (LEDGF): what exactly are the autoantibodies trying to tell us? Arthritis Rheum. 50, 684–688.

Halbert, S.P., Karsh, J., Anken, M., 1981. Studies on autoantibodies to deoxyribonucleic acid and deoxyribonucleoprotein with enzyme-immunoassay (ELISA). J. Lab. Clin. Med. 97, 97–111.

Hanly, J.G., Urowitz, M.B., Siannis, F., Farewell, V., Gordon, C., Bae, S.C., et al., 2008. Autoantibodies and neuropsychiatric events at the time of systemic lupus erythematosus diagnosis: Results from an international inception cohort study. Arthritis Rheum. 58, 843–853.

Hanly, J.G., Su, L., Farewell, V., Fritzler, M.J., 2010. Comparison between multiplex assays for autoantibody detection in systemic lupus erythematosus. J. Immunol. Methods. 358, 75–80.

Hargraves, M.M., Richmond, H., Morton, R., 1948. Presentation of two bone marrow elements: the "tart" cells and the "L.E." cell. Mayo Clin. Proc. 23, 25–28.

Hiemann, R., Buttner, T., Krieger, T., Roggenbuck, D., Sack, U., Conrad, K., 2009. Challenges of automated screening and differentiation of non-organ specific autoantibodies on HEp-2 cells. Autoimmun. Rev. 9, 17–22.

Hijmans, W., Schuit, H.R.E., Mandema, E., Nienhuis, R.L.F., Feltkamp, T.E.W., Holborow, E.J., et al., 1964. Comparative study for the detection of antinuclear factors with the fluorescent antibody technique. Ann. Rheum. Dis. 23, 73–77.

Ho, K.T., Reveille, J.D., 2003. The clinical relevance of autoantibodies in scleroderma. Arthritis Res. Ther. 5, 80–93.

Hofstra, J.M., Beck Jr., L.H., Beck, D.M., Wetzels, J.F., Salant, D.J., 2011. Anti-phospholipase A2 receptor antibodies correlate with clinical status in idiopathic membranous nephropathy. Clin. J. Am. Soc. Nephrol. 6, 1286–1291.

Holborow, E.J., Weir, D.M., Johnson, G.D., 1957. A serum factor in lupus erythematosus with affinity for tissue nuclei. Br. Med. J. 2, 732–734.

Ippolito, A., Wallace, D., Gladman, D., Fortin, P., Urowitz, M., Werth, V., et al., 2011. Autoantibodies in systemic lupus erythematosus: comparison of historical and current assessment of seropositivity. Lupus. 20, 250–255.

Jennette, J.C., Falk, R.J., Andrassy, K., Bacon, P.A., Churg, J., Gross, W.L., et al., 1994. Nomenclature of systemic vasculitides. Arthritis Rheum. 37, 187–192.

Kallenberg, C.G., 2011. Anti-neutrophil cytoplasmic antibody (ANCA)-associated vasculitis: where to go? Clin. Exp. Immunol. 164, 1–3.

Kallenberg, C.G., Wouda, A.A., Hoet, M.H., Van Venrooij, W.J., 1988. Development of connective tissue disease in patients presenting with Raynaud's phenomenon: a six year follow up with emphasis on the predictive value of antinuclear antibodies as detected by immunoblotting. Ann. Rheum. Dis. 47, 634–641.

Kasukawa, R., 1987. Preliminary diagnostic criteria for classification of mixed connective tissue disease. In: Kasukawa, R., Sharp, G.C. (Eds.), Mixed Connective Tissue Disease and Anti-Nuclear Antibodies. Excerpta Medica, Amsterdam, pp. 41–47.

Kavanaugh, A.F., Solomon, D.H., 2002. Guidelines for immunologic laboratory testing in the rheumatic diseases: anti-DNA antibody tests. Arthritis Rheum. 47, 546–555.

Keren, D.F., Nakamura, R.M., 1997. Progress and controversies in autoimmune disease testing. Clin. Lab. Med. 17, 483–497.

Kessenbrock, K., Raijmakers, R., Fritzler, M.J., Mahler, M., 2007. Synthetic peptides: the future of patient management in systemic rheumatic diseases? Curr. Med. Chem. 14, 2831–2838.

Khosroshahi, A., Deshpande, V., Stone, J.H., 2011. The clinical and pathological features of IgG(4)-related disease. Curr. Rheumatol. Rep. 13, 473–481.

Klooster, R., Plomp, J.J., Huijbers, M.G., Niks, E.H., Straasheijm, K.R., Detmers, F.J., et al., 2012. Muscle-specific kinase myasthenia gravis IgG4 autoantibodies cause severe neuromuscular junction dysfunction in mice. Brain. 135, 1081–1101.

Kunkel, H.G., Tan, E.M., 1964. Autoantibodies and disease. Adv. Immunol. 4, 351–372.

Kuwana, M., Kaburaki, J., Okano, Y., Tojo, T., Homma, M., 1994. Clinical and prognostic associations based on serum antinuclear antibodies in Japanese patients with systemic sclerosis. Arthritis Rheum. 37, 75–83.

Leavitt, R.Y., Fauci, A.S., Bloch, D.A., Michel, B.A., Hunder, G., Arend, W.P., et al., 1990. The American College of Rheumatology 1990 criteria for the classification of Wegener's granulomatosis. Arthritis Rheum. 33, 1101–1107.

Liao, K.P., Cai, T., Gainer, V., Goryachev, S., Zeng-treitler, Q., Raychaudhuri, S., et al., 2010. Electronic medical records for discovery research in rheumatoid arthritis. Arthritis Care Res. (Hoboken). 62, 1120–1127.

Luqmani, R.A., Suppiah, R., Grayson, P.C., Merkel, P.A., Watts, R., 2011. Nomenclature and classification of vasculitis—update on the ACR/EULAR diagnosis and classification of vasculitis study (DCVAS). Clin. Exp. Immunol. 164 (Suppl 1), 11–13.

Mahler, M., Fritzler, M.J., 2009. The changing landscape of the clinical value of the PM/Scl autoantibody system. Arthritis Res. Ther. 11, 106.

Mahler, M., Fritzler, M.J., 2010. Epitope specificity and significance in systemic autoimmune diseases. Ann. N.Y. Acad. Sci. 1183, 267–287.

Mahler, M., Kessenbrock, K., Raats, J., Fritzler, M.J., 2004. Technical and clinical evaluation of anti-ribosomal P protein immunoassays. J. Clin. Lab. Anal. 18, 215–223.

Mahler, M., Ngo, J., Schulte-Pelkum, J., Luettich, T., Fritzler, M.J., 2008. Limited reliability of the indirect immunofluorescence technique for the detection of anti-Rib-P antibodies. Arthritis Res. Ther. 10, R131.

Mahler, M., Silverman, E.D., Fritzler, M., 2010. Novel diagnostic and clinical aspects of anti-PCNA antibodies detected by novel detection methods. Lupus. 19, 1527–1533.

Mahler, M., Binder, W.L., Fritzler, M.J., 2011a. Recent advances in peptide resolved diagnostics of systemic autoimmune diseases. In: Conrad, K., Chan, E.K.L., Fritzler, M.J., Humbel, R.L., Meroni, P.L., Shoenfeld, Y. (Eds.), From Prediction to Prevention of Autoimmune Diseases, vol. 7. Pabst Science Publishers, Berlin, pp. 598–625.

Mahler, M., Radice, A., Sinico, R.A., Damoiseaux, J., Seaman, A., Buckmelter, K., et al., 2011b. Performance evaluation of a novel chemiluminescence assay for detection of anti-GBM antibodies: an international multicenter study. Nephrol. Dial. Transplant. 27, 243–252.

Mahler, M., Hanly, J.G., Fritzler, M.J., 2012a. Importance of the dense fine speckled pattern on HEp-2 cells and anti-DFS70 antibodies for the diagnosis of systemic autoimmune diseases. Autoimmun. Rev. 11, 642–645.

Mahler, M., Miyachi, K., Peebles, C., Fritzler, M.J., 2012b. The clinical significance of autoantibodies to the proliferating cell nuclear antigen (PCNA). Autoimmun. Rev. 11, 771–775.

Malaviya, A.N., Gogia, S.B., 2010. Development, implementation and benefits of a rheumatology-specific electronic medical record application with automated display of outcome measures. Int. J Rheum. Dis. 13, 347–360.

Mariz, H.A., Sato, E.I., Barbosa, S.H., Rodrigues, S.H., Dellavance, A., Andrade, L.E., 2011. ANA HEp-2 pattern is a critical parameter for discriminating ANA-positive healthy individuals and patients with autoimmune rheumatic diseases. Arthritis Rheum. 63, 191–200.

Masi, A.T., Rodnan, G.P., Medsger Jr., T., Altman, R.D., D'Angelo, W. A., Fries, J.F., et al., 1980. Preliminary criteria for the classification of systemic sclerosis (scleroderma). Arthritis Rheum. 23, 581–590.

Mehra, S., Walker, J., Patterson, K., Fritzler, M.J., 2013. Autoantibodies in systemic sclerosis. Autoimmun. Rev. 12, 350–354.

Meroni, P.L., Schur, P.H., 2010. ANA screening: an old test with new recommendations. Ann. Rheum. Dis. 69, 1420–1422.

Meroni, P.L., Shoenfeld, Y., 2008. Predictive, protective, orphan autoantibodies: the example of the anti-phospholipid antibodies. Autoimmun. Rev. 7, 585–587.

Mustila, A., Paimela, L., Leirisalo-Repo, M., Huhtala, H., Miettinen, A., 2000. Antineutrophil cytoplasmic antibodies in patients with early rheumatoid arthritis—an early marker of progressive erosive disease. Arthritis Rheum. 43, 1371–1377.

Nakamura, R.M., Tan, E.M., 1977. Recent progress in the study of autoantibodies to nuclear antigens. Human Pathol. 9, 85–91.

Nakamura, R.M., Peebles, C.L., Molden, D.P., Tan, E.M., 1984. Advances in laboratory tests for autoantibodies to nuclear antigens in systemic rheumatic diseases. Lab. Med. 15, 190–198.

Nezlin, R., Mozes, E., 1995. Detection of antigens in immune complexes by a dot blot assay. J. Immunol. Methods. 184, 273–276.

Nirula, A., Glaser, S.M., Kalled, S.L., Taylor, F.R., 2011. What is IgG4? A review of the biology of a unique immunoglobulin subtype. Curr. Opin. Rheumatol. 23, 119–124.

Permin, H., Hørbov, S., Wiik, A., Knudsen, J.V., 1978. Antinuclear antibodies in juvenile chronic arthritis. Acta Paediatr. Scand. 67, 181–185.

Petri, M., Orbai, A.-M., Alarcon, G.S., Gordon, C., Merrill, J.T., Fortin, P.R., et al., 2012. Derivation and validation of the Systemic Lupus International Collaborating Clinics classification criteria for systemic lupus erythematosus. Arthritis Rheum. 64, 2677–2686.

Pincus, T., Mandelin, A.M., Swearingen, C.J., 2009. Flowsheets that include MDHAQ physical function, pain, global, and RAPID3 scores, laboratory tests, and medications to monitor patients with all rheumatic diseases: an electronic database for an electronic medical record. Rheum. Dis. Clin. North Am. 35, 829–842, x–xi.

Plenge, R.M., Bridges Jr., S.L., 2011. Personalized medicine in rheumatoid arthritis: miles to go before we sleep. Arthritis Rheum. 63, 590–593.

Pottel, H., Wiik, A., Locht, H., Gordon, T., Roberts-Thomson, P., Abraham, D., et al., 2004. Clinical optimization and multicenter validation of antigen-specific cut-off values on the INNO-LIA ANA update for the detection of autoantibodies in connective tissue disorders. Clin. Exp. Rheumatol. 22, 579–588.

Reichlin, M., Harley, J.B., 1986. Detection by ELISA of antibodies to small RNA protein particles in SLE patients whose sera lack precipitins. Trans. Assoc. Am. Phys. 99, 161–171.

Reimer, G., Raska, I., Tan, E.M., Scheer, U., 1987. Human autoantibodies: probes for nucleolus structure and function. Virchows Arch. B. 54, 131–143.

Renger, F., Bang, H., Feist, E., Fredenhagen, G., Natusch, A., Backhaus, M., et al., 2010. Immediate determination of ACPA and rheumatoid factor—a novel point of care test for detection of anti-MCV antibodies and rheumatoid factor using a lateral-flow immunoassay. Arthritis Res. Ther. 12, R120.

Reveille, J.D., Solomon, D.H., The American College of Rheumatology Ad hoc Committee on Immunologic Testing Guidelines, 2003. Evidence-based guidelines for the use of immunologic tests: anticentromere, Scl-70, and nucleolar antibodies. Arthritis Rheum. 49, 399–412.

Robinson, W.H., Steinman, L., Utz, P.J., 2002. Proteomics technologies for the study of autoimmune disease. Arthritis Rheum. 46, 885–893.

Rose, N.R., 1996. Foreword—the uses of autoantibodies. In: Peter, J.B., Shoenfeld, Y. (Eds.), Autoantibodies. Elsevier, Amsterdam, pp. xxvii–xxix.

Rose, N.R., 2007. Prediction and prevention of autoimmune disease: a personal perspective. Ann. N.Y. Acad. Sci. 1109, 117–128.

Satoh, M., Vazquez-Del, M.M., Chan, E.K.L., 2009. Clinical interpretation of antinuclear antibody tests in systemic rheumatic diseases. Mod. Rheumatol. 19, 219–228.

Savige, J., Gillis, D., Benson, E., Davies, D., Esnault, V., Falk, R.J., et al., 1999. International consensus statement on testing and reporting of antineutrophil cytoplasmic antibodies (ANCA). Am. J. Clin. Pathol. 111, 507–513.

Schachna, L., Wigley, F.M., Morris, S., Gelber, A.C., Rosen, A., Casciola-Rosen, L., 2002. Recognition of granzyme B-generated autoantigen fragments in scleroderma patients with ischemic digital loss. Arthritis Rheum. 46, 1873–1884.

Scussel-Lonzetti, L., Joyal, F., Raynauld, J.P., Roussin, A., Rich, É., Goulet, J.R., et al., 2002. Predicting mortality in systemic sclerosis—analysis of a cohort of 309 French Canadian patients with emphasis on features at diagnosis as predictive factors for survival. Medicine (Baltimore). 81, 154–167.

Sherer, Y., Shoenfeld, Y., 2007. Autoantibody explosion in lupus—155 different autoantibodies in SLE. Lupus. 16 (Suppl), 42.

Sherer, Y., Gorstein, A., Fritzler, M.J., Shoenfeld, Y., 2004. Autoantibody explosion in systemic lupus erythematosus. Semin. Arthritis Rheum. 34, 501–537.

Shoenfeld, Y., Cervera, R., Haass, M., Kallenberg, C., Khamashta, M., Meroni, P., et al., 2007. EASI—the European Autoimmunity Standardisation Initiative: a new initiative that can contribute to agreed diagnostic models of diagnosing autoimmune disorders throughout Europe. Ann. N.Y. Acad. Sci. 1109, 138–144.

Shovman, O., Gilburd, B., Barzilai, O., Shinar, E., Larida, B., Zandman-Goddard, G., et al., 2005a. Evaluation of the BioPlexTM 2200 ANA screen: analysis of 510 healthy subjects: incidence of natural/predictive autoantibodies. Ann. N.Y. Acad. Sci. 1050, 380–388.

Shovman, O., Gilburd, B., Zandman-Goddard, G., Yehiely, A., Langevitz, P., Shoenfeld, Y., 2005b. Multiplexed AtheNA multi-lyte immunoassay for ANA screening in autoimmune diseases. Autoimmunity. 38, 105–109.

Smolen, J.S., Butcher, B., Fritzler, M.J., Gordon, T., Hardin, J., Kalden, J.R., et al., 1997. Reference sera for antinuclear antibodies. II. Further definition of antibody specificities in international antinuclear antibody reference sera by immunofluorescence and Western immunoblotting. Arthritis Rheum. 40, 413–418.

Sokolove, J., Lindstrom, T.M., Robinson, W.H., 2012. Development and deployment of antigen arrays for investigation of B-cell fine specificity in autoimmune disease. Front. Biosci. (Elite. Ed.). 4, 320–330.

Solomon, D.H., Kavanaugh, A.J., Schur, P.H., 2002. Evidence-based guidelines for the use of immunologic tests: antinuclear antibody testing. Arthritis Rheum. 47, 434–444.

Stinton, L.M., Fritzler, M.J., 2007. A clinical approach to autoantibody testing in systemic autoimmune rheumatic disorders. Autoimmun. Rev. 7, 77–84.

Stinton, L.M., Eystathioy, T., Selak, S., Chan, E.K.L., Fritzler, M.J., 2004. Autoantibodies to protein transport and messenger RNA processing pathways: endosomes, lysosomes, Golgi complex, proteasomes, assemblyosomes, exosomes and GW Bodies. Clin. Immunol. 110, 30–44.

Stinton, L.M., Swain, M., Myers, R.P., Shaheen, A.A., Fritzler, M.J., 2010. Autoantibodies to GW bodies and other autoantigens in primary biliary cirrhosis. Clin. Exp. Immunol. 163, 147–156.

Stone, J.H., Zen, Y., Deshpande, V., 2012. IgG4-related disease. N. Engl. J Med. 366, 539–551.

Stott, D.I., 1989. Immunoblotting and dot blotting. J. Immunol. Methods. 119, 153–187.

Tak, P.P., 2012. A personalized medicine approach to biological treatment of rheumatoid arthritis: a preliminary treatment algorithm. Rheumatology (Oxford). 51, 600–609.

Tan, E.M., 1991. Autoantibodies in pathology and cell biology. Cell. 67, 841–842.

Tan, E.M., Feltkamp, T.E.W., Smolen, J.S., Butcher, B., Dawkins, R., Fritzler, M.J., et al., 1997. Range of antinuclear antibodies in "healthy" individuals. Arthritis Rheum. 40, 1601–1611.

Tan, E.M., Smolen, J., McDougal, J.S., Butcher, B.T., Conn, D., Dawkins, R., et al., 1999. A critical evaluation of enzyme immunoassays for the detection of antinuclear antibodies of defined specificities. I. Precision, sensitivity and specificity. Arthritis Rheum. 42, 455–464.

Targoff, I.N., 2002. Laboratory testing in the diagnosis and management of idiopathic inflammatory myopathies. Rheum. Dis. Clin. North Am. 28, 859–890.

Tonuttia, E., Bassetti, D., Piazza, A., Visentini, D., Poletto, M., Bassetto, F., et al., 2004. Diagnostic accuracy of ELISA methods as an alternative screening test to indirect immunofluorescence for the detection of antinuclear antibodies. Evaluation of five commercial kits. Autoimmunity. 37, 171–176.

van de Vaart, R., Drossaert, C.H., Taal, E., van de Laar, M.A., 2013. Giving rheumatology patients online home access to their electronic medical record (EMR): advantages, drawbacks and preconditions according to care providers. Rheumatol. Int. 33, 2405–2410.

van Eenennaam, H., Vogelzangs, J.H.P., Bisschops, L., Te Boome, L.C.J., Seelig, H.P., Renz, M., et al., 2002. Autoantibodies against small nucleolar ribonucleoprotein complexes and their clinical associations. Clin. Exp. Immunol. 130, 532–540.

Vasiliauskiene, L., Wiik, A., Hoier-Madsen, M., 2001. Prevalence and clinical significance of antikeratin antibodies and other serological markers in Lithuanian patients with rheumatoid arthritis. Ann. Rheum. Dis. 60, 459–466.

Vermeersch, P., De Beeck, K.O., Lauwerys, B.R., Van den Bergh, K., Develter, M., Marien, G., et al., 2009. Antinuclear antibodies directed against proliferating cell nuclear antigen are not specifically associated with systemic lupus erythematosus. Ann. Rheum. Dis. 68, 1791–1793.

Visser, H., Cessie, S., Vos, K., Breedveld, F.C., Hazes, J.M.W., 2002. How to diagnose rheumatoid arthritis early. Arthritis Rheum. 46, 357–365.

Vogt, T.M., Aickin, M., Ahmed, F., Schmidt, M., 2004. The prevention index: using technology to improve quality assessment. Health Serv. Res. 39, 511–530.

von Muhlen, C.A., Tan, E.M., 1995. Autoantibodies in the diagnosis of systemic rheumatic disease. Semin. Arthritis Rheum. 24, 323–358.

Walker, J.G., Fritzler, M.J., 2007. Update on autoantibodies in systemic sclerosis. Curr. Opin. Rheum. 19, 580–591.

Warde, N., 2011. Connective tissue diseases: agonistic autoantibodies: do they have a role in the pathophysiology of SSc? Nat. Rev. Rheum. 7, 71.

Wassermann, V.A., Neisser, A., Bruck, C., 1906. Eine serodiagnostische reaktion bei syphilis. Dtsch. Med. Wochenshrift. 19, 745–746.

Welting, T.J., Raijmakers, R., Pruijn, G.J., 2003. Autoantigenicity of nucleolar complexes. Autoimmun. Rev. 2, 313–321.

Wigley, F.M., Wise, R.A., Miller, R., Needleman, B.W., Spence, R.J., 1992. Anticentromere antibody as a predictor of digital ischemic loss in patients with systemic sclerosis. Arthritis Rheum. 35, 688–693.

Wiik, A., 2001. Methods for the detection of anti-neutrophil cytoplasmic antibodies. Recommendations for clinical use of ANCA serology and laboratory efforts to optimize the informative value of ANCA test results. Springer Semin. Immunopathol. 23, 217–229.

Wiik, A., Lam, K., 2001. Report to the European Commission: on the usability of extended DOORS software for education and training, quality assurance and consensus formation. Deliverable D 09, version 2.1.

Wiik, A., 2003a. Testing for ANA and ANCA: diagnostic value and pitfalls. In: Hochberg, M.C., Silman, A.J., Smolen, J.S., Weinblatt, M.E., Weisman, M.H. (Eds.), Rheumatology, third ed. Mosby, Edinburgh, pp. 215–226.

Wiik, A., Cervera, R., Haass, M., Kallenberg, C., Khamashta, M., Meroni, P.L., et al., 2006. European attempts to set guidelines for improving diagnostics of autoimmune rheumatic disorders. Lupus. 15, 391–396.

Wiik, A.S., 2003b. Appropriateness of autoantibody testing in clinical medicine. Clin. Chim. Acta. 333, 177–180.

Wiik, A.S., Gordon, T.P., Kavanaugh, A.F., Lahita, R.G., Reeves, W., Van Venrooij, W.J., et al., 2004. Cutting edge diagnostics in rheumatology: on the role of patients, clinicians, and laboratory scientists in optimizing the use of autoimmune serology. Arthritis Care Res. 51, 291–298.

Wiik, A.S., Hoier-Madsen, M., Forslid, J., Charles, P., Meyrowitsch, J., 2010. Antinuclear antibodies: A contemporary nomenclature using HEp-2 cells. J. Autoimmun. 35, 276–290.

Wilson, W.A., Gharavi, A.E., Koike, T., Lockshin, M.D., Branch, D.W., Piette, J.-C., et al., 1999. International consensus statement on preliminary classification criteria for definite antiphospholipid syndrome. Arthritis Rheum. 42, 1309–1311.

Yamasaki, Y., Narain, S., Yoshida, H., Hernandez, L., Barker, T., Hahn, P.C., et al., 2007. Autoantibodies to RNA helicase A: a new serologic marker of early lupus. Arthritis Rheum. 56, 596–604.

Chapter 78

Prediction of Autoimmune Disease

George S. Eisenbarth[†], Jennifer Barker, and Roberto Gianani

Barbara Davis Center for Childhood Diabetes, Denver, CO, USA

Chapter Outline

Type 1 Diabetes Mellitus as a Model for Prediction of
Autoimmune Disease   1177
The Pancreatic Pathology in Type 1 Diabetes Mellitus and Islet
Autoimmunity   1177
    Genetics   1179
Laboratory Markers of Autoimmunity (Including Autoantibodies
and T Cell Assays)   1179
    Metabolic Studies   1181
Organ-Specific Autoimmune Diseases   1182
    Thyroid   1182

Addison's Disease   1183
Celiac Disease   1183
Multiple Sclerosis   1184
Non-Organ Specific Disease   1184
    Rheumatoid Arthritis   1184
    Systemic Lupus Erythematosus   1185
Conclusions   1185
Acknowledgments   1186
References   1186

Many autoimmune diseases are chronic in nature with a long asymptomatic preclinical period marked by laboratory abnormalities (e.g., the presence of autoantibodies; Table 78.1) and are associated with particular genetic markers. Therefore, individuals with asymptomatic disease can be identified prior to developing tissue destruction with immunologic and immunogenetic testing. Given the prevalence of autoimmune disorders, immunologic and immunogenetic testing is likely to become an important component of what has been termed "personalized medicine." In this review, we will emphasize studies of endocrine autoimmunity, especially type 1 diabetes (T1D) where techniques for disease prediction have dramatically developed over the past two decades. Disease prevalence and characteristics of the test influence positive and negative value of test results (Table 78.2 and 78.3).

TYPE 1 DIABETES MELLITUS AS A MODEL FOR PREDICTION OF AUTOIMMUNE DISEASE

The chronic disease model for T1D (Figure 78.1) is a useful model for the prediction of T1D. In this model, the mass of insulin-producing pancreatic beta cells is depicted on the

y-axis and time on the x-axis (Eisenbarth, 1986). As the disease progresses, the beta cell mass decreases and markers of autoimmunity such as autoantibodies against islet-specific proteins and islet specific T cells emerge. As the beta cell mass diminishes, metabolic abnormalities develop and ultimately clinical diabetes manifests. Studies can be performed at each step along the way to identify individuals at risk for clinical diabetes. This model, however, could not until recently be verified by the direct observation of pancreatic pathology in individuals with T1D and/or islet autoimmunity. The investigation of the pathogenesis of T1D has been traditionally hindered by the difficult access to the pancreas in affected individuals. Following initial studies of autopsy pancreata, recent initiatives have awakened interest in the pathology of the pancreas in T1D. The JDRF-sponsored nPOD initiative and a similar European study are utilizing the pancreata of organ donors with diabetes and islet autoimmunity to correlate the disease status with morphological changes in the islets of Langerhans. The findings of these studies as they pertain to prediction of T1D are summarized below.

THE PANCREATIC PATHOLOGY IN TYPE 1 DIABETES MELLITUS AND ISLET AUTOIMMUNITY

In T1D there are two fundamental patterns of beta cell pathology, namely pattern A and pattern B, characterized

---

† With their deepest regret the Editors note the death of Dr George Eisenbarth during the composition of this text. The Editors' Preface contains a tribute to his many valued achievements and contributions. The corresponding author is Jennifer Barker.

N. Rose & I. Mackay (Eds): The Autoimmune Diseases, Fifth edition. DOI: http://dx.doi.org/10.1016/B978-0-12-384929-8.00078-2

TABLE 78.1 Representative Disease-associated Autoantibodies

Disease	Autoantibodies
Type 1 diabetes	Islet cell autoantibodies Insulin, GAD65, IA-2
Thyroid disease	Anti-thyroid peroxidase Anti-thyroglobulin
Addison's disease	Anti-21-hydroxylase
Celiac disease	Anti-tissue transglutaminase
Neuromyelitis optica	Anti-aquaporin 4
Rheumatoid arthritis	Rheumatoid factor (IgM anti-IgG) Anti-cyclic citrullinated peptide

TABLE 78.2 Sensitivity, Specificity, and Positive (PPV) and Negative Predictive Value (NPV)

Study	Disease	
	Present	Absent
Positive	A (true positive)	B (False positive)
Negative	C (false negative)	D (True negative)
Sensitivity = A/(A + C)	PPV = A/(A + B)	
Specificity = D/(B + D)	NPV = D/(C + D)	

respectively by the presence or absence of pseudo-atrophic islets (i.e., islets without any residual insulin-positive cells).

In pattern A there is usually complete beta cell loss but in some cases residual beta cells can be found. In particular, approximately 30% of individuals with long-standing T1D have residual beta cells; in these cases the pancreas contains both normal and pseudo-atrophic islets in various proportions in different cases. Islet antibody positivity (as determined by radioassay to the four autoantigens to be described below) is strongly associated with pattern A. In contrast the majority of subjects with pattern B are negative for islet autoantibodies and do not express high-risk DR alleles. The pancreata with pattern A, but not the pancreata with pattern B, contain, in some instances, islets infiltrated by mononuclear cells (insulitis). Thus, it appears that islet autoantibody positivity defines a subset of T1D with autoimmune pathogenesis while autoantibody negativity is probably associated with different etiologies. Therefore, it is likely that the true sensitivity for autoimmune diabetes of islet antibodies is higher than previously thought since in new-onset antibody-negative subjects diabetes might be due to non-autoimmune etiology.

From the above findings it is clear that T1D of autoimmune etiology is associated with pseudo-atrophic islets and insulitis. The ability of islet antibodies to predict the disease likely signifies that the changes seen in the pancreata of subjects with T1D are also present in the pancreata of islet autoantibody-positive prediabetic individuals, in particular subjects positive for more than one antibody (positivity for one antibody has a lower positive predictive value than positivity for multiple antibodies). Data from a Belgian group confirmed these predictions by showing that insulitis is present in organ donors positive for multiple antibodies but absent in single antibody positive. In addition we and others have identified pseudo-atrophic islets in multiple islet antibody-positive subjects (unpublished observation) suggesting that in these individuals there is chronic beta cell destruction before the clinical onset of diabetes. Of note, we have identified a subset of individuals previously classified as having a clinical diagnosis of type 2 diabetes mellitus that display pattern A beta cell pathology and, in some cases, islet antibody positivity. It is likely that these subjects correspond to the group previously classified as LADA (latent-onset diabetes of the adult, see also below).

TABLE 78.3 Effect of Disease Prevalence on Positive (PPV) and Negative Predictive Value (NPV) with Identical Test Specificity (99%) and Sensitivity (90%)

	Low Prevalence (0.3%)				High Prevalence (5%)		
	Disease				Disease		
Test	Present	Absent		Test	Present	Absent	
Positive	270	997	1267	Positive	4500	950	5450
Negative	30	98,703	98,730	Negative	500	94,050	94,550
	300	99,700	100,000		5000	95,000	100,000
PPV	270/1267 = 21.3%			4500/5450 = 82.6%			
NPV	98,703/98,730 = 99.97%			94,050/94,550 = 99.5%			

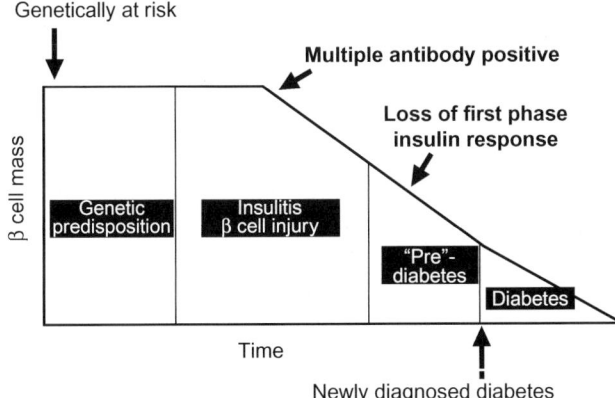

FIGURE 78.1   A model for the natural history of the autoimmunity leading to type 1A diabetes. Individuals who are genetically susceptible to disease are triggered to initiate insulitis or beta cell injury. This is marked by the production of autoantibodies against the pancreas. As loss of beta cell mass continues, metabolic abnormalities such as a loss of first phase insulin response begin and ultimately when enough beta cells are lost, diabetes develops.

As mentioned earlier and discussed more in detail later, positivity for one islet autoantibody has a lower positive predictive value for T1D than positivity for two or more antibodies. This observation has an interesting correlate in the lack of insulitis in single antibody-positive subjects and raises the question of the etiology of single antibody positivity. It is possible that single antibody-positive subjects might have a pathological lesion, which has the potential to result in T cell-mediated islet autoimmunity and T1D but does not necessarily do so in all cases. If this hypothesis is correct, one should be able to detect morphological islet changes in single islet antibody positive but not in control subjects.

Genetics

Although greater than 85% of individuals with T1D do not have a family history of T1D, the risk for diabetes in a first-degree relative of an individual with T1D is approximately 15 times greater than that of individuals from the general population (6% vs. 0.4%) (Tillil and Kobberling, 1987). The major histocompatibility complex (MHC) located on chromosome 6 (6p21.3) is thought to contribute 50% of the genetic risk for T1D (Nerup et al., 1974). Noble et al. (1996) and Erlich et al. (1993) have shown that both DQ and DR alleles have been associated with T1D. HLA haplotypes associated with the highest risk for T1D are DR3, DQ2 (DQA1*0501, DQB1*0201), and DR4, DQ8 (DQA1*0302 DQB1*0302) (Ziegler et al., 1991).

It is estimated that approximately 6% of the population with DR3-DQ2/DR4-DQ8 will develop T1D. However, the risk of diabetes in first-degree relatives with this high-risk HLA genotype is much higher. Approximately 40% of siblings of patients with T1D with DR3-DQ2/DR4-DQ8

will develop T1D. This suggests that other genetic loci within the MHC also contribute to risk of T1D in that relatives with high-risk HLA alleles usually share complete MHC haplotypes. These high-risk genotypes also impact the age at which T1D develops. Approximately 50% of those who develop T1D prior to 5 years of age are heterozygotes for DR3-DQ2/DR4-D8 compared to 2.4% of Colorado newborns (Redondo et al., 2001).

Specific HLA haplotypes protect individuals from disease. Similarly to many studies, Pugliese et al. (1995) have reported that DR2 (DRB1*1501, DQA1*0102, DQB1*0501) and DR7 with DQA1, DQB1*0301 and DRB1*1401 are protective for the development of T1D.

Additional genetic loci such as the insulin gene (Bell et al., 1984; Bennett et al., 1997), CTLA-4 (Lowe et al., 2000; Nistico et al., 1996), and PTPN22 (Bottini, et al., 2004), and more than 50 other loci, have also been associated with T1D.

HLA haplotypes and to a lesser extent insulin gene polymorphisms are the only genetic markers that have been used to identify individuals from the general population at high risk for the development of T1D. Studies such as the Diabetes Autoimmunity Study in the Young (DAISY) in Denver, Colorado, USA (Rewers et al., 1996), and the Finnish Type 1 Diabetes Prediction and Prevention project (DIPP) (Kupila et al., 2001) follow children from the general population who are at high risk for the development of T1D based upon the presence of moderate or high-risk HLA genotypes.

The presence of high-risk HLA genotypes increases the likelihood of T1D by an order of magnitude. In the general population those with the highest-risk HLA haplotypes have a risk for T1D of approximately 6%, compared with a risk of 0.4% in the general population (Tillil and Kobberling, 1987). In first-degree relatives this risk increases from approximately 6% to approximately 40% in those with the highest-risk HLA genotypes. However, risk is not absolute with a significant subset of individuals with high-risk HLA genotypes never developing islet autoimmunity. Further evaluation, including the use of anti-islet autoantibodies, will refine prediction.

LABORATORY MARKERS OF AUTOIMMUNITY (INCLUDING AUTOANTIBODIES AND T CELL ASSAYS)

Since the discovery of islet cell autoantibodies (ICA), detected by incubation of serum with sections of frozen human pancreas (Bottazzo et al., 1980; Lendrum et al., 1975), autoantibodies have been used to identify individuals at risk for T1D. ICA is measured in Juvenile Diabetes Foundation (JDF) units with positive often defined as ≥ 10 JDF units. Bonifacio et al. (1990) and

(Chase et al., 1991) have showed that the risk for diabetes increases as the ICA level increases. In first-degree relatives, the risk for T1D increases from 40% with a low cut-off (≥4 JDF units) to 100% (in one study) with a high cut-off (≥80 JDF units) (Bonifacio et al., 1990). The relationship between level and PPV for diabetes has also been observed in cohorts without an affected first-degree relative (Chase et al., 1991).

The specific antigens of ICA include the glutamic acid decarboxylase (GAD65), the protein tyrosine phosphatase ICA512 (IA-2), and ZnT8. Insulin autoantibodies are not detected with the staining of frozen pancreas. These autoantibodies are the current so-called biochemical autoantibodies. Sensitive and specific radioimmunoassays (RIA) have been developed for autoantibodies to insulin, GAD65 IA-2. More recently, antibodies to Znt8 were discovered and are also used for both the prediction and the diagnosis of diabetes. In particular, antibodies to Znt8 identified a subset at higher diabetes risk in individuals with one antibody to GAD, IA-2, or insulin (Yu et al., 2012).

When ICA is present in the company of biochemical autoantibodies, the risk for T1D increases. Individuals who expressed ICA alone were at a much lower risk for T1D (less than 5%) compared with those positive for ICA and biochemical autoantibodies (66.2%) (MacLaren et al., 1999). This is probably related to higher prevalence of false-positive ICA in subjects without biochemical antibody. Yu et al. (2001) demonstrated that higher levels of ICA are associated with expression of one or more biochemical autoantibodies. Previous reports have described heterogeneity among islet cell antibodies with better predictive value for diabetes in the subset reacting to multiple autoantigens. Therefore, the risk conferred by ICA can also be identified through testing for biochemical autoantibodies.

Life-table analysis has shown that expression of multiple biochemical autoantibodies is associated with a greater risk for T1D (Figure 78.2). Individuals who express three anti-islet autoantibodies are at an approximately 70% risk for T1D after 5 years, compared with 12% for those who express one anti-islet autoantibody (Verge et al., 1996).

A number of population-based prospective studies such as DAISY and the German babyDIAB study have established that islet autoimmunity can appear years before the onset of diabetes and can occur as early as the first year of life. The risk for T1D does not appear to dissipate over time for individuals with multiple autoantibodies. Gardner et al. (1999) followed first-degree relatives with multiple autoantibodies and found a progressive increase in incidence of T1D over time such that at 15 years, 66% had developed diabetes. The development of diabetes did not appear to be decreasing at the end of the study. This has led to the hypothesis that all

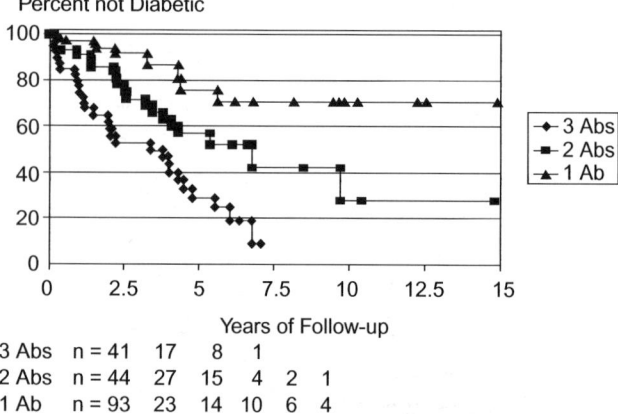

FIGURE 78.2   First-degree relatives of individuals with T1D were followed for development of diabetes. Those relatives who expressed more than two or three autoantibodies were at a greater risk for the development of diabetes compared with those who expressed one autoantibody (Verge et al., 1996).

individuals who express multiple autoantibodies will develop diabetes given enough time. In contrast, the expression of a single biochemical autoantibody is associated with a long-term risk of less than 20% in relatives of patients with T1D. Transient expression of autoantibodies in the DAISY study was not associated with high-risk genotypes or family history of diabetes and the development of T1D (Barker et al., 2004).

LaGasse et al. (2002) have used biochemical autoantibodies to screen school children in Washington State, USA. Approximately 4500 school children were screened, 12 children were found to have two or three positive autoantibodies. Six children developed diabetes during 8-year follow-up. All expressed at least two autoantibodies. None of the children with zero or one autoantibody developed diabetes. This indicates that autoantibodies can be used in a large population to screen for disease.

The DAISY study has identified children with biochemical autoantibodies and followed them for the onset of diabetes. Children diagnosed with this intensive screening program tend to be found at an earlier stage of disease and have less diabetic ketoacidosis (Barker et al., 2004). These children also have lower blood glucose levels at the time of diagnosis (Figure 78.3).

The use of autoantibody assays has identified individuals previously classified as type 2 diabetics as having an autoimmune process associated with a faster progression to insulin dependency compared with autoantibody-negative individuals. Approximately 45% of such adults positive for ICA required insulin at 6 years post onset of diabetes compared to 5% of those with no autoantibodies. This so-called latent autoimmune diabetes of adults (LADA) was analyzed in the UKPDS study. Similarly, Fuchtenbusch et al. (1997) have demonstrated that in women with gestational diabetes,

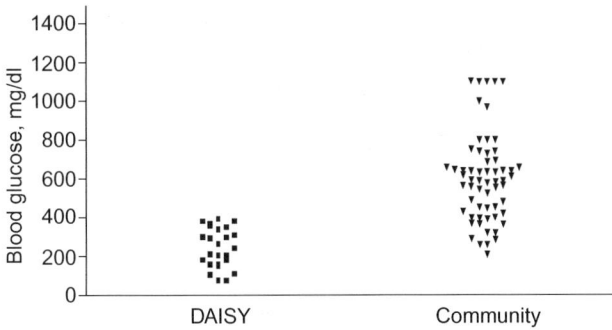

FIGURE 78.3   Blood glucose levels at diagnosis of diabetes in individuals diagnosed with diabetes through an intensive screening program compared with those diagnosed from the community.

the presence of one, two, or three autoantibodies conferred a risk for insulin dependency of 17%, 61%, and 84%, respectively, during follow-up of approximately 2 years. Autoantibodies can be used in adults diagnosed with diabetes as a prognostic factor for insulin dependency.

Multiple international workshops evaluating different assay formats for islet autoantibodies in mouse models of T1D and humans indicate that standard ELISA formats are inadequate in contrast to fluid phase radioassays. For example, ELISA anti-insulin autoantibody assays could detect insulin antibodies following subcutaneous insulin therapy but could not detect pre-diabetic insulin autoantibodies (Greenbaum et al., 1992) (Figure 78.4).

More recently, however, GAD and IA-2 antibody-modified ELISA have achieved sensitivity and specificity equivalent to in-house RIA and an electrochemiluminescence IAA assay was recently reported to be more sensitive than IAA radioassay (Yu et al., 2012).

T1D is known to be a T cell-mediated disease. Autoantibodies are likely only a marker of the autoimmune process and are not themselves directly pathogenic. Therefore, efforts are underway to develop reliable T cell assays for T1D. Tetramer analysis has allowed for the detection of T cells that react to beta cell antigens. Tetramer analysis employs the use of multimeric peptide–MHC complexes to detect T cells. Using this technology, soluble HLA-DR401 or DR404 tetramers with a GAD65 epitope were found to react with T cells of newly diagnosed T1D and individuals at risk for T1D (Reijonen et al., 2002, 2003). In 2011, the Immunology of Diabetes Society conducted two workshops to validate class 1 and class II antigen-specific tetramers. For class I, peripheral blood T cell responses were measured by multiple centers in 35 patients with newly diagnosed T1D using both tetramers and pentamers encompassing epitopes of preproinsulin and GAD. All epitopes were recognized by T1D patients with a prevalence ranging from 5 to 25%.

Class II GAD and proinsulin epitopes were similarly evaluated and found to be positive in at least 74% of patients. Of note, only a minority of patients tested by tetramer and ELISPOT were positive for both assays.

ELISPOT (enzyme linked immunoabsorbent spot) is utilized to monitor CD4$^+$ and CD48$^+$ lymphocyte response to antigens.

In particular, a CD8 T cell response to a peptide of islet amyloid polypeptide (IAPP) has been described (Panagiotopoulos et al., 2003). More recently, French groups have demonstrated reactivity to epitopes of the islet autoantigens Znt8 in 80% of children with T1D but only 18% of controls (Énée et al., 2012). Similarly, Dang and coworkers identified a CD4 Znt8 response in the peripheral blood of patients with T1D (Dang et al., 2011).

Further refinement of both tetramer and ELISPOT are needed for these technologies to significantly contribute to the prediction of T1D.

Metabolic Studies

Metabolic abnormalities begin to appear as the beta cell mass diminishes to the point at which it cannot appropriately respond to a glucose load. An early metabolic abnormality is the loss of the first phase insulin response (FPIR) on the intravenous glucose tolerance test (IVGTT). The FPIR is the sum of the insulin levels at 1 and 3 minutes after an intravenous glucose load. In the presence of islet autoantibodies, levels that are less than the first percentile of age-matched normal controls identify individuals that are at a 50% risk of the development of overt diabetes at 5 years and 90% at 10 years (Bingley et al., 1992; Bleich et al., 1990). This relationship remains true in individuals who are positive for anti-islet autoantibodies (Bleich et al., 1990). In the DIPP study, Keskinen et al., 2002 followed children with multiple anti-islet autoantibodies and showed that they have lower FPIR than children with ICA only (Figure 78.5) and that half of the children with abnormal FPIR developed overt diabetes during the time period of the study. The metabolic state of an individual at risk for T1D is dynamic and beta cell loss may be ongoing, so repeat evaluation is necessary in order to be maximally sensitive. In addition to being able to correctly identify individuals at risk for overt diabetes, an FPIR greater than the 10th percentile has a good negative predictive value. Relatives with FPIR greater than the 10th percentile rarely progress to T1D over a 3-year period. Using the FPIR in addition to autoantibody data led to the development of a model of risk for T1D. In this model, the time remaining before the development of T1D was dependent upon the FPIR and IAA level (Jackson et al., 1988).

The FPIR is not without problems. It is a measure of beta cell function, and thus only an indirect measure of beta cell mass. As such, situations that increase insulin resistance such

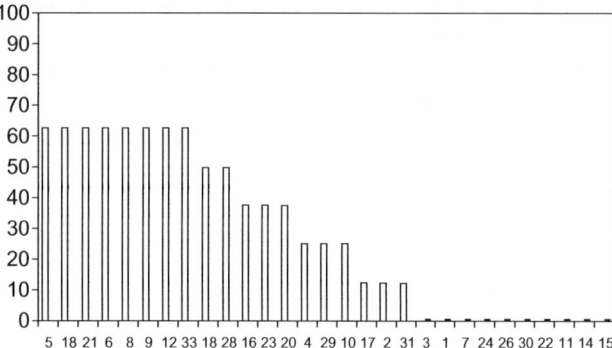

FIGURE 78.4 Percentage of positive IAA (defined as ≥3SD above the mean) healthy individuals who became diabetic (*n* = 8). Numbers along the x-axis indicate different laboratories. Open bars are laboratories using RIA and closed bars are those using ELISA (Greenbaum et al., 1992).

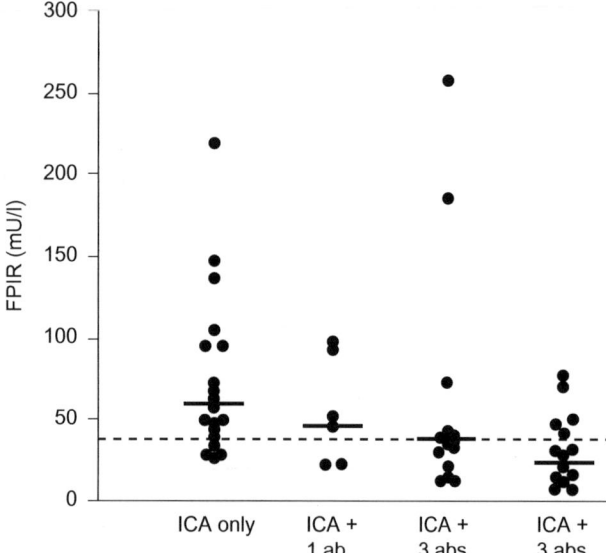

FIGURE 78.5 Level of FPIR is associated with number of positive autoantibodies; children with three autoantibodies expressed the lowest FPIR. The dotted line represents the first percentile in age-matched normal controls (Keskinen et al., 2002).

as puberty and obesity may affect the results. In addition, there is significant intra-subject variability with coefficients of variation ranging between 4 and 36% (Allen et al., 1993; Arslanian et al., 1993; Smith et al., 1988). The timing of loss of FPIR differs in the progression to T1D in different groups. For example, in young children who express autoantibodies, the FPIR may already be lost at the time of first autoantibody expression (Keskinen et al., 2002) and some individuals maintain FPIR into their first year of diagnosis of T1D.

As the beta cell mass continues to diminish, the metabolic abnormalities become more pronounced and may be detected in routine oral glucose tolerance testing, initially with impaired glucose tolerance (glucose 2 hours after oral glucose ≥140 mg/dl and <200 mg/dl). It is of

note that early in the time course of T1D, the metabolic abnormality might not be observed in the fasting state. At this point, the individual is not symptomatic but may rapidly progress to symptomatic diabetes. Useful prognostic metabolic information can be obtained by careful analysis of C-peptide secretion and subclinical abnormalities of glucose incursions of oral glucose tolerance testing (Sosenko et al., 2008).

ORGAN-SPECIFIC AUTOIMMUNE DISEASES

Thyroid

Autoimmune thyroid disease (AIT) manifested as either hypothyroidism or hyperthyroidism is very common in the general population. Approximately 5% of the population is hypothyroid and 1.3% hyperthyroid (Hollowell et al., 2002). AIT occurs at an increased frequency in individuals with T1D (28% (Umpierrez et al., 2003)), Addison's disease (AD) (14−21% (Betterle et al., 2002; Kasperlik-Zaluska et al., 1998; Zelissen et al 1995; Lendrum et al., 1975)), celiac disease (CD) (up to 12% (Ansaldi et al., 2003)), and other autoimmune diseases. Therefore, the first step in prediction requires knowledge of the individual's medical history. Routine screening for thyroid disease is generally recommended in these individuals as there is a high pretest probability of disease and the studies are relatively non-invasive.

Risk for AIT is weakly related to HLA genotypes that vary dependent upon the population. Santamaria et al. (1994) reported that DRB1*0201 increased the risk for AIT in T1D. Kim et al. (2003) reported that DQB1*0401 increased the risk in the Korean diabetic population. DQB1*0302 has been associated with AIT in the Czech diabetic population (Sumnik et al., 2003). DR3 and DR5 have been associated with thyroid autoimmunity in German blood donors (Boehm et al., 1993).

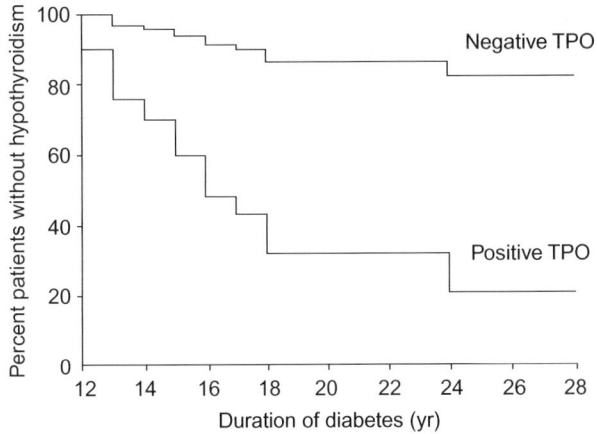

FIGURE 78.6 The development of hypothyroidism in the diabetic population is dependent upon the production of thyroid autoantibodies. Individuals who express TPO are at a much higher risk for hypothyroidism compared with those who do not (Umpierrez et al., 2003).

AIT is accompanied by autoantibodies to thyroid antigens, anti-thyroid peroxidase (TPO), and anti-thyroglobulin (TG) (Vakeva et al., 1992). These autoantibodies are positive in approximately 10% of the general population (Hollowell et al., 2002) and in around 90% of the hypothyroid population (Vakeva et al., 1992). Prospective follow-up by Vanderpump et al. (1995) in the Whickham study has shown that women with positive TPO autoantibodies and normal TSH have a 2.1% per year risk of developing hypothyroidism with an overall risk of 27% of hypothyroidism at 20 years.

In high-risk populations such as T1D, progression to AIT is related to the presence of TPO and TG antibodies, with approximately 80% of T1D positive for TPO antibodies progressing to AIT compared to 15% of those TPO negative (Umpierrez et al., 2003) (Figure 78.6). Of note, individuals with negative TPO autoantibodies still progressed to AIT but at a much lower rate.

Similarly to T1D, in which abnormalities of glucose metabolism identify individuals at a greater risk for clinical diabetes, individuals who have abnormalities of thyroid metabolism are at an increased risk for the development of overt hypothyroidism. Of those with an elevated TSH and normal thyroid hormone, 55% were hypothyroid at 20 years, with a 4.3% yearly incidence.

Screening for thyroid autoimmunity in high-risk populations such as T1D with TPO and/or TG autoantibodies may identify individuals at an increased risk for autoimmune thyroid disease for closer monitoring. The efficacy of this screening has not been fully evaluated.

Addison's Disease

Addison's disease (AD) is an autoimmune endocrine disease resulting in primary adrenal insufficiency. It is a rare disease in the general population, occurring in approximately 1/10,000 individuals. However, it does occur with other autoimmune endocrine diseases including T1D and AIT. The combination of two of the three autoimmune diseases (T1D, AD, and/or AIT) is known as autoimmune polyendocrine syndrome II (APS-II).

Genetic risk for AD is conferred by the major histocompatibility complex (MHC) on chromosome 6. This includes the HLA class II region. AD is associated with DRB1*0404 DQ8 (Yu et al., 1999). Gambelunghe et al. (1999), Park et al. (2002), and Baker et al. (2011) have shown that polymorphisms of other loci within the MHC including HLA-B15 MIC-A are associated with AD both in the diabetic and non-diabetic populations.

AD is accompanied by the production of autoantibodies against the adrenal cortex (Anderson et al., 1957). Winqvist et al. (1992) and Baumann-Antczak et al. (1992) have identified the cytochrome p450 enzyme 21-hydroxylase as the major antigen for these antibodies. Falorni et al. (1997) has shown that 21-hydroxylase autoantibodies are highly sensitive and specific for AD. Reflecting the increased risk for AD in people with T1D, individuals with T1D express adrenal autoantibodies at a rate of 1–2% (Brewer et al., 1997; Peterson et al., 1997; Yu et al., 1999). Recently, the first international serum exchange for the determination of 21-hydroxylase antibodies (Falorni et al., 2011) showed good agreement between participating laboratories but also revealed important discrepancies in individuals' specimens. These results demonstrate the need for an international 21-hydroxylase antibody standardization program.

Formal adrenal function is tested using cortrosyn (ACTH) stimulation. We have recently demonstrated that moderately elevated ACTH is a more useful early indicator of impending AD than 21-hydroxylase AA, PRA, or peak cortisol in the 2 months to 2 years preceding the onset of AD (Baker et al., 2012). Thus annual measurement of ACTH is likely sufficient to monitor individuals with 21-hydroxylase autoantibodies, reserving cortrosyn testing for those with moderately elevated ACTH or Addison's symptoms.

Celiac Disease

Celiac disease (CD) is an autoimmune disease characterized by gluten insensitivity. Symptoms range from malabsorption, diarrhea, and stunted growth to less specific symptoms of fatigue and malaise. Celiac disease can be found in the company of T1D and AIT, occurring in as many as 10% of individuals with T1D (De Vitis et al., 1996) and AIT (Ansaldi et al., 2003).

Celiac disease occurs in association with specific HLA genotypes. In individuals with T1D who are

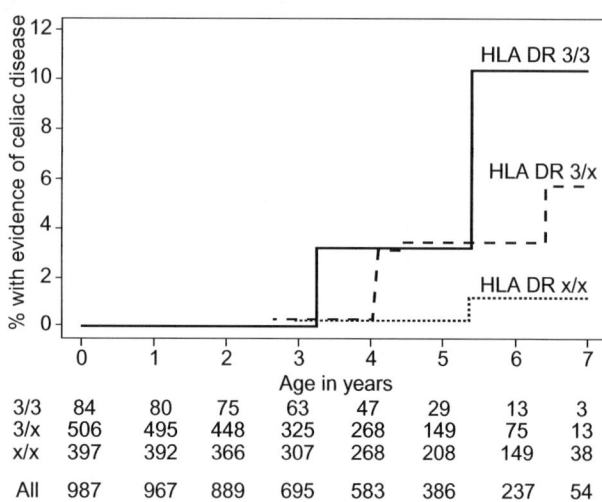

3/3	84	80	75	63	47	29	13	3
3/x	506	495	448	325	268	149	75	13
x/x	397	392	366	307	268	208	149	38
All	987	967	889	695	583	386	237	54

FIGURE 78.7 The production of tissue transglutaminase autoantibodies is highly dependent on the presence of HLA DR3 (Hoffenberg et al., 2003).

homozygous for HLA DQ2, approximately one-third are positive for autoantibodies to tissue transglutaminase (tTG) (Bao et al., 1999). Ninety-five percent of individuals with CD have HLA DQA1*0501, DQB1*0201, compared with 36% of the general population (Hall et al., 1991). DQA1*0501, DQB1*0201 generally occurs with DR3-DQ2 (DQA1*0501DQB1*0201) and DR5, DR7 heterozygotes (DRB1*0701 DQA1*0501). Hoffenberg et al. (2003) have prospectively followed neonates from the general population with the high-risk DR3-DQ2 HLA haplotypes in Denver, Colorado. Children with high-risk haplotypes were enrolled and followed for the development of autoantibodies to tTG. At age 5 years, 3.2% of children DR3/3 homozygous developed positive tTG compared with 3.4% of heterozygotes and 0.3% of children negative for DR3 (Figure 78.7).

Celiac diseasse is associated with the expression of autoantibodies. Autoantibodies against gliadin (IgG and IgA) are sensitive but not specific and therefore have a low positive predictive value (deamidated gliadin autoantibodies are more specific). In contrast, antiendomysial autoantibodies (EMA) are highly sensitive and specific. EMA are detected with indirect immunofluorescence against human umbilical cord. Recently tTG has been identified as the autoantigen of EMA and highly sensitive and specific assays have been developed to detect tTG autoantibodies (Dieterich et al., 1997; Fasano et al., 2001; Gillett et al., 2001). Bonamico and coworkers (Bonamico et al., 2011) have demonstrated the feasibility of large-scale screening of the general population for salivary anti-transglutaminase antibodies as determined by radioassay.

Diagnosis of celiac disease is made by biopsy of the small intestinal mucosa showing the characteristic pathologic changes and confirmed with resolution of these findings on biopsy after institution of a gluten-free diet. Because of the invasiveness of the procedure, biopsy should be performed only in individuals with a high likelihood of being positive. Factors that increase the pretest probability of disease include individuals who are symptomatic of disease and individuals with higher levels of autoantibody as measured by the radioimmunoassay. Liu et al. (2003) showed that higher levels of tTG in a radioimmunoassay had a higher PPV for biopsy. The standard cut-off of 0.05 (99% specificity) had a PPV of 76% compared with 96% with a cut-off of 0.5. In addition, the level of tTG autoantibody has been shown to correlate with severity of findings on biopsy (Liu et al., 2003). Therefore, level of autoantibody can be incorporated in an algorithm to decide whether or not to perform the biopsy. The autoantibody levels also decrease on a gluten-free diet and are used to monitor compliance with therapy.

Multiple Sclerosis

Multiple sclerosis (MS) is a chronic autoimmune disease resulting in neurologic deficits. It occurs in the setting of specific HLA alleles. DRB1*1501 has consistently been shown to predispose to MS (Allen et al., 1994; Laaksonen et al., 2002). In a large group of patients, this has been shown to have a dose effect with two copies of the susceptible haplotype associated with a higher risk of MS compared with one or none. Those individuals who express DRB1*1501 on both HLA DRB1 alleles tend to have a more severe disease course (Barcellos et al., 2003).

Autoantibody determinations in these groups are less well defined compared with the other autoimmune disease discussed. In contrast, a variant of multiple sclerosis termed neuromyelitis optica is strongly associated with autoantibodies reacting with aquaporin 4.

NON-ORGAN SPECIFIC DISEASE

Rheumatoid Arthritis

Rheumatoid arthritis (RA) is a systemic autoimmune disease. It is characterized by joint inflammation ultimately leading to joint destruction and disability. At diagnosis, individuals often show signs of advanced joint destruction. Landewe et al. (2002) have shown that early treatment decreases disease severity. Therefore, the ability to predict disease and diagnosis in individuals early would have high clinical utility.

RA is associated with HLA-DR4 (HLA-DRB1*0401 and DRB1*0404), with the strongest association to DRB1*0404 (Silman and Pearson, 2002).

RA is accompanied by the production of autoantibodies. Rheumatoid factor (RF) and anti-cyclic citrullinated peptide (CCP) autoantibodies are commonly identified. Rheumatoid factor is an IgM (rarely IgG) autoantibody directed against IgG. Citrulline is an amino acid that is generated by post-translation modification of arginine by the enzyme peptidylarginine deiminase (PAD) (Vossenaar et al., 2003). Polymorphisms of the gene PAD4 are associated with RA (Vossenaar et al., 2004). Cyclic citrullinated peptide (CCP) autoantibodies are detected in 80% of patients with RA and are produced within the synovium and may have some impact on disease processes (Suzuki et al., 2003). Molecular modeling has shown that DRB1*0401 binds citrullinated peptides (Hill et al., 2003) and the presence of DRB1*0401 is correlated with autoantibodies to CCP (Goldbach-Mansky et al., 2000). Hill et al. (2003) have associated the genetic risk for RA to the presence of anti-CCP.

RA is thought to have a long preclinical phase that is marked by the presence of autoantibodies without the symptoms of arthritis. Aho et al. (1991) followed over 7000 Finnish individuals over the age of 30 years for the development of RA. Twenty-one individuals developed RA, 15 of whom had positive RF in serum samples prior to the development of disease. Halldórsdóttir et al. (2000) have prospectively determined that persistently positive RF is associated with development of disease. Nielen et al. (2004) retrospectively studied frozen serum samples obtained prior to the diagnosis of RA. Approximately 50% of individuals were positive for either RF or CCP a median of 4.5 years prior to symptom onset compared with approximately 1% of the general population control. The sensitivity of positivity for RF or CCP was 36.5%, with a specificity of 98.1%. The positive predictive value for a high-risk population of either RF or CCP autoantibody positive was 43.8%.

Rantapää-Dahlqvist et al. (2003) showed similar findings. However, the PPV of CCP autoantibodies with an estimated population prevalence of 1% was 16%. Therefore, the majority of individuals positive for these autoantibodies in the general population will not progress to disease and may not be candidates for early therapy. Majka and Holers (2003) have postulated that these autoantibodies may have a better utility in individuals with a high pretest probability of disease such as those with high-risk HLA haplotypes or those with a family history of disease.

New second generation anti-CCP antibody-automated assays have demonstrated a better correlation with clinical RA (Elrefaei et al., 2012) than previous ELISA formats. Despite these advancements, however, a recent large study,

using a combination of anti-CCP antibodies and the American College of Rheumatology 1987 criteria, failed to improve early rheumatoid diagnosis in a community-based very early arthritis cohort (Le Loët et al., 2011).

Systemic Lupus Erythematosus

Systemic lupus erythematosus (SLE) is a systemic autoimmune disease characterized by multi-organ involvement. The disease can have a relapsing—remitting course or become persistent with fulminant organ involvement.

Genetic risk is conferred by HLA class II alleles, in particular DR2 or DR3. In addition C4-null alleles occur in increased frequency in individuals in many ethnic groups (Christiansen et al., 1991).

Autoantibodies are produced in SLE and are characteristic of the disease. However, many of the autoantibodies are also produced in individuals who never develop disease. The anti-nuclear antibody is a good screening test for disease in that 95% of individuals with SLE will be positive for this antibody. However, as much as 5% of the general population will also be positive for this autoantibody, albeit at a low titer. Therefore, it is a sensitive but not specific marker of disease. Anti-double stranded DNA antibodies are more disease specific. Specific autoantibodies and quantification using radioimmunoassays have been associated with disease activity. For example, Yamamoto et al. (2000) described a radioimmunoassay for RNPs and found that in individuals with SLE 44% were positive and there was a correlation with SLE nephritis. The use of combinations of autoantibodies can improve sensitivity and specificity for SLE and levels of autoantibodies can be associated with disease activity scores (Ignat et al., 2003).

CONCLUSIONS

Effective prediction of autoimmune disease requires an understanding of the epidemiological concepts of sensitivity, specificity, PPV, NPV, and Bayes' theorem and, usually, assays with specificities $\geq 99\%$. Although assays and algorithms for T1D prediction are routinely set at this level of specificity, for most rheumatologic disorders immunohistochemical or ELISA assays with lower specificities are standard. It is likely that newer fluid phase methodologies would also improve prediction for these disorders. The use of laboratory studies in populations that are at a high risk for disease, defined by family history or the presence of a high-risk HLA haplotype, may also help improve prognostication for these individuals.

Prediction of disease is especially important when early diagnosis and intervention positively impact the patients. For RA, early treatment modifies the disease course and portends a better outcome in patients. For T1D, the early identification of individuals at risk for disease by positive autoantibodies decreased the hospitalization for ketoacidosis compared with controls (Barker et al., 2004). As effective prevention measures are developed for autoimmune diseases, the ability to correctly identify individuals at a high risk for disease will become more important.

Autoimmune diseases are often accompanied by the production of autoantibodies. Certain characteristics of autoantibody production such as level, affinity, duration of positivity, and epitope recognition may be associated with disease development. Autoantibody assays can be used in a cohort of susceptible individuals to identify people at an increased risk for the development of disease. Autoantibody production can precede the development of disease for many years and some individuals who are autoantibody positive may never develop disease. Therefore, precise prognostication for a single individual is difficult. For T1D, the presence of two or more anti-islet autoantibodies is associated with very high risk of progression.

The presence of one autoimmune disease identifies an individual at a high risk for a second autoimmune disease (Pearce and Leech, 2004). The heightened risk for disease in this group increases the pretest probability of disease. Therefore, using autoantibody assays and/or T cell assays in this group will be more efficacious. A positive result will have a high post-test probability of disease in a single individual.

Many autoimmune diseases are T cell dependent. The development of reliable T cell assays that are sensitive and specific for autoimmune disease will be a major advance in the ability to predict disease. When used in combination with autoantibody assays, the T cell assays may refine our diagnostic ability and improve PPV and NPV.

The use of predictive algorithms that incorporate genetic risk expressed by HLA haplotypes or family history of disease, autoantibody production, and early physiological changes such as abnormal FPIR (T1D), mildly elevated TSH (AIT), or elevated ACTH (AD) will identify individuals at different points along the natural history of disease with increasing risk for disease development. These algorithms can be used to identify individuals who might benefit and be willing to participate in intervention studies and change the course of disease. We believe it is likely that most autoimmune disorders are preceded by a long prodrome and that waiting for clinical presentation can be associated with irreversible morbidity (bone erosions at diagnosis of patients with rheumatoid arthritis, osteoporosis with celiac disease, or presentation with T cell lymphoma) or even mortality (e.g., death from cerebral edema at onset of T1D, or hypotensive crisis of Addison's disease). As the field of "personalized" medicine progresses, utilizing knowledge of personal risk factors (genetic, laboratory, clinical) to guide individual care, we believe that early detection of autoimmune disease risk will be increasingly important and will depend on improved tests as well as the development of preventive therapies.

ACKNOWLEDGMENTS

Research was supported by NIH grants DK 32083, DK 32493, A139213 and S-M01-RR00051 (Clinical Research Centers Program) and Diabetes Endocrine Research Center (P30 DK57516 from NIH; JDF grant 1-1999-679), Children's Diabetes Foundation, Autoimmunity Center of Excellence (U19 A146374) and Autoimmunity Prevention Center (U19 A150864).

REFERENCES

Aho, K., Heliövaara, M., Maatela, J., Tuomi, T., Palosuo, T., 1991. Rheumatoid factors antedating clinical rheumatoid arthritis. J. Rheumatol. 18, 1282–1284.

Allen, H.F., Jeffers, B.W., Klingensmith, G.J., Chase, H.P., 1993. First-phase insulin release in normal children. J. Pediatr. 123, 733–738.

Allen, M., Sandberg-Wollheim, M., Sjögren, K., Erlich, H.A., Petterson, U., Gyllensten, U., 1994. Association of susceptibility to multiple sclerosis in Sweden with HLA class II DRB1 and DQB1 alleles. Hum. Immunol. 39, 41–48.

Anderson, J.R., Goudie, R.B., Gray, K.G., Timbury, G.C., 1957. Autoantibodies in Addison's disease. Lancet. 272, 1123–1124.

Ansaldi, N., Palmas, T., Corrias, A., Barbato, M., D'Altiglia, M.R., Campanozzi, A., et al., 2003. Autoimmune thyroid disease and celiac disease in children. J. Pediatr. Gastroenterol. Nutr. 37, 63–66.

Arslanian, S., Austin, A., 1993. Determinants of first and second phase insulin secretion in healthy adolescents. Pediatr. Res. 3, S74.

Baker, P.R., Baschal, E.E., Fain, P.R., Nanduri, P., Triolo, T.M., Siebert, J.C., et al., 2011. Dominant suppression of Addison's disease associated with HLA-B15. J. Clin. Endocrinol. Metab. 96, 2154–2162.

Baker, P.R., Nanduri, P., Gottlieb, P.A., Yu, L., Klingensmith, G.J., Eisenbarth, G.S., et al., 2012. Predicting the onset of Addison's disease: ACTH, renin, cortisol, and 21-hydroxylase autoantibodies. Clin. Endocrinol. (Oxf). 76, 617–624.

Bao, F., Yu, L., Babu, S., Wang, T., Hoffenberg, E.J., Rewers, M., et al., 1999. One third of HLA DQ2 homozygous patients with type 1 diabetes express celiac disease associated transglutaminase autoantibodies. J. Autoimmun. 13, 143–148.

Barcellos, L.F., Oksenberg, J.R., Begovich, A.B., Martin, E.R., Schmidt, S., Vittinghoff, E., et al., 2003. HLA-DR2 dose effect on susceptibility to multiple sclerosis and influence on disease course. Am. J. Hum. Genet. 72, 710–716.

Barker, J.M., Barriga, K.J., Yu, L., Miao, D., Erlich, H.A., Norris, J.M., et al., 2004. Prediction of autoantibody positivity and progression to type 1 diabetes: Diabetes Autoimmunity Study in the Young (DAISY). J. Clin. Endocrinol. Metab. 89, 3896–3902.

Barker, J.M., Goehrig, S.H., Barriga, K., Hoffman, M., Slover, R., Eisenbarth, G.S., et al., 2004. Clinical characteristics of children diagnosed with type 1 diabetes through intensive screening and follow-up. Diab. Care. 27, 1399–1404.

Baumann-Antczak, A., Wedlock, N., Bednarek, J., Kiso, Y., Krishnan, H., Fowler, S., et al., 1992. Autoimmune Addison's disease and 21-hydroxylase. Lancet. 340, 429–430.

Bell, G.I., Horita, S., Karam, J.H., 1984. A polymorphic locus near the human insulin gene is associated with insulin-dependent diabetes mellitus. Diabetes. 33, 176–183.

Bennet, S.T., Wilson, A.J., Esposito, L., Bouzekri, N., Undlien, D.E., Cucca, F., et al., 1997. Insulin VNTR allele-specific effect in type 1 diabetes depends on identity of untransmitted paternal allele. Nat. Genet. 17, 350–352.

Betterle, C., Dal Pra, C., Mantero, F., Zanchetta, R., 2002. Autoimmune adrenal insufficiency and autoimmune polyendocrine syndromes: autoantibodies, autoantigens, and their applicability in diagnosis and disease prediction. Endocr Rev. 23, 327–364.

Bingley, P.J., Colman, P., Eisenbarth, G.S., Jackson, R.A., McCulloch, D.K., Riley, W.J., et al., 1992. Standardization of IVGTT to predict IDDM. Diab. Care. 15, 1313–1316.

Bleich, D., Jackson, R.A., Soeldner, J.S., Eisenbarth, G.S., 1990. Analysis of metabolic progression to type I diabetes in ICA+ relatives of patients with type I diabetes. Diab. Care. 13, 111–118.

Boehm, B.O., Kühnl, P., Löliger, C., Ketzler-Sasse, U., Holzberger, G., Seidl, S., et al., 1993. HLA-DR3 and HLA-DR5 confer risk for autoantibody positivity against the thyroperoxidase (mic-TPO) antigen in healthy blood donors. Clin. Invest. 71, 221–225.

Bonamico, M., Nenna, R., Montuori, M., Luparia, R.P., Turchetti, A., Mennini, M., et al., 2011. First salivary screening of celiac disease by detection of anti-transglutaminase autoantibody radioimmunoassay in 5000 Italian primary schoolchildren. J. Pediatr Gastroenterol Nutr. 52, 17–20.

Bonifacio, E., Bingley, P.J., Shattock, M., Dean, B.M., Dunger, D., Gale, E.A., et al., 1990. Quantification of islet-cell antibodies and prediction of insulin-dependent diabetes. Lancet. 335, 147–149.

Bottazzo, G.F., Dean, B.M., Gorsuch, A.N., Cudworth, A.G., Doniach, D., 1980. Complement-fixing islet-cell antibodies in type-I diabetes: possible monitors of active beta-cell damage. Lancet. 8179, 668–670.

Bottini, N., Musumeci, L., Alonso, A., Rahmouni, S., Nika, K., Rostamkhani, M., et al., 2004. A functional variant of lymphoid tyrosine phosphatase is associated with type I diabetes. Nat. Genet. 36, 337–338.

Brewer, K.W., Parziale, V.S., Eisenbarth, G.S., 1997. Screening patients with insulin-dependent diabetes mellitus for adrenal insufficiency. N. Engl. J. Med. 337, 202.

Chase, H.P., Garg, S.K., Butler-Simon, N., Klingensmith, G., Norris, L., Ruskey, C.T., et al., 1991. Prediction of the course of pre-type I diabetes. J. Pediatr. 118, 838–841.

Christiansen, F.T., Zhang, W.J., Griffiths, M., Mallal, S.A., Dawkins, R.L., 1991. Major histocompatibility complex (MHC) complement deficiency, ancestral haplotypes and systemic lupus erythematosus (SLE): C4 deficiency explains some but not all of the influence of the MHC. J. Rheumatol. 18, 1350–1358.

Dang, M., Rockell, J., Wagner, R., Wenzlau, J.M., Yu, L., Hutton, J.C., et al., 2011. Human type 1 diabetes is associated with T cell autoimmunity to zinc transporter 8. J. Immunol. 186, 6056–6063.

De Vitis, I., Ghirlanda, G., Gasbarrini, G., 1996. Prevalence of coeliac disease in type I diabetes: a multicentre study. Acta Paediatr. Suppl. 412, 56–57.

Deane, K.D., Norris, J.M., Holers, V.M., 2010. Preclinical rheumatoid arthritis: identification, evaluation, and future directions for investigation. Rheum. Dis. Clin. North Am. 36, 213–241.

Dieterich, W., Ehnis, T., Bauer, M., Donner, P., Volta, U., Riecken, E.O., et al., 1997. Identification of tissue transglutaminase as the autoantigen of celiac disease. Nat. Med. 3, 797–801.

Eisenbarth, G.S., 1986. Type 1 diabetes mellitus. A chronic autoimmune disease. N. Engl. J. Med. 314, 1360–1368.

Elrefaei, M., Boose, K., McGee, M., Tarrant, T.K., Lin, F.C., Fine, J.P., et al., 2012. Second generation automated anti-CCP test better predicts the clinical diagnosis of rheumatoid arthritis. J. Clin. Immunol. 32, 131–137.

Énée, É., Kratzer, R., Arnoux, J.B., Barilleau, E., Hamel, Y., Marchi, C., et al., 2012. ZnT8 is a major CD8 + T cell-recognized autoantigen in pediatric type 1 diabetes. Diabetes. 61, 1779–1784.

Erlich, H.A., Zeidler, A., Chang, J., Shaw, S., Raffel, L.J., Klitz, W., et al., 1993. HLA class II alleles and susceptibility and resistance to insulin dependent diabetes mellitus in Mexican-American families. Nat Genet. 3, 358–364.

Falorni, A., Laureti, S., Nikoshkov, A., Picchio, M.L., Hallengren, B., Vandewalle, C.L., et al., 1997. 21-hydroxylase autoantibodies in adult patients with endocrine autoimmune diseases are highly specific for Addison's disease. Clin. Exp. Immunol. 107, 341–346.

Falorni, A., Chen, S., Zanchetta, R., Yu, L., Tiberti, C., Bacosi, M.L., et al., 2011. Measuring adrenal autoantibody response: interlaboratory concordance in the first international serum exchange for the determination of 21-hydroxylase autoantibodies. Clin. Immunol. 140, 291–299.

Fasano, A., Catassi, C., 2001. Current approaches to diagnosis and treatment of celiac disease: an evolving spectrum. Gastroenterology. 120, 636–651.

Füchtenbusch, M., Ferber, K., Standl, E., Ziegler, A.G., 1997. Prediction of type 1 diabetes postpartum in patients with gestational diabetes mellitus by combined islet cell autoantibody screening: a prospective multicenter study. Diabetes. 46, 1459–1467.

Gambelunghe, G., Falorni, A., Ghaderi, M., Laureti, S., Tortoioli, C., Santeusanio, F., et al., 1999. Microsatellite polymorphism of the MHC class I chain-related (MIC-A and MIC-B) genes marks the risk for autoimmune Addison's disease. J. Clin. Endocrinol. Metab. 84, 3701–3707.

Gardner, S.G., Gale, E.A., Williams, A.J., Gillespie, K.M., Lawrence, K.E., Bottazzo, G.F., et al., 1999. Progression to diabetes in relatives with islet autoantibodies. Is it inevitable? Diab. Care. 22, 2049–2054.

Gillett, P.M., Gillett, H.R., Israel, D.M., Metzger, D.L., Stewart, L., Chanoine, J.P., et al., 2001. High prevalence of celiac disease in patients with type 1 diabetes detected by antibodies to endomysium and tissue transglutaminase. Can. J. Gastroenterol. 15, 297–301.

Goldbach-Mansky, R., Lee, J., McCoy, A., Hoxworth, J., Yarboro, C., Smolen, J.S., et al., 2000. Rheumatoid arthritis associated autoantibodies in patients with synovitis of recent onset. Arthritis Res. 2, 236–243.

Greenbaum, C.J., Palmer, J.P., Nagataki, S., Yamaguchi, Y., Molenaar, J.L., Van Beers, W.A., et al., 1992. Improved specificity of ICA assays in the Fourth International Immunology of Diabetes Serum Exchange Workshop. Diabetes. 41, 1570–1574.

Hall, M.A., et al., 1991. Coeliac disease study. Eleventh International Histocompatibility Workshop 6.5, 722–729.

Halldórsdóttir, H.D., Jónsson, T., Thorsteinsson, J., Valdimarsson, H., 2000. A prospective study on the incidence of rheumatoid arthritis among people with persistent increase of rheumatoid factor. Ann. Rheum. Dis. 59, 149–151.

Hill, J.A., Southwood, S., Sette, A., Jevnikar, A.M., Bell, D.A., Cairns, E., 2003. Cutting edge: the conversion of arginine to citrulline allows for a high-affinity peptide interaction with the rheumatoid arthritis-associated HLA-DRB1*0401 MHC class II molecule. J. Immunol. 171, 538–541.

Hollowell, J.G., Staehling, N.W., Flanders, W.D., Hannon, W.H., Gunter, E.W., Spencer, C.A., et al., 2002. Serum TSH, T(4), and thyroid antibodies in the United States population (1988 to 1994): National Health and Nutrition Examination Survey (NHANES III). J. Clin. Endocrinol. Metab. 87, 489–499.

Hoffenberg, E.J., MacKenzie, T., Barriga, K.J., Eisenbarth, G.S., Bao, F., Haas, J.E., et al., 2003. A prospective study of the incidence of childhood celiac disease. J. Pediatr. 143, 308–314.

Hue, S., Monteiro, R.C., Berrih-Aknin, S., Caillat-Zucman, S., 2003. Potential role of NKG2D/MHC class I-related chain A interaction in intrathymic maturation of single-positive CD8 T cells. J. Immunol. 171, 1909–1917.

Ignat, G.P., Rat, A.C., Sychra, J.J., Vo, J., Varga, J., Teodorescu, M., 2003. Information on diagnosis and management of systemic lupus erythematosus derived from the routine measurement of 8 nuclear autoantibodies. J. Rheumatol. 30, 1761–1769.

Jackson, R.A., Soeldner, J.S., Eisenbarth, G.S., 1988. Predicting insulin-dependent diabetes. Lancet. 8611, 627–628.

Kasperlik-Zaluska, A.A., Czarnocka, B., Czech, W., Walecki, J., Makowska, A.M., Brzeziński, J., et al., 1998. Secondary adrenal insufficiency associated with autoimmune disorders: a report of twenty-five cases. Clin. Endocrinol. (Oxf.) 49, 779–783.

Keskinen, P., Korhonen, S., Kupila, A., Veijola, R., Erkkilä, S., Savolainen, H., et al., 2002. First-phase insulin response in young healthy children at genetic and immunological risk for type I diabetes. Diabetologia 45, 1639–1648.

Kim, E.Y., Shin, C.H., Yang, S.W., 2003. Polymorphisms of HLA class II predispose children and adolescents with type 1 diabetes mellitus to autoimmune thyroid disease. J. Autoimmun. 36, 177–181.

Kupila, A., Muona, P., Simell, T., Arvilommi, P., Savolainen, H., Hämäläinen, A.M., et al., 2001. Feasibility of genetic and immunological prediction of type I diabetes in a population-based birth cohort. Diabetologia. 44, 290–297.

Laaksonen, M., Pastinen, T., Sjöroos, M., Kuokkanen, S., Ruutiainen, J., Sumelahti, M.L., et al., 2002. HLA class II associated risk and protection against multiple sclerosis—a Finnish family study. J. Neuroimmunol. 122, 140–145.

LaGasse, J.M., Brantley, M.S., Leech, N.J., Rowe, R.E., Monks, S., Palmer, J.P., et al., 2002. Successful prospective prediction of type 1 diabetes in schoolchildren through multiple defined autoantibodies: an 8-year follow-up of the Washington State Diabetes Prediction Study. Diab Care. 25, 505–511.

Le Loët, X., Strotz, V., Lequerré, T., Boumier, P., Pouplin, S., Mejjad, O., et al., 2011. Combining anti-cyclic citrullinated peptide with the American College of Rheumatology 1987 criteria failed to improve early rheumatoid arthritis diagnosis in the community-based very early arthritis cohort. Rheumatology. 50, 1901–1907.

Liu, E., Bao, F., Barriga, K., Miao, D., Yu, L., Erlich, H.A., et al., 2003. Fluctuating transglutaminase autoantibodies are related to histologic features of celiac disease. Clin. Gastroenterol. Hepatol. 1, 356–362.

Landewe, R.B., Boers, M., Verhoeven, A.C., Westhovens, R., van de Laar, M.A., Markusse, H.M., et al., 2002. COBRA combination therapy in patients with early rheumatoid arthritis: long-term structural benefits of a brief intervention. Arthritis Rheum. 46, 347–356.

Lendrum, R., Walker, G., Gamble, D.R., 1975. Islet-cell antibodies in juvenile diabetes mellitus of recent onset. Lancet. i, 880–883.

Lowe, R., Graham, J., Sund, G., Kockum, I., Landin-Olsson, M., Schaefer, J.B., et al., 2000. The length of the CTLA-4 microsatellite (AT)N-repeat affects the risk for type 1 diabetes. Diabetes Incidence in Sweden Study Group. Autoimmunity. 32, 173–180.

MacLaren, N., Lan, M., Coutant, R., Schatz, D., Silverstein, J., Muir, A., et al., 1999. Only multiple autoantibodies to islet cells (ICA), insulin, GAD65, IA-2 and IA-2beta predict immune-mediated (Type 1) diabetes in relatives. J. Autoimmun. 12, 279–287.

Majka, D.S., Holers, V.M., 2003. Can we accurately predict the development of rheumatoid arthritis in the preclinical phase? Arthritis Rheum. 48, 2701–2705.

Nerup, J., Platz, P., Andersen, O.O., Christy, M., Lyngsoe, J., Poulsen, J.E., et al., 1974. HL-A antigens and diabetes mellitus. Lancet. 7885, 864–866.

Nielen, M.M., van Schaardenburg, D., Reesink, H.W., van de Stadt, R.J., van der Horst-Bruinsma, I.E., de Koning, M.H., et al., 2004. Specific autoantibodies precede the symptoms of rheumatoid arthritis: a study of serial measurements in blood donors. Arthritis Rheum. 50, 380–386.

Noble, J.A., Valdes, A.M., Cook, M., Klitz, W., Thomson, G., Erlich, H.A., 1996. The role of HLA class II genes in insulin-dependent diabetes mellitus: molecular analysis of 180 Caucasian, multiplex families. Am. J. Hum Genet. 59, 1134–1148.

Nistico, L., Buzzetti, R., Pritchard, L.E., Van der Auwera, B., Giovannini, C., Bosi, E., et al., 1996. The CTLA-4 gene region of chromosome 2q33 is linked to, and associated with, type 1 diabetes. Belgian Diabetes Registry. Hum. Mol. Genet. 5, 1075–1080.

Panagiotopoulos, C., Qin, H., Tan, R., Verchere, C.B., 2003. Identification of a beta-cell-specific HLA class I restricted epitope in type 1 diabetes. Diabetes. 52, 2647–2651.

Pearce, S.H., Leech, N.J., 2004. Toward precise forecasting of autoimmune endocrinopathy. J. Clin. Endocrinol. Metab. 89, 544–547.

Peterson, P., Salmi, H., Hyöty, H., Miettinen, A., Ilonen, J., Reijonen, H., et al., 1997. Steroid 21-hydroxylase autoantibodies in insulin-dependent diabetes mellitus. Childhood Diabetes in Finland (DiMe) Study Group. Clin. Immunol. Immunopathol. 82, 37–42.

Park, Y.S., Sanjeevi, C.B., Robles, D., Yu, L., Rewers, M., Gottlieb, P.A., et al., 2002. Additional association of intra-MHC genes, MICA and D6S273, with Addison's disease. Tissue Antigens. 60, 155–163.

Pugliese, A., Gianani, R., Moromisato, R., Awdeh, Z.L., Alper, C.A., Erlich, H.A., et al., 1995. HLA-DQB1*0602 is associated with dominant protection from diabetes even among islet cell antibody-positive first-degree relatives of patients with IDDM. Diabetes. 44, 608–613.

Rantapää-Dahlqvist, S., de Jong, B.A., Berglin, E., Hallmans, G., Wadell, G., Stenlund, H., et al., 2003. Antibodies against cyclic citrullinated peptide and IgA rheumatoid factor predict the development of rheumatoid arthritis. Arthritis Rheum. 48, 2741–2749.

Redondo, M.J., Fain, P.R., Eisenbarth, G.S., 2001. Genetics of type 1A diabetes. Recent. Prog. Horm.Res. 56, 69—89.

Reijonen, H., Kwok, W.W., Nepom, G.T., 2003. Detection of CD4+ autoreactive T cells in T1D using HLA class II tetramers. Ann. N.Y. Acad. Sci. 1005, 82—87.

Reijonen, H., Novak, E.J., Kochik, S., Heninger, A., Liu, A.W., Kwok, W.W., et al., 2002. Detection of GAD65-specific T-cells by major histocompatibility complex class II tetramers in type 1 diabetic patients and at-risk subjects. Diabetes. 51, 1375—1382.

Rewers, M., Bugawan, T.L., Norris, J.M., Blair, A., Beaty, B., Hoffman, M., et al., 1996. Newborn screening for HLA markers associated with IDDM: diabetes autoimmunity study in the young (DAISY). Diabetologia. 39, 807—812.

Santamaria, P., Barbosa, J.J., Lindstrom, A.L., Lemke, T.A., Goetz, F. C., Rich, S.S., 1994. HLA-DQB1-associated susceptibility that distinguishes Hashimoto's thyroiditis from Graves' disease in type I diabetic patients. J. Clin. Endocrinol. Metab. 78, 878—883.

Silman, A.J., Pearson, J.E., 2002. Epidemiology and genetics of rheumatoid arthritis. Arthritis Res. 4, S265—S272.

Smith, C.P., Tarn, A.C., Thomas, J.M., Overkamp, D., Corakci, A., Savage, M.O., et al., 1988. Between and within subject variation of the first phase insulin response to intravenous glucose. Diabetologia. 31, 123—125.

Sosenko, J.M., Krischer, J.P., Palmer, J.P., Mahon, J., Cowie, C., Greenbaum, C.J., et al., 2008. A risk score for type 1 diabetes derived from autoantibody-positive participants in the diabetes prevention trial-type 1. Diab. Care. 31, 528—533.

Suzuki, A., Yamada, R., Chang, X., Tokuhiro, S., Sawada, T., Suzuki, M., et al., 2003. Functional haplotypes of PADI4, encoding citrullinating enzyme peptidylarginine deiminase 4, are associated with rheumatoid arthritis. Nat Genet. 34, 395—402.

Sumnik, Z., Drevínek, P., Snajderová, M., Kolousková, S., Sedláková, P., Pechová, M., et al., 2003. HLA-DQ polymorphisms modify the risk of thyroid autoimmunity in children with type 1 diabetes mellitus. J. Pediatr. Endocrinol. Metab. 16, 851—858.

Tillil, H., Kobberling, J., 1987. Age-corrected empirical genetic risk estimates for first-degree relatives of IDDM patients. Diabetes. 36, 93—99.

Umpierrez, G.E., Latif, K.A., Murphy, M.B., Lambeth, H.C., Stentz, F., Bush, A., et al., 2003. Thyroid dysfunction in patients with type 1 diabetes: a longitudinal study. Diab. Care. 26, 1181—1185.

Vakeva, A., Kontiainen, S., Miettinen, A., Schlenzka, A., Mäenpää, J., 1992. Thyroid peroxidase antibodies in children with autoimmune thyroiditis. J. Clin. Pathol. 45, 106—109.

Vanderpump, M.P., Tunbridge, W.M., French, J.M., Appleton, D., Bates, D., Clark, F., et al., 1995. The incidence of thyroid disorders in the community: a twenty-year follow-up of the Whickham Survey. Clin. Endocrinol. 43, 55—68.

Verge, C.F., Gianani, R., Kawasaki, E., Yu, L., Pietropaolo, M., Jackson, R.A., et al., 1996. Prediction of type I diabetes in first-degree relatives using a combination of insulin, GAD, and ICA512bdc/IA-2 autoantibodies. Diabetes. 45, 926—933.

Vossenaar, E.R., Zendman, A.J., van Venrooij, W.J., Pruijn, G.J., 2003. PAD, a growing family of citrullinating enzymes: genes, features and involvement in disease. Bioessays. 25, 1106—1118.

Vossenaar, E.R., Zendman, A.J., van Venrooij, W.J., 2004. Citrullination, a possible functional link between susceptibility genes and rheumatoid arthritis. Arthritis Res. Ther. 6, 1—5.

Winqvist, O., Karlsson, F.A., Kämpe, O., 1992. 21-Hydroxylase, a major autoantigen in idiopathic Addison's disease. Lancet. 339, 1559—1562.

Yu, J., Yu, L., Bugawan, T.L., Erlich, H.A., Barriga, K., Hoffman, M., et al., 2000. Transient anti-islet autoantibodies: infrequent occurrence and lack of association with genetic risk factors. J. Clin. Endocrinol. Metab. 85, 2421—2428.

Yu, L., Brewer, K.W., Gates, S., Wu, A., Wang, T., Babu, S.R., et al., 1999. DRB1*04 and DQ alleles: expression of 21-hydroxylase autoantibodies and risk of progression to Addison's disease. J. Clin. Endocrinol. Metab. 84, 328—335.

Yamamoto, A.M., Amoura, Z., Johannet, C., Jeronimo, A.L., Campos, H., Koutouzov, S., et al., 2000. Quantitative radioligand assays using de novo-synthesized recombinant autoantigens in connective tissue diseases: new tools to approach the pathogenic significance of anti-RNP antibodies in rheumatic diseases. Arthritis Rheum. 43, 689—698.

Yu, L., Cuthbertson, D.D., Maclaren, N., Jackson, R., Palmer, J.P., Orban, T., et al., 2001. Expression of GAD65 and islet cell antibody (ICA512) autoantibodies among cytoplasmic ICA + relatives is associated with eligibility for the Diabetes Prevention Trial-Type 1. Diabetes. 2001 (50), 1735—1740.

Yu, L., Boulware, D.C., Beam, C.A., Hutton, J.C., Wenzlau, J.M., Greenbaum, C.J., et al., 2012. Zinc transporter-8 autoantibodies improve prediction of type 1 diabetes in relatives positive for the standard biochemical autoantibodies. Diab. Care. 35, 1213—1218.

Yu, L., Dong, F., Miao, D., Fouts, A.R., Wenzlau, J.M., Steck, A.K., 2013. Proinsulin/Insulin autoantibodies measured with electrochemiluminescent assay are the earliest indicator of prediabetic islet autoimmunity. Diab. Care. 36, 2266—2270.

Zelissen, P.M., Bast, E.J.E.G., Croughs, R.J.M., 1995. Associated autoimmunity in Addison's disease. J. Autoimmun. 8, 121—130.

Ziegler, R., Alper, C.A., Awdeh, Z.L., Castano, L., Brink, S.J., Soeldner, J.S., et al., 1991. Specific association of HLA-DR4 with increased prevalence and level of insulin autoantibodies in first-degree relatives of patients with type1 diabetes. Diabetes. 40, 709—714.

Ziegler, R., Alper, C.A., Awdeh, Z.L., Castano, L., Brink, S.J., Soeldner, J.S., et al., 1991. Specific association of HLA-DR4 with increased prevalence and level of insulin autoantibodies in first-degree relatives of patients with type 1 diabetes. Diabetes. 40, 709—714.

Chapter 79

Prevention of Autoimmune Disease: The Type 1 Diabetes Paradigm

Leonard C. Harrison and John M. Wentworth

Walter & Eliza Hall Institute of Medical Research, Royal Parade, Parkville, Victoria, Australia

Chapter Outline

Introduction	1191	Mucosa-mediated Antigen-specific Tolerance	1200
People at Risk for Type 1 Diabetes	1196	Trials of Islet Autoantigen-specific Vaccination in	
Primary Prevention	1198	Humans	1200
Diet and the Intestinal Environment	1198	Epilogue	1203
Viruses	1199	Acknowledgments	1203
Secondary Prevention	1199	References	1203

INTRODUCTION

Autoimmune disease can be prevented to varying degrees in rodent models housed under standardized experimental conditions, by a range of approaches including autoantigen-specific induction of immune tolerance (reviewed in Faria and Weiner, 1999; Harrison and Hafler, 2000; Krause et al., 2000). However, translation to outbred, free-living human populations remains a major challenge and has not yet met with success. Possible reasons for this are discussed later. No potential therapeutic approach to prevention can be assumed initially to be completely safe and therefore prevention is predicated on the ability to identify, with a high degree of positive prediction, individuals likely to progress to clinical disease. It has been known since the 1980s that disease-associated autoantibodies presage the clinical onset of autoimmune thyroid disease, type 1 diabetes (T1D), systemic lupus, primary biliary cirrhosis, celiac disease, and other autoimmune diseases (reviewed in Leslie et al., 2001; Rose, 2008). However, refinement of autoantibody-based disease prediction by longitudinal studies of genetically susceptible individuals, leading to the selection of participants for prevention trials, has only been accomplished in T1D, partly because of the nature of the disease itself and partly due to the concerted efforts of T1D investigators and their supporters.

T1D is currently the best paradigm for autoimmune disease prevention, and the approaches developed in T1D are applicable to other autoimmune diseases. In T1D, susceptibility to autoimmune-mediated destruction of the insulin-secreting beta cells in the pancreatic islets is polygenic but dominated by genes in the major histocompatibility complex, and (increasingly) enhanced by the environment. In the majority of cases, T1D begins months to years before major loss of β cell function leads to hyperglycemia and symptoms (Figure 79.1). Progress in understanding mechanisms of β cell destruction, the ability to identify individuals at high risk for T1D, and proof-of-principle for preventive therapies in the non-obese diabetic (NOD) mouse model have set the scene for prevention of T1D in humans. Arresting immune-mediated β cell damage is relevant not only to individuals at risk but to those with clinical diabetes, in order to preserve residual β cell function, permit possible β cell regeneration, and prevent recurrent autoimmune disease after therapeutic β cell replacement or regeneration.

Experiments in rodent models have contributed substantially to our understanding of the pathogenesis of T1D and the expectation that it should be preventable (Leiter et al., 1987). The inbred, NOD mouse, the most widely used animal model of T1D, shares many features with human T1D, including polygenic inheritance dominated by genes for antigen-presenting major

N. Rose & I. Mackay (Eds): The Autoimmune Diseases, Fifth edition. DOI: http://dx.doi.org/10.1016/B978-0-12-384929-8.00079-4

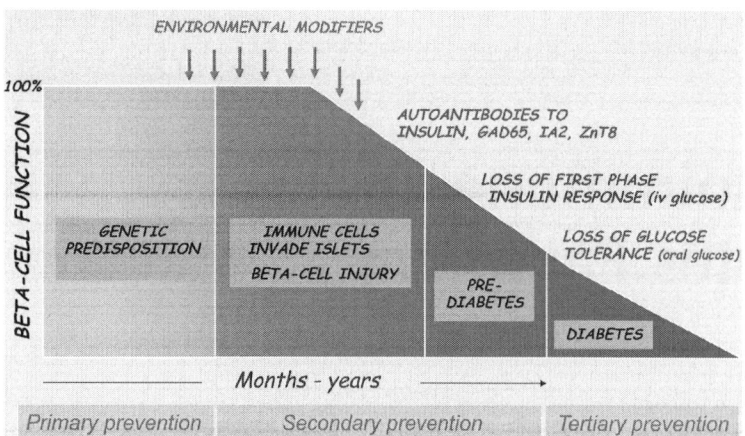

FIGURE 79.1 The natural history of type 1 diabetes.

histocompatibility complex (MHC) and other immune molecules, autoimmunity to insulin and glutamic acid decarboxylase (GAD), transfer of disease by bone marrow, and a protracted preclinical stage (Adorini et al., 2002). Many immune and other interventions reduce the incidence of diabetes in NOD mice (Atkinson and Leiter, 1999), but few totally prevent disease and many are ethically unsuitable in humans. Ideally, the burden of T1D and other autoimmune diseases would be reduced by primary prevention aimed at the environmental factors thought to precipitate disease in genetically at-risk individuals. Recent evidence implicates the contemporary "obesogenic" environment as a risk factor not only for T2D but also T1D (Wentworth et al., 2009). The incidence of T1D is increasing, particularly in overweight individuals with lower risk genes (Fourlanos et al., 2008), and insulin resistance, associated with obesity, is a risk factor for progression to clinical disease in individuals with preclinical islet autoimmunity (Fourlanos et al., 2004). Population-wide strategies to prevent obesity are therefore applicable to the prevention of both T2D and T1D.

Prevention strategies are likely to be most effective early in preclinical autoimmune disease, yet at that time prediction is less exact. Whether to intervene early or later when prediction is more certain but intervention less likely to be effective hinges on the balance of safety and efficacy. Potentially toxic immunosuppressive agents used (for "tertiary prevention") after the clinical presentation of systemic autoimmune diseases such as lupus erythematosus or rheumatoid arthritis could well be effective in stemming islet autoimmunity but are generally ethically unacceptable in asymptomatic individuals, especially children at risk of T1D. On the other hand, other agents such as autoantigens administered to induce immune tolerance, while relatively safe, may be ineffective later in preclinical disease. With the onset of clinical diabetes the safety versus efficacy dilemma is less of an

issue, but the major loss of β cell function and mass at this time militates against efficacy. However, if conventional immunosuppressive agents could decrease the burden of pathogenic, effector T cells at the onset of clinical T1D this may allow induction of efficacious protective immune tolerance, and the potential for β cell recovery and possible regeneration.

Secondary prevention after onset of the autoimmune disease process but before clinical diagnosis and tertiary prevention after diagnosis (or intervention) have received considerable attention. Individuals at high risk for T1D can be identified by the presence of circulating autoantibodies to pancreatic islet autoantigens, allowing for the possibility of secondary prevention. However, the number of candidate agents that meet scientific and ethical criteria for trials in such at-risk individuals is limited, and recruiting these individuals is a major logistical exercise. Consequently, of the many clinical trials undertaken for "prevention" of T1D since the 1980s most have been tertiary trials in individuals with recent-onset T1D. A comprehensive listing of these trials is provided (Table 79.1), in which classification by agent necessitates combining the categories of secondary and tertiary prevention. The primary outcome measure in primary and secondary trials is (the absence of) clinical diabetes; in tertiary trials it is residual β cell function, measured by the increase in plasma C-peptide after either i.v. glucagon or a mixed meal tolerance test. C-peptide is secreted in equimolar proportions to insulin following cleavage of proinsulin in the β cell and is a surrogate for insulin when exogenous insulin or insulin antibodies could interfere with the measurement of endogenous insulin. A number of agents (from azathioprine to cyclosporine to monoclonal antibodies against CD3 and CD20) have been shown to slow the decline of β cell function after diagnosis, but their effect was transient and without ultimate clinical benefit (Table 79.1). Here we will adhere to the strict

TABLE 79.1 Trials for Prevention of T1D

	Participants (n)	Follow-up (months)	Outcome	Reference
Primary Prevention				
Gluten elimination	AR (7)	24	No effect on islet antibody levels.	Hummel et al. (2002)
Cows' milk elimination (trial to reduce IDDM in the genetically at-risk TRIGR)	HLA at-risk infants (230)	120	Reduced incidence of islet autoantibodies; similar incidence of diabetes.	Hummel et al. (2011)
Cows' milk elimination (multicenter TRIGR)	HLA at-risk infants (2159)	120	Ongoing.	Knip et al. (2011)
Secondary and Tertiary Prevention				
Non-Specific Immune Suppression				
Azathioprine (2 mg/kg/day	RD (24)	12	Higher basal and glucagon-stimulated C-peptide, and more remissions.	Harrison et al. (1985)
Cyclosporine (7.5 mg/kg/day)	RD (122)	9	More remissions.	Feutren et al. (1986)
Azathioprine (2 mg/kg/day) + prednisolone (reducing dose)	RD (46)	12	Higher meal-stimulated C-peptide and lower insulin dose.	Silverstein et al. (1988)
Cyclosporine (20 mg/kg/day)	RD (188)	12	Higher glucagon C-peptide and more remissions, especially in recently diagnosed.	Canadian-European Randomized Control Trial Group (1988)
Azathioprine (2 mg/kg/day)	RD (49)	12	Higher meal-stimulated C-peptide.	Cook et al. (1989)
Azathioprine and thymostimulin	RD (45)	12	Higher glucagon-stimulated C-peptide and more remissions.	Moncada et al. (1990)
Cyclosporine	RD (219)	24	Higher meal stimulated C-peptide and more remissions.	Assan et al. (1990)
Cyclosporine (10 mg/kg/day, 4 months)	RD (43)	36	No difference in glucagon-stimulated C-peptide, HbA1C, or insulin dose.	Chase et al. (1990a)
Prednisolone (15 mg/day, 8 months); indomethacin (100 mg/day, 8 months)	RD (25)	24	Lower insulin dose and higher urine C-peptide in prednisolone group.	Secchi et al. (1990)
Cyclosporine (10 mg/kg/day)	RD (23)	12	Higher meal- but not glucagon- or glucose-stimulated C-peptide. No difference in insulin dose.	Skyler and Rabinovitch (1992)
Anti-CD5 mAb/ricin A chain (unblinded)	RD (15)	12	Higher meal-stimulated C-peptide.	Skyler et al. (1993)
Glucocorticoid	RD (32)	12	Higher glucagon-stimulated. C-peptide, but no remissions.	Goday et al. (1993)
Anti-CD4 mAb + glucocorticoid	RD (12)	12	No difference in insulin dose, or islet antibody titers.	Kohnert et al. (1996)
Methotrexate (unblinded)	RD (10)	36	No effect on basal or meal-stimulated C-peptide. Insulin dose higher.	Buckingham and Sandborg (2000)
Anti-CD3 mAb (hOKT3) (unblinded)	RD (18)	12	Increase in meal-stimulated C-peptide in first year. IL-10 detected in serum.	Herold et al. (2002)
Teplizumab (OKT3 (Ala-Ala) anti-CD3 mAb)	RD (42)	24	Improved C-peptide response to mixed meal, lower HbA1c, and reduced insulin dose.	Herold et al. (2005)
CH Agly anti-CD3 mAb	RD (80)	48	Improved C-peptide response to glucose. Clamp/glucagon up to 36 months. Reduced insulin dose with similar HbA1c.	Keymeulen et al. (2005, 2010)

(Continued)

TABLE 79.1 (Continued)

	Participants (n)	Follow-up (months)	Outcome	Reference
Mycophenolate mofetil ± daclizumab (anti-IL-2 receptor mAb) (MMF/DZB)	RD (126)	24	No effect on basal or meal-stimulated C-peptide. Similar HbA1c and insulin dose.	Gottlieb et al. (2010)
Rituximab (anti-CD20 mAb)	RD (87)	12	Increased C-peptide response to mixed meal. Reduced HbA1c and insulin dose.	Pescovitz et al. (2009)
IL-2 + rapamycin	RD (7)	12	Transient decrease in C-peptide response to mixed meal associated with increased numbers of circulating regulatory T cells.	Long et al. (2012)
Abatacept (anti-CTLA-4 mAb)	RD (112)	24	Increased C-peptide response to mixed meal. Reduced HbA1c and insulin dose.	Orban et al. (2011)
Teplizumab (OKT3 (Ala-Ala) anti-CD3 mAb)	RD (516)	12	No difference in HbA1c or insulin dose.	Sherry et al. (2011)
Canakinumab (anti-IL-1 mAb)	RD (69)	12	No effect on mixed meal-stimulated C-peptide	Moran et al. (2013)
Anakinra (IL-1 receptor antagonist)	RD (69)	9	No effect on mixed meal-stimulated C-peptide	Moran et al. (2013)
Teplizumab (OKT3 (Ala-Ala) anti-CD3)	AR (170)	48–72	Ongoing	TrialNet
Non-Specific Immune Stimulation				
BCG vaccine	RD (26)	18	No effect on glucagon-stimulated C-peptide, insulin dose, or HbA1c.	Elliott et al. (1998)
BCG vaccine	RD (94)	24	No effect on mixed meal-stimulated C-peptide, insulin dose, or HbA1c.	Allen et al. (1999)
Q fever vaccine	RD (39)	12	No effect on glucagon-stimulated C-peptide or insulin dose.	Schmidli R (unpublished)
Non-Specific Immune Regulation				
Thymopoietin	RD (32)	6	Lower insulin antibodies and insulin dose. More remissions. No difference in C-peptide or HbA1c.	Giordano et al. (1990)
Gammaglobulin	RD (16)	6	Higher basal C-peptide. Lower insulin dose, unchanged HbA1c.	Panto et al. (1990)
Linomide	RD (63)	12	Lower HbA1c and insulin dose. No difference in glucagon-stimulated C-peptide.	Coutant et al. (1998)
HSP60 p277 peptide (DiaPep)	RD (35)	10	Decrease in glucagon-stimulated C-peptide and insulin dose in placebo but not treated group.	Raz et al. (2001)
1,25-dihydroxy vitamin D3	RD (20)	18	No effect on C-peptide response to a mixed meal or insulin requirement.	Walter et al. (2010)
HSP60 p277 peptide (DiaPep)	RD (146)	12	No effect on C-peptide response to a mixed meal.	Buzzetti et al. (2011)
Antigen-Specific Immune Regulation				
Parenteral insulin (i.v. vs. s.c. 2 weeks)	RD (26)	12	Higher meal-stimulated C-peptide, lower HbA1c.	Shah et al. (1989)
Parenteral (s.c.) insulin	RD (49)	60	Higher glucagon-stimulated C-peptide and improved insulin sensitivity and glycemic control.	Linn et al. (1996)

(Continued)

TABLE 79.1 (Continued)

	Participants (n)	Follow-up (months)	Outcome	Reference
Parenteral insulin (i.v. vs. s.c. 2 weeks)	RD (19)	12	Higher meal and glucagon-stimulated C-peptide and lower HbA1c.	Schnell et al. (1997)
Parenteral (s.c.) insulin	RD (10)		Higher C-peptide response to oral glucose, HbA1C unchanged.	Kobayashi et al. (1996)
Parenteral (s.c.) insulin and sulfonylurea (glipizide)	RD (27)	12	Higher basal and glucagon-stimulated C-peptide, more remissions.	Selam et al. (1993)
Oral insulin	RD (80)	12	No effect on basal C-peptide, HbA1c, insulin dose, or insulin antibodies.	Pozzilli et al. (2000)
Oral insulin	RD (131)	12	No effect on basal, glucagon- or meal-stimulated C-peptide, HbA1c, insulin dose, or islet antibody levels.	Chaillous et al. (2000)
Parenteral (s.c.) insulin	AR (14)	84	Delay in onset of diabetes. No effect on islet antibody levels.	Füchtenbusch et al. (1998)
Parenteral (s.c.) insulin (Diabetes Prevention Trial Type 1—DPT-1)	AR (339)	44	No effect on diabetes development.	Diabetes Prevention Trial-Type 1 Diabetes Study Group (2002)
Intranasal insulin (Melbourne Intranasal Insulin Trial—INIT I)	AR (38)	48	Increased antibody and decreased T cell responses to insulin.	Harrison et al. (2004)
Oral insulin (DPT-1)	AR (372)	52	No effect on diabetes development overall. Post-hoc analysis revealed >4 year delay in diabetes onset in participants with insulin autoantibodies.	Skyler et al. (2005)
Parenteral (s.c.) insulin B chain in incomplete Freund's adjuvant	RD (12)	24	No effect on C-peptide response to mixed meal. Development of sustained insulin-specific antibody and T cell responses.	Orban et al. (2010)
Parenteral (s.c.) insulin B chain 9–23 "altered peptide ligand" NBI-6024-0101 ("Neurocrine")	RD (188)	25	No effect on C-peptide response to mixed meal.	Walter et al. (2009)
Intranasal insulin (Diabetes Prediction and Prevention Project—DIPP)	AR (224)	21	No effect to delay progression to diabetes.	Nanto-Salonen et al. (2008)
Intranasal insulin (Intranasal Insulin Trial II—INIT II)	AR (120)	60	Ongoing.	Harrison, L.C.
Intranasal insulin (Intranasal Insulin Trial III—INIT III)	RD (52)	24	No effect on metabolic parameters. Suppression of T cell responses to insulin and antibody responses to subcutaneous insulin.	Fourlanos et al. (2011)
Parenteral (s.c.) GAD65-alum	RD (47)	6	Increase in fasting and stimulated plasma C-peptide with intermediate dose of 20 micrograms.	Agardh et al. (2005)
Parenteral (s.c.) GAD65-alum	RD (70)	30		Ludvigsson et al. (2008)
Parenteral (s.c.) GAD65-alum	RD (334)	15	Delay in loss of C-peptide secretion, in those treated within 6 months of clinical diagnosis. No effect on metabolic parameters.	Ludvigsson et al. (2012)
Parenteral (s.c.) GAD65-alum	RD (145)	12	No effect on C-peptide response to mixed meal.	Wherrett et al. (2011)
Parenteral (i.m.) proinsulin plasmid DNA	RD (80)	12	Transient improvement in C-peptide response to mixed meal concomitant with a decrease in the CD8 T-cell response to proinsulin.	Roep, B.O.
Parenteral (s.c.) GAD65-alum	AR (50)	60	Ongoing.	Elding Larsson, H.

(Continued)

TABLE 79.1 (Continued)

	Participants (n)	Follow-up (months)	Outcome	Reference
Oral insulin (TrialNet Study TN07)	AR (300–400)	72–96	Ongoing.	TrialNet
β Cell Protection				
Nicotinamide	RD (20)	12	Higher glucagon-stimulated C-peptide at 45 days, then decline. No difference in remissions.	Mendola et al. (1989)
Nicotinamide	RD (23)	9	Higher basal and glucagon-stimulated C-peptide.	Vague et al. (1989)
Nicotinamide	RD (35)	12	No difference in basal or glucagon stimulated C-peptide	Chase et al. (1990b)
Nicotinamide	RD (56)	12	Higher glucagon-stimulated C-peptide in subjects >15 years old.	Pozzilli et al. (1995)
Nicotinamide ± cyclosporine	RD (90)	12	Lower insulin dose. No difference in remissions.	Pozzilli et al. (1994)
Nicotinamide ± parenteral insulin	RD (34)	12	No difference in glucagon-stimulated C-peptide.	Vidal et al. (2000)
Nicotinamide versus vitamin E (no control group)	RD (84)	12	No difference in basal or glucagon-stimulated C-peptide, HbA1c, or insulin dose.	Pozzilli et al. (1997)
Nicotinamide (Deutsche Nicotinamide Intervention Study—DENIS)	AR (55)	36	No effect on diabetes development.	Lampeter et al. (1998)
Nicotinamide (European Nicotinamide Diabetes Intervention Trial—ENDIT)	AR (552)		No effect on diabetes development.	Philips et al. (2002)
Octreotide	RD (20)	12	Higher glucagon-stimulated C-peptide at 6 and 12 months; no difference in HbA1c or insulin dose.	Grunt et al. (1994)
Diazoxide	RD adults (40)	18	Higher basal C-peptide.	Bjork et al. (1996)
Diazoxide	RD children (56)		Higher stimulated C-peptide at 12, not 24, months.	Bjork et al. (2001)
Antioxidants	RD (46)	30	No difference in meal-stimulated C-peptide, insulin dose, or HbA1c.	Ludvigsson et al. (2001)

Abbreviations: AR, islet autoantibody-positive first-degree relative; RD person with recently diagnosed diabetes. Participant numbers are shown in parentheses.

definition of prevention and discuss only studies attempting to prevent clinical T1D. All randomized primary, secondary, and tertiary trials are summarized in Table 79.1, and more recent trials are registered on ClinicalTrials.gov.

Progress in preventing T1D is likely to be incremental, analogous to the evolution of combination treatment regimens for cancer or HIV infection, but more constrained by regulatory considerations. T1D prevention trials have taught us that: treatment will need to begin as early as possible in the preclinical stage; monotherapy is unlikely to be successful; there is a pressing need for mechanistic immune markers, especially of islet autoantigen-reactive T cells, and for non-invasive means of evaluating islet pathology and β cell function.

PEOPLE AT RISK FOR TYPE 1 DIABETES

Neonatal screening for high-risk HLA class II susceptibility genes can identify over half of those destined to develop T1D (Kimpimäki et al., 2001). However, the modest predictive value of genetic testing would only justify a primary intervention that was safe, e.g., diet modification or vaccination. Secondary prevention has focused on first-degree relatives of a T1D proband, who have autoantibodies against one or more islet autoantigens:

insulin, glutamic acid decarboxylase mol. wt. 65,000 isoform (GAD65), tyrosine phosphatase-like insulinoma antigen 2 (IA-2), and zinc transporter 8 (Verge et al., 1996; Bingley et al., 1999; Colman et al., 2000; Harrison, 2001; Wenzlau et al., 2007). A prerequisite for intervention in asymptomatic individuals is a high likelihood of developing clinical disease. Prediction of risk is determined by measuring autoantibody and metabolic markers of T1D (Box 79.1). In young first-degree relatives, the 5-year risk of diabetes is of the order <25%, 25−50%, and >50% if autoantibodies are present to 1, 2, and 3 islet antigens, respectively. For single specificities, autoantibodies to insulin (IAA) are the most predictive. A measure of insulin secretion, first phase insulin response (FPIR) to intravenous glucose, further refines risk prediction. In addition, in autoantibody-positive relatives with normal FPIR, the highest risk was shown to be independently associated with insulin resistance (Fourlanos et al., 2004). This may reflect the increasing incidence of T1D in the "obesogenic" environment and has important implications for lifestyle approaches to prevention. Moreover, stratification of autoantibody-positive individuals based on insulin resistance deserves consideration in the design of prevention trials.

While detection of autoantibodies is fundamental to preclinical diagnosis and disease prediction, about 10% of new-onset T1D patients have no detectable antibodies. Moreover, while first-degree relatives who share susceptibility genes and environmental risk factors have at least a 10-fold higher prevalence of T1D than the background population they represent no more than 15% of people diagnosed with T1D. Identifying the other 85% using available predictive tests is more challenging because the lower prevalence of disease in the general population reduces the predictive value of screening tests compared to relatives (Bayes' theorem). The predictive value of islet autoantibodies in the general population has not been widely investigated but will be important if effective means of secondary prevention are found.

Population heterogeneity is a critical consideration in the design and interpretation of clinical trials. In addition to HLA genes, over 50 genetic loci are associated with classical, juvenile-onset T1D, but very little is known about how they contribute to disease development in different environments, or influence prevention strategies. Although a restricted set of HLA genes is shared among individuals with T1D, HLA-based heterogeneity in T1D progression and age at clinical presentation is well known (Honeyman et al., 1995; Tait et al., 1995). This suggests that T1D comprises disease subtypes and that prevention will most likely require a more "personalized" approach. Indeed, it is known that the natural history of declining β cell function after diagnosis depends on age, HLA status, autoimmune status including number and level of islet autoantibodies, residual β cell function, and insulin resistance (Greenbaum and Harrison, 2003). Inclusion of T1D relatives in secondary prevention trials has been based on age (<40) and islet autoantibodies (≥2), for a predicted 5-year incidence of ≈40%, but more refinement is possible by building subtype analysis into trial design. Up to 10% of adults presenting with diabetes have what appears to be a slowly progressive form of T1D, associated mainly with GAD65 autoantibodies, that initially is non-insulin-requiring (Hagopian et al., 1993; Tuomi et al., 1993; Gottsater et al., 1995; Turner et al., 1997). They have higher residual β cell function at diagnosis than younger patients with classical T1D, which implies a wider and perhaps more penetrable therapeutic window for secondary prevention (Fourlanos et al., 2005).

The "personalized" approach requires new robust surrogate assays of disease mechanisms to identify people most likely to benefit from a specific therapy and allow the design of more practical, cheaper, and efficient boutique trials, rather than larger, expensive trials powered on the endpoint of diabetes. The application of insulin as an immune tolerizing agent in T1D (see below) may afford an example. Considerable evidence implicates insulin as the key, primary autoantigen driving β cell destruction in the NOD mouse, and possibly in children with classic T1D (Narendran et al., 2003). The insulin locus (IDDM2) maps to a variable number of tandem repeats (VNTR) upstream of the proinsulin gene. Long (class III) and short (class I) VNTR alleles are associated, respectively, with lower and higher susceptibility to T1D (Bennett et al., 1995). The length of the VNTR correlates with the level of proinsulin gene transcription in the thymus (Pugliese et al., 1997) and in a peripheral population of myeloid cells (Narendran et al., 2006), and may determine the extent of deletion of proinsulin-specific T cells during their intra-thymic development. The frequency of proinsulin peptide-specific T cells in human blood was reciprocally related to VNTR length (Durinovic-Bello et al., 2010), although an earlier study (Sarugeri et al., 1998) found no association between VNTR allelism and immunity to insulin. Nevertheless, it remains to be determined if IDDM2 VNTR typing would identify individuals most likely to benefit from (pro)insulin-specific immunotherapy.

PRIMARY PREVENTION

Primary prevention targets environmental factors that could precipitate islet autoimmunity in genetically at-risk individuals. The evidence for an etiological role of environment in T1D is persuasive (Wentworth et al., 2009) but will not be detailed here.

Diet and the Intestinal Environment

The hypothesis that early exposure of the infant to cow's milk and/or the lack of breastfeeding predisposes to T1D dates from the 1980s. Two meta-analyses of multiple studies in which T1D prevalence was associated retrospectively with infant feeding revealed only a marginal increase in relative risk (Gerstein, 1994; Norris and Scott, 1996). In the Denver-based Diabetes Autoimmunity Study in the Young (DAISY), infant feeding patterns retrospectively analyzed up to 6 months of age were not related to the development of islet autoantibodies up to 7 years of age (Norris et al., 1996). In the Australian BabyDiab Study (Couper et al., 1999) and the German BabyDiab Study (Hummel et al., 2000), there was no association between infant feeding patterns and the development of islet autoantibodies. Nevertheless, to answer whether cows' milk exposure is a risk, the multi-country Trial to Reduce IDDM in the Genetically at-Risk (TRIGR) was initiated. Newborns with a T1D first-degree relative and with HLA risk alleles, initially exclusively breast-fed, have been randomized to either a casein hydrolysate formula ("Neutramigen") comprising milk proteins of reduced complexity or a conventional cows' milk-based formula until 6 to 8 months of age, and are being followed for 10 years. Initially, casein-based formula was reported to reduce the risk of developing islet autoantibodies (Knip et al., 2010), implying it provided protection against T1D, but TRIGR will not be completed until 2017. Whatever the outcome, it does not mean that milk formula is superior to breast milk for preventing T1D. We sought to reframe the cow's milk hypothesis around mucosal immune function in T1D (Harrison and Honeyman, 1999). The essential role of a normal mucosal immune system in maintaining immune homeostasis is illustrated by the effect of a germ-free versus conventional "dirty" environment on diabetes incidence in NOD mice. The incidence of spontaneous diabetes in NOD mice differs greatly between colonies around the world and appears to be inversely correlated with exposure to microbial infection (Pozzilli et al., 1993). The high incidence of diabetes in NOD mice housed under pathogen-free conditions is reduced by conventional conditions of housing and feeding (Suzuki, 1987; Funda et al., 2005). Under such conditions, bacterial colonization of the intestine is accompanied by maturation of mucosal immune function (Kawaguchi-Miyashita et al., 1996). Emerging evidence indicates that the gut microbiome differs in composition and function between children at risk for T1D and case controls (Brown et al., 2011). Supplementary to the microbiome, breast milk contains growth factors, cytokines and other immunomodulatory agents that promote functional maturation of the intestinal mucosa and mucosal immune system. Breast milk also contains endogenous insulin (Shehadeh et al., 2001), which could induce "oral tolerance" to insulin and so protect against the development of T1D (see below). Thus, rather than cows' milk promoting T1D, human milk could be protective, by immune maturational effects and/or by delivering human insulin to the "tolerogenic" mucosal immune system.

Dietary gluten has also been implicated as an environmental trigger of T1D. Antibodies to wheat gluten proteins are found in a proportion of T1D patients at the time of diagnosis (MacFarlane et al., 2002) and celiac disease and T1D share the HLA risk haplotype A1-B8-DR3-DQ2 and often coexist. In addition, the prevalence of autoimmune diseases, including T1D, in individuals with celiac disease was reported to correlate with duration of exposure to gluten (Ventura et al., 1999). However, in the German BABYDIET Study, delaying the introduction of gluten beyond 12 months of age had no effect on the cumulative incidence of islet autoantibodies or clinical T1D (Hummel et al., 2002). At the population level, compelling evidence links vitamin D deficiency to T1D and other autoimmune diseases. Vitamin D is derived primarily from ultraviolet B light-induced synthesis in the skin and its deficiency is increasingly recognized, not just in populations living furthest from the equator but in people anywhere who avoid sunlight, work and play mainly indoors, are dark-skinned and living in temperate climes, or cover their skin for cultural or religious reasons. The recommended daily allowance of vitamin D has decreased over the past 50 years from 5000 IU to 400 IU (Hypponen et al., 2001). This is the minimum dose required to prevent rickets following adequate prenatal intake but is inadequate for the physiological immune modulating and anti-inflammatory actions of vitamin D (Holick, 2004). Three European studies demonstrated an inverse relationship between vitamin D intake and the incidence of T1D. In a birth cohort study from northern Finland, an area with only 1900 hours' direct sunlight annually and the highest incidence of T1D in the world, T1D status was related to prerecorded data on infants 7−24 months of age given vitamin D in doses below, above, or at the then recommended 2000 IU daily (Hypponen et al., 2001). The 2000 IU dose was associated with a low relative risk of 0.12 (95% CI 0.03−0.47). In a multinational European case-control study, the odds ratio for T1D was significantly reduced in children given vitamin D (EURODIAB Substudy 2 Study Group, 1999). The risk for T1D in Norwegian children was significantly lower if their mothers had taken cod liver oil (a source of vitamin D) during pregnancy (Stene et al., 2000). Randomized controlled trials of vitamin D supplementation in individuals at risk for T1D are required but may never be undertaken given the contemporary public awareness of vitamin D deficiency and the widespread availability of vitamin D.

Viruses

Evidence for viruses in T1D has been reviewed elsewhere (Honeyman, 2005). Viruses could potentially trigger or promote islet autoimmunity in several ways: by directly infecting β cells, infecting the exocrine pancreas with bystander death of β cells, or expressing proteins with sequences that mimic diabetogenic T cell epitopes (molecular mimicry). If a particular virus was clearly implicated, vaccination of children early in life, provided it was safe, should provide protection.

The first virus associated with T1D was rubella (Forrest et al., 1971). Children with congenital rubella born to mothers who contracted rubella early in pregnancy had evidence of infection in the brain, pancreas, and other tissues, and 20% developed insulin-dependent diabetes (Menser et al., 1978). Subsequently, almost twice this proportion of such children were reported to develop islet cell autoantibodies (Ginsberg-Fellner et al., 1985). Children with congenital rubella and ensuing diabetes were noted to have a higher frequency of the T1D susceptibility haplotype HLA-A1-B8-DR3-DQ2 (Menser et al., 1974). Rubella vaccine has virtually eliminated congenital rubella but whether it also represents the first example of primary prevention of T1D is debatable (Gale, 2008). Clearly, other environmental factors are involved because the incidence of T1D has continued to rise. Despite a report of rubella-GAD mimicry (Ou et al., 2000), strengthened by the finding of islet autoantibodies in children infected with rubella virus (Lindberg et al., 1999), there is no evidence from multiple studies (Hummel et al., 2000; DeStefano et al., 2001) that the vaccination with attenuated rubella virus is associated with islet autoimmunity.

Enteroviruses, which commonly infect children, are of ongoing interest in T1D (Honeyman, 2005; Roivainen and Klingel, 2010). Over 70 enterovirus serotypes are recognized with many thousands of strain variants and, except for poliovirus, vaccines are not available. However, if diabetes-associated strains were to be clearly implicated, they would be candidate vaccines for genetically at-risk children.

Strong sequence similarities between T cell epitopes in IA-2 and GAD65 and the VP7 protein of rotavirus in islet antibody-positive relatives (Honeyman et al., 1998) suggested that molecular mimicry with rotavirus might precipitate islet autoimmunity. Rotavirus epidemics occur each winter particularly in kindergartens and are the most common cause of gastroenteritis in children. Rotavirus provides a profound inflammatory stimulus to the gut until sufficient IgA develops, by about 5 years of age. In the Australian BabyDiab Study, rotavirus infections were temporally associated with increases in islet autoantibodies in 24 children before they developed diabetes (Honeyman et al., 2000). It was then shown that rotavirus could infect β cells in islets from mice, pigs, and monkeys (Coulson et al., 2002). A more recent study (Honeyman et al., 2010) found that RV peptides homologous to IA-2 and GAD65 islet autoepitopes were CD4T cell epitopes in the context of HLA DR4, consistent with molecular mimicry. While ubiquitous rotavirus infections could drive cross-reactive immunity to islet autoantigens, this alone is unlikely to be diabetogenic. Mimicry may, however, complement and sustain the immune response to direct infection of β cells. Rotavirus vaccines, initially withdrawn because of safety concerns following cases of intestinal intussusception, are now routinely administered to infants. In countries like Australia where >90% of infants are covered by rotavirus vaccination it will be important to determine if this is associated with a change in the incidence of T1D. As a rider, it should be said that infection by rotavirus or other potentially diabetogenic viruses in a non-inflammatory context, such as during breastfeeding, could conceivably protect against T1D.

SECONDARY PREVENTION

The ideal prevention strategy in autoimmune disease is autoantigen-based immunotherapy, in which an autoantigen is administered to induce protective immune tolerance, also termed "negative vaccination" (Harrison, 2008). The rationale is that autoantigen-driven immunoregulatory mechanisms are physiological and can be boosted or restored to prevent pathological autoimmunity. Approaches include administration of an autoantigen by a "tolerogenic" route (e.g., mucosal), cell type (e.g., resting dendritic cell), mode (e.g., with blockade of costimulation molecules), or form (e.g., as an "altered peptide ligand"), all of which have been shown to prevent or suppress experimental autoimmune diseases in rodents (Faria and Weiner, 1999; Harrison and Hafler, 2000; Krause et al., 2000). Mechanisms encompass deletion and/or induction of anergy in potentially pathogenic effector T or induction of regulatory T cells (iTreg). Autoreactive T cells that are activated strongly by antigen may undergo apoptotic cell death and deletion, while those that survive or respond "partially" may become anergic (von Herrath and Harrison, 2003). Of potential importance clinically is the ability of iTreg generated to specific antigen to exert antigen-non-specific "bystander suppression." Thus, in response to specific antigen iTreg can, by direct cell contact or release of soluble immunosuppressive factors, impair the ability of antigen-presenting dendritic cells to elicit effector T cell responses to any antigen locally at the site of the lesion or in the draining lymph nodes. Bystander suppression does not require that the autoantigen used to induce tolerance is necessarily the major or primary pathogenic autoantigen.

Mucosa-mediated Antigen-specific Tolerance

Most attempts to induce clinical autoantigen-specific tolerance have been mucosa based. Numerous studies have shown that NOD mice can be partially protected from diabetes by mucosal administration of islet autoantigens. Zhang et al. (1991) initially reported protection after oral porcine insulin. Bergerot et al. (1994) then showed that human insulin induced CD4 Treg that could transfer protection to naïve mice. Protection following oral insulin was later found to be associated with decreased expression of IFN-γ-secreting Th1 T cells in the pancreas and pancreatic lymph nodes (Hancock et al., 1995; Ploix et al., 1998). Oral insulin-induced CD4 Treg have also been shown to prevent immune-mediated diabetes induced by lymphocytic choriomeningitis virus (LCMV) infection of mice expressing the viral nucleoprotein of LCMV under control of the rat insulin promoter in their β cells (Homann et al., 1999). The majority of T cells in the islets of oral insulin-treated mice without diabetes were shown to secrete Th2 (IL-4, IL-10) and Th3 (TGF-β) cytokines, in contrast to IFN-γ-secreting Th1 cells in islets of mice developing diabetes. The protective effect of oral insulin was enhanced by simultaneous feeding with IL-10 (Slavin et al., 2001), bacterial component OM-89 (Bellmann et al., 1997; Hartmann et al., 1997), or schistosome egg antigen (Maron et al., 1998), all of which promote Th2 responses. Fusion of insulin to cholera toxin B-subunit (CTB) significantly improved the ability of oral insulin to prevent diabetes (Bergerot et al., 1997). Oral CTB-insulin conjugates in NOD mice induced a shift from a Th1 to a Th2 immunity associated with the induction of regulatory CD4 T cells (Ploix et al., 1999). NOD mice were protected from diabetes by feeding them with potatoes that transgenically express CTB-insulin conjugates (Arakawa et al., 1998). Oral GAD65 has also been shown to suppress diabetes development in NOD mice (Ma et al., 1997). Although it is generally believed that neonates are less susceptible to mucosal tolerance induction, oral administration of insulin, insulin B-chain, or GAD65 peptide during the neonatal period still suppressed diabetes development in NOD mice (Maron et al., 2001). This suggests that mucosal administration of islet autoantigen, e.g., in milk, could be used to treat very young infants at risk of developing T1D.

NOD mice are also protected from diabetes by naso-respiratory administration of islet autoantigens. This route of direct administration to the mucosa avoids antigen degradation in the stomach. When insulin was administered as an aerosol to NOD mice at 8 weeks of age, after the onset of subclinical disease, insulitis and diabetes incidence were both significantly reduced (Harrison et al., 1996). Aerosol insulin induced novel anti-diabetic CD8 $\gamma\delta$ T cells that suppressed the adoptive transfer of diabetes to non-diabetic mice by T cells of diabetic mice. The type of Treg induced by (pro)insulin depends on the route and form of antigen. Naso-respiratory insulin, non-degraded and conformationally intact, induced CD8 $\gamma\delta$ Treg, whereas oral insulin degraded to peptides, or intranasal or oral (pro)insulin peptides, induced CD4 Treg (Hänninen and Harrison, 2000; Martinez et al., 2003). Intranasal administration of the insulin B-chain peptide (aa9-23), an epitope recognized by islet-infiltrating CD4 T cell clones capable of adoptively transferring diabetes to naïve mice, induced CD4 Treg and protected NOD mice from diabetes (Daniel and Wegmann, 1996). A peptide that spans the B-C chain junction in proinsulin also induced CD4 Treg after intranasal administration (Martinez et al., 2003). This peptide, like insulin B9–23, binds to the NOD mouse class II MHC, I-A^{g7} (Harrison et al., 1997), and is a T cell epitope in NOD mice (Chen et al., 2001) and humans at risk for T1D (Rudy et al., 1995). T cell epitope peptides from GAD65 administered intranasally were also protective, and associated with the induction of regulatory CD4 Treg and with reduced IFN-γ responses to GAD65 (Tian et al., 1996). These "proof-of-principle" studies in the NOD mouse indicate that islet autoantigen proteins or peptides are candidate mucosal "vaccines" for prevention of T1D in humans, but this promise remains to be fulfilled (see below).

Trials of Islet Autoantigen-specific Vaccination in Humans

The large multi-center Diabetes Prevention Trial 1 (DPT-1) was launched in the United States in 1994 to determine whether antigen-specific therapy with either systemic or oral insulin would delay or prevent diabetes onset in at-risk first-degree relatives. Previously, intensive systemic insulin therapy had been reported to prolong the "honeymoon phase" after diagnosis (Shah et al., 1989) and a pilot study of prophylactic systemic insulin had suggested that this approach might be of benefit in at-risk relatives (Keller et al., 1993). Whether systemic insulin acted only as a hormone to control blood glucose and "rest" β cells (making them less sensitive to immune attack) or also as an antigen to induce immune tolerance was not clear, and read-outs to identify immune mechanisms were not employed. In DPT-1, low dose systemic insulin (annual intravenous insulin infusions and daily subcutaneous injections) was given to a high-risk group of relatives (>50% risk of diabetes over 5 years), matched with an untreated but closely monitored control group, but it had no effect on diabetes incidence (Diabetes Prevention Trial—Type 1 Diabetes Study Group, 2002). In the subsequent randomized controlled DPT-1 trial of oral insulin, relatives with a 25–50% 5-year risk of diabetes were given 7.5 mg human insulin or placebo daily for a median of 4.3 years. There was no effect overall, but post-trial hypothesis testing revealed a significant delay of approximately 4 years in diabetes onset in participants who were unequivocally positive for insulin autoantibodies at entry (Skyler et al., 2005) (Figure 79.2). That oral insulin only benefited participants with insulin autoimmunity suggests that allelism at the insulin gene susceptibility locus (IDDM2) could determine the immune response not only to endogenous insulin as a target autoantigen but also to oral insulin as a potential therapeutic tool. A follow-up international trial of oral insulin in at-risk relatives using the same 7.5 mg dose is in progress, under the auspices of TrialNet. Ideally, this would have incorporated a higher dose as well since on a body weight basis the 7.5 mg dose equates to only a few micrograms in the mouse, and milligrams of gavaged insulin were required to induce anti-diabetogenic CD4 Treg in NOD mice. Two trials of oral insulin (up to 7.5 mg daily for 12 months) in recently diagnosed patients, attempting tertiary prevention (see below), showed no protective effect on residual β cell function (Chaillous et al., 2000; Pozzilli et al., 2000).

Why have trials of oral insulin in T1D, as well as oral myelin basic protein in multiple sclerosis (Weiner et al., 1993) and oral collagen in rheumatoid arthritis (Trentham et al., 1993; McKown et al., 1999), failed to show clinical effects? The answer is probably for a combination of reasons: selection of subjects with end-stage disease; inadequate dose or bioavailability of the agent, possibly related to the route of administration; co-induction of pathogenic T cells; and genetic heterogeneity. Antigen-specific tolerance on its own is clinically ineffective in end-stage disease. If a balance between pathogenic and protective T cells determines clinical outcome, then antigen-specific tolerance should be most effective in early preclinical disease, or earlier. The question of dose is discussed below. Oral administration may not be optimal for mucosa-mediated tolerance because proteins are degraded after ingestion and the concentration or form of peptide reaching the upper small intestine may be inadequate to induce mucosa-mediated tolerance. Even for a small peptide, mucosal responses occurred after naso-respiratory but not oral administration (Metzler and Wraith, 1993). In the mouse, nasal administration of the model antigen, ovalbumin, elicited antigen-specific T cell responses in cervical, mediastinal, and mesenteric mucosal lymph nodes, whereas oral administration elicited responses only in the mesenteric nodes (Hänninen et al., 2001). Irrespective of route of administration, antigen presentation to the mucosa may be a "double-edged sword" simultaneously inducing both iTreg and pathogenic cytotoxic CD8$^+$ T cells and a clinical effect may not be seen without suppression of the latter, e.g., by transient costimulation blockade with anti-CD40 ligand antibody (Hänninen et al., 2002). Insulin contains potentially pathogenic cytotoxic T cell epitopes but whether mucosal insulin induces cytotoxic CD8$^+$ T cells as well as protective Treg is

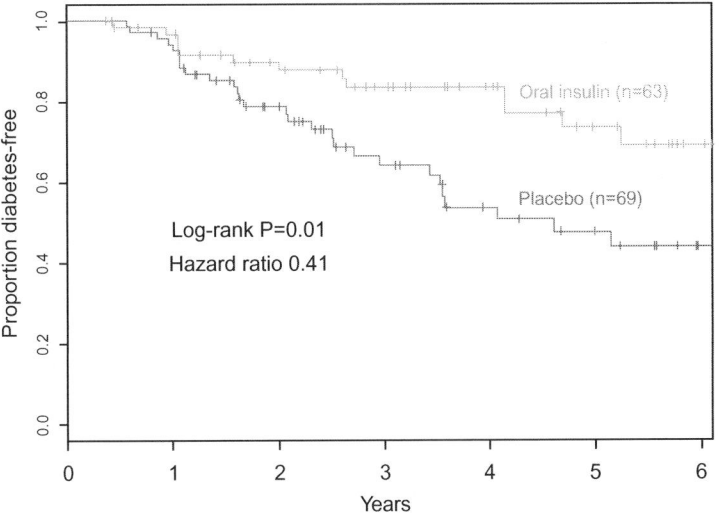

FIGURE 79.2 Oral insulin vaccination delays development of diabetes in at-risk T1D relatives. *Source: Adapted from Skyler et al. 2005.*

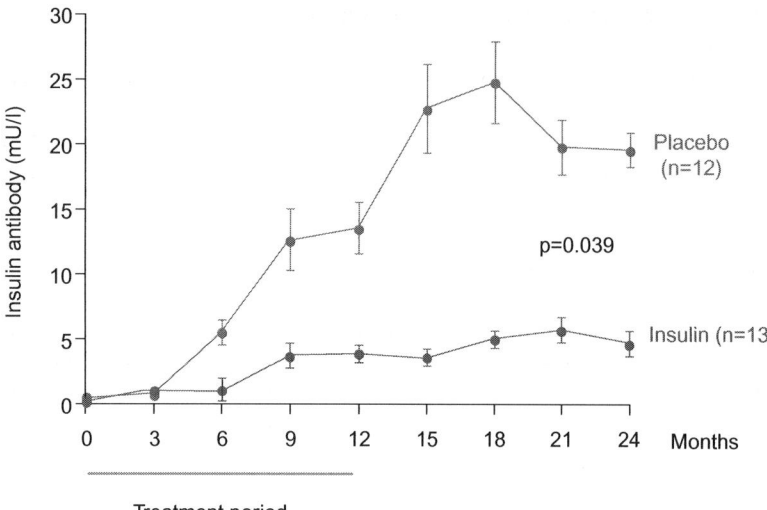

FIGURE 79.3 Nasal insulin vaccination suppresses insulin antibody response to subcutaneous insulin. *Source: Adapted from Fourlanos et al. 2011.*

unknown, but needs to be ascertained. A proinsulin B-C chain peptide that induces CD4[+] Treg in NOD mice is a "combitope" of CD4[+] (I-A[g7]-restricted) and CD8[+] (K[d]-restricte[d]) T cell epitopes, and was significantly more protective after nasal administration when the C-terminal p9 anchor residue for binding to K[d] was delete[d] or mutated (Martinez et al., 2003).

None of the oral autoantigen trials sought evidence for an immune effect and there is a pressing need to evaluate immune responses to mucosal autoantigens in human trials. Without this, it is not clear that the antigen dose used was bioactive/available. How might a response to oral insulin have been assessed? Insulin antibodies are a marker of bioavailability observed after aerosol insulin in NOD mice (Harrison et al., 1996) and intranasal insulin in humans (Harrison et al., 2004). Irrespective of whether or not they are a marker of immunoprotection, induction of insulin antibodies demonstrates that the insulin dose used was bioactive. Insulin autoantibodies are a risk marker for T1D and an increase in insulin antibodies after naso-respiratory insulin seems counterintuitive. However, this is not the case and in both the NOD mouse and humans at risk for T1D naso-respiratory insulin, although associated with a small but significant increase in insulin antibodies, was also associated with a decrease in T cell responses to insulin. This observation is consistent with the earliest descriptions of mucosal tolerance and with later landmark studies in humans using keyhole limpet hemocyanin (KLH) as a model antigen. When KLH was administered nasally to human volunteers it elicited a modest antibody response, but after challenge with subcutaneous KLH both antibody and T cell responses decreased (Waldo et al., 1994). In a recent randomized trial of nasal insulin in people with recent-onset T1D not requiring insulin

treatment at diagnosis, those who received nasal insulin had markedly blunted insulin antibody responses after eventually commencing on subcutaneous insulin treatment (Fourlanos et al., 2011) (Figure 79.3). It will be important to determine if nasal insulin induces insulin-specific regulatory T cells and to demonstrate that nasal insulin like nasal KLH suppresses T cell responses to rechallenge, indicative of T cell tolerance.

The recent evidence for nasal insulin-induced immune tolerance (Fourlanos et al., 2011) cannot be extrapolated to endogenous "autoantigenic" insulin but it provides a mechanistic rationale for randomized trials of nasal insulin vaccination in individuals at risk for T1D. One trial, the T1D Prediction and Prevention Project (DIPP) trial in Finland, has been reported on (Nanto-Salonen et al., 2008); the other, the Type 1 Diabetes Prevention Trial, also known as the Intranasal Insulin Trial II (INIT II) in Australia, New Zealand, and Germany (see stopdiabetes.com.au), is ongoing. In the DIPP trial, nasal insulin (1 U/kg daily) had no effect on progression to diabetes in islet autoantibody-positive children less than 3 years of age. The children were a very high-risk group and many appear to have had borderline β cell function judged by low first phase insulin response to i.v. glucose, suggesting they would have been unlikely to respond. As in the oral insulin trials, markers of immune responses to insulin were not reported. In INIT II, nasal insulin (440 U) or nasal placebo is being administered daily for 7 days and then weekly for a year, with a further 4-year follow-up, in T1D relatives aged 4−30 with autoantibodies to at least two islet antigens ($\approx$ 40% risk of diabetes over 5 years). The primary outcome is diabetes development, secondary outcomes being measures of metabolic and immune function. The insulin dose in INIT II is substantially higher than in the DIPP trial and the participants are older and have less advanced preclinical disease. INIT II aims to complete enrollment by the end of 2013. The question of timing applies even to secondary prevention and antigen-specific vaccination might be most effective before the onset of the disease process. To address this, a trial of oral insulin vaccination in children genetically predisposed to T1D (Pre-POINT trial), with no evidence of underlying islet autoimmunity, has commenced (Achenbach et al., 2008).

In concluding, a few comments on GAD65 vaccination trials are in order. Although GAD65 autoantibodies are a marker of T1D, their singular presence is associated with relatively indolent islet autoimmunity, as seen in latent autoimmune diabetes in adults (LADA) (Fourlanos et al., 2005). Nevertheless, based on evidence that the incidence of diabetes was lowered by systemic GAD65 (Petersen et al., 1994; Tisch et al., 2001) or nasal GAD65 peptides (Tian et al., 1996), a Swedish company, Diamyd P/L, produced recombinant GAD65 and initiated trials of a subcutaneous GAD65-alum (aluminum hydroxide) vaccine (summarized in Table 79.1). Although the initial trials were encouraging, subsequent larger trials failed to substantiate a clinical effect of the vaccine. As discussed above, it is no surprise that the GAD-alum vaccine showed no effect after the onset of clinical diabetes. However, these trials appear to have established the safety of the vaccine and, based on GAD65 antibody responses, its bioactivity, thereby justifying a secondary prevention trial (DIAPREV-IT) of the vaccine in islet autoantibody-positive at-risk children, which is ongoing.

EPILOGUE

Prevention of genetically complex and environmentally shaped autoimmune diseases will require more than a single "magic bullet." Progress towards prevention will occur incrementally and involve a combination of agents tailored to genotype and disease mechanisms, disease stage, and risk status. Environmental agents that precipitate or exacerbate autoimmune disease are likely to be ubiquitous and therefore a single strategy, e.g., vaccination against a specific virus, is unlikely to be the answer. A prerequisite is the identification of at-risk individuals in early life, for which T1D is a paradigm. Prevention strategies must be safe as well as effective. In this regard, autoantigen-specific vaccination as applied in the oral and nasal insulin trials in T1D provide a glimmer of promise. Lessons learnt from the preclinical diagnosis, prediction, and prevention of T1D should be applicable to other autoimmune diseases.

ACKNOWLEDGMENTS

This work was supported by the National Health and Medical Research Council of Australia (Program Grant 516700; Fellowship [LCH] 637301) and made possible through Victorian State Government Operational Infrastructure Support and Australian Government NHMRC IRIIS.

REFERENCES

Achenbach, P., Barker, J., Bonifacio, E., Pre-point Study Group, 2008. Modulating the natural history of type 1 diabetes in children at high genetic risk by mucosal insulin immunization. Curr. Diab. Rep. 8, 87–93.

Adorini, L., Gregori, S., Harrison, L.C., 2002. Understanding autoimmune diabetes: insights from mouse models. Trends. Mol. Med. 8, 31–38.

Agardh, C.D., Cilio, C.M., Lethagen, A., Lynch, K., Leslie, R.D., Palmer, M., et al., 2005. Clinical evidence for the safety of GAD65 immunomodulation in adult-onset autoimmune diabetes. J. Diabetes Complicat. 19, 238–246.

Allen, H.F., Klingensmith, G.J., Jensen, P., Simoes, E., Hayward, A., Chase, H.P., 1999. Effect of Bacillus Calmette-Guerin vaccination on new-onset type 1 diabetes. A randomized clinical study. Diabetes Care. 22, 1703–1707.

Arakawa, T., Yu, J., Chong, D.K., Hough, J., Engen, P.C., Langridge, W.H., 1998. A plant-based cholera toxin B subunit-insulin fusion protein protects against the development of autoimmune diabetes. Nat. Biotechnol. 16, 934–938.

Assan, R., Feutren, G., Sirmai, J., Laborie, C., Boitard, C., Vexiau, P., et al., 1990. Plasma C-peptide levels and clinical remissions in recent-onset type I diabetic patients treated with cyclosporin A and insulin. Diabetes. 39, 768–774.

Atkinson, M.A., Leiter, E.H., 1999. The NOD mouse model of type 1 diabetes: as good as it gets? Nat. Med. 5, 601–604.

Bellmann, K., Kolb, H., Hartmann, B., Rothe, H., Rowsell, P., Rastegar, S., et al., 1997. Intervention in autoimmune diabetes by targeting the gut immune system. Int. J. Immunopharmacol. 19, 573–577.

Bennett, S.T., Lucassen, A.M., Gough, S.C., Powell, E.E., Undlien, D. E., Pritchard, L.E., et al., 1995. Susceptibility to human type 1 diabetes at IDDM2 is determined by tandem repeat variation at the insulin gene minisatellite locus. Nat. Genet. 9, 284–292.

Bergerot, I., Fabien, N., Maguer, V., Thivolet, C., 1994. Oral administration of human insulin to NOD mice generates CD4 + T cells that suppress adoptive transfer of diabetes. J. Autoimmun. 7, 655–663.

Bergerot, I., Ploix, C., Petersen, J., Moulin, V., Rask, C., Fabien, N., et al., 1997. A cholera toxoid-insulin conjugate as an oral vaccine against spontaneous autoimmune diabetes. Proc. Natl. Acad. Sci. U.S.A. 94, 4610–4614.

Bingley, P.J., Williams, A.J., Gale, E.A., 1999. Optimized autoantibody-based risk assessment in family members. Implications for future intervention trials. Diabetes Care. 22, 1796–1801.

Bjork, E., Berne, C., Kampe, O., Wibell, L., Oskarsson, P., Karlsson, F.A., 1996. Diazoxide treatment at onset preserves residual insulin secretion in adults with autoimmune diabetes. Diabetes. 45, 1427–1430.

Bjork, E., Ortqvist, E., Wallensteen, M., Ludvigsson, J., Aman, J., Johansson, C., et al., 2001. Diazoxide treatment at onset in childhood type 1 diabetes. Diabetes. 50, A90.

Brown, C.T., Davis-Richardson, A.G., Giongo, A., Gano, K.A., Crabb, D.B., Mukherjee, N., et al., 2011. Gut microbiome metagenomics analysis suggests a functional model for the development of autoimmunity for type 1 diabetes. PLoS One. 6, e25792.

Buckingham, B.A., Sandborg, C.I., 2000. A randomized trial of methotrexate in newly diagnosed patients with type 1 diabetes mellitus. Clin. Immunol. 96, 86–90.

Buzzetti, R., Cernea, S., Petrone, A., Capizzi, M., Spoletini, M., Zampetti, S., et al., 2011. C-peptide response and HLA genotypes in subjects with recent-onset type 1 diabetes after immunotherapy with DiaPep277: an exploratory study. Diabetes. 60, 3067–3072.

Canadian-European Randomized Control Trial Group, 1988. Cyclosporin-induced remission of IDDM after early intervention. Association of 1 yr of cyclosporin treatment with enhanced insulin secretion. Diabetes. 37, 1574–1582.

Chaillous, L., Lefevre, H., Thivolet, C., Boitard, C., Lahlou, N., Atlan-Gepner, C., et al., 2000. Oral insulin administration and residual beta-cell function in recent-onset type 1 diabetes: a multicentre randomised controlled trial. Diabete Insuline Orale Group. Lancet. 356, 545–549.

Chase, H.P., Butler-Simon, N., Garg, S.K., Hayward, A., Klingensmith, G.J., Hamman, R.F., et al., 1990a. Cyclosporine A for the treatment of new-onset insulin-dependent diabetes mellitus. Pediatrics. 85, 241–245.

Chase, H.P., Butler-Simon, N., Garg, S., McDuffie, M., Hoops, S.L., O'Brien, D., 1990b. A trial of nicotinamide in newly diagnosed patients with type 1 (insulin-dependent) diabetes mellitus. Diabetologia. 33, 444–446.

Chen, W., Bergerot, I., Elliott, J.F., Harrison, L.C., Delovitch, T.L., 2001. Evidence that a peptide spanning the B-C junction of proinsulin is a primary autoantigen epitope in the pathogenesis of type 1 diabetes. J. Immunol. 167, 4926–4935.

Colman, P.G., Steele, C., Couper, J.J., Beresford, S.J., Powell, T., Kewming, K., et al., 2000. Islet autoimmunity in infants with a type I diabetic relative is common but is frequently restricted to one autoantibody. Diabetologia. 43, 203–209.

Cook, J.J., Hudson, I., Harrison, L.C., Dean, B., Colman, P.G., Werther, G.A., et al., 1989. A double-blind controlled trial of azathioprine in children with newly-diagnosed type 1 diabetes. Diabetes. 38, 779–783.

Coulson, B.S., Witterick, P.D., Tan, Y., Hewish, M.J., Mountford, J.N., Harrison, L.C., et al., 2002. Growth of rotaviruses in primary pancreatic cells. J. Virol. 76, 9537–9544.

Couper, J.J., Steele, C., Beresford, S., Powell, T., McCaul, K., Pollard, A., et al., 1999. Lack of association between duration of breast-feeding or introduction of cow's milk and development of islet autoimmunity. Diabetes. 48, 2145–2149.

Coutant, R., Landais, P., Rosilio, M., Johnsen, C., Lahlou, N., Chatelain, P., et al., 1998. Low dose linomide in Type I juvenile diabetes of recent onset: a randomised placebo-controlled double blind trial. Diabetologia. 41, 1040–1046.

Daniel, D., Wegmann, D., 1996. Protection of nonobese diabetic mice from diabetes by intranasal or subcutaneous administration of insulin peptide B-(9–23). Proc. Natl. Acad. Sci. U.S.A. 93, 956–960.

DeStefano, F., Mullooly, J.P., Okoro, C.A., Chen, R.T., Marcy, S.M., Ward, J.I., et al., 2001. Childhood vaccinations, vaccination timing, and risk of type 1 diabetes mellitus. Pediatrics. 108, E112.

Diabetes Prevention Trial-Type 1 Diabetes Study Group, 2002. Effects of insulin in relatives of patients with type 1 diabetes mellitus. N. Engl. J. Med. 346, 1685–1691.

Durinovic-Bello, I., Wu, R.P., Gersuk, V.H., Sanda, S., Shilling, H.G., Nepom, G.T., 2010. Insulin gene VNTR genotype associates with frequency and phenotype of the autoimmune response to proinsulin. Genes Immun. 11, 188–193.

EURODIAB Substudy 2 Study Group, 1999. Vitamin D supplement in early childhood and risk for type I (insulin-dependent) diabetes mellitus. Diabetologia. 42, 51–54.

Elliott, J.F., Marlin, K.L., Couch, R.M., 1998. Effect of bacille Calmette-Guerin vaccination on C-peptide secretion in children newly diagnosed with IDDM. Diabetes Care. 21, 1691–1693.

Faria, A.M., Weiner, H.L., 1999. Oral tolerance: mechanisms and therapeutic applications. Adv. Immunol. 73, 153–164.

Feutren, G., Papoz, L., Assan, R., Vialettes, B., Karsenty, G., Vexiau, P., et al., 1986. Cyclosporin increases the rate and length of remissions in insulin-dependent diabetes of recent onset. Results of a multicentre double-blind trial. Lancet. 2, 119–124.

Forrest, J.M., Menser, M.A., Burgess, J.A., 1971. High frequency of diabetes mellitus in young adults with congenital rubella. Lancet. 2, 332–334.

Fourlanos, S., Narendran, P., Byrnes, G., Colman, P., Harrison, L.C., 2004. Insulin resistance is a risk factor for progression to type 1 diabetes. Diabetologia. 47, 1661–1667.

Fourlanos, S., Dotta, F., Greenbaum, C.K., Palmer, J.P., Rolandsson, O., Colman, P.G., et al., 2005. Latent autoimmune diabetes in adults (LADA) should be less latent. Diabetologia. 48, 2206–2212.

Fourlanos, S., Varney, M., Tait, B.D., Morahan, G., Honeyman, M.C., Colman, P.G., et al., 2008. The rising incidence of type 1 diabetes is accounted for by cases with lower risk HLA genotypes. Diabetes Care. 31, 1546–1549.

Fourlanos, S., Perry, C., Gellert, S.A., Martinuzzi, E., Mallone, R., Butler, J., et al., 2011. Evidence that nasal insulin induces immune tolerance to insulin in adults with autoimmune diabetes. Diabetes. 60, 1237–1245.

Füchtenbusch, M., Rabl, W., Grassl, B., Bachmann, W., Standl, E., Ziegler, A.G., 1998. Delay of type I diabetes in high risk, first degree relatives by parenteral antigen administration: the Schwabing insulin prophylaxis pilot trial. Diabetologia. 41, 536–541.

Funda, D.P., Fundova, P., Harrison, L.C., 2005. Environmental-mucosal interactions in the natural history of type 1 diabetes: the germ-free (GF) NOD mouse model. Ann. N.Y. Acad. Sci. Proceedings of the 7th Scientific Meeting, Immunology of Diabetes Society, Cambridge, UK; 1, 41.

Gale, E.A., 2008. Congenital rubella: citation virus or viral cause of type 1 diabetes? Diabetologia. 51, 1559–1566.

Gerstein, H., 1994. Cow's milk exposure and type 1 diabetes mellitus. Diabetes Care. 17, 13–19.

Ginsberg-Fellner, F., Witt, M.E., Fedun, B., Taub, F., Dobersen, M.J., McEvoy, R.C., et al., 1985. Diabetes mellitus and autoimmunity in patients with the congenital rubella syndrome. Rev. Infect. Dis. 7 (Suppl. 1), S170–S176.

Giordano, C., Panto, F., Amato, M.P., Sapienza, N., Pugliese, A., Galluzzo, A., 1990. Early administration of an immunomodulator and induction of remission in insulin-dependent diabetes mellitus. J. Autoimmun. 3, 611–617.

Goday, A., Pujol-Borrell, R., Fernandez, J., Casamitjana, R., Rios, M., Vilardell, E., et al., 1993. Effects of a short prednisone regime at clinical onset of type 1 diabetes. Diabetes Res. Clin. Pract. 20, 39–46.

Gottlieb, P.A., Quinlan, S., Krause-Steinrauf, H., Greenbaum, C.J., Wilson, D.M., Rodriguez, H., et al., 2010. Failure to preserve beta-cell function with mycophenolate mofetil and daclizumab combined therapy in patients with new-onset type 1 diabetes. Diabetes Care. 33, 826–832.

Gottsater, A., Landin-Olsson, M., Lernmark, A., Fernlund, P., Sundkvist, G., Hagopian, W.A., 1995. Glutamic acid decarboxylase antibody levels predict role of β-cell decline in adult onset diabetes. Diab. Rev. Clin. Prac. 27, 133–140.

Greenbaum, C., Harrison, L.C., 2003. Guidelines for intervention trials in subjects with newly-diagnosed type 1 diabetes. Diabetes. 52, 1059–1065.

Grunt, J.A., al-Hakim, H., Willoughby, L., Howard, C.P., 1994. A randomized trial of a somatostatin analog for preserving beta cell function in children with insulin dependent diabetes mellitus. J. Pediatr. Endocrinol. 7, 331–334.

Hagopian, W.A., Karlsen, A.E., Gottsater, A., Landin-Olsson, M., Grubin, C.E., Sundkvist, G., et al., 1993. Quantitative assay using recombinant human islet glutamic acid decarboxylase (GAD65) shows that 64K autoantibody positivity at onset predicts diabetes type. J. Clin. Invest. 91, 368–374.

Hancock, W.W., Polanski, M., Zhang, J., Blogg, N., Weiner, H.L., 1995. Suppression of insulitis in non-obese diabetic (NOD) mice by oral insulin administration is associated with selective expression of interleukin-4 and -10, transforming growth factor-beta and prostaglandin-E. Am. J. Pathol. 147, 1193–1199.

Hänninen, A., Harrison, L.C., 2000. Gamma delta T cells as mediators of mucosal tolerance: the autoimmune diabetes model. Immunol. Rev. 173, 109–119.

Hänninen, A., Braakhuis, A., Heath, W.R., Harrison, L.C., 2001. Mucosal antigen primes diabetogenic cytotoxic T-lymphocytes regardless of dose or delivery route. Diabetes. 50, 771–775.

Hänninen, A., Martinez, N.R., Davey, G.M., Heath, W.R., Harrison, L.C., 2002. Transient blockade of CD40 ligand dissociates pathogenic from protective mucosal immunity. J. Clin. Invest. 109, 261–267.

Harrison, L.C., 2001. Risk assessment, prediction and prevention of type 1 diabetes. Pediatr. Diabetes. 2, 71–82.

Harrison, L.C., 2008. Vaccination against self to prevent autoimmune disease: the type 1 diabetes model. Immunol. Cell Biol. 89, 139–145.

Harrison, L.C., Hafler, D.A., 2000. Antigen-specific therapy for autoimmune disease. Curr. Opin. Immunol. 12, 704–711.

Harrison, L.C., Honeyman, M.C., 1999. Cow's milk and type 1 diabetes: the real debate is about mucosal immune function. Diabetes. 48, 1501–1507.

Harrison, L.C., Colman, P.G., Dean, B., Baxter, R., Martin, F.I., 1985. Increase in remission rate in newly diagnosed type I diabetic subjects treated with azathioprine. Diabetes. 34, 1306–1308.

Harrison, L.C., Dempsey-Collier, M., Kramer, D.R., Takahashi, K., 1996. Aerosol insulin induces regulatory CD8 gamma delta T cells that prevent murine insulin-dependent diabetes. J. Exp. Med. 184, 2167–2174.

Harrison, L.C., Honeyman, M.C., Trembleau, S., Gregori, S., Gallazzi, F., Augstein, P., et al., 1997. A peptide-binding motif for I-A(g7), the class II major histocompatibility complex (MHC) molecule of NOD and Biozzi AB/H mice. J. Autoimmun. 10, 165–173.

Harrison, L.C., Honeyman, M.C., Steele, C.E., Stone, N.L., Sarugeri, E., Bonifacio, E., et al., 2004. Pancreatic beta-cell function and immune responses to insulin after administration of intranasal insulin to humans at risk for type 1 diabetes. Diabetes Care. 27, 2348–2355.

Hartmann, B., Bellmann, K., Ghiea, I., Kleemann, R., Kolb, H., 1997. Oral insulin for diabetes prevention in NOD mice: potentiation by enhancing Th2 cytokine expression in the gut through bacterial adjuvant. Diabetologia. 40, 902–909.

Herold, K.C., Hagopian, W., Auger, J.A., Poumian-Ruiz, E., Taylor, L., Donaldson, D., et al., 2002. Anti-CD3 monoclonal antibody in new-onset type 1 diabetes mellitus. N. Engl. J. Med. 346, 1692–1698.

Herold, K.C., Gitelman, S.E., Masharani, U., Hagopian, W., Bisikirska, B., Donaldson, D., et al., 2005. A single course of anti-CD3 monoclonal antibody hOKT3gamma1(Ala-Ala) results in improvement in C-peptide responses and clinical parameters for at least 2 years after onset of type 1 diabetes. Diabetes. 54, 1763–1769.

Holick, M.F., 2004. Vitamin D: importance in the prevention of cancers, type 1 diabetes, heart disease, and osteoporosis. Am. J. Clin. Nutr. 79, 362–371.

Homann, D., Dyrberg, T., Petersen, J., Oldstone, M.B., von Herrath, M.G., 1999. Insulin in oral immune "tolerance": a one-amino acid change in the B chain makes the difference. J. Immunol. 163, 1833–1838.

Honeyman, M., 2005. How robust is the evidence for viruses in the induction of type 1 diabetes? Curr Opin. Immunol. 17, 616–623.

Honeyman, M.C., Harrison, L.C., Drummond, B., Colman, P.G., Tait, B.D., 1995. Analysis of families at risk for insulin-dependent diabetes reveals that HLA antigens influence progression to preclinical disease. Mol. Med. 1, 576–582.

Honeyman, M.C., Stone, N.L., Harrison, L.C., 1998. T-cell epitopes in type 1 diabetes autoantigen tyrosine phosphatase IA-2: potential for mimicry with rotavirus and other environmental agents. Mol. Med. 4, 231–239.

Honeyman, M.C., Coulson, B.S., Stone, N.L., Gellert, S.A., Goldwater, P.N., Steele, C.E., et al., 2000. Association between rotavirus infection and pancreatic islet autoimmunity in children at risk of developing type 1 diabetes. Diabetes. 49, 1319–1324.

Honeyman, M.C., Stone, N.L., Falk, B.A., Nepom, G., Harrison, L.C., 2010. Evidence for molecular mimicry between human T cell epitopes in rotavirus and pancreatic islet autoantigens. J. Immunol. 184, 2204–2210.

Hummel, M., Fuchtenbusch, M., Schenker, M., Ziegler, A.G., 2000. No major association of breast-feeding, vaccinations, and childhood viral diseases with early islet autoimmunity in the German BABYDIAB Study. Diabetes Care. 23, 969–974.

Hummel, M., Bonifacio, E., Naserke, H.E., Ziegler, A.G., 2002. Elimination of dietary gluten does not reduce titers of type 1 diabetes-associated autoantibodies in high-risk subjects. Diabetes Care. 25, 1111–1116.

Hummel, S., Pfluger, M., Hummel, M., Bonifacio, E., Ziegler, A.G., 2011. Primary dietary intervention study to reduce the risk of islet autoimmunity in children at increased risk for type 1 diabetes: the BABYDIET study. Diabetes Care. 34, 1301–1305.

Hypponen, E., Laara, E., Reunanen, A., Jarvelin, M.R., Virtanen, S.M., 2001. Intake of vitamin D and risk of type 1 diabetes: a birth-cohort study. Lancet. 358, 1500–1503.

Kawaguchi-Miyashita, M., Shimizu, K., Nanno, M., Shimada, S., Watanabe, T., Koga, Y., et al., 1996. Development and cytolytic function of intestinal intraepithelial T lymphocytes in antigen-minimized mice. Immunology. 89, 268–273.

Keller, R.J., Eisenbarth, G.S., Jackson, R.A., 1993. Insulin prophylaxis in individuals at high risk of type 1 diabetes. Lancet. 341, 927–928.

Keymeulen, B., Vandemeulebroucke, E., Ziegler, A.G., Mathieu, C., Kaufman, L., Hale, G., et al., 2005. Insulin needs after CD3-antibody therapy in new-onset type 1 diabetes. N. Engl. J. Med. 352, 2598–2608.

Keymeulen, B., Walter, M., Mathieu, C., Kaufman, L., Gorus, F., Hilbrands, R., et al., 2010. Four-year metabolic outcome of a randomised controlled CD3-antibody trial in recent-onset type 1 diabetic patients depends on their age and baseline residual beta cell mass. Diabetologia. 53, 614–623.

Kimpimäki, T., Kupila, A., Hämäläinen, A.-M., Kukko, M., Kulmala, P., Savola, K., et al., 2001. The first signs of β-cell autoimmunity appear in infancy in genetically susceptible children from the general population: the Finnish Type 1 Diabetes Prediction and Prevention Study. J. Clin. Endocrinol. Metab. 86, 4782–4788.

Knip, M., Virtanen, S.M., Seppä, K., Ilonen, J., Savilahti, E., Vaarala, O., et al., 2010. Dietary intervention in infancy and later signs of beta-cell autoimmunity. N. Engl. J. Med. 363, 1900–1908.

Knip, M., Virtanen, S.M., Becker, D., Dupre, J., Krischer, J.P., Akerblom, H.K., et al., 2011. Early feeding and risk of type 1 diabetes: experiences from the Trial to Reduce Insulin-dependent Diabetes Mellitus in the Genetically at Risk (TRIGR). Am. J. Clin. Nutr. 94, 1814S–1820S.

Kobayashi, T., Nakanishi, K., Murase, T., Kosaka, K., 1996. Small doses of subcutaneous insulin as a strategy for preventing slowly progressive b-cell failure in islet cell antibody-positive patients with clinical features of NIDDM. Diabetes. 45, 622–626.

Kohnert, K.D., Hehmke, B., Keilacker, H., Ziegler, M., Emmrich, F., Laube, F., et al., 1996. Antibody response to islet autoantigens in anti-CD4/prednisolone immune intervention of type 1 diabetes. Int. J. Clin. Lab. Res. 26, 55–59.

Krause, I., Blank, M., Shoenfeld, Y., 2000. Immunomodulation of experimental autoimmune diseases via oral tolerance. Crit. Rev. Immunol. 20, 1–16.

Lampeter, E.F., Klinghammer, A., Scherbaum, W.A., Heinze, E., Haastert, B., Giani, G., et al., 1998. The Deutsche Nicotinamide Intervention Study: an attempt to prevent type 1 diabetes. DENIS Group. Diabetes. 47, 980–984.

Leiter, E.H., Prochazka, M., Coleman, D.L., 1987. The non-obese diabetic (NOD) mouse. Am. J. Pathol. 128, 380–383.

Leslie, D., Lipsky, P., Notkins, A.B., 2001. Autoantibodies as predictors of disease. J. Clin. Invest. 108, 1417–1422.

Lindberg, B., Ahlfors, K., Carlsson, A., Ericsson, U.B., Landin-Olsson, M., Lernmark, A., et al., 1999. Previous exposure to measles, mumps, and rubella—but not vaccination during adolescence—correlates to the prevalence of pancreatic and thyroid autoantibodies. Pediatrics. 104, e12.

Linn, T., Ortac, K., Laube, H., Federlin, K., 1996. Intensive therapy in adult insulin-dependent diabetes mellitus is associated with improved insulin sensitivity and reserve: a randomized, controlled, prospective study over 5 years in newly diagnosed patients. Metabolism. 45, 1508–1513.

Long, S.A., Rieck, M., Sanda, S., Bollyky, J.B., Samuels, P.L., Goland, R., et al., 2012. Rapamycin/IL-2 combination therapy in patients with type 1 diabetes augments Tregs yet transiently impairs beta-cell function. Diabetes. 61, 2340–2348.

Ludvigsson, J., Samuelsson, U., Johansson, C., Stenhammar, L., 2001. Treatment with antioxidants at onset of type 1 diabetes in children: a randomized, double-blind placebo-controlled study. Diabetes Metab. Res. Rev. 17, 131–136.

Ludvigsson, J., Faresjo, M., Hjorth, M., Axelsson, S., Cheramy, M., Pihl, M., et al., 2008. GAD treatment and insulin secretion in recent-onset type 1 diabetes. N. Engl. J. Med. 359, 1909–1920.

Ludvigsson, J., Krisky, D., Casas, R., Battelino, T., Castano, L., Greening, J., et al., 2012. GAD65 antigen therapy in recently diagnosed type 1 diabetes mellitus. N. Engl. J. Med. 366, 433–442.

Ma, S.W., Zhao, D.L., Yin, Z.Q., Mukherjee, R., Singh, B., Qin, H.Y., et al., 1997. Transgenic plants expressing autoantigens fed to mice to induce oral immune tolerance. Nat. Med. 3, 793–796.

MacFarlane, A.J., Burghardt, K.M., Kelly, J., Simell, T., Simell, O., Altosaar, I., et al., 2002. A type 1 diabetes-related protein from wheat (triticum aestivum): cDNA clone of a wheat storage globulin, Glb1, linked to islet damage. J. Biol. Chem. 278, 54–63.

Maron, R., Palanivel, V., Weiner, H.L., Harn, D.A., 1998. Oral administration of schistosome egg antigens and insulin B-chain generates and enhances Th2-type responses in NOD mice. Clin. Immunol. Immunopathol. 87, 85–92.

Maron, R., Guerau-de-Arellano, M., Zhang, X., Weiner, H.L., 2001. Oral administration of insulin to neonates suppresses spontaneous and cyclophosphamide induced diabetes in the NOD mouse. J. Autoimmun. 16, 21–28.

Martinez, N.R., Augstein, P., Moustakas, A.K., Papadopoulos, G.K., Gregori, S., Adorini, L., et al., 2003. Disabling an integral CTL epitope allows suppression of autoimmune diabetes by intranasal proinsulin peptide. J. Clin. Invest. 111, 1365–1371.

McKown, K.M., Carbone, L.D., Kaplan, S.B., Aelion, J.A., Lohr, K.M., Cremer, M.A., et al., 1999. Lack of efficacy of oral bovine type II collagen added to existing therapy in rheumatoid arthritis. Arthritis Rheum. 42, 1204–1208.

Mendola, G., Casamitjana, R., Gomis, R., 1989. Effect of nicotinamide therapy upon B-cell function in newly diagnosed type 1 (insulin-dependent) diabetic patients. Diabetologia. 32, 160–162.

Menser, M.A., Forrest, J.M., Honeyman, M.C., Burgess, J.A., 1974. Letter: diabetes, HL-A antigens, and congenital rubella. Lancet. 2, 1508–1509.

Menser, M.A., Forrest, J.M., Bransby, R.D., 1978. Rubella infection and diabetes mellitus. Lancet. 1, 57–60.

Metzler, B., Wraith, D.C., 1993. Inhibition of experimental autoimmune encephalomyelitis by inhalation but not oral administration of the encephalitogenic peptide: influence of MHC binding affinity. Int. Immunol. 5, 1159–1165.

Moncada, E., Subira, M.L., Oleaga, A., Goni, F., Sanchez-Ibarrola, A., Monreal, M., et al., 1990. Insulin requirements and residual beta-cell function 12 months after concluding immunotherapy in type I diabetic patients treated with combined azathioprine and thymostimulin administration for one year. J. Autoimmun. 3, 625–638.

Moran, A., Bundy, B., Becker, D., DiMeglio, L.A., Gitelman, S.E., Goland, R., et al., 2013. Interleukin-1 antagonism in type 1 diabetes of recent onset: two multicentre, randomised, double-blind, placebo-controlled trials. Lancet. 381, 1905–1915.

Nanto-Salonen, K., Kupila, A., Simell, S., Siljander, H., Salonsaari, T., Hekkala, A., et al., 2008. Nasal insulin to prevent type 1 diabetes in children with HLA genotypes and autoantibodies conferring increased risk of disease: a double-blind, randomised controlled trial. Lancet. 372, 1746–1755.

Narendran, P., Mannering, S.I., Harrison, L.C., 2003. Proinsulin—a pathogenic autoantigen in type 1 diabetes. Autoimmun. Rev. 2, 204–210.

Narendran, P., Neale, A.M., Lee, B.-H., Ngui, K., Steptoe, R.J., Morahan, G., et al., 2006. Proinsulin is encoded by an RNA splice variant in human blood myeloid cells. Proc. Natl. Acad. Sci. U.S.A. 103, 16430–16435.

Norris, J.M., Scott, F.W., 1996. A meta analysis of infant diet and insulin-dependent diabetes mellitus: do biases play a role. Epidemiology. 7, 87–92.

Norris, J.M., Beaty, B., Klingensmith, G., Yu, L., Hoffman, M., Chase, H.P., et al., 1996. Lack of association between early exposure to cow's milk protein and β cell autoimmunity: Diabetes Autoimmunity Study In the Young (DAISY). JAMA. 276, 609–614.

Orban, T., Farkas, K., Jalahej, H., Kis, J., Treszl, A., Falk, B., et al., 2010. Autoantigen-specific regulatory T cells induced in patients with type 1 diabetes mellitus by insulin B-chain immunotherapy. J. Autoimmun. 34, 408–415.

Orban, T., Bundy, B., Becker, D.J., DiMeglio, L.A., Gitelman, S.E., Goland, R., et al., 2011. Co-stimulation modulation with abatacept in patients with recent-onset type 1 diabetes: a randomised, double-blind, placebo-controlled trial. Lancet. 378, 412–419.

Ou, D., Mitchell, L.A., Metzger, D.L., Gillam, S., Tingle, A.J., 2000. Cross-reactive rubella virus and glutamic acid decarboxylase (65 and 67) protein determinants recognised by T cells of patients with type I diabetes mellitus. Diabetologia. 43, 750–762.

Panto, F., Giordano, C., Amato, M.P., Pugliese, A., Donatelli, M., D'Acquisto, G., et al., 1990. The influence of high dose intravenous immunoglobulins on immunological and metabolic pattern in newly diagnosed type I diabetic patients. J. Autoimmun. 3, 587–592.

Pescovitz, M.D., Greenbaum, C.J., Krause-Steinrauf, H., Becker, D.J., Gitelman, S.E., Goland, R., et al., 2009. Rituximab, B-lymphocyte depletion, and preservation of beta-cell function. N. Engl. J. Med. 361, 2143–2152.

Petersen, J.S., Karlsen, A.E., Markholst, H., Worsaae, A., Dyrberg, T., Michelsen, B., 1994. Neonatal tolerization with glutamic acid decarboxylase but not with bovine serum albumin delays the onset of diabetes in NOD mice. Diabetes. 43, 1478–1484.

Philips, J.C., Scheen, A.J., Le Registre Belge du Diabete, 2002. Infocongress. Study of the prevention of type 1 diabetes with nicotinamide: positive lessons of a negative clinical trial (ENDIT) [Article in French]. Rev. Med. Liege. 57, 672–675.

Ploix, C., Bergerot, I., Fabien, N., Perche, S., Moulin, V., Thivolet, C, 1998. Protection against autoimmune diabetes with oral insulin is associated with the presence of IL-4 type 2 T-cells in the pancreas and pancreatic lymph nodes. Diabetes. 47, 39–44.

Ploix, C., Bergerot, I., Durand, A., Czerkinsky, C., Holmgren, J., Thivolet, C., 1999. Oral administration of cholera toxin B-insulin conjugates protects NOD mice from autoimmune diabetes by inducing CD4 + regulatory T-cells. Diabetes. 48, 2150–2156.

Pozzilli, P., Signore, A., Williams, A.J., Beales, P.E., 1993. NOD mouse colonies around the world—recent facts and figures. Immunol. Today. 14, 193–196.

Pozzilli, P., Visalli, B., Boccuni, M.L., Baroni, M.G., Buzzetti, R., Fioriti, E., et al., 1994. Randomized trial comparing nicotinamide and nicotinamide plus cyclosporin in recent onset insulin-dependent

diabetes (IMDIAB 1). The IMDIAB Study Group. Diabet. Med. 11, 98–104.

Pozzilli, P., Visalli, N., Signore, A., Baroni, M.G., Buzzetti, R., Cavallo, M.G., et al., 1995. Double blind trial of nicotinamide in recent-onset IDDM (the IMDIAB III study). Diabetologia. 38, 848–852.

Pozzilli, P., Visalli, N., Cavallo, M.G., Signore, A., Baroni, M.G., Buzzetti, R., et al., 1997. Vitamin E and nicotinamide have similar effects in maintaining residual beta cell function in recent onset insulin-dependent diabetes (the IMDIAB IV study). Eur. J. Endocrinol. 137, 234–239.

Pozzilli, P., Pitocco, D., Visalli, N., Cavallo, M.G., Buzzetti, R., Crino, A., et al., 2000. No effect of oral insulin on residual beta-cell function in recent-onset type 1 diabetes (the IMDIAB VII). IMDIAB Group. Diabetologia. 43, 1000–1004.

Pugliese, A., Zeller, M., Fernandez Jr., A., Zalcberg, L.J., Bartlett, R.J., Ricordi, C., et al., 1997. The insulin gene is transcribed in the human thymus and transcription levels correlated with allelic variation at the INS VNTR-IDDM2 susceptibility locus for type 1 diabetes. Nat. Genet. 15, 293–297.

Raz, I., Elias, D., Avron, A., Tamir, M., Metzger, M., Cohen, I.R., 2001. Beta-cell function in new-onset type 1 diabetes and immunomodulation with a heat-shock protein peptide (DiaPep277): a randomised, double-blind, phase II trial. Lancet. 358, 1749–1753.

Roivainen, M., Klingel, K., 2010. Virus infections and type 1 diabetes risk. Curr. Diab. Rep. 10, 350–356.

Rose, N.R., 2008. Predictors of autoimmune disease: autoantibodies and beyond. Autoimmunity. 41, 419–428.

Rudy, G., Stone, N., Harrison, L.C., Colman, P.G., McNair, P., Brusic, V., et al., 1995. Similar peptides from two beta-cell autoantigens, proinsulin and glutamic acid decarboxylase, stimulate T cells of individuals at risk for insulin-dependent diabetes. Mol. Med. 1, 625–633.

Sarugeri, E., Dozio, N., Belloni, C., Meschi, F., Pastore, M.R., Bonifacio, E., 1998. Autoimmune responses to the beta cell autoantigen, insulin, and the INS VNTR-IDDM2 locus. Clin. Exp. Immunol. 114, 370–376.

Schnell, O., Eisfelder, B., Standl, E., Ziegler, A.G., 1997. High-dose intravenous insulin infusion versus intensive insulin treatment in newly diagnosed IDDM. Diabetes. 46, 1607–1611.

Secchi, A., Pastore, M.R., Sergi, A., Pontiroli, A.E., Pozza, G., 1990. Prednisone administration in recent onset type I diabetes. J. Autoimmun. 3, 593–600.

Selam, J.L., Woertz, L., Lozano, J., Robinson, M., Chan, E., Charles, M.A., 1993. The use of glipizide combined with intensive insulin treatment for the induction of remissions in new onset adult type I diabetes. Autoimmunity. 16, 281–288.

Shah, S.C., Malone, J.I., Simpson, N.E., 1989. A randomized trial of intensive insulin therapy in newly diagnosed insulin-dependent diabetes mellitus. N. Engl. J. Med. 320, 550–554.

Shehadeh, N., Gelertner, L., Blazer, S., Perlman, R., Etzioni, A., 2001. The importance of insulin content in infant diet: suggestion for a new infant formula period. Acta Pediatr. 90, 93–95.

Sherry, N., Hagopian, W., Ludvigsson, J., Jain, S.M., Wahlen, J., Ferry Jr., R.J., et al., 2011. Teplizumab for treatment of type 1 diabetes (Protégé study): 1-year results from a randomised, placebo-controlled trial. Lancet. 378, 487–497.

Silverstein, J., Maclaren, N., Riley, W., Spillar, R., Radjenovic, D., Johnson, S., 1988. Immunosuppression with azathioprine and prednisone in recent-onset insulin-dependent diabetes mellitus. N. Engl. J. Med. 319, 599—604.

Skyler, J.S., Rabinovitch, A., 1992. Cyclosporine in recent onset type I diabetes mellitus. Effects on islet beta cell function: Miami Cyclosporine Diabetes Study Group. J. Diabetes Complicat. 6, 77—88.

Skyler, J.S., Lorenz, T.J., Schwartz, S., Eisenbarth, G.S., Einhorn, D., Palmer, J.P., et al., 1993. Effects of an anti-CD5 immunoconjugate (CD5-plus) in recent onset type I diabetes mellitus: a preliminary investigation. The CD5 Diabetes Project Team. J. Diabetes Complicat. 7, 224—232.

Skyler, J.S., Krischer, J.P., Wolfsdorf, J., Cowie, C., Palmer, J.P., Greenbaum, C., et al., 2005. Effects of oral insulin in relatives of patients with type 1 diabetes: The Diabetes Prevention Trial—Type 1. Diabetes Care. 28, 1068—1076.

Slavin, A.J., Maron, R., Weiner, H.L., 2001. Mucosal administration of IL-10 enhances oral tolerance in autoimmune encephalomyelitis and diabetes. Int. Immunol. 13, 825—833.

Stene, L.C., Ulriksen, J., Magnus, P., Joner, G., 2000. Use of cod liver oil during pregnancy associated with lower risk of type I diabetes in the offspring. Diabetologia. 43, 1093—1098.

Suzuki, T., 1987. Diabetogenic effects of lymphocyte transfusion on the NOD or NOD nude mouse. In: Rygaard, J., Brunner, N., Graem, N., Spang-Thomson, M. (Eds.), Immune Deficient Animals in Biomedical Research. Basel, Karger, pp. 112—116.

Tait, B.D., Harrison, L.C., Drummond, B., Stewart, V., Varney, M., Honeyman, M.C., 1995. HLA antigens and age at onset of insulin-dependent diabetes. Hum. Immunol. 42, 116—122.

Tian, J., Atkinson, M.A., Clare-Salzler, M., Herschenfeld, A., Forsthuber, T., Lehmann, P.V., et al., 1996. Nasal administration of glutamate decarboxylase (GAD65) peptides induces Th2 responses and prevents murine insulin-dependent diabetes. J. Exp. Med. 183, 1561—1567.

Tisch, R., Wang, B., Weaver, D.J., Liu, B., Bui, T., Arthos, J., et al., 2001. Antigen-specific mediated suppression of beta cell autoimmunity by plasmid DNA vaccination. J. Immunol. 166, 2122—2132.

Trentham, D.A., Dynesius-Trentham, R.A., Orav, E.J., 1993. Effects of oral administration of type II collagen on rheumatoid arthritis. Science. 261, 1727—1730.

Tuomi, T., Groop, L.C., Zimmet, P.Z., Rowley, M.J., Knowles, W., Mackay, I.R., 1993. Antibodies to glutamic acid decarboxylase reveal latent autoimmune diabetes mellitus in adults with a non-insulin-dependent onset of disease. Diabetes. 42, 359—362.

Turner, R., Stratton, I., Horton, V., Manley, S., Zimmet, P., Mackay, I.R., et al., 1997. UKPDS 25: autoantibodies to islet-cell cytoplasm and glutamic acid decarboxylase for prediction of insulin requirement in type 2 diabetes. UK Prospective Diabetes Study Group. Lancet. 350, 1288—1293.

Vague, P., Picq, R., Bernal, M., Lassmann-Vague, V., Vialettes, B., 1989. Effect of nicotinamide treatment on the residual insulin secretion in type 1 (insulin-dependent) diabetic patients. Diabetologia. 32, 316—321.

Ventura, A., Magazzu, G., Greco, L., 1999. Duration of exposure to gluten and risk for autoimmune disorders in patients with celiac disease (SIGEP study group for autoimmune disorders in celiac disease). Gastroenterology. 117, 297—303.

Verge, C.F., Gianani, R., Kawasaki, E., Yu, L., Pietropaolo, M., Jackson, R.A., et al., 1996. Prediction of type I diabetes in first-degree relatives using a combination of insulin, GAD, and ICA512bdc/IA-2 autoantibodies. Diabetes. 45, 926—933.

Vidal, J., Fernandez-Balsells, M., Sesmilo, G., Aguilera, E., Casamitjana, R., Gomis, R., et al., 2000. Effects of nicotinamide and intravenous insulin therapy in newly diagnosed type 1 diabetes. Diabetes Care. 23, 360—364.

von Herrath, M.G., Harrison, L.C., 2003. Antigen-induced regulatory T cells in autoimmunity. Nat. Rev. Immunol. 3, 223—232.

Waldo, F.B., van den Wall Bake, A.W., Mestecky, J., Husby, S., 1994. Suppression of the immune response by nasal immunization. Clin. Immunol. Immunopathol. 72, 30—34.

Walter, M., Philotheou, A., Bonnici, F., Ziegler, A.G., Jimenez, R., NBI-6024 Study Group, 2009. No effect of the altered peptdie ligand NBI-6024 on beta-cell residual function and insulin needs in new-onset type 1 diabetes. Diabetes Care. 32, 2036—2040.

Walter, M., Kaupper, T., Adler, K., Foersch, J., Bonifacio, E., Ziegler, A.G., 2010. No effect of the 1alpha, 25-dihydroxyvitamin D3 on beta-cell residual function and insulin requirement in adults with new-onset type 1 diabetes. Diabetes Care. 33, 1443—1448.

Weiner, H.L., Mackin, G.A., Matsui, M., 1993. Double-blind pilot trial of oral tolerization with myelin antigens in multiple sclerosis. Science. 259, 1321—1324.

Wentworth, J.M., Fourlanos, S., Harrison, L.C., 2009. Deconstructing the stereotypes of diabetes within the modern diabetogenic environment. Nat. Rev. Endocrinol. 5, 483—489.

Wenzlau, J.M., Juhl, K., Yu, L., Moua, O., Sarkar, S.A., Gottlieb, P., et al., 2007. The cation efflux transporter ZnT8 (Slc30A8) is a major autoantigen in human type 1 diabetes. Proc. Natl .Acad Sci. U S A. 2007 Oct 23. 104 (43), 17040—17045.

Wherrett, D.K., Bundy, B., Becker, D.J., DiMeglio, L.A., Gitelman, S.E., Goland, R., et al., 2011. Antigen-based therapy with glutamic acid decarboxylase (GAD) vaccine in patients with recent-onset type 1 diabetes: a randomised double-blind trial. Lancet. 378, 319—327.

Zhang, Z.H., Davidson, L., Eisenbarth, G., Weiner, H.L., 1991. Suppression of diabetes in nonobese diabetic mice by oral administration of porcine insulin. Proc. Natl. Acad. Sci. U.S.A. 88, 10252—10256.

Treatment of Autoimmune Disease: Established Therapies

Bevra H. Hahn and Jennifer K. King

University of California, Los Angeles, Division of Rheumatology, Rehab Center, Los Angeles, CA, USA

Chapter Outline

Principles of Immune Suppression	**1209**	Cyclophosphamide	1214
General Considerations	**1211**	Mycophenolate Mofetil (Cellcept)	1214
Non-Specific Anti-Inflammatory Drugs	**1211**	Azathioprine (Imuran)	1215
NSAIDs	1211	Cyclosporin A	1215
Glucocorticoids	1212	**Other Treatment Options**	**1216**
Established Treatments of Rheumatic Diseases	**1212**	B Cell Suppressive Therapies	1216
Antimalarials	1212	IVIG	1216
Sulfasalazine	1213	**Moving Towards Biological and Molecular Therapies**	**1216**
Leflunomide	1213	**References**	**1217**
Methotrexate	1213		

Rapid advances in immunology and greater understandings of disease etiology and pathogenesis have made the treatment of autoimmune diseases a dynamic and swiftly evolving field. Older, established therapies such as glucocorticoids and non-specific immunosuppressive, chemotherapeutic agents are now being tested against newer, more targeted biologic and molecular therapies. Progress in elucidation of basic mechanisms of autoimmune diseases has led to rapid development of targets on antigen-presenting cells, T/B lymphocytes, cytokines, and costimulatory molecules. In addition, improved measures of defining clinical response and identification of biomarkers reflecting clinical outcomes and prognosis have accelerated the development of treatment options for autoimmune diseases. The goal of this chapter is to review established therapies of autoimmune diseases, with a focus on rheumatic diseases. We will highlight traditional therapies that form the foundation of current clinical practice (see Table 80.1), while laying out a context for which newer biologic and molecular targets are now evolving into the current standard of care (see Chapter 81).

PRINCIPLES OF IMMUNE SUPPRESSION

As with our oncology colleagues, the goals for physicians treating autoimmune diseases are to induce improvement (remission or low disease activity), while arresting irreversible organ damage and minimizing treatment side effects. Although definitive cure and restoration of permanent immunological tolerance would be ideal, most treatments now do not achieve that goal. Treatments are often non-specifically anti-inflammatory and/or immunosuppressive. Thus, the substantive side effects that accompany such treatments require balancing the risks of infection, bone marrow suppression, and other organ toxicity with potential efficacy.

In recent years, the paradigm of "tight control" has emerged, in which goal-directed treatments are based on quantitative and disease-specific measurements that guide providers to rapidly achieve low disease activity or remission. Notably, "tight control" in rheumatoid arthritis (RA) was illustrated in the TICORA study (Grigor et al., 2004) in which 111 patients were randomly assigned to either

N. Rose & I. Mackay (Eds): The Autoimmune Diseases, Fifth edition. DOI: http://dx.doi.org/10.1016/B978-0-12-384929-8.00080-0

TABLE 80.1 Established Immunosuppressives for Autoimmune Diseases

Drug	Primary Mechanism of Action	Side Effects	Indications
Antimalarials	Inhibition of TLR-3/7, raising of lysozyme pH affecting antigen processing	Headache, pruritus, rash, neuropathy, corneal deposition, retinopathy	Systemic lupus erythematosus, rheumatoid arthritis, juvenile idiopathic arthritis, Sjögren's, juvenile dermatomyositis, palindromic rheumatism
Sulfasalazine	Inhibition of prostaglandin synthesis, inhibition of NFκB transcription, reduction of TNF, suppression of B cells	Elevated liver enzymes, leukopenia, agranulocytosis, megaloblastic anemia, GI or CNS side effects	Inflammatory bowel disease (ulcerative colitis), mild rheumatoid arthritis, psoriatic juvenile idiopathic arthritis
Leflunomide	Inhibits dihydroorotate dehydrogenase, affecting *de novo* pyrimidine synthesis	Elevated liver enzymes, diarrhea, rash, hair loss, hypertension, interstitial pneumonitis, class X teratogen	Rheumatoid arthritis
Methotrexate	Inhibits dihydrofolate reductase, interfering with purine and pyrimidine metabolism and amino acid synthesis	Elevated liver enzymes, oral ulcers, diarrhea, mild hair loss, pneumonitis, infections, bone marrow suppression	Rheumatoid arthritis, psoriasis and psoriatic arthritis, seronegative spondyloarthropathies, arthritic manifestations of systemic lupus erythematosus, granulomatosis with polyangiitis, steroid sparing agent
Cyclophosphamide	Alkylating agent that inhibits cell division by cross-linking DNA and reducing DNA synthesis	Infections, bladder toxicity, secondary malignancy, premature ovarian failure, infertility, neutropenia	Systemic lupus erythematosus nephritis or other life-threatening manifestations, transverse myelitis, systemic sclerosis, granulomatosis with polyangiitis, polyarteritis nodosa, rheumatoid vasculitis
Mycophenolate mofetil	Inhibits inosine monophosphate dehydrogenase, affecting *de novo* purine synthesis in activated lymphocytes	Diarrhea, gastrointestinal upset, infection, bone marrow suppression, neoplasia, rash, tremor	Systemic lupus erythematosus nephritis, myasthenia gravis
Azathioprine	Purine antagonist and inhibits synthesis of DNA, RNA, proteins, cellular metabolism	Bone marrow suppression, infection, gastrointestinal upset, nausea, neoplasia	Maintenance therapy for systemic lupus erythematosus nephritis, ulcerative colitis, Crohn's disease, ANCA-positive vasculitis
Cyclosporine	Inhibits transcription of IL-2 production and proliferation of T lymphocytes	Renal toxicity, hypertension, neurologic side effects, skin or lymphoproliferative disorders, significant drug–drug interactions	Refractory ocular and mucocutaneous Behçet's disease, adult systemic lupus membranous nephritis, systemic sclerosis, severe ulcerative colitis, myasthenia gravis; typically not first-line therapy
Rituximab	Anti-CD20 monoclonal antibody against B cells	Infusion reaction, infection, reduced vaccination response, mucocutaneous reactions, malignancy, rare progressive multifocal leukoencephalopathy (PML) due to JC virus	Rheumatoid arthritis, granulomatosis with polyangiitis, microscopic polyangiitis
Belimumab	Inhibits cytokine B lymphocyte stimulator protein (BLys) necessary for B cell proliferation, survival, and differentiation	Nausea, diarrhea, fever, insomnia, depression, leukopenia, angioedema, hypersensitivity	Mild to moderate non-renal or non-central nervous system lupus
IVIG	Interference with Fc receptors, anti-idiotypic antibodies, inhibition of reticuloendothelial clearance	Rate-related infusion reactions, headache, aseptic meningitis, acute renal failure, thrombosis, urticaria, anaphylaxis in IgA-deficient patients	Guillain–Barré syndrome, myasthenia gravis, autoimmune peripheral neuropathies, rheumatic hematologic autoimmune thrombocytopenia, or hemolytic anemia

an intensive or a routine management group. Intensive management consisted of monthly office visits, measurements of disease activity scores (DAS), steroid injections of swollen joints, and every 3-month escalation of treatment by a defined protocol if moderate or high disease activity persisted. In contrast, the routine management group was seen every 3 months, without DAS measurement, and steroid injections and treatment escalation were based on the clinical judgment of the clinician, in contrast to predefined formal targets. After 18 months, patients in the tight control/intensive group showed significantly improved disease activity, physical function, and quality of life, as well as less radiographic progression of arthritis—all at no additional cost compared to routinely managed patients. The BeST study (Goekoop-Ruiterman et al., 2005, 2007) and others (Mottonen et al., 1999; Rantalaiho et al., 2009) similarly illustrated greater remission rates and earlier functional improvement in RA arthritis patients with early, goal-directed therapy emphasizing aggressive treatment to achieve tight control of disease. Given the clear advantages of intensive treatment, the tight control paradigm is reflected in the 2012 update of the American College of Rheumatology's recommendations for the use of disease-modifying antirheumatic drugs and biologics in the treatment of RA (Singh et al., 2012). With greater integration of quantitative measurements and disease activity scores to define targets for treatment remission, goal-directed therapy as demonstrated in RA may serve as a harbinger for tight control treatment algorithms under study in other autoimmune diseases. Already, there is interest in working groups for establishing similarly objective "tight control" measures for seronegative spondyloarthropathies, systemic lupus erythematosus (SLE), and others.

GENERAL CONSIDERATIONS

For many autoimmune disorders, chronic inflammation can lead to a variety of non-specific, constitutional symptoms that include fatigue, muscle pains, weight loss, and/or fever. In fact, 40–80% of patients with systemic lupus erythematosus (SLE, lupus) experience such constitutional symptoms at any one time (Von Feldt, 1995). Furthermore, constitutional symptoms are present in a variety of other disorders such as multiple sclerosis, RA, multisystem autoimmune diseases, and vasculitis. General therapeutic principles focus on treating reversible causes of fatigue, weakness, and weight loss, such as checking for anemia, drug toxicities, and ruling out other potential etiologies such as malignancy, infections, or thyroid/endocrine disorders. Proper muscle conditioning with appropriate aerobic exercise, good sleep management, and pain control may improve symptoms in some

patients. Some studies have shown that stress may induce or exacerbate pre-existing lupus symptoms (Otto & Mackay, 1967; Blumenfield, 1978), in which overall stress reduction may be beneficial (Greco et al., 2004).

In addition, management of precipitating environmental factors such as sun exposure and tobacco smoke is important. UV light in SLE patients induces increased apoptosis in skin cells, thus enhancing self-antigenicity of keratinocytes to express self-antigens on their surface that may stimulate an inflammatory response and autoantibody production leading to photosensitivity, cutaneous SLE, and/or generalized flares (Jones, 1992; Casciola-Rosen et al., 1994). Furthermore, genetically prone RA patients that carry an epitope in the hypervariable region of the HLA-DR chain, known as the "shared epitope," have a higher risk of developing RA if they smoke cigarettes (Padyukov et al., 2004). The relative risk for development of RA in current smokers is 2.3–5.6-fold higher than for non-smokers. In another study, the relative risk for developing RA was 20-fold higher in those with two alleles of the shared epitope, a smoking history, and anti-cyclic citrullinated peptide (anti-CCP) antibodies (Klareskog et al., 2006). Smoking may also increase disease severity (Saag et al., 1997; Wolfe, 2000). The mechanism of interaction between smoking and the shared epitope may primarily affect citrullination of proteins in inflamed synovial tissue. The association between smoking and RA was most robust in patients with anti-CCP autoantibodies detected in blood (Klareskog et al., 2006). Studies have shown an association with smoking and development of autoantibodies, such as ANA (Regius et al., 1988). Smoking may also be associated with increased risk for development of SLE (Ghaussy et al., 2001) and Crohn's disease, although it may lessen the risk of developing ulcerative colitis (Tobin et al., 1987; Mahid et al., 2006). Hence, simple but important lifestyle changes such as reducing sun exposure (for SLE) and avoiding tobacco (for RA, SLE, and Crohn's disease) are important therapeutic considerations in management of autoimmune diseases.

NON-SPECIFIC ANTI-INFLAMMATORY DRUGS

NSAIDs

Non-steroidal anti-inflammatory drugs are widely used throughout the world either over the counter or via prescription. All major NSAID classes share the common mechanism of inhibiting cyclooxygenase, which metabolizes arachidonic acid to cyclic endoperoxidases to form prostaglandins. Prostaglandins' role in inflammation includes induction of swelling, erythema, neutrophil trafficking, changes in vascular permeability, and inhibition of apoptosis (Lu et al., 1995; Harris, 2002). In addition, other non-prostaglandin mechanisms include NSAID inhibition of nuclear factor kappa B (NFκB)-dependent transcription (Amin et al., 1995), thus decreasing nitric oxide that normally may lead to increased vascular permeability and immune cell trafficking. NSAIDs are used commonly in multisystem autoimmune diseases to treat constitutional symptoms, fever, arthritis, serositis, and headache. The potential adverse effects of NSAIDs often limit their use, particularly induction of gastritis (often with bleeding), reduced glomerular blood flow, hypertension, peripheral edema, and the association of high doses with increased risk for myocardial infarction (Solomon, 2012). Thus, for safety concerns, they are recommended most commonly for as-needed rather than continual use.

Glucocorticoids

Glucocorticoids (GC) have a broad range of anti-inflammatory and immunosuppressive effects on both the innate and adaptive immune system. GC bind to an intracellular receptor, where they can directly affect gene transcription, resulting in inhibition of production of inflammatory cytokines, and effects on post-translational mRNA stability. Anti-inflammatory effects include downregulation of nitric oxide synthesis resulting in reduced blood vessel permeability, decreased leukocyte migration to peripheral tissues, inhibition of inflammatory mediators such as eicosanoids, inhibition of collagenases, and suppression of inflammatory cytokines. Effects of GC on immune cells include inhibition of signaling for T cell activation and IL-2 synthesis, downregulation of antigen-presenting cells via blockade of costimulatory molecules, immune deviation toward Th2 cytokines, and induction of T cell apoptosis (Kirouka, 2007). GC are often used to control acute manifestations of inflammatory and autoimmune disorders, dosed on a mg/kg basis depending on the severity of the disease. Typical dosing regimens may be divided as follows from most potent to least: (1) pulse intravenous (IV) therapy with methylprednisolone 500−1000 mg per day, (2) very high-dose oral GC at 1−2 mg/kg/day prednisone or equivalent, (3) high-dose oral GC at 0.6−1 mg/kg/day prednisone or equivalent, (4) medium-dose GC at 0.125−0.5 mg/kg/day prednisone or equivalent, or (5) low-dose GC at <0.125 mg/kg/day prednisone or equivalent (King and Hahn, 2007). Organ threatening manifestations of disease in SLE, dermatomyositis, large and small vessel vasculitis, and multiple sclerosis often require pulse IV steroids as part of the initial induction therapy for acute flare control.

ESTABLISHED TREATMENTS OF RHEUMATIC DISEASES

Antimalarials

Antimalarial medications such as hydroxychloroquine, chloroquine, and quinacrine can be used to treat mild to moderate manifestations of SLE or RA and other rheumatic disorders. Various mechanisms of action may contribute to their utility in immune modulation, including (1) inhibition of activation of intracellular Toll-like receptor (TLR)-3 and TLR-7, (2) blockade of antigen processing by raising intracytoplasmic pH in lysozymes with resultant decreased lymphocyte proliferation, autoantibody production, and NK cell activity, and (3) inhibition of formation of immune complexes (Fox, 1993; Fox and Kang, 1993; Kyburz et al., 2006). In addition, anti-inflammatory effects include inhibition of phospholipases, prostaglandins, blockade of superoxide secretion, suppression of destructive proteolytic enzymes by synoviocytes, and blockade of UV light to protect keratinocytes from increased antigenicity (Wallace, 2007). Hormonal actions may impair insulin release, anti-proliferative effects may inhibit graft versus host disease, and intercalation with DNA may block synthesis to allow degradation of ribosomal RNA (Wallace, 2007). Hydroxychloroquine and chloroquine can also inhibit platelet aggregation and adhesion (Ernst et al., 1984; Jancinova et al., 1994; Edwards et al., 1997), adding to their utility for SLE patients with coexisting anti-phospholipid syndrome and/or platelet abnormalities.

In SLE, antimalarials are most useful in treating constitutional symptoms, skin lesions, and arthritis, and for prevention of disease flare. In addition, the 2007 LUMINA trial illustrated an association between hydroxychloroquine and improved survival (Alarcon et al., 2007). Pregnant mothers with anti-Ro may use hydroxychloroquine to reduce risk of antibody-associated cardiac neonatal lupus (Izmirly et al., 2010). In RA, antimalarials are typically used in combination with other disease modifying agents, such as methotrexate or sulfasalazine. A large observational study indicated reduced risk of diabetes mellitus among patients who were taking hydroxychloroquine for RA compared to those not taking the medication (Wasko et al., 2007). Antimalarials may also decrease antibody levels in Sjögren's syndrome, as well as improve sicca symptoms by inhibiting glandular cholinesterase (Dawson et al., 2005). Hydroxychloroquine has also been used in systemic onset juvenile idiopathic arthritis (Still's disease), juvenile dermatomyositis, and palindromic rheumatism. One study found that the use of antimalarials in palindromic rheumatism patients was associated with a 20% decreased risk of progression to RA or other connective tissue disease (Gonzalez-Lopez et al., 2000). Side effects vary with specific antimalarials (in general the highest risk of important adverse effects is associated with chloroquine). These side effects include neuromuscular and cardiac toxicity, skin changes (particularly hyperpigmentation with all, and yellow discoloration with quinacrine), aplastic anemia (quinacrine), and rare ocular effects, including macular damage. Regular ocular screening of patients treated for more than 6 months with chloroquine or hydroxychloroquine is recommended (Marmor et al., 2011).

Sulfasalazine

Sulfasalazine (azulfidine) was originally proposed for use in RA, although ultimately great benefit was seen in treatment for inflammatory bowel disease (IBD). After oral ingestion, the majority of the intact drug reaches the large intestine and is reduced to sulfapyridine and 5-aminosalicylic acid (5-ASA). For IBD, and specifically ulcerative colitis (UC), 5-ASA acts locally in the colon to decrease inflammatory responses via inhibition of prostaglandin synthesis. Sulfasalazine is effective for maintaining remission in ulcerative colitis (Dissanayake and Truelove, 1973; Mulder et al., 1988). Interestingly, in contrast to UC, the active metabolite in RA patients is sulfapyridine, although the exact mechanism of action has not been clearly identified. Studies involving RA patients taking sulfapyridine (and not 5-ASA) have been linked to improvement of disease parameters with decreases in erythrocyte sedimentation rate and C-reactive protein (Pullar et al., 1985; Taggart et al., 1986). In addition, studies suggest that the parent sulfasalazine drug inhibited NFκB transcription, may inhibit tumor necrosis factor-alpha in macrophages by inducing apoptosis, and may suppress B cell function (Wahl et al., 1998; Rodenburg et al., 2000; Hirohata et al., 2002; Lee et al., 2004). In RA, sulfasalazine is often used in combination therapy with other disease modifying antirheumatic drug (DMARDs) for optimal treatment. Adverse effects include elevated liver function tests, leukopenia, agranulocytosis, megaloblastic anemia, and gastrointestinal or central nervous system effects.

Leflunomide

Leflunomide (LF) is an oral medication that, once absorbed, is metabolized into its active form known as teriflunomide. The main mechanism of action of teriflunomide is to inhibit the mitochondrial enzyme dihydroorotate dehydrogenase (DHODH), which is an enzyme involved in the *de novo* pyridmidine synthesis pathway of ribonucleotide uridine monophosphate pyrimidine (rUMP). Disruption of DHODH prevents activated lymphocytes from moving from the G1 to S phase (Fox,

1998). In addition, the immunomodulatory effects of LF are broad, including inhibition of leukocyte adhesion to endothelial cells and infiltration into synovium, which may be of particular importance in RA (Dimitrijevic and Bartlett, 1996; Salmi et al., 1997; Grisar et al., 2004). In addition, LF preferentially inhibits memory self-reactive lymphocytes, affects dendritic cell antigen presentation, and blocks NFκB activation (Zhang et al., 1997; Manna and Aggarwal, 1999;). LF blocks protein tyrosine kinases Jak1 and Jak3, which affect T cell stimulation via IL-2 receptor activation (Siemasko et al., 1998). LF may also increase the production of transforming growth factor (TGF) beta, which is a known anti-inflammatory cytokine (Cao et al., 1996). Common side effects include diarrhea, rash, hair loss, and elevated liver enzymes. Less common side effects include hypertension, interstitial pneumonitis, leukopenia, hematologic toxicities, and peripheral neuropathy. LF is contraindicated in pregnant and nursing women and in patients with pre-existing liver disease.

Leflunomide is approved by the United States Food and Drug Administration for the treatment of RA. In RA, trials have demonstrated efficacy of LF as monotherapy, with comparable outcomes to those of methotrexate or sulfasalazine monotherapy (Smolen et al., 1999; Emery et al., 2000). In lupus, a controlled trial in patients with mild to moderate disease activity showed benefit of LF treatment after 6 months of treatment compared to placebo (Tam et al., 2004). Other trials have shown efficacy in psoriatic arthritis, juvenile polyarthritis, and resistant dermatomyositis, but not ankylosing spondylitis.

Methotrexate

Methotrexate (MTX) is a folate antagonist that has been used effectively in a variety of autoimmune conditions. Competitive binding blocks the enzyme dihydrofolate reductase from reducing dihydrofolic acid to folinic acid, the active intracellular metabolite involved in purine/pyrimidine metabolism and amino acid/polyamine synthesis. However, at the doses used in rheumatic conditions, which are often lower than in oncologic chemotherapeutic regimens, the exact mechanism of action is uncertain. Animal models suggest that methotrexate increases extracellular concentrations of adenosine in inflammatory tissue, which has anti-inflammatory effects via dephosphorylation of adenine nucleotides (Cronstein, 1996; Morabito et al., 1998). Other possible mechanisms include inhibition of DNA methylation necessary for cell proliferation, induction of apoptosis of activated peripheral T cells, regulation of IL-1β, increased IL-10 synthesis, inhibition of leukotriene B2 formation and cyclooxygenase-2, and interference with neutrophil function (Cronstein, 1996; Genestier et al., 1998; Mello et al., 2000; Seitz et al., 2001). Methotrexate can be taken orally, subcutaneously, or intramuscularly. Side effects include elevation of liver enzymes, especially when concurrently ingesting alcohol, oral ulcers, post-ingestion nausea, diarrhea, and hair loss. More severe complications include pneumonitis, infections due to immune suppression, bone marrow suppression, and hepatic fibrosis. Folic or folinic acid is often used as supplementation to reduce hematologic and other side effects, although folinic acid may interfere with efficacy. Pregnancy should be avoided, as MTX is a known teratogen.

Methotrexate is used in a variety of rheumatic conditions, most prominently in RA, but also in psoriasis/psoriatic arthritis, peripheral joint disease in seronegative spondyloarthropathies, SLE, granulomatosis with polyangiitis (formerly called Wegener's granulomatosis), and other large vessel vasculitides. Barring contraindications or allergy, methotrexate can be considered one of the cornerstones of disease modifying antirheumatic drugs (DMARDs) for the treatment of RA. Studies have shown both short-term and long-term efficacy in RA disease measurements, such as joint pain and swelling, quality of life, objective laboratory markers of inflammation, and radiologic progression of disease (Weinblatt et al., 1992, 1994; Rich et al., 1999), as well as possible improvement in survival (Choi et al., 2002). Methotrexate can be used in monotherapy, but more often in combination therapy with the regimens of (1) sulfasalazine and hydroxychloroquine (O'Dell et al., 1996), or (2) anti-tumor necrosis factor (anti-TNF) inhibitors for greatest efficacy (Lipsky et al., 2000). Numerous trials have demonstrated the value of methotrexate in combination therapy on disease activity measures, reduction of radiographic progression, and functionality. Methotrexate is often used in other disorders to treat peripheral joint arthritis symptoms, such as in psoriasis, seronegative spondylarthritis disorders, and joint manifestations in lupus patients. In vasculitides such as granulomatosis with polyangiitis, oral methotrexate can be used as initial therapy for non-organ threatening, non-renal disease, although its use is associated with a higher relapse rate compared to cyclophosphamide. Thus, methotrexate is a reasonable alternative for patients who cannot tolerate other more toxic (but more effective) treatment regimens (De Groot et al., 2005; Mukhtyar et al., 2009). In addition, methotrexate may be used as a steroid-sparing agent in the large vessel vasculitis in giant cell arteritis, although there is conflicting evidence of its efficacy in this setting (Jover et al., 2001; Hoffman et al., 2002).

Cyclophosphamide

Cyclophosphamide (CYC) is a potent alkylating agent, used most often to treat life-threatening or organ-threatening manifestations of autoimmune and inflammatory diseases.

It can be administered orally or intravenously, and is metabolized by the liver mitochondrial P-450 enzyme into several active metabolites with both therapeutic and toxic effects. CYC has direct effects on DNA resulting in cell death, and modulates T cell activation (McCune and Fox, 1989; Fox and McCune, 1994). The significant side effects often limit more widespread use, and include an increased risk for opportunistic infections such as *Pneumocystis jiroveci* pneumonia and fungal infections, bladder toxicity with hemorrhagic cystitis and carcinoma of the bladder, neutropenia, increased risk of infertility or premature ovarian failure, and development of malignancy. Short-term therapeutic use of CYC aims for rapid control of the underlying inflammatory process (over a period of a few weeks to months), while seeking replacement of CYC when possible with an acceptable alternative to avoid the significant long-term toxicities.

Cyclophosphamide has been used effectively in the treatment of lupus nephritis, interstitial lung disease in multisystem autoimmune disease, and medium and small vessel vasculitis. In patients with severe lupus nephritis, initial landmark trials from the National Institute of Health demonstrated the superiority of monthly high-dose IV CYC ($500-1000$ mg/m^2) for 6 months, followed by two quarterly pulses with glucocorticoids, versus glucocorticoid therapy alone in preserving renal function (Austin et al., 1986; Boumpas et al., 1992; Gourley et al., 1996; Illei et al., 2001). Subsequent studies have investigated the role of low-dose CYC regimens (500 mg IV every 2 weeks $\times$ 6) and found this regimen compared to the higher dose CYC produces similar rates of renal remission in European patients—for up to 10 years (Houssiau et al., 2002, 2010b). It is not known whether the low-dose regimen is effective in African Americans, Asians, or Latinos with lupus nephritis. Small studies suggest a role for CYC in treatment of central nervous system manifestations of SLE, such as transverse myelitis (Barile and Lavalle, 1992; Neuwelt et al., 1995; Kovacs et al., 2000) (see Chapter 57). CYC has also demonstrated stabilization of pulmonary function, dyspnea, skin thickening, and health-related quality of life in patients with symptomatic systemic sclerosis-related interstitial lung disease (Tashkin et al., 2006). Systemic vasculitides such as granulomatosis with polyangiitis, microscopic polyangiitis, rheumatoid vasculitis, polyarteritis nodosa, and autoimmune-associated mononeuritis multiplex are other indications for CYC in which significant clinical improvement and/or survival benefits have been shown (Stone, 2010).

Mycophenolate Mofetil (Cellcept)

Mycophenolate mofetil (MMF) was used initially in the 1990s for the prevention of allograft rejection in renal transplantation. In the past decade, MMF has been shown to be an effective therapy in both induction and maintenance of improvement in SLE nephritis, thus allowing for use of an alternative regimen to cyclophosphamide. MMF reversibly inhibits the enzyme inosine monophosphate dehydrogenase, which is necessary for *de novo* purine synthesis in activated lymphocytes. Blockade with MMF results in reduced T and B cell proliferation, less antibody production, induction of apoptosis of activated T lymphocytes, and hindrance of production and function of adhesion molecules important for lymphocyte migration to inflammatory tissues (Allison and Eugui, 2000). Side effects include diarrhea, nausea, gastrointestinal upset, infections, bone marrow toxicity, neoplasia, and rash. MMF compared to CYC is less likely to cause alopecia and amenorrhea, but rates of infection, serious infection, and death are similar with the two treatments (Touma et al., 2011).

The use of MMF has profoundly changed the outcomes and therapeutic landscape in induction therapy of improvement in diffuse proliferative and membranous serious SLE-related glomerulonephritis. Initial studies in Chinese patients suggested that MMF was an effective alternative to CYC (Chan et al., 2000; Hu et al., 2002). Subsequent clinical trials compared cyclophosphamide to MMF. A recent international, randomized controlled trial (ALMS trial) of 370 SLE patients with active nephritis compared MMF (2–3 g/day) to IV CYC (0.5–1 g/m^2) monthly for 6 months. This induction therapy showed similar efficacy between the two treatments (Appel et al., 2009). Interestingly, however, proportions of African Americans and Latino Americans responding to cyclophosphamide were lower compared to Caucasians and Asians, whereas responses in all four racial groups to MMF were similar (Isenberg et al., 2010). A subsequent meta-analysis similarly confirmed MMF and CYC to be equivalent in efficacy and side effect profiles (Touma et al., 2011), although MMF was not superior to CYC as suggested by an earlier randomized but not blinded clinical trial (Ginzler et al., 2005). A follow-up analysis from the ALMS trial examining non-renal lupus activity in the same nephritis patients showed similar efficacy between MMF and CYC on non-renal manifestations, thus suggesting MMF as a reasonable alternative to CYC for renal and non-renal SLE (Ginzler et al., 2010). Furthermore, in addition to the above trials demonstrating MMF's utility in induction therapy in SLE, a recent study has demonstrated MMF's superiority in safety and efficacy in maintenance therapy for SLE nephritis compared to CYC (Contreras et al., 2004) and azathioprine (Dooley et al., 2011). The American College of Rheumatology's 2012 recently updated guidelines for treatment and management of classes III, IV, and V glomerulonephritis reflect the current state of the art regarding use of MMF (Hahn et al., 2012). MMF has also been used as a steroid-sparing agent for the treatment of other rheumatic

diseases, and for the treatment of autoimmune hepatitis (see Chapter 61). The US FDA has not approved either cyclophosphamide or mycophenolate mofetil (or the active metabolite of MMF, myfortic acid) for treatment of lupus nephritis or other manifestations of SLE, but all are widely used in the United States for serious or life-threatening SLE.

Azathioprine (Imuran)

Azathioprine (AZA) is a pro-drug that is metabolized to its active component 6-mercaptopurine (6-MP), a purine antagonist that inhibits DNA synthesis and lymphocyte proliferation. Intracellular metabolism of 6-MP results in decreased numbers of circulating lymphocytes, IL-2 secretion, and immunoglobulin production (Wilke, 2010). It is approved by the US Food and Drug Administration for prevention of renal transplant rejection and the treatment of rheumatoid arthritis; however, off-label use is common for maintenance of improvement in lupus nephritis and inflammatory bowel disease, or as a steroid-sparing agent. Adverse effects include nausea, vomiting, bone marrow suppression, increased risk of infection, and malignancy. Individuals with a homozygous genetic polymorphism of the enzyme thiopurine methyltransferase (TPMT) that reduces the metabolism of AZA may be at greater risk for AZA toxicity. Some authorities recommend checking for this genetic polymorphism prior to initiation of therapy. A number of studies have shown efficacy of AZA over placebo in the treatment of RA (Urowitz et al., 1973; Cade et al., 1976; Woodland et al., 1981), although more recent combination therapies of methotrexate plus biologics or other DMARDs are in wider use. In addition, AZA can be used for effective maintenance therapy in lupus nephritis (Contreras et al., 2004; Houssiau et al., 2010a), ulcerative colitis and Crohn's bowel disease (Timmer et al., 2007; Prefontaine et al., 2009), ANCA-positive vasculitis (Pagnoux et al., 2008), and autoimmune hepatitis (see Chapter 61).

Cyclosporin A

Cyclosporin A (CSA) is a cyclic peptide of 11 amino acids that binds with high affinity to cyclophilins, which competitively bind to calcineurin. This leads to inhibition of translocation of transcription factors, NF-AT, thus reducing transcription of early cytokine genes that encode IL-2, TNF-α, interferon-γ, IL-3, IL-4, CD40, and granulocyte-macrophage colony-stimulating factor (Schreiber and Crabtree, 1992; Wiederrecht et al., 1993; Timmerman et al., 1996). Furthermore, CSA interferes with antigen presentation by antigen-presenting cells. The ultimate net effect is reduction of lymphocyte proliferation. CSA is metabolized by the cytochrome P450 3A4 liver enzymes and has a variety of drug—drug interactions that may interfere with blood concentration levels, thus requiring monitoring of CSA levels. Side effects include renal toxicity, hypertension, neurologic side effects such as tremor, encephalopathy, increased risk of skin or lymphoproliferative malignancies, and heightened risk for infection. However, unlike many alkylating agents and purine antagonists, CSA lacks clinically significant bone marrow suppression. CSA has been used in a variety of established and suspected autoimmune disorders, including RA, psoriatic arthritis, ocular and mucocutaneous Behçet's disease, adult lupus membranous nephritis, systemic sclerosis, atopic dermatitis, severe ulcerative colitis, pemphigus vulgaris, and myasthenia gravis (Magee, 2012). However, concern over long-term side effects, especially of renal toxicity, hypertension, and a myriad of drug interactions, has limited utility in chronic autoimmune diseases, except in patients who have failed more conventional therapies. Tacrolimus, another oral medication that inhibits T lymphocyte activation similarly to cyclosporine, is used widely for prevention of allograft rejection. Because its potential adverse effects are slightly less than those of cyclosporine, it is being used for some autoimmune diseases and is being studied in systemic lupus erythematosus, RA, and autoimmune hepatitis (Li et al., 2012).

OTHER TREATMENT OPTIONS

B Cell Suppressive Therapies

Targeting autoreactive B cells or B cell maturation signals has become successful therapy for autoimmune rheumatic conditions, and will be discussed briefly here and in further detail in Chapter 81. The use of rituximab, a chimeric anti-CD20 monoclonal antibody, causes depletion of B cells via various mechanisms, including Fc gamma receptor-mediated antibody-dependent cytotoxicity, antibody-dependent complement-mediated cell lysis, and B cell apoptosis (Cragg et al., 2005). Rituximab has shown efficacy and is FDA approved for treatment of RA, granulomatosis with polyangiitis, and microscopic polyangiitis. In particular, there is recent excitement over results of the RAVE trial in patients with ANCA(+) vasculitis, which shows that rituximab is an effective and safer alternative to cyclophosphamide, especially in patients with relapsing disease (Stone et al., 2010). However, further studies with long-term data are necessary before drawing definitive conclusions regarding the superiority of rituxan over standard of care cyclophosphamide (Jones et al., 2010), but current results are promising. Of note, rituximab was not shown to be superior to placebo for treatment of SLE patients with active disease (renal or non-renal) who were receiving GC plus

hydroxychloroquine plus an immunosuppressive drug (Merrill et al., 2010; Rovin et al., 2012). Depletion of maturing B cells by inhibition of the cytokine B lymphocyte stimulator protein (BLyS, BAFF), which induces B cell proliferation, survival, and differentiation into plasma cells, has been met with great excitement. In 2011, belimumab, a fully humanized monoclonal antibody that targets BlyS, and hence decreases the availability of BlyS to activate B lymphocytes, became the first drug in 50 years to be approved for the treatment of non-renal and non-central nervous system lupus disease (Furie et al., 2011; Navarra et al., 2011; Hahn, 2013). Of note, belimumab is meant for lupus patients who are anti-nuclear antibody or anti-double stranded DNA positive, and interestingly showed less response in African American patients. A recent study showed that responses are durable for a 4-year period—the follow-up period of the study (Merrill et al., 2012). Ongoing studies will test the efficacy of belimumab over the long term in patients with lupus nephritis and possibly in those with vasculitis.

IVIG

The use of intravenous immune globulin (IVIG) in autoimmune diseases has several possible mechanisms of action, including interference with Fc receptors on effector cells, anti-idiotypic antibody activity against serum autoantibodies, inhibition of reticuloendothelial clearance of antibody-covered platelets via Fc receptors, and regulation of expression of proinflammatory cytokines and adhesion molecules in inflammatory states (Silvergleid, 2011). In addition, other effects of IVIG include solubilization and clearance of immune complexes, altered T cell subsets, and increased T regulatory cells. IVIG is found to be useful in the autoimmune demyelinating Guillain—Barré syndrome, myasthenia gravis, autoimmune peripheral neuropathies, rheumatic hematologic conditions such as autoimmune thrombocytopenia or hemolytic anemia, and antibody-mediated CNS diseases resulting from interference with neurotransmitter function (see Chapter 57). Small studies have also shown that IVIG is a reasonable second-line therapy for refractory dermatomyositis or polymyositis (Dalakas et al., 1993; Cherin et al., 2002). Adverse effects of IVIG treatment include allergic reactions, including anaphylaxis (particularly in males who are IgA deficient), headache, aseptic meningitis, thrombosis, and nausea.

MOVING TOWARDS BIOLOGICAL AND MOLECULAR THERAPIES

Over the past few decades, progressive advancement in our understandings of immunopathogenesis has led to a significant expansion of potential therapeutic targets. This scientific progress has ushered in widespread use of new biologic and molecular treatments specifically targeting B and T cells, costimulation and signal transduction molecules, maturation factors, cytokines, and Toll-like receptors on antigen-presenting cells. For example, anti-TNF therapy is now routinely used in rheumatoid arthritis and seronegative spondyloarthritides, as monotherapy or in combination therapy with traditional DMARDs as mentioned above (Singh et al., 2012). Such new therapeutic targets are the subject of the next chapter, and continue to improve the standard treatments and outcomes for many autoimmune diseases.

REFERENCES

Alarcon, G.S., Mcgwin, G., Bertoli, A.M., Fessler, B.J., Calvo-Alen, J., Bastian, H.M., et al., 2007. Effect of hydroxychloroquine on the survival of patients with systemic lupus erythematosus: data from LUMINA, a multiethnic US cohort (LUMINA L). Ann. Rheum. Dis. 66, 1168–1172.

Allison, A.C., Eugui, E.M., 2000. Mycophenolate mofetil and its mechanisms of action. Immunopharmacology. 47, 85–118.

Amin, A.R., Vyas, P., Attur, M., Leszczynska-Piziak, J., Patel, I.R., Weissmann, G., et al., 1995. The mode of action of aspirin-like drugs: effect on inducible nitric oxide synthase. Proc. Natl. Acad. Sci. USA. 92, 7926–7930.

Appel, G.B., Contreras, G., Dooley, M.A., Ginzler, E.M., Isenberg, D., Jayne, D., et al., 2009. Mycophenolate mofetil versus cyclophosphamide for induction treatment of lupus nephritis. J. Am. Soc. Nephrol. 20, 1103–1112.

Austin III, H.A., Klippel, J.H., Balow, J.E., Le Riche, N.G., Steinberg, A.D., Plotz, P.H., et al., 1986. Therapy of lupus nephritis. Controlled trial of prednisone and cytotoxic drugs. N. Engl. J. Med. 314, 614–619.

Barile, L., Lavalle, C., 1992. Transverse myelitis in systemic lupus erythematosus—the effect of IV pulse methylprednisolone and cyclophosphamide. J. Rheumatol. 19, 370–372.

Blumenfield, M., 1978. Psychological aspects of systemic lupus erythematosus. Prim. Care. 5, 159–171.

Boumpas, D.T., Austin III, H.A., Vaughn, E.M., Klippel, J.H., Steinberg, A.D., Yarboro, C.H., et al., 1992. Controlled trial of pulse methylprednisolone versus two regimens of pulse cyclophosphamide in severe lupus nephritis. Lancet. 340, 741–745.

Cade, R., Stein, G., Pickering, M., Schlein, E., Spooner, G., 1976. Low dose, long-term treatment of rheumatoid arthritis with azathioprine. South. Med. J. 69, 388–392.

Cao, W.W., Kao, P.N., Aoki, Y., Xu, J.C., Shorthouse, R.A., Morris, R.E., 1996. A novel mechanism of action of the immunomodulatory drug, leflunomide: augmentation of the immunosuppressive cytokine, TGF-beta 1, and suppression of the immunostimulatory cytokine, IL-2. Transplant. Proc. 28, 3079–3080.

Casciola-Rosen, L.A., Anhalt, G., Rosen, A., 1994. Autoantigens targeted in systemic lupus erythematosus are clustered in two populations of surface structures on apoptotic keratinocytes. J. Exp. Med. 179, 1317–1330.

Chan, T.M., Li, F.K., Tang, C.S., Wong, R.W., Fang, G.X., Ji, Y.L., et al., 2000. Efficacy of mycophenolate mofetil in patients with diffuse proliferative lupus nephritis. Hong Kong-Guangzhou Nephrology Study Group. N. Engl. J. Med. 343, 1156–1162.

Cherin, P., Pelletier, S., Teixeira, A., Laforet, P., Genereau, T., Simon, A., et al., 2002. Results and long-term followup of intravenous immunoglobulin infusions in chronic, refractory polymyositis: an open study with thirty-five adult patients. Arthritis Rheum. 46, 467–474.

Choi, H.K., Hernan, M.A., Seeger, J.D., Robins, J.M., Wolfe, F., 2002. Methotrexate and mortality in patients with rheumatoid arthritis: a prospective study. Lancet. 359, 1173–1177.

Contreras, G., Pardo, V., Leclercq, B., Lenz, O., Tozman, E., O'Nan, P., et al., 2004. Sequential therapies for proliferative lupus nephritis. N. Engl. J. Med. 350, 971–980.

Cragg, M.S., Walshe, C.A., Ivanov, A.O., Glennie, M.J., 2005. The biology of CD20 and its potential as a target for mAb therapy. Curr. Dir. Autoimmun. 8, 140–174.

Cronstein, B.N., 1996. Molecular therapeutics. Methotrexate and its mechanism of action. Arthritis Rheum. 39, 1951–1960.

Dalakas, M.C., Illa, I., Dambrosia, J.M., Soueidan, S.A., Stein, D.P., Otero, C., et al., 1993. A controlled trial of high-dose intravenous immune globulin infusions as treatment for dermatomyositis. N. Engl. J. Med. 329, 1993–2000.

Dawson, L.J., Caulfield, V.L., Stanbury, J.B., Field, A.E., Christmas, S.E., Smith, P.M., 2005. Hydroxychloroquine therapy in patients with primary Sjogren's syndrome may improve salivary gland hypofunction by inhibition of glandular cholinesterase. Rheumatology (Oxford). 44, 449–455.

De Groot, K., Rasmussen, N., Bacon, P.A., Tervaert, J.W., Feighery, C., Gregorini, G., et al., 2005. Randomized trial of cyclophosphamide versus methotrexate for induction of remission in early systemic antineutrophil cytoplasmic antibody-associated vasculitis. Arthritis Rheum. 52, 2461–2469.

Dimitrijevic, M., Bartlett, R.R., 1996. Leflunomide, a novel immunomodulating drug, inhibits homotypic adhesion of mononuclear cells in rheumatoid arthritis. Transplant. Proc. 28, 3086–3087.

Dissanayake, A.S., Truelove, S.C., 1973. A controlled therapeutic trial of long-term maintenance treatment of ulcerative colitis with sulphazalazine (Salazopyrin). Gut. 14, 923–926.

Dooley, M.A., Jayne, D., Ginzler, E.M., Isenberg, D., Olsen, N.J., Wofsy, D., et al., 2011. Mycophenolate versus azathioprine as maintenance therapy for lupus nephritis. N. Engl. J. Med. 365, 1886–1895.

Edwards, M.H., Pierangeli, S., Liu, X., Barker, J.H., Anderson, G., Harris, E.N., 1997. Hydroxychloroquine reverses thrombogenic properties of antiphospholipid antibodies in mice. Circulation. 96, 4380–4384.

Emery, P., Breedveld, F.C., Lemmel, E.M., Kaltwasser, J.P., Dawes, P.T., Gomor, B., et al., 2000. A comparison of the efficacy and safety of leflunomide and methotrexate for the treatment of rheumatoid arthritis. Rheumatology (Oxford). 39, 655–665.

Ernst, E., Rose, M., Lee, R., 1984. Modification of transoperative changes in blood fluidity by hydroxychloroquine: a possible explanation for the drug's antithrombotic effect. Pharmatherapeutica. 4, 48–52.

Fox, D.A., McCune, W.J., 1994. Immunosuppressive drug therapy of systemic lupus erythematosus. Rheum. Dis. Clin. North Am. 20, 265–299.

Fox, R.I., 1993. Mechanism of action of hydroxychloroquine as an anti-rheumatic drug. Semin. Arthritis Rheum. 23, 82–91.

Fox, R.I., 1998. Mechanism of action of leflunomide in rheumatoid arthritis. J. Rheumatol. Suppl. 53, 20–26.

Fox, R.I., Kang, H.I., 1993. Mechanism of action of antimalarial drugs: inhibition of antigen processing and presentation. Lupus. 2 (Suppl. 1), S9–S12.

Furie, R., Petri, M., Zamani, O., Cervera, R., Wallace, D.J., Tegzova, D., et al., 2011. A phase III, randomized, placebo-controlled study of belimumab, a monoclonal antibody that inhibits B lymphocyte stimulator, in patients with systemic lupus erythematosus. Arthritis Rheum. 63, 3918–3930.

Genestier, L., Paillot, R., Fournel, S., Ferraro, C., Miossec, P., Revillard, J.P., 1998. Immunosuppressive properties of methotrexate: apoptosis and clonal deletion of activated peripheral T cells. J. Clin. Invest. 102, 322–328.

Ghaussy, N.O., Sibbitt Jr., W.L., Qualls, C.R., 2001. Cigarette smoking, alcohol consumption, and the risk of systemic lupus erythematosus: a case-control study. J. Rheumatol. 28, 2449–2453.

Ginzler, E.M., Dooley, M.A., Aranow, C., Kim, M.Y., Buyon, J., Merrill, J.T., et al., 2005. Mycophenolate mofetil or intravenous cyclophosphamide for lupus nephritis. N. Engl. J. Med. 353, 2219–2228.

Ginzler, E.M., Wofsy, D., Isenberg, D., Gordon, C., Lisk, L., Dooley, M.A., 2010. Nonrenal disease activity following mycophenolate mofetil or intravenous cyclophosphamide as induction treatment for lupus nephritis: findings in a multicenter, prospective, randomized, open-label, parallel-group clinical trial. Arthritis Rheum. 62, 211–221.

Goekoop-Ruiterman, Y.P., De Vries-Bouwstra, J.K., Allaart, C.F., Van Zeben, D., Kerstens, P.J., Hazes, J.M., et al., 2005. Clinical and radiographic outcomes of four different treatment strategies in patients with early rheumatoid arthritis (the BeSt study): a randomized, controlled trial. Arthritis Rheum. 52, 3381–3390.

Goekoop-Ruiterman, Y.P., De Vries-Bouwstra, J.K., Allaart, C.F., Van Zeben, D., Kerstens, P.J., Hazes, J.M., et al., 2007. Comparison of treatment strategies in early rheumatoid arthritis: a randomized trial. Ann. Intern. Med. 146, 406–415.

Gonzalez-Lopez, L., Gamez-Nava, J.I., Jhangri, G., Russell, A.S., Suarez-Almazor, M.E., 2000. Decreased progression to rheumatoid arthritis or other connective tissue diseases in patients with palindromic rheumatism treated with antimalarials. J. Rheumatol. 27, 41–46.

Gourley, M.F., Austin III, H.A., Scott, D., Yarboro, C.H., Vaughan, E.M., Muir, J., et al., 1996. Methylprednisolone and cyclophosphamide, alone or in combination, in patients with lupus nephritis. A randomized, controlled trial. Ann. Intern. Med. 125, 549–557.

Greco, C.M., Rudy, T.E., Manzi, S., 2004. Effects of a stress-reduction program on psychological function, pain, and physical function of systemic lupus erythematosus patients: a randomized controlled trial. Arthritis Rheum. 51, 625–634.

Grigor, C., Capell, H., Stirling, A., McMahon, A.D., Lock, P., Vallance, R., et al., 2004. Effect of a treatment strategy of tight control for rheumatoid arthritis (the TICORA study): a single-blind randomised controlled trial. Lancet. 364, 263–269.

Grisar, J., Aringer, M., Koller, M.D., Stummvoll, G.H., Eselbock, D., Zwolfer, B., et al., 2004. Leflunomide inhibits transendothelial migration of peripheral blood mononuclear cells. Ann. Rheum. Dis. 63, 1632–1637.

Hahn, B.H., 2013. Belimumab for systemic lupus erythematosus. N. Engl. J. Med. 368, 1528–1535.

Hahn, B.H., McMahon, M.A., Wilkinson, A., Wallace, W.D., Daikh, D.I., Fitzgerald, J.D., et al., 2012. American College of Rheumatology guidelines for screening, treatment, and management of lupus nephritis. Arthritis Care Res. (Hoboken). 64, 797–808.

Harris Jr., R.C., 2002. Cyclooxygenase-2 inhibition and renal physiology. Am. J. Cardiol. 89, 10D–17D.

Hirohata, S., Ohshima, N., Yanagida, T., Aramaki, K., 2002. Regulation of human B cell function by sulfasalazine and its metabolites. Int. Immunopharmacol. 2, 631–640.

Hoffman, G.S., Cid, M.C., Hellmann, D.B., Guillevin, L., Stone, J.H., Schousboe, J., et al., 2002. A multicenter, randomized, double-blind, placebo-controlled trial of adjuvant methotrexate treatment for giant cell arteritis. Arthritis Rheum. 46, 1309–1318.

Houssiau, F.A., Vasconcelos, C., D'Cruz, D., Sebastiani, G.D., Garrido Ed Ede, R., Danieli, M.G., et al., 2002. Immunosuppressive therapy in lupus nephritis: the Euro-Lupus Nephritis Trial, a randomized trial of low-dose versus high-dose intravenous cyclophosphamide. Arthritis Rheum. 46, 2121–2131.

Houssiau, F.A., D'Cruz, D., Sangle, S., Remy, P., Vasconcelos, C., Petrovic, R., et al., 2010a. Azathioprine versus mycophenolate mofetil for long-term immunosuppression in lupus nephritis: results from the MAINTAIN Nephritis Trial. Ann. Rheum. Dis. 69, 2083–2089.

Houssiau, F.A., Vasconcelos, C., D'Cruz, D., Sebastiani, G.D., De Ramon Garrido, E., Danieli, M.G., et al., 2010b. The 10-year follow-up data of the Euro-Lupus Nephritis Trial comparing low-dose and high-dose intravenous cyclophosphamide. Ann. Rheum. Dis. 69, 61–64.

Hu, W., Liu, Z., Chen, H., Tang, Z., Wang, Q., Shen, K., et al., 2002. Mycophenolate mofetil vs cyclophosphamide therapy for patients with diffuse proliferative lupus nephritis. Chin. Med. J. (Engl). 115, 705–709.

Illei, G.G., Austin, H.A., Crane, M., Collins, L., Gourley, M.F., Yarboro, C.H., et al., 2001. Combination therapy with pulse cyclophosphamide plus pulse methylprednisolone improves long-term renal outcome without adding toxicity in patients with lupus nephritis. Ann. Intern. Med. 135, 248–257.

Isenberg, D., Appel, G.B., Contreras, G., Dooley, M.A., Ginzler, E.M., Jayne, D., et al., 2010. Influence of race/ethnicity on response to lupus nephritis treatment: the ALMS study. Rheumatology (Oxford). 49, 128–140.

Izmirly, P.M., Kim, M.Y., Llanos, C., Le, P.U., Guerra, M.M., Askanase, A.D., et al., 2010. Evaluation of the risk of anti-SSA/Ro-SSB/La antibody-associated cardiac manifestations of neonatal lupus in fetuses of mothers with systemic lupus erythematosus exposed to hydroxychloroquine. Ann. Rheum. Dis. 69, 1827–1830.

Jancinova, V., Nosal, R., Petrikova, M., 1994. On the inhibitory effect of chloroquine on blood platelet aggregation. Thromb. Res. 74, 495–504.

Jones, R.B., Tervaert, J.W., Hauser, T., Luqmani, R., Morgan, M.D., Peh, C.A., et al., 2010. Rituximab versus cyclophosphamide in ANCA-associated renal vasculitis. N. Engl. J. Med. 363, 211–220.

Jones, S.K., 1992. Ultraviolet radiation (UVR) induces cell-surface Ro/SSA antigen expression by human keratinocytes in vitro: a possible mechanism for the UVR induction of cutaneous lupus lesions. Br. J. Dermatol. 126, 546–553.

Jover, J.A., Hernandez-Garcia, C., Morado, I.C., Vargas, E., Banares, A., Fernandez-Gutierrez, B., 2001. Combined treatment of giant-cell arteritis with methotrexate and prednisone: a randomized, double-blind, placebo controlled trial. Ann. Intern. Med. 134, 106–114.

King, J.K., Hahn, B.H., 2007. Systemic lupus erythematosus: modern strategies for management: a moving target. Best Pract. Res. Clin. Rheumatol. 21, 971–987.

Kirouka, B.D., 2007. Systemic glucocorticoid therapy in systemic lupus erythematosus. In: Wallace, D.J. (Ed.), Dubois' Lupus Erythematosus, seventh ed. Lippincott Williams and Wilkins, Philadelphia.

Klareskog, L., Stolt, P., Lundberg, K., Kallberg, H., Bengtsson, C., Grunewald, J., et al., 2006. A new model for an etiology of rheumatoid arthritis: smoking may trigger HLA-DR (shared epitope)-restricted immune reactions to autoantigens modified by citrullination. Arthritis Rheum. 54, 38–46.

Kovacs, B., Lafferty, T.L., Brent, L.H., Dehoratius, R.J., 2000. Transverse myelopathy in systemic lupus erythematosus: an analysis of 14 cases and review of the literature. Ann. Rheum. Dis. 59, 120–124.

Kyburz, D., Brentano, F., Gay, S., 2006. Mode of action of hydroxychloroquine in RA—evidence of an inhibitory effect on toll-like receptor signaling. Nat. Clin. Pract. Rheumatol. 2, 458–459.

Lee, C.K., Lee, E.Y., Chung, S.M., Mun, S.H., Yoo, B., Moon, H.B., 2004. Effects of disease-modifying antirheumatic drugs and antiinflammatory cytokines on human osteoclastogenesis through interaction with receptor activator of nuclear factor kappaB, osteoprotegerin, and receptor activator of nuclear factor kappaB ligand. Arthritis Rheum. 50, 3831–3843.

Li, X., Ren, H., Zhang, Z., Zhang, W., Wu, X., Xu, Y., et al., 2012. Mycophenolate mofetil or tacrolimus compared with intravenous cyhclophosphamide in the induction treatment for active lupus nephritis. Nephrol. Dial. Transplant. 27, 1467–1472.

Lipsky, P.E., Van Der Heijde, D.M., St. Clair, E.W., Furst, D.E., Breedveld, F.C., Kalden, J.R., et al., 2000. Infliximab and methotrexate in the treatment of rheumatoid arthritis. Anti-Tumor Necrosis Factor Trial in Rheumatoid Arthritis with Concomitant Therapy Study Group. N. Engl. J. Med. 343, 1594–1602.

Lu, X., Xie, W., Reed, D., Bradshaw, W.S., Simmons, D.L., 1995. Nonsteroidal antiinflammatory drugs cause apoptosis and induce cyclooxygenases in chicken embryo fibroblasts. Proc. Natl. Acad. Sci. USA. 92, 7961–7965.

Magee, C., 2012. Pharmacology and side effects of cyclosporine and tacrolimus: Furst, D.E., Romain, P.L., (Eds.), UpToDate (www.uptodate.com).

Mahid, S.S., Minor, K.S., Soto, R.E., Hornung, C.A., Galandiuk, S., 2006. Smoking and inflammatory bowel disease: a meta-analysis. Mayo. Clin. Proc. 81, 1462–1471.

Manna, S.K., Aggarwal, B.B., 1999. Immunosuppressive leflunomide metabolite (A77 1726) blocks TNF-dependent nuclear factor-kappa B activation and gene expression. J. Immunol. 162, 2095–2102.

Marmor, M.F., Kelner, U., Timothy, Y., Lai, M.D., Lyons, J.S., Mieler, W.F., 2011. Revised recommendations on screening for chloroquine and hyddroxychloroquine retinopathy. Opthalmol. 112, 415–422.

McCune, W.J., Fox, D., 1989. Intravenous cyclophosphamide therapy of severe SLE. Rheum. Dis. Clin. North Am. 15, 455–477.

Mello, S.B., Barros, D.M., Silva, A.S., Laurindo, I.M., Novaes, G.S., 2000. Methotrexate as a preferential cyclooxygenase 2 inhibitor in whole blood of patients with rheumatoid arthritis. Rheumatology (Oxford). 39, 533–536.

Merrill, J.T., Neuwelt, C.M., Wallace, D.J., Shanahan, J.C., Latinis, K.M., Oates, J.C., et al., 2010. Efficacy and safety of rituximab in moderately-to-severely active systemic lupus erythematosus: the randomized, double-blind, phase II/III systemic lupus erythematosus evaluation of rituximab trial. Arthritis Rheum. 62, 222–233.

Merrill, J.T., Ginzler, E.M., Wallace, D.J., McKay, J.D., Lisse, J.R., Aranow, C., et al., 2012. Long-term safety profile of belimumab plus standard therapy in patients with systemic lupus erythematosus. Arthritis Rheum. 64, 3364–3373.

Morabito, L., Montesinos, M.C., Schreibman, D.M., Balter, L., Thompson, L.F., Resta, R., et al., 1998. Methotrexate and sulfasalazine promote adenosine release by a mechanism that requires ecto-5'-nucleotidase-mediated conversion of adenine nucleotides. J. Clin. Invest. 101, 295–300.

Mottonen, T., Hannonen, P., Leirisalo-Repo, M., Nissila, M., Kautiainen, H., Korpela, M., et al., 1999. Comparison of combination therapy with single-drug therapy in early rheumatoid arthritis: a randomised trial. FIN-RACo trial group. Lancet. 353, 1568–1573.

Mukhtyar, C., Guillevin, L., Cid, M.C., Dasgupta, B., De Groot, K., Gross, W., et al., 2009. EULAR recommendations for the management of primary small and medium vessel vasculitis. Ann. Rheum. Dis. 68, 310–317.

Mulder, C.J., Tytgat, G.N., Weterman, I.T., Dekker, W., Blok, P., Schrijver, M., et al., 1988. Double-blind comparison of slow-release 5-aminosalicylate and sulfasalazine in remission maintenance in ulcerative colitis. Gastroenterology. 95, 1449–1453.

Navarra, S.V., Guzman, R.M., Gallacher, A.E., Hall, S., Levy, R.A., Jimenez, R.E., et al., 2011. Efficacy and safety of belimumab in patients with active systemic lupus erythematosus: a randomised, placebo-controlled, phase 3 trial. Lancet. 377, 721–731.

Neuwelt, C.M., Lacks, S., Kaye, B.R., Ellman, J.B., Borenstein, D.G., 1995. Role of intravenous cyclophosphamide in the treatment of severe neuropsychiatric systemic lupus erythematosus. Am. J. Med. 98, 32–41.

O'Dell, J.R., Haire, C.E., Erikson, N., Drymalski, W., Palmer, W., Eckhoff, P.J., et al., 1996. Treatment of rheumatoid arthritis with methotrexate alone, sulfasalazine and hydroxychloroquine, or a combination of all three medications. N. Engl. J. Med. 334, 1287–1291.

Otto, R., Mackay, I.R., 1967. Psycho-social and emotional disturbance in systemic lupus erythematosus. Med. J. Aust. 2, 488–493.

Padyukov, L., Silva, C., Stolt, P., Alfredsson, L., Klareskog, L., 2004. A gene-environment interaction between smoking and shared epitope genes in HLA-DR provides a high risk of seropositive rheumatoid arthritis. Arthritis Rheum. 50, 3085–3092.

Pagnoux, C., Mahr, A., Hamidou, M.A., Boffa, J.J., Ruivard, M., Ducroix, J.P., et al., 2008. Azathioprine or methotrexate maintenance for ANCA-associated vasculitis. N. Engl. J. Med. 359, 2790–2803.

Prefontaine, E., Sutherland, L.R., MacDonald, J.K., Cepoiu, M., 2009. Azathioprine or 6-mercaptopurine for maintenance of remission in Crohn's disease. Cochrane Database Syst. Rev. CD000067.

Pullar, T., Hunter, J.A., Capell, H.A., 1985. Which component of sulphasalazine is active in rheumatoid arthritis? Br. Med. J. (Clin. Res. Ed.). 290, 1535–1538.

Rantalaiho, V., Korpela, M., Hannonen, P., Kautiainen, H., Jarvenpaa, S., Leirisalo-Repo, M., et al., 2009. The good initial response to therapy with a combination of traditional disease-modifying antirheumatic drugs is sustained over time: the eleven-year results of the Finnish rheumatoid arthritis combination therapy trial. Arthritis Rheum. 60, 1222−1231.

Regius, O., Lengyel, E., Borzsonyi, L., Beregi, E., 1988. The effect of smoking on the presence of antinuclear antibodies and on the morphology of lymphocytes in aged subjects. Z. Gerontol. 21, 161−163.

Rich, E., Moreland, L.W., Alarcon, G.S., 1999. Paucity of radiographic progression in rheumatoid arthritis treated with methotrexate as the first disease modifying antirheumatic drug. J. Rheumatol. 26, 259−261.

Rodenburg, R.J., Ganga, A., Van Lent, P.L., Van De Putte, L.B., Van Venrooij, W.J., 2000. The antiinflammatory drug sulfasalazine inhibits tumor necrosis factor alpha expression in macrophages by inducing apoptosis. Arthritis Rheum. 43, 1941−1950.

Rovin, B.H., Furie, R., Latinis, K., Looney, R.J., Fervenza, F.C., Sanchez-Guerrero, J., et al., 2012. Efficacy and safety of rituximab in patients with active proliferative lupus nephritis: the Lupus Nephritis Assessment with Rituximab study. Arthritis Rheum. 64, 1215−1226.

Saag, K.G., Cerhan, J.R., Kolluri, S., Ohashi, K., Hunninghake, G.W., Schwartz, D.A., 1997. Cigarette smoking and rheumatoid arthritis severity. Ann. Rheum. Dis. 56, 463−469.

Salmi, M., Rajala, P., Jalkanen, S., 1997. Homing of mucosal leukocytes to joints. Distinct endothelial ligands in synovium mediate leukocyte-subtype specific adhesion. J. Clin. Invest. 99, 2165−2172.

Schreiber, S.L., Crabtree, G.R., 1992. The mechanism of action of cyclosporin A and FK506. Immunol. Today. 13, 136−142.

Seitz, M., Zwicker, M., Wider, B., 2001. Enhanced in vitro induced production of interleukin 10 by peripheral blood mononuclear cells in rheumatoid arthritis is associated with clinical response to methotrexate treatment. J. Rheumatol. 28, 496−501.

Siemasko, K., Chong, A.S., Jack, H.M., Gong, H., Williams, J.W., Finnegan, A., 1998. Inhibition of JAK3 and STAT6 tyrosine phosphorylation by the immunosuppressive drug leflunomide leads to a block in IgG1 production. J. Immunol. 160, 1581−1588.

Silvergleid, A.J., Berger, M., 2011. General principles in the use of immune globulin: Schrier, S.L., Stiehm, E.R., Tirnauer, J.S., Feldweg, A.M. (Eds), UpToDate (www.uptodate.com).

Singh, J.A., Furst, D.E., Bharat, A., Curtis, J.R., Kavanaugh, A.F., Kremer, J.M., et al., 2012. 2012 update of the 2008 American College of Rheumatology recommendations for the use of disease-modifying antirheumatic drugs and biologic agents in the treatment of rheumatoid arthritis. Arthritis Care Res. (Hoboken). 64, 625−639.

Smolen, J.S., Kalden, J.R., Scott, D.L., Rozman, B., Kvien, T.K., Larsen, A., et al., 1999. Efficacy and safety of leflunomide compared with placebo and sulphasalazine in active rheumatoid arthritis: a double-blind, randomised, multicentre trial. European Leflunomide Study Group. Lancet. 353, 259−266.

Solomon, D., 2012. Nonselective NSAIDs: overview of adverse effects: Furst, D.E., Romain, P.L. (Eds) UpToDate (www.uptodate.com).

Stone, J.H., 2010. General principles of the use of cyclophosphamide in rheumatic and renal disease: Furst, D.E., Ramirez, M.P. (Eds) UpToDate (www.uptodate.com).

Stone, J.H., Merkel, P.A., Spiera, R., Seo, P., Langford, C.A., Hoffman, G.S., et al., 2010. Rituximab versus cyclophosphamide for ANCA-associated vasculitis. N. Engl. J. Med. 363, 221−232.

Taggart, A.J., Neumann, V.C., Hill, J., Astbury, C., Le Gallez, P., Dixon, J.S., 1986. 5-Aminosalicylic acid or sulphapyridine. Which is the active moiety of sulphasalazine in rheumatoid arthritis? Drugs. 32 (Suppl. 1), 27−34.

Tam, L.S., Li, E.K., Wong, C.K., Lam, C.W., Szeto, C.C., 2004. Double-blind, randomized, placebo-controlled pilot study of leflunomide in systemic lupus erythematosus. Lupus. 13, 601−604.

Tashkin, D.P., Elashoff, R., Clements, P.J., Goldin, J., Roth, M.D., Furst, D.E., et al., 2006. Cyclophosphamide versus placebo in scleroderma lung disease. N. Engl. J. Med. 354, 2655−2666.

Timmer, A., McDonald, J.W., MacDonald, J.K., 2007. Azathioprine and 6-mercaptopurine for maintenance of remission in ulcerative colitis. Cochrane Database Syst. Rev. CD000478.

Timmerman, L.A., Clipstone, N.A., Ho, S.N., Northrop, J.P., Crabtree, G.R., 1996. Rapid shuttling of NF-AT in discrimination of Ca2 + signals and immunosuppression. Nature. 383, 837−840.

Tobin, M.V., Logan, R.F., Langman, M.J., Mcconnell, R.B., Gilmore, I.T., 1987. Cigarette smoking and inflammatory bowel disease. Gastroenterology. 93, 316−321.

Touma, Z., Gladman, D.D., Urowitz, M.B., Beyene, J., Uleryk, E.M., Shah, P.S., 2011. Mycophenolate mofetil for induction treatment of lupus nephritis: a systematic review and metaanalysis. J. Rheumatol. 38, 69−78.

Urowitz, M.B., Gordon, D.A., Smythe, H.A., Pruzanski, W., Ogryzio, M.A., 1973. Azathioprine in rheumatoid arthritis. A double-blind, cross over study. Arthritis Rheum. 16, 411−418.

Von Feldt, J.M., 1995. Systemic lupus erythematosus. Recognizing its various presentations. Postgrad. Med. 97, 79, 83, 86.

Wahl, C., Liptay, S., Adler, G., Schmid, R.M., 1998. Sulfasalazine: a potent and specific inhibitor of nuclear factor kappa B. J. Clin. Invest. 101, 1163−1174.

Wallace, D., 2007. Antimalarial therapies. In: Wallace, D.J. (Ed.), Dubois' Lupus Erythematosus. Lippincot Williams and Wilkins, Philadelphia.

Wasko, M.C., Hubert, H.B., Lingala, V.B., Elliott, J.R., Luggen, M.E., Fries, J.F., et al., 2007. Hydroxychloroquine and risk of diabetes in patients with rheumatoid arthritis. JAMA. 298, 187−193.

Weinblatt, M.E., Weissman, B.N., Holdsworth, D.E., Fraser, P.A., Maier, A.L., Falchuk, K.R., et al., 1992. Long-term prospective study of methotrexate in the treatment of rheumatoid arthritis. 84-month update. Arthritis Rheum. 35, 129−137.

Weinblatt, M.E., Kaplan, H., Germain, B.F., Block, S., Solomon, S.D., Merriman, R.C., et al., 1994. Methotrexate in rheumatoid arthritis. A five-year prospective multicenter study. Arthritis Rheum. 37, 1492−1498.

Wiederrecht, G., Lam, E., Hung, S., Martin, M., Sigal, N., 1993. The mechanism of action of FK-506 and cyclosporin A. Ann. N.Y. Acad. Sci. 696, 9−19.

Wilke, W.S., 2010. Pharmacology and side effects of azathioprine when used in rheumatic disease: Furst, D.E., Romain, P.L. (Eds) UpToDate (www.uptodate.com).

Wolfe, F., 2000. The effect of smoking on clinical, laboratory, and radiographic status in rheumatoid arthritis. J. Rheumatol. 27, 630−637.

Woodland, J., Chaput De Saintonge, D.M., Evans, S.J., Sharman, V.L., Currey, H.L., 1981. Azathioprine in rheumatoid arthritis: double-blind study of full versus half doses versus placebo. Ann. Rheum. Dis. 40, 355−359.

Zhang, X., Brunner, T., Carter, L., Dutton, R.W., Rogers, P., Bradley, L., et al., 1997. Unequal death in T helper cell (Th)1 and Th2 effectors: Th1, but not Th2, effectors undergo rapid Fas/FasL-mediated apoptosis. J. Exp. Med. 185, 1837−1849.

Chapter 81

Treatment of Autoimmune Disease: Biological and Molecular Therapies

Lucienne Chatenoud

Université Paris Descartes, Sorbonne Paris Cité, Paris, France, INSERM U1013, Hôpital Necker-Enfants Malades, Paris, France

Chapter Contents

Introduction	1221	Other Soluble Receptors and Protein Fusion	
The Therapeutic Armamentarium Derived from		Conjugates	1232
Biotechnology	1221	Soluble Autoantigens	1232
Monoclonal Antibodies (mAbs)	1221	Bone Marrow Transplantation	1232
The Problem of Sensitization can be Partly Overcome		Cell Therapy and Gene Therapy	1234
with Humanized and Human mAbs	1222	Cell Therapy	1234
Further Opportunities are Offered by Genetic		Gene Therapy	1235
Engineering	1222	Perspectives for the Future	1235
Main Targets	1223	References	1235

INTRODUCTION

Autoimmune diseases represent a major therapeutic challenge. In many cases, the disease is severe enough to significantly reduce longevity. In other cases, the disease causes major handicaps and discomfort that justify the usage of aggressive treatments generating their own hazards. In the past treatments were mainly palliative (substitutive), anti-inflammatory, or immunosuppressive without any specificity for the pathogenic mechanisms of the disease.

Over the last two decades modern technologies have made new agents available, in particular monoclonal antibodies directed to key immune cell receptors or cytokines, which have created a true revolution with major advancements in the treatment of rheumatoid arthritis, multiple sclerosis, psoriasis, or systemic lupus erythematosus. Our aim is to review these treatments with particular emphasis on the experimental background and the numerous and diversified animal models that led to their discovery and development as well as on the salient results which established them in the clinical arena. In addition, we will also present strategies that are still in development but that may, in a not too distant future, fill

important gaps. In particular, an ambitious goal is that of inducing or, in the case of established autoimmune diseases, restoring immune tolerance to target autoantigens. This may be defined operationally as the possibility to harness the pathologic immune response following a short-term treatment while keeping intact the capacity of the host to respond normally to exogenous antigens. Restoration of self-tolerance has the major advantage of avoiding the side effects linked to chronic immunosuppression and, most importantly, of providing a real cure for the disease.

Last but not least, it will be interesting to present how lessons drawn from the development of novel therapeutic strategies in one particular autoimmune disease may be translated into beneficial therapies for other autoimmune conditions.

THE THERAPEUTIC ARMAMENTARIUM DERIVED FROM BIOTECHNOLOGY

Monoclonal Antibodies (mAbs)

Murine monoclonal antibodies (mAbs) produced by mouse or rat hybridomas (Kohler and Milstein, 1975)

N. Rose & I. Mackay (Eds): The Autoimmune Diseases, Fifth edition. DOI: http://dx.doi.org/10.1016/B978-0-12-384929-8.00081-2

specific for immune cell receptors were introduced in clinical practice more than 30 years ago and their use initially developed in the field of solid organ transplantation. Two major side effects, namely the sensitization against the xenogeneic molecule and the cytokine releasing potential observed with some particular specificities, explain why the use of rodent mAbs remained initially mostly confined to transplantation with only very few attempts in autoimmunity. The advent of human mAbs that are less immunogenic and better tolerated has completely changed the picture and allowed a more widespread use of these interesting therapeutic tools. In fact, at variance with conventional immunosuppressants, some mAbs specific for relevant lymphocyte receptors are unique in their capacity to induce, under adequate circumstances, immune tolerance to soluble proteins, foreign tissue alloantigens, and autoantigens.

Conventional chemicals mostly act through removal and/or the functional inhibition of their targets. In contrast, mAbs display a wide spectrum of pharmacological and biological activities highly relevant to their capacity to "reprogram" the immune system. Thus, depending on their fine specificity, mAbs will remove target cells, inhibit or block the functional capacity of the target without depleting it, neutralize major cytokines, and/or serve as receptor agonists triggering activation signals for specialized T cell subsets, e.g., regulatory T cells (Sakaguchi, 2000; Bach, 2003).

The Problem of Sensitization can be Partly Overcome with Humanized and Human mAbs

The repeated administration of murine mAbs invariably triggered a humoral immune response of which the main clinical consequence was the neutralization of the antibody's therapeutic activity. Interestingly, this was not a global anti-mouse or anti-rat response; it was very restricted in its specificity with essentially anti-isotypic and anti-idiotypic antibodies being produced (Benjamin et al., 1986; Chatenoud et al., 1986a,b). Anti-idiotypic antibodies that compete with the therapeutic antibody for antigen binding represent the neutralizing component of the response while anti-isotypic antibodies are mostly non-neutralizing (Baudrihaye et al., 1984). Another peculiarity of this humoral response is its oligoclonality (Chatenoud et al., 1986b) which explains that, at variance with what is observed in patients immunized to polyclonal anti-lymphocyte globulins, serum sickness was a rare consequence of sensitization to mAbs since the amount of immune complexes formed would be insufficient to elicit a generalized reaction. Anti-monoclonal IgE responses associated with symptoms of anaphylaxis were reported but remained a very uncommon observation (Abramowicz et al., 1992, 1996).

Until humanized mAbs or, more recently, fully human antibodies became available, the only way to cope with the problem of sensitization was to associate adequate doses of chemical immunosuppressants (Hricik et al., 1990). Two types of humanized antibodies have been derived from molecular engineering. Chimeric mAbs express intact rodent variable regions linked to human immunoglobulin constant domains (Elliott et al., 1994a). In fully reshaped or complementarity determining region (CDR)-grafted antibodies, the rodent hypervariable regions interacting with the antigen (i.e., CDRs) are included within human heavy and light chain immunoglobulin frameworks (Riechmann et al., 1988).

Humanized mAbs have significantly reduced, though not totally avoided, the risk of deleterious anti-idiotypic responses. The clinical data available indicate that both chimeric and reshaped humanized mAbs may be immunogenic when administered alone, without associated immunosuppressants, after a single or repeated antibody course (Elliott et al., 1994b; Herold et al., 2002; Keymeulen et al., 2005). It has been the general experience that, as for murine antibodies, combining low doses of chemical immunosuppressants is an efficient way to overcome such sensitization (Nashan et al., 1997; Vincenti et al., 1998; Feldmann, 2002).

Fully human mAbs, which already entered clinical practice, have been produced by different means. First, mice have been invalidated for the expression of endogenous (mouse) immunoglobulin genes and concurrently made transgenic for sufficient human constant and variable immunoglobulin-encoding sequences to provide for antibody diversity; B cells from these immunized mice produce human antibodies that can be used in conventional fusions to obtain hybridomas yielding high-affinity mAbs derived from *in vivo* antigen-driven selection. Second, there is a fully *in vitro* approach using cDNA libraries expressed on filamentous phages to derive high-affinity antibodies to a wide variety of antigens, including those for which the conventional hybridoma technology fails due to poor immunogenicity (Marks et al., 1991). Third, human–mouse chimeras can be established using normal mice irradiated and reconstituted with bone marrow cells from immunodeficient (SCID) mice; after human lymphocytes from presensitized donors are inoculated, these mice are boosted with the antigen of interest, and sensitized human B cells recovered and used for conventional fusions (Lubin et al., 1994).

Further Opportunities are Offered by Genetic Engineering

Engineering Fc Regions of mAbs to Avoid Side Effects and Prolong Half-life

Antibody engineering allows the design of tailor-made antibodies to fit at best therapeutic indications.

Antibodies expressing human Fc portions have a significantly prolonged half-life. In addition, the choice of the human Fc portion will influence the antibody effector capacities, i.e., its activity in terms of complement fixation, opsonisation, and antibody-dependent cell cytotoxicity (ADCC). Furthermore, in the case of CD3 antibodies, humanization can circumvent problems due to their intrinsic mitogenic and cytokine-releasing capacity that leads *in vivo* to a "flu-like" syndrome. This syndrome was regularly observed with murine CD3 mAbs such as OKT3, and although transient it represented a major and troublesome side effect that totally precluded the use of CD3 mAbs for indications other than organ transplantation (Abramowicz et al., 1989; Chatenoud et al., 1990; Chatenoud, 2003). This mitogenic capacity is linked to the ability of the Fc portion of CD3 mAbs to interact with monocyte Fc receptors (Chatenoud, 2003). Thus "non-mitogenic" CD3 antibodies were obtained by inserting adequate mutations into the Fc domains to hamper Fc receptor binding (Bolt et al., 1993; Alegre et al., 1994; Chatenoud, 2003). Clinical use of two different Fc mutated CD3 mAbs, teplizumab (OKT3γ1Ala-Ala) and otelixizumab (ChAglyCD3), in autoimmunity and transplantation, confirmed that their use was free of major side effects (Friend et al., 1999; Woodle et al., 1999; Herold et al., 2002; Hering et al., 2004; Keymeulen et al., 2005; Sherry et al., 2011).

Engineering Variable Regions of mAbs to Increase Affinity

In case the affinity of a given mAb is too low for *in vivo* use, phage display technology is an interesting approach to generate an improved fully human reagent with no requirement for prior immunization or use of hybridoma technology. Phage display can be used to mimic artificially the processes used *in vivo* by the immune system to obtain high-affinity antibodies. This has been achieved by shuffling the heavy or light chains by random or directed mutagenesis of CDR (Barbas et al., 1994), as done by error-prone polymerase chain reaction (PCR) (Gram et al., 1992). Using such artificial affinity maturation of phage antibody repertoires, affinities of mAbs in the nanomolar to picomolar range have been generated that are perfectly suitable for therapeutic use (Barbas, 1995; Foote and Eisen, 1995).

Main Targets

T Cell Antigens

CD3 Antibodies The story of CD3 mAbs is paradoxical and remarkable. They were the first therapeutic antibody introduced in clinical practice in 1981, about 4 years before the molecular complexities and the key functional role of the CD3 molecule were discovered (Clevers et al., 1988). The OKT3 mAb, a mouse IgG2a (Kung et al., 1979), was initially used to treat and prevent renal allograft rejection (Cosimi et al., 1981a; Vigeral et al., 1986; Debure et al., 1988). This occurred without much *in vivo* preclinical data available due to the tight species specificity of anti-T cell mAbs in general and CD3 antibodies in particular. Chimpanzees are the only non-human primates harboring T lymphocytes cross-reacting with mAbs to human CD3. In addition, antibodies to mouse CD3 were difficult to produce, the first one being characterized by Leo et al. in 1987 (Leo et al., 1987). During the 1980s controlled studies clearly demonstrated that mAb OKT3 was a potent immunosuppressant very efficient at reversing early acute renal allograft rejection episodes (Cosimi et al., 1981b; Ortho Multicenter Transplant Study Group, 1985), an indication for which this mAb was rapidly licensed both in the USA and Europe. Through the study of OKT3-treated patients an enormous body of knowledge was gained on the mode of action of murine anti-T cell monoclonals and their side effects, well illustrated by over 3000 manuscripts published on the topic. These studies have been invaluable for the design of more refined approaches especially using humanized mAbs. Over the last 10 years, as other immunosuppressants developed, the use of OKT3 was progressively abandoned, essentially because of its cytokine releasing potential (Cosimi, 1987; Abramowicz et al., 1989; Chatenoud et al., 1989, 1990).

CD3 mAbs used *in vitro* in functional studies and *in vivo*, both in the experimental and the clinical setting, are specific for the ε chain of the CD3 complex. The experimental work conducted in different rat and mouse models suggested that, more than simply depressing all immune responses, CD3 mAbs could also induce immune tolerance to both alloantigens and autoantigens (Hayward and Shreiber, 1989; Nicolls et al., 1993; Plain et al., 1999; You et al., 2012; Goto et al., 2013) and, perhaps more impressively, could restore self-tolerance in established autoimmunity (Chatenoud et al., 1994, 1997; Belghith et al., 2003; Chatenoud, 2003). Based on these data, CD3 mAbs have again entered the clinical arena but now as well-tolerated humanized non-mitogenic mAbs (Bolt et al., 1993; Alegre et al., 1994) used not only in transplantation, but also in autoimmunity in protocols aimed at antigen-specific long-term effects rather than just immunosuppression.

CD3 mAbs and Autoimmune Diabetes Trials have been conducted using anti-CD3 to treat patients with recent-onset type 1 diabetes based on our earlier data on diabetes-prone non-obese diabetic (NOD) mice. Short-term (5 days) treatment of overtly diabetic NOD mice with low doses (5−20 μg/day) of CD3 mAbs, in either their mitogenic (whole 145 2C11) or non-mitogenic version (F(ab')2 fragments of 145 2C11), induces disease remission by restoring self-tolerance (Chatenoud et al., 1994, 1997; Belghith et al., 2003; Chatenoud, 2003). The effect is long-lasting and specific to β cell autoantigens (Chatenoud et al., 1994, 1997). Immune mechanisms mediating this tolerogenic capacity evolve in two distinct consecutive phases (Chatenoud, 2003, 2010; Chatenoud and Bluestone, 2007). The first induction phase coincides with antibody administration and results in clearing of insulitis, explaining the rapid return to normoglycemia, with a transient Th2 polarization which is irrelevant to the long-term effect since there is prolonged remission of disease after anti-CD3 treatment of IL-4 deficient NOD mice (NOD IL-4$^{-/-}$) (Belghith et al., 2003; Chatenoud, 2003). The second maintenance phase results in upregulation and/or appearance of specialized subsets of CD4$^+$CD25$^+$ and CD4$^+$CD62L$^+$ regulatory T cells that mediate transferable active tolerance, and that effectively control pathogenic effector cells as shown by co-transfer experiments in immunodeficient NOD SCID mice (Chatenoud et al., 1994, 2001; Belghith et al., 2003). The proportions of regulatory CD4$^+$CD25$^+$ T cells increase in pancreatic and mesenteric lymph nodes of anti-CD3-treated tolerant mice (Belghith et al., 2003). Interestingly, CD4$^+$CD25$^+$ regulatory T cells induced by anti-CD3 may not be derived exclusively from conventional natural regulatory CD4$^+$CD25$^+$FoxP3$^+$ T cells but also, and perhaps even essentially so, from peripheral CD4$^+$CD25$^-$ precursors that differentiate into adaptive regulatory T cells (Belghith et al., 2003; You et al., 2007). In fact, CD3-specific mAb treatment induces diabetes remission also in NOD mice deficient for the costimulation molecule CD28 (NOD CD28$^{-/-}$), t are devoid of the thymic natural suppressor CD4$^+$CD25$^+$ population (Belghith et al., 2003). Also important, the immunoregulatory cytokine TGF-β appears to be a key player in this T cell-mediated regulation although its precise role, whether a mediator of regulation or a growth and/or differentiation factor for regulatory T cells, is not yet determined. Thus, CD4$^+$ T cells from mice tolerant after CD3 mAb treatment consistently produce high levels of TGF-β, and *in vivo* neutralization of TGF-β after injection of specific mAbs fully prevents anti-CD3-specific-induced remission (Belghith et al., 2003; Kuhn et al., 2011).

Clinical trials have been conducted to ascertain adequate modalities that will reproduce this remarkable effect. Results from an open trial using teplizumab (OKT3γ1 Ala-Ala) in patients that present recent-onset type 1 diabetes were very encouraging (Herold et al., 2002, 2005). Thus, at 1 year after a short-term treatment, a significant preservation of the β cell mass was observed in treated patients compared with controls (Herold et al., 2002, 2005). The results of a European multicentric

randomized placebo-controlled trial using the otelixizumab (ChAglyCD3) mAb, also in autoimmune type 1 diabetes, which we conducted in collaboration with diabetology centers in Belgium (Belgium Diabetes Registry; Clinical coordinator Prof. B. Keymeulen) and Germany (Prof. A. Ziegler, Munich), fully confirmed the expectations. In fact, results obtained at 18 months of follow-up showed not only a significant preservation of the β cell mass in otelixizumab- versus placebo-treated patients but also an impressive decrease in the insulin needs that lasted for up to 4 years after the end of the short course treatment (Keymeulen et al., 2005, 2010).

Based on these results, Phase III trials were launched by two biotech companies in association with large pharmaceutical companies using designs that were quite different from that of the previous Phase II studies. The Phase III study using teplizumab (MacroGenics/Eli Lilly trial) had a composite end-point chosen arbitrarily (i.e., insulin requirement ≤0.5 units/kg/day and HbA1c ≤6.5%) that had not been previously validated in a controlled trial and which seemed to be an unfortunate choice (Bach, 2011; Sherry et al., 2011). The Phase III trial using otelixizumab (Tolerx/GlaxoSmithKline trial) used a reduced dose with the aim of reducing side effects. This dose, which has not been validated for efficacy in a proper Phase II placebo-controlled study, was 16 times lower than the one used in the successful Phase II academic trial (3.1 mg compared to 48 mg). Negative results reported in press releases for both studies caused great discouragement in the diabetes community (see MacroGenics, 2010; GlaxoSmithKline, 2011).

Importantly, a post-hoc analysis of the data from the teplizumab study was performed using the conventional end-points validated by all previous trials in the field, namely C-peptide production and insulin needs, which evidenced a significant therapeutic effect (Sherry et al., 2011). A better response was observed in patients presenting the highest stimulated C-peptide at inclusion and in children. The response was dose dependent, i.e., only observed in patients receiving the higher dose tested of 17 mg (cumulated equivalent for a 70 kg individual) (Sherry et al., 2011; Daifotis et al., 2013).

Efforts to lead at least one of the two CD3 antibodies on the market continue. It is indeed so far the only product that has shown a prolonged therapeutic activity following a short treatment thereby suggesting that it induces an "operational" restoration of immune tolerance. Time will tell if these promising results can be extended to other autoimmune diseases.

For the sake of completeness we may mention before closing that interesting data have also been reported using teplizumab in psoriatic arthritis (Utset et al., 2002). Finally, a fully human CD3 mAb, NI-004, was used in a Phase I study to treat patients with moderate to severe

Crohn's disease with encouraging results (van der Woude et al., 2010).

CD4 Antibodies The tolerogenic capacity of CD4 mAbs in mice was highlighted from the outset, since at variance with other xenogeneic mAbs, anti-CD4 did not elicit the usual anti-globulin response (Benjamin and Waldmann, 1986; Gutstein et al., 1986). In addition, humoral responses to foreign soluble protein antigens were specifically inhibited if delivery was under the cover of brief treatment with anti-CD4. The effect was obtained with both depleting and non-depleting CD4 antibodies, and it could be maintained long term merely by repeating antigen administration at regular intervals in absence of any further anti-CD4 treatment. Importantly, identical results were obtained in non-human primates using a humanized mAb specific for human CD4 and cross-reacting with monkey cells (Winsor-Hines et al., 2004). In this system CD4$^+$ T cells, but not B cells, were rendered tolerant and effectively transferred such tolerance to naïve hosts. The single caveat is that only high CD4 mAb dosages are tolerogenic. In the mouse anti-CD4 affords tolerance also to alloantigens (anti-CD4 mAbs are effective alone in the case of cardiac or islet allografts but must be combined with anti-CD8 mAbs in the case of skin allografts) and also often in the case of autoantigens (Wofsy and Seaman, 1987; Shizuru et al., 1988; Qin et al., 1993; Bushell et al., 1995, 2003; Waldmann and Cobbold, 2001; Cobbold et al., 2003). Effective treatment of an ongoing autoimmune disease was demonstrated for murine lupus in NZB/NZW F1 mice (Wofsy and Seaman, 1987), and in established diabetes in NOD mice (Maki et al., 1992), but only when using depleting CD4 antibodies.

The first pilot trials that used mouse mAbs to human CD4 were applied to patients presenting long-standing rheumatoid arthritis (RA), psoriasis, inflammatory bowel disease, and uveitis (Goldberg et al., 1990, 1991; Emmrich et al., 1991; Horneff et al., 1991; Reiter et al., 1991; Wendling et al., 1991; Morel et al., 1992; Bachelez et al., 1998). In these trials partial and short-term disappearance of circulating CD4$^+$ cells was observed, together with coating of CD4$^+$ T cells and dose-dependent saturation of CD4 binding sites (Goldberg et al., 1990, 1991; Emmrich et al., 1991; Horneff et al., 1991; Reiter et al., 1991; Wendling et al., 1991; Morel et al., 1992; Bachelez et al., 1998). Results in terms of therapeutic effectiveness were encouraging but short-lasting, and were obscured by the anti-globulin response which rapidly developed and prompted trials using humanized CD4 mAbs (Goldberg et al., 1990, 1991; Emmrich et al., 1991; Horneff et al., 1991; Reiter et al., 1991; Wendling et al., 1991; Morel et al., 1992).

The chimeric cM-T412 mAb (human IgG1), a depleting anti-human CD4 mAb, was used in RA with encouraging results in open studies, especially with high cumulative doses, ranging from 350 to 700 mg (Moreland et al., 1993; Van Der Lubbe et al., 1993, 1994); these results, however, were not confirmed in a large randomized double-blind placebo-controlled study (Van Der Lubbe et al., 1995). Mild sensitization was reported in a majority of the patients (Moreland et al., 1993; Van Der Lubbe et al., 1993, 1994). Of major concern was the persisting CD4$^+$ cell depletion observed with mAb cM-T412, up to 60% from baseline for over 18−30 months (Moreland et al., 1994), contrary to what had initially been reported with the parental mouse M-T151 anti-CD4 mAb (Reiter et al., 1991). Apoptosis could mediate, at least in part, this massive depletion (Choy et al., 1993). The disappointing clinical results in ongoing RA are not necessarily surprising, since they are fully in keeping with preclinical data. In fact, in collagen-induced arthritis, a murine model for human RA, anti-CD4 in contrast to mAbs to TNF, to be discussed below, were effective for prevention but not for treatment of ongoing disease (Marinova-Mutafchieva et al., 2000). The cM-T412 mAb has also been used in patients with multiple sclerosis, but here again without any evident clinical benefit (van Oosten et al., 1997).

The non-depleting humanized mAb to CD4, OKT4cdr4A (the CDR-grafted version of OKT4A), was used in patients with severe psoriasis; one open pilot study and a placebo-controlled one were conducted, with promising data (Bachelez et al., 1998; Gottlieb et al., 2000).

Results from open pilot studies suggested that CD4 mAb therapy, especially in combination with antibodies to CD52, could be effective in treating severe forms of vasculitis (Mathieson et al., 1990; Lockwood et al., 1993).

It is fair to conclude with anti-CD4 mAbs by pointing out that their development was seriously hampered by non-scientific considerations linked to patenting and marketing, explaining the incredible gap between the wealth of experimental data accrued and the paucity of controlled clinical trials conducted. It is hoped that CD4 antibodies will someday "revive" and be made available for trials especially designed on the lessons drawn from preclinical studies.

CD25 Antibodies CD25, the α-chain of the IL-2 receptor, is expressed on activated T cells (Waldmann, 1989), which explains the interest in it as a therapeutic target. Experimental data suggested an immunosuppressive capacity of anti-CD25 that significantly delayed rejection of heart allografts in the mouse (Kirkman et al., 1985) and of renal allografts in non-human primates (Reed et al., 1989). In autoimmunity, anti-CD25 mAb prevented onset of collagen-induced arthritis (Banerjee et al., 1988), insulitis, and diabetes in NOD mice (Kelley et al., 1988) and lupus nephritis in NZB/NZW F1 mice (Kelley et al., 1988). In diabetes-prone Bio Breeding (BB) rats there was reversal of established disease after treatment with anti-CD25 and low-dose cyclosporine (Hahn et al., 1987).

In the clinic mouse mAbs to human CD25 were effective for prevention but not for reversal of renal allograft rejection (Soulillou et al., 1990; Kirkman et al., 1991; Kriaa et al., 1993). By the late 1990s two humanized mAbs to CD25, one chimeric (basiliximab/Simulect®) and one CDR grafted (daclizumab/Zenapax®), were shown to be well tolerated and effective as part of induction regimens to prevent organ allograft rejection, and were approved for use as induction therapies in organ transplantation (Nashan et al., 1997; Vincenti et al., 1998; Waldmann and O'Shea, 1998; Bumgardner et al., 2001). Moreover humanized CD25 antibodies appear beneficial for treatment of some severe autoimmune diseases, uveitis in particular (Nussenblatt et al., 1999, 2003, 2005; Yeh et al., 2008).

The use of anti-CD25 was tested for the treatment of multiple sclerosis in a series of non-randomized pilot studies which showed efficacy of daclizumab administered alone or in combination with interferon (IFN)-β (Bielekova et al., 2004, 2009). These results were confirmed in a multicenter Phase II study including 230 patients (Wynn et al., 2010). The addition of daclizumab to IFN-β for maintenance therapy in patients with recurrent/relapsing disease significantly reduced the number of new brain lesions or the progression of existing ones as assessed by magnetic resonance imaging (MRI) when compared to IFN-β monotherapy. Daclizumab was withdrawn from the market in 2009 for commercial reasons, leaving basiliximab as the only available agent.

Last but not least, none of the studies supports a tolerance promoting activity of anti-CD25 perhaps because CD25 is also expressed on a subset of T cells endowed with regulatory/suppressor capacities that are critical in maintaining immune tolerance (Sakaguchi, 2004). Thus elimination or inhibition of the functional capacity of this subset using CD25 mAbs might be counterproductive if the aim is tolerance induction.

Targeting Costimulatory Pathways

The CD28/CD80, 86 (B7.1, B7.2) Pathway Delivery of activation signals through the T cell receptor/CD3 pathway is insufficient to activate naïve T cells. Costimulation signals are required that are transduced through the specialized receptor, CD28, that interacts with its specific ligands CD80 (B7.1) and CD86 (B7.2) at the surface of the antigen-presenting cell (APC). Fusion proteins have been produced using the cytotoxic T

lymphocyte-associated antigen-4 (CTLA-4, CD152) molecule that is homologous to CD28 and expressed on T cells following activation (Linsley et al., 1991). CTLA-4 is also constitutively expressed on the specialized regulatory/suppressor T cell subset $CD4^+CD25^+$ (Read et al., 2000; Takahashi et al., 2000).

Abatacept (CTLA-4Ig) is a fusion protein including the extracellular domain of CTLA-4 combined with the Fc domain of human IgG1 (Linsley et al., 1992), and shows higher avidity for CD80 than CD86. Treatment *in vivo* with CTLA-4Ig effectively blocked immune responses to alloantigens (Lin et al., 1993; Lakkis et al., 1997; Onodera et al., 1997), xenoantigens (Lenschow et al., 1992), and autoantigens. Thus, in NZB/NZW mice treatment with CTLA-4Ig blocked autoantibody production and prolonged mouse half-life (Finck et al., 1994). Mostly CTLA-4Ig was more effective for preventing than reversing established immune responses and generally a robust and long-standing tolerance was not the general rule. Belatacept (LEA29Y) is a CTLA-4Ig derived molecule with two amino acid mutations which confer higher avidity for both CD80 and CD86. This explains why LEA29Y is more potent *in vitro* than CTLA-4Ig.

In the clinic, in a Phase I open-label study on 43 patients with psoriasis, abatacept resulted in >50% sustained (>6 months) improvement in disease activity in 46% of patients (Abrams et al., 1999). Promising results were also obtained in rheumatoid arthritis, according to double-blind placebo-controlled studies using abatacept or belatacept alone (Moreland et al., 2002) or abatacept combined with methotrexate (Kremer et al., 2003, 2005). This explains why abatacept (Orencia®) was first approved by the Food and Drug Administration (FDA) in 2005 for the treatment of rheumatoid arthritis. Abatacept was also tested in a multicenter, double-blind, randomized controlled trial, including patients aged 6–45 years recently diagnosed with type 1 diabetes (Orban et al., 2011). The difference between groups was present throughout the trial, with an estimated delay in C-peptide reduction with abatacept of about 10 months. A decrease in insulin needs was also reported which, however, was noted only for the first 12 months of treatment (Orban et al., 2011). A longer follow-up is needed to assess if, and if yes for how long, the effect is maintained after treatment cessation. Indeed, relevant data in the mouse question the ability of CTLA-4Ig if administered alone to favor immune tolerance thus promoting a long-lasting therapeutic effect. First, regulatory T cells are dependent on CD28 for their thymic development and their survival at the periphery (Salomon et al., 2000). As a consequence, treatment with CTLA-4Ig drastically reduces regulatory T cells and may therefore exacerbate autoimmunity (Salomon et al., 2000). Second, it has been well established that CD28–CD80 (B7) interactions are more relevant for the stimulation of naïve than of memory T cells (Bluestone et al., 2006) thereby questioning the real effectiveness of CTLA-4Ig in advanced stages of type 1 diabetes.

Presently, belatacept has been validated and approved in transplantation as part of the immunosuppression maintenance regimens to avoid the use of calcineurin inhibitors cyclosporin A (CSA) and FK-506 (Vincenti et al., 2005; Bluestone et al., 2006; Wojciechowski and Vincenti, 2011).

The CD40/CD40 Ligand (CD40L) Pathway

CD40 is a member of the TNF receptor superfamily and is constitutively expressed by various cell types including B lymphocytes and antigen-presenting cells. CD40 interacts with CD154 (CD40L), a member of the TNF superfamily expressed at the surface of activated T lymphocytes, activated mast cells, and basophils, and also on activated human and primate platelets. The CD40/CD154 costimulation pathway is essential for both T–B and T–T cooperation. CD40/CD154 interactions lead to germinal center formation and immunoglobulin class switching. Severe immunodeficiency is caused by disruption of this pathway due to gene knockout in mice, or somatic mutations in humans. Initial studies in the mouse and in non-human primates using *in vivo* administration of antibodies to CD154, either alone or in combination with CTLA-4Ig, showed great promise to prolong fully mismatched allograft survival and prevent autoimmune diseases (Larsen et al., 1996; Larsen and Pearson, 1997; Kirk et al., 1999; Bagenstose et al., 2005; Komura et al., 2008), albeit rapidly tempered when the first clinical trials in renal allograft recipients and in patients with systemic lupus erythematosus showed severe thromboembolic events (Kawai et al., 2000; Boumpas et al., 2003; Robles-Carrillo et al., 2010) with one of the mAbs used (humanized 5C8). While such events were not observed with the IDEC-131 mAb, this proved ineffective in patients with SLE (Davis et al., 2001; Kalunian et al., 2002). However, interesting results were observed in immune thrombocytopenic purpura that were confirmed in subsequent studies using either humanized 5C8 or IDEC131 (Kuwana et al., 2004; Patel et al., 2008).

The thromboembolic events were related to the expression of CD40L on activated platelets; there are also data showing that immune complexes of CD40L and humanized anti-CD40L antibodies may induce thrombosis through binding to the human FcγRIIa IgG receptor on platelets. Treatments which prevent this side effect have been described which may open new possibilities (Kawai et al., 2000, 2004; Law and Grewal, 2009). Finally, it has also been proposed that antibodies to CD40L could act by depleting activated T cells rather than blocking costimulation, which would also open novel perspectives especially in established autoimmunity (Monk et al., 2003).

Adhesion Molecules

The Alpha-4 Integrin VLA-4

Integrins are adhesion molecules of fundamental importance to the recruitment of leukocytes in inflammation. The alpha4beta1 integrin VLA-4 is a leukocyte ligand for endothelial vascular cell adhesion molecule-1 (VCAM-1), fibronectin, and osteopontin. The interaction between VLA-4 at the surface of activated lymphocytes and monocytes with its ligand VCAM-1 is essential for cell migration into inflamed parenchyma. Promising data in experimental models of blockade of VLA-4 prompted use of a specific humanized monoclonal antibody (natalizumab, Tysabri®) in randomized placebo-controlled trials, first in multiple sclerosis (Miller et al., 2003). In 213 patients with relapsing–remitting or relapsing secondary progressive multiple sclerosis given natalizumab or placebo every 28 days for 6 months, there was a marked reduction in the number of new brain lesions (gadolinium-enhanced magnetic resonance imaging) in treated patients (Miller et al., 2003).

The same antibody was applied in Crohn's disease (Ghosh et al., 2003). Similarly, in 248 patients with moderate to severe Crohn's disease, two infusions of mAb given 4 weeks apart induced higher remission rates than did placebo and significant improvement in the Crohn's Disease Activity Index, together with improved quality of life (Ghosh et al., 2003). Unfortunately reports indicated that chronic administration of this antibody gave rise to the risk of opportunistic brain infection caused by the JC virus that temporarily stopped the use of natalizumab (Kleinschmidt-DeMasters and Tyler, 2005; Langer-Gould et al., 2005). The first two cases were observed in multiple sclerosis patients receiving natalizumab associated with IFN-β for more than 2 years. The third reported case affected a patient with Crohn's disease treated with natalizumab alone.

An interesting debate has developed in the literature, following the description of these cases, which highlighted that other immunomodulatory biologic agents including rituximab (anti-CD20), efalizumab (anti-CD11a), and TNF blockers (both anti-TNF mABs such as infliximab and the soluble TNF receptor etanercept) could elicit the same adverse effect (Mohan et al., 2001; Goldberg et al., 2002; Kothary et al., 2011). Thus, already in 2001, nearly 20 instances of clinical signs of demyelination had been reported in patients with inflammatory arthritis treated with infliximab or etanercept (Mohan et al., 2001). A brain biopsy in one of them showed that there was in fact no demyelination but authentic progressive multifocal leukoencephalopathy (PML) (Roos and Ostor, 2006).

Concerning natalizumab, in 2006 a panel of experts assessed 3417 patients with multiple sclerosis, Crohn's disease, or RA, who had received the antibody for an average of 17 months, and did not identify additional cases of PML (Yousry et al., 2006). Given the beneficial effect of the antibody on the progression of multiple sclerosis, this reassuring assessment led to the antibody being reintroduced. However, since the reintroduction of natalizumab, as many as 102 new cases of PML have been reported (Tavazzi et al., 2011). The incidence of PML appears related to the duration of treatment, with a peak incidence of 2.41 cases per 1000 patients treated for 2 years or more. The benefit/risk ratio of the drug being regarded as positive, natalizumab remains a therapeutic option of interest in multiple sclerosis and Crohn's disease, subject, however, to strict patient selection and follow-up (Fontoura, 2010; Ford et al., 2011; Iaffaldano et al., 2011).

Leukocyte Function-associated Antigen (LFA)-1 A humanized mAb, efalizumab (Raptiva®), specific for the CD11a subunit of LFA-1, has been tested in psoriasis. When administered subcutaneously once a week, improvement was observed within 2—4 weeks, and lasted for up to 2 years (Leonardi, 2004). Results from three randomized, placebo-controlled trials in patients exhibiting moderate to severe plaque psoriasis likewise showed promising results (Menter et al., 2004); here the follow-up lasted for 12 weeks as a double-blind trial and there was an additional 12 weeks of extended treatment phase (Menter et al., 2004). Based on these results efalizumab was approved in 2003 by the FDA for this indication. However, in 2009, it was withdrawn from the European and North American market due to three cases of PML out of a total of 46,000 treated patients and based on a benefit/risk ratio considered as unfavorable (Korman et al., 2009; Tavazzi et al., 2011).

B Cell Antigens (CD20)

Rituximab is a human—mouse chimeric mAb, specific for the CD20 B cell antigen, which causes rapid depletion of B lymphocytes. Rituximab was approved in the United States in 1997 and in Europe in 1998 (MabThera®) to treat severe refractory CD20-positive non-Hodgkin's B cell lymphoma. The use of anti-CD20 has been extended to first-line therapy and maintenance therapy in lymphoma, for stem-cell transplantation procedures and also for a variety of autoimmune disorders, including RA, immune thrombocytopenic purpura, autoimmune hemolytic anemia, systemic lupus erythematosus, vasculitis, dermatomyositis, multiple sclerosis, and type 1 diabetes (De Vita et al., 2002; Leandro et al., 2002; Silverman and

Weisman, 2003; Looney et al., 2004a,b; Rastetter et al., 2004; Pescovitz et al., 2009).

Among these there are indications that are obvious since the physiopathology of the disease involves pathogenic autoantibodies and therefore it seems appropriate to destroy the B cells producing these autoantibodies. The surprise was that in some of these indications, such as systemic lupus erythematosus, the effectiveness of CD20 antibody was rather disappointing compared to the very encouraging results observed in multiple sclerosis or type 1 diabetes, two conditions wherein pathogenic T cells and not autoantibodies are regarded as the main actors. At a fundamental level, these results highlight the pathogenic role of B lymphocytes not only as antibody-producing cells but also as antigen-presenting cells, and which hitherto had been considered of marginal importance in some of these autoimmune diseases.

In systemic lupus erythematosus, a first report, further supported by a series of off-label trials, described that B cell depletion was successfully obtained in patients using rituximab and that disease remission could be achieved (Leandro et al., 2005). However, two multicenter randomized placebo-controlled trials, one in patients with moderate to severe non-renal disease and the other in proliferative lupus nephritis, did not confirm such benefit (Merrill et al., 2010; Rovin et al., 2012). The reasons which may explain such a discrepancy are numerous and have been recently critically reviewed by Furtado and Isenberg (Furtado and Isenberg, 2013).

The quest to find agents that will better and more efficaciously target B cells continues. Among other B cell-directed antibodies that have been or are being tested are ocrelizumab (anti-CD20) (Cang et al., 2012) and epratuzumab (anti-CD22). In addition, major hope is focused on antibodies blocking factors that sustain B cell differentiation and/or activation such as belimumab (Benlysta®), a monoclonal antibody to BLyS/BAFF, which was tested in two Phase III studies and was recently approved by the FDA to treat systemic lupus erythematosus (Navarra et al., 2011). In combination with standard therapies belimumab achieved improvement in both disease remission and time to flare with, in addition, a good safety profile.

New molecules that achieve B cell depletion/blockade have been recently introduced and include inhibitors of survival factors. Among these atacicept is a recombinant molecule (formerly referred to as TACI-Ig) coupling a human Fc fragment and soluble TACI that is the receptor for the cytokines BlyS/BAFF (B lymphocyte stimulator) and APRIL (a proliferation-inducing ligand) (Ginzler et al., 2012).

In RA, Phase II randomized, double-blind, placebo-controlled trials showed that treatment with anti-CD20 was safe and led to major and sustained clinical responses (Edwards et al., 2004; Emery et al., 2006). Results were confirmed and, as a consequence, led to the licensing of the drug in 2006 for this indication. In the USA rituximab is indicated for treatment of patients with moderate to severe disease who have failed other disease modifying anti-rheumatic drugs and at least one TNF inhibitor always in conjunction with methotrexate. Indeed, the efficacy and the duration of the benefit are significantly more pronounced when rituximab is combined with methotrexate (Tak et al., 2012). In Europe rituximab is approved for severe disease.

In multiple sclerosis, a Phase II trial showed that a single course of rituximab reduced inflammatory brain lesions and clinical relapses (Hauser et al., 2008). Presently the question is whether rituximab will be developed further in this indication or if second generation CD20 antibodies such as ocrelizumab (Cang et al., 2012), which is currently being tested in Phase II studies, will be selected instead for marketing.

In type 1 diabetes compelling evidence has been accumulated to demonstrate that the pivotal role of B lymphocytes is due to their capacity to act as autoantigen-presenting cells. Indeed, NOD mice expressing a genetic invalidation for the gene encoding the µ immunoglobulin chain are devoid of B cells and are fully protected from disease (Serreze et al., 1996). Based on this rationale CD20 antibodies were tested almost in parallel in the NOD mouse and in clinical trials. Due to lack of available anti-mouse CD20 antibodies, transgenic NOD mice expressing the human CD20 on B cells were used (Hu et al., 2007). Treatment of these mice with a single cycle of an anti-human CD20 monoclonal antibody temporarily depleted B cells and significantly reduced and delayed the onset of diabetes. Furthermore, disease could be reversed in about one-third of overtly diabetic mice (Hu et al., 2007). In patients presenting recent-onset type 1 diabetes, rituximab administered on days 1, 8, 15, and 22 of study showed a significant effect on β cell function at 1 year of follow-up (Pescovitz et al., 2009). The level of C-peptide was significantly higher in the rituximab group compared to the placebo group. The rituximab group also had significantly lower HbA1c levels and required less insulin. Unfortunately, the effect was not long-lasting as immune tolerance was not induced. Moreover, immunological monitoring studies showed a significant yet reversible incapacity of treated patients to mount efficient antibody responses for several months after treatment, linked to the deep and prolonged B cell depletion observed. However, this trial was considered important as it paves the way to the combination of therapies targeting T and B cells (Hu et al., 2013).

Leukocyte Antigens (CD52)

Antibodies to CD52 target a small (12 amino acids) glycosylphosphatidylinositol (GPI)-anchored protein of undefined function expressed at the surface of human B and T cells and monocyte/macrophages. Anti CD52 mAbs are highly depleting and have potent efficacy in long-term acceptance of organ allografts and maintaining remission in established and otherwise intractable autoimmune diseases, notably multiple sclerosis, vasculitis, and rheumatoid arthritis (Mathieson et al., 1990; Lockwood et al., 1993, 1996; Calne et al., 1999).

The first rat mAb to CD52, Campath-1H, was characterized in 1983. A fully reshaped humanized version, Campath-1H (human IgG1), was derived by genetic engineering (Riechmann et al., 1988) and is marketed as alemtuzumab (Lemtrada®). Its depleting capacity has led to its extensive use *in vivo* to treat $CD52^+$ hematologic malignancies, and *in vitro* to purge bone marrow transplants to prevent graft versus host (GVH) disease. Upon the first injection, Campath-1H triggers an acute self-limited cytokine release that causes a transient flu-like syndrome.

Campath-1H has been given to patients with rheumatoid arthritis, 50% of whom, after 3 and 6 months, showed improvement in the Paulus score (Isaacs et al., 1992). Campath-1H also proved very effective in severe systemic small vessel vasculitis in which the pathogenesis depends mainly on T cell-mediated mechanisms (Mathieson et al., 1990; Lockwood et al., 1993, 1996). The long-term remissions that were obtained when combining antibodies to CD52 and CD4 were particularly impressive (Mathieson et al., 1990; Lockwood et al., 1993, 1996).

Results with anti-CD52 in multiple sclerosis were also very promising and the drug has been recently approved for this indication (Moreau et al., 1994; Coles et al., 1999a,b). The initial trials included patients with long-standing relapsing/remitting multiple sclerosis unresponsive to conventional treatments. Long-term follow-up showed a marked decrease in the appearance of new lesions in the central nervous system as assessed by MRI scanning that correlated with the persisting and significant depletion of peripheral $CD4^+$ T lymphocytes (Moreau et al., 1994; Coles et al., 1999a,b, 2004). These results were confirmed in Phase II studies including one that showed the superiority of alemtuzumab compared to IFN-β monotherapy (CAMMS223 Trial Investigators et al., 2008). Phase III trials have been completed and alemtuzumab has been approved for treatment of relapsing/remitting multiple sclerosis (Cohen et al., 2012).

Treatment with alemtuzumab elicits some side effects including a long-lasting profound lymphopenia (which, importantly, is not associated with increased rate of opportunistic infections) and a cytokine release syndrome after the first injection (which may be prevented by corticosteroids), and a neutralizing anti-idiotypic immunization is observed in a significant proportion of patients. Another more unexpected side effect was the development of autoimmune disorders, particularly autoimmune thyroiditis (in up to 30% of patients with multiple sclerosis) or more rarely autoimmune cytopenias (Coles et al., 1999b; CAMMS223 Trial Investigators et al., 2008; Walsh et al., 2008; Jones et al., 2009). In one of the trials in multiple sclerosis several cases (2.8%) of idiopathic thrombocytopenic purpura have been reported (CAMMS223 Trial Investigators et al., 2008; Cuker et al., 2011). The occurrence of these complications is independent of the therapeutic effect of the antibody, but appears to be related to treatment-induced lymphopenia. Interesting data suggest that these autoimmune manifestations occur in patients in whom homeostatic cell proliferation following depletion induced by the antibody is more important. This phenomenon is dependent on IL-21, a cytokine for which circulating levels are increased before treatment in patients who will develop the post-treatment autoimmune manifestations. Therefore it has been proposed to use IL-21 pretreatment levels to serve as a predictive parameter to identify patients at risk of this type of side effect (Jones et al., 2009).

In conclusion, alemtuzumab appears to be a treatment of choice in relapsing/remitting multiple sclerosis and also for severe autoimmune diseases refractory to other treatment.

Cytokines

Blocking TNF Pathways Humanized mAbs to TNF proved a major breakthrough in the treatment of rheumatoid arthritis, consequent on the pioneering experimental and clinical work of Feldmann and Maini (Elliott et al., 1994a; Feldmann, 2002). The seminal finding was that neutralizing antibodies to TNF significantly decreased the production of most of the proinflammatory cytokines, i.e., IL-1, IL-6, IL-8, GM-CSF, normally produced in *in vitro* cultures of cells that infiltrate synovial membranes in RA (Brennan et al., 1989; Brennan and Feldmann, 1992; Feldmann, 2002). The relevance of this finding to events *in vivo* was validated in mice that express a human TNF transgene and develop a form of chronic arthritis fully preventable by mAbs to TNF (Brennan and Feldmann, 1992; Feldmann, 2002). In addition, in collagen-induced arthritis, neutralizing antibodies to murine TNF given at onset of disease decreased the severity of objective and histopathological features (swollen joints and bone erosions) (Piguet et al., 1992; Williams et al., 1992, 1994). An unexpected but potentially relevant observation was that, in established arthritis, combination of a suboptimal dose of anti-TNF (which had no significant effect *per se*) with anti-CD4 greatly improved joint inflammation and helped heal paw swelling and bone erosions (Williams et al., 1994; Marinova-Mutafchieva et al., 2000). Thus

neutralizing inflammation, as with anti-TNF, effectively "sensitizes'" the immune system to T cell-directed immuno-intervention: this could be relevant to various autoimmune diseases other than RA.

The first randomized placebo-controlled, double-blind study showing effectiveness of the chimeric neutralizing antibody to TNF, cA2 [human IgG1, now termed infliximab (Remicade®)] in long-standing rheumatoid arthritis was reported in 1994 (Elliott et al., 1994a); there was significant therapeutic benefit lasting for several weeks after the end of treatment. Some patients with relapse of RA underwent two or more courses of treatment; the mean duration of remissions progressively diminished due to sensitization to the mAb (Elliott et al., 1994b). In further studies, anti-TNF was combined with methotrexate thus avoiding sensitization and obtaining longer-lasting remissions (Maini et al., 1998; Feldmann and Maini, 2001; Feldmann, 2002). Data from a Phase III trial showed that anti-TNF arrested joint damage in more than 50% of patients; the effect was noted by 6 months after beginning of treatment and lasted for the 2 years of the study (Maini et al., 1999; Lipsky et al., 2000). Infliximab was thus approved for use, in combination with methotrexate, both in the USA and Europe.

Given these results with infliximab, other biologic agents against TNF were developed. Another chimeric anti-TNF mAb named CDP571 also was clinically effective (Rankin et al., 1995), as were two fusion proteins linking the TNF receptor molecules p55 or p75 to a human IgG constant region (lenercept and etanercept/Enbrel®, respectively) (Moreland et al., 1996, 1997; Furst et al., 2003). However, only etanercept was actively developed in the clinic and became approved. Other interesting candidates are on the way, one being the fully human D2E7 antibody (adalimumab), which has shown efficacy in Phase II and III trials (Kempeni, 1999; den Broeder et al., 2002).

Also mAbs to TNF were used successfully in severe Crohn's disease and have been approved for this use (Van Dullemen et al., 1995; Present et al., 1999). Although the pathophysiology of Crohn's disease remains unclear (see Chapter 60), inflammatory cytokines are significantly involved (Van Deventer, 1997). The therapeutic benefit derived from anti-TNF treatment correlated with a decreased production of IFN-γ by mononuclear cells infiltrating the lamina propria of the colon (Plevy et al., 1997). Interestingly, at variance with what is observed in RA, TNF receptor fusion proteins were not effective in Crohn's disease.

Subsequently, data from trials using anti-TNF in juvenile arthritis (Lovell et al., 2000), ankylosing spondylitis (Brandt et al., 2000), psoriatic arthritis (Mease et al., 2000), and psoriasis have been published (Chaudhari et al., 2001).

One adverse effect reported, especially in patients undergoing repeated treatments with infliximab, was the increased incidence of tuberculosis (at both pulmonary and extra-pulmonary sites) (Keane et al., 2001; Gomez-Reino et al., 2003). This is one reason why combination therapy with drugs aimed at neutralizing TNF and IL-1 has been recently disallowed by the FDA. Other side effects that have been related to TNF blockers include the induction of autoantibodies and the occurrence of non-Hodgkin's lymphoma (Brown et al., 2002; Wolfe and Michaud, 2004). Autoantibody formation is commonly seen in patients receiving prolonged treatment with infliximab (Louis et al., 2003; Caramaschi et al., 2006). These include anti-nuclear antibodies, anti-Sm, anti-RNP, and in a few cases anti-double stranded DNA autoantibodies; their presence is usually not associated with clinical signs of systemic autoimmune rheumatic disease. Concerning the occurrence of lymphoma, Wolfe and Michaud reported an extensive study on 18,572 patients with RA who were enrolled in the National Data Bank for Rheumatic Diseases (Wolfe and Michaud, 2004). The overall standardized incidence ratio for lymphoma in RA patients not receiving methotrexate or biologics was 1.0 (95% confidence interval [95% CI] 0.4–2.5), 2.9 (95% CI 1.7–4.9) in patients treated with TNF blockers, 2.6 (95% CI 1.4–4.5) in patients receiving infliximab (with or without etanercept), and 3.8 (95% CI 1.9–7.5) in patients receiving etanercept, with or without infliximab (Wolfe and Michaud, 2004). The authors concluded that current data are insufficient to firmly establish a causal relationship because lymphomas are increased in RA independently from the treatment. Although the risk appears higher when TNF blockers are administered, differences between therapies are slight, and confidence intervals for treatment groups overlap.

There is no doubt that the story of anti-TNF antibodies in RA is a beautiful one that constituted a real revolution in the field (Taylor and Feldmann, 2009).

Antibodies to Interferon (IFN)-γ Treatment with antibodies to IFN-γ has been attempted in several experimental autoimmune diseases on the rationale that the central effects of IFN-γ in Th1-mediated immune responses include macrophage activation and upregulation of major histocompatibility complex molecules. mAbs to IFN-γ successfully prevented autoimmune diabetes in BB rats and NOD mice (Nicoletti et al., 1990; Debray-Sachs et al., 1991). In (NZBxNZW) F1 mice, anti-IFN-γ treatment when started early (by 4 months of age) delayed the onset of glomerulonephritis and significantly prolonged survival; anti-IFN-γ appeared to act by inhibiting production of anti-DNA autoantibodies rather than affecting immune complex formation.

In patients with RA a randomized double-blind trial compared the effectiveness of treatment with anti-IFN-γ vs. anti-TNF or placebo (Sigidin et al., 2001). Promising data were obtained which, unfortunately, are still awaiting confirmation.

Fontolizumab, a human anti-IFN-γ antibody, was tested for the treatment of Crohn's disease (Hommes, 2006; Reinisch, 2006; Reinisch et al., 2010). The first trials showed a therapeutic efficacy of antibodies after two infusions 4 weeks apart (Hommes, 2006; Reinisch, 2006). In contrast, a Phase II controlled study did not show efficacy at 4 weeks after a single infusion of the antibody, followed by three monthly subcutaneous injections (Reinisch et al., 2010). However, the significant decrease in C-reactive protein (CRP) observed in all patients and the higher proportion of partial or complete remissions seen in the subgroup of patients who received the highest doses of subcutaneous antibody leaves room for substantial improvements in the protocol design which may ameliorate the outcome.

Antibodies to Interleukin (IL)-12 (p40) Interleukin (IL)-12 promotes the differentiation of helper Th1 lymphocytes that are IFN-γ and IL-2 producers. Interleukin 12 is constituted by the p40 and p35 subunits. The p40 subunit is shared by another cytokine, IL-23 (p40/p19), which participates in the differentiation of Th17 cells. The importance of the IL-12/IFN-γ and IL-23/IL-17 pathways in the pathophysiology of psoriasis, multiple sclerosis, and Crohn's disease fostered the development of antibodies directed to the p40 subunit which could therefore inhibit both IL-12 and IL-23 (D'Elios et al., 2010; Damsker et al., 2010). Ustekinumab, a human anti-p40 antibody, proved successful in psoriasis, psoriatic arthritis, and Crohn's disease, but not in multiple sclerosis.

In psoriasis the efficacy of ustekinumab (Stelara®) is clear according to three Phase III clinical trials (Tsai et al., 2011; McInnes et al., 2013) and the clinical response is accompanied by significant improvement in quality of life. The drug was approved in the United States and in Europe for this indication. Another important Phase III clinical trial demonstrated the superior efficacy of ustekinumab (regardless of dosing regimen) in psoriasis compared with high-dose etanercept at week 12 (Griffiths et al., 2010). Long-term efficacy has been demonstrated over 3 and even up to 5 years with a good safety profile (Kimball et al., 2012; Kumar et al., 2013). Ustekinumab is also beneficial in psoriatic arthritis according to Phase II and III clinical trials, providing further guidance on management of concurrent disease (McInnes et al., 2013).

In Crohn's disease recent results from a randomized placebo-controlled trial on 526 patients showed that ustekinumab induces a high rate of remission in patients with moderate to severe disease resistant to TNF blockers (Sandborn et al., 2008, 2012).

In multiple sclerosis, and challenging data supporting a major role of IL-12 and IL-17 pathways in this disease, treatment did not reduce the cumulative number of MRI-identifiable lesions (Segal et al., 2008).

Antibodies to Interleukin (IL)-6 In the 1990s, IL-6 had been identified as the key growth factor for plasma cells and multiple myeloma B cells. Circulating levels of IL-6 and soluble receptor for IL-6 are used as prognostic parameters in this lymphoproliferative disease. These observations have stimulated the clinical use of IL-6 neutralizing antibodies which proved effective in inhibiting tumor growth. However, a major problem was that IL-6/anti-IL-6 complexes were not eliminated, which, in fact, prolonged the half-life of the cytokine (Lu et al., 1992). This difficulty was overcome by targeting the IL-6 receptor (IL-6R) by development of the humanized antibody tocilizumab.

Tocilizumab (Actemra®) was approved by the FDA for refractory rheumatoid arthritis in 2010 and for systemic juvenile arthritis in 2011. The antibody is also used in Castleman's disease.

In rheumatoid arthritis tocilizumab induces rapid and sustained improvement including normalization of indices of inflammation (CRP), a reduction of radiological joint damage, and inhibition of B cell hyperactivity (Emery et al., 2008; Karsdal et al., 2012).

Other Soluble Receptors and Protein Fusion Conjugates

The use of soluble receptors to TNF and CTLA-4Ig is discussed above and also in Chapter 36. Another human fusion protein, alefacept, was developed by coupling LFA-3 to human IgG1 to provide an agent that binds to CD2 on T lymphocytes. In controlled multicenter studies, this agent was used weekly in chronic plaque psoriasis for one or two 12-week courses. The drug was well tolerated, and a minimal 75% reduction of the disease score (PASI index) was observed 2 weeks from the last dose, lasting for 7 months (Krueger, 2003; Lebwohl et al., 2003). Alefacept (Amevive®) was approved by the FDA in 2003 for this indication.

Two recent meta-analyses have compared the safety profile and efficacy of various biological agents used for the treatment of psoriasis (Brimhall et al., 2008; Kimball et al., 2012). Results showed that alefacept was less effective than efalizumab, etanercept, or infliximab in terms of reduction in PASI scores. Based on these data alefacept was withdrawn from the market.

A recombinant human IL-1 receptor antagonist (IL-1Ra), anakinra, has been tested in severe rheumatic diseases with encouraging results in patients with systemic juvenile arthritis resistant to other drugs (Verbsky and White, 2004). Favorable data were also reported in refractory SLE (Moosig et al., 2004). In RA large placebo-controlled trials including international multicenter studies demonstrated the safety of the drug as well as sustained clinical improvement (Nuki et al., 2002; Fleischmann et al., 2003) and, importantly, IL-1Ra significantly reduced radiologic progression of bone erosions (Jiang et al., 2000).

Atacicept, the recombinant soluble fully human recombinant fusion protein described above, inhibits B cell-stimulating factors APRIL and BLyS/BAFF. These cytokines are members of the TNF superfamily and potentiate B cell survival and antibody production. Levels of BLyS and APRIL are increased in patients with SLE which explains why trials are under way to test the effectiveness of atacicept in SLE and also in RA (Bracewell et al., 2009; Looney, 2010; Furtado and Isenberg, 2013).

SOLUBLE AUTOANTIGENS

Immunological tolerance to a wide spectrum of antigens (and autoantigens) can be induced by parenteral, nasal, or oral delivery of a soluble antigen. This approach has proven to be successful in several animal models of autoimmunity, either spontaneous or experimentally induced by immunization against autoantigens. Thus the onset of diabetes in NOD mice can be prevented by administration: of insulin or GAD using various routes of administration s.c., i.v., nasal, or oral. Similarly, experimental autoimmune encephalomyelitis (EAE) is preventable by administration of the soluble myelin antigen which is ultimately used to induce the disease.

The details of the underlying mechanisms are the subject of another chapter (see Chapter 79), but mention can be made that autoantigen-induced tolerance, whether using proteins, peptides or altered peptide ligands, is beset by a number of obstacles. These include limitation of the treatment to early disease stages; loss of therapeutic effectiveness as disease progresses; a long lag time to achieve efficacy, which may represent a problem in the case of acute autoimmune responses; risk of disease acceleration by triggering rather than downregulating the autoimmune response; and sensitization with potential risks of anaphylaxis and/or production of neutralizing antibodies leading to serious problems when the autoantigen molecule, e.g., insulin, is physiologically relevant.

BONE MARROW TRANSPLANTATION

Autoimmune diseases include genetic components expressed in the lymphoid and macrophage lineages and thus qualify as stem cell disorders (Ikehara et al., 1990).

Hence patients with serious autoimmune diseases can be considered for high-dose immunosuppression followed by hematopoietic stem cell transplantation (HSCT) (Marmont et al., 1997; Tyndall et al., 1997; Ikehara, 1998). This strategy was initially based on clinical observations in patients with malignancies and concurrent autoimmune diseases (McAllister et al., 1997) as well as results of HSCT in experimental models (Karussis et al., 1992, 1993; van Bekkum, 1998). The latter showed that all types of HSCT, whether allogeneic, syngeneic, or autologous, may induce high remission rates provided adequate conditioning regimens are administered. For example, excellent results were obtained in murine models of spontaneous autoimmunity such as autoimmune diabetes in the NOD mouse or BB rat, and lupus in (NZBxNZW) F1 mice (Ikehara et al., 1985). The mechanisms involve both central and peripheral chimerism. Although successful, the strategy is, however, hardly applicable in humans, due to the hazards associated with conditioning regimens and potential GVH disease.

More attention has been given in serious autoimmune diseases to transplantation of autologous bone marrow-derived stem cells, with the initial aims to induce very deep immunosuppression by reason of the protection afforded by bone marrow cell reconstitution, to reduce the disease activity, or even provide a cure. Other modes of action may be operative, such as the resetting of immunoregulatory circuits. Thus regulatory T cells may recover before effector cells, or benefit may come from the initial elimination of the latter. There is also the possibly useful role of G-CSF (granulocyte-colony stimulating factor), usually administered pre-transplant to mobilize stem cells, or post-transplant to accelerate reconstitution. G-CSF could be beneficial by downregulating effector cells as shown for NOD mice (Kared et al., 2005) and mice with EAE (Zavala et al., 2002).

The First International Symposium on Haemopoietic Stem Cell Therapy in autoimmune diseases took place in 1996 (Tyndall et al., 1997), and inaugurated collaborations including publication by the European Group for Blood and Marrow Transplantation (EBMT), the European League Against Rheumatism (EULAR), and the European Charcot Foundation of consensus reports of guidelines for autologous HSCT in autoimmune diseases, and reports by participating centers on their results to the EBMT registry. These recommendations have recently been updated (Daikeler et al., 2011). In addition, a record compiled by the EBMT has been established so that all centers performing this procedure can cumulate and compare their results. A similar registry was created in North America (Center for International Blood and Marrow Transplant Research, CIBMTR). To date, the estimation is that more than 3000 patients with autoimmune diseases have received hematopoietic stem cells.

The source of the stem cell transplant is mostly mobilized cells from peripheral blood, as these appear to afford a faster and more complete recovery compared with bone marrow-derived stem cells. Mobilization of blood stem cells is performed using cyclophosphamide in combination with hematopoietic growth factors, G-CSF alone, or combined with GM-CSF. According to different studies, the grafts are either purged of mature T cells, which may contain autoreactive effectors, by selection of CD34$^+$ cells with or without additional mAb-dependent T cell depletion, or are not manipulated. Pre-transplant conditioning regimens, for which the aim is to ablate as completely as possible the diseased (autoreactive) component of the immune system, include chemotherapy-based regimens, such as BEAM (BCNU, etoposide, cytosine arabinoside, melphalan), cyclophosphamide with or without antilymphocyte globulins and with or without other drugs, or total body irradiation and busulfan (Daikeler et al., 2011).

Phase I/II studies have been reported in a wide range of autoimmune diseases, including multiple sclerosis, systemic sclerosis (scleroderma), SLE, rheumatoid arthritis, Crohn's disease, and type 1 diabetes. A recent retrospective analysis in 900 patients who received a first autologous bone marrow transplant indicates an overall 5-year survival rate of 85% and a disease-free survival rate of 43% (Farge et al., 2010). Reports provide a conspectus of results on HSCT in rheumatic diseases and multiple sclerosis.

Farge et al. reported on 57 patients with systemic sclerosis in European Phase I–II studies from 1996 up to 2002 with a response in two-thirds of these over a follow-up of 36 months, which was durable and with an "acceptable" morbidity/mortality risk (Farge et al., 2004). At 5 years, the probability of progression was 48% and the projected survival was 72% (Farge et al., 2004). Despite proven toxicity and a significant risk of early mortality, these results and those obtained in other pilot studies justified the performance of larger trials: three prospective studies and randomized controlled studies have been launched. The results of one of these have been reported: in 10 patients with diffuse systemic sclerosis, including lung or visceral disease who received an autologous stem cell transplant, significant clinical improvement was observed in all cases after 1 year of follow-up whereas there was sustained disease progression in 8/9 "control" patients treated with monthly courses of cyclophosphamide (Burt et al., 2011). The two other multicenter studies are in progress.

Since 1996 several hundred patients with multiple sclerosis have received an autologous bone marrow transplant. The first studies performed in patients with severe disease with significant functional disability allowed assessment of risk/safety ratio but not of efficacy. Subsequently, with the implementation of the procedure in patients with less severe disease, significant clinical benefit was observed in some groups of patients, including those with aggressive recurrent/relapsing forms of the disease (Atkins, 2010). In addition, a better selection of patients along with an increasing expertise of the centers involved resulted in a reduction of treatment-related mortality, estimated at 1.3% between 2001 and 2007 (Mancardi and Saccardi, 2008). One of the first multicenter studies included 85 patients who showed a retrospective probability of survival without relapse at 3 years of 74% for primary progressive, 78% for secondary or recurrent/progressive relapsing forms, and 89% in younger patients (under 40 years of age) (Fassas et al., 2002). In a Phase I/II study on 21 patients with severe recurrent/relapsing forms not responding to IFN-β, none of the patients showed any signs of disease progression after a follow-up of 24 to 48 months, and clinical improvement was observed in 81% of cases with no treatment-related mortality (Burt et al., 2009). The long-term data of another Phase I/II trial started in 1995 and including 35 patients have been recently reported (Daikeler et al., 2011). The survival disease-free rate at 15 years was 44% for patients enrolled with active MRI-evident neurological damage but only 10% for patients without active lesions. These results and those from the retrospective analysis of data from the EBMT registry indicate that autologous bone marrow transplantation is an option only in patients with severe and active multiple sclerosis unresponsive to other treatments (Daikeler et al., 2011).

Patients with severe SLE received an autologous stem cell transplantation. Two major studies reported a disease-free survival rate at 5 years of 50% (Jayne et al., 2004; Burt et al., 2011). The transplant not only induced an improvement in serological markers of disease activity but also a prolonged remission (at least 5 years) of lung damage and of the associated antiphospholipid syndrome. Treatment-related mortality was 4–12%. It should be noted that the EBMT registry data indicate a greater frequency of severe infections in patients with SLE receiving transplants compared to other groups of patients (39% vs. 22%) (Farge et al., 2010).

Before the introduction of biological therapies (monoclonal antibodies or fusion proteins blocking TNF), rheumatoid arthritis was one of the first indications for autologous stem cell transplantation. The procedure was well tolerated and induced good clinical responses (Van Laar and Tyndall, 2003), with best results in seronegative disease. Currently, given the progress with TNF blockers and other new biological therapies, autologous stem cell transplants have become rare (Moore et al., 2002; Snowden et al., 2004, 2008; Verburg et al., 2005).

New indications for autologous stem cell transplantation have recently been explored, as in refractory celiac disease at high risk of developing lymphoma, and type 1 diabetes. In the first instance, 18 patients with refractory celiac disease were selected; 13 received a stem cell transplant that induced clinical and biological improvement (Al-toma et al., 2007; Tack et al., 2010). The advantage of this strategy is suggested by the fact that the five enrolled "control" patients who did not receive a transplant all succumbed to T cell lymphoma.

In type 1 diabetes a prospective study included 23 patients (aged 13–31 years) (Couri et al., 2009). Hematopoietic stem cells were mobilized with cyclophosphamide and GCSF, collected by leukapheresis and cryopreserved. The cells were injected intravenously after conditioning with cyclophosphamide and rabbit antithymocyte globulin. During the long-term follow-up 20/23 were weaned from insulin treatment. Of these, 12 patients were insulin independent for 14–52 months showing stimulated C-peptide response levels significantly greater than pretreatment values. Eventually all became insulin dependent again. In terms of side effects, two patients developed bilateral nosocomial pneumonia, three developed late endocrine dysfunction, and nine developed oligospermia. Thus this therapy may afford disease remission with, in about 50% of patients, insulin independency for 1–4 years. However, the type of conditioning regimen required is quite heavy, similar to that used in life-threatening autoimmune diseases. Considering the risk/benefit ratio it is difficult to recommend such a strategy for wide application in type 1 diabetes even limited to adolescents and adults. For obvious reasons it is inappropriate for use in children.

CELL THERAPY AND GENE THERAPY

Cell Therapy

The culture *in vitro* of specialized subsets of immune cells that can be reinfused into a subject with an autoimmune disease is another emerging therapy that has benefited from experience with tumor immunology. Two cell types in particular have elicited interest: tolerogenic dendritic cells and regulatory T cells.

Dendritic cells are normally potent stimulators of immune responses but, when appropriately manipulated *in vitro*, express powerful tolerogenic properties shown by suppression *in vivo* of alloimmune and autoimmune responses. Several factors influence this tolerogenic capacity of dendritic cells, including the precise subset of dendritic cell considered, and their degree of differentiation/maturation: immature or "semi-mature" dendritic cells are tolerogenic whereas mature dendritic cells are immunogenic (see Chapter 12). Several *in vitro* procedures have been described to derive tolerogenic dendritic cells, including treatment with CTLA-4Ig (Lu et al., 1999), IL-10 (Takayama et al., 1998), vitamin D3 (Adorini, 2004), or TGF-β (Alard et al., 2004).

The cellular and molecular mechanisms that drive the modulatory capacity of such tolerizing dendritic cells vary, depending on the model studied, and although at best only partly understood, these mechanisms mostly rely on a capacity to initiate states of peripheral tolerance: anergy, immune deviation, or induction of regulatory T cells.

The culture of regulatory T cells is another option. According to recent data, *in vitro* expanded CD25$^+$ regulatory T cells were highly effective in reversing established diabetes in NOD mice (Bluestone and Tang, 2004; Tang et al., 2004; Fischbach et al., 2013).

Gene Therapy

It is tempting to treat autoimmune diseases by administration of immunoregulatory cytokines according to data from experimental models, including IL-4 and IL-10 in NOD mice (Rapoport et al., 1993; Goudy et al., 2001) and IL-10 in rats with EAE (Rott et al., 1994), clinical application remains problematic, perhaps except for IL-10 in Crohn's disease (Tilg et al., 2002). Gene therapy has successfully been used in several settings in animal models. Transduction with genes for regulatory cytokines, notably IL-4 (Yamamoto et al., 2001), IL-10 (Moritani et al., 1996), and TGF-β (Piccirillo et al., 1998) protects mice from autoimmune diabetes (NOD), and also from EAE (Tarner et al., 2003). In some cases, immune cells were transduced, with the idea that these cells would deliver the cytokine *in situ* after they had homed to the affected target organ (Yamamoto et al., 2001; Tarner et al., 2003). It has also been possible to inhibit the progression of advanced diabetes in NOD mice by genetic induction of large amounts of an ICAM-1 fusion protein (Bertry-Coussot et al., 2002).

The difficulties associated with clinical application of gene therapy are considerable. These include the selection of an efficacious and safe vector, long-term maintenance of the expression of the transduced gene, difficulties in controlling the amount of protein produced with risks of uncontrollable hyperproduction, and uncertainty about the site of delivery of the expressed protein (see Bottino et al., 2003 for review). Ingenious procedures are being developed in genetic diseases, and in cancer, where the need for gene therapy is urgent. Perhaps only when the problems are solved in these settings will gene therapy become applicable to human autoimmune diseases. Meanwhile use should be encouraged in animal models of autoimmunity to provide original information on disease mechanisms and prepare for future clinical applications.

There are as yet early experimental studies aiming at promoting target cell reconstitution, applicable to islet cells in diabetes, by antecedent administration of precursor cells and subsequent genetic manipulation to commit them to the β cell lineage. There is a double caveat: the intrinsic difficulty of the procedure, and the likelihood of relapse of the autoimmune process on newly generated cells (Bottino et al., 2003).

PERSPECTIVES FOR THE FUTURE

In addition to policies based on disease severity (risk/benefit ratio), the overall policy will vary according to the phases of progression of a particular autoimmune disease and perceptions of urgency at its onset. When there is urgency, as pertains in recently diagnosed type 1 diabetes or multiple sclerosis, the hope is that the autoimmune destruction can be halted before irreversible lesions develop. Currently, patients with type 1 diabetes are not given immunotherapy because of the availability of a substitutive treatment with insulin, but an anti-T cell mAb, of which the most promising is anti-CD3, is an attractive approach: anti-CD3 acts rapidly and the effect is long-lasting after a short therapeutic course (Herold et al., 2002; Keymeulen et al., 2005; Sherry et al., 2011).

When inflammation is the more prominent feature, interest turns to the new anti-inflammatory protocols exemplified by mAbs to TNF or IL-1 RA. However, these agents that counter inflammation have relatively short-term effects and may come to supplement rather than replace other approaches discussed above, notably in rheumatoid arthritis.

When an autoimmune disease exposes the patient to a risk of major morbidity, examples being multiple sclerosis, severe SLE, vasculitis, or rapidly progressing systemic juvenile arthritis, high-risk treatments must be considered such as potent biological agents, high-dose non-specific chemical immunosuppression, or even autologous bone marrow transplantation.

As a conclusion, it is hoped—if not anticipated—that emergent therapies based on the progress of biotechnology, including gene and cell therapy, will progressively complement and perhaps replace conventional treatments. The rapidity with which anti-TNF antibodies have become accessible to patients with rheumatoid arthritis and Crohn's disease is most encouraging. Nevertheless, there are still numerous problems concerning the development and evaluation of the various drugs being studied. The multitude of these drugs and their potential clinical applications are remarkable.

Major efforts should be made to identify the best applications and promote their development for the benefit of patients beyond commercial constraints.

REFERENCES

Abramowicz, D., Crusiaux, A., Goldman, M., 1992. Anaphylactic shock after retreatment with OKT3 monoclonal antibody. N. Engl. J. Med. 327, 736.

Abramowicz, D., Crusiaux, A., Niaudet, P., Kreis, H., Chatenoud, L., Goldman, M., 1996. The IgE humoral response in OKT3-treated patients—incidence and fine specificity. Transplantation. 61, 577–581.

Abramowicz, D., Schandene, L., Goldman, M., Crusiaux, A., Vereerstraeten, P., De Pauw, L., et al., 1989. Release of tumor necrosis factor, interleukin-2, and gamma-interferon in serum after injection of OKT3 monoclonal antibody in kidney transplant recipients. Transplantation. 47, 606–608.

Abrams, J.R., Lebwohl, M.G., Guzzo, C.A., Jegasothy, B.V., Goldfarb, M.T., Goffe, B.S., et al., 1999. CTLA4Ig-mediated blockade of T-cell costimulation in patients with psoriasis vulgaris. J. Clin. Invest. 103, 1243–1252.

Adorini, L., 2004. Tolerogenic dendritic cells induced by vitamin D receptor ligands enhance regulatory T cells inhibiting allograft rejection and autoimmune diseases. Kidney Int. 65, 1538.

Al-toma, A., Visser, O.J., van Roessel, H.M., von Blomberg, B.M., Verbeek, W.H., Scholten, P.E., et al., 2007. Autologous hematopoietic stem cell transplantation in refractory celiac disease with aberrant T cells. Blood. 109, 2243–2249.

Alard, P., Clark, S.L., Kosiewicz, M.M., 2004. Mechanisms of tolerance induced by TGF beta-treated APC: CD4 regulatory T cells prevent the induction of the immune response possibly through a mechanism involving TGF beta. Eur. J. Immunol. 34, 1021–1030.

Alegre, M.L., Peterson, L.J., Xu, D., Sattar, H.A., Jeyarajah, D.R., Kowalkowski, K., et al., 1994. A non-activating "humanized" anti-CD3 monoclonal antibody retains immunosuppressive properties in vivo. Transplantation. 57, 1537–1543.

Atkins, H., 2010. Hematopoietic SCT for the treatment of multiple sclerosis. Bone Marrow Transplant. 45, 1671–1681.

Bach, J.F., 2003. Regulatory T cells under scrutiny. Nat. Rev. Immunol. 3, 189–198.

Bach, J.F., 2011. Anti-CD3 antibodies for type 1 diabetes: beyond expectations. Lancet. 378, 459–460.

Bachelez, H., Flageul, B., Dubertret, L., Fraitag, S., Grossman, R., Brousse, N., et al., 1998. Treatment of recalcitrant plaque psoriasis with a humanized non-depleting antibody to CD4. J. Autoimmun. 11, 53–62.

Bagenstose, L.M., Agarwal, R.K., Silver, P.B., Harlan, D.M., Hoffmann, S.C., Kampen, R.L., et al., 2005. Disruption of CD40/CD40-ligand interactions in a retinal autoimmunity model results in protection without tolerance. J. Immunol. 175, 124–130.

Banerjee, S., Wei, B.Y., Hillman, K., Luthra, H.S., David, C.S., 1988. Immunosuppression of collagen-induced arthritis in mice with an anti-IL-2 receptor antibody. J. Immunol. 141, 1150–1154.

Barbas III, C.F., 1995. Synthetic human antibodies. Nat. Med. 1, 837–839.

Barbas III, C.F., Hu, D., Dunlop, N., Sawyer, L., Cababa, D., Hendry, R.M., et al., 1994. In vitro evolution of a neutralizing human antibody to human immunodeficiency virus type 1 to enhance affinity and broaden strain cross-reactivity. Proc. Natl. Acad. Sci. USA. 91, 3809–3813.

Baudrihaye, M.F., Chatenoud, L., Kreis, H., Goldstein, G., Bach, J.F., 1984. Unusually restricted anti-isotype human immune response to OKT3 monoclonal antibody. Eur. J. Immunol. 14, 686–691.

Belghith, M., Bluestone, J.A., Barriot, S., Megret, J., Bach, J.F., Chatenoud, L., 2003. TGF-beta-dependent mechanisms mediate restoration of self-tolerance induced by antibodies to CD3 in overt autoimmune diabetes. Nat. Med. 9, 1202–1208.

Benjamin, R.J., Waldmann, H., 1986. Induction of tolerance by monoclonal antibody therapy. Nature. 320, 449–451.

Benjamin, R.J., Cobbold, S.P., Clark, M.R., Waldmann, H., 1986. Tolerance to rat monoclonal antibodies. Implications for serotherapy. J. Exp. Med. 163, 1539–1552.

Bertry-Coussot, L., Lucas, B., Danel, C., Halbwachs-Mecarelli, L., Bach, J.F., Chatenoud, L., et al., 2002. Long-term reversal of established autoimmunity upon transient blockade of the LFA-1/intercellular adhesion molecule-1 pathway. J. Immunol. 168, 3641–3648.

Bielekova, B., Richert, N., Howard, T., Blevins, G., Markovic-Plese, S., McCartin, J., et al., 2004. Humanized anti-CD25 (daclizumab) inhibits disease activity in multiple sclerosis patients failing to respond to interferon beta. Proc. Natl. Acad. Sci. USA. 101, 8705–8708.

Bielekova, B., Howard, T., Packer, A.N., Richert, N., Blevins, G., Ohayon, J., et al., 2009. Effect of anti-CD25 antibody daclizumab in the inhibition of inflammation and stabilization of disease progression in multiple sclerosis. Arch. Neurol. 66, 483–489.

Bluestone, J.A., Tang, Q., 2004. Therapeutic vaccination using CD4 + CD25 + antigen-specific regulatory T cells. Proc. Natl. Acad. Sci. USA. 101 (Suppl. 2), 14622–14626.

Bluestone, J.A., St. Clair, E.W., Turka, L.A., 2006. CTLA4Ig: bridging the basic immunology with clinical application. Immunity. 24, 233–238.

Bolt, S., Routledge, E., Lloyd, I., Chatenoud, L., Pope, H., Gorman, S.D., et al., 1993. The generation of a humanized, non-mitogenic CD3 monoclonal antibody which retains in vitro immunosuppressive properties. Eur. J. Immunol. 23, 403–411.

Bottino, R., Lemarchand, P., Trucco, M., Giannoukakis, N., 2003. Gene- and cell-based therapeutics for type I diabetes mellitus. Gene Ther. 10, 875–889.

Boumpas, D.T., Furie, R., Manzi, S., Illei, G.G., Wallace, D.J., Balow, J.E., et al., 2003. A short course of BG9588 (anti-CD40 ligand antibody) improves serologic activity and decreases hematuria in patients with proliferative lupus glomerulonephritis. Arthritis Rheum. 48, 719–727.

Bracewell, C., Isaacs, J.D., Emery, P., Ng, W.F., 2009. Ataciept, a novel B cell-targeting biological therapy for the treatment of rheumatoid arthritis. Expert Opin. Biol. Ther. 9, 909–919.

Brandt, J., Haibel, H., Cornely, D., Golder, W., Gonzalez, J., Reddig, J., et al., 2000. Successful treatment of active ankylosing spondylitis with the anti-tumor necrosis factor alpha monoclonal antibody infliximab. Arthritis Rheum. 43, 1346–1352.

Brennan, F.M., Feldmann, M., 1992. Cytokines in autoimmunity. Curr. Opin. Immunol. 4, 754–759.

Brimhall, A.K., King, L.N., Licciardone, J.C., Jacobe, H., Menter, A., 2008. Safety and efficacy of alefacept, efalizumab, etanercept and infliximab in treating moderate to severe plaque psoriasis: a meta-analysis of randomized controlled trials. Br. J. Dermatol. 159, 274–285.

Brown, S.L., Greene, M.H., Gershon, S.K., Edwards, E.T., Braun, M.M., 2002. Tumor necrosis factor antagonist therapy and lymphoma development: twenty-six cases reported to the Food and Drug Administration. Arthritis Rheum. 46, 3151–3158.

Bumgardner, G.L., Hardie, I., Johnson, R.W., Lin, A., Nashan, B., Pescovitz, M.D., et al., 2001. Results of 3-year phase III clinical trials with daclizumab prophylaxis for prevention of acute rejection after renal transplantation. Transplantation. 72, 839–845.

Burt, R.K., Loh, Y., Cohen, B., Stefoski, D., Balabanov, R., Katsamakis, G., et al., 2009. Autologous non-myeloablative haemopoietic stem cell transplantation in relapsing-remitting multiple sclerosis: a phase I/II study. Lancet Neurol. 8, 244–253.

Burt, R.K., Shah, S.J., Dill, K., Grant, T., Gheorghiade, M., Schroeder, J., et al., 2011. Autologous non-myeloablative haemopoietic stem-cell transplantation compared with pulse cyclophosphamide once per month for systemic sclerosis (ASSIST): an open-label, randomised phase 2 trial. Lancet. 378, 498–506.

Bushell, A., Karim, M., Kingsley, C.I., Wood, K.J., 2003. Pretransplant blood transfusion without additional immunotherapy generates CD25 + CD4 + regulatory T cells: a potential explanation for the blood-transfusion effect. Transplantation. 76, 449–455.

Bushell, A., Morris, P.J., Wood, K.J., 1995. Transplantation tolerance induced by antigen pretreatment and depleting anti-CD4 antibody depends on CD4 + T cell regulation during the induction phase of the response. Eur. J. Immunol. 25, 2643–2649.

Calne, R., Moffatt, S.D., Friend, P.J., Jamieson, N.V., Bradley, J.A., Hale, G., et al., 1999. Campath IH allows low-dose cyclosporine monotherapy in 31 cadaveric renal allograft recipients. Transplantation. 68, 1613–1616.

CAMMS223 Trial Investigators, Coles, A.J., Compston, D.A., Selmaj, K.W., Lake, S.L., Moran, S., et al., 2008. Alemtuzumab vs. interferon beta-1a in early multiple sclerosis. N. Engl. J. Med. 359, 1786–1801.

Cang, S., Mukhi, N., Wang, K., Liu, D., 2012. Novel CD20 monoclonal antibodies for lymphoma therapy. J. Hematol. Oncol. 5, 64.

Caramaschi, P., Biasi, D., Colombatti, M., Pieropan, S., Martinelli, N., Carletto, A., et al., 2006. Anti-TNFalpha therapy in rheumatoid arthritis and autoimmunity. Rheumatol. Int. 26, 209–214.

Chatenoud, L., 1986. The immune response against therapeutic mono-clonal antibodies. Immunol. Today. 7, 367–368.

Chatenoud, L., 2003. CD3-specific antibody-induced active tolerance: from bench to bedside. Nat. Rev. Immunol. 3, 123–132.

Chatenoud, L., 2010. Immune therapy for type 1 diabetes mellitus—what is unique about anti-CD3 antibodies?. Nat. Rev. Endocrinol. 6, 149–157.

Chatenoud, L., Bluestone, J.A., 2007. CD3-specific antibodies: a portal to the treatment of autoimmunity. Nat. Rev. Immunol. 7, 622–632.

Chatenoud, L., Baudrihaye, M.F., Chkoff, N., Kreis, H., Goldstein, G., Bach, J.F., 1986a. Restriction of the human in vivo immune response against the mouse monoclonal antibody OKT3. J. Immunol. 137, 830–838.

Chatenoud, L., Jonker, M., Villemain, F., Goldstein, G., Bach, J.F., 1986b. The human immune response to the OKT3 monoclonal anti-body is oligoclonal. Science. 232, 1406–1408.

Chatenoud, L., Ferran, C., Reuter, A., Legendre, C., Gevaert, Y., Kreis, H., et al., 1989. Systemic reaction to the anti-T-cell monoclonal antibody OKT3 in relation to serum levels of tumor necrosis factor and interferon-gamma. N. Engl. J. Med. 320, 1420–1421.

Chatenoud, L., Ferran, C., Legendre, C., Thouard, I., Merite, S., Reuter, A., et al., 1990. In vivo cell activation following OKT3 administration. Systemic cytokine release and modulation by corticosteroids. Transplantation. 49, 697–702.

Chatenoud, L., Primo, J., Bach, J.F., 1997. CD3 antibody-induced domi-nant self tolerance in overtly diabetic NOD mice. J. Immunol. 158, 2947–2954.

Chatenoud, L., Salomon, B., Bluestone, J.A., 2001. Suppressor T cells—they're back and critical for regulation of autoimmunity! Immunol. Rev. 182, 149–163.

Chatenoud, L., Thervet, E., Primo, J., Bach, J.F., 1994. Anti-CD3 antibody induces long-term remission of overt autoimmunity in nonobese diabetic mice. Proc. Natl. Acad. Sci. USA. 91, 123–127.

Chaudhari, U., Romano, P., Mulcahy, L.D., Dooley, L.T., Baker, D.G., Gottlieb, A.B., 2001. Efficacy and safety of infliximab monotherapy for plaque-type psoriasis: a randomised trial. Lancet. 357, 1842–1847.

Choy, E.H., Adjaye, J., Forrest, L., Kingsley, G.H., Panayi, G.S., 1993. Chimaeric anti-CD4 monoclonal antibody cross-linked by monocyte Fc gamma receptor mediates apoptosis of human CD4 lymphocytes. Eur. J. Immunol. 23, 2676–2681.

Clevers, H., Alarcon, B., Wileman, T., Terhorst, C., 1988. The T cell receptor/CD3 complex: a dynamic protein ensemble. Annu. Rev. Immunol. 6, 629–662.

Cobbold, S.P., Adams, E., Graca, L., Waldmann, H., 2003. Serial analy-sis of gene expression provides new insights into regulatory T cells. Semin. Immunol. 15, 209–214.

Cohen, J.A., Coles, A.J., Arnold, D.L., Confavreux, C., Fox, E.J., Hartung, H.P., et al., 2012. Alemtuzumab versus interferon beta 1a as first-line treatment for patients with relapsing-remitting multiple sclerosis: a randomised controlled phase 3 trial. Lancet. 380, 1819–1828.

Coles, A., Deans, J., Compston, A., 2004. Campath-1H treatment of multiple sclerosis: lessons from the bedside for the bench. Clin. Neurol. Neurosurg. 106, 270–274.

Coles, A.J., Wing, M.G., Molyneux, P., Paolillo, A., Davie, C.M., Hale, G., et al., 1999a. Monoclonal antibody treatment exposes three mechanisms underlying the clinical course of multiple sclerosis. Ann. Neurol. 46, 296–304.

Coles, A.J., Wing, M.G., Smith, S., Corradu, F., Greer, S., Taylor, C., et al., 1999b. Pulsed monoclonal antibody treatment and autoimmune thyroid disease in multiple sclerosis. Lancet. 354, 1691–1695.

Cosimi, A.B., 1987. Clinical development of Orthoclone OKT3. Transplant. Proc. 19, 7–16.

Cosimi, A.B., Burton, R.C., Colvin, R.B., Goldstein, G., Delmonico, F. L., Laquaglia, M.P., et al., 1981a. Treatment of acute renal allograft rejection with OKT3 monoclonal antibody. Transplantation. 32, 535–539.

Cosimi, A.B., Colvin, R.B., Burton, R.C., Rubin, R.H., Goldstein, G., Kung, P.C., et al., 1981b. Use of monoclonal antibodies to T-cell subsets for immunologic monitoring and treatment in recipients of renal allografts. N. Engl. J. Med. 305, 308–314.

Couri, C.E., Oliveira, M.C., Stracieri, A.B., Moraes, D.A., Pieroni, F., Barros, G.M., et al., 2009. C-peptide levels and insulin indepen-dence following autologous nonmyeloablative hematopoietic stem cell transplantation in newly diagnosed type 1 diabetes mellitus. JAMA. 301, 1573–1579.

Cuker, A., Coles, A.J., Sullivan, H., Fox, E., Goldberg, M., Oyuela, P., et al., 2011. A distinctive form of immune thrombocytopenia in a phase 2 study of alemtuzumab for the treatment of relapsing-remitting multiple sclerosis. Blood. 118, 6299–6305.

D'Elios, M.M., Del Prete, G., Amedei, A., 2010. Targeting IL-23 in human diseases. Expert Opin. Ther. Targets. 14, 759–774.

Daifotis, A.G., Koenig, S., Chatenoud, L., Herold, K.C., 2013. Anti-CD3 clinical trials in type 1 diabetes mellitus. Clin. Immunol. 13, S1521–S6616.

Daikeler, T., Labopin, M., Di Gioia, M., Abinun, M., Alexander, T., Miniati, I., et al., 2011. Secondary autoimmune diseases occurring after HSCT for an autoimmune disease: a retrospective study of the EBMT Autoimmune Disease Working Party. Blood. 118, 1693–1698.

Damsker, J.M., Hansen, A.M., Caspi, R.R., 2010. Th1 and Th17 cells: adversaries and collaborators. Ann. N.Y. Acad. Sci. 1183, 211–221.

Davis Jr., J.C., Totoritis, M.C., Rosenberg, J., Sklenar, T.A., Wofsy, D., 2001. Phase I clinical trial of a monoclonal antibody against CD40-ligand (IDEC-131) in patients with systemic lupus erythematosus. J. Rheumatol. 28, 95–101.

De Vita, S., Zaja, F., Sacco, S., De Candia, A., Fanin, R., Ferraccioli, G., 2002. Efficacy of selective B cell blockade in the treatment of rheumatoid arthritis: evidence for a pathogenetic role of B cells. Arthritis Rheum. 46, 2029–2033.

Debray-Sachs, M., Carnaud, C., Boitard, C., Cohen, H., Gresser, I., Bedossa, P., et al., 1991. Prevention of diabetes in NOD mice treated with antibody to murine IFN gamma. J. Autoimmun. 4, 237–248.

Debure, A., Chkoff, N., Chatenoud, L., Lacombe, M., Campos, H., Noel, L.H., et al., 1988. One-month prophylactic use of OKT3 in cadaver kidney transplant recipients. Transplantation. 45, 546–553.

den Broeder, A., van de Putte, L., Rau, R., Schattenkirchner, M., Van Riel, P., Sander, O., et al., 2002. A single dose, placebo controlled study of the fully human anti-tumor necrosis factor-alpha antibody adalimumab (D2E7) in patients with rheumatoid arthritis. J. Rheumatol. 29, 2288–2298.

Edwards, J.C., Szczepanski, L., Szechinski, J., Filipowicz-Sosnowska, A., Emery, P., Close, D.R., et al., 2004. Efficacy of B-cell-targeted therapy with rituximab in patients with rheumatoid arthritis. N. Engl. J. Med. 350, 2572–2581.

Elliott, M.J., Maini, R.N., Feldmann, M., Kalden, J.R., Antoni, C., Smolen, J.S., et al., 1994a. Randomised double-blind comparison of chimeric monoclonal antibody to tumour necrosis factor alpha (cA2) versus placebo in rheumatoid arthritis. Lancet. 344, 1105–1110.

Elliott, M.J., Maini, R.N., Feldmann, M., Long-Fox, A., Charles, P., Bijl, H., et al., 1994b. Repeated therapy with monoclonal antibody to tumour necrosis factor alpha (cA2) in patients with rheumatoid arthritis. Lancet. 344, 1125–1127.

Emery, P., Fleischmann, R., Filipowicz-Sosnowska, A., Schechtman, J., Szczepanski, L., Kavanaugh, A., et al., 2006. The efficacy and safety of rituximab in patients with active rheumatoid arthritis despite methotrexate treatment: results of a phase IIB randomized, double-blind, placebo-controlled, dose-ranging trial. Arthritis Rheum. 54, 1390–1400.

Emery, P., Keystone, E., Tony, H.P., Cantagrel, A., van Vollenhoven, R., Sanchez, A., et al., 2008. IL-6 receptor inhibition with tocilizumab improves treatment outcomes in patients with rheumatoid arthritis refractory to anti-tumour necrosis factor biologicals: results from a 24-week multicentre randomised placebo-controlled trial. Ann. Rheum. Dis. 67, 1516–1523.

Emmrich, J., Seyfarth, M., Fleig, W.E., Emmrich, F., 1991. Treatment of inflammatory bowel disease with anti-CD4 monoclonal antibody. Lancet. 338, 570–571.

Farge, D., Labopin, M., Tyndall, A., Fassas, A., Mancardi, G.L., Van Laar, J., et al., 2010. Autologous hematopoietic stem cell transplantation for autoimmune diseases: an observational study on 12 years' experience from the European Group for Blood and Marrow Transplantation Working Party on Autoimmune Diseases. Haematologica. 95, 284–292.

Farge, D., Passweg, J., van Laar, J.M., Marjanovic, Z., Besenthal, C., Finke, J., et al., 2004. Autologous stem cell transplantation in the treatment of systemic sclerosis: report from the EBMT/EULAR Registry. Ann. Rheum. Dis. 63, 974–981.

Fassas, A., Passweg, J.R., Anagnostopoulos, A., Kazis, A., Kozak, T., Havrdova, E., et al., 2002. Hematopoietic stem cell transplantation for multiple sclerosis. A retrospective multicenter study. J. Neurol. 249, 1088–1097.

Feldmann, M., 2002. Development of anti-TNF therapy for rheumatoid arthritis. Nat. Rev. Immunol. 2, 364–371.

Feldmann, M., Maini, T., 2001. Anti-TNF alpha therapy of rheumatoid arthritis: what have we learned? Annu. Rev. Immunol. 19, 163–196.

Finck, B.K., Linsley, P.S., Wofsy, D., 1994. Treatment of murine lupus with CTLA4Ig. Science. 265, 1225–1227.

Fischbach, M.A., Bluestone, J.A., Lim, W.A., 2013. Cell-based therapeutics: the next pillar of medicine. Sci. Transl. Med. 5, 177–179.

Fleischmann, R.M., Schechtman, J., Bennett, R., Handel, M.L., Burmester, G.R., Tesser, J., et al., 2003. Anakinra, a recombinant human interleukin-1 receptor antagonist (r-metHuIL-1ra), in patients with rheumatoid arthritis: a large, international, multicenter, placebo-controlled trial. Arthritis Rheum. 48, 927–934.

Fontoura, P., 2010. Monoclonal antibody therapy in multiple sclerosis: paradigm shifts and emerging challenges. MAbs. 2, 670–681.

Foote, J., Eisen, H.N., 1995. Kinetic and affinity limits on antibodies produced during immune responses. Proc. Natl. Acad. Sci. USA. 92, 1254–1256.

Ford, A.C., Sandborn, W.J., Khan, K.J., Hanauer, S.B., Talley, N.J., Moayyedi, P., 2011. Efficacy of biological therapies in inflammatory bowel disease: systematic review and meta-analysis. Am. J. Gastroenterol. 106, 644–659.

Friend, P.J., Hale, G., Chatenoud, L., Rebello, P., Bradley, J., Thiru, S., et al., 1999. Phase I study of an engineered aglycosylated humanized CD3 antibody in renal transplant rejection. Transplantation. 68, 1632–1637.

Furst, D.E., Weisman, M., Paulus, H.E., Bulpitt, K., Weinblatt, M., Polisson, R., et al., 2003. Intravenous human recombinant tumor necrosis factor receptor p55-Fc IgG1 fusion protein, Ro 45-2081 (lenercept): results of a dose-finding study in rheumatoid arthritis. J. Rheumatol. 30, 2123–2126.

Furtado, J., Isenberg, D.A., 2013. B cell elimination in systemic lupus erythematosus. Clin. Immunol. 146, 90–103.

Ghosh, S., Goldin, E., Gordon, F.H., Malchow, H.A., Rask-Madsen, J., Rutgeerts, P., et al., 2003. Natalizumab for active Crohn's disease. N. Engl. J. Med. 348, 24–32.

Ginzler, E.M., Wax, S., Rajeswaran, A., Copt, S., Hillson, J., Ramos, E., et al., 2012. Atacicept in combination with MMF and corticosteroids in lupus nephritis: results of a prematurely terminated trial. Arthritis Res. Ther. 14, R33.

GlaxoSmithKline, 2011. Press Release: GlaxoSmithKline and Tolerx announce phase III DEFEND-1 study of otelixizumab in type 1 diabetes did not meet its primary endpoint. Available from: <http://us.gsk.com/html/media-news/pressreleases/2011/2011_pressrelease_10039.htm>.

Goldberg, D., Chatenoud, L., Morel, P., Boitard, C., Revillard, J.P., Bertoye, P., et al., 1990. Preliminary trial of an anti-CD4 monoclonal antibody (MoAb) in rheumatoid arthritis (RA). Arthritis Rheum. 33, S153.

Goldberg, D., Morel, P., Chatenoud, L., Boitard, C., Menkes, C.J., Bertoye, P.H., et al., 1991. Immunological effects of high dose administration of anti-CD4 antibody in rheumatoid arthritis patients. J. Autoimmun. 4, 617–630.

Goldberg, S.L., Pecora, A.L., Alter, R.S., Kroll, M.S., Rowley, S.D., Waintraub, S.E., et al., 2002. Unusual viral infections (progressive multifocal leukoencephalopathy and cytomegalovirus disease) after high-dose chemotherapy with autologous blood stem cell rescue and peritransplantation rituximab. Blood. 99, 1486–1488.

Gomez-Reino, J.J., Carmona, L., Valverde, V.R., Mola, E.M., Montero, M.D., 2003. Treatment of rheumatoid arthritis with tumor necrosis factor inhibitors may predispose to significant increase in tuberculosis risk: a multicenter active-surveillance report. Arthritis Rheum. 48, 2122–2127.

Goto, R., You, S., Zaitsu, M., Chatenoud, L., Wood, K.J., 2013. Delayed anti-CD3 therapy results in depletion of alloreactive T cells and the dominance of Foxp3(+) CD4(+) graft infiltrating cells. Am. J. Transplant. 13, 1655–1664.

Gottlieb, A.B., Lebwohl, M., Shirin, S., Sherr, A., Gilleaudeau, P., Singer, G., et al., 2000. Anti-CD4 monoclonal antibody treatment of moderate to severe psoriasis vulgaris: results of a pilot, multicenter, multiple-dose, placebo-controlled study. J. Am. Acad. Dermatol. 43, 595–604.

Goudy, K., Song, S., Wasserfall, C., Zhang, Y.C., Kapturczak, M., Muir, A., et al., 2001. Adeno-associated virus vector-mediated IL-10 gene delivery prevents type 1 diabetes in NOD mice. Proc. Natl. Acad. Sci. USA. 98, 13913–13918.

Gram, H., Marconi, L.A., Barbas III, C.F., Collet, T.A., Lerner, R.A., Kang, A.S., 1992. In vitro selection and affinity maturation of antibodies from a naive combinatorial immunoglobulin library. Proc. Natl. Acad. Sci. USA. 89, 3576–3580.

Griffiths, C.E., Strober, B.E., van de Kerkhof, P., Ho, V., Fidelus-Gort, R., Yeilding, N., et al., 2010. Comparison of ustekinumab and etanercept for moderate-to-severe psoriasis.. N. Engl. J. Med. 362, 118–128.

Gutstein, N.L., Seaman, W.E., Scott, J.H., Wofsy, D., 1986. Induction of immune tolerance by administration of monoclonal antibody to L3T4. J. Immunol. 137, 1127–1132.

Hahn, H.J., Lucke, S., Kloting, I., Volk, H.D., Baehr, R.V., Diamantstein, T., 1987. Curing BB rats of freshly manifested diabetes by short-term treatment with a combination of a monoclonal anti-interleukin 2 receptor antibody and a subtherapeutic dose of cyclosporin A. Eur. J. Immunol. 17, 1075–1078.

Hauser, S.L., Waubant, E., Arnold, D.L., Vollmer, T., Antel, J., Fox, R. J., et al., 2008. B-cell depletion with rituximab in relapsing-remitting multiple sclerosis. N. Engl. J. Med. 358, 676–688.

Hayward, A.R., Shreiber, M., 1989. Neonatal injection of CD3 antibody into nonobese diabetic mice reduces the incidence of insulitis and diabetes. J. Immunol. 143, 1555–1559.

Hering, B.J., Kandaswamy, R., Harmon, J.V., Ansite, J.D., Clemmings, S.M., Sakai, T., et al., 2004. Transplantation of cultured islets from two-layer preserved pancreases in type 1 diabetes with anti-CD3 antibody. Am. J. Transplant. 4, 390–401.

Herold, K.C., Gitelman, S.E., Masharani, U., Hagopian, W., Bisikirska, B., Donaldson, D., et al., 2005. A single course of anti-CD3 monoclonal antibody hOKT3gamma1(Ala-Ala) results in improvement in C-peptide responses and clinical parameters for at least 2 years after onset of type 1 diabetes. Diabetes. 54, 1763–1769.

Herold, K.C., Hagopian, W., Auger, J.A., Poumian Ruiz, E., Taylor, L., Donaldson, D., et al., 2002. Anti-CD3 monoclonal antibody in new-onset type 1 diabetes mellitus. N. Engl. J. Med. 346, 1692–1698.

Hommes, D.W., Mikhajlova, T.L., Stoinov, S., Stimac, D., Vucelic, B., Lonovics, J., et al., 2006. Fontolizumab, a humanised anti-interferon-gamma antibody, demonstrates safety and potential clinical activity in patients with moderate-to-severe Crohn's disease. Gut. 55, 1131–1137.

Horneff, G., Burmester, G.R., Emmrich, F., Kalden, J.R., 1991. Treatment of rheumatoid arthritis with an anti-CD4 monoclonal antibody. Arthritis Rheum. 34, 129–140.

Hricik, D.E., Mayes, J.T., Schulak, J.A., 1990. Inhibition of anti-OKT3 antibody generation by cyclosporine—results of a prospective randomized trial. Transplantation. 50, 237–240.

Hu, C., Ding, H., Zhang, X., Wong, F.S., Wen, L., 2013. Combination treatment with anti-CD20 and oral anti-CD3 prevents and reverses autoimmune diabetes. Diabetes. 62, 2849–2858.

Hu, C.Y., Rodriguez-Pinto, D., Du, W., Ahuja, A., Henegariu, O., Wong, F.S., et al., 2007. Treatment with CD20-specific antibody prevents and reverses autoimmune diabetes in mice. J. Clin. Invest. 117, 3857–3867.

Iaffaldano, P., Lucchese, G., Trojano, M., 2011. Treating multiple sclerosis with natalizumab. Expert Rev. Neurother. 11, 1683–1692.

Ikehara, S., 1998. Bone marrow transplantation for autoimmune diseases. Acta Haematol. 99, 116–132.

Ikehara, S., Kawamura, M., Takao, F., Inaba, M., Yasumizu, R., Than, S., et al., 1990. Organ-specific and systemic autoimmune diseases originate from defects in hematopoietic stem cells. Proc. Natl. Acad. Sci. USA. 87, 8341–8344.

Ikehara, S., Ohtsuki, H., Good, R.A., Asamoto, H., Nakamura, T., Sekita, K., et al., 1985. Prevention of type I diabetes in nonobese diabetic mice by allogenic bone marrow transplantation. Proc. Natl. Acad. Sci. USA. 82, 7743–7747.

Isaacs, J.D., Watts, R.A., Hazleman, B.L., Hale, G., Keogan, M.T., Cobbold, S.P., et al., 1992. Humanised monoclonal antibody therapy for rheumatoid arthritis. Lancet. 340, 748–752.

Jayne, D., Passweg, J., Marmont, A., Farge, D., Zhao, X., Arnold, R., et al., 2004. Autologous stem cell transplantation for systemic lupus erythematosus. Lupus. 13, 168–176.

Jiang, Y., Genant, H.K., Watt, I., Cobby, M., Bresnihan, B., Aitchison, R., et al., 2000. A multicenter, double-blind, dose-ranging, randomized, placebo-controlled study of recombinant human interleukin-1 receptor antagonist in patients with rheumatoid arthritis: radiologic progression and correlation of Genant and Larsen scores. Arthritis Rheum. 43, 1001–1009.

Jones, J.L., Phuah, C.L., Cox, A.L., Thompson, S.A., Ban, M., Shawcross, J., et al., 2009. IL-21 drives secondary autoimmunity in patients with multiple sclerosis, following therapeutic lymphocyte depletion with alemtuzumab (Campath-1H). J. Clin. Invest. 119, 2052–2061.

Kalunian, K.C., Davis Jr., J.C., Merrill, J.T., Totoritis, M.C., Wofsy, D., 2002. Treatment of systemic lupus erythematosus by inhibition of T cell costimulation with anti-CD154: a randomized, double-blind, placebo-controlled trial. Arthritis Rheum. 46, 3251–3258.

Kared, H., Adle-Biassette, A., Bach, J.-F., Chatenoud, L., Zavala, F., 2005. G-CSF treatment prevents diabetes in NOD mice by recruiting plasmacytoid dendritic cells and functional CD4 + CD25 + regulatory T cells. Diabetes. 54, 78–84.

Karsdal, M.A., Schett, G., Emery, P., Harari, O., Byrjalsen, I., Kenwright, A., et al., 2012. IL-6 receptor inhibition positively modulates bone balance in rheumatoid arthritis patients with an inadequate response to anti-tumor necrosis factor therapy: biochemical marker analysis of bone metabolism in the tocilizumab RADIATE study (NCT00106522). Semin. Arthritis Rheum. 42, 131–139.

Karussis, D.M., Slavin, S., Lehmann, D., Mizrachi-koll, R., Abramsky, O., Ben-Nun, A., 1992. Prevention of experimental autoimmune encephalomyelitis and induction of tolerance with acute immunosuppression followed by syngeneic bone marrow transplantation. J. Immunol. 148, 1693–1698.

Karussis, D.M., Vourka-Karussis, U., Lehmann, D., Ovadia, H., Mizrachi-Koll, R., Ben-Nun, A., et al., 1993. Prevention and reversal of adoptively transferred, chronic relapsing experimental autoimmune encephalomyelitis with a single high dose cytoreductive treatment followed by syngeneic bone marrow transplantation. J. Clin. Invest. 92, 765–772.

Kawai, T., Andrews, D., Colvin, R.B., Sachs, D.H., Cosimi, A.B., 2000. Thromboembolic complications after treatment with monoclonal antibody against CD40 ligand. Nat. Med. 6, 114.

Kawai, T., Sogawa, H., Boskovic, S., Abrahamian, G., Smith, R.N., Wee, S.L., et al., 2004. CD154 blockade for induction of mixed chimerism and prolonged renal allograft survival in nonhuman primates. Am. J. Transplant. 4, 1391–1398.

Keane, J., Gershon, S., Wise, R.P., Mirabile-Levens, E., Kasznica, J., Schwieterman, W.D., et al., 2001. Tuberculosis associated with infliximab, a tumor necrosis factor alpha-neutralizing agent. N. Engl. J. Med. 345, 1098–1104.

Kelley, V.E., Gaulton, G.N., Hattori, M., Ikegami, H., Eisenbarth, G., Strom, T.B., 1988. Anti-interleukin 2 receptor antibody suppresses murine diabetic insulitis and lupus nephritis. J. Immunol. 140, 59–61.

Kempeni, J., 1999. Preliminary results of early clinical trials with the fully human anti-TNFalpha monoclonal antibody D2E7. Ann. Rheum. Dis. 58 (Suppl. 1), 70–72.

Keymeulen, B., Walter, M., Mathieu, C., Kaufman, L., Gorus, F., Hilbrands, R., et al., 2010. Four-year metabolic outcome of a randomised controlled CD3-antibody trial in recent-onset type 1 diabetic patients depends on their age and baseline residual beta cell mass. Diabetologia. 53, 614–623.

Keymeulen, B., Vandemeulebroucke, E., Ziegler, A.G., Mathieu, C., Kaufman, L., Hale, G., et al., 2005. Insulin needs after CD3-antibody therapy in new-onset type 1 diabetes. N. Engl. J. Med. 352, 2598–2608.

Kimball, A.B., Gordon, K.B., Fakharzadeh, S., Yeilding, N., Szapary, P. O., Schenkel, B., et al., 2012. Long-term efficacy of ustekinumab in patients with moderate-to-severe psoriasis: results from the PHOENIX 1 trial through up to 3 years. Br. J. Dermatol. 166, 861–872.

Kirk, A.D., Burkly, L.C., Batty, D.S., Baumgartner, R.E., Berning, J.D., Buchanan, K., et al., 1999. Treatment with humanized monoclonal antibody against CD154 prevents acute renal allograft rejection in nonhuman primates. Nat. Med. 5, 686–693.

Kirkman, R.L., Barrett, L.V., Gaulton, G.N., Kelley, V.E., Ythier, A., Strom, T.B., 1985. Administration of an anti-interleukin 2 receptor monoclonal antibody prolongs cardiac allograft survival in mice. J. Exp. Med. 162, 358–362.

Kirkman, R.L., Shapiro, M.E., Carpenter, C.B., Mckay, D.B., Milford, E.L., Ramos, E.L., et al., 1991. A randomized prospective trial of anti-Tac monoclonal antibody in human renal transplantation. Transplantation. 51, 107–113.

Kleinschmidt-DeMasters, B.K., Tyler, K.L., 2005. Progressive multifocal leukoencephalopathy complicating treatment with natalizumab and interferon beta-1a for multiple sclerosis. N. Engl. J. Med. 353, 369–374.

Kohler, G., Milstein, C., 1975. Continuous cultures of fused cells secreting antibody of predefined specificity. Nature. 256, 495–497.

Komura, K., Fujimoto, M., Yanaba, K., Matsushita, T., Matsushita, Y., Horikawa, M., et al., 2008. Blockade of CD40/CD40 ligand interactions attenuates skin fibrosis and autoimmunity in the tight-skin mouse. Ann. Rheum. Dis. 67, 867–872.

Korman, B.D., Tyler, K.L., Korman, N.J., 2009. Progressive multifocal leukoencephalopathy, efalizumab, and immunosuppression: a cautionary tale for dermatologists. Arch. Dermatol. 145, 937–942.

Kothary, N., Diak, I.L., Brinker, A., Bezabeh, S., Avigan, M., Dal Pan, G., 2011. Progressive multifocal leukoencephalopathy associated with efalizumab use in psoriasis patients. J. Am. Acad. Dermatol. 65, 546–551.

Kremer, J.M., Dougados, M., Emery, P., Durez, P., Sibilia, J., Shergy, W., et al., 2005. Treatment of rheumatoid arthritis with the selective costimulation modulator abatacept: twelve-month results of a phase iib, double-blind, randomized, placebo-controlled trial. Arthritis Rheum. 52, 2263–2271.

Kremer, J.M., Westhovens, R., Leon, M., Di Giorgio, E., Alten, R., Steinfeld, S., et al., 2003. Treatment of rheumatoid arthritis by selective inhibition of T-cell activation with fusion protein CTLA4Ig. N. Engl. J. Med. 349, 1907–1915.

Kriaa, F., Hiesse, C., Alard, P., Lantz, O., Noury, J., Charpentier, B., et al., 1993. Prophylactic use of the anti-IL-2 receptor monoclonal antibody LO-Tact-1 in cadaveric renal transplantation: results of a randomized study. Transplant. Proc. 25, 817–819.

Krueger, G.G., 2003. Clinical response to alefacept: results of a phase 3 study of intravenous administration of alefacept in patients with chronic plaque psoriasis. J. Eur. Acad. Dermatol. Venereol. 17 (Suppl. 2), 17–24.

Kuhn, C., You, S., Valette, F., Hale, G., van Endert, P., Bach, J.F., et al., 2011. Human CD3 transgenic mice: preclinical testing of antibodies promoting immune tolerance. Sci. Transl. Med. 3, 68ra10.

Kumar, N., Narang, K., Cressey, B.D., Gottlieb, A.B., 2013. Long-term safety of ustekinumab for psoriasis. Expert Opin. Drug. Saf. Jun. 8, [Epub ahead of print].

Kung, P., Goldstein, G., Reinherz, E.L., Schlossman, S.F., 1979. Monoclonal antibodies defining distinctive human T cell surface antigens. Science. 206, 347–349.

Kuwana, M., Nomura, S., Fujimura, K., Nagasawa, T., Muto, Y., Kurata, Y., et al., 2004. Effect of a single injection of humanized anti-CD154 monoclonal antibody on the platelet-specific autoimmune response in patients with immune thrombocytopenic purpura. Blood. 103, 1229–1236.

Lakkis, F.G., Konieczny, B.T., Saleem, S., Baddoura, F.K., Linsley, P. S., Alexander, D.Z., et al., 1997. Blocking the CD28-B7 T cell costimulation pathway induces long term cardiac allograft acceptance in the absence of IL-4. J. Immunol. 158, 2443–2448.

Langer-Gould, A., Atlas, S.W., Green, A.J., Bollen, A.W., Pelletier, D., 2005. Progressive multifocal leukoencephalopathy in a patient treated with natalizumab. N. Engl. J. Med. 353, 375–381.

Larsen, C.P., Elwood, E.T., Alexander, D.Z., Ritchie, S.C., Hendrix, R., Tuckerburden, C., et al., 1996. Long-term acceptance of skin and cardiac allografts after blocking CD40 and CD28 pathways. Nature. 381, 434–438.

Larsen, C.P., Pearson, T.C., 1997. The CD40 pathway in allograft rejection, acceptance, and tolerance. Curr. Opin. Immunol. 9, 641–647.

Law, C.L., Grewal, I.S., 2009. Therapeutic interventions targeting CD40L (CD154) and CD40: the opportunities and challenges. Adv. Exp. Med. Biol. 647, 8–36.

Leandro, M.J., Cambridge, G., Edwards, J.C., Ehrenstein, M.R., Isenberg, D.A., 2005. B-cell depletion in the treatment of patients with systemic lupus erythematosus: a longitudinal analysis of 24 patients. Rheumatology (Oxford). 44, 1542–1545.

Leandro, M.J., Edwards, J.C., Cambridge, G., 2002. Clinical outcome in 22 patients with rheumatoid arthritis treated with B lymphocyte depletion. Ann. Rheum. Dis. 61, 883–888.

Lebwohl, M., Christophers, E., Langley, R., Ortonne, J.P., Roberts, J., Griffiths, C.E., 2003. An international, randomized, double-blind, placebo-controlled phase 3 trial of intramuscular alefacept in patients with chronic plaque psoriasis. Arch. Dermatol. 139, 719–727.

Lenschow, D.J., Zeng, Y., Thistlethwaite, J.R., Montag, A., Brady, W., Gibson, M.G., et al., 1992. Long-term survival of xenogeneic pancreatic islet grafts induced by CTLA4Ig. Science. 257, 789–792.

Leo, O., Foo, M., Sachs, D.H., Samelson, L.E., Bluestone, J.A., 1987. Identification of a monoclonal antibody specific for a murine T3 polypeptide. Proc. Natl. Acad. Sci. USA. 84, 1374–1378.

Leonardi, C.L., 2004. Efalizumab in the treatment of psoriasis. Dermatol. Ther. 17, 393–400.

Lin, H., Bolling, S.F., Linsley, P.S., Wei, R.Q., Gordon, D., Thompson, C.B., et al., 1993. Long-term acceptance of major histocompatibility complex mismatched cardiac allografts induced by CTLA4Ig plus donor-specific transfusion. J. Exp. Med. 178, 1801–1806.

Linsley, P.S., Brady, W., Urnes, M., Grosmaire, L.S., Damle, N.K., Ledbetter, J.A., 1991. CTLA-4 is a second receptor for the B cell activation antigen B7. J. Exp. Med. 174, 561–569.

Linsley, P.S., Wallace, P.M., Johnson, J., Gibson, M.G., Greene, J.L., Ledbetter, J.A., et al., 1992. Immunosuppression in vivo by a soluble form of the CTLA-4 T cell activation molecule. Science. 257, 792–795.

Lipsky, P.E., van der Heijde, D.M., St. Clair, E.W., Furst, D.E., Breedveld, F.C., Kalden, J.R., et al., 2000. Infliximab and methotrexate in the treatment of rheumatoid arthritis. Anti-Tumor Necrosis Factor Trial in Rheumatoid Arthritis with Concomitant Therapy Study Group. N. Engl. J. Med. 343, 1594–1602.

Lockwood, C.M., Thiru, S., Isaacs, J.D., Hale, G., Waldmann, H., 1993. Long-term remission of intractable systemic vasculitis with monoclonal antibody therapy. Lancet. 341, 1620–1622.

Lockwood, C.M., Thiru, S., Stewart, S., Hale, G., Isaacs, J., Wraight, P., et al., 1996. Reatment of refractory Wegener's granulomatosis with humanized monoclonal antibodies. QJM. 89, 903–912.

Looney, R.J., 2010. B cell-targeted therapies for systemic lupus erythematosus: an update on clinical trial data. Drugs. 70, 529–540.

Looney, R.J., Anolik, J., Sanz, I., 2004a. B lymphocytes in systemic lupus erythematosus: lessons from therapy targeting B cells. Lupus. 13, 381–390.

Looney, R.J., Anolik, J.H., Campbell, D., Felgar, R.E., Young, F., Arend, L.J., et al., 2004b. B cell depletion as a novel treatment for systemic lupus erythematosus: a phase I/II dose-escalation trial of rituximab. Arthritis Rheum. 50, 2580–2589.

Louis, M., Rauch, J., Armstrong, M., Fitzcharles, M.A., 2003. Induction of autoantibodies during prolonged treatment with infliximab. J. Rheumatol. 30, 2557–2562.

Lovell, D.J., Giannini, E.H., Reiff, A., Cawkwell, G.D., Silverman, E.D., Nocton, J.J., et al., 2000. Etanercept in children with polyarticular juvenile rheumatoid arthritis. Pediatric Rheumatology Collaborative Study Group. N. Engl. J. Med. 342, 763–769.

Lu, Z.Y., Brochier, J., Wijdenes, J., Brailly, H., Bataille, R., Klein, B., 1992. High amounts of circulating interleukin (IL)-6 in the form of monomeric immune complexes during anti-IL-6 therapy. Towards a new methodology for measuring overall cytokine production in human in vivo. Eur. J. Immunol. 22, 2819–2824.

Lu, L., Lee, W.C., Takayama, T., Qian, S., Gambotto, A., Robbins, P.D., et al., 1999. Genetic engineering of dendritic cells to express immunosuppressive molecules (viral IL-10, TGF-beta, and CTLA4Ig). J. Leukoc. Biol. 66, 293–296.

Lubin, I., Segall, H., Marcus, H., David, M., Kulova, L., Steinitz, M., et al., 1994. Engraftment of human peripheral blood lymphocytes in normal strains of mice. Blood. 83, 2368–2381.

MacroGenics, 2010. Press Release: MacroGenics and Lilly Announce Pivotal Clinical Trial of Teplizumab Did Not Meet Primary Efficacy Endpoint. Available at: <http://www.macrogenics.com/press_releases-284.html>.

Maini, R., St. Clair, E.W., Breedveld, F., Furst, D., Kalden, J., Weisman, M., et al., 1999. Infliximab (chimeric anti-tumour necrosis factor alpha monoclonal antibody) versus placebo in rheumatoid arthritis patients receiving concomitant methotrexate: a randomised phase III trial. ATTRACT Study Group. Lancet. 354, 1932–1939.

Maini, R.N., Breedveld, F.C., Kalden, J.R., Smolen, J.S., Davis, D., Macfarlane, J.D., et al., 1998. Therapeutic efficacy of multiple intravenous infusions of anti-tumor necrosis factor alpha monoclonal antibody combined with low-dose weekly methotrexate in rheumatoid arthritis. Arthritis Rheum. 41, 1552–1563.

Maki, T., Ichikawa, T., Blanco, R., Porter, J., 1992. Long-term abrogation of autoimmune diabetes in nonobese diabetic mice by immunotherapy with anti-lymphocyte serum. Proc. Natl. Acad. Sci. USA. 89, 3434–3438.

Mancardi, G., Saccardi, R., 2008. Autologous haematopoietic stem-cell transplantation in multiple sclerosis. Lancet Neurol. 7, 626–636.

Marinova-Mutafchieva, L., Williams, R.O., Mauri, C., Mason, L.J., Walmsley, M.J., Taylor, P.C., et al., 2000. A comparative study into the mechanisms of action of anti-tumor necrosis factor alpha, anti-CD4, and combined anti-tumor necrosis factor alpha/anti-CD4 treatment in early collagen-induced arthritis. Arthritis Rheum. 43, 638–644.

Marks, J.D., Hoogenboom, H.R., Bonnert, T.P., McCafferty, J., Griffiths, A.D., Winter, G., 1991. By-passing immunization. Human antibodies from V-gene libraries displayed on phage. J. Mol. Biol. 222, 581–597.

Marmont, A.M., Van Lint, M.T., Gualandi, F., Bacigalupo, A., 1997. Autologous marrow stem cell transplantation for severe systemic lupus erythematosus of long duration. Lupus. 6, 545–548.

Mathieson, P.W., Cobbold, S.P., Hale, G., Clark, M.R., Oliveira, D.B., Lockwood, C.M., et al., 1990. Monoclonal-antibody therapy in systemic vasculitis. N. Engl. J. Med. 323, 250–254.

McAllister, L.D., Beatty, P.G., Rose, J., 1997. Allogeneic bone marrow transplant for chronic myelogenous leukemia in a patient with multiple sclerosis. Bone Marrow Transplant. 19, 395–397.

McInnes, I.B., Kavanaugh, A., Gottlieb, A.B., Puig, L., Rahman, P., Ritchlin, C., et al., 2013. Efficacy and safety of ustekinumab in patients with active psoriatic arthritis: 1 year results of the phase 3, multicentre, double-blind, placebo-controlled PSUMMIT 1 trial. Lancet. S0140–S6736, 60594–2.

Mease, P.J., Goffe, B.S., Metz, J., VanderStoep, A., Finck, B., Burge, D. J., 2000. Etanercept in the treatment of psoriatic arthritis and psoriasis: a randomised trial. Lancet. 356, 385–390.

Menter, A., Kosinski, M., Bresnahan, B.W., Papp, K.A., Ware Jr., J.E., 2004. Impact of efalizumab on psoriasis-specific patient-reported outcomes. Results from three randomized, placebo-controlled clinical trials of moderate to severe plaque psoriasis. J. Drugs Dermatol. 3, 27–38.

Merrill, J.T., Neuwelt, C.M., Wallace, D.J., Shanahan, J.C., Latinis, K.M., Oates, J.C., et al., 2010. Efficacy and safety of rituximab in moderately-to-severely active systemic lupus erythematosus: the randomized, double-blind, phase II/III systemic lupus erythematosus evaluation of rituximab trial. Arthritis Rheum. 62, 222–233.

Miller, D.H., Khan, O.A., Sheremata, W.A., Blumhardt, L.D., Rice, G. P., Libonati, M.A., et al., 2003. A controlled trial of natalizumab for relapsing multiple sclerosis. N. Engl. J. Med. 348, 15–23.

Mohan, N., Edwards, E.T., Cupps, T.R., Oliverio, P.J., Sandberg, G., Crayton, H., et al., 2001. Demyelination occurring during anti-tumor necrosis factor alpha therapy for inflammatory arthritides. Arthritis Rheum. 44, 2862–2869.

Monk, N.J., Hargreaves, R.E., Marsh, J.E., Farrar, C.A., Sacks, S.H., Millrain, M., et al., 2003. Fc-dependent depletion of activated T cells occurs through CD40L-specific antibody rather than costimulation blockade. Nat. Med. 9, 1275–1280.

Moore, J., Brooks, P., Milliken, S., Biggs, J., Ma, D., Handel, M., et al., 2002. A pilot randomized trial comparing CD34-selected versus unmanipulated hemopoietic stem cell transplantation for severe, refractory rheumatoid arthritis. Arthritis Rheum. 46, 2301–2309.

Moosig, F., Zeuner, R., Renk, C., Schroder, J.O., 2004. IL-1RA in refractory systemic lupus erythematosus. Lupus. 13, 605–606.

Moreau, T., Thorpe, J., Miller, D., Moseley, I., Hale, G., Waldmann, H., et al., 1994. Reliminary evidence from magnetic resonance imaging for reduction in disease activity after lymphocyte depletion in multiple sclerosis. Lancet. 344, 298–301.

Morel, P., Revillard, J.P., Nicolas, J.F., Wijdenes, J., Rizova, H., Thivolet, J., 1992. Anti-CD4 monoclonal antibody therapy in severe psoriasis. J. Autoimmun. 5, 465–477.

Moreland, L.W., Alten, R., Van den Bosch, F., Appelboom, T., Leon, M., Emery, P., et al., 2002. Costimulatory blockade in patients with rheumatoid arthritis: a pilot, dose-finding, double-blind, placebo-controlled clinical trial evaluating CTLA-4Ig and LEA29Y eighty-five days after the first infusion. Arthritis Rheum. 46, 1470–1479.

Moreland, L.W., Baumgartner, S.W., Schiff, M.H., Tindall, E.A., Fleischmann, R.M., Weaver, A.L., et al., 1997. Treatment of rheumatoid arthritis with a recombinant human tumor necrosis factor receptor (p75)-Fc fusion protein. N. Engl. J. Med. 337, 141–147.

Moreland, L.W., Bucy, R.P., Tilden, A., Pratt, P.W., Lobuglio, A.F., Khazaeli, M., et al., 1993. Use of a chimeric monoclonal anti-CD4 antibody in patients with refractory rheumatoid arthritis. Arthritis Rheum. 36, 307–318.

Moreland, L.W., Margolies, G., Heck Jr., L.W., Saway, A., Blosch, C., Hanna, R., et al., 1996. Recombinant soluble tumor necrosis factor receptor (p80) fusion protein: toxicity and dose finding trial in refractory rheumatoid arthritis. J. Rheumatol. 23, 1849–1855.

Moreland, L.W., Pratt, P.W., Bucy, R.P., Jackson, B.S., Feldman, J.W., Koopman, W.J., 1994. Treatment of refractory rheumatoid arthritis with a chimeric anti-CD4 monoclonal antibody. Long-term followup of CD4 + T cell counts. Arthritis Rheum. 37, 834–838.

Moritani, M., Yoshimoto, K., Ii, S., Kondo, M., Iwahana, H., Yamaoka, T., et al., 1996. Prevention of adoptively transferred diabetes in non-obese diabetic mice with IL-10-transduced islet-specific Th1 lymphocytes. A gene therapy model for autoimmune diabetes. J. Clin. Invest. 98, 1851–1859.

Nashan, B., Moore, R., Amlot, P., Schmidt, A.G., Abeywickrama, K., Soulillou, J.P., 1997. Randomised trial of basiliximab versus placebo for control of acute cellular rejection in renal allograft recipients. CHIB 201 International Study Group. Lancet. 350, 1193–1198.

Navarra, S.V., Guzman, R.M., Gallacher, A.E., Hall, S., Levy, R.A., Jimenez, R.E., et al., 2011. Efficacy and safety of belimumab in patients with active systemic lupus erythematosus: a randomised, placebo-controlled, phase 3 trial. Lancet. 377, 721–731.

Nicoletti, F., Meroni, P.L., Landolfo, S., Gariglio, M., Guzzardi, S., Barcellini, W., et al., 1990. Prevention of diabetes in BB/Wor rats treated with monoclonal antibodies to interferon-gamma. Lancet. 336, 319.

Nicolls, M.R., Aversa, G.G., Pearce, N.W., Spinelli, A., Berger, M.F., Gurley, K.E., et al., 1993. Induction of long-term specific tolerance to allografts in rats by therapy with an anti-CD3-like monoclonal antibody. Transplantation. 55, 459–468.

Nuki, G., Bresnihan, B., Bear, M.B., McCabe, D., 2002. Long-term safety and maintenance of clinical improvement following treatment with ana-kinra (recombinant human interleukin-1 receptor antagonist) in patients with rheumatoid arthritis: extension phase of a randomized, double-blind, placebo-controlled trial. Arthritis Rheum. 46, 2838–2846.

Nussenblatt, R.B., Fortin, E., Schiffman, R., Rizzo, L., Smith, J., Van Veldhuisen, P., et al., 1999. Treatment of noninfectious intermediate and posterior uveitis with the humanized anti-Tac mAb: a phase I/II clinical trial. Proc. Natl. Acad. Sci. USA. 96, 7462–7466.

Nussenblatt, R.B., Peterson, J.S., Foster, C.S., Rao, N.A., See, R.F., Letko, E., et al., 2005. Initial evaluation of subcutaneous daclizumab treatments for noninfectious uveitis: a multicenter noncomparative interventional case series. Ophthalmology. 112, 764–770.

Nussenblatt, R.B., Thompson, D.J., Li, Z., Chan, C.C., Peterson, J.S., Robinson, R.R., et al., 2003. Humanized anti-interleukin-2 (IL-2) receptor alpha therapy: long-term results in uveitis patients and preliminary safety and activity data for establishing parameters for subcutaneous administration. J. Autoimmun. 21, 283–293.

Onodera, K., Chandraker, A., Schaub, M., Stadlbauer, T.H., Korom, S., Peach, R., et al., 1997. CD28-B7 T cell costimulatory blockade by CTLA4Ig in sensitized rat recipients: induction of transplantation tolerance in association with depressed cell-mediated and humoral immune responses. J. Immunol. 159, 1711–1717.

Orban, T., Bundy, B., Becker, D.J., DiMeglio, L.A., Gitelman, S.E., Goland, R., et al., 2011. Co-stimulation modulation with abatacept in patients with recent-onset type 1 diabetes: a randomised, double-blind, placebo-controlled trial. Lancet. 378, 412–419.

Ortho Multicenter Transplant Study Group, 1985. A randomized clinical trial of OKT3 monoclonal antibody for acute rejection of cadaveric renal transplants. N. Engl. J. Med. 313, 337–342.

Patel, V.L., Schwartz, J., Bussel, J.B., 2008. The effect of anti-CD40 ligand in immune thrombocytopenic purpura. Br. J. Haematol. 141, 545–548.

Pescovitz, M.D., Greenbaum, C.J., Krause-Steinrauf, H., Becker, D.J., Gitelman, S.E., Goland, R., et al., 2009. Rituximab, B-lymphocyte depletion, and preservation of beta-cell function. N. Engl. J. Med. 361, 2143–2152.

Piccirillo, C.A., Chang, Y., Prud'homme, G.J., 1998. TGF-beta1 somatic gene therapy prevents autoimmune disease in nonobese diabetic mice. J. Immunol. 161, 3950–3956.

Piguet, P.F., Grau, G.E., Vesin, C., Loetscher, H., Gentz, R., Lesslauer, W., 1992. Evolution of collagen arthritis in mice is arrested by treatment with anti-tumour necrosis factor (TNF) antibody or a recombinant soluble TNF receptor. Immunology. 77, 510–514.

Plain, K.M., Chen, J., Merten, S., He, X.Y., Hall, B.M., 1999. Induction of specific tolerance to allografts in rats by therapy with non-mitogenic, non-depleting anti-CD3 monoclonal antibody: association with TH2 cytokines not anergy. Transplantation. 67, 605–613.

Plevy, S.E., Landers, C.J., Prehn, J., Carramanzana, N.M., Deem, R.L., Shealy, D., et al., 1997. A role for TNF-alpha and mucosal T helper-1 cytokines in the pathogenesis of Crohn's disease. J. Immunol. 159, 6276–6282.

Present, D.H., Rutgeerts, P., Targan, S., Hanauer, S.B., Mayer, L., van Hogezand, R.A., et al., 1999. Infliximab for the treatment of fistulas in patients with Crohn's disease. N. Engl. J. Med. 340, 1398–1405.

Qin, S., Cobbold, S.P., Pope, H., Elliott, J., Kioussis, D., Davies, J., et al., 1993. "Infectious" transplantation tolerance. Science. 259, 974–977.

Rankin, E.C., Choy, E.H., Kassimos, D., Kingsley, G.H., Sopwith, A.M., Isenberg, D.A., et al., 1995. The therapeutic effects of an engineered human anti-tumour necrosis factor alpha antibody (CDP571) in rheumatoid arthritis. Br. J. Rheumatol. 34, 334–342.

Rapoport, M.J., Jaramillo, A., Zipris, D., Lazarus, A.H., Serreze, D.V., Leiter, E.H., et al., 1993. Interleukin 4 reverses T cell proliferative unresponsiveness and prevents the onset of diabetes in nonobese diabetic mice. J. Exp. Med. 178, 87–99.

Rastetter, W., Molina, A., White, C.A., 2004. Rituximab: expanding role in therapy for lymphomas and autoimmune diseases. Annu. Rev. Med. 55, 477–503.

Read, S., Malmstrom, V., Powrie, F., 2000. Cytotoxic T lymphocyte-associated antigen 4 plays an essential role in the function of CD25 (+)CD4(+) regulatory cells that control intestinal inflammation. J. Exp. Med. 192, 295–302.

Reed, M.H., Shapiro, M.E., Strom, T.B., Milford, E.L., Carpenter, C.B., Weinberg, D.S., et al., 1989. Prolongation of primate renal allograft survival by anti-Tac, an anti-human IL-2 receptor monoclonal antibody. Transplantation. 47, 55–59.

Reinisch, W., de Villiers, W., Bene, L., Simon, L., Racz, I., Katz, S., et al., 2010. Fontolizumab in moderate to severe Crohn's disease: a phase 2, randomized, double-blind, placebo-controlled, multiple-dose study. Inflamm. Bowel Dis. 16, 233–242.

Reinisch, W., Hommes, D.W., Van Assche, G., Colombel, J.F., Gendre, J.P., Oldenburg, B., et al., 2006. A dose-escalating, placebo-controlled, double-blind, single-dose and multi-dose, safety and tolerability study of fontolizumab, a humanised anti-interferon-gamma antibody, in patients with moderate-to-severe Crohn's disease. Gut. 55, 1138–1144.

Reiter, C., Kakavand, B., Rieber, E.P., Schattenkirchner, M., Riethmuller, G., Kruger, K., 1991. Treatment of rheumatoid arthritis with monoclonal CD4 antibody M-T151. Clinical results and immunopharmacologic effects in an open study, including repeated administration. Arthritis Rheum. 34, 525–536.

Riechmann, L., Clark, M., Waldmann, H., Winter, G., 1988. Reshaping human antibodies for therapy. Nature. 332, 323–327.

Robles-Carrillo, L., Meyer, T., Hatfield, M., Desai, H., Davila, M., Langer, F., et al., 2010. Anti-CD40L immune complexes potently activate platelets in vitro and cause thrombosis in FCGR2A transgenic mice. J. Immunol. 185, 1577–1583.

Roos, J.C., Ostor, A.J., 2006. Anti-tumor necrosis factor alpha therapy and the risk of JC virus infection. Arthritis Rheum. 54, 381–382.

Rott, O., Fleischer, B., Cash, E., 1994. Interleukin-10 prevents experimental allergic encephalomyelitis in rats. Eur. J. Immunol. 24, 1434–1440.

Rovin, B.H., Furie, R., Latinis, K., Fervenza, F.C., Sanchez-Guerrero, J., Maciuca, R., et al., 2012. LUNAR Investigator Group. Efficacy and safety of rituximab in patients with active proliferative lupus nephritis: the Lupus Nephritis Assessment with Rituximab study. Arthritis Rheum. 64, 1215–1226.

Sakaguchi, S., 2000. Regulatory T cells: key controllers of immunologic self-tolerance. Cell. 101, 455–458.

Sakaguchi, S., 2004. Naturally arising CD4 + regulatory T cells for immunologic self-tolerance and negative control of immune responses. Annu. Rev. Immunol. 22, 531–562.

Salomon, B., Lenschow, D.J., Rhee, L., Ashourian, N., Singh, B., Sharpe, A., et al., 2000. B7/CD28 Costimulation is essential for the homeostasis of the CD4 + CD25 + immunoregulatory T cells that control autoimmune diabetes. Immunity. 12, 431–440.

Sandborn, W.J., Feagan, B.G., Fedorak, R.N., Scherl, E., Fleisher, M.R., Katz, S., et al., 2008. A randomized trial of ustekinumab, a human interleukin-12/23 monoclonal antibody, in patients with moderate-to-severe Crohn's disease. Gastroenterology. 135, 1130–1141.

Sandborn, W.J., Gasink, C., Gao, L.L., Blank, M.A., Johanns, J., Guzzo, C., et al., 2012. Ustekinumab induction and maintenance therapy in refractory Crohn's disease. N. Engl. J. Med. 367, 1519–1528.

Segal, B.M., Constantinescu, C.S., Raychaudhuri, A., Kim, L., Fidelus-Gort, R., Kasper, L.H., et al., 2008. Repeated subcutaneous injections of IL12/23 p40 neutralising antibody, ustekinumab, in patients with relapsing-remitting multiple sclerosis: a phase II, double-blind, placebo-controlled, randomised, dose-ranging study. Lancet Neurol. 7, 796–804.

Serreze, D.V., Chapman, H.D., Varnum, D.S., Hanson, M.S., Reifsnyder, P.C., Richard, S.D., et al., 1996. B lymphocytes are essential for the initiation of T cell-mediated autoimmune diabetes: analysis of a new "speed congenic" stock of NOD.Ig mu(null) mice. J. Exp. Med. 184, 2049–2053.

Sherry, N., Hagopian, W., Ludvigsson, J., Jain, S.M., Wahlen, J., Ferry Jr., R.J., et al., 2011. Teplizumab for treatment of type 1 diabetes (Protege study): 1-year results from a randomised, placebo-controlled trial. Lancet. 378, 487–497.

Shizuru, J.A., Taylor-Edwards, C., Banks, B.A., Gregory, A.K., Fathman, C.G., 1988. Immunotherapy of the nonobese diabetic mouse: treatment with an antibody to T-helper lymphocytes. Science. 240, 659–662.

Sigidin, Y.A., Loukina, G.V., Skurkovich, B., Skurkovich, S., 2001. Randomized, double-blind trial of anti-interferon-gamma antibodies in rheumatoid arthritis. Scand. J. Rheumatol. 30, 203–207.

Silverman, G.J., Weisman, S., 2003. Rituximab therapy and autoimmune disorders: prospects for anti-B cell therapy. Arthritis Rheum. 48, 1484–1492.

Snowden, J.A., Kapoor, S., Wilson, A.G., 2008. Stem cell transplantation in rheumatoid arthritis. Autoimmunity. 41, 625–631.

Snowden, J.A., Passweg, J., Moore, J.J., Milliken, S., Cannell, P., Van Laar, J., et al., 2004. Autologous hemopoietic stem cell transplantation in severe rheumatoid arthritis: a report from the EBMT and ABMTR. J. Rheumatol. 31, 482–488.

Soulillou, J.P., Cantarovich, D., Le Mauff, B., Giral, M., Robillard, N., Hourmant, M., et al., 1990. Randomized controlled trial of a monoclonal antibody against the interleukin-2 receptor (33B3.1) as compared with rabbit antithymocyte globulin for prophylaxis against rejection of renal allografts. N. Engl. J. Med. 322, 1175–1182.

Tack, G.J., Wondergem, M.J., Al-Toma, A., Verbeek, W.H., Schmittel, A., Machado, M.V., et al., 2010. Auto-SCT in refractory celiac disease type II patients unresponsive to cladribine therapy. Bone Marrow Transplant. 46, 840–846.

Tak, P.P., Rigby, W., Rubbert-Roth, A., Peterfy, C., van Vollenhoven, R.F., Stohl, W., et al., 2012. Sustained inhibition of progressive joint damage with rituximab plus methotrexate in early active rheumatoid arthritis: 2-year results from the randomised controlled trial IMAGE. Ann. Rheum. Dis. 71, 351–357.

Takahashi, T., Tagami, T., Yamazaki, S., Uede, T., Shimizu, J., Sakaguchi, N., et al., 2000. Immunologic self-tolerance maintained by CD25(+)CD4(+) regulatory T cells constitutively expressing cytotoxic T lymphocyte-associated antigen 4. J. Exp. Med. 192, 303–310.

Takayama, T., Nishioka, Y., Lu, L., Lotze, M.T., Tahara, H., Thomson, A.W., 1998. Retroviral delivery of viral interleukin-10 into myeloid dendritic cells markedly inhibits their allostimulatory activity and promotes the induction of T-cell hyporesponsiveness. Transplantation. 66, 1567–1574.

Tang, Q., Henriksen, K.J., Bi, M., Finger, E.B., Szot, G., Ye, J., et al., 2004. In vitro-expanded antigen-specific regulatory T cells suppress autoimmune diabetes. J. Exp. Med. 199, 1455–1465.

Tarner, I.H., Slavin, A.J., McBride, J., Levicnik, A., Smith, R., Nolan, G.P., et al., 2003. Treatment of autoimmune disease by adoptive cellular gene therapy. Ann. N.Y. Acad. Sci. 998, 512–519.

Tavazzi, E., Ferrante, P., Khalili, K., 2011. Progressive multifocal leukoencephalopathy: an unexpected complication of modern therapeutic monoclonal antibody therapies. Clin. Microbiol. Infect. 17, 1776–1780.

Taylor, P.C., Feldmann, M., 2009. Anti-TNF biologic agents: still the therapy of choice for rheumatoid arthritis. Nat. Rev. Rheumatol. 5, 578–582.

Tilg, H., van Montfrans, C., van den Ende, A., Kaser, A., van Deventer, S.J., Schreiber, S., et al., 2002. Treatment of Crohn's disease with recombinant human interleukin 10 induces the proinflammatory cytokine interferon gamma. Gut. 50, 191–195.

Tsai, T.F., Ho, J.C., Song, M., Szapary, P., Guzzo, C., Shen, Y.K., et al., 2011. Efficacy and safety of ustekinumab for the treatment of moderate-to-severe psoriasis: a phase III, randomized, placebo-controlled trial in Taiwanese and Korean patients (PEARL). J. Dermatol. Sci. 63, 154–163.

Tyndall, A., Black, C., Finke, J., Winkler, J., Mertlesmann, R., Peter, H. H., et al., 1997. Treatment of systemic sclerosis with autologous haemopoietic stem cell transplantation. Lancet. 349, 254.

Utset, T.O., Auger, J.A., Peace, D., Zivin, R.A., Xu, D., Jolliffe, L., et al., 2002. Modified anti-CD3 therapy in psoriatic arthritis: a phase I/II clinical trial. J. Rheumatol. 29, 1907–1913.

van Bekkum, D.W., 1998. New opportunities for the treatment of severe autoimmune diseases: bone marrow transplantation. Clin. Immunol. Immunopathol. 89, 1–10.

Van Der Lubbe, P.A., Dijkmans, B.A., Markusse, H.M., Nassander, U., Breedveld, F.C., 1995. A randomized, double-blind, placebo-controlled study of CD4 monoclonal antibody therapy in early rheumatoid arthritis. Arthritis Rheum. 38, 1097–1106.

Van Der Lubbe, P.A., Reiter, C., Breedveld, F.C., Kruger, K., Schattenkirchner, M., Sanders, M.E., et al., 1993. Chimeric CD4 monoclonal antibody cM-T412 as a therapeutic approach to rheumatoid arthritis. Arthritis Rheum. 36, 1375–1379.

Van Der Lubbe, P.A., Reiter, C., Miltenburg, A.M., Kruger, K., De Ruyter, A.N., Rieber, E.P., et al., 1994. Treatment of rheumatoid arthritis with a chimeric CD4 monoclonal antibody (cM-T412): immunopharmacological aspects and mechanisms of action. Scand. J. Immunol. 39, 286–294.

van der Woude, C.J., Stokkers, P., van Bodegraven, A.A., Van Assche, G., Hebzda, Z., Paradowski, L., et al., 2010. Phase I, double-blind, randomized, placebo-controlled, dose-escalation study of NI-0401 (a fully human anti-CD3 monoclonal antibody) in patients with moderate to severe active Crohn's disease. Inflamm. Bowel Dis. 16, 1708–1716.

Van Deventer, S.J., 1997. Tumour necrosis factor and Crohn's disease. Gut. 40, 443–448.

Van Dullemen, H.M., Van Deventer, S.J., Hommes, D.W., Bijl, H.A., Jansen, J., Tytgat, G.N., et al., 1995. Treatment of Crohn's disease with anti-tumor necrosis factor chimeric monoclonal antibody (cA2). Gastroenterology. 109, 129–135.

Van Laar, J.M., Tyndall, A., 2003. Intense immunosuppression and stem-cell transplantation for patients with severe rheumatic autoimmune disease: a review. Cancer Control. 10, 57–65.

van Oosten, B.W., Lai, M., Hodgkinson, S., Barkhof, F., Miller, D.H., Moseley, I.F., et al., 1997. Treatment of multiple sclerosis with the monoclonal anti-CD4 antibody cM-T412: results of a randomized, double-blind, placebo-controlled, MR-monitored phase II trial. Neurology. 49, 351–357.

Verbsky, J.W., White, A.J., 2004. Effective use of the recombinant interleukin 1 receptor antagonist anakinra in therapy resistant systemic onset juvenile rheumatoid arthritis. J. Rheumatol. 31, 2071–2075.

Verburg, R.J., Sont, J.K., van Laar, J.M., 2005. Reduction of joint damage in severe rheumatoid arthritis by high-dose chemotherapy and autologous stem cell transplantation. Arthritis Rheum. 52, 421–424.

Vigeral, P., Chkoff, N., Chatenoud, L., Campos, H., Lacombe, M., Droz, D., et al., 1986. Prophylactic use of OKT3 monoclonal antibody in cadaver kidney recipients. Utilization of OKT3 as the sole immunosuppressive agent. Transplantation. 41, 730–733.

Vincenti, F., Kirkman, R., Light, S., Bumgardner, G., Pescovitz, M., Halloran, P., et al., 1998. Interleukin-2-receptor blockade with daclizumab to prevent acute rejection in renal transplantation. Daclizumab Triple Therapy Study Group. N. Engl. J. Med. 338, 161–165.

Vincenti, F., Larsen, C., Durrbach, A., Wekerle, T., Nashan, B., Blancho, G., et al., 2005. Costimulation blockade with belatacept in renal transplantation. N. Engl. J. Med. 353, 770–781.

Waldmann, H., Cobbold, S., 2001. Regulating the immune response to transplants: a role for CD4 + regulatory cells. Immunity. 14, 399–406.

Waldmann, T.A., 1989. The multi-subunit interleukin-2 receptor. Annu. Rev. Biochem. 58, 875–911.

Waldmann, T.A., O'Shea, J., 1998. The use of antibodies against the IL-2 receptor in transplantation. Curr. Opin. Immunol. 10, 507–512.

Walsh, M., Chaudhry, A., Jayne, D., 2008. Long-term follow-up of relapsing/refractory anti-neutrophil cytoplasm antibody associated vasculitis treated with the lymphocyte depleting antibody alemtuzumab (CAMPATH-1H). Ann. Rheum. Dis. 67, 1322–1327.

Wendling, D., Wijdenes, J., Racadot, E., Morel-Fourrier, B., 1991. Therapeutic use of monoclonal anti-CD4 antibody in rheumatoid arthritis. J. Rheumatol. 18, 325–327.

Williams, R.O., Feldmann, M., Maini, R.N., 1992. Anti-tumor necrosis factor ameliorates joint disease in murine collagen-induced arthritis. Proc. Natl. Acad. Sci. USA. 89, 9784–9788.

Williams, R.O., Mason, L.J., Feldmann, M., Maini, R.N., 1994. Synergy between anti-CD4 and anti-tumor necrosis factor in the amelioration of established collagen-induced arthritis. Proc. Natl. Acad. Sci. USA. 91, 2762–2766.

Winsor-Hines, D., Merrill, C., O'Mahony, M., Rao, P.E., Cobbold, S.P., Waldmann, H., et al., 2004. Induction of immunological tolerance/hyporesponsiveness in baboons with a nondepleting CD4 antibody. J. Immunol. 173, 4715–4723.

Wofsy, D., Seaman, W.E., 1987. Reversal of advanced murine lupus in NZB/NZW F1 mice by treatment with monoclonal antibody to L3T4. J. Immunol. 138, 3247–3253.

Wojciechowski, D., Vincenti, F., 2011. Challenges and opportunities in targeting the costimulation pathway in solid organ transplantation. Semin. Immunol. 23, 157–164.

Wolfe, F., Michaud, K., 2004. Lymphoma in rheumatoid arthritis: the effect of methotrexate and anti-tumor necrosis factor therapy in 18,572 patients. Arthritis Rheum. 50, 1740–1751.

Woodle, E.S., Xu, D., Zivin, R.A., Auger, J., Charette, J., O'Laughlin, R., et al., 1999. Phase I trial of a humanized, Fc receptor nonbinding OKT3 antibody, huOKT3gamma1(Ala-Ala) in the treatment of acute renal allograft rejection. Transplantation. 68, 608–616.

Wynn, D., Kaufman, M., Montalban, X., Vollmer, T., Simon, J., Elkins, J., et al., 2010. Daclizumab in active relapsing multiple sclerosis (CHOICE study): a phase 2, randomised, double-blind, placebo-controlled, add-on trial with interferon beta. Lancet Neurol. 9, 381–390.

Yamamoto, A.M., Chernajovsky, Y., Lepault, F., Podhajcer, O., Feldmann, M., Bach, J.F., et al., 2001. The activity of immunoregulatory T cells mediating active tolerance is potentiated in nonobese diabetic mice by an IL-4-based retroviral gene therapy. J. Immunol. 166, 4973–4980.

Yeh, S., Wroblewski, K., Buggage, R., Li, Z., Kurup, S.K., Sen, H.N., et al., 2008. High-dose humanized anti-IL-2 receptor alpha antibody (daclizumab) for the treatment of active, non-infectious uveitis. J. Autoimmun. 31, 91–97.

You, S., Leforban, B., Garcia, C., Bach, J.F., Bluestone, J.A., Chatenoud, L., 2007. Adaptive TGF-beta-dependent regulatory T cells control autoimmune diabetes and are a privileged target of anti-CD3 antibody treatment. Proc. Natl. Acad. Sci. USA. 104, 6335–6340.

You, S., Zuber, J., Kuhn, C., Baas, M., Valette, F., Sauvaget, V., et al., 2012. Induction of allograft tolerance by monoclonal CD3 antibodies: a matter of timing. Am. J. Transplant. 12, 2909–2919.

Yousry, T.A., Major, E.O., Ryschkewitsch, C., Fahle, G., Fischer, S., Hou, J., et al., 2006. Evaluation of patients treated with natalizumab for progressive multifocal leukoencephalopathy. N. Engl. J. Med. 354, 924–933.

Zavala, F., Abad, S., Ezine, S., Taupin, V., Masson, A., Bach, J.F., 2002. G-CSF therapy of ongoing experimental allergic encephalomyelitis via chemokine- and cytokine-based immune deviation. J. Immunol. 168, 2011–2019.

Note: Page numbers followed by "*f*", "*t*" and "*b*"refer to figures, tables and box, respectively.

A

AA-type amyloidosis, 41−42, 44
Abatacept, 149, 533
Absent in melanoma 2 (AIM2)-like receptors (ALRs), 166
Acetylation, 23−24
Acetylcholine receptors (AChR), 777
Acquired hemolytic anemia, 15−16
Acquired thrombotic thrombocytopenic purpura (aTTP), 713
　incidence of, 713
　Von Willebrand antigen and activity, 713
Acquired von Willebrand disease (avWD), 722
Activation-induced cytidine deaminase (AID), 64
Activation of immune system
　antigen-presenting cells (APCs), 20
　B cells, 20
　dendritic cells (DCs), 20
　IL-1, IL-6 and IL-12 inhibition, 20
　innate immune response, 19−20
　major histocompatibility complex (MHC), 20
　mature T cells, 20
　self-reactive T and B lymphocytes, 24−25
　T cells, 20
Acute inflammatory demyelinating polyradiculoneuropathy, 758
Acute motor and sensory neuropathy (AMSAN), 759
Acute motor axonal neuropathy (AMAN), 758−759
Adaptive immune system, 4−5, 40, 54t, 58−66
　B cells, role of, 62−63
　immunoglobulin antibodies, 63−64
　secondary lymphoid tissues, 64−66
　T cells, role of, 59−60
　　functional activities, 60−61
Addison, Thomas, 587, 605
Addison's disease (AD), 605−606, 1183
　associated with HLA DRB1*03, 609
　autoantigen of, 608
　autoimmune, 588−589
　　adrenal glands, imaging of, 596
　　autoimmune regulator (AIRE) gene, role of, 591
　　clinical manifestations, 595
　　clinical presentations of autoimmune adrenalitis number, 597t
　　clinical signs and symptoms, 596−597

computed tomography (CT) studies, 596
　DEHA (dehydroepiandrosterone), 598
　diagnosis, 595−596
　different clinical presentations of, 596−597
　dual-release hydrocortisone tablet, 598
　general biochemical indices, 595
　genetic predisposition of, 591
　hormonal tests, 595−596
　24-hour urinary free-cortisol test, 597
　imaging studies, 596
　incidence of osteoporosis, 599
　levels of ACTH and, 595−596
　measurement of disease activity, 594
　MHC class I chain-related A (MIC-A), role of, 591
　mineralocorticoid replacement, 598
　natural history, 594−595
　nuclear magnetic resonance (NMR) studies, 596
　prevalence of ACA, 592
　rate of mortality of, 598−599
　risk of, 594
　risk of adrenal crisis, 598
　stages, 594, 595t
　steroid doses during surgery and medical procedures, 598
　subcutaneous cortisol infusion, 598
　therapy, 597−599
autoimmune thyroid disease and/or type 1 diabetes, 607−608
cell-mediated immunity, 591
epidemiology of, 588−589
frequency of, 589
general prevalence of, 589
idiopathic, 591−592
specific markers for onset of, 612−613
therapy
　hydrocortisone, 613
　replacement therapy, 613
tuberculosis, 588−589
Y85C mutation, 609
Adhesion molecules, 297−299, 298t
　atherosclerosis, 1057−1058
　clinical applications, 304−306
　multistep adhesion cascade, 300f, 302−303
　　naïve T cell homing and dendritic cell interactions, 302−303
　primary sclerosing cholangitis (PSC), 931
　as targets for treatment of inflammatory, 305t

Adrenals, anatomy and physiology of, 587−588
　adrenal cortex, 588
　feedback mechanism, 588
　zona fasciculata, 588
　zona glomerulosa, 588, 594
　zona reticularis, 588
Advisory Committee on Immunization Practices, 290
Agrin, 777
AIRE genes, 5, 1007, 1150−1151
　for autoimmunity, 22
Alarmins, 239
Alexine, 12
Alopecia areata (AA)
　antibody markers in, 974
　autoimmune features, 972−973
　clinical, pathologic, and epidemiologic features, 971−972
　genetics of, 973
　major susceptibility genes, 973t
　pathologic effector mechanisms, 973
　in vivo and *in vitro* models, 973
　　C3H/HeJ mouse, 973
　　xenograft mouse model, 973
Alpha-4 integrin, 1227−1228
Amphiphysin I, 824−825
Amyloid A protein, 58
ANCA-associated vasculitis (AAV), 1069
　animal models, 1076
　autoantibodies, 1077−1078
　autoimmune pathogenesis, 1074−1075
　clinical, epidemiologic, and pathologic features, 1073−1074
　environmental influences, 1075−1076
　genetic features, 1075
　pathologic effector mechanisms, 1076−1077
Anergic B cells, 153−154
Animal models
　advantanges, 437−438
　alopecia areata (AA), 973
　antigen-specific tolerization strategies, evaluation of, 436
　aplastic anemia, 687−688
　autoimmune adrenalitis (AA), 590−591
　　induced immunity, 590
　　spontatneous, 590−591
　autoimmune gastritis, 625f
　autoimmune hemolytic anemia (AIHA), 650
　　C3HeB/FeJ mice, 650
　　New Zealand Black (NZB) mouse, 650

Animal models (*Continued*)
    autoimmune hepatitis (AIH), 897–898
    autoimmune hypophysitis, 640
    autoimmune lymphoproliferative syndrome
        (ALPS), 704–705
    autoimmune pancreatitis, 942
    autoimmune polyglandular (polyendocrine)
        syndromes (APS), 611–612
        AIRE-deficient mice, 611
        Bio-breeding (BB) rat, 611
        non-obese diabetes (NOD) mouse, 611
        spontaneous animal models, 611
        thymectomy, 611–612
    autoimmune (type 1) diabetes/autoimmune
        diabetes mellitus (AI-DM), 581–582
        LEW.1AR1-iddm rat, 581–582
        non-obese diabetes (NOD) mouse,
            581–582
        wild bank voles (*Myodes glareolus*),
            581–582
    based on cells function, 442–444
        autoimmune gastritis, 443
        BDC2.5 CD4 T cell clone, 442
        CD45Rb transfer model for autoimmune
            colitis, 442–443
        IBD, 442–443
        MBP-LCMV-Ag transgenic mice, 443
        multiple sclerosis, 442
        type 1 diabetes, 442
    bullous pemphigoid (BP), 963–964
    BXSB mice, 422
    celiac disease, 861
    of celiac disease, 375–376
    challenges using, 264–270
    chronic inflammatory demyelinating
        polyradiculoneuropathy (CIDP),
        768–769
    of contact hypersensitivity (CHS), 113
    cryoglobulinemic vasculitis, 1080
    cryptogenic organizing pneumonia (COP),
        1113
    disadvantages, 437–438
    experimental autoimmune orchitis (EAO) of
        ovary, 1013–1015
    experimental autoimmune thyroiditis
        resulting from immune modulation,
        561–562
    genetically manipulated models of systemic
        autoimmunity, 423–427
        clearance and recycle of dead cells,
            426–427
        complement system, 426
        cytokines, 425–426
        innate immune cell signaling, 427
        lymphocyte activation molecules,
            423–424
        ubiquitination-protein ligases, 424–425
    genetic knockout mouse, 436
    Graves' disease (hashitoxicosis), 566–567
        AKR/N mice, 566
        BALB/c mice, 566
        transgenic mice expressing human TSH-R
            A subunit, 566
    Guillain–Barré syndrome, 763

HLA-A2 transgenic NOD mice, 435–436
HLA-B27 transgenic mice, 366–367
HLA-DR transgenic mice, 374–375
humanized, 372–376
    collagen-induced arthritis, 373–374
ICOS deficient mouse, 436
for identifying autoaggressive T-cell
    specificities, 435–436
idiopathic pulmonary fibrosis, 1113
IgA vasculitis, 1081
IL-12-p35-deficient animals, 71
immune-mediated inner ear disease
    (IMIED), 810–811
immune therapies, developing of, 436
immune thrombocytopenia (ITP), 668
immunization-induced thyroiditis, 561
induced autoimmune disease, 268–269
induced lupus models with iNKT cell
    deficiency, 116
infection-induced autoimmunity, 270
MRL mouse strain, 422
of MS, 71
of multiple sclerosis (MS), 374–375
myocarditis, 1040–1042
NZB (New Zealand Black, H-2^d) mouse,
    422
ocular disease, 798
of organ-specific autoimmunity, 435–444
    comparison of models and humans, 444
    development of T cell-driven, 440, 441*f*
    encephalomyelitis (EAE) model, 440
    genetically engineered, 439
    induced models, 439–440, 443–444
    multiple sclerosis, 444
    non-obese diabetic (NOD) mouse,
        438–439
    RIP-LCMV, 439–440
    RIP-OVA, 439–440
    type 1 diabetes, 444
    virus-infected models, 440
pathogen-induced murine models, 266*t*
pemphigus foliaceus, 961
pemphigus vulgaris (PV), 959
pernicious anemia, 624–625
    A23 TCR transgenic mice, 624
    A51 TCR transgenic mice, 624
    BALB/c mice, 624
    C57BL/6 mice, 624
    C3H/He mice, 624
polyarteritis nodosa, 1071
primary biliary cirrhosis, 916–917, 918*t*
primary sclerosing cholangitis (PSC), 930
protein/peptide and adjuvant-triggered,
    440–442
    autoimmune uveitis, 442
    multiple sclerosis, 440
    myasthenia gravis, 441–442
    streptozotocin (STZ)-induced diabetes,
        442
    thyroid-specific autoimmunity, 440–441
psoriasis
    mouse models, 980–981
    transplantation models, 981
rheumathic heart disease (RHD), 1027–1028

rheumatic fever (RF), 1027–1028
RIP-LCMV diabetes model, 436
spontaneous autoimmune disease, 269
spontaneous models of lupus, 421–423
spontaneous thyroiditis, 562
of systemic autoimmunity, 427–428, 429*t*
of systemic sclerosis (SSc), 467*t*
    Fra2-transgenic mice, 469
    growth factor-induced fibrosis model of,
        468
    murine models of bleomycin-induced
        fibrosis, 468
    Scl-GvHD models, 468
    tight skin mice (Tsk) type 1 and type 2
        (Tsk1 and Tsk2) mice, 468
    TβRIIΔk mice, 469
    UCD200 chickens, 467–468
    Wnt-10b-transgenic mice, 469
TCR avidity, 436
Th1 cells, role in immunopathology, 71
Th1 cytokine-mediated mouse colitis
    models, 115
transgenic expression of IL-4, 71
for type 1 diabetes, 376
    nonobese diabetic (NOD) mouse model,
        435–436
    type 1 diabetes (T1D), 1191–1192
for understanding complexity of organ-
    specific autoimmunity, 436–437
vitiligo, 976–977
WASP deficient mice, 406
Ankylosing spondylitis, 24, 73, 366, 793–794
    aberrant bone formation in, 542–543
        wnt antagonists, role in, 542–543
    cytokines, role of, 542
    immune response in, 542
ANNA-3, 825
ANNA-2 (anti-Ri), 825
Anti-AMPAR, 822
Antibody-dependent cellular cytotoxicity
    (ADCC), 56, 63
Antibody production defects, 406–411
    common variable immunodeficiency
        (CVID), 406–408
    immunodeficiency with hyper-IgM (HIGM)
        syndrome, 409–411
    selective IgA deficiency, 408–409
    X-linked agammaglobulinemia (XLA), 406
Anti-α cell receptors, 12–13
Anticoagulant (bleeding) diseases, 714–722
    antibodies
        against fibrinogen or fibrin, 714
        to thrombin and prothrombin, 714–716
    autoimmune inhibitors
        to factor V, 716–717
        to factor VII, 717
        to factor VIII, 717–720
        to factor IX, 720
        to factor X, 720
        to factor XI, 720–721
        to factor XII, 721
        to factor XIII, 721–722
        T cell epitopes, 719
        von Willebrand Factor (vWF), 722

Anti-cyclic citrullinated protein (CCP), 22
Anti-GABA-B-R, 822
Anti-GAD65, 824
Antigen presenting cells (APCs), 20, 29–30, 71, 161
  in giant cell arteritis (GCA), 1092–1093
  scavenger, 71
Antigen receptors, 59f
Antigen-specific therapies, 31
Antigen-specific T-lymphocytes, 40
Antigen-specific Tregs, 28–29
Anti-inflammatory therapy, 31
Anti-MAG paraproteinemic demyelinating peripheral neuropathy (anti-MAG PDPN), 768
Antimalarial medications, 1212–1213
Antineutrophil cytoplasmic antibody, 204
Antineutrophil-cytoplasmic-autoantibody, 993
Anti-PCA-1, 826
Antiphospholipid syndrome (APS), 206, 456–457, 712
  antiphospholipid antibodies (aPL) in, 481, 484–485
    anti-b2GPI antibodies, 487
    cellular interactions, 487–488
    mechanisms of, 486–489
    thrombophilic properties, 487–488
  b2GPI–anti-b2GPI complex in, 485
  classical clinical criterion, 481
    Sydney Consensus Statement, 482t
  clinical spectrum of, 482–484
    cardiac involvement, 483–484
    catastrophic antiphospholipid syndrome (CAPS), 484
    hematologic changes, 483
    neurological manifestations, 483
    obstetric complications, 482
    pulmonary manifestation, 484
    renal dysfunction, 484
    skin manifestations, 483
    thrombotic events, 482–483
    valve abnormalities, 483–484
  complement system in, 489
  determination of, 481
  neurological manifestations, 488–489
  "non-criteria" aPL, 485–486
    antiphosphatidylethanolamine (aPE), 486
    antiphosphatidylserine (anti-PS), 486
    antiprothrombin antibodies (anti-PT), 486
    IgA subtype, 485
    low-level aPL, 486
    phosphatidylserine/prothrombin (aPS/PT), 486
  obstetric expressions of, 488
  presence of anti-cardiolipin or anti-B2GPI, 481
  serological criterion, 481
  seronegative, 486
  treatment of, 489–490
Anti-Scl-70, 471
Aphthous ulcers, 41–42, 45
APLAID, 47
Aplastic anemia
  animal models, 687–688

associated with drugs, 686
autoimmune features, 687
clinical, pathologic, and epidemiologic features, 685–687
and clonality, 690–691
diagnosis, 686
disease severity in, 686
environmental features, 687
fluorescent in situ hybridization (FISH) analysis, 685–686
genetic abnormalities, 685
  DKC1, 685
  hTERC gene mutation, 685
historic background, 685
pathogenic mechanisms, 687
population-based case-control study of, 686
therapy for, 688–689
  alemtuzumab, 689
  bone marrow transplantation (BMT), 688–689
  cyclophosphamide, 687–688
  cyclosporine (CSA), 689
  fludarabine, 688
  hATG/CSA regimen, 689
  high-dose cyclophosphamide without BMT, 689–690
  immunosuppressive therapy, 689
  mycophenolate, 689
T lymphocytes, role of, 687
Apoptosis, 245–246, 695
  apoptotic cells
    anti-inflammatory effects of, 251
    as sources of autoantigen, 247
  autoimmune diseases, 998–999
  in autoimmunity, 246–248
  clearance of dead cells, 249–251
    "find-me" signals, 249
    phosphatidylserine, 249–250
  defective, 246
  excessive, 247
  history, 245
  in lymphocytes, 695–696
  signaling pathways to, 696f
Apoptotic cell morphology, 246
Apotopes, 247–248
AQP4 proteins, 820–821
Aquaporin-4 (AQP4) antibodies, 817–818
Aquaporins, 810
Arthralgia, 41–42
Arthritis, 41–42
Arthritis with IBD, 538
Arthritogenic peptide hypothesis, 538–539
Aryl hydrocarbon receptor (AhR), 72–73
Asthma, 110–111
Atacicept, 458
Ataxia, 45, 818
Atg5–Atg12–Atg16 complex, 257–258
Atg12–Atg5 complex associates, 257–258
Atherosclerosis, 46, 108–110
  activation sites, 1056–1057
  adaptive immunity in, 1054–1056
    B lymphocytes, 1055–1056
    CD8 T lymphocytes, 1055
    Foxp3 regulatory CD4+ T cells, 1055

innate-like B1a cells, 1056
Th1 CD4 T cells, 1054
Th2 CD4+ T cells, 1054
Th17 CD4+ T cells, 1054–1055
adhesion molecules in, 1057–1058
autoantigens, 1050–1051
  β2 glycoprotein 1 (β2-GP1), 1050–1051
  heat shock protein 60 (HSP60), 1050
  oxidized low-density lipoprotein (OxLDL), 1050
BAFF blocking reagents, 1060–1061
B7/CD28 family, role of, 1057
B cell homing in, 1059
canakinumab therapy, 1060–1061
cellular components involved in pathogenesis, 1052t
dendritic cells (DCs), role in, 1057
development of inflammatory lesions, 1049–1050
endothelial cells, role of, 1056
innate immunity in, 1051–1054
  macrophages, 1051–1053
  mast cells, 1054
  neutrophils, 1053–1054
  NK cells, 1053
  NKT cell, 1053
leukocyte recruitment, 1057–1058
methotrexate therapy, 1060–1061
monocyte homing in, 1058–1059
mouse models of, 1050
smooth muscle cells (SMC), role of, 1056
statins for, 1060–1061
T cell homing in, 1059
TLR2 expression, 1057
TNF/TNF receptor family, role of, 1057
vaccination strategies, 1059–1060
Autoantibodies against cytokines in humans, 1142–1143
  in APECED, 1151–1152
  erythropoietin, 1144
  granulocyte-macrophage colony stimulating factor (GM-CSF), 1143, 1146–1147
    B cell tolerance, 1149
    impact, 1143–1144
    pathogenic monoclonal autoantibodies, 1147
    preferred V-gene usage, 1147
    somatic mutations, 1148
  IFN-γ, 1144
  IL-1α, 1142, 1145
  IL-6, 1142–1143, 1145
  IL-8, 1145
  IL-17A, IL-17F, and IL-22, 1144
  inhibitory activity, 1147–1148
  opportunistic infections with a thymoma, 1144
  osteoprotegerin, 1144–1145
  response to a B cell epitope, 1148–1149
  T cell tolerance, 1150–1152
  therapeutic benefits, 1145
  TNF, 1142
  type 1 and type II interferon, 1142

Autoantibody, 14—15, 311, 312t
assays and technologies for testing,
1165—1166
clinical interpretation, 1166—1167
clinical practice guidelines (CPG),
1167
standardization and quality assurance,
1170
formation, 1152—1153
laboratory reports, electronic medical
records, and cost analysis, 1167—1170
spectrum of, 1163—1165
used in diagnosis of autoimmune diseases,
1164t
Autoantibody detection
addressable laser bead immunoassays
(ALBIA), 1162
contemporary and emerging technologies,
1163t
enzyme linked immunoassays (ELISA),
1162
line immunoassays (LIA), 1162
Autoantibody-mediated tissue damage, 21
Autoantigens, 5, 30
Autocytotoxins, 13
Autoimmune Addison's disease (AD),
588—589
adrenal glands, imaging of, 596
autoimmune regulator (AIRE) gene, role of,
591
clinical manifestations, 595
clinical presentations of autoimmune
adrenalitis number, 597t
clinical signs and symptoms, 596—597
computed tomography (CT) studies, 596
diagnosis, 595—596
different clinical presentations of,
596—597
general biochemical indices, 595
genetic predisposition of, 591
incidence of osteoporosis, 599
levels of ACTH and, 595—596
measurement of disease activity, 594
MHC class I chain-related A (MIC-A), role
of, 591
natural history, 594—595
prevalence of ACA, 592
rate of mortality of, 598—599
risk of, 594
adrenal crisis, 598
stages, 594, 595t
tests
hormonal tests, 595—596
24-hour urinary free-cortisol test, 597
imaging studies, 596
nuclear magnetic resonance (NMR)
studies, 596
therapy, 597—599
DEHA (dehydroepiandrosterone), 598
dual-release hydrocortisone tablet, 598
mineralocorticoid replacement, 598
steroid doses during surgery and medical
procedures, 598
subcutaneous cortisol infusion, 598

Autoimmune adrenalitis (AA)
animal models, 590—591
induced immunity, 590
spontaneous, 590—591
epidemiology of, 588—589
histopathology, 589—590
diffuse lymphocytic adrenalitis, 590
focal lymphocytic adrenalitis, 589—590
immunologic studies, 591—594
adrenal autoantigens, identification of,
592—593
adrenal cortical antibodies (ACA),
591—592
autoantibody-binding sites on 21-OH, 593
cell-mediated immunity, 591
genetic predisposition of, 591
21-OH, identification of, 592—593
21-OHAbs determinations, 593
steroidogenic autoantigens, identification
of, 593—594
steroid-producing cell antibodies (StCA),
592
Autoimmune blistering diseases, 957t
Autoimmune bullous diseases, 955
hemidesmosomal plaque, 956
hemidesmosomes, 956
lamina lucida in, 956
mortality rate, 966
pemphigus foliaceus, 960—962
pemphigus vulgaris (PV), 956—960
treatment, 965—966
azathioprine, 966
corticosteroids, 966
cyclophosphamide, 966
dapsone, 966
methotrexate, 966
mycophenolate mofetil, 966
prednisone, 966
Autoimmune diseases, 3, 5
animal models of, 20—21, 30
antigens, role of, 27—28
anti-self-reactivity of, 21
association of MHC polymorphisms with,
22—23
autoantibodies and their antigens, role of,
993—994
central tolerance and, 24—25
characteristics of, 993
defining, 21
epidemiological data, 277t
incidence data, 278t
features of
adaptive immune system, 20—21
innate immune response, 19—20
flares and remissions during, 30
genetic component
association of MHC polymorphisms, 22
epigenetic alterations association, 23—24
GWAS Studies, 22—24
multiple susceptibility loci, 22—24
single gene defects, 22
high-throughput technologies, role in
understanding of, 31
hormones and, 24

IL-1, IL-6 and IL-12 inhibition, 20
of kidney, 994—1000
ANCA epitope specificity, 996—997
anti-GBM autoantibodies, 996—997
antigenic alterations of "self" proteins,
997—999
apoptosis, 998—999
autoreactive T and B cells, role of,
994—996
environmental factors, 999
hexamer structure, 997—998
hyperactivity of Fc-FcR pathway, 997
microbial infections, 999—1000
molecular mimicry, 1000
neutrophil extracellular traps (NETs), 1000
protein tyrosine phosphatase-N22
(PTPN22), role of, 999
neutralization of high mobility group protein
B1 (HMGB1), 20
pathogenicity of, 21
peripheral tolerance and, 25
polymorphisms in autoantigens and, 27
prevalence of, 21
reductionist principle of isolating a single
variable, 8
regulatory lymphocytes, role of, 28—29
self-antigen drives of, 27
steps leading to human, 7
tissue damages, mechanisms of, 29—30
Toll-like receptor (TLR) signaling, 19—20
treatment of, 30—31
triggers of, 25—26
Autoimmune gastritis, 619. See also Pernicious
anemia
autoantibodies associated with, 622—623, 626
environmental triggers for, 626—627
mouse model of, 625f
Autoimmune hemolytic anemia (AIHA), 23,
666
animal models, 650
C3HeB/FeJ mice, 650
New Zealand Black (NZB) mouse, 650
NZB mice, 656
rat RBC immunization of mice, 656
B cells and tolerance, 655—656
cause of hemolysis in, 652
classification of, 649, 650t
clinical features, 653—654
concurrent neoplastic disease with, 655
drugs, effect of, 655
etiology of, 654—655
gender and age, 655
genetic predisposition, 654—655
historical background, 649
infectious agents, role of, 655
laboratory diagnosis of, 654
mechanisms of RBC destruction, 650—653
changes in glycosylation, 652
cold reactive anti-RBC autoantibodies,
650—651
RBC autoantigens in, 653, 653t
warm reactive antibodies, 651
warm reactive IgG anti-RBC
autoantibodies, 651—652

Rh-specific Treg cells, 656
T helper (Th) cell and tolerance, 656
    Rh autoantigen-specific effector Th cells,
        656
treatment, 654
    corticosteroids, 654
    cyclophosphamide, 654
    cytotoxic drugs, 654
    prednisolone, 654
    rituximab, 654
    splenectomy, 654
Autoimmune hemophilia A (aHA)
    clinical presentation, 717−718
    genetic factors in, 719
    T cell epitopes in, 719
    treatment, 719−720
        combination with cyclophosphamide, 719
        corticosteroids, 719
        desmopressin, 719
        immunosuppressive therapy, 719
        ivIG, 719
        modified-Bonn−Malmö protocol, 719
        rituximab, 719
Autoimmune hepatitis (AIH)
    AIH type 1, 889−890, 896
    AIH type 2, 889−890
        prevalence, 892
    animal models, 897−898
    autoantibodies, role of, 893−896
        anti-LC1, 896
        anti-LKM1, 894−896
        anti-LKM3 antibodies, 894−896
        antimitochondrial antibody (AMA), 893
        anti-SLA, 896
        SMA, 893−894
    autoimmune disorders, incidence of, 890
    autoimmune features, 892−893
    clinical features, 890−891
    criteria for diagnosis, 891t
    defined, 889
    diagnosis of, 890
    diagnostic system, 891
    epidemiologic features, 892
    epidemiology, 890−891
    genetic features, 896−897
        AIRE1 mutation, 897
        HLA association, 896
    histological feature of, 891
    International Autoimmune Hepatitis Group
        Revised Diagnostic Scoring System,
        891t
    pathological features, 891−892
    pathologic effector mechanisms, 898−900
        CD8⁺ T cells and impaired T cell
            suppressor function, 899−900
        putative mechanisms of autoimmune liver
            damage, 898
        Th17 cells, 899
    PSC-AIH, 928
    sex ratio, 890
    treatment and outcome, 900−903
        calcineurin inhibitors, 901
        combination of budesonide and
            azathioprine, 901

combination of predniso(lo)ne and
    azathioprine, 900
cyclosporin, 901
CYP2D6-specific Tregs, 902
duration, 902
infliximab, 901−902
liver transplantation, 902
long-term immunosuppressive treatment,
    901
mycophenolate mofetil, 901−902
rituximab, 901−902
tacrolimus, 901
Autoimmune hypophysitis
    animal models, 640
    anterior and posterior lobe, involvement of,
        634
    autoantigens, 639
    autoimmune features, 639
    body of literature, 634−635
        published cases of, 635t
    classification of, 633
    classification of sellar masses, 638t
    clinical presentation, 635−637
    common symptoms, 635
        cavernous sinus, 635
        defective production of anterior pituitary
            hormones, 635−636
        defects of growth hormone, 635−636
        deficit of posterior pituitary, 637
        headache, 635
        hypoadrenalism, 635−636
        prolactin deficiency, 635−636
        visual disturbances, 635
    definition, 633
    diagnosis, 641
        MRI features, 641
    epidemiology, 634−635
    genetic and environmental influences, 640
    granulomatous hypophysitis, 637−638
    historical background, 633−634
    hypophysitis secondary to CTLA-4
        blockade, 634−635, 642−644
        clinical trials, 643t
    IgG4 plasmacytic hypophysitis, 638
    lymphocytic adenohypophysitis (LAH),
        633−635
    lymphocytic hypophysitis, 637
    necrotizing hypophysitis, 639
    outcome of treatment, 642
    pathological features, 637−639
    posterior lobe and infundibulum,
        involvement of, 634
    primary and secondary hypophysitis, 633
    primary hypophysitis, 637, 642−643
    T and B lymphocytes, role of, 637
    treatment of, 641−642
        azathioprine, 641
        cyclosporine, 641
        glucocorticoids, 641
        hormone replacement, 642
        ipilimumab, 642
        methotrexate, 641
        pituitary surgery, 641−642
        prednisolone, 641

rituximab, 641
stereotactic radiotherapy, 642
surgery, 641−642
xanthomatous hypophysitis, 638
Autoimmune/inflammatory syndrome induced
    by adjuvants(ASIA), 1127−1128
Autoimmune leucopenia, 677
Autoimmune lymphoproliferative syndrome
    (ALPS), 22, 414, 667, 695−696
    autoantibodies in, 698−699
    autoimmune peripheral destruction in, 696
    biomarkers, 707
    classification and distribution of different
        categories of patients, 697t
    clinical and laboratory features of, 698
    clinical and pathological features, 696−697
        FAS pathway of apoptosis, 696−697
    clinical presentation, 697−698
    diagnostic criteria for, 697b
    differential diagnoses, 698b
    genetic features, 702
        CASP10 mutations, 703−704
        FASLG mutations, 703−704
        mutations in FAS (TNFRSF6) gene,
            702−703, 703f
        somatic mutations in FAS, 703
    hepatosplenomegaly in, 698
    imaging studies, 699
    initial presentation of, 697−698
    laboratory evaluation, 698−699
        complete blood count (CBC), 698−699
        Coombs direct antiglobulin test (DAT),
            698−699
        lymph node biopsy, 699
        molecular genetic testing of FAS
            (TNFRSF6), Fas Ligand (TNFSF6), and
            caspase-10 genes (CASP10), 699
        serum levels of vitamin B12, IL-10,
            698−699
    lymphadenopathy in, 698
    malignant transformation of lymphocytes,
        698
    mortality rate, 700
    multilineage cytopenias in, 696
    nonmalignant lymphadenopathy in, 696
    pathogenic effector mechanisms, 705
    prognosis and outcome, 700
        determinants of prognosis, 700
    related disorders
        caspase-8 deficiency state (CEDS),
            700−702
        FADD deficiency, 701−702
        RAS-associated autoimmune
            lymphoproliferative disorder (RALD),
            702
    splenomegaly in, 696
    treatment, 699−700
        algorithm, 701f
        azathioprine, 699
        corticosteroids, 699
        cyclosporine, 699
        hydroxychloroquine, 699
        methylprednisolone for AIHA and ITP,
            700

Autoimmune lymphoproliferative syndrome
(ALPS) (*Continued*)
mycophenolate mofetil, 699
penicillin V for pneumococcal sepsis, 700
sirolimus, 700
spleen guards, 699–700
vaccination, 700
in vivo and *in vitro* models of disease,
704–705
lymphoproliferation (lpr) mouse strains,
704
Autoimmune myopathies
association of malignancy with myositis, 551
association of myositis and cancer, 548–549
autoantibodies, association of, 549–551
HMG coA reductase autoantibodies,
550–551
myositis-specific, 549–550
autoantigens, expression of, 551–552
GrB-mediated cleavage, 552
MDA5 and Ro52, 552
characteristic pathology, 548
clinical and pathological descriptions,
547–548
definining, 547
dermatomyositis (DM), 547
epidemiology, 548–549
immune effector pathways, 552
immune-mediated necrotizing myopathy
(IMNM), 547–548
inclusion body myositis (IBM), 547
mechanisms of, 551–552
polymyositis (PM), 547
skin manifestations, 548
therapy of, 552–553
Autoimmune neutropenia
in acquired immune deficiency syndrome
(AIDS), 680
clinical and pathologic features, 677–678
differential diagnosis, 679–680
drug-induced, 680
genetic forms of, 680
historical background, 677
of infancy (AINI), 678
neutrophil counts, 678
laboratory diagnosis, 680–681
mechanism of cell destruction, 680
neutrophil agglutination reaction, 681
neutrophil-specific antigens, role of, 678
primary
in adolescents and adults, 678
neutrophil-specific antigens in, 678–679
secondary, 679
treatment, 681
gammaglobulin, 681
G-CSF, 681
steroids, 681
Autoimmune orchitis
associated with viral infection, 1009, 1012
in dark mink, 1008
in day 3 thymectomized (d3tx) mice, 1009
in Lewis rat with transgenic human HLA
B27/β2m, 1008
post-vasectomy, 1008

Autoimmune pancreatitis
animal models, 942
autoimmune features, 940–941
B cell-activating factor (BAFF) and, 942
clinical features, 938–939
epidemiologic features, 940
extra-pancreatic lesions in, 939
genetic and environmental factors, 941–942
Helicobactor pylori infection and, 942–943
historic background, 937–938
immunological markers, 944
laboratory tests, 938
misdiagnosis of pancreatic cancer, 938–939
pathological features, 939–940
pathological mechanisms, 942–944
serum IgG4 elevation, 941
symptoms, 938
treatment and outcome, 944
ultrasound and radioimage findings, 938
Autoimmune-polyendocrinopathy-candidiasis-
ectodermal-dystrophy (APECED), 22,
412–413, 606, 897
Autoimmune polyglandular (polyendocrine)
syndromes (APS), 596, 1012
animal models, 611–612
AIRE-deficient mice, 611
Bio-breeding (BB) rat, 611
non-obese diabetes (NOD) mouse, 611
spontaneous, 611
thymectomy, 611–612
APS-1, 605
autoimmune regulator *(AIRE)* gene,
608–610
autoimmunity in, 612
genetic features, 608–610
hypoparathyroidism, 613
type 1 IFN and Th17 cytokines in, 612
APS-2, 605
AIRE gene polymorphisms in, 610
associated HLA Alleles and non-HLA
genes, 609–610, 609*t*
autoantibodies, 608
classical definition of, 607–608
cytotoxic T lymphocyte-associated protein
4 *(CTLA-4)* gene, 610
prevalence of, 607–608
risk of autoimmune disorders, 607–608
APS-3, 608
APS-4, 608
autoimmune features, 608
adrenocortical cell antibodies (ACC-Ab),
role of, 608
NACHT leucine-rich-repeat protein 5
(NALP5), 608
organ-specific self antigens, 608
P450c21 antibodies, 608
steroid producing cells (StC-Ab), role of,
608
tryptophan hydroxylase, 608
type 1 interferon (IFN) antibodies, 608
clinical classification of, 596*b*
clinical pathologic and epidemiologic
features, 606–608
environmental factors, 610

historic background, 605
immunologic markers in diagnosis, 612–613
pathogenic mechanisms, 612
adrenalitis in, 612
autoreactive T cells in, 612
CD4$^+$ T cells, role of, 612
CD8$^+$ T cells, role of, 612
endocrine glands in, 612
T cell-mediated autoimmunity, 612
treatment and outcome, 613
amphotericin B, 613
calciferol sterols, 613
fluconazole, 613
fludrocortisone, 613
itraconazole, 613
ketoconazole, 613
Autoimmune polyglandular syndrome type 2,
639
Autoimmune regulator (AIRE) gene, 605
Autoimmune regulator (AIRE) protein, 59–60
Autoimmune response, evolution of, 3–4
Autoimmune skin diseases, 206
Autoimmune thyroid disease (ATD), 498,
855–856, 1182–1183
Autoimmune thyroiditis
atrophic thyroiditis (primary myxedema),
557
autoantibodies, 558–559, 563
autoantibodies against T4 and T3, 559
T cell responses, 559–560
thyroglobulin (TG), 558–559
thyroid peroxidase (TPO), 559
TSH-receptor (TSH-R) blocking
antibodies, 559
clinical, pathologic, and epidemiologic
features, 557–558
pathological changes in, 558
clinical features of myxedema, 557
degree of fibrosis, 558
environmental influences, 560–561
dietary iodine-induced injury, 561
pregnancy, 560–561
radioactive substances, 561
role of infection, 561
smoking, 561
genetic factors, 560
germinal center formation, 558
goitrous (Hashimoto's) thyroiditis, 557–558
historic background, 557
non-iatrogenic hypothyroidism, 557–558
pathologic effector mechanisms, 562–563
antibody-mediated injury, 562–563
T cell-mediated injury, 562–563
TSH-R blocking antibodies, function of,
562
reference ranges
serum IgG4 levels, 558
thyroid stimulating hormone (TSH) levels,
557
thyroxine (T4) levels, 557
transient neonatal hypothyroidism, 562
treatment and outcome, 563–564
types, 558*t*
in vivo models, 561–562

experimental autoimmune thyroiditis resulting from immune modulation, 561—562
immunization-induced thyroiditis, 561
spontaneous thyroiditis, 562
Autoimmune-triggered tissue injury, 19—20
Autoimmune (type 1) diabetes/autoimmune diabetes mellitus (AI-DM)
autoantibodies, 582
autoimmune features, 580
basis of diagnosis and classification of, 577t
clinical pathological features, 575—577
definition, 575
Diabetes Autoantibody (DASP) and Islet Autoantibody (IASP) Standardization Programs, 582
epidemiologic features, 577—578
genetic factors, 578—579, 579t
IILA-DR-DQ alleles, 578
non-HLA factors, 578—579
involvement of immune cells in, 576—577
nomenclature used to describe, 576t
pathological feature of, 576—577
pathologic effector mechanisms, 580—581
antigen-presenting cells (APCs), 581
triggering autoimmunity, 580—581
in vivo and in vitro models, 581—582
LEW.1AR1-iddm rat, 581—582
non-obese diabetes (NOD) mouse, 581—582
wild bank voles (Myodes glareolus), 581—582
Autoimmunity, 8—9
B lymphocyte activating factor (BAFF), 154—155
contemporary view of, 14—15
"Dark Ages" of, 15t
gut microbiota and, 29
tonic signaling and, 154
Autoinflammation
definition, 40
historical perspective, 39—40
IL-1-related disease with, 41
mechanisms in, 40—41, 42f
molecular pathology and features, 43t
spectrum of, 40, 41f
Autoinflammatory component in common diseases, 46
Autoinflammatory diseases, 4, 208
Autoinflammatory syndrome, 39
Autonomic neuropathy, 846, 1128—1129
Autophagy, 167
chaperone-mediated (CMA), 257
defined, 257
in innate immunity, 258
in lymphocyte development and activation, 258—259
pathways, 257—258
in regulating T cell development and activation, 259
in tolerance and autoimmunity, 260
Autophagy-related (Atg) proteins, 257—258
Autoreactive T cells, 269
Azathioprine (AZA), 641, 699, 770, 900—901, 966, 1215

B

BAFF receptor (BAFF-R), 154, 500
Basophils, 53
basic biology, 206—207
in immune diseases, 207—208
in autoinflammatory diseases, 208
IgE in systemic autoimmune diseases, 207
in lupus nephritis, 207—208
in rheumatoid arthritis, 208
role in immunity, 206—207
Batten disease, 1133
B-cell activating factor (BAFF), 425, 500, 669
in autoimmune pancreatitis, 942
autoimmunity, 154—155
in SjS and SLE, 500
B cell antigens (CD20), 1228—1229
B cell lymphomas, 498
B cell receptors (BCR)
basic understanding, 148b
pre-B cell receptor (pre-BCR), 137—138
B cells, 4, 57
activation of, 147—148
antigen-triggered, 147, 149
high affinity class-switched antibody and, 150
immediate consequences of, 148
interaction with helper T cells, 148—149
secondary signals for, 148
activation of immune system, 20
anergic, 153—154
autoantigen-mediated selection of immature, 141f
autoantigen-sensitive, 136—137
in autoimmune hemolytic anemia (AIHA), 655—656
autoreactive, 24—25, 151—154
BAFF interaction and, 24—25
clonal deletion, 151—153
cytokine production, 155
development and functions, 62—63
development of, 131—132
tonic signaling in, 154
follicular, 132
"ignorant" autoreactive, 151
immunocompetence, 24—25
intraepithelial, 132—133
in juvenile idiopathic arthritis (JIA), 532
in lymphoid organs, 149—150
memory, 133—134
receptor editing, 151—153
regulatory, 155—156
response to antigenic stimulation, 21
in sexual dimorphism, 320
sIgM⁺, 139—140
systemic lupus erythematosus (SLE), role in, 451
T cell interactions, 148—149
cell surface molecules involved in, 148—149
cytokines involved in, 149
tolerance, 140—142, 151—154
anergy, 153
antibody-independent activity, 155—156
autoreactive BCR and, 151

clonal deletion, 151—153
defective receptor editing, 153
receptor editing, 151—153
B cell suppressive therapies, 1216
Behçet's disease, 794—795, 820
Belimumab, 458
BENTA disease, 706—707
Bilateral immune-mediated Ménière's disease, 805
clinical features, 806
expression of cochlin, 808—809
genetic susceptibility, 810
Birdshot retinopathy, 1129
Bleomycin-induced fibrosis, 466
B lineage cells, 134
B lymphocytes, 131
development of, 134
antigen-independent, 134—136
in fetal liver, omentum, and bone marrow, 134
B lymphocyte survival factor (BLyS), 154—155
B lymphoid chronic lymphocytic leukemia (B-CLL), 706—707
B lymphopoiesis, 134
Bone marrow (BM) disorder, 664
Bone marrow transplantation (BMT), 685, 688—689, 1232—1234
related complications, 688
from unrelated donors, 688—689
Borrelia burgdorferi, 105
Bovine collagen implants, 290—291
Brainstem encephalitis, 846
Bullous pemphigoid (BP)
anti-BP180 autoantibodies, 964
autoantibodies in, 963
BP230 antigen, 963
BP180 (BPAG2) antigen, 963
clinical, pathologic, and epidemiologic features, 963
genetics, 963
HLA association, 963
pathologic effector mechanisms, 964
T cell activation, 963
in vivo and in vitro models, 963—964
Burnet, Macfarlane, 15
Burnet's Clonal Selection Theory, 16
Bystander activation, 268

C

Caenorhabditis elegans, 245
Candida albicans, 72—74
Candidal esophagitis, 606
Candidiasis, 605—606
CANDLE, 47
Carboxy-terminal leucine-rich repeats, 166
Cardiac APS, 483—484
CARD15 (NOD-2) gene, 23
Caspase-8 deficiency state (CEDS), 700—702
pathogenic effector mechanisms, 706
Caspase recruitment (CARD), 166
Caspases, 695
Caspr2, 824

Catastrophic antiphospholipid syndrome (CAPS), 484
C3bBb, 57–58
C5 convertase (C3bBb3b), 220
CD3 antibodies, 1223–1225
CD4 antibodies, 1225
CD4 cells, 59–60
CD4 lymphocytes, 61
CD8 cells, 59–60
CD25 antibodies, 1225–1226
CD28/CD80 antibodies, 1226–1227
CD40/CD40 ligand (CD40L) pathway, 1227
CD45 phosphatase, 60
CD80, 26
CD80/CD86 costimulatory molecules, 57
CD86, 26
Celiac disease, 855, 1183–1184
  animal models, 861
  autoantibodies, role of, 857–859
    anti-TG2 antibodies, 858
    IgA antiendomysium antibodies (EMA), 857
  autoreactive intraepithelial lymphocytes (IELs), role of, 859
  clinical features and associated disorders, 855–856
  effector mechanisms, 864
  environmental influences, 860
    climate, 860
    gliadin proteins, 860
    gluten protein, 860
  epidemiology, 856–857
  genetic predisposition, 859–860
  historical achievements in study of, 856b
  HLA association, 859
  intestinal lesion in, 856, 858f
    stages, 857f
  non-celiac gluten sensitivity, 856
  non-HLA genes in, 859–860
  pathogenic mechanisms, 861–864
    disease-associated HLA-DQ molecules, 862–864
    gluten-reactive CD4+ T Cells, 861
    mucosal antigen-presenting cells, 864
    role of the TG2 enzyme, 861–862
  serology, 864–865
  staining of immune complexes, 865
  treatment and outcome, 865
    challenges, 865–866
    enzyme supplementation, 865–866
    gluten-free diet, 865–866
    prolyl endopeptidases, 865–866
    TG2 inhibitors, 865–866
Cell therapy, 1234–1235
Chediak–Higashi syndrome, 680
Chemoattractant cytokines, 239
Chemoattractant receptors, 299–302, 301t
  clinical applications, 304–306
  as targets for treatment of inflammatory, 305t
Chemokines, 239
Chemotactic cytokines (chemokines), 54–56
Cholinergic anti-inflammatory pathway, 20

Chronic ataxic neuropathy with ophthalmoplegia, M-protein, and anti-disialosyl antibodies (CANOMAD), 767
Chronic enterocolitis. See Inflammatory bowel disease (IBD)
Chronic granulomatous disease (CGD), 411
Chronic inflammatory demyelinating polyradiculoneuropathy (CIDP), 766–770
  animal models, 768–769
  environmental influences, 768
  epidemiology and clinical features, 766–767
    multifocal-acquired demyelinating sensory and motor neuropathy (MADSAM), 767
    multifocal-acquired sensory and motor neuropathy (MASAM), 767
    multifocal motor neuropathy with conduction block (MMNCB), 766–767
    paraproteinemic demyelinating peripheral neuropathy, 767
  features of autoimmunity, 768
  history, 766
  immunogenetic features, 768
  pathogenic mechanisms, 769
  treatment and outcome, 769–770
    azathioprine, 770
    Campath-1H (alemtuzemab), 769–770
    ciclosporin, 770
    fingolimod, 769–770
    immunosuppressive drugs, 769–770
    interferon-β1a, 769–770
    IVIG, 769–770
    mycophenolate, 770
    plasma exchange, 769–770
    rituximab, 770
    steroids, 769–770
Chronic mucocutaneous candidiasis, 606
  Th17 cells, role of, 606
Chronic urticaria (CU)
  autoantibody markers, 984
    histamine-releasing IgG autoantibodies, 983–984
    mast cells, 983–984
  autoimmune features, 982–983
  clinical, pathologic, and epidemiologic features, 982
  genetic features, 983
  pathologic effector mechanisms, 983–984
  in vivo and in vitro models, 983
Churg–Strauss syndrome (CSS), 204, 1069
  eosinophils in, 209–210
Chymase (MCT), 56
Cicatricial pemphigoid (CP), 964–965
CINCA, 43–44
C1 inhibitor (C1 inh), 220
Citrobacter, 72
C-Jun/activator protein 1 (AP-1), 44
Classic hereditary autoinflammatory syndrome, 41–45
Class switching, 150
CMaf gene, 73

CNS diseases with autoantibodies to intracellular antigens, 824–826
Coagulation cascade, 711
Cogan's syndrome, 807–808
  DEP1/CD148, role of, 807
  inner ear pathology, 807
  morbidity in, 807
  putative autoantigen targets in, 809t
Cogan syndrome, 793–794
Colchicine, 44
Collagen-induced arthritis (CIA), 71
Combined immune deficiencies (CID), 404–405
Common variable immunodeficiency (CVID), 406–408, 666–667, 679
Complementarity determining regions (CDRs), 63
Complement cascades, 313
Complement system, 57–58, 58f, 217–219
  anaphylatoxins triggering by, 58
  in antiphospholipid syndrome (APS), 489
  biological effects of activation, 220–221
  complement activation pathways, 217–219
    alternative pathway, 219
    classical, 218
    lectin pathway (LP), 218–219
    membrane attack complex (MAC), 219
  complement regulatory proteins, 58
  components of, 57–58
  control of activation, 219–220
    fluid phase regulator, 220
    membrane-bound regulators, 220
  involvement in autoimmune diseases, 221–224
    autoimmune hemolytic anemia (AIHA), 221–222
    complement-mediated cytotoxicity, 223
    experimental autoimmune myasthenia gravis (EAMG), 223
    Graves' disease (GD), 224
    Guillain–Barré syndrome (GBS), 223
    Hashimoto's thyroiditis (HT), 224
    hemolytic uremic syndrome (HUS), 222–223
    ischemia/reperfusion injury (IRI), 224
    myasthenia gravis (MG), 223
    paroxysmal noctural hemoglobinuria (PNH), 221–222
    partial lipodystrophy (PLD), 222
    pernicious anemia (PA), 224
    retinal pigment epithelium (RPE), 223
    rheumatoid arthritis (RA), 223
    Sjögren's syndrome, 224
    systemic lupus erythematosus (SLE), 222
    thrombotic thrombocytopenic purpura (TTP), 222–223
  potent immunologic activities of, 57–58
  sequential enzyme reactions of, 57–58
Complete Freund's adjuvant (CFA), 269–270, 277
Contact hypersensitivity (CHS), 113
Convertase (C3bBb), 220
Craniopharyngioma, 633
C-reactive protein (CRP), 58, 251

CREST syndrome, 453, 463–464
Crohn's disease, 23, 72–73, 115, 163, 167,
    793–794, 874–875, 1231–1232
Cryoglobulinemic vasculitis
    animal models, 1080
    autoantibodies, 1080
    autoimmune pathogenesis, 1079
    clinical, epidemiologic, and pathologic
        features, 1079
    genetic features and environmental
        influences, 1079–1080
    pathologic effector mechanisms, 1080
Cryopyrin-associated periodic syndrome
    (CAPS), 40, 43–44
Cryptogenic organizing pneumonia (COP),
    1105
    animal model, 1113
    autoimmune features, 1109–1110
    clinical, epidemiologic, and pathologic
        features, 1106–1107
    genetic features, 1112
    history, 1105–1106
    pathologic effector mechanisms, 1113–1116
    treatment and outcome, 1116
Csf2 gene, 73
C-terminal leucine-rich repeats (LRRs), 166
CTLA-4, 23
CTLA4-Ig fusion protein, 149
CTLA-4Ig therapy, 436
C-type lectin receptors (CLR), 263–264
Currie, Alastair, 245
Curzio, Carlo, 463
Cyclophosphamide (CYC), 654, 687,
    689–690, 719, 800, 844, 966,
    1116–1117, 1214
Cyclosporine A (CSA), 1215–1216
Cystic fibrosis, 1012
Cystitis, interstitial, 1129–1130
Cytokines
    chemoattractant, 239
    class II receptors, 235–236
        type III interferons λ, 236
        type II interferons γ, 235–236
        type I interferons α and β, 235
    effector, 315–316, 316t
    history of, 229
    immunity and, 230–232
    immunosuppressive, 239
    non-interferon members, 236
    receptor subsets, 232–235
        βc chain subset, 233
        common γc chain subset, 232–233
        gp130 receptor chain, 233–234
        p35 or p40 ligand chain, 234–235
        Th17, 235
Cytotoxic T cells, 314
Cytotoxic T lymphocytes, 61f

D

Damage-associated molecular patterns
    (DAMPs), 56–57
Darwin, Charles, 3
Deamidation, 372
Defensins, 54–56

Deimination, 371–372
Dendritic cells (DCs), 53–57, 59–61, 161
    activation of, 176
    activation of immune system, 20
    antigen processing by, 175–176
    in Crohn's disease (CrD), 182
    and cytokine production, 70
    ex vivo manipulation of, 182–183
    immunosuppression by, 57
    immunotherapy, 182
    in inflammatory bowel diseases (IBD), 182
    mouse, 176–178
        PPRs of, 177t
        thymus, 179
    pattern recognition receptors (PRRs), 176
        in mouse, 177t
    role in limiting immune responses, 57
    subsets, 176
        human, 180
        in human skin, 180–181
        tolerance and, 179–180
    in systemic lupus erythematosus (SLE), 181
    targeting in autoimmune disease, 182–183
    in ulcerative colitis (UC), 182
Denkkollektiv, 11
Dermatitis herpetiformis (DH), 965
Dermatologic APS, 483
Dermopathy, 568
Diabetes, 20. See also Type 1 diabetes (T1D)
Diffuse lymphocytic adrenalitis, 590
DiGeorge syndrome (DGS), 405
Dilated cardiomyopathy (DCM), 1035–1037
    animal models, 1040–1042
    genetic features, 1039
    pathogenic mechanisms, 1040–1042
    tests for
        immunoassay of antibodies, 1038
        immunofluorescence tests, 1037–1038
        immunologic assessment of biopsies,
            1038–1039
        Western immunoblot analysis, 1037–1038
    treatment for, 1043–1044
Direct antibody-mediated disease, 311–312
Disease-modifying antirheumatic drugs
    (DMARDs), 281
Docking protein 7 (Dok-7), 777
DQA1*0501, 22
DQ allele, 22
DQB1*0302, 22
Drug-induced pemphigus, 962
Dyserythropoiesis, 686
Dyskeratosis congenita (DKC), 685

E

Early complement component deficiency,
    411–412
Effector mechanisms, 311
Efferocytosis, 249
Ehrlich, Paul, 12–13, 685
Encephalitis with antibodies to N-methyl-d-
    aspartate receptor (NMDAR), 821
Endocrinopathies, 606–607
Endometriosis, 1130–1131
Enthesitis-related arthritis, 526–527

Environmental agents, role in autoimmunity,
    283
    evidence for, 284–285, 284b
    identification of risk factors, 292b
    identifying and defining, 285–286, 286t
    infectious agents, 369–370
    mechanisms for developing autoimmune
        diseases, 291
    non-infectious environmental exposures,
        286–291
        drugs, 286–288, 287t
        foods, 289–290
        heavy metals, 290
        implants, 290–291
        microchimerism, 290
        occupational exposures, 288, 288t
        stressful life events, 291
        tobacco smoke, 290
Eosinophilia–myalgia syndrome, 466
Eosinophilic granulomatosis with polyangiitis
    (EGPA), 1069
Eosinophils, 53–56, 637
    basic biology, 208
    in Churg–Strauss syndrome (CSS),
        209–210
    immunity, role in, 208
Epidermolysis bullosa acquisita (EBA),
    965
Epigenetic alterations, 23–24
Epigenetics
    acetylation, 383
    ANCA-associated vasculitis, 391
    arginine methylation, 383–384
    deacetylation, 383
    DNA methylation, 382
    epigenetic code, 382
    epigenetic therapy, 394–396
        generation of regulatory T cells, 396
        histone deacetylase inhibitors, 395
        targeting DNA methylation, 395
    histone acetyltransferases (HATs), 383
    histone methylation, 383
    histone post-translational modifications
        (PTMs), 382–383
    of immune tolerance, 384–386
        regulators of tolerant T cells, 384–385
    microRNA (miRNA), 384
    modifications, 382–384
    multiple sclerosis (MS), 393–394
        acetylation homeostasis, deregulation of,
            394
        DNA hypomethylation, 393–394
        neo-epitopes, generation of, 393
    regulatory T cells (Tregs)
        CpG DNA methylation and, 385
        epigenetic modulation of, 386
        histone acetylation on development and
            function of, 385–386
    rheumatoid arthritis (RA), 389–390
    Sjögren's syndrome (SS), 390–391
    stability, 384
    systemic lupus erythematosus (SLE),
        386–389
        DNA methylation and, 386–387

Epigenetics (*Continued*)
 epigenetic disruption of B Cell tolerance,
   388–389
 histone acetylation in, 388
 systemic sclerosis (SSc), 390
 type 1 diabetes (T1D), 391–393
   chromatin remodeling and histone
     acetylation, 392
   genome-wide DNA methylation profiling,
     392
   histone deacetylase inhibitors, 392–393
 ubiquitination, 384
Epilepsy, 1131
Episcleritis, 793–794
Epratuzumab, 458
Epstein–Barr virus (EBV) infection, 259, 344,
   466, 512–513, 531, 742
Erythrocytes, 53, 57
Estrogen receptor, 24
Etanercept, 45, 800, 1117
Eustachius, Bartolomeo, 587
Evans syndrome (ES), 666
Exotoxins, 14
Experimental autoimmune adrenalitis (EAA),
   590
Experimental autoimmune disease of the testis,
   1008–1011
Experimental autoimmune encephalitis (EAE),
   166
Experimental autoimmune encephalomyelitis
   (EAE), 71–74
Experimental autoimmune orchitis (EAO),
   1008
 induced by immunization with testis antigen
   in adjuvant, 1009–1011
 of ovary, 1013–1015
Experimental autoimmune uveitis (EAU), 71,
   793, 798
Ex-Tregs, 74–75

F

FADD deficiency, 701–702
Familial Cold Autoinflammatory Syndrome
   (FCAS), 43–44
Familial Mediterranean fever (FMF), 44
FAS-dependent extrinsic apoptotic pathway,
   414
Fas-expressing cell, 22
Fas/fas ligand interactions, 163
FAS ligand (FASL), 414
Fas protein, 22
Fatigue syndrome, 1131–1132
Fcε receptors (FcεRI), 56
FcRIIB, 28
Felty's syndrome, 679
Fingolimod, 304
Fleck, Ludwik, 11
Focal lymphocytic adrenalitis, 589–590
Folate deficiency, 1132
Follicular B cells, 132
Follicular dendritic cells (FDC), 57, 149
Follicular T helper cells (TFH), 77–78
 activation of Bcl6 and, 77
 differentiation, 77

 expression of SAP and SLAM, 77
 subtypes of, 77
 upregulation of CXCR5, 77
Foods, 289–290
FoxP3 deficiency, 22
Freund's adjuvant, 15–16
Freund's complete adjuvant (FCA), 440

G

Gene therapy, 1235
Genetic studies of autoimmunity
 gene linkage studies, 347–351
   CD25, 348
   of combined datasets and limits of linkage
     analyses, 348–349
   CTLA4, 347–348
   diabetes susceptibility loci, 348
   in lupus, 349–351
   in multiple sclerosis, 349
   racial heterogeneity in lupus inheritance,
     350–351
   STAT4, 350
   TNFR1, TNFR2, LTBR, 350
   type 1 diabetes, 347–349
 genome wide association studies, 351–355
   BLK gene, 355
   CD6 gene, 354
   CD25 gene, 352
   CD40 gene, 353
   CD58 gene, 353
   CD69 gene, 352
   CYP27B1 gene, 353
   IFIH1, 351–352
   IL2 and IL21 cytokine genes, 352
   IL12B gene, 354
   IL10 gene, 352
   IL7R gene, 352–353
   IRF8 gene, 353
   ITGAM gene, 354
   in lupus, 354–355
   of multiple sclerosis, 352–354
   PHRF1 gene, 355
   TNFRSF1A gene, 353
   of type 1 diabetes, 351–352
 HLA association with autoimmunity,
   347
 human leukocyte antigen (HLA) complex,
   343–347
   C4A and C4B genes, 345
   C2 complement component, 345–346
   C1q deficiency, 346
   FCGR2A, FCGR3A, FCGR3B, 346
   INS gene, 343–344
   IRF5, 346
   lupus, 345–346
   multiple sclerosis (MS), 344–345
   PTPN22 gene, 344
   TNF genes, 345
   type 1 diabetes, 343–344
 mechanisms of complement and Fc
   associations with autoimmunity,
   346–347
 molecular mechanisms, 355–356
 multiple sclerosis (MS), 342

 systemic lupus erythematosus (SLE, lupus),
   342–343
 type 1 (autoimmune) diabetes (T1D), 342
Genome-wide association scans (GWAS), 22
Germ-free (GF) environment
 effect on experimental diseases, 331–333
   experimental allergic encephalomyelitis
     (EAE), 332
   experimental arthritis, 332
   germ-free NOD mice, 331–332
   lupus disease in NZB mice, 332–333
 raising animals in, 331, 337
Germinal centers (GC), 64–66, 65f, 150
Germinoma, 633
Giant cell arteritis (GCA), 1087–1096
 CD4$^+$ T cells, role of, 1093
 clinical manifestations of, 1089–1090
 clinical profile in, 1089t
 cranial, 1089–1090
 epidemiology, 1089–1090
 genetic features, 1091
 historic background, 1088
 HLA class II-associated with, 1091
 hyperplastic intima, 1094
 inflammation of medium-sized arteries in,
   1090
 macrophages in, 1093–1094
 pathogenic mechanisms, 1091–1092
 physiological role of adventitial DCs, 1093
 principal features of, 1088t
 systemic inflammatory component of,
   1094–1095
 T cells and antigen-presenting cells in,
   1092–1093
 Toll-like receptors, 1092–1093
 treatment, monitoring, and outcome,
   1095–1096
   corticosteroids, 1095
   prednisolone, 1095
 vascular lesion in, 1091
 vasculitic component of, 1090, 1094
Glucksmann, Alfred, 245
Glucocorticoids (GC), 641, 1212
Glucose-6-phosphoisomerase (G6PI), 515–516
Glutamic acid decarboxylase, 5
Glycine receptor (GlyR), 822–823
Glycosyl-phosphatidylinositol (GPI), 221–222
Gottron's papules, 548
G protein-coupled receptor (GPR), 8
Granulocyte-macrophage colony-stimulating
   factor (GMCSF), 62–63
Granulomatosis with polyangiitis (GPA),
   1069
Granulomatous hypophysitis, 637–638
Graves' disease, 23, 558, 609–610, 679
 autoantibodies, 568
   TG and TPO antibodies, 568
   TSAb or TBII levels, 568
 autoimmune features, 565
   T cell responses, 565
   thyroglobulin, 565
   TPO autoantibodies, 565
   TSH-R stimulating antibodies (TSAb),
     565

clinical, pathologic and epidemiologic
  features, 564—565
environmental factors, 566
  cytokine treatment, 566
  infections, role of, 566
  major life events, impact of, 566
  smoking impact, 566
genetic features, 565—566
  HLA genes, role of, 565—566
  polymorphisms in the *TSH-R* gene, 566
historic background, 564
in vivo models, 566—567
  AKR/N mice, 566
  BALB/c mice, 566
  transgenic mice expressing human TSH-R
    A subunit, 566
pathologic effector mechanisms, 567—568,
  567f
treatment and outcome, 568
  carbimazole, 568
  methimazole, 568
  propylthiouracil, 568
  radioiodine, 568
  radioiodine treatment, 568
  thyroidectomy, 568
Group 1 metabotropic glutamate receptors, 822
Guanylate-binding protein 5 (GBP5), 166
Guillain—Barré syndrome, 329, 757
  activated T cells, 764—765
  animal models, 763
  autoimmune features, 759—762
    anti-ganglioside antibodies in, 759—761
    functional effects of antibodies, 761—762
    gangliosides in peripheral nerve, 761
    molecular mimicry, 759
  cellular and humoral immune elements, 765
  cellular mechanisms, 763—765
  clinical features and subtypes of, 758—759
    acute inflammatory demyelinating
      polyradiculoneuropathy, 758
    acute motor and sensory neuropathy
      (AMSAN), 759
    acute motor axonal neuropathy (AMAN),
      758—759
    Miller Fisher or Fisher Syndrome (FS),
      759
  environmental effects, 762
    Campylobacter jejuni, 762
    respiratory tract infection, 762
  epidemiology, 758
  genetic aspects, 765—766
  historical background, 757—758
  macrophages, role of, 765
  treatment and outcomes, 766
Gynecological tumors, 847

H

Hashimoto's disease, 15—16
Hashimoto's thyroiditis, 633—634, 639
Heat shock proteins, 56—57
Heavy metals, 290
Helminths, 56
Helper T cells, 61
Hematologic APS, 483

Hematopoietic cell developments, 134
Hematopoietic stem cells (HSCs), 53
Hemophagocytic lymphohistiocytosis (HLH),
  531
  familial FHLH, 531
  reactive (ReHLH), 531
Hepatitis/aplastic anemia syndrome, 686—687
Hepatosplenomegaly, 45
Hereditary autoinflammatory disorders, 41—45
  CAPS, 43—44
  common phenotype, 41—42
  familial Mediterranean fever (FMF), 44
  HOIL mutations, disease due to, 47—48
  hyperimmunoglobulinemia D and periodic
    fever (HIDS), 45
  inflammasome activation of IL-1β, 43—44
  PLCg2 deficiency, 47
  proteasome defects, 47
  rare, 46—48
  TRAPS, 44—45
Hereditary periodic fever syndromes, 39,
  41—42
Herpes gestationis (HG), 964
High-affinity IgG antibodies, 21
High endothelial venules (HEV), 64
High-titer autoantibodies, 40
Histamine, 56
Histone code, 382
Histone deacetylases (HDACs), 382
Histone post-translational modifications
  (PTMs), 382—383
Homeostasis, 3—4
  restoring of, 7—8
Horror autotoxicus, 12—13
Horvitz, Robert, 245
Human autoimmune ovarian disease, 1015
Human leukocyte antigens (HLA), 23,
  365—366
  Addison's disease (AD), 609
  autoimmune hepatitis (AIH), 896
  autoimmune polyglandular (polyendocrine)
    syndromes (APS), 609—610
  bullous pemphigoid (BP), 963
  celiac disease, 859
  class II molecules, 366, 369
    association with autoimmune diseases,
      368—369
    modulation of cytokine networks, 376
  class I molecules, 365—366
  giant cell arteritis (GCA), 1091
  HLA-B27, 366—368
    AIDS and, 367
    associated diseases, 794—795
    evolution and, 368
    NK cells and, 367—368
    peptide binding and, 367
    transgenic mice, 366—367
  HLA-DR transgenic mice, 374—375
  myasthenia gravis, 780t
  non-susceptible HLA alleles, 374
  pemphigus foliaceus, 961
  pemphigus vulgaris (PV), 959
  primary biliary cirrhosis, 915
  rheumathic heart disease (RHD), 1025

rheumatic fever (RF), 1025
  spondyloarthritis (SpA), 538—540
3-hydroxyl-3-methylglutaryl-coenzyme A
  (HMG-CoA) reductase, 45
Hydroxyl radicals, 54—56
Hyper-IgD syndrome (HIDS), 40, 208
Hyperimmunoglobulinemia D and periodic
  fever (HIDS), 45
Hyperprolactinemia, 637
Hypertrophic pachymeningitis, 946
Hypochlorous acid, 54—56
Hypoparathyroidism, 605—607
Hypopyon, 794—795

I

Idiopathic male infertility, 1011—1012
Idiopathic pulmonary alveolar proteinosis
  (IPAP), 1143—1144
Idiopathic pulmonary fibrosis (IPF), 1105
  animal models, 1113
  autoantibodies associated with, 1111t
  autoimmune features, 1110—1112
  clinical, epidemiologic, and pathologic
    features, 1107—1109
  genetic features, 1111t
  history, 1105—1106
  pathologic effector mechanisms, 1114—1116
  treatment and outcome, 1116—1117
    anti-fibrotic agents, 1117
    azathioprine, 1117
    colchicine, 1117
    corticosteroids, 1116
    cyclophosphamide, 1116—1117
    cyclosporine A, 1117
    cytotoxic agents, 1116—1117
    etanercept, 1117
    interferon γ-1b, 1117
    lung transplantation, 1117
    pirfenidone, 1117
IFN-γ, 71, 1231
IFN-beta therapy, 444
IgA pemphigus, 962—963
IgA vasculitis
  animal models, 1081
  autoantibodies, 1081—1082
  autoimmune pathogenesis, 1081
  clinical, epidemiologic, and pathologic
    features, 1080—1081
  genetic features and environmental
    influences, 1081
  pathologic effector mechanisms, 1081
IgE antibodies, 63
IgG4 plasmacytic hypophysitis, 638
IgG4-related disease
  clinical features, 945
  comprehensive clinical diagnostic criteria,
    947t
  definition, 944—945
  diagnostic criteria, 947
  epidemiology, 945
  gastrointestinal disease, 947
  historical background, 945
  hypertrophic pachymeningitis, 946
  hypophysitis, 946

IgG4-related disease (*Continued*)
  kidney disease, 946
  lacrimal and salivary gland lesions, 945
  liver disease, 946
  lung disease, 945–946
  pathological findings, 947
  prostate disease, 947
  retroperitoneal fibrosis, 946
  sclerosing cholangitis, 946
  thyroid disease, 946–947
  treatment, 947–948
IgL chains, 138–139
IgM B cell receptor (BCR), 62
IL-1 receptor antagonist (IL-1Ra), 40–41, 161
Il10 gene, 73
IL17F gene, 72
IL17RA gene, 72
IL23R, 73
IL-36 receptor antagonist, 46
Immune complex disease, 11, 312
Immune-mediated inner ear disease (IMIED),
      805
  animal models, 810–811
  associated with primary vasculitides,
      807–808
  associated with systemic autoimmune
      diseases, 806–807
  clinical features, 805–806
  criteria to assess, 806
  evidence of autoimmunity, 808–809
  putative autoantigen targets in, 809*t*
  treatment, 811
Immune response, 3
  defective downregulation of, 28
  gut microbiota and, 29
  IL-1, IL-6 and IL-12 inhibition, 20
  pathogenic autoreactivity associated with
      tissue damage, 21
  regulatory lymphocytes, role of, 28–29
Immune system, 3–4
  activation of, 26–27
  adaptive, 4–5
  innate, 4
Immune thrombocytopenia (ITP)
  acute, 663
  adults, epidemiology and clinical
      presentation in, 665
    bleeding risk, 665
    fatal hemorrhage risk, 665
    incidence of, 665
    initial manifestation, 665
    rate of comorbidities, 45
    in women, 665
  anomalies of megakaryopoiesis, 669
  anti-GP IIb/IIIa and/or anti-GP Ib/IX
      specificity, 670–671
  antiplatelet antibodies on
      megakaryocytopoiesis, effect of, 670
  autoantibodies, 670–671
  autoimmune markers in primary,
      665–666
    antinuclear antibodies, 665–666
    antiphospholipid antibodies (aPLs), 665
    antithyroid antibodies, 666

  autoimmune lymphoproliferative
      syndrome, 667
  common variable immunodeficiency
      (CVID), 666–667
  primary immunodeficiencies, 666–667
  Velocardiofacial/DiGeorge syndrome, 667
  Wiskott–Aldrich syndrome (WAS), 667
central and peripheral pathogenesis of, 671*f*
children, epidemiology and clinical
      presentation in, 664–665
  cause of death, 664–665
  due to viral infections, 664
  peak age of presentation, 664
  prognosis, 664–665
chronic, 663, 665
common in SLE, 666
diagnosis, 664
  blood group Rh(D) typing, 664
  detection of *Helicobacter pylori* (HP)
      infection, 664
  differential diagnosis, 664*t*
  direct antiglobulin test (DAT), 664
  serologic evaluation for HIV and HCV
      infection, 664
family-based, 667
general features and definitions, 663
genetic markers of, 667–668
infection-associated, 670
  molecular mimicry, 670
pathogenesis of, 663
pathologic effector mechanisms,
      668–670
  antibody-mediated platelet destruction,
      668–669
  antigen-presenting cells (APCs), role of,
      668
  B cell activating factor (BAFF), role of,
      669
  CD4$^+$ Th cells, role of, 668–669
  T cell-mediated cytotoxicity and NK cell
      activity, 669
persistent, 663
platelet production in chronic, 669–670
serum levels of thrombopoietin (TPO),
      669–670
severe, 663
in vivo models, 668
Immune tolerance, 87
Immunobiology, 15–16
Immunochemistry, 14–15
Immunocompetent lymphocytes, 21
Immunodeficiency with hyper-IgM (HIGM)
      syndrome, 409–411
Immunodysregulation, polyendocrinopathy,
      enteropathy, X-linked (IPEX)
      syndrome, 413–414
Immunologic homeostasis, 5
Immunologic self, 5
Immunology
  earliest discoveries in, 11
  shift to immunochemistry, 14–15
Immunoproteasomes, 47
Immunoreceptor tyrosine-based activation
      motifs (ITAMs), 60

Immunoreceptor tyrosine-based inhibitory
      motifs (ITIMs), 154
Immunosuppression, 29
  dendritic cells (DCs), 57
Immunosuppressive cytokines, 239
Immunosuppressive therapy, 689, 719,
      769–770, 901, 976, 1043, 1098–1099,
      1210*t*
  principles, 1209–1211
Implants, 290–291
Indirect immunofluorescence (IIF), 1161–1162
Induced Tregs (iTregs), 94–96
Infectious triggers of autoimmunity
  autoimmune CNS demyelinating disease,
      270
  bystander activation, 268
  emerging mechanism of, 268–269
  pathogen-induced murine models, 266*t*
  potential mechanisms of, 264–269, 265*f*
    molecular mimicry, 264–268
  in priming of autoreactive immune
      responses, 263–264
  reciprocal relationships of pathogen-derived
      mechanisms, 269
  virus pathogens, 267*t*
Inflammasomes, 40–41, 54–56, 55*f*
Inflammatory bowel disease (IBD), 19–20,
      111, 236, 248, 925
  adaptive immunity, 877–878
  age of onset, 874
  antigen-presenting cells (APCs), 877
  biomarkers, 878–879
    C-reactive protein (CRP), 879
    fecal, 878–879
    lactoferrin, 878–879
    serologic, 879
  CARD15 (NOD-2) gene and, 23
  differential diagnosis, 874*t*
  disease presentation, 874–875
  environmental factors, 874
  epidemiology, 874
  epithelial barrier and innate immunity, 877
  genetics, 875–876, 876*t*
    ATG16L1, 876
    CARD9, 876
    IL-23/IL-12 pathway, 876
    NOD2 (CARD15), 875–876
    non-overlapping susceptibility loci, 875
    role for autophagy, 876
  history, 873–874
  host–microbial interactions, 878
  immunopathogenesis, 876–878
  luminal bacterial composition, 878
  MALT in, 876–877
  pathology, 875
  prevalence of pANCA and ASCA positivity,
      878*t*
  PSC-, 926
  smoking and, 874
  Th1, role of, 71
  treatment of, 879–882
    adalimumab (Humira), 880
    aminosalicylates, 879
    anti-TNF antibody therapies, 880–881

certolizumab pegol (cimzia), 881
corticosteroids, 879–880
cyclosporine, 880
infliximab, 880
inhibitors of leukocyte infiltration, 881
methotrexate, 880
MLN0002, 881
natalizumab (Tysabri), 881
sargramostin, 881
surgery, 881–882
thiopurines, 880
visilizumab, 881
Treg frequency in, 76
Inflammatory chemokines, 302
Inflammatory lesions in arteries, 46
Infliximab, 436, 504–505
Innate immune defects, 411–412
chronic granulomatous disease (CGD), 411
early complement component deficiency,
411–412
toll-like receptor 3 (TLR3) polymorphism
and, 412
Innate immune response, 19–20, 40, 53, 54t
activation of, 19–20
secondary, 19–20
cellular components in, 54–57
soluble mediators, 57–58
in systemic lupus, 19–20
Innate immune system, 4, 39
Insulin-dependent diabetes, 23
Interleukin-1 receptor family (IL-1R), 166
Interleukins
IL-1β, 40–41
in CAPS, 41
direct effect of signaling, 44
inflammasome activation of, 43–44
role in gout, 46
in type 2 diabetes, 46
IL-1/TLR family of receptors, 237–238
IL-2, 23
IL-6, 233–234, 316, 1232
IL-10, 29–30
IL-21, 23
IL-23, 71
IL-12 cytokine family, 234, 1231–1232
IL-17 dysregulation, 46
IL-17 receptors, 316
Interphotoreceptor retinoid-binding protein
(IRBP), 793
Intestinal microbiome, 330–331
changes over lifetime, 330
composition and genotyping techniques, 330
environment and, 330–331
hygiene hypothesis, 334–336
autoimmune diabetes, onset of, 335
prevention of insulin-dependent diabetes
in NOD mice, 335–336
prevention of type 1 diabetes, 335–336
reduction in diversity, 337
Intracellular nucleic acid sensors, 166
Intraepithelial B cells, 132–133
Intraepithelial lymphocytes (IEL), 64
Intraocular inflammation, 13
Intravenous immune globulin (IVIG), 1216

Invariant NKT (iNKT) cells, 104
activation of, 105, 117–118
"altered-self" for, 105
beneficial role of, 113–116, 114t
Crohn's disease, 115
diabetes, 113–115
multiple sclerosis (MS), 115
systemic lupus erythematosus (SLE),
115–116
CD1d-reactive subset of, 107t
cell-mediated influence on immune
response, 116–117
cytokine production, 106
detrimental role of, 108–113, 109t
asthma, 110–111
atherosclerosis, 108–110
inflammatory bowel disease (IBD), 111
primary biliary cirrhosis (PBC), 111
rheumatoid arthritis (RA), 111–112
skin disorders, 112–113
ulcerative colitis, 111
distribution, 104–105, 108
downstream effects, 106
effector/memory phenotype, 104
kinds of, 106–107
in non-obese diabetic (NOD) mice, 113–115
technical problems, 107–108
Iridocyclitis, 533
Ischemia/reperfusion injury, 248
Isoprenoids, 45

J
JASL, 47
JC virus-induced progressive multifocal
leukoencephalopathy (PML), 304
JMP, 47
Jun N-terminal kinase (JNK), 166
Juvenile idiopathic arthritis (JIA), 793–794
B cells, role of, 532
clinical features, 525–528
age at onset, 526t
sex ratio, 526t
systemic arthritis, 525–526
enthesitis-related arthritis, 526–527
epidemiology, 525
etiology, 528–532
FoxP3+ Treg cells, role of, 532
ILAR classification, 527–528
IL-17+ T cells, role of, 532
inflammatory synovitis in, 532
life-threatening complications, 525–526
oligoarthritis, 527, 531–532
pathogenesis, 528–532
psoriatic arthritis, 527
rheumatoid factor-negative polyarthritis, 527
rheumatoid factor (RF)-positive rheumatoid
arthritis, 526
SF CD4:CD8 ratio in, 532
systemic, 526, 528–531
Th1/Th17 phenotype, role of, 532
treatment of, 532–533
anti-TNF agents, 533
cyclosporine, 533
glucocorticoid eye drops, 533

intra-articular triamcinolone hexacetonide
joint injections, 533
methotrexate (MTX), 533
safety profile of biological agents, 533
undifferentiated arthritis, 527

K
Kastner, Daniel, 40
Kawasaki's disease
animal models, 1072
autoantibodies, 1073
autoimmune pathogenesis, 1072
clinical, epidemiologic, and pathologic
features, 1071–1072
conventional therapy for, 1072
genetic features and environmental
influences, 1072
Keratinocytes, 25–26
Kerr, John F., 245
Klebsiella pneumoniae, 72
Koebner phenomenon, 27–28
Kostmann's syndrome, 680
Kuhn, Thomas, 11
Küpffer cells, 57

L
Lambert–Eaton myasthenic syndrome
(LEMS), 785–786, 847–848
clinical features of, 786
epidemiology, 786
etiology, 786
investigation, 786
pathophysiology, 786
symptomatic treatment, 786
3,4-diaminopyridine, 786
IVIG, 786
plasma exchange, 786
rituximab, 786
treatment, 786
Landsteiner, Karl, 12
Langerhans cells (LCs), 180–181
Lectin pathway, 57–58
Leflunomide (LF), 1213
Lens autoantibodies, 13
Lens-induced inflammatory disease, 13–14
Leucine-rich repeats (LRRs), 166
Leukocitidin, 677
Leukocyte antigens (CD52), 1229–1230
Leukocyte function-associated antigen (LFA)-1
A, 1228
Leukocytoclastic vasculitis, 504–505
Leukotrienes, 56
LFA-1 (lymphocyte function-associated
antigen-1), 64
LGI1, 823–824
Libman–Sacks endocarditis, 456–457
Lichen sclerosis, 1132–1133
Linear IgA disease (LAD), 965
Linear ubiquitin chain assembly complex
(LUBAC), 47
Lipodystrophy, 46–47
Lipopolysaccharides, 151
Listeria monocytogenes, 70

Liver transplantation (LT), 902, 926, 932–933
Low-affinity IgM antibodies, 21
Low density lipoprotein receptor-related
    protein 4 (Lrp4), 777
LOX-1, 251
L-selectin, 64
Lupus autoimmunity, 247
Lupus erythematosus (LE) cell phenomenon,
    889–890
Lyme disease, 793–794
Lymphadenopathy, 41–42, 45
Lymphochoriomeningitis virus (LCMV), 87
Lymphocyte activating factor (LAF), 229–230
Lymphocyte-dependent autoimmune disease,
    69
Lymphocyte development, 134
Lymphocyte homeostasis, 695
Lymphocytes, 4–5, 59–60, 64. See also B
    cells; T cells
    antigen recognition by, 54f
Lymphocytic hypophysitis, 637
Lymphocytic infundibulo-neurohypophysitis
    (LINH), 634
Lymphocytic mastitis, 1133
Lymphodrek, 230
Lymphoid chemokines, 302
Lymphoid follicles, 64
Lymphokines, 229–230
Lymphopenia, 483
Lymphoplasmacytic sclerosing pancreatitis
    (LPSP), 937–938
Lyn, 207–208
Lysosomal-associated membrane protein 2a
    (LAMP-2a) transporter, 257
Lysozyme, 54–56

M

Macroautophagy, 257, 259
Macrophage activating activity (MAF),
    229–230
Macrophage activation syndrome (MAS),
    525–526, 530–531
Macrophage receptor with collagenous
    structure (MARCO), 164–165
Macrophages, 30, 53–56, 59–61, 187–188,
    313, 637
    in adaptive immunity and tolerance, 168
    antigen generation, 169
    C-type lectin receptors, 165
    and cytokine production, 70
    endocytosis, role in, 166–167
    Fc and complement receptors, 163–164
    functions and their role in autoimmune
        disease, 170t
    homeostatic clearance of cell debris, 169
    interactions with T and B lymphocytes,
        167–168
    maintenance and homeostasis, 165
    modulation of activation, 169–171
    NLR family of receptors and, 166
    origin and distribution of, 162–163
    phagocytosis, role in, 166–167
    receptor recognition of endogenous ligands,
        165

recognition, sensing, and responses,
    163–166
role in innate immunity, 161
scavenger receptors, 164–165
sensing, role in, 166
splenic, 57
Major histocompatibility complex (MHC), 20,
    365–368
autoimmunity and, 366
Ma1/Ma2 (Ma and Ta) autoantigens, 825–826
Mannose binding protein (MBP), 57–58
Marchiafava–Micheli syndrome, 221–222
Mast cells, 53–56, 314
Medawar, Peter, 15
MEFV gene mutation, 44
Megakaryocytes, 53
Melanoma-associated retinopathy (MAR), 847
Memory B cells, 133–134
Mendelian-inherited fever syndromes, 40
Mental retardation, 45
Metabolic–genetic storage diseases, 1133
Metchnikoff, Ilya, 11
Methotrexate (MTX), 1213–1214
Methylation, 23–24
Mevalonate, 45
Mevalonate kinase deficiency (MKD), 45
Mevalonic aciduria (MA), 45
MHC class I and MHC class II molecules,
    59–60
Microautophagy, 257
Microbiome composition and autoimmune
    diseases, 333
    rheumatoid arthritis (RA), 333
    type I diabetes, 333
Microchimerism, 290, 467
Microscopic polyangiitis (MPA), 204, 1069
Migration inhibitory factors (MIF), 229–230
Miller Fisher/Fisher Syndrome (FS), 759
Monoclonal antibodies (MAbs), 1221–1232
Monoclonal autoantibodies, 1146–1149
Monocytes, 53–56, 313
    heterogeneity, 162f
    origin and distribution of, 162–163
    relationship to myeloid-derived classical DC,
        163
Morgenroth, Julius, 12
Movement disorders, 1133–1134
Muckle–Wells syndrome (MWS), 43–44, 810
Mucosa-associated lymphoid tissue (MALT),
    64
    lymphomas, 498
Mucosal associated invariant T (MAIT) cells,
    104
Mucosal NKT (mNKT), 104
Multiple autoimmune syndromes (MAS), 596
Multiple sclerosis (MS), 22, 115, 393–394,
    1184
    acetylation homeostasis, deregulation of, 394
    alleles identified in, 740
    animal model of, 374–375
    autoantigen-specific T cells, 745
    central nervous system (CNS) involvement,
        735, 737
    clinical features, 736–738

clinically definite multiple sclerosis
    (CDMS), 736
clinically isolated syndromes (CIS), 736
DNA hypomethylation, 393–394
environmental factors, 740–742
epidemiology, 739–742
Epstein–Barr virus (EBV) infection and,
    742
gadolinium-enhancing lesions in, 72
genetic factors, 739–740, 741f
genome-wide association studies (GWAS),
    739–740
historic background, 735–736
imaging studies, 737–738
immune dysregulation in, 744–745
immune pathogenesis, 742–745
    T cell pathogenesis, 743–744
immunologic markers, 738
    anti-PLP autoantibodies, 738
    CSF anti-MBP, 738
    CSF anti-MOG, 738
    CSF OCBs, 738
    myelin basic protein (MBP), 738
    tau protein, 738
meningeal ectopic B Cell follicles, 745
neo-epitopes, generation of, 393
pathological examination, 738–739
    axonal reduction and acute damage, 739
    chronic-inactive plaque, 739
    demyelination, 739
    hypertrophic astrocytes and mild astroglial
        scarring, 739
    inflammation in lesions, 738–739
    inflammatory cell profile of active lesions,
        739
    plaques, 738–739
pathophysiology of, 743f
primary progressive MS (PPMS), 737
primary progressive multiple sclerosis
    (PPMS), 736
remitting multiple sclerosis (RRMS), 736
role of DQ molecules in predisposition, 375
secondary progressive multiple sclerosis
    (SPMS), 736–737
signs and symptoms, 736
Th1 and Th2 cells, role of, 744
therapeutic approaches, 745–749
    Avonex, 746–747
    Betaseron, 746–747
    dimethyl fumarate, 748–749
    disease modifying therapy (DMT), 745
    FDA approved, 746t
    fingolimod, 748
    glatiramer acetate, 747
    interferons, 746–747
    β-Interferon therapy, 747
    mitoxantrone, 748
    natalizumab, 747
    teriflunomide, 748
vitamin D and, 742
Multipotent progenitors (MPPs), 53
Multistep navigation, 299–302
Muscle-specific kinase (MuSK), 777
Myalgia, 41–42

Myasthenia gravis, 621–622
  AChR, MuSK and Lrp4, role of, 778–779
  age at onset, 780t
  antibodies in, 782–783
    AChR antibodies, 782–783
    MuSK antibodies, 782
  antibody status, 780t
  CD4$^+$ T lymphocytes, role of, 784–785
  childhood onset AChRab$^+$, 780–781
  cholinesterase inhibitors and, 780
  clinical heterogeneity, 780–782
  diagnosis, 780
  epidemiology, 779
  etiology, 779–780
  general aspects, 780
  history, 778t
  HLA association, 780t
  late onset AChRab$^+$, 781
  MuSK antibody-positive, 781
  neonatal, 781–782
  pathogenic mechanisms, 783–784
    AChR and MuSK antibodies, pathogenicity of, 783
    AChR antibody-positive, 783
    MuSK antibody-positive, 784
  serological testing, 782
  thymic pathology, 780t
  thymoma-associated, 781
  thymus and, 785
Mycobacterium tuberculosis, 70
Mycophenolate mofetil (MMF), 1214–1215
Mycoplasma pneumoniae infection, 655
MyD88 ("myeloid differentiation primary response protein 88"), 166
Myelin-associated antigens, 71
Myelin-associated glycoprotein (MAG), 757
Myelitis, 846
Myelodysplastic syndromes (MDS), 163, 664, 686
Myeloid-derived dendritic cells (DC), 187–188
Myeloperoxidase, 204
Myocarditis
  animal models, 1040–1042
  autoimmune features, 1037–1039
    circulating antibodies, 1037
  classic description of, 1033
  clinical, pathologic, and epidemiologic features, 1033–1037
    classification scheme for, 1034t
    clinical diagnosis of, 1034
    Dallas criteria, 1034–1035
    histologic forms of, 1035
    immunoperoxidase staining, 1035
  environmental features, 1039–1040
  genetic features, 1039
  pathogenic mechanisms, 1040–1042
  tests for
    immunoassay of antibodies, 1038
    immunofluorescence tests, 1037–1038
    immunologic assessment of biopsies, 1038–1039
    Western immunoblot analysis, 1037–1038
  treatment for, 1043–1044

azathiaprine, 1043
immunosuppressive therapy, 1043
prednisone, 1043

N

N-acetylglucosaminyl-phosphatidol, 221–222
Nailfold capillaroscopy, 464
Nakajo–Nishimura syndrome (NNS), 47
Narcolepsy, 1134
Natalizumab (Tysabri), 304, 747, 881
National Vaccine Injury Compensation Program, 290
Natural killer (NK) cells, 4, 53–56, 61
  activating receptors of, 56f
Natural killer T (NKT) cells, 314
  adhesion to target cells, 190–191
  autoimmunity and, 193–195
    genetics, 194–195
    impaired cytotoxic function, 193–194
  cell receptor signaling, 190–193
  cell responses, 190–191
  chemokine and cytokine production, 192–193
  on cytokines, 187–188
  cytolytic granule exocytosis, 192
  development, 188–189
  differentiation, 188–189
  effector functions, 190–193
  functional responses, 189–190
  invariant NKT (iNKT) cells, 104
  molecular detection system, 187–188
  phenotype and tissue localization of, 189
  role in promoting perforin-containing granule polarization, 191–192
  specificity and signaling of human, 191t
  terms, 103–104
  type I, 104
  type II, 104
  type III, 104
Necroptosis, 248
Necrosis, 248–249
  necrotic cells
    immuno-stimulatory effects of, 251–252
    receptors for, 251
Necrotic cell death, 56
Necrotizing arteritis, 1067–1069
Necrotizing hypophysitis, 639
Neomycin phosphotransferase II (NeoR), 259
NETosis, 201–202, 248
Neurological APS, 483
Neurological syndromes of autoimmune causation, 818
  ataxia, 818
  autoimmune encephalitis, 818
  epilepsy, 818
  psychiatric disorders, 818
  spinal myelitis, 818
  stiff person syndrome, 818
Neuromuscular junction (NMJ), 777–778
  development of, 777
  ion channel targets for autoantibodies at, 779f
  postsynaptic membrane in, 777

Neuromuscular transmission, 779
Neuromyelitis optica (NMO), 820
Neuronal nuclear antigens (NNA), 825
Neutropenia, 483
Neutrophil extracellular traps (NETs), 54–56, 201–202
  antimicrobial peptides of, 202b
Neutrophils, 53–56, 201–206, 313, 637
  basic biology, 201–202
  entry during an inflammatory response, 55f
  pathogenic role in autoimmune diseases, 202–206
    antiphospholipid syndrome, 206
    autoimmune skin diseases, 206
    primary Sjögren syndrome, 206
    rheumatoid arthritis, 205
    systemic lupus erythematosus, 202–204
    systemic sclerosis, 206
    systemic vasculitides, 204–205
  role in immunity, 201–202
NF-κB, 44
Nitric oxide, 54–56
NLRP3 gene, 43–44
NLRP3 inflammasome, 40–41, 44
  in atherosclerosis, 46
  in gout, 46
NLRP3 protein, 43–44
NOD-like receptors (NLRs), 56–57, 166
NOMID, 43–44
Non-Hodgkin lymphoma (NHL), 498
Non-phagocytic basophils, 54–56
Non-steroidal anti-inflammatory drugs (NSAIDs), 538, 1211–1212
Nucleotide-binding and oligomerization domain (NOD)-like receptors (NLRs), 263–264
Nucleotide-binding and oligomerization (NACHT) domain, 166

O

Obstetric APS, 482
Occupational exposures, 288, 288t
Ocrelizumab, 458
Ocular disease
  animal models, 798
  autoimmune features, 796–797
  clinical features, 793–795
  epidemiologic features, 795–796
  episcleritis, 793–794
  genetic factors, 797–798
  historical background, 793
  hormonal influences, 797
  human leukocyte antigens, role of, 798t
  immunologic markers, 799–800
  intermediate uveitis, 795
  ocular immune system, 799
  panuveitis, 795
  pathogenic mechanisms, 798–799
  pathologic features, 795
  posterior uveitis, 795
  scleritis, 793–794
  tissue damage, 799
  treatment and outcomes, 800–801
    adalimumab, 800

Ocular disease (*Continued*)
  azathioprine, 800
  chlorambucil, 800
  corticosteroids, 800
  cyclophosphamide, 800
  cyclosporine, 800
  daclizumab, 800
  dexamethasone, 800
  etanercept, 800
  fluocinolone acetonide, 800
  infliximab, 800
  long-term steroid therapy, 800
  methotrexate, 800
  mycophenolate mofetil, 800
  rapamycin, 800
  rituximab, 800
  steroid implants, 800
  tacrolimus, 800
  therapeutic guidelines, 800–801
Osteoarthritis (OA), 527, 1134–1135
Owen, Ray, 15, 87

P

Pancreatic islet autoantigen, 5
Paraneoplastic cerebellar degeneration (PCD),
    844
Paraneoplastic encephalomyelitis (PEM), 845
Paraneoplastic limbic encephalitis (LE),
    845–846
Paraneoplastic optic neuropathy, 847
Paraneoplastic pemphigus (PNP), 962
Paraneoplastic syndromes, 836*b*
  antibodies, role of, 838–844, 839*t*
    anti-amphiphysin, 842–843
    anti-CRMP5 (anti-CV2), 842
    anti-ganglionic neuronal acetylcholine
        receptor, 843
    anti-glutamic acid decarboxylase (anti-
        GAD65), 843
    anti-Hu antibody, 838–840
    anti-Ma antibodies, 841
    anti-N methyl-D-aspartate receptor (anti-
        NMDAR), 843
    anti-Ri (ANNA2), 840–841
    anti-Tr antibody, 842
    anti-voltage-gated potassium channel, 844
    anti-Yo antibody, 841–842
    ion channel, 843–844
    synaptic/cell surface antibodies, 842–843
  diagnosis of, 837–838
    neurologic syndromes, 837*b*
  neurologic syndromes, 835–836
  pathogenesis of, 836–837, 836*t*
  Purkinje cell and, 835
  treatment of, 844, 845*t*
    corticosteroids, 844
    cyclophosphamide, 844
    rituximab, 844
    tacrolimus, 844
  vision loss and, 847
Parathyroid disease, 1135–1136
Parkinson's disease, 248
Paroxysmal cold hemoglobinuria (PKH), 11,
    13

Parthanatos, 248–249
  in autoimmunity, 249
Pasteur, Louis, 11
Pasteur's rabies vaccine, 440
Pathogen-associated molecular patterns
    (PAMPS), 25–26, 263–264
Pathogenic autoreactivity associated with tissue
    damage, 21
Pathogens of protective effect, 335–336
  strength, 336–337
Pattern recognition receptors (PRRs), 4, 176,
    263–264
  in mouse, 177*t*
PCA-2, 826
PCA-Tr autoantibodies, 824
Pediatric autoimmune neuropsychiatric
    disorder associated with streptococcal
    infections (PANDAS), 1133–1134
Pemphigoid gestationis (PG), 964
Pemphigus foliaceus, 960–962
  autoantibodies, 960–961
    anti-Dsg1 antibodies, 961
  CD4$^+$ T cell lines, 961
  classic form of, 960
  clinical features, 960
  environmental factors, 961–962
  epidemiologic features, 960
  genetic features, 961
  HLA alleles, 961
  IgG4 autoantibodies, 961
  pathologic effector mechanisms, 961
  pathologic features, 960
  T cell activation, 961
  in vivo and *in vitro* models, 961
Pemphigus vulgaris (PV), 956–960
  clinical features, 956
  Dsg1 and Dsg3, role of, 958
  Dsg3-specific T cells, 959
  epidemiologic features, 956
  genetic features, 959
  HLA alleles, 959
  IgG autoantibodies, 956–958
  pathological features, 956
  pathologic effector mechanisms, 959–960
    autoantibodies, 959–960
  T cell activation, 958–959
  Th1/Th2 cells in, 958–959
  in vivo and *in vitro* models, 959
    active immunization model, 959
    autoantibody passive transfer model, 959
Peptidylargenine deiminase (PAD), 259–260
Perez, Charles, 245
Periodic fever with aphthous stomatitis,
    pharyngitis, and cervical adenitis
    (PFAPA), 46
Peripheral blood mononuclear cells (PBMCs),
    41
Peripheral tolerance, 25, 90–97
  impact of dendritic cells (DC), 91–93
    resting DCs, 92–93
  mechanism of, 93–96
    anergy, 94
    clonal deletion, 93–94
    ignorance, 94

induced Tregs (iTregs), 94–96
  negative regulatory mechanisms that
      impact tolerance, 96
tissue antigens, expression of, 96–97
Pernicious anemia, 619
  associated diseases, 621–622
    Hashimoto's thyroiditis, 621–622
    insulin-dependent type 1 diabetes mellitus,
        621–622
    Lambert–Eaton syndrome, 621–622
    myasthenia gravis, 621–622
    premature graying of hair, 621–622
    primary Addison's disease, 621–622
    primary hypoparathyroidism, 621–622
    primary ovarian failure, 621–622
    thyrotoxicosis, 621–622
    vitiligo, 621–622
  autoantibodies associated with, 622–623,
      626
  autoimmune endocrinopathies and, 621–622
  with autoimmune thyroid diseases, 619
  clinical, pathologic, and epidemiologic
      features, 620–622
    age of onset, 620
    evolution of gastric atrophy, 621
    gastric parietal cell antibody, role of,
        621
    precursor stem cells, role of, 621
    risk of developing gastric cancer, 620
    type A gastritis, 620–621
    vitamin B12 deficiency, 620
  genetic features, 623–624
  H$^+$/K$^+$ ATPase activity, 622–623, 622*f*
  in vivo and *in vitro* models, 624–625
    A23 TCR transgenic mice, 624
    A51 TCR transgenic mice, 624
    BALB/c mice, 624
    C57BL/6 mice, 624
    C3H/He mice, 624
  pathologic effector mechanisms, 626
    CD4$^+$ T cells, 626
    Th1- and Th2-type cytokines, 626
  T cell immunity
    CD4$^+$ and CD8$^+$ T cells, 623
  treatment
    azathioprine, 621
    corticosteroids, 621
    vitamin B12 replacement, 627
Peyer's patches, 64, 302–303, 878
Pfeiffer, Richard, 12
Phagocytic cells, 54–56
Phagocytosis, 54–56
Phosphatidylserine, 56
Pirquet, Clemens von, 11
Pituitary adenomas, 633
PLAID, 47
Plasmacytoid DC (PDC), 163, 187–188
Platelet-activating factor, 56
PLCγ2-related phenotypes, 47
Pneumococcal pneumonia, 40
PNMA proteins, 826
POEMS syndrome, 767
Poly(ADP-ribosyl)ation of nuclear proteins,
    248–249

Polyarteritis nodosa, 793–795
  animal models, 1071
  autoantibody markers, 1071
  autoimmune pathogenesis, 1070
  clinical, epidemiologic, and pathologic
    features, 1070
  genetic features and environmental
    influences, 1070–1071
  pathologic effector mechanisms, 1071
Polygenic or acquired autoinflammatory
    disorders, 46
Polyglandular autoimmune syndrome (PAS)
    type 1, 606
Polymyositis, 793–794
Polypeptide J (joining) chain, 63
Porphyromonas gingivalis, 679
Post-translational modifications in
    autoimmunity, 371–372
  deamidation, 372
  deimination, 371–372
Pre-B cell receptor (pre-BCR), 137–138
Pre-BII cells, 138
Premature ovarian insufficiency (POI), 1015
Primary antiphospholipid syndrome, 806
Primary biliary cirrhosis (PBC), 111
  animal models, 916–917, 918t
    dominant negative TGF-βreceptor II mice,
      916–917
    NOD.c3c4 congenic mice, 916–917
    scurfy mice, 916–917
    xenobiotic-immunized models, 916–917
  autoantibodies, 918–919
  autoimmune pathogenesis for, 913–914
    antinuclear antibodies (ANA), 914
    2-oxoacid dehydrogenase complexes (2-
      OADCs), 914
  clinical features, 910
  diagnosis, 909
  environmental influences, 916
    infectious agents, 916
    xenobiotics, 916, 917t
  epidemiology, 910–912
  epigenetic effects, 915
  familial, 914–915
  fetal microchimerism, 916
  genome-wide association studies (GWAS),
    915
  history, 909
  HLA association, 915
  natural history, 910–912
  pathologic effector mechanisms, 917–918
  pathology, 910
  population-based epidemiological studies, 912t
  prevalence, 911t
  progression of, 911
  risk factors, 913b
  treatment
    azathioprine, 913
    colchicine, 913
    cyclosporin, 913
    OLT, 913
    penicillamine, 913
    ursodeoxycholic acid (UDCA), 913
  X chromosome genes, role of, 916

Primary hemostasis, 711
Primary hypophysitis, 637, 642–643
Primary sclerosing cholangitis (PSC)
  adhesion molecules, 931
  animal models, 930
  associated malignancies, 929
    cholangiocarcinoma (CCA), 929
    colorectal neoplasia, 929
    gallbladder neoplasia, 929
    hepatocellular carcinoma, 929
  autoantibodies, 931
  autoimmune features, 932
  bacterial translocation in, 930–931
  biliary strictures in, 926
  biochemical features, 926–927
  cholangiography, 927
  cirrhosis and, 926
  development of death or liver
    transplantation, 926
  diagnosis, 926–927
  epidemiologic features, 925
  etiology of, 930
  genetics, 929–930
  histologic findings, 927
  IBD, 926
  innate system, 930–931
  lithocholic acid (LCA), role of, 931–932
  liver–gut axis, 931
  lymphocyte homing, 931
  natural history and clinical features, 926
  pathogen-associated molecular patterns,
    930–931
  pathogenic mechanisms, 930–932
  pediatric, 927–928
  progressive cholestasis and, 926
  PSC-AIH, 928
  risk factors, 925
  small duct, 927–928
  subtypes, 927–928
  T cells, role of, 931
  therapies for, 932–933
    endoscopic therapy, 932
    liver transplantation, 932–933
    UDCA, 932
  transporter defects and bile acids, 931–932
Primary Sjögren syndrome
  pathogenic role of neutrophils, 206
Probiotics and autoimmune disease, 333–334
  effect of probiotic mixtures, 334
  Lactobacillus johnsonii N6.2, 334
  Pediococcus acidilactici, 334
Procoagulant thrombotic diseases, 712–714
  ADAMTS13 and thrombotic events,
    713–714
    deficiency non-inhibitory antibodies,
      713–714
  autoantibodies, 712–713
    IgG and IgM autoantibodies, 713
    to protein S, 712–713
Proinflammatory apoptotic debris, 19–20
Prostaglandins, 56
Prostate disease, 947
Prostatitis, 1136–1137
Proteases, 54–56

Proteinase 3, 204
Protein isoprenylation, 45
PSMB8, 47
Psoriasis, 23, 46, 72–73, 206
  animal models
    mouse models, 980–981
    transplantation models, 981
    in vitro, 981
  autoantibody markers, 981–982
  autoimmune basis for, 978–980
  autoimmune features, 978–980
  classification, 979t
  clinical, pathologic, and epidemiologic
    features, 978
  genetic features, 980
  pathogenetic mechanism, 981
  signals of, 980t
Psoriatic arthritis, 527, 538
PSTAT3, 71–72
Ptpn22, 23
Pulmonary APS, 484
Purkinje cell antigen-1 (PCA-1; Yo), 826
Purpura, 1069–1070
Pyrexins, 229
Pyrin (PYD), 44, 166

R
RAG-dependent recombination, 4
Rapsyn, 777
RAS-associated autoimmune
    lymphoproliferative disorder (RALD),
    702, 704–707
  pathogenic effector mechanisms, 705–706
Rathke's cleft cyst, 633
Raynaud's phenomenon, 456–457, 496,
    504–505
Reactive arthritis, 22, 538
Recombination signal sequence (RSS)
    nucleotide motifs, 59
Regulatory T cells (Tregs), 155, 443f
  antigen-specific, 28–29
  CD45Rb transfer model for autoimmune
    colitis, 442–443
  CpG DNA methylation and, 385
  effector T cell responses, 75–76
  epigenetic modulation of, 386
  ex-Tregs, 74–75
  Foxp3 expression and, 74–75
  histone acetylation on development and
    function of, 385–386
  periphery (pTregs), 75
  Th17 cells, reciprocal relationship with,
    72–73
  thymus (tTregs), 75
  upregulation of Tbet, 76
Reiter syndrome, 793–794
Relapsing polychondritis (RP), 1136
Renal APS, 484
Reproductive hormones, link with immune
    system, 321–323
  androgens, 322–323
  estrogens, 321–322
  progesterone, 322
Retinal S-antigen, 793

Rheumathic heart disease (RHD)
 autoantibodies as markers, 1029–1030
 autoimmune features, 1024
 genetic polymorphism associated with, 1026t
 genetic predisposition, 1024–1027
 HLA association, 1025
 pathologic effector mechanisms, 1028–1029
 T cells activation, 1029
Rheumatic fever (RF), 26
 adaptive immune response, 1025–1027
 autoantibodies as markers, 1029–1030
  cardiac myosin, 1030
  N-acetyl β-D-glucosamine, 1029–1030
 autoimmune features, 1024
 clinical, pathologic, and epidemiologic
   features, 1023–1024
 genetic polymorphism associated with, 1026t
 genetic predisposition, 1024–1027
  CTLA4 genes, 1027
  DRB1, DRB3, DQB1 DQA1 genes, 1027
  FcγRIIA gene, 1025
  Ficolin gene, 1025
  IL-10 gene, 1027
  IL-1Ra gene, 1027
  MBL2 gene, 1024–1025
  single nucleotide polymorphisms (SNPs),
    1027
  TGF-B1 gene, 1027
  TLR-2 gene, 1025
  TNF-α gene, 1027
 HLA association, 1025
 in vivo and in vitro models, 1027–1028
 incidence of ARF, 1024
 innate immune response, 1024–1025
 pathologic effector mechanisms,
   1028–1029
 polyarthritis and carditis manifestations in,
   1023
 Streptococcus pyogenes, role of, 1024
 Sydenham's chorea in, 1023
Rheumatoid arthritis (RA), 20, 22, 25–26, 72,
   111–112, 333, 389–390, 679,
   1184–1185
 activated phenotype of RASFs, 389–390
 affected joints, 511–512
 autoantibodies, 517–519
  anticitrullinated-protein antibodies
    (ACPA), 517–519
  citrullinated antigens, 517–519
 autoimmune features, 512–514
  citrullinated peptides, 513, 515
  rheumatoid factor (RF), 512–513
 basophils, role of, 208
 causes of, 511
 clinical characteristics of, 511–512
 collagen-induced arthritis, animal model,
   373–374
 complement system, involvement of, 223
 environmental factors, role of, 511
 epidemiologic features, 511–512
 genetic features, 514–515
  HLA-DRB1 alleles, 514
   human leucocyte antigen (HLA)-DRw4,
     514

 major histocompatibility complex (MHC)
   class II gene, 514
  PTPN22 gene, 514–515
  signal transducers and activators of
    transcription (STATs), 515
  SNPs, 515
  tumor necrosis factor, alpha-induced
    protein 3 (TNFAIP3) genes, 515
 HLA-DQ6 alleles associated with, 374
 hyperacetylation and hypoacetylation in, 389
 in vivo models, 515–516
  adjuvants, 515
  cellular immune responses, 515
  collagen-induced arthritis (CIA), 515
  IL-1 receptor antagonist (IL-1ra)
    deficiency, 516
  KRN mouse model, 515–516
  "non-immune" models, 516
  SKG model, 515–516
  transgenic T cell receptor (TCR) mouse,
    515–516
 miRNAs, role of, 390
 pathogenic role of neutrophils, 205
 pathologic effector mechanisms, 516–517
  antigen presenting cells (APC), role of,
    516
  bone destruction, 517
  cartilage damage, 516–517
  fibroblast-like synovial cells (FLS), role
    of, 516
  osteoclast differentiation and activation,
    517
  Th1 and Th17 cells, role of, 516
  T or B cell activation, 516–517
 Porphyromonas gingivalis (P. gingivalis)
   and, 370
 small ubiquitin-like modifiers (SUMOs),
   role of, 390
 Th1, role of, 71
Rheumatoid factor-negative polyarthritis, 527
Rheumatoid factor (RF)-positive rheumatoid
   arthritis, 526
RIG-I helicase receptor (RLR), 166
(RIG-I)-like helicases (RLH), 263–264
RIG-like helicases, 166
Rituximab, 458, 1228–1229
RORβt, 71–72

S

Salmonella infection, 105
Sandhoff disease, 1133
Sarcoidosis, 793–795, 819, 1137
Schmidt syndrome, 605
Schwachman–Diamond syndrome, 680
Scleritis, 793–794
Scleroderma
 clinical features, 463–464
 history, 463
Secondary hemostasis, 711
Selective IgA deficiency, 408–409
Self-peptide–self-MHC complexes, 24
Self-reactive CD4+ T helper cells (Th), 69–70
Sensorineural hearing loss, 806–807
Serositis, 41–42

Serpin G1, 220
Serum amyloid P (SAP), 251
Severe aplastic anemia (SAA), 686
Severe combined immunodeficiency (SCID),
   403–404
Severe congenital neutropenias (SCN), 680
Sex hormones, role in autoimmune disease,
   24
Sexual dimorphism
 consequences for autoimmunity of, 324–325
 defined, 319
 differences between male and female, 320t
  environmental effects, 324
 in immune system, 319–321
 sex chromosome, relation with, 319,
   323–324
  X chromosome, 323
  Y chromosome, 323–324
Shared epitope, 22
Shrinkage necrosis, 245
Siglec-1, 165–166
Siglec1 (CD169), 167
Silicone implants, 291
Single nucleotide polymorphisms (SNPs), 22
Sjögren's syndrome (SS), 390–391, 679, 806,
   819–820, 855–856
 autoantibodies in, 502
 BAFF gene, 500
 B cell hyperactivity, 495
 clinical features, 496–498
  endocrine involvement, 498
  gastrointestinal and hepatobiliary
    manifestations, 497
  local manifestations, 496
  lymphoproliferative disease, 498
  musculoskeletal manifestations, 496
  neuropsychiatric involvement, 497–498
  psychopathological features and distinct
    personality traits, 497–498
  Raynaud's phenomenon, 496
  renal involvement, 497
  respiratory tract involvement, 496
  salivary and lachrymal glands,
    manifestation in, 496
  systemic manifestations, 496–498
  vasculitis, 497
 coexisting SLE and, 498
 diagnosis and differential diagnosis of, 498
 environmental factors, role of, 495–496,
   503–504
  hormonal factors, 503–504
  stress, 503
  viruses, 503
 epigenetic mechanisms, 503
 etiopathogenesis, 502–504
 European American Consensus Group
   Criteria, 500b
 exocrine gland destruction, 504
  apoptosis, 504
  aquaporins, 504
  neurotransmission, 504
 genetics of, 502–503
 immunopathology, 498–502
  B lymphocytes, role of, 499

cellular populations—cytokine production, 498—502
  dendritic cells (DCs), role of, 499—500
  epithelial cells, role of, 500—502
  macrophages, role of, 499—500
  salivary gland epithelium, 500—502
  T lymphocytes, role of, 498—499
lymphocytic infiltration of exocrine in, 495
principal target of, 495—496
secondary, 498
structural abnormalities, 504
  basal membrane, disorganization of, 504
  changes in tight junctions, 504
therapy of, 504—505
  cevimeline, 504—505
  corticosteroids, 504—505
  cytotoxic drugs, 504—505
  dental treatment, 504—505
  eye lubricants, 504—505
  hydroxychloroquine, 504—505
  non-steroidal anti-inflammatory drugs, 504—505
  pilcarpine, 504—505
  vaginal lubricants, 504—505
Skin disorders, 112—113
SLAM protein, 77
Small vessel vasculitis, 1069—1070
Soluble TNF receptor (sTNFR), 45
Somatic hypermutation (SHM), 150
Somatic mutation, 24
Specific pathogen-free (SPF) animals, 337
Sperm granuloma, 1012
Sphingomonas spp., 105
Spondyloarthritis (SpA)
  arthritis with IBD, 538
  bacterial trigger, 541
  clinical manifestations, 537—538
    back pain, 537
  cytokines, role of, 541
    in ankylosing spondylitis, 542
  definition, 537—538
  HLA-B27, role of, 538—540
    arthritogenic peptide hypothesis, 538—539
    misfolded hypothesis, 539—540
  male-to-female ratio, 537
  non-MHC genes *ERAP1* and *IL23R*, role of, 540
  prevalence, 537
  psoriatic arthritis, 538
  reactive arthritis, 538
  treatment of
    corticosteroids, 538
    disease-modifying antirheumatic drugs (DMARDs), 538
    non-steroidal anti-inflammatory drugs (NSAIDs), 538
Spondyloarthropathies, 366—368
Spontaneous autoimmune thyroiditis, 562
Staphylococcus aureus, 72—74
Stiff person syndrome, 818, 847
Still's disease, 526
Streptococcal-related rheumatic carditis, 1133—1134
Stressful life events, 291

Subacute cutaneous lupus (SCLE), 457—458
Subacute sensory neuronopathy, 846
Sulfasalazine (azulfidine), 1213
Sulston, John, 245
Superoxide anions, 54—56
Sydenham's chorea, 1133—1134
Sympathetic ophthalmia, 13, 15—16
Syndrome of sensorineural hearing loss (SNHL), 805
  in adult patients, 805
  animal models, 809—811
  autoimmune vestibulo-cochlear disorders, 805
  bilateral immune-mediated Ménière's disease, 805
  causes of, 805
  clinical features, 805—806
  evidence of autoimmunity, 808—809
  genetic susceptibility, 810
  idiopathic progressive bilateral SNHL, 805
  proteins responsible for, 809
  sudden SNHL, 805
  treatment, 811
    antioxidants, 811
    biological agents, 811
    cochlear implantation, 811
    hematopoietic stem cell transplantation, 811
    heparin, 811
    methylprednisolone, 811
    prednisolone, 811
    steroid, 811
Systemic immunopathic disorders with encephalitis and myelitis, 818—820
Systemic inflammation, 41—42
Systemic JIA (sJIA), 526, 528—531
  genetics, 528, 529*t*
  growth impairment, 529—530
  interleukin-1 (IL-1), role of, 530
  interleukin-6 (IL-6), role of, 528—530
  interleukin-18 (IL-18), role of, 530
  macrophage activation syndrome (MAS), 530—531
  proinflammatory mediators, 528
Systemic lupus erythematosus (SLE), 20, 22, 76, 115—116, 248, 281, 386—389, 679, 793—795, 806, 817—819, 998—999, 1185
  arthritis of, 454—455
  associated autoantibodies, 25—26
  autoantibodies associated with, 452—453, 453*t*
  classification criteria for, 453*b*
  commonly affected organs and tissues, 451
  deforming arthritis of Jaccoud in, 454—455
  diagnosis of, 453—454
  DNA methylation and, 386—387
    miRNA control, 387—388
  environmental epigenetics in, 388
  epidemiology, 452
  epigenetic disruption of B Cell tolerance, 388—389
  general symptoms, 453
  genetics, 452

histone acetylation in, 388
immune thrombocytopenia (ITP) in, 666
measurement of disease activity, 454—458
  acute cutaneous lupus, 457—458
  anticlotting factor antibodies in, 457
  autoimmune hemolytic anemia, 457
  BILAG-2004, 454
  BILAG-2004 index, 454
  cardiac involvement, 456—457
  dermatological changes, 457—458
  eye involvement, 458
  hematologic changes, 457
  lupus anticoagulants in, 457
  manifestation of gastrointestinal lupus, 458
  musculoskeletal changes, 454—455
  neuropsychiatric manifestations, 455—456
  optic neuritis, 458
  papilledema, 458
  parenchymal lung involvement, 457
  renal involvement, 455
  retinal vein occlusion, 458
  retinopathy, 458
  SELENA-SLEDAI index, 454
  sicca syndrome, 458
  Sjögren's syndrome, 458
  subacute cutaneous lupus (SCLE), 457—458
  sub-cutaneous lupus, 457—458
pathogenesis, 451
pathogenic role of neutrophils, 202—204
  low-density granulocytes in, 203
  NETosis in, 203—204, 203*f*
  neutropenia and abnormal neutrophil function, 202—203
  neutrophils and organ damage in, 204
T and B cells, roles of, 451
therapies for, 458
type I interferons and, 27—28
Systemic sclerosis (SSc), 206, 390, 463—464
  animal models of, 467—469, 467*t*
    Fra2-transgenic mice, 469
    growth factor-induced fibrosis model of, 468
    murine models of bleomycin-induced fibrosis, 468
    Scl-GvHD models, 468
    tight skin mice (Tsk) type 1 and type 2 (Tsk1 and Tsk2) mice, 468
    TβRIIΔk mice, 469
    UCD200 chickens, 467—468
    Wnt-10b-transgenic mice, 469
  atrophy, 464
  autoimmune features and immunologic markers in, 465—466
    anticentromere antibodies (ACA), 465—466
    antifibrillin-1 antibodies, 465
    antifibroblast antibodies, 465
    antihistone antibodies (AHA), 466
    anti-polymyositis/scleroderma (anti-PM-Scl) antibodies, 466
    anti-Th/To antibodies, 466

Systemic sclerosis (SSc) (*Continued*)
  diagnostic and prognostic antibodies, 465–466
    potential pathogenetic antibodies, 465
    RNA polymerases (anti-RNAP antibodies) I, II, and III, 466
  early symptoms of, 464
  endothelial cell (EC) injury and apoptosis, 464
  environmental factors, 466–467
  epidemiologic features, 464–465
  epidermis of long-standing, 464
  fibrosis in, 472–473
    collagens involved, 472
    TGF-β, role of, 473
    upregulation of ECM production, 472
  gastrointestinal (GI) complications, 464
  genetic features, 466
  immunological abnormalities, 470–472
    autoantibodies, 471
    B cells, role of, 471
    chemokines, 472
    cytokines, 472
    T cells, role of, 470
  inflammatory cell infiltration, 464
  pathogenic mechanisms, 469–473
    cellular abnormalities, 470
    cytokine abnormalities, 470
    microvascular EC injury and apoptosis, 469–470
    platelet activation, 469–470
    vascular endothelial growth factor (VEGF), role of, 470
    vasculopathy, 469–470
  pathologic features, 464
  spectrum of changes of affected skin, 464
  tissue fibrosis, 464
Systemic vasculitides
  pathogenic role of neutrophils, 204–205
    in ANCA-associated vasculitis, 205
    neutrophils and vasculitic organ damage, 204–205

T

Takayasu's arteritis (TA)
  clinical manifestations of, 1089–1090
  clinical spectrum in, 1097*t*
  corticosteroid monotherapy, 1099
  genetic features, 1098
  histomorphologic findings, 1096
  historic background, 1096
  imaging modalities, 1097–1098
  immunosuppressive therapy, 1098–1099
  inflammatory infiltration in, 1096
  pathogenic mechanisms, 1098
Target-organ antigen, 24
T-bet, 70, 73–74
TCDD, 72–73
T cell developmental defects, 403–406
  combined immune deficiencies (CID), 404–405
  DiGeorge syndrome (DGS), 405

  severe combined immunodeficiency (SCID), 403–404
  Wiskott–Aldrich syndrome (WAS), 405–406
T cell differentiation, 23–24
T cell lymphopenia, 25
T cell receptor (TCR) with a peptide–MHC complex, 26, 60–61
T cells
  αβ, 59–61
  γδ, 59–61
  activation
    cytokine expression, 27
    epitopes of self-antigen and, 27
    by foreign-peptide–self-MHC complex, 26
    viral infection and, 71
  activation of immune system, 20
  antiself reactive, 24
  autoimmune thyroiditis, 559–560
  B Cell interactions, 148–149
  bullous pemphigoid (BP), 963
  CD4$^+$, 60, 74–76
  CD8$^+$, 60
  CD25$^+$, 74
  development, 59–60
  "double positive," 59–60
  effector, 303–306
  functional activities, 60–61
  in giant cell arteritis (GCA), 1092–1093
  helper, 61
  independent antibody responses, 150–151
  mediated cytotoxicity, 61
  microvascular determinants of recruitment, 297
  migratory routes of, 299*f*
  in pemphigus foliaceus, 961
  in pemphigus vulgaris (PV), 958–959
  peripheral, 26
  primary sclerosing cholangitis (PSC), 931
  response to antigenic stimulation, 21
  in sexual dimorphism, 320
  subpopulations, 62*f*
  systemic lupus erythematosus (SLE), role in, 451
  in thymus, 368–369
  trafficking of regulatory, 303
Terminal deoxynucleotidyl transferase (TdT), 59, 62
TGF-β, 71–72, 316
Th1 cells, 70–71, 303
  differentiation, 70
  IFN-γ production, 70
  IL-12 and, 70
  imbalance between Th1/Th2 subsets, 71
  immune responses to extracellular pathogens, 70
  role in inflammation and autoimmune pathology, 71
Th17 cells, 71–74, 303, 314–315
  differentiation, 71–72, 74
  discovery and differentiation, 71–72
  function, 72
  IFN-γ production, 73–74

  IL-10 and, 73
  IL-23 and, 73–74
  lineage-specific transcription factor, 71–72
  pathogenicity and plasticity, 73–74
  reciprocal relationship with Tregs, 72–73
  regulation in the intestine, 74
  signature cytokines IL-17A and IL-17F, 72
  specific chemokine receptor CCR6, 71–72
  survival/expansion of pathogenic, 73
  tissue inflammation and neutrophil recruitment, role in, 72
  transcriptional program, 73
Theile's murine encephalomyelitis virus (TMEV), 440
T helper cells (Th)
  in autoimmune hemolytic anemia (AIHA), 656
  effector, 314–315, 315*t*
  effector mechanisms, 69–70
  generation and function of, 70*f*
  self-reactive CD4$^+$, 69–70
  Th1 cells, 70–71, 303
    differentiation, 70
    IFN-γ production, 70
    IL-12 and, 70
    imbalance between Th1/Th2 subsets, 71
    immune responses to extracellular pathogens, 70
    role in inflammation and autoimmune pathology, 71
  Th2 cells, 78, 303
    role in eosinophil recruitment and mast cell activation, 78
  Th9 cells, 78
  Th17 cells, 71–74, 303, 314–315
    differentiation, 71–72, 74
    discovery and differentiation, 71–72
    function, 72
    IFN-γ production, 73–74
    IL-10 and, 73
    IL-23 and, 73–74
    lineage-specific transcription factor, 71–72
    pathogenicity and plasticity, 73–74
    reciprocal relationship with Tregs, 72–73
    regulation in the intestine, 74
    signature cytokines IL-17A and IL-17F, 72
    specific chemokine receptor CCR6, 71–72
    survival/expansion of pathogenic, 73
    tissue inflammation and neutrophil recruitment, role in, 72
    transcriptional program, 73
Threshold hypothesis, 439–440
Thrombotic APS, 482–483
Thromboxanes, 56
Thymic epithelial cells, 59–60
Thymic tolerance, 87–90
  expression of tissue restricted antigens, 90
  mechanisms of, 88–90
    anergy, 89
    clonal deletion, 88–89
    development of regulatory T cells, 89–90
  thymocyte development, 87–88, 88*f*

Thyroglobulin, 5
Thyroid-associated ophthalmopathy, 568
    corticosteroid therapy, 568
    glycosaminoglycan release, 568
T-independent antigens, 64–66, 151
TIR-domain containing adaptor protein
    (TIRAP/Mal), 166
T lymphocytes, 59
TNF inhibitors, 30–31
TNF receptor-associated periodic syndrome
    (TRAPS), 39
TNFR mutations, 45
TNFRSF1A, 44–45
Tobacco smoke, 290
    autoimmunity and, 370
    inflammatory bowel disease (IBD) and,
        874
Toll-interleukin-1 receptor (TIR)-domain-
    containing adaptor inducing IFN-β, 166
Toll-like receptor adaptor molecule (TRAM),
    166
Toll-like receptors (TLRs), 56–57, 161–162,
    263–264, 275–276
    activation
        IL-1β, 40–41
Tonic signaling
    autoimmunity and, 154
    in B cells, 154
Tourette syndrome, 1133–1134
Toxic-oil syndrome, 466
Treponema pallidum, 13–14
Trypanasoma cruzi, 321
Tryptophan-depleting enzyme indoleamine 2,3-
    dioxygenase, 57
Tschopp, Jurg, 40–41
Tumor necrosis factor (TNF), 236–237
Type A gastritis, 620–621
Type 2 diabetes mellitus, 46
Type 1 diabetes (T1D), 333, 391–393
    animal models, 1191–1192
    chromatin remodeling and histone
        acetylation, 392
    genome-wide DNA methylation profiling,
        392
    histone deacetylase inhibitors, 392–393
    islet autoantigen-specific vaccination in
        humans, 1200–1203
        GAD65 vaccination trials, 1203

Intranasal Insulin Trial II (INIT II),
    1202–1203
    oral autoantigen trials, 1202
laboratory markers of autoimmunity,
    1179–1182
metabolic abnormalities, 1181–1182
mucosa-mediated antigen-specific tolerance,
    1200
pathogenesis of, 1191–1192
people at risk for, 1196–1197
prediction of, 1177
    genetics, 1179
    islet autoimmunity, 1177–1179
    pancreatic pathology, 1177–1179
primary prevention, 1198–1199
    diet and the intestinal environment,
        1198–1199
secondary prevention, 1199–1203
trials for prevention of, 1193t
viruses in, 1199
Type 1 T regulatory (Tr1) cells, 76–77
    IL-10 production, 76

U

Uhlenhuth, Paul, 13
Ulcerative colitis, 111, 793–794, 875
Undifferentiated arthritis, 527
Uric acid, 56–57
Ustekinumab, 72
Uveitis, 72
Uveitogenic antigens, 793

V

Vaccines, 40, 290
    beneficial effects, 275
    certainty and unceratainty about, 280
    challenges using animal models, 277–279
    historical associations, 276–277
    human papillomavirus (HPV) vaccine, 276
    practical approach, 279–281
    theoretical concerns, 276
Vasculitides, 1068b
    of large and medium-sized blood vessels,
        1087
Vasectomy, 1012
V(D)J genes, 64
Velocardiofacial/DiGeorge syndrome, 667

Vitamin D deficiency and autoimmune
    diseases, 370–371
Vitiligo
    activated cytotoxic T cells, 975
    atypical cases of, 975
    autoantibodies in, 977–978
    autoimmune basis of, 975–976
    classification, 974t
    clinical, pathologic, and epidemiologic
        features, 974–975
    depigmentation, 976
    genetic features, 976
    immune mechanism in, 976
    immunosuppressive drugs for, 976
    lymphocyte-mediated destruction of
        melanocytes, 976
    pathogenetic mechanism, 977
    races and geographic areas, 975
    in vivo and in vitro models, 976–977
VLA-4 Integrins, 1227–1228
Vogt–Koyanagi–Harada syndrome, 795
Voltage-gated calcium channels (VGCC), 777
Voltage-gated potassium channels (VGKC),
    777, 817–818, 823
Voltage-gated sodium channels (VGSC), 777

W

Wallace, Alfred Russel, 3
Wassermann antibody, 13–14
Wassermann test, 14
Wegener's granulomatosis, 639, 793–795,
    1069
West Nile Virus (WNV), 269
"White-dot syndromes," 795
Wiskott–Aldrich syndrome (WAS), 667
Witebsky, Ernest, 14–15
Wyllie, Andrew, 245

X

Xanthomatous hypophysitis, 638
X chromosome, 24
X-linked agammaglobulinemia (XLA), 406
XX chromosome, 24

Z

ZAP70, 26

CPI Antony Rowe
Eastbourne, UK
May 26, 2015